O9-ABE-281

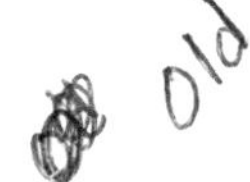

Fundamentals of Diagnostic Radiology

Third Edition

Fundamentals of Diagnostic Radiology

Third Edition

EDITORS

WILLIAM E. BRANT, MD, FACR

Professor of Radiology
Director, ThoracoAbdominal Division
Department of Radiology
University of Virginia Health System
Charlottesville, Virginia

CLYDE A. HELMS, MD

Professor of Radiology and Surgery
Chief, Division of Musculoskeletal Radiology
Department of Radiology
Duke University Medical Center
Durham, North Carolina

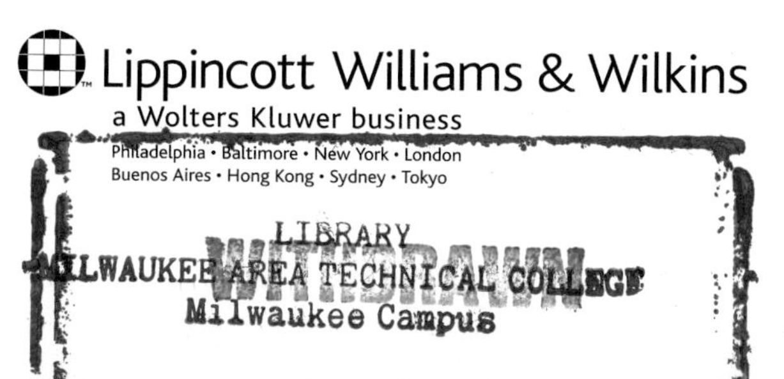

Lippincott Williams & Wilkins
a Wolters Kluwer business
Philadelphia • Baltimore • New York • London
Buenos Aires • Hong Kong • Sydney • Tokyo

Acquisitions Editor: Lisa McAllister
Developmental Editor: Rebecca Barroso
Managing Editor: Kerry Barrett
Marketing Manager: Angela Panetta
Project Manager: Nicole Walz
Senior Manufacturing Manager: Benjamin Rivera
Design Coordinator: Risa Clow
Cover Designer: Wanda Espana
Production Services: TechBooks
Printer: Maple-Vail

530 Walnut Street
Philadelphia, PA 19106 USA
LWW.com

Printed in the USA

Library of Congress Cataloging-in-Publication Data

Fundamentals of diagnostic radiology / [edited by] William E. Brant and Clyde A. Helms.—3rd ed.
p. ; cm.
Includes bibliographical references and index.
ISBN 0-7817-6135-2 (hardcover version) – ISBN 0-7817-6518-8 (paperback version) (alk. paper)
1. Diagnosis, Radioscopic. 2. Diagnostic imaging. I. Brant, William E.
II. Helms, Clyde A. III. Title.
[DNLM: 1. Diagnostic Imaging. WN 180 F981 2006]
RC78.F86 2006
616.07′57—dc22 2006011195

Care has been taken to confirm the accuracy of the information presented and to describe generally accepted practices. However, the authors, editors, and publisher are not responsible for errors or omissions or for any consequences from application of the information in this book and make no warranty, expressed or implied, with respect to the currency, completeness, or accuracy of the contents of the publication. Application of this information in a particular situation remains the professional responsibility of the practitioner.

The authors, editors, and publisher have exerted every effort to ensure that drug selection and dosage set forth in this text are in accordance with current recommendations and practice at the time of publication. However, in view of ongoing research, changes in government regulations, and the constant flow of information relating to drug therapy and drug reactions, the reader is urged to check the package insert for each drug for any change in indications and dosage and for added warnings and precautions. This is particularly important when the recommended agent is a new or infrequently employed drug.

Some drugs and medical devices presented in this publication have Food and Drug Administration (FDA) clearance for limited use in restricted research settings. It is the responsibility of the health care provider to ascertain the FDA status of each drug or device planned for use in their clinical practice.

To purchase additional copies of this book, call our costomer service department at (800) 638-3030 or fax orders to (301) 223-2320. International customers should call (301) 223-2300.

Visit Lippincott Williams & Wilkins on the Internet: http://www.LWW.com. Lippincott Williams & Wilkins customer service representatives are available from 8:30 am to 6:00 pm, EST, Monday through Friday, for telephone access.

10 9 8 7 6 5 4 3 2 1

I dedicate this book to my wife, Barbara, my true companion and the love of my life and to my expanding family: Dan and Lindsay, Ryan and Tiffany, Jonathan Allen, Rachel and Rob, Jake and Dilara, Dan and Debra, and our precious grandchildren, Evan Edward, Finley Matthew, and Danielle Marion.

—WEB

To my wife, Nancy Marie Major, and to our son, Austin Michael.

—CAH

CONTENTS

Foreword *xi*
Preface *xiii*
Contributors *xv*
List of Universal Abbreviations *xix*

SECTION I: BASIC PRINCIPLES *1*

1 **Diagnostic Imaging Methods** *3*
William E. Brant

SECTION II: NEURORADIOLOGY *27*

Section Editor: Erik H.L. Gaensler

2 **Introduction to Brain Imaging** *29*
David J. Seidenwurm

3 **Craniofacial Trauma** *55*
Robert M. Barr, Alisa D. Gean, and Tuong H. Le

4 **Cerebrovascular Disease** *86*
Howard A. Rowley

5 **Central Nervous System Neoplasms and Tumor like Masses** *122*
Kelly K. Koeller

6 **Central Nervous System Infections** *156*
Walter L. Olsen

7 **White Matter and Neurodegenerative Diseases** *184*
Jerome A. Barakos

8 **Pediatric Neuroimaging** *213*
Todd E. Lempert and Erik H.L. Gaensler

9 **Head and Neck Imaging** *241*
Jerome A. Barakos

10 **Nondegenerative Diseases of the Spine** *271*
Erik H.L. Gaensler

11 **Lumbar Spine: Disk Disease and Stenosis** *322*
Clyde A. Helms

SECTION III: PULMONARY *333*

Section Editor: Jeffrey S. Klein

12 **Methods of Examination, Normal Anatomy, and Radiographic Findings of Chest Disease** *335*
Santiago Miró and Jeffrey S. Klein

13 **Mediastinum and Hila** *389*
Jeffrey S. Klein

14 **Pulmonary Vascular Disease** *417*
Jeffrey S. Klein

15 **Pulmonary Neoplasms** *433*
Jeffrey S. Klein

16 **Pulmonary Infection** *460*
Timothy J. Higgins and Jeffrey S. Klein

17 **Diffuse Lung Disease** *479*
Jeffrey S. Klein

18 **Airways Disease** *511*
Jeffrey S. Klein

19 **Pleura, Chest Wall, Diaphragm, and Miscellaneous Chest Disorders** *527*
Jeffrey S. Klein

SECTION IV: BREAST RADIOLOGY *563*

20 **Breast Imaging** *565*
Karen K. Lindfors and Huong T. Le-Petross

SECTION V: CARDIAC RADIOLOGY *601*

Section Editor: David K. Shelton

21 **Cardiac Anatomy, Physiology, and Imaging Methods** *603*
David K. Shelton

22 **Cardiac Imaging in Acquired Diseases** *629*
David K. Shelton

23 **Cardiac MRI** *652*
Christopher M. Kramer

SECTION VI: VASCULAR AND INTERVENTIONAL RADIOLOGY *669*

Section Editor: Tony P. Smith

24 Thoracic Aorta, Pulmonary Arteries, and Peripheral Vascular Disorders *671*
Michael J. Miller, Jr. and Tony P. Smith

25 Abdominal Arteries, Venous System, and Non-vascular Intervention *700*
Michael J. Miller, Jr. and Tony P. Smith

SECTION VII: GASTROINTESTINAL TRACT *731*

26 Abdomen and Pelvis *733*
William E. Brant

27 Liver, Biliary Tree, and Gallbladder *756*
William E. Brant

28 Pancreas and Spleen *782*
William E. Brant

29 Pharynx and Esophagus *798*
William E. Brant

30 Stomach and Duodenum *816*
William E. Brant

31 Mesenteric Small Bowel *832*
William E. Brant

32 Colon and Appendix *848*
William E. Brant

SECTION VIII: GENITOURINARY TRACT *865*

33 Adrenal Glands and Kidneys *867*
William E. Brant

34 Pelvicaliceal System, Ureters, Bladder, and Urethra *887*
William E. Brant

35 Genital Tract: Radiographic Imaging and MR *909*
William E. Brant

SECTION IX: ULTRASONOGRAPHY *925*

36 Abdomen Ultrasound *927*
William E. Brant

37 Genital Tract and Bladder Ultrasound *954*
William E. Brant

38 Obstetric Ultrasound *976*
William E. Brant

39 Chest, Thyroid, Parathyroid, and Neonatal Brain Ultrasound *1002*
William E. Brant

40 Vascular Ultrasound *1019*
Raymond S. Dougherty and William E. Brant

SECTION X: MUSCULOSKELETAL RADIOLOGY *1061*

41 Benign Cystic Bone Lesions *1063*
Clyde A. Helms

42 Malignant Bone and Soft Tissue Tumors *1086*
Clyde A. Helms

43 Skeletal Trauma *1102*
Clyde A. Helms

44 Arthritis *1132*
Clyde A. Helms

45 Metabolic Bone Disease *1156*
Clyde A. Helms

46 Skeletal "Don't Touch" Lesions *1168*
Clyde A. Helms

47 Miscellaneous Bone Lesions *1183*
Clyde A. Helms

48 Magnetic Resonance Imaging of the Knee *1192*
Clyde A. Helms

49 Magnetic Resonance Imaging of the Shoulder *1205*
Clyde A. Helms

50 Magnetic Resonance Imaging of the Foot and Ankle *1214*
Clyde A. Helms

SECTION XI: PEDIATRIC RADIOLOGY *1225*

51 **Pediatric Chest** *1227*
Susan D. John and Leonard E. Swischuk

52 **Pediatric Abdomen and Pelvis** *1277*
Susan D. John and Leonard E. Swischuk

SECTION XII: NUCLEAR RADIOLOGY *1329*

Section Editor: David K. Shelton

53 **Introduction to Nuclear Radiology** *1331*
David K. Shelton

54 **Essential Science of Nuclear Radiology** *1336*
Ramsey D. Badawi, Linda A. Kroger, and Jerrold T. Bushberg

55 **Skeletal System Scintigraphy** *1357*
David K. Shelton and Michael F. Hartshorne

56 **Pulmonary Scintigraphy** *1371*
David K. Shelton and Rhonda A. Wyatt

57 **Cardiovascular System Scintigraphy** *1383*
David K. Shelton and Michael F. Hartshorne

58 **Endocrine Gland Scintigraphy** *1400*
Marc G. Cote

59 **Gastrointestinal, Liver/Spleen, and Hepatobiliary Scintigraphy** *1412*
David K. Shelton and Michael F. Hartshorne

60 **Genitourinary System Scintigraphy** *1424*
Mike McBiles and Peter W. Blue

61 **Scintigraphic Diagnosis of Inflammation and Infection** *1436*
Christopher J. Palestro and Charito Love

62 **Molecular Imaging of Tumors** *1452*
James H. Timmons

63 **Central Nervous System Scintigraphy** *1468*
David H. Lewis and Vivek Manchanda

64 **Positron Emission Tomography** *1483*
Bijan Bijan, David K. Shelton, and William E. Brant

Index *1521*

FOREWORD

Congratulations to Drs. Brant and Helms for updating their classic and outstanding textbook, *Fundamentals of Diagnostic Radiology,* in this third edition. For many years, this textbook has served as a basic overview of diagnostic imaging for medical students, radiology residents, and others in the medical field. The third edition comes in two different formats: a single hardcover edition as previously published and a new four-volume soft-cover edition that can be carried around easily as one rotates on different services. The third edition retains many of the previous authors; however, chapters on chest, bones, and joints; the gastrointestinal tract; ultrasound; breast imaging; and pediatrics all have major revisions, and new authors have written chapters on cardiovascular and vascular/interventional radiology as well as on nuclear medicine.

The third edition continues the strong legacy of past editions, emphasizing the fundamentals of diagnostic imaging. Two new chapters on cardiac imaging and PET-CT are appropriately added to update these new imaging topics. Basic chapters have also been expanded to include topics such as virtual colonoscopy, the use of CT in the evaluation of renal stones, CT of abdominal trauma, and pulmonary complications of bone marrow transplants. To complete newer topics the authors have included global infectious diseases such as SARS and anthrax.

This complete textbook will continue to be basic reading for diagnostic radiology residents, serving as a review as they prepare for written and oral boards. It is also a great textbook for medical students and those practitioners who want a concise reference textbook of diagnostic imaging for their offices.

I commend Drs. Brant and Helms for this updated third edition of their outstanding textbook, *Fundamentals of Diagnostic Imaging,* as did Drs. Keats and Ravin before me in their forewords to the previous editions.

One of an academician's rewards is watching one's previous residents/coworkers excel in academic radiology. I have personally followed Drs. Brant and Helms as they rose through academics, Bill first as one of my residents and Clyde as a teacher and coworker. Thanks to these two superb teachers of radiology for their outstanding textbook.

Alfred B. Watson, Jr., MD, MPH

PREFACE TO THE THIRD EDITION

We are happy and proud to offer a third edition of our *Fundamentals of Diagnostic Radiology* text. We cherish the fact that so many radiology residents around the country continue to use our text as we had originally intended—as a first read for beginning residents and as a concise but comprehensive review text for preparation for American Board of Radiology written and oral examinations. We are particularly pleased that most of our authors from our original text published in 1994 have returned to contribute to this edition. In 1992 as we conceived the notion of writing this text we deliberately chose authors who were very junior faculty or fresh out of their fellowship training to identify what is fundamental and important to the student of radiology. Now more than a decade later these same authors are leaders in the teaching of radiology, serving as department chairs, division chiefs, professors, and senior radiologists. All have kept pace with what is fundamental and important in learning the rapidly progressing specialty of diagnostic imaging. Dr. Erik Gaensler has returned to organize his expert group of neuroradiologists writing the Neuroradiology section. These include Kelly Koeller, the former chairman of Radiologic Pathology at the Armed Forces Institute of Pathology and currently associate professor of radiology at the Mayo Clinic; Alisa Gean, a leading expert in brain trauma imaging; and Howard Rowley, the Chief of Neuroradiology at the University of Wisconsin. Dr. Susan John, the primary author of our pediatric radiology chapters, is now the Chair of the Department of Diagnostic and Interventional Imaging at the University of Texas–Houston Medical School. Susan is the first woman to chair a major department at her institution. Dr. David K. Shelton, Professor of Radiology and Chief of the Nuclear Medicine division at the University of California–Davis was essential in reorganizing and authoring the Nuclear Radiology section. Without his commitment and fine work we would have been in deep trouble completing this revision. He made a major contribution as the section editor for Cardiac Radiology as well. Jeffrey Klein again contributed the entire chest radiology section, covering the topics so vital to diagnostic radiology. Tony Smith and Michael Miller have provided a stellar rewrite of the entire Vascular and Interventional Radiology section.

Our new edition features a revised organization to keep pace with the dynamics of the American Board of Radiology examinations. In addition to our introductory chapter, we have the 11 sections matching the categories of the oral board examination. Cardiac Radiology and Vascular and Interventional Radiology are now separate sections. We have added a chapter dedicated to the expanding use of Cardiac MR. We have added a chapter on Positron Emission Tomography and PET-CT to match the rapid expansion of this combined imaging modality. All chapters feature updated and added illustrations to match our reputation as pictorialists. We have added descriptions of renal stone CT, abdominal trauma CT, CT and MR urography, the imaging of anthrax and severe acute respiratory distress syndrome (SARS), the pulmonary complications of bone marrow transplant, breast MR, and many more topics of current interest. We have striven in every case to keep to our goals of being fundamental and comprehensive while concise. Growth in the size of our book parallels growth in the scope of our field. We have learned that many residents with shoulders strained by its weight have taken our book to their local copy shop and had it rebound into manageable soft-cover sections. Our publisher has agreed to offer the current edition with a four-volume soft cover option in addition to our original single-volume hardcover text.

We offer our thanks to the many individuals in addition to our authors who have contributed mightily to the text's completion. Kerry Barrett, Managing Editor, and Lisa McAllister, Executive Editor, at Lippincott Williams & Wilkins, have guided this edition from inception to completion. Barbara Stabb and her team at TechBooks in York, Pennsylvania, provided outstanding book production services. Most of all we thank the many residents, fellows, medical students, and faculty colleagues with whom we have worked and who have challenged us as teachers and radiologists.

William E. Brant, MD, FACR
Clyde A. Helms, MD

CONTRIBUTORS

Ramsey D. Badawi, PhD
Assistant Professor of Radiology
University of California, Davis
Senior PET Physicist
Department of Radiology
University of California, Davis Medical Center
Sacramento, California

Jerome A. Barakos, MD
Assistant Clinical Professor
Department of Radiology, Neuroradiology Section
University of California, San Francisco
Director of Neuroimaging
Department of Radiology
California Pacific Medical Center
San Francisco, California

Robert M. Barr, MD
Mecklenburg Radiology Associates, P.A.
Presbyterian Hospital
Charlotte, North Carolina

Bijan Bijan, MD
Assistant Professor of Diagnostic Radiology and Nuclear Medicine
Department of Cross-Sectional Body Imaging/MRI and Nuclear Medicine/PET Divisions
University of California, Davis Medical Center
Sacramento, California
Director of Radiology
MRI Department
Elk Grove Diagnostic Imaging–MRI Medical Center
Elk Grove, California

Peter W. Blue, MD
Professor of Radiology
University of South Carolina School of Medicine
Columbia, South Carolina
Chief, Nuclear Medicine Service
Moncrief Army Community Hospital
Fort Jackson, South Carolina

William E. Brant, MD, FACR
Professor of Radiology
Director, ThoracoAbdominal Division
Department of Radiology
University of Virginia Health System
Charlottesville, Virginia

Jerrold T. Bushberg, PhD, DABMP
Clinical Professor
Department of Radiology
University of California, Davis
School of Medicine
Sacramento, California

Marc G. Cote, DO, FACP
Chief, Department of Radiology
Nuclear Medicine Consultant to the Office of the Army Surgeon General
Madigan Army Medical Center
Tacoma, Washington

Raymond S. Dougherty, MD
Associate Clinical Professor
Residency Program Director
Diagnostic Radiologist, Division of Abdominal Imaging
Department of Radiology
University of California, Davis Medical Center
Sacramento, California

Erik H.L. Gaensler, MD
Associate Clinical Professor
Department of Radiology
University of California, San Francisco
San Francisco, California

Alisa D. Gean, MD
Professor of Radiology, Neurology, and Neurosurgery
University of California, San Francisco
Chief of Neuroradiology
San Francisco General Hospital
San Francisco, California

Michael F. Hartshorne, MD
Professor of Radiology
University of New Mexico School of Medicine
Staff Radiologist
University of New Mexico Hospital
Albuquerque, New Mexico

Clyde A. Helms, MD
Professor of Radiology and Surgery
Chief, Division of Musculoskeletal Radiology
Department of Radiology
Duke University Medical Center
Durham, North Carolina

Timothy J. Higgins, MD
Clinical Instructor of Radiology
University of Vermant College of Medicine
Resident in Radiology
Fletcher Allen Health Care
Burlington, Vermant

Susan D. John, MD, FACR
Professor and Chair, Diagnostic and Interventional Imaging
University of Texas Health Science Center
Chair, Imaging Services
Memorial Hermann Children's Hospital
Houston, Texas

Jeffrey S. Klein, MD
Professor of Radiology
University of Vermont College of Medicine
Chief of Thoracic Radiology
Fletcher Allen Health Care
Burlington, Vermont

Kelly K. Koeller, MD, FACR
Associate Professor of Radiology
Mayo Clinic
Rochester, Minnesota

Christopher M. Kramer, MD
Professor of Radiology and Medicine
Associate Chief, Cardiovascular Division
Department of Medicine
University of Virginia Health System
Charlottesville, Virginia

Linda A. Kroger, MS
Radiation Safety Officer
University of California, Davis Health System
Sacramento, California

Tuong H. Le, MD, PhD
Assistant Clinical Professor
Department of Radiology
San Francisco General Hospital
University of California
San Francisco, California

Todd E. Lempert, MD
Chief, Diagnostic and Interventional Neuroradiology
Mission Hospital
Mission Viejo, California

Huong T. Le-Petross, MD, FRCPS
Assistant Professor of Radiology
Radiologist, Breast Imaging Section
The University of Texas M.D. Anderson Cancer Center
Houston, Texas

David H. Lewis, MD
Associate Professor of Radiology
University of Washington School of Medicine
Director of Nuclear Medicine
Harborview Medical Center
Seattle, Washington

Karen K. Lindfors, MD, MPH
Professor of Clinical Radiology
Chief of Breast Imaging
University of California, Davis School of Medicine
Sacramento, California

Charito Love, MD
Research Scientist
Division of Nuclear Medicine
Long Island Jewish Medical Center
New Hyde Park, New York

Vivek Manchanda, MD
Chief Resident
Nuclear Medicine Division
Department of Radiology
University of Washington
Seattle, Washington

Mike McBiles, MD
Staff Radiologist
Saratoga Hospital
Saratoga Springs, New York

Michael J. Miller, Jr., MD
Associate in Department of Interventional Radiology
Duke University Medical Center
Durham, North Carolina

Santiago Miró, BSc, MD
Assistant Professor of Radiology
Université Laval, Quebec, QC, Canada
Attending Radiologist, Cardio-thoracic Section Hôpital Laval, Quebec, QC, Canada

Walter L. Olsen, MD
Assistant Clinical Professor of Radiology
University of California, San Diego
Radiologist, San Diego Diagnostic Radiology Medical Group
San Diego, California

Christopher J. Palestro, MD
Professor of Nuclear Medicine and Radiology
Albert Einstein College of Medicine
Bronx, New York
Chief, Division of Nuclear Medicine
Long Island Jewish Medical Center
New Hyde Park, New York

Howard A. Rowley, MA, MD
Chief of Neuroradiology
Joseph Sackett Professor of Radiology
Associate Professor of Radiology, Neurology, and Neurosurgery
University of Wisconsin
Madison, Wisconsin

David J. Seidenwurm, MD
Chair, Diagnostic Division
Radiological Associates of Sacramento
Neuroradiologist, Diagnostic Imaging and Radiation Oncology
Sutter Medical Center
Sacramento, California

David K. Shelton, MD
Professor, Nuclear Medicine and Radiology
Chief, Nuclear Medicine
University of California, Davis Medical Center
Sacramento, California

Tony P. Smith, MD
Professor of Radiology
Chief, Division of Interventional Radiology
Department of Radiology
Duke University Medical Center
Durham, North Carolina

Leonard E. Swischuk, MD
Chairman and Professor of Radiology
University of Texas Medical Branch
Galveston, Texas

James H. Timmons, MD, PhD
Radiology Consultants PLC
Director, Nuclear Medicine and PET
Department of Radiology
Battle Creek Health Systems
Battle Creek, Michigan

Rhonda A. Wyatt, MD
Chief of Nuclear Medicine
Department of Radiology
MD Imaging
Redding, California

LIST OF UNIVERSAL ABBREVIATIONS

AIDS	Acquired immunodeficiency syndrome
ARDS	Acute respiratory distress syndrome
CNS	Central nervous system
CT	Computed tomography
CSF	Cerebrospinal fluid
FDG PET	Fluorodeoxyglucose positron emission tomography
GI	Gastrointestinal
GRE	Gradient recalled echo (MR sequence)
HIV	Human immunodeficiency virus
HRCT	High resolution computed tomography (Lungs)
IV	Intravenous
LA	Left atrium
LV	Left ventricle
MR	Magnetic resonance imaging
PA	Pulmonary artery
PET	Positron emission tomography
PET-CT	Positron emission tomography-computed tomography
SPECT	Single-photon emission computed tomography
STIR	Short TI inversion recovery (MR sequence)
RA	Right atrium
RV	Right ventricle
T1WI	T1-weighted image
T2WI	T2-weighted image
TE	Time of echo (for MR sequences)
TR	Time of repetition (for MR sequences)
US	Ultrasound

SECTION I

Basic Principles

Chapter 1

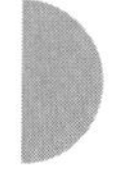

Diagnostic Imaging Methods

William E. Brant

Conventional Radiography

Cross-Sectional Imaging Techniques
- Computed Tomography
- Magnetic Resonance Imaging
- Ultrasonography

Radiographic Contrast Agents
- Iodinated Contrast Agents
- Magnetic Resonance Imaging Intravascular Contrast Agents
- Gastrointestinal Contrast Agents
- Ultrasound Intravascular Contrast Agents

Diagnostic radiology is a dynamic specialty that continues to undergo rapid change with ongoing advancements in technology. Not only has the number of imaging methods increased, but each method continues to undergo improvement and refinement of its use in medical diagnosis. This chapter reviews the basics of the major diagnostic imaging methods and provides the basic principles of image interpretation for each method. Contrast agents commonly used in diagnostic radiology are also discussed. The basics of nuclear radiology are discussed in later chapters.

CONVENTIONAL RADIOGRAPHY

Conventional radiographic examination of the human body dates back to the genesis of diagnostic radiology in 1895, when Wilhelm Roentgen produced the first x-ray film image of his wife's hand. Conventional radiography remains fundamental to the practice of diagnostic imaging.

Image Generation. X-rays are a form of radiant energy that is similar in many ways to visible light. X-rays differ from visible light in that they have a very short wavelength and are able to penetrate many substances that are opaque to light. The x-ray beam is produced by bombarding a tungsten target with an electron beam within an x-ray tube (1).

Film Radiography. Conventional film radiography utilizes a screen-film system within a film cassette as the x-ray detector. As x-rays pass through the human body, they are attenuated by interaction with body tissues (absorption and scatter) and produce an image pattern on film that is recognizable as human anatomy. X-rays that are transmitted through the patient bombard a fluorescent particle–coated screen within the film cassette, causing a photochemical interaction that emits light rays, which expose photographic film within the cassette (Fig. 1.1). The film is removed from the cassette and developed by an automated chemical film processor. The final product is an x-ray image of the patient's anatomy on a film (Fig. 1.2).

Computed radiography (CR) is a filmless system that eliminates chemical processing and provides digital radiographic images. CR substitutes a phosphor imaging plate for the film screen cassette (2). The same gantry, x-ray tube, and exposure control systems used in conventional radiography are utilized for CR. The phosphor-coated imaging plate interacts with x-rays transmitted through the patient to capture a latent image. The phosphor plate is placed within a reading device that scans the plate with a helium-neon laser, emitting light, which is then captured by a photomultiplier tube and processed into a digital image. The digital image is transferred to a computerized picture archiving and communication system (PACS). The PACS stores and transmits digital images via computer networks to give physicians and health care providers in many locations simultaneous instant access to the diagnostic images.

Digital radiography (DR) provides a film-free and cassette-free system for capturing x-ray images in digital format. DR substitutes a fixed electronic detector or charge-coupled device for the film screen cassette or phosphor imaging plate. Direct readout detectors produce an immediate DR image. Most DR detectors are installed in a fixed gantry, limiting the ability of the system to obtain

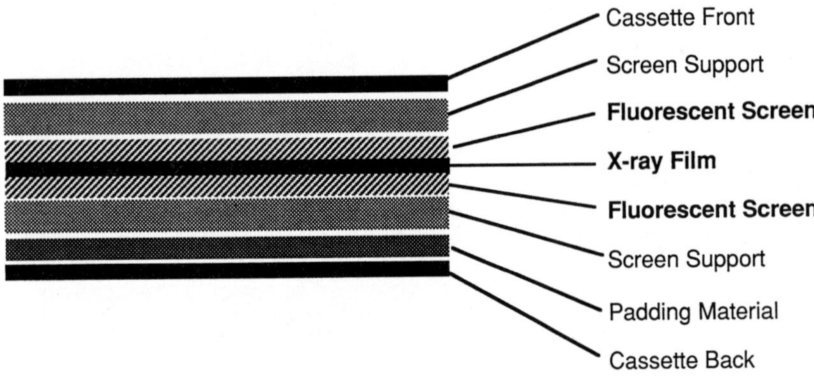

FIGURE 1.1. **X-ray Film Cassette.** Diagram demonstrating a sheet of x-ray film between two fluorescent screens within a light-proof cassette.

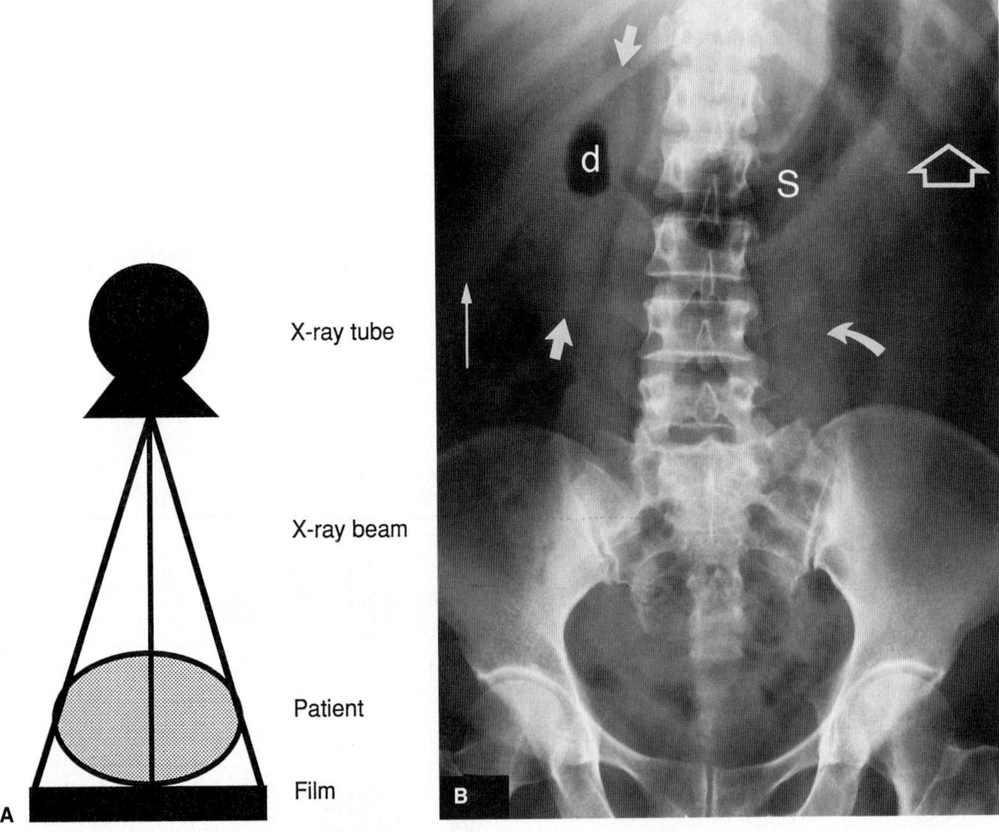

FIGURE 1.2. **Conventional Radiography. A.** Diagram of an x-ray tube producing x-rays that pass through the patient and expose the radiographic film. For digital radiography, a phosphor imaging plate or fixed electronic detector takes the place of the film cassette. **B.** Supine AP radiograph of the abdomen reveals the patient's anatomy because anatomic structures differ in their capacity to attenuate x-rays that pass through the patient. The stomach (S) and duodenum (d) are visualized because air in the lumen is of different radiographic density than the soft tissues that surround the GI tract. The right kidney (*between short straight arrows*), edge of the liver (*long straight arrow*), edge of the spleen (*open arrow*), and the left psoas muscle (*curved arrow*) are visualized because fat outlines the soft tissue density of these structures. The bones of the spine, pelvis, and hips are clearly seen through the soft tissues because of their high radiographic density.

images portably at the patient's bedside. CR is generally used for that purpose in a digital imaging department. Direct digital image capture is particularly useful for angiography, because it provides rapid digital image subtraction, and for fluoroscopy, because it captures video images with low, continuous levels of radiation.

Conventional tomography provides radiographic images of slices of a living patient. This is done by simultaneously moving both the x-ray tube and the x-ray detector around a pivot point centered in the patient in the plane of the anatomic structures to be studied (Fig. 1.3). Structures above and below the focal plane are blurred by the motion of the tube and detector. Objects within the focal plane are visualized with improved detail as a result of the blurring of the overlying and underlying structures. The motion of the x-ray tube and detector may be linear, circular, elliptic, spiral, or hypocycloid. Tomography is a useful adjunct to conventional radiographs in situations in which improved detail is needed for diagnosis. However, with the proliferation and wide availability of cross-sectional imaging, the use of conventional tomography is currently quite limited.

Fluoroscopy enables real-time radiographic visualization of moving anatomic structures. A continuous x-ray beam passes through the patient and falls onto a fluorescing screen (Fig. 1.4). The faint light pattern emitted by the fluorescing screen is amplified electronically by an image intensifier, and the image is displayed on a television monitor and recorded digitally as a single image or series of images for real-time viewing (i.e., a movie or "cinefluoroscopy"). Fluoroscopy is extremely useful to evaluate motion such as GI peristalsis, movement of the diaphragm with respiration, and cardiac action. Fluoroscopy is also used to perform and monitor continuously radiographic procedures, such as barium studies and catheter placements. Video and static fluoroscopic images are routinely stored in digital format on a PACS.

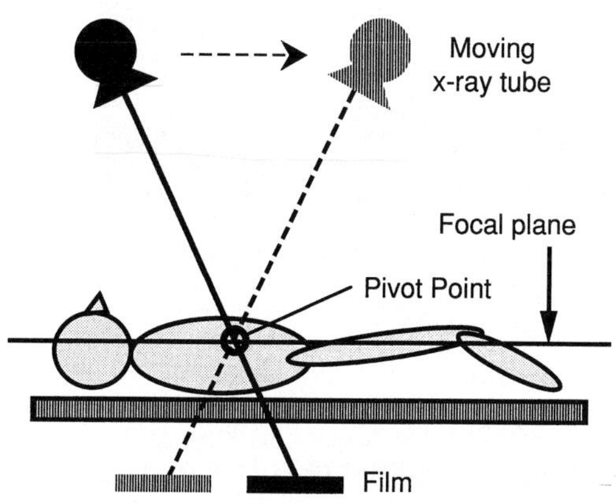

FIGURE 1.3. **Conventional Tomography.** In this technique, the x-ray tube and film simultaneously move about a pivot point at the level of the desired focal plane. Anatomic structures within the focal plane remain in sharp focus, whereas the structures above and below the focal plane are blurred by the motion of the tube and film.

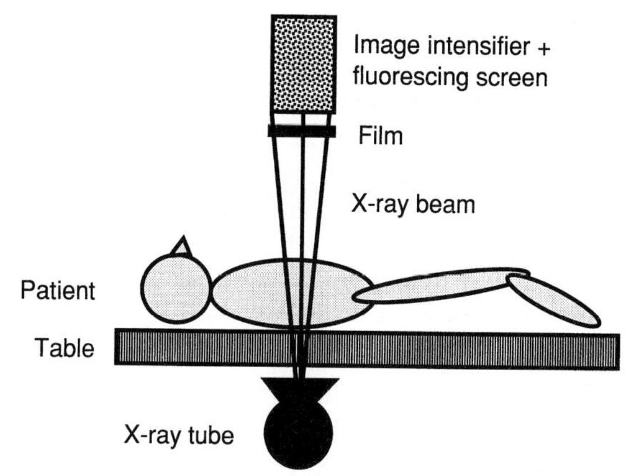

FIGURE 1.4. **Fluoroscopy.** This diagram of a fluoroscopic unit illustrates the x-ray tube located beneath the patient examination table and the fluorescing screen with the image intensifier positioned above the patient. Amplification of the faint fluorescing image by the image intensifier allows the radiation exposure to the patient to be kept at low levels during fluoroscopy. The real-time fluoroscopic images are viewed on a television monitor and may be recorded on videotape. Radiographs are obtained by digital image capture or by placing a film cassette between the patient and the image intensifier and exposing the image receptor with a brief pulse of radiation.

Conventional angiography involves the opacification of blood vessels by intravascular injection of iodinated contrast agents. Conventional arteriography uses small flexible catheters that are placed in the arterial system, usually via puncture of the femoral artery in the groin. With the use of fluoroscopy for guidance, catheters of various sizes and shapes can be manipulated selectively into virtually every major artery. Contrast injection is performed by hand or by mechanical injector and is accompanied by timed rapid-sequence filming or digital computer acquisition (DR) of the fluoroscopic image. The result is a timed series of images depicting contrast flow through the injected artery and the tissues that the artery supplies. Conventional venography is performed by contrast injection of veins via distal puncture or selective catheterization.

Naming Radiographic Views. Most radiographic views are named on the basis of the way that the x-ray beam passes through the patient. A posteroanterior (PA) chest radiograph is one in which the x-ray beam passes through the back of the patient and exits through the front of the patient to expose an x-ray detector positioned against the patient's chest. An anteroposterior (AP) chest radiograph is exposed by an x-ray beam passing through the patient from front to back. A craniocaudad (CC) mammogram is produced by passing a beam through the breast in a vertical (cranial to caudad) direction, with the patient standing or sitting. Views are additionally named by identifying the position of the patient. Erect, supine, or prone views may be specified. A right lateral decubitus view of the chest is exposed with a horizontal x-ray beam passing through the chest of a patient lying on his or her right side. Radiographs taken during fluoroscopy are named on the basis of the patient's position relative to the fluoroscopic table, because the x-ray tube is positioned beneath the table. A right posterior oblique (RPO) view is obtained with the patient lying with the right side of his or her back against the table and the left side elevated away from the table. The x-ray beam generated by the x-ray tube located beneath the table passes through the patient to the x-ray cassette or detector located above the patient.

Principles of Interpretation. Conventional radiographs demonstrate five basic radiographic densities: air, fat, soft tissue, bone, and metal (or x-ray contrast agents). Air attenuates very little of the x-ray beam, allowing nearly the full force of the beam to blacken the image. Bone, metal, and radiographic contrast agents attenuate a large proportion of the x-ray beam, allowing very little radiation through to blacken the image. Thus, bone, metallic objects, and structures opacified by x-ray contrast agents appear white on radiographs. Fat and soft tissues attenuate intermediate amounts of the x-ray beam, resulting in proportional degrees of image blackening (shades of gray). Thick structures attenuate more radiation than thin structures of the same composition. Anatomic structures are seen on radiographs when they are outlined in whole or in part by tissues of different x-ray attenuation. Air in the lung outlines pulmonary vascular structures, producing a detailed pattern of the lung parenchyma (Fig. 1.5). Fat within the abdomen outlines the margins of the liver, spleen, and kidneys, allowing their visualization (Fig. 1.2B). The high density of bones enables visualization of bone details through overlying soft tissues. Metallic objects such as surgical clips are usually clearly seen because they highly attenuate the x-ray beam. Radiographic contrast agents are suspensions of iodine and barium compounds that highly attenuate the x-ray beam and are used to outline anatomic structures. Disease states may obscure normally visualized anatomic structures by silhouetting their outline. For example, pneumonia in the right middle lobe of the lung replaces air in the alveoli with fluid and silhouettes the right heart border (Fig. 1.6). Nancy Major provides an excellent text on the basics of radiographic interpretation (3).

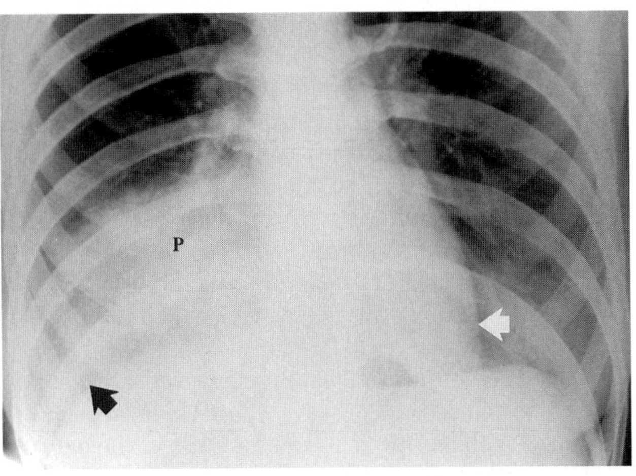

FIGURE 1.6. **Right Middle Lobe and Left Lower Lobe Pneumonia.** PA erect chest radiograph demonstrates pneumonia (P) in the right middle lobe replacing air density in the lung with soft tissue density and silhouetting the right heart border. The dome of the right hemidiaphragm (*black arrow*) is defined by air in the normal right lower lobe and remains visible through the right middle lobe infiltrate. The left heart border (*white arrow*), defined by air in the lingula, remains well defined despite infiltrate in the left lower lobe.

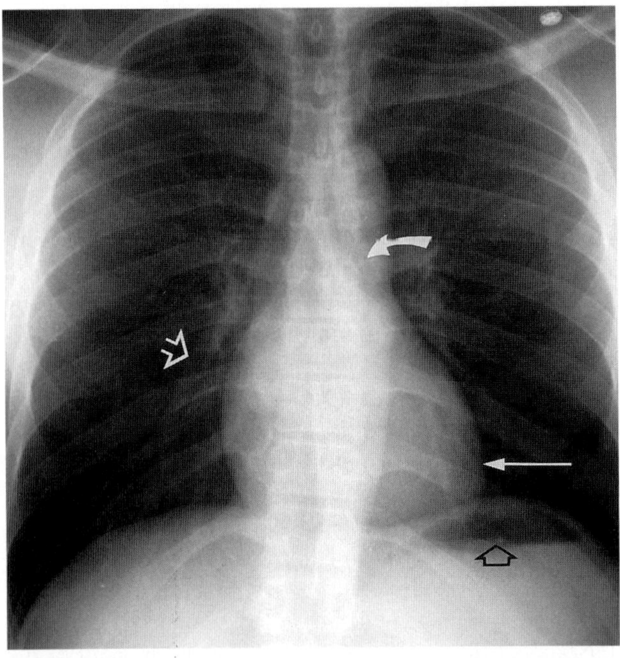

FIGURE 1.5. **Erect PA Chest Radiograph.** The pulmonary arteries (*white open arrow*) are seen in the lung because the vessels are outlined by air in alveoli. The left cardiac border (*long arrow*) is crisply defined by the adjacent air-filled lung. The left main bronchus (*curved arrow*) is seen because its air-filled lumen is surrounded by soft tissue of the mediastinum. An air-fluid level (*open black arrow*) in the stomach confirms the erect position of the patient during exposure of the radiograph.

CROSS-SECTIONAL IMAGING TECHNIQUES

CT, MR, and US are techniques that produce cross-sectional images of the body. All three interrogate a three-dimensional volume or slice of patient tissue to produce a two-dimensional image. The resulting image is made up of a matrix of picture elements (*pixels*), each of which

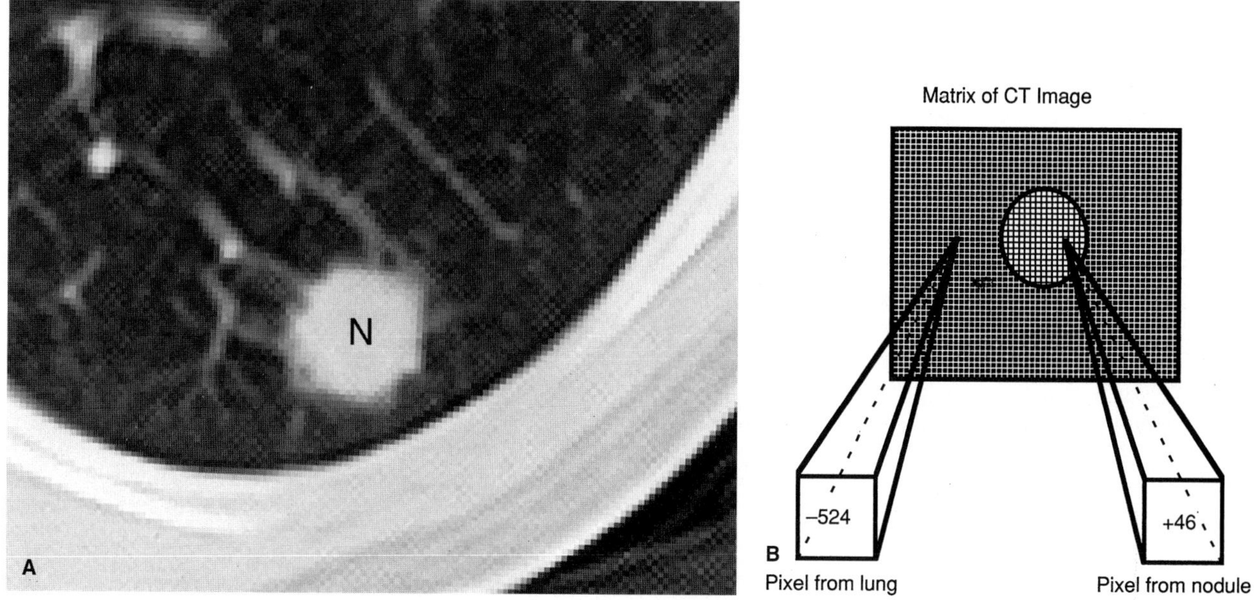

FIGURE 1.7. **Image Matrix. A.** Magnified CT image of a pulmonary nodule (N). The pixels that make up the image are evident as tiny squares within the image. The window width is set at 2,000 H with a window level of 600 H to accentuate visualization of the white soft tissue nodule on a background of gray, air-filled lung. **B.** Diagram of the matrix that constitutes the CT image. A pixel from the air-filled lung with a calculated CT number of 524 H is gray, whereas a pixel from the soft tissue nodule with a calculated CT number of +46 H is white.

represents a volume element (*voxel*) of patient tissue. The tissue composition of the voxel is averaged (*volume averaged*) for display as a pixel. CT and MR assign a numeric value to each picture element in the matrix. The matrix of picture elements that make up each image is usually between 128 × 256 (32,768 pixels) and 560 × 560 (313,600 pixels) and is determined by the specified acquisition parameters (Fig. 1.7).

To produce an anatomic image, shades of gray are assigned to ranges of pixel values. For example, 16 shades of gray may be divided over a *window width* of 320 pixel values (Fig. 1.8). Groups of 20 pixel values are each assigned one of the 16 gray shades. The middle gray shade is assigned to the pixel values centered on a selected *window level.* Pixels with values greater than the upper limit of the window width are displayed white, and pixels with values less than the lower limit of the window width are displayed black. To analyze optimally all of the anatomic information of any particular slice, the image is viewed at different window-width and window-level settings, which are optimized for bone, air-filled lung, soft tissue, and so forth (Fig. 1.9).

The digital images obtained by CT, MR, and US examination are ideal for storage and access on PACS. Current PACSs allow a broad range of image manipulation during viewing and interpretation of images. Among the features that can be used are interactive alterations in window width and window level, magnification, fusing of images from different modalities, reformatting serial images in different anatomic planes, creation of three-dimensional reconstructions, and marking of key images that summarize major findings.

Computed Tomography

CT uses a computer to reconstruct mathematically a cross-sectional image of the body from measurements of x-ray transmission through thin slices of patient tissue. CT displays each imaged slice separately, without the superimposition of blurred structures that is seen with conventional tomography. A narrow, well-collimated beam of x-rays is generated on one side of the patient (Fig. 1.10). The x-ray beam is attenuated by absorption and scatter as it passes through the patient. Sensitive detectors on the opposite side of the patient measure x-ray transmission through the slice. These measurements are systematically repeated many times from different directions while the x-ray tube is pulsed as it rotates 360° around the patient. CT numbers are assigned to each pixel in the image by a computer algorithm that uses as data these measurements of transmitted x-rays. CT pixel numbers are proportional to the difference in average x-ray attenuation of the tissue within the voxel and that of water. A Hounsfield unit (H) scale, named for Sir Godfrey N. Hounsfield, the inventor of CT, is used. Water is assigned a value of 0 H, with the scale extending from 1,024 H for air to +3,000 to 4,000 H for

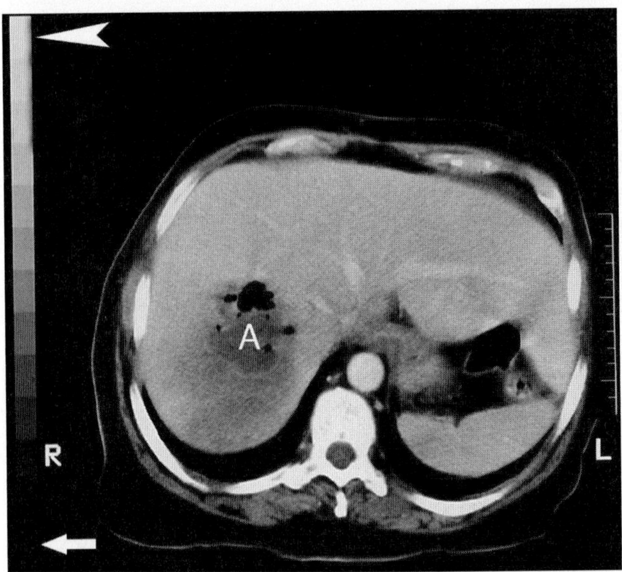

FIGURE 1.8. **Gray Scale.** A CT image of the abdomen includes a gray scale along its left edge. Each individual pixel in the CT image is assigned a shade of gray, depending on its calculated CT number (H unit) and the window width and window level selected by the CT operator. Pure white (*arrowhead*) and pure black (*arrow*) are at the top and bottom of the gray scale. Along the right side of the CT image is a centimeter scale that can be used to measure the size of objects in the image. *R* indicates the patient's right side, and *L* indicates the patient's left side. Cross-sectional images in the transverse plane are routinely viewed from "below," as if standing at the patient's feet. This orientation allows easy correlation with plain-film radiographs, which are routinely viewed as if facing the patient with the patient's right side to the viewer's left. This patient has an abscess (A) in the liver.

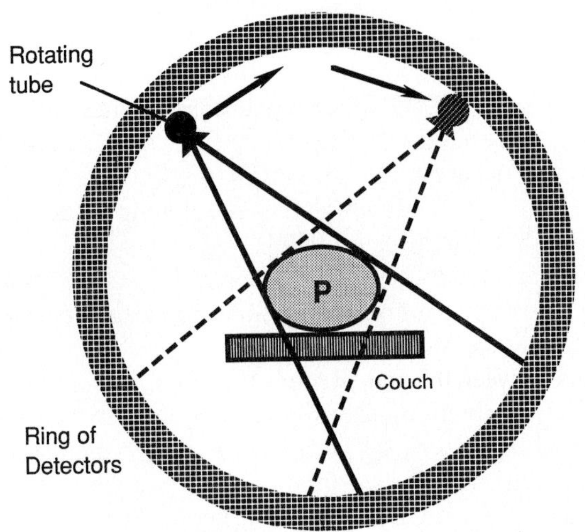

FIGURE 1.10. **Computed Tomography.** Diagram of a CT scanner. The patient (P) is placed on an examination couch within the core of the CT unit. An x-ray tube rotates 360° around the patient, producing pulses of radiation that pass through the patient. Transmitted x-rays are detected by a circumferential bank of radiation detectors. X-ray transmission data are sent to a computer, which uses an assigned algorithm to calculate the matrix of CT numbers used to produce the anatomic cross-sectional image. With the helical CT scan technique, the patient couch moves the patient continuously through the rotating x-ray beam. In MDCT, multiple image slices are obtained simultaneously as the patient is moved through the scanner.

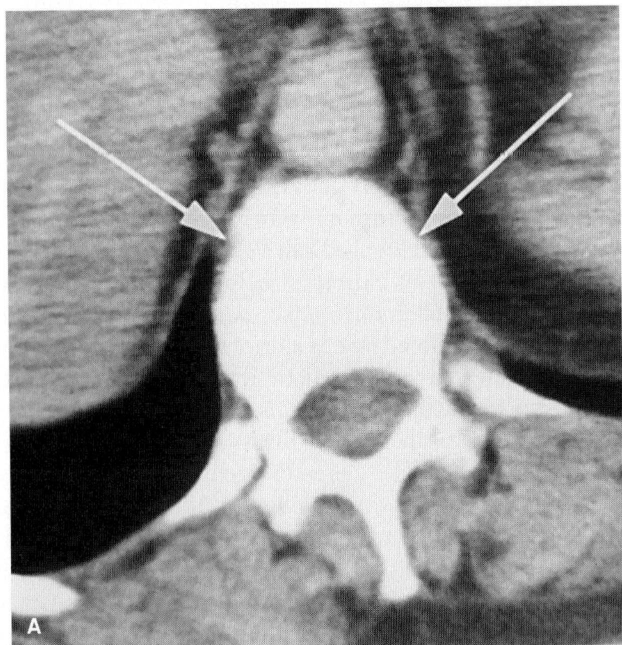

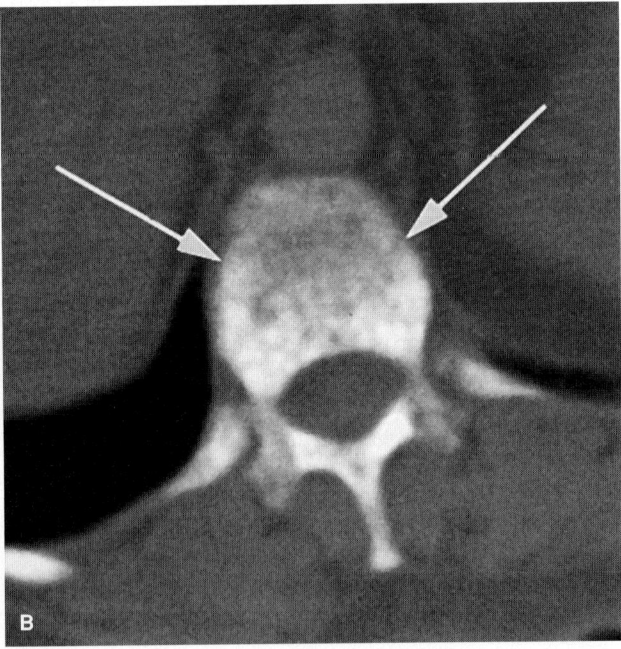

FIGURE 1.9. **CT Windows. A.** A CT image of the upper abdomen photographed with "soft tissue windows" (window width = 482 H, window level = 14 H) portrays a thoracic vertebra (*arrows*) entirely white with no bone detail. **B.** The same CT image re-photographed with "bone windows" (window width = 2,000 H, window level = 400 H) demonstrates destructive changes in the vertebral body (*arrows*) owing to metastatic lung carcinoma.

very dense bone. H units are not absolute values but, rather, are relative values that may vary from one CT system to another. In general, bone is +400 to +1,000 H, soft tissue is +40 to +80 H, fat is −60 to −100 H, lung tissue is −400 to −600 H, and air is −1,000 H.

Voxel dimensions are determined by the computer algorithm chosen for reconstruction and the thickness of the scanned slice. Most CT units allow slice thickness specifications between 0.5 and 10 mm. Data for an individual slice, 360° tube rotation, are routinely acquired in 1 s or less. The advantages of CT compared with MR include rapid scan acquisition, superior bone detail, and demonstration of calcifications. CT scanning is generally limited to the axial plane; however, images may be reformatted in sagittal, coronal, or oblique planes or as three-dimensional images.

Conventional CT (nonhelical) obtains image data one slice at a time (4). The patient holds his or her breath, a slice is taken, the patient breathes, the table moves, and the sequence is repeated. This technique requires at least two to three times the total scanning time of helical CT for any given patient scan volume, making optimization of scanning during maximum contrast more difficult. Minor changes in lung volume with each breath-hold may make substantial changes in the chest and abdomen anatomy scanned, resulting in "skip" areas. More recent conventional scanners can simulate helical scanning by the "cluster" technique. Several sequential scans are obtained during a single breath-hold.

Helical CT, also called *spiral CT,* is performed by moving the patient table at a constant speed through the CT gantry while scanning continuously with an x-ray tube rotating around the patient. A continuous volume of image data is acquired during a single breath-hold. This technique dramatically improves the speed of image acquisition, enables scanning during optimal contrast opacification, and eliminates artifacts caused by misregistration and variations in patient breathing. The entire liver may be scanned in a single breath-hold; the entire abdomen and pelvis, in two to three breath-holds, all during the first 60 to 90 seconds of intravenous contrast administration. Volume acquisition enables retrospective reconstruction of multiple overlapping slices, improving visualization of small lesions and making high-detail three-dimensional CT angiography possible (Fig. 1.11) (5).

Multidetector helical CT (MDCT) is the latest technical advance in CT imaging; it utilizes the principles of the helical scanner but incorporates multiple rows of detector rings (6). This allows the acquisition of multiple slices per tube rotation, increasing the area of the patient that can be covered in a given time by the x-ray beam. Available systems have moved from two slices to 64 slices, which covers 40 mm of patient length for each 1-second or less rotation of the tube. Prototype 256-detector scanners are being developed. The key advantage of MDCT is speed. MDCT is five to eight times faster than single-slice helical CT. For body scanning, 1-mm slices can be obtained creating isotropic voxels (1 × 1 × 1 mm), allowing image reconstruction in any anatomic plane without loss of resolution (4). Broad area coverage allows for high-detail CT angiography and "virtual" CT colonoscopy and bronchoscopy. A disadvantage of MDCT is radiation dose, which can be three to five times higher with MDCT than with single-slice CT.

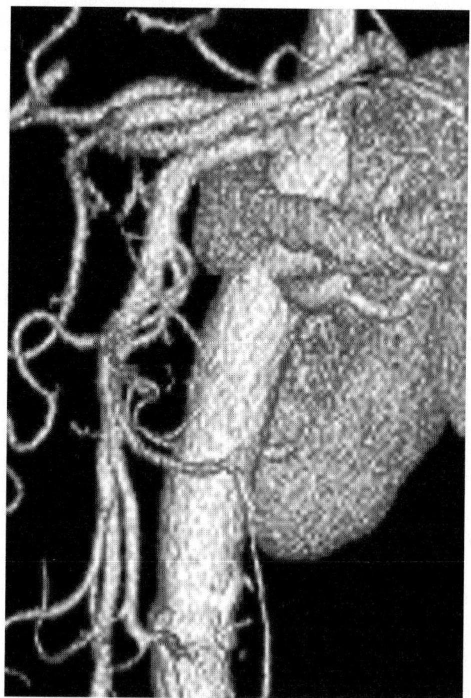

FIGURE 1.11. **CT Angiogram.** A three-dimensional, shaded surface display, angiogram image of the aorta and its branches was created from a series of axial plane MDCT images obtained during rapid bolus IV contrast agent administration. Contrast enhancement greatly increases the CT numbers of the arteries and kidneys and allows removal of structures with lower CT density from the image by "thresholding." Only pixels with CT numbers higher than a specified threshold value are displayed. Computer algorithms create a "virtual" three-dimensional image from data provided by many overlapping axial slices. The three-dimensional image can be rotated and viewed from any desired angle. "Shading," simulating light cast from a remote light source, enhances the three-dimensional visual effect.

Radiation Dose in CT. As the diagnostic capability of CT expands dramatically, so does its utilization. Unfortunately, the technologic advances in CT carry a price of increased radiation exposure to each patient imaged (7,8). CT now accounts for more than 40% of all radiation exposure to patients from diagnostic imaging. There may be as many as 65 million CT examinations performed each year in the United States and as many as 260 million CTs performed yearly worldwide. Many (up to 11%) of these examinations are performed on infants and children, who are more susceptible to the adverse effects of radiation. These considerations mandate a responsibility for the radiologist and the ordering physician to limit CT to definitive indications; provide dose-efficient CT imaging protocols; offer alternative imaging techniques, especially for young children, who are at the greatest risk from radiation; work with manufacturers to limit radiation dose; and educate patients and health care providers about the potential risks of low-dose radiation.

Contrast Administration in CT. Intravenous iodine-based contrast agents are administered in CT to enhance density differences between lesions and surrounding parenchyma, to demonstrate vascular anatomy and vessel patency, and to characterize lesions by their patterns of contrast enhancement. Optimal use of intravenous contrast depends upon the anatomy, physiology, and pathology of the organ of interest. In the brain, the normal blood-brain barrier of tight neural capillary endothelial junctions prevents access of contrast into the neural extravascular space. Defects in the blood-brain barrier associated with tumors, stroke, infection, and other lesions enable contrast accumulation within abnormal tissue, improving its visibility. In nonneural tissues, the capillary endothelium has loose junctions, enabling free access of contrast into the extravascular space. Contrast administration and the timing of CT scanning must be carefully planned to optimize differences in enhancement patterns between lesions and normal tissues. For example, most liver tumors are supplied predominantly by the hepatic artery, whereas the liver parenchyma is supplied predominantly by the portal vein (about 70%), with a lesser contribution from the hepatic artery (about 30%). Contrast given by bolus injection into a peripheral arm vein will arrive earliest in the hepatic artery and enhance (that is, increase the CT density of) many tumors to a greater extent than the liver parenchyma. Maximal enhancement of the liver parenchyma is delayed 1 to 2 minutes until the contrast has circulated through the intestinal tract and returned to the liver via the portal vein. Differentiation of tumor and parenchyma by contrast enhancement can thus be maximized by administration of an IV bolus of contrast and by performing rapid CT scanning of the liver in the first 1 to 2 minutes following contrast administration. Helical CT is ideal for this early and rapid scanning of the liver. Oral or rectal contrast is generally required to opacify the bowel for CT scans of the abdomen and pelvis. Bowel without intraluminal contrast may be difficult to differentiate from tumors, lymph nodes, and hematomas.

CT Artifacts. *Artifacts* are components of the image that do not faithfully reproduce actual anatomic structures because of distortion, addition, or deletion of information. Artifacts degrade the image and may cause errors in diagnosis (9).

Volume averaging is present in every CT image and must always be considered in image interpretation. The displayed two-dimensional image is created from data obtained and *averaged* from a three-dimensional volume of patient tissue. Slices above and below the image that is being interpreted must be examined for sources of volume averaging that may be misinterpreted as pathology.

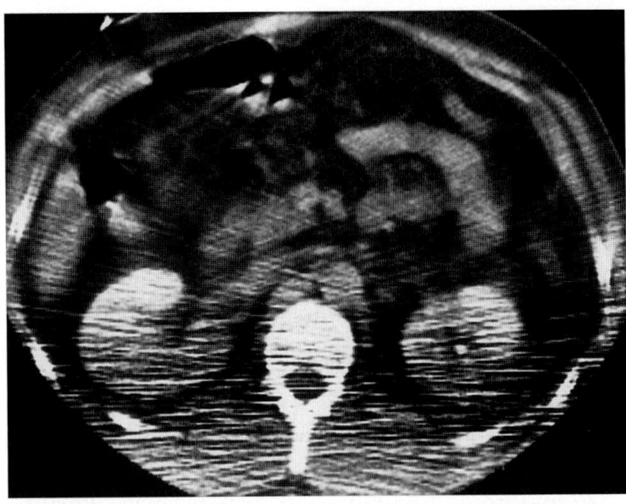

FIGURE 1.12. **Beam-Hardening Artifact.** A CT image of the abdomen is severely degraded by a beam-hardening artifact that produces dark streaks across the lower half of the image. The artifact was caused by marked attenuation of the x-ray beam by the patient's arms, which were kept at his sides owing to injury.

A beam-hardening artifact results from greater attenuation of low-energy x-ray photons than high-energy x-ray photons as they pass through tissue. The mean energy of the x-ray beam is increased (the beam is "hardened"), resulting in less attenuation at the end of the beam than at its beginning. Beam-hardening errors are seen as areas or streaks of low density (Fig. 1.12) extending from structures of high x-ray attenuation, such as the petrous bones, shoulders, and hips.

A *motion artifact* results when structures move to different positions during image acquisition. Motion occurs as a result of voluntary or involuntary patient movement, breathing, heartbeat, vessel pulsation, or peristalsis. Motion is demonstrated in the image as prominent streaks from high- to low-density interfaces or as blurred or duplicated images (Fig. 1.13).

Streak artifacts emanate from high-density sharp-edged objects, such as vascular clips and dental fillings (Fig. 1.14). Reconstruction algorithms cannot handle the extreme differences in x-ray attenuation between very dense objects and adjacent tissue.

Principles of CT Interpretation. Like all imaging analysis, CT interpretation is based on an organized and comprehensive approach. CT images are viewed in sequential anatomic order, with each slice examined with reference to slices above and below. The radiologist must seek to develop a three-dimensional concept of the anatomy and pathology displayed. The study must be interpreted with reference to the scan parameters, slice thickness and

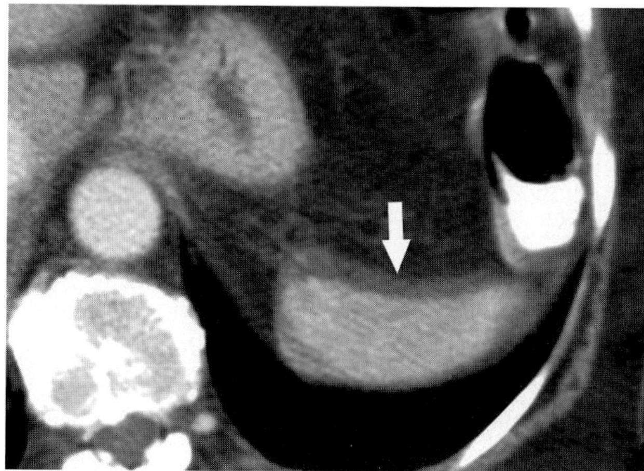

FIGURE 1.13. **Motion Artifact.** Breathing motion during image acquisition duplicates the margin (*arrow*) of the spleen, simulating a subcapsular hematoma in this patient, who was imaged because of abdominal trauma.

spacing, administration of contrast, and artifacts. Images are oriented so that the observer is looking at the patient from below. The patient's right side is oriented on the left side of the image. Optimal bone detail is viewed at "bone windows," generally a window width of 2,000 H and a window level of 400 to 600 H. Lungs are viewed at "lung windows," with a window width of 1,000 to 2,000 H and window levels of about 500 to 600 H. Soft tissues are examined at a window width of 400 to 500 H and window level 20 to 40 H. Narrow windows (width of 100 to 150 H, level of 70 to 80 H) increase image contrast and aid in the detection of subtle liver and spleen lesions. PACS workstation viewing allows the interpreter to actively change window width and level settings to optimize visualization of anatomic structures.

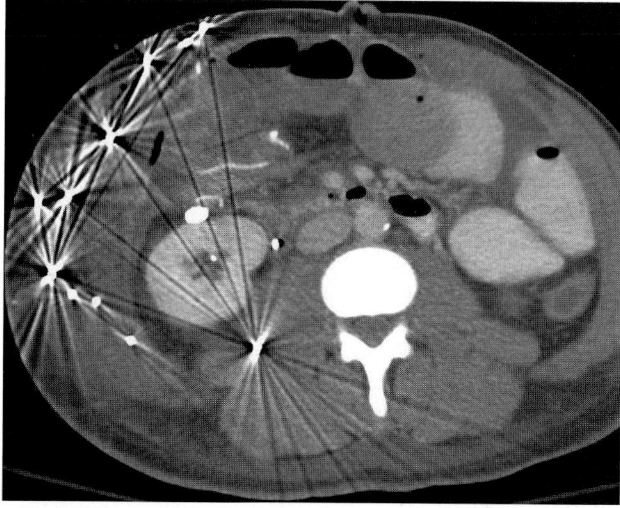

FIGURE 1.14. **Streak Artifact.** Shotgun pellets produce a severe streak artifact on this CT image.

Magnetic Resonance Imaging

MR is a technique that produces tomographic images by means of magnetic fields and radio waves. Although CT evaluates only a single tissue parameter—x-ray attenuation—MR analyzes multiple tissue characteristics, including hydrogen (proton) density, T1 and T2 relaxation times of tissue, and blood flow within tissue. The soft tissue contrast provided by MR is substantially better than for any other imaging modality. Differences in the density of protons available to contribute to the MR signal discriminate one tissue from another. Most tissues can be differentiated by significant differences in their characteristic T1 and T2 relaxation times. T1 and T2 are features of the three-dimensional molecular environment that surrounds each proton in the tissue imaged. T1 is a measure of a proton's ability to exchange energy with its surrounding chemical matrix. It is a measure of how quickly a tissue can become magnetized. T2 conveys how quickly a given tissue loses its magnetization. Blood flow has a complex effect on the MR signal that may decrease or increase signal intensity within blood vessels.

The complex physics of MR is beyond the scope of this book. In the simplest terms, MR is based on the ability of a small number of protons within the body to absorb and emit radio wave energy when the body is placed within a strong magnetic field. Different tissues absorb and release radio wave energy at different, detectable, and characteristic rates. MR scans are obtained by placing the patient in a static magnetic field 0.02 to 4 tesla (T) in strength, depending on the particular MR unit used. Low–field strength systems (<0.1 T), midfield systems (0.1 to 1.0 T), and high-field systems (1.5 and 3.0 T) each have their own advantages and disadvantages. The choice of unit for imaging is based on preference and local availability. A small number of tissue protons in the patient align with the main magnetic field and are subsequently displaced from their alignment by application of radiofrequency (RF) gradients. When the RF gradient is terminated, the displaced protons realign with the main magnetic field, releasing a small pulse of energy that is detected, localized, and then processed by a computer algorithm similar to that used in CT to produce a cross-sectional tomographic anatomic image. Slice location is determined by application of a slice selection gradient of gradually increasing intensity along the z axis. The small energy pulses released by tissue protons are further localized by "frequency encoding" in one direction (x axis) and "phase encoding" in the other direction (y axis). Images can be obtained in any anatomic plane by adjusting the orientation of the x axis, y axis, and z axis magnetic field gradients. Because the MR signal is very weak, prolonged imaging time is often required for

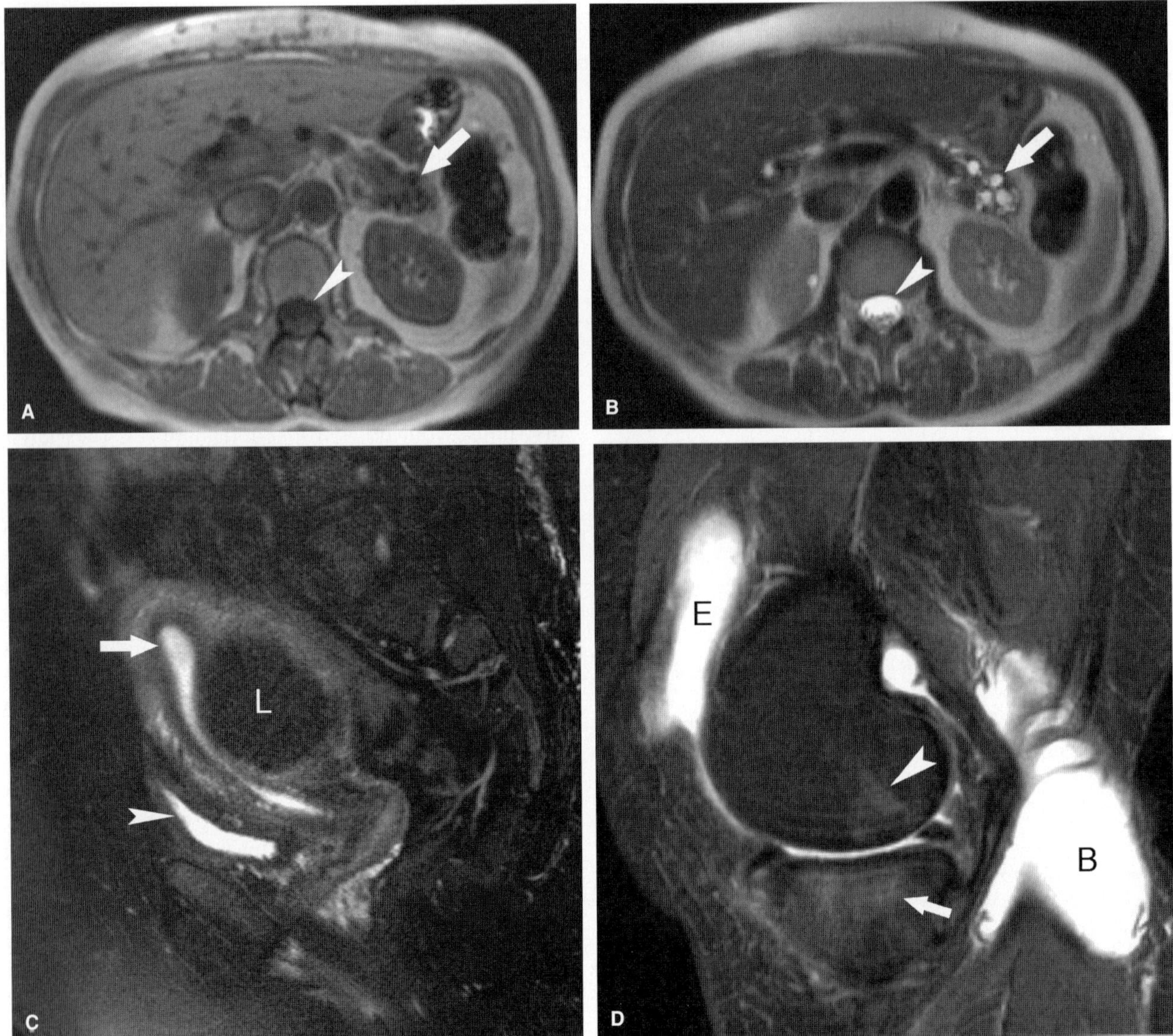

FIGURE 1.15. **MR Sequences.** Gradient recall in-phase T1WI **(A)** and HASTE T2WI **(B)**, taken at the same slice location, demonstrates dark signal in free water on the T1WI and bright signal of free water on the T2WI. Note the improved conspicuity of the cystic lesion (*arrows*) of the pancreas on the T2WI compared to the T1WI. The CSF (*arrowheads*) in the spinal canal also shows marked increase in signal on the T2WI. **C.** Sagittal TSE T2WI with fat saturation shows a low-signal leiomyoma (L) and bright signal from fluid in the endometrial canal (*arrow*) and from urine in the bladder (*arrowhead*). Note the lack of signal from fat as compared to **B,** the T2WI without fat saturation. **D.** Sagittal plane STIR image of the knee accentuates bright signal from free water in the knee effusion (E), Baker's cyst (B), and bone bruise edema in the femoral condyle (*arrowhead*) and tibial plateau (*arrow*).

optimal images. Standard spin-echo sequences produce a batch of images in 10 to 20 minutes. Rather than obtaining data for each image one slice at a time, many spin-echo MR sequences obtain data for all slices in the imaged tissue volume throughout the entire imaging time. Thus, motion caused by breathing and cardiac and vascular pulsation may degrade the image substantially. MR has advanced to rapid-imaging breath-hold techniques using GRE, echo train, and echo-planar sequences. Continuing technologic improvements are making MR acquisition times comparable to those for CT.

Present MR technology relies on a variety of MR sequence techniques, with many variations used by different MR manufacturers (Fig. 1.15). Acronyms rule (10).

Spin-echo (SE) pulse sequences produce standard T1WIs, T2WIs, and proton density–weighted images. T1WIs emphasize differences in the T1 relaxation times between tissues. T1WIs usually provide the best anatomic detail and are good for identifying fat, subacute hemorrhage, and proteinaceous fluids. T2WIs emphasize differences in the T2 relaxation times of tissues and usually provide the most sensitive detection of edema and pathologic lesions. Proton density–weighted images accentuate proton density differences in tissues and are most useful in brain imaging.

Two major components of MR instrument settings selected by the operator for SE sequences are *time of repetition* (TR) and *time of echo* (TE). TR is the time between administered RF pulses, or the time provided for protons to align with the main magnetic field. TE is the time provided for absorbed radio wave energy to be released and detected). Spin-echo T1WIs are obtained by selecting short TR (≤500 ms) and short TE (≤20-ms) settings. Spin-echo T2WIs use a long TR (≥2000 ms) and long TE (≥70 ms). Proton density–weighted images use a long TR (2,000 to 3,000 ms) and a short TE (25 to 30 ms) to minimize T1 and T2 effects and accentuate hydrogen-density differences in tissues.

Multiple spin-echo sequences, also known as echo train, rapid-acquisition relaxation-enhanced (RARE), fast spin-echo (FSE), or turbo spin-echo (TSE) sequences, significantly reduce image acquisition time. Signal intensity is less than with SE sequences, and image blurring occurs. Fat is bright on T2WIs, impairing detection of pathology, such as edema in fat adjacent to an inflammatory process. Addition of fat-suppression techniques counters this effect. Fast low-angle acquisition with relaxation enhancement (FLARE) and half-Fourier acquisition single-shot turbo spin-echo (HASTE) are variations of this technique.

Inversion recovery (IR) pulse sequences are used mainly to emphasize differences in T1 relaxation times of tissues. A delay time, the *time of inversion* (TI) is added to the TE, and TR instrument settings selected by the operator. Standard IR sequences, which use a long TI, produce T1WIs. Tissues with short T1 times yield a brighter signal. *Short TI inversion recovery* (STIR) sequences are the most commonly used. This sequence achieves additive T1-weighted, T2-weighted, and proton density–weighted contrast to increase lesion conspicuity. With STIR sequences, all tissues with short T1 relaxation times, including fat, are suppressed, whereas tissues with high water content, including many pathologic lesions, are accentuated, yielding a bright signal on a dark background of nulled short-T1 tissue. STIR images more closely resemble strongly T2WIs.

Gradient-recalled echo pulse sequences are used to perform fast MR and MR angiography. Rapid image sequences are particularly useful in body MR to minimize motion artifact of breathing, heartbeat, vessel pulsation, and bowel peristalsis. Partial "flip angles" of less than 90° are used to decrease the time to signal recovery. Signal intensity arising from T2 relaxation characteristics of tissue is strongly affected by imperfections in the magnetic field on GRE images. Magnetization decay time with GRE imaging is termed T2* ("T2 star") and is much shorter than the "true" T2 decay times seen with SE imaging. GRE images are characteristically low in image contrast, have prominent artifacts, and demonstrate flowing blood with bright signal. T1-, T2-, T2*-, and proton density–image weighting are determined by the combination of flip angle, TR, and TE settings. Fast GRE techniques include fast low-angle shot (FLASH), gradient-recalled acquisition in steady state (GRASS), and true fast imaging with steady-state precession (FISP), snapshot FLASH, rapid acquisition with gradient echo (RAGE), and magnetization-prepared RAGE (MPRAGE).

Echo-planar imaging is a fast MR technique that can produce single-slice images in 20 ms and multislice studies in 20 s. All spatial encoding information is obtained after a single RF excitation, compared with the multiple RF excitations separated by TR intervals that are required for conventional MR. Motion artifacts are reduced, and moving structures can be "freeze-frame" imaged. Special hardware is required for echo-planar imaging, but standard SE, GRE, and IR pulse sequences can be obtained. Echo-planar imaging overcomes many of the time and motion limitations of conventional MR and enables expansion of MR to new areas such as blood perfusion and cortical activation of the brain.

Fat-suppression techniques are used in MR to detect the presence of fat or to suppress signal from fat to enhance detection of pathology (tumor invasion into fat or edema in fat) (11). The *fat-saturation* technique suppresses large amounts of fat and is optimal for suppressing macroscopic fat within fat cells (Fig. 1.15C). This technique is highly sensitive to magnetic field inhomogeneity and misregistration artifacts and does not work well with low-field magnets. A saturation pulse at the resonance frequency of fat is applied to each slice. The technique is specific for fat and can be used effectively with contrast-enhanced images. IR provides global homogeneous fat suppression but suppresses all tissues with very short T1, including tissue enhanced by administration of intravenous gadolinium, mucoid tissue, hemorrhage, and proteinaceous fluid (Fig. 1.15D). It can be used with low-field magnets and is insensitive to inhomogeneities in the magnetic field. *Opposed-phase MR* is fast, reliable, and optimal for detection of small amounts of fat, such as intracellular fat in adrenal adenomas and fatty-infiltrated liver (Fig. 1.16). Resonance frequency of water is different (faster than) that of fat. *In-phase* (IP) images add signal from fat and water. *Opposed-phase* (or *out-of-phase* [OP]) images subtract water signal from fat signal. Adipose tissue contains abundant fat and little water, so the signal is minimally reduced on OP images. However, tissues with low fat content but high water content (e.g., adrenal adenomas) show a prominent loss of signal on OP images compared to IP images. The obvious limitation is that opposed-phase MR does not suppress signal from adipose tissue.

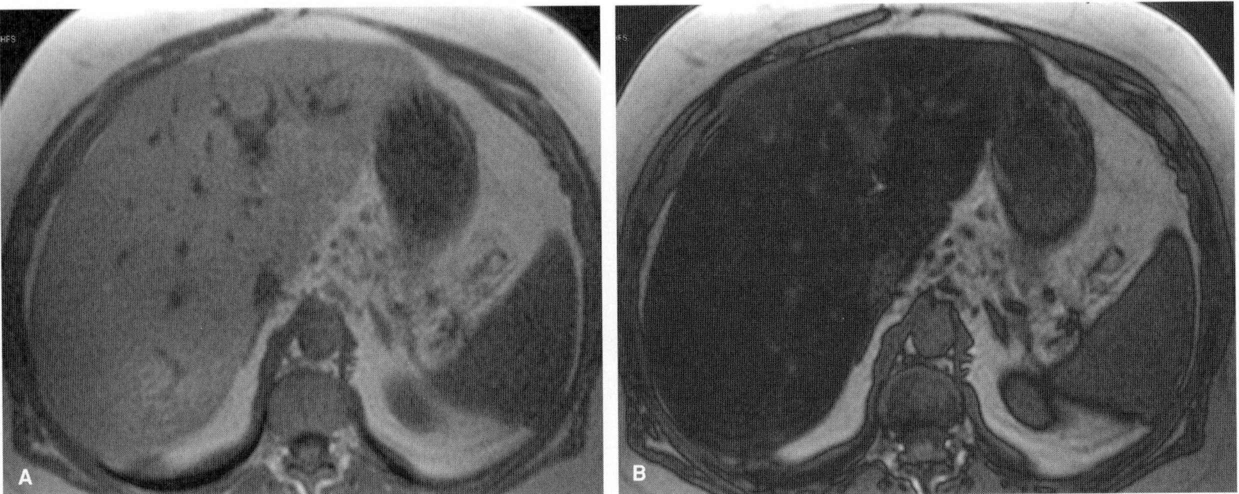

FIGURE 1.16. Opposed Phase Fat-Suppression Technique. Compare the IP image of the liver **(A)** with the OP image of the liver **(B).** The dramatic darkening of the liver on the OP image is indicative of diffuse fatty infiltration. The signal from fat within hepatocytes is subtracted from the total signal, including fat and water on the IP image.

Advantages of MR. Among the advantages of MR are its outstanding soft tissue contrast resolution, its ability to provide images in any anatomic plane, and the absence of ionizing radiation. MR is limited in its ability to demonstrate dense bone detail or calcifications, involves long imaging times for many pulse sequences, possesses limited spatial resolution compared with CT, has limited availability in some geographic areas, and is expensive. Because of the physically confining space for the patient within the magnet, a number of patients experience symptoms of claustrophobia and require sedation or are simply unable to tolerate MR scanning. "Open" magnet design aids in the MR imaging of very large and claustrophobic patients, but these units are generally of lower field strength and lack the resolution of the high-field strength "tube" magnets.

Contrast Administration in MR. Gadolinium chelates are used, similar to the use of iodinated contrast agents in CT, to identify regions of disruption of the blood-brain barrier, to enhance organs to accentuate pathology (Fig. 1.17), and to document patterns of lesion enhancement. Gadolinium is a rare-earth heavy metal ion with paramagnetic effect that shortens the T1 and T2 relaxation times of hydrogen nuclei within its local magnetic field. Gadolinium is essential to providing high-quality MR angiographic studies by enhancing the signal differences between blood vessels and surrounding tissues. At recommended doses,

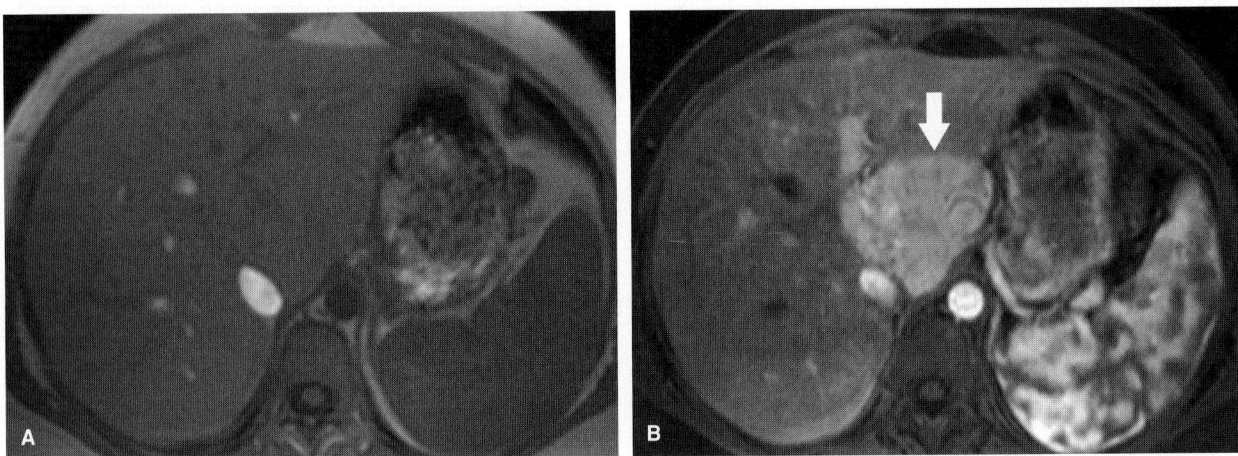

FIGURE 1.17. Contrast Administration in MR. Intravenous administration of gadolinium chelate dramatically increases the conspicuity of the liver mass on an early post-contrast image **(B),** compared to a noncontrast image **(A).** The mottled enhancement of the spleen is caused by the relatively slow diffusion of contrast through the splenic sinusoids.

gadolinium shortens T1 to a much greater extent than it shortens T2. Increases in signal intensity resulting from T1 shortening attributable to concentrations of gadolinium are best seen on T1WI. However, when very high tissue concentration is reached, such as in the renal collecting system, T2 shortening causes a significant loss of signal intensity that is best seen on T2WIs.

Safety Considerations. MR is contraindicated in patients who have electrically, magnetically, or mechanically activated implants, including cardiac pacemakers, insulin pumps, cochlear implants, neurostimulators, bone-growth stimulators, and implantable drug infusion pumps (12,13). Patients with intracardiac pacing wires or Swan-Ganz catheters are at risk for RF current–induced cardiac fibrillation and burns. Ferromagnetic implants, such as cerebral aneurysm clips, vascular clips, and skin staples, are at risk for movement and dislodgment, burns, and induced electrical currents. Bullets, shrapnel, and metallic fragments may move and cause additional injury or become projectiles in the magnetic field. Metal workers and patients with a history of penetrating eye injuries should be screened with radiographs of the orbits to detect intraocular metallic foreign bodies that may dislodge, tear the retina, and cause blindness. A number of implants have been confirmed to be safe for MR, including nonferromagnetic vascular clips and staples and orthopaedic devices composed of nonferromagnetic materials. Prosthetic heart valves with metal components and stainless steel Greenfield filters are considered safe because the in vivo forces affecting them are stronger than the deflecting forces of the electromagnetic field. No convincing body of evidence indicates that short-term exposure to the electromagnetic fields of MR harms a developing fetus, although it is not possible to prove that MR is absolutely safe during pregnancy. Pregnant patients can be scanned, provided the study is medically indicated.

MR Artifacts. Artifacts are intrinsic to MR and must be recognized to avoid mistaking them for disease (14).

A *magnetic susceptibility artifact* is caused by focal distortions in the main magnetic field resulting from the presence of ferromagnetic objects such as orthopaedic devices, surgical clips and wire, dentures, and metallic foreign bodies in the patient. The artifact is seen as areas of signal void at the location of the metal implant (Fig. 1.18), often with a rim of increased intensity and a distortion of the image in the vicinity.

Motion artifacts are common in MR because of the long image acquisition time. Random motion produces blurring of the image. Periodic motion, such as that caused by pulsating blood vessels, causes ghosts of the moving structures (Fig. 1.19). Motion artifacts are most visible along the phase-encoded direction. Swapping phase- and frequency-encoded directions may make the artifacts less bothersome.

Chemical shift misregistration occurs at interfaces between fat and water. Protons bound in lipid molecules experience a slightly lower magnetic influence than protons in water when exposed to an externally applied gradient magnetic field, resulting in misregistration of signal location. The artifact is seen as a line of high signal intensity on one side of the fat-water interface and a line of signal void at the opposite side of the fat-water interface

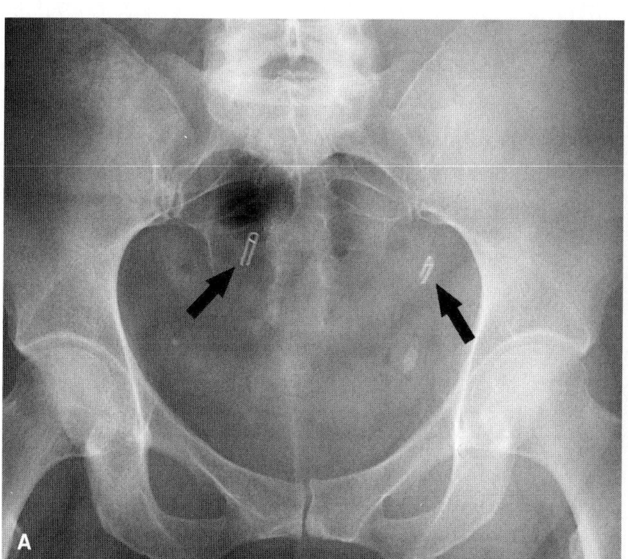

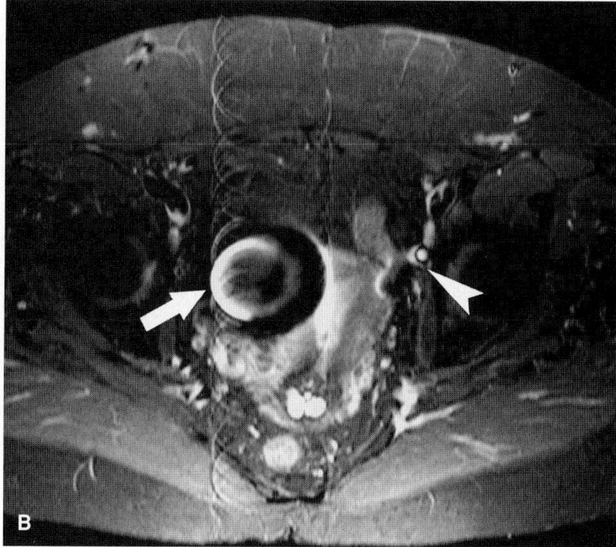

FIGURE 1.18. **Magnetic Susceptibility Artifact.** Radiograph of the pelvis **(A)** and axial plane T2WI **(B)** in the same patient show the artifact (*white arrow, white arrowhead*) produced by metallic clips (*black arrows*) used for tubal ligation. The dramatic increase in artifact on the right side (*white arrow*) as compared to the left side (*white arrowhead*) is caused by proximity of the right-sided clip to a blood vessel, which created a pulsatile motion of the clip.

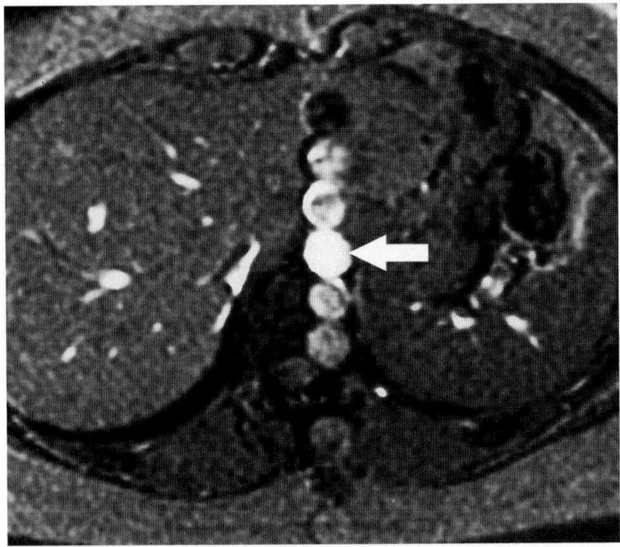

FIGURE 1.19. **Motion Artifact.** Pulsations of the aorta (*arrow*) produce numerous ghosts of the aorta in the phase-encoded direction. Swapping the phase-encoded direction with the frequency-encoded direction will enable evaluation of the left lobe of the liver.

(Fig. 1.20). Evaluation of the bladder wall and renal margins is difficult in the presence of this artifact.

Truncation errors occur adjacent to sharp boundaries between tissues of markedly different contrast. This artifact is attributable to inherent errors in the Fourier transform technique of image reconstruction. The artifact appears as regularly spaced, alternating, parallel bands of bright and dark signal. It may simulate a syrinx of the spinal cord or a meniscal tear in the knee.

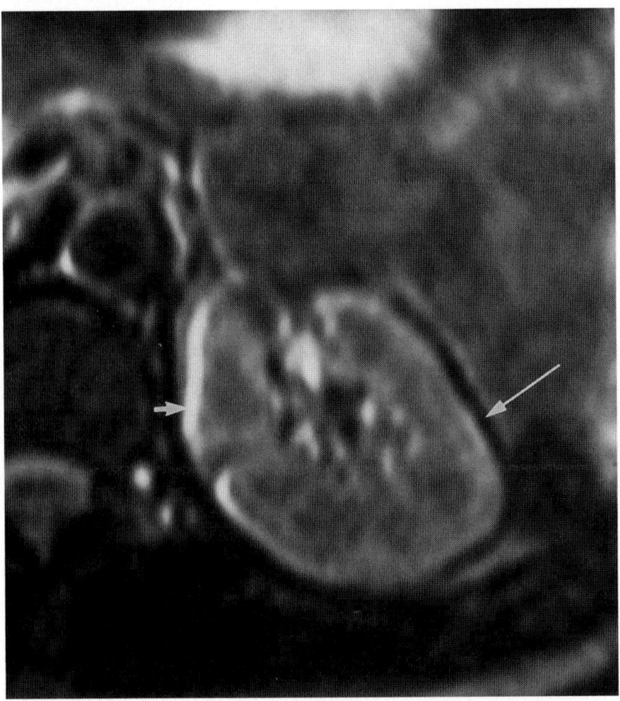

FIGURE 1.20. **Chemical Shift Artifact.** Chemical shift misregistration between fat and kidney tissue produces a high-density band (*short arrow*) on the medial aspect of the left kidney and a low-density band (*long arrow*) on its lateral aspect.

Aliasing, or an image wraparound artifact, occurs when anatomy outside the designated field of view but within the image plane is mismapped onto the opposite side of the image, for instance, on a midline sagittal brain MR, the patient's nose may be artifactually displayed over the area of the posterior fossa. Aliasing may be eliminated by increasing the field of view (at the expense of loss of image resolution) or by increasing the number of phase-encoding steps outside the field of view (oversampling).

Principles of MR Interpretation. Outstanding soft tissue contrast is obtained in MR by designing imaging sequences that accentuate differences in T1 and T2 tissue relaxation times. Sequences that accentuate differences in proton density are fruitful in brain imaging but are generally less useful for extracranial soft tissue imaging, in which proton density differences are small. Interpretation of MR depends on a clear understanding of the biophysical basis of MR tissue contrast. Water is the major source of the MR signal in tissues other than fat. Mineral-rich structures, such as bone and calculi, and collagenous tissues, such as ligaments, tendons, fibrocartilage, and tissue fibrosis, are low in water content and lack mobile protons to produce an MR signal. These tissues are low in signal intensity on all MR sequences. Water in tissue exists in at least two physical states: *free water* with unrestricted motion and *bound water* with restricted motion owing to hydrogen bonding with proteins. Free water is found mainly in extracellular fluid, whereas bound water is found mainly in intracellular fluid. Intracellular water is both bound and free and is in a condition of rapid exchange between the two states.

Free Water. Free water has long T1 and T2 relaxation times, resulting in low signal intensity on T1WIs and high signal intensity on T2WIs (Table 1.1). Organs with abundant extracellular fluid—and therefore large amounts of free water—include the kidneys (urine); ovaries and thyroid (fluid-filled follicles); spleen and penis (stagnant

TABLE 1.1 Rules of MR Soft Tissue Contrast

T1-Weighted Images		
Short T1	→	High signal
Long T1	→	Low signal
T2-Weighted Images		
Short T2	→	Low signal
Long T2	→	High signal

blood); and prostate, testes, and seminal vesicles (fluid in tubules) (Table 1.2). Edema is an increase in extracellular fluid and tends to have the effect of prolonging T1 and T2 relaxation times in affected tissues. Most neoplastic tissues have an increase in extracellular fluid as well as an increase in the proportion of intracellular free water, resulting in tumor visualization with bright signal intensity on T2WIs. In organs such as the kidney that are also rich in extracellular or free water, neoplasms may appear isointense or hypointense compared with the bright normal parenchyma on T2WIs. Neoplasms that are hypocellular or fibrotic appear dark on T2WIs because fibrous tissue dominates their signal characteristics. Simple cysts, cerebrospinal fluid, urine in the bladder, and bile in the gallbladder all reflect the signal characteristics of free water.

Proteinaceous Fluids. The addition of protein to free water has the effect of shortening the T1 relaxation time, thus brightening the signal on T1WIs. T2 relaxation is also shortened, but the T1 shortening effect is dominant even on T2WIs. Therefore, proteinaceous fluid collections remain bright on T2WIs. Proteinaceous fluids include synovial fluid, complicated cysts, abscesses, many pathologic fluid collections, and necrotic areas within tumors.

Soft Tissues. Soft tissues that have a predominance of intracellular bound water have shorter T1 and T2 times than do tissues with large amounts of extracellular water. These tissues, which include the liver, pancreas, adrenal glands, and muscle, have intermediate signal intensities on both T1WIs and T2WIs. Intracellular protein synthesis shortens T1 even more; therefore, muscle, because it is less active in protein synthesis, is lower in signal intensity on T1WIs than are organs with more active protein synthesis. Benign tumors with a predominance of normal cells, such as focal nodular hyperplasia in the liver, tend to remain isointense with their surrounding normal parenchyma on all imaging sequences. Hyaline cartilage has a predominance of extracellular water, but the water is extensively bound to a mucopolysaccharide matrix. Its signal characteristics resemble cellular soft tissues, and it is intermediate in strength on most imaging sequences.

Fat. Protons in fat are bound to hydrophobic intermediate-sized molecules and exchange energy efficiently within their chemical environment. T1 relaxation time is short, resulting in a bright signal on T1WIs. T2 of fat is shorter than T2 of water, resulting in lower signal intensity for fat, relative to water, on strongly T2WIs. On images with lesser degrees of T2 weighting, T1 effect predominates and fat appears isointense or slightly hyperintense compared with water. Specialized fat-saturation imaging sequences may be used to reduce the signal intensity of fat and enhance the visibility of edema and pathologic processes within fat. STIR sequences suppress signals from all tissues with short T1 times, including fat.

Flowing Blood. The MR signal of slow-moving blood, such as in the spleen, venous plexuses, and cavernous hemangiomas, is dominated by the large amount of extracellular water present, resulting in low signal on T1WIs and high signal on T2WIs. Higher-velocity blood flow, however, alters the MR signal in complex ways, depending on multiple factors. Protons may move out of the imaging plane between RF absorption and RF release, resulting in high-velocity signal loss. Alternatively, blood may be replaced by fully magnetized blood from outside of the image volume, resulting in flow-related enhancement. Flow-related enhancement predominates in GRE imaging, resulting in bright signal intensity ("white blood") for flowing blood, whereas high-velocity signal loss predominates in spin-echo imaging, resulting in signal void ("black blood") in areas of flowing blood.

TABLE 1.2 MR of Tissues and Body Fluids

Tissue/Body Fluid	*Examples*	*T1WI Signal*	*T2WI Signal*
Gas	Air in lung, gas in bowel	Absent	Absent
Mineral-rich tissue	Cortical bone, calculi	Absent	Absent
Collagenous tissue	Ligaments, tendons, fibrocartilage, scar tissue	Low	Low
Fat	Adipose tissue, fatty bone marrow	High	Intermediate to high
High bound water tissue	Liver, pancreas, adrenal, muscle, hyaline cartilage	Low	Low to intermediate
High free water tissue	Kidney, testes, prostate, seminal vesicles, ovary, thyroid, spleen, penis, simple cysts, bladder, gallbladder, edema, urine, bile, CSF	Low	High
Proteinaceous fluid	Complicated cysts, abscess, synovial fluid, nucleus pulposis	Intermediate	High

Modified from Mitchell DG, Burk DL Jr, Vinitski S, Rifkin MD. The biophysical basis of tissue contrast in extracranial MR imaging. AJR Am J Roentgenol 1987;149:831–837.

TABLE 1.3 MR of Hemorrhage

Age	Dominant Component	T1WI Signal	T2WI Signal
Hyperacute (<1 day)			
Arterial	Free water + oxyhemoglobin	Low	High
Venous	Free water + deoxyhemoglobin	Low	Less bright than arterial hemorrhage
Acute (1–6 days)	Deoxyhemoglobin	Low	Low
Chronic (>7 days)	Methemoglobin		
	Intracellular	High	Low
	Extracellular	High	High
Scar	Hemosiderin	Low	Low

Modified from Mitchell DG, Burk DL Jr, Vinitski S, Rifkin MD. The biophysical basis of tissue contrast in extracranial MR imaging. AJR Am J Roentgenol 1987;149:831–837.

Hemorrhage. MR of hemorrhage depends on the age of the hemorrhage, the physical and oxidative state of hemoglobin, the location of the hemorrhage, and whether the source of hemorrhage was arterial or venous (Table 1.3) (15). Hemorrhage in the first few hours (hyperacute) is high in free water and thus has low signal on T1WIs and high signal on T2WIs. Immediately following intraparenchymal arterial hemorrhage, red blood cells are saturated with oxygen and contain oxyhemoglobin, which is not paramagnetic and has little effect on the MR signal from surrounding water protons. Hemorrhage from a venous source contains deoxyhemoglobin, which is paramagnetic and does affect signal from surrounding water protons. Intracellular deoxyhemoglobin selectively shortens T2, reducing signal intensity on T2WIs. Thus, acute hemorrhage from a venous source is not as bright on T2WIs as is acute hemorrhage from an arterial source. Within a few hours, red blood cells, from either arterial or venous sources, desaturate and contain predominantly deoxyhemoglobin. The most hypoxic and desaturated portions of the hematoma have the lowest signal. A dark hematoma at this stage is often surrounded by high intensity owing to encircling serum and edema. By approximately 1 week, intracellular deoxyhemoglobin is converted to intracellular methemoglobin beginning at the periphery of the clot. Intracellular methemoglobin is paramagnetic but has restricted motion and is heterogeneous in distribution, shortening T1 and selectively shortening T2, resulting in high signal on T1WIs and low signal on T2WIs. Lysis of red blood cells at 1 week to 1 month increases access of methemoglobin to water molecules, enhancing the T1 shortening effect. T1 shortening predominates over T2 shortening even on T2WIs, resulting in high signal on both T1WIs and T2WIs. The more dilute the concentration of extracellular methemoglobin (the more water that is present), the higher the signal intensity on T2WIs. Areas of low signal intensity on T2WIs correspond to retracted clot with intact red cell membranes.

At approximately the same time as lysis of red blood cells is occurring centrally within the clot, releasing free methemoglobin, hemosiderin is being ingested by macrophages at the periphery of the clot. Hemosiderin is highly paramagnetic, but water insolubility precludes close interaction with water, thus restricting T1 shortening. Limited motion of hemosiderin in its intracellular location causes local inhomogeneous magnetic susceptibility and T2 shortening. The result is low signal on both T1WIs and T2WIs. Edema surrounding the hypointense band of hemosiderin produces a concentric outer rim of hyperintensity as long as edema is present. Hemosiderin-laden macrophages quickly enter the bloodstream, removing hemosiderin from hematoma in nonneural tissues and in areas of the brain where the blood-brain barrier is destroyed, such as in areas of hemorrhage into a tumor. Where the blood-brain barrier is quickly repaired, the hemosiderin may remain in brain tissue for long periods and be seen as an area of persisting low intensity. Differentiation of hematoma from other tissues generally requires at least two pulse sequences. Different areas of the hematoma may show signal intensity effects dominated by components that are in differing stages of evolution.

Ultrasonography

US imaging is performed with the pulse-echo technique (Fig. 1.21) (16–18). The US transducer converts electrical energy to a brief pulse of high-frequency sound energy that is transmitted into patient tissues (19). The US transducer then becomes a receiver, detecting echoes of sound energy reflected from tissue. The depth of any particular echo is determined by measuring the round trip time of flight for the transmitted pulse and the returning echo and by calculating the depth of the reflecting tissue interface by assuming an average speed of sound in tissue of 1,540 m/s. The US instrument assumes that all returning echoes originate from along the line of sight of the transmitted pulse. The composite image is produced by interrogating tissue in the field of view with multiple closely spaced US pulses. The shape and appearance of the resulting image depend on the design of the particular transducer used

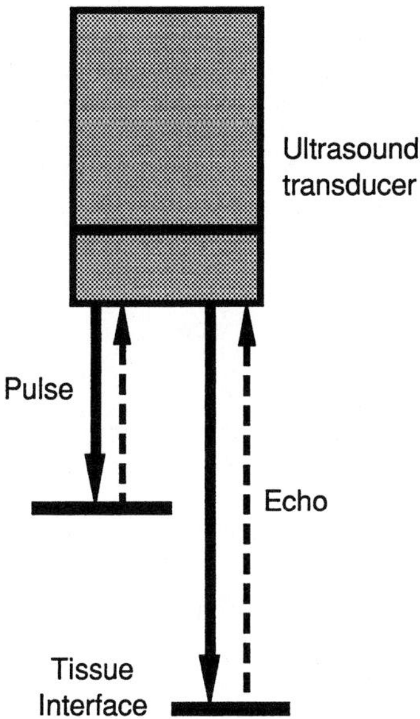

FIGURE 1.21. **US Pulse-Echo Technique.** The US transducer transmits a brief pulse of US energy into tissue. The transmitted US pulse encounters tissue interfaces that reflect a portion of the US beam back to the transducer. The depth of the tissue interface is determined by the round trip time of flight for the transmitted pulse and the returning echo, assuming an average speed of 1,540 m/s for sound transmission in human tissue.

(Fig. 1.22). Modern US units operate sufficiently quickly to produce nearly real-time images of moving patient tissue, enabling assessment of respiratory and cardiac movement, vascular pulsations, peristalsis, and the moving fetus. Most medical imaging is performed using US transducers that produce sound pulses in the frequency range of 1 to 10 MHz. Higher-frequency transducers (5 to 10 MHz) yield the greatest spatial resolution but are restricted by limited penetration. Lower-frequency transducers (1 to 3.5 MHz) enable better penetration of tissues but at the cost of poorer resolution. High-frequency transducers are routinely used for endoluminal applications; examination of superficial structures such as thyroid, breast, and testes; and examination of infants, children, and small adults. Lower-frequency transducers are used for most abdominal, pelvic, and obstetric applications.

US examinations are performed by applying the US transducer directly onto the patient's skin using a water-soluble gel as a coupling agent to ensure good contact and transmission of the US beam. Images may be produced in any anatomic plane by adjusting the orientation and angulation of the transducer and the position of the patient. The standard orthogonal planes—axial, sagittal, and coronal—provide the easiest recognition of anatomy but may not be optimal for demonstration of all anatomic structures. The quality of all US examinations depends heavily on the skill and diligence of the sonographer. US examinations generally provide the most diagnostic information when they are directed at solving a particular clinical problem.

Visualization of anatomic structures by US is limited by bone and by gas-containing structures such as bowel and lung. Sound energy is nearly completely absorbed at interfaces between soft tissue and bone, causing an acoustic shadow with limited visualization of structures deep to the bone surface. Soft tissue–gas interfaces cause nearly complete reflection of the sound beam, preventing visualization of deeper structures. Optimal visualization of many organs is performed through "acoustic windows" that allow adequate sound transmission. The liver is imaged through the windows of the intercostal spaces. The pancreas is visualized through the window of the left lobe of the liver. Pelvic organs are examined through the urine-filled bladder, which displaces the gas-filled bowel out of the pelvis. US visualization of structures in the chest depends on finding windows between bone and air-filled lung. US examination may also be limited by surgical wounds, dressings, and skin lesions, which preclude firm transducer contact with the skin. Endoluminal techniques obviate many of the problems of surface scanning. Endovaginal transducers allow close and highly detailed visualization of the uterus and ovaries without intervening tissues. Endorectal transducers enable intimate examination of the prostate gland and rectum.

Doppler US is an important adjunct to real-time gray-scale imaging. The Doppler effect is a shift in the frequency of returning echoes, compared with the transmitted pulse, caused by reflection of the sound wave from a moving object. In medical imaging, the moving objects of interest are red blood cells in flowing blood. If blood flow is relatively away from the face of the transducer, the echo frequency is shifted lower. If blood flow is relatively toward the face of the transducer, the echo frequency is shifted higher. The amount of frequency shift is proportional to the relative velocity of the red blood cells.

Doppler US can detect not only the presence of blood flow but can also determine its direction and velocity. The Doppler frequency shift is in the audible range, producing a sound of blood flow that has additional diagnostic value. *Pulsed Doppler* uses a Doppler sample volume that is time-gated to interrogate only a select volume of patient tissue for the Doppler shift. *Duplex Doppler* combines real-time gray-scale imaging with pulsed Doppler to enable accurate placement of the Doppler sample volume in visualized blood vessels or specific areas of interest. *Color Doppler* combines gray scale and color-coded Doppler information in a single image. Stationary tissue with echoes having no Doppler shift are displayed in shades of gray, whereas blood flow and moving tissue, which produce echoes with a detectable Doppler shift, are displayed in color. Blood flow relatively toward the transducer face is usually displayed in shades of red, whereas blood flow relatively away from the transducer face is displayed in shades of blue. Lighter

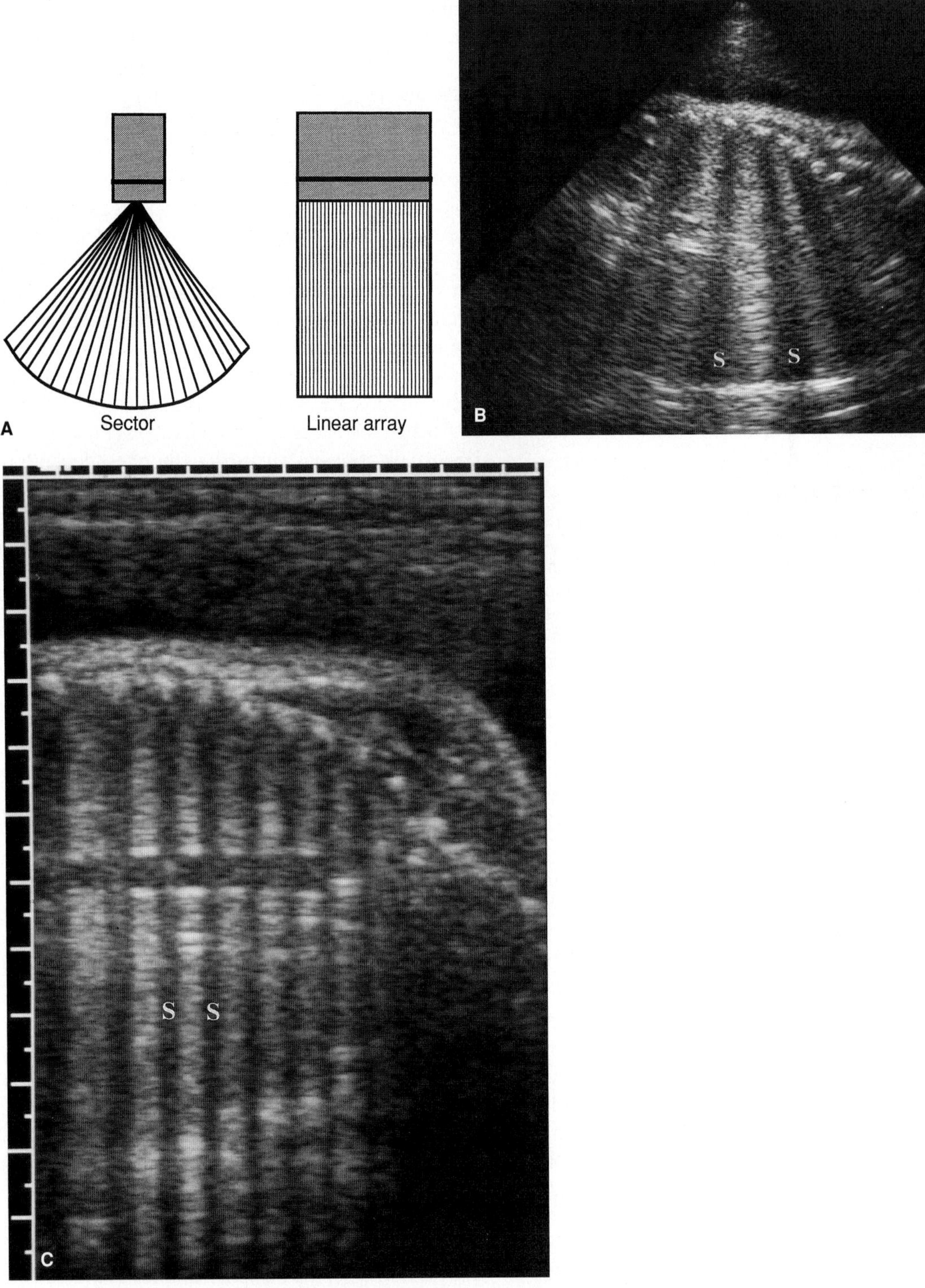

FIGURE 1.22. **Sector Versus Linear Array US Transducers. A.** Diagram of the diverging US beams transmitted by a sector transducer *(left)* and the parallel US beams transmitted by a linear array transducer *(right)*. Sector transducers have the advantage of wider field of view in the far field, whereas linear array transducers have a wider field of view in the near field. **B.** Sector transducer image of a fetus shows prominent shadowing (S) from the fetal ribs. Note how the width of the shadows expands with increasing depth because of the diverging US beams. **C.** Linear array transducer image of the same fetus shows parallel nonwidening shadows (S) from the fetal ribs. Note the improved visualization in the near field.

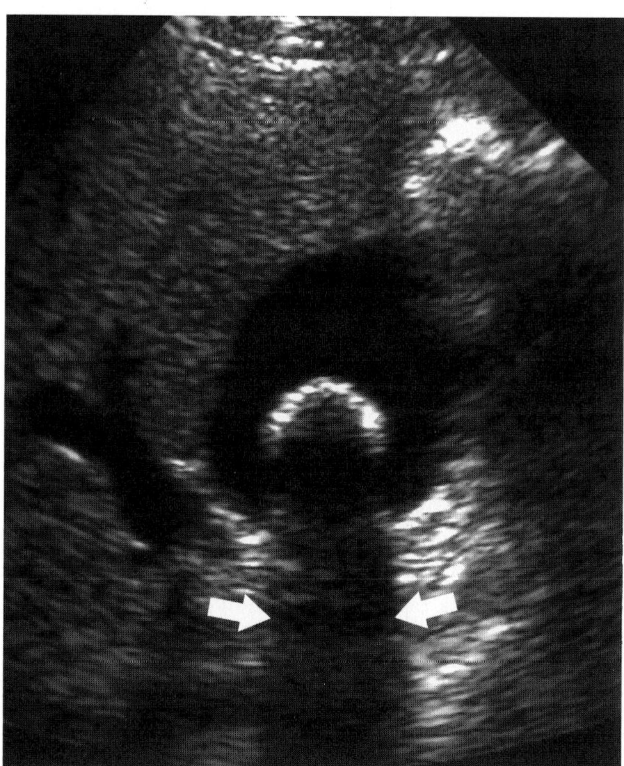

FIGURE 1.23. **Acoustic Shadowing.** A gallstone within the gallbladder produces a dark acoustic shadow (*arrows*) by absorption of the US beam. Demonstration of acoustic shadowing is important in the US detection of biliary and renal calculi.

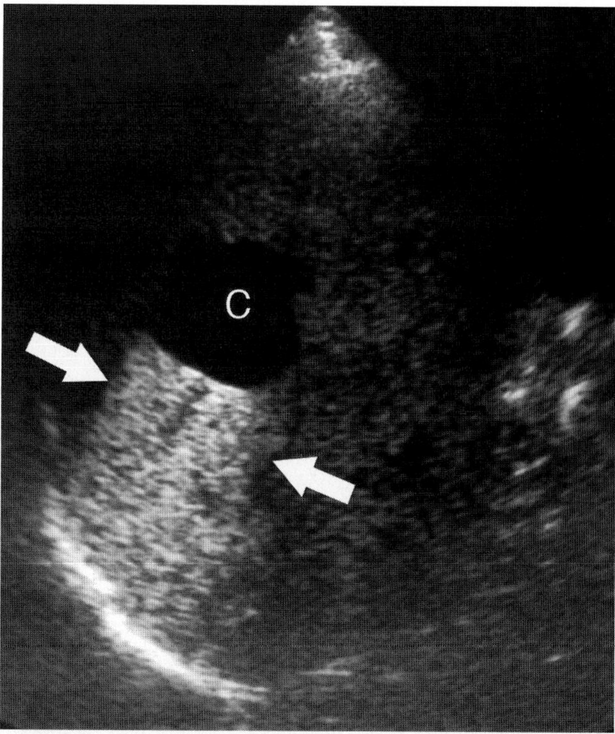

FIGURE 1.24. **Acoustic Enhancement.** US image of a cyst (C) in the liver demonstrates acoustic enhancement (*arrows*) as a band of bright echoes deep to the cyst.

shades of color imply higher flow velocities. Doppler US is discussed in further detail in Chapter 40.

US Artifacts. Artifacts are extremely common in US imaging and must be recognized to avoid diagnostic errors (20). Some artifacts, such as acoustic shadowing, are diagnostically useful.

Acoustic shadowing is produced by nearly complete absorption or reflection of the US beam, obscuring deeper tissue structures. Acoustic shadows are produced by gallstones (Fig. 1.23), urinary tract stones, bone, metallic objects, and gas bubbles. The presence of acoustic shadowing aids in the identification of all types of calculi.

Acoustic enhancement refers to the increased intensity of echoes deep to structures that transmit sound exceptionally well, such as cysts (Fig. 1.24), fluid-filled bladder and gallbladder, and some solid masses, such as lymphoma-replaced lymph nodes. The presence of acoustic enhancement aids in the identification of cystic masses.

Reverberation artifacts are caused by repeated reflections between strong acoustic reflectors. Returning echoes are re-reflected into tissues, producing multiple echoes of the same structures that are portrayed on the image progressively deeper in tissue because of the prolonged time of flight of echoes that eventually return to the transducer. A reverberation artifact is seen as repeating bands of echoes of progressively decreasing intensity at regularly spaced intervals.

Mirror-image artifacts are common when examining the upper abdomen and diaphragm. Multipath reflection from the strong sound reflection produced by the air-filled lung surface above the curving diaphragm results in depiction of liver or spleen tissue patterns both below and above the diaphragm (Fig. 1.25).

The *ring down,* or *comet tail,* artifact is seen as a pattern of tapering bright echoes trailing from small bright reflectors such as air bubbles and cholesterol crystals. The artifact may be the result of vibrations of the reflector or of multiple short-path reverberations.

Principles of US Interpretation. Interpretation of US examination is best performed by the radiologist who has studied the images produced by the sonographer and who, with transducer in hand, has personally examined the patient. US in the hands of a skilled physician is a dynamic extension of physical examination. The examining physician has the opportunity to query the patient regarding current and past symptoms, previous surgery, and pertinent medical history. Suspected masses can be palpated, as well as examined by US. Artifacts are more easily differentiated from true components of the image during real-time examination. Active examination enables rapid assessment of

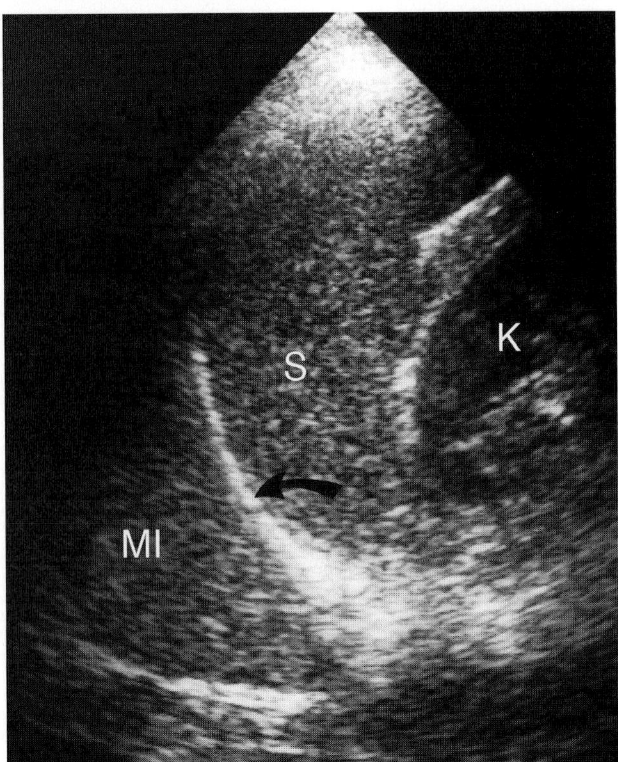

FIGURE 1.25. **Mirror-Image Artifact.** Longitudinal image of the left upper quadrant of the abdomen demonstrates the spleen (S), diaphragm (*arrow*), and artifactual mirror image (*MI*) of the spleen above the diaphragm. K, left kidney.

three-dimensional anatomic relationships. The real-time US examination yields thousands of images within a few minutes. The static recorded images serve only to document the dynamic real-time examination. All questions of interpretation should be answered by active sonographic examination.

Fluid-containing structures such as cysts, dilated calyces and ureters, and the distended bladder and gallbladder characteristically demonstrate well-defined walls, an absence of internal echoes, and distal acoustic enhancement. Solid tissue demonstrates a speckled pattern of tissue texture with definable blood vessels. Fat is usually highly echogenic, whereas solid organs such as the liver, pancreas, and kidney demonstrate lower degrees of echogenicity. Lesions within or arising from organs demonstrate mass effect with alteration of organ contour and displacement of blood vessels and with alteration in tissue texture. Lesions of lower echogenicity (lower-intensity echoes) than surrounding parenchyma are termed *hypoechoic*, and lesions of greater echogenicity (higher-intensity echoes) than surrounding parenchyma are called *hyperechoic*. The term *anechoic* refers to the complete absence of echoes, such as within simple cysts. Cystic structures that contain echogenic fluid such as blood, pus, or mucin may cause confusion in the sonographic differentiation of cystic and solid lesions. Echogenic cystic structures demonstrate an absence of internal blood vessels, fluid-fluid layering, shifting contents with transducer compression or change in patient position, and well-defined walls. Acoustic enhancement might or might not be present.

RADIOGRAPHIC CONTRAST AGENTS

Iodinated Contrast Agents

Water-soluble contrast agents, which consist of molecules containing atoms of iodine, are used extensively for intravascular applications in CT, urography, and angiography, and for arthrography, cystography, fistulography, and opacification of the lumen of the GI tract (21). With the ever-expanding use of CT, the number of patients exposed to iodinated contrast agents continues to increase. Fortunately, the risk of adverse reaction is low, but real risk is inherent in their use. The administration of any contrast agent, regardless of dose or route of administration, carries a finite risk of mild to life-threatening reaction. Older, cheaper, high-osmolar ionic agents have been replaced in most applications by newer but more expensive, low-osmolar agents because of safety considerations.

Ionic contrast agents (high-osmolality contrast agents) have been considered safe and effective for more than 70 years. All iodinated contrast agents have a chemical structure that is based on a benzene ring containing three iodine atoms. Ionic media are acid salts that dissociate in water into an iodine-containing, negatively charged anion (diatrizoate, iothalamate) and a positively charged cation (sodium or meglumine). To achieve a sufficient concentration of iodine for radiographic visualization, ionic agents are markedly hypertonic (approximately six times the osmolality of plasma). High osmolality and viscosity can cause significant hemodynamic, cardiac, and subjective effects, including vasodilatation, heat, pain, osmotic diuresis, and decreased myocardial contractility. Following IV injection, contrast media are distributed quickly into the extracellular space. Excretion is by renal glomerular filtration. Vicarious excretion through the liver, biliary system, and intestinal tract occurs when renal function is impaired.

Nonionic contrast agents (low-osmolality contrast agents) have an osmolality reduced to one to three times that of blood, resulting in a significant decrease in the already low incidence of adverse reactions. Reduction in osmolality is achieved by making compounds that are nonionic monomers (iopamidol [Isovue], iohexol [Omnipaque], ioversol [Optiray]); nonionic dimers (iodixanol [Visipaque], ioxilan [Oxilan]); or monoacidic dimers (ioxaglate [Hexabrix]). Iodixanol is iso-osmolar with plasma (22). Reduced osmolality results in less hemodynamic alteration on contrast injection. Nonionic contrast agents continue to be significantly more expensive than ionic contrast agents.

Adverse side effects are uncommon, ranging from 5% to 12% of intravascular injections with ionic agents to 1% to 3% with nonionic lower-osmolality agents (21). The precise pathophysiology of adverse reactions to contrast agents is unknown. However, an increasing body of evidence suggests that a true allergic reaction mediated by immunoglobulin E is a likely precipitating event. Triggering of mast cells to release histamine is related to severe reactions. Accurate prediction of contrast reactions is not possible, but patients with a history of allergy, asthma, or previous contrast reaction are clearly at higher risk. Cardiovascular effects are more common and more severe in patients with cardiac disease.

Mild adverse effects are most common. Nausea, vomiting, urticaria, feeling of warmth with injection, and pain at the injection site occur with greater frequency following injection of ionic agents and are related to their higher osmolality. Most mild reactions do not require treatment. Patients should be observed for 20 to 30 minutes to ensure that the reaction does not become more severe.

Moderate reactions are not life threatening but commonly require treatment for symptoms. Patients with severe hives, vasovagal reactions, bronchospasm, and mild laryngeal edema should be monitored until symptoms resolve. Diphenhydramine is effective for relief of symptomatic hives. Beta-agonist inhalers help with bronchospasm, and epinephrine is indicated for laryngeal spasm. Leg elevation is indicated for vasovagal reactions and hypotension.

Severe, potentially life-threatening side effects nearly always occur within the first 20 minutes following intravascular injection. These are rare but should be recognized and treated immediately. The risk of death precipitated by intravenous injection of iodinated contrast is estimated at 1 in 130,000 (23). Severe bronchospasm or severe laryngeal edema may progress to loss of consciousness, seizures, and cardiac arrest. Complete cardiovascular collapse requires life-support equipment and immediate cardiopulmonary resuscitation. Cardiotoxic effects include hypotension, dysrhythmias, and precipitation of acute congestive heart failure.

Local adverse effects. Venous thrombosis may occur as a result of endothelial damage precipitated by intravenous infusion of contrast. Extravasation of contrast at the injection site is associated with pain, edema, skin slough, or deeper tissue necrosis. If extravasation occurs, the affected limb should be elevated. Warm compresses may help with absorption of the contrast agent, while cold compresses seem more effective at reducing pain at the injection site.

Contrast-induced nephropathy, defined as acute renal failure occurring within 48 hours of contrast agent administration, is a significant source of morbidity related to the expanded use of contrast-enhanced imaging (24,25). Serum creatinine levels rise in the first 24 hours following contrast administration, peak at 3 to 5 days, and usually return to baseline by 10 to 14 days. Some patients are left with permanent renal damage. Oliguric renal failure with 24-hour urine volume <400 mL may occur. The incidence of contrast-induced nephropathy, defined as >25% increase in serum creatinine within 5 days, is approximately 2% in the general population but considerably higher in high-risk populations. The most prominent risk factors are diabetes and chronic renal insufficiency. The incidence of contrast-induced nephropathy is 9% to 40% in diabetics with mild to moderate renal insufficiency and 50% to 90% in diabetics with severe renal insufficiency. Adequate hydration is essential in the prevention of contrast-induced nephropathy. Patients should be encouraged to drink several liters of fluid over the 12 to 24 hours before and after intravascular contrast administration. Administration of N-acetylcysteine and use of iodixanol (Visipaque) appear to be somewhat effective in preventing contrast-induced nephropathy. N-acetylcysteine is given orally (600 mg twice daily the day before and on the day of contrast administration) or IV (150 mg/kg in 500 mL of normal saline over 30 minutes prior to the examination and 50 mg/kg in 500 mL of normal saline over 4 hours after the examination). The benefit of use of iodixanol is suggested by several studies but remains to be proven.

Patients on chronic dialysis are at risk for adverse effect of the osmotic load of contrast and its direct toxicity on the heart. Because contrast agents are readily cleared from the blood by dialysis, dialysis on the same day as contrast administration is prudent.

Metformin (Glucophage) is an oral antihyperglycemic agent used to treat Type 2 diabetes mellitus. It may precipitate potentially fatal lactic acidosis in the presence of renal impairment. The U.S. Food and Drug Administration recommends temporarily withholding metformin in patients receiving iodinated contrast agents for radiographic studies. Metformin should be discontinued for 48 hours after contrast administration and reinstated only after renal function has been reevaluated and found to be normal (21). Withholding metformin is not necessary following gadolinium administration in the smaller doses used for MR. If gadolinium is used in large doses for conventional angiography, metformin should be withheld for 48 hours.

Patients at high risk for adverse reactions should be identified (21). The need for contrast administration should be reassessed with consideration of diagnostic alternatives. If contrast is to be administered the patient should be adequately hydrated. Premedication should be considered. Risk factors include the following: (*1*) previous history of adverse reaction to contrast agents administered intravascularly (sensation of heat, flushing, or a single episode of nausea or vomiting does not increase the risk); (*2*) a clear history of asthma or allergies (atopic individuals; a history of specific allergies to shellfish or iodine is not reliable as a predictor of contrast reaction); (*3*) known cardiac dysfunction, including severe congestive heart failure, severe arrhythmias, unstable angina, recent myocardial infarction, or pulmonary hypertension; (*4*) renal insufficiency, especially in patients with diabetes; (*5*) sickle cell disease; (*6*) multiple myeloma; (*7*) age over 55 years.

Premedication regimens have been proven to decrease, but not eliminate, the frequency of contrast reactions. Two regimens listed by the American College of Radiology (21) are:

1. Prednisone 50 mg orally taken at 13, 7, and 1 hour prior to contrast administration. Diphenhydramine 50 mg orally, IV, or intramuscularly at 1 hour prior to contrast. Use nonionic low-osmolality agent.
2. Methylprednisolone 32 mg orally at 12 and 2 hours prior to contrast administration. Use of diphenhydramine is optional. Nonionic low-osmolality agent should be used.

Magnetic Resonance Imaging Intravascular Contrast Agents

Gadolinium chelates are the most commonly used MR contrast agents. They enhance tissue on MR by paramagnetic effect produced by the presence of gadolinium within the molecule. Available agents include ionic contrast agents (gadopentetate dimeglumine Magnevist and gadobenate dimeglumine [MultiHance]) and nonionic agents (gadodiamide [Omniscan], gadoteridol [ProHance], and gadoversetamide [OptiMark]). The agents differ primarily in osmolality and viscosity. Their distribution and elimination are very similar to the water-soluble, iodine-based contrast agents used in CT. Gadolinium chelates are injected intravenously, diffuse rapidly into the extracellular fluid and blood pool spaces, and are excreted by glomerular filtration. Approximately 80% of the injected dose is excreted within 3 hours. MR imaging is usually performed immediately after injection.

Adverse reactions to gadolinium agents administered at the 0.1 to 0.2 mmol/kg doses used for MR are quite uncommon (0.07% to 2.4%) (21). Mild reactions of nausea, vomiting, headache, warmth or coldness at the injection site, paresthesias, dizziness, or itching are most common. Life-threatening reactions are rare (<0.01%). Gadolinium has no nephrotoxicity at doses used for MR. Since gadolinium agents are radiodense, they have been recommended for use in conventional angiography in patients with renal impairment or history of severe reaction to iodinated agents.

Gastrointestinal Contrast Agents

Barium sulfate is the standard opaque contrast agent for routine fluoroscopic contrast studies of the upper and lower GI tract. Current formulations provide excellent coating of the GI mucosa. "Thin," more fluid suspensions are used for single-contrast studies, whereas "thick," more viscous suspensions coat the mucosa for double-contrast examinations. Barium preparations are remarkably well tolerated. Aspiration of barium rarely causes a clinical problem. Small amounts are cleared from the lungs within hours; however, huge amounts may result in pneumonia. Suspected allergic reactions, including hives, respiratory arrest, and anaphylaxis, have been reported rarely; allergic reactions to the latex used in enema balloons and rectal examination gloves are more common than reactions to the barium products themselves. The major risk from the use of barium sulfate is barium peritonitis resulting from the spill of barium into the peritoneal cavity as a result of perforations of the GI tract. Barium deposits act as foreign bodies, inducing fibrin deposition and massive ascites. Bacterial contamination from intestinal contents can lead to sepsis, shock, and death in up to 50% of patients.

Gas Agents. Air and carbon dioxide gas are effective and inexpensive contrast agents for both CT and fluoroscopic studies. A number of effervescent powders, granules, and tablets that release carbon dioxide on contact with water are routinely used. These preparations are excellent for distending the stomach for CT or barium studies. Injection of air directly into the GI tract via a nasogastric or enema tube may be used to distend the stomach or colon.

Water-soluble iodinated contrast media opacify the bowel lumen by passive filling, rather than mucosal coating, and are considered by most radiologists to be inferior to barium agents for routine fluoroscopic GI studies. Because of the high mortality associated with barium peritonitis, however, water-soluble agents are indicated when GI tract perforation is suspected. Water-soluble agents are quickly reabsorbed through the peritoneal surface if a perforation is present. Dilute solutions (2% to 5%) of ionic agents are routinely used in CT to opacify the GI tract. Ionic contrast agents stimulate intestinal peristalsis, which promotes faster opacification of the distal bowel on CT and may be useful in the postoperative patient with ileus. The major risk of oral water-soluble agents is aspiration, which causes chemical pneumonitis. Low-osmolar agents may be safer and are preferred when aspiration is deemed a risk. Large volumes of hypertonic water-soluble agents in the GI tract draw water into the gut and may result in hypovolemia, shock, and even death, especially in infants and debilitated adults.

Ultrasound Intravascular Contrast Agents

US contrast agents are now available to improve US characterization of tissue and lesion vascularity, similar to the use of intravascular contrast agents in CT and MR (26). US contrast agents consist of microbubbles of air or perfluorocarbon gas encased within a thin shell made of protein, lipid, or polymers. Their size—slightly smaller than red blood cells—keeps the microbubbles within the vascular system and allows them to flow through the pulmonary circulation to the systemic circulation following peripheral intravenous injection. The contrast thus acts as a blood pool agent. The gas diffuses through its shell, resulting in disappearance of the microbubbles with a half-life in blood of a few minutes. No adverse bioeffects of the agents have been reported. Currently available agents include galactose-palmitic acid (Levovist), albumin microspheres (Optison), and perflutren lipid microspheres (Definity). A variety of US imaging techniques, some requiring additional software or hardware, are utilized for contrast agent imaging. These include power and spectral Doppler, harmonic imaging, and pulse-inversion imaging. The microbubbles interact with the imaging technique, oscillate at a resonant frequency, and can be made to abruptly disrupt to improve the signal from the contrast agent. Imaging is performed in arterial and venous phases. Contrast washout or sustained enhancement of lesions can be assessed.

REFERENCES

1. Bushberg JT, Seibert JA, Leidholdt EMJ, Boone JM. The Essential Physics of Medical Imaging. 2nd ed. Baltimore: Lippincott Williams & Wilkins, 2001.
2. Seibert JA. Considerations for selecting a digital radiography system. J Am Coll Radiol 2005;2: 287–290.
3. Major N. Practical Approach to Radiology [In press]. Philadelphia: Elsevier, 2005.
4. Mahesh M. Search for isotropic resolution in CT from conventional through multiple row detector. RadioGraphics 2002;22:949–962.
5. Cody DD. Image processing in CT. RadioGraphics 2002;22:1255–1268.
6. Rydberg J, Buckwalter KA, Caldemeyer KS, et al. Multisection CT: scanning techniques and clinical applications. RadioGraphics 2000;20:1787–1806.
7. McNitt-Gray MF. Radiation dose in CT. RadioGraphics 2002;22: 1541–1553.
8. Frush DP, Applegate K. Computed tomography and radiation: understanding the issues. J Am Coll Radiol 2004;1:113–119.
9. Barrett JF, Keat N. Artifacts in CT: recognition and avoidance. RadioGraphics 2004;24:1679–1691.
10. Brown MA, Semelka RC. MR imaging abbreviations, definitions, and descriptions: a review. Radiology 1999;213:647–662.
11. Delfault EM, Beltran J, Johnson G, et al. Fat suppression in MR imaging: techniques and pitfalls. RadioGraphics 1999;19:373–382.
12. Kanal E, Borgstede JP, Barkovich AJ, et al. American College of Radiology white paper on MR safety. AJR Am J Roentgenol 2002;178:1335–1347.
13. Kanal E, Borgstede JP, Barkovich AJ, et al. American College of Radiology white paper on MR safety: 2004 update and revisions. AJR Am J Roentgenol 2004;182:1111–1114.
14. Arena L, Morehouse HT, Safir J. MR imaging artifacts that simulate disease: how to recognize and eliminate them. RadioGraphics 1995;15:1373–1394.
15. Mitchell DG, Burk DL Jr, Vinitski S, Rifkin MD. The biophysical basis of tissue contrast in extracranial MR imaging. AJR Am J Roentgenol 1987:831–837.
16. Brant WE. The Core Curriculum: Ultrasound. Philadelphia: Lippincott Williams & Wilkins, 2001:524.
17. Goldstein A. Overview of the physics of US. RadioGraphics 1993;13:701–704.
18. Ziskin MC. Fundamental physics of ultrasound and its propagation in tissue. RadioGraphics 1993;13:705–709.
19. Hangiandreou NJ. B-mode US: basic concepts and new technology. RadioGraphics 2003;23:1019–1033.
20. Keogh CF, Cooperberg PL. Is it real or is it an artifact. Ultrasound Q 2001;17:201–210.
21. American College of Radiology Committee on Drugs and Contrast Media. Manual on Contrast Media. 5th ed. Reston, VA: American College of Radiology, 2004.
22. Association of University Radiologists. Abstracts from the Contrast Media Research Symposium. Acad Radiol 2005;12:S2–S85.
23. Bettmann MA, Heeren T, Greenfield A, et al. Adverse events with radiographic contrast agents: results of the SCVIR contrast agent registry. Radiology 1997;203:611–620.
24. Gleeson TG, Bulugahapitiya S. Contrast-induced nephropathy. AJR Am J Roentgenol 2004;183:1673–1689.
25. Ashley JB, Millward SF. Contrast agent-induced nephropathy: a simple way to identify patients with preexisting renal insufficiency. AJR Am J Roentgenol 2003;181:451–454.
26. Brannigan M, Burns PN, Wilson SR. Blood flow patterns in focal liver lesions at microbubble-enhanced US. RadioGraphics 2004;24:921–935.

SECTION II

Neuroradiology

Section Editor:
Erik H.L. Gaensler

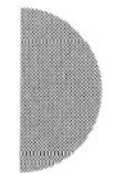

Chapter 2

Introduction to Brain Imaging

David J. Seidenwurm

Looking at the Brain

Current Neuroimaging Options

Imaging Strategy for Common Clinical Syndromes

Analysis of the Abnormality

This chapter provides an atlas of neuroanatomy and a discussion of the principles of brain imaging and interpretation. Brain anatomy is shown on CT in axial plane (Figs. 2.1 to 2.4) and on MR in T2-weighted axial plane (Figs. 2.5 to 2.17) and T1-weighted coronal plane (Figs. 2.18 to 2.27) images. Figures 2.28 to 2.36 are examples of specialized high-resolution MR brain imaging.

LOOKING AT THE BRAIN

A few simple principles can be employed to insure that no neurosurgical emergency is missed, even on a first cursory look at an emergency CT scan at midnight.

Midline. The middle of the patient's brain should be in the middle of the patient's head and the two sides of the brain should look alike (Figs. 2.1 to 2.4). While there are important functional asymmetries between the right and left hemispheres, the anatomic differences are subtle and play no role in clinical neuroradiology. Any shift of midline structures is presumed to represent a mass lesion on the side from which the midline is displaced. For practical purposes, there are no "sucking" brain wounds that draw the midline toward themselves. If the interventricular septum and third ventricle are located in the midline, no subfalcine herniation is present (Fig. 2.1).

Symmetry of the brain is the key to radiologic evaluation. Only experience teaches how much asymmetry is within the range of normal variation. Generally, the sulcal pattern should be symmetric. The sulci on one side are the same size as the corresponding sulci on the other. The anterior interhemispheric fissure should be visualized (Figs. 2.1 and 2.5). Loss of sulci may result from compression owing to mass or opacification of CSF following subarachnoid hemorrhage or, less commonly, meningitis or spreading of a CSF-borne tumor. The sulci extend to the inner table of the skull. In older patients, some atrophy is normal. Significant medial displacement of the sulci may represent compression resulting from an extracerebral fluid collection, such as a subdural or epidural hematoma. Because these may be bilateral and similar in density to the brain, care needs to be taken in evaluating the periphery of the brain.

Basal Cisterns. More subtle, but more important, signs of intracranial mass include distortion of the CSF spaces of the posterior fossa and base of the brain. The key structures here are the quadrigeminal plate cistern and the suprasellar cistern (Figs. 2.2 to 2.4, 2.10, 2.11, 2.19). Because these CSF spaces are traversed by important neural structures, careful attention to these regions is essential. The quadrigeminal plate cistern in the axial plane has the appearance of a symmetric smile (Figs. 2.2 and 2.3). Any asymmetry must be suspect, and abnormality of this cistern may represent rotation of the brain stem resulting from transtentorial herniation, effacement of the cistern on account of cerebellar or brainstem mass, or opacification of the cistern as in subarachnoid hemorrhage.

The suprasellar cistern looks like a pentagon or the Jewish star, depending upon the angulation of the scan through it (Figs. 2.3, 2.4, 2.10, 2.11). The five corners of the pentagon are the interhemispheric fissure anteriorly, the sylvian cisterns anterolaterally, and the ambient cisterns posterolaterally. The sixth point of the Jewish star is in the interpeduncular fossa posteriorly. The cistern has the density of CSF and the structure is symmetric. The anatomic continuations of the cistern are the same

(*text continues on page 44*)

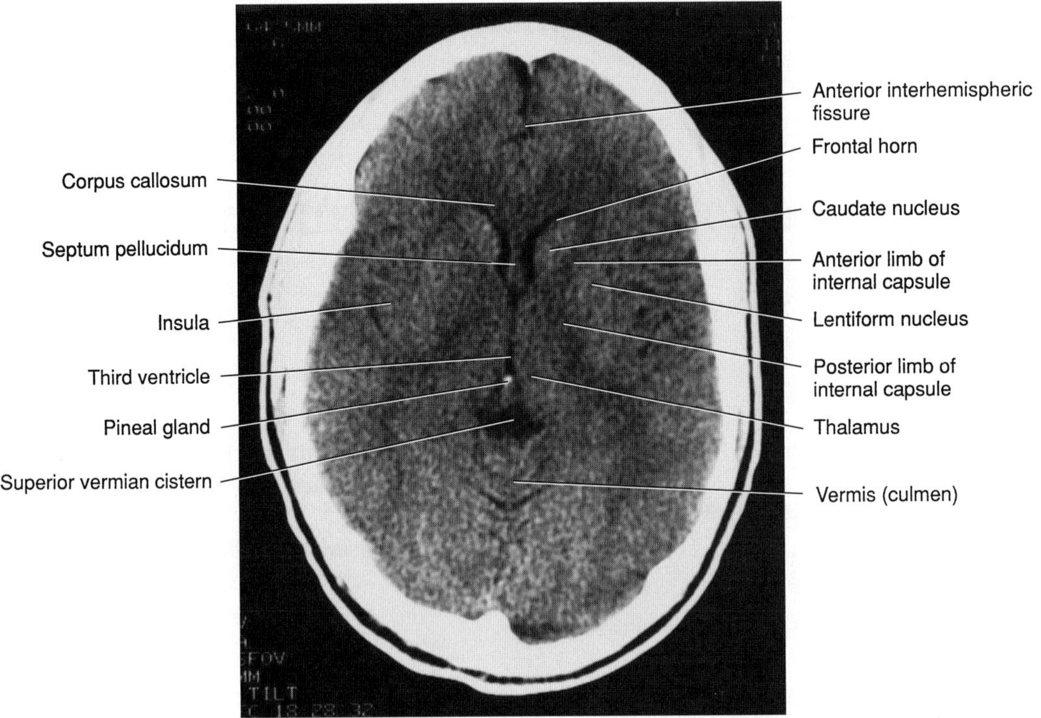

FIGURE 2.1. **Brain CT.** Without intravenous contrast, axial plane through the third ventricle.

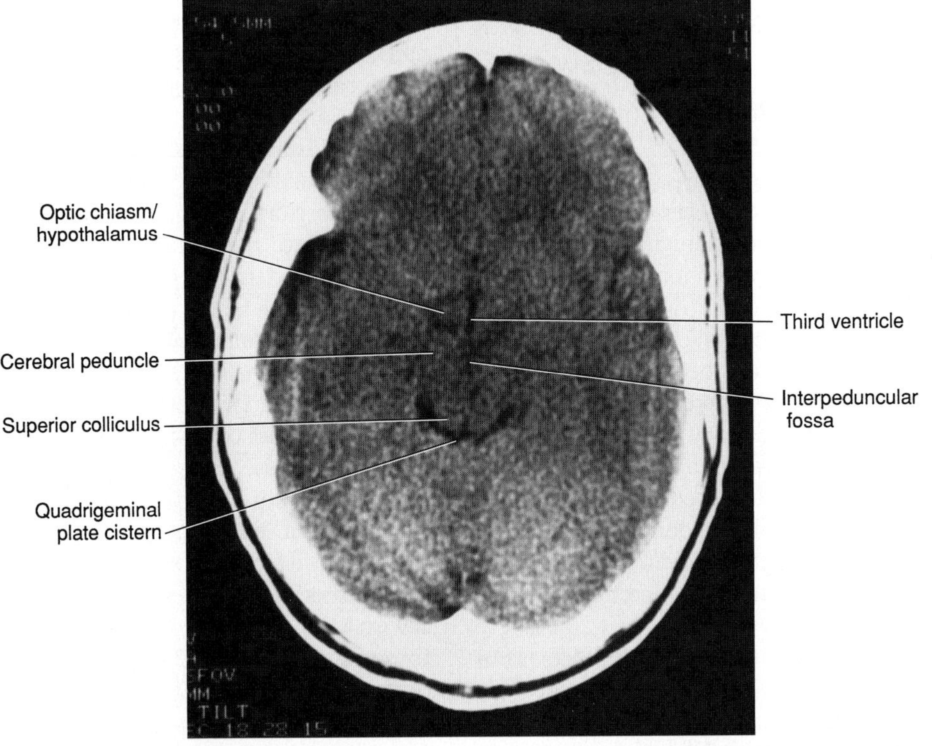

FIGURE 2.2. **Brain CT.** Without intravenous contrast, axial plane through the quadrigeminal plate cistern.

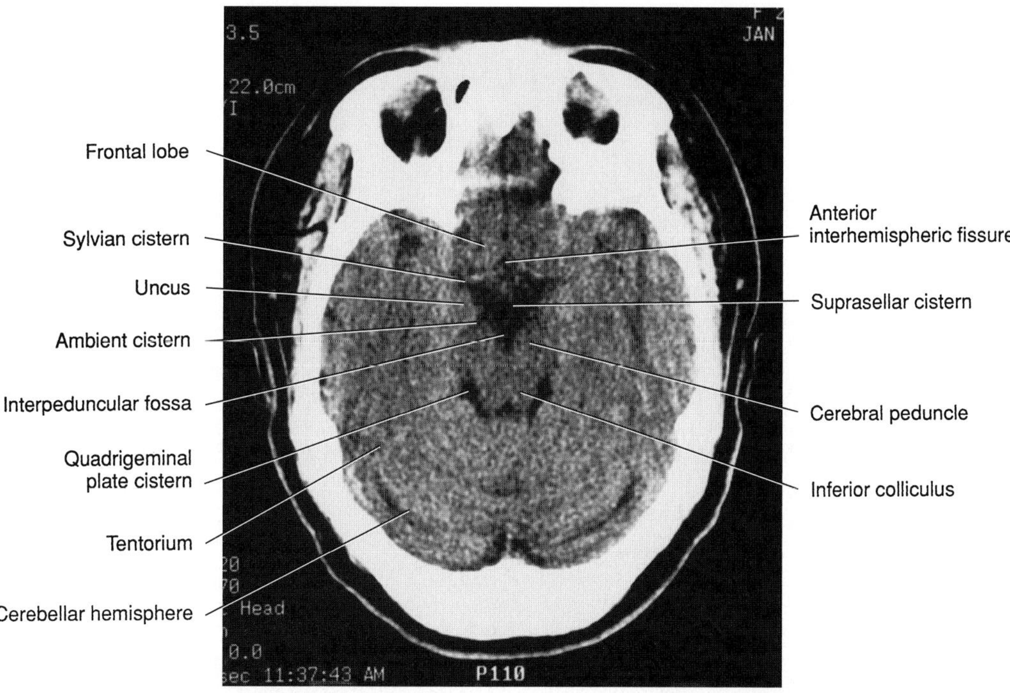

FIGURE 2.3. **Brain CT.** Without intravenous contrast, axial plane through the suprasellar cistern.

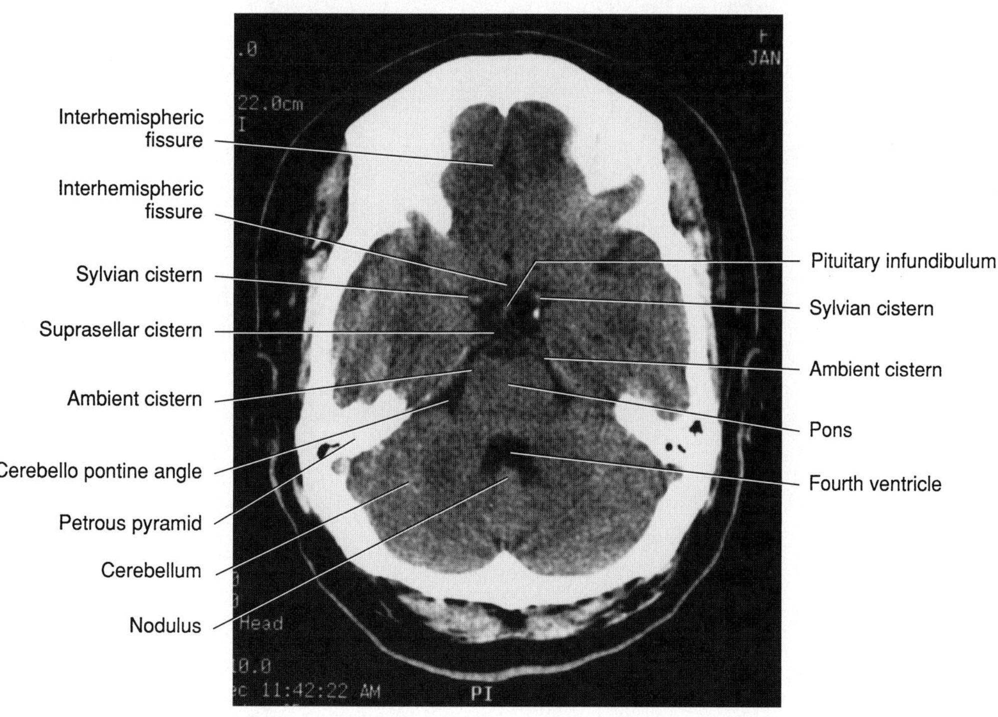

FIGURE 2.4. **Brain CT.** Without intravenous contrast, axial plane through the pons and fourth ventricle.

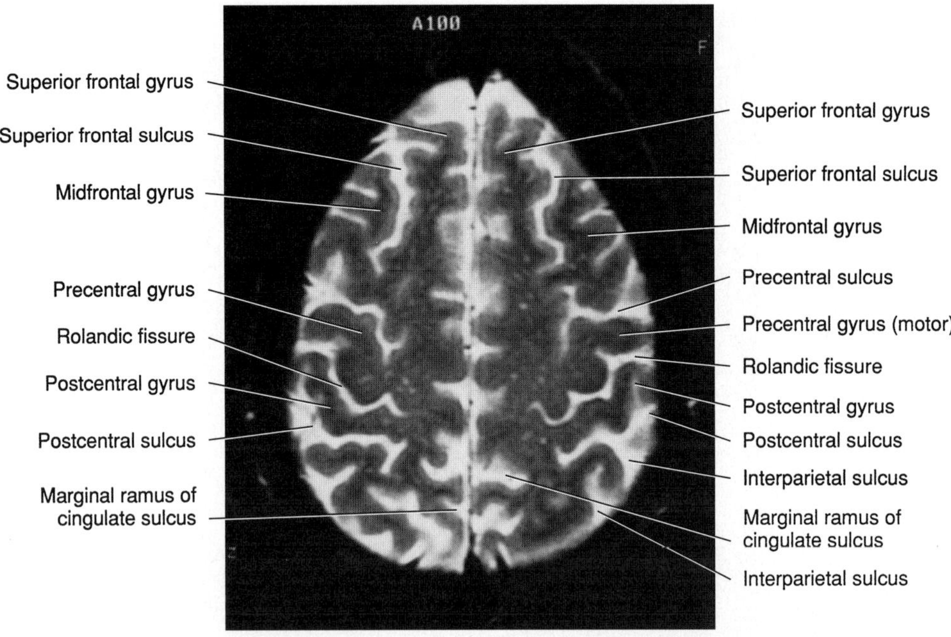

FIGURE 2.5. **Brain MR.** T2-weighted, axial plane through the cerebral hemispheres.

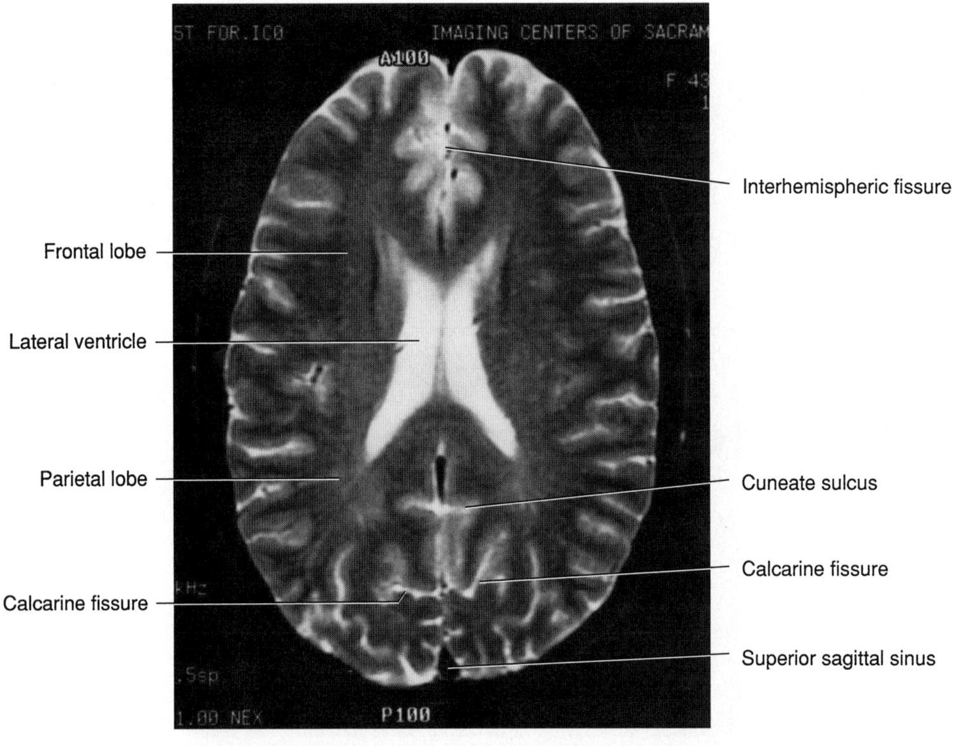

FIGURE 2.6. **Brain MR.** T2-weighted, axial plane through the body of the lateral ventricles.

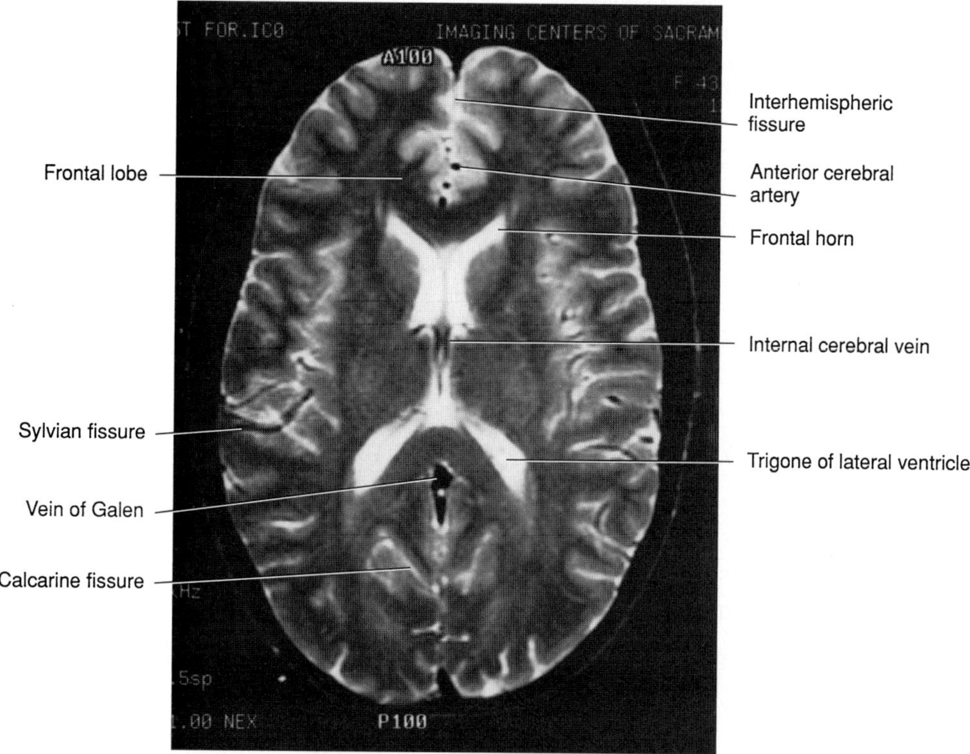

FIGURE 2.7. **Brain MR.** T2-weighted, axial plane through level of the internal cerebral veins.

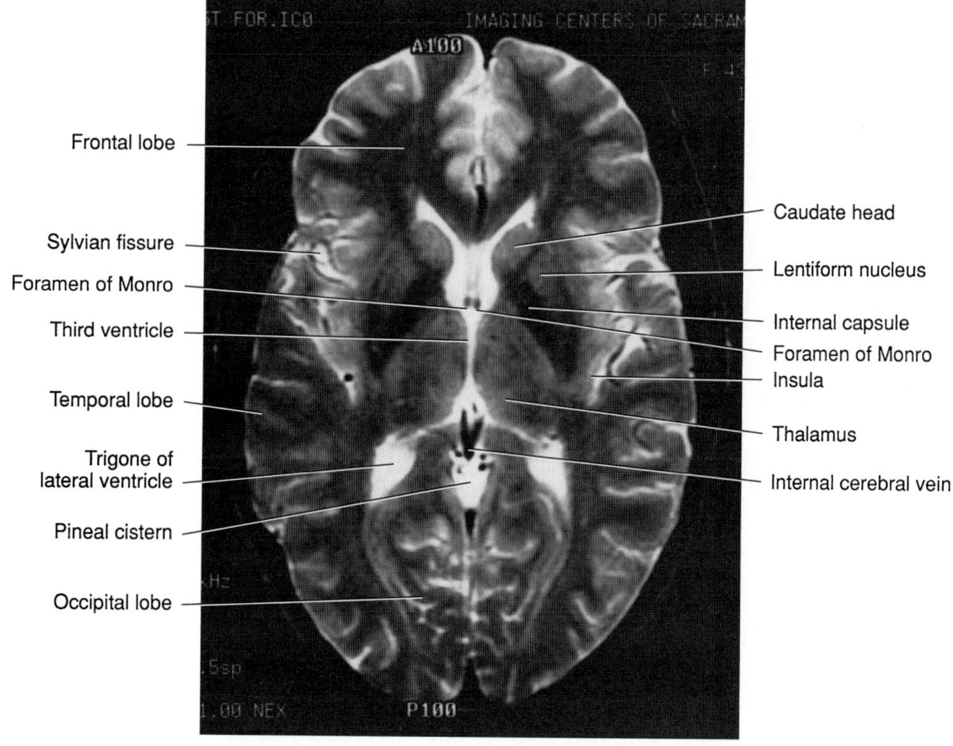

FIGURE 2.8. **Brain MR.** T2-weighted, axial plane through foramina of Monro and third ventricle.

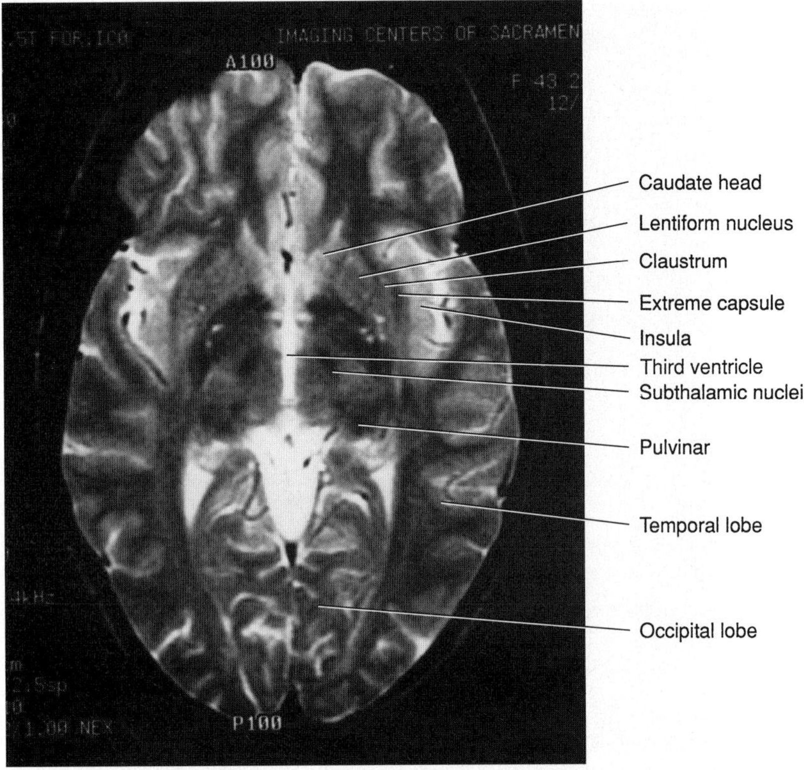

FIGURE 2.9. **Brain MR.** T2-weighted, axial plane through third ventricle.

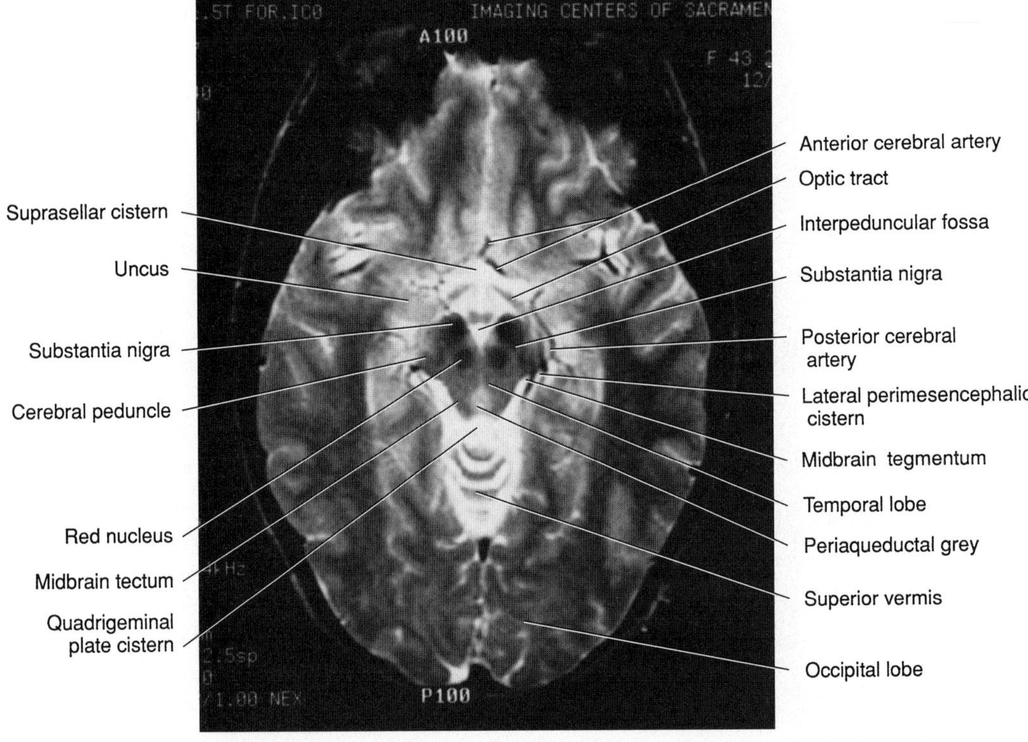

FIGURE 2.10. **Brain MR.** T2-weighted, axial plane through midbrain and suprasellar cistern.

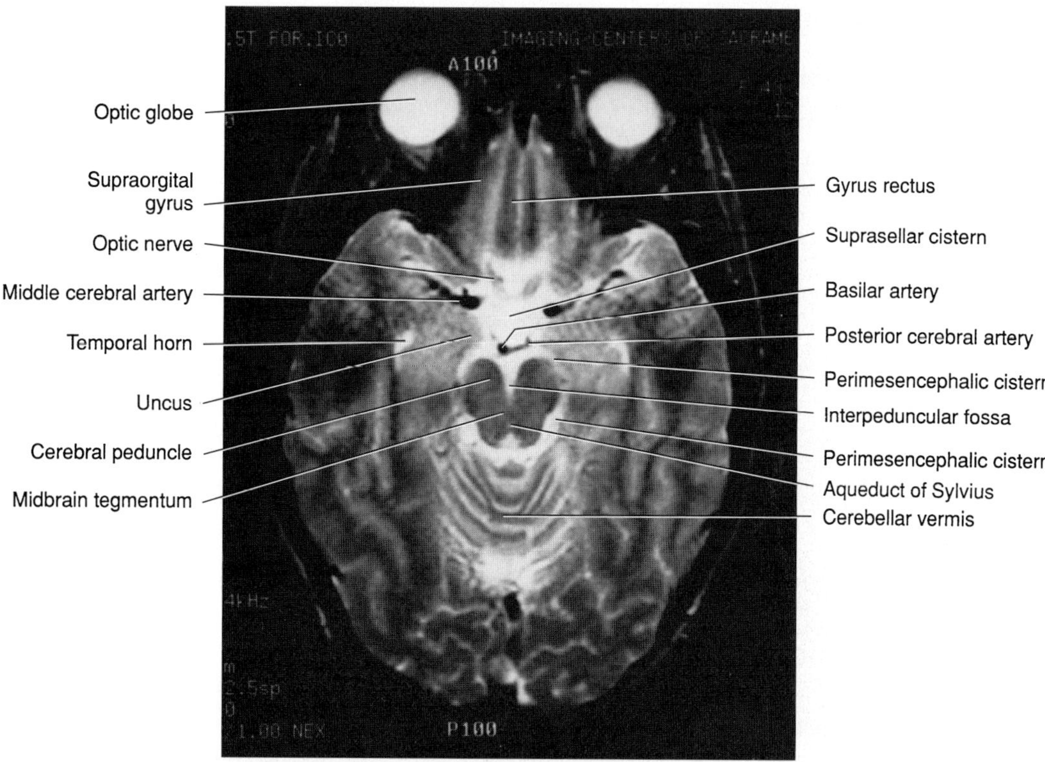

FIGURE 2.11. **Brain MR.** T2-weighted, axial plane through midbrain, vermis, and suprasellar cistern.

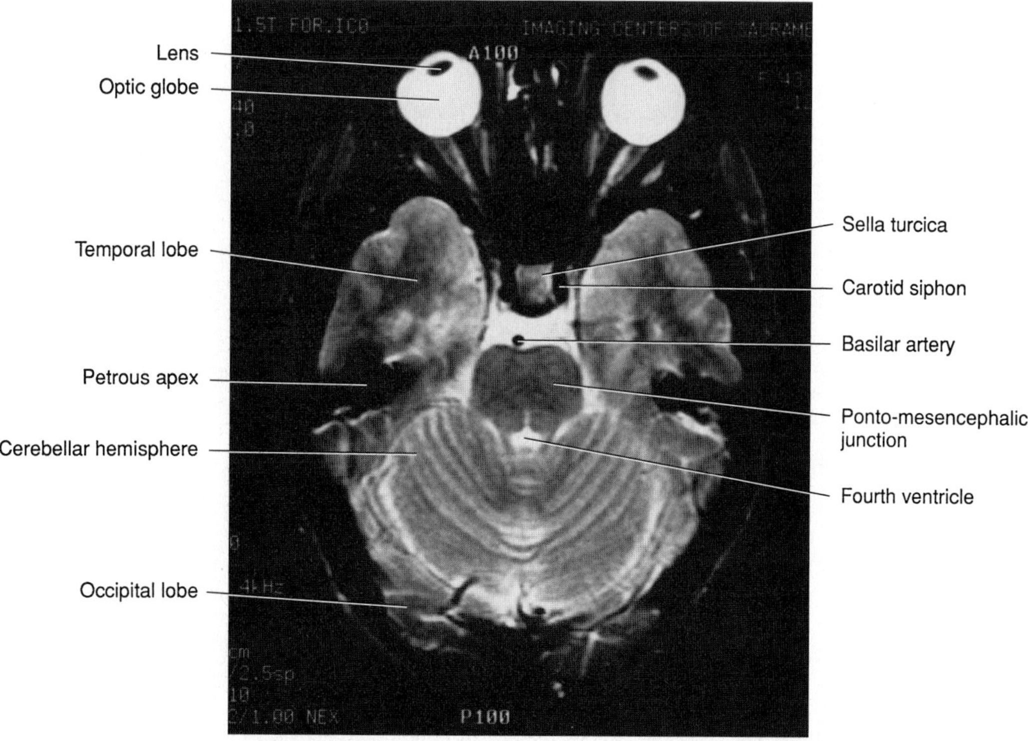

FIGURE 2.12. **Brain MR.** T2-weighted, axial plane through pontomesencephalic junction.

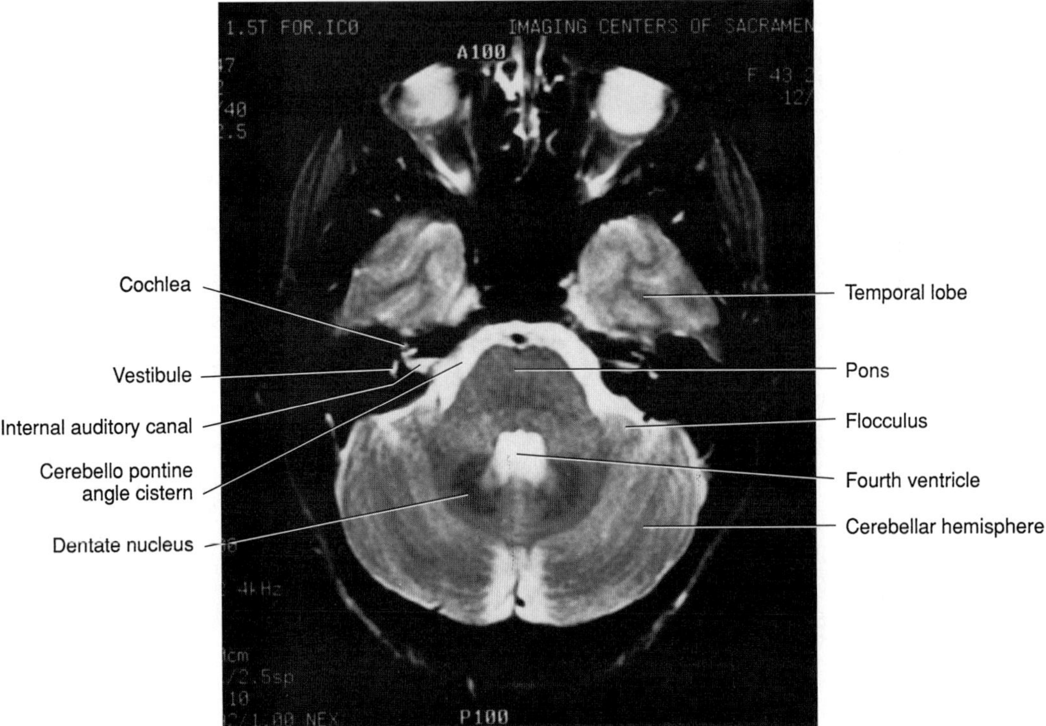

FIGURE 2.13. **Brain MR.** T2-weighted, axial plane through fourth ventricle.

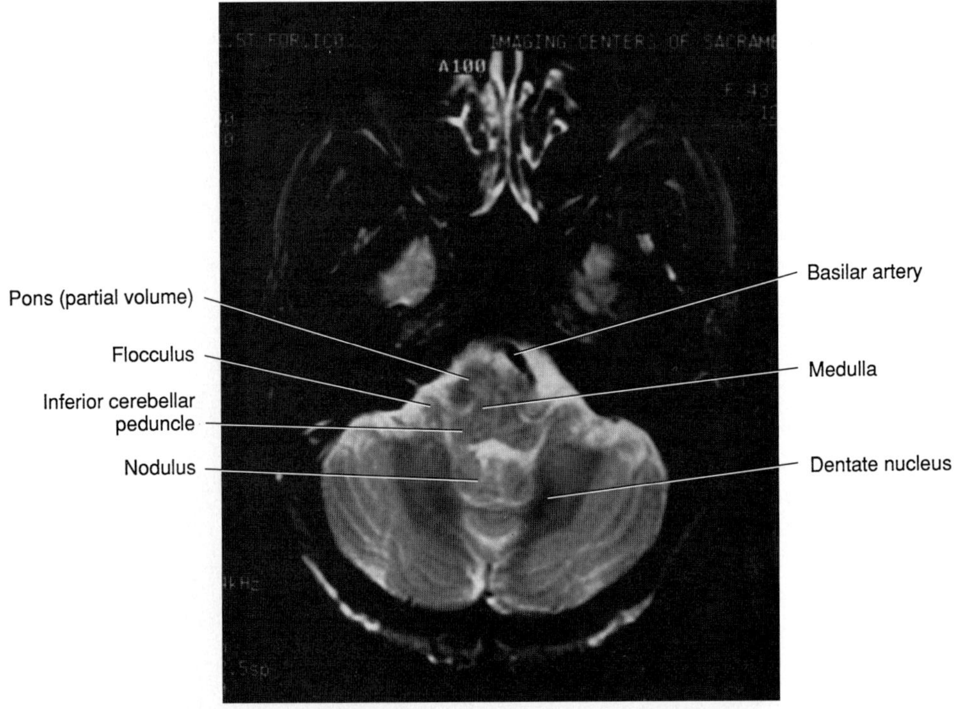

FIGURE 2.14. **Brain MR.** T2-weighted, axial plane through medulla.

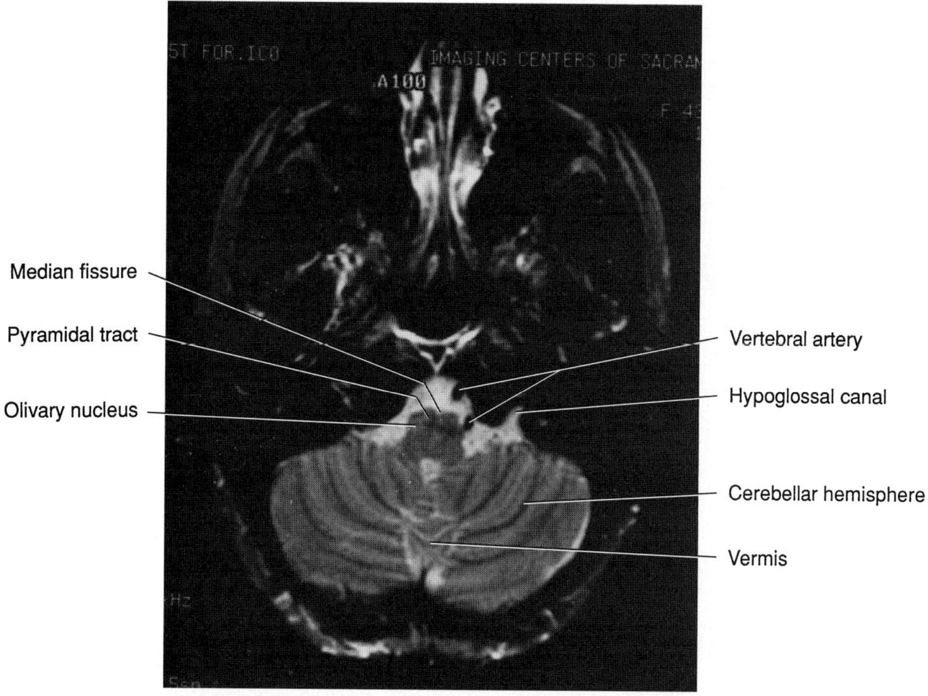

FIGURE 2.15. **Brain MR.** T2-weighted, axial plane through the cerebellar vermis.

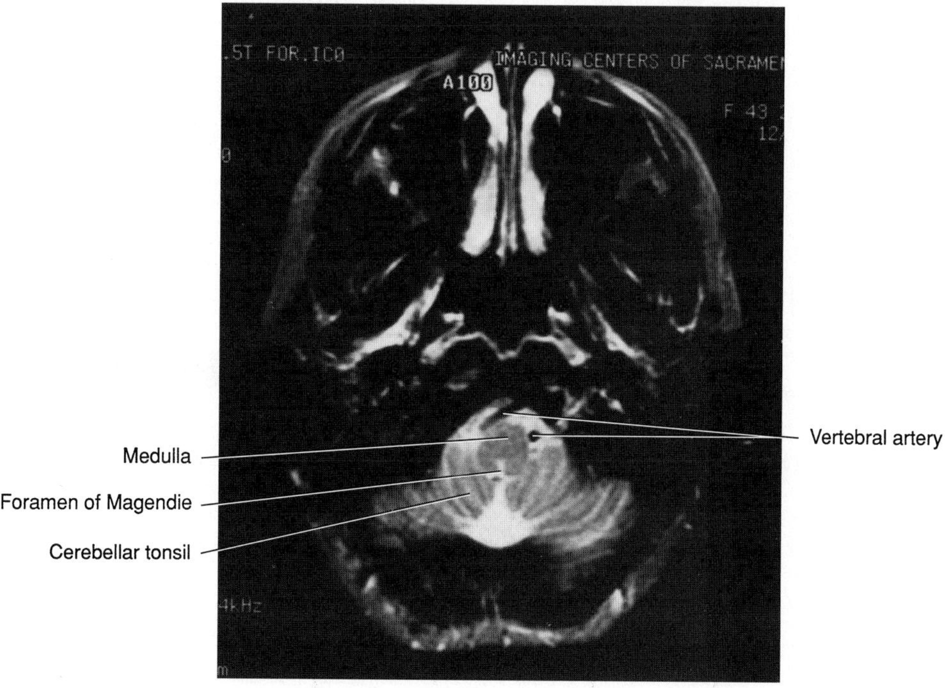

FIGURE 2.16. **Brain MR.** T2-weighted, axial plane through foramen of Magendie.

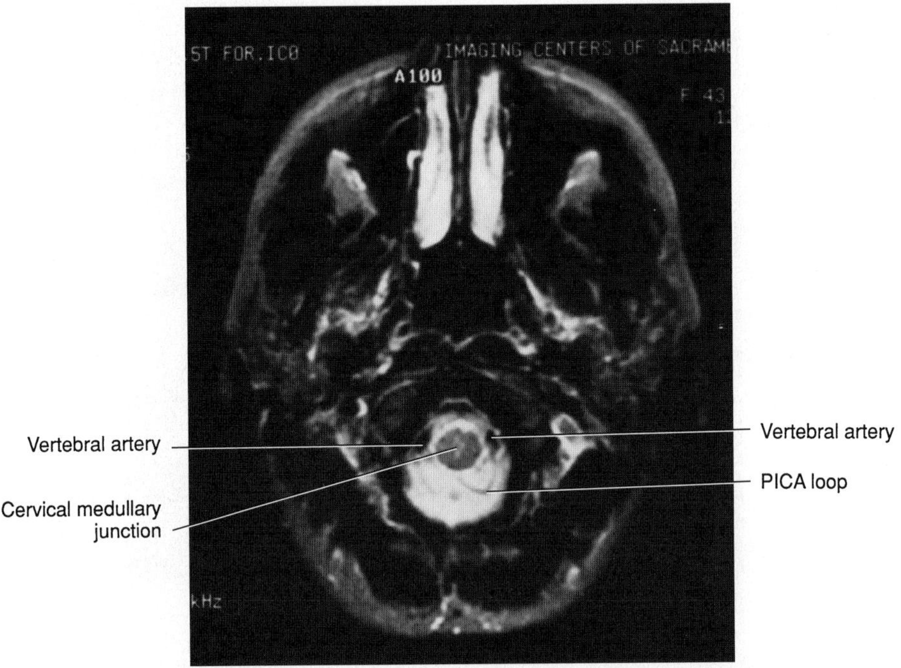

FIGURE 2.17. **Brain MR.** T2-weighted, axial plane through cervical medullary junction.

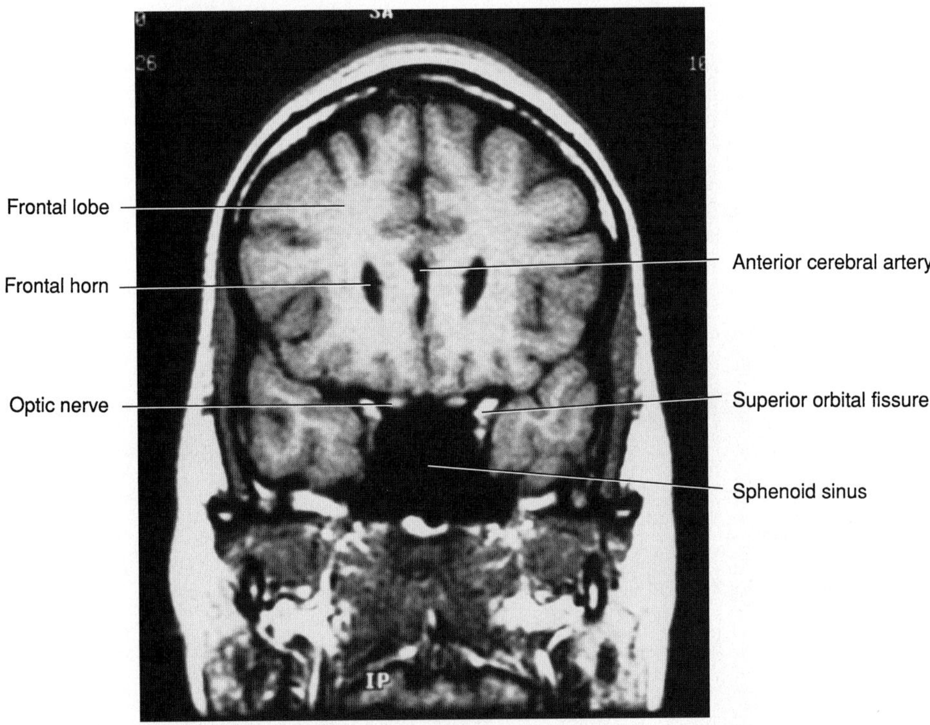

FIGURE 2.18. **Brain MR.** T1-weighted, coronal plane through frontal lobes.

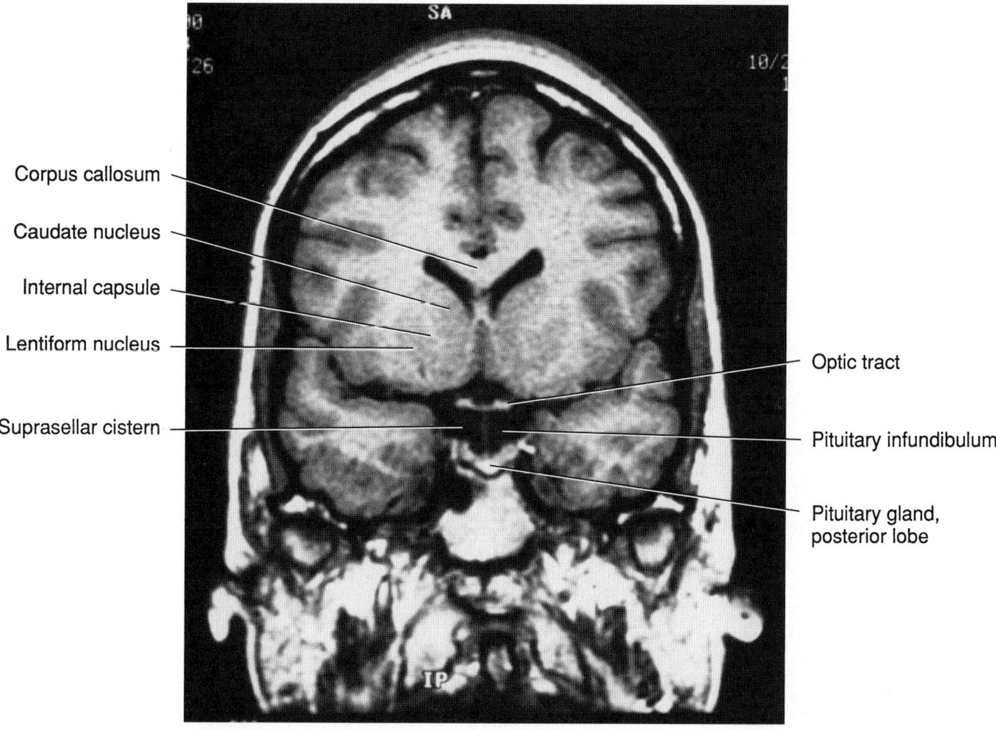

FIGURE 2.19. **Brain MR.** T1-weighted, coronal plane through pituitary infundibulum.

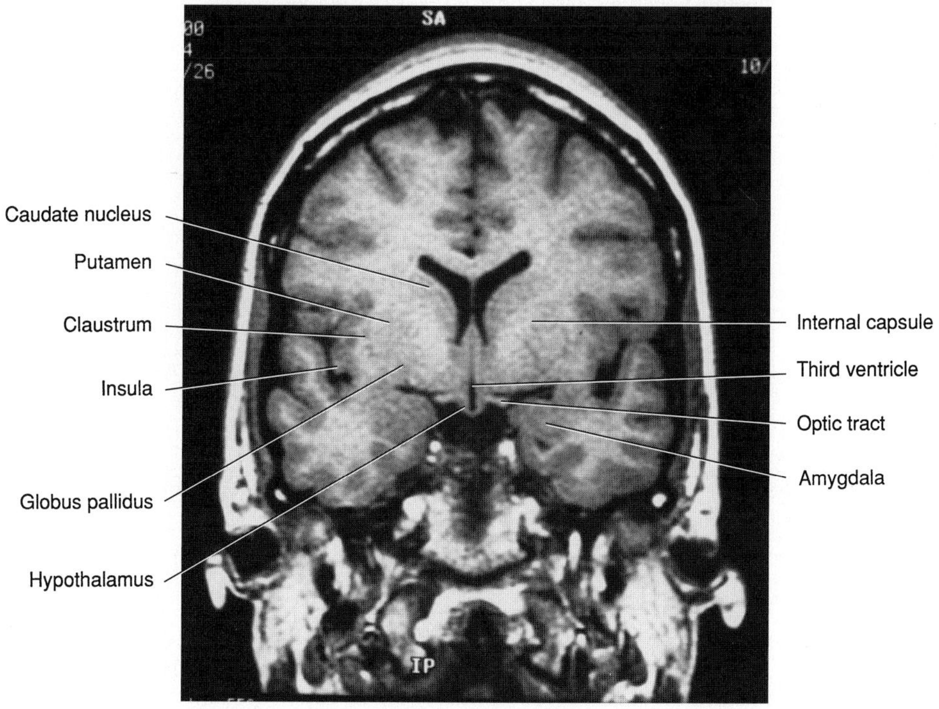

FIGURE 2.20. **Brain MR.** T1-weighted, coronal plane through optic tracts.

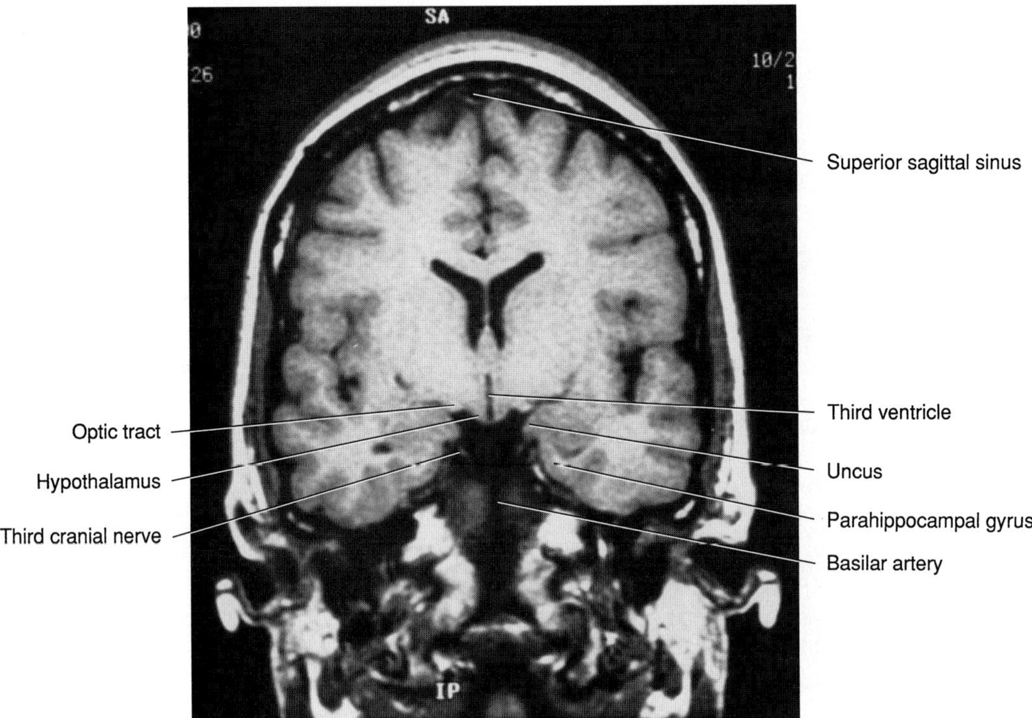

FIGURE 2.21. **Brain MR.** T1-weighted, coronal plane through uncus.

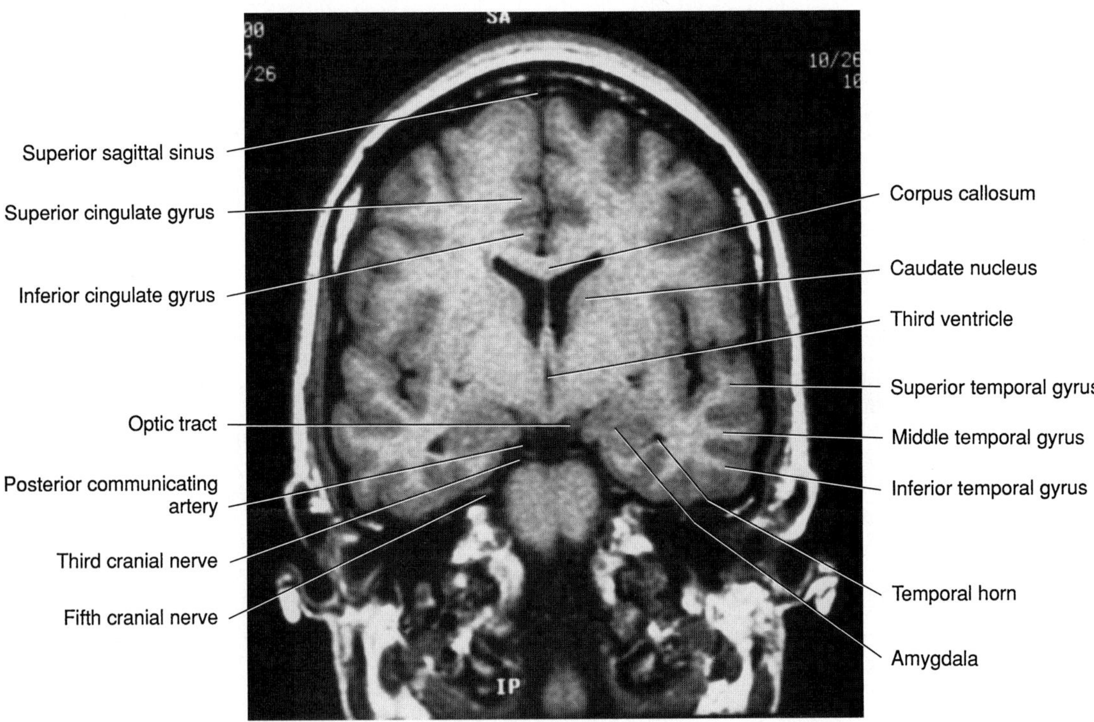

FIGURE 2.22. **Brain MR.** T1-weighted, coronal plane through anterior third ventricle.

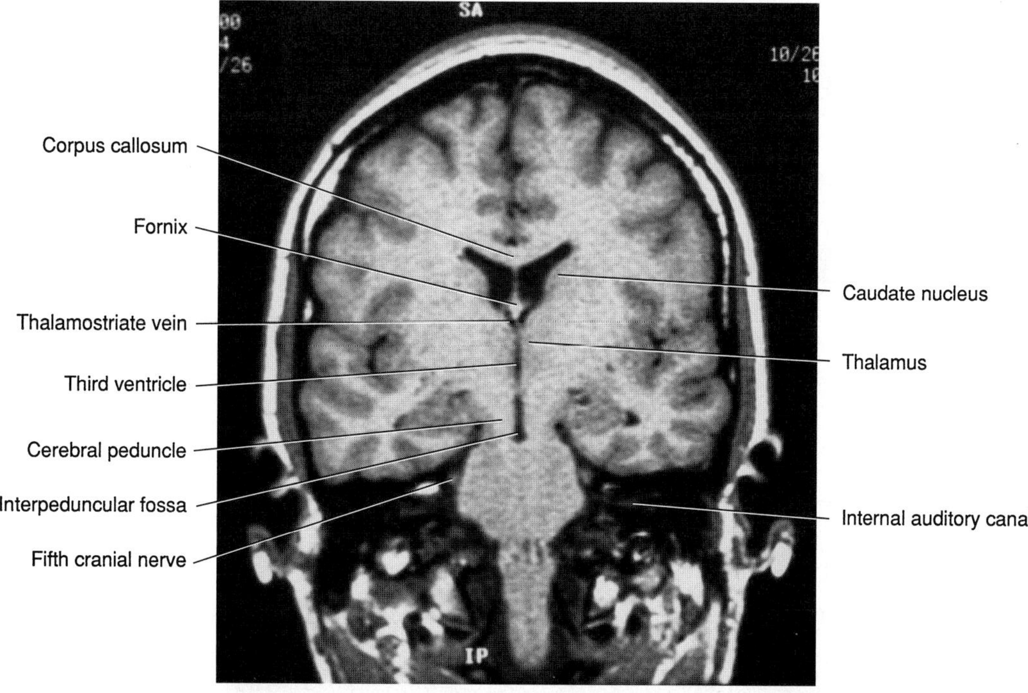

FIGURE 2.23. **Brain MR.** T1-weighted, coronal plane through third ventricle.

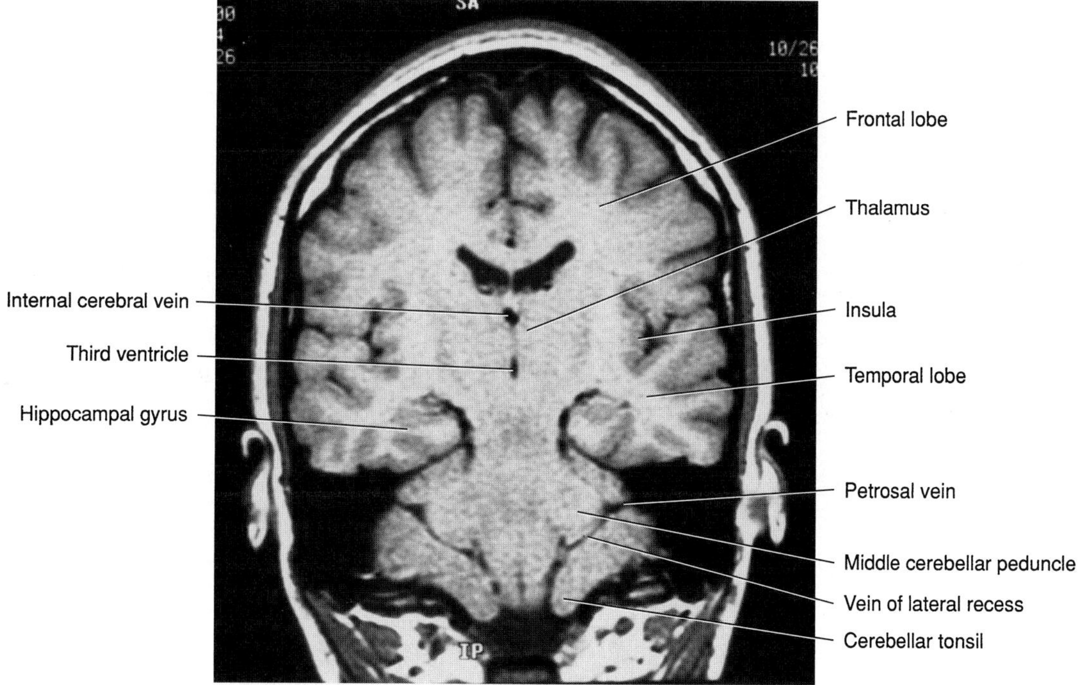

FIGURE 2.24. **Brain MR.** T1-weighted, coronal plane through middle cerebellar peduncle.

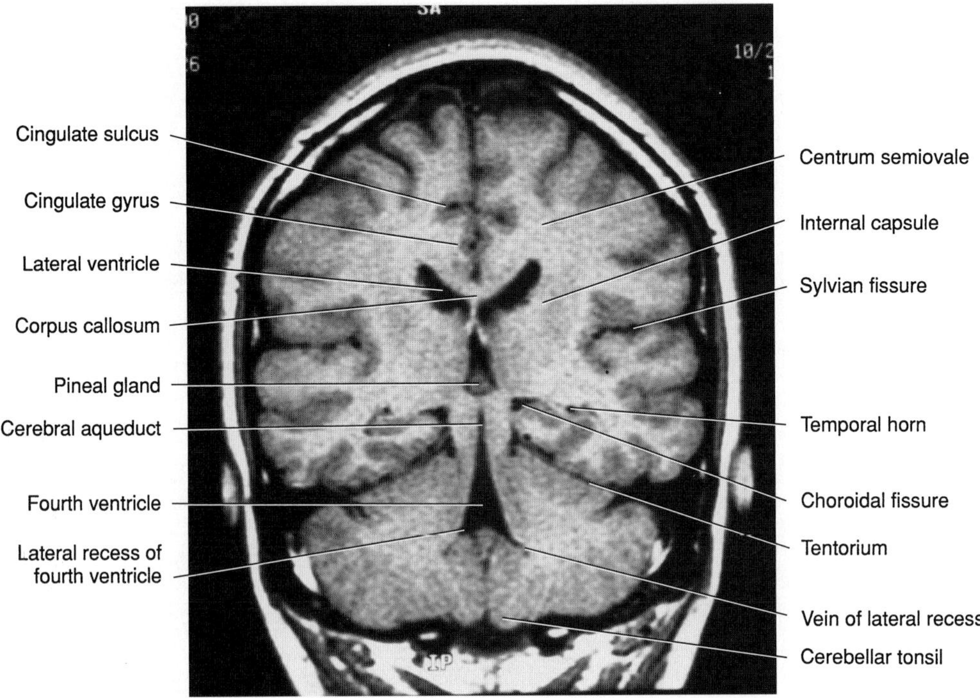

FIGURE 2.25. **Brain MR.** T1-weighted, coronal plane through cerebral aqueduct.

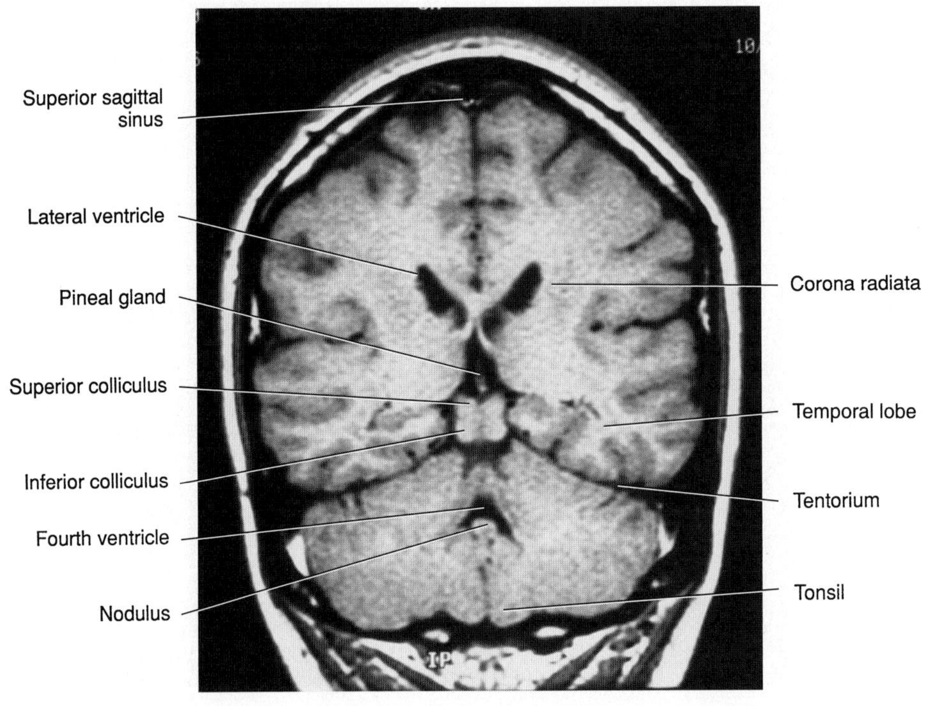

FIGURE 2.26. **Brain MR.** T1-weighted, coronal plane through fourth ventricle.

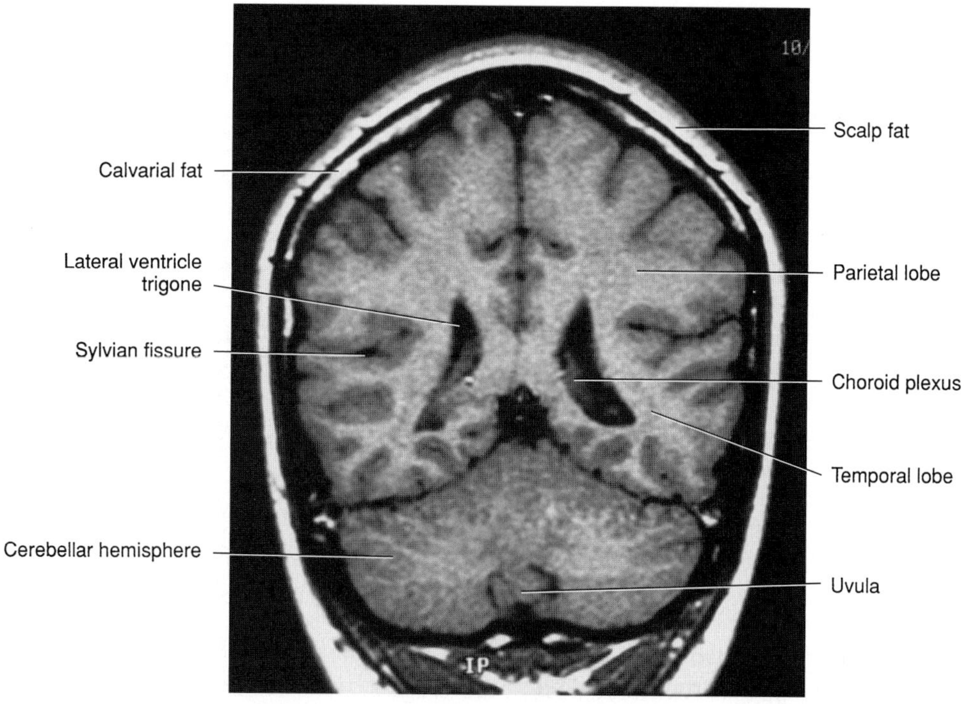

FIGURE 2.27. **Brain MR.** T1-weighted, coronal plane through trigones of lateral ventricles.

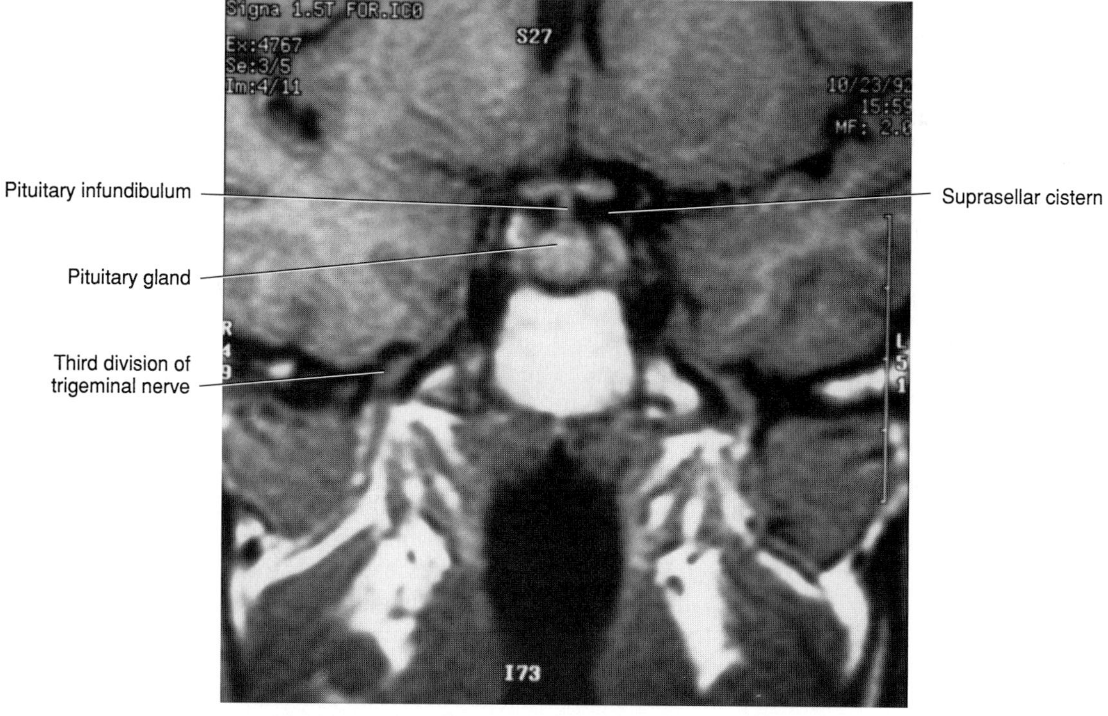

FIGURE 2.28. **Brain MR.** T1-weighted, coronal plane through pituitary gland.

density as CSF. Significant asymmetry may be a result of uncal herniation. Central mass may be the result of a sellar or suprasellar tumor. Opacification of the cistern may be the result of subarachnoid hemorrhage or meningitis.

Ventricles. The final structure that must be evaluated in a quick review of a brain scan is the ventricular system. It is best to start with the fourth ventricle in the posterior fossa, because it is the hardest to see on CT scanning (Fig. 2.4). Asymmetry or shift of the fourth ventricle may be the only sign of significant intracranial masses. Because of the shape of the fourth ventricle, some asymmetry in appearance may reflect the patient's position in the scanner.

The overall size of the ventricular system is assessed next (Figs. 2.1, 2.2, 2.4, and 2.6 to 2.16). Enlargement of the lateral ventricles and third ventricle in the setting of headache, or with signs of intracranial mass, may represent hydrocephalus, a potentially fatal yet easily treatable condition. Hydrocephalus is distinguished from enlargement of the ventricular system as the result of atrophy by a discrepancy in the degree of ventricular and sulcal enlargement, and by a characteristic pattern of frontal horn and temporal horn enlargement and a round appearance of the anterior portion of the third ventricle.

Emergency CT Checklist. When confronted with a CT scan under emergency conditions, radiologists must ask themselves these five questions.

1. Is the middle of the brain in the middle of the head?
2. Do the two sides of the brain look alike?
3. Can you see the smile and the pentagon or Jewish star?
4. Is the fourth ventricle in the midline and more or less symmetrical?
5. Are the lateral ventricles huge, with effaced sulci?

If a radiologist can give the right answers to these five questions, there is no neurosurgical emergency. This approach leaves many important diagnoses unmade, but the diseases are either untreatable or treatment can safely be delayed several hours. It is important to note that thrombolysis candidates require close scrutiny of the basal ganglia and cortex for signs of early ischemia. When stroke triage is performed, specialized imaging techniques such as perfusion CT and CT angiography (CTA) supplement the initial screening CT. In an increasing number of centers, MR stroke triage is performed, provided that the clinical suspicion of intracranial hemorrhage is very low and no contraindication to MR is known.

Midline Structures. The anatomy of the midline of the brain is extremely complex, and because the structures are not duplicated, principles of symmetry cannot be applied. The midline anatomy must be learned in detail. There are three prime areas to study.

Suprasellar Region. The first is the suprasellar and sellar region. On virtually every MR examination it is possible to localize the sella turcica, the pituitary gland, pituitary infundibulum, optic chiasm, anterior third ventricle, mammillary bodies, and anterior interhemispheric fissure. Important vascular structures are also seen in this region. The tip of the basilar artery and the posterior cerebral arteries are seen posteriorly, and the anterior cerebral arteries are visualized anterior and superior to the sella (Fig. 2.10). The anterior cerebral arteries travel in the interhemispheric fissure. Slightly off the midline, the "s" shaped carotid siphons (Fig. 2.10) and the posterior communicating arteries are visualized. Parallel to the course of the posterior communicating artery, we frequently see the third cranial nerve (Fig. 2.29). In the parasagittal location, near the optic chiasm, we see the optic nerve anteriorly and the optic tract posteriorly (Figs. 2.10, 2.11, and 2.29 to 2.31).

Pineal Region. The next important region to study in the midline is the pineal region (Figs. 2.1, 2.8 to 2.11, 2.30, and 2.31). It is crucial to identify the midbrain, the midbrain tegmentum, (frequently with a small lucency representing the decussation of the superior cerebellar peduncle), the aqueduct of Sylvius, the midbrain tectum with superior and inferior colliculi, the pineal gland, and the superior cerebellar vermian lobules. If the precentral cerebellar vein can be seen in the superior vermian cistern, a mass here is unlikely.

Craniocervical Junction. Historically, the craniocervical junction (Figs. 2.17 and 2.32) was a relative blind spot to the neuroradiologist, but this is no longer true, so it is particularly important to study this region. The anterior arch of C1, the odontoid process, and the cervical occipital ligaments are seen anteriorly. The sharp inferior edge of the clivus marks the anterior lip of the foramen magnum. The posterior lip is marked by the cortical margin of the occipital bone. The cerebellar tonsils should project no more than 3 mm below a line drawn between the anterior and posterior lips of the foramen magnum. The obex, the most posterior projection of the dorsal medulla, should lie above this imaginary line. The only structures visible at this level within the calvarium and spinal canal are the cervical medullary junction and a tiny bit of cerebellar tonsilar tissue. Any other soft tissue in this location is pathologic.

CURRENT NEUROIMAGING OPTIONS

With the bewildering and ever-increasing array of examinations available for imaging the brain, it seems a hopeless task to decide which of them is best for a given clinical situation. To make matters easier, we can eliminate two from the start. Plain radiography is useless in patient management and is only of value in the documentation of fracture for medical/legal reasons. Nuclear medicine brain scans are useful in certain specialized settings, such as medically refractory epilepsy and dementia, in which PET scans play important roles (see Chapter 64). We still must decide between CT, MR, US, and angiography in the evaluation of the acute neurologic patient.

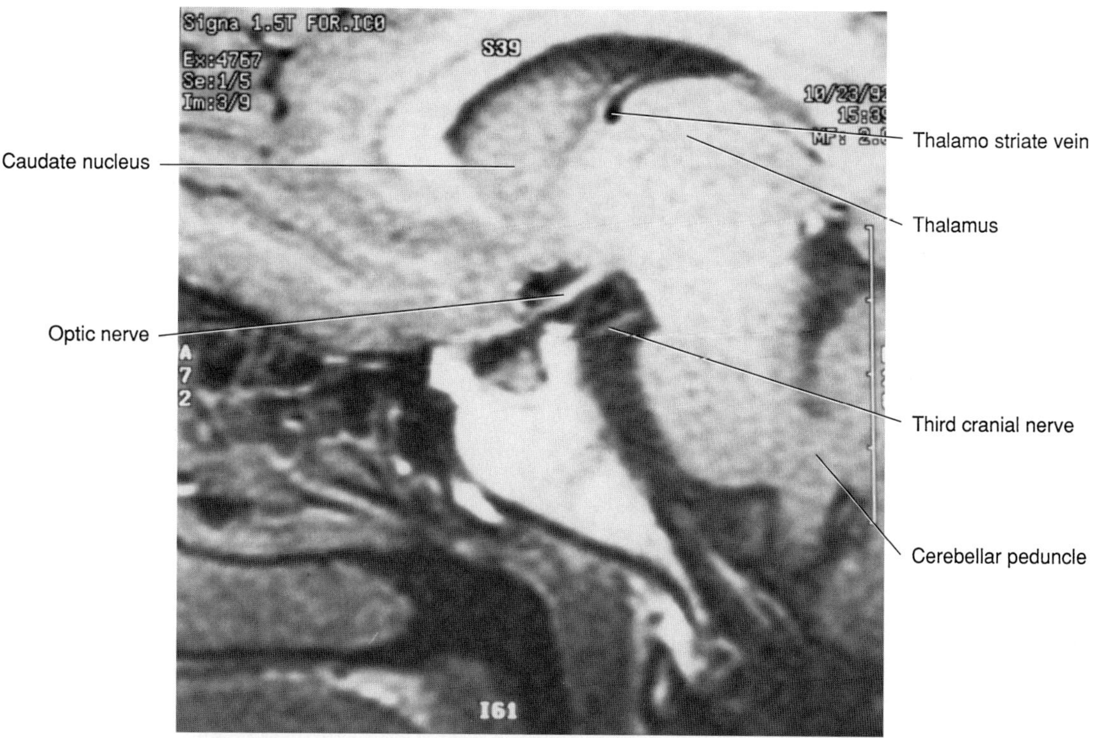

FIGURE 2.29. **Brain MR.** T1-weighted, sagittal plane through optic nerve.

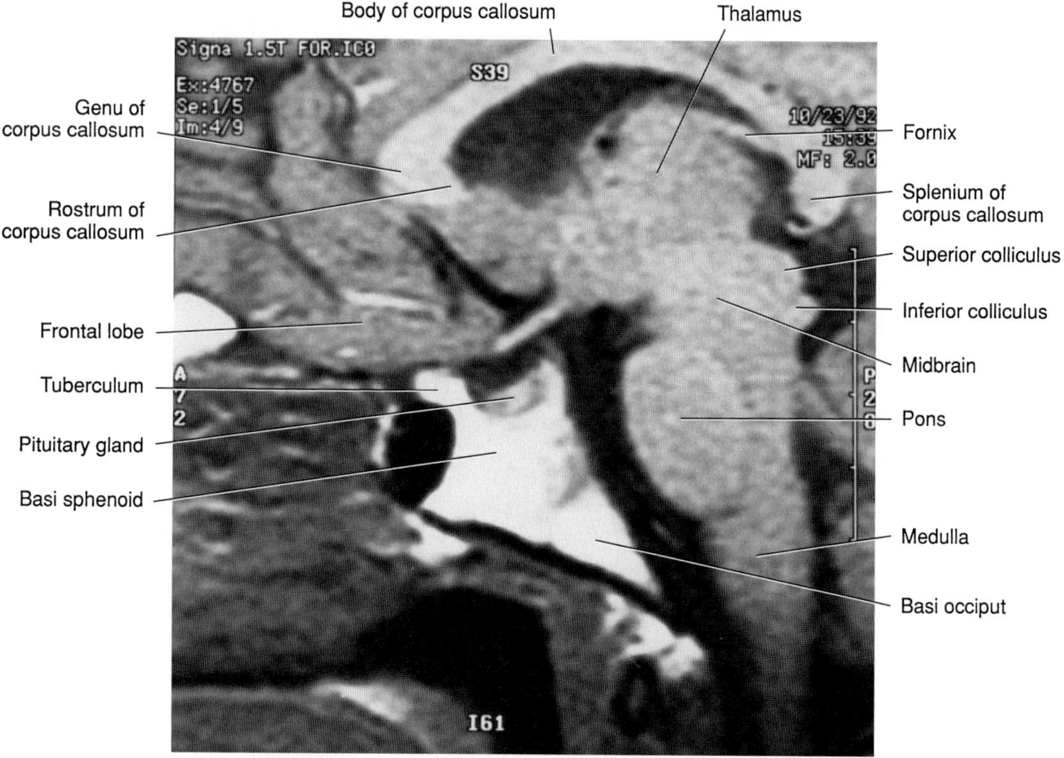

FIGURE 2.30. **Brain MR.** T1-weighted, sagittal plane through parasellar region.

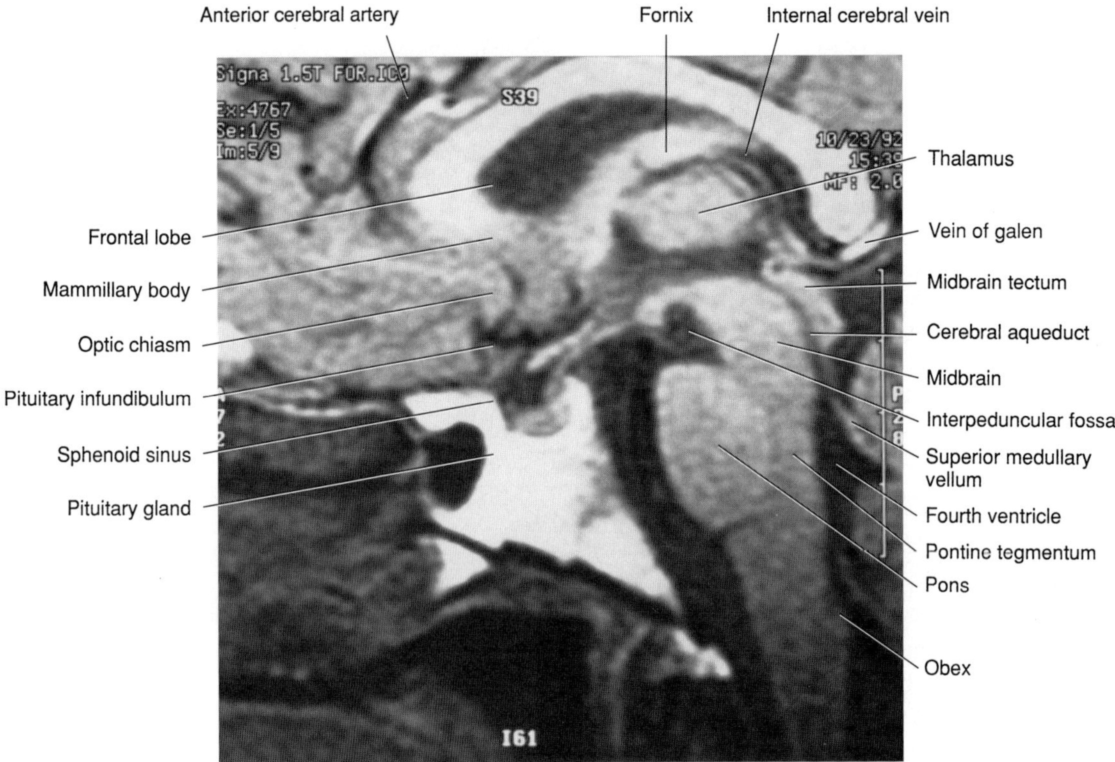

FIGURE 2.31. **Brain MR.** T1-weighted, sagittal midline plane through pituitary infundibulum.

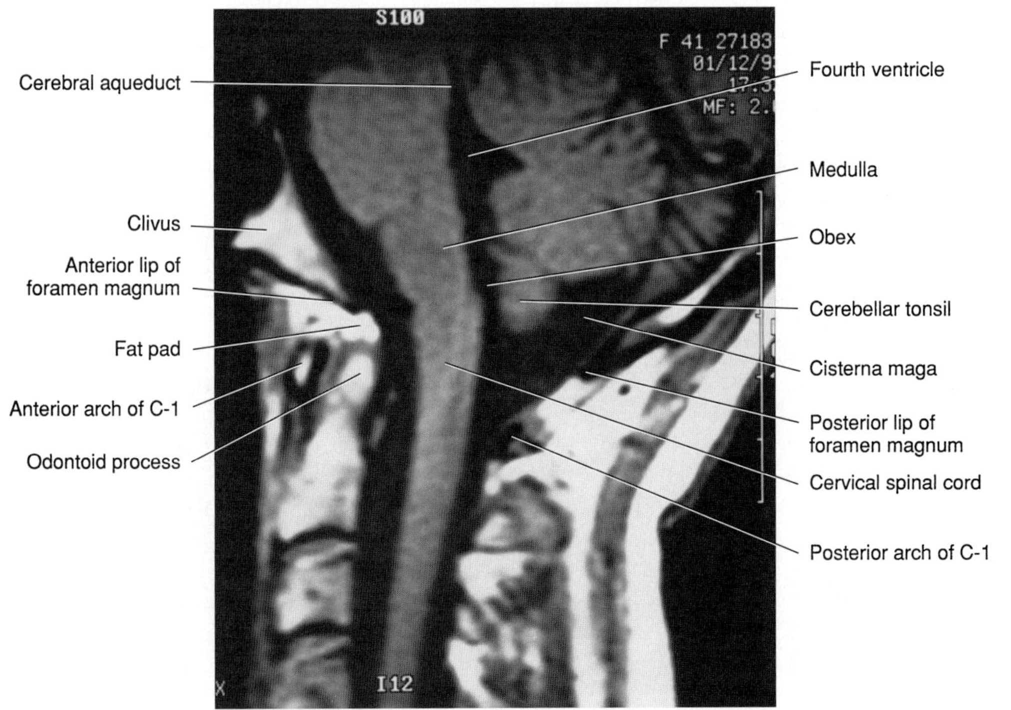

FIGURE 2.32. **Brain MR.** T1-weighted, sagittal plane through craniocervical junction.

The radiologist also needs to decide whether to give intravenous contrast material and which special CT and MR techniques to employ. Angiography is used in the acute setting based upon the appropriate combination of CT, MR, and clinical findings. US may be used as the first test in infants, or for evaluation of the carotids, or with transcranial techniques for evaluation of the intracranial vessels after initial imaging triage. Therefore, the only contenders for the "first test" for the brain are MR and CT. A standard MR examination generally consists of a T1WI, a T2WI, and fluid-attenuated inversion recovery (FLAIR) or "proton density" images and may be supplemented by T1WIs with gadolinium-based contrast agents. A standard CT examination consists of axial images reviewed at brain and bone windows and may be supplemented by repeat images with intravenous iodinated contrast.

As a general rule in brain imaging, CT is performed for acute neurologic illness and MR for the more chronic and subacute cases. That is, if the onset of neurologic symptoms referable to the brain was within 48 hours, start with a CT. If the problem is older than 3 days, start with an MR. If the CT or MR suggest a primary vascular lesion, such as an arteriovenous malformation (AVM) or aneurysm, do a catheter angiogram or MR or CT angiogram. If the CT or MR suggests tumor, give contrast. If the CT or MR fails to demonstrate an acute infarct and the symptoms suggest a transient ischemic attack or stroke, do a carotid Doppler US, or MR angiography (MRA) or CTA. Don't use intravenous iodinated contrast for CT in the acute setting unless brain abscess or tumor is a strong consideration or if needed for your stroke triage protocol. Give gadolinium for MR whenever there is a clinical finding that suggests a specific neurologic localization, a seizure, or a strong history of cancer or infectious disease. Exceptions to these general guidelines are few. Follow the rules and you'll be doing the right thing in the majority of cases. Sometimes an MR will be required to clarify a questionable finding on CT. Also, remember that some patients are simply too sick to study easily with MR. These include multisystem trauma patients or those who require assisted ventilation. Patients who cannot hold still, such as children or highly agitated adults, must be sedated for MR. Sedation carries its own set of risks, which must be weighed carefully, and properly trained personnel and appropriate monitoring are essential.

MR spectroscopy, MR and CT angiography and perfusion techniques, and MR diffusion techniques are now routine in neuroradiology practice.

Proton MR spectroscopy shows the distribution of brain metabolites based upon the chemical shift of the protons within them, which is a property determined by the chemical environment of the protons in question. This is the form of magnetic resonance analysis you learned in organic chemistry! In practice, three normal metabolites are the most interesting: choline, which is a marker for cell membranes and hence a marker for cellular density; N-acetyl aspartate (NAA), which is a compound found only in neurons and therefore a marker of neuronal density; and creatine, which is evenly distributed in many types of cells and serves as a reference standard.

Choline may be considered a tumor marker. If an intracranial mass is indeterminate with respect to etiology, elevation of the choline-to-creatine ratio may help to distinguish radiation necrosis from recurrent tumor or infection. Another use of the choline peak is tumor grading. Since the prognosis of a primary brain tumor is determined by the highest histologic grade of tissue within it, and histologic grade correlates with choline-to-creatine ratio, biopsy of the site with the highest choline-to-creatine ratio is likely to reflect the histologic grade of the tumor. Biopsy targeted by MR spectroscopy will better reflect the true nature of the lesion. This rule is not perfect; for example, if the choline peak is sky high, think of a meningioma.

A decrease in the NAA-to-creatine ratio is seen in a variety of conditions that are associated with neuronal death. Focally decreased NAA is seen in mesial temporal sclerosis and infarcts. Global depletion of NAA can be seen in multiple sclerosis and dementing diseases such as Alzheimer's disease (AD), which also demonstrates elevated myoinositol. Any space-occupying mass that replaces brain will also have a small NAA peak. Abscesses and metastatic lesions will have lower NAA-to-creatine ratios than primary brain tumors, which tend to infiltrate rather than replace brain. Markedly elevated NAA levels are seen in Canavan's disease as a result of a specific defect in the enzyme that metabolizes it. The NAA accumulates, producing a distinct spectroscopic pattern.

Elevated levels of abnormal metabolites are sometimes present in the brain. A nonspecific necrosis peak is seen in malignant tumors, infections, and some active demyelinating lesions. A characteristic doublet peak of lactic acid can help make the diagnosis of ischemia. This has been useful in infants with suspected hypoxemic ischemic encephalopathy. This may also aid in diagnosis of mitochondrial encephalopathies.

Noninvasive angiographic techniques are now routinely used. CTA depends upon the rapid bolus injection of iodinated contrast, rapid imaging with a multidetector spiral CT, and rapid data processing to produce clinically useful images of the cerebral vessels. Two major classes of images are produced with these studies: relatively thick cross-sectional images using maximum intensity projection (MIP) and shaded three-dimensional surface renderings. Because reconstruction techniques are time consuming, bone is hard to distinguish from vessels, and venous contamination can be problematic, it is best to go where the climate suits your clothes when interpreting CTA. Look at the MIP images most likely to answer your clinical question and remember that CTA is a problem-solving technique rather than a screening method. In subarachnoid hemorrhage, use the sagittal MIP for the carotid ophthalmic aneurysm, the posterior communicating artery (Pcomm) and the posterior inferior cerebellar artery (PICA) origin, the coronal MIP for the anterior communicating artery (Acomm), carotid "T" and basilar tip, and the axial MIP for the Acomm and Pcomm. Remember that the middle cerebral artery (MCA) is a relative blind spot so it must be inspected carefully on all images. Once an aneurysm is found, the shaded surface renderings are invaluable in treatment planning, especially in determining the configuration of the neck and sizing the aneurysm for coil selection. In suspected infarct, use the symptoms as a guide and carefully follow the appropriate vessels to an abrupt halt or significant narrowing. A vessel segment ought to reside completely within the MIP volume to be analyzed accurately. Be careful not to misinterpret a vessel leaving the slice as an obstruction or one curving partly outside the slice as a stenosis. Confirm the degree of stenosis by viewing the vessel in cross section.

MRA is harder to obtain but easier to read. There is inherently greater contrast between the vessel and the surrounding tissues. MRA depends upon the phenomenon of *flow-related enhancement,* in which moving spins behave differently than stationary spins. Images are created by choosing parameters that increase the signal of the flowing blood. First-pass gadolinium-enhanced MRA provides superior quality images that enhance diagnostic confidence but not necessarily accuracy. Both source images and MIP reconstructions of user-defined volumes are reviewed. Separate images of the anterior and posterior cerebral circulations are performed and the right and left carotid systems are viewed separately. Because the vessels are viewed in isolation, the conspicuity of aneurysms and other vascular lesions is excellent, though artifacts resulting from patient motion, in-plane vascular flow, and susceptibility artifacts can be problematic. MRA is most useful when patients are not acutely ill. Intracranial vascular stenoses and aneurysms are reliable depicted. Both MRA and CTA are very useful extracranially as well.

Diffusion-weighted MR imaging (also called simply ***diffusion-weighted imaging*** [DWI]) has greatly enhanced the ability of MRI to diagnose cerebral infarct early and accurately. This technique exploits the phenomenon of diffusion, which is related to Brownian motion at the molecular level. DWI takes advantage of the fact that intracellular water molecules are much more limited in their movement than extracellular ones, because they quickly bump into the cell membrane that contains them. The more restricted the movement of water, the brighter it will be on DWI sequences. In stroke, ischemic areas tend to swell following osmosis of free water into the dying cells, and these areas become bright on DWI as a result of the increased ratio of intracellular to extracellular water. This change on DWI precedes changes on T2 and FLAIR, making DWI a key sequence in the early detection of stroke. CSF contains the least restricted water in the brain and will be dark on DWI. Low signal on DWI therefore distinguishes arachnoid cysts from intracranial epidermoid cysts.

Tumor, trauma, and infection can have an ambiguous appearance on DWI, as both intracellular and extracellular water may increase. Fortunately, the T2 effects of extracellular edema can be accounted for and "subtracted" out using apparent diffusion coefficient (ADC) maps. Please refer to the examples in Chapter 4, as a picture is worth a thousand words in understanding this complicated and powerful tool that has become routine part of daily practice. Some evidence suggests restricted diffusion in multiple sclerosis and brain abscess.

The diffusion phenomenon has also been exploited to map white matter tracts for surgical treatment planning and other purposes. This tool, *tensor diffusion imaging* (TDI), exploits the fact that within elongated cell processes such as axons, water can diffuse more freely "down the tube" than "sideways," allowing for "tractography." MR and CT perfusion techniques are extremely useful for the depiction of regions of relatively diminished flow in ischemic cerebral tissue and perfusion. Most MR perfusion scans rely on a first-pass bolus gadolinium injection, during which the brain is imaged sequentially. Because the gadolinium is paramagnetic, the signal on highly T2*-weighted images is decreased in a manner proportional to perfusion. The abnormally perfused brain does not demonstrate this flow-related phenomenon as much or as soon. In the acute stroke patient, a delay of the time to peak that is greater than 6 seconds strongly suggests ischemia. Other perfusion parameters are also employed. CT perfusion relies on the principle that perfused areas of the brain will attenuate the x-ray beam more than the ischemic brain during an iodinated contrast injection. This is because more of the contrast agent will reach the normal brain sooner than it will reach the abnormal brain. Sequential scans are performed, and the time to peak enhancement and other parameters can be calculated. Delayed arrival of contrast and transit of contrast documents ischemia, and other parameters may predict infarct.

MR perfusion techniques also play an important role in the management of primary brain tumors by predicting the most malignant portion of the tumor, which determines the biologic nature of the lesion and the patient's prognosis. Increased relative cerebral blood volume within a tumor appears to correlate with tumor angiogenesis and hence tumor grade. Areas of increasing abnormality on perfusion-weighted MR examinations correlate well with areas of increasing malignancy. Biopsy and treatment guided by these images promise to improve prognosis and outcome in patients with astrocytoma and other brain tumors.

Functional MR imaging (FMRI) refers to studies of the brain using blood oxygen level–dependent imaging (BOLD). These images rely upon the fact that deoxyhemoglobin produces changes in magnetic susceptibility that

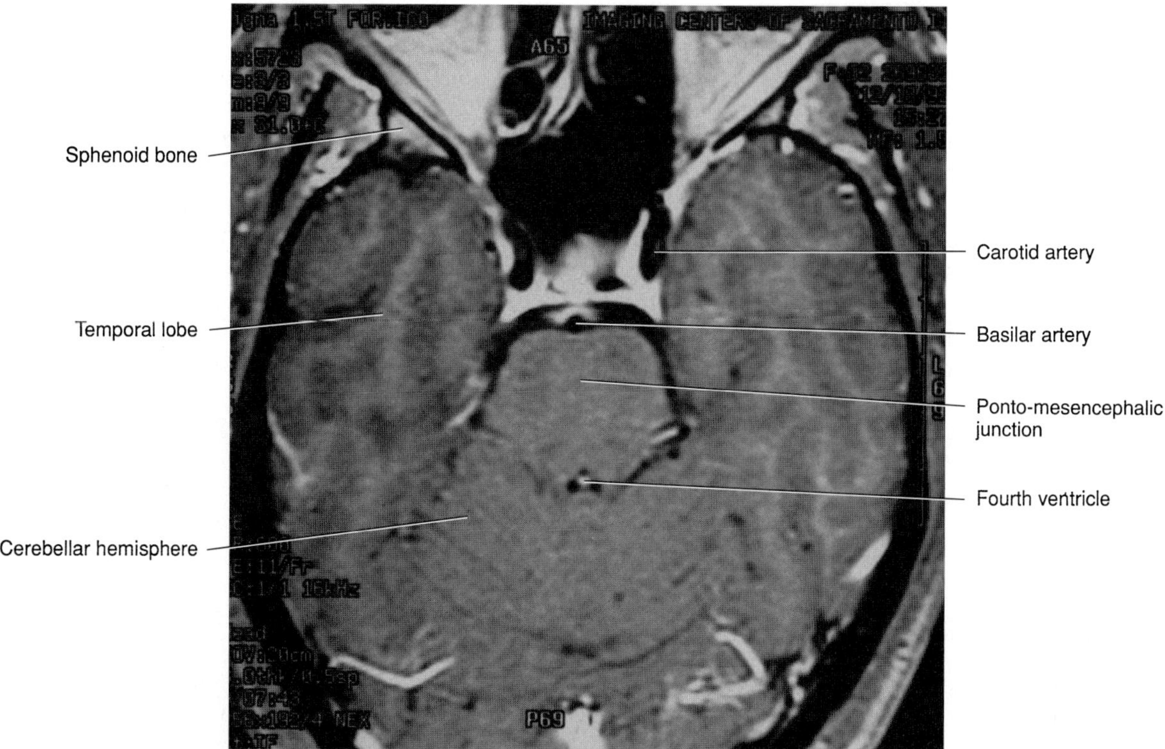

FIGURE 2.33. **Brain MR.** T1-weighted, gadolinium-enhanced, axial plane, through pontomesencephalic junction.

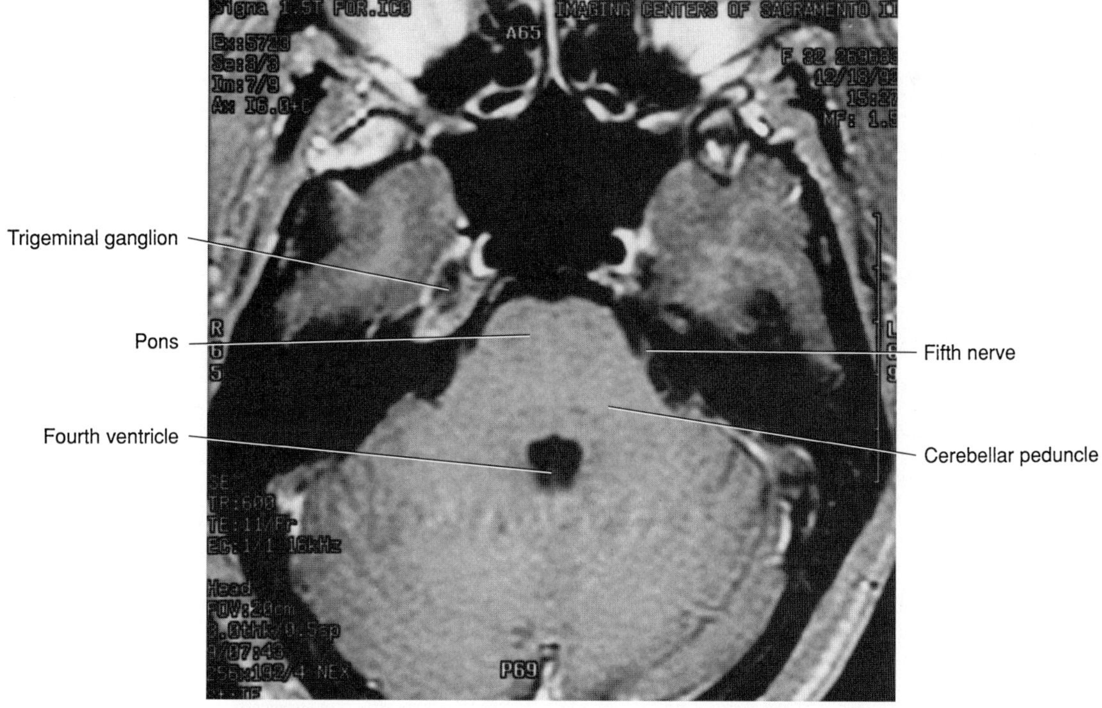

FIGURE 2.34. **Brain MR.** T1-weighted, gadolinium-enhanced, axial plane, through fourth ventricle and fifth cranial nerve.

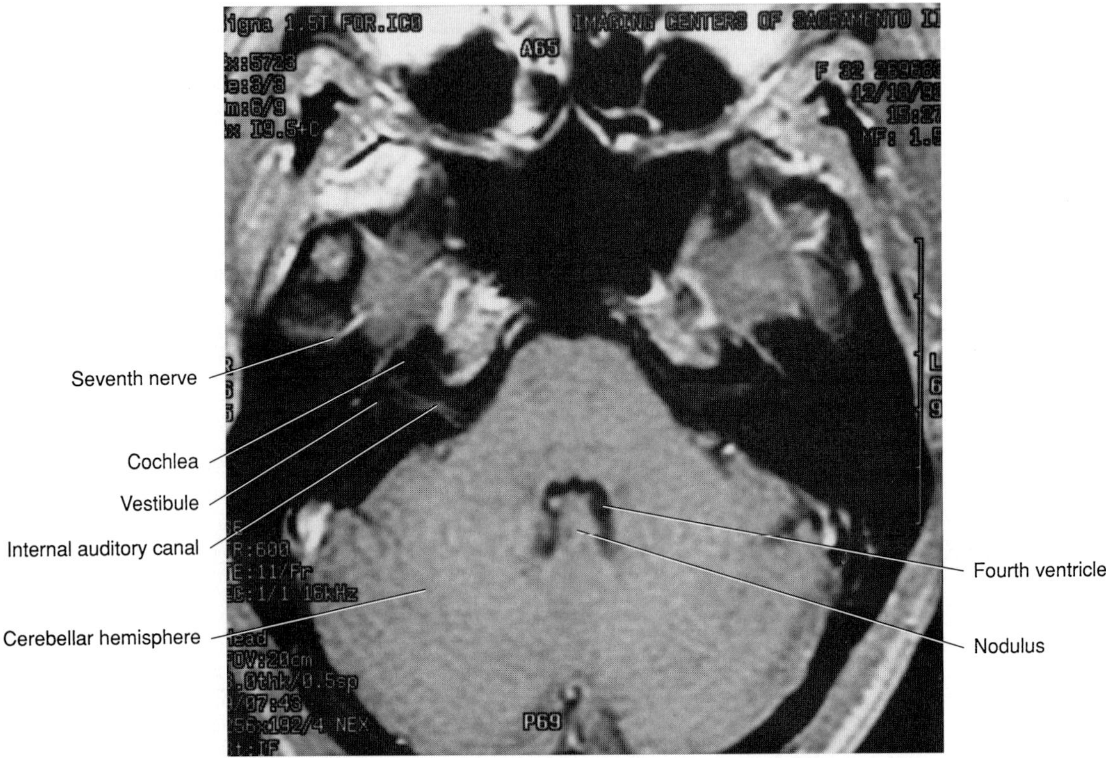

FIGURE 2.35. **Brain MR.** T1-weighted, axial plane through internal auditory canal.

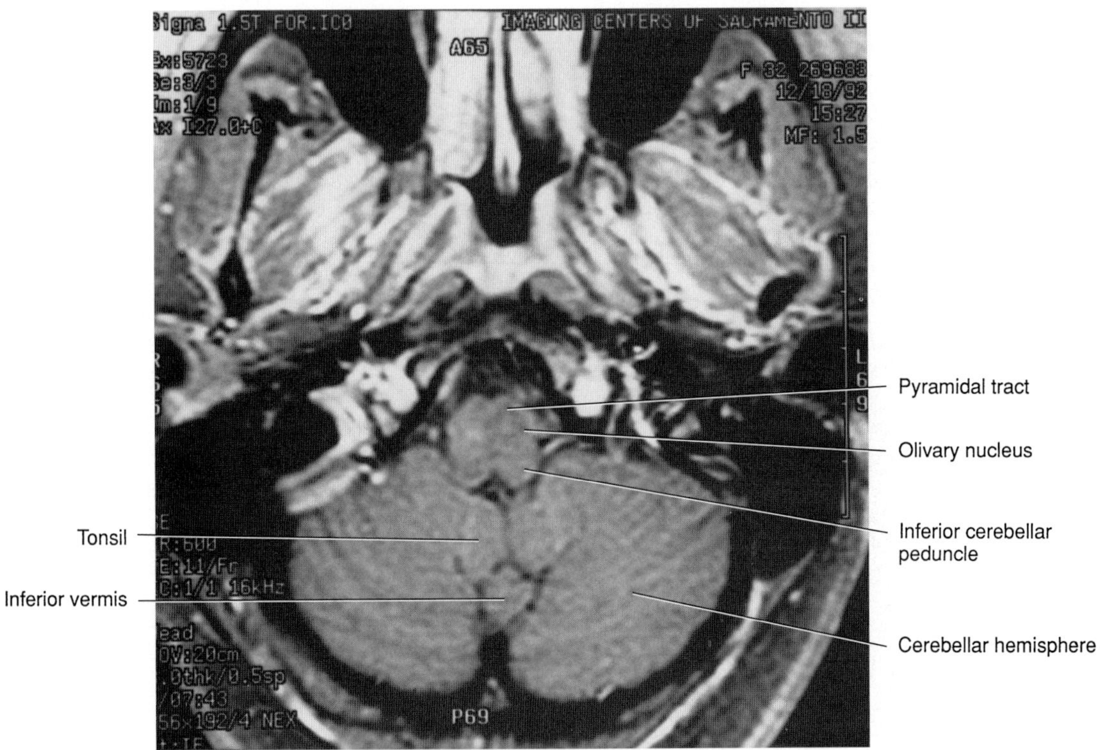

FIGURE 2.36. **Brain MR.** T1-weighted, axial plane through medulla.

are proportional to the metabolic activity in a given brain structure. Some controversy persists as to the exact nature of the BOLD signal change, but it is known to correlate well with neuronal activity. By comparing images captured during sensory stimulation, motor activity, or a higher cortical task with those obtained while the patient is in a resting or control condition, one can create images highlighting the area or areas of the brain that are responsible for the brain function in question. Reliable localization of motor and language functions assists in planning surgery for epilepsy, brain tumors, and arteriovenous malformations. fMRI has become an essential technique for basic neurobehavioral and neurophysiologic research. The potential for this powerful technique has only begun to be explored.

IMAGING STRATEGY FOR COMMON CLINICAL SYNDROMES

While an almost infinite variety of clinical symptoms may be related to the CNS, most patients can be divided into a limited number of categories (Table 2.1).

Acute trauma patients have perhaps the most dramatic presentation. A noncontrast enhanced CT scan is preferred, because CT can be obtained quickly and on virtually any patient. Furthermore, CT scanners are almost universally available in hospital emergency rooms. The most important abnormalities to be detected are extracerebral hematomas. These lesions produce devastating neurologic symptoms that can be completely reversed if treated early. Intracerebral contusions are of secondary interest because they are more difficult to treat surgically, and the results of treatment are less encouraging.

Stroke. Noncontrast CT scan is the preferred initial imaging study. The majority of strokes are bland infarcts, and in the acute phase the CT scan is normal or nearly normal. In these patients we search for evidence of hemorrhage. A cerebral hematoma presenting as a stroke suggests hypertensive encephalopathy or amyloid angiopathy, depending upon the distribution of the lesion and the age of the patient. Subarachnoid hemorrhage requires further workup by MR and/or angiography to search for an aneurysm or AVM. If no hemorrhage is seen, a bland infarct is presumed to be present but, as yet, occult to CT scanning. The absence of hemorrhage visible on CT allows the clinician to perform anticoagulation or thrombolytic therapy to prevent progression or even reverse the neurologic deficit.

Prethrombolytic Evaluation. Recent developments in stroke therapy require further attention to the examination of patients considered for acute thrombolysis, because hemorrhagic complications are more common when early signs of large infarcts are present on the initial CT or, by inference, MR. Loss of gray/white distinction, low attenuation in the basal ganglia, and poor definition of the insula on CT may contraindicate thrombolytic therapy.

In some centers, stroke triage is performed to evaluate the potential for salvaging an ischemic brain. The point is to distinguish brain that is irreversibly damaged from that which is merely temporarily starved for blood flow, and to visualize the offending vascular lesion directly. Local factors determine whether CT or MR is preferred. MR is clearly superior in depicting irreversible infarct sooner and provides an enormous amount of useful physiologic data relatively rapidly, and gadolinium contrast is safer than iodinated contrast. CT, however, is more readily available within the stroke treatment time window, is almost never contraindicated, detects virtually all acute hemorrhage, and provides almost all of the information potentially available with MRI rapidly and safely.

CT techniques rely on the usually valid inference that visible parenchymal changes are irreversible, and that, conversely, some areas of diminished blood flow might be saved if the plain CT appears normal. A CT perfusion study demonstrating asymmetry corresponding to clinical symptoms may thus define an "ischemic penumbra" if one mentally subtracts the abnormal plain CT volume from the abnormally perfused volume of brain. One can compare multiple perfusion parameter maps to refine this assessment. Relative cerebral blood volume appears to correlate

TABLE 2.1 Preferred Initial Imaging Study by Clinical Presentations

Clinical Presentation	CT Without Contrast	CT With Contrast	MR Without Contrast	MR With Contrast
Trauma	XX			
Stroke	XX			
Seizure	X	X	X	XX
Infection	X	X	X	XX
Cancer	X	X	X	XX
Acute headache	XX			
Chronic headache			XX	
Dementia			XX	
Coma	XX			

XX, best study; X, acceptable study (depends on circumstances).

with infarct, allowing a mismatch between perfusion time and volume to suggest the ischemic penumbra. A quick CTA can show the vascular occlusion directly.

MR techniques can be used similarly. Highly T2-weighted sequences are used to exclude hemorrhage, diffusion-weighted imaging defines infarcted tissue, and perfusion scans show areas of diminished blood flow. By subtracting the volume of abnormal diffusion from the volume of abnormal perfusion, the area of "diffusion-perfusion mismatch" representing the penumbra of potentially salvageable brain is defined. MRA defines the vascular lesion directly.

Use these techniques cautiously, validate them in your institution with the stroke team, and remember to keep your protocol as simple as possible. Keep in mind that the exclusion of hemorrhage in this population is critical and the data that support MR for this purpose are still controversial. Remember also that no treatment for stroke has been approved on the basis of these advanced imaging techniques.

Seizure patients present interesting problems for the radiologist. If it is the patient's first seizure, an intracranial tumor, infection, or other acute process must be excluded. For this reason, contrast-enhanced MR or contrast-enhanced CT is the preferred approach. If the patient is in the immediate postictal state, or if a residual neurologic deficit is present at the time of imaging, a noncontrast CT scan should be obtained as the first study.

If the seizure disorder is chronic, and particularly if it is refractory to medical therapy, then a detailed MR examination, including high-resolution coronal images of the medial temporal lobes and other clinically suspected abnormal brain structures, is performed.

Infection and Cancer. In any patient in whom infectious disease or cancer is a consideration, contrast-enhanced MR is the preferred study. Parenchymal tumor or metastatic disease will be demonstrated with this study, and contrast-enhanced MR has the advantage of depicting meningeal disease much better than any other imaging modality. In some centers and under certain clinical conditions, contrast-enhanced CT is performed rather than MR. It is difficult to quantify the clinical impact of this choice of imaging strategy. It can be justified on grounds of economic cost and considerable clinical experience.

Headache is a frequent indication for imaging of the brain. Patients with severe acute headaches should be imaged with noncontrast head CT. Acute severe headaches may be the result of subarachnoid hemorrhage, acute hydrocephalus, or an enlarging intracranial mass. The chronic headache patient is generally evaluated by MR scanning. If the headache is not accompanied by local neurologic symptoms, a noncontrast MR scan is usually sufficient. However, if the headache is associated with focal neurologic complaints, then gadolinium-enhanced MR scanning is indicated. When chronic headache is the sole presenting complaint, the yield of imaging is low.

Coma. It is crucial to distinguish between a patient with an acute confusional state or coma and a patient who is chronically demented. The comatose or acutely confused patient should be imaged to detect an intracranial hemorrhage. These patients are studied urgently with noncontrast CT. However, the majority of patients who present in this manner will not have an acute structural lesion of the brain. Many will be comatose owing to metabolic abnormalities of the brain. An acute infarct may be present, but this may be invisible on CT, particularly in the brainstem.

Dementia. The chronic dementia patient is generally studied by noncontrast MR as a screening examination for large frontal masses, hydrocephalus, and other treatable abnormalities that may cause a clinical picture that is indistinguishable from AD. MR may also demonstrate small-vessel ischemic changes in the cerebral white matter and small infarcts, which also may clinically mimic AD. If these findings are not present, and the clinical picture is correct, the clinician may offer a diagnosis of AD. PET studies may play a role in assessing prognosis and guiding therapy, especially in the clinical setting of mild cognitive impairment.

ANALYSIS OF THE ABNORMALITY

When an abnormality is detected, the goal of the radiologist is to categorize the finding and, if possible, make a specific diagnosis. Given the large number and relatively infrequent specific findings of neurologic diseases, it is essential to adopt a systematic analytic method to narrow the range of differential diagnostic possibilities. Armed with an amalgam of basic clinical, anatomic, and pathologic knowledge, we can create such a system.

The central question in lesion analysis is the presence of mass or atrophy. Once the brain has completed its development, any injury resulting in tissue loss is permanent. While functional recovery can occur, tissue loss is virtually never restored. Whenever focal or diffuse tissue loss is identified, a strong inference is drawn that the lesion is permanent and untreatable. On the other hand, if the brain is expanded, with normal structures displaced away from the lesion, the lesion is probably active and potentially treatable. Therefore, the urgency for specific diagnosis is greater.

Mass. The concept of mass effect is an essential starting point. A mass is recognized by displacement of normal structures away from the abnormality. The term *mass* is used in a sense that differs somewhat from our understanding of mass in physics, where the central feature of mass is its gravitational affect. The term *mass* in neuroradiology is employed in the sense of an object occupying space. Since two solid objects cannot coexist in the same space, the mass displaces normal cerebral structures away from it. The normal midline structures may be shifted contralateral to the mass. The sulci adjacent to the mass may be effaced, since the CSF in the sulci is displaced by the mass. Similarly, ipsilateral ventricular structures may be compressed by a mass, rendering the ipsilateral ventricle smaller than the contralateral ventricle. These specific points might be summarized by the question: Is there too much tissue within the skull?

Atrophy. Conversely, an atrophic lesion is recognized by widening of the ipsilateral sulci or enlargement of the ventricle adjacent to the lesion. We may ask the question: Is there too little brain? It is important to note that we have not listed shift of the midline toward the side of the lesion as a sign of atrophy. Shift ipsilateral to an atrophic lesion is very unusual and is only seen commonly in congenital hemiatrophy. Even if a complete hemispherectomy is performed, shift of the midline toward the side of the hemispherectomy defect is almost always a sign of mass in the remaining cerebral hemisphere or an extra axial mass compressing it.

When a pattern of diffuse cerebral atrophy is encountered, the first question we must ask is: What is the patient's age? If the patient is over 65 and has normal cognitive function, a diagnosis of age-appropriate cerebral atrophy can be made. Experience teaches us the range of normal to be expected for each age group. If the patient is demented, a diagnosis of AD may be made on clinical grounds. It has been recently suggested that specific neuroradiologic features of AD exist, such as focal atrophy of the hippocampal regions of the medial temporal lobe, but this has yet to be confirmed prospectively with sufficient reliability. PET scanning may sometimes be useful in this setting. If the patient is below 65 years of age, a large number of relatively rare conditions (discussed in Chapter 7) must be considered.

Reversible Atrophy. It is most important for the radiologist to consider the three common causes of reversible cerebral atrophy. They are related to dehydration and starvation. Patients with Addison's disease or other causes of dehydration or abnormal fluid balance may occasionally present with a CT picture of atrophy. With treatment, a more normal appearance of the brain can be restored. Nutritional causes of reversible cerebral atrophy exist in anorexia nervosa and bulimia. The relative contribution of dehydration and starvation in these conditions is difficult to determine. Alcoholism may also occasionally result in reversible "cerebral atrophy." Although the neurotoxic effects of alcohol are not reversible, it has been hypothesized that the accompanying nutritional deficiencies may be corrected, restoring a more normal appearance to the brain on imaging studies.

Mass Lesion: Intra-axial or Extra-axial. Should a mass be identified, the first question we must ask is: Is the mass *intra-axial,* within the brain and expanding it, or *extra-axial,* outside the brain and compressing it? This distinction is usually obvious, but in some cases it is very difficult. Intra-axial masses are more dangerous to the patient and less easily treated than extra-axial masses. Therefore, we prefer to orient our approach to detect extra-axial masses reliably. Intra-axial masses are, most commonly, metastases, intracranial hemorrhages, primary intracranial tumors such as glioblastoma, and brain abscesses. Extra-axial masses are, most commonly, subdural or epidural hematomas, meningiomas, neuromas, and dermoid or epidermoid cysts.

To distinguish an intra-axial from an extra-axial mass, concentrate on the margins of the mass. Just as the beach is more interesting than the open sea, the interface between the mass and the surrounding brain is more interesting than the center of the mass. Extra-axial masses generally possess a broad dural surface. In contrast, intra-axial masses are surrounded completely by brain. In the posterior fossa, the most reliable sign of an extra-axial mass is widening of the ipsilateral subarachnoid space. The cerebellum and brainstem are displaced away from the bony margins of the calvarium by the mass. In contrast, intra-axial masses demonstrate a narrow ipsilateral subarachnoid space. In the supratentorial compartment, we evaluate a mass somewhat differently. With an intra-axial mass, the gyri are expanded and the CSF spaces are compressed. The CSF spaces adjacent to an extra-axial mass, on the other hand, become larger as we approach the mass.

With the multiplanar capability of MR we are frequently able to visualize direct displacement of the brain away from the dura by an extra-axial mass. When gadolinium is administered, extra-axial masses frequently show dural enhancement, whereas this is less common with intra-axial masses. Extra-axial masses tend to enhance homogeneously, e.g., meningioma or neuroma, or not at all, e.g., extracerebral hematomas and cysts. Intra-axial lesions tend to enhance in a ringlike or irregular fashion. In general, intra-axial masses have more surrounding edema than extra-axial masses of the same size.

Solitary or Multiple. Once a mass is identified and its location within or outside the brain is established, the next question we ask is: Is this a solitary lesion, or are there multiple lesions? The implication is that a single lesion is more likely to be the result of isolated primary cerebral disease and that multiple lesions are more likely to be manifestations of widespread or systemic diseases. A single ring-enhancing lesion within the brain may suggest a glioblastoma. Multiple ring-enhancing lesions within the brain more likely represent metastases or abscesses. If a single infarct is identified, it is likely to be caused by a lesion within the carotid circulation ipsilateral to the lesion. If multiple infarcts are seen, they may represent border zone infarcts resulting from global hypoperfusion or they may be a result of a cardiac source of emboli.

Gray Matter or White Matter. If a lesion within the brain is primarily manifest by lucency on CT or increased signal on the T2-weighted MR, the most important question is whether the lesion involves gray matter, white matter, or both. Diseases primarily involving white matter without mass effect are attributable to a wide array of causes (see Chapter 7). Lesions involving gray matter are usually a result of infarct, trauma, or encephalitis. If the lesion has mass effect, these conditions are likely acute. If the lesion is atrophic, it is likely chronic.

If the white matter is exclusively involved and the lesion is expansile, a pattern of edema is most likely present. Usually this will represent vasogenic edema caused by an intracerebral mass. The frondlike pattern of white matter extension and mass effect is typical. This form of edema results from disturbances in tight capillary junctions that occur in association with cerebral tumors, abscesses, or hematomas. This type of edema tends to progress relatively slowly and persist over time. If there is relatively more edema compared to the size of the lesion, a tumor or abscess is considered to be more likely than a hematoma.

If there is white matter expansion and increased T2 signal on MR or lucency on CT with gray matter involvement, cytotoxic edema is present. Cytotoxic edema results from increased tissue water content following the neuropathologic response to cell death. In these cases, infarct, trauma, or encephalitis should be considered. This is called the *gray matter pattern.*

Lesion Distribution. When a gray matter pattern is identified, the distribution of the gray matter abnormality allows us to distinguish among infarct, trauma, and encephalitis. Infarcts are distributed according to vascular patterns described in Chapter 4. For example, if a wedge-shaped lesion involves the opercula of the sylvian fissure and the underlying white matter and basal ganglia, a diagnosis of middle cerebral artery territory infarct is made. Similarly, if the medial aspect of the cerebral hemisphere anteriorly and over the convexity is involved, an anterior cerebral infarct is diagnosed. If the area of involvement falls between two major vascular territories, a border zone or "watershed" infarct is likely. With multiple border zone infarcts, global hypoperfusion because of cardiac arrest must be suspected. If the deep gray matter structures bilaterally are involved, pure anoxia owing to carbon monoxide poisoning or respiratory arrest should be considered. These pure patterns are somewhat idealized, because hypoxemia and ischemia are frequently associated.

Traumatic lesions are also distributed in a characteristic fashion (see Chapter 3). Because of the transmission of forces through the brain and the relationship of the brain to the surrounding skull, traumatic lesions tend to occur at the orbital frontal and frontal polar regions, the temporal poles, and the occipital poles in acceleration/deceleration injuries. A direct blow produces injury beneath the site of blow and opposite the site. The lesion opposite the blow is called the *contra-coup injury*. Penetrating brain wounds are distributed according to the path of the missile or the location of the trauma.

Herpes simplex encephalitis is also distributed in a characteristic fashion. This disease spreads from the oral and nasal mucosa to the trigeminal and olfactory ganglion cells and then transdurally to the brain. The most common locations for involvement are *(1)* the medial temporal lobes adjacent to the trigeminal ganglia and *(2)* the orbital frontal regions adjacent to the olfactory bulbs. Other forms of encephalitis are less common and are diagnosed by typical clinical presentation, characteristic CSF findings, cultures, and mixed gray and white matter pattern of involvement at other sites.

Contrast Enhancement. The next question we ask about a cerebral abnormality is whether or not it is associated with abnormal contrast enhancement. Enhancement of the brain parenchyma means that the blood-brain barrier has broken down and that the process is biologically active. In the astrocytoma tumor line, an increase in enhancement correlates with higher tumor grade. However, enhancement does not imply malignancy. Infarcts, hemorrhages, abscesses, and encephalitis all can demonstrate contrast enhancement. However, in these nonneoplastic processes, enhancement appears only in the acute phase and resolves with time.

Signal Intensity or Attenuation Pattern. You will note that we have saved patterns of signal intensity for last. These patterns are specific to the imaging modality or MR pulse sequence employed and are therefore the least generally applicable and to a great extent the least reliable radiologic findings. Knowledge of the physical basis for imaging with CT and MR is necessary to understand the pattern of signal intensities within the brain. However, as a starting point, one need only know that if an abnormality is white on CT or white on T1 MR or black on T2 MR, hemorrhage must be considered. Also, if the brain is as bright as a light bulb on diffusion-weighted MR images, infarct is suggested. This topic is discussed extensively elsewhere.

SUGGESTED READINGS

Atlas S, ed. Magnetic Resonance Imaging of the Brain and Spine. Philadelphia: Lippincott Williams & Wilkins, 2002.

Brodal P. The Central Nervous System: Structure and Function. 1st ed. New York: Oxford University Press, 1992.

Burger PC. Surgical Pathology of the Nervous System and Its Coverings. New York: Churchill-Livingstone, 2002.

Davis RL, Robertson DM. Textbook of Neuropathology. 3rd ed. Baltimore, MD: Williams & Wilkins, 1997.

DeGroot J. Correlative Neuroanatomy. 21st ed. Norwalk, CT: Appleton & Lange, 1991.

Escourolle R, Poirier J, Gray F. Manual of Basic Neuropathology. 4th ed. London: Butterworth-Heinemann, 2003.

Grossman RI, Yousem DM. Neuroradiology: The Requisites. St. Louis: Mosby, 2003.

Osborn A. Diagnostic Imaging: Brain. Salt Lake City: AMIRSYS, 2004.

Plum F, Posner JB. The Diagnosis of Stupor and Coma. 3rd ed. Philadelphia: FA Davis, 1980.

Sox HC, Blatt MA, Higgins MC, Marton KI. Medical Decision Making. Boston: Butterworths, 1988.

Von Kummer R, Bozzao L, Manalfe C. Early CT Diagnosis of Hemispheric Brain Infarction. Berlin: Springer, 1995.

Chapter 3

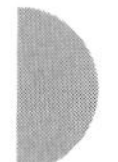

Craniofacial Trauma

Robert M. Barr, Alisa D. Gean, and Tuong H. Le

Head Trauma
Primary Head Injury: Extra-axial
Primary Head Injury: Intra-axial
Secondary Head Injury
Brainstem Injury
Penetrating Trauma
Predicting Outcome After Acute Head Trauma
Child Abuse

Facial Trauma

HEAD TRAUMA

Imaging Strategy. *CT.* Imaging of acute head trauma is performed to detect treatable lesions before secondary neurologic damage occurs. Currently, this is best performed by CT for several reasons: it is quick, widely available, and highly accurate in the detection of acute intra-axial and extra-axial hemorrhage, as well as skull, temporal bone, facial, and orbital fractures. Monitoring equipment is easily accommodated. CT images must be reviewed using multiple windows. A narrow window width is used to evaluate the brain, whereas a slightly wider window width is used to exaggerate contrast between extra-axial collections and the adjacent skull, and a very wide window is used to evaluate the skull itself (see Figs. 3.1, 3.6). Contiguous 5-mm sections through the brain provide sufficient detail and can be obtained with modern scanners in less than 15 minutes. Thinner sections are used to evaluate the orbits, facial skeleton, and skull base. IV contrast media is not used in the acute setting because it may mimic or mask underlying hemorrhage.

When CT is performed in unconscious patients with severe head injury, it may be wise to include routine coverage of the craniocervical junction. A study by Link et al. (1) found that 18% of these patients had fractures of C1, C2, or the occipital condyles and that roughly half of all fractures were missed by plain radiographs.

MR has traditionally been less desirable than CT in the acute setting because of the longer examination times, difficulty in managing life support and other monitoring equipment, and inferior demonstration of bone detail. MR, however, has been shown to be comparable or superior to CT in the detection of acute epidural and subdural hematomas and nonhemorrhagic brain injury (2,3). MR is also more sensitive to brainstem injury and, especially with fluid-attentuated inversion recovery (FLAIR) and gradient-echo pulse sequences, to acute, subacute, and chronic hemorrhage (4,5). Diffusion-weighted and diffusion tensor imaging have improved detection of both acute and chronic neuronal injury (6–9). In the majority of cases, MR is the modality of choice for patients with subacute and chronic head injury and is recommended for patients with acute head trauma when neurologic findings are unexplained by CT. MR is also more accurate in predicting long-term prognosis. With the development of parallel imaging, faster sequences, improved monitoring equipment, and greater scanner availability, MR will continue to play an increasing role in the evaluation of acute head trauma.

Skull Films. Unfortunately, plain films continue to be used in evaluating patients with acute head trauma, despite abundant evidence that they are not helpful (10–12). Patients who are judged to be at low risk for intracranial injury on the basis of a careful history and physical examination should be observed, and patients at high risk should be imaged by CT. Plain films virtually never demonstrate significant findings in the low-risk group and are inadequate to characterize or exclude intracranial injury in the high-risk group. Further, the absence of skull fractures on plain films clearly does not exclude significant intracranial injury. In fact, in one large autopsy series of patients with fatal head injuries, only 75% had skull fractures (13). The decision to obtain a head CT in the setting of trauma must be based on clinical grounds. Skull films are poor predictors of significant intracranial pathology and should not be used either to prevent or encourage further diagnostic evaluation.

Scalp Injury. When interpreting CT scans for head trauma, it is helpful to begin by examining the extracranial structures for evidence of scalp injury or radiopaque foreign bodies. Scalp soft tissue swelling is often the only reliable evidence of the site of impact. The subgaleal hematoma is the most common manifestation of scalp injury and can be recognized on CT or MR as focal soft tissue swelling of the scalp located beneath the subcutaneous fibrofatty tissue and above the temporalis muscle and calvarium.

Skull Fractures. Nondisplaced linear fractures of the calvarium are the most common type of skull fracture. They may be difficult to detect on CT scans, especially when the fracture plane is parallel to the plane of section. Fortunately, isolated linear skull fractures do not require treatment. Surgical management is usually indicated for depressed and compound skull fractures, both of which are seen better on CT scans than on plain films (Fig. 3.1). Depressed fractures are frequently associated with an underlying contusion. Intracranial air ("pneumocephalus") may be seen with compound skull fractures or fractures involving the paranasal sinuses. Thin-section CT using a bone algorithm is the best method to evaluate fractures in critical areas, such as the skull base, orbit, or facial bones. Thin sections can also be helpful to evaluate the degree of comminution and depression of bone fragments.

Temporal Bone Fractures. Thin-section, high-resolution CT scanning has led to a dramatic improvement in the ability to detect and characterize temporal bone fractures. Patients with fractures of the temporal bone may present with deafness, facial nerve palsies, vertigo, dizziness, or nystagmus. Clinical symptoms are often masked in the presence of other serious injuries. Physical signs of temporal bone fracture include hemotympanum, CSF otorrhea, and ecchymosis over the mastoid process ("Battle's sign"). Temporal bone fractures may be first suspected on standard head CT scans performed to exclude intracranial injury. Findings such as opacification of the mastoid air cells, fluid in the middle ear cavity, pneumocephalus, or occasionally pneumolabyrinth, should raise the suspicion of a temporal bone fracture. Optimal evaluation of a suspected temporal bone fracture requires thin-section (1 to 1.5 mm) axial and direct coronal CT imaging using a bone algorithm. With multidetector CT, thinner-section axial imaging can be performed, and coronal reformats may be adequate for interpretation.

Fractures of the temporal bone can be classified as longitudinal or transverse depending on their orientation relative to the long axis of the petrous bone. If the fracture parallels the long axis of the petrous pyramid, it is termed a "longitudinal" fracture; fractures perpendicular to the long axis of the petrous bone are termed "transverse" fractures. "Mixed" fracture types also occur.

The longitudinal temporal bone fracture (Fig. 3.2) represents 70% to 90% of temporal bone fractures (14). It

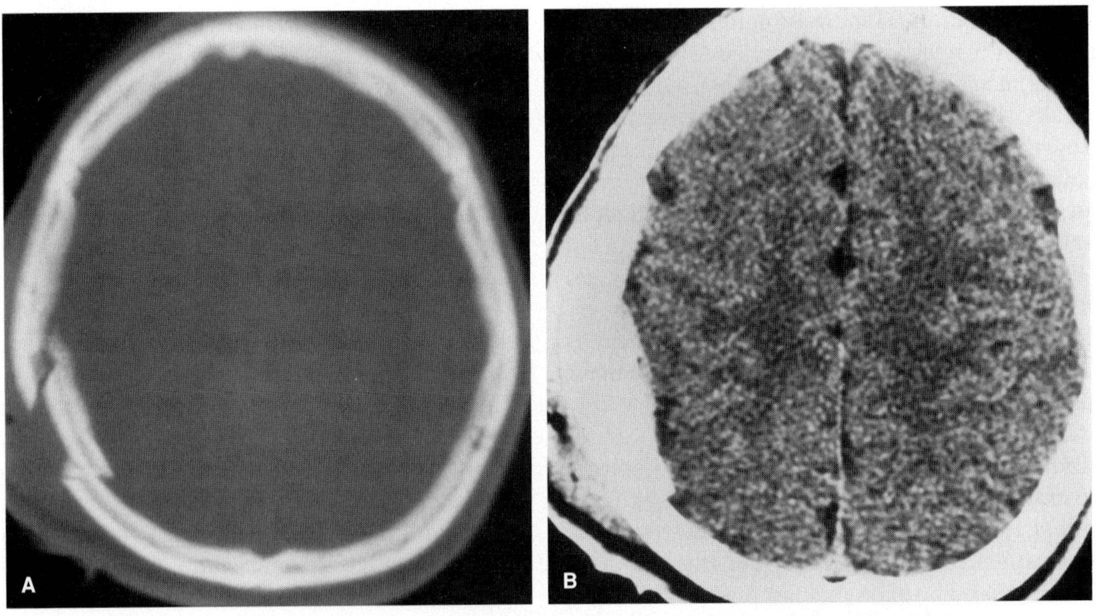

FIGURE 3.1. **Depressed Skull Fracture. A.** Axial CT scan demonstrates a right parietal depressed skull fracture with overlying soft tissue swelling. The fracture is well seen when a wide window is used to enhance contrast between bone and soft tissue. **B.** The narrower window demonstrates excellent contrast between gray and white matter but fails to show the fracture. A small extra-axial hematoma is seen in the right parietal area.

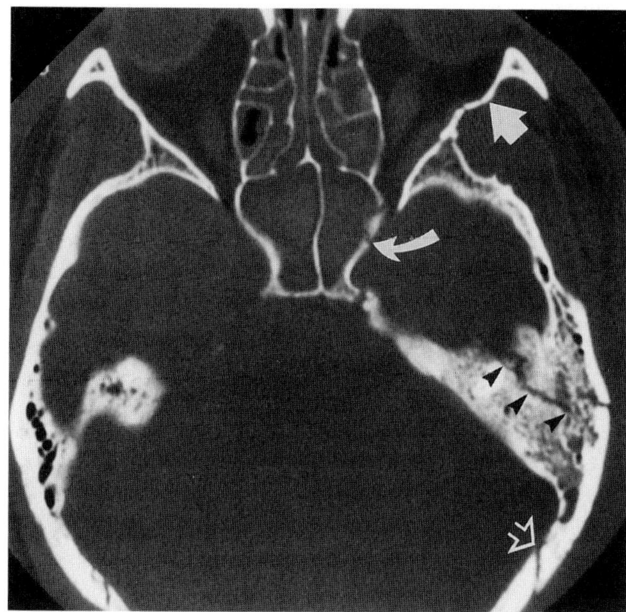

FIGURE 3.2. **Longitudinal Temporal Bone Fracture.** Axial CT scan shows a longitudinal left temporal bone fracture (*arrowheads*) with opacification of the mastoid air cells. Diastasis of the left lambdoid suture (*open arrow*) and fractures of the sphenoid sinus (*curved arrow*) and left lateral orbital wall (*arrow*) are also present. (Reprinted with permission from Gean AD. Imaging of Head Trauma. Philadelphia: Lippincott Williams & Wilkins; 1994:63.)

results from a blow to the side of the head. Complications include conductive hearing loss, dislocation or fracture of the ossicles, and CSF otorhinorrhea. Facial nerve palsy may occur, but it is often delayed and incomplete. Sensorineural hearing loss is uncommon.

The transverse temporal bone fracture usually results from a blow to the occiput or frontal region. Complications are usually more severe and include sensorineural hearing loss, severe vertigo, nystagmus, and perilymphatic fistula. Facial palsy is seen in 30% to 50% of these cases and is often complete (14). Transverse fractures may also involve the carotid canal or jugular foramen, causing injury to the carotid artery or jugular vein.

Mixed or complex temporal bone fractures represent approximately 10% of temporal bone fractures. They involve a combination of fracture planes and generally follow severe crushing blows to the skull. Patients with mixed temporal bone fractures have a high incidence of associated intracranial injury.

Classification of Head Injury. Traumatic head injury can be divided into primary and secondary forms. Primary lesions are those that occur as a direct result of a blow to the head. Secondary lesions occur as a consequence of primary lesions, usually as a result of mass effect or vascular compromise. Secondary lesions are often preventable, whereas primary injuries, by definition, have already occurred by the time the patient arrives in the emergency department.

Primary lesions include epidural, subdural, subarachnoid, and intraventricular hemorrhage, as well as diffuse axonal injury (DAI), cortical contusions, intracerebral hematomas, and subcortical gray matter injury. Direct injury to the cerebral vasculature is another type of primary lesion.

Secondary lesions include cerebral swelling, brain herniation, hydrocephalus, ischemia or infarction, CSF leak, leptomeningeal cyst, and encephalomalacia.

Brainstem injury, which is also divided into primary and secondary forms, is discussed later in this chapter.

Primary Head Injury: Extra-axial

Epidural hematomas are usually arterial in origin and often result from a skull fracture that disrupts the middle meningeal artery. The developing hematoma strips the dura from the inner table of the skull, forming an ovoid mass that displaces the adjacent brain. They may occur from stretching or tearing of meningeal arteries without an associated fracture, especially in children. Overall, skull fractures are seen in 85% to 95% of cases. In approximately a third of patients with an epidural hematoma, neurologic deterioration occurs after a lucid interval (15).

Most epidural hematomas are temporal or temporoparietal in location, although frontal and occipital hematomas can also occur. Venous epidural hematomas are less common than arterial epidurals and tend to occur at the vertex, posterior fossa, or anterior aspect of the middle cranial fossa. Venous epidural hematomas usually occur as a result of disrupted dural venous sinuses.

On CT, acute epidural hematomas appear as well-defined, high-attenuation lenticular or biconvex extra-axial collections (Fig. 3.3). Associated mass effect with sulcal effacement and midline shift is frequently seen. Bone windows usually demonstrate an overlying linear skull fracture. Because epidural hematomas exist in the potential space between the dura and inner table of the skull, they usually will not cross cranial sutures, where the periosteal layer of the dura is firmly attached (Fig. 3.4). Near the vertex, however, the periosteum forms the outer wall of the sagittal sinus and is less tightly adherent to the sagittal suture. Therefore, vertex epidurals, which are usually of venous origin from disruption of the sagittal sinus, can cross the midline. Occasionally, an acute epidural hematoma will appear heterogeneous, containing irregular areas of lower attenuation. This finding may indicate active extravasation of fresh unclotted blood into the collection and warrants immediate surgical attention.

Subdural hematomas are typically venous in origin, resulting from stretching or tearing of cortical veins that traverse the subdural space en route to the dural sinuses. They may also result from disruption of penetrating branches of

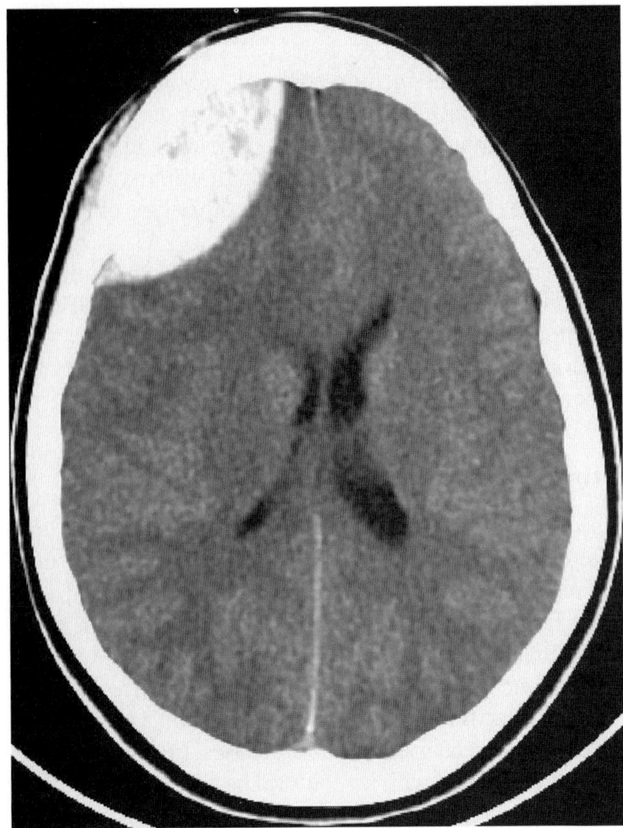

FIGURE 3.3. **Epidural Hematoma.** Axial CT scan demonstrates a biconvex, high-attenuation, extra-axial collection causing mass effect on the right frontal lobe and mild midline shift (subfalcial herniation). Note how the epidural hematoma does not extend beyond the right coronal suture.

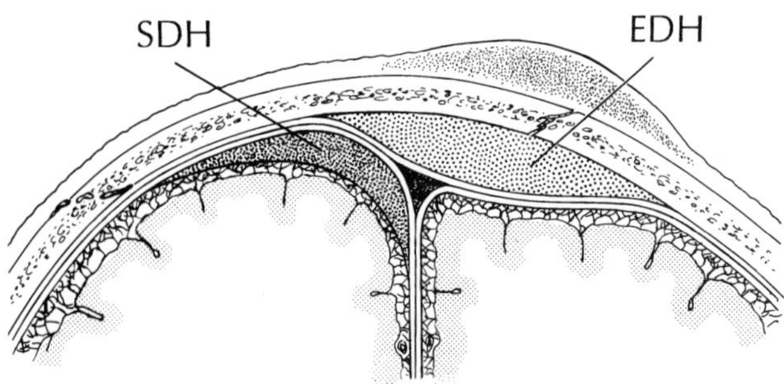

FIGURE 3.4. **Epidural Versus Subdural Hematoma.** Axial diagram of the brain surface in the frontal region demonstrates the characteristic locations of the epidural hematoma (EDH) compared with the subdural hematoma (SDH). Note how the EDH is located above the outer dural layer and the SDH is located beneath the inner dural layer. Only the EDH can cross the falx cerebri. (Reprinted with permission from Gean AD. Imaging of Head Trauma. Philadelphia: Lippincott Williams & Wilkins; 1994:76.)

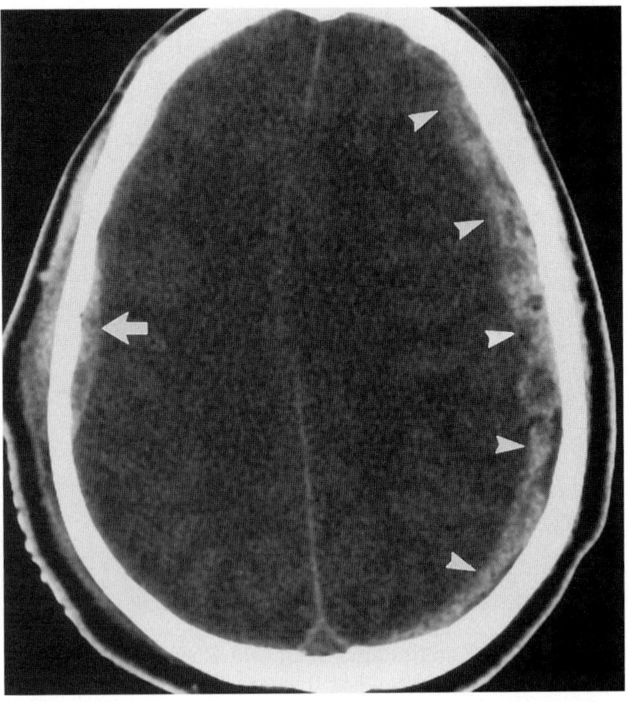

FIGURE 3.5. **Left Subdural and Right Epidural Hematomas.** Axial CT scan demonstrates a crescent-shaped high-attenuation collection extending along the entire left hemisphere consistent with a subdural hematoma (*arrowheads*). Compare the appearance with that of a small epidural hematoma seen on the right (*arrow*), where overlying scalp soft tissue swelling is also present. (Reprinted with permission from Gean AD. Imaging of Head Trauma. Philadelphia: Lippincott Williams & Wilkins; 1994:120.)

superficial cerebral arteries. Because the inner dural layer and arachnoid are not as firmly attached as the structures that make up the epidural space, the subdural hematoma typically extends over a much larger area than the epidural hematoma. Patients with a subdural hematoma commonly present after acute deceleration injury from a motor vehicle accident or fall. The same mechanism can cause cortical contusions and DAI, which are frequently seen in association with acute subdural hematomas.

On axial CT, acute subdural hematomas appear as crescent-shaped extra-axial collections of high attenuation (Fig. 3.5). Small subdural hematomas may be masked by adjacent cortical bone when viewed on a narrow window width but will be apparent with an intermediate window width (Fig. 3.6). Most subdural hematomas are supratentorial, located along the convexity. They are also frequently seen along the falx and tentorium. Because dural reflections form the falx cerebri and tentorium, subdural collections will not cross these structures (see Fig. 3.4). Unlike epidural hematomas, subdural hematomas can cross sutural margins and, in fact, are frequently seen layering along the entire hemispheric convexity from the anterior falx to

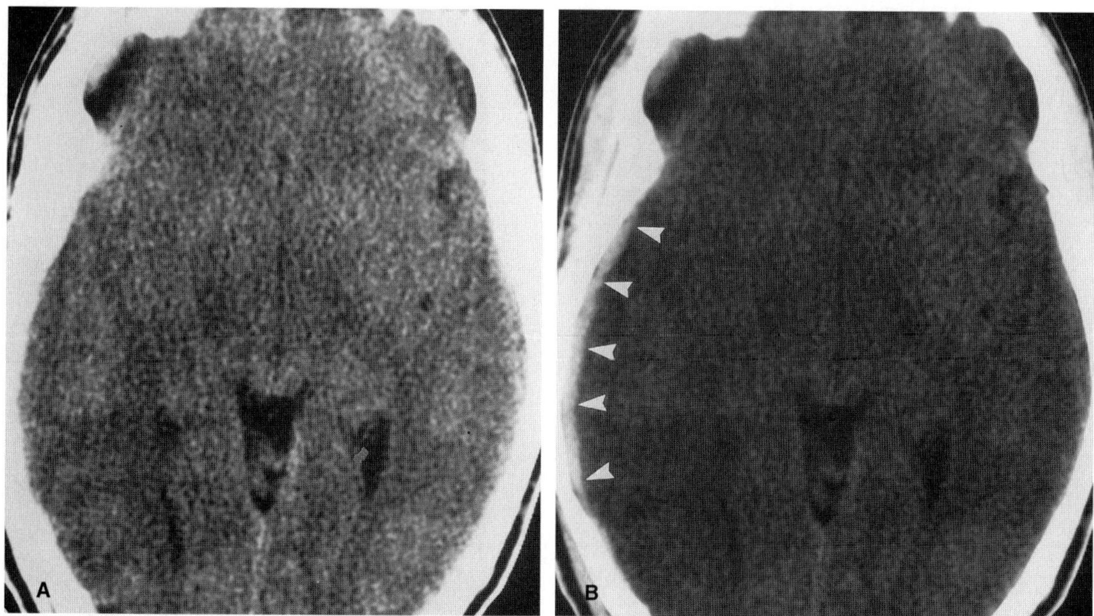

FIGURE 3.6. **Subdural Hematoma Seen on Intermediate Window Only.** A small right temporal subdural hematoma is masked on the CT that used a narrow window **(A)** but is clearly seen **(B)** (*arrowheads*) with an intermediate (or subdural) window.

the posterior falx. Diffuse swelling of the underlying hemisphere is common with subdural hematomas. Because of this, there may be more mass effect than would be expected by the size of the collection, and there may be little or no reduction in midline shift after evacuation of a hemispheric subdural hematoma.

The CT appearance of subdural hematomas changes with time. The density of an acute subdural hematoma initially increases because of clot retraction. By the time most acute subdural hematomas are imaged, the collection is hyperdense, measuring 50 to 60 H, relative to normal brain, which measures 18 to 30 H. The density will then progressively decrease as protein degradation occurs within the hematoma. Occasionally, acute subdural blood may be isodense or hypodense in patients with severe anemia or active extravasation ("hyperacute" subdural hematoma). Rebleeding during evolution of a subdural hematoma causes a heterogeneous appearance from the mixture of fresh blood and partially liquefied hematoma (Fig. 3.7). A sediment level or "hematocrit effect" may be seen either from rebleeding or in patients with clotting disorders (Fig. 3.8). Chronic subdural hematomas have low attenuation values, similar to those of CSF (Fig. 3.9). On noncontrast CT scans, it can be difficult to distinguish them from prominent subarachnoid space secondary to cerebral atrophy. Contrast enhancement can help by demonstrating an enhancing capsule or displaced cortical veins.

During the transition from acute to chronic subdural hematomas, an isodense phase occurs, usually between several days and 3 weeks after the acute event. Although the subdural hematoma itself is less conspicuous during this isodense phase, there are indirect signs on a noncontrast CT scan that should lead to the correct diagnosis. These include effacement of sulci, displacement of cortex with white matter "buckling," and midline shift (Fig. 3.10).

The MR appearance of subdural hematomas depends on the biochemical state of hemoglobin, which varies with the age of the hematoma (see Chapter 4). Acute subdural hematomas are isointense to brain on T1WIs and hypointense on T2WIs. MR is particularly helpful during the subacute phase, when the subdural hematoma may be isodense or hypodense on CT scans. T1WIs will demonstrate high signal intensity caused by the presence of methemoglobin in the subdural collection. This high signal clearly distinguishes subdural hematomas from most nonhemorrhagic fluid collections. MR also reveals that subacute subdural hematomas frequently have a lentiform or biconvex appearance when seen in the coronal plane (Fig. 3.11), rather than the crescent-shaped appearance that is characteristic on axial CT scans. The multiplanar capability of MR scanning is helpful in identifying small convexities and vertex hematomas that might not be detected on axial CT scans because of the similar attenuation of the adjacent bone.

Subarachnoid hemorrhage is common in head injury but is rarely large enough to cause a significant mass effect. It results from the disruption of small subarachnoid vessels or direct extension into the subarachnoid space by a contusion or hematoma. On CT, subarachnoid hemorrhage

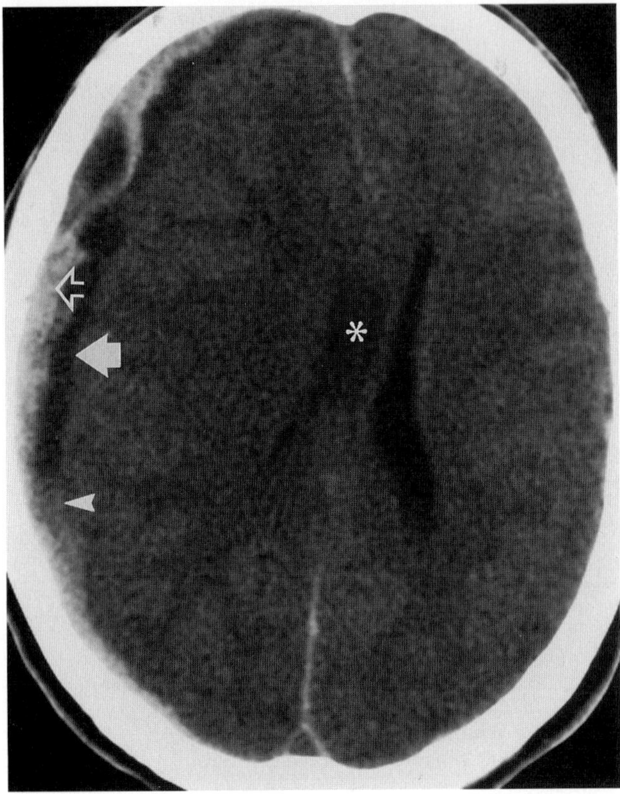

FIGURE 3.7. **Acute and Chronic Subdural Hematoma.** Axial CT scan demonstrates the heterogeneous appearance of superimposed acute and chronic subdural hematomas. The higher-attenuation material (*open arrow*) represents fresh bleeding into a chronic, low-attenuation subdural hematoma (*closed arrow*). Layering of acute blood products is seen in the posterior aspect of the collection (*arrowhead*). Midline shift or "subfalcial herniation" is also present, evidenced by displacement of the right lateral ventricle (*asterisk*) across the midline.

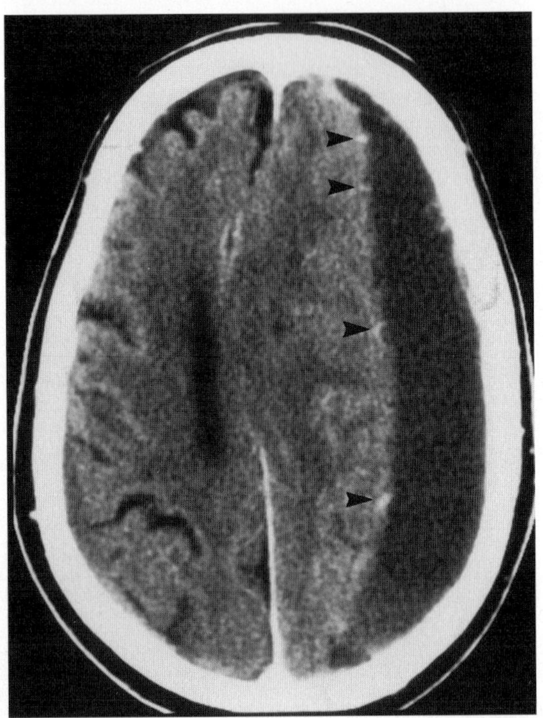

FIGURE 3.9. **Chronic Subdural Hematoma.** Contrast-enhanced CT scan shows a large water-density left subdural collection consistent with a chronic subdural hematoma. There is considerable mass effect with midline shift. Displaced cortical veins can be seen along the brain surface *(arrowheads)*. (Reprinted with permission from Gean AD. Imaging of Head Trauma. Philadelphia: Lippincott Williams & Wilkins; 1994:96.)

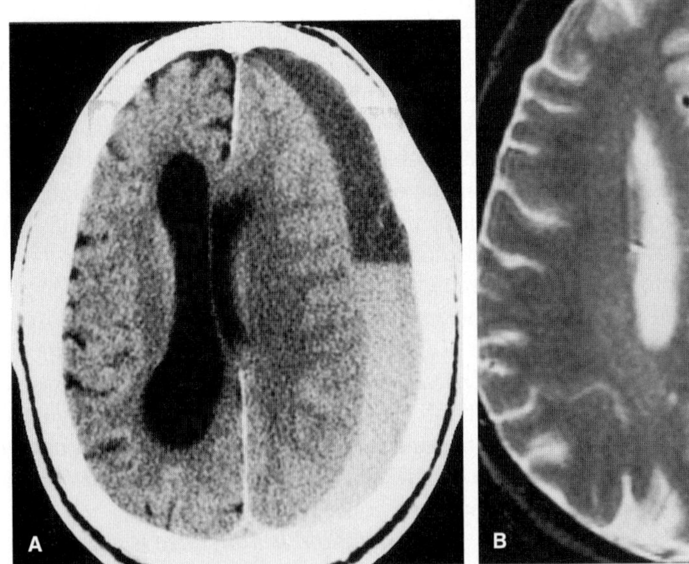

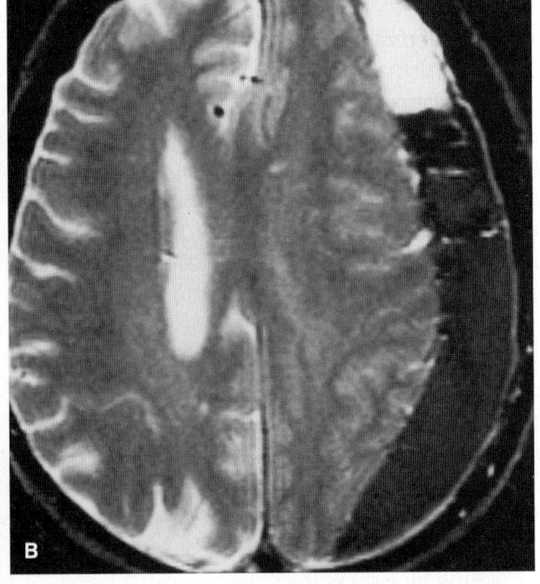

FIGURE 3.8. **Subdural Hematomas With Hematocrit Effect.** A CT scan **(A)** and T2-WI **(B)** in two different patients show large left hemispheric subdural hematomas with fluid–fluid levels, known as the hematocrit effect. This appearance can be seen in patients with clotting disorders or in patients with rebleeding into an older subdural collection. (Reprinted with permission from Gean AD. Imaging of Head Trauma. Philadelphia: Lippincott Williams & Wilkins; 1994:89, 95.)

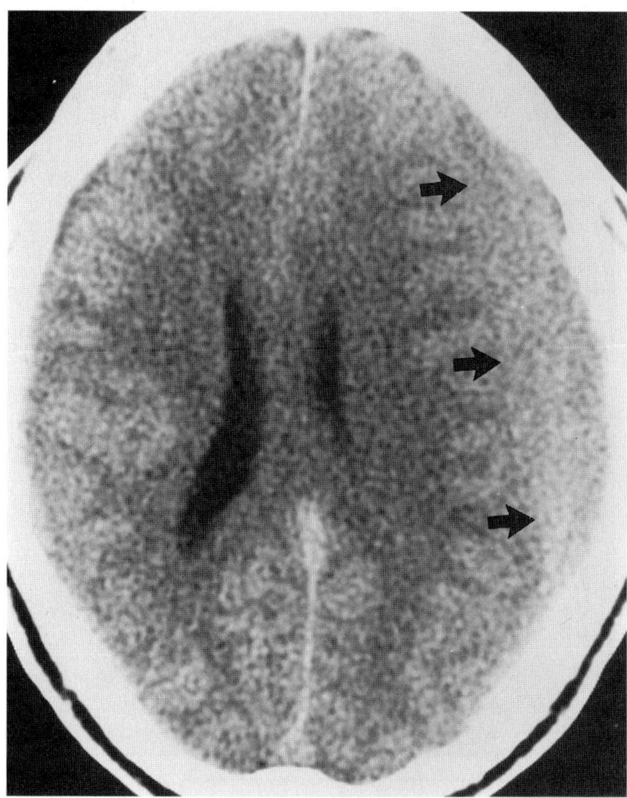

FIGURE 3.10. Subacute Subdural Hematoma on CT. Noncontrast CT scan shows an isodense left subdural hematoma with displacement of the underlying cortex (*arrows*), compression of the lateral ventricle, and mild midline shift.

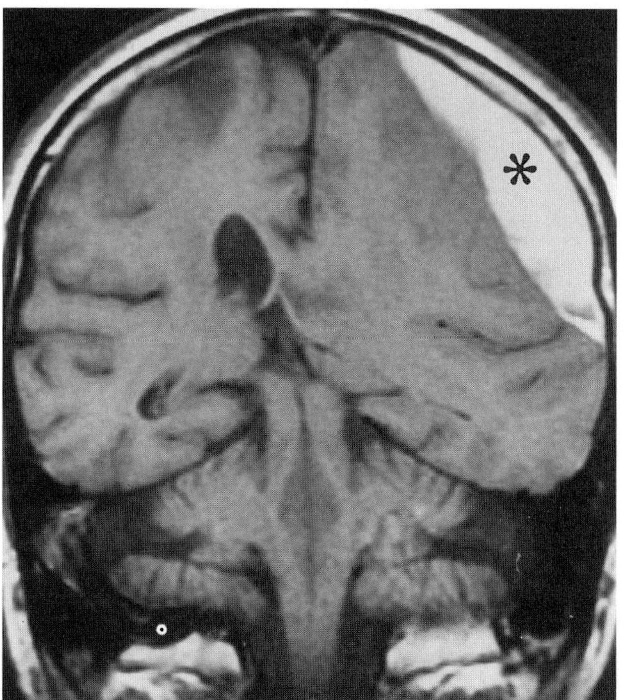

FIGURE 3.11. Subacute Subdural Hematoma on MR. Noncontrast coronal T1WI shows a well-defined, uniform, hyperintense extra-axial collection (*asterisk*) with associated mass effect on the left cerebral hemisphere. This represents a subacute subdural hematoma. The increased signal intensity on a T1-weighted sequence is attributable to methemoglobin. Subdural hematomas can appear crescent-shaped in the axial plane and biconvex in the coronal plane.

appears as linear areas of high attenuation within the cisterns and sulci (Fig. 3.12). Subarachnoid collections along the convexity or tentorium can be differentiated from subdural hematomas by their extension into adjacent sulci. Occasionally, the only finding is apparent effacement of sulci when the sulci are filled with small amounts of blood. In patients who are found unconscious after an unwitnessed event, detection of subarachnoid hemorrhage may indicate a ruptured aneurysm, rather than trauma, as the primary cause. In such cases, contrast-enhanced CT angiography and/or conventional catheter angiography needs to be considered.

Hyperacute subarachnoid hemorrhage may be more difficult to detect on conventional MR than it is on CT scans, because it can be isointense to brain parenchyma on T1W and T2W images. However, FLAIR has been shown to be more sensitive than CT in detecting acute subarachnoid hemorrhage in an animal model, especially when a high volume (1 to 2 mL) is present (5). Subacute subarachnoid hemorrhage may be better appreciated on MR because of its high signal intensity at a time when the blood is isointense to CSF on CT. Chronic hemorrhage on MR scans may show hemosiderin staining in the subarachnoid space, which appears as areas of markedly decreased signal intensity on T1- and T2-weighted sequences ("superficial hemosiderosis"). Subarachnoid hemorrhage may lead to subsequent hydrocephalus by impaired CSF resorption at the level of the arachnoid villi.

Intraventricular hemorrhage is commonly seen in patients with head injuries and can occur by several mechanisms. First, it can result from rotationally induced tearing of subependymal veins on the surface of the ventricles. Another mechanism is by direct extension of a parenchymal hematoma into the ventricular system. Third, intraventricular blood can result from retrograde flow of subarachnoid hemorrhage into the ventricular system through the fourth ventricular outflow foramina. Patients with intraventricular hemorrhage are at risk for subsequent hydrocephalus by obstruction, at the level of either the aqueduct or the arachnoid villi.

On CT, intraventricular hemorrhage appears as hyperdense material, layering dependently within the ventricular system (see Fig. 3.17b). Tiny collections of increased density layering in the occipital horns may be the only clue to intraventricular hemorrhage.

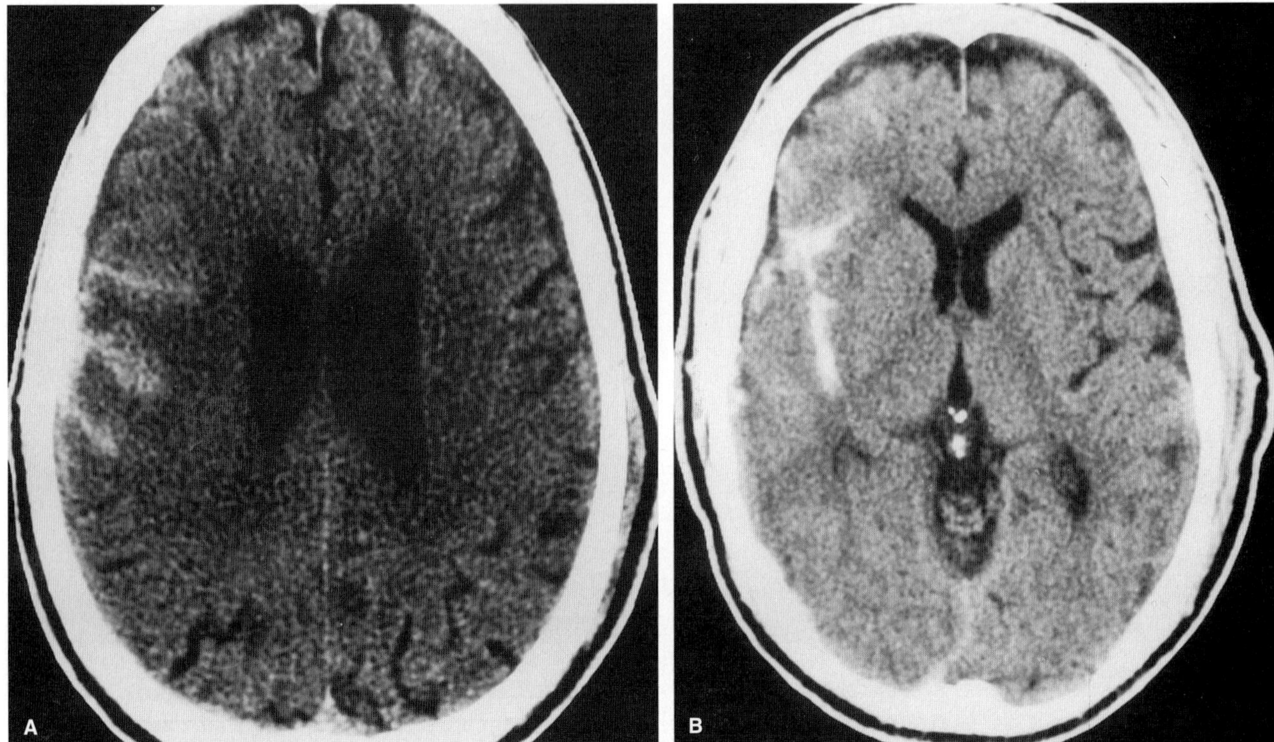

FIGURE 3.12. **Subarachnoid Hemorrhage.** Noncontrast axial CT scans in two different patients demonstrate high-attenuation material within the sulci **(A)** and right sylvian fissure **(B)** consistent with subarachnoid hemorrhage. (Reprinted with permission from Gean AD. Imaging of Head Trauma. Philadelphia: Lippincott Williams & Wilkins; 1994:130, 131.)

Primary Head Injury: Intra-axial

Diffuse axonal injury (DAI) is one of the most common types of primary neuronal injury in patients with severe head trauma. As the name implies, DAI is characterized by widespread disruption of axons that occurs at the time of an acceleration or deceleration injury. The affected areas of the brain may be distant from the site of direct impact; in fact, direct impact is not necessary to cause this type of injury.

The incidence of DAI was likely underestimated until recently because of the difficulty in visualizing these lesions on existing imaging studies as well as on histologic specimens. DAI is much better seen by MR than CT. This factor accounts to a large degree for the increased success of MR at explaining neurologic deficits after trauma and in predicting long-term outcome. Though MR has improved the detection of DAI in patients who have suffered head trauma, the incidence of this form of injury is probably still underestimated. Newer imaging methods, such as diffusion-weighted and diffusion tensor imaging with three-dimensional (3D) tractography, have shown potential in improving the detection of white matter injury in both acute and chronic DAI (6–9,16).

Patients with DAI are most commonly injured in high-speed motor vehicle accidents. These lesions have not been seen as a consequence of simple falls, such as when a patient falls from the standing position. Loss of consciousness typically starts immediately after the injury and is more severe than in patients with cortical contusions or hematomas.

CT findings in DAI can be subtle or absent. Only approximately 20% of lesions contain sufficient hemorrhage to be visible on CT scans, accounting for the low sensitivity of this modality. Most common is the finding of small, petechial hemorrhages at the gray–white junction of the cerebral hemispheres or corpus callosum (Fig. 3.13). Ill-defined areas of decreased attenuation on CT may occasionally be seen with nonhemorrhagic lesions.

On MR, nonhemorrhagic DAI lesions appear as small foci of increased signal on T2WIs (T2 prolongation) within the white matter (Fig. 3.14). The lesions tend to be multiple, with as many as 15 to 20 lesions seen in patients with severe head injury. If seen on T1WIs, they appear as subtle areas of decreased intensity. Petechial hemorrhage causes a central hypointensity on T2WIs and hyperintensity on T1WIs within a few days as a result of intracellular methemoglobin. The conspicuity of DAI on MR diminishes over weeks to months as the damaged axons degenerate and the edema resolves. Residual findings might include nonspecific atrophy or hemosiderin staining, which can persist for years and is especially obvious on gradient-echo sequences (Fig. 3.15).

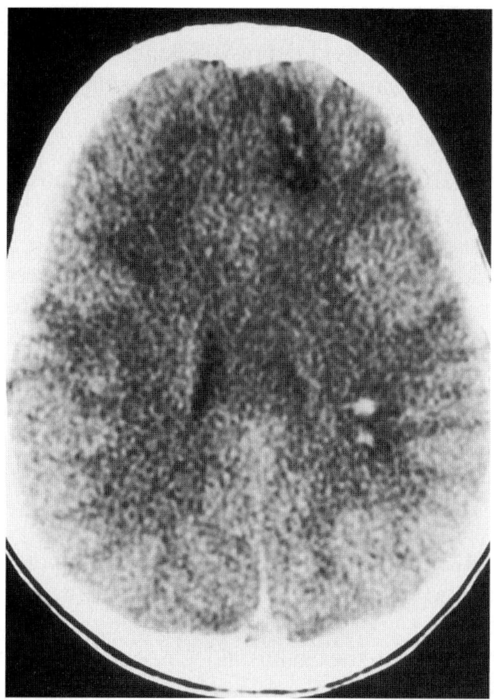

FIGURE 3.13. **The CT Appearance of DAI.** Noncontrast CT scan shows punctuate, high-attenuation foci with surrounding edema in the left frontal and parietal white matter consistent with hemorrhagic DAI. Additional lesions could be seen at other levels.

DAI is seen in characteristic locations that correlate with the severity of the trauma. Patients with the mildest forms of injury have lesions confined to the frontal and temporal white matter, near the gray–white junction. The lesions typically involve the parasagittal regions of the frontal lobes and periventricular regions of the temporal lobes. Patients with more severe trauma have DAI involving lobar white matter as well as the corpus callosum, especially the posterior body and splenium (Fig. 3.16). The corpus callosum accounts for approximately 20% of all DAI lesions (15). Initially thought to be caused by direct impact from the falx, injury to the corpus callosum, as shown by experimental work (17), is most commonly caused by rotational shear forces, like all forms of DAI. The corpus callosum may be particularly susceptible to DAI because the falx prevents displacement of the cerebral hemispheres. DAI of the corpus callosum is almost always seen in association with lesions in the lobar white matter. DAI in the most severe cases involves the dorsolateral aspect of the midbrain and upper pons, in addition to the lobar white matter and corpus callosum (see "Brainstem Injury").

Cortical contusions are areas of focal brain injury primarily involving superficial gray matter. Patients with cortical contusions are much less likely to have loss of consciousness at the time of injury than are patients with DAI. Contusions are also associated with a better prognosis than

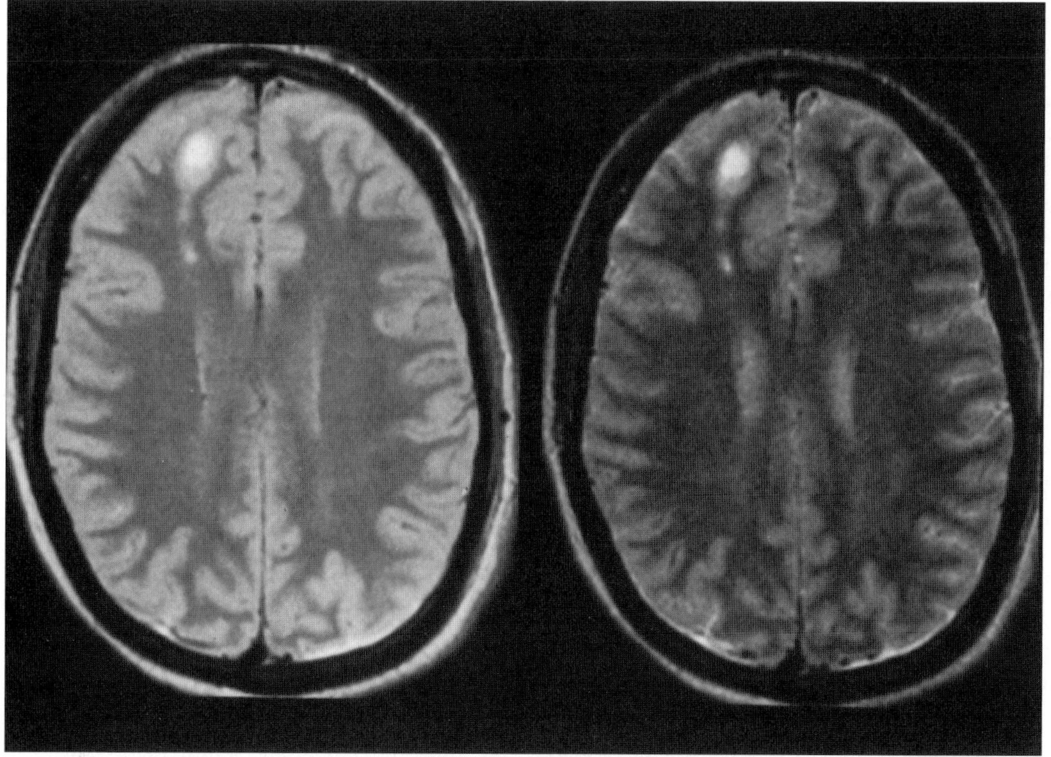

FIGURE 3.14. **The MR Appearance of Acute DAI.** Proton-density (*left*) and T2-weighted (*right*) MR images show several adjacent foci of high signal, representing DAI in the right frontal parasagittal white matter. (Reprinted with permission from Gean AD. Imaging of Head Trauma. Philadelphia: Lippincott Williams & Wilkins; 1994:225.)

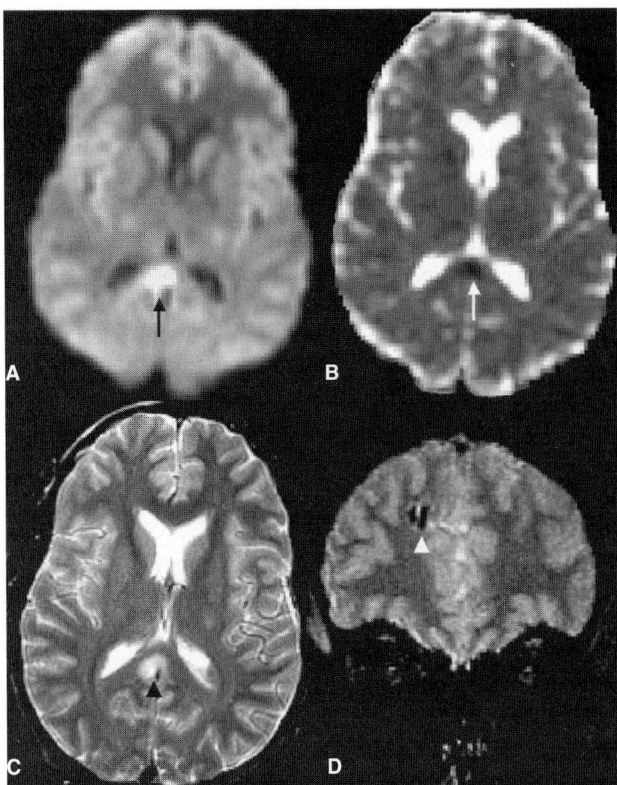

FIGURE 3.15. **The Appearance of Acute DAI on Diffusion-Weighted MR.** **(A)** Combined diffusion-weighted (DW) and **(B)** apparent diffusion coefficient (ADC) MR images from a patient who fell down nine steps show a focus of high signal on the combined DW image (*white arrow*) and dark signal on the ADC image (*black arrow*) within the splenium of the corpus callosum. Note that the extent of ADC abnormality is smaller than signal abnormality on the combined DW image. The reduced ADC represents the true area of acute cytotoxic injury, while the bright signal area on the combined DW image also has contribution from vasogenic edema (T2 prolongation). The T2 abnormality that appears on the combined DW image without the corresponding ADC abnormality has been termed 'T2 shinethrough.' **(C)** The T2 abnormality can be appreciated on the spin-echo T2WI (*black arrowhead*). **(D)** This patient also has findings of hemorrhagic DAI involving the peripheral gray–white junction in the right frontal lobe (*white arrowhead*). (Reprinted with permission from Le TH, et al. Diffusion tensor imaging with three-dimensional fiber tractography of traumatic axonal shearing injury: an imaging correlate for the posterior callosal "disconnection" syndrome: Case Report. Neurosurgery 2005;56(1):E195–201.)

DAI. They are very common in patients with severe head trauma and are usually well seen on CT scans. Contusions characteristically occur near bony protuberances of the skull and skull base. They tend to be multiple and bilateral and are more commonly hemorrhagic than DAI. Common sites are the temporal lobes above the petrous bone or posterior to the greater sphenoid wing, and the frontal lobes above the cribriform plate, the planum sphenoidale, and the lesser sphenoid wing (Fig. 3.17a). Less than 10% of lesions involve the cerebellum (18). Contusions can also occur at the margins of depressed skull fractures.

The CT appearance of cortical contusions characteristically varies with the age of the lesion. Many nonhemorrhagic lesions are initially poorly seen but become more obvious during the first week because of associated edema. Hemorrhagic lesions are seen as foci of high attenuation within superficial gray matter (Fig. 3.17b). These may be surrounded by larger areas of low attenuation secondary to surrounding edema. During the first week, the characteristic CT pattern of mixed areas of hypodensity and hyperdensity ("salt and pepper" pattern) becomes more apparent. Occasionally, surgical decompression of the contused brain is required to alleviate severe mass effect. Areas of prior contusion can often be recognized as foci of encephalomalacia within the same characteristic locations just described.

On MR, contusions appear as poorly marginated areas of increased signal on proton density and T2-weighted sequences. They are recognized because of their characteristic distribution in the frontal and temporal lobes and often have a "gyral" morphology. Hemorrhage causes heterogeneous signal intensity that varies depending on the age of the lesion (Fig. 3.18). Hemosiderin staining from hemorrhage of any cause leads to markedly decreased signal intensity on a T2WI, especially at higher field strengths. This signal loss can persist indefinitely as a marker of prior hemorrhage.

Intracerebral Hematoma. Occasionally, intraparenchymal hemorrhage is seen that is not necessarily associated with cortical contusion but rather represents shear-induced hemorrhage from the rupture of small intraparenchymal blood vessels. This lesion is known simply as an *intracerebral hematoma.* Intracerebral hematomas tend to have less surrounding edema than cortical contusions because they represent bleeding into areas of relatively normal brain. Most intracerebral hematomas are located in the frontotemporal white matter, although they have also been described in the basal ganglia. They are often associated with skull fractures and other primary neuronal lesions, including contusions and DAI. In the absence of other significant lesions, patients with intracerebral hematomas can remain lucid after their injury. When symptoms develop, they commonly result from the mass effect associated with an expanding hematoma. Intracerebral hematomas can also present late secondary to delayed hemorrhage, which is another cause of clinical deterioration during the first several days after head trauma (Fig. 3.19).

Subcortical gray matter injury is an uncommon manifestation of primary intra-axial injury and is seen as multiple petechial hemorrhages primarily affecting the basal ganglia and thalamus. These represent microscopic perivascular collections of blood that may result from disruption of multiple small perforating vessels.

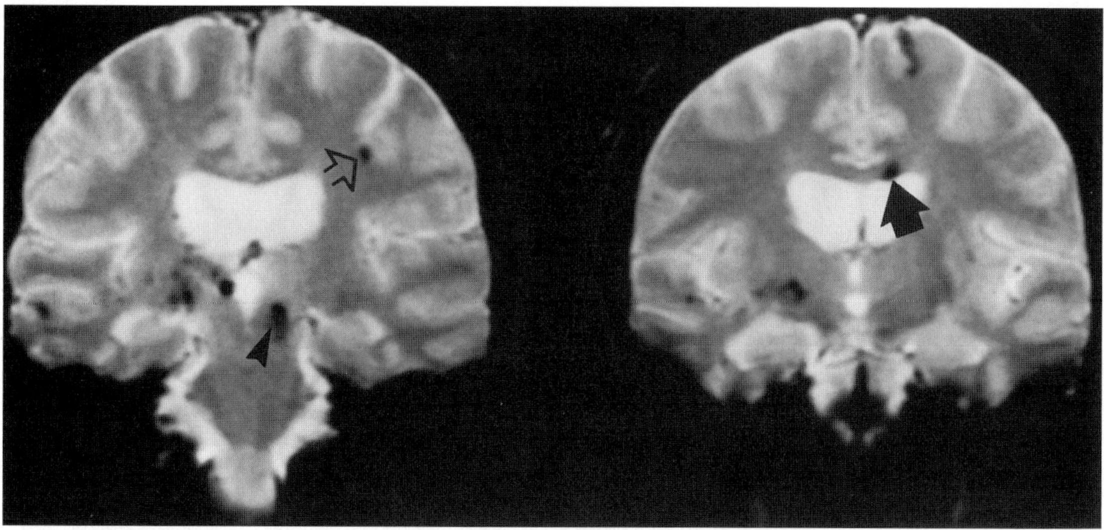

FIGURE 3.16. **The MR Appearance of Chronic DAI.** Coronal gradient-echo images in a patient with a history of prior severe head trauma demonstrate numerous hypointense foci in a distribution characteristic of DAI, including the gray–white junction (*open arrow*), corpus callosum (*closed arrow*), and cerebral peduncle (*arrowhead*). Evidence of remote hemorrhage is especially conspicuous on gradient-echo sequences. (Reprinted with permission from Gean AD. Imaging of Head Trauma. Philadelphia: Lippincott Williams & Wilkins; 1994:235.)

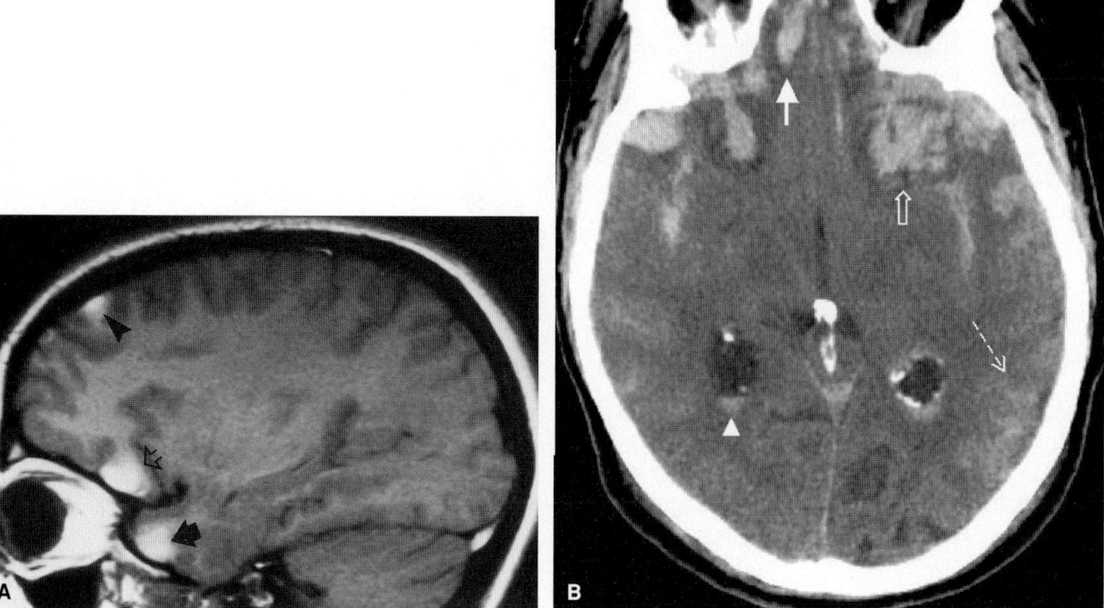

FIGURE 3.17. **The MR and CT Appearance of Cortical Contusion. A.** Sagittal T1WI demonstrates multiple peripheral areas of increased signal intensity involving the inferior frontal (*open arrow*), anterior temporal (*closed arrow*), and superior frontal lobes (*arrowhead*) consistent with subacute hemorrhage from cortical contusion. (Reprinted with permission from Gean AD. Imaging of Head Trauma. Philadelphia: Lippincott Williams & Wilkins; 1994:151.) **B.** Noncontrast CT scan reveals high-attenuation lesions involving the bilateral inferior frontal (*open arrow*) and anterior temporal (*closed arrow*) gray matter, consistent with hemorrhagic cortical contusions. The patient also has high-attenuation fluid within the lateral ventricles (*arrowhead*), consistent with intraventricular hemorrhage, and diffuse high-attenuation fluid within the bilateral subarachnoid spaces of the temporal lobe (*broken arrow*), consistent with subarachnoid hemorrhages.

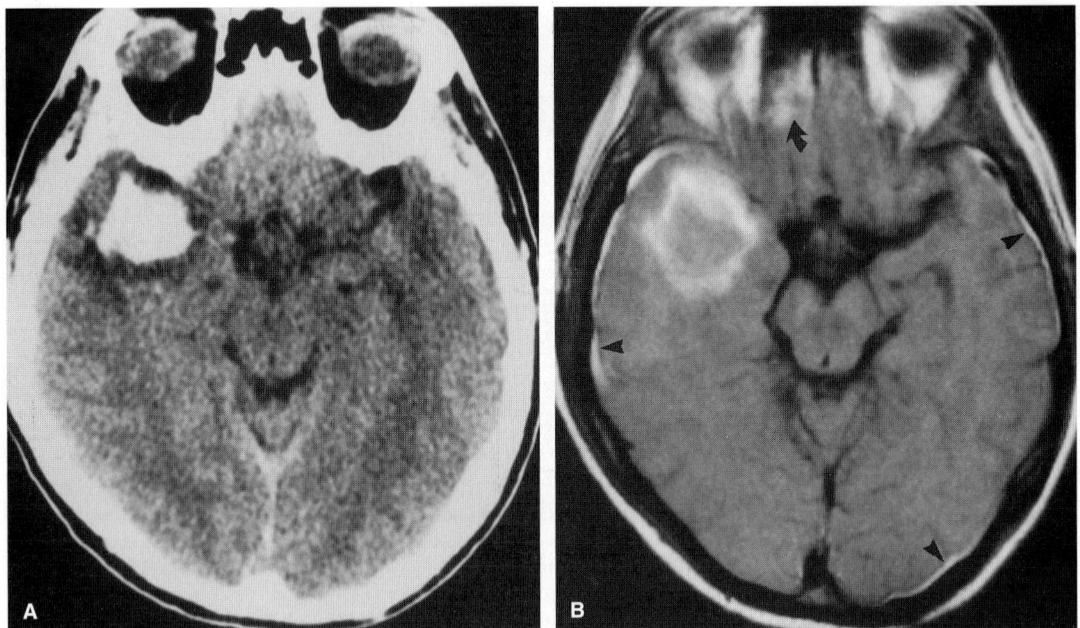

FIGURE 3.18. **Intracerebral Hematoma. A.** Axial CT scan demonstrates a high-attenuation mass within the right temporal lobe. **B.** The corresponding T1WI demonstrates a central region of isointensity consistent with acute hemorrhage (deoxyhemoglobin). The surrounding high signal intensity rim represents the conversion to methemoglobin that begins to form at the periphery of a hematoma. High signal in the inferior right frontal lobe (*curved arrow*) represents an associated frontal contusion. A small amount of subdural blood is also present bilaterally and is hyperintense (*arrowheads*).

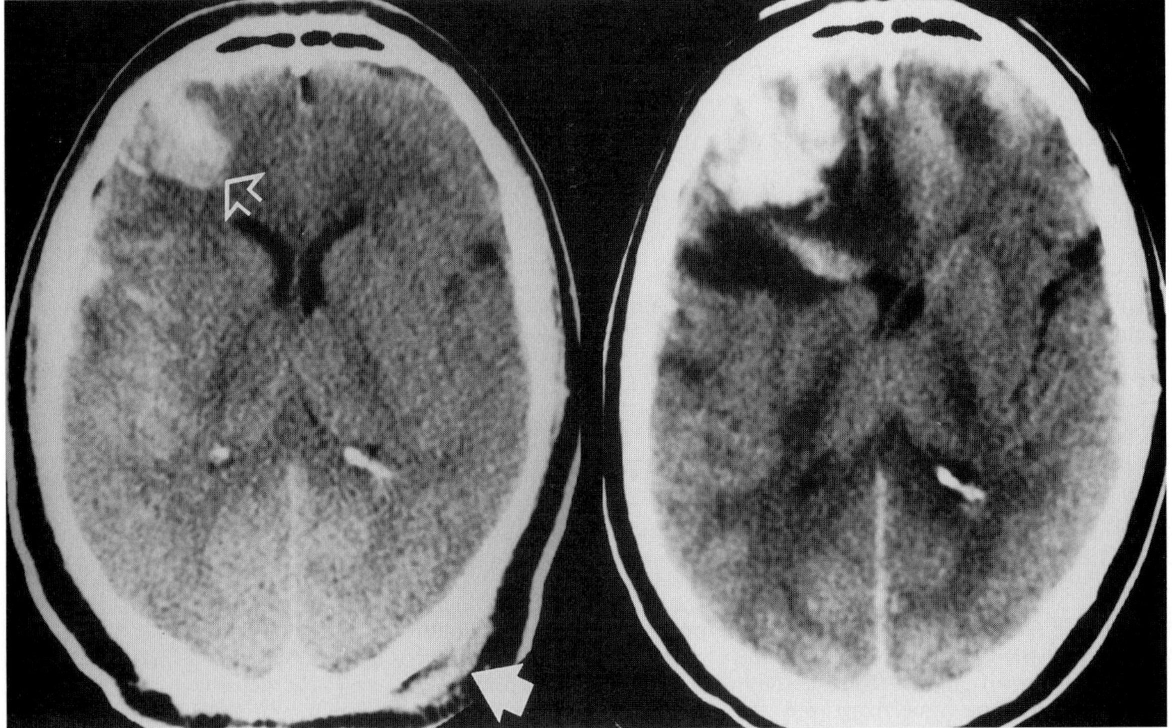

FIGURE 3.19. **Delayed Hemorrhage.** Admission CT scan (*left*) shows a small right frontal hematoma without significant mass effect (*open arrow*). Left parietal soft tissue swelling indicates the site of impact (*closed arrow*). A follow-up CT scan (*right*) was performed when the patient's clinical condition deteriorated, and it demonstrates a marked increase in the size of the hematoma with increased edema, mass effect, and compression of the ipsilateral frontal horn.

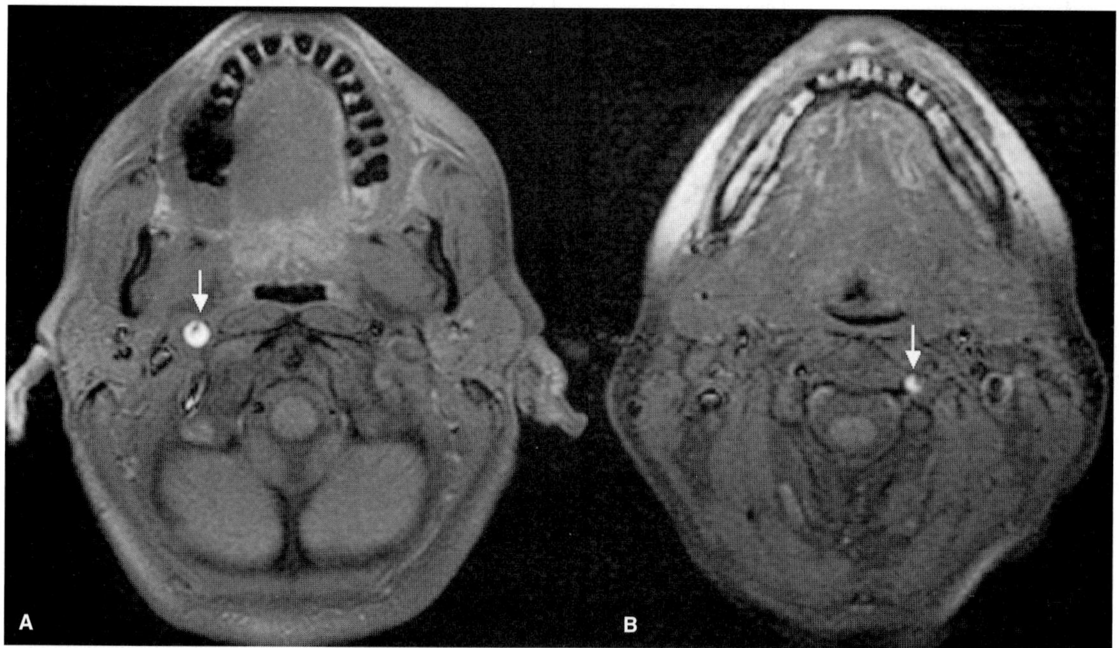

FIGURE 3.20. **The MR Appearance of Carotid and Vertebral Artery Dissection. A.** T1WI with fat suppression demonstrates an acute dissection of the right internal carotid artery with surrounding intramural hematoma which appears as high T1 signal (*arrow*). **B.** Image from the same patient also demonstrates crescentic high T1 signal of the left vertebral artery (*arrow*), again representing an intramural hematoma from an acute dissection.

These lesions are typically seen following severe head trauma.

Vascular injuries as causes of intra-axial and extra-axial hematomas were discussed previously. Other types of traumatic vascular injury include arterial dissection or occlusion, pseudoaneurysm formation, and the acquired arteriovenous fistula. Arterial injury commonly accompanies fractures of the base of the skull. The internal carotid is the most often injured artery, especially at sites of fixation. These include its entrance to the carotid canal at the base of the petrous bone and its exit from the cavernous sinus below the anterior clinoid process.

MR findings of vascular injury include the presence of an intramural hematoma (best seen on a T1WI with fat suppression, Fig. 3.20) or intimal flap with dissection, or the absence of normal vascular flow void with occlusion. An associated parenchymal infarction might also be seen. There is a potential role for MR angiography in evaluating patients with suspected traumatic vascular injury. Conventional angiograms are usually needed to confirm and delineate dissections and may also show spasm or pseudoaneurysm formation in injuries to the vessel wall.

A *carotid cavernous fistula* (CCF) is a communication between the cavernous portion of the internal carotid artery and the surrounding venous plexus. The lesion typically follows a full-thickness arterial injury, resulting in venous engorgement of the cavernous sinus and its draining tributaries (e.g., the ipsilateral superior ophthalmic vein and inferior petrosal sinus). Findings may be bilateral, because venous channels connect the cavernous sinuses. A CCF most often results from severe head injury. Skull base fractures, especially those involving the sphenoid bone, indicate patients at increased risk for associated cavernous carotid injury. The CCF may also result from ruptured cavernous carotid aneurysms. On MR, the CCF may manifest as an enlarged superior ophthalmic vein, a cavernous sinus, and petrosal sinus flow voids. There may be evidence of proptosis, swelling of the preseptal soft tissues, and enlargement of the extraocular musculature. Diagnosis usually requires selective carotid angiography with rapid filming to demonstrate the site of communication (Fig. 3.21). On occasion, patients present with findings weeks or months after the initial trauma.

Dural fistulas are also associated with trauma. For example, they may be caused by laceration of the middle meningeal artery with resultant formation of a fistula connecting the meningeal artery to the meningeal vein. Drainage via meningeal veins prevents formation of an epidural hematoma. Patients may be asymptomatic or present with nonspecific complaints, including tinnitus.

Mechanisms of Primary Head Injuries. Early research suggested that head injuries could be explained by areas of parenchymal compression and rarefaction caused by direct impact. Many authors still use the terms *coup* and *contrecoup* to describe intracranial lesions that characteristically occur on and opposite to, respectively, the side of a blow to the head. However, Gentry and others have questioned the use of these terms, which they

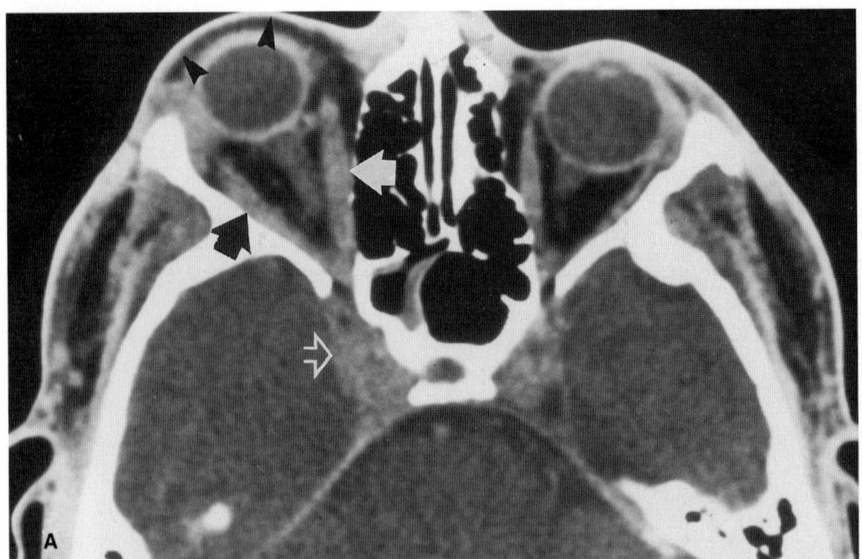

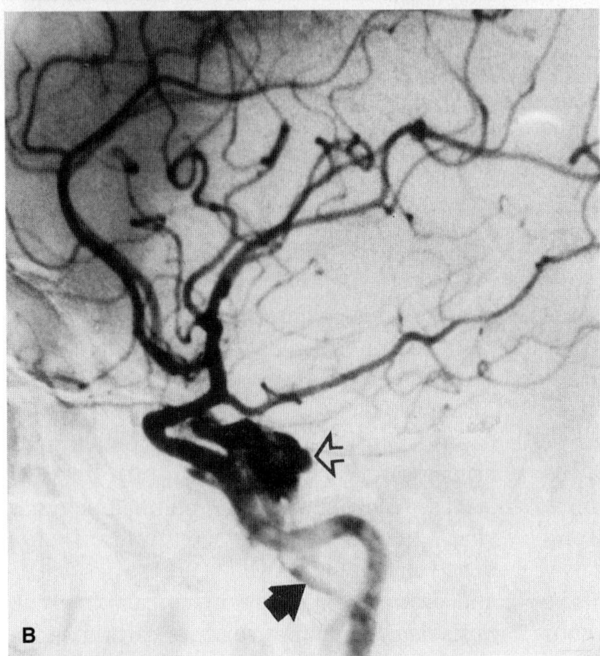

FIGURE 3.21. **Carotid Cavernous Fistula. A.** CT scan shows fullness in the right cavernous sinus (*open arrow*) and right proptosis, with swelling of the extraocular muscles (*closed arrows*) and preseptal soft tissues (*arrowheads*). **B.** Internal carotid angiogram in a different patient shows abnormal opacification of the cavernous sinus (*open arrow*) and jugular vein (*closed arrow*) during the arterial phase. (Reprinted with permission from Gean AD. Imaging of Head Trauma. Philadelphia: Lippincott Williams & Wilkins; 1994:349.)

feel incorrectly imply that neuronal injury is caused by compression and rarefaction strains subsequent to direct impact. Gennarelli et al. have shown in a primate model that all major types of intra-axial lesions, as well as subdural hematomas, can be produced purely by rotational acceleration of the head without direct impact. Only skull fractures and epidural hematomas require a physical blow to the head. Rotational acceleration causes damage by shear forces, rather than by compression-rarefaction strain. Compression-rarefaction strain is not felt to play a significant role in most head injuries.

The character of the accelerational force influences the type of injury produced. Cortical contusions and intracranial hematosis are more severe when the period of acceleration or deceleration is very short, whereas DAI and gliding contusions are associated with a longer acceleration or deceleration injury. Thus, DAI is more common in motor vehicle accidents, while contusions and hematomas are more frequent in falls.

Secondary Head Injury

Diffuse cerebral swelling is a common manifestation of head trauma. It may occur either because of an increase in cerebral blood volume *(hyperemia)* or an increase in tissue fluid content *(cerebral edema)*. Both conditions lead to generalized mass effect, with effacement of sulci, suprasellar and quadrigeminal plate cisterns, and compression of the ventricular system. Effacement of the brainstem cisterns indicates severe mass effect and may herald impending transtentorial herniation.

Cerebral swelling from hyperemia is most commonly seen in children and adolescents. The pathogenesis is poorly understood but appears to be the result of loss of normal cerebral autoregulation. Hyperemia is recognized on CT as ill-defined mass effect, effacement of sulci, and normal attenuation of brain. Acute subdural hematomas are often associated with unilateral swelling of the ipsilateral hemisphere.

Diffuse cerebral edema occurs secondary to tissue hypoxia. Because of the increase in tissue fluid, edema causes decreased attenuation on CT images, with loss of gray–white differentiation. The cerebellum and brainstem are usually spared and may appear hyperdense relative to the cerebral hemispheres (Fig. 3.22). Often, the falx and cerebral vessels appear dense, mimicking acute subarachnoid hemorrhage. Focal areas of edema are frequently seen in association with cortical contusions and may contribute significantly to mass effect.

Brain Herniation. Several forms of herniation are seen secondary to mass effect produced by primary intracranial injury. These are not specific for head trauma and can be seen secondary to mass effect produced by other causes as well, including intracranial hemorrhage, infarction, or neoplasm (Fig. 3.23).

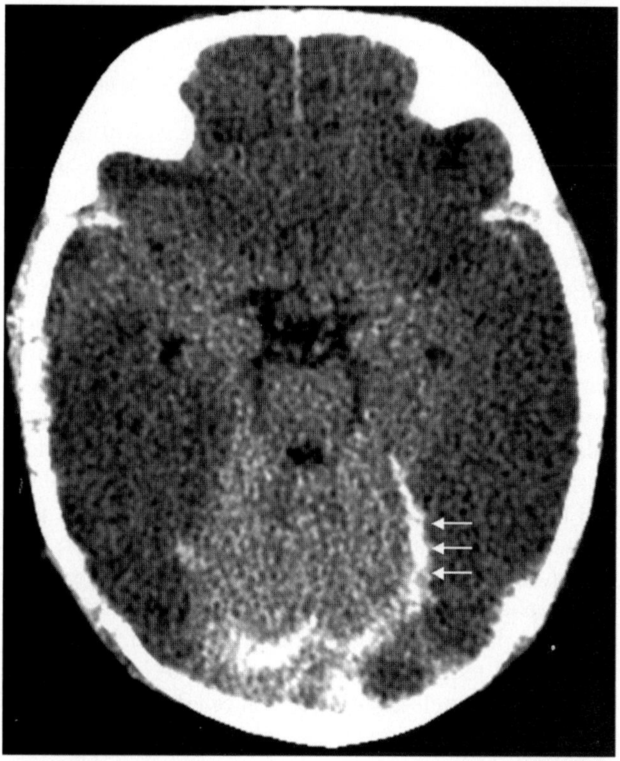

FIGURE 3.22. **Diffuse Cerebral Edema.** Noncontrast CT scan in an infant with diffuse cerebral edema following strangulation. There is a diffuse decrease in attenuation of the cerebral hemispheres with loss of gray–white differentiation. Sparing of the brainstem and cerebellum causes these structures to appear dense relative to the rest of the brain. Subdural hematomas are noted overlying the tentorium (*arrows*).

Subfalcial herniation, in which the cingulate gyrus is displaced across the midline under the falx cerebri, is the most common form of brain herniation (see Fig. 3.7). Compression of the adjacent lateral ventricle may be seen on CT scans, as well as enlargement of the contralateral ventricle from obstruction at the level of the foramen of Monro. Both anterior cerebral arteries (ACAs) may be displaced to the contralateral side. These patients are at risk of ACA infarction in the distribution of the callosomarginal branch of the ACA, where it becomes trapped against the falx.

Uncal herniation, in which the medial aspect of the temporal lobe is displaced medially over the free margin of the tentorium, is also common (Fig. 3.23). Uncal herniation causes focal effacement of the ambient cistern and the lateral aspect of the suprasellar cistern. Rarely, displacement of the brainstem causes compression of the contralateral cerebral peduncle against the tentorial margin, resulting in peduncular hemorrhage or infarction. The focal impression on the cerebral peduncle is known as Kernohan's notch. Mass effect on the third cranial nerve and compression of the contralateral cerebral peduncle cause a recognizable clinical syndrome characterized by a blown pupil with ipsilateral hemiparesis.

Transtentorial Herniation. The brain can herniate either downward or upward across the tentorium. Descending transtentorial herniation is recognized by effacement of the suprasellar and perimesencephalic cisterns. Pineal calcification, usually seen at about the same level as calcified choroid plexus in the trigones of the lateral ventricles, is displaced inferiorly. Large posterior fossa hematomas can cause ascending transtentorial herniation, in which the vermis and portions of the cerebellar hemispheres can herniate through the tentorial incisura. This is much less common than descending transtentorial herniation. Posterior fossa hematomas can also cause herniation of the cerebellar tonsils downward through the foramen magnum. Finally, external herniation can occur in which swelling or mass effect causes the brain to herniate through a calvarial defect. This can be posttraumatic or occur at the time of craniotomy and prevent closure of the skull flap.

Hydrocephalus can occur after subarachnoid or intraventricular hemorrhage as a result of either impaired CSF reabsorption at the level of the arachnoid granulations or obstruction at the level of the aqueduct or fourth ventricular outflow foramina. Mass effect from cerebral swelling or an adjacent hematoma can also cause hydrocephalus by compression of the aqueduct or outflow foramina of the fourth ventricle. Asymmetric lateral ventricular dilatation can be produced by compression of the foramen of Monro.

Ischemia or Infarction. Posttraumatic ischemia or infarction can result from raised intracranial pressure, embolization from a vascular dissection, or direct mass effect

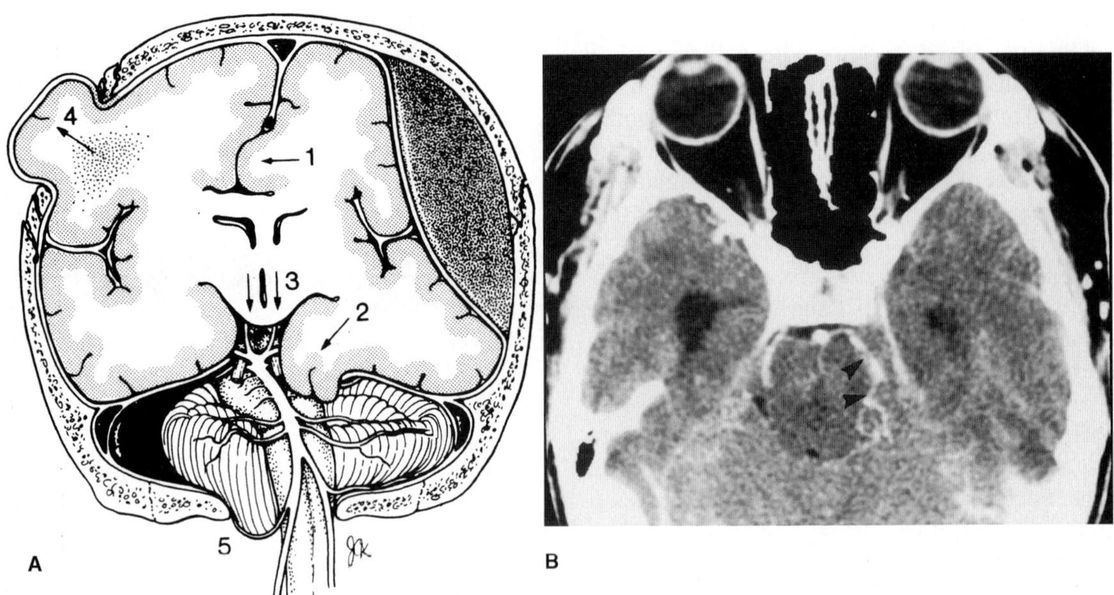

FIGURE 3.23. **Brain Herniation. A.** Diagram of the major types of brain herniation. 1, subfalcial herniation; 2, uncal herniation; 3, descending transtentorial herniation; 4, external herniation; 5, tonsillar herniation. (Reprinted with permission from Gean AD. Imaging of Head Trauma. Philadelphia: Lippincott Williams & Wilkins; 1994:264.) **B.** Uncal herniation. Contrast-enhanced CT scan shows compression of the left aspect of the brainstem, displacement of the left posterior cerebral artery (PCA) (*arrowheads*), and effacement of the ambient and crural cisterns. The temporal horns of the lateral ventricles are dilated, indicating obstructive hydrocephalus. Compression of the PCA during uncal herniation can lead to a PCA infarct. (Reprinted with permission from Gean AD. Imaging of Head Trauma. Philadelphia: Lippincott Williams & Wilkins; 1994:273.)

on cerebral vasculature from brain herniation or an overlying extra-axial collection. In addition, patients may suffer diffuse ischemic damage from acute reduction in cerebral blood flow or from hypoxemia secondary to respiratory arrest or status epilepticus. Patterns of infarction from focal mass effect include anterior cerebral artery infarction from subfalcial herniation, posterior cerebral artery infarction from uncal herniation, and posterior inferior communicating artery infarction from tonsillar herniation. Ischemia or infarction secondary to globally reduced cerebral perfusion tends to occur in characteristic "watershed zones" and is not specific for trauma (see Chapter 4).

CSF leak requires a dural tear and can occur after calvarial or skull base fractures. CSF rhinorrhea occurs subsequent to fractures in which a communication develops between the subarachnoid space and the paranasal sinuses or middle ear cavity. CSF otorrhea occurs when a communication between the subarachnoid space and middle ear occurs in association with disruption of the tympanic membrane. CSF leaks can be difficult to localize and can lead to recurrent meningeal infection. Radionuclide cisternography is highly sensitive for the presence of CSF extravasation; however, CT scanning with intrathecal contrast is required for detailed anatomic localization of the defect (Fig. 3.24).

Leptomeningeal cyst or "growing fracture" is caused by a traumatic tear in the dura, which allows an outpouching of arachnoid to occur at the site of a suture or skull fracture. This leads to progressive, slow widening of the skull defect or suture, presumably as a result of CSF pulsations. The leptomeningeal cyst appears as a lytic skull defect on CT or plain skull films, which can enlarge over time.

Encephalomalacia. Focal encephalomalacia consists of tissue loss with surrounding gliosis and is a frequent manifestation of remote head injury. It may be asymptomatic or serve as a potential seizure focus. CT demonstrates fairly well-defined areas of low attenuation, with volume loss. There may be dilation of adjacent portions of the ventricular system (Fig. 3.25). Encephalomalacia will follow CSF signal on MR sequences, except for gliosis, which appears as increased signal intensity on both proton-density and T2-weighted images. The appearance of encephalomalacia is not specific for posttraumatic injury, but the locations are characteristic: anteroinferior frontal and temporal lobes. Focal volume loss along the white matter tracts associated with cell death is known as wallerian degeneration and may be seen on CT and especially MR studies.

Brainstem Injury

Primary. The most common form of primary brainstem injury is DAI, which affects the dorsolateral aspect of the midbrain and upper pons (Fig. 3.26). The superior cerebellar peduncles and the medial lemnisci are

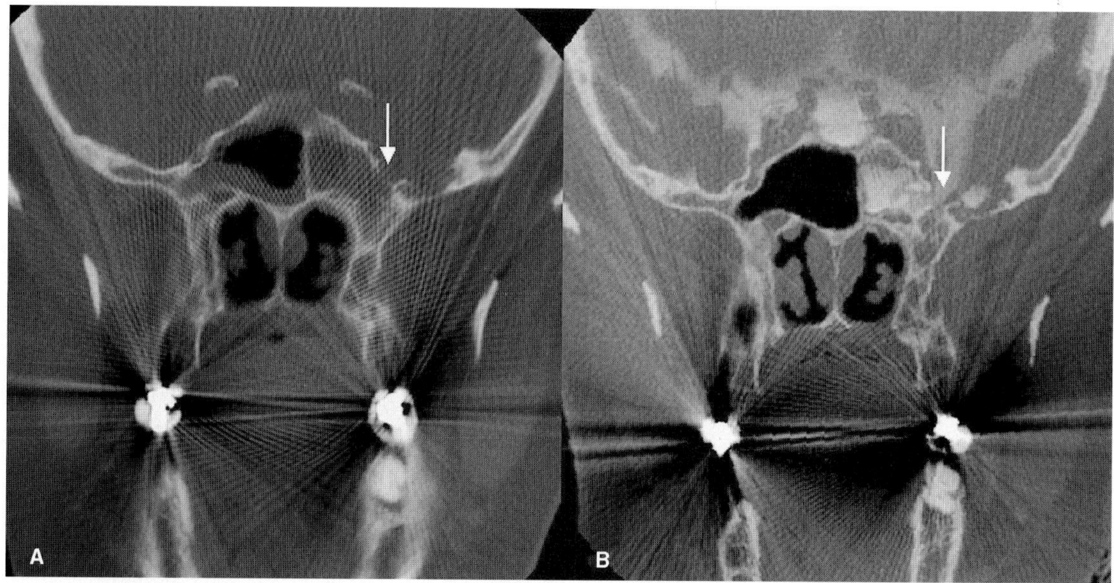

FIGURE 3.24. **CSF Leak. A.** Coronal CT image with bone window of the paranasal sinuses in a patient with chronic sinusitis and CSF leak demonstrates periosteal mucosal thickening of the sphenoid sinuses. A defect of the left superolateral wall of the sphenoid sinus is seen (*arrow*). **B.** Follow-up imaging with intrathecal contrast demonstrates contrast extravasation into the left sphenoid sinus through the defect of the left superolateral wall (*arrow*). The exact cause of the bony defect in this patient is unknown.

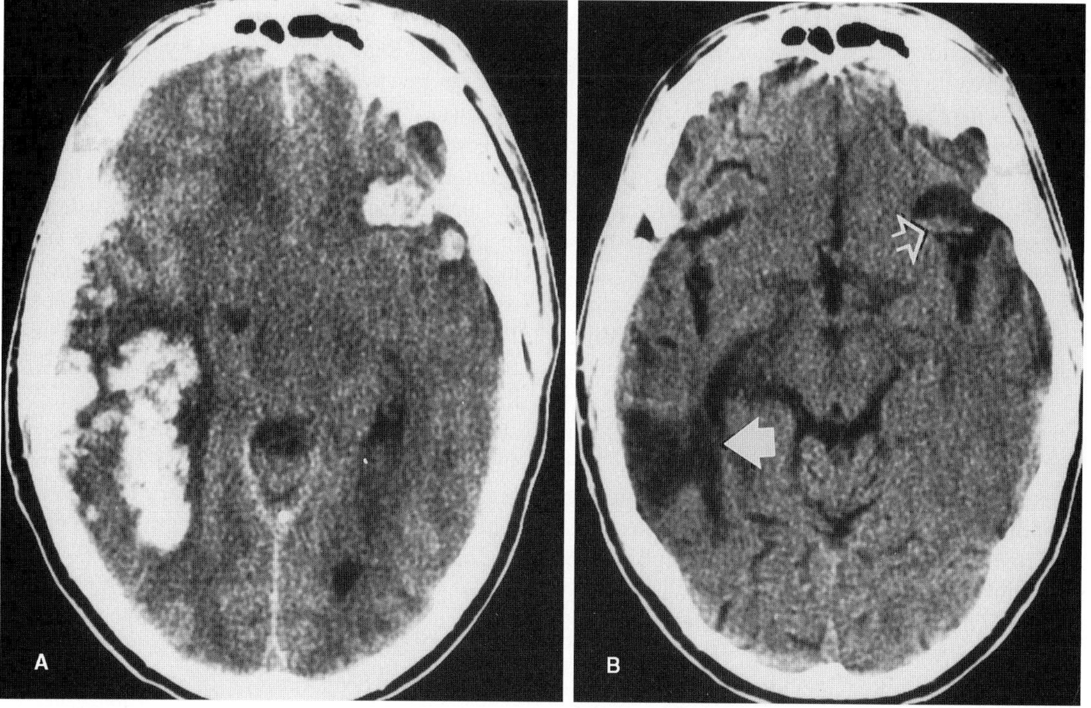

FIGURE 3.25. **Posttraumatic Encephalomalacia.** Admission **(A)** and follow-up **(B)** scans in a patient with severe head trauma show the interval development of left frontal (*open arrow*) and right posterior temporal (*closed arrow*) encephalomalacia in the same locations as the initial intracerebral hematomas. (Reprinted with permission from Gean AD. Imaging of Head Trauma. Philadelphia: Lippincott Williams & Wilkins; 1994:507.)

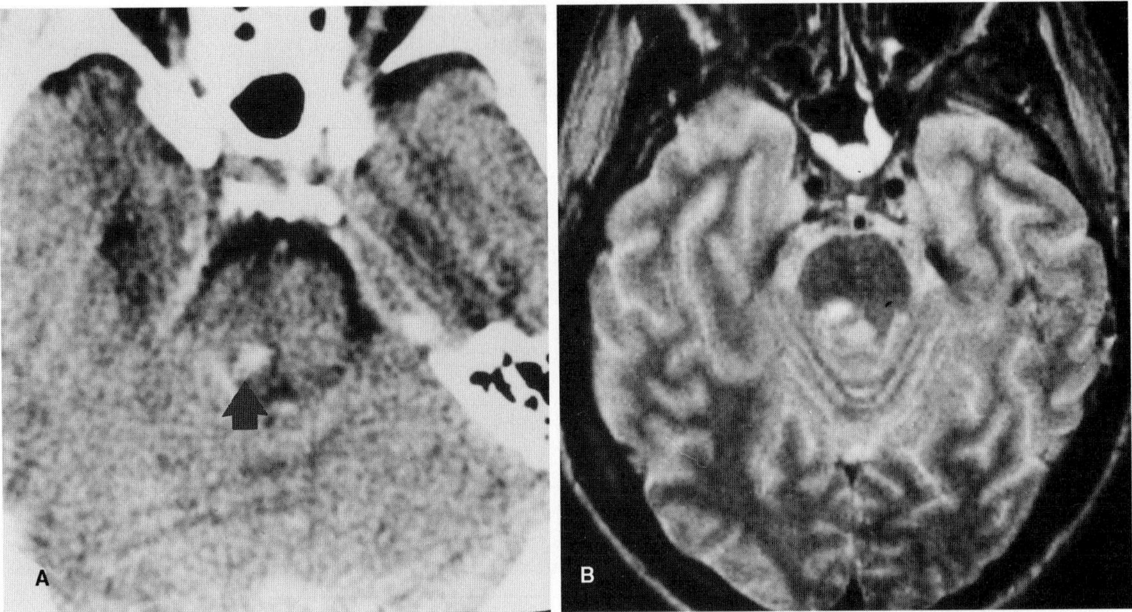

FIGURE 3.26. **Brainstem DAI. A.** Noncontrast CT scan shows a punctate focus of increased attenuation representing focal hemorrhage from DAI of the brainstem (*arrow*). Note the characteristic location in the dorsolateral aspect of the brainstem. **B.** T2WI in a different patient shows a hyperintense lesion in a similar location.

particularly vulnerable. Both the location and lack of sufficient amounts of hemorrhage make this lesion difficult to diagnose on CT scans. Brainstem DAI is nearly always seen in association with lesions of the frontal or temporal white matter and corpus callosum. This distinguishes brainstem DAI from a rare form of primary injury caused by direct impact of the free margin of the tentorium on the brainstem. Primary brainstem injury may also occur in the form of multiple petechial hemorrhages in the periaqueductal regions of the rostral brainstem (see previous discussion on subcortical gray matter injury). They are not associated with DAI, although they occur in a similar distribution. This form of injury represents disruption of penetrating brainstem blood vessels by shear strain and carries a grim prognosis.

An extremely rare form of indirect primary brainstem injury is the pontomedullary separation or rent. As the name implies, this represents a tear in the ventral surface of the brainstem at the junction of the pons and medulla. There is a spectrum of severity ranging from a small tear to complete avulsion of the brainstem. Pontomedullary separation can occur without associated diffuse cerebral injury. This lesion is usually fatal.

Secondary brainstem injury includes infarction, hemorrhage, or compression of the brainstem as a result of adjacent or systemic pathology. Brainstem infarction from hypotension-induced cerebral hypoperfusion is usually seen in conjunction with supratentorial ischemic injury. The brainstem may be relatively spared in hypoxic injury. Mechanical compression of the brainstem usually occurs in the setting of uncal herniation. There may be visible displacement or a change in the overall shape of the brainstem as a result of the mass effect. Neurologic injury caused by brainstem compression may be reversible in the absence of intrinsic brainstem lesions.

Brainstem lesions that occur as a result of downward herniation, hypoxia, or ischemia usually involve the ventral or ventrolateral aspect of the brainstem, in contrast to primary brainstem lesions, which are most common in the dorsolateral aspect of the brainstem. A characteristic secondary brainstem lesion is the Duret hemorrhage. This is a midline hematoma in the tegmentum of the rostral pons and midbrain seen in association with descending transtentorial herniation. It is believed to result from stretching or tearing of penetrating arteries as the brainstem is caudally displaced (Fig. 3.27). The brainstem infarct is another type of secondary brainstem injury that typically occurs in the central tegmentum of the pons and midbrain.

Penetrating Trauma

Unlike blunt head trauma, in which diffuse injury often occurs secondary to acceleration-induced shear strain, in penetrating injury the damage is defined by the trajectory of the object. Penetrating sharp objects such as knives or glass cause tissue laceration along their course, with resultant bleeding or infarction from vascular injury. Plain films or CT can be used to confirm and localize radiopaque

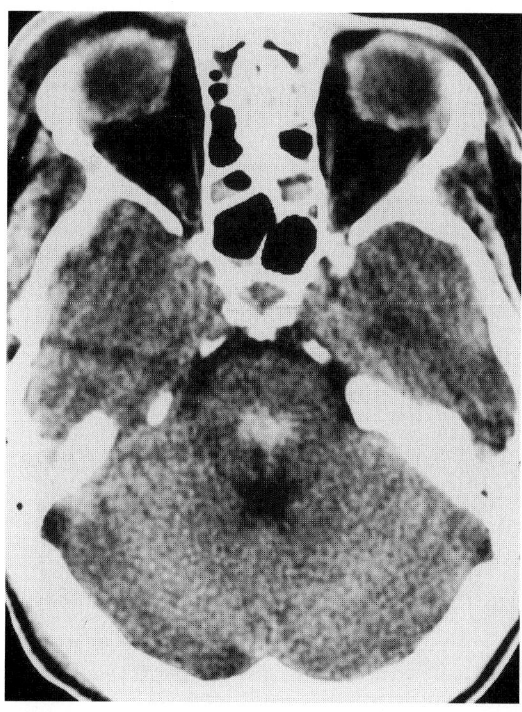

FIGURE 3.27. **Duret Hemorrhage.** Noncontrast CT scan performed 24 hours after severe head trauma shows a midline pontine hemorrhage. This type of secondary brainstem injury, known as the Duret hemorrhage, occurs in association with downward transtentorial herniation and can be distinguished from most primary brainstem injuries by its midline location (compare with Fig. 3.26). (Reprinted with permission from Gean AD. Imaging of Head Trauma. Philadelphia: Lippincott Williams & Wilkins; 1994:282.)

intracranial foreign bodies. Leaded glass and metal are hyperdense on CT scans, whereas wood is hypodense.

Gunshot wounds are among the most common causes of penetrating head trauma. They can cause the type of injuries seen in nonpenetrating trauma as well, because significant blunt force occurs from the bullet's impact on the skull. Metallic foreign bodies such as bullet fragments often cause a significant streak artifact, which can obscure underlying injury. Tilting the CT gantry to change the plane of section helps minimize this artifact. The entry and exit sites can often be distinguished by the direction of beveling of the calvarial defect or from the pattern of calvarial fracture. The bullet path can often be recognized on CT as a linear hemorrhagic strip (Fig. 3.28). Gunshot wounds in which the bullet crosses the midline or in which small fragments are seen displaced from the main bullet are associated with a poorer prognosis.

Additional complications of penetrating injury are caused by associated skull fractures and dural lacerations with resultant pneumocephalus, CSF leaks, and infection. Fragments of bone, skin, or hair that may be driven intracranially also increase the risk of subsequent abscess formation.

Predicting Outcome After Acute Head Trauma

The Glasgow coma scale (GCS), which stratifies patients with acute head trauma based on clinical findings, including level of consciousness, brainstem reflexes, and response to pain, helps standardize assessment of the severity of injury (Table 3.1). Mild head injury refers to a GCS score of 13 to 15, moderate head injury refers to a GCS score of 9 to 12, and severe head injury is defined as a GCS score of 8 or below. Although there is a direct correlation between the initial GCS score and subsequent morbidity and mortality, the GCS is limited in its ability to predict long-term outcome. Likewise, CT findings, although they are valuable in identifying injuries requiring acute intervention, do not correlate well with prognosis. There is growing evidence, however, that MR will be helpful in determining a patient's prognosis after severe head injury (9,18,19). This reflects the advantage of MR over CT in detecting brainstem injury and DAI. MR studies have shown good correlation between initial GCS and the number and distribution of DAI lesions. Numerous DAI lesions and the presence of DAI in the corpus callosum or brainstem are associated with more severe clinical findings and low initial scores on the GCS. Perhaps more important is the finding that the number of DAI lesions and the presence of brainstem injury or corpus callosum DAI are associated with poor long-term outcome (18). The number of cortical contusions is not related to outcome, except in cases with significant mass effect. There is also a poor correlation between the presence of an isolated epidural or subdural hematoma and long-term outcome, unless transtentorial herniation is also present.

Child Abuse

Nonaccidental trauma accounts for at least 80% of deaths from head trauma in children younger than 2 years of age (20). It is important to consider the possibility of child abuse and to recognize the characteristic features of these suspected cases.

Skull fractures represent the second most common skeletal injury in child abuse (the most common is long bone fracture). They are only found in approximately 50% of children with intracranial injuries from abuse (21,22). In patients with suspected intracranial injury, CT should be the initial imaging study. Skull films are rarely indicated, except perhaps for documentation of cranial injury in neurologically intact children with suspected child abuse.

Subdural hematomas are the most commonly recognized intracranial complication from child abuse. The association of subdural hematomas and retinal hemorrhages in children with metaphyseal long bone fractures was described as "whiplash shaken injury" by Caffey in 1946 (23). The mechanism was thought to be one of violent shaking,

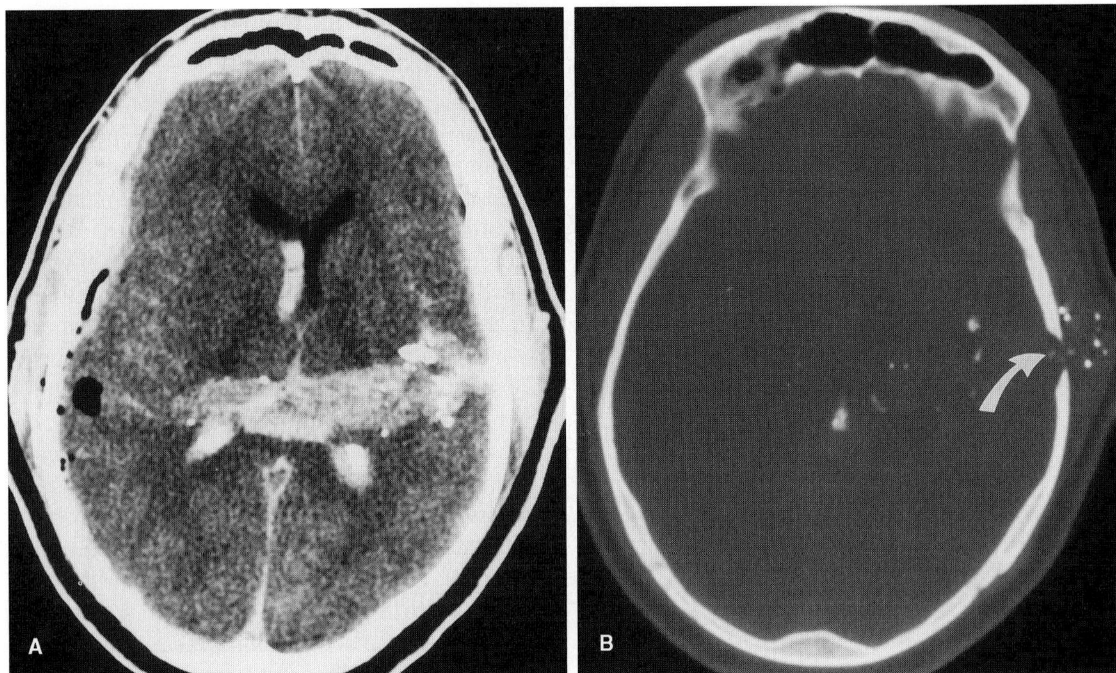

FIGURE 3.28. **Gunshot Wound. A.** Noncontrast CT scan shows hemorrhage delineating the bullet's path in this despondent southpaw. There is associated intraventricular and subarachnoid hemorrhage as well as pneumocephalus and a right subdural hematoma. **B.** Bone window shows the typical beveled entry site (*arrow*) and scattered bullet fragments along the trajectory. (Reprinted with permission from Gean AD. Imaging of Head Trauma. Philadelphia: Lippincott Williams & Wilkins; 1994:193.)

with generation of rotational and shear forces intracranially because of the weak neck musculature. The mechanism might include impact against a soft object such as a mattress, which has been shown experimentally (24) to increase the forces produced into the range that could cause coma, subdural hematomas, and primary brain injury, leading to the term *shaken impact injury.*

Subdural hematomas in child abuse often are found in the posterior interhemispheric fissure. These are seen on CT as hyperdense collections with a flat medial border along the falx and an irregular convex lateral border. Subdural hematomas may also be found along the convexity, over the tentorial surface, at the skull base, or in the posterior fossa (see Fig. 3.22). Occasionally, low-density extra-axial fluid collections are seen in infants without any clear precipitating trauma or infection. These most often represent dilated CSF spaces, known as "benign enlargement of the subarachnoid space of infancy," but can mimic chronic subdural hematomas. They occur in neurologically intact infants 3 to 6 months of age who present with enlarging head circumference. In this setting, they require no treatment and usually regress by age 2. An old term for this condition, "external hydrocephalus," has been abandoned by many because it fails to convey the benign nature of the condition. Epidural hematomas are not frequently seen in child abuse.

TABLE 3.1 The Glasgow Coma Scale

Eye Opening	*Best Motor*	*Best Verbal*
4 - spontaneous	6 - obeys	5 - oriented
3 - to voice	5 - localizes	4 - confused
2 - to pain	4 - withdraws	3 - inappropriate words
1 - none	3 - abnormal flexion	2 - incomprehensible words
	2 - extensure posturing	1 - nothing
	1 - flaccid	

The total score is the sum of the scores in each category.

The most common intra-axial manifestation of head injury related to child abuse is diffuse brain swelling. The initial swelling is believed to be caused by vasodilation associated with loss of autoregulation. At this stage, the injury may be reversible, despite dramatic findings on CT. CT scans show global effacement of the subarachnoid space and compressed ventricles. As the brain becomes edematous, the normal attenuation of gray and white matter may appear indistinguishable or even reversed. The cerebral hemispheres will demonstrate diffusely decreased attenuation. The brainstem, cerebellum, and possibly deep gray matter structures may be spared (see Fig. 3.22). Cerebral edema in the setting of shaking injury can also occur secondary to respiratory depression, apnea, and hypoxia. The other manifestations of intra-axial injury previously

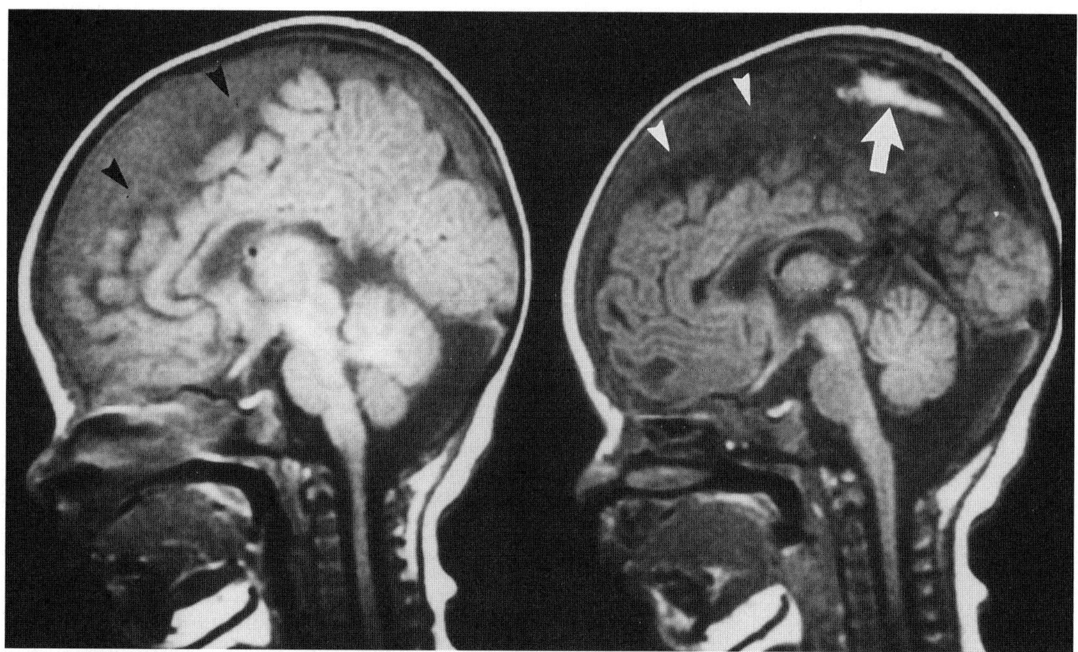

FIGURE 3.29. **Subacute and Chronic Interhemispheric Subdural Hematomas.** Midline sagittal and parasagittal T1WIs in a child demonstrate a low signal intensity chronic subdural hematoma (*arrowheads*) and superimposed high signal intensity subacute hematoma (*arrow*). The presence of intracranial injury of different ages is strong presumptive evidence of child abuse. The appearance is not pathognomonic for child abuse, however, because subdural hematomas do have a propensity to rebleed.

described in this chapter may also be seen in child abuse, including DAI and brainstem injury. Cortical contusions occur but are considered less common, possibly because the inner surface of the skull is relatively smooth in children. In infants, head trauma may lead to tears at the gray–white junction, especially in the frontal and temporal lobes.

Multiple injuries of various ages also strongly suggest child abuse. Chronic sequelae of head injury in children include chronic subdural collections (which may occasionally calcify), global cerebral atrophy, and encephalomalacia. Although CT is the modality of choice for the evaluation of acute head injury in children, MR can help identify subdural collections of various ages or hemosiderin deposits from prior hemorrhages (Fig. 3.29). The ability of MR to identify these remote intracranial hemorrhages makes it an important tool in the evaluation of suspected child abuse. In some centers, it has been proposed as a necessary complement to the skeletal series. MR is also recommended when patients are clinically stable after head injury to help determine the full extent of injury and prognosis.

FACIAL TRAUMA

Imaging Strategy. *Plain Films.* Many facial fractures can often be diagnosed by plain films alone and need no further imaging. Four views are usually adequate in the plain-film evaluation of acute facial trauma: the Caldwell view, a shallow Waters view, a cross-table lateral view, and a submental vertex view. When patients are acutely injured and unable to undergo upright imaging, the Caldwell and Waters views can be obtained supine in the anteroposterior projection. Films obtained in the posteroanterior projection provide better bone detail and less magnification and may be helpful if the initial films are difficult to interpret. The lateral and submental vertex views are both obtained with a horizontal beam, thus enabling the detection of air–fluid levels.

CT is indicated when the clinical or plain-film findings suggest complex facial fractures or complications such as extraocular muscle entrapment or optic nerve impingement. Patients with facial fractures frequently have concurrent intracranial injury, especially victims of motor vehicle accidents. Imaging of the potential intracranial injury takes precedence in the acute management of these patients. If CT of the facial bones is required in patients suspected of concurrent intracranial injury, it is usually performed after CT imaging of the brain or delayed several days until the patient is clinically stable.

Either 1-mm or overlapping 3-mm sections are usually obtained through the facial bones in the axial plane using a bone algorithm. Depending on pitch and rotational speed, the overlapping sections can be reconstructed to thinner sections. The field of view should extend from the orbital roof to the superior alveolar ridge. The frontal sinus or

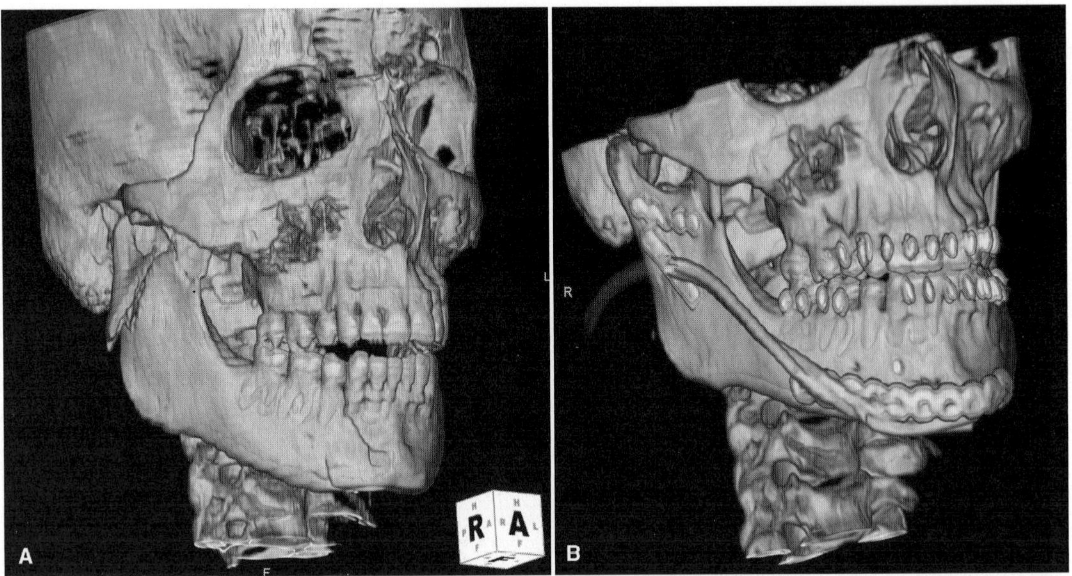

FIGURE 3.30. **Three-Dimensional Reconstruction for Preoperative Planning. A.** Preoperative 3D reconstruction from a facial CT demonstrates right mandibular condylar (*arrow*) and comminuted parasymphyseal (*arrowhead*) fractures. **B.** Postoperative 3D reconstructed image shows interval plate fixation of both fractures (*arrows*).

maxillary dentition can be included if fractures are suspected in these areas. The mandible should be included when maxillary alveolar or palatal fractures are seen because of the high incidence of associated mandibular fractures in this setting. A standard algorithm with soft tissue windows can be used to evaluate potential nonosseous injury, especially in the orbits. If there is no concern for a cervical spine injury, patients can also undergo scans in the direct coronal plane for better visualization of the orbital floors, palate, and floor of the anterior cranial fossa. Coronal reformations of axial or helical acquisitions may be used when patients are unable to tolerate direct coronal scanning. Contrast is unnecessary except in the rare circumstance in which vascular injury is being considered. Occasionally, 3D reconstruction may be used for planning preoperative repair of displaced or comminuted facial fractures (Fig 3.30).

MR. The facial bones are difficult to visualize on MR scanning because they and the adjacent aerated sinuses are relatively void of signal. CT is the preferred modality for cross-sectional evaluation of facial injuries, primarily because it provides excellent bone detail. MR may be useful for injuries to orbital contents, including the optic nerve, the globe, and the extraocular muscles. It is also useful for assessing potential vascular complications, such as arterial dissections, pseudoaneurysms, and arteriovenous fistulas, and it is the best way to evaluate trauma to the temporomandibular joint.

Angiography may be indicated when clinical or radiographic evidence suggests a vascular injury. Vascular injuries are more frequent with penetrating trauma, such as that occurring from gunshot or stab wounds. Fractures that extend through the carotid canal also predispose to vascular injury and may require angiographic evaluation.

Soft Tissue Findings. Indirect signs of facial injury on plain films can help provide objective evidence of trauma, localize the site of impact, and direct attention to areas of potential bony injury. Soft tissue swelling is the most commonly seen plain-film finding in facial trauma. It may help localize the site of impact but does not necessarily indicate associated facial fractures or other more severe injury.

Paranasal sinus opacification suggests the presence of an associated fracture, particularly when air–fluid levels are seen. Fluid levels are most commonly seen in the maxillary sinus but may also be seen in the frontal or sphenoid sinuses. The ethmoids may become opacified with acute hemorrhage but are less likely to demonstrate fluid levels on plain films, probably because they contain internal septa.

Air in the soft tissues is also suggestive of associated fractures, depending on location. Orbital emphysema is most commonly caused by fracture of the thin medial orbital wall. Orbital floor blowout fractures can also cause orbital emphysema (Fig. 3.31).

Occasionally, facial films reveal important findings unrelated to fracture of the facial bones. For example, the films should be scrutinized for the presence of foreign bodies that may not be clinically apparent. The craniocervical junction and upper cervical spine should be examined when included on the film. Nasopharyngeal and prevertebral soft tissue swelling can indicate hemorrhage from

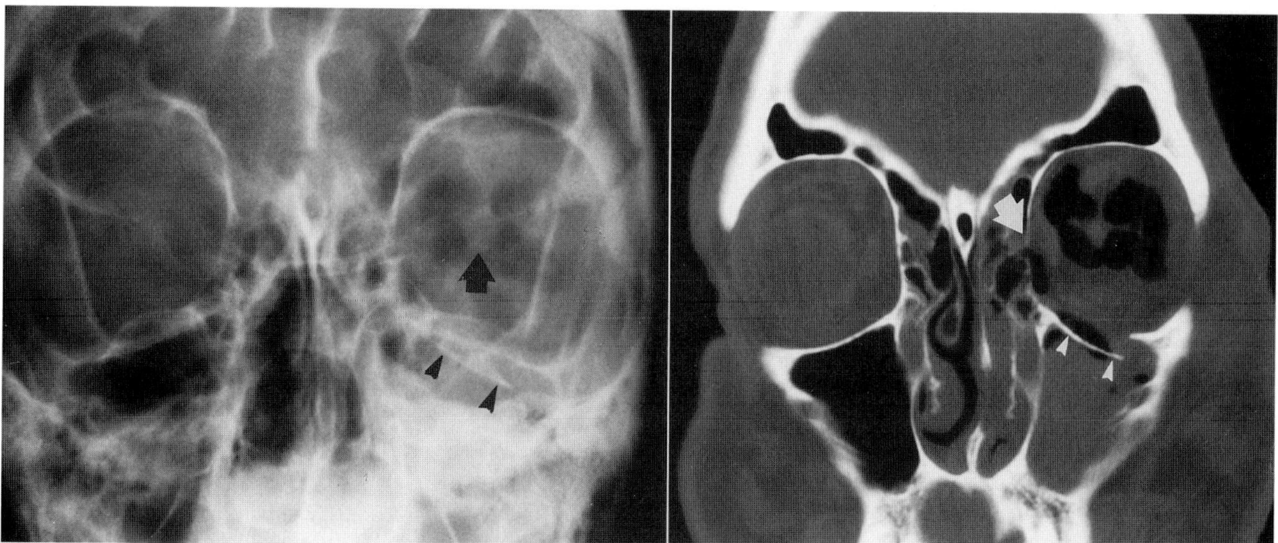

FIGURE 3.31. **Orbital Injuries. A.** Orbital emphysema on plain film. Air in the left orbit can be seen outlining the optic nerve (*arrow*) in this shallow Waters view. An ipsilateral orbital floor fracture is also evident (*arrowheads*). **B.** Orbital floor blowout fracture on CT scan. Direct coronal CT scan from the same patient shows a depressed left orbital floor fracture (*arrowheads*) with opacification of the ipsilateral maxillary sinus. Orbital air can be seen outlining the optic nerve. A subtle medial wall fracture is also present (*arrow*), which likely accounts for the large amount of orbital emphysema in this case.

cervical or skull base fractures. Pneumocephalus or depressed skull fractures are also occasionally seen. Rarely, a shift of pineal calcification can be detected, indicating the presence of intracranial mass effect. Although plain films are usually no longer indicated for evaluation of head trauma, it still pays to remain alert to indirect manifestations of head trauma when reviewing facial films.

Nasal Fractures. Nasal bone fractures are the most common fractures of the facial skeleton. They can occur as an isolated injury or in association with other facial fractures. Nasal trauma frequently results in a depressed fracture of one of the paired nasal bones, without associated ethmoidal injury. An anterior blow can fracture both nasal bones as well as the nasal septum. Associated fractures of the frontal process of the maxilla can be seen. Cartilaginous nasal injury cannot be diagnosed radiographically.

Nasal fractures are usually clinically evident and do not require radiologic diagnosis. Films of the nasal bone may document injury but are generally not useful for patient management and are often unnecessary. Fractures of the nasal bone may be transverse or longitudinal. Longitudinal fractures can be confused with the nasomaxillary suture and nasociliary grooves, which have the same orientation. Transverse fractures of the nasal bone are more common and are easily detected because they are oriented perpendicular to the normal suture line.

When films are obtained, remember to look for fractures of the anterior nasal spine of the maxilla, which may be associated with nasal fractures. One potentially serious injury that can be suggested on plain films or CT is a septal hematoma. Trauma to the septal cartilage may lead to hematoma formation between the perichondrium and cartilage, which can cause cartilage necrosis by disrupting the vascular supply. An organized hematoma can also cause difficulty in breathing and may predispose to septal abscess formation.

Maxillary and Paranasal Sinus Fractures. Fracture of the maxillary alveolus is the most common isolated maxillary fracture. It frequently results from a blow to the chin that drives the teeth of the mandible into the maxillary dental arch. These fractures are usually demonstrated by dental films or panoramic (Panorex) radiographs, but can be seen on CT if the scan is extended inferior to the level of the palate. Associated fractures of the mandible are common with this form of injury, as predicted by the mechanism.

Fractures of the palatine process of the maxilla and horizontal plate of the palatine bone commonly occur in the sagittal plane near the midline (Fig. 3.32). Palatine fractures may also be seen in association with complex fractures of the midface.

The most common isolated sinus fracture involves the anterolateral wall of the maxillary antrum. The fracture may be seen directly or may be suspected by the finding of a maxillary sinus fluid level in the setting of acute trauma.

Isolated frontal sinus fractures can also occur and may be more serious if they extend intracranially. Frontal sinus fractures may be linear or comminuted and depressed. Open (compound) frontal sinus fractures involve the

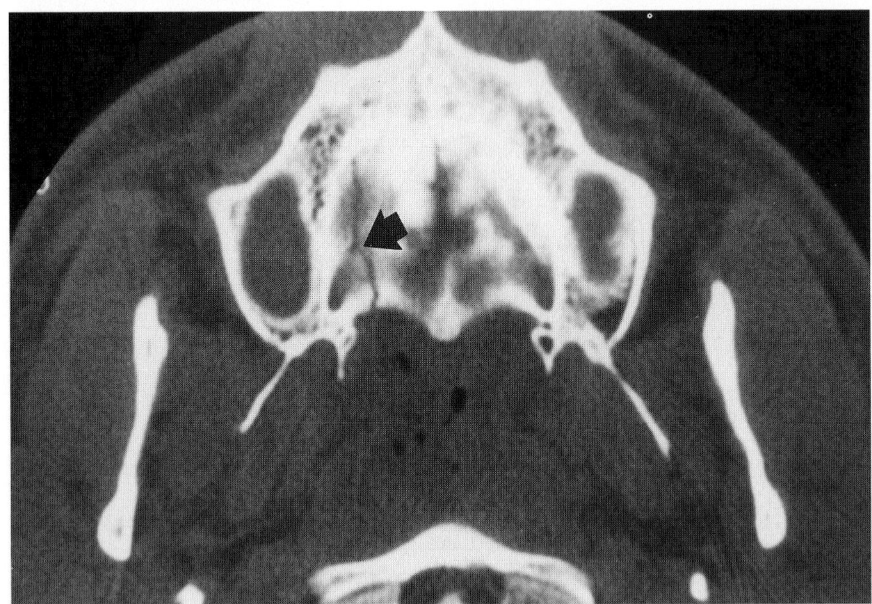

FIGURE 3.32. **Palate Fracture.** Axial CT scan demonstrates a nondisplaced right palatine fracture in the characteristic parasagittal location (*arrow*). (Reprinted with permission from Gean AD. Imaging of Head Trauma. Philadelphia: Lippincott Williams & Wilkins; 1994:439.)

posterior sinus wall (Fig. 3.33). These can lead to CSF rhinorrhea and recurrent meningitis or intracerebral abscess formation. Pneumocephalus may be seen in association with these fractures. Fractures of the medial wall and superior rim of the orbit frequently involve the frontal sinus.

Fractures of the sphenoid sinus are often seen in association with fractures of the orbital roof, nasoethmoid complex, midface, or temporal bone. Nondisplaced sphenoid sinus fractures may be subtle on CT. Angiography should be considered if there is a suspicion of associated vascular injury involving the cavernous portion of the internal carotid artery.

Orbital Trauma. *Fractures.* The orbit is involved in a number of facial fractures, including the tripod, Le Fort, and nasoethmoidal complex fractures. Isolated orbital wall fractures usually involve either the medial wall or orbital floor. Medial wall fractures are detected on plain films by the presence of orbital emphysema and opacification of the adjacent ethmoid air cells. Medial wall fractures can be directly visualized well with axial or coronal CT scans. Bone displacement is usually minimal, and muscle entrapment is unusual.

Orbital floor fractures are usually linear when seen in association with other facial fractures. These are rarely associated with entrapment. Comminuted orbital floor fractures, or blowout fractures, may be seen as an isolated injury and result from a direct blow to the eye. Intraorbital pressure is acutely increased and relieved by fracture through the orbital floor (Fig. 3.34). The orbital rim remains intact in pure blowout fractures. Blowout fractures

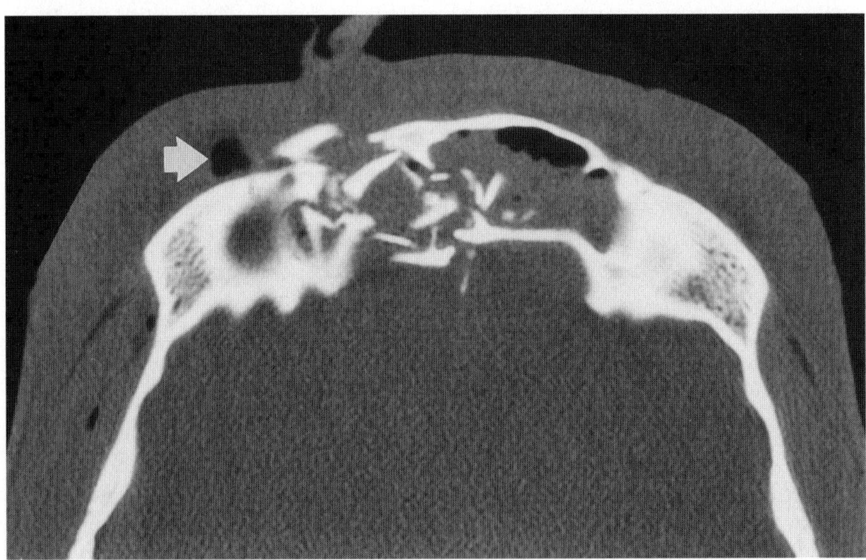

FIGURE 3.33. **"Open" Frontal Sinus Fracture.** Noncontrast CT scan demonstrates a severely comminuted fracture involving both walls of the frontal sinus (open fracture). The frontal sinus is opacified and subcutaneous air is present (*arrow*). Open fractures are prone to CSF leakage and meningitis or intracerebral abscess formation. (Reprinted with permission from Gean AD. Imaging of Head Trauma. Philadelphia: Lippincott Williams & Wilkins; 1994:46.)

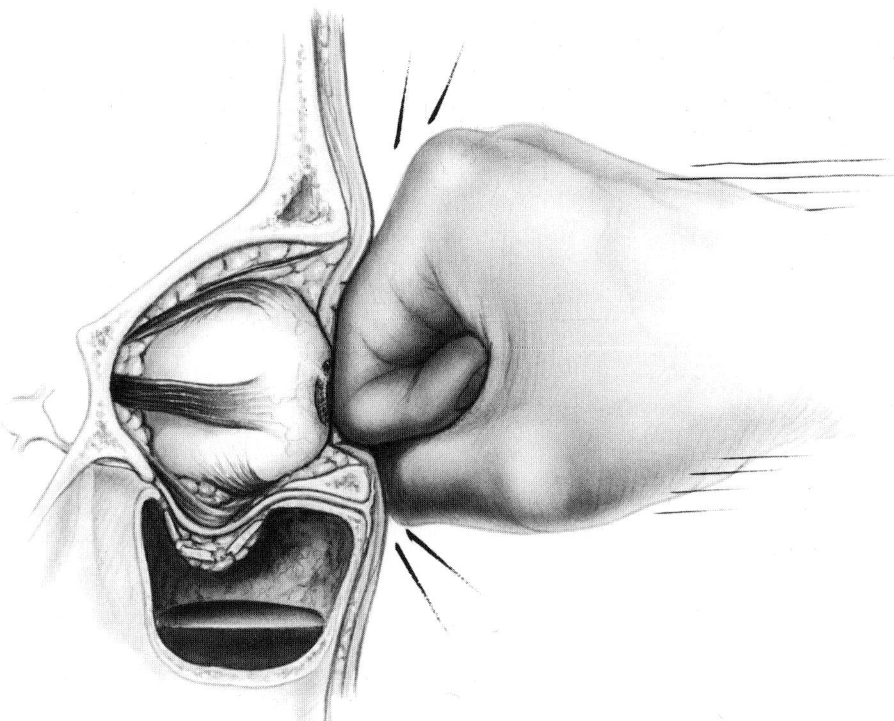

FIGURE 3.34. **Diagram of Orbital Floor Blowout Fracture.** Sudden increase in intraocular pressure from a direct blow to the eye can lead to a comminuted fracture of the orbital floor, with herniation of orbital contents into the maxillary sinus. A fluid level in the sinus is often seen acutely secondary to bleeding. (Reprinted with permission from Gean AD. Imaging of Head Trauma. Philadelphia: Lippincott Williams & Wilkins; 1994:478.)

are often associated with herniation of orbital contents through the fracture. When the inferior rectus muscle is compromised, patients will experience persistent vertical diplopia. Mild or transient diplopia can occur simply as a result of periorbital edema or hemorrhage. Rarely, fragments from an orbital floor fracture buckle upward into the orbit, an injury referred to as a "blow-in" fracture.

Plain-film findings suggestive of orbital floor blowout fractures include orbital emphysema, a fluid level in the ipsilateral maxillary sinus, indistinct orbital floor on Waters view, and soft tissue representing prolapsed orbital contents in the superior aspect of the maxillary sinus (Fig. 3.35). A bony spicule may be seen in the antrum, representing the inferiorly displaced fracture fragment. Blowout

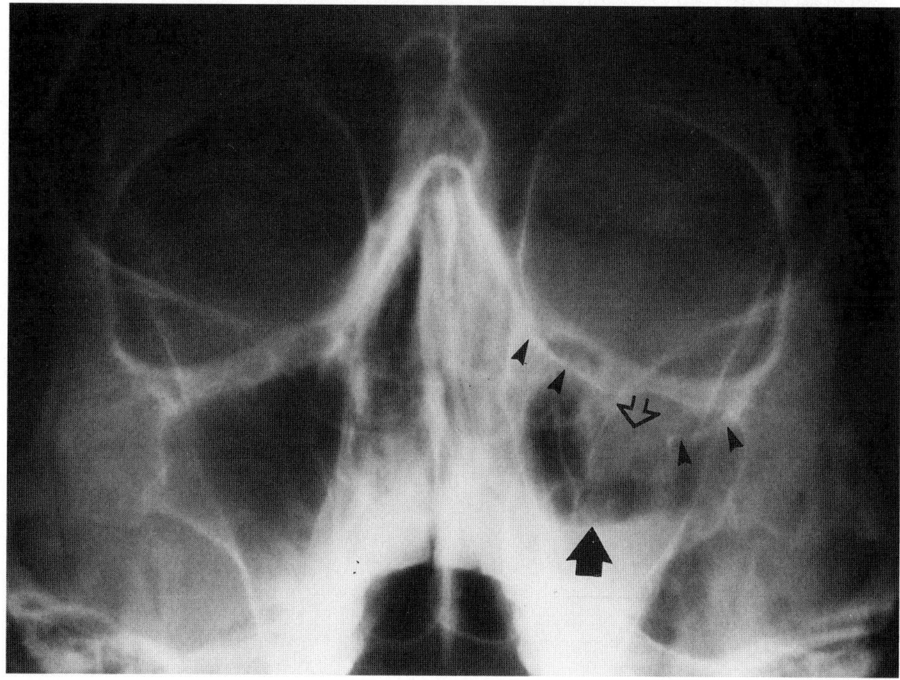

FIGURE 3.35. **Orbital Floor Blowout Fracture on Plain Film.** Waters view shows the major findings associated with an orbital floor blowout injury: disruption of the orbital floor (*arrowheads*), soft tissue mass in the superior aspect of the maxillary sinus (*open arrow*), and a maxillary sinus fluid level (*closed arrow*). (Reprinted with permission from Gean AD. Imaging of Head Trauma. Philadelphia: Lippincott Williams & Wilkins; 1994:478.)

fractures are best seen on direct coronal CT images (see Fig. 3.31b). These should be obtained with the patient lying prone. In the supine position, fluid and debris in the maxillary antrum will layer against the orbital floor and could obscure soft tissue that is herniated through the fracture.

Soft Tissue Injury. Penetrating foreign bodies such as bullets, metal fragments, glass, or other sharp objects account for a significant amount of traumatic injury to the orbit. Thin-section CT is the method of choice for confirming the presence and localization of foreign bodies (Fig. 3.36). CT can usually clearly define the relationship of bone fragments or foreign bodies to critical structures such as the optic nerve, globe, or extraocular muscles (Fig. 3.37). MR carries a potential risk of further injury by causing motion of intraocular ferromagnetic metal.

Traumatic optic neuropathy is seen in a significant number of patients with severe head trauma and occasionally occurs in patients with relatively minor deceleration injury. Damage may be maximal initially, with unilateral blindness or decreased acuity, or may worsen in the first few days after the injury. When delayed worsening occurs, secondary optic nerve compression from edema or hemorrhage in the optic nerve sheath should be considered. Imaging studies, particularly CT scans, are indicated to detect fractures through the optic canal or orbital apex. Rarely, displaced fractures are responsible for direct injury to the optic nerve sheath. More commonly, these fractures are nondisplaced but serve as evidence of severe stress transmitted to the orbital apex. Primary optic nerve injury may occur as a result of deceleration strain causing damage to the delicate meningeal vessels or direct neural disruption. Secondary optic nerve injury may occur as a result of swelling of the optic nerve within the rigid bony canal, with subsequent mechanical compression and vascular compromise.

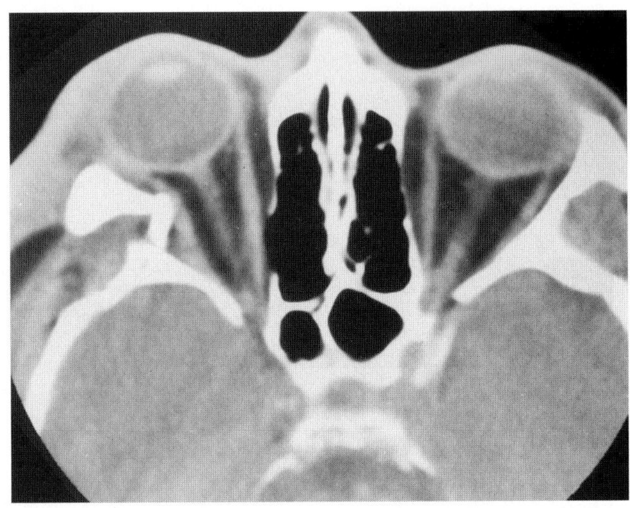

FIGURE 3.37. **Lateral Orbital Wall Fracture With Impingement of Lateral Rectus Muscle.** Noncontrast CT scan precisely localizes the site and degree of impingement on the right lateral rectus muscle in this patient with a comminuted fracture involving the zygomaticofrontal suture.

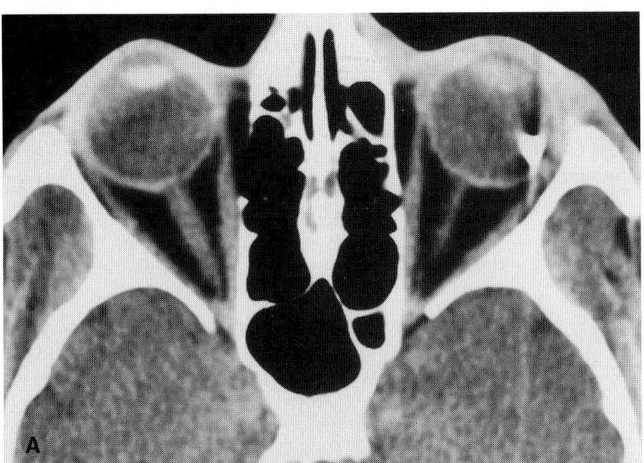

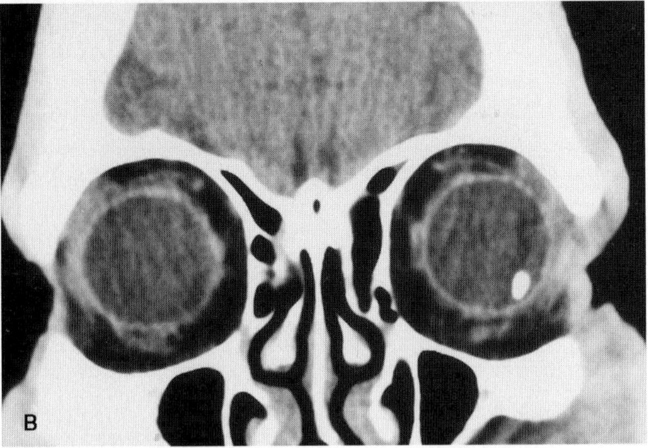

FIGURE 3.36. **Intraocular Metallic Foreign Body.** Axial **(A)** and coronal **(B)** CT scans confirm the presence of a metallic foreign body in the left globe.

Fractures of the Zygoma. The zygoma, or "cheekbone," is one of the most common sites of injury in fractures that involve multiple facial bones. Zygomatic arch fractures may occur as an isolated finding or as part of a zygomaticomaxillary complex ("tripod," "quadripod," or "trimalar") fracture. Comminution and depression are frequently seen with zygomatic arch fractures. On plain films, the zygomatic arch is best evaluated on the submental vertex view (Fig. 3.38). Deformity of the arch is a frequent finding in populations with a high incidence of facial trauma, and clinical examination may be required to differentiate acute from chronic injury.

Zygomaticomaxillary complex fractures usually result from a blow to the face. The zygoma articulates with the frontal, maxillary, sphenoid, and temporal bones. Fractures are somewhat variable but typically involve the zygomatic arch, zygomaticofrontal suture, infraorbital rim, orbital floor, lateral wall of the maxillary sinus, and lateral wall of the orbit. Injury to the infraorbital nerve is

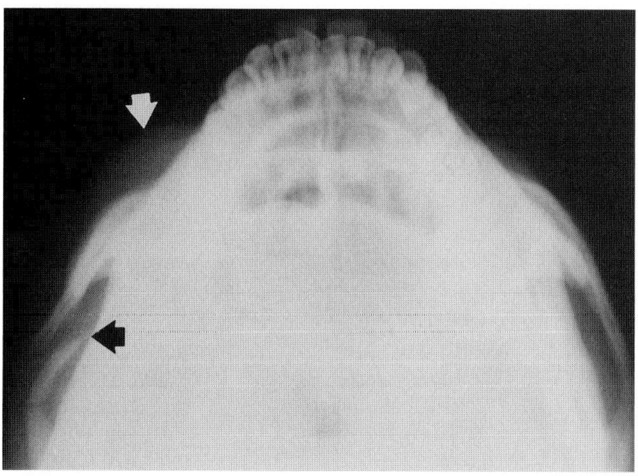

FIGURE 3.38. Right Zygomatic Arch Fracture. Submental vertex view shows a comminuted, depressed right zygomatic arch fracture (*black arrow*). Soft tissue swelling anterior to the body of the zygoma is also seen (*white arrow*). (Reprinted with permission from Gean AD. Imaging of Head Trauma. Philadelphia: Lippincott Williams & Wilkins; 1994:448.)

common secondary to fracture of the infraorbital rim at the infraorbital foramen. Diastasis of the zygomaticofrontal suture may injure the lateral canthal ligament or suspensory ligaments of the globe. Many of the fractures associated with this injury can be seen on both plain films and CT scans (Fig. 3.39). Associated findings on plain films include opacification of the ipsilateral maxillary antrum and posterior displacement of the body of the zygoma on the submental vertex view with overlying soft-tissue swelling.

Fractures of the Midface (Le Fort Fractures). Complex fractures of the facial bones are frequently classified according to the method of Le Fort, who developed his theory by inflicting facial trauma on cadavers and analyzing the results. He described three general patterns of fractures that differ in location of the fracture plane across the face (Fig. 3.40) (25). The three Le Fort fractures initially described are bilateral processes. All involve the pterygoid plates, which help anchor the facial bones to the skull. Although there is great variability in complex facial fractures, and the classic Le Fort injuries are rarely seen in their pure form, they remain a convenient way to categorize and describe basic patterns of injury. Frequently, similar patterns of injury are seen on one side only and are known as "hemi–Le Forts." Combinations also occur, such as a Le Fort I pattern on one side and a Le Fort II pattern on the other.

Le Fort I or "floating palate" fracture is a horizontal fracture through the maxillary sinuses. It extends through the nasal septum and walls of the maxillary sinuses into the inferior aspect of the pterygoid plates. The fracture plane is parallel to the plane of axial CT images but is recognized

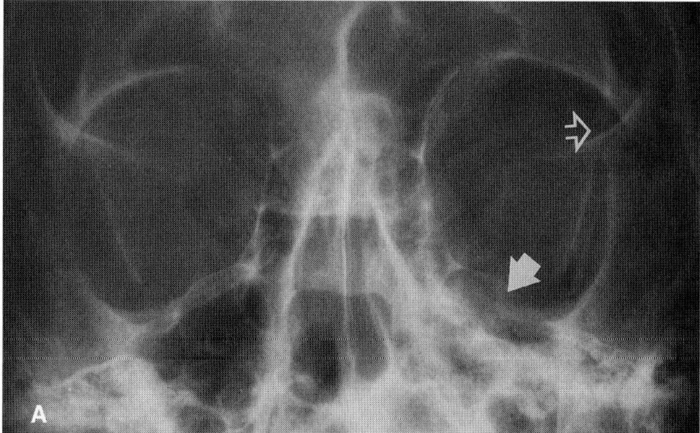

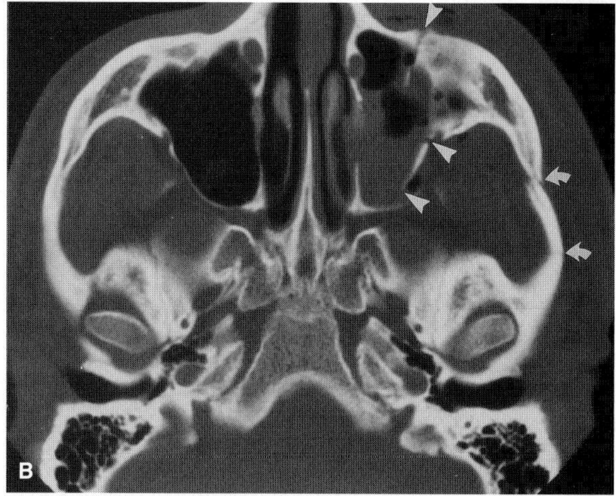

FIGURE 3.39. Zygomaticomaxillary Complex Fracture. A. Plain film shows diastasis of the left zygomaticofrontal suture (*open arrow*) and disruption of the orbital floor (*closed arrow*). An associated zygomatic arch fracture was seen on submental vertex view (not shown). **B.** A CT scan in a different patient shows comminuted left zygomatic arch fracture (*curved arrows*), with fractures of the anterior and posterolateral walls of the maxillary sinus (*arrowheads*). Associated signs of acute injury include soft tissue swelling and partial opacification of the maxillary sinus. (Reprinted with permission from Gean AD. Imaging of Head Trauma. Philadelphia: Lippincott Williams & Wilkins; 1994:452.)

by the fracture of all walls of both maxillary sinuses (Fig. 3.41). It is well seen in the coronal plane. There may be an associated midpalatal or maxillary split fracture. The Le Fort I fracture is more often seen in the pure form than either the Le Fort II or Le Fort III fractures. It occasionally may be accompanied by a unilateral zygomaticomaxillary complex fracture.

Le Fort II or "pyramidal" fracture describes a fracture through the medial orbital and lateral maxillary walls. It begins at the bridge of the nose and extends in a pyramidal fashion through the nasal septum; frontal process of the maxilla; medial wall of the orbit; inferior orbital rim; superior, lateral, and posterior walls of the maxillary antrum; and midportion of the pterygoid plates. The zygomatic arch and lateral orbital walls are left intact. The Le Fort II is usually associated with posterior displacement

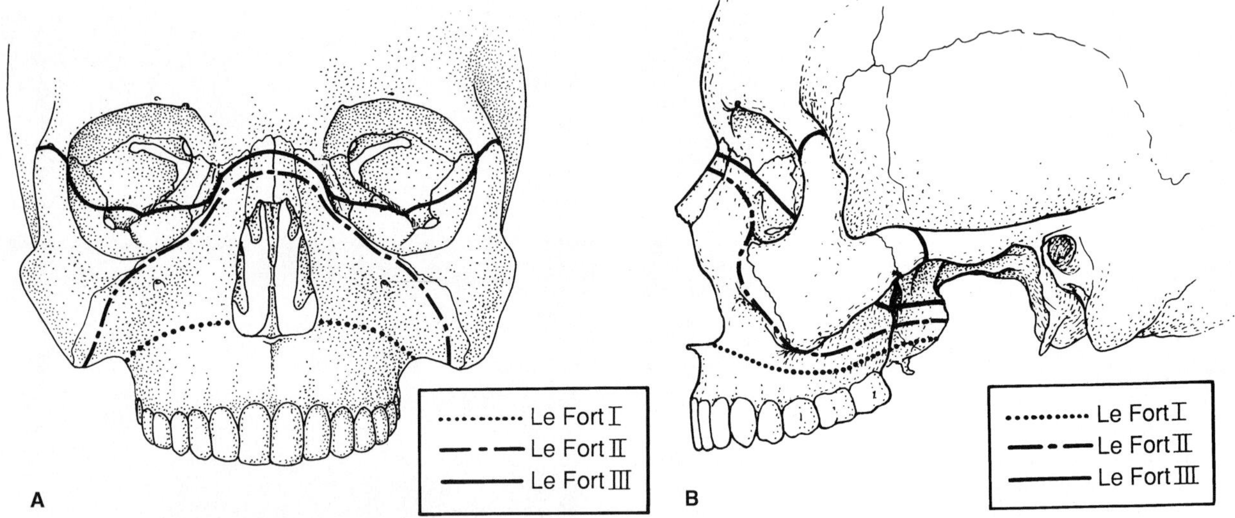

FIGURE 3.40. **Diagram of Le Fort Fractures.** Frontal **(A)** and lateral **(B)** projections demonstrate the patterns of facial fractures as originally described by Le Fort. (Reprinted with permission from Gean AD. Imaging of Head Trauma. Philadelphia: Lippincott Williams & Wilkins; 1994:454.)

of the facial bones, resulting in a "dish-face" deformity and malocclusion. The infraorbital nerve is frequently injured. Le Fort II fractures are rarely seen in the pure form.

Le Fort III fracture, or "craniofacial dysjunction," is a horizontally oriented fracture through the orbits. It begins near the nasofrontal suture and extends posteriorly to involve the nasal septum, medial and lateral orbital walls, zygomatic arch, and base (superior aspect) of the pterygoid plates. Patients with a Le Fort III fracture also have dish-face deformity and malocclusion. Injury to the infraorbital nerve is less commonly seen with Le Fort III than with Le Fort II fractures. A recognizable feature on plain films is the elongated appearance of the orbits on Waters and Caldwell views.

When interpreting CT scans obtained for facial trauma, it is probably best to describe the specific bones that are fractured on either side of the face. When appropriate, the Le Fort injury that best describes the distribution of fractures may also be used to categorize complex fractures.

Nasoethmoidal Fractures. Nasoethmoidal complex injuries describe the constellation of findings seen as a result of a blow to the midface between the eyes. This term encompasses a wide variety of different fracture complexes

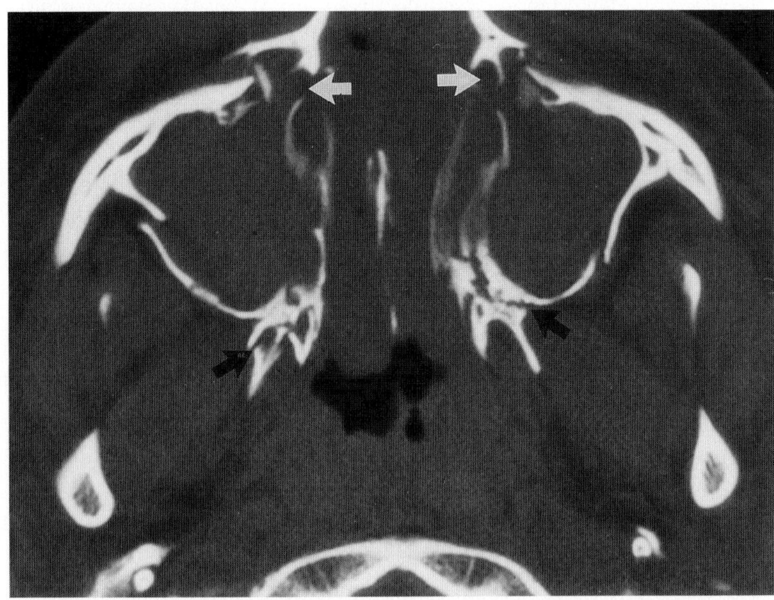

FIGURE 3.41. **Le Fort I Fracture.** Axial CT scan demonstrates comminuted fractures involving all walls of both maxillary sinuses, with associated fractures through the pterygoid plates (*black arrows*). Both nasolacrimal ducts are also disrupted (*white arrows*). Both maxillary antra are completely opacified. (Reprinted with permission from Gean AD. Imaging of Head Trauma. Philadelphia: Lippincott Williams & Wilkins; 1994:456.)

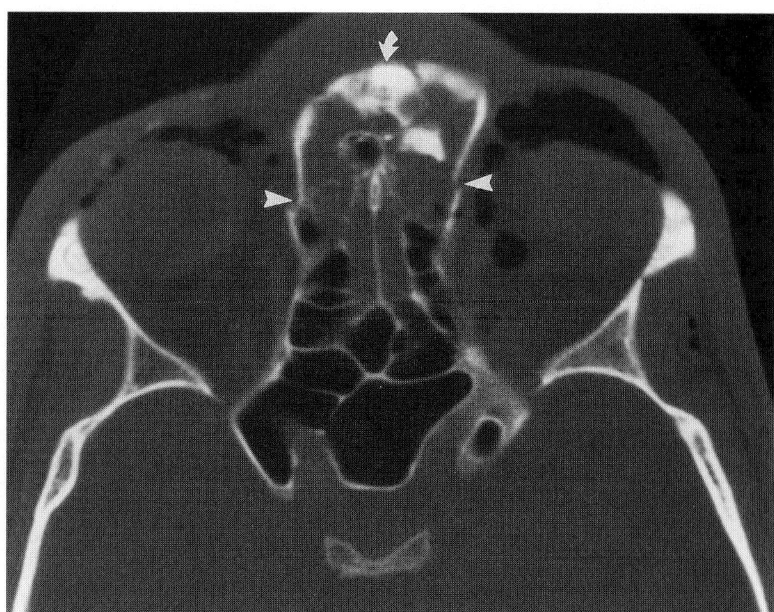

FIGURE 3.42. **Nasoethmoidal Complex Fracture.** Axial CT scan demonstrates a depressed fracture involving the root of the nose (*curved arrow*) and anterior ethmoids. Bilateral fractures of the medial orbital walls are also present (*arrowheads*) with bilateral orbital emphysema.

that are best described by listing the specific fractures seen on CT scans. These injuries may include fractures of the lamina papyracea; inferior, medial, and supraorbital rims; frontal or ethmoid sinuses; orbital roofs; nasal bone and frontal process of the maxilla; and sphenoid bone (Fig. 3.42). These fractures have also been called *orbitoethmoid* or *nasoethmoid–orbital fractures* because of the importance of the often associated orbital injuries. There may be associated fractures of the skull base and clivus. Other findings include orbital and intracranial air, opacification of the ethmoid and frontal sinuses, and depression of the midface. Nasoethmoidal fractures can be suspected on plain films when the lateral view shows posterior displacement of nasion. Thin-section CT helps evaluate the extent of the injury and helps localize bony fragments that might encroach on the optic nerve or canal.

Complications of nasoethmoidal complex fractures depend on the location and extent of injury. Patients with fractures involving the floor of the anterior cranial fossa are prone to develop CSF leaks because of the high frequency of associated dural lacerations. The olfactory nerves are frequently injured when fractures extend to the cribriform plate. As mentioned earlier, orbital injuries are often seen as a component of nasoethmoid fractures. The globes or optic nerves may be damaged by displaced medial orbital wall fracture fragments.

Mandibular fractures are extremely common in patients with maxillofacial injury. Plain films are used in

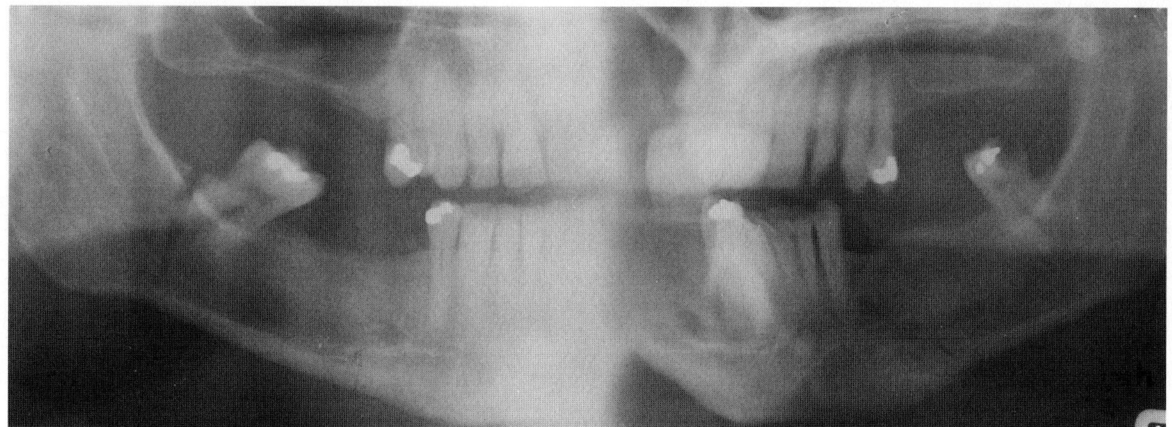

FIGURE 3.43. **Panorex Radiograph With Bilateral Mandibular Fractures.** Fractures of the left mandibular angle (extending into the root of a molar tooth) and right horizontal ramus are both clearly seen on single panoramic film. (Reprinted with permission from Gean AD. Imaging of Head Trauma. Philadelphia: Lippincott Williams & Wilkins; 1994:431.)

the initial evaluation of patients with suspected mandibular injury. The mandibular series includes posteroanterior, lateral, Towne, and bilateral oblique projections. CT or Panorex films can also be used to evaluate mandibular injury (Fig. 3.43).

Mandibular fractures can be considered either simple or compound. Simple fractures are most common in the ramus and condyle and do not communicate externally or with the mouth. Compound fractures are those that communicate internally through a tooth socket or externally through a laceration (Fig. 3.44). Fractures of the body of the mandible are almost always compound fractures. Pathologic mandibular fractures can occur at sites of infection or neoplasm. Mandibular fractures are frequently multiple or bilateral, and such fractures often involve the condyle (Fig. 3.45). Subcondylar fractures may be recognized on plain films by the "cortical ring" sign, a well-corticated density seen above the condylar neck on lateral views because of the horizontal axis of the fragment. A common pattern of injury is a unilateral condylar fracture with a contralateral fracture of the mandibular angle. The mandibular angle is also the most common site of isolated injury. Fractures of the ramus and coronoid processes are rare. Fractures through the symphysis or parasymphyseal region are common but difficult to diagnose on plain films because of the obliquity of the fracture plane.

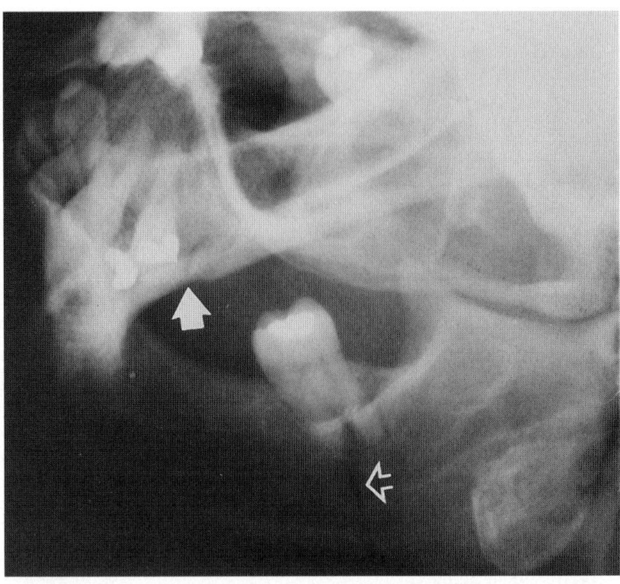

FIGURE 3.44. **Compound Fracture of the Mandible.** Oblique view of the mandible demonstrates a posterior ramus fracture extending through the adjacent tooth socket (*open arrow*). A contralateral fracture of the horizontal ramus is also present (*closed arrow*). (Reprinted with permission from Gean AD. Imaging of Head Trauma. Philadelphia: Lippincott Williams & Wilkins; 1994:467.)

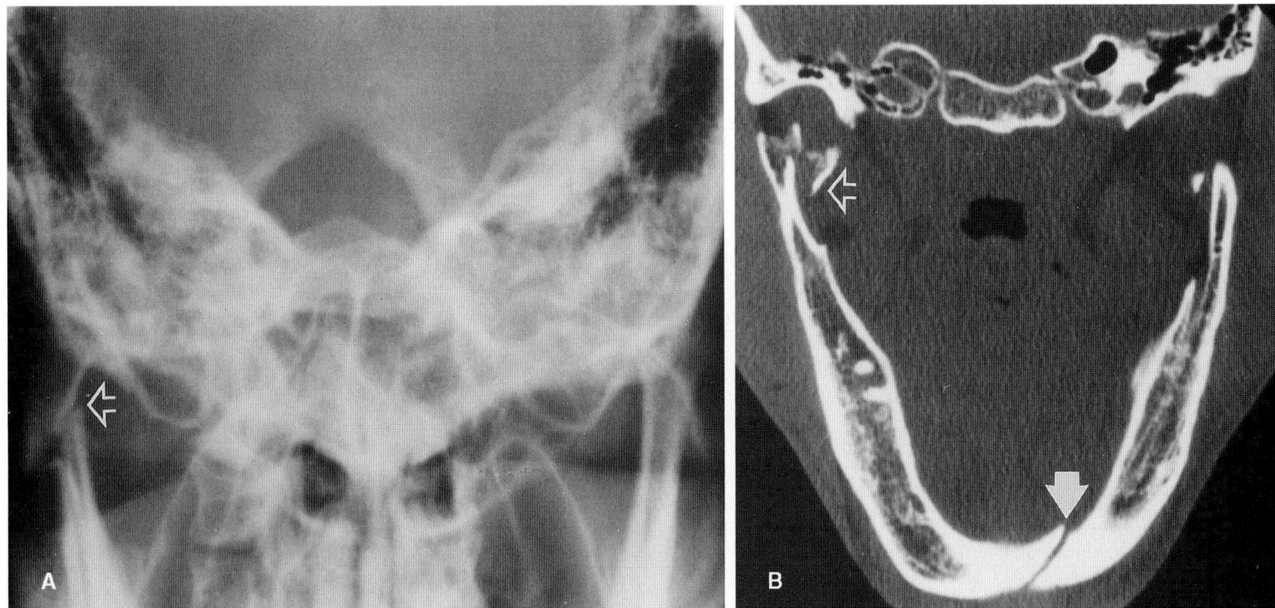

FIGURE 3.45. **Mandibular Condylar Fracture. A.** Plain film (Towne projection) shows a displaced right subcondylar fracture (*open arrow*). **B.** Axial CT in a different patient shows a right condylar fracture (*open arrow*) and an associated parasymphyseal fracture (*closed arrow*). The latter fracture is easily missed on plain films because of the oblique fracture plane. (Reprinted with permission from Gean AD. Imaging of Head Trauma. Philadelphia: Lippincott Williams & Wilkins; 1994:464.)

Fractures involving the dentoalveolar complex are also often missed on mandibular series and require intraoral dental films or CT for evaluation. Bilateral fractures through the mandibular body or comminuted fractures can lead to airway obstruction from posterior displacement of the tongue and free mandibular fragment.

SUGGESTED READINGS

Intracranial Injury

Eelkema EA, Hecht ST, Horton JA. Head trauma. In: Latchaw RE, ed. MR and CT Imaging of the Head, Neck, and Spine. 2nd ed. St. Louis: CV Mosby, 1991:203–265.

Gean AD. Imaging of Head Trauma. New York: Raven Press,1994.

Cranial and Skull Base Injury

Davidson HC. Imaging of the temporal bone. Neuroimaging Clin North Am 2004;14(4):721–760.

Holland BA, Brant-Zawadzki M. High-resolution CT of temporal bone trauma. AJNR Am J Neuroradiol 1984;5:291–295.

Head Trauma in Child Abuse

Merten DF, Radkowski MA, Leonidas JC. The abused child: a radiological reappraisal. Radiology 1983;146:377–381.

Petitti N, Williams DW III. CT and MR imaging of nonaccidental pediatric head trauma. Acad Radiol 1998;5(3):215–223.

Sato Y, Smith WL. Head injury in child abuse. Neuroimaging Clin North Am 1991;1:475–492.

Facial Trauma

DelBalso AM, Hall RE. Mandibular and dentoalveolar fractures. Neuroimaging Clin North Am 1991;1:285–303.

Kassel EE, Gruss JS. Imaging of midfacial fractures. Neuroimaging Clin North Am 1991;1:259–283.

Som PM, Brandwein MS. Sinonasal facial fractures and postoperative findings. In: Som PM, Curtin HD, eds. Head and Neck Imaging. 4th ed. St. Louis: CV Mosby, 2003:374–438.

REFERENCES

1. Link TM, Schuierer G, Hufendiek A, et al. Substantial head trauma: value of routine CT examination of the cervicocranium. Radiology 1995;196:741–745.
2. Gentry LR, Godersky JC, Thompson B, et al. Prospective comparative study of intermediate-field MR and CT in the evaluation of closed head trauma. AJR Am J Roentgenol 1988;150:673–682.
3. Orrison WW, Gentry LR, Stimac GK, et al. Blinded comparison of cranial CT and MR in closed head injury evaluation. AJNR Am J Neuroradiol 1995;15:351–356.
4. Noguchi K, Ogawa T, Seto H, et al. Subacute and chronic subarachnoid hemorrhage: diagnosis with fluid-attenuated inversion-recovery MR imaging. Radiology 1997;203(1):257–262.
5. Woodcock RJ Jr, Short J, Do HM, et al. Imaging of acute subarachnoid hemorrhage with a fluid-attenuated inversion recovery sequence in an animal model: comparison with non-contrast-enhanced CT. AJNR Am J Neuroradiol 2001;22(9):1698–1703.
6. Alsop DC, Murai H, Detre JA, McIntosh TK, Smith DH. Detection of acute pathologic changes following experimental traumatic brain injury using diffusion-weighted magnetic resonance imaging. J Neurotrauma 1996;13:515–521.
7. Liu AY, Maldjian JA, Bagley, LJ, et al. Traumatic brain injury: diffusion-weighted MR imaging findings. AJNR Am J Neuroradiol 1999;20:1636–1641.
8. Arfanakis K, Haughton VM, Carew JD, et al. Diffusion tensor MR imaging in diffuse axonal injury. AJNR Am J Neuroradiol 2002;23(5):794–802.
9. Huisman TA, Schwamm LH, Schaefer PW, et al. Diffusion tensor imaging as potential biomarker of white matter injury in diffuse axonal injury. AJNR Am J Neuroradiol 2004;25(3):370–376.
10. Masters SJ. Evaluation of head trauma: efficacy of skull films. AJR Am J Roentgenol 1980;135:539–547.
11. Bell RS, Loop JW. The utility and futility of radiographic skull examination for trauma. N Engl J Med 1971;284:236–239.
12. Hackney DB. Skull radiography in the evaluation of acute head trauma: a survey of current practice. Radiology 1991;181:711–714.
13. Adams JH. Pathology of nonmissile head injury. Neuroimaging Clin North Am 1991;1:397–410.
14. Gentry LR. Temporal bone trauma. Neuroimaging Clin North Am 1991;1:319–340.
15. Gentry LR. Imaging of closed head injury. Radiology 1994;191:1–17.
16. Le TH, Mukherjee P, Henry RG, et al. Diffusion tensor imaging with three-dimensional fiber tractography of traumatic axonal shearing injury: an imaging correlate for the posterior callosal "disconnection" syndrome. Neurosurgery 2005;56(1):E195–201.
17. Gennarelli TA, Thibault LE, Adams JH, et al. Diffuse axonal injury and traumatic coma in the primate. In: Dacey RG Jr, Winn HR, Rimel RW, et al, eds. Trauma of the Central Nervous System. New York: Raven Press, 1985:169–193.
18. Gentry LR. Head trauma. In: Atlas SW, ed. Magnetic Resonance Imaging of the Brain and Spine. 2nd ed. Philadelphia: Lippincott Williams & Wilkins, 1996;611–647.
19. Shanmuganathan K, Gullapallo RP, Mirvis SE, et al. Whole brain apparent diffusion coeffiecient in traumatic brain injury: correlation with Glasgow Scale score. AJNR Am J Neuroradiol 2004;25(4): 539–544.
20. Bruce DA, Zimmerman RA. Shaken impact syndrome. Pediatr Ann 1989;18:482–494.
21. Merten DF, Osborne DRS, Radkowski AM. Craniocerebral trauma in the child abuse syndrome: radiological observations. Pediatr Radiol 1984;14:272–277.
22. Zimmerman RA, Bilaniuk LT. Pediatric head trauma. Neuroimaging Clin North Am 1994;4:349–366.
23. Caffey J. Multiple fractures in the long bones of infants suffering from chronic subdural hematoma. AJR Am J Roentgenol 1946;56: 163–173.
24. Duhaime AC, Gennarelli TA, Thibault LE, et al. The shaken baby syndrome. A clinical, pathological, and biomechanical study. J Neurosurg 1987;66:409–415.
25. Le Fort R. Etude experimental sur les fractures de la machoire superieure, parts I, II, III. Rev Chir (Paris) 1901;23:208–227.

Chapter 4

Cerebrovascular Disease

Howard A. Rowley

ISCHEMIC STROKE
Pathophysiologic Basis for Imaging Changes
Hemorrhagic Transformation of Infarction
Use of Contrast in Ischemic Stroke
Pattern Recognition in Ischemic Stroke
Anterior (Carotid) Circulation
Posterior (Vertebrobasilar) Circulation
Watershed (Border Zone) Infarction
Small-Vessel Ischemia
Venous Infarction

HEMORRHAGE
Imaging of Hemorrhage
Subarachnoid Hemorrhage
Parenchymal Hemorrhage
Primary Hemorrhage Versus Hemorrhagic Neoplasm
Primary Hemorrhage Versus Hemorrhagic Transformation of Infarction

Stroke is a clinical term applied to any abrupt nontraumatic brain insult—literally "a blow from an unseen hand." Strokes are caused by either brain infarction (75%) or hemorrhage (25%) and must be distinguished from other conditions that cause abrupt neurologic deficits. *Infarction* is a permanent injury that occurs when tissue perfusion is decreased long enough to cause necrosis, typically as the result of occlusion of the feeding artery. *Transient ischemic attacks* (TIAs) are defined as transient neurologic symptoms or signs lasting less than 24 hours, which may serve as a "warning sign" of an infarction occurring in the next few weeks or months. TIAs are often caused by temporary occlusion of a feeding artery. *Hemorrhage* is seen when blood ruptures through the arterial wall, spilling into the surrounding parenchyma, subarachnoid space, or ventricles.

Stroke is the third leading cause of death in the United States and a major source of long-term disability among survivors. The approach to treatment of ischemic stroke has been largely preventative or supportive in the past, but approval of IV thrombolysis for acute stroke and neuroprotective drug development have made rapid imaging and intervention a critical part of stroke management. The patient with hemorrhage may harbor an aneurysm, vascular malformation, or other condition, and each condition involves important differences in treatment options. The radiologist plays a critical role in the triage and evaluation of all stroke patients. Selection of the proper imaging technique, recognition of early ischemic changes, differentiation of stroke from other brain disorders, and recognition of important stroke subtypes can have a significant impact on therapy and outcome.

This chapter reviews the pathophysiology of stroke, the time course of findings on CT and MR, patterns of arterial and venous occlusions, and overall radiologic approach to evaluation of the stroke patient.

ISCHEMIC STROKE

Etiology. Despite our best clinical efforts, no clear source is ever identified in up to a quarter of patients with brain infarction. Among those with an established mechanism, about two thirds of infarcts are caused by thrombi and one third are caused by emboli. Thrombi are formed at sites of abnormal vascular endothelium, typically over an area of atherosclerotic plaque or ulcer. A large-artery thrombosis in the neck may or may not cause distal infarction, depending on the time course of occlusion and available collateral supply. Small-vessel thrombi frequently occur in end arteries of the brain, accounting for about one fifth of infarcts ("lacunes"). Emboli may arise from the heart, aortic arch, carotid arteries, or vertebral arteries, causing infarction by distal migration and occlusion. There is obviously overlap between the thrombotic and embolic groups, since the majority of emboli begin as thrombi somewhere more

TABLE 4.1 Differential Diagnosis of Ischemic Stroke by Age

Pediatric	*Young Adult*	*Elderly*
Congenital heart disease	Cardiac emboli	Atherosclerosis
Blood dyscrasias	Atherosclerosis	Cardiac emboli
Meningitis	Drug abuse	Coagulopathy
Arterial dissection	Arterial dissection	Amyloid
Trauma	Coagulopathy	Vasculitis
ECMO	Vasculitis	Venous thrombosis
Venous thrombosis	Venous thrombosis	

ECMO, extracorporeal membrane oxygenation.

proximal in the cardiovascular tree (hence the practical term "thromboembolic disease"). Vasculitis, vasospasm, coagulopathies, global hypoperfusion, and venous thrombosis each account for 5% or fewer of acute strokes, but are important to recognize because of differing treatment and prognosis. A patient's age, medical history, and type of stroke seen will help establish the major etiologic considerations (Table 4.1).

Pathophysiologic Basis for Imaging Changes

Brain Metabolism and Selective Vulnerability. Neurons lead a precarious life. The brain consumes 20% of the total cardiac output to maintain its minute-to-minute delivery of glucose and oxygen. Because the brain holds no significant long-term energy stores (e.g., glycogen, fat), disruption of blood flow for even a few minutes will lead to neuronal death. The extent of injury depends on both the duration and degree of ischemia. Minor reduction in perfusion is initially compensated for by increased extraction of substrate, but injury becomes inevitable below a critical flow threshold (10 to 20 mL/100 g tissue/min vs. normal 55 mL/100 g/min).

Certain cell types and neuroanatomic regions show selective vulnerability to ischemic injury. Gray matter normally receives 3 to 4 times more blood flow than white matter and is therefore more likely to suffer under conditions of oligemia. Some subsets of neurons (e.g., cerebellar Purkinje cells, hippocampal CA-1 neurons) are injured more readily than others, possibly because of their greater concentrations of receptors for excitatory amino acids. The slower-metabolizing capillary endothelial cells and white matter oligodendrocytes are more resistant to ischemia than gray matter but will also die when deprived of nutrients. Cells served by penetrating end arteries or those residing in the watershed zone between major territories have no alternate route for perfusion and are therefore more prone to infarction. Damage will likely be more severe in a patient with an incomplete circle of Willis than in one with a complete arterial collateral pathway.

Imaging Findings in Acute Ischemia. Ischemia causes a cascade of cellular level events leading to the gross pathologic changes detected in clinical imaging. Failure of membrane pumps permits efflux of potassium ions (K^+) and simultaneous influx of calcium ions (Ca^{2+}), sodium ions (Na^+), and water. This leads to cellular ("cytotoxic") edema, observed clinically as increased water content in the affected region. *Changes in brain water are key to understanding signs of infarction by CT and MR.* Even a small increase in water content causes characteristic decreased attenuation on CT, low signal on T1WIs, and high signal on T2- and diffusion-weighted MR. This edema peaks 3 to 7 days postinfarction and is maximal in the gray matter. A smaller component of vasogenic edema also develops as the more resistant capillary endothelial cells lose integrity. (In contrast, tumor-associated edema is primarily vasogenic and preferentially affects the white matter; see Chapter 5.)

Careful inspection of CT and MR images captured within minutes to a few hours after vessel occlusion can give clues to ischemic injury, even before gross tissue edema or mass effect are seen. These "hyperacute" signs primarily relate to morphologic changes in the vessels rather than density or signal changes in the parenchyma. On CT, the actual thrombus may occasionally be seen in larger intracranial branches, resulting in the "hyperdense artery sign" (Fig. 4.1). On MR, the normal black signal of flowing blood within the lumen ("flow void") is immediately lost and may be replaced by abnormal signal representing clotting or slow flow (Fig. 4.2). Loss of the flow void is best seen acutely in the large vessels (carotid siphon, vertebrobasilar vessels, middle cerebral artery [MCA] branches). Dissolution of clot and improved collateral flow may occur within the first few days, leading to re-establishment of flow void on follow-up MR exams.

Acute MCA Ischemia on CT: Insular Ribbon and Lentiform Nucleus Edema. CT scans done within 6 hours of MCA occlusion will commonly exhibit the "insular ribbon sign," a subtle but important blurring of the gray–white layers of the insula caused by early edema (Fig. 4.3). Early edema may also be most conspicuous in the putamen in proximal middle cerebral artery occlusions (lentiform nucleus edema sign). MR exams in the first few hours may show a similar loss of gray–white borders and slight crowding of sulci in areas destined to undergo infarction. However, the most sensitive imaging sequence for detection of brain ischemia is diffusion-weighted MR imaging (DWI), which may turn positive minutes after infarction begins, well before a CT would show even subtle signs. Hyperintense signal on DWIs ("light-bulb sign") precedes T2 hyperintensity, which typically develops at 6 to 12 hours postictal. (Fig. 4.4).

CT Screening for Thrombolysis. Careful but rapid interpretation of CT scans is particularly important in patients who are candidates for thrombolytic drug

(text continues on page 90)

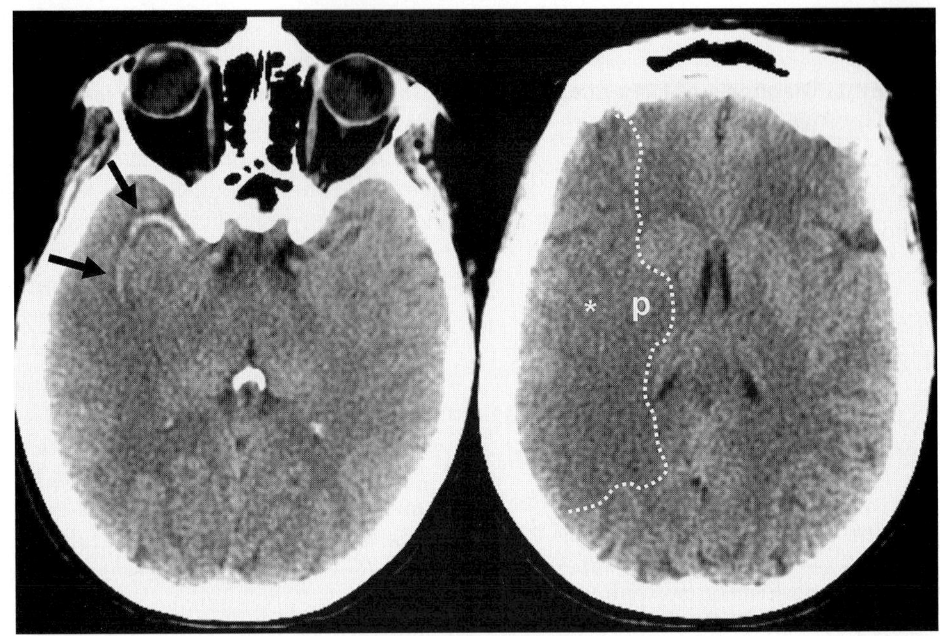

FIGURE 4.1. **Hyperdense Artery Sign and Early Edema on CT.** Three hours postocclusion, high density is seen in the proximal right middle cerebral artery (MCA) (*arrows*). Acute thrombus fills the lumen. Low attenuation and loss of gray–white distinction are seen in the insula (*asterisk*), posterior putamen (P), and majority of the MCA cortex (within dashed lines).

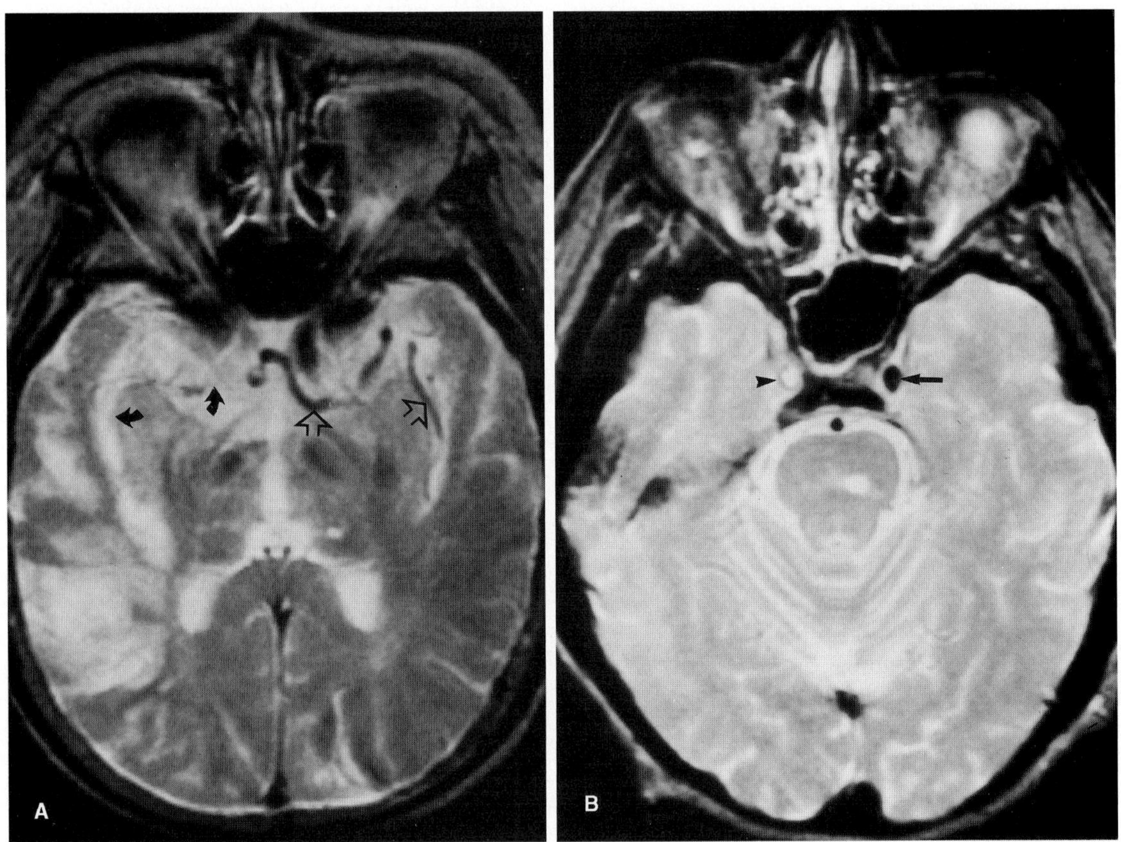

FIGURE 4.2. **Loss of Flow Void. A.** Six hours after right internal carotid occlusion, there is a loss of vascular flow voids in the internal carotid and middle cerebral artery branches (*arrows*) compared with the patent left side (*open arrows*). Hyperintensity is developing in the right posterior sylvian region, indicative of early edema on this T2WI. **B.** A section below shows complete occlusion of the right internal carotid artery in its cavernous segment (*arrowhead*), with normal flow void preserved on the left (*arrow*). An older lacune in the pons is also seen.

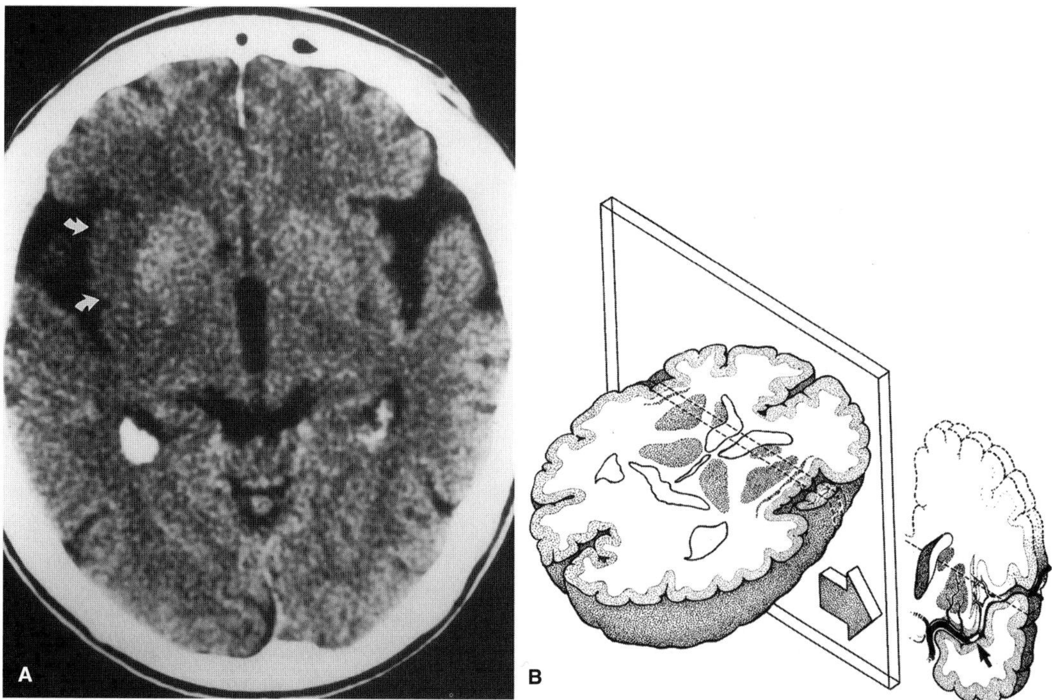

FIGURE 4.3. **Insular Ribbon Sign. A.** A noncontrast CT done 4 hours after right middle cerebral artery (MCA) occlusion shows decreased attenuation and loss of gray–white borders in the right insular region (*arrows*). **B.** Diagram of the insula in transverse and coronal planes. The insular cortex, claustrum, and extreme capsule are infarcted due to occlusion of the MCA (*arrow*) beyond the lateral lenticulostriate vessels. (From Truwit CL, et al. Loss of the insular ribbon: another early CT sign of acute middle cerebral artery infarction. Radiology 1990;176:801–806; used with permission.)

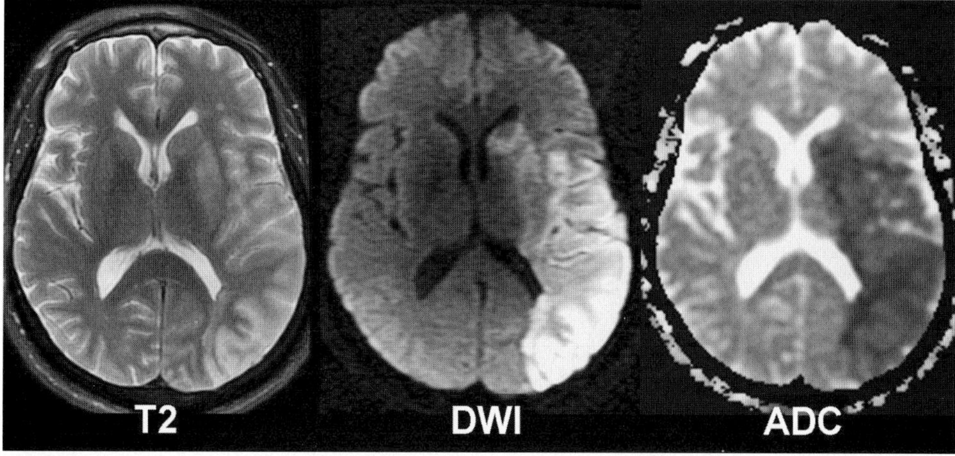

FIGURE 4.4. **Edema in Early Ischemia.** This patient was found unresponsive with unknown time of symptom onset. Edema is detected as high signal intensity and mild sulcal effacement in the left middle cerebral artery territory on T2W transverse images. Hyperintensity on the diffusion-weighted image (DWI) and hypointensity on the apparent diffusion coefficient (ADC) map are characteristic of cytotoxic edema in acute ischemia. Note preferential gray matter involvement during early ischemia. These images suggest the stroke is approximately 4 to 8 hours old.

treatment (e.g., tissue plasminogen activator [tPA]). Administration of intravenous tPA within 3 hours of stroke onset has been reported to improve neurologic outcome, provided that rigid inclusion and exclusion treatment criteria are met. A screening CT is examined to exclude patients with brain hemorrhage, masses, or other structural abnormalities that contraindicate thrombolysis. Patients with extensive edema on their initial CT scan may be at particularly high risk for reperfusion hemorrhage, so these patients should be excluded from thrombolytic treatment. Although universal guidelines are not agreed upon, patients with edema affecting more than one third of the MCA territory should generally be excluded. More subtle baseline changes, such as an isolated insular ribbon sign or limited lentiform nucleus edema alone, are not considered contraindications for thrombolysis. Current work suggests that perfusion-sensitive CT and MR techniques may also prove useful in identifying ischemic but still salvageable tissue (ischemic penumbra) to help guide selection of patients for acute treatment beyond 3 hours. The treatment window of opportunity may also widen beyond 3 hours as intra-arterial interventions and neuroprotective drugs are introduced in clinical use.

Diffusion-Weighted MR in Acute Ischemia. DWI uses a novel form of MR tissue contrast to noninvasively detect ischemic changes within minutes of stroke onset. DWIs are acquired by applying a strong gradient pair that sensitizes the images to microscopic (brownian) water motion. Brain water diffusion rates fall rapidly during acute ischemia, recovering to normal over days or weeks in infarcted tissues. Because random water motion is slowed down in areas of acute ischemia, the early infarct stands out as bright signal on DWIs, compared to dark signal (dephasing) in the normal areas. Acute stroke patients may show clear DWI changes hours before any abnormality can be seen on spin-echo T2WIs (Fig. 4.5). This can also be a useful way to distinguish new ischemic areas (high signal on DWIs) from older lesions (normal or low signal on DWIs). Via a series of different diffusion gradient strengths, the process may also be quantified in an apparent diffusion coefficient (ADC). The ADC reflects "pure" diffusion behavior, free of any underlying T2 contributions ("shine through" or "dark through"). DWI acquisition is facilitated using echo-planar MR systems, with their inherently faster, stronger gradients and rapid digitization equipment.

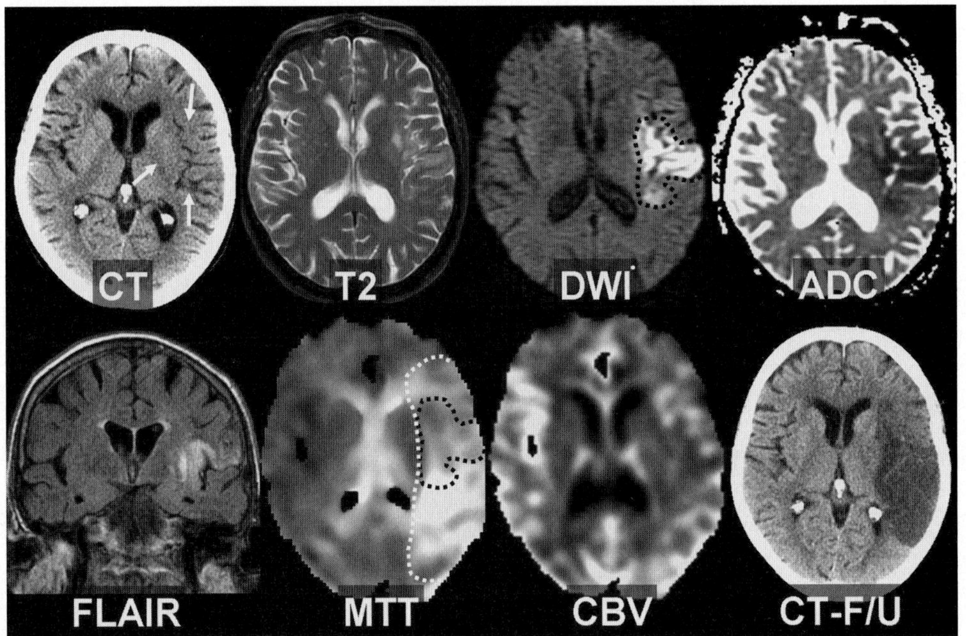

FIGURE 4.5. **Diffusion-Perfusion Mismatch in Acute Ischemia.** This 86-year-old woman with a history of atrial fibrillation developed sudden right hemiplegia and aphasia. The noncontrast CT shows subtle low attenuation in the left putamen, insula, and sylvian cortex (*arrows*). On the T2WI, the cortical gray matter shows mild edema, confirmed to represent cytotoxic edema on the diffusion-weighted image (DWI) and the apparent diffusion coefficient (ADC). Fluid-attenuated inversion recovery (FLAIR) shows cortical edema and stasis in the left middle cerebral artery. Perfusion-weighted images (mean transit time [MTT] and cerebral blood volume [CBV]) show a larger area at risk, extending into the parietal lobe (MTT defect in white dashes; DWI lesion superimposed in black dashes). The hypoperfused tissue not yet infarcted is considered tissue at risk, or the ischemic penumbra. Diffusion lesions tend to "grow into" severe surrounding perfusion lesions if untreated. The follow-up CT (CT-F/U) shows extension of infarction into the penumbral tissue identified by MTT.

FLuid-Attenuated Inversion Recovery (FLAIR) in Ischemia. FLAIR allows heavy T2 weighting of the parenchyma while simultaneously suppressing free water signal from the CSF. These techniques increase the conspicuity of T2 changes in ischemia. FLAIR is not inherently better than T2 MR for early detection of ischemia, but it may be particularly helpful in detecting small lesions in the cortex and for exclusion of acute subarachnoid hemorrhage.

Subacute and Chronic Ischemia. In the subacute phase, edema leads to mass effect, ranging from slight sulcal effacement to marked midline shift with brain herniation, depending on the size and location of infarct. These changes peak at 3 to 7 days, with progressive brain softening (encephalomalacia) ensuing thereafter. One potential imaging pitfall, the "fogging effect," may be encountered on CTs obtained during the second week after infarction, while edema and mass effect are subsiding. At this stage, decrease in edema and accumulation of proteins from cell lysis balance one another such that brain morphology and density in the injured region can appear nearly normal by CT. Fogging effects are much less of a problem on MR because of its greater tissue sensitivity, particularly when contrast is used (Fig. 4.6). Edema or mass effect that persists beyond 1 month effectively rules out simple ischemia and should raise the possibility of recurrent infarction or an underlying tumor.

In the weeks and months following infarction, macrophages remove dead tissue, leaving a small amount of gliotic scar and encephalomalacia behind. CSF takes up the space previously occupied by brain. The affected corticospinal tract atrophies (wallerian degeneration), leading to a shrunken appearance of the ipsilateral cerebral peduncle. If hemorrhage accompanied the infarct, hemosiderin may be seen grossly or detected as signal hypointensity by T2WIs. Widening of adjacent sulci and "ex vacuo" dilatation of the ventricle occurs adjacent to the infarcted area (Fig. 4.7).

Hemorrhagic Transformation of Infarction

Reperfusion into infarcted capillary beds may lead secondarily to gross or microscopic hemorrhage, seen in up to half of infarcts. In most cases this takes the form of microscopic leakage (diapedesis) of red blood cells, but on rare occasions a frank hematoma will form. Physical disruption of the capillary endothelial cells, loss of

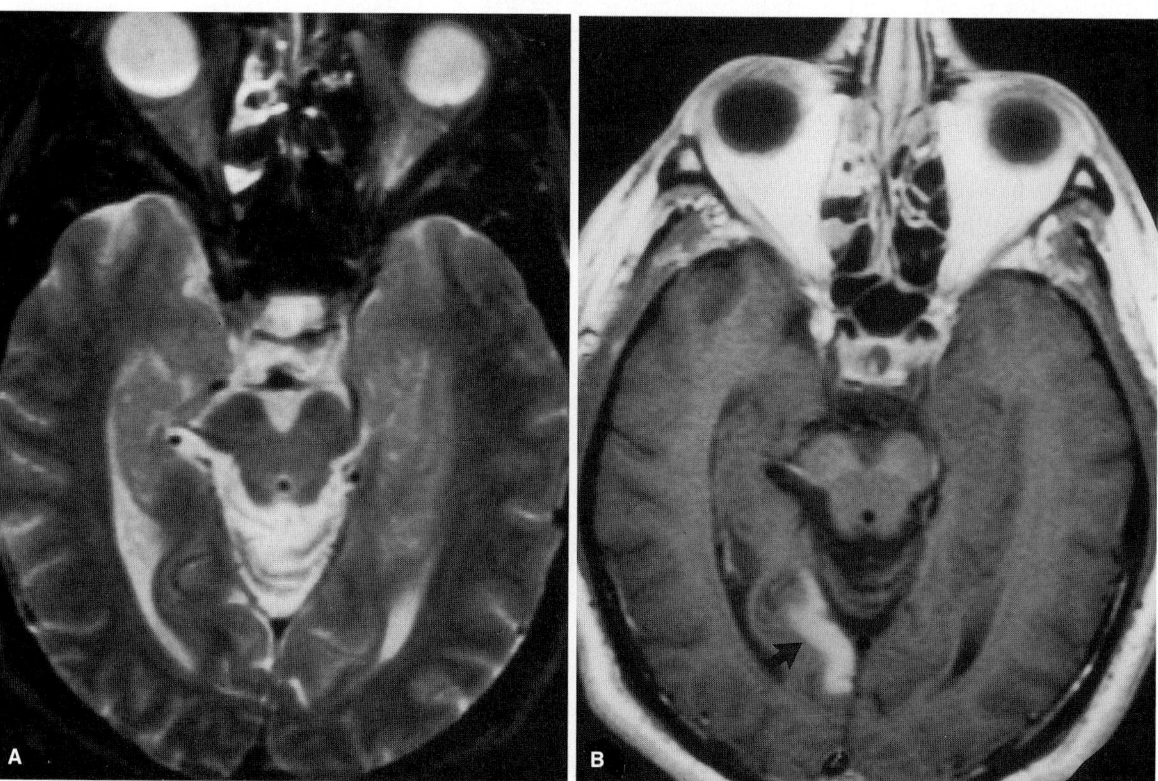

FIGURE 4.6. **Fogging Effect in Subacute Infarction.** As edema and mass effect subside, but before development of atrophy, infarcts may be inconspicuous on unenhanced CT or MR. **A.** The T2WI is essentially normal in the occipital regions 13 days after right posterior cerebral artery infarction. **B.** T1WI after gadolinium administration shows enhancement of the infarcted deep right occipital cortex (*arrow.*)

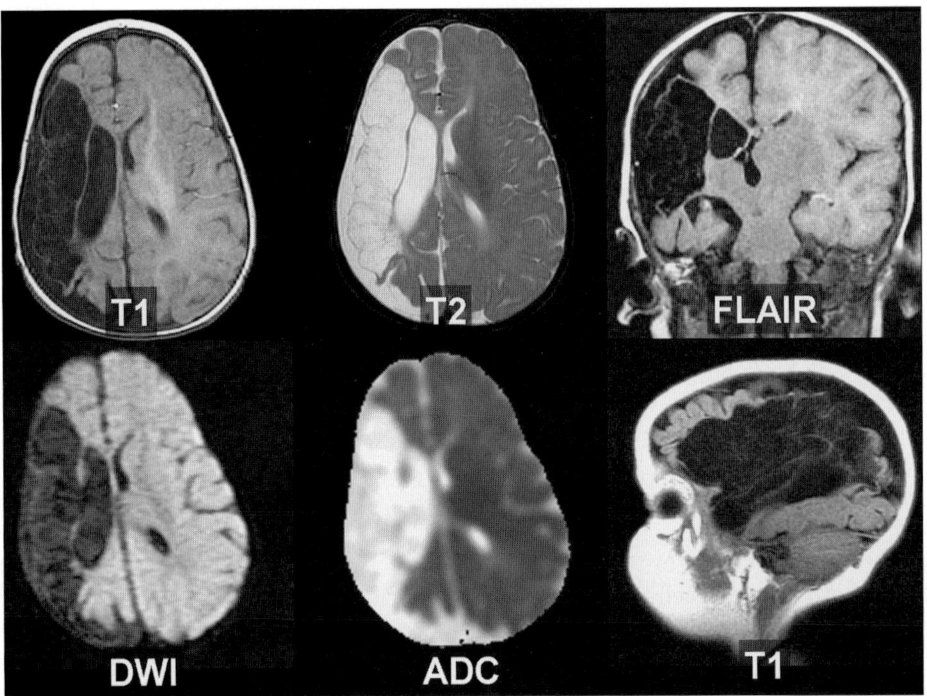

FIGURE 4.7. Chronic Infarction. Cystic encephalomalacia is present in the right middle cerebral artery territory on a MR of a 7-month-old with neonatal infarction. Note cystic changes approaching CSF on all sequences, including diffusion-weighted (DWI) and apparent diffusion coefficient (ADC), with minimal gliosis. There is volume loss with widening of the ipsilateral ventricle (ex vacuo dilatation).

vascular autoregulation, and anticoagulation or use of thrombolytics may all contribute to the development of these hemorrhages. Patients may develop headaches at the time of bleeding but commonly have no new symptoms, presumably because the hemorrhage occurs within brain areas that are already dead or dysfunctional. Hemorrhagic infarction is confined to the territory of the infarcted vessel, whereas primary hemorrhage does not necessarily respect vascular boundaries. Intraventricular extension is uncommonly seen with hemorrhagic transformation and should raise the possibility of another process (such as hypertensive bleed or a ruptured arteriovenous malformation [AVM]).

The peak time for hemorrhagic transformation is at about 1 to 2 weeks postinfarction. It is usually manifested as a serpiginous line of petechial blood following the gyral contours of the infarcted cortex. These dots of hemorrhage are often patchy and discontinuous. On CT a faint line of high attenuation is observed, and on MR bright signal is seen along the affected gyrus on the unenhanced T1WI because of methemoglobin (Fig. 4.8.A). (Alternate explanations for this bright signal have been offered,

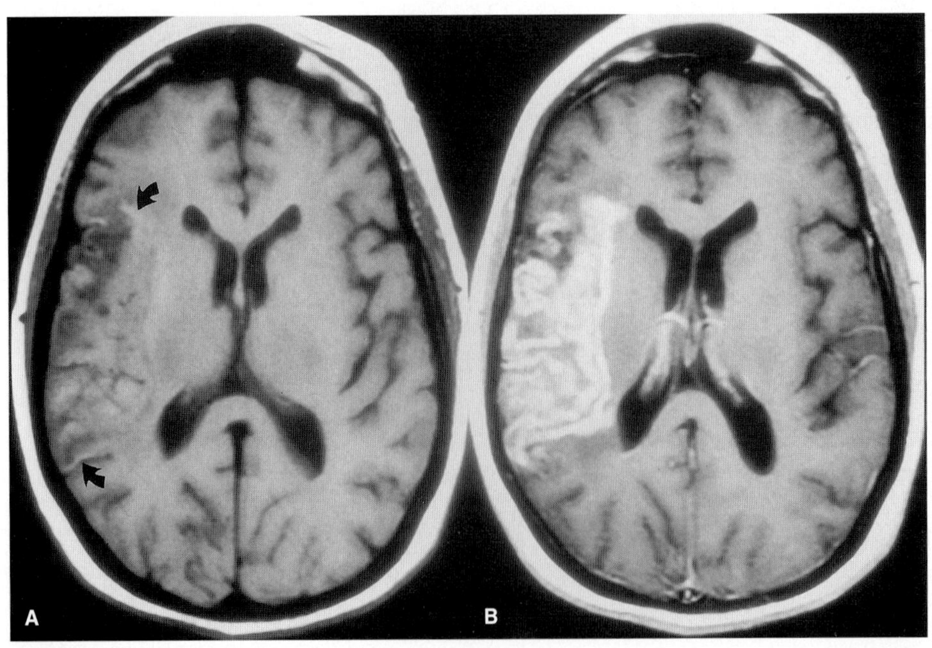

FIGURE 4.8. Petechial Hemorrhage and Gyral Enhancement in Subacute Infarction. A. Precontrast T1WI shows mild effacement of sulci in the right middle cerebral artery territory. A few subtle areas of bright signal intensity scattered along the cortex indicate areas of petechial hemorrhage or laminar necrosis (*arrows*). **B.** Postcontrast T1WI demonstrates marked gyral enhancement, a hallmark of subacute infarction.

including laminar necrosis or calcification related to infarction; the practical point is to recognize this appearance as a feature of ischemia.) The petechial gyral pattern is not seen in primary brain hemorrhage and can be helpful in confirming the underlying ischemic etiology of a suspicious lesion. This is considered a normal part of the evolution of an infarct. Management in the presence of petechial hemorrhage is controversial, but many neurologists continue anticoagulation if there is a well-documented embolic source.

More extensive hemorrhagic transformation of the infarcted tissue may lead to the formation of a gross parenchymal hematoma. Here, the blood does not conform to a gyrus and may form a clot that is indistinguishable from a primary hematoma. Large cortical infarcts are at somewhat higher risk for this type of change, compared with limited cortical or subcortical lesions. Catastrophic hemorrhagic transformation can also follow thrombolysis, particularly when treatment is delayed or the baseline CT shows extensive edema. In contrast to the petechial gyral transformation described above, gross parenchymal hematomas tend to occur earlier and are more commonly associated with clinical deterioration. Confluent hematomas seen on infarct follow-up studies should be reported promptly since anticoagulation therapy is contraindicated, even when the finding is incidental.

Use of Contrast in Ischemic Stroke

CT Contrast. *A noncontrast CT remains the radiologic exam of choice for emergency assessment of suspected acute stroke.* An unenhanced study is necessary to help triage the patient. It serves to rule out hemorrhage, may define patterns and extent of ischemic injury, shows areas of abnormal vascular calcification (e.g., giant aneurysms), and excludes mass lesions. This is important first-line information needed by the clinician faced with determining the need for lumbar puncture, vascular surgery, anticoagulation, thrombolysis, cardiac evaluation, or other therapies. However, all acute stroke CTs should be reviewed on a scanning console or a picture archiving and communication system, because the unenhanced study may rarely show the need for intravenous contrast. A nonstroke lesion such as a tumor, abscess, or an isodense subdural hematoma might be suspected on the noncontrast exam and then be shown to better advantage with contrast.

Older studies had suggested that contrast is contraindicated in brain infarction. They cited a slightly increased risk of seizures and other untoward CNS effects, presumably caused by a toxic effect of the contrast as it leaks through the abnormal blood-brain barrier. Most of these data, however, were based on studies that used ionic contrast media. Recent CT protocols have safely used contrast, not only to exclude tumor or infection but also to evaluate vessels (CT angiography) and blood delivery (CT perfusion).

An intact blood-brain barrier normally excludes contrast from the brain. Leakage of macromolecular contrast agents through damaged vessels leads to local accumulation of iodine, seen as high attenuation (enhancement) of infarcted parenchyma. Breakdown of the blood-brain barrier underlies both hemorrhagic transformation and contrast enhancement of infarctions. Not surprisingly, then, these processes are seen at roughly the same time and often in combination. As with petechial gyral hemorrhage, a gyral pattern of enhancement (by CT or MR) is highly specific evidence of an underlying infarction. CT-detected enhancement of infarcted brain parenchyma typically begins at about 1 week, peaks at 7 to 14 days, often assumes a gyral pattern, and is less commonly observed in subcortical regions (Fig. 4.8.B). Enhancement is seen in about half of patients during the 1st week and in about two thirds of patients between weeks 1 and 4. As gliosis ensues and the blood-brain barrier is repaired, enhancement fades and then resolves by 3 months.

MR Contrast. Most of the comments regarding the strategy, pathophysiology, and enhancement patterns for CT also generally hold true for contrast in MR. Intravenous gadolinium contrast agents are very well tolerated by stroke patients and may give valuable information not readily available from the noncontrast MR. Stasis of gadolinium within vessels or leakage of contrast through an abnormal blood-brain barrier will shorten T1 relaxation of adjacent protons, leading to hyperintensity (enhancement) on T1WIs. As with CT, a noncontrast MR sequence is mandatory before contrast is given, since enhancement and subacute blood both appear hyperintense on T1WIs. (This will be discussed in the "Hemorrhage" section.) An intravenous bolus of contrast may also be captured dynamically using rapid imaging techniques to produce a family of perfusion-weighted images to help identify ischemic regions.

Intravascular enhancement on MR is commonly seen in the infarcted territory during the first week. This may be caused by slow flow or vasodilatation leading to stasis of gadolinium, likely in both arteries and veins. The intravascular enhancement pattern may be detected within minutes of vessel occlusion, is seen in a majority of cortical infarcts at 1 to 3 days, and resolves by 10 days. The proximal trunks of more distally occluded arteries and leptomeningeal cortical channels are most prominently involved (Fig. 4.9). The area of vascular enhancement may extend beyond the T2 hyperintensity, possibly indicating recruitment of collateral supply at the ischemic border. Meningeal enhancement, which attends meningitis, and dural enhancement seen postoperatively can superficially resemble intravascular enhancement, but the distinction should be obvious on clinical grounds. MR intravascular enhancement helps identify early strokes, indicates ongoing slow flow, and has no obvious CT counterpart.

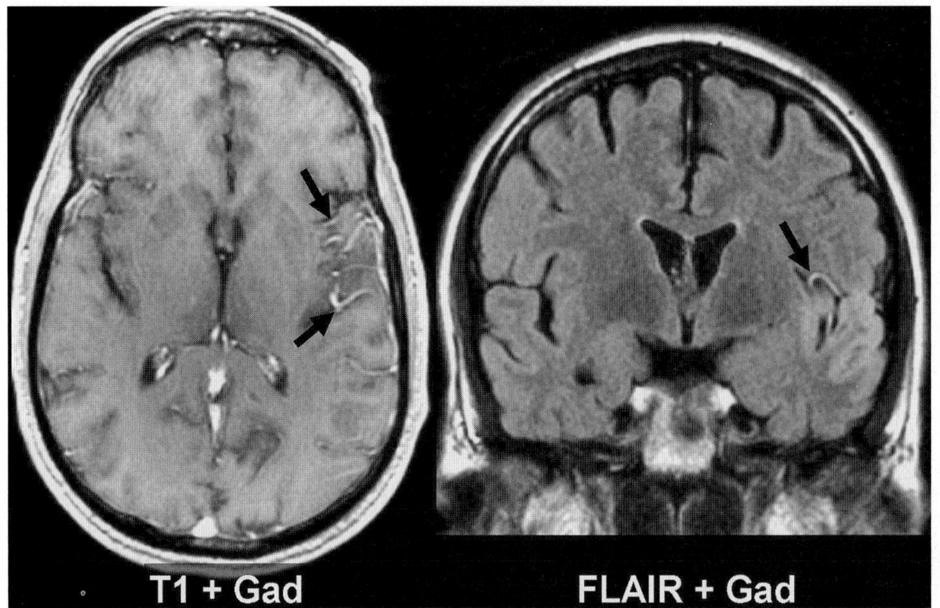

FIGURE 4.9. **Intravascular Stasis and Enhancement in Acute Infarction.** Postcontrast T1 and fluid-attenuated inversion-recovery (FLAIR) images in acute left middle cerebral artery (MCA) infarction. Mild sulcal effacement and prominent enhancement of sylvian branches of the MCA (*arrows*) are evident on T1. As seen here, FLAIR can show similar vascular signs of stasis, either before or after contrast. Intravascular enhancement is typically seen only during the first 10 days after stroke.

MR parenchymal enhancement occurs in a similar pattern to that seen on CT (and with the same time course seen by nuclear medicine infarct scans of the past). It may occur as early as day 1, but more typically begins after the first week, a time when intravascular enhancement is waning (Fig. 4.10). Reperfusion after thrombolysis can lead to early enhancement. Virtually all cortical infarcts enhance on MR at 2 weeks. Elster has summarized this in his "Rule of Threes": MR parenchymal enhancement peaks at 3 days to 3 weeks and resolves by 3 months.

The imaging time courses for CT and MR examinations in brain infarction are summarized in Table 4.2.

Pattern Recognition in Ischemic Stroke

Familiarity with the major vascular territories can help distinguish between infarction and other pathologic processes. The clinical time course and localization should be consistent with the imaging findings, and all should correspond to a known vascular distribution. Stroke localization is not necessarily synonymous with "focal." An ischemic event may cause a pattern of damage that is diffuse (hypoxic-ischemic injury); multifocal (vasculitis, emboli); or focal (single embolism or thrombus). The vessels causing stroke may be large or small, and they may be on either the arterial or venous side. There is no such thing as a "funny" stroke; if it doesn't fit a vascular territory, then the differential diagnosis changes (Fig. 4.11).

The relation of vascular anatomy to functional neuroanatomy is at the heart of clinical/radiologic correlation in stroke. Classically, strokes and TIAs are divided into anterior (carotid territory) or posterior (vertebrobasilar territory) events. Patients with anterior circulation ischemia have been shown to benefit from carotid endarterectomy when the carotid is narrowed by at least 70% compared to its normal diameter. Surgery has not been proven beneficial for patients with lesser degrees of carotid stenosis or for those with posterior territory TIAs, who therefore usually receive medical therapy (e.g., anticoagulation). Ischemia in the carotid territory may cause visual changes,

TABLE 4.2 Imaging Time Course After Brain Infarction

Time	*CT*	*MR*
Minutes	No changes	Absent flow void Arterial enhancement (days 1–10) DWI: high signal
2–6 hours	Hyperdense artery sign Insular ribbon sign	Brain swelling (T1) Subtle T2 hyperintensity
6–12 hours	Sulcal effacement ± Decreased attenuation	T2 hyperintensity
12–24 hours	Decreased attenuation	T1 hypointensity
3–7 days	Maximal swelling	Maximal swelling
3–21 days	Gyral enhancement (peak: 7–14 days)	Gyral enhancement (peak: 3–21 days) Petechial methemoglobin
30–90 days	Encephalomalacia Loss of enhancement Resolution of petechial blood	Encephalomalacia Loss of enhancement Resolution of petechial blood

DWI, diffusion-weighted imaging.

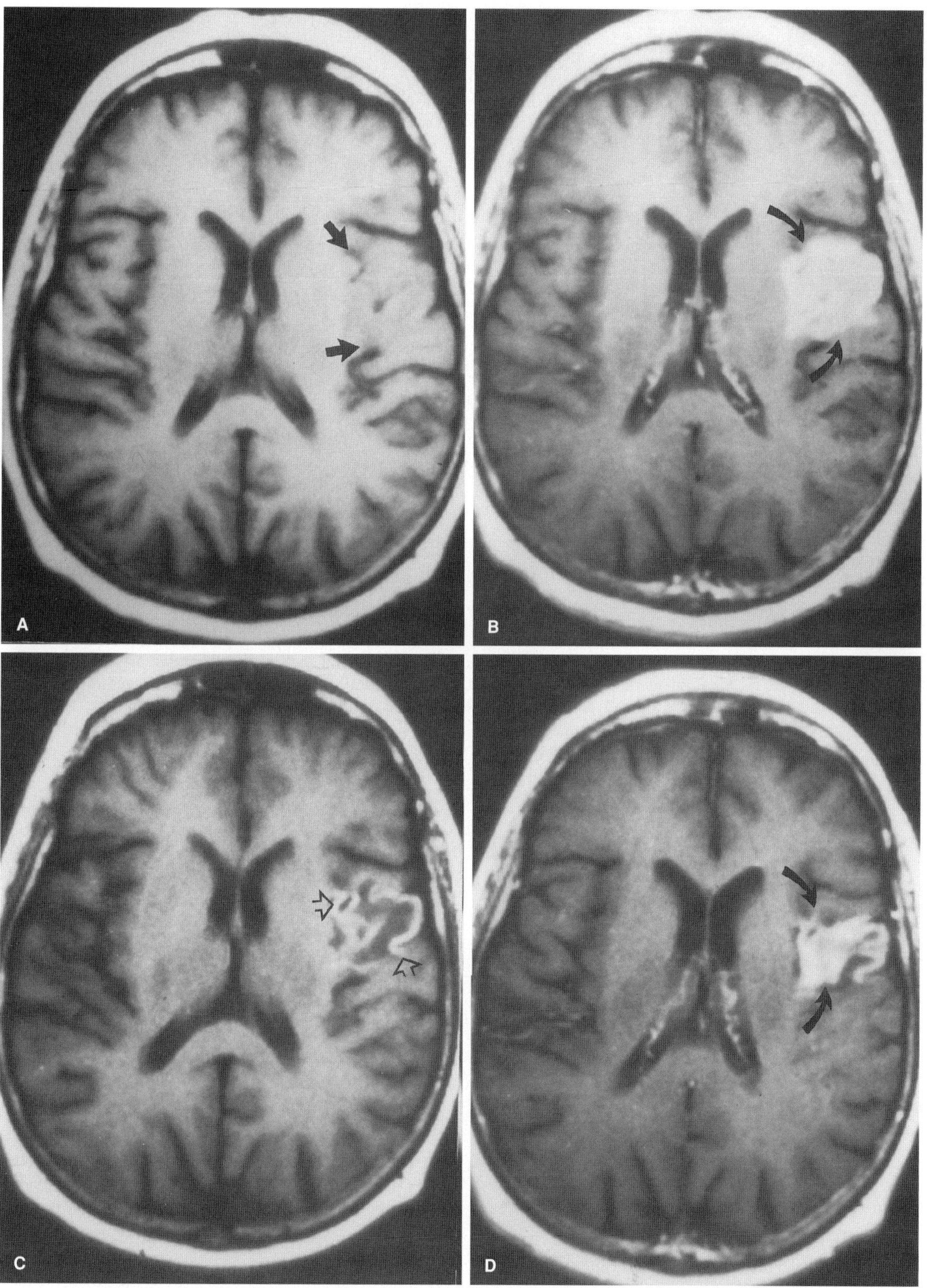

FIGURE 4.10. **Evolution of Petechial Hemorrhage and Parenchymal Enhancement.** Precontrast and postcontrast T1WIs in left sylvian cortical infarction. The acute studies **(A** and **B)** show nonhemorrhagic swelling (*straight arrows*) with prominent cortical enhancement (**B,** *curved arrows*). At the 2-month follow-up **(C** and **D)** petechial hemorrhage (*open arrows*) and decreasing parenchymal enhancement (**D,** *curved arrows*) are seen. Parenchymal enhancement resolved by 3 months.

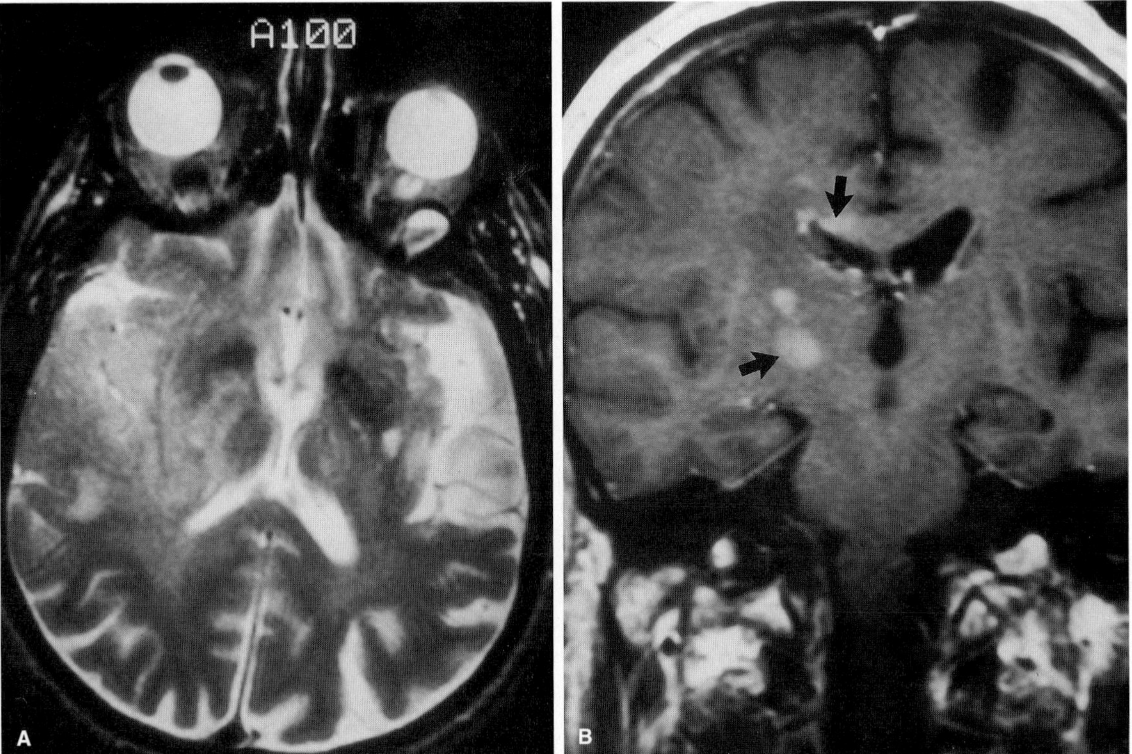

FIGURE 4.11. **Glioblastoma Mimicking a Stroke. A.** T2W axial section shows edema primarily in the right middle cerebral artery territory, but with additional involvement of the medial temporal lobe, thalamus, and periatrial regions. **B.** Postcontrast coronal T1WI shows patchy, nodular areas of enhancement in the basal ganglia and periventricular regions (*arrows*). Even with a strong clinical history for strokelike onset, the nonvascular distribution and atypical enhancement pattern effectively exclude underlying infarction. When in doubt, follow-up imaging studies will usually clarify the diagnosis.

aphasia, or sensorimotor deficits caused by retinal, cortical, or subcortical damage. Vertebrobasilar strokes are more likely to cause syncope, ataxia, cranial nerve findings, homonymous visual field deficits, and facial symptoms opposite those of the body. A given deficit can be predicted from the known functional topography of the cortex and its connections through the internal capsule (Fig. 4.12).

The patterns of injury observed after occlusion of large arteries in the anterior and posterior circulations, small arteries in any region, and of the dural venous channels are reviewed in turn.

Anterior (Carotid) Circulation

Internal Carotid Artery (ICA). Thromboembolic disease in the ICA may cause TIAs or infarction in its MCA or anterior cerebral artery (ACA) branches or in the watershed zone between them. Embolic occlusion of the ophthalmic branch of the ICA may cause transient monocular blindness (amaurosis fugax). Observation of any of these patterns should prompt imaging of the carotid arteries. The extent and distribution of ischemia observed depend on the time course of occlusion, degree of oligemia, and available collateral supply. Complete carotid occlusions are occasionally found in asymptomatic patients with a well-developed collateral supply.

Atherosclerotic disease near the carotid bifurcation is responsible for the majority of ischemic events in the ICA territory. Arterial dissection, trauma, fibromuscular dysplasia, tumor encasement, prior neck radiotherapy, and connective tissue diseases may also cause significant carotid narrowing (Fig. 4.13). Hemodynamic effects begin to be seen when there is $>80\%$ reduction in area or $>60\%$ decrease in diameter. Lesions causing less severe narrowing may nonetheless become symptomatic when they serve as a nidus for thrombus formation or are unmasked by hypotension. Studies have shown a clear benefit of endarterectomy in symptomatic patients with $>70\%$ stenosis but not for those with $<30\%$ narrowing. In many centers, carotid stents are now used in place of surgery, especially for high-risk patients.

Noninvasive screening of the carotid arteries may be achieved with either US, MR angiography (MRA), or CT angiography (CTA). The choice of modality depends on the abilities of the available personnel and equipment.

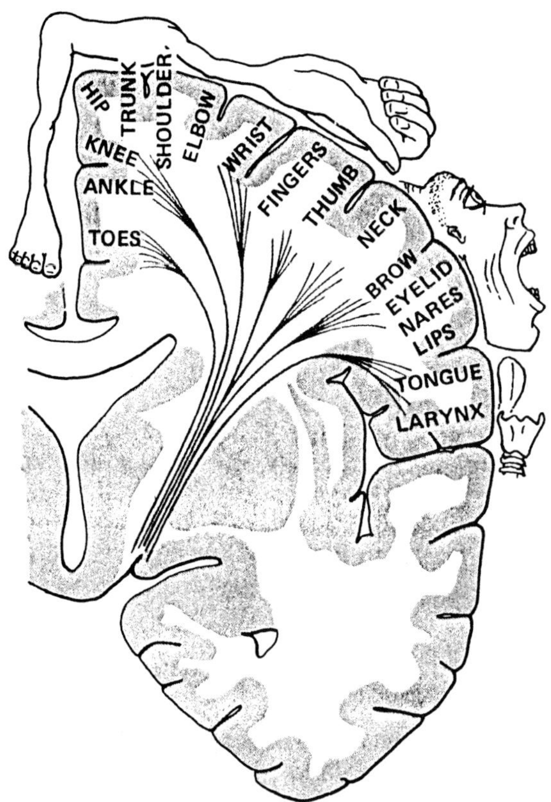

FIGURE 4.12. **Homunculus.** A coronal section through the precentral (motor) cortex depicts the topographic representation of the opposite side of the body. The face and hand areas are served by the middle cerebral artery territory, the leg by the anterior cerebral artery. (From Gilman S, Winans SS. Manter & Gatz's Essentials of Clinical Neuroanatomy & Neurophysiology. 6th ed. Philadelphia: Davis, 1982; used with permission.)

Sensitivity and specificity are as high as 85% to 90% for each of these techniques. These methods noninvasively identify patients with hemodynamically significant disease who might then be referred for conventional angiography or directly to intervention. US is the most commonly employed screening exam in most centers. It has the advantage of portability and generally lower costs, and it can be performed in patients with contraindications to MR/MRA. US is more operator-dependent than MRA and is unable to reliably assess portions of the distal ICA near the skull base. CTA provides excellent visualization from the arch to the intracranial circulation, but at the small risk of contrast toxicity and radiation exposure. MRA can evaluate the entire course of the carotid and may be quickly performed in conjunction with the patient's brain MR study. It is a particularly good method for screening pediatric or elderly patients in whom conventional angiography may be technically more difficult.

Selective common carotid angiography remains the gold standard for preprocedure carotid artery evaluation but is being replaced by noninvasive studies in many centers. The study should cover the entire ICA, including the cervical and cranial portions. Evaluation of the surgically inaccessible cranial segments (petrous, cavernous, and supraclinoid) is necessary to exclude high-grade intracranial stenoses or "tandem" lesions that might contraindicate endarterectomy.

Anterior Cerebral Artery. The terminal bifurcation of the ICA is into the ACA and MCA (Fig. 4.14). The ACA is divided into three subgroups: *medial lenticulostriate* branches serve the rostral portions of the basal ganglia, *pericallosal* branches supply the corpus callosum, and *hemispheric* branches serve the medial aspects of the frontal and parietal lobes (Fig. 4.15). About 5% of infarcts involve the ACA.

The medial lenticulostriate branches penetrate the anterior perforating substance to give variable supply to the anteroinferior aspect of the internal capsule, putamen, globus pallidus, caudate head, and portions of the hypothalamus and optic chiasm. The largest of these vessels supplies the caudate head/anterior internal capsule region and is recognized as the recurrent artery of Heubner. Infarction in the medial lenticulostriate territory may cause problems with speech production (motor aphasia), facial weakness, and disturbances in mood and judgment.

Above the takeoff of the lenticulostriate branches, the ACAs are interconnected by the anterior communicating artery. Each ACA ascends further, giving off branches to the frontal pole (orbitofrontal and frontopolar arteries).The ACAs terminate as a bifurcation into the (lower) pericallosal and (upper) callosomarginal branches. These arteries run parallel to the corpus callosum from front to back, supplying the medial cortex of the frontal and parietal lobes. As its name would imply, the pericallosal artery courses around and feeds the corpus callosum. ACA branching patterns are quite variable from one patient to the next, with about 10% having only one pericallosal branch that supplies both hemispheres—an "azygos" ACA (Fig. 4.16).

Unilateral damage in the ACA hemispheric branches will cause preferential leg weakness on the opposite side of the body (Table 4.3). Bilateral ACA infarctions lead to incontinence and an awake but apathetic state known as akinetic mutism. Infarction of the corpus callosum can cause a variety of interhemispheric disconnection syndromes.

Middle Cerebral Artery. The MCA supplies more brain tissue than any other intracranial vessel and is host to almost two thirds of infarcts. Its offspring are the *lateral lenticulostriate branches,* which supply most of the basal ganglia region, and the *hemispheric branches,* which serve the lateral cerebral surface (Figs. 4.4, 4.17).

The lateral lenticulostriate branches arise from the proximal MCA as numerous small perforating end arteries distributed to the putamen, lateral globus pallidus, superior half of the internal capsule and adjacent corona radiata, and majority of the caudate. Isolated vascular lesions of the globus pallidus or putamen are commonly

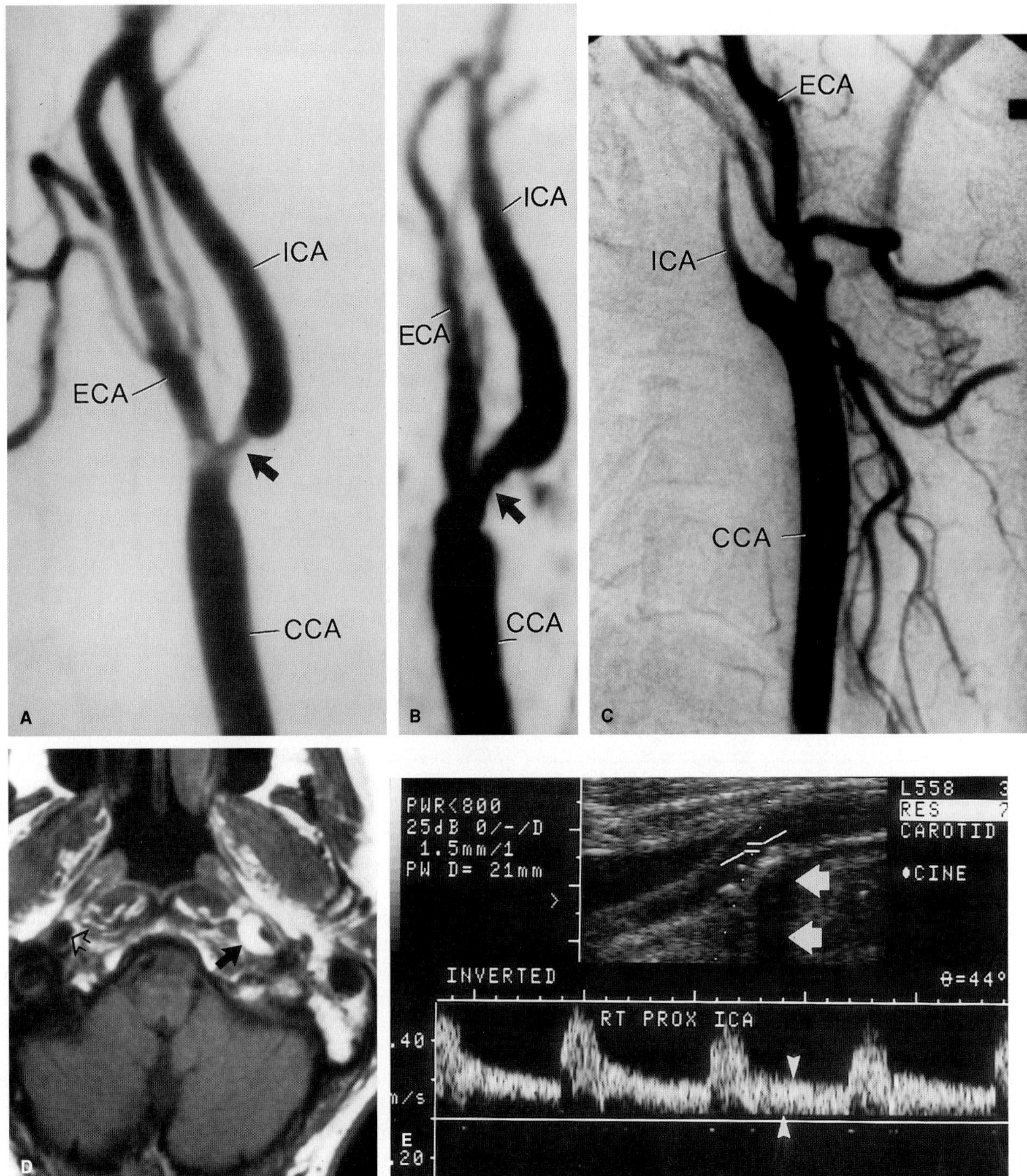

FIGURE 4.13. **Carotid Disease. A.** Atherosclerosis. Lateral view of the carotid bifurcation by conventional digital subtraction angiography. The diameter of the proximal internal carotid artery (ICA) (*arrow*) is reduced approximately 60% compared with its normal caliber above. CCA, common carotid artery; ECA, external carotid artery and its branches. **B.** Atherosclerosis. Lateral maximum intensity projection from a two-dimensional time-of-flight MR angiogram in the same patient shows a very similar pattern of flow-related enhancement. **C.** Carotid dissection with a tapering occlusion in the ICA just above the bifurcation. **D.** T1WI of carotid dissection in another patient shows the "mural crescent sign" indicative of intramural thrombus in the petrous portion of the left ICA (*arrow*). Note the normal caliber flow void and scant amounts of fat surrounding the normal right ICA (*open arrow*). **E.** Carotid US shows calcified plaque with acoustic shadowing (*arrows*), vessel narrowing, and spectral broadening (*between arrowheads*) in a case of atherosclerosis. **F.** and **G.** CTA of carotid dissection with pseudoaneurysm. Source images **(F)** show a flap (*White arrows*) between the narrowed native lumen and the medially-situated pseudoaneurysm. Thick-slab two-dimensional reconstructions **(G)** show a normal carotid bifurcation and distal cervical "wind-sock" pseudoaneurysm (*black arrow*).

(*Continued*)

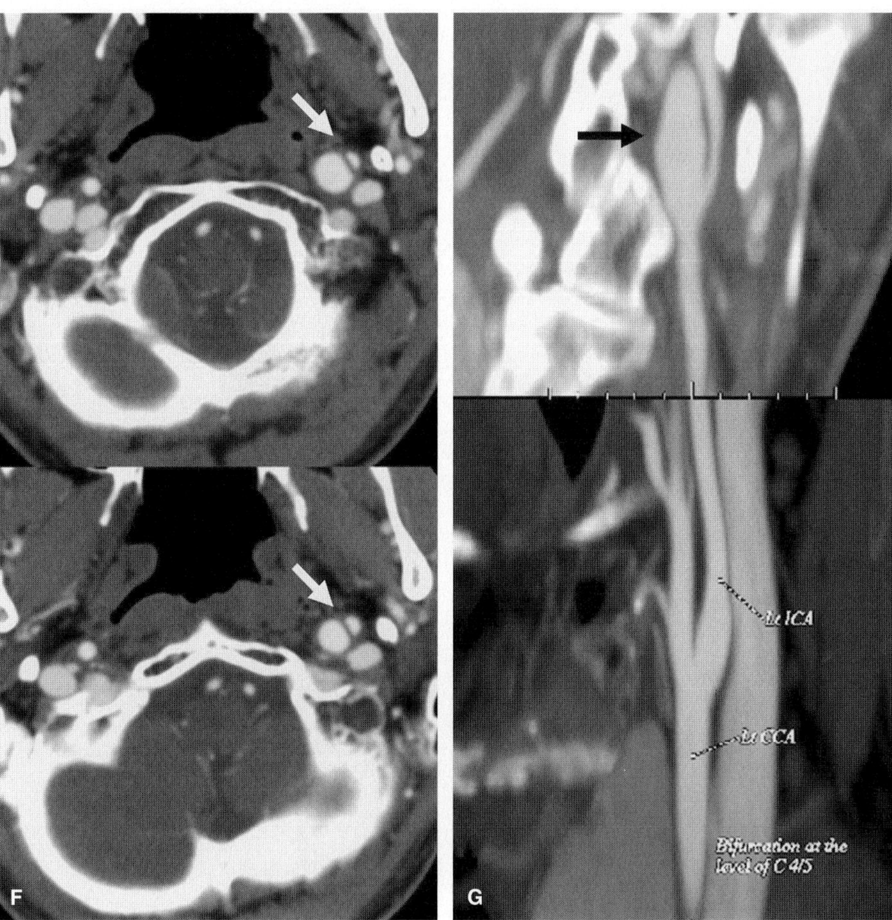

FIGURE 4.13. *(Continued)*

asymptomatic or may affect contralateral muscle tone and motor control. Lesions of the internal capsule or corona radiata may cause pure or mixed sensory and motor deficits on the opposite side of the body. Interruption of visual connections to the lateral geniculate nucleus results in a subtle type of contralateral homonymous hemianopsia. Rarely, the arcuate fasciculus pathway from the Wernicke to the Broca speech areas may be selectively infarcted, leading to a conduction aphasia (inability to repeat or read aloud, despite preserved comprehension and fluency).

The MCA loops laterally through the insula, where it bifurcates or trifurcates into its major cortical branches (Fig. 4.14A). The insula itself is supplied by hemispheric branches, not by the lateral lenticulostriate branches. When the proximal MCA is occluded, this insular region is furthest from any potential collateral supply, probably explaining the early appearance of the edema that gives rise to the "insular ribbon sign" (Fig. 4.3). The anterior hemispheric branches of the MCA supply the anterolateral tip of the temporal lobe (anterior temporal artery), the frontal lobe (operculofrontal arteries), and the motor and sensory strips (central sulcus arteries). Posterior hemispheric branches of the MCA supply the parietal lobe behind the sensory strip (posterior parietal artery), the posterolateral parietal and lateral occipital lobes (angular artery), and the majority of the temporal lobe (posterior temporal artery).

Occlusion of the rostral MCA branches of the dominant hemisphere will cause a motor (Broca) aphasia in which comprehension remains intact. Posterior branches in the dominant hemisphere supply the Wernicke area and cause a receptive aphasia when occluded. Posterior temporal branch occlusion may interrupt visual radiations, causing contralateral homonymous field defects. Involvement of either hemisphere's precentral gyrus (motor strip) will produce contralateral weakness that affects the face and arm more than the leg (Fig. 4.12). Contralateral cortical sensory loss occurs when the primary or association sensory cortex behind the central sulcus is affected. In the nondominant right hemisphere, posterior MCA infarcts commonly cause bizarre impairment in visuospatial abilities and sometimes neglect (or nonrecognition) of the left body. Complete occlusion of the MCA beyond the lenticulostriate branches causes a combination of these deficits: contralateral face and arm hemiparesis, field defect, and either neglect or global aphasia, depending on which hemisphere is affected. Leg weakness may also be seen when the MCA

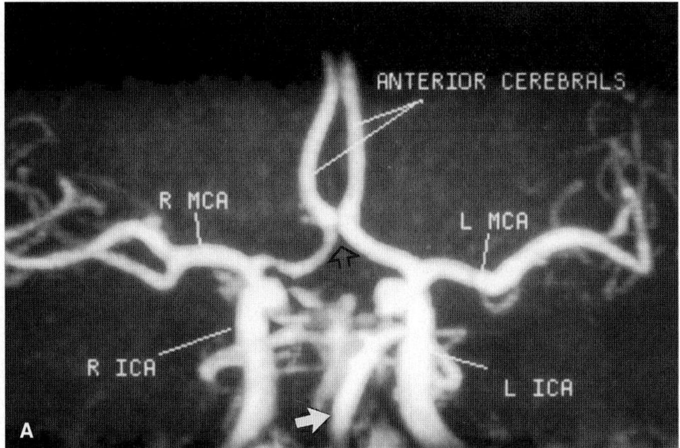

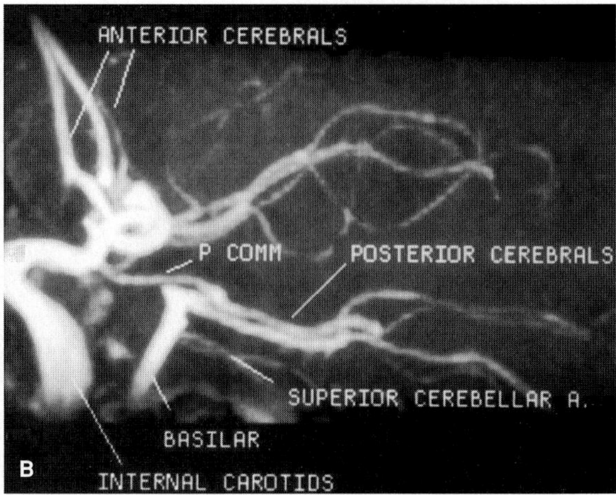

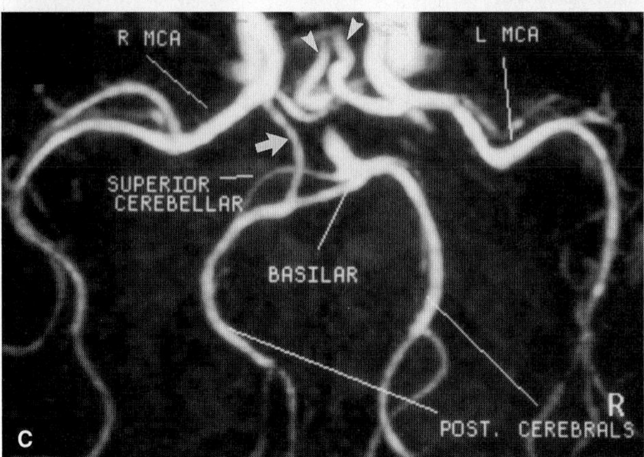

FIGURE 4.14. **MR Angiography of the Normal Circle of Willis and Its Branches. A.** The anterior (coronal) projection depicts the normal internal carotid arteries (ICA) with bifurcation into the anterior cerebral artery and middle cerebral artery intracranial branches. The basilar artery and cerebellar branches project below (*arrow*). The anterior communicating artery is very short in this patient (*open arrow*). **B.** Lateral projection shows a single large posterior communicating artery (P COMM) connecting the anterior to posterior circulations. The superior cerebellar and posterior cerebral branches of the basilar artery are clearly shown. **C.** Submentovertex projection outlines the relationship of the major vessels to the circle of Willis. We are looking "down the barrel" of the ICAs and basilar artery. A single posterior communicating artery is again seen (*arrow*); the opposite side is likely hypoplastic. The anterior cerebrals project between the ICAs (*arrowheads*).

stem is occluded, because of internal capsule involvement. These relationships are summarized in Table 4.3.

Posterior (Vertebrobasilar) Circulation

Vertebral Arteries. The vertebral arteries usually originate from the subclavian arteries, ascend straight upward in the transverse foramina of C6–C3, turn sharply through the C2–C1 foramen magnum levels, and unite anterior to the low medulla to form the basilar artery (Fig. 4.18). Atherosclerotic narrowing commonly affects the vertebral arteries at their origins and may affect the basilar artery over variable lengths. Narrowing of the cervical portion of the vertebrals may be caused by compressive uncovertebral osteophytes. Rapid head turning (e.g., motor vehicle accidents) may stretch the vertebral arteries at the C1–C2 level, leading to arterial dissection. Any of these conditions may cause vertebrobasilar ischemia via thrombotic or embolic mechanisms. Anticoagulation and antiplatelet agents remain the mainstay of treatment for vertebrobasilar ischemia. Angioplasty and stenting are sometimes feasible for correction of atherosclerotic lesions but are usually reserved for severe medically refractory cases.

Basilar Artery. The basilar artery is formed by the union of the two vertebral arteries. As it ascends between the clivus and the brainstem, it sends large branches to the cerebellum and smaller perforating vessels to the brainstem. The basilar ends at its bifurcation into the posterior cerebral arteries, just above the tentorium cerebelli. Occlusion of the basilar artery itself is usually

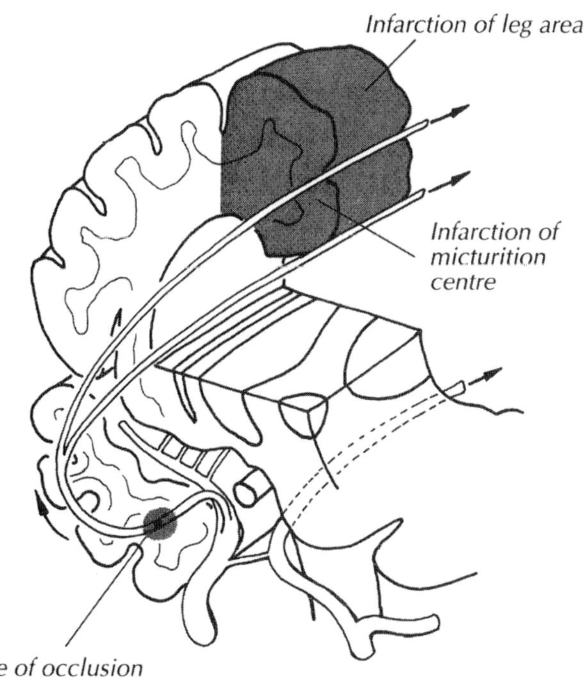

FIGURE 4.15. **Anterior Cerebral Artery (ACA) Occlusion.** An ACA occlusion causes infarction of the paramedian frontal cortex responsible for motor and sensory function of the opposite leg (*stippled area*). If the occlusion is bilateral, incontinence and akinetic mutism may also be seen. (From Patten J. Neurological Differential Diagnosis. New York: Springer, 1996; used with permission.)

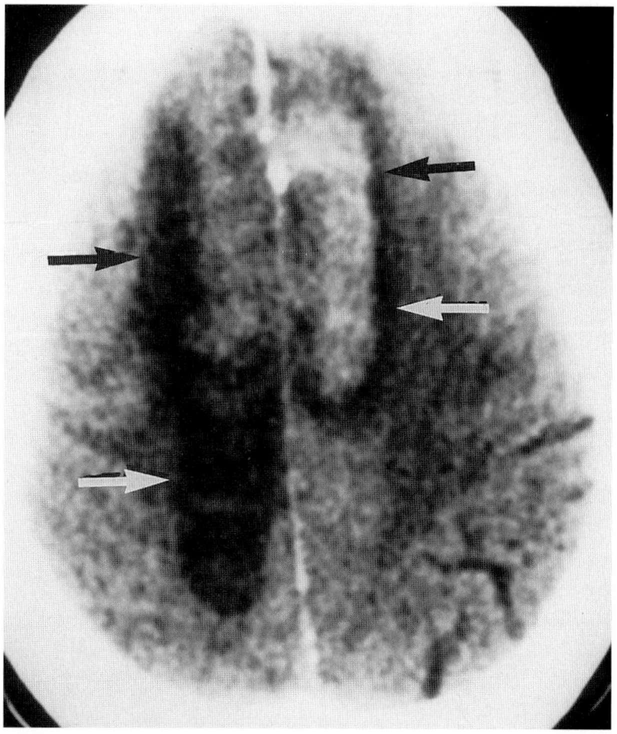

FIGURE 4.16. **Hemorrhagic Infarction.** Hemorrhagic infarction in a bilateral anterior cerebral artery (ACA) distribution (*arrows*) shown by noncontrast CT. This was an embolic stroke, presumably occluding an azygos ACA.

rapidly fatal, owing to infarction of respiratory and cardiac centers in the medulla. Occlusion of the perforating end arteries from the basilar artery causes focal brainstem infarction, which is usually manifested as cranial nerve dysfunction, ataxia, somnolence, and crossed motor or sensory deficits. These lesions characteristically respect the midline of the brainstem and often extend to the ventral surface (Fig. 4.19). Metabolic disturbances (e.g., central pontine myelinolysis) and hypertensive hemorrhages (most commonly in the pons) tend to be more centrally or diffusely located. Large or multiple lesions in the pons can cause a nightmarish syndrome of quadriparesis with intact cognition—the "locked in" state.

Posterior Cerebral Artery (PCA). The basilar artery ends at its bifurcation into the PCAs at the midbrain level, just above the tentorial hiatus. The major branches of the PCA include the midbrain and thalamic *perforating vessels*, the *posterior choroidal arteries*, and the *cortical branches* to the medial temporal and occipital lobes (Fig. 4.20). Ten percent to 15% of infarcts occur in the PCA territory.

The proximal segments of the PCAs sweep posterolaterally around the midbrain, giving off small perforating branches to the mesencephalon and thalamus along the way. Midbrain infarction causes loss of the pupillary light responses, impaired upgaze, and somnolence, caused by damage of the quadrigeminal plate, third cranial nerve nuclei, and reticular activating formation, respectively. Proximal PCA perforators also supply the majority of the thalamus and sometimes portions of the posterior limb of the internal capsule. Thalamic infarction may cause a variety of disturbances, but contralateral sensory loss is the most common problem.

The posterior choroidal arteries arise from the proximal PCA to supply the choroid plexus of the third and lateral ventricles, pineal gland, and regions contiguous with the third ventricle. Isolated posterior choroid infarctions are rare because of their rich collateral supply through the choroid plexus. PCA cortical branches supply the inferomedial temporal lobe (inferior temporal arteries), superior occipital gyrus (parieto-occipital artery), and visual cortex of the occipital lobes (calcarine artery) (Fig. 4.21). Hemispheric PCA occlusions are usually caused by an embolic source. Inferomedial temporal infarction may cause memory deficits, which are severe when bilateral. Loss of the primary visual cortex causes complete loss of vision in the opposite visual field (homonymous hemianopsia).

In about 20% of patients, one or both of the proximal PCA segments may be hypoplastic or absent. In these cases, flow is derived from the ICA system via a prominent

TABLE 4.3 Functional Vascular Anatomy*

Vessel	Branch	Side	Deficit/Syndrome
ACA	Hemispheric	Either	Leg weakness
		Both	Incontinence, akinetic mutism
	Medial lenticulostriates	Either	Facial weakness
		Left	Dysarthria ± motor aphasia
MCA	Hemispheric	Either	Face and arm >leg weakness
		Left	Motor aphasia (anterior lesion)
			Receptive aphasia (posterior lesion)
			Global aphasia (total MCA)
			Neglect syndromes
		Right	Visulospatial dysfunction
	Lateral lenticulostriates	Either	Variable lacunar syndromes
PCA	Hemispheric	Either	Hemianopsia
		Both	Cortical blindness
			Memory deficits
	Thalamoperforators	Either	Somnolence
			Sensory disturbances
Cerebellar	PICA, AICA, or SCA	Either	Ataxia, vertigo, vomiting
			Coma if mass effect
			± brainstem deficits
Watershed	ACA/MCA/PCA	Either	Man-in-a-barrel syndrome
		Bilateral	Severe memory problems

*Assumes left hemisphere language dominance.
PICA, posterior inferior cerebellar artery; AICA, anterior inferior cerebellar artery; SCA, superior cerebellar artery; ACA, anterior cerebral artery; MCA, middle cerebral artery; PCA, posterior cerebral artery.

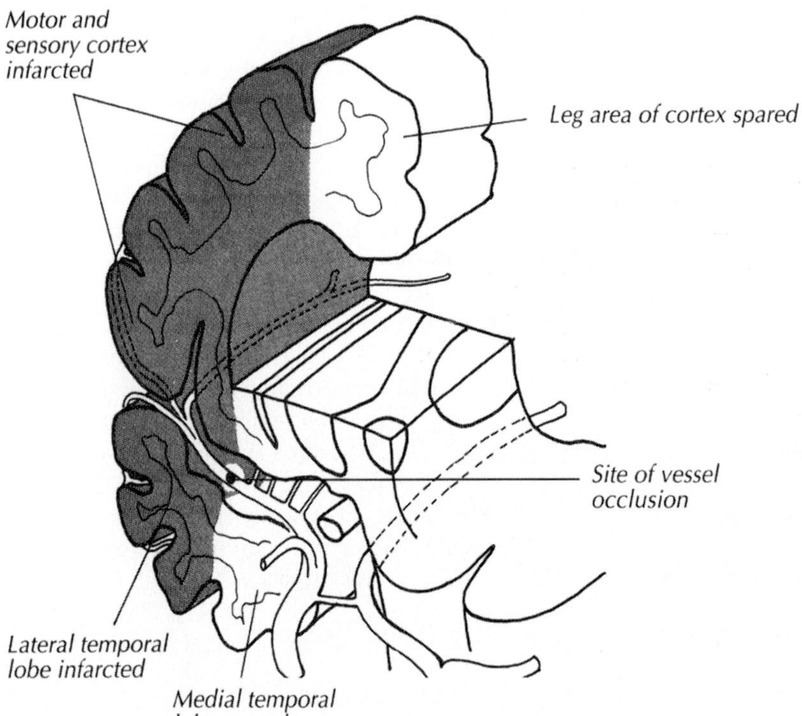

FIGURE 4.17. **Middle Cerebral Artery (MCA) Occlusion.** An MCA occlusion distal to the lateral lenticulostriate branches causes infarction of the motor and sensory cortex of the arm and face (*stippled area*). More proximal occlusion will also affect the internal capsule, potentially adding leg deficits. (From Patten J. Neurological Differential Diagnosis. New York: Springer, 1996; used with permission.)

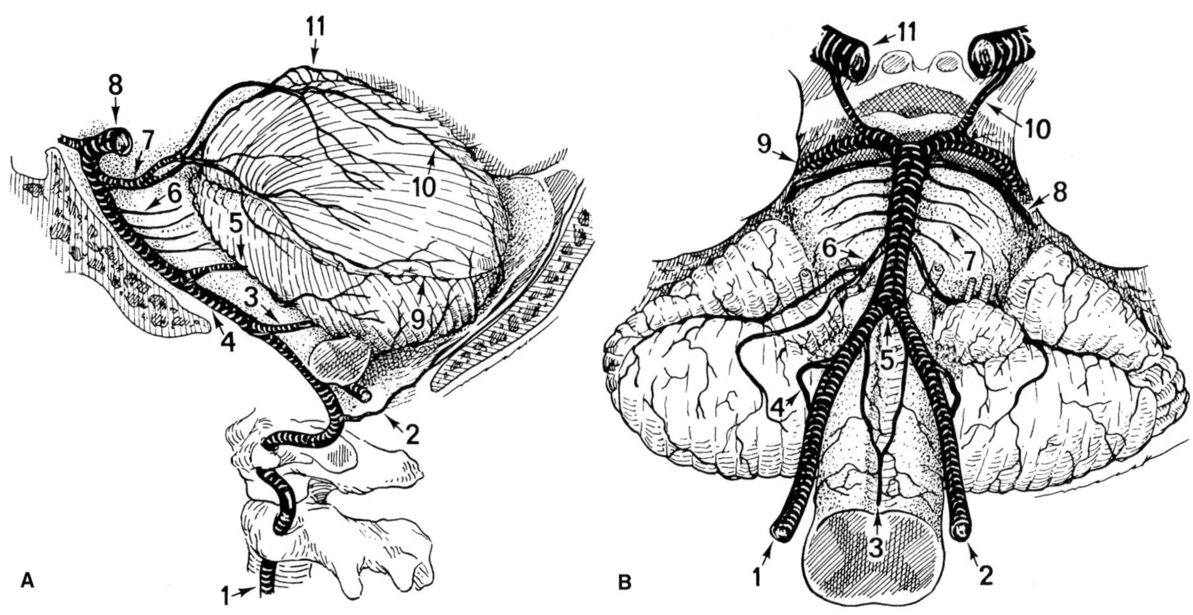

FIGURE 4.18. **Vertebrobasilar Arteries. A.** Lateral view. 1, left vertebral; 2, posterior meningeal; 3, posterior inferior cerebellar (PICA); 4, basilar; 5, anterior inferior cerebellar (AICA); 6, pontine perforators; 7, superior cerebellar (SCA); 8, posterior cerebral (PCA); 9, branches of the SCA and AICA in the horizontal fissure of the cerebellum; 10, SCA hemispheric branches; 11, superior vermian branches. **B.** Anterior view. 1, right vertebral; 2, left vertebral; 3, anterior spinal; 4, PICA; 5, basilar; 6, AICA; 7, pontine; 8, SCA; 9, PCA; 10, posterior communicating; 11, internal carotid artery. (From Osborn AG. Introduction to Cerebral Angiography. Philadelphia: Harper & Row, 1980; used with permission.)

posterior communicating artery. This is commonly referred to as "fetal origin" of the PCA, since embryologically the PCA develops with the ICA. Because this is a fairly common variation, both vertebral and carotid disease should be considered when evaluating PCA infarctions.

Cerebellar Arteries. Headache, vertigo, nausea, vomiting, and ipsilateral ataxia are the hallmarks of cerebellar stroke; 85% are ischemic and 15% are primary hemorrhages. Clinically, it is difficult to distinguish which cerebellar subterritory is involved and whether the stroke derives from infarction or hemorrhage. *Because of clinical urgency, acute evaluation of suspected cerebellar strokes should be performed by CT.* Cerebellar hemorrhages and any infarctions with significant mass effect are neurosurgical emergencies requiring posterior fossa decompression. Multiplanar MR is preferred for evaluation beyond the acute phase, since beam-hardening artifacts degrade posterior fossa images on CT.

Although deficits related to the cerebellar territories are hard to distinguish clinically, it is important to recognize characteristic distributions to elucidate stroke mechanisms. The correct order of cerebellar branches going from top to bottom can be remembered using the acronym *SAP*: the *s*uperior, *a*nterior inferior, and *p*osterior inferior cerebellar arteries (Fig. 4.18).

Superior Cerebellar Arteries (SCA). The upper parts of the cerebellum are supplied by the SCA. These arise from the distal basilar artery as the last large branches

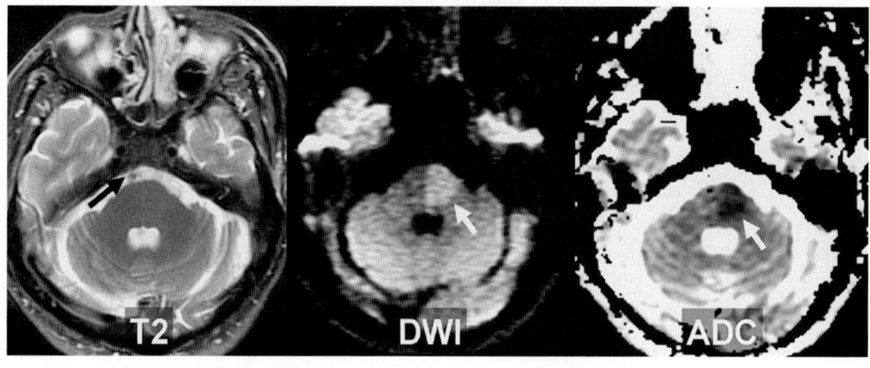

FIGURE 4.19. **Acute Brainstem Infarction.** Although T2 appears normal in the pons, the diffusion-weighted image (DWI) and the apparent diffusion coefficient (ADC) map show a left paramedian pontine infarct (*white arrows*), which respects the midline. Note lack of normal flow void in the basilar artery on T2 (*black arrow*) caused by focal atherosclerosis.

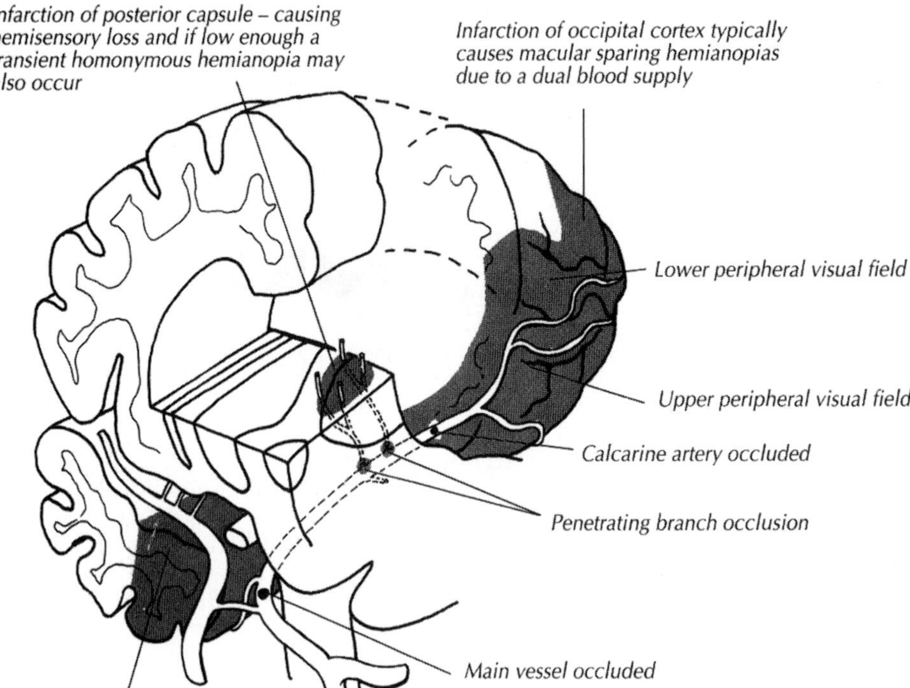

FIGURE 4.20. **Posterior Cerebral Artery (PCA) Occlusion.** A PCA occlusion results in syndromes of memory impairment, opposite visual field loss, and sometimes hemisensory deficits. (From Patten J. Neurological Differential Diagnosis. New York: Springer, 1996; used with permission.)

beneath the tentorium cerebelli. The SCA territory includes the superior vermis, middle and superior cerebellar peduncles, and superolateral aspects of the cerebellar hemispheres (i.e., the "roof" of the cerebellum). Most SCA infarcts are embolic.

Anterior Inferior Cerebellar Arteries (AICA). These arteries arise from the proximal basilar to supply the anteromedial cerebellum and sometimes part of the middle cerebellar peduncle. The AICA is usually the smallest of the three major cerebellar hemisphere branches. Occlusion commonly causes ipsilateral limb ataxia, nausea, vomiting, dizziness, and headache.

Posterior Inferior Cerebellar Arteries (PICA). The bottom of the cerebellum is supplied by the PICA. The PICA is the first major intracranial branch of the vertebrobasilar system, usually arising from the distal vertebral artery 1 to 2 cm below the basilar origin. Its territory is variable but often includes the dorsolateral medulla, inferior vermis, and posterolateral cerebellar hemisphere. The PICA maintains a reciprocal relation with the AICA above it: If the PICA is large, then the ipsilateral AICA is usually small, and vice versa. This arrangement is sometimes referred to as the *AICA-PICA loop.* The PICA is usually the largest cerebellar hemispheric branch and the most commonly infarcted. Occlusions may occur from extension of a vertebral dissection that began at the C1–C2 level (Fig. 4.22). If only the cerebellar hemisphere is affected, ipsilateral limb ataxia, nausea, vomiting, dizziness, and headache are seen, just

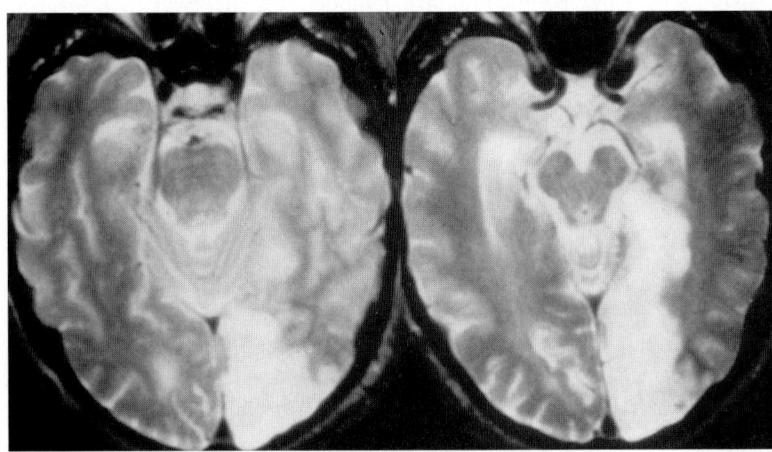

FIGURE 4.21. **Posterior Cerebral Artery Infarction.** Adjacent T2WIs show involvement of the left occipital lobe and medial temporal lobe. The patient presented with a dense right homonymous visual field defect.

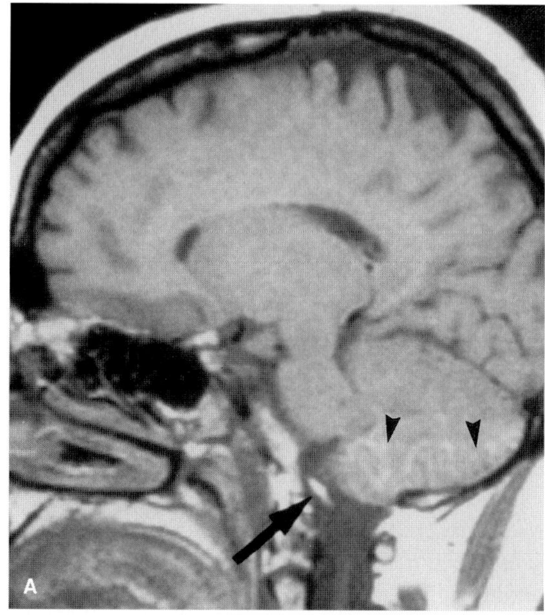
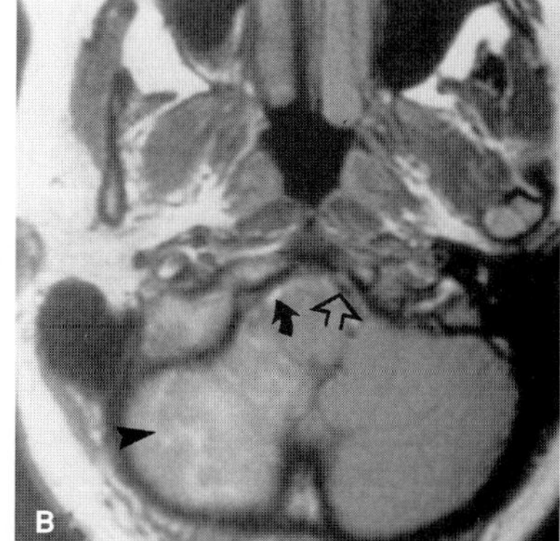
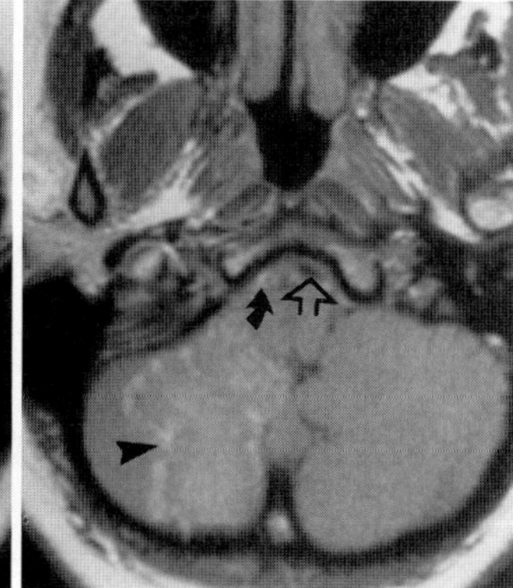

FIGURE 4.22. **Vertebral Dissection With Posterior Inferior Cerebellar Artery (PICA) Infarction.** This patient developed neck pain and ataxia following a skiing accident. Sagittal **(A)** and transverse **(B)** T1WIs without contrast show high signal in the occluded right vertebral artery (*closed arrows*) with preserved flow void in the left vertebral artery (*open arrows*). Hemorrhagic infarction is seen in the right PICA territory (*arrowheads*).

as for AICA infarcts. Involvement of the medulla in PICA infarction adds elements of Wallenberg syndrome, including ataxia, facial numbness, Horner syndrome, dysphagia, and dysarthria.

Watershed (Border Zone) Infarction

An episode of transient global hypoperfusion may result in bilateral infarctions in the watershed regions between arterial territories (also referred to as the *border zones*). Typical triggering events include cardiac arrest, massive bleeding, anaphylaxis, and surgery under general anesthesia. The border zones are regions perfused by terminal branches of two adjacent arterial territories (Fig. 4.23). When flow in one or both of the parent vessels falls below a critical level, the brain tissue in the watershed zone is the first to suffer. Unilateral watershed damage may be seen when carotid occlusion or stenosis is unmasked by global hypotension. Images show a string of small deep white matter lesions ("rosary bead sign") or damage extending out from the "corners" of the lateral ventricles on higher sections (Fig. 4.24). Characteristic clinical findings include weakness isolated to the upper arms ("man-in-a-barrel syndrome"), cortical blindness, and memory loss.

Small-Vessel Ischemia

Lacunes are small subcortical infarcts that may occur in any territory. They account for about 15% to 20% of all strokes. Lacunes are the cavities (literally, "little lakes"; 2 to 5 mm^3) left in the brain as the result of occlusion of a penetrating artery, causing infarction and ensuing encephalomalacia. Patients usually have a history of longstanding hypertension, which leads to lipohyalinosis of the vessels and eventual thrombosis. TIAs precede the stroke in 60% of cases, and a stuttering course is common in the first 2 days. Pure motor or sensory syndromes may occur with these small lesions. Characteristic locations include the lenticular nucleus (37%), pons (16%), thalamus (14%), caudate (10%), and internal capsule/corona radiata (10%) (Fig. 4.25).

Internal capsule lacunes are an especially important subset of lacunes because they are quite common and cause characteristic syndromes. Axonal projections to and from the cortex must funnel through the internal capsule and brainstem, where even tiny lacunes may cause major deficits. The internal capsule receives its supply from multiple small perforating arteries at the base of the brain, all of which are common sites for lacunar infarction and hypertensive hemorrhages. Its contributors include the ACA and MCA lenticulostriate branches, the ICA anterior choroidal branch, and the PCA thalamogeniculate branches. Isolated lesions of the anterior limb interrupt connections of the anterior frontal lobe, but are usually clinically silent. Beginning at the genu and working back, the capsule carries corticobulbar, *h*ead, *a*rm, and then *l*eg fibers in a somatotopically organized fashion (Fig. 4.26). (Our little homunculus man, *HAL*, stands in the posterior limb with his head at the genu, reclining with his head directed medially as he enters the cerebral peduncle.) Lesions in the posterior limb are clinically most important because they may cause severe sensory, motor, or mixed deficits. Lesions at the genu may disrupt speech production or swallowing but generally become apparent only when bilateral.

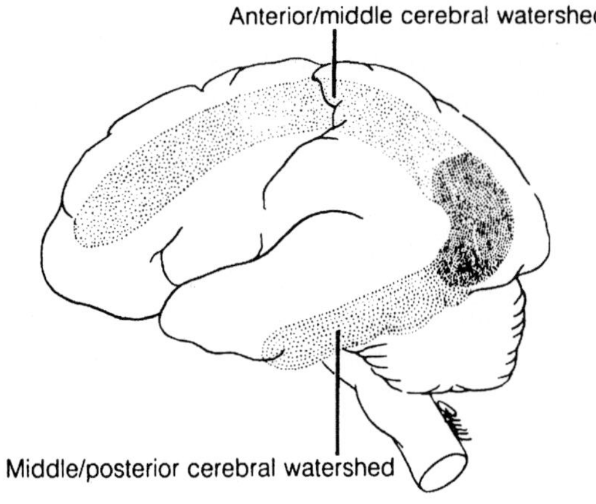

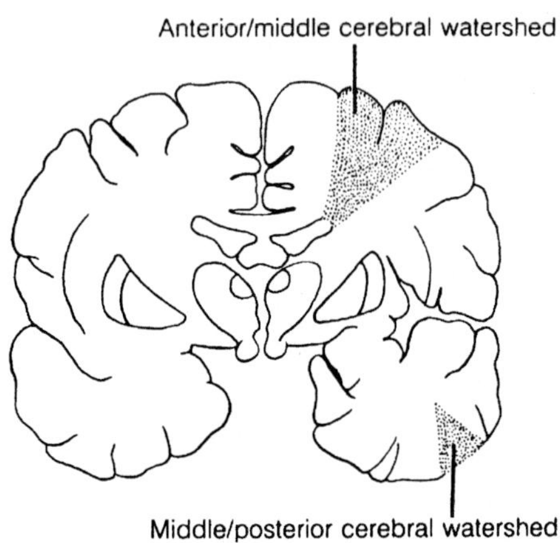

FIGURE 4.23. **Watershed Ischemia.** Stippled brain areas are served by terminal branches of adjacent parent arteries. The watershed zones are at highest risk of infarction when flow is reduced in one or both carotids. (From Simon RP, Aminoff MJ, Greenberg DA, eds. Clinical Neurology. Norwalk, CT: Appleton & Lange, 1989; used with permission.)

Lacunes Versus Perivascular Spaces. "Etat lacunaire" refers to a state of multiple lacunar infarctions. The term is still used in the literature and should be distinguished from the term "etat crible," which refers to the enlarged perivascular spaces (Virchow-Robin spaces) that may develop around perforating vessels (Fig. 4.27). These normal spaces may simulate lacunes but have no associated neurologic deficit or other clinical relevance. By definition, Virchow-Robin spaces should follow CSF intensity on all MR sequences, have no associated mass effect, and occur along the path of a penetrating vessel. Common locations include the medial temporal lobes and inferior third of the putamen and thalamus. Occasionally they may be seen along the course of small medullary veins near the vertex. Most perivascular spaces seen on MR are between 1 and 3 mm in diameter, but some may be 5 mm or larger. Enlarged perivascular spaces are observed as a normal variant in all age groups (Fig. 4.28). Both increasing size and frequency are noted with increasing age.

Small-Vessel Ischemic Changes. Small foci of T2 hyperintensity are commonly seen scattered throughout the brains of older patients, with or without clinical symptoms. These "UBOs" (unidentified bright objects) can cause considerable consternation. They are commonly associated with patchy or diffuse T2 hyperintensity in the centrum semiovale (Fig. 4.28). Pages could be filled with different authors' terms for related processes: small-vessel ischemic disease, senescent change, Binswanger disease, multi-infarct dementia, and leukoaraiosis, to name a few. There is no consensus on when these imaging changes should be considered abnormal, and when they simply represent a normal part of the aging process. At one end of the spectrum are patients who have collected enough tiny infarcts over the years to impair brain function. Individually or in small numbers, these are presumably asymptomatic, but in aggregate they lead to a multi-infarct dementia picture. At the other end of the spectrum are perfectly healthy patients who have presumably developed a speck of gliosis or occlusion of an inconsequential tiny vessel as a normal part of aging. The clinical findings must determine which patients with small-vessel ischemic changes need further workup.

Vasculitis. Patchy inflammatory changes in arterial walls may lead to either large-vessel or small-vessel stroke. Vasculitis may be triggered by autoimmune disorders; drug exposure (heroin, amphetamines); polyarteritis nodosa; and idiopathic processes (e.g., giant cell arteritis). Vasculitic infarcts are often scattered across multiple vascular territories and therefore may produce atypical patterns of damage. Varying stages of inflammation, necrosis, fibrosis, and aneurysms may be seen simultaneously.

Cases of suspected vasculitis are evaluated by conventional angiography, which provides the highest possible resolution. Views of the intracranial circulation and the external carotid artery are reviewed in search of irregular focal narrowing. Positive sites may then be selected for biopsy confirmation. Sometimes the vessels affected are so small that the angiogram is normal. In these cases, skin, nerve, muscle, or random temporal artery biopsy may be required to make the diagnosis. Diagnostic confirmation is important, since many of the vasculitides respond to steroids or cytotoxic drugs.

Venous Infarction

Venous occlusion is an uncommon but important cause of stroke. Characteristically, venous infarcts occur in younger

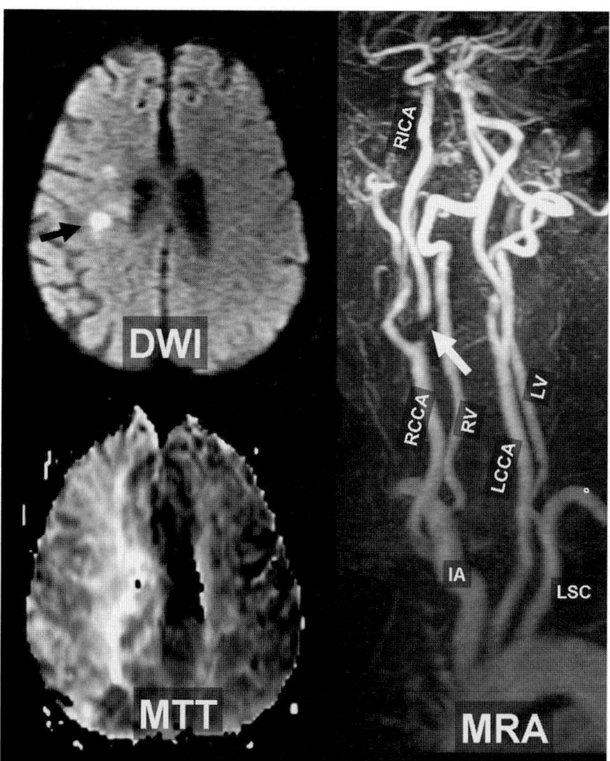

FIGURE 4.24. **Watershed Infarctions.** This patient presented with left body "shaking limb" transient ischemic attacks. The diffusion-weighted image (DWI) shows a cluster of lesions in the right corona radiata (*black arrow*). The mean transit time (MTT) maps indicate long transit times for the entire hemisphere, particularly the deep watershed zones (whiter colors = longer times). Gadolinium-enhanced MR angiogram (MRA) shows fairly normal great vessel origins, but a critical stenosis of the proximal right internal carotid artery with a flow gap (*white arrow*). Mechanisms leading watershed ischemia are debated, but may include distal emboli, local thrombosis caused by slow flow, and hemodynamic causes.

patients, who present with headache, sudden focal deficits, and often seizures. Predisposing factors include hypercoagulable states; pregnancy; infection (spread from contiguous scalp, face, middle ear, or sinus); dehydration; meningitis; and direct invasion by tumor. Although the arterial supply is intact, blockage of the outflow leads to stasis, deoxygenation of blood, and neuronal death. Continued perfusion into damaged, occluded vessels frequently leads to hemorrhage. Any dural sinus or cortical vein may be affected, but the most common are transverse (lateral), superior sagittal, and cavernous sinus occlusions.

A pattern of hemorrhagic infarction in the deep cortical or subcortical regions is usually present. These lesions tend to be rounded and may spare some overlying cortex, as opposed to the classic wedge-shaped arterial occlusions that grow larger toward the surface (Fig. 4.29). Venous infarctions may also be suspected when there is an apparent infarct that does not conform to a known arterial territory.

The venous clot responsible may be seen indirectly as a filling defect in the superior sagittal sinus on contrast-enhanced CT, i.e., the "empty delta" sign (Fig. 4.30). The empty delta sign is usually present 1 to 4 weeks after sinus occlusion, but it may not be seen in the acute and chronic phases of the disease. Small venous occlusions are not reliably detected by CT. An appearance that mimics the empty delta sign has also been described in up to 10% of normal patients when CT scanning is delayed for more than 30 minutes after contrast infusion. This is probably a result of differential blood pool clearance and dural absorption of contrast, effectively highlighting the dural margins of a normal venous sinus.

A combination of spin-echo MR and MR venography probably provides the best imaging evaluation for dural sinus occlusion. On MR, venous sinus thrombosis is suspected when venous flow voids are lost and confirmed when an actual clot is observed (Fig. 4.29). Normal but

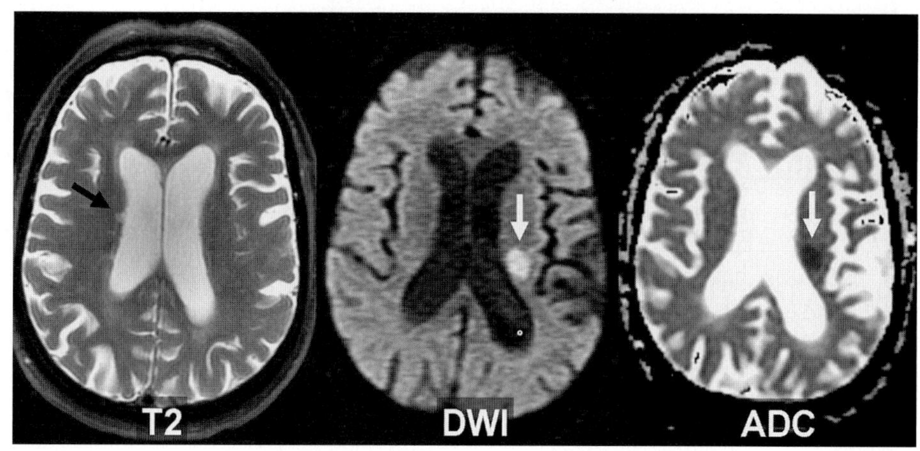

FIGURE 4.25. **Old Versus New Lacunes Distinguished by T2 and Diffusion-Weighted Imaging (DWI).** This patient presented with a pure motor stroke. T2 shows a small old lacune in the right periventricular white matter (*black arrow*) and age-related periatrial white matter changes. The cytotoxic edema of the acute infarct is seen only on DWI and apparent diffusion coefficient (ADC) maps (*white arrows*). DWI in an acute infarct may remain hyperintense for about a month and evolves toward more waterlike signal thereafter.

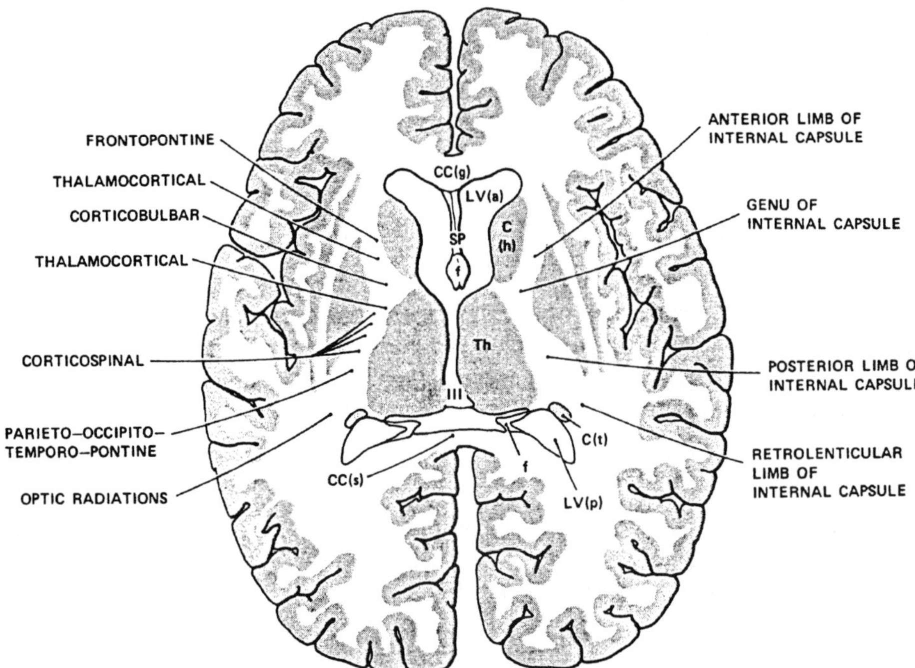

FIGURE 4.26. **Somatotopy of the Internal Capsule.** Transverse diagram showing the main parts of the internal capsule (labeled on the right) and major fiber tracts passing through it (labeled on the left). CC(g), genu of the corpus callosum; CC(s), splenium of the corpus callosum; C(h), caudate head; C(t), caudate tail; f, fornix; LV(a), anterior horn of the lateral ventricle; LV(p), posterior horn of the lateral ventricle; SP, septum pellucidum; Th, thalamus; III, third ventricle. (From Gilman S, Winans SS. Manter & Gatz's Essentials of Clinical Neuroanatomy & Neurophysiology. 6th Ed. Philadelphia: Davis, 1982; used with permission.)

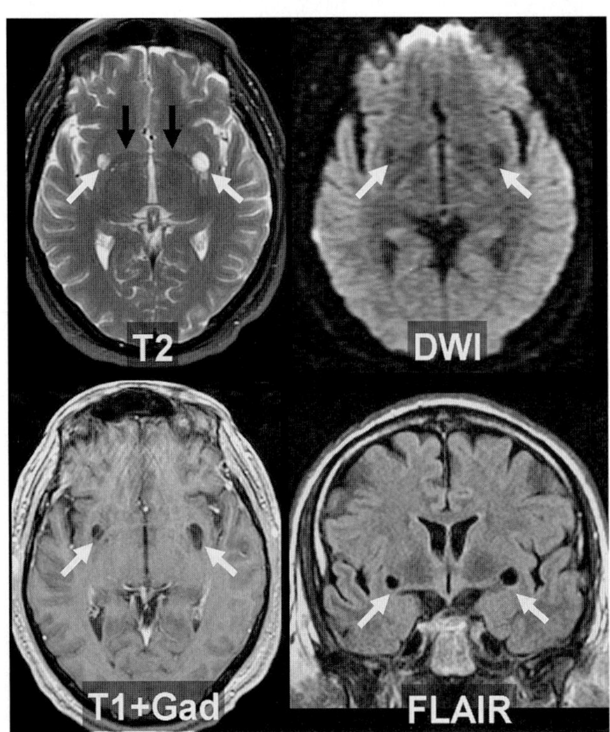

FIGURE 4.27. **Virchow-Robin Spaces.** All sequences show enlarged but normal perivascular spaces (*white arrows*) that exactly follow CSF intensity. There is no mass effect, and the patient had no symptoms referable to this region. These spaces are commonly seen at the ends of the anterior commissure ("black mustache," *black arrows*) in the anterior inferior basal ganglia. They should not be mistaken for lacunes, which typically show diffusion-weighted image (DWI) hyperintensity acutely and signs of gliosis on fluid-attenuated inversion recovery (FLAIR) chronically. Gad, gadolinium contrast.

slowly flowing blood can sometimes cause high signal within veins, a potential MR pitfall in the diagnosis of venous occlusion. MR venography can be very helpful in equivocal cases. Whole-brain CTA protocols, modified to add a slightly longer scan delay after injection, also offer excellent noninvasive evaluation of venous disease. Conventional angiography is now reserved mostly for difficult diagnostic cases or when endovascular intervention is considered.

HEMORRHAGE

Hemorrhage occurs when an artery or vein ruptures, allowing blood to burst forth into the brain parenchyma or subarachnoid spaces. Although mixed patterns occur, hemorrhages are most conveniently divided into *subarachnoid* and *parenchymal* categories. Imaging studies are critical in determining the source of bleeding and in showing any associated complications. The location and pattern of hemorrhage help predict the identity of the underlying lesion and direct further workup.

Imaging of Hemorrhage

Hemorrhages are detected by increased attenuation on CT and complex signal patterns related to iron oxidation on MR. In both cases, the formation of "clot," which has far less serum and (therefore less water) than whole blood, also plays a role in the imaging findings. *A noncontrast CT remains the test of choice for emergency evaluation of suspected hemorrhage.* Although acute blood can

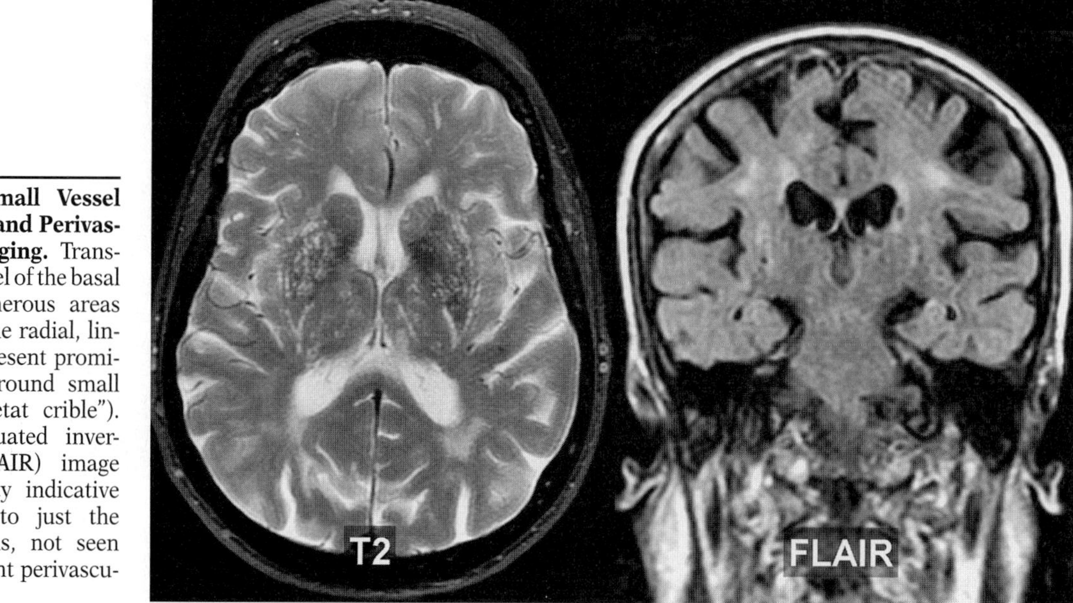

FIGURE 4.28. **Small Vessel Ischemic Changes and Perivascular Spaces in Aging.** Transverse T2WI at the level of the basal ganglia shows numerous areas of hyperintensity. The radial, linear areas likely represent prominent CSF spaces around small medullary veins ("etat crible"). Coronal fluid-attenuated inversion recovery (FLAIR) image shows hyperintensity indicative of gliosis limited to just the old ischemic lesions, not seen around the prominent perivascular spaces.

sometimes be challenging to detect on routine MR, sensitivity is excellent when FLAIR is used for subarachnoid hemorrhage and gradient-echo T2* sequences are used for parenchymal bleeding. MR is better than CT for detection and characterization of subacute or chronic hemorrhage (Fig. 4.31).

The MR signal generated by blood depends on a complex interplay of hematocrit, oxygen content, type of hemoglobin and chemical state of its iron-containing moieties, tissue pH, protein content of any clot formed, and the integrity of red blood cell membranes. Dominant among these mechanisms is the oxidation state and location of iron species related to hemoglobin. Oxygenated hemoglobin is sequentially converted to deoxyhemoglobin, methemoglobin, and then hemosiderin over time. The magnetic properties of the resultant degradation products change the MR relaxation rates of adjacent protons, allowing the hemorrhage to be detected. A small halo of surrounding edema is common in the subacute phase of parenchymal bleeds, sometimes making interpretation of signal changes quite complex. High-field scanners and gradient-echo sequences tend to improve conspicuity of subacute and chronic blood products. The general pattern of MR signal changes seen over time on a 1.5-Tesla magnet is summarized in Table 4.4 and in Fig. 4.32. Individual cases may, of course, vary somewhat from these simplified guidelines because of the multiple factors involved.

An examination of the physical chemistry involved will help us understand the complicated signal changes seen during the evolution of a hemorrhage. To change the signal characteristics of a tissue, hemorrhage must affect T1 or T2 relaxation. The sequential oxidation products of hemoglobin accomplish this because of changes in both magnetic properties and in molecular conformation. Iron within hemorrhage breakdown products changes the effective local magnetic field, a process known as *magnetic susceptibility*. This change in field is translated into an alteration in signal intensity because of acceleration or slowing of T1 and T2 relaxation rates. Changes in T1 relaxation occur only within a very short range (measured in angstroms), while T2 effects can be seen millimeters away.

Under normal conditions, circulating red blood cells contain a mixture of both oxyhemoglobin and deoxyhemoglobin. During transit through the capillary bed, tissues extract oxygen according to metabolic needs, converting oxyhemoglobin to deoxyhemoglobin in the process. Neither of these forms have much detectable effect on T1 signal intensity in clinical images, but they may be distinguished by their opposite effects on T2WIs. *Oxyhemoglobin* is a diamagnetic compound containing ferrous (Fe^{+2}) ions, detected as *high signal intensity* on T2WIs (particularly first echo). Deoxyhemoglobin also contains Fe^{+2} ions but is a paramagnetic substance. The magnetic susceptibility of deoxyhemoglobin causes accelerated dephasing of spins on T2 or T2*W images (e.g., gradient-recalled echo sequences), which results in signal loss. *Deoxyhemoglobin* is therefore *hypointense* on heavily T2WIs. These patterns of altered T2 signal are occasionally encountered on clinical images of acute hemorrhage. These same magnetic susceptibility effects, related to the balance of blood oxygenation, form the basis for clinical functional MR mapping methods (brain regions activated by a task recruit more blood flow and oxyhemoglobin, detected as a focal *increase* in T2* signal).

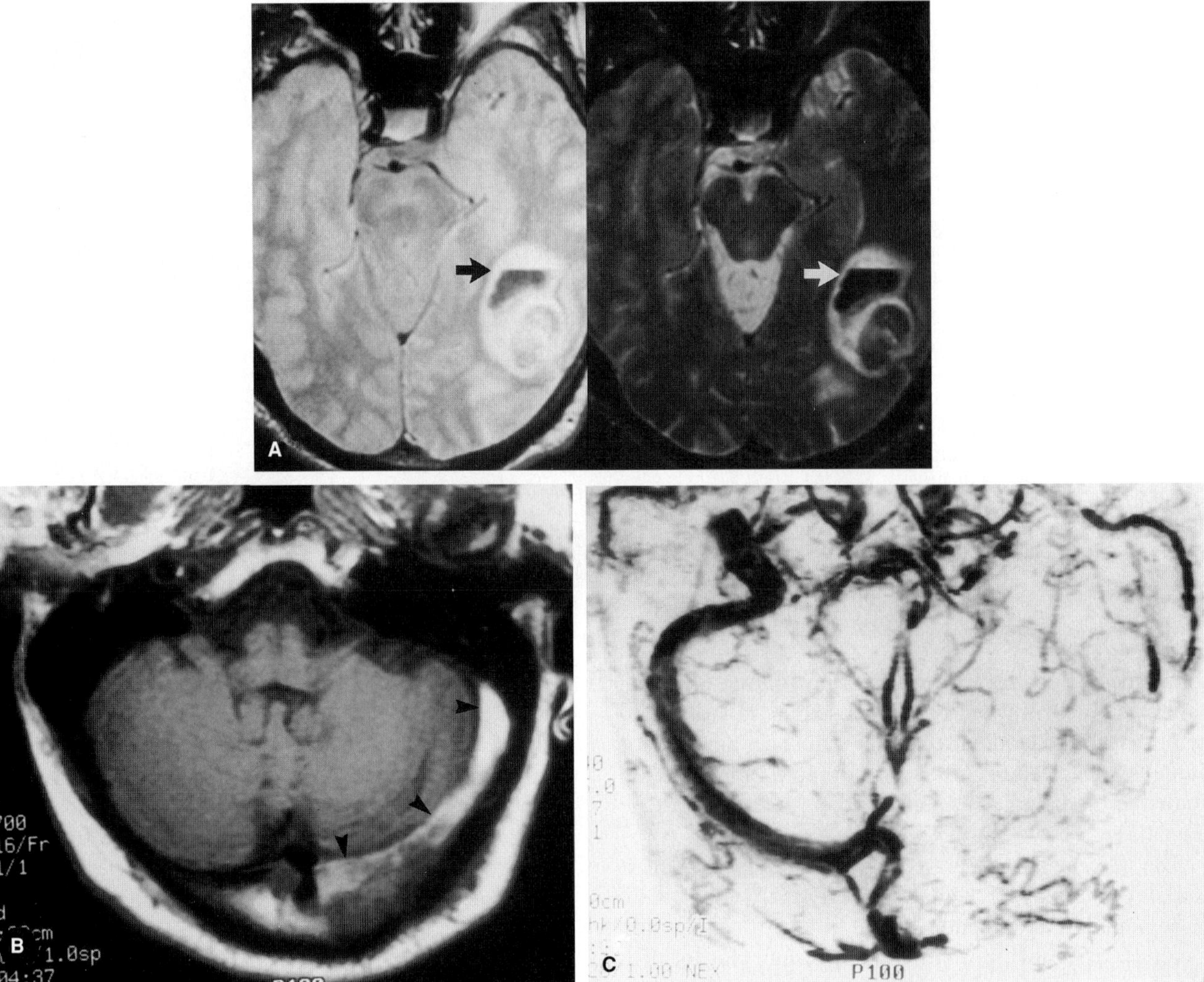

FIGURE 4.29. **Transverse Sinus Occlusion With Venous Infarction. A.** This patient presented with headache and new focal seizures. First- and second-echo T2WIs show hemorrhage deep in the left posterior temporal region with layering of blood clot—the "hematocrit effect" (*arrow*). Signal intensities suggest a dependent layer of intracellular methemoglobin or deoxyhemoglobin with a supernatant of extracellular methemoglobin. A small amount of edema surrounds the hematoma. **B.** Transverse noncontrast T1WI through the posterior fossa shows hyperintensity in the left transverse sinus (*arrowheads*), consistent with thrombus containing methemoglobin. **C.** Submentovertex projection from a two-dimensional time-of-flight MR angiogram confirms normal flow on the right but lack of flow in the left transverse sinus.

When hemorrhage occurs, oxyhemoglobin is converted to deoxyhemoglobin at a rate dependent on local pH and oxygen tension. This takes place over hours for parenchymal hematomas but can be delayed considerably when oxygen-containing CSF surrounds subarachnoid blood. This may explain why acute subarachnoid blood is relatively difficult to detect by routine MR but is readily detectable with FLAIR imaging (signal in bloody CSF is not suppressed). In parenchymal or extra-axial hematomas, further oxidation of deoxyhemoglobin leads to formation of methemoglobin, a ferric (Fe^{+3}) paramagnetic substance. This occurs over several days or longer—parallel in time course to lysis of red blood cells.

Methemoglobin causes a marked acceleration in T1 relaxation, leading to bright signal on T1WIs (Fig. 4.8A). This T1 shortening occurs with both intracellular and extracellular methemoglobin. The influence of methemoglobin on T2 relaxation is more complicated and depends on whether it is intracellular or extracellular. Thus, methemoglobin contained within intact red cells is able to set up local field gradients between the cell and the protons outside; this magnetic susceptibility leads to signal loss on T2WIs. After cell lysis, methemoglobin is dispersed throughout the

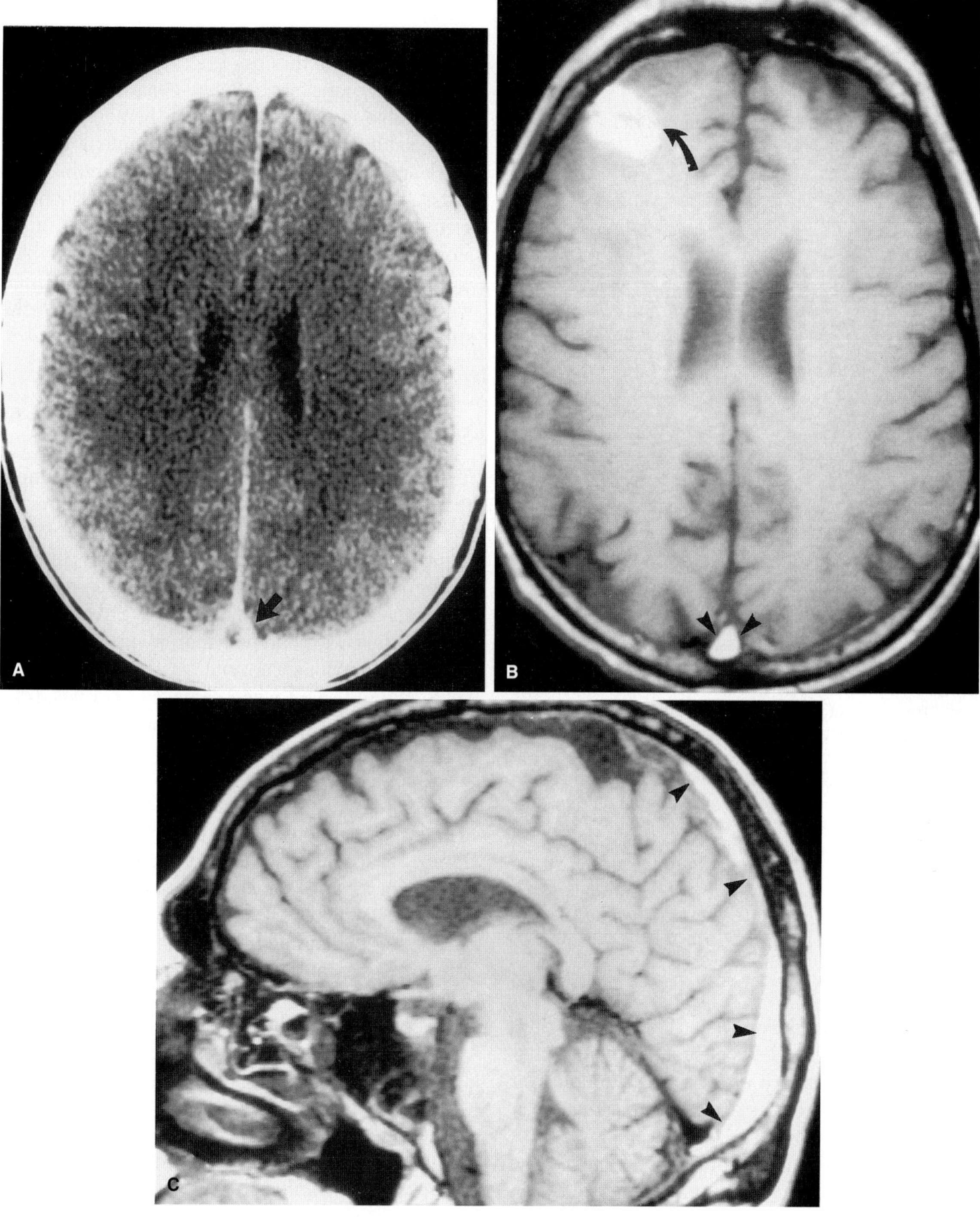

FIGURE 4.30. **Superior Sagittal Sinus Thrombosis With Hemorrhagic Infarction.** This patient was on chemotherapy for lymphoma when he developed headache and was found to have papilledema. Venous occlusion was probably caused by dehydration. **A.** The initial contrast-enhanced CT shows a filling defect in the sagittal sinus—the "empty delta" sign (*arrow*). No hemorrhage was detected. He was treated with anticoagulants but presented 1 week later with worsening headaches. **B.** Follow-up axial noncontrast T1 MR shows high signal with mass effect in the right frontal lobe, indicative of hemorrhagic infarction (*curved arrow*). The normal flow void of the superior sagittal sinus has been replaced by high-signal clot (*arrowheads*). Hyperintense blood on T1 indicates presence of methemoglobin. **C.** Sagittal T1 image confirms clot in the superior sagittal sinus (*arrowheads*).

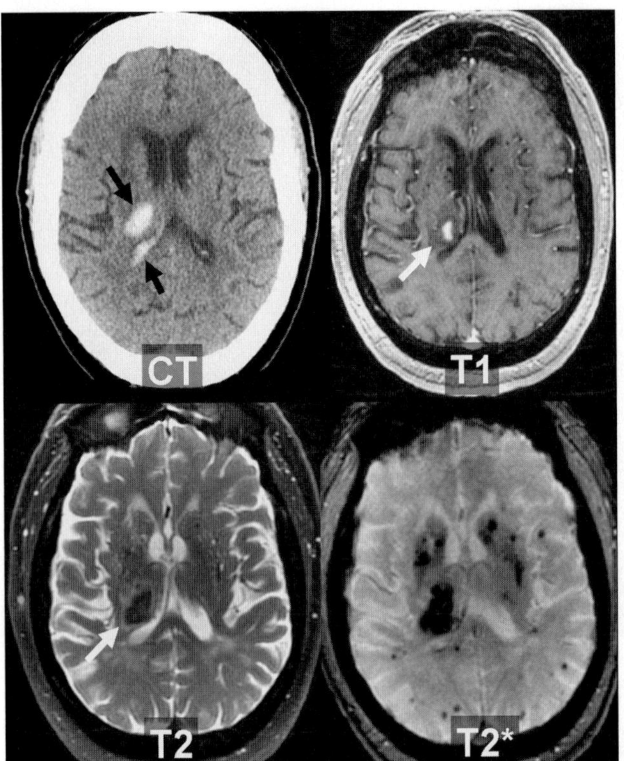

FIGURE 4.31. **CT Versus MR in Parenchymal Hemorrhage Caused by Amyloid Angiopathy.** CT shows an acute right thalamic hematoma with extension into the occipital horn of the right lateral ventricle (*black arrows*). T1 and routine fast spin-echo T2 also show focal clot (*white arrows*), with central methemoglobin (bright on T1, dark on T2) and peripheral deoxyhemoglobin (isointense on T1, dark on T2). A gradient-recalled T2* image shows innumerable additional small lesions related to susceptibility effects in old hemosiderin. While the CT shows the acute lesion most easily, including the intraventricular component, the MR with T2* sequences more fully characterizes the blood products and is necessary to make the diagnosis of amyloid.

tissue water, the gradient is lost, and T2 relaxation similar to that for CSF is seen. T2WIs of subacute hematomas therefore show a "hematocrit effect": a dependent layer of intact cells exhibiting dark signal and a plasma supernatant showing bright signal (Fig. 4.29A).

Further oxidation of hemoglobin and breakdown of the globin molecule lead to accumulation of hemosiderin in the lysosomes of macrophages. Hemosiderin causes the gross rust-colored stain at the edges of an old hematoma seen at surgery or autopsy, even years after the event. This is a paramagnetic ferric (Fe^{+3}) –containing substance that is insoluble in water. As a result, hemosiderin shows no appreciable T1 effects but very prominent T2 shortening (dark signal) because of magnetic susceptibility (T2*) effects. An area of remote hemorrhage will commonly be seen as atrophy alone on CT or T1WIs, but a dark rim along the cleft on a T2WI implicates a prior bleed. Occasionally, large or recurrent subarachnoid hemorrhages will lead to diffuse hemosiderin deposition on the brain surface, a condition known as *superficial hemosiderosis* (or *superficial siderosis*).

Subarachnoid Hemorrhage

The subarachnoid space is the CSF-lined compartment that surrounds the blood vessels and communicates with the ventricular system. Subarachnoid hemorrhage (SAH) is most commonly the result of aneurysm rupture. AVMs of the brain or spinal cord and vascular malformations involving the dura may also cause SAH but usually in combination with parenchymal or subdural bleeding, respectively. Previously normal vessels may rupture into the subarachnoid space when damaged by drugs, trauma, or dissection. SAH may also occasionally be seen in patients with marked thrombocytopenia or other severe coagulopathies.

Patients with aneurysms may develop symptoms attributable to either bleeding or local mass effect. Sudden, severe headache is the most common symptom of aneurysm rupture, sometimes described by patients as the worst headache of their life. Unruptured aneurysms or aneurysms with limited surrounding hemorrhage may also develop significant mass effect, with or without headache. Classic presentations in this regard are the unilateral third nerve palsy caused by a posterior communicating artery aneurysm, cavernous sinus syndrome caused by an internal carotid artery/parasellar aneurysm, and optic chiasmal syndrome (bitemporal field defect) caused by an anterior communicating artery aneurysm.

A patient who presents with SAH is very likely to harbor a ruptured congenital (berry) aneurysm (Fig. 4.33). One

TABLE 4.4 Evolution of Hemorrhage by MR

Time	*RBCs*	*Hemoglobin State*	*T1 Signal*	*T2 Signal*
<1 day	Intact	Oxyhemoglobin	Iso/dark	Bright
0–2 days	Intact	Deoxyhemoglobin	Iso/dark	Dark
2–14 days	Intact	Methemoglobin (intracellular)	Bright	Dark
10–21 days	Lysed	Methemoglobin (extracellular)	Bright	Bright
≥21 days	Lysed	Hemosiderin/ferritin	Iso/dark	Dark

RBCs, Red blood cells.

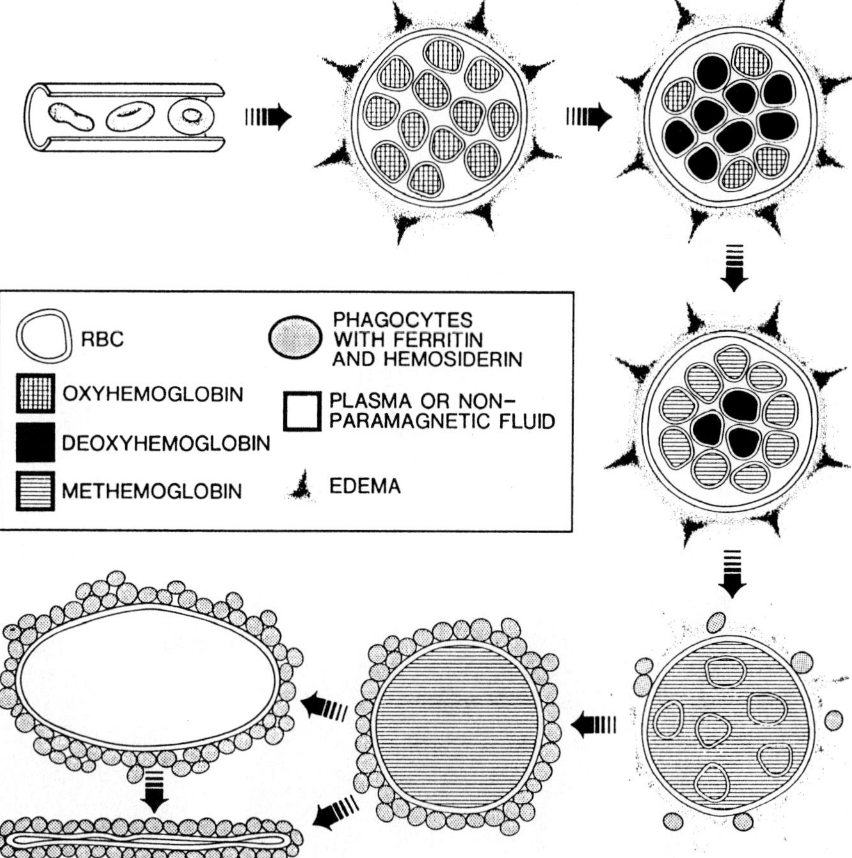

FIGURE 4.32. **Biochemical Evolution of Hemorrhage.** Within minutes of hemorrhage, a hematoma consists of intact red blood cells (RBC) containing oxyhemoglobin. Over several hours, the clot begins to retract and the hemoglobin is oxidized from oxyhemoglobin to deoxyhemoglobin to methemoglobin. Methemoglobin tends to form in a ring that converges from the periphery to the center over time. Red cells lyse, releasing methemoglobin into the surrounding fluid. Macrophages break down the iron products into hemosiderin and ferritin, leaving a stain at the periphery of older hematomas. (From Atlas SW. Magnetic Resonance Imaging of the Brain and Spine. New York: Raven Press, 1991; used with permission.)

percent to 2% of the population has aneurysms, thought to occur because of a congenital absence of the arterial media. Probably many of these aneurysms remain asymptomatic, but those larger than 3 to 5 mm are at increased risk for rupture. Berry aneurysms often occur near branch points of the circle of Willis. About 85% sprout from the anterior part of the circle of Willis, while 15% arise in the vertebrobasilar territory. Common locations include the anterior communicating (33%), middle cerebral (30%), posterior communicating (25%), and basilar (10%) arteries. Less commonly, the ophthalmic artery, cavernous ICA, or PICA are to blame. When distal branch aneurysms are seen, an episode of prior trauma or systemic infection should be considered (e.g., bacterial endocarditis with "mycotic" aneurysm). Other conditions associated with aneurysms include atherosclerosis, fibromuscular disease, and polycystic kidney disease. Management depends on the clinical situation and the location and size of the aneurysm. Treatment options include surgical clipping, interventional endovascular coil embolization, and combinations of the two (Fig. 4.34).

Even large acute SAHs easily seen with CT may be entirely missed on routine spin-echo MR. CT is more than 90% sensitive for the detection of acute SAH, probably because of the increased density of clotted blood. The use of FLAIR sequences on MR can improve conspicuity of acute blood, but CT is still considered the imaging method of choice when clinical findings suggest the possibility of SAH (Fig. 4.34). SAHs may be quite difficult to detect, even by CT, when the patient's hematocrit is low, the amount of hemorrhage is small, or there is a delay in scanning. In these cases, detection of red blood cells or xanthochromia by lumbar puncture may be the only way to confirm a suspected SAH. The most sensitive places to look for SAH on CT are the dependent portions of the subarachnoid space where gravity causes the blood to settle: the interpeduncular fossa and the far posterior aspects of the occipital horns (Fig. 4.35). Prompt scanning is important, because dissolution of subarachnoid blood reduces CT sensitivity to 66% by day 3.

About 15% to 20% of patients with subarachnoid bleeding will have multiple aneurysms. Because of this multiplicity, a CTA or "four-vessel" angiogram is needed on the initial evaluation. Sometimes special views or maneuvers are needed to visualize the offending aneurysm (e.g., opposite common carotid compression to fill the anterior communicating artery). When multiple aneurysms are present, the one that is largest or most irregular, has focal mass effect, is intra-aneurysmal, or shows a change

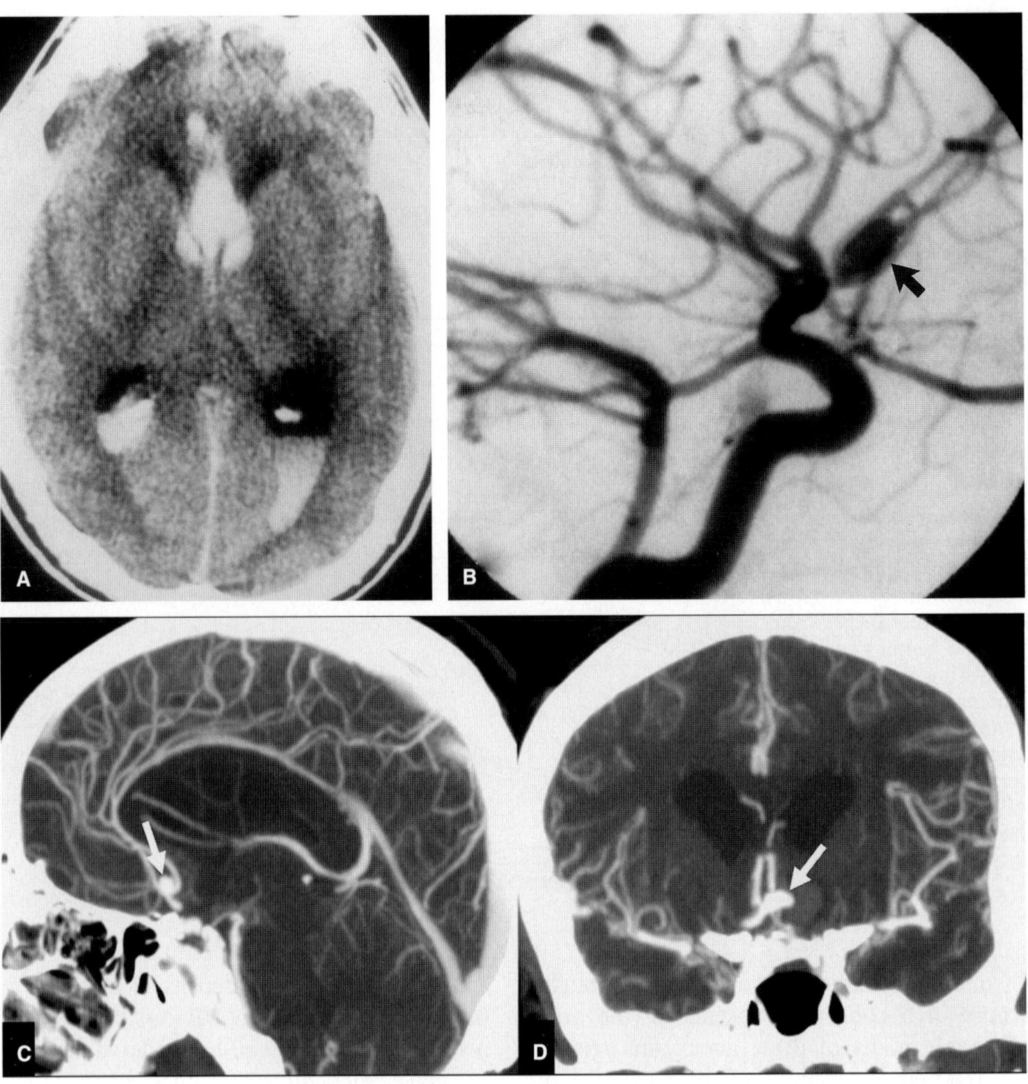

FIGURE 4.33. **Ruptured Anterior Communicating Artery Aneurysms. A.** This 21-year-old man collapsed immediately after snorting a line of cocaine. Noncontrast CT shows blood in the interhemispheric fissure and in the dependent portions of the lateral ventricles. Blood in the ventricles, cisterns, or layered in the sulci is subarachnoid by definition. **B.** Lateral view from a digital subtraction angiogram demonstrates a large anterior communicating artery aneurysm (*arrow*). Over half of drug abusers with intracranial hemorrhage will be found to have an underlying aneurysm or arteriovenous malformation. **C.** and **D.** CT angiograms from a similar case showing a ruptured aneurysm (*white arrows*) in sagittal **(C)** and coronal **(D)** thick two-dimensional reconstructions.

on serial exams is likely to be the culprit. CTA has become an important front line screening tool for emergent evaluation of SAH and in some centers has largely replaced diagnostic angiography. MRA is not yet of proven reliability for the primary workup of a patient presenting with SAH. The combination of MR and MRA probably detects the vast majority of aneurysms greater than 3 mm, making it a reasonable elective screening tool for some at-risk patients (strong family histories, polycystic kidney disease, etc.).

The location of blood in the subarachnoid spaces is imperfectly correlated with the location of a ruptured aneurysm, as subarachnoid blood can layer dependently. Sometimes a parenchymal clot will surround the site of hemorrhage, or thrombus may be seen in the aneurysm itself. When the routine screening CT shows SAH, CTA can be performed immediately to find aneurysms while the patient is still on the scanner. Within a few days, a focus of methemoglobin may sometimes pinpoint the bleeding site on MR. Unless there has been a massive SAH or

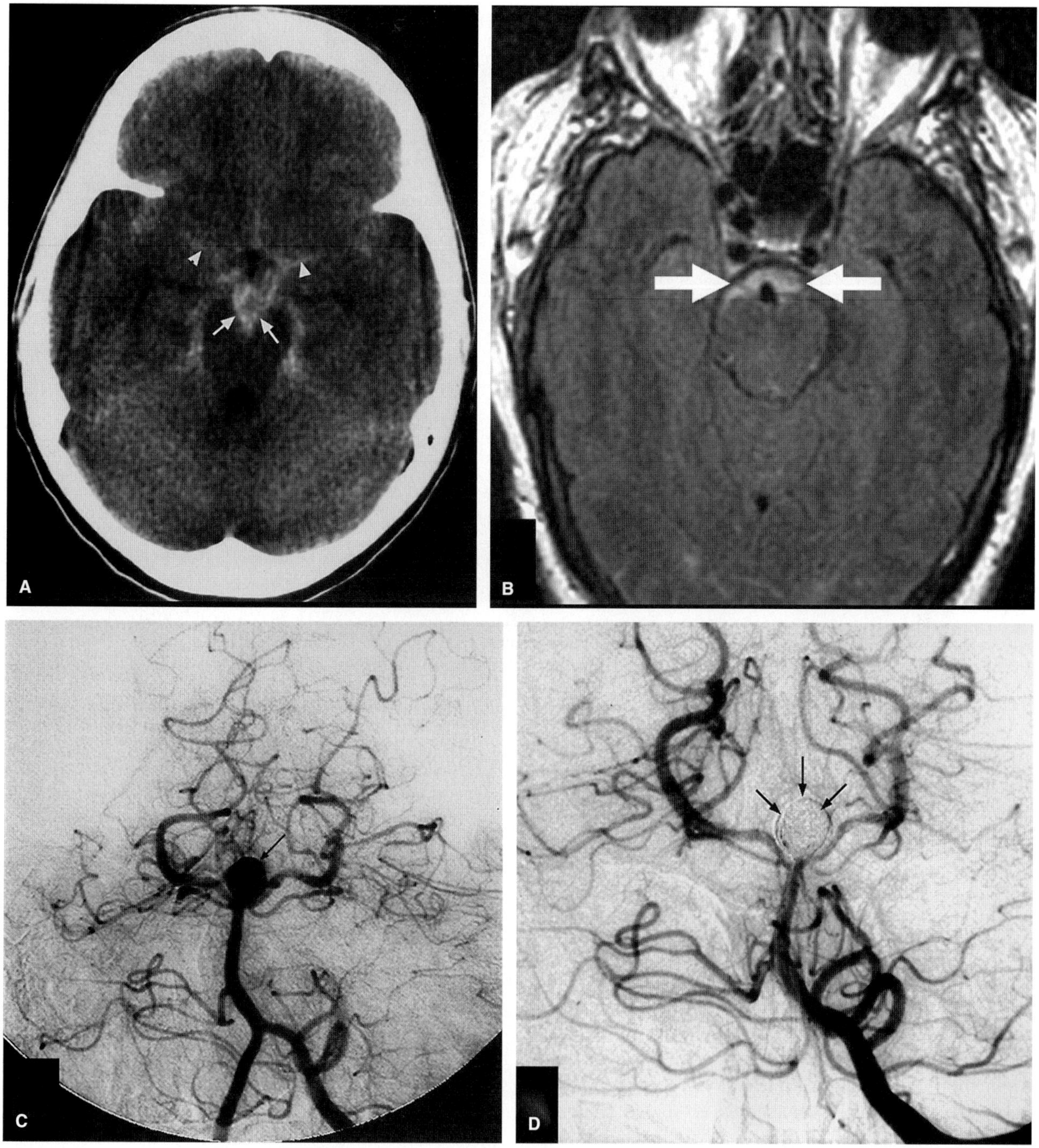

FIGURE 4.34. **Endovascular Coil Treatment of a Basilar Tip Aneurysm.** This 36-year-old patient presented with a severe headache. **A.** A noncontrast CT shows prominent subarachnoid hemorrhage in the interpeduncular fossa (*arrows*) and throughout the basilar cisterns (*arrowheads*). **B.** Subarachnoid hemorrhage is commonly missed on routine MR sequences, but is easily visible on a T2 fluid-attenuated inversion-recovery image (*white arrows*). **C.** Angiogram, frontal view of a left vertebral injection shows a basilar tip aneurysm (*arrow*). **D.** Angiogram following endovascular placement of electrolytically detachable platinum coils shows obliteration of the aneurysm (*arrows*) with preservation of adjacent arterial branches.

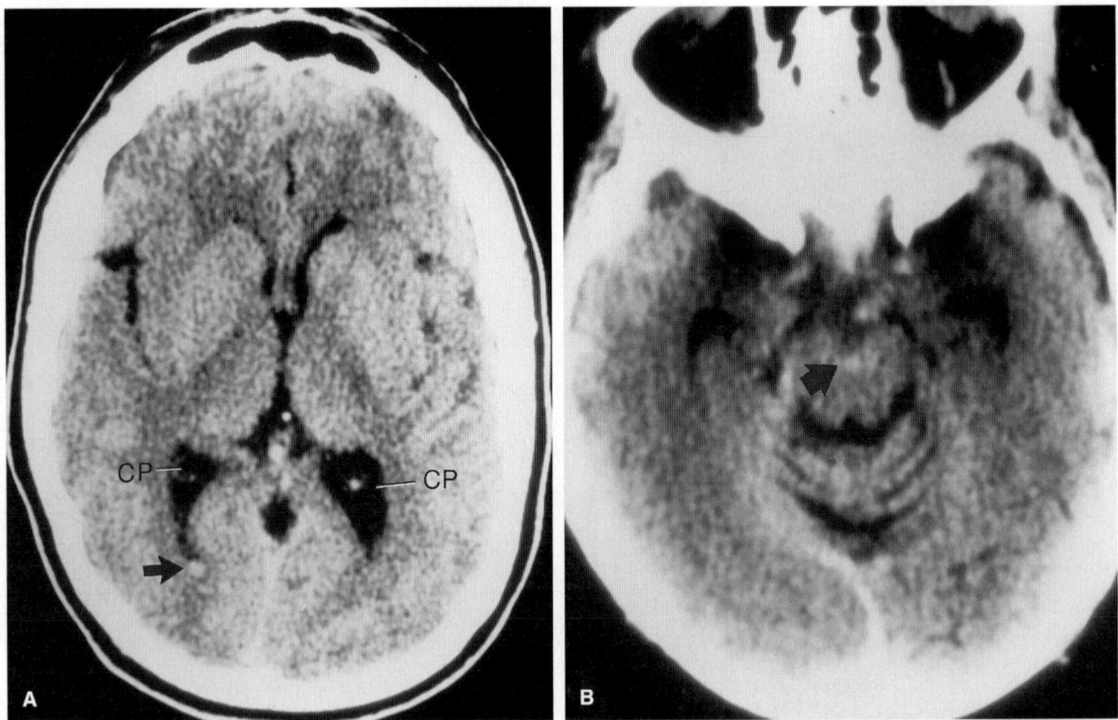

FIGURE 4.35. **Subtle Subarachnoid Hemorrhage (SAH) by CT.** The most sensitive areas for detecting SAH are the dependent parts of the occipital horns (**A,** *arrow*) and the interpeduncular fossa (**B**, *arrow*). The choroid plexus at the atrium of the lateral ventricle (**A,** CP) normally appears dense because of calcification or enhancement. The nondependent location of the choroid differentiates it from hemorrhage.

rebleeding, subarachnoid blood is generally inconspicuous on CT at 1 week.

Evaluation and management of aneurysmal SAH have changed considerably over the past 10 years as a result of wider application of CTA and endovascular coil embolization. While aneurysms that are easily accessible surgically can still be well treated by traditional open clipping, endovascular coiling has been shown to have lower morbidity and mortality overall. Early clipping or coiling allows more aggressive treatment for vasospasm, a much-feared complication seen beginning a few days after SAH. These considerations have led many centers to screen all acute SAHs using diagnostic CTA, followed by angiography for complex cases or those expected to proceed to coil intervention. Two- and three-dimensional CTA reconstructions of aneurysms can help select and plan either open surgical or endovascular procedures.

Follow-up studies are an integral part of SAH evaluation. The initial or subsequent CT may show communicating hydrocephalus requiring a ventriculostomy or shunt. Episodes of possible rebleeding are evaluated with noncontrast CT. Infarcts may also be seen in patients with elevated intracranial pressure or vasospasm and are the main pathologic finding in patients whose condition continues to deteriorate after the initial SAH. Posttreatment angiography is used to assess adequacy of clip placement and to rule out vasospasm. Angiography or MRA can be used to follow coiled aneurysms.

Parenchymal Hemorrhage

Primary intraparenchymal hemorrhage occurs as a result of bleeding directly into the brain substance. Traumatic hemorrhages are not included in this section; they are discussed in Chapter 3. Parenchymal bleeds generally have a higher initial mortality than infarcts, but on recovery they show fewer deficits than a similar-sized infarct. This is because hemorrhage tends to tear through and displace brain tissue but can be resorbed. A similar-sized infarct is made up of dead rather than merely displaced neurons. The main differential considerations are hypertensive hemorrhage, vascular malformations, drug effects, amyloid angiopathy, and bloody tumors.

Hypertensive hemorrhages are seen in the putamen (35% to 50%), the subcortical white matter (30%), the cerebellum (15%), the thalamus (10% to 15%), and the pons (5% to 10%) (Fig. 4.36). As with lacunes, lipohyalinosis of vessels is thought to be the primary predisposing pathologic feature, although miliary aneurysms in the vessel wall may also play a role. Small hypertensive hemorrhages

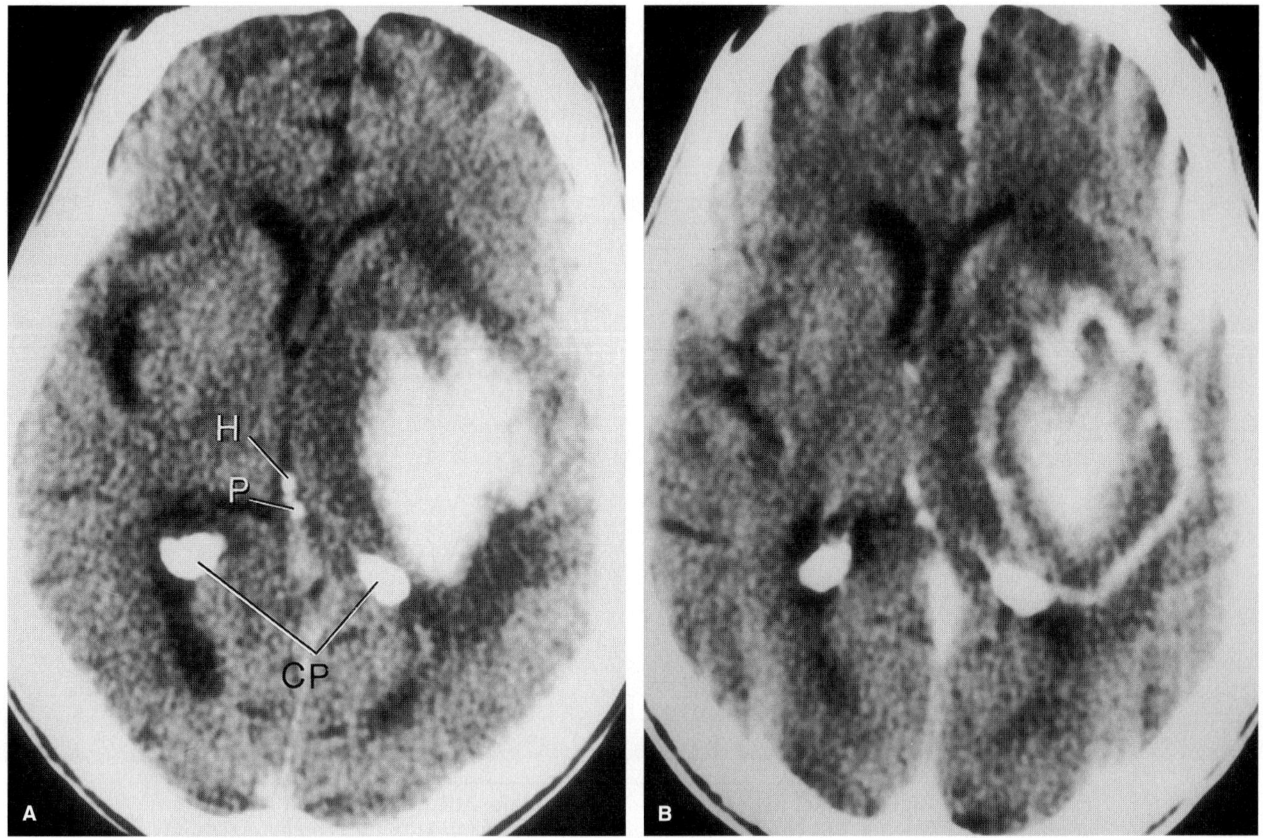

FIGURE 4.36. **Hypertensive Putaminal Hemorrhage With Enhancement at 10 Days.** The precontrast study **(A)** shows a large hematoma centered in the left putamen. Dense calcification of the choroid plexus (CP), pineal (P), and habenula (H) should not be mistaken for intraventricular extension. Moderate mass effect and a small amount of surrounding edema are evident. A ring of enhancement surrounds this benign hematoma **(B),** likely because of a vascular capsule. Resolving infarcts and hemorrhages normally show enhancement at the subacute phase.

may resolve with few deficits. Bleeds in the posterior fossa, those with a large amount of mass effect, or those that extend into the ventricular system have a relatively poor prognosis.

Vascular malformations are encountered far less frequently than hypertension but are a cause of hemorrhage that must be ruled out, especially in young patients. Vascular malformations develop following a congenitally abnormal vascular connection that may enlarge over time. The relative frequency of vascular malformations as a cause of intracranial hemorrhage is about 5%. There are four main subtypes: AVMs, cavernous malformations, telangiectasias, and venous malformations.

Arteriovenous malformations are the most common type of brain vascular malformation. AVMs are an abnormal tangle of arteries directly connected to veins without an intervening capillary network. About 80% to 90% are supratentorial, but any area may be affected. Most patients present with hemorrhage or seizures. AVMs have a 2% to 3% annual risk of bleeding, but the risk may double or triple in the first year after an initial bleed. Treatment depends on the age of the patient, symptoms, and philosophy of the attending physicians. Embolization, surgery, and radiotherapy all may play a role.

Unruptured AVMs typically appear as a jumble of enlarged vessels without mass effect (Fig. 4.37). Noncontrast CT will show a mixed-attenuation lesion, sometimes with evidence of calcification. MR demonstrates flow voids or complex flow patterns, sometimes leading to artifacts in the phase-encoding direction. T2W or T2*W images may show dark signal intensity related to the AVM, a sign of prior hemorrhage with hemosiderin deposition. Intravenous contrast usually results in marked enhancement and therefore increased conspicuity of the AVM on both CT and MR studies. Feeding arteries and draining veins may show impressive enlargement well beyond the center (nidus) of the AVM. About 10% of AVMs will develop an associated aneurysm, generally on a feeding artery. Angiography remains the definitive method for evaluation of the anatomy and dynamic flow patterns of AVMs.

AVMs can be difficult to detect soon after hemorrhage. Occasionally, the AVM will obliterate itself at the time

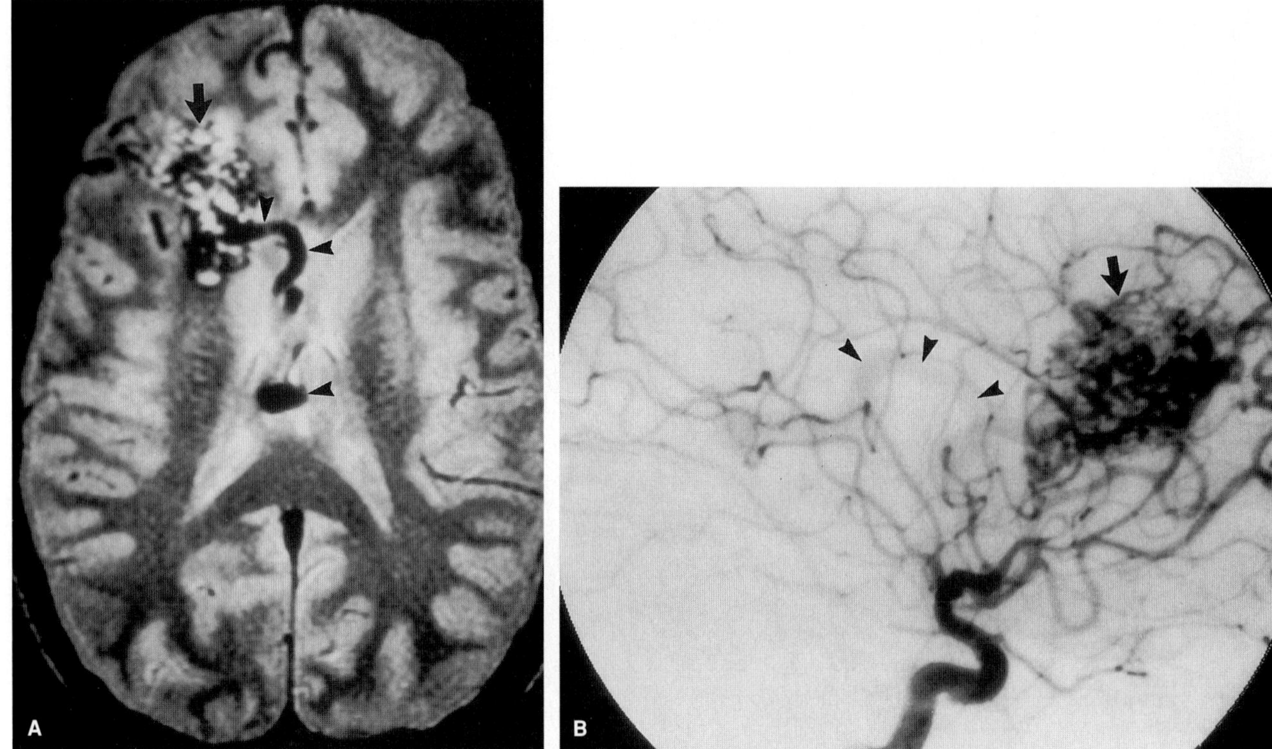

FIGURE 4.37. **Right Frontal Arteriovenous Malformation.** MR was performed because of headaches. **A.** Transverse T2WI shows a large right frontal lesion (*arrow*) with a complex mixture of hyperintensity and hypointensity caused by turbulent flow. A tortuous flow void headed toward the midline indicates a large draining vein (*arrowheads*). **B.** Digital subtraction angiography in the lateral projection (internal carotid artery injection) depicts the large frontal nidus (*arrow*) and tortuous draining vein (*arrowheads*).

of rupture, but more commonly the resultant hematoma compresses and obscures many of the remaining vessels. Contrast studies may identify an enhancing portion of a vascular malformation adjacent to a hemorrhage. Normally, acute hemorrhage will not take up contrast unless there is an associated vascular malformation. A subacute hematoma of any cause may enhance because of a surrounding vascular capsule and should not be mistaken for an AVM (Fig. 4.36).

Cavernous malformations are thin-walled sinusoidal vessels (neither arteries nor veins) that may present with seizures or small parenchymal hemorrhages. These lesions may be asymptomatic and can occur on a familial basis. CT scans and angiography are usually normal. MR will show a reticulated, often enhancing lesion with dark rim (hemosiderin) on T2.

Venous malformations (also called *developmental venous anomalies* or *venous angiomas*) are congenitally anomalous veins that drain normal brain. They are seen in 1% to 2% of patients studied by contrast MR but may easily be missed on CT or noncontrast MR. The classic appearance is of an enlarged enhancing stellate venous complex that extends to the ventricular or cortical surface. The contrast-enhanced MR appearance is usually diagnostic, such that angiography is rarely needed. Although these may bleed, treatment is somewhat controversial because they are commonly seen in asymptomatic patients and are often the only venous drainage for a brain region.

Telangiectasias are dilated capillary-sized vessels and are usually diagnosed at autopsy. These are generally small, solitary lesions found incidentally by MR. No treatment is necessary.

Occult Cerebrovascular Malformations. CT and MR cannot always reliably distinguish among these subtypes of small, angiographically occult ("cryptic") vascular malformations. The generic term *occult cerebrovascular malformation* is used to describe telangiectasias, cavernous malformations, and small thrombosed AVMs. Occult cerebrovascular malformations are usually inconspicuous on CT but may be detected as a small area of calcification. On MR, an occult cerebrovascular malformation should be suspected when focal heterogeneous signal (acute/subacute blood) is seen with a surrounding ring of hypointensity (hemosiderin) (Fig. 4.38). Venous malformations may provide drainage for occult cerebrovascular malformations, but no feeding vessels should be seen.

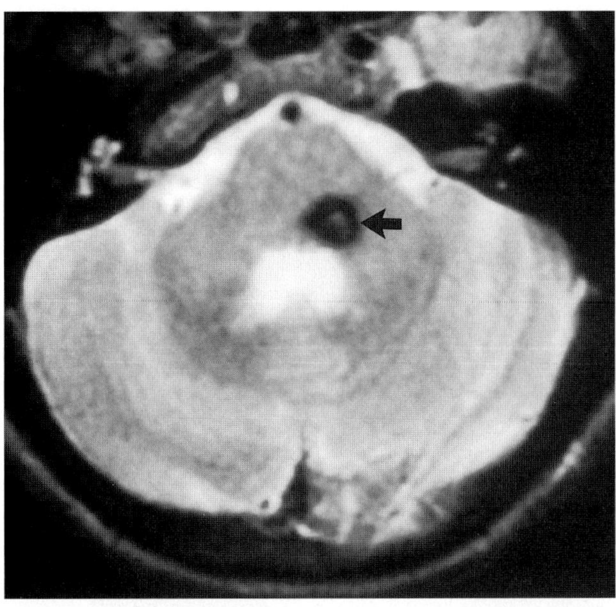

FIGURE 4.38. **Pontine Occult Cerebrovascular Malformation.** T2 transverse image showing a focal rim of marked hypointensity with slight central hyperintensity (*arrow*). The rim indicates ferritin or hemosiderin deposition, and the core represents subacute blood products or abnormal parenchyma related to the anomalous vessels.

Unless it has recently ruptured, an occult cerebrovascular malformation should show no mass effect or edema. If all these criteria are met, conventional angiography may be unnecessary.

Hemorrhage Caused by Coagulopathies. Intracranial hemorrhage may also occur because of blood dyscrasias. Chronic oral anticoagulation increases by eightfold the risk of intracranial hemorrhage. The association is particularly true when the coagulation parameters are extended beyond the recommended therapeutic range.

Drug-Associated Hemorrhage. Sympathomimetic drugs seem to provide an effective (if unintended) stress test for the presence of brain vascular anomalies (Fig. 4.33). Drugs such as amphetamines and cocaine have been commonly associated with intracranial hemorrhage. Symptoms develop within minutes to hours following use of the drug. The genesis may be related to transient hypertension or arteritis-like vascular change similar to periarteritis nodosa. Up to 50% of drug abusers who suffer an intracranial hemorrhage have a demonstrable underlying structural cause, such as an aneurysm or AVM.

Amyloid angiopathy or "congophilic" angiopathy is an increasingly recognized cause of intracranial hemorrhage and is frequently lobar in nature. It is characterized by amyloid deposits in the media and adventitia of medium size and small cortical leptomeningeal arteries. It is not associated with systemic vascular amyloidosis. This angiopathy characteristically affects elderly individuals. Autopsy incidence rises steeply, ranging from 8% in the seventh decade to 22% to 35% in the eighth decade, 40% in the ninth decade, and 58% in persons older than 90. It is rarely seen in patients younger than 55. Cerebral amyloid angiopathy is associated with progressive senile dementia in about 30% of cases. Systemic hypertension is common in this age group but is not directly related to cerebral amyloid angiopathy. Widespread, multifocal involvement can be seen in some cases, particularly when T2*W MR sequences are used to make old hemorrhages more conspicuous. Amyloid angiopathy should come to mind when an elderly, frequently demented patient presents with new or recurrent superficial hemorrhages. Pre-existing amyloid "microbleeds" may also be an underlying source for some cases of postthrombolytic hemorrhage.

Primary Hemorrhage Versus Hemorrhagic Neoplasm

Intracranial tumors are an uncommon but well-recognized cause of intracranial hemorrhage. They account for 1% to 2% of bleeds in autopsy series and as many as 6% to 10% in clinical radiologic series. Tumor necrosis, vascular invasion, and neovascularity may contribute to the pathogenesis of hemorrhagic neoplasms. Glioblastomas are the most common primary brain tumors to hemorrhage, while in the metastatic category, bronchogenic carcinoma, thyroid, melanoma, choriocarcinoma, and renal cell carcinoma often bleed (Fig. 4.39).

It may be possible to distinguish between a hemorrhagic neoplasm and a primary (benign) intracranial hemorrhage based on the MR findings. Intratumoral bleeds tend to be more complex and heterogeneous than benign hematomas. The expected evolution of blood products is commonly delayed with tumors, possibly because of profound intratumoral hypoxia. If a patient is scanned during the acute phase, lack of enhancement beyond the hematoma strongly supports a primary intracranial hemorrhage. If there is an enhancing component, then lesions such as tumor or AVM must be considered. In the subacute phase, however, a resolving hematoma may develop a thin

TABLE 4.5 Features of Benign Versus Malignant Intracranial Hemorrhage

Sign	*Benign*	*Malignant*
Evolution of blood products	Peripheral to central	Irregular, complex
Hemosiderin rim	Complete	Delayed, incomplete
Surrounding edema	Minimal/mild	Moderate/severe
Acute enhancement patterns	Minimal (unless AVM)	Moderate/severe

AVM, arteriovenous malformation.

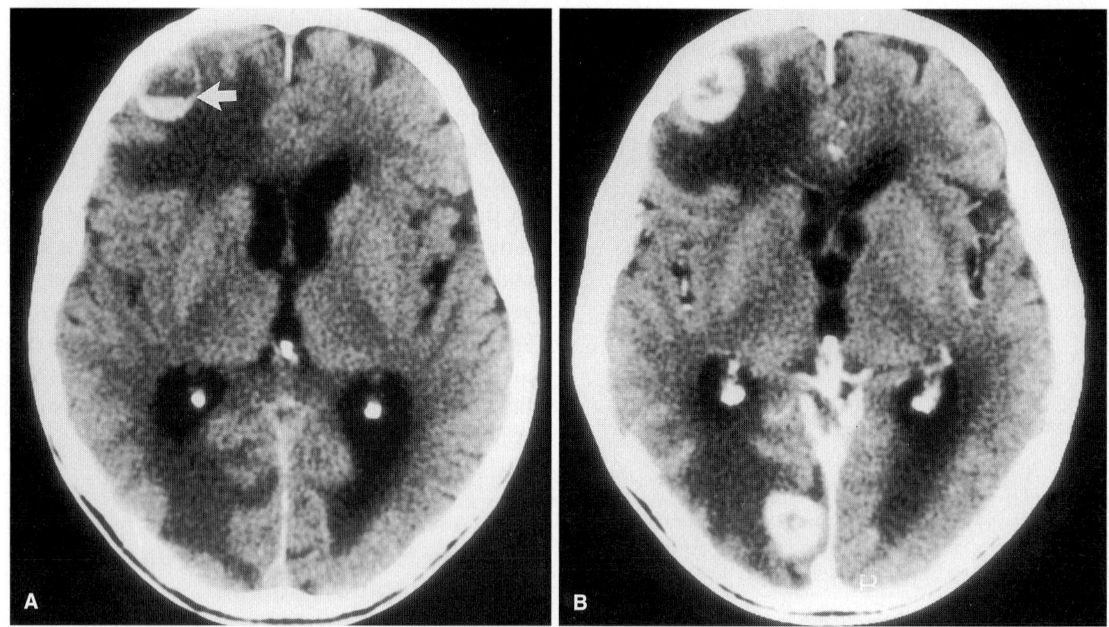

FIGURE 4.39. **Hemorrhagic Metastases.** This patient with oat cell carcinoma of the lung presented with new-onset seizures. The precontrast CT **(A)** shows a rounded bloody mass in the right frontal lobe with a "hematocrit" layer (*arrow*). Marked white matter edema surrounds this lesion and is also seen in the right occipital lobe. Postcontrast scan **(B)** shows irregular ring enhancement of the bloody lesion, and a second discrete focus is identified in the occipital lobe. The degree of surrounding edema, the focal and irregular enhancement, and the nonvascular distribution implicate metastases and not stroke.

area of ring enhancement of its own (Fig. 4.36). Both acute hemorrhage and hemorrhagic neoplasms may cause an edematous reaction, although with tumors, edema is more predominant. In a benign intracranial hypertensive bleed, the edema should begin to substantially resolve within a week, while in the presence of a neoplasm it should persist. With a resolving benign hematoma, a fully circumferential hemosiderin ring begins to develop at about 2 to 3 weeks on MR. In the hematoma associated with tumor, this hemosiderin ring may be absent or incomplete. These useful differential features are summarized in Table 4.5. Sometimes when the findings are ambiguous, a follow-up exam in 3 to 6 weeks will clarify the diagnosis, avoiding the need for a biopsy.

Primary Hemorrhage Versus Hemorrhagic Transformation of Infarction

As discussed in the ischemia section, it may also be difficult to distinguish between primary intracranial hemorrhage and hemorrhagic infarction. In hemorrhagic infarction, arterial occlusion causes infarction of the parent vessel itself, along with its brain territory. If clot dissolution occurs or if collateral flow ensues, blood may then be extruded from the damaged vessel wall. Hemorrhagic infarctions therefore tend to be in classic vascular distributions and infrequently show much mass effect. They are less confluent than hematomas and usually exhibit some degree of contrast enhancement, since breakdown of the blood-brain barrier is present by definition. They are not associated with intraventricular blood, which may accompany a primary bleed. Primary hemorrhage is characterized by disruption of the blood vessel wall, leading to extravasation of blood into the surrounding tissues, sometimes at a distance from the damaged vessel. Unlike hemorrhagic infarcts, primary hemorrhages may therefore cross vascular boundaries.

SUGGESTED READINGS

Butcher KS. Refining the perfusion-diffusion mismatch hypothesis. Stroke 2005;36:1153–1159.

Chalela JA, Kang DW, Luby M, et al. Early magnetic resonance imaging findings in patients receiving tissue plasminogen activator predict outcome: insights into the pathophysiology of acute stroke in the thrombolysis era. Ann Neurol 2004;55:105–112.

Davis SM, Donnan GA, Butcher KS, Parsons M. Selection of thrombolytic therapy beyond 3 h using magnetic resonance imaging. Curr Opin Neurol 2005;18:47–52.

Derdeyn CP, Videen TO, Yundt KD, et al. Variability of cerebral blood volume and oxygen extraction: stages of cerebral haemodynamic impairment revisited. Brain 2002;125:595–607.

Eastwood JD, Lev MH, Wintermark M, et al. Correlation of early dynamic CT perfusion imaging with whole-brain MR diffusion and perfusion imaging in acute hemispheric stroke. AJNR Am J Neuroradiol 2003;24:1869–1875.

Elster AD, Moody DM. Early cerebral infarction: gadopentetate dimeglumine enhancement. Radiology 1990;177:627–632.
Furlan A, Higashida R, Wechsler L, et al. Intra-arterial prourokinase for acute ischemic stroke. The PROACT II study: a randomized controlled trial. Prolyse in Acute Cerebral Thromboembolism. JAMA 1999;282:2003–2011.
Group NS. Tissue plasminogen activator for acute ischemic stroke. The National Institute of Neurological Disorders and Stroke rt-PA Stroke Study Group. N Engl J Med 1995;333:1581–1587.
Hacke W. Association of outcome with early stroke treatment pooled analysis of ATLANTIS, ECASS, and NINDS rt-PA stroke trials. Lancet 2004;363:768–774.
Hacke W, Albers G, Al-Rawi Y, et al. The Desmoteplase in Acute Ischemic Stroke Trial (DIAS): a phase II MRI-based 9-hour window acute stroke thrombolysis trial with intravenous desmoteplase. Stroke 2005;36: 66–73.
Kidwell CS, Chalela JA, Saver JL, et al. Comparison of MRI and CT for detection of acute intracerebral hemorrhage. JAMA 2004;292:1823–1830.
Kliendorfer D. Eligibility for recombinant tissue plasminogen activator in acute ischemia stroke. Stroke 2004;35:e27–e29.
Latchaw RE, Yonas H, Hunter GJ, et al. Guidelines and recommendations for perfusion imaging in cerebral ischemia: a scientific statement for healthcare professionals by the writing group on perfusion imaging, from the Council on Cardiovascular Radiology of the American Heart Association. Stroke 2003;34:1084–1104.
Lev MH, Segal AZ, Farkas J, et al. Utility of perfusion-weighted CT imaging in acute middle cerebral artery stroke treated with intra-arterial thrombolysis: prediction of final infarct volume and clinical outcome. Stroke 2001;32:2021–2028.
Molyneux AJ, Kerr RS, Yu LM, et al. International subarachnoid aneurysm trial (ISAT) of neurosurgical clipping versus endovascular coiling in 2143 patients with ruptured intracranial aneurysms: a randomised comparison of effects on survival, dependency, seizures, rebleeding, subgroups, and aneurysm occlusion. Lancet 2005;366: 809–817.
Roberts TP, Rowley HA. Diffusion weighted magnetic resonance imaging in stroke. Eur J Radiol 2003;45:185–194.
Rowley HA, Roberts TP. Clinical perspectives in perfusion: neuroradiologic applications. Top Magn Reson Imaging 2004;15:28–40.
Schaefer PW. Assessing tissue viability with MR diffusion and perfusion imaging. AJNR Am J Neuroradiol 2003;24:436–443.
Sunshine JL. CT, MR imaging, and MR angiography in the evaluation of patients with acute stroke. J Vasc Interv Radiol 2004;15:S47–55.
von Kummer R. Early major ischemic changes on computed tomography should preclude use of tissue plasminogen activator. Stroke 2003;34:820–821.

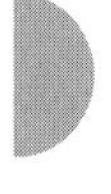

Chapter 5

Central Nervous System Neoplasms and Tumorlike Masses

Kelly K. Koeller

Clinical Presentation

Approach to Radiographic Abnormality

Imaging Protocol

Appearance of Tumors

The Postoperative Patient

The Follow-up Scan

Specific Neoplasms
- Intra-axial Tumors: Glial
- Intra-axial Tumors: Nonglial and Mixed Glial
- Posterior Fossa Tumors
- Extra-axial Tumors
- Intraventricular Tumors
- Pineal Region Masses
- Sellar Masses
- Nerve Sheath Tumors
- Masses of Maldevelopmental Origin

Although neoplasms of the CNS are rare, these lesions garner exceptional interest because of the dramatic and sometimes catastrophic alteration they induce in the lives of affected patients. The overall annual incidence is approximately 20,000 new cases in the United States. Most (80% to 85%) occur in those older than 15 years of age, most commonly (70%) in the supratentorial compartment. Metastatic lesions comprise about 30% of all CNS neoplasms in this age group. In contrast, tumors that arise in those younger than 15 years of age tend to be located in the posterior fossa (70%) and metastatic disease during childhood is rare. In terms of prevalence, CNS tumors are second only to leukemia during the childhood years.

While CNS neoplasms are classically categorized by neuropathologists according to their cell of origin, analysis of these lesions on imaging studies is perhaps best approached with regard to their anatomic location. This chapter will consider a broad spectrum of CNS tumors and tumorlike masses defined not only by their histologic composition but also grouped according to their common locations and consideration of the appropriate differential diagnosis.

Classification. The original classification scheme proposed by Bailey and Cushing in the 1920s serves as the foundation for the histological categorization of all brain tumors currently proposed by the World Health Organization (WHO). Basically, the WHO classification scheme recognizes seven major categories based on the cell of origin (Table 5.1). These include tumors of neuroepithelial cells (primarily glial cells composed of astrocytes, oligodendrocytes, ependymal cells, and choroid plexus); tumors of the nerve sheath (composed of Schwann cells and fibroblasts); tumors of the meninges (composed of meningothelial, mesenchymal, and melanocytic tumors); tumors of lymphoproliferative cells; tumors of germ cell origin; tumors of the sella; and metastatic disease. Each of these cells of origin give rise to a particular tumor type.

The cell of origin directly impacts on tumor nomenclature. If the cellular composition is primarily astrocytes, then the tumor is called an *astrocytoma*. If the majority of the cells are oligodendroglial, then it is termed an *oligodendroglioma*, and so on. The brain itself is predominantly composed of neuroepithelial cells, and hence the most common tumor type is derived from this cell line. In addition to the glial cells, other cells found in the group include those of neuronal, mixed neuronal-glial, neuroblastic, pineal parenchymal, and embryonal cell types. Although the neuron is the most common cell type overall in the brain, mature neurons do not divide and thus cannot produce neoplastic growth. Therefore, most (40% to

TABLE 5.1 Intracranial Neoplasms and Their Cells of Origins

Type of Cell	*Neoplasm*
Glial cells	
Astrocyte	Astrocytoma
Oligodendrocyte	Oligodendroglioma
Ependyma	Ependymoma
Choroid plexus	Choroid plexus tumors
Nonglial cells	
Nerve sheath cells	
Schwann cells	Schwannoma
Fibroblasts/Schwann cells	Neurofibroma
Mesenchymal cells	
Meninges	Meningioma
Blood vessels	Hemangioblastoma
Bone	Osteocartilaginous tumors, sarcoma
Lymphocytes, leukocytes	Primary
	Lymphoma
	Langerhans cell histiocytosis
	Leukemia, myeloma (both rare)
	Secondary
	Lymphoma
	Myeloma
	Leukemia
Germ cells	Germinoma
	Teratomatous types (embryonal carcinoma, yolk sac tumor, teratoma, choriocarcinoma)
Other neuroepithelial cells	Craniopharyngioma
	Rathke's cleft cyst
Endoderm, mesoderm, ectoderm elements	Epidermoid/dermoid
	Lipoma
	Hamartoma

50%) tumors of the brain itself are gliomas. Because they arise from the brain parenchyma itself, these tumors are virtually always intra-axial in location.

Because most nonglial tumors do not arise from neuroepithelial tissue in the brain parenchyma, they are overwhelmingly located outside of the brain proper, i.e., along the coverings of the brain or within the ventricular system. Tumors arising from these "outside" locations are therefore referred to as *extra-axial* tumors. These concepts of *intra-axial* and *extra-axial* are critical to the correct interpretation of cross-sectional CNS imaging studies. In general, the histologic composition of these tumors is directly linked with the location of the tumor.

CLINICAL PRESENTATION

The clinical presentation of a CNS neoplasm is almost always related to increased intracranial pressure, seizure activity, or a focal neurologic deficit.

Subfalcine Herniation. The falx is a very tough, fibrous structure that is very resistant to any sort of displacement. When a mass is located in certain key locations or is of sufficient size, portions of the brain itself may be pushed across the midline or through dural openings. This displacement of the brain is called *herniation,* and many types have been defined according to the brain structure that is most affected. *Subfalcine* (or *cingulate*) herniation is the most common type of herniation and occurs when the cingulate gyrus is displaced under the margin of the interhemispheric falx. Even if the cingulate gyrus is not displaced underneath the falx, significant general midline shift is considered to be present if the shift is 3 mm or greater.

Uncal and Central Herniation. The uncus represents the hooked extremity of the parahippocampal formation of the medial temporal lobe. Uncal herniation often compromises the many tracts running through the brainstem as well as the cranial nerves, particularly the oculomotor (III) nerve, causing an ipsilateral pupillary dilation (or "blown pupil"). On imaging studies, effacement of the ambient cistern and contralateral hydrocephalus are the hallmarks of uncal herniation. Central herniation is the result of either downward or upward displacement of the brainstem through the tentorial incisura. It most commonly results from bilateral or midline supratentorial masses that cause complete obliteration of the cisternal spaces. Elongation of the brainstem in the anteroposterior axis and narrowing in the transverse axis is seen on axial images.

Hydrocephalus. The mass effect of an intracranial neoplasm may be sufficient by itself to produce increased intracranial pressure or hydrocephalus secondary to obstruction of the flow of CSF as it circulates through the ventricles and into the subarachnoid space. The increased pressure is associated with a classic clinical triad of headaches, nausea/vomiting, and papilledema (caused by partial obstruction of the venous outflow from the optic nerve). These features may occur at any time during the course of the brain tumor. In addition, altered mental status (particularly with bifrontal lobe tumors) or alterations in equilibrium (commonly seen in cerebellar or eighth cranial nerve tumors) may be present. Intracranial neoplasms usually present with an indolent course marked by progressive headache and focal neurologic deficit, but they may also present abruptly.

APPROACH TO RADIOGRAPHIC ABNORMALITY

The detection of an intracranial abnormality on any imaging study should immediately provoke three questions.

Mass? By far the most important question to ask is, "Is it a mass?" It is important to consider that abnormal attenuation on CT or signal intensity on MR does not necessarily equate to a "mass," which must have mass effect. In other words, it must displace normal brain structures. Many diseases may produce mass effect and therefore qualify as a "mass." However, all tumors by their very nature should have mass effect.

If mass effect is not seen on an imaging study, the abnormality is highly unlikely to represent a tumor. Differentiation of a small neoplasm from a small infarct may be very difficult in some cases. While the clinical presentation may allow differentiation, advanced MR imaging techniques, especially diffusion-weighted imaging (DWI), perfusion imaging, and MR spectroscopy (MRS), may also play an essential role in the assessment of such circumstances. If these studies are not available, a follow-up conventional imaging study (preferably with MR imaging) in 3 weeks' time may be helpful. Virtually all infarcts will be smaller in size by 3 weeks after clinical presentation. If the lesion is the same size or larger at 3 weeks, a neoplasm should be favored. Also, as detailed in Chapter 4, a subacute infarct will often show signs of subtle hemorrhage. Obviously, because the treatments for tumor and infarct are dramatically different, the distinction between a tumor and an infarct is critical for appropriate clinical management of the patient.

Intra-axial or Extra-axial? Once a mass has been determined, the next important question to ask is, "Is the mass intra-axial or extra-axial?" As presented earlier, an intra-axial mass is a mass that is of the brain itself (i.e., it arises from the brain parenchyma). An extra-axial mass refers to everything outside the brain (arachnoid, meninges, dural sinuses, skull, etc.). The ventricular system is also considered extra-axial. Determining the intra-axial or extra-axial location of a mass is crucial to formulating an appropriate differential diagnosis. Extra-axial lesions are characterized by "white matter buckling" or inward compression of the white matter (often with thinning of the fronds of the white matter) and maintenance of the gray matter–white matter interface (Fig. 5.1). In contradistinction, an intra-axial mass expands the white matter, thickens its fronds, and blurs the gray matter–white matter interface. However, white matter buckling is not foolproof in differentiating extra-axial from intra-axial lesions. Where extensive white matter edema is present, no buckling of the white matter may occur. Therefore, while the "white matter buckling" sign is helpful when present, its absence does not necessarily indicate that a lesion is intra-axial.

Tumor Margin? A third question often posed is, "Where is the tumor margin?" The histologic examination of a typical brain tumor actually provides the answer. On microscopic analysis, every glioma and practically every intra-axial neoplasm lack a capsule, and therefore it is possible for neoplastic cells to migrate far from the apparent center of the tumor. The consequence is that there is no distinct margin for an intra-axial neoplasm. Therefore, determining the margin is not possible on microscopy and certainly is not possible by cross-sectional imaging. Treat-

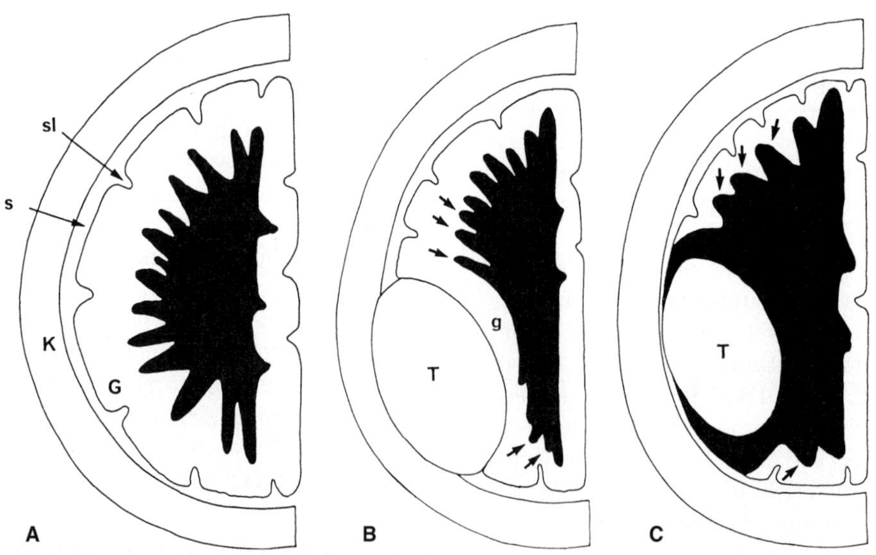

FIGURE 5.1. **Extra- Versus Intra-axial Locations for Intracranial Lesions.** The presence of "white matter buckling" may provide a valuable clue in determining whether an intracranial mass is intra-axial or extra-axial in location. **A.** Diagrammatic representation of normal axial image at level of centrum semiovale. Fronds of white matter (black area) insinuate themselves into cortical gray matter (G). s, subarachnoid space; sl, sulcus. **B.** Extra-axial tumor (T) crowds fronds of white matter producing white matter buckling. g, gray matter. **C.** Intra-axial tumor (T) expands white matter, thickening white matter fronds. Tumor is bathed by white matter edema. (Reprinted with permission from George AE, Russell EJ, and Kricheff II. White matter buckling: CT sign of extra-axial intracranial mass. AJNR Am J Neuroradiol 1980;1:425–430.)

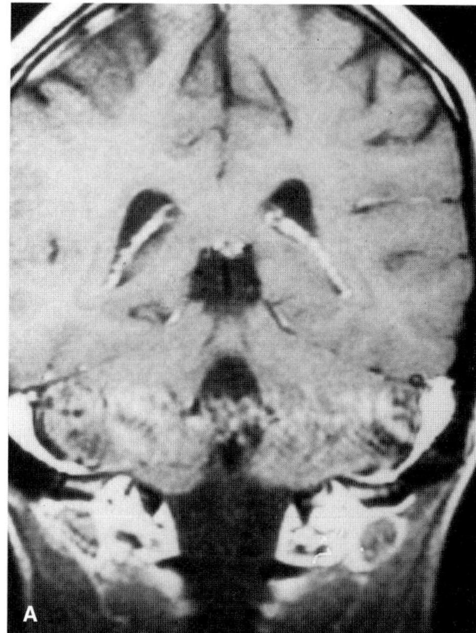

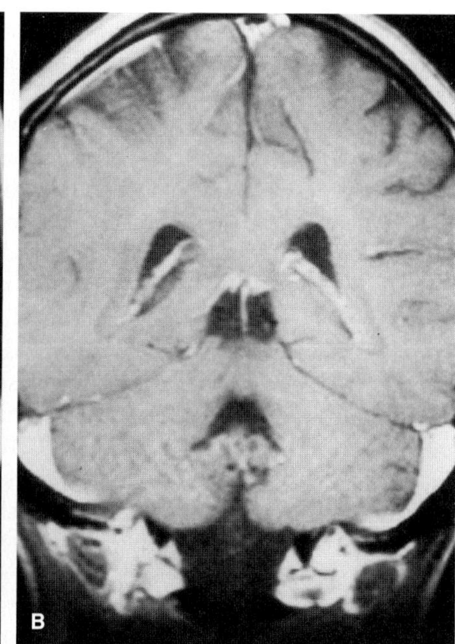

FIGURE 5.2. **Flow Compensation in Posterior Fossa Imaging.** Postcontrast images show the improvement in visualization of posterior fossa structures by employing the flow compensation technique. **A.** Without flow compensation. A significant phase artifact generated from the enhancing dural sinuses degrades the image. **B.** With flow compensation. The image is markedly improved.

ment is typically directed to the entire region of abnormal hyperintensity on T2WIs, not just the region described by enhancement on the T1-weighted postcontrast sequence. MRS is valuable in identifying areas of spread in regions with normal T2 signal.

Trying to make a histologic diagnosis from an MR or CT scan is fraught with hazard. However, it is possible to render an intelligent analysis of the mass, including assessment of signal intensities and enhancement characteristics of the mass, and to present an accurate differential diagnosis whenever one encounters a mass suspected of being a CNS tumor on an imaging study.

IMAGING PROTOCOL

Imaging evaluation of intracranial neoplasms is best conducted by MR, which is far superior to CT because of its multiplanar capability, increased contrast resolution, and lack of ionizing radiation. CT is superior to MR in the assessment of calcification, although the use of GRE sequences increases the sensitivity of the latter technique to calcification. CT is invaluable for the evaluation of bony abnormalities, such as erosion of the skull base.

MR. A basic MR evaluation of a patient suspected of having an intracranial neoplasm includes a sagittal T1-weighted sequence followed by an axial T2-weighted sequence. Fluid-attenuated inversion recovery (FLAIR) imaging is utilized for improved visualization of abnormal signal intensity involving the periventricular and peripheral regions. An unenhanced T1-weighted sequence is performed to allow distinction between inherent T1 shortening, such as in hemorrhage, and contrast enhancement. Depending on the location of the tumor, either the axial or the coronal plane is selected for this sequence. For temporal lobe and midline lesions, the coronal plane often provides the best delineation of the tumor. To assist neurosurgical and radiation oncologic planning, all three orthogonal imaging planes should be obtained following the administration of contrast. Performance of all of these sequences can be easily completed within 45 minutes on 1.5-tesla MR units. Improved contrast and signal-to-noise resolution are gained with studies performed on 3-tesla units using different scanning parameters. Implementing gradient-moment nulling (flow-compensating) techniques facilitates evaluation of the posterior fossa by decreasing phase artifact generated by the dural sinuses (Fig. 5.2). Advanced MR techniques such as MRS, DWI, perfusion imaging, and metabolic imaging may also be of value in many cases.

APPEARANCE OF TUMORS

The cross-sectional imaging appearance of CNS tumors varies with their cellular composition and the presence or absence of hemorrhage and calcification. On CT, intra-axial neoplasms will typically appear as hypodense masses with a variable amount of surrounding white matter edema, the area of which roughly correlates with the biologic behavior of the tumor. On MR, the mass is usually dark on T1 (T1 prolongation) and bright on T2 (T2 prolongation), with variable surrounding vasogenic edema. The presence of calcification within the tumor usually produces marked hypointensity on T1WIs and T2WIs. Occasionally, because of the surface area of the crystals producing T1 shortening, calcification may appear bright on a T1WI.

Nontumoral Hemorrhage. The appearance of intracranial parenchymal hemorrhage usually depends on the age of the blood. In hyperacute (less than 6 hours) hemorrhage, the predominant oxyhemoglobin will produce T1 and T2 prolongation (dark on T1, bright on T2). When the hemorrhage has been present for 6 to 24 hours, the effect of deoxyhemoglobin predominates and the lesion has mild T1 prolongation (dark on T1WIs) and moderate T2 shortening (darker on T2WIs). After 3 to 4 days, methemoglobin begins to predominate, first being intracellular, producing T1 and T2 shortening (bright on T1WIs, dark on T2WIs), and then, as the red blood cells begin to lyse, becoming extracellular where the lesion has T1 shortening and T2 prolongation (bright on both T1WIs and T2WIs). In chronic hemorrhages (older than 10 to 14 days), hemosiderin appears, producing a rim of extreme T2 shortening. This peripheral, markedly hypointense rim occurs because of migrating macrophages, which carry the hemosiderin to the periphery of the hemorrhage. On CT, acute hemorrhage (less than 1 week old) has increased attenuation (hyperdensity) compared to normal brain tissue. By 1 to 3 weeks after the hemorrhage, the signal becomes isodense compared to the normal brain parenchyma. After 3 weeks, the focus of hemorrhage is hypodense to brain parenchyma, simulating the attenuation of CSF. This evolution of blood breakdown products is illustrated in detail in Chapter 4.

Tumoral Hemorrhage. The appearance of intratumoral hemorrhage reflects the heterogeneous nature of the tumor and is quite different than benign parenchymal hemorrhage. Intratumoral hemorrhage is often intermittent, producing a heterogeneous mixture of the various blood breakdown products just described. In addition, hemorrhage may occur in cystic or necrotic portions of the tumor, creating blood–blood or fluid–blood levels. Debris from the necrotic mass will also contribute to this heterogeneous mixture. Normal deoxyhemoglobin evolution is delayed, such that it will persist for longer than the usual 3 to 4 days after hemorrhage. The typical hemosiderin ring does not form with intratumoral hemorrhage, probably as a result of interference with the migration of the macrophages by viable tumor at the margins. In cases where there is confusion about the nature of an intracranial hemorrhage, the presence of a nonhemorrhagic mass adjacent to the hemorrhage, the persistence of T2 prolongation (most likely representing edema or tumor itself), and mass effect all suggest intratumoral hemorrhage instead of a simple parenchymal hematoma. Gadolinium administration is often helpful in these cases, because benign hematomas should not have as significant an enhancing rim as those from tumors.

Hemorrhagic Neoplasms. Because of their high vascularity, certain neoplasms are noted for their propensity to hemorrhage. Choriocarcinoma among primary tumors and metastases from melanoma, thyroid carcinoma, and renal carcinoma show this characteristic. In the setting of multiple hemorrhagic lesions within the brain, these tumors should be considered. Multiple cryptic arteriovenous malformations, occurring either de novo or secondary to radiation therapy, can have a similar appearance, with the exception of surrounding vasogenic edema.

T1 Shortening. In addition to hemorrhage, two other entities may produce focal T1 shortening on MR scans. Fat within lipomas or dermoids produces marked T1 shortening and intermediate signal on T2WIs following the signal intensity of subcutaneous fat. The presence of chemical shift artifact on T2WIs associated with such a lesion helps to confirm the presence of fat. Melanin, as seen in melanotic melanoma, also follows the same signal intensities as fat on T1WIs and T2WIs.

Hyperdense Neoplasms. Tumors of high cellular density—usually those with small cells such as lymphoma, pineoblastoma, neuroblastoma, or medulloblastoma—are usually hyperdense compared to brain tissue on CT. In addition, metastases from melanoma, lung carcinoma, colon carcinoma, and breast carcinoma may be hyperdense. On MR, these same tumors are typically hypointense on T2WIs, with the appearance presumably being related to a high nucleus:cytoplasm ratio of the tumor cells, which produces less free water and thus less T2 prolongation. On occasion, isointensity or hyperintensity may be seen because of heterogeneity of the tumor matrix.

Enhancement. Contrast enhancement, whether from iodinated contrast agents used in CT or paramagnetic gadolinium agents used in MR, occurs based on one primary factor: breakdown of the blood–brain barrier. Unlike nonneural endothelium, the endothelium of the cerebral capillaries allows the passage of only small molecules through their tight junctions and narrow intercellular gaps. The macromolecules that make up contrast agents are too large to pass this barrier under normal circumstances. The blood–brain barrier breaks down in many pathologic states, including intra-axial tumors (either primary or metastatic), inflammatory diseases, subacute infarcts, postoperative gliosis, and radiation necrosis. However, some tumors, particularly low-grade neoplasms, will not show enhancement, presumably because they form new capillaries that are quite similar to the native cerebral capillaries, with the blood–brain barrier left intact. More biologically aggressive, high-grade neoplasms tend to have fenestrated capillaries that allow the passage of contrast media and consequently show image enhancement. However, the fact that a lesion enhances only means that there is breakdown of the blood–brain barrier, and the presence or absence of enhancement cannot be used to categorically state that a lesion is low-grade or high-grade (Fig. 5.3). In addition, some specialized areas of the brain, such as the choroid plexus, pituitary and pineal glands, tuber cinereum, and area postrema, have no blood–brain barrier and will normally enhance after administration of a contrast agent.

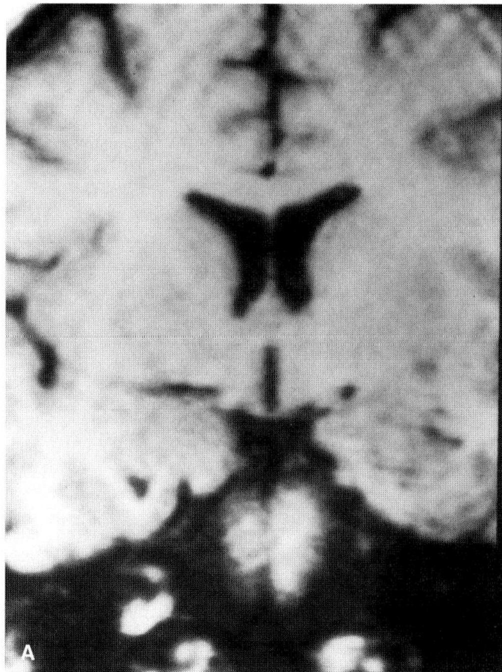

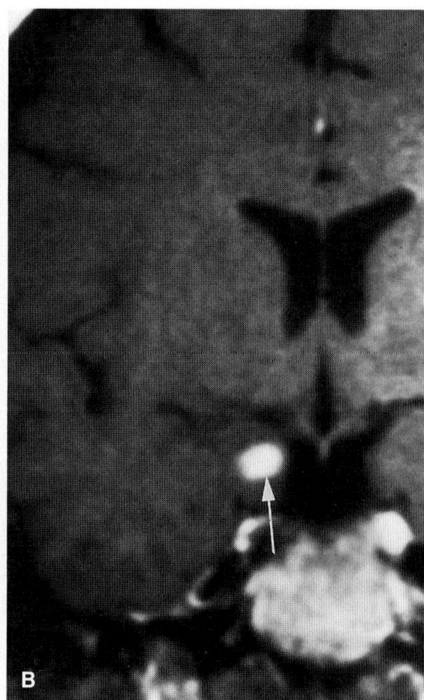

FIGURE 5.3. **Enhancement: Low-Grade or High-Grade Tumor?** Young adult woman with long history of medically refractory seizures. Intense enhancement (*arrow*) of temporal lobe lesion pathologically proven to be a ganglioglioma, a low-grade neoplasm.

THE POSTOPERATIVE PATIENT

In the evaluation of the postoperative brain tumor patient, timing is of the essence. Ideally, these patients should have an MR scan performed within 72 hours after surgery to serve as a baseline scan for future follow-up. Granulation tissue, which occurs in all neurosurgical postoperative patients, takes about 72 hours to fully develop and enhances after administration of contrast. Once formed, this tissue in the operative site and dura may persist for weeks to months. Because most malignant brain tumors have at least some enhancement, the presence of enhancement on a study performed during this 72-hour window can be interpreted as being enhancement secondary to residual tumor and not to granulation tissue. After 72 hours, it is practically impossible to make this distinction by this method alone.

Safety. Postoperative neurosurgical patients are often not ideal candidates for scanning in an MR unit, and proper monitoring of vital signs to assure their safety is paramount. If the appropriate monitoring and life-support equipment (e.g., shielded pulse oximeter and oxygen) and personnel are not available to safely perform an MR study, a monitored contrast-enhanced CT should be substituted.

THE FOLLOW-UP SCAN

Many malignant tumors will be treated by a combination of chemotherapy and radiation therapy following surgical debulking. Typical radiation doses are in the range of 50 to 54 Gy, most often delivered in fractionated doses (about 1.8 Gy each visit) over several weeks' time. As a consequence, radiation injury in the white matter occurs in two forms: diffuse white matter injury and radiation necrosis.

Despite the widespread involvement seen in diffuse white matter injury, most patients do not have any neurologic deficits. A "geographic distribution" of white matter hyperintensity on a T2WI conforming to the selected radiation ports is typical for diffuse white matter radiation injury and should not be misinterpreted as vasogenic edema from the tumor. Virtually all patients following whole-brain or large-volume radiation will demonstrate this pattern of involvement 6 months or more after the therapy is completed. Affected areas do not enhance on postcontrast imaging. Distinction from a brain tumor is seldom a problem in the setting of diffuse white matter injury.

In contrast, the much less commonly seen radiation necrosis is virtually indistinguishable from that of recurrent tumor on CT or conventional MR images, because both usually have mass effect and enhancement. Clinically, patients with radiation necrosis often present with focal neurologic deficits. However, MRS, DWI, perfusion imaging, and metabolic imaging (PET or SPECT-thallium studies) are useful in making this distinction. While radiation necrosis may have an elevated lactate peak on MRS secondary to necrosis, the elevated choline peak and depressed n-acetyl aspartate (NAA) peak are usually absent (Fig. 5.4). Affected areas are composed of heavily necrotic tissue. Consequently, restricted water diffusion is typical on DWI and corresponding apparent diffusion coefficient map images. In contrast, the overwhelming majority of brain tumors do not cause restricted water diffusion and

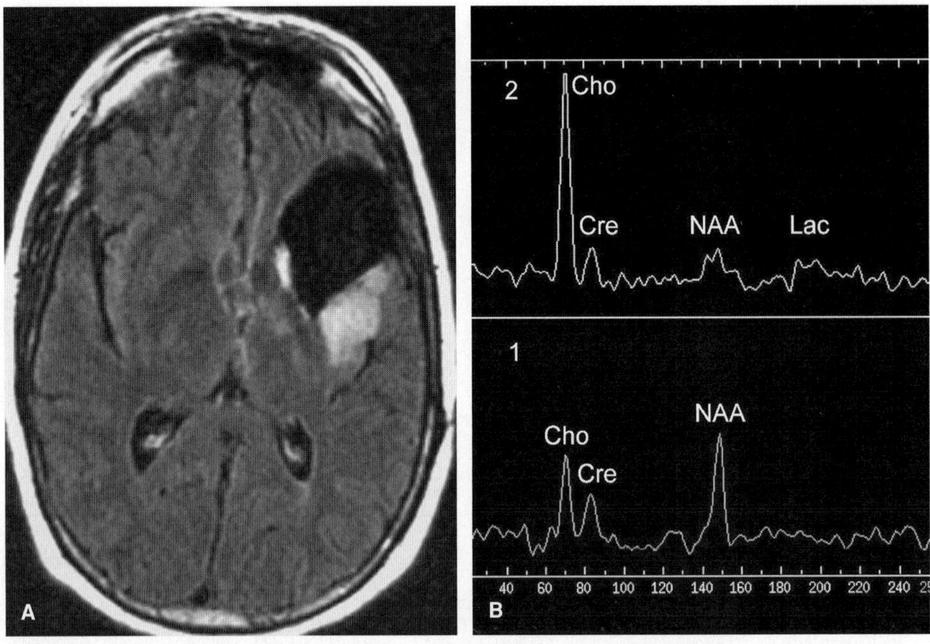

FIGURE 5.4. **Recurrent Tumor or Radiation Necrosis? A.** Axial FLAIR image shows heterogeneous mass with cystlike component anteriorly and hyperintense soft tissue portion along its posterior margin. **B.** MRS evaluation with region of interest (ROI) of normal brain (1) shows n-acetyl aspartate (NAA) peak larger than either choline (Cho) or creatine (Cre) peaks. MRS with ROI of the posterior soft tissue portion (2) shows a markedly elevated choline peak and depressed NAA peak. Slight elevation of lactate is also seen. This pattern is not consistent with radiation necrosis, which would be expected to have a prominent lactate peak and a normal choline peak. Instead, this pattern is more consistent with a neoplasm, which was confirmed histologically as a recurrent oligodendroglioma. (Case courtesy of Howard Rowley, MD)

will not be hyperintense on DWI. Similarly, while absence of increased perfusion is noted in radiation necrosis, many tumors demonstrate elevated local blood flow on perfusion imaging. With metabolic imaging, radiation necrosis shows normal to decreased metabolic activity, while recurrent tumor is usually increased, especially if the original tumor was high-grade (e.g., WHO grade III or IV; see "Astrocytomas" section). Distinguishing between recurrent tumor and radiation necrosis using metabolic imaging is less accurate if the original brain tumor was WHO grade I or II.

SPECIFIC NEOPLASMS

It is difficult, in many circumstances, to suggest a specific *histologic* diagnosis based on the imaging characteristics alone. However, when other factors are taken into account, such as the location of these tumors (intra-axial, extra-axial, intraventricular, sellar region, pineal region) and clinical information (age, gender, endocrinologic data, etc.), the differential diagnosis can be limited to just a few possibilities and sometimes a single most likely entity. Some intracranial tumors have a definite predilection for one gender and are listed in Table 5.2.

Intra-axial Tumors: Glial

Gliomas, derived from glial cells, account for 40% to 50% of all primary CNS neoplasms. Most of these tumors are histologically regarded as astrocytomas and oligodendrogliomas.

Astrocytomas account for 70% of all gliomas. These neoplasms are graded according to five histologic features: cellularity, mitotic activity, pleomorphism, necrosis, and endothelial proliferation. Four grades are currently recognized. The grade I tumors are generally well-circumscribed on imaging and gross pathologic inspection. The pilocytic

TABLE 5.2 Tumor Predominance by Gender

Females	*Males*
Meningioma (4:1)	Pineal germinoma (10:1)
Neurofibroma	Pineal parenchymal tumor (4:1 to 7:1)
Pineocytoma	Medulloblastoma (3:1)
Pituitary tumor	Glioblastoma multiforme (3:2)
	Choroid plexus papilloma (2:1)
	CNS lymphoma
	Hamartoma of the tuber cinereum

astrocytoma and subependymal giant cell astrocytoma are the prototypical examples of this tumor type. A diffuse astrocytoma lacking the well-circumscribed morphology seen in the grade I tumors but with a low degree of cellularity, mitotic activity, and pleomorphism characterizes the grade II tumors. Specifically, these tumors lack necrosis and endothelial proliferation. Grade III tumors, termed *anaplastic astrocytoma*, demonstrate increased amounts of cellularity, mitoses, and pleomorphism on histology. The most malignant form (WHO grade IV) of an astrocytoma, the *glioblastoma multiforme* (GBM), has marked amounts of cellularity, mitotic activity, and pleomorphism (as the name *multiforme* would imply). However, in contrast to the other types described, extensive necrosis and endothelial proliferation are prominent features of this tumor. All glial tumors lack a capsule and therefore have at least the potential to spread throughout the CNS. Still, the lower-grade (WHO grade I and II) astrocytomas and the higher-grade (WHO grade III and IV) astrocytomas are associated with certain distinct clinical and morphologic features that emphasize the differences in prognosis for patients with these tumors.

Lower-Grade Tumors. Since the lower-grade WHO I and WHO II astrocytomas are usually very slow-growing and exhibit such nonaggressive behavior, patients with these tumors often do well with surgical resection alone. Prognosis for these tumors is measured in terms of years. These astrocytomas tend to occur in younger patients, usually children and adults 20 to 40 years old. They are usually well-demarcated tumors without necrosis or neovascularity, rarely hemorrhage, and are often cystic. They show calcification in 20% of cases and rarely have surrounding edema. On CT, they are hypodense with little or no enhancement. On MR, compared to gray matter, they are hypointense on T1WIs, hyperintense on T2WIs, and show minimal enhancement (Fig. 5.5).

Higher-Grade Tumors. In contrast to the lower-grade astrocytomas, the higher-grade astrocytomas tend to occur in patients older than 40 years of age. These tumors are poorly delineated microscopically, although they may appear well-circumscribed grossly. Necrosis, hemorrhage, and neovascularity are common, particularly in the GBM. Surrounding white matter edema is very common (Table 5.3). On CT, they are typically heterogeneous. On MR they are isointense to hypointense compared to gray matter on T1WIs and hyperintense on T2WIs. A ringlike pattern on postcontrast imaging may be seen (Fig. 5.6).

Pathology. Astrocytomas may demonstrate a paradox in their gross appearances. The well-differentiated low-grade astrocytomas are frequently ill-defined, as they insinuate themselves through the neurons and other supporting cells that make up the "scaffold" of the brain parenchyma, whereas the highly malignant GBM is macroscopically better circumscribed. In truth, all astrocytomas are poorly circumscribed upon microscopic examination.

Spread. Gliomas spread from their native site by one of four ways. They may spread via the white matter tracts, such as the corona radiata, corticospinal tracts, corpus callosum, and hippocampal commissures. They may spread by way of either natural passages, such as the perivascular (Virchow-Robin) spaces, or along the subpial or subependymal surfaces. Finally, tumors may also rarely spread across the meninges.

Glioblastoma multiforme (GBM), the most malignant form of an astrocytoma, is also the most common type of glioma. The peak age of incidence is 45 to 55 years old, with men slightly more often affected. The deep white matter of the frontal lobe, the largest lobe in the brain, is the most common location, followed by the temporal lobe and the basal ganglia.

Imaging. The cross-sectional imaging appearance reflects the pattern of necrosis, hemorrhage, and neovascularity seen microscopically. The classic appearance on either CT or MR is an expansile mass with central necrosis, ring enhancement, and a large surrounding region of vasogenic edema. On noncontrast CT, the tumor is typically heterogeneous and lobulated, with marked surrounding white matter edema. Calcification may be seen occasionally. Necrosis and hemorrhage are common. The most common hemorrhagic neoplasms in the brain are GBM, metastasis, and oligodendroglioma (Table 5.4). On MR, the tumor nidus commonly shows T1 and T2 prolongation (dark on T1WIs, bright on T2WIs) compared to gray matter (Fig. 5.6). Because of cellular debris from the necrosis, the signal intensity of these cystlike areas is usually slightly different from that of CSF. Reflective of the endothelial proliferation seen histologically, the tumor tends to be highly vascular. Multiple markedly hypointense holes representing flow voids may occasionally be seen.

Ring Enhancement. On contrast-enhanced CT and MR, more than 90% of all GBMs will show at least some enhancement, usually in an irregular, occasionally nodular, ringlike pattern. Many other lesions can present with ring-enhancing masses. A convenient method to remember these is with the mnemonic *MAGIC DR* (Table 5.5). The first three entities (metastasis, abscess, and glioma) are by far the most common causes of this appearance and are listed in order of frequency. The "irregular ring" enhancement of a neoplasm is often distinct from the typical "smooth ring" seen in cerebral abscesses (compare Fig. 5.6 with Fig. 6.3A). Furthermore, an abscess rim typically is hyperintense on T1WIs and hypointense on T2WIs—features not commonly seen in tumors.

"Butterfly Glioma." GBM is one of two entities (CNS lymphoma is the other) that commonly may have bihemispheric spread through the corpus callosum with involvement of both frontal lobes. Because the imaging appearance somewhat resembles the wings of a butterfly, such masses are commonly referred to as "butterfly gliomas." It is important to recognize that abnormal signal intensity

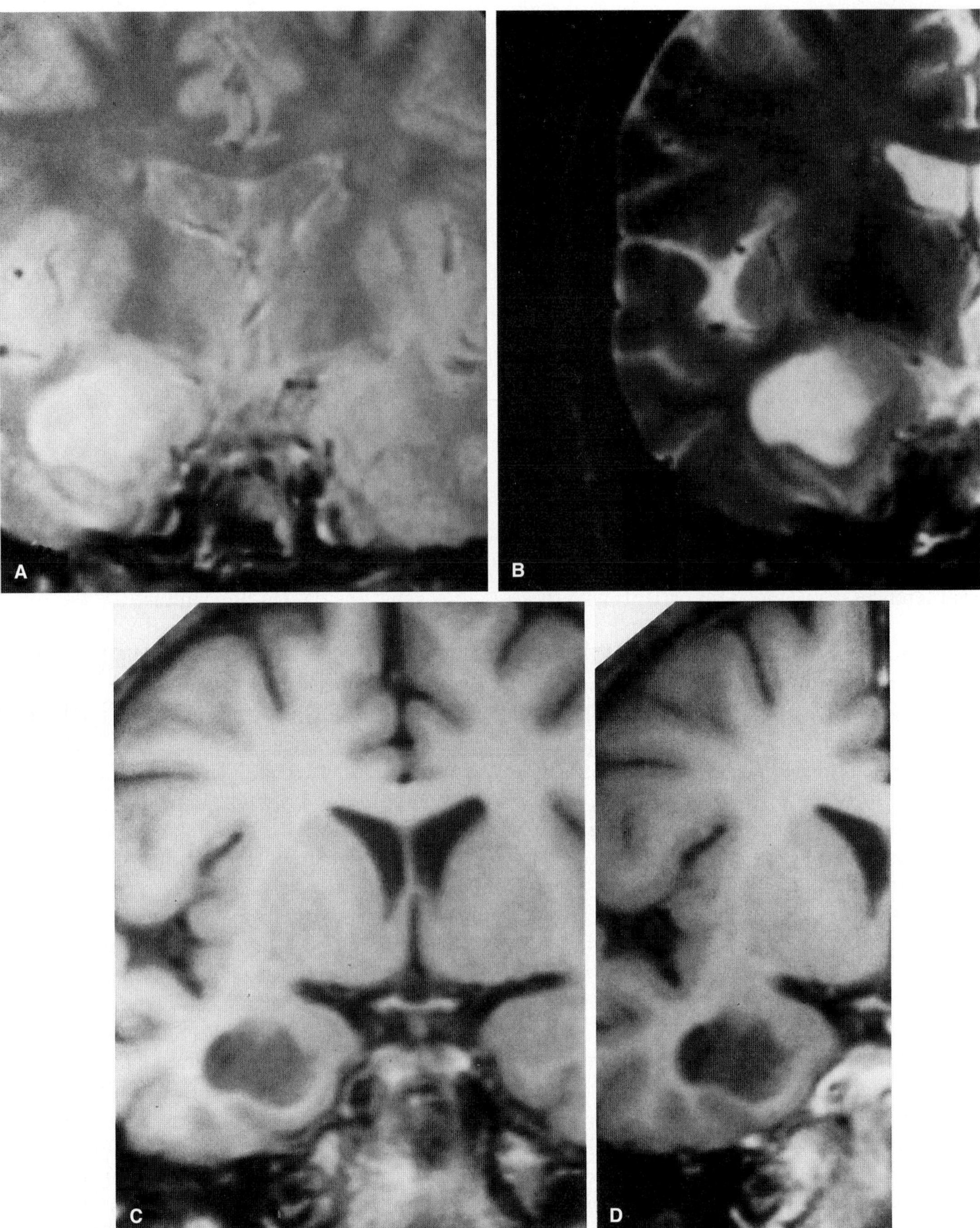

FIGURE 5.5. **Typical Appearance of Low-Grade Astrocytoma. A.** and **B.** Hyperintense well-defined temporal lobe mass on T2WIs. Precontrast **(C)** and postcontrast **(D)** T1WIs show hypointense mass without enhancement.

within the corpus callosum is secondary to the disease process itself and does not simply represent vasogenic edema. This is because the callosal fibers and projection fibers of the internal capsule are packed so tightly together that edema fluid cannot be conducted through them. Therefore, if a neoplasm is suspected, any T2 hyperintensity seen in the corpus callosum or internal capsule must be considered secondary to neoplastic spread and not a consequence of vasogenic edema. Other diseases, ranging from infection to demyelinating disease, may also involve the corpus callosum and produce the "butterfly glioma" appearance.

Treatment and Prognosis. Surgical resection, chemotherapy, and radiation therapy are standard treatments for patients with such tumors. Reduction in size, in association with some symptomatic improvement, is typically noted. Treated lesions are often extensively necrotic and calcified.

TABLE 5.3 Intra-axial Lesions With Marked Surrounding Edema

Metastasis	Radiation necrosis
Abscess	Hematoma (mild)
Glioblastoma multiforme	

However, usually within 1 year after surgery, the tumor frequently recurs. Therefore, the prognosis for these patients is much worse compared to those with the lower-grade astrocytomas. Patients with a GBM carry a dismal prognosis, with only a 2% survival rate at 3 years. New treatment modalities, such as gamma-knife surgery and more advanced chemotherapy protocols, are under constant evaluation in hopes of improving the poor outlook for affected patients.

Lower-grade astrocytomas are characterized by slow growth and are associated with a longer clinical course. Patients often have productive lives for many years following diagnosis. These tumors account for 20% to 30% of all gliomas. Men are slightly more frequently affected, and the peak incidence is between 30 and 40 years old. In children, they tend to occur along the optic pathways, hypothalamus, and near/in the third ventricle. In adults, the lesions are usually located in the cerebral hemispheres.

TABLE 5.4 Hemorrhagic Tumors

Glioblastoma multiforme: most common overall
Metastasis: second most common overall
- Renal cell carcinoma
- Thyroid carcinoma
- Choriocarcinoma
- Melanoma

Oligodendroglioma: second most common primary tumor

Pathology. Lower-grade astrocytomas are pathologically divided into the *fibrillary astrocytoma* (WHO grade II), the *pilocytic astrocytoma* (WHO grade I), and the *subependymal giant cell astrocytoma* (WHO grade I). The pilocytic astrocytoma will be discussed separately in the

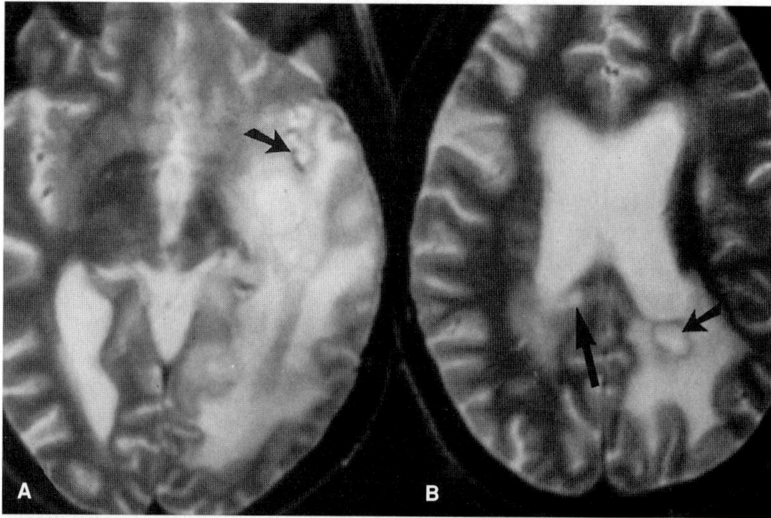

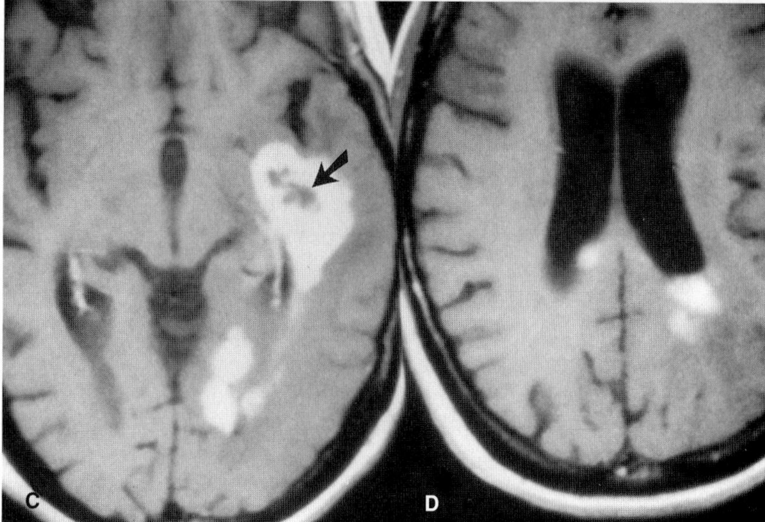

FIGURE 5.6. **Glioblastoma Multiforme. A.** and **B.** Axial T2WIs showing large areas of hyperintensity, predominantly in the left cerebral hemisphere. Note dark rim lesions (*small arrows*) of the anterior left temporal lobe and the left posterior periventricular area. Also note the abnormal hyperintensity (*large arrow*) extending across splenium of corpus callosum. **C.** and **D.** Postcontrast T1WIs through same levels as in **A** and **B** show multiple enhancing lesions corresponding to areas of T2 hyperintensity. The central area of hypointensity (*arrow*) within the left temporal lesion was proven pathologically to be necrosis, characteristic of glioblastoma multiforme.

TABLE 5.5 Ring-Enhancing Lesions ("MAGIC DR")

***M**etastasis*
***A**bscess*
***G**lioblastoma multiforme*
***I**nfarct (subacute phase)*
***C**ontusion*
***D**emyelinating disease*
***R**esolving hematoma, radiation necrosis*

"Posterior Fossa Tumors" section. *Gemistocytic astrocytoma* (WHO grade II) and *protoplasmic astrocytoma* (WHO grade II) are rare variants of the fibrillary form. The *pleomorphic xanthoastrocytoma* (WHO grade II) is a distinct clinicopathologic entity, primarily seen in adolescents and young adults, and is characterized by a heterogeneous mass with a soft tissue component located peripherally along the meningocerebral interface. It is believed that approximately 10% of all lower-grade astrocytomas will degenerate into a more aggressive WHO grade III or IV tumor.

Imaging. On CT and MR, these lesions generally have variable amounts of surrounding vasogenic edema and variable enhancement. Fewer than 50% will show enhancement in any portion of the mass. They may not be apparent on either noncontrast or contrast-enhanced CT and, rarely, may not even have any abnormal T2 hyperintensity. Calcification (25% of cases) and hemorrhage may be present, but necrosis does not occur. The tumors are usually poorly marginated, with mild mass effect (Fig. 5.5). The variable appearance may occasionally make distinction from an acute infarct difficult. In such circumstances, further evaluation with advanced MR techniques (e.g., DWI) may aid in establishing the correct diagnosis.

Treatment and Prognosis. Surgical resection is the primary therapeutic approach, with chemotherapy and radiation therapy used according to histologic grade and by experimental protocol. Recurrence is much less common compared to the GBM, and patients with these tumors enjoy a corresponding better outlook, with a mean survival time of 6 to 8 years.

Gliomatosis cerebri is a rare neuroepithelial neoplasm of unknown origin that is the result of widespread infiltration of neoplastic cells (probably astrocytes) in varying degrees of differentiation. By definition, at least three lobes of the brain are involved. Despite the diffuse involvement of the brain seen pathologically and on imaging studies, the clinical symptoms are often mild. Peak incidence is between 40 and 50 years of age, but it may occur at any time of life. Frequently, the lesion appears to smolder for weeks to years before erupting into a full-blown GBM or anaplastic astrocytoma. Radiotherapy may temporarily improve the radiologic appearance and improve clinical symptoms. The long-term prognosis is poor, with a less than 30% survival rate at 3 years.

Imaging. There are two basic imaging appearances of gliomatosis cerebri: diffuse involvement of the cerebral white matter without a mass, or one with a discrete mass. In the former, the CT appearance of gliomatosis cerebri is almost always normal, as the lesions are isodense to normal brain parenchyma and do not enhance. MR plays an important role in establishing this diagnosis, particularly in assessing the diffuse involvement of the brain. Involved regions are characterized by diffuse T1 and T2 prolongation throughout the white matter and gray matter, particularly the centrum semiovale, hypothalamus, basal ganglia, and thalamus. The relative lack of mass effect in this form of the disease is striking. Distinction between the gray matter and white matter is often lost. Enhancement is typically absent unless a distinct mass is present. This appearance may be quite similar to that seen in the progressive multifocal leukoencephalopathy that occurs in immunocompromised patients.

The second imaging appearance includes all of the features described above with the addition of a focal mass, which in most circumstances represents a WHO grade III or higher lesion. Evaluation with MRS is helpful in identifying the more biologically aggressive regions and directing potential sites for surgical biopsy.

Oligodendroglioma accounts for 5% to 18% of all gliomas (about 4% of all intracranial neoplasms). It is more common in adults, with a peak age of 30 to 50 years old. Children are affected in about 6% of cases. The tumor is supratentorial in 85% of cases and most commonly (50% to 65% of the time) located in the frontal lobe. The tumor usually grows slowly and, on microscopy, shows calcification in 100% of cases, with hemorrhage and cysts occurring in about 20% of cases. Hematogenous or subarachnoid spread is uncommon. Accordingly, the tumor warrants a WHO grade II designation. However, the postoperative survival rates for patients with this tumor are quite variable and disappointing, with 38% to 75% survival at 5 years and 20% to 60% survival at 10 years.

Frequently, the tumor is combined with elements of astrocytes and is accordingly labeled as a *mixed glioma* (e.g., oligoastrocytoma).

Imaging. Oligodendroglioma is most commonly located in the frontal lobes and often extends to the cortex, where it may erode the calvarium. On CT, calcification is reported in about 70% of cases, compared to about 25% of astrocytomas (Fig. 5.7). However, since the astrocytoma is so much more common than the oligodendroglioma, a calcified tumor in the brain is more likely to be an astrocytoma rather than an oligodendroglioma (Table 5.6). On MR, it is usually hypointense on T1WIs and hyperintense on T2WIs compared to gray matter. Surrounding vasogenic edema is seen in only about one third of cases. Following contrast administration, about 66% of these tumors show some enhancement, although the degree of enhancement is variable. The appearance in an adult of a heterogeneous

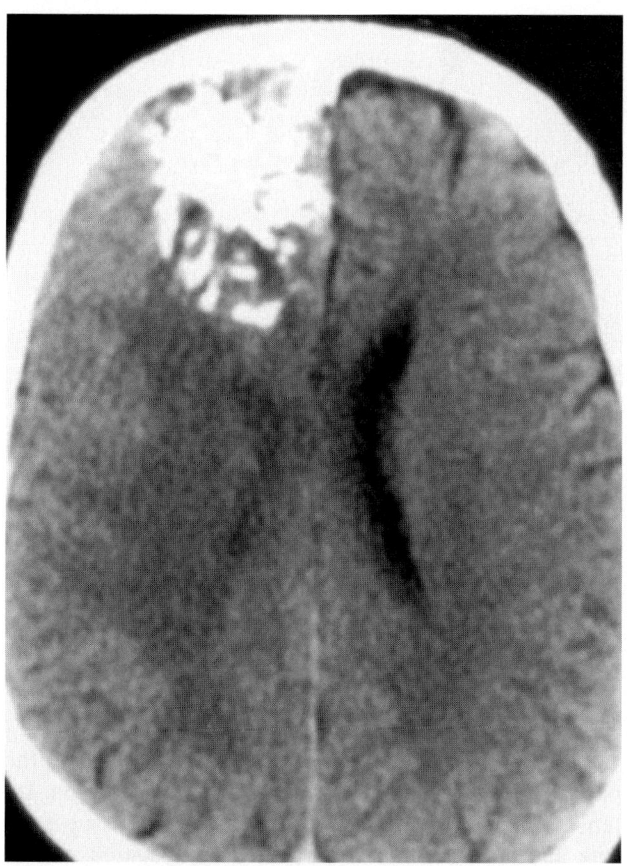

FIGURE 5.7. **Oligodendroglioma.** Axial CT shows heavily calcified mass of the right frontal lobe extending to the cortical margin.

calcified mass within the periphery of a frontal lobe with calvarial erosion and relative absence of edema should suggest the diagnosis of an oligodendroglioma. Variant forms include *oligoastrocytoma* and *anaplastic oligodendroglioma*. While the imaging appearance of the former is practically indistinguishable from that of oligodendroglioma, the latter tumor may mimic the appearance of a GBM.

Intra-axial Tumors: Nonglial and Mixed Glial

Primary CNS Lymphoma. The incidence and demographics of primary CNS lymphoma have changed dramatically as a consequence of the increasing population of immunocompromised patients, particularly those with AIDS. Once considered extremely rare as a primary neoplasm, this tumor (almost always a B-cell non-Hodgkin lymphoma) is now the fourth most common primary CNS neoplasm (following GBM, meningioma, and low-grade astrocytoma). There are some predictions that it will become the most common primary CNS neoplasm by the year 2010. Confusion, lethargy, and memory loss are common clinical symptoms. Interestingly, the tumor is exquisitely sensitive to steroid therapy and radiotherapy initially, only to rebound with a vengeance. This has led some to coin the phrase *ghost tumor* to describe this response. Consequently, it has been advocated to withhold steroid therapy prior to neurosurgical biopsy, because steroid treatment may interfere with accurate histologic interpretation. Recent therapeutic advances have led to some multi-year survivals.

Imaging. CNS lymphoma is composed of small blue cells with a high nucleus-to-cytoplasm ratio packed tightly together in the perivascular (Virchow-Robin) spaces. This histology directly correlates with the classic imaging appearance of hyperdensity on noncontrast CT and hypointensity on T2WIs, which is often contrasted with surrounding vasogenic edema. Another helpful clue is the tendency of lymphoma to be located either adjacent to the ventricular system or along the leptomeninges. At least some enhancement is seen in virtually all lesions. In immunocompromised patients, the imaging appearance changes to reflect the increased predilection for necrosis and multifocality (Fig. 5.8). Most lesions (85%) are supratentorial, with about 10% occurring in the cerebellum. Calcification and hemorrhage are rare. Subependymal spread is common, and bihemispheric involvement via the corpus callosum (the "butterfly glioma" pattern) may be seen.

Differentiating from Toxoplasmosis. In contrast to CNS lymphoma, toxoplasmosis is not associated with subependymal spread and, because it is an abscess, is more likely to be located within the gray matter–white matter junction or within the basal ganglia. Ringlike enhancement is typical on postcontrast imaging and, in some cases, may show a highly characteristic enhancing mural nodule. PET and SPECT-thallium scans, DWI, and MRS may differentiate between primary CNS lymphoma and toxoplasmosis. When these modalities are not available, an empiric trial of anti-*Toxoplasma* therapy for 3 weeks may be utilized. If the lesions do not regress in size, a presumption is made that the lesion is not toxoplasmosis, and a stereotactic biopsy may be performed to secure the diagnosis. Other considerations in the differential diagnosis include metastasis and focal cerebritis.

Ganglioglioma and Gangliocytoma. As its name implies, *ganglioglioma* is composed of both glial cells and differentiated neurons (ganglion cells). In contrast, *gangliocytoma* and *ganglioneuroma* are pure neuronal tumors without a glial component. Both ganglioglioma and gangliocytoma account for about 1% of all intracranial

TABLE 5.6 Calcified Glial Tumors: "Old Elephants Age Gracefully," in Order of Frequency

Oligodendroglioma
Ependymoma
Astrocytoma
Glioblastoma multiforme

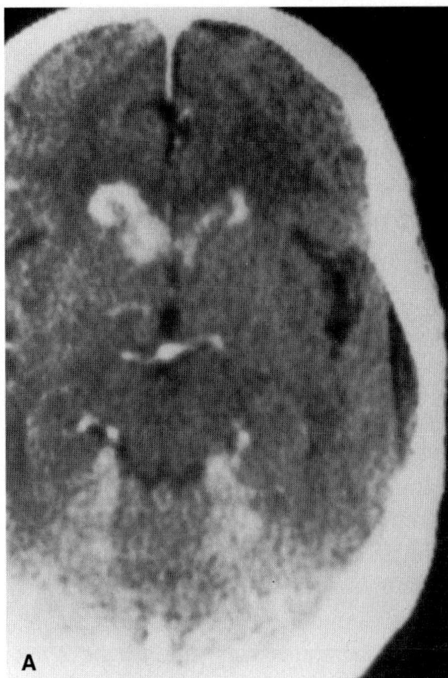

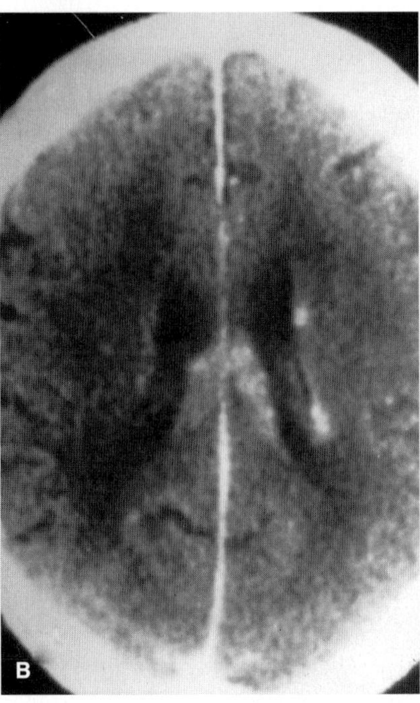

FIGURE 5.8. **CNS Lymphoma.** A 69-year-old immunocompromised man with altered mental status of a progressive nature. Postcontrast axial CT scans show multiple areas of enhancement in a predominantly periventricular distribution. Involvement of the genu of the corpus callosum and subependymal spread (within the frontal horns) are also seen.

neoplasms and are relatively low-grade neoplasms associated with a good prognosis. While they may occur at any time of life, most (80%) occur in patients younger than 30 years of age. Males are slightly more commonly affected. Reflective of their slow growth, the clinical presentation is often with long-standing symptoms, typically in the form of focal seizures or hypothalamic dysfunction, depending on their location. Ganglioglioma is the most common tumor seen in patients with chronic temporal lobe epilepsy. While the temporal lobe is the most common location, they may occur anywhere, even within the spinal cord. The floor of the third ventricle is the most common location of the gangliocytoma.

Imaging. On CT, these tumors are most often hypodense or isodense, well-circumscribed lesions with little associated mass effect or surrounding edema. A peripheral location and calcification (35%) are frequent features of gangliogliomas. The tumors may or may not enhance on postcontrast imaging. On MR, they are usually hypointense to isointense relative to gray matter on T1WIs and almost always hyperintense to gray matter on T2WIs. The imaging appearance is not specific and may be mimicked by lower-grade astrocytoma, oligodendroglioma, and dysembryoplastic neuroepithelial tumor (Fig. 5.3).

Desmoplastic Infantile Ganglioglioma. This rare variant of ganglioglioma manifests as a very large heterogeneous mass and is almost always seen in the first year of life. Boys are affected twice as often as girls. A rapidly expanding head circumference is the most common clinical finding. The typical imaging appearance is a large peripheral heterogeneous mass with both cystlike and solid components. The solid soft tissue region is almost always located along the meningocerebral interface, similar to the pattern seen in the pleomorphic xanthoastrocytoma. Intense enhancement of this "desmoplastic" soft tissue is the rule. Because of adherence of the desmoplastic tissue to the dura, surgical resection is often difficult and the overall prognosis is guarded.

Dysembryoplastic Neuroepithelial Tumor. Originally described in 1988, dysembryoplastic neuroepithelial tumor (DNT) is the most common tumor associated with medically refractory partial complex seizures. Most patients are between 10 and 30 years old, and neurologic deficits are not common. The overall prognosis for patients is excellent even if only partial resection of the tumor is attained. Tumors are identified histologically by the presence of cortical dysplasia and an oligodendroglial pattern ("specific glioneuronal unit"). Accordingly, the tumor is peripheral in location, as it almost always involves the cortical gray matter. Some lesions may produce a "soap bubble" appearance with exophytic extension beyond the normal cortical gray matter margin. Pressure erosion effects in the adjacent skull may be seen in such cases. Calcification occurs in only about 5% of cases, much less than noted in gangliogliomas. Corresponding to its WHO grade I classification, surrounding vasogenic edema is almost always absent. Enhancement is variable.

Supratentorial primitive neuroectodermal tumor (S-PNET) is primarily noted in the early childhood period, with a mean age of presentation at 5 years. Males are more commonly affected. Along with teratoma, the S-PNET is one of the most common congenital intracranial neoplasms (Table 5.7). Patients typically present with symptoms of increased intracranial pressure or seizures. Overall, the tumor is associated with a poorer prognosis

TABLE 5.7 Congenital Brain Tumors in Infants Younger Than 60 Days Old

Teratoma: most common (one third to one half of all tumors), two thirds are supratentorial
Primitive neuroectodermal tumors: curvilinear, sparse calcification
Astrocytoma
Choroid plexus papilloma
Ependymoma
Medulloepithelioma
Germinoma
Angioblastic meningioma
Ganglioglioma

(34% 5-year survival rate) compared to the medulloblastoma (85%).

Pathology. S-PNET is believed to arise from bipotential precursor cells of the germinal matrix with the ability to differentiate along either glial or neuronal cell lines. Because similar histology is also seen in other tumors (notably, medulloblastoma, ependymoblastoma, pineoblastoma, and retinoblastoma), some authorities have proposed that all of these tumors should be considered PNETs. However, the majority opinion of the latest WHO classification considers all of these tumors as separate clinicopathologic entities and restricts the use of the term *PNET* to a small group of embryonal tumors within the cerebral hemispheres or suprasellar region.

Imaging. The most common cross-sectional imaging appearance is a large well-demarcated heterogeneous mass with both solid and cystlike areas within the deep cerebral white matter. A periventricular or intraventricular location with hydrocephalus is common. On CT, calcification is very common (50% to 70% of cases). Regions of necrosis and hemorrhage are also common. Surrounding vasogenic edema is variable. The solid nonhemorrhagic portions of the tumor are usually hypointense on T1WIs and isointense to hypointense on T2WIs compared to gray matter. These regions enhance on postcontrast imaging.

Metastasis to the CNS from extracranial sites accounts for about one third of all intracranial neoplasms. Metastases may be intra-axial (most commonly from lung, breast, melanoma, and colon carcinomas); within the subarachnoid spaces; extra-axial; dural (most commonly, breast carcinoma, lymphoma, prostate carcinoma, lung carcinoma, and neuroblastoma); or skull (Table 5.8). They may occur at any age but most frequently present in older age groups, often with seizures or focal deficits. Clinically silent metastases are most common in patients with oat cell carcinoma, lung carcinoma (especially adenocarcinoma), and melanoma.

Most (80% to 85%) metastatic lesions occur supratentorially, with the exception of renal cell carcinoma, which has a predilection for the posterior fossa. While most metastases are multiple, up to 30% are solitary (with melanoma, lung carcinoma, and breast carcinoma the most likely primaries). About 10% of metastases are hemorrhagic and are especially common in melanoma, thyroid carcinoma, and renal cell carcinoma (Fig. 5.9).

TABLE 5.8 Most Common Metastases to the CNS

Intra-axial	*Extra-axial*	*Hemorrhagic*
Lung carcinoma	Breast carcinoma	Melanoma
Breast carcinoma	Prostate carcinoma	Renal carcinoma
Melanoma	Lung carcinoma	Thyroid carcinoma
Colon carcinoma	Neuroblastoma	Choriocarcinoma

Imaging. The classic appearance of metastatic spread on CT or MR is one of multiple foci located at the gray matter–white matter junction, hypodense on CT, hypointense on T1WIs, and variable signal intensity on T2WIs, with marked vasogenic edema surrounding each lesion. Upon contrast administration, there is intense enhancement, which is variable in its form (ring or nodular) (Fig. 5.10). Postcontrast MR is especially helpful in the detection of cortically based lesions, which do not demonstrate much edema in the surrounding parenchyma (presumably because of a lack of interstitial tissue). Triple-dose gadolinium MR studies may reveal additional lesions when only a single lesion is evident on a single-dose study. This may be an important patient management consideration, because a patient with a single metastasis may be treated by surgical resection whereas one with multiple lesions is more commonly treated by radiotherapy or chemotherapy.

Leptomeningeal Spread. Leptomeningeal carcinomatosis is the result of leptomeningeal spread by primary CNS malignancies, extracranial adenocarcinoma (especially of lung or breast origin), leukemia, or lymphoma. Characterized by basilar cistern involvement, patients commonly present with cranial nerve palsies. Not surprisingly, its imaging appearance may exactly mimic that of meningitis. Postcontrast MR is the imaging modality of choice and detection is enhanced using fat suppression, FLAIR, or magnetization transfer techniques. The presence of hydrocephalus in a patient with a known malignancy should raise the possibility of this diagnosis.

Skull Lesions. As with metastases to the spinal vertebral bodies, those that arise in the skull may be obscured if only contrast-enhanced T1WIs are reviewed. For this reason, noncontrast T1WIs should always be obtained in cases of suspected skull metastasis. Inversion recovery images and fat-suppressed T2WIs are other MR sequences of value. While CT with bone windows is superior in detecting subtle bone erosion, MR is superior in evaluating epidural and intracranial extension of skull metastasis.

Posterior Fossa Tumors

The posterior fossa is the most common site for intracranial neoplasms in the pediatric population. Medulloblastoma and cerebellar astrocytoma account for about two

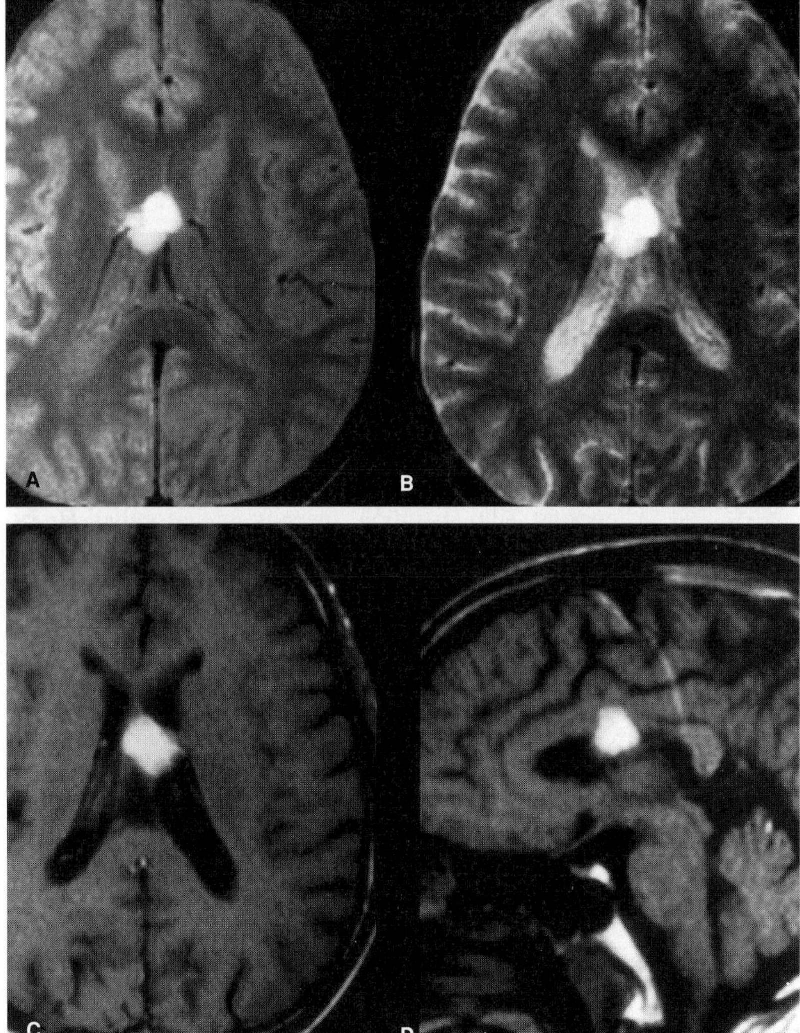

FIGURE 5.9. **Thyroid Metastasis.** Adult woman with florid pulmonary metastases (not shown) from thyroid carcinoma and recent onset of headaches. Axial T2WIs (**A,** first echo; **B,** second echo) show hyperintense mass of corpus callosum body. Hyperintensity persists on axial **(C)** and sagittal **(D)** T1WIs (without contrast), confirming the hemorrhagic nature of the lesion. Metastases from renal cell carcinoma, choriocarcinoma, and melanoma are the most common to hemorrhage. Among primary tumors, glioblastoma multiforme and oligodendroglioma are the most common to do so.

thirds of all posterior fossa neoplasms in children, with ependymoma and brainstem glioma composing the remaining third (Table 5.9). The hemangioblastoma is the most common primary cerebellar neoplasm in the adult population. Symptoms related to cerebellar dysfunction (ataxia, nausea, vomiting, etc.) or cranial nerve deficits dominate the clinical picture of patients with these lesions.

Medulloblastoma is the most common pediatric CNS malignancy and, along with the pilocytic astrocytoma, the most common pediatric posterior fossa tumor. Most cases manifest before 10 years of age, with peak incidence between 4 and 8 years. A smaller peak is also seen between 15 and 35 years of age, and the tumor may occasionally manifest well into the older adult ages. Males are more commonly affected (60%). A brief clinical presentation of less than 3 months is typical and usually includes headache, vomiting, and truncal ataxia. The vast majority (85%) arise from the cerebellar vermis. Extension into the adjacent fourth ventricle and subsequent development of hydrocephalus is common. When the tumor arises in older children and adults, it tends to be located more laterally within the cerebellar hemisphere. Accordingly, the tumor is believed to arise from undifferentiated bipotential precursor cells, which are located in the cerebellar midline early in life and then migrate more laterally with advancing age. Medulloblastoma is a highly malignant neoplasm (WHO grade IV) with rapid growth. Subarachnoid CSF spread is common (33%) at the time of diagnosis.

Imaging. Most medulloblastomas manifest as solid, hyperdense masses on CT. Cystic change or necrosis occurs in up to 60% of cases and calcification is noted in 20%. Hemorrhage is rare. The single most reliable way to differentiate a medulloblastoma from an astrocytoma on cross-sectional imaging studies is to utilize a noncontrast CT scan; the astrocytoma will usually be hypodense and the medulloblastoma will almost never be hypodense. The

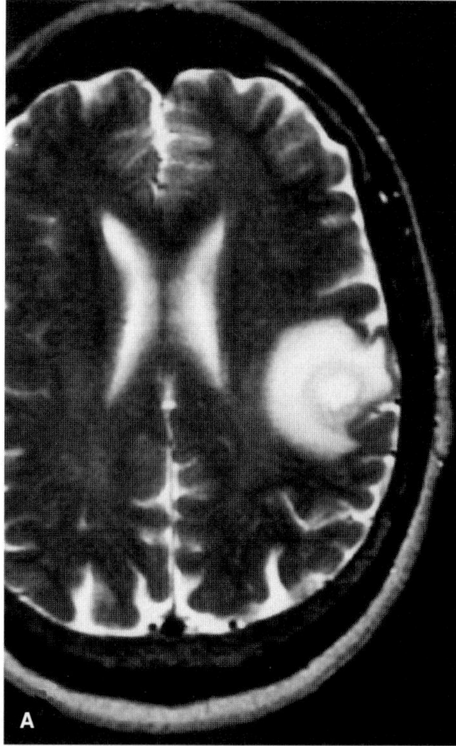

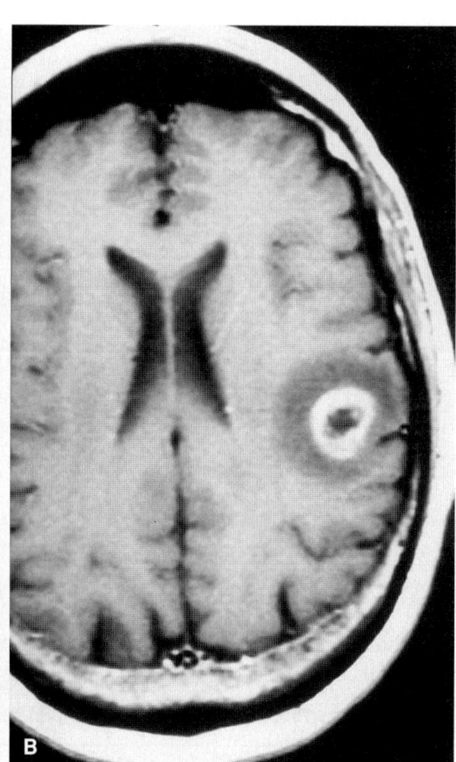

FIGURE 5.10. **Cerebral Metastasis.** Axial T2WI **(A)** shows prominent T2 prolongation consistent with vasogenic edema surrounding a lesion within the left posterior frontal lobe. Note the mildly hypointense ring representing the margin of the mass. Postcontrast axial T1WI **(B)** shows intense ring enhancement with a central hypointense area. The irregular shape of the rim (compared with the usual smooth wall of an abscess) is a clue to the true nature of this lung metastasis.

combination of falcine calcification and medulloblastoma has been linked with nevoid basal cell carcinoma.

On MR, the tumor is usually isointense to hypointense compared to white matter on T1WIs and has a more variable appearance on T2WIs, probably reflecting the varying nucleus-to-cytoplasm ratio. Surrounding vasogenic edema is almost always present. Blurring of the cerebellar folia on the midline sagittal MR image can be a helpful differentiating feature and reflects the infiltrative nature of these neoplasms. Following administration of contrast, the tumor demonstrates intense although usually heterogeneous enhancement (Fig. 5.11). Cerebellopontine angle involvement is rare. MRS evaluation has revealed elevated choline, reduced NAA, reduced creatine, and occasionally elevated lipid and lactic acid peaks.

TABLE 5.9 Posterior Fossa Masses in Children

Tumor	*Location*	*Appearance*
Medulloblastoma	Cerebellar vermis (85%)	Hyperdense on CT Hypointense on T1WIs Variable on T2WIs
Pilocytic astrocytoma	Cerebellar vermis, hemisphere	Cystic, with solid mural nodule that enhances intensely
Ependymoma	Fourth ventricle	Foraminal extension Heterogeneous on CT and MR Intense but heterogeneous enhancement
Brainstem glioma	Brainstem	Expansile brainstem Isodense to hypodense on CT Hypointense on T1WIs Hyperintense on T2WIs

Treatment. Surgical resection, chemotherapy, and radiation therapy are the primary means of treatment for patients with a medulloblastoma. CSF metastases are commonly found in the ventricular system, at the operative site, and in the thecal sac of the spinal canal. The presence of such lesions is associated with a poorer prognosis. Postcontrast MR imaging plays a pivotal role in demonstrating metastatic spread as brightly enhancing foci in these locations. It is particularly important that postcontrast MR evaluation of the spinal canal be performed preoperatively. Postoperative granulation tissue and hemorrhagic debris interferes with the accurate detection of "drop" metastases during the first 6 to 8 weeks after surgery, thereby delaying appropriate therapy and potentially threatening survival. Systemic metastasis may occur in about 5% of cases, with bone being the most common site (77%).

Pilocytic astrocytoma is the most common pediatric CNS tumor and is virtually as common as the medulloblastoma among all tumors arising in the posterior fossa. The

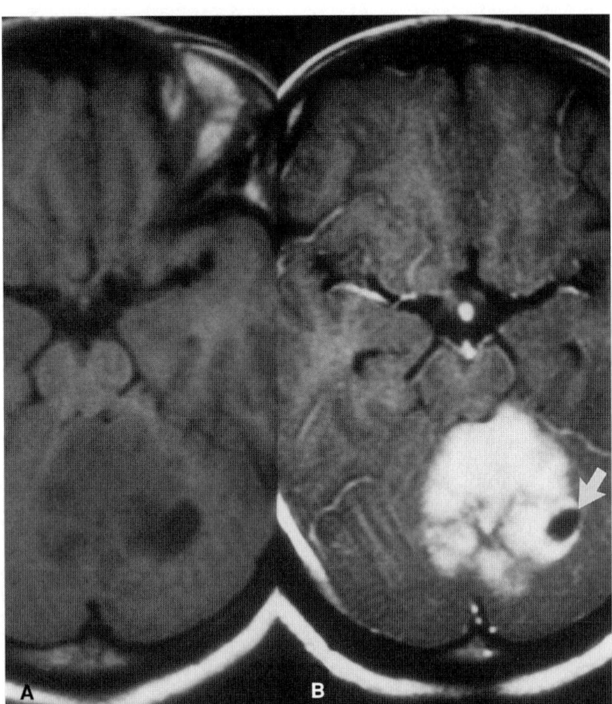

FIGURE 5.11. **Medulloblastoma.** Axial T1W precontrast **(A)** and postcontrast **(B)** images demonstrate a fairly well-circumscribed and intensely enhancing posterior fossa mass that lies in the region of the vermis and extends slightly into the left cerebellar hemisphere. The well-defined area of hypointensity (*arrow*) along the left lateral margin of enhancing mass represents a cyst, a not uncommon feature of these tumors.

most common location is the cerebellum (60%), and the tumor accounts for 85% of all cerebellar astrocytomas. Other common locations include the optic pathways and hypothalamus. Most patients present before 20 years of age and the clinical presentation is typically of several months' duration. Headache, vomiting, gait disturbance, blurred vision, diplopia, and neck pain are common symptoms when the tumor arises in the cerebellum. Pilocytic astrocytoma is the most common tumor seen in neurofibromatosis type 1 (NF1) and is present in 15% to 21% of all NF1 patients, usually in sites other than the cerebellum. The tumor is regarded as WHO grade I.

Imaging. There are two basic imaging manifestations of pilocytic astrocytoma. About 66% are cystlike with an enhancing mural nodule. The cyst wall may or may not enhance. The other third of cases manifest as solid masses with or without a necrotic center. Calcification occurs in 20% of cases, usually in the solid tumor types. Hemorrhage is rare. On CT, they present as a well-demarcated vermian or hemispheric mass, with the solid portion being isodense or hypodense to brain tissue. On MR, they are isointense to hypointense compared to gray matter on T1WIs and hyperintense compared to gray matter on T2WIs. The cystic portion usually contains proteinaceous fluid and therefore does not exactly follow the signal intensity of CSF. On noncontrast MR, one should exercise caution in ascribing hypointensity on T1WIs and hyperintensity on T2WIs within a mass as "cystic." Truly cystic lesions can only be confidently identified by the presence of fluid–fluid levels or wave pulsation phenomenon. Surrounding vasogenic edema is rare. The mural nodule of the cystic forms enhances intensely, while the solid component of the noncystic forms enhances to some degree but is more variable in intensity (Fig. 5.12).

Differential Diagnosis. The appearance of a cystic cerebellar mass with an enhancing mural nodule should suggest two possible diagnoses, and the best discriminator between the two is the patient's age. Pilocytic astrocytoma occurs much more commonly in children, with a peak age of birth to 9 years. In contrast, the peak age of presentation for a hemangioblastoma is 35 years. This tumor is the

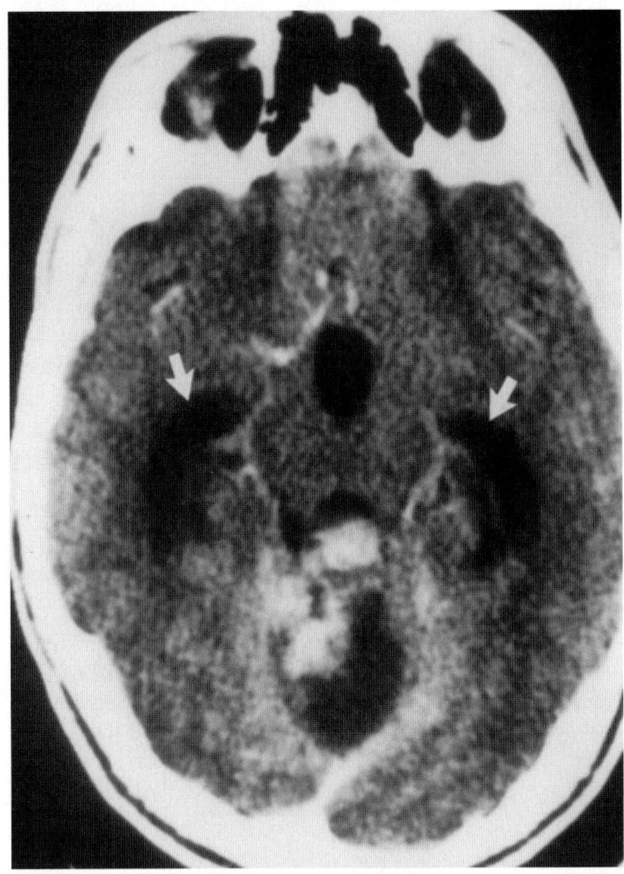

FIGURE 5.12. **Pilocytic Astrocytoma.** Axial postcontrast CT scan shows a heterogeneous posterior fossa mass with both cystic and solid enhancing components. Hydrocephalus, as evidenced by the dilated temporal horns (*arrows*), is also present. Hemangioblastomas may also appear as cystic posterior fossa masses with mural nodules. Age of the patient is a useful discriminator between pilocytic astrocytomas (peak age, 9 years) and hemangioblastomas (peak age, 35 years).

most common *primary* cerebellar neoplasm of the posterior fossa in adults, but metastasis is the most common cerebellar adult neoplasm overall. Other possible cerebellar lesions include infection (especially toxoplasmosis) and other cystic gliomas.

Ependymoma accounts for about 3% to 9% of all neuroepithelial neoplasms and most commonly manifests in children and adolescents. The tumor arises from the ependymal cells that line the ventricular system and the central canal of the spinal cord. Not surprisingly, the tumor is most commonly seen as an intraventricular or spinal cord mass. In children, 60% to 70% occur within the posterior fossa, with 70% of those centered within the fourth ventricle. Curiously, there is a predilection of the tumor to originate within the brain itself (i.e., intra-axial) instead of the ventricular system when it arises supratentorially. Symptoms are insidious at onset and are related to increased intraventricular pressure from obstruction of CSF flow.

Pathology. Ependymoma is a moderately cellular tumor with fairly low biologic behavior and is considered WHO grade II. When it arises in the fourth ventricle, this soft and pliable tumor frequently extends through the foramina of Luschka or Magendie into the cerebellopontine angle. Calcification occurs in 40% to 80% of cases. Subarachnoid seeding is rare, and its presence should suggest the possibility of a malignant ependymoma. When the tumor arises in the fourth ventricle, gross total resection is difficult to attain, leading to increased recurrence and decreased survival. Overall 5-year survival is about 60%. Several variant forms (cellular, papillary, clear cell, tanycytic, and anaplastic) have been identified.

Imaging. On CT, these tumors are isodense with a mixture of calcification, cystic change, and even hemorrhage, producing an overall heterogeneous appearance. This pattern is also seen on MR, where they are isointense compared to gray matter on T1WIs and hyperintense to gray matter on T2WIs. Following contrast, there is heterogeneous enhancement of the solid component. Extraventricular extension from the fourth ventricle through the adjacent foramina is highly characteristic (Fig. 5.13). Choroid plexus papilloma may demonstrate a similar appearance. Postoperative MR evaluation with contrast is important to exclude residual disease, which carries a poorer prognosis.

Brainstem glioma accounts for about 15% of all pediatric CNS neoplasms. There is no gender predilection and the peak incidence is between 3 and 10 years of age. The overwhelming majority of such tumors are astrocytomas; they range the entire WHO classification but most often are WHO grade I or II lesions. Regardless of the grade, the tumor infiltrates through the normal tracts and produces expansile enlargement of the brainstem, causing cranial nerve palsies, pyramidal tract signs, and ataxia as a consequence. Because of the numerous critical structures (e.g., cranial nerve nuclei) located within this region, the prognosis for patients with a brainstem glioma is guarded (10% to 30% 5-year survival). Chemotherapy and radiation therapy, rather than surgery, are the main treatment options. The tumor is difficult to treat and nearly always recurs within 2 years after completion of therapy.

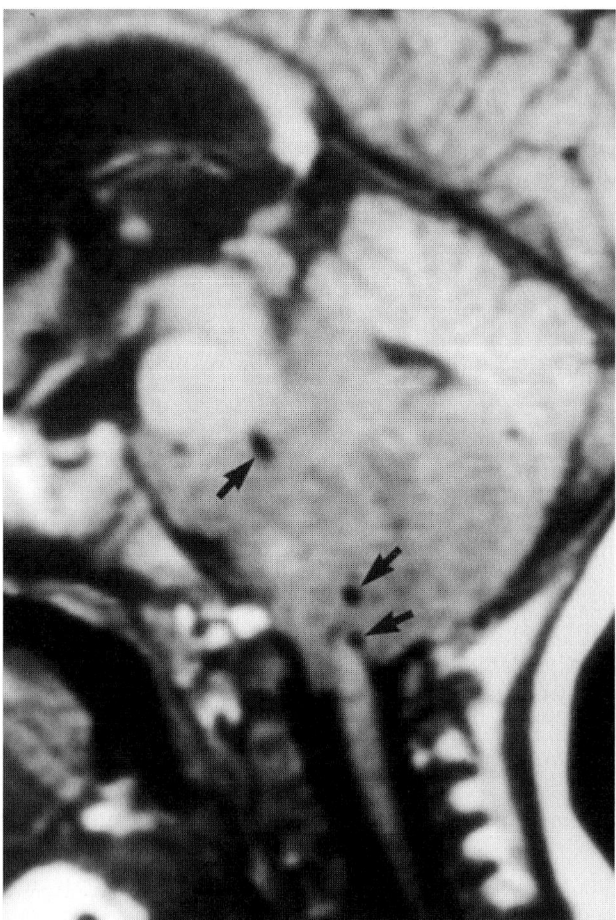

FIGURE 5.13. **Ependymoma.** Sagittal noncontrast T1WI in 4-year-old patient with ataxia. A lobulated mass extends inferiorly through the foramen magnum. The mass also extended through the foramen of Luschka (not shown). The tumor is centered within the fourth ventricle, with only a small portion of the fourth ventricle still visible at the superior margin of the mass. The dark holes (*arrows*) contained within the mass represent vessels surrounded by this soft tumor.

Key Features. Detection of a brainstem glioma may be difficult. Three imaging features are helpful in suggesting the diagnosis. First, exophytic growth into the adjacent cisternal spaces occurs in about 60% of cases. Second, if the ventral portion of the pons extends beyond the anterior margin of the basilar artery, then abnormal enlargement of the pons is present. In addition to brainstem glioma, diagnostic considerations include encephalitis, tuberculoma, acute disseminated encephalomyelitis, infarction, resolving hematoma, and vascular malformation. The presence of blood breakdown products on MR makes detection of one of the vascular causes fairly straightforward. However, encephalitis and tuberculoma cannot be distinguished from a brainstem glioma based on imaging characteristics alone. Third, alteration of the normal fourth ventricle contour provides a useful clue. The floor of the fourth ventricle may be flattened, the ventricle itself may be displaced posteriorly, and the ventricle may be rotated if there is involvement of the lateral recesses. In cases in which the tumor grows exophytically into the cerebellar hemispheres, it may mimic a cerebellar astrocytoma. Occasionally, a brainstem glioma may involve not only the pons (the most common site) but also the medulla and even the cervical cord. When a brainstem glioma extends through the foramen magnum, it may resemble an ependymoma. However, ependymomas are separate from the brainstem and typically enhance more vigorously than brainstem gliomas.

Imaging. On CT, brainstem gliomas manifests as a focal, hypodense to isodense expansion of the brainstem, with extremely variable enhancement that may change with time. Although the degree of enhancement does not reliably correlate with the grade of the tumor, the presence of calcification within the mass implicates a lower-grade tumor. On MR, typical prolongation of T1 and T2 is seen (Fig. 5.14). T2WIs are best to assess the true extent of the tumor, because the signal hyperintensity of the tumor contrasts sharply with the relatively low signal of normal white matter. Because of the slow growth of these tumors, hydrocephalus is not usually seen. Hemorrhages or cysts occur in about 25% of cases.

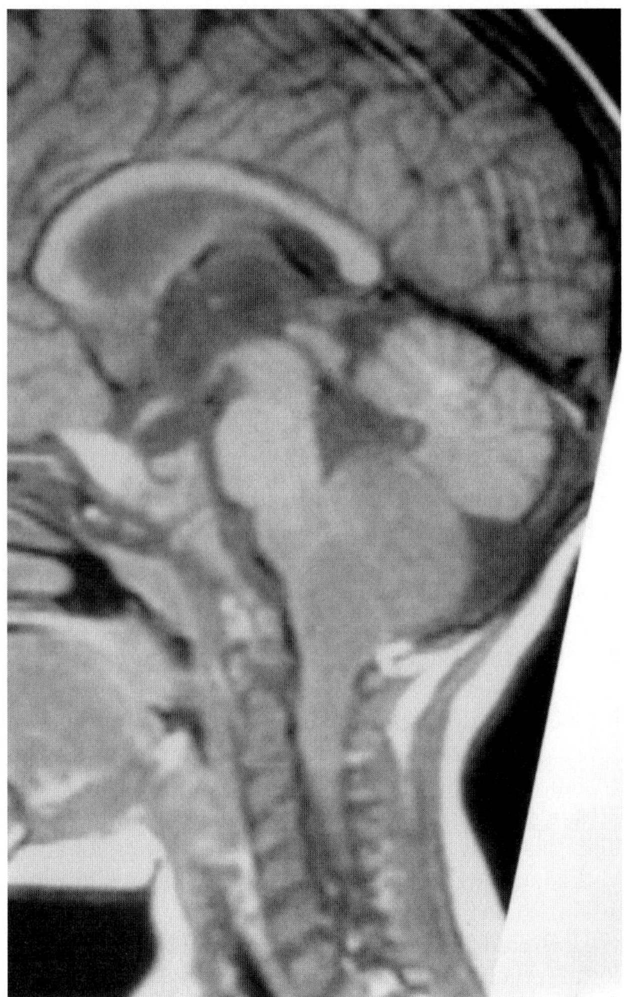

FIGURE 5.14. **Brainstem Glioma.** Midline sagittal T1WI in a young child with progressive ataxia. The large mass, slightly hypointense to the normal surrounding brainstem, has a large exophytic component and involves the upper cervical cord as well.

Capillary hemangioblastomas are benign neoplasms of endothelial origin. They are most common in young and middle-aged adults and are the most common primary cerebellar neoplasm in the adult population. Approximately 4% to 20% occur as part of the von Hippel-Lindau syndrome (discussed in Chapter 8), in which case they are often multiple. They occur most often in the cerebellar hemispheres; other sites of involvement include the spinal cord (especially the cervical portion), medulla, and even the cerebral hemispheres (very rare). Because they contain no capsule, recurrence is common if only partial resection is performed.

Imaging. The classic appearance is a well-defined cystic mass with an intensely enhancing mural nodule (60% of cases). Because the tumor nidus receives its blood supply from the pia mater, the nodule (which represents the tumor itself) is always superficial in location. Up to 40% are entirely solid and have a nonspecific imaging appearance. Calcification is very rare. On MR, they manifest as cystlike masses with hypointensity on T1WIs and hyperintensity on T2WIs compared to gray matter. Surrounding edema may be present. Serpiginous flow voids within the nodule may be seen in some cases. In the less common presentation of a solid mass, the margins are usually ill-defined, and occasionally hemorrhage is present. Because of the highly vascular nature of the nodule, intense enhancement is the rule (Fig. 5.15). If CT or MR is negative in highly clinically suspicious cases, angiography may be helpful in revealing small (less than 1 cm) lesions.

Dysplastic Cerebellar Gangliocytoma (Lhermitte-Duclos Disease). Although believed to represent a hamartoma and not a true neoplasm by WHO standards, the imaging appearance of a dysplastic cerebellar gangliocytoma is similar to that of many neoplasms arising in this region. The disease carries the eponym of the two physicians credited with identifying the index case in 1920. Half of all patients with the disease also have Cowden disease, an autosomal dominant phacomatosis associated with colonic polyps, cutaneous tumors, meningioma, and glioma, as well as thyroid and breast neoplasms. The CT appearance is often normal. The classic feature seen on MR imaging is a "striated" cerebellar mass on both T1WIs and T2WIs

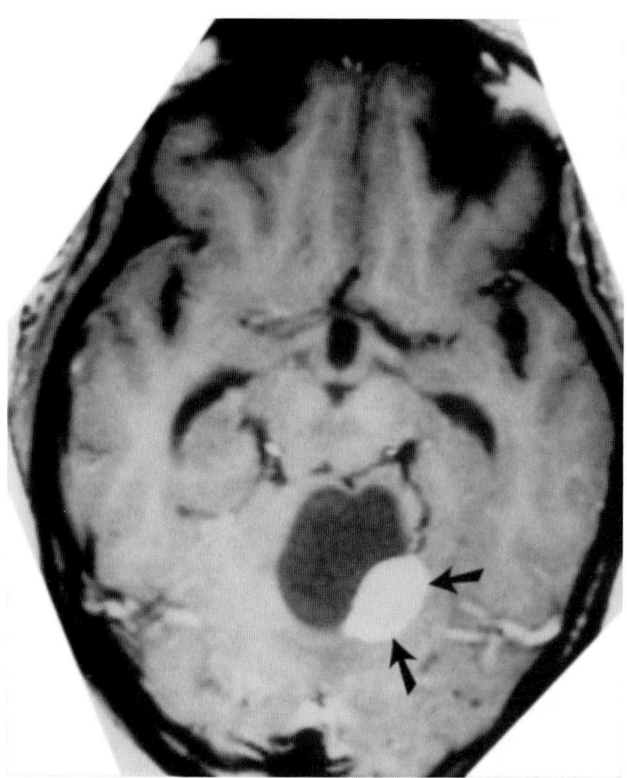

FIGURE 5.15. **Hemangioblastoma.** Classic appearance on postcontrast axial T1WI of a cystlike posterior fossa mass with intensely enhancing mural nodule (*arrow*), which represents the tumor itself.

with minimal surrounding vasogenic edema and no enhancement on postcontrast studies.

Atypical teratoid/rhabdoid tumor (ATRT) shares biologic and histologic features with the malignant rhabdoid tumor of the kidney. It accounts for about 2% of all pediatric CNS tumors, and most patients are less than 5 years of age at the time of presentation. The tumor is highly malignant and classified as WHO grade IV. About half of all tumors arise in the posterior fossa. While it often mimics the appearance of a medulloblastoma, ATRT frequently extends into the adjacent cerebellopontine cistern, a feature rarely associated with a medulloblastoma.

Extra-axial Tumors

Meningioma is by far the most common extra-axial neoplasm of adults and accounts for 15% of all intracranial neoplasms, second only to gliomas in overall prevalence. The peak age of presentation is 50 to 60 years of age. For both intracranial (2:1) and intraspinal (4:1) meningiomas, women are more commonly affected. Because the tumor is hormonally sensitive, it may increase in size during pregnancy. Multiple tumors (up to 9% of all cases) are associated with neurofibromatosis. The tumor is rare in children without this phacomatosis. Most meningiomas have benign biologic activity and grow slowly, most frequently found in parasagittal or convexity locations (50%). Other locations include the sphenoid wing (20%), the olfactory groove/planum sphenoidale (10%), the parasellar region (10%), and a wide range of miscellaneous locations (10%), such as the ventricles (the most common site in children), the tentorium, and the optic nerve sheath. About 2% to 3% are intraspinal, with the thoracic spine the most common location.

Pathology. Meningioma arises from arachnoid cap, cells with some probable contribution from dural fibroblasts and pial cells. It is believed that intraventricular meningiomas arise from arachnoidal cap cell rests that are buried within the choroid plexus. There are 15 types of meningioma identified in the WHO classification scheme, nine of which are considered WHO grade I, three as WHO grade II, and three as WHO grade III tumors. Despite these histologic distinctions, only two basic shapes are noted on imaging studies: globular and en plaque. Malignant variants of meningiomas are rare, occurring in about 1% of cases. It is not possible to reliably distinguish malignant from nonmalignant meningiomas based on imaging characteristics alone.

Imaging. Meningiomas present some of the most classic radiologic findings of any disease process. Even on plain skull films, these tumors can be suspected by the findings of focal sclerosis, prominent dural grooves from enlarged middle meningeal arteries, and calcification. On CT, a well-defined hyperdense (85%) mass with variable surrounding edema and intense and homogeneous enhancement on postcontrast studies is highly characteristic (Fig. 5.16). Hyperostosis of the adjacent inner table is noted about 40% of the time. Calcification is seen in 10% to 20% of cases.

On MR, the tumor is typically isointense to hypointense to gray matter on T1WIs and isointense to hyperintense to gray matter on T2WIs. Hyperintensity on a T2WI almost always correlates with the angiomatous type of meningioma. Heterogeneity is the rule because of the presence of cysts, vessels, or calcification. Often, there may be a hypointense rim around the tumor. Prominent pial blood vessel flow voids are frequent (80%) and provide evidence of the extra-axial nature of the tumor. CSF clefts around the margin of the tumor also confirm the extra-axial location in 80% of cases. A key imaging feature is the broad dural base of these extra-axial masses. While adjacent dural thickening (the "dural tail") is common (seen in 60% of cases), it is not specific for a meningioma and does not necessarily indicate involvement by meningioma tumor cells.

Special attention should be given to possible involvement of the dural sinuses, as this finding is an important neurosurgical consideration. Any diminution in the caliber of a dural sinus adjacent to a meningioma is highly suspicious for involvement. Further evaluation with MR angiography or conventional angiography should be pursued to confirm this finding.

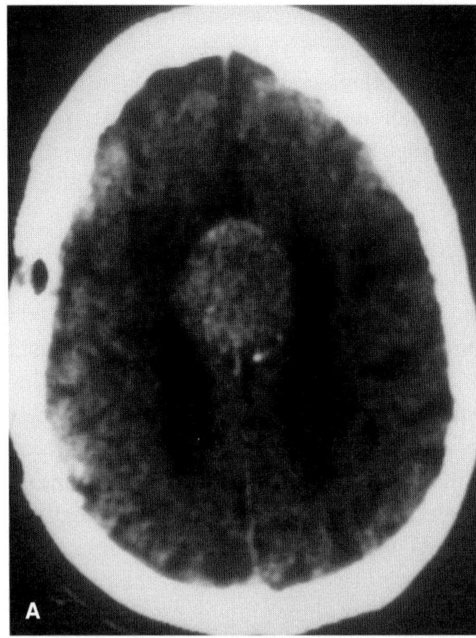

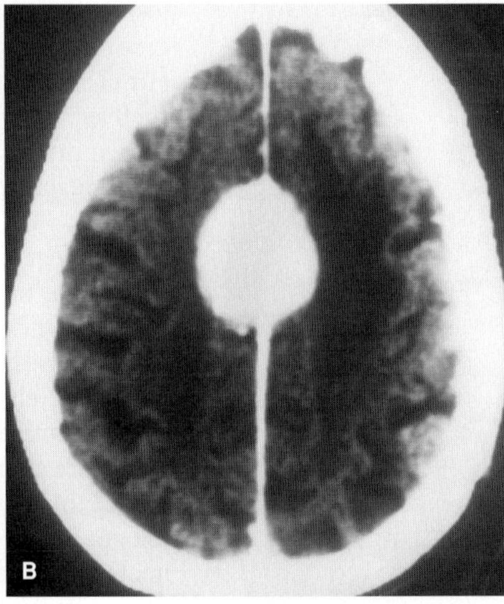

FIGURE 5.16. **Meningioma.** Precontrast **(A)** and postcontrast **(B)** CT images of falcine meningioma. On the precontrast study, the mass is hyperdense to normal brain parenchyma. With contrast, there is intense enhancement. Half of all meningiomas occur parasagittally or along the convexity.

Angiographically, meningiomas manifest several classic findings. During the arterial phase, there is a radial arrangement of the vessels, with an early dense tumor blush that persists well into the venous phase (Fig. 5.17). In addition, enlarged dural vessels and arteriovenous shunting may be noted. Meningeal branches, most commonly the middle meningeal artery, from the external carotid circulation are the primary supply to this tumor. The anterior meningeal artery (arising from the ophthalmic arteries) and posterior meningeal artery (arising from the vertebral arteries) also provide blood supply to these tumors. Preoperative embolization of these vessels often facilitates neurosurgical resection.

Hemangiopericytoma. Previously considered as "angioblastic meningioma," the hemangiopericytoma is now recognized as a distinct clinicopathologic entity. This rare tumor has a peak incidence at 30 to 50 years and arises from modified pericapillary smooth muscle cells (pericytes of Zimmerman). Unlike most meningiomas, the tumor is associated with an aggressive biologic behavior and a high recurrence rate and shows a predilection for late distant metastasis. The overall imaging appearance is often very similar to that of a meningioma, with a few exceptions. Hemangiopericytomas show a propensity (33% of cases) for a narrow base of attachment to the dura, instead of the broad dural base seen in the vast majority of meningiomas.

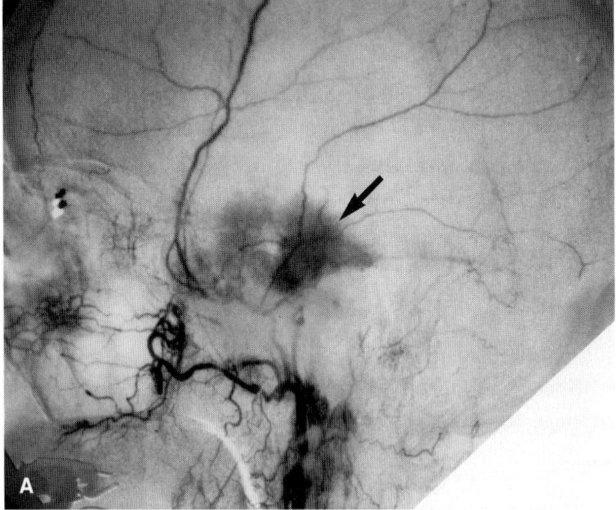

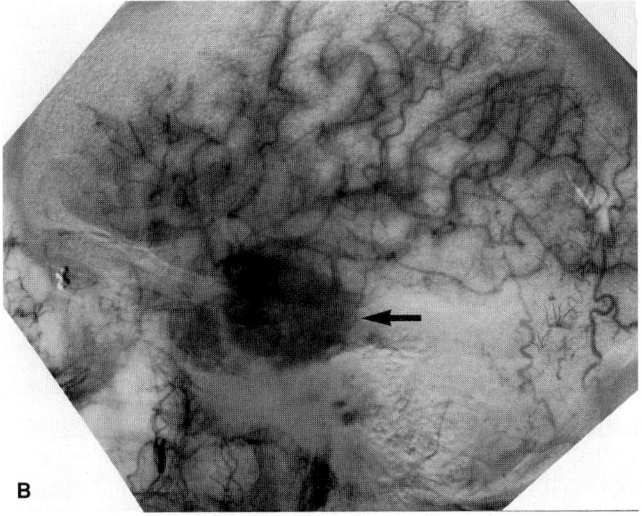

FIGURE 5.17. **Meningioma on Angiogram.** Selective external carotid injection. **(A)** demonstrates early blush (*arrow*) on arterial phase. **(B)** Persistent staining is evident on venous phase.

The tumor is also typically multilobulated instead of being "hemispheric," as commonly seen in meningiomas. Bone destruction is much more commonly noted in hemangiopericytomas than meningiomas. Calcification and hyperostosis are not common features.

Secondary CNS Lymphoma. Involvement of the brain by systemic lymphoma is rare and much less common than primary CNS lymphoma. When it occurs, it much more commonly involves the leptomeninges. Distinguishing between this tumor and meningioma is often not possible, as the imaging appearance may exactly mimic the latter.

Metastasis. Dural metastasis is the most common form of extra-axial spread, seen in 18% of autopsy series. When symptoms occur, they are most often secondary to compression of the brain parenchyma or development of a dural venous sinus thrombosis. Skull lesions, usually secondary to breast, lung, prostate, or renal carcinoma, give rise to epidural metastases. Subdural lesions are believed to result from hematogenous spread and, in the case of spinal lesions, spread from pelvic tumors by way of the Batson venous plexus. Both epidural and subdural metastases typically have a biconvex shape but may be distinguished by the presence of adjacent skull involvement in the presence of an epidural location.

Intraventricular Tumors

Intraventricular masses are easy to visualize on cross-sectional imaging studies because they stand out in comparison to the density or signal intensity of CSF. Ependymomas are most common in the fourth ventricle and are described in detail in the "Posterior Fossa Tumors" section. Central neurocytomas, subependymomas, subependymal giant cell astrocytomas, and other astrocytomas are more common in the body and anterior portion of the lateral ventricle. In contrast, choroid plexus papilloma, choroid plexus carcinoma, meningioma, and metastasis are more common in the posterior portion of the lateral ventricle. The most common atrial mass in an adult is a meningioma. Lung carcinoma and renal cell carcinoma are the most common primary tumors to spread to the ventricle, where the choroid plexus, the most highly vascular part of the ventricular system, is the favored site. While it is not a tumor, a colloid cyst is an important consideration for masses in the anterosuperior portion of the third ventricle. A list of the most common intraventricular masses in order of frequency is provided in Table 5.10. A differential diagnosis for lateral ventricular tumors based on the location and the age of the patient is given in Table 5.11.

TABLE 5.10 Intraventricular Masses

Choroid plexus papilloma (24%)
Choroid plexus carcinoma (2%)
Ependymoma (18%)
Subependymoma (11%)
Central neurocytoma (10%)
Subependymal giant cell astrocytoma (6%)
All other astrocytomas (9%)
Meningioma (6%)
Colloid cyst (4%)
Metastasis (2%)

Choroid Plexus Papilloma and Carcinoma. Choroid plexus papilloma accounts for only about 0.5% of all intracranial neoplasms overall but is very common in the pediatric age group. The tumor is most commonly seen in the lateral ventricle, especially in children. When it arises in the fourth ventricle (the second most common location), there is equal prevalence throughout the first five decades of life. The clinical presentation of choroid plexus papilloma is often related to the presence of increased intracranial pressure and hydrocephalus, which occur because of marked increase production of CSF by the tumor, impaired CSF resorption (secondary to tumoral hemorrhage), and CSF obstruction (secondary to the shear bulk of the mass). The tumor is fairly bland from a biologic perspective and is regarded as a WHO grade I lesion. About 20% of cases

TABLE 5.11 Most Common Lateral Ventricle Masses, by Location and Age

Age (yr)	*Foramen of Monro*	*Body*	*Trigone*
0–10		Primitive neuroectodermal tumor Teratoma Choroid plexus papilloma	Choroid plexus papilloma
10–40	Subependymal giant cell astrocytoma Pilocytic astrocytoma	Ependymoma Pilocytic astrocytoma Central neurocytoma	
>40		Subependymoma	Meningioma Metastasis

Adapted from Jelinek J, Smirniotopoulos JG, Parisi JE, et al. Lateral ventricular neoplasms of the brain: differential diagnosis based on clinical, CT, and MR findings. AJNR Am J Neuroradiol 1990;11:567–574.

occur as a choroid plexus carcinoma (WHO grade III), with the vast majority of these cases seen in young children.

Imaging. On CT, these are well-defined masses that are isodense to hyperdense compared to normal brain and typically are multilobulated (Fig. 5.18). Engulfment of the glomus of the choroid plexus is reported to be a distinguishing feature. Choroid plexus calcification in the first decade of life is atypical and suggests the possibility of a choroid plexus papilloma. On MR, they are isointense compared to gray matter on T1WIs and hyperintense compared to gray matter on T2WIs. These highly vascular tumors enhance markedly. Carcinomatous degeneration is suggested by heterogeneity or parenchymal invasion into the adjacent brain.

Both tumors may show subarachnoid spread. The prognosis for a patient with a choroid plexus papilloma is quite favorable if the mass is resected early, before irreversible damage secondary to hydrocephalus or repeated hemorrhage has occurred. The prognosis for those with a choroid plexus carcinoma is more guarded.

Central neurocytoma is a tumor of neuroepithelial lineage arising from the septum pellucidum or the ventricular wall. Half of these originate in the lateral ventricle near the foramen of Monro and about 10% are bilateral. Nearly 20% involve the third ventricle. Rarely, they may arise elsewhere in the brain or spinal cord, in which case they are termed *extraventricular central neurocytoma*. Most patients (75%) are between 20 and 40 years of age and present with brief symptoms related to increased intracranial pressure. The histologic features are remarkably similar to that of an oligodendroglioma, which can lead to diagnostic confusion; many central neurocytomas were initially mistaken as intraventricular oligodendrogliomas. It is now known that the latter is actually quite rare and less common than the central neurocytoma, a WHO grade II lesion.

Imaging. The tumor is characterized by a well-circumscribed lobulated mass within the lateral or third ventricles in most cases. Overall hyperdensity is seen on CT, although cystic changes and calcification are both common. On MR, the tumor is hyperintense on both T1WIs and T2WIs compared to white matter. The areas of cystic change are typically numerous and give the mass a "Swiss cheese" morphology. Enhancement is usually intense and diffuse on postcontrast imaging (Fig 5.19).

Subependymoma. Immediately underneath the ependymal lining of the ventricular system lies a thin subependymal glial layer. A tumor that arises from this region is termed *subependymoma* and classified as WHO grade I. Many patients are completely asymptomatic. When symptoms do occur, they are often related to hydrocephalus (80%) or focal neurologic deficits (25%). Rarely, the tumor may bleed, leading to subarachnoid hemorrhage. Most occur in patients older than 40 years of age, in contrast to the younger ages seen in the central neurocytoma. Slightly more than half arise in the fourth ventricle, with about 45% located in the lateral ventricle. On CT and MR, the tumor manifests as a well-circumscribed lobulated intraventricular mass. It is usually isodense to hypodense on CT, with frequent calcification (33%) and cystic degeneration (20%). Hypointensity on T1WIs and hyperintensity on T2WIs are seen on MR. The vast majority show at least some enhancement, although generally the enhancement is not as diffuse as that seen in central neurocytoma.

Subependymal giant cell astrocytoma has a strong association with tuberous sclerosis, occurring in up to 10%

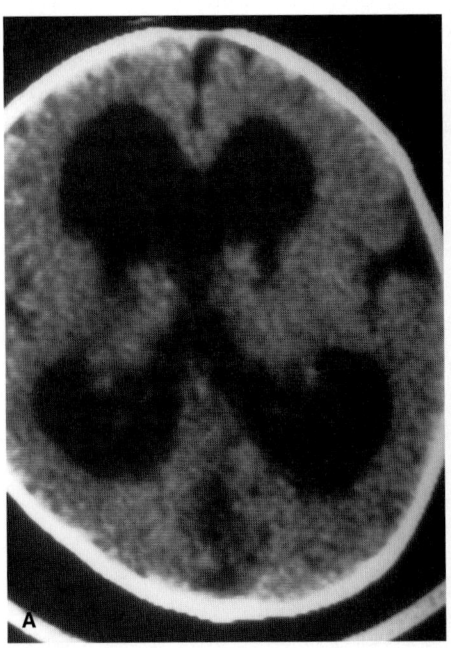

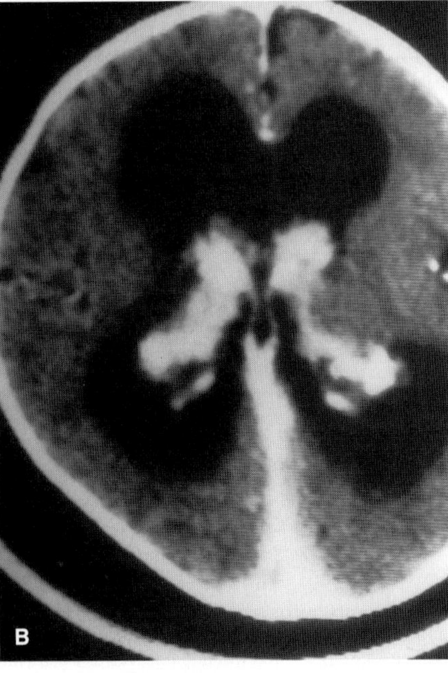

***FIGURE 5.18.* Choroid Plexus Papilloma.** Precontrast **(A)** and postcontrast **(B)** CT scans. Note the enlarged ventricles and extremely prominent choroid plexus formation bilaterally. Hydrocephalus results from increased production of CSF and decreased resorption secondary to proteinaceous debris and hemorrhage.

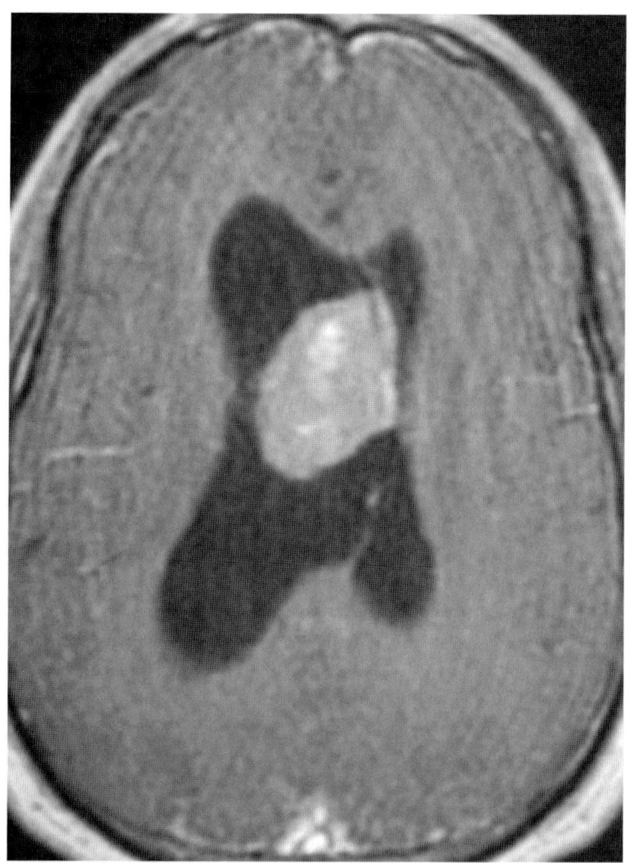

FIGURE 5.19. **Central Neurocytoma.** Postcontrast axial T1WI shows intense diffuse enhancement of an intraventricular mass arising from the septum pellucidum.

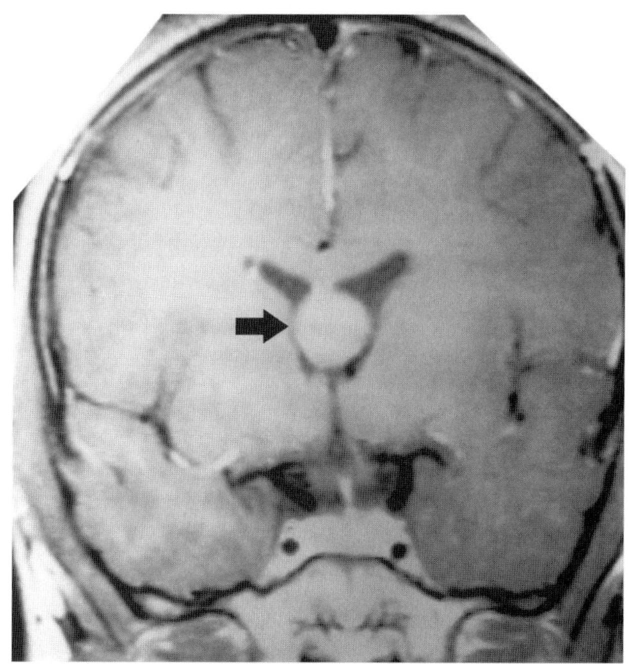

FIGURE 5.20. **Colloid Cyst.** Coronal T1WI shows the typical appearance and characteristic location in the third ventricle (*arrow*).

of patients. It is extremely rare in patients who do not have this syndrome. Any mass discovered in the region of the foramen of Monro in a young patient should provoke investigation for other manifestations of tuberous sclerosis, including subependymal and cortical hamartomas. The tumor is benign (WHO grade I) and slow-growing, with calcification a common feature. Because of its location within the foramen of Monro, it almost always produces some degree of hydrocephalus. On MR, it is typically isointense to slightly hyperintense to gray matter on T1WIs and hyperintense to gray matter on T2WIs, with some heterogeneity noted because of the calcification. Intense enhancement is the rule on postcontrast imaging. Tuberous sclerosis is discussed in greater detail in Chapter 8, which discusses pediatric neuroimaging.

Colloid cyst. While not a true neoplasm, the colloid cyst may mimic such lesions and characteristically occurs in the anterosuperior portion of the third ventricle near the foramen of Monro. It accounts for 2% of all intracranial masses, yet is important because of its propensity to cause acute hydrocephalus as a consequence of foraminal obstruction. The classic presentation is that of acute onset of a severe headache, which can be reproduced by the patient tilting the head forward (Brun phenomenon). Occasional fatalities have been reported.

Pathology. Some colloid cysts are entirely cystic, while others have a heterogeneous composition of old hemorrhage, cholesterol crystals, and various ions. Many lesions have an epithelial lining similar to that of the respiratory mucosa.

Imaging. The imaging appearance is variable. On CT, almost all are hyperdense to brain tissue. On MR, extremely variable signal intensity is seen on both T1WIs and T2WIs (Fig. 5.20). While rim enhancement has been seen in up to 40%, solid enhancement is definitely not a feature of this lesion and should provoke consideration of a different diagnosis. Other lesions that occur in the anterosuperior portion of the third ventricle are listed in Table 5.12.

TABLE 5.12 Masses of the Anterosuperior Third Ventricle

Colloid cyst
Meningioma
Choroid plexus papilloma
Hamartoma
Glioma
Vascular lesion
Granulomatous disease

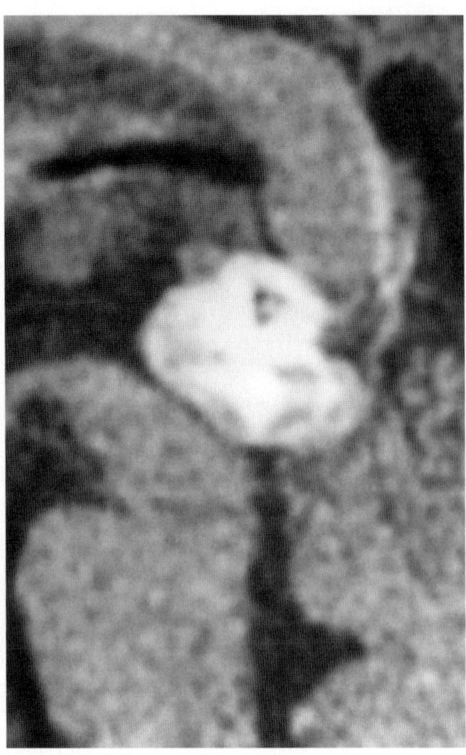

FIGURE 5.21. **Pineal Germinoma.** Postcontrast sagittal T1WI in young adult male with onset of Parinaud syndrome. The lobulated pineal mass shows heterogeneous enhancement. It is not possible to distinguish pineal germinomas from pineal parenchymal tumors on the basis of an imaging study alone.

Pineal Region Masses

Germ cell tumors constitute the most common type of neoplasm of the pineal region, accounting for 60% of all pineal masses (Fig. 5.21). Pineal parenchymal tumors such as pineoblastoma (malignant) and pineocytoma (benign) compose about 15% of these masses. The remaining 26% are divided among glioma (from adjacent brain parenchyma), meningioma (from the tentorium) (Fig. 5.22), and miscellaneous lesions such as arachnoid cyst, vein of Galen malformation, lipoma, and pineal cyst (Table 5.13). No distinction can be made on imaging studies between germinomas and pineal parenchymal tumors. However, a calcified pineal mass in a female patient is more likely to be secondary to a pineocytoma, whereas in a male patient, this same appearance is more likely to be caused by a germinoma. When calcification in the pineal region exceeds 1 cm in size, a pathologic pineal process should be suspected.

The size and location of the mass are important imaging characteristics for preoperative planning. If a lesion does not contain a large supratentorial component, the preferred infratentorial approach may be performed.

Germ cell tumors are well-defined, usually midline masses occurring most commonly (65%) in the pineal region, where they account for about 60% of all pineal masses. Germinoma is by far the most common intracranial germ cell tumor and also occurs in the suprasellar region (35%). It is most commonly seen in children and young adults, with a peak incidence around the age of puberty. CSF dissemination is common. Histologically, the germinoma is similar to testicular seminoma and ovarian dysgerminoma. For those arising in the pineal region, male

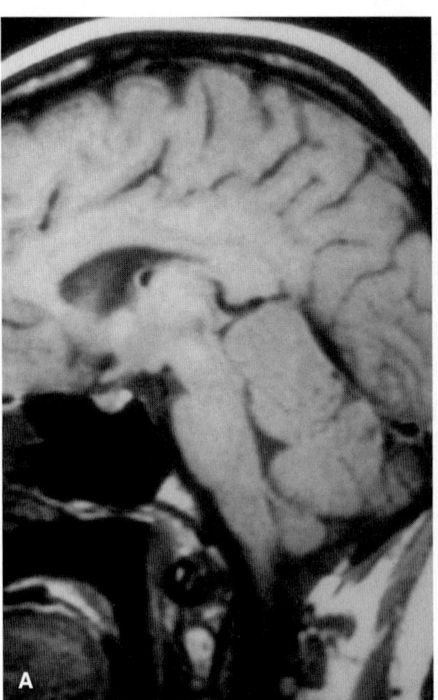

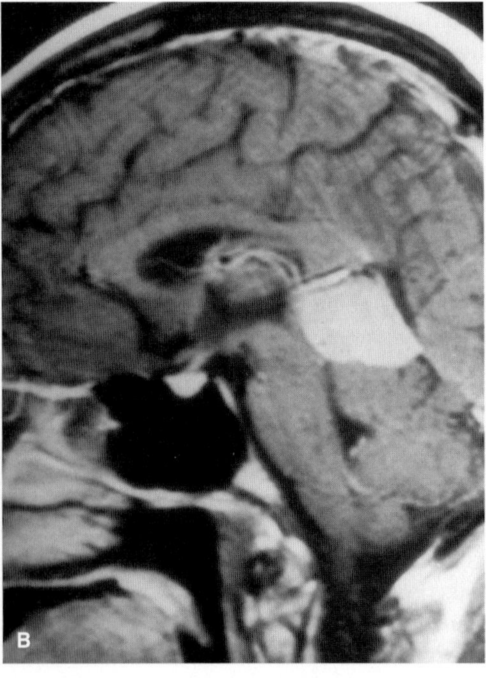

FIGURE 5.22. **Tentorial Meningioma.** Midline sagittal precontrast **(A)** and postcontrast **(B)** T1WIs of dura-based, intensely enhancing mass compressing the superior portion of the cerebellum and the tectum. The pineal gland itself is not evident; it is most likely severely flattened by the expanding meningioma.

TABLE 5.13 Pineal Region Masses

Germ Cell Tumors (60%)	*Pineal Parenchymal Tumors (14%)*	*Others*
Germinoma	Pineocytoma	Pineal cyst
Teratoma	Pineoblastoma	Glioma
Embryonal carcinoma		Meningioma (tentorial)
Endodermal sinus tumor		Vein of Galen malformation
Choriocarcinoma		Arachnoid cyst
		Lipoma

patients are much more commonly affected than female patients (10:1). Clinical presentation is related to compression by the mass on the sylvian aqueduct, producing hydrocephalus, or to compression of the superior colliculus, producing Parinaud syndrome (paralysis of upward gaze). For those arising in the suprasellar region, there is no gender predilection. Because of compression of the optic chiasm and infundibulum, symptoms related to hypothalamic dysfunction (emotional disturbance, diabetes insipidus, precocious puberty, etc.) and visual changes are common.

Imaging. In both the pineal and suprasellar regions, germinoma typically manifests as a isodense to hyperdense well-circumscribed mass on CT. "Engulfment" of the normal physiologic calcification is a distinguishing feature of germinomas from the "exploded" appearance most commonly seen in pineal parenchymal tumors. On MR, nonspecific hypointensity on T1WIs and hyperintensity on T2WIs is common. Occasionally, hypointensity on a T2WI may be seen and favors a germinoma instead of a pineal parenchymal tumor. Intense enhancement on either CT or MR is the rule (Fig. 5.21). In the final analysis, there are no discriminating factors on imaging studies between pineal parenchymal tumors and germinomas that allow accurate differentiation.

Other Germ Cell Tumors. Teratoma, embryonal carcinoma, choriocarcinoma, and endodermal sinus tumor compose the remainder of the germ cell tumors and are all much less common than germinomas. Most teratomas occur at an earlier age than germinomas and have a variable radiographic appearance and biologic behavior. In addition to the pineal region (the most common location), the tumor also arises in the third ventricle and posterior fossa. Because it is composed of all three germ cell lines, it is usually extremely heterogeneous on CT and MR, with a mixture of fat, calcification, and cysts. Hydrocephalus is frequently noted and enhancement is variable. Detection of a midline heterogeneous mass in a child should suggest this diagnosis.

Embryonal carcinoma, choriocarcinoma, and endodermal sinus tumor are highly malignant types of germ cell tumors. All are frequently hemorrhagic but have no specific radiographic features. Alpha-fetoprotein (AFP) may be elevated in embryonal cell carcinoma, teratoma, or choriocarcinoma. Human chorionic gonadotropin (HCG) may be elevated in choriocarcinoma or teratoma. Germinomas are not associated with elevated HCG or AFP levels. Microneurosurgical and stereotactic techniques allow relatively safe biopsy of suspicious pineal masses for more accurate histologic confirmation of the diagnosis.

Pineocytoma and pineoblastoma are true pineal parenchymal tumors that account for 14% of all pineal masses.

Pineoblastoma. The pineoblastoma is histologically and radiographically similar to medulloblastoma and has been categorized as part of the PNET "family" by some neuropathologists. It occurs primarily in young children, although it may be seen in patients up to 30 years of age. The tumor is rarely well-circumscribed, often demonstrating a lobular contour, local invasion, and frequent calcification. Intratumoral hemorrhage is rare. Similar to other PNETs, CSF spread is common. The tumor is highly malignant and classified as a WHO grade IV tumor. Rarely, it may occur in combination with bilateral retinoblastomas to constitute the so-called "trilateral retinoblastoma."

Pineocytoma. The pineocytoma is most commonly seen in adults, although there is a broad age range for presentation. It is also usually well demarcated, noninvasive, and slow growing. Often calcified, it rarely metastasizes. On either CT or MR, the pineocytoma cannot be reliably differentiated from either pineal germinoma or pineoblastoma.

Imaging. Both types of pineal parenchymal tumors are isodense to hyperdense on CT. On MR, they are usually isointense to hypointense on T1WIs. There is much variability in signal intensity of these tumors on T2WIs, with most being isointense to hyperintense to gray matter. Both the native tumor and its metastases enhance intensely with contrast.

Pineal cysts are common (about 40% in autopsy series) and have internal signal intensity similar to that of CSF. The lack of CSF pulsation may cause slightly higher signal on T1WIs and on T2WIs. No enhancement of the cyst itself is seen and no internal architecture is noted. If the cyst is eccentric to the pineal gland itself, it may be difficult to differentiate this lesion from a small pineal neoplasm. Slight flattening of the superior colliculus may be seen, but the cysts do not cause Parinaud syndrome or hydrocephalus. Intracystic hemorrhage is rare.

Sellar Masses

Pituitary adenomas account for about 10% to 15% of all intracranial tumors and constitute the most common sellar masses by far, being five times more common than craniopharyngiomas and Rathke cleft cysts. Based on their size, they are considered either microadenomas (10 mm or smaller) or macroadenomas (>10 mm). In general, about 75% of adenomas are hormonally active and most of these will be microadenomas. The other 25% are nonsecreting adenomas and most of these will be macroadenomas. Because of the general topographic relationship of the secretory cells within the pituitary gland, attention may be focused on particular regions of the gland, depending on the presenting clinical signs and symptoms and laboratory findings. Prolactinomas and growth hormone (GH)–secreting adenomas are more commonly located within the lateral aspects of the gland. Adenomas with secretion of adrenocorticotropic hormone (ACTH), thyroid-stimulating hormone, or follicle-stimulating hormone/luteinizing hormone are more common in the central region of the gland. Clinical symptoms are related to the type of hormone secreted. For instance, ACTH-producing tumors produce Cushing disease, and GH-producing tumors produce acromegaly in adults and gigantism in children. Prolactinomas are the most common (40% to 50%) of the secreting adenomas and are marked clinically by amenorrhea, galactorrhea, or impotence. A serum prolactin level of >150 ng/mL almost always indicates a prolactinoma and levels >1,000 ng/mL herald invasion into the cavernous sinus (normal prolactin levels are <20 ng/mL).

Imaging. MR is the imaging modality of choice to detect pituitary tumors. Microadenomas are usually best detected on coronal T1WIs as focal areas of hypointensity (on noncontrast studies) compared to the rest of the pituitary gland (Fig. 5.23). Occasionally, they may be isointense or even hyperintense on noncontrast studies. Other associated features include deviation of the infundibulum, asymmetric convexity of the pituitary gland, and mild downsloping of the roof of the sphenoid sinus. In general, administration of gadolinium contrast increases the conspicuity of these often small neoplasms, which are revealed as hypointense foci within the gland on immediate postcontrast scans or as hyperintense foci on delayed imaging (about 30 minutes postinjection). The use of narrow window levels is essential to optimally visualize these small lesions. Macroadenomas are never a problem to visualize on MR. When they are heterogeneous because of cyst formation or hemorrhage (Fig. 5.24), and differentiation from a craniopharyngioma or parasellar meningioma is difficult, the use of contrast may be helpful (Fig. 5.25). Macroadenomas most commonly manifest because of optic chiasm or nerve compression, hydrocephalus, cranial nerve palsies, or anterior pituitary dysfunction. These lesions are isointense to gray matter on T1WIs and characteristically produce "draping" of the optic chiasm over the top of the tumor. Invasion of the cavernous sinus can only be accurately determined when there is tumor tissue between the internal carotid artery flow void and the lateral wall of the cavernous sinus.

Craniopharyngioma and Rathke cleft cyst arise from squamous epithelial remnants of the anterior lobe of the pituitary gland, with the craniopharyngiomas derived from the pars tuberalis and Rathke cleft cyst arising from the pars intermedia. However, whereas Rathke cleft cysts are usually asymptomatic (seen in up to 33% of autopsies), craniopharyngiomas are frequently symptomatic because of their larger size. Symptoms related to increased intracranial pressure, optic nerve or chiasm compression, or hypothalamic dysfunction are common. Craniopharyngioma is the most common suprasellar mass in the pediatric population. In addition to showing a peak incidence between 5 and 10 years of age, the tumor is associated with a second peak, seen between the ages of 50 and 60 years. Most craniopharyngiomas involve both intrasellar and suprasellar compartments (70%), 20% are intrasellar only,

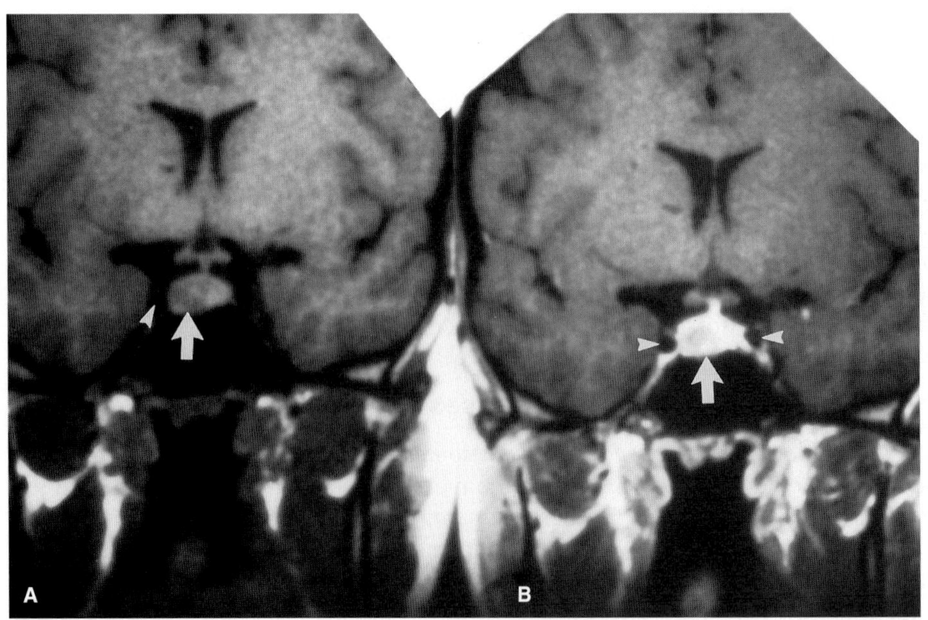

FIGURE 5.23. **Pituitary Microadenoma. A.** Precontrast thin-section coronal T1WI through the sella in patient with elevated prolactin levels shows prominent right aspect of gland with slight hypointensity (*arrow*) compared to the normal pituitary gland on the left. Downsloping of the sphenoid roof is also seen. **B.** With contrast, the lesion is slightly more conspicuous, measuring 8 mm in transverse diameter. Note the normal flow voids (*arrowheads*) of the internal carotid arteries and normal enhancement of the cavernous sinuses.

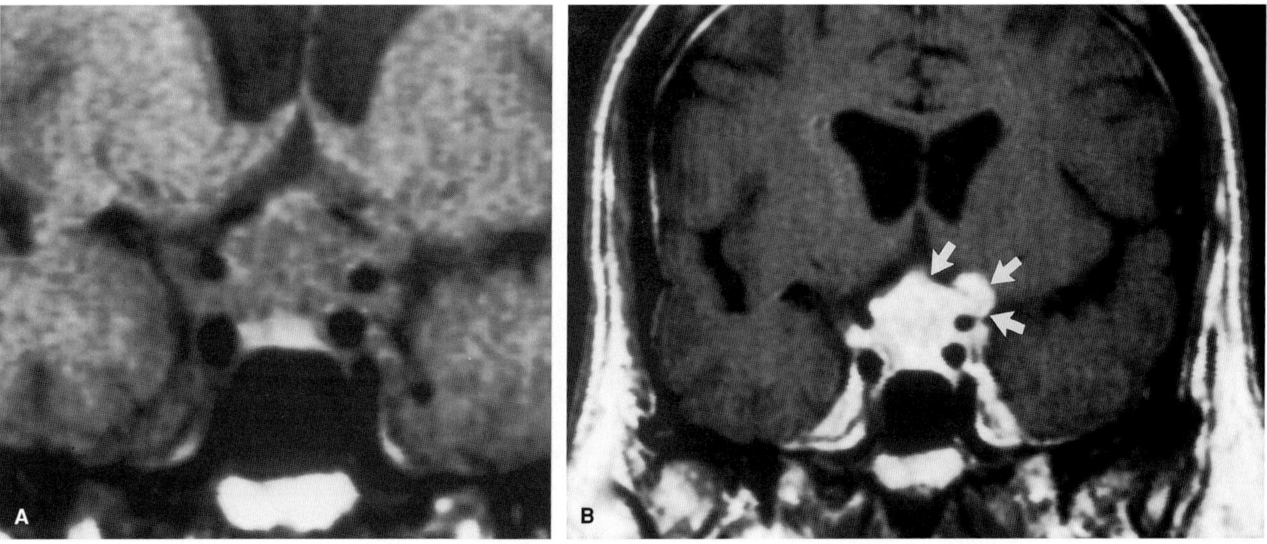

FIGURE 5.24. **Pituitary Macroadenoma.** Coronal T1WIs without **(A)** and with **(B)** contrast show an enhancing mass (*arrow*) extending beyond the lateral margin of the cavernous sinus and flow voids of the left internal carotid artery.

and 10% are purely extrasellar. Solid and cystic components are typical, with the fluid of the cyst often containing cholesterol crystals and grossly having the appearance of "crankcase oil."

Imaging. On CT, the classic appearance of a craniopharyngioma is a large cystlike sellar/suprasellar mass with an enhancing rim and evidence of some calcification. In children, calcification is seen in up to 80% of cases (compared to 40% for adult cases). On MR, because of the presence of the liquid cholesterol, the classic finding of hyperintensity on T1WIs and T2WIs, corresponding to the cystic portion, is most common (Fig. 5.26). However, some craniopharyngiomas do not contain fluid but instead will have a solid nodule that may be completely calcified. Enhancement of the rim and any soft tissue component is noted.

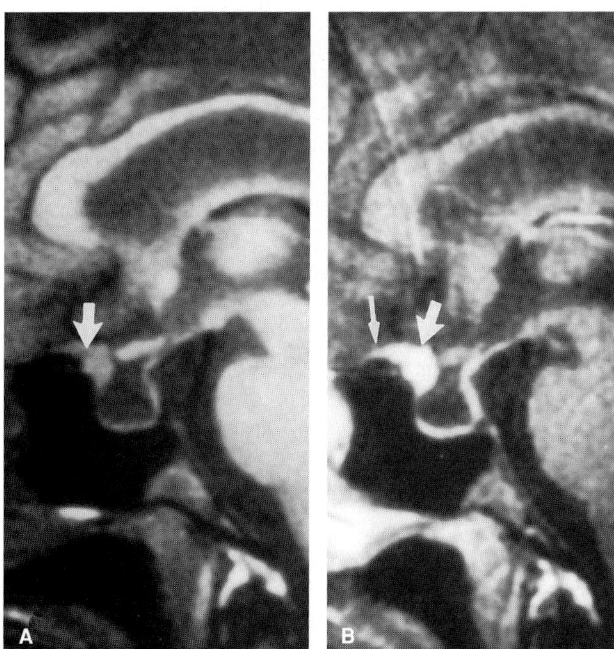

FIGURE 5.25. **Tuberculum Sella Meningioma.** Suprasellar enhancing mass (*arrows*) in the region of the tuberculum sella with extension along the planum sphenoidale (*small arrow*), a highly characteristic feature of parasellar meningiomas.

Rathke's cleft cyst is either purely intrasellar (66%) or intrasellar and suprasellar (33%). The cyst contents are variable. Most commonly, a mucoid fluid fills the cyst. Less commonly, serous fluid or desquamated cellular debris occupies the cyst. Because of this variability, the cyst may be hyperintense on T1WIs and T2WIs, appearing identical to a craniopharyngioma, or it may be isointense to hypointense on either sequence because of cellular debris mimicking the appearance of a solid nodule. Compared to craniopharyngiomas, Rathke cleft cysts rarely show peripheral enhancement. A complete differential diagnosis (and long-standing mnemonic) for suprasellar masses is outlined in Table 5.14.

Nerve Sheath Tumors

There are three types of nerve sheath tumors: *schwannoma* (also known as neurilemoma or neurinoma), *neurofibroma,* and *malignant nerve sheath tumor,* which is quite rare and will not be discussed.

Schwannoma arises from Schwann cells that form the myelin sheaths of axons. The tumor is focal and encapsulated and affects the cranial nerves, most often the vestibulocochlear (VIII) and trigeminal (V) nerves. Cystic degeneration is common, especially in larger lesions, and may be accompanied by hemorrhage in 5% of cases.

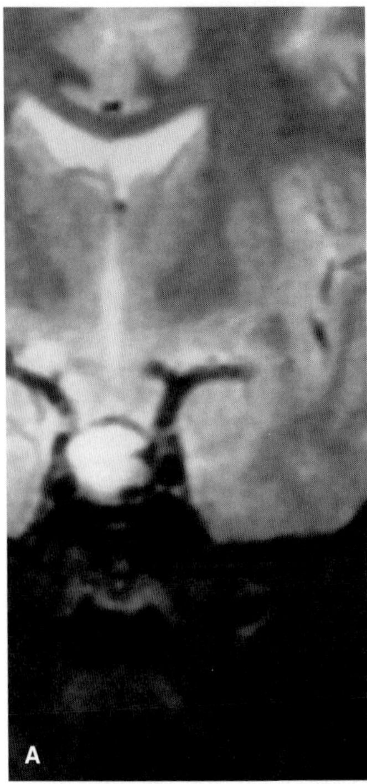

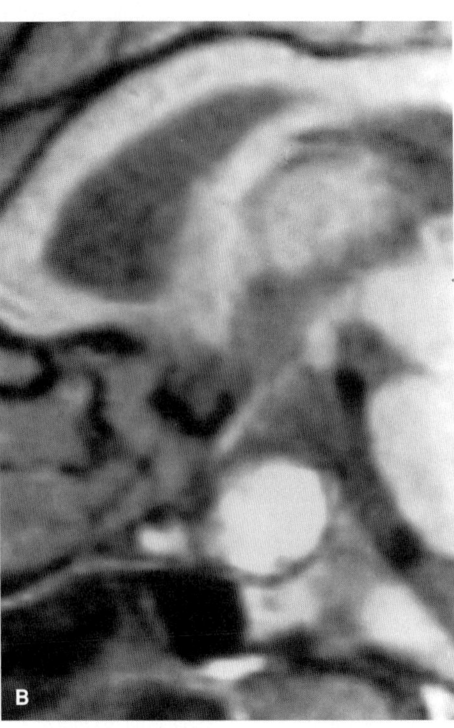

FIGURE 5.26. **Craniopharyngioma. A.** Coronal T2WI through the sella in a patient with mild visual symptoms. A hyperintense intrasellar mass (*arrow*) with suprasellar component is seen. **B.** Sagittal T1WI shows hyperintense signal (*arrow*) that is maintained, consistent with the presence of liquid cholesterol that is characteristic of these tumors.

Comprising about 8% of all intracranial neoplasms, it is more commonly seen in adults. Symptoms depend on the cranial nerve involved. Depending on the size and location, hydrocephalus, brainstem compression, or neuropathy may be present.

On CT, schwannoma is usually isodense to hypodense. On MR, thin-section (<3-mm) axial and coronal T1WI images through the basal cisterns are ideal to exclude this neoplasm, which demonstrates hypointensity to gray matter on T1WIs and hyperintensity to gray matter on T2WIs. Intense enhancement is seen on post-contrast images. The larger a schwannoma is, the more likely it is to show heterogeneity because of cystic degeneration or hemorrhage.

Vestibular schwannoma typically arises from the vestibular division of the eighth cranial nerve within the internal auditory canal and produces ipsilateral sensorineural hearing loss. Patients may first detect the presence of such a tumor by noticing a difference in speech perception between each ear while using the telephone. The tumor may be completely intracanalicular, or it may extend into the adjacent cerebellopontine cistern. Expansion of the canal is an imaging hallmark. The presence of bilateral vestibular schwannomas is one of the diagnostic criteria for neurofibromatosis type 2. Thin-section T2-weighted fast spin-echo images are useful in screening patients suspected of having a vestibular schwannoma. Differentiation from a cerebellopontine meningioma may be difficult. The single most helpful imaging feature is extension of the enhancement along the course of the seventh and eighth nerves, seen in about 80% of vestibular schwannomas (Fig. 5.27). Meningiomas very rarely demonstrate this feature and frequently will have a "dural tail" (Fig. 5.28). A precontrast, fat-suppressed sequence is ideal to detect the unlikely intracanalicular lipoma. Other cerebellopontine angle lesions include epidermoid (Fig. 5.29) and schwannoma arising from other cranial nerves nearby. A mnemonic for cerebellopontine angle lesions is given in Table 5.15.

TABLE 5.14 Suprasellar Masses ("SATCHMO")

Sella (pituitary) tumor, sarcoid
Aneurysm, ***a***rachnoid cyst
Teratoma
Craniopharyngioma
Hypothalamic glioma, ***h***amartoma of tuber cinereum, ***h***istiocytosis
Meningioma
Optic nerve glioma

Trigeminal schwannoma can be identified by its location within the pontine cistern at the midpons level, between the trigeminal ganglion located in the Meckel cavity (just posterolateral to the cavernous sinus) and the brainstem (Fig. 5.30). Extension through the ganglion and into the foramen ovale, foramen rotundum, or superior orbital fissure may be seen. Less commonly, schwannoma may also involve cranial nerves IX to XI.

Neurofibroma, on the other hand, arises from fibroblasts and Schwann cells, is usually fusiform, and involves the cutaneous exiting spinal nerves. It is rarely cystic or hemorrhagic. Neurofibroma, which is rarely solitary, is more commonly seen in the spine as part of neurofibromatosis types 1 and 2. Affected patients most commonly present with multiple radiculopathies or signs and

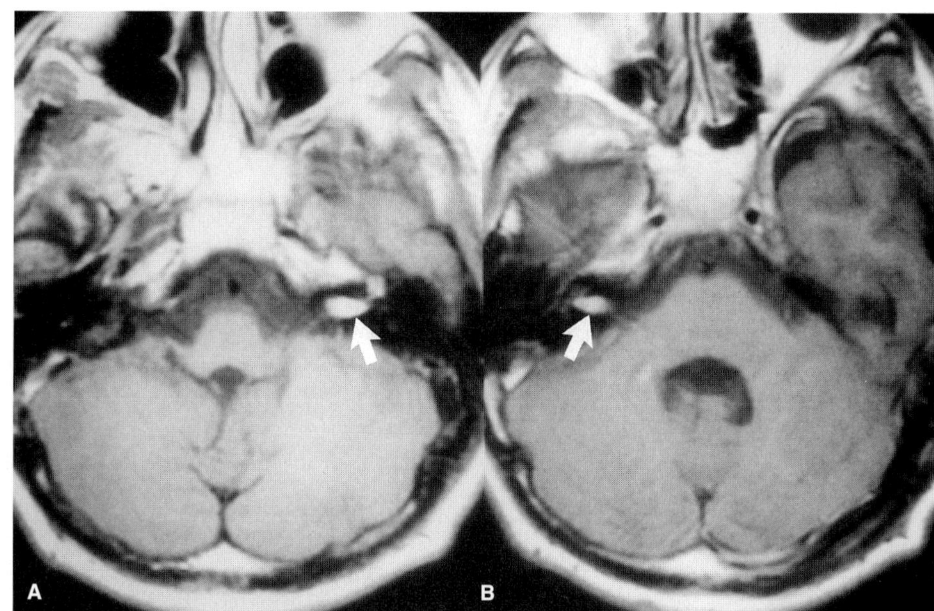

FIGURE 5.27. **Vestibular Schwannoma. A.** and **B.** Postcontrast axial T1WIs showing bilateral intracanalicular acoustic schwannomas (*arrows*) in patient with neurofibromatosis type 2. Extension into the internal acoustic canal and lack of a broad dural base differentiate this entity from meningioma.

symptoms related to cord compression. The tumor is discussed in greater detail in Chapter 8, which discusses pediatric neuroimaging.

Masses of Maldevelopmental Origin

Epidermoid and dermoid are uncommon congenital masses that result from enclosure of ectodermal elements when the neural tube closes. Epidermoids account for about 1% of all intracranial neoplasms, whereas dermoids, as intracranial masses, are much less common. Both are benign and characterized by slow growth. The peak age of incidence is 40 to 50 years old for epidermoids and 20 to 30 years old for dermoids. Both lesions are lined by squamous epithelium and produce large amounts of keratin. The key histologic distinction between an epidermoid and a dermoid is that the dermoid contains a "pilosebaceous unit" (composed of skin, hair follicles, and dermal appendages), while the epidermoid does not. Epidermoids are most often located off the midline at the skull base (i.e., cerebellopontine cistern, parasellar, or the posterior fossa) while dermoids are characteristically midline masses, most common at the inferior vermis or at the vallecula. Epidermoids are commonly tightly adherent to and compress adjacent structures, most commonly the cranial nerves. Symptoms from dermoids are usually secondary to obstruction of CSF pathways, chemical meningitis (secondary to rupture of the dermoid), or infection if associated with a sinus tract. A comparison of epidermoids and dermoids is provided in Table 5.16.

Imaging. On imaging studies, the differing compositions of the two lesions produce different signal intensities. Epidermoids are well-circumscribed, lobulated soft tissue masses that, because of the presence of solid cholesterol and/or CSF within the interstices of the tumor, most commonly have signal intensities on both CT and MR that follow that of CSF (hypodense on CT, hypointense on T1WIs, and hyperintense on T2WIs) (Fig. 5.29). Rim enhancement secondary to the presence of granulation tissue may be seen following contrast administration. On occasion, epidermoids contain enough liquid cholesterol (similar to craniopharyngioma) to produce T1 shortening

TABLE 5.15 Cerebellopontine Masses ("AMEN")

Lesion	*T1WIs (Compared to Gray Matter)*	*T2WIs (Compared to Gray Matter)*	*Gadolinium Enhancement*
Acoustic (vestibular) schwannoma (80%)	Hypo	Hyper	Yes
Meningioma (11%)	Iso to hypo	Iso to hyper	Yes
Ependymoma (4%)	Hypo	Hyper	Yes
Neuroepithelial cyst (arachnoid, epidermoid) (5%)	CSF	CSF	No

Hypo, hypointense relative to gray matter; hyper, hyperintense relative to gray matter; Iso, isointense relative to gray matter; CSF, follows signal CSF.

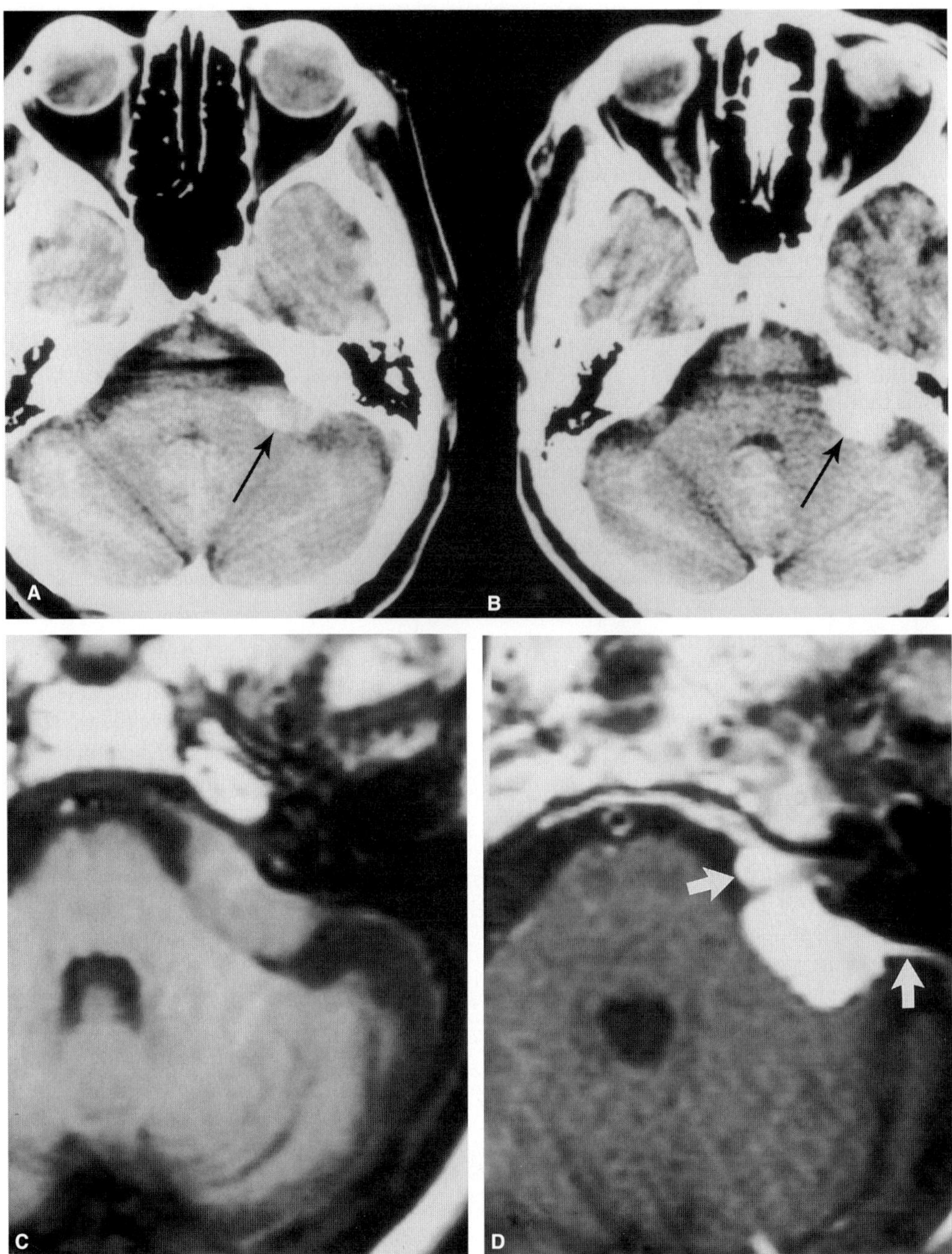

FIGURE 5.28. **Cerebellopontine Meningioma.** Noncontrast **(A)** and postcontrast **(B)** CT scans show left cerebellopontine mass (*arrows*), which intensely enhances. Noncontrast **(C)** and postcontrast **(D)** T1WIs show extra-axial lesion with broad dural base and intense enhancement. There is no extension along the neurovascular bundle of internal acoustic canal. Note the dural tails (*arrows*) extending anteriorly and posteriorly within the cerebellopontine angle.

(hyperintensity) of the mass. The primary differential diagnosis is an arachnoid cyst. DWI is very useful in distinguishing between these lesions, because the epidermoid is hyperintense compared to CSF, while the arachnoid cyst is isointense.

Dermoids, on the other hand, typically have signal characteristics that follow that of fat (low density on CT, hyperintense on T1WIs, with signal suppression on fat-suppressed images) (Fig. 5.31). They do not enhance unless infected. Heterogeneity of the mass may be seen because of calcification and other soft tissue components. The presence of a fat–fluid level is practically pathognomonic. If no heterogeneity is present, it may be difficult to distinguish a dermoid from a lipoma. Occasionally, dermoids may

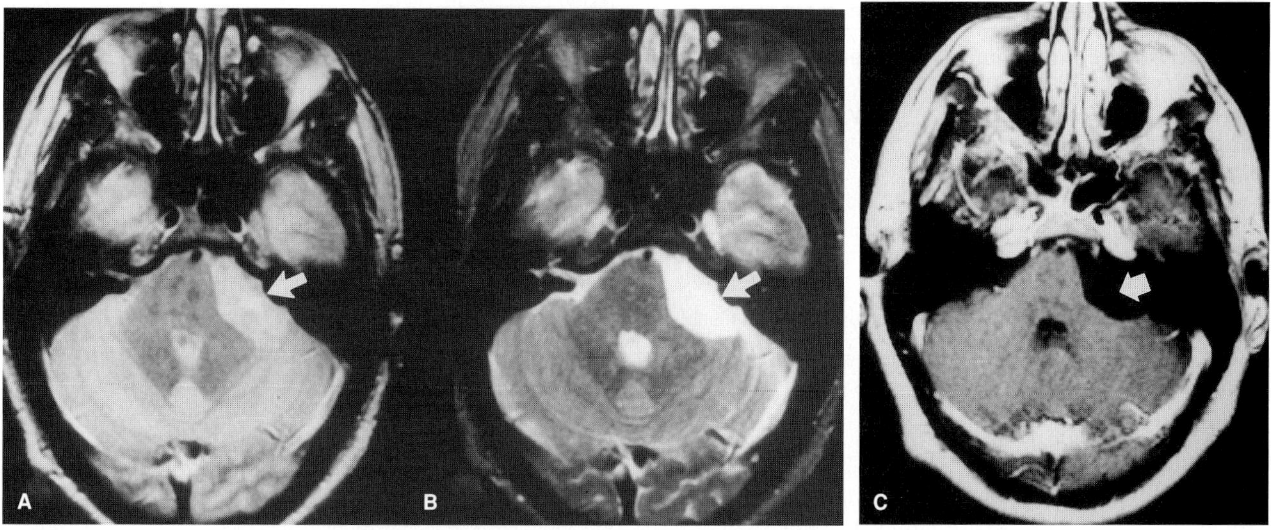

FIGURE 5.29. **Epidermoid.** Axial T2WIs (**A,** first echo; **B,** second echo) show left cerebellopontine angle mass (*arrows*) that closely follows signal intensity of CSF. Postcontrast T1WI **(C)** shows no enhancement of the extra-axial mass (*arrow*), which again has signal intensity similar to that of CSF.

rupture into the subarachnoid space, producing chemical meningitis and manifesting as multiple foci of T1 shortening. In the presence of an intracranial dermoid, the nasofrontal and occipital regions of the scalp should be evaluated to detect a sinus tract.

Intracranial lipomas are usually asymptomatic and incidental findings on imaging studies. These masses occur at all ages and are most common in the interhemispheric falx (often associated with agenesis of the corpus callosum), quadrigeminal plate, and suprasellar regions. Lipomas are thought to arise from incomplete resorption of the meninx primitiva as it develops into the subarachnoid space (Fig. 5.32). They have low density on CT but occasionally contain calcification. On MR, they exhibit T1 hyperintensity, following the signal intensity of subcutaneous fat. No enhancement is seen. The presence of either chemical shift artifact or signal suppression on a fat-saturated T1WI establishes the diagnosis. Lipomas are associated

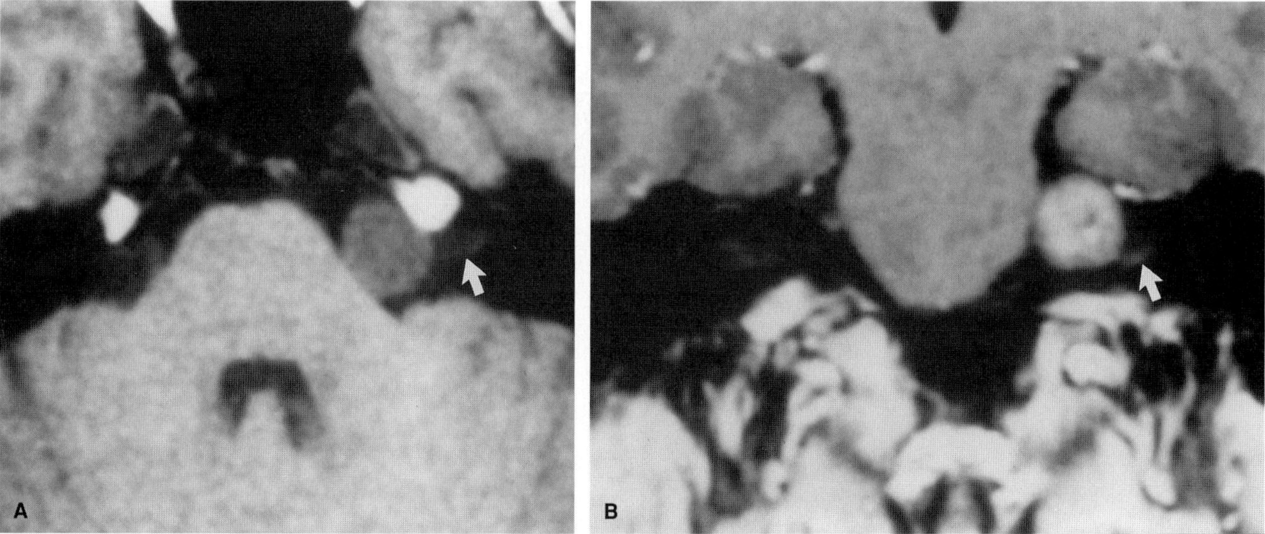

FIGURE 5.30. **Trigeminal Schwannoma. A.** Axial T1WI in a patient with dizziness shows an isointense mass in cisternal space near vicinity of internal auditory canal. Note the portion of seventh and eighth nerve complex (*arrow*) displaced by mass. **B.** Postcontrast coronal T1WI shows homogeneous enhancement. Again, note that the seventh and eighth nerve complex (*arrow*) is displaced by this schwannoma from the trigeminal nerve.

TABLE 5.16 Epidermoid Versus Dermoid

Characteristic	*Epidermoid*	*Dermoid*
Frequency	Common	Uncommon
Peak age	40 to 50 yr	20 to 30 yr
Germ Cells	Ectoderm	Ectoderm and mesoderm
Location	Off midline (cerebellopontine cistern, parasellar, posterior fossa)	Midline (pericerebellar, suprasellar)
Imaging	Follows CSF most commonly, lobulated, peripheral enhancement, hyperintense on DWI	Typical "fat" attenuation or signal

with blood vessels and cranial nerves. The presence of either a flow void or a cranial nerve traversing the mass assures the diagnosis of a lipoma and effectively excludes a dermoid.

Arachnoid cysts account for about 1% of all intracranial masses and are congenital in nature. "Secondary" or "acquired arachnoid cysts" are in reality leptomeningeal cysts resulting from a prior inflammatory process (meningitis, hemorrhage, etc.). True arachnoid cysts are created by secretion of CSF from the cells lining the cyst and are therefore intra-arachnoidal. They are most commonly (50%) seen in the middle cranial fossa, where they may be quite large. Other sites include the frontal convexity, the suprasellar and quadrigeminal cisterns, and the posterior fossa. If they attain sufficient size to obstruct CSF flow or compress the brain, they may become symptomatic.

Imaging. Arachnoid cysts follow the attenuation/signal intensity pattern of CSF on CT and MR. Remodeling of the adjacent bone may be seen. Hemorrhage may occur after trauma or spontaneously. Unless infection is present, no enhancement is noted. In contrast to the hyperintensity seen with epidermoids, arachnoid cysts do not show evidence of water restriction on DWI. Differentiation from an enlarged cisterna magna is possible on cisternography, with immediate filling with iodinated contrast of the cisterna magna compared to no or delayed filling of the arachnoid cyst.

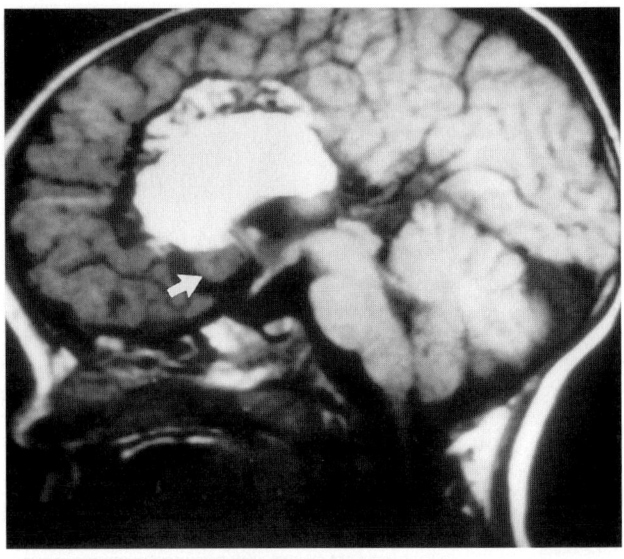

FIGURE 5.32. **Lipoma With Agenesis of Corpus Callosum.** Sagittal T1WI shows large hyperintense midline mass. The development of a lipoma in this location prevents normal development of the corpus callosum. Note that only a portion of the genu (*arrow*) is present, while the remaining structures of the corpus callosum are absent.

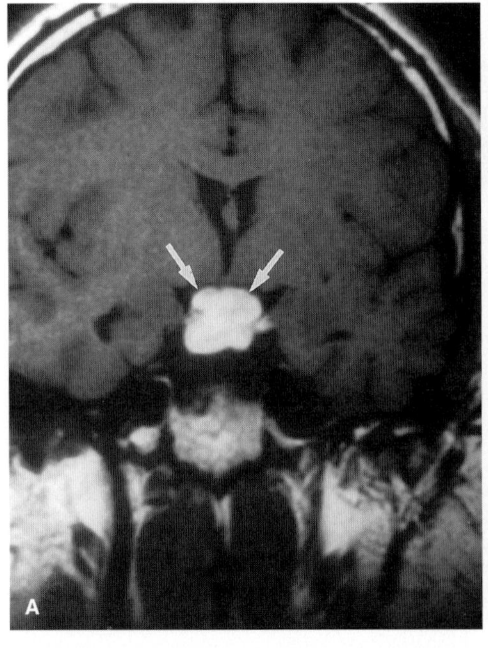

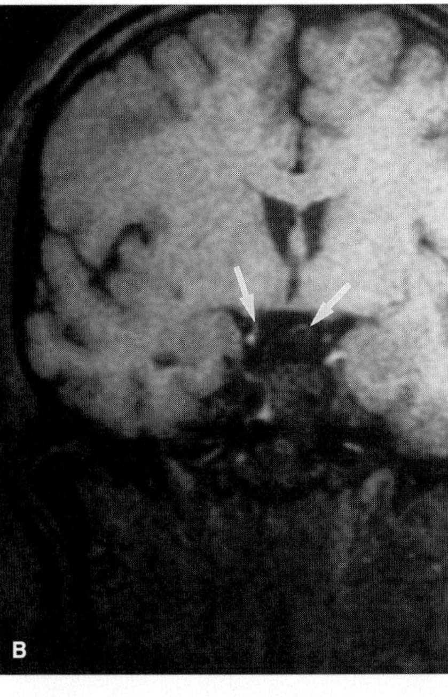

FIGURE 5.31. **Dermoid Tumor.** Coronal T1WI **(A)** shows a hyperintense suprasellar mass (*arrow*). When a fat-suppression technique is used **(B),** the signal of the dermoid becomes isointense, following the signal of subcutaneous fat, confirming the nature of the lesion.

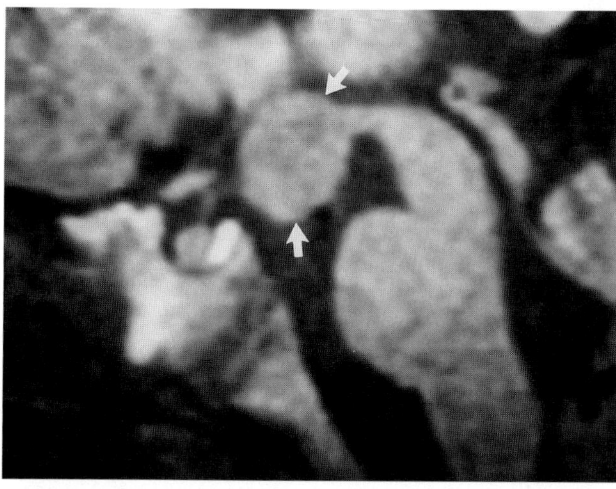

FIGURE 5.33. **Hamartoma of Tuber Cinereum.** This lesion was found in a young adult with diabetes insipidus. Hamartomas may vary in size, from 1 to 2 mm to larger lesions such as this one (*arrows*).

Hamartoma of the tuber cinereum is a rare congenital malformation of normal neuronal tissue in an abnormal location that is more common in boys presenting with precocious puberty, gelastic seizures, developmental delay, and hyperactivity. The mass is well circumscribed, round or oval in shape, and centered in the region of the tuber cinereum (at the base of the infundibulum). It does not calcify or hemorrhage. On CT and MR, it has essentially the same signal intensity as brain tissue and does not enhance (Fig. 5.33). Along with the characteristic location, a stalk connecting the mass with the tuber cinereum or mamillary bodies cinches the diagnosis.

SUGGESTED READINGS

Bendszus M, Warmuth-Metz M, Klein R, et al. MR spectroscopy in gliomatosis cerebri. AJNR Am J Neuroradiol 2000;21:375–380.

Buetow PC, Smirniotopoulos JG, Done S. Congenital brain tumors: a review of 45 cases. AJNR Am J Neuroradiol 1990;11:793–799.

Burger PC. Malignant astrocytic neoplasms: classification, pathologic anatomy, and response to therapy. Semin Oncol 1986;13:16–26.

Castillo M, Davis PC, Takei Y, Hoffman JCJ. Intracranial ganglioglioma: MR, CT, and clinical findings in 18 patients. AJNR Am J Neuroradiol 1990;11:109–114.

Coates TL, Hinshaw DB, Peckman N, et al. Pediatric choroid plexus neoplasms: MR, CT, and pathologic correlation. Radiology 1989;173: 81–88.

Davis PC, Wichman RD, Takei Y, Hoffman JCJ. Primary cerebral neuroblastoma: CT and MR findings in 12 cases. AJNR Am J Neuroradiol 1990;11:115–120.

Dina TS. Primary central nervous lymphoma versus toxoplasmosis in AIDS. Radiology 1991;179:823–828.

Edwards MSB, Hudgins RJ, Wilson CB, et al. Pineal region tumors in children. J Neurosurg 1988;68:689–697.

Galassi W, Phuttharak W, Hesselink JR, Healy JF, Dietrich RB, Imbesi SG. Intracranial meningeal disease: comparison of contrast-enhanced MR imaging with fluid-attenuated inversion recovery and fat-suppressed T1-weighted sequences. AJNR Am J Neuroradiol 2005;26:553–559.

Ganti SR, Hilal SK, Stein BM, et al. CT of pineal region tumors. AJR Am J Radiol 1986;146:451–458.

Gao P-Y, Osborn AG, Smirniotopoulos JG, Harris CP. Epidermoid tumor of the cerebellopontine angle. AJNR Am J Neuroradiol 1992;13:863–872.

George AE, Russell EJ, Kricheff II. White matter buckling: CT sign of extra-axial intracranial mass. AJNR Am J Neuroradiol 1980;1:425–430.

Goldsher D, Litt AW, Pinto RS, et al. Dural "tail" associated with meningiomas on Gd-DTPA-enhanced MR images: characteristics, differential diagnostic value, and possible implications for treatment. Radiology 1990;176:447–450.

Hahn F, Gurney J. CT signs of central descending transtentorial herniation. AJNR Am J Neuroradiol 1985;6:844–845.

Haimes AB, Zimmerman RD, Morgello S. MR imaging of brain abscess. AJNR Am J Neuroradiol 1989;10:279–291.

Hanna SL, Langston JW, Parham DM, Douglass EC. Primary malignant rhabdoid tumor of the brain: clinical, imaging, and pathologic findings. AJNR Am J Neuroradiol 1993;14:107–115.

Henkelman RM, Watts JF, Kucharczyk W. High signal intensity in MR images of calcified brain tissue. Radiology 1991;179:199–206.

Hochberg FH, Miller DC. Primary central nervous system lymphoma. J Neurosurg 1988;68:835–853.

Kahn D, Follett KA, Bushnell DL, et al. Diagnosis of recurrent brain tumor: value of 201TI SPECT vs. 18F-fluorodeoxyglucose PET. AJR Am J Radiol 1994;163:1459–1465.

Kelly PJ, Daumas-Duport C, Scheithauer BW, et al. Stereotactic histologic correlation of CT- and MR-defined abnormalities in patients with glial neoplasms. Mayo Clin Proc 1987;62:450–459.

Kirsch C, Smirniotopoulos JG, Koeller KK. Colloid cysts: radiologic-pathologic correlation with review of the Armed Forces Institiute of Pathology (AFIP) experience and world literature. Int J Neuroradiol 1997;3:460–469.

Kleihues P, Cavenee WK, eds. Pathology and Genetics of Tumours of the Nervous System. Lyon, France: IARC Press, 2000.

Koeller KK, Dillon WP. MR appearance of dysembryoplastic neuroepithelial tumors (DNT). AJNR Am J Neuroradiol 1992;1319–1325.

Koeller KK, Henry JM. Superficial gliomas: radiologic-pathologic correlation. Radiographics 2001;21:1533–1556.

Koeller KK, Rushing EJ. Medulloblastoma: a comprehensive review with radiologic-pathologic correlation. Radiographics 2003;23:1613–1637.

Koeller KK, Rushing EJ. Pilocytic astrocytoma: radiologic-pathologic correlation. Radiographics 2004;24:1693–1708.

Koeller KK, Sandberg GD. Cerebral intraventricular neoplasms: radiologic-pathologic correlation. Radiographics 2002;22:1473–1505.

Koeller KK, Smirniotopoulos JG, Jones RV. Primary central nervous system lymphoma: radiologic-pathologic correlation. Radiographics 1997;17:1497–1526.

Lee SR, Sanches J, Mark AS, et al. Posterior fossa hemangioblastomas: MR imaging. Radiology 1989;171:463–468.

Lee Y-Y, Tassel PV. Intracranial oligodendrogliomas: imaging findings in 35 untreated cases. AJNR Am J Neuroradiol 1989;10: 119–127.

Olson EM, Tien RD, Chamberlain MC. Osseous metastasis in medulloblastoma: MRI findings in an unusual case. Clin Imaging 1991;15: 286–289.

Sage MR. Blood-brain barrier: Phenomenon of increasing importance to the imaging clinician. AJR Am J Radiol 1982;138:887–898.

So YT, Beckstead JH, Davis RL. Primary central nervous system lymphoma in acquired immune deficiency syndrome: a clinical and pathological study. Ann Neurol 1986;20:566–572.

Spagnoli MV, Grossman RI, Packer RJ, et al. Magnetic resonance imaging determination of gliomatosis cerebri. Neuroradiology 1987;29:15–18.

Sze G, Milano E, Johnson C, Heier L. Detection of brain metastasis: comparison of contrast-enhanced MR with unenhanced MR and enhanced CT. AJNR Am J Neuroradiol 1990;11:785–791.

Tokumaru A, O'uchi T, Eguchi T, et al. Prominent meningeal enhancement adjacent to meningioma on Gd-DTPA-enhanced MR images: histopathologic correlation. Radiology 1990;175:431–433.

Valk PE, Dillon WP. Radiation injury of the brain. AJNR Am J Neuroradiol 1991;12:45–62.

Waggenspack GA, Guinto FCJ. MR and CT of masses of the anterosuperior third ventricle. AJNR Am J Neuroradiol 1989;10:105–110.

Yuh WTC, Engelken JD, Muhonen MG, et al. Experience with high-dose MR imaging in the evaluation of brain metastasis. AJNR Am J Neuroradiol 1992;13:335–345.

Chapter 6

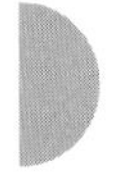

Central Nervous System Infections

Walter L. Olsen

Parenchymal Infections
- Pyogenic Cerebritis and Abscess
- Mycobacterial Infections
- Fungal Infections
- Parasitic Infections
- Spirochete Infections
- Viral Infections

Extra-axial Infections
- Meningitis
- Subdural and Epidural Infections

Acquired Immunodeficiency Syndrome

CNS infections commonly require evaluation by radiologists. Because these infections often have dire neurologic consequences, early diagnosis and management are crucial. CT and MR have significantly aided this effort. For example, prior to CT, pyogenic abscesses of the brain carried a 30% to 70% mortality rate. The mortality rate has dropped to less than 5% in recent years, largely because of the ability of cross-sectional imaging to accurately diagnose the abscess and monitor the efficacy of treatment. MR is usually the imaging modality of choice in the evaluation of CNS infection, because of its improved sensitivity. However, because both CT and MR are highly accurate, the choice of modality often depends on the clinical situation. Gravely ill patients are often better evaluated by CT, which is faster, less susceptible to patient motion artifact, and permits closer patient monitoring. MR is generally preferable in the clinically stable patient.

PARENCHYMAL INFECTIONS

Pyogenic Cerebritis and Abscess

Pyogenic infections of the brain may develop by direct extension following trauma, surgery, sinusitis, dental infections, or otomastoiditis. Hematogenous infections occur even more frequently, especially in patients with lung infections, endocarditis, or congenital heart disease. Anaerobic bacteria are the most common organisms overall. Infection with *Staphylococcus aureus* is common after surgery or trauma. Gram-negative rod, pneumococcal, streptococcal, listerial, nocardial, and actinomycotic infections also occur with some frequency. With infections resulting from hematogenous spread, the frontal and parietal lobes (middle cerebral artery distribution) are most commonly involved, with the abscess centered at the gray–white junction. The frontal lobes are most commonly affected with spread of sinus infections. The temporal lobe or cerebellum is involved in patients with spread from otomastoiditis.

Clinical symptoms in patients with pyogenic brain infections may be mild or severe. Usually there is headache. There may be varying degrees of lethargy, obtundation, nausea, vomiting, and fever. Fever is absent more than 50% of the time. Meningeal signs are present in only 30% of patients. Focal neurologic deficits, papilledema, nuchal rigidity, and seizures often develop rapidly, over the course of a few days. This is in distinction to tumors, where these symptoms usually develop more slowly. There is often, but not invariably, an elevated white blood cell count. CSF findings are often nonspecific and are usually not obtained because of the risk of lumbar puncture in the setting of a brain mass.

Pathologically, there are four stages of evolution of a brain abscess, which correlate with the imaging findings.

Early Cerebritis. Within the first few days of infection, the infected portion of brain is swollen and edematous. Areas of necrosis are filled with polymorphonuclear leukocytes, lymphocytes, and plasma cells. Organisms are present in both the center and the periphery of the lesion, which has ill-defined margins. CT scans may be normal or show an area of low density (Fig. 6.1A). There may be mild mass effect and patchy areas of enhancement within the lesion. On MR the lesion shows increased signal on proton density images, fluid-attenuated inversion recovery (FLAIR) images, and T2WIs, with low intensity or isointensity on T1WIs (Figs. 6.1B, C). Enhancement with gadolinium is inconstant at this stage. Use of high-dose (0.3-mmoL/kg) gadolinium and/or magnetization transfer will increase the likelihood of detecting enhancement. A ring of enhancement is not present at this stage,

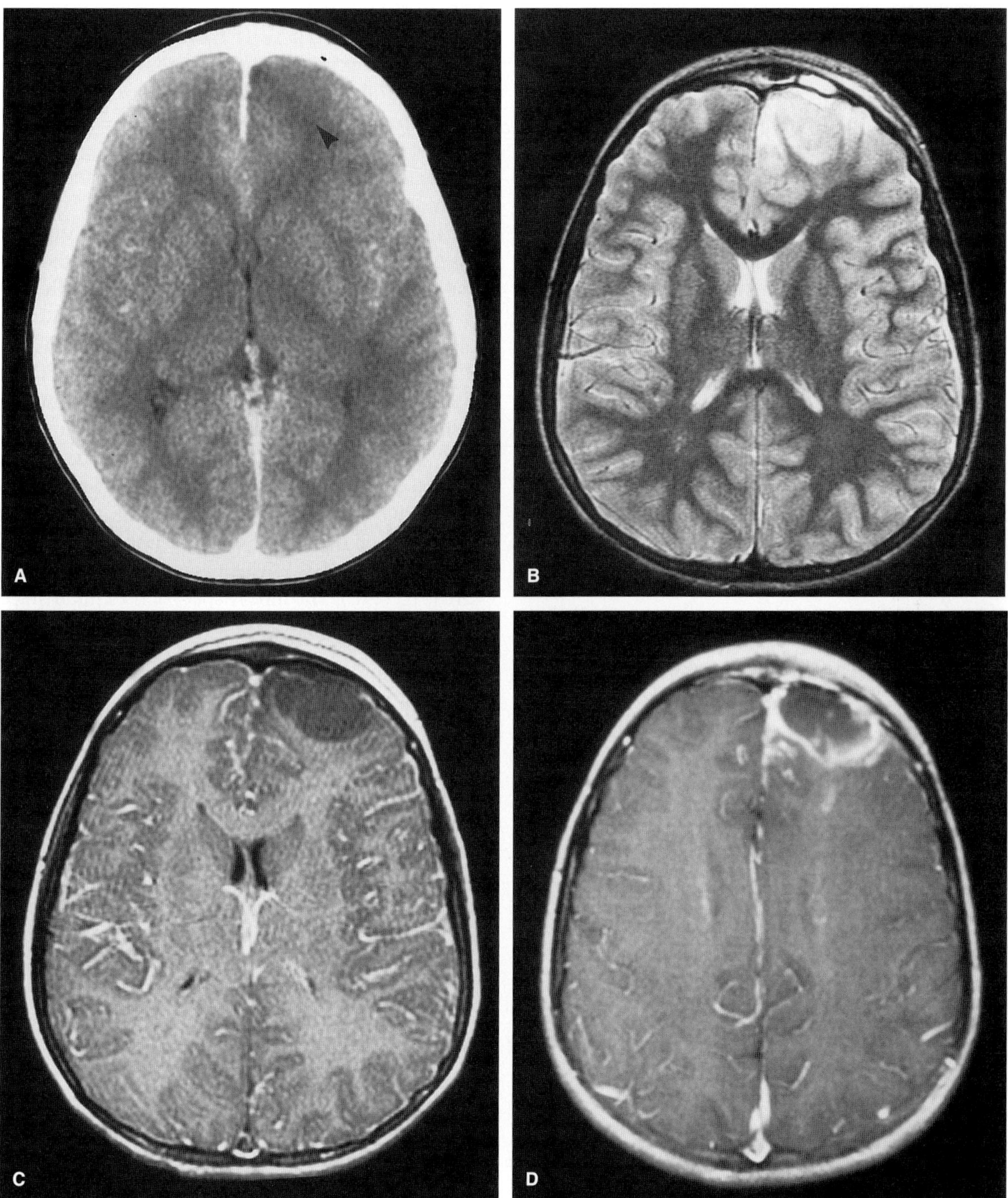

FIGURE 6.1. **Early Cerebritis. A.** Contrast CT scan shows a subtle area of decreased density in the left frontal lobe (*arrowhead*). **B.** T2WI obtained the next day shows high signal intensity in the left frontal lobe and left frontal sinusitis. **C.** Gadolinium-enhanced T1WI shows low signal intensity without enhancement, consistent with early cerebritis. **D.** Two weeks later, a T1W, gadolinium-enhanced scan shows a ring-enhancing abscess.

distinguishing it from the later three stages. Unfortunately, these imaging features are nonspecific and can be seen with tumors or infarcts. The clinical features are therefore most important in making the correct diagnosis. If the diagnosis can be made at this stage, nonsurgical treatment with antibiotics is often effective.

Late cerebritis occurs within 1 or 2 weeks of infection. Central necrosis is increased, with fewer organisms detected pathologically. There is vascular proliferation at the periphery of the lesion, with more inflammatory cells, which represents the brain's effort to contain the infection. Not surprisingly, this results in thick, irregular contrast enhancement at the edges of the lesion on imaging studies (Fig. 6.2). Centrally, there is increased signal on FLAIR images and T2WIs. Diffusion-weighted imaging (DWI) may show some increased signal within the center of the lesion. Vasogenic edema is seen outside the enhancing rim at this stage as well. Delayed scans may show central filling in with contrast. No discrete, low-signal capsule is evident on T2WIs, in distinction to some mature abscesses. This stage can also be treated effectively with antibiotic therapy, but distinguishing late cerebritis from an early abscess or tumor can be difficult, and surgery is often performed.

Early Capsule. Within 2 weeks, the infection is walled off as a capsule of collagen and reticulin forms in the inflammatory, vascular margin of the infection. Macrophages, phagocytes, and neutrophils are also present in the capsule. The necrotic center contains very few organisms. Contrast-enhanced CT and MR scans show a well defined rim of enhancement (Fig. 6.1D). The rim tends to be low in signal on T2WIs. Centrally there is necrosis (low density on CT, low signal on T1WIs, and high signal on intermediate images, FLAIR images, and T2WIs). Prominent surrounding vasogenic edema is usually present. There is increased signal centrally on DWI, which is very helpful in distinguishing abscesses from necrotic tumors, which are not usually bright on diffusion.

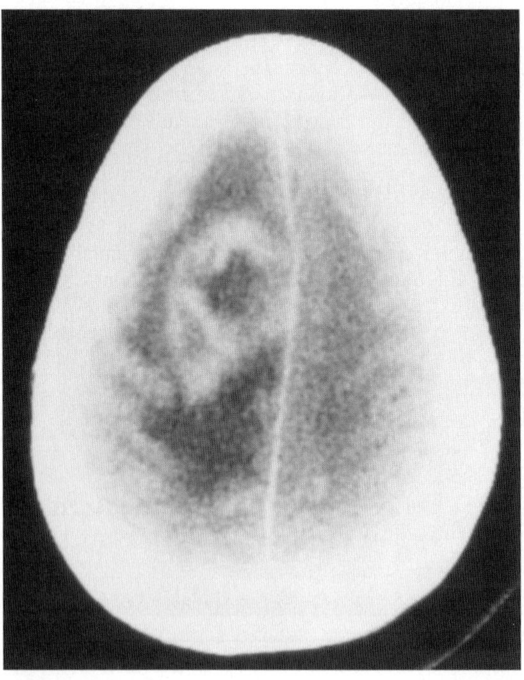

FIGURE 6.2. **Late Cerebritis.** This contrast-enhanced CT scan demonstrates irregular enhancement peripherally and low density centrally. There is surrounding low-density vasogenic edema. This is typical of the late cerebritis stage of pyogenic infection.

Late Capsule. In the late capsule stage, the rim of enhancement becomes even better defined and thin, reflecting more complete collagen in the abscess wall (Fig. 6.3). Multiloculation is common. The capsule often exhibits characteristic MR features that are helpful diagnostically at this stage. On T1WIs, the capsule is usually isointense or hyperintense to white matter, and on T2WIs it is usually hypointense to white matter (Fig. 6.4A, B) These signal characteristics suggest paramagnetic T1 and T2 shortening, similar to that seen in hematoma evolution (see Chapter 4). However, hemorrhage is not often found pathologically, and the paramagnetic effects may be secondary to the presence of free radicals produced by macrophages in the capsule. In any case, the MR appearance of the capsule is fairly specific for abscess. There is marked increased signal centrally on DWI, which is a very helpful imaging feature (Fig. 6.4C). The inner aspect of the enhancing capsule is often (about 50% of the time) thinner than the peripheral aspect (Figs. 6.3C, 6.4D). This reflects decreased blood supply and fibroblast migration centrally compared with cortically. This thin medial rim predisposes to intraventricular rupture, with resulting ependymitis/ventriculitis (Fig. 6.3C). CT or MR scans reveal enhancement of the ependymal lining of the ventricle and sometimes abnormal density/signal intensity of the intraventricular CSF.

A solitary abscess is usually treated surgically. Often, stereotactic needle aspiration, followed by antibiotic therapy, is performed, especially if the abscess is in an eloquent area of the brain. If there is significant mass effect, or if the lesion is in a relatively "safe" area, a formal drainage or resection is performed. If there are multiple abscesses, or if the patient is at high surgical risk, antibiotic therapy alone is used. Imaging studies should be performed frequently (about once a week) to monitor the efficacy of treatment and to assess for complications such as ventriculitis, infarction, or hydrocephalus.

The differential diagnosis of pyogenic abscess includes tumor and resolving hematoma. The clinical features, combined with the appearance of central high signal on DWI, thin enhancing rim (thinnest medially), much edema, and paramagnetic effects in the capsule (with no blood products centrally), should strongly suggest a brain abscess.

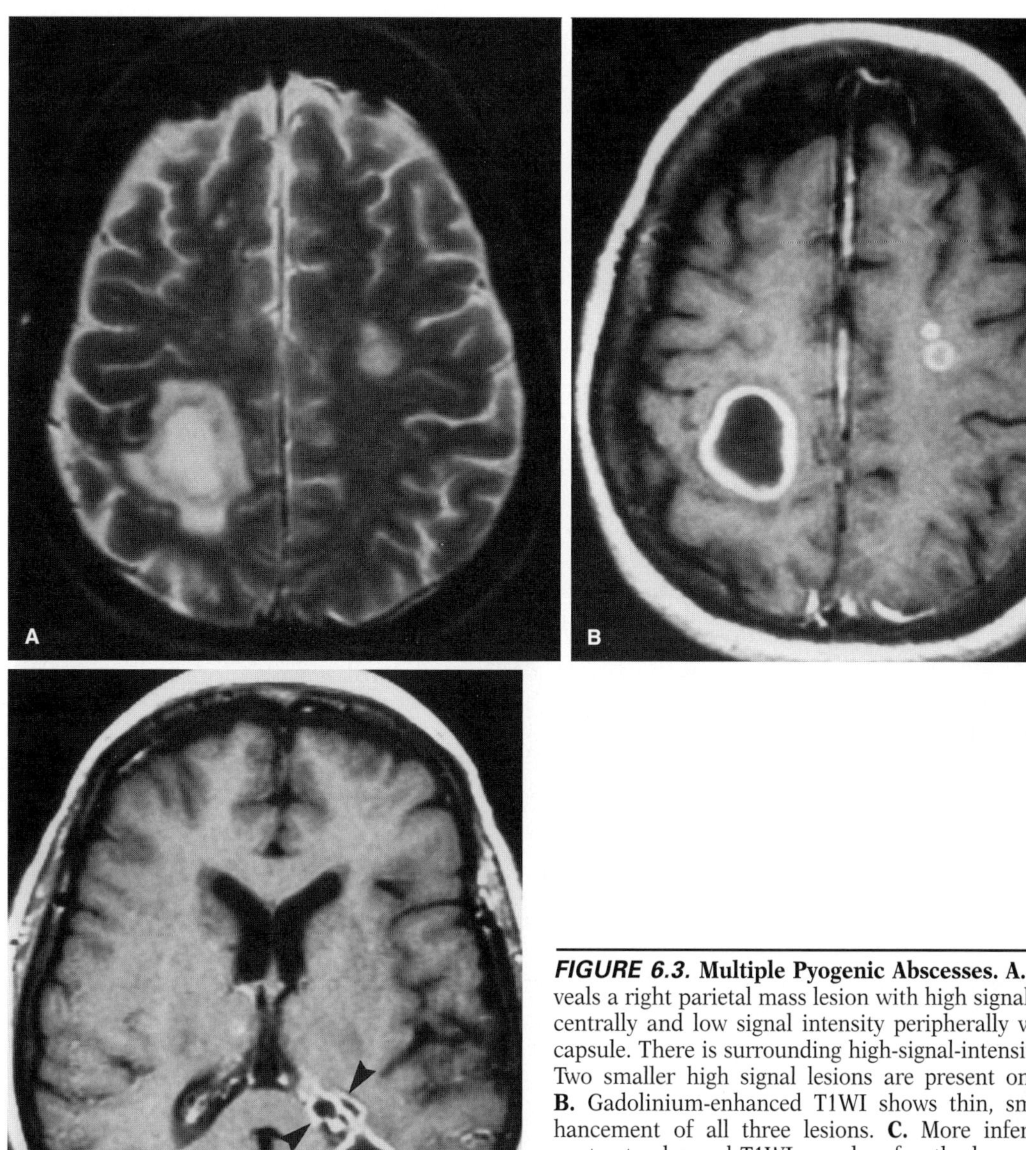

FIGURE 6.3. **Multiple Pyogenic Abscesses. A.** T2WI reveals a right parietal mass lesion with high signal intensity centrally and low signal intensity peripherally within the capsule. There is surrounding high-signal-intensity edema. Two smaller high signal lesions are present on the left. **B.** Gadolinium-enhanced T1WI shows thin, smooth enhancement of all three lesions. **C.** More inferiorly, the contrast-enhanced T1WI reveals a fourth abscess that has extended into the atrium of the left lateral ventricle (*arrowheads*). The enhancement pattern and intraventricular extension favor the diagnosis of abscess over tumor. These lesions proved to be abscesses that cultured anaerobic streptococci. (Case courtesy of Dr. Vincent Burke, Atherton, California.)

Septic Embolus. Infections that begin with a septic embolus may not have the typical appearance of an abscess. The embolus frequently causes an infarct that dominates the imaging findings. Depending on the size of the embolus, there may be a small rounded area of enhancement or a larger, wedge-shaped cortical infarct. As with other embolic infarcts, hemorrhage may occur. Because the nonviable, infarcted tissue has a poor blood supply, a typical capsule may not form. A thicker, more irregular ring of enhancement that persists within an area of infarction should suggest the diagnosis. Septic emboli may lead to mycotic aneurysm formation, which can result in intraparenchymal or subarachnoid hemorrhage.

Listeria monocytogenes is an anaerobic gram-positive bacillus that primarily infects immunocompromised patients. The organism can cause meningitis, meningoencephalitis, and abscesses. Listerial rhombencephalitis involves the brainstem and cerebellum. MR scans reveal areas of abnormal signal and enhancement in the brainstem and cerebellar white matter tracts. The appearance is similar to that of acute disseminated encephalomyelitis (see "Viral Infections"). Occasionally, otherwise healthy patients may develop this infection.

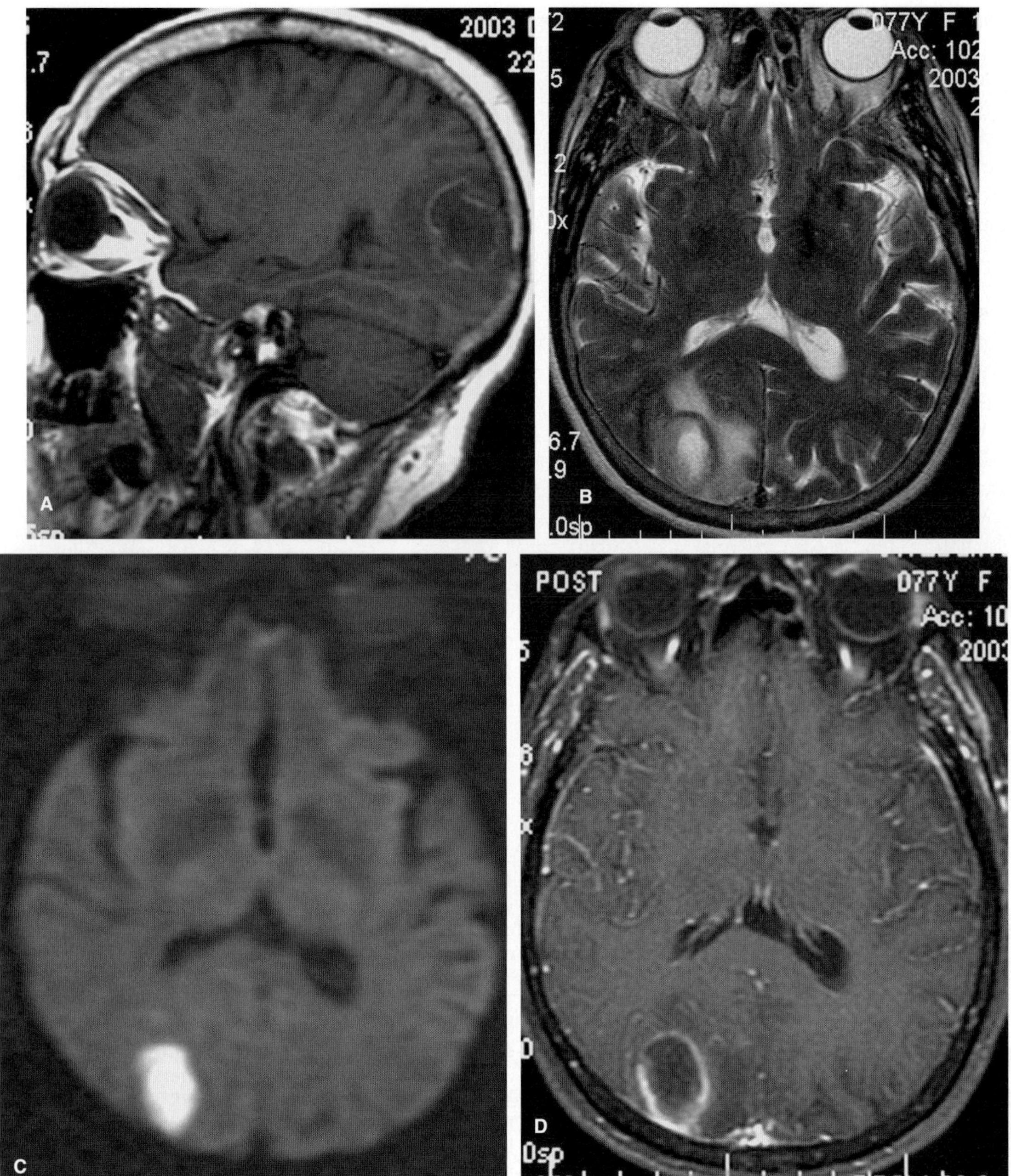

FIGURE 6.4. **Pyogenic Cerebral Abscess.** This case illustrates most of the classic features of a cerebral abscess. **A.** T1W sagittal scan shows high signal in the rim of the abscess as a result of paramagnetic T1 shortening. **B.** T2WI shows low signal in the rim from T2 shortening with high signal centrally and significant surrounding edema. **C.** Diffusion-weighted scan shows increased signal centrally, a characteristic feature of abscesses that is usually not seen with necrotic tumors. **D.** Postcontrast T1WI shows enhancement of the rim that is thinnest medially, as is often the case with abscesses.

Mycobacterial Infections

The most common form of CNS mycobacterial infection is tuberculous meningitis, which will be discussed later in this chapter. Focal mycobacterial infection of the brain occurs in two forms: tuberculoma and abscess. A tuberculoma is a granuloma with central caseous necrosis. A tuberculous abscess has characteristics similar to those of a pyogenic abscess, but it develops in patients with impaired T-cell immunity.

Tuberculoma. In the early 1900s, one third of all brain mass lesions in England were tuberculomas. Because of improved prevention and treatment, these lesions are now unusual in industrialized countries. In developing areas of the world, however, tuberculomas account for 15% to 30% of brain masses. Approximately 5% to 10% of patients with tuberculosis develop CNS disease. There is a predilection for the extremes of age: children and the elderly. The infection spreads to the brain hematogenously from the lungs. In developed countries, tuberculomas usually result from reactivation of quiescent disease, although only 50% of patients have a known history of previous tuberculosis. Most lesions in adults are supratentorial, involving the frontal or parietal lobes. Sixty percent of tuberculomas in children are in the posterior fossa, usually the cerebellum. Multiple lesions are common. Most tuberculomas are not associated with tuberculous meningitis. Clinical features include headache, seizures, papilledema, and focal neurologic signs. Fever is seen only rarely. The CSF is almost always abnormal, showing elevated protein and reduced glucose. An abnormal chest radiograph is present in up to 50% of patients. These lesions can be treated medically if there are characteristic clinical and imaging features. Surgery is often performed when the diagnosis is in doubt, for medical treatment failures, and for large lesions.

Noncontrast CT scans show one or more isodense or slightly hyperdense nodules or small mass lesions. Multiple lesions are present about 50% of the time. The center of the tuberculoma is usually denser than the fluidlike center of a pyogenic abscess because of caseous necrosis. A "target" appearance, with a central calcification surrounded by rim enhancement, is an uncommon but helpful finding, strongly suggesting the diagnosis. Calcification is present in fewer than 5% of cases at the initial diagnosis but is commonly seen with treatment as the lesions resolve. With MR, tuberculomas may be high or low in signal intensity with T2WIs, depending upon the size of the lesion and the water content of the caseous necrosis. (Fig. 6.5A) The wall of the tuberculoma is often low in signal on T2WIs. There is significant enhancement after gadolinium administration, with a solid nodular or thick ring-shaped appearance (Fig. 6.5B). There may or may not be increased signal on DWI, unlike bacterial infections, which usually show restricted diffusion (Fig. 6.5C). Surrounding edema is often mild. The differential diagnosis includes tumor, pyogenic abscess, fungal and parasitic infections, and sarcoidosis.

Tuberculous abscess is a rare complication seen primarily in immunocompromised patients. Abnormal T-cell

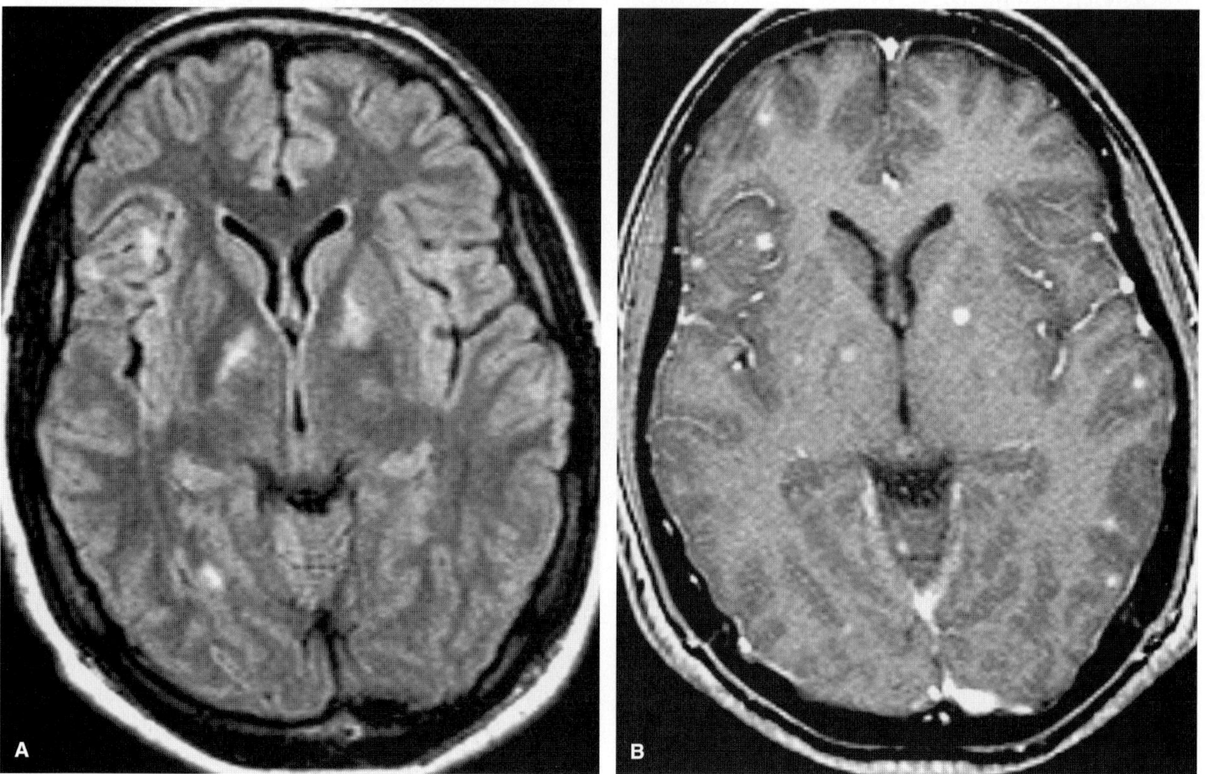

FIGURE 6.5. **Multiple Tuberculomas. A.** Fluid-attenuated inversion recovery (FLAIR) axial scan shows multiple small areas of increased signal without significant edema bilaterally. **B.** Postcontrast T1W axial scan shows multiple small enhancing nodules. **C.** There is no abnormal restricted diffusion on this DWI axial scan. The appearance of tuberculomas on diffusion-weighted imaging (DWI) is variable, unlike pyogenic infections, which almost always show restricted diffusion (bright on DWI).

function prevents the normal host response of tuberculoma formation with caseous necrosis. Symptoms develop more rapidly than with tuberculomas. The imaging features are similar to that seen with pyogenic abscesses. The lesions are often large and multiloculated, in distinction to tuberculomas. Prominent edema and mass effect also distinguish tuberculous abscess from tuberculoma. Atypical mycobacterial infections are also more common in immunocompromised patients.

Fungal Infections

Fungal infections of the CNS can be grouped into endemic and cosmopolitan categories. *Endemic* fungal infections are geographically restricted. They can occur in both immunocompetent and immunosuppressed patients. *Cosmopolitan* fungal infections occur worldwide, usually in immunosuppressed patients, infants, the elderly or chronically ill, with the exception of cryptococcosis, which also occurs in patients with normal immunity.

Endemic Fungal Infections. The most common endemic fungal infections in the United States are coccidioidomycosis, North American blastomycosis, and histoplasmosis. These infections usually manifest as granulomatous meningitis, as will be discussed. Focal parenchymal lesions are unusual. CNS involvement is a manifestation of disseminated infection, with hematogenous spread, usually from pulmonary disease.

Coccidioidomycosis occurs in the southwestern United States. The spores are inhaled, with outbreaks occurring after groundbreaking for construction projects. Most infected patients are asymptomatic or have mild respiratory symptoms. Less than 1% of patients develop disseminated infection and meningitis. Focal parenchymal granulomas are rare.

Blastomycosis occurs in the Ohio and Mississippi River valleys. CNS involvement occurs in 6% to 33% of disseminated cases. Meningitis is the most frequent presentation, but parenchymal abscesses and granulomas occur more frequently than with coccidioidomycosis. Epidural granulomas and abscesses also occur in the head and spine, usually from direct extension from bone infection. Up to 40% of focal brain lesions are multiple.

Histoplasmosis is usually a benign, asymptomatic infection, occurring in the Midwest and southern United States. Dissemination is unusual, and only a small percent of disseminated cases involve the CNS. Meningitis is most common, but multiple or solitary granulomas may occur. Abscesses are unusual.

As seen with CT or MR, most fungal granulomas are small and show solid or thick rim enhancement (Fig. 6.6). Fungal abscesses (as sometimes seen with blastomycosis) have an appearance similar to that of the pyogenic abscesses that were described earlier. Meningeal enhancement from meningitis is a common accompanying feature. Hydrocephalus is also common, especially with coccidioidomycosis.

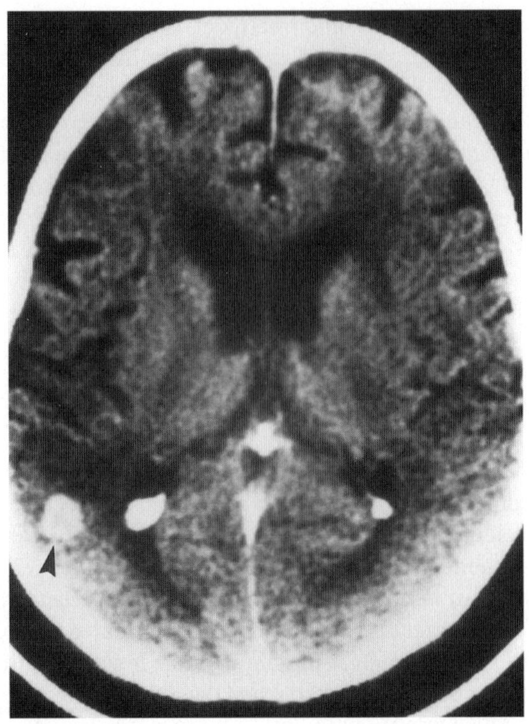

FIGURE 6.6. **Histoplasmosis Granuloma.** This patient had disseminated histoplasmosis with several lesions in the brain and spine. This contrast-enhanced CT scan shows a solidly enhancing lesion near the atrium of the right lateral ventricle (*arrowhead*). Most fungal granulomas are small and show either solid or thick rim enhancement. (Case courtesy of Dr. J. R. Jinkins, San Antonio, Texas.)

Cosmopolitan Fungal Infections. The most common cosmopolitan fungal infections are cryptococcosis, aspergillosis, mucormycosis, and candidiasis. These infections also usually present as meningitis, but focal parenchymal lesions are fairly common.

Aspergillosis involves the CNS in 60% to 70% of patients with disseminated disease. The infection may arise from hematogenous spread or by direct extension from an infected paranasal sinus, leading to meningitis or meningoencephalitis. Parenchymal disease usually takes the form of an abscess. Granulomas are unusual. The abscesses are often multiple and show irregular ring enhancement (Fig. 6.7). Subcortical or cortical infarcts and hemorrhage from blood vessel invasion may occur. The mortality rate with invasive intracerebral aspergillosis is greater than 85%.

Mucormycosis. Mucor invades the brain usually by direct extension from the sinuses, nose, or oral cavity, but hematogenous spread also occurs. Almost all patients are diabetic or otherwise immunocompromised. The mortality rate in treated diabetic patients is 65% to 75% and is

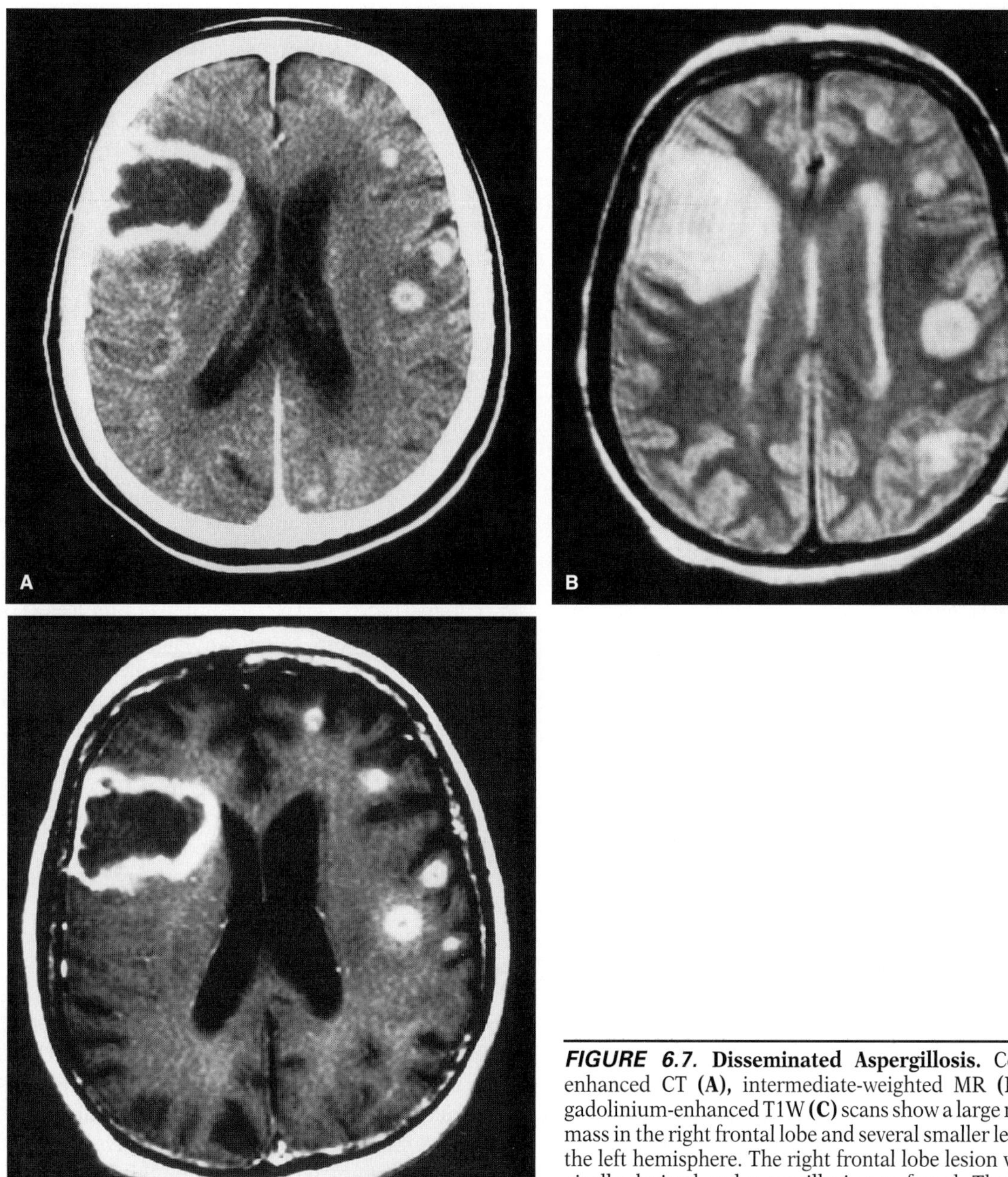

FIGURE 6.7. **Disseminated Aspergillosis.** Contrast-enhanced CT **(A)**, intermediate-weighted MR **(B)**, and gadolinium-enhanced T1W **(C)** scans show a large necrotic mass in the right frontal lobe and several smaller lesions in the left hemisphere. The right frontal lobe lesion was surgically drained and aspergillosis was found. The patient was a poorly controlled diabetic.

worse in immunocompromised patients. Like aspergillosis, mucormycosis tends to invade blood vessels. Imaging studies in patients with CNS mucormycosis will reveal single or multiple mass lesions with varying degrees of peripheral enhancement. The amount of enhancement depends upon the compromised host's ability to fight the infection. Surrounding edema is variable in amount. Smaller lesions will show a solid enhancement pattern. The lesions are often in the base of the brain, adjacent to diseased sinuses. Infarcts, intra-axial or extra-axial hemorrhage, and meningeal enhancement can be seen with CT or MR. A lesion with peripheral enhancement, cortical sparing, and a nonvascular distribution is more likely to be a mucormycotic abscess than an infarct, but often it is difficult to distinguish the two.

Candidiasis usually causes meningitis, but granulomas and small abscesses may occur. Spread to the CNS is usually hematogenous from the lungs or GI. In cases of CNS candidiasis, meningeal enhancement or multiple small enhancing granulomas or microabscesses are usually seen. Infarcts, hydrocephalus, and large abscesses may also be identified.

Cryptococcosis is the most frequently reported CNS fungal infection. It occurs in patients with normal immune function in about 50% of cases. This is also an extremely common infection in patients with AIDS, as will be discussed later in this chapter. Infection of the CNS occurs via hematogenous spread from the lungs. Serologies and CSF studies are valuable in making the diagnosis: about 90% of patients have antigen in the CSF and/or antibody in the serum. The usual manifestation is meningitis. Granulomas can occur and are usually multiple. Abscesses are less common. CT scans in patients with cryptococcosis are usually normal, reflecting relatively mild meningeal involvement in most cases. Mass lesions are seen in about 10% of cases. Cryptococcomas are shown as small, usually multiple, solid-enhancing, peripheral parenchymal nodules. Calcifications within a granuloma are occasionally seen. With the improved sensitivity of MR, meningeal and parenchymal lesions are seen more frequently than with CT. Leptomeningeal nodules are often only seen on T1W, contrast-enhanced MR as multiple tiny enhancing lesions near the basal cisternae and sulci. Diffuse meningeal enhancement is unusual. Granulomas may show either solid or ring enhancement.

Another characteristic cryptococcal lesion is the gelatinous pseudocyst. This is a cystic lesion, usually in the basal ganglia, representing enlarged Virchow-Robin spaces filled with the organism. These lesions are usually found only in immunocompromised patients (see Fig. 6.33). Viewed on CT, gelatinous pseudocysts are smooth, round, low-density masses in the basal ganglia which show no contrast enhancement. They are usually better seen with MR than with CT, as lesions are nearly isointense with CSF on all sequences that do not enhance.

Parasitic Infections

Parasitic infections are common throughout much of the developing world but are relatively uncommon in the industrialized nations. The most common infections likely to be encountered in the United States are cysticercosis, echinococcosis, toxoplasmosis, and rarely amebiasis. CNS involvement in malaria, trypanosomiasis, paragonimiasis, sparganosis, and schistosomiasis is rarely encountered in the United States and will not be discussed.

Cysticercosis is caused by the larvae of the pork tapeworm *Taenia solium*. Infestation occurs via the fecal-oral route. When larvae are ingested, intestinal disease results, and eggs are released into the bowel stream. The life cycle can be completed if the eggs are ingested by the pig but not by humans. In this situation, the eggs form oncospheres (primary larvae), which hatch in the intestine and are hematogenously distributed throughout the body and form cysticerci (secondary larvae). The cysticerci cannot develop further in humans and they eventually die. Cysticerci that reach the CNS may infest the parenchyma, meninges, ventricles, or spine. This disease is fairly frequently encountered in the southwestern United States in Latin American immigrants. Seizures occur in more than 90% of patients. Cysticercosis is the most common cause of seizures in Latin America. Encephalitic symptoms are also common. Treatment is with anticysticercus drugs such as praziquantel and albendazole.

Parenchymal cysticercosis is the most common type. Early in the infestation, during the tissue invasion stage, CT or MR scans show edema and/or nodular enhancement. Later, the viable cysts appear as small (usually 1 cm or less), solitary or multiple rounded lesions that are low density on CT and isointense to CSF on MR (Fig. 6.8). The lesions are usually peripherally distributed near the gray–white junction or in the gray matter. A small marginal nodule representing the scolex is sometimes seen (Figs. 6.8B and 6.9). There is usually no enhancement or edema at this vesicular stage. When the cyst dies, the fluid within it leaks into the surrounding brain, causing inflammation. This produces clinical symptoms of an acute encephalitis, which may be severe, depending on the number of lesions. Imaging studies now reveal ring-enhancing lesions with surrounding edema (Fig. 6.9). The cyst fluid is of increased density on CT and increased signal compared with CSF on T1W and T2W MR. As the dead cyst degenerates, it becomes smaller, showing nodular enhancement, and then calcifies. CT scans at this late stage show small, peripheral calcifications, with no edema or enhancement (Fig. 6.10). With MR, the calcifications are best seen on T2W or T2*W GRE images, but they are better demonstrated by CT. Imaging with CT or MR is useful in staging and monitoring treatment. Once the cyst has degenerated, further drug therapy is not warranted.

Intraventricular cysticercosis is similar to the parenchymal variety in pathogenesis and appearance (Fig. 6.11). The cysts are usually isodense and isointense to CSF, making them difficult to visualize. MR is superior to CT for imaging, as subtle signal changes and lack of CSF pulsations within the cyst makes them more visible. Enhancement may or may not be present, depending on the stage of disease, similar to the parenchymal form. The cysts may obstruct the foramen of Monro, the third ventricle, or the cerebral aqueduct, resulting in hydrocephalus. If acute hydrocephalus occurs, death may rapidly ensue. Ventriculitis occurs if the cyst ruptures.

Meningeal infestation is known as *meningobasal* (because the basal cisterns are most frequently involved) or *racemose* (Latin for "clusters") cysticercosis. The cysts lack a scolex but may grow by proliferation of the cyst wall. The cysts may grow in grapelike clusters (Figs. 6.12, 6.13) or conform to the shape of the cistern. No mural nodules or calcifications are seen. CT scans show CSF-density cysts in the basal cisterns. MR reveals cysts that are isointense with CSF, often with mural enhancement or diffuse meningeal enhancement. Hydrocephalus is commonly observed.

Spinal cysticercosis is usually intradural, but can be either intramedullary or extramedullary. Intramedullary

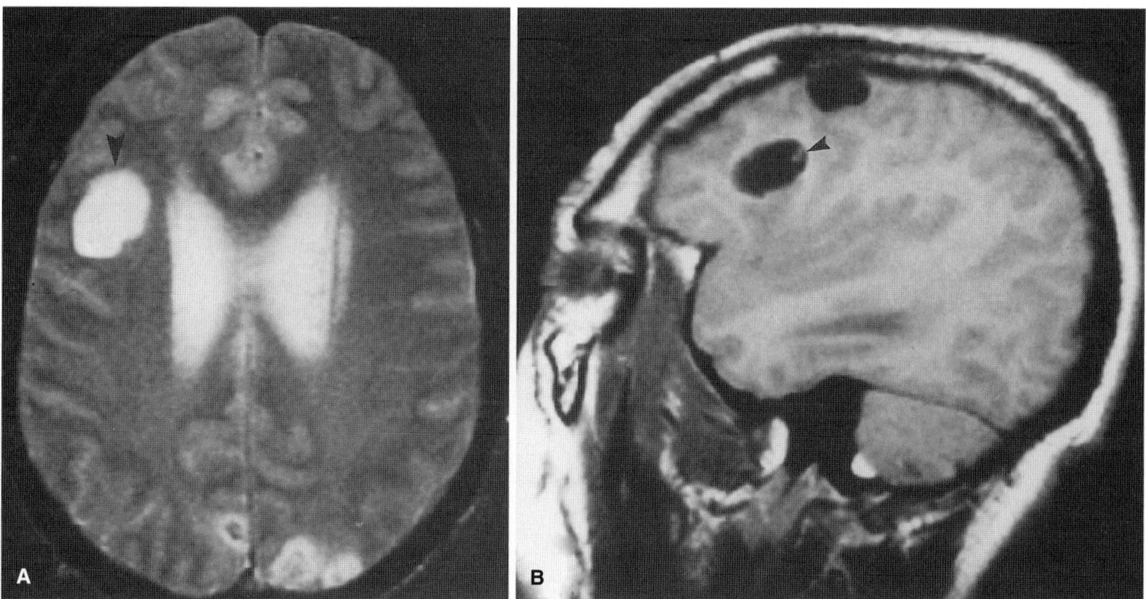

FIGURE 6.8. **Cysticercosis. A.** T2WI shows a right frontal lesion isointense with CSF (*arrowhead*). There is no surrounding edema, indicating that this is early in the course of the disease. Three smaller lesions are present posteriorly. **B.** The T1W parasagittal image in the same patient shows two cysticercal cysts that are isointense with CSF. A scolex is visible in one of the cysts (*arrowhead*).

lesions are best seen with MR as solid or ring-enhancing cord lesions, similar to that seen in the brain parenchyma. Extramedullary cysts are analogous to the racemose form and, like most spinal pathology, are also best evaluated with MR.

Echinococcosis, also known as hydatid disease, occurs in South America, Africa, Central Europe, the Middle East, and rarely in the southwestern United States. The etiologic agent is the dog tapeworm, and humans are intermediate hosts. Hydatid cysts are most frequently present in the lung and liver, but the brain is involved in 1% to 4% of cases. The cysts are usually solitary, unilocular, large, round, and smoothly marginated. They are most often supratentorial, in the middle cerebral artery territory. There may rarely be mural calcification. With CT, the fluid within the cyst is usually isodense with CSF. There is usually no surrounding edema or abnormal contrast enhancement, unless the cyst has ruptured, leading to an inflammatory reaction. With MR, the lesions are usually nearly isointense with CSF.

Toxoplasmosis is caused by the protozoa *Toxoplasma gondii*, which occurs worldwide. The disease may be either congenital or acquired. The acquired form is seen primarily in immunocompromised patients and is very common in AIDS patients, as will be discussed later. The congenital form results when a pregnant woman eats poorly cooked meat or is infected by a cat. A diffuse encephalitis of the fetal brain ensues, usually causing severe destruction. The infant is usually born with microcephaly (Fig. 6.14), chorioretinitis, and mental retardation. Imaging studies reveal atrophy, dilated ventricles, and calcifications. The calcifications occur in the periventricular white matter, basal ganglia and cerebral hemispheres. This is in distinction to congenital cytomegalovirus (CMV), in which the calcifications are usually periventricular only.

Amebic meningoencephalitis is sometimes seen in the southern United States. The amebae enter the nasal cavity of patients swimming in infested freshwater ponds or pools. There is direct extension through the cribriform plate to the brain. Severe meningoencephalitis results and is usually fatal. Imaging studies often underestimate the severity of the disease. Early in the infection, there may be meningeal and/or gray matter enhancement. Later, there is diffuse cerebral edema. There are a few reports of single or multiple, ring-enhancing or solid-enhancing lesions with surrounding edema in patients with amebic brain abscesses. Amebic abscesses are more common in immunosuppressed patients.

Spirochete Infections

Neurosyphilis develops in about 5% of patients who are not treated for the primary infection. Involvement of the CNS usually occurs in the secondary or tertiary stages. Because of effective antibiotic therapy, the disease is rare. However, there has been a significant increase in incidence since the AIDS epidemic. Neurosyphilis is more likely to develop in HIV-infected patients, and the neurologic symptoms occur after a shorter latency period than

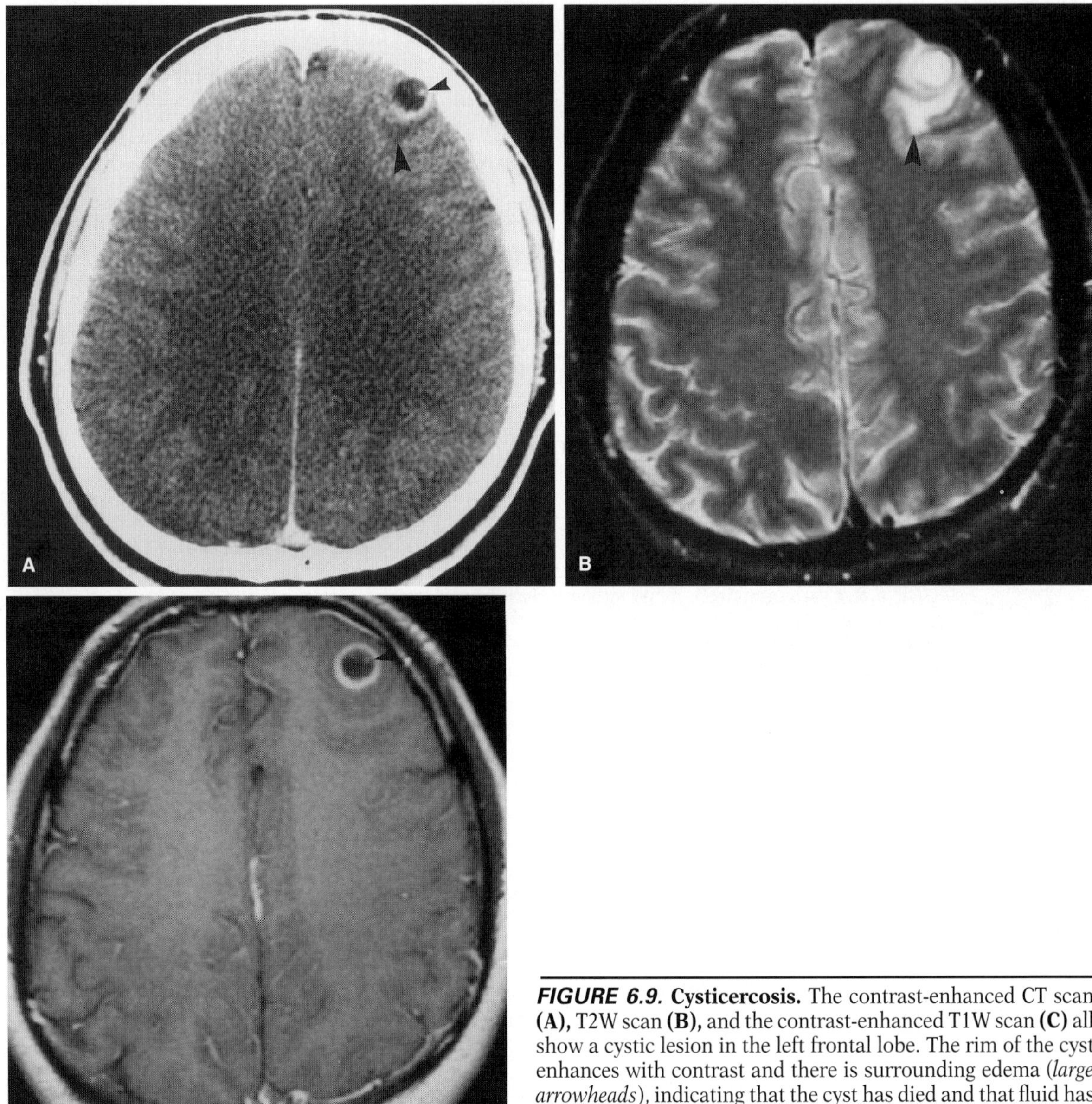

FIGURE 6.9. **Cysticercosis.** The contrast-enhanced CT scan **(A),** T2W scan **(B),** and the contrast-enhanced T1W scan **(C)** all show a cystic lesion in the left frontal lobe. The rim of the cyst enhances with contrast and there is surrounding edema (*large arrowheads*), indicating that the cyst has died and that fluid has leaked out, inciting an inflammatory response. The scolex is visible (*small arrowheads*).

in uninfected patients. Patients with neurosyphilis are usually asymptomatic. Symptomatic patients may have an aseptic meningitis, tabes dorsalis, general paresis, or meningovascular disease. Imaging studies are usually normal in patients with tabes dorsalis, but rarely gummas are found. These usually appear as small enhancing nodules at the surface of the brain, with adjacent meningeal enhancement. Meningovascular syphilis presents as an acute stroke syndrome or a subacute illness with a variety of symptoms. Pathologically, there is thickening of the meninges and a medium to large vessel arteritis. Imaging studies reveal small infarcts of the basal ganglia, white matter, cerebral cortex, or cerebellum (Fig. 6.15A). The infarcts may exhibit patchy or gyriform enhancement, which is best seen with MR. Meningeal enhancement is unusual, but cranial nerve enhancement in patients with syphilitic cranial neuritis has been described. Angiography in patients with meningovascular neurosyphilis reveals multiple segmental constrictions and/or occlusions of large and medium arteries, including the distal internal carotid, anterior cerebral, middle cerebral, posterior cerebral, and distal basilar arteries (Fig. 6.15B).

Lyme disease is a multisystem spirochete infection caused by *Borrelia burgdorferi*. It is found worldwide in deer, mice, raccoons, and birds. It is spread to humans via ticks, especially the deer tick. The disease occurs most frequently on the East Coast, but may occur anywhere in the United States. The disease begins as a flulike illness,

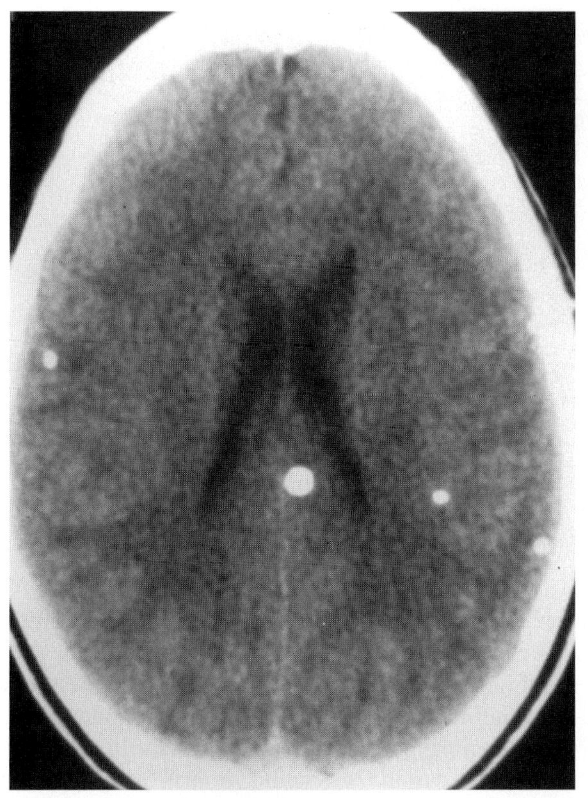

FIGURE 6.10. **Late-Stage Cysticercosis.** This unenhanced CT scan shows multiple calcifications in the gray matter and gray–white junction, which are typical of old cysticercosis.

with a rash and an expanding skin lesion at the tick bite site. In a small percentage of patients, cardiac, arthritic, or neurologic symptoms develop. Neurologic abnormalities are found in 10% to 15% of patients. A variety of symptoms, including peripheral and cranial neuropathies, radiculopathies, myelopathies, encephalitis, meningitis, pain syndromes, cognitive disorders, and movement disorders, have been reported. Treatment with antibiotics and corticosteroids may have variable results. MR is the modality of choice for imaging these patients. In patients with cranial neuritis, MR scans may show thick, enhancing cranial nerves. Cranial nerves III to VIII can be involved, with the facial nerve most commonly affected. In patients with parenchymal CNS Lyme disease, MR scans show multiple small white matter lesions, similar to that seen with multiple sclerosis. The lesions can be found in the supratentorial and infratentorial white matter tracts. The lesions often enhance with contrast in a nodular or ring pattern, depending on the size. There may be meningeal enhancement. The differential diagnosis includes multiple sclerosis and other demyelinating processes.

Viral Infections

The most common viral infections of the CNS include CMV, herpes simplex, varicella zoster, and HIV. Rubella was once a devastating fetal viral infection

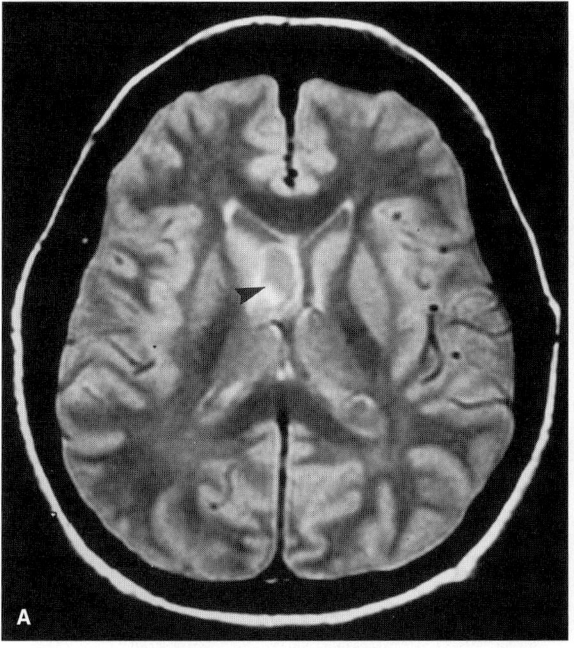

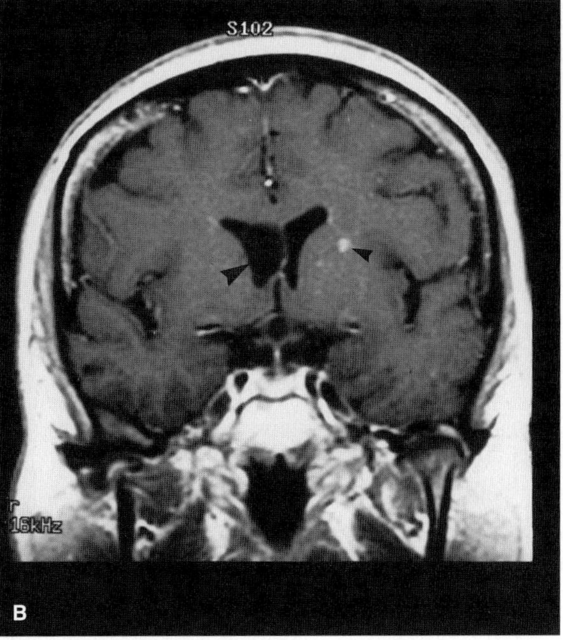

FIGURE 6.11. **Intraventricular Cysticercosis.** Intermediate-weighted axial **(A)** and gadolinium-enhanced T1W coronal **(B)** scans show a cystic mass in the frontal horn of the right lateral ventricle (*large arrowheads*). The lesion is of slightly increased signal intensity compared with CSF in the ventricle. The scolex is of high signal intensity in the posterior aspect of the cyst in **(A)**. There is also a small parenchymal lesion in the left basal ganglia (*small arrowhead*).

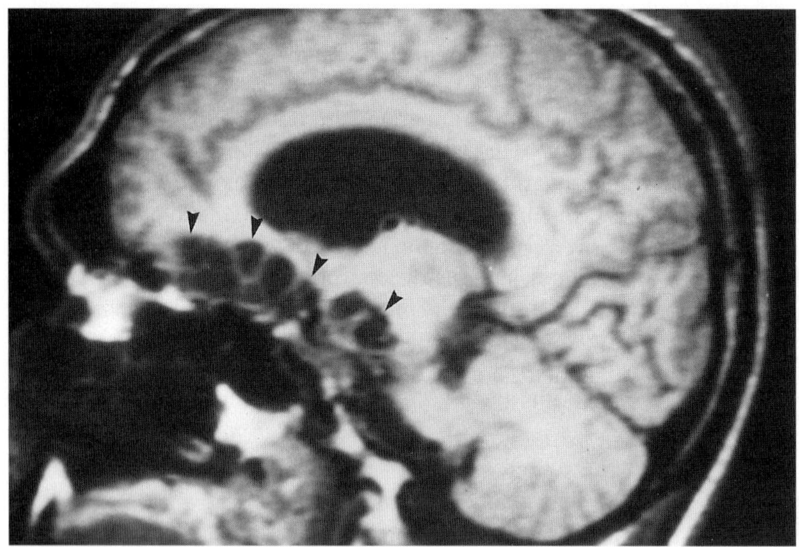

FIGURE 6.12. **Subarachnoid (Racemose) Cysticercosis.** There are multiple cysts in a grapelike cluster in the basal cisterns on this parasagittal T1WI (*arrowheads*). These cysts lack a scolex but grow by proliferation of the cyst wall.

but is now uncommon because of widespread immunization.

Cytomegalovirus is a DNA virus in the herpesvirus family. It causes symptomatic CNS disease primarily through congenital transmission. Maternal CMV infection results in transplacental transmission to the fetus in 30% to 50% of cases and symptomatic disease in 5%. Symptomatic neonates may have hepatosplenomegaly, jaundice, cerebral involvement (psychomotor retardation), chorioretinitis, and deafness. Mental retardation and deafness are present in 20% of cases. The intracranial manifestations of congenital CMV infection largely depend upon the time of infection during gestation. Infection in the first trimester results in necrosis in the germinal matrix, resulting in migrational anomalies. MR scans may show a spectrum of abnormalities, including agyria, polymicrogyria, and focal

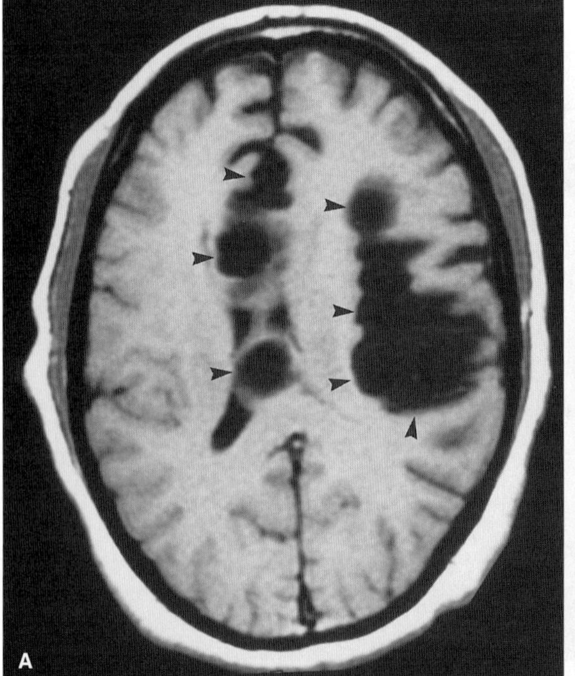

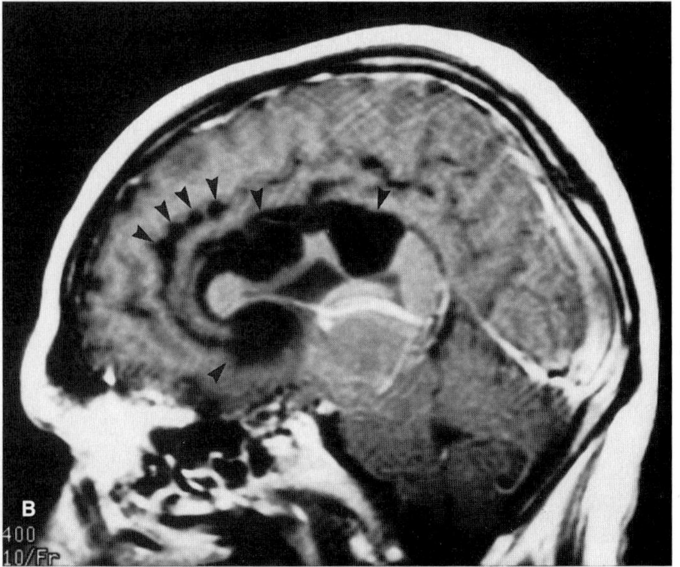

FIGURE 6.13. **Subarachnoid (Racemose) Cysticercosis.** T1W axial **(A)** and gadolinium-enhanced T1W sagittal **(B)** scans show multiple nonenhancing cysts (*arrowheads*) in the left sylvian fissure, callosal sulcus, and cingulate sulcus. The corpus callosum is markedly distorted by the cysts.

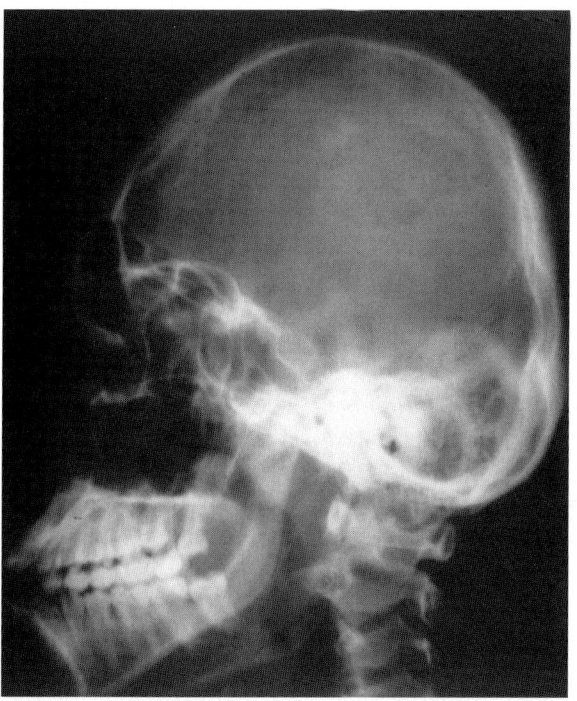

FIGURE 6.14. **Microcephaly.** A lateral skull film shows a small cranial vault, as can be seen in congenital toxoplasmosis or other TORCH (*T*oxoplasmosis; *O*ther, which includes syphilis; *R*ubella; *C*ytomegalovirus; and *H*erpes) infections.

cortical dysplasia. Delayed myelination and cerebellar hypoplasia are also common findings. Patients infected later during gestation may have a normal gyral pattern, but delayed myelination and periventricular white matter lesions are often seen. The most common finding with CT scanning is periventricular calcification (Fig. 6.16). These are detected better with CT than MR. There are usually no calcifications of the basal ganglia or cortices, as is seen in congenital toxoplasmosis. Parenchymal atrophy and ventriculomegaly are common. The disease has been diagnosed in utero with obstetric US. Periventricular hyperechoic calcifications, preceded by hypoechoic periventricular ringlike zones, are characteristic findings. CMV infection in adults is unusual, except in immunosuppressed patients. This will be discussed in the AIDS section.

Herpes simplex encephalitis occurs most frequently in neonates. The infant is usually infected during descent through the birth canal when the mother has genital (type 2) herpes. Occasionally there is transplacental transmission before delivery, but this usually results in spontaneous abortion. The infection causes a severe encephalitis, which is either fatal or has severe neurologic consequences. The patient usually presents with seizures in the second to fourth week of life. If the patient survives, varying degrees of microcephaly, mental

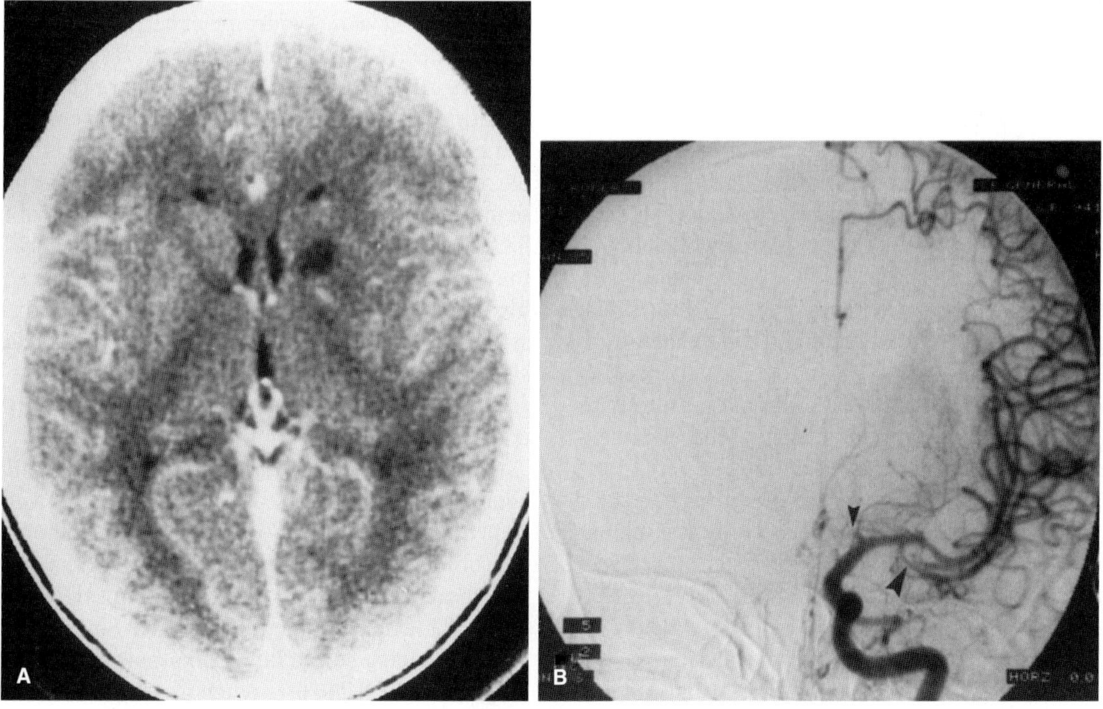

FIGURE 6.15. **Meningovascular Syphilis. A.** Contrast-enhanced CT scan reveals a small infarct in the left striate nucleus in this 21-year-old man with meningovascular syphilis. **B.** A left internal carotid arteriogram in the frontal projection on another patient with meningovascular syphilis shows occlusion of the left anterior cerebral artery (*small arrowhead*) and narrowing of branches of the left middle cerebral artery (*large arrowhead*). Both patients improved with penicillin therapy.

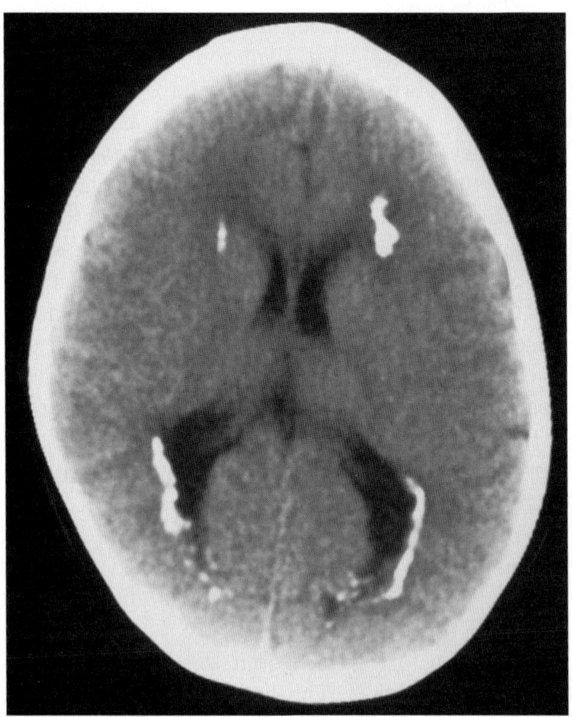

FIGURE 6.16. **Congenital Cytomegalovirus Infection.** A noncontrast CT scan shows multiple periventricular high density calcifications. The calcifications in congenital cytomegalovirus infection tend to be periventricular only, as in this case. With congenital toxoplasmosis, calcifications may be found throughout the brain.

retardation, microphthalmia, enlarged ventricles, intracranial calcifications, and multicystic encephalomalacia may occur. Early in the course of the encephalitis, CT scans may reveal diffuse brain swelling or bilateral patchy areas of decreased density in the cerebral white matter and cortex, with relative sparing of the basal ganglia, thalami, and posterior fossa structures (Fig. 6.17A). Cranial sonography will show areas of increased echogenicity corresponding to these low-density zones. The low-density lesions progress to areas of necrosis, which are sometimes hemorrhagic and may eventually calcify. Multicystic encephalomalacia is the end result. Increased density in the cortical gray matter is characteristic during this late stage (Fig. 6.17B). With MR there is decreased gray–white matter contrast early in the infection, reflecting gray matter edema. Later, there is decreased signal on T2WIs within the thinned cortical gray matter.

In adults, herpes simplex infection may cause encephalitis or cranial neuritis. The infection usually is secondary to reactivation of latent herpes simplex type 1. Patients with herpes encephalitis present with the gradual onset of personality changes, dysphasia, and focal neurologic deficits. Seizures and coma may occur. An inconstant but characteristic electroencephalographic finding is a localized spiked and slow wave pattern. Early diagnosis is crucial, because there is a greater than 70% mortality rate in untreated patients. Unfortunately, CSF studies are often negative. Treatment is with acyclovir, which significantly reduces mortality, but many survivors have permanent deficits. CT scans show a poorly defined area of decreased density in one or both temporal lobes (Figs. 6.18, 6.19A). The predilection for the temporal lobes is because the virus is usually latent within the gasserian ganglion. The frontal lobes may also be involved. The insular cortex is often involved, but the adjacent putamen is usually spared. There is usually swelling with mass effect. Streaky enhancement is variable. The CT findings are not usually seen before the fifth day of symptoms. With MR, the findings may be identified somewhat sooner. There is a nonspecific pattern of increased signal on the intermediate, FLAIR, and T2W images in the temporal and/or frontal lobe(s) with sparing of the putamen. This increased signal is best seen on a FLAIR sequence (Fig. 6.19B, C). Increased signal on DWI has been reported. Early on, meningeal enhancement may be seen. Later, there may be parenchymal enhancement or evidence of hemorrhage. The differential diagnosis includes middle cerebral artery infarct (which will often involve the putamen, unlike herpes), early bacterial cerebritis, and other types of viral encephalitis.

Varicella zoster rarely causes an encephalitis that is similar to that caused by herpes simplex. Another unusual manifestation is the syndrome of herpes zoster ophthalmicus and delayed contralateral hemiparesis caused by cerebral angiitis. In this syndrome, there are cerebral infarcts resulting from large and medium vessel angiitis on the same side as ophthalmic zoster skin manifestations. Imaging studies show typical infarcts, and angiography shows segmental areas of narrowing and/or beading of the arteries. Herpes zoster may also cause cranial neuritis, which may involve any of the cranial nerves. The most commonly involved is the facial nerve, resulting in the Ramsay Hunt syndrome. Clinically, there is ear pain and facial paralysis, accompanied by a vesicular eruption about the ear. CT scans are usually normal, but MR may reveal increased contrast enhancement of the facial nerve.

Acute disseminated encephalomyelitis (ADEM) is an acute demyelinating disease that occurs after a viral infection, following a vaccination, or sometimes spontaneously. It probably has an autoimmune basis; organisms are not isolated from brain tissue. Symptoms develop acutely: fever, headache, and meningeal signs. Seizures, focal neurologic deficits, stupor, and coma may develop. The mortality rate is 10% to 20%. When treated early with steroids, most patients make a full recovery. T2WIs and FLAIR imaging are much more sensitive than CT in identifying lesions of increased signal intensity in the white matter (Fig. 6.20). The brainstem, cerebellum, and basal ganglia are often involved. Optic neuritis is also common. The

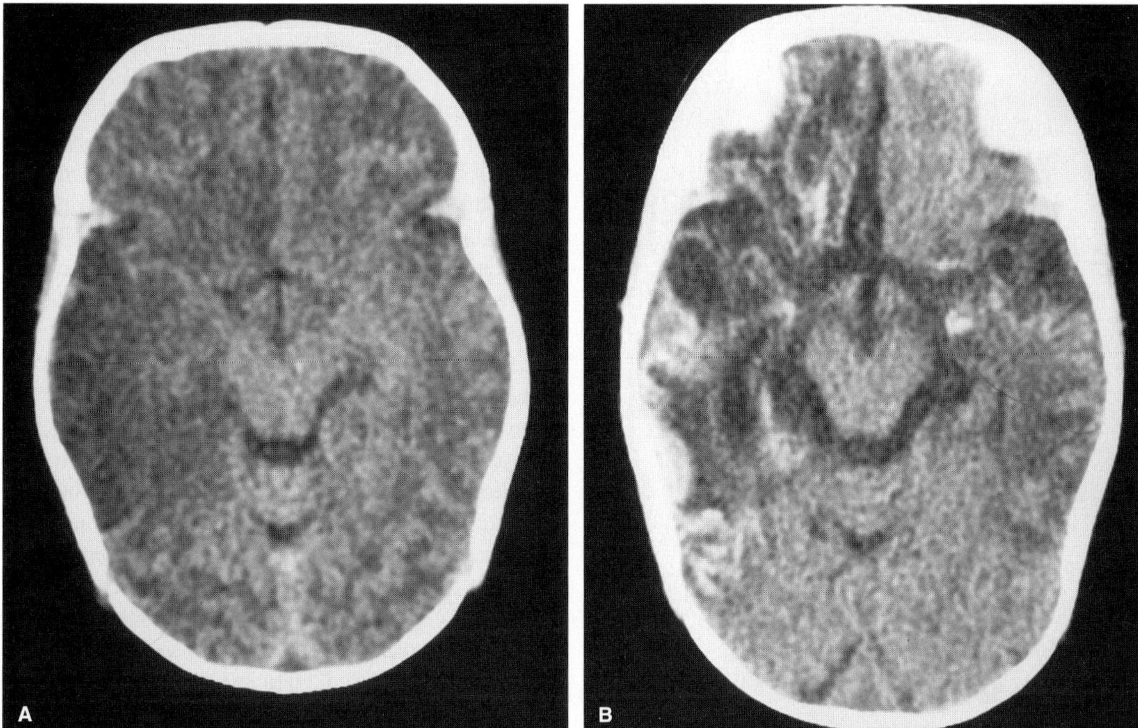

FIGURE 6.17. **Neonatal Herpes. A.** There is low density and swelling in the right temporal lobe, and to a lesser extent in the frontal and left temporal lobes, on the noncontrast CT scan of this 2-week-old child with herpes type 2 infection in the acute stage. **B.** Three weeks later, the noncontrast CT scan on this same infant reveals multiple areas of cystic encephalomalacia and widespread gray matter calcification, which are typical of late-stage neonatal herpes infection.

lesions are usually multiple, but few in number. Sometimes there is solid or ring enhancement of the lesions. The appearance is similar to that seen in multiple sclerosis, but with a monophasic clinical course. The lesions regress with successful treatment, correlating with clinical improvement. Acute hemorrhagic leukoencephalitis is a severe variant of ADEM that is often fatal. Pathologically, there is perivascular hemorrhagic necrosis, primarily in the centrum semiovale. The major imaging feature is a rapid progression of white matter lesions over the course of a few days.

Subacute sclerosing panencephalitis is caused by a variant of the measles virus. It typically occurs in children and young adults who had measles before age 2, after a 6- to 10-year asymptomatic period. The disease causes progressive dementia, seizures, and paralysis, leading to death. There is no treatment. Imaging studies initially reveal focal lesions in the gray matter and subcortical white matter. Later, there are periventricular white matter lesions that may enhance. In the late stages there is usually profound cortical atrophy.

Progressive multifocal leukoencephalopathy (PML) is a demyelinating disease caused by a papova virus (the JC virus—not to be confused with the Creutzfeldt-Jakob agent, which is a prion). It occurs only in immunosuppressed patients and has an increased incidence in patients with AIDS, as will be discussed.

Encephalitis can be caused by a variety of viruses not already discussed, including flaviviruses (arboviruses), Epstein-Barr virus, mumps, measles, rubella, and enteroviruses. Rickettsia (Rocky Mountain spotted fever) and mycoplasma pneumoniae may also produce encephalitis. In the United States, St. Louis, California, western equine, and eastern equine encephalitis are caused by flavivirus infection. Japanese encephalitis is a flaviviral encephalitis found in Asia. Bilateral thalamic and basal ganglia lesions are typical of this disease. A related virus causes West Nile fever, which has an increasing incidence in the United States. This is a mosquito-borne infection that results in a meningoencephalitis of variable clinical severity. As with Japanese encephalitis, MR shows increased signal on T2WIs in the thalami and basal ganglia (Fig. 6.21). Rasmussen encephalitis is a devastating disease of childhood, most likely of viral etiology. There are intractable seizures and progressive neurologic deficits. The disease usually affects one cerebral hemisphere. Imaging studies show severe atrophy of the involved hemisphere. PET scans show the hemisphere to be hypometabolic.

Creutzfeldt-Jakob disease of the sporadic type (sCJD) is caused by a transmissible protein called a *prion* or

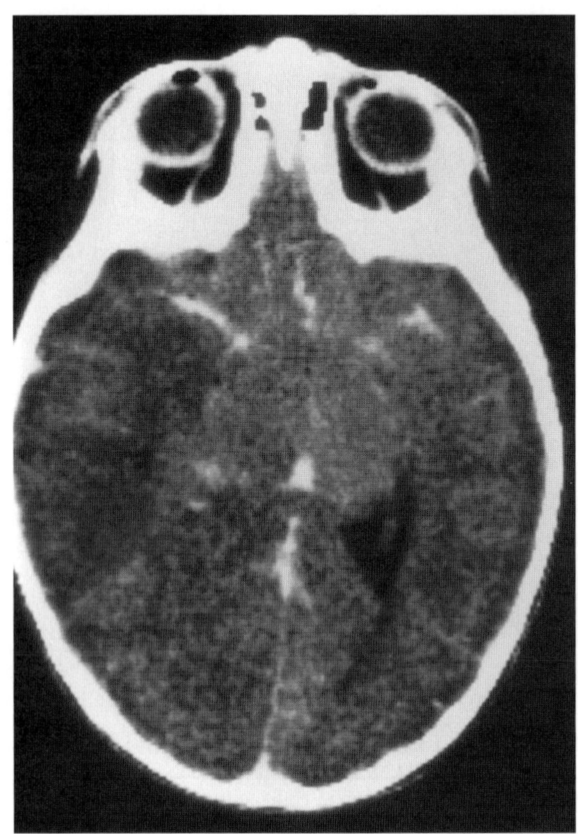

FIGURE 6.18. **Adult Herpes Encephalitis.** Both temporal lobes are of low density and appear swollen, especially on the right, on this contrast-enhanced CT scan. The appearance is similar to cerebral infarcts, but the clinical presentation is usually different.

slow virus. Clinically, there is rapidly progressive dementia, ataxia, and myoclonus, leading to death. Conventional MR scans are often normal early in the disease. DWI frequently demonstrates increased signal in the cerebral cortex and basal ganglia in early cases. Atrophy and increased signal in the cortex and basal ganglia on FLAIR and T2W images develop as the disease progresses.

Variant Creutzfeldt-Jakob disease (vCJD) is linked to bovine spongiform encephalopathy in cows. Most cases have occurred in the United Kingdom. This prion infection is transmitted to humans who eat infected beef. The clinical features are similar to sCJD. MR scans usually show characteristic findings of increased T2 signal in the pulvinar (posterior) nuclei of the thalamus.

EXTRA-AXIAL INFECTIONS

Meningitis

Meningitis can be caused by bacteria, mycobacteria, fungi, parasites, and viruses. Bacterial meningitis is caused by *Haemophilus influenzae* (in children), *Neisseria meningitidis* (in teens and young adults), and *Streptococcus pneumoniae* (in older adults) in over 80% of cases. *Escherichia coli*, group B streptococcus, and *Listeria monocytogenes*occur commonly in neonates. The bacteria most commonly enter the meninges during a systemic bacteremia but can spread directly from infected sinuses or after surgery or trauma. Patients present with a relatively acute onset of fever, a stiff neck, and headache, followed by a decline in mental status. CSF studies are usually diagnostic, and imaging studies are generally not required. CT scans may be performed in the emergency setting in acutely comatose patients or in patients with a nonspecific headache but are usually normal (Fig 6.22A). The inflammatory exudate caused by the meningitis may occasionally produce high density within the subarachnoid spaces, similar to that seen in subarachnoid hemorrhage.

The increased density is often more pronounced in the peripheral sulci than in the basal cisterns, unlike most cases of aneurysmal bleeding. Diffuse cerebral edema is sometimes seen (Fig. 6.22B). If contrast is given, there may or may not be meningeal enhancement. CT and MR are more often used later in the course of meningitis, when there are suspected complications such as hydrocephalus, cerebritis/abscess, ventriculitis, and venous or arterial infarctions. The hydrocephalus that may develop is usually of the communicating type, reflecting decreased function of the arachnoid villi in absorbing CSF. Subdural effusions may be seen in infants, especially with *H influenza* meningitis. With CT and MR, subdural effusions appear as thin collections along the surface of the brain that are isodense/isointense with CSF (Fig. 6.23). These sterile effusions can be identified with cranial sonography in infants. Echogenic sulci, ventriculomegaly, and abnormal parenchymal echogenicity have also been reported in infants with bacterial meningitis, imaged with US (Fig. 6.22C).

Tuberculous meningitis is the most common form of CNS tuberculosis. It is usually caused by *Mycobacterium tuberculosis*, but atypical mycobacteria, such as *M avium-intracellulare* can cause meningitis in AIDS patients. Tuberculous meningitis has a predilection for infants and children but is seen in all age groups. The disease spreads to the meninges hematogenously from the lungs, but the chest radiograph is normal in 40% to 75% of patients. The tuberculin skin test is also frequently negative. Clinically there is usually a subacute or insidious onset of headache, malaise, weakness, apathy, or focal neurologic findings. Imaging studies will show enhancing, thickened meninges, especially near the base of the brain (Fig. 6.24), unlike bacterial meningitis, where the peripheral meninges are more often involved. The often marked thickening of the meninges also distinguishes tuberculous and other granulomatous meningitides from pyogenic meningitis. The thick exudate in the basal cisterns may extend into the Virchow-Robin spaces, causing a vasculitis. This frequently leads to infarcts, which are better detected with MR than with CT.

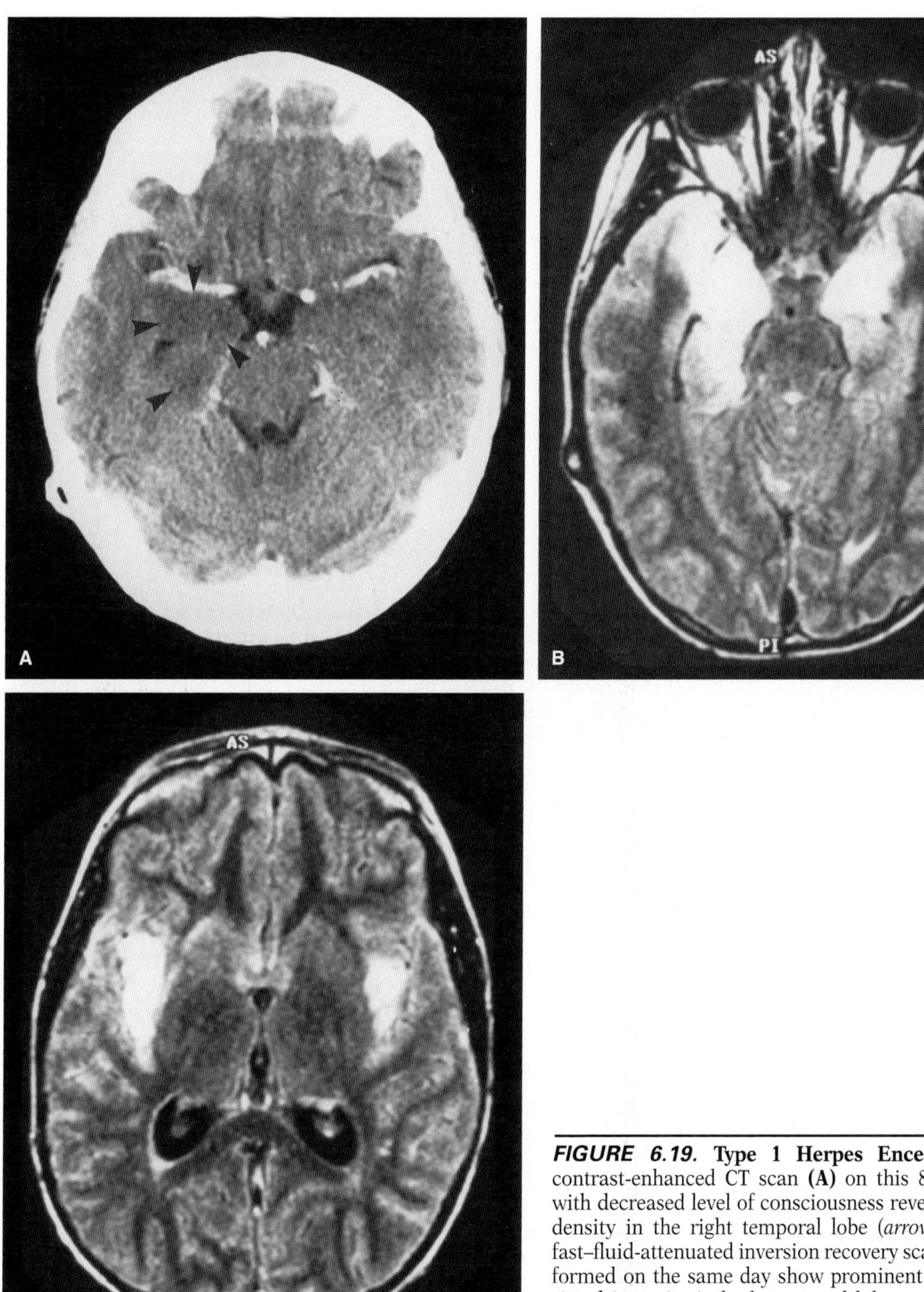

FIGURE 6.19. **Type 1 Herpes Encephalitis.** The contrast-enhanced CT scan **(A)** on this 8-year-old boy with decreased level of consciousness reveals subtle low density in the right temporal lobe (*arrowheads*). T2W fast–fluid-attenuated inversion recovery scans **(B, C)** performed on the same day show prominent areas of high signal intensity in both temporal lobes with sparing of the putamina. This case illustrates why MR is the imaging modality of choice when herpes encephalitis is suspected.

Communicating hydrocephalus is another relatively common complication.

The differential diagnosis of tuberculous meningitis includes fungal meningitis, racemose cysticercosis, sarcoidosis, and carcinomatous meningitis.

Fungal meningitis usually causes thick meningeal enhancement in the basal cisterns, as with tuberculosis (Fig. 6.25). Enhancement is variable with cryptococcosis, depending on the immune status of the patient. Hydrocephalus is common, but infarcts and extension of fungal meningitis into the brain occur less frequently than with tuberculous or pyogenic meningitis (except in cases of aspergillosis and mucormycosis).

Racemose cysticercosis may show thick meningeal enhancement, but cystic lesions in the cisterns are also frequently found (see Figs 6.12, 6.13).

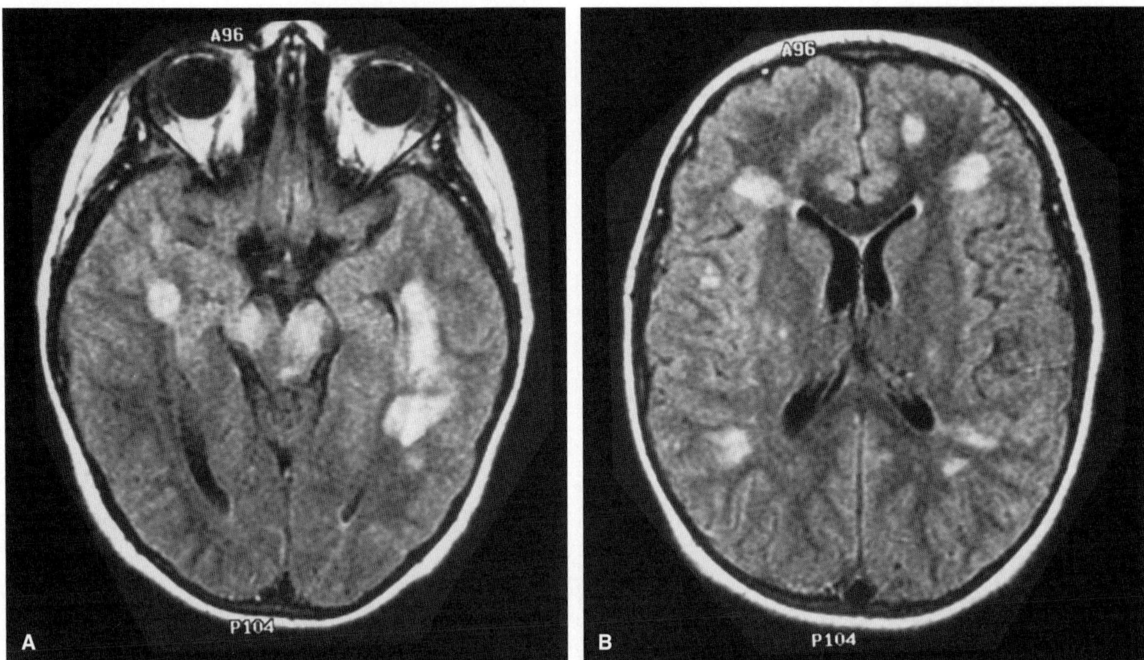

FIGURE 6.20. **Acute Disseminated Encephalomyelitis (ADEM).** The T2W fast–fluid-attenuated inversion recovery (FLAIR) scans **(A, B)** show multiple areas of high signal intensity in the cerebral white matter and midbrain. FLAIR sequences are extremely sensitive for detecting white matter lesions. This 8-year-old child recovered fully after steroid therapy.

Sarcoidosis involves the CNS in up to 14% of patients at autopsy, but causes neurologic symptoms only rarely. It primarily affects the leptomeninges, so that abnormal meningeal enhancement is seen with CT or MR. Focal parenchymal enhancing mass lesions or nonenhancing small white matter lesions may also be seen.

Viral meningitis is caused most commonly by the enteroviruses but can be caused by mumps, togaviruses, herpes simplex, lymphocytic choriomeningitis virus, and HIV. Most patients do not require treatment and neurologic deficits are uncommon. Imaging studies are typically normal.

Subdural and Epidural Infections

Extra-axial pyogenic infections may also involve the epidural or subdural spaces. An epidural abscess may be caused by penetrating injuries, surgery, sinusitis, mastoiditis, orbital infection, or, rarely, hematogenous spread. CT scans show an inwardly convex, extra-axial collection with increased density compared to CSF (Fig. 6.26). The inner margin usually enhances with contrast. There may be adjacent sinusitis or skull abnormalities. MR is more sensitive in demonstrating these lesions and can do so in multiple planes. The strong dural attachments prevent rapid expansion of epidural abscesses. However, a subdural empyema may spread rapidly throughout the subdural space and is acutely life threatening. Cortical venous thrombosis resulting in venous infarcts is a common result of these infections. Subdural empyemas are caused by the same conditions that produce epidural abscesses. Both CT and MR can demonstrate these subdural collections, which usually have enhancing inner margins (Fig. 6.27A, B). MR is more sensitive in showing smaller lesions because of the problem of partial volume averaging with the calvarium on CT. MR is also better at detecting venous thrombosis and venous infarcts. Subdural empyemas show increased signal on DWI, distinguishing them from subdural effusions (Fig. 6.27C).

Mild, smooth dural, or meningeal enhancement may be seen after brain surgery and in patients with a ventriculostomy tube, especially with MR (Fig. 6.28). The enhancement can persist for years and should be considered benign in this clinical setting. It most likely reflects a chemical meningitis resulting from perioperative hemorrhage. Intracranial hypotension from a spontaneous or iatrogenic CSF leak also results in smooth dural thickening and enhancement.

ACQUIRED IMMUNODEFICIENCY SYNDROME

The CNS is a common site of involvement in patients with AIDS. The incidence of CNS involvement has decreased since the introduction of highly active antiretroviral therapy (HAART), yet up to two thirds of AIDS patients

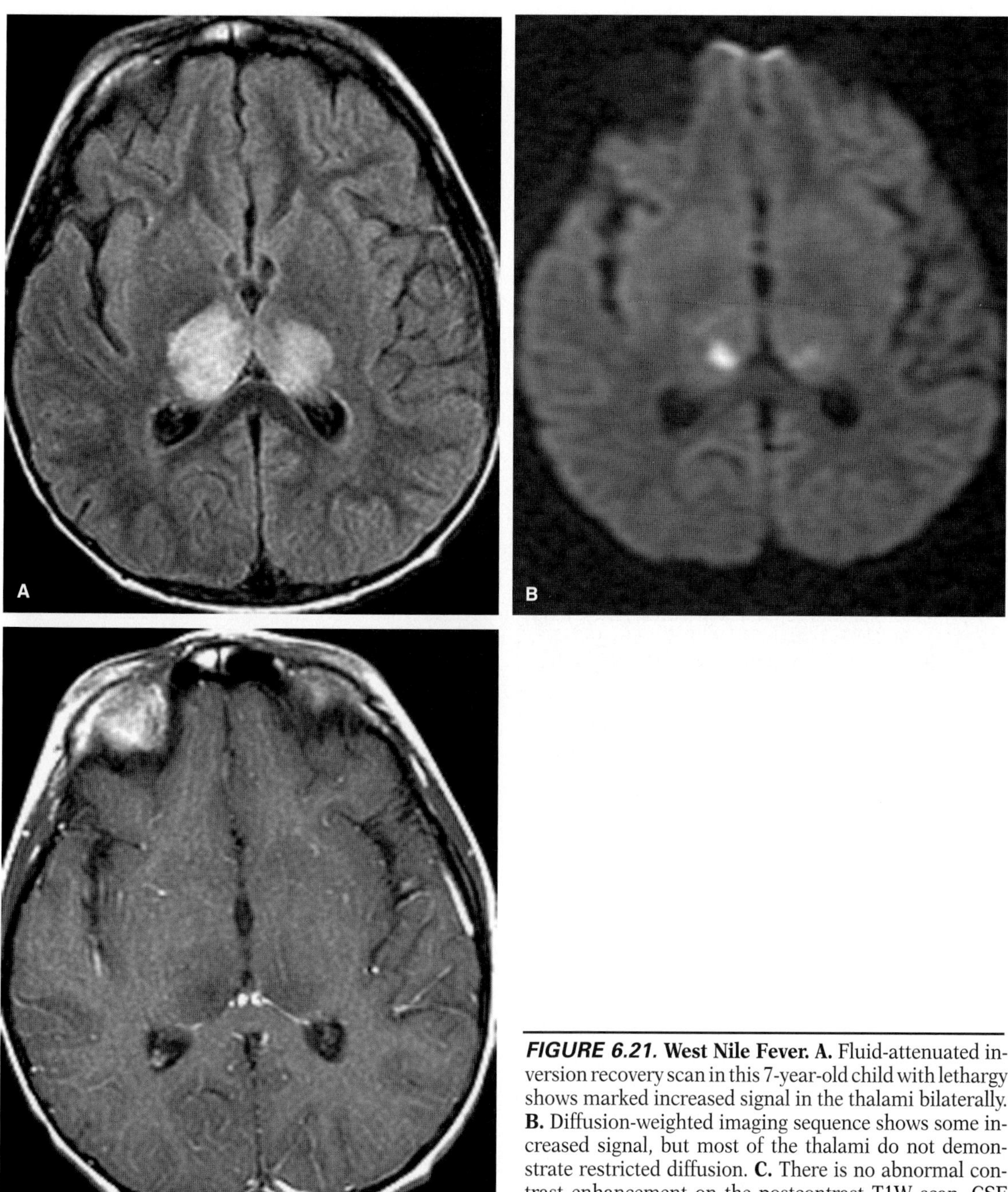

FIGURE 6.21. **West Nile Fever. A.** Fluid-attenuated inversion recovery scan in this 7-year-old child with lethargy shows marked increased signal in the thalami bilaterally. **B.** Diffusion-weighted imaging sequence shows some increased signal, but most of the thalami do not demonstrate restricted diffusion. **C.** There is no abnormal contrast enhancement on the postcontrast T1W scan. CSF studies were positive for the virus that causes West Nile Fever.

develop some kind of CNS disease. A variety of infections and neoplasms may be diagnosed in these patients. The most common infections include HIV encephalopathy; toxoplasmosis, cryptococcosis, and other fungal infections; CMV and Herpes meningoencephalitis; mycobacterial infection; PML; and meningovascular syphilis. Primary CNS lymphoma is by far the most common tumor, but metastatic lymphoma, gliomas, and rarely Kaposi sarcoma may also occur.

HIV Encephalopathy. The etiologic agent in AIDS, HIV is neurotropic, infecting the brain in up to 90% of patients at autopsy. Clinical symptoms of brain involvement by HIV occur in a minority of these patients. Pathologically, HIV infection results in vacuolation of the white matter, with areas of demyelination and multinucleated giant cells. The centrum semiovale is involved most severely, but all white matter tracts, including the brainstem and cerebellum, may be affected. The cortical gray matter is

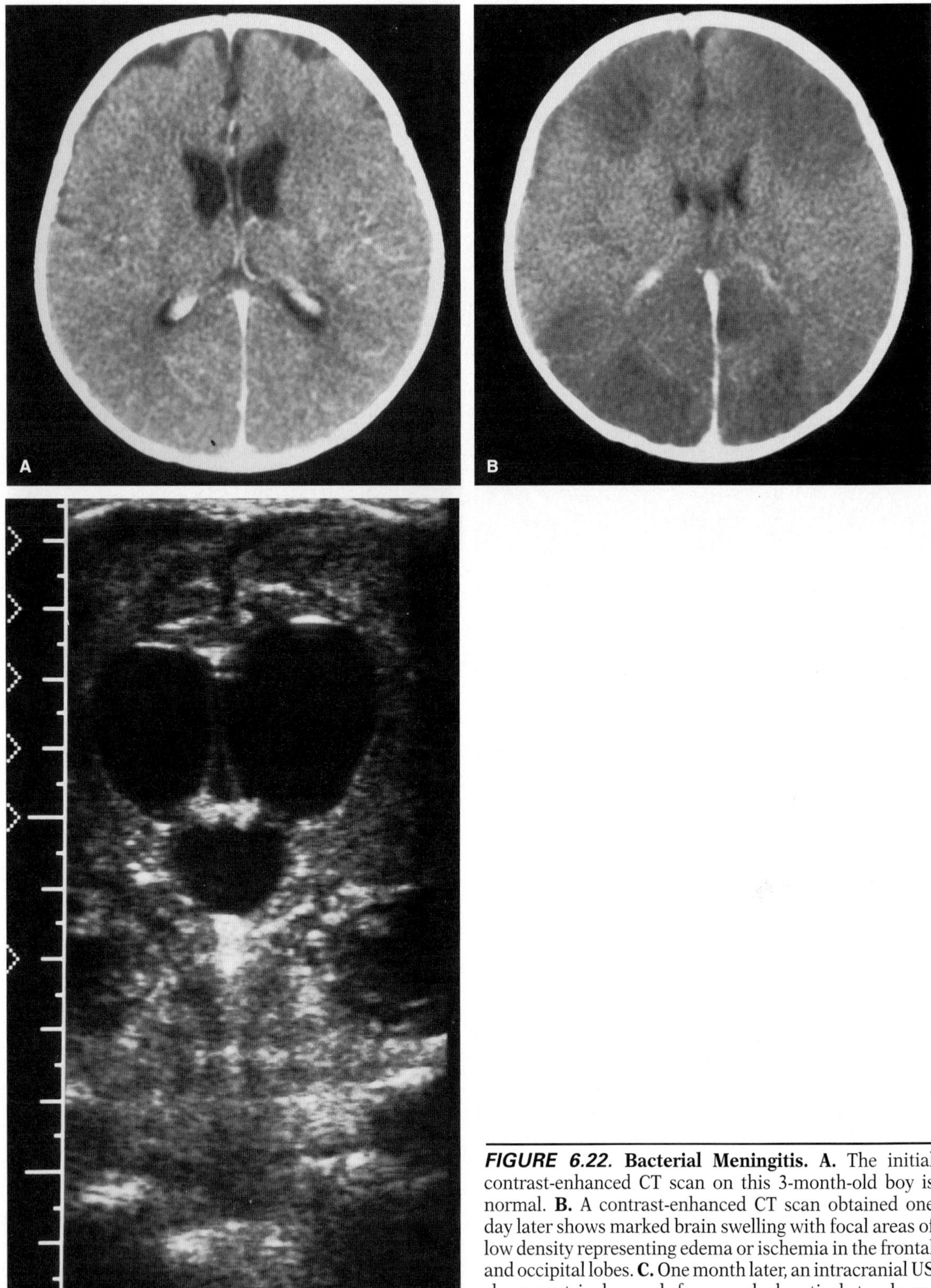

FIGURE 6.22. **Bacterial Meningitis. A.** The initial contrast-enhanced CT scan on this 3-month-old boy is normal. **B.** A contrast-enhanced CT scan obtained one day later shows marked brain swelling with focal areas of low density representing edema or ischemia in the frontal and occipital lobes. **C.** One month later, an intracranial US shows ventriculomegaly from marked cortical atrophy resulting from widespread cortical destruction.

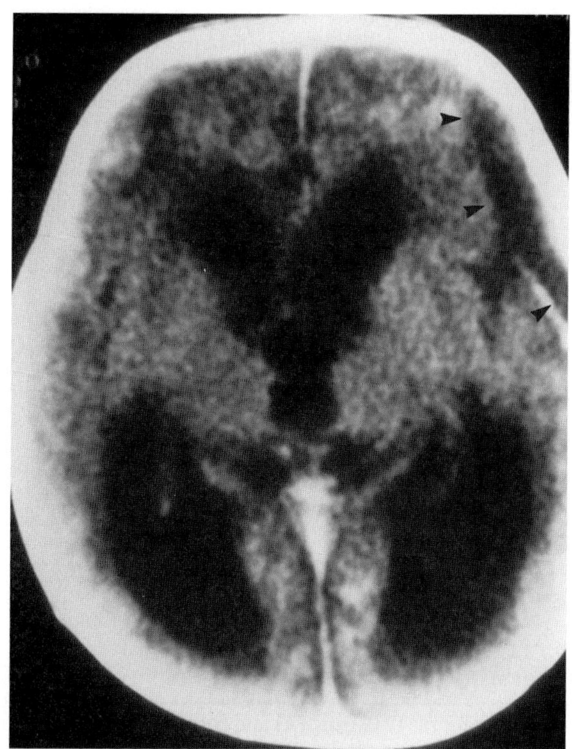

FIGURE 6.23. **Subdural Effusion.** A contrast-enhanced CT scan on this 6-year-old with *Haemophilus influenzae* meningitis reveals a subdural collection nearly isodense with CSF (*arrowheads*). Subdural effusions are common with *H influenzae* meningitis. There is also enlargement of the lateral and third ventricles because of communicating hydrocephalus, which is a common complication of meningitis.

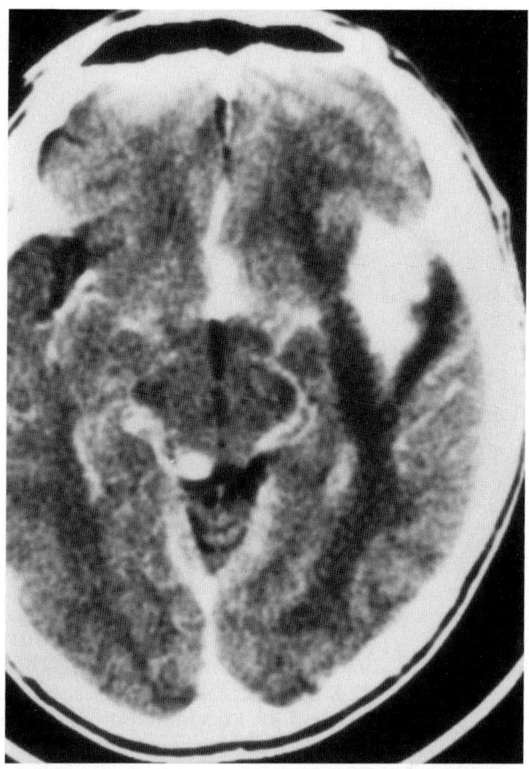

FIGURE 6.24. **Tuberculous Meningitis.** Contrast-enhanced CT scan shows marked abnormal contrast enhancement in the left sylvian fissure, interhemispheric fissure, ambient cistern, and along the tentorium. This thick, irregular enhancement in the basal cisterns is typical of a pachymeningitis such as tuberculosis or fungal meningitis. CT scans in patients with bacterial meningitis are usually normal or may reveal subtle increased density or enhancement in the peripheral sulci.

usually spared. Clinically, patients with HIV encephalitis may develop a subcortical dementia with cognitive, behavioral, and motor deterioration. This is known as AIDS dementia complex (ADC), which occurs in about 7% to 15% of AIDS patients. Infants and children with HIV encephalitis exhibit loss of developmental milestones, apathy, failure of brain growth, and spastic paraparesis. This is the most common form of CNS disease in pediatric patients with AIDS, in whom opportunistic infections and CNS tumors are unusual.

Diffuse atrophy is the most common manifestation of HIV infection of the brain on neuroimaging studies (Fig. 6.29). This is largely central atrophy, reflecting the predominant white matter involvement. White matter lesions are also commonly seen in patients with ADC. MR is significantly more sensitive than CT for detecting these abnormalities. A diffuse pattern of increased signal in the deep white matter or multiple small punctate white matter lesions on T2WIs are the most common findings. The punctate lesions do not correlate well with symptoms. The lesions do not exhibit mass effect or abnormal contrast enhancement.

The most severe cases of HIV encephalopathy show extensive bilateral areas of abnormal signal throughout the periventricular white matter, brainstem, and cerebellum (Fig. 6.30). A decreased n-acetyl aspartate (NAA) peak is often found in the affected white matter with MR spectroscopy. Such severe involvement usually correlates with symptoms of ADC. The clinical and imaging abnormalities often respond to treatment with HAART. In infants and children with HIV infection, atrophy is the most common observation, followed by calcifications in the basal ganglia. White matter calcifications and low-density lesions are also sometimes seen.

Toxoplasmosis is the most common opportunistic CNS infection in AIDS, occurring in about 13% to 33% of patients with CNS complications. It occurs in patients with CD4 counts below 100 cells/mm^3. *T gondii* is an obligate intracellular protozoan that is ubiquitous throughout the world, causing subclinical or mild infection in a large percentage of the population. In AIDS, CNS toxoplasmosis results from reactivation of the previously acquired infection. A necrotizing encephalitis usually results, with the formation of thin-walled abscesses. Patients present clinically with headache, fever, lethargy, decreased level of consciousness, and focal signs, which initially can be

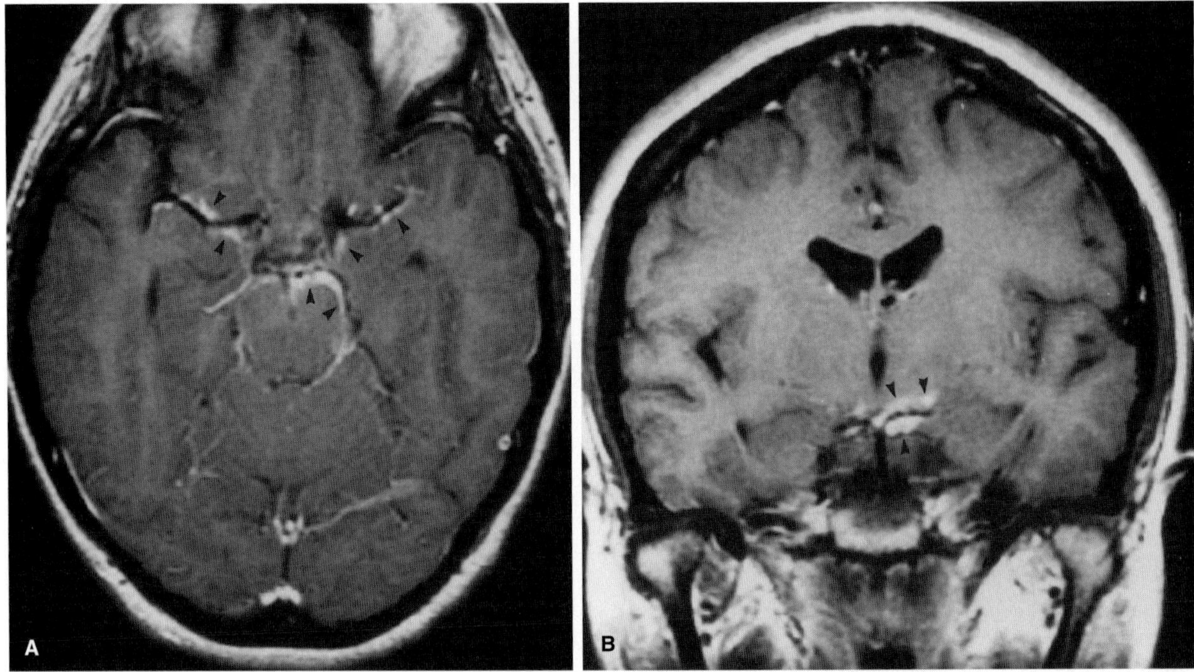

FIGURE 6.25. **Coccidioidomycosis Meningitis.** Contrast-enhanced, T1W axial **(A)** and coronal **(B)** scans reveal abnormal enhancement of the meninges in the basal cisterns (*arrowheads*).

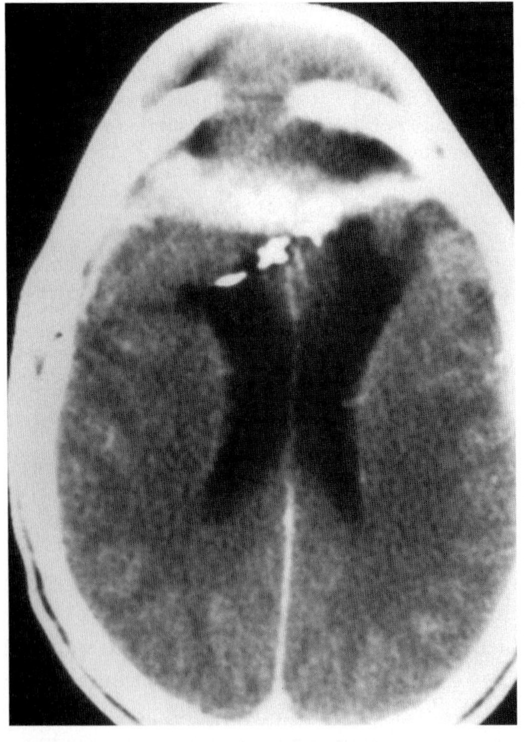

FIGURE 6.26. **Epidural Abscess.** This patient had a penetrating injury to the frontal bone several months prior to this contrast-enhanced CT scan. There is medium-density pus extending through the calvarial defect into the epidural space. The inner margin enhances markedly. Surgical clips are present near the frontal horn of the right lateral ventricle.

confused with the subacute encephalitis of HIV infection. Neuroimaging studies are therefore crucial in patient management.

The typical appearance of CNS toxoplasmosis is that of multiple enhancing mass lesions with surrounding vasogenic edema (Figs. 6.31, 6.32). The lesions are usually relatively small—between 1 and 4 cm in diameter. Larger lesions usually exhibit ring enhancement, while smaller lesions are usually solid. The lesions are usually of increased signal on precontrast T2WIs. Unlike bacterial abscesses, toxoplasmosis lesions are not high in signal on DWI. The basal ganglia are a favored site, but white matter and cortical lesions are also common. The main differential consideration is primary CNS lymphoma, which will be discussed later. A clinical and imaging response to antitoxoplasmosis antibiotics will usually distinguish between toxoplasmosis and lymphoma in most cases (Fig. 6.32). Biopsy is usually reserved for atypical cases or when there is no response to antibiotics. Other infections or tumors may occasionally mimic toxoplasmosis but are unusual. Fungal, mycobacterial, and amebic abscesses have been described. Bacterial abscesses are rare in AIDS patients.

Fungal Meningitis. Although fungal abscesses and granulomas are unusual, fungal meningitis is a common complication of AIDS, occurring in 5% to 15% of patients. Cryptococcosis is the most common fungal infection. Meningitis is usually mild because of the diminished inflammatory response of the immunocompromised host. Therefore, there is usually little or no enhancement of the meninges, and imaging studies are usually normal. The

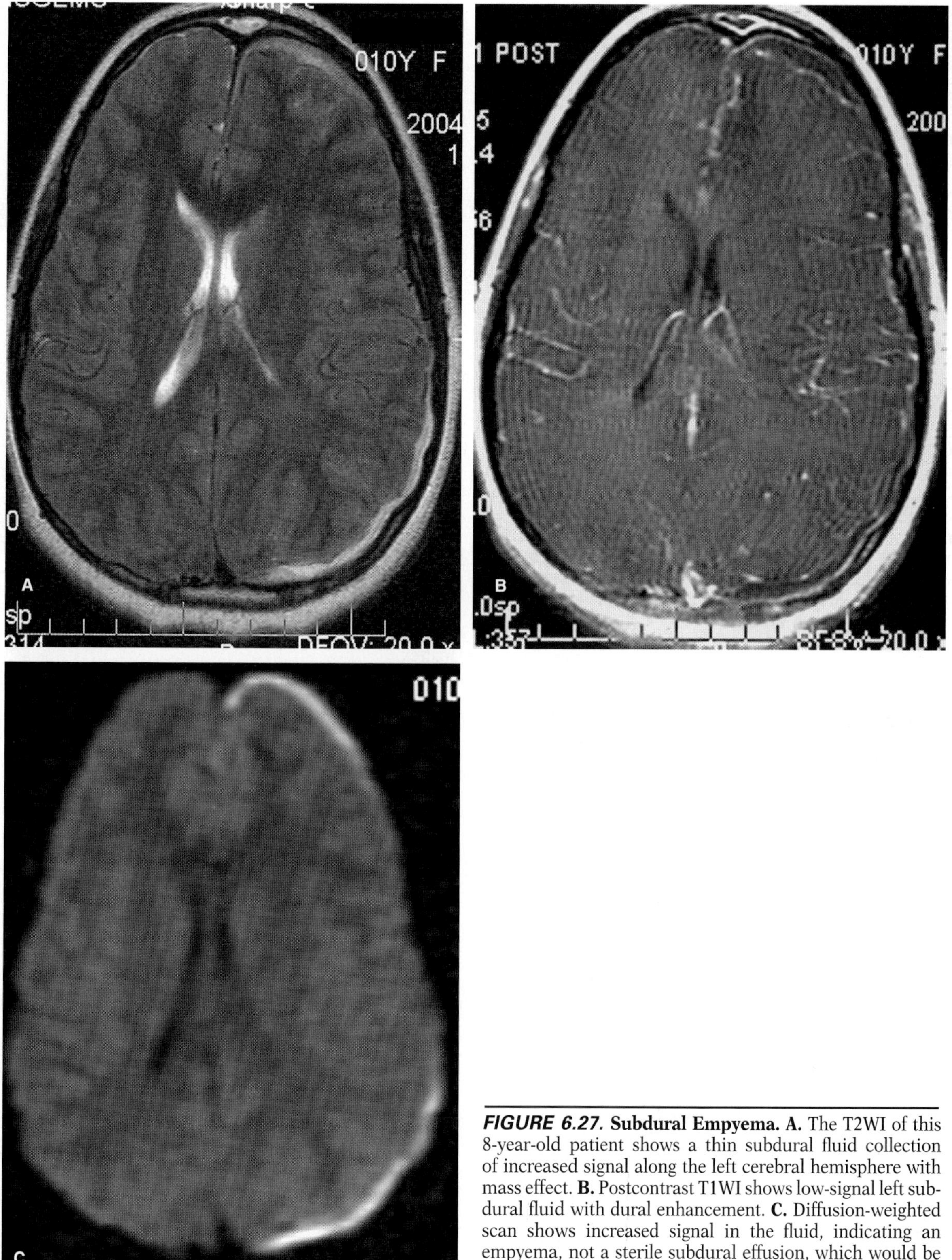

FIGURE 6.27. **Subdural Empyema. A.** The T2WI of this 8-year-old patient shows a thin subdural fluid collection of increased signal along the left cerebral hemisphere with mass effect. **B.** Postcontrast T1WI shows low-signal left subdural fluid with dural enhancement. **C.** Diffusion-weighted scan shows increased signal in the fluid, indicating an empyema, not a sterile subdural effusion, which would be dark on this sequence.

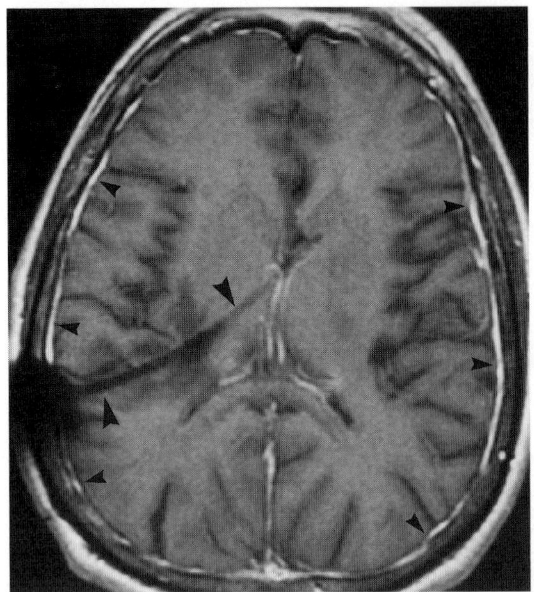

FIGURE 6.28. **Benign Postoperative Meningeal Enhancement.** Several years after brain surgery, this T1W, contrast-enhanced MR scan reveals smooth but definitely abnormal enhancement of the dura (*small arrowheads*). There were no signs of infection or tumor recurrence. A ventricular shunt tube is seen on the right side (*large arrowheads*).

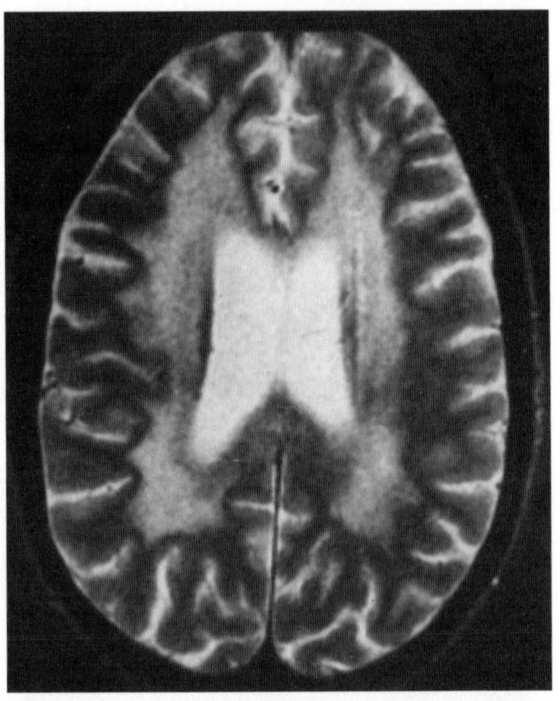

FIGURE 6.30. **HIV Encephalopathy.** This young patient clinically had the AIDS dementia complex. The T2WI shows widespread abnormal high signal in the periventricular white matter.

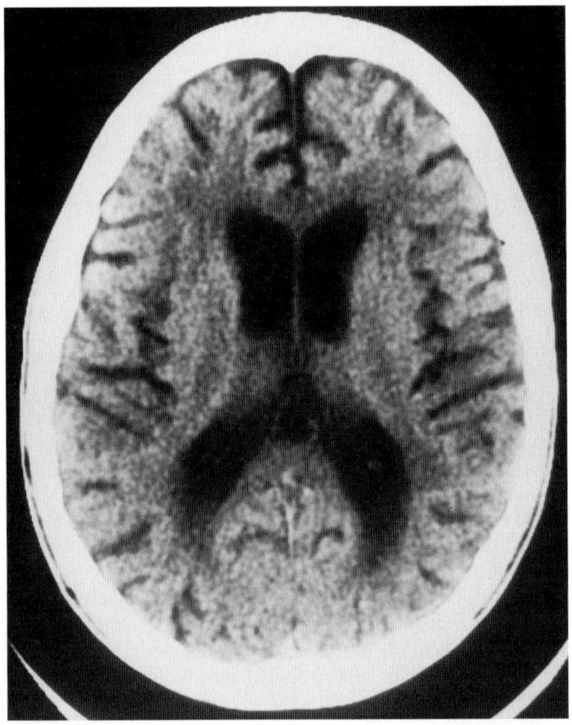

FIGURE 6.29. **AIDS-Related Atrophy.** A noncontrast CT scan reveals enlarged ventricles and sulci in this 24-year-old patient with AIDS. This is the most common abnormality found on brain imaging of patients with AIDS. It often correlates with the AIDS dementia complex.

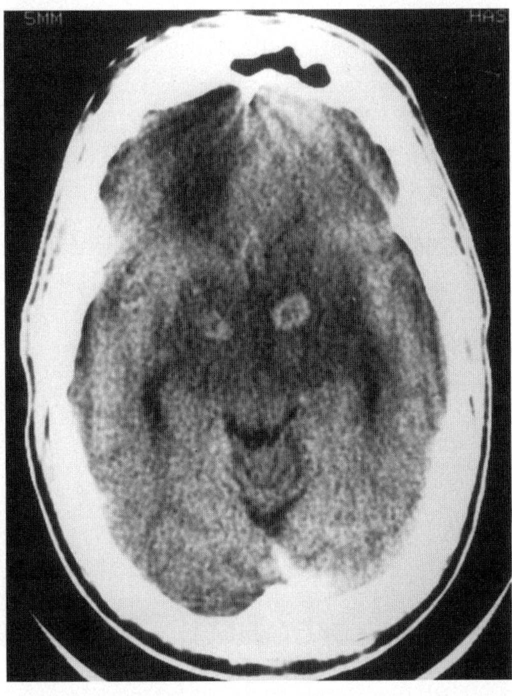

FIGURE 6.31. **Toxoplasmosis.** A contrast-enhanced CT scan reveals bilateral ring-enhancing lesions in the basal ganglia of this patient with AIDS. There is marked surrounding low-density edema. The basal ganglia are a common site for toxoplasmosis.

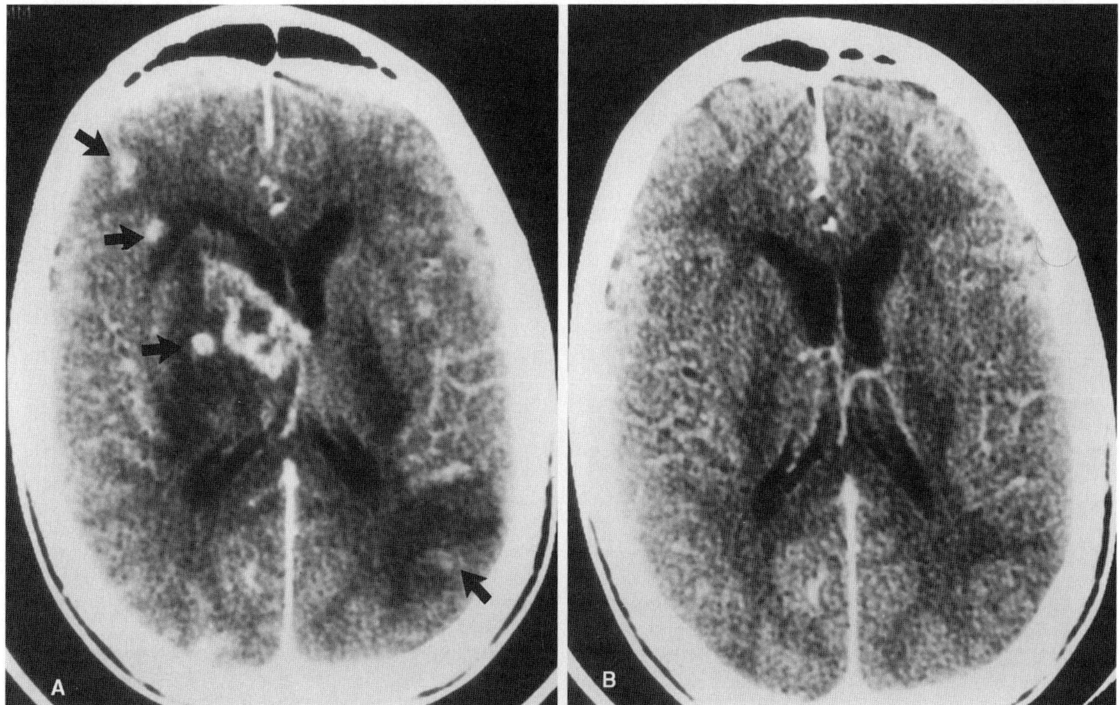

FIGURE 6.32. **Toxoplasmosis. A.** A contrast-enhanced CT scan shows a large right basal ganglia–enhancing mass and several other small enhancing lesions (*arrows*). The small size and multiplicity of the lesions favor toxoplasmosis over lymphoma. **B.** Following 2 weeks of antibiotic therapy, the contrast-enhanced CT scan reveals complete resolution of the lesions, typical for toxoplasmosis.

diagnosis is made when there are elevated cryptococcal antigen titers in the serum and CSF.

As already mentioned, cryptococcosis may sometimes present as dilated Virchow-Robin spaces filled with cryptococcus organisms, known as *gelatinous pseudocysts*. These cysts appear as rounded, smoothly marginated lesions in the basal ganglia that are nearly isodense and isointense to CSF (Fig. 6.33). There is no enhancement following contrast administration, which distinguishes these lesions from toxoplasmosis. Enhancing cryptococcomas are rare.

Progressive multifocal leukoencephalopathy is an infection of immunosuppressed patients caused by reactivation of a papova virus (the JC virus). The incidence of PML in AIDS patients is approximately 8%. It can also occur in other immunosuppressed patients, such as transplant recipients and leukemics, but it does not occur in patients with normal immunity. The infection causes demyelination and necrosis, primarily involving white matter. Clinical symptoms include changes in mental status, blindness, aphasia, hemiparesis, ataxia, and other focal findings. There is a progressive course to death within months, although treatment with HAART significantly prolongs survival. In non-AIDS immunosuppressed patients, PML has a predilection for the occipital lobes, but in AIDS patients, any part of the brain may be involved. MR reveals focal lesions of increased signal on FLAIR and T2W images and decreased signal on T1WIs within the subcortical and deep white matter (Fig. 6.34). CT shows white matter lesions of decreased density. The lesions may be solitary or multifocal. Mass effect and contrast enhancement are almost always absent, which are important distinguishing features. Rarely, both gray and white matter or the basal ganglia are involved, simulating an infarct. The main differential diagnosis in the setting of AIDS is that of HIV encephalitis. Unlike PML, HIV encephalitis is usually more diffuse and less intense on T2WIs, and does not extend to the gray–white junction.

Viral Infection. CMV infection is a common CNS infection in AIDS patients pathologically but does not usually result in frank tissue necrosis and is usually subclinical. There are many cases of pathologically proven CMV brain infection with normal CT and MR scans. CMV meningoencephalitis is occasionally imaged as areas of increased signal on T2WIs in the periventricular white matter. Subependymal contrast enhancement, if present, is a valuable diagnostic sign. Rarely, CMV will present as a ring-enhancing mass. Herpes virus and varicella virus infections are also only occasionally imaged. In AIDS patients, these viral infections often have a more benign clinical course and imaging appearance because of a diminished immune response.

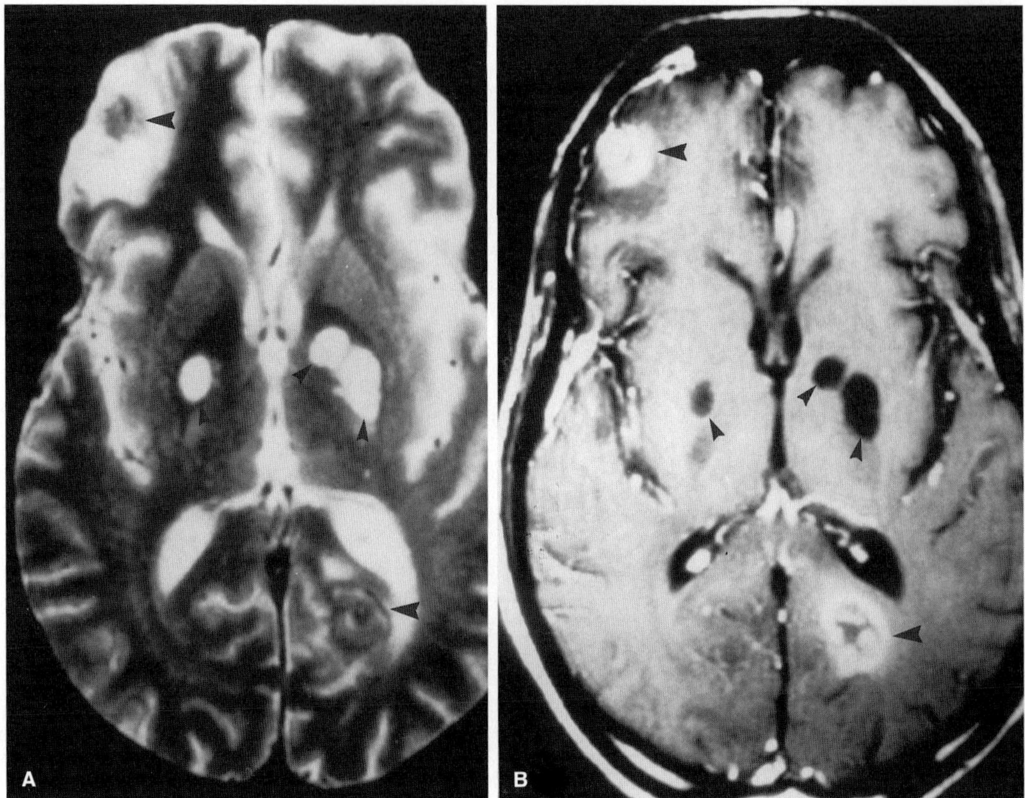

FIGURE 6.33. **Cryptococcosis and Toxoplasmosis. A.** T2WI reveals multiple rounded lesions that are isointense to CSF in the basal ganglia (*small arrowheads*). There is no surrounding edema. Darker lesions with surrounding edema are present in the right frontal and left occipital areas (*large arrowheads*). **B.** A contrast-enhanced T1WI again reveals the basal ganglia lesions to be isointense with CSF (*small arrowheads*). There is no contrast enhancement. The appearance of these lesions is typical of gelatinous pseudocysts of cryptococcosis. These lesions represent dilated Virchow-Robin spaces filled with cryptococcus organisms. The right frontal and left occipital lesions do enhance with contrast (*large arrowheads*), as is typical of toxoplasmosis.

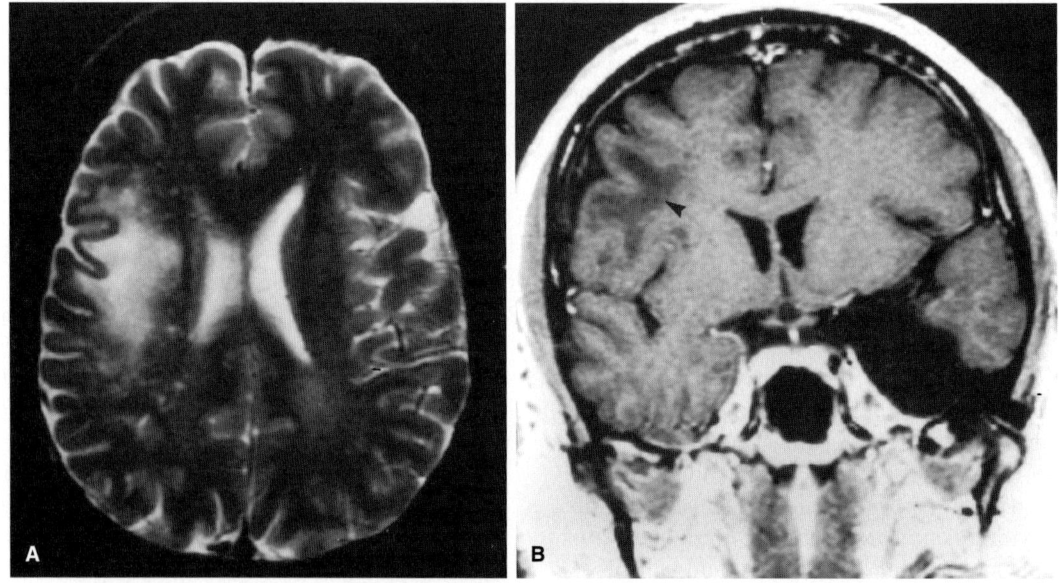

FIGURE 6.34. **Progressive Multifocal Leukoencephalopathy (PML). A.** There is an area of abnormal high signal intensity in the right corona radiata on this T2WI. There is no significant mass effect. **B.** On the contrast-enhanced T1WI, the lesion is of low signal intensity (*arrowhead*), and does not enhance. These are typical features of PML, which was proven with biopsy in this patient with AIDS. Incidentally, a left temporal arachnoid cyst can be noted.

Intracranial mycobacterial infections occur in a small percentage of AIDS patients. Most of these patients are intravenous drug abusers with pulmonary tuberculosis. Chest radiographs are positive in about 65% of cases. There is a very high mortality rate (nearly 80%) in these patients. Most patients present with meningitis. Imaging studies in these patients reveal communicating hydrocephalus and/or meningeal enhancement. Tuberculomas occur in about 25% of patients with HIV-related CNS tuberculosis, but tuberculous abscesses are less common. Tuberculomas are usually smaller and have less edema than tuberculous abscesses.

Primary CNS lymphoma is by far the most common intracranial tumor in AIDS. Up to 6% of AIDS patients will develop this tumor. It is the main differential diagnostic consideration along with toxoplasmosis when a mass lesion is found in patients with AIDS. Patients present with symptoms of a space-occupying lesion, as with toxoplasmosis. Solitary or multiple enhancing mass lesions are found with neuroimaging studies (Fig. 6.35). The lesions are usually centrally located within the deep white matter or basal ganglia, but cortical lesions also occur. There may be subependymal spread or extension across the corpus callosum, which do not usually occur with toxoplasmosis. With MR imaging, there is variable signal intensity, with areas of low or high signal on T2WIs and isosignal or low signal on T1WIs. With CT, the lesions are often isodense with gray matter. The lesions almost always enhance with contrast in either a ring or solid pattern. The imaging appearance is often indistinguishable from that of toxoplasmosis. The main distinguishing features are size and number. Toxoplasmosis is more frequently multiple, and the lesions are usually smaller than with lymphoma. Isointensity with white matter on T2WIs and diffuse, homogeneous contrast enhancement favor lymphoma. High signal on T2WIs (often with a low signal rim) and ring enhancement following contrast administration favor toxoplasmosis. MR spectroscopy shows increased choline and decreased NAA with lymphoma, while toxoplasmosis shows decreased choline and NAA with increased lipid and lactate. Toxoplasmosis is also more common than lymphoma and responds to antibiotic therapy.

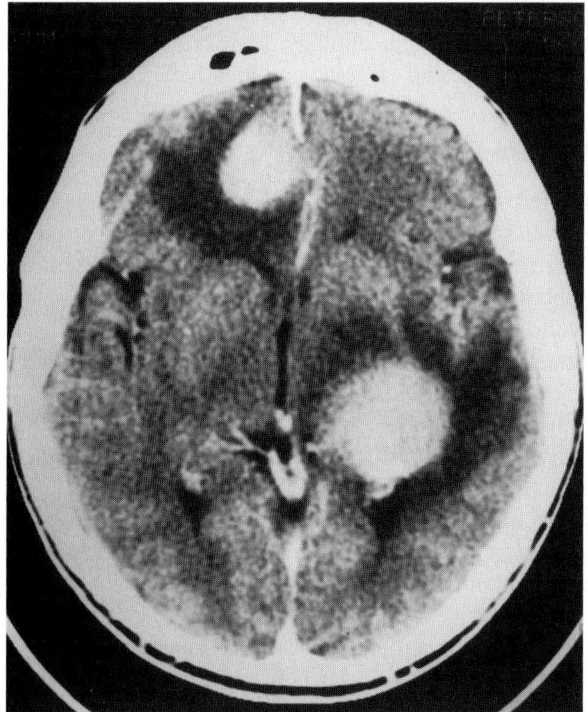

FIGURE 6.35. **Primary CNS Lymphoma.** There are two solidly enhancing mass lesions with surrounding edema on this CT scan of a patient with AIDS. The relatively large size and solid enhancement pattern are more suggestive of lymphoma than toxoplasmosis, as was proven in this case.

SUGGESTED READINGS

Barkovich AJ, Lindan CE. Congenital cytomegalovirus infection of the brain: imaging analysis and embryologic considerations. AJNR Am J Neuroradiol 1994;15:703–715.

Brightbill TC, Ihmeidan IH, Donovan Post MJ, Berger JR, Katz DA. Neurosyphilis in HIV-positive and HIV-negative patients: neuroimaging findings. AJNR Am J Neuroradiol 1995;16:703–711.

Collie DA, Summers DM, Ironside JW, et al. Diagnosing variant Creutzfeldt-Jakob disease with the pulvinar sign: MR imaging findings in 86 neuropathologically confirmed cases. AJNR Am J Neuroradiol 2003;24:1560–1569.

Dumas JL, Visy JM, Belin C, Gaston A, Goldlust D, Dumas M. Parenchymal neurocysticercosis: follow-up and staging by MRI. Neuroradiology 1997;39:12–18.

Lai PH, Ho JT, Chen WL, et al. Brain abscess and necrotic brain tumor: discrimination with proton MR spectroscopy and diffusion-weighted imaging. AJNR Am J Neuroradiol 2002;23:1369–1377.

Lim CCT, Sitoh YY, Hui F, et al. Nipah viral encephalitis or Japanese encephalitis? MR findings in a new zoonotic disease. AJNR Am J Neuroradiol 2000;21:455–461.

Mader I, Stock KW, Ettlin T, Probst A. Acute disseminated encephalomyelitis: MR and CT features. AJNR Am J Neuroradiol 1996; 17:104–109.

Mishra AM, Gupta RK, Jaggi RS, et al. Role of diffusion-weighted imaging and in vivo proton magnetic resonance spectroscopy in the differential diagnosis of ring-enhancing intracranial cystic mass lesions. J Comput Assist Tomogr 2004;28:540–547.

Rosas H, Wippold FJ II. West Nile virus: case report with MR imaging findings. AJNR Am J Neuroradiol 2003;24:1376–1378.

Sibtain NA, Chinn RJS. Imaging of the central nervous system in HIV infection. Imaging 2002;14:48–59.

Stadnik TW, Demaerel P, Luypaert RR, et al. Imaging tutorial: differential diagnosis of bright lesions on diffusion-weighted MR images [erratum Radiographics 2003;23:686]. Radiographics 2003;23:e7.

Thurnher MM, Schindler EG, Thurnher SA, Pernerstorfer-Schon H, Kleibl-Popov C, Rieger A. Highly active antiretroviral therapy for patients with AIDS dementia complex: effect on MR imaging findings and clinical course. AJNR Am J Neuroradiol 2000;21:670–678.

Tien RD, Chu PK, Hesselink JR, Duberg A, Wiley C. Intracranial cryptococcosis in immunocompromised patients: CT and MR findings in 29 cases. AJNR Am J Neuroradiol 1991;12:283–289.

Ukisu R, Kushihashi T, Kitanosono T, et al. Serial diffusion-weighted MRI of Creutzfeldt-Jakob disease. AJR Am J Radiol 2005;184:560–566.

Whiteman M, Espinoza L, Donovan Post MJ, Bell MD, Falcone S. Central nervous system tuberculosis in HIV-infected patients: clinical and radiographic findings. AJNR Am J Neuroradiol 1995;16:1319–1327.

Wong AM, Zimmerman RA, Simon EM, Pollock AN, Bilaniuk LT. Diffusion-weighted MR imaging of subdural empyemas in children. AJNR Am J Neuroradiol 2004;25:1016–1021.

Chapter 7

White Matter and Neurodegenerative Diseases

Jerome A. Barakos

Demyelinating Diseases
Primary Demyelination
Ischemic Demyelination
Infection-related Demyelination
Toxic and Metabolic Demyelination

Dysmyelinating Diseases

Cerebrospinal Fluid Dynamics

Neurodegenerative Disorders

In contrast to gray matter, which contains neuronal cell bodies, white matter is composed of the long processes of these neurons. The axonal processes are wrapped by myelin sheaths, and it is the lipid composition of these sheaths for which white matter is named. In this chapter, a host of diseases characterized by the involvement of white matter is described. This is followed by a discussion of hydrocephalus and neurodegenerative disorders.

The marked sensitivity of T2WIs allows white matter lesions to be readily detected. The difficulty that confronts the radiologist is that a wide gamut of diseases may involve the white matter, and these lesions are often nonspecific in nature. An understanding of these white matter diseases, their clinical features, and parenchymal patterns of involvement is important in enabling the radiologist to generate a useful differential diagnostic list.

Cerebral white matter diseases are classified into two broad categories: demyelinating and dysmyelinating. *Demyelination* is an acquired disorder that affects normal myelin. The vast majority of white matter diseases, especially in the adult, fall into this category and are the principal focus of this chapter. In contrast, *dysmyelination* is an inherited disorder affecting the formation or maintenance of myelin, and thus is typically encountered in the pediatric population. Dysmyelination is rare and is discussed later in this chapter.

DEMYELINATING DISEASES

Demyelinating disease can be divided into four main categories based on etiology: (*1*) primary, (*2*) ischemic, (*3*) infectious, and (*4*) toxic and metabolic (Table 7.1).

Primary Demyelination

Multiple sclerosis (MS) is the classic example of a primary demyelinating disease. MS is a disease characterized by immune dysfunction in the production of abnormal immunoglobulins and T cells, which are activated against myelin and mediate the damage associated with the disease. MS is a chronic, relapsing, often disabling disease affecting more than a quarter of a million people in the United States alone. The age of onset is between 20 and 40 years, with only 10% of cases presenting in individuals older than 50. There is a female predominance of almost two to one. Although several environmental factors have been associated with MS, such as higher geographic latitudes and upper socioeconomic status, the etiology of MS remains unclear.

Establishing a diagnosis of MS is challenging, because no specific examination, laboratory test, or physical finding is unequivocally diagnostic or pathognomonic of this disorder. Making a diagnosis of MS is portentous, as there are significant implications on many aspects of one's life, including eligibility for health insurance. However,

TABLE 7.1 Classification of White Matter Diseases

Primary demyelination
Multiple sclerosis
Ischemic demyelination
Deep white matter infarcts
Lacunar infarcts
Vasculitis (including sarcoidosis and lupus)
Dissection
Thromboembolic infarcts
Migrainous ischemia
Moyamoya disease
Postanoxia
Infection-related demyelination
Progressive multifocal leukoencephalopathy
HIV encephalopathy
Acute disseminated encephalomyelitis
Subacute sclerosing panencephalitis
Lyme disease
Neurosyphilis
Toxic and metabolic demyelination
Central pontine myelinolysis
Marchiafava-Bignami disease
Wernicke-Korsakoff syndrome
Radiation injury
Necrotizing leukoencephalopathy
Dysmyelination (inherited white matter disease)
Metachromatic leukodystrophy
Adrenal leukodystrophy
Leigh disease
Alexander disease

establishing the diagnosis is important because promising therapies are available, including β-interferon and antineoplastic drugs. These agents suppress the activity of the T cells, B cells, and macrophages that are thought to lead the attack on the myelin sheath.

The classic clinical definition of MS is multiple CNS lesions separated in both time and space. Patients may present with virtually any neurologic deficit, but they most commonly present with limb weakness, paresthesia, vertigo, and visual or urinary disturbances. Important characteristics of MS symptoms are their multiplicity and tendency to vary over time. The clinical course of MS is characterized by unpredictable relapses and remissions of symptoms. The diagnosis can be supported with clinical studies, which include visual, somatosensory, or motor-evoked potentials and analysis of CSF for oligoclonal banding, immunoglobulin G index, and presence of myelin basic protein. Histopathologically, active MS lesions represent areas of selective destruction of myelin sheaths and perivenular inflammation, with relative sparing of the underlying axons. These lesions may occur throughout the white matter of the CNS, including the spinal cord. The inflammatory demyelination interrupts nerve conduction and nerve function, producing the symptoms of MS. Note that histopathologically, the inflammation is a key differentiating feature between MS and other white matter conditions, such as osmotic myelinolysis (central pontine and extrapontine myelinolysis) and posterior reversible encephalopathy syndrome (PRE), which lack inflammatory changes.

MR is the most sensitive indicator in the detection of MS plaques, but imaging findings alone should never be considered diagnostic. In clinically confirmed cases of MS, MR typically demonstrates lesions in more than 90% of

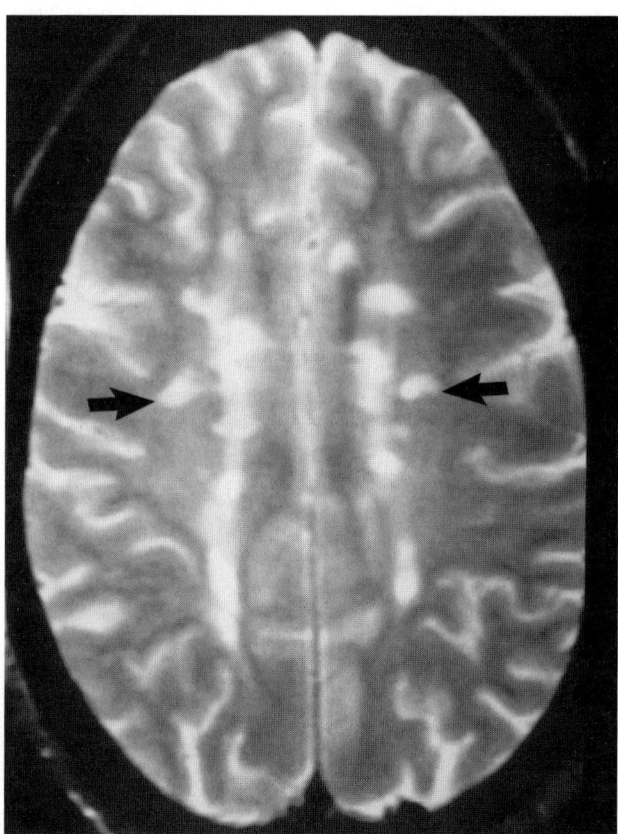

FIGURE 7.1. **Multiple Sclerosis.** T2WI of a 26-year-old woman with MS demonstrates a cluster of periventricular white matter lesions. These lesions are ovoid, and many are perpendicular to the long axis of the ventricles (perivenular in location, referred to as Dawson's fingers) (*arrows*). Although the periventricular lesions are very suggestive of MS, these lesions are nonspecific and must be correlated with clinical examination and other clinical studies (visual, somatosensory, or motor-evoked potentials, and analysis of CSF for oligoclonal banding and immunoglobulin G index) before confirming a diagnosis of MS. These lesions may be indistinguishable from other demyelinating conditions, such as acute disseminated encephalomyelitis, Lyme disease, and autoimmune/connective tissue disorders such as systemic lupus erythematosus.

cases. This compares with far less than 50% for CT and 70% to 85% for laboratory tests such as brainstem-evoked potentials and CSF oligoclonal bands. Nevertheless, the ultimate diagnosis rests with the careful combination of clinical symptoms, history, and clinical testing, including MR imaging.

A variety of T2WI techniques have been described for optimizing the detection of white matter lesions, including conventional spin-echo (SE) imaging, fast SE (FSE), short tau inversion recovery (STIR), and fluid-attenuated inversion recovery (FLAIR) sequences. As the name suggests, FLAIR imaging has the advantage of providing heavy T2 weighting while suppressing signal from CSF. As such, FLAIR images provide improved lesion conspicuity of periventricular lesions, which may be obscured by the bright signal of CSF on SE or FSE T2WIs. Comparative studies have demonstrated that FLAIR imaging provides the best visualization of supratentorial white matter lesions. However, the FLAIR sequence may have mild limitations when imaging the posterior fossa and spine, partly because of pulsation artifacts.

MS plaques are typically round or ovoid, with a periventricular or subcortical location (Fig. 7.1). Lesions are bright on T2WIs, reflecting active inflammation or chronic scarring, and only a fraction of MS plaques will demonstrate contrast enhancement. Lesions that enhance are thought to reflect new lesions with active demyelination and disruption of the blood–brain barrier (Fig. 7.2). In older lesions, without residual inflammatory reaction, abnormal high signal on T2WIs persists, reflecting residual scarring. Within the CNS, cells can mount only a limited response to neuronal injury. This scarring typically manifests as a focal proliferation of astroglia at the site of injury, termed *gliosis*. In severe cases of MS, actual loss of neuronal tissue may occur and the white matter lesions may actually have dark signal on T1WIs, often referred to as the "dark lesions" of MS. These lesions are prognostically significant, since they reflect actual loss of underlying neuronal tissue rather than simple demyelination. Additionally, in chronic cases of MS, there is diffuse loss of deep cerebral white matter, with associated thinning of the corpus callosum and potential ex vacuo ventriculomegaly.

MS lesions are nonspecific, and many of the diseases and conditions discussed in this chapter may have a similar appearance. Patients with migraines are especially challenging, because both their symptoms and imaging findings may closely mimic those of MS. A pattern that is suggestive of MS is one of periventricular lesions that are ovoid and aligned perpendicular to the long axis of the ventricles. This pattern is the result of the alignment of the lesions along the perivenular spaces. Additional characteristic features include lesions along the callosal septal interface, as well as lesions that are confluent in nature and greater than 6 mm in diameter with a periventricular location (Fig. 7.3).

In addition to the periventricular white matter, the cerebellar and cerebral peduncles as well as the corpus callosum, medulla, and spinal cord can be involved in MS (Fig. 7.4). Ischemic changes are rare in these locations; as a result, if periventricular lesions are accompanied by lesions in any of these areas, this dramatically increases the specificity for the diagnosis of MS. For example, because ischemic changes rarely involve the medulla and cerebellar/cerebral peduncles, the presence of posterior fossa lesions is a useful differential diagnostic factor in suggesting

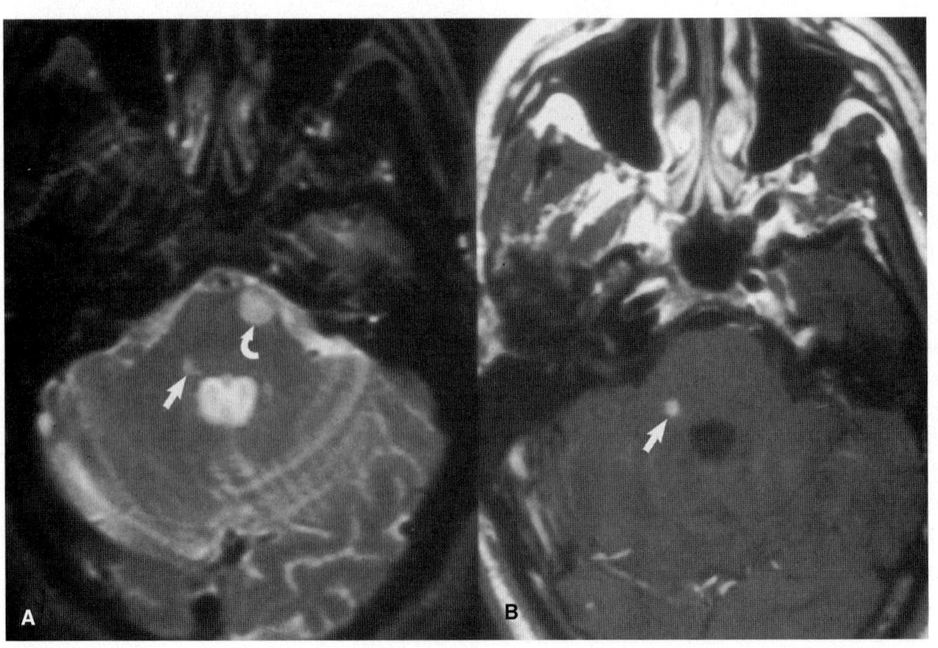

FIGURE 7.2. **Multiple Sclerosis With Lesion Enhancement.** Images of a 28-year-old woman with a recent flareup in clinical symptoms. Axial fast spin-echo T2W **(A)** and gadolinium-enhanced T1W **(B)** images reveal interval development (compared to prior MR exam performed 6 months earlier) of a new contrast-enhancing lesion within the right brachium pontis (*arrow*). The larger left anterior pontine lesion (*curved arrow*) is unchanged when compared to the earlier exam and fails to enhance. Contrast enhancement is reflective of actively demyelinating lesions and can be used to assess disease activity.

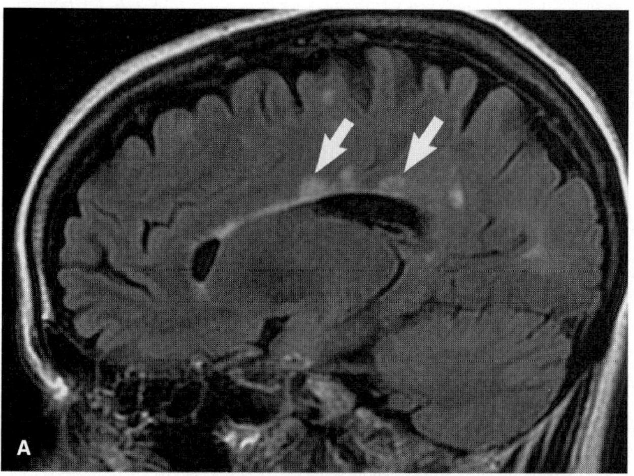

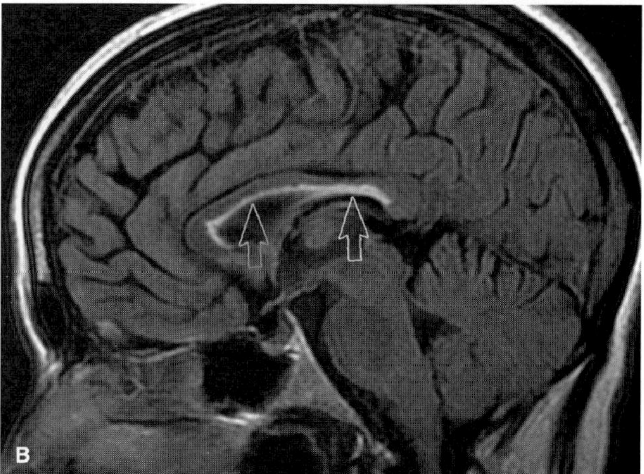

FIGURE 7.3. **Multiple Sclerosis With Callosal–Septal Involvement.** Sagittal fluid-attenuated inversion recovery images show lesions located along the ventricular ependymal surface (*arrows*) as well as along the callosal–septal interface (*open arrows*), which are very characteristic for MS. The callosal–septal interface refers to the region where the septum pellucidum contacts the undersurface of the corpus callosum.

MS. This is particularly important in patients older than 50 years, because it is difficult to decide whether multifocal white matter lesions are the result of ischemia or a demyelinating process. Additional concepts for making this distinction are discussed in the next subsection.

MS lesions may also present as a large, conglomerate, deep white matter mass that can be mistaken for a neoplasm (Fig. 7.5). A characteristic finding in these conglomerate MS plaques is that they often demonstrate a peripheral crescentic rim of contrast enhancement, which

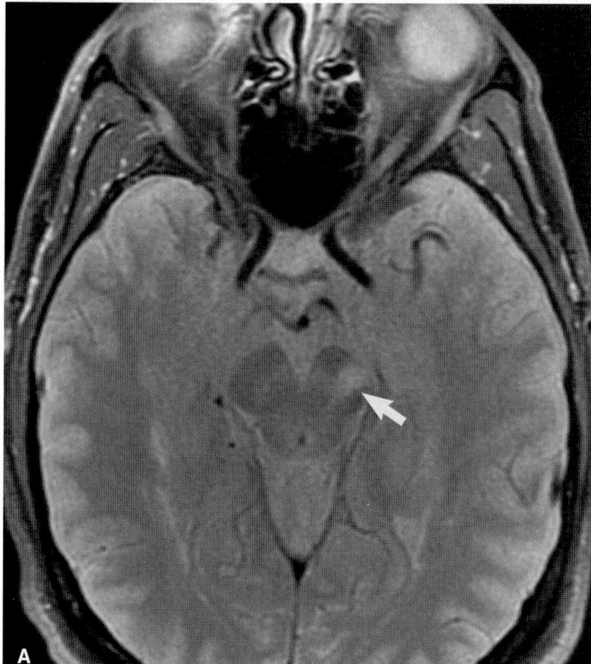

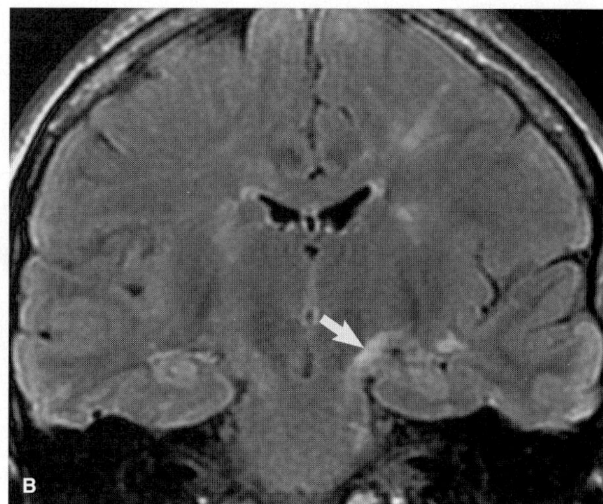

FIGURE 7.4. **Multiple Sclerosis With Brainstem Involvement.** MR images of a 31-year-old male with a history of right-sided weakness and sensory changes. Axial proton density–weighted image **(A)** and coronal fluid-attenuated inversion recovery image **(B)** reveal a lesion involving the left corticospinal tracts at the level of the midbrain (cerebral peduncle) (*arrow*). Lesions within the medulla and cerebellar/cerebral peduncles are quite characteristic for MS and serve to support this diagnosis when supratentorial lesions appear nonspecific in nature.

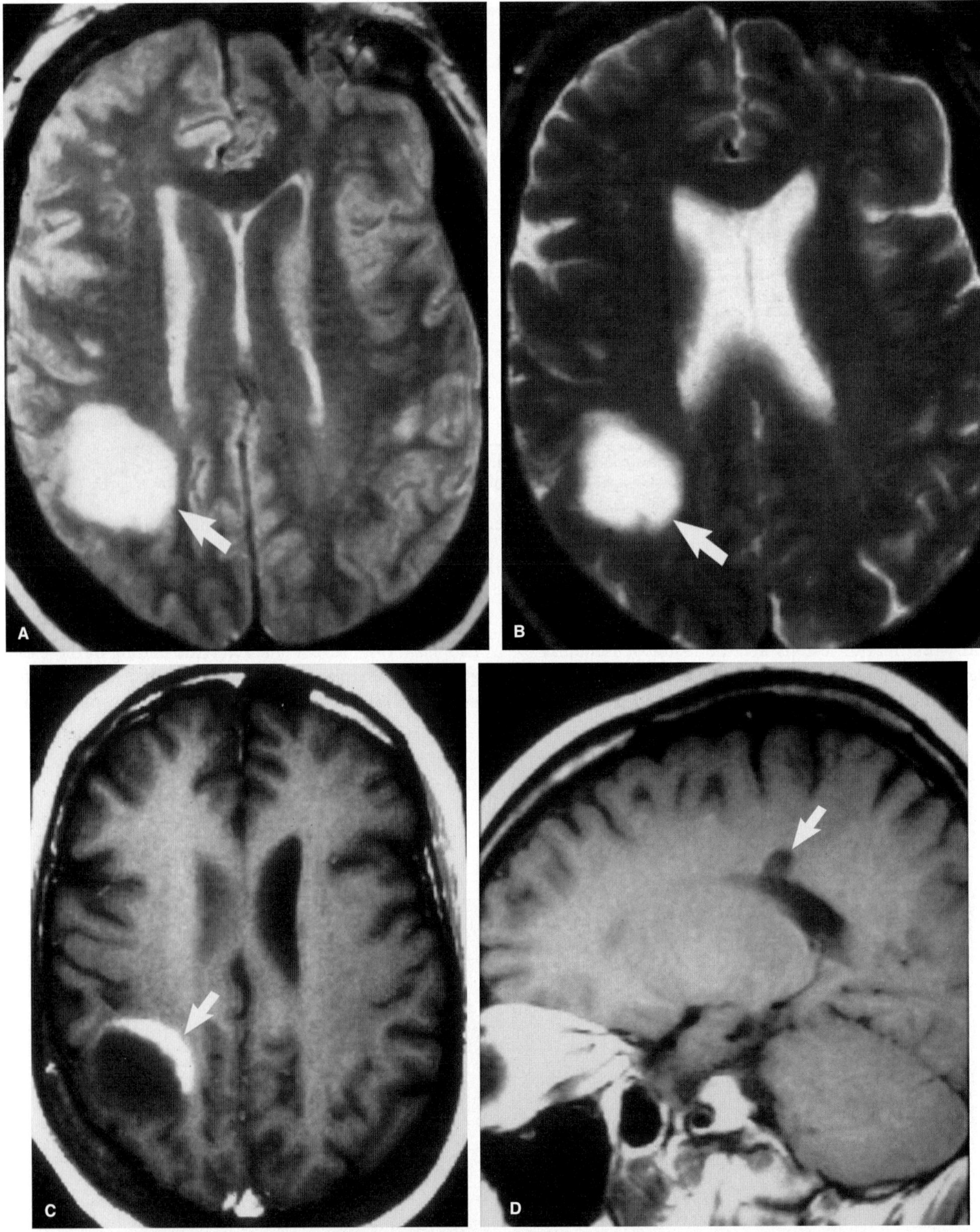

FIGURE 7.5. **Tumefactive Multiple Sclerosis.** Images from a 32-year-old woman presenting with transient bouts of left hemiparesis, as well as depression and fatigue. Proton density weighted image (PDWI) **(A),** T2WI **(B),** and postgadolinium T1WI **(C)** reveal a large right parietal mass with a peripheral rim of enhancement (*arrow*). This lesion could easily be mistaken for a neoplasm or progressive multifocal leukoencephalopathy and undergo biopsy. The sagittal T1WI **(D)** demonstrates the presence of a characteristic periependymal lesion (*arrow*), suggesting the diagnosis of MS. These are the "dark lesions" of MS, which are of greater concern than simple demyelinating plaques, because they represent actual neuronal loss. The diagnosis of MS was confirmed with additional clinical testing, including evoked potentials and CSF oligoclonal bands.

represents the advancing region of active demyelination. Detecting this pattern of enhancement, and searching carefully for other more characteristic periventricular lesions, are helpful in distinguishing a giant MS plaque from a neoplasm.

The spinal cord may also be involved with MS, and whenever a focal abnormality of the spinal cord is detected, a demyelinating MS plaque must be in the differential diagnosis. Demyelinating plaques may have mild mass effect as well as contrast enhancement, thus mimicking a neoplasm. The majority of spinal cord MS lesions (70% to 80%) will have associated plaques in the brain. In the setting of a cord lesion, performing an MR scan of the head may confirm the diagnosis, thus avoiding a spinal cord biopsy (see Chapter 10).

Ischemic Demyelination

Although MR imaging is extremely sensitive in the detection of white matter lesions, a major difficulty in arriving at a diagnosis is that white matter lesions are often nonspecific. Thus, distinguishing MS lesions from other white matter lesions can be difficult. The most commonly encountered white matter lesions are ischemic in origin.

Age-Related Demyelination. Small-vessel ischemic changes within the deep cerebral white matter are seen with such frequency in the older population (>60 years) that they are considered a normal part of aging. This represents an arteriosclerotic vasculopathy of the penetrating cerebral arteries. The deep white matter is more susceptible to ischemic injury than gray matter, because it is supplied by long, small-caliber penetrating end arteries, without significant collateral supply. In contrast, cortical gray matter, as well as parts of the brainstem such as the midbrain and medulla, have robust collateral blood supply, thus minimizing the risk of ischemia. The deep penetrating vessels supplying the white matter become narrowed by arteriosclerosis and lipohyalin deposits. The result is the formation of small ischemic lesions, primarily involving the deep cerebral and periventricular white matter as well as the basal ganglia (Fig. 7.6). The cortex, subcortical "U" fibers, central corpus callosum, medulla, midbrain, and cerebellar peduncles are usually spared because of their dual blood supply, which decreases their vulnerability to hypoperfusion. As previously described, if lesions are identified in these locations, a cause other than ischemia should be entertained.

Histologically, areas of infarction demonstrate axonal atrophy with diminished myelin. Early neuropathologists noted the areas of paleness associated with these changes and coined the term "myelin pallor." These white matter changes have received many names over the years, including leukoaraiosis, microangiopathic leukoencephalopathy, and subcortical arteriosclerotic encephalopathy. None of these terms are very satisfying, as they do not accurately reflect all the changes observed histologically and overstate the clinical significance of these lesions. A more appropriate term may simply be "age-related white matter changes." These small ischemic white matter lesions are often asymptomatic, and clinical correlation is always required before a diagnosis of subcortical arteriosclerotic encephalopathy or multi-infarct dementia (Binswanger disease) is made. The white matter infarcts just described differ from lacunar infarcts. Lacunae refer to small infarcts (5 to 10 mm) occurring within the basal ganglia, typically the upper two thirds of the putamina. Both lacunar and deep white matter infarcts have similar etiologies and are the result of disease involving the deep penetrating arteries.

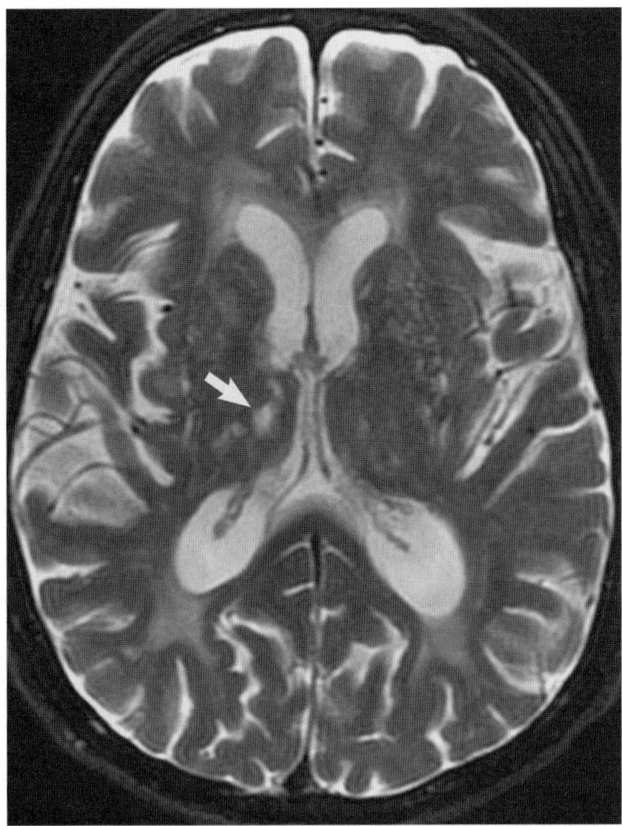

FIGURE 7.6. **Ischemic Demyelination.** This 72-year-old woman presented with forgetfulness. Axial fast spin-echo T2WI reveals diffuse patchy lesions throughout the subcortical and deep white matter. These lesions are in keeping with ischemic demyelination of the deep white matter, with several old lacunar infarcts of the basal ganglia (*arrow*). Note the ex vacuo ventriculomegaly resulting from loss of deep cerebral white matter.

Differentiating white matter lesions related to ischemic changes from MS lesions can be difficult, especially in the older patient. This is important because 10% of patients who present with MS are older than 50 years of age.

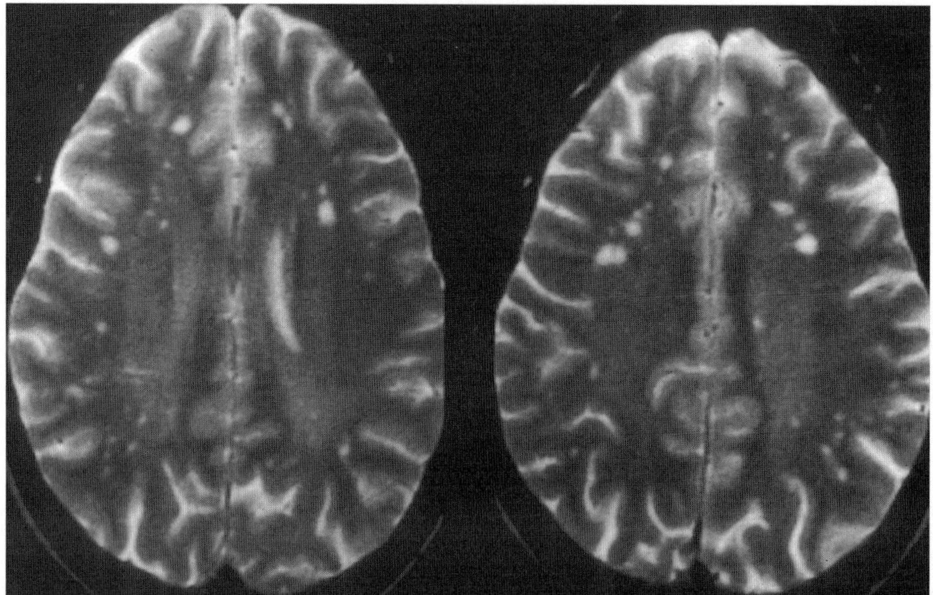

FIGURE 7.7. **Antiphospholipid Antibody Syndrome.** This 32-year-old woman presented with headaches and a history of several miscarriages. T2WIs demonstrated scattered focal subcortical and deep white matter lesions. Although these lesions are nonspecific, serum testing revealed elevated circulating pathogenic immunoglobulins/antibodies specifically targeting DNA and other nuclear constituents collectively termed antibodies to nuclear antigens, e.g., lupus anticoagulants and anticardiolipin antibodies. This represents an immune complex disease referred to as antiphospholipid antibody syndrome.

Clinical testing and history are helpful. Additionally, deep white matter infarcts tend to spare the subcortical arcuate fibers and the corpus callosum, both of which can be involved with MS. Involvement of the callosal–septal interface is quite specific for MS.

Nonspecific punctuate white matter lesions (small bright lesions on T2WIs) are more prominent in any patient with a vasculopathy, whether related to atherosclerosis (age, hypertension, diabetes, hyperlipidemia, coronary artery disease); hypercoagulable conditions; or vasculitis (lupus, sarcoid, polyarteritis nodosa, Behçet syndrome). In younger individuals with punctuate white matter lesions, hypercoagulable states, as well as embolic and vasculitic etiologies, figure prominently (Figs. 7.7, 7.8, 7.9). Hypercoagulable conditions include a diverse set of diseases with the common theme of increased risk of microvascular thrombotic disease. Serum testing can be used to evaluate for the presence of these disease conditions, which include homocystinemia, antiphospholipid syndrome, Factor V Leiden, prothrombin gene mutation, and deficiencies of natural proteins that prevent clotting (the anticoagulant proteins such as antithrombin, protein C, and protein S deficiencies). A classic case presentation is that of a young adult female with prior miscarriages presenting with headaches/migraines and ischemic white matter changes. These findings are suggestive of antiphospholipid syndrome (a.k.a. phospholipid antibody syndrome), where circulating antiphospholipid antibodies (cardiolipin or lupus anticoagulant antibodies) lead to a hypercoagulable state with resultant white matter and ischemic changes.

In the young adult population presenting with small white matter lesions, in addition to hypercoagulable conditions and migrainous ischemia, consider cardiogenic embolic etiologies. An echocardiogram plays an important role in the evaluation of a potential patent foramen ovale

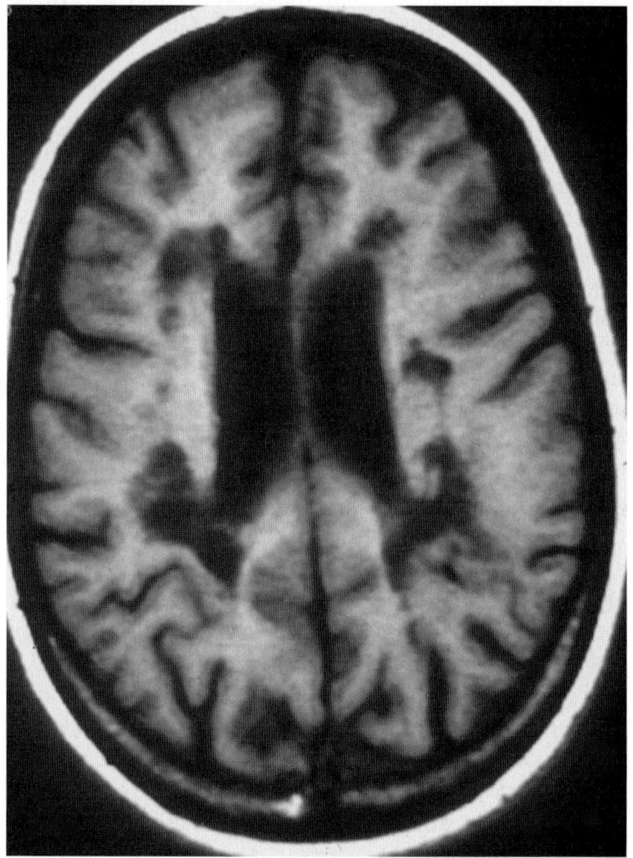

FIGURE 7.8. **Lupus Cerebritis.** Image from a 38-year-old woman presenting with cognitive deficits and history of a connective tissue disorder. The T1WI demonstrates numerous dark periventricular lesions with striking loss of deep white matter and associated ex vacuo ventriculomegaly. These dark lesions represent underlying axonal loss with neuronal dropout, reflecting a more severe stage of white matter disease. These findings are characteristic of any severe or long-standing white matter disease such as chronic MS, or as in this case, chronic lupus cerebritis.

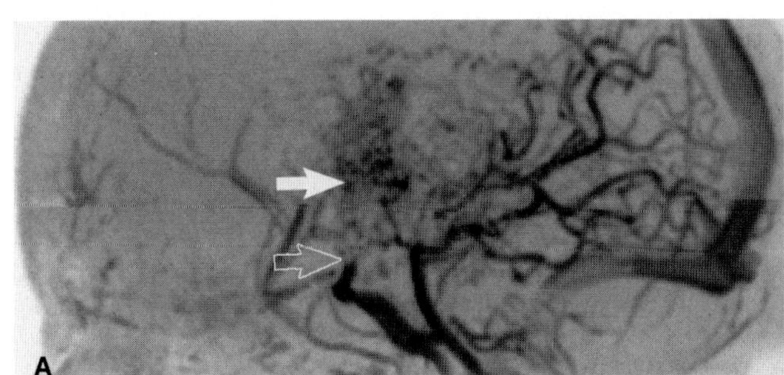

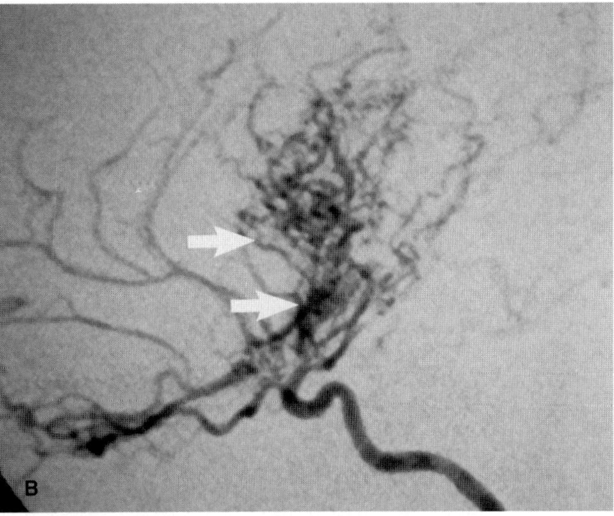

FIGURE 7.9. **Moyamoya Disease.** Six-year-old boy presents with episodes of focal motor weakness. T2WI (not shown) showed multiple scattered subcortical white matter T2 hyperintensities. MR angiography **(A)** and conventional angiography **(B)** reveal marked stenosis of the supraclinoid internal carotid vasculature (*open arrow*), with a dramatic proliferation of tiny collateral vessels (*arrows*) presenting as a "puff of smoke" (the literal Japanese translation of *moyamoya*). The cause of this vascular disorder is unknown but can be treated with various external to internal vascular bypass surgeries such as encephaloduroarteriosynangiosis. MR angiography plays a useful role in assessing the patency of these shunts once surgically completed.

or valvular vegetation. In many normal children and young adults, subcortical lesions and periventricular hyperintensities are common; they are reported to be present in these locations in 6% and 74%, respectively, of the young normal population. Commonly these punctuate foci of white matter T2 hyperintensity will have no known etiology despite evaluation for all the conditions outlined above. In this setting, these lesions are simply the gliotic residue of a remote unspecified insult, usually an immune-mediated postviral condition.

Ependymitis granularis is a normal anatomic finding that may mimic pathology. Ependymitis granularis consists of an area of high signal on a T2WI along the tips of the frontal horns (Fig. 7.10). These foci of signal range in width from several millimeters to a centimeter. Histologic studies of this subependymal area reveal a loose network of axons with low myelin count. This porous ependyma allows transependymal flow of CSF, resulting in a focal area of T2 prolongation. Unfortunately, this entity has been given a name that sounds more like a disease entity than a simple histologic observation. Similarly, with the use of FLAIR imaging, a region of periventricular T2 hyperintensity can be noted about the ventricular trigones as a normal finding. With age, prominent periventricular T2 hyperintensity may be noted along the entire length of the lateral ventricles as a normal finding, and this may be referred to as *senescent periventricular hyperintensity.*

Prominent perivascular spaces can also mimic deep white matter or lacunar infarcts. As blood vessels penetrate into the brain parenchyma, they are enveloped by CSF and a thin sheath of pia. These CSF-filled perivascular clefts are called Virchow-Robin spaces and present as punctate foci of high signal on T2WIs (Fig. 7.11). They are typically located in the centrum semiovale (high cerebral hemispheric white matter) and the lower basal ganglia at the level of the anterior commissure, where the lenticulostriate arteries enter the brain parenchyma. These perivascular spaces are typically 1 to 2 mm in diameter but can be considerably larger. They can be seen as a normal variant at any age but become more prominent with increasing age as atrophy occurs.

An important means for differentiating a periventricular space from a parenchymal lesion is the use of the proton density–weighted (first-echo T2W) or FLAIR images. On the proton density–weighted sequence, CSF has similar signal intensity as white matter. A perivascular space is composed of CSF and will parallel CSF signal intensity on all sequences (i.e., isointense to brain parenchyma on proton density sequences). In contrast, ischemic lesions, unless cavitated with cystic change, will be bright on the proton density sequence as a result of the presence of associated gliosis. Both a deep infarct and a perivascular space will be bright on the second-echo T2WI, but only the infarct will remain bright on the first-echo image. Similarly, on a FLAIR image, because fluid signal is attenuated, only true parenchymal lesions with gliosis will yield abnormal signal. On occasion, however, a small amount of persistent T2 hyperintensity can be associated with

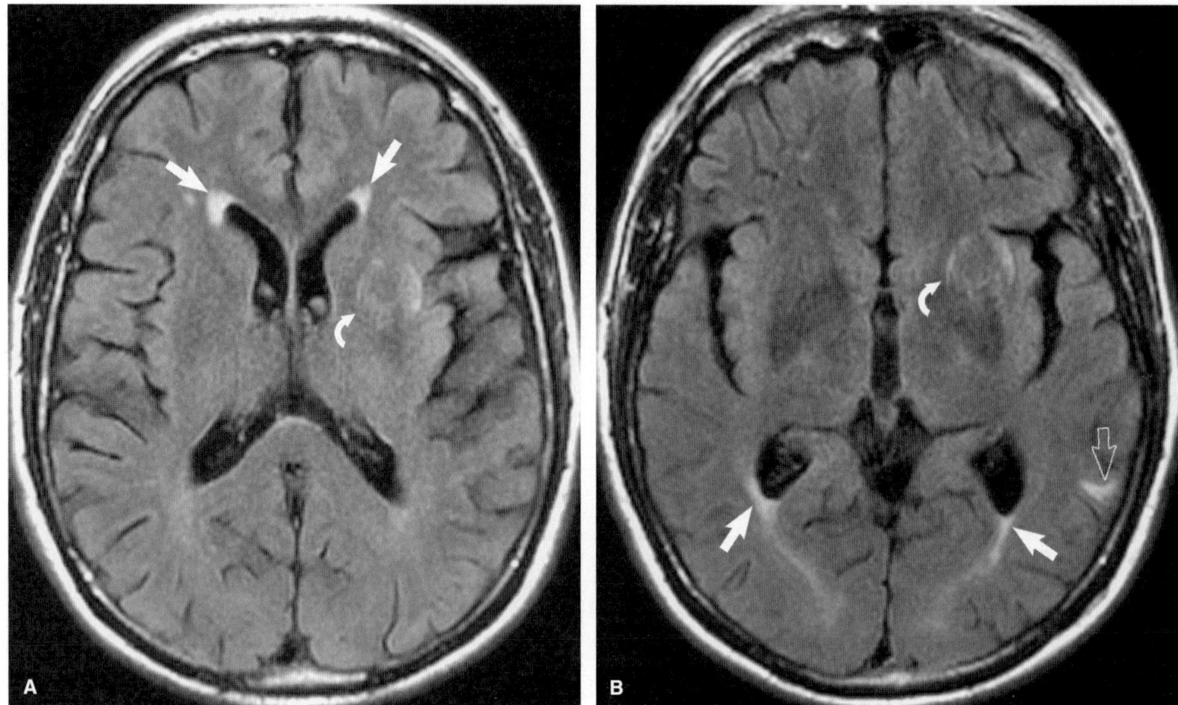

FIGURE 7.10. **Ependymitis Granularis (Normal Finding). A.** and **B.** Axial fluid-attenuated inversion recovery images in a 42-year-old man presenting with headaches. The periventricular hyperintensity noted about the tips of the frontal and occipital ventricular horns is a normal finding (*arrows*). These areas of periependymal hyperintensity may be exacerbated by any process that results in underlying white matter disease. Note the circular artifact located within the left basal ganglia; it is related to magnetic susceptibility artifact from the patient's orthodontic braces (*curved arrow*). One should be aware of artifacts that may mimic pathologic lesions, especially flow and magnetic susceptibility artifacts that can give rise to lesions that are not necessarily contiguous to the cause of the artifact. **B.** Incidental note is made of a small focus of subcortical hyperintensity along the left temporoparietal lobe related to a site of posttraumatic gliosis (*open arrow*).

perivascular spaces on the proton density or FLAIR sequences. An additional differentiating feature between giant perivascular spaces and lacunae is location. Lacunar infarcts tend to occur in the upper two thirds of the corpus striatum because they reflect end-arteriole infarcts in the distal vascular distribution. In contrast, periventricular spaces are typically smaller, bilateral, and often symmetric within the inferior third of the striatum, where the vessels enter the anterior perforated substance.

FIGURE 7.11. **Virchow-Robin Spaces.** Small punctuate foci of water signal are noted within the centrum semiovale **(A)** and basal ganglia **(B),** consistent with perivascular (PV) spaces. These spaces penetrate the brain parenchyma and reflect PV extensions of the pia mater that accompany the arteries entering and the veins emerging from the cerebral cortex. These PV spaces are almost imperceptible on the proton density–weighted image **(C),** which help confirm their identity as water, rather than white matter ischemic gliotic lesions. Although PV spaces are typically 1 to 2 mm in diameter, they can be considerably larger. Large PV spaces (about 0.5 to 1 cm) are occasionally noted within the caudal aspect of the basal ganglia and referred to as giant PV spaces. Coronal T1WI **(D)** and fast spin-echo T2WI **(E)** in a 38-year-old man demonstrate well-rounded, left-sided cysts along the course of the lenticulostriate arteries as they enter the basal ganglia through the anterior perforated substance (*arrow*). An old cavitated lacunar infarction may have a similar appearance but would be distinctly unusual in the inferior portion of the striatum. Note that lacunar infarcts are the result of vessel occlusion and thus occur along the distal extent of the lenticulostriate arteries; therefore, they tend to be located more superiorly within the basal ganglia. Additionally, lacunar infarcts may have associated gliotic T2 hyperintensity on proton density and fluid-attenuated inversion recovery images, a finding not seen with giant PV spaces.

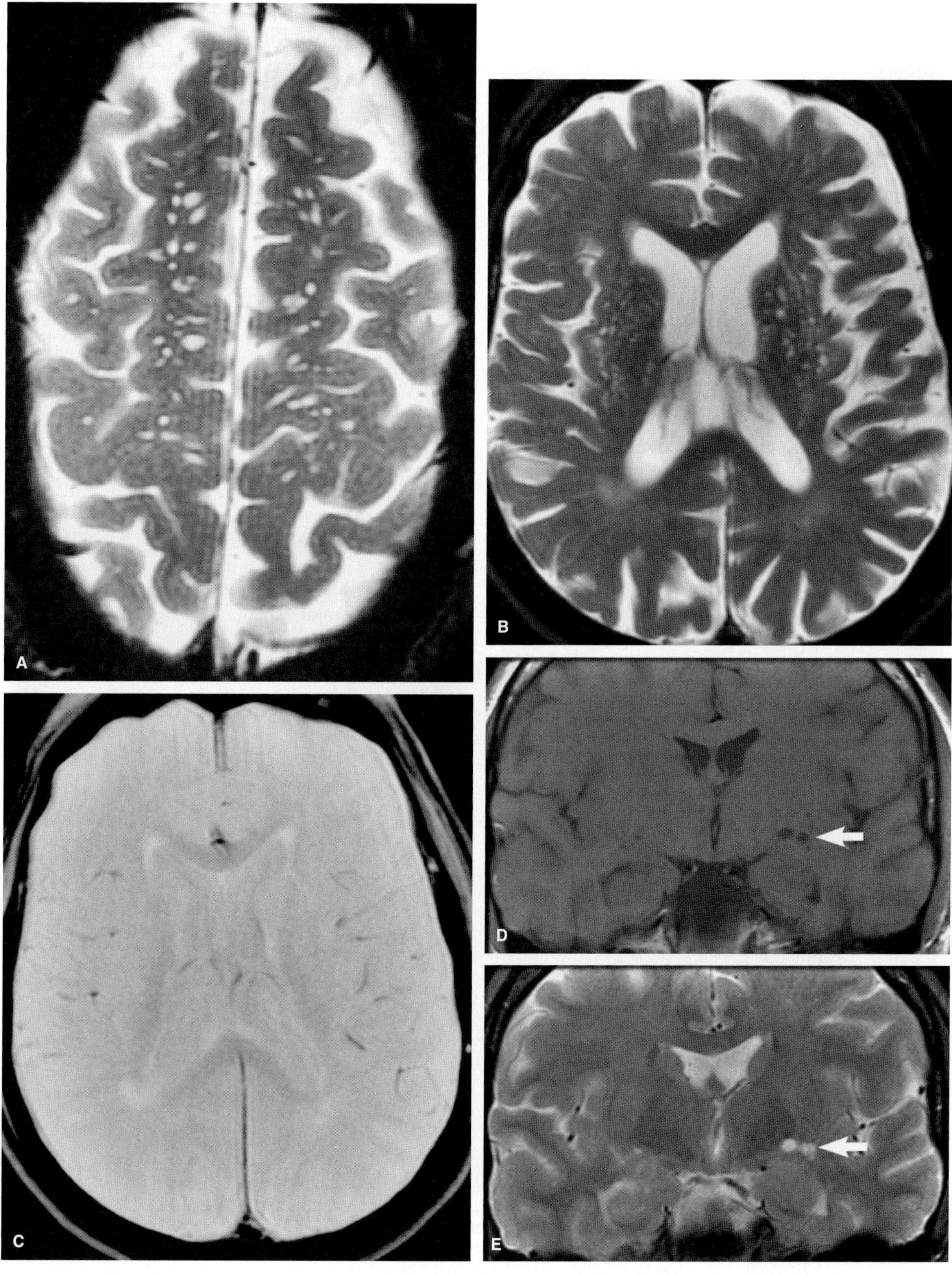
A
B
C
D
E

Infection-related Demyelination

Various infectious agents may result in white matter disease, either directly or indirectly, and most commonly are viral. Some of the more common agents are described here. For further discussion of virus-induced white matter pathology, see Chapter 6.

Progressive multifocal leukoencephalopathy (PML) is seen with increasing frequency because of the growing number of AIDS patients. PML represents a reactivation of a latent JC polyoma virus. This opportunistic infection is usually seen in severely immunocompromised patients with very low T-cell counts, particularly individuals with AIDS, lymphoma, organ transplantation, and disseminated malignancies. The JC virus infects oligodendrocytes, which are the axonal support cells that generate the myelin sheath. As a result, damage to the oligodendrocytes results in widespread demyelination. PML typically involves the deep cerebral white matter, with subcortical U-fiber involvement, but spares the cortex and deep gray matter (Fig. 7.12). Lesions are characterized by a lack of mass effect, contrast enhancement, and hemorrhage and are typically located in the parietooccipital region. These lesions progress rapidly and coalesce into larger confluent asymmetric areas. Although most lesions involve supratentorial white matter, gray matter and infratentorial involvement (cerebellum and brainstem) are not uncommon. PML is relentlessly progressive, with death typically ensuing within several months from the time of initial diagnosis.

HIV Encephalopathy. HIV involvement of the brain presents as a subacute encephalitis, referred to as *AIDS dementia complex* or *diffuse HIV encephalopathy*. This is characterized clinically by a progressive dementia without focal neurologic signs. HIV encephalopathy does not appear to be the result of a direct infection of the neurons or macroglia (i.e., CNS support cells, astrocytes, oligodendrocytes). Instead, the active HIV infection develops in the microglia (brain macrophages). The cytokines and excitatory compounds that are produced as a result of this infection have a toxic effect on adjacent neurons.

HIV encephalopathy most often results in mild cerebral atrophy without a focal abnormality. Occasionally, HIV encephalopathy causes focal or diffuse white matter hyperintensities on T2WIs. Typically, HIV white matter involvement presents as subtle, diffuse T2 hyperintensity that often is bilateral and relatively symmetric (Fig. 7.13). This supratentorial white matter signal abnormality is ill defined and often involves a large area, in contrast to the dense lesions that are characteristic of PML. HIV encephalopathy can also present with more

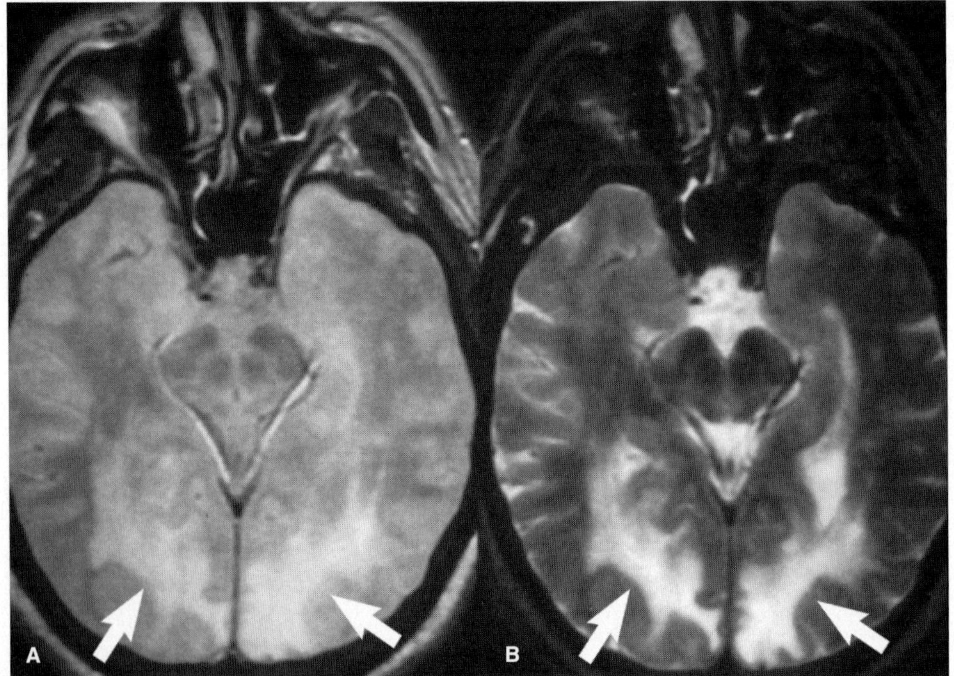

FIGURE 7.12. **Progressive Multifocal Leukoencephalopathy.** A 32-year-old HIV-positive man presents with cognitive deterioration and weakness. Proton density weighted image (PDWI) **(A)** and T2WI **(B)** reveal large confluent areas of T2 hyperintensity in the subcortical white matter of the parietooccipital lobes (*arrows*). Characteristic features of this demyelinating process include minimal mass effect, despite the large size of these patchy white matter lesions, and essentially no contrast enhancement or hemorrhage. A very low T-cell count reflecting an immunocompromised status is key to the diagnosis. In an immunocompetent patient, differential diagnostic considerations would include posterior reversible encephalopathy syndrome, which can have an identical imaging appearance.

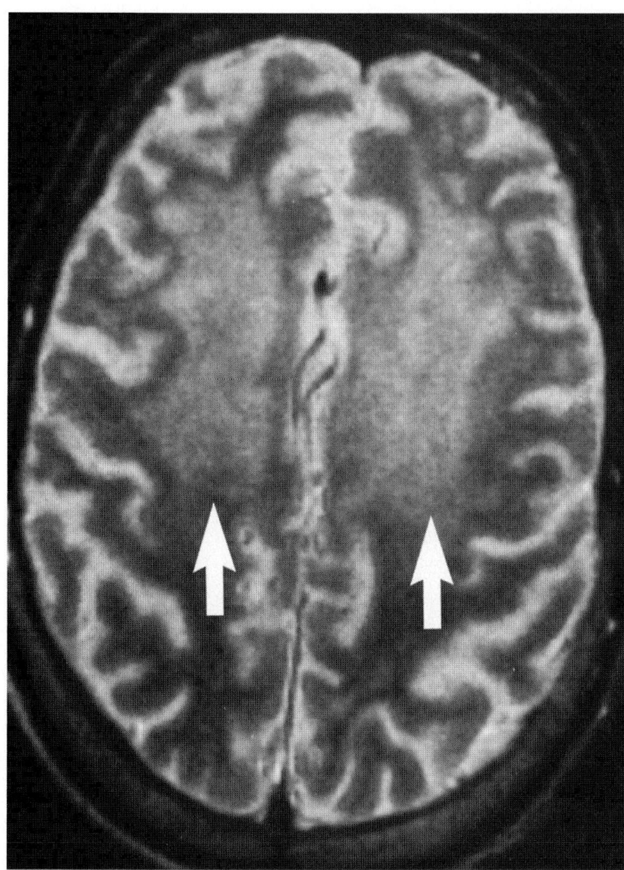

FIGURE 7.13. **HIV Encephalopathy.** T2WI of a 27-year-old man demonstrates diffuse hazy hyperintensity of the deep cerebral white matter (*arrows*), as well as cortical atrophy. Note how this hazy T2 hyperintensity differs from the dense confluent lesions of progressive multifocal leukoencephalopathy shown in Figure 7.12.

focal punctate lesions. HIV lesions do not demonstrate contrast enhancement.

Demyelination may also occur as an indirect result of a viral infection. Specifically, demyelination may follow a viral illness, the result of a virus-induced autoimmune response to white matter.

Acute disseminated encephalomyelitis (ADEM), a postinfectious and postvaccinal encephalomyelitis, typically occurs after a viral illness or vaccination, with measles, rubella, varicella, and mumps being the most common agents. This condition is considered an immune-mediated inflammatory demyelinating disease, but sometimes it has no recognized antecedent infection or inciting malady.

It is theorized that the body's antiviral immune reaction cross-reacts with myelin sheaths, resulting in an acute, aggressive form of demyelination. This unintended antiviral response against myelin is a result of shared molecular homology between viral proteins and normal human CNS proteins. Recall that oligodendrocytes are responsible for the formation and maintenance of the myelin sheaths, and their damage results in demyelination.

Demyelinating lesions associated with ADEM typically begin approximately 2 weeks after a viral infection with the abrupt clinical onset of neurologic symptoms, which include decreased levels of consciousness varying from lethargy to coma; convulsions; multifocal neurologic symptoms such as hemiparesis, paraparesis, and tetraparesis; cranial nerve palsies; movement disorders; and seizures. In the majority of cases, there is spontaneous resolution of symptoms, but permanent sequelae can be seen in up to 25% of patients, with some even progressing to death. Although ADEM occurs most commonly in children, persons of any age can be affected. Lesions primarily involve white matter, but gray matter may also be affected. MR imaging demonstrates multifocal or confluent white matter lesions similar to those of MS (Fig 7.14). A differential feature is that ADEM is a monophasic illness, unlike MS, which has a remitting and relapsing course. This is a feature often useful in differentiating ADEM from MS. Specifically, if the majority of the identified white matter lesions enhance, this suggests a monophasic demyelinating process (i.e., ADEM).

Subacute sclerosing panencephalitis represents a reactivated, slowly progressive infection caused by the measles virus. Children between the ages of 5 and 12 years who have had measles, usually before the age of 3, are typically affected. MR demonstrates patchy areas of periventricular demyelination as well as lesions of the basal ganglia. The disease course is variable and may be rapidly progressive or protracted.

Herpes encephalitis is the most common fatal encephalitis. Although this condition is also discussed in Chapter 6, its importance warrants repetition. The form of herpes encephalitis that we will discuss occurs in children and adults and is caused by herpes simplex virus (HSV) type 1 (oral herpes); this is in contrast to neonatal herpes encephalitis, which is caused by herpes simplex virus 2 (genital herpes). Presenting symptomology may be nonspecific, such as headache, fever, mental deterioration, and seizures. As a result of this variable clinical presentation, diagnosis may be difficult. This emphasizes the crucial role of the radiologist in entertaining this diagnosis when appropriate imaging findings are noted. Antiviral treatment is simple and effective, but failure to treat yields 100% mortality. Although the diagnosis may be confirmed by polymerase chain reaction detection of herpes DNA in CSF, therapy must be instituted prior to the return of this test result.

HSV type 1 has a particular predilection for the limbic system, with localization of infection to temporal lobes, insular cortex, subfrontal area, and cingulate gyri (Fig. 7.15). The limbic system is responsible for integration of emotion, memory, and complex behavior, and involvement of these structures accounts for some of the behavioral symptoms at presentation. Imaging reveals primarily T2 hyperintensity of the involved cortex and subcortical structures presenting as an encephalitis with variable contrast

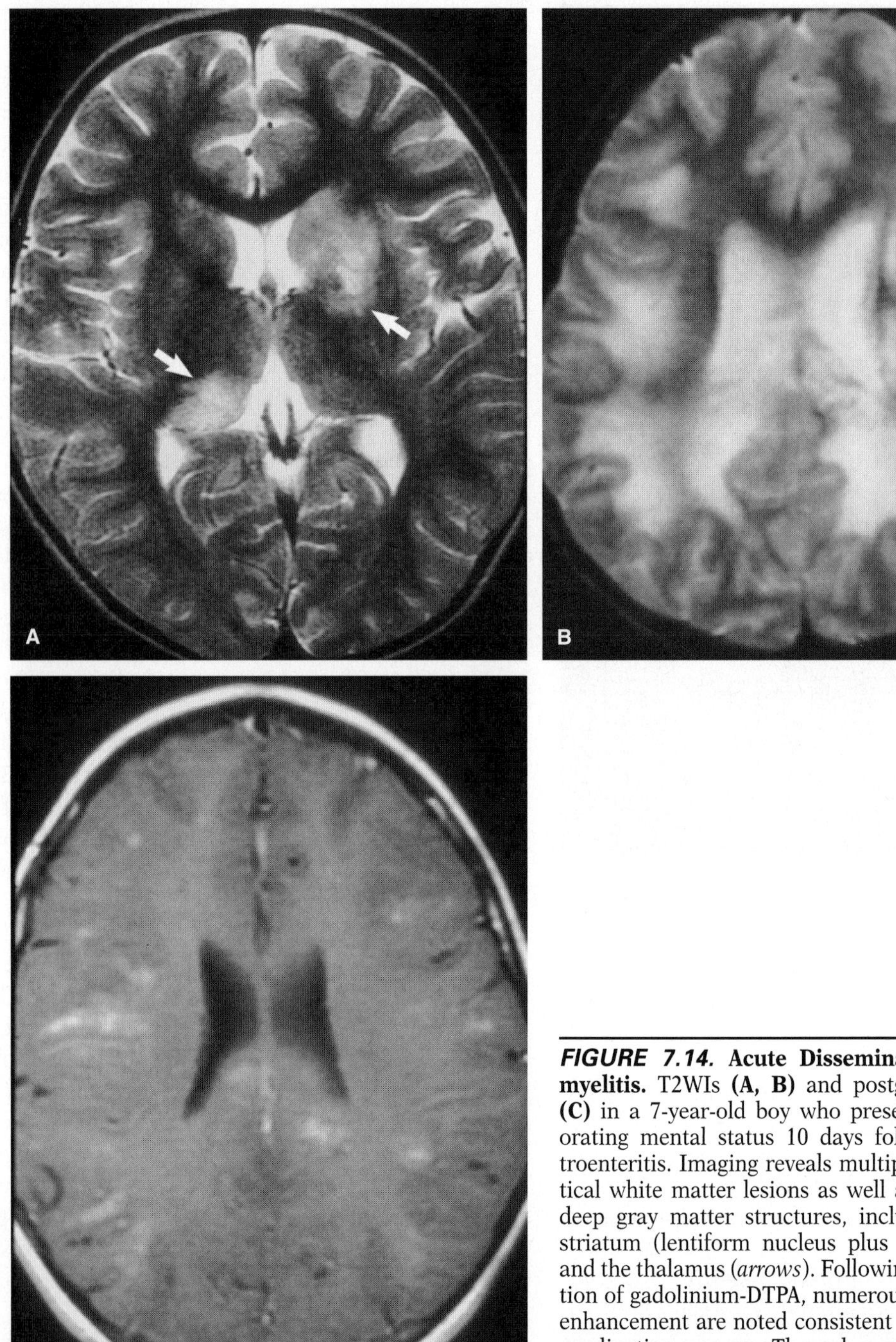

FIGURE 7.14. **Acute Disseminated Encephalomyelitis.** T2WIs **(A, B)** and postgadolinium T1WI **(C)** in a 7-year-old boy who presented with deteriorating mental status 10 days following viral gastroenteritis. Imaging reveals multiple patchy subcortical white matter lesions as well as involvement of deep gray matter structures, including the corpus striatum (lentiform nucleus plus caudate nucleus) and the thalamus (*arrows*). Following the administration of gadolinium-DTPA, numerous punctate foci of enhancement are noted consistent with an acute demyelinating process. The enhancement of most lesions is suggestive of a monophasic demyelinating process. The patient improved after treatment with steroids.

enhancement. Initially, herpes encephalitis is usually unilateral; however, sequential bilateral involvement is highly suggestive of the disease. Histopathologically, herpes infection is a fulminant necrotizing meningoencephalitis associated with edema, necrosis, hemorrhage, and eventually encephalomalacia. As a result, hemorrhage within the area of involved parenchyma is strongly supportive of this diagnosis.

Toxic and Metabolic Demyelination

Central pontine myelinolysis (CPM) is a disorder that results in characteristic demyelination of the central pons. This is most commonly seen in patients with electrolyte abnormalities, particularly involving hyponatremia, that are rapidly corrected, giving rise to the term "osmotic demyelination syndrome." This condition occurs most commonly

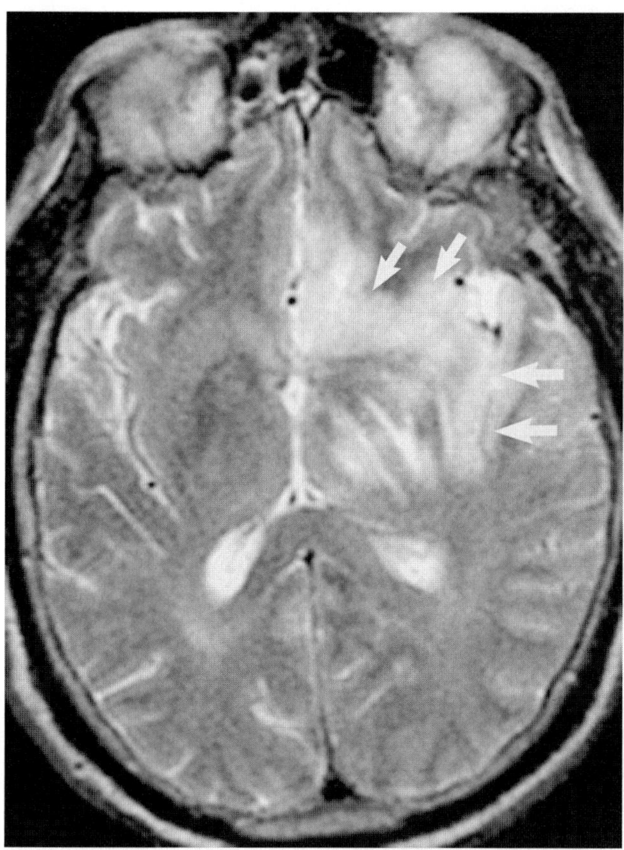

FIGURE 7.15. **Herpes Encephalitis.** T2WI of a 31-year-old man who presented with behavioral disturbance and new-onset seizures. MR demonstrates diffuse hyperintensity of the right insular cortex, and the adjacent orbitofrontal and temporal lobes are characteristic for herpes encephalitis (*arrows*). The radiologist must have a low threshold for considering this diagnosis when signal abnormality of the temporal lobes, insular cortex, or cingulate gyrus is noted, as failure of treatment results in 100% mortality.

in children and alcoholics with malnutrition. Occasionally, cases have been associated with diabetes, leukemia, transplant recipients, chronically debilitated patients, and others with conditions resulting in chronic malnutrition. The clinical course is classically described as biphasic, beginning with a generalized encephalopathy caused by the hyponatremia, which usually transiently improves following initial correction of sodium. This is followed by a second neurologic syndrome, which occurs 2 to 3 days following correction or overcorrection of hyponatremia caused by myelinolysis. This latter phase is classically characterized by a rapidly evolving corticospinal syndrome with quadriplegia, acute changes in mental status, and a "locked-in" state in which the patient is mute, unable to move, and occasionally comatose. Patients tend to be extremely ill and often have a very poor prognosis.

The pathophysiology of CPM relates to a disturbance in the physiologic balance of osmoles in the brain. Oligodendroglial cells are most susceptible to CPM-related osmotic stresses, with the distribution of CPM changes paralleling the distribution of oligodendroglial cells within the central pons, thalamus, globus pallidus, putamen, lateral geniculate body, and other extrapontine sites. The mechanism of myelinolysis remains to be completely elucidated, but it appears to be distinct from a demyelinating process like that of MS, in which an inflammatory response predominates. CPM is characterized by intramyelinitic splitting, vacuolization, and rupture of myelin sheaths, presumably because of osmotic effects. However, there is preservation of neurons and axons. Note that there is no inflammatory reaction associated with osmotic demyelination, differentiating this process from MS, which is characterized by marked perivascular inflammation. MR characteristically demonstrates abnormal high signal on T2WI, corresponding to the regions of central pontine demyelination (Fig. 7.16). Additionally, extrapontine sites of involvement have been described in this condition, including the white matter of the cerebellum, thalamus, globus pallidus, putamen, and lateral geniculate body, giving rise to the term extrapontine myelinolysis.

Posterior reversible encephalopathy syndrome (PRE) is a condition characterized by signal changes within the brain parenchyma, primarily involving the posterior vascular distribution. This condition has also been referred to as *reversible posterior leukoencephalopathy syndrome*. Patients present with headache, seizures, visual changes, and altered mental status, with MR revealing symmetric areas of bilateral subcortical and cortical vasogenic edema within the parietooccipital lobes (Fig. 7.17>). The leading theory regarding the etiology of this condition is a temporary failure of the autoregulatory capabilities of the cerebral vessels, leading to hyperperfusion, breakdown of the blood–brain barrier, and consequent vasogenic edema, but no acute ischemic changes. Autoregulation maintains a constant blood flow to the brain, despite systemic blood pressure alterations, but this can be overcome at a "breakthrough" point, at which point the increased systemic blood pressure is transmitted to the brain, resulting in brain hyperperfusion. This increased perfusion pressure is sufficient to overcome the blood–brain barrier, allowing extravasation of fluid, macromolecules, and even red blood cells into the brain parenchyma. The preferential involvement of the parietal and occipital lobes is thought to be related to the relatively poor sympathetic innervation of the posterior circulation.

A very diverse set of conditions leads to this characteristic clinical and radiologic presentation, including treatment with cyclosporin A or tacrolimus (FK506), acute renal failure/uremia, hemolytic uremic syndrome, eclampsia, thrombotic thrombocytopenia purpura, and treatment with a wide variety of chemotherapeutic agents, including interferon. This suggests a final common etiologic pathway involving either endothelial injury, elevated blood

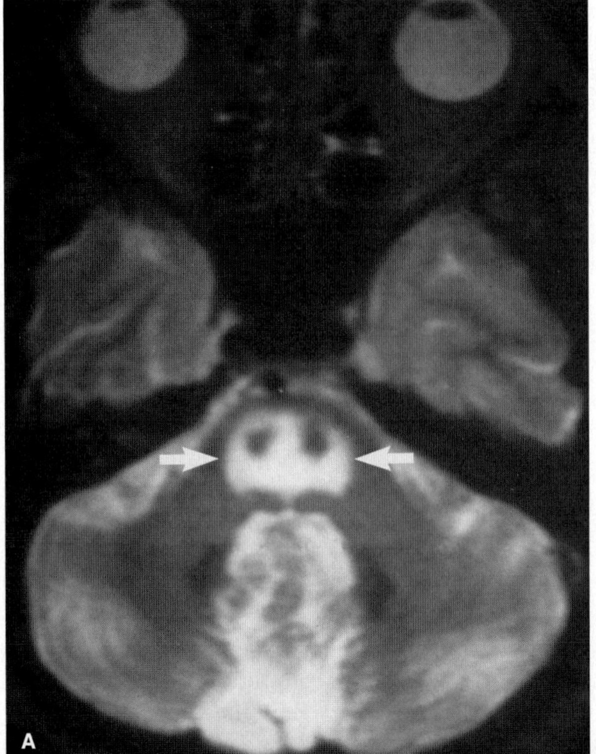

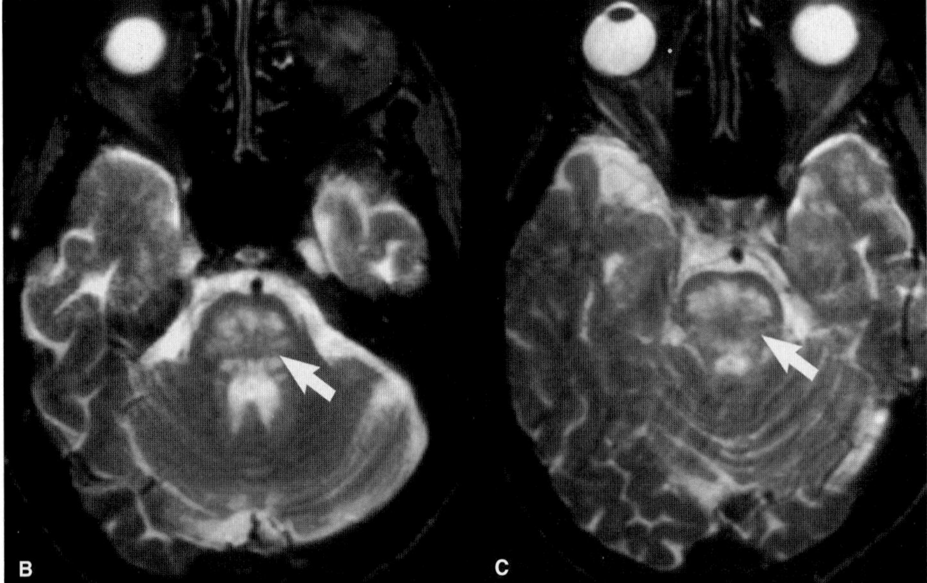

FIGURE 7.16. **Central Pontine Myelinolysis (CPM).** A 52-year-old alcoholic was admitted with a serum sodium of 110 mEq/mL. After rapid normalization of sodium, the patient became comatose. The T2WI **(A)** demonstrates well-defined intense high signal within the basis pontis (*arrows*). Often, the central corticospinal tracts remain preserved, giving rise to this characteristic appearance of two rounded areas of spared central pontine tracts. Note that CPM should be differentiated from ischemic demyelination, as both conditions may have T2 hyperintensity within the basis pontis. **B.** and **C.** A 72-year-old man presented with progressive confusion and known vasculopathy related to longstanding hypertension and diabetes, without evidence of osmotic or electrolyte disturbance. The T2WIs reveal diffuse patchy T2 hyperintensity of the basis pontis (*arrows*). Given the clinical history, this finding is consistent with small vessel ischemic changes within the pons rather than CPM. Statistically speaking, hyperintensity within the pons will be more often related to ischemic demyelination than CPM, simply because of the relative frequency of ischemic pathology. However, clinical history will allow easy differentiation between these conditions.

pressure, or a combination of these factors. Associated clinical conditions presumably contribute to this physiologic effect by cytotoxic effects on the vascular endothelium (endotoxins), causing increasing capillary permeability that allows this process to occur at near normal blood pressures, or by inducing or exacerbating hypertension. Hypertension is commonly associated with PRE but may be relatively mild and is not universally present, especially in the setting of immunosuppression. Note that this condition is not always reversible and may occasionally result in hemorrhagic infarctions.

Marchiafava-Bignami disease is a rare form of demyelination seen most frequently in alcoholics. This condition was first described in Italian red wine drinkers, but it has since been reported with other types of alcohol use as well as in nonalcoholics. The disease is characterized by demyelination involving the central fibers (medial zone) of the corpus callosum, although other white matter tracts may be involved, including the anterior and posterior commissures, the centrum semiovale, and the middle cerebral peduncles. This is felt to reflect a form of osmotic demyelination, as discussed earlier in extrapontine myelinolysis.

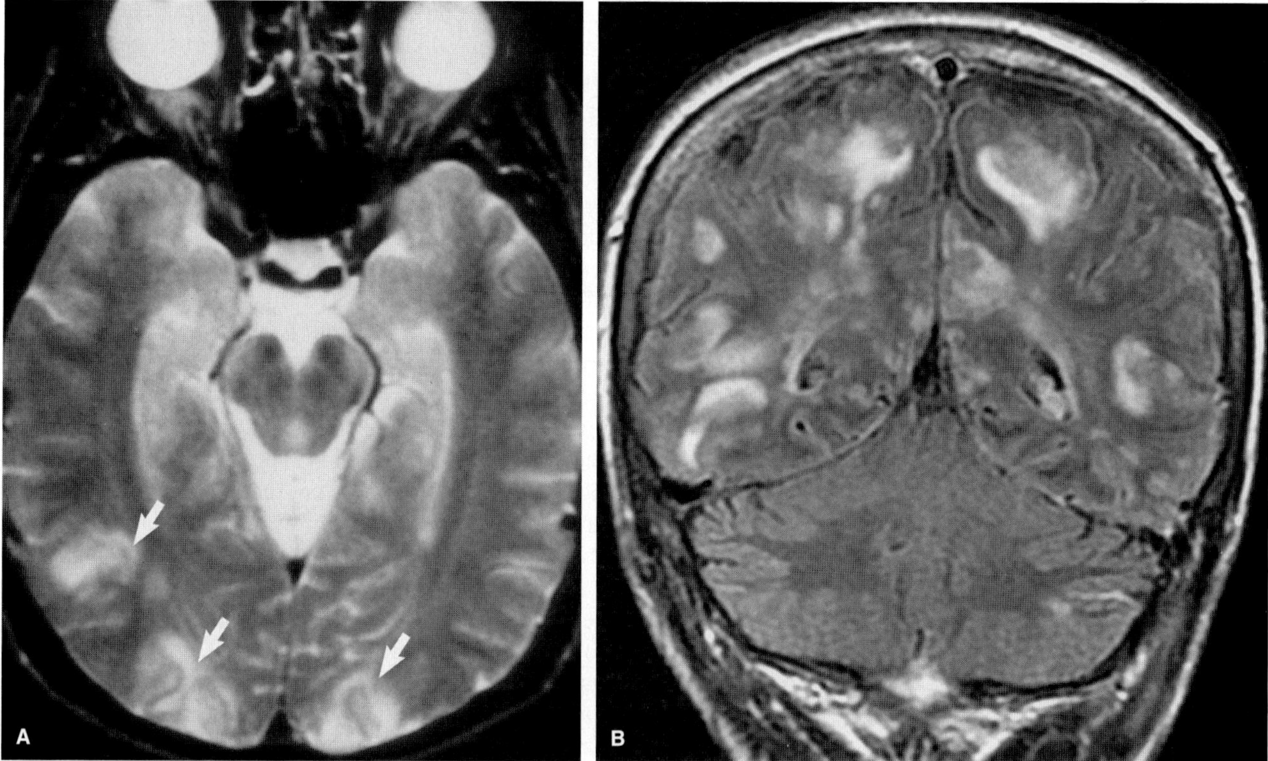

FIGURE 7.17. **Posterior Reversible Encephalopathy Syndrome (PRES).** A 43-year-old transplant patient who was being treated with cyclosporine presented with visual disturbances and confusion. Axial **(A)** and coronal **(B)** T2WIs reveal patchy areas of cortically based signal abnormality within the parietooccipital lobes (*arrows*), corresponding to the posterior vascular distribution. These findings are in keeping with dysfunction of vascular permeability, the result of a combination of endothelial toxicity and elevated blood pressure. Both clinical symptoms and imaging findings resolved after the cyclosporine doses were reduced.

Onset is usually insidious, with the most common symptom being nonspecific dementia.

Wernicke encephalopathy and Korsakoff syndrome are metabolic disorders caused by thiamine (B1 vitamin) deficiency secondary to poor oral intake in severe chronic alcoholics (most common association), hematologic malignancies, or recurrent vomiting in pregnant patients. In fact, this condition may occur in many different non-alcohol-related pathologic conditions that share the common denominator of malnutrition. In general, there is a good clinical response to thiamine administration. Classically, Wernicke encephalopathy is characterized by the clinical triad of acute onset of ocular movement abnormalities, ataxia, and confusion. Korsakoff, a Russian psychiatrist, described the disturbance of memory in long-term alcoholics. Therefore, if persistent learning and memory deficits are present in patients with Wernicke encephalopathy, the symptom complex is termed Wernicke-Korsakoff syndrome.

In the acute stage of this disease, MR may reveal T2 hyperintensity or contrast enhancement of the mamillary bodies, basal ganglia, thalamus, and brainstem, with periaqueductal involvement. In contrast, the chronic stage may show atrophy of the mamillary bodies, midbrain tegmentum, as well as dilatation of the third ventricle. Except for the mamillary body involvement, these findings are very similar to Leigh disease, which supports the notion that enzymatic deregulation in Leigh disease is tied in some fashion to thiamine metabolism.

Radiation Leukoencephalitis. Radiation may result in damage to the white matter secondary to a radiation-induced vasculopathy. Radiation leukoencephalitis usually follows a cumulative dose in excess of 40 Gy delivered to the brain and occurs 6 to 9 months after treatment. Findings consist of areas of abnormal high signal on T2WIs, typically involving confluent areas of white matter extending to involve the subcortical U fibers in the distribution of the irradiated brain (Fig. 7.18). Note that this represents an indirect effect of radiation on the brain and results from an arteritis (endothelial hypertrophy, medial hyalinization, and fibrosis) involving small arteries and arterioles.

Radiation Necrosis and Radiation Arteritis. In contrast to the rather benign nature of radiation leukoencephalitis, radiation necrosis and radiation arteritis are major hazards related to CNS radiation. Both of these radiation effects are strongly dose related and are less

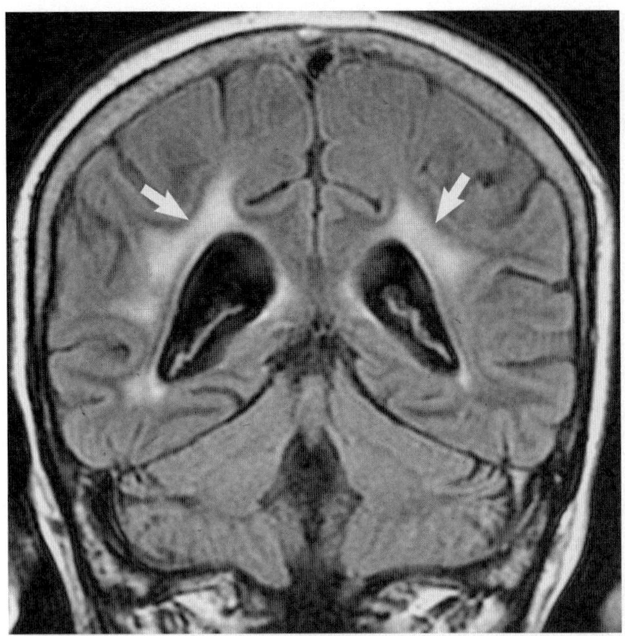

FIGURE 7.18. **Radiation Leukoencephalopathy.** MR of a 62-year-old woman obtained 1 year after whole brain radiation for metastatic breast carcinoma to the brain shows a delayed neurologic sequelae of radiotherapy. Coronal fluid-attenuated inversion recovery image reveals confluent areas of high signal involving the periventricular white matter (*arrows*). This finding may be associated with loss of deep cerebral white matter with concomitant ex vacuo ventriculomegaly, as noted in this case. Although this condition may result in some degree of neurocognitive deficits, this patient was entirely asymptomatic and was simply returning for a routine follow-up examination.

commonly seen today because of greater fractionation of CNS radiation doses. Radiation necrosis may occur several weeks to years after radiation, but it most commonly occurs between 6 and 24 months after radiation. Radiation necrosis is rarely noted at less than 6 months after treatment unless gamma knife is employed (Fig. 7.19). Note that gamma knife is an ablative procedure designed to destroy targeted tissue and thus may more easily incite frank radiation necrosis. This is in contrast to radiation therapy, which is not ablative in nature. Radiation necrosis can be progressive and fatal. Radiation necrosis typically presents as an enhancing lesion with mass effect and ring enhancement or as multiple foci of enhancement, mimicking recurrent neoplasm. Radiation may also induce telangiectasia within the radiation field, which may appear similar to cryptic vascular malformations.

Radiation necrosis is found most commonly in or near the irradiated tumor bed, but it sometimes is more remote from the tumor bed. It is theorized that the partially injured brain parenchyma within and adjacent to the tumor bed is more susceptible to radiation injury, thus accounting for the distribution of radiation necrosis. After resection of a brain neoplasm and subsequent radiation therapy, it can be very difficult to differentiate tumor recurrence from radiation-associated necrosis, because both conditions may continue to grow and demonstrate imaging features characteristic of neoplasm, i.e., lesion growth, irregular ring enhancement, edema, and mass effect (Fig. 7.20). If during serial scanning a lesion within the treated tumor bed stabilizes and regresses, this is obviously radiation necrosis, but if the lesion progresses, differentiation between tumor and radiation necrosis is difficult. PET and MR spectroscopy (MRS) are valuable in distinguishing between tumor recurrence and radiation necrosis. With PET scanning, a short-lived radioactive isotope (e.g., ^{18}F fluorodeoxyglucose) that decays by emitting a positron, is combined with glucose, a metabolically active molecule. This tracer mimics glucose and is taken up and retained by tissues with higher than normal metabolic activity, such as tumor recurrence. This is in contrast to radiation necrosis, which is not metabolically active (Fig. 7.21).

Proton (hydrogen) MRS imaging characterizes the metabolite profiles of tumoral and nontumoral brain lesions. This biochemical information helps distinguish areas of tumor recurrence from areas of radiation necrosis. Major brain metabolites include choline (Cho), creatine (Cr), and n-acetylaspartate (NAA) (located at 3.2, 3.0, and 2.0 ppm, respectively). Choline reflects cellular density and proliferation, and is often elevated with tumor. Creatine is a normal cellular metabolite and is often stable in a variety of disease conditions. Thus creatine is often used as a denominator in calculating choline and NAA ratios (Cho/Cr and NAA/Cr), which corrects for individual variation and allows for comparison between individual subjects. NAA is a neuronal marker and reflects neuronal density. Loss of the NAA signal is consistent with neuronal loss or damage, which can be seen in a wide variety of disease conditions, including radiation necrosis and even MS.

Large vessels included within the radiation port may undergo radiation-induced endothelial hypertrophy, medial hyalinization, and fibrosis. The net result is a progressive vascular narrowing that may be obliterative in nature. This often involves the cavernous and supraclinoid portions of the carotid arteries in children who have undergone irradiation of the parasellar region for treatment of tumors, for example, craniopharyngiomas or optic and hypothalamic gliomas. The near complete obliteration of the supraclinoid carotid arteries results in cerebral and striatal ischemic changes. Occasionally, there may be a compensatory proliferation of lenticulostriate collaterals. When performing angiography, these collateral vessels present with a blush, which in Japan has been referred to as *Moyamoya,* meaning "puff of smoke." Moyamoya disease classically refers to a supraclinoid obliterative arteriopathy that occurs primarily in children and is idiopathic in nature (Fig. 7.8).

When methotrexate chemotherapy (intrathecal or systemic) is administered in combination with CNS radiation,

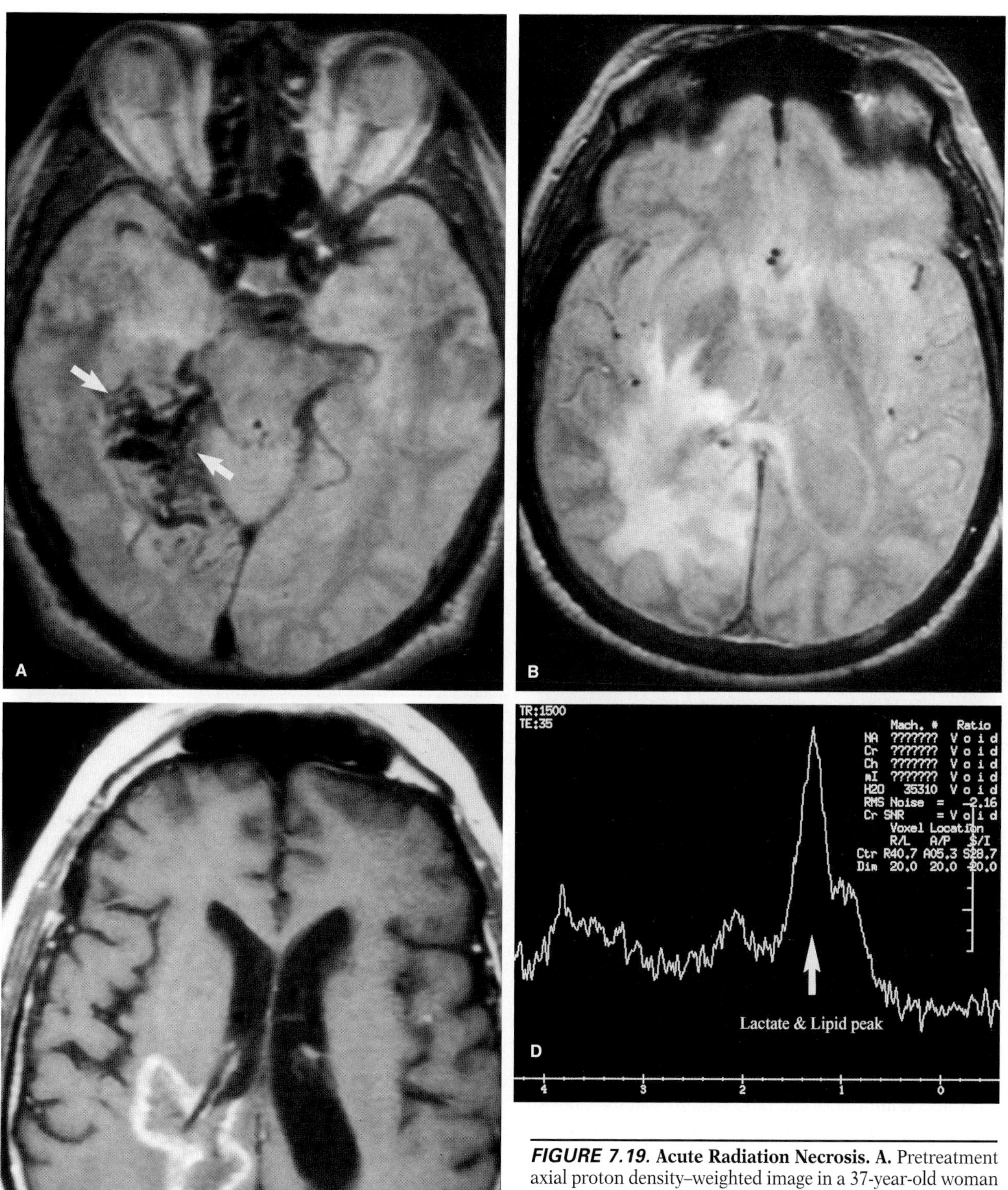

FIGURE 7.19. **Acute Radiation Necrosis. A.** Pretreatment axial proton density–weighted image in a 37-year-old woman with a deep temporoparietal arteriovascular malformation (*arrows*). **B.** and **C.** Less than 6 months after treatment with gamma knife radiation, the patient returned with marked vasogenic edema and contrast enhancement, consistent with radiation necrosis. Note that without clinical history, these imaging findings are indistinguishable from a neoplastic or infectious process. **D.** MR spectroscopy of the lesion reveals marked elevation of lactate and lipids (0.9 to 1.3 ppm), with reductions of all other major metabolites (choline, creatine, and N-acetylaspartate).

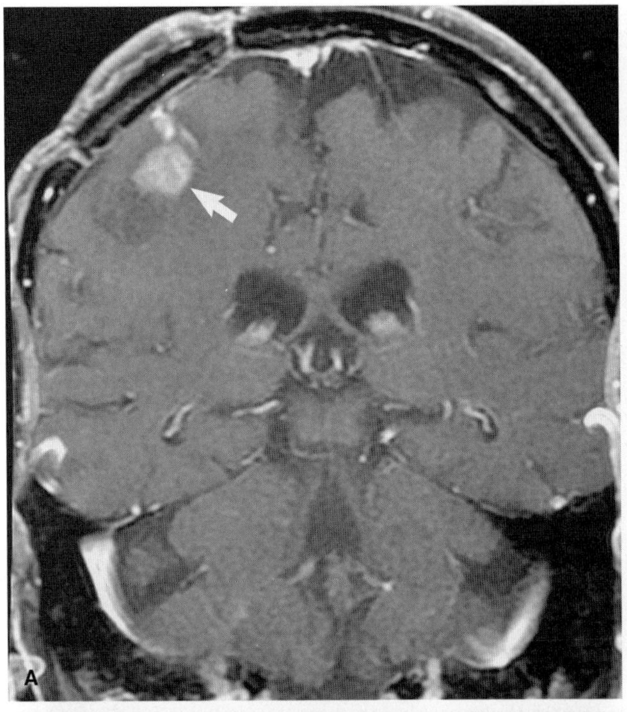

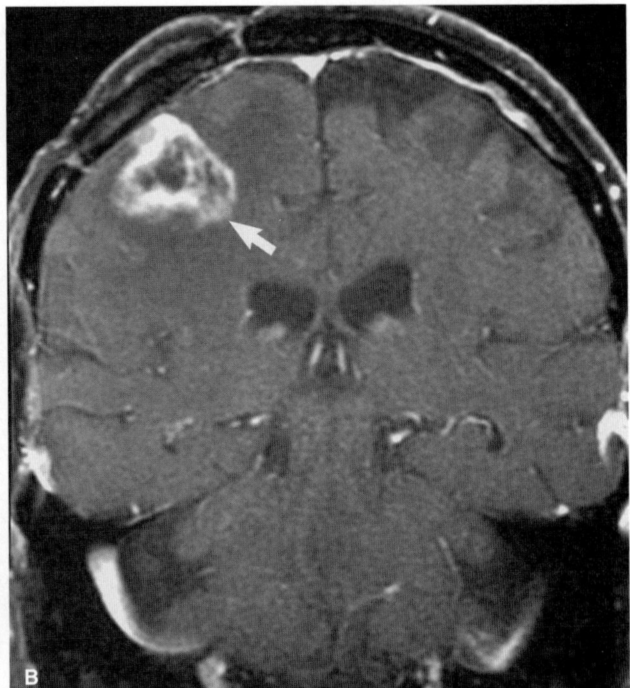

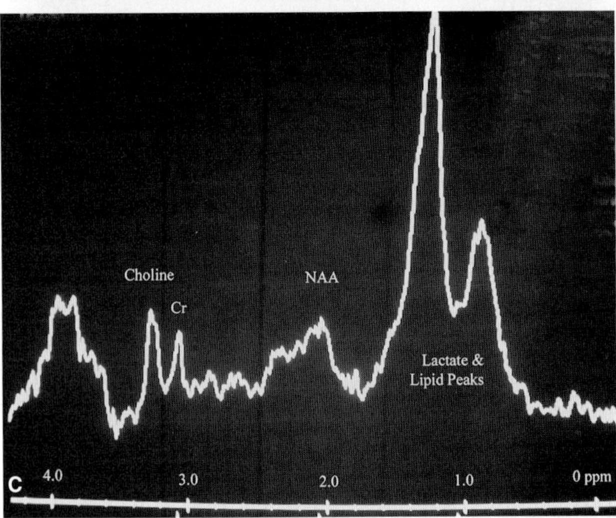

FIGURE 7.20. **Radiation Necrosis.** This 47-year-old man presented at 6 months **(A)** and 8 months **(B)** after resection and irradiation of a high right frontoparietal glioma. Coronal gadolinium-enhanced T1WI reveals interval appearance **(A)** and progression **(B)** of a ring-enhancing mass lesion within the operative bed (*arrows*). Despite this ominous appearance, this lesion revealed no radioisotope uptake on ^{18}F-2-fluoro-2-d-deoxyglucose PET. **C.** MR spectroscopy (MRS) of the lesion reveals marked elevation of lactate and lipids (0.9 to 1.3 ppm) with reduction in all other major metabolites (choline, creatine, and N-acetylaspartate). Both PET and MRS confirm the diagnosis of radiation necrosis. Serial MR scanning performed at 3-month intervals revealed a slowly regressing lesion that resolved by the 24-month follow-up study.

these agents may have a synergistic effect in causing marked white matter abnormalities. It is theorized that low-dose radiation alters the blood–brain barrier, allowing increased penetration of methotrexate to neurotoxic levels. This has been noted most frequently in children being treated for leukemia, and two specific conditions have been described. The first has been called *mineralizing microangiopathy*, which is seen in up to one third of these children. This results in diffuse destructive changes to the brain characterized by symmetric corticomedullary junction and basal ganglia calcifications. There is also diffuse signal abnormality throughout the white matter. A more serious but less common complication of combined radiation and methotrexate therapy is called *necrotizing leukoencephalopathy*. This process results in widespread damage to the white matter, consisting of demyelination, necrosis, and gliosis. MR reveals large, diffuse, confluent areas of white matter signal abnormality with cortical sparing. Clinically, these children may have symptoms ranging from slight reductions in cognitive function to progressive dementia, seizures, hemiplegia, and coma.

DYSMYELINATING DISEASES

The disease processes that have been described up until this point are demyelinating, as they represent the destruction of normal myelin. In contrast, the *dysmyelinating* conditions, also referred to as leukodystrophies, are disorders in which myelin is abnormally formed or

TABLE 7.2 Dysmyelinating Diseases

Disease	Head Size	Age of Onset (yr)	White Matter Involvement	Gray Matter Involvement
Metachromatic leukodystrophy	Normal	Infantile form: 1–2 Juvenile form: 5–7	Diffusely affected	None
Adrenoleukodystrophy	Normal	5–10	Symmetric occipital and splenium of corpus callosum	None
Leigh disease	Normal	<5	Focal areas of subcortical white matter	Basal ganglia and periaqueductal gray
Alexander disease	Normal to large	≤1	Frontal	None
Canavan disease	Normal to large	≤1	Diffusely affected	Vacuolization of cortical gray matter

cannot be maintained in its normal state because of an inherited enzymatic or metabolic disorder. Although most of these conditions are not treatable, establishing a diagnosis is valuable in providing a prognosis and enables parental genetic counseling. These conditions are characterized by the progressive destruction of myelin owing to the accumulation of various catabolites, depending on the specific enzyme deficiency. Children often present clinically with progressive mental and motor deterioration. Radiographically, these diseases present with diffuse white matter lesions that are very similar to one another; however, some distinguishing features do exist (Table 7.2). The radiologist may play an important role in the diagnosis of these conditions, because astute interpretation of abnormal imaging findings may allow them to be the first physician to suggest the possibility of a metabolic disease. Factors that are helpful in differentiation between the leukodystrophies include the age of onset and the pattern of white matter involvement. Ultimately, serum biochemical and enzymatic analyses allow a specific diagnosis to be made. Dysmyelinating diseases are rather uncommon, and we will focus on a few of the classic conditions.

Metachromatic leukodystrophy is the most common of the leukodystrophies. It is transmitted by an autosomal recessive pattern and is the result of a deficiency of the enzyme arylsulfatase A. The most common type is an infantile form that becomes apparent at approximately 2 years of age with gait disorder and mental deterioration. There is steady disease progression, with death occurring within 5 years of the time of onset. MR demonstrates progressive symmetric areas of nonspecific white matter involvement with sparing of the subcortical U fibers. Imaging findings are typically nonspecific.

Adrenal leukodystrophy is a sex-linked recessive condition (peroxisomal enzyme deficiency) occurring only in boys. Typical age of onset is between 5 and 10 years of age. As the name implies, these patients often have symptoms related to the adrenal gland, such as adrenal insufficiency or abnormal skin pigmentation. Adrenal leukodystrophy has a striking predilection for the visual and auditory pathways, presenting with symmetric involvement of the periatrial white matter with extension into the splenium of the corpus callosum (Fig. 7.22). The predilection for periatrial involvement results in early extension to the medial and lateral geniculate nuclei, which represent relays for the auditory and visual pathways, respectively. This accounts for the early presentation of visual and auditory symptomatology in these children.

Leigh disease, also called subacute necrotizing encephalomyelopathy, is a mitochondrial enzyme defect that commonly manifests in infancy or childhood (usually younger than 5 years). Leigh disease has histopathologic findings similar to those of Wernicke encephalopathy (metabolic disorder caused by thiamine [B1 vitamin] deficiency secondary to poor oral intake in chronic alcoholics); hence the suspicion that it is related to an inborn defect in thiamine metabolism. Clinical findings are extremely variable and often nonspecific. Symmetric focal necrotic lesions are found in the basal ganglia and thalamus as well as in the subcortical white matter (Fig. 7.23). Lesions may also extend into the midbrain, medulla, and posterior columns of the spinal cord. A characteristic finding is involvement of the periaqueductal gray matter. In contrast to Wernicke encephalopathy, there is sparing of the mamillary bodies. In the same family of mitochondrial disorders are two additional encephalopathies, which have the acronyms MELAS (mitochondrial myelopathy, encephalopathy, lactic acidosis, and strokelike episodes) and MERRF (myoclonic epilepsy and ragged-red fibers). These inherited mitochondrial abnormalities are caused by point mutations of mitochondrial DNA or mitochondrial RNA and represent progressive neurodegenerative disorders characterized clinically by strokes, strokelike events, nausea, vomiting, encephalopathy, seizures, short stature, headaches, muscle weakness, exercise intolerance, neurosensory hearing loss, and myopathy.

Alexander and Canavan diseases are the rarest of the leukodystrophies and may appear as early as the first few weeks of life. Patients often have an enlarged brain

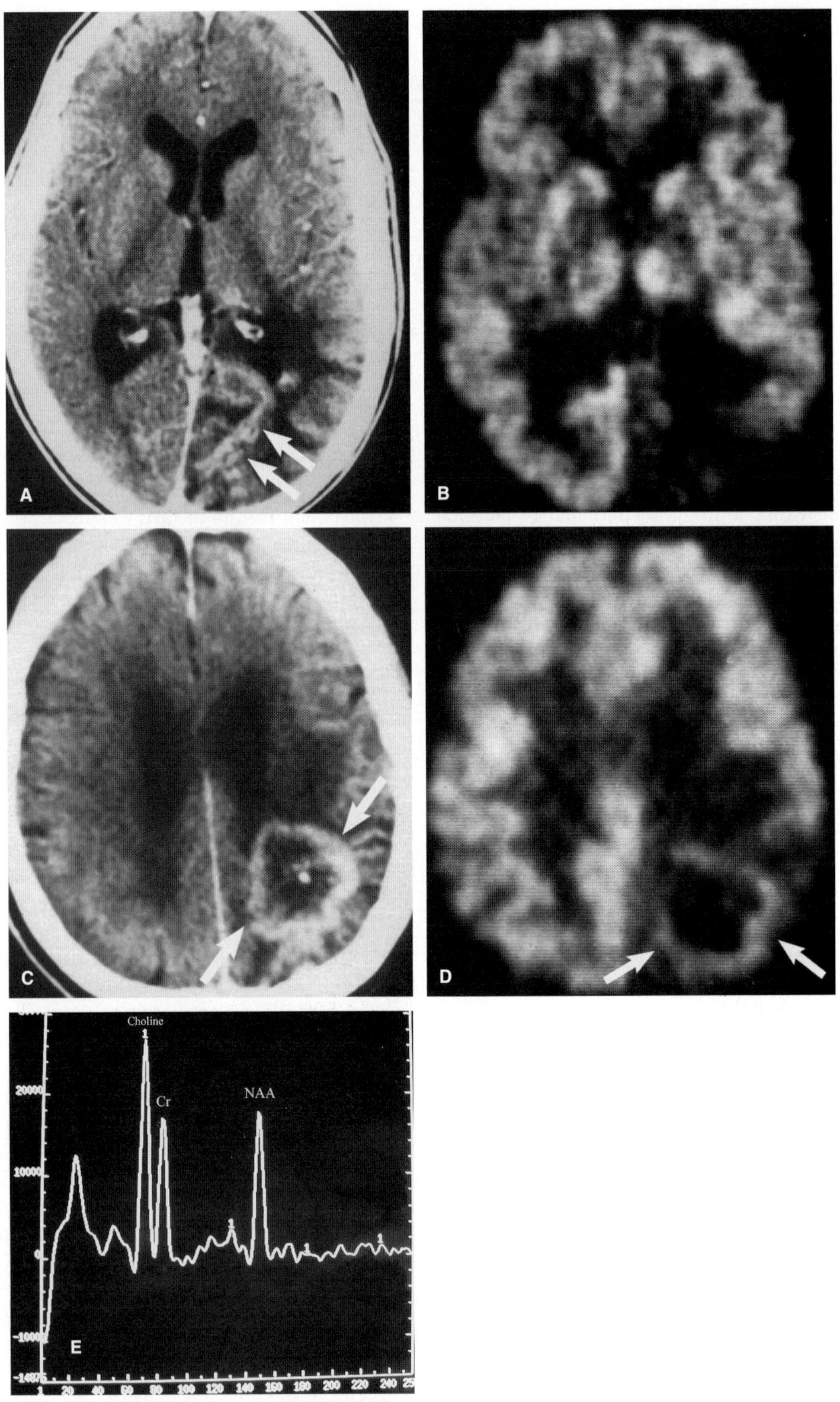
A
B
C
D
Choline
Cr
NAA
E

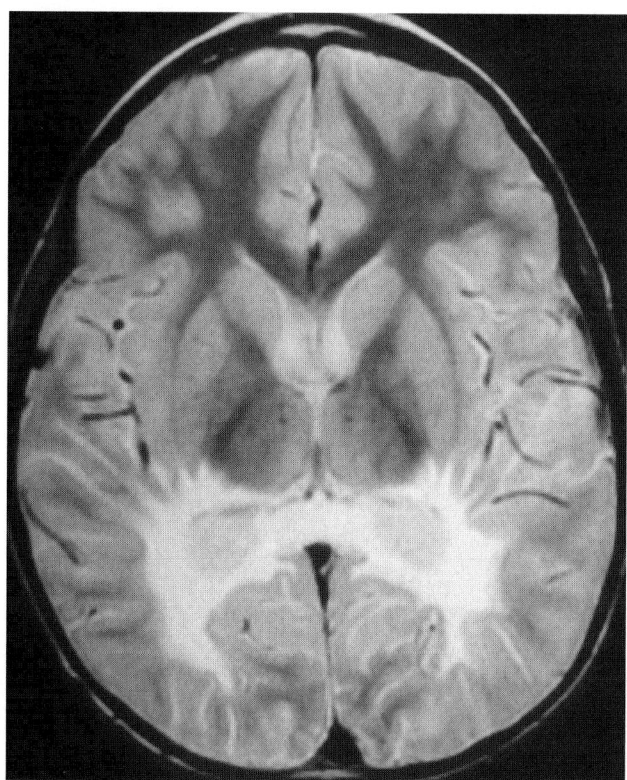

FIGURE 7.22. **Adrenal Leukodystrophy.** MR of a 5-year-old boy who presented with gradual gait disturbance, hearing and visual symptoms, and adrenal insufficiency. Axial T2WI reveals high signal within the periatrial and occipital white matter extending into the splenium of the corpus callosum as well as the region of the medial and lateral geniculate bodies, accounting for the patient's hearing and visual symptoms, respectively.

and have macrocephaly on examination. Typically, these patients present with seizures, spasticity, and delayed developmental milestones. In Alexander disease, white matter lesions often begin in the frontal white matter and progress posteriorly (Fig. 7.24). Canavan disease is caused by a deficiency of the enzyme aspartoacylase, which leads to the buildup of NAA in the brain and subsequent myelin destruction. This results in a pathognomonic MR spectra consisting of a giant NAA peak.

CEREBROSPINAL FLUID DYNAMICS

In patients with acute hydrocephalus, transependymal flow of CSF may mimic periventricular white matter disease. CSF is produced predominantly by the choroid plexus of the lateral, third, and fourth ventricles. CSF flows from the lateral ventricles into the third ventricle through the foramina of Monro and then by way of the cerebral aqueduct into the fourth ventricle. The CSF leaves the ventricular system via the lateral and medial fourth ventricular foramina (the foramina of Luschka and Magendie, respectively). CSF then travels through the basilar cisterns and over the surfaces of the cerebral hemispheres. The principal site of absorption is into the venous circulation through the arachnoid villi, which project into the dural sinuses, primarily the superior sagittal sinus. Although the principal routes of CSF production and absorption are as outlined, a significant amount of CSF may be both produced and reabsorbed via the ependymal lining of the ventricles. This transependymal flow of CSF can become an important means of CSF reabsorption during ventricular obstruction.

Hydrocephalus is caused by an obstruction of the CSF circulatory pathway and is classified into two principal types: noncommunicating and communicating. *Noncommunicating hydrocephalus* refers to an obstruction occurring within the ventricular system that prevents CSF from exiting the ventricles (Fig. 7.25). In contrast, with *communicating hydrocephalus,* the level of obstruction is beyond the ventricular system, located instead within the subarachnoid space. CSF is able to exit the ventricular system but fails to undergo normal resorption by the arachnoid villi. In theory, with communicating hydrocephalus, most of the ventricular system is enlarged, whereas with noncommunicating hydrocephalus, dilation occurs up to the point of obstruction. The fourth ventricle often does not dilate because of the relatively confined nature of the posterior fossa and thus cannot be used as a reliable means by which to differentiate communicating from noncommunicating hydrocephalus. Communicating hydrocephalus will commonly demonstrate supratentorial ventriculomegaly, with a fourth ventricle that appears normal. Although dilation of the fourth ventricle is suggestive of communicating

FIGURE 7.21. **Radiation Necrosis Versus Tumor Recurrence.** Contrast-enhanced CT and PET (^{18}F-2-fluoro-2-d-deoxyglucose) scans. **A.** CT reveals a new linear area of enhancement within the tumor bed 10 months after surgery and focal irradiation for a high-grade glioma (*arrows*). **B.** The PET scan demonstrates no significant activity in this area, suggesting that the enhancement represents radiation necrosis. **C.** A CT of a different patient 6 months after surgery and focal irradiation for a high-grade glioma reveals a focus of ring enhancement (*arrows*). **D.** The PET scan reveals increased metabolic activity in this region, suggesting recurrent tumor. **E.** This finding is confirmed on the representative single-voxel MR spectroscopy, performed in the area of enhancement, which demonstrates an elevated choline peak (largest peak), with reduced creatine and N-acetylaspartate levels (next peaks, respectively, moving from left to right).

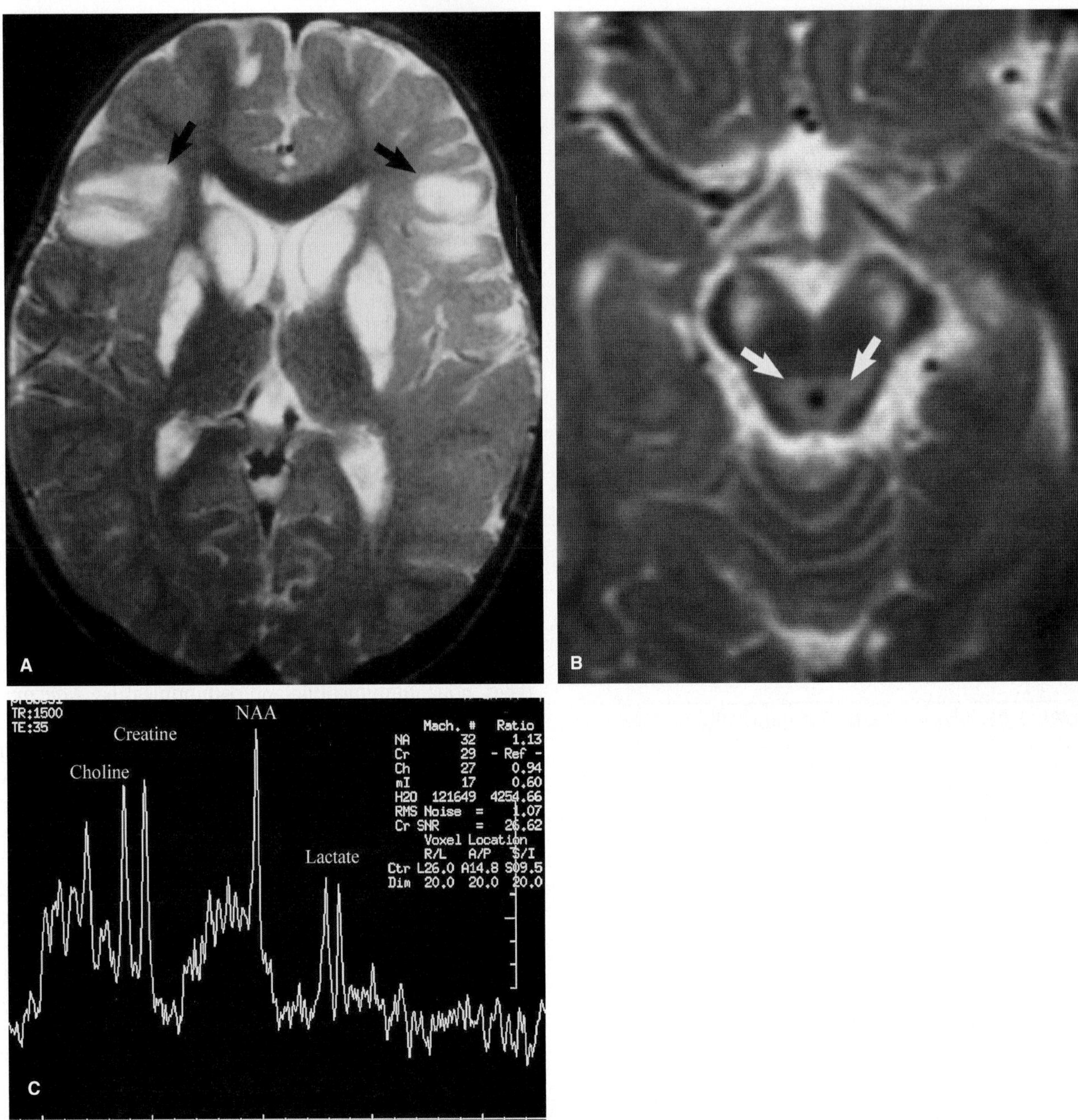

FIGURE 7.23. **Leigh Disease.** Leigh disease (mitochondrial enzyme defect) in a 3-year-old patient presenting with progressive hypotonia and seizures. **A.** T2WI demonstrates a wide spectrum of gray and white matter lesions reported in Leigh disease, including basal ganglia (globus pallidus, putamen, caudate); brainstem (midbrain and periaqueductal gray); and subcortical white matter involvement (*arrows*). **B.** Involvement of the periaqueductal gray matter (*arrows*) is quite characteristic for either Leigh disease or Wernicke syndrome. Both conditions are associated with thiamine deficiency; the former is related to mitochondrial enzymatic deficiencies involved with the metabolism of thiamine, and in the latter, it is nutritional. A differentiating feature is involvement of the mamillary bodies in Wernicke syndrome, which is absent in Leigh disease. **C.** MR spectroscopy reveals an elevated lactate peak at 1.3 ppm, which supports the diagnosis of Leigh disease. Mitochondrial enzyme deficiencies associated with Leigh disease include pyruvate dehydrogenase complex, pyruvate carboxylase, and electron transport chain, which result in elevated blood, CSF and CNS lactate, and pyruvate levels.

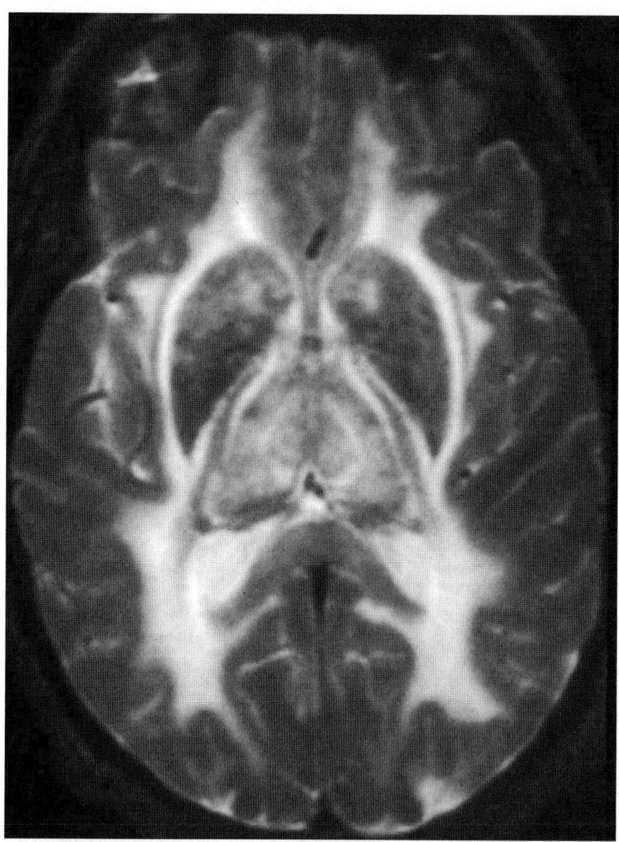

FIGURE 7.24. **Canavan Disease.** A 12-month-old child presented with progressive spastic quadriparesis and macrocephaly. Axial T2WI reveals diffuse high signal extending throughout the cerebral white matter. This is a nonspecific finding that could reflect an advanced stage of any of the leukodystrophies. However, if MR spectroscopy were to reveal markedly elevated N-acetylaspartate (NAA), this would be diagnostic of a deficiency of the enzyme aspartoacylase (Canavan disease), which leads to the buildup of NAA in the brain and subsequent myelin destruction.

hydrocephalus, it is not a reliable sign, because obstruction at the outlet foramina of the fourth ventricle (Luschka and Magendie) may result in a similar appearance.

In assessing for the presence of hydrocephalus, specific attention should be directed to the third ventricle and the temporal ventricular horns. Convex bowing of the lateral walls and inferior recesses of the third ventricle is characteristic for hydrocephalus. As with fourth ventricular enlargement, however, this finding is seldom present. A far more sensitive indicator of hydrocephalus is enlargement of the temporal horns. The temporal horns sometimes will demonstrate enlargement, even before lateral ventricular involvement is evident. Bowing and stretching of the corpus callosum, easily detected on the sagittal images, is an additional finding that is suggestive of hydrocephalus.

Ex Vacuo Ventriculomegaly. A distinction must be made between hydrocephalus and ex vacuo ventriculomegaly. The latter represents an enlarged ventricular system that is simply the result of parenchymal atrophy. With atrophy, the loss of brain matter results in prominence of all CSF spaces, both the cerebral sulci as well as the ventricles. In contrast, with hydrocephalus the ventricles are enlarged out of proportion to the sulci. The third ventricle and temporal ventricular horns are particularly helpful in making this distinction. Both of these ventricular spaces are surrounded by tissue that is not typically subject to significant atrophy. The third ventricle is surrounded by the thalamus (gray matter), and there is a relative paucity of white matter within the temporal lobes. This is in contrast to the large amount of white matter surrounding the lateral ventricles, which may atrophy. Enlargement of the third ventricle, with bowing of its lateral and inferior recesses as well as temporal horn enlargement, suggests hydrocephalus.

Subarachnoid hemorrhage and meningitis are the most frequent causes of acute hydrocephalus and may result in either communicating or noncommunicating hydrocephalus, with obstruction at any level of the ventricular system, the basilar cisterns, or the arachnoid villi. The obstruction is caused by adhesions and inflammation, and no obstructing mass is typically detected. Noncommunicating hydrocephalus can be the result of either an acquired or a congenital obstructive process. Benign congenital webs may form across the cerebral aqueduct, resulting in aqueductal stenosis. Additionally, the Chiari and Dandy-Walker malformations are believed to represent adhesions occurring during CNS development, at the outlet foramina of the fourth ventricle and posterior fossa. A variety of neoplasms may result in obstructive hydrocephalus, often in very characteristic locations. Colloid cysts typically block the anterior third ventricle, pineal tumors and tectal gliomas obstruct the aqueduct, and ependymomas and medulloblastomas interrupt CSF flow at the level of the fourth ventricle. Whenever hydrocephalus is detected, it is important to inspect the ventricles for an obstructing mass. A location that should be specifically evaluated is the cerebral aqueduct. On routine axial and sagittal images, a normal pulsatile flow void should be detected; otherwise, the diagnosis of aqueductal stenosis should be considered.

The duration of hydrocephalus affects the imaging findings. In acute hydrocephalus, there is insufficient time for compensatory mechanisms, and a striking amount of transependymal CSF flow will be noted. This results in a dramatic accumulation of high signal in the periventricular white matter on T2WIs. In chronic forms of hydrocephalus, compensatory mechanisms of CNS production and resorption have occurred and the degree of transependymal flow is minimal.

Normal pressure hydrocephalus (NPH) is a chronic, low-level form of hydrocephalus. The classic clinical triad is dementia, gait disturbance, and urinary incontinence. In this condition, the CSF pressure is within normal limits,

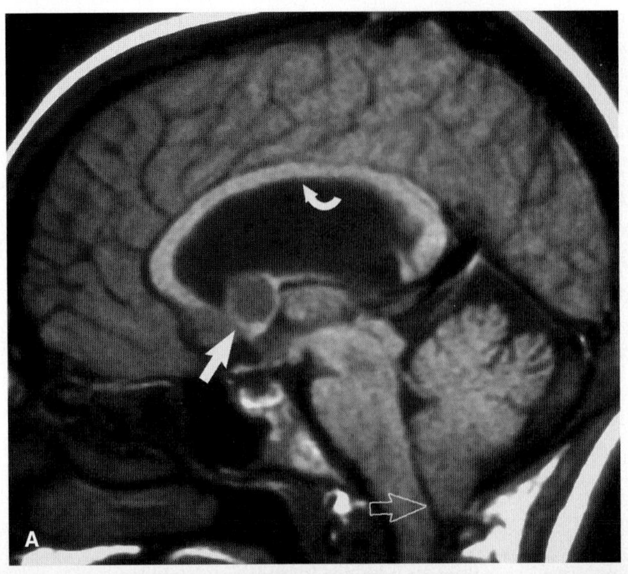

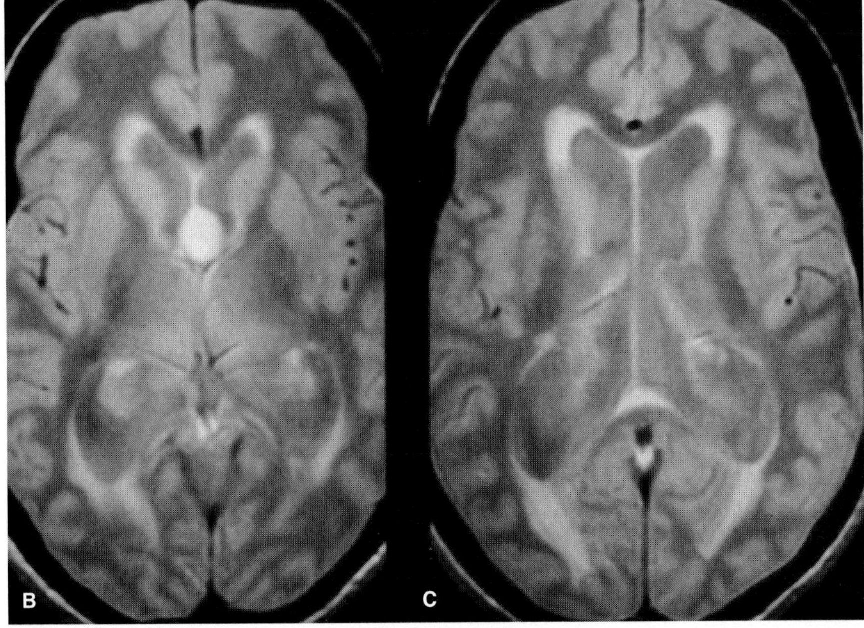

FIGURE 7.25. **Hydrocephalus.** Images of a 36-year-old woman who presented with postural headaches. **A.** Sagittal T1WI reveals an obstructing mass within the roof of the third ventricle consistent with a colloid cyst (*arrow*). Pressure changes reflective of hydrocephalous are noted, including upward bowing of the corpus callosum (*curved arrow*) as well as tonsillar ectopia (*open arrow*). **B.** and **C.** Axial PDWIs reveal dilated ventricles with periventricular hyperintensity consistent with transependymal flow of CSF.

but a slight gradient exists between the ventricular system and the subarachnoid space because of an incomplete subarachnoid CSF block. This most commonly results from a previous subarachnoid hemorrhage or meningeal infection. The result is diffuse ventriculomegaly that is out of proportion to the degree of sulcal prominence. Differentiating mild hydrocephalus from atrophic ventriculomegaly can be very difficult. Studies suggest that MR CSF velocity and stroke volume calculations can be used to predict which patients may have favorable response to ventriculoperitoneal shunting. In addition to cross-sectional studies, radioisotope studies may be of value. The classic findings on radioisotope cisternogram are early entry of the radiopharmaceutical into the lateral ventricles, with persistence at 24 and 48 hours, and considerable delay in the ascent to the parasagittal region. Differentiating NPH from atrophic ventriculomegaly can be very difficult, and unfortunately, no imaging study is definitive in making this diagnosis. NPH is not a radiographic diagnosis, and close correlation of clinical and imaging findings is required to establish the diagnosis. The definitive diagnosis of NPH is made on demonstrating clinical improvement following ventricular shunting.

NEURODEGENERATIVE DISORDERS

Neurodegenerative disorders frequently have no known cause and result in progressive neurologic deterioration that is faster than expected given the patient's age.

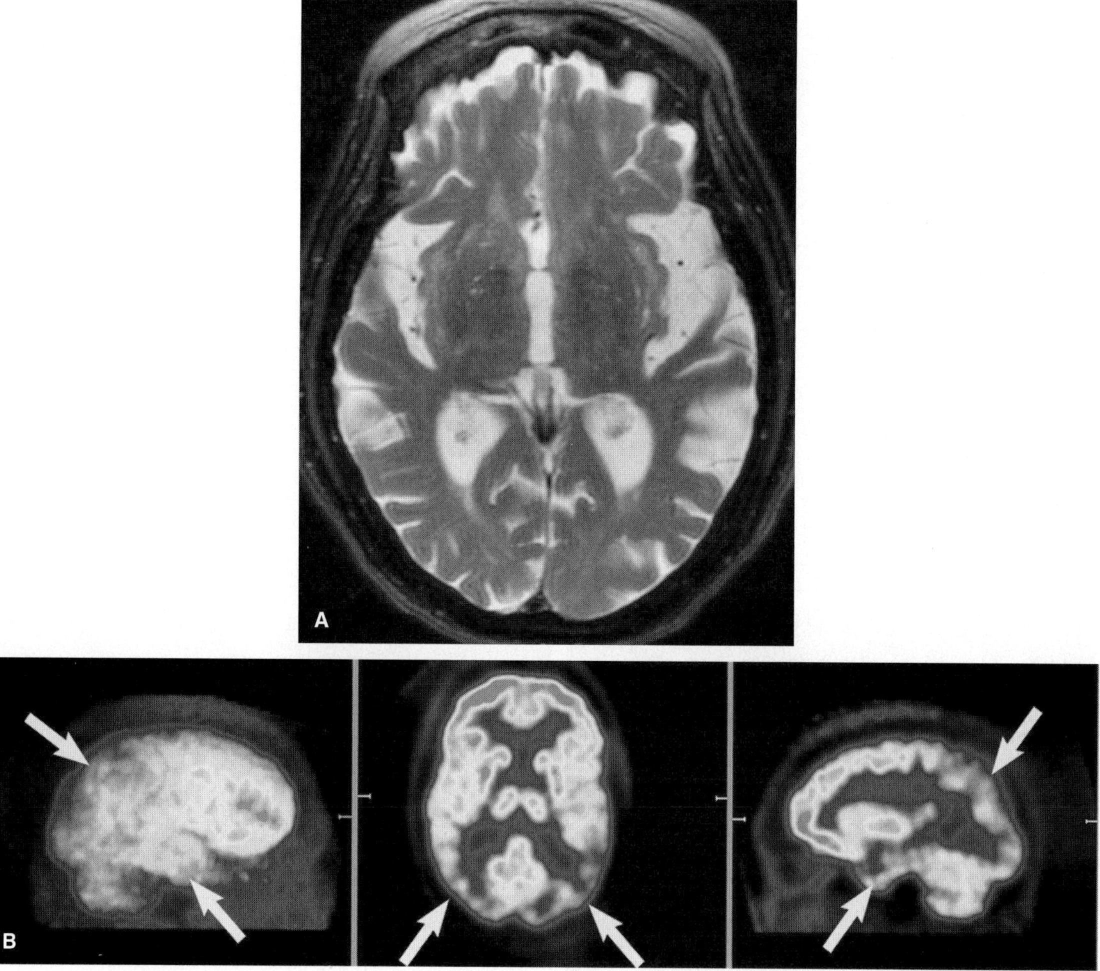

FIGURE 7.26. **Alzheimer Disease (AD).** Axial fast spin-echo T2WI **(A)** in a 60-year-old man with early dementia reveals prominent parietotemporal atrophy and minimal white matter ischemic disease. AD is a neurodegenerative disorder and the most common cause of dementia. Imaging is relatively nonspecific in the diagnosis of AD, but the presence of parietotemporal cortical atrophy with a paucity of white matter ischemic changes supports the diagnosis of a neurodegenerative disease rather than ischemic or multi-infarct dementia. **B.** Three PET images (lateral volumetric summated image, axial, and sagittal) from the same patient reveal metabolic reductions throughout the parietotemporal lobes (*arrows*) corresponding to the MR findings and characteristic for AD.

Alzheimer disease (AD) is the most common neurodegenerative disease and the most common cause of dementia. It is estimated that in the United States alone there are about 4 million people with this disorder. The number of those affected by AD is rapidly increasing as the world's population ages. It is estimated that by the year 2050, the number of people with AD will increase threefold, to about 60 million worldwide, with about 14 million in the United States alone. Although the cause of AD is not clear, histopathologically the disease is characterized by two abnormal structures in the brain: *neuritic plaques* and *neurofibrillary tangles*. Neuritic plaques are composed of tortuous neuritic processes surrounding a central amyloid core, which consists primarily of a small peptide known as β-amyloid, derived from a larger amyloid precursor protein. Neurofibrillary tangles contain an abnormal tau protein that is associated with microtubules. Both plaques and tangles seem to interfere with normal neuronal functioning.

Neuroimaging studies of patients with AD demonstrate diffuse atrophy, with a predilection for the hippocampal formation, temporal lobes, and parietotemporal cortices. As a result, enlargement of the temporal horns, suprasellar cisterns, and sylvian fissures may be useful in discriminating AD from normal age-related atrophy (Fig. 7.26). A variety of functional imaging modalities (PET as well as perfusion MR with regional cerebral blood flow calculations) are being used to diagnosis and differentiate AD from senescent dementia. PET may play an important role in diagnosis and treating AD; specifically, ^{18}F-labelled PET

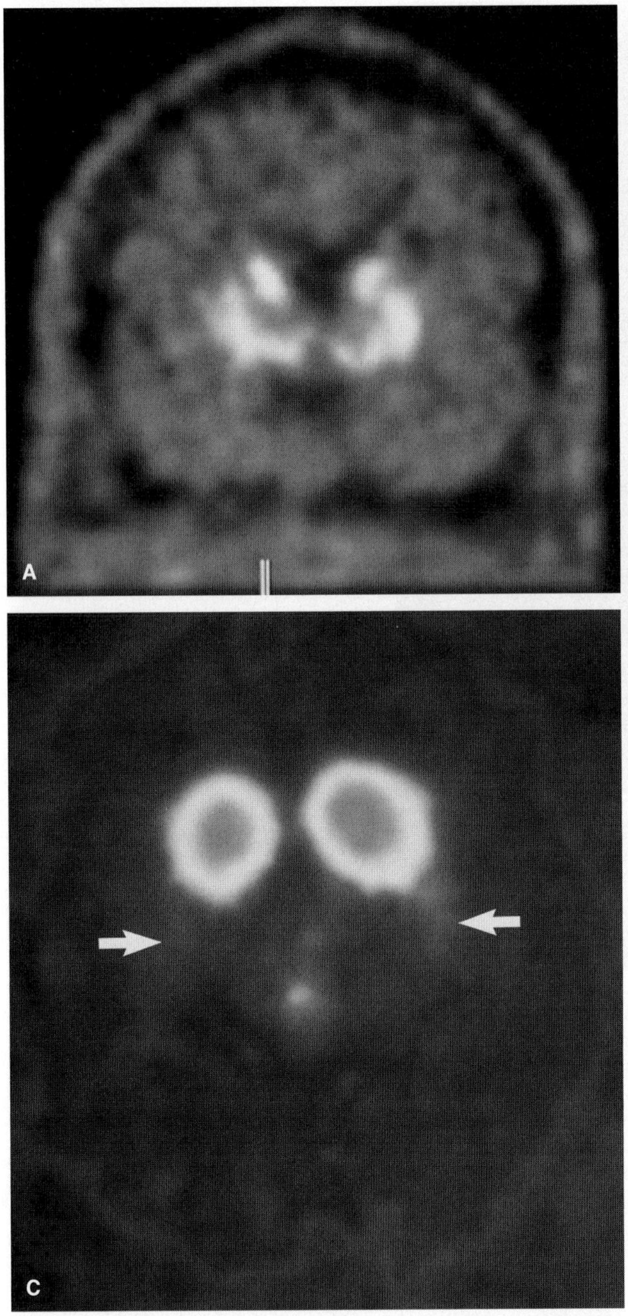

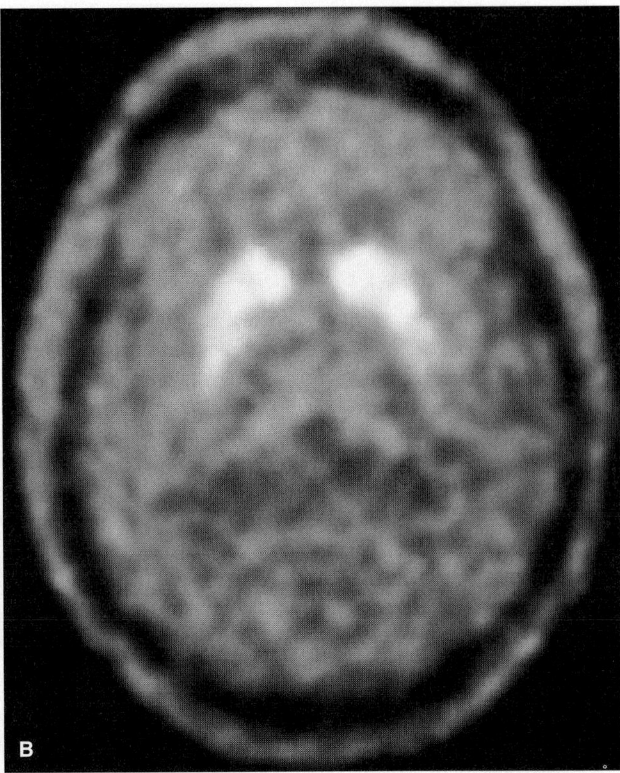

FIGURE 7.27. ^{18}**F-Labelled Levodopa (DOPA) PET Scan.** A 52-year-old man was misdiagnosed with early-onset Parkinson disease. **A.** and **B.** Images from ^{18}F-DOPA PET scanning reveal a normal distribution of dopamine receptors, with expected uptake in the caudate head and putamen. With Parkinson disease there is loss of uptake in the putamen. As a result of this study, the correct diagnosis of essential tremor was made. **C.** A 63-year-old man presented with clinical symptoms that were nondiagnostic for Parkinson disease. ^{18}F-DOPA PET scan reveals loss of uptake in the putamen (*arrows*), consistent with Parkinson disease, which allowed a definitive diagnosis to be made.

ligands (specific for AD-related proteins) may allow for the early detection of this disease as well as help to identify treatments by evaluating the early response to drugs, far before any changes in clinical symptoms would be evident.

Parkinson disease is the most common basal ganglia disorder and one of the leading causes of neurologic disability in individuals older than age 60. This disease is characterized clinically by tremor, muscular rigidity, and loss of postural reflexes. About 25% of Parkinson patients also develop dementia. Parkinsonism results from a deficiency of the neurotransmitter dopamine caused by dysfunction of the dopaminergic neuronal system, specifically the pars compacta of the substantia nigra. The loss of these nerve cells results in a decreased concentration of endogenous striatal dopamine, and after approximately 80% of these cells die, the patient begins to develop symptoms. MR imaging is relatively insensitive in the detection of this loss of tissue, but it can be used to image patients with movement disorders to exclude other underlying pathologies, such as stroke or tumor. MR may occasionally reveal thinning of the pars compacta. The substantia nigra is made of the pars compacta (high signal intensity band on T2WIs) posteriorly, which is sandwiched between the pars

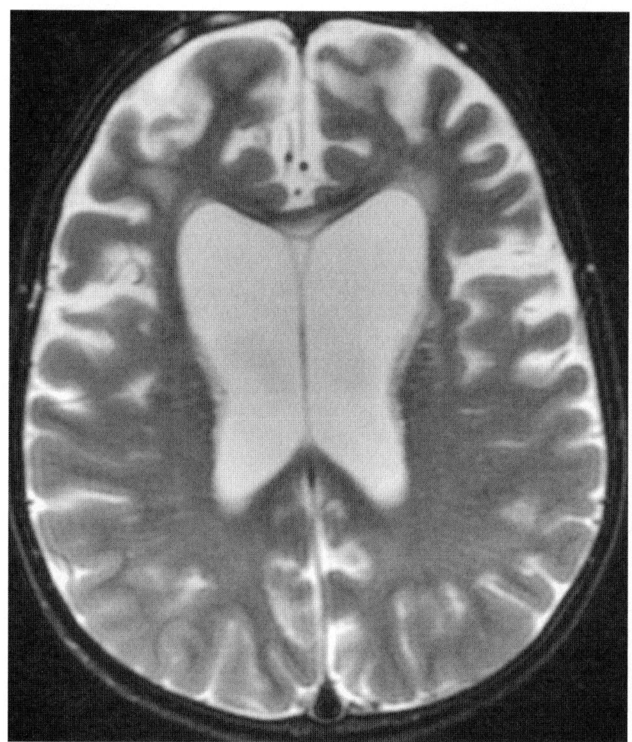

FIGURE 7.28. **Huntington Disease.** Axial fast spin-echo T2WI in a 51-year-old woman who presented with movement and behavioral disorders, with familial history of similar presentation in her father. The striking caudate head atrophy results in characteristic enlargement of the frontal horns. This condition is a movement disorder that is autosomal dominant with full penetrance, with typical onset in the fifth decade of life.

reticularis anteriorly and the red nuclei posteriorly. With thinning of the pars compacta, the high signal intensity band between the pars reticularis and the red nuclei is lost. However, this finding is only occasionally noted in very severe forms of the disease. In contrast, PET is a more sensitive tool in the study of diseases of the dopaminergic system. Specifically, ^{18}F-labelled PET ligands have been developed for imaging the postsynaptic dopamine D1 and D2 receptor system. The involvement of this receptor system in numerous brain disorders such as schizophrenia, Parkinson disease, and other movement disorders has prompted an intense research in this field. With ^{18}F-labelled levodopa (DOPA), Parkinson patients show a characteristic deficit in putaminal DOPA uptake (Fig. 7.27). The symptoms of Parkinson disease can sometimes be alleviated by treatment with levodopa, which increases the amount of dopamine that is endogenously synthesized, facilitating the activity of the remaining dopaminergic neurons. A variety of parkinsonian syndromes exist, including Parkinson disease, progressive supranuclear palsy, and striatonigral degeneration. Idiopathic Parkinson disease is referred to as *paralysis agitans* and affects 2% to 3% of the population at some time during their life.

The following are degenerative diseases of the extrapyramidal nuclei.

Huntington disease is a progressive hereditary disorder that appears in the fourth and fifth decades of life. This disease is characterized by a movement disorder (typically choreoathetosis), dementia, and emotional disturbance. Huntington disease is inherited in an autosomal dominant pattern with complete penetrance. Although neuroimaging studies demonstrate diffuse cortical atrophy, the caudate nucleus and putamen are most severely affected. Atrophy of the caudate nucleus results in characteristic enlargement of the frontal horns, which take on a heart-shape configuration (Fig. 7.28).

Wilson disease, also known as hepatolenticular degeneration, is an inborn error of copper metabolism that is associated with hepatic cirrhosis and degenerative changes of the basal ganglia. A deficiency of ceruloplasmin (serum transport protein of copper) results in deposition of toxic levels of copper in various organs. Patients present with

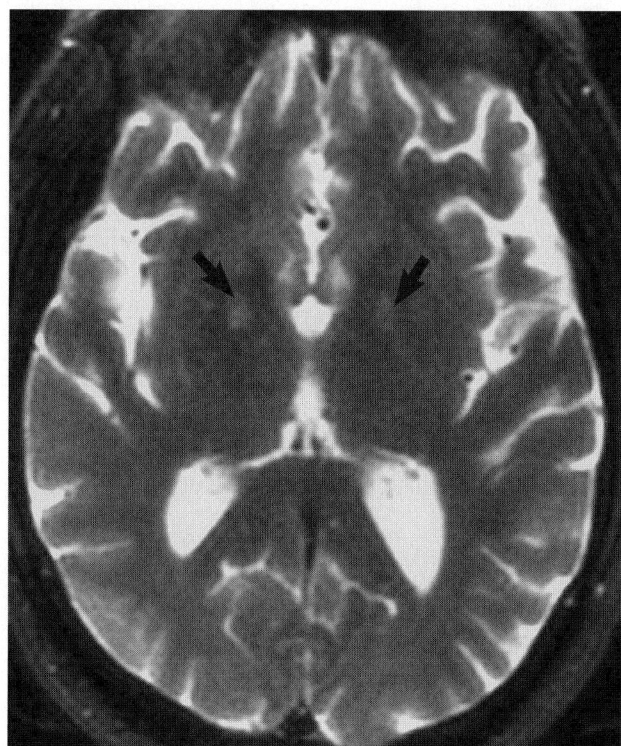

FIGURE 7.29. **Carbon Monoxide Toxicity.** This 35-year-old man presented with confusion following carbon monoxide exposure during recreational boating. Bilateral hyperintense lesions of the globus pallidus are noted (*arrows*). Bilateral lesions of the basal ganglia can be seen in a variety of insults, including methanol toxicity (putaminal); metabolic conditions such as Wilson disease (hepatolenticular degeneration, a disorder of copper metabolism); Hallervorden-Spatz disease (iron deposition within the globus pallidus); and mitochondrial disorders (Leigh disease and Kearns-Sayre syndrome).

varied neurologic and psychiatric findings, including dystonia, tremor, and rigidity. The Kayser-Fleischer ring, an intracorneal deposit of copper, is virtually diagnostic of the disease when present (75% of cases). MR findings include diffuse atrophy with signal abnormalities involving the deep gray matter nuclei and deep white matter.

In addition to these neurodegenerative diseases, abnormalities of the basal ganglia can have a wide range of causes. Toxins such as carbon monoxide or methanol poisoning may result in signal abnormalities of the basal ganglia, characteristically the globus pallidus and putamen, respectively (Fig. 7.29). Also, infectious conditions such as West Nile Virus (WNV) and Creutzfeldt-Jakob disease (CJD) may present with areas of signal abnormality within the basal ganglia. Both of these conditions have become of great concern recently, given their increased incidence and unusual modes of transmission (WNV via mosquitoes and CJD via consumption of infected beef products). T1 shortening (high signal on T1WIs) has been described within the basal ganglia and brainstem, associated with hepatic dysfunction, such as hepatic encephalopathy as well as hyperalimentation. The cause of these findings has not been fully determined. Occasionally, faint calcification of the basal ganglia may also appear as high signal on T1WIs. This is the result of the hydration layer effect, where water molecules that are adjacent to the calcification have reduced relaxation times. This same effect causes T1 shortening with proteinaceous fluids. As a result, any condition that results in subtle calcifications within the basal ganglia may demonstrate T1 shortening within the basal ganglia.

SUGGESTED READINGS

Ali M, Safriel Y, Sohi J, et al. West Nile virus infection: MR imaging findings in the nervous system. AJNR Am J Neuroradiol 2005;26:289–297.

Brubaker LM, Smith JK, Lee YZ, et al. Hemodynamic and permeability changes in posterior reversible encephalopathy syndrome measured by dynamic susceptibility perfusion-weighted MR Imaging. AJNR Am J Neuroradiol 2005;26:825–830.

Collie DA, Summers DM, Sellar RJ, et al. Diagnosing variant Creutzfeldt-Jakob disease with the pulvinar sign: MR imaging findings in 86 neuropathologically confirmed Cases. AJNR Am J Neuroradiol 2003;24:1560–1569.

de Leeuw FE, de Groot JC, Achten E, et al. Prevalence of cerebral white matter lesions in elderly people: a population-based magnetic resonance imaging study—the Rotterdam Scan Study. J Neurol Neurosurg Psychiatry 2001;70:9–14.

Di Rocco M, Biancheri R, Rossi A, Filocamo M, Tortori-Donati P. Genetic disorders affecting white matter in the pediatric age [review]. Am J Med Genet B Neuropsychiatr Genet 2004 Aug 15;129(1):85–93.

Garg RK. Acute disseminated encephalomyelitis [review]. Postgrad Med J 2003;79(927):11–17.

Grossman RI, McGowan JC. Perspectives on multiple sclerosis [review]. AJNR Am J Neuroradiol 1998;19:1251–1265.

Gupta VK. White matter hyperintensities: pearls and pitfalls in interpretation of MRI abnormalities. Stroke 2004 Dec;35(12):2756–2757.

Hustinx R, Pourdehnad M, Kaschten B, Alavi A. PET imaging for differentiating recurrent brain tumor from radiation necrosis [review]. Radiol Clin North Am 2005 Jan;43(1):35–47.

Kantarci K, Jack CR Jr. Neuroimaging in Alzheimer disease: an evidence-based review [review]. Neuroimaging Clin North Am 2003 May;13(2):197–209.

Lakhkar BN, Aggarwal M, John JR. MRI in white matter diseases—clinicoradiological correlation. Ind J Radiol Imag 2002;12(1):43–50.

Lampl C, Yazdi K. Central pontine myelinolysis [review]. Eur Neurol 2002;47(1):3–10.

Lamy C, Oppenheim C, Meder JF, Mas JL. Neuroimaging in posterior reversible encephalopathy syndrome [review]. J Neuroimaging 2004 Apr;14(2):89–96.

Martin RJ. Central pontine and extrapontine myelinolysis: the osmotic demyelination syndromes [review]. J Neurol Neurosurg Psychiatry 2004 Sep;75(suppl 3):iii22–28.

Petrella JR, Coleman RE, Doraiswamy PM. Neuroimaging and early diagnosis of Alzheimer disease: a look to the future [review]. Radiology 2003 Feb;226(2):315–336.

Poser CM, Brinar VV. Diagnostic criteria for multiple sclerosis: an historical review. Clin Neurol Neurosurg 2004 Jun;106(3):147–158.

Sakamoto S, Ishii K, Hosaka K, et al. Detectability of hypometabolic regions in mild Alzheimer disease: function of time after the injection of 2-[fluorine 18]-fluoro-2-deoxy-d-glucose. AJNR Am J Neuroradiol 2005 Apr;26:843–847.

Scheid R, Preul C, Gruber O, Wiggins C, von Cramon DY. Diffuse axonal injury associated with chronic traumatic brain injury: evidence from T2*-weighted gradient-echo imaging at 3 T. AJNR Am J Neuroradiol 2003 Jun–Jul;24(6):1049–1056.

Scroop R, Sage MR, Voyvodic F, Kat E. Radiographic imaging procedures in the diagnosis of the major central neuropathological consequences of alcohol abuse [review]. Australas Radiol 2002 Jun;46(2):146–153.

Stott VL, Hurrell MA, Anderson TJ. Reversible posterior leukoencephalopathy syndrome: a misnomer reviewed. Intern Med J 2005 Feb;35(2):83–90.

Swartz RH, Kern RZ. Migraine is associated with magnetic resonance imaging white matter abnormalities: a meta-analysis [review]. Arch Neurol. 2004 Sep;61(9):1366–1368.

Chapter 8

Pediatric Neuroimaging

Todd E. Lempert and Erik H.L. Gaensler

Normal Patterns of Myelination

Hypoxic Ischemic Encephalopathy
Hypoxic Ischemic Injury and the Premature Infant
Profound Versus Partial Hypoxic Ischemic Brain Injury

Congenital Lesions

Migration Anomalies

The Phakomatoses

Specific areas of neuroimaging are sufficiently different between the pediatric and adult populations to warrant a separate discussion. These pediatric-specific topics include normal patterns of myelination, hypoxic ischemic brain injury, congenital lesions, migration anomalies, and phakomatoses (neurocutaneous syndromes). Congenital white matter diseases are discussed in Chapter 7, and spine anomalies are covered in Chapter 10.

MR has established itself as the procedure of choice for pediatric neuroimaging, although specific situations for which CT and US remain advantageous will be described. MR scanners are designed to image adult patients, and special arrangements must be made to accommodate the pediatric population. Sedation is usually required for children under 6 years of age, and pediatric sedation protocols should be performed in conjunction with the pediatric medicine service. For imaging of neonates, sedation may not be necessary, but careful coordination between the clinical and imaging staff is essential to ensure patient safety and optional imaging. Imaging of ill neonates requires MR-compatible support systems to providing heat, oxygen, IV drugs, monitoring, etc.

NORMAL PATTERNS OF MYELINATION

Any discussion of pediatric neuroimaging should begin with normal myelination as a frame of reference. T1WIs and T2WIs allow evaluation and staging of the myelination process. T1WIs provide a detailed view of actively myelinating structures in the first 8 months of life. Areas that become myelinated stand out as high signal on T1WIs against a background of low-signal-intensity unmyelinated white matter. This is because the myelin sheath (a lipid) is hydrophobic; therefore, myelinated white matter has a decreased amount of water—the source of mobile hydrogen protons, which form the basis of the MR signal. As a memory aid, recall that myelinated white matter (because of the lipid myelin sheath) parallels the signal intensity of lipid (fat) on T1W and conventional spin-echo T2W sequences.

Heavily weighted T2 images (long time of repetition/time of echo = 3,000/120) are recommended for the age range of 0 to 12 months. The water content of the infant brain is high, and heavily T2WIs are needed to discriminate between many brain structures that have similarly long T2 relaxation times. The myelination landmarks given in Table 8.1 are based on sequences performed at 1.5 Tesla. Other field strength magnets may show differing timetables of signal change with respect to the patient's age. It is important to compare "apples to apples," so clinicians must select scanners and sequences consistently for a given child so that meaningful comparisons can be made.

Evaluation of every pediatric brain MR image should begin with an assessment of myelin development. This important step will help determine the presence or absence of myelination delay and provide a framework for interpretation of suspected neuropathology.

As described above, T1WIs are useful for assessing myelination in the first 8 months; thereafter the T2WIs become more important. In general, myelination proceeds from dorsal to ventral, from caudad to cephalad, and

TABLE 8.1 Myelination Landmarks by Age

Age (Months)	Location/Appearance
Newborn	Dorsal brainstem, ventrolateral thalamus, lentiform nucleus, central corticospinal tracts: high signal on T1WIs Posterior limb internal capsule posterior portion: low signal on T2WIs
3	Anterior limb internal capsule: high signal on T1WIs Cerebellar white matter: high signal on T1WIs
4	Splenium of corpus callosum: high signal on T1WIs Centrum semiovale: high signal on T1WIs
6	Genu of corpus callosum: high signal on T1WIs Splenium of corpus callosum: low signal on T2WIs
8	Subcortical white matter: high signal on T1WIs Genu: low signal on T2WIs
11	Anterior limb internal capsule: low signal on T2WIs
14	Occipital white matter: low signal on T2WIs
16	Frontal white matter: low signal on T2WIs
18	Adult appearance except for terminal myelination zones (periatrial and adjacent to frontal horns)
24	Dark white matter on T2 (some minimal high-signal areas may persist peripherally—if in doubt, do a follow-up scan)

from central to peripheral. At birth, MR shows ongoing myelination of the dorsal lentiform nucleus, lateral geniculate nucleus, dorsal brainstem, cerebellar peduncles, ventrolateral thalamus, posterior limb of the internal capsule, and corticospinal tract extending into the perirolandic (precentral and postcentral) white matter (Fig. 8.1).

The anterior limb of the internal capsule should develop high signal intensity on T1WIs by 3 months (Fig. 8.2). The corpus callosum provides the next set of landmarks, with the splenium becoming bright on T1WIs by 4 months and the genu by 6 months. At 6 months, the splenium becomes low signal intensity on T2WIs, but the unmyelinated peripheral white matter remains high signal (Fig. 8.3). With growth, the deep white matter gradually assumes the adult low signal intensity on T2WIs, with some high signal intensity persisting in the terminal myelination zones on T2WIs (Figs. 8.4, 8.5).

One way to help remember the stages of myelination is that myelination parallels developmental landmarks. Newborns can breathe and have function of the motor components of the cranial nerves—all medullary and pontine tracts. Motor functions that allow the child to roll over, crawl, and stand develop in the first year, paralleling the myelination of the internal capsule. Higher cortical functions such as speech are the last to appear, tracking with the maturation of the hemispheric white matter in the second year of life.

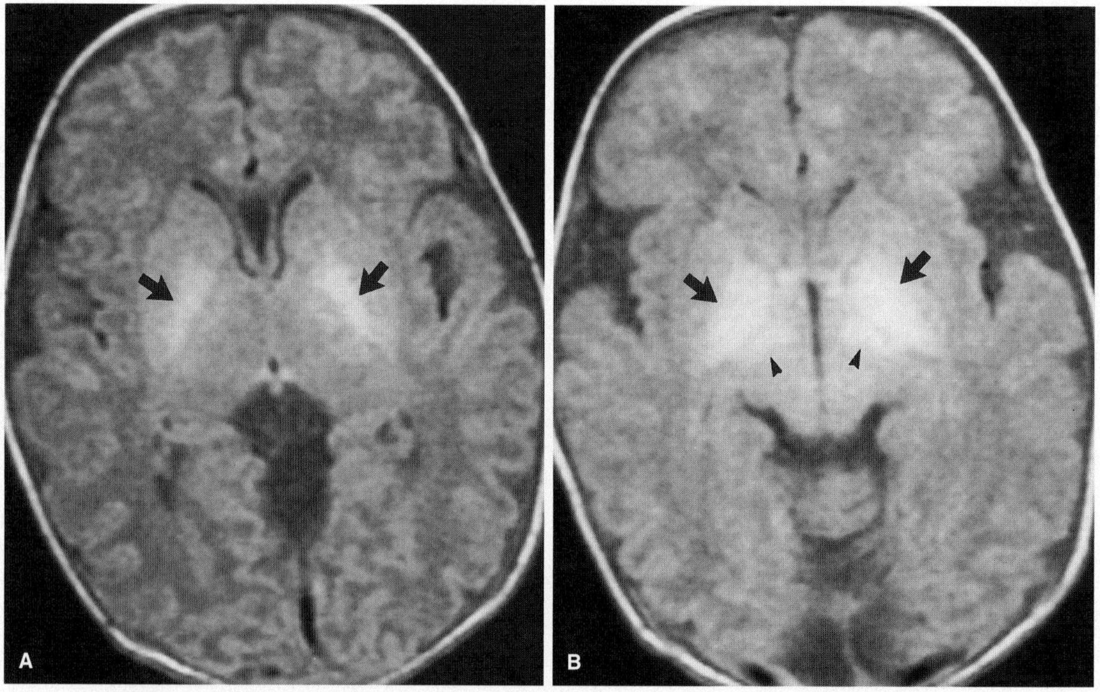

FIGURE 8.1. **Normal Myelination in a Newborn.** T1WI of a newborn infant. **A.** The level of the internal capsule shows normal high signal intensity of the posterior limb of the internal capsule (*arrows*). Note the absence of high signal intensity in the anterior limb. **B.** At a slightly lower level, the ventral lateral thalamus (*arrowheads*) and lentiform nuclei (*arrows*) are high signal intensity, consistent with myelination in these areas present at birth.

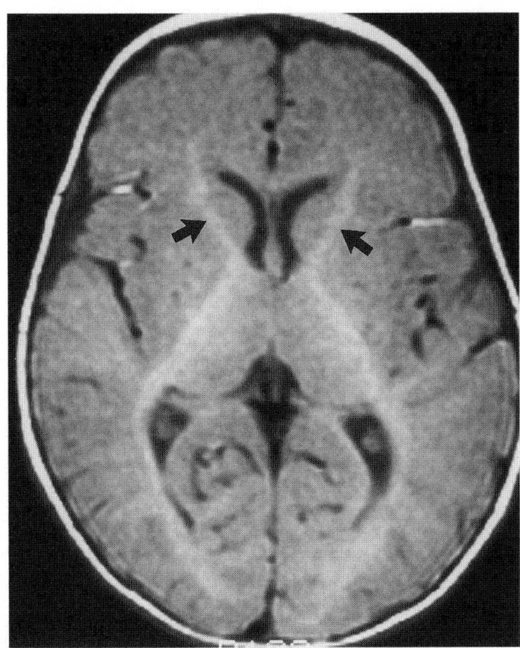

FIGURE 8.2. **Normal Myelination at 3 Months.** Axial T1WI of a 3-month old infant. The level of the internal capsule shows extension of high signal into the anterior limb of the internal capsule, reflecting progressive myelination of this region (*arrows*).

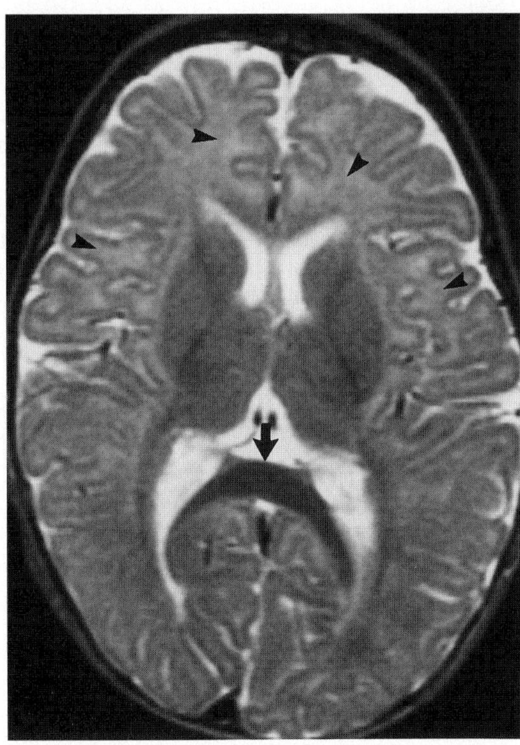

FIGURE 8.3. **Normal Myelination at 6 Months.** Axial T2WI of a 6-month-old infant at the level of the corpus callosum. The splenium of the corpus callosum is low signal intensity (*arrow*), but the unmyelinated deep and superficial cerebral white matter is high signal intensity (*arrowheads*).

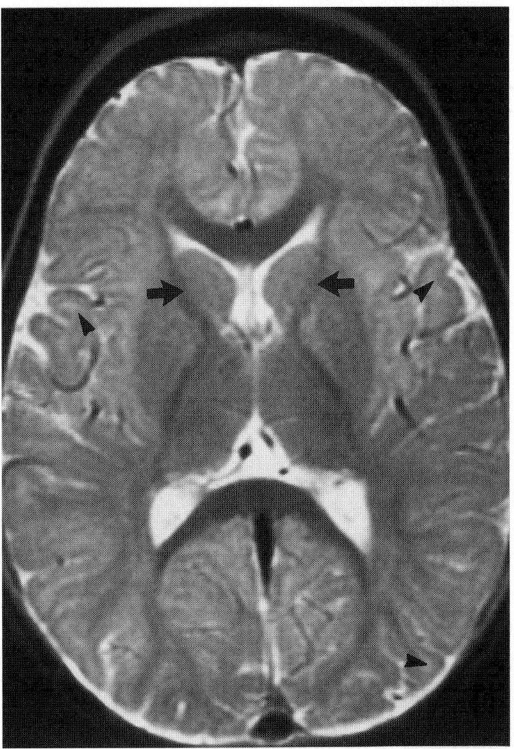

FIGURE 8.4. **Normal Myelination at 11 Months.** Axial T2WI of an 11-month-old infant at the level of the atria of the lateral ventricles. Note that the anterior limb of the internal capsule is now low signal (*arrows*). There has been progressive myelination of central white matter (low signal) but the subcortical white matter (*arrowheads*) is still unmyelinated and high signal intensity.

Delayed Myelination. The differential diagnosis of delayed myelination is broad, including in utero insults (hypoxia/ischemia, infection, toxins, coagulopathies, etc.); metabolic/nutritional disorders; and leukodystrophy, such as Pelizaeus-Merzbacher disease. (Refer to Chapter 7 for further discussion of the leukodystrophies.) Delayed myelination also shows excellent correlation with clinical measures of developmental delay.

In utero insults have been shown to cause delayed myelination in both premature and full-term neonates. Look for other findings of hypoxic ischemic encephalopathy (HIE) in conjunction with myelination delay. Nutritional deficiencies caused by poor diet or malabsorption syndromes cause myelination delay because of an inadequate supply of myelin precursors. Similarly, inborn errors of metabolism (amino and organic acidopathies) cause delayed myelination.

Pelizaeus-Merzbacher Disease is a rare X-linked leukodystrophy, mentioned here because MR demonstrates an arrest of myelin development, usually in the neonatal period. It can mimic other etiologies of delayed myelination because it shows lack only of myelin formation, rather than myelin formation followed by destruction (typical

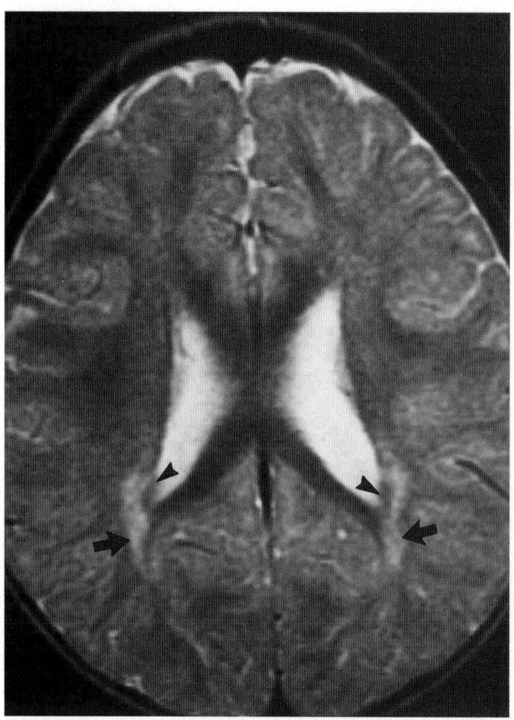

FIGURE 8.5. **Normal Myelination at 18 Months.** Axial T2WI of a normal 18-month-old infant. The process of normal myelination is essentially complete except for terminal myelination zones, which show persistent high signal (*arrows*) in the periatrial region. A thin hypointense band of white matter separates the terminal myelination zone from the atrial margin (*arrowheads*). Note that terminal myelination zones are usually "fuzzier" in appearance. Moral of the story: be careful about calling periventricular leukomalacia in patients who are not yet fully myelinated.

of most other leukodystrophies). A follow-up scan can be helpful in detecting a pattern of arrested myelination such as Pelizaeus-Merzbacher disease.

A large percentage of cases of myelination delay have no known cause but are related to a clinical diagnosis of developmental delay (developmental function <80% of expected for chronologic age). If a particular MR scan shows myelination delay (corrected for prematurity), a careful search for additional clues may yield a diagnosis (e.g., periventricular calcifications indicative of TORCH [*T*oxoplasmosis; *O*ther, which includes syphilis; *R*ubella; *C*ytomegalovirus; and *H*erpes] infection).

HYPOXIC ISCHEMIC ENCEPHALOPATHY

HIE refers to damage to the brain from hypoxia/ischemia occurring in utero or around the time of delivery. Many factors may predispose an infant to hypoxic injury, including in utero conditions such as infection, intrauterine growth retardation, inheritable and metabolic derangements, hypoglycemia, etc., which are entirely unrelated to the birthing process. Additionally, a wide variety of conditions (infection, inborn errors of metabolism, etc.) may mimic the imaging findings of HIE, and careful correlation with clinical history is needed. As a result, it is important to understand that the imaging findings of HIE are not indicative of any wrongdoing by the obstetrician.

Unfortunately, HIE is not uncommon in the pediatric population, with each pediatric center seeing multiple cases annually. As neonatologists learn how to save younger and younger fetuses, more cases will be seen, because ischemic brain injury is related to prematurity and its inherent complications. Knowledge of brain development and the reproducible patterns of brain damage can help answer questions about the severity of the insult and the timing of the injury. Patterns of brain injury can be divided into first and second trimester, late third trimester and perinatal, and postnatal. These patterns are summarized in Table 8.2.

The first and second trimesters of embryonic growth are characterized by rapid development of key brain structures. Hypoxic ischemic insults to the developing brain at this time are often severe and may arrest or alter further brain development. These changes may be global, as is seen in hydranencephaly, or more focal.

Hydranencephaly represents ischemic infarction of both cerebral hemispheres and is believed to be caused

TABLE 8.2 Imaging of Hypoxic Ischemic Brain Injury

Time	*Deep Gray*	*Cortex*	*Other*
First trimester	Spared	Cortical irregularity Hydranencephaly	
<26 weeks	Spared	Spared	Periatrial injury No gliosis Ex vacuo enlargement
>28 weeks	Spared	Spared	Periatrial gliosis: high signal on T2WIs
Term	Spared	Watershed infarcts Ulegyria	Variable deep, superficial white matter gliosis and atrophy Myelination delay Injury to hippocampus, pons

by early compromise of both carotid arteries with preservation of the posterior circulation. Hypercoagulable states, placental issues, and severe in utero infections have all been implicated. The pattern of destruction is characterized by little or no supratentorial brain tissue (Fig. 8.6). Severe hydrocephalus can mimic this appearance, but a thin "rind" of cortical gray matter is usually preserved. In hydranencephaly, no such "rind" is seen. There is usually complete infarction of all supratentorial cerebral tissues in the vascular distribution of the carotid arteries, with preservation of the thalami and cerebellum, which are supplied by the vertebral arteries.

Prenatal HIE. The classic theory is that ischemic injuries correlate with the location of arterial border zones—areas that are uniquely sensitive to watershed infarction. These border zones, in general, move centrifugally (outward) as the brain develops. In the first trimester and early second trimester, these zones start in the immediate periventricular region. By the late second trimester and early third trimester they move outward, into more peripheral white matter and cortical gray matter. Recently, infectious, autoregulatory, and metabolic mechanisms of periventricular white matter injury have challenged the "shifting vascular border zone" hypothesis.

Regardless of etiology, when the areas of peritrigonal white matter are injured, they undergo neuronal loss and cystic cavitary atrophy. Over time these cysts are incorporated into the ventricular wall, and the ventricles expand because of ex vacuo enlargement. The resulting atrial margin is often crenulated where necrotic periventricular white matter cysts have been incorporated. This characteristic enlargement of the ventricular atria is called *colpocephaly,* while the entire process referring to the damage and loss of the deep periventricular white matter is termed *periventricular leukomalacia.* The fetal brain under 26 weeks of age does not mount a significant glial or scarring response. As a result, a fetus less than 26 weeks of age does not exhibit T2 hyperintensity in the areas of white matter damage (Fig. 8.7). In contrast, if there is evidence of T2 hyperintensity in the damaged deep periventricular white matter, this suggests the injury occurred while the fetus was able to mount a glial response, i.e., after 26 weeks of age.

Periventricular Leukomalacia (PVL). After 26 weeks, the brain responds to HIE by gliosis in the periatrial region. *Gliosis* refers to the reaction of the brain to injury, much as fibrosis or scarring is the universal reaction to injury in the remainder of the body. Because neurons do not regenerate, it is up to the glial cells to react to the damage. The end stage of injury to the periventricular white matter is termed *leukomalacia*—literally "softening of the white matter." This damage is best seen on proton density–weighted images. PVL can be differentiated from the normal peritrigonal terminal myelination zones by noting an extension of high signal on T2WIs to the ventricular margin. This is caused by a loss of the normal thin myelinated white matter roof (tapetum) of the atrium of the lateral ventricle. Periatrial white matter thinning and atrial enlargement are also evident (Fig. 8.8).

In the late third trimester and perinatal period, there is continuing centrifugal extension of the arterial border zones sensitive to watershed infarction. Infants born at term who sustain insults during this period will demonstrate infarcts in the peripheral white matter and cortex (Fig. 8.9). Watershed infarctions occur at border zone regions between arterial distributions of major cerebral vessels (see Chapter 4).

The important border zones are (*1*) in the parasagittal cerebrum, between the anterior and middle cerebral arteries, which leads to an appearance of bilateral infarcts in the paramedian cortex and subsequent gliosis of subcortical white matter; and (*2*) the posterior convexity, between the anterior, middle, and posterior cerebral arteries, is another important border zone. Hypoxic ischemic injury shows bilateral parieto-occipital watershed infarcts. Also important is (*3*) the medial surface between the anterior and posterior cerebral arteries. A remodeling of subcortical infarcts occurring in the depths of sulci that spare the overlying gyri in any of these areas may lead to a characteristic pattern of mushroom-shaped gyri called *ulegyria.* The brainstem may be affected with selective neuronal loss of cranial nerve nuclei or neurons of the pons (pontosubicular necrosis). The Purkinje cells of the cerebellum also appear to be sensitive to HIE, as are the hippocampi.

Term infants with HIE can also demonstrate gliosis of affected periventricular white matter, ex vacuo ventricular enlargement, and resulting apposition of sulci to the ventricular surface because of white matter loss, a pattern seen with PVL. Associated sequelae of HIE include delayed myelination and thinning of large white matter tracts such as the corpus callosum. Tapering off of the size of the splenium of the corpus callosum on sagittal images is a good clue that PVL is present (Fig. 8.8).

Remember, term infants will primarily show peripheral damage corresponding to peripheral border zones. Periatrial damage, white mater loss, and delayed myelination are associated findings. Thus, the patterns of in utero HIE can be correlated with gestational age (Table 8.2).

Hypoxic Ischemic Injury and the Premature Infant

Premature infants present special challenges, and clinicians often image the brains of infants that are developmentally immature. The first step is to note the degree of prematurity and subtract the intervening time interval. For example, if we image an infant who is 2 months old, but was delivered 2 months premature, we should expect to see the appearance of a newborn term infant. Premature

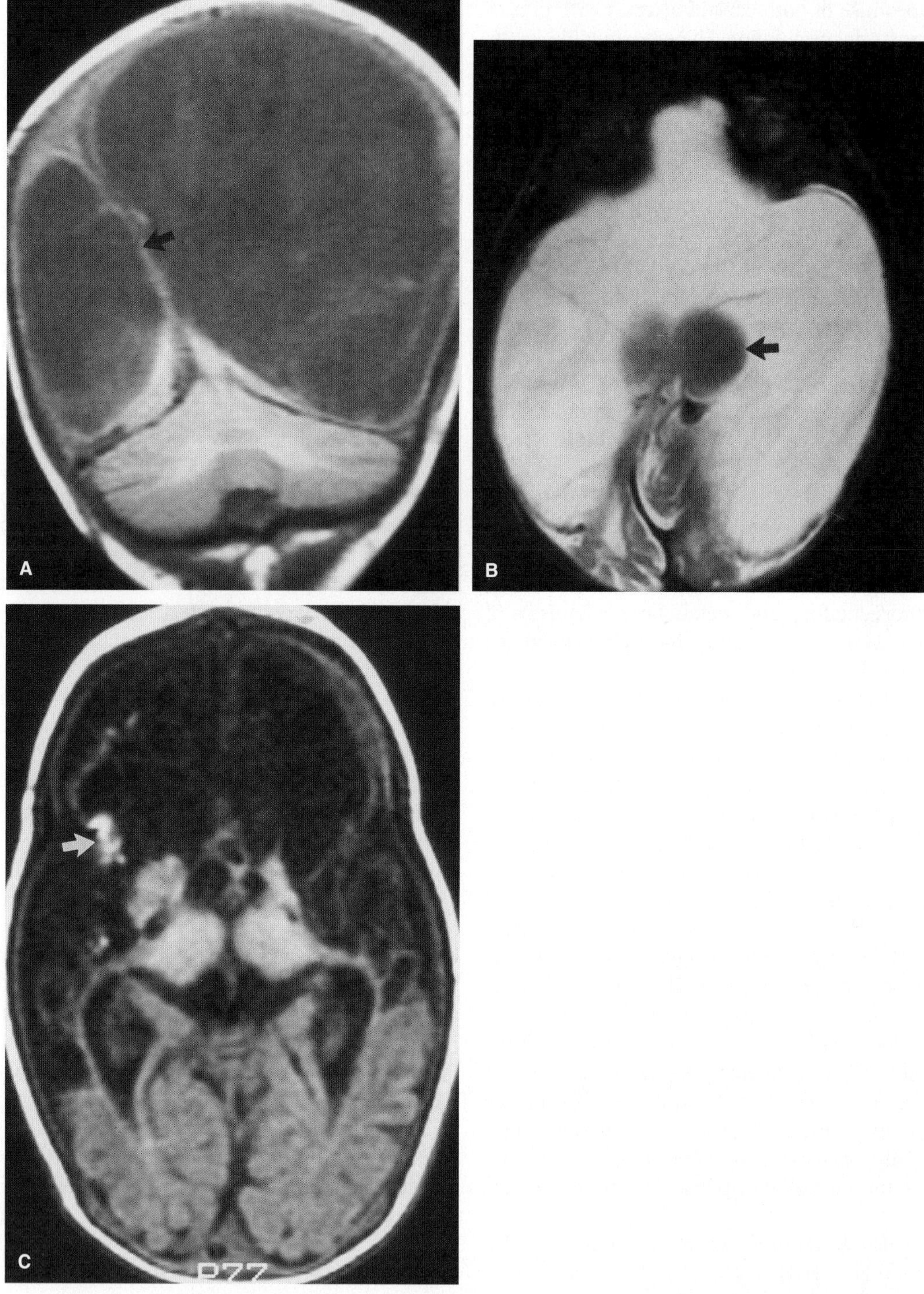

FIGURE 8.6. **Hydranencephaly. A.** Coronal T1WI. Hydranencephaly reflects varying degrees of infarction of both cerebral hemispheres. Note that the anterior circulation is completely infarcted, with only a thin rim of leptomeningeal connective tissue (no cortex). Some cerebral tissue supplied by the posterior circulation has been spared. The presence of the falx (*arrow*) excludes holoprosencephaly as the diagnosis. **B.** Axial T2WI of the same case. Note that the brainstem is preserved (*arrow*). **C.** Axial T1WI of a different case with similar findings to the hydranencephaly case seen in **A.** and **B.** Note that there is some sparing of the posterior temporal lobes. The presence of punctate foci of high signal (*arrow*) reflecting dystrophic calcification indicate that the initial insult was an in utero infection, probably of the TORCH group (*T*oxoplasma; *O*ther, which includes syphilis; *R*ubella, *C*ytomegalovirus; and *H*erpes; see Chapter 6). This case illustrates the common final pathway of early severe in utero brain destruction, whether the inciting event was ischemic or infectious.

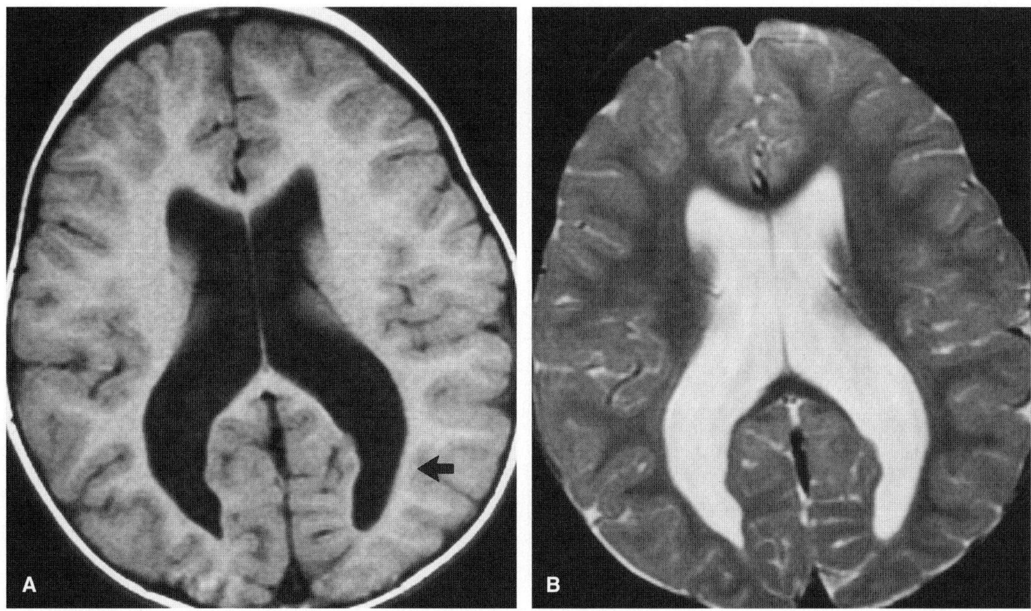

FIGURE 8.7. **Hypoxic Ischemic Injury at Less Than 26 Weeks Gestation. A.** Axial T1WI of a child who sustained a hypoxic ischemic injury at less than 26 weeks of gestation, resulting in injury to the periatrial white matter. This is reflected in the ex vacuo enlargement of the atria of the lateral ventricles. The severe periatrial white matter thinning has resulted in close apposition of a sulcus to the ventricular margin (*arrow*). **B.** The lack of periventricular gliosis is consistent with an insult occurring at 26 weeks of gestation or less.

infants sometimes show delayed myelination, however, because extrauterine life places many severe stresses on the developmentally immature brain, with oxygenation and nutrition being particular challenges. Premature infants still have periventricular border zones that are sensitive to HIE. Damage to the periventricular regions leading to varying degrees of PVL is common in premature infants. In severe cases, white matter undergoes cystic necrosis and subsequently becomes incorporated into the margins of the ventricle.

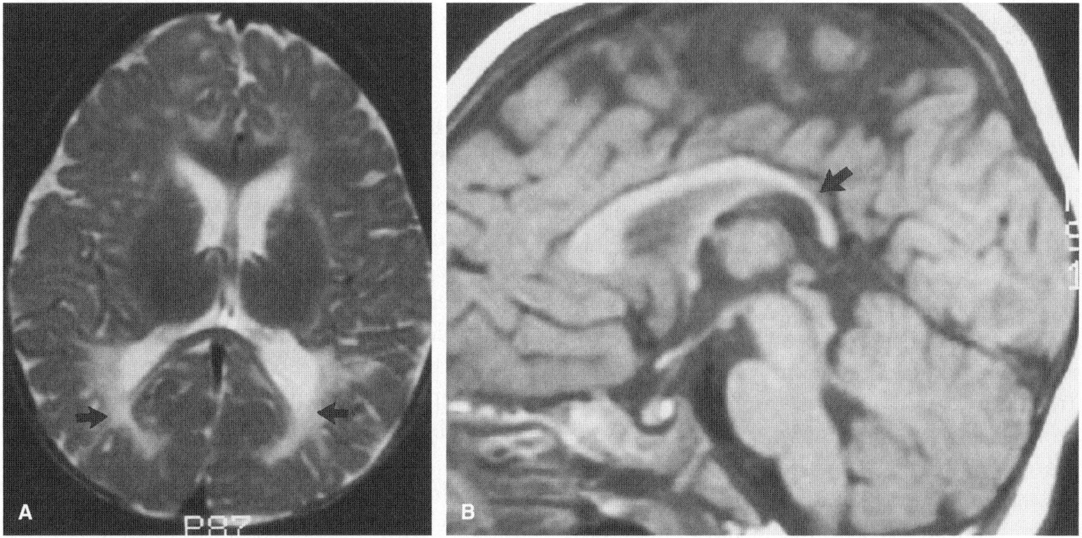

FIGURE 8.8. **Periventricular Leukomalacia. A.** Axial T2WI of a child who sustained an in utero hypoxic ischemic injury later than 26 weeks of gestation, resulting in periventricular leukomalacia. Note the high signal intensity caused by gliosis in the periatrial region (*arrows*) that extends to the ventricular margin. **B.** Hypoxic ischemic injury causes white matter injury and subsequent white matter loss, as evidenced by thinning of the posterior corpus callosum (*arrow*) on this sagittal T1WI.

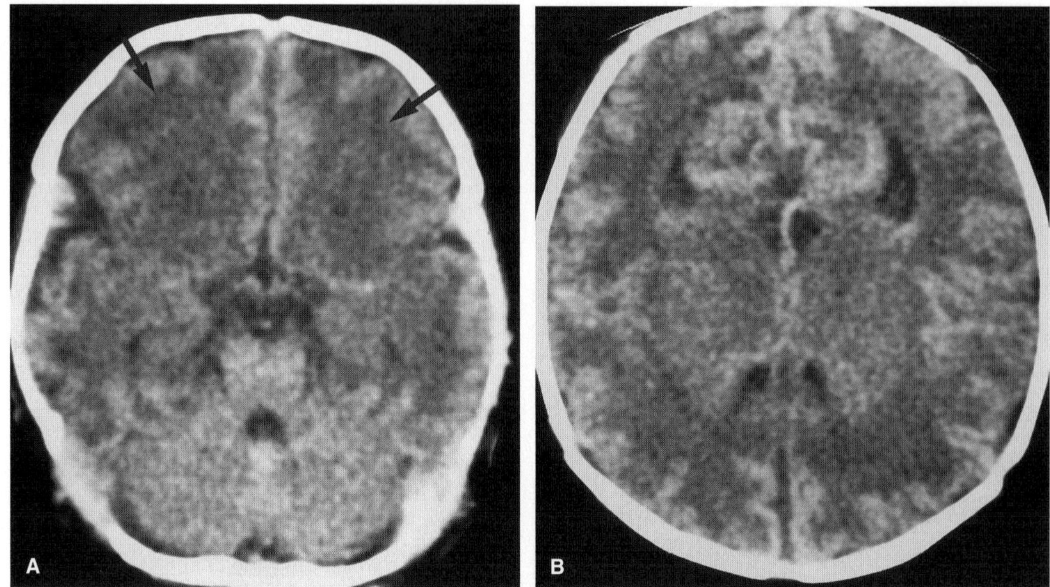

FIGURE 8.9. **Prolonged Hypoxic Ischemic Injury on CT.** This 2-day-old infant sustained a prolonged hypoxic ischemic injury. **A.** CT scan obtained soon after the event demonstrates diffuse low attenuation of the supratentorial brain, especially in the subcortical white matter (*arrows*), because of edema. The clue to the severe nature of the injury is the relative "white" appearance of the cerebellum. The cerebellum is more resistant to ischemia than the supratentorial brain. **B.** Axial image at the level of the basal ganglia shows generalized diminished attenuation of the basal ganglia caused by edema. Note the indistinctness of the posterior limbs of the internal capsule relative to the thalamus and lentiform nucleus. This is subtle evidence for injury to the ventrolateral thalamus. Follow-up scans taken at 1 month demonstrated severe postischemic injury and encephalomalacia to the supratentorial cortex, lentiform nucleus, and thalamus.

Germinal Matrix Hemorrhage. The germinal matrix, a zone of proliferating, richly vascularized neuroectodermal cells, is also exquisitely sensitive to injury. The response of this region to disturbances in cardiorespiratory function, whether caused by apnea, hypoxia, acidosis, bradycardia, unstable blood pressure, or impaired cerebral blood flow autoregulation, leads to rupture and hemorrhage of fragile blood vessels within the germinal matrix. Premature infants at risk for germinal matrix hemorrhage are best evaluated by serial neonatal neurosonography, which is reviewed in Chapter 39. Isolated acute germinal matrix hemorrhage, termed grade I subependymal hemorrhage, has the sonographic appearance of an echogenic focus directly anterior to the caudothalamic groove (see Fig. 39.22). In time, the hemorrhage either disappears entirely or evolves into a subependymal cyst. Bleeding may occur in the germinal matrix alone, dissect into the parenchyma, or rupture into the ventricle (see Fig. 39.23).

Term infants rarely suffer subependymal hemorrhage, since developmentally, their germinal matrix has involuted and their arterial border zones have moved peripherally. This leads to a number of useful rules:

1. Isolated periventricular leukomalacia in the term infant is only rarely caused by birth-related hypoxic ischemic events.
2. Gliosis in the periatrial region (seen best on proton-density scans) is caused by injury to the developing brain at 28 weeks gestational age or older.
3. Ex vacuo atrial enlargement without gliosis reflects injury prior to 26 weeks.

Profound Versus Partial Hypoxic Ischemic Brain Injury

Differing injury patterns can be detected by MR, which distinguishes between term infants subjected to severe hypoxic ischemic insults and those with milder or partial episodes of hypoxia. Examples of profound hypoxic ischemic events include full cardiorespiratory arrest and complete placental abruption. The MR appearance will vary depending on the age of the patient and whether the injury is evaluated acutely, subacutely, or in the chronic phase.

Profound perinatal HIE tends to damage central brain areas with relative sparing of the cerebral cortex. Evaluated acutely (immediate to 3 days) by CT, these infants may show injury to deep gray matter structures (basal ganglia and thalamus) with relative cortical sparing. In newborn infants, this may lead to the peculiar appearance of deep gray matter structures becoming isodense

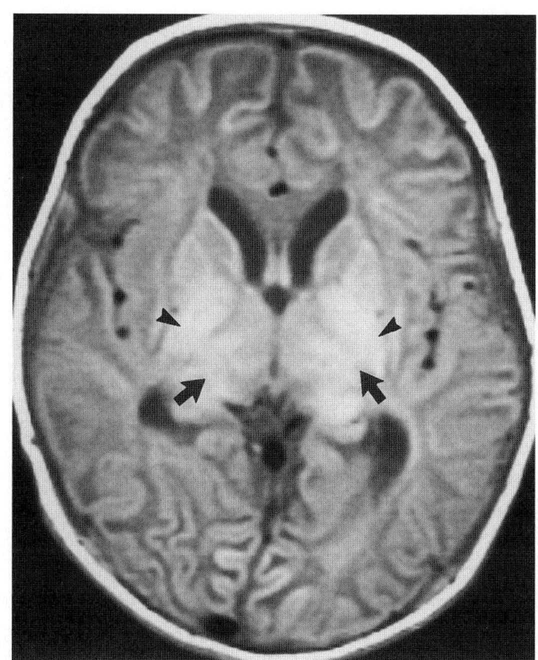

FIGURE 8.10. **Profound Perinatal Hypoxic Ischemic Encephalopathy: Acute.** Axial T1WI of a term infant evaluated acutely by MR. Mottled high signal intensity is seen in the posterolateral lentiform nuclei (*arrowheads*) and ventrolateral thalami (*arrows*). These high-signal-intensity areas most likely represent blood breakdown products.

to surrounding white matter, a very subtle abnormality (Fig. 8.9).

Profound HIE in the perinatal period evaluated acutely (up to 3 weeks) by MR will show mottled, globular high signal on T1WIs in the basal ganglia (posterolateral lentiform nuclei) and the ventral/lateral thalami (Fig. 8.10). These same areas show mottled low signal intensity on T2WIs. The signal intensity abnormalities may reflect hemorrhagic byproducts. Additionally, similar signal intensity abnormalities may be present in the tegmentum of the midbrain, lateral geniculate nuclei, and hippocampi (Fig. 8.11).

Cortical damage in the "hyperacute" phase is often missed on spin-echo images. T2WIs taken in the first few days may show apparently normal cortex and subjacent white matter. Careful inspection of proton density–weighted images is useful in identifying cortical edema, which results in loss of the gray–white matter interface, indicative of injury. Diffusion-weighted imaging (DWI), discussed in detail in Chapter 4, is extremely helpful in detecting early ischemic damage in neonates (Fig 8.12). Spectroscopy (to look for an elevated lactate peak) is also very useful in this early window and is probably the earliest and most sensitive indicator of ischemic injury (Fig 8.12).

In the subacute period (3 weeks to 3 months), the signal intensity of damaged basal ganglia may be variable on T2WIs. Damage to the cortex and white matter

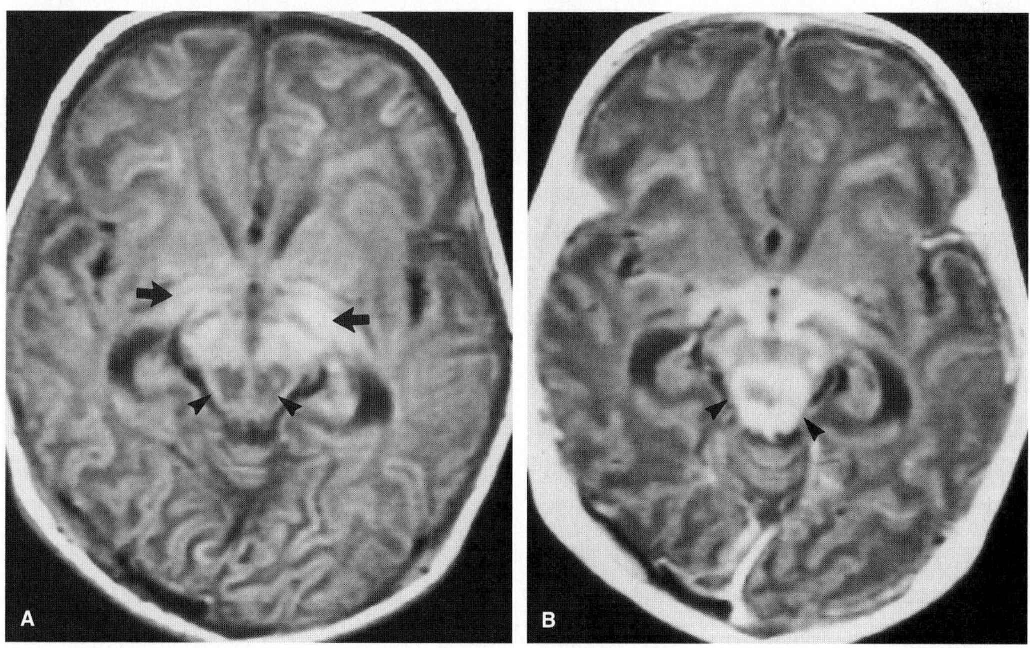

FIGURE 8.11. **Profound Perinatal Hypoxic Ischemic Encephalopathy: Acute. A.** T1WI at the level of the midbrain (same case as in Fig. 8.10). Mottled high signal intensity is seen in the lateral geniculate nuclei (*arrows*), and abnormal low signal is seen in the midbrain tegmentum (*arrowheads*). The actively myelinating regions such as the midbrain tegmentum are particularly susceptible to injury. **B.** Axial T1WI following gadolinium administration shows breakdown of the blood-brain barrier caused by ischemia in the midbrain tegmentum (*arrowheads*).

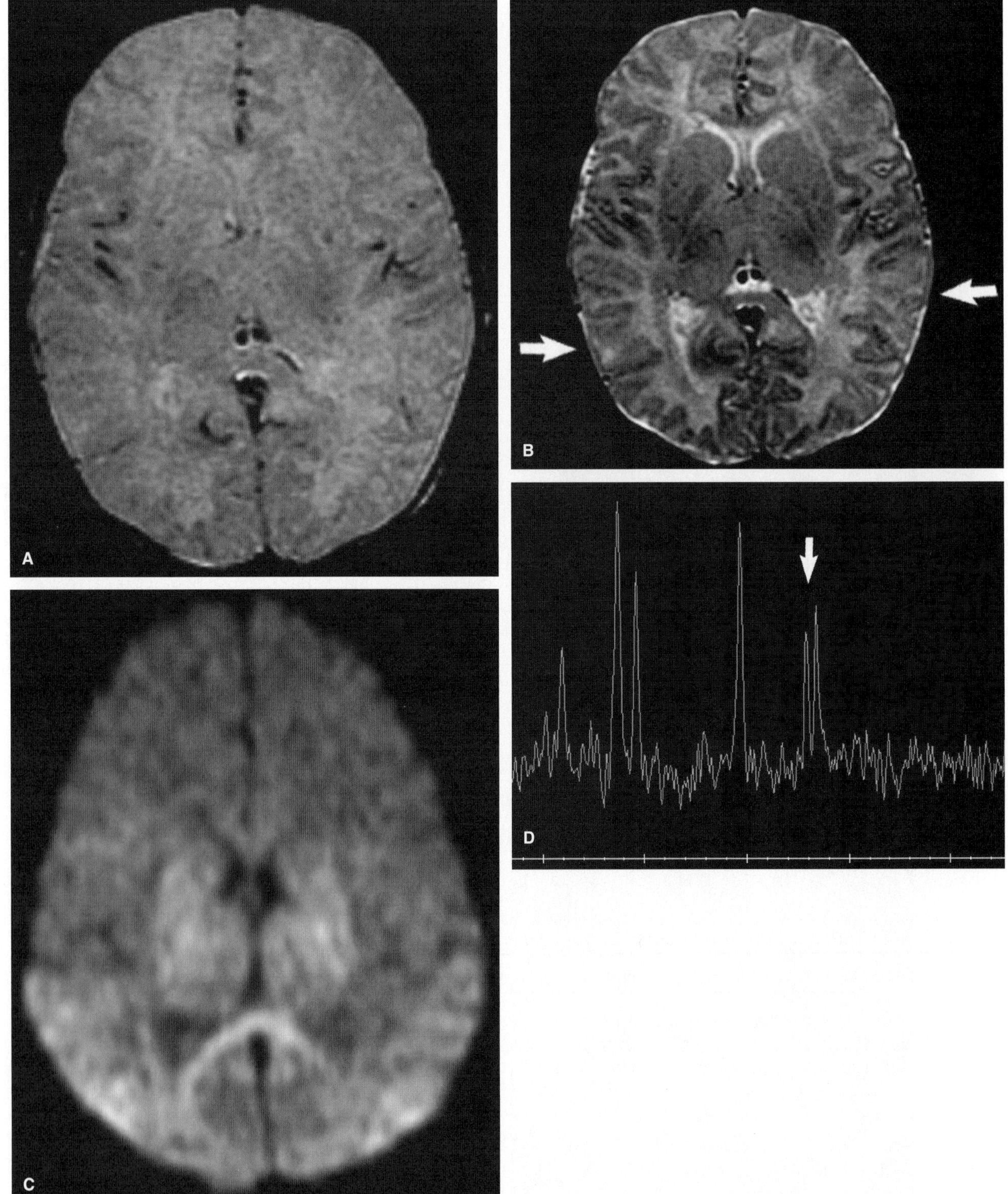

FIGURE 8.12. **Perinatal Hypoxic Ischemic Injury. A**. Proton-density-weighted image shows loss of gray–white differentiation throughout the brain. **B.** T2WI image shows cortical involvement (*arrows*). **C.** Diffusion-weighted image shows reduced diffusion in the posterior watershed regions bilaterally. **D.** MR spectroscopy through the basal ganglia shows elevation of the lipid/lactate peak (*arrow*).

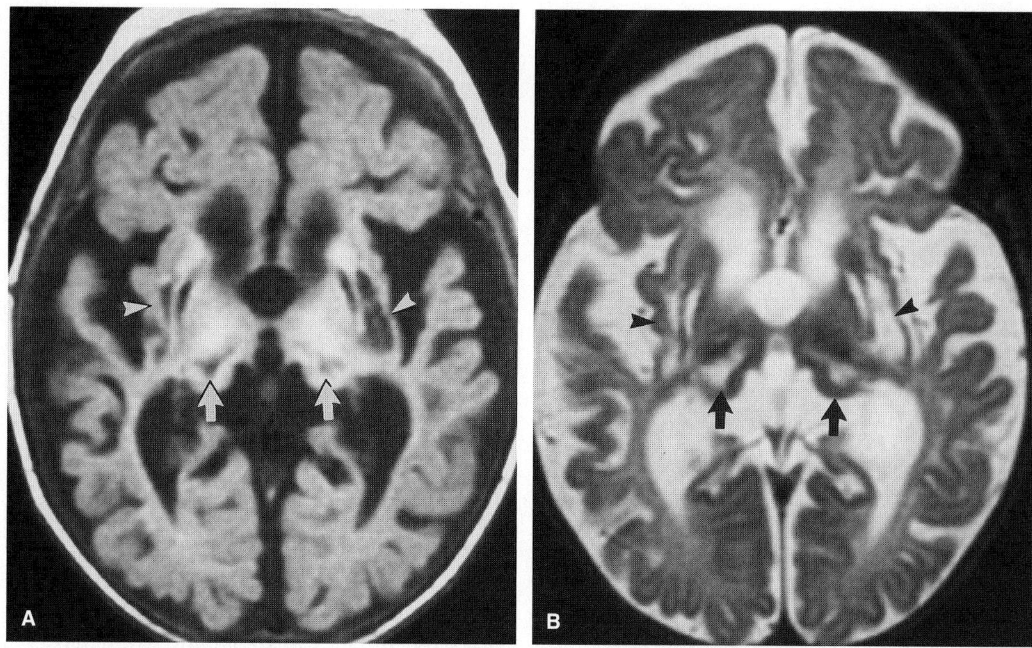

FIGURE 8.13. **Profound Perinatal Hypoxic Ischemic Encephalopathy: Chronic.** Profound perinatal hypoxic ischemic encephalopathy in a term infant evaluated chronically shows the evolving changes on MR. **A.** T1WI shows neuronal loss in the posterolateral lentiform (*arrowheads*) and ventrolateral thalami (*arrows*). Marked periatrial white matter atrophy is also seen. **B.** T2WI shows high signal intensity in the posterolateral lentiform (*arrowheads*) and ventrolateral thalami (*arrows*) caused by neuronal loss and gliosis.

becomes more evident. Profound HIE in the perinatal period evaluated chronically (>3 months) predominantly shows evolving injury to central gray matter: the posterolateral lentiform nuclei and the ventral/lateral thalami. The small area of cortex involved is the perirolandic cortex (precentral and postcentral gyri). The affected areas evaluated chronically have evolved in their appearance because of atrophy and gliosis (high signal on T2WIs) (Fig. 8.13). Table 8.3 summarizes the imaging findings in profound perinatal hypoxic ischemic brain injury.

The basal ganglia regions are also extremely sensitive to toxic and metabolic processes and will exhibit a relatively nonspecific response to these nonhypoxic insults as well (Fig. 8.14).

TABLE 8.3 Imaging of Profound Perinatal Hypoxic Ischemic Injury

Time	*Deep Gray (PLL, VLT)*	*Cortex*	*Other*
Acute	Isodense to white matter on CT Mottled high signal on T1WIs Mottled low signal on T2WIs	Normal—may see blurred gray–white junction on protein density images	Both areas may show increased signal on diffusion-weighted images and elevated lactate peaks on MR spectroscopy
Subacute	Variable signal on T1WIs and T2WIs	Perirolandic cortex: high signal on T1WIs, low signal on T2WIs	Atrophy: hippocampi, lateral geniculate, midbrain tegmentum Deep, superficial perirolandic white matter gliosis and atrophy, high signal on T2WIs, variable myelination delay
Chronic	High signal on T2WIs	Perirolandic cortex: high signal on T2WIs Thinned gyri, atrophy	Atrophy: hippocampi, lateral geniculate, midbrain tegmentum Deep, superficial perirolandic white matter gliosis and atrophy, high signal on T2WIs, variable myelination delay

Adapted from Barkovich AJ. MR and CT evaluation of profound neonatal and infantile asphyxia. AJNR Am J Neuroradiol 1992;13:959–972; used with permission.
PLL, posterolateral lentiform; VLT, ventrolateral thalamus.

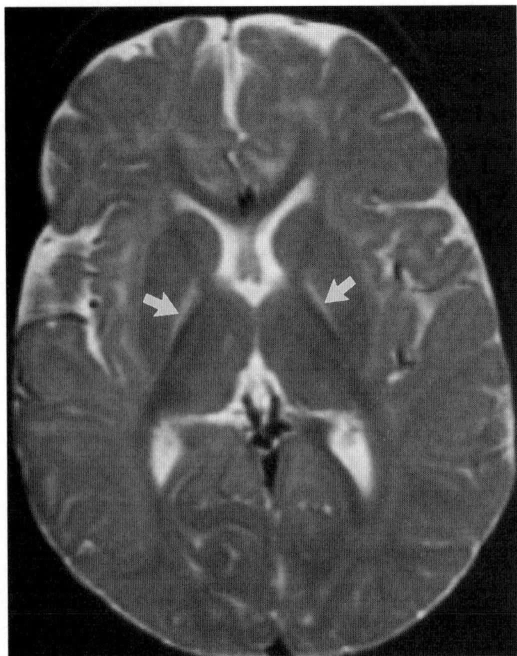

FIGURE 8.14. **Nonhypoxic Ischemic Encephalopathy (HIE) Basal Ganglia Injury.** Axial T2WI of a child at the level of the basal ganglia. A wide variety of metabolic and inflammatory insults can affect the basal ganglia. In this case, neonatal kernicterus has damaged the basal ganglia (globus pallidus) (*arrows*) and the subthalamic nuclei (not shown), a somewhat different pattern than in HIE. This case illustrates the relatively nonspecific response of the basal ganglia to nonhypoxic ischemic injury.

Profound postnatal HIE tends to injure a much larger proportion of cerebral cortex, with relative sparing of the perirolandic cortex. Postnatal HIE damages the corpus striatum (globus pallidus, putamen, caudate) and tends to spare the thalamus (Table 8.4).

Partial perinatal HIE. Partial or milder hypoxic ischemic events in the perinatal period, such as a nuchal cord, tend to spare central brain areas and will damage more peripheral gray matter. This is because the "diving reflex" redistributes blood to the basal ganglia, brainstem, and cerebellum. These peripheral infarcts are often located in watershed zones, as previously described. The peripheral infarcts will often progress over time to petechial gyral hemorrhage and eventually to areas of cortical thinning. Marked diminution and high signal on T2WIs of the subcortical and deep white matter are also seen.

TABLE 8.4 Imaging of Profound Postnatal Hypoxic Ischemic Injury

Deep Gray Matter	*Cortex*	*Other*
Damage to corpus striatum: high signal on T2WIs Relative sparing of thalami	Majority of cortex injured: high signal on T2WIs Relative sparing of perirolandic cortex Thinned gyri	Atrophy: hippocampi, lateral geniculate

Adapted from Barkovich AJ. MR and CT evaluation of profound neonatal and infantile asphyxia. AJNR Am J Neuroradiol 1992;13:959–972; used with permission.

Acute hypoxic ischemic damage can be difficult to discern in newborn infants. Some helpful hints follow:

1. Unmyelinated white matter is bright on T2WIs, making infarcts less apparent—it is like looking for watery areas in an ocean. Fluid-attenuated inversion-recovery sequences are not helpful, but DWI is very useful. MR spectroscopy has become the most sensitive tool, as lactate elevation may be the only abnormal finding, particularly early on (Fig. 8.12).
2. T1WIs can be a source of confusion. Do not confuse normal active myelination (basal ganglia, thalami, cerebral peduncles, perirolandic white matter) with the petechial hemorrhage caused by profound HIE. Petechial hemorrhage occurs in the putamina and thalami as punctate clumps on T1WIs and as blurred normal margins between the posterior limb of the internal capsule and the thalamus on T2WIs. Subtle punctate hyperintensity of a gyrus may indicate petechial hemorrhage on T1WIs.
3. Cytotoxic cerebral edema is better seen on CT than on T2WIs. CT is still a useful tool and is far easier to obtain than MR. Diffusion imaging has done much to solve this problem but is sometimes tricky to obtain (Fig 8.12).
4. After 24 to 72 hours, an extremely useful sign of infarction is the loss of normal gray matter hypointensity amidst a sea of hyperintense (unmyelinated) white matter on T2WIs.

Severe HIE in the perinatal period imaged acutely may show a global pattern of injury, with severe low density of the cerebral hemispheres caused by diffuse edema. The cerebellum is relatively resistant to injury, leading to the "white cerebellum" sign (Fig. 8.9). This CT sign shows a normal cerebellum appearing relatively white against a background of edematous supratentorial brain. MR is relatively insensitive to signs of edema in infants, and CT is still the preferred modality for assessing supratentorial brain edema. An MR correlate to this CT finding is the "dark cerebellum" sign on T2WIs. The normal cerebellum appears uniformly dark compared with the relatively hyperintense edematous supratentorial brain.

Summary. The developing brain shows continually shifting areas of brain vulnerability to HIE and changing brain response. A general knowledge of these regions and an understanding of the brain's response to damage are necessary to sort out differing patterns of brain injury. US is the best modality for demonstrating germinal matrix hemorrhage. CT is useful in demonstrating early signs of brain edema and hemorrhage. MR is able to demonstrate many of the characteristic conditions associated with HIE, including selective neuronal loss, watershed infarction, selective thalamic and basal ganglia necrosis, pontosubicular necrosis, hippocampal necrosis, PVL, white matter thinning, and delayed myelination. MR spectroscopy with evaluation of the lactate peak is the most sensitive early indicator of significant ischemic damage.

CONGENITAL LESIONS

Congenital lesions cannot be lumped into convenient categories by appearance. Most are unique in their appearance. Some of the entities that share common features are grouped together.

Septo-optic dysplasia (SOD) is defined as hypoplasia of the optic nerves with complete or partial absence of the septum pellucidum. The absence of the septum pellucidum results in a characteristic squared-off appearance of the frontal horns. There is also variable hypoplasia of the optic nerves, which may be limited to the optic disks, sparing the optic nerves. A fundoscopic examination of the optic nerves is often a helpful correlate (Fig. 8.15). There is more to SOD than the name alone suggests. Endocrine abnormalities are common (related to hypothalamic–pituitary axis abnormalities with reduction in growth hormone), and migration anomalies and periventricular cysts are also seen. Some find it easiest to consider SOD as part of the spectrum of holoprosencephaly, representing the mildest form of the continuum.

Holoprosencephaly is a spectrum of disorders related to failed cleavage of the developing brain. Holoprosencephaly also presents with orbital hypotelorism and varying degrees of facial dysmorphism.

Alobar holoprosencephaly is a severe malformation with a dismal prognosis. This type of holoprosencephaly is distinctive, consisting of an anterior rind of brain tissue and a monoventricle, which communicates with a dorsal cyst. The thalami are fused and the septum pellucidum, corpus callosum, and falx are absent (Fig. 8.16).

Alobar holoprosencephaly only really needs to be discriminated from two other entities: hydranencephaly (Fig. 8.6), which represents bilateral in utero cerebral hemisphere infarction, and severe hydrocephalus, with secondary pressure atrophy of the septum pellucidum. A reliable discriminating sign of alobar holoprosencephaly are the tips of the upside-down U-shaped mantle of brain tissue. These ends of the "U" are known as the hippocampal ridges and are best seen in the axial plane.

Semilobar holoprosencephaly is less severe and shows partial fusion of the hemispheres. The corpus callosum and the septum pellucidum are absent or dysgenic. There is a high association with migration anomalies (abnormalities of cortical development) (Fig. 8.17). The posterior portion of the interhemispheric fissure and falx are usually formed in cases of semilobar holoprosencephaly.

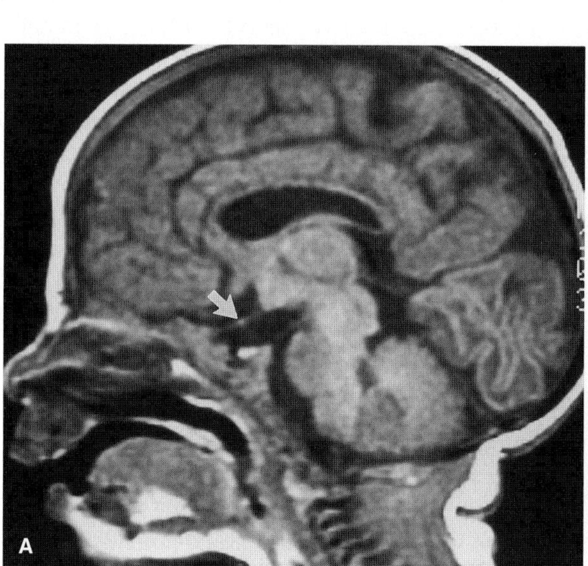

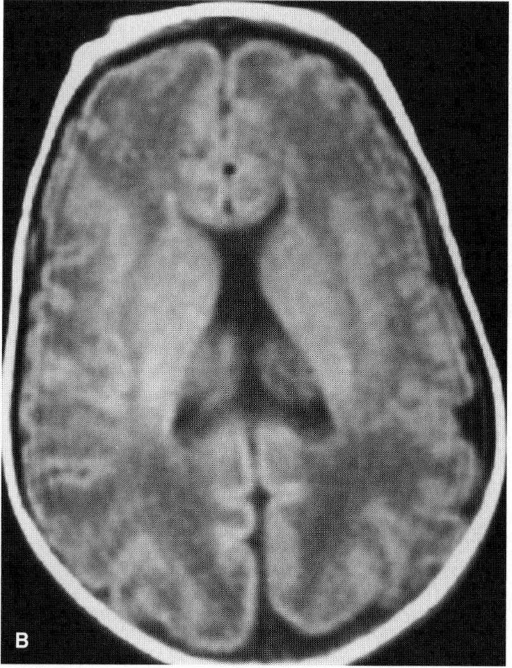

FIGURE 8.15. **Septo-optic Dysplasia. A.** Sagittal T1WI shows a hypoplastic optic nerve (*arrow*), an inconstant finding on MR imaging of septo-optic dysplasia. **B.** Axial T1WI shows absence of the septum pellucidum, which is characteristic of septo-optic dysplasia.

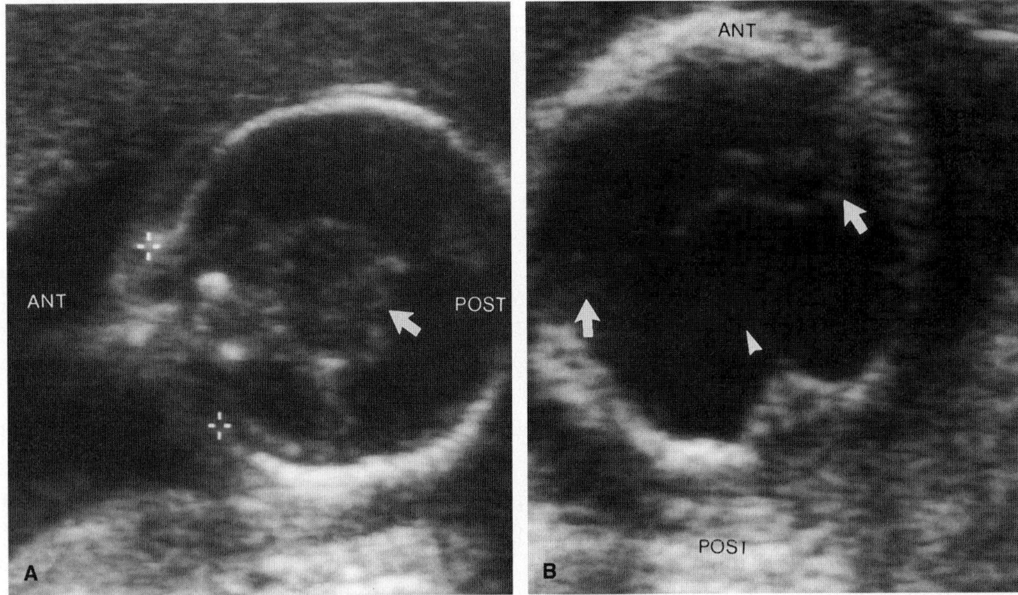

FIGURE 8.16. **Alobar Holoprosencephaly. A.** An axial obstetrical US through the fetal brain demonstrates the in utero appearance of alobar holoprosencephaly. This severe disorder consists of a monoventricle, with absence of the septum pellucidum, corpus callosum, and falx. The thalami are fused (*arrow*). The white markers are placed at the orbits to measure the degree of hypotelorism. **B.** An axial image at a slightly higher level shows the posterior tips of the mantle of cerebral tissue, termed hippocampal ridges (*arrows*), that are characteristic of holoprosencephaly. This mantle is displaced forward within the calvaria by the posterior monoventricle. The monoventricle communicates with the CSF space called the dorsal sac (*arrowhead*).

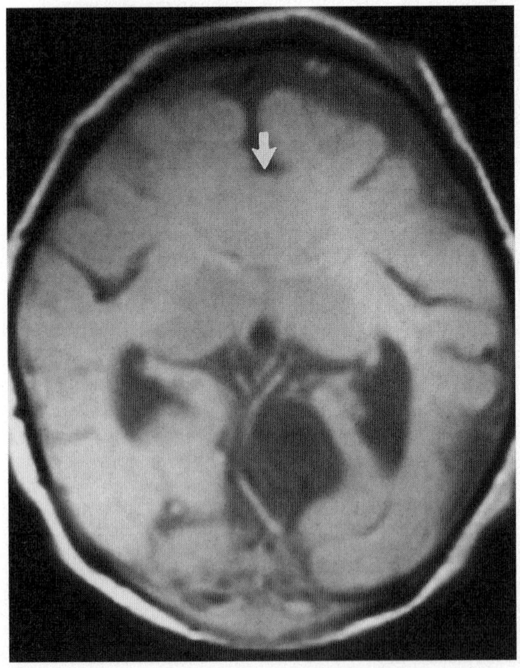

FIGURE 8.17. **Semilobar Holoprosencephaly.** An MR image of semilobar holoprosencephaly shows partial fusion of the anterior cerebral hemispheres (*arrow*).

Lobar holoprosencephaly is characterized by a relatively normal-appearing brain. Typically, there is partial absence of a frontal interhemispheric fissure. The absent septum pellucidum and the relatively normal brain give this entity an overlap with SOD. The body and splenium of the corpus callosum are usually present, with the genu and rostrum absent (dysgenic corpus callosum).

The absence of the septum pellucidum is a constant helpful feature of the holoprosencephalies. Any portion of a visible septum pellucidum excludes holoprosencephaly and should prompt consideration of severe hydrocephalus or agenesis of the corpus callosum. Remember, absence of the septum pellucidum is strongly associated with other malformations, including anomalies of the face and cerebral cortex (schizencephaly, polymicrogyria, and pachygyria). Coronal T1 images are extremely helpful in demonstrating a narrow portion of hemisphere fusion, confirming the diagnosis of holoprosencephaly.

Agenesis of the Corpus Callosum. The corpus callosum forms from front to back and myelinates from back to front. Following these principles, partial agenesis of the corpus callosum will result in formation of the genu and anterior body and absence of the posterior body and splenium.

Two conditions deviate from the typical callosal agenesis appearance. Both secondary destruction of the corpus callosum and holoprosencephaly can result in nonsequential segments of absent callosum. The resultant dysgenic callosal pattern thus yields valuable clues regarding brain development and a correct diagnosis. For example, a callosum that is missing *only* a genu segment may indicate an insult to the brain after development of the corpus callosum, or it may point to lobar holoprosencephaly (if the septum is absent), which exhibits disorganized callosal development.

The imaging appearance of callosal dysgenesis is variable, ranging from complete to partial absence of callosal tissue. Concomitant with the absence of the corpus callosum is failure of eversion of the cingulate gyrus, with lack of cingulate sulcus formation. The medial hemispheric sulci extend to the third ventricle, which on a sagittal image results in a radial, spoke-wheel appearance of the gyri along the interhemispheric fissure. Without the supporting deep white matter fibers, there is alteration in the configuration of the ventricles, with the frontal horns taking on a "steer-horn" appearance in the coronal plane and a "racing car" appearance in the axial plane (Fig. 8.18). This is the result of redirection of longitudinal callosal fibers (Probst bundles) along the medial ventricular walls. Additionally, because of the redirection of the Probst bundles and decrease in posterior white matter, there is dilation of the occipital horns, called *colpocephaly*. Interhemispheric cysts may be seen, frequently in communication with the third ventricle.

It is important to describe a potential pitfall in interpretation. Occasionally, callosal hypogenesis will be accompanied by relative prominence of the hippocampal commissure. The hippocampal commissure should not be mistaken for the splenium, erroneously signaling "atypical callosal hypogenesis" or callosal dysgenesis.

Lipomas of the corpus callosum have imaging criteria that are similar to other intracranial lipomas in other locations. Lipomas are felt to represent congenital abnormalities and show high signal intensity on T1WIs, which suppresses with the use of fat-saturation imaging. Occasionally these lesions may be misinterpreted as interhemispheric hemorrhage or fat within the interhemispheric falx. If you are reading any scan suspicious for lipoma in any location (and fat-saturation images were mistakenly not obtained), look for chemical shift artifact along the frequency encoding direction of the scan. This is a second sign that can confirm the presence of fat.

Lipomas do not cause mass effect, and vessels course through these lesions unperturbed, reflecting their development basis, as they occur because of the persistence of the meninx primitiva. Lipomas of the corpus callosum are occasionally associated with callosal anomalies (Fig. 8.19).

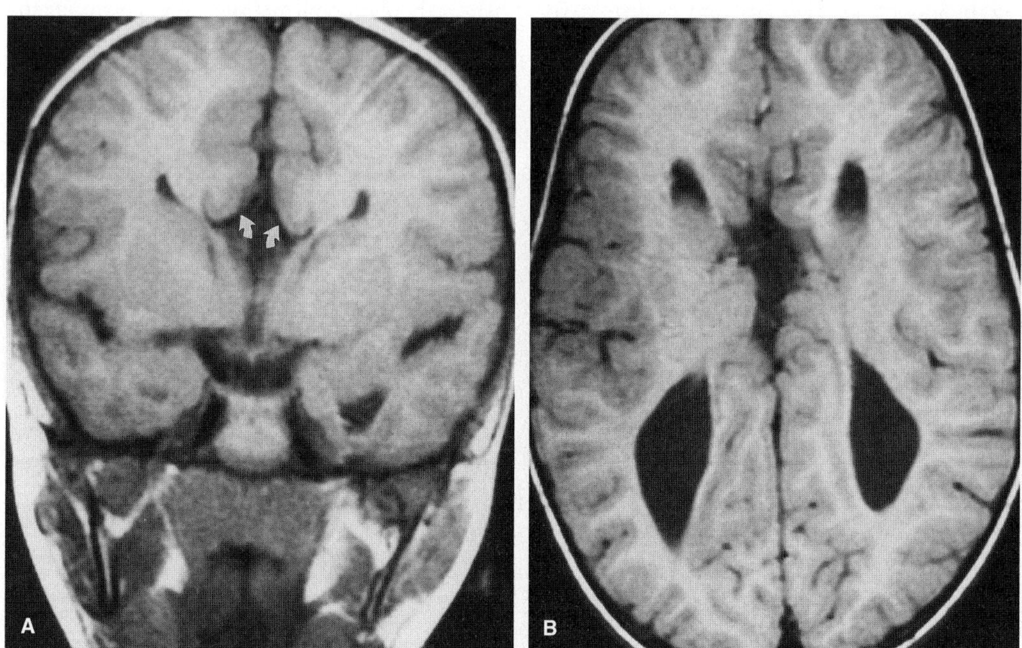

FIGURE 8.18. **Agenesis of the Corpus Callosum. A.** Coronal T1WI shows a "steer-horn" shape of the frontal horns of the lateral ventricle. There is absence of the midline corpus callosal tissue and cingulate sulcus (*arrows*). **B.** Axial T1WI of the same case showing the "racing car" configuration of the ventricles. The frontal horns look like the front wheels and the atria of the lateral ventricles look like the larger rear tires on a racing car. In the US literature, this has been described as the "parallel ventricle" sign.

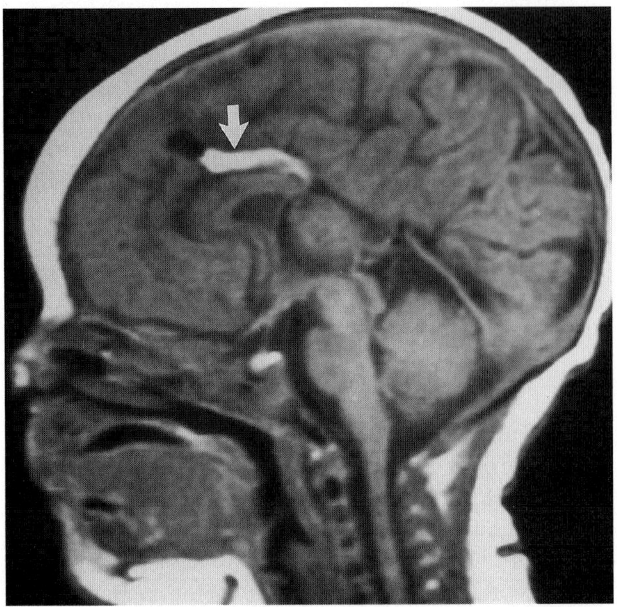

FIGURE 8.19. **Lipoma of the Corpus Callosum.** Sagittal T1WI shows a high-signal-intensity lipoma of the corpus callosum (*arrow*) with accompanying hypogenesis of the posterior body and splenium of the corpus callosum.

Other common locations of intracranial lipomas include the pericallosal interhemispheric fissure, quadrigeminal plate, and suprasellar cisterns. Less common locations include the cerebellopontine angle, sylvian fissure, cerebellar vermis (Fig. 8.20), and the lamina terminalis. Beware of fat globules that are "floating" in the CSF spaces, particularly those rising to the anterior horns of the lateral ventricles. This is a sign of a ruptured dermoid (see Chapter 5).

Cephaloceles represent the failure of the skull and dura to close over the brain, leading to a herniation of intracranial contents through the defect. *Meningoceles* reflect herniation of the leptomeninges alone, while *encephaloceles* are associated with herniation of brain and leptomeninges. Occipital encephaloceles are the most common. Other locations include the frontoethmoidal, parietal, and sphenoidal regions. The brain remaining inside the calvaria is typically stretched and distorted toward the defect. Frontoethmoidal encephaloceles are associated with craniofacial anomalies (including hypertelorism) and a higher incidence of callosal abnormalities (Figs. 8.21, 8.22). Nasal dermoids are a more benign part of this spectrum but require evaluation with sagittal T2WIs to insure there is no potential for CSF leak developing with resection.

Sphenoid encephaloceles are often occult and present as a nasopharyngeal mass that contains variable amounts of herniated third ventricle, hypothalamus, and optic chiasm.

MIGRATION ANOMALIES

This group of disorders reflects varying patterns of arrested migration as neurons attempt to travel from the subependymal regions (i.e., germinal matrix) toward the brain surface. Many of the discrete layers of the cortex are formed by directed migration of specific neurons from the germinal matrix outward along radial-glial fibers,

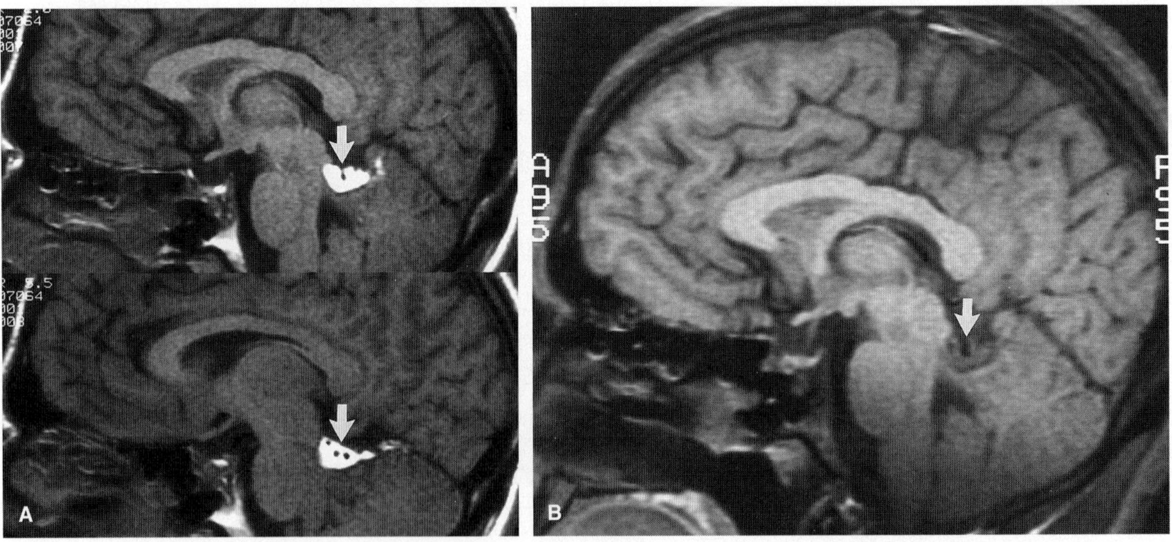

FIGURE 8.20. **Lipoma of the Cerebellar Vermis. A.** Sagittal T1WI shows a lipoma of the superior vermis (*arrows*). Note that a vessel courses through the lipoma unperturbed. **B.** A fat-saturation T1WI shows the suppression of fat signal from the image, confirming the diagnosis of lipoma (*arrow*).

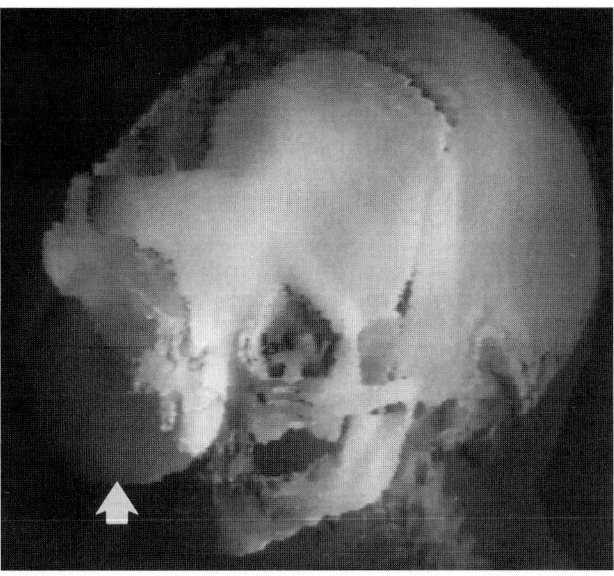

FIGURE 8.21. **Frontal Encephalocele.** A three-dimensional reformatted CT image of a dramatic frontal encephalocele shows a calvarial defect and a soft tissue sac (*arrow*) herniating out through the defect.

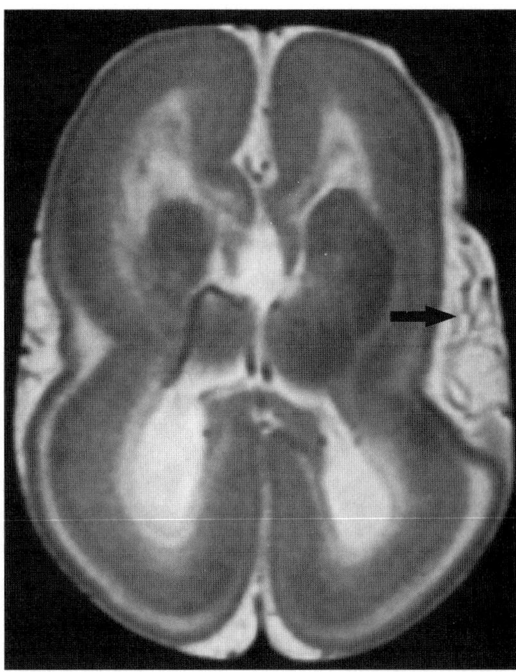

FIGURE 8.23. **Lissencephaly.** Axial T2WI of lissencephaly. The brain has a smooth agyric appearance with an abnormally thickened multilayered cortex. The anomalous cortical venous drainage pattern is also seen (*arrow*).

which serve as a scaffolding for the movement of neurons. If neurons destined to become cortical gray matter end up in the wrong place because of arrested migration, they can become foci of seizure activity.

Lissencephaly and pachygria/agyria complex are synonymous terms for the most severe disorder in this spectrum: absence of gyri. The lack of sulcation gives a smooth hourglass appearance to the brain. The cortex is abnormally thick (Fig. 8.23) and multilayered. The terms "classic," "type I," and "X-linked" lissencephaly are interchangeable and refer to a pattern of arrested neuronal migration in which only four cortical layers are present, with band heterotopias. The premature infant's brain can mimic the appearance of lissencephaly. However, the history of prematurity and a cortex of normal thickness distinguish the premature infant.

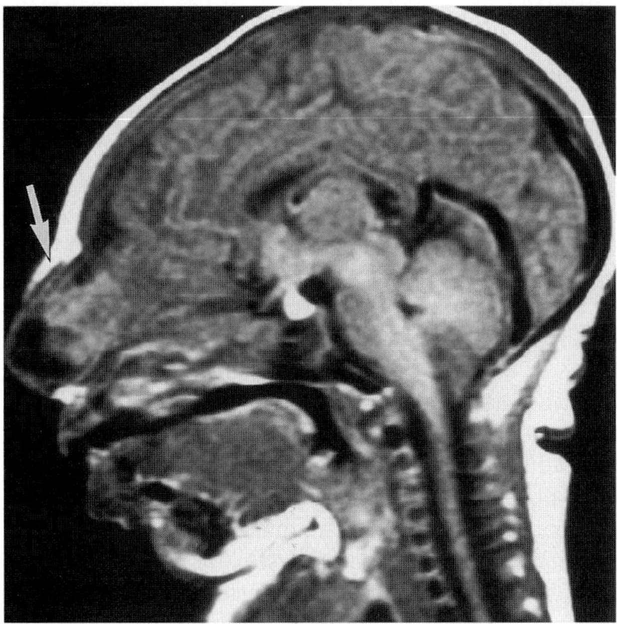

FIGURE 8.22. **Frontal Encephalocele.** T1WI of a frontal encephalocele shows herniation of brain and meninges through the defect (*arrow*).

Polymicrogyria and pachygria are both milder disorders of neuronal migration than agyria. They can appear similar, although with high-resolution thin-section MR, the differences are more easily detected. Strictly speaking, pachygyria is an incomplete lissencephaly, and polymicrogyria is a cortical dysplasia. Pachygyria is seen as broad, thick gyri with shallow sulci. Polymicrogyria is characterized by a thick mantle of gray matter with multiple small gyri. Underlying white matter gliosis in polymicrogyria can sometimes help differentiate it from pachygyria. In both polymicrogyria and pachygyria, the normal interdigitating fingers of subcortical white matter are absent.

These anomalies produce an abnormally thickened cortex with little or no sulcation, but in distinction to lissencephaly, they are more focal (Figs. 8.24, 8.25). Cortical dysplasias also show anomalous cortical venous drainage, which should not be confused with the abnormal

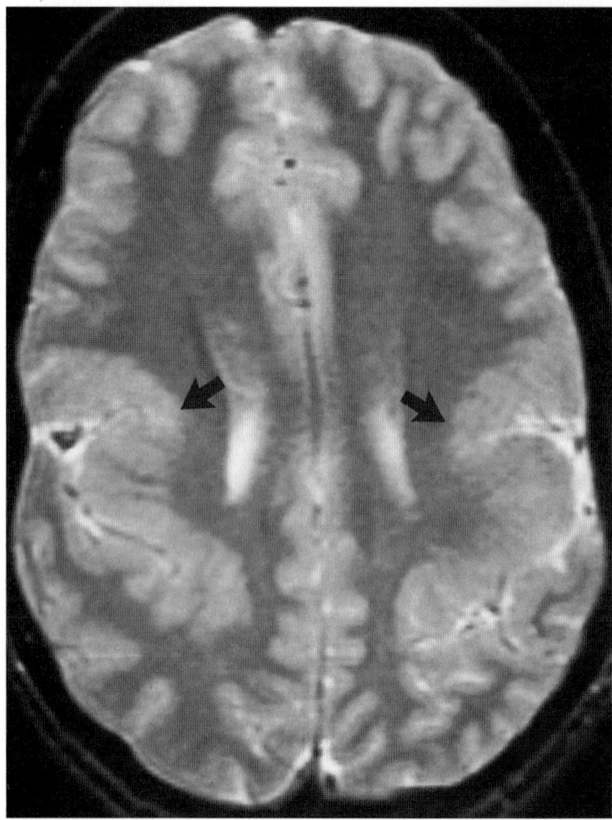

FIGURE 8.24. **Polymicrogyria.** Bilateral areas of focal cortical thickening with deep clefting are seen in both hemispheres in this case of polymicrogyria (*arrows*).

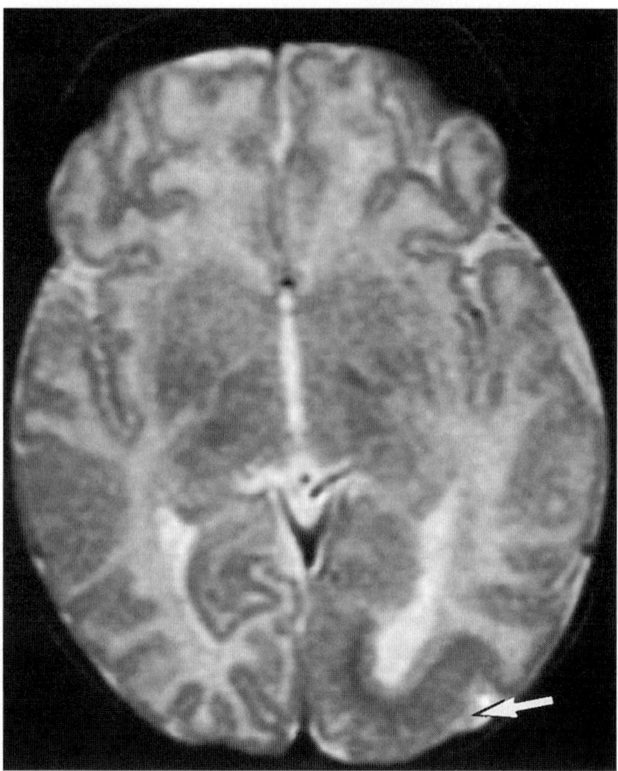

FIGURE 8.25. **Pachygyria.** A more focal area of smooth cortical thickening is seen in this more subtle case of focal pachygyria (*arrow*).

vessels seen in arteriovenous malformations. Other associated anomalies are common, including heterotopic gray matter, schizencephaly, and callosal hypogenesis. Sometimes an entire hemisphere may be enlarged and composed of polymicrogyric and pachygyric changes. This condition is called *hemimegalencephaly* and may be associated with various syndromes, such as neurofibromatosis.

Heterotopic Gray Matter. As neurons migrate from the germinal matrix to the overlying cerebral cortex, their journey may be disrupted, resulting in trapped nests of gray matter deep within the brain. These islands of gray matter can be seen anywhere between the ependymal surface and the subcortical white matter and are called *heterotopic gray matter.* Heterotopic gray matter appears isointense to normal gray matter on all imaging sequences. These lesions do not enhance with gadolinium and do not calcify (Fig. 8.26). The only significant mimics of heterotopic gray matter are the lesions seen in tuberous sclerosis, which do calcify. Most heterotopic gray matter is nodular, although band or laminar heterotopias can be seen. A band heterotopia presents as a smooth layer of gray matter within the subcortical white matter, resulting in a double cortex appearance. This condition is typically associated with severe seizure disorders and significant developmental delay.

Schizencephaly represents an abnormality of neuronal migration resulting in gray matter–lined clefts that deeply invaginate the brain. The etiology of this condition is felt to be an in utero insult or expression of a genetic factor during the sixth week of gestation that damages the germinal matrix and impedes neural migration. These clefts often extend from the ventricular ependymal surface to the pial cortical surface, giving rise to a pial-ependymal seam, which communicates with the ventricle. Clefts that do not extend to the ventricle are simply focal cortical dysplasias, also known as polymicrogyric clefts. Schizencephaly is frequently associated with other migrational anomalies, such as cortical dysplasias and heterotopic gray matter. Multiple imaging planes are often necessary to optimally visualize these clefts and migrational anomalies. The clefts are described as being either "open lip" or "closed lip" in appearance (Fig 8.27), depending on whether the walls of the clefts are wide open or apposed, respectively. A large open-lipped schizencephalic cleft may look like a zone of encephalomalacia that communicates with the ventricle, referred to as *porencephaly*. These two conditions are easily differentiated; schizencephalic clefts are lined by gray matter, whereas porencephalic cysts are lined by a thin layer of white matter.

All children with migration anomalies can present with seizures. When imaging a child for seizures, MR should

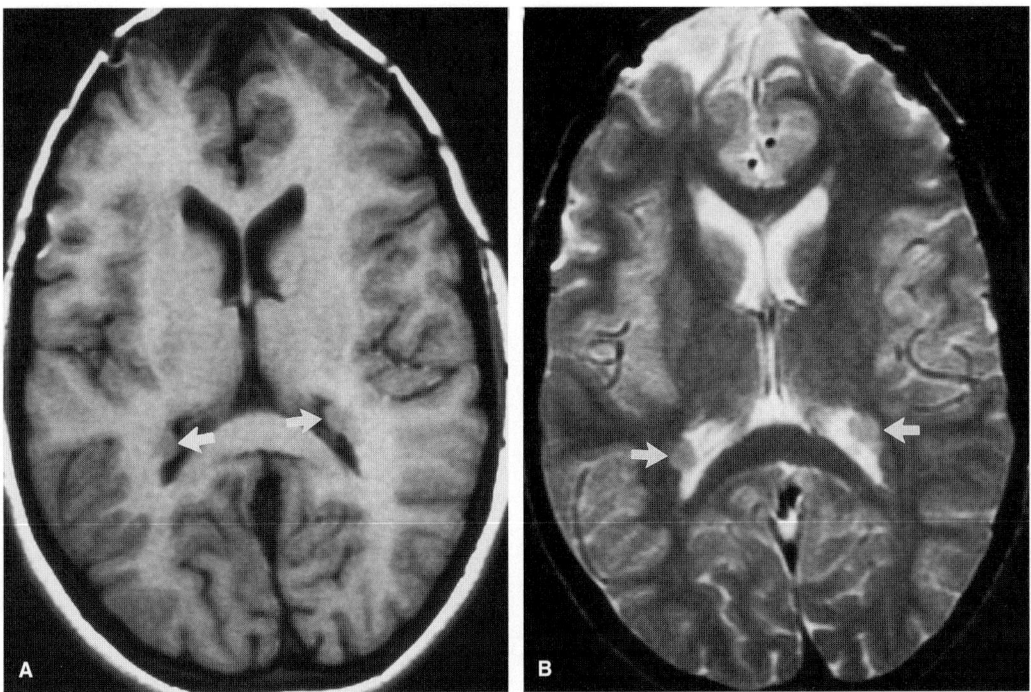

FIGURE 8.26. **Heterotopic Gray Matter. A.** T1WI demonstrates heterotopic gray matter (*arrows*) along the ependymal surface of the ventricle. Damage to the frontal lobes was secondary to trauma. **B.** A T2WI obtained at the same level shows the heterotopic nodules that parallel gray matter signal in all sequences (*arrows*).

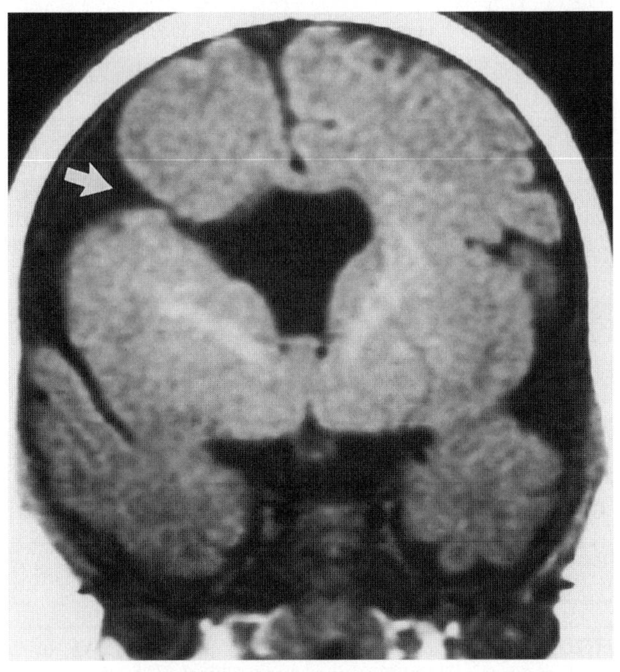

FIGURE 8.27. **Schizencephaly.** An open-lip schizencephaly is seen on this coronal T1WI. The cleft is lined by thickened polymicrogyric gray matter (*arrow*).

include high-resolution, thin-section T1 and T2W sequences, performed in numerous imaging planes in search of suspicious-looking thickened or polymicrogyric cortex.

Chiari malformations refer to a group of disorders that represent congenital hindbrain abnormalities. Four types of Chiari malformations are described in the literature, and we will focus on the two most commonly encountered. Types I and II Chiari malformations involve the brain and spine.

Chiari II malformations are the serious neural tube disorders that are screened for in maternal prenatal US and alpha-fetoprotein programs. Starting from the head down, the key abnormalities are described.

Supratentorial Brain. Nearly all patients will present with hydrocephalus. Most cases show partial or complete agenesis of the corpus callosum. The falx cerebri is often fenestrated, resulting in herniation of individual gyri across midline. The massa intermedia (midline rounded mass of gray matter connecting the thalami on sagittal images) is enlarged. The posterior cingulate gyrus is often dysplastic.

Posterior Fossa. Most of the hindbrain findings in Chiari II malformation derive from a diminutive posterior fossa, with brain structures squeezed superiorly, inferiorly, and anteriorly. The cerebellum is squeezed up against the tentorium, down through the foramen magnum (tonsillar herniation), and forward around the brainstem. The fourth

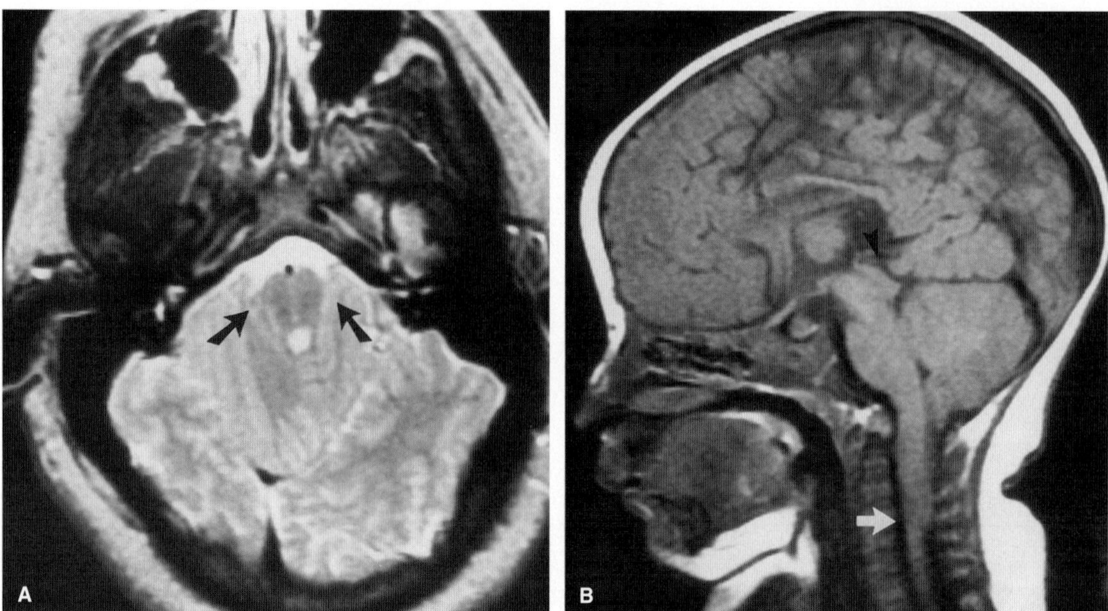

FIGURE 8.28. **Chiari II Malformation. A.** Axial T1WI of a Chiari II malformation demonstrates how the small posterior fossa squeezes the cerebellum around the brainstem (*arrows*). **B.** Sagittal T1WI shows breaking of the tectum (*arrowhead*) and downward displacement of the cerebellar tonsils. A cervicomedullary kink is identified (*arrow*).

ventricle is squeezed into a small vertical slit. The pons and medulla are also squeezed inferiorly, and with fixed attachments of the upper cervical spinal cord, so a cervicomedullary kink often develops as the medulla buckles downward (Fig. 8.28).

Spine. Most Chiari II malformations present with myelomeningocele. A myelomeningocele represents a failure to close the caudal end of the neural tube during development. This splayed open neural tube also fails to induce a dural or bony covering (Fig. 8.29). Please refer to Fig. 10.55 for a review of the spectrum of spinal dysraphism.

Chiari I malformations consist of cerebellar tonsillar ectopia (tonsils extend >5 mm below the foramen magnum). Although patients may be asymptomatic, alterations of CSF dynamics at the level of the foramen magnum are believed to give rise to cervical spinal cord syrinx in some patients (Fig. 8.30). For this reason, the exact number of millimeters of downward extension of the cerebellar tonsils is less important than the degree of crowding of the foramen magnum. Chiari II malformations are associated with cord syrinx (Fig. 8.31).

Cystic Lesions of the Posterior Fossa. A simple working classification of cystic posterior fossa malformations is to consider them within the spectrum of Dandy-Walker malformations.

Dandy-Walker Malformations. In distinction to Chiari malformations, Dandy-Walker malformations are characterized by a large posterior fossa with a high tentorial insertion. The posterior fossa is filled by a cystically

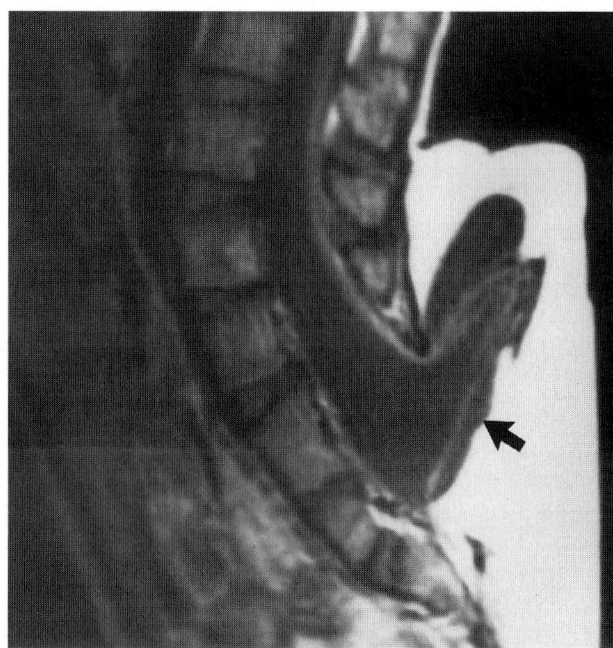

FIGURE 8.29. **Myelomeningocele.** Sagittal T1WI of a myelomeningocele in a patient with Chiari II malformation. The myelomeningocele sac (*arrow*) contains neural tissue and meninges and protrudes through the dysraphic posterior elements of the lumbar spine.

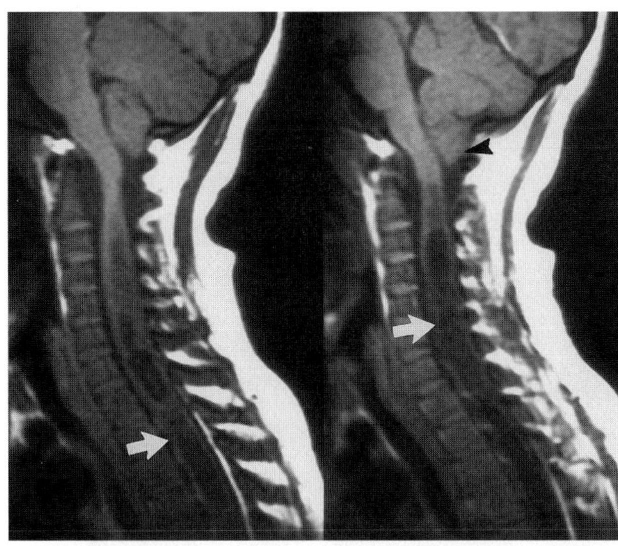

FIGURE 8.30. **Chiari I Malformation: Syrinx.** Altered CSF flow dynamics around the foramen magnum from tonsillar ectopia (*arrowhead*) in this Chiari I malformation patient have resulted in cervical cord syrinx (*arrows*).

dilated fourth ventricle that exerts mass effect (Fig. 8.32). Hypoplasia or absence of the cerebellar vermis and cerebellar hemispheres are associated findings. Hydrocephalus is also common in this disorder, as is callosal hypogenesis. From this definition follow the less severe entities within the spectrum: Dandy-Walker variant and mega cisterna magna, both of which may have a normal position of the torcula.

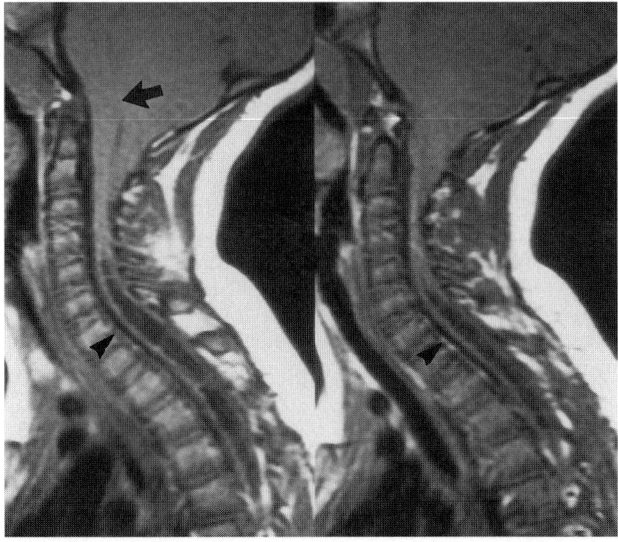

FIGURE 8.31. **Chiari II Malformation: Syrinx.** Sagittal T1WIs show features of Chiari II malformation with syrinx formation in the cervical cord (*arrowheads*). Note the more crowded appearance of the posterior fossa as compared with the Chiari I malformation shown in Fig. 8.30. The cisterna magna is obliterated, and the fourth ventricle (*arrow*) is effaced.

Dandy-Walker variant shows a normal-sized posterior fossa and hypoplasia or absence of the vermis and cerebellar hemispheres but no significant mass effect. ***Mega cisterna magna*** shows a normal-sized posterior fossa and relatively normal cerebellar hemispheres and vermis. It is characterized by a prominent cisterna magna CSF space without mass effect. Mega cisterna magna exerts no mass effect, in distinction from retrocerebellar arachnoid cysts and epidermoid neoplasms. These mass lesions cause an inward convex bowing of brain tissue at their interface, and long-standing masses will cause smooth erosion of the inner table of the skull (see Chapter 5).

THE PHAKOMATOSES

The phakomatoses are a group of hereditary syndromes of the neuroectodermal system that are grouped together because they all share neurologic and cutaneous manifestations.

Neurofibromatosis is divided into type 1 (NF-1, known as von Recklinghausen disease), with characteristic neurocutaneous manifestations, and neurofibromatosis

TABLE 8.5 Neurofibromatosis: Type 1 (NF-1) Versus Type 2 (NF-2)

	NF-1 (von Recklinghausen Syndrome)	*NF-2**
Epidemiology		
Incidence	1 in 4,000	1 in 50,000
Age at presentation	Childhood	Young adult
Affected chromosome	17	22*
CNS findings		
Vestibular schwannomas	No	Yes*
Meningiomas	No	Yes
Spinal glial tumors	No	Yes
Altered signal in white matter	Yes	No
Altered signal in basal ganglia	Yes	No
Dural ectasia	Yes	No
Optic & other gliomas	Yes	Yes
Skeletal findings		
Sphenoid dysplasia	Yes	No
Thinning long bone cortex (ribbon ribs)	Yes	No
Other findings		
Plexiform neurofibromas	Yes	No
Café au lait spots	Typically six or more	Rare
Iris hamartomas (Lisch nodules)	Yes	No
Vascular stenoses	Yes	No

*For NF-2, use the number 2 as your mnemonic: NF-2 patients typically have 2 (bilateral) acoustic schwannomas and an abnormal chromosome 22.

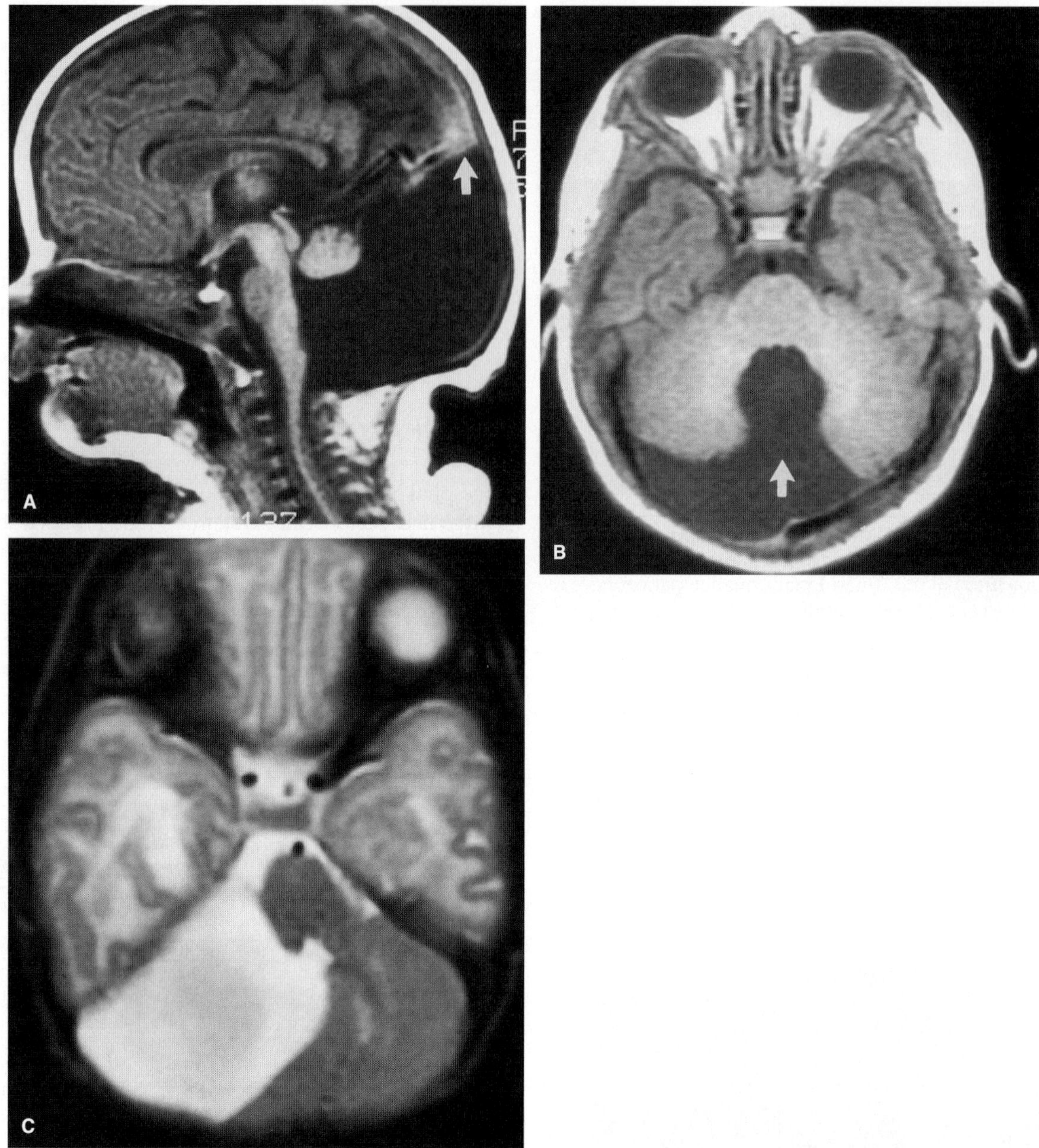

FIGURE 8.32. **Dandy-Walker Malformation. A.** Dandy-Walker malformation characteristically demonstrates a cystic dilated fourth ventricle and vermian agenesis, as demonstrated on this sagittal T1WI. The posterior fossa is enlarged, as seen by a high torcular insertion (*arrow*). **B.** Axial T1WI shows the cystically dilated fourth ventricle (*arrow*). **C.** This case demonstrates some of the features of Dandy-Walker malformation, but there is also asymmetric hypoplasia of the right cerebellar hemisphere.

type 2 (NF-2), which has very few, if any neurocutaneous lesions (Table 8.5). Note that NF-1 is one of the most common inherited CNS disorders, where as NF-2 is about one tenth as common.

Neurofibromatosis type 1 is characterized by skin lesions (café au lait spots), neurofibromas, and ocular findings. The findings in the brain consist of tumors and nonneoplastic lesions in the white matter and globus pallidus. NF-1 is associated with a high incidence of gliomas, with the optic pathways most commonly affected. A typical tumor causes fusiform enlargement of the optic nerve (Fig. 8.33). However, the chiasm, optic tracts, and optic radiations can also become involved. Some optic pathway gliomas are intensely enhancing, but this is not a predictor of histologic grade, a topic covered in detail in Chapter 5. Parenchymal involvement along optic pathways is seen

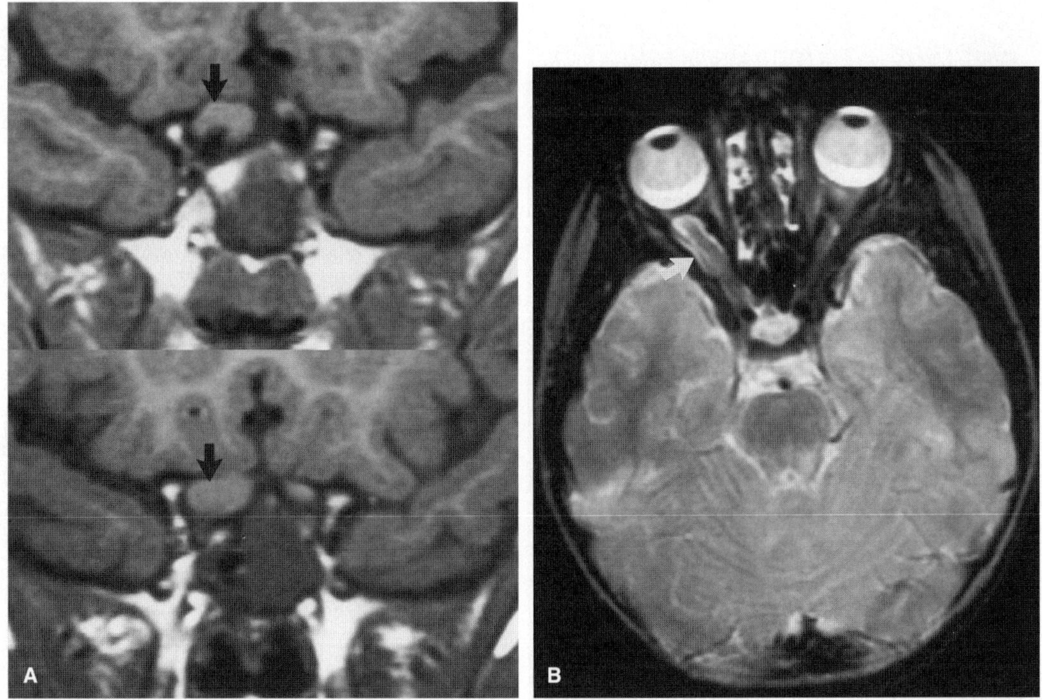

FIGURE 8.33. **Neurofibromatosis: Optic Glioma. A.** Optic nerve gliomas in a neurofibromatosis type I case are fusiform enlargements of the nerve on thin-section coronal T1WIs (*arrows*). **B.** Axial T2WI at the mid-orbit level shows the fusiform enlargement of the right optic nerve (*arrow*).

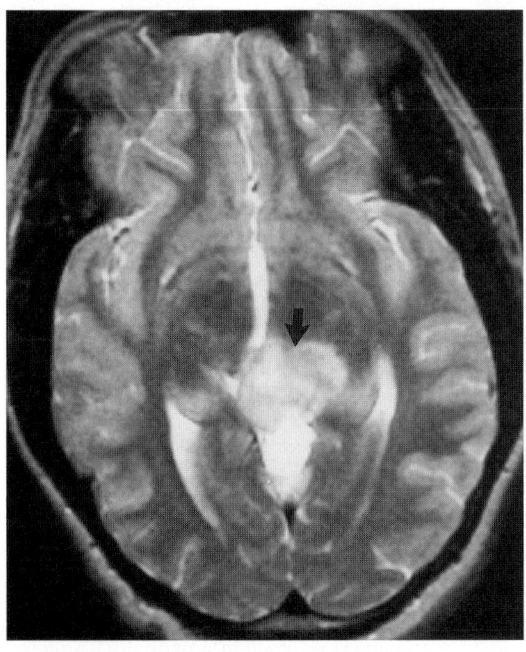

FIGURE 8.34. **Neurofibromatosis: Glioma.** Axial T2WI shows an exophytic tectal glioma (*arrow*) in this patient with neurofibromatosis type I.

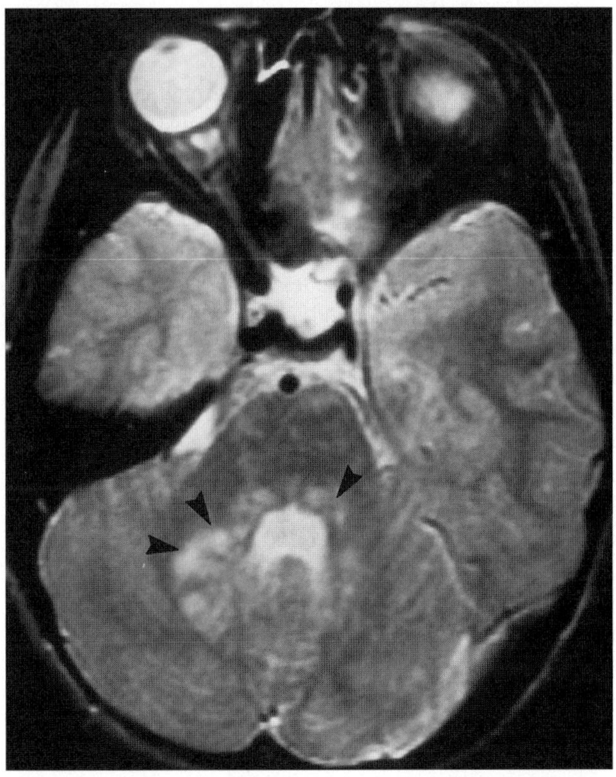

FIGURE 8.35. **Neurofibromatosis: Nonneoplastic Lesions.** T2WI of patient with neurofibromatosis type I shows multifocal area of hyperintense signal in both middle cerebellar peduncles (*arrowheads*).

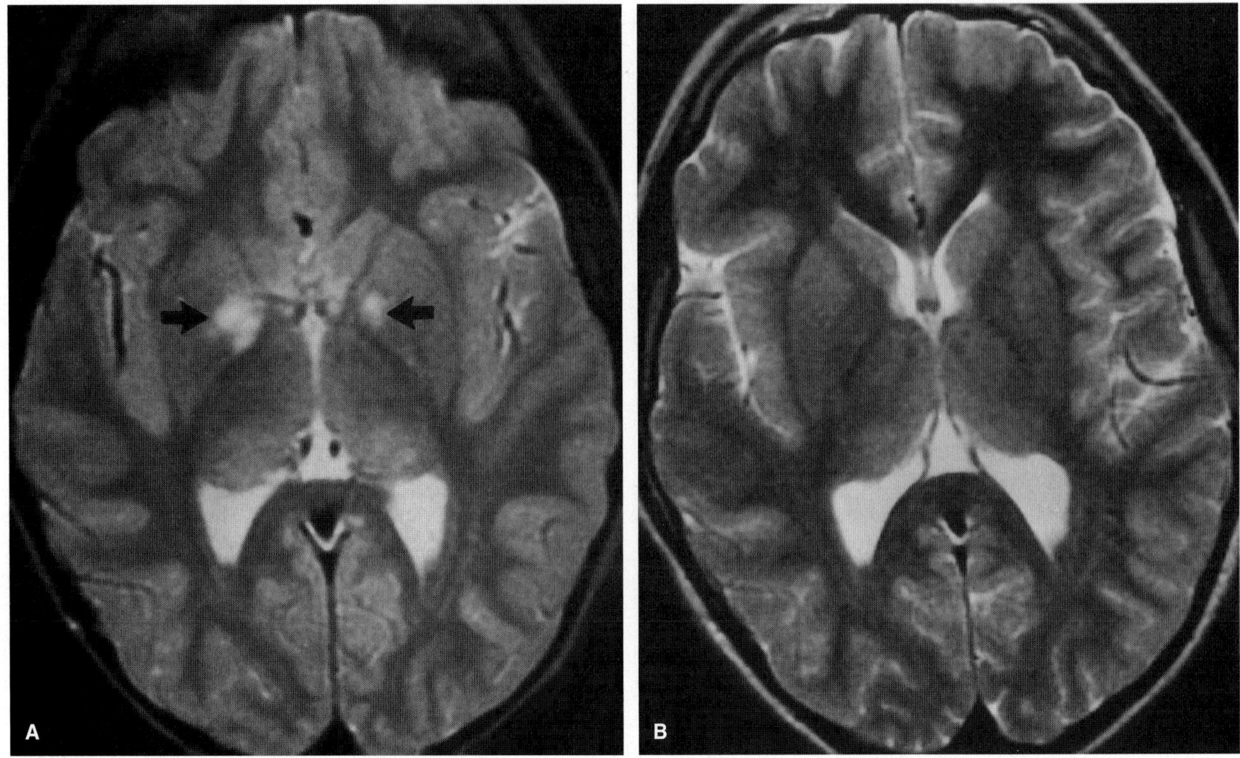

FIGURE 8.36. **Neurofibromatosis: Nonneoplastic Lesions. A.** Hyperintense foci on T2WI are seen in the basal ganglia in this patient with neurofibromatosis type 1 (*arrows*). **B.** The lesions are seen to regress on a 4-year follow-up scan.

as hyperintense signal on T2WIs. Parenchymal gliomas may also occur in the cerebellum, brainstem, and cerebrum (Fig. 8.34).

Hyperintense foci in the deep cerebral and cerebellar white matter are commonly seen on T2WIs. The etiology of these lesions is uncertain but is suggestive of benign myelin vacuolization. These lesions wax and wane when analyzed over serial scans, do not cause mass effect, and do not enhance (Figs. 8.35, 8.36). In general, these lesions tend to regress with increasing age. Lesion progression in a child more than 10 years old warrants close follow-up to rule out neoplastic transformation. Significant enlargement, new mass effect, and gadolinium enhancement may herald degeneration into gliomas. The globus pallidi may also exhibit abnormal hyperintense signal on both T1WIs and T2WIs.

NF-1 has other manifestations. These include plexiform neurofibromas (ropelike masses of neural tissue in subcutaneous soft tissues); vascular lesions (aneurysms, vascular ectasias, stenoses, moyamoya disease); spinal lesions (neurofibromas, meningoceles, scoliosis); and osseous lesions (sphenoid bone/lambdoid suture dysplasia, pseudoarthrosis, rib abnormalities).

Neurofibromatosis type 2 differs considerably from NF-1. The classic feature of NF-2 is bilateral acoustic

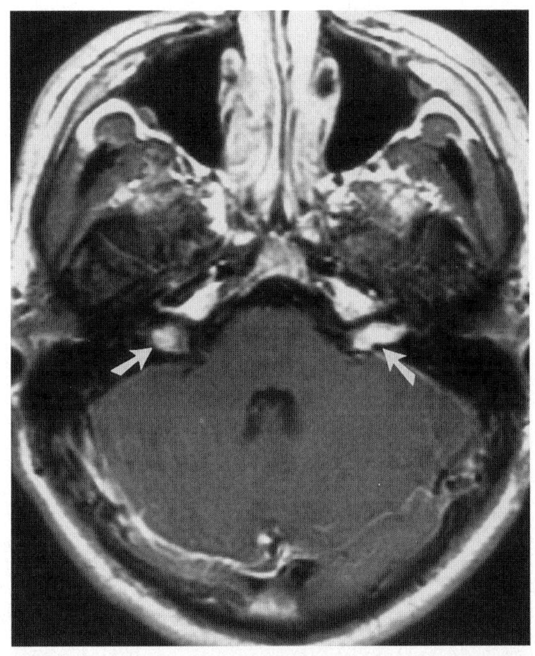

FIGURE 8.37. **Neurofibromatosis Type 2.** Axial T1W post–gadolinium administration image in a patient with neurofibromatosis type 2 shows bilateral enhancing acoustic schwannomas of the eighth cranial nerves (*arrows*).

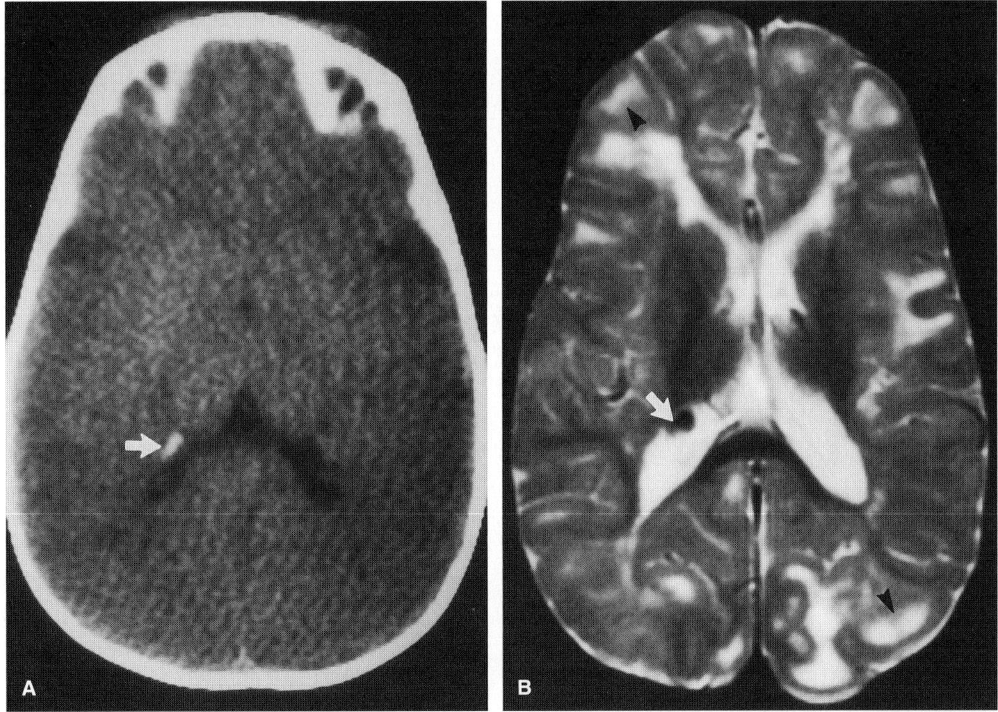

FIGURE 8.38. **Tuberous Sclerosis. A.** An axial slice from a CT scan in a patient with tuberous sclerosis shows a single calcified ependymal tuber (*arrow*). **B.** T2WI shows the same ependymal tuber seen on the CT scan. The tuber is seen as low-signal-intensity nodule (*arrow*). The subcortical tubers are also well demonstrated (*arrowheads*).

neuromas (the modern term for which is vestibular schwannoma; see Chapter 5). These patients often have meningiomas and schwannomas involving other cranial nerves, with cranial nerve V the second most common site for schwannomas in patients with NF-2 (Fig. 8.37). NF-2 also has spinal manifestations, which include meningiomas, ependymomas, and nerve sheath tumors (both schwannomas and neurofibromas).

Tuberous sclerosis is another distinctive neurocutaneous disorder. The skin lesions are adenoma sebaceum and ash-leaf spots. Brain lesions consist of subependymal hamartomas and cortical tubers (Fig. 8.38). Some of the

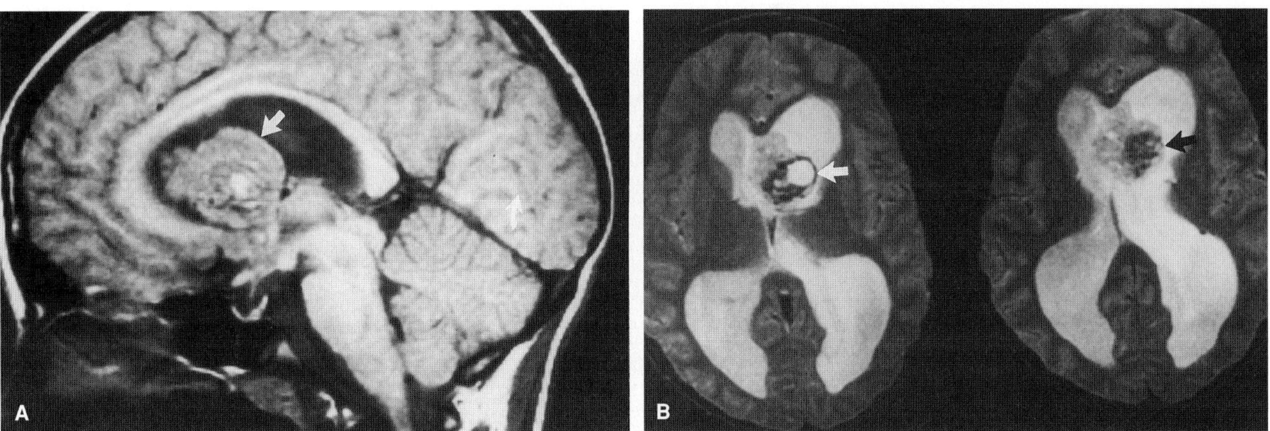

FIGURE 8.39. **Tuberous Sclerosis. A.** In another case of tuberous sclerosis, the sagittal T1WI demonstrates a giant cell astrocytoma arising in the region of the foramen of Monro (*arrow*). **B.** Axial T2WIs of a giant cell astrocytoma with concomitant hydrocephalus. The lesion (*arrows*) is heterogeneous signal intensity.

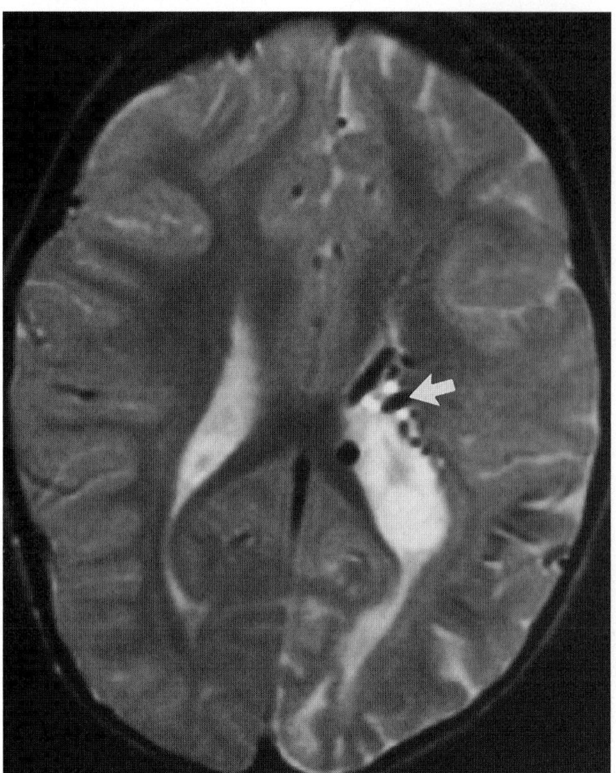

FIGURE 8.40. **Sturge-Weber Syndrome.** Axial T2WI illustrates the dilated ependymal veins seen in Sturge-Weber syndrome. The veins (*arrow*) are serpentine flow voids bordering the ependymal surface of the ventricle.

subependymal nodules near the foramen of Monro can enlarge, cause mass effect, and invade brain tissue. Locally aggressive nodules are called subependymal "giant cell astrocytomas," are typically located at the foramina of Monro, and may lead to hydrocephalus (Fig. 8.39).

Both cortical and subependymal lesions can undergo age-dependent calcification. Subependymal nodules represent hamartomas, and before calcification they tend to parallel white matter signal on MR images. Subependymal nodules are distinct from heterotopic gray matter in both their signal characteristics and tendency to calcify. Calcified nodules may be isointense or hyperintense on T1WIs. Enhancement of nodules at the foramen of Monro does not determine malignant transformation to a giant cell astrocytoma; rather, look for brain invasion to make this distinction. Cortical tubers are usually hypointense on T1WIs and hyperintense on T2WIs, and they may calcify.

Sturge-Weber Syndrome, or encephalotrigeminal angiomatosis, features angiomatous lesions of the skin and meninges. The facial lesion (a skin angioma called a port-wine nevus) appears in the ophthalmic division of the fifth cranial nerve. The pathologic entity seen in the brain is pial angiomatosis. These pial angiomas undergo age-dependent calcification and appear on CT scans as gyral cortical calcifications. The pial angiomatosis results in chronic ischemia of the gray matter, leading to gyral atrophy and underlying gliosis.

Another sequela of pial angiomatosis is alteration of normal superficial cortical venous drainage with concomitant enlargement of deep and subependymal veins (Fig. 8.40). These dilated subependymal veins can mimic arteriovenous malformations. Gadolinium enhancement can reveal the full extent of pial angiomatosis and is helpful in cases where calcific atrophic changes have not yet occurred (Fig. 8.41). Young children may show subtle hypointensity of the underlying white matter on T2WIs without calcification of the cortex. Ipsilateral choroid plexus hypertrophy is another feature of this entity (Fig. 8.42). The gradient-recalled echo technique should be used on MR images to accentuate the presence of calcium (Fig. 8.43).

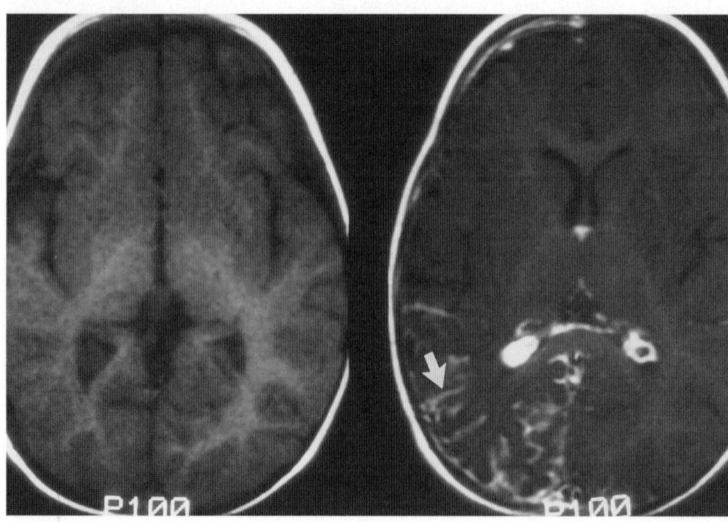

FIGURE 8.41. **Sturge-Weber Syndrome.** A young patient with Sturge-Weber syndrome with before (*left*) and after (*right*) gadolinium T1WI demonstrating the full extent of pial angiomatosis (*arrow*). Gadolinium may be particularly useful in younger patients who do not yet demonstrate cortical calcifications.

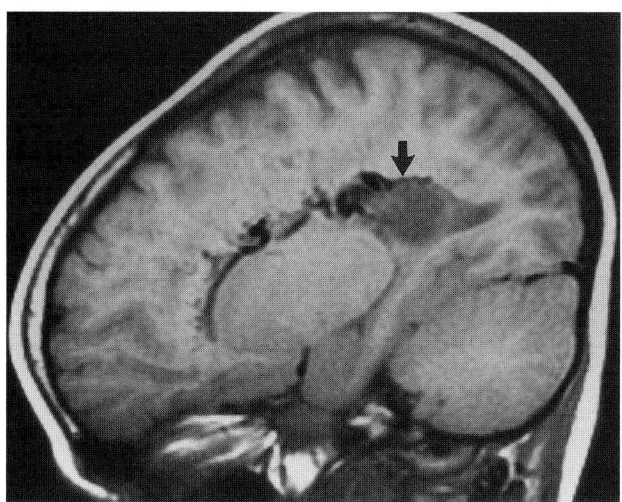

FIGURE 8.42. **Sturge-Weber Syndrome.** Sagittal T1WI of a patient with Sturge-Weber syndrome shows ipsilateral choroid plexus hypertrophy (*arrow*).

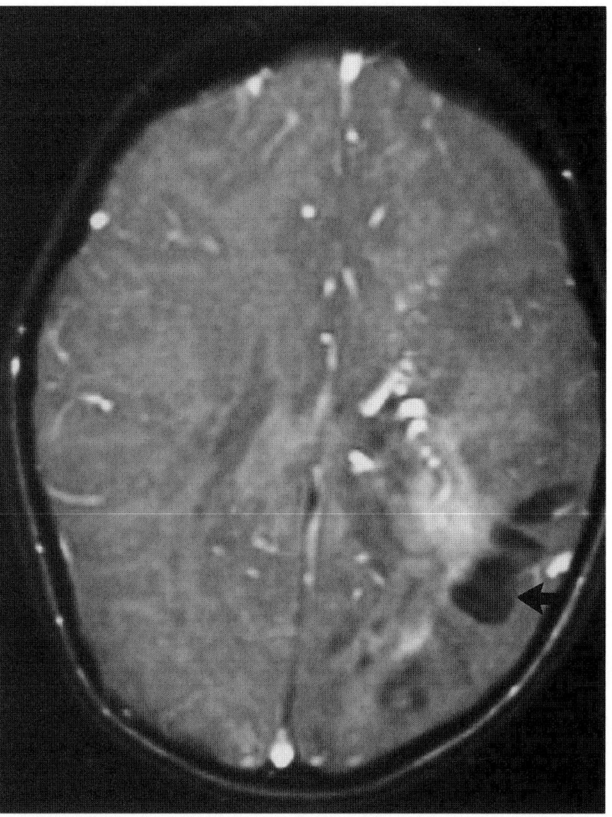

FIGURE 8.43. **Sturge-Weber Syndrome.** Gradient-recalled echo image accentuates the magnetic susceptibility artifact associated with the cortical calcifications (*arrow*) of Sturge-Weber syndrome.

Von Hippel-Lindau Syndrome is an inherited disorder consisting of retinal angiomas and cerebellar and spinal hemangioblastomas. Hemangioblastomas are considered benign neoplasms (see Chapter 5), and the presence of multifocal spinal cord nodules near the pia-arachnoid surface represents multicentric tumors, not drop metastasis.

Characteristic features of cerebellar hemangioblastomas include a well-circumscribed cystic lesion with an enhancing mural nodule. Other appearances include solid tumors, solid masses with central cysts, and a cyst alone (Figs. 8.44, 8.45). Another helpful finding is a large blood vessel leading to the nodule. The small multifocal

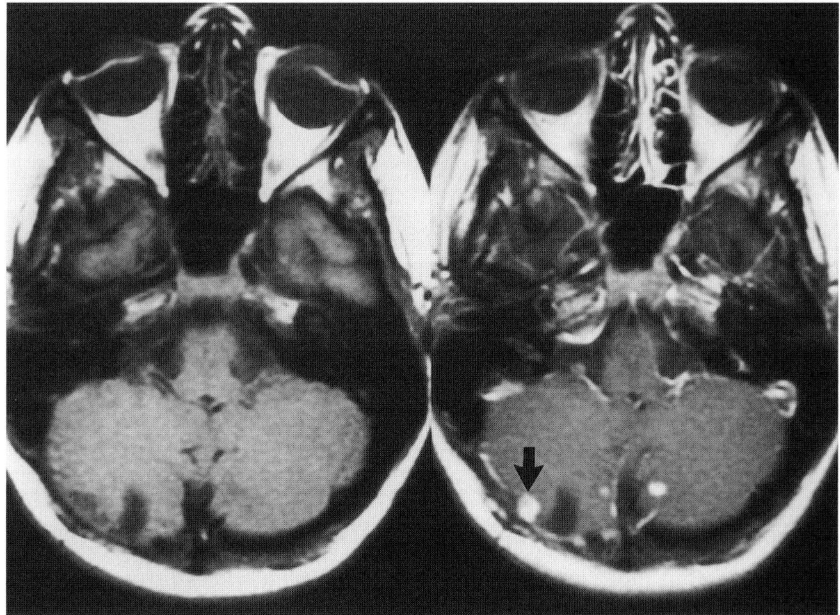

FIGURE 8.44. **Von Hippel-Lindau Syndrome.** Axial T1WIs in a patient with von Hippel-Lindau syndrome. The left image is pre–gadolinium injection and the right image is post–gadolinium injection. Some of the lesions are cystic, and one of the enhancing foci (*arrow*) was seen to represent a mural nodule on a lower image.

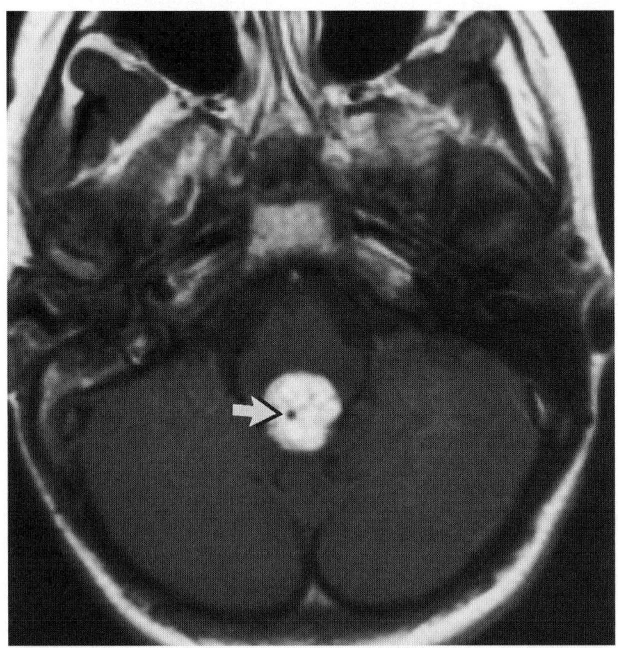

FIGURE 8.45. **Von Hippel-Lindau Syndrome.** Von Hippel-Lindau syndrome has a variable appearance, as demonstrated in this case of a solid enhancing mass in the fourth ventricle. A central speck of hypointensity represents a blood vessel (*arrow*).

hemangioblastoma nodules are seen near the pial surface of the cerebellum or spinal cord.

Although they are considered benign neoplasms, recurrence rates of up to 25% are reported. These vascular lesions are prone to sudden spontaneous hemorrhage. Gadolinium-enhanced MR imaging is the examination of choice for preoperative evaluation. Other associations with von Hippel-Lindau syndrome include renal cell carcinoma, along with angiomas of the liver and kidney.

SUGGESTED READINGS

Barkovich AJ. Pediatric Neuroimaging. 4th ed. Philadelphia: Lippincott Williams & Wilkins, 2005.

Barkovich AJ. MR and CT evaluation of profound neonatal and infantile asphyxia. AJNR Am J Neuroradiol 1992;13:959–972.

Barkovich AJ, Raybaud CJ. Malformations of cortical development. Neuroimaging Clin North Am 2004;41:401–423.

Barkovich AJ, Hajnal BL, Vigneron D, et al. Prediction of neuromotor outcome in perinatal asphyxia: evaluation of MR scoring systems. AJNR Am J Neuroradiol 1998;19:143–149.

Brodsky MC, Glasier CM. Optic nerve hypoplasia: clinical significance of associated central nervous system abnormalities on magnetic resonance imaging. Arch Ophthalmol 1993;111:66–74.

Glass, RB, Fernbach SK, Norton KI, et al. The infant skull: a vault of information. Radiographics 2004;24:507–522.

Hunt RW, Neil JJ, Coleman LT, et al. Apparent diffusion coefficient in the posterior limb of the internal capsule predicts outcome after perinatal asphyxia. Pediatrics 2004;114:999–1002.

Inder TE, Huppi PS, Warfield S, et al. Periventricular white matter injury in the premature neonate is followed by reduced cerebral cortex gray matter volume at term. Ann Neurol 1999;46:755–760.

McLone DG, Dias MS. The Chiari II malformation: cause and impact. Childs Nerv Syst 2003;19:540–550.

Ment LR, Bada HS, Barnes P, et al. Practice parameter: neuroimaging of the neonate. Neurology 2002;58:1726–1738.

Nelson MD Jr, Maher K, Gilles FH. A different approach to cysts of the posterior fossa. Pediatr Radiol 2004;34:720–732.

Simon EM, et al. The middle interhemispheric variant of holoprosencephaly. AJNR Am J Neuroradiol 2002;23:151–156.

Smirniotopoulos JG, Murphy FM. The phakomatoses. AJNR Am J Neuroradiol 1992;13:725–746.

Truwit CL, Lempert TE. Pediatric Neuroimaging: A Casebook Approach. Piedmont, CA: DPS Press, 1991.

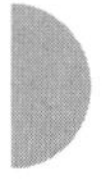

Chapter 9

Head and Neck Imaging

Jerome A. Barakos

Paranasal Sinuses and Nasal Cavity

Skull Base
Tumors of the Skull Base
Temporal Bone

Suprahyoid Head and Neck
Superficial Mucosal Space
Parapharyngeal Space
Carotid Space
Parotid Space
Masticator Space
Retropharyngeal Space
Prevertebral Space
Trans-spatial Diseases

Lymph Nodes

Orbit

Congenital Lesions

Head and neck is a term used collectively to describe the extracranial structures, including the sinonasal cavity, skull base, pharynx, oral cavity, larynx, neck, orbit, and temporal bone. The head and neck region encompasses a tremendous spectrum of tissues in a compact space, with almost every organ system represented, including the digestive, respiratory, nervous, osseous, and vascular systems. Because of this anatomic complexity, the head and neck region is an area approached with considerable trepidation. However, accurate assessment of this area can be accomplished by understanding both the normal anatomy and the scope of pathologic entities that may occur. We will begin our discussion by considering lesions of the paranasal sinuses and nasal cavity. This will be followed by a review of the skull base, the deep spaces of the neck, the lymph nodes, the orbits, and finally congenital head and neck lesions.

Imaging Methods. Both multislice helical CT and MR can provide exquisite imaging of the normal and pathologic anatomy of the head and neck. Although each modality has advantages and disadvantages, the decision on whether to use CT versus MR for each individual case is often based on considering which technique the patient is more likely to tolerate. For example, if a patient has difficulty handling their oral secretions because of prior head and neck surgery, particularly following tracheotomy or partial glossectomy, they may have significant hardship lying still for the time required for MR scanning. In such cases, the rapid imaging time of multislice helical CT is more likely to yield a study unmarred by motion artifact. Because calcification is better depicted with CT, this is the modality of choice when looking for obstructing salivary ductal calculi (sialoliths) or for the detection of fractures. In contrast, MR provides outstanding sensitivity for the discrimination of soft tissues and often better demonstrates the full extent of pathology. At the same time, the superior tissue contrast discrimination of MR allows for enhanced diagnostic specificity. The direct multiplanar capability of MR may also provide for improved evaluation of pathologic entities. For example, because of the horizontal orientation of the palate, floor of the mouth, and skull base, sagittal and coronal imaging are invaluable in optimally assessing these areas.

Positron Emission Tomography (PET). The advent of PET imaging has had a profound effect on the evaluation of head and neck malignancies. In combination with either MR or CT imaging, PET has greatly increased the sensitivity and specificity in the evaluation of primary as well as recurrent malignancies. PET is a functional imaging modality based upon the distribution of a glucose analogue radioisotope (^{18}F-fluorodeoxyglucose). Pathologic conditions that have an affinity for glucose will take up this

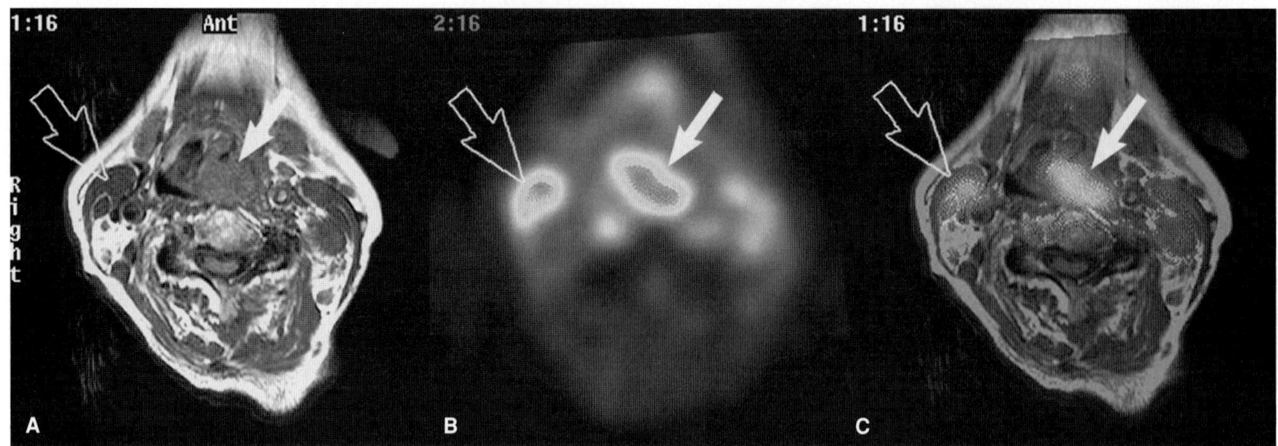

FIGURE 9.1. **(Color Plates) Positron Emission Tomography (PET). A.** Axial T1WI of a 77-year-old man who presented with a large right hypopharyngeal malignancy (*solid arrow*) and extensive ipsilateral necrotic adenopathy (not shown). As expected, histology reflected a squamous cell carcinoma, the most common malignancy arising from the head and neck mucosal surfaces. PET **(B)** and fused MR/PET **(C)** scans confirm the abnormal radioisotope accumulation within the hypopharyngeal malignancy (*solid arrows*). However, the PET study demonstrates an abnormality of the right sternocleidomastoid muscle that was not suspected on MR imaging (*open arrows*). This proved to be a diffuse infiltrative metastatic focus of the right sternocleidomastoid muscle. This case demonstrates the value and increased specificity of combining functional/physiologic imaging (PET) with morphologic imaging (MR).

isotope at a greater rate than normal surrounding tissues and thus be identifiable as areas of abnormality (Fig. 9.1).

Lesions found on PET scan are characterized by a standardized uptake value (SUV). The SUV refers to the relative radioactivity of a particular lesion when standardized to the injection dose and adjusted for body weight. As a result, the SUV is an absolute value that can be compared from patient to patient and exam to exam. In general, an SUV of greater than 3.0 is considered pathologic, but there are many caveats. A wide variety of nonmalignant conditions may give rise to an elevated SUV, most notably infection and postoperative changes. Additionally, some neoplasms have poor glucose affinity, resulting in a low SUV. PET alone may be highly sensitive, but it is not very specific. The true benefit of PET is realized when its physiologic/functional information is combined with the high-spatial-resolution morphologic information of CT and MR. In summary, combining PET findings with CT and/or MR results in a marked increase in specificity, making this combination a powerful diagnostic tool.

PARANASAL SINUSES AND NASAL CAVITY

Sinusitis. Inflammatory disease is the most common pathology involving the paranasal sinuses and nasal cavity. Mild mucosal thickening, primarily within the maxillary and ethmoid sinuses, is common, even in asymptomatic individuals. In contrast, acute sinusitis is characterized by the presence of air–fluid levels or foamy-appearing sinus secretions and is typically caused by a viral upper respiratory tract infection (Fig. 9.2). In chronic sinusitis, changes include mucoperiosteal thickening as well as osseous thickening of the sinus walls. Soft tissue findings suggestive of sinusitis are best detected on T2WIs, as they are often high in signal. An exception is chronic sinus secretions that have become so desiccated that they yield no signal and may mimic an aerated sinus. These sinus concretions and the bony wall thickening associated with chronic sinusitis are most easily appreciated on CT.

Endoscopic sinonasal surgery, used for the evaluation and treatment of inflammatory sinonasal disease, is being performed with increasing frequency. Direct coronal sinus CT provides exquisite definition of sinonasal anatomy and provides pre-endoscopic sinus assessment (Fig. 9.3). Knowledge of the anatomy of the lateral wall of the nasal cavity and routes of mucociliary drainage of the paranasal sinuses is critical to understanding patterns of inflammatory sinonasal disease. A major area of mucociliary drainage is the middle meatus, known as the *ostiomeatal unit.* It is important to note that disease limited to the infundibulum of the maxillary ostium will result in isolated obstruction of the maxillary sinus. In contrast, a lesion located in the hiatus semilunaris (middle meatus) results in combined obstruction of the ipsilateral maxillary sinus, anterior and middle ethmoid air cells, and the frontal sinus. This combined pattern of sinonasal disease has been described as the "ostiomeatal pattern" of obstruction. This pattern is significant because it indicates that one's

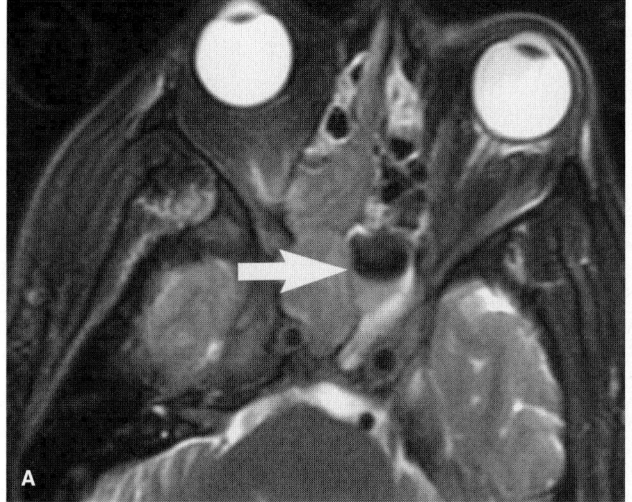

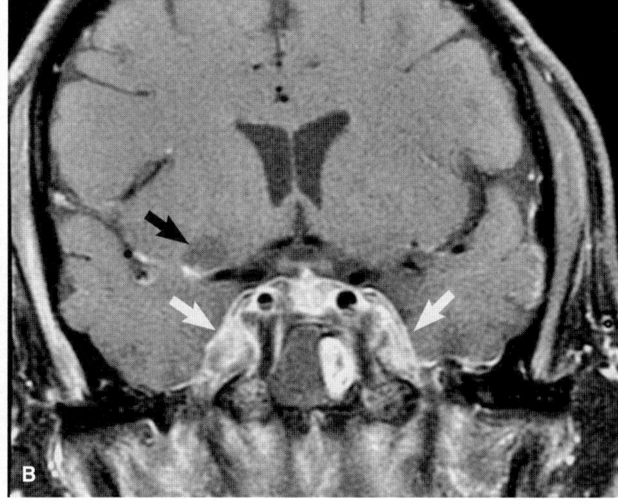

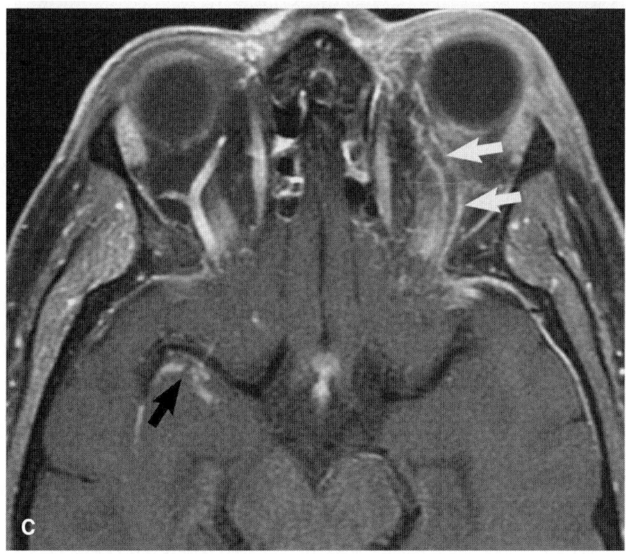

FIGURE 9.2. **Acute Sinusitis With Cavernous Sinus Thrombosis. A.** Axial T2WI of a 27-year-old man who presented with a rapidly progressive sinusitis. The right sphenoid and ethmoid sinuses are opacified, with an air–fluid level within the left sphenoid sinus (*arrow*). Sphenoid sinusitis is of great clinical concern as it may easily extend intracranially owing to the presence of valveless veins. Coronal T1WI **(B)** and axial fat-saturated T1WI with gadolinium contrast **(C).** The patient's clinical condition deteriorated rapidly as the infection extended into the cavernous sinus, with resultant cavernous sinus and left superior ophthalmic vein thrombosis. The cavernous sinus thrombosis is characterized by the marked enlargement of the sinuses (*arrows,* **B**), while frank thrombus is visualized within the left superior ophthalmic vein (*arrows,* **C**). Differential diagnostic conditions would include a carotid-cavernous fistula and Tolosa-Hunt syndrome (an idiopathic nongranulomatous inflammatory condition of the cavernous sinus). Note the parenchymal abscess forming along the right middle cerebral artery cistern (*black arrows*).

attention should be directed to identifying the offending lesion within the hiatus semilunaris, rather than simply describing the presence of diffuse sinus disease.

Several common complications are associated with sinusitis, including inflammatory polyps, mucous retention cysts, mucoceles, and most importantly cavernous sinus thrombosis.

Inflammatory Polyps. Chronic inflammation leads to mucosal hyperplasia, which results in mucosal redundancy and polyp formation. Most often these polyps blend imperceptibly with the mucoperiosteal thickening and cannot be clearly differentiated. When an antral polyp expands to the point where it prolapses through the sinus ostium, it is referred to as an *antrochoanal* polyp. Although these polyps may not be associated with chronic sinusitis, they are similar to inflammatory polyps in that they represent areas of reactive mucosal thickening. Their characteristic appearance is that of a soft tissue mass extending from the maxillary sinus to fill the ipsilateral nasal cavity and nasopharynx. Often, the ostium of the maxillary sinus will be enlarged secondary to the mass effect of the polyp. The importance in recognizing such a lesion is that if it is surgically snared as if it were a nasal polyp, without regard for its antral stalk, it will recur.

Mucous retention cysts simply represent obstructed mucous glands within the mucosal lining. These lesions have a characteristic rounded appearance, measuring one to several centimeters in diameter, with the maxillary sinus being most commonly involved. These lesions are commonly recognized in asymptomatic individuals.

Mucocele is similar to a retention cyst, but instead of a single mucous gland becoming obstructed, the entire sinus is obstructed. This typically occurs because of a mass obstructing the draining sinus ostium. The characteristic feature of a mucocele is frank expansion of the sinus with associated sinus wall bony thinning and remodeling. The frontal sinus is the sinus most commonly affected, but any sinus may be involved (Fig. 9.4). If the mucocele becomes

B: ETHMOID BULLA
mm: MIDDLE MEATUS
m : MIDDLE TURBINATE
u: UNCINATE PROCESS
im: INFERIOR MEATUS
it: INFERIOR TURBINATE
M: MAXILLARY SINUS
S: NASAL SEPTUM
***: HIATUS SEMILUNARIS
- - -: INFUNDIBULUM
→: MUCOCILIARY CLEARANCE OF THE MAXILLARY SINUS

FIGURE 9.3. **Ostiomeatal Unit (OMU).** Line drawing in coronal plane demonstrates the anatomy of the OMU. Lines with arrows show the normal route of mucociliary clearance. Infundibular (*dashed line*) and OMU (*solid line*) patterns of obstruction are shown. Coronal CT far surpasses plain sinus films in evaluating problems of the OMU for potential relief through endoscopic surgery. B, ethmoid bulla; M, maxillary sinus; u, uncinate process; mt, middle turbinate; mm, middle meatus; im, inferior meatus; it, inferior turbinate; S, nasal septum. (Reprinted with permission. From Babbel RW, Harnsberger HR, Sonkens J, Hunt S. Recurring patterns of inflammatory sinonasal disease demonstrated on screening sinus CT. AJNR Am J Neuroradiol 1992;13:903–912.)

infected, it demonstrates peripheral enhancement and is referred to as a *mucopyocele*.

Inverting Papilloma. A variety of papillomas occur within the nasal cavity, but most attention has focused on the inverting papilloma. These papillomas are named based on their histologic appearance. In this condition, the neoplastic nasal epithelium inverts and grows into the underlying mucosa. These papillomas are not believed to be associated with allergy or chronic infection because they are almost invariably unilateral in location. Inverting

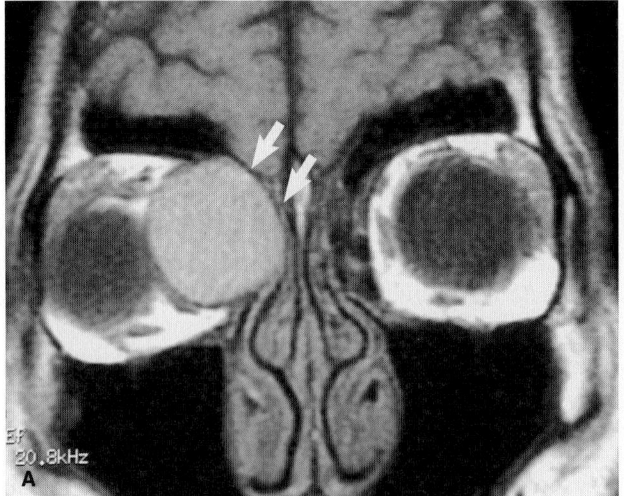

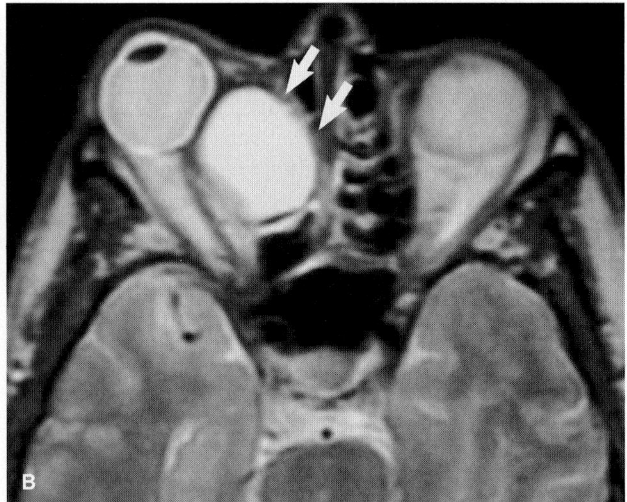

FIGURE 9.4. **Sinus Mucocele. A.** Coronal T1WI. **B.** Axial T2WI. Patient presented with proptosis, resulting from mass effect from an ethmoid sinus mucocele (*arrows*). A mucocele results from chronic obstruction of a paranasal sinus that becomes blocked and converted into a fluid-filled cyst. Over time this lesion may expand, eroding bone and resulting in proptosis. Differential diagnostic considerations would include a dermoid cyst, which would be characterized by the presence of fat (see Fig. 9.36).

papillomas occur exclusively on the lateral nasal wall, centered on the hiatus semilunaris. Because of their increased association with squamous cell carcinoma, it is recommended that these lesions be surgically resected with wide mucosal margins.

Juvenile nasopharyngeal angiofibromas are typically seen in male adolescents presenting with epistaxis. The tumor arises from fibrovascular stroma of the nasal wall adjacent to the sphenopalatine foramen. This is a benign tumor that can be very locally aggressive. In an adolescent male presenting with a nasal mass and epistaxis, it is important to have a high clinical suspicion for this lesion, because life-threatening hemorrhage may result if a biopsy or limited resection is attempted. The tumor characteristically fills the nasopharynx and bows the posterior wall of the maxillary sinus forward. In fact, the retromaxillary pterygopalatine fossa location is a hallmark feature that should elicit this diagnosis for consideration. Juvenile nasopharyngeal angiofibromas enhance markedly with contrast administration, differentiating them from the rarer lymphangioma. Preoperatively, interventional radiology may play a role in embolization of these lesions, making them less vascular and facilitating surgical resection.

Malignancies. The tissues within the paranasal sinuses and nasal cavity that give rise to malignancies include squamous epithelium, lymphoid tissue, and minor salivary glands. The corresponding malignancies are therefore squamous cell carcinoma, lymphoma, and minor salivary tumors. Because the entire upper aerodigestive tract is lined with squamous epithelium, it follows that *squamous cell carcinoma* is the most common malignancy (80% to 90%) of not only the paranasal sinuses and nasal cavity, but of the entire head and neck. Squamous cell carcinoma of the sinuses is often clinically silent until it is quite advanced. Early symptoms are usually related to obstructive sinusitis. Imaging findings consist of an opacified sinus with associated bony wall destruction. These findings are nonspecific and do not allow differentiation from non-Hodgkin lymphoma or a minor salivary gland malignancy. The presence of constitutional symptoms with prominent head and neck or systemic adenopathy suggests lymphoma, particularly in a child or young adult.

Minor salivary glands are dispersed throughout the upper aerodigestive tract but are most highly concentrated in the palate. Any of these minor salivary glands found throughout the head and neck may give rise to salivary neoplasms. In contrast to parotid gland salivary neoplasms, the majority of which are benign, most minor salivary neoplasms are malignant. The most common salivary malignancies include adenoid cystic carcinoma, adenocarcinoma, and mucoepidermoid carcinoma.

An *esthesioneuroblastoma* is an additional malignancy that should be mentioned when describing lesions of the nasal cavity. The esthesioneuroblastoma is a tumor that arises from the neurosensory receptor cells of the olfactory nerve and mucosa. Thus, this lesion may originate anywhere from the cribriform plate to the turbinates. This tumor is often quite destructive by the time of diagnosis and is found high within the nasal vault (Fig. 9.5). Involvement of the cribriform plate with extension into the anterior cranial fossa is not uncommon with esthesioneuroblastoma and should suggest this lesion.

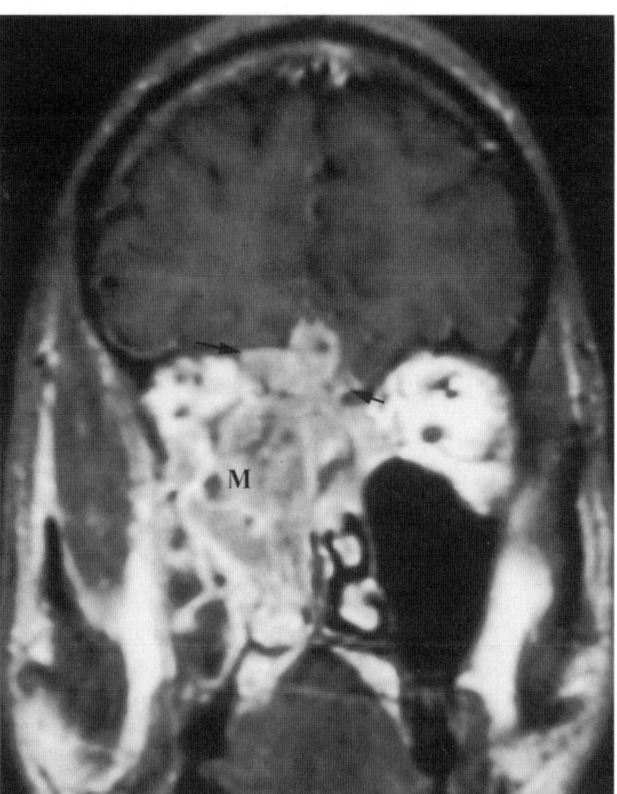

FIGURE 9.5. **Esthesioneuroblastoma.** Coronal fat-suppressed postgadolinium T1WI. A large destructive mass (M) in the nasal cavity extends through the cribriform plate into the anterior cranial fossa (*arrows*). This degree of frank bony destruction is unusual for squamous cell carcinoma and lymphoma, but characteristic for esthesioneuroblastoma.

In assessing the size and extent of sinonasal cavity pathology, it is often difficult to differentiate the offending lesion from associated obstructed sinus secretions. In such instances, heavily T2W sequences are of value, because in general, sinus secretions will be brighter than the malignancy, which is often isointense with respect to muscle.

SKULL BASE

The skull base extends from the nose anteriorly to the occipital protuberance posteriorly and is composed of five bones: the ethmoid, sphenoid, occipital, temporal, and frontal bones. The skull base contains many foramina through which both vessels and nerves pass. Because the skull base has an undulating surface with a horizontal orientation, coronal or sagittal images are valuable in its evaluation.

Tumors of the Skull Base

Tumors may arise that are intrinsic to the skull base. Additionally, an extrinsic lesion may extend to involve the skull base either from above or below. Any lesion from the paranasal sinuses and nasal cavity already described may extend to involve the skull base. Other lesions that may extend to involve the skull base include paragangliomas, neural sheath tumors (schwannoma and neurofibroma), and meningiomas. Although various primary malignant neoplasms of the skull base are described in the following, most malignant lesions of the skull base are metastatic in origin.

Primary malignant neoplasms are relatively uncommon, comprising only about 2% to 3% of skull base tumors. The three most common primary malignant tumors are chordoma, chondrosarcoma, and osteogenic sarcoma. *Chordoma* is a bone neoplasm that arises from remnants of the primitive notochord. Classically, this lesion will present as a destructive midline mass centered in the clivus. These tumors may be found anywhere along the craniospinal axis; typically 35% of lesions involve the clivus, 50% the sacrum, and 15% the vertebral bodies. Radiographically, this lesion is characterized as a midline destructive bony lesion with predilection for the sphenooccipital synchondrosis. On a sagittal image, the sphenooccipital synchondrosis is occasionally seen as a horizontal line in the midclivus, midway between sella and basion (tip of clivus). *Chondrosarcomas* are malignant tumors that develop from cartilage. Because the skull base is preformed in cartilage, there is a predilection for chondrosarcoma to involve the skull base. A preferred site of origin is parasellar in location, at the petroclival junction. *Osteogenic sarcoma* is typically the result of prior radiation therapy or malignant transformation of Paget disease.

Although a central destructive clival lesion is characteristic for chordoma and a paraclival destructive bony lesion is suggestive of chondrosarcoma, our differential diagnostic list includes several other bony lesions. The skull base, like any bone, may be affected by metastases, myeloma, plasmacytoma, fibrous dysplasia, and Paget disease. As with any bony lesion, CT helps to differentiate among these diagnostic possibilities. For example, fibrous dysplasia will reveal a smooth, ground-glass appearance on CT, while Paget disease will demonstrate trabecular coarsening, and neither of these conditions will reveal bony destruction.

Lesions of the jugular foramen are most commonly paragangliomas and are discussed under the heading "Carotid Space." These patients commonly present with pulsatile tinnitus and a conductive hearing loss. These tumors are best initially evaluated with CT. If extension into the jugular fossa is identified, MR is valuable in defining the full extent of the lesion. CT often demonstrates "motheaten" destruction of the bone surrounding the jugular fossa, with MR revealing the typical heterogeneous "salt and pepper" signal related to numerous flow voids. Malignant tumors are often indistinguishable from paragangliomas on CT, but most fail to demonstrate flow voids on MR. Other lesions of the jugular fossa include schwannomas (arising from cranial nerves IX to XI) and meningiomas. These lesions cause a smooth expansion of the jugular foramen with marked enhancement. Additionally, schwannomas may demonstrate cystic components.

Temporal Bone

Although a thorough discussion of the temporal bone is beyond the scope of this chapter, we will focus on some highlights. The most common diseases involving the temporal bone are inflammatory in nature and include cholesteatomas. Eustachian tube dysfunction with resultant decreased intratympanic pressure is believed to be the principal defect responsible for inflammatory disease of the middle ear and mastoid.

Cholesteatoma is an epidermoid cyst composed of desquamating stratified squamous epithelium. These cysts enlarge because of the progressive accumulation of epithelial debris within their lumen. They may be either congenital (2%) or acquired (98%). Congenital cholesteatomas originate from epithelial rests within or adjacent to the temporal bone. Acquired cholesteatomas originate from the stratified squamous epithelium of the tympanic membrane. These begin as localized tympanic membrane retraction pockets. The diagnosis of a cholesteatoma is based on the detection of a soft tissue mass within the middle ear cavity, typically with associated bony erosion. The superior portion of the tympanic membrane (pars flaccida) retracts easily and is the most common site for formation of an acquired cholesteatoma. Cholesteatomas arising in this area originate within the Prussak space (superior recess of the tympanic membrane), which is located medial to the pars flaccida between the scutum and the neck of the malleus. Thus, a finding of soft tissue in this region with subtle erosion of the scutum and medial displacement of the ossicles is characteristic of a cholesteatoma. Note that when fluid or inflammatory pathology is present, such as with otitis media, these changes cannot be differentiated from cholesteatoma because they have similar densities.

Although most cholesteatomas can be easily diagnosed otoscopically, the clinician cannot judge the size and full extent of the lesion. As a result, CT plays an important role in determining the size of the lesion, as well as the status of the ossicles, the labyrinth, the tegmen, and the facial nerve. MR has a limited role in the evaluation of erosive lesions of the temporal bone, because the lack of landmarks does not allow localization of the process and it gives no information concerning the status of the ossicles and other bony structures.

Cholesterol granuloma, also known as *giant cholesterol cyst,* is a type of granulation tissue that may involve the petrous apex. These lesions represent petrous apex air cells that have become partially obstructed and are filled with cholesterol debris and hemorrhagic fluid. Because of their hemorrhagic components, these lesions are characterized by high signal on both T1WIs and T2WIs. When faced with an opacified petrous apex, differential diagnostic considerations include: retained fluid secretions (parallels signal intensity of fluid, dark T1, bright T2, and no enhancement); petrous apicitis (parallels signal intensity of abscess, dark T1, bright T2, and ring enhancement); and nonaerated petrous apex (parallels signal intensity of fatty bone marrow, bright T1, dark T2, and no enhancement).

SUPRAHYOID HEAD AND NECK

When a patient presents with a head and neck mass, the age of presentation is an important consideration when establishing a differential diagnostic list. In the pediatric age group, the majority of lesions (>90%) will be benign and consist of a variety of congenital or inflammatory entities (see "Congenital Lesions"). If a malignancy is encountered, it will most likely be a lymphoma (e.g., Burkitt lymphoma if rapid growth is noted) or rhabdomyosarcoma. In sharp contrast, when an adult presents with a head and neck mass (excluding thyroid lesions), the vast majority of lesions (>90%) will be malignant (Fig. 9.6). In the younger adult (20 to 40 years), the most common malignancy will be lymphoma (Fig. 9.7), and in adults older than 40 years, the most common neck mass will be nodal metastases.

The suprahyoid head and neck is traditionally divided into compartments that include the nasopharynx, oropharynx, and oral cavity. An understanding of the division between these spaces is essential to accurately determine and describe the full extent of mucosal lesions.

The term *nasopharynx* is frequently misused as a nonspecific term to describe any area in the upper aerodigestive tract. In fact, the nasopharynx refers to a very specific portion of the pharynx. The nasopharynx lies above the oropharynx and is divided from the oropharynx by a horizontal line drawn along the hard and soft palates. Posteriorly the nasopharynx is bounded by the pharyngeal constrictor muscles, and anteriorly it is bounded by the nasal cavity at the nasal choana (paired funnel-shaped openings between the nasal cavity and the nasopharynx). Below the hard palate lie the *oral cavity* and *oropharynx.* These two areas are divided by a ring of structures that includes the circumvallate papillae (located along the

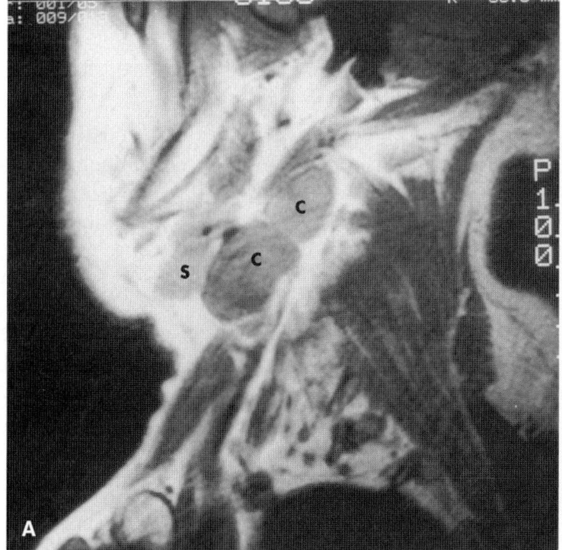

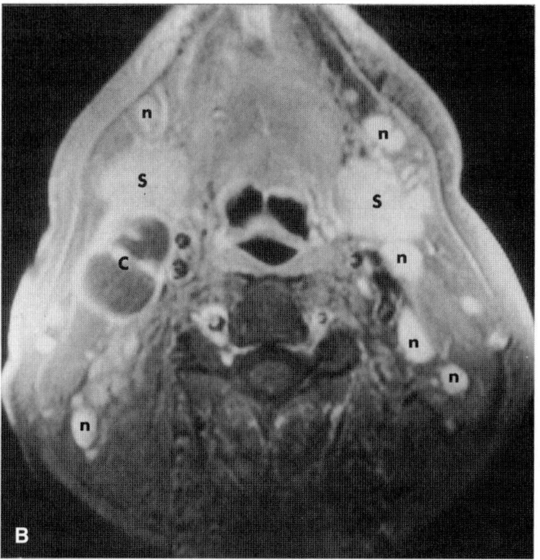

FIGURE 9.6. **Squamous Cell Carcinoma: Cystic Nodal Metastasis. A.** Sagittal T1WI. **B.** Axial postgadolinium fat-suppressed T1WI. This 43-year-old patient was referred for a "branchial cleft cyst." Patient had a 6-month history of a right-sided neck mass that would swell during upper respiratory tract infections. Images reveal a multiseptated cystic lesion (c) in the right jugular nodal chain. On biopsy, this proved to be a squamous cell, cystic nodal metastasis. Although this lesion may appear similar to a branchial cleft cyst, the presence of multiple additional nodes (n) is unusual. A branchial cleft cyst may exhibit a thickened wall with septations, depending on current or previous infections. S, submandibular glands. Note that the jugulodigastric node is easily identified by its characteristic location; situated immediately posterior to the submandibular gland.

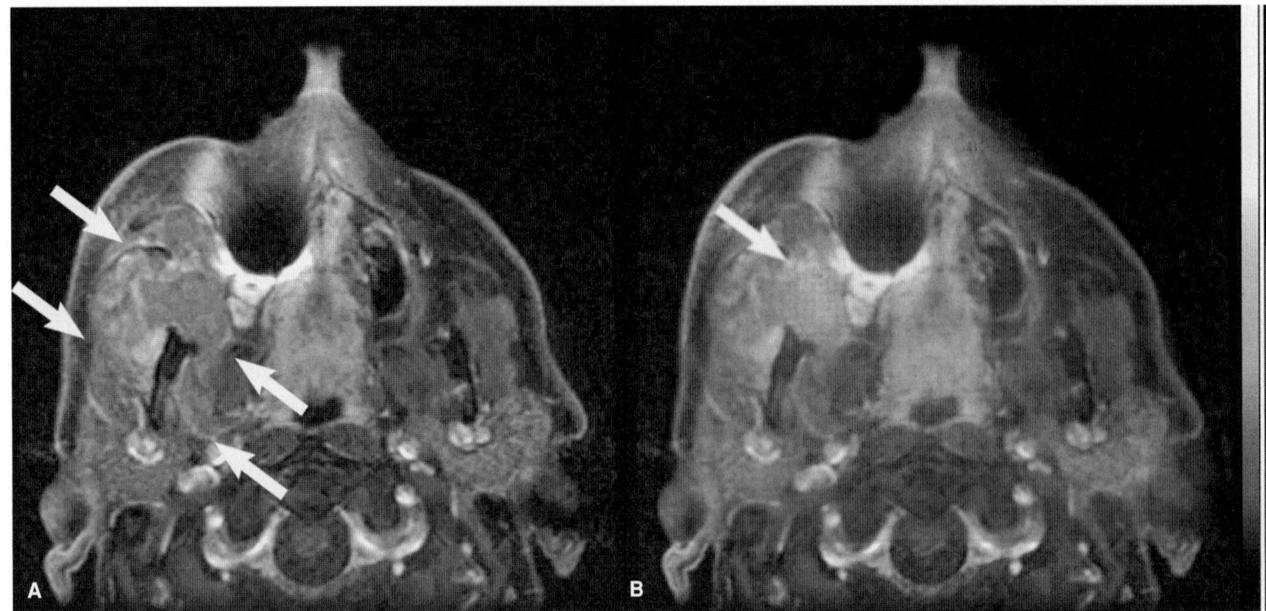

FIGURE 9.7. **(Color Plates) Non-Hodgkin Lymphoma of the Masticator Space. A.** Axial T1WI. **B.** Corresponding fused MR/PET scan. A 21-year-old man presented with a diffusely infiltrating mass of the right masticator space (*arrows*). Although MR reveals a diffusely infiltrating lesion, PET demonstrates that only a focal portion of the lesions is glucose avid (*arrow*). This helped direct the biopsy to the most metabolically active portion of the lesion, increasing the likelihood that a pathologic diagnosis could be made. Much of the remaining infiltrative change of the masticator space proved to be reactive in nature, without frank tumor. This case highlights the improved specificity that results from combining morphologic imaging (MR/CT) with physiologic (PET) imaging.

posterior aspect of the tongue), the tonsillar pillars, and the soft palate.

These traditional compartments (nasopharynx, oropharynx, and oral cavity) are important for describing the spread of superficial, mucosa-based lesions. In contrast to this division, multiple facial planes divide the deep head and neck into spaces that form true compartments. It is important to realize that these deep spaces are unrelated to the traditional division of the head and neck and traverse the neck without regard to the traditional divisions. Therefore, when describing deep head and neck lesions, the traditional pharyngeal subdivisions are of limited value. Most radiologists have adapted a spatial approach to the head and neck, described as follows and popularized by Harnsberger.

The deep anatomy of the head and neck is subdivided by layers of the deep cervical fascia into the following spaces: *(1)* superficial mucosal, *(2)* parapharyngeal, *(3)* carotid, *(4)* parotid, *(5)* masticator, *(6)* retropharyngeal, and *(7)* prevertebral. When evaluating a patient with pathology in the deep head and neck, it is important to determine within which space the pathology lies. Because only a limited number of structures are located within each compartment, these are the structures from which pathology will arise. Therefore, only specific pathology will be found within these separate fascial spaces, markedly limiting the differential diagnosis. For example, the principal structures within the parotid space are the parotid gland and parotid lymph nodes. Consequently, if a parotid space mass is identified, the diagnosis is primarily limited to either a parotid tumor or nodal disease. Each of these seven spaces will be reviewed in detail (Table 9.1). Note that although this spatial division is popular with radiologists, surgeons and otolaryngologists occasionally use different terms, e.g., "retrostyloid space" instead of "carotid space."

Superficial Mucosal Space

The superficial mucosal space includes all structures on the airway side of the pharyngobasilar fascia. The principal constituent of this space is the mucosa of the upper aerodigestive tract, which consists of squamous epithelium, submucosal lymphatics, and hundreds of minor salivary glands. The pharyngobasilar fascia represents the superior aponeurosis of the superior pharyngeal constrictor muscle, which inserts into the skull base. This tough fascia separates the mucosal space from the surrounding parapharyngeal space. Lesions originating within the superficial mucosal space may invade deep to the mucosal surface, resulting first in lateral displacement and then obliteration of the parapharyngeal space. However,

TABLE 9.1 Deep Compartments of the Head and Neck

Compartment	Contents	Pathology
Mucosal	Squamous mucosa Lymphoid tissue (adenoids, lingual tonsils) Minor salivary glands	Nasopharyngeal carcinoma Squamous cell carcinoma Lymphoma Minor salivary gland tumors Juvenile angiofibroma Rhabdomyosarcoma
Parapharyngeal	Fat Trigeminal nerve (V3) Internal maxillary artery Ascending pharyngeal artery	Minor salivary gland tumor Lipoma Cellulitis/abscess Schwannoma
Parotid	Parotid gland Intraparotid lymph nodes Facial nerve (VII) External carotid artery Retromandibular vein	Salivary gland tumors Metastatic adenopathy Lymphoma Parotid cysts
Carotid	Cranial nerves IX–XII Sympathetic nerves Jugular chain nodes Carotid artery Jugular vein	Schwannoma Neurofibroma Paraganglionoma Metastatic adenopathy Lymphoma Cellulitis/abscess Meningioma
Masticator	Muscles of mastication Ramus and body of mandible Inferior alveolar nerve	Odontogenic abscess Osteomyelitis Direct spread of squamous cell carcinoma Lymphoma Minor salivary tumor Sarcoma of muscle or bone
Retropharyngeal	Lymph nodes (lateral and medial retropharyngeal) Fat	Metastatic adenopathy Lymphoma
Prevertebral	Cervical vertebrae Prevertebral muscles Paraspinal muscles Phrenic nerve	Abscess/cellulitis Osseous metastases Chordoma Osteomyelitis Cellulitis Abscess

For further discussion see Harnsberger, et al. Diagnostic Imaging: Head and Neck. Salt Lake City, UT: AMIRSYS, 2004.

many early lesions that begin within the mucosal space present as only mild mucosal irregularities or asymmetries (Fig. 9.8). This space is easily evaluated by the clinician and thus the radiologist should have a low threshold for suggesting the presence of abnormalities within this space. In children, there is frequently prominent adenoidal tissue that fills the nasopharynx. Even in adults, following an upper respiratory infection, prominent mucosal tissue may be noted; this is of little concern as long as there is no invasion of deep facial places and no associated adenopathy (Fig. 9.9).

Benign Lesions. The most common benign lesions arising in the mucosal space are Tornwaldt cysts and lesions related to minor salivary gland tissue. *Tornwaldt cysts* are found in the midline and have high intensity on T2WIs (Fig. 9.10). They are believed to be remnants of notochordal tissue aberrantly located in the nasopharynx and have an incidence of approximately 1% to 2% in normal patients. Lesions arising from minor salivary glands include retention cysts and benign neoplasms. *Retention cysts* represent obstructed glands similar to those found within the paranasal sinuses. The most common benign neoplasm is the benign mixed-cell tumor (pleomorphic adenoma). Both of these lesions present as well-circumscribed, rounded lesions that have high signal intensity on T2WIs.

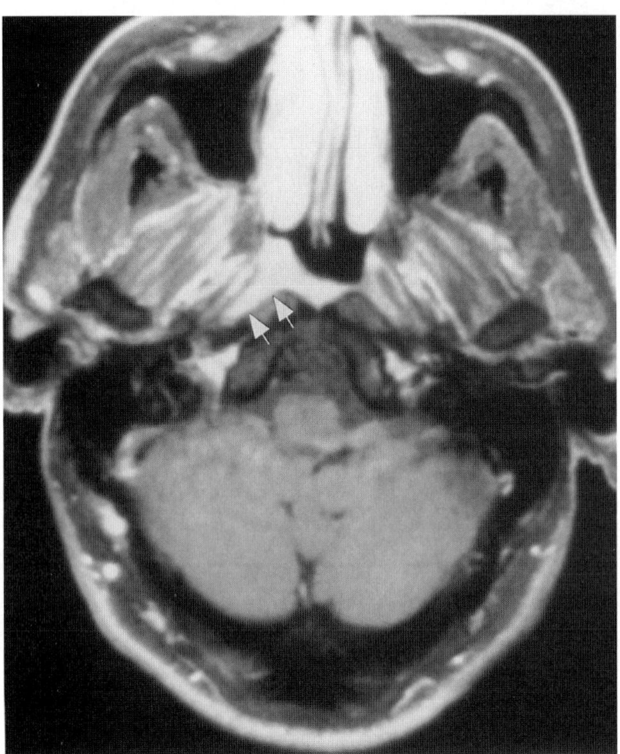

FIGURE 9.8. **Squamous Cell Carcinoma.** Axial postgadolinium fat-suppressed T1WI through the level of the nasopharynx. Contrast-enhancing soft tissue fills the right fossa of Rosenmüller (*arrows*). Although this lesion does not obviously invade the underlying parapharyngeal tissues, submandibular nodal metastases were present. This example underscores the point that even mild asymmetries of the mucosal space may represent a malignancy, and careful correlation with physical examination should be suggested by the radiologist.

Malignant Lesions. The most common malignant neoplasms of the mucosal space are squamous cell carcinoma, non-Hodgkin lymphoma, and minor salivary gland malignancies; of these, squamous cell carcinoma is by far the most common. Unfortunately, these malignancies all appear similar on CT and MR. Initially there is mass effect, often associated with lateral compression or obliteration of the parapharyngeal space, followed by invasion of the skull base. An early triad of radiographic findings consists of *(1)* superficial nasopharyngeal mucosal asymmetry, *(2)* ipsilateral retropharyngeal adenopathy, and *(3)* mastoid opacification. Mastoid opacification is an important early warning sign (Fig. 9.11). Mastoid opacification is easily detected on T2WIs and suggests potential dysfunction of the eustachian tube, frequently the result of tumor infiltration of the tensor veli palatini muscles. This finding directs the radiologist to carefully evaluate the mucosa of the nasopharynx. Note that both the nasopharynx and the mastoid air cells are included on every head CT and MR scan, and these areas should not be overlooked on routine head imaging.

Fat-suppressed, fast spin-echo (FSE) T2, and contrast-enhanced imaging are useful in detecting and defining the extent of pathology. Additionally, these sequences allow the detection of subtle perineural spread of neoplasms, particularly along cranial nerves extending into the skull base. This is particularly important with adenoid cystic carcinoma, which has a marked propensity for perineural spread and is the most common minor salivary gland malignancy (Fig. 9.12).

Squamous cell carcinoma is the most common malignancy of the upper aerodigestive tract. However, a particular variant of squamous cell carcinoma occurs within the nasopharynx and is termed *nasopharyngeal carcinoma.* Nasopharyngeal carcinoma has several unique histologic features that distinguish it from squamous cell carcinoma. Although squamous cell carcinoma is common in the Caucasian population, nasopharyngeal carcinoma is not, with an incidence of about 1 in 100,000 people per year. This is in contrast to rates that are 20 times higher in Asia, particularly in southern regions of China. Although smoking and alcohol abuse are often associated with squamous cell carcinoma, they have no causal association with nasopharyngeal carcinoma. However, both environmental and genetic factors do appear to play a role in the genesis of nasopharyngeal carcinoma. Specifically, immunoglobulin-A antibodies to the Epstein-Barr virus have been associated with nasopharyngeal carcinoma.

Lymphoma involving the mucosa cannot be differentiated by imaging from squamous cell or minor salivary gland carcinoma. However, non-Hodgkin lymphoma frequently has systemic manifestations, with extranodal and extralymphatic sites of involvement that are atypical for these other malignancies. Thus, the presence of a mucosal mass in association with bulky supraclavicular and mediastinal adenopathy as well as splenomegaly would be suggestive of lymphoma.

Parapharyngeal Space

The parapharyngeal space is a triangular, fat-filled compartment that extends from the skull base to the submandibular gland region. It is located at the center of the surrounding spaces and is compressed or infiltrated in a characteristic fashion by masses originating from the various spaces. The primary importance of the parapharyngeal space is that it serves as an important landmark of mass effect in the deep face. When a lesion occurs in any of the four surrounding spaces, there will be characteristic impressions on the parapharyngeal fat space, which will suggest the space of tumor origin.

The parapharyngeal space is surrounded by the carotid space posteriorly, the parotid space laterally, the masticator space anteriorly, and the superficial mucosal space medially. Therefore, the parapharyngeal space will be compressed on its medial surface by masses originating

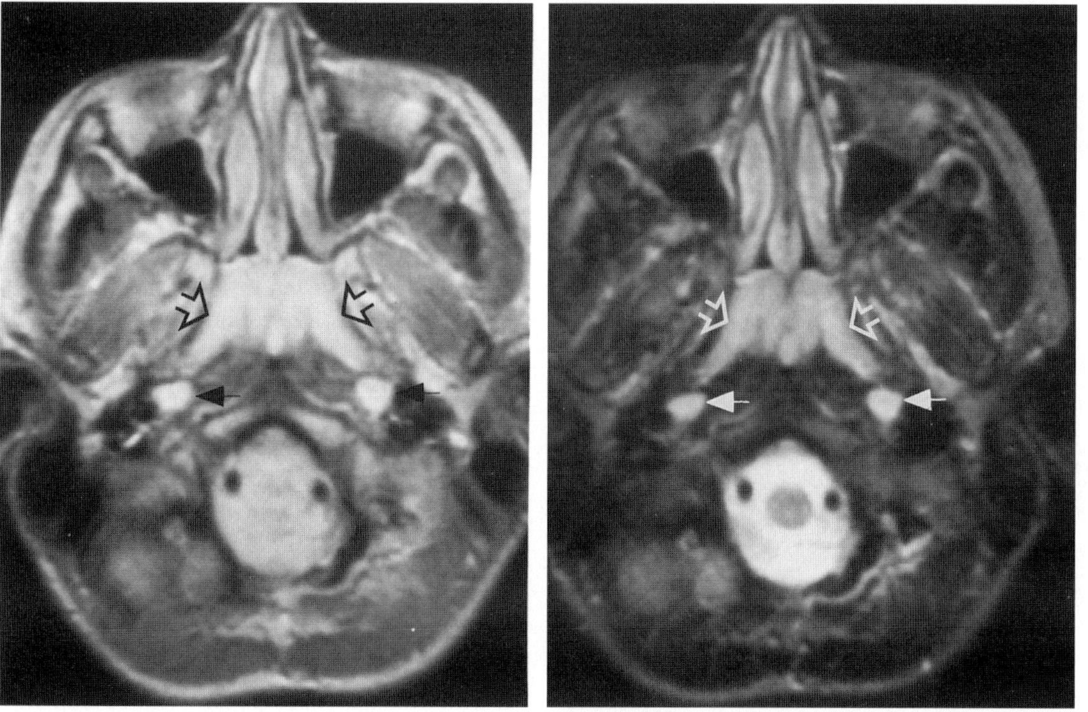

FIGURE 9.9. **Adenoidal Hypertrophy.** Axial first-echo and second-echo T2 images in a 5-year-old child. Prominent adenoidal tissue (*open arrows*) fills the nasopharynx, expanding the fossa of Rosenmüller bilaterally. Additionally, lateral pharyngeal nodes (*arrowheads*) are clearly visualized. These findings are typical for a child. The age of the patient and the symmetry are in keeping with normal findings.

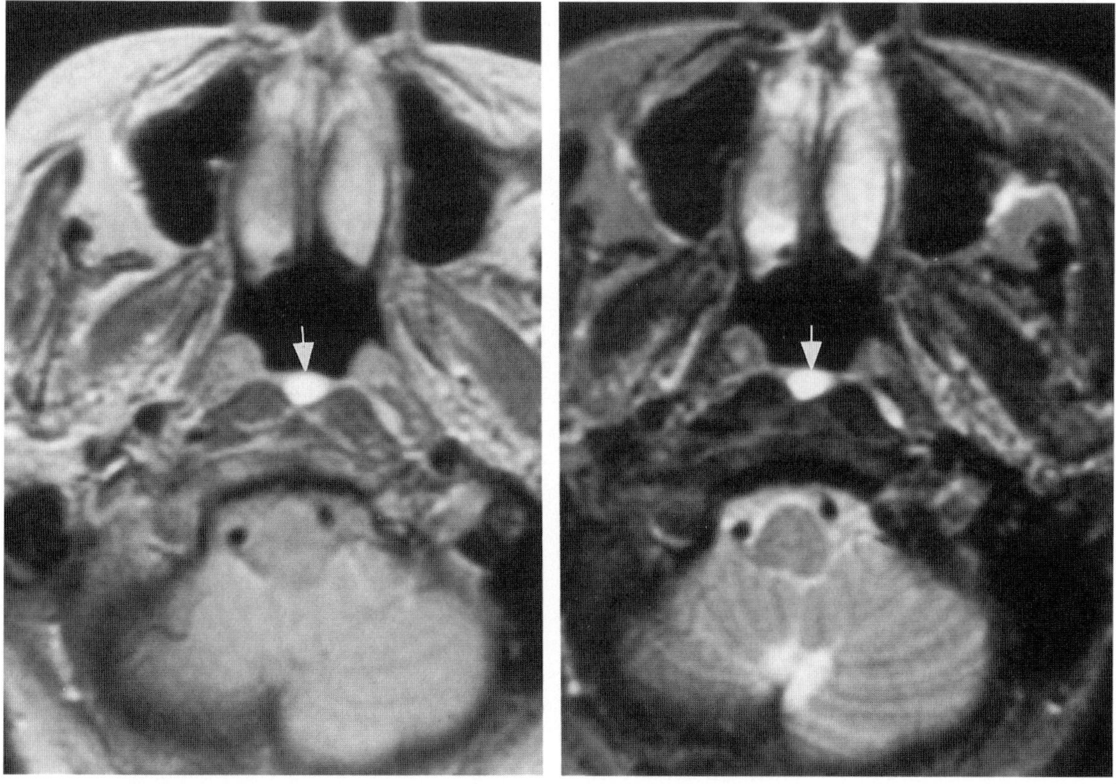

FIGURE 9.10. **Tornwaldt Cyst.** Axial first-echo and second-echo T2WIs. A high-signal-intensity lesion appears in the superficial mucosa (*arrows*). This midline location is characteristic of a Tornwaldt cyst, a remnant of the primitive notochord, and is found in 1% to 2% of the normal population.

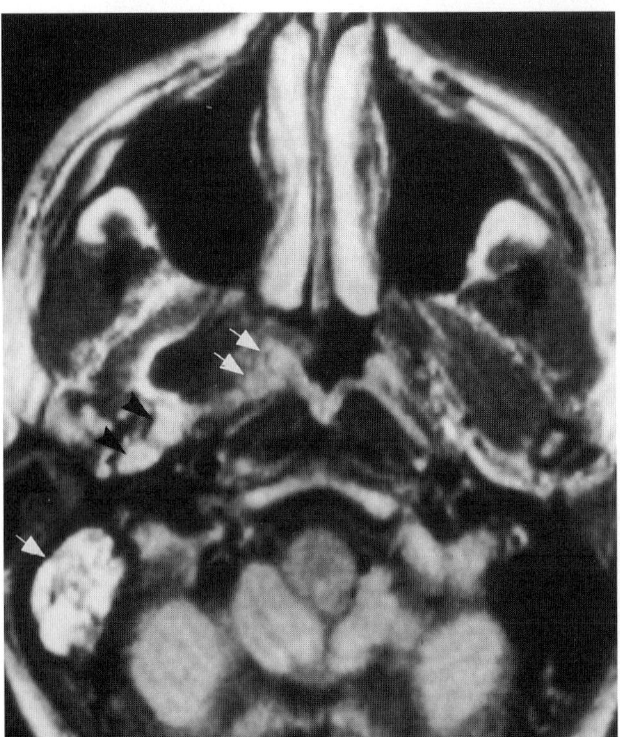

FIGURE 9.11. **Nasopharyngeal Malignancy.** Axial post-gadolinium T1WI. The triad of nasopharyngeal malignancy consists of (*1*) mucosal mass (*double white arrows*) of the lateral nasopharynx (fossa of Rosenmüller), (*2*) lateral retropharyngeal nodes (*arrowheads*), and (*3*) mastoid opacification (*white arrow*). Mastoid opacification is the result of dysfunction of the eustachian tube, and should always prompt search for the offending nasopharyngeal mass.

from the mucosal surface, displaced anteriorly by carotid sheath masses, displaced medially by parotid masses, and displaced posteriorly and medially by masses within the masticator space. Thus, by assessing the location and displacement pattern of the parapharyngeal space, one can assign a space of origin to a deep facial mass (Fig. 9.13).

Carotid Space

Masses of the carotid space deviate the parapharyngeal space anteriorly and will separate or anteriorly displace the carotid and jugular vein. They sometimes displace the styloid process anteriorly, which narrows the stylomandibular notch (the space between the styloid process and the mandible). This is a characteristic feature that distinguishes these lesions from deep parotid space lesions, which widen the stylomandibular notch.

Pseudomasses. When evaluating carotid space tumors, there are several pseudomasses of the carotid space that must be taken into account. These pseudomasses are vascular variants that may be mistaken for masses both clinically and radiographically. Asymmetry of the internal jugular veins is the most common variation in the vascular anatomy of the neck. Marked asymmetry between the size of the left and right jugular veins is common, with the right vein typically being the larger of the two. Additionally, the jugular veins may demonstrate considerable variability in the degree of signal within their lumina, ranging from bright to signal void. The intraluminal bright regions should not be mistaken for thrombosis. It is important to follow the signal on serial images to visualize the tubular nature, thus confirming that the signal represents vasculature; otherwise it may easily be mistaken for adenopathy. Tortuosity of the carotid artery may present as a submucosal pulsatile mass in the pharynx. This variation, which is frequently seen in the elderly, is easily detected on CT or MR and obviates the need for further diagnostic workup unless a posttraumatic aneurysm is suspected.

Tumors. Most carotid space masses are benign neoplasms that arise from nerves located within the carotid sheath. The most common lesions are *paragangliomas* (also called *chemodectomas*) and nerve sheath tumors such as *schwannomas* and *neurofibromas*. Paragangliomas are vascular tumors that arise from neural crest cell derivatives. These lesions are named according to the nerves from which they arise and their location of origin. When arising from the carotid body, at the carotid bifurcation, paragangliomas are called *carotid body tumors* (Fig. 9.14). Paragangliomas may also arise from the ganglion of the vagus nerve (glomus vagale tumors), along the jugular ganglion of the vagus nerve (glomus jugulare tumors), and around the Arnold and Jacobson nerves in the middle ear (glomus tympanicum tumors). Despite the use of different names, the imaging features and histology remain the same.

Clinically, patients with paragangliomas present with a painless, slowly progressive neck mass that may be pulsatile with an associated bruit. Because these lesions are located within the carotid sheath, there are often associated slowly progressive cranial neuropathies (cranial nerves IX to XII) (Fig. 9.15). Paragangliomas are often multiple (5% to 10%) and, in familial cases, are multiple 25% to 33% of the time. Therefore, if a lesion is detected, it is essential to look for others.

Angiographically, paragangliomas are very vascular, with a strong blush in the capillary phase. Treatment often consists of surgical resection. Interventional radiology plays an important role in permitting preoperative embolization, thus reducing blood loss during surgery. On CT and MR scanning, paragangliomas and neuromas are both densely enhancing and are typically indistinguishable. In contrast, on MR, paragangliomas are characterized by multiple flow voids and prominent enhancement, but neuromas usually do not demonstrate flow voids and can be cystic (Fig. 9.16). These features reflect the typically more vascular nature of paragangliomas. Note that these findings are not pathognomonic for paragangliomas, because very vascular schwannomas may also, on occasion, have associated flow voids.

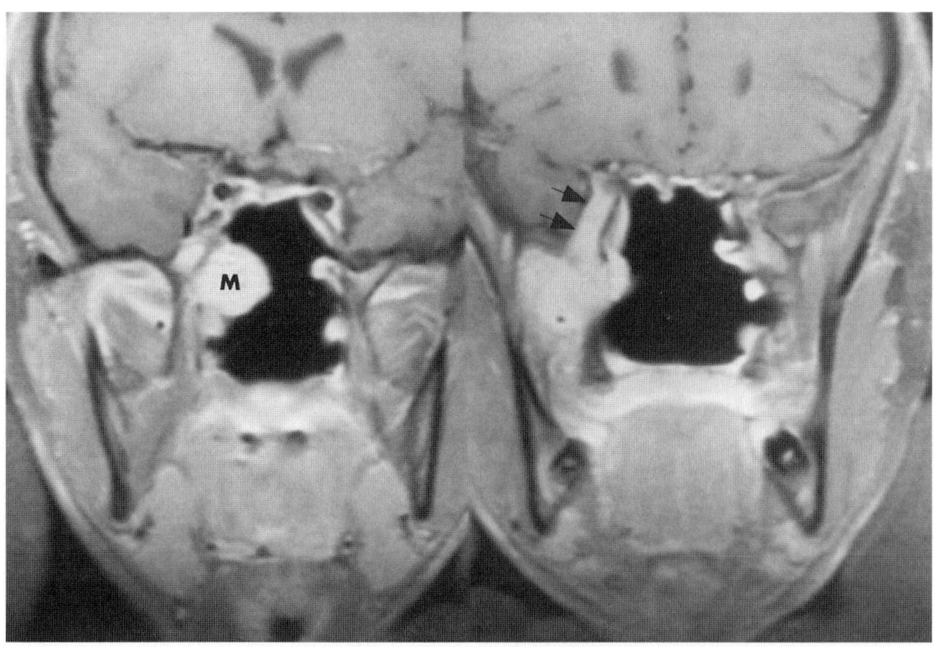

FIGURE 9.12. **Recurrent Adenoid Cystic Carcinoma.** Coronal postgadolinium fat-suppressed T1WIs of a 50-year-old patient after resection of nasal septum and turbinates for adenoid cystic carcinoma. A recurrent mass (M) extends into the right pterygopalatine fossa (*arrows*). Adenoid cystic carcinoma has a marked propensity for perineural spread, which allows the tumor to extend rapidly into noncontiguous spaces. Once the tumor enters the pterygopalatine fossa, it may extend into the orbit via the inferior orbital foramen, into the cavernous sinus via the foramen rotundum, and into the infratemporal fossa via the pterygomaxillary fissure. Once in the cavernous sinus, the tumor can travel back along the cisternal portion of the trigeminal nerve into the brain stem.

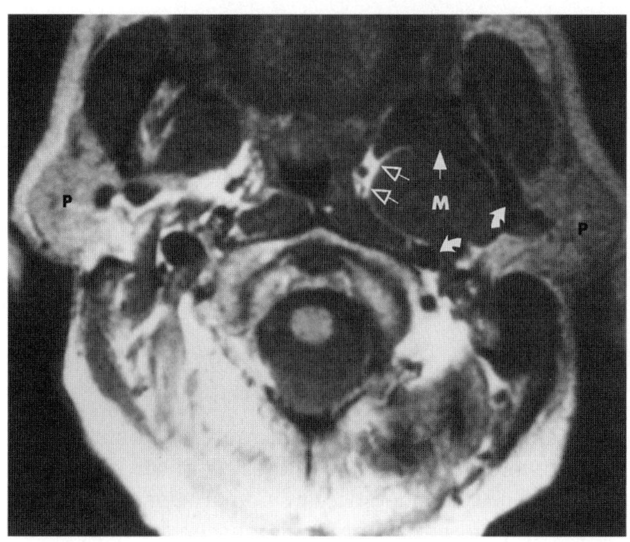

FIGURE 9.13. **Parotid Benign Mixed-Cell Adenoma (Pleomorphic Adenoma).** Axial T1WI through the level of the oropharynx. A mass (M) displaces the parapharyngeal space medially (*open white arrows*) and the masticator space anteriorly (*white arrow*). The stylomandibular notch from the carotid space to the mandible (*curved arrows*) is widened, characteristic of a deep lobe parotid lesion. Conversely, a lesion originating from the carotid space would result in narrowing of the stylomandibular notch. The lesion is sharply demarcated from the normal parotid tissue (P).

Schwannomas are encapsulated tumors that arise from nerve sheath coverings and do not infiltrate the substance of the nerve. Within the carotid space, schwannomas often arise from the vagus nerve and present as benign neck masses. Schwannomas may occasionally show cystic change and necrosis. In contrast to schwannomas, neurofibromas are not encapsulated and usually occur as multiple lesions that permeate the substance of the nerve fibers.

Lymph nodes are a common source of pathology within the carotid space. In fact, the principal malignancy of the carotid space is squamous cell nodal metastasis (Fig. 9.17). The deep cervical jugular nodal chain is located within the carotid space and serves as the final common efferent pathway of lymphatic drainage from the head and neck. As such, any pathology of the head and neck (metastases, lymphoma, infection, benign hyperplasia) will typically involve the jugular nodal chain and be found within the carotid space.

Parotid Space

Masses arising from the deep lobe of the parotid gland will deviate the parapharyngeal space medially. Unlike carotid space masses, deep parotid masses push the styloid process and carotid vessels posteriorly. This results in

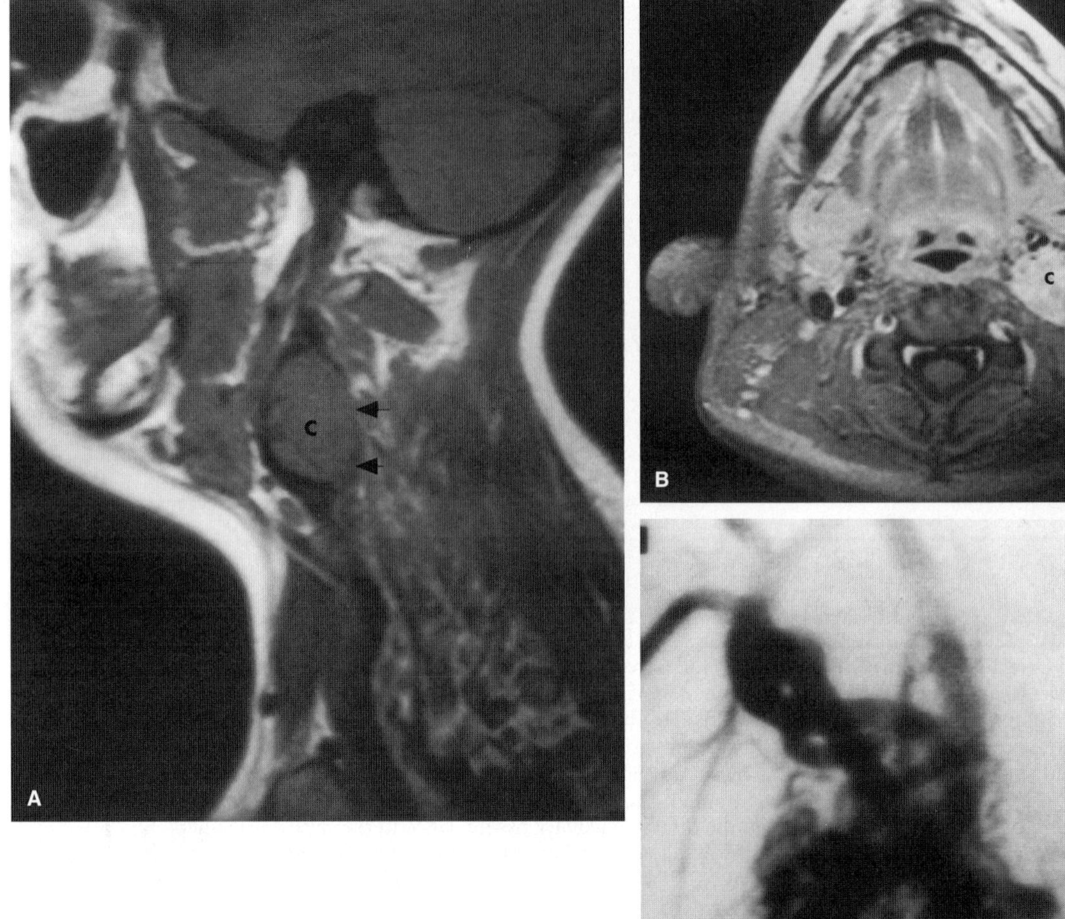

FIGURE 9.14. **Carotid Body Tumor.** Sagittal T1WI **(A),** axial postgadolinium fat-suppressed T1WI **(B),** and angiogram **(C).** A vascular mass located between the carotid bifurcation, with splaying of the internal and external carotid arteries, is characteristic of a carotid body tumor (c). The multiple flow voids in the axial image supports the diagnosis of a paraganglioma. The angiogram confirms the marked vascularity of this lesion. Angiography is helpful in providing preoperative embolization, which makes the lesion less vascular and easier to remove surgically.

characteristic widening of the stylomastoid foramen (Fig. 9.13). The structures within the parotid space that may give rise to pathology include the parotid gland and lymph nodes. The parotid gland is the only salivary gland with lymph nodes contained within its capsule. This reflects the embryogenesis of the parotid gland, the late encapsulation of which results in the presence of 10 to 20 nodes within the gland parenchyma (Fig. 9.18). Consequently, pathology of the parotid space includes salivary gland tumors and nodal disease.

Parotid Tumors. Most parotid tumors are benign (80%), and most of these are benign mixed-cell tumors (pleomorphic adenomas). The second most common benign salivary gland tumor is the Warthin tumor. Malignant tumors, which account for 20% of all parotid lesions, include adenocystic carcinoma, adenocarcinoma, squamous cell carcinoma, and mucoepidermoid carcinoma. MR and CT imaging cannot with certainty differentiate benign from malignant disease. Both may present as well-circumscribed lesions. Tumor homogeneity, indistinct margins, and signal intensity are poor predictors of histology. Nevertheless, benign pleomorphic adenomas are typically well circumscribed and very bright on T2WIs and demonstrate heterogeneous enhancement (Fig. 9.19). Both CT and MR are useful in portraying the relationship of a tumor to surrounding normal anatomy and can demonstrate

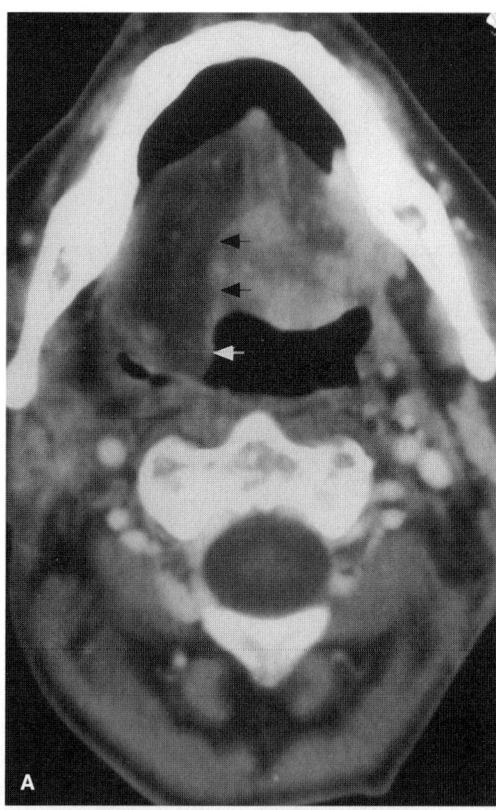

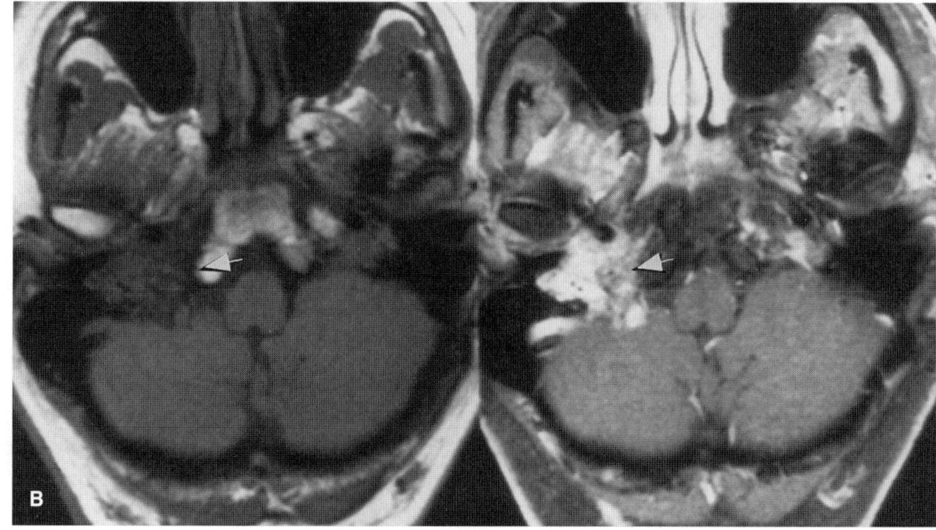

FIGURE 9.15. **Glomus Jugulare Tumor. A.** Axial contrast-enhanced CT. Fatty atrophy of the right tongue (hypoglossal nerve palsy) (*black arrows*) and patulousness of the right oropharynx (vagus nerve palsy) (*white arrow*) are evident. Dysfunction of multiple lower cranial nerves suggests involvement of the skull base, where cranial nerves IX through XII arise in close proximity. **B.** Axial T1WIs with fat suppression, pregadolinium (*left*) and postgadolinium (*right*). A contrast-enhancing mass (*arrows*) extending through the right jugular foramen into the posterior fossa is indicative of glomus jugulare tumor.

the location and extent of a parotid mass before biopsy. A feature predictive of malignancy is infiltration into deep neck structures, such as the masticator or parapharyngeal space. Clinical involvement of the facial nerve is another ominous finding suggestive of malignancy.

The presence of multiple lesions within the parotid space may be seen with several conditions, including either inflammatory or malignant adenopathy. Another possibility is the Warthin tumor (benign salivary gland tumor), which is multiple 10% of the time and more common in men. Parotid cysts have been seen in collagen vascular disease (Sjögren syndrome) and also described in patients with AIDS (Fig. 9.20). These parotid cysts, also known as lymphoepithelial cysts, are believed to be the result of partial obstruction of the terminal ducts by surrounding lymphocytic infiltration.

Masticator Space

The masticator space is formed by a superficial layer of the deep cervical fascia that surrounds the muscles of mastication and the mandible. It extends from the angle of the

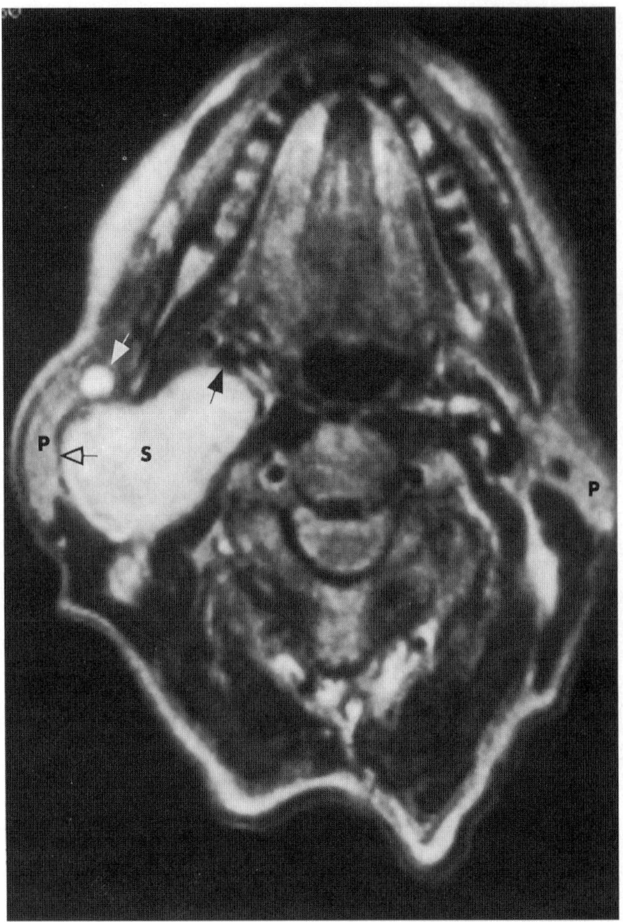

FIGURE 9.16. **Schwannoma.** Axial T2WI through the floor of the mouth. The patient presented with a painless neck mass. A homogeneous mass (S) displaces the carotid space anteriorly (*black arrow*) and the parotid space (P) laterally (*open arrow*). Anterior displacement of the carotid artery is characteristic of a carotid space mass. The lack of associated flow voids suggests that this lesion is a nerve sheath tumor, i.e., schwannoma of the vagus nerve, as opposed to a paraganglioma. High signal within the right retromandibular vein (*white arrow*) is a result of partial compression. Normal flow void is seen in the opposite retromandibular vein.

mandible superiorly to the skull base and over the temporalis muscle. The muscles of mastication include the temporalis, the medial and lateral pterygoid, and the masseter. In addition, branches of the trigeminal nerve and the internal maxillary artery are located within this space. Masses in the masticator space displace the parapharyngeal space medially and posteriorly.

Most masses of the masticator space are infectious in origin. They usually result from either dental caries or dental extraction. A mass will often surround the mandible and may extend superiorly along the temporalis muscle. Additionally, pseudotumors of the masticator space are common and include accessory parotid glands as well as marked muscle hypertrophy resulting from bruxism. Occasionally, an accessory parotid gland may occur along the anterior surface of the masseter muscle and can be mistaken for a mass. Asymmetry of the muscles of mastication may result from unilateral atrophy, owing to compromise of the mandibular division of the fifth cranial nerve (V3). This is most commonly seen in patients with head and neck neoplasms with perineural extension along the trigeminal nerve.

Primary malignancies of the masticator space are very uncommon. Malignancies of this space most often result from the extension of oropharyngeal or tongue base squamous cell carcinoma to involve the muscles of mastication (Fig. 9.21). In addition, tumor or infection from oropharyngeal or nasopharyngeal lesions may spread along the third division of the fifth cranial nerve, allowing the tumor to ascend through the foramen ovale into the cavernous sinus (Fig. 9.22). From this location, a tumor may extend posteriorly along the cisternal portion of the trigeminal nerve to the brainstem. Primary malignancies of the masticator space include sarcomas arising from muscle, chondroid, or nerve elements. In addition, sarcomas of the bone such as osteosarcoma and Ewing sarcoma may be seen. Non-Hodgkin lymphoma will occasionally involve the mandible or extraosseous soft tissues of the masticator space (Fig. 9.7).

Retropharyngeal Space

The retropharyngeal space is a potential space that lies posterior to the superficial mucosal space and pharyngeal constrictor muscles and anterior to the prevertebral space. A mass within this space results in characteristic posterior displacement of the prevertebral muscles. The fascial planes in this area are complex but can be considered as forming a single compartment for simplicity. This space is significant because it serves as a potential conduit for the spread of tumor or infection from the pharynx to the mediastinum (Fig. 9.23). In contrast to the carotid and parotid spaces, in which inflammatory disease and metastases account for a minority of lesions, most lesions of the retropharyngeal space are a result of infection or nodal malignancy. This space is most often involved with nodal malignancy because of lymphoma or metastatic head and neck squamous cell carcinoma. These tumors frequently affect the retropharyngeal nodes, which are divided into a medial and lateral group. The lateral retropharyngeal nodes, also known as nodes of Rouviere, are normal when seen in younger patients but must be viewed with suspicion in individuals older than 30 years. In addition, head and neck infections may sometimes extend into the retropharyngeal space via lymphatics. Because the retropharyngeal space may serve as a conduit, spreading infection into the mediastinum, this space has also been referred to as the "danger space." Neck infections are most often the result of tonsillitis, dental disease, trauma, endocarditis, and

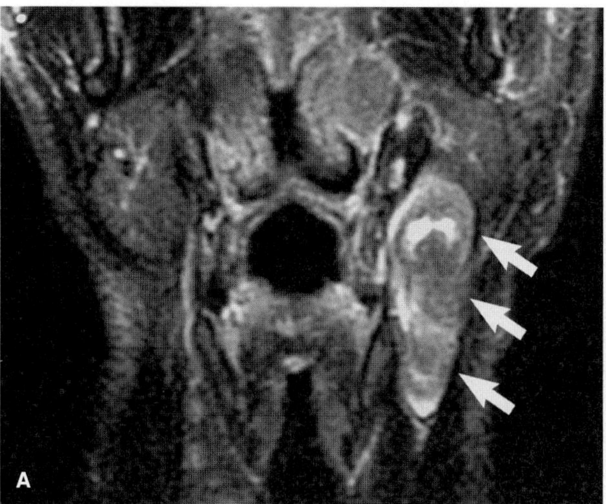

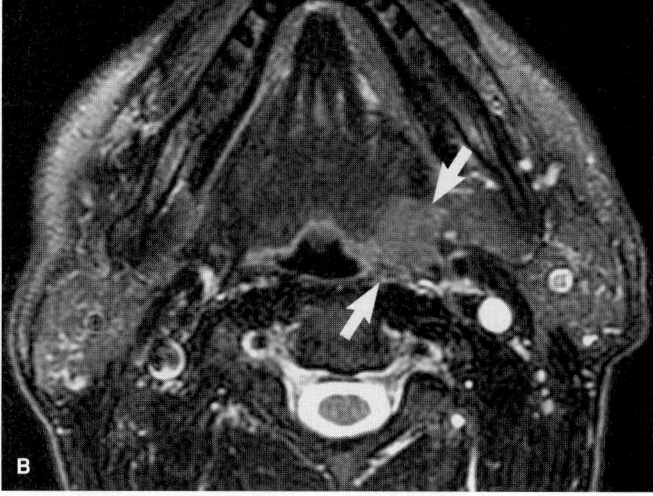

FIGURE 9.17. **Carotid Space Mass (Jugular Chain Adenopathy).** This 68-year-old man presented with a left neck mass. **A.** Coronal T2WI reveals left deep jugular chain lymph nodes (*arrows*), with foci of high signal, indicating necrosis. The presence of abnormal adenopathy must initiate a search for the primary lesion, which is most commonly a mucosa-based squamous cell carcinoma. **B.** Axial T2WI reveals the primary lesion, consisting of a tonsillar squamous cell carcinoma (*arrows*).

systemic infections such as tuberculosis. With the advent of antibiotics, infections occur much less commonly but are often seen in immunosuppressed patients. On routine T1WIs and T2WIs it can be difficult to differentiate an abscess from cellulitis, as both can be isointense to muscle on T1 and hyperintense on T2. Gadolinium is of value in making this differentiation, as an abscess will demonstrate a rim of contrast enhancement surrounding a liquefied center.

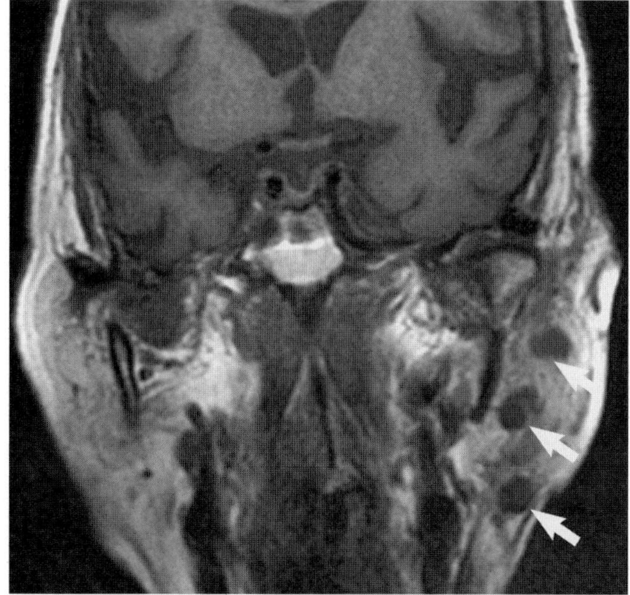

FIGURE 9.18. **Metastatic Lymph Nodes Within the Parotid Gland Capsule.** This 79-year-old man presented with left parotid swelling. Coronal T1WI reveals several enlarged nodes within the left parotid gland (*arrows*). The parotid gland serves as the drainage pathway for the posterior auricular scalp and is characterized by its fatty signal intensity. The finding of parotid nodes initiated a search for ipsilateral pathology, which revealed a retroauricular scalp angiosarcoma.

Prevertebral Space

The prevertebral space is formed by the prevertebral fascia, which surrounds the prevertebral muscles. Masses of the prevertebral space displace the prevertebral muscles anteriorly. This allows prevertebral lesions to be easily differentiated from retropharyngeal processes, which will displace these muscles posteriorly. The structures that give rise to most pathologies in this space are the cervical vertebral bodies. Any process that involves the vertebral bodies, such as tumor (metastasis, chordoma, etc.) or osteomyelitis, may extend anteriorly to involve this space.

Trans-spatial Diseases

Occasionally, masses may not be localized to one of the spaces described above. Such masses are often secondary to lesions involving anatomic structures that normally traverse spaces of the head and neck, e.g., lymphatics, nerves, and vessels. Examples include the following three categories: (*1*) lymphatic masses (lymphangioma); (*2*) neural masses (neurofibroma, schwannoma, perineural spread of tumor); and (*3*) vascular masses (hemangioma). Differentiation between these subtypes can occasionally be made by virtue of signal intensity characteristics. For instance, neurofibromas may have a characteristic low-intensity center on T1 and often involve more than one

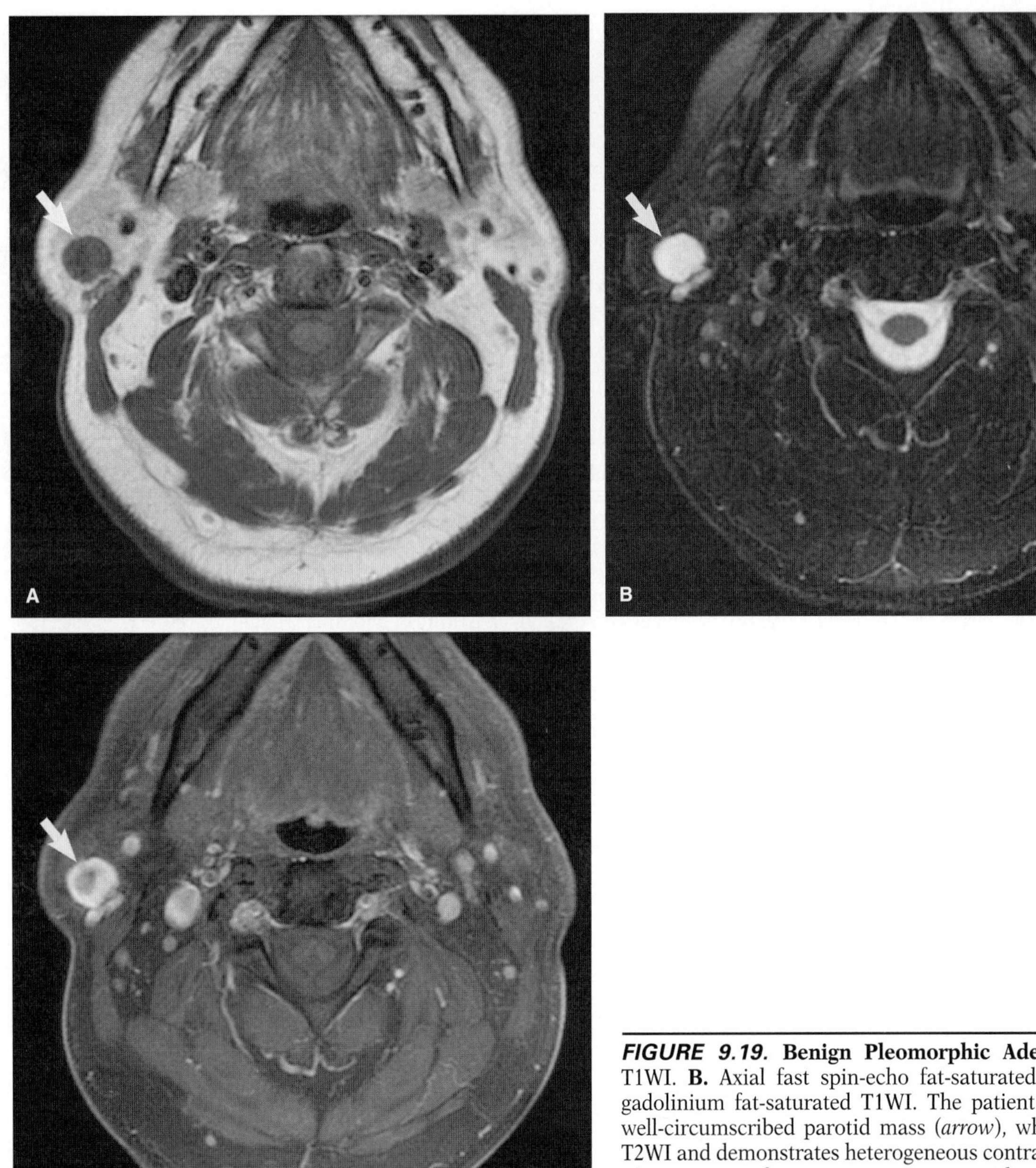

FIGURE 9.19. **Benign Pleomorphic Adenoma. A.** Axial T1WI. **B.** Axial fast spin-echo fat-saturated T2WI. **C.** Post-gadolinium fat-saturated T1WI. The patient presents with a well-circumscribed parotid mass (*arrow*), which is bright on T2WI and demonstrates heterogeneous contrast enhancement. These imaging features are consistent with a benign pleomorphic ademona, which is the most common parotid lesion, accounting for 80% of all benign parotid tumors.

peripheral nerve. This is distinctly different from both lymphatic and vascular masses. Lymphangiomas and hemangiomas are congenital abnormalities that look quite similar on MR. Both entities have increased signal intensity on T2WIs and are infiltrative. Hemangiomas may have phleboliths, which may be easily detected on CT (Fig. 9.24). Lymphangiomas tend to have heterogeneous signal intensity with evidence of blood degradation products. Both entities should be considered in a patient with a history of chronic facial swelling and who shows CT or MR evidence of an infiltrative process that traverses several spaces.

Perineural Disease. Perineural spread of disease allows tumor or infection to gain access into noncontiguous spaces of the head and neck. The complex system of cranial nerves coursing through the skull base serves as a conduit for the spread of tumor and infection. Fungal infections (Fig. 9.22), squamous cell carcinoma, and adenoid cystic carcinoma have a particular proclivity for perineural spread of disease, which serves as a hallmark of these diseases. If a patient with a known head and neck primary neoplasm or immunocompromised status (susceptible to fungal infections) presents with facial numbness or dysesthesias, this is highly suggestive of perineural spread of

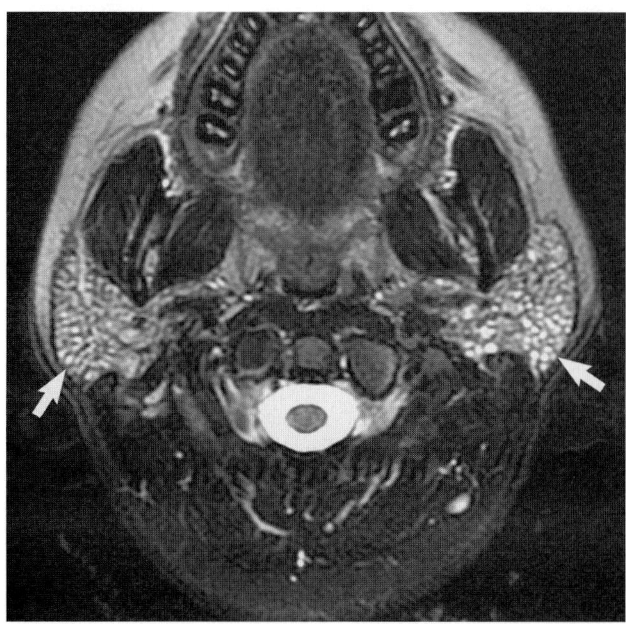

FIGURE 9.20. **Benign Lymphoepithelial Cysts in Sjögren Syndrome.** Axial T2WI. The 27-year-old woman presented with parotid swelling and complaints of dry eyes and mouth and was diagnosed with Sjögren syndrome, a chronic autoimmune disorder. MR reveals innumerable tiny parotid cysts, reflecting the lymphocytic infiltration of the exocrine glands, which causes lymphatic obstruction and cyst formation (*arrows*). Parotid cysts (benign lymphoepithelial cysts) can be seen in a variety of conditions with lymphocytic infiltration, including AIDS.

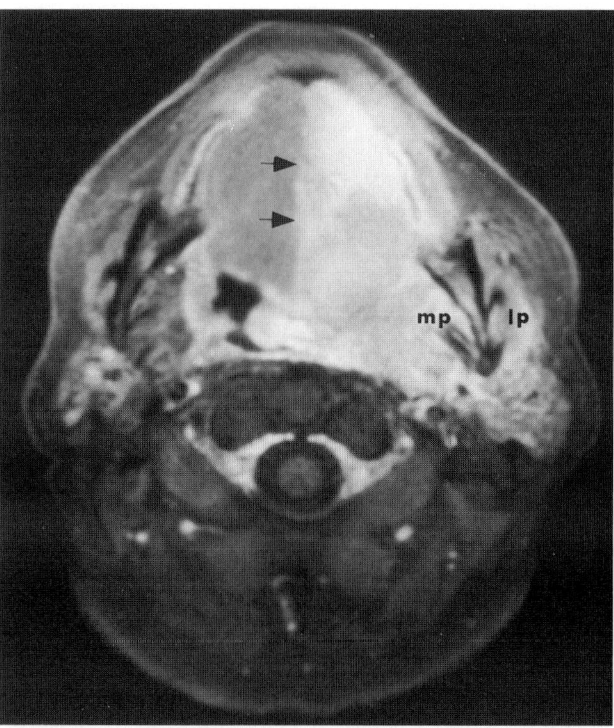

FIGURE 9.21. **Squamous Cell Carcinoma of the Tongue.** Axial postgadolinium fat-suppressed T1WI through the level of the oropharynx. A left tongue base squamous cell carcinoma extends posteriorly along the oropharyngeal wall into the masticator space. Malignancies of the masticator space are most frequently the result of the direct posterior extension of oropharyngeal squamous cell carcinoma. In this example, the left half of the tongue (*arrows*) is diffusely enhancing, indicating denervation myositis, due to involvement of the hypoglossal nerve. Later, the muscles will atrophy and become replaced by fat. mp, medial pterygoid muscle; lp, lateral pterygoid muscle.

disease, and careful attention must be paid to imaging of the cranial nerves of the skull base (Fig. 9.25).

LYMPH NODES

Once a primary neoplasm of the head and neck is detected, the assessment of lymph nodes is a vital part of tumor staging. The presence of a single ipsilateral malignant node reduces the patient's expected survival by 50%, with extracapsular nodal extension reducing survival by an additional 25%. Thus, the detection of nodal disease is critical for both prognosis and therapy. CT, MR, and PET all play a vital role in the staging of head and neck neoplasms, because clinically, it is difficult to determine the full size of the primary neoplasm and its associated nodal extension. At least 15% of malignant nodes are clinically occult because of their deep location (e.g., retropharyngeal nodes) and thus are not palpable by the clinician. The overall error rate in assessing the presence of adenopathy by palpation is between 25% and 33%. Thus, PET combined with either CT or MR is vital in obtaining the most accurate pretreatment planning information.

There are at least 10 major lymph node groups in the head and neck. Knowledge of the location of these cervical lymph node chains and the usual modes of spread of head and neck disease is essential for successful analysis of CT and MR scans. We will focus on the principal lymph node group of the neck: the internal jugular chain. The internal jugular nodal chain serves as the final common afferent pathway for lymphatic drainage of the entire head and neck. This nodal chain follows the oblique course of the jugular vein beneath and adjacent to the anterior border of the sternocleidomastoid muscle. The jugulodigastric node is the highest node of the internal jugular chain. It is located where the posterior belly of the digastric muscle crosses this chain, near the level of the hyoid bone. The jugulodigastric lymph node is immediately posterior to the submandibular gland and provides lymphatic drainage from the tonsil, oral cavity, pharynx, and submandibular nodes.

The jugulodigastric node and submandibular nodes may normally measure up to 1.5 cm in diameter; in contrast, all other nodes of the head and neck are considered abnormal if larger than 1.0 cm. When an enlarged node

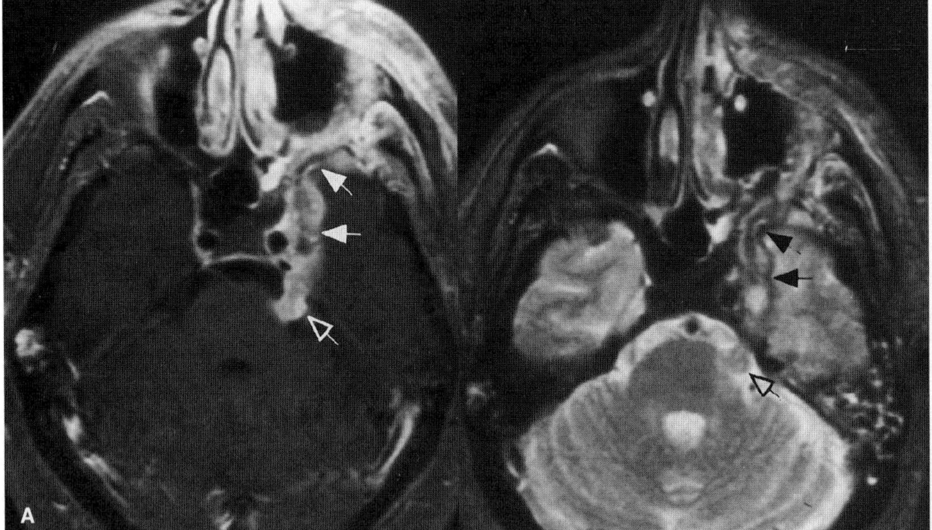

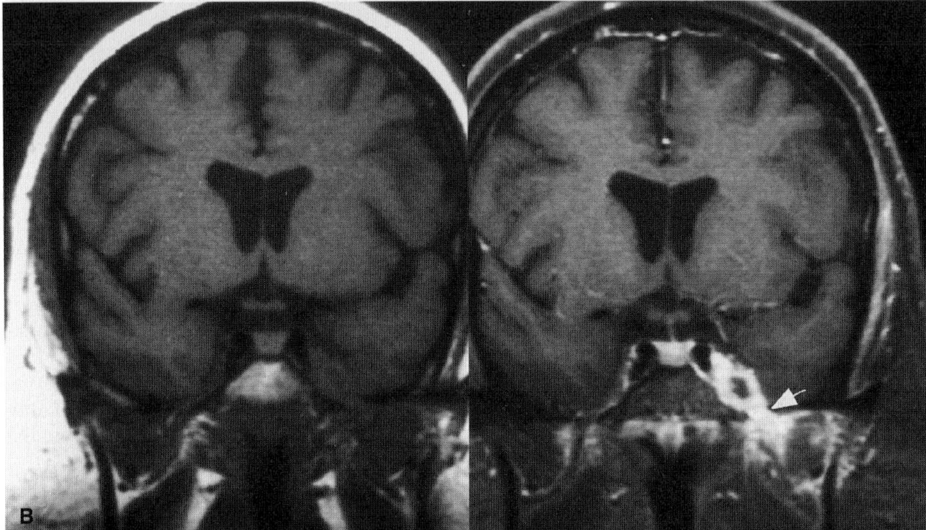

FIGURE 9.22. **Perineural Spread of Disease: Mucormycosis Infection.** A 32-year-old man presented in diabetic ketoacidosis, with left facial numbness. Perineural spread of disease is noted extending from the anterior cheek all the way to the cavernous sinus and brainstem. Perineural spread of a neoplasm, such as adenoid cystic carcinoma or squamous carcinoma, would have an identical imaging appearance. **A.** Axial postgadolinium fat-suppressed T1WI (*left*) and T2WI (*right*) through the level of the nasopharynx. Soft tissue infiltration involves the left malleolar soft tissues, and extends along the maxillary division of the trigeminal nerve (V2) (*arrows*) into the cavernous sinus. From the cavernous sinus, contrast-enhancing tissue extends along the cisternal portion of the trigeminal nerve (*open arrows*) to the brainstem. **B.** Coronal T1WIs, pregadolinium (*left*) and postgadolinium (*right*) with fat suppression. Contrast enhancement is seen filling the cavernous sinus and extending through the foramen ovale (*arrow*) into the masticator space along the mandibular division of the trigeminal nerve (V3).

is encountered on CT or MR, differentiation between a benign reactive node and a malignant one can be difficult. Several features that suggest malignancy are (*1*) peripheral nodal enhancement with central necrosis, (*2*) extracapsular spread with infiltration of adjacent tissues, and (*3*) a matted conglomerate mass of nodes. Nodal size itself is a less reliable indicator of malignancy, but it is used because the other more reliable differentiating features are frequently not present. If size criteria alone are used, approximately 70% of enlarged nodes are secondary to metastatic disease and 30% are caused by benign reactive hyperplasia. Note that the features described as characteristic for malignancy are the same as those for infection, and the two cannot be differentiated by imaging. Fortunately, this distinction is often easily made clinically.

PET scanning plays a vital role in the staging of any head and neck malignancy. Because metastatic nodes, regardless of size, are typically very glucose avid, PET provides exquisite sensitivity and specificity in the detection of cervical metastatic nodal disease. A lymph node that appears normal by size criteria on MR or CT may in fact be malignant if hot on PET scan (Fig. 9.26). The converse is also true; an enlarged lymph node on MR or CT may in fact be benign reactive in nature, if cold on PET.

Lymph nodes can be accurately detected with either multislice helical CT or MR, and the decision regarding which technique to use should be based upon the imaging the patient is most likely to tolerate. Head and neck oncology patients often have respiratory and swallowing issues that prevent them from keeping sufficiently still for satisfactory MR scans. In contrast, multislice CT provides for rapid thin-section imaging of the neck with minimal motion artifact. With MR imaging, lymph nodes are well visualized on fat-suppressed FSE T2WIs, as well as precontrast T1WIs and postcontrast fat-suppressed T1WIs. Normal lymph nodes demonstrate homogeneous signal

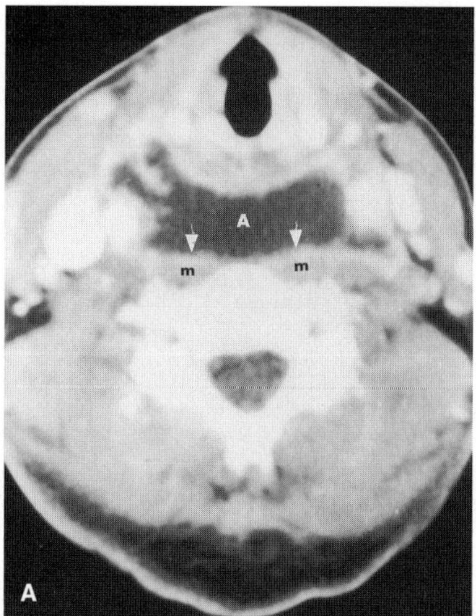

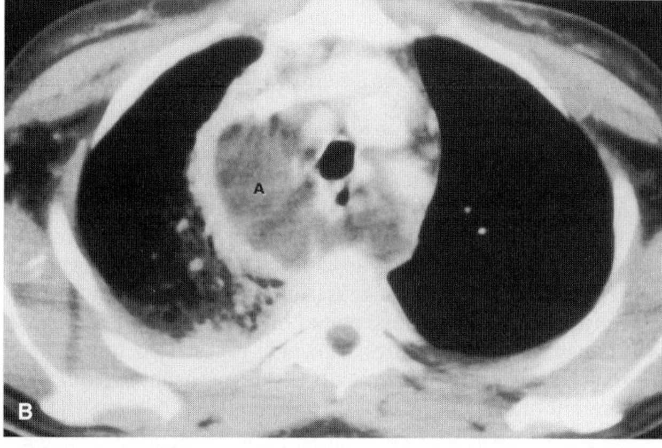

FIGURE 9.23. **Retropharyngeal Abscess.** Axial postcontrast CT through the level of the larynx **(A)** and the upper mediastinum **(B).** A large fluid collection (*A*) extends from the retropharyngeal space into the upper mediastinum. The posterior displacement of the prevertebral muscles (m) (*arrows*) identifies this collection as being retropharyngeal as opposed to prevertebral.

intensity, whether on precontrast or postcontrast T1WIs or T2WIs. Any heterogeneity in signal, especially in the presence of cystic change or necrosis, is consistent with metastatic disease (Fig. 9.6). Note that a fatty central hilus is a normal finding. Shape is also a differentiating feature, as a rounded shape suggests neoplastic nodal infiltration with associated nodal expansion. In contrast, if a node is enlarged but maintains its normal reniform configuration, it more likely reflects benign reactive change rather than metastatic disease.

ORBIT

Both CT and MR are valuable for imaging of the orbit; each has distinct merits. When evaluating for calcification, such as in retinoblastoma in a child with leukocoria or for bony fracture following trauma, CT is the modality of choice. MR, on the other hand, with its multiplanar capability and superior soft tissue discrimination, has proven to be of tremendous value in orbital imaging. For most orbital abnormalities, including evaluation of the visual pathways, MR is the procedure of choice.

Knowledge of the contents of the various orbital spaces provides insight into the naturally occurring lesions that develop within each area. The retrobulbar space contains both the extraconal and the intraconal spaces, which are separated by the muscle cone or "annulus of Zinn." This muscle cone is formed by the extraocular muscles (superior, inferior, medial, and lateral rectus; superior oblique; and levator palpebrae superior) and a fibrous septum. Together these structures form a cone with its base at the posterior of the globe and its apex at the superior orbital fissure. When identifying an intraconal lesion, an essential issue is whether the lesion arises from the optic nerve sheath complex or is extrinsic to it. The optic nerve sheath complex is composed of the optic nerve and the surrounding perioptic nerve sheath. The optic nerve is an extension of the brain enveloped by CSF and leptomeninges, which form the optic nerve sheath. Therefore, the CSF space that envelops the optic nerve is continuous with the intracranial subarachnoid space. If a lesion arises from the optic nerve sheath complex, the most common lesion is either an optic nerve glioma or optic sheath meningioma.

Optic nerve glioma is the most common tumor of the optic nerve and typically occurs during the first decade of life (Fig. 9.27). There is a high association with neurofibromatosis type 1, particularly when there is bilateral optic nerve involvement. Histologically, these lesions are low-grade pilocytic astrocytomas. The characteristic imaging finding is that of enlargement of the optic nerve sheath complex. The enlarged sheath complex may be tubular, fusiform, or eccentric with kinking. Some optic nerve gliomas have extensive associated thickening of the perioptic meninges. Histologically, this reflects peritumoral-reactive meningeal change, which has been termed *arachnoidal hyperplasia* or *gliomatosis*. This finding is often seen in patients with neurofibromatosis.

Optic sheath meningiomas arise from hemangioendothelial cells of the arachnoid layer of the optic nerve sheath. These lesions assume a circular configuration and grow in a linear fashion along the optic nerve. Optic sheath meningiomas demonstrate a characteristic "tram track" pattern of linear contrast enhancement, because the nerve sheath enhances, rather than the nerve itself. MR easily displays any tumor extension along the optic nerve sheath through the orbital apex (Fig. 9.28). In contrast to optic nerve gliomas, meningiomas may invade and grow through the dura, resulting in an irregular and asymmetric appearance. Additionally, optic sheath meningiomas may be extensively calcified, whereas optic nerve gliomas rarely have any calcification. In patients with sarcoidosis,

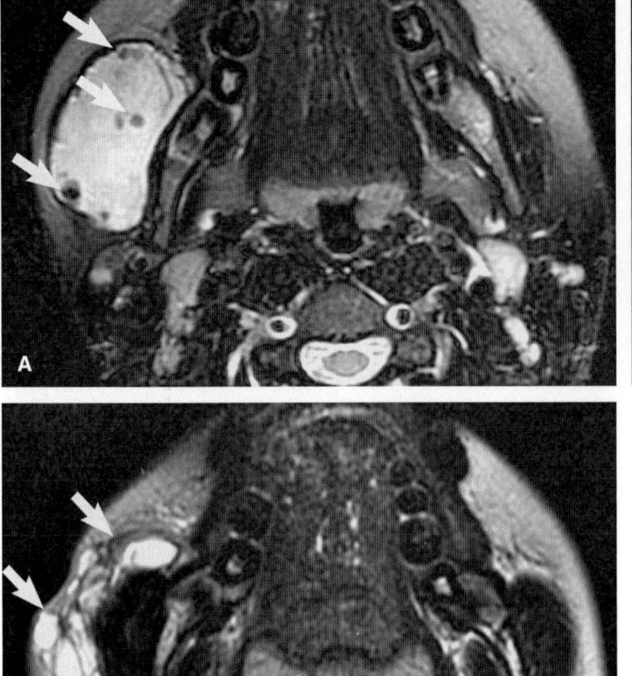

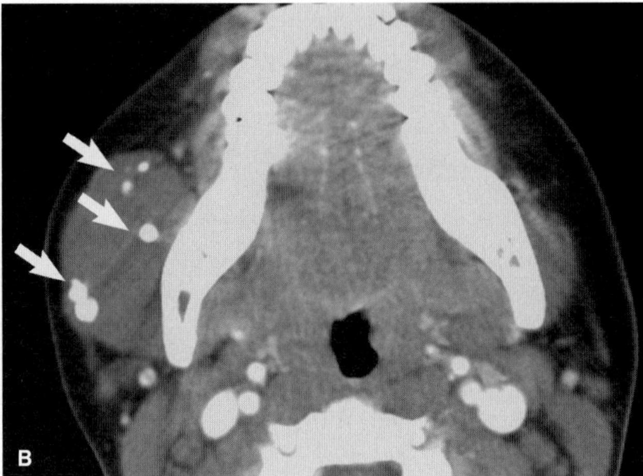

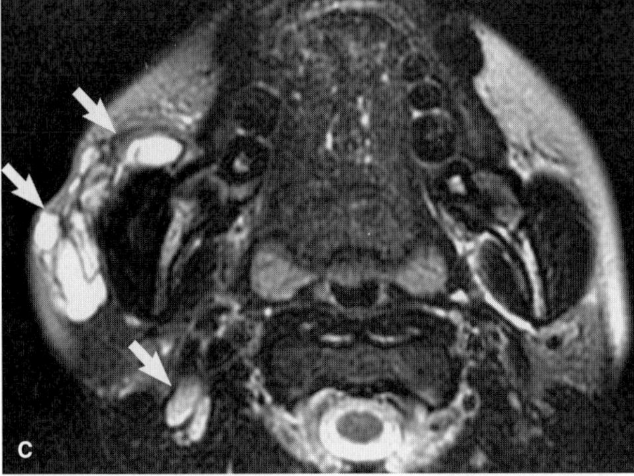

FIGURE 9.24. **Hemangioma.** Patient presented with a facial mass which demonstrates high signal on T2WI **(A)** with punctuate foci of signal void (*arrows*). On CT **(B),** these foci of low T2 signal prove to be phleboliths (*arrows*), which is essentially pathognomonic of the diagnosis of hemangioma. In another patient with a similar clinical presentation, a T2WI **(C)** reveals a multilobulated and multiseptated high-signal-intensity lesion with imaging characteristics also consistent with hemangioma (*arrows*). Lymphangiomas may be indistinguishable from this lesion, but often have fluid–fluid levels related to hemorrhage.

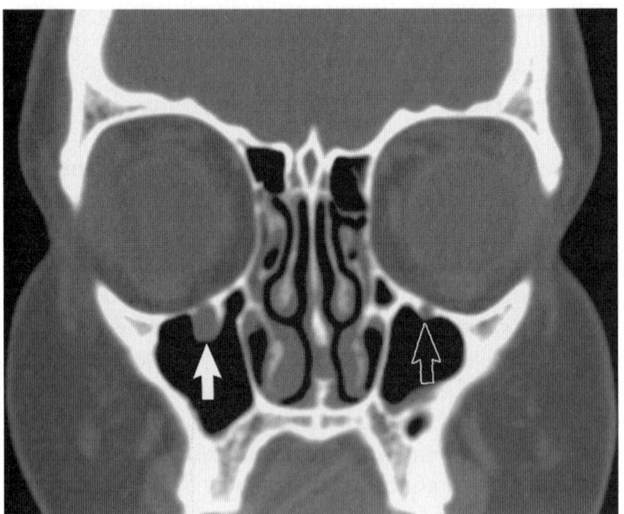

FIGURE 9.25. **Perineural Spread of Tumor.** This 18-year-old woman was recent postresection of a right cheek melanoma with clean histologic margins. However, a CT was performed following persistent maxillary division paresthesias. Coronal plane image reveals abnormal enlargement of the maxillary nerve within the infraorbital canal (*solid arrow*), which extended back to the pterygopalatine fossa. Focal nerve biopsy revealed perineural spread of melanoma. Compare to normal infraorbital nerve and canal (*open arrow*).

leukemia or lymphoma, cellular infiltrates may deposit within the perioptic nerve sheath CSF space. In such cases, contrast enhancement of the perioptic nerve sheath space may mimic the "tram track" appearance of a nerve sheath meningioma. An important differential diagnostic consideration for enhancement of the optic nerve sheath is optic neuritis. In contrast to the conditions just mentioned, which demonstrate enhancement of the optic nerve sheath (i.e., peripheral optic nerve enhancement), optic neuritis demonstrates abnormal T2 hyperintensity and contrast enhancement as a result of inflammation of the optic nerve itself (Fig. 9.29). Optic neuritis presents with an acute visual deficit, often described as "blurring" of vision, and can be the first sign of multiple sclerosis (MS). Approximately 20% of patients with MS initially present with an episode of optic neuritis. In fact, of patients with isolated optic neuritis, approximately 50% eventually are diagnosed with MS.

Vascular Lesions. A variety of vascular lesions may develop in the orbit. The four lesions we will consider include capillary hemangioma, lymphangioma, cavernous hemangioma, and varix. These lesions are readily distinguished by a combination of imaging and clinical findings, including the patient's age (see Table 9.2). *Capillary hemangiomas*

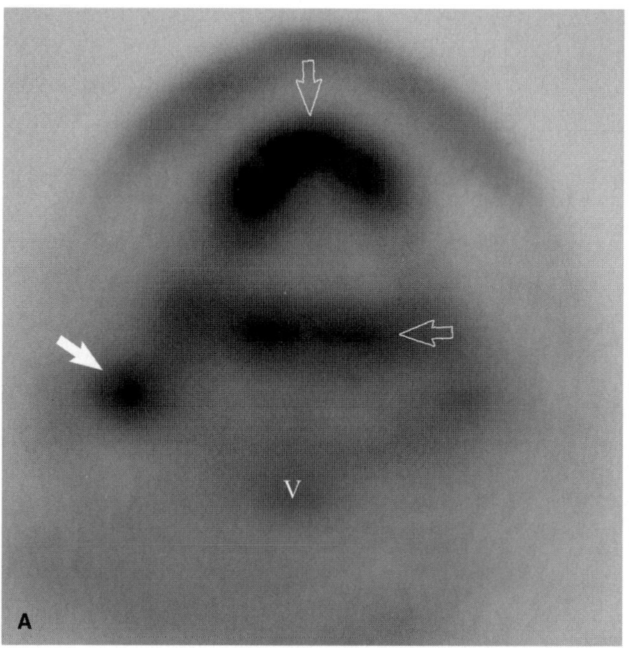

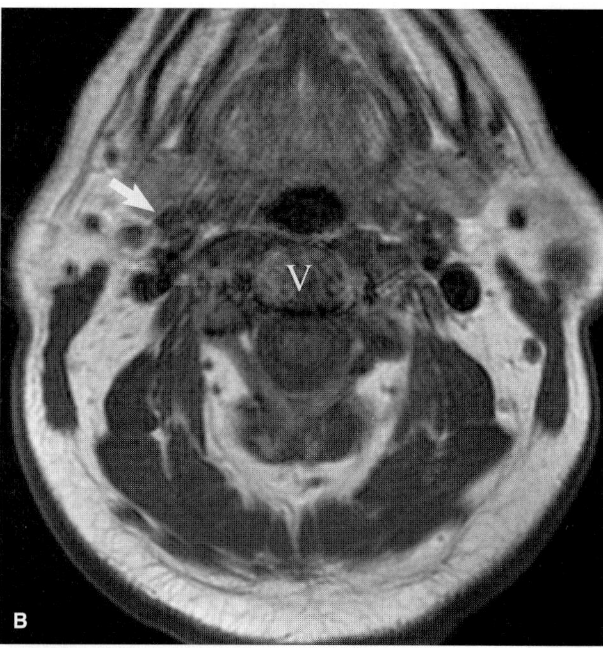

FIGURE 9.26. **Metastatic Lymph Node That Appeared Normal Based on MR Size Criteria.** This 68-year-old man presented with a right nasopharyngeal carcinoma, which appeared localized without significant cervical adenopathy. However, a PET scan **(A)** revealed a focus of abnormal uptake (*arrow*) in a lymph node, which appeared normal on MR. Note incidental uptake in the lingual salivary glands and tongue base lymphoidal tissue on the PET scan (*open arrows*). **B.** This lymph node (*arrow*) appears morphologically benign on MR, but was proven metastatic disease on modified radical neck dissection. V, vertebral body.

develop in infants (younger than 1 year) and are diagnosed within the first weeks of life. Although these lesions may grow rapidly in size, they typically plateau during the first year or two then regress spontaneously. On imaging studies, a capillary hemangioma appears as an infiltrative soft tissue complex, often with multiple vascular flow voids. In contrast, *lymphangiomas* are one of the most common orbital tumors of childhood and occur in an older group of children (3 to 15 years). Lymphangiomas are characterized by their propensity to bleed, and they often contain blood degradation products. An acute hemorrhage may result in marked expansion of the lesion with sudden proptosis (Fig. 9.30). MR reveals a multiloculated, lobular mass with characteristic signal heterogeneity caused by blood degradation products (Fig. 9.31). The older age of presentation, combined with the characteristic heterogeneous signal related to blood products, allows differentiation from the capillary hemangiomas. *Cavernous hemangiomas* are one of the most common orbital masses in adults. In contrast to the other vascular lesions of the orbit, hemangiomas are characterized as a sharply circumscribed, rounded mass (Fig. 9.32). These lesions demonstrate diffuse enhancement, sometimes with a mottled pattern. The venous *varix* is an enormously dilated vein that is characterized by its marked change in size with the Valsalva maneuver.

Superior ophthalmic vein is well visualized on MR studies. Pathology includes thrombosis and enlargement. Thrombosis often occurs in conjunction with cavernous sinus thrombosis and presents as loss of the normal flow void, with signal intensity related to the age of the thrombus. Enlargement of the superior ophthalmic vein may also be seen with cavernous carotid fistulas (Fig. 9.33). Cavernous carotid fistulas represent direct or indirect communication between the internal carotid artery and the venous cavernous sinus. These are either spontaneous or posttraumatic, and patients may present with pulsating exophthalmos and bruit.

Pseudotumor and lymphoma are two important orbital lesions that may present with similar imaging findings. Idiopathic inflammatory pseudotumor is a poorly characterized condition that results from an inflammatory lymphocytic infiltrate. This is the most common cause of an intraorbital mass lesion in the adult population. Pseudotumor is often rapidly developing and presents with painful proptosis, chemosis, and ophthalmoplegia. In contrast, lymphoma tends to present with painless proptosis. Lymphoma is the third most common adult orbital mass lesion, following pseudotumor and cavernous hemangioma. On imaging studies, both lymphoma and pseudotumor appear as diffusely infiltrating lesions capable of involving and extending into any retrobulbar structures (Fig. 9.34). Several reports have suggested that T2 shortening of the tumor (dark on T2) is suggestive of pseudotumor. Nevertheless, the distinction between these two entities frequently

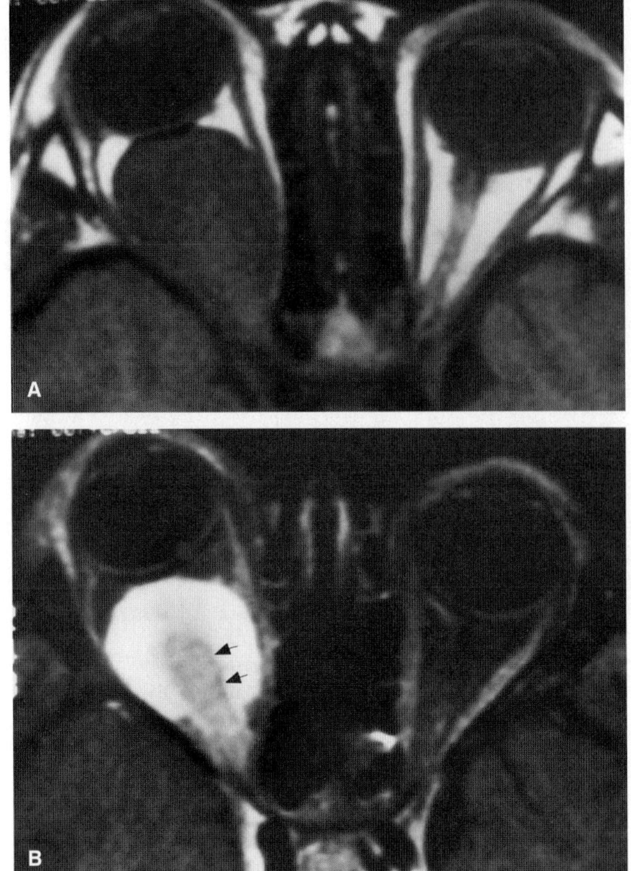

FIGURE 9.27. Optic Nerve Glioma. Axial pregadolinium **(A)** and postgadolinium **(B)** fat-suppressed T1WIs through the orbits. A large mass involves the right optic nerve. Following the administration of contrast, the enlarged optic nerve (*arrows*) is visible coursing through markedly thickened optic sheath soft tissue. This soft tissue represents arachnoidal hyperplasia, a finding associated with optic gliomas in patients with neurofibromatosis.

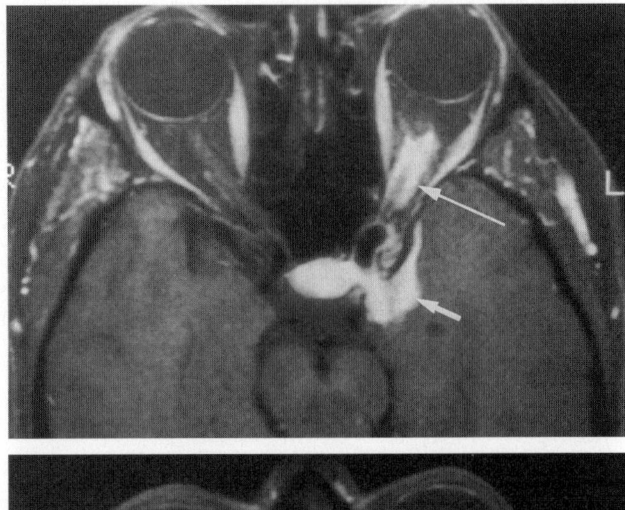

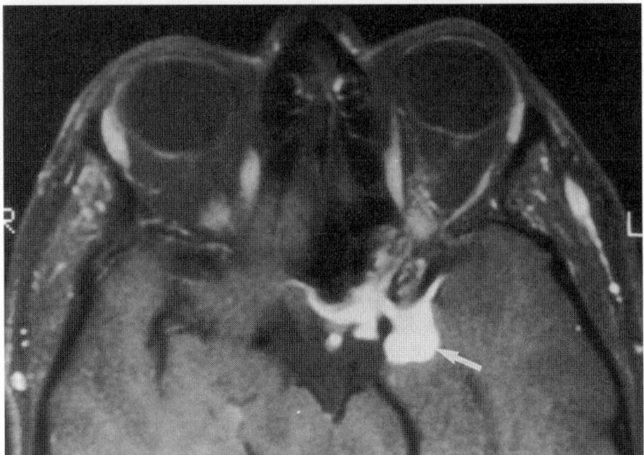

FIGURE 9.28. Optic Sheath Meningioma. Axial postgadolinium fat-suppression T1WI through the orbits. "Tram track" enhancement involves the left optic nerve sheath (*long arrow*), and a tumor (*short arrows*) extends into the middle cranial fossa. The "tram track" enhancement and the dural tail within the middle cranial fossa are characteristic of a meningioma.

remains very difficult clinically, radiographically, and even histopathologically.

It is reported that a trial dose of steroids may be valuable in differentiating these two entities. Steroids are reported to have a lasting effect, eliminating a pseudotumor lesion. However, the cytolytic effect of steroids on lymphoma may also have a similar but short-lived response that may initially be confounding. Additionally, when a diffusely infiltrative mass is encountered in a young child anywhere in the head and neck region, including the orbits, rhabdomyosarcoma should be a consideration.

Thyroid ophthalmopathy (Graves disease) is a common lesion and is the most frequent cause of unilateral or bilateral proptosis in adults. This condition is the result of an inflammatory infiltration of the orbital muscles and orbital connective tissues. Most patients will have clinical or laboratory evidence of hyperthyroidism, but 10% will not; these are referred to as "euthyroid ophthalmopathy." Imaging findings consist of enlargement of the extraocular muscles with sparing of the tendinous attachments to the globe (Fig. 9.35). This is in contrast to pseudotumor, which typically involves the muscle attachments to the globe. The muscles involved, in decreasing order of frequency, are the ***i***nferior, ***m***edial, ***s***uperior, and ***l***ateral rectus (pneumonic "***I'm slow***" reminds one of the order of muscle involvement and the typical orbital symptoms of Grave disease, namely lid lag and limitation in orbital movement). Eighty percent of patients have bilateral muscle involvement. In some cases of thyroid ophthalmopathy, the extraocular muscles may be normal, and exophthalmos is the result of increased retrobulbar fat.

Lacrimal Gland. The extraconal space primarily contains fat and the lacrimal gland. However, many lesions

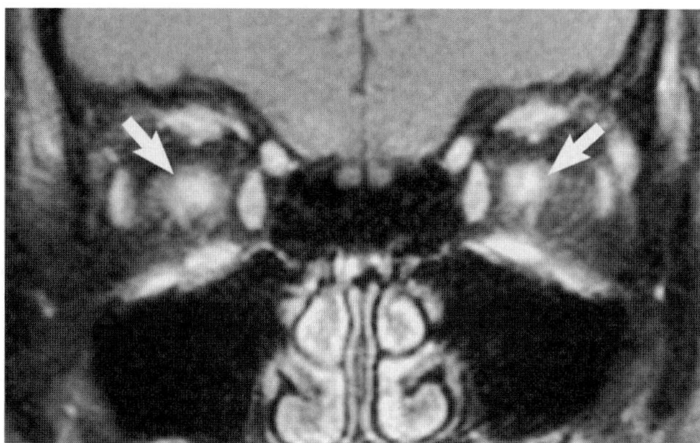

FIGURE 9.29. **Optic Neuritis.** This 23-year-old woman presented with bilateral loss of vision. Coronal fat-saturated T1WI postgadolinium administration reveals marked enhancement of both optic nerves characteristic of optic neuritis (*arrows*), which often heralds the onset of multiple sclerosis. Optic neuritis reflects a demyelinating often related to multiple sclerosis; however, other etiologies include demyelination or inflammation secondary to infections related to sinusitis, tuberculosis, and viral agents such as herpes and cytomegalovirus, or as a complication of radiation therapy.

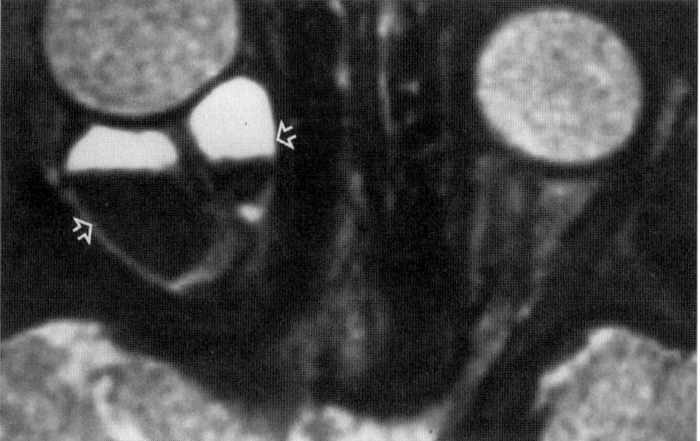

FIGURE 9.30. **Lymphangioma.** Axial T2WI reveals a cystic retrobulbar lesion (*arrows*) with a hematocrit effect (serum layered above red blood cells). Hemorrhage into a lesion is a characteristic feature of lymphangiomas and may be responsible for the rapid development of proptosis.

involving the extraconal space are the result of tumor or inflammation extending from surrounding structures. These may include most of the lesions described earlier, as well as sinus-related inflammation. In contrast, lesions arising from within the extraconal space are primarily lacrimal in origin. Lesions of the lacrimal gland are very nonspecific, but can be divided into inflammatory types (e.g., sarcoidosis, Sjögren syndrome) and neoplastic types. Neoplasms of the lacrimal gland include epithelial and lymphoid tumors. Epithelial tumors are any of the lesions that arise from the salivary glands, such as benign mixed-cell tumor or adenoid cystic carcinoma. Lymphoid tumors include lymphoma and pseudotumor. Although none of these lesions have specific imaging findings, dermoid is one lesion that does have a characteristic finding, consisting of a fat–fluid level (Fig. 9.36).

TABLE 9.2 Vascular Orbital Lesions

Lesion	*Age*	*Imaging Features*	*Morphology*
Capillary hemangioma	<1 yr	Flow voids	Infiltrative lesion
Lymphangioma	3–15 yr	Blood products	Multiloculated, lobular mass
Cavernous hemangioma	Adults	Well-circumscribed mass	Rounded mass
Varix	Any age	Dilated vein, may enlarge with Valsalva maneuver	Vascular structure

Globe. A variety of lesions may involve the globe, and as usual, clinical history is vital in arriving at a useful differential diagnosis. In the pediatric age group, retinoblastoma is the most common primary ocular malignancy and presents characteristically with leukocoria (white pupillary reflex) and a calcified ocular mass (Fig. 9.37). Other conditions are rare and include developmental abnormalities (persistent hyperplastic primary vitreous tumor and Coats disease), acquired retinal lesions (retinopathy of prematurity), and infection (primarily endophthalmitis secondary to *Toxocara canis*). Note that although retinopathy of prematurity and persistent hyperplastic primary vitreous tumour may be bilateral, Coats disease and ocular toxocariasis are almost always unilateral. In the adult, common ocular pathology includes retinal and choroidal detachment, uveal melanoma, and metastasis.

CONGENITAL LESIONS

In children, neck masses tend to be benign, including both congenital (thyroglossal duct cysts, branchial cleft cysts, and lymphangiomas/cystic hygromas) and inflammatory lesions. When malignancy is entertained, the most common lesion in the pediatric age group is lymphoma, followed by rhabdomyosarcoma.

Thyroglossal duct cysts account for about 90% of congenital neck lesions and usually are found in children but may be seen in adults. The thyroglossal duct represents an epithelium-lined tract along which the primordial thyroid gland migrates. This tubular structure originates from the foramen cecum (at the tongue base), extends anterior to the thyrohyoid membrane and strap muscles, and ends at the level of the thyroid isthmus. The duct normally involutes by 8 to 10 weeks of gestation. Because the duct

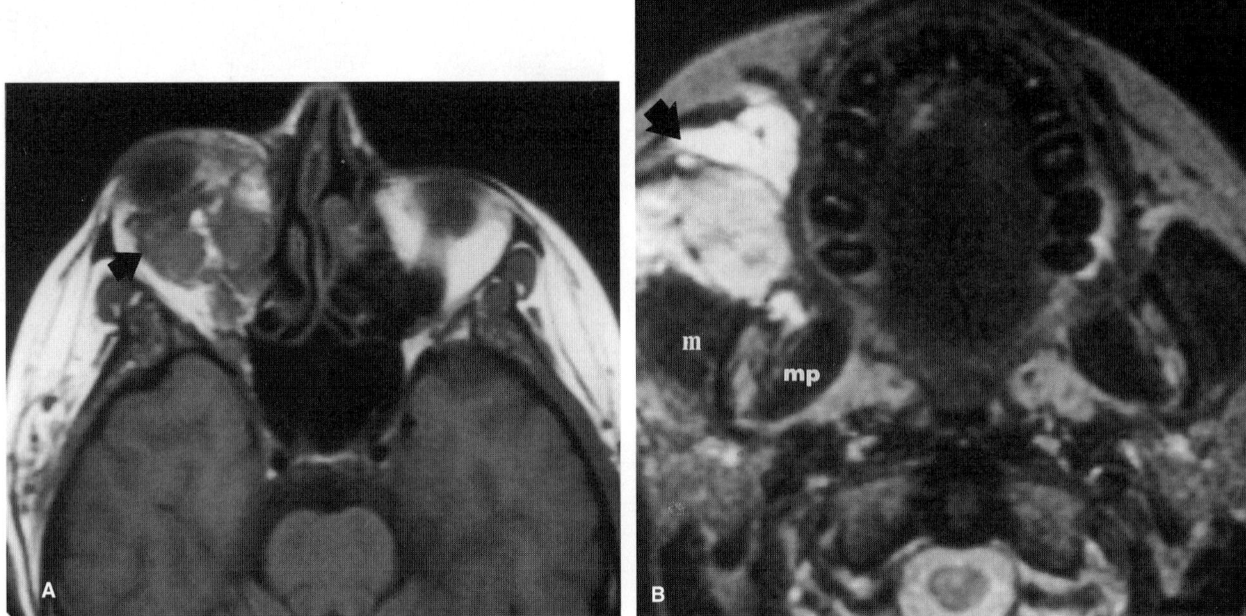

FIGURE 9.31. **Lymphangioma.** Axial T1WI **(A)** through the orbit and T2WI **(B)** through the midface. A heterogeneous lesion (*arrows*) extends from the right orbit through the inferior orbital fissure into the masticator space. The heterogeneous signal of this lesion, as well as its tendency to extend across fascial spaces, is characteristic for lymphangioma. *m*, masseter muscle; *mp*, medial pterygoid muscle.

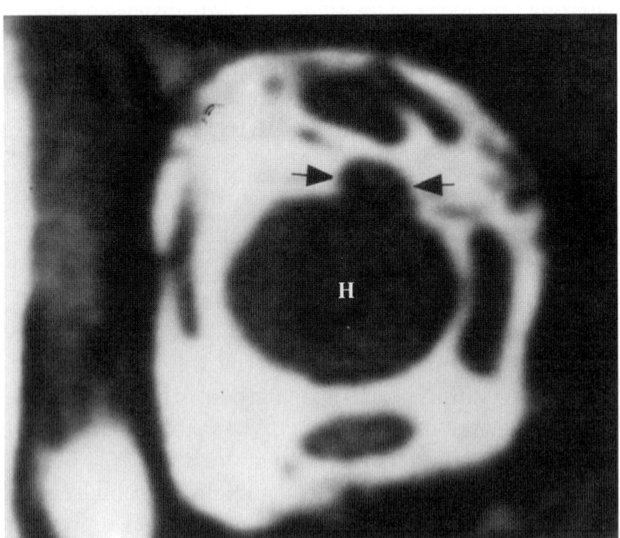

FIGURE 9.32. **Cavernous Hemangioma.** Coronal T1WI through the midorbit. A well-circumscribed retrobulbar mass (H) is identified. The optic nerve is clearly separate from the mass (*arrows*). The well-circumscribed nature of this mass is characteristic of a cavernous hemangioma, the most common orbital mass in adults.

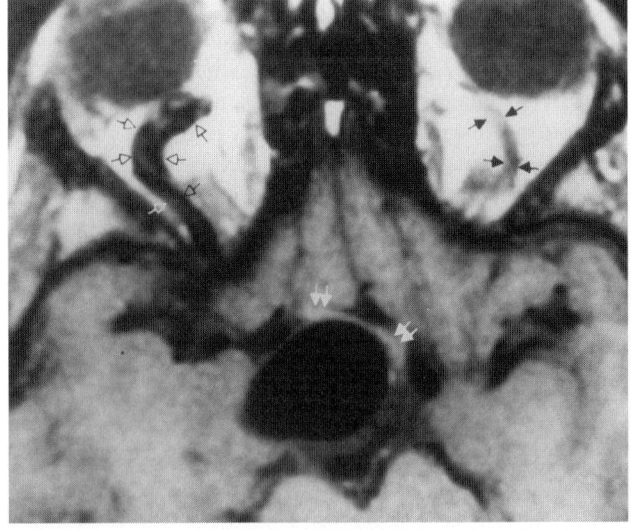

FIGURE 9.33. **Carotid Cavernous Fistula.** Axial T1WI through the superior orbit. Following a remote head injury, this patient presented with right chemosis. A large flow void is identified within the right cavernous sinus (*white arrows*). The right superior ophthalmic vein is abnormally dilated (*open arrows*), but the left vein is normal (*black arrows*). Dilatation of the superior ophthalmic vein is an important clue to the presence of a carotid cavernous fistula.

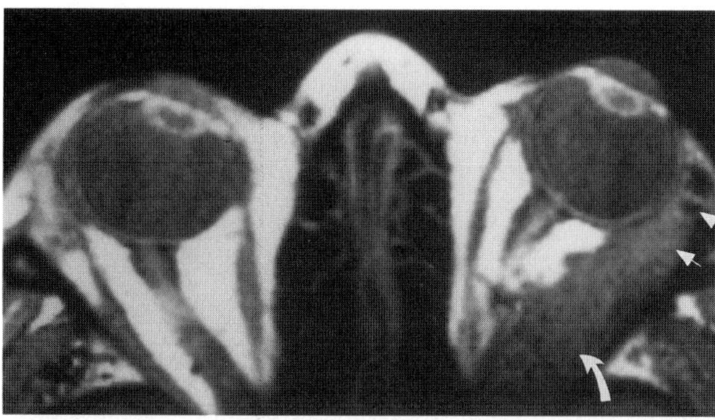

FIGURE 9.34. **Pseudotumor.** Axial T1WI through the orbits. A diffusely infiltrating lesion (*curved arrow*) extends throughout the lateral rectus muscle, including involvement of its tendinous insertion on the globe (*short arrows*). This feature distinguishes pseudotumor from thyroid ophthalmopathy, in which the muscle insertion is spared.

is lined with secretory epithelium, any portion of the thyroglossal duct that fails to involute may give rise to a cyst or sinus tract. Additionally, thyroid glandular tissue can arrest anywhere along the course of the thyroglossal duct, giving rise to ectopic thyroid tissue. Seventy-five percent of thyroglossal duct cysts are midline, and most are located at or below the level of the hyoid bone in the region of the thyrohyoid membrane. In fact, thyroglossal duct cysts are the most common midline neck mass.

Surgery is the treatment of choice for these lesions because they may become infected. These lesions tend to recur if incompletely resected. Therefore, sagittal MR is ideal for determining the full extent of the lesion prior to surgery. On CT and MR, these lesions appear as cystic masses with

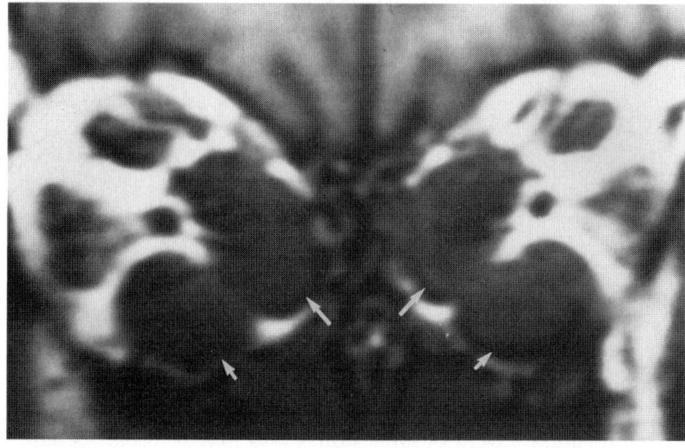

FIGURE 9.35. **Thyroid Ophthalmopathy.** Coronal T1WI through the midorbits. Marked extraocular muscle enlargement is identified, involving primarily the medial (*long arrows*) and inferior (*short arrows*) rectus muscles. Thyroid ophthalmopathy is the most common cause of proptosis in the adult. Severe muscle hypertrophy may result in orbital apex compression and loss of vision.

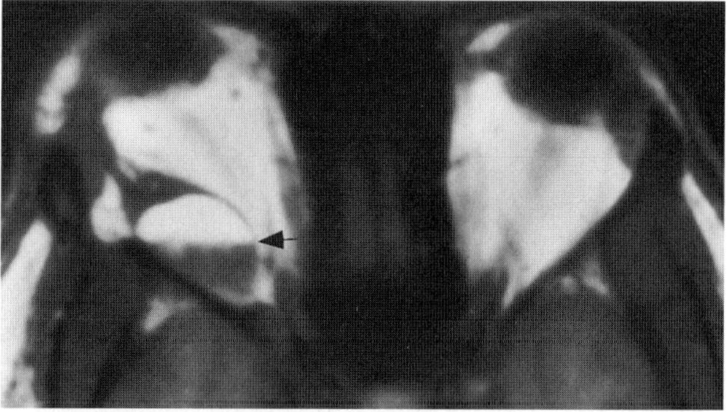

FIGURE 9.36. **Dermoid.** Axial T1WI. A well-circumscribed mass in the lateral orbit demonstrates a fat–fluid level (*arrow*) characteristic for a dermoid.

a uniformly thin peripheral rim of capsular enhancement, with occasional septations (Fig. 9.38). Differential diagnostic considerations include necrotic anterior cervical nodes, thrombosed anterior jugular vein, abscess, or obstructed laryngocele. A laryngocele represents an abnormal dilatation of the appendix of the laryngeal ventricle. The laryngeal ventricle separates the false and true cords and anteriorly ends in a blind pouch termed the appendix. The laryngocele develops as a consequence of chronically increased intraglottic pressure, as may be seen in musicians (wind instruments), glass blowers, or excessive coughers. Laryngoceles are classified as internal, external, or mixed, according to their relation to the thyrohyoid membrane. When these lesions are confined to the larynx, they are called internal, but when they protrude above the thyroid cartilage and through the thyrohyoid membrane, they are termed external and typically present as a lateral neck mass near the hyoid bone (Fig. 9.39). Most commonly, laryngoceles have portions that are both in and outside of the thyrohyoid membrane and are called mixed. Laryngoceles that develop without a known predisposing factor should raise the suspicion of an underlying neoplasm obstructing the laryngeal ventricle.

Branchial Cleft Cysts. The structures of the face and neck are derived from the branchial cleft apparatus, which consists of six branchial arches. A branchial cleft cyst, sinus, or fistula may develop if there is failure of the cervical sinus or pouch remnants to regress. Although branchial abnormalities can arise from any of the pouches, the majority (95%) arise from the second branchial cleft. The course of the second branchial cleft begins at the base of the tonsillar fossa and extends between the internal and external carotid arteries. Thus, second branchial cleft cysts are typically found along this pathway, anterior to the middle portion of the sternocleidomastoid muscle and lateral to the internal jugular vein at the level of the carotid bifurcation. The usual clinical presentation is that of a painless neck mass along the anterior border of the

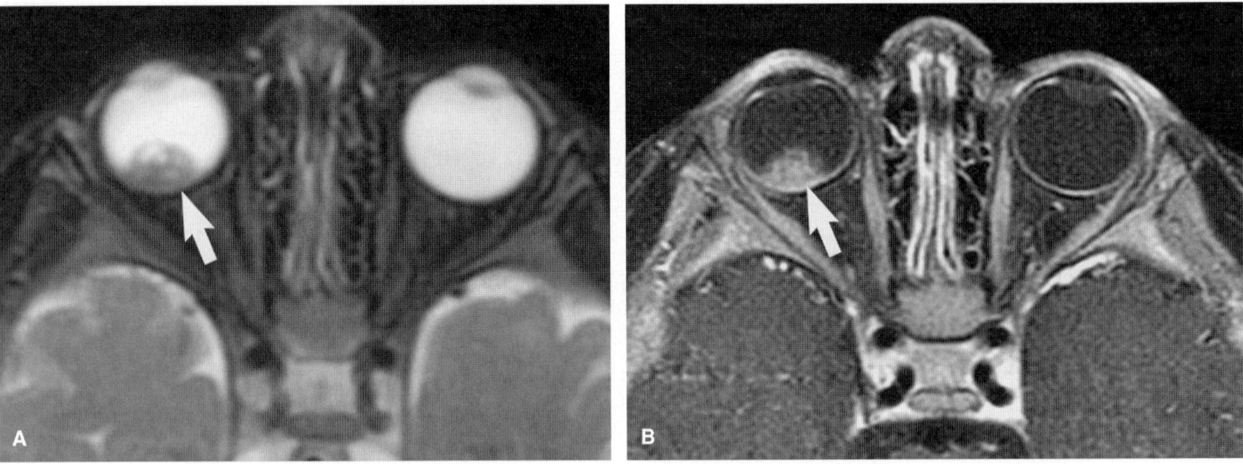

FIGURE 9.37. **Retinoblastoma.** The most common primary ocular malignancy of childhood is retinoblastoma. An 18-month-old infant presented with leukocoria (white pupillary reflex). Axial T2WI **(A)** and postgadolinium T1WI **(B)** reveal an ocular mass confined to the globe without extraocular extension or optic nerve infiltration (*arrow*). MR and CT play an important preoperative role allowing accurate characterization of the full extent of the lesion.

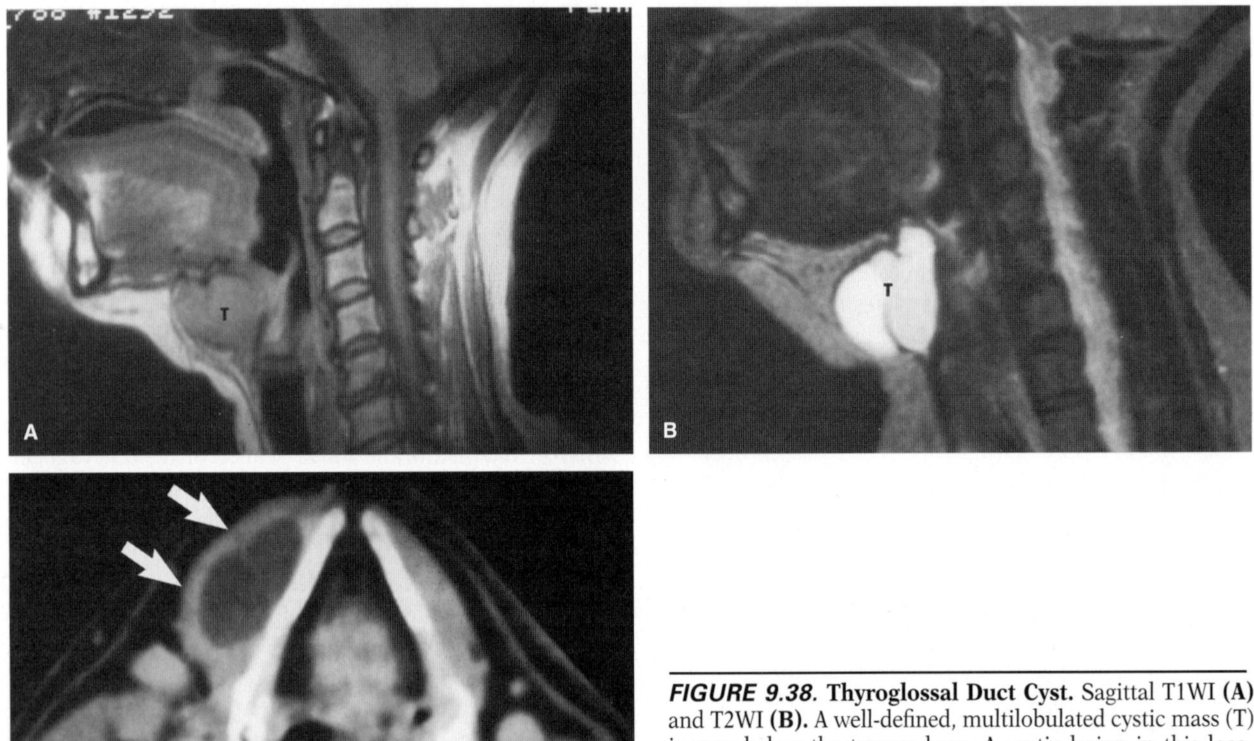

FIGURE 9.38. **Thyroglossal Duct Cyst.** Sagittal T1WI **(A)** and T2WI **(B).** A well-defined, multilobulated cystic mass (T) is seen below the tongue base. A cystic lesion in this location is highly suggestive of a remnant of the thyroglossal duct. Imaging in the sagittal plane is important in defining the full craniocaudal extent of the lesion. **C.** CT in a different patient. The thyroglossal duct cyst (*arrows*) may be embedded within the strap musculature of the neck. Although most commonly midline, they are off midline in 25% of cases. Differential diagnostic considerations include necrotic anterior cervical node, thrombosed anterior jugular vein, or abscess.

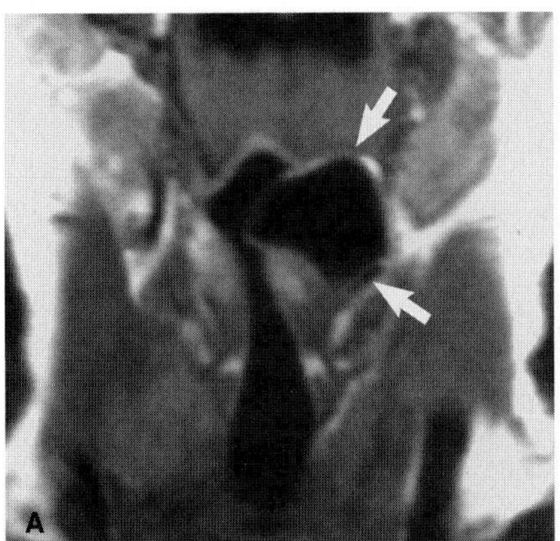

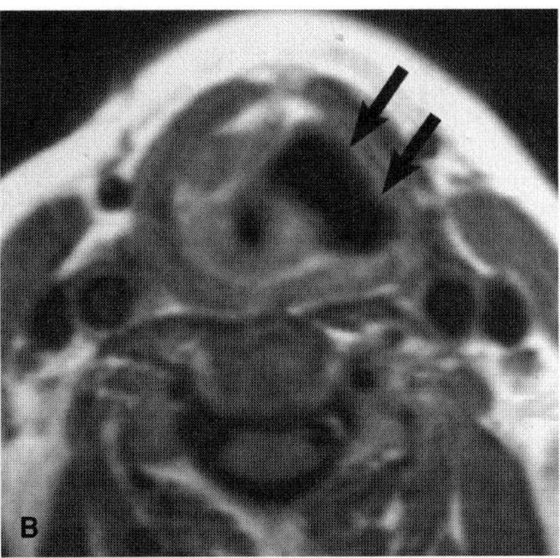

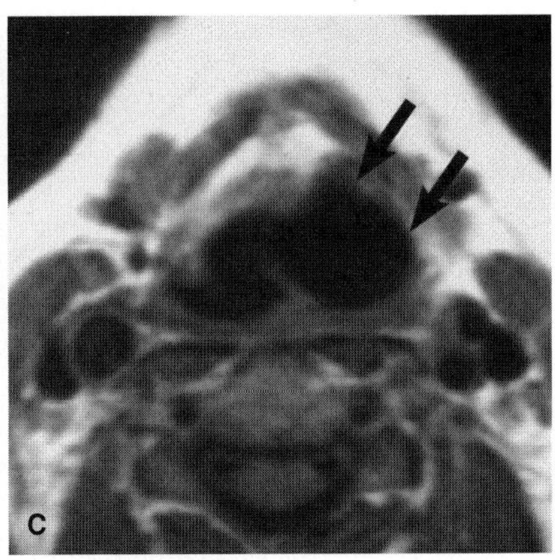

FIGURE 9.39. **Laryngocele.** A trumpet player presented with mild left neck fullness. Coronal **(A)** and axial **(B, C)** T1WIs reveal an air-filled mass associated with the larynx consistent with a laryngocele (*arrows*). These lesions may be fluid filled and mimic a neck abscess or thyroglossal duct cyst. Diagnostic features of the laryngocele are that they communicate with the laryngeal ventricle and are found deep to the strap muscles. In contrast, thyroglossal duct cysts are either superficial or embedded within the strap muscles.

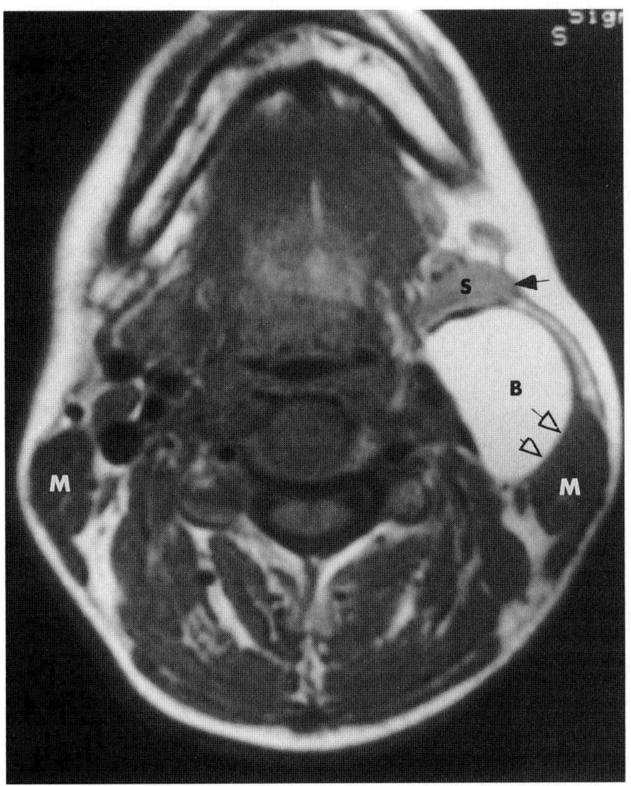

FIGURE 9.40. **Branchial Cleft Cyst.** Axial T1WI through the floor of mouth. A well-rounded, noninfiltrating lesion (B) is seen anterior to the left sternocleidomastoid muscle (*M*), which is displaced posteriorly (*open arrows*). The submandibular gland (*S*) is displaced anteriorly (*arrow*). This lesion is at the level of the carotid bifurcation. This combination of features is characteristic of a branchial cleft cyst. Branchial cleft cysts may display high signal on the T1WI, the result of T1 shortening effect owing to proteinaceous fluid. Differential diagnostic considerations would include necrotic cervical adenopathy. This is especially true in adults, in whom a neck mass is much more likely to be a malignancy rather than a congenital lesion.

sternocleidomastoid muscle, presenting during the first to third decade. These lesions tend to vary in size over time, often enlarging with upper respiratory tract infections.

Branchial cleft cysts are readily identified on CT and MR as well-circumscribed cystic lesions. Wall thickness, irregularity, and enhancement are related to active or prior infections. With MR, the T1W signal characteristics of the cyst may be either hypointense or hyperintense (Figs. 9.40, 9.41). This signal variability is related to proteinaceous cyst contents. Differential diagnostic considerations include necrotic nodes, abscesses, cystic neural lesions, and thrombosed vessels.

Lymphangiomas are congenital malformations of the lymphatic channels. These lesions are benign and nonencapsulated. Histologically, they are classified as capillary, cavernous, or cystic. Any of these histologic types can be found in a given lesion, but the preponderance of a certain type dictates how the lesion is classified. The capillary lymphangiomas are composed of capillary-size, thin-walled lymphatic channels. In contrast, cavernous lymphangiomas are composed of moderately dilated lymphatics with a fibrous adventitia. Cystic hygromas represent enormously dilated lymphatic channels.

The lymphatic system develops from primitive embryonic lymph sacs that are in turn derived from the venous system. If these sacs fail to communicate with the venous system, they dilate as they accumulate lymphatic fluid. Thus, lymphangiomas represent sequestrations of the primitive embryonic lymph sacs. If this defect is localized, the result is an isolated cystic hygroma. However, extensive defects in this lymphovenous communication are incompatible with life and result in fetal hydrops. Various congenital malformation syndromes occur in association with fetal cystic hygromas, including Turner syndrome,

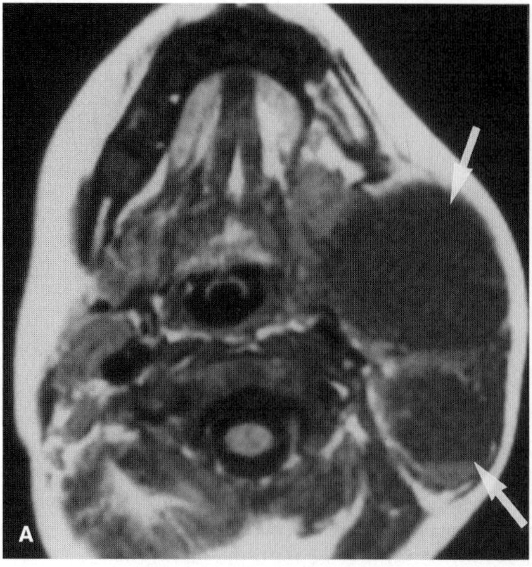

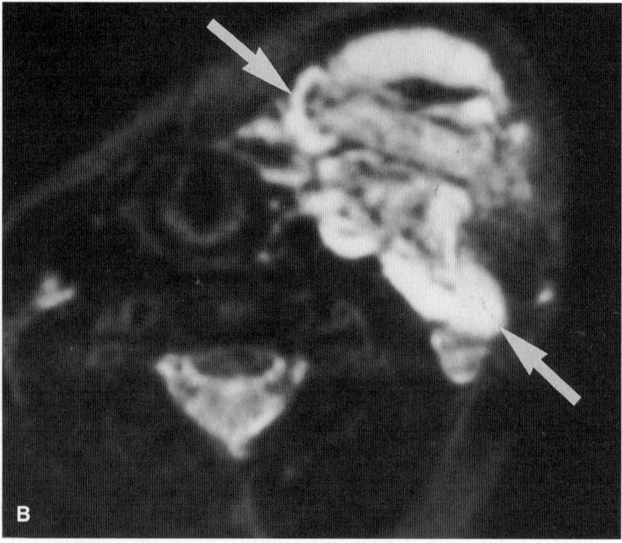

FIGURE 9.41. **Cystic Hygroma.** Axial T1WI at the level of the floor of the mouth **(A)** and T2WI at the level of the larynx **(B)** of a 2-month-old infant. A multiloculated lesion (*arrows*) extends within the soft tissues of the anterior neck. The trans-spatial nature of this lesion and its heterogeneous T2 signal is characteristic of a cystic hygroma or lymphangioma.

fetal alcohol syndrome, Noonan syndrome, and several chromosomal aneuploidies. Most lymphangiomas present by 2 years of age (90%), with 50% presenting at the time of birth. This early presentation reflects that the time of greatest lymphatic development occurs in the first 2 years of life.

Lymphangiomas and cystic hygromas appear as painless compressible neck masses that, if large enough, will transilluminate. The lesions commonly occur in the posterior triangle of the neck. On imaging studies, these lesions are multiloculated cystic masses with septations (Fig. 9.40); they also have a propensity to hemorrhage into themselves. This may result in a dramatic, acute increase in the size of the lesion. On imaging studies, one can expect a hemorrhage–fluid level or heterogeneous signal characteristics associated with blood degradation products. Because these lesions are easily compressible, they tend not to displace adjacent soft tissue structures, and this may prove a helpful differentiating feature from other cystic lesions, such as necrotic lymph nodes.

SUGGESTED READINGS

Babbel RW, Harnsberger HR, Sonkens J, et al. Recurring patterns of inflammatory sinonasal disease demonstrated on screening sinus CT. AJNR Am J Neuroradiol 1992;13:903–912.

Di Martino E, Nowak B, Hassam H, at al. Diagnosis and staging of head and neck cancer: a comparison of modern imaging modalities (positron emission tomography, computed tomography, color-coded duplex sonography) with panendoscopic and histopathologic findings. Arch Otolaryngol Head Neck Surg 2000;126:1457–1461.

Dillon WP. Head and neck imaging [review]. AJNR Am J Neuroradiol 2000 Jan;21:25–28.

Fischbein NJ, Noworolski SM, Henry RG, et al. Assessment of metastatic cervical adenopathy using dynamic contrast-enhanced MR imaging. AJNR Am J Neuroradiol 2003 Mar;24:301–311.

Harnsberger HR, et al. Diagnostic Imaging: Head and Neck. Salt Lake City, UT: AMIRSYS, 2004.

Harnsberger HR. Handbook of Head and Neck Imaging. St. Louis: Mosby, 1995.

Hudgins PA, Kingdom TT, Weissler MC, et al. Selective neck dissection: CT and MR imaging findings. AJNR Am J Neuroradiol 2005 May;26:1174–1177.

Koeller KK, Alamo L, Adair CF, Smirniotopoulos JG. Congenital cystic masses of the neck: radiologic-pathologic correlation [erratum in Radiographics 1999;19:282]. Radiographics 1999;19:121–146.

Kapoor V, Fukui MB, McCook BM. Role of 18FFDG PET/CT in the treatment of head and neck cancers: post-therapy evaluation and pitfalls. AJR Am J Roentgenol 2005 Feb 1;184(2):589–597.

Lapela M, Eigtved A, Jyrkkio S, et al. Experience in qualitative and quantitative FDG PET in follow-up of patients with suspected recurrence from head and neck cancer. Eur J Cancer 2000;36:858–867.

Li P, Zhuang H, Mozley PD, et al. Evaluation of recurrent squamous cell carcinoma of the head and neck with FDG positron emission tomography. Clin Nucl Med 2001;26:131–135.

Lell M, Baum U, Greess H, et al. Head and neck tumors: imaging recurrent tumor and post-therapeutic changes with CT and MRI. Eur J Radiol 2000;33:239–247.

Moritz JD, Ludwig A, Oestmann JW. Contrast-enhanced color Doppler sonography for evaluation of enlarged cervical lymph nodes in head and neck tumors. AJR Am J Roentgenol 2000;174:1279–1284.

Mukherji SK. Head and Neck MR imaging. Neuroimaging Clin N Am 2004 Nov;14(4):xi.

Muller-Forell WS. Imaging of Orbital and Visual Pathway Pathology. New York, NY: Springer-Verlag, 2002.

Chang PC, Fischbein NJ, McCalmont TH, et al. Perineural spread of malignant melanoma of the head and neck: clinical and imaging features. AJNR Am J Neuroradiol 2004 Jan;25:5–11.

Rao AB, Koeller KK, Adair CF. From the archives of the AFIP: Paragangliomas of the head and neck: radiologic-pathologic correlation [review]. Radiographics 1999;19:1605–1632.

Som PM, Curtin HD. Head and Neck Imaging. St. Louis: Mosby, 2002.

Mukherji SK, Wolf GT. Evaluation of head and neck squamous cell carcinoma after treatment. AJNR Am J Neuroradiol 2003 Oct;24:1743–1746.

Taylor RJ, Wahl RL, Sharma PK, et al. Sentinel node localization in oral cavity and oropharynx squamous cell cancer. Arch Otolaryngol Head Neck Surg 2001;127:970–974.

Chapter 10

Nondegenerative Diseases of the Spine

Erik H.L. Gaensler

Common Clinical Syndromes
Imaging Methods

Inflammation

Infection
Pyogenic Infections
Nonpyogenic Infections

Neoplasms
Intramedullary Masses
Intradural/Extramedullary Masses
Extradural Masses

Vascular Diseases

Congenital Malformations

Trauma

This chapter focuses on nondegenerative diseases of the spinal cord, meninges, and paraspinous soft tissues and is divided into sections covering inflammation, infection, neoplasms, vascular diseases, congenital malformations, and trauma (1–5). The spine is composed of vertebrae, which house the spinal cord and proximal spinal nerves, and thereby represents a "border zone" between the CNS and the musculoskeletal system (this is true politically as well as anatomically—with both neurosurgeons and orthopaedic surgeons claiming the spine as their province). Disk degeneration and spinal stenosis are covered in Chapter 11. Primary osseous tumors involving the vertebrae are covered in Section X.

Common Clinical Syndromes

The clinical syndromes produced by degenerative disease and nondegenerative disease can be indistinguishable. Patients with spine disorders present with focal or diffuse back pain, radiculopathy, or myelopathy. Focal back pain without neurologic compromise or fever is not usually an emergency and is an epidemic in our society, with tremendous implications in terms of lost productivity. Focal back pain can be caused by a wide variety of both degenerative and nondegenerative processes. In the low back, the causes most commonly are orthopaedic, such as muscle and ligament strain, facet joint disease, or discogenic disease that does not compromise the nerve roots. However, vertebral metastases or infectious discitis may also cause focal back pain. Because degenerative disease of the spine is far more common than nondegenerative disease, nondegenerative processes may initially be overlooked, with disastrous consequences. Therefore, a good clinical history that specifically addresses any previous cancers or ongoing fevers and chills is crucial in raising the suspicion for a nondegenerative process. When history and physical findings are nonspecific, as often is the case, imaging procedures become central to the diagnosis.

In patients with spinal neurologic findings, an attempt should be made to distinguish between the clinical syndromes of myelopathy and radiculopathy, because they differ in significant respects, including degree of urgency. Important distinctions between radiculopathy and myelopathy are summarized in Table 10.1.

Myelopathy results from compromise of the spinal cord itself, owing to mechanical compression, intrinsic lesions, or inflammatory processes loosely grouped under the term "myelitis." Classic symptoms include bladder and bowel incontinence, spasticity, weakness, and ataxia. With cord compression, a clear motor or sensory spinal cord "level" may develop, and knowledge of this level is helpful in focusing the imaging examination. However, the lesion may be several vertebral bodies higher than the apparent dermatomal sensory level, particularly in the thoracic

TABLE 10.1 Myelopathy Versus Radiculopathy

	Myelopathy	*Radiculopathy*
Cause	Spinal cord compromise	Spinal nerve compromise
Typical disease processes	Extramedullary disease: cord compression caused by epidural mass effect Cervical spinal stenosis Intramedullary disease: tumor, inflammation, AVMs, SDAVFs	Osteophytic spurring (especially cervical spine) Disk herniations Lumbar spinal stenosis Extramedullary and paraspinous tumors and inflammatory processes compromising nerve roots
Neurologic findings	Ataxia Bowel and bladder incontinence Babinski sign	Weakness and diminished reflexes in specific muscle groups; dermatomal sensory deficits
Accuracy of clinical localization	Often poor; lesion may be several levels higher than anticipated	Usually quite good
Urgency for imaging (of acute presentations)	High—little recovery expected with deficits untreated >24 hr	Low—short delay for conservative treatment usually entails little risk
Preferred imaging modality	MR has no substitute as the initial screening exam	MR, although CT with intrathecal contrast is still excellent, particularly in cervical spine

AVM, arteriovenous malformation; SDAVF, spinal dural arteriovenous fistula.

region. Myelopathy often presents without a clear sensory level, and complete screening of the cord from the cervicomedullary junction to the conus may be required.

The spinal cord, like the brain, has limited healing powers. In fact, the spinal cord in many respects is less tolerant of injury than the brain. A small benign mass, such as a 2-cm epidural hematoma or meningioma, may permanently damage the cord because of the small diameter of the spinal canal. However, a similar-sized mass may be asymptomatic within the voluminous calvaria. The "plasticity" of the brain, whereby remaining cortex can assume the function of injured areas through a complex network of redundant neurons, is well documented, particularly in younger patients. The spinal cord, which consists mostly of long linear axonal tracts, has far less plasticity. After 24 hours of acute cord compression, little hope may remain for significant recovery of function. Therefore, acute myelopathy is an emergency in which the radiologist should do everything to facilitate prompt imaging.

Radiculopathy generally results from impingement of the spinal nerves, either within the spinal canal, lateral recess, or neural foramen, or along the extraforaminal course of the nerve. This compromise, typically because of mass effect, results in specific dermatomal sensory deficits and/or muscle group weakness. These are outlined in any neurology or physical diagnosis text and are worth knowing. The most common causes of pain and neurologic deficit are disk herniations and spinal stenosis and, in the cervical spine, uncovertebral joint spurring. Of course, malignant and infectious processes compromise spinal nerves but overall are less common. The peripheral nervous system, unlike the CNS, has significant ability to withstand injury and to regenerate. Therefore, pure radicular symptoms, although at times they are excruciatingly painful, rarely represent a surgical emergency. Extensive epidural neoplasms and infections may present with mixed myelopathic and radicular signs. These patients must be imaged with the urgency of a pure cord syndrome.

Imaging Methods

Plain radiographs of the spine were once the initial test in every spine evaluation, but with newer techniques, this is no longer logical or cost effective. Radiographs continue to be useful for ruling out trauma to the vertebral column and other acute screening settings. Plain films and fluoroscopy are indispensable for correct localization in the operating room. Radiographs have a great deal of useful information to offer when evaluating degenerative processes, particularly with extensive osteophyte formation in the cervical spine. Flexion and extension plain films used to be the only dynamic imaging technique for assessment of spine stability. MR now also can be done in flexion and extension, which can be useful in evaluating cord compression that is positional (see Fig. 10.8).

In nondegenerative disease, careful attention should be paid to the integrity of the vertebral bodies and pedicles, which are frequent sites of metastases. However, plain films cannot detect early infiltrative changes in the marrow space, which are easily seen on MR. The classic radiographic findings of widened interpedicular distance with tumors and midline bony spurs with diastematomyelia are rarely seen except on board examinations.

Myelography. The indications for plain film myelography alone are limited. Myelography today is almost always done in conjunction with CT (see following). Indications include complex postoperative cases and patients in whom MR is contraindicated because of MR-incompatible implanted devices. *Ionic contrast agents are absolutely contraindicated for myelography* because they can result in severe inflammation, seizures, arachnoiditis, and even death. Always personally inspect the vial of contrast you are using, and fill the syringe yourself.

The recommended dosage of nonionic contrast in adults depends on the region to be studied, the size of the patient, and the size of the thecal sac. A convenient and conservative rule of thumb in adults is not to exceed 3 g of intrathecal iodine, which works out to 17 mL of 180 mg/mL, 12.5 mL of 240 mg/mL, or 10 mL of 300 mg/mL (these are three standard concentrations). In general, lumbar myelography should be performed using contrast media with a concentration between 180 and 240 mg/mL, and cervical and/or thoracic myelography should be performed with concentrations of 200 to 300 mg/mL. The smaller the area of the subarachnoid space, the denser the contrast must be for good plain films. Plain films and fluoroscopic spot films, however, are becoming increasingly superfluous with the dramatic improvements in multiplanar CT reconstructions.

Myelography begins with a lumbar puncture, with the patient in prone position under fluoroscopy. The preferred puncture site depends on the clinical findings, but is usually the midlumbar region, inferior to the posterior elements of L2 or L3. This injection level will avoid most disk herniations and spinal stenosis, which are usually worse at lower levels, and the conus, which in adults lies between the T12–L1 and L1–L2 disk spaces. Care should be taken to place the needle near the midline to reduce the chances of an extra-arachnoid injection or spearing of an exiting nerve root. Contrast should be injected only after spontaneous CSF backflow is established. The complications of poor needle placement include subdural and epidural injection. Examples of these complications are well illustrated in older neuroradiology textbooks. If there is doubt as to where the contrast is going, stop, take frontal and lateral spot films, and examine them carefully. Avoid any air bubbles in the tubing system, as they can cause filling defects, which are easily confused with drop metastases. If tumor or infection is suspected, collect adequate CSF for chemistry, cultures, and cytology if this has not already been done. For routine degenerative cases, CSF examination has not proved worthwhile.

C1–C2 punctures are rarely required and are inherently more dangerous than lumbar injection, as direct injury to the cord or a low-lying posterior inferior cerebellar artery loop can occur. The puncture is best done under lateral fluoroscopy, with the needle placed in the posterior third of the spinal canal between C1 and C2. Classic indications include known blocks caudally or the need for dense opacification of the cervical and upper thoracic spinal canal for plain films. Today, one of the rare good reasons for a C1–C2 puncture would be complete spine block in the midthoracic region identified by lumbar myelography, with the need to define the upper extent of the block—in a patient with a pacemaker (thus precluding MR). If the pacemaker were not an issue, MR would be the study of choice. MR is far quicker, more comfortable, and, most important, safer for the patient. Even if there is no technical complication with a myelogram, patients with spine block can deteriorate from the subtle fluid and pressure shifts that inevitably accompany needle placement in the subarachnoid space, a syndrome known as "spinal coning." The multiple steps in the evaluation of spine block by plain film myelography followed by CT are shown in Fig. 10.1. Contrast this with the simplicity and elegance of MR, as shown in Fig. 10.2. In oncologic cases, MR has the additional benefit of excellent evaluation of the marrow space—which is not available with CT.

Space-occupying lesions of the spinal canal are classified according to their location as intramedullary, intradural-extramedullary, or extradural. This distinction can be made on myelography, as well as on CT and MR, and is critical in formulating a differential diagnosis. Intramedullary lesions are usually confined to the spinal cord itself but may be exophytic. Extramedullary lesions are by definition outside the cord, but may be either intradural or extradural. A summary of the radiologic appearance and differential diagnosis for each lesion location is outlined in Table 10.2. Remember that the lesion must be seen in at least two (and preferably three) 90° orthogonal planes, since large intradural lesions may simulate an extradural mass on any single view. Similarly, bilateral extradural disease can flatten the cord, increasing its apparent anteroposterior dimension in sagittal view and thereby giving the false impression of an intramedullary mass (Fig. 10.3). Correlation with axial imaging is invaluable in this regard. Also remember that lateral lesions, such as lateral disk herniations, may be completely missed by myelography. In almost all cases today, a CT is performed after myelography.

CT. The decline of plain film myelography for degenerative disease was initially because of CT, especially CT with intrathecal contrast, which is superior to myelography in diagnostic accuracy. However, CT has largely been replaced by MR for most screening examinations of the spine, except for acute trauma. Low-dose CT myelography remains the gold standard in cases where the limits of the thecal sac or nerve root sleeves need to be precisely defined, such as in complex postoperative states. Small leptomeningeal (drop) metastases can be identified (see Fig. 10.34); however, MR with gadolinium has replaced CT myelography as the initial screening examination for drop metastases (see Figs 10.33, 10.35).

CT is far less effective than MR in depicting intramedullary diseases of the spinal cord, such as primary tumors, myelitis, and syringohydromyelia. For example,

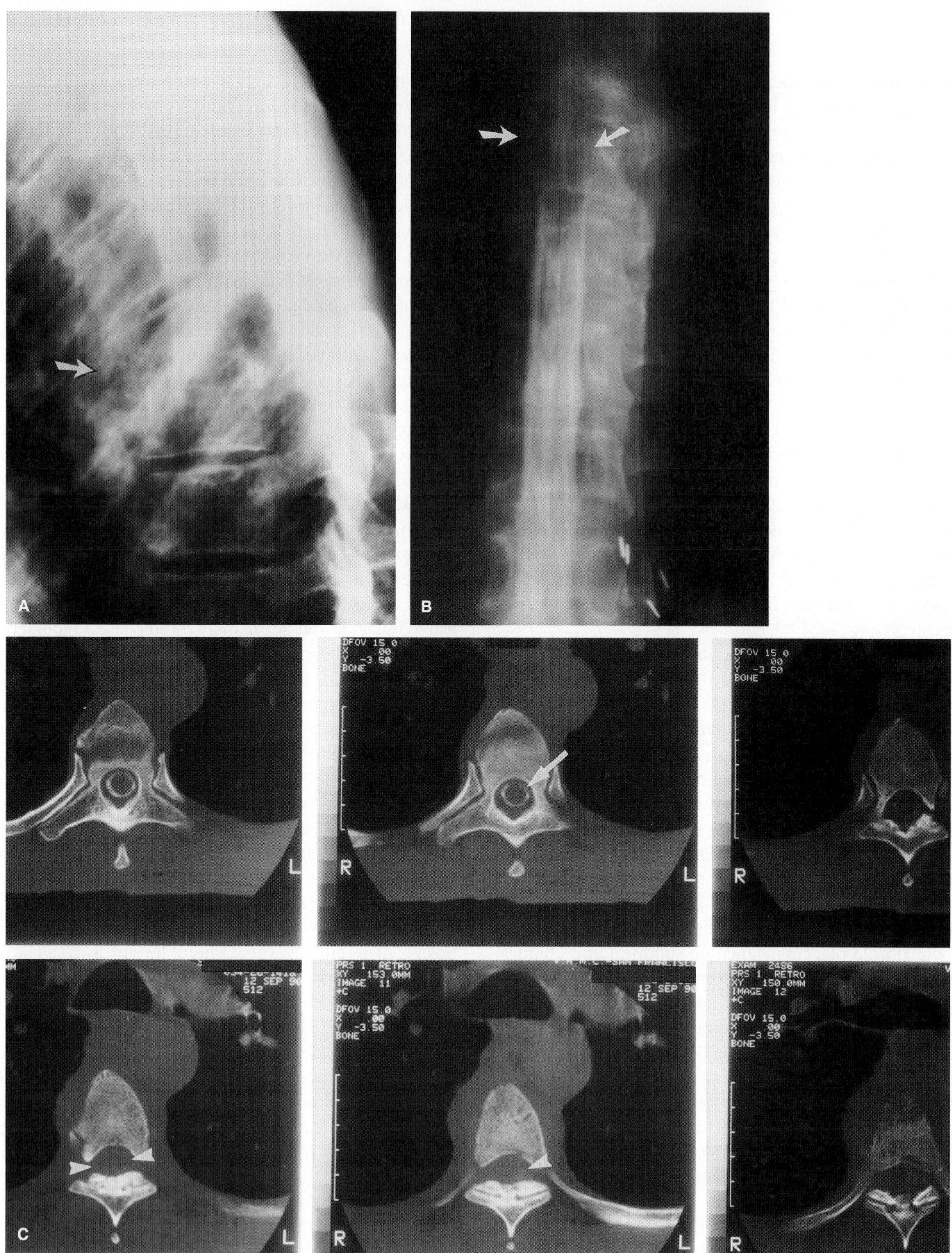

FIGURE 10.1. **Acute Cord Compression.** Middle-aged patient with acute myelopathy and midthoracic back pain, worked up the "old-fashioned" way, as the patient had a pacemaker. **A.** Plain film obtained in the emergency department shows compression fracture of a midthoracic vertebra (*arrow*). **B.** Lumbar myelogram shows complete block to contrast in the midthoracic vertebrae (*arrows*). A portable C-arm fluoroscope then had to be obtained to do a C1–C2 puncture, followed by a cervical and upper thoracic myelogram (not shown). **C.** Upper thoracic CT myelogram images show gradual effacement of the subarachnoid space (*arrow*), which disappears at site of the block (*arrowheads*) (*Continued*).

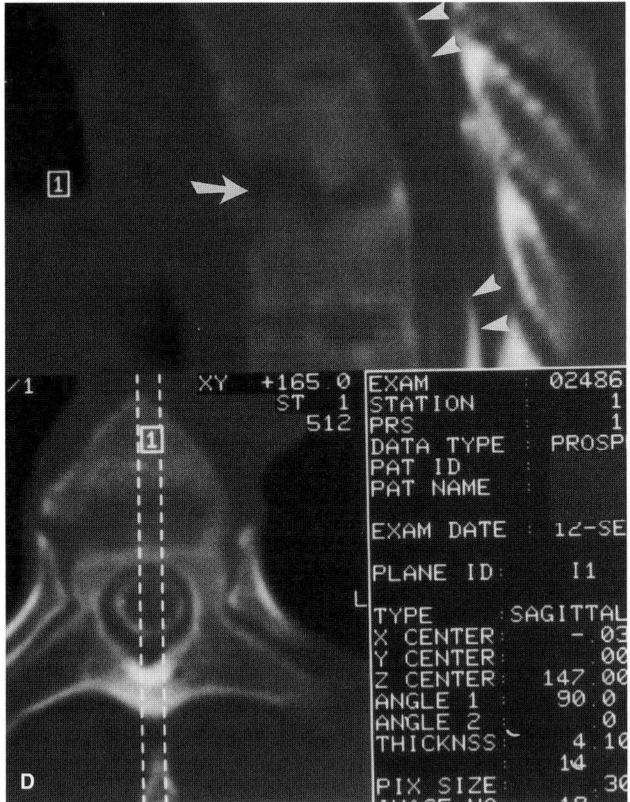

FIGURE 10.1. (*Continued*) **D.** Sagittal reconstruction enables assessment of the entire process in a single image, showing cord compression centered around an abnormal disk space (*arrow*), consistent with infection, which was proven at laminectomy. Note the gradual effacement of the subarachnoid space (*arrowheads*).

a nonexpansile multiple sclerosis (MS) plaque will escape detection on any imaging examination except MR.

MR has done for the spinal canal what CT did for the calvaria, allowing for the first time a noninvasive "look inside." Therefore, it is the examination of choice for any disorder of the spine resulting in myelopathy. The key to the success of MR has been its superior soft tissue contrast (including the ability to evaluate the marrow compartment), multiplanar capabilities, noninvasiveness, and high sensitivity to gadolinium enhancement.

MR scanning techniques for the spine continue to improve, and with the wide variety of imaging systems available, it makes little sense to recommend specific protocols in a general text. A few general guidelines follow. Surface coils are an absolute must to obtain an adequate signal-to-noise ratio in most systems. Motion-suppression techniques, such as anterior radiofrequency saturation bands, gradient moment nulling, and cardiac/respiratory gating, are critical to reduce motion artifact. Fast spin-echo (FSE) sequences have replaced conventional spin echo for spine work, with great time saving and little cost when only degenerative disease is present. The FSE technique, however, is poor for marrow evaluation, but this can be overcome by using fat saturation with the T2WI, a technique widely used in musculoskeletal MR to search for marrow edema. Short time inversion recovery (STIR) probably offers the highest sensitivity for marrow space edema. Fast inversion recovery techniques compete with T2 FSE with fat saturation as the optimal marrow-screening exam (see Figs 10.37, 10.43).

Gradient-echo images are poor for marrow space evaluation because of susceptibility effects from the bony trabeculae and are of little utility in evaluating nondegenerative spinal disease, except when searching for blood

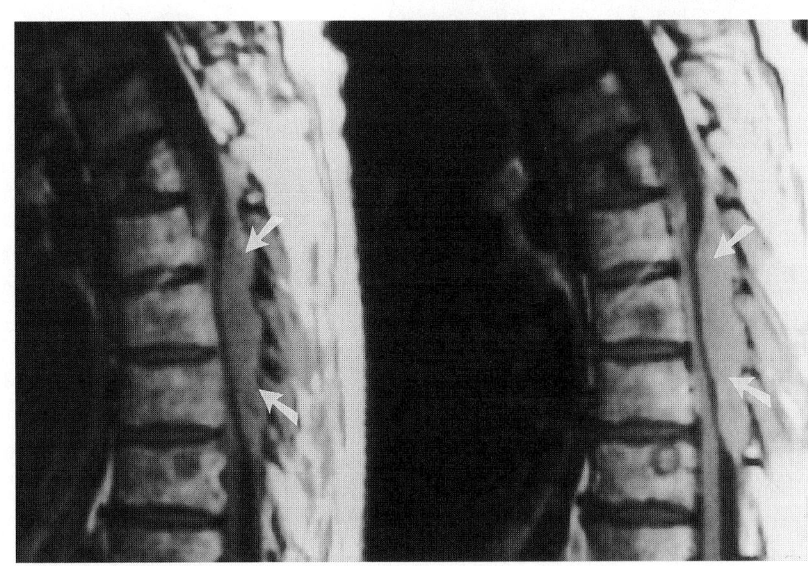

FIGURE 10.2. **Acute Cord Compression: MR.** Evaluation of thoracic cord compression the easy way (compare with Fig. 10.1). A middle-aged patient presented to a physician's office with acute myelopathy. This emergency MR using T1 and T2 sagittal and axial sequences took 20 minutes, was completely noninvasive, and gave excellent detail of the marrow space, unavailable on CT. The epidural soft tissue mass (*arrows*) proved to be lymphoma.

TABLE 10.2 Differential Diagnosis of Spinal Lesions by Location

LOCATION AND IMAGING APPEARANCE

DIFFERENTIAL DIAGNOSIS

A. INTRADURAL INTRAMEDULLARY

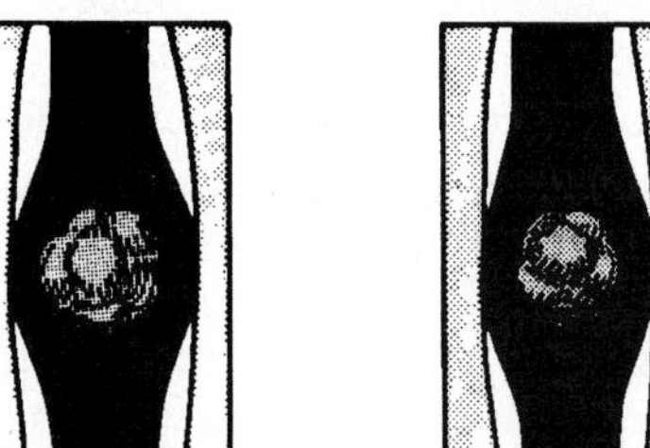
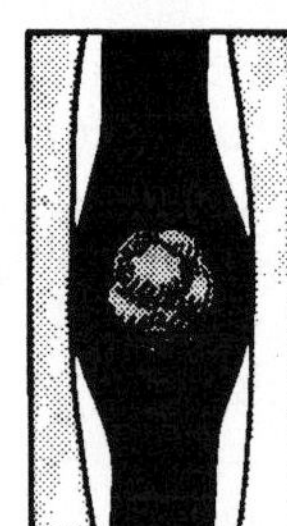
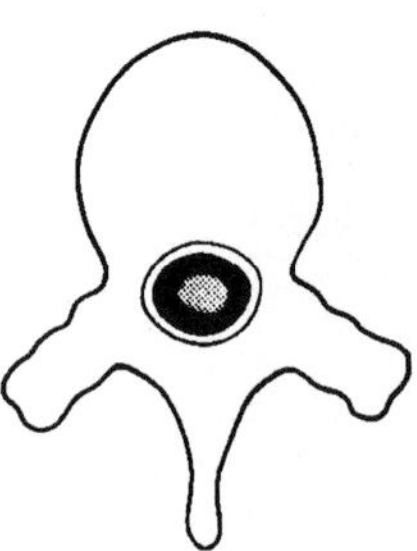

Ependymoma
Astrocytoma
Hemanigioblastoma
Lipoma/(Epi)dermoid
Syringohydromyelia
Intramedullary AVM
Rare site: met/abscess

Cord appears widened in all views. The CSF space appears thinned on all sides in all views.

B. INTRADURAL EXTRAMEDULLARY

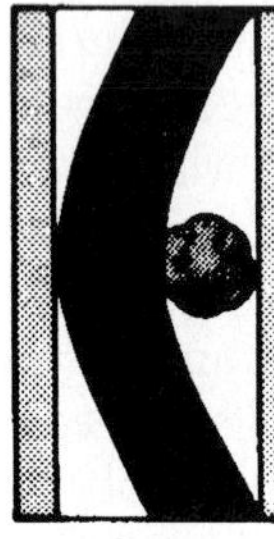
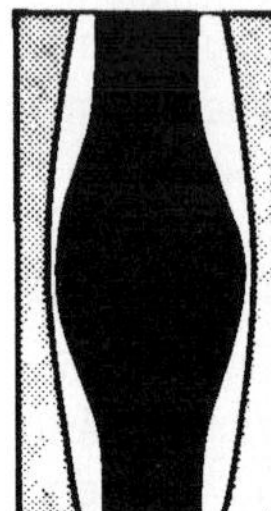
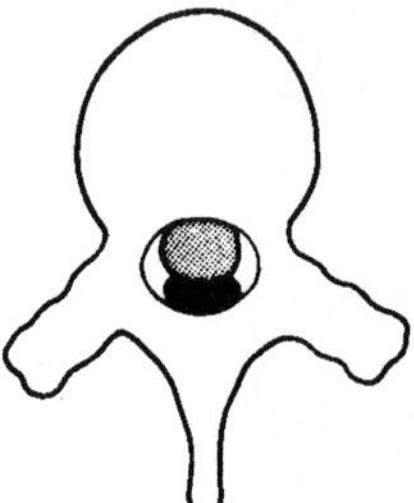

DIFFERENTIAL DIAGNOSIS

Meningioma
Schwannoma/neurinoma
Neurofibroma
Hemangiopericytoma
Lipoma/(Epi)dermoid
Arachnoid cyst/adhesion
Drop/leptomeningeal met
Veins (extramedullary AVM)

The contrast/CSF forms acute angles with the mass (which may have a dural attachment—"marble on the carpet"). This results in a "meniscus" around the mass and a widened contrast column between the cord and the mass on one side, with effacement of the CSF on the other.

C. EXTRADURAL

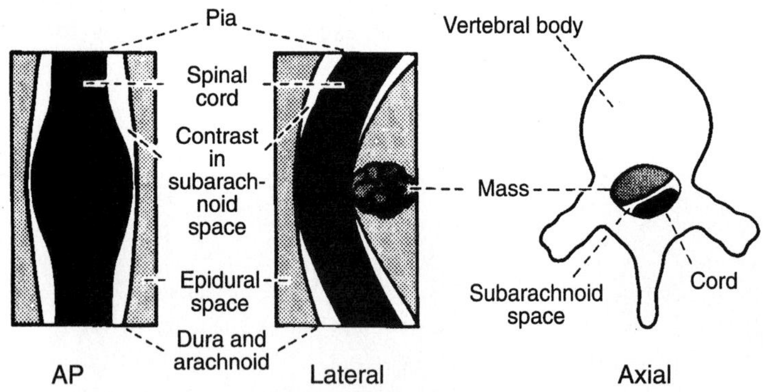

DIFFERENTIAL DIAGNOSIS

Degenerative
- Herniated disc
- Synovial cyst
- Osteophyte
- Rheumatoid pannus

Nondegenerative
- Metastasis
- Abscess
- Hematoma
- 1° tumor expansion or invasion
- Epidural lipomatosis

The dura and the sac will be displaced together, away from the mass. The CSF angles around the mass will be obtuse with a "marble under the carpet" appearance. The cord may be widened in one plane by pressure from the mass, with contrast material thinned on both sides of the cord.

AP, anteroposterior; AVM, arteriovenous malformation; met, metastasis.
Adapted with permission from Latchaw RE, ed. MR and CT of the Head, Neck, and Spine. 2nd ed. St. Louis: Mosby, 1991.

breakdown products (see Fig. 10.65). Ultra thin-section imaging (<1 mm) without interslice gaps is now performed with three-dimensional Fourier transformation and rivals CT for thin-slice profiles, critical in the cervical spine for examination of the foramina.

Other pitfalls with spinal MR include motion sensitivity, imprecise detection of calcium, and occasional false-negative results with contrast examinations. Despite motion compensation techniques, both physiologic motion and patient movement remain problematic.

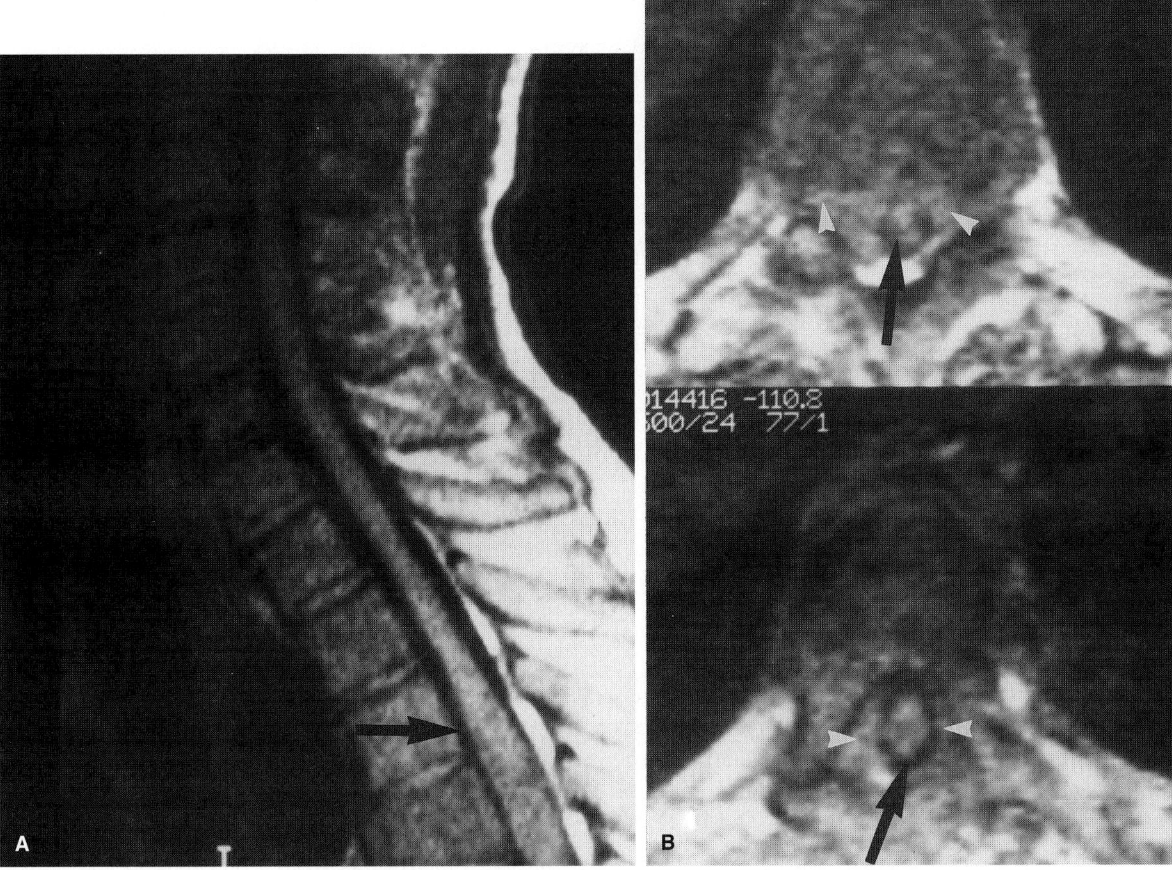

FIGURE 10.3. **Extramedullary Tumor.** This patient presented with myelopathy with an upper thoracic sensory level. **A.** On this midline sagittal image, the spinal cord appears widened (*arrow*), suggestive of an intramedullary lesion. The patient was unable to remain still for additional images. **B.** Subsequent repeat imaging in the axial plain shows that extramedullary tumor (*arrowheads*) has flattened the cord (*arrow*) from its sides, increasing its anteroposterior dimensions and giving the spurious impression of an intramedullary expansile process on the midline sagittal images. The moral is the same as on plain films: always look at pathology in two (preferable 90° opposed) orthogonal planes.

Both exaggerate osseous encroachment of the spinal canal and neural foramina, because far more movement occurs during the 4 to 8 minutes it may take to do a three-dimensional Fourier transformation cervical spine axial image than a 20-ms CT slice. Spin-echo MR techniques are generally inferior to CT in the detection of subtle calcification. This may be important in defining small osteophytic spurs or ossification of the posterior longitudinal ligament, identifying retropulsed bone fragments following trauma, or characterizing calcification in tumors. Gradient-recalled techniques may overestimate the size of calcific structures, because of susceptibility effects. Gadolinium is essential in the evaluation of infection and intrathecal metastases but may obscure vertebral metastases by making them isointense with surrounding marrow fat (Fig. 10.4), a problem solved by using fat saturation. Also, it is difficult to evaluate hemorrhage on postcontrast images. Always obtain a precontrast T1 "scout" image to avoid these latter two pitfalls.

Diffusion imaging can help distinguish between vertebral body metastases and compression fractures, as tumor areas show diffusion restriction as compared to fracture zones. Diffusion and perfusion studies of vertebral tumors are not routinely performed, however, because needle biopsy is relatively straightforward. There is great promise for diffusion, perfusion, and spectroscopy techniques for intramedullary disease, as the spinal cord represents a "brain" in miniature. Research in this area, however, has lagged work in the brain for two reasons. The small size of the spinal cord makes MR sampling more difficult, and intramedullary lesions are rarer than brain lesions. There are already case reports of diffusion restriction in spinal cord stroke, and there is great promise

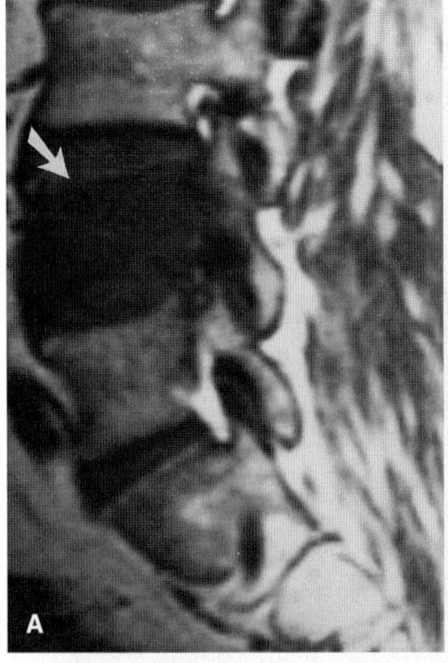

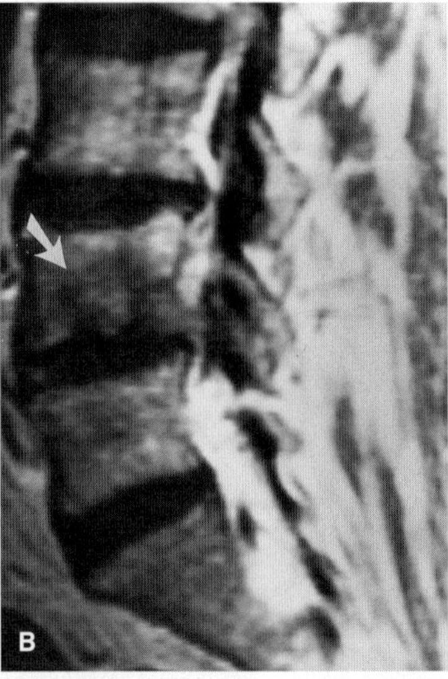

FIGURE 10.4. **Gadolinium-Enhanced Imaging Potential Pitfalls. A.** Infiltration of the entire L4 vertebral body (*arrow*) on this unenhanced lumbar MR is readily apparent. **B.** After contrast administration, the area involved with metastatic tumor (*arrow*) has enhanced to isointensity with the remaining normal vertebrae and is far less conspicuous. The lesion still could be visualized with fat saturation or short time inversion recovery techniques, despite the gadolinium, but why do things the hard way? Moral: always obtain a precontrast image when using gadolinium in the spine (or use fat saturation if it is too late).

for diffusion tensor imaging in evaluating the long axonal tracts of the cord.

Spinal angiography is technically demanding, dangerous in untrained hands, and difficult to interpret. There is no reliable spinal version of the circle of Willis allowing collateral flow from multiple sources, although some variable interconnected vascular arcades exist. Therefore, an inadvertent catheter-induced complication can have tragic consequences. Excellent texts exist on spinal angiography, but this area has increasingly become the province of interventional neuroradiologists, who can both diagnose and often treat spinal arteriovenous malformations—the main indication for spinal angiography.

Nuclear medicine bone scans are unique in their ability to screen the entire skeleton for metastases in one sitting. When abnormal vertebral uptake is noted, however, plain films may fail to show the abnormality. MR is more often used instead because it demonstrates early marrow space infiltration and can rule out spinal cord compression. Bone scans are highly sensitive but quite nonspecific, because both degenerative and nondegenerative processes will show increased uptake. When such patients are referred for MR, it is critical to be aware of the bone scan findings to protocol the examination appropriately. Bone scans and PET scans are discussed further in the nuclear medicine chapters.

US has limited applications in the spine, because in adults the posterior elements obscure the potential acoustic window. However, in neonates the unossified posterior elements provide a window through which spinal anomalies can be evaluated, and excellent work has been done in this highly specialized area. Once the laminae have been removed surgically, intraoperative US has proven to be an excellent tool for the evaluation of the spinal cord for tumor, syrinx, and other intramedullary processes, minimizing the need for cord exploration.

INFLAMMATION

This section focuses on inflammatory diseases that cause myelopathy, principally through direct involvement of the spinal cord (6–12). The mechanism of many of these disorders is not fully understood, and they are sometimes lumped under the term "myelitis." Myelitis may be focal or diffuse. When both clinical and pathologic findings are confined to distinct level(s), the term "transverse myelitis" may be used. It must be recognized that this is not really a specific disease but rather a category of diseases, and few agree on exactly what processes should be lumped under "transverse myelitis." In practice, it is better to carefully describe the imaging findings, and give a differential diagnosis, than to invoke such nonspecific terms in MR reports.

Multiple sclerosis is the most common spinal cord "inflammatory" disorder, and the most common cause of intramedullary lesions seen on MR. The epidemiology and pathophysiology of MS are reviewed in detail in Chapter 7. Multiple sclerosis of the brain and spinal cord are similar in terms of patient profile, with the hallmark of the disease being multiple neurologic deficits separated both anatomically and temporally. While imaging can be helpful, the diagnosis ultimately rests on clinical grounds. When spinal MS predominates, it tends to follow a progressive clinical course, as opposed to the relapsing/remitting pattern that is more characteristic with brain involvement. The majority of MS patients have mixed presentations, with both brain and spinal cord involvement. Spinal cord disease is isolated in fewer than 20% of cases. Two thirds of spinal MS lesions occur in the cervical region.

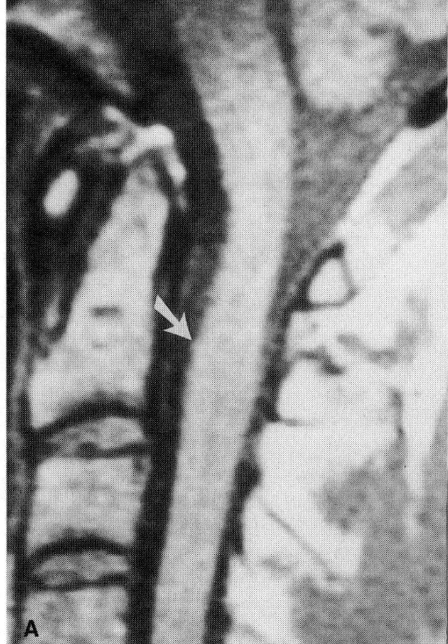

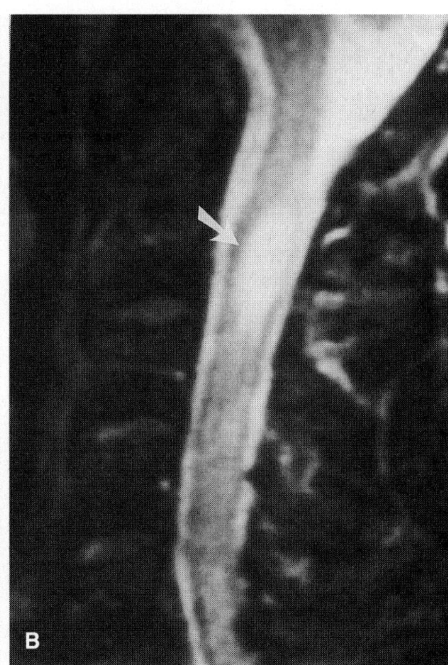

FIGURE 10.5. **Multiple Sclerosis.** A solitary lesion (*arrow*) shows subtle cord expansion on a T1WI **(A)** and **(B)** becomes bright on the T2WI because of edema. Differential considerations included an intramedullary tumor, and the diagnosis of MS was supported by the confirmation of concomitant periventricular lesions classic for MS on brain MR.

The best screening study is a sagittal T2W or STIR series, in which MS plaques appear as areas of increased signal intensity. Usually there is no significant change in cord diameter, which is why cord MS plaques were typically occult myelographically. Occasionally, there may be subtle cord expansion in the acute phase because of edema, (Fig. 10.5) and "burnt out" MS plaques can present as myelomalacia (literally "cord softening" or atrophy). Cord plaques, unlike brain plaques, may not be visible as areas of hypointensity on T1WIs.

As in the brain, plaque enhancement correlates with acute lesion activity (Fig. 10.6). Because the white matter is on the "outside" of the cord, MS plaques tend to be peripheral (Fig 10.6B). However, edema and enhancement can extend into the central gray matter as well, probably because of perivenular inflammatory changes. Differentiation of a solitary plaque from a glial tumor may be difficult, although MS plaques typically are shorter than two vertebral segments in length and involve less than half the cross-sectional area of the cord. When a mysterious bright intramedullary lesion is seen on a T2WI (Fig 10.5B), the next step should be MR of the brain to search for concomitant MS plaques. The brain and spinal cord are composed of the same tissue types, are physically connected, and share the CSF. Therefore, a good general rule is that, when presented with any diffuse spinal process, either intramedullary or leptomeningeal, the clinician should remember to look "upstairs," because the same process may be involving the brain and its coverings.

Lupus Erythematosus. Other CNS inflammatory processes are seen in both the brain and spinal cord. A classic example is systemic lupus erythematosus (SLE), where a necrotizing arteritis leads to cord ischemia and injury. Antibodies may also damage neuronal elements directly. The spinal cord will show diffuse areas of increased signal intensity with cord swelling on T2WIs. SLE "lesions" have less well-defined margins than the discrete plaques of MS and may involve four to five vertebral body segments (Fig. 10.7). Lupus of the cord may show dramatic improvement on MR after corticosteroids. MS plaques, in contrast, represent areas of focal myelin destruction, and although the symptoms improve with corticosteroids, the MR findings improve less dramatically.

Rheumatoid arthritis (RA) is another "collagen-vascular" disease that can compromise the spinal cord, although the mechanisms are different. Focal inflammatory changes, termed "pannus," destroy the transverse ligament of C1, allowing the odontoid to slide posteriorly relative to C1 and compressing the cord, particularly in flexion (Fig. 10.8B). Therefore, the neurologic injury in RA is caused by atlantoaxial instability rather a primary intramedullary lesion. The instability leads to intermittent cord compression, which in time leads to myelomalacia. Sixty percent of RA patients have cervical spine findings, and frank atlantoaxial instability is seen in 5%. Patients with spinal RA typically will have involvement in their hands and elsewhere. This is a useful discriminator, as a soft tissue mass at the C1–C2 articulation with instability does not necessarily imply RA. A fibrous pseudotumor may occur in the same location with os odontoideum and can develop in response to any chronically unstable spinal anatomy, including an ununited type 1 dens fracture.

Radiation myelitis is similar to radiation injury to the brain (see Chapter 7). Peak incidence occurs roughly 6 to 18 months after initial treatment, with affected areas demonstrating increased signal intensity on T2WIs, with

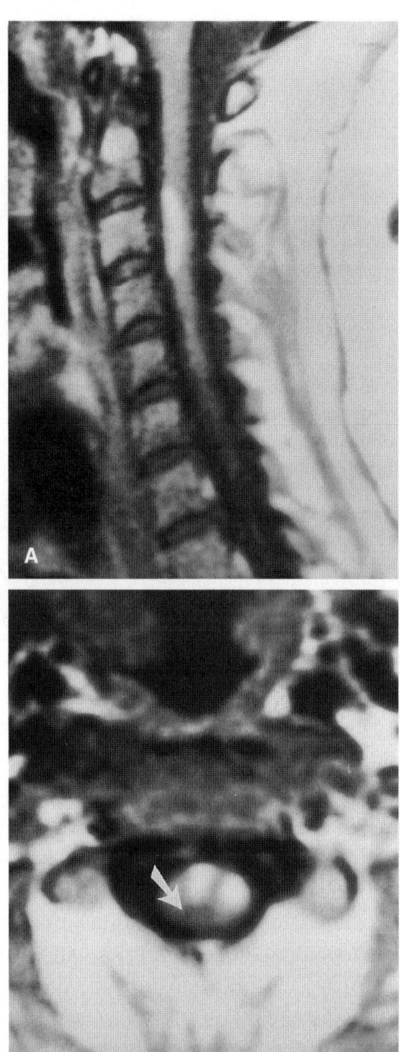

FIGURE 10.6. **Multiple Sclerosis.** Considerable swelling and enhancement of the spinal cord is noted on these postcontrast sagittal **(A)** and axial **(B)** images. Note how the central gray matter (*arrow*) is displaced posteriorly by the inflammatory changes in the anterior white matter.

variable enhancement (Fig. 10.9). Radiation myelitis can lead to paralysis, and fear of this complication is usually the limiting factor in radiotherapy for vertebral body metastases. Radiation has a very characteristic effect on the vertebral bodies. The normal erythropoietic marrow is destroyed and replaced by fat, making the vertebrae very homogeneously bright on T1WIs (Figs. 10.9, 10.10). In growing children, cellular repopulation of the vertebral marrow may occur, with stunted growth of the affected vertebrae because of radiation injury to the epiphyses being the main finding (Fig. 10.10).

Acute viral illnesses are associated with myelitis in a number of ways, some of which are well described, and others, which are still poorly understood. The polio virus causes direct injury to the anterior horn cells. Herpes zoster is invisible to imaging when latent, but cord swelling and enhancement have been reported with acute shingles outbreaks, appearing at spinal levels corresponding to the dermatologic outbreak. Measles provokes an autoimmune reaction that can damage the cord, which has been studied experimentally as a model for MS, and is termed *subacute sclerosing panencephalitis*. Acute disseminated encephalomyelitis (ADEM; see Chapter 7) is a monophasic postviral syndrome that also affects spinal cord, as the term "encephalomyelitis" suggests.

These patients typically have sudden high fevers (presumably viral in origin), followed within 4 weeks by rapid onset of motor, sensory, and usually autonomic dysfunction, referable to a specific spinal cord level. Many neurologists reserve the catch-all term "transverse myelitis" for this clinical presentation, which may be caused by an autoimmune process. The imaging findings typically are a focal area of cord swelling with high signal on T2WIs, with variable enhancement. It is difficult not to draw comparisons with Guillain-Barré syndrome (also known as acute inflammatory polyradiculoneuropathy). By whatever name, this is a progressive ascending motor weakness that affects more than one limb but involves peripheral nerves rather than the spinal cord. Guillain-Barré has been seen after vaccinations and evolves over a maximum of 4 weeks. Often the spinal nerves enhance (Fig 10.11), although this finding is nonspecific and can be seen in infections and neoplasms involving the CSF pathways and even is occasionally present in disk disease.

Myelopathy is seen in AIDS patients, with vacuolar changes in the spinal cord. This appears to be a direct effect of HIV itself, rather than concomitant infections or a postinfectious syndrome. The role of MR in AIDS myelopathy is more to exclude other treatable conditions, such as unsuspected cord compression, than to make a highly specific diagnosis.

Neurosarcoidosis. Inflammatory conditions involving pia and arachnoid have a similar differential diagnosis whether they involve cerebral or spinal leptomeninges. A classic example is neurosarcoidosis, which can present as diffuse leptomeningeal granulomatous nodules, which typically enhance (Fig. 10.12). This appearance is similar to that of carcinomatous (see Fig 10.35) and mycobacterial meningitis (see Fig. 10.20), and the distinction must be made on clinical grounds. Sarcoid can also present with intramedullary or vertebral body granulomatous changes.

Arachnoiditis. One "physical agent" that causes leptomeningeal irritation is Pantopaque (iodophenylundecylic acid), which was once used in myelography. Keep this complication in mind in patients whose plain spine films show the telltale pearly white beads of residual Pantopaque. On MR, these droplets appear bright on T1WI

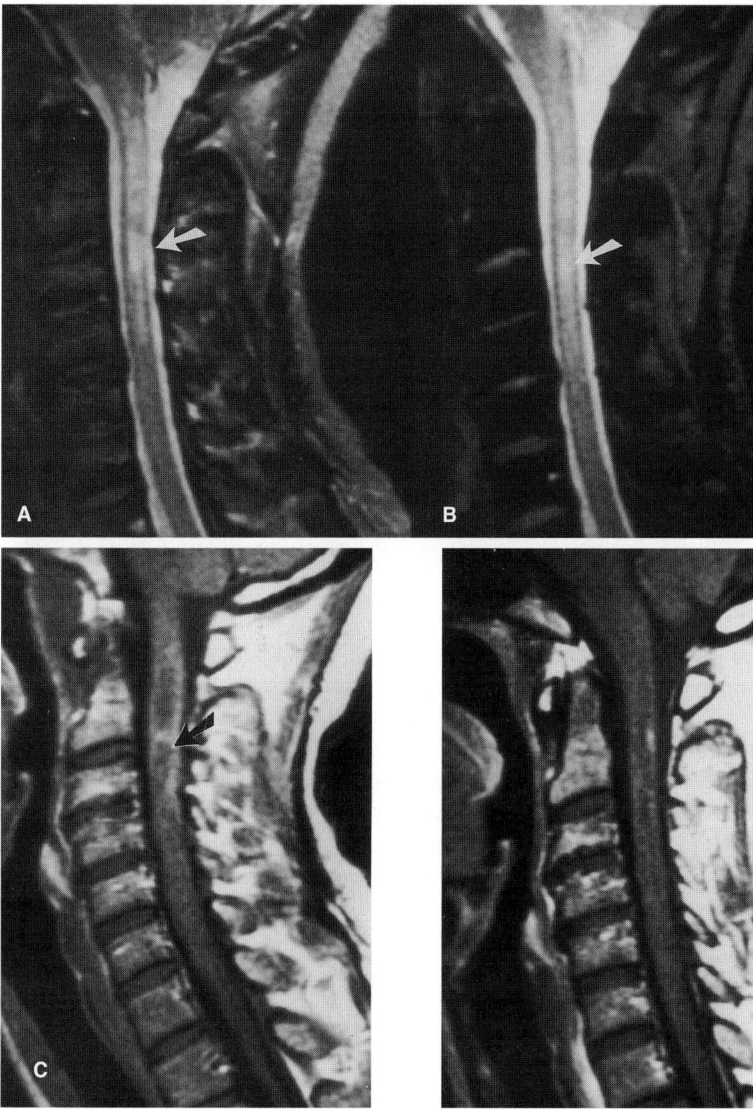

FIGURE 10.7. **Systemic Lupus Erythematosus.** MR in a 40-year-old patient with new myelopathy. The spinal cord shows ill-defined areas of edema on **(A)** a T2WI and **(B)** a gradient-echo image (*arrows*). Postcontrast images **(C)** show mild enhancement (*arrow*). The brain was free of abnormalities.

because of their lipid content. Today, the most common causes of arachnoiditis remain iatrogenic, including inflammation after spine surgery, spinal anesthesia, or spine "injection" procedures such as epidural nerve blocks. In arachnoiditis, the normally free-layering lumbar roots become adherent to each other or to the peripheral wall of the thecal sac, giving the sac a "bald" appearance on myelography or T2WIs.

The remaining list of "inflammatory" conditions of the spinal cord is long and parallels the differential considerations in the brain. Chemotherapy and other toxins, metabolic disorders, electrical burns, and lightning are physical factors that can injure the cord. Deficiencies in vitamins such as B12 and folate, while not strictly inflammatory, can cause degeneration of the posterior columns. Much of the damage that occurs in spinal cord trauma is not caused by the mechanical forces but by the inflammatory reaction that follows.

INFECTION

Infections involving the spine can be classified according to the causative organism or according to their anatomic location. Both approaches are useful. Certain infections, such as pediatric pyogenic meningitis, are so dramatic in their presentation that there is little need for imaging, with emergent lumbar puncture and CSF analysis serving as the cornerstone of diagnosis. Other processes, such as fungal osteomyelitis in the immunocompromised cancer patient, can be quite subtle, and imaging plays a crucial (if not always successful) role in differentiating spinal infection from tumor (13–16). Evaluation of the pathologic vertebral body is a constant challenge, and the many "rules of thumb" sprinkled throughout this chapter are summarized in Table 10.3.

In most spine infections, the organism is seeded via the arterial route. As is the case with most bacteremia, the

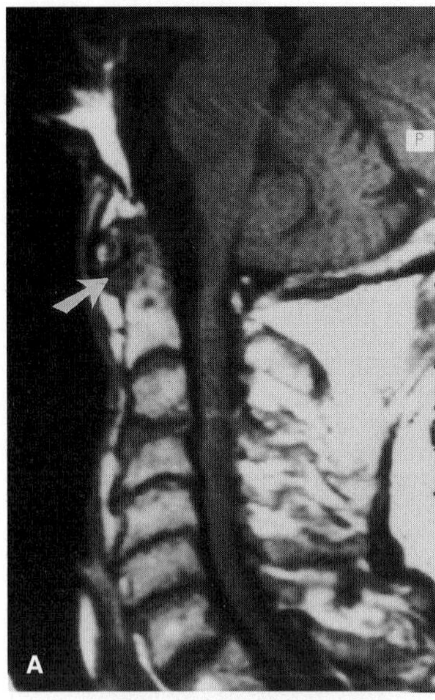

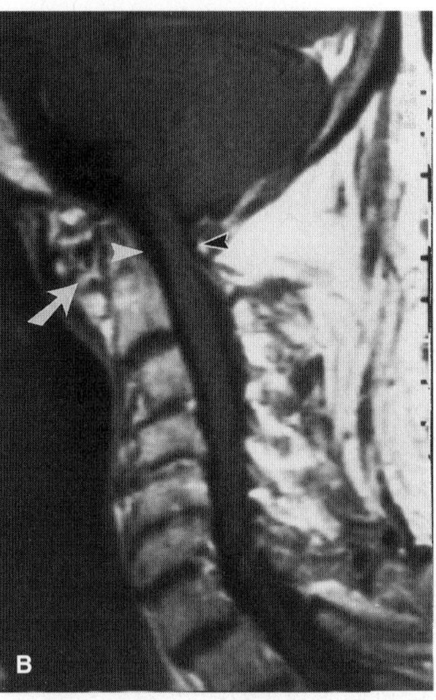

FIGURE 10.8. **Rheumatoid Arthritis. A.** This elderly patient had myelopathy caused by atlantoaxial instability secondary to pannus (*arrow*), which has destroyed the transverse ligament of C1. In extension, no cord impingement is seen. **B.** In flexion, the dens has borderline mass effect on the cord (*arrowheads*). The pannus enhances vigorously with contrast (*arrow*).

source of the organism is usually the skin, GI tract, or lungs. Exceptions are children with spinal dysraphism or immediate postoperative patients, where a direct portal for infection exists.

Osteomyelitis/Discitis. In adults the disk itself has a relatively poor blood supply, so primary infection is rare. In children, however, arteries penetrate the growing disk, providing a direct route for hematogenous primary infection. Once these vessels have involuted, the most common spinal site of hematogenous infectious "seeding" is the vertebral body, particularly the portions near the endplates, which have the richest blood supply. Vertebral osteomyelitis then develops (Fig. 10.13),with loss of marrow signal on T1WIs and endplate definition. As pyogenic infection breaks through the endplate into the disk, discitis ensues, with inevitable infection of the adjacent vertebral body.

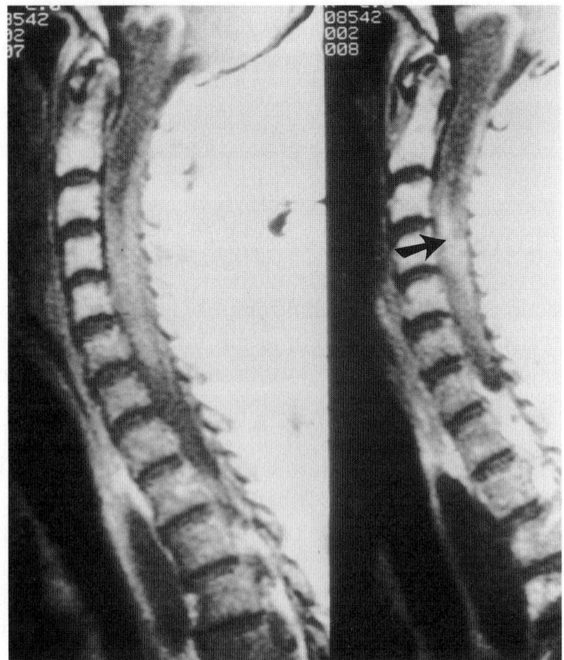

FIGURE 10.9. **Radiation Myelitis.** Intramedullary enhancement (*arrow*) is noted in this patient who received radiation therapy to the neck. Note also the increased signal in the marrow of the vertebrae secondary to radiation.

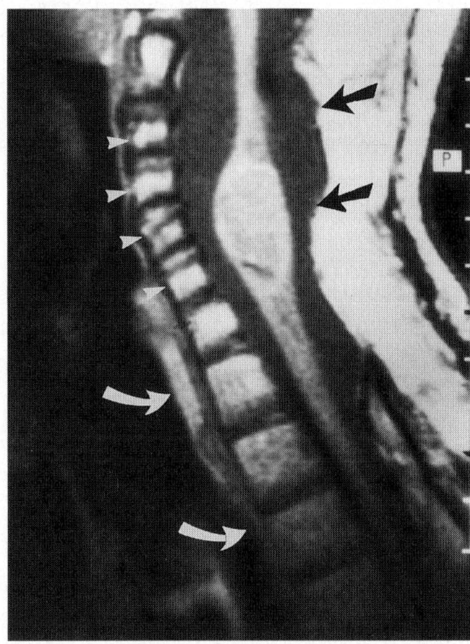

FIGURE 10.10. **Radiation Effect.** This child underwent laminectomy (*arrows*) and radiation for an intramedullary astrocytoma. Note the growth retardation of the vertebrae within the x-ray therapy field (*arrowheads*), as compared with vertebrae left outside the field (*curved arrows*). The epiphyseal plates of vertebrae, like any other rapidly dividing tissue, are highly sensitive to radiation injury.

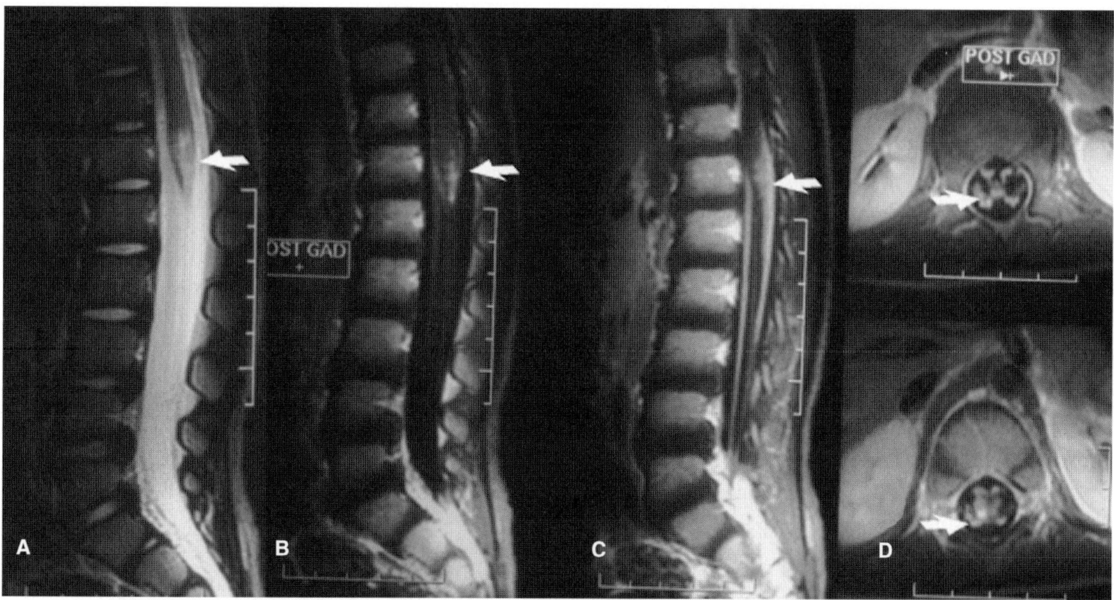

FIGURE 10.11. **Guillain-Barré or Acute Inflammatory Demyelinating Polyradiculopathy.** This toilet-trained 3-year-old suffered acute ataxia and loss of bowel control after a diarrheal illness. **A.** T2WI shows conus edema (*arrows*). **B.** to **D.** T1 postcontrast images show intense enhancement of the conus and spinal nerves (*arrows*). The patient recovered fully in 6 to 8 weeks.

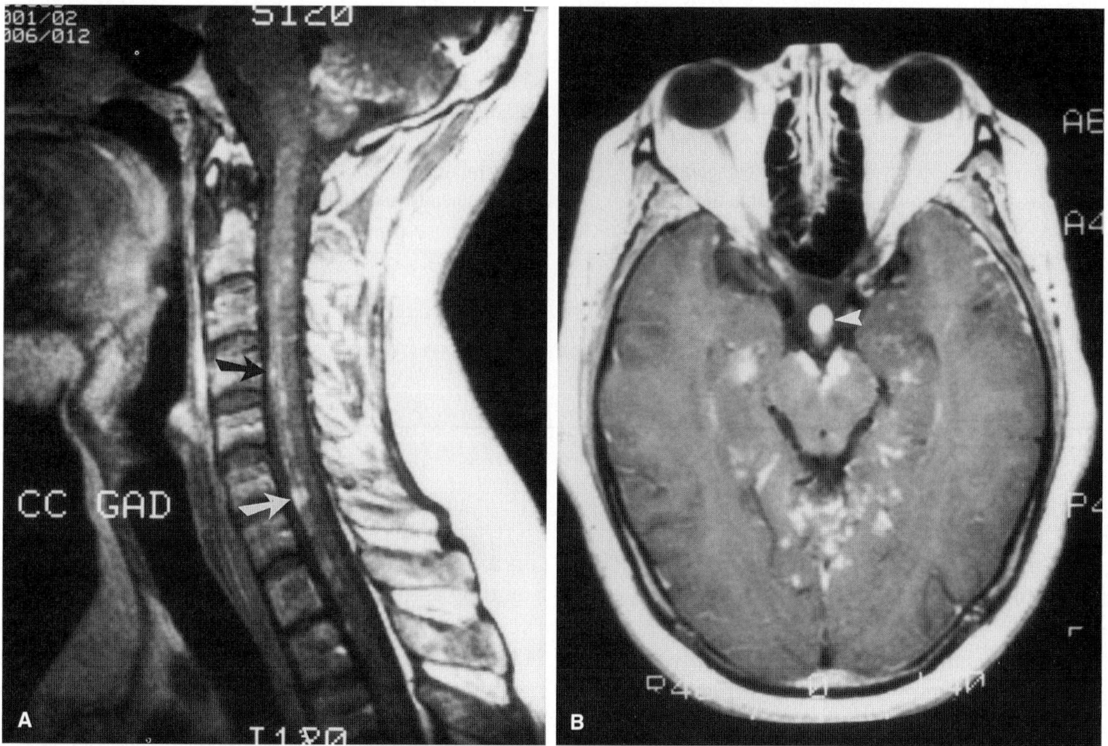

FIGURE 10.12. **Neurosarcoidosis. A.** Multiple nodular enhancing areas are seen involving both the leptomeninges and the peripheral cord (*arrows*). **B.** A concomitant scan of the brain reveals similar findings involving leptomeninges, as well as the pituitary stalk (*arrowhead*). Accumulation of granulation tissue in this region is the source of the "suprasellar mass" associated with sarcoid.

TABLE 10.3 Imaging Evaluation of the Pathologically Collapsed Vertebral Body

Criteria	*Infection*	*Neoplasm*	*Osteoporosis*
Number of vertebrae affected, and pattern	Single vertebral involvement is rare Usually at least two vertebrae around an affected disk (pyogenic) or intact disk with subligamentous spread (tuberculosis or fungus)	Isolated or noncontiguous involvement common	Typically several vertebra show loss of height, to varying degrees
Portions of vertebra affected	Destruction greatest at endplates Posterior elements relatively spared Abnormal marrow signal centered around disk in osteomyelitis/discitis complex	Irregular vertebral body involvement Pedicles typically affected Entire vertebra often infiltrated	Anterior "wedge" deformity of the vertebral body Posterior elements spared Portions of vertebral body retain normal marrow, even with acute compression fracture
Marrow signal	Decreased on T1 Increased on T2 Normal diffusion	Decreased on T1 Increased on T2 Restricted diffusion caused by "marrow packing"	T1 and T2 normal (unless acute fracture) Diffusion may be increased at the fracture plane
Disk integrity	Pyogenic: disk involved and enhances Nonpyogenic: disk spared	Disks typically spared (prostate cancer an exception)	Disks spared
Epidural component (if present)	Granulation tissue (best seen postgadolinium) extends several levels above and below the affected vertebrae	Focal mass usually only at level of affected vertebra(e) Lymphoma an exception, with more extensive epidural mass	Rare, unless acute fracture with hematoma or retropulsion of fragments
Caveats	Discogenic vertebral sclerosis can mimic the osteomyelitis complex on T1W images (but not on enhanced scans)	Gadolinium enhancement may obscure metastases by reducing their conspicuity relative to fat	Acute compression fractures show marrow edema and can be difficult to distinguish from pathologic fracture (although posterior elements are usually spared) Follow-up scan in 3 to 6 months helps make the distinction

This creates an osteomyelitis/discitis complex that has been termed "pyogenic spondylodiscitis" (Fig. 10.14). This pattern is highly suggestive of infection and unusual with neoplasms (Table 10.3). The epidural space can also be seeded hematogenously, but more often is involved by direct extension. After the disk and epidural space are involved, extension into the paraspinous soft tissues, such as the psoas muscle, often occurs.

Epidural Abscess. Many epidural infections do not have the well-encapsulated "liquid" collections we associate with abscesses elsewhere in the body and technically are better termed "epidural phlegmon." The dura presents a relative barrier to infection, so infections tend to spread in a craniocaudal fashion within the epidural space, extending as many as three to four interspaces away from the vertebral abnormality, which is unusual with neoplasms (Table 10.3). Epidural abscesses have little room to expand axially, given the confines of the spinal canal, and can lead to cord compression (Fig. 10.15). The majority are posterior in location, and lower thoracic and lumbar sites are most common.

Subdural empyemas are rare and tend to be associated with surgery or other violation of the dura. This is fortunate, because subdural infections could rapidly spread

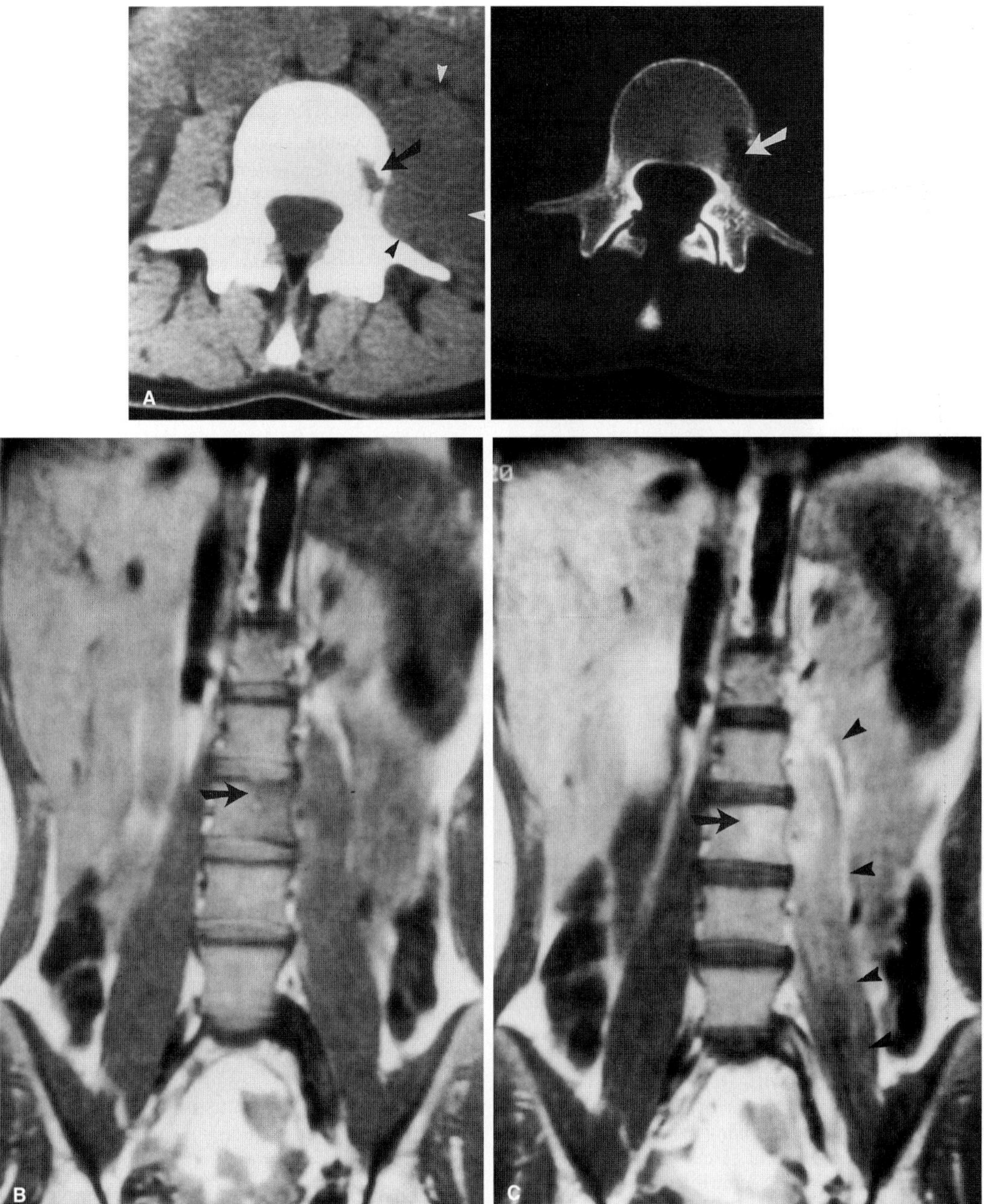

FIGURE 10.13. **Early Osteomyelitis.** This young athlete developed back pain and a slightly elevated sedimentation rate, with negative blood cultures, negative plain films, and a bone scan showing increased uptake at L3. **A.** CTs filmed with different windows show a destructive process within the vertebral body (*arrow*), which extends into the left psoas muscle (*arrowheads*), which is enlarged. **B.** Coronal unenhanced T1WI shows decreased signal intensity within the left-sided marrow space of L3, consistent with edema (*arrow*). **C.** Postcontrast T1WI shows marked enhancement within the affected portion of L3 (*arrow*) and the left psoas (*arrowheads*), which is enlarged and enhances all the way into the pelvis. This pattern would be unusual for a tumor. Biopsy yielded *Streptococcus aureus*. The disks appear spared, which is atypical for *S aureus*. Note how well the coronal plane shows both the spine and paraspinous tissues over a large area. This plane is underutilized but is very effective in imaging of paraspinous processes.

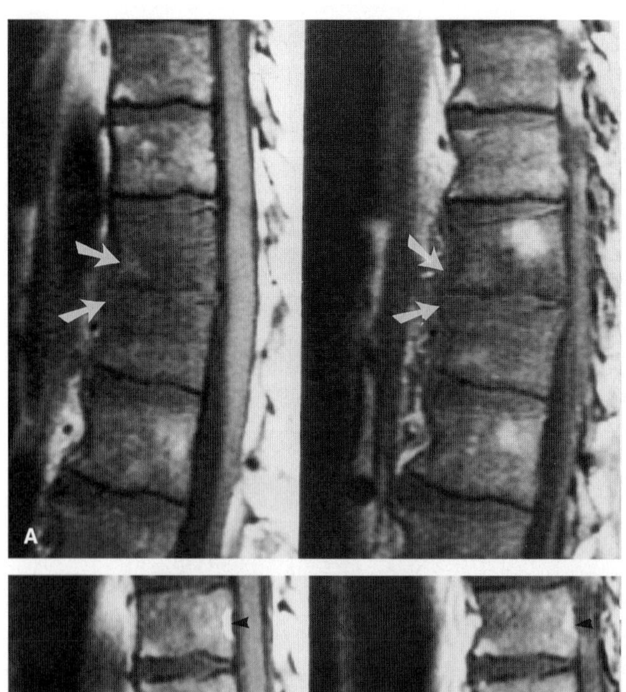

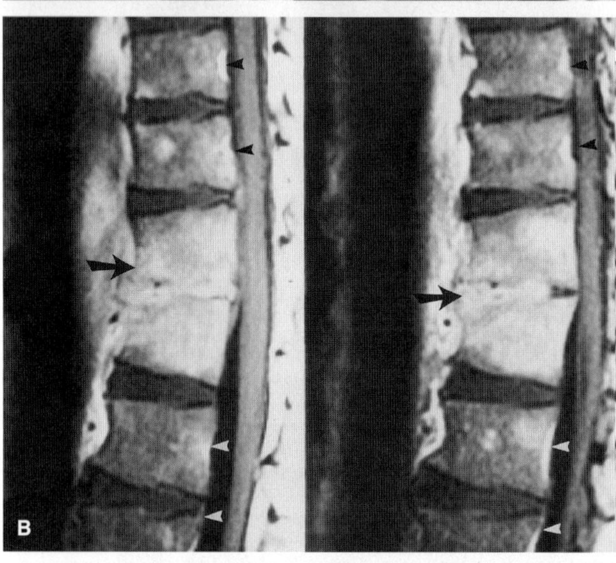

FIGURE 10.14. **Osteomyelitis With Discitis. A.** T1W sagittal images show decreased signal in a pair of vertebral body endplates (*arrows*) centered around an abnormal disk. **B.** The disk (*arrow*) enhances intensely, confirming discitis. This "osteomyelitis/discitis complex" is classic for pyogenic infection and virtually rules out neoplasm. Note the basivertebral venous plexus (*arrowheads*), which normally becomes bright after gadolinium because of normal venous enhancement. This basivertebral plexus enhancement confirms that gadolinium was given, much as nasal mucosal enhancement does in the head. Enhanced basivertebral veins should not be mistaken for epidural infection or tumor.

through the arachnoid layer, resulting in meningitis. Infection of the subarachnoid space is termed *meningitis* whether it is in the brain or spinal canal. Indeed, the theory of a lumbar puncture is that there is continuous mixing of the CSF, with the fluid in the lumbar recesses being representative of the fluid bathing the brain. The clinical presentation of meningitis is discussed in detail in Chapter 6. Meningitis typically is caused by direct hematogenous seeding of the CSF, rather than contiguous spread of adjacent vertebral infection, unless there is a disruption of the leptomeninges on a congenital or acquired basis. Postcontrast MR is the most sensitive imaging examination for meningitis in both the brain and the spine, but the finding of leptomeningeal enhancement often appears relatively late in the infection's course and sometimes not at all. Therefore, *a negative enhanced MR does not exclude meningitis—and should never delay or be a substitute for a lumbar puncture.*

Spinal cord abscesses are rare and are usually the result of direct seeding of the cord from overwhelming sepsis. Given the difficulty of myelography in an acutely ill patient and the relative insensitivity of the technique for small intramedullary lesions, the imaging literature on this topic is sketchy, with most data from autopsy reports. MR allows a direct look inside the cord in these patients. Spinal cord pyogenic abscesses, not surprisingly, appear similar to those in the brain: bright on T2WIs, with rim enhancement (Fig. 10.16).

Plain films cannot identify a spinal infection unless some disk or bone destruction has occurred, which may take 4 to 8 weeks, with the earliest sign being erosion of the vertebral endplates. Because older patients often have significant loss of vertebral body and disk height because of degenerative processes, evaluation of plain films in the setting of suspected infection is difficult, even following months of symptoms. Late in the infectious course, the endplates may become sclerotic as healing occurs, sometimes leading to fusion across the obliterated disk space. Radionuclide bone scans can turn positive in infection far sooner than plain films, but they suffer from the same ambiguity: degenerative and nondegenerative processes can look the same. Indium-labeled white cell studies and gallium scans are more specific for infection, but they are relatively insensitive for small foci of vertebral osteomyelitis.

CT is useful for paraspinous disease, such as psoas infection, which may be associated with vertebral osteomyelitis and epidural abscess (Fig. 10.13). However, CT does not show the contents of the spinal canal adequately unless intrathecal contrast is used. MR can demonstrate the initial replacement of the fatty marrow by osteomyelitis and has therefore become the preferred technique of examination. Gadolinium-enhanced images are extremely helpful in confirming discitis. When evaluating the extent of epidural involvement, fat suppression is a useful adjunct, as the epidural fat is inherently bright (Fig. 10.17).

Pyogenic Infections

Staphylococcus aureus is by far the most common cause of spine infection in adults, followed by gram-negative bacteria, particularly *Escherichia coli, Pseudomonas,* and *Klebsiella*. *Salmonella* is seen in association with sickle cell

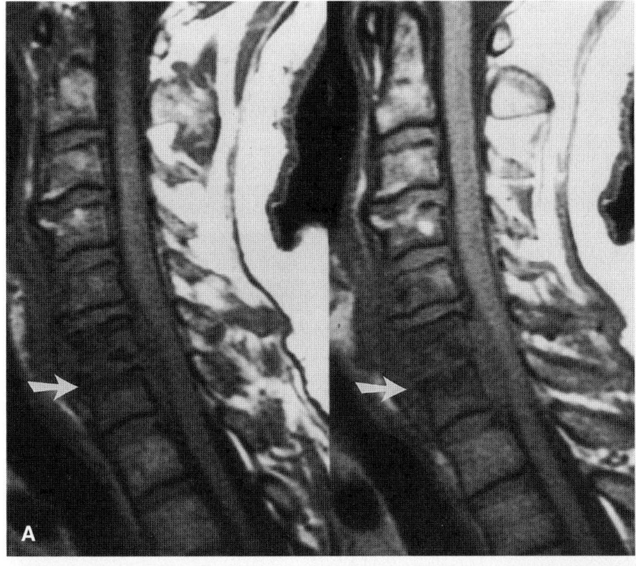

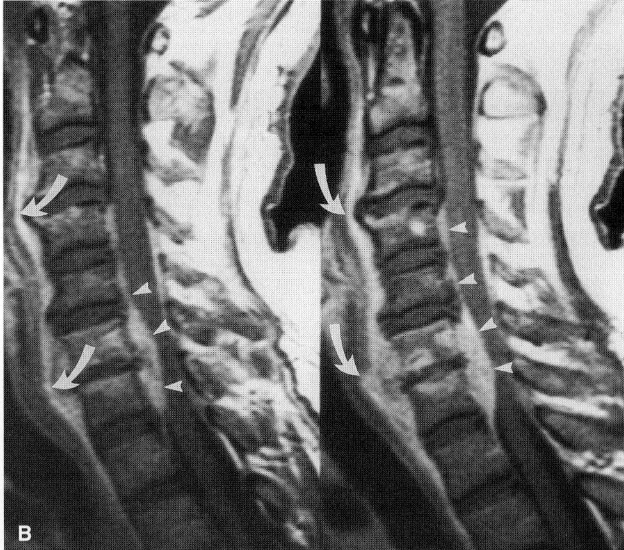

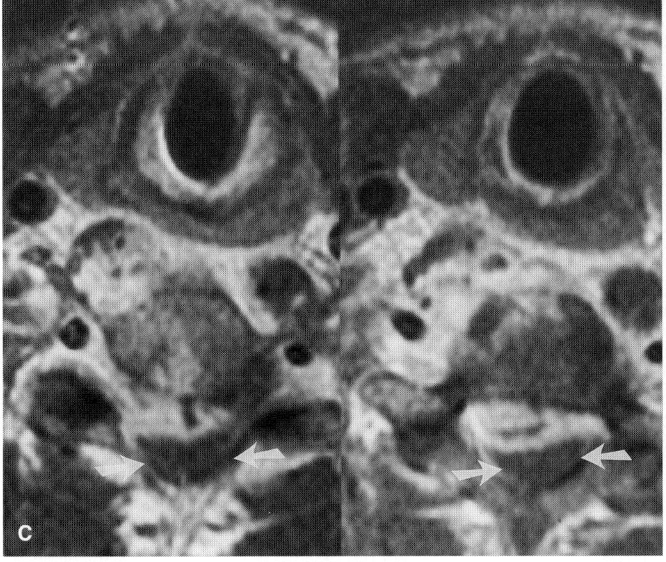

FIGURE 10.15. **Osteomyelitis With Discitis and Epidural Abscess.** T1W sagittal images before **(A)** and after **(B)** contrast show an osteomyelitis-discitis complex centered around an abnormal enhancing disk (*straight arrows*). Considerable enhancing tissue is seen within the epidural space (*arrowheads*) as well as anterior to the spine, involving the anterior longitudinal ligament (*curved arrows*). Ligamentous involvement extending several vertebral bodies away from the area of infiltrated marrow favors infection and is unusual for metastatic tumor. **C.** Axial images confirm compression of the cord (*arrows*).

disease. As already mentioned, the vertebrae are seeded hematogenously in most cases, resulting in osteomyelitis that then spreads to the disk space and adjacent vertebral body. This process typically results in severe back pain that, unlike degenerative conditions, is unrelieved by any positional maneuvers. Fevers, chills, leukocytosis, and an elevated sedimentation rate may be present. However, the early and haphazard use of antibiotics for any "malaise" may mask these findings. Blood cultures are often negative, mandating disk biopsy. Disk aspirates have a low yield after antibiotics have been initiated, and are best obtained pretreatment.

S aureus produces enzymes that rapidly "digest" disks. This has led to the plain film "pearl" that destruction of the disk space implies pyogenic infection. Tuberculous spondylitis, in contrast, often spares the disk. On MR *Staphylococcus* infections can be detected as early as the isolated osteomyelitis phase, as marrow edema with enhancement, well before any discitis has developed (Fig. 10.13). Once the infection has broken through to the disk, intense contrast enhancement confirms the discitis (Fig. 10.14) and usually shows subligamentous spread to the vertebra on the other side of the disk. Infection can travel along the anterior and posterior longitudinal ligaments, extending several vertebral body levels away from the affected disk. As the infection progresses, epidural involvement, with or without pathologic fracturing of the vertebra, can lead to cord compression (Fig. 10.15). Epidural infection can have a variable appearance, ranging from rounded rim-enhancing areas, which yield frank pus at surgery, to more oblong stretches of thickened granulation tissue.

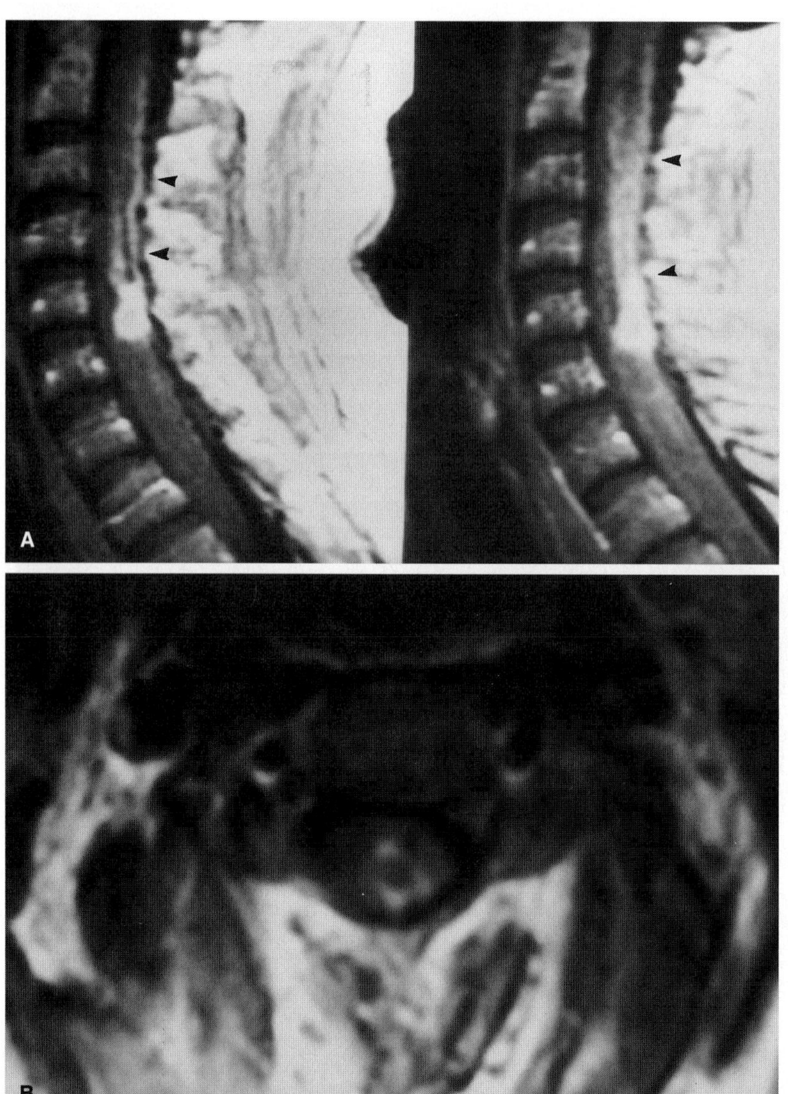

FIGURE 10.16. **Spinal Cord Abscess. (A)** Sagittal and **(B)** axial enhanced images through the cervical spine show intramedullary enhancement in this patient with overwhelming sepsis, who developed myelopathy. Laminectomy (*arrowheads*) and biopsy revealed abscess.

Nonpyogenic Infections

The most important nonpyogenic infections of the spine are tuberculosis (TB) and fungal diseases. These disorders present a diagnostic challenge for several reasons. First, they typically have an indolent course and do not present with the acute pain and leukocytosis that are the hallmark of pyogenic infections. Second, the population most at risk for nonpyogenic infections, aside from certain endemic areas, is the immunosuppressed. Patients who are immunocompromised because of chemotherapy are at risk for metastases from their primary tumor, and AIDS patients are at risk for lymphoma involving the spine. In both settings, therefore, a pathologic fracture with mild epidural mass effect could represent either infection or neoplasm. The dichotomy of the potential treatments—antibiotics versus radiation—mandates a definitive diagnosis, often requiring biopsy. Sometimes, however, the radiologist can steer the workup in such a way that invasiveness of this biopsy is minimized or can detect findings so characteristic of a given disease that biopsy is not necessary (Table 10.3). Figure 10.18 illustrates such a case as it evolved, from plain films to CT and finally to MR.

TB of the spine, or Pott disease, causes slow collapse of one or usually more vertebral bodies, which spread underneath the longitudinal ligaments (Fig. 10.19). The result is an acute kyphotic or "gibbus" deformity. This angulation, coupled with epidural granulation tissue and bony fragments, can lead to cord compression. Unlike pyogenic infections, the disks can be preserved. In late-stage spinal TB, large paraspinal abscesses without severe pain or frank pus are common, leading to the expression "cold abscess." (Fig. 10.19D). As with other extrapulmonary TB, the chest film may be unrevealing, with the source being a primary lung lesion that is clinically silent. Unfortunately, the incidence of tuberculous spondylitis, as with other forms of TB, is on

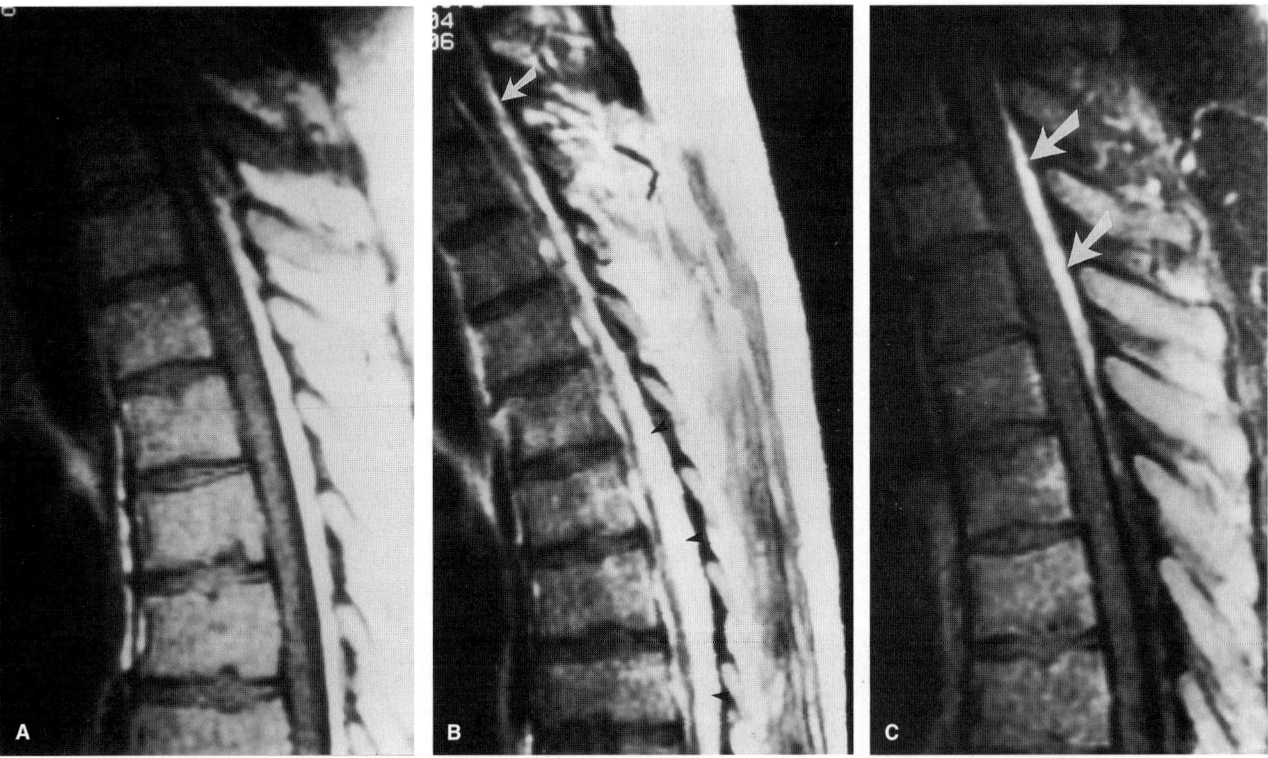

FIGURE 10.17. **Value of Fat Suppression on MR in Epidural Abscess. A.** Unenhanced T1W sagittal images are unremarkable in this immunosuppressed patient with infrascapular back pain. **B.** Postcontrast images, slightly motion-blurred and off midline, show enhancement posterior to the upper thoracic cord, where there is little epidural fat (*arrow*). However, in the middle and lower thoracic spine it is difficult to distinguish enhancement from normal epidural fat (*arrowheads*). **C.** Fat suppression images reveal the true extent of the epidural abscess (*arrows*).

the rise, with new strains with multiple drug resistances. In many parts of the developing world, TB is the most common cause of vertebral body infection, with the majority of cases seen in patients under the age of 20. TB can also affect the meninges of the spine, causing an intense pachymeningitis that enhances dramatically (Fig. 10.20). Brucellosis can present as granulomatous osteomyelitis of the spine that can be difficult to distinguish from TB. Both are acid-fast bacilli, which may cause caseating granulomas.

Fungal infections can be particularly difficult to differentiate from malignant processes, with the classic problem being *Candida* and *Aspergillus* in the oncology patient. Coccidioidomycosis and blastomycosis have specific endemic areas, but with widespread travel, geographic borders have less meaning. Coccidioidomycosis (Fig. 10.18) is common in the southwestern United States, and blastomycosis is more common in the southeast. Both are common in Africa and South America, with some variation in strains. Another distinction is that coccidioidomycosis, like TB, spares the disks, whereas blastomycosis, like actinomycosis, can destroy the disks and the ribs. *Cryptococcus*, usually associated with meningitis, also affects the vertebrae, with well-defined osteolytic changes.

Other infectious agents can occasionally involve the spine. Cysticercosis can involve the CSF pathways at any point and has been described in the lumbar recesses. Intramedullary toxoplasmosis has been described in AIDS patients. *Echinococcus* will occasionally affect the vertebral bodies. Viral and postviral syndromes are discussed in the "Inflammation" section.

NEOPLASMS

MR is unique in its ability to detect nonexpansile tumors of the spinal cord, and it is the only reliable noninvasive method for detection of tumors within the spinal canal that do not affect bone. When formulating the differential diagnosis for a spinal tumor, it is important to establish the location of the lesion as intramedullary, intradural extramedullary, or extradural, as described previously under "Myelography" and in Table 10.2. After the "compartment" is determined, consider the patient's age when ranking the lesions occurring in that compartment, in order of likelihood (16–21). In children, 38% of symptomatic spinal canal lesions are developmental. Meningiomas constitute

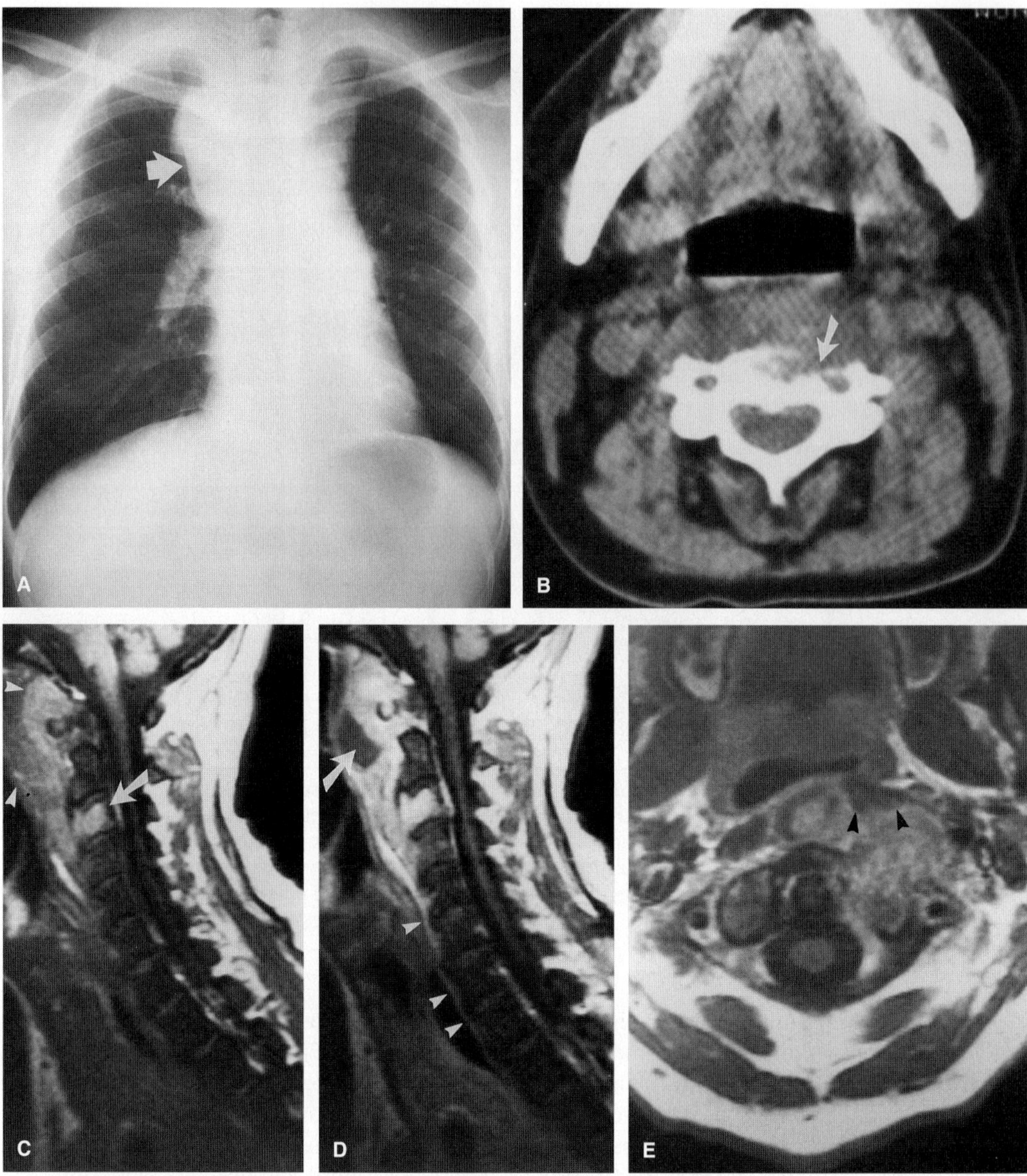

FIGURE 10.18. **Coccidioidomycosis Osteomyelitis With Prevertebral Abscess.** This 26-year-old patient presented with 3 months of fevers, weight loss, and chills. **A.** Chest film shows an anterior mediastinal mass (*arrow*) suspicious for lymphoma. **B.** A CT confirmed mediastinal adenopathy and showed destructive changes in C3 (*arrow*) that are atypical for lymphoma. **C.** T1W image shows abnormal low signal in all of the cervical vertebrae caused by anemia of chronic disease, likely accompanied by increased marrow iron. The C3 vertebral body (*arrow*) is infiltrated with fluid. In a normal patient it would be the darkest vertebral body; here it is the brightest. An anterior mass (*arrowheads*) is noted in the prevertebral space. **D.** After contrast injection, the prevertebral mass (*arrow*) shows central low signal, consistent with necrosis or abscess. Note the dense enhancement of the anterior longitudinal ligament (*arrowheads*) well into the lower cervical spine, suggestive of infection. This proved to be "reactivated" coccidioidomycosis in a patient who was HIV positive. In retrospect, the chest film **(A)** shows lung and hilar calcifications from the initial infection. **E.** Axial image proves that the mass is in the prevertebral space rather than the retropharyngeal space, as the longus colli muscle (*arrowheads*) is displaced forward.

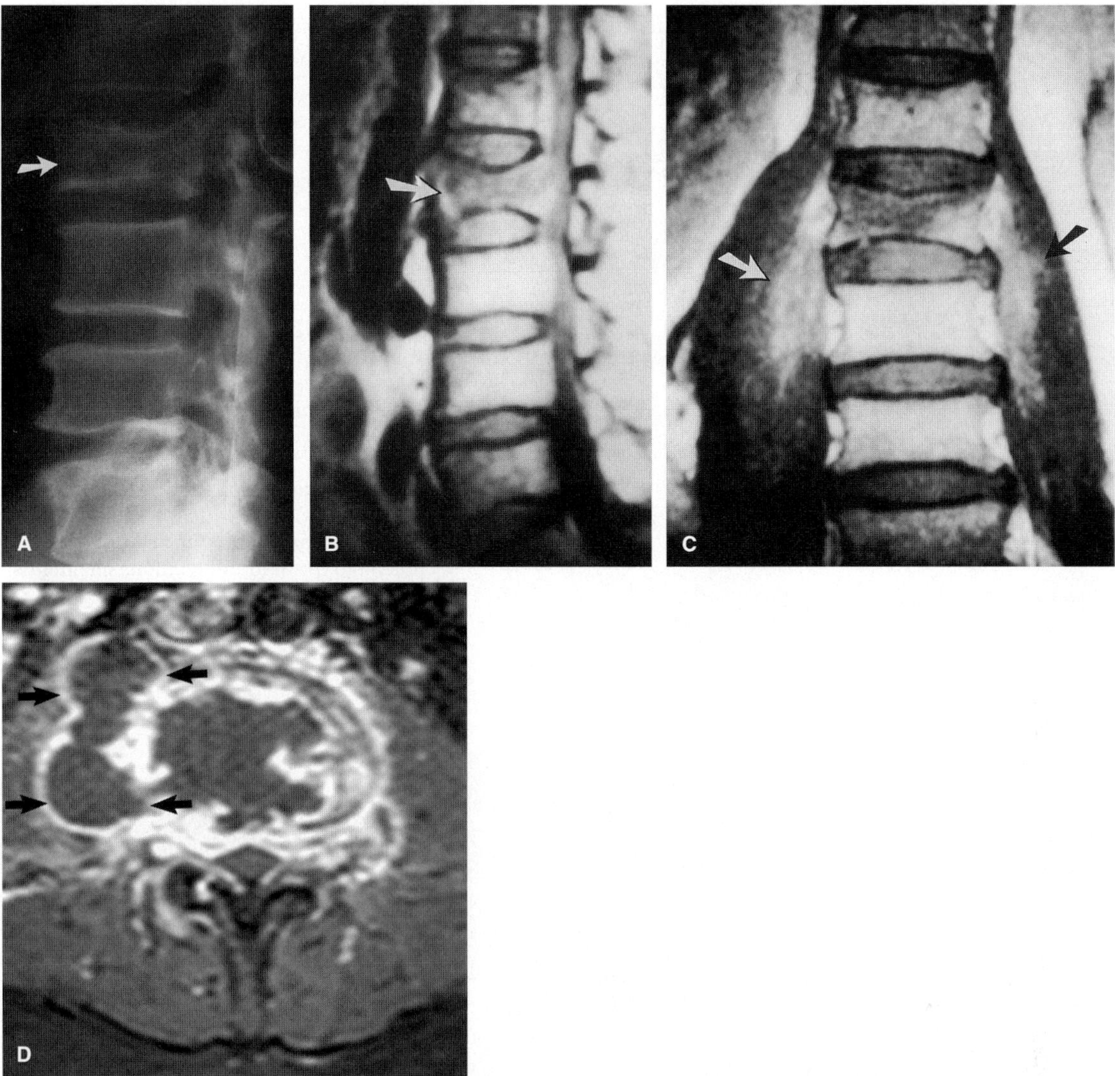

FIGURE 10.19. **Tuberculous Osteomyelitis (Pott Disease). A.** Plain film shows loss of height of L2 (*arrow*), with subtle sclerotic changes. **B.** Enhanced T1WI shows abnormal marrow throughout L2 (*arrow*) consistent with a pathologic fracture, making neoplasm or infection prime suspects. Acute compression fractures usually show anterior "wedging," and chronic compression fractures have normal marrow. **C.** Coronal enhanced images reveal bilateral psoas infiltration (*arrows*) but normal disks, consistent with a nonpyogenic infection such as tuberculosis. Contrast this with the disk involvement seen in Fig. 10.14. Metastatic tumor rarely infiltrates the psoas in such a diffuse fashion. **D.** Another patient with more chronic spinal tuberculosis with a "cold abscess" in the right psoas muscle (*arrows*).

25% of all intraspinal lesions in adults but are rare in children. These figures exclude vertebral metastases, which are the most common neoplastic condition involving the adult spine. MR is also an excellent tool for evaluating these osseous metastases (Fig. 10.21). Signal alterations from tumor infiltration within the normally bright marrow fat on T1WIs usually precede any bony changes detectable on plain film or CT, and MR is probably the earliest reliable method (aside from bone marrow biopsy) for detecting the presence of metastatic disease in the spine. Technetium bone scanning, however, remains the most cost-effective tool for whole-body screening.

Intramedullary Masses

The classic plain film finding of an intramedullary mass—widening of the interpedicular distance caused by slow expansile forces—is seen in fewer than 10% of cases. Plain CT is not useful for intramedullary tumors, because bony changes are relatively rare. Even with intrathecal contrast,

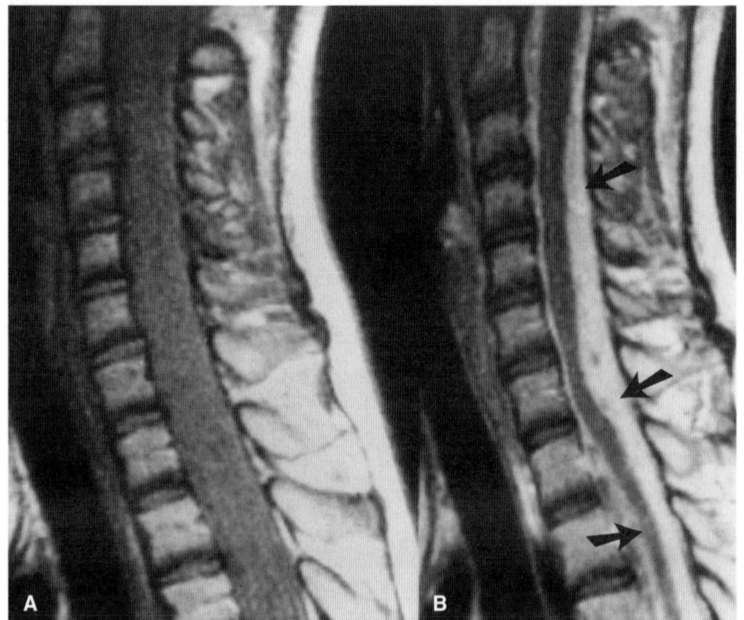

FIGURE 10.20. **Tuberculous Meningitis. A.** Sagittal unenhanced T1 image through the cervical spine shows relatively homogenous signal intensity tissue filling the spinal canal, making it difficult to decide whether the process is intramedullary or extramedullary. **B.** Postcontrast image demonstrates enhancing granulation tissue filling the subarachnoid space (*arrows*). This patient had similar pachymeningitis surrounding the brain, yet was surprisingly intact clinically, typical for tuberculous meningitis, which is less angioinvasive and consequently less destructive than pyogenic meningitis.

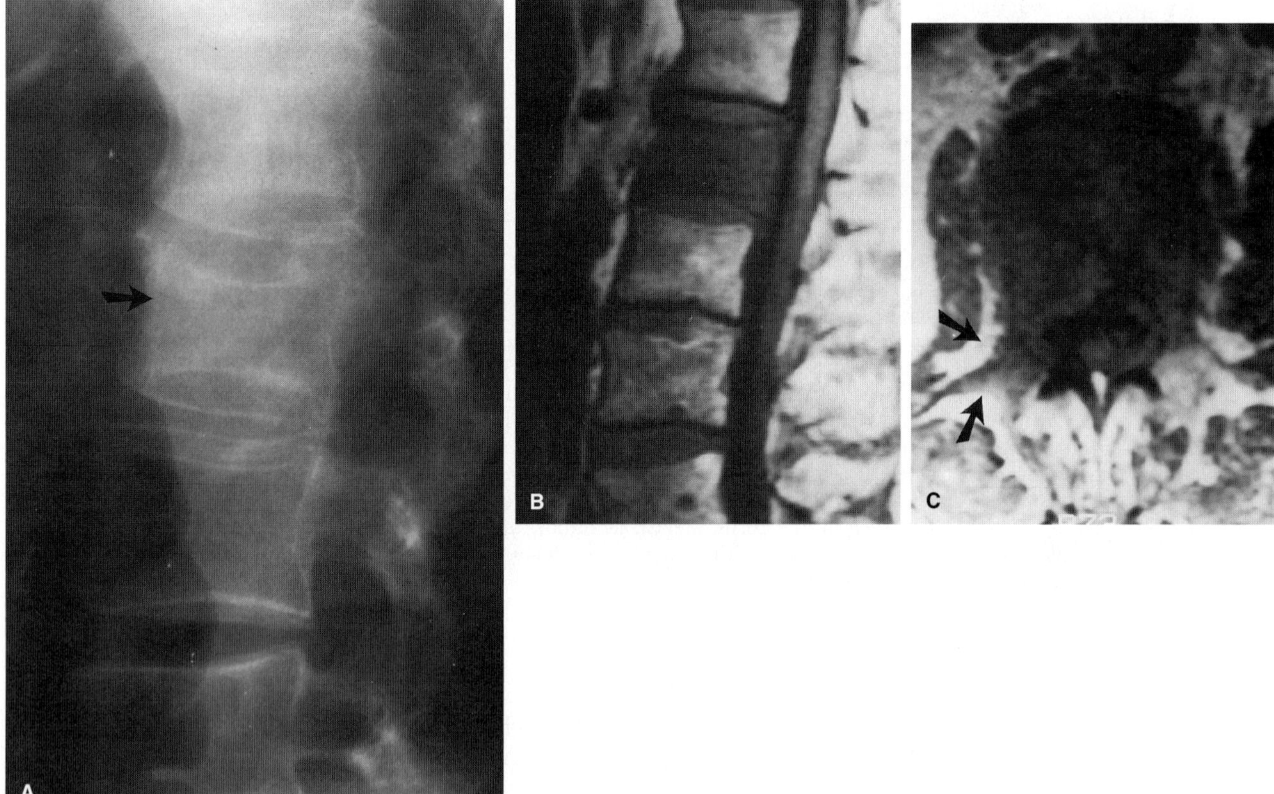

FIGURE 10.21. **Prostate Metastasis. A.** Plain film in this elderly man with acute lower back pain reveals a compression deformity at L1 (*arrow*), which could represent either a benign or pathologic compression fracture. Sagittal **(B)** and axial **(C)** T1WIs reveal infiltration of the entire vertebral body marrow space, including the right pedicle (*arrows*), a pattern that is highly indicative of metastasis. Biopsy revealed prostate carcinoma.

the crucial internal details of the cord are not visualized. MR is clearly the study of choice.

Astrocytomas and ependymomas are the two most common primary intramedullary tumors, but the distinction between them is difficult to make on imaging grounds alone. Both are expansile, low in signal intensity on T1WIs, and bright on T2WIs, with variable enhancement. Both have an increased incidence in neurofibromatosis. While some guidelines, based on involvement of the entire cord diameter and longer cord segments (favors astrocytoma) and presence of cysts and hemorrhage (favors ependymoma), have been proposed to distinguish between the two types of tumors, in any single case they are rarely a substitute for biopsy. Gadolinium contrast is useful to identify the tumor nidus as well as to document spread of tumor along CSF pathways.

Hemangioblastomas, on the other hand, are very distinctive, with a focal vascular blush at their nidus, with angiographic signs being virtually pathognomonic. Syringomyelia, while not a neoplasm, presents as an intramedullary mass on plain film myelogram and is therefore traditionally included in this gamut. Abscesses (Fig. 10.16), metastases (Fig. 10.10), lipomas (see Fig. 10.58), and teratomas will present on rare occasions as intramedullary masses.

Ependymomas are the most common spinal cord tumor in adults. They can be divided into the cellular (intramedullary) and myxopapillary (filum terminale) types. Spinal ependymomas are genetically and epidemiologically different from intracranial types. Peak incidence is in the fourth decade, with a male predominance. These slow-growing neoplasms arise from ependymal cells lining the central canal of the cord or cell rests along the filum. Histologically, these tumors are usually benign, but a complete curative excision may be impossible with the intramedullary types. Associated hemorrhage can be seen, especially on MR, and cystic areas are common (Fig. 10.22). The filum terminale ependymomas are also known as myxopapillary ependymomas on account of their unique histology, and because of their location, a reasonably specific diagnosis can be made on imaging. Myxopapillary ependymomas often can be excised completely, particularly if they are well encapsulated (Fig. 10.23).

Astrocytoma. Most (75%) astrocytomas occur in the cervical and upper to midthoracic cord, and presentation in the conus is rarer than with ependymomas. Fusiform cord widening, hyperintensity on T2WIs, and contrast enhancement often extend over several vertebral body segments (Fig. 10.24). They generally have a lower histologic grade than astrocytomas in the brain. As in the brain, there

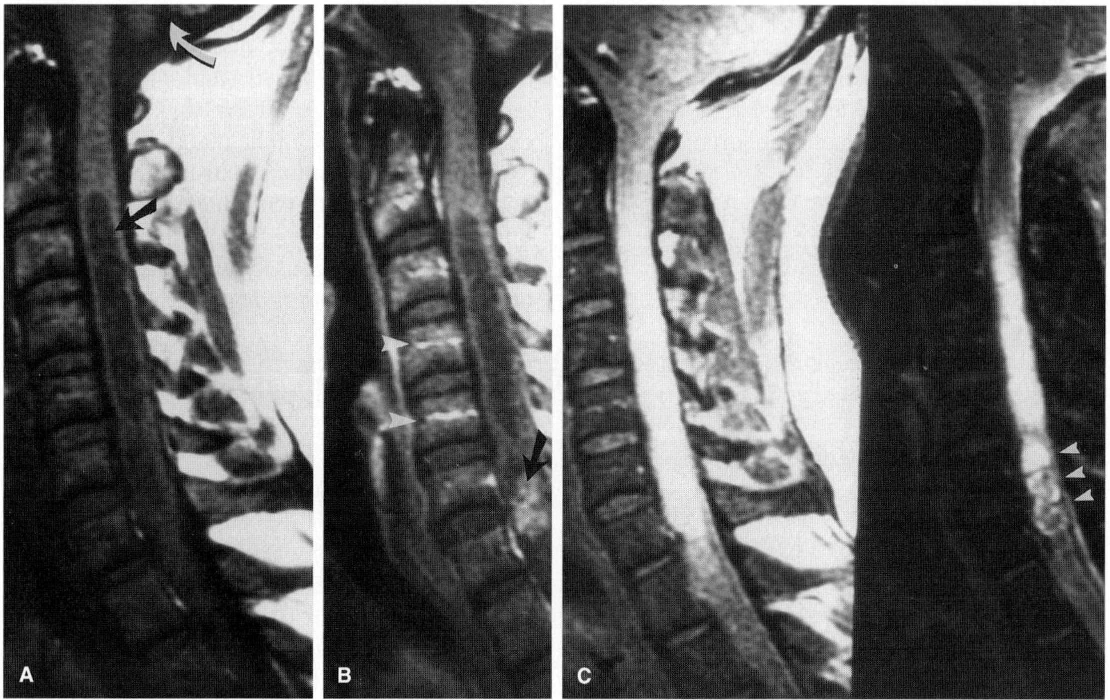

FIGURE 10.22. **Ependymoma. A.** T1WI shows a cavity (*arrow*) within the cervical cord, but the cerebellar tonsils (*curved arrow*) are in the normal position, so this cannot be a Chiari I malformation (contrast with Fig. 10.26). **B.** Postcontrast image shows an enhancing nodule (*arrow*) at the lower pole of the intramedullary cavity. Note the normal enhancement of the basivertebral plexus (*arrowheads*). **C.** T2WIs show blood breakdown products at the lower end of the cavity (*arrowheads*), suggestive of hemorrhage within the tumor.

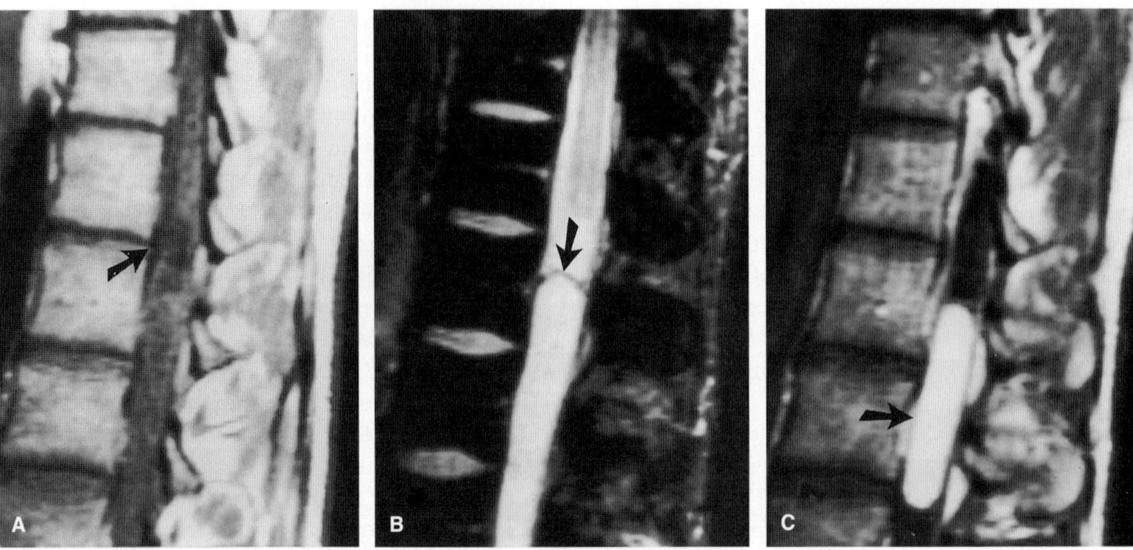

FIGURE 10.23. **Myxopapillary Ependymoma of the Filum Terminale. A.** This 29-year-old patient presented with lower extremity radicular complaints. T1W sagittal image shows an irregular appearance to the conus (*arrow*) and surrounding CSF, but no distinct mass. **B.** Sagittal gradient refocused echo image demonstrates a low signal "rim" (*arrow*), suggesting an intraspinal mass. **C.** Postcontrast image confirms an enhancing encapsulated intraspinal mass (*arrow*) abutting the conus. A complete resection was performed and the patient has done well. When myelography was the only technique for examining the lumbar spinal canal, a "conus shot" was mandatory to rule tumors (like this one) that can mimic disk disease in presentation.

is considerable histologic variability, and the unusual variants, such as protoplasmic astrocytoma, can involve the spinal cord over a considerable length. Astrocytomas are the most common spinal cord tumor in children, with peak incidence in the third decade, younger than for ependymomas. They may be exophytic, and at times may even appear largely extramedullary. Brainstem gliomas will sometimes extend through the medulla into the rostral cervical spine.

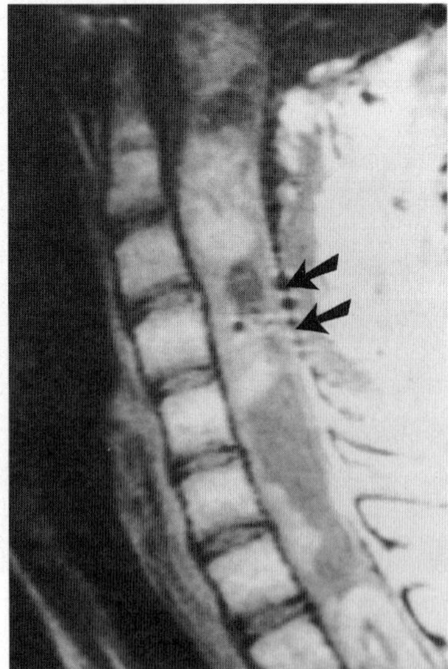

FIGURE 10.24. **Astrocytoma.** Astrocytoma of the cervical spine in a child with neurofibromatosis type 1. The patient had undergone a laminectomy (*arrows*) in an attempt at decompression.

Hemangioblastomas occur in the spine as well as the posterior fossa. Both types have a high association with Von Hippel-Lindau syndrome. These rare tumors, with their characteristic densely enhancing nidus, represent 2% of intraspinal neoplasms. Forty percent are extramedullary and 20% are multiple. The nidus shows vascular hypertrophy and may be mistaken for an arteriovenous malformation (AVM). However, intramedullary AVMs do not typically show a related cyst or cord expansion (compare Figs. 10.25 and 10.49).

Syringohydromyelia. *Hydromyelia* refers to dilation of the central canal of the spinal cord, which is lined by ependyma. *Syringomyelia*, on the other hand, is a cavity outside the central canal that is lined by glial cells. Distinction between these two conditions is difficult on imaging studies, given that the lining of the cavity cannot be examined histologically. The generic term covering either—"syringohydromyelia"—is a bit of a tongue twister, and the abbreviated "syrinx" is often used for both conditions. The etiology of a syrinx can be developmental, such as in the Arnold-Chiari malformations (see Chapter 8). However, trauma and tumors, as well as inflammatory and ischemic conditions, can also lead to a syrinx.

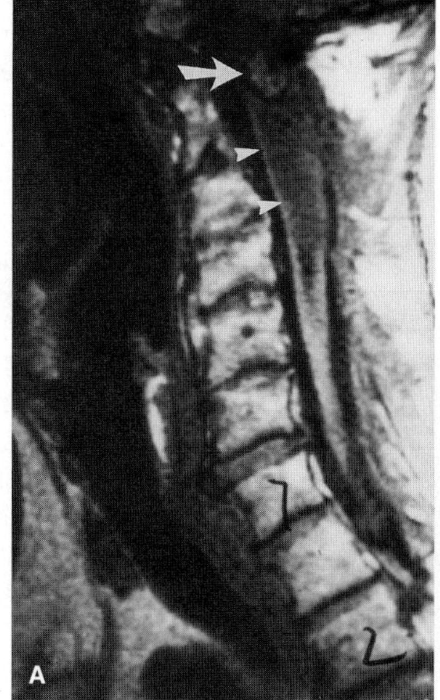

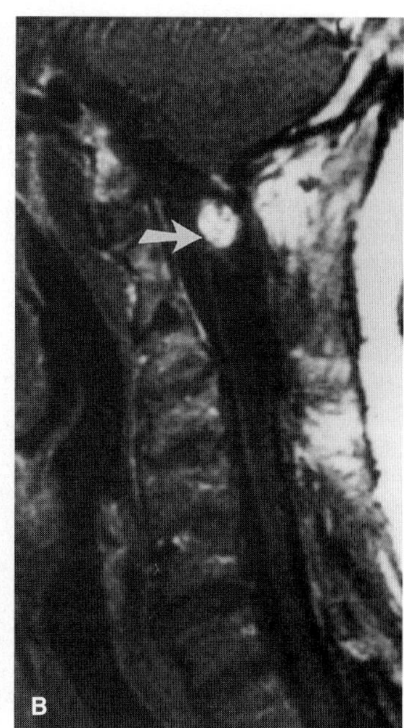

FIGURE 10.25. **Hemangioblastoma. A.** Sagittal T1WI shows expansion of the upper cervical cord caused by a low-signal central mass (*arrow*), which has a darker inferior component suggestive of a cyst (*arrowheads*). This cavity must be investigated further, as it lacks sharp margins and does not follow CSF signal (compare to Fig. 10.26). **B.** Postcontrast image shows an intensely enhancing nodule (*arrow*) at the level of the foramen magnum, classic for a hemangioblastoma. (Courtesy of Dr William P. Dillon, University of California, San Francisco.)

The preferred imaging method is T1WIs in the sagittal and axial planes, along with sagittal T2WIs. Be aware that high signal truncation (Gibbs) artifacts can superimpose themselves over the cord, mimicking a syrinx. A syrinx cavity should have very well-defined margins, and its contents should follow CSF signal intensity. Always suspect tumor as a cause of unexplained syrinx. Unless definite benign etiology is apparent, such as prior history of cord contusion or the low cerebellar tonsils of a Chiari I malformation (Fig. 10.26), give gadolinium to search for a tumor nidus. If the syrinx borders are indistinct and the signal is brighter than CSF on T1WIs and darker than CSF on T2WIs, you may be dealing with severe central cord edema. It is critical to establish the full extent of the cavity for potential shunting, so if on a cervical spine examination, a cord cavity extends into the thoracic spine, follow it down, or the patient will inevitably need to return to complete the examination. With CT myelography, contrast often enters into a syrinx cavity with delayed images. Occasionally, this technique is useful in establishing the degree to which a cord cavity communicates with the CSF.

Intradural/Extramedullary Masses

Meningioma is the most common intradural tumor in the thoracic region and represents roughly 25% of all adult intraspinal tumors. Most (80%) occur in women, with an average age of 45. Multiple meningiomas, as in the brain, raise the question of neurofibromatosis. The usual location is extramedullary/intradural, although there can be an extradural component. Dense calcification can occur, as in the brain (Fig. 10.27). CT and MR characteristics are similar to that of intracranial meningiomas, with dense homogenous enhancement and broad dural tails (Fig. 10.28). The main differential consideration is usually schwannoma, which often will extend out through a neural foramen, and lacks a broad dural base. Schwannomas are less well vascularized than meningiomas and may undergo cystic necrosis.

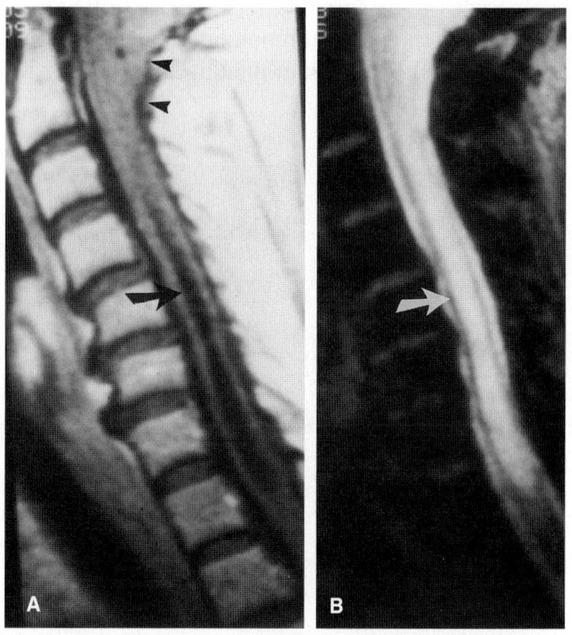

FIGURE 10.26. **Syrinx. A.** T1WI. **B.** T2WI. This intramedullary lesion (*arrow*) shows the classic features of a benign syrinx: The margins of the intramedullary cavity are sharp and the intramedullary contents follow CSF signals on all sequences. The cause of the syrinx—the low cerebellar tonsils of the Chiari malformation (*arrowheads*)—is also seen.

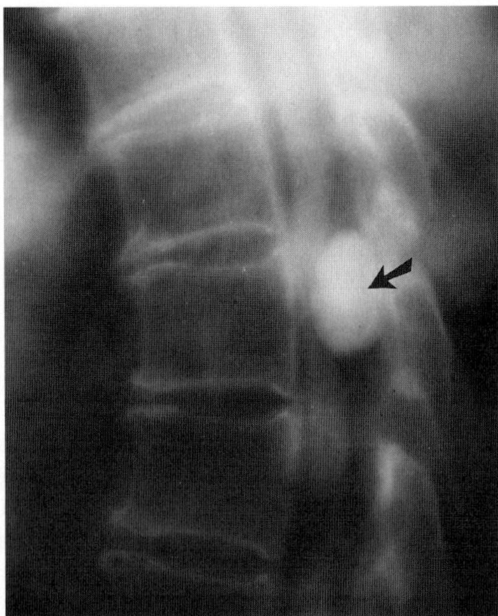

FIGURE 10.27. **Meningioma.** This myelogram was performed using air as contrast, a "pneumomyelogram." A densely calcified dorsal intradural extramedullary mass (*arrow*) seen indenting the cord proved to be a meningioma. Schwannomas rarely calcify to this extent. (Courtesy of Dr Van Halbach, University of California, San Francisco.)

Nerve sheath tumors include schwannoma (also known as neurinoma, neurolemmoma, neuroma) and neurofibromas. *Schwannoma* is the preferred term, because pathologically these tumors are composed of Schwann cells. They are the most common intraspinal mass, comprising 29% of the total. Schwannomas usually originate from the dorsal sensory nerve roots, but they remain encapsulated and extrinsic to the nerve, causing symptoms by mass effect. Most are solitary and sporadic, with a peak presentation in the fifth decade, although with MR more are being discovered as incidental findings in younger patients (Fig. 10.29). Extension into the neural foramen is a frequent finding, especially in the cervical and thoracic regions. Part of the tumor will be intraspinal, and part will be extraspinal, with the waist at the often-expanded neural foramen, giving the classic "dumbbell" appearance (Fig. 10.30). In the lumbar region, schwannomas tend to remain within the dural sac (Fig. 10.29).

Spinal neurofibromas are associated with neurofibromatosis (NF) type 1 and its chromosome 17 abnormalities. NF-2, which is related to an abnormality of chromosome 22, is associated with multiple meningiomas and schwannomas but not neurofibromas. Spinal neurofibromas can have a plexiform configuration, extending out through multiple adjacent neural foramina (Fig. 10.31). Pathologically, neurofibromas (unlike schwannomas) contain collagen and myxoid tissue, infiltrate the nerve without encapsulated margins, and have a malignant potential. Unlike schwannomas, neurofibromas rarely show cystic degeneration or internal hemorrhage. Radiographically, however, these two types of nerve sheath tumors are often indistinguishable. Both can be intradural or extradural in location. In patients with NF-1, look for the additional imaging findings of kyphoscoliosis, rib dysplasia (ribbon ribs), and scalloping of the posterior vertebral body caused by dural ectasia (Fig. 10.32). As in the brain, both schwannomas and neurofibromas enhance. Heterogeneous enhancement with areas of low signal is more

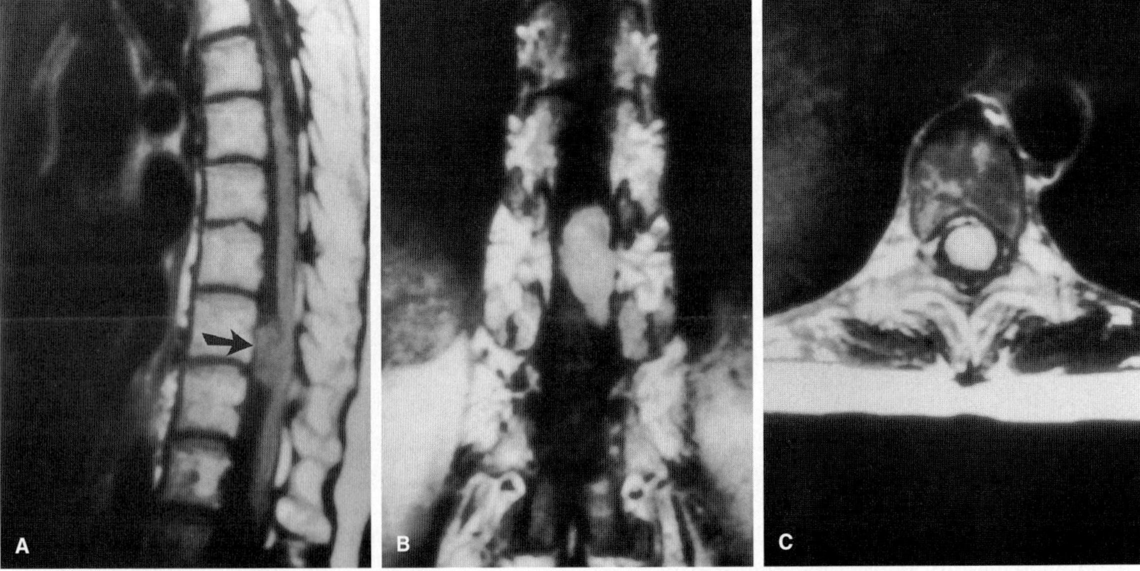

FIGURE 10.28. **Meningioma. A.** Sagittal T1WI shows a well-defined anterior extradural intraspinal mass with a broad dural base (*arrow*). Coronal **(B)** and axial **(C)** images show severe cord compression and the dense enhancement characteristic of meningioma.

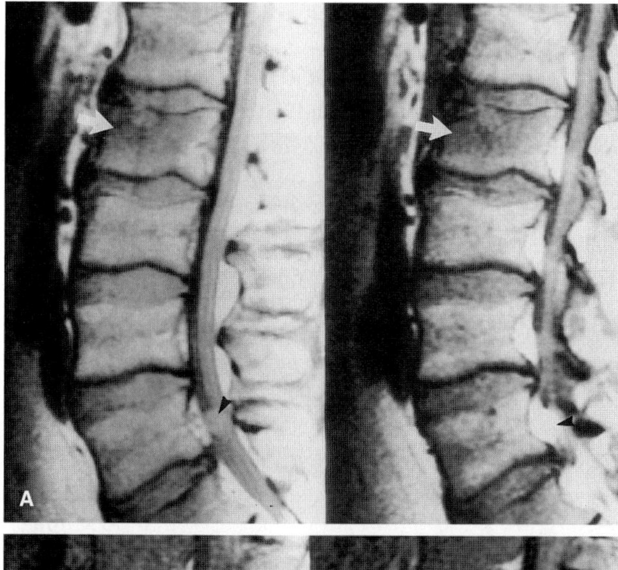

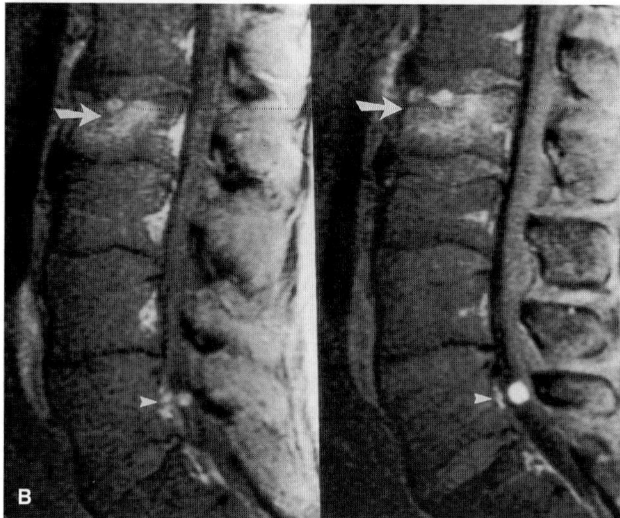

FIGURE 10.29. **Schwannoma. A.** This patient had acute focal back pain after an accident, resulting in an acute compression fracture of the superior aspect of L2, which shows marrow edema (*arrow*). A small intraspinal mass was also noted at L5 (*arrowhead*). **B.** This lesion enhanced with contrast (*arrowhead*). This was unchanged on follow-up examination and likely represents a small schwannoma. Note enhancement of the L2 compression fracture (*arrow*), which is highlighted on this fat-saturation image.

characteristic of a neurofibroma. The cutaneous stigmata of neurofibromatosis, such as café-au-lait spots, help confirm the diagnosis.

Intrathecal (Drop) Metastases. The classic cause of spinal intradural/extramedullary metastases is subarachnoid seeding of primary CNS tumors, such as posterior fossa medulloblastomas, ependymomas, and pineal region neoplasms. Tumor cells in the posterior fossa exfoliate into the CSF and "drop" down into the spinal canal, implant on the pia, and grow into small nodules, giving rise to the term "drop metastases" (Fig. 10.33). However, any tumor spreading via the CSF pathways of the brain can involve the spinal leptomeninges. Solid tumors, such as breast and lung carcinoma, can metastasize to the subarachnoid space. Leukemia, which will be discussed below, probably has the highest rate of infiltration of the meninges of any non-CNS tumor. These leptomeningeal metastases can cause considerable inflammation, and patients can present with signs of meningeal irritation, leading to the term "carcinomatous meningitis." Systemic lymphoma (particularly T-cell lymphomas) and carcinomas can also spread to the CSF pathways.

Leptomeningeal metastases classically appear as multiple intradural nodules, causing filling defects on myelography (Fig. 10.34) or CT myelograms. MR with gadolinium enhancement is now the preferred method for screening, as it is noninvasive (Fig. 10.35). Sometimes thin, smooth sheets of intrathecal tumor cells, described by pathologists as "sugar coating" of the cord and roots, will be difficult to detect on myelograms because there is no discrete mass. The differential diagnosis of thickened leptomeninges (pachymeningitis) includes carcinomatous and infectious meningitis, postinfectious states such as Guillain-Barré syndrome, and inflammatory arachnoiditis in the postoperative patient. In the immunocompromised patient, diffuse leptomeningeal enhancement requires CSF analysis to distinguish between tumor and infection.

Blood in the subarachnoid space may be bright on T1WIs, and in the immediate postoperative period it is essential to obtain pre–gadolinium injection images to ensure that trace methemoglobin is not mistaken for enhancing drop metastases. Subarachnoid and subdural blood in the spinal canal can cause leptomeningeal irritation and enhancement, further confusing the postoperative "rule out drop metastasis" scan. These problems are easily avoided by obtaining a *preoperative* enhanced MR scan of the spine in any patient at risk for spinal drop metastases, such as a child with medulloblastoma. Once such a child has been sedated and contrast given for the brain, a complete spinal scan will only take another 15 minutes or so; this will save a lot of consternation postoperatively, when the case requires staging for adjunctive chemotherapy and radiation.

Extradural Masses

Metastases. Neoplasm is the second most common cause of extradural mass, after disk herniations and other degenerative processes; however, in immunosuppressed patients and in certain parts of the world, infections may outnumber neoplasms as a source of extradural mass effect. Primary vertebral tumors such as chordomas, giant cell tumors, hemangiomas, and sarcomas behave like any other extradural mass in terms of myelographic findings and must be kept in the differential diagnosis. The most

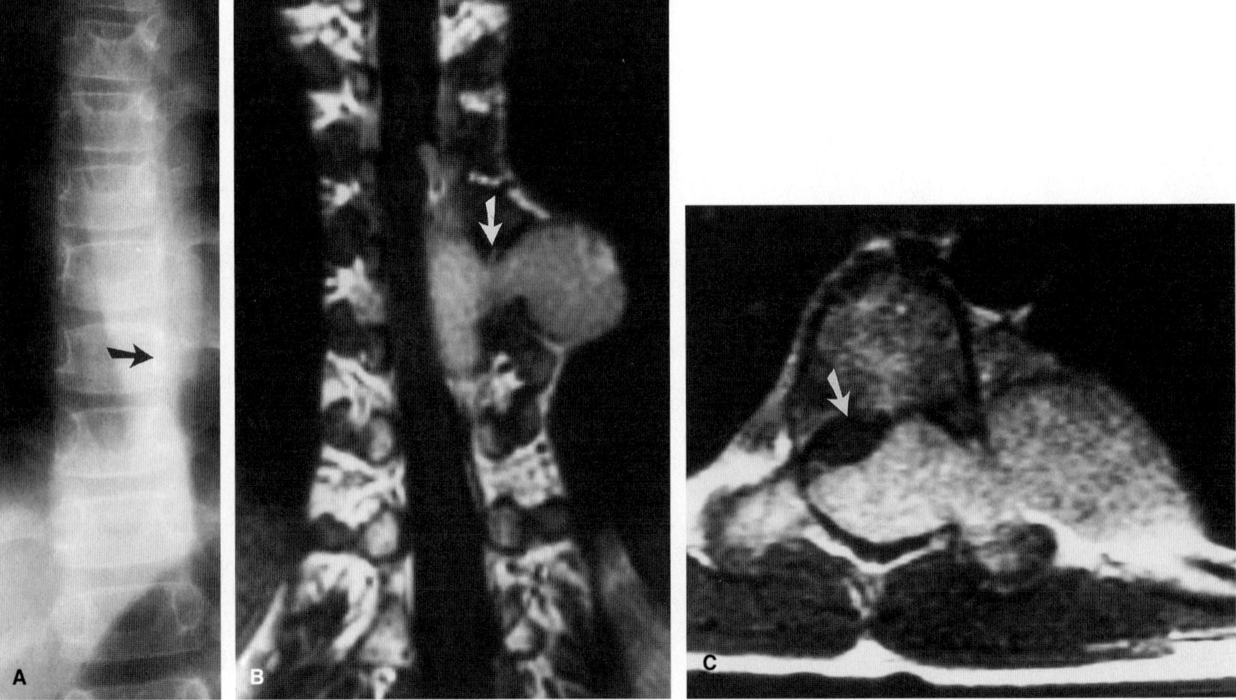

FIGURE 10.30. **"Dumbbell" Schwannoma. A.** Plain thoracic anteroposterior film shows erosion of a left-sided pedicle (*arrow*). **B.** Coronal T1WI demonstrates a huge neurofibroma with both intraspinal and extraspinal components in the classic dumbbell configuration with the waist at the neural foramen (*arrow*). **C.** Axial image is helpful in identifying the position of the spinal cord (*arrow*) and in assessing the degree of cord compression.

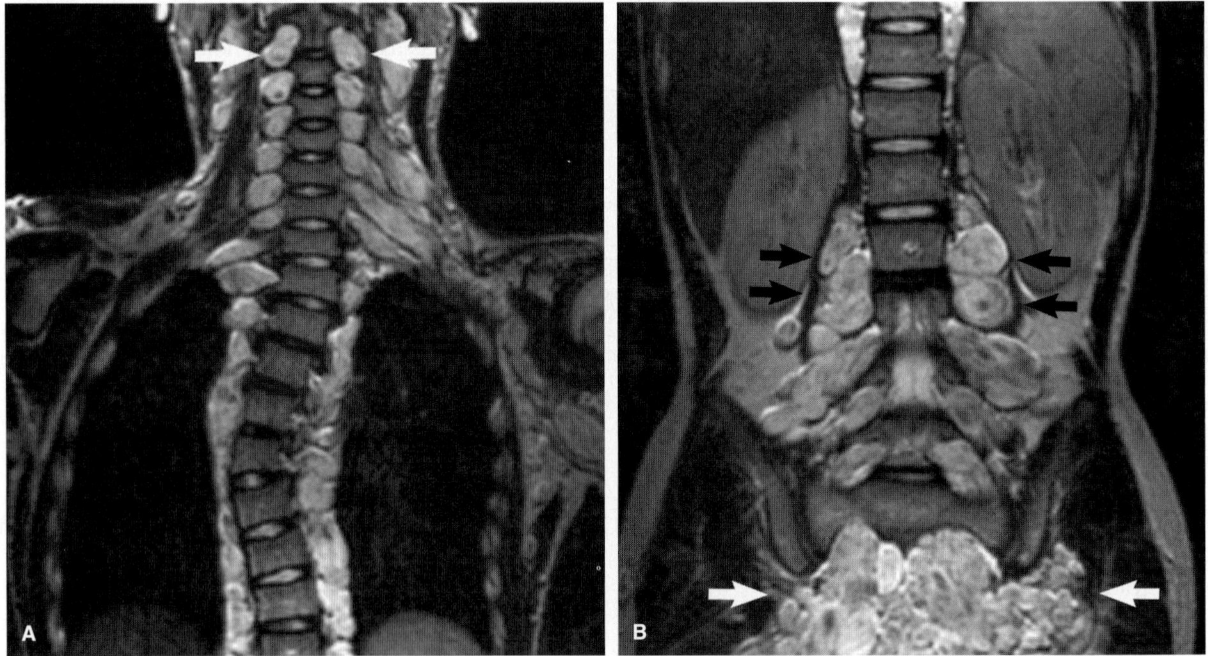

FIGURE 10.31. **Neurofibromatosis Type 1. A.** The thoracic spine shows foraminal masses at every level, beginning at C2–C3 (*arrows*). These neurofibromas have resulted in scoliosis, a frequent finding in neurofibromatosis type 1. **B.** Lumbar postcontrast coronal images reveal multiple enhancing masses, consistent with neurofibromas, which extend out the neural foramina (*black arrows*), creating a large conglomerate pelvic mass, consistent with a plexiform neurofibroma (*white arrows*).

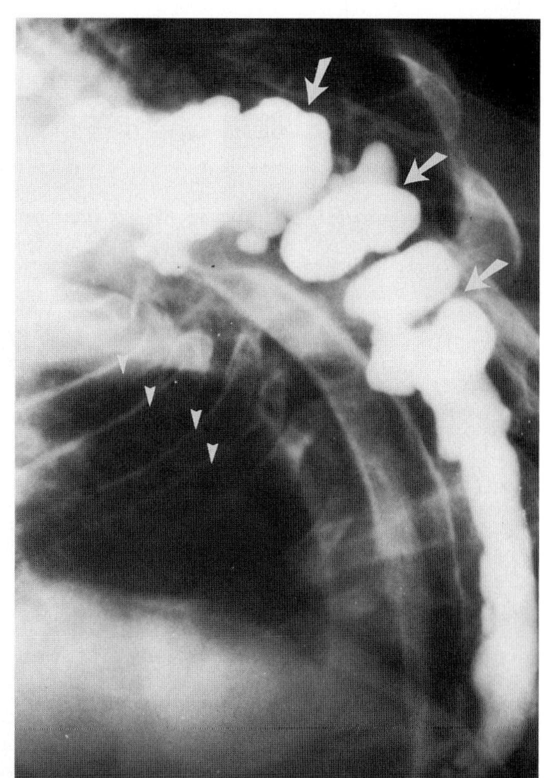

FIGURE 10.32. **Neurofibromatosis.** Myelogram shows severe dural ectasia caused by neurofibromatosis (*arrows*). Note also the "ribbon ribs" (*arrowheads*).

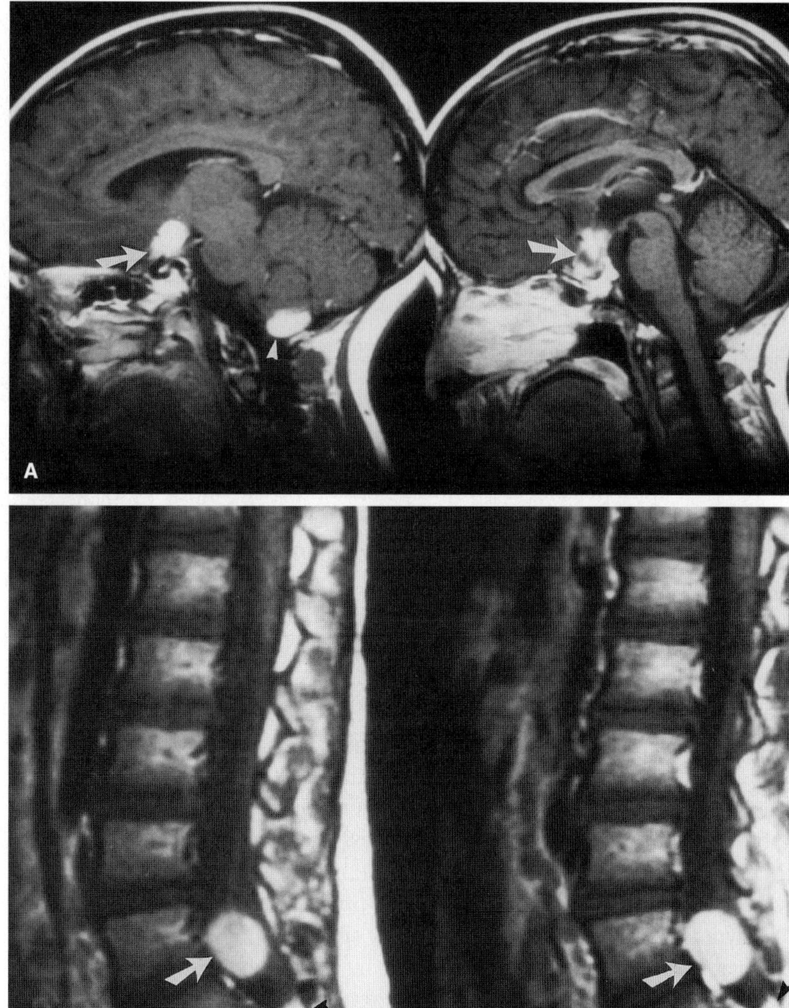

FIGURE 10.33. **CNS Drop Metastases. A.** Sagittal enhanced midline T1WIs through the brain show a suprasellar juvenile pilocytic astrocytoma (*arrow*), with a metastasis that has reached the cerebellar tonsils via the CSF (*arrowhead*). **B.** Sagittal enhanced lumbar T1WIs show a large intra-arachnoid metastatic nodule posterior to L5 (*arrow*). High-signal tissue is also seen posterior to S2 (*arrowheads*). If it were clinically necessary to confirm that this sacral area represents tumor rather than epidural fat, fat-saturation images would be useful.

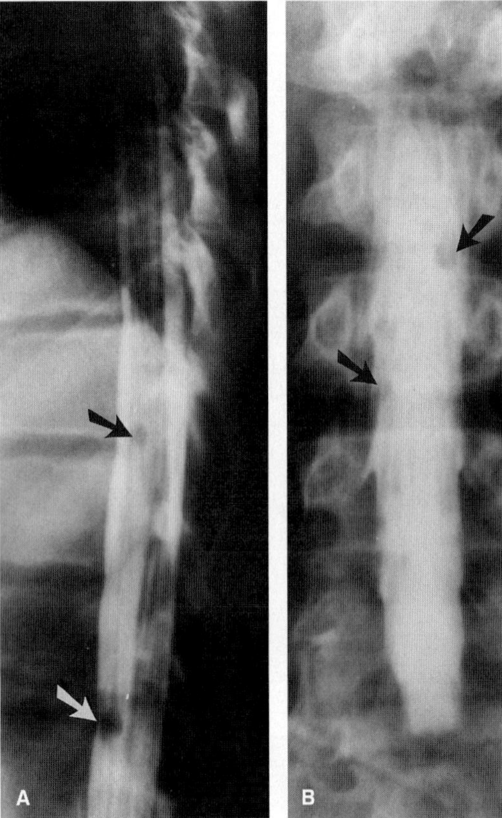

FIGURE 10.34. **Intrathecal Metastases.** Lateral **(A)** and anteroposterior **(B)** myelographic images show multiple nodular filling defects within the subarachnoid space (*arrows*), consistent with nodular leptomeningeal metastases, in this case of lung carcinoma.

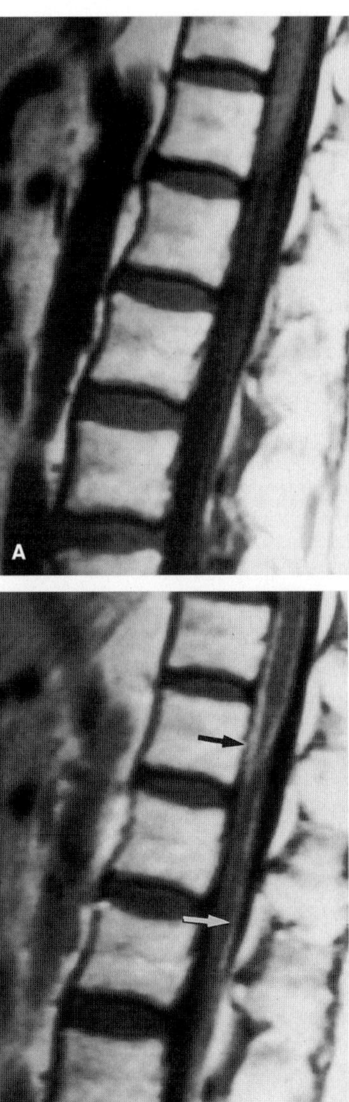

FIGURE 10.35. **Carcinomatous Meningitis. A.** Sagittal unenhanced T1WI in this breast cancer patient is unremarkable. **B.** Enhanced image through the conus shows fine sheets of enhancing tumor coating the distal cord and cauda equina (*arrows*). This thin diffuse "cake frosting" type of leptomeningeal tumor involvement may be hard to detect myelographically.

common extradural neoplasm, however, is metastatic spread of solid tumors, such as breast, lung, and prostate carcinoma. Most metastases, like infection, reach the vertebrae via arterial seeding, although prostate carcinoma may preferentially ascend to the lumbar region via the Batson venous plexus. The vertebral marrow space, like the liver and the lungs, "filters" a great deal of blood and is a fertile ground for metastatic deposits.

As these deposits grow, they replace normal marrow, which contains considerable fat and is bright on T1WIs. Metastases therefore appear as low signal areas on T1WIs or high signal areas on T2WIs, because of their higher water content versus fat. Prostate cancer and other densely sclerotic metastases can be somewhat confusing on MR, unless one appreciates that areas of intensely sclerotic bone may be dark on all sequences. Historically, unenhanced T1WIs were the mainstay of vertebral body evaluation, but today newer sequences that provide different T2 effects are more sensitive for marrow space pathology. Fast versions of STIR and T2 FSE with fat saturation are ideal for increasing the conspicuity of abnormal marrow (Fig. 10.36; see Fig. 10.43). As with other metastases, neovascularity develops to supply the expanding mass of intravertebral tumor cells, which is why vertebral metastases can enhance intensely, although this may reduce their conspicuity against background fat (Fig. 10.4), unless fat saturation is used. With gradient-refocused images, the metastases should also be bright, but susceptibility effects from the bony trabeculae reduce their conspicuity, making these sequences less useful.

Diffusion-weighted imaging (DWI) showed great promise in initial studies (17). In theory, malignant

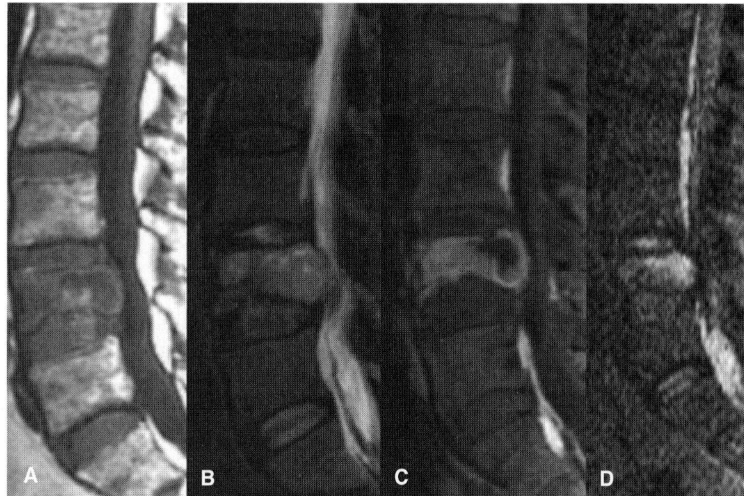

FIGURE 10.36. **Restricted Diffusion Within a Vertebral Metastasis. A.** T1WI shows complete infiltration of the marrow of L4, with mild retropulsion of the posterior portion of the vertebra into the spinal canal. **B.** T2WI image shows increased signal, as expected. **C.** Diffuse enhancement after gadolinium administration. **D.** Diffusion-weighted image shows increased signal. This is caused by restricted diffusion of water, which is predominantly intracellular, within the tumor cells packing the marrow space.

compression fractures will be bright on DWI because of the restriction of water in the infiltrating tumor cells (Fig. 10.37); therefore such effect is absent with benign and osteoporotic fractures, where extracellular water may be increased. Unfortunately, infiltrated vertebrae can show areas of both tumor (decreased apparent diffusion coefficient) and "pathologic" fracture (increased apparent diffusion coefficient), confusing the picture.

Once tumor has infiltrated the cortex, spread to the epidural space can occur, which along with compression fractures may lead to cord compromise. Certain signs (summarized in Table 10.3) help determine whether a compression fracture is caused by infection or tumor or is merely secondary to osteoporosis (Fig. 10.38). In general, metastases differ from pyogenic infection in that they involve the vertebrae diffusely but not contiguously, sparing the disks, with epidural mass and enhancement limited to the levels of the pathologic vertebrae (Fig. 10.39). Marked involvement of the pedicles is another sign of neoplasm (Fig. 10.40). Exceptions include disk-sparing nonpyogenic infections, such as TB, and lymphoma, which may have extensive epidural infiltration.

Direct Extension of Paraspinous Tumor. Retroperitoneal and mediastinal tumors can invade the vertebral column and spinal canal by direct extension. Neuroblastoma and its relatives ganglioneuroma and ganglioneuroblastoma arise from primitive paraspinous neural remnants that are similar to fetal neuroblasts. These tumors frequently involve the spinal canal, infiltrating through the neural foramina (Figs. 10.41, 10.42). Any paraspinous tumor can do likewise, including lymphomas, apical lung (Pancoast) tumors, and a variety of retroperitoneal and mediastinal carcinomas and sarcomas.

Hematologic malignancies affecting the spine include leukemia, myeloma, and lymphoma. Leukemias change the appearance of the vertebrae in the characteristic

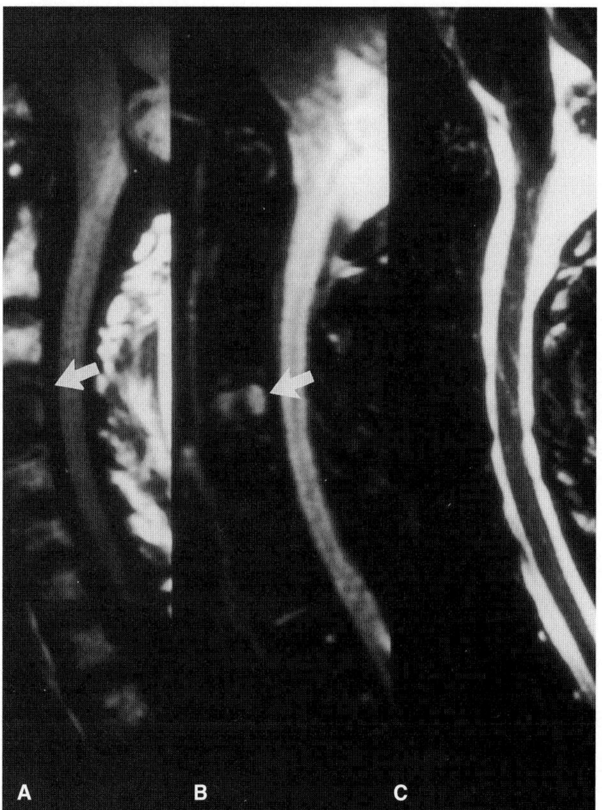

FIGURE 10.37. **Value of Inversion Recovery in the Evaluation of Metastases.** This patient has breast carcinoma. **A.** Vertebrae C2 and C3 are bright, consistent with radiation; C4 (*arrow*) is quite dark, raising the question of metastasis; C5 and below are intermediate in signal and may or may not be normal. **B.** This short time inversion recovery image shows high signal, consistent with metastasis limited to C4 (*arrow*). **C.** Fast spin-echo sequence with T2 weighting shows little useful information on the marrow, one of the shortcomings of this technique. (Courtesy of Dr Rahul Mehta, Stanford, CA.)

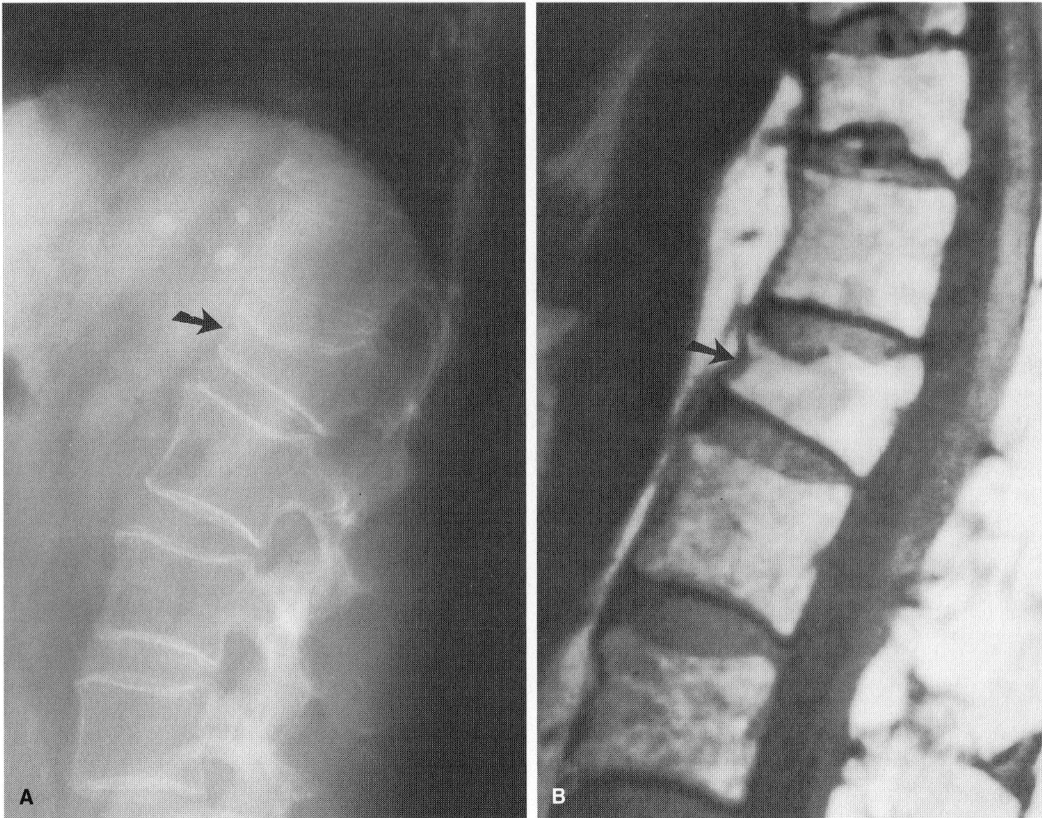

FIGURE 10.38. **Benign Compression Fracture. A.** Plain films show a compression fracture of L1 (*arrow*). The vertebral body shows a classic wedge deformity, with greater loss of height anteriorly than posteriorly and intact pedicles on the anteroposterior view (not shown). This configuration is suggestive of a benign compression fracture. **B.** T1 sagittal MR shows normal marrow signal in the affected vertebra (*arrow*), confirming a benign cause of the compression fracture, such as osteoporosis.

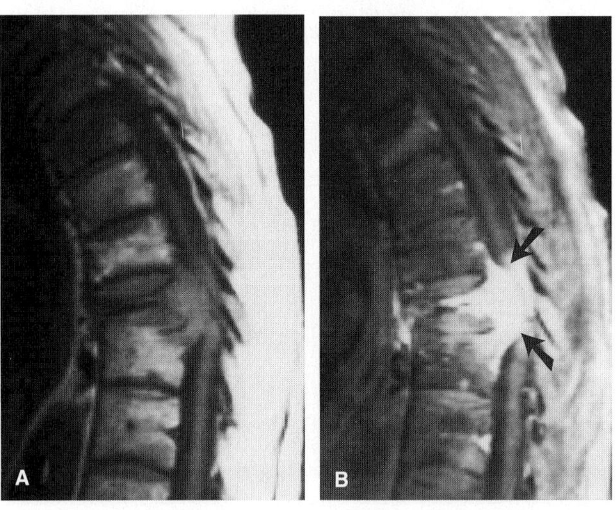

FIGURE 10.39. **Metastatic Lung Carcinoma With Pathologic Fracture. A.** Precontrast image shows many of the features of metastatic involvement, such as complete infiltration of the affected vertebra and disk sparing. **B.** Postcontrast image demonstrates that the epidural involvement (*arrows*) is largely limited to the level of the affected vertebra, and there is no multisegment enhancement of the anterior and posterior longitudinal ligaments, as is often seen in infection. Contrast this case with Fig. 10.15, which shows a typical epidural abscess.

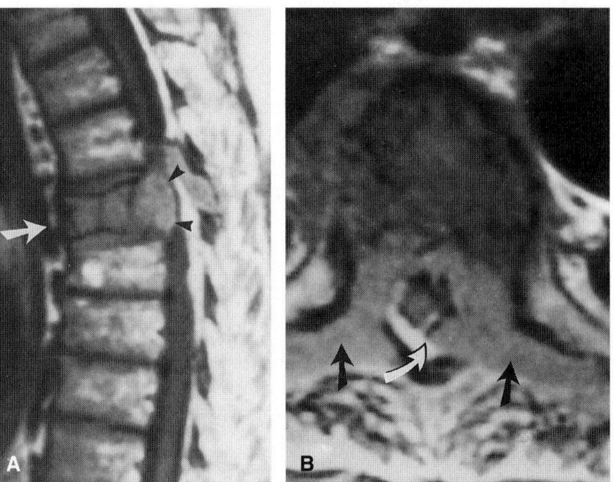

FIGURE 10.40. **Multiple Myeloma.** Sagittal **(A)** and axial **(B)** MR images show several features associated with neoplastic infiltration in a midthoracic vertebra (*large arrow*). The affected vertebra is completely involved, the disks are spared, and the epidural mass (*arrowheads*) is limited to the level of the affected vertebra. The pedicles and lamina are infiltrated and expanded (*small black arrows*) and the epidural fat (*curved arrow*) is displaced rather than infiltrated. None of these signs alone confirms a neoplastic process, but taken together, they are highly suggestive of metastatic tumor.

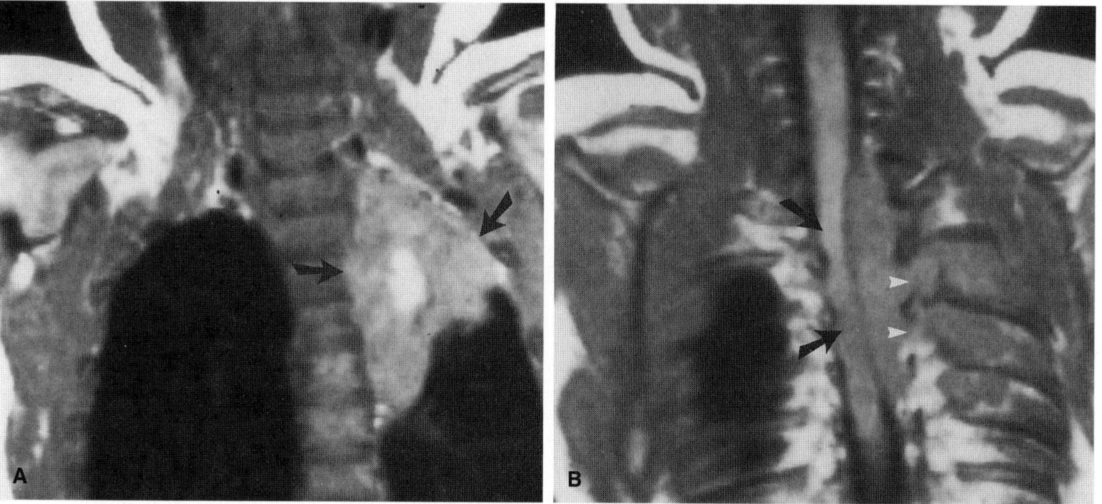

FIGURE 10.41. **Neuroblastoma. A.** This patient presented with flaccidity of the lower extremities and an apical paraspinous chest mass (*arrows*). **B.** The myelopathy is easily explained by cord compression (*arrows*) caused by the neuroblastoma infiltrating into the spinal canal via multiple neural foramina (*arrowheads*).

fashion of diffuse, even replacement of the marrow with tumor (Fig. 10.43; see also Fig. 10.67). Solid leukemic infiltrates, or chloromas, can involve the epidural space and cause cord compression. Studies have been performed by tracking the MR appearance of the marrow in these patients through induction chemotherapy, radiation, bone marrow transplantation, and repopulation with normal marrow cells, which are referenced and worth reviewing when evaluating such cases (Fig. 10.44) (20).

Multiple myeloma can present as a diffuse and homogeneous low signal in the spine on T1WIs but more typically shows multiple focal defects (Fig 10.40). Solitary plasmacytomas are in the differential diagnosis for vertebral plana (totally collapsed vertebral body), along with eosinophilic granuloma, leukemia and severe osteoporosis (22). Technetium bone scans may miss myeloma lesions, which are often relatively "indolent" metabolically. This has made MR spine "screening" of myeloma patents a useful practice.

Myelofibrosis will present as very dark marrow space on T1WIs and remains dark on T2WIs since there is "dry" fibrous tissue rather than "wet" tumor replacing the

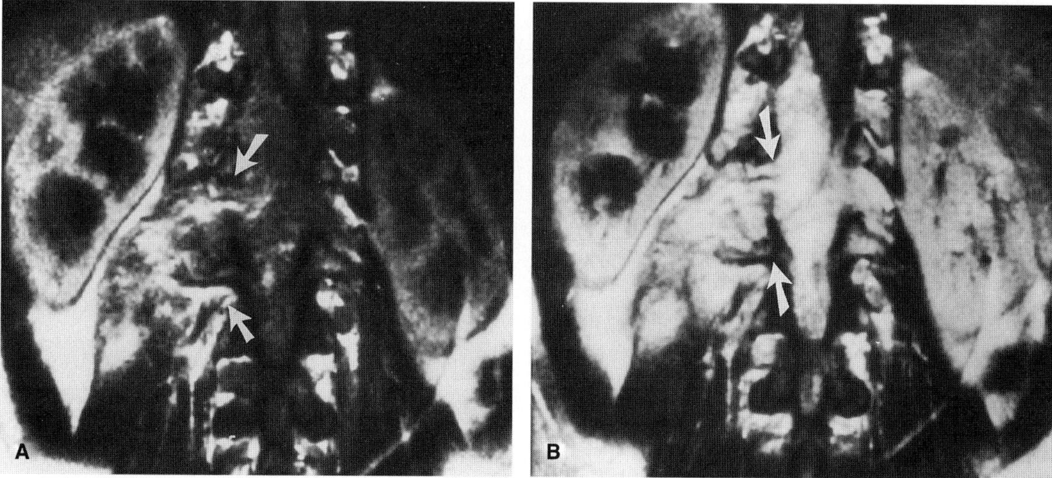

FIGURE 10.42. **Ganglioneuroblastoma. A.** This tumor is believed to represent a more "mature" or differentiated form of tumor of the sympathetic nervous system than neuroblastoma. It shares a similar paraspinous distribution and tendency to dumbbell into the spinal canal (*arrows*) via the neural foramina. **B.** Note the diffuse enhancement with gadolinium.

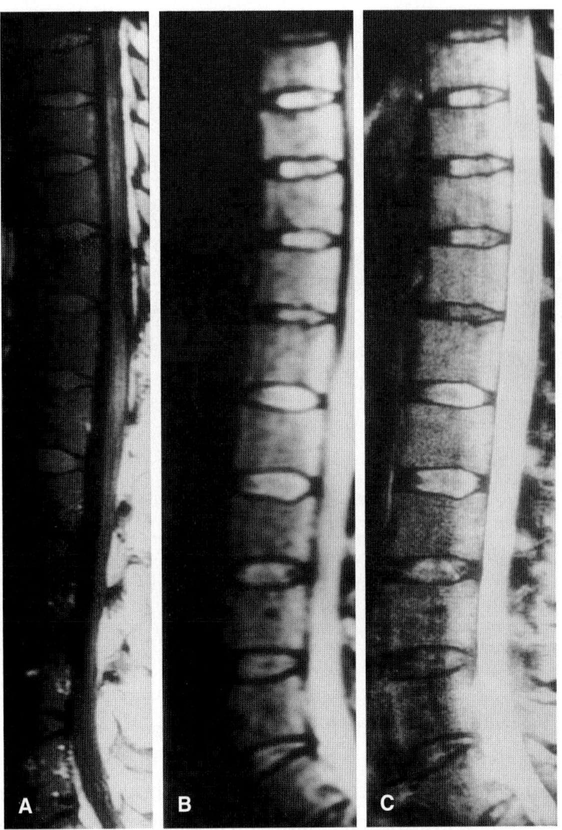

FIGURE 10.43. **Three MR Techniques for Evaluating the Marrow in Leukemia. A.** T1WI shows diffuse homogenous infiltration of the marrow, which is dark, as leukemic cells, high in water content, have replaced the normal marrow fat. Normal marrow should be brighter than the disks on T1W spin-echo images. **B.** Short time inversion-recovery (STIR) technique makes this "watery" marrow bright. **C.** "Fast inversion recovery" produces the same effect as conventional STIR in a fraction of the time. (Courtesy of Dr Rahul Mehta, Stanford, CA.)

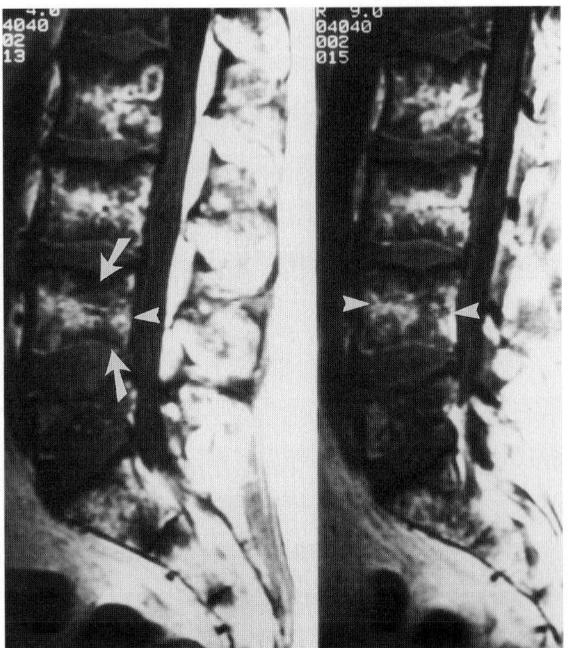

FIGURE 10.44. **Bone Marrow Transplantation.** Marrow repopulation is occurring in this patient after bone marrow transplantation. The new hematopoietic marrow, dark on T1WIs, has settled in the areas of the vertebrae adjacent to the endplates (*arrow*), probably because of the rich arterial supply to these regions. The centers of the vertebrae (*arrowheads*) show less new active marrow ingrowth and more fat, and consequently, is bright on T1WIz.

marrow (Fig. 10.45). Patients with hemoglobinopathies, such as sickle cell disease, may have areas of extramedullary hematopoiesis, which are often paraspinous, and can infiltrate into the spinal canal, causing cord compression.

Lymphoma is another "hematologic" tumor, with protean imaging manifestations that can serve (and have served) as the topic for an entire monograph. Non-Hodgkin and B-cell types predominate in the CNS. More than 30% of systemic lymphomas have skeletal manifestations, and spinal involvement is usually secondary rather than primary. Tumor masses may be intraspinal, paraspinal, or both (extradural > intradural > intramedullary). Cord compression is a common presenting symptom (Fig. 10.46). The epidural and paraspinous masses are usually more extensive than metastatic disease from solid tumors and can mimic the appearance of epidural infection. Lymphomas involving the mediastinum and retroperitoneum

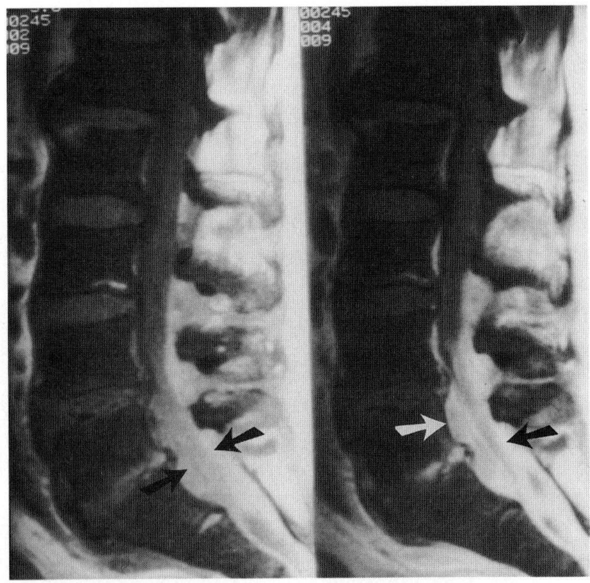

FIGURE 10.45. **Myelofibrosis.** This patient has very dark marrow compartment on these enhanced T1WIs because of myelofibrosis, which has replaced the normal erythropoietic marrow. The marrow remained dark on T2WIs, as there is no increased water in this marrow condition. Note the enhancing epidural abscess (*arrows*).

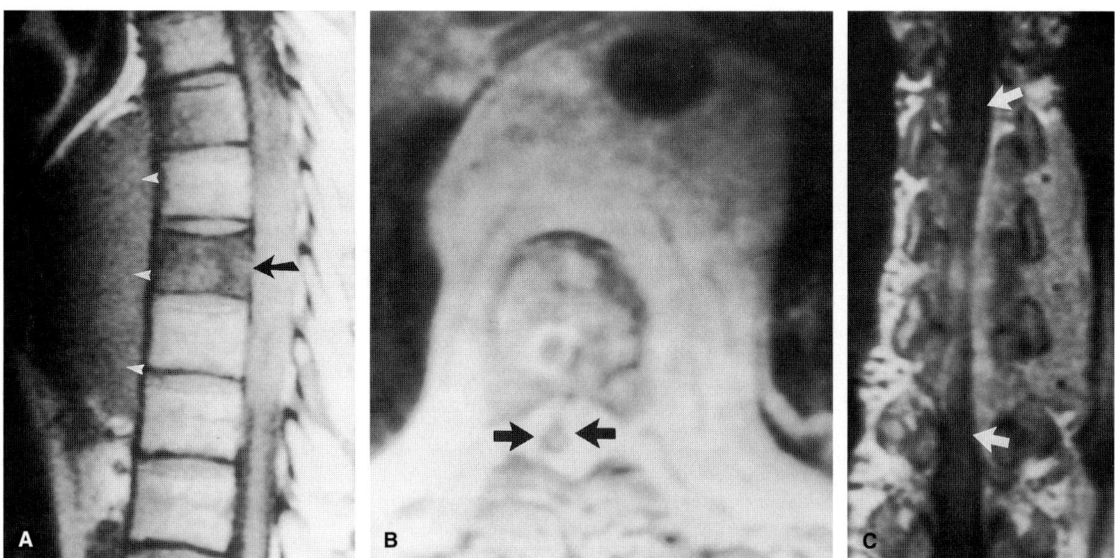

FIGURE 10.46. **Lymphoma. A.** Sagittal T1WI shows a large posterior mediastinal mass (*arrowheads*), with infiltration of a midthoracic vertebral body (*arrow*). **B.** Axial image shows the cord (*arrow*) and the degree of compression. **C.** A coronal image nicely shows the craniocaudal extent of spinal canal compromise (*arrows*). Lymphoma adjacent to the spine is always a threat for cord compression.

can insidiously invade the spinal canal via the neural foramina. Given that CT remains the dominant technique for following lymphoma in the chest and abdomen, subtle intraspinous extension can easily be missed, and any lymphoma patient with back pain should be evaluated by MR (Fig. 10.47).

VASCULAR DISEASES

Spinal Cord Infarction. Vascular diseases of the spine and spinal cord can be divided into cord infarctions and vascular malformations. Spinal "strokes" are quite rare in comparison with cerebrovascular accidents. The classic scenario is a patient who becomes paralyzed after major thoracic surgery, such as repair of a thoracic aortic aneurysm (23). The affected segments of the cord will appear bright on T2WIs and DWIs, with enhancement, similar to a brain infarct, followed by the development of myelomalacia. The spinal gray matter in an infarct will enhance to a greater degree than the white matter, as is the case in the brain (Fig. 10.48) (24). These findings were difficult to assess prior to the advent of MR, when the diagnosis was generally made solely on clinical grounds. Obviously, when a patient in the recovery room after aortic surgery is paraplegic, it does not require great insight to consider a cord infarct. More subtle, however, are cases where atherosclerotic disease or severe degenerative disease leads to thromboembolic cord infarctions, and infarcts must be considered in the differential of unexplained myelopathy.

Spinal AVM. Spinal stroke can also be related to spinal AVMs. These lesions are an area of growing interest for two reasons. First, the development of superselective, interventional neural-angiographic and microsurgical techniques has led to improved understanding and treatment of the lesions. Second, MR has allowed widespread screening of patients with unexplained myelopathy, leading to the discovery of more patients with spinal AVMs.

"Arteriovenous malformation" is used here as a generic term to cover any abnormal vascular complex; this necessarily violates a number of rather complicated spinal AVM classification systems, where true AVMs represent a specific subtype. For a deeper discussion, the excellent article by Rosenblum et al is recommended (25). For a first pass at this topic, it is worth going back to the initial question one should ask about any spinal lesion: Is the location intramedullary, intradural/extramedullary, or extradural? While an oversimplification, this approach provides a good initial analysis of spinal AVMs.

Intramedullary AVMs have a congenital "nidus" of abnormal vessels within the cord substance that causes symptoms by hemorrhage or ischemia because of steal phenomenon. These typically present in young patients with hemorrhage, leading to acute paraparesis. Some are high flow, with visible signal voids within the cord substance (Fig. 10.49). Others escape detection even with angiography and are similar to cavernous vascular malformations in the brain. MR is the primary means for their identification (Fig. 10.50).

Extramedullary AVMs are located in the pia or the dura. When in the dura, they can be as far lateral from the cord

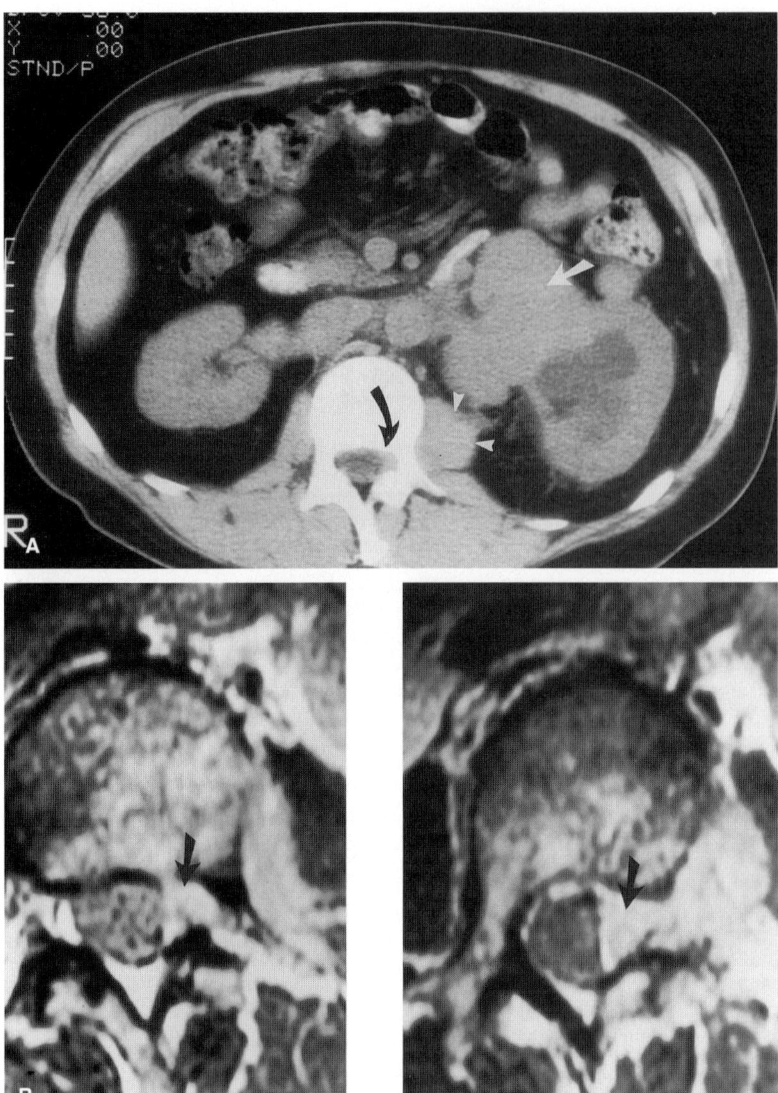

FIGURE 10.47. **Lymphoma Infiltrating the Spinal Canal: Difficulty of CT Visualization. A.** This patient with lymphoma was imaged for new back pain. Left renal involvement is obvious (*white arrow*), and left psoas infiltration is also noted (*arrowhead*). Spinal canal involvement (*curved arrow*), even in retrospect, is equivocal. **B.** The MR images clearly demonstrate involvement of the spinal canal (*arrows*). Any time a patient with paraspinous tumor presents with back pain, MR is the study of choice.

as the nerve root sleeves. The lesion is typically an arteriovenous fistula—a direct connection between an artery and vein without an intervening nidus of congenitally abnormal vasculature (26). The direct arterial inflow into the local venous system through the fistula, undamped by the resistance of a capillary bed, raises pressure within the coronal venous plexus draining the spinal cord, which is valveless (Fig. 10.51). Spinal dural arteriovenous fistulas (SDAVFs) cause symptoms through venous hypertension and congestion of the cord with edema. This edema can be detected on MR as increased signal on T2WIs, typically within an enlarged conus (see Fig. 10.53A), which often enhances. The reason for cord enhancement in SDAVFs is not fully understood, but it probably results from breakdown of the blood-brain barrier because of either chronic infarction or some sort of capillary leak phenomenon secondary to venous hypertension. Regardless of the explanation, enhancement of the cord with SDAVFs is yet another reason why a postcontrast scan should be obtained in any patient with unexplained myelopathy.

The dilated vessels of the coronal venous plexus sometimes can be visualized by MR, but this is quite technique dependent. With older imaging systems, normal CSF flow created tubular flow voids that mimicked vessels, leading to false-positive examinations (Fig. 10.52). Now, various motion-suppression techniques have reduced this problem, and the sensitivity of MR for these small veins has improved (27). In the face of an equivocal MR, an alternate examination, short of spinal angiography, has been supine thoracic high-dose plain film myelography. The dilated veins of the coronal venous plexus appear as serpentine filling defects in the dorsal subarachnoid space on myelography (Fig. 10.53B). An additional advantage of myelography is the potential to identify the primary arterialized vein fed by the fistula, a landmark that can greatly facilitate the angiographer's search for the arterial supply

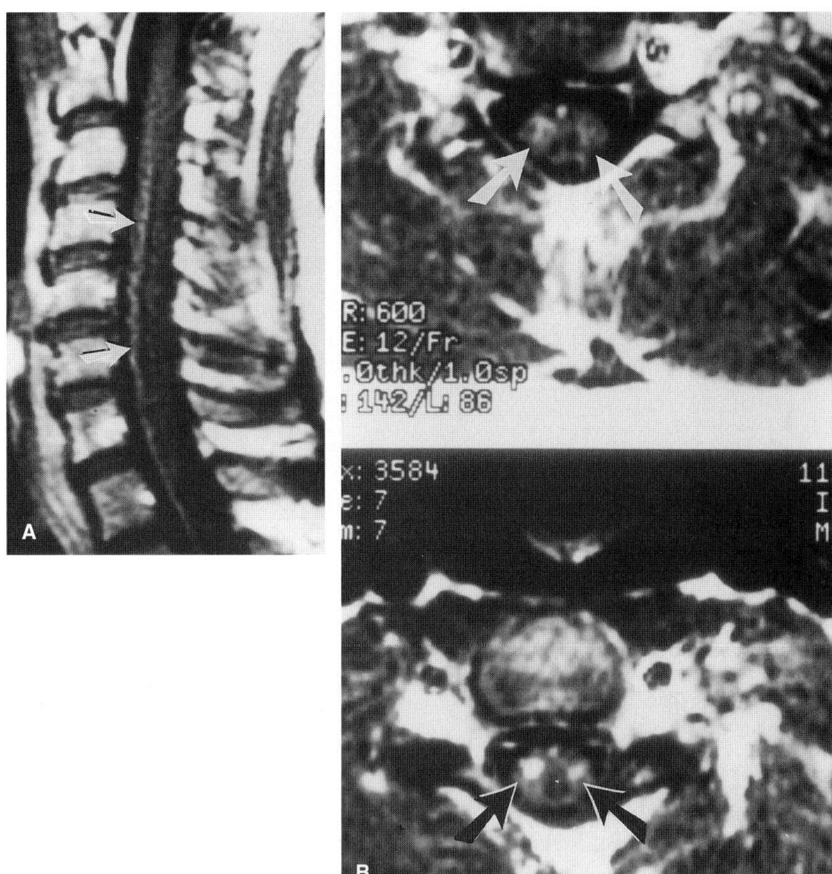

FIGURE 10.48. **Spinal Stroke.** This patient, who presented with acute myelopathy, has increased signal in the cervical cord seen on T2WIs. Postcontrast sagittal **(A)** and **(B)** axial images show enhancement of the central gray matter (*arrows*), a finding highly suggestive of infarct.

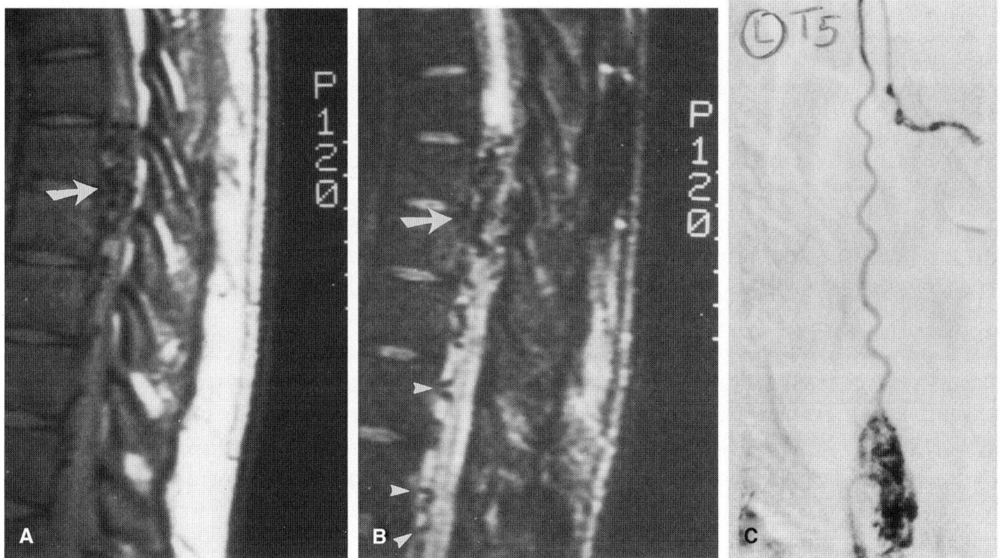

FIGURE 10.49. **Intramedullary Arteriovenous Malformation (AVM).** Sagittal proton density **(A)** and T2W **(B)** images show multiple serpentine signal voids within the midthoracic spinal cord (*arrow*), consistent with an intramedullary AVM. A long draining vessel is also noted in the subarachnoid space (*arrowheads*). **C.** Spinal angiogram injecting the left T5 intercostal artery confirms the MR findings. (Courtesy of Dr Grant Hieshima, University of California, San Francisco.)

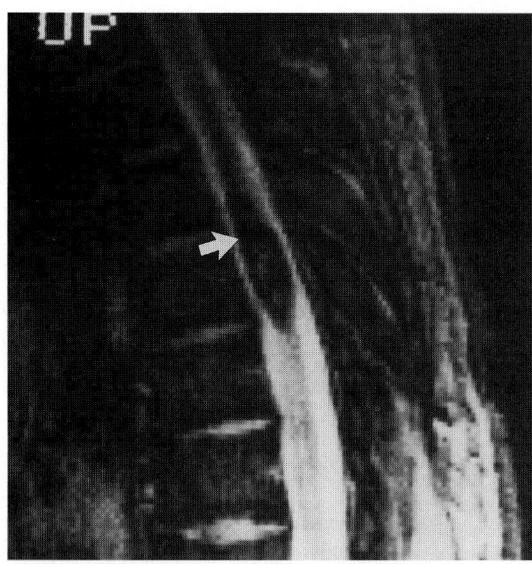

FIGURE 10.50. **Occult Vascular Malformation.** An intramedullary area of decreased signal was present on all sequences but was most prominent on this gradient series (*arrow*). No abnormal vessels were seen on MR or angiography, consistent with an occult vascular malformation, which was confirmed surgically.

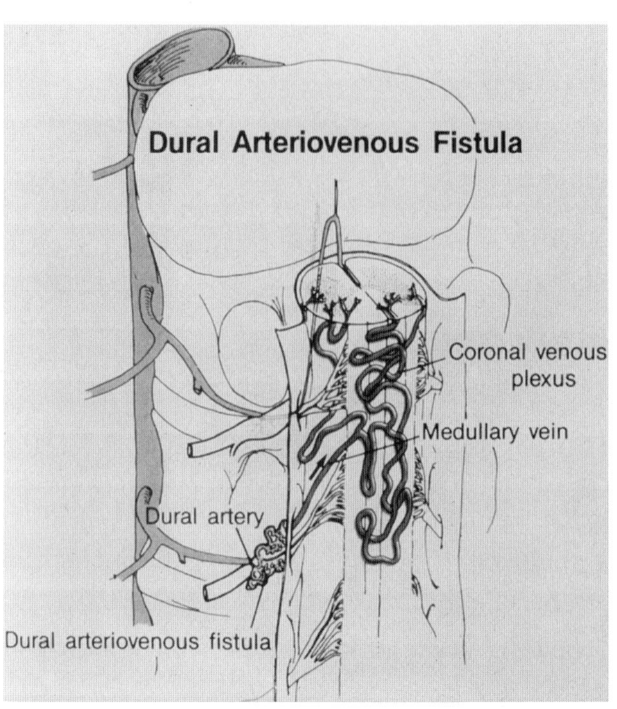

FIGURE 10.51. **Anatomy of a Spinal Dural Arteriovenous Fistula.** The fistula is an abnormal direct connection between an artery and a vein in the dura of the nerve root sleeve. The fistula results in reversal of flow in the draining vein (*arrow*), which in turn feeds the coronal venous plexus with arterial blood under high pressure. The coronal venous plexus dilates, becoming visible to imaging studies, and the cord then has difficulty draining its blood because of this fistula-induced venous hypertension and becomes edematous and bright on T2WIs (see Fig. 10.53). (From Rosenblum B, Oldfield EH, Doppman JL, et al (25), page 796; used with permission.)

to fistula (Fig. 10.53C). Nowadays, focused MR angiography is increasingly successful in depicting dilated spinal veins and even predicting the level of the fistula (28), reducing the iodinated contrast load needed in subsequent catheter angiography.

CONGENITAL MALFORMATIONS

MR has become the primary method for investigation of children born with neural axis defects, whether they involve the brain or the spine. Pediatric brain malformations, along with the combined brain and spine malformation of the Chiari II syndrome, are discussed in detail in Chapter 8 (see Figs. 8.30, 8.31, 8.33). The Chiari I syndrome was mentioned in the discussion of syringohydromyelia (see Fig. 8.32). This section briefly addresses the remaining range of congenital spine problems, emphasizing those that are not immediately apparent at birth and may present in adulthood. A reading of Barkovich is recommended for a more complete discussion of these disorders, which easily are as complex as the remaining topics of this chapter combined (29).

In the spine, neural tube defects that are open or have associated dermal defects are usually detected by prenatal US or at birth. Anomalies of neural tube closure where the covering skin is intact are subtler. They range from asymptomatic nonfusion of the posterior elements (spina bifida occulta) to severe cord tethering with spinal lipomas (Fig. 10.54). A picture is worth a thousand words in understanding the range of presentations of spinal dysraphism, and Fig. 10.55, adapted from Barkovich's text, serves as an introduction to this complex topic (29). It is worth remembering that developmental lesions are the most common cause of pediatric intraspinal masses, and T1WIs are preferred for evaluating fine anatomic detail as well as the fat components that are seen in many of these disorders. The standard pediatric spine examination for congenital anomalies, therefore, includes T1W sagittal and axial images; T2WIs are less critical. If there is a "sacral dimple" or other skin defect, tape a marker (such as a vitamin E capsule) over it to insure that the defect is identifiable on the scan.

Tethered Cord. When the cord is truly tethered, the conus will be low in position, particularly as growth occurs. Before describing the conus as low in position, the clinician must recall that the conus in a newborn is normally at L2 and typically ascends by one to two vertebral segments as the child grows. It can be difficult to determine the exact position of the conus, as the roots of the

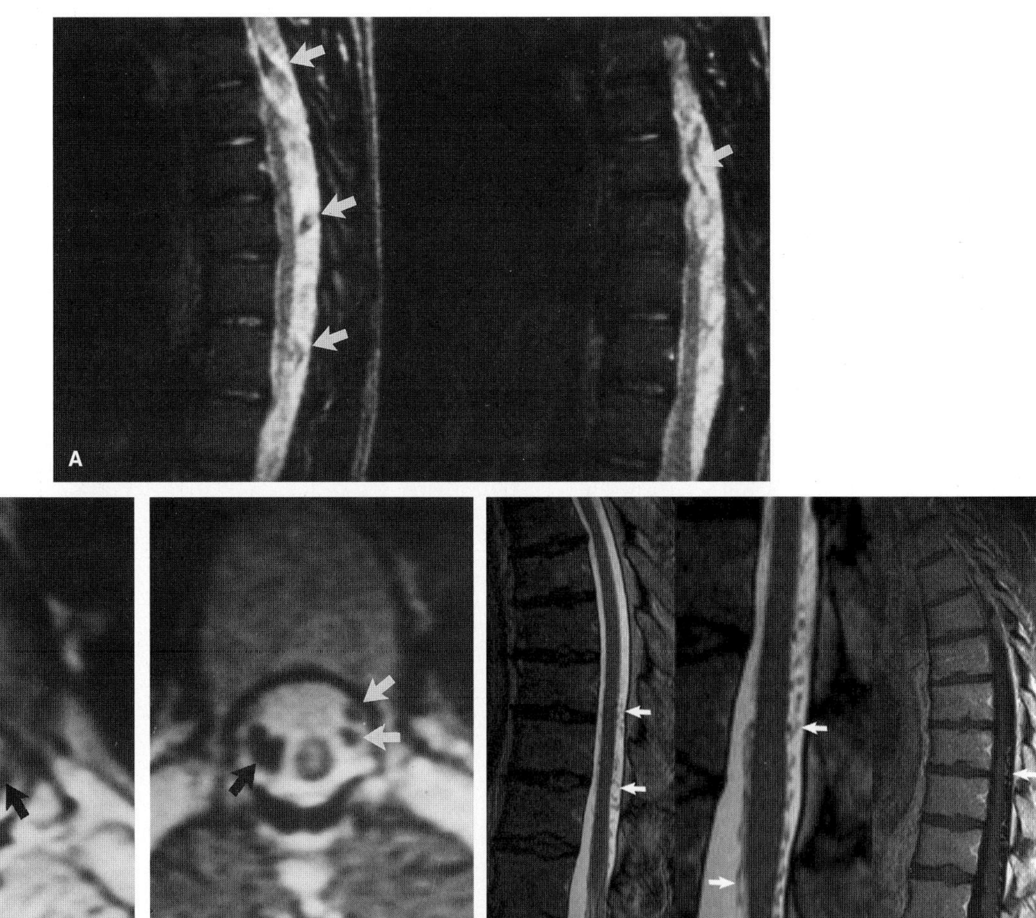

FIGURE 10.52. **False-Positive Versus True-Positive Findings of Dilated Spinal Veins. A.** Sagittal T2WIs show multiple large tubular signal voids in the subarachnoid space (*arrows*), without cord edema. **B.** Axial images show flow voids that are most prominent in the lateral aspects of the spinal canal (*arrows*), areas of maximal velocity of CSF pulsation. All of the signal voids seen here are caused by CSF pulsation rather than abnormal vessels in the subarachnoid space. The scan was repeated with cardiac gating and these "abnormalities" disappeared. **Second Patient: C.** T2W1 sagittal image shows dilated serpentine flow voids arrows in the subarachnoid space. **D.** Detail of an adjacent slice shows abnormal vessels both dorsal and ventral to the spinal cord (*arrows*). **E.** Postgadolinium image shows enhancement of the coronal venous plexus (*arrows*). Note that flow artifacts will not enhance, so contrast helps make this distinction. A spinal dural arteriovenous fistula was found at angiography. (Courtesy of Dr Christopher Dowd, San Francisco, CA.)

cauda equina, when tethered, form a taut mass in the posterior lumbar canal, obscuring the conus/cauda junction (Fig. 10.56). Not every lumbar intradural fatty deposit implies pathologic tethering, and small fibrolipomas of the filum terminale may be noted on MR examinations in patients with normal conus position and no symptoms of cord tethering (Fig. 10.57). A cohort of these patients needs to be followed throughout their lives before such fibrolipomas can be dismissed as incidental, since symptoms of cord tethering occasionally can present well into adulthood.

Intramedullary lipomas can be seen in patients with normal or bifid spinal canals and, as with brain lipomas, may be discovered incidentally. These are usually thoracic, more common in males, and, when symptomatic, present with myelopathy in young adulthood (Fig. 10.58). If any cysts, hemorrhage, or debris are seen in association with the fat, a teratoma should be suspected. Dermoid and epidermoid tumors occur intraspinally, with imaging characteristics similar to their presentations in the brain. Both may be associated with dorsal dermal sinus tracts. "Implantation epidermoid" can occur as rare complication of

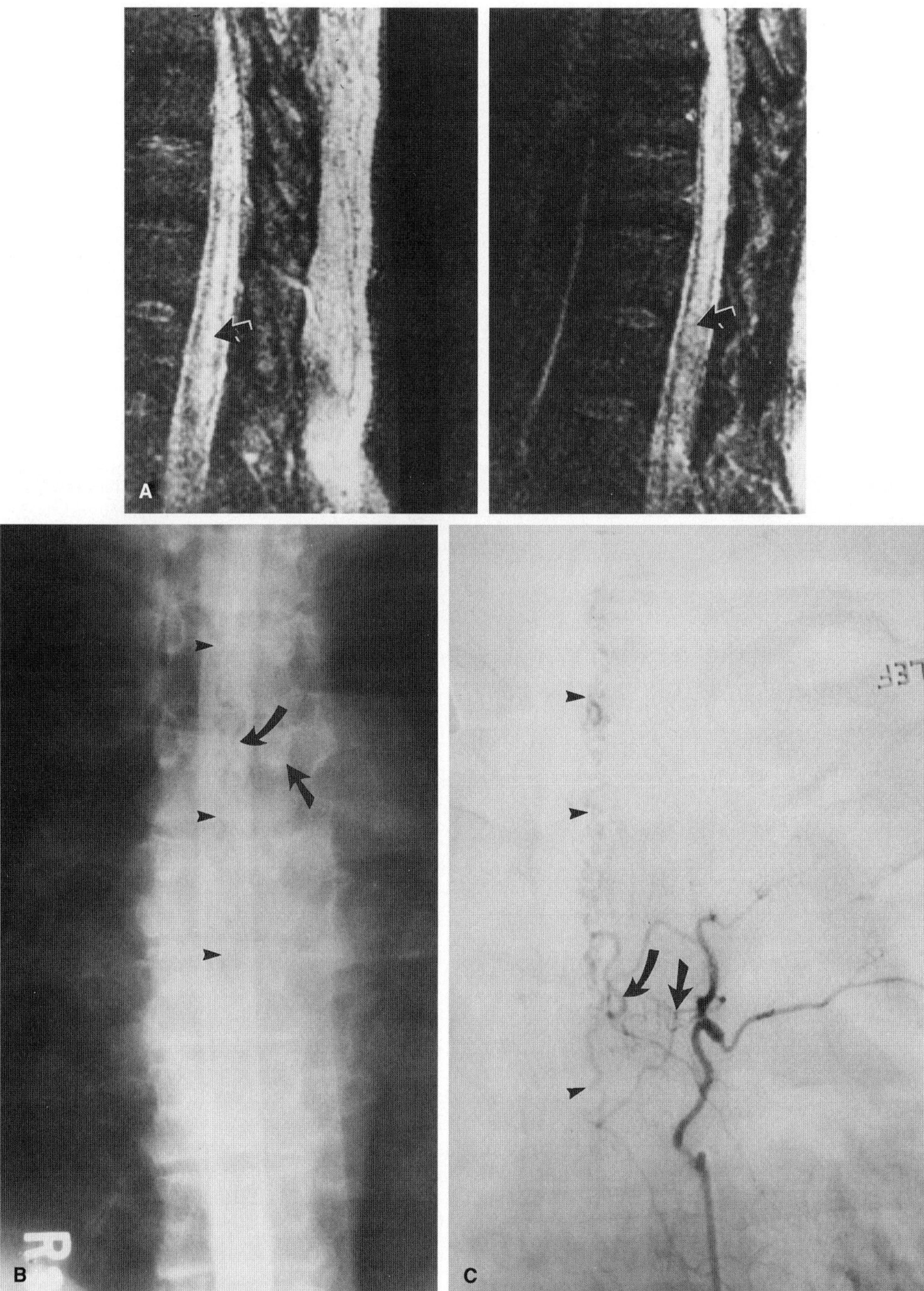

FIGURE 10.53. **Spinal Dural Arteriovenous Fistula. A.** This 45-year-old patient had progressive myelopathy, and this T2W series showed increased signal in the conus (*arrow*), consistent with edema. MR was equivocal for abnormal vessels in the subarachnoid space. **B.** A supine thoracic myelogram demonstrates abnormal vessels causing filling defects in the contrast column posterior to the cord (*arrowheads*). The largest vessel (*curved arrow*) appears to exit the spinal canal just below the left T5 pedicle (*arrow*) and represents the arterialized vein fed by the fistula. The myelogram, therefore, suggests a promising site to begin spinal angiography. **C.** A spinal angiogram demonstrates the dural fistula (*straight arrow*) and the arterialized vein with reversal of flow (*curved arrow*) that has led to dilation of the entire coronal venous plexus (*arrowheads*). Note how the subarachnoid vessels seen on the angiogram and myelogram are superimposable. Compare to the diagram shown in Fig. 10.51.

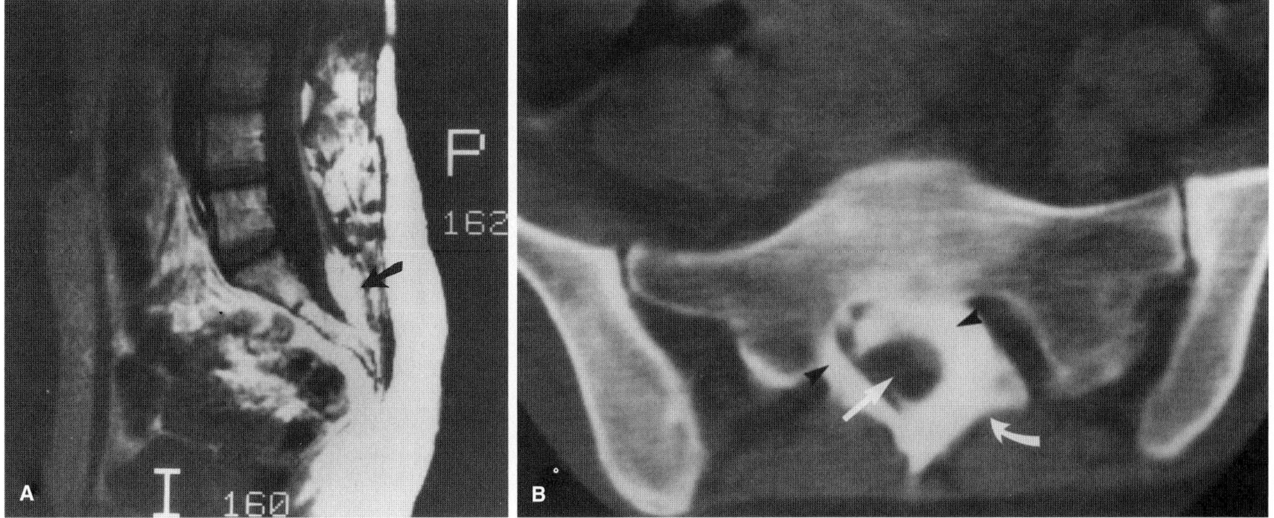

FIGURE 10.54. **Spinal Lipoma. A.** Sagittal T1WI shows a dorsal intraspinal lipoma (*arrow*) at S1. **B.** An axial CT myelogram demonstrates that the distal lipoma (*arrow*) is intrathecal, surrounded by enhanced CSF (*arrowheads*), with an incomplete posterior sacrum (*curved arrow*), consistent with spinal dysraphism. This defect is illustrated schematically in Fig. 10.55A.

lumbar puncture, which is why the needle bevel must be kept in place during a lumbar puncture. Intraspinal teratomas are a distinct entity from sacrococcygeal teratoma, a pediatric lesion with a high malignant potential that is often associated with other anomalies.

Caudal Regression Syndrome. A number of other sacral anomalies have been grouped under the term "caudal regression syndrome," where the distal spine and sacrum may be hypoplastic or absent and the conus has a blunted appearance (Fig. 10.59). Caudal regression is believed to be caused by an insult to the mesoderm during the fourth gestational week, and associated cardiac and renal anomalies are common. There is a high association with maternal diabetes. However, subtle forms, such as partial sacral agenesis, may not be discovered until adulthood. The distal spine is also the site of a number of CSF-filled, arachnoid-lined cystic lesions with associated bony deformity, ranging from small perineural (Tarlov) cysts (Fig. 10.60) to huge anterior sacral meningoceles. The latter is distinct from a posterior meningocele, which, like a myelomeningocele, results from failure of neural tube closure rather than leptomeningeal diverticulation.

Arachnoid cysts in the spine present as masses that are relatively isointense to CSF (Fig. 10.61). As in the brain, the primary differential diagnostic consideration is an epidermoid. Also as in the brain, spinal epidermoids are easily differentiated from arachnoid cysts: they show reduced diffusion and thus are bright on DWIs.

Scoliosis. Many unsuspected spinal abnormalities present as curvature of the spine, or *scoliosis*. Most adolescents with curvature of the spine have idiopathic scoliosis, but when the onset is earlier or more severe, or plain scoliosis films show a vertebral anomaly (Fig. 10.62), MR is indicated to rule out an intraspinal abnormality. These cases are collectively known as "congenital scoliosis," and the primary cause, such as cord tethering, must be addressed before the spine undergoes mechanical straightening. Diastematomyelia is one of the most dramatic disorders in this category (Fig. 10.63). The spinal cord is "split" into two hemicords by a sagittal bony or cartilaginous spur. Each hemicord has a dorsal and ventral horn and a central canal. Most occur in the lower thoracic region and are accompanied by vertebral segmentation abnormalities. Syrinx develops in 50% of cases. "Split notochord syndrome" is the cause, and there is a spectrum of severity, ranging from a single dural tube with a fibrous band, to two separate bony canals.

TRAUMA

In the acute trauma patient, the spine must be evaluated immediately to rule out fractures. Unstable fractures can compromise the diameter of the spinal canal, leading to cord compression and paralysis. Plain films, therefore, have been the study of choice in the emergency department, because they can be obtained quickly and inexpensively without significant interruption of other resuscitation efforts. Recent data show that plain films are perfectly adequate in low-risk cases (30). After severe trauma, a modern helical CT of the cervical spine takes just a few extra seconds beyond the mandatory head CT. Subtle lesions, such as fractures of the foramen transversaria (which houses the vertebral artery), can be missed

(*text continues on p. 317*)

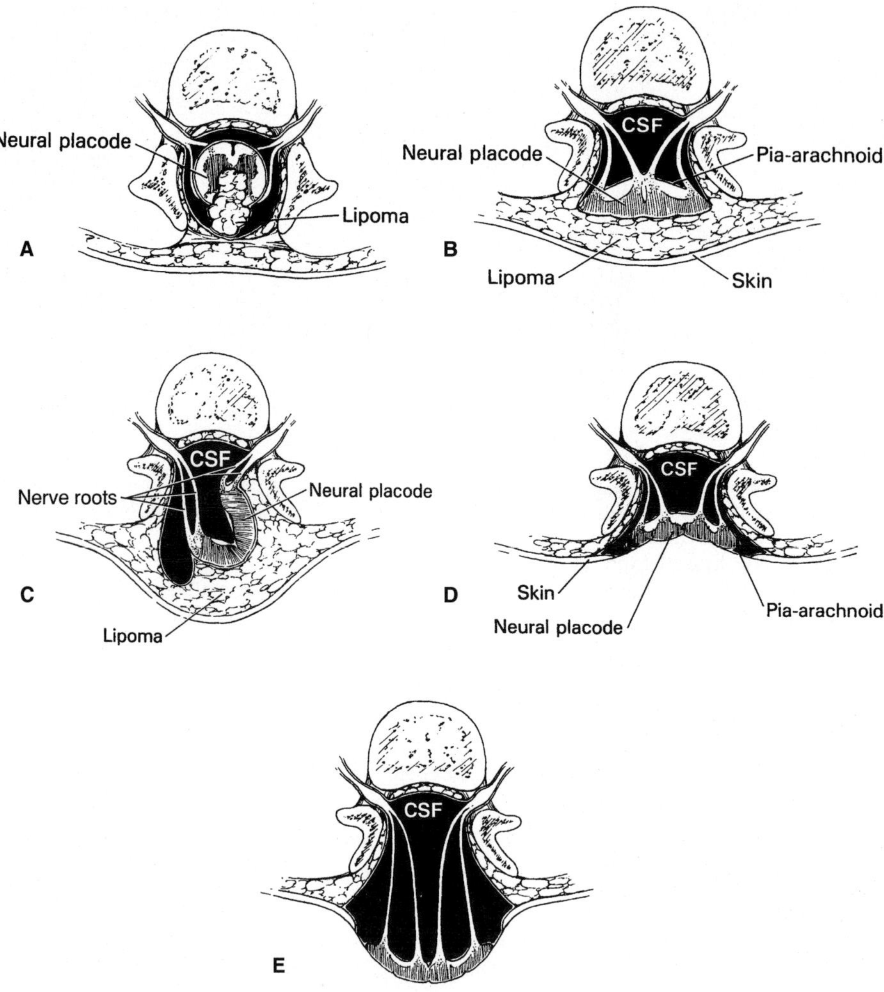

FIGURE 10.55. **Spinal Dysraphism.** This series of drawings from Barkovich's text (29) nicely illustrates the range of appearances of spinal dysraphism. In all of these conditions, there has been failure of the lips of the neural folds to close in the midline dorsally, forming a tube. The incompletely fused plaque of neural tissue is referred to as the neural "placode." When the placode is covered by intact skin and subcutaneous fat, without dorsal herniation of neural tissue, the defect **(A** and **B)** may be overlooked in examination of the newborn, giving rise to the term "occult spinal dysraphism." **A.** Spinal lipoma. The dorsal spinal cord has failed to close, with an intradural lipoma situated between the lips of the unfused placode. MR and CT appearances of this defect are shown in Fig. 10.54. **B.** Lipomyelocele. The dorsal dura is incomplete. The subarachnoid space lies ventral to the placode, which is covered by pia and arachnoid on its internal surface. The subcutaneous fat is contiguous with a lipoma, which is adherent to the dorsal surface of the placode. **C.** Lipomyelomeningocele. This is similar to the lipomyelocele **(B),** except there the subarachnoid space is dilated, causing the placode to bulge posteriorly. In this drawing, the lipoma is asymmetric and extends into the canal on the left, rotating the placode and causing discrepancy in the length of the nerve roots, which complicates surgical repair. Lipomyelomeningoceles are seen in conjunction with rostral craniospinal abnormalities in the Chiari II malformation, illustrated in Figs. 8.31 and 8.33. **D.** Myelocele. The neural placode is contiguous with the skin and will be obvious on newborn examination. The ventral aspect of the placode has the same anatomy as the lipomyelocele. **E.** Meningomyelocele. The ventral subarachnoid space is dilated, displacing the placode posteriorly (as in lipomyelomeningocele). Otherwise, the defect is identical to a myelocele. (From Barkovich AJ [29], pages 709–724; used with permission.)

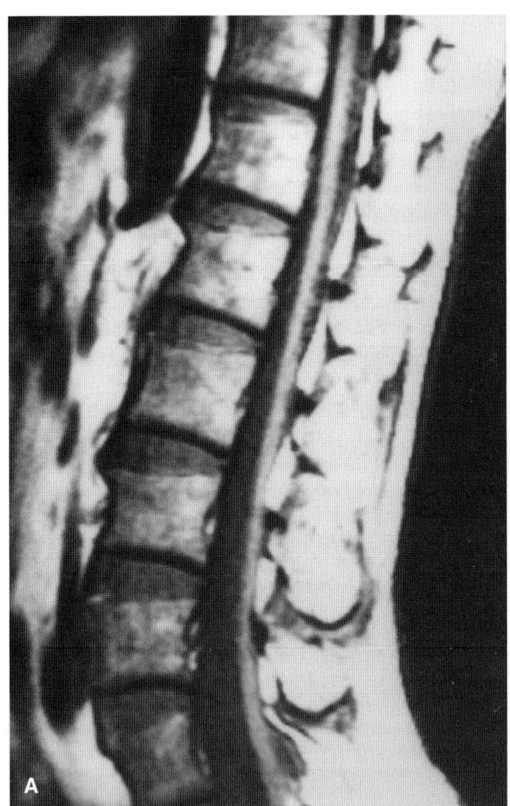

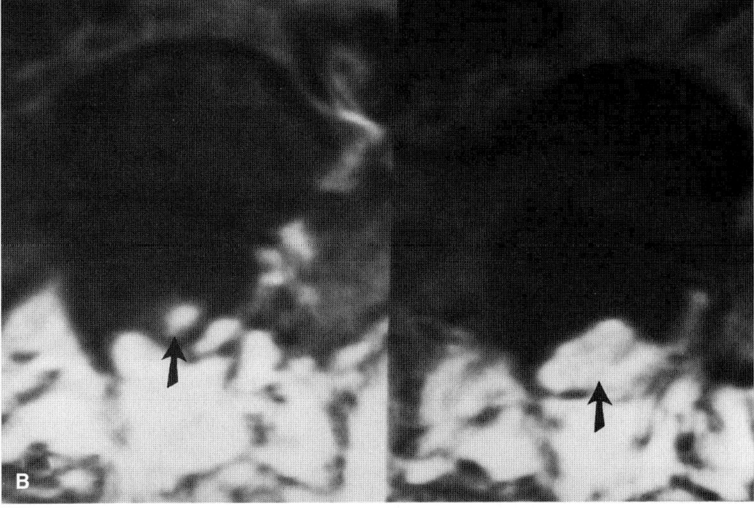

FIGURE 10.56. **Adult Cord Tethering.** This young adult presented with a gait disorder. **A.** It is difficult to be certain of the position of the conus in sagittal images because of the clumping of the roots posteriorly, but it is definitely very low. **B.** Axial T1WIs demonstrate spinal dysraphism with a lipoma (*arrows*), consistent with cord tethering.

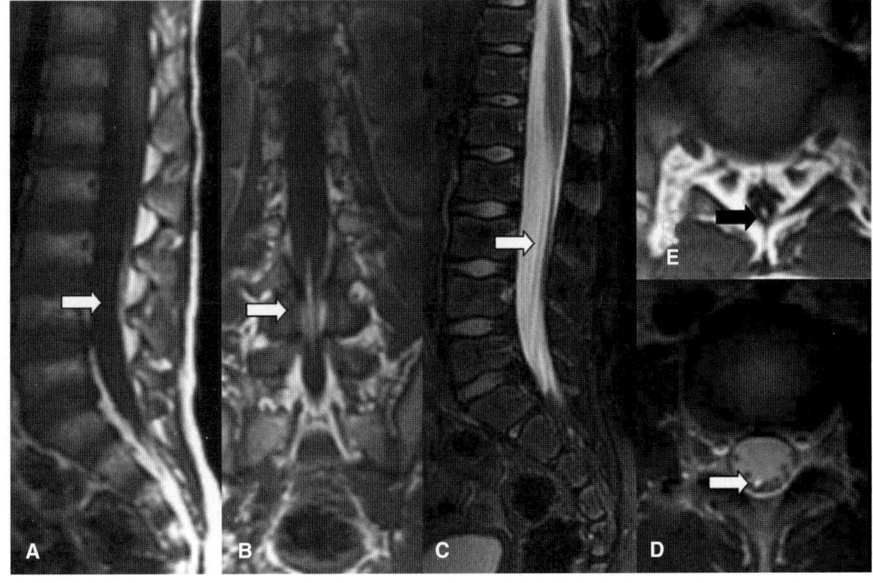

FIGURE 10.57. **Fibrolipoma of the Filum Terminale. A.** and **B.** Sagittal and coronal T1WIs show that the conus is normal in position, with the filum terminale showing high signal consistent with fat (*arrows*). **C.** Sagittal T2WI shows low signal, confirming fat; a T1WI with fat saturation could be used in the same way (*arrow*). **D.** and **E.** Axial T1WI and T2WI confirm the intrathecal position of the thickened fatty filum (*arrows*).

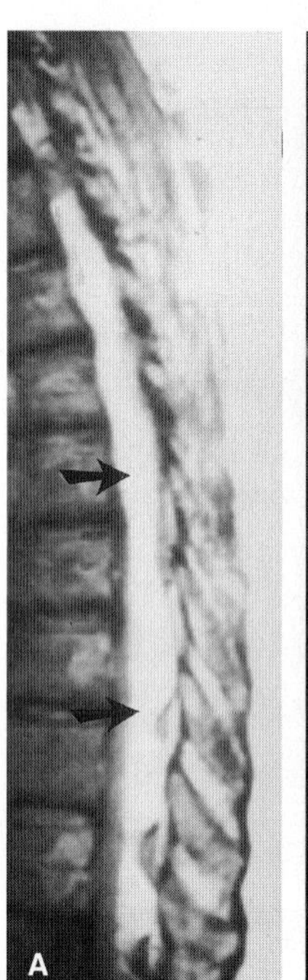

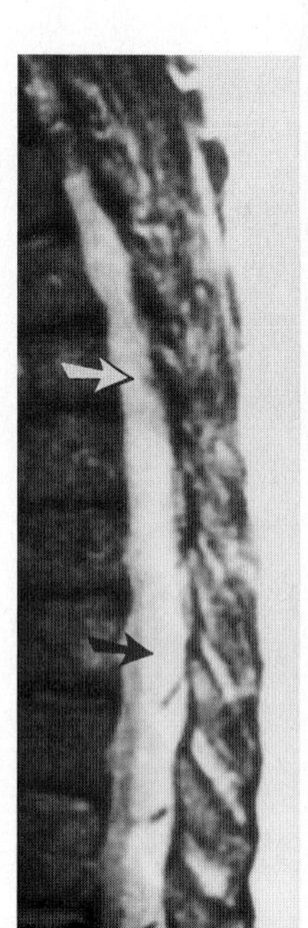

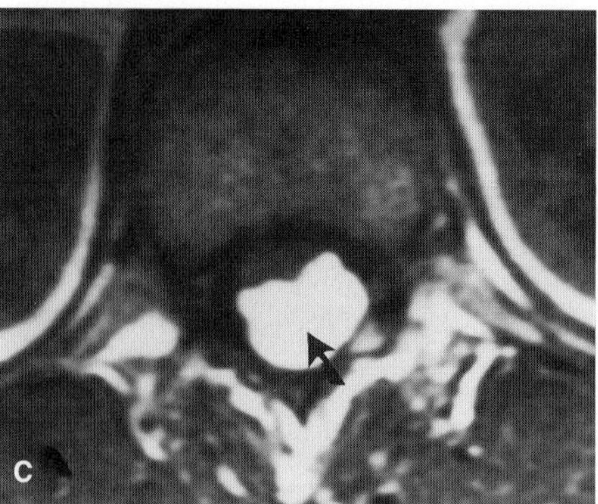

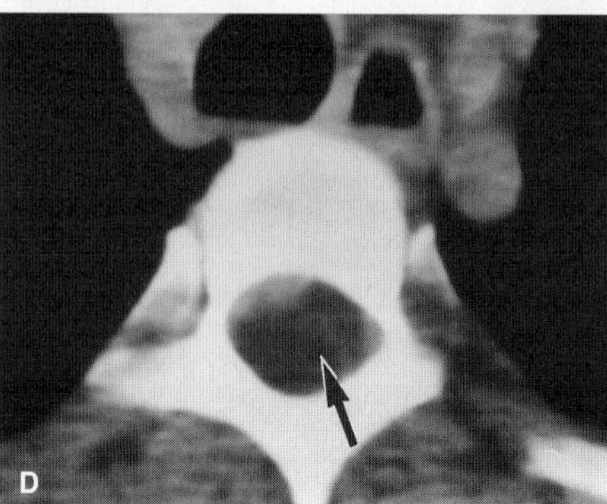

FIGURE 10.58. **Intrathecal Lipoma Noted Incidentally After Trauma. A.** Sagittal T1WI shows a high-signal intraspinal mass (*arrows*), which appears to be intramedullary. Possible diagnoses include lipoma and hemorrhage in the methemoglobin state. A fat-saturated T1WI would be ideal for making this distinction. **B.** T2WI shows relative signal drop-off within the mass (*arrows*), which would be more consistent with fat than methemoglobin. **C.** Axial T1WI shows the lipoma (*arrow*) is central within the canal and is probably intramedullary. **D.** The CT demonstrates a low-attenuation mass, confirming a lipoma (*arrow*).

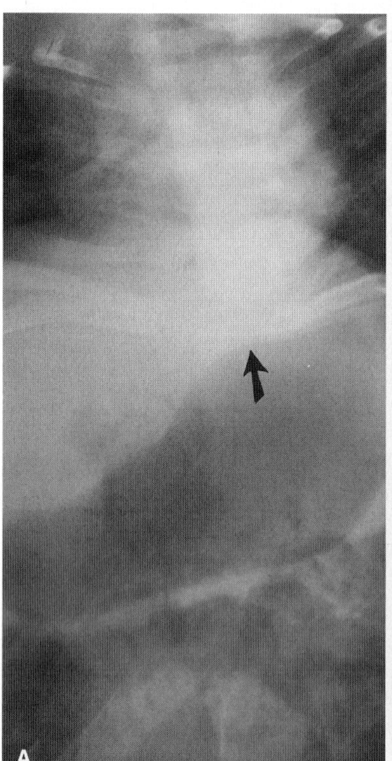

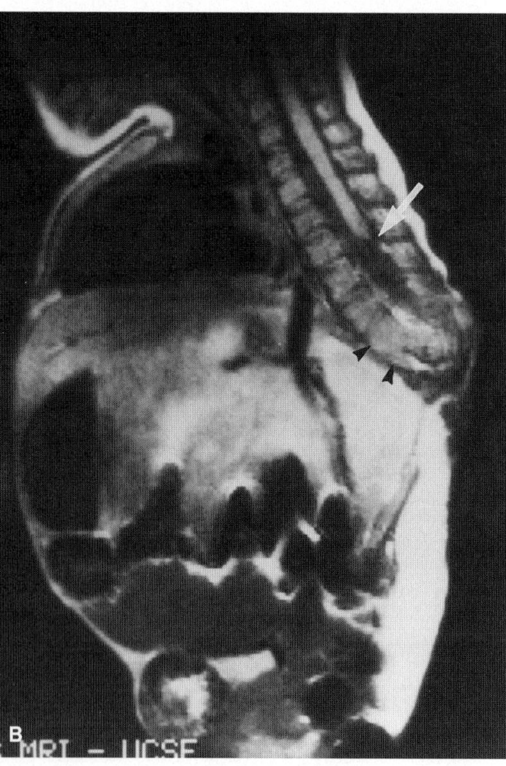

FIGURE 10.59. **Severe Caudal Regression Syndrome. A.** Plain film of the abdomen shows absence of the spinal column below T8 (*arrow*). **B.** Sagittal T1WI shows a characteristic blunted appearance of the distal cord (*arrow*) and fusion of the caudal vertebrae (*arrowheads*), the lowest of which is dysplastic. (From Barkovich AJ [29], page 242; used with permission.)

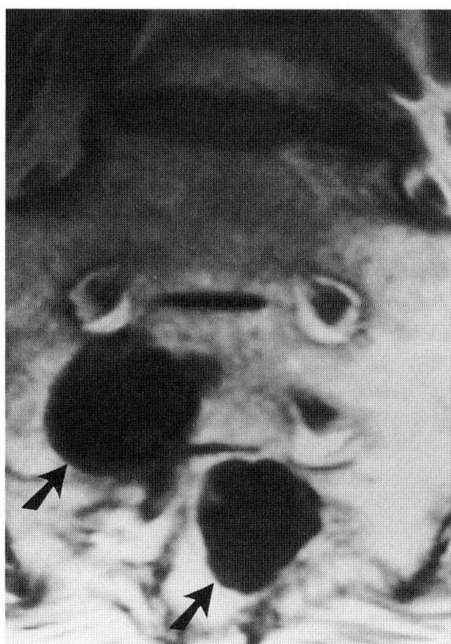

FIGURE 10.60. **Sacral Cysts.** Leptomeningeal-lined sacral cysts have been classified many different ways. The spectrum includes intrasacral meningoceles, anterior sacral meningoceles, and perineural (Tarlov) cysts (*arrows*), shown here in this T1WI through the sacrum. These are often asymptomatic, but they can result in radicular compression.

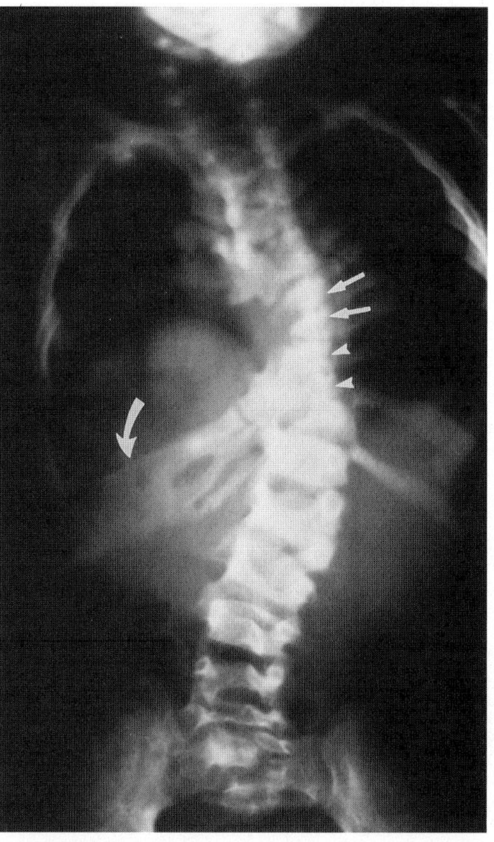

FIGURE 10.62. **Congenital Scoliosis.** This plain film shows hemivertebrae (*arrows*), block vertebrae (*arrowheads*), and fused ribs (*curved arrow*), leaving no doubt that this is congenital rather than idiopathic scoliosis. An MR would be valuable to evaluate the spinal cord for position and possible mass effect.

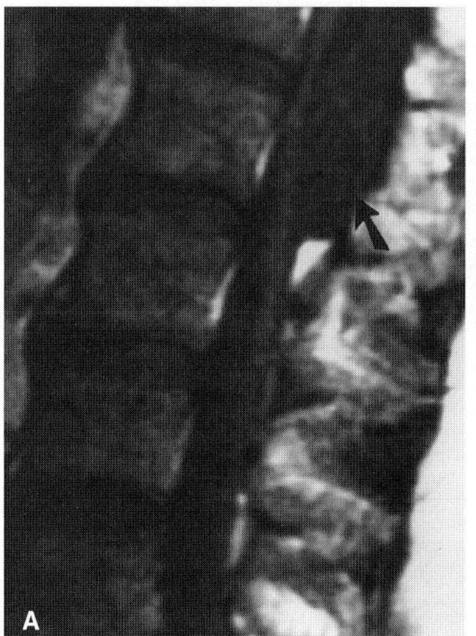

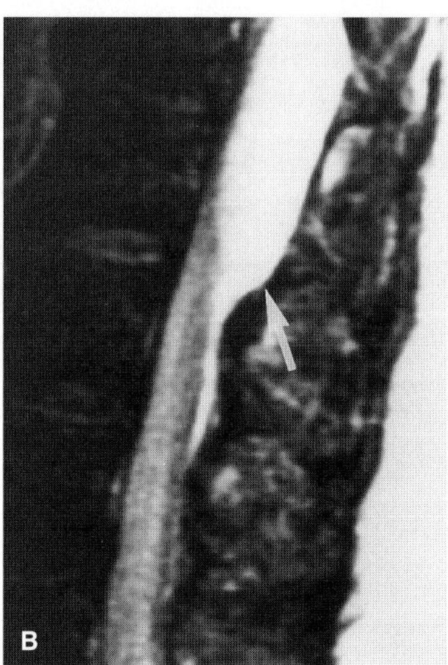

FIGURE 10.61. **Arachnoid Cyst. A.** Sagittal T1WI shows a mass isointense to CSF (*arrow*) posterior to the proximal cauda equina, displacing it forward. **B.** This mass becomes brighter than the remainder of the CSF on the T2WI (*arrow*). This proved to be an arachnoid cyst. These can be congenital or related to prior inflammation or injury. Epidermoid is the main differential consideration.

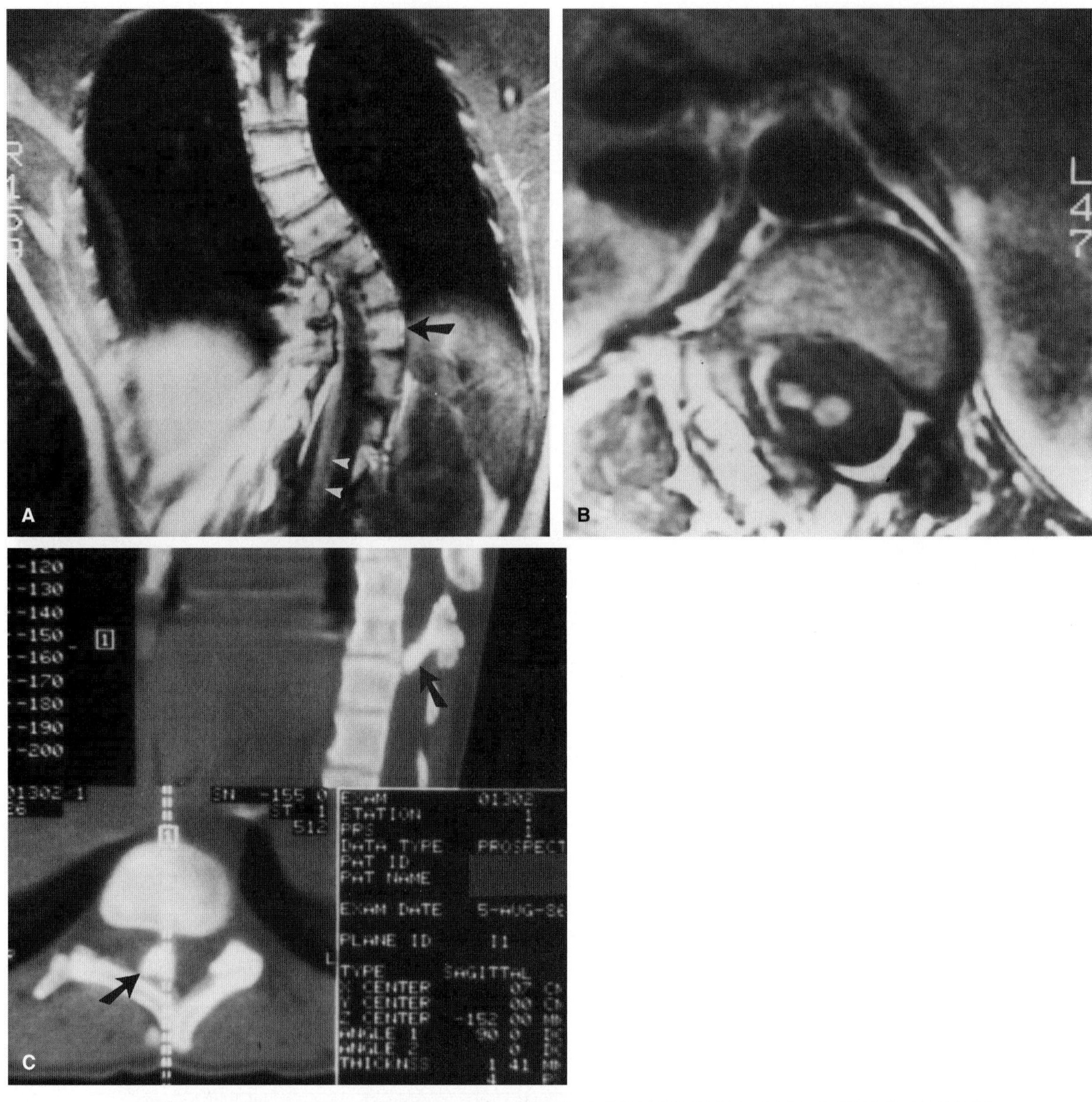

FIGURE 10.63. **Diastematomyelia.** This 15-year-old patient with progressive scoliosis, despite bracing, was a candidate for surgery. Plain films had been unrevealing. **A.** Coronal MR shows the levoscoliosis with its apex (*arrow*) near the thoracolumbar junction. Distal to this apex, the cord appears to be separated into two distinct parallel portions (*arrowheads*). **B.** Axial image confirms a split cord, or diastematomyelia. MR is not good at assessing bony content of the midline fibrocartilaginous spur. **C.** CT scan and sagittal reconstruction on a similar patient confirm a dense, bony midline spur (*arrows*). This spur was also visible on plain film.

on plain films. When complex spine fractures are seen on plain films, CT studies are very helpful to define the relationship of the bone fragments. Spine fractures and their evaluation are critical topics for radiology residents and others responsible for emergency radiology to master (see Chapter 43).

Some discussion, however, is needed concerning the immediate and delayed consequences of vertebral trauma to the spinal cord and spinal nerves, which cannot properly be evaluated on plain films or with noncontrast CT. These include cord contusion, epidural hematoma (and their sequelae, such as myelomalacia and syringohydromyelia), and nerve root avulsion (30–33).

Cord Contusion. The spinal cord, like the brain, lies suspended in a bath of CSF, contained by arachnoid membranes, dura, and bone. The cord, again like the brain, is subject to significant impact against its surrounding bony suit of armor during abrupt acceleration and deceleration. In the brain, contusions appear at the site of a blow and 180° opposite, in the classic coup–contrecoup pattern. Certain bony sites, such as the planum sphenoidale, tend to traumatize adjacent brain because of their irregular contour. In the spine, contusions usually occur at sites of fractures, secondary to bony impingement and cord compression (Fig. 10.64). However, spinal cord contusions may occur in the absence of spinal fractures following hyperflexion or hyperextension, resulting in myelopathy (Fig. 10.65). The anterior and posterior spinal ligaments must be examined carefully for edema, representing either partial or complete tears, with risk of future instability.

The presence of spinal cord edema, and particularly cord hemorrhage, has been established as a poor prognostic factor in spinal cord injury patients evaluated by MR. Therefore, T2* or gradient-echo images are a critical portion of any MR protocol for spine trauma. Certain types of injury, such as sudden distraction forces along the long axis of the spine, can lead to cord avulsion (Fig. 10.66).

If the spinal cord is injured, myelomalacia results and further changes can occur because of CSF flow patterns. An area of myelomalacia can enlarge with CSF entry, particularly if the adhesions disturb CSF flow, and evolve into a posttraumatic syrinx. The expanding syrinx can cause further neurologic deficit and require shunting.

Epidural Hematoma. As in the head, extra-axial or, more appropriately, "extramedullary" hematomas can follow trauma, with certain important distinctions. Subdural hematomas are rare in the spine (and usually related to coagulopathies (Fig. 10.67), while epidural hematomas are far more common. The reverse is true in the calvaria, as discussed in Chapter 3.

This distinction can be explained by differences in venous anatomy between the skull and the spine, as the majority of posttraumatic bleeding is venous. In the bony calvaria, the dura is functionally the periosteum, with no potential space between the dura and bone for low-pressure venous blood to accumulate. It takes bleeding under arterial pressure to create an epidural hematoma by stripping the dura away from the inner table. In the spine, the dura is separated from the bone by epidural fat. In the ventral spinal canal, the epidural space also contains a rich plexus of veins that drains the vertebral bodies. Trauma, with or without vertebral fracture, can tear these veins, resulting in an epidural hematoma. These hematomas grow with time, leading to cord compression in the setting of normal plain films. CT may detect these epidural hematomas in the lumbar spine, where there is some fat to provide contrast, but generally will not demonstrate an epidural hematoma in the cervical or thoracic spine unless intrathecal contrast is given. MR is the study of choice, given its ability to image the contents of the spinal canal noninvasively and depict the products of blood breakdown (Fig. 10.68).

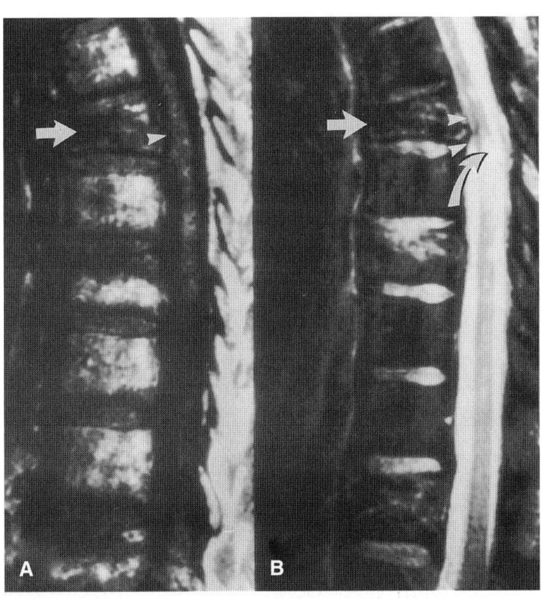

FIGURE 10.64. **Spinal Contusion. A.** Compression fracture (*arrow*) with narrowing of the spinal canal (*arrowheads*) caused by retropulsed bony fragments. **B.** Intramedullary edema (*curved arrow*), seen on this T2WI, is a poor prognostic factor in this setting. The presence of a hematoma is associated with an even poorer outcome. Fortunately, none is evident.

Nerve Root Avulsion. Most of these traumatic complications have been discussed in terms of their effects on the spinal cord. It should be remembered that epidural hematomas and contusions can also affect nerve roots and result in radicular complaints. An additional form of direct trauma to the spinal nerve roots is avulsion from their connection to the cord. In the spinal canal, the most common site for root avulsion is the cervical spine, probably because of its wide range of motion during accidents. The roots serving the brachial plexus and upper extremities are typically affected, with obvious neurologic deficits. Birth trauma, typically traction on the shoulder, is one of the classic causes of nerve root avulsion at the cervicothoracic

(*text continues on p. 320*)

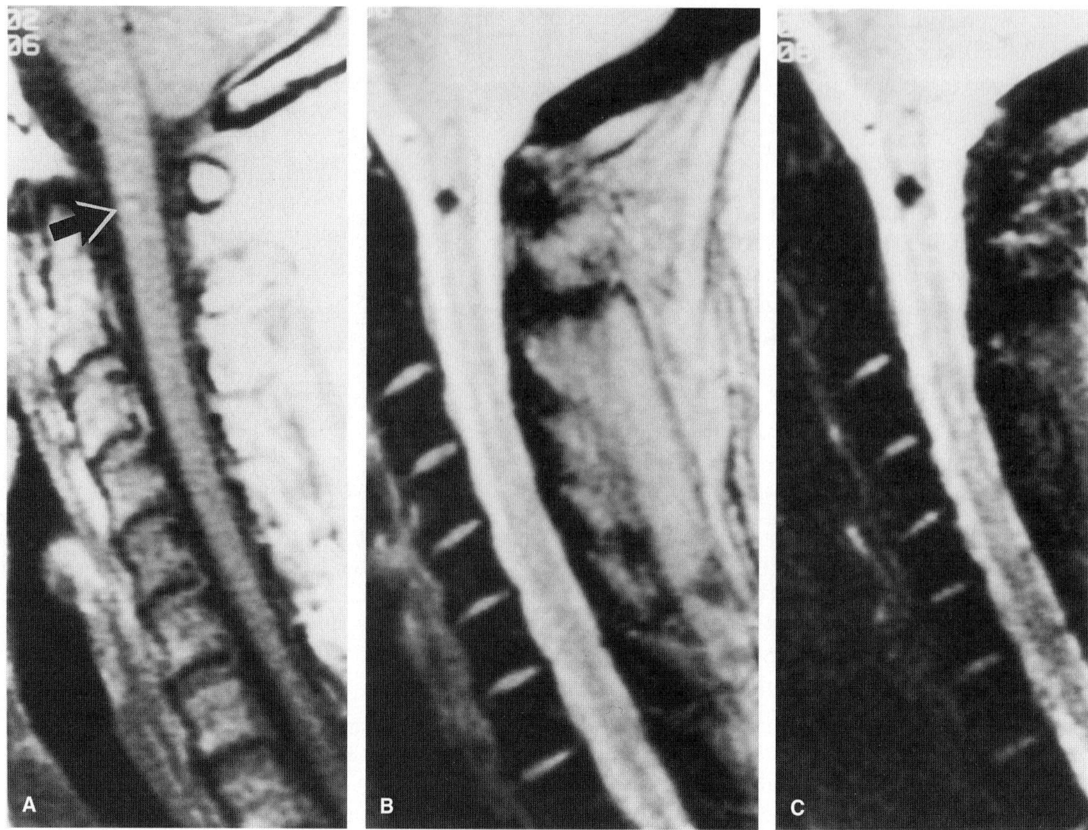

FIGURE 10.65. **Cord Hematoma. A.** Sagittal T1WI shows a tiny focus of methemoglobin with a dark rim (*arrow*) in the cord posterior to the dens. The dark rim "blooms" on the first **(B)** and second **(C)** echoes of the gradient refocused sequence, consistent with hemosiderin.

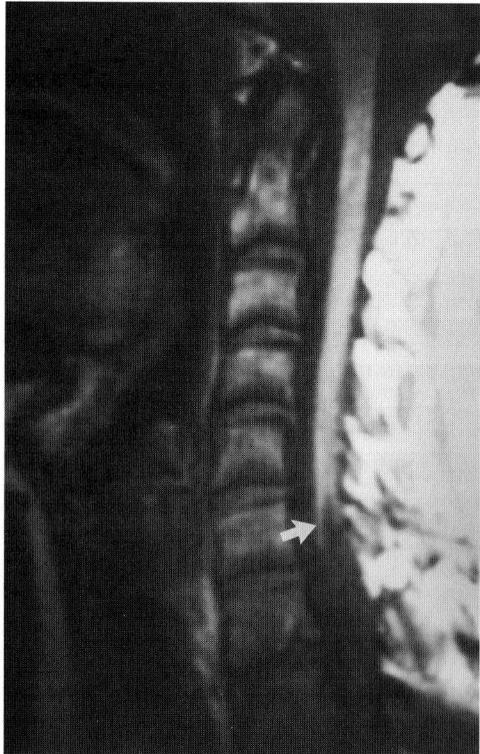

FIGURE 10.66. **Cord Avulsion.** The junction of the cervical and thoracic cord is a weak point where tearing can occur in injuries that stretch the cord (*arrow*).

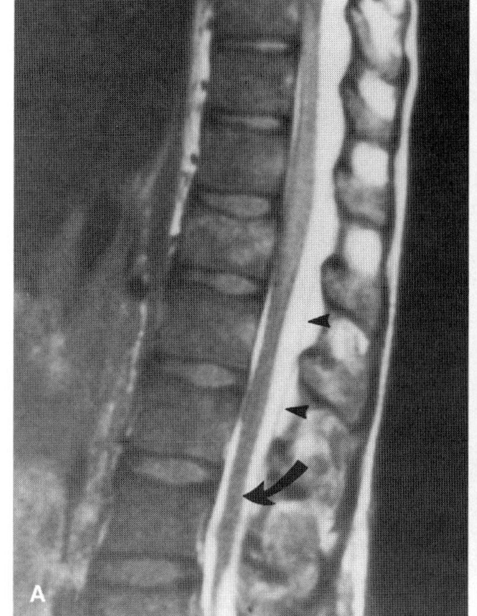

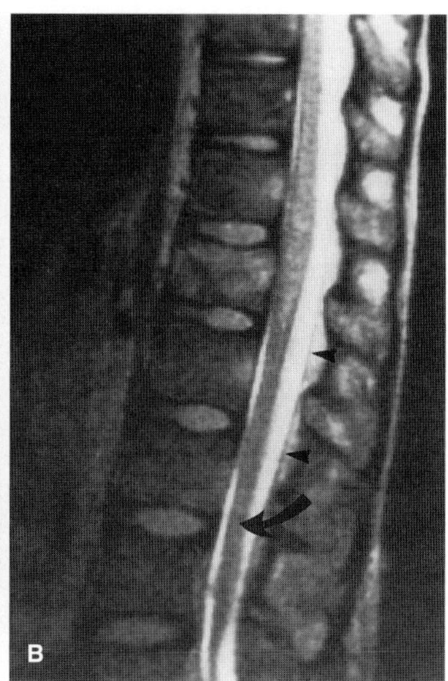

FIGURE 10.67. **Spinal Hematoma.** A spinal subdural hematoma (*arrows*) occurred spontaneously in this thrombocytopenic leukemia patient. Note the low marrow signal, which is consistent with leukemia, and the constriction of the thecal sac (*curved arrow*) by the hematoma. The hematoma is difficult to distinguish from epidural fat (*arrowheads*) on the T1WI **(A)** but becomes more obvious as the epidural fat darkens on the T2WI **(B)**.

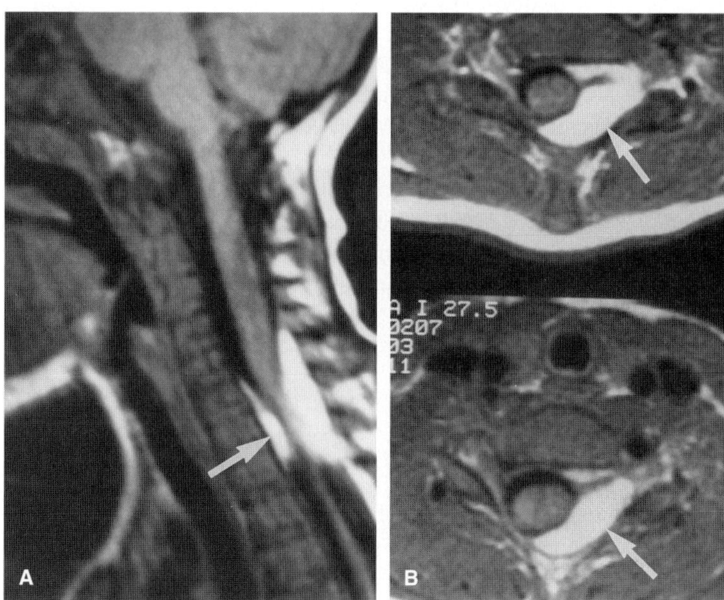

FIGURE 10.68. **Epidural Hematoma.** T1 sagittal **(A)** and axial **(B)** images show a bright epidural mass (*arrows*) consistent with a hematoma in the methemoglobin stage. An epidural hematoma can occur in the face of normal plain films and must be suspected if there is neurologic compromise.

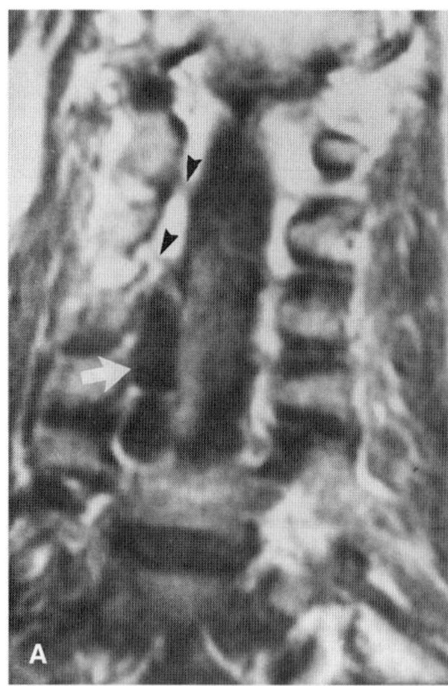

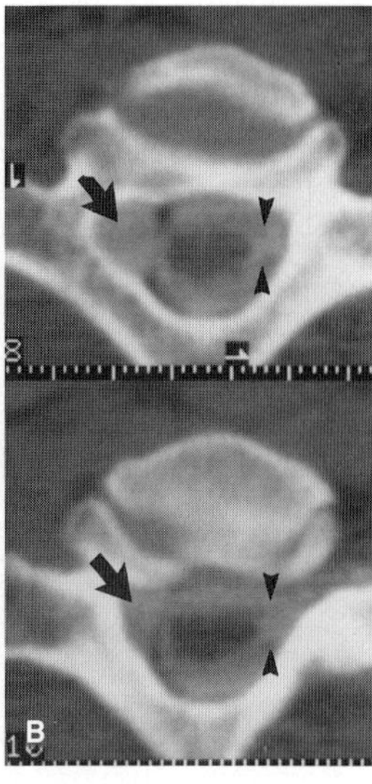

FIGURE 10.69. **Nerve Root Avulsion. A.** Coronal T1 image shows a low signal collection in the right epidural space in the midcervical spine (*arrow*), consistent with CSF that has leaked through avulsed nerve root sleeves. Intact spinal nerves (*arrowheads*) are seen in the upper cervical canal bilaterally, traversing through the normal epidural fat. **B.** CT myelograms confirm the absence of the right-sided nerve roots and the CSF leak (*arrow*). Note the normal roots on the left outlined by myelographic contrast (*arrowheads*).

junction. This can result in an Erb palsy on the affected side—the shoulder will be adducted and internally rotated, the elbow extended and pronated, and the wrist flexed, all because of injury to the C5, C6, and C7 roots. The clinical diagnosis can be confirmed by MR or CT myelography. Typically, CSF will leak out into the epidural space through the rent in the arachnoid and dura from the missing nerve, as can be seen in Fig. 10.69. The thoracic spinal nerves (other than T1) and nerves of the lumbar cauda equina rarely undergo avulsion. Given the small field of view needed, thin (1 to 2 mm), highly T2W axial images give excellent detail and can be reconstructed into "MR myelograms," much like MR angiograms.

While MR is often not practical in the acute setting, it has become a superb noninvasive tool for evaluating the neurologic complications of trauma. MR has increased our understanding of spinal cord injury and facilitates prediction of long-term outcome.

REFERENCES

1. Atlas S, ed. Magnetic Resonance Imaging of the Brain and Spine. 3rd ed. Philadelphia: Lippincott Williams & Wilkins, 2002.
2. Enzmann DR, DeLaPaz RL, Rubin JB, eds. Magnetic Resonance of the Spine. St. Louis: Mosby, 1990.
3. Ramsay RG. Teaching Atlas of Spine Imaging. New York: Thieme, 1999.
4. Modic MT, Masaryk TM, Ross JS. Magnetic Resonance Imaging of the Spine. St. Louis: Mosby, 1994.
5. Ross JS, Brant-Zawadski M, Moore KR, et al. Diagnostic Imaging: Spine. Salt Lake City: AMIRSYS, 2004.
6. Tartaglino LM, Friedman DP, Flanders AE. Multiple sclerosis in the spinal cord: MR appearance and correlation with clinical parameters. Radiology 1995;195:725–732.
7. Reijnierse M, Dijkmans BA, Hansen B, et al. Neurologic dysfunction in patients with rheumatoid arthritis of the cervical spine. Predictive value of clinical, radiographic and MR imaging parameters. Eur Radiol 2001;11:467–473.
8. Provenzale JM, Barboriak DP, Gaensler EHL, et al. Lupus-related myelitis: Serial MR findings. AJNR Am J Neuroradiol 1994;15:1911–1917.
9. Byun WM, Park WK, Park BH, et al. Guillain-Barré syndrome: MR imaging findings of the spine in eight patients. Radiology 1998;208:137–141.
10. Ross JS. Magnetic resonance imaging of the postoperative spine. Semin Musculoskelet Radiol 2000;4:281–291.
11. Quencer RM, Post MJD. Spinal cord lesions in patients with AIDS. Neuroimaging Clin North Am 1997;7:359–373.
12. Wang PY, Shen WC, Jan JS. Serial MRI changes in radiation myelopathy. Neuroradiology 1995;37:374–377.
13. Ledermann HP, Schweitzer ME, Morrison WB, et al. MR imaging findings in spinal infections: rules or myths? Radiology 2003;228:506–514.
14. Post MJD, Sze G, Quencer RM, et al. Gadolinium-enhanced MR in spinal infection. J Comput Assist Tomogr 1990;14:721–729.
15. Smith AS, Weinstein MA, Mizushima A, et al. MR imaging characteristics of tuberculous spondylitis vs. vertebral osteomyelitis. AJNR Am J Neuroradiol 1989;10:619–625.
16. Koeller KK, Rosenblum RS, Morrison AL. Neoplasms of the spinal cord and filum terminale: radiologic-pathologic correlation. Radiographics 2000;20:1721–1749.
17. Baur A, Dietrich O, Reiser M. Diffusion-weighted imaging of the spinal column. Neuroimaging Clin North Am 2002;12:147–160.
18. Bourgouin PM, Lesage J, Fontaine S. A pattern approach to the differential diagnosis of intramedullary spinal cord lesions on MR imaging. Am J Roentgenol 1998;170:1645–1649.
19. Egelhoff JC, Bates DJ, Ross JS, et al. Spinal MR findings in neurofibromatosis types 1 and 2. AJNR Am J Neuroradiol 1992;13:1071–1077.
20. Stevens SK, Moore SG, Amylon MD. Repopulation of marrow after transplantation: MR imaging with pathologic correlation. Radiology 1990;175:213–218.
21. Yuh WTC, Zachar CK, Barloon TJ, et al. Vertebral compression fractures: distinction between benign and malignant causes with MR imaging. Radiology 1989;172:215–218.
22. Cuenod CA, Laredo JD, Chevret S, et al. Acute vertebral collapse due to osteoporosis or malignancy: appearance on unenhanced and gadolinium-enhanced MR images. Radiology 1996;199:541–549.
23. Mawad ME, Rivera V, Crawford S, et al. Spinal cord ischemia after the resection of thoracoabdominal aneurysms: MR findings in 24 patients. AJNR Am J Neuroradiol 1990;11:987–991.
24. Friedman DP, Flanders AE. Enhancement of gray matter in anterior spinal infarction. AJNR Am J Neuroradiol 1992;13:983–985.
25. Rosenblum B, Oldfield EH, Doppman JL, et al. Spinal arteriovenous malformations: a comparison of dural arteriovenous fistulas and intradural AVMs in 81 patients. J Neurosurg 1987;67:795–802.

26. Ernst RJ, Gaskill-Shipley M, Tomsik TA, et al. Cervical myelopathy associated with intracranial dural arteriovenous fistula: MR findings before and after treatment. AJNR Am J Neuroradiol 1997;18:1330–1334.
27. Luetmer PH, Lane JI, Gilbertson JR, et al. Preangiographic evaluation of spinal dural arteriovenous fistulas with elliptic centric contrast-enhanced MR angiography and effect on radiation dose and volume of iodinated contrast material. AJNR Am J Neuroradiol 2005;26:711–718.
28. Saraf-Lavi E, Bowen BC, Quencer RM, et al. Detection of spinal dural arteriovenous fistulae with MR imaging and contrast enhanced-enhanced MR angiography: sensitivity, specificity, and prediction of vertebral level. AJNR Am J Neuroradiol 2002;23:858–867.
29. Barkovich AJ. Congenital anomalies of the spine. In: Barkovich AJ, ed. Pediatric Neuroimaging. Philadelphia: Lippincott Williams & Wilkins, 2005:704–762.
30. Silberstien M, Tress BM, Hennessy O. Delayed neurologic deterioration in the patient with spine trauma: role of MR imaging. AJNR Am J Neuroradiol 1992;13:1373–1381.
31. Nguyen GK, Clark R. Adequacy of plain radiography in the diagnosis of cervical spine injuries. Emerg Radiol 2004 Nov 26.
32. Flanders AE, Spetell CM, Tartaglino LM. Forecasting motor recovery after cervical cord injury: value of MR imaging. Radiology 1996;201:649–655.
33. Gasparotti R, Ferraresi S, Pinelli L, et al. Three-dimensional MR myelography of traumatic injuries of the brachial plexus. AJNR Am J Neuroradiol 1997;18:1733–1742.

Chapter 11

Lumbar Spine: Disk Disease and Stenosis

Clyde A. Helms

Imaging Methods
Disk Disease
Spinal Stenosis
Postoperative Changes
Bony Abnormalities

Imaging Methods

Imaging the lumbar spine for disk disease and stenosis has evolved in the past 20 years from predominantly myelography-oriented examinations to plain CT and MR examinations. Multiple studies have shown that myelography is not as accurate as CT or MR (1–3), yet myelography continues to be performed. Little justification exists for using a lumbar myelogram to determine disk disease or stenosis in this era.

Although few differences between CT and MR have been noted concerning diagnostic accuracy in the lumbar spine, MR will give more information and a more complete anatomic depiction than will CT. For example, MR can determine whether a disk is degenerated by showing loss of signal on T2WIs (Fig. 11.1). CT cannot provide this information. Whether or not this is useful information remains to be proven.

To achieve a high degree of accuracy, the proper imaging protocols must be observed. With CT scans, thin-section (3- to 5-mm) axial images should be obtained from the midbody of L3 to the midbody of S1 in a contiguous manner, i.e., no skip areas or gaps should be present (Fig. 11.2). One of the leading causes of failed back surgery is missed free fragments. Skip areas will often allow a free fragment to remain undiagnosed. Angling the gantry parallel to the endplates is not necessary, and image reformations are not helpful in the routine evaluation of disk disease and stenosis.

The MR imaging protocol is similar to that of CT, in that thin-section axial images should be obtained from the midbody of L3 to the midbody of S1 (Fig. 11.3). Angling of the plane of imaging to be parallel to the endplates is not necessary, and contiguous images without skip areas are considered mandatory. Even though sagittal images will be obtained, free fragments and areas of stenosis

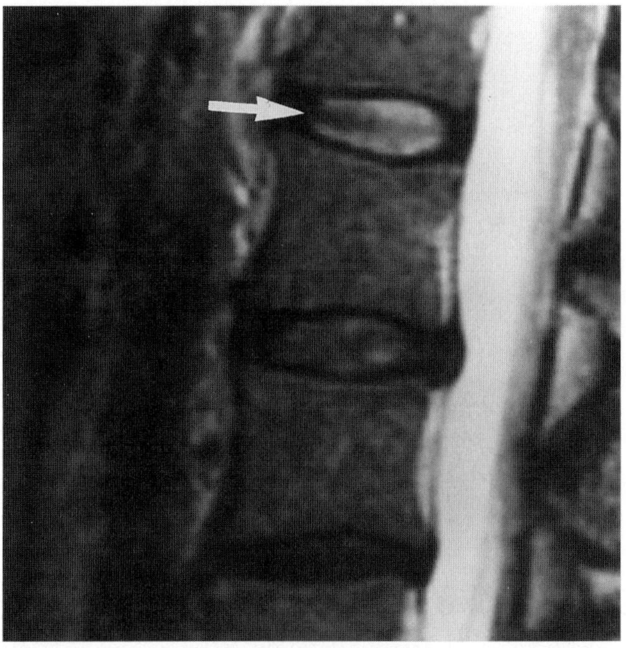

FIGURE 11.1. **Desiccated Disk.** A sagittal T2WI (TR, 4,000; TE, 102) shows the L2-L3 and L3-L4 disks to be abnormally low in signal, indicating disk dessication and degeneration. Compare with the normal L1-L2 disk (*arrow*), which has high signal.

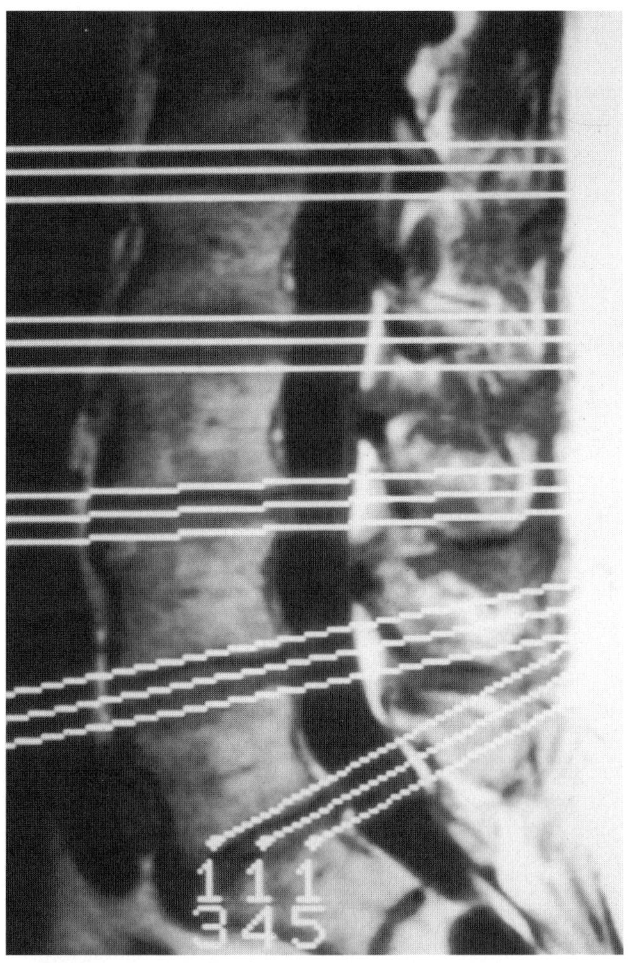

FIGURE 11.2. **Inadequate Technique: Skip Areas.** This MR scout film has cursors placed through the disk spaces. This allows large gaps or skip areas that can result in missed free fragments of disks.

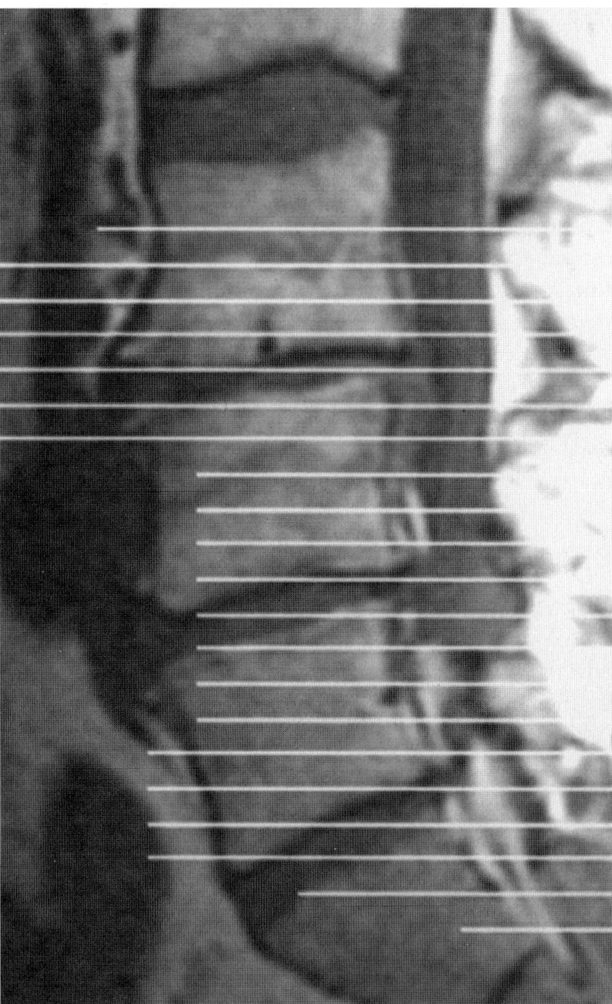

FIGURE 11.3. **Proper MR Technique.** This MR scout, with cursors placed contiguously from the body of L3 to S1, allows complete coverage of the lower lumbar spine in the axial plane.

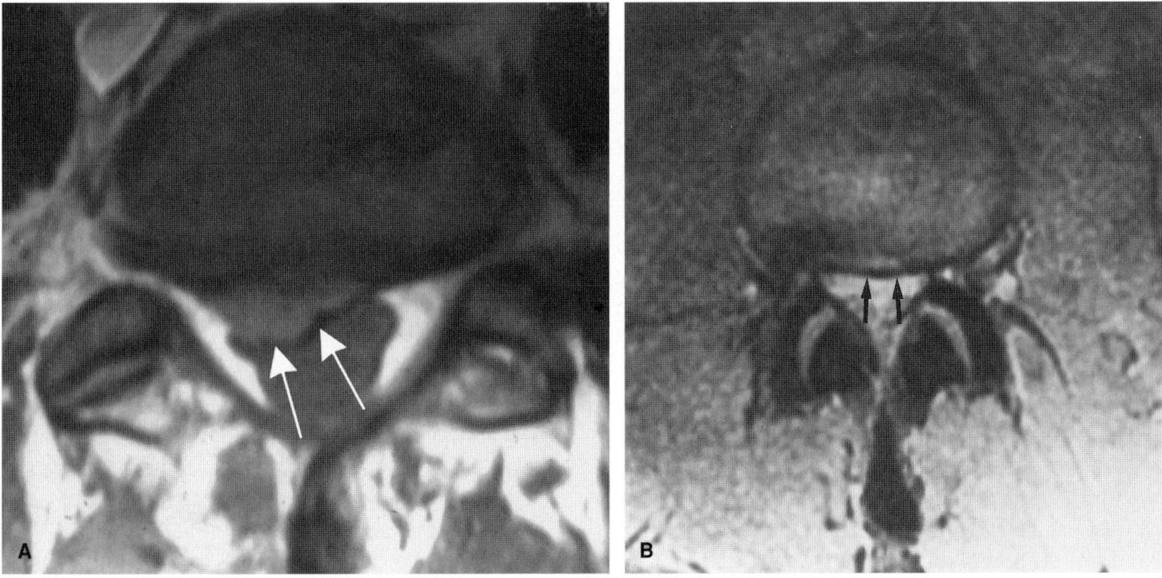

FIGURE 11.4. **Disk Protrusions.** Axial images show focal **(A)** (*arrows*) and broad-based **(B)** disk protrusions (*arrows*). Because both are showing impression of the thecal sac, they could each cause symptoms.

are often seen on axial images to better advantage than on sagittal images. Other entities that can be overlooked if gaps are present in the axial imaging protocol include conjoined nerve roots, pars defects (spondylolysis), and lateral recess stenosis. These entities occur cephalad or caudal to the vertebral body, away from the disk level; thus, axial images limited to the disk level will not show them, and they may not be conspicuous on the sagittal images.

Both T1WIs (or proton density–weighted images) and T2WI (or T2*WI) should be obtained in the sagittal and the axial planes. Attempting to shorten the study by foregoing one of the sequences is not recommended.

Disk Disease

Disk Protrusions. Terminology plays a large role in how radiologists describe disk bulges or protrusions. Since the advent of CT in the 1970s, disk bulges have been described by their morphology. A broad-based disk bulge has been said to be a *bulging annulus fibrosus,* and a focal disk bulge is a *herniated nucleus pulposus.* These interpretations are no more than 90% accurate. More significantly, most surgeons are not concerned with the name applied to a disk bulge; they do not treat a bulging annulus differently than a herniated nucleus pulposus. They treat the patient's symptoms and have to decide whether the disk bulge is responsible for those symptoms. Most surgeons are satisfied with the terms "bulge" or "protrusion." Up to 50% of the asymptomatic population have disk protrusions (4); hence, evidence of a disk bulge on CT or MR does not mean it is clinically significant.

Both CT and MR have a high degree of accuracy in delineating disk protrusions and showing whether neural tissue is impressed (Fig. 11.4). MR can also show whether annular fibers of the disk are disrupted by noting high signal on T2WIs, which disrupts the annulus. This has been termed a "high intensity zone" (HIZ) (Fig. 11.5). Although CT cannot be used to diagnose annular tears clinicians treat them the same way they treat protrusions (annular fibers intact).

Free Fragments. A type of disk protrusion that is critical to diagnose is the free fragment or sequestration. Missing free fragments is one of the most common causes of failed back surgery (5). The preoperative diagnosis of a free fragment contraindicates chymopapain, percutaneous discectomy, and, for many surgeons, microdiscectomy. At the very least, the presence of a free fragment means the surgeon must explore more cephalad or caudally during the surgery to remove the free fragment. Because free fragments can be very difficult to diagnose clinically, imaging is critical in the evaluation of the spine for any patient contemplating surgery. At times it can be difficult to ascertain whether a disk that has extruded is still attached to the parent disk or is really "free." If disk material is above or below the level of the disk space, whether it is attached really does not matter. Chymopapain and percutaneous discectomy would still be contraindicated, and many surgeons would not perform or, at the very least, would modify a microdiscectomy. The key element is recognizing that disk material is present away from the level of the disk space.

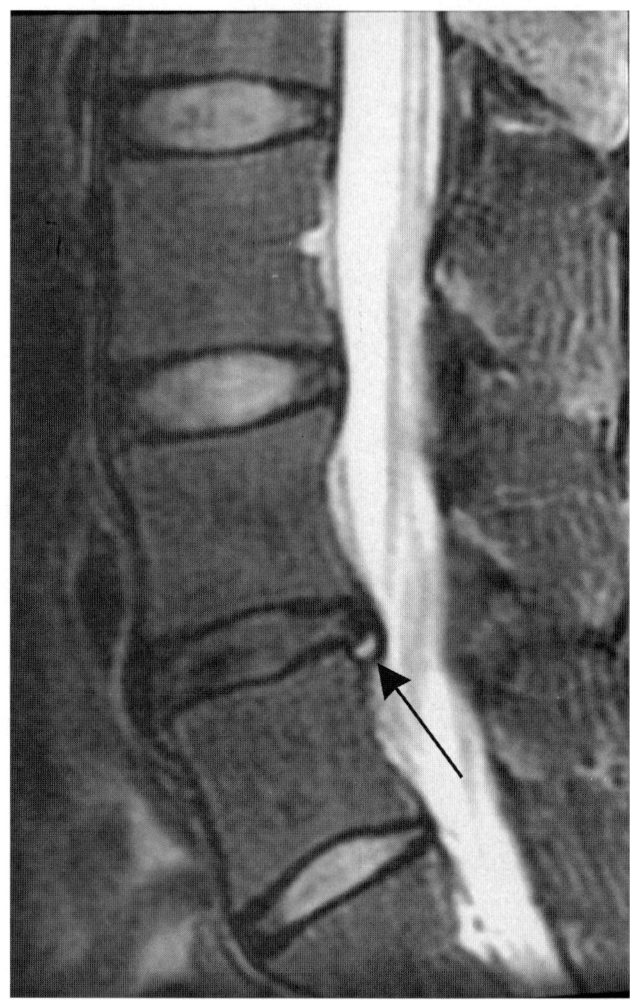

FIGURE 11.5. **Annular Tear.** This sagittal fast spin-echo T2 image shows a focus of increased signal (*arrow*) in the annulus, which is called a high intensity zone (HIZ) and indicates an annular tear.

Free fragments are diagnosed on CT by the presence of soft tissue density with a higher attenuation value than that of the thecal sac, which is located away from the disk space. A conjoined root (a normal variant of two roots exiting the thecal sac together; seen in 1% to 3% of the population [6]) (Fig. 11.6) or a Tarlov cyst (a normal variant referring to a dilated nerve root sleeve) can have a similar appearance to a free fragment, but these will have

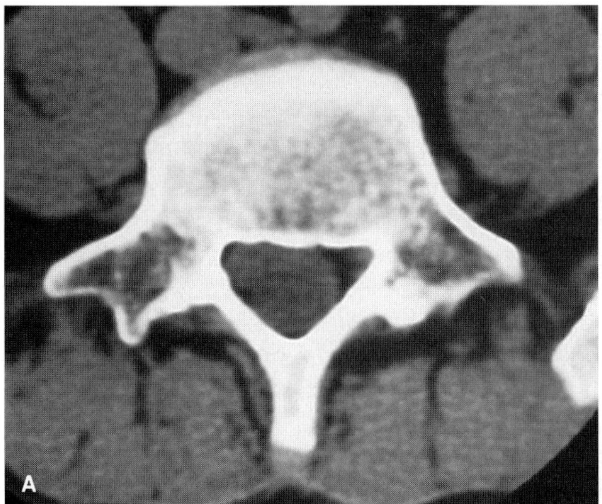

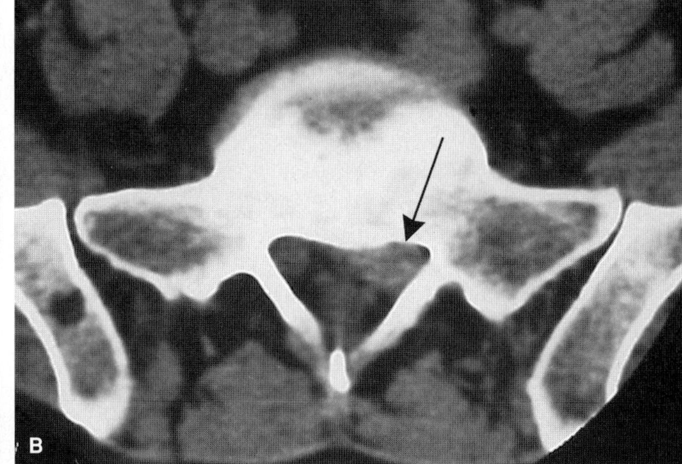

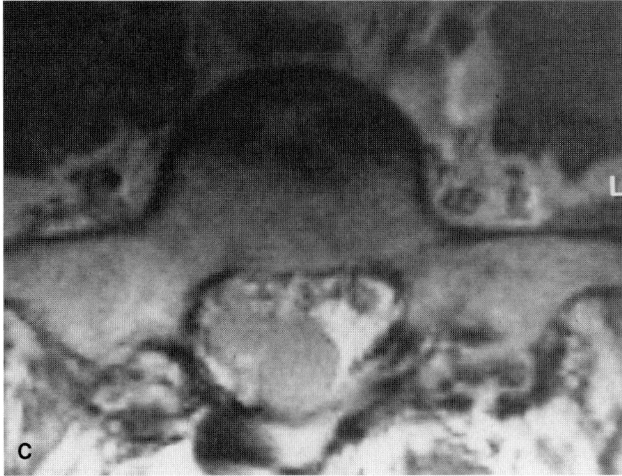

FIGURE 11.6. **Conjoined Root and Free Fragment. A.** A soft tissue mass is seen in the right L5 lateral recess, which has CT attenuation values that are identical to those of the thecal sac. This is a conjoined nerve root. **B.** In the same patient, a soft tissue mass is present in the left S1 lateral recess (*arrow*), which has a density greater than that of the adjacent thecal sac. This is a free fragment. **C.** An axial proton density–weighted MR image shows a mass in the right lateral recess that had signal characteristics identical to that of the thecal sac on all sequences. This is a conjoined nerve root. A free fragment would not have signal identical to that of the thecal sac on all sequences.

attenuation values similar to that of the thecal sac. A conjoined root has a characteristic appearance on MR (Fig. 11.6C). Free fragments are diagnosed on MR by noting disk material that has moved away from the disk space (Fig. 11.7). Free fragments migrate either cephalad or caudally, with no documented preference (7). It is imperative to obtain contiguous axial images without large skip areas or gaps when imaging with both CT and MR to avoid missing free fragments.

Lateral Disks. Disks will occasionally protrude in a lateral direction, causing the nerve root that has already exited the central canal to be stretched (Fig. 11.8). Although not common (<5% of cases), these disks are frequently overlooked and are known to be a source of failed back surgery (8). Because they affect the already exited root, they can clinically mimic symptoms of disk protrusion from one level more cephalad (Fig. 11.9). For example, in a patient who has multilevel disk disease and symptoms referable to the L3-L4 disk, the disk protrusion is usually a posterior bulge that impresses the L4 nerve root. However, a lateral disk at L4-L5 could impress the L4 nerve root and cause the same symptoms. If not noticed, surgery could be performed at the L3-L4 disk, which is the wrong level. Notifying the surgeon that the disk is lateral to the neuro foramen is also important, because a standard surgical approach through the lamina might not allow removal of a lateral disk. Lateral disks are best identified on axial images. Sagittal images will often show a lateral disk occluding a neuro foramen, but many times a lateral disk will not extend into the foramen and the sagittal images will appear normal.

SPINAL STENOSIS

By definition, *spinal stenosis* is encroachment of the bony or soft tissue structures in the spine on one or more of the neural elements, with resulting symptoms. This definition does not typically apply if the narrowing is solely from a disk bulge. It is classically divided into congenital

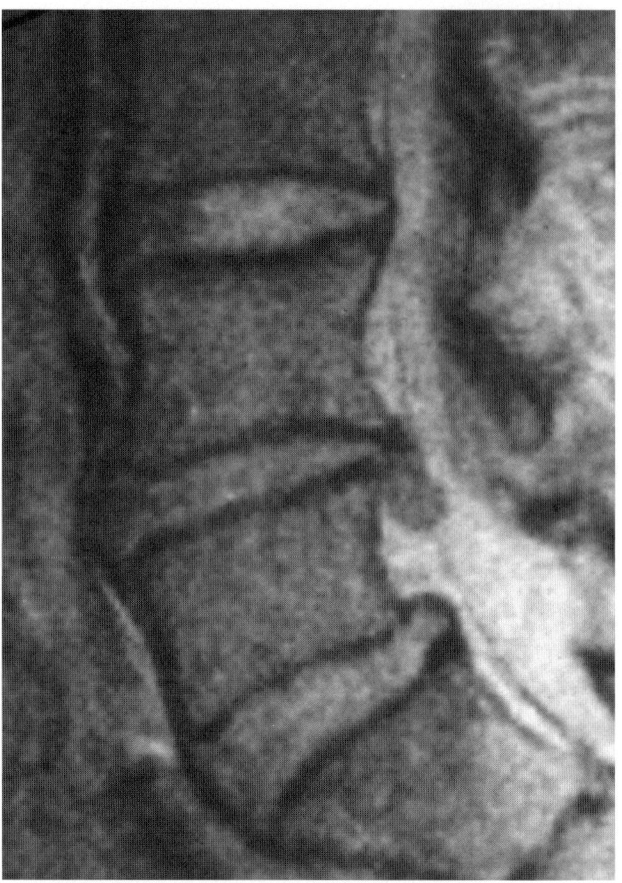

FIGURE 11.7. **Free Fragment.** A sagittal T2WI shows disk material extending caudally from the L4-L5 disk space. This is a large free fragment or sequestration.

and acquired types; however, even the most severe forms of congenital stenosis do not cause symptoms unless a component of acquired stenosis (usually degenerative disease of the facets and the disks) is present. A more useful classification of stenosis is on an anatomic basis: central canal, neuroforaminal, and lateral recess. One must realize that stenosis and disk disease are often present concomitantly, and clinically differentiating between the two can be challenging. As with disk disease, any imaging findings must be matched with clinical findings. It is not unusual to have a patient with stenosis that appears severe on images but who is asymptomatic.

Central Canal Stenosis. Although measurements were once considered very useful in the determination of central canal stenosis, they are no longer considered a valid indicator of disease. Instead, simply noting whether the thecal sac is compressed or round will reliably determine central canal stenosis (Fig. 11.10). A subjective assessment as to whether the compression (usually in an anteroposterior direction) is mild, moderate, or severe is all that is necessary for evaluating the central canal.

The most common cause of central canal stenosis is degenerative disease of the facets, with bony hypertrophy that encroaches on the central canal (Fig. 11.11). This is also the most common cause of lateral recess stenosis. When the facets undergo degenerative joint disease (DJD), they often have some slippage, which results in buckling of the ligamentum flavum. This has been termed *ligamentum flavum hypertrophy* and is a common cause of central canal stenosis (Fig. 11.12). Frequently, mild disk bulging is associated with minimal facet hypertrophy and ligamentum flavum hypertrophy. This combination can result in severe focal central canal stenosis. Both CT and MR will show these bony and soft tissue changes. Less common causes of central canal stenosis include bony overgrowth from Paget disease, achondroplasia, posttraumatic changes, and severe spondylolisthesis.

Neuroforaminal Stenosis. DJD of the facet with bony hypertrophy is the most common cause of neuroforaminal stenosis; however, encroachment on the nerve root in the neuro foramen can be seen with free disk fragments, postoperative scar, and from a lateral disk protrusion. The neuro foramina are best evaluated on axial images just cephalad to the disk space. The disk space lies at the inferior portion of the neuro foramen, and the exiting nerve root lies in the superior or cephalad portion of the neuro foramen. Although the neuro foramen can be seen clearly on sagittal MR images (Fig. 11.8A), care must be taken to evaluate the entire neuro foramen and not just the 4 or 5 mm shown in one sagittal image.

Lateral Recess Stenosis. The lateral recesses are the bony canals in which the nerve roots lie after they leave the thecal sac and before they enter the neuro foramen. Hypertrophy of the superior articular facet from DJD is the most common cause of encroachment on the lateral recesses (Fig. 11.11); however, as with the neuro foramen, disk fragments and postoperative scar can cause nerve root impingement.

Spondylolysis and Spondylolisthesis. Defects in the bony pars interarticularis (spondylolysis) are found in up to 10% of asymptomatic individuals, yet they can be a source of low back pain and instability. Prior to disk surgery or other back surgery, the identification of any spondylolysis is imperative. Because spondylolysis can mimic back pain from other pathology, it must be assessed preoperatively. If necessary, it can then be surgically addressed. Failure to note and evaluate spondylolysis is a known source of failed back surgery. CT is superior to MR imaging at identifying spondylolysis (9). Although MR will show spondylolysis defects, these defects can sometimes be very difficult to see. Spondylolysis is identified on axial images through the midvertebral body as a break in the normally intact bony ring of the lamina (Fig. 11.13). Hence, a protocol that does not include an axial cut through the middle of each vertebral body may overlook spondylolysis defects.

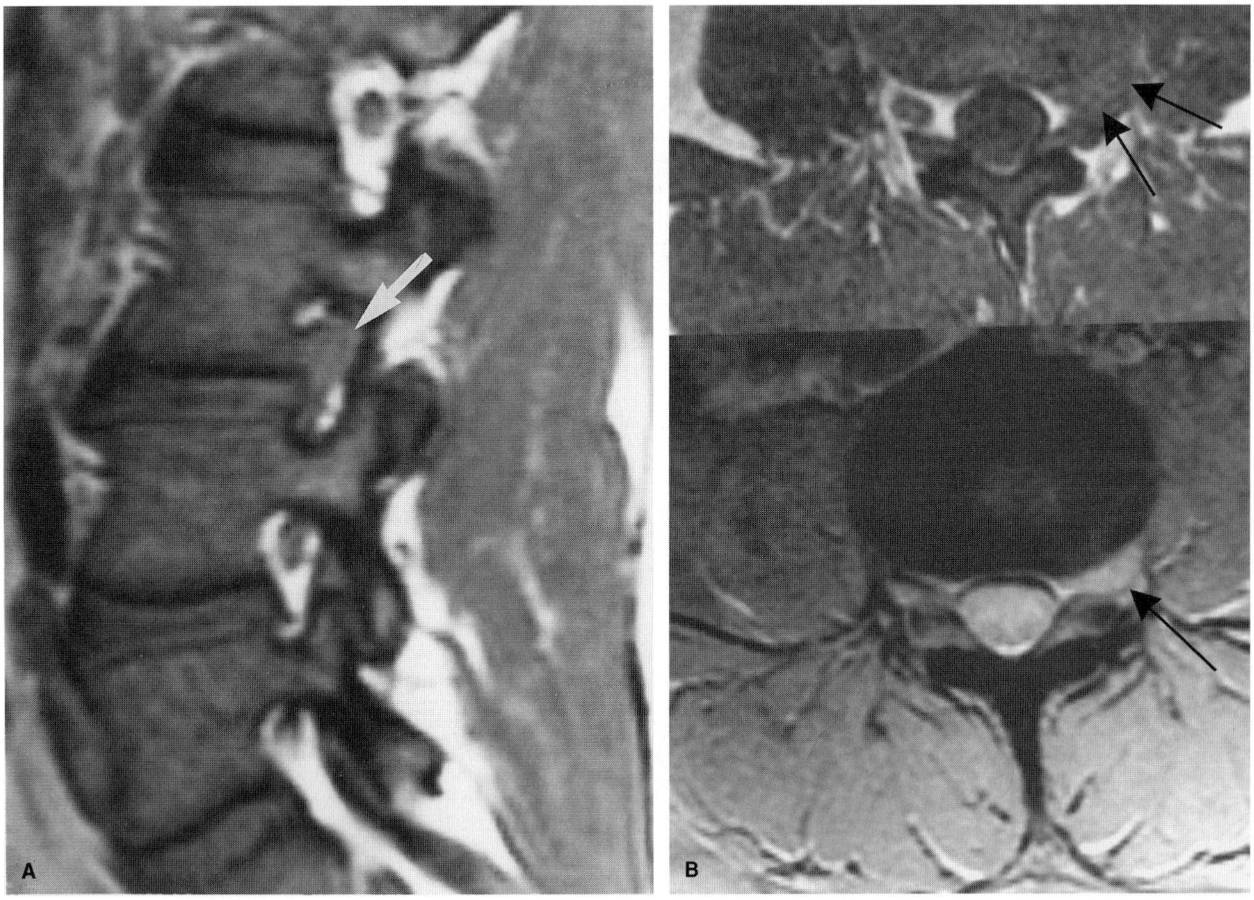

FIGURE 11.8. Lateral Disk (MR). A. A sagittal T1WI (TR, 600; TE, 30) through the left neuro foramen shows a low signal structure in the L4 neuro foramen (*arrow*), which is a lateral disk protrusion. **B.** Axial T1W (*upper*) (TR, 600; TE, 30) and T2* images (*lower*) (TR, 600; TE, 30; 30°) show the lateral disk (*arrows*) in the left neuro foramen.

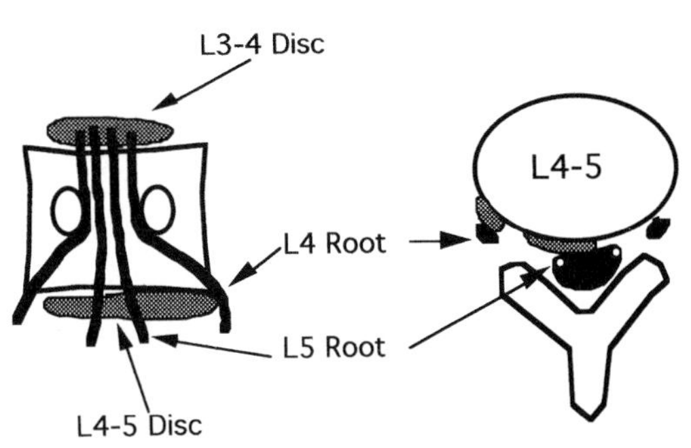

FIGURE 11.9. Schematic of Lateral Disk. This schematic illustrates how a posterior L4-L5 disk protrusion affects the L5 nerve root, yet a lateral L4-L5 disk affects the L4 root.

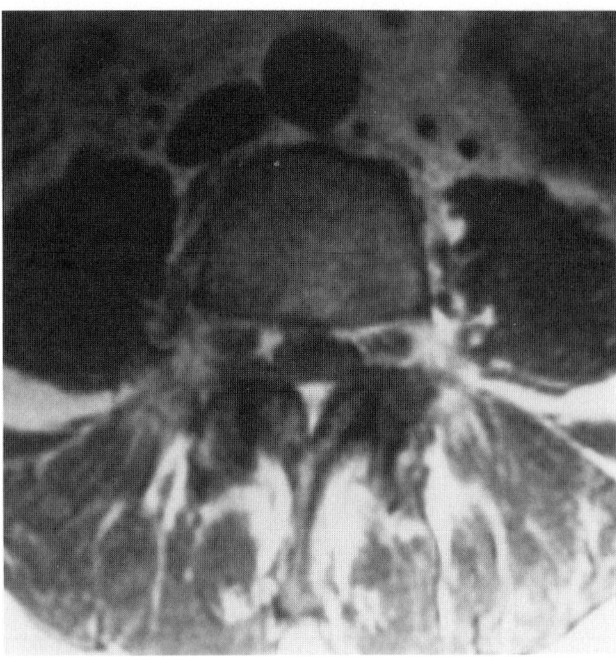

FIGURE 11.10. Central Canal Stenosis. An axial T1WI demonstrates absence of the normally round thecal sac caused by central canal stenosis. This represents mild central canal stenosis and may or may not be a source of symptoms.

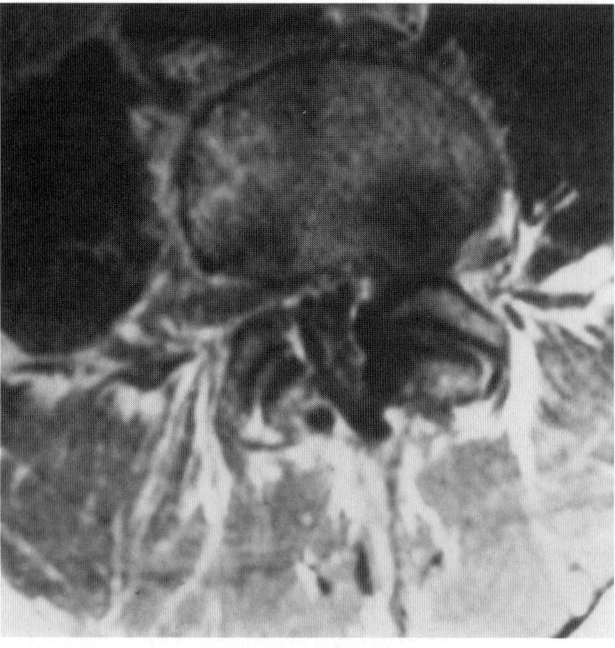

FIGURE 11.11. **Facet Hypertrophy Causing Stenosis.** This axial T1WI shows marked left-sided facet degenerative disease with hypertrophy of the facets, causing lateral recess and central canal stenosis.

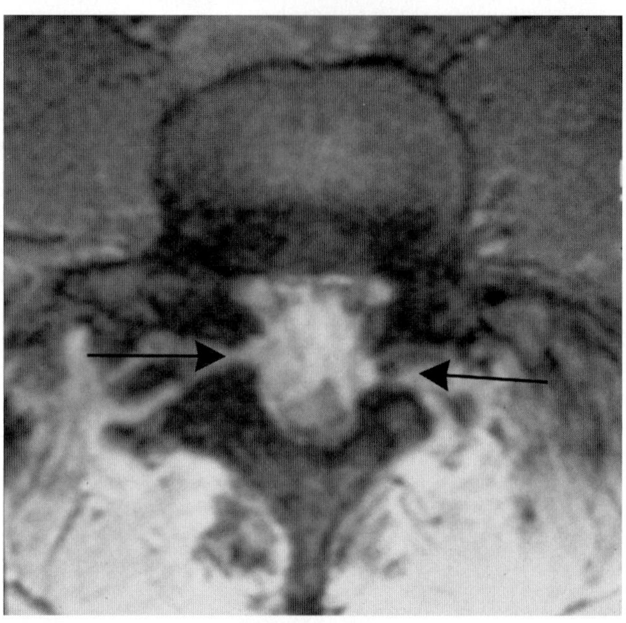

FIGURE 11.13. **Spondylolysis.** An axial T2WI through the mid-vertebral body reveals a break in the bony laminae bilaterally (*arrows*), which indicates spondylolysis. An axial cut through the pedicles should have an intact bony ring around the central canal.

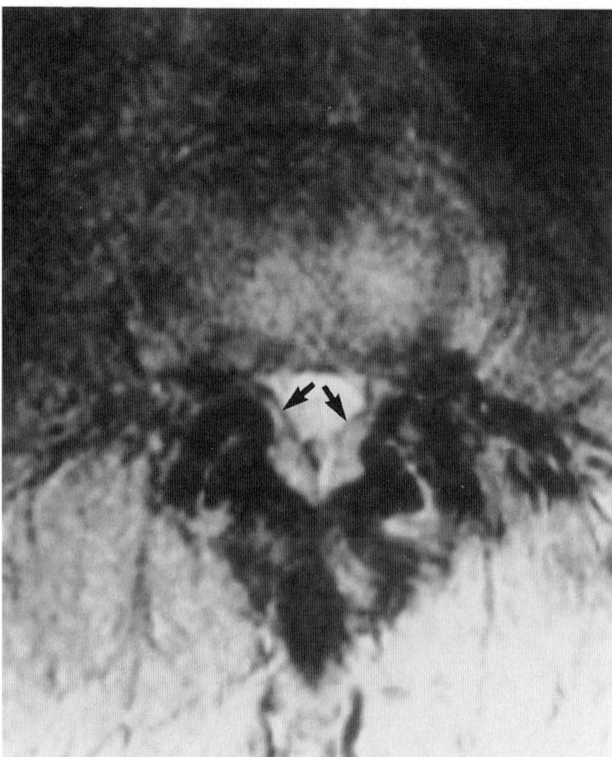

FIGURE 11.12. **Ligamentum Flavum Hypertrophy.** Inward bulging of the ligamentum flavum (*arrows*) is shown on this axial T2WI. Central canal stenosis from ligamentum flavum hypertrophy is common.

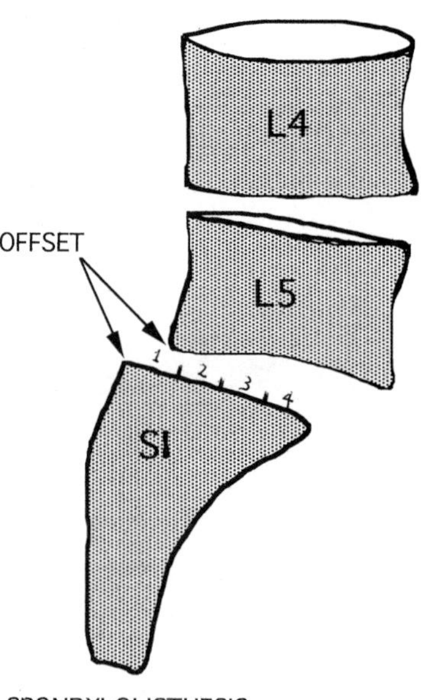

FIGURE 11.14. **Schematic of the Spondylolisthesis Grading Scale.** This schematic shows the grading scale used to gauge the degree of spondylolisthesis. This example would be a grade 1 spondylolisthesis, because the posterior edge of the slipped L5 vertebral body lies above the first quadrant of the S1 vertebral body.

Spondylolisthesis (forward slippage of one vertebral body on a lower one) occurs from either slippage of two vertebral bodies following bilateral spondylolysis or from DJD of the facets with slippage of the facets. Bilateral spondylolysis can result in a large amount of slippage, but facet DJD will usually result in only minimal slippage. If spondylolisthesis is severe, the result can be central canal stenosis, neuroforaminal stenosis, or both. A grading scale that is widely used to describe the degree of spondylolisthesis is the Meyerding grading scale. The more caudal vertebral body is divided into fourths, and the posterior corner of the more cephalad vertebral body is marked at the position where it has slipped forward. If it has slipped forward only into the first quarter of the more caudal vertebral body, it is a grade 1 spondylolisthesis; slippage into the second quarter is a grade 2, and so on (Fig. 11.14).

POSTOPERATIVE CHANGES

Failed back surgery is unfortunately common. It has many causes, including inadequate surgery (e.g., missed free disk fragments), postoperative scarring, failure of bone grafting for fusion, and recurrent disk protrusion. CT is useful in evaluating bone grafts, but it is not reliable for differentiating postoperative scar from disk material. However, MR has been particularly useful in distinguishing scar from disk material (10).

The use of intravenous gadolinium will allow virtual certainty in distinguishing scar tissue from a disk. Scar tissue will enhance following administration of gadolinium, whereas disk material will have only minimal peripheral enhancement, presumably owing to inflammation (Fig. 11.15).

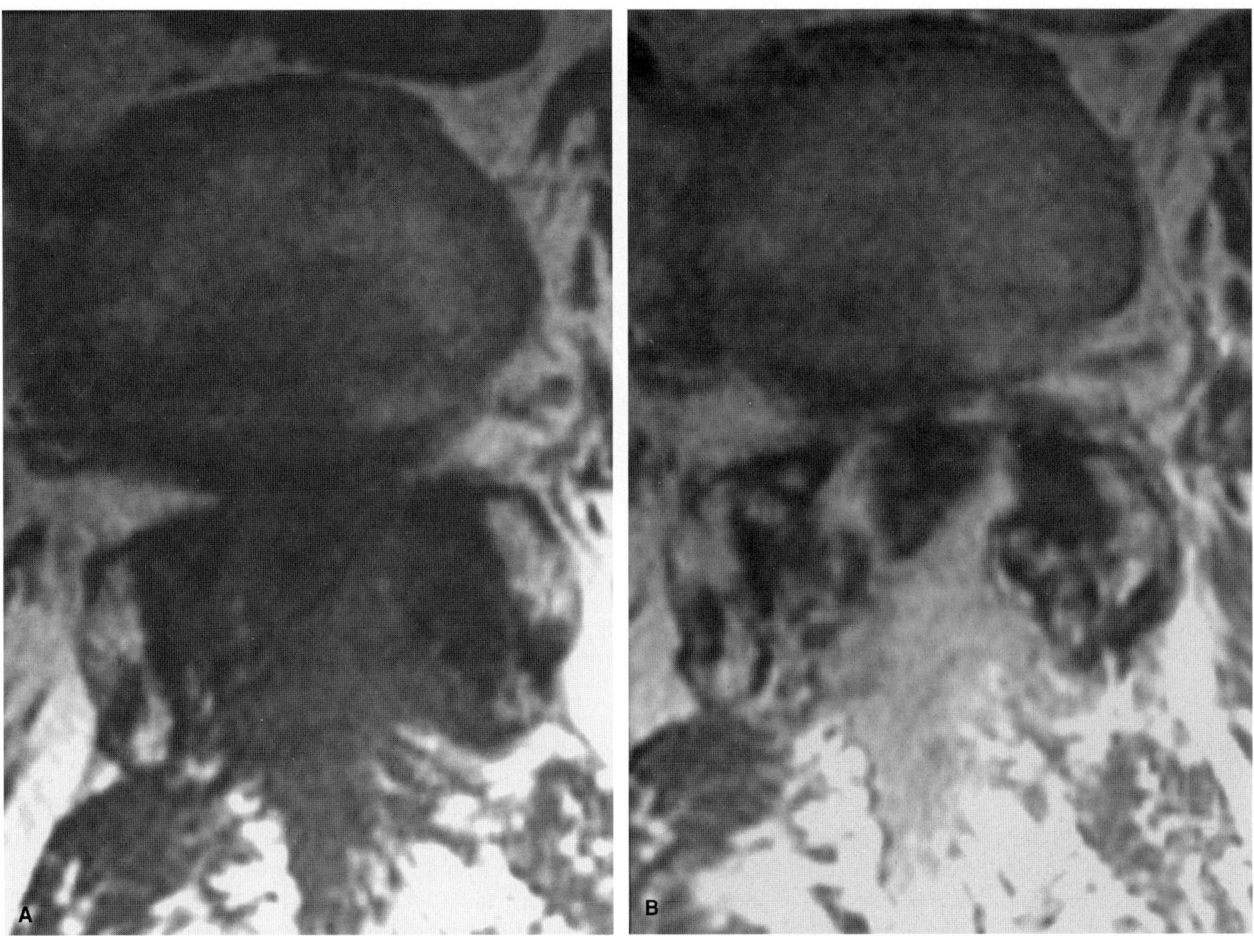

FIGURE 11.15. **Postoperative Scar Enhancement With Gadolinium. A.** Axial T1WI shows scar tissue surrounding the thecal sac, making evaluation for recurrent disk protrusion difficult. **B.** Axial T1WI through the same level following administration of gadolinium–diethylenetriamine pentaacetic acid (Gd-DTPA) intravenously shows enhancement of the scar tissue surrounding the thecal sac. No significant disk protrusion can be identified.

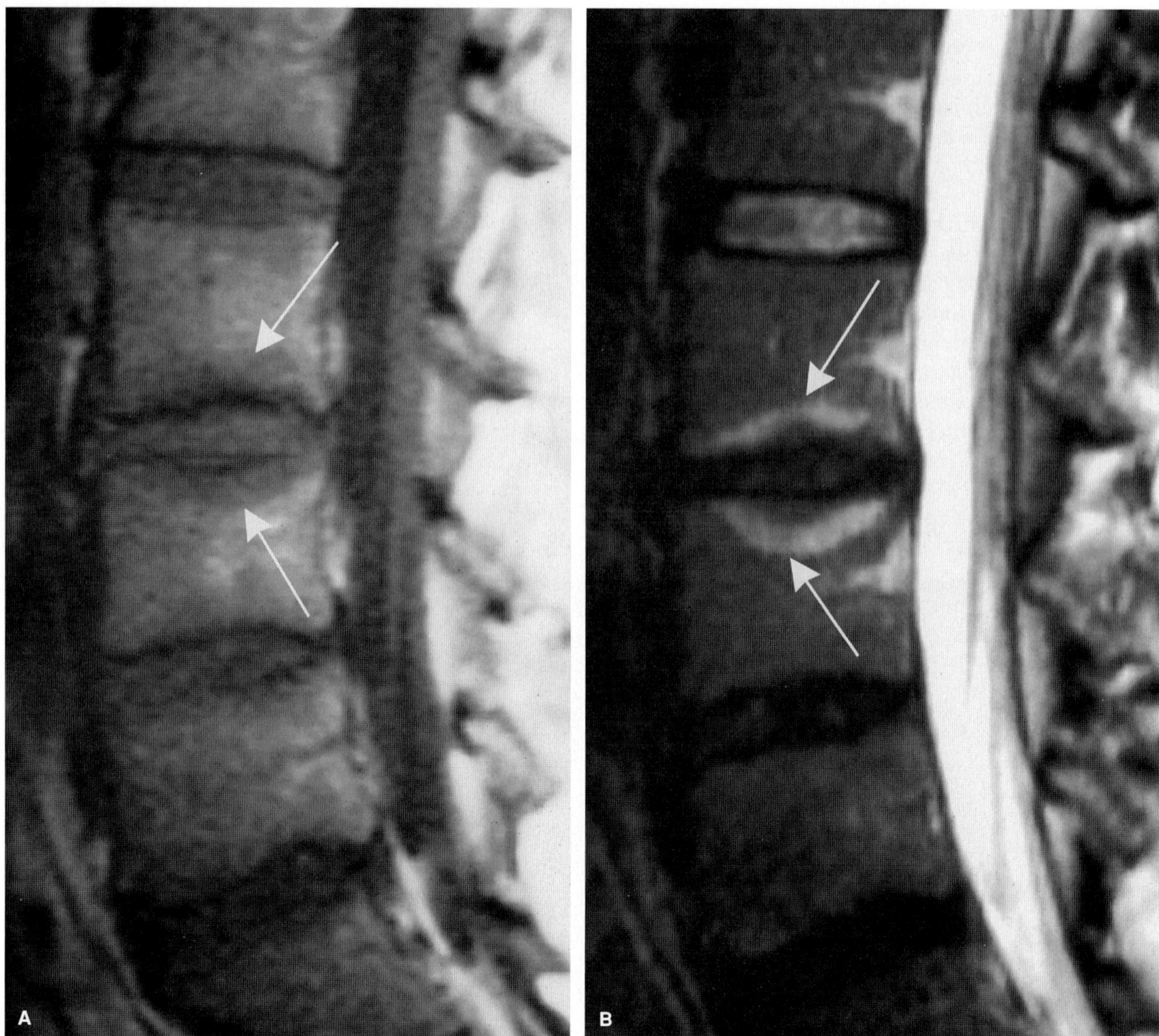

FIGURE 11.16. **Type 1 Marrow Changes. A.** Sagittal T1WI in a patient with degenerative disk disease at L3-L4 shows faint bands of low signal parallel to the L3-L4 endplates (*arrows*). **B.** Sagittal fast spin-echo T2WI with fat suppression shows bands of high signal adjacent to the L3-L4 endplates (*arrows*). This represents granulation tissue seen with degenerative disk disease and has been called type 1 marrow change. It can be differentiated from a disk infection by the low signal of the disk on the T2WI.

BONY ABNORMALITIES

Parallel bands of high or low signal adjacent to the vertebral body endplates are often seen with MR imaging in association with degenerative disk disease. The most common appearance is of high-signal bands on T1WIs that remain high on T2WIs. This represents fatty marrow conversion. It was seen in 16% of cases in the first report in the literature (1) and was termed type 2. Type 1 changes are seen as low-signal bands parallel to the endplates on T1WIs that get brighter on T2WIs (Fig. 11.16). This represents an inflammatory or granulomatous response to degenerative disk disease. Type 2 changes were reported in 4% of cases, and these must be distinguished from disk space infection. In disk space infection, the disk should be bright on the T2WI (Fig. 11.17); for a degenerative disk to have high signal on a T2WI is unusual. Type 3 changes are parallel bands of low signal adjacent to the endplates on both T1WIs and T2WIs. Type 3 changes represent bony sclerosis and can be seen on plain films.

MR imaging and CT have changed diagnostic imaging of the lumbar spine from a painful, invasive study

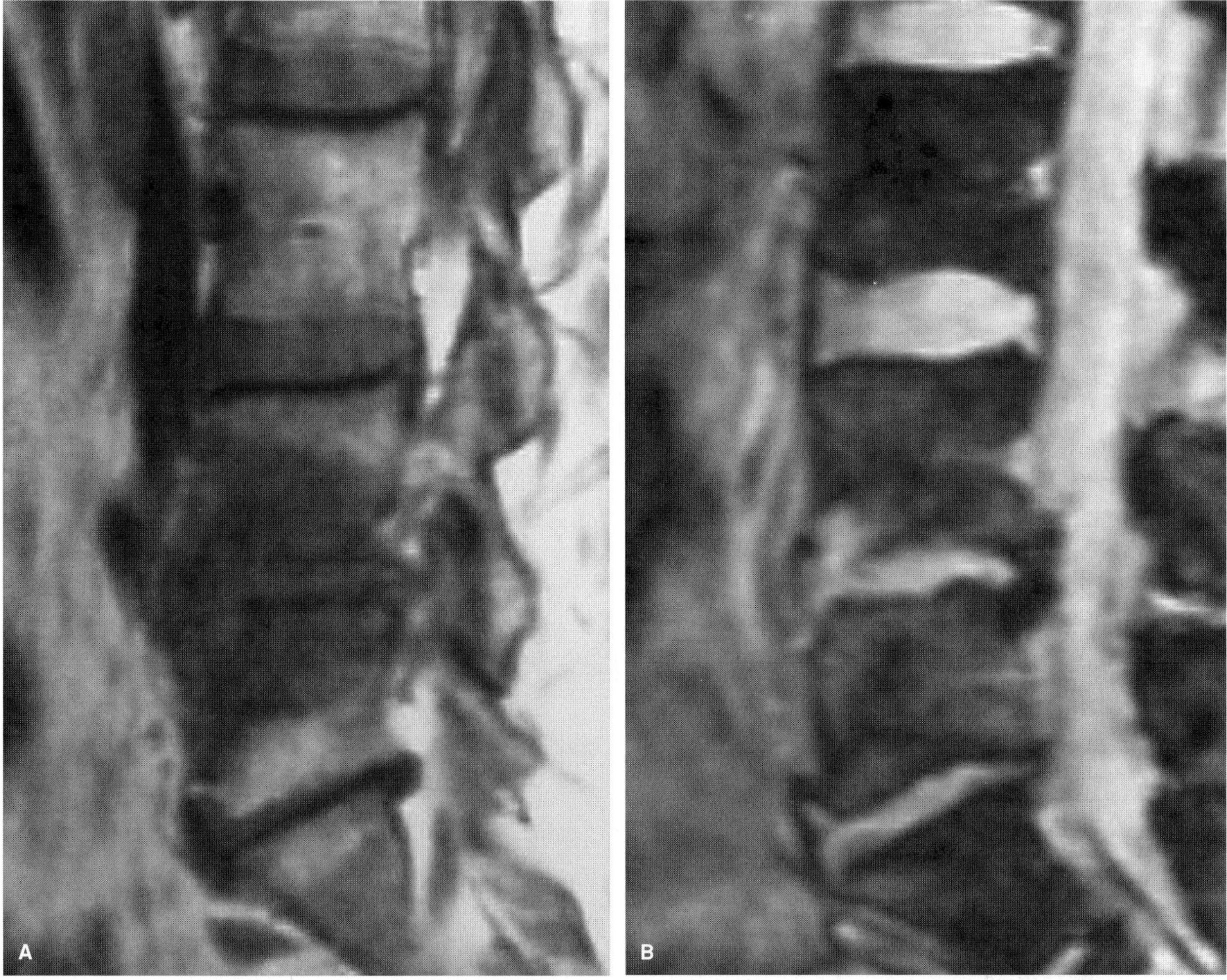

FIGURE 11.17. **Disk Infection. A.** Sagittal T1WI shows bands of low signal in the vertebral bodies adjacent to the L4-L5 endplates. **B.** On a T2W (gradient-echo) image the vertebral body/endplate signal increase is faintly seen, as it is a gradient-echo sequence. However, note the high signal in the disk, which makes this consistent with a disk infection rather than a type 2 signal of a degenerative disk.

to a highly accurate, noninvasive study that provides a more complete anatomic depiction than with plain films or myelography.

REFERENCES

1. Modic M, Masaryk T, Ross J, et al. Imaging of degenerative disk disease. Radiology 1988;168:177–186.
2. Hesselink J. Spine imaging: history, achievements, remaining frontiers. AJR Am J Roentgenol 1988;150:1223–1230.
3. Sartoris DJ, Resnick D. Computed tomography of the spine: an update and review. CRC Crit Rev Diagn Imaging 1987;27:271–296.
4. Jensen MC, Brant-Zawadzki MN, Obuchowski N, et al. Magnetic resonance imaging of the lumbar spine in people without back pain. N Engl J Med 1994;331(2):69–73.
5. Onik G, Mooney V, Maroon J, et al. Automated percutaneous discectomy: a prospective multi-institutional study. Neurosurgery 1990;26:228–233.
6. Helms CA, Dorwart RH, Gray M. The CT appearance of conjoined nerve roots and differentiation from a herniated nucleus pulposus. Radiology 1982;144:803–807.
7. Masaryk T, Ross J, Modic M, et al. High-resolution MR imaging of sequestered lumbar intervertebral disks. AJR Am J Roentgenol 1988;150:1155–1162.
8. Winter DDB, Munk PL, Helms CA, et al. CT and MR of lateral disc herniation: typical appearance and pitfalls of interpretation. Can Assoc Radiol 1989;40:256–259.
9. Grenier N, Kressel HY, Schiebler ML, et al. Isthmic spondylolysis of the lumbar spine: MR imaging at 1.5 T. Radiology 1989;170:489–494.
10. Ross J, Masaryk T, Schrader M, et al. MR imaging of the postoperative spine: assessment with gadopentetate dimeglumine. AJR Am J Roentgenol 1990;155:867–872.

SECTION III

Pulmonary

Section Editor: Jeffrey S. Klein

Methods of Examination, Normal Anatomy, and Radiographic Findings of Chest Disease

Santiago Miró and Jeffrey S. Klein

Imaging Modalities

Normal Lung Anatomy
- Posteroanterior Chest Radiograph
- Lateral Chest Radiograph
- Anatomy of the Normal Mediastinum and Thoracic Inlet
- Normal Hilar Anatomy
- Pleural Anatomy
- Chest Wall Anatomy
- Anatomy of the Diaphragm

Radiographic Findings in Chest Disease
- Pulmonary Opacity
- Pulmonary Lucency
- Mediastinal Masses
- Mediastinal Widening
- Pneumomediastinum and Pneumopericardium
- Hilar Disease
- Pleural Effusion
- Pneumothorax
- Localized Pleural Thickening
- Diffuse Pleural Thickening
- Pleural and Extrapleural Lesions
- Chest Wall Lesions
- Diaphragm

There are many imaging techniques available to the radiologist for the evaluation of thoracic disease (1). The decision about which imaging procedures to perform depends upon many factors, the most important of which are the availability of various modalities and the type of information sought. Although conventional radiographs of the chest still constitute 25% to 35% of the volume of any general radiology department, there has been a steady decline in favor of CT, despite the considerable increase in radiation to the patient. The recent years have seen near disappearance of diagnostic thoracic vascular interventions, thanks to CT and MR. The recent advent of multichannel, parallel MR imaging might allow for gradual replacement of CT for thoracic vascular diagnostics. Although the imaging algorithm for specific problems may seem relatively straightforward, medical judgment should be preferred. For example, a thin-section CT showing a suspicious solitary pulmonary nodule might be followed directly by a thoracotomy, or rather, in selected patients, by transthoracic needle biopsy. This type of flexible approach will often streamline the diagnostic workup and ultimately lead to better patient care.

Imaging Modalities

Conventional Chest Radiography. Posteroanterior (PA) and lateral chest radiographs are the mainstays of thoracic imaging. Conventional radiographs should be performed as the initial imaging study in all patients with thoracic disease. These films are obtained in most radiology departments on a dedicated chest unit capable of obtaining radiographs with a focus-to-film distance of 6 feet, a high kilovoltage-potential (140-kVp) technique, a grid to reduce scatter, and a phototimer to control the length of exposure (2).

The recognition of proper radiographic technique on frontal radiographs involves assessment of four basic features: *penetration, rotation, inspiration,* and *motion*. Proper penetration is present when there is faint visualization of the intervertebral disk spaces of the thoracic spine and

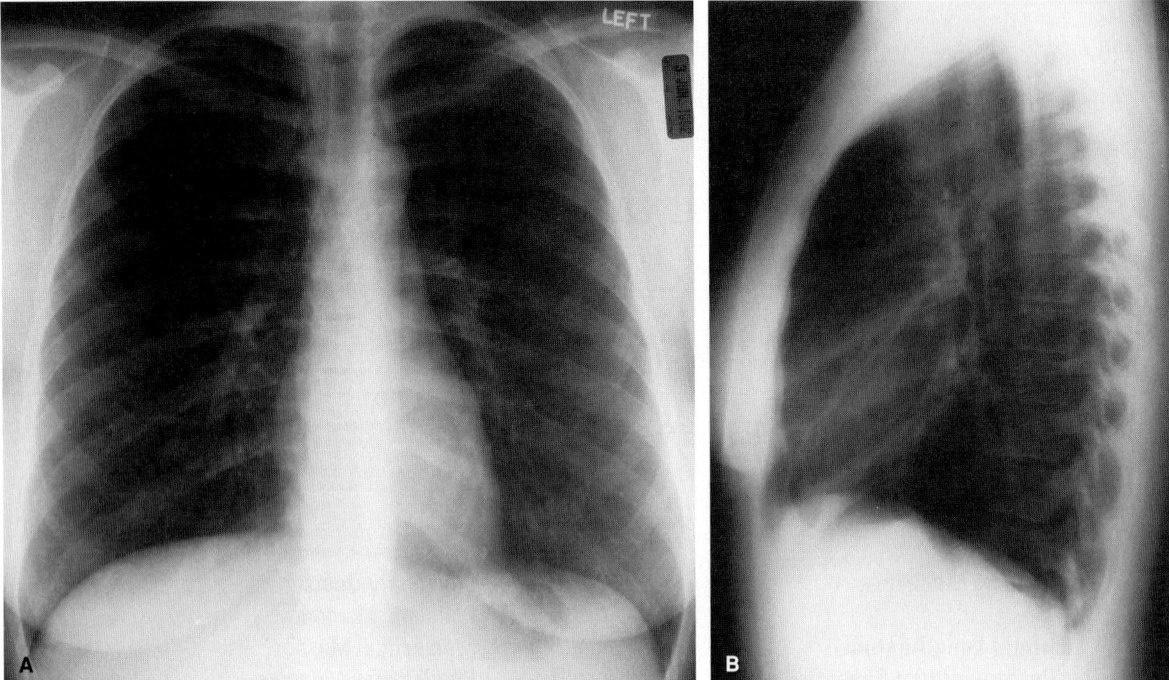

FIGURE 12.1. **Normal PA (A) and Lateral (B) Radiographs of the Chest.**

discrete branching vessels can be identified through the cardiac shadow and the diaphragms. Rotation is assessed by noting the relationship between a vertical line drawn midway between the medial cortical margins of the clavicular heads and one drawn vertically through the spinous processes of the thoracic vertebrae. Superimposition of these lines (the former in the midline anteriorly and the latter in the midline posteriorly) indicates a properly positioned, nonrotated patient. An appropriate deep inspiration in a normal individual is present when the apex of the right hemidiaphragm is visible below the tenth posterior rib. Finally, the cardiac margin, diaphragm, and pulmonary vessels should be sharply marginated in a completely still patient who has suspended respiration during the radiographic exposure (Fig. 12.1).

Portable Radiography. Portable anteroposterior (AP) radiographs are obtained when patients cannot be safely mobilized (3). Portable radiographs help monitor a patient's cardiopulmonary status; assess the position of various monitoring and life support tubes, lines, and catheters; and detect complications related to the use of these devices.

There are technical and patient-related compromises as well as inherent physiologic changes with portable bedside radiography. The limited maximal kilovoltage potential of portable units requires longer exposures to penetrate cardiomediastinal structures, which results in greater motion artifact. Because critically ill patients are difficult to position for portable radiographs, the patient is often rotated. Inaccuracies in directing the x-ray beam perpendicular to the patient lead to kyphotic or lordotic radiographs. The short focus-to-film distance (typically 40 inches) and AP technique result in magnification of intrathoracic structures. For instance, the apparent cardiac diameter increases by 15% to 20%, bringing the upper limit of normal for the cardiothoracic ratio from 50% on a PA radiograph to 57% on an AP. Physiologically, the supine position of critically ill patients elevates the diaphragm, thus compressing lower lobes and decreasing lung volumes. The normal gravitational effect evens out the blood flow between upper and lower zones in supine patients, which makes assessment of pulmonary venous hypertension difficult. The increase in systemic venous return to the heart produces a widening of the upper mediastinum or "vascular pedicle." The gravitational layering of free-flowing fluid may hide small effusions. Similarly, a pneumothorax may be difficult to detect because free intrapleural air rises to a nondependent position, producing a subtle anteromedial or inferior radiolucency. A device called the *inclinometer* has been developed that accurately records the position of the bedridden patient from supine to completely upright. This device, which clips onto the portable film cassette, gives an accurate estimate of the patient's position at the time of the radiograph, which helps assess the distribution of pulmonary blood flow, pleural effusions, and pneumothorax.

Digital or Analog? The main advantages of digital chest radiography are superior contrast resolution and the availability of the image on any computer monitor through a PACS (Picture Archiving and Communication System). Contrast levels and windows can be adjusted to enhance visualization of various regions in the chest or compensate partly for faulty exposure. Although digital images have poorer spatial resolution than their analog counterparts, these benefits render the system appealing.

Special Techniques. A *lateral decubitus* radiograph is obtained with a horizontal x-ray beam while the patient lies in the decubitus position. It is used to detect small effusions, to characterize free-flowing effusions on the decubitus side, or to detect a small pneumothorax on the contralateral side. As little as 5 mL of fluid (Fig. 12.2) or 15 mL of air can be demonstrated by this view. Normally, the downside diaphragm assumes a higher position than the upside one. Air trapping can be demonstrated in the dependent lung in patients with a check valve bronchial obstruction who are unable to cooperate for inspiratory/expiratory radiographs or chest fluoroscopy.

An *expiratory radiograph*obtained at residual volume (end of maximal forced expiration) can detect focal or diffuse air trapping and eases detection of a small pneumothorax. In the absence of a direct communication between the pleura and the bronchi, the volume of air in the pleural space remains stable, whereas the volume of air in the lung parenchyma decreases. Because the lung is also displaced away from the chest wall, the visceral pleural line becomes more visible.

An *apical lordotic view* improves visualization of the lung apices, which are obscured on routine PA radiographs by the clavicles and first costochondral junctions. Caudocephalad angulation of the tube projects these anterior bony structures superiorly, providing an unimpeded view of the apices. This view enhances the visualization of middle lobe atelectasis by placing the inferiorly displaced minor fissure in tangent with the x-ray beam and by increasing the AP thickness of the atelectatic middle lobe.

Chest fluoroscopy is used mainly to assess chest dynamics on patients with suspected diaphragmatic paralysis. Although it has been widely abandoned to the benefit of CT, fluoroscopy can still often bring the same answers as CT at a fraction of the radiation exposure: evaluation of a nodular opacity seen on only one view, evaluation of apparent pseudotumor images caused by vertebral lamina, osteophytes, vertebral transverse processes, healed rib fractures, skin lesions, nipples, or other external objects.

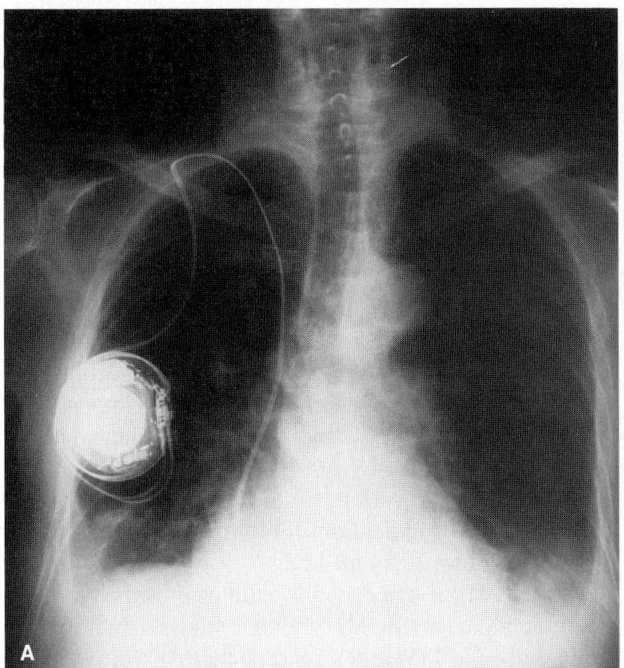

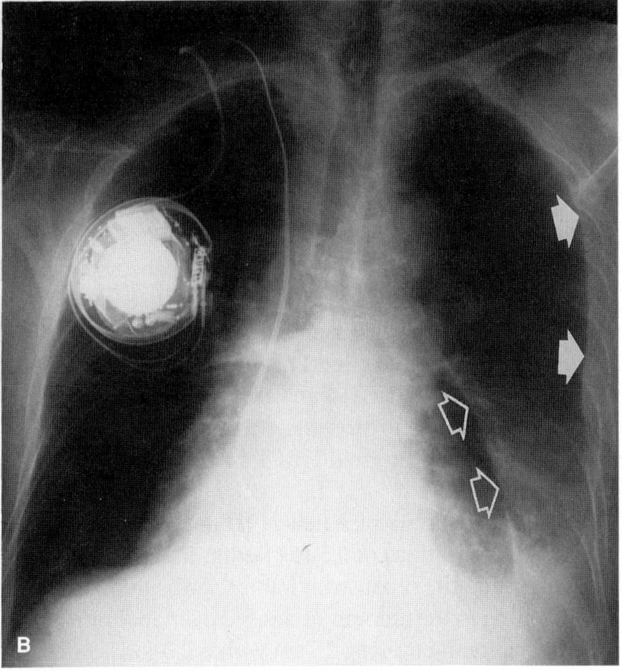

FIGURE 12.2. **Lateral Decubitus Film for the Detection of Pleural Effusion.** An upright radiograph **(A)** in a patient recovering from pulmonary edema shows blunting of both lateral costophrenic sulci. A left lateral decubitus film **(B)** demonstrates free-flowing effusion laterally on the down side (*solid arrows*) and within the lateral aspect of an incomplete oblique fissure (*open arrows*). Note the clearing of fluid from the right lateral costophrenic sulcus with the patient in the opposite decubitus position, with fluid layering medially along the mediastinal pleural surface.

CT and HRCT. Thoracic chest CTs can be acquired either in an incremental "stop, acquire, and go" mode, such as for HRCTs, or in a helical mode, whereby acquisition occurs while the patient translates through the gantry on the CT scan table. The latter allows single breath-hold scans with optimal contrast enhancement, without the respiratory misregistration inherent in incremental scanning. Multidetector scanners now allow for full chest coverage with collimation as narrow as 1.0 mm in approximately 20 seconds. Cardiac gating on such scanners can eliminate pulsation artifacts, for example, in the ascending aorta, and also allows for diagnostic evaluation of the heart, at a threefold or fourfold increase in radiation dose (4). Scans without contrast are usually performed for evaluation or follow-up of parenchymal disease. Iodinated contrast material is administered for mediastinal mass or cancer staging evaluation, systemic or pulmonary arterial evaluation, or for cardiac studies.

The field of view for image reconstruction is determined by measuring the widest transverse diameter, as seen on the CT scout view. An edge-enhancing computer reconstruction algorithm ("bone" or "sharp" algorithm) improves the spatial resolution of parenchymal structures and is used for all types of thoracic CT scans. Most frequently, the image is reconstructed in a 512 × 512 matrix size. Matrix sizes up to 1,024 × 1,024 are now available, but studies would be needed to assess whether there is any diagnostic benefit to this fourfold increase in image size. Although images can still be filmed using a laser camera, PACS workstation viewing offers the possibility to modify window width (WW) and window level (WL) as needed. Routine settings for CT display of mediastinal structures are WW = 400 and WL = 40 and for the lungs are WW = 1,500 and WL = –700.

HRCT technique involves incremental thinly collimated scans (1.0 to 1.5 mm) obtained at evenly spaced intervals through the thorax for the evaluation of diffuse bronchial or parenchymal lung disease. Image acquisition time is limited to minimize the effects of respiratory and cardiac motion. Expiratory HRCT scans are useful for the detection of air trapping in patients with small airways disease. Normal and abnormal HRCT findings are reviewed in Chapter 17.

The volume of data of a helical CT is acquired with a thickness (collimation) of 0.5 to 10 mm, and the user can then determine the reconstruction interval, which is chosen according to the amount of desired overlap. For example, a helical scan covering 25 cm with a 2.0-mm collimation can be reconstructed with a 2.0-mm interval, yielding 125 contiguous images with no overlap, but could also be reconstructed at a 1.25-mm interval, yielding 200 images, each of which overlaps the following image by 0.75 mm (4).

The major advantages of CT are its superior contrast resolution and cross-sectional display format. Superior contrast resolution allows for the differentiation of calcium, soft tissue, and fat within lung nodules or mediastinal structures. Intravenous enhancement improves contrast within structures or masses, as well as within blood vessels (e.g., pulmonary emboli, aortic dissection). The cross-sectional display eliminates the superimposition of structures and allows visualization of parenchymal nodules as small as 2 mm.

The clinical indications for thoracic CT will vary among institutions. The indications for thoracic CT and HRCT are shown in Tables 12.1 and 12.2.

TABLE 12.1 Indications for Thoracic CT

Indication	*Example*
Evaluation of an abnormality identified on conventional radiographs	Densitometry of a solitary pulmonary nodule Localization and characterization of a hilar or mediastinal mass
Staging of lung cancer	Assessment of extent of the primary tumor and the relationship of the tumor to the pleura, chest wall, airways, and mediastinum Detection of hilar and mediastinal lymph node enlargement
Detection of occult pulmonary metastases	Extrathoracic malignancies with a propensity to metastasize to the lung (osteogenic sarcoma, breast and renal cell carcinoma).
Detection of mediastinal nodes	Lymphoma, metastases Infections
Distinction of empyema from lung abscess	Contrast-enhanced CT can usually distinguish a peripheral lung abscess from loculated empyema
Detection of central pulmonary embolism	Angio-CT with high injection rate, thin collimation, and precise contrast bolus timing
Detection and evaluation of aortic disease: aneurysm, dissection, intramural hematoma, aortitis, trauma	Detection and localization of extent, including aortic branch involvement

MR. As MR usage expands, studies must be tailored to the individual patient. Morphologic studies usually require only spin-echo T1W and T2W sequences in the axial plane. Coronal and sagittal planes are used in selected cases. Mass evaluation might benefit from fat-suppressed sequences such as STIR, or from gadolinium-enhanced sequences. Angiographic acquisitions are most often performed with GRE volumetric acquisitions. Cardiac sequences benefit from cardiac-gated balanced steady-state free precession

TABLE 12.2 Indications for Thoracic HRCT

Indication	*Example*
Solitary pulmonary nodule	Breath-hold volumetric exam with thin collimation for accurate density determination without respiratory misregistration
Detection of lung disease in a patient with pulmonary symptoms or abnormal pulmonary function studies and a normal or equivocal chest film	Emphysema Extrinsic allergic alveolitis Small airways disease Immunocompromised patient
Evaluation of diffusely abnormal chest film	
A baseline for evaluation of patients with chronic diffuse infiltrative lung disease for follow-up changes with therapy	Cystic fibrosis Sarcoidosis Interstitial lung disease Histiocytosis X Adult respiratory distress syndrome
To determine approach (type and location) of biopsy	Bronchoscopy versus VATS or needle biopsy

VATS = video assisted thoracic surgery

(SSFP) techniques. Respiratory motion is minimized by performing rapid single breath-hold acquisitions or by using respiratory compensation techniques. The latest generation of multichannel scanners with parallel imaging and faster gradients show promise in evaluation of embolic disease, without the radiation cost of multidetector CTs (5).

The major advantages of MR are the superior contrast resolution between tumor and fat, the ability to characterize tissues based on T1 and T2 relaxation times, the ability to scan in direct sagittal and coronal planes, and the lack of need for intravenous iodinated contrast (6). In addition, the ability to obtain images along the long axis of the aorta and the advent of cine-MR techniques have made MR the primary modality for the imaging of most congenital and acquired thoracic vascular disorders. Direct coronal scans are of benefit in imaging regions that lie within the axial plane and are therefore difficult to depict on CT. For this reason, superior sulcus tumors, subcarinal and aortopulmonary window lesions, and certain hilar masses are better depicted by MR than CT. MR is superior to CT in the diagnosis of chest wall or mediastinal invasion because of the high contrast between tumor and chest wall fat and musculature and tumor and mediastinal fat, respectively. The characterization of tissues by their T1 and T2 relaxation times allows for the diagnosis of fluid-filled cysts, hemorrhage, and hematoma formation. The ability to distinguish tumor from fibrosis,

TABLE 12.3 Indications for MR of the Thorax

Evaluation of aortic disease in stable patients:
 Dissection, aneurysm, intramural hematoma, aortitis
Assessment of superior sulcus tumors
Evaluation of mediastinal, vascular, and chest wall invasion of lung cancer
Staging of lung cancer patients unable to receive intravenous iodinated contrast
Evaluation of posterior mediastinal masses

based on their T1 and T2 relaxation times, has proven particularly useful in the follow-up of patients irradiated for Hodgkin disease. MR is currently unable to distinguish benign masses from malignant masses or lymph nodes.

The major disadvantages of thoracic MR scanning are the limited spatial resolution, the inability to detect calcium, and the difficulties in imaging the pulmonary parenchyma. MR is also more time-consuming and expensive than CT. These factors, along with the ability of CT to provide superior or equivalent information in most situations, have limited the use of thoracic MR for most noncardiovascular thoracic disorders. The primary indications for thoracic MR are listed in Table 12.3.

PET. PET utilizing fluorodeoxyglucose (FDG) is an imaging modality based on the metabolic activity of neoplastic and inflammatory tissues and therefore can be considered complementary to the anatomic information provided by chest radiography and CT (1). The role of PET in oncologic diagnosis and staging has developed gradually over the past decade. There is a growing published experience of whole-body PET in the evaluation of patients with malignancy, particularly bronchogenic carcinoma, and of thoracic PET for the evaluation of the solitary pulmonary nodule.

US. Transthoracic US is now commonly used for the detection, characterization, and sampling of pleural, peripheral parenchymal, and mediastinal lesions (see Chapter 39). The aspiration of small pleural effusions visualized on real-time US is preferable to blind thoracentesis. Similarly, sampling of visible pleural masses in patients with malignant effusions can diminish the number of negative pleural biopsies. The aspiration of pleural-based masses and abscesses can be safely performed by US-guided needle placement into the lesion through the point of contact between the mass and pleura. Large anterior mediastinal masses that have a broad area of contact with the parasternal chest wall may be biopsied without transgressing the lung.

Real-time US can also confirm phrenic nerve paralysis without the use of ionizing radiation. It also easily detects subpulmonic and subphrenic fluid collections, which may cause diaphragmatic elevation.

Ventilation/Perfusion Lung Scanning. The nuclear medicine examinations utilized in the evaluation of noncardiac thoracic disease are ventilation/perfusion (V/Q) lung scintigraphy (see Chapter 56) and gallium scintigraphy. V/Q scanning is used almost exclusively for the diagnosis of pulmonary embolism, although quantitative VQ imaging may be useful in the planning of bullectomy, lung volume reduction surgery for emphysema, and lung transplantation. Gallium-67 scanning of the chest is used in the detection of pulmonary infection (e.g., *Pneumocystis carinii* pneumonia in a patient with a normal radiograph) or inflammation (e.g., disease activity in idiopathic pulmonary fibrosis) and in the evaluation of suspected sarcoidosis.

Diagnostic arteriography has mainly been replaced by angio-CT. Pulmonary angiograms are only performed in cases where angio-CT is suboptimal or equivocal.

Thanks to the newer scanners and to the improvement of three-dimensional (3D) rendering tools, thoracic aortography has also been largely replaced by CT, MR, or US. On occasion, an equivocal diagnosis of an aortic laceration following blunt chest trauma can be resolved with this technique. Inflammatory changes of infectious aortitis are also better imaged with MR or CT.

Active bleeding through a bronchial artery is still best addressed by bronchial arteriography, as an active bleeding site is often difficult to pinpoint. When massive or recurrent hemoptysis occur, most commonly from bronchiectasis, neoplasm, or mycetoma, arteriography and embolization can be performed in the same setting.

Transthoracic needle biopsy guided by CT, fluoroscopy, or US is a diagnostic technique utilized in selected patients with pulmonary, pleural, or mediastinal lesions (7).

Percutaneous catheter drainage of intrathoracic air or fluid collections, performed by imaging-guided placement of small-bore multihole catheters, is used for the treatment of empyema, pneumothorax, malignant pleural effusion, and other intrathoracic fluid collections (3).

NORMAL LUNG ANATOMY

Tracheobronchial Tree (Fig. 12.3). The trachea is a hollow cylinder composed of a series of C-shaped cartilaginous rings. The rings are completed posteriorly by a flat band of muscle and connective tissue called the *posterior tracheal membrane.* The tracheal mucosa consists of pseudostratified, ciliated columnar epithelium, which contains scattered neuroendocrine (APUD) cells. The submucosa contains cartilage, smooth muscle, and seromucous glands. The left lateral wall of the distal trachea is indented by the transverse portion of the aortic arch.

The trachea is approximately 12 cm long in adults, with an upper limit of normal coronal tracheal diameter of 25 mm in men and 21 mm in women. In cross section, the trachea is oval or horseshoe-shaped, with a coronal-to-sagittal diameter ratio of 0.6:1.0. A narrowing of the coronal diameter producing a coronal/sagittal ratio of <0.6 is termed a *saber sheath trachea* and is seen in patients with chronic obstructive pulmonary disease.

On chest radiographs, the trachea is seen as a vertically oriented cylindric lucency extending from the cricoid cartilage superiorly to the main bronchi inferiorly. A slight tracheal deviation to the right after entering the thorax can be a normal radiographic finding. The interface of the right upper lobe (RUL) with the right lateral tracheal wall is called the *right paratracheal stripe* (Fig. 12.4A). This stripe should be uniformly smooth and should not exceed 4 mm in width; thickening or nodularity reflects disease in any of the component tissues, including medial tracking pleural effusion. The left lateral wall is surrounded by mediastinal vessels and fat and is not normally visible radiographically. The posterior trachea can be visualized on the lateral chest (Fig. 12.4B). The presence of air in the esophagus produces the tracheoesophageal stripe, which represents the combined thickness of the tracheal and esophageal walls and intervening fat. This stripe should measure less than 5 mm; thickening is most commonly seen with esophageal carcinoma.

The bronchial system exhibits a branching pattern of asymmetric dichotomy, with the daughter bronchi of a parent bronchus varying in diameter, length, and the number of divisions. The bronchial generation "n" indicates the number of divisions since the trachea, which bears generation number 1 (8). The main bronchi arise from the trachea at the carina, with the right bronchus forming a more obtuse angle with the long axis of the trachea. The right main bronchus is considerably shorter than the left main bronchus (mean lengths of 2.2 cm and 5 cm, respectively). The tracheal and main, lobar, and segmental bronchial anatomy are easily seen on CT (Fig. 12.5). Bronchi on end can be seen as a ring shadow on chest radiographs. Bronchi gradually lose their cartilaginous support between generations 1 and 12 to 15. Once this happens, these 1- to 3-mm airways are called *bronchioles* (9). Bronchioles bearing alveoli on their walls are termed *respiratory bronchioles*. The latter divide into alveolar ducts and alveolar sacs. The airway just before the first respiratory bronchiole is the *terminal bronchiole*. It is the smallest bronchiole without respiratory exchange structures. In average, a total of 21 to 25 generations are found between the trachea and the alveoli.

Lobar and Segmental Anatomy (Fig. 12.6). The lungs are divided by the *interlobar fissures,* which are invaginations of the visceral pleura. On the right, the minor fissure

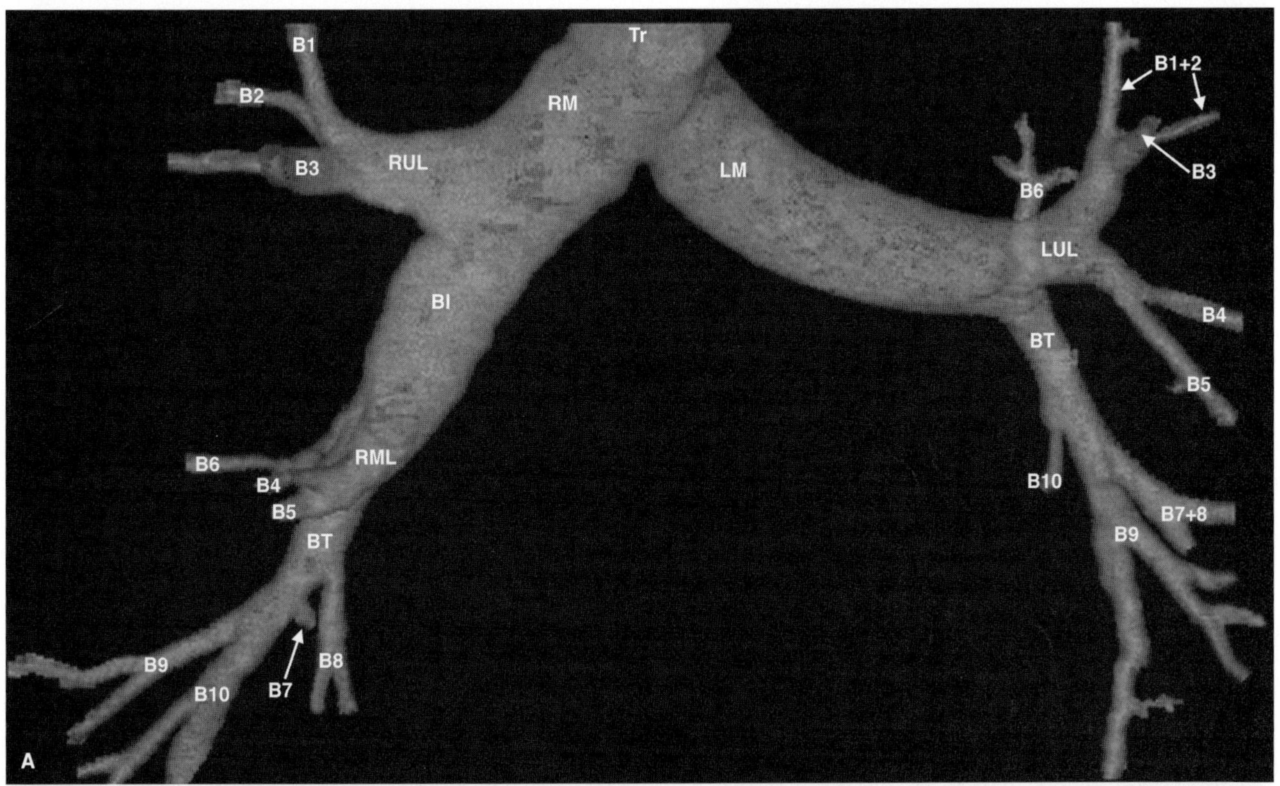

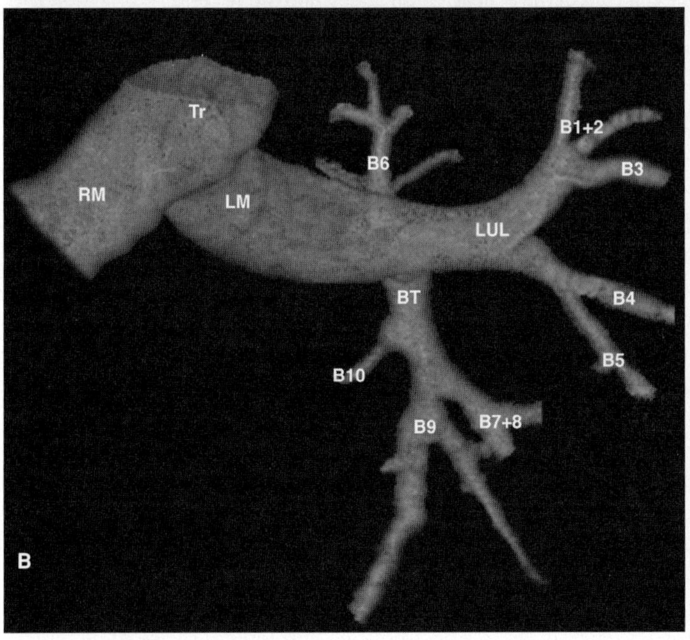

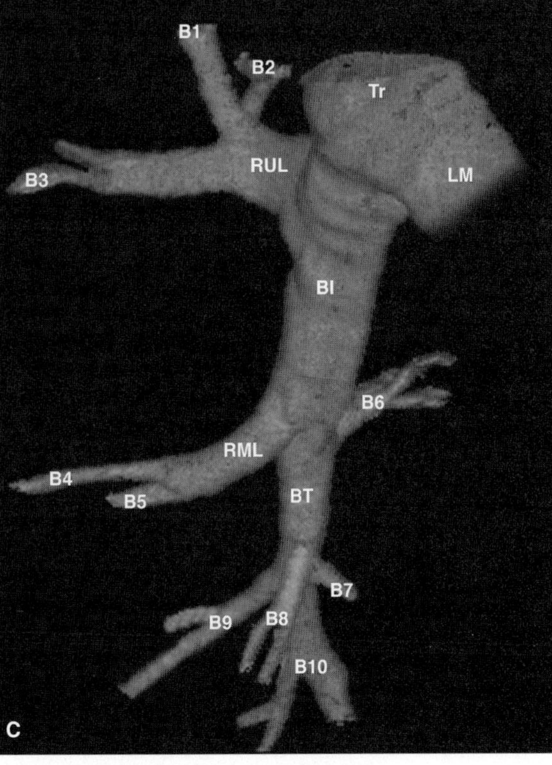

FIGURE 12.3. **Prevailing Pattern of Segmental Bronchi.** Virtual bronchography three-dimensional rendered images of the usual bronchial anatomy. **A.** Left and right bronchial tree. **B.** Oblique view of the left bronchial tree. **C.** Oblique view of the right bronchial tree. Tr, trachea; RUL, right upper lobe; LUL, left upper lobe; RM, right main bronchus; LM, left main bronchus; BT, left lower lobe basal trunk; RML, right middle lobe; B1, apical (upper lobe); B2, posterior (upper lobe); B3, anterior (upper lobe); B4, lateral (middle lobe) and superior (lingula); B5, medial (middle lobe) and inferior (lingula); B6, superior (lower lobe); B7, medial basilar (lower lobe); B8, anterior (lower lobe); B9, lateral basilar (lower lobe); B10, posterior (lower lobe).

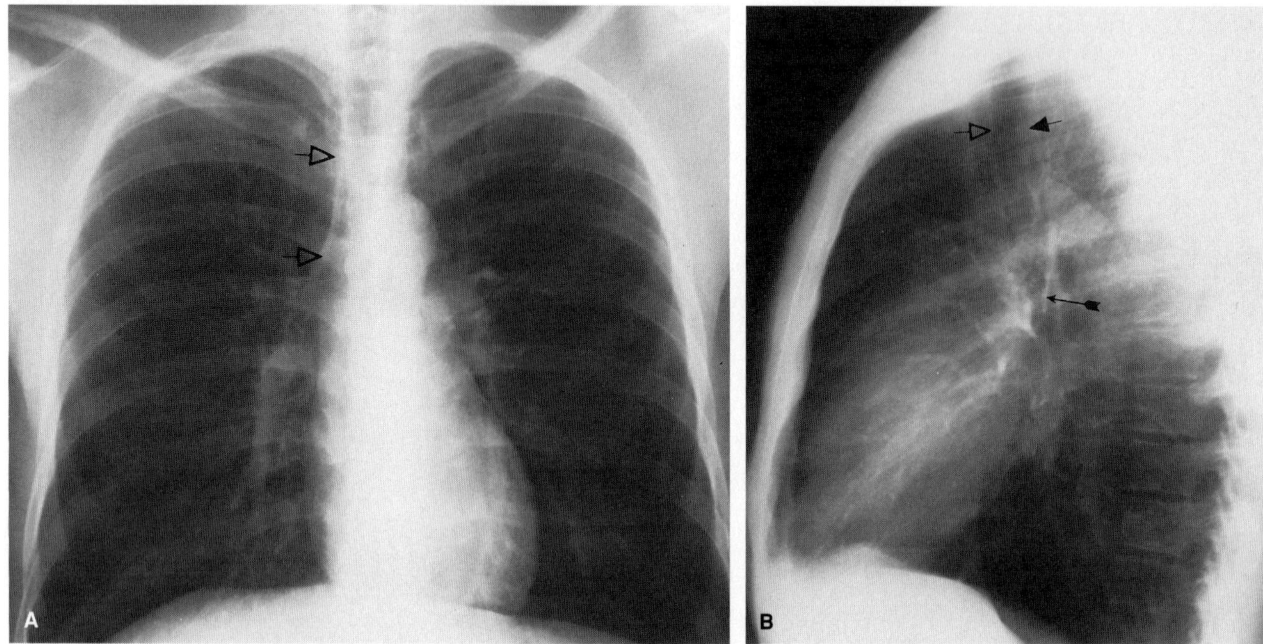

FIGURE 12.4. **Trachea. A.** The right paratracheal stripe (*open arrows*) is composed of the right lateral tracheal wall, a small amount of mediastinal fat, paratracheal lymph nodes, and the visceral and parietal pleural layers of the right upper lobe. **B.** Left lateral chest film shows the anterior (*open arrow*) and posterior (*short solid arrow*) walls of the trachea. The posterior wall of the bronchus intermedius (*long solid arrow*) is readily visible on lateral radiographs as it crosses the end-on view of the left upper lobe bronchus. Because these structures are central, their relationship tends to remain even on rotated films. This is easily seen on CT (see Fig 12.5B, image 3).

separates the middle from the upper lobe. The major fissure separates the lower lobe from the upper lobe superiorly and from the middle lobe inferiorly. The upper lobe bronchus and its artery, arising from the truncus anterior, branch into three segmental branches: anterior, apical, and posterior. The middle lobe bronchus arises from the intermediate bronchus and divides into medial and lateral segmental branches, with its blood supplied by a branch of the right interlobar pulmonary artery. The right lower lobe (RLL) is supplied by the RLL bronchus and pulmonary artery. It is subdivided into a superior segment and four basal segments: anterior, lateral, posterior, and medial.

The left lung is divided into upper and lower lobes by the left major fissure. The left upper lobe (LUL) is analogous to the combined right upper and middle lobes. The LUL is subdivided into four segments: anterior, apicoposterior, and the superior and inferior lingular segments. Arterial supply to the anterior and apicoposterior segments parallels the bronchi and is via branches of the upper division of the left main pulmonary artery. The superior and inferior lingular arteries are proximal branches of the left interlobar pulmonary artery, analogous to the middle lobe's blood supply. The left lower lobe (LLL) has a superior segment and three basal segments: anteromedial, lateral, and posterior.

Respiratory Portion of Lung. The respiratory bronchioles contain a few alveoli along their walls and give rise to the gas-exchanging units of the lung: the *alveolar ducts* and the *alveolar sacs*. The pulmonary alveolus is lined by two types of epithelial cells (pneumocytes). Type 1 pneumocytes are flattened squamous cells covering 95% of the alveolar surface area and are invisible by light microscopy. These cells are incapable of mitosis or repair. The rarer type 2 pneumocytes are cuboidal cells, which are visible under light microscopy and are capable of mitosis. Type 2 pneumocytes are the source of new type 1 pneumocytes and provide a mechanism for repair following alveolar damage. These cells are also thought to be the source of alveolar surfactant, a phospholipid that lowers the surface tension of alveolar walls and prevents alveolar collapse at low lung volumes.

Pulmonary subsegmental anatomy is discussed in Chapter 17, along with the HRCT description of these anatomic structures.

Fissures. The interlobar pulmonary fissures represent invaginations of the visceral pleura deep into the substance of the lung (Fig. 12.6) (10). These fissures may completely or incompletely separate the lobes from one another. An incomplete fissure has important consequences regarding interlobar spread of parenchymal consolidation, collateral air drift in patients with lobar bronchial obstruction,

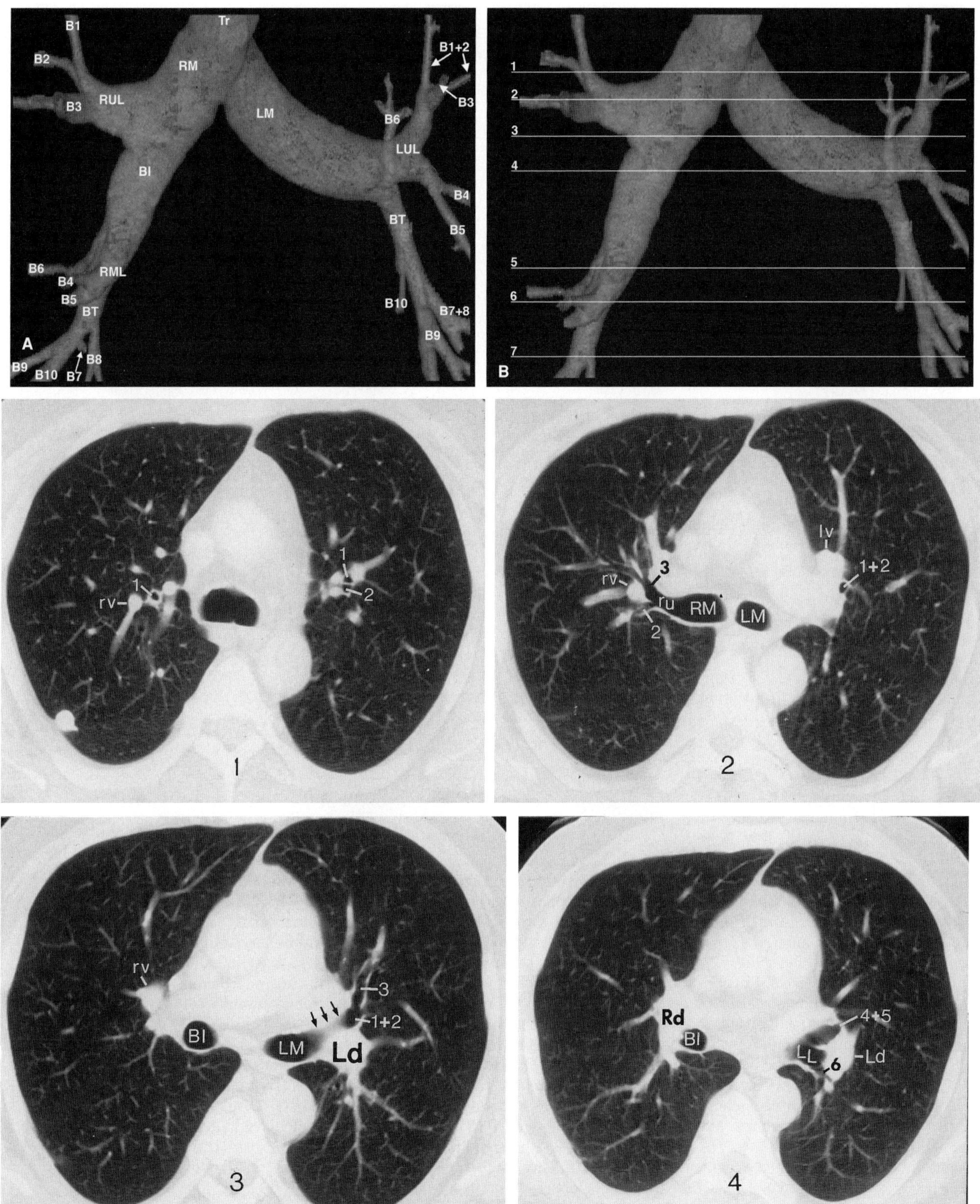

FIGURE 12.5. **Tracheobronchial and Hilar Anatomy. A.** Three-dimensional volume-rendered virtual bronchographic view of the bronchial tree. Tr, trachea; RM, right main bronchus; LM, left main bronchus; RUL, right upper lobe; RML, right middle lobe; LUL, left upper lobe; BI, bronchus intermedius; BT, basal trunk. **B.** Levels of the CT images depicting the bronchial and hilar anatomy. *(continued)*

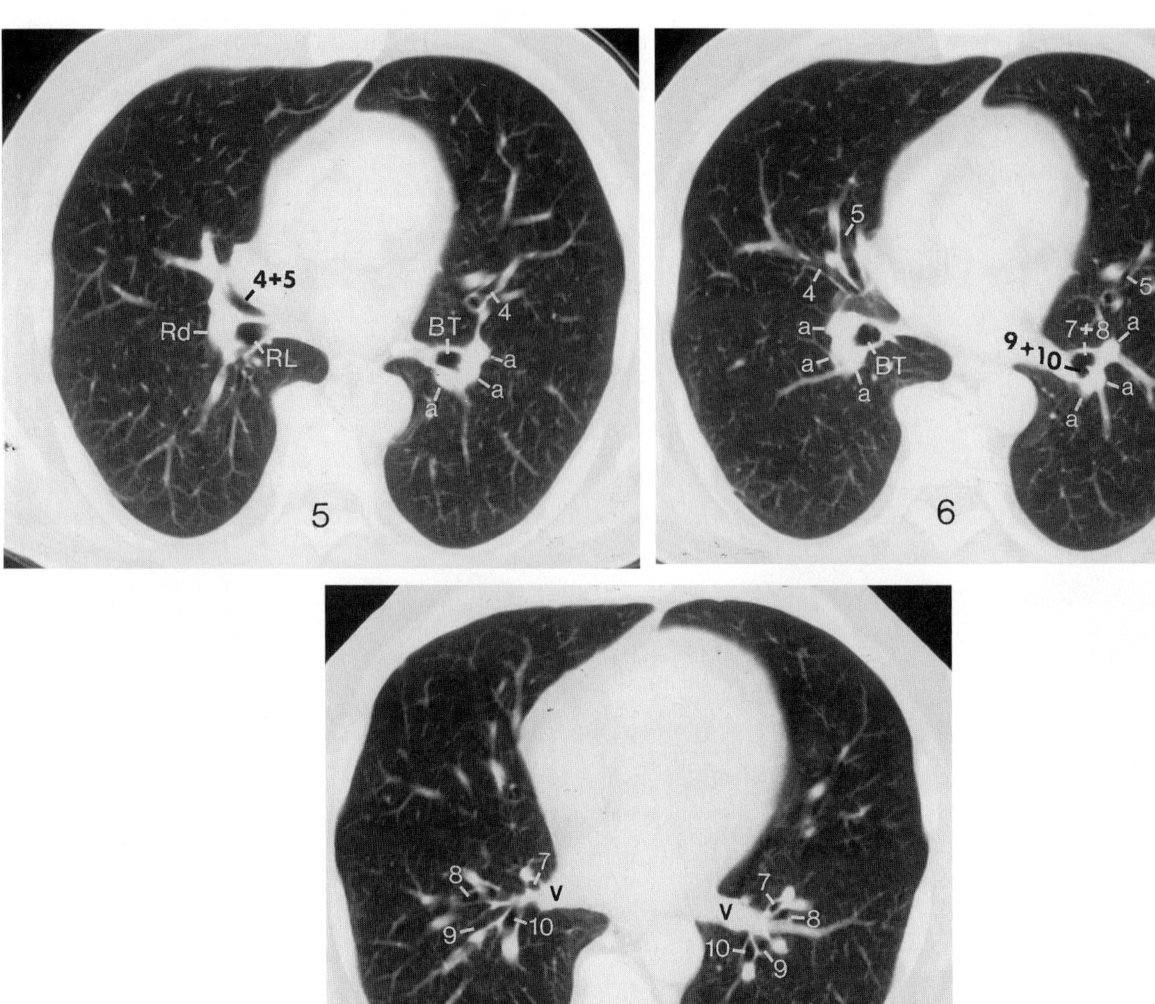

FIGURE 12.5. (*Continued*) **1. Level of tracheal carina.** Right apical bronchus (1); right superior posterior pulmonary vein (rv); left apicoposterior bronchus (1 and 2 on the left). **2. Level of right upper lobe bronchus.** Right main bronchus (RM); right upper lobe bronchus (ru); right upper lobe anterior (3) and posterior (2) segmental bronchi; right superior pulmonary vein (rv); left main bronchus (LM); left apicoposterior segmental bronchus (1+2); left superior pulmonary vein (lv). **3. Level of left upper lobe bronchus, superior division.** Bronchus intermedius (BI), with its posterior border at the level of the left main (LM); right superior pulmonary vein (rv); superior division of left upper lobe bronchus (*small arrows*); left upper lobe anterior (3) and apicoposterior (1+2) segmental bronchi; left descending pulmonary artery (Ld). **4. Level of left upper lobe bronchus, inferior (lingular) division.** Bronchus intermedius (BI); right descending pulmonary artery (Rd); lingular bronchus (4+5); left lower lobe bronchus (LL); left lower lobe superior segmental bronchus (6); left descending pulmonary artery (Ld). **5. Level of middle lobe bronchus.** Middle lobe bronchus (4+5); right lower lobe bronchus (RL); right descending pulmonary artery (Rd); lingular superior segmental bronchus (4); left lower lobe basal trunk (BT); left lower lobe segmental arteries (a). **6. Level of lower lobe basal trunks.** Lateral (4) and medial (5) segmental bronchi of the middle lobe; right lower lobe basal trunk (BT); right lower lobe basal segmental arteries (a, on right); lingular segmental bronchus (5); left lower lobe anteromedial segmental bronchus (7+8); left lower lobe lateral and posterior basal segmental bronchi (9+10); left lower lobe basal segmental arteries (a, on left).**7. Level of basal segmental bronchi.** Right lower lobe medial (7, on right), anterior (8, on right), lateral (9, on right), and posterior (10, on right) basal segmental bronchi; right inferior pulmonary vein (v, on right); left lower lobe medial (7, on left), anterior (8, on left), lateral (9, on left), and posterior (10, on left) basal segmental bronchi; left inferior pulmonary vein (v, on left).

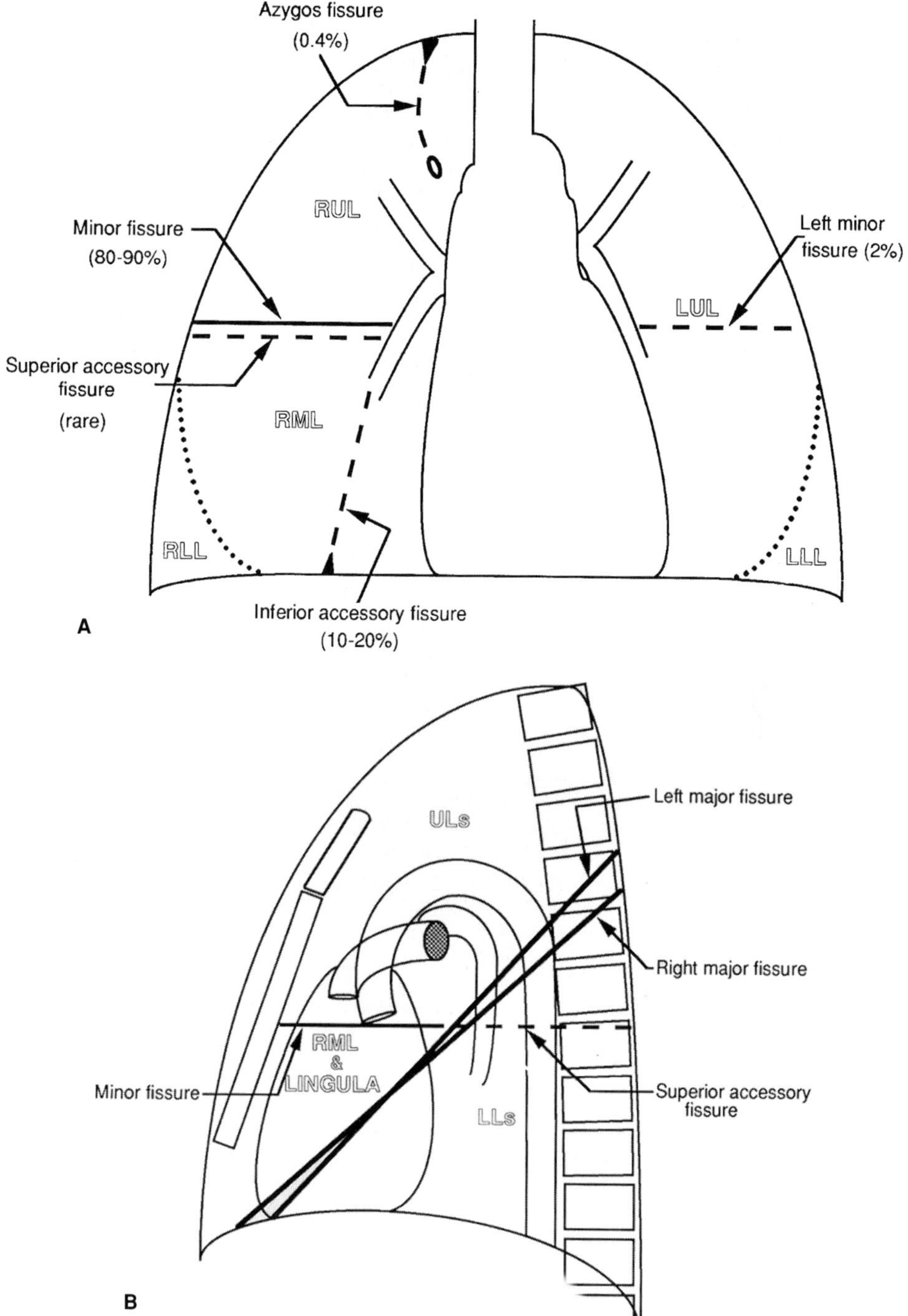

FIGURE 12.6. **Normal Lobar and Fissural Anatomy. A.** Frontal view. **B.** Lateral view. RUL, right upper lobe; LUL, left upper lobe; RML, right middle lobe; RLL, right lower lobe; LLL, left lower lobe; ULs, upper lobes; LLs, lower lobes.

and the appearance of pleural effusion in the supine patient. The fissures are well delineated on CT or HRCT (Fig. 12.7).

In most individuals, there are two interlobar fissures on the right and one on the left. The fissures are complete laterally and incomplete medially, fusing with the adjacent lobe. The *minor fissure* is complete in about 25% of individuals but fuses with the RUL in about 50%. The inferior fissure of the right middle lobe (RML) is well developed and there is very little fusion between the RML and the RLL. This oblique fissure is complete in less than 35% of individuals, with fusion between the lobes most common along the posteromedial portion of the fissure. The *left major fissure* is similar to the *right major fissure,* with fusion along the posterior aspect in approximately 35% of individuals.

The major and minor fissures are best visualized on lateral radiographs. Variable portions of the major fissures

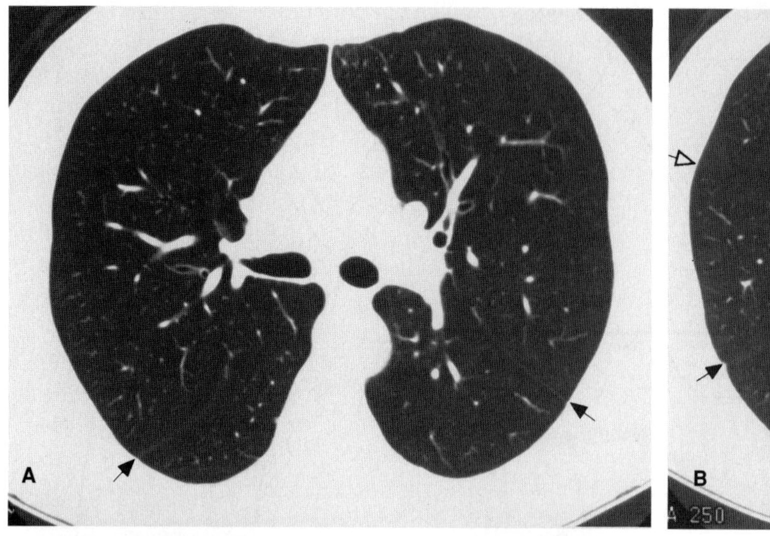

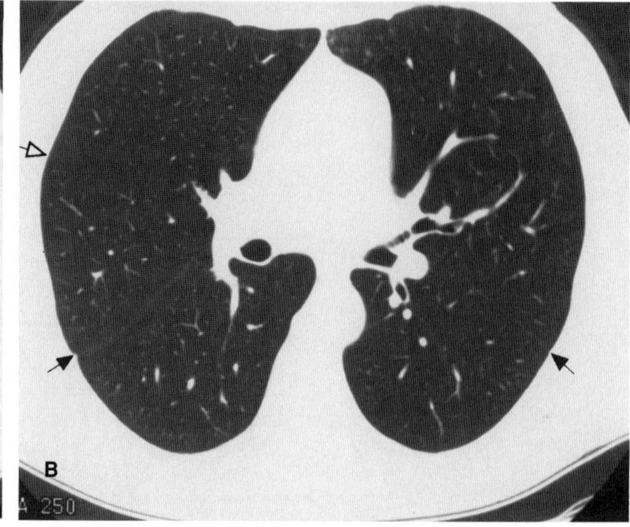

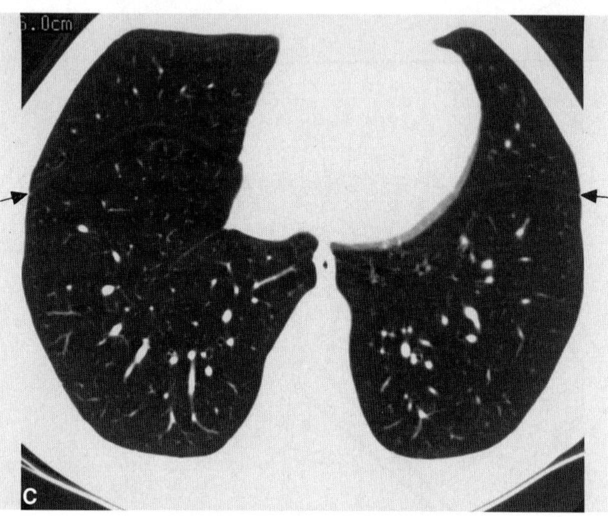

FIGURE 12.7. **Fissural Anatomy on HRCT.** The oblique fissures appear as thin curvilinear lines (*solid arrows*) concave anteriorly in the upper thorax **(A)**, flat lines in the midthorax **(B)**, and convex anterior lines in the lower chest **(C).** The apex of the domed minor fissure is seen as an avascular zone in the midthorax (*open arrow* in **B**).

are seen as obliquely oriented, thin white lines coursing anteroinferiorly from posterior to anterior. The left major fissure usually begins more superiorly and has a slightly more vertical course than the right major fissure. At their points of contact with the diaphragm or chest wall, the fissures often have a triangular configuration, with the apex of the triangle pointing toward the fissure. This appearance is the result of the presence of a small amount of fat within the distal aspect of the fissure. Although the major fissures are not usually visualized on frontal radiographs because of their oblique course relative to the x-ray beam, occasional extrapleural fat infiltration along their superolateral aspect can give rise to a curvilinear edge in the upper thorax. The minor fissure projects at the level of the right fourth rib and is seen as a thin undulating line on frontal radiographs in approximately 50% of individuals. On a lateral radiograph, the minor fissure is often seen as a thin curvilinear line with a convex superior margin. Not uncommonly, the posterior aspect of the minor fissure extends posterior to the margin of the right major fissure. This is because the minor fissure abuts the entire convexity of the anterior lower lobe, but the major fissure interface is caused by the crest of the convexity.

The *inferior accessory fissure* is the most common accessory fissure and is found in approximately 10% to 20% of individuals. This fissure, which separates the medial basal from the remaining basal segments of the lower lobe, is often incomplete (Fig. 12.6). It may be seen on frontal radiographs as a thin curvilinear line extending superiorly from the medial third of the hemidiaphragm toward the lower hilum. The inferior accessory fissure has been misidentified as the inferior pulmonary ligament (invisible on normal chest radiographs) and is responsible for the juxtaphrenic peak described in upper lobe volume loss. A small triangle of extrapleural fat, seen at its point of insertion on the diaphragm, helps identify the inferior accessory fissure. An inferior accessory fissure can be seen on CT scans through the lower thorax, where it is identified

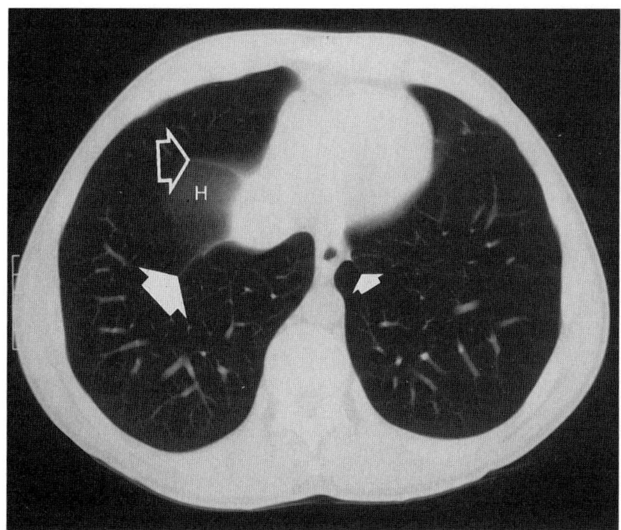

FIGURE 12.8. **Inferior Pulmonary and Pericardiophrenic Ligaments.** A CT scan just above the diaphragm demonstrates a thin line (*small solid arrow*) extending posterolaterally at the level of the esophagus that represents the sublobar septum extending to the inferior pulmonary ligament. On the right, a curvilinear line (*large solid arrow*) extending from just lateral to the inferior vena cava represents the right pericardiophrenic ligament containing branches of the phrenic nerve and pericardiophrenic vessels. More anteriorly, a thin line (*open arrow*) is seen just above the apex of the right hemidiaphragm (H), which represents fat within the inferior aspect of the major fissure.

as a curvilinear line extending anterolaterally from just in front of the inferior pulmonary ligament toward the major fissure.

The *azygos fissure* is seen in 0.5% of individuals (Fig. 12.6). It is composed of four layers of pleura (two visceral, two parietal) and represents an invagination of the right apical pleura by the azygos vein, which has incompletely migrated to its normal position at the right tracheobronchial angle. The azygos fissure appears as a vertical curvilinear line, convex laterally, which extends inferiorly from the lung apex and ends in a teardrop, which is the azygos vein. The significance of this fissure lies in its ability to limit the spread of apical segmental consolidation to the azygos lobe (that portion of the apical segment delineated by the azygos fissure) and in excluding pneumothorax from the apical portion of the pleural space.

The *superior accessory fissure* separates the superior segment from the basal segments of the lower lobe. On the right side it may be distinguished from the minor fissure on lateral radiographs, because it extends posteriorly from the major fissure to the chest wall.

The *left minor fissure* is a rarely seen normal variant that separates the lingula from the remaining portions of the upper lobe.

Ligaments. The *inferior pulmonary ligament* is a sheet of connective tissue that extends from the hilum superiorly to a level at or just above the hemidiaphragm. Thus, it comprises fused visceral and parietal pleura and binds the lower lobe to the mediastinum and runs alongside the esophagus. The ligament contains the inferior pulmonary vein superiorly and a variable number of lymph nodes. The inferior pulmonary ligament is sometimes seen on CT scans through the lower thorax as a small laterally directed beak of mediastinal pleura adjacent to the esophagus (Fig. 12.8). The tethering effect of this ligament on the lower lobe accounts for the medial location and triangular appearance of lower lobe collapse. The ligament may also act as a barrier to the spread of pleural and mediastinal fluid and may marginate medial pleural or mediastinal air collections to produce a characteristic appearance on radiographs.

The *sublobar septum* (Fig. 12.8) has been mistaken for the inferior pulmonary ligament. It is a linear structure seen on CT near the inferior pulmonary ligament extending into the lung from the mediastinal pleura.

The *pericardiophrenic ligament* is a triangular density extending toward the lung that is seen along the posterior aspect of the right heart border on lung windows on chest CT (Fig. 12.8). It represents a reflection of pleura over the inferior portion of the phrenic nerve and pericardiophrenic vessels. It is distinguished from the sublobar septum by its more anterior location and by its characteristic ramifications as branches of the nerve and vessel reflect over the hemidiaphragm.

Pulmonary Arteries (Fig. 12.9A-C) (11). The pulmonary artery is an elastic artery that arises from the right ventricle approximately the 1:00 position relative to the ascending aorta. These two structures then rotate from right to left until the pulmonary artery lies at the 5:00 position. The left pulmonary artery is a direct continuation of the main pulmonary artery. The right artery branches just below the carina, with an angle close to 90°. Within the left hilum, the artery envelopes the upper margin of the left main bronchus, at which point it divides into the upper and lower lobe arteries. The arch formed by the left lower lobe artery over the left hilar bronchi (i.e., the bronchus is hypoarterial) is easily seen on the lateral view. On the other hand, the right pulmonary artery courses laterally and anterior to the main bronchus. The right artery divides within the pericardium into the truncus anterior and interlobar arteries. In contradistinction to the left side, the right interlobar artery courses anterolateral to the bronchus (i.e., the bronchus is epi arterial). The different spatial relationships are essential when determining bronchial and pulmonary situs. At the same level that the bronchi lose their cartilage and become bronchioles, the elastic arteries lose their elastic lamina and become muscular arteries. Thickening of the alveolocapillary membrane from edema fluid or

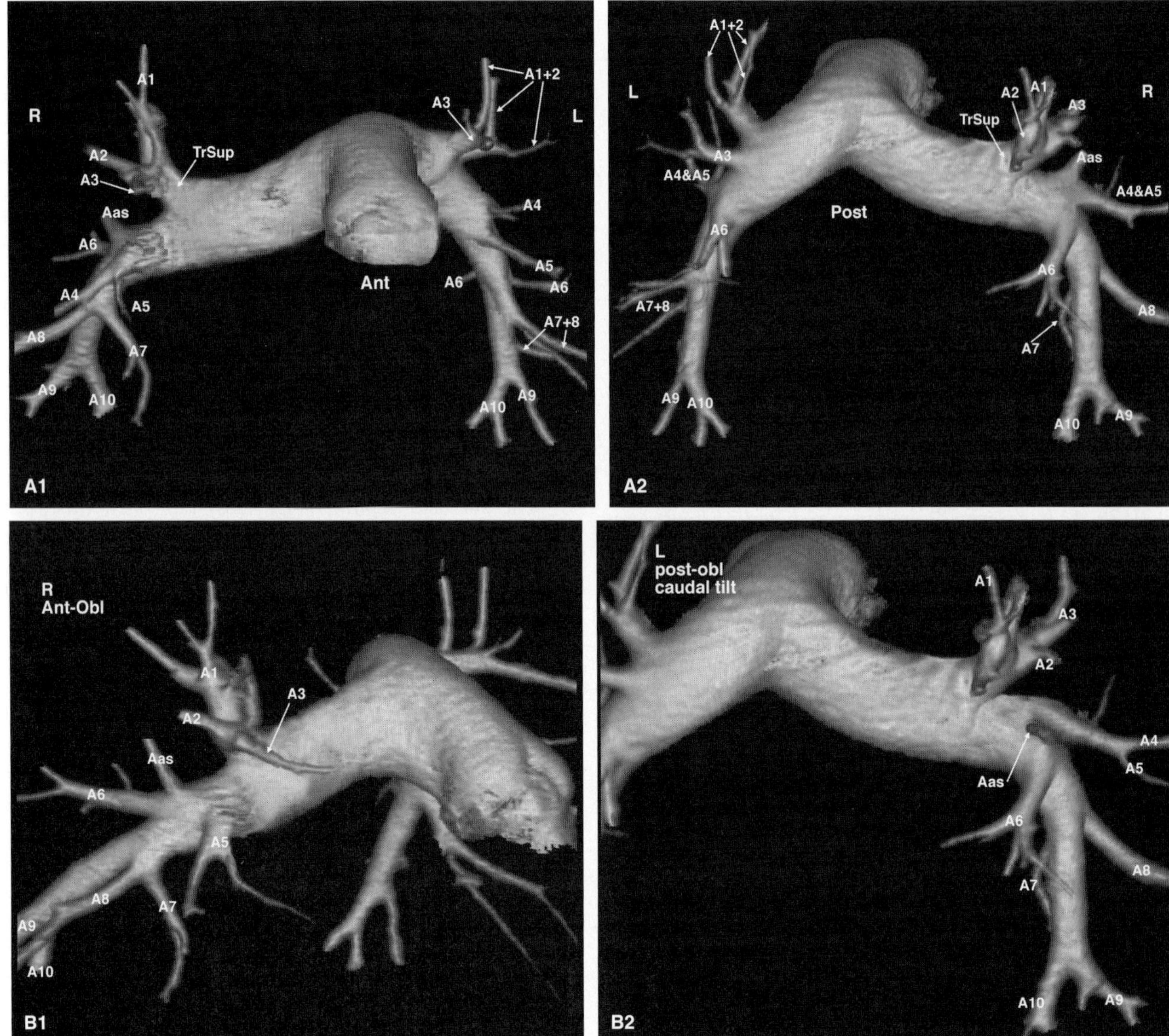

FIGURE 12.9. **Prevailing Pattern of Segmental Arteries and Venous Returns.** Three-dimensional volume-rendered images of the pulmonary arterial system in different views depict the most usual arterial anatomy. The branches of the right and left pulmonary arteries accompany and divide in parallel with the corresponding bronchi. **A.** Left and right pulmonary arteries, (1) anterior view; (2) posterior view. **B.** Right pulmonary artery, (1) anterior view; (2) posterior view. **C.** Left pulmonary artery, (1) anterior view; (2) posterior view. TrSup, truncus superior; A1, apical (upper lobe); A2, posterior (upper lobe); A3, anterior (upper lobe); A4, lateral (middle lobe) and superior (lingula); A5, medial (middle lobe) and inferior (lingula); A6, superior (lower lobe); A7, medial basal (lower lobe); A8, anterior basal (lower lobe); A9, lateral basal (lower lobe); A10, posterior basal (lower lobe). Note that the right upper lobe receives an accessory branch from the proximal right interlobar pulmonary artery (Aas). **D.** Left atrium and venous returns, (1) anterior view; (2) posterior view. Three-dimensional volume-rendered images of the left atrium and venous returns depict the most usual venous return anatomy. Significantly more variation exists than in the bronchial/arterial systems. Although only the main returns are depicted here, the reader will find an extensive discussion in Yamashita (11). RSup, Right superior venous return; LSup, left superior venous return; RInf, right inferior venous return; LInf, left inferior venous return. Several branches can join the left atrium separate from their lobar venous return. The most common ones are RSup (RML), right middle lobe branch of the RSup; LInf(SupSeg) and RInf(SupSeg), branches from the superior segments of the lower lobes. Lapp, Left atrial appendage; MV, mitral valve plane.

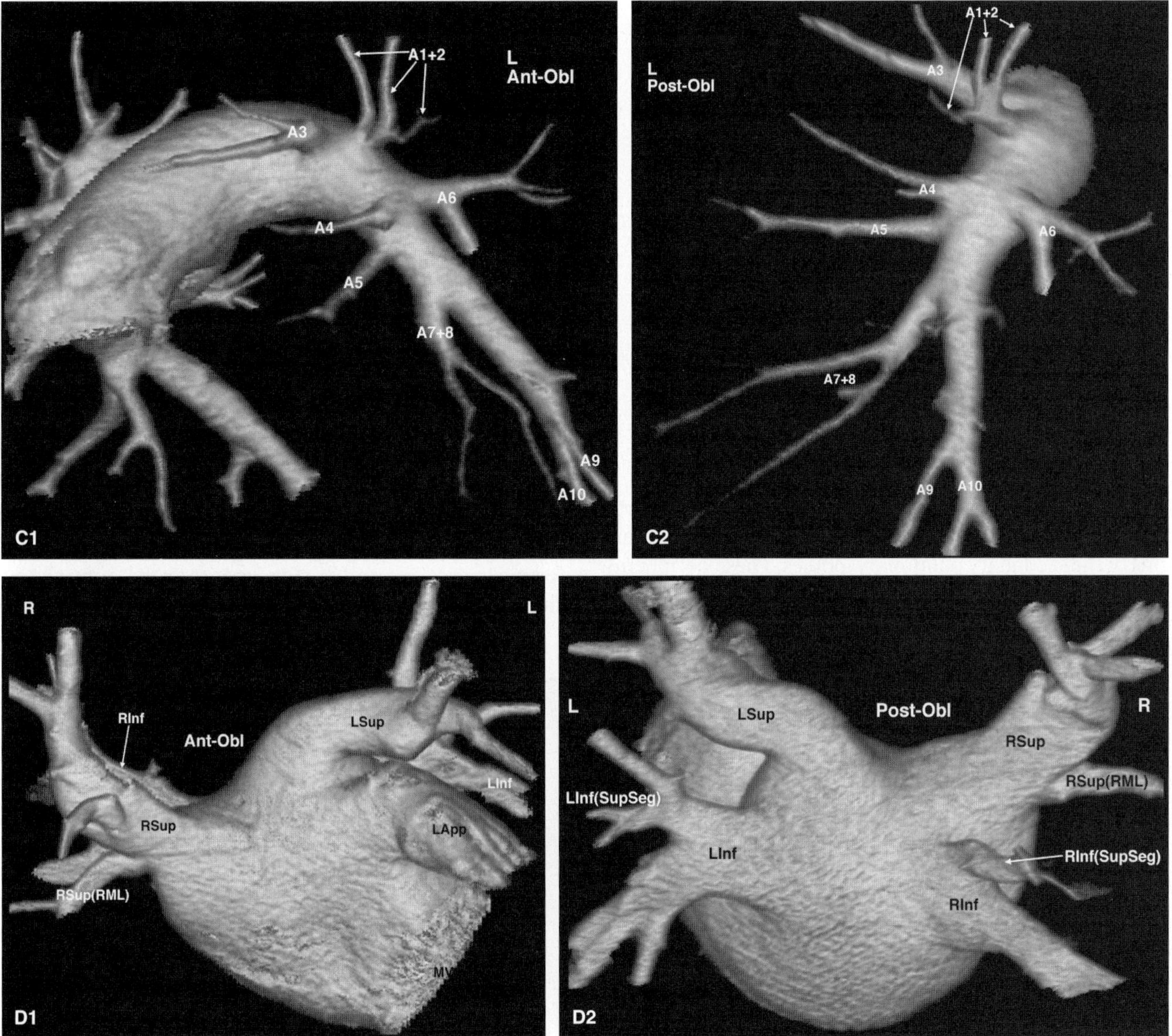

FIGURE 12.9. (*Continued*)

fibrosis impedes gas exchange and results in dyspnea and hypoxemia.

Bronchial arteries are the primary nutrient vessels of the lung. They supply blood to the bronchial walls to the level of the terminal bronchioles. In addition, several mediastinal structures receive a variable amount of blood supply from the bronchial circulation. These include the tracheal wall, middle third of the esophagus, visceral pleura, mediastinal lymph nodes, vagus nerve, pericardium, and thymus.

The bronchial arteries usually arise from the proximal descending thoracic aorta at the level of the carina but may show significant variability. Most commonly there are one right-sided and two left-sided arteries. The right bronchial artery usually arises from the posterolateral wall of the aorta in common with an intercostal artery as an intercostobronchial trunk. The left bronchial arteries arise individually from the anterolateral aorta or, rarely, from an intercostal artery. Approximately two thirds of the blood from the bronchial arterial system returns to the pulmonary venous system via the bronchial veins (a small right-to-left shunt). The remaining blood, which includes veins draining the large bronchi, tracheal bifurcation, and mediastinum, drains into the azygos or hemiazygos systems.

Pulmonary veins (Fig. 12.9D) arise within the interlobular septa from the alveolar and visceral pleural capillaries. The veins travel in connective tissue envelopes that are separate from the bronchoarterial trunks. The pulmonary veins, which may number from three to eight, drain into the left atrium.

Pulmonary lymphatics help clear fluid and particulate matter from the pulmonary interstitium. There are two major lymphatic pathways in the lung and pleura. The visceral pleural lymphatics, which reside in the vascular

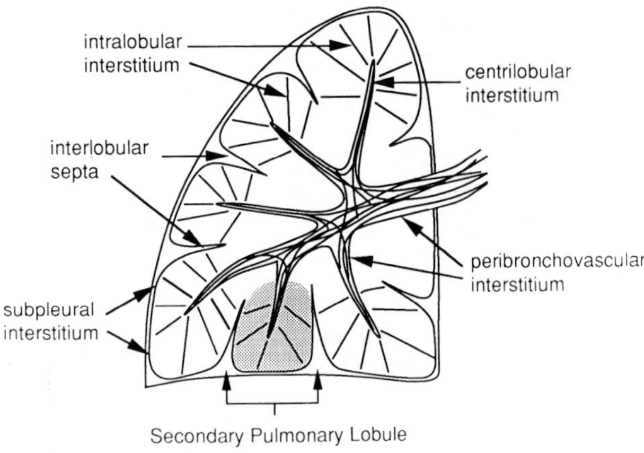

FIGURE 12.10. **Diagram of the Pulmonary Interstitium.**

(innermost) layer of the visceral pleura, form a network over the surface of the lung that roughly parallels the margins of the secondary pulmonary lobules. These peripheral lymphatics penetrate the lung to course centrally within interlobular septa, along with the pulmonary veins, toward the hilum. The parenchymal lymphatics originate in proximity to the alveolar septa ("juxta-alveolar lymphatics") and course centrally with the bronchoarterial bundle. The perivenous and bronchoarterial lymphatics communicate via obliquely oriented lymphatics located within the central regions of the lung. These perivenous lymphatics and their surrounding connective tissue, when distended by fluid, account for the radiographic appearance of Kerley A lines.

Pulmonary interstitium is the scaffolding of the lung and as such provides support for the airways and pulmonary vessels (Fig. 12.10) (10). It begins within the hilum and extends peripherally to the visceral pleura. The interstitial compartment that extends from the mediastinum and envelopes the bronchovascular bundles is termed the *axial interstitium*. The axial fiber system continues distally as the *centrilobular interstitium* along with the arterioles, capillaries, and bronchioles to provide support for the air-exchanging portions of the lung. The *subpleural interstitium* and interlobular septa are parts of the *peripheral interstitium,* which divides secondary pulmonary lobules. The pulmonary veins and lymphatics lie within the peripheral interstitium. The *intralobular interstitium* is a thin network of fibers that bridges the gap between the centrilobular and peripheral compartments.

Edema involving the axial interstitium is recognized radiographically as peribronchial cuffing. Pathologic involvement of the intralobular interstitium is difficult to discern radiographically, but may account for some cases of so-called "ground-glass" opacity on chest radiographs and HRCT scans. Thickening of portions of this interstitium are occasionally seen as intralobular lines on HRCT. Radiographically, edema of the peripheral and subpleural interstitium accounts for Kerley B lines (or interlobular lines on HRCT) and "thickened" fissures on chest radiographs.

Posteroanterior Chest Radiograph

A firm knowledge of the normal anatomy displayed on the frontal (usually PA) chest radiograph is key to detecting and localizing pathologic conditions and to avoid mistaking normal structures for pathologic findings.

Soft tissues of the chest wall consist of the skin, subcutaneous fat, and muscles. The lateral edges of the sternocleidomastoid muscles are readily visible in most patients. The visualization of normal fat in the supraclavicular fossae and the companion shadows of skin and subcutaneous fat paralleling the clavicles helps exclude mass, adenopathy, or edema in this region. The inferolateral edge of the pectoralis major muscle is normally seen curving toward the axilla. Both breast shadows should be evaluated routinely to detect evidence of prior mastectomy or distorting mass. The soft tissues lateral to the bony thorax should be smooth, symmetric, homogeneous densities.

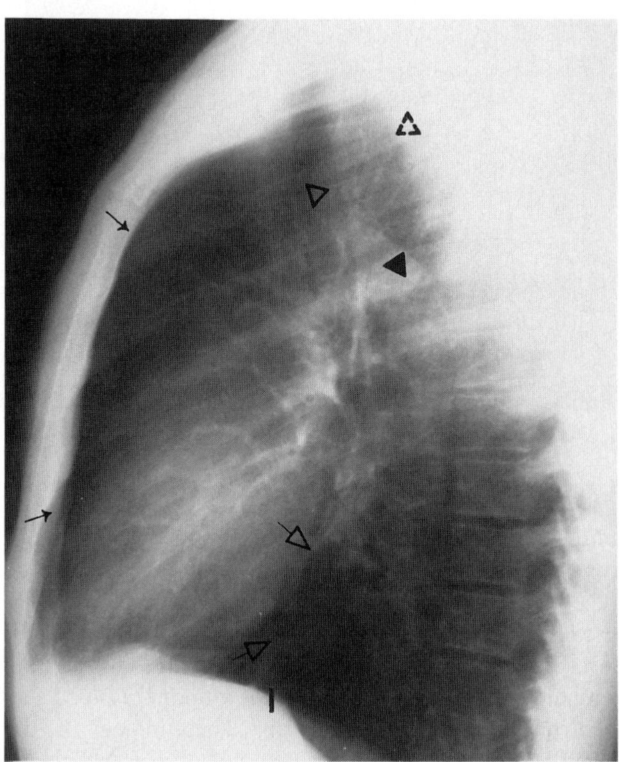

FIGURE 12.11. **Radiolucent Spaces on Lateral Chest Radiographs.** The retrosternal space is demarcated anteriorly by the posterior margin of the sternum (*small arrows*) and the heart and ascending aorta posteriorly and accounts for the anterior junction line seen on frontal radiographs. The retrotracheal triangle is marginated by the posterior wall of the trachea anteriorly (*open triangle*), the spine posteriorly (*broken triangle*), and the aortic arch inferiorly (*solid triangle*). The retrocardiac space is demarcated anteriorly by the posterior cardiac margin (*upper open arrow*) and the inferior vena cava (*I, lower open arrow*).

Bones. The thoracic spine, ribs and costal cartilages, clavicles, and scapulae are routinely visible on frontal chest radiographs. The bodies of the thoracic vertebrae should be vertically aligned, with endplates, pedicles, and spinous processes visualized. Twelve pairs of symmetric ribs should be seen; the upper ribs have smooth superior and inferior cortical margins, while the middle and lower ribs have flanged inferior cortices where the intercostal neurovascular bundles run. Cervical ribs are identified in approximately 2% of individuals and may be associated with symptoms of thoracic outlet syndrome. Companion shadows paralleling the inferior margins of the first and second ribs represent extrapleural fat, which may be abundant in obese individuals. Costal cartilage calcification is seen in a majority of adults, increases in prevalence with advancing age, and can add multiple shadows to the PA view. Men typically show calcification at the upper and lower margins, while the majority of women develop central cartilaginous calcification.

Lung–Lung Interfaces. A familiarity with the normal mediastinal interfaces is key to the interpretation of frontal chest radiographs (2). The lung–mediastinal interfaces are seen as sharp edges where the lung and adjacent pleura reflect off of various mediastinal structures. The lung–lung interfaces as seen on frontal radiographs relate directly to the space available in three regions viewed on the lateral film: the retrosternal space, the retrotracheal triangle, and the retrocardiac space (Fig. 12.11).

The retrosternal airspace reflects contact of the anterosuperior aspect of the upper lobes (Fig. 12.11). On frontal radiographs the *anterior junction line* is seen as a thin vertical line that overlies the thoracic spine (Fig. 12.12). The anterior junction anatomy is an inferior extension of the upper lobe reflections off the innominate veins, with the latter producing an inverted V-shaped retromanubrial opacity. The anterior junction line often disappears after sternotomy, or when abundant anterior mediastinal fat precludes retrosternal contact of the upper lobes.

A second potential lung–lung interface is seen on the lateral chest radiograph as the *retrotracheal triangle,* a radiolucent region representing contact of the posterosuperior portions of the upper lobes (Fig. 12.11). If the retrotracheal space available is small, only a right paraesophageal interface is visualized on the PA view (Fig. 12.13). If the space is large, a posterior junction line is seen (Figs. 12.12, 12.13) (Table 12.4).

The third potential lung–lung interface occurs in the *retrocardiac space* (Fig. 12.11). If that space is large, the azygoesophageal recess of the RLL can abut the preaortic recess of the left lower lobe to produce an inferior *posterior junction line* (Fig. 12.13).

Lung–Mediastinal Interfaces (Table 12.5). The right lateral margin of the superior vena cava is commonly seen as a straight or slightly concave interface with the RUL extending from the level of the clavicle to the superior margin of the right atrium. Prominence or convexity of the

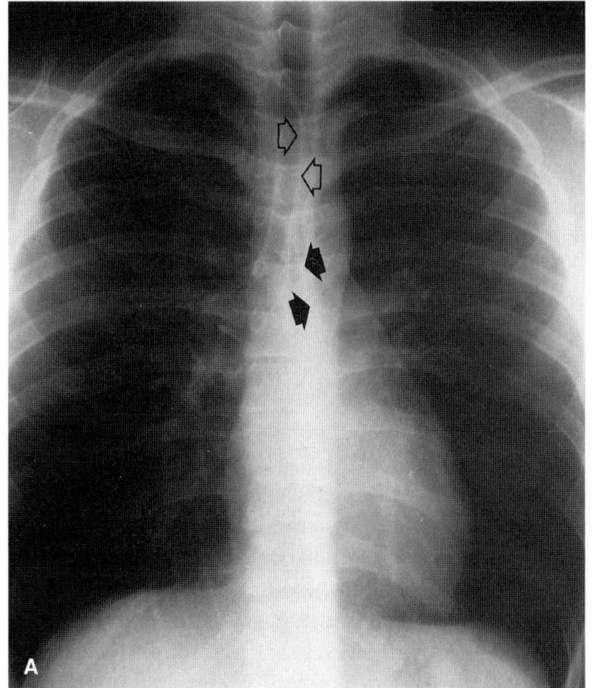

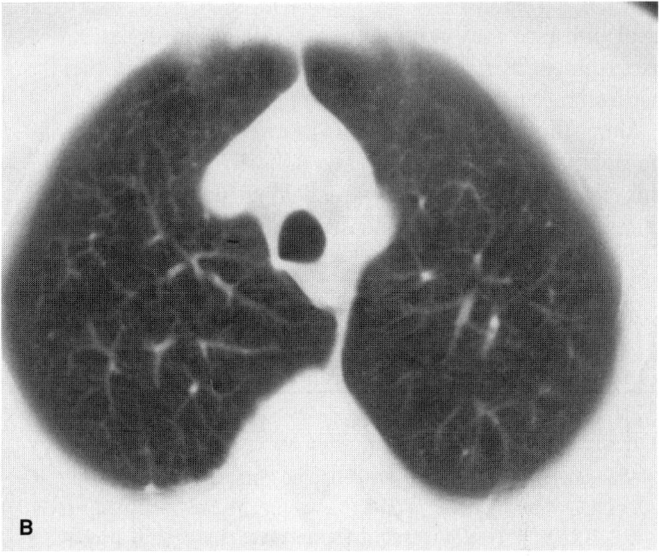

FIGURE 12.12. **Anterior and Posterior Junction Lines. A.** A posteroanterior chest film shows both anterior (*solid arrows*) and posterior (*open arrows*) junction lines. **B.** CT through the upper thorax in another patient shows the anterior junction line in the retrosternal space, while the posterior junction line lies in the retrotracheal space.

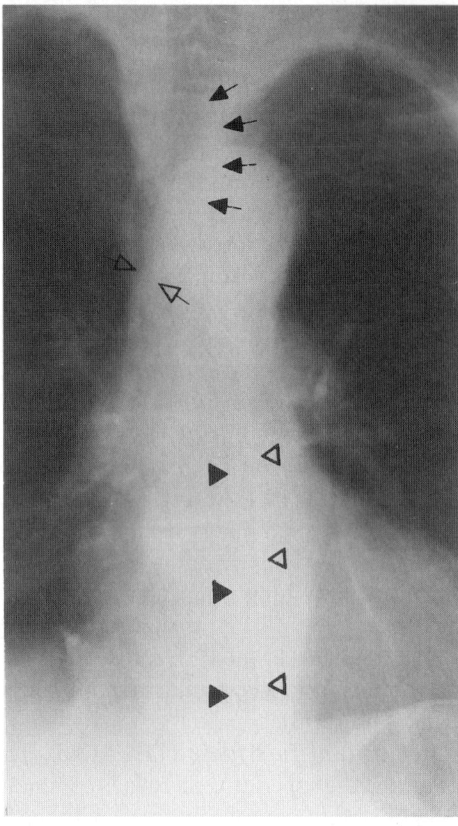

FIGURE 12.13. **Lung–Lung Interfaces on a Frontal Radiograph.** Coned down view of a PA film shows the right paraesophageal interface (*solid arrows*). The azygos arch (*open arrows*) separates the supra-azygos lung from the infra-azygos lung, which creates the azygoesophageal recess interface (*solid triangles*). The retrocardiac left lung creates the preaortic recess interface (*open triangles*).

caval interface may represent caval dilatation or lateral displacement by a dilated or tortuous aortic arch or other mediastinal mass.

Along the right upper mediastinum, the RUL contacts the right lateral tracheal wall in a majority of individuals. This produces the right paratracheal stripe (Fig. 12.4A). The thickness of this line, measured above the level of the azygos vein, should not exceed 4 mm. Thickening or nodularity of the paratracheal stripe is seen in abnormalities of the tissues comprising the strip, including tracheal tumors, paratracheal lymph node enlargement, and right pleural effusion (Fig. 12.2).

TABLE 12.4 Anterior and Posterior Junction Lines

Line	*Features*
Anterior junction line	Obliquely oriented from right superior to left inferior Extends from upper sternum to base of heart
Posterior junction line	Vertically oriented in the midline Extends from upper thoracic spine to level of azygos and aortic arches

TABLE 12.5 Normal Lung–Mediastinal Interfaces

Right-sided	Right paraesophageal interface Superior vena cava/right paratracheal stripe Anterior arch of the azygos vein Right paraspinal interface Azygoesophageal recess Lateral margin of right atrium Confluence of right pulmonary veins (right border of left atrium) Lateral margin of inferior vena cava
Left-sided	Lateral margin of left subclavian artery Transverse aortic arch Left superior intercostal vein ("aortic nipple") Aortopulmonary window interface Aortopulmonary interface Lateral margin of main pulmonary artery Preaortic recess Left paraspinal interface Left atrial appendage Left ventricle Epipericardial fat pad

The arch of the azygos vein separates the right paraesophageal from the upper azygos esophageal space (Fig. 12.13). The measurement should be made through the midpoint of the azygos arch perpendicular to the right main bronchus. Supine positioning or performance of the Müller maneuver (forced inspiration against a closed glottis) will increase azygos venous diameter. In general, a diameter of >10 mm on a PA radiograph should raise the possibility of mass, adenopathy, or dilatation of the azygos vein; the latter may be seen with right heart failure, obstruction of venous return to the heart, or a congenital venous anomaly such as azygos continuation of the inferior vena cava. An increase in diameter of the azygos vein from prior comparable radiographs is more important than the actual measurement.

The *azygoesophageal recess* interface is a vertically oriented interface overlying the thoracic spine. (Fig. 12.13). While normally straight or concave in contour, the middle third of the interface may have a slight rightward convexity at the level of the right inferior pulmonary veins. Convexity of the superior third of the interface should suggest subcarinal lymph node enlargement or a mass. Convexity of the middle third of this recess is usually a result of the confluence of right pulmonary veins or the right border of the left atrium. Left atrial dilatation will enlarge and laterally displace this interface, producing a double-density interface composed of the right lateral borders of both the right and the left atria. Convexity of the inferior third is most commonly due to a sliding hiatal hernia.

Occasionally a tortuous descending aorta or enlarged paraesophageal lymph nodes can cause this recess to be convex to the right in its lower third. When air is present in the distal portion of the esophagus and the azygoesophageal recess interfaces with the right lateral wall of the esophagus, a line (the right inferior esophagopleural stripe) rather than an edge is seen.

The *paraspinal interface* is a straight, vertical interface extending the length of the right hemithorax and represents contact of the right lung with a small amount of tissue lateral to the thoracic spine. It is inconsistently visualized on the right side. A focal convexity of this interface suggests spinal or paraspinal disease.

The right heart projects just to the right of the lateral margin of the thoracic spine on a normal PA radiograph (Fig. 12.11). This portion of the heart is the lateral margin of the right atrium, which creates a smooth convex interface with the medial segment of the middle lobe. Individuals with pectus excavatum have leftward cardiac displacement and may not demonstrate this interface. In patients with right atrial dilatation, this interface may extend well into the right lung.

The right lateral border of the inferior vena cava may be seen at the level of the right hemidiaphragm as a concave lateral interface. The inferior vena caval interface is best visualized on lateral radiographs (Fig. 12.11). This interface may be absent in patients with azygos continuation of the inferior vena cava.

In the uppermost portion of the left mediastinum, one or more interfaces may be recognized cephalad to the aortic arch. The interface most often visualized is the subclavian artery (Fig. 12.14). It is unusual for the LUL to interface with the left lateral wall of the trachea to form the left paratracheal stripe, because the subclavian artery and adjacent fat usually intervene.

The transverse portion of the aortic arch ("aortic knob") creates a small convex indentation on the left lung in normal individuals (Fig. 12.14). As the aorta elongates and dilates with age, this interface projects more laterally, and lung may be seen to encircle a greater circumference of the knob.

In approximately 5% of individuals, the left superior intercostal vein may be seen on frontal radiographs as a rounded or triangular opacity that focally indents the lung immediately superolateral to the aortic arch. This density, termed the "aortic nipple" (Fig 12.15), represents the superior intercostal vein as it arches anteriorly from its paraspinal position around the aortic arch to drain into the posterior aspect of the left innominate vein. This structure, which normally measures <5 mm, may enlarge with elevation of right atrial pressure or with congenital or acquired obstruction of venous return to the right heart.

Immediately inferior to the aortic arch, the LUL contacts the mediastinum to produce the *aortopulmonary*

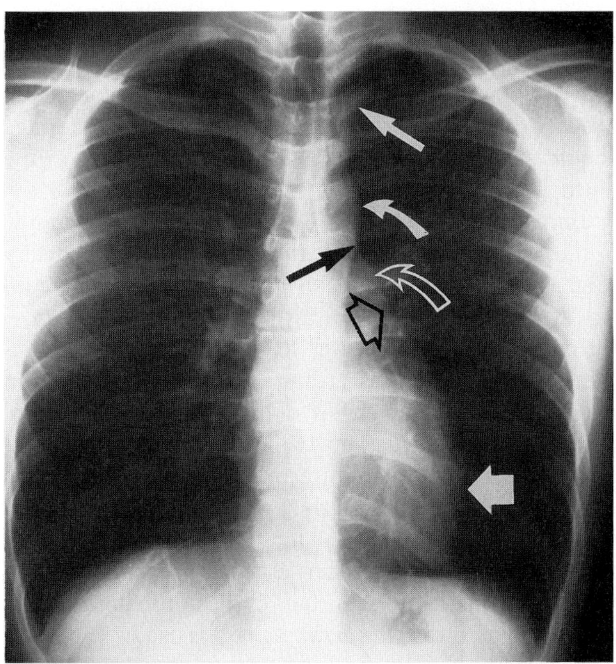

FIGURE 12.14. **Lung–Mediastinal Interfaces, Left Side.** Posteroanterior chest radiograph shows the normal contours along the left mediastinum (from superior to inferior): left subclavian artery (*long straight white arrow*), aortic knob (*curved white arrow*), aortopulmonary window (*straight black arrow*), main pulmonary artery (*curved open white arrow*), left atrial appendage (*open black arrow*), and left ventricle (*solid white arrow*).

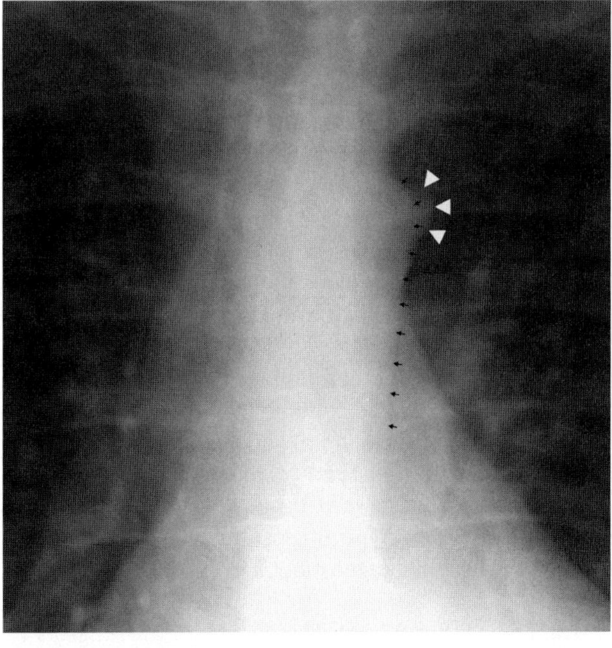

FIGURE 12.15. **Aortic Nipple.** The contour of the "aortic nipple" is formed by the left superior intercostal vein (*white arrowheads*). The small black arrows denote the contour of the aortic knob.

window interface (Fig. 12.14). This interface is usually straight or concave toward the lung; the latter appearance is seen with a tortuous aorta, emphysema, or congenital absence of the left pericardium. A convex lateral interface should suggest mass or lymph node enlargement in the aortopulmonary window.

Immediately inferior to the aortopulmonary window is the left lateral border of the main pulmonary artery (Fig. 12.14). The interface of this structure may be convex, straight, or concave toward the lung. Enlargement of the main pulmonary artery is seen as an idiopathic condition in young women, as a result of poststenotic dilatation in valvular pulmonic stenosis, or in conditions where there is increased flow or pressure in the pulmonary arterial system, such as left-to-right intracardiac shunts.

The preaortic recess interface is seen in a small percentage of normal individuals as a reflection of the LLL with the esophagus anterior to the descending aorta, extending vertically from the undersurface of the aortic knob a variable distance toward the diaphragm. It is usually etched in black (negative Mach effect).

The left paraspinal interface represents the reflection of the left lung off the paraspinal soft tissues, which largely consist of fat but also contain the sympathetic chain, proximal intercostal vessels, intercostal lymph nodes, and hemiazygos and accessory hemiazygos veins. The left paraspinal interface, which is etched in white (positive Mach effect), is seen in a majority of individuals, in contrast to the right paraspinal interface. Neurogenic tumors, hematoma, paraspinal abscess, lipomatosis, and medial pleural effusion can cause lateral displacement of this interface.

The left atrial appendage forms a concave interface immediately below the main pulmonary artery (Fig. 12.14). Straightening or convexity of this interface used to be seen commonly in rheumatic mitral valve disease but may be seen in patients with left atrial enlargement of any cause.

The left ventricle comprises most of the left heart border. A gentle convex margin with the lingula is normal (Fig. 12.14). Abnormalities of the left ventricular contour will be discussed in detail in the section on cardiovascular disease.

Fat adjacent to the cardiac apex may create a focal bulge in the left cardiac contour that obscures the heart border at the left cardiophrenic angle. This epipericardial fat pad is usually unilateral or more prominent on the left and is most often seen in obese patients and those on corticosteroids. A typical appearance on the lateral radiograph is usually diagnostic; CT is helpful in equivocal cases.

The Lungs (Fig. 12.14). The opacity of the lungs as visualized radiographically is attributable solely to the presence of the pulmonary vasculature and enveloping interstitial structures. The arteries are solid cylinders branching along the airways. Both gradually diminish in caliber as they divide. Bronchi smaller than subsegmental are not visible radiographically. The pulmonary veins can often be traced horizontally to the left atrium, whereas the arteries can be followed to their hilar origin, which lies more cephalad than the left atrium. The effects of gravity explain the predominance of vasculature in an upright patient, as well as isodistribution of vessels in the supine patient. The normal dark gray opacity of the upper lungs increases inferiorly in women as a result of summation of overlying breast tissue, or in men with prominent pectoralis muscles. The opacity of the lung may be increased by processes that render the interstitium or airspaces opaque or decreased by any process associated with diminished blood flow to the lung or destruction of parenchymal structures.

Diaphragm. The diaphragm is the major inspiratory muscle comprised of muscular origins along the costal margins and insertions into the membranous dome. The right hemidiaphragm overlies the liver, and the left hemidiaphragm overlies the stomach and spleen. On frontal radiographs exposed in deep inspiration, the apex of the right hemidiaphragm typically lies at the level of the sixth anterior rib, approximately one half interspace above the apex of the left hemidiaphragm (Fig. 12.14). A scalloped appearance to the hemidiaphragm is not uncommon. Focal bulges in the diaphragmatic contour are usually a result of acquired diaphragmatic eventration (thinning).

Upper Abdomen. Portions of the liver, spleen, and gastric fundus are routinely visualized on most frontal chest radiographs. Abnormalities of abdominal situs may be identified by noting the location and appearance of the liver, stomach, and spleen. Enlargement of the liver may cause right diaphragmatic elevation and right lateral compression of the stomach. Intrahepatic air may be seen within the biliary tree, portal vein, or a hepatic abscess. Calcified hepatic lesions or calcified gallstones overlying the lower portion of the liver may be visible. A mass arising within the gastric fundus can occasionally be seen as a soft tissue opacity protruding into a gas-filled gastric lumen. Splenomegaly may be identified by noting a soft tissue mass in the left upper quadrant that displaces the stomach bubble anteromedially and the splenic flexure of the colon inferiorly.

Lateral Chest Radiograph

The normal lateral chest film is a challenge because of summation of the right hemithorax over the left (Fig. 12.1). However, knowledge of normal lateral radiographic anatomy can greatly aid in detection and localization of parenchymal and cardiomediastinal processes (12,13).

Soft Tissues. Air outlining the anterior axillary folds may render the anterior edges of these skin folds visible overlying the superior aspect of the thorax. The edges are seen as bilateral opacities that are concave anteriorly and can be followed through the level of the thoracic inlet to merge with the soft tissues of the arms.

Bones. The anterior margins of the scapulae project as oblique straight edges overlying the superior and posterior aspects of the thorax, often over the retrotracheal triangle. The anterior and posterior cortical margins of the thoracic vertebral bodies should be aligned, forming a gradual kyphosis.

Lung Interfaces. The retrotracheal (or Raider) triangle is bordered by the posterior border of the trachea/esophagus, the anterior border of the spine, and the top of the aortic arch (Fig. 12.11). Masses and air-space disease near the apices, retrotracheal masses (e.g., aberrant subclavian artery or posterior thyroid goiter), or esophageal masses may produce an abnormal opacity in this region.

If the descending aorta is tortuous, its posterior margin and occasionally its anterior margin may be followed for varying distances, depending upon where the aorta returns to a prespinal position to traverse the aortic hiatus and enter the abdomen. Rarely, the superior margin of the arch of the azygos vein is visible projecting over the lower aspect of the aortic arch. In certain individuals, the posterior edges of the innominate or left subclavian arteries may be visible in relation to the tracheal air column.

The appearance of the retrosternal space depends upon the shape of the sternum and the amount of anterior mediastinal fat. On well-penetrated lateral radiographs, the body of the sternum is readily visible (Fig. 12.11). A thin retrosternal stripe from a small amount of fat immediately behind the body of the sternum is usually seen. Sternal fracture, infection, tumor, or prior sternotomy can distort or thicken this stripe. Enlargement of internal mammary arteries (e.g., coarctation of the aorta) or lymph nodes (typically with lymphoma or metastatic breast carcinoma) produces masses seen projecting through the concavities between the costal cartilages. Inferiorly, the left lung may be excluded from contacting the anteromedial chest wall by a round or triangular opacity, which represents the cardiac apex and adjacent extrapleural fat. This impression on the anterior surface of the lingula has been termed the *cardiac incisura* and should not be mistaken for a mass. CT will prove helpful in equivocal cases. A mass arising within the anterior mediastinum may not be visible on a PA view but will usually encroach on this retrosternal clear space.

The anterior pericardium can be identified separately from the myocardium in 20% of subjects. This thin line represents the pericardial layers between the epicardial and pericardial fat. Nodularity or thickness >2.0 mm suggests disease or effusion.

The posterior aspect of the inferior vena cava is visible in a majority of individuals as a concave posterior or straight edge that is visible at the posteroinferior cardiac margin, just above the diaphragm (Fig. 12.11). In the pediatric population, its absence often concurs with cardiac abnormalities.

The hemidiaphragms appear as parallel domed structures on lateral radiographs (Fig. 12.1). The posterior portion lies at a more inferior level than the anterior portion, creating a deep posterior costophrenic sulcus and a shallow anterior sulcus. There are several methods of distinguishing the right from the left hemidiaphragm on the lateral view. The anterior left hemidiaphragm is obliterated (silhouetted) by the cardiac contact, whereas the right hemidiaphragm is seen in its entire anteroposterior course. On a well-positioned left lateral chest radiograph, with the right side of the thorax farther from the x-ray cassette than the left, the right anterior and posterior costophrenic sulci should project beyond the corresponding left-sided sulci as a result of x-ray beam divergence. Identification of the right and left costophrenic sulci allows identification of the corresponding hemidiaphragms. The presence of air in the stomach or splenic flexure projecting above one hemidiaphragm and below another identifies the more cephalad structure as the left hemidiaphragm. Occasionally, when the right and left major fissures are distinguishable (the left is more vertically oriented than the right), following a major fissure to its point of contact with the diaphragm will allow identification of that hemidiaphragm.

Anatomy of the Normal Mediastinum and Thoracic Inlet

The mediastinum is a narrow, vertically oriented structure that resides between the medial parietal pleural layers of the lungs. It contains central cardiovascular, tracheobronchial structures and the esophagus enveloped in fat with intermixed lymph nodes (Fig. 12.16) (Table 12.6) (14). The thoracic inlet structures are best depicted by CT and MR (Fig 12.17A). Several schemes have been described to divide the mediastinum into separate compartments. We will use an anatomic method, in which a line drawn through the sternal angle anteriorly and fourth thoracic intervertebral space posteriorly divides the mediastinum into superior and inferior compartments. The inferior mediastinum is further subdivided into anterior, middle, and posterior compartments. This division of the mediastinum is purely arbitrary, as there are no true anatomic boundaries between the three compartments. However, by using the most easily recognizable mediastinal structure—the heart—as the focal point, the relationship of mediastinal masses to the heart allows for simple and consistent compartmentalization. Furthermore, this division of the mediastinum corresponds to easily recognizable regions seen on the lateral chest radiograph. A minor variation of the anatomic method, in which there is no superior and inferior division and the anterior, middle, and posterior compartments extend vertically from the thoracic inlet

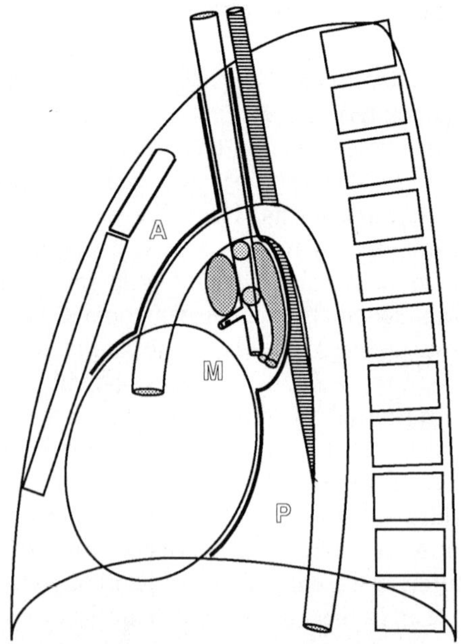

FIGURE 12.16. **Mediastinal Compartments as Defined on Lateral View.** A, Anterior mediastinum; M, middle mediastinum; P, posterior mediastinum.

TABLE 12.6 Contents of the Thoracic Inlet and Mediastinum

Compartment	*Contents*
Thoracic inlet	Thymus
	Confluence of right and left internal jugular and subclavian veins
	Right and left carotid arteries
	Right and left subclavian arteries
	Trachea
	Esophagus
	Prevertebral fascia
	Phrenic, vagus, recurrent laryngeal nerves
	Muscles
Anterior mediastinum	Internal mammary vessels
	Internal mammary and prevascular lymph nodes
	Thymus
Middle mediastinum	Heart and pericardium
	Ascending and transverse aorta
	Main and proximal right and left pulmonary arteries
	Confluence of pulmonary veins
	Superior and inferior vena cava
	Trachea and main bronchi
	Lymph nodes and fat within mediastinal spaces
Posterior mediastinum	Descending aorta
	Esophagus
	Azygos and hemiazygos veins
	Thoracic duct
	Sympathetic ganglia and intercostal nerves
	Lymph nodes

superiorly to the diaphragm inferiorly, is most practical to radiologists and is used here (Fig. 12.16). Within each compartment are readily identifiable structures and a number of spaces, in free communication with one another, which contain fat and lymph nodes. The structures and spaces native to each compartment and their normal appearance are reviewed here.

Anterior Mediastinum. The anterior (prevascular) mediastinal compartment includes all structures behind the sternum and anterior to the heart and great vessels, plus the internal mammary vessels and lymph nodes, thymus, and the brachiocephalic veins (Table 12.6). The internal mammary vessels reside within the parasternal fat and lie on either side of the sternum. Normal lymph nodes accompany the vessels but are not routinely visualized on CT. The interface of the retrosternal space with the anterior portion of the right and left lungs may be visualized on lateral chest radiographs (see the section "Lateral Chest Radiograph"). The thymus is a triangular or bilobed structure that is maximal in size at puberty and then undergoes gradual fatty involution. In most individuals over the age of 35, the thymus is predominantly fatty, with little or no intermixed glandular (soft tissue) component (Fig. 12.17A). The margins of the gland in an adult should be flat or concave toward the lung. The left lobe is commonly larger than the right. Anatomically, the thymus lies in the prevascular space, which is continuous with the retrosternal space anteriorly. It lies immediately anterior to the superior vena cava, aortic arch and great vessels, the main pulmonary artery, and, more inferiorly, the heart. The prevascular space generally retains the triangular configuration of the involuted thymus. Normal lymph nodes may be visible on CT within the fat of the prevascular space. Beginning at the level of the aortic arch in most individuals, the anterior portion of the prevascular space tapers to form a thin, vertically oriented linear density that represents the anterior junction line. The right and left brachiocephalic veins occupy the posterior aspect of the prevascular space at the level of the root of the great vessels. The right brachiocephalic vein is seen on CT as a round density owing to its vertical orientation, while the crossing left brachiocephalic vein appears oval or tubular in configuration.

Middle Mediastinum. The middle (vascular) mediastinal compartment comprises the pericardium and its contents, the aortic arch and proximal great arteries, the central pulmonary arteries and veins, the trachea and main bronchi, and lymph nodes (Table 12.6). The hila may be considered as extensions of the middle mediastinal compartment. The phrenic and vagus nerves are not visible on CT scans, but run together in the space between the subclavian arteries and brachiocephalic veins. The recurrent laryngeal nerves lie on each side within the tracheoesophageal groove. Four middle mediastinal spaces surrounding the trachea and carina can be distinguished

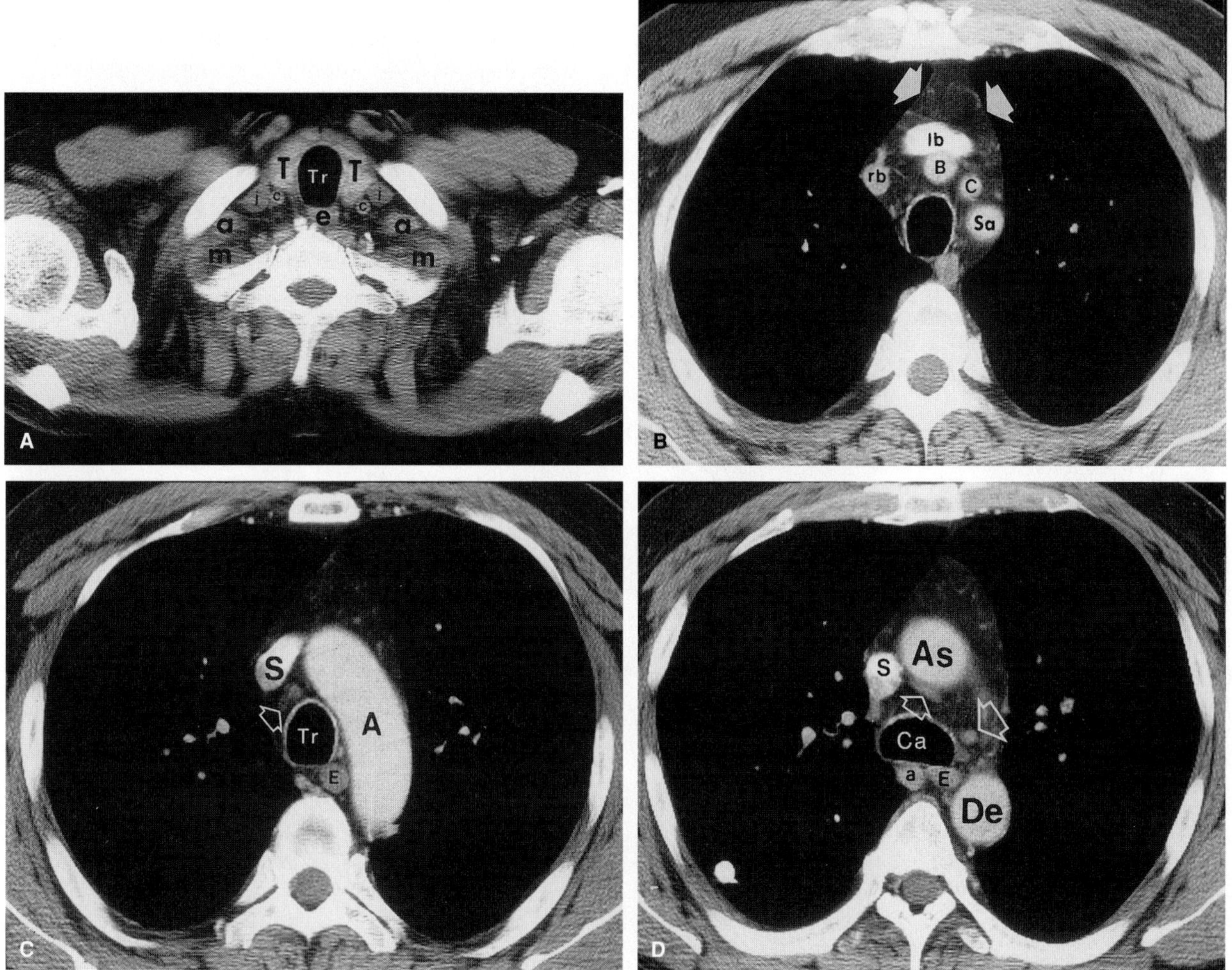

FIGURE 12.17. **Normal Mediastinal Anatomy on CT. A. Thoracic inlet.** Tr, trachea; t, thyroid; e, esophagus; j, internal jugular vein; c, common carotid artery; a, anterior scalene muscle; m, middle scalene muscle. **B. Supra-aortic level.** CT scan demonstrates the triangular appearance of the fatty thymus (*arrows*) occupying the anterior mediastinum. lb, Left brachiocephalic vein; rb, right brachiocephalic vein; B, brachiocephalic artery; C, common carotid artery; Sa, left subclavian artery. **C. Aortic arch level.** Four main structures are identified at this level: A, aortic arch; S, superior vena cava; Tr, trachea; E, esophagus. Normal-sized lymph nodes are seen in the retrocaval, pretracheal space (*open arrow*). **D. Aortopulmonary window level.** The aortopulmonary window contains fat and small lymph nodes (*large open arrow*). The retro-aortic portion of the superior pericardial recess is seen as a crescent-shaped fluid-filled structure (*small open arrow*). As, ascending aorta; De, descending aorta; S, superior vena cava; Ca, tracheal carina; a, azygos vein; E, esophagus. (*continued*)

(Fig. 12.17C). The *right paratracheal space,* containing lymph nodes and a small amount of fat, appears as the right paratracheal stripe on PA views. This space extends from the thoracic inlet superiorly to the azygos vein inferiorly. The *pretracheal space* is seen between the trachea posteriorly and the posterior margin of the ascending aorta anteriorly and is contiguous with the precarinal space inferiorly. It contains fat, lymph nodes, and the retroaortic portion of the superior pericardial recess and is the anatomic route used during routine transcervical mediastinoscopy. The *retrotracheal space* varies in AP dimension, depending upon the degree of invagination of the RUL behind the upper trachea. To the left of the trachea lies the *aortopulmonary window.* The borders of the aortopulmonary window are: the aortic arch superiorly; the left pulmonary artery inferiorly; the distal trachea, left main bronchus, and esophagus medially; the mediastinal pleural surface of the left upper lobe laterally; the posterior surface of the ascending aorta anteriorly; and the anterior surface of the proximal descending aorta posteriorly.

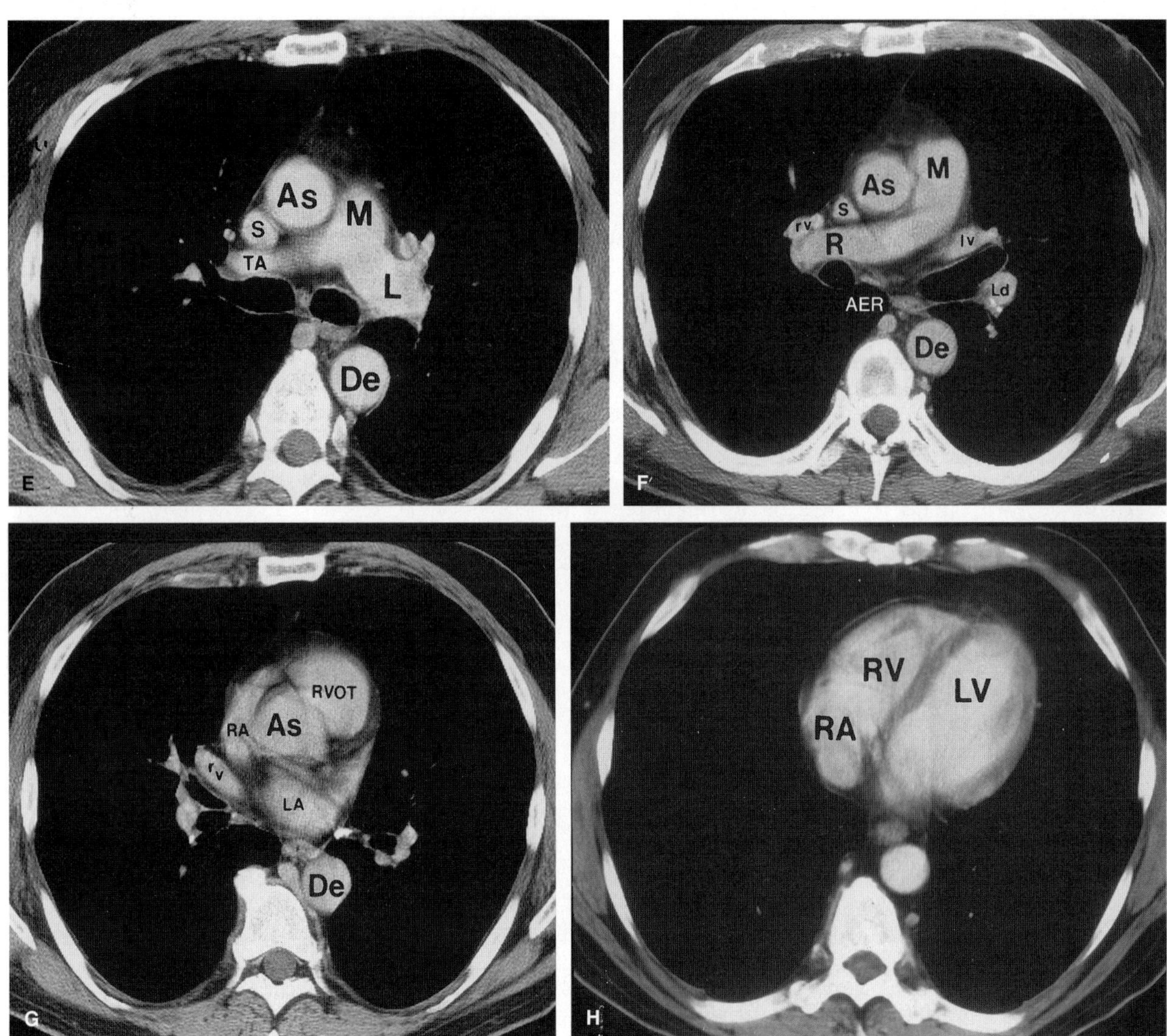

FIGURE 12.17. *(Continued)* **E. Main and left pulmonary artery level.** As, ascending aorta; S, superior vena cava; De, descending aorta, M, main pulmonary artery; L, left pulmonary artery; TA, truncus anterior branch of right pulmonary artery. **F. Right pulmonary artery and azygoesophageal recess level.** M, main pulmonary artery; R, right pulmonary artery; As, ascending aorta; De, descending aorta; S, superior vena cava; rv, right superior pulmonary veins; lv, left superior pulmonary veins; Ld, left descending pulmonary artery; AER, azygoesophageal recess. **G. Right ventricular outflow tract/atrial appendages.** RVOT, Right ventricular outflow tract; RA, right atrium; LA, left atrium; rv, right superior pulmonary vein; As, ascending aorta; De, descending aorta. **H. Ventricles and intraventricular septum.** RA, right atrium; RV, right ventricle; LV, left ventricle.

This space contains fat, lymph nodes, the ligamentum arteriosum, and the left recurrent laryngeal nerve.

Continuing inferiorly, the main and left pulmonary arteries occupy the left anterolateral portion of the middle mediastinum (Fig. 12.17D). The tracheal carina forms the posterior margin of the middle mediastinum. The RUL bronchus is seen just below the tracheal carina. More inferiorly, the right pulmonary artery is seen coursing toward the right and slightly posteriorly, just behind the ascending aorta and anterior to the bronchus intermedius (Fig. 12.17E). The subcarinal space is outlined posteriorly by air in the azygoesophageal recess and anteriorly by the posterior aspect of the transverse right pulmonary artery. The left superior pulmonary vein lies immediately anterior to the left main and upper lobe bronchi.

The main pulmonary artery can be followed inferiorly to the level of the outflow tract of the right ventricle. At this level, the right and left atrial appendages and the top of the left atrium proper may be seen (Fig. 12.17F). Also at this level, the right superior pulmonary vein lies anterior to the middle lobe bronchus, which in turn lies immediately anterior to the RLL bronchus. Inferiorly, the right atrium proper, right ventricle, and left ventricle are identified (Fig. 12.17G).

ATS Nodal Stations. To provide greater uniformity in the nodal staging of bronchogenic carcinoma and thereby help guide diagnostic and therapeutic efforts in this disease, the American Thoracic Society (ATS) has devised a standard classification scheme for mediastinal lymph nodes (see Fig. 13.8).

Posterior Mediastinum. The posterior (postvascular) mediastinal compartment lies behind the pericardium and includes the esophagus, the descending aorta, the azygos and hemiazygos veins, the thoracic duct, and the intercostal and autonomic nerves (Table 12.5). The esophagus lies posterior or posterolateral to the trachea, from the level of the thoracic inlet superiorly to the tracheal carina inferiorly. From the thoracic inlet to the level of the aortic arch, the right and left upper lobes of the lungs meet behind the esophagus and anterior to the spine to form the narrow posterior junction line seen on CT scans through the upper thorax and appearing as a vertical line through the tracheal air column on frontal radiographs. The esophagus then maintains a constant relationship with the descending thoracic aorta, usually lying anteromedial to the aorta (Figs. 12.17, 12.18) down to the level of the aortic hiatus, where the aorta is in a direct prevertebral position while the esophagus crosses the aorta anteriorly to exit the thorax via the esophageal hiatus. There are lymph nodes about the descending aorta that are not normally visible. The descending aorta lies anterolateral to the thoracic spine at the level of the aortopulmonary window. In young adults, the aorta maintains this position to the level of the aortic hiatus of the diaphragm, where it lies directly in the midline. In older patients and those with a tortuous or dilated aorta, the vessel lies more laterally and protrudes into the LLL as it descends, carrying the esophagus with it before returning to a midline position at the level of the aortic hiatus. The azygos and hemiazygos veins lie on the right and left sides, respectively, posterolateral to the descending aorta within a fat-containing space that contains the thoracic duct and the sympathetic chains (normally not visible) and small lymph nodes (Fig. 12.18). Inferiorly, this space is continuous with the retrocrural space and laterally with the paraspinal space, which contains the intercostal arteries, veins, and lymph nodes.

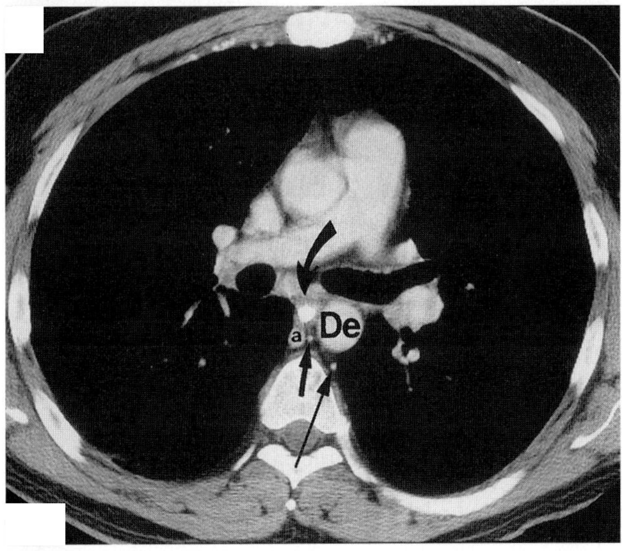

FIGURE 12.18. **Posterior Mediastinal Anatomy.** A CT scan shows a contrast-filled esophagus (*curved arrow*) anteromedial to the proximal descending aorta (De). Also visible within the posterior mediastinum are the azygos vein (a), hemiazygos vein (*long arrow*), and thoracic duct (*short arrow*).

Normal Hilar Anatomy

Frontal View. The hilum represents the junction of the lung with the mediastinum and is composed of upper lobe pulmonary veins and branches of the pulmonary artery and corresponding bronchi (Fig. 12.19). These are all enveloped by small amounts of fat, with intermixed lymph nodes.

The shape of the right hilum on frontal radiographs has been likened to a sideways V, with the opening pointing rightward (Fig. 12.19A, B). The upper portion of the V is composed primarily of the truncus anterior and the posterior division of the right superior pulmonary vein. The right interlobar artery forms the lower half of the V, as it descends lateral to the bronchus intermedius. The right inferior pulmonary vein crosses the lower right hilar shadow but does not contribute to its opacity (Fig. 12.19A).

On CT, the upper portion of the right hilum is composed of the right superior pulmonary vein, truncus anterior division of the right pulmonary artery, and the RUL bronchus. The RUL pulmonary vein courses vertically, anterolateral to the truncus anterior (Figs. 12.5B, 12.17D–F). Here again, the epi-arterial position of the bronchus can be recognized. The lower portion of the right hilum is composed of the right descending (or interlobar) pulmonary artery laterally and the bronchus intermedius and proximal RLL bronchus medially (Fig. 12.17E, F).

The upper left hilar shadow is composed centrally of the distal left main pulmonary artery and, more peripherally, of one or more branches of its LUL division and the posterior division of the left superior pulmonary vein (Fig. 12.19). The left pulmonary artery and left descending artery arch over the left mainstem bronchus and are thus named *hypo-arterial.* The descending artery then forms the

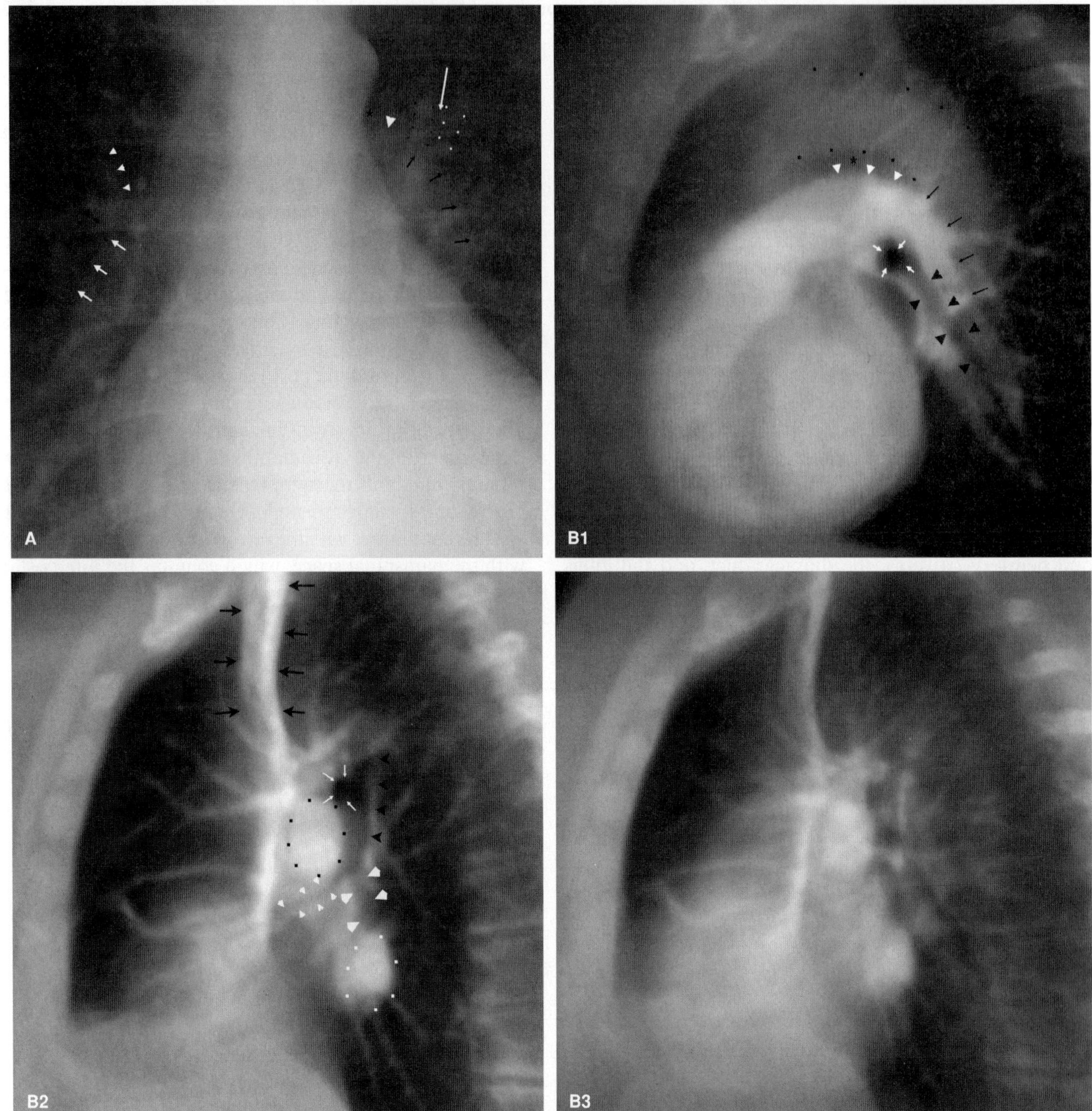

FIGURE 12.19. **Normal Frontal and Lateral Hilar Anatomy. A.** Cone-down frontal view. **Right hilum:** *Short white arrows,* border of the interlobar artery; *small black arrowheads,* right superior pulmonary vein; *small white arrowheads,* truncus anterior. The lucency between these (*long black arrow*) is from the apical segmental bronchus. **Left hilum:** *Large white arrowhead,* left pulmonary artery; *short black arrows,* border of the left descending pulmonary artery; *black dots,* left superior pulmonary vein; *white dots,* left upper lobe artery; *long white arrow,* apicoposterior segmental bronchus. The asterisk is in the AP window. **B.** Using two-dimensional imaging techniques, one can gain adequate insight of the complex lateral hilar anatomy. This view shows a 50-mm average sagittal projection over the hila of a contrast CT with 3-mm collimation reconstructed at 2-mm. **(1)** The left hilum. *Small white arrows* outline the left upper lobe bronchus; *small black arrowheads* border the left lower lobe bronchus; *long black arrows* delineate the left descending artery; AP window (*asterisk*) lies between the inferior border of the aorta (lined with *small black dots*) and the left pulmonary artery (*white arrowheads*). **(2)** The right hilum. Note the relationship between the right upper lobe bronchus (*small white arrows*) and the right pulmonary artery (*black dots*). *Black arrowheads* indicate the posterior border of the bronchus intermedius; *small white arrowheads* line the middle lobe bronchus; *large white arrowheads* outline the right lower lobe bronchus; *white dots* line the right lower venous return; *black arrows* delineate the superior vena cava (SVC). The differential density is the result of the heavier contrast layering along the posterior aspect of the vessel in a supine acquisition. **(3)** Two-dimensional average merge of **(1)** and **(2)**. Using the data from **(1)** and **(2)**, note the relationship between the different structures described above.

lower portion of the left hilar shadow as it descends behind the left heart.

On CT of the upper left hilum, the left superior pulmonary vein courses anterior to the left pulmonary artery and, more inferiorly, anterior to the LUL bronchus to empty into the superolateral aspect of the left atrium (Fig. 12.17D–F). The left pulmonary artery arches posteriorly, superiorly, and to the left, over the left main and upper lobe bronchi (thus being hypo-arterial), to bifurcate into upper and lower lobe arteries (Fig. 12.17D, E). The lower portion of the left hilum is composed of the left descending artery, which lies posterolateral to the LLL bronchus (Fig. 12.17E). The left inferior pulmonary vein courses horizontally at a level slightly behind that of the right inferior vein to empty into the left atrium, just medial to the left basal trunk bronchus.

As seen on frontal radiographs, the right and left pulmonary arteries comprise the predominant portion of the hilar opacity, with the superior pulmonary veins, lobar bronchi, bronchopulmonary lymph nodes, and a small amount of fat contributing little to the overall hilar density (Fig. 12.19A). In over 90% of normal individuals, the left hilar shadow is higher than the right. This is because the left pulmonary artery, which comprises the predominant portion of the left hilar shadow, ascends over the left main and upper lobe bronchus, whereas the right pulmonary artery lies inferior to the RUL bronchus. In the remainder of individuals, the right and left hila lie at the same level; a right hilum that lies above the left suggests volume loss in the right upper or left lower lobe.

Left Lateral View. On a true lateral radiograph, the right and left hilar shadows are not completely superimposed and comprise a combination of the right and left pulmonary arteries and the superior pulmonary veins (Fig. 12.19C, D). The anterior aspect of the hilar shadow is composed of the transverse portion of the right pulmonary artery, which produces a vertically oriented oval opacity projecting immediately anterior to the bronchus intermedius. The confluence of right superior pulmonary veins overlaps the lower portion of the right pulmonary artery and contributes to its opacity. Superiorly and posteriorly, the comma-shaped left pulmonary artery passes above and behind the round or oval lucency representing the horizontally oriented LUL bronchus summating on a portion of the left mainstem bronchus, and then descends behind the LLL bronchus. The confluence of left superior pulmonary veins, which lies behind the level of the right superior pulmonary vein, creates an opacity that occupies the posteroinferior aspect of the composite hilar shadow. The avascular aspect of the composite hilar shadow, inferior to the shadow of the right pulmonary artery and veins and anterior to the descending left pulmonary artery and left superior vein, is called the *inferior hilar window.* This region is roughly triangular in shape, with its apex at the junction of the LUL and LLL bronchi and its base directed anteriorly and inferiorly. The RML and lingular veins cross the inferior hilar window, but because of their small size, they do not contribute significant opacity to this area.

The vascular structures of the composite hilar shadow are suspended around the central bronchi (Fig. 12.19). Beginning superiorly, the RUL bronchus is seen in approximately 50% of individuals as an end-on, round lucency at the upper margin of the composite hilar shadow. Recognition of this bronchus, when not visible on prior radiographs, should suggest a mass or lymph node enlargement about the bronchus. The posterior wall of the bronchus intermedius is a thin vertical line, 2 mm or thinner, extending inferiorly from the posterior aspect of the RUL bronchus. The line is seen in 95% of patients and extends inferiorly to bisect the end-on lucency of the LUL bronchus on a lateral film. This structure is rendered visible because air within the intermediate bronchus anteriorly and lung within the azygoesophageal recess posteriorly outlines its posterior wall. Thickening or nodularity of this line is seen in bronchogenic carcinoma, pulmonary edema, or enlargement of azygoesophageal recess lymph nodes. The LUL bronchus, which is seen in 75% of individuals, lies no more than 4 cm directly inferior to the RUL bronchus. This bronchus is visualized with greater frequency than the RUL bronchus because it is outlined by the left pulmonary artery and by other mediastinal structures, while the RUL bronchus is contacted only by the right main pulmonary artery anteroinferiorly and the azygos arch superiorly. The projection of the posterior wall of the bronchus intermedius over the LUL bronchus also helps identify the LUL bronchus. Below the oval lucency of the latter, the basal trunk of the LLL bronchus can sometimes be identified, with its anterior wall visible as a white line, outlined by air in the bronchial lumen and air in the lung. The LLL bronchus is seen immediately below and continuous with the horizontal LUL bronchus.

The appearance of the hila changes with a slight degree of rotation. If on a left lateral radiograph, the patient is rotated slightly right side back and left side forward, the more posteriorly positioned left pulmonary artery will be summated on the more anterior right main pulmonary artery, and the hila are termed "closed." If on the other hand, the rotation is slightly left side back and right side forward, the left pulmonary artery is further separated from the right and the hila are termed "open." If the patient is in a true lateral position, the beam divergence will magnify the right-sided structures and simulate minimal "closing" of the hila. The relationship of the right-sided bronchus intermedius to the round hole of the end-on LUL bronchus can be helpful in evaluating differences in rotation between serial lateral views on the same patient. Analyzing this normal hilar relationship is helpful in determining the side of the posterior costophrenic sulcus if the ribs are not completely superimposed.

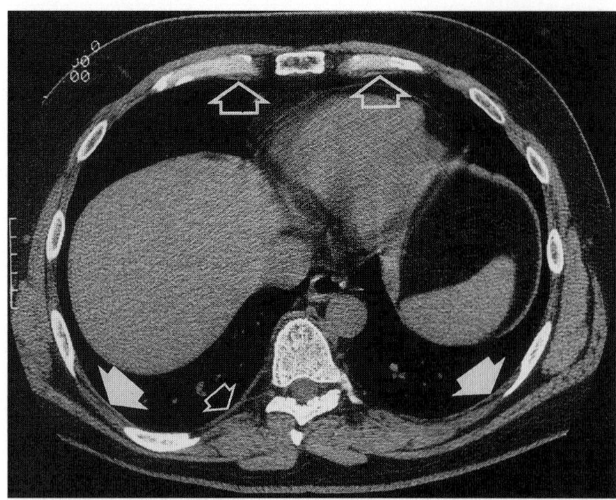

FIGURE 12.20. **HRCT of the Pleura.** HRCT scan through the lung bases demonstrates normal intercostal stripes (*solid arrows*) that are separated from the intercostal muscles by a layer of fat. An intercostal vein (*small open arrow*) is seen in the paravertebral region. Anteriorly, the transverse thoracic muscles (*large open arrows*) line the parasternal pleural surface.

Pleural Anatomy

The pleura is a serosal membrane that envelops the lung and lines the costal surface, diaphragm, and mediastinum (15). It is composed of two layers, the visceral and the parietal pleura, that join at the hilum. Blood supply to the parietal pleura is via the systemic circulation, while the visceral pleura is supplied by the pulmonary circulation. The parietal pleura is contiguous with the chest wall and diaphragm and therefore extends deep posteriorly into the costophrenic sulci, while the visceral pleura is adherent to the surface of the lung. The pleural space is a potential space between the two pleural layers and normally contains a small amount of fluid (<5 mL) that reduces friction during breathing.

The normal costal, diaphragmatic, and mediastinal pleura is not visible on plain radiographs or CT. On HRCT, a 1- to 2-mm stripe may be seen lining the intercostal spaces between adjacent ribs (Fig. 12.20). This "intercostal stripe" represents the combination of the two pleural layers, the endothoracic fascia, and the innermost intercostal muscle (Fig. 12.21). Internal to the ribs, the normal pleura is not seen and the inner cortex of rib appears to contact the lung. The presence of soft tissue density between the inner rib and the lung, best appreciated on HRCT studies, indicates pleural thickening. The innermost intercostal muscle is anatomically absent in the paravertebral area, and if a thin line is visible between the lung and paravertebral fat or rib, it represents a combination of the two pleural surfaces and the endothoracic fascia.

Chest Wall Anatomy

The radiographic anatomy of the soft tissues and bony structures of the chest wall were discussed in the section on the normal frontal radiograph. CT provides detailed anatomic information about the normal chest wall and axillae. A detailed knowledge of normal cross-sectional chest wall and axillary anatomy is key to accurate localization and characterization of disease processes. Chest wall anatomy as seen on CT at six representative levels is shown in Fig. 12.22.

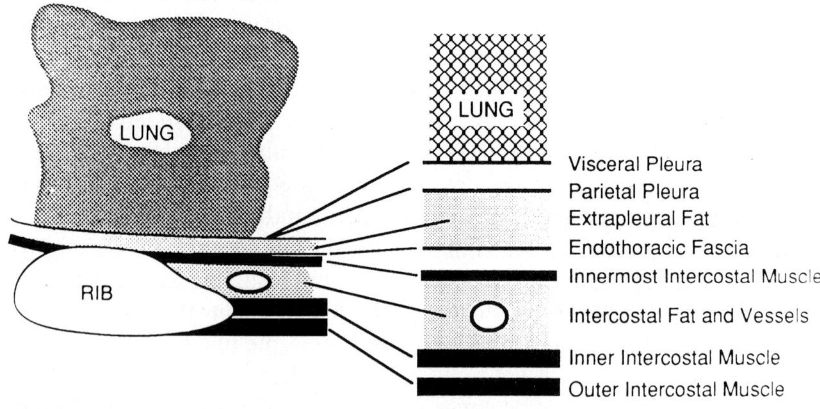

FIGURE 12.21. **Normal Pleural and Chest Wall Anatomy.** The visceral pleura is 0.1 to 0.2 mm thick and is composed of a single layer of mesothelial cells and its associated fibroelastic fascia, called the subpleural interstitium, that is part of the peripheral interstitial network. The parietal pleura is 0.1 mm thick and is composed of a single layer of mesothelial cells lining a loose connective tissue layer containing systemic capillaries, lymphatic vessels, and sensory nerves. Outside the parietal pleura is the fibroelastic endothoracic fascia, which is separated from the pleura by a thin layer of extrapleural fat. The endothoracic fascia lines the ribs and intercostal muscles.

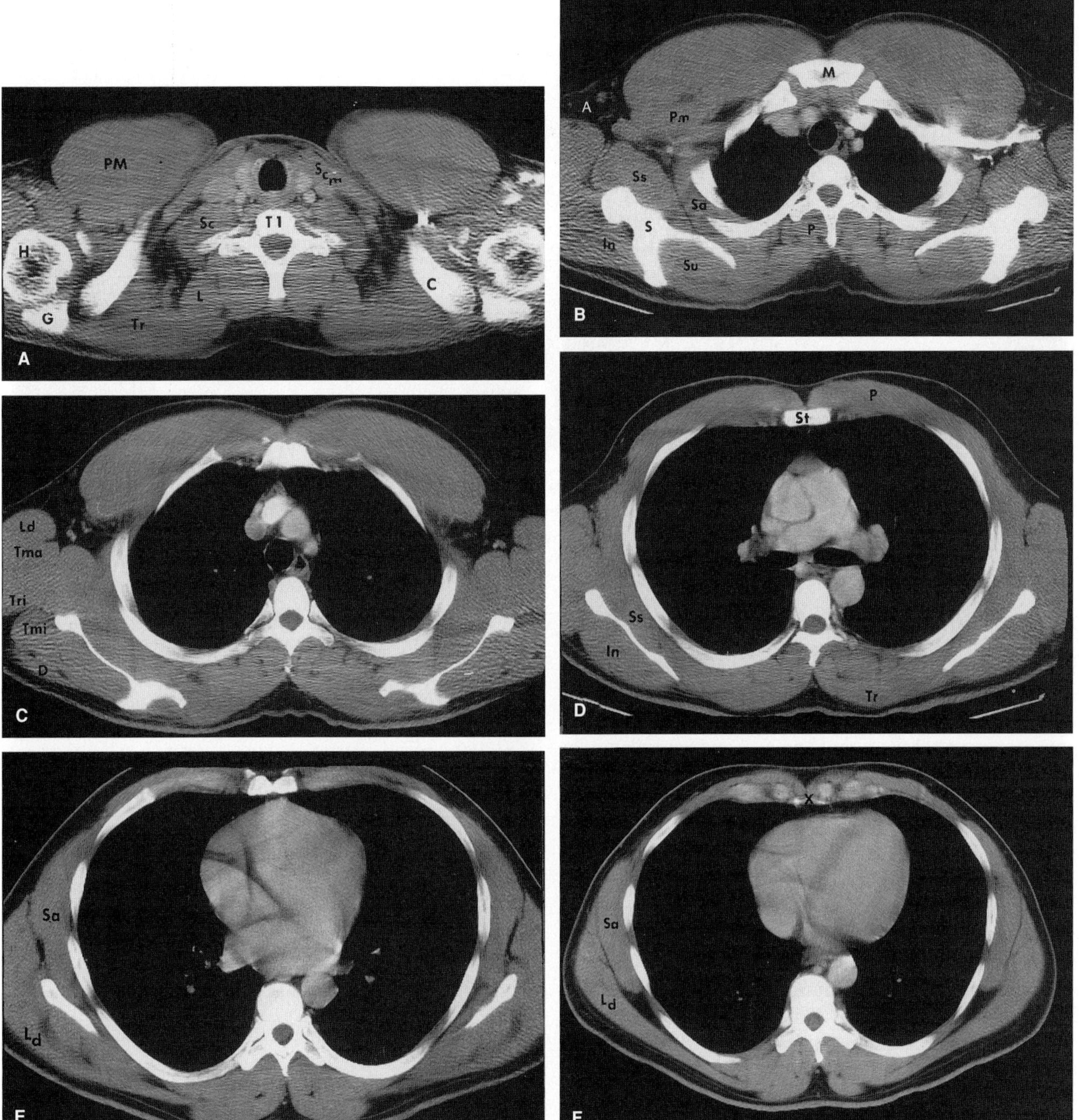

FIGURE 12.22. **Normal Chest Wall Anatomy on CT. A. Level of the thoracic inlet.** PM, pectoralis major muscle; Tr, trapezius muscle; L, levator scapulae muscle; Sc, scalene muscle; Scm, sternocleidomastoid muscle; H, humeral head; G, glenoid; C, distal clavicle; T1, first thoracic vertebral body. **B. Level of the axillary vessels.** Pm, pectoralis minor muscle; Sa, serratus anterior muscle; Su, supraspinatus muscle; In, infraspinatus muscle; Ss, subscapularis muscle; P, paraspinal muscles; M, manubrium of the sternum; S, body of the scapula; A, axilla with normal lymph nodes. **C. Level of the sternomanubrial joint.** Ld, latissimus dorsi muscle; Tma, teres major muscle; Tri, long head of the triceps muscle; Tmi, teres minor muscle; D, deltoid muscle. **D. Level of the body of the sternum.** P, pectoralis muscles; Ss, subscapularis muscle; In, infraspinatus muscle; Tr, trapezius muscle; St, body of the sternum. **E. Level of tip of scapula.** Ld, Latissimus dorsi muscle; Sa, serratus anterior muscle. **F. Level of the xiphoid process.** Ld, latissimus dorsi muscle; Sa, serratus anterior muscle; X, xiphoid process of the sternum.

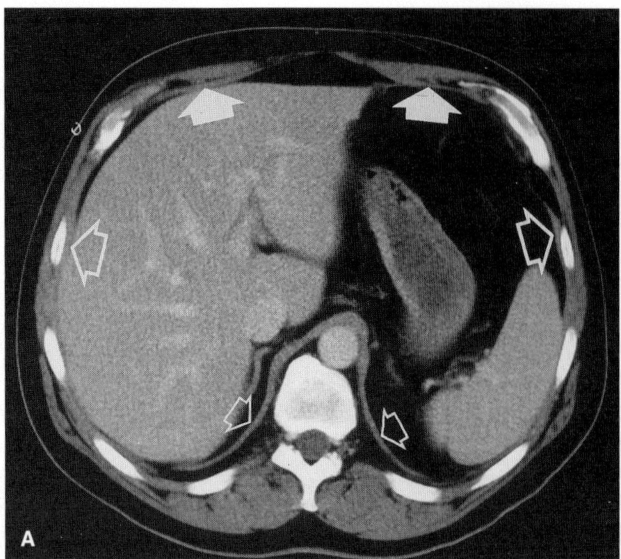

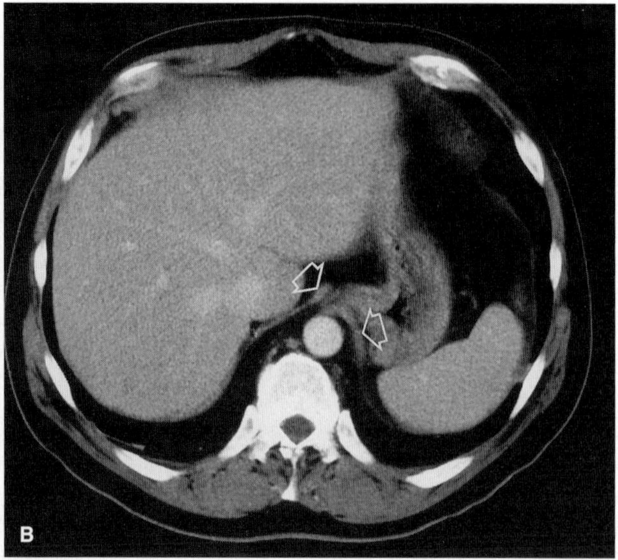

FIGURE 12.23. **Normal Anatomy of the Diaphragm on CT. A.** A scan through the upper abdomen demonstrates the crura of the diaphragm posteriorly (*small open arrows*), the costal origins of the diaphragm laterally (*large open arrows*), and the costal cartilaginous origins anterolaterally (*solid arrows*). **B.** More inferiorly, the esophageal hiatus is seen between the crura (*open arrows*).

Anatomy of the Diaphragm

The diaphragm is composed of striated muscle and a large central tendon separating the thoracic and abdominal cavities. The diaphragmatic muscle arises anteriorly from the posterior aspect of the xiphoid process and anterolaterally, laterally, and posterolaterally from the sixth to the twelfth costal cartilages and ribs. The diaphragmatic crura originate from the upper lumbar vertebrae and course to the posterior aspect of the central tendon. They have no direct action on the rib cage (Fig. 12.23). The diaphragm has three normal openings and two potential gaps. The *aortic hiatus* lies in the midline, immediately behind the diaphragmatic crura and anterior to the twelfth thoracic vertebral body. The aorta, thoracic duct, and azygos and hemiazygos veins traverse this opening. The *esophageal hiatus* usually lies slightly to the left of midline, cephalad to the aortic hiatus, and transmits the esophagus and vagus nerves. The inferior vena cava pierces the central tendon of the diaphragm at the level of the eighth thoracic intervertebral disk space. The foramina of Morgagni are triangular gaps in the muscles of the anteromedial diaphragm. This cleft is normally occupied by fat and the internal mammary vessels; it is a site of potential intrathoracic herniation of abdominal contents. The foramina of Bochdalek are defects in the closure of the posterolateral diaphragm at the junction of the pleuroperitoneal membrane with the transverse septum. Hernias through the foramina of Morgagni and Bochdalek are discussed in Chapter 19.

On CT scans, the domes of the diaphragms appear as rounded opacities on either side of the chest at the level of the base of the heart. In some patients scanned on deep inspiration, the diaphragm has an undulating or nodular appearance from contraction of slips of diaphragmatic muscle. This appearance is seen with increasing frequency in older patients, and is more common on the left than the right. Posteriorly, the superior aspects of the diaphragmatic crura are seen. The crura are curvilinear opacities that arise from the upper two to three lumbar vertebrae. Their associated esophageal and aortic openings within the bundles of the crura are well visualized on CT (Fig. 12.23). Continuing inferiorly into the upper abdomen, the inferior aspects of the diaphragmatic crura may have a rounded appearance in cross section and should not be mistaken for enlarged retrocrural lymph nodes. Review of contiguous CT images will allow for proper identification of these structures.

RADIOGRAPHIC FINDINGS IN CHEST DISEASE

Parenchymal lung disease can be divided into those processes that produce an abnormal increase in the density of all or a portion of the lung on chest radiographs (pulmonary opacity) and those that produce an abnormal decrease in lung density (pulmonary lucency). The normal density of the lungs is a result of the relative proportion of air to soft tissue (blood or parenchyma) in a ratio of 11 to 1. Therefore, it stands to reason that processes that increase the relative amount of soft tissue will create a significant decrease in this ratio and be more easily discernible

TABLE 12.7 Patterns of Parenchymal Opacity

Type	*Example*
Airspace (alveolar) filling	Pneumococcal pneumonia
Interstitial opacities	
Reticular/linear	Idiopathic pulmonary fibrosis
Reticulonodular	Sarcoidosis
Branching	Allergic bronchopulmonary aspergillosis
Nodular	
Miliary (<2 mm)	Miliary tuberculosis
Micronodule (2–7 mm)	Acute hypersensitivity pneumonitis
Nodule (7–30 mm)	Metastatic disease, granuloma
Mass (>30 mm)	Bronchogenic carcinoma
Atelectasis	Endobronchial neoplasm

than diffuse processes, which destroy blood vessels and parenchyma and cause little change in this ratio, thereby producing only small decreases in overall lung density. CT, by virtue of its superior contrast resolution, is more sensitive than plain radiography to subtle decreases in overall radiographic density.

Abnormal pulmonary opacities may be classified into airspace-filling opacities, opacity resulting from atelectasis, interstitial opacities, nodular or masslike opacities, and branching opacities (Table 12.7). These patterns have been shown to accurately represent pulmonary pathologic processes in correlative radiographic–pathologic studies, and are a practical means of generating a differential diagnosis based on the known patterns of parenchymal involvement in a wide variety of pulmonary diseases.

Pulmonary Opacity

Airspace Disease. Radiographic findings of airspace disease are listed in Table 12.8. Airspace patterns of opacity develop when the air normally present within the terminal airspaces of the lung is replaced by material of soft tissue density, such as blood, transudate, exudate, or neoplastic cells. A segmental distribution of disease may be seen in a process such as pneumococcal pneumonia, which begins in the terminal airspaces and spreads from involved to uninvolved airspaces via interalveolar channels (pores of Kohn) and channels bridging preterminal bronchioles with alveoli (canals of Lambert). Initially, the opacity is poorly marginated, because the airspace-filling process extends in an irregular fashion to involve adjacent airspaces, creating an irregular interface with the x-ray beam. Not uncommonly, airspace nodules, which are poorly marginated, rounded opacities 6 to 8 mm in diameter, may be seen at the leading edge of an airspace-filling process. These nodules represent filling of acini or other sublobular structures and are most often seen in diffuse alveolar pulmonary edema and transbronchial spread of cavitary tuberculosis.

A characteristic of airspace-filling processes is the tendency of airspace shadows to coalesce as they extend through the lung (16). When the airspaces are rendered opaque by the presence of intra-alveolar cellular material and fluid, the normally aerated bronchi become visible as tubular lucencies called *air bronchograms* (Fig. 12.24). Occasionally, small intraacinous bronchi or groups of uninvolved alveoli may be visible within an airspace nodule as air bronchiolograms or air alveolograms, respectively. Rarely, severe interstitial disease encroaching upon the airspaces may produce an air bronchogram; this is most typically seen in "alveolar" sarcoid. When the airspace-filling process extends to the interlobar fissure, it is seen as a sharply marginated lobar opacity.

TABLE 12.8 Radiographic Characteristics of Airspace Disease

Lobar or segmental distribution
Poorly marginated
Airspace nodules
Tendency to coalesce
Air bronchograms
Bat's wing (butterfly) distribution
Rapidly changing over time

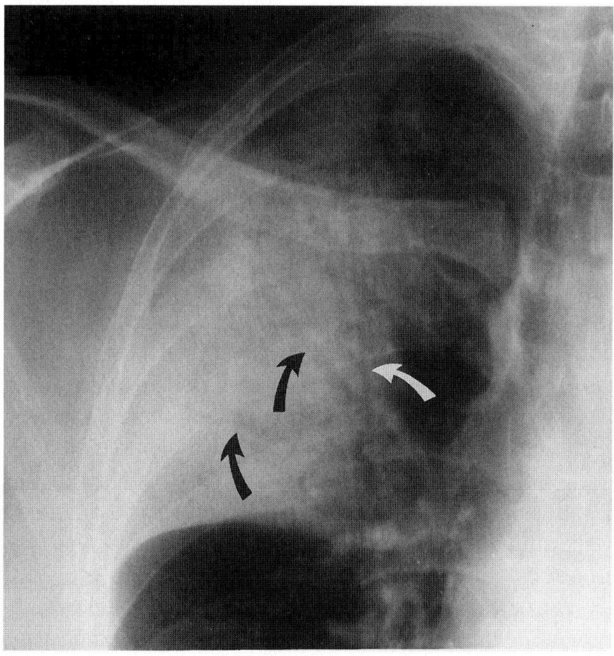

FIGURE 12.24. **Air Bronchograms in Airspace Disease.** Cone-down view of the right upper lobe in a patient with pneumococcal pneumonia shows homogeneous lobar airspace disease delineated inferiorly by the minor fissure. Note the presence of air bronchograms (*arrows*) within the opacified lobe.

TABLE 12.9 Diffuse Confluent Airspace Opacities: Differential Diagnosis

Type	*Example*
Pulmonary edema	Cardiogenic
	Fluid overload/renal failure
	Noncardiogenic (ARDS) (see Table 14.2)
Pneumonia	*Pneumocystis carinii*
	Gram-negative bacteria
	Influenza
	Fungi
	Histoplasmosis
	Aspergillosis
Hemorrhage	See Table 14.3
Neoplasm	Bronchoalveolar cell carcinoma
	Lymphoma
Alveolar proteinosis	Acute silica inhalation
	Lymphoma
	Leukemia
	AIDS

A pattern of parenchymal opacity that reliably represents an airspace-filling process is the "bat's wing" or "butterfly" pattern of disease. In this pattern, dense opacities occupy the central regions of lung and extend laterally to abruptly marginate before reaching the peripheral portions of the lung; hence the term "bat's wing" (see Fig. 14.2). To date, there is no explanation for this distribution of disease, which appears almost exclusively in patients with pulmonary edema or hemorrhage. Another feature of airspace-filling processes is the tendency to rapidly change in appearance over short intervals of time. The development or resolution of parenchymal opacities within hours usually indicates an airspace-filling process; prominent exceptions include atelectasis and interstitial pulmonary edema. The differential diagnosis of diffuse confluent airspace opacities is reviewed in Table 12.9.

The CT and HRCT findings of airspace disease are similar to those described on plain chest radiographs. These are: (*1*) lobar, segmental, and/or lobular distribution of disease; (*2*) poorly marginated opacities that tend to coalesce; (*3*) airspace nodules; and (*4*) air bronchograms. A lobar or segmental distribution of disease is easily appreciated on cross-sectional imaging. CT and HRCT are further capable of showing individually opacified lobules, termed a "patchwork quilt" appearance, which is seen in many airspace processes, most classically bronchopneumonia (see Fig. 17.3). Coalescence of opacities, commonly seen in pulmonary edema and pneumonia, is best assessed on serial CT studies. With isolated airspace disease, the interlobular septa are normal or obscured. As with plain films, the presence of airspace nodules provides further evidence of an airspace process. On HRCT studies, these nodules are usually seen within the peribronchiolar (centrilobular) region of the pulmonary lobule. Air bronchograms or bronchiolograms are usually better appreciated on CT and HRCT than on plain radiographs owing to superior contrast resolution and the cross-sectional nature of CT. This is particularly true in those regions of the lung where bronchi course in the transverse plane (anterior segments of upper lobes, middle lobe and lingula, and superior segments of the lower lobes).

Atelectasis literally means "incomplete expansion." It is used to describe any condition in which there is loss of lung volume, and it is usually but not invariably associated with an increase in radiographic density. There are four basic mechanisms of atelectasis (Table 12.10) (17).

The most common form of atelectasis is *obstructive* or *resorptive atelectasis* and is secondary to complete endobronchial obstruction of a lobar bronchus with resorption of gas distally. Incomplete bronchial obstruction more often produces air trapping from a check-valve effect rather than atelectasis, because air enters but cannot exit the lung. Complete obstruction of a central bronchus may not produce atelectasis if collateral airflow to the obstructed lung (via pores of Kohn, canals of Lambert, or incomplete interlobar fissures) allows the lung to remain inflated. An obstructed lobe or lung containing 100% oxygen, as may be seen in some mechanically ventilated patients, will collapse more rapidly (sometimes within minutes) than lung containing ambient air. This is the result of the rapid absorption of oxygen from the alveolar spaces into the alveolar capillaries. Bronchogenic carcinoma, foreign bodies, mucous plugs, and malpositioned endotracheal tubes are the most common causes of endobronchial obstruction and secondary resorptive atelectasis.

Passive or *relaxation atelectasis* results from the mass effect of an air or fluid collection within the pleural space on the subjacent lung. Since the natural tendency of the lung is to collapse when dissociated from the chest wall, pleural collections will produce atelectasis. The degree of atelectasis depends upon the size of the pleural collection and upon the compliance of the lung and visceral pleura. A large pleural or chest wall mass or an elevated diaphragm can also produce passive atelectasis. *Compressive atelectasis*

TABLE 12.10 Types of Pulmonary Atelectasis

Type	*Example*
Obstructive (resorptive)	Bronchogenic carcinoma (endobronchial)
Passive (relaxation)	Pleural effusion
	Pneumothorax
Compressive	Bulla
Cicatricial	Post–primary tuberculosis
	Radiation fibrosis
Adhesive	Respiratory distress syndrome of the newborn

is a form of passive atelectasis in which an intrapulmonary mass compresses adjacent lung parenchyma; common causes include bullae, abscesses, and tumors.

Processes resulting in parenchymal fibrosis reduce alveolar volume and produce *cicatricial atelectasis*. Localized cicatricial atelectasis is most often seen in association with chronic upper lobe fibronodular tuberculosis. The radiographic appearance is that of severe lobar volume loss with scarring, bronchiectasis, and compensatory hyperinflation of the adjacent lung. Diffuse cicatricial atelectasis is seen in interstitial fibrosis of any etiology. An overall increase in lung density, with reticular opacities and diminished lung volumes, is characteristic of this condition.

Adhesive atelectasis occurs in association with surfactant deficiency. Type 2 pneumocytes, the cells responsible for surfactant production, may be injured as a result of general anesthesia, ischemia, or radiation. Surfactant deficiency causes increased alveolar surface tension and results in diffuse alveolar collapse and volume loss. Radiographs show a diminution in lung volume, which may be associated with an increase in density.

Lobar Atelectasis. The only direct radiographic finding of lobar atelectasis is the displacement of an interlobar fissure (Table 12.11) (18). There are several indirect findings of atelectasis, most of which reflect attempts to compensate for the volume loss (Fig. 12.25). Diminished aeration results in increased density in the affected portion of lung, plus bronchovascular crowding. Ipsilateral shift of the trachea, heart, or mediastinum and hilar structures is a common finding in lobar atelectasis. Shift of the entire mediastinum is typical of collapse of an entire lung. Compensatory hyperinflation represents an attempt by the remaining normal lung to partially fill the space lost by the affected lung. This mechanism usually develops with chronic volume loss and is not seen in acute collapse. It is seen as increased lucency with attenuation of pulmonary vascular markings. In complete lung or upper lobe atelectasis, the contralateral upper lobe may herniate across the midline, bowing the anterior junction line toward the affected side. A characteristic but seldom seen plain radiographic finding of compensatory hyperinflation is the "shifting granuloma," in which a preexisting granuloma in an adjacent aerated lung changes position as it moves toward the collapsed lobe. In chronic atelectasis of a lung, a decrease in size of the hemithorax with approximation of the ribs may be seen. The absence of an air bronchogram helps distinguish resorptive lobar atelectasis from lobar pneumonia, particularly if the atelectatic lobe is only slightly diminished in volume. A triangular configuration with the apex at the pulmonary hilum is common to all types of lobar atelectasis. The fissure bordering the collapse typically assumes a concave configuration. Complete lobar atelectasis can easily be missed on PA and lateral radiographs but is easily appreciated on CT.

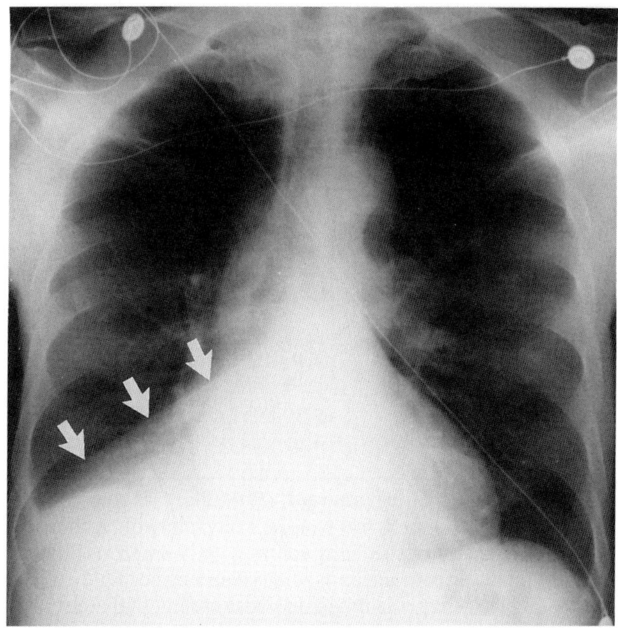

FIGURE 12.25. **Lobar Atelectasis.** Upright frontal chest radiograph in a postoperative patient with right lower lobe atelectasis shows a homogeneous triangular opacity in the right lower lung that partially obscures the right hemidiaphragm. The upper margin of the collapsed lobe is marginated by the inferiorly displaced major fissure (*arrows*). Bronchoscopy retrieved a mucous plug from the right lower lobe bronchus, and the lobe subsequently re-expanded.

TABLE 12.11 Radiographic Signs in Lobar Atelectasis

Direct Signs	*Indirect Signs*
Displacement of interlobar fissure	Increased density of atelectatic lung
	Bronchovascular crowding
	Ipsilateral diaphragm elevation
	Ipsilateral tracheal/cardiac/mediastinal shift
	Hilar elevation (upper lobe atelectasis) or depression (lower lobe atelectasis)
	Compensatory hyperinflation of other lobe(s)
	Shifting granuloma
	Ipsilateral small hemithorax
	Ipsilateral rib space narrowing

Segmental Atelectasis. Atelectasis of one or several segments of a lobe is difficult to determine on plain radiographs. The appearance ranges from a thin linear opacity to a wedge-shaped opacity that does not abut an interlobar fissure. Segmental atelectasis is better appreciated on CT.

Subsegmental (Platelike) Atelectasis. Bandlike linear opacities representing linear atelectasis are commonly associated with hypoventilation. This is seen in patients with pleuritic chest pain, postoperative patients, or patients

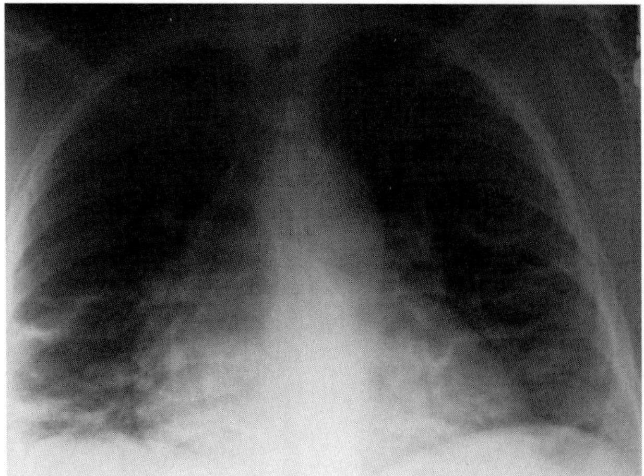

FIGURE 12.26. **Subsegmental (Platelike) Atelectasis. A.** Frontal chest radiograph in a woman 1 day following a cholecystectomy shows diminished lung volumes and numerous bilateral middle and lower zone linear opacities coursing perpendicular to the costal pleura, representing areas of subsegmental atelectasis. **B.** The opacities resolved within several days.

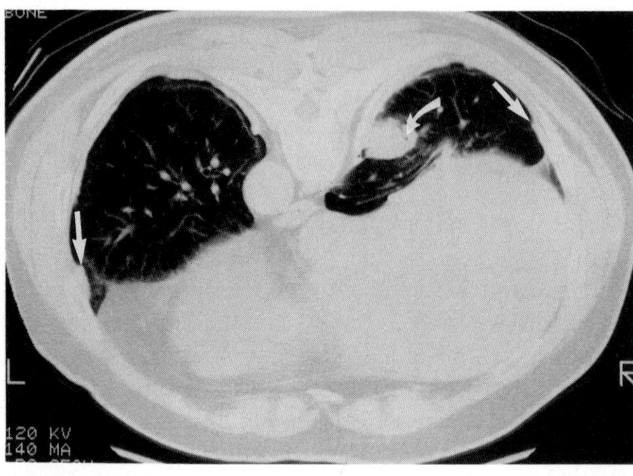

FIGURE 12.27. **Round Atelectasis.** Prone CT scan through the lung bases in a patient with asbestos-related pleural disease and rounded atelectasis shows a triangular opacity in the posteromedial right lower lobe associated with pleural thickening. Note the bronchus at the apex of the triangle (*curved arrow*). Bilateral pleural plaques are also evident (*straight arrows*).

with massive hepatosplenomegaly or ascites. Subsegmental atelectasis tends to occur at the lung bases. The linear shadows are 2 to 10 cm in length and are typically oriented perpendicular to the costal pleura (Fig. 12.26). Pathologically, these areas of linear collapse are deep to invaginations of visceral pleura formed by incomplete fissures or scars.

Rounded Atelectasis. This is an uncommon form of atelectasis in which the collapsed lung forms a round mass in the lower lobe. This condition is most closely associated with asbestos-related pleural disease but may be seen in any condition associated with an exudative (proteinaceous) pleural effusion. The process develops when pleural adhesions form in the resolving phase of a pleural effusion and cause the adjacent lung to roll up into a ball as it reexpands. The round opacity is most often found along the inferior and posterior costal pleural surfaces adjacent to an area of pleural fibrosis or plaque formation. Plain radiographs reveal a well-defined, pleural-based mass between 2 and 7 cm adjacent to an area of pleural thickening in the lower lung. The identification of a curvilinear bronchovascular bundle or "comet tail" entering the anterior inferior margin of the mass, as seen on lateral radiographs or tomograms, is characteristic. The CT appearance of round atelectasis is characteristic (Fig. 12.27). The round or wedge-shaped mass forms an acute angle with the pleura and is seen adjacent to an area of pleural thickening, usually in the inferior and posterior thorax. The "comet tail" of vessels and bronchi is seen curving between the hilum and the apex of the mass. The atelectatic lung enhances following intravenous contrast administration. When the characteristic CT findings are seen in a patient with a known history of pleural disease, the appearance is diagnostic and no further evaluation is necessary. However, if any of the above criteria are not satisfied, the lesion should be biopsied to exclude malignancy.

Right Upper Lobe Atelectasis (Fig. 12.28A) (19). In RUL atelectasis, the lung collapses superiorly and medially, with superomedial displacement of the minor fissure and anteromedial displacement of the upper half of the major fissure, producing a right upper paramediastinal density on frontal radiographs, which can obliterate the normal right paratracheal stripe and azygos vein. A central convex mass will prevent part of the usual fissure concavity. This appearance produces the S sign of Golden. The trachea is deviated toward the right, and the right hilum and hemidiaphragm are elevated. "Tenting" or "peaking" of the diaphragm is occasionally seen and represents fat within the inferior aspect of a stretched inferior accessory fissure. Compensatory hyperinflation of the middle and lower lobes may be seen in chronic atelectasis, and the LUL may herniate across the midline anteriorly toward the right. Scarring from tuberculosis, endobronchial tumor, and mucous plugging are common causes of RUL atelectasis.

Left upper lobe/lingular atelectasis (Fig. 12.28B) has a different appearance from RUL atelectasis because of the absence of a minor fissure. The LUL collapses anteriorly, maintaining a broad area of contact with the anterior costal pleural surface. The major fissure shifts anteriorly and is seen marginating a long, narrow band of increased opacity paralleling the anterior chest wall on lateral radiographs. Diagnosis on frontal radiographs may be difficult. There is a veil of increased opacity over the left upper thorax, which can obliterate the aortic knob, AP window, and

(*text continues on page 373*)

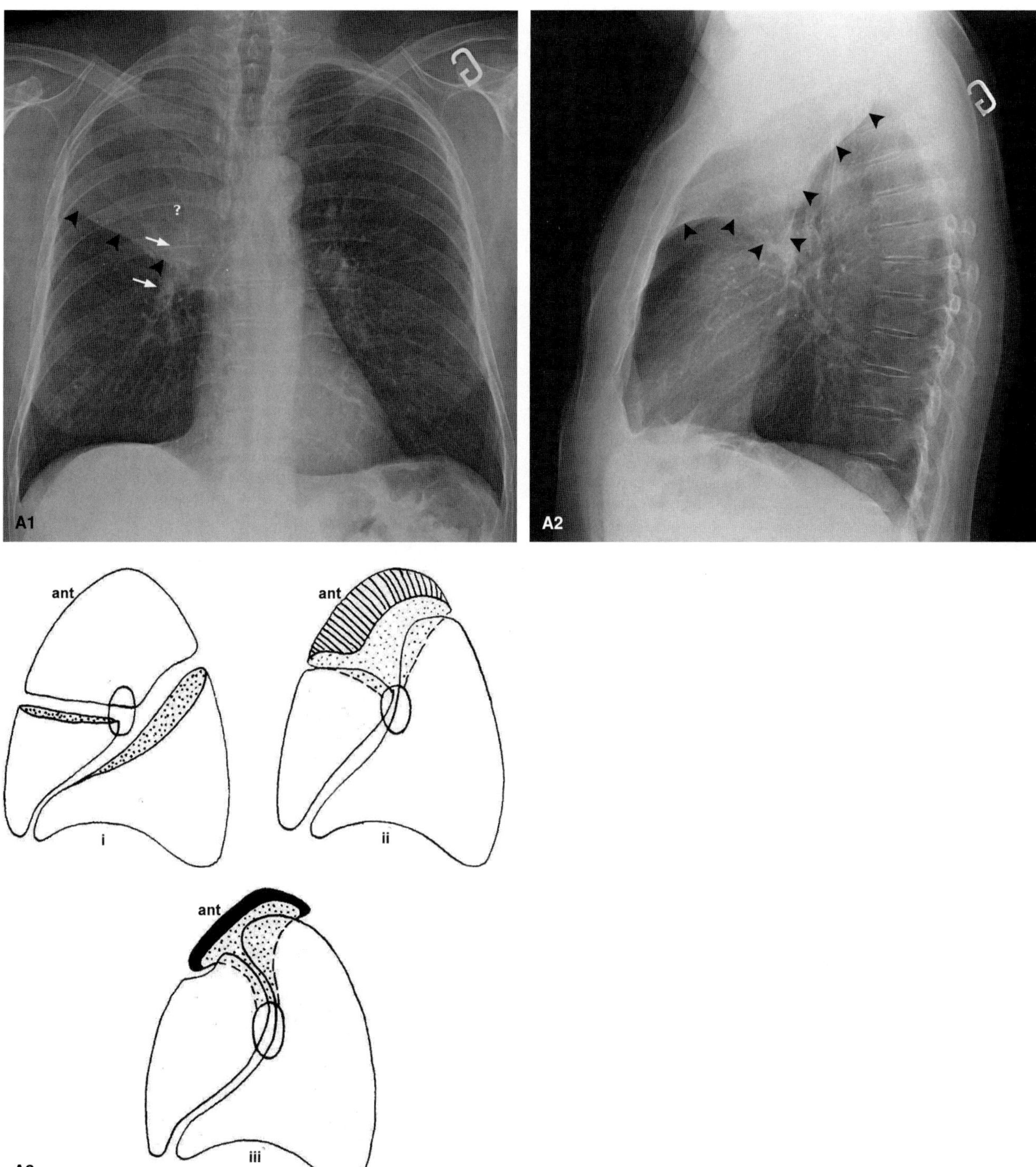

FIGURE 12.28. **Lobar Atelectasis, PA, Lateral, and Schematic Representations. A. Right upper lobe.** *Black arrowheads* outline the elevated and bowed minor fissure; *black arrows* outline the right major fissure, as in diagram **ii.** Note the elevated right hilum, with the *white arrows* showing the interlobar artery, and the silhouetting of the normal contours of the SVC and upper hilum (*white question mark*). The significant density is caused by mucus retention within the atelectatic lobe (courtesy of Dr. Louise Samson). (*continued*)

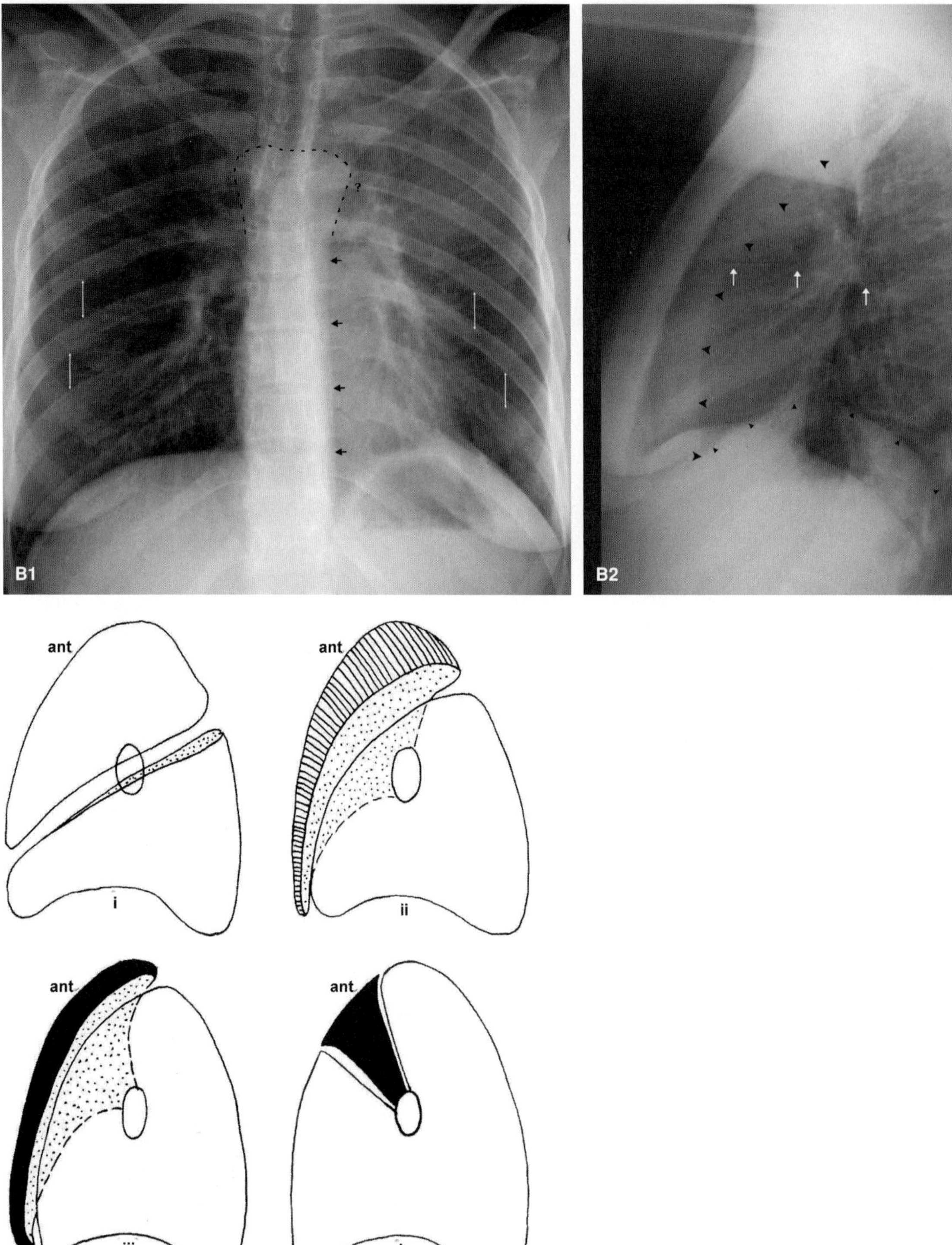

FIGURE 12.28. (*Continued*) **B. Left upper lobe (LUL).** *Large black arrowheads* outline the major fissure, as in diagram **iii,** reaching down to the slightly elevated left hemidiaphragm (*small black arrowheads*). The nondisplaced right minor fissure demonstrates this is a left-sided process. On the posteroanterior view, we note the diffuse opacity of the LUL. Note that the contours of the aortic knob and anteroposterior window are silhouetted (*black question mark*) and that the LUL bronchus is retracted superiorly (*white arrowheads*). The *black broken line* outlines the manubrium, not to be mistaken for the aortic knob. The *small black arrows* outline the descending aorta, which remains visible in LUL atelectasis. The congruent *white double arrows* (pair "a" and pair "b") show the narrowing of the rib cage from the volume loss. (*continued*)

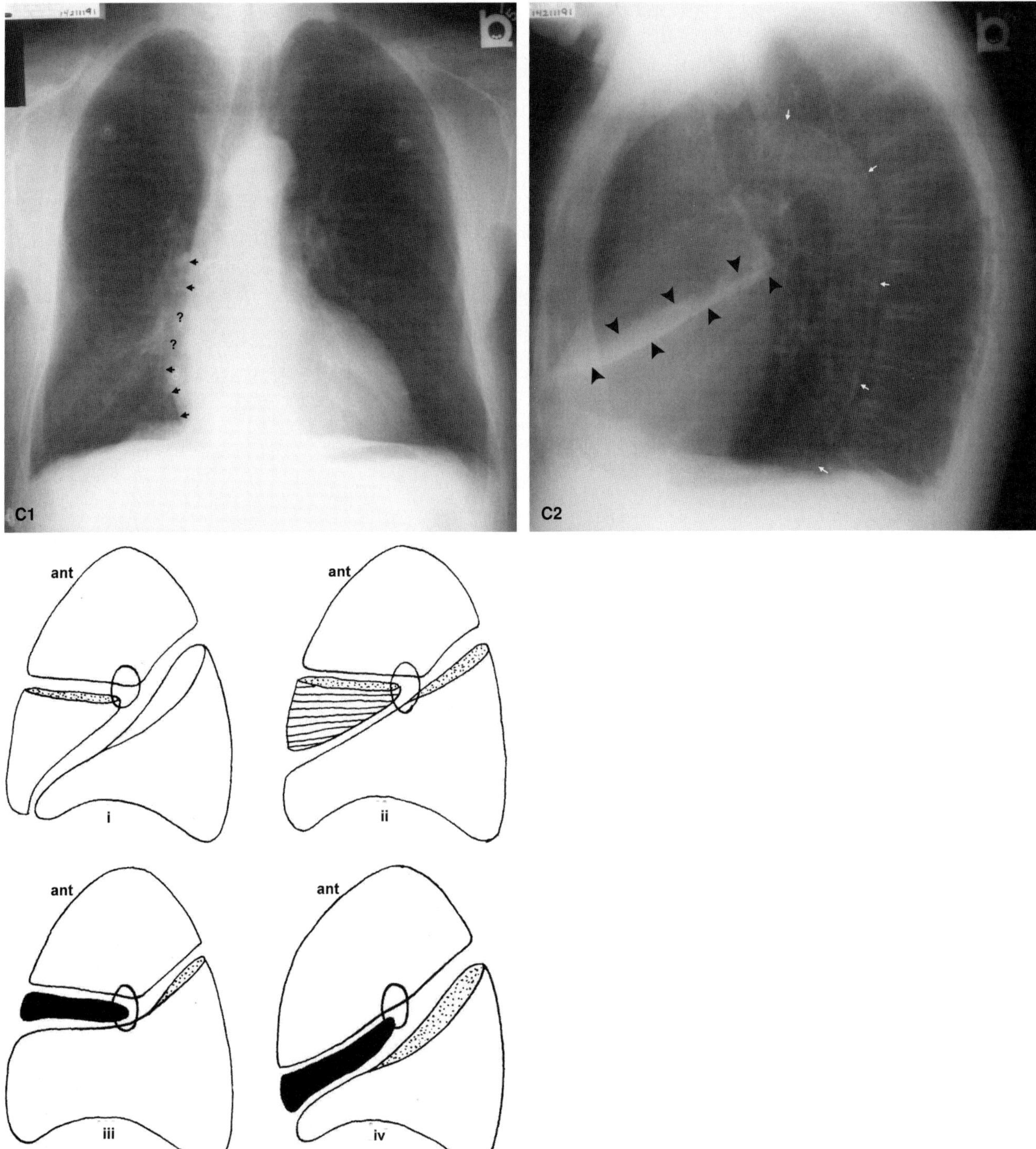

FIGURE 12.28. *(Continued)* **C. Right middle lobe.** On the lateral view, the *black arrowheads* outline the upper and lower edges of the minor fissure, as in diagram **iv.** On the posteroanterior view, we note that the mid-cardiac of the right mediastinal contour (*small black arrows*) is silhouetted (*black question marks*). (*continued*)

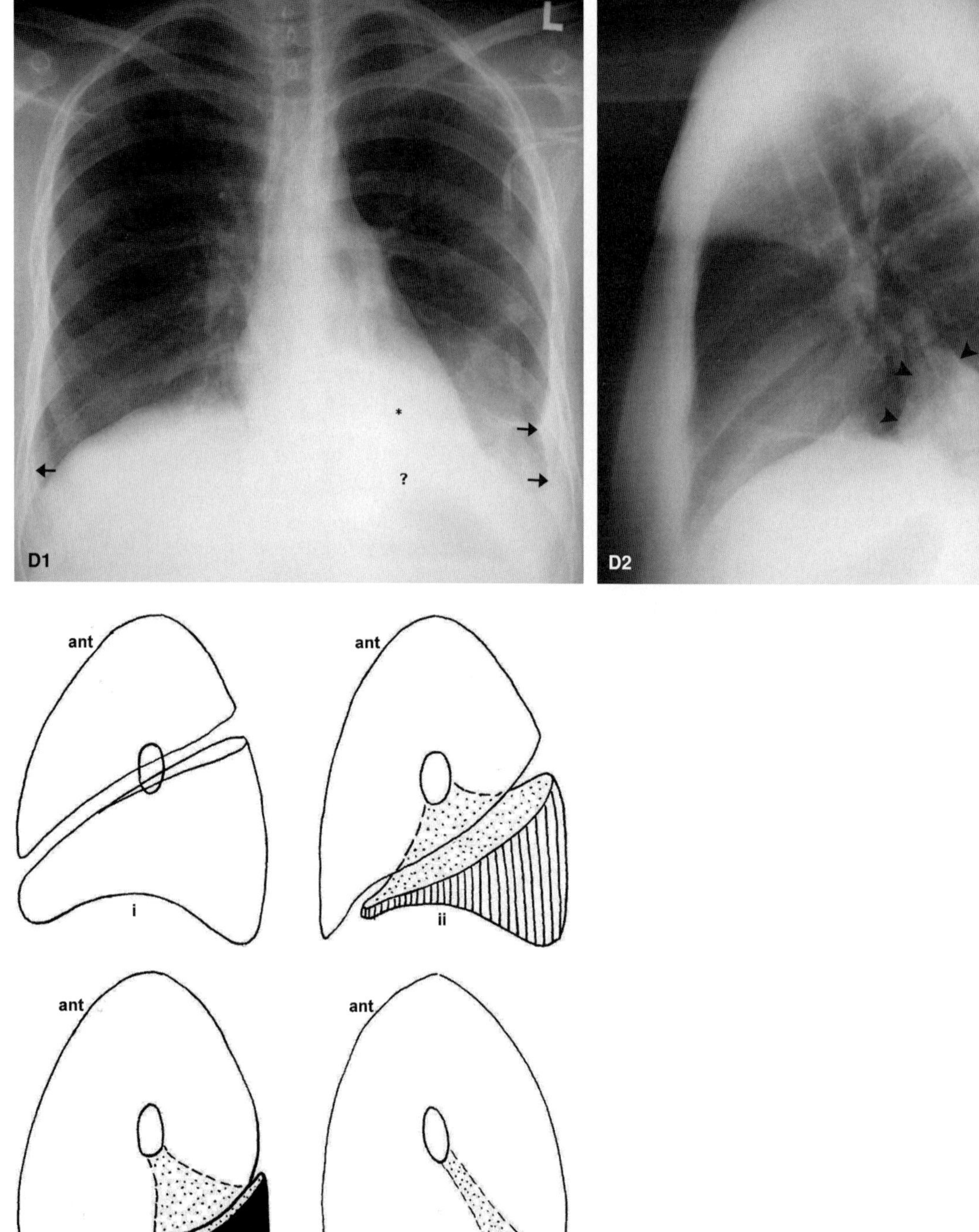

FIGURE 12.28. (*Continued*) **D. Right and left middle lobes.** Both lower lobes collapse in a similar fashion. In this example of left lower lobe atelectasis with effusions (*black arrows*), note how the major fissure (*large black arrowheads*) outlines the atelectatic lobe (*asterisk*), as depicted on diagram **iii.** The contour of the left hemidiaphragm is lost (*question mark*). The inferior displacement of the hilum demonstrates volume loss: note the vertical migration of the left mainstem bronchus (*small black arrows*), and the contour of the left descending pulmonary artery (*white arrowheads*). (Diagrams from Reed (19); used with permission from RSNA.)

left upper cardiac margin. The apex of the left hemithorax remains lucent as a result of hyperinflation of the superior segment of the LLL. Leftward tracheal displacement, hilar and diaphragmatic elevation, and leftward bulging of the anterior junction line from an overinflated RUL are additional clues to the diagnosis. An uncommon finding on the frontal radiograph in LUL atelectasis is a crescent of air ("Luftsichel") along the left upper mediastinum, which represents a portion of the overinflated superior segment of the LLL interposed between the aortic arch medially and the collapsed upper lobe laterally (see Fig. 15.9). Postinflammatory cicatrization and endobronchial tumor are the most common causes of LUL atelectasis.

Middle lobe atelectasis (Fig. 12.28C) displaces the minor fissure inferiorly and the major fissure superiorly. Because of the minimal thickness of the collapsed middle lobe and the oblique orientation of the inferiorly displaced minor fissure, the detection of middle lobe atelectasis on frontal radiographs is difficult. The only finding on frontal radiographs may be a vague density over the right lower lung, with obscuration of the right heart margin. The lateral radiograph shows a typical triangular density, with its apex at the hilum. A lordotic frontal radiograph, which projects the minor fissure tangent to the frontal x-ray beam, will depict the atelectatic middle lobe as a triangular opacity, which is sharply marginated superiorly by the minor fissure, with its apex directed laterally. Middle lobe atelectasis is most often cicatricial and follows middle lobe infection with secondary fibrosis and bronchiectasis.

Right Lower Lobe Atelectasis (Fig. 12.28D). The RLL collapses toward the lower mediastinum owing to the tethering effect of the inferior pulmonary ligament. This results in inferior displacement of the upper half of the major fissure and posterior displacement of the lower half, producing a triangular opacity in the right lower paravertebral space that obscures the medial right hemidiaphragm on frontal radiographs (Fig. 12.25). The lateral margin of this triangular opacity is formed by the displaced major fissure. The right hemidiaphragm may be elevated. The right interlobar pulmonary artery is obscured within the opaque collapsed lower lobe, a finding that helps distinguish the triangular opacity of RLL atelectasis from a medial pleural effusion, which tends to displace the interlobar artery laterally rather than obscure it. On lateral radiographs, a vague triangular opacity with its apex at the hilum and its base over the posterior portion of the right hemidiaphragm and posterior costophrenic sulcus may be seen. Mucous plugs, foreign bodies, and endobronchial tumors are the most common etiologic agents.

Left lower lobe atelectasis (Fig. 12.28D) is similar in appearance to atelectasis of the RLL. A triangular opacity in the left lower paramediastinal region, with loss of the medial retrocardiac diaphragmatic outline, is seen on frontal radiographs. In addition, the left hilum is displaced inferiorly and the interlobar artery is obscured. The diaphragm may be elevated and the heart shifted toward the left. Compensatory hyperinflation of the LUL may be seen. The LLL commonly is atelectatic in patients with large hearts and in postoperative patients, particularly those who have had coronary bypass surgery.

Combined middle and right lower lobe atelectases may be seen with obstruction of the bronchus intermedius by a mucous plug or tumor. The radiographic appearance on the frontal radiograph is characteristic, with a homogeneous triangular opacity sharply marginated superiorly by the depressed minor fissure and obscuration both of the right heart border and the right hemidiaphragm. Cardiac and mediastinal shift toward the right is common.

Collapse of an entire lung is most often seen with obstructing masses in the main bronchus. The lung is opacified, with an absence of air bronchograms. The trachea and heart are shifted toward the side of collapse, with herniation of the contralateral anteromedial lung across the midline to widen the retrosternal space on lateral radiographs and bulge the anterior junction line on frontal radiographs. The chest wall may show approximation of the ribs in chronic collapse. Compensatory diaphragmatic elevation in left lung atelectasis may be recognized by noting superior displacement of the gastric air bubble or splenic flexure of the colon.

Interstitial Disease. Interstitial opacities are produced by processes that thicken the interstitial compartments of the lung. Water, blood, tumor, cells, fibrous tissue, or any combination of these may render the interstitial space visible on radiographs. Interstitial opacities are usually divided into reticular, reticulonodular, nodular, and linear patterns on plain radiographs (Fig. 12.29) (Table 12.12) (20,21). The predominant pattern of opacity produced by an interstitial process depends upon the nature of the underlying disease and the portion of the interstitium affected.

Reticular pattern refers to a network of curvilinear opacities that usually involves the lungs diffusely. The subdivision of reticular opacities into fine, medium, and coarse opacities refers to the size of the lucent spaces created by these intersecting curvilinear opacities (Fig. 12.29). A fine reticular pattern, also known as a "ground-glass pattern," is seen in processes that thicken or line the parenchymal interstitium of the lung to produce a fine network of lines with intervening lucent spaces on the order of 1 to 2 mm in diameter. Diseases that most commonly produce this appearance include interstitial pulmonary edema and usual interstitial pneumonitis. Medium reticulation, also termed "honeycombing," refers to reticular interstitial opacities where the intervening spaces are 3 to 10 mm in diameter. This pattern is most commonly seen in pulmonary fibrosis involving the parenchymal and peripheral interstitial spaces. Coarse reticular opacities with spaces greater

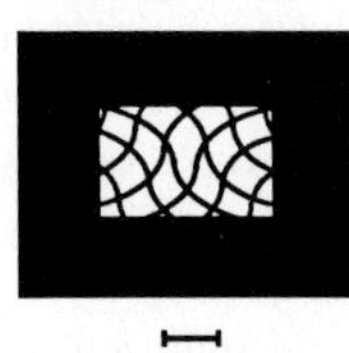
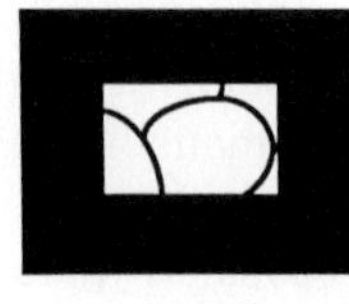
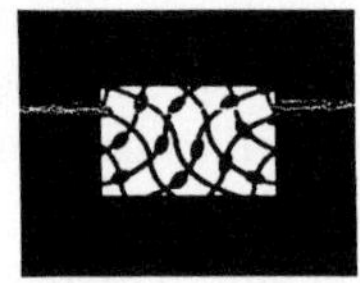

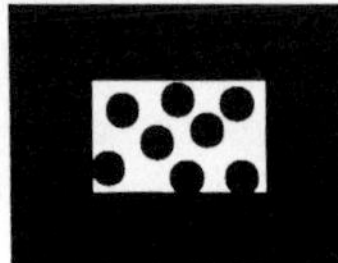
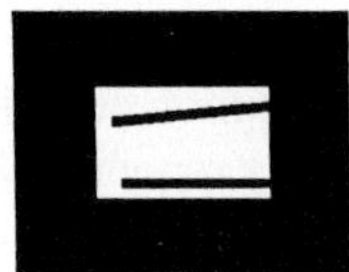

FIGURE 12.29. **Patterns of Interstitial Opacity on Chest Radiographs.**

than 1 cm in diameter are seen most commonly in diseases that produce cystic spaces as a result of parenchymal destruction. The most common interstitial diseases associated with coarse reticulation are idiopathic pulmonary fibrosis, sarcoidosis, and Langerhans cell histiocytosis of the lung.

Nodular opacities represent small rounded lesions within the pulmonary interstitium. In contrast to airspace nodules, interstitial nodules are homogeneous (they lack air bronchiolograms or air alveolograms) and well defined, as their margins are sharp and they are surrounded by normally aerated lung. In addition, unlike airspace nodules, which tend to be uniform in diameter (approximately 8 mm), these opacities can be divided into miliary opacities (<2 mm), micronodules (2 to 7 mm), nodules (7 to 30 mm), or masses (>30 mm). A micronodular or miliary pattern is seen predominantly in granulomatous processes (e.g., miliary tuberculosis or histoplasmosis)

TABLE 12.12 Patterns of Pulmonary Opacities

Predominantly linear	
Chronic interstitial edema	
Lymphangitic carcinomatosis	
Interstitial fibrosis of any etiology	
Predominantly reticular: acute	
Edema	Heart failure
	Fluid overload
	Nephropathy
Infection	Viral
	Mycoplasma
	Pneumocystis carinii
	Malaria
Drug reactions	
Predominantly reticular: chronic	
Postinfectious scarring	Tuberculosis (postprimary)
	Histoplasmosis (chronic)
	Coccidioidomycosis (chronic)
	Pneumocystis carinii
Chronic interstitial edema	Mitral valve disease
Collagen vascular disease	Rheumatoid lung
	Scleroderma
	Dermatomyositis/polymyositis
	Ankylosing spondylitis
	Mixed connective tissue disease
	Idiopathic pulmonary hemorrhage
Granulomatous disease	Sarcoidosis
	Eosinophilic granuloma
Neoplasm	Lymphangitic carcinomatosis
	Lymphoma and lymphocytic disorders
	Lymphocytic interstitial pneumonitis
Inhalational	Asbestosis
	Silicosis and coal worker's pneumoconiosis
	Hypersensitivity pneumonitis (chronic phase)
	Chronic aspiration
Drug reaction	Nitrofurantoin
	Chemotherapeutic agents
	Amiodarone
	Radiation pneumonitis (chronic)
Idiopathic	Idiopathic pulmonary fibrosis
	Lymphangioleiomyomatosis
	Tuberous sclerosis
	Neurofibromatosis
	Amyloidosis (alveolar septal form)
Predominantly nodular	
Infection	Mycobacteria
	Tuberculosis
	Nontuberculous mycobacteria
	Fungi
	Histoplasmosis
	Blastomycosis
	Coccidioidomycosis
	Cryptococcosis
	Virus
	Varicella (healed)
	Bacterial
	Septic emboli
	Parasites

(*continued*)

TABLE 12.12 Patterns of Pulmonary Opacities (Continued)

Inhalation diseases	Inorganic (pneumoconiosis)
	Silicosis* and coal worker's pneumoconiosis*
	Berylliosis*
	Siderosis
	Heavy metal dust
	Talcosis
	Organic
	Hypersensitivity pneumonitis
	Toxic inhalants
	Isocyanates
Granulomatous disease	Sarcoidosis*
	Langerhans cell histiocytosis (early)
Vascular	Arteriovenous malformation
	Vasculitis
	Wegener
	Lymphomatoid granulomatosis
	Systemic lupus erythematosus
Neoplasm	
Primary	Synchronous bronchogenic carcinoma
Metastatic	Lymphoma*
	Hodgkin
	Non-Hodgkin
	Bronchogenic carcinoma*
	Thyroid carcinoma
	Renal cell carcinoma*
	Breast carcinoma*
	Melanoma
	Choriocarcinoma
	Osteogenic carcinoma
Idiopathic	Alveolar microlithiasis
	Amyloidosis (nodular form)

*These entities can also present as reticulonodular disease.
Adapted from Reed (21); information used with permission.

(see Fig. 16.9), hematogenous pulmonary metastases (most commonly thyroid and renal cell carcinoma), and pneumoconioses (silicosis) (see Fig. 17.10). Nodules and masses are most often seen in metastatic disease to the lung.

Reticulonodular opacities may be produced by the overlap of numerous reticular shadows or by the presence of both nodular and reticular opacities. Although this appearance appears to be frequent on radiographs, only a few diseases actually show reticulonodular involvement on pathology specimens. Silicosis, sarcoidosis, and lymphangitic carcinomatosis are diseases that may give rise to true reticulonodular opacities.

Linear patterns of interstitial opacities are seen in processes that thicken the axial (bronchovascular) or peripheral interstitium of the lung. Because the axial interstitium surrounds the bronchovascular structures, thickening of this compartment produces parallel linear opacities radiating from the hila when visualized in length or peribronchial "cuffs" when viewed end-on. A central distribution of linear interstitial disease is most often seen with interstitial pulmonary edema or "increased markings" emphysema. This pattern of interstitial disease may be impossible to distinguish from airways diseases, such as bronchiectasis and asthma, which primarily thicken the walls of airways. Thickening of the peripheral interstitium of the lung produces linear opacities that are either 2 to 6 cm long, <1-mm-thick lines that are obliquely oriented and course through the substance of the lung toward the hila (Kerley A lines) or shorter (1 to 2 cm) thin lines that are peripheral and course perpendicular to and contact the pleural surface (Kerley B lines). Kerley A lines correspond to thickening of connective tissue sheets within the lung, which contain lymphatic communications between the perivenous and bronchoarterial lymphatics, while Kerley B lines represent thickened peripheral subpleural interlobular septa (see Fig. 14.1) (22). A linear pattern of disease is seen in pulmonary edema, lymphangitic carcinomatosis, and acute viral or atypical bacterial pneumonia. The HRCT findings of interstitial lung disease are reviewed in Chapter 17.

Pulmonary nodule refers to a discrete rounded opacity within the lung measuring less than 3 cm in diameter. A round opacity greater than 3 cm in diameter is termed a *pulmonary mass*. A solitary pulmonary nodule presents a common diagnostic dilemma that will be discussed in a subsequent section.

Mucoid Impaction. Branching tubular opacities that are distinguished from normal vascular shadows invariably represent mucus-filled, dilated bronchi and are termed *bronchoceles* or *mucoid impactions*. Their appearance has been likened to that of a gloved finger or the shape of the letters V or Y, depending upon the length of airway and number of branches involved. When in a central perihilar location, these bronchoceles are a result of nonobstructive bronchiectasis, as in cystic fibrosis or allergic bronchopulmonary aspergillosis, or of postobstructive bronchiectasis distal to an endobronchial tumor or a congenitally atretic bronchus. In the latter condition, a typical location—immediately distal to the expected location of the apical segmental bronchus and a hyperlucent segment or lobe distal to the bronchocele owing to collateral air drift—should suggest the diagnosis. Peripheral bronchoceles are most often seen in cystic fibrosis and posttuberculous bronchiectasis.

Pulmonary Lucency

Abnormal lucency of the lung may be localized or diffuse (Table 12.13) (21). Focal radiolucent lesions of the lung include cavities, cysts, bullae, blebs, and pneumatoceles (Fig. 12.30). These lesions are usually recognized by identification of the wall that marginates the lucent lesion.

Cavities form when a pulmonary mass undergoes necrosis and communicates with an airway, leading to gas within

TABLE 12.13 Causes of Pulmonary Lucency

Localized	Cavity
	Cyst
	Bulla
	Bleb
	Pneumatocele
Diffuse	Technical factors
Unilateral	Grid cutoff
	Patient rotation
	Extrapulmonary disorder
	Soft tissue abnormalities
	Absent pectoralis muscle
	Mastectomy
	Contralateral pleural effusion/thickening
	Pneumothorax
	Pulmonary disease
	Diminished pulmonary blood flow
	Hypoplastic lung/pulmonary artery
	Obstruction of pulmonary artery
	Pulmonary embolism
	Mediastinal/hilar tumor
	Fibrosing mediastinitis
	Diminished pulmonary blood flow and hyperinflation
	Lobar atelectasis/resection
	Swyer-James syndrome
	Endobronchial tumor/foreign body producing a check-valve effect
Bilateral	Technical factors
	Overpenetrated radiograph
	Diminished pulmonary blood flow
	Congenital pulmonary outflow obstruction
	Mediastinal tumor
	Pulmonary arterial hypertension
	Chronic thromboembolic disease
	Fibrosing mediastinitis
	Diminished pulmonary blood flow and hyperinflation
	Emphysema
	Asthma

Adapted from Reed (21); information used with permission.

its center. The wall of a cavity is usually irregular or lobulated and, by definition, is greater than 1 mm thick. Lung abscess and necrotic neoplasm are the most common cavitary pulmonary lesions. A *bulla* is a gas collection within the pulmonary parenchyma that is >1 cm in diameter and has a thin wall <1 mm thick. It represents a focal area of parenchymal destruction (emphysema) and may contain fibrous strands, residual blood vessels, or alveolar septa. An *air cyst* is any well-circumscribed intrapulmonary gas collection with a smooth thin wall >1 mm thick. While some of these lesions will have a true epithelial lining (bronchogenic cyst that communicates with a bronchus), most do not and likely represent postinflammatory or posttraumatic lesions (23). A *bleb* is a collection of gas <1 cm in size within the layers of the visceral pleura. It is usually found in the apical portion of the lung. These small gas collections are not seen on plain radiographs but may be visualized on chest CT, where they are indistinguishable from paraseptal emphysema. Rupture of an apical bleb can lead to spontaneous pneumothorax. *Pneumatoceles* are thin-walled, gas-containing structures that represent distended airspaces distal to a check-valve obstruction of a bronchus or bronchiole, most commonly secondary to staphylococcal pneumonia. A *traumatic air cyst* results from pulmonary laceration following blunt trauma. These lesions generally resolve within 4 to 6 months. *Bronchiectatic cysts* are usually multiple, rounded, thin-walled lucencies found in clusters in the lower lobes, and represent saccular dilatations of airways in varicose or cystic bronchiectasis.

Unilateral pulmonary hyperlucency must be distinguished from differences in lung density resulting from technical factors or overlying soft tissue abnormalities. Grid cutoff from a combination of lateral and near or far focus-grid decentering may lead to a graduated increase in density across the width of the chest film, simulating unilateral hyperlucency. Rotation of the patient will produce an increase in density over the lung rotated away from the film cassette. Congenital absence of the pectoralis muscle (Poland syndrome) or mastectomy can produce apparent hyperlucency.

True unilateral hyperlucent lung is a result of decreased blood flow to the lung. Diminished blood flow may result from a primary vascular abnormality, shunting of blood away from a lung that traps air, or a combination of the two. Hypoplasia of the right or left pulmonary artery produces a lung that is hyperlucent and diminished in size. A similar appearance may be produced by lobar resection or atelectasis, where the remaining lobe or lung hyperinflates to accommodate the hemithorax, thereby attenuating pulmonary vessels and producing hyperlucency. Pulmonary arterial obstruction may be secondary to extrinsic compression or invasion by a hilar mass or to pulmonary embolism. A check-valve effect from an endobronchial tumor or foreign body can produce air trapping, resulting in shunting of blood and unilateral hyperlucency. The Swyer-James syndrome or unilateral hyperlucent lung is a condition that follows adenoviral infection during infancy (see Fig. 18.16). An asymmetric obliterative bronchiolitis with severe air trapping on expiration and secondary unilateral pulmonary artery hypoplasia produces the hyperlucency in this condition. Finally, asymmetric involvement of lung by emphysema can produce a hyperlucent lung; this is most common with severe bullous disease.

Bilateral hyperlucent lungs may be simulated by an overpenetrated film or by a thin patient. As with unilateral hyperlucency, true bilateral hyperlucent lungs are the result of diminished pulmonary blood flow. This may be the result of congenital pulmonary stenosis, most commonly

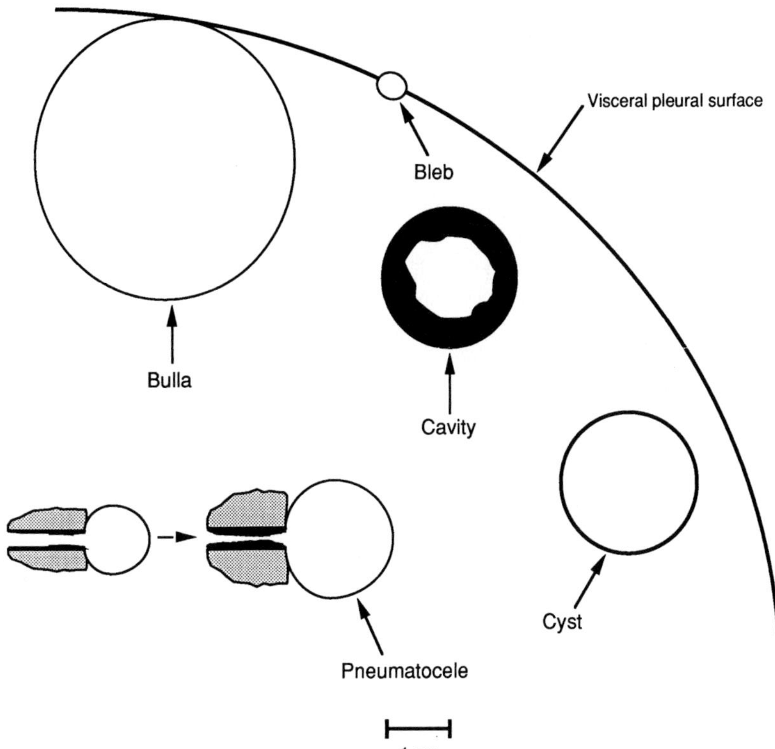

FIGURE 12.30. **Focal Lucent Pulmonary Lesions.**

associated with the tetralogy of Fallot, or secondary to an acquired obstruction of the pulmonary circulation, as in pulmonary arterial hypertension or chronic thromboembolic disease. Pulmonary emphysema results in hyperinflation with air trapping on expiration, destruction of the pulmonary microvasculature, and attenuation of lobar and segmental vessels, thereby producing bilateral hyperlucency (24). Asthma produces transient air trapping and diffuse bilateral vascular attenuation, resulting in both hyperinflation and hyperlucency.

Mediastinal Masses

Mediastinal masses are recognized on frontal radiographs by the presence of a soft tissue density that causes obliteration or displacement of the mediastinal contours or interfaces. The lung–mass interface typically is well defined laterally, where it is convex with the adjacent lung, and it creates obtuse angles with the lung at its superior and inferior margins. This latter characteristic is diagnostic of an extrapulmonary lesion, whether intramediastinal or pleural. Lateral displacement of the trachea or heart may be seen with large mediastinal masses, sometimes first recognized by displacement of an indwelling endotracheal tube, nasogastric tube, or intravascular catheter. The presence of calcification, fat, or, rarely, a fat–fluid level (as in a cystic teratoma) can limit the differential diagnosis of a mediastinal mass.

Virtually every patient with a mediastinal mass will have thoracic CT or MR performed, with US usually limited to evaluation of vascular masses and for real-time imaging guidance during transthoracic needle biopsy.

The vascular origin of a mediastinal mass is readily apparent on contrast-enhanced CT, MR, and, occasionally, transthoracic or transesophageal US. The recognition of fat within a mediastinal mass on CT or MR limits the differential diagnosis to a small number of entities, including diaphragmatic hernia, lipoma, teratoma, epicardial fat pad, and thymolipoma. A fat–fluid level is virtually diagnostic of a mature teratoma. Although calcification is occasionally detected radiographically within mediastinal masses, CT is considerably more sensitive and provides more specific characterization of the calcification. The presence of coarse calcification within an anterior mediastinal mass should suggest the diagnosis of a teratoma (especially if a tooth is seen) or thymoma (coarse calcification). Curvilinear rimlike calcification should suggest a cyst or aneurysm. Conversely, the presence of calcification within an untreated mediastinal mass virtually excludes the diagnosis of lymphoma.

Frontal and lateral chest radiographs usually localize a mediastinal mass to a structure within the anterior, middle, or posterior mediastinal compartments (see Chapter 13). For instance, if the contours of a lesion are outlined by air and seen above the clavicles, then the lesion must be in the posterior mediastinum. Conversely, if the contours of a

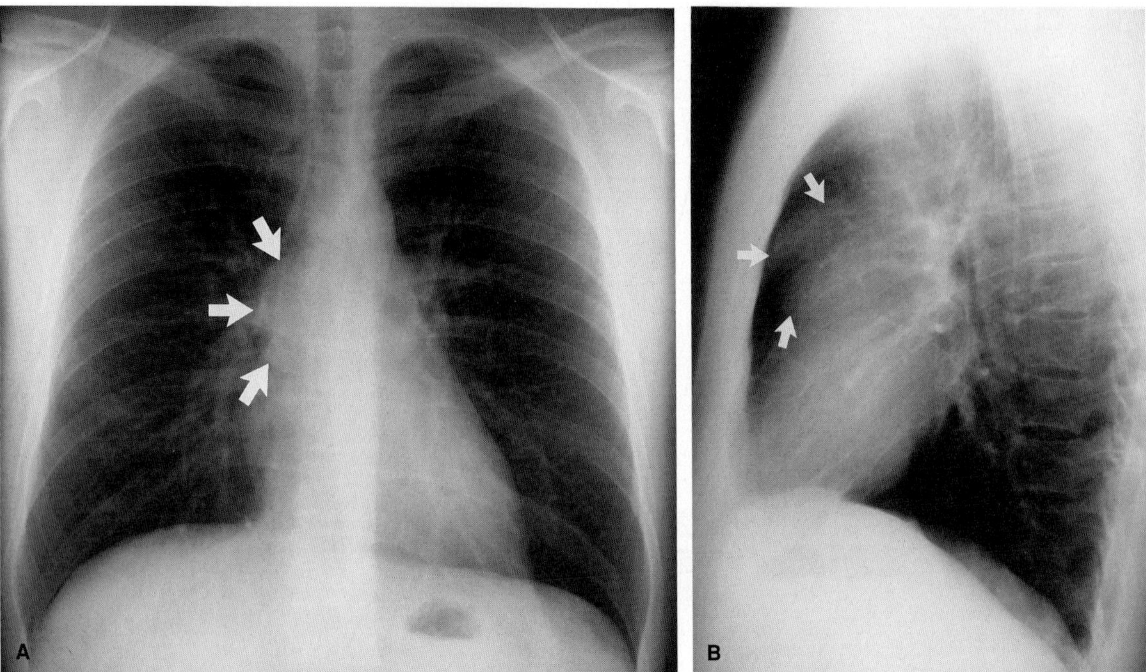

FIGURE 12.31. **Anterior Mediastinal Mass Resulting From Seminoma.** Frontal **(A)** and lateral **(B)** chest radiographs in a 35-year-old man with a history of cough and fatigue demonstrate a lobulated mass (*arrows*) in the right anterior mediastinum. A CT-guided biopsy showed seminoma.

lesion are lost at the thoracic inlet level, it must be anterior. Obviously, CT and MR provide more precise information regarding structures involved by the mass. This not only helps narrow the differential diagnosis but is key in guiding further diagnostic procedures (Fig. 12.31). For example, a posterior mediastinal mass intimately related to the esophagus may best be evaluated by esophagoscopy and transesophageal biopsy, while a subcarinal mass is best approached by bronchoscopy and transcarinal needle aspiration biopsy.

Mediastinal Widening

Mediastinal widening is described as a smooth, uniform increase in the transverse diameter of the mediastinum on frontal chest radiographs. True mediastinal disease is often difficult to distinguish from technical factors, including AP technique, supine positioning, and rotation. Clues to the presence of disease include change in mediastinal width from prior frontal radiographs, mass effect on adjacent mediastinal structures (tracheal deviation or displacement of an indwelling nasogastric tube or central venous catheter), increased density of the mediastinum, and obscuration of the normal mediastinal contours, most specifically the aortic knob and paratracheal stripe. While normal measurements have been developed for mediastinal width, there is such great individual variability that absolute measurements are somewhat useless.

Pneumomediastinum and Pneumopericardium

The diagnosis of *pneumomediastinum* is usually made by findings on conventional radiographs. Small amounts of extraluminal air appear as linear or curvilinear lucencies lining anatomic structures within the mediastinal contours (see Fig. 13.20). Larger collections may be seen outlining the cardiac silhouette, mediastinal vessels, tracheobronchial tree, or esophagus. The most common finding is air outlining the left heart border, where a curvilinear lucency representing pneumomediastinum is paralleled by a thin curvilinear opacity representing the combined thickness of the visceral and parietal pleura of the lingula. Another sign of pneumomediastinum is the "continuous diaphragm" sign, in which air dissects between the pericardium above and central diaphragm below to allow visualization of the central portion of the diaphragm in contiguity with the right and left hemidiaphragms, each of which is outlined by air in the lower lobes, respectively. While this sign is fairly specific for pneumomediastinum, pneumopericardium may produce a similar finding. Small amounts of mediastinal air are often more easily appreciated on the lateral film, with air outlining the aortic root or main or central pulmonary arteries.

Pneumomediastinum should be distinguished from three entities that may mimic some of the radiographic findings and have significantly different etiologies and

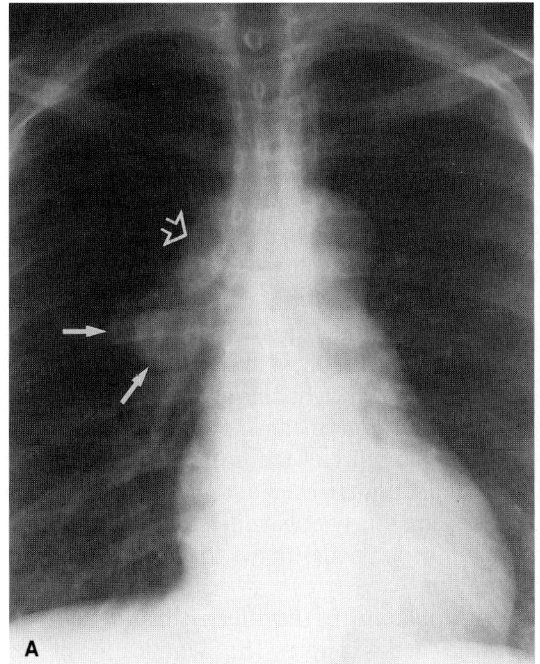

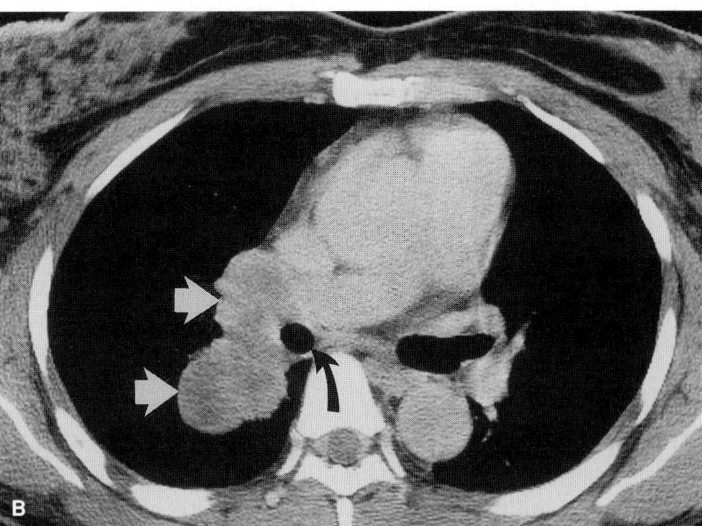

FIGURE 12.32. **Hilar Lymph Node Enlargement. A.** A posteroanterior radiograph in a 49-year-old woman with metastatic renal cell carcinoma demonstrates a lobulated enlargement and increased density of the right hilum (*solid arrows*) with concomitant paratracheal lymph node enlargement (*open arrow*). **B.** A CT scan through the hila shows the lobulated soft tissue mass (*short arrows*) within the right hilum surrounding the bronchus intermedius (*curved arrow*).

therapeutic implications: pneumopericardium, medial pneumothorax, and Mach bands. Air in the pericardial sac is limited by the normal pericardial reflections and extends superiorly to the proximal ascending aorta and main pulmonary artery. Additionally, pneumopericardium is often secondary to an infectious process with associated pericardial fluid and thickening, which will produce an air–fluid level on horizontal beam radiographs. Air within the pericardial sac will rise to a nondependent position on decubitus positioning, unlike mediastinal air, which is not mobile. The differentiation of pneumomediastinum from a medial pneumothorax is also aided by decubitus views, because pleural air will rise nondependently along the lateral pleural space. In contrast to pneumothorax, pneumomediastinum may be seen to outline intramediastinal structures (pulmonary artery, trachea) and is often bilateral. However, the distinction between pneumomediastinum and pneumothorax may be impossible, and the two conditions often coexist, particularly in the neonatal period. Paramediastinal lucent bands created by Mach effect are easily distinguished from pneumomediastinum. The lateral margin of lucent Mach bands consists of lung parenchyma, as opposed to the thin pleural line seen with mediastinal air. These bands represent an optical illusion (caused by a retinal reinforcement response [25]) that disappears when the interface between mediastinal soft tissues and lung is covered.

Hilar Disease

Signs of enlarged bronchopulmonary lymph nodes or hilar mass on frontal chest radiographs include hilar enlargement, increased hilar density, lobulation of the hilar contour, and distortion of central bronchi (26). An abnormal hilum is most easily appreciated by comparison with the contralateral hilum and by review of prior chest radiographs (Fig. 12.32). CT will often show a left hilar mass that is not evident on routine radiographs. On the right, the normally sharp right hilar angle, formed by the intersection of the lower lateral aspect of the right superior pulmonary vein with the upper lateral aspect of the right interlobar pulmonary artery, is often distorted or obscured by a right hilar mass. An increase in density of the hilar shadow is seen with a hilar mass that lies primarily anterior or posterior to the normal hilar vascular shadows. In such patients, the enlarged hilar nodes will produce an increase in density on frontal views and a lobulated appearance when viewed in profile on a lateral radiograph.

When an abnormally dense hilum is noted, the relationship between the vessels and the density must be assessed. A density through which the normal hilar vessels (interlobar artery, upper lobe arteries, left descending artery) can be seen constitutes a "hilum overlay" sign, which indicates a mass superimposed on the hilum. Conversely, vascular structures that converge only as far as the lateral margin of the increased hilar density indicate enlargement of intrahilar vascular structures (the "hilum convergence" sign). The lateral radiograph or a CT will clarify the abnormality. In patients with small lung volumes or exaggerated kyphosis, a mass in the lower right hilum on frontal radiographs may be simulated by the end-on projection of a horizontally oriented right interlobar artery. Comparison with prior radiographs will usually resolve the matter, with CT reserved for equivocal cases.

Tumors involving the lobar bronchi or bronchus intermedius may produce luminal narrowing of the bronchi with enlargement of the hilar shadow. Occasionally, an endobronchial mass produces an abrupt cutoff of the bronchial air column, which is associated with lobar atelectasis or obstructive pneumonitis. In a small percentage of normal individuals, the right or left anterior segment, upper lobe bronchi are visualized as end-on ring shadows at the superolateral margin of the hila. The presence of a soft tissue density greater than 5 mm in thickness lateral to an anterior segmental bronchus is suspicious for mass or adenopathy in this region; the posterior division of the superior vein that lies immediately lateral to the anterior segmental bronchus should not exceed this thickness. Abnormal thickening of the walls of the main or lobar bronchi is a prominent feature of hilar abnormality on lateral chest films.

Enlargement of the right or left hilar shadow from pulmonary artery dilatation is produced by increased flow or increased pressure in the pulmonary arterial circulation. Pulmonary artery dilatation is usually assessed by measurement of the right interlobar pulmonary artery on PA radiographs. The margins of this vessel are readily visible, with the lateral margin outlined by air in the lower lobe and the medial margin outlined by air in the bronchus intermedius. The upper limit of normal for the transverse diameter of the proximal right interlobar artery, as measured on a PA radiograph at a level immediately lateral to the proximal portion of the bronchus intermedius, is 17 mm in men and 15 mm in women (see Fig. 14.14).

The lateral radiograph can confirm the impression of hilar abnormality seen on frontal radiographs and may demonstrate a mass when the frontal radiograph is normal. Hilar masses that lie predominantly anterior or posterior to the hilar vessels are best visualized on the lateral view. Because the lateral radiograph is a composite of both hilar shadows, the cumulative density of bilateral hilar masses may produce a significant increase in the normal density of the composite shadow, which is more easily appreciated on a lateral than on a frontal view.

The radiographic findings of a hilar mass on lateral radiographs are an abnormal size of or a lobulated contour to the normal vascular shadows, the presence of soft tissue in a region that is normally radiolucent, an increase in density of the composite hilar shadow, and abnormalities of the central bronchi. An increase in the size and density of the composite hilar shadow is best appreciated by comparison with prior radiographs, as is usually seen with bilateral hilar lymph node enlargement from sarcoidosis. Hilar lymph node enlargement produces lobulation of the normally smooth outlines of the right and left main pulmonary arteries. There are additional findings unique to the lateral radiograph that suggest the presence of a hilar mass and may allow lateralization of the hilar abnormality. Because the RUL bronchus is visualized on the lateral radiograph in only a minority of individuals, visualization of the RUL bronchial lumen, particularly if it was invisible on a prior lateral radiograph, is strong evidence of mass or adenopathy in the upper right hilum. A lobulated posterior wall of the bronchus intermedius, or a thickness >3 mm, indicates an abnormality of the bronchus (bronchitis or bronchogenic carcinoma), edema of the axial interstitium (pulmonary edema or, lymphangitic carcinomatosis), or enlargement of lymph nodes in the posterior aspect of the lower right hilum.

The normal anatomy of the inferior hilar window was reviewed earlier in this chapter. The identification of a soft tissue mass >1 cm in diameter within this radiolucent region is an accurate indicator of unilateral or bilateral hilar mass. Occasionally, the silhouetting of the anterior wall of the LLL bronchus, recognized as a concave anterior curvilinear structure contiguous with the anterior aspect of the LUL bronchus, allows lateralization of a mass to the left lower hilum (Fig. 12.33). The added opacity of a mass within the normally radiolucent inferior hilar window produces an oval opacity to the composite hilar shadow on lateral radiographs.

On a lateral radiograph, enlargement of pulmonary arteries is assessed by measuring the left descending pulmonary artery as it arches over the left mainstem/LUL bronchus at a 2:00 position (Fig 12.19B).

Helical CT is the most sensitive method of detecting and localizing enlarged hilar (bronchopulmonary) lymph nodes and masses. Although contrast enhancement is almost never necessary to assess mediastinal nodes, it simplifies identification of enlarged vascular structures or nonenhancing hilar nodes (defined as nodes that exceed 10 mm in short-axis diameter) or masses. Hilar masses are seen on axial or coronal spin-echo MR as round masses of low or intermediate signal intensity, in distinction to the signal void of flowing blood within the hilar vessels or of air in the bronchi. Coronal MR may be superior to CT in the detection of enlarged hilar lymph nodes because it displays the hilar vessels, which are oriented in the cephalocaudad direction, in length rather than in cross section. Displacement or distortion of the hilar vessels provides indirect evidence of hilar disease. Tumor invasion of a branch of the pulmonary artery or vein within the hilum produces a filling defect within the vessel on contrast-enhanced CT or intraluminal signal on MR. The density characteristics of hilar masses on CT can help provide important information

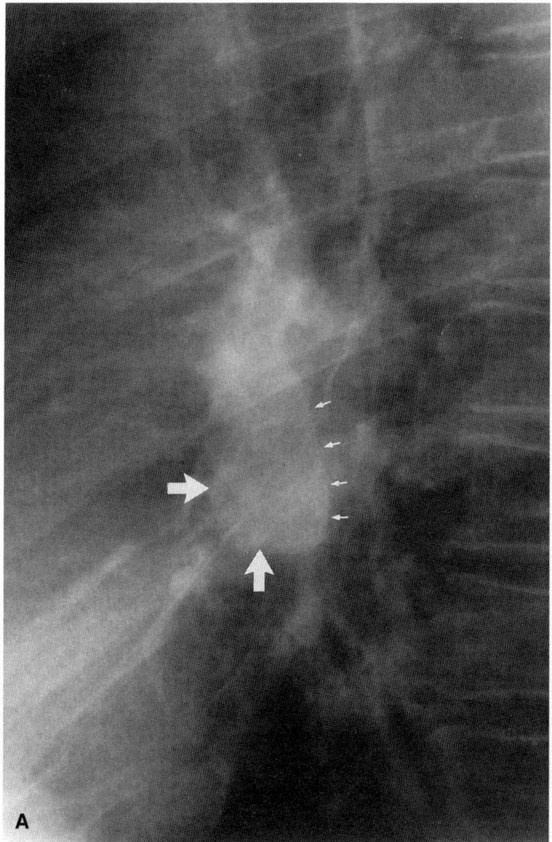

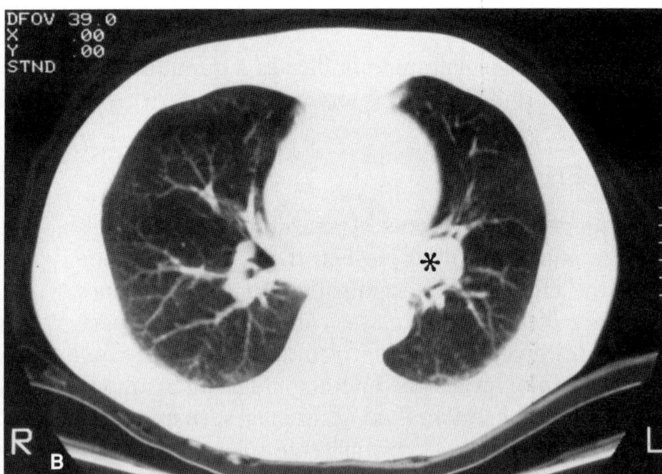

FIGURE 12.33. Hilar Mass Within the Inferior Hilar Window. A. A cone-down view of a lateral radiograph in a patient subsequently found to have a plasmacytoma of the left hilum shows a mass (*large arrows*) within the inferior hilar window obliterating the anterior wall of the left lower lobe bronchus (*small arrows*). **B.** A CT scan through the lower hila confirms the presence of a left hilar mass (*asterisk*).

for differential diagnosis; for example, a round, cystic hilar mass with imperceptible walls in an asymptomatic young person is typical of a bronchogenic cyst.

Enlarged hilar lymph nodes can be detected by CT without the use of intravenous contrast. A detailed knowledge of the normal hilar vascular and bronchial anatomy, as seen on CT, is necessary for the identification of subtle hilar contour abnormalities. In those portions of the hilum where lung directly contacts a wall of a bronchus, thickening or lobulation of the normal thin linear shadow of the bronchial wall indicates hilar abnormality. This is particularly well seen where the RLL and LLL contact the posterior walls of the bronchus intermedius and the LUL bronchus, respectively (Fig. 12.34). Lymph node enlargement in these regions is obscured on frontal radiographs by the overlying cardiac and hilar vascular shadows. CT is more sensitive than plain radiographs or MR for the detection of soft tissue masses within lobar or proximal segmental bronchi. In most patients with an endobronchial mass, a large extraluminal component produces a radiographically visible hilar soft tissue mass and obstructive atelectasis.

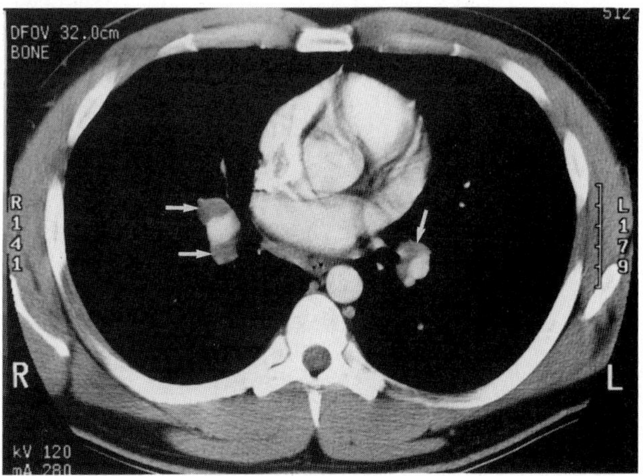

FIGURE 12.34. Enlarged Hilar Nodes on CT. Enhanced CT in a patient with biopsy-proven sarcoidosis demonstrates bilateral hilar lymph node enlargement (*arrows*).

Enlarged hilar lymph nodes may have different appearances on CT. Enlargement of discrete lymph nodes, most commonly seen in sarcoidosis, appears as multiple distinct round masses (Fig. 12.34). When tumor or an inflammatory process extends through the nodal capsule to involve contiguous nodes, a single large mass of confluent lymph nodes is produced that may be difficult to distinguish from a primary hilar bronchogenic carcinoma. This latter appearance is most often seen in hilar nodal metastases from small cell carcinoma of the lung or lymphoma (see Fig. 15.10). As in enlargement of mediastinal lymph nodes, the CT density of enlarged hilar nodes can provide clues to the diagnosis (see Table 13.5).

An abnormally small hilum indicates a diminution in the size of the right or left pulmonary artery.

Pleural Effusion

The radiographic appearance of pleural effusions depends upon the amount of fluid present, the patient's position during the radiographic examination, and the presence or absence of adhesions between the visceral and parietal pleura. Small amounts of pleural fluid initially collect between the lower lobe and diaphragm in a subpulmonic location. As more fluid accumulates, it spills into the posterior and lateral costophrenic sulci. A moderate amount of pleural fluid (>175 mL) in the erect patient will have a characteristic appearance on the frontal radiograph, with a homogeneous lower zone opacity seen in the lateral costophrenic sulcus with a concave interface toward the lung. This concave margin, known as a *pleural meniscus,* appears higher laterally than medially on frontal radiographs because the lateral aspect of the effusion, which surrounds the costal surface of the lung, is tangent to the frontal x-ray beam. Similarly, the meniscus of pleural fluid as seen on lateral radiographs peaks anteriorly and posteriorly (Fig. 12.35) (27).

In patients with suspected pleural effusion, a lateral decubitus film with the affected side down is the most sensitive technique to detect small amounts of fluid. With this technique, pleural fluid collections as small as 5 mL may be seen layering between the lung and lateral chest wall. While a moderate-size, free-flowing collection should be obvious on upright radiographs, a large pleural effusion can cause passive atelectasis of the entire lung, producing an opaque hemithorax. It may be difficult to distinguish the latter condition from collapse of an entire lung. While a massive effusion should produce contralateral mediastinal shift, a collapsed lung without pleural effusion will show shift toward the opaque side. In some patients, CT or US may be necessary to distinguish pleural fluid from collapsed lung.

CT is quite sensitive in the detection of free pleural fluid. On axial scans, pleural fluid layers posteriorly with a characteristic meniscoid appearance and has a CT attenuation value of 0 to 20 H. Small effusions may be difficult to

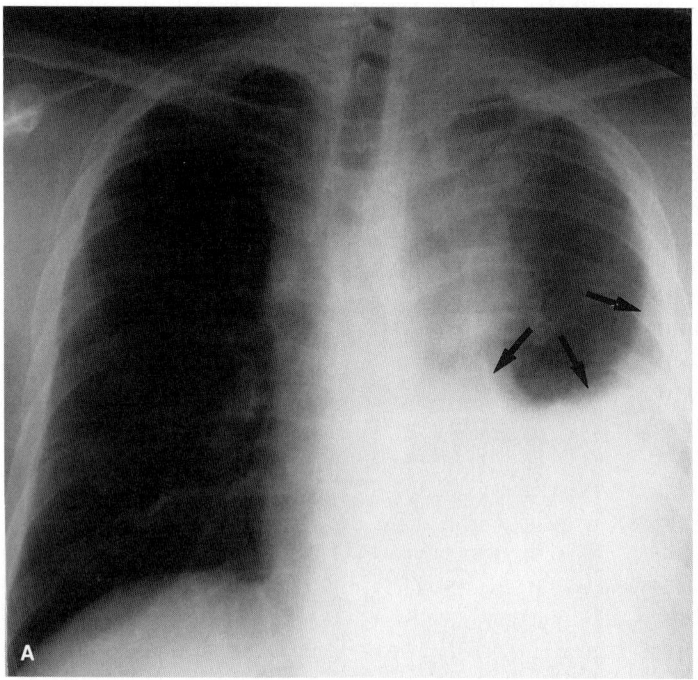

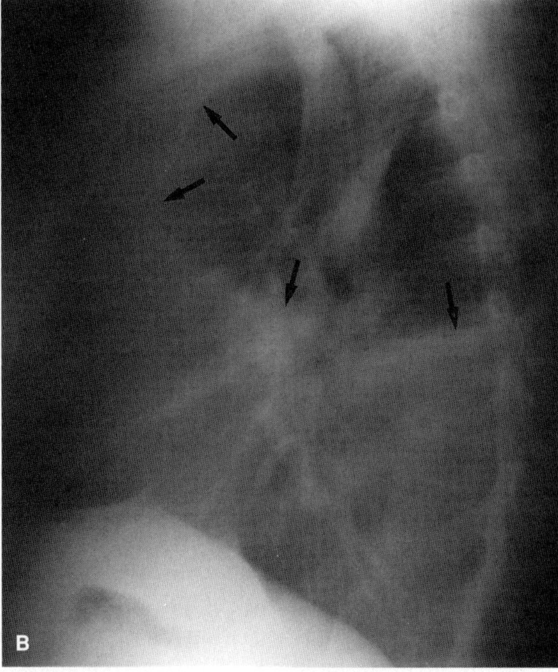

FIGURE 12.35. **Pleural Effusion on Chest Radiographs.** Posteroanterior **(A)** and lateral **(B)** chest radiographs demonstrate the typical meniscoid appearance (*arrows*) in a patient with a left pleural effusion resulting from mediastinal Hodgkin lymphoma.

differentiate from pleural thickening, fibrosis, or dependent atelectasis, and decubitus scans are useful in making this distinction. The pleural and peritoneal spaces are oriented in the axial plane at the level of the diaphragm. This may cause some difficulty in localizing the fluid to one or both spaces. Fluid in either the pleural or peritoneal space can displace the liver and spleen medially, away from the chest wall. A key to distinguishing ascites from pleural fluid on axial CT scans is to observe the relationship of the fluid to the diaphragmatic crus. Pleural fluid in the posterior costophrenic sulcus will lie posteromedial to the diaphragm and displace the crus laterally. In contrast, peritoneal fluid lies within the confines of the diaphragm and therefore will displace the crus medially. Another useful distinguishing feature is the quality of the interface of the fluid with the liver or spleen. Intraperitoneal fluid will show a distinct, sharp interface with the liver and spleen as it directly contacts these organs, whereas pleural effusions will have a hazy, indistinct interface with these viscera because of the interposed hemidiaphragms. Because the peritoneal space does not extend posterior to the bare area of the liver, right-sided fluid extending posteromedially must be pleural. A large effusion will allow the inferior edge of the adjacent atelectatic lower lobe to float in the fluid, creating a curvilinear opacity that can be misinterpreted as the diaphragm separating pleural fluid from ascites. This "pseudodiaphragm" is recognized as a broad band that does not extend far laterally or anteriorly and is contiguous superiorly with an atelectatic lung containing air bronchograms (Fig. 12.36). US is particularly useful in detecting free flowing pleural effusions, which are usually seen as anechoic collections at the base of the pleural space surrounding atelectatic lung (see Chapter 39).

Pleural fluid may become loculated between the pleural layers to produce an appearance indistinguishable from that of a pleural mass. Fluid loculated within the costal pleural layers appears as a vertically oriented elliptical opacity with a broad area of contact with the chest wall, producing a sharp, convex interface with the lung when viewed in tangent. CT is commonly utilized to detect and localize loculated pleural fluid collections. The characteristic finding is a sharply marginated lenticular mass of fluid attenuation conforming to the concavity of the chest wall that forms obtuse angles at its edges and compresses and displaces the subjacent lung. Multiple fluid locules can mimic pleural metastases or malignant mesothelioma radiographically; CT or US can confirm the fluid characteristics of these pleural "masses."

Pleural fluid may extend into the interlobar fissures, producing characteristic findings. Free fluid within the minor fissure is usually seen as smooth, symmetric thickening on a frontal radiograph. Fluid within the major fissure is normally not visible on frontal radiographs, as the fissures are viewed en face. An exception is fluid extending into the lateral aspect of an incomplete major fissure, which produces a curvilinear density extending from the inferolateral to the superomedial aspect of the lung. Fluid loculated between the leaves of visceral pleura within an interlobar fissure results in an elliptic opacity oriented along the length of the fissure. These loculated collections of pleural fluid are termed "pseudotumors" and are most often seen within the minor fissure on frontal radiographs in patients with congestive heart failure. The tendency for these opacities to disappear rapidly with diuresis has led to the term "vanishing lung tumor." Although a characteristic appearance on plain radiographs is usually sufficient for diagnosis, the CT demonstration of a localized fluid collection in the expected location of the major or minor fissure is confirmatory.

An uncommon appearance of pleural effusion is seen when fluid accumulates between the lower lobe and diaphragm and is termed a *subpulmonic* effusion. While small amounts of pleural fluid normally accumulate in this location, it is uncommon for larger effusions to remain subpulmonic without spilling into the posterior and lateral costophrenic sulci. A subpulmonic effusion may be difficult to appreciate on upright chest radiographs, because the fluid collection mimics an elevated hemidiaphragm. Clues to its presence on frontal radiographs include: apparent and new elevation of the diaphragm, lateral peaking of the hemidiaphragm that is accentuated on expiration, a minor fissure that is close to the diaphragm (right-sided effusions), and an increased separation of the gastric air bubble from the base of the lung (left-sided effusions). Despite the atypical subpulmonic accumulation of fluid with the patient upright, the effusion will layer dependently on lateral decubitus radiographs (Fig. 12.37).

The radiographic detection of pleural effusion in the supine patient can be difficult because fluid accumulates in a dependent location posteriorly. The most common finding is a hazy opacification of the affected hemithorax with obscuration of the hemidiaphragm and blunting of the lateral costophrenic angle. Fluid extending over the apex of the lung may produce a soft tissue cap with a concave interface inferiorly, while medial fluid may cause an apparent mediastinal widening.

Pneumothorax

The classic radiographic finding of pneumothorax on upright chest films is visualization of the visceral pleura as a curvilinear line that parallels the chest wall, separating the partially collapsed lung centrally from pleural air peripherally (Fig. 12.38). An expiratory radiograph aids in the detection of a small pneumothorax by increasing the volume of intrapleural air relative to lung, thereby displacing the visceral pleural reflection away from the chest wall and by exaggerating the differences in density of pneumothorax (black) to lung (gray) at the end of expiration. In a small

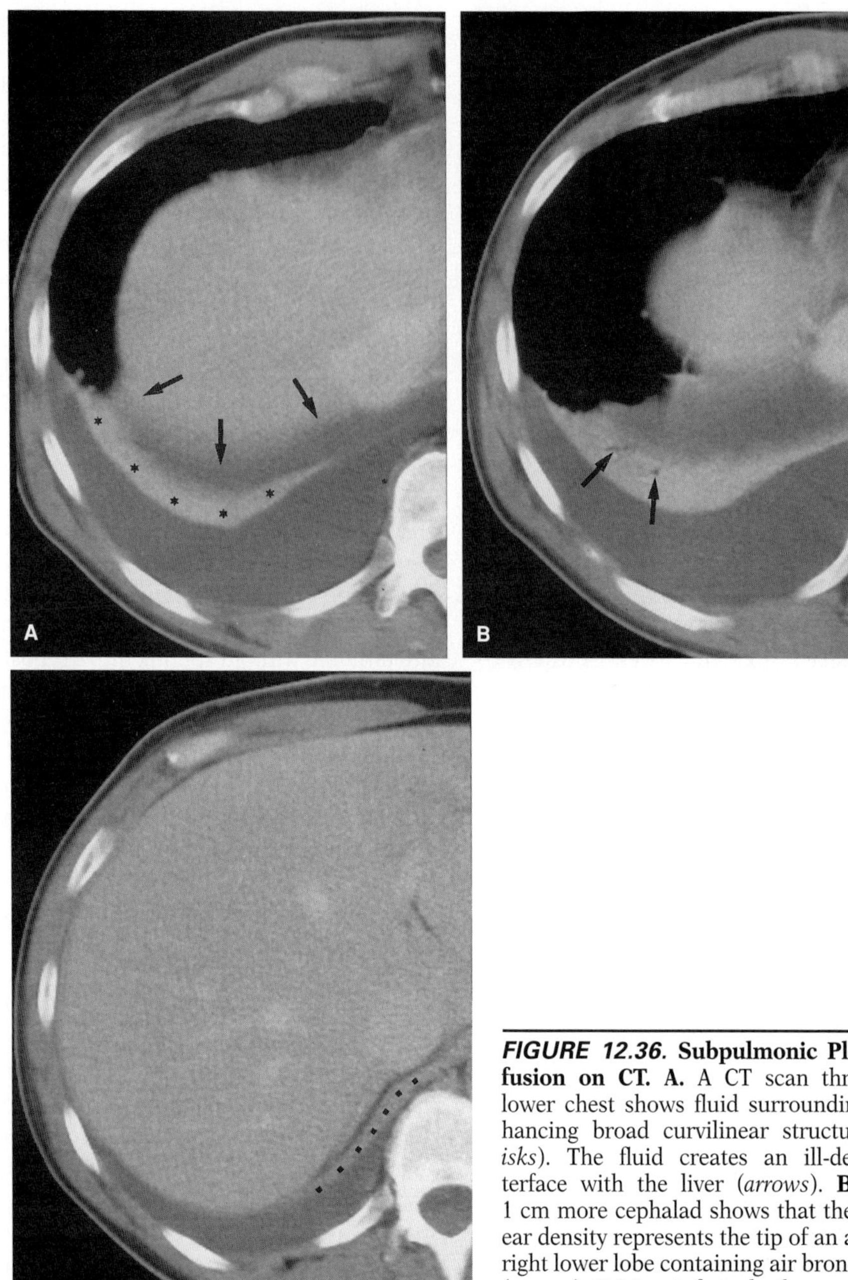

FIGURE 12.36. **Subpulmonic Pleural Effusion on CT. A.** A CT scan through the lower chest shows fluid surrounding an enhancing broad curvilinear structure (*asterisks*). The fluid creates an ill-defined interface with the liver (*arrows*). **B.** A scan 1 cm more cephalad shows that the curvilinear density represents the tip of an atelectatic right lower lobe containing air bronchograms (*arrows*). **C.** More inferiorly, the crus of the diaphragm (*dotted structure*) is displaced laterally by posteromedial pleural fluid.

percentage of patients, a pneumothorax will be visible only on a lateral or decubitus film or a frontal radiograph obtained in full inspiration. This suggests that when there is a strong clinical suspicion of pneumothorax and the frontal expiratory radiograph is normal, a lateral or inspiratory film may be beneficial for proper diagnosis.

The detection of a pneumothorax is difficult when chest films are obtained in the supine position. Approximately 30% of pneumothoraces imaged on supine radiographs go undetected. Because many portable radiographs are obtained with the patient supine, the recognition of a pneumothorax on a supine film is particularly important in the critically ill patient, who is at high risk from iatrogenic trauma or barotrauma. In a supine patient, the most nondependent portion of the pleural space is anterior or anteromedial. Small pneumothoraces will initially collect in these regions and will fail to produce a visible pleural line. The affected hemithorax may appear hyperlucent. Anteromedial air may sharpen the borders of mediastinal soft tissue structures, resulting in improved visualization of the

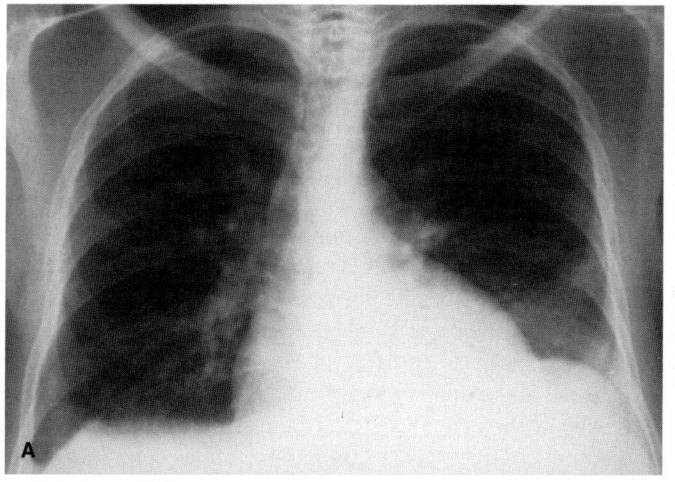

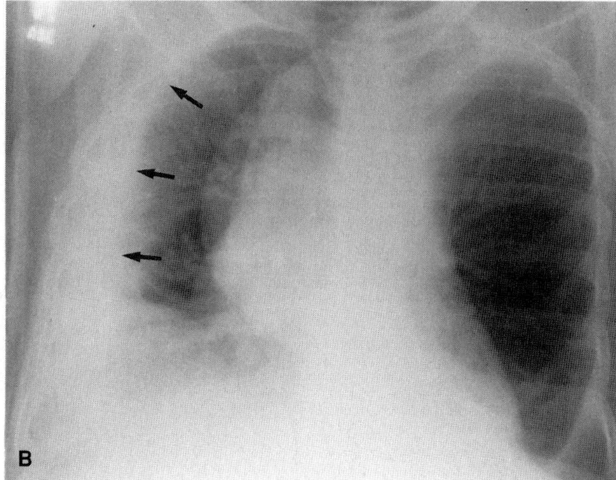

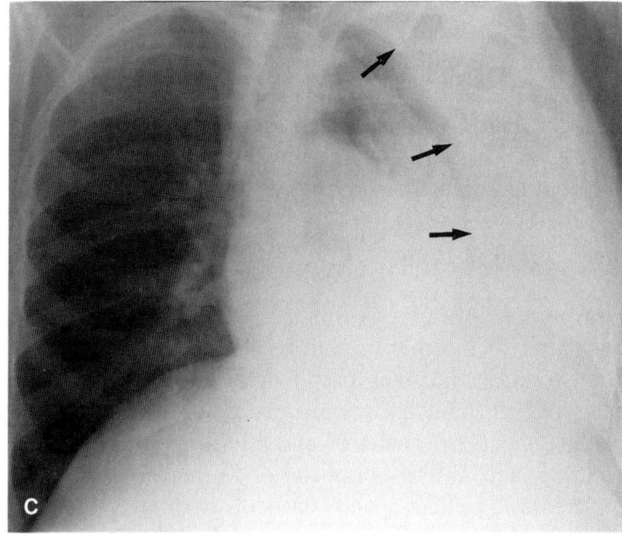

FIGURE 12.37. **Bilateral Subpulmonic Pleural Effusions. A.** An upright posteroanterior radiograph in a 41-year-old woman with ascites demonstrates apparent elevation of both hemidiaphragms. Right **(B)** and left **(C)** decubitus films demonstrate dependent layering of the subpulmonic pleural fluid (*arrows*).

cardiac margin and aortic knob. The lateral costophrenic sulcus may appear abnormally deep and hyperlucent, a finding known as the "deep sulcus" sign. Visualization of the anterior costophrenic sulcus owing to air anteriorly and inferiorly produces the "double diaphragm" sign, as the dome and anterior portions of the diaphragm are outlined by lung and pleural air, respectively. When an anterior pneumothorax is suspected on a supine radiograph, an upright film, lateral decubitus film with the affected side up, or CT scan should be obtained (Fig. 12.39).

Subpulmonic pneumothoraces are rare. Radiographically, a localized area of hyperlucency is seen inferiorly, with the visceral pleural line paralleling the hemidiaphragm. Loculated pneumothoraces develop as the result of adhesions between visceral and parietal pleura and may be found anywhere in the pleural space. CT is often necessary for diagnosis.

Several entities produce a curvilinear line or interface or hyperlucency on chest radiographs and must be distinguished from a pneumothorax. Skin folds resulting from the compression of redundant skin by the radiographic cassette can produce a curvilinear interface that simulates the visceral pleural line. A skin fold produces an edge or interface with atmospheric air, in distinction to the visceral pleural line seen in a pneumothorax. The interface produced by a skin fold rarely continues over the lung apex and is often seen to extend beyond the chest wall. Pulmonary vascular opacities may be followed peripheral to the skin fold interface. Bullae may simulate pneumothorax by producing localized or unilateral hyperlucency. They are marginated by thin curvilinear walls that are concave rather than convex to the chest wall. The distinction of pneumothorax from bullous disease may be difficult but is usually evident by the clinical presentation. However, since this distinction has important therapeutic implications, certain patients may require CT.

CT is more sensitive than conventional radiographs in the detection of pneumothorax because of its cross-sectional nature and superior contrast resolution. The CT demonstration of linear parenchymal bands of tissue traversing large avascular areas helps distinguish bullae from loculated pneumothoraces. CT may be used to

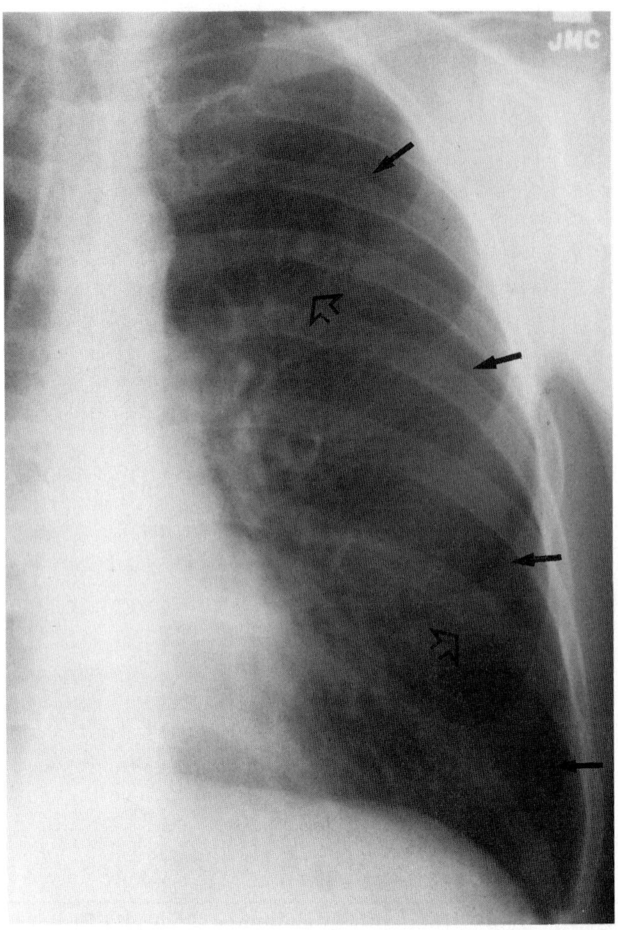

FIGURE 12.38. **The Visceral Pleural Line in Pneumothorax.** A cone-down view of an upright posteroanterior radiograph in a patient with a spontaneous pneumothorax demonstrates a curvilinear visceral pleural line (*solid arrows*) separating the lung medially from the chest wall laterally. Note the presence of thin-walled cysts (*open arrows*) from *Coccidioides* infection, which are most likely responsible for the pneumothorax.

detect and drain loculated pneumothoraces in critically ill patients.

Localized Pleural Thickening

Localized pleural thickening is seen as a flat, smooth, slightly raised soft tissue opacity extending over one or two intercostal spaces that displaces the lung from the innermost cortical margin of the ribs when viewed in tangent. Localized pleural thickening viewed en face is usually undetectable radiographically because the lesion does not significantly attenuate the x-ray beam and does not present a raised edge to be recognized as a distinct opacity. An exception is the presence of pleural calcification, which can usually be recognized as discrete thin linear or curvilinear calcific opacities paralleling the inner surface of the ribs when viewed end-on or as geographic areas of increased density with round or lobulated borders when viewed en face. Focal areas of pleural fibrosis are best appreciated on conventional and high-resolution CT scans, where they are easily distinguished from deposits of subpleural fat by their density.

There are two additional radiographic findings that mimic the appearance of focal pleural thickening. The apical cap is a curvilinear subpleural opacity <5 mm thick with a sharp or slightly irregular inferior margin which represents nonspecific fibrosis of the apical lung and adjacent visceral pleura. While it is usually bilateral and symmetric, slight asymmetry in thickness is common. Any growth of the opacity, significant asymmetry, inferior convexity of the opacity, rib destruction, or symptoms should prompt a CT or MR examination followed by biopsy to exclude an apical neoplasm (Pancoast or superior sulcus tumor). The companion shadows of the inferior aspects of the first and second ribs are smooth apical linear opacities that parallel the lower cortical margins of the first two ribs and represent the pleural layers and subpleural fat viewed in tangent. These are most prominent in obese individuals and should not be mistaken for pleural fibrosis.

Diffuse Pleural Thickening

Fibrothorax appears as a thin, smooth band of soft tissue with a sharp internal margin seen immediately beneath and parallel to the inner margin of the ribs and intercostal spaces. It is usually unilateral and extends over large areas of the dependent (posterior and inferior) portions of the pleural space. Anterior or posterior costal pleural thickening creates a veillike opacity without sharp margins when viewed en face on frontal radiographs. Blunting of the lateral costophrenic sulcus may be seen on frontal radiographs, while sparing of the posterior costophrenic sulcus and an absence of layering fluid on decubitus positioning help distinguish pleural fibrosis from a small effusion. Fibrothorax tends to spare the interlobar fissures and mediastinal pleura. CT and HRCT are more sensitive than conventional radiographs in the detection of pleural thickening. The diminished volume of the affected hemithorax seen with extensive fibrothorax is more easily appreciated on axial CT images than on frontal radiographs (see Fig. 19.9). CT and HRCT provide an unimpeded view of the underlying lung in patients with diffuse pleural thickening, allowing detection of associated interstitial pulmonary fibrosis. This is important in evaluating patients with suspected asbestosis and in assessing the extent of pulmonary disease in patients being considered for pleurectomy.

Pleural and Extrapleural Lesions

The shape and margins of a peripheral opacity as seen on conventional radiographs help define the opacity as parenchymal, pleural, or extrapleural. Pleural masses form

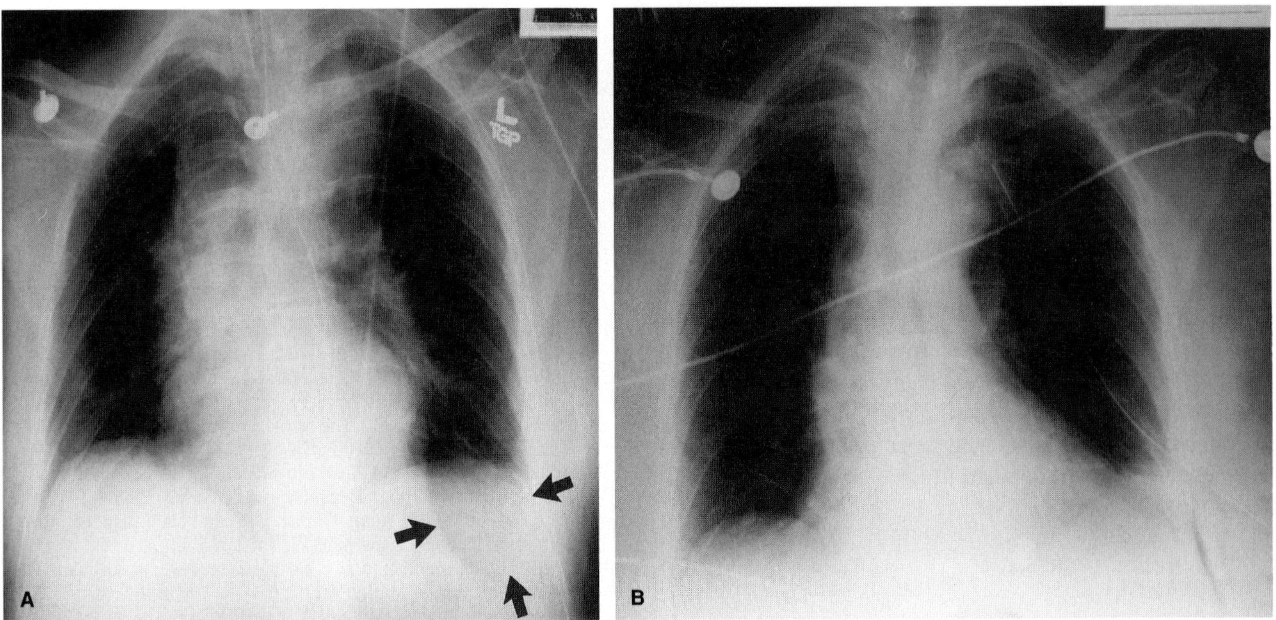

FIGURE 12.39. **Deep Sulcus Sign in Supine Patient With Pneumothorax. A.** A supine chest film obtained following placement of a left internal jugular central venous catheter shows a deep sulcus sign at the left base (*arrows*), representative of a pneumothorax. **B.** Film obtained after placement of a left thoracostomy tube shows that the deep sulcus sign has resolved.

obtuse angles with the adjacent normal pleura, in distinction to peripheral lung lesions, which usually contact the normal pleura at acute angles. Pleural and extrapleural masses are usually vertically oriented elliptic opacities. Pleural lesions tend to have smooth, well-defined margins as they compress normal lung. These smooth margins are best appreciated on radiographic projections with the x-ray beam tangent to the interface between the mass and the lung. Another feature of pleural lesions is the clarity of the margin of the lesion on frontal and lateral radiographs; a mass sharply outlined by lung on one view but poorly marginated on the orthogonal view should suggest a pleural or extrapleural process. In contrast, intraparenchymal lesions are surrounded by air and will have similar margins on both views. Pleural lesions, unlike parenchymal lesions, do not change position with respiratory motion. Lung disease is often confined to a lobe, while pleural disease may extend across fissures. Pedunculated pleural lesions such as fibromas are rare but can present with radiographic features of both pleural and parenchymal lesions.

Despite the aforementioned features, the distinction of pleural from peripheral parenchymal lesions may be difficult. This distinction has important diagnostic implications; while parenchymal processes are best evaluated by examination of expectorated sputum or by bronchoscopy, pleural lesions will require thoracentesis or pleural biopsy. CT is often used to help distinguish between pleural and parenchymal disease (see Chapter 19). A peripheral lesion that is completely surrounded by lung on CT is intraparenchymal, with the exception being the rare pleural lesion arising within an interlobar fissure. Peripheral lung masses generally have irregular margins and may contain air bronchograms. Those parenchymal lesions that contact the pleura will form acute angles with the chest wall, as on plain films. The CT appearance of pleural and extrapleural or chest wall lesions are similar. Both pleural and extrapleural lesions are sharply defined and form obtuse angles with the chest wall (see Fig. 19.10); rib destruction or subcutaneous mass are the only findings that localize an extrapulmonary lesion to the chest wall. When a peripheral parenchymal lesion invades the pleura, determining the origin of the mass may be impossible. CT can further characterize peripheral lesions by their density; a smooth fatty mass is almost certainly a pleural lipoma (see Fig. 19.10), whereas a homogeneous pleural or extrapleural soft tissue mass is most likely a fibroma or neurogenic tumor (see Fig. 19.11). The signal intensity on T1W and T2W spin-echo MR images may be useful in the characterization of focal pleural masses. On T1WIs and T2WIs, loculated fluid collections will show homogeneous low and high signal respectively. Lipomas will show homogeneous high signal intensity on T1WI and intermediate signal intensity on T2WI, while fibromas are typically of intermediate and high signal intensity, respectively, as a result of the high cellularity of these tumors.

Chest Wall Lesions

Chest wall lesions become evident radiographically when (*1*) they extend into the thorax and become outlined by displaced lung, (*2*) there is bone displacement or destruction by the mass, or (*3*) they protrude externally from the skin surface to be outlined by air in the atmosphere. CT, MR, and US are all useful in assessing the characteristics of chest wall lesions. While CT and MR are most useful in determining the extent of intrathoracic involvement by chest wall lesions, US is the least expensive and simplest method of characterizing the nature of palpable chest wall lesions, particularly if they are thought to be vascular or cystic in nature. The radiographic findings of chest wall lesions related to specific bony or soft tissue components of the chest wall are detailed in the section on chest wall disease in Chapter 19.

Diaphragm

Radiographic findings of diaphragmatic disorders include elevation and depression of the diaphragm and abnormalities of diaphragmatic contour. The diagnostic considerations of diaphragmatic disease are reviewed in Chapter 19.

REFERENCES

1. Wilkinson GA, Fraser RG. Roentgenography of the chest. Appl Radiol 1975;4:41–53.
2. Ravin CE, Chotas HG. Chest radiography. Radiology 1997;204:593–600.
3. Wandtke JC. Bedside chest radiography. Radiology 1994;192:282–284.
4. Prokop M, Galanski M, van der Molen AJ, Schaefer-Prokop CM. Spiral and Multislice Computed Tomography of the Body. 1st ed. Thieme, 2003:109–160.
5. Bogaert J, Dymarkowski S, Taylor AM. Clinical Cardiac MRI. 1st ed. Berlin: Springer, 2005:1–31.
6. Webb WR, Sostman HD. MR imaging of thoracic disease: clinical uses. Radiology 1992;182:621–630.
7. Westcott JL. Percutaneous transthoracic biopsy. Radiology 1988;169: 593–601.
8. Horsfield K, Cumming G. Morphology of the bronchial tree in man. J Appl Physiol 1968;24:373–383.
9. Vanpeperstraete F. The cartilaginous skeleton of the bronchial tree. Adv Anat Embryol Cell Biol 1974;48:1–15.
10. Raasch BN, Carsky EW, Lane EJ, et al. Radiographic anatomy of the interlobar fissures: a study of 100 specimens. AJR Am J Roentgenol 1982;138:1043–1049.
11. Yamashita H. Roentgenologic Anatomy of the Lung. 1st ed. Tokyo: Igaku-Shoin, 1978.
12. Proto AV, Speckman JM. The left lateral radiograph of the chest 1. Med Radiogr Photogr 1979;55:30–74.
13. Proto AV, Speckman JM. The left lateral radiograph of the chest 2. Med Radiogr Photogr 1980;56:38–64.
14. Heitzman R. The Mediastinum: Radiologic Correlations with Anatomy and Pathology. Berlin: Springer-Verlag, 1988:311–349.
15. Im JG, Webb WR, Rosen A, Gamsu G. Costal pleura: appearances at high-resolution CT. Radiology 1989;171:125–131.
16. Felson B. The roentgen diagnosis of disseminated pulmonary alveolar diseases. Semin Radiol 1967;2:3.
17. Fraser RS, Colman N, Müller NL, Paré PD. Diseases of the Chest. 4th ed. Philadelphia: Saunders, 1999:534–560.
18. Proto AV, Tocino I. Radiographic manifestations of lobar collapse. Semin Roentgenol 1980;15:117–173.
19. Lubert M, Krause GR. Patterns of lobar collapse as observed radiographically. Radiology 1951;56:165–172.
20. Felson B. Disseminated interstitial diseases of the lung. Ann Radiol 1966;9:325.
21. Reed JC. Plain Film Patterns and Differential Diagnosis. 5th ed. St Louis: Mosby, 2003.
22. Kerley P. Radiology in heart disease. Br Med J 1933;2:594–597.
23. Godwin JD, Webb WR, Savoca CJ, et al. Multiple thin-walled cystic lesions of the lung. AJR Am J Roentgenol 1980;135:593–604.
24. Simon G. Radiology and emphysema. Clin Radiol 1964;15:293–306.
25. Lane EJ, Proto AV, Philips TW. Mach bands and density perception. Radiology 1976;121:9–13.
26. Mller NL, Webb WR. Imaging of the pulmonary hila. Invest Radiol 1985;20:661–671.
27. Raasch BN, Carsky EW, Lane EJ, et al. Pleural effusion: explanation of some typical appearances. AJR Am J Roentgenol 1982;139:899–904.

Chapter 13

Mediastinum and Hila

Jeffrey S. Klein

Mediastinal Masses
Thoracic Inlet Masses
Anterior Mediastinal Masses
Middle Mediastinal Masses
Posterior Mediastinal Masses

Diffuse Mediastinal Disease

The Hila
Unilateral Hilar Enlargement
Bilateral Hilar Enlargement
Small Hila

This chapter will review the radiologic approach to mediastinal masses, diffuse mediastinal disease, and hilar abnormalities.

MEDIASTINAL MASSES

Localized mediastinal abnormalities are common diagnostic challenges for the radiologist. Patients with mediastinal masses tend to present in one of two fashions: with symptoms related to local mass effect or invasion of adjacent mediastinal structures (stridor in a patient with thyroid goiter), or incidentally with an abnormality on a routine chest radiograph. Occasionally, a mediastinal mass is discovered in the course of an evaluation for known malignancy (e.g., a patient with non-Hodgkin lymphoma) or for a condition such as myasthenia gravis, in which there is an association with thymoma. Multidetector-row CT (MDCT) and MR are the primary cross-sectional modalities used to evaluate mediastinal masses, with PET useful to assess response of mediastinal tumors to therapy, particularly lymphoma, and to distinguish residual or recurrent tumor from fibrosis (Table 13.1).

For the purposes of the following discussion, the mediastinum is divided into superior (thoracic inlet) and inferior components, with the inferior mediastinum subdivided into anterior, middle, and posterior compartments, as described in Chapter 12.

Thoracic Inlet Masses

The thoracic inlet is the region of the upper thorax marginated by the first rib and represents the junction between the neck and thorax. Masses in this region commonly present as neck masses or with symptoms of upper airway obstruction resulting from tracheal compression. Thyroid masses, lymphomatous nodes, and lymphangiomas are the most common thoracic inlet masses (Table 13.2).

Thyroid Masses. In a small percentage of patients with a cervical thyroid goiter, a thyroid carcinoma, or an enlarged gland from thyroiditis, extension of the thyroid through the thoracic inlet into the superior mediastinum may occur. These lesions are usually discovered as incidental findings on chest radiographs; a minority of patients will present with complaints of dyspnea or dysphagia as a result of tracheal or esophageal compression by the mass. Thyroid goiters arising from the lower pole of the thyroid or the thyroid isthmus can enter the superior mediastinum anterior to the trachea (80% of cases) or to the right and posterolateral to the trachea (20% of cases).

On chest radiographs, an anterosuperior mediastinal mass typically deviates the trachea laterally and either posteriorly (anterior masses) or anteriorly (posterior masses). Coarse, clumped calcifications are common in thyroid goiters. Radioiodine studies should be performed as the initial imaging procedure, although false-negative results do occur. CT usually shows characteristic findings: (*1*) well-defined margins, (*2*) continuity of the mass with the cervical thyroid, (*3*) coarse calcifications, (*4*) cystic or necrotic areas, (*5*) baseline high CT attenuation (because of intrinsic iodine content), and (*6*) intense enhancement (>25 H) as a result of the hypervascularity of most thyroid masses and prolonged enhancement (resulting from active uptake of iodine from contrast media) following intravenous

TABLE 13.1 Utility of MDCT, MR, and PET in the Evaluation of Mediastinal Masses

Indication for Study	*Modalities*
Confirming the presence of a mass versus tortuous vascular structures	MDCT = MR
Localization of mass to anterior, middle, or posterior compartment	MDCT = MR
Suspected aneurysm or vascular anomaly	MDCT = MR
Tissue characterization of mass	
Detection of fluid	MDCT = MR = US (for anterior masses or periesophageal masses)
Detection of calcium	CT
Distinction of tumor from fibrosis	PET>MR>CT
Relationship to adjacent structures	
Vascular invasion	MDCT = MR
Tracheal involvement	MDCT > MR
Involvement of spinal canal	MR > MDCT
Thoracic inlet lesions	MR = MDCT
Contraindication to iodinated contrast	MR > MDCT
Percutaneous biopsy of mediastinal mass	CT US for anterior mediastinal masses

MDCT, multidetector-row CT.

contrast administration (Fig. 13.1) (1). MR is useful in depicting the longitudinal extension of thyroid goiters without the use of intravenous contrast.

Parathyroid Masses. In approximately 2% of patients, the parathyroid glands fail to separate from the thymus in the neck and descend with the gland into the anterosuperior mediastinum. These glands can be found near the thoracic inlet in or about the thymus. This becomes important in the small percentage of patients with persistent clinical and biochemical evidence of hyperparathyroidism following routine neck exploration and parathyroidectomy. Most of these ectopic parathyroidlesions are small (<3 cm) adenomas; rarely, they represent hyperplastic glands or parathyroid carcinoma. When US and nuclear medicine studies have failed to localize a lesion in the neck, CT, MR, or technetium[99] sestamibi scanning may be useful in detecting mediastinal lesions (Fig. 13.2).

Lymphangiomas. These uncommon masses are tumors comprised of dilated lymphatic channels. The cystic or cavernous form (cystic hygroma) is most commonly discovered in infancy and is often associated with chromosomal abnormalities, including Turner syndrome and trisomies 13, 18, and 21. In infants, these lesions tend to extend from the neck into the anterior mediastinum; less commonly they may arise primarily within the anterior mediastinum in older patients. Histologically, these tumors are composed of cystic spaces lined by epithelium and contain clear, straw-colored fluid. Although these lesions are benign histologically, they tend to insinuate themselves between vascular structures and the trachea. This makes complete surgical resection of lymphangiomas difficult, and they frequently recur. CT demonstrates a well-defined cystic mass within the thoracic inlet or superior mediastinum. MR typically shows a mass of high signal intensity on T2WIs because of the fluid content.

TABLE 13.2 Thoracic Inlet Masses

Thyroid mass	Goiter Malignancy Thyromegaly resulting from thyroiditis
Parathyroid mass	Hyperplasia Adenoma Carcinoma
Lymph node mass	Lymphoma Hodgkin Non-Hodgkin Metastases Inflammatory Tuberculosis
Lymphangioma	

Anterior Mediastinal Masses

A number of neoplasms and nonneoplastic conditions arise in the anterior mediastinum and produce anterior mediastinal masses. These include thymic neoplasms, lymphoma, germ cell neoplasms, and primary mesenchymal tumors (Table 13.3).

Thymomas or ***thymic epithelial neoplasms*** are the second most common primary mediastinal neoplasms in adults after lymphoma. These lesions are neoplasms that arise from thymic epithelium and contain varying numbers of intermixed lymphocytes. The traditional classification of these tumors is into *thymomas,* which are histologically benign but may be either encapsulated (noninvasive) or invasive, and *thymic carcinomas*, in which the epithelial component shows signs of frank malignancy. The World Health Organization has recently reclassified these neoplasms based upon the morphology of the epithelial component and the ratio of epithelial cells to lymphocytes. The classification system divides these neoplasms into types A, AB, B1, B2, B3, and C, with a spectrum of histologic changes ranging from the classic encapsulated thymoma (A), which has a favorable prognosis, to thymic carcinoma (C), which generally carries a poor prognosis (2).

The average age at diagnosis of thymoma is 45 to 50; these lesions are rare in patients under the age of 20. While most often associated with myasthenia gravis, thymoma has been associated with other autoimmune diseases, such

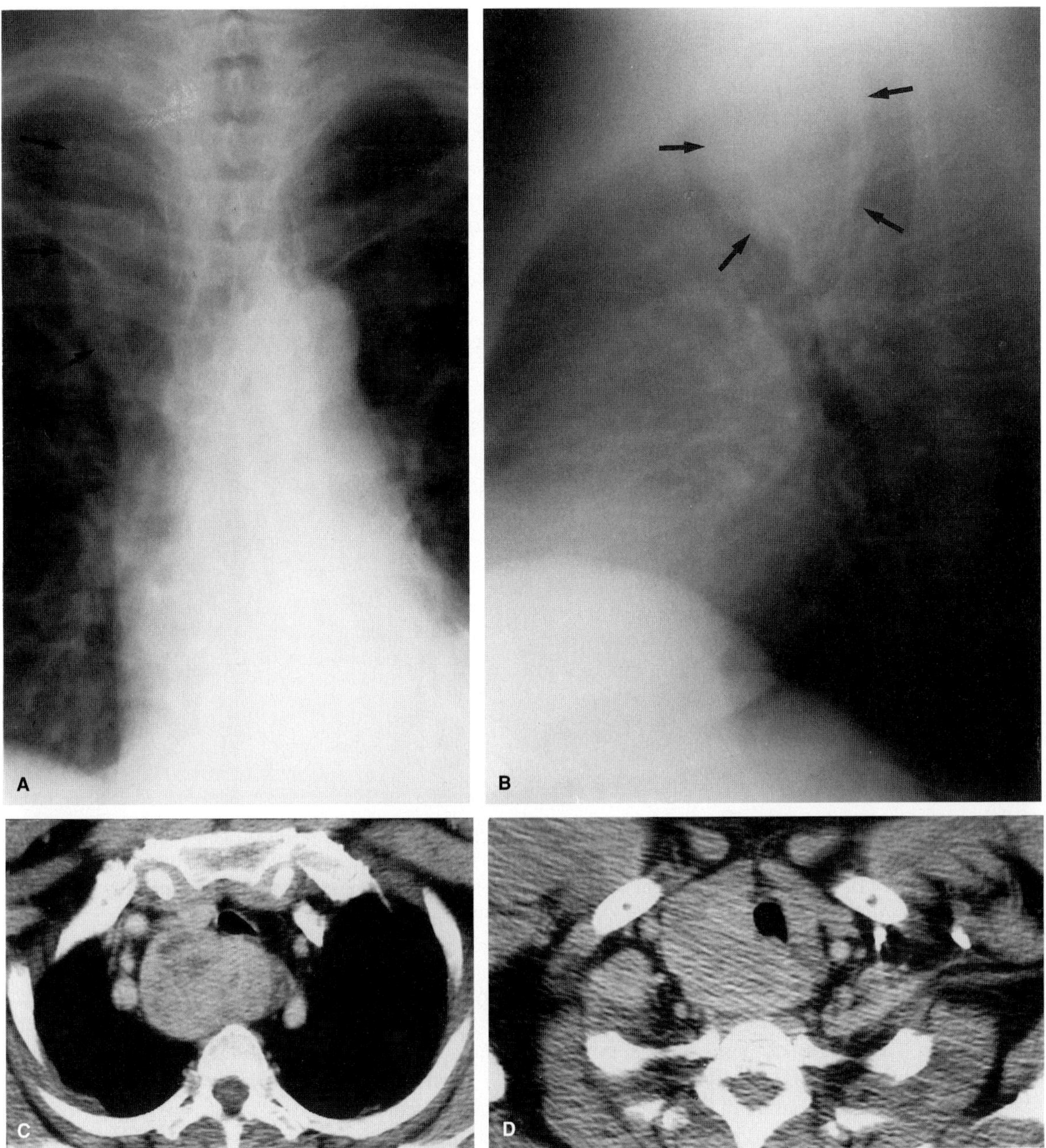

FIGURE 13.1. **Thyroid Goiter.** Posteroanterior **(A)** and lateral **(B)** radiographs show a right superior mediastinal mass (*arrows*) compressing the trachea from the posterior. **C.** Contrast-enhanced CT at the level of the sternoclavicular joints shows inhomogeneous increased attenuation and enlargement of the thyroid gland that extends retrotracheally. **D.** More superiorly, the mass is contiguous with the right lobe of an enlarged gland.

as pure red cell aplasia, Graves disease, Sjögren syndrome, and hypogammaglobulinemia. Of patients with myasthenia gravis, 10% to 28% have a thymoma, while a larger percentage of patients with thymoma (30% to 54%) have or will develop myasthenia.

On chest radiographs, thymomas are seen as round or oval, smooth or lobulated soft tissue masses arising near the origin of the great vessels at the base of the heart (Fig. 13.3) (2). CT is best for characterizing thymomas and detecting local invasion preoperatively. As a result of their firm consistency, thymomas characteristically maintain their shape where they contact the sternum anteriorly and heart and great vessels posteriorly. Compared to type A tumors, higher-grade thymomas, particularly types B3 and C, tend to show larger size, more irregular margins, heterogeneous enhancement, regions of necrosis,

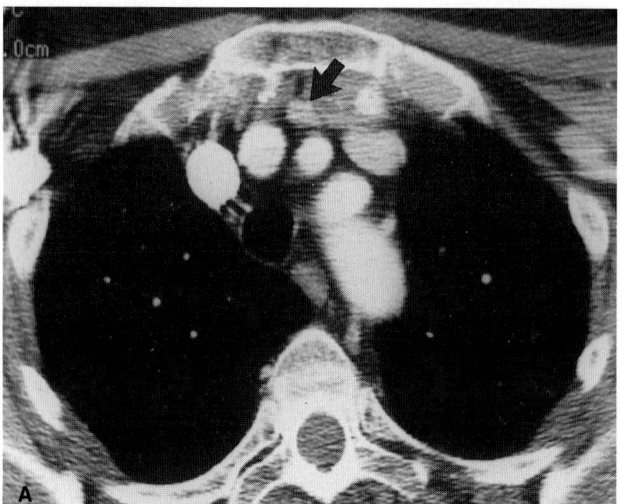

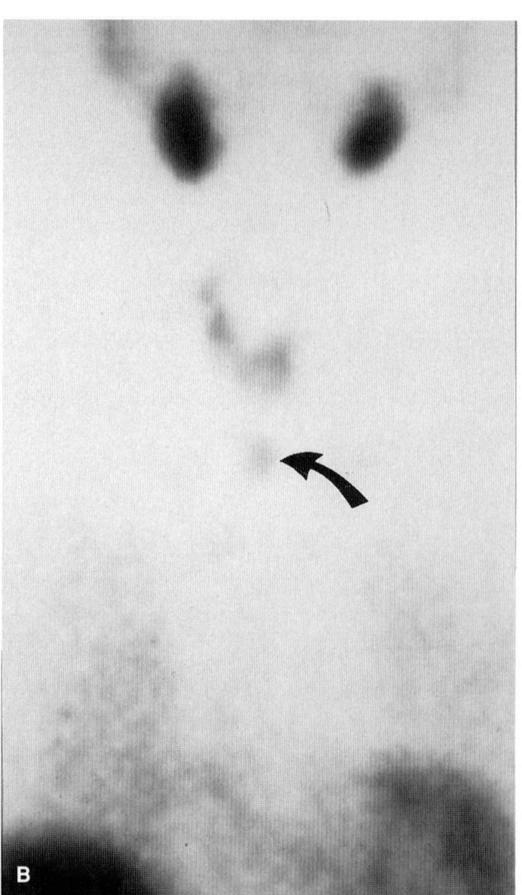

FIGURE 13.2. **Ectopic Parathyroid Adenoma. A.** In a patient with recurrent hyperparathyroidism after parathyroidectomy, an enhanced CT shows a prevascular mediastinal nodule (*arrow*). **B.** Technetium[99] sestamibi scan shows a focal area of increased activity in the superior mediastinum (*arrow*) corresponding to the nodule on CT.

mediastinal nodal metastases, and calcification. Invasion of tumor through the thymic capsule is present in 33% to 50% of patients. In the majority of these patients, this determination cannot be made by CT or MR and may even be difficult to determine on examination of the resected specimen. Local invasion of pleura, lung, pericardium, chest wall, diaphragm, and great vessels occurs in decreasing order of frequency in 10% to 15% of patients. Contiguity of a thymoma with the adjacent chest wall or mediastinal structures cannot be used as reliable evidence of invasion of these structures. Drop metastases to dependent portions of the pleural space are a recognized route of spread of thymoma that has invaded the pleura. Extrathoracic metastases are rare, although transdiaphragmatic spread of a pleural tumor into the retroperitoneum has been described. For these reasons, it is important to image the entire thorax and upper abdomen in any patient with suspected invasive disease.

In patients with myasthenia gravis who are being evaluated for thymoma, CT can demonstrate tumors that are invisible on conventional radiographs. However, very small thymic tumors may not be distinguishable from a normal or hyperplastic gland with CT, particularly in younger patients with a large amount of residual thymic tissue.

Thymic cysts may be congenital or acquired. Congenital unilocular thymic cysts are rare lesions that represent remnants of the thymopharyngeal duct and contain thin or gelatinous fluid. They are characterized histologically by an epithelial lining, with thymic tissue in the cyst wall, which distinguishes thymic cysts histologically from other congenital cystic lesions within the anterior mediastinum. Acquired multilocular thymic cysts are postinflammatory in nature and have been associated with AIDS, prior radiation or surgery, and autoimmune conditions such as Sjögren syndrome, myasthenia gravis, and aplastic anemia; in these latter conditions, clinical and radiologic distinction of multilocular thymic cyst from thymoma may be difficult; in fact, the two conditions can coexist. Large cysts will be evident as soft tissue masses on conventional radiographs, and CT or MR will demonstrate the cystic nature of the lesion. If the distinction between a true thymic cyst, cystic degeneration of a thymoma or lymphoma, a germ

TABLE 13.3 Anterior Mediastinal Masses

Thymic masses	Thymoma
	Thymic cyst
	Thymolipoma
	Thymic hyperplasia
	Thymic neuroendocrine tumors
	Thymic carcinoma
	Thymic lymphoma
Lymphoma	Hodgkin
	Non-Hodgkin
Germ cell neoplasms	Teratoma (benign or malignant)
	Seminoma
	Embryonal cell carcinoma
	Endodermal sinus tumor
	Choriocarcinoma
Thyroid mass	Goiter
	Tumor
	Adenoma
	Carcinoma
	Thyroiditis
Ectopic parathyroid mass	Hyperplasia
	Adenoma
	Carcinoma
Mesenchymal tumor	Lipoma
	Hemangioma
	Leiomyoma
	Liposarcoma
	Angiosarcoma

cell neoplasm, or lymphangioma is impossible on clinical and radiologic grounds, the lesion should be biopsied or resected.

Thymolipoma is a rare, benign thymic neoplasm that consists primarily of fat with intermixed rests of normal thymic tissue. These masses are asymptomatic and therefore are typically large when first detected. Chest radiographs show a large anterior mediastinal mass that, because of its pliable nature, tends to envelope the heart and diaphragm. CT demonstrates a fatty mass with interspersed soft tissue densities. Resection is curative.

Thymic Carcinoid. Neuroendocrine tumors of the thymus are rare malignant neoplasms believed to arise from thymic cells of neural crest origin (amine precursor uptake and decarboxylation [APUD] or Kulchitsky cells). The most common histologic type is carcinoid tumor, which, as with similar lesions arising within the bronchi, ranges in differentiation and behavior from typical carcinoid to atypical carcinoid to small cell carcinoma. Approximately 40% of patients have Cushing syndrome as a result of adrenocorticotropic hormone secretion by the tumor; these patients tend to have smaller lesions at time of diagnosis since they present early with signs of corticosteroid excess. The carcinoid syndrome is uncommon. This lesion is indistinguishable from thymoma on plain radiographs and CT scans.

Thymic hyperplasia is defined as enlargement of a thymus that is normal on gross and histologic examination. This rare entity occurs primarily in children as a rebound effect in response to an antecedent stress, discontinuation

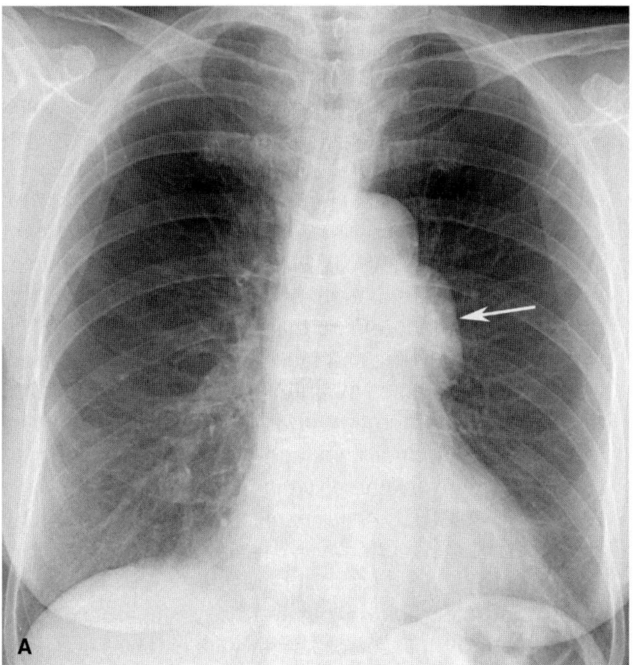

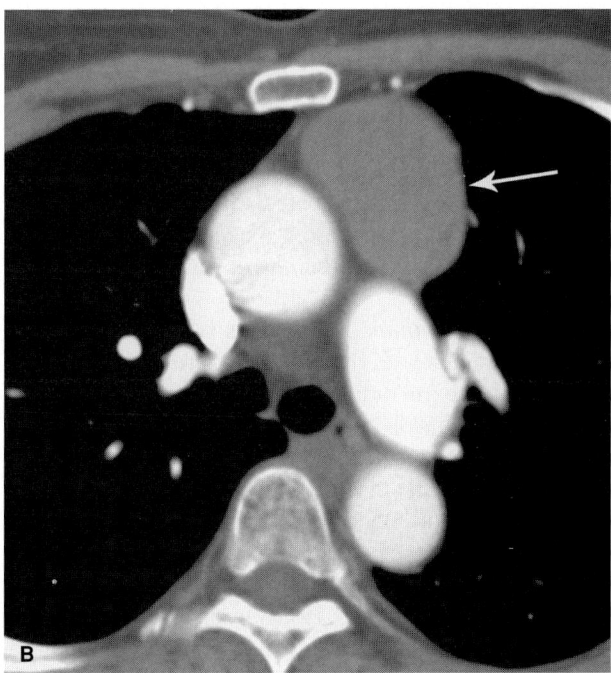

FIGURE 13.3. **Thymoma. A.** Posteroanterior chest radiograph reveals a left mediastinal mass (*arrow*). **B.** CT confirms a solid anterior mediastinal mass (*arrow*). Biopsy revealed a thymoma.

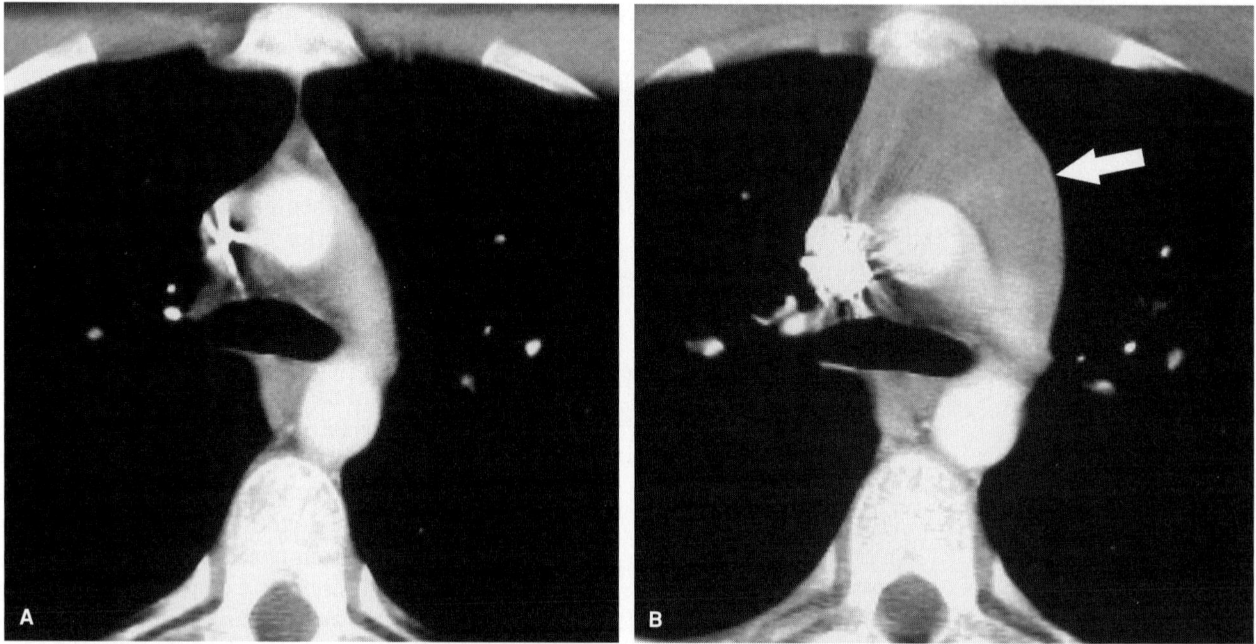

FIGURE 13.4. **Thymic Hyperplasia. A.** Enhanced CT in a 12-year-old undergoing chemotherapy for rhabdomyosarcoma shows virtual absence of thymic tissue. **B.** Scan 3 months following completion of chemotherapy shows uniform enlargement of thymus (*arrow*), reflecting rebound hyperplasia.

of chemotherapy, or treatment of hypercortisolism. An association with Graves disease has also been noted. The term *thymic hyperplasia* has been used incorrectly to describe the histologic findings of lymphoid follicular hyperplasia of the thymus, found in 60% of patients with myasthenia gravis. In contrast to most cases of true thymic hyperplasia, lymphoid hyperplasia does not produce thymic enlargement. Most patients with thymic hyperplasia have normal or diffusely enlarged glands on CT (Fig. 13.4); occasionally thymic hyperplasia will present as a mass that is radiographically indistinguishable from thymoma. Most cases can be resolved by noting a decrease in size on follow-up studies, thereby obviating the need for biopsy.

Thymic Lymphoma. The thymus is involved in 40% to 50% of patients with the nodular sclerosing subtype of Hodgkin disease. Its radiographic appearance is indistinguishable from that of other solid neoplasms arising within the thymus. The presence of lymph node enlargement in other portions of the mediastinum or anterior chest wall involvement should suggest the diagnosis.

Lymphoma—either Hodgkin disease or non-Hodgkin lymphoma (NHL)—is the most common primary mediastinal neoplasm in adults. Hodgkin disease involves the thorax in 85% of patients at the time of presentation. The majority (90%) of patients with intrathoracic involvement have mediastinal lymph node enlargement; this most commonly involves the anterior mediastinal and hilar nodal groups. The anterior mediastinum is the most frequent site of a localized nodal mass in patients with Hodgkin disease, particularly those with the nodular sclerosing type (Fig. 13.5). Isolated enlargement of mediastinal or hilar nodes outside the anterior mediastinum should suggest an alternative diagnosis. Only 25% of patients with Hodgkin lymphoma have disease limited to the mediastinum at the time of diagnosis. NHL involves the thorax in approximately 40% of patients at presentation. In contrast to Hodgkin disease, only 50% of patients with NHL and intrathoracic disease have mediastinal nodal involvement, and only 10% of NHL patients have disease that is limited to the mediastinum. Of the various subtypes of NHL that present with mediastinal masses, lymphoblastic lymphoma and diffuse large B-cell lymphoma are the most common (Fig. 13.6). Lymphoma involving a single mediastinal or hilar nodal group is much more common in NHL than in Hodgkin disease. NHL most commonly involves middle mediastinal and hilar lymph nodes; juxtaphrenic and posterior mediastinal nodal involvement is uncommon but is seen almost exclusively in NHL. Patterns of pulmonary parenchymal involvement in lymphoma are discussed in Chapter 15.

While Hodgkin disease spreads in a fairly predictable pattern from one nodal group to an adjacent group, NHL is felt to be a multifocal disorder in which patterns of involvement are unpredictable. Localized intrathoracic Hodgkin disease is usually treated with radiation therapy, with 90% response rates. More widespread Hodgkin disease and

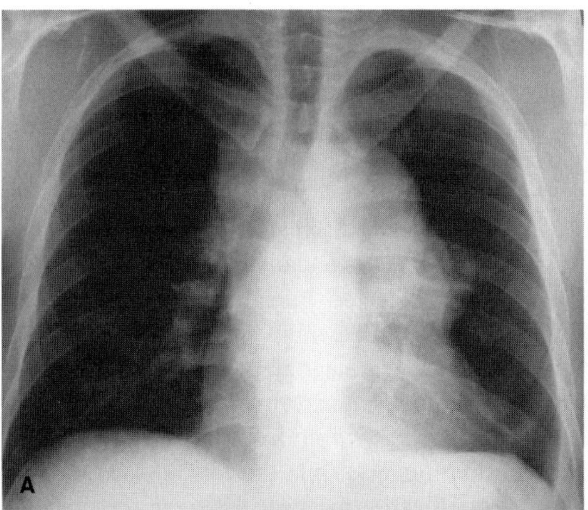

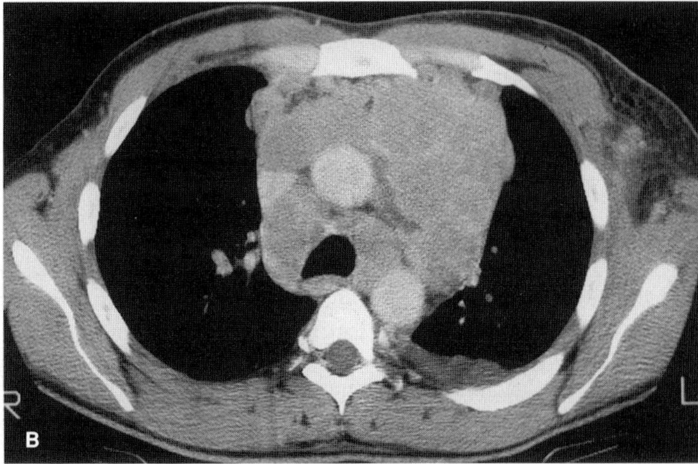

FIGURE 13.5. **Hodgkin Lymphoma. A.** Posteroanterior chest radiograph in a 35-year-old man shows a large, lobulated mediastinal mass. **B.** Contrast-enhanced CT at the level of the aortic arch shows bulky anterior and middle mediastinal lymphadenopathy.

NHL are treated with chemotherapy, with better response rates for Hodgkin disease than for NHL.

On conventional radiographs, lymphoma involving the anterior mediastinum is indistinguishable from thymoma or germ cell neoplasm and presents as a lobulated mass projecting to one or both sides (Fig. 13.5). Calcification in untreated lymphoma is extremely uncommon, and its presence within an anterior mediastinal mass should suggest another diagnosis. Involvement of other lymph nodes in the mediastinum or hila makes lymphoma more likely. An enlarged spleen displacing the gastric air bubble medially, seen in the upper abdominal portion of the frontal chest film, provides an additional clue to the diagnosis.

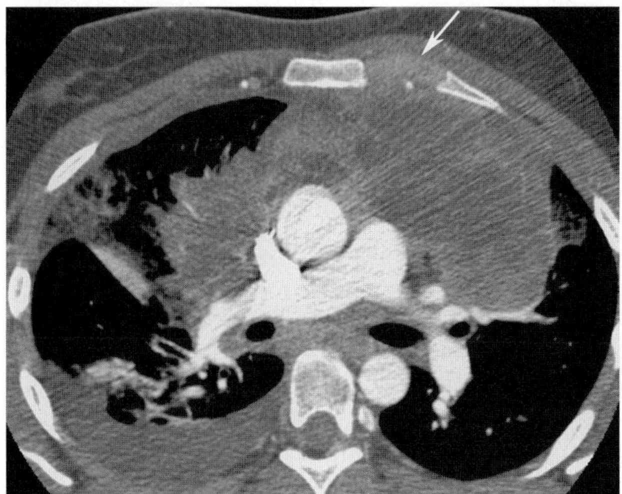

FIGURE 13.6. **Non-Hodgkin Lymphoma, Diffuse Large B-cell Type.** Enhanced CT scan in a 34-year-old woman shows a large anterior mediastinal mass with mixed attenuation invading right upper lobe and anterior chest wall (*arrow*) with associated right pleural effusion. Core needle biopsy showed diffuse large B-cell lymphoma.

CT is performed in virtually all patients with lymphoma. The advantages of chest CT include the ability to better characterize and localize masses seen on chest radiographs; detection of subradiographic sites of involvement that can alter disease staging, prognosis, and therapy; guidance for transthoracic or open biopsy; the ability to monitor response to therapy; and detection of relapse. The appearance of nodal involvement in lymphoma varies; most commonly, discrete enlarged solid lymph nodes or conglomerate masses of nodes are seen (Fig. 13.5B). Central necrosis, seen in 20% of patients, has no prognostic significance. Nodal calcification is rare in the absence of previous mediastinal radiation or systemic chemotherapy. Parenchymal involvement is usually the result of direct extranodal extension of a tumor from hilar nodes along the bronchovascular lymphatics; this is better appreciated on axial CT images than on chest radiographs (3). Likewise, a tumor extending from the mediastinum to the pericardium, subpleural space, and chest wall is best appreciated on CT or MR. On MR, untreated lymphoma appears as a mass of uniform low signal intensity on T1WIs and uniform high signal intensity or intermixed areas of low and high signal intensity on T2WIs. The areas of low signal intensity on T2WIs of untreated patients may be a result of foci of fibrotic tissue in nodular sclerosing Hodgkin disease.

CT, MR, gallium scintigraphy, and fluorodeoxyglucose (FDG) PET have been used to monitor the response of lymphoma to therapy. While CT can accurately assess tumor regression and detect relapse within nodal groups outside the treated region, the ability to distinguish residual tumor from sterilized fibrotic masses is limited. Residual soft tissue masses have been reported in up to

50% of patients, most commonly with nodular sclerosing Hodgkin disease, and are more common when the pretreatment mass is large. Some patients with residual masses on CT or MR will have tumor recurrence within 6 to 12 months after the completion of therapy. In general, the appearance of high-signal-intensity regions on T2WIs more than 6 months after treatment should suggest recurrence. Radionuclide scintigraphy with gallium-67, particularly SPECT, has been largely replaced by FDG-PET in the initial diagnosis and staging of thoracic lymphoma. PET is clearly superior to CT or MR in distinguishing recurrent tumor from fibrosis in both Hodgkin disease and NHL (4).

Germ cell neoplasms, which include teratoma, seminoma, choriocarcinoma, endodermal sinus tumor, and embryonal cell carcinoma, arise from collections of primitive germ cells that arrest in the anterior mediastinum on their journey to the gonads during embryologic development. Since they are histologically indistinguishable from germ cell tumors arising in the testes and ovaries, the diagnosis of a primary malignant mediastinal germ cell neoplasm requires exclusion of a primary gonadal tumor as a source of mediastinal metastases. A key in distinguishing primary from metastatic mediastinal germ cell neoplasm is the presence of retroperitoneal lymph node involvement in metastatic gonadal tumors.

The most common benign mediastinal germ cell neoplasm is teratoma, comprising 60% to 70% of mediastinal germ cell neoplasms (5). Teratomas may be cystic or solid. Cystic or mature teratoma is the most common type of teratoma seen in the mediastinum. In contrast to a dermoid cyst, which is an ovarian neoplasm containing only elements derived from the ectodermal germinal layer, a cystic teratoma of the mediastinum commonly contains tissues of ectodermal, mesodermal, and endodermal origins. For this reason, it is inaccurate to use the term "dermoid cyst" to describe cystic mediastinal germ cell neoplasms. Solid teratomas are usually malignant. Most germ cell neoplasms are detected in patients in the third or fourth decade of life. While benign tumors have a slight female preponderance (female/male, 60%/40%), malignant tumors are seen almost exclusively in men.

Radiographically, these tumors have a distribution similar to that of thymomas. While the majority are located in the anterior mediastinum, up to 10% are found in the posterior mediastinum. Benign lesions are often round or oval and smooth in contour; an irregular, lobulated, or ill-defined margin suggests malignancy. Calcification is present in 33% to 50% of tumors but is nonspecific unless in the form of a tooth. On CT, benign teratomas are usually cystic and may contain soft tissue, bone, teeth, fat, or, rarely, fat–fluid levels. Seminoma, choriocarcinoma, and endodermal sinus (yolk sac) tumors are malignant lesions seen primarily in young men. Seminoma is the most common malignant germ cell neoplasm, accounting for 30% of these tumors. The radiographic findings are nonspecific. CT typically shows a large lobulated soft tissue mass that may contain areas of hemorrhage, calcification, or necrosis (Fig. 13.7). Elevated serum levels of α-fetoprotein or

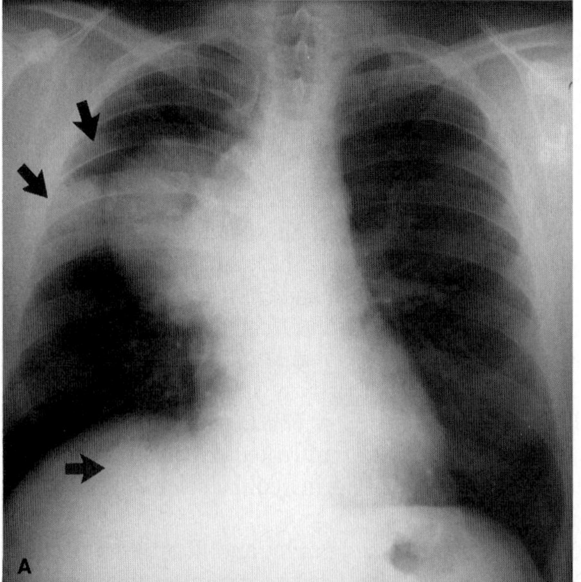

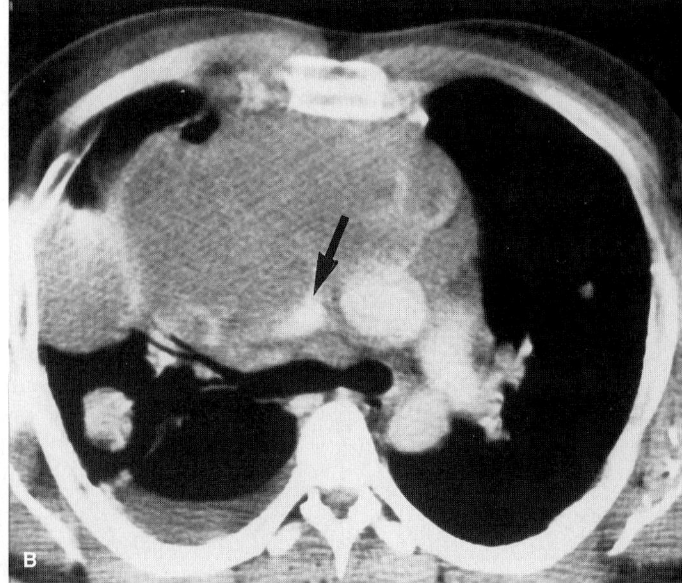

FIGURE 13.7. **Malignant Germ Cell Tumor. A.** Posteroanterior chest radiograph in a 38-year-old man reveals a right mediastinal mass with discrete right lung nodules (*arrows*). **B.** Contrast-enhanced CT demonstrates a large anterior mediastinal mass invading the superior vena cava (*arrow*) with right lung nodules and a small pleural effusion. CT-guided biopsy showed choriocarcinoma.

human chorionic gonadotropin are helpful in the diagnosis of suspected malignant mediastinal germ cell neoplasm, while clinical and CT evidence of gynecomastia is an additional clue.

Thyroid Masses. While masses arising from the thyroid can present as anterior and superior mediastinal masses, these lesions are best considered as thoracic inlet masses, as discussed earlier.

Mesenchymal Tumors. Benign and malignant tumors arising from the fibrous, fatty, muscular, or vascular tissues of the mediastinum may present as mediastinal masses, most commonly in the anterior mediastinum. Lipomas can occur in any location in the mediastinum but are most often anterior. The diagnosis is made by recognition of a well-defined mass of uniform fatty attenuation (under –50 H). The presence of soft tissue elements should raise the possibility of a thymolipoma or liposarcoma; the latter may show evidence of invasion of adjacent structures at the time of diagnosis. Fat within a mature teratoma or transdiaphragmatic herniation of omental fat is usually easily distinguished from a lipoma.

Hemangiomas are benign tumors composed of vascular channels and may be associated with the syndrome of hereditary hemorrhagic telangiectasia. A pathognomonic sign on chest radiographs is the recognition of phleboliths within a smooth or lobulated soft tissue mass. Angiosarcomas are rare malignant vascular neoplasms that are indistinguishable from other invasive neoplasms arising within the anterior mediastinum.

Leiomyomas are rare benign neoplasms that arise from smooth muscle within the mediastinum. Similarly, fibromas and mesenchymomas (tumors that contain more than one mesenchymal element) can appear as anterior mediastinal masses.

Middle Mediastinal Masses

Lymph Node Enlargement and Masses (Table 13.4). Most middle mediastinal lymph node masses are malignant, representing metastases from bronchogenic carcinoma, extrathoracic malignancy, or lymphoma (6). Benign causes of middle mediastinal lymph node enlargement include sarcoidosis, mycobacterial and fungal infection, angiofollicular lymph node hyperplasia (Castleman disease), and angioimmunoblastic lymphadenopathy.

On plain radiographs, several findings suggest that a middle mediastinal mass represents lymph node enlargement. The presence of multiple bilateral mediastinal masses that distort the lung/mediastinal interface is relatively specific for lymph node enlargement. Solitary masses resulting from lymph node enlargement tend to be elongated and lobulated rather than spherical, since usually more than a single node in a vertical chain of nodes is involved. Occasionally, calcification can be detected within enlarged lymph nodes on plain radiographs; CT is more sensitive in detecting nodal calcification and its distribution within lymph nodes.

TABLE 13.4 Middle Mediastinal Masses

Lymph node masses	Malignancy
	Bronchogenic carcinoma
	Lymphoma
	Leukemia
	Kaposi sarcoma
	Extrathoracic malignancy
	Head and neck tumors (squamous cell carcinoma of skin, larynx; thyroid carcinoma)
	Genitourinary tumors (renal cell carcinoma, seminoma)
	Breast carcinoma
	Melanoma
	Infection
	Bacteria
	Anaerobic lung abscess
	Anthrax
	Plague
	Tularemia
	Tuberculosis
	Fungi
	Histoplasmosis
	Coccidioidomycosis
	Cryptococcosis
	Viral infection
	Measles
	Mononucleosis
	Idiopathic
	Sarcoidosis
	Castleman disease
	Angioimmunoblastic lymphadenopathy
Foregut and mesothelial cysts	Bronchogenic cyst
	Pericardial cyst
Tracheal and central bronchial neoplasms	Malignant
	Carcinoid tumor (bronchi)
	Adenoid cystic carcinoma (trachea)
	Squamous cell carcinoma
Diaphragmatic hernias	Foramen of Morgagni hernia
	Traumatic hernia
Vascular lesions	Arterial
	Double arch/right arch
	Tortuous innominate/subclavian artery
	Aneurysm of the aortic arch
	Venous
	Dilated azygos vein
	Dilated hemiazygos vein
	Dilated SVC
	Left-sided SVC
	Dilated left superior intercostal vein
	Dilatation of the main pulmonary artery

SVC, superior vena cava.

One of the prime indications for performing thoracic CT is to detect the presence of enlarged mediastinal lymph nodes. CT is most often obtained to confirm an abnormal

TABLE 13.5 Density of Mediastinal/Hilar Nodes on CT

Calcification	
Central	Mycobacteria
	Fungus
Peripheral (eggshell)	Silicosis
	Sarcoidosis
Hypervascular	Carcinoid tumor/small cell carcinoma
	Kaposi sarcoma
	Metastases
	Renal cell carcinoma
	Thyroid carcinoma
	Castleman disease
Necrosis	Mycobacteria
	Fungus
	Metastases
	Squamous cell carcinoma
	Seminoma
	Lymphoma

chest radiographic finding or to evaluate a patient with suspected mediastinal disease despite normal radiographs (a patient with a suspicious solitary pulmonary nodule or with cervical Hodgkin disease). The ability of CT to image in the axial plane and its inherent high contrast resolution allow for the recognition of abnormally enlarged lymph nodes that would not be evident on chest radiographs. In general, abnormal lymph nodes are seen as round or oval soft tissue masses that measure >1.0 cm in their short axis diameter. Although CT is unable to distinguish between benign inflammatory nodes and those involved by malignancy based upon size criteria alone, CT can provide useful information about the internal density of the nodes (Table 13.5).

A standardized classification system for hilar and mediastinal lymph nodes has recently been advanced by the American Thoracic Society (Fig.13.8) (7). This scheme correlates with easily identifiable CT and anatomic landmarks and is most important when reporting lymph node enlargement in patients with bronchogenic carcinoma.

MR is as sensitive as CT in detecting enlarged mediastinal lymph nodes. Advantages of MR include the absence of iodinated contrast, easy distinction between vascular and soft tissue structures, exquisite contrast resolution between mediastinal nodes and fat on T1W sequences, and the ability to image in the direct coronal or sagittal plane. The latter feature is an advantage in those mediastinal regions that parallel the axial plane (subcarinal space, aortopulmonary window) and therefore tend to suffer from partial volume averaging effects on CT. The major disadvantages of MR at present are the inability to detect nodal calcification and limited spatial resolution; the latter can result in an inability to distinguish between a group of normal size nodes and a single enlarged node, thereby leading to false-positive results.

In addition to the detection and characterization of enlarged mediastinal nodes, CT can help guide diagnostic nodal tissue sampling. This is usually most helpful in the setting of suspected bronchogenic carcinoma, where accurate staging of mediastinal nodal disease is important for prognostic purposes and treatment planning. The recognition of enlarged subcarinal or pretracheal nodes on CT may suggest biopsy via transcarinal Wang needle or mediastinoscopy, respectively.

As mentioned above, mediastinal lymph node enlargement is common in Hodgkin disease and NHL. Lymphoma accounts for 20% of all mediastinal neoplasms in adults, and most patients with intrathoracic lymphoma have concomitant extrathoracic disease. In most patients, the nodal enlargement is bilateral but asymmetric. Nodular sclerosing Hodgkin disease commonly results in lymph node enlargement, predominantly within the anterior mediastinum and thymus. Isolated posterior nodal enlargement is usually seen only in patients with NHL.

Leukemia, particularly the T-lymphocytic varieties, can cause intrathoracic lymph node enlargement. The lymph node enlargement is usually confined to the middle mediastinal and hilar nodes.

The most common source of metastases to middle mediastinal nodes is bronchogenic carcinoma. In the majority of patients, symptoms or plain radiographic findings suggest the presence of a primary tumor in the lung. In a small percentage of patients, particularly those with small cell carcinoma, the primary carcinoma may be inconspicuous or invisible on plain radiographs, with nodal metastases being the only visible abnormality. Lymph node enlargement is often unilateral on the side of the visible pulmonary or hilar abnormality. Paratracheal and aorticopulmonary nodes are most commonly involved. Since the accuracy of CT in predicting the presence or absence of mediastinal lymph node metastases is approximately 60% to 70%, PET—and in particular integrated CT/PET—should be performed in most patients with bronchogenic carcinoma. A more thorough discussion of mediastinal nodal involvement in bronchogenic carcinoma may be found in Chapter 15.

Lymph node metastases from extrathoracic malignancies can result in mediastinal node enlargement, either with or without concomitant pulmonary metastases. These mediastinal nodal metastases may result from inferior extension of neck masses (thyroid carcinoma, head and neck tumors); extension along lymphatic channels from below the diaphragm (testicular or renal cell carcinoma, GI malignancies); or hematogenous extension (breast carcinoma, melanoma, Kaposi sarcoma) (8).

Mediastinal lymph node enlargement is very common in patients with sarcoidosis, occurring in 60% to 90% of patients at some stage of their disease. Nodal enlargement is typically bilateral and symmetric and involves the hila as well as the mediastinum (Fig. 13.9); this usually

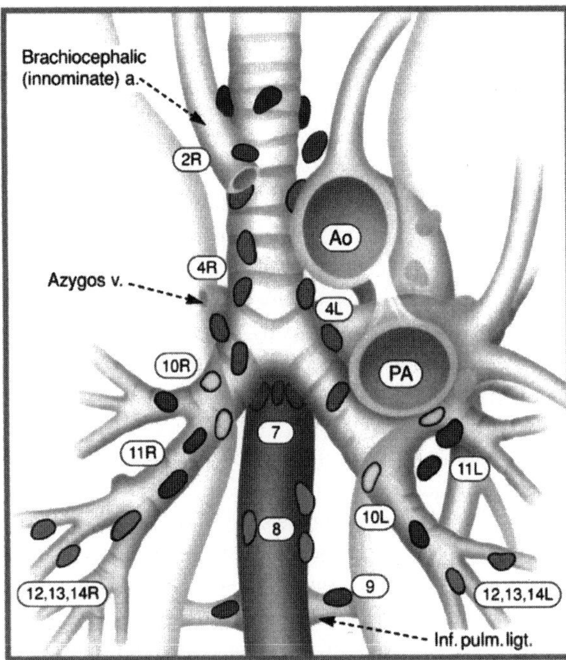

Superior Mediastinal Nodes

- 1 Highest Mediastinal
- 2 Upper Paratracheal
- 3 Pre-vascular and Retrotracheal
- 4 Lower Paratracheal (including Azygos Nodes)

N_2 = single digit, ipsilateral
N_3 = single digit, contralateral or supraclavicular

Aortic Nodes

- 5 Subaortic (A-P window)
- 6 Para-aortic (ascending aorta or phrenic)

Inferior Mediastinal Nodes

- 7 Subcarinal
- 8 Paraesophageal (below carina)
- 9 Pulmonary Ligament

N_1 Nodes

- 10 Hilar
- 11 Interlobar
- 12 Lobar
- 13 Segmental
- 14 Subsegmental

(Mountain/Dresler modifications from Naruke/ATS-LCSG Map)

FIGURE 13.8. **American Thoracic Society Nodal Stations.** Ao, aorta; PA, pulmonary artery. From Mountain CF, Dresler CM. Regional lymph node classification for lung cancer staging. Chest 1997;111:1718–1723; reprinted with permission.

allows for differentiation of sarcoidosis from lymphoma and metastatic disease. In sarcoidosis, the enlarged nodes produce a lobulated appearance on chest radiographs and CT, because the enlarged nodes do not coalesce. This is in contrast to lymphoma and nodal metastases, in which the intranodal tumor extends through the nodal capsule to form conglomerate enlarged nodal masses. Right and left paratracheal lymph nodes are typically involved; anterior or posterior mediastinal nodal enlargement has been described with greater frequency recently, probably as a

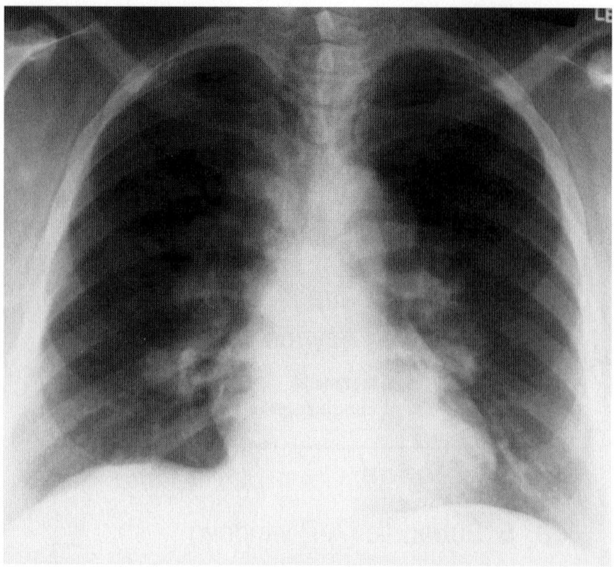

FIGURE 13.9. **Lymphadenopathy in Sarcoidosis.** Posteroanterior radiograph in a 56-year-old woman with sarcoidosis reveals discrete hilar, paratracheal, and aortopulmonary window lymphadenopathy.

result of the improved sensitivity of CT for detecting nodal involvement in these regions.

A variety of infections, most commonly histoplasmosis, coccidioidomycosis, cryptococcosis, and tuberculosis, can cause mediastinal nodal enlargement (Fig. 13.10). Typically these patients have parenchymal opacities on chest radiographs, but isolated lymph node enlargement may be seen, particularly in children and young adults. Bacterial infections such as anthrax, bubonic plague, and tularemia are uncommon causes of lymph node enlargement. Typically, there will be symptoms and signs of acute infection, and chest radiographs will show evidence of pneumonia. Bacterial lung abscesses also may be associated with reactive lymph node enlargement. Hilar and mediastinal lymph nodes may be enlarged in patients with measles pneumonia and infectious mononucleosis.

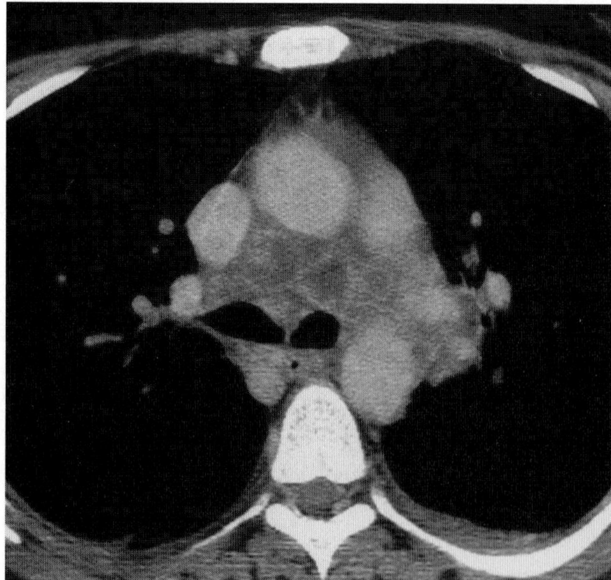

FIGURE 13.10. **Tuberculous Lymphadenopathy.** Contrast-enhanced CT at the level of the tracheal carina demonstrates enlarged precarinal and left peribronchial lymph nodes with central necrosis and peripheral enhancement. Material obtained by mediastinoscopy revealed *Mycobacterium tuberculosis*.

Angiofollicular lymph node hyperplasia (Castleman disease) is characterized by enlargement of hilar and mediastinal lymph nodes, predominantly in the middle and posterior mediastinal compartments. In the more common hyaline vascular type, the disease is localized to one lymph node region and presents as an asymptomatic mediastinal soft tissue mass. Histologically, there is replacement of normal nodal architecture with multiple germinal centers and multiple small vessels with hyalinized walls that course perpendicularly toward the germinal centers to give a characteristic "lollipop" appearance on light microscopy. The vascular nature of these masses accounts for the intense enhancement seen on contrast-enhanced CT or angiography. Calcification within these masses has been described. These lesions are cured by resection.

Angioimmunoblastic lymphadenopathy is a rare disorder seen in older adults; it is characterized by constitutional symptoms, lymphadenopathy, hepatosplenomegaly, and skin rash. Hemolytic anemia and hypergammaglobulinemia may be seen. Histologically, the enlarged nodes contain a chronic inflammatory infiltrate and are hypervascular. Chest radiographs and CT show hilar and mediastinal lymph node enlargement that are indistinguishable from other etiologies. As with Castleman disease, the vascular nature of the involved lymph nodes accounts for the contrast enhancement seen on CT. These patients manifest signs of immunodeficiency similar to those associated with AIDS, with one third developing high-grade lymphoma and many succumbing to opportunistic infections such as *Pneumocystis carinii* pneumonia and cytomegalovirus inclusion disease.

Foregut and mesothelial cysts are common mediastinal lesions that typically present as asymptomatic masses on routine chest radiographs in young adults. CT and MR show findings characteristic of the cystic nature of these lesions.

Congenital *bronchogenic cysts* result from anomalous budding of the tracheobronchial tree during development. To be characterized as bronchogenic in origin, the wall of the cyst must be lined by a respiratory epithelium with pseudostratified columnar cells and contain seromucous glands; some may contain cartilage and smooth muscle within their walls. It is often difficult to distinguish between bronchogenic and enteric cysts based on their location and pathologic appearance; the term *foregut cyst* has been used to describe those lesions that cannot be specifically characterized. The majority of bronchogenic cysts

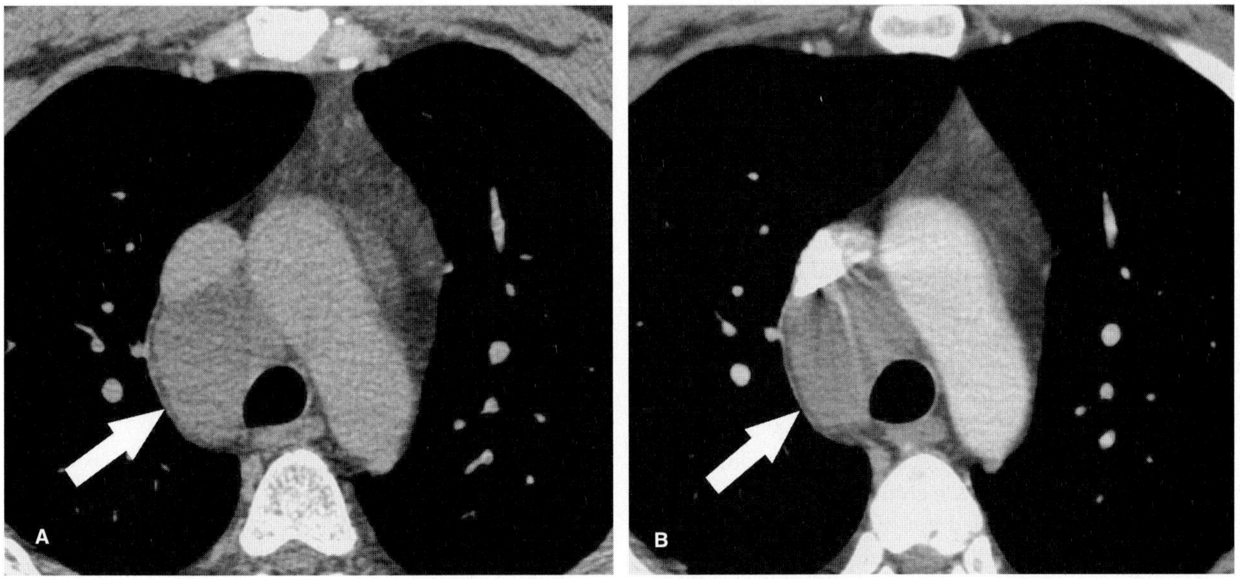

FIGURE 13.11. **Bronchogenic Cyst.** Unenhanced **(A)** and enhanced **(B)** CT scans in a 38-year-old man demonstrate a smooth, low-attenuation paratracheal mass (*arrows*) that fails to enhance, consistent with a bronchogenic cyst.

(80% to 90%) arise within the mediastinum in the vicinity of the tracheal carina. Most mediastinal lesions are asymptomatic; occasionally, compression of the tracheobronchial tree or esophagus may produce dyspnea, wheezing, or dysphagia. Rarely, mediastinal cysts become secondarily infected after communication with the airway or esophagus, or they cause symptomatic compression after rapid enlargement following hemorrhage. Bronchogenic cysts are seen as soft tissue masses in the subcarinal or right paratracheal space on frontal chest radiographs; less common sites of involvement include the hilum, posterior mediastinum, and periesophageal region. They appear as a single smooth, round, or elliptic mass; a minority are lobulated in contour. CT is the method of choice for the diagnosis of a mediastinal cyst. If a well-defined, thin-walled mass of fluid density (0 to 10 H) is seen that fails to enhance following intravenous contrast administration, it can be assumed to represent a benign cyst (Fig. 13.11) (9). High CT numbers (>40 H) suggesting a solid mass can be seen when the cyst is filled with mucoid material, milk of calcium, or blood. Calcification of the cyst wall has been described but is uncommon. MR shows characteristic low signal intensity on T1WIs and high signal intensity on T2WIs. The presence of proteinaceous material within the cyst will shorten T1 relaxation times, yielding high signal intensity on T1WIs. In many patients, resection is required for definitive diagnosis. Both transbronchoscopic and percutaneous needle aspiration and drainage have been used successfully for the diagnosis and treatment of these lesions.

Pericardial cysts arise from the parietal pericardium and contain clear serous fluid surrounded by a layer of mesothelial cells. Most often, they arise in the anterior cardiophrenic angles, with right-sided lesions being twice as common as left-sided lesions; approximately 20% arise more superiorly within the mediastinum. These lesions usually present as incidental asymptomatic round or oval masses in the cardiophrenic angle (Fig. 13.12). Their pliable nature can be demonstrated with a change in patient position. CT typically shows a unilocular cystic mass

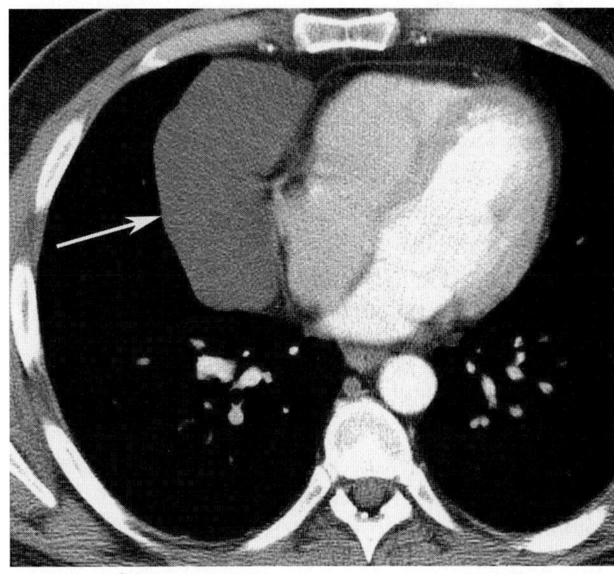

FIGURE 13.12. **Pericardial Cyst.** Enhanced CT scan through heart shows a smooth, sharply marginated, low-attenuation mass (*arrow*) in the right cardiophrenic angle, consistent with a pericardial cyst.

adjacent to the heart; MR or US via a subxiphoid approach shows findings characteristic of a simple cyst. As with bronchogenic cysts, there have been reports of cysts with high attenuation on CT that on resection are found to be filled with proteinaceous or mucoid material.

Tracheal and central bronchial masses commonly produce upper airway symptoms with obstructive pneumonitis and atelectasis and rarely present as asymptomatic mediastinal masses. Occasionally, central airway masses present as radiographic abnormalities when they distort the tracheal air column or mediastinal contour. These masses are discussed in Chapter 18.

Diaphragmatic hernias, which may present as pericardiac masses, are discussed in Chapter 19.

Vascular Lesions. Congenital or acquired anomalies of the heart and great vessels are common middle mediastinal masses and are discussed in Chapter 14.

Neurogenic Lesions. Rarely, a neurofibroma arising from the phrenic nerve may present as a middle mediastinal juxtacardiac mass.

Posterior Mediastinal Masses

Neurogenic Tumors (Table 13.6). Posterior mediastinal masses arising from neural elements are classified by their tissue of origin. Three groups have been recognized: (*1*) tumors arising from intercostal nerves (neurofibroma, schwannoma); (*2*) sympathetic ganglia (ganglioneuroma, ganglioneuroblastoma, and neuroblastoma); and (*3*) paraganglionic cells (chemodectoma, pheochromocytoma). Tumors in each of these three groups may be benign or malignant neoplasms (5). Although neurogenic tumors can occur at any age, they are most common in young patients. Neuroblastoma and ganglioneuroma are most common in children, whereas neurofibroma and schwannoma affect adults more frequently.

Histologically, both neurofibroma and schwannoma are comprised of spindle cells that arise from the Schwann cell. While neurofibroma is an encapsulated tumor that contains interspersed neurons, schwannoma is not encapsulated and contains no neuronal elements. Both tumors are more common in patients with neurofibromatosis. Multiple lesions in the mediastinum, particularly bilateral apicoposterior masses, are virtually diagnostic of neurofibromatosis. A small percentage of schwannomas (10%) are locally invasive (malignant schwannoma).

Radiographically, intercostal nerve tumors appear as round or oval paravertebral soft tissue masses. CT shows a smooth or lobulated paraspinal soft tissue mass, which may erode the adjacent vertebral body or rib. CT demonstration of tumor extension from the paravertebral space into the spinal canal via an enlarged intervertebral foramen is characteristic of a "dumbbell" neurofibroma. MR is the modality of choice for imaging a suspected neurofibroma. In addition to the occasional demonstration

TABLE 13.6 Posterior Mediastinal Masses

Neurogenic tumors	Peripheral (intercostal) nerves
	Neurofibroma
	Schwannoma
	Sympathetic ganglia
	Ganglioneuroma
	Ganglioneuroblastoma
	Neuroblastoma
	Paraganglion cells
	Chemodectoma
	Pheochromocytoma
Esophageal lesions	Duplication (enteric) cyst
	Diverticulum
	Neoplasm
	Leiomyoma
	Squamous cell carcinoma
	Esophageal dilatation
	Achalasia
	Scleroderma
	Peptic stricture
	Carcinoma
	Paraesophageal varices
	Hiatal hernia
	Sliding
	Paraesophageal
Foregut cysts	Enteric
	Neurenteric
Vertebral lesion	Trauma
	Paraspinal hematoma
	Infection
	Paraspinal abscess
	Tuberculosis
	Staphylococcus
	Tumor
	Metastases (bronchogenic, breast, renal cell carcinoma)
	Multiple myeloma
	Lymphoma
	Degenerative disease (osteophytosis)
	Extramedullary hematopoiesis
Lateral thoracic meningocele	
Pancreatic pseudocyst	

of both intra- and extra-spinal canal components, MR of neurofibromas shows typical high signal intensity on T2WIs.

Tumors that arise from the sympathetic ganglia represent a continuum from the histologically benign ganglioneuroma found in adolescents and young adults to the highly malignant neuroblastoma seen almost exclusively in children under the age of 5. These tumors generally present as elongated, vertically oriented paravertebral soft tissue masses with a broad area of contact with the posterior mediastinum (Figs. 13.13, 13.14). These findings may help distinguish these lesions from neurofibromas, which

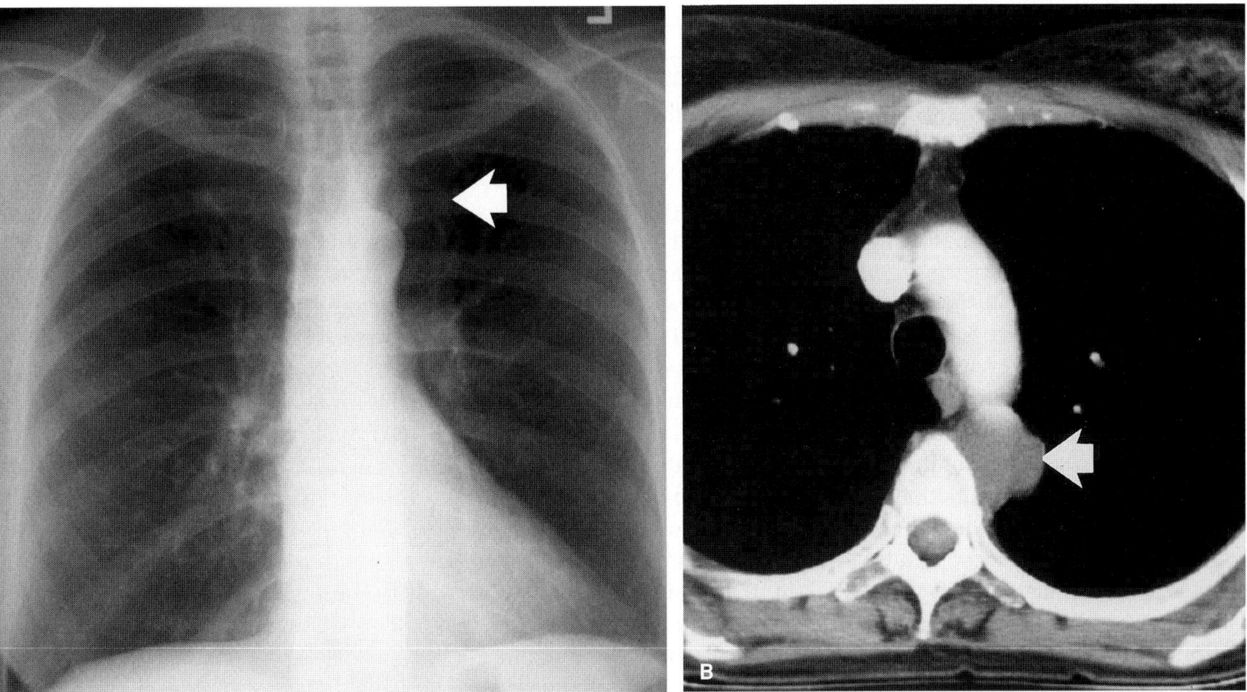

FIGURE 13.13. **Neurofibroma. A.** Frontal chest radiograph shows a left upper mediastinal mass (*arrow*). **B.** Contrast-enhanced CT confirms the presence of a left paravertebral soft tissue mass (*arrow*). Surgical resection confirmed a neurofibroma.

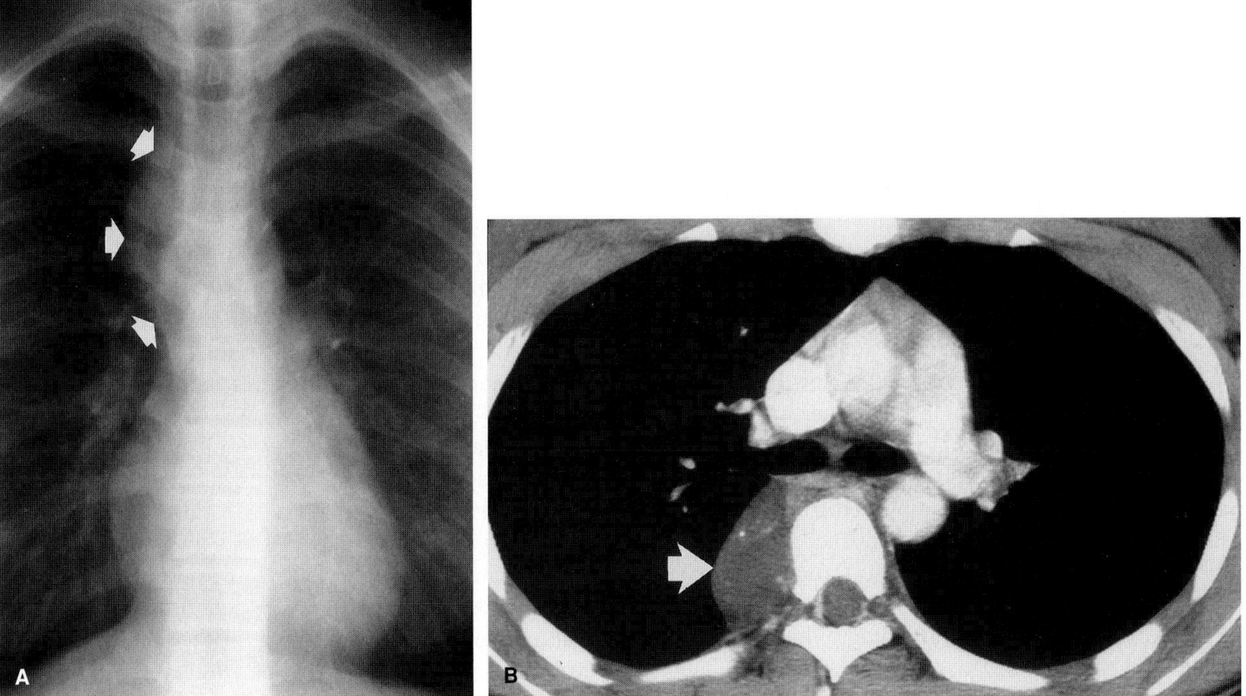

FIGURE 13.14. **Ganglioneuroma. A.** Posteroanterior radiograph in a 15-year-old woman reveals an oval, vertically oriented, right-sided mediastinal mass (*arrows*). **B.** Contrast-enhanced CT shows a low-attenuation posterior mediastinal mass (*arrow*) with calcification. This was surgically proven to be ganglioneuroma.

usually maintain an acute angle with the vertebral column and posterior mediastinum and therefore tend to show sharp superior and inferior margins on lateral chest radiographs. Large masses may erode vertebral bodies or ribs. Calcification, seen in up to 25% of cases, is a helpful diagnostic feature of these tumors but does not help distinguish benign from malignant neoplasms. Because these tumors often produce catecholamines, urinary levels of vanillylmandelic acid or metanephrines, which are byproducts of catecholamine metabolism, may be elevated. Prognosis depends upon the histologic features of the tumor and the patient's age and extent of disease at the time of diagnosis.

Paragangliomas are tumors that arise in the aorticopulmonary paraganglia of the middle mediastinum or the aorticosympathetic ganglia of the posterior mediastinum. They are divided into nonfunctioning neoplasms (chemodectomas), which occur almost exclusively in or about the aortopulmonary window, and functioning neoplasms (pheochromocytomas), which are found in the posterior sympathetic chain or in or about the heart or pericardium. Approximately 2% of all pheochromocytomas arise in the mediastinum. The posterior mediastinum is the site of fewer than 25% of mediastinal paragangliomas, with the majority arising in the anterior or middle mediastinum. Radiographically, these tumors are indistinguishable from other neurogenic tumors. However, most patients have hypertension and biochemical evidence of excess catecholamine production. CT and angiography demonstrate hypervascular masses; radionuclide iodine-131-meta-iodobenzylguanidine (MIBG) scanning is diagnostic in functioning tumors.

Esophageal Lesions. Because most of the intrathoracic esophagus is intimately associated with the thoracic spine and descending thoracic aorta, lesions in the middle or distal third of the esophagus may present as posterior mediastinal masses. Common presenting symptoms include dysphagia and aspiration pneumonia, although many patients are asymptomatic.

The majority of esophageal neoplasms, excluding lesions that arise at the esophagogastric junction, are squamous cell carcinomas. Unlike benign neoplasms of the posterior mediastinum, these lesions, when seen on chest radiographs, are rarely asymptomatic. Typically these patients have a history of dysphagia and significant weight loss. Difficulty in detecting asymptomatic lesions and the absence of a serosa account for the advanced stage of most esophageal carcinoma at presentation and a 5-year survival rate of less than 20%. Most patients with esophageal carcinoma have abnormal plain radiographic findings, including an abnormal azygoesophageal interface, widening of the mediastinum (resulting from the tumor itself or a dilated esophagus proximal to the obstructing lesion), abnormal thickening of the tracheoesophageal stripe, and tracheal deviation and compression. The diagnosis is usually made on barium esophagram and confirmed by endoscopic biopsy. CT scanning has proved accurate for staging esophageal carcinoma: findings include an intraluminal mass; thickening of the esophageal wall; loss of fat planes between the esophagus and adjacent mediastinal structures (usually the trachea, with upper esophageal lesions, and the descending aorta, with lower esophageal lesions); and evidence of nodal and distant metastases.

Several benign esophageal neoplasms, including leiomyoma, fibroma, and lipoma, can present as smooth, solitary mediastinal masses projecting laterally from the posterior mediastinum on frontal chest radiographs. They generally involve the lower third of the esophagus from the level of the subcarinal space to the esophageal hiatus. Initial evaluation is with barium studies, which show a smooth, broad-based mass forming obtuse margins with the esophageal wall. CT demonstrates a smooth, well-defined soft tissue mass adjacent to the esophagus without obstruction. The absence of esophageal dilatation above the mass helps distinguish benign tumors from carcinoma.

Pulsion diverticula arising at the cervicothoracic esophageal junction or distal esophagus are false diverticula representing mucosal outpouchings through defects in the muscular layer of the esophagus. A large proximal pulsion diverticulum (Zenker) may extend through the thoracic inlet and appear as a retroesophageal superior mediastinal mass containing an air–fluid level on upright chest radiographs. A distal pulsion diverticulum appears as a juxtadiaphragmatic mass with an air–fluid level projecting to the right of midline. Barium swallow is diagnostic.

A dilated esophagus resulting from functional (achalasia, scleroderma) or anatomic (stricture, carcinoma) obstruction may produce a mass that courses vertically over the length of the mediastinum, projecting toward the right side on frontal chest radiographs. An air–fluid level on upright films is usually present. A completely air-filled, dilated esophagus appears as a thin curvilinear line along the medial right thorax, because the right lateral wall of the esophagus is outlined by intraluminal air medially and the right lung laterally. Barium study or CT will confirm the diagnosis of a dilated esophagus; determination of the cause of obstruction often requires endoscopy or esophageal manometry.

Esophageal varices may produce a round or lobulated retrocardiac mass in patients with portal hypertension. The diagnosis is usually made by endoscopic recognition of submucosal varices involving the distal esophagus. The varices are readily recognized on contrast CT, MR, or portal venography.

A common cause of a mass in the posteroinferior mediastinum is a hiatal hernia. This results from a separation of the superior margins of the diaphragmatic crura and stretching of the phrenicoesophageal ligament. The stomach is by far the most common structure in the hernia sac; the gastric cardia (sliding hernia) or fundus (paraesophageal hernia) may be involved. Rarely, omental fat, ascitic fluid, or a pancreatic pseudocyst herniates through the esophageal hiatus into the mediastinum. The characteristic location at the esophageal hiatus and the presence of a rounded density containing an air or air–fluid level on upright films are diagnostic. Barium swallow or a CT scan will confirm the diagnosis (see Fig. 19.25).

Enteric/Neurenteric Cysts. Enteric cysts are fluid-filled masses lined by enteric epithelium. Esophageal cysts usually arise intramurally or immediately adjacent to the esophagus. When an enteric cyst has a persistent communication with the spinal canal (canal of Kovalevski) and is associated with congenital defects of the thoracic spine (anterior spina bifida, hemivertebrae, or butterfly vertebrae), it is termed a *neurenteric cyst*. CT or MR can confirm the cystic nature of these masses (Fig. 13.15). If the cyst communicates with the GI tract, it may contain air or an air–fluid level or opacify with contrast during an upper GI series.

Vertebral Abnormalities. A variety of conditions that affect the thoracic spine may manifest as posterior mediastinal masses. These lesions typically produce lateral deviation of the paraspinal reflection on frontal radiographs. Often, the bony origin of these lesions is not obvious on initial examination, making distinction from neurogenic tumors and other posterior mediastinal masses difficult.

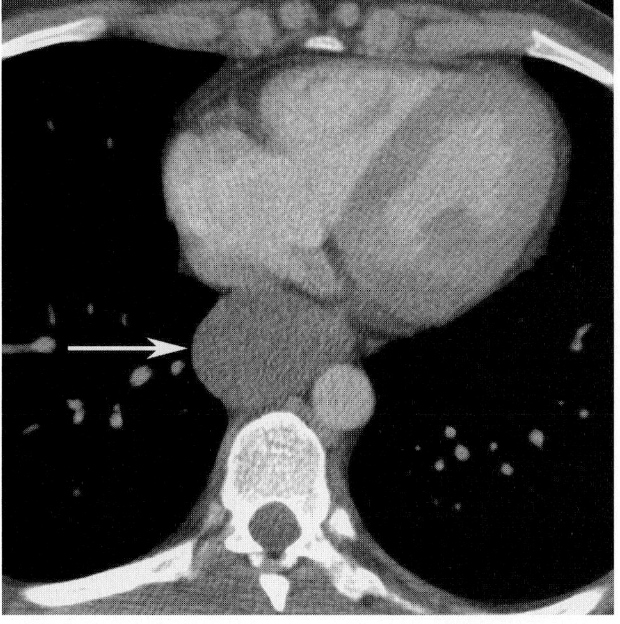

FIGURE 13.15. **Esophageal Duplication Cyst.** Enhanced CT in an 18-year-old man with a posterior mediastinal mass on chest radiography (not shown) demonstrates a low-attenuation right paraesophageal mass (*arrow*), consistent with an esophageal duplication cyst.

Neoplastic, infectious, metabolic, traumatic, or degenerative processes of the thoracic spine may produce a paraspinal mass by one of four mechanisms: (*1*) expansion of vertebral body or posterior elements (multiple myeloma, aneurysmal bone cyst); (*2*) extraosseous extension of infection, tumor, or marrow elements (infectious spondylitis, metastatic carcinoma, extramedullary hematopoiesis, respectively); (*3*) pathologic fracture and paraspinal hematoma formation (any destructive neoplastic or inflammatory process, trauma); or (*4*) protrusion of degenerative osteophytes. Neoplastic processes are usually easily identified by expansion and destruction of vertebral bodies, with sparing of intervertebral disks. Bronchogenic, breast, or renal cell carcinoma are the most common primary sites of thoracic spinal metastases. Infectious spondylitis is distinguished from neoplastic processes by the presence of a paravertebral mass centered at the point of maximal bone destruction. In patients with a paravertebral abscess secondary to tuberculosis or bacterial infection, narrowing of the adjacent disk space and destruction of vertebral endplates are important clues to the diagnosis. Extramedullary hematopoiesis is seen almost exclusively in conditions associated with ineffective production or excessive destruction of erythrocytes, such as thalassemia major, congenital spherocytosis, and sickle cell anemia. It is recognized by noting expansion of the medullary space and cyst formation within long bones, ribs, and vertebral bodies, with associated lobulated paraspinal soft tissue masses. These masses, which represent hyperplastic bone marrow that has extruded from the vertebral bodies and posterior ribs, are typically seen in the lower thoracic and upper lumbar region. Traumatic injuries to the thoracic spine are usually obvious from the patient's history and recognition of spine fracture on conventional and CT studies of the spine. Degenerative disk disease may produce a localized paraspinal mass on frontal radiographs. Well-penetrated films will show the characteristic inferolaterally projecting osteophytes at the level of the mass, which are most commonly right-sided because of the inhibitory effect of the pulsating descending aorta on left-sided osteophyte formation.

Lateral thoracic meningoceles represent an anomalous herniation of the spinal meninges through an intervertebral foramen, resulting in a paravertebral soft tissue mass. Most meningoceles are discovered in middle-aged patients as asymptomatic masses. They are slightly more common on the right, and are multiple in 10% of cases. There is a high association between lateral thoracic meningoceles and neurofibromatosis. A meningocele is the most common posterior mediastinal mass in

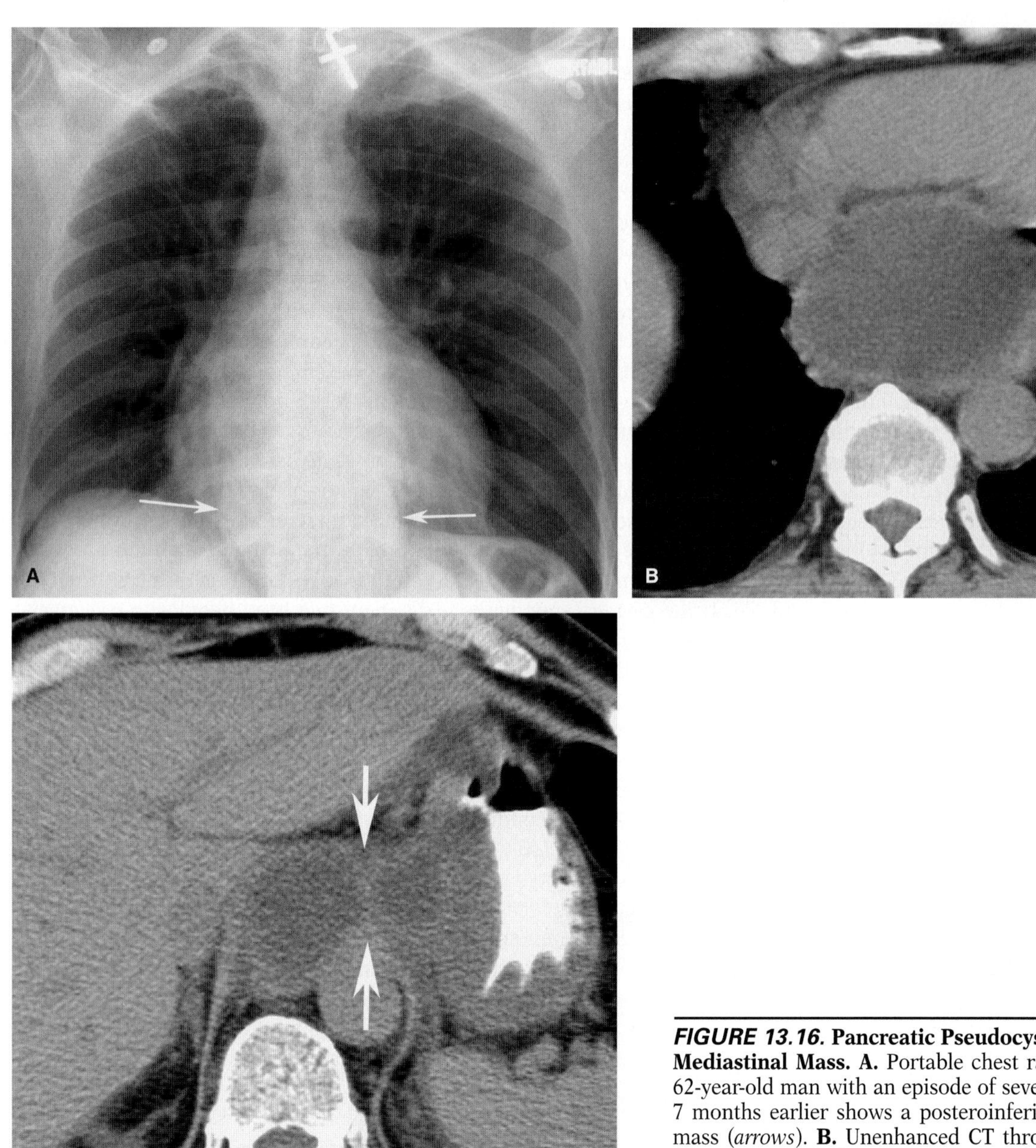

FIGURE 13.16. **Pancreatic Pseudocyst as Posterior Mediastinal Mass. A.** Portable chest radiograph in a 62-year-old man with an episode of severe pancreatitis 7 months earlier shows a posteroinferior mediastinal mass (*arrows*). **B.** Unenhanced CT through the lower chest shows a thick-walled cystic posterior mediastinal mass. **C.** Scan through the upper abdomen shows communication of the abdominal and thoracic components of the pseudocyst (*arrows*) via the esophageal hiatus.

patients with neurofibromatosis; conversely, approximately two thirds of patients with meningoceles have neurofibromatosis. Chest radiographs typically reveal a round, well-defined paraspinal mass that is indistinguishable from a neurofibroma. Additional clues to the diagnosis include rib erosion, enlargement of the adjacent neural foramen, vertebral anomalies, or kyphoscoliosis. When a lateral meningocele is associated with kyphoscoliosis, it is usually found at the apex of the scoliotic curve on the convex side. MR demonstration of a herniated subarachnoid space is the diagnostic technique of choice; conventional or CT myelography, which demonstrates filling of the meningocele with contrast, is reserved for equivocal cases.

Miscellaneous Conditions. A pancreatic pseudocyst rarely produces a posterior mediastinal mass by extending cephalad from the retroperitoneum through the esophageal or aortic hiatus of the diaphragm. The diagnosis relies on CT demonstration of continuity of a predominantly cystic mass with its retroperitoneal portion

(Fig. 13.16). The presence of a left pleural effusion is a further clue to the diagnosis. Hernias through the foramen of Bochdalek, which produce a posterior mediastinal mass, are discussed in Chapter 19.

Rarely, malignant lymph node enlargement may produce a recognizable paraspinal mass. This is most often seen in NHL and metastatic lung cancer; other mediastinal or extrathoracic sites of involvement are invariably present.

Despite the advances in detection and characterization of mediastinal masses with cross-sectional imaging, most patients will require tissue sampling for definitive diagnosis. However, the radiologist can use the information provided by CT or MR to help limit the differential diagnosis and thereby guide the appropriate evaluation and treatment. In a large percentage of cases, when tissue sampling is required, it can be accomplished by CT- or US-guided transthoracic biopsy.

DIFFUSE MEDIASTINAL DISEASE

The differential diagnosis of diffuse widening of the mediastinum is reviewed in Table 13.7.

TABLE 13.7 Diffuse Mediastinal Widening

Smooth	Mediastinal lipomatosis
	Malignant infiltration
	Lymphoma
	Small cell carcinoma
	Adenocarcinoma
	Mediastinal hemorrhage
	Arterial bleeding
	Traumatic aortic arch/great vessel laceration
	Aneurysmal rupture
	Venous bleeding
	SVC/right atrial laceration
	Mediastinitis
	Acute (suppurative)
	Chronic (sclerosing)
	Histoplasmosis
	Tuberculosis
	Idiopathic
Lobulated	Lymph node enlargement (see Table 14.4)
	Thymic mass (see Table 13.3)
	Germ cell neoplasm (see Table 13.3)
	Vascular lesions
	Tortuosity of great vessels
	SVC occlusion (dilated venous collaterals)
	Malignancy
	Sclerosing mediastinitis
	Catheter-induced thrombosis
	Neurofibromatosis

SVC, superior vena cava.

Mediastinal infection is an uncommon condition that may be divided into acute and chronic forms based upon etiology, clinical features, and radiologic findings. The distinction between acute and chronic infection is important because there are considerable differences in treatment and prognosis.

Acute mediastinitis is caused by bacterial infection that most often develops following esophageal perforation or is a complication of cardiothoracic surgery. Esophageal perforation may complicate esophageal instrumentation (e.g., endoscopy, biopsy, dilatation, or stent placement); penetrating chest trauma; esophageal carcinoma; foreign body or corrosive ingestion; or vomiting. Spontaneous esophageal perforation following prolonged vomiting is termed *Boerhaave syndrome*. In this condition, a vertical tear occurs along the left posterolateral wall of the distal esophagus, just above the esophagogastric junction, leading to signs and symptoms of acute mediastinitis. Less commonly, acute mediastinitis may develop from intramediastinal extension of infection in the neck, retropharyngeal space, lungs, pleural space, pericardium, or spine.

The clinical presentation of acute mediastinitis is usually dramatic and is characterized by severe retrosternal chest pain, fever, chills, and dysphagia, often accompanied by evidence of septic shock. Physical examination may reveal findings associated with pneumomediastinum, with subcutaneous emphysema in the neck and an apical, systolic crunching sound on chest auscultation (Hamman sign).

The most common chest radiographic findings are widening of the superior mediastinum in 66% of patients and pleural effusion in 50% of patients. Specific findings such as mediastinal air or air–fluid levels are less common. When mediastinitis occurs in association with Boerhaave syndrome, pneumoperitoneum and left hydropneumothorax may be seen.

When esophageal perforation is suspected, an esophagram should be performed to detect leakage of contrast into the mediastinum and to localize the exact site of perforation. In a patient not at risk for aspiration, a water-soluble contrast agent is administered initially. Once gross contrast extravasation has been excluded, barium is then given for superior radiographic detail. The sensitivity of the esophagram for detecting contrast leakage is highest when the study is obtained within 24 hours of the perforation.

MDCT is the radiologic study of choice for the diagnosis of acute mediastinitis (10). CT findings include extra luminal gas, bulging of the mediastinal contours, and focal or diffuse soft tissue infiltration of mediastinal fat. Localized fluid collections suggest focal abscess formation. Associated findings include mediastinal venous thrombosis, pneumothorax, pleural effusion or empyema, subphrenic abscess, and vertebral osteomyelitis.

While the clinical and radiographic diagnosis of mediastinitis is often straightforward, it may be difficult in postoperative patients who have undergone recent median sternotomy. In these patients, infiltration of mediastinal fat and focal air or fluid collections may be normal findings on postoperative CT scans performed days to weeks following the removal of intraoperatively placed mediastinal drains. In such patients, the progression of findings on follow-up CT scans will correctly identify the majority of those with postoperative mediastinal infection.

The prognosis for patients with acute mediastinitis varies with the underlying etiology and the extent of mediastinal involvement at the time of diagnosis. Esophageal perforation is associated with the poorest outcome, with a mortality approaching 50%. A delay in diagnosis and treatment of the mediastinal infection of greater than 24 hours is associated with a significant increase in overall morbidity and mortality.

In addition to its sensitivity in the diagnosis of mediastinitis, CT can be used to guide treatment and predict outcome. Those patients with evidence of extensive mediastinal infection, seen on CT as diffuse infiltration of the mediastinal fat without evidence of abscess formation, have a mortality approaching 50%. In contrast, patients with discrete mediastinal abscesses that are amenable to surgical or percutaneous drainage, or with small localized abscesses that are amenable to antibiotic therapy alone, have a more favorable prognosis. In addition, patients with mediastinal abscesses and contiguous empyema or subphrenic abscess may respond favorably to drainage of these extramediastinal collections.

Chronic Sclerosing (Fibrosing) Mediastinitis. The hallmarks of chronic sclerosing mediastinitis are chronic inflammatory changes and mediastinal fibrosis. The most common cause of this rare condition is granulomatous infection, usually secondary to *Histoplasma capsulatum.* Tuberculous infection, radiation therapy, and drugs (methysergide) are less common causes. Idiopathic mediastinal fibrosis, which is probably an autoimmune process, is related to fibrosis in other regions, including the retroperitoneum, intraorbital fat, and thyroid gland.

Several theories have been advanced to explain the pathogenesis of sclerosing mediastinitis owing to histoplasmosis. The most widely accepted theory suggests that affected patients develop an idiosyncratic hypersensitivity response to a fungal antigen that "leaks" from infected mediastinal lymph nodes.

Clinically, this condition occurs in adults and presents with a variety of symptoms, depending upon the extent of fibrosis and the mediastinal structures compromised by the fibrotic process. The superior vena cava (SVC) is the most commonly affected structure, with involvement in over 75% of symptomatic patients. The SVC syndrome manifests with headache, epistaxis, cyanosis, jugular venous distention, and edema of the face, neck, and upper extremities. The most serious and potentially fatal manifestation of sclerosing mediastinitis is obstruction of the central pulmonary veins, which produces pulmonary edema that may mimic severe mitral stenosis. Patients with involvement of the tracheobronchial tree may have cough, dyspnea, wheezing, hemoptysis, and obstructive pneumonitis. Dysphagia or hematemesis can be seen with esophageal involvement. Less commonly, pulmonary arterial hypertension and cor pulmonale can develop from narrowing of the pulmonary arteries.

The most common finding noted on chest radiographs is asymmetric lobulated widening of the upper mediastinum, most often on the right. When the process is secondary to granulomatous infection, enlarged calcified lymph nodes may be seen. Narrowing of the tracheobronchial tree may be evident. The sequelae of vascular involvement may be seen, including oligemia from pulmonary arterial compression or venous hypertension and pulmonary edema from involvement of the central pulmonary veins. Postobstructive atelectasis or consolidation may also be seen.

CT is the modality of choice for the diagnosis and assessment of chronic sclerosing mediastinitis. Enlarged lymph nodes with calcification are the most common finding (Fig. 13.17). The fibrotic infiltration of the mediastinal fat that is characteristic of this condition is seen as abnormal soft tissue density replacing the normal mediastinal fat with obliteration of the normal mediastinal interfaces. CT delineates the degree of involvement of the mediastinal vessels, trachea, and central bronchi. In patients with significant SVC involvement, collateral venous channels within the mediastinum and chest wall are well demonstrated.

MR is superior to CT for the assessment of vascular involvement. The ability to examine the mediastinal vessels in both the axial and coronal planes without the need for intravenous contrast helps detect vascular compromise. A significant disadvantage of MR is its inability to detect nodal calcification, a finding that is key to the diagnosis. For this reason, MR is most often utilized as an adjunct to CT when findings of vascular involvement are equivocal.

A definitive diagnosis of chronic sclerosing mediastinitis and the establishment of the underlying etiology are difficult. Skin tests for histoplasmosis and tuberculosis may add additional information but are usually not helpful. The precise diagnosis, and more important the distinction from infiltrating malignancy, usually requires biopsy.

Mediastinal Hemorrhage. Injury to mediastinal vessels resulting from blunt or penetrating thoracic trauma is the most common cause of mediastinal hemorrhage. Blunt chest trauma most often occurs in the setting of a motor

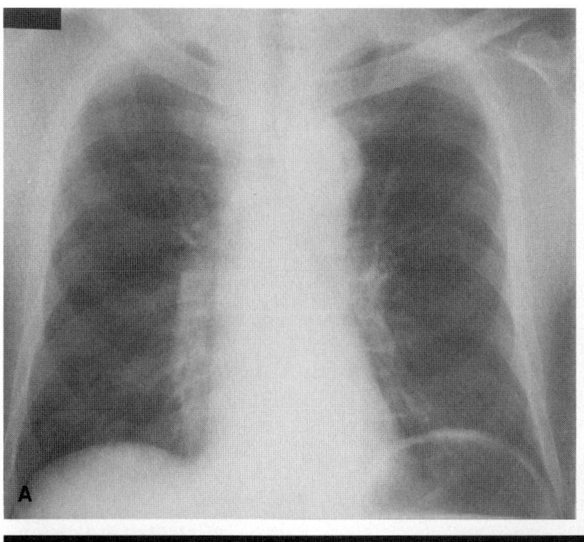

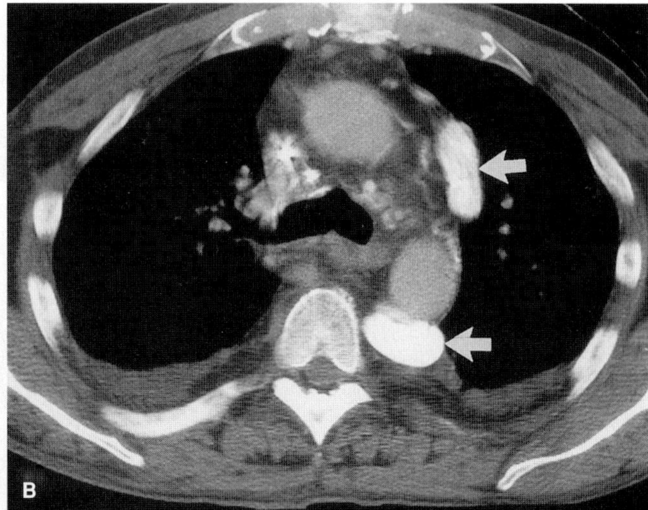

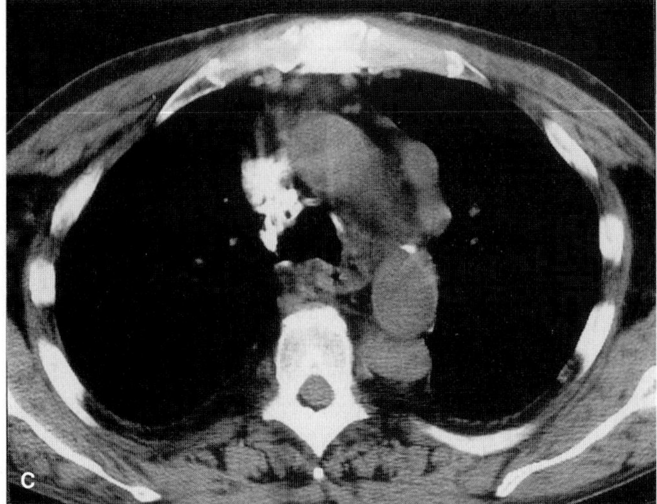

FIGURE 13.17. **Sclerosing Mediastinitis From Histoplasmosis. A.** Posteroanterior chest film in an asymptomatic 68-year-old man shows lobulated widening of the upper mediastinum. **B.** Contrast-enhanced CT reveals marked dilatation of the left superior intercostal vein (*arrows*), high-attenuation material in and around the superior vena cava, and numerous collaterals within the mediastinal fat. **C.** A noncontrast scan at approximately the same level reveals mediastinal calcification obliterating the superior vena cava. The patient was a former resident of Ohio where histoplasmosis is endemic.

vehicle accident, when rapid deceleration and thoracic cage compression produce shearing effects at the aortic isthmus. Iatrogenic trauma, usually from attempts at central line placement, can also cause mediastinal hemorrhage. Spontaneous hemorrhage may develop in patients with a coagulopathy, or with aortic rupture from aneurysm or dissection. Chronic hemodialysis, radiation vasculitis, and bleeding into a mediastinal mass are rare causes of mediastinal hemorrhage.

In the nontraumatic setting, the symptoms and signs of mediastinal hemorrhage are often mild or absent. The patient may complain of retrosternal chest pain radiating toward the back. Rarely, SVC compression may result in the SVC syndrome. Extension of blood from the mediastinum superiorly into the retropharyngeal space may result in neck stiffness, odynophagia, or stridor.

The main radiographic finding in mediastinal hemorrhage of any cause is a focal or diffuse widening of the mediastinum that obscures the normal mediastinal contours (11). In mediastinal hemorrhage, the mediastinum develops a flat or slightly convex outward contour, unlike the round, lobulated, or irregular contour seen with enlarged lymph nodes or a localized mediastinal mass. Blood extending from the mediastinum into the pleural or extrapleural space produces a free-flowing effusion or a loculated extrapleural collection, respectively. Rarely, extension of blood into the lungs via the bronchovascular interstitium produces interstitial opacities that mimic pulmonary edema. Serial radiographs may show rapid changes in mediastinal or pleural fluid collections in patients with persistent hemorrhage. CT demonstrates abnormal soft tissue within the mediastinum that obliterates the normal interfaces between the mediastinal fat, the vessels, and the airways (Fig. 13.18). Freshly clotted blood is high in attenuation and is usually easily appreciated on helical CT. CT is also superior to plain radiography in

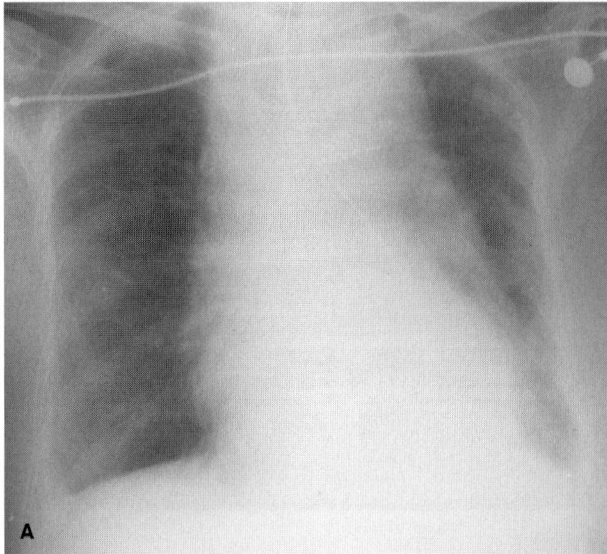

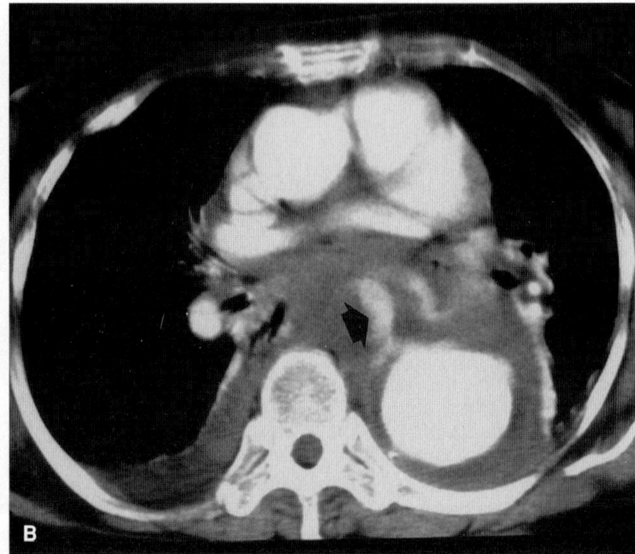

FIGURE 13.18. **Mediastinal Hematoma From Ruptured Thoracic Aortic Aneurysm. A.** Portable chest radiograph in an 83-year-old woman with chest pain shows marked mediastinal widening. **B.** Contrast-enhanced CT demonstrates aneurysmal dilatation of the descending aorta, with active extravasation (*arrow*) into a large mediastinal hematoma. The patient was not a surgical candidate and expired shortly after the study.

demonstrating the extramediastinal extent of hemorrhage and is useful in demonstrating associated thoracic injuries in patients following blunt chest trauma.

Mediastinal lipomatosis is a benign, asymptomatic condition characterized by excessive deposition of fat in the mediastinum. Predisposing conditions include obesity, Cushing disease, and corticosteroid therapy. However, this entity is unassociated with identifiable conditions in approximately 50% of patients.

On conventional radiographs, the most common finding is smooth, symmetric widening of the superior mediastinum. If the amount of fat deposition is marked, the mediastinum may show lobulated margins. Unlike mediastinal tumor infiltration or hemorrhage, which usually cause tracheal deviation or narrowing, the trachea remains at midline in mediastinal lipomatosis. Fat may also accumulate in the paraspinal regions, chest wall, and cardiophrenic angles; the latter produces enlargement of the epipericardial fat pads that is a clue to the proper diagnosis.

CT provides a definitive diagnosis by demonstrating abundant, homogeneous, unencapsulated fat that bulges the mediastinal contours (Fig. 13.19). Displacement or compression of mediastinal structures, particularly the trachea, is notable by its absence. Heterogeneity within the fat suggests other primary or superimposed conditions, such as neoplastic infiltration, infection, hemorrhage, or fibrosis.

Multiple symmetric lipomatosis is a rare entity that resembles simple mediastinal lipomatosis radiographically. The distinction between these two conditions is made by the distribution of abnormal fat and mass effect on mediastinal structures. In multiple symmetric lipomatosis, the cardiophrenic angles, paraspinal areas, and the anterior mediastinum are spared; periscapular lipomas may also be seen. The trachea is often compressed or displaced by fat in patients with this condition, whereas this is not seen in simple lipomatosis.

Malignancy. Malignant involvement of the mediastinum is typically seen as discrete masses or lymph node enlargement. Rarely, diffuse soft tissue infiltration of the mediastinal fat may occur, either alone or in association with focal lesions. Plain radiographs are nonspecific, usually demonstrating mediastinal widening. CT shows soft tissue infiltration of the normal mediastinal fat and obliteration of the normal tissue planes. This pattern is most common with extracapsular spread of lymphoma or small cell carcinoma of the lung. The latter disease has a high propensity to invade mediastinal structures and therefore may present with symptoms of airway obstruction or SVC syndrome.

Pneumomediastinum is the presence of extraluminal gas within the mediastinum. Possible sources of such gas include the lungs, trachea, central bronchi, esophagus, and extension of gas from the neck or abdomen (Table 13.8) (Fig. 13.20) (12).

Air from the lungs is the most common source of pneumomediastinum. The mechanism of pneumomediastinum formation involves a sudden rise in intrathoracic and intra-alveolar pressure that leads to alveolar rupture. The

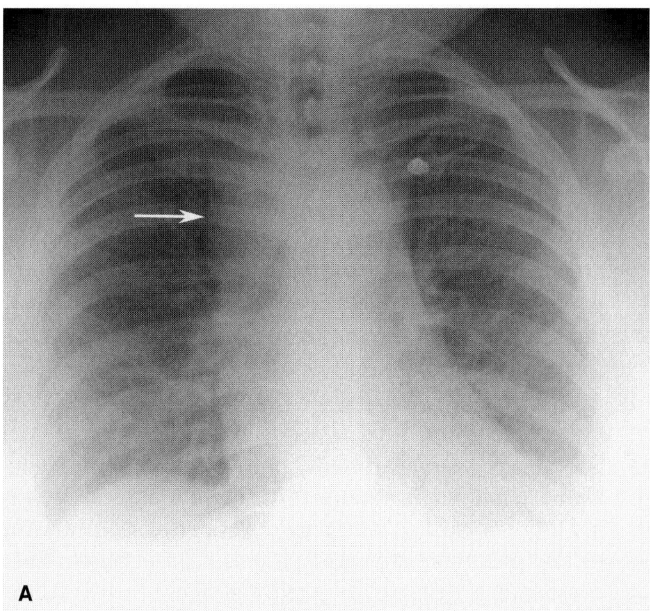

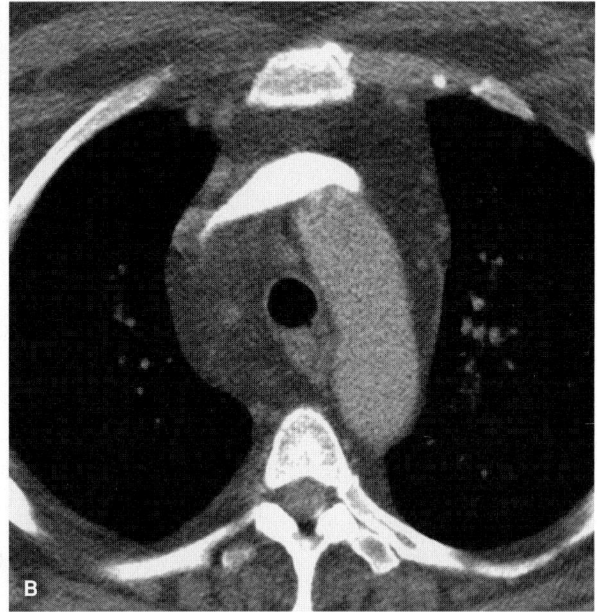

FIGURE 13.19. **Mediastinal Lipomatosis. A.** Frontal chest radiograph shows a widened superior mediastinum, particularly on the right (*arrow*). **B.** Unenhanced CT at the level of the aortic arch shows abundant mediastinal fat, responsible for the mediastinal widening.

extra-alveolar air first collects within the bronchovascular interstitium and then dissects centrally to the hilum and mediastinum (the Macklin effect). Less commonly, the air may dissect peripherally toward the subpleural interstitium and rupture through the visceral pleura to produce a pneumothorax.

Pneumomediastinum most commonly complicates mechanical ventilation in patients with ARDS, because the combination of positive pressure ventilation and abnormally stiff lungs predisposes to alveolar rupture. Spontaneous pneumomediastinum can occur with deep inspiratory or Valsalva maneuvers during strenuous exercise, childbirth, weightlifting, and inhalation of drugs such as marijuana, nitrous oxide, and crack cocaine. Patients with asthma are prone to pneumomediastinum; this is related to the airways obstruction that characterizes this disease. Prolonged vomiting from any cause may lead to intrathoracic pressures that are sufficiently high to produce pneumomediastinum. In patients with diabetic ketoacidosis, the increased respiratory effort that accompanies attempts at correcting the underlying metabolic acidosis can lead to pneumomediastinum. Blunt chest trauma can result in pneumomediastinum as a result of an abrupt increase in intra-alveolar pressure and shearing forces affecting the alveolar walls.

Pneumomediastinum arising from the tracheobronchial tree or esophagus usually is a result of traumatic disruption of these structures. The marked shearing forces that develop with blunt trauma may lead to fracture of the trachea or mainstem bronchi. Penetrating trauma to the tracheobronchial tree is usually iatrogenic and may follow endotracheal intubation, bronchoscopy, or tracheostomy. Rarely, neoplasms or inflammatory lesions (e.g., tuberculosis) may erode through the tracheal wall and into the peritracheal fat. Esophageal rupture is most often spontaneous, usually in the setting of severe, prolonged vomiting (Boerhaave syndrome). In addition to pneumomediastinum, a left hydropneumothorax and

TABLE 13.8 Pneumomediastinum

Intrathoracic source	Alveoli
	Valsalva maneuver
	Positive pressure ventilation
	Esophagus
	Boerhaave syndrome
	Endoscopic interventions (biopsy, dilatation, sclerotherapy)
	Carcinoma
	Tracheobronchial tree
	Bronchial stump dehiscence
	Tracheobronchial laceration
	Fistula formation
	Tracheal/esophageal malignancy
	Infection (tuberculosis, histoplasmosis)
Extrathoracic source	Recent sternotomy/thoracotomy
	Pneumoperitoneum/pneumoretroperitoneum
	Subcutaneous emphysema in neck
	Stab wound
	Laryngeal fracture

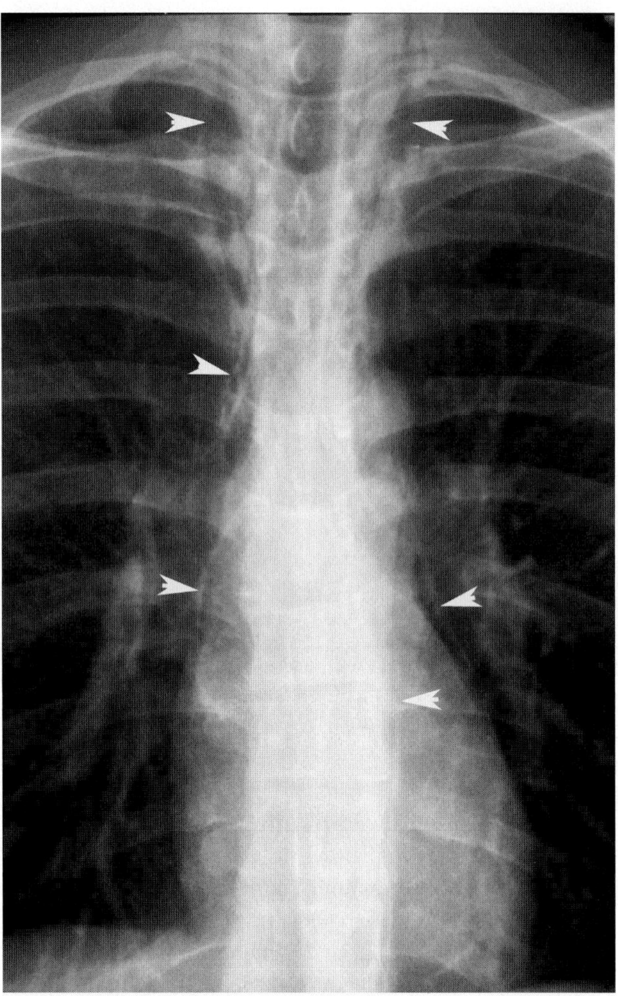

FIGURE 13.20. **Pneumomediastinum.** Cone-down view of a patient with spontaneous pneumomediastinum shows vertically oriented lucencies (*arrowheads*) outlining the aorta, esophagus, and heart and extending into the thoracic inlet superiorly.

pneumoperitoneum may be present in this condition. Spontaneous esophageal rupture may occur during childbirth, during a severe asthmatic episode, or with blunt chest trauma. Endoscopic procedures, stent placement, esophageal dilatation, corrosive ingestion, and carcinoma may lead to esophageal perforation. Mediastinal gas may be produced by bacterial organisms in acute mediastinitis.

Air within the soft tissues of the neck from penetrating trauma or laryngeal fracture may lead to pneumomediastinum by extending inferiorly through the retropharyngeal and prevertebral spaces, or along the sheaths of the great vessels. Deep space infections in the neck can spread along the same fascial planes and lead to mediastinitis. The term *Ludwig angina* describes the substernal chest pain caused by the intramediastinal extension of such infections. Rarely, pneumomediastinum develops as air dissects superiorly from the retroperitoneum through the aortic hiatus or from the peritoneal cavity along the internal mammary vascular sheaths.

The symptoms associated with pneumomediastinum vary with the underlying etiology, extent of mediastinal air, and presence of mediastinitis. Mediastinal air without infection is generally asymptomatic and does not require treatment. In some patients with spontaneous pneumomediastinum, there may be substernal, pleuritic-type chest pain of sudden onset that can be related to a specific inciting incident, such as vomiting or the Valsalva maneuver. Dyspnea may be present. In adults, mediastinal air under pressure usually escapes into the neck, producing crepitus over the neck, supraclavicular regions, and chest wall. Rarely, mediastinal air under pressure may produce a tension pneumomediastinum in which the clinical findings are those of cardiac tamponade. Patients with mediastinitis and pneumomediastinum are usually seriously ill with chest pain, high fevers, dyspnea, and signs of sepsis. The radiographic findings of pneumomediastinum are reviewed in Chapter 12.

THE HILA

Hilar abnormalities are first appreciated on conventional posteroanterior and lateral chest radiographs. CT and MR are used to confirm and characterize hilar masses or to detect subradiographic involvement of the hila; the latter most often in patients with bronchogenic carcinoma.

Unilateral Hilar Enlargement

Malignancy (Table 13.9). A hilar mass usually represents bronchogenic carcinoma or confluent lymph node metastases (Fig. 13.21). Unilateral hilar enlargement may be the presenting radiographic feature of squamous cell carcinoma, where the hilar mass represents the central extension of an endobronchial tumor from its origin within a segmental bronchus. Concomitant hilar lymph node involvement may contribute to hilar enlargement in some of these patients. Approximately 20% of patients with squamous cell carcinoma have a hilar mass on chest radiograph. In contrast, patients with adenocarcinoma and large cell carcinoma more commonly present with a peripheral pulmonary nodule or mass. In many patients, the hilar mass may be obscured by adjacent lung collapse or obstructive pneumonitis.

Unilateral hilar enlargement resulting from metastatic lymph node involvement is most often seen in small cell carcinoma. The propensity of this tumor for early invasion of the bronchial submucosa and peribronchial lymphatics accounts for the high incidence of widespread hematogenous and hilar and mediastinal lymph node metastases

TABLE 13.9 Unilateral Hilar Enlargement

Lymph node enlargement	
Malignancy	Bronchogenic carcinoma
	Lymph node metastases
	Bronchogenic carcinoma
	Head and neck malignancy
	Squamous cell carcinoma of skin, larynx
	Thyroid carcinoma
	Breast carcinoma
	Melanoma
	Genitourinary malignancy
	Renal cell carcinoma
	Testicular neoplasm
	Lymphoma
Infection	Tuberculosis
	Histoplasmosis
	Coccidioidomycosis
	Pneumonic plague
	Tularemia
	Anaerobic lung abscess
	Measles
	Mononucleosis
Pulmonary artery enlargement	Valvular pulmonic stenosis
	Pulmonary artery aneurysm
	Infection
	Tuberculosis (Rasmussen aneurysm)
	Left-to-right shunts
	Patent ductus arteriosis
	Atrial and ventricular septal defects
	Arteritis (see below)
	Tetralogy of Fallot
	Central pulmonary embolus
	Chronic thromboembolic disease
	Pulmonary arteritis
	Behçet disease
	Hughes-Stovin syndrome
	Takayasu arteritis
Cyst	Bronchogenic cyst

at the time of diagnosis. Plain film evidence of enlarged hilar lymph nodes resulting from metastases from adenocarcinoma of lung or large cell carcinoma are seen in only 10% to 15% of patients. Contrast-enhanced CT or MR is more sensitive for detecting enlarged hilar nodes and should be performed in all patients to guide further staging procedures and for proper preoperative or treatment planning.

Metastases to hilar and mediastinal lymph nodes from extrathoracic malignancies are uncommon, occurring in approximately 2% of patients. The malignancies that are most often associated with intrathoracic nodal metastases are genitourinary (renal and testicular); head and neck (skin, larynx, and thyroid); breast; and melanoma (7). In renal cell carcinoma and seminoma, lymphatic spread of tumor to retroperitoneal nodes and up the thoracic duct to the posterior mediastinum is the mode of spread to thoracic nodes. Although there is no direct communication between the thoracic duct and anterior mediastinal lymph nodes, reflux of tumor emboli through incompetent valves may allow tumor spread to hilar, paratracheal, and intraparenchymal lymphatics. Head and neck tumors reach the mediastinum via lymphatic spread from cervical lymph nodes. Intrathoracic nodal metastases from breast carcinoma are often seen late in the course of disease, often years after the initial diagnosis. Malignant melanoma is the extrathoracic neoplasm with the highest incidence of intrathoracic nodal metastases; patients with nodal disease will almost invariably have radiographic evidence of parenchymal metastases.

Although 75% of patients presenting with Hodgkin lymphoma have evidence of intrathoracic lymph node enlargement, isolated unilateral hilar lymph node enlargement is uncommon. The thoracic manifestations in NHL differ in primary pulmonary lymphoma, versus lymphoma that primarily involves extrathoracic sites with secondary pulmonary involvement. Thoracic involvement in primary pulmonary lymphoma is largely limited to parenchymal and pleural disease, whereas secondary pulmonary lymphoma generally manifests as intrathoracic lymph node enlargement, with 35% showing hilar or middle mediastinal lymph node enlargement and some presenting as an isolated finding.

Infection. Unilateral hilar or mediastinal lymph node enlargement is a characteristic feature in primary pulmonary tuberculosis in distinction to postprimary tuberculosis; an exception is the severely immunocompromised patient with AIDS. Isolated lymph node enlargement as a manifestation of primary tuberculosis is more common in children than in adults. There is almost always concomitant parenchymal disease in immunocompetent patients with lymph node enlargement. Fungal infections such as histoplasmosis and coccidioidomycosis may present with hilar lymph node enlargement, typically associated with patchy or lobar airspace consolidation in the ipsilateral lung. A variety of bacterial infections have been associated with unilateral hilar lymph node enlargement, including plague, tularemia, and anaerobic lung abscess. A characteristic finding in patients with pneumonic plague is the detection on unenhanced CT of increased attenuation within hilar and mediastinal nodes that drain regions of parenchymal involvement owing to intranodal hemorrhage. Tularemia (*Francisella tularensis*) causes parenchymal consolidation in association with hilar lymph node enlargement and pleural effusion.

The viral infections most commonly associated with hilar lymph node enlargement are infectious mononucleosis and measles pneumonia. The thorax is infrequently involved in mononucleosis, but hilar lymph node

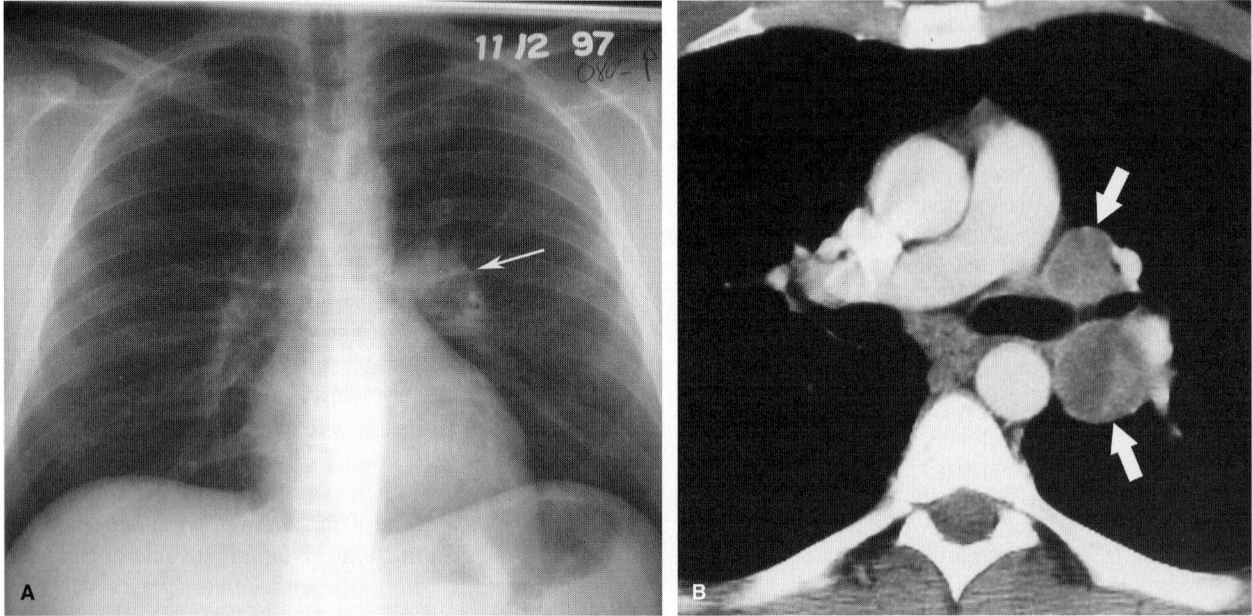

FIGURE 13.21. **Hilar Nodal Metastases From Melanoma. A.** Posteroanterior radiograph in a patient with melanoma shows left hilar enlargement (*arrow*). **B.** Enhanced CT scan shows enlarged left hilar lymph nodes (*arrows*) from metastatic disease.

enlargement is the most common manifestation of intrathoracic disease. Lymph node enlargement may accompany the reticular interstitial opacities of typical measles pneumonia, or it may be associated with nodular, segmental, or lobar opacities and pleural effusion in atypical measles pneumonia.

Pulmonary Artery Enlargement. Although unilateral hilar enlargement is most often the result of a mass or enlarged lymph nodes, abnormal enlargement of the right or left pulmonary artery may cause hilar prominence (Fig. 13.22). Vascular disorders that produce unilateral pulmonary artery enlargement include poststenotic

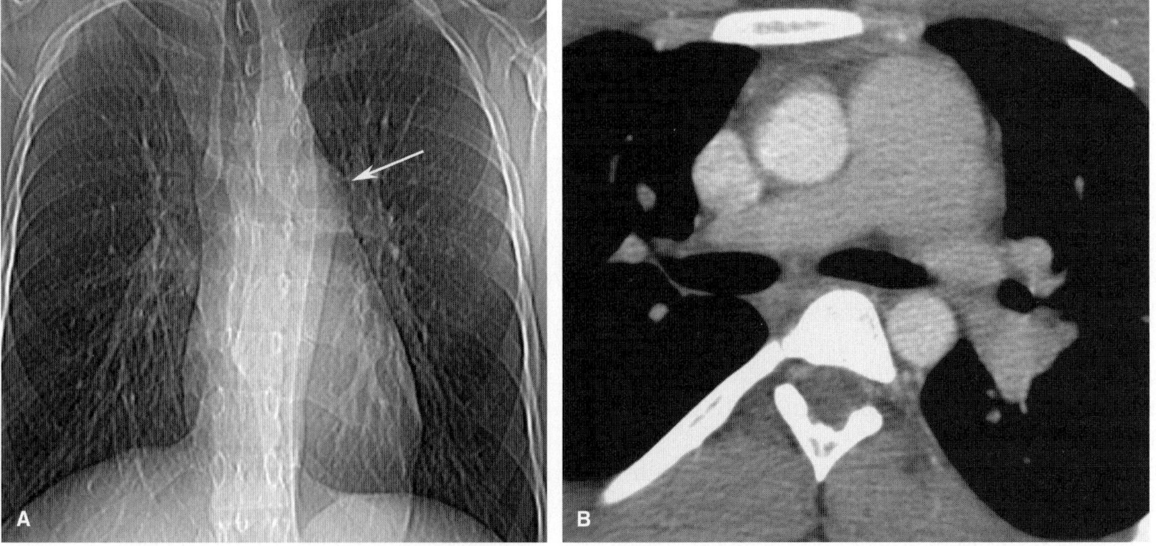

FIGURE 13.22. **Unilateral Hilar Enlargement From Idiopathic Dilatation of the Pulmonary Artery. A.** Scout view from chest CT shows abnormal convexity in the region of the main pulmonary artery (*arrow*). Note thoracic scoliosis. **B.** Enhanced CT scan shows dilated main pulmonary artery with normal right and left pulmonary arteries. Physical examination and echocardiogram showed no evidence of pulmonic valve disease.

dilatation from valvular or postvalvular pulmonic stenosis, pulmonary artery aneurysms, and distension of the pulmonary artery by thrombus or tumor. Patients with congenital valvular pulmonic stenosis may develop poststenotic dilatation or aneurysms of the main and left pulmonary arteries from the jet effect of blood upon these vessels. Rarely, stenoses resulting from pulmonary artery vasculitis, congenital rubella, or Williams syndrome may lead to poststenotic dilatation of a pulmonary artery. Aneurysms of the central pulmonary arteries are usually associated with congenital heart disease, such as pulmonic stenosis and left-to-right shunts from ventricular septal defect and patent ductus arteriosis. Rare vasculitides such as Behçet disease and Hughes-Stovins syndrome may present with pulmonary artery aneurysms. A large pulmonary embolus lodging in the proximal portion of a pulmonary artery may cause proximal dilatation. Obviously, these patients are symptomatic and will show characteristic findings on perfusion lung scan, helical CT, and pulmonary arteriography.

Bronchogenic cyst is an uncommon cause of a hilar mass. CT and MR will show a round, smooth, thin-walled cyst, usually found in an asymptomatic young adult. Because the hilum is an unusual location for a bronchogenic cyst, and distinction from a necrotic tumor or lymph node mass cannot be made radiographically, these lesions should be biopsied or removed.

Bilateral Hilar Enlargement

Bilateral hilar enlargement is the result of enlargement of either the hilar lymph nodes or the central pulmonary arteries (Table 13.10).

Malignancy. The malignancies producing bilateral hilar lymph node enlargement are similar to those producing unilateral enlargement. In distinction to unilateral nodal enlargement, metastases are uncommon causes of bilateral hilar nodal enlargement. The most frequent solid tumors producing bilateral hilar disease are small cell carcinoma of the lung and malignant melanoma.

TABLE 13.10 Bilateral Hilar Enlargement

Lymph node enlargement	Malignancy (see Table 13.2)
	Infection (see Table 13.2)
	Inflammatory disease
	Sarcoidosis
	Berylliosis
	Angioimmunoblastic lymphadenopathy
	Inhalational disease
	Silicosis
Pulmonary artery enlargement	Pulmonary arterial hypertension
	Left-to-right intracardiac shunt
	High output state
	Anemia
	Thyrotoxicosis
	Cystic fibrosis

Bilateral hilar lymph node involvement by lymphoma is more common in Hodgkin disease than NHL. Hilar involvement is virtually never seen without concomitant anterior mediastinal nodal enlargement in Hodgkin disease, whereas NHL may produce isolated hilar disease.

The most common chest radiographic manifestation of leukemic involvement of the thorax is hilar and mediastinal lymph node enlargement; it is seen in up to 25% of patients. Lymph node enlargement is much more common in the lymphocytic than the myelogenous form, particularly in chronic lymphocytic leukemia.

Infection. Mediastinal and hilar lymph node enlargement from infection is most often seen in tuberculous and fungal infection with histoplasmosis and coccidioidomycosis. In these diseases, the lymph node enlargement may be unilateral or bilateral. With bilateral disease, the enlargement is asymmetric in distinction to sarcoidosis, which is typically symmetric. Bacterial infection from *Bacillus anthracis* (anthrax) and *Yersinia pestis* (plague) may produce bilateral hilar enlargement. In anthrax infection, the lymph node enlargement is often associated with patchy airspace opacities in the lower lobes. The bubonic form of plague may produce marked hilar and mediastinal adenopathy without pneumonia. Recurrent bacterial infection complicating cystic fibrosis is often associated with bilateral hilar lymph node enlargement, and distinction from pulmonary artery enlargement owing to pulmonary hypertension may be difficult.

Sarcoidosis is associated with bilateral hilar lymph node enlargement in 80% of patients. Most of these patients have concomitant paratracheal lymph node enlargement, and nearly half have concomitant radiographic parenchymal disease. The pattern of lymph node involvement in sarcoidosis has been termed the 1-2-3 sign, with 1 = right paratracheal, 2 = right hilar, and 3 = left hilar lymph node enlargement (Fig. 13.9; see Fig. 17.25). The enlarged nodes produce symmetric, lobulated hilar masses on plain film, since the enlarged nodes remain separate. In 20% of patients, the involved lymph nodes will calcify; usually the calcifications are punctate in appearance, but occasionally peripheral "eggshell" calcification is seen. In some patients, the involved nodes can be seen to enhance after contrast administration on CT. In the majority of patients, the enlarged nodes resolve within 2 years of discovery; in a small percentage, the nodes remain enlarged for many years.

Berylliosis and Silicosis. The hilar and mediastinal lymph node enlargement of chronic berylliosis is radiographically indistinguishable from that of sarcoidosis. Similarly, silicosis can produce hilar and mediastinal lymph node enlargement; eggshell calcification of hilar nodes is highly suggestive of this entity, although

TABLE 13.11 Small Hilum (Hila)

Unilateral	Absence or hypoplasia of the pulmonary artery
	Hypoplastic or hypogenetic lung
	Swyer-James syndrome
	Lobar atelectasis
	Lobar resection
	Compression/invasion of the pulmonary artery
	Cyst
	Neoplasm
	Fibrosing mediastinitis
Bilateral	Emphysema
	Obstruction to pulmonary flow
	Fibrosing mediastinitis
	Tetralogy of Fallot
	Valvular pulmonic stenosis
	Ebstein anomaly

peripheral nodal calcification may also be seen with sarcoidosis, histoplasmosis, or amyloidosis.

Bilateral pulmonary artery enlargement is seen with increased flow or increased resistance in the pulmonary circulation. The conditions associated with bilateral pulmonary arterial enlargement are reviewed in Chapter 14.

Small Hila

Bilaterally small hila (Table 13.11) can be seen in some adults with severe pulmonary overinflation from emphysema or in those with diminished pulmonary blood flow due to congenital pulmonary outflow obstruction (tetralogy of Fallot, Ebstein anomaly).

The most common causes of a small hilum are atelectasis and resection of a portion of lung, which leave a small residual hilar artery supplying the remaining lobe or lobes. Hypoplasia of the pulmonary artery, often with associated abnormalities of the ipsilateral lung (hypogenetic lung syndrome, Swyer-James syndrome), is another cause of a small hilum. Less commonly, invasion of the proximal pulmonary artery by mediastinal tumor, or obstruction of the pulmonary artery on account of fibrosing mediastinitis, can produce a diminutive hilar shadow. In any patient in whom a small hilum is a new radiographic finding, a CT scan should be performed to assess the mediastinum for central obstructing lesions. The left hilum can appear small in patients in whom the hilar shadow is obscured by the upper left heart margin or by fat in the region of the aortopulmonic interface. In these cases, the lateral radiograph will usually show a left pulmonary artery of normal size.

REFERENCES

1. Glazer GM, Axel L, Moss AA. CT diagnosis of mediastinal thyroid. AJR Am J Roentgenol 1992;138:495–498.
2. Tomiyama N, Johkoh T, Mihara N, et al. Using the World Health Organization classification of thymic epithelial neoplasms to describe CT findings. AJR Am J Roentgenol 2002;179:881–886.
3. Uffmann M, Schaefer-Prokop C. Radiological diagnostics of Hodgkin and non-Hodgkin lymphomas of the thorax. Radiologe 2004;44:444–456.
4. Zinzani PL, Magagnoli M, Chierchietti F, et al. The role of positron emission tomography (PET) in the management of lymphoma patients. Ann Oncol 1999;10:1181–1184.
5. Strollo DC, Rosado-de-Christenson ML, Jett JR. Primary mediastinal tumors. Part 1: tumors of the anterior mediastinum. Chest 1997; 112(2):511–522.
6. Strollo DC, Rosado-de-Christenson ML, Jett JR. Primary mediastinal tumors. Part 2: tumors of the middle and posterior mediastinum. Chest 1997;112(5):1344–1357.
7. Mountain CF, Dresler CM. Regional lymph node classification for lung cancer. Chest 1997;111:1718–1723.
8. McLoud TC, Kalisher L, Stark P, et al. Intrathoracic lymph node metastases from extrathoracic neoplasm. AJR Am J Roentgenol 1978;131:403–407.
9. McAdams HP, Kirejczyk WM, Rosado-de-Christenson ML, Matsumoto S. Bronchogenic cyst: imaging features with clinical and histopathologic correlation. Radiology 2000;217:441–446.
10. Carrol CL, Jeffrey RB, Federle MP, et al. CT evaluation of mediastinal infections. J Comput Assist Tomogr 1989;11:449–454.
11. Woodring JH, Loh FK, Kryscio RJ. Mediastinal hemorrhage: an evaluation of radiographic manifestations. Radiology 1984;151: 15–21.
12. Gray JM, Hanson GC. Mediastinal emphysema: etiology, diagnosis, and treatment. Thorax 1966;21:325–332.

Chapter 14

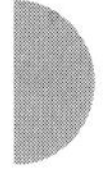

Pulmonary Vascular Disease

Jeffrey S. Klein

Pulmonary Edema
Pulmonary Hemorrhage
Pulmonary Embolism
Pulmonary Arterial Hypertension

Pulmonary Edema

Basic Principles. Under normal conditions, the interstitial space of the lung is kept dry by pulmonary lymphatics located within the axial and peripheral interstitium of the lung. The lymphatics drain the small amounts of transudated fluid that enters the interstitial spaces as an ultrafiltrate of plasma. Because there are no lymphatic structures immediately within the alveolar walls (parenchymal interstitium), filtered interstitial fluid is drawn to the lymphatics by a pressure gradient from the alveolar interstitium to the axial and peripheral interstitium. When the rate of fluid accumulation in the interstitium exceeds the lymphatic drainage capabilities of the lung, fluid accumulates first within the interstitial space. As the amount of extravascular fluid increases, fluid accumulates in the corners of the alveolar spaces. Progressive fluid accumulation eventually produces flooding of the alveolar spaces, resulting in airspace pulmonary edema. While interstitial edema may leave the gas-exchanging properties of the lung unaffected, flooding of the alveolar spaces leads to impaired oxygen and carbon dioxide exchange.

Excess fluid accumulation in the lung is caused by one of three basic mechanisms. The most common mechanism involves a change in the normal Starling forces that govern fluid movement in the lung. Because normal fluid movement is determined by the differences in hydrostatic and oncotic pressure between the pulmonary capillaries and surrounding alveolar interstitium, an imbalance in these forces may lead to pulmonary edema. Pulmonary edema is most commonly the result of increased capillary hydrostatic pressure from left heart failure, although diminished plasma oncotic pressure or diminished interstitial hydrostatic pressure may be contributing factors. Another mechanism involves an absence or obstruction of the normal pulmonary lymphatics, which leads to the excess accumulation of interstitial fluid. Third, a wide variety of disorders can injure the capillary endothelium and alveolar epithelium, producing an increase in capillary permeability that allows protein-rich fluid to escape from the capillaries and into the pulmonary interstitium.

Radiographic findings in pulmonary edema can be divided into interstitial and airspace components. The radiographic appearance of interstitial pulmonary edema is attributed to thickening of the various components of the interstitial spaces by fluid (1). Thickening of the axial interstitium results in the loss of definition of the intrapulmonary vascular shadows, peribronchial cuffing, and tram tracking. Edema within alveolar septa is not discernible as discrete opacities but produces a ground-glass opacification in the perihilar and lower lung zones—regions in which fluid tends to accumulate in the early phases of edema. Involvement of peripheral and subpleural interstitial structures produces Kerley lines and subpleural edema. Kerley A and B lines represent thickening of central connective tissue septa and peripheral interlobular septa, respectively, while Kerley C lines represent a network of thickened interlobular septa (Fig. 14.1). Subpleural edema is the accumulation of fluid within the innermost (interstitial) layer of the visceral pleura and is best seen on the lateral radiograph as smooth thickening of the interlobar fissures. The radiographic changes of interstitial pulmonary edema may progress to those of airspace edema or, if successfully treated, resolve within 12 to 24 hours.

Airspace pulmonary edema develops when progressive fluid accumulates in the interstitial spaces and spills into

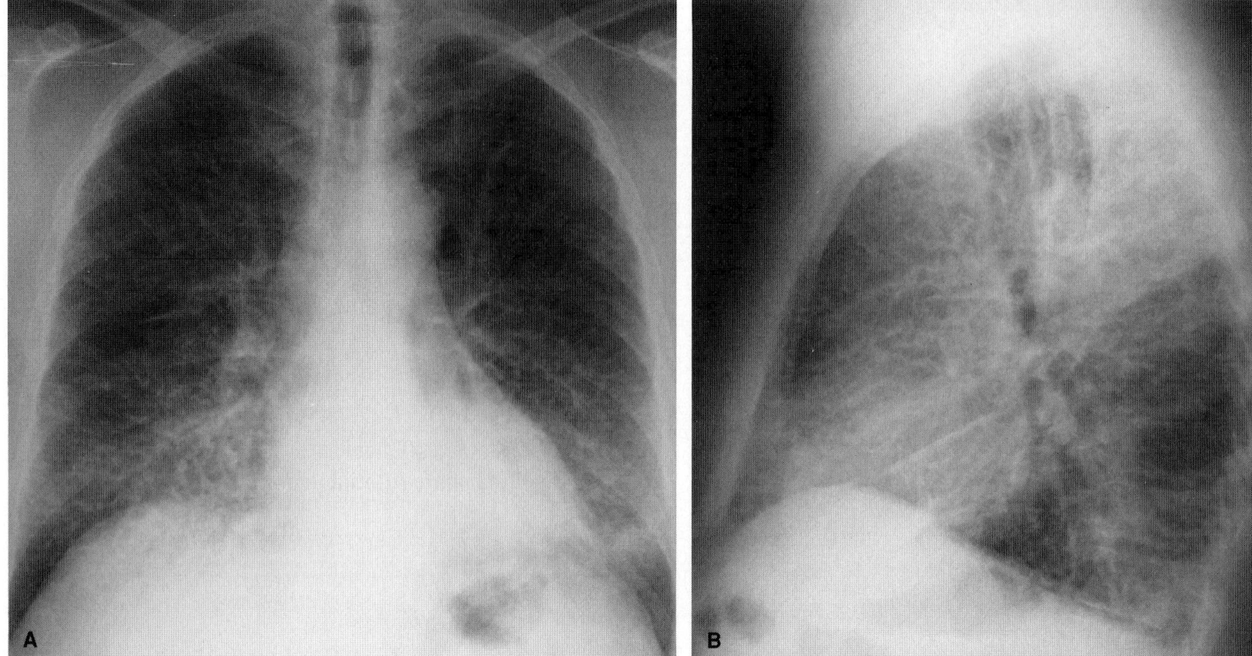

FIGURE 14.1. Interstitial Pulmonary Edema Caused by Cardiac Disease. Posteroanterior **(A)** and lateral **(B)** chest films in a 65-year-old man with an anterior wall myocardial infarction shows bilateral linear opacities (Kerley A, B, and C lines) representing interstitial pulmonary edema. Note the prominence of upper lobe vessels, indicating concomitant pulmonary venous hypertension.

the alveoli. The chest radiograph typically shows symmetric bilateral airspace opacities that are confluent and predominate in the mid and lower lung zones. Airspace nodules and the findings of interstitial edema (Kerley B lines and subpleural edema) may be seen peripherally. An uncommon form of airspace pulmonary edema, seen most commonly in left heart failure or renal failure, is the "bat's wing" or "butterfly" distribution of disease. In this situation, the airspace opacification is sharply confined to the central, parahilar regions of lung, with sparing of the peripheral or subpleural regions (Fig. 14.2). The reason for this distribution of edema is unknown. As with interstitial edema, the airspace opacities of alveolar edema tend to change rapidly, often within hours. The differential diagnosis of diffuse airspace opacities has been reviewed (see Table 12.9).

Although not commonly used to evaluate the patient with pulmonary edema, CT and HRCT demonstrate fairly characteristic findings in this disorder (2). Thickening of subpleural, septal, and bronchovascular structures are well depicted on HRCT. Mild parenchymal edema produces a ground-glass pattern around the hila (Fig. 14.3). Early alveolar edema is seen as centrilobular airspace nodules surrounding the arteries within the lobular core, while severe alveolar edema produces dense perihilar airspace opacification. Cardiomegaly, pulmonary venous distention, and pleural effusions are associated findings in cardiogenic or fluid overload edema.

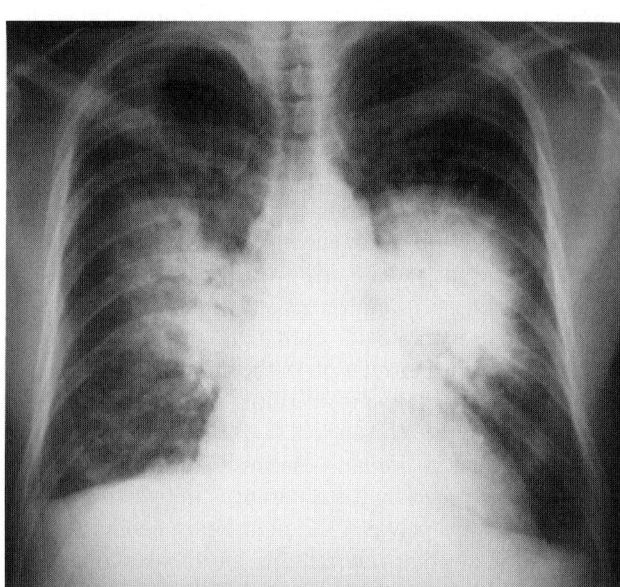

FIGURE 14.2. Perihilar "Bat's Wing" Pulmonary Edema. Frontal chest radiograph in a 32-year-old man with dilated cardiomyopathy reveals dense bilateral perihilar airspace opacification resulting from pulmonary edema.

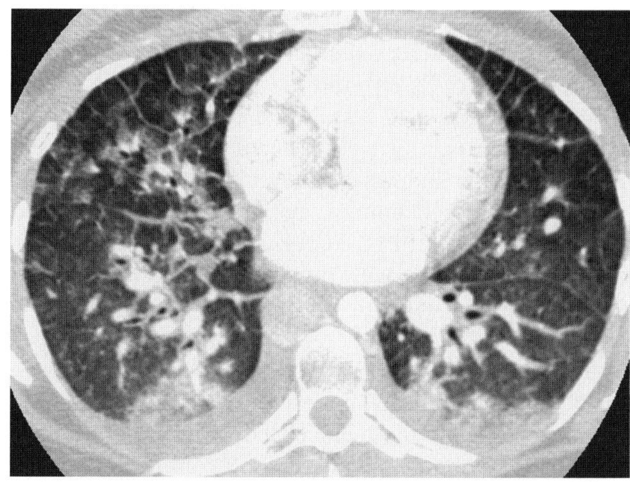

FIGURE 14.3. **Thin-Section CT of Interstitial Pulmonary Edema.** Thin-section CT in a 28-year-old woman with postpartum cardiomyopathy shows characteristic findings of interstitial edema: interlobular septal thickening, peribronchial cuffing, and ground-glass and airspace opacities. Note the associated findings of congestive heart failure, with pulmonary vascular engorgement and bilateral pleural effusions.

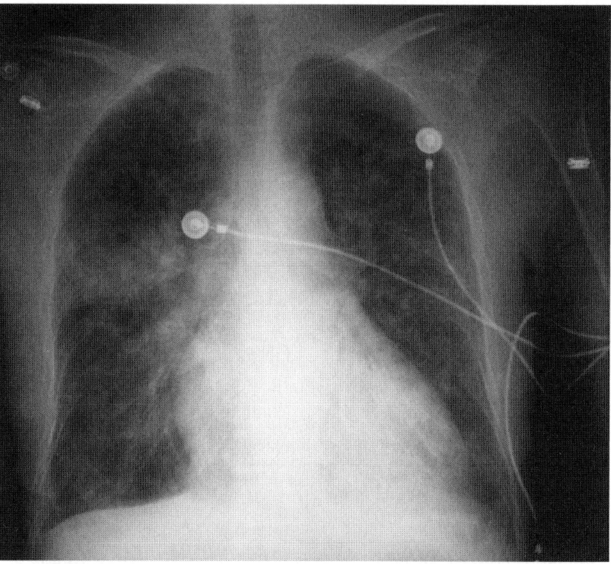

FIGURE 14.4. **Interstitial and Right Upper Lung Pulmonary Edema.** In a 64-year-old woman with unstable angina and mitral regurgitation on echocardiography, posteroanterior chest radiograph shows diffuse interstitial pulmonary edema with localized right upper lobe airspace opacification, the latter secondary to ischemic mitral valvular dysfunction.

Atypical Radiographic Appearances. Several conditions may give rise to atypical radiographic appearances of pulmonary edema. Because the distribution of edema is affected by gravity, it is not surprising that edema fluid accumulates posteriorly or unilaterally in patients maintaining a prolonged supine or decubitus position, respectively. The diagnosis of unilateral edema is suggested by typical radiographic and clinical findings of pulmonary edema in one lung that resolve rapidly or redistribute with changes in patient positioning. Another cause of asymmetric or unilateral pulmonary edema is an interruption in the blood supply to one lung. This may be seen in pulmonary artery hypoplasia or in an acquired obstruction to pulmonary arterial blood flow, such as central pulmonary embolus or extrinsic compression of the pulmonary artery from tumor or fibrosis. In these conditions, the lung with diminished pulmonary blood flow is "protected" from the transudation of fluid and the development of pulmonary edema. Bronchogenic carcinoma, lymphoma, or other causes of unilateral lymph node enlargement can impede normal lymphatic drainage and predispose to unilateral pulmonary edema. Similarly, unilateral pulmonary venous obstruction from tumor or fibrosing mediastinitis will predispose to edema on the affected side. Unilateral pulmonary edema may develop in the lung that is re-expanded by the rapid evacuation of a large pleural fluid collection or pneumothorax. This is known as *re-expansion pulmonary edema* and is discussed in a subsequent section.

Alveolar pulmonary edema localized to the right upper lung may be seen in patients with severe mitral regurgitation. Edema formation is likely the result of preferential regurgitant flow of blood into the right upper lobe pulmonary vein across the superiorly and posteriorly oriented mitral valve. These patients will usually have typical radiographic findings of interstitial edema elsewhere in the lungs (Fig. 14.4).

Patients with pulmonary emphysema may have unusual appearances of alveolar edema. Areas of bullae, most commonly in the apical portions of the lungs, are spared from the development of alveolar edema because the pulmonary blood flow to these regions has already been obliterated by the emphysematous process. These emphysematous regions within adjacent areas of airspace opacification can simulate cavity formation and may be difficult to distinguish radiographically from necrotizing pneumonia or pneumatocele formation. Comparison with previous radiographs and correlation with the clinical course will aid in the proper diagnosis.

Hydrostatic pulmonary edema (normal capillary permeability) is the most common form of pulmonary edema. Patients with acute or chronic renal failure may develop pulmonary edema because of increased pulmonary capillary hydrostatic pressure. The elevated hydrostatic pressure is caused by a combination of hypervolemia and LV dysfunction, with resultant pulmonary venous and capillary hypertension. Volume overload without renal failure may also produce pulmonary edema by a hydrostatic mechanism. Decreased capillary oncotic pressure, present in patients with hypoalbuminemia secondary to the nephrotic syndrome or liver failure, is not considered to be an independent risk factor for the development of pulmonary edema but is a cofactor in several conditions.

TABLE 14.1 Causes of Pulmonary Venous Hypertension and Pulmonary Edema

Obstruction to LV outflow	Aortic coarctation Aortic stenosis Hypoplastic left heart syndrome
LV failure	
Mitral valve disease	Mitral stenosis Mitral insufficiency
LA myxoma	
Cor triatriatum	
Obstruction of pulmonary veins	
Central pulmonary veins	Fibrosing mediastinitis Pulmonary vein stenosis Pulmonary venous thrombosis
Intrapulmonary veins	Pulmonary venoocclusive disease

Hydrostatic pulmonary edema is usually caused by pulmonary venous hypertension secondary to congestive heart failure. Thus, identification of the radiographic findings of pulmonary venous hypertension and pulmonary edema will provide the diagnosis. The majority of these patients will have LV failure or mitral valve disease. A list of the causes of mechanical or functional obstruction to pulmonary venous return is found in Table 14.1.

The radiographic findings of pulmonary venous hypertension are enlargement of pulmonary veins and redistribution of pulmonary blood flow to the upper lung zones (1). Pulmonary venous enlargement is seen as progressive dilatation of horizontally oriented pulmonary veins on serial chest radiographs. The redistribution of pulmonary blood flow results from lower zone pulmonary venous constriction and increased resistance to lower zone blood flow, with resultant preferential flow through upper lobe vessels. Therefore, in pulmonary venous hypertension in the upright patient, the upper zone vessels are as large as or larger in diameter than the lower zone vessels. This is the opposite of the normal appearance, in which the lower zone vessels are larger than the upper zone vessels as the result of the normal gravitational effects on pulmonary blood flow. It should be noted that there are conditions other than pulmonary venous hypertension in which there is distention of upper zone pulmonary vessels, including left-right shunts and basilar lung disease. The association of upper zone vascular prominence with findings of LV failure (cardiomegaly, pulmonary edema, and pleural effusion) usually allows for the correct diagnosis.

The sequence of events following the development of pulmonary venous hypertension has been studied in patients with acute cardiac decompensation following myocardial infarction. Several studies have correlated the radiographic findings of pulmonary venous hypertension in the erect patient with measurements of pulmonary capillary wedge pressure (PCWP) using flow-directed balloon occlusion (i.e., Swan-Ganz) catheters. When PCWP is normal (8 to 12 mm Hg), the chest radiograph is normal. Mild elevation of PCWP (12 to 18 mm Hg) produces constriction of lower lobe vessels and enlargement of upper lobe vessels. Progressive elevation of PCWP (19 to 25 mm Hg) leads to the findings of interstitial pulmonary edema: loss of vascular definition, peribronchial cuffing, and Kerley lines (Fig. 14.1). PCWP above 25 mm Hg produces alveolar filling with radiographic findings of bilateral airspace opacities in the perihilar and lower lung zones.

The causes of pulmonary venous hypertension may be divided radiographically into those associated with a normal heart size and those associated with cardiomegaly. A severe, long-standing obstruction to LV outflow (e.g., aortic stenosis) is usually associated with a normal heart size unless the LV has failed. Chronic left ventricular failure is invariably associated with cardiomegaly, although acute LV decompensation, as in acute myocardial infarction or acute aortic regurgitation, may show a normal heart size. Obstruction or incompetence at the level of the mitral valve (e.g., mitral stenosis or regurgitation, left atrial myxoma) may only show left atrial enlargement without ventricular dilatation. Obstruction of the central pulmonary veins (i.e., fibrosing mediastinitis, pulmonary vein thrombosis) is usually associated with the radiographic findings of pulmonary venous hypertension and pulmonary edema with a normal heart size. Intrapulmonary venous obstruction (i.e., pulmonary venoocclusive disease) may show only pulmonary edema, but often the diagnosis is delayed until pulmonary arterial hypertension (PAH) has developed (Table 14.1).

Increased Capillary Permeability Edema. Rapidly progressive respiratory compromise caused by leakage of protein-rich edema fluid into the lung, resulting from damage to the pulmonary microcirculation, may develop as a complication of a variety of systemic conditions. When respiratory failure develops as a result of this condition and is associated with increased lung stiffness (noncompliance) it is termed ARDS (for *acute respiratory distress syndrome*) (3). The edema associated with this syndrome is called *lung injury* or *increased capillary permeability edema,* as compared to the normal alveolocapillary permeability of hydrostatic edema. A long list of pulmonary and nonpulmonary disorders have been associated with increased-permeability edema (Table 14.2) ; the most common are shock, severe trauma, burns, sepsis, narcotic overdose, and pancreatitis. Although the precise pathogenesis of capillary permeability edema has yet to be completely elucidated, current evidence suggests that recruitment and activation of neutrophils in the lung with release of enzymes and oxygen radicals are key factors in the development of capillary endothelial damage.

The pathologic changes associated with ARDS are those of diffuse alveolar damage and are common to all

TABLE 14.2 Etiologies of Increased Permeability Pulmonary Edema

Septicemia	Gram-negative bacteria
Shock	
Major surgery	
Burns	
Acute pancreatitis	
Disseminated intravascular coagulation	
Drugs	Narcotics Heroin Crack cocaine Aspirin
Inhalation of noxious fumes	Nitrogen dioxide (silo-filler's disease) Hydrocarbons Smoke Chlorine Phosgene
Aspiration of fluid	Fresh or salt water near drowning Gastric fluid aspiration (Mendelson syndrome)
Fat embolism	
Amniotic fluid embolism	

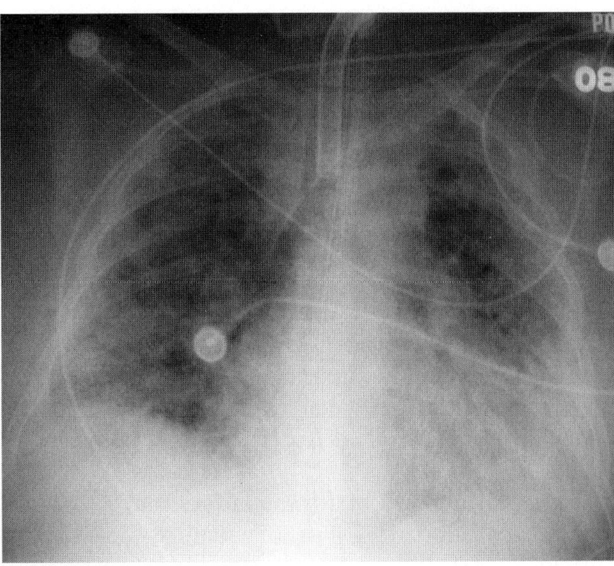

FIGURE 14.5. **Increased Permeability (Lung Injury) Edema in ARDS.** Portable chest radiograph in a 46-year-old woman with severe pancreatitis and respiratory failure reveals bilateral airspace opacification with a somewhat peripheral distribution, representing diffuse alveolar damage and permeability edema.

patients regardless of the underlying etiology. Within 12 to 24 hours following the initial insult (stage 1 ARDS), damage to capillary endothelium produces engorged capillaries and proteinaceous interstitial edema. Within the first week (stage 2), the injury to type 1 pneumocytes leads to the flooding of alveoli with edema fluid and proteinaceous and cellular debris, which form hyaline membranes lining the distal airways and alveoli. In stage 3 ARDS, type 2 pneumocytes proliferate in an attempt to reline the denuded alveolar surfaces, and fibroblastic tissue proliferates within the airspaces. This fibroblastic tissue may resolve and leave minimal scarring or—particularly in those with severe disease and long-standing oxygen requirements—result in extensive interstitial fibrosis.

Radiographically, ARDS follows a predictable pattern. Chest radiographs become abnormal by 12 to 24 hours following the onset of dyspnea and demonstrate patchy peripheral airspace opacities (Fig. 14.5) (2). These opacities coalesce over the next several days to produce confluent bilateral airspace opacities with air bronchograms. Radiographic improvement in the opacities may be seen within the first week, but this is often caused by the effects of increasing positive pressure ventilation rather than true histologic improvement. After 1 week, the airspace opacities gradually give way to a coarse reticulonodular pattern that may resolve over the course of several months or remain unchanged, in which case the pattern represents irreversible pulmonary fibrosis (i.e., honeycombing). Pneumonia complicating ARDS is difficult to diagnose radiographically, but it should be suspected when a focal area of airspace opacification or a significant pleural effusion develops during the course of the disease. Likewise, the superimposition of LV failure may be impossible to recognize but is suggested by rapid clinical and radiographic deterioration associated with changes in measured PCWP and edema fluid protein content. Pneumomediastinum and pneumothorax may result as a complication of positive pressure ventilation to stiff lungs and should be sought on portable chest radiographs.

Radiographic Distinction of Hydrostatic From Increased Capillary Permeability Edema. Beyond identifying the presence of pulmonary edema, the ability to distinguish between types of pulmonary edema has significant diagnostic and therapeutic import. Measurements of PCWP and transbronchial sampling of pulmonary edema fluid are techniques that accurately distinguish hydrostatic from increased capillary permeability edema. In hydrostatic edema, PCWP measurements are elevated and a protein-poor transudative edema fluid is present, while in increased-permeability edema, there is a normal PCWP and proteinaceous edema fluid is seen. Milne and colleagues have described the findings on the chest radiograph that can be used to distinguish cardiac and overhydration edema from increased capillary permeability edema (3). In pulmonary edema associated with chronic cardiac failure, the heart is usually enlarged and displays an inverted (redistributed) pulmonary blood flow pattern. The distribution of edema is even from central to peripheral over the lower lung zones. The vascular pedicle, which represents the mediastinal width at the level of the superior vena cava and left subclavian artery, is widened

(>53 mm on posteroanterior [PA] radiograph), reflecting increased circulating blood volume. Lung volumes are diminished because of decreased pulmonary compliance from edema. Peribronchial cuffing, Kerley lines, and pleural effusions represent interstitial and intrapleural transudation of fluid, respectively.

Overhydration or renal failure edema has some features in common with chronic cardiac failure and may be indistinguishable radiographically. Capillary permeability edema can sometimes be distinguished from hydrostatic edema. A more peripheral distribution of edema with a normal heart size and normal vascular pedicle width, the latter indicating normal circulating blood volume, are findings typical of increased capillary permeability edema.

It should be noted that some factors may render radiographic distinction of types of pulmonary edema difficult. Radiographs of supine patients will make evaluation of pulmonary blood flow distribution and vascular pedicle width difficult. The presence of severe alveolar edema will obscure underlying vascular markings. Many patients with capillary permeability edema will be overhydrated in attempts to maintain circulating blood volume, producing complex radiographic findings.

Neurogenic pulmonary edema following head trauma, seizure, or increased intracranial pressure is a complex phenomenon that appears to involve both hydrostatic and increased permeability mechanisms. Massive sympathetic discharge from the brain in these conditions produces systemic vasoconstriction and increased venous return, with resultant increase in LV diastolic pressure and hydrostatic pulmonary edema. However, the finding of protein-rich edema fluid and normal PCWP in some patients suggests that increased permeability may be a contributing factor.

High-altitude pulmonary edema develops in certain individuals after rapid ascent to altitudes above 3,500 m. Edema typically develops within 48 to 72 hours of ascent and appears to reflect a varied individual response to hypoxemia, in which scattered areas of pulmonary arterial spasm result in transient PAH. This produces an overflow of blood at high pressure to uninvolved areas, resulting in damage to the capillary endothelium and increased permeability edema that is patchy in distribution. Rapid resolution usually occurs within 24 to 48 hours after the administration of supplemental oxygen or a return to sea level.

Re-expansion Pulmonary Edema. Rapid re-expansion of a lung after collapse lasting greater than 48 hours may result in the development of unilateral pulmonary edema. Marked increases in negative pleural pressure following pleural tube placement, impaired pulmonary lymphatic drainage following prolonged lung collapse, and ischemia-induced surfactant deficiency resulting in the need for high negative pleural pressure to re-expand the collapsed lung are proposed mechanisms. Recent evidence points toward prolonged collapse producing ischemia and hypoxemia within the lung, which promotes anaerobic metabolism and formation of free radicals. Reperfusion of the lung upon re-expansion then leads to lung injury and permeability edema. Gradual re-expansion of the lung by slow removal of pleural air or fluid over a 24- to 48-hour period and administration of supplemental oxygen helps limit the incidence and severity of this complication.

Acute Upper Airway Obstruction. Pulmonary edema may be seen during or immediately after treatment of acute upper airway obstruction. The proposed mechanism involves the creation of markedly negative intrathoracic pressure by attempts to inspire against an extrathoracic airway obstruction, producing transudation of fluid into the lung. There are no distinguishing radiographic features.

Amniotic Fluid Embolism. A severe and often fatal form of pulmonary edema may develop in a pregnant woman when amniotic fluid gains access to the systemic circulation during labor. There is an association of this entity with fetal distress and demise, because the mucin within fetal meconium plays a key role in the pathogenesis of this disorder. Embolic obstruction of the pulmonary vasculature by mucin and fetal squames within the amniotic fluid leads to sudden PAH and cor pulmonale with decreased cardiac output and pulmonary edema. An anaphylactoid reaction and disseminated intravascular coagulopathy (DIC) from factors within the amniotic fluid contribute to the shock state. Radiographically, there are bilateral confluent airspace opacities indistinguishable from pulmonary edema of other etiologies. In severe cases, there is secondary enlargement of the central pulmonary arteries and right heart as a manifestation of cor pulmonale. The diagnosis can be confirmed by identification of fetal squames and mucin in blood samples obtained from indwelling pulmonary artery catheters.

Fat Embolism. The embolization of marrow fat to the lung is a common complication occurring 24 to 72 hours after the fracture of a long bone (e.g., femur). Within the lung, the fat is hydrolyzed to its component fatty acids, causing increased pulmonary capillary permeability and hemorrhagic pulmonary edema. Radiographically and on CT, confluent ground-glass and airspace opacities are seen (Fig. 14.6). The diagnosis is made by recognizing findings of systemic fat embolism (petechial rash, CNS depression) and pulmonary changes in the appropriate time period following trauma. Most patients have a mild course with minimal respiratory compromise, while a minority will develop progressive respiratory failure leading to death.

Pulmonary Hemorrhage

Hemorrhage or hemorrhagic edema of the lung can result from trauma; bleeding diathesis; infections (invasive aspergillosis, mucormycosis, *Pseudomonas*, influenza); drugs (penicillamine); pulmonary embolism; fat

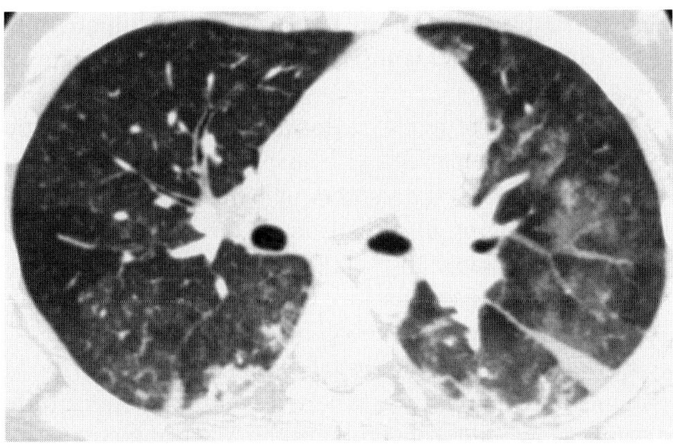

FIGURE 14.6. **Fat Embolism Producing Permeability Edema.** CT in an 18-year-old man with dyspnea and hypoxemia 48 hours after intramedullary rod placement for a femoral fracture shows asymmetric ground-glass and airspace opacities with small left pleural effusion.

embolism; ARDS; and autoimmune diseases (Table 14.3) (4). The autoimmune diseases that can cause pulmonary hemorrhage include Goodpasture syndrome, idiopathic pulmonary hemorrhage, Wegener granulomatosis, systemic lupus erythematosus, rheumatoid arthritis, and polyarteritis nodosa.

Goodpasture syndrome is an autoimmune disease characterized by damage to the alveolar and renal glomerular basement membranes by a cytotoxic antibody. The antibody is directed primarily against renal glomerular basement membrane and cross-reacts with alveolar basement membrane to produce the renal injury and pulmonary hemorrhage characteristic of this disorder. Young adult men are most commonly affected and present with cough, hemoptysis, dyspnea, and fatigue. The pulmonary complaints usually precede clinical evidence of renal failure. Chest films show bilateral coalescent airspace opacities that are radiographically indistinguishable from those of pulmonary edema (Fig. 14.7). Within several days, the airspace opacities resolve, giving rise to reticular opacities in the same distribution. Complete radiographic resolution is seen within 2 weeks, except in those with recurrent episodes of hemorrhage, in whom the reticular opacities persist and represent pulmonary fibrosis. The diagnosis is made by immunofluorescent studies of renal or lung tissue, which show a smooth wavy line of fluorescent staining along the basement membrane. The overall prognosis is poor, although the use of immunosuppressive drugs and plasmapheresis has improved survival.

TABLE 14.3 Causes of Pulmonary Hemorrhage

Spontaneous	Thrombocytopenia
	Hemophilia
	Anticoagulant therapy
Trauma	Pulmonary contusion
Embolic disease	Pulmonary embolism
	Fat embolism
Vasculitis	Autoimmune
	Goodpasture syndrome
	Idiopathic pulmonary hemorrhage
	Wegener granulomatosis
	Infectious
	Gram-negative bacteria
	Influenza
	Aspergillosis
	Mucormycosis
Drugs	Penicillamine

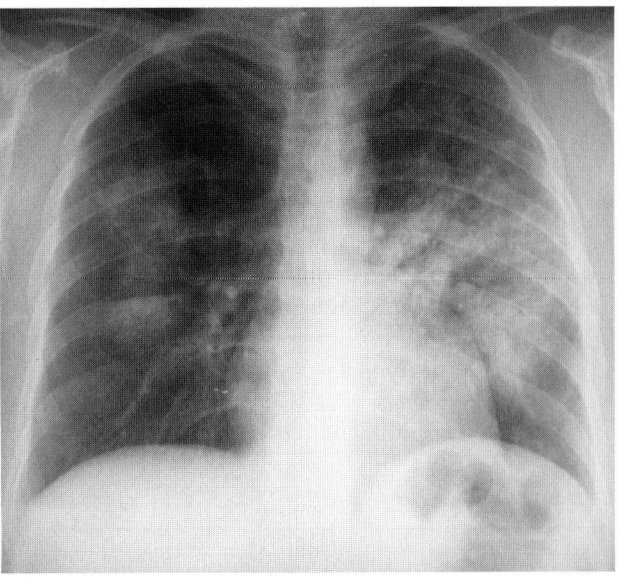

FIGURE 14.7. **Pulmonary Hemorrhage in Goodpasture Syndrome.** Posteroanterior chest film in a patient with Goodpasture syndrome shows asymmetric bilateral airspace disease presenting intra-alveolar blood.

Idiopathic Pulmonary Hemorrhage. The pulmonary manifestations of idiopathic pulmonary hemorrhage are clinically and radiographically indistinguishable from those of Goodpasture syndrome. In distinction to Goodpasture syndrome, this disorder is most common in children, with an equal sex distribution. The diagnosis is one of exclusion and is suggested when pulmonary hemorrhage and anemia are found in a patient with normal renal function and urinalysis and an absence of antiglomerular basement membrane antibodies.

Other Vasculitides. Wegener granulomatosis, systemic lupus erythematosus, rheumatoid arthritis, and polyarteritis nodosa are autoimmune disorders associated with a systemic immune complex vasculitis (5). The development of pulmonary hemorrhage in these diseases is secondary to small vessel pulmonary arteritis and capillaritis, which result in spontaneous hemorrhage. The pulmonary manifestations of these diseases are discussed in subsequent sections.

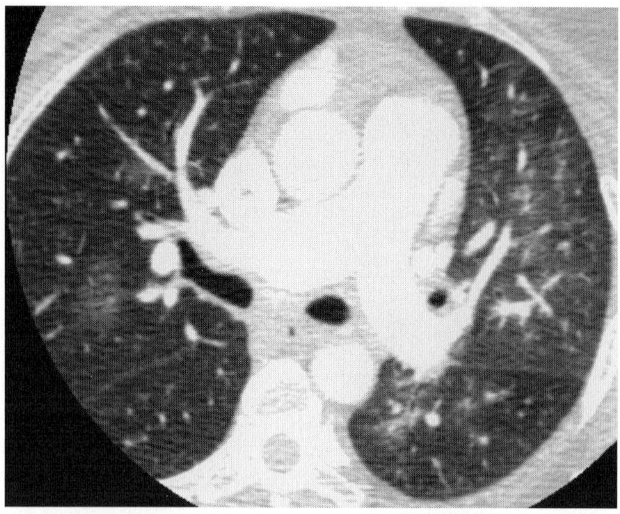

FIGURE 14.8. **CT of Pulmonary Hemorrhage.** Thin-section CT in a 46-year-old woman with hemoptysis 1 day after initiation of prophylactic anticoagulation for radiofrequency ablation of atrial fibrillation shows asymmetric bilateral perihilar ground-glass opacities, reflecting alveolar hemorrhage.

Differentiation of pulmonary hemorrhage from pulmonary edema or pneumonia may be difficult, particularly because many causes of pulmonary edema and pneumonia may have a significant hemorrhagic component. The rapid development of airspace opacities associated with a dropping hematocrit and hemoptysis should suggest the diagnosis (Fig. 14.8). Hemoptysis, however, is not always present. Associated renal disease, hematuria, or findings of a collagen vascular disorder or systemic vasculitis may provide additional clues. The distinction of pulmonary hemorrhage from pneumonia is made by the absence of fever or purulent sputum and the finding of a normal or elevated carbon monoxide–diffusing capacity. This latter determination is directly related to the volume of gas-exchanging intravascular and extravascular intrapulmonary red blood cells and is therefore elevated in pulmonary hemorrhage or hemorrhagic edema but decreased in pneumonia. The presence of hemosiderin-laden macrophages in sputum, bronchoalveolar lavage fluid, or tissue specimens is evidence of chronic or recurrent intrapulmonary hemorrhage. A rapid radiographic improvement of the airspace opacities in pulmonary hemorrhage is common and may aid in diagnosis.

Pulmonary Embolism

Pulmonary embolism (PE) is a common cause of acute chest symptoms. While it is associated with significant morbidity and mortality, treatment with anticoagulation can significantly reduce the likelihood of recurrent emboli that might result in chronic thromboembolic pulmonary hypertension or death. Since anticoagulation has associated morbidity, particularly in elderly and debilitated patients, an accurate diagnosis of the presence or absence of PE is necessary.

The radiologist plays a central role in the diagnostic evaluation of the patient with suspected PE. This section will briefly review the aspects of patient evaluation not related to imaging and then detail the various imaging modalities available to the radiologist. A practical algorithm that serves as a useful guide to the workup of each patient with suspected PE will be provided.

Clinical and Laboratory Findings. The majority of patients with PE have a variety of symptoms, including dyspnea (84%), pleuritic chest pain (74%), anxiety (59%), and cough (53%). However, in certain groups of patients at high risk for PE, asymptomatic embolization is known to occur. Physical examination may reveal tachypnea (respiratory rate >16/min), rales, and a prominent pulmonary component of the second heart sound. Unfortunately, these findings are entirely nonspecific. Only a minority of patients presenting to an emergency department with pleuritic chest pain will be found to have PE.

The main laboratory test obtained in patients with suspected pulmonary embolism is a plasma D-dimer level. D-dimer is a degradation product of fibrin and is a very sensitive indicator of the presence of venous thrombosis. Enzyme-linked immunosorbent assay D-dimer measurements have a sensitivity for deep venous thrombosis (DVT) of 98% to 100%, and therefore a normal value will effectively exclude the possibility of DVT and PE, particularly when the clinical probability for PE is low.

Radiologic Evaluation. A number of imaging techniques are routinely employed in the evaluation of the patient with suspected PE. These include the chest radiograph, ventilation/perfusion (V/Q) lung scintigraphy, helical CT angiography, and conventional pulmonary angiography. Noninvasive methods of imaging DVTs include compression and Doppler ultrasound of the legs, lower-extremity indirect CT venography, and magnetic resonance venography of the extremities and pelvis. The relatively noninvasive nature and high accuracy of these techniques to diagnose DVT and an increasing familiarity with their performance and interpretation among radiologists has led to their widespread use in the workup of PE. A practical algorithm for the radiologic evaluation of PE is shown in Fig. 14.9.

Chest radiography is the first examination obtained in all patients with suspected PE. Although the majority of patients with PE will have abnormal radiographs, a significant percentage of patients will have normal chest radiographs. The radiographic findings include cardiac, pulmonary arterial, parenchymal, pleural, and diaphragmatic changes (6).

Cardiac, or more precisely right heart enlargement, is an uncommon finding seen with massive or extensive PE producing cor pulmonale. Enlargement of the central

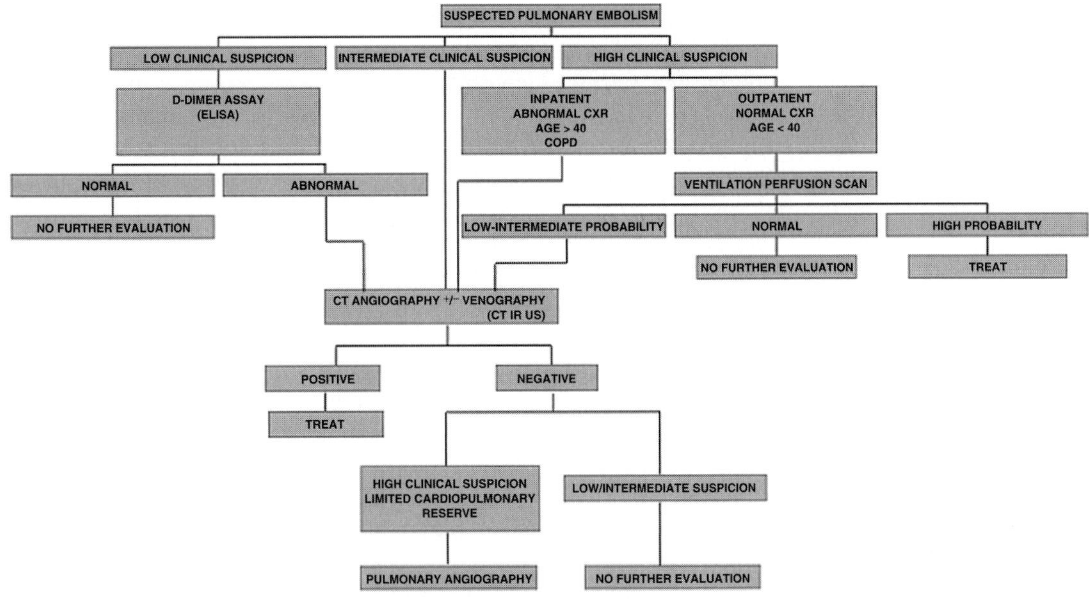

FIGURE 14.9. **Algorithm for the Radiologic Evaluation of Pulmonary Thromboembolism.** PE, pulmonary embolism.

pulmonary arteries from PAH may also be seen but is more commonly a late sequela of chronic thromboembolic disease. The most common radiographic findings in PE without infarction are localized peripheral oligemia with or without distended proximal vessels (Westermark sign) and peripheral airspace opacification or linear atelectasis. The airspace opacification represents localized pulmonary hemorrhage produced by bronchial and pulmonary venous collateral flow to the obstructed region and is seen with peripheral but not central emboli. Volume loss in the lower lung from adhesive atelectasis caused by ischemic injury to type 2 pneumocytes and secondary surfactant deficiency may produce diaphragmatic elevation and the development of linear atelectasis.

Less than 10% of all PEs result in lung infarction. Collateral bronchial arterial and retrograde pulmonary venous flow prevent infarction in most patients. The distinction between embolism without and with infarction is usually impossible radiographically and is of limited importance, as treatment is identical. Infarction from embolism occurs with greater frequency in patients with underlying heart failure because of their limited collateral bronchial arterial flow to the ischemic region. In PEs with infarction, the cardiac, pulmonary arterial, and peripheral vascular changes are indistinguishable from those seen in embolism without infarction. Radiographic features that suggest infarction include the presence of a small pleural effusion and the development of a pleura-based wedge-shaped opacity (Hampton hump). This opacity, typically found in the posterior or lateral costophrenic sulcus of the lung, is wedge-shaped, homogeneous, and lacks air bronchograms. The blunted apex of the wedge points toward the occluded feeding vessel, while the base is against the pleural surface. This wedge-shaped opacity is often obscured by surrounding areas of hemorrhage in the early phases following infarction and becomes more obvious with time as the peripheral areas of hemorrhage resolve. A distinction between PE with and without infarction is usually made by noting changes in the radiographic opacities with time. In embolism without infarction, the airspace opacities should resolve completely within 7 to 10 days, while infarcts resolve over the course of several weeks or months and usually leave a residual linear parenchymal scar and/or localized pleural thickening.

None of the aforementioned radiographic findings, either alone or in combination, are useful in making a firm diagnosis of PE. Conversely, a completely normal radiograph may be seen in up to 40% of patients with emboli. The prime utility of the chest radiograph in the evaluation of PE is in the detection of conditions that mimic PE clinically, such as pneumonia or pneumothorax, and as an aid to the interpretation of the ventilation/perfusion lung scan.

Ventilation/Perfusion (V/Q) Lung Scintigraphy. The intravenous administration of macroaggregates of albumin radiolabeled with technetium (Tc-99m) has given the radiologist a noninvasive method of assessing the patency of the pulmonary circulation. The sensitivity of this technique allows for the confident exclusion of PE when a technically adequate perfusion scan is normal. The addition of ventilation scanning increases the specificity of an abnormal perfusion scan and is always performed in conjunction with the perfusion scan when possible.

Perfusion lung scanning is performed by intravenous injection of 5 mCi of Tc-99m macroaggregated albumin with the patient supine (see Chapter 56). Images are then obtained in eight projections: anteroposterior, PA, right and left lateral, and right and left anterior and posterior oblique views. If perfusion abnormalities are present, a ventilation scan utilizing krypton-81m, xenon-133, or aerosolized Tc-99m diethylenetriamine pentaacetic acid (DTPA) is then performed. The use of krypton-81m and Tc-99m DTPA allows for comparable oblique projections identical to the perfusion scan. Perfusion defects can then be characterized as ventilation/perfusion matches (absent ventilation/absent perfusion) or mismatches (normal ventilation/absent perfusion). Ventilation/perfusion mismatch is the hallmark of PE.

Although V/Q scanning is commonly used in the evaluation of the patient with suspected PE, there are limitations to its utility for the diagnosis of PE. First, only a minority of patients (27% in the Prospective Investigation of Pulmonary Embolism Diagnosis [PIOPED] study) undergoing V/Q studies will have either a normal or high-probability study, a result that clinicians can confidently rely upon to guide treatment decisions (5). Second, there is significant interobserver variability in the interpretation of V/Q studies. Finally, there are few well-constructed prospective studies evaluating the accuracy of various patterns of V/Q abnormality in predicting the likelihood of PE.

Several diagnostic schemes have been proposed to assign a probability of PE (as determined by pulmonary angiography) given specific combinations of ventilation, perfusion, and concurrent chest radiographic findings. The V/Q scan interpretation categories published with the results of the PIOPED study have become the standard for radiologists interpreting V/Q studies. A normal V/Q scan effectively excludes PE because of the high sensitivity of the test. A high-probability scan, particularly in a patient with a strong clinical suspicion for embolic disease, can be confidently treated for PE. Patients with intermediate or indeterminate (because of extensive obstructive lung disease) probability scans have a 30% to 40% incidence of PE. Likewise, those with a low-probability V/Q scan and a high clinical suspicion for PE should have further noninvasive imaging of the deep venous system or pulmonary arteries. See Chapter 56 for an expanded discussion of pulmonary scintigraphy.

Despite its limitations, V/Q scanning can provide useful information and remains a useful noninvasive screening modality for detecting PE. Although uncommon, a normal perfusion study excludes embolism, whereas a high-probability V/Q study, in the appropriate clinical setting, allows for a confident enough diagnosis of PE to initiate anticoagulant therapy. Currently, its role in the evaluation of PE is primarily limited to those patients with a high likelihood of having a diagnostic result (i.e., normal or high probability); such patients are generally young individuals with normal chest radiographs and no history of chronic obstructive pulmonary disease.

Helical CT Pulmonary Angiography. Dynamic CT angiography of the pulmonary arteries (CTPA) using multidetector CT (MDCT) has proven accurate in the detection of PE (7). Contiguous or overlapping 1- to 2-mm scans through the entire thorax during injection of 80 to 120 mL of 300 to 350 mg I(iodine)/mL nonionic contrast injected through an 18-gauge or larger intravenous catheter allows routine dense opacification of second- and third-order subsegmental pulmonary arteries. Scans must be interpreted on workstations in a paging or cine mode to allow efficient review and accurate interpretation of the large data sets produced by the current 16- to 64-channel MDCT scanners.

Emboli are recognized as intraluminal filling defects (Fig. 14.10) or nonopacified vessels with a convex filling toward the proximal lumen. Secondary findings that can be seen on CT include peripheral oligemia (Westermark sign), pleura-based wedge-shaped consolidation reflecting peripheral hemorrhage or infarct (Fig. 14.11), linear atelectasis, and pleural effusion. The detection of a high-attenuation thrombus in the pulmonary arteries on unenhanced CT in patients with PE has been rarely described. Common diagnostic pitfalls in the detection of PE on CTPA include motion artifact, streak artifact from dense contrast or catheters, partial volume averaging of obliquely oriented vessels, prominent hilar lymphoid tissue, poorly opacified pulmonary veins, mucus-filled bronchi, and regional areas of increased pulmonary arterial resistance from consolidation or atelectasis, all of which can simulate intraluminal arterial filling defects.

At present MDCT is widely considered the first-line diagnostic modality for the evaluation of suspected PE.

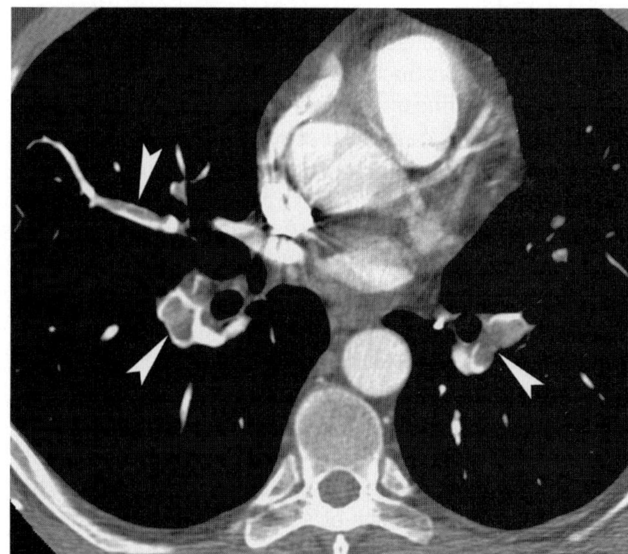

FIGURE 14.10. **Pulmonary Embolism on CT Angiography.** CT pulmonary angiogram in a 47-year-old man demonstrates filling defects (*arrowheads*) within the middle lobe and both lower lobe pulmonary arteries, representing pulmonary emboli.

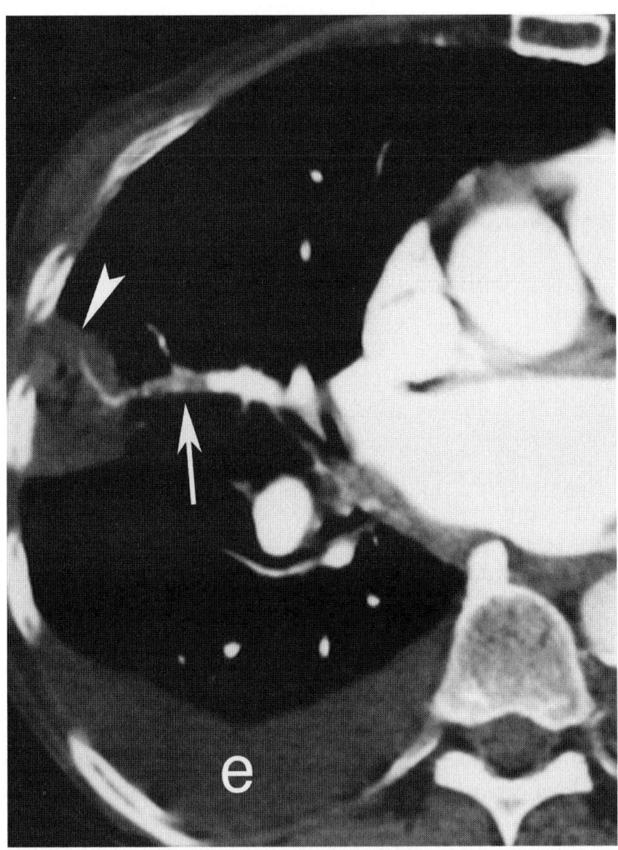

FIGURE 14.11. **Pulmonary Infarct (Hampton Hump).** Enhanced CT scan in a patient with pulmonary infarction shows a smooth, eccentrically cavitated, pleura-based mass (*arrowhead*) representing an infarct, with the thrombus visible as a filling defect (*arrow*) in the lateral segment middle lobe pulmonary artery. An associated right pleural effusion (e) is a common finding in pulmonary infarction.

Confident detection of a discrete intraluminal filling defect is highly specific for PE. Conversely, multiple studies have shown that the negative predictive value of a good-quality CTPA for PE is greater than 95%. For these reasons, only those patients at high risk for significant morbidity or mortality from recurrent PE (i.e., patients with severe chronic obstructive pulmonary disease or cor pulmonale) should be considered for conventional angiography following a negative or inconclusive CT study; the latter occurs in approximately 5% of patients referred for CTPA, a percentage similar to that of nondiagnostic pulmonary arteriograms.

Although the ability to detect small emboli has improved significantly with MDCT (Fig. 14.12), the main limitation of CTPA remains the reliable detection of small (subsegmental) emboli, although the frequency and clinical significance of such emboli is the subject of significant debate. In addition to the detection of emboli, up to two thirds of patients with acute chest symptoms who are studied with CTPA to exclude PE have an alternative diagnosis suggested by findings detected on CT, something not possible with techniques that only evaluate the pulmonary vasculature such as perfusion scintigraphy, MR angiography, and conventional angiography.

Pulmonary angiography has traditionally been considered to be the gold standard in the diagnosis of PE (8). Digital subtraction angiography is the technique selectively utilized when a definitive diagnosis of PE or DVT cannot be achieved by less invasive means. This study, which requires right heart and pulmonary arterial catheterization with selective injection of nonionic contrast, can be performed safely in a majority of patients. The accuracy of pulmonary arteriography in the diagnosis of PE is high. Based upon clinical follow-up of patients with negative studies, the sensitivity of pulmonary angiography is 98% to 99%, although as with CTPA, the accuracy for the detection of subsegmental PE is closer to 66%.

PE is diagnosed on pulmonary angiography when an intraluminal filling defect or the trailing end of an occluding thrombus is outlined by contrast (Fig. 14.13). Secondary signs, including a prolonged arterial phase, diminished peripheral perfusion, and delay in the venous phase, are nonspecific and are not used to diagnose PE. Once a thrombus is unequivocally identified, the study is terminated. The only exception would be a patient who is considered a candidate for surgical thrombectomy or thrombolytic therapy, where precise knowledge of the laterality, location, and extent of the thrombus is required.

The overall complication rate of pulmonary angiography is 2% to 5% and can be divided into those related to contrast administration and those secondary to cardiac catheterization and injection of intrapulmonary arterial contrast. Mortality from pulmonary angiography is less than 0.5% and is usually related to sudden RV failure from transient elevation of pulmonary artery pressure secondary to contrast injection. Death from pulmonary angiography is seen almost exclusively in critically ill patients and those with preexisting severe PAH (pulmonary artery systolic pressure >70 mm Hg) or RV dysfunction (RV end diastolic pressure >20 mm Hg). However, there is no significant increase in the incidence of major, nonfatal reactions in patients with PAH. In addition, the majority of patients with severe RV dysfunction have uneventful studies. When one considers the added safety of selective contrast injections using nonionic contrast agents and the high mortality of untreated PE in this population, pulmonary angiography should be performed in these patients when indicated.

Noninvasive Imaging for Deep Venous Thrombosis. The use of noninvasive techniques for the diagnosis of DVT has altered the conventional approach to the evaluation of pulmonary thromboembolic disease (see Chapter 40). Because 90% of PEs arise from the lower extremities, and because the treatment for proximal (i.e., above-the-knee)

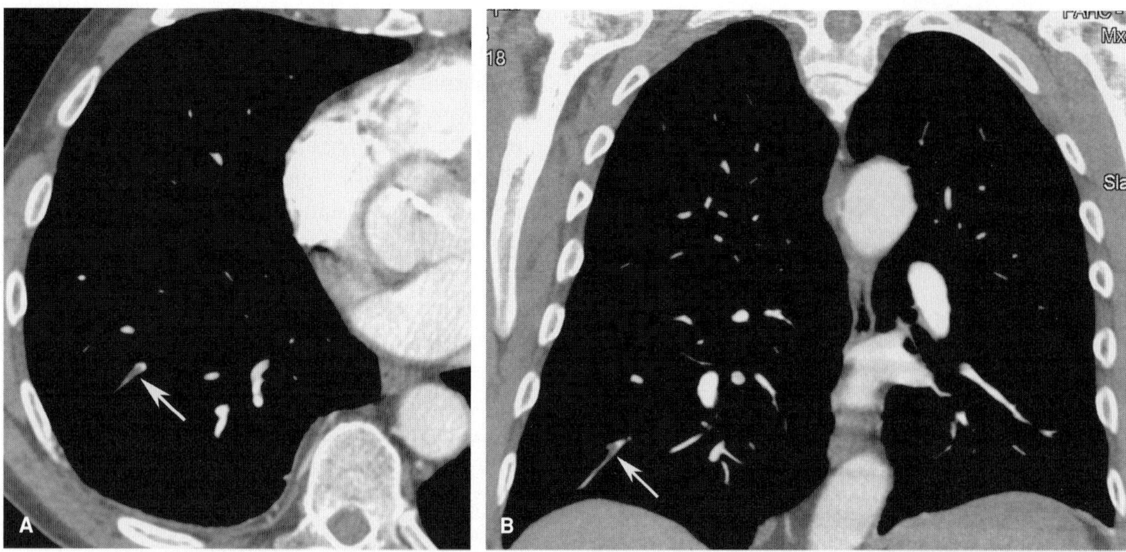

FIGURE 14.12. **Subsegmental Pulmonary Embolism on Isotropic Multidetector CT (MDCT).** Axial **(A)** and coronal reconstructed CT **(B)** on CT angiography from a 40-slice MDCT scanner show an isolated subsegmental embolus to a branch of the right lower lobe lateral basal segmental artery (*arrows*).

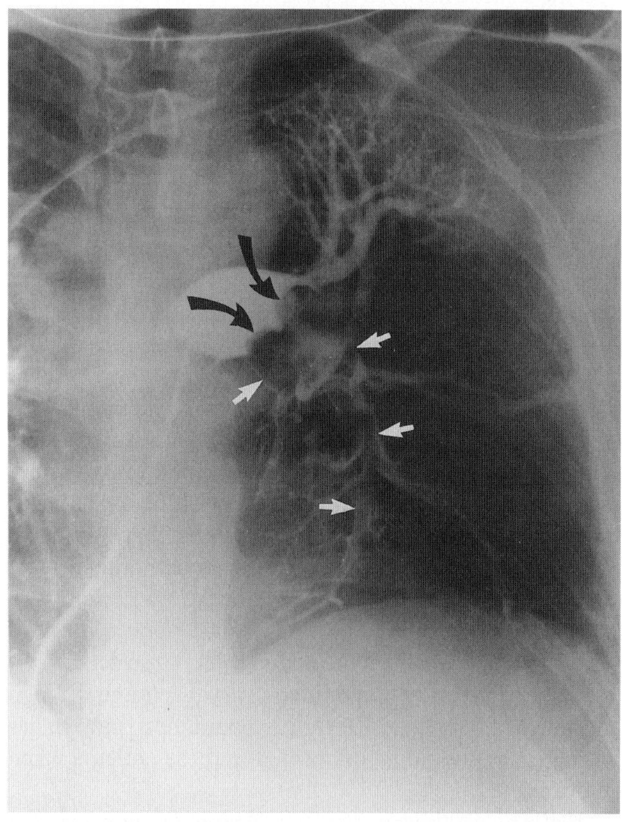

FIGURE 14.13. **Pulmonary Embolism on Pulmonary Arteriogram.** A frontal radiograph from a left pulmonary arteriogram reveals a large intraluminal filling defect within the main and left interlobar pulmonary artery, diagnostic of pulmonary embolism. Note the typical meniscus of contrast outlining the trailing edge of the thrombus (*curved black arrows*) and a rim of contrast around the body of the thrombus (*small white arrows*).

DVT is identical to that for proven PE, a confident diagnosis of proximal DVT can provide an endpoint in patient evaluation for thromboembolic disease.

When performed by skilled personnel, compression US has a sensitivity of 90% to 95% and a specificity of 95% to 98% for the diagnosis of acute DVT when compared to contrast venography. False-negative studies occur when DVT is limited to the calf or pelvis, or in patients with duplicated deep venous systems. False-positive studies are seen most often in patients with prior DVT. In addition to providing an accurate diagnosis of the presence of DVT, US offers the advantage of imaging the nonvenous structures in the leg, allowing the radiologist to diagnose conditions that may simulate DVT clinically, such as Baker cysts, enlarged lymph nodes, pseudoaneurysms, and pelvic masses compressing the iliac vein.

Although accurate for the diagnosis of proximal DVT, a negative compression US study does not exclude PE. Thus, patients with a negative US study should undergo evaluation of the pulmonary arteries with CT or conventional angiography.

Indirect CT venography (CTV), typically performed after contrast injection has been administered for CTPA, has been utilized to allow detection of thigh and pelvic DVT. Axial or helical scans performed from the popliteal fossa to the diaphragm obtained approximately 3 minutes after the initiation of contrast injection for CTPA have been shown in preliminary studies to have a high accuracy in the detection of proximal lower-extremity and pelvic DVT. The addition of CTV to CTPA can provide incremental information for the diagnosis of venous thromboembolic disease, particularly when a proximal DVT is detected in a patient with a poor quality, equivocal, or negative CTPA study.

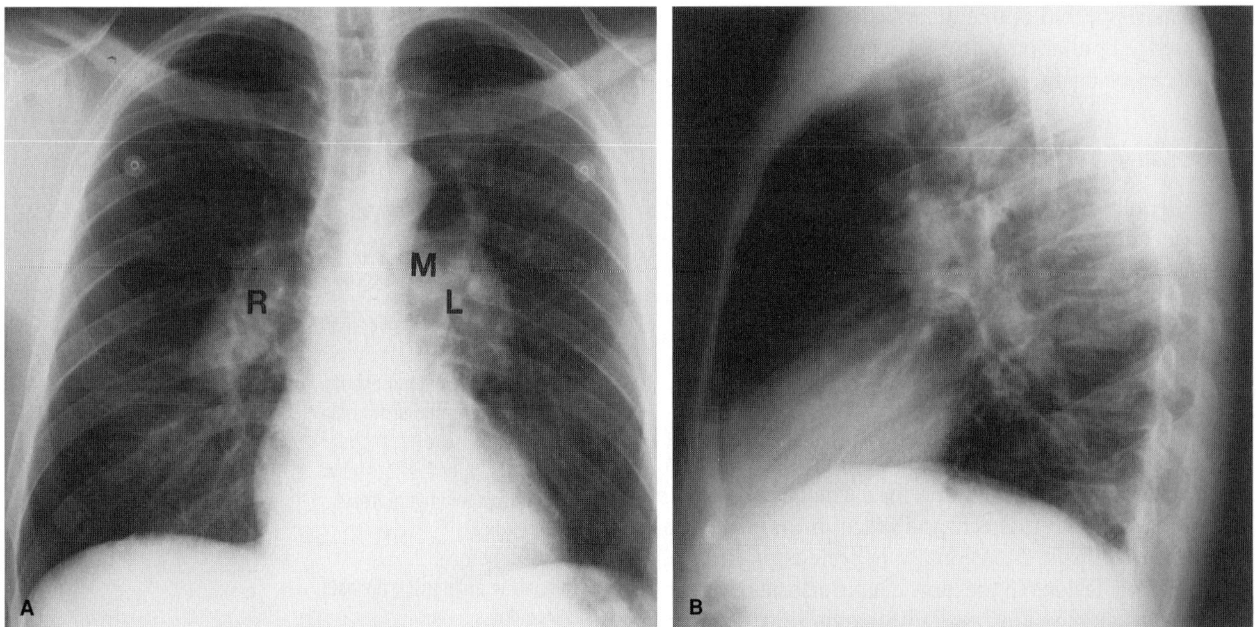

FIGURE 14.14. **Pulmonary Arterial Hypertension.** Posteroanterior **(A)** and lateral **(B)** chest radiographs in a 32-year-old woman with pulmonary hypertension from chronic pulmonary thromboembolic disease show enlarged main (M), right (R), and left (L) pulmonary arteries with diminutive peripheral vessels.

MR venography and radionuclide scintigraphy can be used to detect DVT but are not used routinely in clinical practice for this purpose.

Nonthrombotic pulmonary embolism can occur rarely. The most commonly described conditions are (*1*) air embolism, usually as a result of air within a venous catheter or air injected during contrast-enhanced CT; (*2*) macroscopic fat embolism following long bone fracture, with pulmonary embolization of marrow elements; (*3*) methylmethacrylate embolization complicating vertebroplasty; and (*4*) radioactive seed implant embolization from prostate brachytherapy.

Pulmonary tumor emboli can develop in a small percentage of patients with malignancies such as bronchoalveolar cell carcinoma, breast cancer, hepatoma, and GI malignancies. These tumor emboli may lead to significant respiratory symptoms because of occlusion of small vessels. Imaging features are uncommon but include central pulmonary arterial dilation and enlarged, nodular peripheral pulmonary artery branches on thin-section CT.

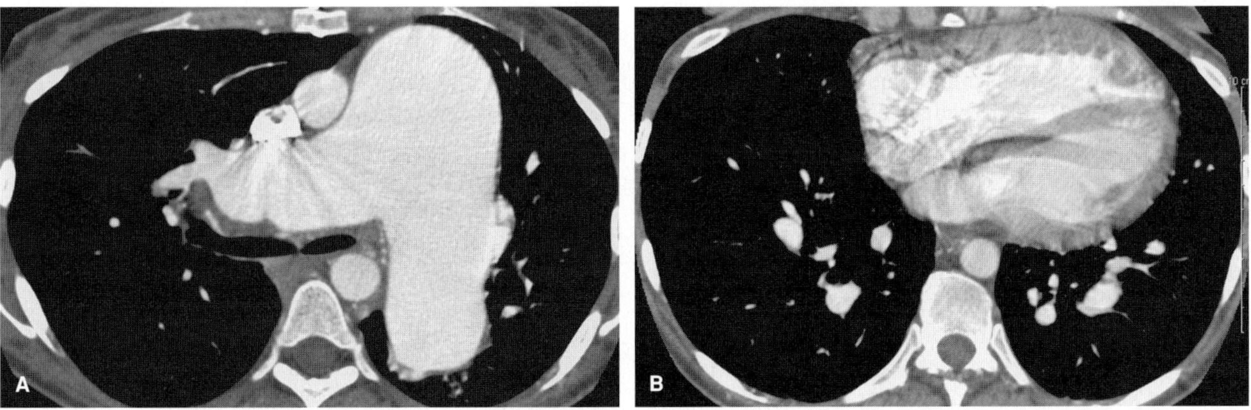

FIGURE 14.15. **Eisenmenger Syndrome.** Pulmonary arterial hypertension from left-to-right shunt resulting from atrial septal defect. Enhanced CT scan in a 49-year-old woman with prior repair of an atrial septal defect **(A)** shows massive dilatation of the main, right, and left pulmonary arteries, reflecting pulmonary arterial hypertension. Scan at the level of the heart **(B)** shows right ventricular hypertrophy and dilatation as a result of pulmonary hypertension.

In patients suspected of this disorder, aspiration cytology from a wedged pulmonary arterial occlusion (Swan-Ganz) catheter can be useful for diagnosis.

Pulmonary Arterial Hypertension

PAH is defined as a systolic pressure in the pulmonary artery exceeding 30 mm Hg, measured either directly, by catheterization of the pulmonary artery, or estimated by echocardiography. The diagnosis of PAH is usually evident from the clinical history, physical findings, and appearance on chest radiographs. The typical radiographic findings of PAH are enlarged main and hilar pulmonary arteries that taper rapidly toward the lung periphery (Fig. 14.14). Associated enlargement of the RV, seen on lateral radiographs as prominence of the anterosuperior cardiac margin with obliteration of the retrosternal airspace, is an additional clue to the diagnosis. Occasionally, hypertension-induced atherosclerotic lesions in the large elastic arteries can produce mural calcifications on radiographs or CT, a rare finding that is specific for PAH. A useful measurement for enlargement of the central pulmonary arteries, usually indicating PAH in the absence of a left-to-right shunt, is a transverse diameter of the proximal interlobar pulmonary artery on PA chest radiograph that exceeds 16 mm. Another specific indicator of PAH is a transverse measurement of the main pulmonary artery on CT or MR that exceeds 28.6 mm. However, a normal measurement of the main or right interlobar pulmonary artery does not exclude PAH, as patients with mild or even moderate elevation of pulmonary artery pressure may have normal-size arteries. Those patients with long-standing PAH will develop RV hypertrophy, with eventual RV dilatation and failure ("cor pulmonale"). In addition, MR may also demonstrate intraluminal signal during the early diastolic phase of the cardiac cycle, a finding indicative of turbulent flow caused by the increased vascular resistance that is sometimes seen with marked elevation of pulmonary artery pressure.

In addition to PAH, enlargement of the central pulmonary arteries may be seen in conditions associated with increased flow through the pulmonary circulation. This occurs in patients with a high cardiac output, such as anemia, thyrotoxicosis, or those with left-to-right shunts. The latter includes atrial and ventricular septal defects, patent ductus arteriosus, and partial anomalous pulmonary venous return. Early in the course of left-to-right shunts, the pulmonary artery pressure is normal or slightly elevated, because pulmonary vascular resistance drops to compensate for the increased flow. In these patients, there is enlargement of both central and peripheral pulmonary arteries, producing "shunt vascularity" on chest radiographs. Later, usually in young adulthood, the muscular pulmonary arterioles develop medial hyperplasia and intimal fibrosis, with resultant increased pulmonary vascular resistance (Fig. 14.15). When this occurs, the chest radiograph demonstrates findings typical of PAH that are indistinguishable from PAH caused by other etiologies.

TABLE 14.4 Causes of Pulmonary Arterial Hypertension

Pulmonary venous hypertension
Left heart disease
LV failure
Mitral valve disease
Obstruction of pulmonary venous return
Fibrosing mediastinitis
Cor triatriatum
LA myxoma
Pulmonary venoocclusive disease (pulmonary capillary hemangiomatosis)
Lung disease/chronic hypoxemia
Emphysema/chronic bronchitis
Cystic lung disease
Langerhans cell histiocytosis
Lymphangioleiomyomatosis
Cystic fibrosis
Interstitial fibrosis
Idiopathic pulmonary fibrosis
Sarcoidosis
Radiation fibrosis (rare)
Small airways disease
Constrictive bronchiolitis
Hypoventilation
Obesity
Chest wall deformity (kyphoscoliosis)
Pulmonary arterial disease
Left-to-right shunt (Eisenmenger syndrome)
ASD
VSD
PDA
Partial anomalous pulmonary venous return
Primary pulmonary hypertension (plexogenic pulmonary arteriopathy)
Pulmonary vasculitis
Connective tissue disease
HIV infection
Drugs (fenfluramine, dexfenfluramine, "fen-phen")
Chronic pulmonary thromboembolic disease

ASD = atrial septal defect.
VSD = ventricular septal defect.
PDA = patent ductus arterious.

An increase in resistance to pulmonary blood flow is the most common cause of PAH (Table 14.4). The disorders producing increased pulmonary vascular resistance are pulmonary venous hypertension, parenchymal lung disease, chest wall deformity, diffuse pleural fibrosis, pulmonary arterial disease, and idiopathic pulmonary vascular disease. The most common cause of chronic elevation of pulmonary venous pressure is mitral stenosis, although any impedance to pulmonary venous return to the left heart can produce venous hypertension. Less common entities in this group include chronic LV failure, atrial

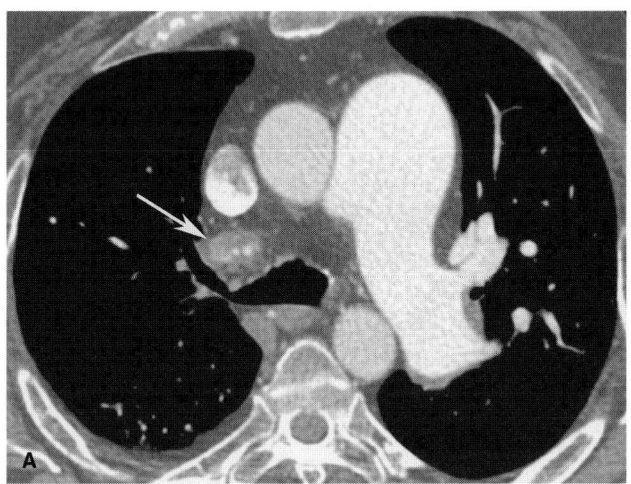

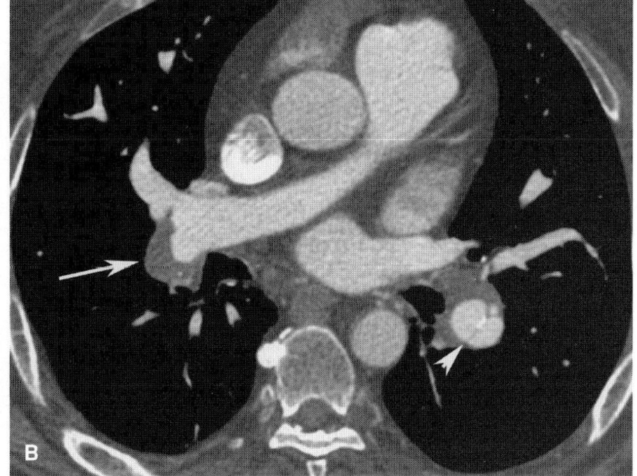

FIGURE 14.16. **Chronic Thromboembolic Pulmonary Hypertension.** Enhanced CT scan at the level of the main pulmonary artery **(A)** shows dilated main and left pulmonary arteries, with thrombosis of the truncus anterior branch of the right pulmonary artery (*arrow*). At the level of the hila **(B)**, there is an eccentric filling defect (*arrow*) in the right interlobar artery and a weblike filling defect (*arrowhead*) containing calcification in the left interlobar artery. These findings are characteristic of chronic unresolved emboli.

myxoma, cor triatriatum, and pulmonary vein stenosis or occlusion. In addition to the characteristic pulmonary arterial changes of PAH, patients may show LV dilatation in LV failure or LA enlargement in mitral stenosis or cor triatriatum. The radiographic signs of pulmonary venous hypertension and pulmonary edema may be seen early in the course of these disorders but are often absent by the time PAH has developed.

Parenchymal lung disease, particularly centrilobular emphysema and diffuse interstitial fibrosis, are common causes of PAH. The mechanisms by which these disorders produce increased vascular resistance include chronic hypoxemia and reflex vasoconstriction and the development of irreversible changes in pulmonary arteriolar caliber, with widespread obliteration of the pulmonary vascular bed. The radiographic findings of emphysema and interstitial fibrosis are usually evident on plain radiographs by the time PAH has developed.

Chronic hypoxemia from alveolar hypoventilation is the likely mechanism for PAH that complicates pleural fibrosis, kyphoscoliosis, and the obesity-hypoventilation syndrome. Pleural thickening and kyphoscoliosis are readily evident radiographically. The obesity-hypoventilation (obstructive sleep apnea) syndrome is usually associated with marked truncal obesity and lungs that are diminished in volume (mostly owing to diaphragmatic elevation) but are normal in appearance.

Disorders of the pulmonary arteries that produce PAH include chronic PEs, vasculitis, and pulmonary arteriopathy resulting from long-standing increased pulmonary blood flow from left-to-right shunt. Occlusion of lobar and segmental vessels producing PAH can result from failure of pulmonary thromboemboli to lyse or completely recanalize (Fig. 14.16). Rarely, pulmonary vasculitis resulting from diseases such as rheumatoid lung disease or Takayasu arteritis can produce obliteration of the pulmonary vasculature and lead to PAH.

The diagnosis of large vessel thromboembolic pulmonary hypertension is usually made by echocardiography, which provides an indirect estimate of pulmonary artery pressure. CT angiographic findings of chronic thromboembolic pulmonary hypertension (CTPH) correlate with conventional angiographic findings and include focal stenoses, bandlike or weblike filling defects, and eccentric wall thickening. Lung windows in patients with CTPH classically demonstrate a pattern of mosaic attenuation, with the hyperlucent regions demonstrating attenuated vascular markings (mosaic oligemia) as compared to areas of increased attenuation that result from hyperemia from intact pulmonary artery branches.

Idiopathic or *primary pulmonary hypertension* encompasses diseases of the pulmonary arterioles and venules that are not attributable to other etiologies and have characteristic histologic findings. *Plexogenic pulmonary arteriopathy, recurrent microscopic PE,* and *pulmonary venoocclusive disease* (PVOD) are the three diseases that comprise this category. Plexogenic pulmonary arteriopathy is a disease of young women in whom medial hypertrophy and intimal fibrosis obliterate the muscular arteries. Dilated vascular channels within the periphery of the obliterated vessel produce the plexogenic lesions seen on biopsy in virtually all patients with this disease. Progressive dyspnea and fatigue develop with characteristic physical findings of PAH and cor pulmonale. In plexogenic pulmonary arteriopathy, pulmonary perfusion scans typically show normal perfusion or small, nonsegmental peripheral perfusion defects, allowing distinction from large-vessel thromboembolic disease. Microembolic disease is clinically and radiographically indistinguishable from plexogenic arteriopathy. In this entity, plexogenic lesions within arterioles are absent. Perfusion scans are more likely to show small perfusion defects in this disorder. The presence of small microemboli histologically is not a distinguishing feature, because in situ thrombosis within diseased arterioles can have a similar appearance. In PVOD, the obliteration of small intrapulmonary venules results in interstitial pulmonary edema. A condition related to PVOD is *pulmonary capillary hemangiomatosis* (PCH), which is characterized by the proliferation of capillaries throughout the pulmonary interstitium, resulting in venular obstruction. The transmission of increased pressure to the arterial side leads to medial hypertrophy and obliteration of vessel lumina with resultant arterial hypertension. Chest radiographs often show interstitial or airspace pulmonary edema with a normal heart size. Perfusion lung scanning is usually normal or shows small peripheral nonsegmental defects. The combination of pulmonary edema with a normal heart size, absent findings for pulmonary venous hypertension, normal PCWP, and the insidious onset of dyspnea should suggest this diagnosis rather than left heart failure, mitral valve disease, or large-vessel pulmonary venous occlusion. Thin-section CT features of PVOD and PCH are those of pulmonary venous hypertension and include interlobular septal thickening, centrilobular nodular ground-glass opacities, and pleural effusions (9). A definitive diagnosis can only be made by characteristic findings on open lung biopsy. The prognosis is universally poor, with most patients succumbing to their disease within 2 years of diagnosis.

REFERENCES

1. Pistolesi M, Miniati M, Milne ENC, et al. The chest roentgenogram in pulmonary edema. Clin Chest Med 1985;6:315–344.
2. Ketai L, Godwin D. A new view of pulmonary edema and acute respiratory distress syndrome. J Thorac Imaging 1998;13:147–171.
3. Milne ENC, Pistolesi M, Miniati M, et al. The radiologic distinction of cardiogenic and noncardiogenic edema. AJR Am J Roentgenol 1985;144:879–894.
4. Albelda SM, Gefter WB, Epstein DM, et al. Diffuse pulmonary hemorrhage: a review and classification. Radiology 1985;154:289–297.
5. The PIOPED investigators. Value of the ventilation/perfusion scan in acute pulmonary embolism: results of the prospective investigation of pulmonary embolism diagnosis (PIOPED). JAMA 1990;263:2753–2759.
6. Buckner CB, Walker CW, Purnell GL. Pulmonary embolism: chest radiographic abnormalities. J Thorac Imaging 1989;4:23–27.
7. Schoepf UJ, Costello P. CT angiography for diagnosis of pulmonary embolism: state of the art. Radiology 2004;230:329–337.
8. Stein PD, Athanasoulis C, Alavi A, et al. Complications and validity of pulmonary angiography in acute pulmonary embolism. Circulation 1992;85:462–468.
9. Hansell DM. Small-vessel diseases of the Lung: CT-Pathologic correlates. Radiology 2002;225:639–653.

Chapter 15

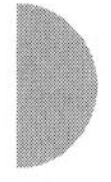

Pulmonary Neoplasms

Jeffrey S. Klein

The Solitary Pulmonary Nodule
Lesions Presenting as SPNs

Bronchogenic Carcinoma
Cytologic and Pathologic Features
Radiologic Staging of Lung Cancer

Tracheal and Bronchial Masses

Metastatic Disease to the Thorax

Nonepithelial Parenchymal Malignancies and Neoplastic-Like Conditions

THE SOLITARY PULMONARY NODULE

The radiologic evaluation of a solitary pulmonary nodule (SPN) is one of the most common and most difficult diagnostic dilemmas in thoracic radiology (1). The prevalence of SPNs has increased recently as a result of the growing use of chest CT—specifically its use to screen for occult lung cancer. Before embarking on a detailed diagnostic evaluation of an SPN, one must determine whether the nodular opacity seen on the chest radiograph is real or artifactual. If the opacity is judged to represent a real lesion, the radiologist must then determine whether it is an SPN. First, is the lesion truly solitary? Not uncommonly, a dominant pulmonary nodule on chest radiographs is associated with smaller nodules or nodules that are obscured by the heart or the hemidiaphragms. A careful search on posteroanterior (PA) and lateral chest radiographs will identify most of these patients, although CT may be necessary to identify additional nodules not seen on chest radiographs. Multiple pulmonary nodules of similar size and appearance are almost always metastases or granulomas and require an evaluation that differs from that for a solitary lesion.

Second, is the lesion intrapulmonary? Intrapulmonary lesions are discrete opacities that are completely circumscribed by aerated lung on both frontal and lateral radiographs. A pleural or mediastinal lesion may be outlined by lung when it projects inward. However, the base of the lesion, which forms obtuse angles with the lung, is not outlined by lung when it arises from the pleura or mediastinum. Skin lesions and chest wall lesions, including bone islands and healing rib fractures, can also mimic intrapulmonary nodules. Some skin lesions are circumscribed by air, but a careful physical examination of the patient, usually following the chest radiograph, will reveal the surface lesion responsible for the "nodule" seen on chest film. One of the most troublesome skin "lesions" to distinguish from a true pulmonary nodule is the nipple shadow. This is usually readily identified by performing chest films with nipple markers. Occasionally, chest fluoroscopy or CT will be necessary for confident localization of a nodular opacity seen on conventional radiographs.

Finally, is the lesion a nodule? A nodule is a discrete round or oval opacity 4 to 30 mm in diameter; linear or angular opacities are not nodules and represent scars or areas of linear atelectasis. Three-dimensional analysis of the shape of an SPN on volumetric CT can help distinguish flat scars from true SPNs. When a focal opacity is seen in the lung apices, an apical lordotic film or CT scan may be necessary to distinguish a linear from a nodular opacity. A round opacity greater than 3 cm in diameter is termed a mass. Because the majority of lung masses in patients over the age of 35 represent bronchogenic carcinoma, these lesions are not considered SPNs.

Once an SPN has been identified, the radiologist should initiate a series of investigations to determine whether the nodule is definitely benign or suspicious for malignancy (i.e., indeterminate). This stepwise approach is summarized in Fig. 15.1.

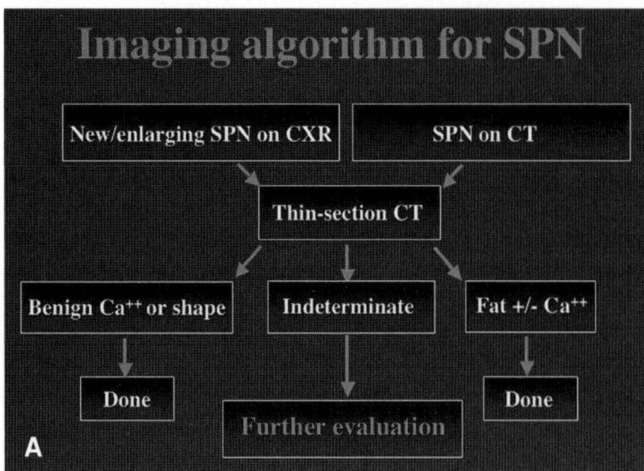

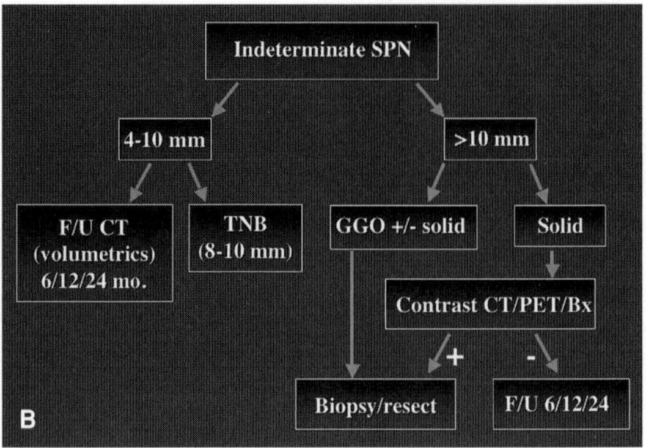

FIGURE 15.1. **Imaging Algorithm for the Solitary Pulmonary Nodule.** SPN, solitary pulmonary nodule; Ca^{++}, calcification; TNB, transthoracic needle biopsy; CXR, chest x-ray; GGO, ground-glass opacity; Bx, biopsy; F/U, follow-up.

Clinical Factors. Before considering the radiologic characteristics used to distinguish benign from indeterminate nodules, several important clinical factors may be helpful in making this distinction. In a patient under the age of 35, particularly a nonsmoker without a history of malignancy, an SPN is invariably a granuloma, hamartoma, or inflammatory lesion. These nodules can be followed with plain radiographs to confirm their benign nature. Patients over the age of 35, particularly those who are current or recent cigarette smokers, have a significant incidence of malignant SPNs: approximately 50% of noncalcified SPNs in patients over 50 years of age are malignant at thoracotomy. Therefore, as a rule, an SPN in a patient over 35 years of age should never be followed radiographically without tissue confirmation unless a benign pattern of calcification or the presence of intralesional fat is identified on radiographs or HRCT, or there has been radiographically documented lack of growth over a minimum of 2 years. There are exceptions to this rule: a history of cigarette smoking, asbestos exposure, or both raises the level of concern for malignancy in a patient with an SPN. Alternatively, if the patient is from an area where histoplasmosis or tuberculosis is endemic, the likelihood of a granuloma is greater; in such patients, a conservative approach may be warranted. Finally, the finding of an SPN in a patient with an extrathoracic malignancy raises the possibility of a solitary pulmonary metastasis. If the lung is the sole site of metastatic disease, distinguishing between a primary bronchogenic carcinoma and a pulmonary metastasis is usually not important, as many surgeons will resect a solitary pulmonary metastasis. An SPN that arises more than 2 years after the diagnosis of an extrathoracic malignancy is almost always a primary lung tumor rather than a metastasis; breast carcinoma and melanoma are notable exceptions to this rule.

Growth Pattern. Pulmonary malignancies grow at a relatively predictable rate. The growth rate of an SPN is usually expressed as the *doubling time,* or the time it takes for a nodule to double its volume. For a sphere, this corresponds to a 25% increase in diameter. Although some benign lesions (mostly hamartomas and histoplasmomas) may exhibit a growth rate similar to that of malignant lesions, the absence of growth or an extraordinarily slow or rapid rate of growth is reliable evidence that an SPN is benign. Studies have shown that bronchogenic carcinoma has a doubling time of between 1 month and 2 years. Therefore, a doubling time of less than 1 month or greater than 2 years reliably characterizes a lesion as benign. Infectious lesions and rapidly growing metastases from choriocarcinoma, seminoma, or osteogenic sarcoma comprise the majority of rapidly growing solitary nodules, while lack of growth or a doubling time exceeding 2 years is seen in hamartomas and histoplasmomas. However, there are exceptions to this rule. Giant cell carcinoma, a subtype of large cell carcinoma, and pulmonary carcinosarcomas and blastomas may have a doubling time of less than 1 month. Even more common pulmonary malignancies, such as the occasional adenocarcinoma or carcinoid tumors, may have a doubling time of greater than 2 years. Any malignancy that hemorrhages into its substance will appear to enlarge rapidly. There are two important caveats to using the growth rate of an SPN to determine benignity. The first is that the growth rate of an SPN that is not visible on prior radiographs cannot be estimated, since noncalcified nodules less than 1 cm in diameter are not usually visible on conventional radiographs. Most important, with few exceptions, a patient over the age of 35 with a noncalcified SPN should not be evaluated prospectively to determine benignity by following the growth rate on serial chest radiographs. The assessment of growth rate to determine benignity should only be used retrospectively in comparing the size of an SPN with prior radiographs from at least 2 years previously.

In patients with clinical and imaging characteristics suggesting a probably benign SPN, particularly for lesions <10 mm diameter, multidetector CT (MDCT) analysis of nodule volume appears to provide a noninvasive method of assessing nodule growth and determining which lesions require biopsy or resection. Preliminary studies have shown that this technique is more accurate than cross-sectional measurements in determining nodule volume and distinguishing between growing malignant SPNs and stable benign lesions. If a decision is made to simply follow an SPN radiologically, either because of an overwhelming likelihood of benignity or because the patient cannot tolerate an invasive diagnostic procedure, the lesion should be followed by chest radiographs or limited thin-section CT at 3 to 6 months, 12 months, and 24 months following initial detection.

Size. Although size does not reliably discriminate benign from malignant SPNs, the larger the lesion, the greater the likelihood of malignancy. Masses exceeding 4 cm in diameter are usually malignant. However, the converse does not hold true; many pulmonary malignancies are less than 2 cm in diameter at the time of diagnosis, particularly if detected by screening chest CT.

Margin (Border) Characteristics. The appearance of the edge of an SPN is a helpful sign in determining the nature of the lesion. The edge characteristics are best evaluated on thin-section CT, as this technique is considerably more accurate than plain radiographs. A round, smoothly marginated nodule is most likely a granuloma or hamartoma, although a rare primary pulmonary malignancy such as a carcinoid tumor, adenocarcinoma, or a solitary metastasis may have a perfectly smooth margin. A notched or lobulated margin is strongly suggestive but not diagnostic of malignancy. Pathologic examination has shown that the lobulated edge of a malignant nodule represents mounds of tumor extending into the adjacent lung. A spiculated margin is highly suspicious for malignancy (Fig. 15.2). The term *corona radiata* has been used to describe this appearance, in which linear densities radiate from the edge of a nodule into the adjacent lung. Pathologically, these linear radiations represent reoriented connective tissue (interlobular) septa drawn into the tumor by the cicatrizing (scarring) nature of many malignant lung tumors. Tumor extension from the nodule, or fibrosis and edema of these connective tissue septa, may thicken these linear densities. However, it has been shown that spiculation is not specific for malignancy, because benign processes that produce cicatrization can have an identical appearance. Benign lesions that may show a spiculated margin include lipoid pneumonia, organizing pneumonia, tuberculomas, and the mass lesions of progressive massive fibrosis in complicated silicosis. A peripherally situated pulmonary nodule may contact the costal pleura or interlobar fissure via a linear opacity known as a "pleural tail." As with the corona radiata, the recognition of this line, while suggestive of malignancy (particularly bronchioloalveolar cell carcinoma), is not specific and may be seen in peripheral granulomas.

There are additional characteristics of the border of an SPN that help identify the nature of the lesion. The presence of small "satellite" nodules around the periphery of a dominant nodule is strongly suggestive of benign disease, particularly granulomatous infection. The identification of feeding and draining vessels emanating from the hilar aspect of an SPN is pathognomonic of a pulmonary arteriovenous malformation (AVM). Contrast-enhanced helical CT scanning through the nodule or MR is diagnostic. A posttraumatic pulmonary artery pseudoaneurysm will show marked contrast enhancement and contiguity with the feeding artery on CT. The presence of a halo of ground-glass opacity encircling an SPN in an immunocompromised, neutropenic patient should suggest the diagnosis of invasive pulmonary aspergillosis. Finally, a nodule or mass adjacent to an area of pleural thickening, with a "comet tail" of bronchi and vessels entering the hilar aspect of the mass, and associated with lobar volume loss is characteristic of round atelectasis.

Density. The internal density of an SPN is probably the single most important factor in characterizing the lesion as benign or indeterminate. In general, lesions that are calcified are benign. There are five patterns of calcification that reliably indicate the benignity of an SPN (Fig. 15.3). These patterns can be identified on plain chest radiographs, but thin-section CT is often necessary to detect and characterize the calcification. *Complete* or *central calcification* within an SPN is specific for a healed granuloma from tuberculosis or histoplasmosis. *Concentric* or *laminated calcification* indicates a granuloma and allows confident exclusion of neoplasm. *Popcorn calcification* within a nodule is diagnostic of a pulmonary hamartoma in which the cartilaginous component has calcified.

It is important to remember that calcification within an SPN is synonymous with a benign lesion only if the calcification follows one of the four patterns of benign calcification shown in Fig. 15.3. Approximately 10% of malignant nodules contain calcification on CT. A bronchogenic carcinoma that arises in an area of previous granulomatous infection may engulf a preexisting calcified granuloma as it enlarges. In this situation, the calcification will be eccentric in the nodule, allowing distinction from a centrally calcified granuloma. Malignant pulmonary neoplasms may demonstrate small or microscopic foci of calcification, particularly adenocarcinomas that produce mucin or psammoma bodies. The rare solitary pulmonary metastasis from osteosarcoma or chondrosarcoma may contain calcium, but the diagnosis in these patients will usually be obvious clinically.

The identification of fat within an SPN is diagnostic of a pulmonary hamartoma (Fig. 15.4). A discussion of the radiographic and CT features of a pulmonary hamartoma can be found in the section "Lesions Presenting as SPNs."

It is important to remember that not all SPNs can be reliably characterized by their internal attenuation characteristics. A nodule with a diameter greater than 3 cm, those showing lobulated or spiculated margins,

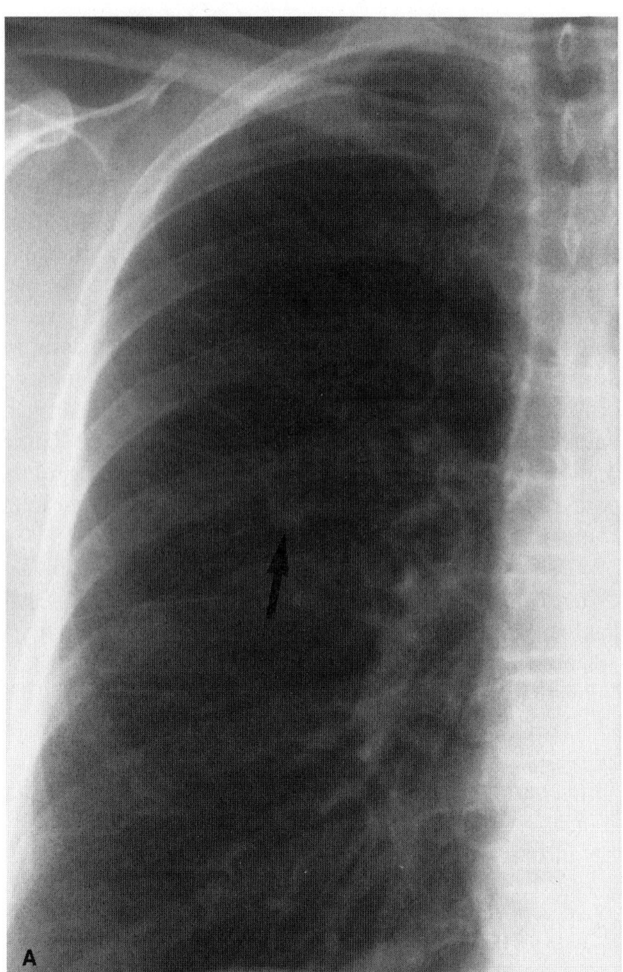

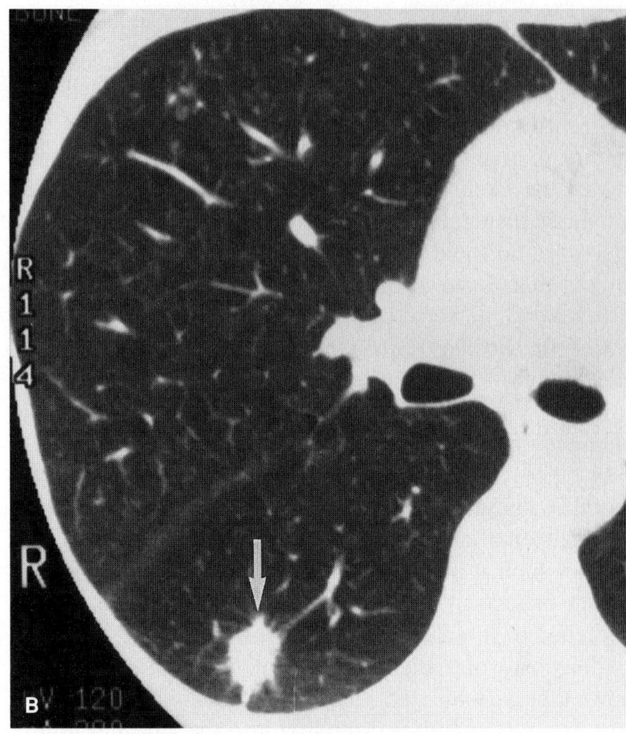

FIGURE 15.2. **Adenocarcinoma Presenting as Solitary Pulmonary Nodule. A.** Cone-down view of posteroanterior radiograph shows nodule in the right mid-lung (*arrow*). **B.** Thin-section CT shows 12-mm nodule with spiculated margins (*arrow*) in the superior segment of the right lower lobe. Transthoracic needle biopsy revealed adenocarcinoma.

thick-walled cavitary lesions, or those showing mixed soft tissue and ground-glass attenuation have a high likelihood of malignancy, regardless of internal density. Likewise, the demonstration of an air bronchogram, bubbly lucencies, or mixed solid/ground-glass attenuation within an SPN is highly suspicious for adenocarcinoma, particularly bronchioloalveolar cell subtypes. Such SPNs, along with those small, well-defined solid lesions lacking benign calcification or fat on HRCT or marginal characteristics of granulomas or AVMs are suspicious enough for malignancy to be considered indeterminate.

Contrast-Enhanced CT and PET. Several studies have demonstrated the utility of dynamic, contrast-enhanced CT in the evaluation of SPNs, with virtually all malignant lesions demonstrating an increase in attenuation of greater than 15 H after contrast administration (Fig. 15.5) (2). Therefore, lack of significant (>15 H) enhancement of a solid nodule 6 to 30 mm in diameter after intravenous iodinated contrast effectively excludes malignancy (sensitivity = 98%).

PET using fluorine-18-labeled fluorodeoxyglucose (FDG) has shown a high accuracy in the distinction between benign and malignant SPNs (Fig. 15.6) (3). For lesions >10 mm diameter, the sensitivity and specificity of FDG-PET is 97%, with a specificity of 78%, mostly as a result of inflammatory lesions such as active granulomas that are FDG-avid. False-negative PET studies are seen in patients with lesions <10 mm diameter and metabolically hypoactive lesions such as carcinoid tumor and bronchoalveolar cell carcinoma.

Management Decisions (Fig. 15.1). Patients with indeterminate SPNs should have either close radiologic follow-up or undergo transthoracic biopsy or resection. When the lesion is very likely to be malignant, it is reasonable to forgo biopsy and proceed directly to thoracotomy and resection. However, there are several reasons to

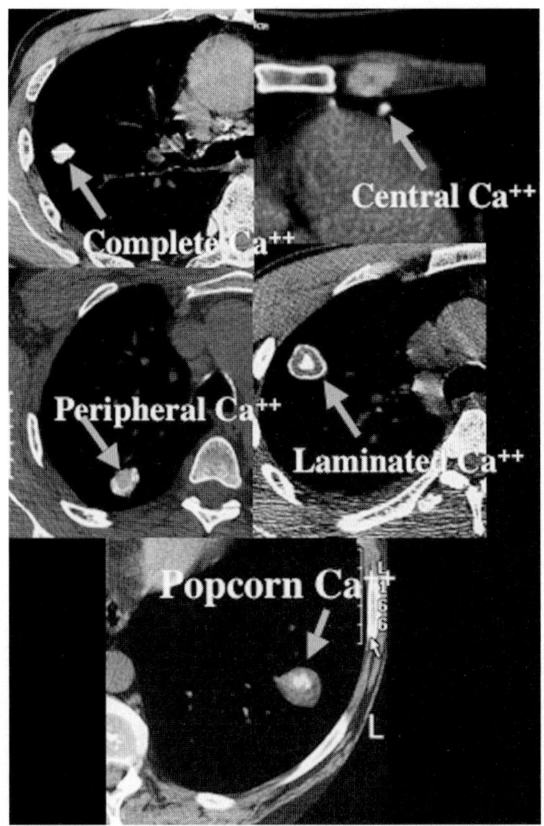

FIGURE 15.3. **Benign Patterns of Calcification Within a Solitary Pulmonary Nodule.**

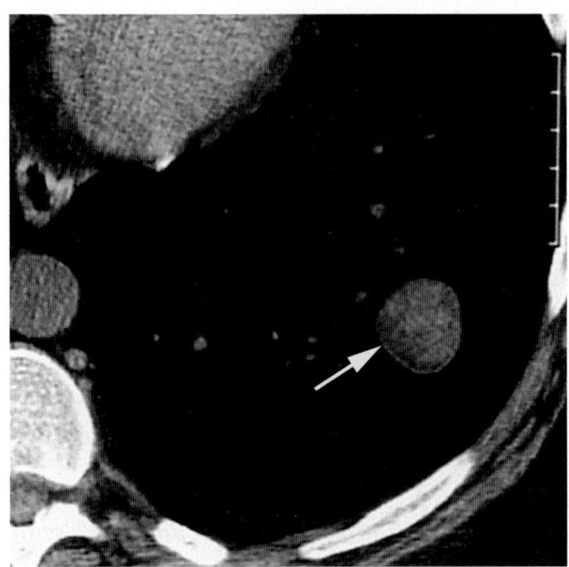

FIGURE 15.4. **Fat in Pulmonary Hamartoma.** Cone-down view of unenhanced thin-section CT through left lower lobe nodule shows fat in medial aspect of lesion (*arrow*), diagnostic of a hamartoma.

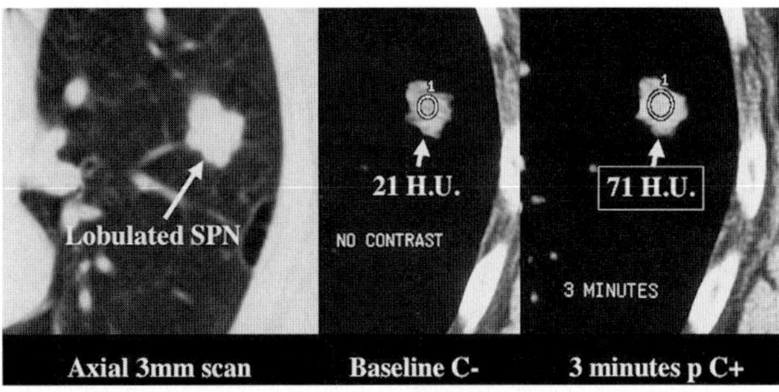

FIGURE 15.5. **Contrast CT in Malignant Solitary Pulmonary Nodule.** Thin-collimation (3-mm) CT scans through left upper lobe nodule in a 62-year-old woman with biopsy-proven lung cancer shows a lobulated contour with positive enhancement of 50 H after contrast administration.

perform a preoperative biopsy on an indeterminate SPN. The primary reason to biopsy an indeterminate SPN is to make the diagnosis of a benign lesion, thereby avoiding an unnecessary thoracoscopy or thoracotomy. This would most benefit the patient with a reasonable likelihood of having a benign lesion. Factors suggesting benignity include: age under 35, nonsmoker, patient from an area endemic for tuberculosis or histoplasmosis, nodule <2 cm with smooth margins, and a doubling time of less than 30 days or greater than 2 years. The other major indication for the biopsy of an indeterminate SPN is a patient with limited pulmonary reserve who is a poor surgical candidate for pulmonary resection. In these patients, a biopsy can provide a diagnosis and guide nonoperative therapy. Because most SPNs are peripherally situated in the lung, transthoracic needle biopsy (TNB) is the procedure of choice for tissue sampling. Peripheral lesions requiring biopsy that are too small for successful transthoracic needle biopsy (i.e., lesions <5 mm diameter) can be sampled with video-assisted thoracoscopic surgery (VATS). Patients with SPNs that are

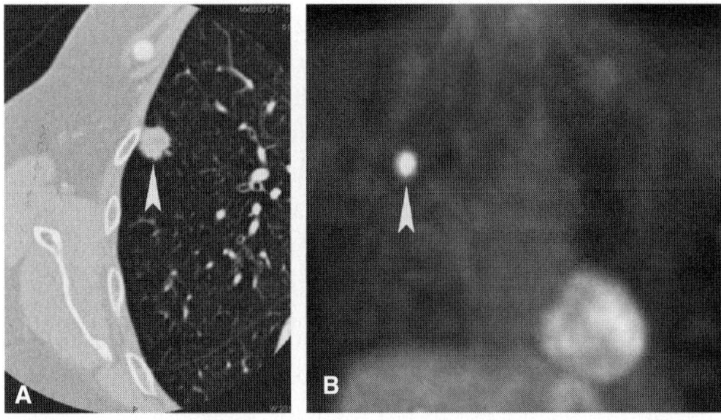

FIGURE 15.6. **Positive PET Scan in Malignant Solitary Pulmonary Nodule. A.** Cone-down thin-section CT of right upper lobe in a 72-year-old man shows a peripheral speculated SPN (*arrowhead*). **B.** Coronal maximum intensity projection of PET demonstrates marked increased uptake in the lesion (*arrowhead*). Biopsy showed a squamous cell carcinoma.

centrally situated, with a large bronchus entering the lesion, should undergo transbronchoscopic biopsy.

An SPN that is judged to be benign based on patient age, growth rate, presence of benign calcification, or those with a specific benign diagnosis provided by TNB should be followed with radiographs or CT for a minimum of 2 and preferably 3 years to confirm their benign nature. The radiographic follow-up consists of PA and lateral chest radiographs or limited thin-section CT at 6-month intervals.

Lesions Presenting as SPNs

The differential diagnosis of an SPN is shown in Table 15.1. In addition to bronchogenic carcinoma (particularly adenocarcinoma) and granulomas (e.g., tuberculosis and histoplasmosis), there are a number of entities that may produce an SPN. Many of these entities are discussed elsewhere in the text.

Carcinoid Tumors. While carcinoid tumors may present as SPNs, the majority (80%) are central endobronchial lesions that present with atelectasis or obstructive pneumonitis. A detailed discussion of carcinoid tumors can be found in the section on malignant pulmonary neoplasms.

Pulmonary hamartoma is a benign neoplasm composed of an abnormal arrangement of the mesenchymal and epithelial elements found in normal lung. Histologically, these lesions contain cartilage surrounded by fibrous connective tissue, with variable amounts of fat, smooth muscle, and seromucous glands; calcification and ossification are seen in 30%. These tumors are seen most commonly in the fourth and fifth decades of life. Approximately 90% of hamartomas arise within the pulmonary parenchyma, accounting for approximately 5% of all SPNs.

These lesions usually present as incidental findings on chest radiographs. While the diagnosis is often suggested on plain radiographs, CT is obtained in most patients. A confident diagnosis of hamartoma can be made when HRCT shows a nodule <2.5 cm in diameter demonstrating a smooth or lobulated border and containing focal fat. Calcification, when present, is in the form of multiple clumps of calcium dispersed throughout the lesion ("popcorn" calcification) (Fig. 15.7). As a rule, hamartomas that contain calcium also contain fat. While hamartomas tend to grow slowly, the presence of characteristic HRCT findings allows for observation alone. Rapid growth, pulmonary symptoms, or a size >2.5 cm warrants transthoracic biopsy or resection.

Non-Hodgkin Lymphoma. Primary pulmonary lymphoma arising from the bronchus-associated lymphoid tissue (BALT) are low-grade B-cell lymphomas that present in adults in their 50s. The most common radiographic finding is an SPN or focal airspace opacity (Fig. 15.8). The diagnosis is made by immunohistochemistry and flow cytometry of resected specimens or of aspirated cells obtained by TNB.

TABLE 15.1 Solitary Pulmonary Nodule or Mass

Neoplasm	Bronchogenic carcinoma
	Hamartoma
	Bronchial adenoma
	Granular cell myoblastoma
	Mesenchymal neoplasms
	Leiomyoma/leiomyosarcoma
	Fibroma
	Lipoma
	Neurofibroma
	Lymphoma
	Solitary metastasis
	Colon carcinoma
Infection	Septic embolus
	Staphylococcus
	Round pneumonia
	Pneumococcus
	Legionella
	Nocardia
	Fungi
	Lung abscess
	Infectious granuloma
	Tuberculosis
	Histoplasmosis
	Coccidioidomycosis
	Cryptococcosis
	Parasitic
	Echinococcal cyst
	Amebic abscess
Collagen vascular disease	Necrobiotic nodule (rheumatoid lung)
	Wegener granulomatosis
Vascular	Infarct
	Arteriovenous malformation
	Pulmonary artery aneurysm
	Hematoma
Airways	Congenital foregut malformations
	Bronchogenic cyst
	Sequestration
	Mucocele
	Infected bulla
Miscellaneous	Amyloidoma
	Round atelectasis

Granular cell myoblastoma is a benign neoplasm arising from neural elements in the central airways or parenchyma. The skin is the most common site for these tumors. These tumors may present as SPNs or as endobronchial masses.

Leiomyoma/Leiomyosarcoma, Fibroma, Neurofibroma. Arising from the smooth muscle of the airways or pulmonary vessels, leiomyomas and leiomyosarcomas are rare neoplasms that present as endobronchial or intrapulmonary lesions with equal frequency. Radiographically, the parenchymal lesions are sharply marginated, smooth

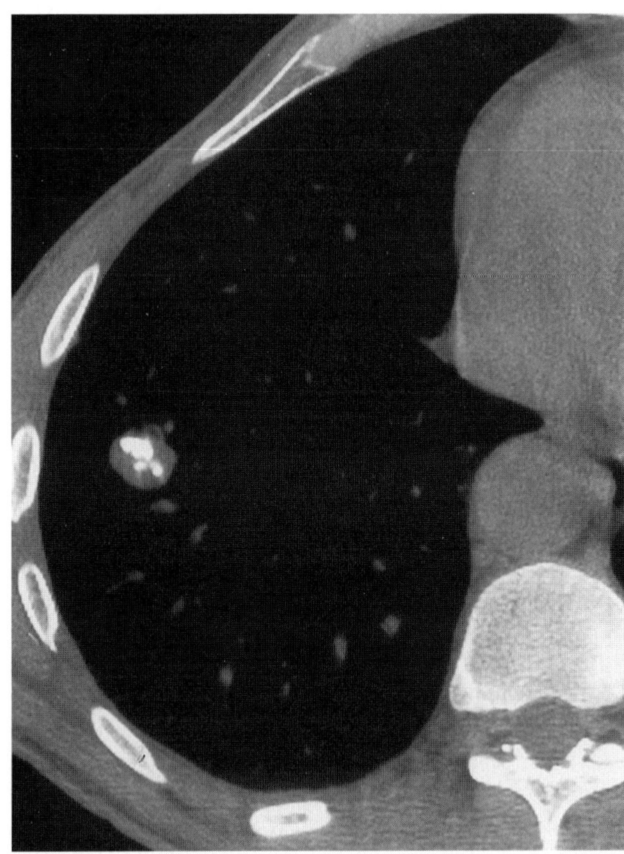

FIGURE 15.7. **Hamartoma.** Thin-section CT shows a smoothly marginated nodule containing coarse "popcorn" calcifications typical of a pulmonary hamartoma.

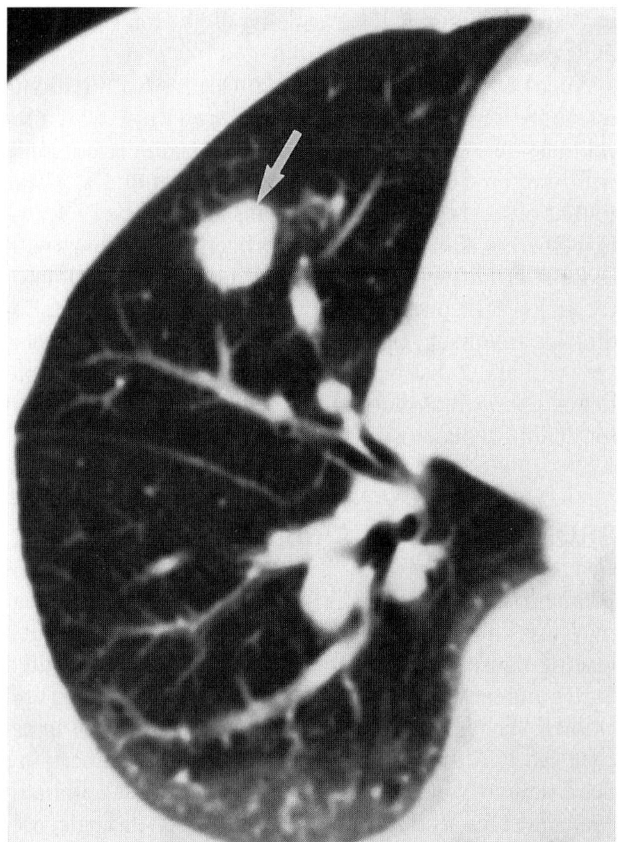

FIGURE 15.8. **Non-Hodgkin Lymphoma Presenting as a Solitary Pulmonary Nodule.** CT scan in a 73-year-old patient with carcinoma of the breast shows a smoothly marginated 2-cm nodule (*arrow*) in the middle lobe. A diagnosis of low-grade non-Hodgkin lymphoma (lymphoma of the bronchus-associated lymphoid tissue, or BALToma) was made by transthoracic needle biopsy.

or lobulated nodules or masses. The histologic distinction of benign from malignant lesions is difficult. Similarly, fibromas and neurofibromas appearing as SPNs lack distinguishing radiographic features.

Lipomas are rare intrapulmonary lesions that arise more commonly within the tracheobronchial tree to produce atelectasis. The demonstration of fat attenuation on CT is diagnostic.

Hemangiopericytoma is a connective tissue tumor that arises within the lung from the pericyte, a cell associated with the arteriolar and capillary endothelium. On chest radiographs, these lesions are seen as SPNs and are indistinguishable from bronchogenic carcinoma.

Plasma cell granuloma (inflammatory pseudotumor) of lung refers to a localized chronic inflammatory response to an unknown agent in the lung. It is characterized histologically by an abundance of plasma cells. There are no distinguishing radiographic features.

Lipoid Pneumonia. The inadvertent aspiration of mineral oils ingested by elderly patients to treat constipation may produce a localized pulmonary lesion. Patients with gastroesophageal reflux or disordered swallowing mechanisms are at particular risk. Radiographically, a focal area of airspace opacification or a solid mass may be seen in the lower lobes. A spiculated appearance to the edge of the mass is not uncommon, as the oil may produce a chronic inflammatory reaction in the surrounding lung that leads to fibrosis. While CT can demonstrate fat within the lesion, most patients with the masslike form of this entity require resection for definitive diagnosis (see Fig. 19-34).

Bronchogenic Cyst. Fluid-filled cystic lesions of the lung may produce an SPN. Intrapulmonary bronchogenic cysts are uncommon causes of SPNs; 90% of these lesions are found in the middle mediastinum. The characteristic finding is a sharply marginated cyst on CT or MR in a young patient, although distinction from an infected bulla, solitary echinococcal cyst, mucocele, or thin-walled lung abscess may be impossible. Superinfection of a lung bulla may produce an SPN or mass. In such patients, the radiographic or CT appearance of an intraparenchymal air–fluid level within a thin-walled localized air collection (usually in an upper lobe), with typical bullous changes in other portions of lung, usually allows for the proper diagnosis.

Focal Organizing Pneumonia. Occasionally, patients who have a resolving pneumonia or even those with a focal mass–like form of cryptogenic organizing pneumonia will have an SPN detected on radiographs or CT. These lesions often show irregular margins and may be PET positive, thereby showing a significant overlap of findings with those of bronchogenic carcinoma. Sometimes a history of recent lower respiratory tract infection will be present. Radiologic follow-up, perhaps after empiric antibiotic therapy, will allow distinction from malignancy in most patients, although a minority will require surgical resection for definitive diagnosis.

BRONCHOGENIC CARCINOMA

Bronchogenic carcinoma is one of several neoplasms that may arise within the lung (Table 15.2). It is now the leading cause of death from malignancy in the United States and most industrialized countries for both men and women, having surpassed breast cancer in women in recent years. Although survival rates for lung cancer are poor, radiology plays a central role in diagnosis and management. This section will review the key pathologic, epidemiologic, and radiologic features of bronchogenic carcinoma with an emphasis on the radiologic staging of this disease.

TABLE 15.2 Pulmonary Neoplasms

Benign
Epithelial
Squamous cell papilloma
Pleomorphic adenoma (benign mixed tumor)
Mesenchymal
Hamartoma
Lipoma
Neurofibroma
Leiomyoma
Granular cell myoblastoma
Hemangiopericytoma
Malignant
Epithelial
Bronchogenic carcinoma
Carcinoid tumor
Bronchial gland carcinoma
Mucoepidermoid carcinoma
Adenoid cystic carcinoma (cylindroma)
Epithelial/mesenchymal
Pulmonary blastoma
Carcinosarcoma
Lymphoid
Non-Hodgkin lymphoma
Hodgkin lymphoma

Cytologic and Pathologic Features

Bronchogenic carcinoma is a malignant neoplasm that arises from the bronchial or alveolar epithelium. Ninety-nine percent of malignant epithelial neoplasms of the lung arise from the bronchi or lung, while fewer than 0.5% arise from the trachea. Bronchogenic carcinoma is divided into four main histologic subtypes based on their gross and microscopic features: adenocarcinoma, squamous cell carcinoma, small cell carcinoma, and large cell carcinoma (Table 15.3).

Adenocarcinoma is the most common type of lung cancer, accounting for approximately one third of all bronchogenic carcinomas. It is the most common subtype of lung cancer in nonsmokers. Whereas these tumors were once found to occur overwhelmingly in the lung periphery, they are now found in the central portions of the lungs in about one fourth of cases. These tumors arise from the bronchiolar or alveolar epithelium and have an irregular or spiculated appearance where they invade adjacent lung. Fibrosis in and about the tumor is common. These gross features usually produce an ill-defined pulmonary nodule or central mass on chest radiographs (Fig. 15.2). Histologically, adenocarcinoma demonstrates gland formation and mucin production. A subtype of adenocarcinoma, *bronchioloalveolar cell carcinoma* (BAC), has unique pathologic features. This tumor is characterized by growth along preexisting bronchiolar and alveolar walls ("lepidic growth") without invasion or distortion of these structures. When localized, BAC appears as a solitary pulmonary nodule or as a focal area of ground-glass opacity on CT scans. Diffuse disease, which represents either multifocal origin of disease or transbronchial spread of tumor, may present as airspace opacification simulating pneumonia or as diffuse bilateral nodular airspace opacities.

Squamous cell carcinoma is the second most common subtype of bronchogenic carcinoma, accounting for approximately one fourth of all cases. This tumor arises centrally within a lobar or segmental bronchus. Grossly, these tumors are polypoid masses that grow into the bronchial lumen while simultaneously invading the bronchial wall. The central location and endobronchial component of the tumor account for the presenting symptoms of cough and hemoptysis and for the common radiographic findings of a hilar mass with or without obstructive pneumonitis or atelectasis (Fig. 15.9). Central necrosis is common in large tumors; cavitation may be seen if communication has occurred between the central portion of the mass and the bronchial lumen. Histologically, squamous cell carcinoma is characterized by invasion of the bronchial wall by nests of malignant cells with abundant cytoplasm. The formation of keratin pearls and intercellular bridges, seen in well-differentiated tumors, is specific for this tumor.

Small cell carcinoma accounts for 25% of bronchogenic carcinomas and arises centrally within main or

TABLE 15.3 Subtypes of Bronchogenic Carcinoma

Type	Incidence	Radiologic Features	Treatment	Five-Year Survival
Adenocarcinoma	35%	Peripheral nodule Peripheral mass	I–IIIa = surgery IV = XRT/chemo	17%
Squamous cell	25%	Hilar mass Atelectasis	I–IIIa = surgery IV = XRT/chemo	15%
Small cell	25%	Hilar mass Mediastinal mass	Chemotherapy	5%
Large cell	15%	Large peripheral mass	I–IIIa = surgery IV = XRT/chemo	11%

XRT, radiation therapy.

lobar bronchi. These tumors are the most malignant neoplasms arising from bronchial neuroendocrine (Kulchitsky) cells and are alternatively referred to as Kulchitsky cell cancers or KCC-3. Typical carcinoid tumors (KCC-1) represent the least malignant type, and atypical carcinoid tumors (KCC-2) are intermediate in aggressiveness. Small cell carcinomas exhibit a small endobronchial component, invading the bronchial wall and peribronchial tissues early in the course of disease. This produces a hilar or mediastinal mass with extrinsic bronchial compression and obstruction. Invasion of the submucosal and peribronchial lymphatics leads to local lymph node enlargement (Fig. 15.10) and hematogenous dissemination, which are almost invariable at the time of presentation. Microscopically, these malignant cells are tightly clustered, with nuclei molded together because of the scant amount of cytoplasm. This lesion is distinguished from carcinoid tumor histologically by the presence of mitoses. Electron

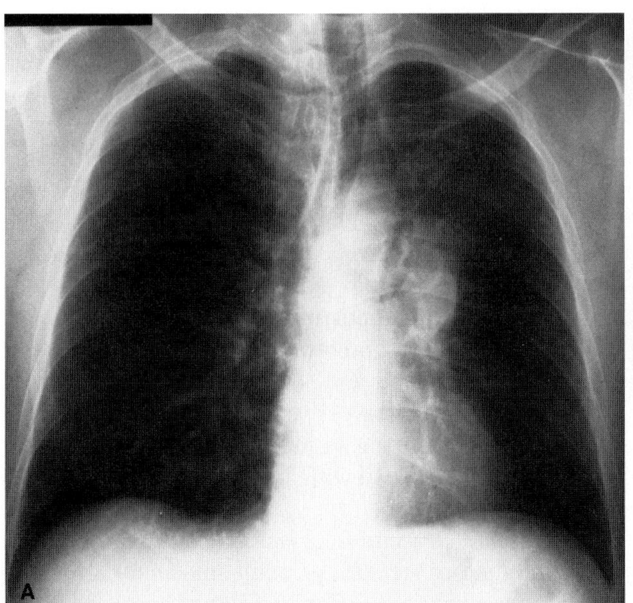

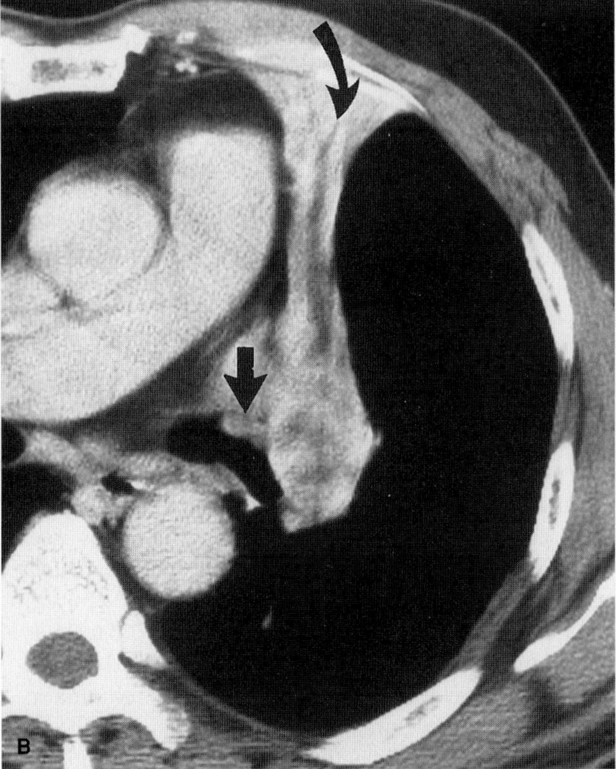

FIGURE 15.9. **Squamous Cell Carcinoma. A.** Posteroanterior chest film in a 58-year-old male smoker with hemoptysis shows a left hilar mass with left upper lobe atelectasis. **B.** Enhanced CT scan shows the left hilar mass occluding the left upper lobe bronchus with an endobronchial component (*straight arrow*). Note the presence of mucus bronchograms within the atelectatic lung (*curved arrow*).

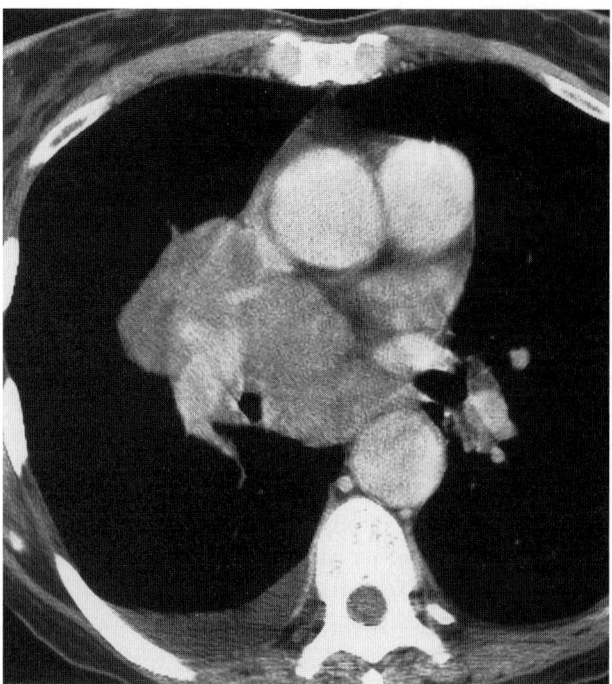

FIGURE 15.10. **Small Cell Carcinoma.** CT scan at the level of the bronchus intermedius demonstrates a large mass in the right hilum invading the middle mediastinum and subcarinal region. Cytologic examination of the associated right pleural effusion revealed small cell carcinoma.

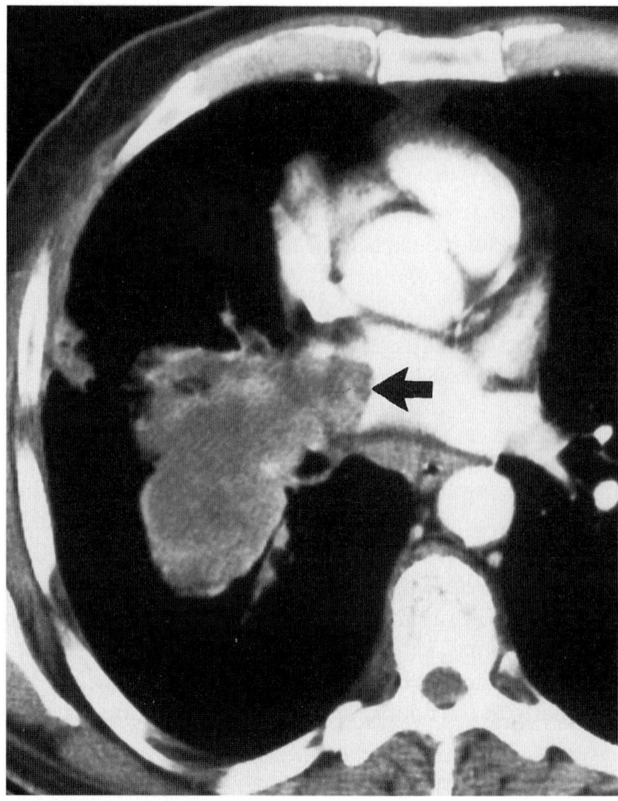

FIGURE 15.11. **Large Cell Carcinoma.** CT scan in a 53-year-old man reveals a right lung mass extending to the right hilum and invading the left atrium (*arrow*). CT-guided transthoracic biopsy showed large cell carcinoma.

microscopy demonstrates the presence of intracytoplasmic neurosecretory granules.

Large cell carcinoma accounts for 15% of bronchogenic carcinomas and is occasionally diagnosed when a non–small cell bronchogenic carcinoma lacks the histologic characteristics of squamous cell carcinoma or adenocarcinoma. Histologic features include large cells with abundant cytoplasm and prominent nucleoli. This tumor tends to arise peripherally as a solitary mass and is often large at the time of presentation (Fig. 15.11).

Epidemiology. The majority of patients with bronchogenic carcinoma are cigarette smokers who are over 40 years of age. Men are most commonly affected, although the percentage of female lung cancer patients has risen steadily in parallel with the increased prevalence of heavy cigarette smoking among women. The overall 5-year survival rate for all patients with lung cancer is 10% to 15%.

In addition to cigarette smoke, well-recognized risk factors for the development of bronchogenic carcinoma include asbestos exposure, previous Hodgkin lymphoma, radon exposure, viral infection, and diffuse interstitial or localized lung fibrosis. Cigarette smoke is by far the leading cause of lung cancer, with approximately 87% of cases attributed to smoking. The relationship between cigarette smoke and bronchogenic carcinoma is irrefutable, with the intensity of smoking (number of pack-years) showing the greatest positive correlation with development rates of malignancy. Lung cancer is uncommon in nonsmokers, and cigarette smoking is associated with a 10- to 30-fold increase in the incidence of bronchogenic carcinoma as compared to nonsmokers. Cessation of smoking decreases the risk of developing lung cancer, with the greatest decline found in those with the longest smoking cessation interval. Carcinogens in cigarette smoke produce cellular atypia and squamous metaplasia of the bronchiolar epithelium that may precede malignant transformation. Small cell carcinoma and squamous cell carcinoma are the two histologic subtypes with the strongest association with cigarette smoking in men, while cigarette smoking in women is associated with an increased incidence of all histologic subtypes.

A subset of cigarette smokers is at particular risk of developing lung cancer. Young adult smokers with bullous lung disease tend to develop their lung cancers at an earlier age than the general population of smokers. Proposed theories include greater susceptibility of the lining of the bulla to metaplastic transformation and impaired ventilation within the bulla leading to prolonged exposure to the carcinogens in cigarette smoke.

Asbestos exposure is associated with an increased incidence of bronchogenic carcinoma, malignant pleural mesothelioma, laryngeal carcinoma, and esophagogastric carcinoma. Bronchogenic carcinoma may follow prolonged exposure (usually 20 years or greater in duration) from the mining or processing of asbestos fibers. A long latency period from the initial asbestos exposure, generally 35 years or longer, is necessary for the development of bronchogenic carcinoma. While asbestos exposure alone is associated with a fourfold increase in the incidence of bronchogenic carcinoma, concomitant cigarette smoking, perhaps by acting as a cocarcinogen, is associated with a 40- to 50-fold increase in the incidence as compared to the nonexposed, nonsmoking individual.

Patients previously treated for mediastinal Hodgkin disease with radiation, chemotherapy, or a combination of the two have an eightfold increase in lung cancer beginning 10 years after treatment. Exposure to inhaled radioactive material, particularly radon, is associated with the development of small cell carcinoma of lung 20 years or more after the exposure.

The link between viral infection and bronchogenic carcinoma comes chiefly from the study of jaagsiekte, a disease of sheep that closely resembles bronchioloalveolar cell carcinoma of the lung in humans. This disease is caused by a retroviral infection, leading to speculation that a similar pathogenesis exists in humans with this subtype of adenocarcinoma.

It has been suggested that local lung scarring as a result of inflammation or infarction can induce the development of a "scar carcinoma," most commonly adenocarcinoma. Because adenocarcinoma can produce fibrous tissue, it is unclear whether the "scar" is the result or the cause of the carcinoma. Nevertheless, there are patients in whom a focal scar can be identified on prior radiographs in the region of a carcinoma. Diffuse interstitial fibrosis in patients with scleroderma has been associated with an increased incidence of bronchogenic carcinoma, particularly bronchioloalveolar cell carcinoma. Similarly, adenocarcinoma occurs with greater than expected frequency in patients with interstitial fibrosis associated with rheumatoid lung disease.

Radiographic findings in bronchogenic carcinoma depend on the subtype of cancer (4) and the stage of disease at the time of diagnosis. The two most common findings are an SPN (size between 2 mm and 3 cm) or mass (3 cm or larger in size) and a hilar mass with or without bronchial obstruction. All cell types can present with a pulmonary nodule. Because squamous and small cell carcinoma arise from the central bronchi, the majority of these types of bronchogenic carcinoma produce a hilar mass. The hilar mass represents either the extraluminal portion of the bronchial tumor or hilar lymph node enlargement from metastatic disease. Extension of the hilar lesion into the mediastinum or the presence of mediastinal nodal metastases can produce a smooth or lobulated mediastinal mass. Marked mediastinal nodal enlargement producing a lobulated mediastinal contour is characteristic of small cell carcinoma. Extensive replacement of the mediastinal fat by either primary tumor or extracapsular nodal extension may produce diffuse mediastinal widening, with loss of the mediastinal fat planes and compression or invasion of the trachea or central bronchi, esophagus, and mediastinal vascular structures, as seen on contrast-enhanced CT or MR.

Obstruction of the bronchial lumen by the endobronchial component of a tumor can result in several different radiographic findings. The most common finding is resorptive atelectasis or obstructive pneumonitis of lung distal to the obstructing lesion. Resorptive atelectasis is recognized by the classic findings of lobar or whole lung collapse, whereas obstructive pneumonitis results in minimal or no atelectasis or occasionally an increase in the volume of the affected portion of lung. An abnormal increase in lobar or whole lung volume is recognized radiographically by a bulging interlobar fissure marginating the obstructed lobe or by mediastinal shift, respectively, and is termed "drowned lung." Occasionally, the mass producing the lobar atelectasis creates a central convexity in the normally concave contour of the collapsed lobe, producing the S sign of Golden (Fig. 15.9). Most commonly, the opacity of the obstructed lung obscures the underlying central lesion. The lung with obstructive pneumonitis is not infected but rather shows a chronic inflammatory infiltrate and alveolar filling with lipid-laden macrophages; the latter finding accounts for the descriptive terms "golden" or "endogenous lipoid pneumonia."

Additional radiographic features of atelectasis that should suggest obstruction by tumor include obliteration of the main or proximal lobar bronchial air column, hilar mass, combined middle and lower lobe atelectasis, and atelectasis or opacification that persists beyond 3 to 4 weeks. CT confirms the presence of lobar atelectasis and typically demonstrates mucus bronchograms within the lung distal to the obstructing lesion (Fig. 15.9). The central mass is readily distinguished from vascular structures, with narrowing or occlusion of the bronchial lumen best seen on images viewed at lung windows. The central tumor is usually distinguished from atelectatic lung by the contrast between the perfused but nonventilated enhancing lung and the low-attenuation, nonenhancing central mass. An uncommon manifestation of bronchial obstruction by bronchogenic carcinoma is the development of mucoid impaction (mucocele). This represents mucus within dilated segmental bronchi distal to the obstructing neoplasm. The appearance has been likened to a gloved hand, with the dilated bronchi representing the fingers of the glove. Radiographic visualization of the mucocele requires collateral ventilation to the obstructed lobe or segment.

Tumors that arise from the bronchiolar or alveolar epithelium—namely, adenocarcinoma and large cell

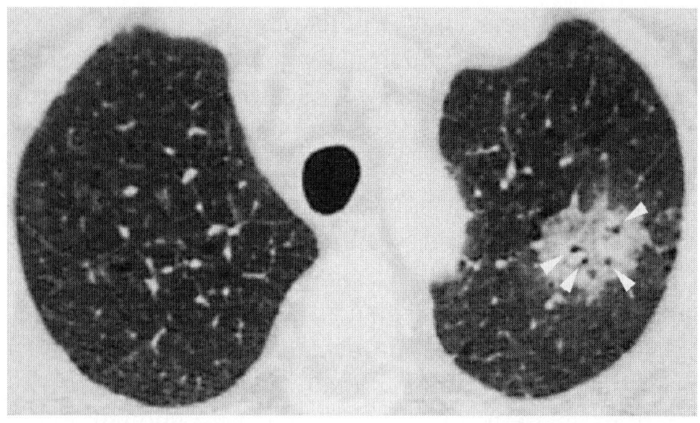

FIGURE 15.12. **Bronchioloalveolar Cell Carcinoma.** Thin-section CT in a 57-year-old woman shows a left upper lobe nodule containing cystic lucencies (*arrowheads*) and mixed solid/ground-glass attenuation. Biopsy proved bronchioloalveolar cell carcinoma.

carcinoma—commonly produce an SPN or mass on chest radiography. The radiographic evaluation of the SPN, in particular the size, growth rate, shape, margins, and internal density, has been reviewed in detail earlier in this chapter. A notched, lobulated, or spiculated margin to the nodule is common in bronchogenic carcinoma (Fig. 15.2). The radially spiculated appearance of a peripheral nodule has been termed "corona radiata." While it was initially thought to be pathognomonic for malignancy, the finding of a corona radiata is nonspecific and can be seen in granulomas. The edge characteristics of an SPN are best appreciated on thin-section HRCT images through the lesion.

Cavitation of solitary malignant nodules is uncommon. The walls of cavitating neoplasms tend to be thicker and more nodular than those of inflammatory lesions. The presence of air bronchograms or bubbly lucencies within a nodule or mass or mixed solid/ground-glass attenuation is highly suggestive of an adenocarcinoma, particularly bronchioloalveolar cell carcinoma (Fig. 15.12). Eccentric calcification within nodules may represent dystrophic calcification of necrotic regions, granulomas engulfed by an enlarging tumor, or calcification of mucin or psammoma bodies secreted by tumor cells in adenocarcinomas.

The size and growth pattern of an SPN are important characteristics. Masses >3 cm in diameter seen in adults over 35 years of age are overwhelmingly malignant. The volume-doubling time (equivalent to a 25% increase in diameter) for a malignant nodule usually ranges from 1 month (some squamous cell and large cell carcinomas) to 4 years (certain bronchioloalveolar cell carcinomas).

Pancoast (superior sulcus) tumor is a peripheral neoplasm arising in that portion of the lung apex indented superiorly by the subclavian artery. Although they can be of any cell type, the majority of these lesions are squamous cell carcinomas or adenocarcinomas. The presenting symptoms are related to invasion of adjacent structures, with arm pain and muscular atrophy attributable to brachial plexus involvement, Horner syndrome from involvement of the sympathetic chain, and shoulder pain from chest wall invasion (Fig. 15.13). The chest radiographic finding of an apical density may be mistaken for a pleuroparenchymal fibrous cap, which is a common finding in older individuals. Apical thickness exceeding 5 mm, asymmetry of the apical opacities of >5 mm, enlargement on serial radiographs, or evidence of rib destruction should prompt further evaluation with helical CT or MR. The presence of a mass with an inferior convex margin toward the lung and/or the presence of rib or vertebral body destruction are uncommon plain film findings. MDCT demonstrates the apical region to better advantage and is best for determining the extent of chest wall and vertebral invasion. Coronal and sagittal MR is useful for determining the relationship of the mass to the subclavian artery, brachial plexus, and spinal canal (Fig. 15.13).

Airspace opacification caused by bronchogenic carcinoma is an uncommon radiographic finding in the absence of an obstructing endobronchial lesion. BAC may produce airspace opacification as malignant cells grow along the preexisting parenchymal lattice while producing large amounts of mucus. The majority (60% to 90%) of BACs are localized and appear as SPNs. CT often shows air-filled bronchi within the lesion and a pleural tail extending from the tumor toward the pleural surface. The diffuse form may present as lobar or multilobar airspace opacification or as diffuse bilateral airspace nodules. These latter appearances may be indistinguishable from pneumonia or edema, although the clinical findings, chronicity of the process, and cytologic examination of sputum and bronchoalveolar lavage specimens should provide the correct diagnosis. The production of copious amounts of mucus by these tumors may be an occasional clinical feature. An additional finding on contrast-enhanced CT in patients with the diffuse form of BAC is the so-called "CT angiogram" sign within consolidated areas (Fig. 15.14). In these patients, filling of the airspaces with mucoid material produced by the malignant cells creates low-density airspace opacification surrounding the enhanced pulmonary arteries that traverses the consolidated regions. However, the CT angiogram sign is not specific for BAC and may be seen in other airspace-filling diseases, including lymphoma and lipoid pneumonia.

Superior vena cava (SVC) syndrome results from obstruction of the SVC from compression or invasion by mediastinal tumor, particularly small cell carcinoma or lymphoma. Lung cancer is the most common cause of SVC syndrome.

A malignant pleural effusion is an exudative fluid collection in a patient with proven malignancy that shows malignant cytology on thoracentesis or tumor on pleural biopsy. Although the presence of a pleural effusion in patients with bronchogenic carcinoma is associated with

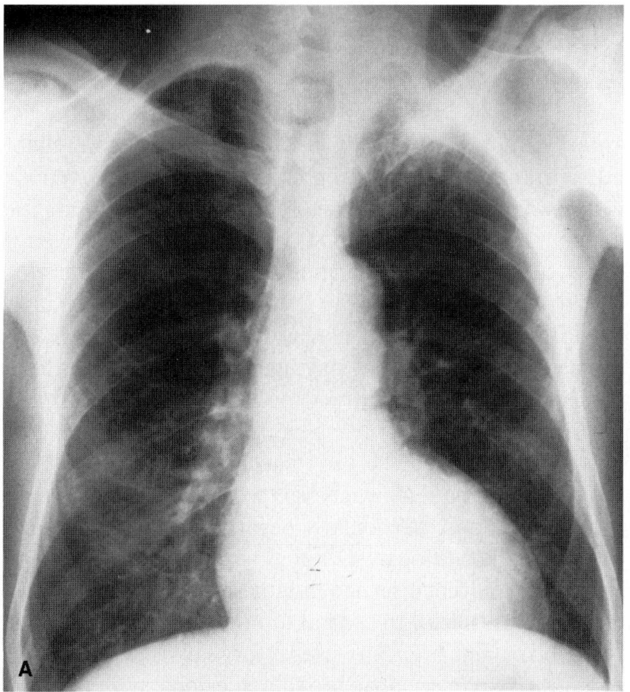

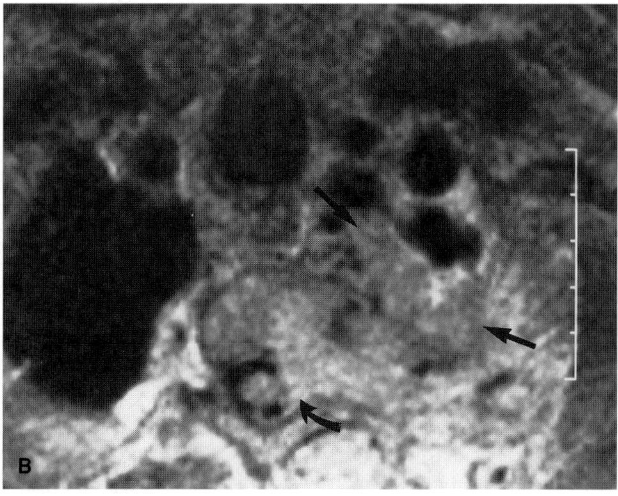

FIGURE 15.13. **Superior Sulcus (Pancoast) Tumor. A.** Posteroanterior chest film in a 56-year-old man with left shoulder and back pain reveals a left apical opacity. **B.** T1WI through the lung apices shows a left apical mass (*straight arrows*) with invasion of the spinal canal (*curved arrow*). Biopsy showed squamous cell carcinoma.

a poor prognosis, it is not synonymous with malignant pleural involvement, because central lymphatic obstruction and postobstructive infection can produce benign effusions in patients with malignancy. Smooth or lobulated pleural thickening or a discrete pleural mass suggests malignant pleural involvement. Contrast-enhanced CT may demonstrate pleural thickening or mass obscured by pleural fluid on plain radiographs. The utility of CT in the diagnosis of pleural and chest wall invasion is discussed in the section on lung cancer staging. Chest wall invasion is detected radiographically by the presence of an extrathoracic soft tissue mass or rib destruction. CT is more sensitive in detecting subtle bone destruction, while MR is better for detecting invasion of chest wall fat or muscle, particularly in superior sulcus tumors. Diaphragmatic elevation and paralysis may be seen with malignant invasion of the phrenic nerve. Progressive enlargement of the cardiac silhouette may be seen in patients with a malignant pericardial effusion; echocardiography and pericardiocentesis are diagnostic.

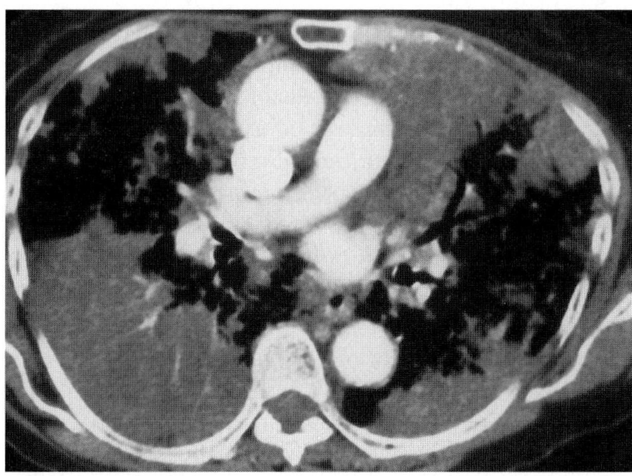

FIGURE 15.14. **Bronchioloalveolar Cell Carcinoma as Airspace Consolidation.** Enhanced CT scan in an 82-year-old woman with progressive dyspnea shows bilateral low-attenuation airspace opacification with visible pulmonary vessels ("CT angiogram sign"). Examination of sputum cytology showed bronchioloalveolar cell carcinoma.

Lymphangitic carcinomatosis represents invasion of the lymphatic channels of the lung by tumor. Invasion of lymphatics or neoplastic involvement of hilar and mediastinal nodes leads to retrograde (centrifugal) lymphatic flow with dilatation of lymphatic channels, interstitial deposits of tumor, and fibrosis. Radiographically, the typical findings are linear and reticulonodular opacities with peribronchial cuffing and subpleural edema or pleural effusion. In bronchogenic carcinoma, invasion and obstruction of lymphatics at the site of tumor may produce a segmental or lobar distribution of opacities. Lymphangitic spread to hilar and mediastinal lymph nodes produces unilateral lymph node enlargement with interstitial opacities, while hematogenous dissemination of tumor to the pulmonary capillaries

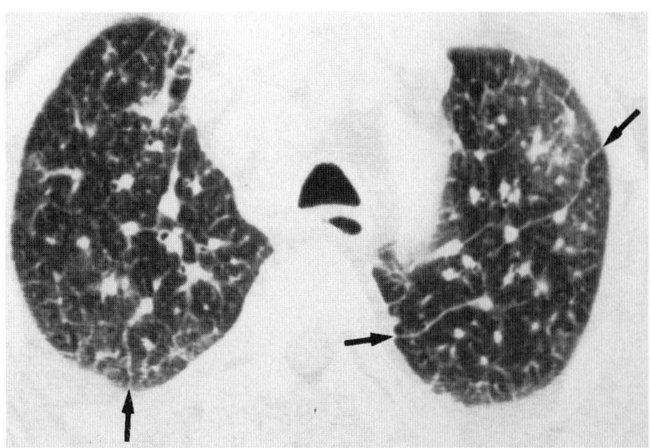

FIGURE 15.15. **Lymphangitic Carcinomatosis.** High-resolution CT through the upper lobes in a patient with colon carcinoma shows smooth and nodular thickening of the interlobular septa (*arrows*) representing lymphangitic carcinomatosis. The diagnosis was confirmed by transbronchial biopsy.

with secondary lymphatic invasion leads to bilateral interstitial abnormalities. Unilateral or asymmetric involvement of the lungs by lymphangitic tumor suggests lung cancer rather than an extrapulmonary site (Fig. 15.15; see Fig. 17.4). HRCT best demonstrates the characteristic smooth or beaded thickening of the interlobular septa and bronchovascular interstitium.

Diagnostic Evaluation. While prevention of lung cancer is the best and most cost-effective solution to the problem of lung cancer mortality, this is not achievable as long as the addictive habit of cigarette smoking is not entirely eliminated. Early detection and treatment have the potential to improve survival rates from this deadly disease. Screening with periodic chest radiographs in high-risk patients has not been shown to be effective because chest radiographs only detect lesions exceeding 1 cm in diameter. As a result of its cross-sectional format and volumetric data acquisition, MDCT is capable of routinely detecting lesions as small as 1 to 2 mm in diameter. Several nonrandomized studies have demonstrated promising results for cancer detection using low-dose spiral CT acquisition techniques. The potential drawback of increased radiation exposure with CT as compared to chest radiography for lung cancer screening has been minimized by reducing exposure factors (30 to 50 mA versus 120 mA). The higher cost of CT versus conventional radiography remains an obstacle to widespread screening. However, cost savings from early diagnosis and treatment is an additional benefit of screening high-risk patients.

FDG-PET scans have been shown to have a very high sensitivity and moderately high specificity in detecting malignant tumors. FDG is a glucose precursor that is incorporated into metabolically active cells but is not further metabolized. Because malignant tumors have a higher rate of glucose metabolism than most benign processes, increased FDG uptake is suggestive of malignancy. The current threshold for lung cancer detection appears to be a lesion size of 1 cm. This technique is not limited to primary tumor detection. PET scans using FDG can reliably discriminate between malignant and benign lymph nodes exceeding 1 cm in diameter. Sensitivities and specificities of approximately 90% and 80%, respectively, have been reported for lymph node staging using this technique (5). In particular, integrated PET-CT has improved the accuracy of PET imaging of lung cancer and should be considered in all patients for nodal staging. This is in contrast to CT and MR, where the accuracy for lymph node metastases is 60% to 70%.

Efforts to diagnose lung cancer should also attempt to stage the patient whenever possible so that management decisions, particularly regarding resectability, can be made expeditiously. Cytologic examination of sputum or bronchoalveolar lavage fluid is simple and inexpensive and is most useful in central tumors. Bronchoscopy with endobronchial biopsy is useful for the visualization and biopsy of main or lobar bronchial lesions, with bronchoscopically guided transcarinal Wang needle biopsy used to sample subcarinal masses. Endoscopic ultrasound has recently proven useful in mediastinal nodal sampling of periesophageal lymph nodes in patients with lung cancer. CT- or fluoroscopically guided transthoracic biopsy of peripheral masses can establish a diagnosis in over 90% of patients with lung cancer. Radiologically guided sampling of hilar or mediastinal masses in patients with negative bronchoscopic examinations can provide material for cancer diagnosis and staging. Where available, FDG-PET scans may complement CT and MR scans and decrease the need for more invasive staging procedures.

CT is obtained in all patients with possible bronchogenic carcinoma to guide efforts at tissue sampling. The detection of distal lesions in the adrenal gland, liver, or bones with biopsy of accessible lesions can provide both diagnostic and staging information. The relationship of the tumor to the central airways determines the utility of transbronchoscopic endobronchial or endotracheal biopsy, while the detection of large subcarinal nodes can direct transcarinal biopsy with a Wang needle. The pleura may be evaluated for thickening, masses, or effusions, suggesting that thoracentesis or closed pleural biopsy is the appropriate initial diagnostic procedure. Thoracotomy with resection of a peripheral lesion is appropriate for suspicious solitary lesions lacking clinical or CT evidence of unresectable nodal, mediastinal, pleural, or extrathoracic metastases. In some cases, patients with peripheral lesions may benefit from more limited surgery using VATS. Radiology may occasionally play a role in VATS by guiding placement of localizing needles and wires preoperatively using CT or intraoperative sonographic guidance.

Radiologic Staging of Lung Cancer

The primary role of the radiologist in imaging the patient with bronchogenic carcinoma is to determine the anatomic extent or stage of the tumor (6). This has prognostic importance and determines the resectability of the lesion. In patients with small cell carcinoma, which is almost invariably not a surgically curable disease, patients are divided into two groups: those with disease limited to one hemithorax (limited disease) and those with contralateral lung or extrathoracic spread (extensive disease). The staging of non–small cell bronchogenic carcinoma is based on the extent of the primary tumor (T), the presence of nodal involvement (N), and evidence of distant metastases (M). Using this TNM classification, lung cancer is divided into four stages. This TNM scheme has recently been modified (Table 15.4) (7). The major distinction in lung cancer staging is the division of patients with stage I to IIIa (resectable) from those with stage IIIb and IV (unresectable) disease (Table 15.5). Stage IIIa disease represents T3 disease (i.e., localized tumor invasion of the pleura, chest wall, diaphragm, or pericardium or tumor extending into the proximal main bronchus with sparing of the tracheal carina) associated with ipsilateral hilar nodal involvement (N1) or a T1 or T2 lesion associated with mediastinal or subcarinal nodal involvement (N2). The surgical techniques used for stage IIIa disease include en bloc resection of locally invaded chest wall, pleura, or pericardium; resection of proximal main bronchial tumors by resecting distal trachea and reimplanting the contralateral main bronchus into the proximal trachea; and mediastinal and subcarinal lymph node dissection with resection of the lung. Stage IIIb disease represents invasion of tracheal carina, mediastinum, major cardiovascular structures, esophagus, or vertebral body (T4); separate tumor nodules in the same lobe (T4); malignant pleural effusion (T4); or contralateral hilar, mediastinal, scalene, or supraclavicular nodal involvement (N3). The presence of distant metastases or separate tumor nodules in different lobes is classified as M1 or stage IV disease.

TABLE 15.4 TNM Classification of Lung Cancer

Primary Tumor (T)	
Tx	Malignant cells in sputum without identifiable tumor
T0	No evidence of primary tumor
T1	Tumor <3.0 cm in diameter, surrounded by lung or visceral pleura, arising distal to a main bronchus
T2	Tumor >3.0 cm in diameter; any tumor invading the visceral pleura; any tumor with atelectasis or obstructive pneumonitis of less than an entire lung; tumor must be >2 cm from the tracheal carina
T3	Any tumor with localized chest wall, diaphragmatic, mediastinal pleural, or pericardial invasion; the tumor may be <2 cm from the carina but cannot involve the carina
T4	Any tumor that invades the mediastinum or vital mediastinal structures including the heart, great vessels, trachea, carina, or vertebral body; separate tumor nodules in the same lobe; presence of a malignant pleural effusion
Nodal metastases (N)	
N0	No evidence of nodal metastases
N1	Metastasis to ipsilateral peribronchial or hilar nodes, including involvement by contiguous spread of tumor
N2	Metastasis to ipsilateral mediastinal or subcarinal nodes
N3	Metastasis to contralateral mediastinal or hilar nodes or scalene or supraclavicular nodes
Distant metastases (M)	
M0	No evidence of distant metastases
M1	Distant metastases; separate tumor nodules in different lobes

TABLE 15.5 Clinical Staging of Lung Cancer Based on TNM Classification

Stage	TNM
Ia	T1 N0 M0
Ib	T2 N0 M0
IIa	T1 N1 M0
IIb	T2 N1 M0
	T3 N0 M0
IIIa	T1 or T2 N2 M0
	T3 N1 or N2 M0
IIIb	Any T N3 M0
	T4 Any N M0
IV	Any T Any N M1

Primary Tumor (T). *Chest Wall Invasion.* Tumors invading the chest wall (including the superior pulmonary sulcus), diaphragm, mediastinal pleura, pericardium, or proximal main bronchus are considered resectable by many surgeons and are classified as T3 lesions (Fig. 15.16). In patients with superior sulcus tumors, vertebral body or mediastinal invasion or involvement of the brachial plexus or subclavian artery above the lung apex precludes surgical resection. Lower grade superior sulcus tumors can be treated by local irradiation followed by en bloc resection of the tumor and chest wall with reasonable survival rates.

Rib destruction or presence of an extrathoracic soft tissue mass are the only plain film findings specific for chest wall invasion; pleural thickening adjacent to a lung mass is nonspecific and need not indicate chest wall invasion. The CT diagnosis of chest wall invasion can be difficult, although CT should be obtained if this is suspected. CT findings suggestive of chest wall invasion are obtuse angles at the point of contact of the tumor and pleura, >3 cm of contact between tumor and pleura, pleural thickening adjacent to the mass, and infiltration of extrapleural fat. Extrathoracic extension of the mass or rib destruction are specific but insensitive CT findings for chest wall invasion (Fig. 15.16). Additional techniques that have been described to assess parietal pleural invasion by tumor include assessment of respiratory movement on dynamic expiratory CT and the use of diagnostic pneumothorax.

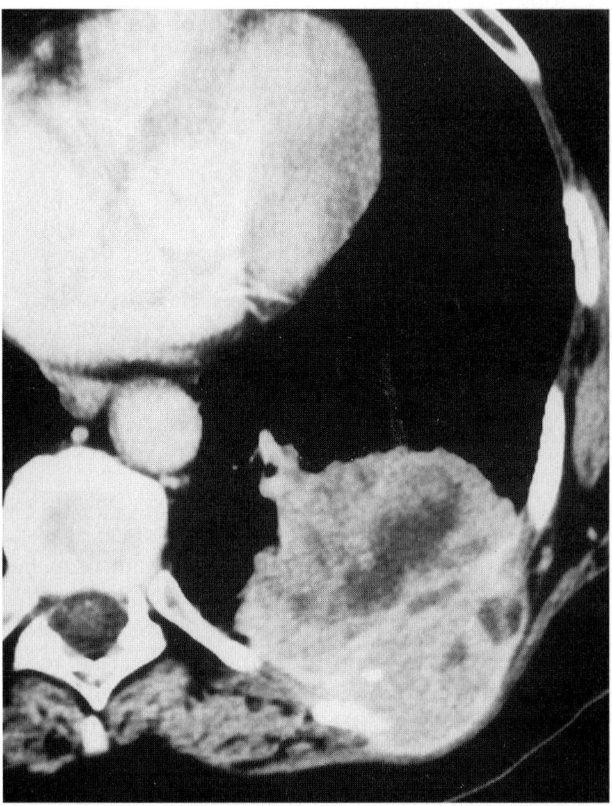

FIGURE 15.16. **T3 Tumor With Localized Chest Wall Invasion.** A CT scan through a large left lower lobe adenocarcinoma shows invasion of the posterior chest wall. A portion of the chest wall was removed en bloc with the tumor.

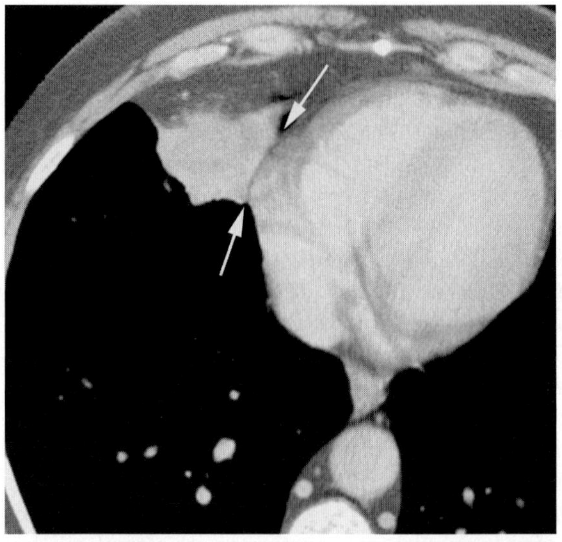

FIGURE 15.17. **CT to Assess Mediastinal Invasion of Lung Cancer.** In a patient with a medial segment, middle lobe, non–small cell carcinoma, CT shows a fat plane (*arrows*) between the lesion and the heart. Surgical resection confirmed the absence of pericardial or mediastinal invasion.

MR is equal to CT in its ability to diagnose chest wall invasion. T2WIs show excellent contrast between tumor and chest wall muscle and fat and are used in selected cases to detect chest wall invasion. MR also detects early obliteration of the high-signal extrapleural fat that may be an early finding in chest wall invasion. Coronal MR images are useful in superior sulcus tumors to determine chest wall, brachial plexus, or subclavian artery involvement.

Mediastinal Invasion. Tumor invasion of the mediastinum with involvement of the heart, great vessels, trachea, or esophagus (T4 tumor) precludes resection. Localized invasion of the mediastinal pleura or pericardium (T3 tumor) does not prevent resection, although extensive invasion with replacement of mediastinal fat does.

On conventional radiographs, a mediastinal mass, mediastinal widening, or diaphragmatic elevation (from phrenic nerve involvement) suggests invasion. As with the diagnosis of chest wall invasion, CT demonstration of tumor mass in contiguity with the mediastinal pleura or thickening of the mediastinal pleura does not necessarily indicate mediastinal extension or unresectability. However, a significant mediastinal mass that is contiguous with a lung tumor, compresses mediastinal vessels or esophagus, or replaces mediastinal fat strongly suggests this diagnosis. Other findings that may suggest mediastinal invasion include: (*1*) obliteration of the fat plane adjacent to the descending aorta or other mediastinal vessels, (*2*) tumor contacting more than one fourth of the circumference of the aortic wall, or (*3*) tumor contacting more than 3 cm of the mediastinum. If none of these findings are present, the tumor is potentially resectable, even though 29% of resectable lesions lacking any of these findings are found to invade the mediastinum locally (Fig. 15.17) (8).

As with CT, MR is incapable of accurately demonstrating mediastinal pleural invasion or minimal invasion of mediastinal fat. Mediastinal invasion can be diagnosed with a reasonable degree of accuracy when there is significant obliteration of fat planes or compression or displacement of mediastinal vessels. In one study, MR was found to be significantly more accurate than CT in diagnosing mediastinal invasion, but this result was based on a small number of patients who had invasion, and the study predated the advent of isotropic MDCT (8). Other studies have shown no significant advantage of MR over CT for this purpose. MR is occasionally performed when vascular invasion is suspected and is likely more accurate than CT in this regard.

Central Airway Involvement. Tumors that extend into a main bronchus within 2 cm of the tracheal carina (T3 tumors) are resectable. Although tracheal carinal involvement (T4 tumor) (Fig. 15.18) can be treated by carinal resection with end-to-side anastomosis of the remaining bronchus to the tracheal stump ("sleeve pneumonectomy"), most surgeons would consider this an unresectable tumor. Although plain films can occasionally demonstrate

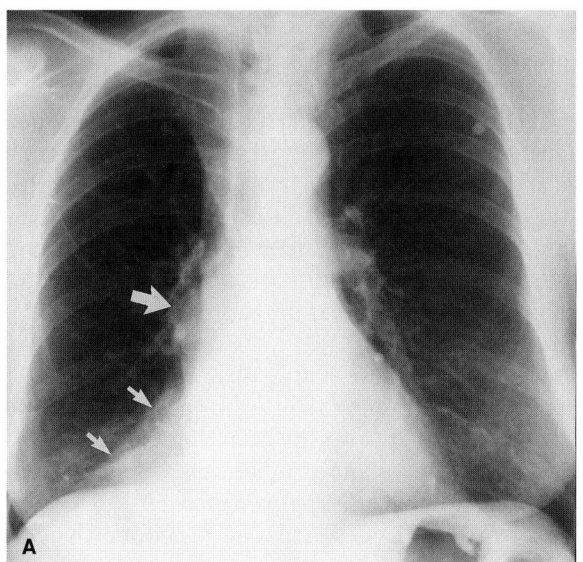

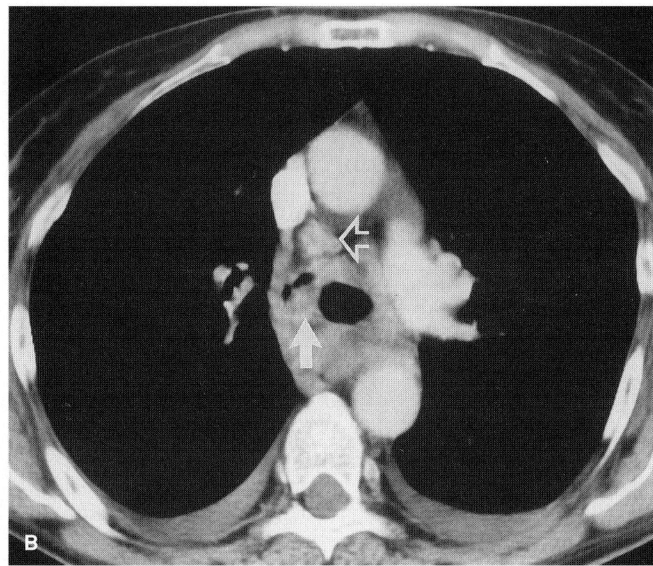

FIGURE 15.18. **Tracheal Carinal Involvement in Squamous Cell Carcinoma. A.** A frontal chest radiograph in a middle-aged woman with hemoptysis shows a mass in the lower right hilum (*large arrow*) with right lower lobe atelectasis (*small arrows*). **B.** A CT scan demonstrates a mass surrounding the main bronchi, with irregular narrowing of the right main bronchial lumen and infiltration of the tracheal carina (*arrow*). An enlarged precarinal lymph node (*open arrow*) and small bilateral pleural effusions are also seen. Bronchoscopy revealed invasion of the tracheal carina by squamous cell carcinoma.

a mass within the main bronchus or trachea, CT is more accurate in assessing the relationship of the mass to the tracheal carina (Fig. 15.18B). However, CT is known to underestimate the mucosal or submucosal extent of tumor as seen bronchoscopically. Therefore, any patient with a central lesion should undergo bronchoscopy to determine the proximal extent of the tumor, unless CT shows obvious carinal or tracheal invasion.

Multiple Tumor Nodules in the Same Lobe. The recent update to the International Staging System for non-small cell lung cancer classifies cases of satellite tumor nodules in the same lobe as the primary tumor as T4 disease, based on prognosis. Despite their IIIb categorization, most patients with multiple nodules in the same lobe and absent nodal or distant metastases will undergo attempts at curative resection.

Pleural Effusion. Malignant pleural effusion (T4 tumor) precludes curative resection of a tumor. In a patient with bronchogenic carcinoma, pleural effusion can occur for a variety of reasons, including pleural invasion, obstructive pneumonia, and lymphatic or pulmonary venous obstruction by tumor. Although the presence of effusion associated with lung cancer indicates a poor prognosis, only those patients with tumor cells in the pleural fluid or on pleural biopsy are considered unresectable. Other patients with effusion are considered to have "resectable" lesions, despite their poor prognosis. Usually plain radiographs, including decubitus films, are sufficient to diagnosis a pleural effusion. Thoracentesis with cytologic examination and/or pleural biopsy is necessary for definitive diagnosis of malignant pleural involvement. Pleural thickening >1 cm, lobulated pleural thickening, or circumferential pleural thickening (i.e., involvement of the mediastinal pleura) on CT or MR strongly suggests pleural invasion (Fig. 15.19). While PET can be useful in characterizing pleural effusions in patients with lung cancer as malignant, caution is advised in patients who have undergone prior pleurodesis, as focal plaques from intrapleural talc administration can be FDG avid on PET.

Lymph Node Metastases (N). Selected patients with ipsilateral mediastinal or subcarinal node metastases are classified as N2 and are considered potentially resectable. However, patients with N2 nodal disease (i.e., stage IIIa lung cancer) have a significantly worse prognosis as compared to patients classified with stage IIIa disease because of a T3 lesion. Those patients with N2 disease from nonbulky intracapsular nodal metastases limited to one mediastinal nodal station have the best 5-year survival rates following extensive mediastinal nodal dissection. Contralateral hilar or mediastinal, supraclavicular or infraclavicular nodal metastases represent N3 disease and are unresectable (Fig. 15.20).

The detection of a large mediastinal mass on chest radiograph in a patient with lung cancer requires mediastinoscopic or transthoracic biopsy confirmation of tumor invasion before deeming the patient unresectable. A

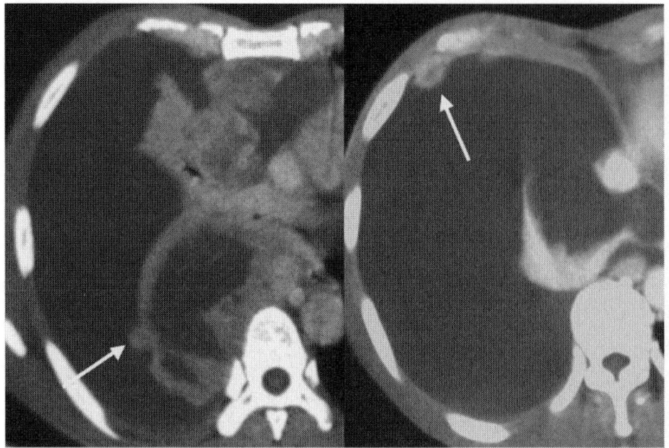

FIGURE 15.19. **Pleural Metastases (T4) in Bronchogenic Carcinoma.** CT images through the lower chest in a patient with a large right lower lobe tumor show a large pleural effusion with discrete pleural nodules (*arrows*) representing pleural metastases.

normal chest radiograph or the suggestion of hilar or mediastinal adenopathy should prompt a chest CT to assess the status of the lymph nodes. No single measurement allows completely accurate distinction of normal from malignant nodes. This is because malignant involvement does not always enlarge the lymph node (producing false-negative findings and reducing sensitivity), while enlarged nodes in patients with lung cancer may represent reactive hyperplasia rather than tumor replacement (producing false-positive findings and reducing specificity). If a small nodal diameter (5 mm) is used as the dividing point between benign and malignant, sensitivity will be excellent but specificity will be low. However, choosing a large nodal diameter (2 cm) increases specificity but decreases sensitivity. Most radiologists use a short-axis nodal diameter of 1 cm because this value achieves the best compromise of sensitivity and specificity.

Recent studies have shown that CT is relatively inaccurate in determining the nodal status of the patient with lung cancer. Both sensitivity and specificity for nodal metastases, when a short-axis diameter of 1 cm or greater is used as abnormal, are approximately 60% to 65% on a patient-by-patient basis and may be even lower when looking at individual nodal stations (9). Although CT cannot be considered accurate enough to determine with certainty whether or not mediastinal lymph nodes are involved by tumor, it can provide information of value in guiding invasive staging procedures such as mediastinoscopy, transcarinal Wang biopsy, endoscopic US–guided biopsy, and transthoracic or open biopsy. As discussed earlier, PET—particularly integrated PET-CT—provides superior accuracy in nodal staging of lung cancer (10).

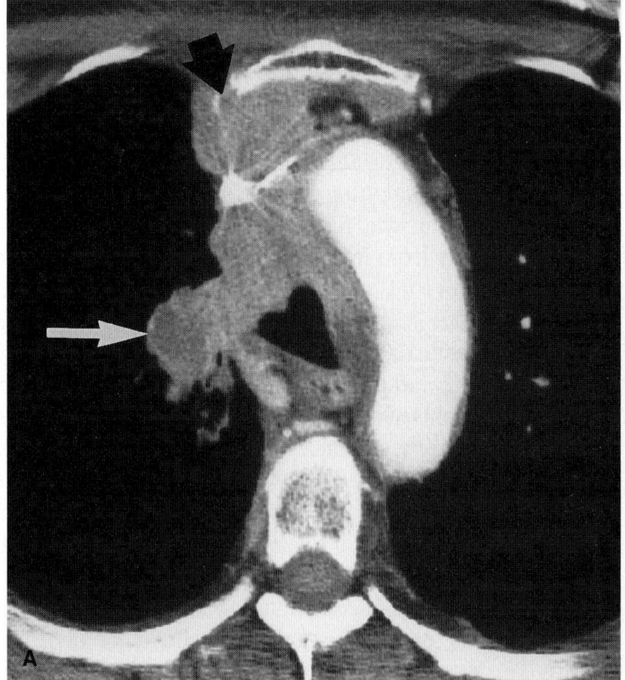

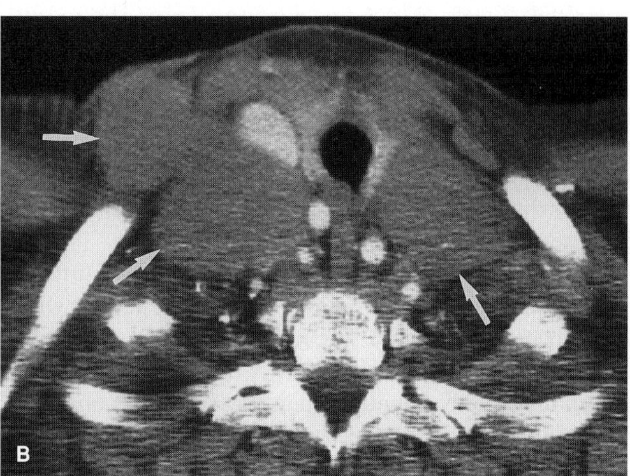

FIGURE 15.20. **N3 Nodal Metastases in Bronchogenic Carcinoma. A.** CT scan through the aortic arch in a 57-year-old man shows a right hilar mass (*white arrow*) invading the distal trachea and mediastinal fat (T4 tumor). There are enlarged prevascular lymph nodes (N2) (*black arrow*). **B.** Scan at the supraclavicular level shows marked bilateral supraclavicular lymphadenopathy (*arrows*) representing N3 disease.

In select institutions, mediastinoscopy complements CT in the nodal staging of lung cancer. Most patients with enlarged mediastinal nodes on CT that are accessible to transcervical mediastinoscopy (pretracheal, anterior subcarinal, and right tracheobronchial nodes) should have mediastinoscopy and biopsy. The decision of whether patients with negative CT studies for nodal enlargement should undergo mediastinoscopy depends on the local surgical practice. In patients with small, peripheral lung nodules, mediastinal metastases are uncommon, and thoracotomy may be warranted without prior CT or mediastinoscopy, but this remains controversial. Patients with borderline pulmonary function benefit most from mediastinoscopy, because a positive mediastinoscopic biopsy almost certainly precludes any attempt at resection.

The accuracy of MR is equal to that of CT in the diagnosis of mediastinal lymph node metastases, although it is rarely used for this purpose alone. There are specific advantages and disadvantages of MR in characterizing mediastinal lymph nodes. Clusters of normal-size nodes may be mistaken for a single enlarged nodal mass because of the limited spatial resolution of MR. MR is incapable of demonstrating calcification within nodes, which is diagnostic of benign lymph node disease. Aortopulmonary window and subcarinal nodes are nicely demonstrated on coronal MR images, although coronal reconstructions from MDCT can demonstrate enlarged nodes in these regions with equal efficacy.

Metastatic Disease (M). Each patient with proven lung cancer should be carefully evaluated for the presence of distant metastases (M1). Unequivocal evidence of metastases can obviate an unnecessary thoracotomy. Common sites of extrathoracic spread in patients with lung cancer include lymph nodes, liver, adrenal gland, bone, and brain. Metastases to lobes outside the primary lobe or to the other lung, although intrathoracic, are also considered M1 disease. Involvement of these sites probably represents hematogenous spread of tumor from the lung.

CT of the chest and upper abdomen is part of the initial evaluation in virtually all patients evaluated for bronchogenic carcinoma. This is adequate for assessing the liver, spleen, adrenal glands, and upper abdominal lymph nodes for evidence of metastases. US or MR may be used to distinguish soft tissue hepatic masses from incidental cysts. Technetium-99m-methylene diphosphonate radionuclide bone scanning or whole-body FDG-PET imaging is used to detect bone metastases, with preliminary studies suggesting that PET is as sensitive but more specific than bone scanning (7). Plain films are obtained to assess specific foci of abnormally increased bone tracer uptake or to evaluate localized bone pain.

Imaging of the brain is routinely performed in patients with symptoms or signs suggesting intracranial metastases. This usually involves MR or contrast-enhanced head CT. Head scanning in patients without clinical evidence of CNS involvement is somewhat more controversial. Because virtually all patients with isolated or asymptomatic brain metastases are found to have adenocarcinoma or large cell carcinoma, patients with these subtypes of bronchogenic carcinoma should have head CT scans, regardless of the clinical findings, to identify silent metastases. Patients with positive findings can be spared an unnecessary thoracotomy.

Approximately 60% to 65% of patients with small cell carcinoma have metastatic disease at the time of diagnosis. Because it is likely that all patients with small cell carcinoma have gross or microscopic metastatic foci at presentation, these patients are generally not candidates for curative surgical resection. However, accurate staging of these patients for extrathoracic involvement determines prognosis and allows for proper assessment of response to chemotherapy. An additional reason for extrathoracic staging of small cell carcinoma is the ability to manage localized bone or soft tissue involvement with radiation or resection.

Adrenal masses are seen in approximately 10% of patients undergoing staging CT examinations for bronchogenic carcinoma. However, approximately 5% of normal individuals are known to have benign adrenal cortical adenomas. In fact, isolated adrenal masses in patients with non–small cell bronchogenic carcinoma are twice as likely to be adenomas than metastases. In many patients, the adrenal mass is the only extrathoracic site of abnormality, making accurate diagnosis of the adrenal mass crucial in determining management.

Methods used to distinguish adenomas from malignant (primary or metastatic) adrenal lesions include CT, chemical-shift MR, FDG-PET, and fine-needle aspiration biopsy (see Chapter 33). The combined ability of unenhanced CT to detect lipid-rich adenomas ($\leq$10 H) and delayed enhanced CT to detect lipid-poor adenomas ($\geq$60% relative washout at 15 minutes) has been utilized with high accuracy to distinguish between adenomas and malignant adrenal lesions (Fig. 15.21). Chemical-shift MR is rarely used nowadays to characterize adrenal lesions. PET has a sensitivity approaching 100% for detecting adrenal metastases, such that a negative study effectively excludes this possibility. However, adenomas can be FDG avid and produce false-positive studies; therefore, isolated, FDG-positive adrenal lesions may require biopsy for definitive characterization.

TRACHEAL AND BRONCHIAL MASSES

Tracheal Neoplasms. Intratracheal masses may be divided into neoplastic (11) and nonneoplastic masses. Primary tracheal tumors are rare; however, 90% of all primary tracheal tumors in adults are malignant. The majority of primary tracheal malignancies arise from

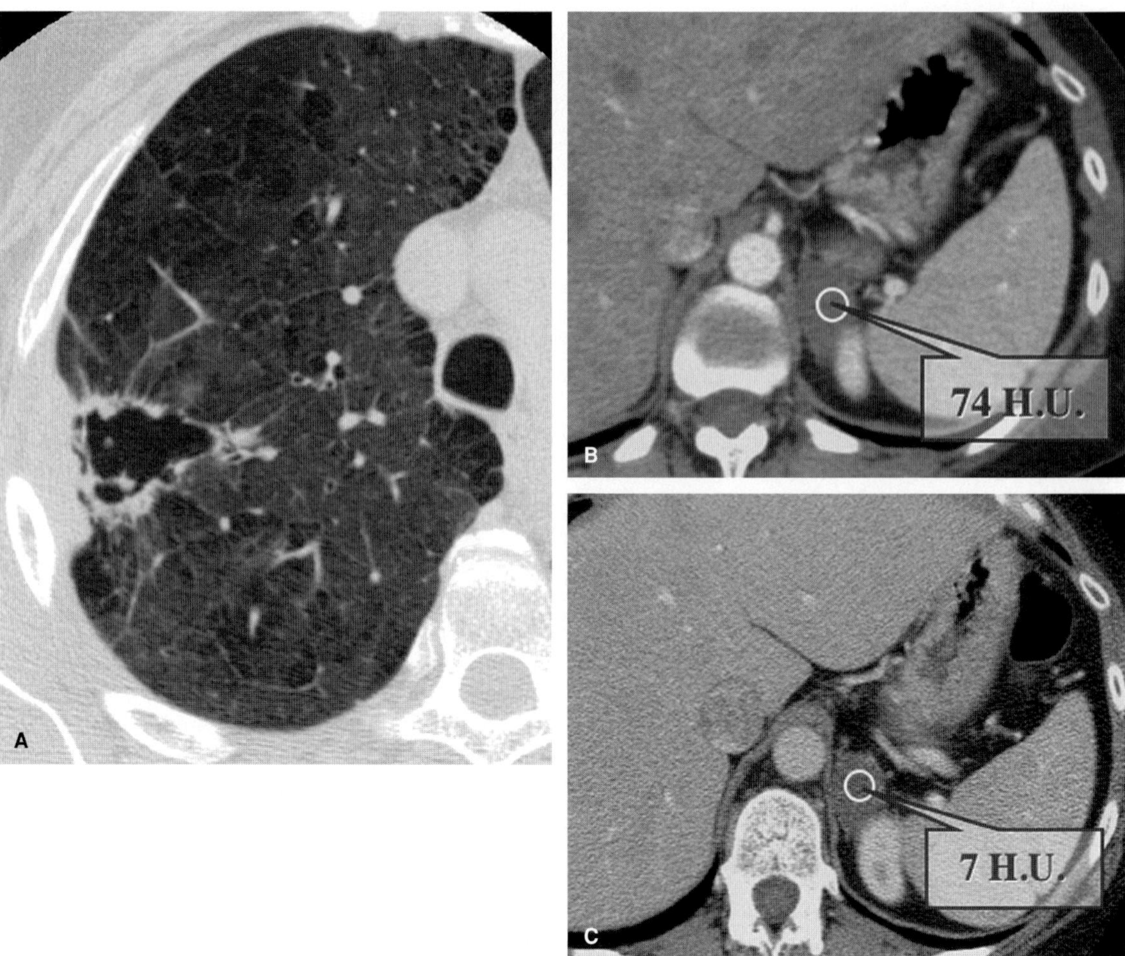

FIGURE 15.21. **Adrenal Mass Characterization by Delayed Enhanced CT.** In a patient with a cavitary right upper lobe cancer **(A),** dynamic enhanced scan **(B),** and 10-minute delayed enhanced **(C)** scans show a washout percentage of 90% ([74 – 7]/74 × 100), which is indicative of an adenoma.

tracheal epithelium or mucous glands (90%); the remainder arise from the mesenchymal elements of the tracheal wall (10%). Squamous cell carcinoma is the most common primary tracheal malignancy, accounting for at least 50% of all malignant tracheal neoplasms (Fig. 15.22). These tumors affect middle-aged male smokers and are associated with laryngeal, bronchogenic, or esophageal malignancies in up to 25% of cases. The majority arise in the distal trachea within 3 to 4 cm of the tracheal carina, with the cervical trachea the next most common site. Cough, hemoptysis, dyspnea, and wheezing are common presenting symptoms. Patients may be mistakenly treated for asthma before the correct diagnosis is made. Adenoid cystic carcinoma (formerly called cylindroma) is a malignant neoplasm that arises from the tracheal salivary glands and accounts for 40% of primary tracheal malignancies. This neoplasm tends to involve the posterolateral wall of the distal two thirds of the trachea or main or lobar bronchi.

The diagnosis of a primary tracheal malignancy is rarely made prospectively on chest radiographs, although well-penetrated radiographs can demonstrate distortion of the tracheal air column by a mass. CT typically shows a lobulated or irregular soft tissue mass that eccentrically narrows the tracheal lumen and has a variable extraluminal component (Fig. 15.22B). Masses >2 cm in diameter are likely to be malignant, while those <2 cm are more likely benign. Calcification is uncommon. Resectability of these lesions depends on the length of tracheal involvement and the extent of mediastinal invasion at the time of diagnosis. CT is particularly well suited for determining mediastinal involvement and has become the modality of choice for imaging tracheal neoplasms. The prognosis in patients with squamous cell carcinoma is poor, as up to 50% of patients have mediastinal extension of tumor at the time of diagnosis. While adenoid cystic carcinoma has a better prognosis, these slow-growing lesions are locally invasive with a tendency toward late recurrence and metastases.

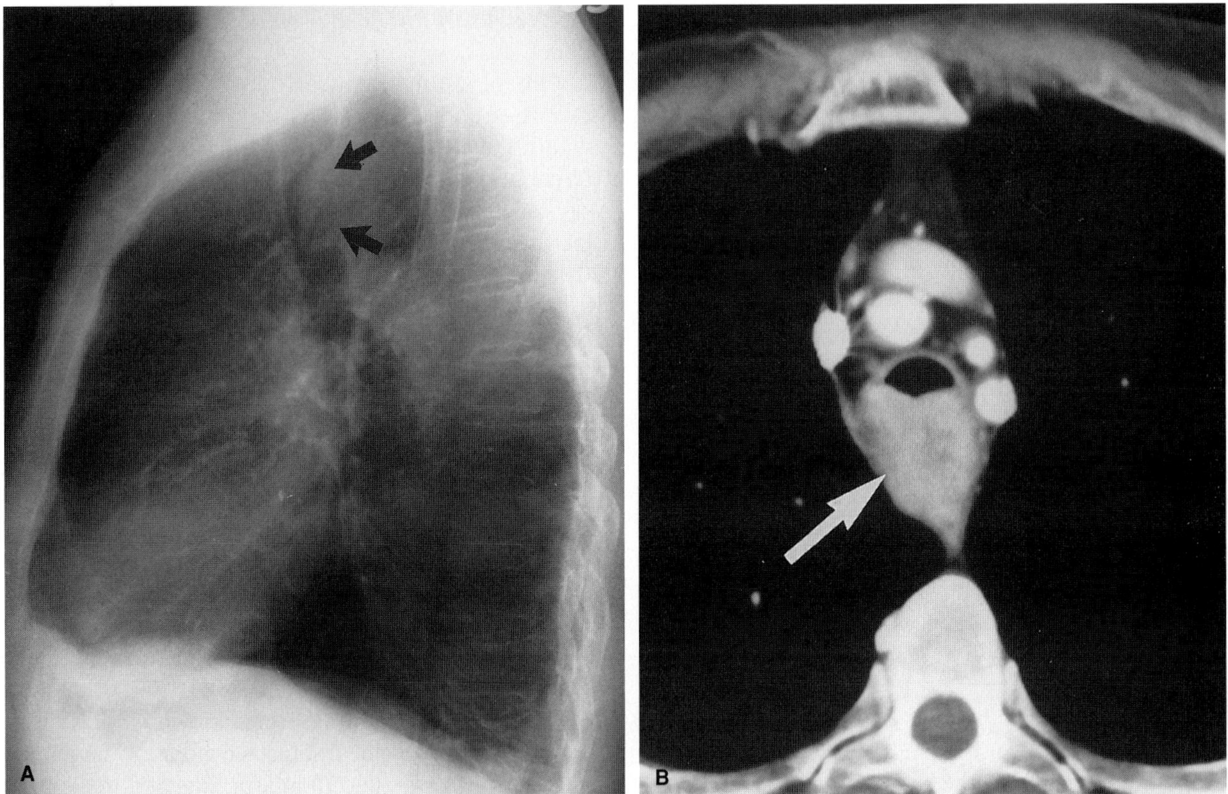

FIGURE 15.22. **Squamous Cell Carcinoma of the Trachea. A.** Lateral chest radiograph in a 68-year-old man shows a mass in the mid-trachea (*arrows*). **B.** CT scan demonstrates an enhancing mass (*arrow*) in the posterior trachea with narrowing of the tracheal lumen. Bronchoscopic biopsy showed squamous cell carcinoma.

A variety of other lesions comprise the remainder of primary tracheal malignancies and include mucoepidermoid carcinoma, carcinoid tumor, adenocarcinoma, lymphoma, small cell carcinoma, leiomyosarcoma, fibrosarcoma, and chondrosarcoma. Chondrosarcoma arises from tracheal cartilage and is identified by the presence of calcified chondroid matrix within the tumor. The trachea may be secondarily involved by malignancy, either by direct invasion or by hematogenous spread. Laryngeal carcinoma may extend below the vocal cords to involve the cervical trachea. There is also a tendency for tumor to recur at the tracheostomy site in patients who have undergone total laryngectomies for carcinoma. Papillary and follicular carcinoma are the most common types of thyroid malignancy to invade the trachea. Squamous cell carcinoma of the upper third of the esophagus can invade the posterior tracheal wall and may produce a tracheoesophageal fistula. Bronchogenic carcinoma may involve the trachea by direct proximal extension from central bronchi, by extranodal spread of tumor from metastatic pretracheal or paratracheal lymph nodes, or by direct invasion of large right upper lobe tumors. CT is best at demonstrating tumor invasion of the tracheal wall and the extent of intraluminal mass. The extrathoracic primary tumors that are most often associated with hematogenous endotracheal metastases are carcinomas of the breast, kidney, and colon and melanoma. These lesions may appear on CT as irregular thickening of the tracheal wall or as well-defined, localized masses that are indistinguishable from benign tracheal tumors.

Chondroma, fibroma, squamous cell papilloma (Fig. 15.23), hemangioma, and granular cell myoblastoma are the most common benign tracheal tumors in adults. A *chondroma* arises from the tracheal cartilage and produces a well-circumscribed endoluminal mass. CT may demonstrate stippled cartilaginous calcification within the mass. *Fibromas* are sessile or pedunculated fibrous masses arising in the cervical trachea. *Squamous cell papilloma* is a mucosal lesion caused by infection with human papilloma virus. This disease typically produces multiple laryngeal masses in children born to women with venereal warts (condylomata acuminata). The trachea, bronchi, and lungs may become involved over time. These lesions usually regress by adolescence and therefore are uncommon causes of a solitary tracheal lesion in adults. *Hemangiomas* are seen in the cervical trachea almost exclusively in infants and young children; they appear as focal masses on CT. *Granular cell myoblastoma* is a neoplasm that arises

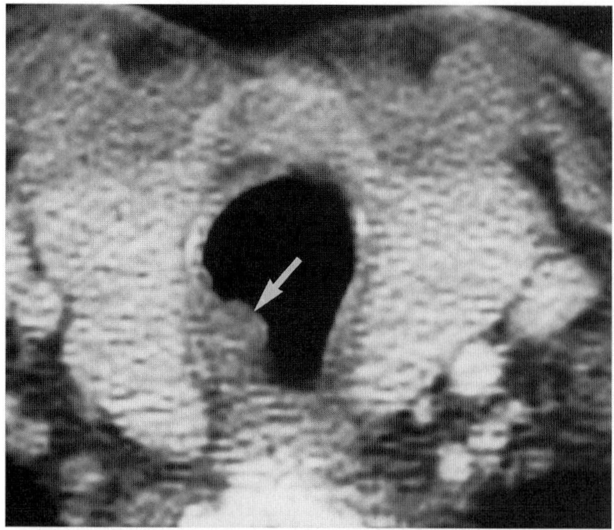

FIGURE 15.23. **Squamous Cell Papilloma.** Magnified view of a CT scan at the level of the thyroid in a 48-year-old man with laryngotracheal papillomatosis shows a mural nodule (*arrow*) along the right posterolateral wall of the trachea, representing a squamous cell papilloma.

from neural elements in the tracheal or bronchial wall. These lesions usually involve the cervical trachea or main bronchi. CT shows a broad-based or pedunculated soft tissue mass that may invade the tracheal wall. This neoplasm has a tendency toward local recurrence.

Nonneoplastic intratracheal masses from ectopic intratracheal thyroid or thymic tissue have been reported and are radiographically indistinguishable from intratracheal neoplasms. Intratracheal thyroid is seen in women with extratracheal goiters. The intratracheal tissue is likewise goitrous and most commonly found in the posterolateral wall of the cervical trachea, although any portion of the trachea may be involved. Mucus plugs may appear as intratracheal masses in patients with excess sputum production or diminished clearance mechanisms. They are typically low-attenuation masses on CT that change position or disappear after an effective cough.

Primary malignant neoplasms of the central bronchi include carcinoma, carcinoid tumor, and bronchial gland tumors (adenoid cystic carcinoma and mucoepidermoid carcinoma). Carcinoid and bronchial gland tumors account for approximately 1% of all tracheobronchial neoplasms; 90% of these lesions arise in a bronchus or lung, while the remainder arise within the trachea. Carcinoid tumor accounts for nearly 90%, adenoid cystic carcinoma 8%, and mucoepidermoid 2% of these lesions. However, adenoid cystic carcinoma accounts for 90% and carcinoid 10% of all malignant tracheal neoplasms excluding bronchogenic carcinoma. The use of the term "bronchial adenoma" to describe these lesions is misleading because these are malignant tumors that tend to locally invade and metastasize to regional lymph nodes.

Carcinoid tumors arise from neuroendocrine (amine precursor uptake and decarboxylation or Kulchitsky) cells within the airways. There is a spectrum of histologic differentiation and malignant behavior in tumors of Kulchitsky cell origin, ranging from the low-grade malignant typical carcinoid (KCC-1) to atypical carcinoid (KCC-2) to the highly malignant small cell carcinoma (KCC-3). Eighty percent of bronchial carcinoid tumors arise within central bronchi, and patients present with cough, dyspnea, wheezing, recurrent episodes of atelectasis or pneumonia, or hemoptysis (Fig. 15.24). The hemoptysis may be massive and is attributable to the highly vascular nature of these lesions. The average age at diagnosis is 50. Histologically, these tumors show sheets or trabeculae of uniform cells separated by a fibrovascular stroma. The cells may contain intracytoplasmic inclusions; immunohistochemistry will reveal a variety of neuroendocrine products, including serotonin, vasoactive intestinal polypeptide, adrenocorticotropic hormone, and antidiuretic hormone. Carcinoid syndrome is seen in fewer than 3% of cases.

Radiologically, central bronchial carcinoids present with atelectasis or pneumonia secondary to large airway obstruction. A hyperlucent lobe or lung of diminished volume may result from incomplete obstruction or collateral airflow with reflex hypoxic vasoconstriction; this finding is also rarely seen in bronchogenic carcinoma. Carcinoids

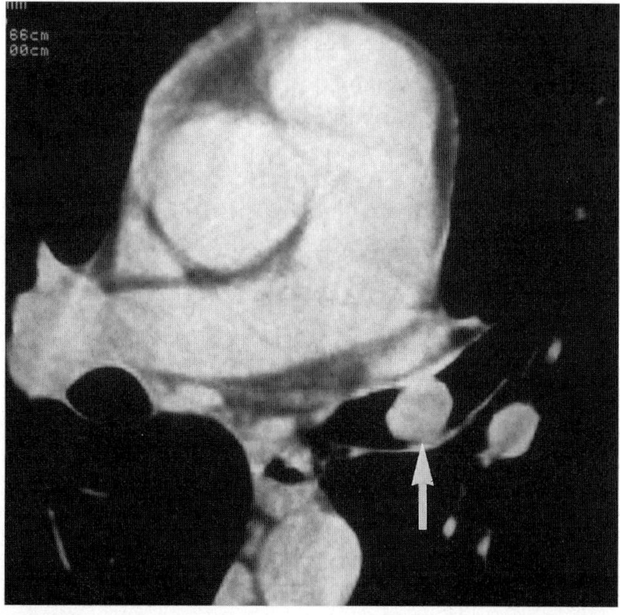

FIGURE 15.24. **Bronchial Carcinoid.** CT scan through the left upper lobe bronchus in a 35-year-old man shows a smooth endoluminal mass (*arrow*) at the junction of the left main and upper lobe bronchi. Bronchoscopic biopsy showed carcinoid tumor, which required a left pneumonectomy for curative resection.

arising within the lung have a propensity to involve the right upper and middle lobes and appear as well-defined smooth or lobulated nodules or masses. Calcification or ossification is seen in 10% of pathologic specimens but is rarely visualized on plain radiographs. CT is ideally suited to demonstrate the relationship of the mass to the central airways. The typical appearance on CT is a smooth or lobulated soft tissue mass within a main or lobar bronchus (Fig. 15.24). The presence of a small intraluminal and large extraluminal soft tissue component has given rise to the descriptive term "iceberg tumor." Atypical carcinoids tend to have more irregular margins and inhomogeneous contrast enhancement and are much more likely to be associated with hilar and mediastinal lymph node metastases. In some cases, the presence of small punctate peripheral calcifications or marked contrast enhancement on CT may allow distinction from bronchogenic carcinoma.

The prognosis for patients with typical bronchial carcinoid is excellent, with a 5-year survival rate of 90%. Regional lymph node metastases, seen in approximately 5% of operative specimens, lower the 5-year survival rate to 70%. Atypical carcinoids are associated with metastases in up to 70% of cases, although these may appear many years after discovery of the primary tumor. The 5-year survival rate in these patients is less than 50%.

Pulmonary hamartoma is a benign neoplasm comprised of disorganized epithelial and mesenchymal elements normally found in the bronchus or lung. Histologically, these lesions contain cartilage surrounded by fibrous connective tissue, with variable amounts of fat, smooth muscle, and seromucous glands; calcification and ossification are seen in 30% of cases. Ninety percent of these lesions arise within the pulmonary parenchyma; fewer than 10% are endobronchial. Endobronchial hamartomas are usually pedunculated lesions with fatty centers covered by fibrous tissue that contain little cartilage. Patients are usually diagnosed in the fifth decade. Central bronchial hamartomas present with cough or upper airway obstruction. CT shows a soft tissue mass that is usually indistinguishable from a bronchial carcinoid.

METASTATIC DISEASE TO THE THORAX

The spread of extrapulmonary neoplasm to the lung may occur by direct invasion of the pulmonary parenchyma or as a result of hematogenous dissemination, with the latter mechanism much more common (12). Rarely, a tumor can disseminate throughout the lungs via the tracheobronchial tree, as in laryngotracheal papillomatosis and some cases of bronchioloalveolar cell carcinoma. Transpleural spread of tumor can be seen in cases of invasive thymoma.

Direct invasion of the lung may occur with mediastinal, pleural, or chest wall malignancies. The most common mediastinal malignancies to invade the lung are esophageal carcinoma, lymphoma, and malignant germ cell tumors, or any malignancy metastasizing to mediastinal or hilar lymph nodes. Malignant mesothelioma and metastases to the pleura or chest wall can extend through the pleura to invade the adjacent lung.

Hematogenous metastases to the lung may be seen with any tumor that gains access to the SVC, inferior vena cava, or thoracic duct, because the pulmonary artery is the final common pathway for these channels. Although only a minority of tumor emboli survive within the pulmonary interstitium, those that do produce one of two morphologic and radiographic appearances: pulmonary nodules or lymphangitic carcinomatosis.

Pulmonary nodules are the most common manifestation of hematogenous metastases to the lung. They are most commonly seen in carcinomas of the lung, breast, kidney, thyroid, colon, uterus, and head and neck. Although most patients have multiple nodules, metastases can present as SPNs. SPNs caused by metastasis are typically smooth in contour, while primary bronchogenic tumors tend to be lobulated or spiculated. The likelihood that an SPN represents a solitary metastasis in a patient with a synchronous extrathoracic malignancy is slightly less than 50%, while SPNs in patients with prior malignancies are almost always primary bronchogenic tumors or granulomas. However, the site of the primary tumor may affect the likelihood that an SPN is a metastasis. Carcinoma of the rectosigmoid colon, osteogenic sarcoma, renal cell carcinoma, and melanoma are more likely to result in solitary pulmonary metastases. It should be cautioned that what may appear as a solitary metastasis on plain radiographs may be only one of multiple pulmonary nodules as shown by chest CT.

Nodular pulmonary metastases are usually smooth or lobulated lesions that are found in greater numbers in the peripheral portions of the lower lobes because of the greater pulmonary blood flow to these regions. Helical CT is the modality of choice for the evaluation of pulmonary metastases because it is considerably more sensitive than plain radiographs, conventional whole lung tomography, and incremental CT in detecting lung nodules. There are no characteristic features of nodular metastases that allow distinction among different primary neoplasms. Similarly, the distinction between metastases and granulomas is usually impossible, although there are three findings on CT that may help in this regard. First, the demonstration of a feeding vessel entering the central aspect of a well-defined peripheral pulmonary nodule strongly suggests hematogenous metastases; however, this may be seen in other bloodborne pulmonary processes such as pulmonary infarcts and septic emboli. Second, the demonstration of calcification within multiple pulmonary nodules, in the absence of a history of a primary bone-forming neoplasm such as osteogenic sarcoma or chondrosarcoma, is diagnostic of granulomas. Although primary mucinous adenocarcinomas of the colon and ovary may rarely produce

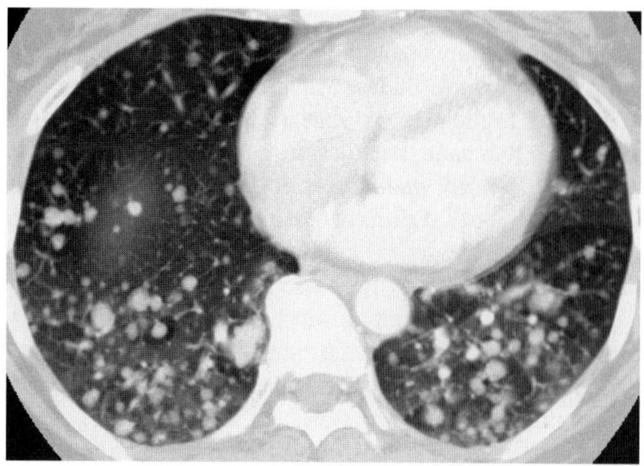

FIGURE 15.25. **Nodular Pulmonary Metastases.** CT scan through the lower lobes in a 50-year-old woman with metastatic papillary carcinoma of the thyroid shows multiple smooth nodules, reflecting hematogenous pulmonary metastases.

calcification within pulmonary metastases, these microscopic calcifications are usually too small to be detected, even on CT. Finally, in patients with miliary nodular opacities, the presence of one or more larger nodules interspersed with uniformly sized miliary nodules is highly suggestive of metastases from melanoma or carcinoma of the lung, thyroid (Fig. 15.25), or kidney.

The diagnosis of nodular pulmonary metastases is usually presumptive. It is based on the demonstration of multiple pulmonary nodules in a patient with a known malignancy that has a propensity for lung metastases who lacks evidence of a granulomatous process. In some patients, particularly those with SPNs and no evidence of additional sites of metastases, or those with a history of a prior localized malignancy, a biopsy of the nodule should be performed. Although most patients with extrathoracic malignancy who have malignant SPNs have primary bronchogenic carcinoma, patients with an SPN and a history of melanoma, seminoma, or sarcoma are more likely to have a solitary metastasis. In selected patients, resection of a solitary pulmonary metastasis or several peripheral metastases may be undertaken. CT is the best imaging modality to follow the response of metastases to chemotherapy, with resolution of nodules indicating a positive response. An important caveat is that persistent nodular opacities representing sterilized tumor deposits may be seen following successful treatment of metastatic choriocarcinoma or seminoma. In these patients, follow-up CT scans will demonstrate a lack of growth of these "sterile" nodules.

Lymphangitic Carcinomatosis (LC). While direct parenchymal lymphatic invasion and obstruction of hilar and mediastinal lymph nodes by bronchogenic carcinoma is the most common cause of unilateral LC, extrapulmonary malignancies may invade pulmonary lymphatics after hematogenous dissemination to both lungs to produce interstitial deposits of tumor. In LC, the tumor cells invade the lymphatics within the peribronchovascular and peripheral interstitium, resulting in lymphatic dilatation, interstitial edema, and fibrosis. The most common extrathoracic malignancies to produce LC are carcinomas of the breast, stomach, pancreas, and prostate. Occasionally, LC will present in a patient without a known primary malignancy. Most patients with LC have slowly progressive dyspnea and a nonproductive cough.

The chest radiographic findings in LC complicating extrathoracic malignancy correlate with the involvement of the peribronchovascular and peripheral interstitium seen pathologically. Peribronchial cuffing and linear opacities, particularly Kerley B lines, are characteristically seen. Coarse reticulonodular opacities may also be present. Concomitant hilar and mediastinal lymph node enlargement need not be present.

The predominant HRCT findings in lymphangitic carcinomatosis are thickening of interlobular septa and the subpleural interstitium (Fig. 15.15, see Fig. 17-4). While nodular thickening of the septa, reflecting tumor nodules, is characteristic of LC, it is seen in only a minority of patients. The thickened septal lines do not distort the pulmonary lobule, a feature that helps distinguish LC from interstitial fibrosis, which characteristically distorts the normal lobular shape. Visibility of the intralobular bronchioles or prominence of the centrilobular vessel is frequently seen, as is thickening of the peribronchovascular interstitium within the central (parahilar) portions of the lung. The findings may be unilateral or even limited to one lobe, particularly when LC occurs secondary to bronchogenic carcinoma. Because most patients with LC have pathologic involvement of the peribronchovascular interstitium, the diagnosis is best made by transbronchial biopsy. In a patient with the appropriate history, the HRCT appearance of lymphangitic spread may be specific enough to obviate the need for transbronchial biopsy. Occasionally, the HRCT study will demonstrate the typical findings of LC when the conventional radiograph is normal or equivocal.

NONEPITHELIAL PARENCHYMAL MALIGNANCIES AND NEOPLASTIC-LIKE CONDITIONS

Lymphoma. Parenchymal involvement in Hodgkin disease is two to three times more common than in non-Hodgkin lymphoma. Parenchymal abnormalities in Hodgkin lymphoma usually produce linear and coarse reticulonodular opacities that extend directly into the lung from enlarged hilar lymph nodes. Extensive areas of parenchymal involvement can produce masslike opacities and areas of airspace opacification. Atelectasis in Hodgkin disease is rarely caused by extrinsic nodal compression of the bronchi, but rather develops from an obstructing endobronchial tumor. Extension into the subpleural lymphatics may produce subpleural plaques or masses that are visible only by CT. While parenchymal involvement in Hodgkin disease does not occur in the absence of hilar and mediastinal nodal disease (excluding patients who have undergone mediastinal irradiation), non-Hodgkin lymphoma may involve the parenchyma without concomitant nodal disease in up to 50%. The parenchymal involvement most often appears as masses or airspace opacities (Fig. 15.8); the latter may simulate lobar pneumonia. Coarse reticulonodular or tree-in-bud opacities are uncommon, and rarely, an SPN is the sole manifestation of intrathoracic disease. Most cases of primary pulmonary non-Hodgkin lymphoma arise from the BALT and represent low-grade B-cell lymphomas.

Nodular Lymphoid Hyperplasia. This entity, previously termed *pseudolymphoma*, is used to describe a localized nonneoplastic reactive proliferation of lymphocytes in the lung. Histologically, the distinction from well-differentiated lymphoma may be difficult; the demonstration of a polyclonal population of lymphocytes with multiple germinal centers and the absence of lymph node enlargement are necessary for the diagnosis. This condition produces a sharply marginated pulmonary nodule or mass. The mass may contain air bronchograms as alveoli are compressed by large numbers of interstitial lymphocytes. Nodular lymphoid hyperplasia is usually associated with a good prognosis, although it may develop into lymphoma in patients with Sjögren syndrome.

Lymphocytic interstitial pneumonitis or diffuse lymphoid hyperplasia is an infiltration of the pulmonary interstitium by mature lymphocytes that is histologically indistinguishable from nodular lymphoid hyperplasia. Patients with Sjögren syndrome, hypogammaglobulinemia, multicentric Castleman disease and AIDS are at particular risk for this condition. Radiographically, a predominantly lower lobe reticulonodular and linear pattern of disease is seen, often with intermixed areas of airspace opacification. CT findings include diffuse ground-glass opacity, poorly defined centrilobular nodules, and thin-walled cysts (Fig. 15.26); lymph node enlargement may be an associated finding. Some patients with this disorder develop frank pulmonary lymphoma or interstitial fibrosis; others resolve with the administration of corticosteroid treatment. In children with AIDS, the course of lymphocytic interstitial pneumonitis is often indolent.

Posttransplant lymphoproliferative disorder represents a spectrum of entities ranging from benign polyclonal lymphoid proliferation to aggressive non-Hodgkin lymphoma that develop in a small percentage of transplant patients, with lung transplant recipients most commonly affected. Infection with Epstein-Barr virus is responsible for most cases. The disease often presents with extranodal disease, with the lung commonly involved. The most common imaging finding is that of solitary or multiple sharply

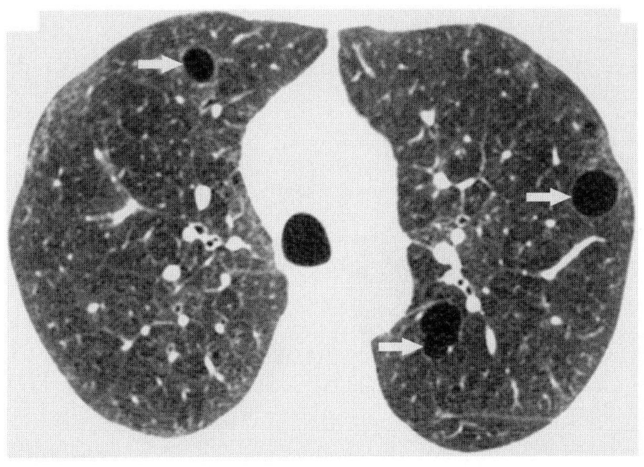

FIGURE 15.26. **Lymphocytic Interstitial Pneumonitis.** CT scan through the upper lobes in a 52-year-old man with AIDS shows characteristic ground-glass opacity with thin-walled cysts (*arrows*), indicative of lymphocytic interstitial pneumonitis.

marginated nodules or masses. Treatment varies, but for indolent forms of disease, reduction in immunosuppression is effective.

Lymphomatoid granulomatosis was originally thought to represent a distinct histologic entity but has recently been reclassified as a form of pulmonary lymphoma. Histologically, there are multiple round nodules containing lymphocytes that infiltrate small vessels to produce an obliterative vasculitis. These findings are similar to Wegener granulomatosis, although well-formed granulomas are rare in lymphomatoid granulomatosis. CNS and skin involvement are common, but renal failure is not present. Radiographically, there are multiple nodular opacities with a lower lobe predilection. Cavitation is common and results from ischemic necrosis. This condition is a lymphatic malignancy and is treated with chemotherapy. The prognosis is poor, with 50% of patients developing frank lymphoma. The overall 5-year survival rate is approximately 20%.

Leukemia. While leukemic involvement of the lung is found in approximately one third of patients at autopsy, clinical or radiographic evidence of parenchymal infiltration is uncommon during life. The majority of pulmonary disease in leukemic patients is caused by pneumonia complicating immunosuppression, edema from cardiac disease, or hemorrhage owing to thrombocytopenia. Parenchymal involvement in leukemia usually takes the form of interstitial infiltration by leukemic cells, with resultant peribronchial cuffing and reticulonodular opacities on chest radiograph. Focal accumulation of leukemic cells can produce a chloroma and the radiographic appearance of an SPN. An unusual pulmonary manifestation of leukemia is *pulmonary leukostasis*, which is seen in acute leukemia or those in blast crisis in whom the peripheral white blood cell count exceeds 100,000 to 200,000/cm^3. In

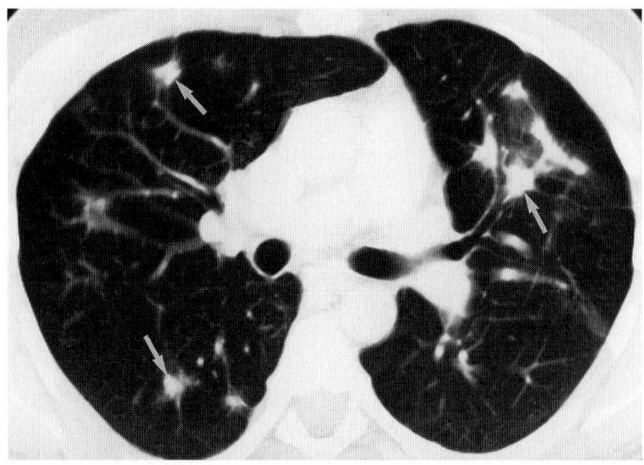

FIGURE 15.27. **Kaposi Sarcoma.** CT scan in a 41-year-old man with AIDS and cutaneous lesions reveals bilateral irregularly marginated nodules (*arrows*) with a peribronchovascular distribution. The presence of pulmonary involvement with Kaposi sarcoma was confirmed by bronchoscopy.

this condition, the white cell blasts clump within the pulmonary microvasculature to produce dyspnea. Approximately half of affected patients have normal radiographs, while the remainder demonstrate a diffuse reticulonodular pattern of disease.

Kaposi sarcoma (KS) of the lung is a common complication of AIDS. Pulmonary involvement almost invariably follows skin, oropharyngeal, and/or visceral involvement. The histologic features are characteristic: clusters of spindle cells with numerous mitotic figures are separated by thin-walled vascular channels containing red blood cells. The tumor involves the tracheobronchial mucosa and the peribronchovascular, alveolar, and subpleural interstitium of the lung. KS produces small to medium, poorly marginated nodular and coarse linear opacities that extend from the hilum into the mid-lung and lower lung. CT shows the typical peribronchovascular location of the opacities and may demonstrate air bronchograms traversing masslike areas of confluent disease (Fig. 15.27). A bloody pleural effusion is present in up to 50% of patients; this is attributed to lesions within the subpleural interstitium of the lung. Hilar and mediastinal lymph node enlargement is found in 20% of patients. Important diagnostic features of pulmonary KS are the slow rate of progression of disease (usually over many months) and the absence of fever or pulmonary symptoms despite extensive parenchymal disease. Bleeding from endobronchial or parenchymal lesions may produce focal or diffuse airspace opacities that are difficult to distinguish from complicating bacterial pneumonia or *Pneumocystis carinii* infection.

The diagnosis of pulmonary KS is usually made indirectly, by the visualization of typical endobronchial lesions in a patient with characteristic chest radiographic findings. Combined thallium and gallium lung scanning has been used successfully to distinguish KS from pneumonia and non-Hodgkin lymphoma. While pneumonia is both

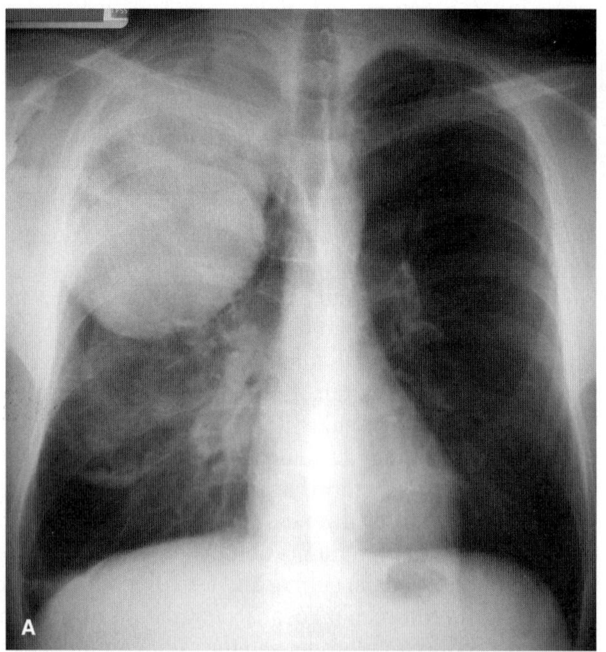

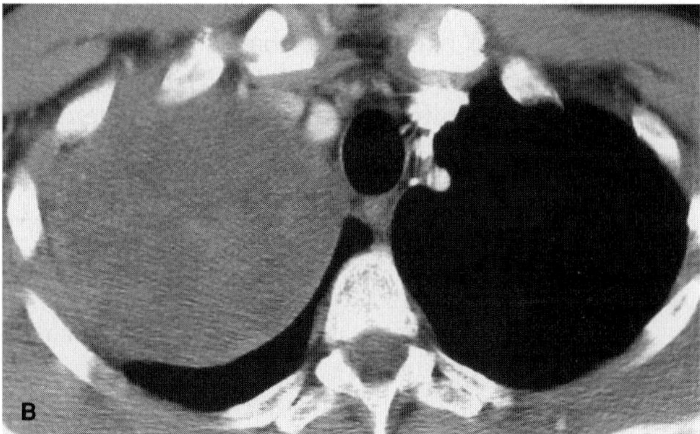

FIGURE 15.28. **Pulmonary Blastoma. A.** Posteroanterior radiograph in a 29-year-old man with hemoptysis shows a large right upper lobe mass. **B.** Enhanced CT shows a large mass that occupies much of the right upper lobe. Pathologic examination of the pneumonectomy specimen revealed pulmonary blastoma.

gallium and thallium avid, lymphoma is gallium avid only and KS is thallium avid only.

Pulmonary blastoma is a rare malignant tumor affecting children and young adults. The tumors are comprised of both mesenchymal and glandular elements of lung, with an appearance that simulates fetal lung at 10 to 16 weeks' gestation. Those tumors composed predominantly of glandular elements are also called *fetal adenocarcinomas*, while tumors with malignant mesenchyme alone are referred to as *cystic and pleuropulmonary blastomas of childhood*. Tumors with mixed malignant epithelial and mesenchymal components are termed *biphasic blastomas*. Pulmonary blastomas are difficult to distinguish histologically from carcinosarcomas. These tumors tend to be extremely large at presentation (Fig. 15.28). Diagnosis is made by resection of the lesion. The prognosis is poor because many lesions have metastasized at the time of diagnosis.

REFERENCES

1. Leef JL III, Klein JS. The solitary pulmonary nodule. Radiol Clin North Am 2002;40:123–143.
2. Swensen SJ, Viggiano RW, Midthun DE, et al. Lung nodule enhancement at CT: multicenter study. Radiology 2000;214:73–80.
3. Gould MK, Maclean CC, Kuschner WG, Rydzak CE, Owens DK. Accuracy of positron emission tomography for diagnosis of pulmonary nodules and mass lesions: a meta-analysis. JAMA 2001;285: 914–924.
4. Neoplasms of the lungs, airways, and pleura. In: Hansell DM, Armstrong P, Lynch DA, McAdams HP. Imaging of Diseases of the Chest. 4th ed. Philadelphia, PA: Elsevier Mosby, 2005:788–797.
5. Gould MK, Kuschner WG, Rydzak CE, et al. Test performance of positron emission tomography and computed tomography for mediastinal staging in patients with non-small-cell lung cancer. Ann Intern Med 2003;139:879–892.
6. Ravenel JG. Lung cancer staging. Semin Roentgenol 2004;39:373–385.
7. Marom EM, McAdams HP, Erasmus JJ, et al. Staging non-small cell lung cancer with whole-body PET. Radiology 1999;212:803–809.
8. Glazer HS, Kaiser LR, Anderson DJ, et al. Indeterminate mediastinal invasion in bronchogenic carcinoma: CT evaluation. Radiology 1989;173:37–42.
9. McLoud TC, Bourgouin PM, Greenberg RW, et al. Bronchogenic carcinoma: analysis of staging in the mediastinum with CT by correlative lymph node mapping and sampling. Radiology 1992;182:319–323.
10. Lardinois D, Weder W, Hany TF, et al. Staging of non-small-cell lung cancer with integrated positron emission tomography and computed tomography. N Engl J Med 2004;25:2500–2507.
11. Weber AL, Grillo HC. Tracheal tumors: a radiological, clinical, and pathological evaluation of 84 cases. Radiol Clin North Am 1978;16:227–246.
12. Neoplasms of the lungs, airways, and pleura. In: Hansell DM, Armstrong P, Lynch DA, McAdams HP. Imaging of Diseases of the Chest. 4th ed. Philadelphia, PA: Elsevier Mosby, 2005:864–872.

Chapter 16

Pulmonary Infection

Timothy J. Higgins and Jeffrey S. Klein

Infection in the Normal Host
Bacterial Pneumonia
Viral Pneumonia
Fungal Pneumonia
Parasitic Infection

Infection in the Immunocompromised Host and in Aids

INFECTION IN THE NORMAL HOST

The bronchopulmonary system is open to the atmosphere and therefore is relatively accessible to airborne microorganisms. Multiple host defense mechanisms exist at the level of the pharynx, trachea, and central bronchi. When these mechanisms fail, pathogenic organisms can penetrate to the small distal bronchi and the pulmonary parenchyma. Once the invading organisms penetrate the parenchyma, there is activation of both the cellular and humoral immune systems. This response may manifest clinically and radiographically as pneumonia, and in a normal host will often lead to eradication or at least suppression of the infecting organisms. If the immune response is impaired, a lower respiratory tract infection may lead to a very severe illness and often death, despite appropriate antibiotic therapy.

Mechanisms of Disease and Radiographic Patterns. Microorganisms responsible for producing pneumonia enter the lung and cause infection by three potential routes: via the tracheobronchial tree, via the pulmonary vasculature, or via direct spread from infection in the mediastinum, chest wall, or upper abdomen.

Infection via the tracheobronchial tree is generally secondary to inhalation or aspiration of infectious microorganisms and can be divided into three subtypes based on gross pathologic appearance and radiographic patterns: lobar pneumonia, lobular or bronchopneumonia, and interstitial pneumonia. As will be discussed in later sections, certain organisms will typically produce one of these three patterns, although there may be considerable overlap.

Lobar pneumonia is typical of pneumococcal pulmonary infection. In this pattern of disease, the inflammatory exudate begins within the distal airspaces. The inflammatory process spreads via the pores of Kohn and canals of Lambert to produce nonsegmental consolidation. If untreated, the inflammation may eventually involve an entire lobe (Fig. 16.1). Because the airways are usually spared, air bronchograms are common and significant volume loss is unusual (see Table 12.7).

Bronchopneumonia is the most common pattern of disease and is most typical of staphylococcal pneumonia. In the early stages of bronchopneumonia, the inflammation is centered primarily in and around lobular bronchi. As the inflammation progresses, exudative fluid extends peripherally along the bronchus to involve the entire pulmonary lobule. Radiographically, multifocal opacities that are roughly lobular in configuration produce a "patchwork quilt" appearance because of the interspersion of normal and diseased lobules (Fig. 16.2). While bronchopneumonia is the most common cause of multifocal patchy airspace opacities, there is a broad list of differential diagnostic considerations (see Table 12.9). Exudate within the bronchi accounts for the absence of air bronchograms in bronchopneumonia. With coalescence of affected areas, the pattern may resemble lobar pneumonia.

In interstitial pneumonia, seen in viral and mycoplasma infection, there is inflammatory thickening of bronchial and bronchiolar walls and the pulmonary interstitium. This results in a radiographic pattern of airways thickening and reticulonodular opacities (see Table 12.12). Air bronchograms are absent because the alveolar spaces

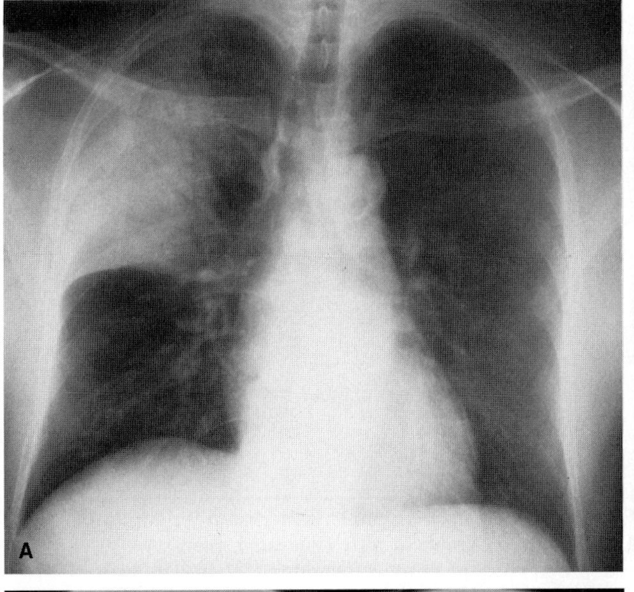

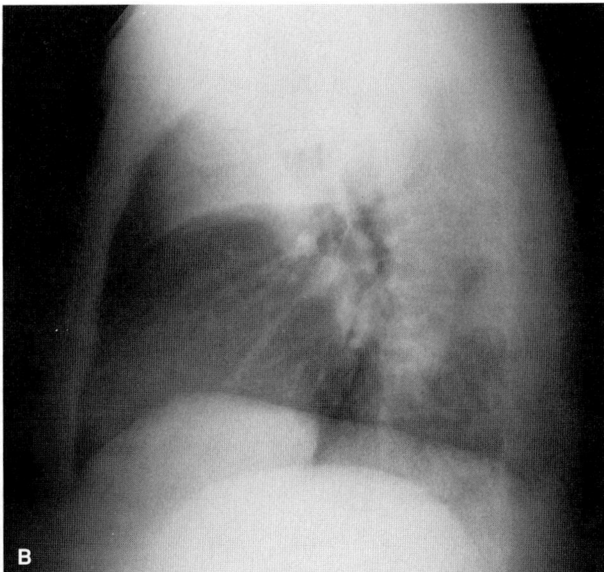

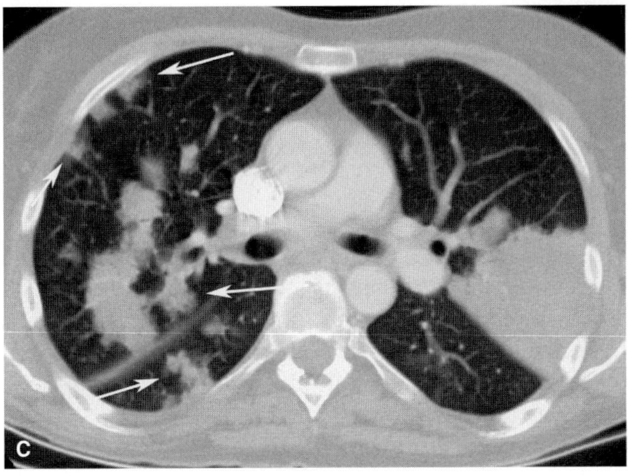

FIGURE 16.1. **Pneumococcal Pneumonia.** Posteroanterior **(A)** and lateral **(B)** radiographs in a 57-year-old man with fever, chills, and productive cough demonstrate airspace opacification in the right upper lobe with air bronchograms. Sputum culture was positive for *Streptococcus pneumonia*. CT scan in another patient with pneumococcal pneumonia **(C)** shows dense multifocal segmental airspace opacification in the upper lobes. Note the lobular pattern of consolidation in the right upper lobe and superior segment of the right lower lobe (*arrows*), reflecting bronchopneumonia.

remain aerated. Segmental and subsegmental atelectasis from small airways obstruction is common.

The spread of infection to the lung via the pulmonary vasculature usually occurs in the setting of systemic sepsis. The pattern of parenchymal involvement is patchy and bilateral. The lung bases are most severely involved, because blood flow is greatest in the dependent portions of the lungs. Pulmonary infection from direct spread usually results in a localized parenchymal process adjacent to an extrapulmonary source of infection. If an organism causes extensive parenchymal necrosis, abscess formation may result.

Bacterial Pneumonia

Gram-Positive Bacteria

***Streptococcus pneumoniae* (pneumococcus).** *S pneumoniae* is a gram-positive organism that may cause infection in healthy individuals but is much more commonly seen in the elderly, alcoholics, and other compromised hosts. Patients with sickle cell disease or who have undergone splenectomy are at particular risk for severe pneumococcal pneumonia.

Pneumococcal pneumonia tends to begin in the lower lobes or the posterior segments of the upper lobes. Initially there is involvement of the terminal airways, but rather than remaining localized to this site, there is rapid development of an airspace inflammatory exudate. The spread of infection to contiguous airspaces via interalveolar connections accounts for the nonsegmental distribution and homogeneity of the resultant consolidation.

The typical radiographic appearance of acute pneumococcal pneumonia is lobar consolidation (Fig. 16.1). Air bronchograms are usually evident. Cavitation in pneumococcal pneumonia is rare, with the exception of infections caused by serotype 3. Uncomplicated parapneumonic effusion or empyema may be seen in up to 50% of patients. With appropriate therapy, complete clearing may be seen in 10 to 14 days. In older patients or those

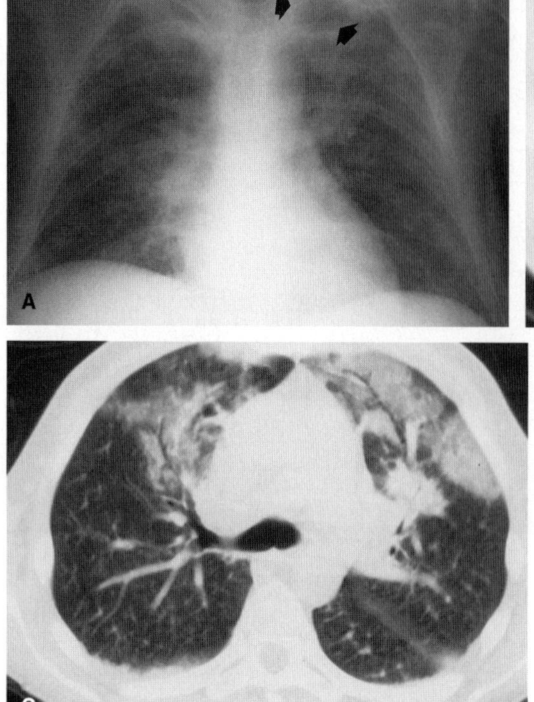

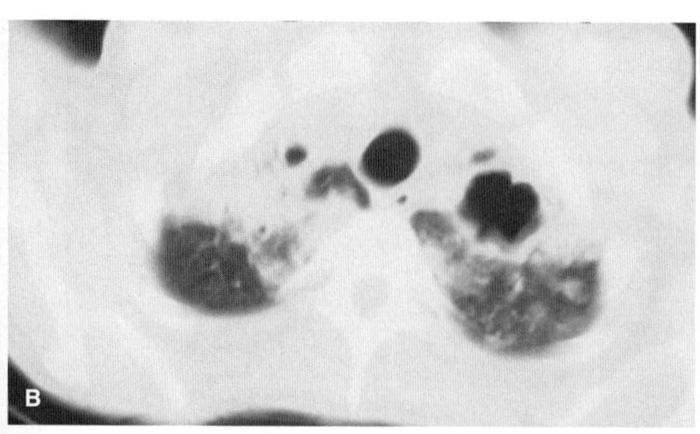

FIGURE 16.2. ***Pseudomonas aeruginosa*** **Pneumonia.** **A.** Frontal radiograph in an HIV-positive man with fever and progressive respiratory symptoms shows multifocal airspace opacities with dense apical opacification with cavitation (*arrows*). **B.** A CT scan through the apices shows airspace opacification with left apical cavitation. **C.** A scan at the level of the tracheal carina shows airspace disease in the anterior segments of right and left upper lobes with sparing of the dependent portions of lung. Bronchoscopy revealed *Pseudomonas*.

with underlying disease, complete resolution may take 8 to 10 weeks.

Patients with pneumococcal pneumonia occasionally present with atypical radiographic patterns of disease (1). Patchy lobular opacities similar to those seen with bronchopneumonia (Fig. 16.1C) or rarely, a reticulonodular pattern may be seen. In some patients, the atypical appearance may relate to the presence of preexisting lung disease (e.g., emphysema), partial treatment, or an impaired immune response (e.g., AIDS). In children, pneumococcal pneumonia may present as a spherical opacity ("round pneumonia") simulating a parenchymal mass.

Staphylococcus aureus pneumonia is most common in hospitalized and debilitated patients. It may also develop following hematogenous spread to the lung in patients with endocarditis or indwelling catheters and intravenous drug users. Community-acquired infection may complicate influenza or other viral pneumonias.

S aureus typically produces a bronchopneumonia and appears radiographically as patchy opacities (Fig. 16.3). In severe cases, the opacities may become confluent to produce lobar opacification. Because the inflammatory exudate fills the airways, air bronchograms are rarely seen. In adults, the process is often bilateral and may be complicated by abscess formation in 25% to 75% of patients. In patients who develop pulmonary infection from hematogenous seeding, one sees multiple bilateral poorly defined nodular opacities that eventually become more sharply defined and cavitate. Parapneumonic effusion and empyema are common. Pneumatocele formation is common in children and may lead to pneumothorax. Pneumatoceles may be distinguished from abscesses by their thin walls, rapid change in size, and tendency to develop during the late phase of infection.

Streptococcus pyogenes. Acute streptococcal pneumonia is rarely seen today, though it can occasionally complicate viral infection or streptococcal pharyngitis. Its radiographic appearance is similar to that of staphylococcal pneumonia, with lobular or segmental lower lobe opacities. The process may be complicated by abscess formation and cavitation; empyema is relatively common.

Bacillus anthracis. Anthrax is caused by a sporulating gram-positive bacillus that is distributed worldwide. Naturally occurring inhalational anthrax is rare; however, anthrax has been used as an agent of bioterrorism in the United States. The primary radiographic manifestations of inhalational anthrax are related to the underlying pathology of hemorrhagic lymphadenitis and mediastinitis accompanied by hemorrhagic pleural effusions. Conventional radiographs demonstrate mediastinal widening, hilar enlargement, and often pleural effusion. Frank areas of consolidation are not usually present, but peribronchial opacities may be seen. CT scans of recent bioterrorism victims, performed in 2001 without intravenous contrast, demonstrated high-attenuation lymphadenopathy and pleural effusions secondary to hemorrhage. CT scans may show extensive adenopathy in the setting of

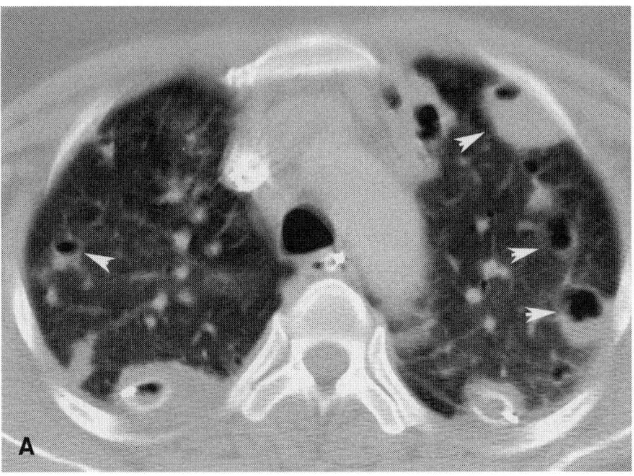

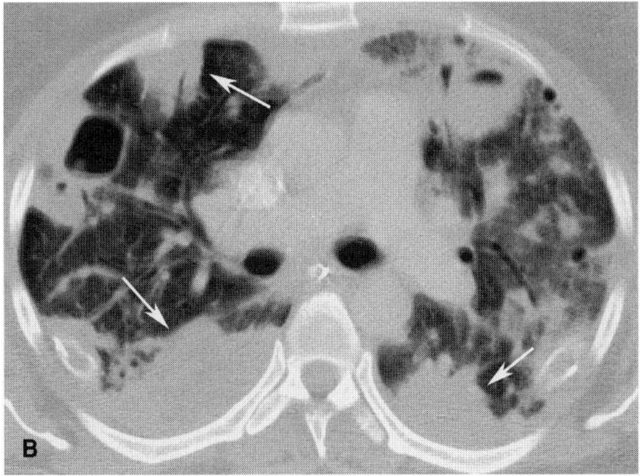

FIGURE 16.3. ***Staphylococcus aureus* Pneumonia.** CT scans at the top of the aortic arch **(A)** and central pulmonary arteries **(B)** show a combination of abscess and cavity formation (*arrowheads*) and lobular consolidation (*arrows*). Sputum cultures showed *S aureus* pneumonia.

normal radiographs and should be obtained if the suspicion of anthrax is high (2).

Gram-Negative Bacteria

Gram-negative bacteria are increasingly important causes of pneumonia in hospitalized patients, accounting for over 50% of nosocomial pulmonary infections. While gram-negative organisms may be isolated from only a small percentage of healthy individuals, the isolation rate in hospitalized and severely ill patients ranges from 40% to 75%. The organisms most often responsible for pneumonia include members of the Enterobacteriaceae family (*Klebsiella*, *Escherichia coli*, *Proteus*); *Pseudomonas aeruginosa*; *Haemophilus influenzae*; and *Legionella pneumophila* (3).

The radiographic appearance of gram-negative bacterial pneumonia varies from small ill-defined nodules to patchy areas of opacification that may become confluent and resemble lobar pneumonia. Involvement is usually bilateral and multifocal, and the lower lobes are most frequently affected. Abscess formation and cavitation are relatively common. Parapneumonic effusion is common and is often complicated by empyema formation.

Klebsiella pneumoniae. *Klebsiella* pneumonia occurs predominantly in older alcoholic men and debilitated hospitalized patients. Radiographically it appears as a homogeneous lobar opacification containing air bronchograms. Three features help distinguish it radiographically from pneumococcal pneumonia: (*1*) the volume of the involved lobe may be increased by the exuberant inflammatory exudate, producing a bulging interlobar fissure; (*2*) an abscess may develop, with cavity formation, which is uncommon in pneumococcal pneumonia; and (*3*) the incidence of pleural effusion and empyema is higher. Pulmonary gangrene may be seen but is uncommon.

Haemophilus influenzae. In adults, *H influenzae* infection is most common in patients with chronic obstructive pulmonary disease (COPD), alcoholism, diabetes mellitus, and those with an anatomic or functional splenectomy. It most often causes bronchitis, although it may extend to produce bilateral lower lobe bronchopneumonia.

Pseudomonas aeruginosa pneumonia most often affects debilitated patients, particularly those requiring mechanical ventilation. There is a high mortality rate associated with the disease. The radiographic pattern of parenchymal involvement depends upon the method by which the organisms reach the lung. Patchy opacities with abscess formation, which mimic staphylococcal pneumonia, are common when the infection reaches the lung via the tracheobronchial tree (Fig. 16.2). Diffuse, bilateral, ill-defined nodular opacities usually reflect hematogenous dissemination. Pleural effusions are common and are usually small.

Legionella pneumophila. Legionnaires disease is caused by infection with *L pneumophila*, a gram-negative bacillus commonly found in air conditioning and humidifier systems. This infection tends to affect older men. Community-acquired infection is seen in patients with COPD or malignancy, while nosocomial infection primarily affects immunocompromised patients or those with renal failure or malignancy.

The characteristic radiographic pattern is airspace opacification, which is initially peripheral and sublobar. In some patients, the airspace opacities appear as a round pneumonia. The infection progresses to lobar or multilobar involvement despite the initiation of antibiotic therapy. At the peak of disease, the parenchymal involvement is usually bilateral. Pleural effusions are seen in approximately 30% of patients. Cavitation is not seen except in the immunocompromised patient (Fig. 16.4). The radiographic resolution of pneumonia is often prolonged and may lag behind symptomatic improvement.

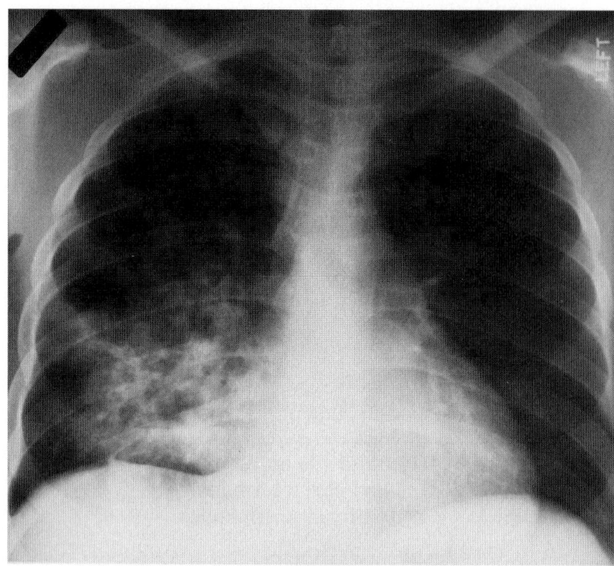

FIGURE 16.4. ***Legionella*** **Pneumonia in an Immunocompromised Patient.** Frontal chest radiograph in a 35-year-old man with AIDS demonstrates a middle lobe airspace opacification with areas of cavitation. Bronchoscopy showed *L pneumophila* pneumonia.

Anaerobic Bacterial Infection

The majority of anaerobic lung infections arise from aspiration of infected oropharyngeal contents (4). Approximately 25% of patients give a history of impaired consciousness, and many are alcoholic. The most common organisms responsible are the gram-negative bacilli *Bacteroides* and *Fusobacterium*, although the majority of pulmonary infections are polymicrobial. All anaerobic pulmonary infections produce a similar radiographic appearance. The distribution of parenchymal opacities reflects the gravitational flow of aspirated material. When aspiration occurs in the supine position, it is the posterior segments of the upper lobes and superior segments of the lower lobes that are predominantly involved, whereas aspiration in the erect position leads to involvement of basal segments of the lower lobes. The typical radiographic appearance is peripheral lobular and segmental airspace opacities. Cavitation within areas of consolidation is relatively common, and discrete lung abscesses may be seen in up to 50% of patients. Hilar and/or mediastinal lymph node enlargement may be seen in those with lung abscesses. Empyema, with or without bronchopleural fistula formation, is a common complication and is seen in up to 50% of patients.

Atypical Bacterial Infections

Actinomycosis. *Actinomyces israelii* is an anaerobic gram-positive filamentous bacterium that is a normal inhabitant of the human oropharynx. It causes disease when it gains access to devitalized or infected tissues that facilitate its growth. Actinomycosis most commonly follows dental extractions, manifesting as mandibular osteomyelitis or a soft tissue abscess. The lungs may be infected by aspiration of infectious oral debris or, less commonly, by direct extension from the primary site of disease.

The radiographic pattern of actinomycosis is often indistinguishable from that of nocardiosis. Findings consist of nonsegmental airspace opacities in the periphery of the lower lobes. In some cases, the infection manifests as a localized masslike opacity that mimics bronchogenic carcinoma. If therapy is not instituted, a lung abscess may develop. Thoracic actinomycosis is characterized by its ability to spread to contiguous tissues without regard for normal anatomic barriers. Extension into the pleura will cause empyema, while chest wall involvement is characterized by osteomyelitis of the ribs and chest wall abscess. Involvement of the ribs is seen as wavy periosteal reaction or lytic rib destruction (5). If the pleuropulmonary disease becomes chronic, extensive fibrosis may be seen. Rarely, the disease is disseminated and a miliary pattern is seen.

Mycoplasma display both bacterial and viral characteristics and are considered as a separate group. They are probably the most common atypical pneumonia and account for 10% to 30% of all community-acquired pneumonia. Affected patients usually have a subacute illness of 2 to 3 weeks' duration. Symptoms include fever, nonproductive cough, headache, and malaise. Unusual physical findings include bullous myringitis and rash.

In the early stages of infection, interstitial inflammation leads to a fine reticular pattern on the chest radiograph. This may progress to patchy segmental airspace opacities (Fig. 16.5), which may coalesce to produce lobar consolidation. CT of mycoplasma pneumonia usually appears as patchy airspace opacities with a tree-in-bud appearance that reflects infectious bronchiolitis (Fig. 16.6). The process is often unilateral and tends to involve the lower lobes. Pleural effusion may be seen in the consolidative form of disease and occurs most commonly in children. Lymph node enlargement is uncommon but may be seen in children. Radiographic resolution may require 4 to 6 weeks.

Mycobacterial Infections

Mycobacterium tuberculosis is an aerobic acid-fast bacillus. Two principal forms of tuberculous pulmonary disease are recognized clinically and radiographically: primary tuberculosis (TB) and "reactivation" or postprimary disease. The inflammatory response to *M tuberculosis* differs from the normal response to bacterial organisms in that it involves cell-mediated immunity (delayed hypersensitivity). Initially, droplet nuclei laden with bacilli are inhaled and implant in a subpleural location. In most

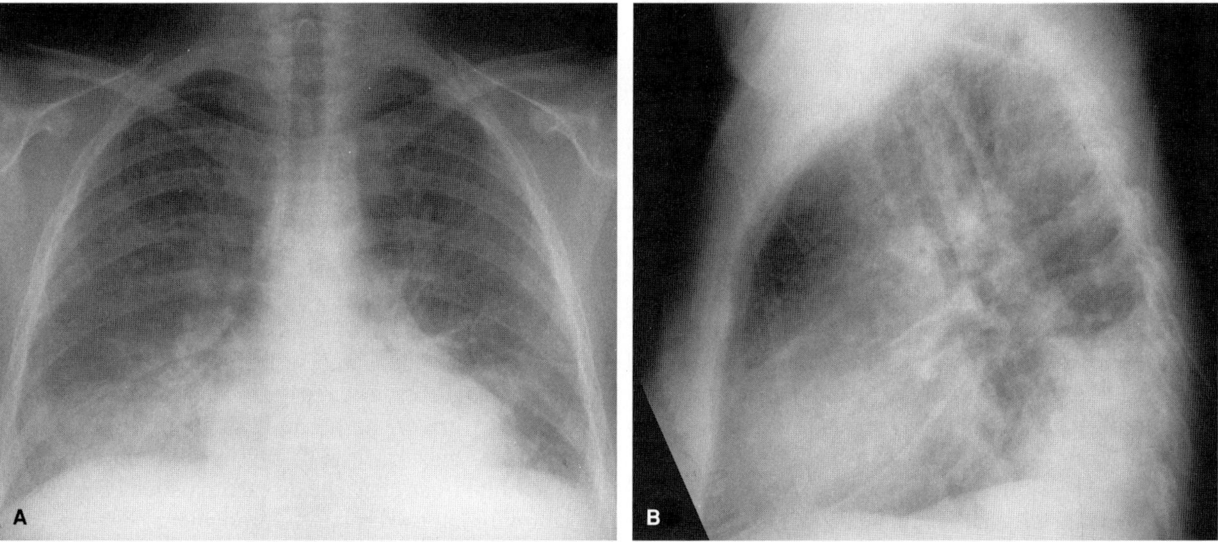

FIGURE 16.5. ***Mycoplasma* Pneumonia.** Posteroanterior **(A)** and lateral **(B)** radiographs in a 21-year-old woman demonstrate mixed diffuse interstitial and bibasilar airspace opacities. Immunofluorescent staining of induced sputum samples revealed *M pneumoniae*.

patients, the bacilli are phagocytized and killed by alveolar macrophages. If the bacilli overcome the immune response of the host, an inflammatory focus is established. The macrophages are then transformed into epithelioid cells, which aggregate to form granulomas. The granulomas are usually well-formed by 1 to 3 weeks, coinciding with the development of delayed hypersensitivity. The granulomas typically demonstrate central caseous necrosis, thereby distinguishing them from the granulomas seen in sarcoidosis. Inflammation and enlargement of draining hilar and mediastinal lymph nodes is common in primary disease, particularly in children and immunocompromised patients.

In primary infection, the parenchymal disease and adenopathy may completely resolve, or there may be a residual focus of scarring or calcification. In some situations, usually in infants under the age of 1 year, local parenchymal disease progresses and is termed *progressive primary TB*. More commonly, the disease will be contained by the granulomatous response and recur years later (reactivation or postprimary TB) in the setting of weakened host defenses from aging, alcoholism, diabetes, cancer, or HIV infection. Postprimary TB develops under the influence of hypersensitivity, with caseous necrosis seen histologically.

Primary tuberculosis has classically been a disease of childhood, although the incidence of primary disease has

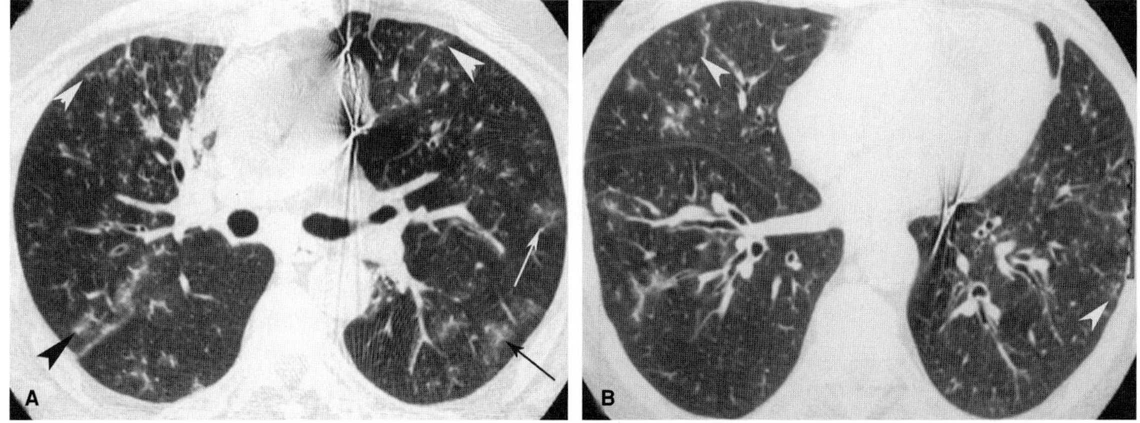

FIGURE 16.6. **CT of *Mycoplasma* Pneumonia.** Thin-section CT scans through the upper **(A)** and lower **(B)** lungs in a patient with mycoplasma pneumonia show patchy ground-glass opacities (*arrows*) with scattered tree-in-bud opacities (*arrowheads*).

increased because of the HIV epidemic. Most patients with primary TB are asymptomatic and have no radiographic sequelae of infection. In some patients a Ranke complex, consisting of a calcified parenchymal focus (the Ghon lesion) and nodal calcification, is seen. If the patient is symptomatic, a nonspecific focal pneumonitis occurs and is seen as small, ill-defined areas of segmental or lobar opacification (Fig. 16.7). The parenchymal consolidation may mimic a bacterial pneumonia, but the clinical and radiographic course is much more indolent. Cavitation is relatively uncommon in the immunocompetent patient (6). The pulmonary focus may resolve completely or persist as a Ghon lesion or a Ranke complex. *Tuberculomas* are discrete nodular opacities that may develop in primary TB but are much more common in postprimary disease. Unilateral pleural effusions are seen in 25% of cases and are usually associated with parenchymal disease. If a tuberculous empyema develops, it may break through the parietal pleura to form an extrapleural collection (empyema necessitatis). Unilateral hilar or mediastinal lymph node enlargement is common, particularly in children, and may be the sole radiographic manifestation of infection. Bilateral hilar or mediastinal lymph node enlargement may be seen, but this is uncommon and is almost invariably asymmetric in distinction to lymph node enlargement in sarcoidosis. During the primary tuberculous infection, there is hematogenous dissemination of the organism to regions with a high partial pressure of oxygen; these include the lung apices, renal medullae, and bone marrow. These microscopic foci are clinically silent and serve as a source of reactivation disease.

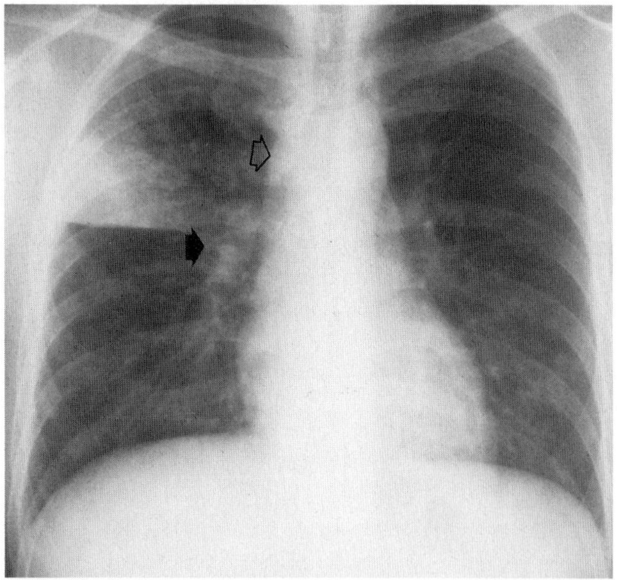

FIGURE 16.7. **Primary Tuberculosis.** A posteroanterior chest radiograph in a 32-year-old homeless man shows airspace disease within the anterior segment of the right upper lobe, with right hilar (*solid arrow*) and paratracheal (*open arrow*) lymph node enlargement. Sputum stains and cultures revealed *Mycobacterium tuberculosis*.

Postprimary TB patients often present with cough and constitutional symptoms, including chills, night sweats, and weight loss. Reactivation tends to occur in the apical and posterior segments of the upper lobes and the superior segments of the lower lobes. Ill-defined patchy and nodular opacities are commonly seen. Cavitation is an important radiographic feature of postprimary infection and usually indicates active and transmissible disease (Fig. 16.8). The cavitary focus may lead to transbronchial spread of organisms and result in a multifocal bronchopneumonia. Erosion of a cavitary focus into a branch of the pulmonary artery can produce an aneurysm (Rasmussen aneurysm) and cause hemoptysis. With appropriate antimicrobial treatment, the disease is usually controlled by a granulomatous response. Parenchymal healing is associated with fibrosis, bronchiectasis, and volume loss (cicatrizing atelectasis) in the upper lobes.

There are several late complications of pulmonary TB. Interstitial fibrosis can cause pulmonary insufficiency and secondary pulmonary arterial hypertension. Hemoptysis may be secondary to bronchiectasis, mycetoma formation in an old tuberculous cavity, or erosion of a calcified peribronchial lymph node (broncholith) into a bronchus. Bronchostenosis is a result of healed endobronchial TB.

Miliary TB may complicate either primary or reactivation disease. It results from hematogenous dissemination of tubercle bacilli and produces diffuse bilateral 2- to 3-mm pulmonary nodules (Fig. 16.9). Miliary disease is associated with a high mortality and requires prompt therapy.

Atypical Mycobacterial Infection. There are several nontuberculous mycobacteria that may cause pulmonary disease (7). The most common organisms responsible for pulmonary disease are *Mycobacterium avium-intracellulare* (MAI) or *M kansasii*. Disease in nonimmunocompromised patients typically affects patients with underlying COPD. The radiographic features are often indistinguishable from those of reactivation TB, with chronic fibrocavitary opacities involving the upper lobes. While cavitation is common, pleural effusion, lymph node enlargement, and miliary spread are distinctly unusual. A second pattern of disease with MAI has recently been described in middle-aged and elderly women, with small peribronchial nodules and bronchiectasis seen in a middle lobe and lingular distribution (Fig. 16.10). Although the disease caused by nontuberculous mycobacteria tends to be more indolent than that seen with *M tuberculosis*, it is often difficult to treat effectively.

Viral Pneumonia

Viruses are a major cause of upper respiratory tract and airways infection, although pneumonia is relatively uncommon. The diagnosis of viral pneumonia is often one

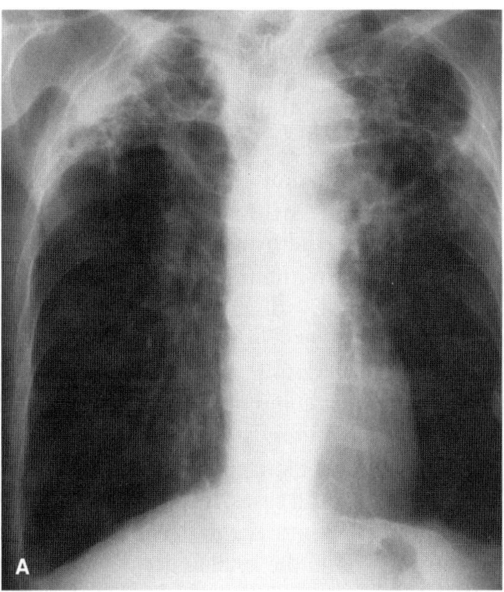

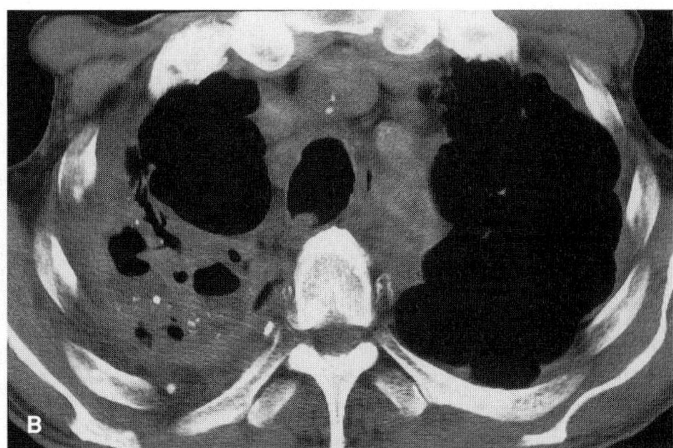

FIGURE 16.8. **Postprimary (Reactivation) Tuberculosis. A.** Frontal chest film in a 69-year-old Asian immigrant with a cough and severe wasting reveals hyperinflation with marked fibrotic and cavitary disease in the upper lobes with severe volume loss. **B.** A CT scan through the lung apices demonstrates consolidative and cavitary changes with air–fluid levels and pleural and parenchymal calcifications. Sputum cultures were positive for *Mycobacterium tuberculosis*.

of exclusion. Chest radiographic features are nonspecific and usually demonstrate a pattern of bronchopneumonia or interstitial opacities (8). Resolution is usually complete, but permanent sequelae may be seen, including bronchiectasis, bronchiolitis obliterans (which may produce a unilateral hyperlucent lung or Swyer-James syndrome), and interstitial fibrosis.

Influenza. In adults, the most common cause of viral pneumonia is influenza. Outbreaks of influenza can occur in pandemics, epidemics, or sporadically. In most patients the disease is confined to the upper respiratory tract, but in elderly persons, those with underlying cardiopulmonary disease or immunocompromise, and pregnant women, a severe hemorrhagic pneumonia may develop. In adults with influenzal pneumonia, there is often bilateral lower lobe patchy airspace opacification. In children, a diffuse interstitial reticulonodular pattern is more commonly seen. Bacterial superinfection with *Streptococcus* or *Staphylococcus* organisms contributes to a fulminating course that may result in death. The development of lobar consolidation, pleural effusion, or cavitation suggests bacterial superinfection.

Respiratory syncytial virus and ***parainfluenza virus*** are common causes of epidemic viral pneumonia in children. When seen in adults, the disease is usually in the setting of a debilitated or immunocompromised patient (Fig. 16.11). Findings are similar to other viral pneumonias: patchy airspace opacities, bronchial wall thickening, and tree-in-bud opacities.

Varicella-zoster, which causes chickenpox and shingles, may produce a severe pneumonia in adults. Patients on immunosuppressive therapy or with lymphoma are at greatest risk. Chest radiographs characteristically show diffuse bilateral ill-defined nodular opacities 5 to 10 mm in diameter. These opacities usually resolve completely, although in some patients they involute and calcify to produce innumerable small (2 to 3 mm) calcified nodules (Fig. 16.12).

Adenovirus is a frequent cause of upper and, occasionally, lower respiratory tract infection. Overinflation and bronchopneumonia accompanied by lobar atelectasis are the most frequent radiographic manifestations of adenovirus pneumonia; however, adenovirus in children may present as lobar or segmental consolidation.

SARS-Associated Coronavirus (SARS-CoV). Severe Acute Respiratory Syndrome (SARS) is a recently described respiratory illness caused by a new coronavirus not previously seen in humans, SARS-CoV. The disease appears to have originated in southern China and rapidly spread to other areas of the world, causing over 8,000 reported cases in late 2002 and early 2003. The clinical symptoms and signs as well as the radiographic manifestations of SARS are nonspecific. Unilateral or bilateral areas of airspace opacity are seen on initial radiographs in the majority of affected patients. The opacities are typically peripheral and lower zone in location, progressively involving the central lungs. Occasionally, initial radiographs are negative; CT demonstrates areas of ground-glass opacity

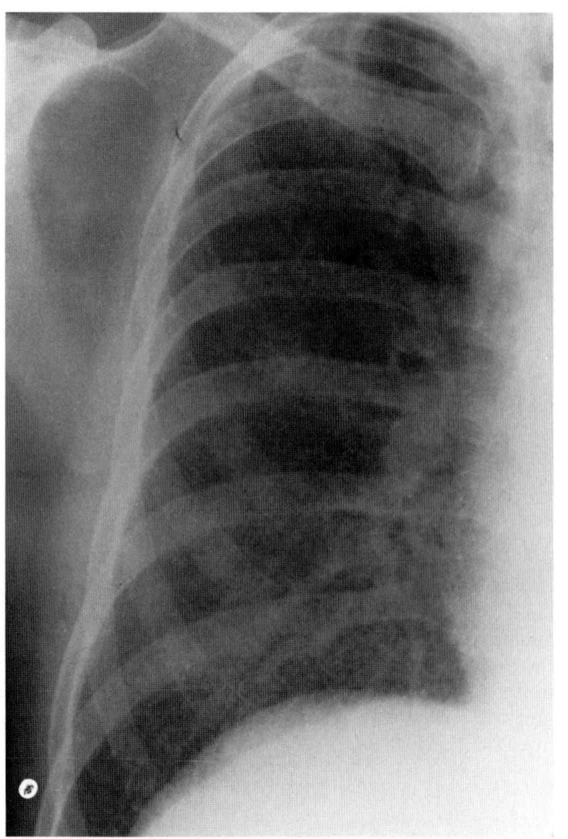

FIGURE 16.9. **Miliary Tuberculosis.** A cone-down view of a frontal radiograph demonstrates innumerable micronodular opacities characteristic of micronodular (miliary) interstitial disease. Transbronchial biopsy demonstrated caseating granulomas containing acid-fast bacilli.

and/or consolidation (9). Lymphadenopathy and pleural effusions are not characteristic.

Fungal Pneumonia

Fungal infections are now seen with increased frequency because of an increase in the incidence of disease caused by pathogenic fungi in healthy hosts and the emergence of opportunistic species in immunocompromised hosts. Fungi can cause pulmonary disease by several mechanisms. Some fungi, including *Histoplasma capsulatum, Coccidioides immitis*, and *Blastomyces dermatitidis,* are primary pathogens and most commonly infect normal hosts (10). Other fungi, most notably *Aspergillus, Candida*, and *Cryptococcus*, are opportunistic pathogens in immunocompromised individuals. In all cases, the fungi elicit a necrotizing granulomatous reaction. The high mortality of untreated invasive infection and the availability of effective antifungal therapy with intravenous amphotericin B and the oral azoles (e.g., fluconazole, itraconazole) has made the early and accurate diagnosis of fungal infection imperative. A number of serologic assays (complement fixation, immunodiffusion) and histologic methods are available for the accurate diagnosis of fungal infection.

Histoplasmosis. *H capsulatum* is endemic to certain areas of North America, most notably the Ohio, Mississippi, and St. Lawrence River valleys and Mexico. The overwhelming majority (95% to 99%) of infections by *H capsulatum* are asymptomatic. A routine chest film demonstrating multiple well-defined calcified nodules less than 1 cm in size, with or without calcified hilar or mediastinal lymph nodes, may be the only indication of prior infection.

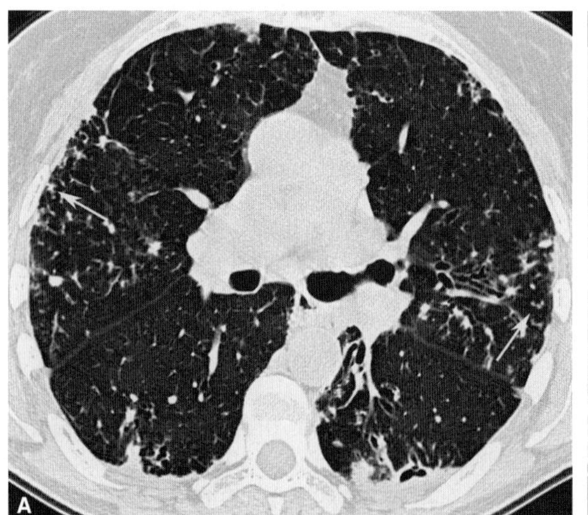

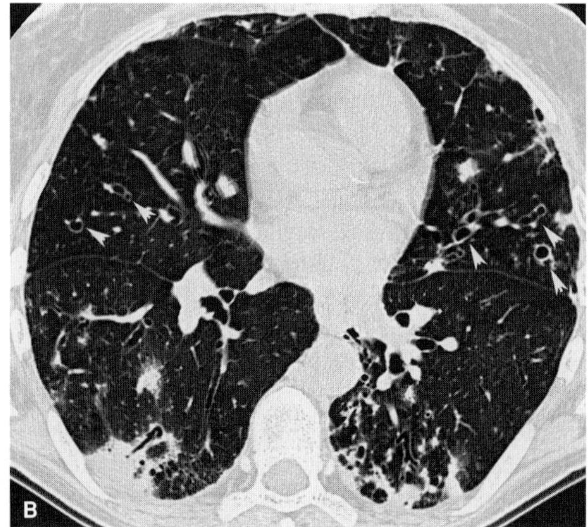

FIGURE 16.10. ***Mycobacterium avium-intracellulare*** **(MAI) Infection.** Thin-section CT scans through mid-lungs **(A)** and lower **(B)** lungs in a patient with MAI pulmonary infection show bronchiectasis (*arrowheads*), scattered nodules, and tree-in-bud (*arrows*).

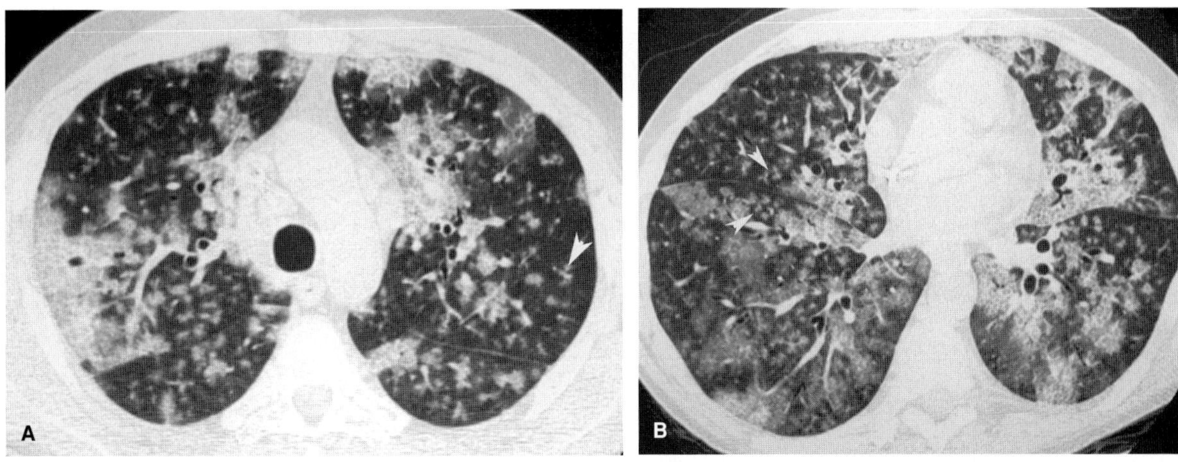

FIGURE 16.11. **Parainfluenza Virus Pneumonia.** CT through upper lungs **(A)** and mid-lungs **(B)** in a patient with acute myelogenous leukemia (AML) shows striking bronchopneumonia and bronchiolitis (*arrowheads*). Parainfluenza virus was isolated from bronchoalveolar lavage fluid.

Acute histoplasma infection most often presents with the abrupt onset of flulike symptoms. The chest radiograph in such patients may be normal or may show nonspecific changes, including subsegmental airspace opacities with or without associated hilar lymph enlargement. If the patient inhales a large inoculum of organisms, widespread, fairly discrete nodular opacities 3 to 4 mm in diameter are seen with hilar adenopathy. Alternatively, acute histoplasmosis may result in a solitary, sharply defined nodular opacity, <3 cm in diameter, termed a *histoplasmoma*. Histoplasmomas are most common in the lower lobes and frequently calcify.

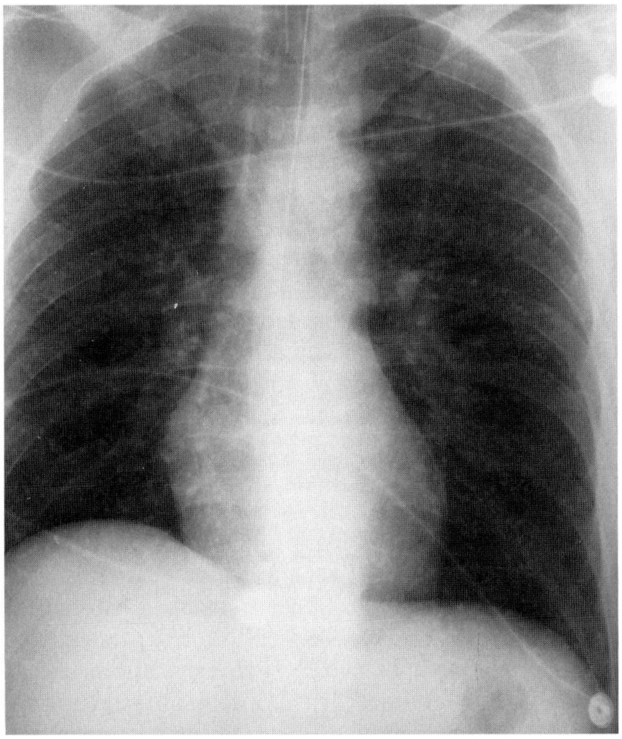

H capsulatum can also cause chronic pulmonary disease, usually in patients with underlying emphysema. Unilateral or bilateral upper lobe cicatrizing atelectasis with marked hilar retraction may mimic the radiographic findings seen in postprimary TB. Similarly, chronic upper lobe fibrocavitary disease may be seen. Involvement of the mediastinum by chronic granulomatous inflammation may lead to fibrosing mediastinitis, while endobronchial disease can produce bronchostenosis.

Asymptomatic blood-borne dissemination of *H capsulatum* is common, as judged by the frequency of calcified splenic granulomas in residents of endemic areas. Clinically apparent disseminated histoplasmosis, however, is extremely rare and is usually seen in infants or immunocompromised adults. The chest film most commonly shows widespread 2- to 3-mm nodules that are indistinguishable from those of miliary TB, though reticular opacities and patchy areas of consolidations may also be seen.

Coccidioidomycosis. *Coccidioides immitis* is endemic to the southwestern United States and the San Joaquin Valley of California. There are four types of clinical and radiographic coccidioidal pulmonary infection: acute, persistent, chronic progressive, and disseminated coccidioidomycosis. Acute coccidioidomycosis develops in 40% of infected adults. These patients develop a self-limiting viral-type illness, which is referred to as "valley fever" when associated with erythema nodosum and arthralgias. The chest radiograph may be normal or show focal or

FIGURE 16.12. **Healed Varicella Pneumonia.** Frontal chest radiograph in a 38-year-old man shows multiple small calcified nodules representing healed varicella pneumonia.

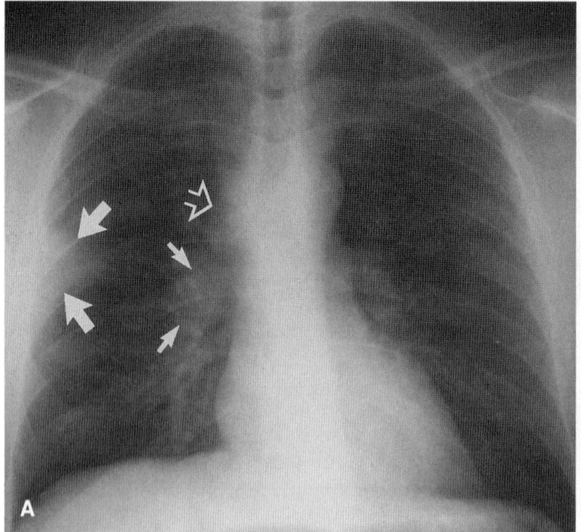

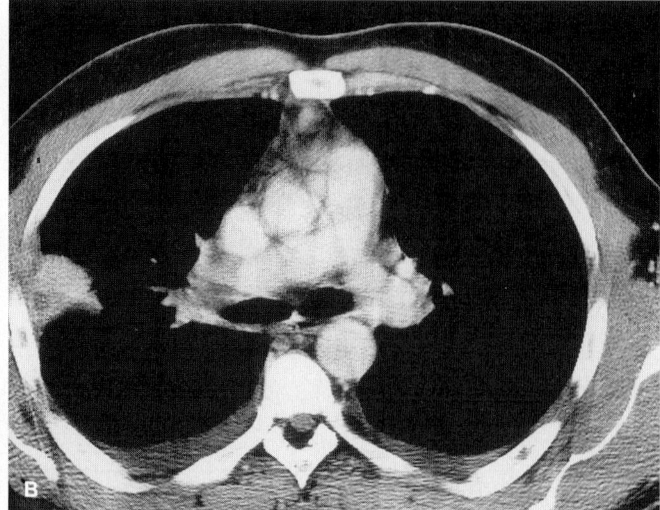

FIGURE 16.13. **Primary *Coccidioides* Infection. A.** Frontal radiograph in a 42-year-old man reveals a pleura-based, wedge-shaped opacity in the peripheral portion of the right upper lobe (*large arrows*) with enlarged right hilar (*small arrows*) and paratracheal (*open arrow*) nodes. **B.** A CT scan confirms the presence of right hilar nodal enlargement and shows a small focus of necrosis within the parenchymal lesion. Fluoroscopically guided transthoracic biopsy of the peripheral lung lesion revealed coccidioidomycosis.

multifocal segmental airspace opacities that resolve over several months. Hilar and mediastinal adenopathy and pleural effusions may be seen in association with parenchymal disease (Fig. 16.13).

Patients whose symptoms or radiographic abnormalities persist beyond 6 to 8 weeks are considered to have persistent coccidioidomycosis. The radiographic features of persistent pulmonary disease include coccidioidal nodules or masses (coccidioidomas), persistent areas of consolidation, and miliary nodules. Coccidioidal nodules are areas of round pneumonia, usually located in the subpleural regions of the upper lobes. These nodules tend to cavitate rapidly and produce characteristic thin-walled cavities. In chronic progressive disease, upper lobe fibrocavitary disease similar to postprimary TB and histoplasmosis is seen. Disseminated (miliary) coccidioidomycosis is relatively rare and usually affects immunocompromised patients and non-Caucasians (Fig. 16.14).

Blastomycosis. North American blastomycosis, caused by *B dermatitidis,* is a chronic systemic disease primarily affecting the lungs and skin. Its geographic distribution overlaps that of histoplasmosis but extends farther to the east and north. The pulmonary infection is often asymptomatic. Symptomatic infection resembles that of an acute bacterial pneumonia. The radiographic findings in pulmonary blastomycosis are nonspecific. The most common manifestation of disease is homogeneous nonsegmental airspace opacification with a propensity for the upper lobes. A less common presentation is single or multiple masses, which cavitate in 15% of cases. Pulmonary masses tend to occur in patients with prolonged symptoms (>1 month) and may mimic bronchogenic carcinoma. A third pattern of disease is diffuse reticulonodular opacities. Pleural effusion and lymph node enlargement are uncommon. A disseminated miliary form may be seen in immunocompromised hosts.

Aspergillus species are responsible for a spectrum of pulmonary diseases in humans. These include aspergilloma or mycetoma formation within preexisting cavities, semi-invasive (chronic necrotizing) aspergillosis in patients with mildly impaired immunity, invasive pulmonary aspergillosis in the neutropenic lymphoma or leukemia patient, and allergic bronchopulmonary aspergillosis in the hyperimmune patient.

An aspergilloma (mycetoma, fungus ball) is a ball of hyphae, mucus, and cellular debris that colonizes a preexisting bulla or a parenchymal cavity created by some other pathogen or destructive process. Invasion into adjacent lung parenchyma does not occur unless host defense mechanisms are compromised. The mycetoma is usually asymptomatic, but may cause hemoptysis, which may be massive (>350 mL/24 hours). An aspergilloma is seen as a solid round mass within an upper lobe cavity, with an "air crescent" separating the mycetoma from the cavity wall (Fig. 16.15). The mycetoma is usually free within the cavity and can be seen to roll dependently on decubitus radiographs or CT. Progressive apical pleural thickening adjacent to a cavity is a common radiographic finding and should prompt a search for a complicating mycetoma. Semi-invasive and invasive aspergillosis are discussed later in this chapter, while allergic bronchopulmonary aspergillosis is reviewed in Chapter 18.

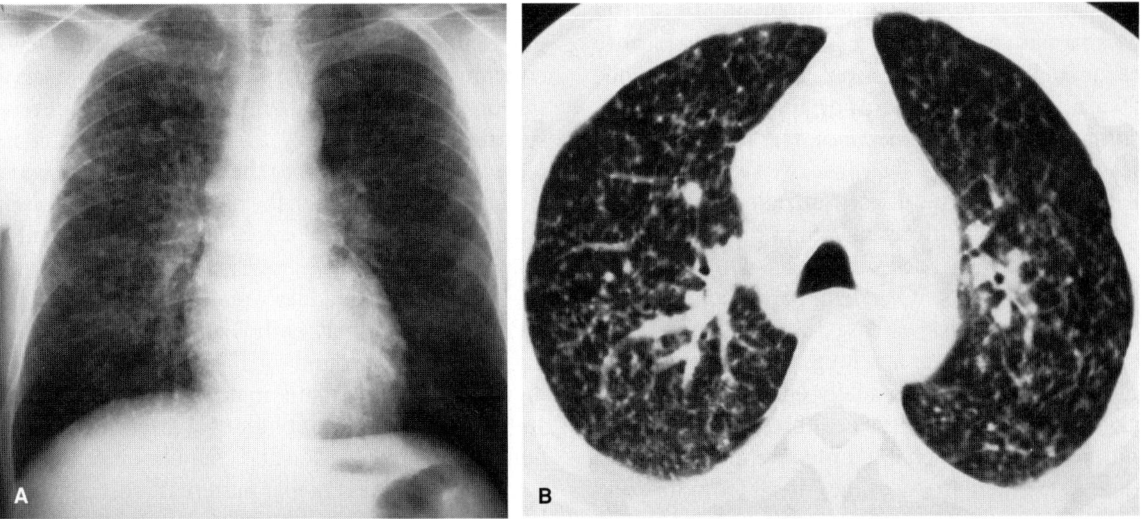

FIGURE 16.14. **Disseminated (Miliary) Coccidioidomycosis. A.** Frontal radiograph in a 42-year-old patient with AIDS shows miliary nodulation with enlarged hilar and mediastinal nodes. **B.** CT confirms the presence of diffuse nodular and reticular opacities. Transbronchial biopsy showed *Coccidioides* infection.

Parasitic Infection

Parasitic infections of the lung are relatively uncommon in the United States. However, increases in travel to countries where parasites are endemic, the immigration of people from these regions to the United States, and growing numbers of immunocompromised patients require a familiarity with these infections. In general, parasitic diseases of the thorax are manifested by either a direct invasion of lungs and pleura or, less commonly, a hypersensitivity reaction (11).

Amebiasis. Symptomatic infection with *Entamoeba histolytica* is usually confined to the GI tract and liver. If the infection remains confined to the subphrenic space, a right pleural effusion and basilar atelectasis may result from local diaphragmatic inflammation. The most common method of pleuropulmonary involvement by amebiasis is by the direct intrathoracic extension of infection

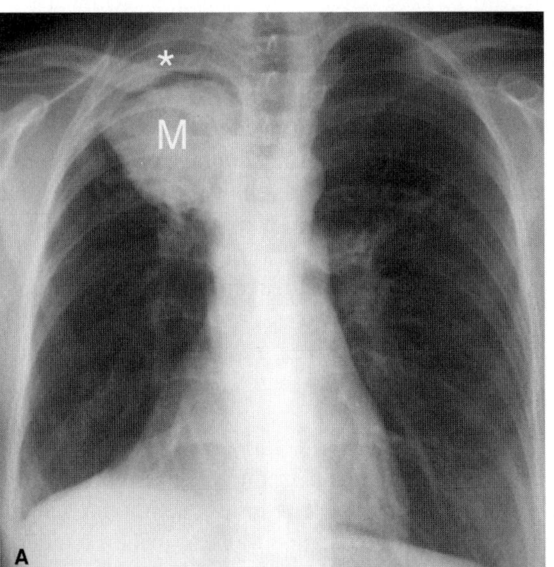

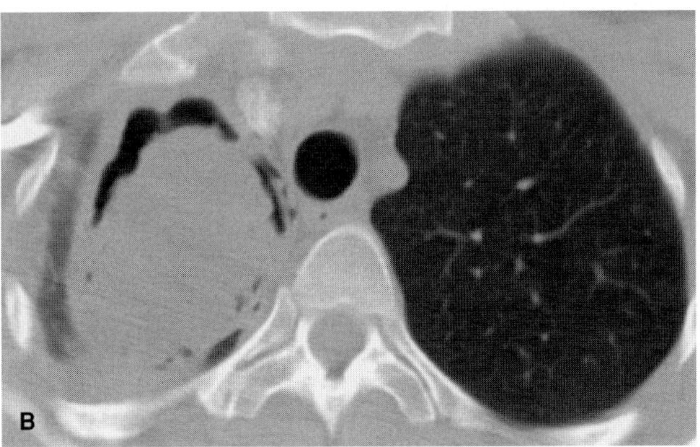

FIGURE 16.15. **Aspergilloma. A.** Posteroanterior chest radiograph in a 32-year-old woman with prior tuberculosis and recent hemoptysis shows a mass (M) in the right upper lung capped by a crescent of air with adjacent apical pleural thickening (*asterisk*). **B.** CT scan shows a mass representing a mycetoma within a preexisting cavity. Sputum showed heavy *Aspergillus*.

from a hepatic abscess. This transdiaphragmatic spread of organisms may extend into the right pleural space to produce an empyema or may involve the right lower lobe to produce an amebic pneumonia or lung abscess.

Hydatid Disease (Echinococcosis) of the Lung. *Echinococcus granulosus* is the cause of most cases of human hydatid disease. The disease is endemic in sheep-raising areas and is relatively uncommon in the United States. Dogs are the usual definitive hosts, with sheep acting as intermediate hosts. When a human becomes an accidental intermediate host, disease may result. The larval organisms travel to the liver and lungs and, if they survive host defenses, encyst and gradually enlarge. Pulmonary echinococcal cysts are composed of three layers: an exocyst (chitinous layer), which is a protective membrane; an inner endocyst, which produces the "daughter cysts"; and a surrounding capsule of compressed, fibrotic lung known as the pericyst.

Pulmonary echinococcal cysts characteristically present as well-circumscribed, spherical soft tissue masses. In distinction to hepatic cysts, lung cysts do not have calcified walls. The cysts range in size from 1 to 20 cm, with a predilection for the lower lobes and the right side. While most cysts remain asymptomatic, patients may present when the cyst develops a communication with the bronchial tree. If the pericyst ruptures, a thin crescent of air will be seen around the periphery of the cyst, producing the "meniscus" or "crescent" sign. If the cyst itself ruptures, the contents of the cyst are expelled into the airways, producing an air–fluid level. On occasion, the cyst wall may be seen crumpled and floating within an uncollapsed pericyst, producing the pathognomonic "sign of the camalote" or "water lily" sign. Rarely, a cyst will rupture into the pleural space, producing a large pleural effusion.

Paragonimiasis results from infection with the lung fluke *Paragonimus westermani*. The organism is found predominantly in eastern Asia and is usually acquired by eating raw crabs or snails. Infestation of the lung may be asymptomatic, or a patient may present with cough, hemoptysis, dyspnea, and fever. In 20% of affected patients, the chest radiograph is normal. The most common radiographic finding is multiple cysts with variable wall thickness. These cystic opacities may become confluent and are often associated with focal atelectasis and subsegmental consolidation. Dense linear opacities representing the burrows of the organisms may be identified. Because the flukes penetrate the pleura, effusions are common and may be massive.

Schistosomiasis. Human schistosomiasis is caused by three blood flukes: *Schistosoma mansoni*, *S japonicum*, and *S haematobium*. It is one of the most important parasitic infestations of humans worldwide, although it is rarely acquired in the United States. The life cycle of the fluke is complex, with human infestation acquired through contact with infested water. The larvae penetrate the skin or oropharyngeal mucosa and travel via the venous circulation to the pulmonary capillaries. As the larvae pass through the lungs, an allergic response may develop, presenting radiographically as transient airspace opacities (eosinophilic pneumonia) that resolve spontaneously. The larvae then pass through the pulmonary capillaries into the systemic circulation. *S japonicum* and *S mansoni* eventually migrate to the mesenteric venules, while *S haematobium* migrates to bladder venules. The mature flukes produce ova, which may embolize to the lungs, where they implant in and around small pulmonary arterioles. The organism induces granulomatous inflammation and fibrosis, which leads to an obliterative arteriolitis, resulting in pulmonary hypertension and cor pulmonale. Radiographically, a diffuse fine reticular pattern is most commonly seen in association with dilatation of the central pulmonary arteries. Small nodular opacities resembling miliary TB may be seen as granulomata forming around ova.

INFECTION IN THE IMMUNOCOMPROMISED HOST AND IN AIDS

Immunocompromise is defined as a decrease in the normal host defense mechanisms that fight infection. Immunocompromised patients include those with HIV infection, underlying hematologic malignancy, and individuals receiving chemotherapeutic and immunosuppressive therapy. The types of pulmonary infection seen in the immunocompromised patient depend on the specific defect(s) in host defense mechanisms. While the majority of pulmonary complications in immunocompromised patients are infectious in nature, noninfectious complications of disease can account for up to 25% of lung disease in this population. The accurate identification of the predominant radiographic pattern of abnormality in the immunocompromised patient helps limit the differential diagnostic considerations (Tables 16.1, 16.2) (12). With the advent of highly active antiretroviral therapy (HAART) and effective prophylaxis, the incidence of opportunistic infection in HIV/AIDS has decreased dramatically. Bacterial respiratory infections now account for most pulmonary infections in individuals living with HIV in the developed world (13,14).

Bacterial Pneumonia. Bacteria are the most common cause of pneumonia in immunocompromised hosts. In HIV-infected patients, bacterial pneumonia may occur early in the course of infection and has an incidence six times that seen in the normal population. The occurrence of two or more episodes of bacterial pneumonia within 1 year is categorized as an AIDS-defining illness for patients with HIV infection. The most common organisms causing pneumonia in HIV patients are *S pneumoniae*,

TABLE 16.1 Radiographic Patterns of Abnormality in Non-HIV Immunocompromised Patients

Pattern	*Potential Etiology*
Lobar/segmental consolidation	Gram-negative bacteria Gram-positive bacteria *Legionella*
Nodules ± cavitation	Fungi *Aspergillus* species *Coccidioides immitis* *Cryptococcus neoformans* *Mucor* species *Nocardia asteroides* *Legionella micdadei* Neoplasm Other
Diffuse lung disease	*Pneumocystis jiroveci* Viral pneumonia Fungi *Toxoplasma gondii* *Strongyloides stercoralis* Drug reaction Hemorrhage Radiation pneumonitis Nonspecific interstitial pneumonia (NSIP) Lymphangitic carcinomatosis

Modified from McLoud and Naidich (12); material used with permission.

TABLE 16.2 Radiographic Patterns of Abnormality in AIDS Patients

Pattern	*Potential Etiology*
Normal	*Pneumocystis jiroveci* pneumonia (PCP) Tuberculosis or fungal infection Nonspecific interstitial pneumonia (NSIP)
Focal lung disease	Bacterial pneumonia PCP Mycobacterial/fungal infection Non-Hodgkin lymphoma
Diffuse lung disease	PCP PCP + other infection (cytomegalovirus, *Mycobacterium avium-intracellulare*, miliary tuberculosis, fungus) *Mycobacterium tuberculosis* Fungal infection NSIP Lymphocytic interstitial pneumonia (LIP) Kaposi sarcoma
Nodules	Non-Hodgkin lymphoma Kaposi sarcoma Septic emboli Mycobacterial/fungal infection
Adenopathy	Mycobacterial or fungal infection Kaposi sarcoma Non-Hodgkin lymphoma PCP (uncommon)
Pleural effusion	Kaposi sarcoma Mycobacterial/fungal infection Non-Hodgkin lymphoma Pyogenic empyema PCP (uncommon)

Modified from McLoud and Naidich (12); material used with permission.

H influenzae, S aureus, E coli, and *P aeruginosa*. Uncommon causes of bacterial pneumonia in the AIDS population include *Nocardia asteroides, Rhodococcus equi, Bartonella henselae,* and *B quintana* (bacillary angiomatosis). In the non-HIV immunocompromised patient, *S aureus* and gram-negative aerobes including *Klebsiella, Proteus, E coli, Pseudomonas, Enterobacter,* and *Serratia* are the most common bacterial pathogens. Bacterial pneumonia is characterized by focal segmental or lobar airspace opacities. Cavitation is more frequent in the immunocompromised population than in normal individuals and may occur as multiple microabscesses. Multilobar involvement and diffuse pneumonia may occur and are distinctly unusual in normal individuals. Pleural effusions and empyema are uncommon (13).

Renal transplant recipients and patients on high-dose corticosteroids are at increased risk of pneumonia caused by *Legionella pneumophila* and *L micdadei* (Pittsburgh agent). *L pneumophila* causes multilobar focal areas of consolidation, sometimes with cavitation and pleural effusion. The Pittsburgh agent causes a characteristic appearance of multiple, well-circumscribed, centrally cavitating nodules.

Nocardia is a gram-positive, branching, filamentous bacillus that is weakly acid fast. *N asteroides* is the most important cause of pulmonary disease. It is usually an opportunistic infection in patients on immunosuppressive therapy, those with lymphoma or leukemia, and patients with alveolar proteinosis. The most frequent radiographic presentation is a homogeneous, nonsegmental airspace opacity or a mass. Cavitation is frequent (Fig. 16.16). Infection may extend into the pleural space and chest wall to produce empyema and osteomyelitis, respectively. Hilar lymph nodes may be enlarged. Treatment is with sulfur antibiotics.

Tuberculosis. The incidence of TB has increased considerably since the onset of the AIDS epidemic. Most cases are caused by reactivation of previously acquired disease. The diagnosis of TB in immunocompromised hosts is complicated because skin reactivity and sputum analysis are less sensitive in immunocompromised hosts and the yield of bronchoalveolar lavage is decreased in this patient population. The chest radiographic findings depend on the stage of HIV infection and the degree of immune dysfunction, which can be estimated by the CD4 count. In

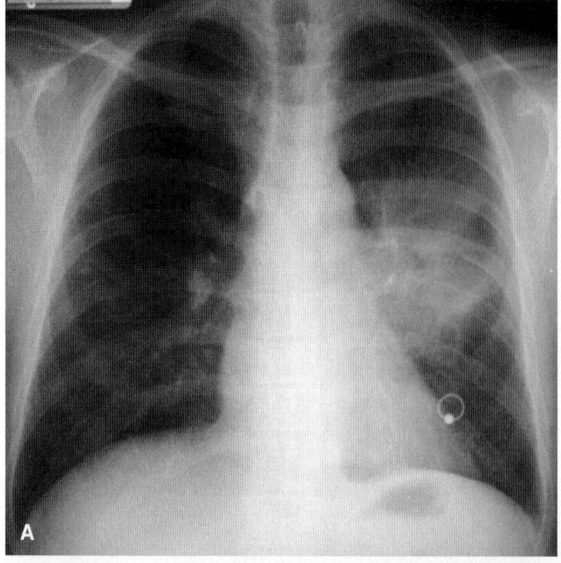

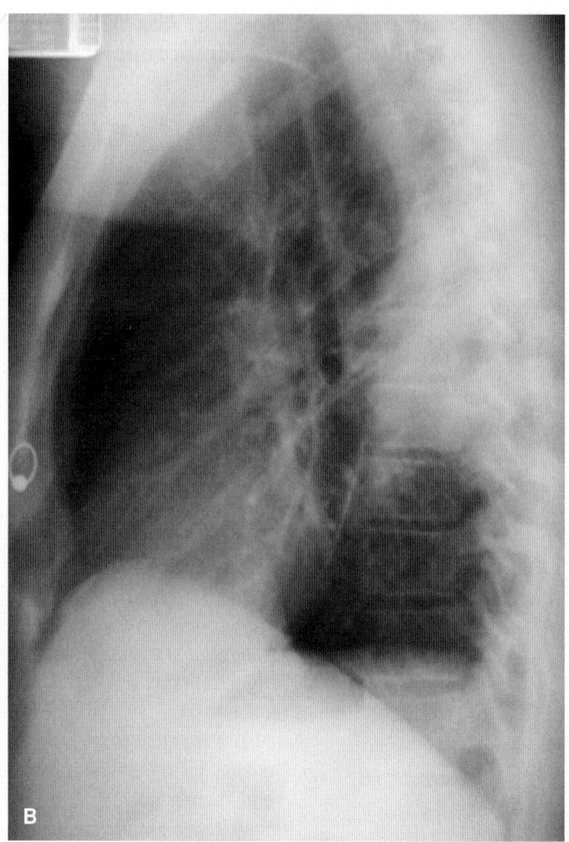

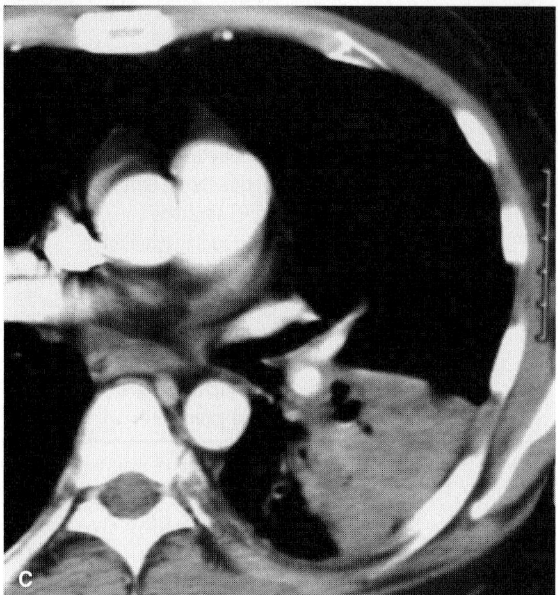

FIGURE 16.16. **Nocardiosis.** Posteroanterior **(A)** and lateral **(B)** chest radiographs in a 34-year-old man with AIDS show airspace opacification in the superior segment of the left lower lobe. CT **(C)** shows consolidation with cavitation. Sputum stain and culture showed Nocardia infection.

the early stages of AIDS (CD4 >200 cells/mm^3), a postprimary pattern of upper lobe fibrocavitary disease indistinguishable from that seen in the immunocompetent patient is most common. Later in the course of AIDS (CD4 50 to 200 cells/mm^3), the radiographic features most often associated with primary disease are seen and include lobar consolidation, mediastinal and hilar lymphadenopathy, and pleural effusion (6). Rim-enhancing nodes with central necrosis on CT scans are a characteristic finding and should strongly suggest TB in a patient with AIDS. In advanced AIDS (CD4 <50 cells/mm^3), the radiographic findings are atypical and are characterized by diffuse reticular or nodular (miliary) opacities.

Mycobacterium avium-intracellulare (MAI) infection is the most common non-tuberculous mycobacterial infection in AIDS patients. The disease primarily affects the GI tract, but disseminated disease can involve the chest. Lymphadenopathy is the major radiographic manifestation, but nonspecific focal airspace opacity or diffuse nodular opacities may be seen. Infection by *M kansasii* may produce a pattern identical to that of postprimary TB.

Viral pneumonia is uncommon in AIDS and other immunocompromised patients with defects in cell-mediated immunity (Fig. 16.11).

Cytomegalovirus is a common cause of viral pneumonia in patients with impaired cell-mediated immunity, specifically renal transplant recipients and lymphoma. It is an uncommon cause of pneumonia in the AIDS population. Chest radiographs show diffuse bilateral reticular or nodular opacities in the lower lobes.

Aspergillosis. Invasive aspergillus infection usually occurs in severely immunocompromised patients with neutropenia, most commonly those with leukemia or those receiving chemotherapy or corticosteroids. It occurs less frequently in AIDS patients, usually in the terminal stages of disease. The radiographic manifestations range from large nodular opacities to diffuse parenchymal consolidation (Fig. 16.17). The organism tends to invade blood vessels, causing infarction. Much of the observed opacity represents hemorrhage and edema. If pleural effusion develops, it usually indicates empyema. Cavitation, in the form of an air crescent, is not usually evident on chest films early in the course of disease, but it characteristically develops when the patient's complement of circulating neutrophils returns to a normal level. CT, particularly HRCT, is useful for the early diagnosis of invasive aspergillosis. The demonstration of a zone of relative decreased attenuation surrounding a dense, masslike opacity has been termed the "CT halo sign" and is relatively specific for invasive aspergillosis in a neutropenic patient (Fig. 16.18). The halo represents a region of edema and hemorrhage where an air crescent will develop, separating the region of infected, necrotic lung from normal parenchyma.

Semi-invasive aspergillosis is an unusual form of *Aspergillus* pulmonary infection seen in patients with mild degrees of immunosuppression. The organism invades previously diseased lung tissue, producing slowly progressive airspace opacification or chronic cavitary disease.

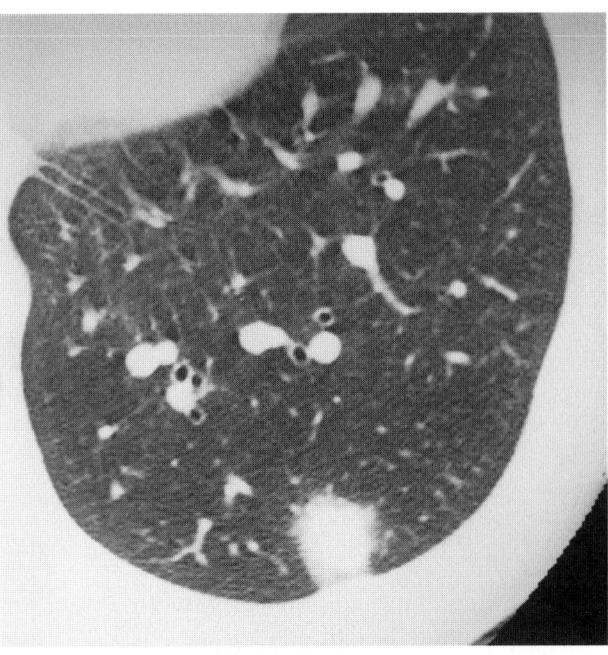

FIGURE 16.18. **HRCT of Invasive Aspergillosis (the "CT Halo" Sign).** Cone-down view of an HRCT through the left lower lobe in a patient receiving high-dose corticosteroid therapy shows a nodule with a halo of ground-glass opacity, characteristic of invasive aspergillosis.

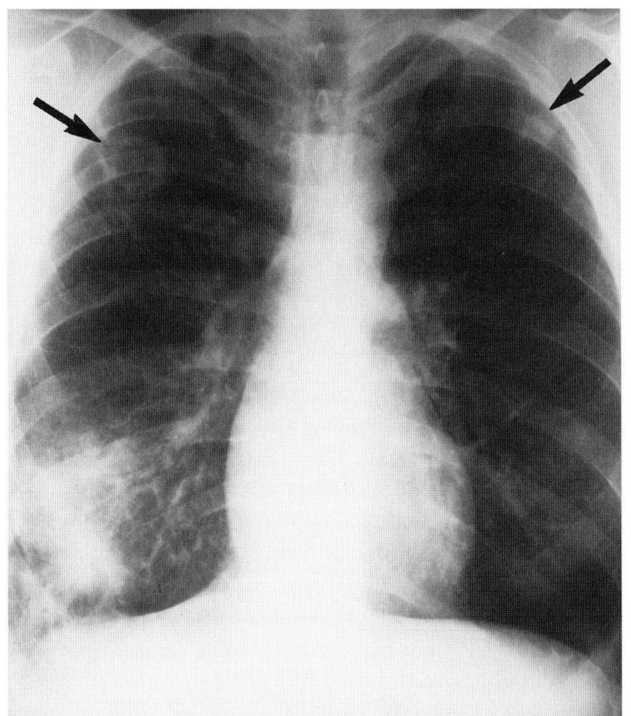

FIGURE 16.17. **Invasive Aspergillosis.** Posteroanterior radiograph in an immunocompromised patient with *Aspergillus* infection reveals right lower lobe opacification and bilateral upper lobe nodules with cavitation (*arrows*).

Coccidioidomycosis in AIDS and other immunocompromised hosts is usually manifested by disseminated infection rather than the localized granulomatous disease seen in normal hosts. Pulmonary involvement is usually diffuse and produces miliary nodules, diffuse nodules, or reticulonodular opacities (Fig. 16.14). Hilar and mediastinal lymphadenopathy and pleural effusions are uncommon.

Cryptococcosis. *Cryptococcus neoformans* is a budding yeast commonly found in soil and bird droppings. *Cryptococcus* is the most common cause of fungal infection in the AIDS population but can affect any immunocompromised patient. In some patients, particularly those with AIDS, the organism disseminates from its portal of entry in the lung to involve the CNS, bones, and mucocutaneous tissues. Meningitis is the most serious consequence of infection. There are several chest radiographic patterns of disease: single or multiple nodules or masses (mimicking bronchogenic carcinoma) (Fig. 16.19), single or multiple patchy airspace opacities, and multiple small nodules (mimicking miliary TB). Cavitation, lymphadenopathy, and pleural effusion are more commonly seen in AIDS patients than in normal hosts.

Candidiasis. *Candida albicans* is an unusual cause of pneumonia in the immunocompromised patient. Patients

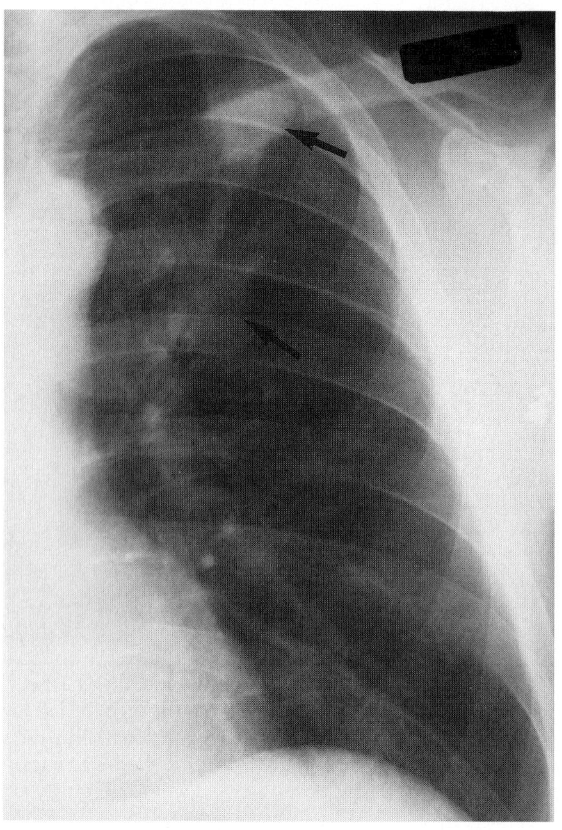

FIGURE 16.19. ***Cryptococcus*** **in AIDS.** Cone-down view of the left upper lobe in a 45-year-old AIDS patient shows two left upper lobe nodules (*arrows*). Stains of a transthoracic needle biopsy aspirate showed cryptococcal pneumonia.

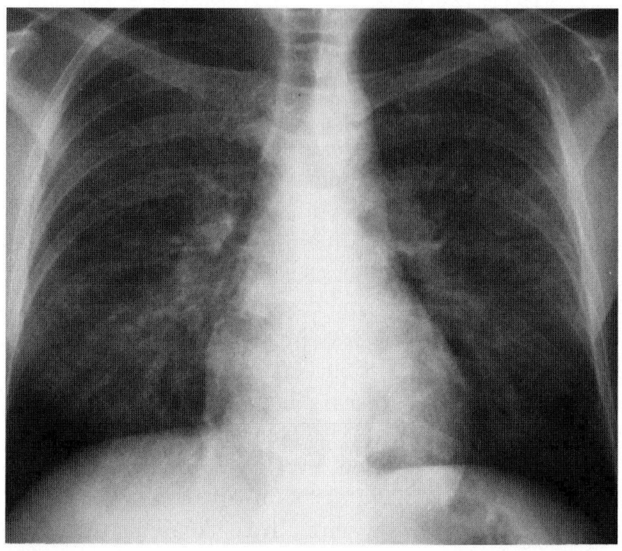

FIGURE 16.20. ***Pneumocystis jiroveci*** **Pneumonia.** Frontal radiograph in a 36-year-old man with HIV infection shows bilateral symmetric fine reticular or ground-glass opacities. Stains of induced sputum revealed *P jiroveci*.

with severe neutropenia caused by lymphoma or leukemia in the late stages of disease are most susceptible. The diagnosis is often difficult because *Candida* is a common colonizer in immunocompromised patients and its presence is often associated with other opportunistic infections. Chest radiographs in patients with *Candida* pneumonia show diffuse, bilateral, nonsegmental airspace or interstitial opacities. Miliary nodules may be seen, but cavitation, adenopathy, and pleural effusion are uncommon features.

Mucormycosis is a rare cause of pneumonia in immunocompromised patients with lymphoma, leukemia, or diabetes. Pulmonary infection is commonly accompanied by paranasal sinus infection, which may extend to involve the brain or meninges. Chest radiographic appearances include a solitary nodule or mass or focal airspace opacity, which may cavitate. Pleural effusion is uncommon.

Pneumocystis jiroveci Pneumonia. *P jiroveci* (formerly *P carinii*) is a fungus commonly found in human lungs, although clinically significant pneumonia is seen only in immunocompromised individuals. *P jiroveci* pneumonia (PCP) is most common in AIDS patients, usually in the late stages of HIV infection (CD4 <200 cells/mm^3) (15). With the advent of HAART, the incidence of PCP has decreased significantly in the developed world. PCP still occurs in patients with HIV infection who are undiagnosed, not taking or responding to HAART, and those failing or not taking prophylaxis with trimethoprim sulfamethoxazole. Despite HAART and prophylaxis, PCP remains the most common AIDS-defining opportunistic infection. Organ transplant recipients on immunosuppressive drugs (particularly corticosteroids) and patients with lymphoreticular malignancies are also at increased risk for infection.

The chest radiograph may be normal in the early phase of disease. In such patients, gallium scanning or HRCT of the lung may provide evidence of subradiographic disease. As the disease progresses, a fine reticular or ground-glass pattern develops, particularly in the parahilar regions (Fig. 16.20). Progressive disease leads to confluent symmetric airspace opacification. Pleural effusion or lymph node enlargement is distinctly uncommon (<5%) and should suggest an alternative or additional diagnosis. The diagnosis of PCP in AIDS is made by methenamine silver staining of induced sputum samples or bronchoalveolar lavage fluid specimens.

Several atypical radiographic features of PCP have been described. PCP may manifest as single or multiple pulmonary nodules, simulating fungal infection or such malignancies as Kaposi sarcoma. Thin-walled cysts or pneumatoceles may develop during the course of disease and are responsible for an increased incidence of spontaneous pneumothorax, complicating PCP (Fig. 16.21). Patients receiving prophylaxis with inhaled aerosolized pentamidine

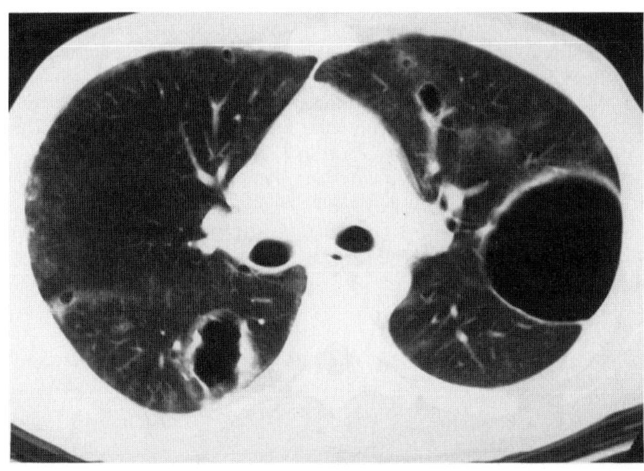

FIGURE 16.21. **Lung Cysts in *Pneumocystis jiroveci* Pneumonia.** CT in a patient with documented *P jiroveci* pneumonia shows scattered areas of ground-glass opacity with variably sized thin-walled cysts. Note the subpleural location of the large left upper lobe cyst.

TABLE 16.3 Pulmonary Complications in Bone Marrow Transplant Recipients

Time Period	*Complication*
Neutropenic phase (0–30 days)	Pulmonary edema Alveolar hemorrhage Fungal infection Drug reaction
Early phase (30–100 days)	Fungal infection Drug reaction Cytomegalovirus infection Upper respiratory virus infection Idiopathic pneumonia Acute graft-versus-host disease
Late phase (>100 days)	Bronchiolitis obliterans Bronchiolitis obliterans–organizing pneumonia Chronic graft-versus-host disease Upper respiratory virus (to 6 months) Idiopathic pneumonia (to 6 months)

Modified from Gosselin and Adams (16); material used with permission.

are prone to develop predominantly upper lobe PCP, which simulates postprimary TB. Rare cases of miliary PCP simulating TB or disseminated fungal infection have been reported. Patients receiving systemic prophylaxis with cotrimoxazole are also at risk for extrapulmonary *Pneumocystis* infection. Systemic *Pneumocystis* infection generally involves the liver, spleen, kidney, and lymph nodes, and appears on CT or US as microabscesses or punctate calcifications.

Toxoplasmosis. *Toxoplasma gondii* is an obligate intracellular protozoan whose definitive host is the cat. Humans acquire the organism by ingestion of material contaminated by oocyst-containing stool. It has been estimated that toxoplasmosis exists in a chronic asymptomatic form in 50% of the population of the United States. Disease can be recognized in four clinicopathologic forms: congenital, ocular, lymphatic, and generalized. Pulmonary involvement is usually seen in the generalized form of the disease, which affects immunocompromised hosts, including those with AIDS, organ transplant recipients, and patients with leukemia or lymphoma.

The radiographic findings in pulmonary toxoplasmosis include diffuse reticular opacities that resemble those of acute viral pneumonia. Less commonly, airspace opacities with air bronchograms may be seen. Hilar and mediastinal lymph node enlargement is common, while pleural effusion is rare. With generalized disease, most often seen in patients with AIDS, diffuse bilateral small nodular opacities may be seen.

Bone marrow transplant (BMT) recipients have a high (40% to 60%) incidence of pulmonary complications. Because of the predictable course of immune suppression, a timeline of expected pulmonary complications can be constructed to help narrow the differential diagnosis for radiographic abnormalities in patients following BMT. The time following BMT can be divided into three phases: the neutropenic phase, the early phase, and the late phase. The neutropenic phase lasts for approximately the first 30 days, followed by the early phase (from 30 to 100 days), and finally the late phase (more than 100 days post-BMT). Complications can be infectious or noninfectious and are detailed according to time of presentation in Table 16.3 (16).

REFERENCES

1. Kantor HG. Many radiologic faces of pneumococcal pneumonia. AJR Am J Roentgenol 1981;137:1213–1220.
2. Krol CM, Uszynski M, Dillon EH, et al. Dynamic CT features of inhalational anthrax infection. AJR Am J Roentgenol 2002;178:1063–1066.
3. Pierce AK, Sandford JP. Aerobic gram-negative bacillary pneumonias: state of the art. Am Rev Respir Dis 1974;110:647–658.
4. Bartlett JG, Finegold SM. Anaerobic infections of the lung and pleural space. Am Rev Respir Dis 1974;110:56–77.
5. Kwong JS, Muller NL, Godwin JD, et al. Thoracic actinomycosis: CT findings in eight patients. Radiology 1992;183:189–192.
6. Leung AL. Pulmonary tuberculosis: the essentials. Radiology 1999;210:307–322.
7. Contreras MA, Cheung OT, Sanders DE, et al. Pulmonary infection with nontuberculous mycobacteria. Am Rev Respir Dis 1988;137: 149–152.
8. Kim EA, Lee KS, Primack SL, Yoon HK, et al. Viral pneumonias in adults: radiologic and pathologic findings. Radiographics 2002;22: S137–S149.
9. Antonio GE, Wong KT, Hui DS, et al. Imaging of severe acute respiratory syndrome in Hong Kong. AJR Am J Roentgenol 2003;181:11–17.
10. Bhalla M, McLoud TC. Pulmonary Infections in the Normal Host. In: McCloud TC (ed). Thoracic Radiology. St. Louis: Mosby, 1998: 122–130.

11. Martinez S, Restrepo S, Carrillo J, Betancourt S, et al. Thoracic manifestations of tropical parasitic infections: a pictorial review. Radiographics 2005;25:135–155.
12. McLoud TC, Naidich DP. Thoracic disease in the immunocompromised patient. Radiol Clin North Am 1992;30:525–554.
13. Brecher CW, Aviram G, Boiselle P. CT and radiography of bacterial respiratory infections in AIDS patients. AJR Am J Roentgenol 2003;180:1203–1209.
14. Shah RM, Kaji AV, Ostrum BJ, Friedman AC. Interpretation of chest radiographs in AIDS patients: usefulness of CD4 lymphocyte counts. Radiographics 1997;17:47–58.
15. Morris A, Lundgren JD, Masur H, et al. Current epidemiology of *Pneumocystis* pneumonia. Emerg Infect Dis 2004;10:1713–1720.
16. Gosselin M, Adams R. Pulmonary complications in bone marrow transplantation. J Thorac Imaging 2002;17:132–144.

Chapter 17

Diffuse Lung Disease

Jeffrey S. Klein

HRCT of the Pulmonary Interstitium
HRCT Signs of Disease

Chronic Interstitial Lung Disease
Chronic Interstitial Pulmonary Edema
Connective Tissue Disease
Idiopathic Chronic Interstitial Pneumonias
Other Chronic Interstitial Lung Diseases

Inhalational Disease
Pneumoconiosis
Hypersensitivity Pneumonitis

Granulomatous Diseases
Sarcoidosis
Berylliosis
Langerhans Cell Histiocytosis of Lung
Wegener Granulomatosis

Eosinophilic Lung Disease
Idiopathic Eosinophilic Lung Disease
Eosinophilic Lung Disease of Identifiable Etiology
Eosinophilic Lung Disease Associated with Autoimmune Diseases

Miscellaneous Disorders

Diffuse lung disease represents a broad spectrum of disorders that primarily affect the pulmonary interstitium (Table 17.1). These diseases present in a variety of manners, most typically with symptoms of progressive dyspnea. However, some patients present with minimal or no symptoms and interstitial lung disease is discovered either incidentally or during radiologic screening for interstitial disease associated with collagen vascular disease. Restrictive lung disease and hypoxemia on pulmonary function tests are characteristically present. The radiographic findings produced by interstitial disease are reviewed in Chapter 12. HRCT has revolutionized the diagnosis of interstitial lung disease, and its role in the evaluation of interstitial disease is detailed in this chapter.

HRCT OF THE PULMONARY INTERSTITIUM

Normal Anatomy. HRCT provides the most direct radiographic method for assessment of the pulmonary interstitium. The general utility of HRCT in the evaluation of chronic interstitial lung disease is outlined in Table 17.2 (1). The pulmonary interstitium is the scaffolding of the lung, providing support for the airways, gas-exchanging units, and vascular structures. It is a continuous network of connective tissue fibers that begins at the lung hilum and extends peripherally to the visceral pleura (see Fig. 12.10). The central interstitial compartment extending from the mediastinum peripherally and enveloping the bronchovascular bundles is termed the *axial* or *bronchovascular interstitium*. The axial interstitium is contiguous with the interstitium surrounding the small centrilobular arteriole and bronchiole within the secondary pulmonary lobule, where it is called the *centrilobular interstitium*. The most peripheral component of the interstitium is the *subpleural* or *peripheral interstitium,* which lies between the visceral pleura and the lung surface. Invaginations of the subpleural interstitium into the lung parenchyma form the borders of the secondary pulmonary lobules and represent the interlobular septa. Extending between the centrilobular interstitium within the lobular core and the interlobular septal/subpleural interstitium in the lobular periphery is a fine network of connective tissue fibers that support the alveolar spaces called the *intralobular, parenchymal,* or *alveolar interstitium.*

The secondary pulmonary lobule is defined as that subsegment of lung supplied by three to five terminal bronchioles and separated from adjacent secondary lobules by intervening connective tissue (interlobular septa) (Fig. 17.1).

TABLE 17.1 The Alphabet Soup of Interstitial Lung Disease

Abbreviation	*Disease*
AIP	Acute interstitial pneumonia
BOOP	Bronchiolitis obliterans with organizing pneumonia
COP	Cryptogenic organizing pneumonia
CWP	Coal worker's pneumoconiosis
DIP	Desquamative interstitial pneumonia
EG	Eosinophilic granuloma
IPF	Idiopathic pulmonary fibrosis
LIP	Lymphocytic interstitial pneumonitis
LAM	Lymphangioleiomyomatosis
LCH	Langerhans cell histiocytosis
NF	Neurofibromatosis
NSIP	Nonspecific interstitial pneumonia
PAP	Pulmonary alveolar proteinosis
PMF	Progressive massive fibrosis
RB-ILD	Respiratory bronchiolitis–associated interstitial lung disease
SLE	Systemic lupus erythematosus
TS	Tuberous sclerosis
UIP	Usual interstitial pneumonia

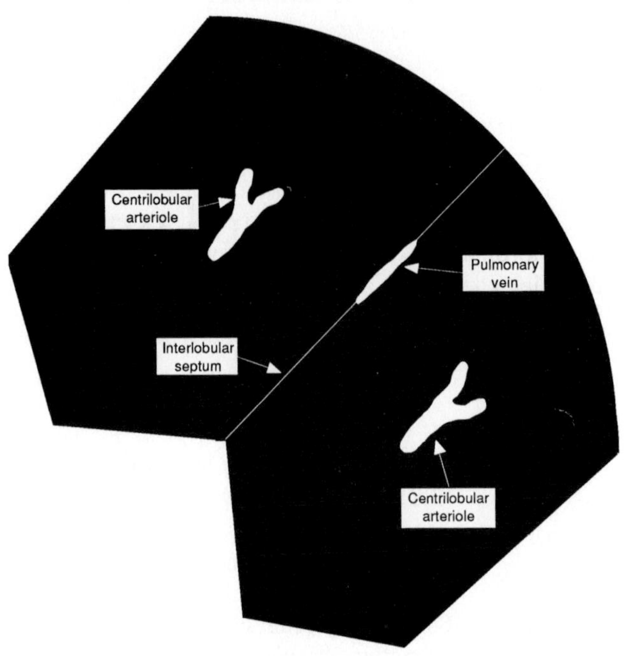

FIGURE 17.1. **Diagram of the Normal Secondary Pulmonary Lobule.**

Each terminal bronchiole further subdivides into respiratory bronchioles, alveolar ducts, alveolar sacs, and alveoli. The unit of lung subtended from a single terminal bronchiole is called a *pulmonary acinus*. The centrilobular artery and preterminal bronchiole are located in the center of the secondary lobule. Pulmonary veins and lymphatics run at the margins of lobules within the interlobular septa, with lymphatics and connective tissue found within the contiguous subpleural interstitium. The secondary pulmonary lobule is typically polyhedral in shape, with each side ranging from 1.0 to 2.5 cm in length. The interlobular septa are most prominent over the periphery of the lung, where they are readily seen on HRCT. At the surface of the lung, these septa are short structures that course perpendicular to the pleural surface and completely separate adjacent lobules. Within the parahilar portions of the lung, the interlobular septa are longer and more obliquely oriented and incompletely marginate the secondary lobules.

Normal HRCT Findings. HRCT can demonstrate much of the normal anatomy of the secondary pulmonary lobule. Interlobular septa are normally 0.1 mm thick and can be seen in the lung periphery, particularly along the anterior and mediastinal pleural surfaces (Fig. 17.2). Centrilobular arteries (1 mm in diameter) are V- or Y-shaped structures on HRCT seen within 5 to 10 mm of the pleural surface. Normal intralobular (0.7 mm) and acinar

TABLE 17.2 Utility of HRCT in the Evaluation of Chronic Interstitial Lung Disease

1. Detection of clinically suspected parenchymal abnormality when the chest radiograph is normal or shows questionable abnormality
2. Characterization of parenchymal abnormalities
3. Biopsy planning:
   Determination of route for biopsy, i.e., transbronchial, open lung or bronchoalveolar lavage
   Targeting biopsy to area(s) of active disease, avoiding areas of end-stage fibrosis
4. Monitoring of response to therapy or progression of disease

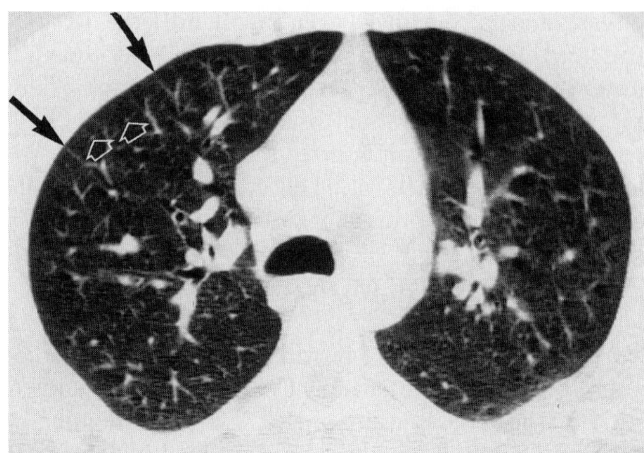

FIGURE 17.2. **HRCT of Normal Lobular Anatomy.** Normal interlobular septa (*solid black arrows*) and centrilobular arteries (*open white arrows*) are clearly visible.

(0.3 to 0.5 mm) arteries are commonly seen. Normal airways are visible only to within 3 cm of the pleura. The centrilobular bronchiole, with a diameter of 1 mm and a wall thickness of 0.15 mm, is not normally visible on HRCT. Pulmonary veins (0.5 cm) are occasionally seen as linear or dotlike structures within 1 to 2 cm of the pleura and, when visible, indicate the locations of interlobular septa. The peribronchovascular, centrilobular, and intralobular interstitial compartments are not normally visible on HRCT.

HRCT Signs of Disease

The signs of interstitial lung disease on HRCT are illustrated in Fig. 17.3, and their differential diagnosis is listed in Table 17.3 (1).

Interlobular (Septal) Lines. Septal thickening is most often seen as thin, short, 1- to 2-cm lines oriented perpendicular to and intersecting the costal pleura. These lines are best visualized in the subpleural and juxtadiaphragmatic regions of the lung, where they outline the

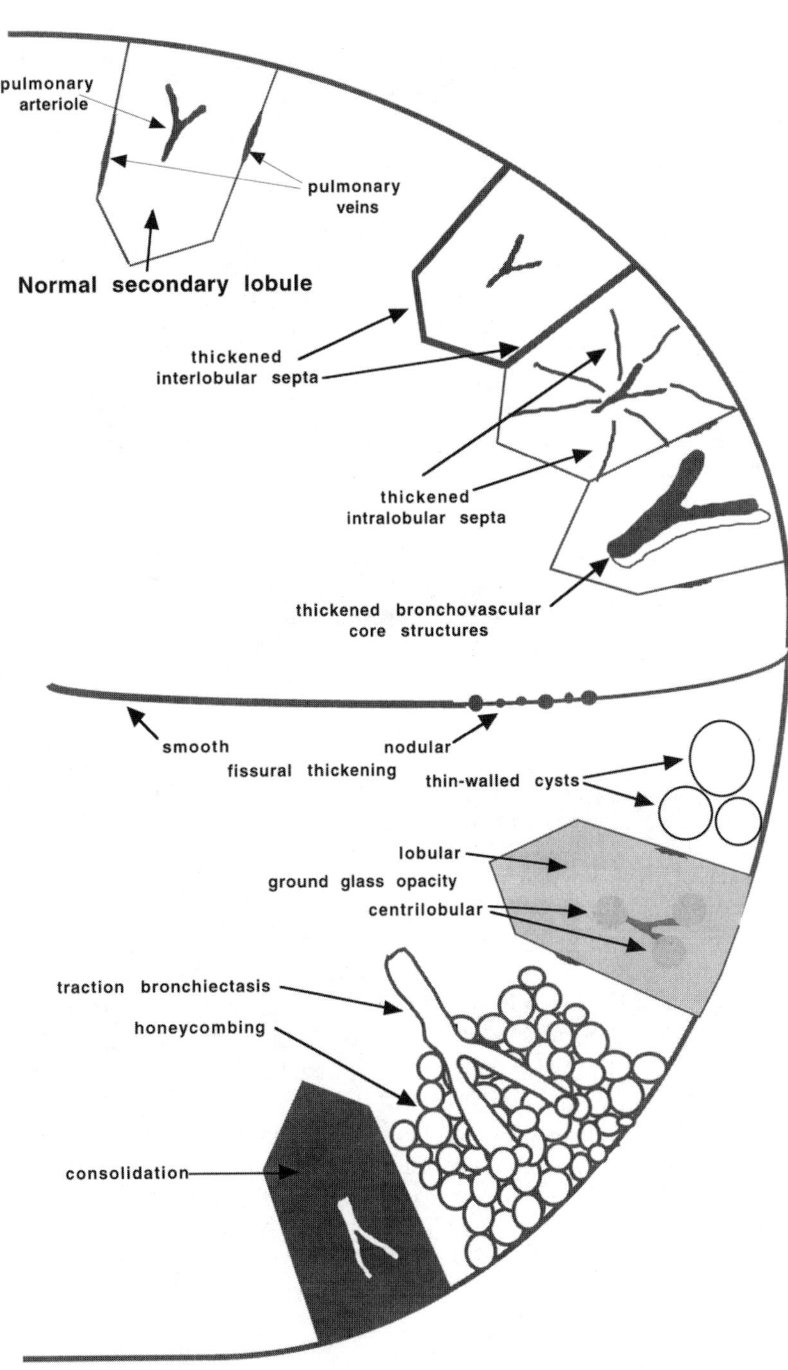

FIGURE 17.3. **HRCT Findings in Interstitial Lung Disease.** Reprinted with permission from The Radiologist, Baltimore: Williams and Wilkins, 1998.

TABLE 17.3 Differential Diagnostic HRCT Features in Interstitial Lung Disease

HRCT Finding	Differential Diagnosis	HRCT Finding	Differential Diagnosis
Interlobular (septal) lines	Interstitial edema Lymphangitic carcinomatosis Sarcoidosis Idiopathic pulmonary fibrosis (IPF) (and other forms of usual interstitial pneumonia [UIP])		Neurofibromatosis (pneumatocele) (emphysema)
		Irregular lung interfaces	Pulmonary edema IPF (UIP) Sarcoidosis
		Micronodules, random distribution	Miliary tuberculosis or histoplasmosis Hematogenous metastases Silicosis/coal worker's pneumoconiosis (CWP) EG
Intralobular lines	IPF (UIP) Asbestosis Alveolar proteinosis Hypersensitivity pneumonitis (chronic)		
"Thickened" fissures	Pulmonary edema Sarcoidosis Lymphangitic carcinomatosis	Micronodules, perilymphatic distribution	Sarcoidosis Lymphangitic carcinomatosis Silicosis/CWP
Peribronchovascular interstitial thickening	Pulmonary edema (smooth) Sarcoidosis (nodular) Lymphangitic carcinomatosis (smooth or nodular)	Ground-glass opacities	UIP Desquamative interstitial pneumonia Acute interstitial pneumonia (AIP) Hypersensitivity pneumonitis
Centrilobular nodules	Hypersensitivity pneumonitis Bronchiolitis obliterans with organizing pneumonia (BOOP)/cryptogenic organizing pneumonia (COP) Respiratory bronchiolitis–associated interstitial lung disease (RB-ILD)		BOOP/COP RB-ILD Hemorrhage Pneumocystis jiroveci pneumonia Cytomegalovirus pneumonia Alveolar proteinosis
Subpleural lines	Asbestosis IPF (UIP)	Architectural distortion Traction bronchiectasis	IPF/UIP Sarcoidosis Silicosis/CWP
Parenchymal bands	Asbestosis IPF (UIP) Sarcoidosis	Conglomerate mass	Sarcoidosis Silicosis CWP Radiation fibrosis
Honeycombing	IPF (UIP) Asbestosis Hypersensitivity pneumonitis (chronic) Sarcoidosis	Consolidation	BOOP/COP Sarcoidosis
Thin-walled cysts	Eosinophilic granuloma (EG) Lymphangioleiomyomatosis Tuberous sclerosis		AIP UIP

anterior and posterior margins of secondary lobules. In the central regions of the lung, the thickened septa can completely envelope lobules to produce polygonal structures. Although septa can be seen in normal individuals, these lines are thicker (>1 mm) and more numerous in patients with diseases primarily affecting the interlobular interstitium, such as interstitial pulmonary edema, idiopathic pulmonary fibrosis, and lymphangitic carcinomatosis (Fig. 17.4). Interlobular lines on HRCT are the equivalent of Kerley B lines seen in the inferolateral portions of the lungs on frontal radiographs. Within the central regions of the lung, long (2 to 6 cm) linear opacities representing obliquely oriented connective tissue septa can be seen, which are the equivalent of radiographic Kerley A lines.

Intralobular Lines. In some patients, a lattice of fine lines is seen within the central portion of the pulmonary lobule radiating out toward the thickened lobular borders to produce a "spoke-and-wheel" or "spiderweb" appearance. These lines are not normally visible on HRCT and represent thickening of the intralobular or parenchymal interstitium. Intralobular lines usually represent fibrosis and are most commonly seen in idiopathic pulmonary fibrosis (IPF) and other forms of usual interstitial pneumonia (UIP). However, intralobular lines can also be seen in other infiltrative diseases such as pulmonary alveolar proteinosis (PAP).

"Thickened" Fissures. The apparent thickening of interlobar fissures in patients with interstitial lung disease is usually a direct extension of the thickening of interlobular septa to involve the subpleural interstitium of the lung. While such a process normally involves all pleural surfaces equally, the "thickening" is usually best appreciated on the fissures, where two layers of visceral pleura—and therefore two layers of subpleural

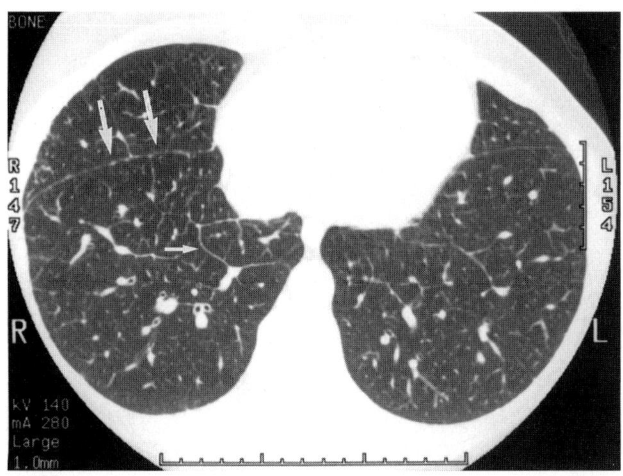

FIGURE 17.4. **Interlobular Septal Lines in Lymphangitic Carcinomatosis.** An HRCT scan through the upper lobes in a patient with lymphangitic carcinomatosis shows thickened interlobular septa (*small arrow*). Note the presence of nodular fissural thickening (*large arrows*), another common finding in this entity.

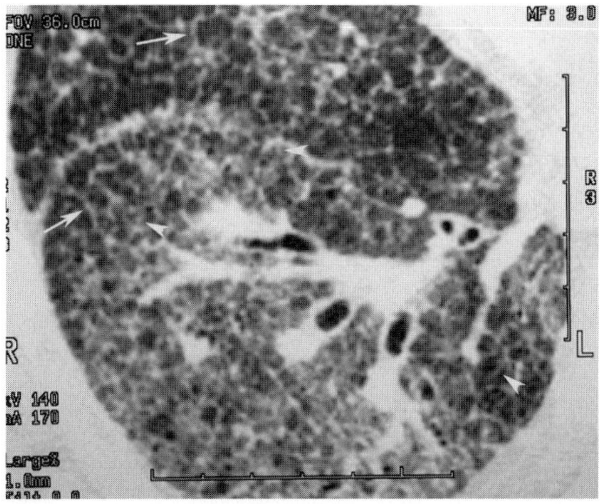

FIGURE 17.5. **Intralobular Lines in Idiopathic Pulmonary Fibrosis (IPF).** A targeted HRCT through the right lower lobe in a patient with IPF shows thickening of intralobular (*long arrows*) and interlobular (*arrowheads*) lines associated with ground-glass opacity.

interstitium—are seen outlined on either side by aerated lung. The fissural thickening can be smooth or nodular. Smooth fissural thickening is virtually indistinguishable from a small amount of pleural fluid within the fissure and is most commonly seen with pulmonary edema. Nodular fissural thickening is commonly seen in sarcoidosis and lymphangitic carcinomatosis (Fig. 17.4), where the nodules lie within the subpleural lymphatics.

Thickened bronchovascular structures of the lung result from thickening of the peribronchovascular interstitium. This produces apparent enlargement of perihilar vascular structures and thickening of bronchial walls, which is the HRCT equivalent of peribronchial cuffing and tram tracking seen radiographically. While pulmonary edema causes smooth thickening of the peribronchovascular interstitium, nodular or irregular thickening can be seen in sarcoidosis or UIP (Fig. 17.5). Lymphangitic carcinomatosis can result in either smooth or irregular peribronchovascular thickening, although the former is more common (Fig. 17.6).

Centrilobular (Lobular Core) Abnormalities. Thickening of the axial interstitium within the lobular core produces an abnormal prominence of the "dotlike" or branching centrilobular arteriole. Diseases that commonly produce this appearance include pulmonary edema, lymphangitic carcinomatosis, and UIP. The centrilobular bronchiole is not normally seen on HRCT but may be rendered visible as a result of luminal dilatation or thickening of the centrilobular interstitium. Small airways disease can produce centrilobular bronchiolar abnormalities, which are seen on HRCT as fluid-filled dilated branching Y-shaped structures that produce a "tree-in-bud" appearance. Ill-defined centrilobular nodules represent disease of the bronchiole and adjacent parenchyma and can be seen in subacute hypersensitivity pneumonitis (Fig. 17.7), cryptogenic organizing pneumonia (COP), and other disorders.

Subpleural Lines. These 5- to 10-cm-long curvilinear opacities are found within 1 cm of the pleura and parallel the chest wall. They are most frequent in the posterior portions of the lower lobes and remain unchanged on prone scans. This finding, which probably represents an early phase of lung fibrosis, should be distinguished from a similar line that is seen as a result of atelectasis in the

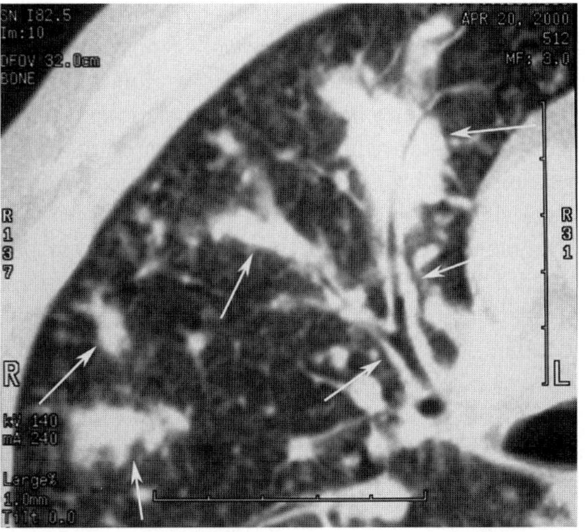

FIGURE 17.6. **Thickened Bronchovascular Structures in Lymphangitic Carcinomatosis.** In a patient with lymphangitic carcinomatosis, an HRCT shows both smooth and nodular thickening of the bronchovascular structures (*arrows*) that represents lymphatic tumor surrounding the axial interstitium.

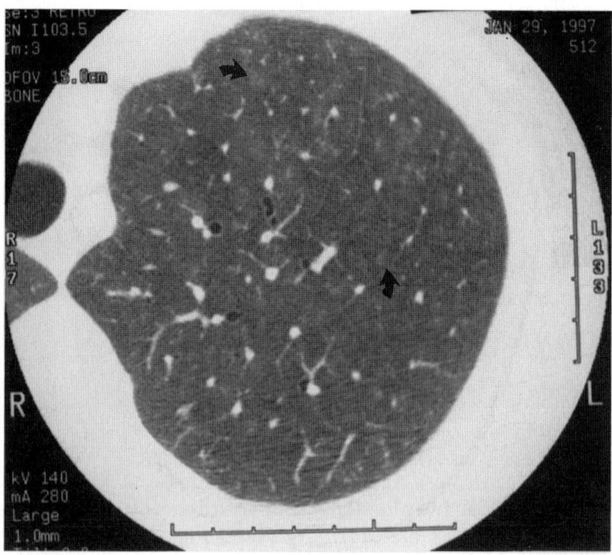

FIGURE 17.7. **Centrilobular Ground-Glass Nodules in Subacute Hypersensitivity Pneumonitis.** HRCT shows the typical poorly defined centrilobular nodules (*arrows*) of subacute hypersensitivity pneumonitis ("bird-fancier's lung").

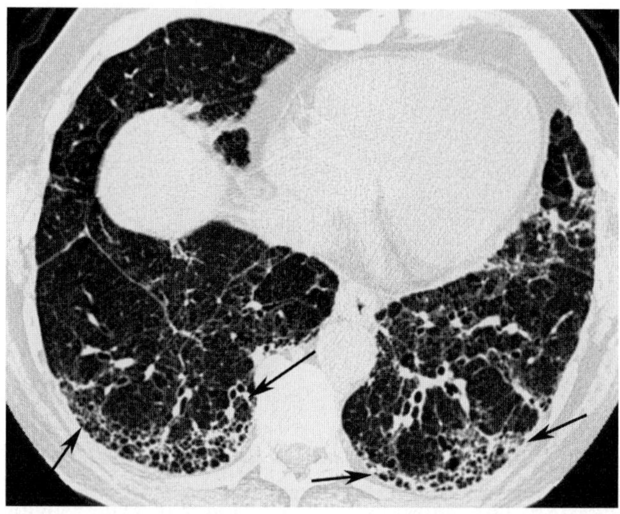

FIGURE 17.8. **Honeycomb Lung in Idiopathic Pulmonary Fibrosis.** HRCT in a patient with IPF shows peripheral honeycombing (*arrows*) indicative of end-stage pulmonary fibrosis.

dependent portion of the lungs in normal individuals. Subpleural lines are most often seen in patients with asbestosis and, less commonly, IPF.

Parenchymal bands are nontapering linear opacities, 2 to 5 cm in length, that extend from the lung to contact the pleural surface. These fibrotic bands can be distinguished from vessels and thickened septa by their length, thickness, course, absence of branching, and their association with regional parenchymal distortion. Parenchymal bands are usually seen in asbestosis, IPF, and sarcoidosis.

Honeycombing, seen as small (6 to 10 mm) cystic spaces with thick (1 to 3 mm) walls, most often in the posterior subpleural regions of the lower lobes, represents end-stage pulmonary fibrosis of various etiologies. Pathologically, the cysts are lined by bronchiolar epithelium and are the result of bronchiolectasis. Most patients show additional signs of interstitial disease, including thickened interlobular and intralobular lines, parenchymal bands, irregularity of lung interfaces, and areas of ground-glass opacification. Honeycombing is frequently seen in IPF (and other forms of UIP) (Fig. 17.8), chronic hypersensitivity pneumonitis, and occasionally sarcoidosis.

Thin-walled cysts are a common manifestation of late stages of Langerhans cell histiocytosis of lung (LCH) and lymphangioleiomyomatosis (LAM). These cysts are slightly larger in diameter (10 mm) than honeycomb cysts, are more uniform in size, and have thinner walls. Honeycomb cysts usually have shared walls, while the cysts of LCH and LAM do not. The cysts of LCH and LAM are usually evenly distributed from central to peripheral portions of the upper lobes (Fig. 17.9), with or without lower lobe involvement, while honeycombing tends to occur in the subpleural regions of the lower lobes. While normal lung may be found in the intervening spaces between the cysts of LCH and LAM, honeycombing uniformly destroys lung and produces distortion of lung interfaces and traction bronchiectasis, features not found in eosinophilic granulomatosis (EG) and LAM.

Irregularity of Lung Interfaces. A common HRCT sign of interstitial disease, irregularity of the normally smooth interface between the bronchovascular bundles and the surrounding lung reflects edema or fibrosis of the axial interstitium or infiltration by granulomas (Fig. 17.6) or tumor. Similarly, irregularity of the interface between fissures or pleural surfaces and adjacent lung indicates

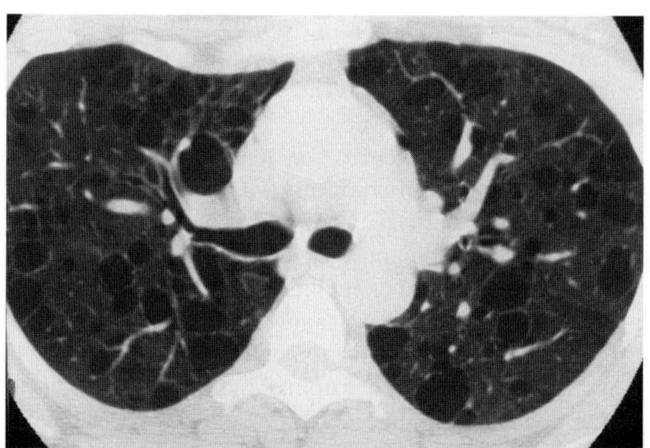

FIGURE 17.9. **Thin-Walled Cysts in Lymphangioleiomyomatosis (LAM).** An HRCT of a patient with LAM shows multiple, variably sized, round, thin-walled cysts.

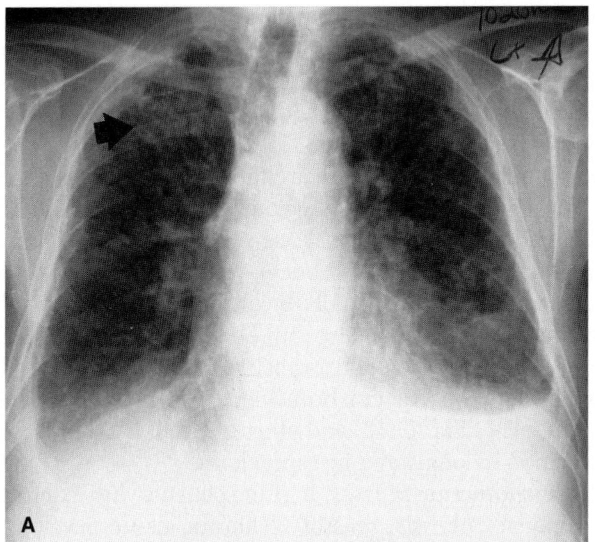

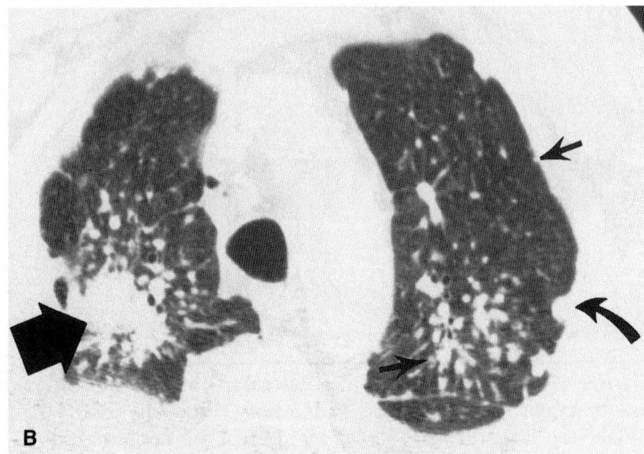

FIGURE 17.10. **Nodules and a Conglomerate Mass in Silicosis. A.** Posteroanterior radiograph of a 79-year-old patient with silicosis shows diffuse nodules as well as a conglomerate mass in the right upper lobe (*arrow*). **B.** HRCT scan through the upper lobes shows peribronchovascular and subpleural micronodules (*small arrows*), larger nodules (*curved arrow*), and a conglomerate mass representing progressive massive fibrosis in the right upper lobe (*large arrow*). The pleural effusions are caused by concomitant congestive heart failure.

peripheral interstitial disease. Pulmonary edema, IPF, and sarcoidosis are the most common causes of irregular lung interfaces.

Micronodules. These 1- to 3-mm, sharply marginated, round opacities seen on HRCT represent conglomerates of granulomas or tumor cells within the interstitium. These are most often seen in sarcoidosis, EG, silicosis (Fig. 17.10), miliary tuberculosis (TB) or histoplasmosis, metastatic adenocarcinoma, and lymphangitic carcinomatosis. They may be seen along the central bronchovascular structures (sarcoidosis, EG); within interlobular septa or subpleural interstitium (sarcoidosis, lymphangitic carcinomatosis, silicosis); or within the substance of the pulmonary lobules (metastatic adenocarcinoma, miliary granulomatous infection). Nodules predominating in the peribronchovascular, interlobular, and subpleural regions—those portions of the interstitium where the lymphatics lie—are said to have a "perilymphatic" distribution. Because it may be difficult to distinguish vertically oriented small upper and lower lobe vessels from interstitial nodules on HRCT, contiguous, thick (10 mm) scans are often helpful.

Ground-Glass or Hazy Increased Density. Multifocal areas of increased density can sometimes be identified in patients with diffuse interstitial lung disease. These regions, which often respect lobular borders, are distinguished from typical airspace opacification by their granular appearance with maintained visibility of pulmonary vessels and the absence of air bronchograms. These opacities are most often produced by thickening of the alveolar septa, with or without lining of the alveolar spaces by inflammatory exudate or fluid. Diseases commonly associated with this appearance include desquamative interstitial pneumonia (DIP), *Pneumocystis jiroveci* (formerly *P carinii*) pneumonia, acute hypersensitivity pneumonitis (Fig. 17.11), nonspecific interstitial pneumonia (NSIP), and interstitial pulmonary edema. The ground-glass densities are occasionally confined to the immediate centrilobular regions of the pulmonary lobules, where they appear as fuzzy nodular densities that outline the normally invisible centrilobular bronchiole (Fig. 17.7). This

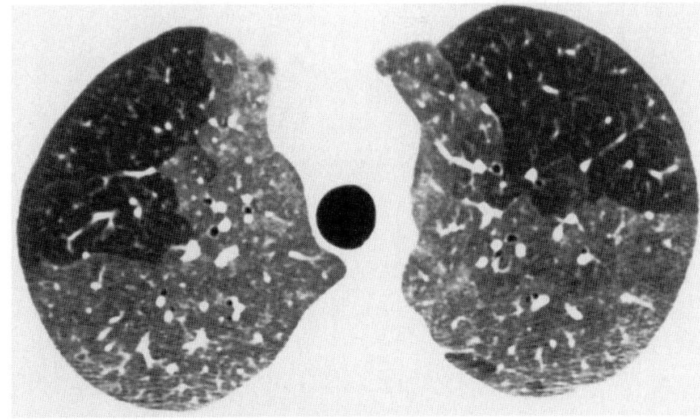

FIGURE 17.11. **Ground-Glass Opacity in Acute Hypersensitivity Pneumonitis.** An HRCT through the upper lobes shows confluent ground-glass opacity in a patient with hypersensitivity pneumonitis. Note that the pulmonary vessels are still visible within the areas of abnormality.

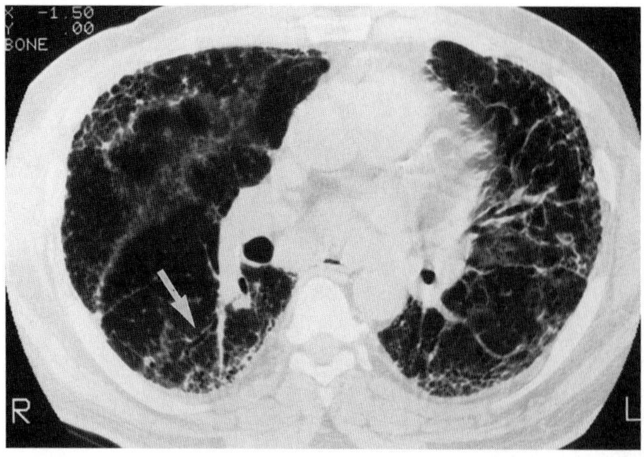

FIGURE 17.12. **Architectural Distortion and Traction Bronchiectasis in Idiopathic Pulmonary Fibrosis.** HRCT through the lower lobes shows peripheral honeycombing, traction bronchiectasis (*arrow*), and resultant architectural distortion.

reflects involvement of the peribronchovascular interstitium and surrounding alveoli by an inflammatory process and is seen in hypersensitivity pneumonitis, COP, and panbronchiolitis. The presence of ground-glass opacities is important because it often implies an active inflammatory process or edema that is reversible and warrants aggressive treatment. However, ground-glass abnormality associated with a predominant pattern of honeycombing can represent microscopic pulmonary fibrosis.

Architectural Distortion and Traction Bronchiectasis. Processes that result in extensive parenchymal fibrosis can distort the normal architecture of the lung, creating irregularities of the lung–mediastinal, lung–pleural, and lung–vascular interfaces. Parenchymal distortion is often better appreciated on HRCT than on plain radiographs. Sarcoidosis and UIP (Fig. 17.12) are the diseases most commonly associated with architectural distortion.

A finding commonly associated with architectural distortion is *traction bronchiectasis*, in which fibrosis causes traction on the walls of bronchi, resulting in irregular dilatation. While this usually involves segmental and subsegmental bronchi, it also can be seen at the intralobular level, where traction bronchiolectasis contributes to honeycombing. Traction bronchiectasis is most commonly seen in IPF (Fig. 17.12) and other forms of UIP but is also common in long-standing sarcoidosis.

Conglomerate Masses. In some patients with extensive pulmonary fibrosis, masses of fibrotic tissue develop in the parahilar regions of the upper lobes, often associated with peripheral bullae. On CT and HRCT, these masses are seen to contain crowded vessels and dilated bronchi. These conglomerate masses are most often seen in patients with end-stage sarcoidosis but can occur in complicated silicosis with progressive massive fibrosis (PMF) (Fig. 17.10) or radiation fibrosis following treatment of Hodgkin lymphoma or lung cancer. A similar finding is seen rarely in intravenous drug users when a granulomatous fibrosis results as a response to intravenous talc or starch mixed with narcotics.

Consolidation refers to increased lung density that obscures underlying blood vessels; air bronchograms are commonly present. This finding can be seen with any

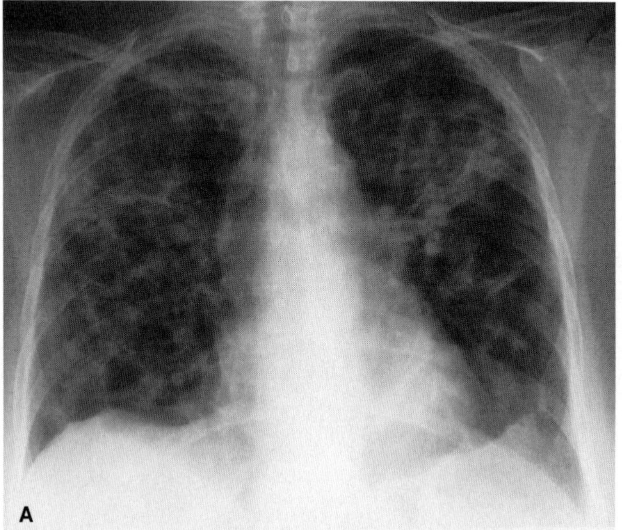

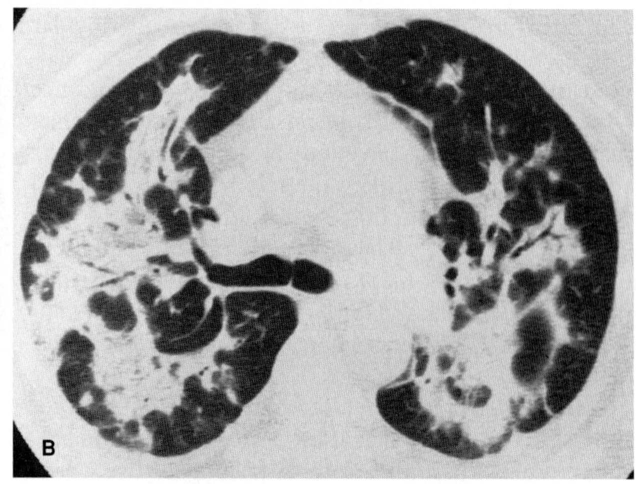

FIGURE 17.13. **Consolidation in Cryptogenic Organizing Pneumonia (COP). A.** Posteroanterior radiograph in a 53-year-old patient with fever, dyspnea, and a dry cough shows patchy consolidation and diminished lung volumes. **B.** HRCT scan shows multifocal areas of consolidation in a peribronchial distribution. Note air bronchograms with mild bronchial dilatation within the consolidated areas. An open lung biopsy showed COP.

TABLE 17.4 Differential Diagnostic Features in Chronic Interstitial Lung Disease

Finding	*Differential Diagnosis*
Upper zone distribution	Tuberculosis (postprimary)
	Chronic fungal infection
	Histoplasmosis
	Coccidioidomycosis
	Sarcoidosis
	Eosinophilic granuloma
	Silicosis
	Ankylosing spondylitis
	Hypersensitivity pneumonitis (chronic)
	Radiation fibrosis from treatment of head and neck malignancy
Lower zone distribution	Idiopathic pulmonary fibrosis
	Asbestosis
	Rheumatoid lung
	Scleroderma
	Neurofibromatosis
	Dermatomyositis/polymyositis
	Chronic aspiration
Normal or increased lung volumes	Sarcoidosis
	Eosinophilic granuloma
	Lymphangioleiomyomatosis
	Tuberous sclerosis
	Interstitial disease superimposed on emphysema
Honeycombing	Idiopathic pulmonary fibrosis
	Sarcoidosis
	Eosinophilic granuloma
	Rheumatoid lung
	Scleroderma
	Pneumoconiosis
	Hypersensitivity pneumonitis
	Chronic aspiration
	Radiation fibrosis
Miliary nodules	Tuberculosis
	Fungi
	Histoplasmosis
	Coccidioidomycosis
	Cryptococcosis
	Silicosis
	Metastases
	Thyroid carcinoma
	Renal cell carcinoma
	Bronchogenic carcinoma
	Melanoma
	Choriocarcinoma
	Sarcoidosis
	Eosinophilic granuloma
Hilar/mediastinal lymph node enlargement	Sarcoidosis
	Lymphangitic carcinomatosis
	Lymphoma
	Hematogenous metastases
	Tuberculosis
	Fungal infection
	Silicosis
Pleural disease	Asbestosis (plaques)
	Lymphangitic carcinomatosis (effusion)
	Rheumatoid lung disease (effusion/thickening)
	Lymphangioleiomyomatosis (chylous effusion)
Abnormalities of soft tissues and bony thorax	Skin nodules
	Neurofibromatosis
	Subcutaneous calcifications
	Dermatomyositis
	Scleroderma
	Erosion of distal clavicles
	Rheumatoid lung
	Scleroderma
	Rib lesions
	Ribbon ribs/erosion of inferior rib margins
	Neurofibromatosis
	Erosion of superior margins
	Rheumatoid lung
	Scleroderma
	Kyphoscoliosis
	Neurofibromatosis
	Lytic bone lesions
	Metastases
	Eosinophilic granuloma

airspace-filling process (Fig. 17.13) but occasionally occurs in interstitial diseases such as UIP and sarcoidosis.

CHRONIC INTERSTITIAL LUNG DISEASE

Chronic interstitial lung disease usually results from diffuse inflammatory processes that primarily affect the axial and parenchymal interstitium of the lung. A wide variety of disease processes can result in diffuse damage to the pulmonary interstitium (2). Careful evaluation of all available radiologic studies and correlation with clinical findings and laboratory data are essential to the accurate diagnosis of chronic interstitial lung disease (Table 17.4). However, the majority of patients with interstitial lung disease will require histologic examination of lung tissue for definitive diagnosis.

Chronic Interstitial Pulmonary Edema

Chronic elevation of pulmonary venous pressure may lead to increased interstitial markings on plain radiographs. The interstitial thickening is caused by distention of pulmonary lymphatics and chronic interstitial edema, which may lead to fibrosis. This is seen most commonly in patients with long-standing mitral stenosis or LV failure. Radiographically, peribronchial cuffing, tram tracking, poor definition of vascular markings, and linear or reticular opacities may be seen. Redistribution of blood flow to the upper lobes, a manifestation of pulmonary venous hypertension, and prominence of the fissures caused by subpleural edema and fibrosis are concomitant findings. Honeycombing is not a feature of chronic pulmonary venous hypertension; its presence in a patient with cardiac disease should suggest another cause of pulmonary fibrosis (e.g., amiodarone lung toxicity).

Connective Tissue Disease

These disorders are associated with immunologically mediated inflammation and damage to connective tissues throughout the body. The most common thoracic manifestations of this group of heterogeneous disorders are vasculitis and interstitial fibrosis, although the pleura, chest wall, diaphragm, and heart may also be affected (3).

Rheumatoid Lung Disease (Table 17.5). Rheumatoid arthritis produces a chronic arthritis of peripheral joints. Extra-articular manifestations are seen in up to 75% of patients. In contrast to the disease as a whole, which is more common in women, pulmonary involvement is more common in men. The pleuropulmonary manifestations of rheumatoid disease typically follow the onset of joint disease and tend to be seen in patients with high serum rheumatoid factor titers and eosinophilia. However, in up to 15% of patients, pleuropulmonary involvement precedes the joint disease.

The most common radiographic manifestation of parenchymal lung involvement is an interstitial pneumonitis and fibrosis, which histologically is a form of UIP. This begins as an alveolitis (inflammation of the alveolar interstitium) that is seen radiographically as fine reticular or ground-glass opacities with a lower zone predominance. There is gradual progression to end-stage pulmonary fibrosis with the development of a bibasilar medium or coarse reticular or reticulonodular pattern (honeycombing) (Fig. 17.14). HRCT is more sensitive in detecting the earliest parenchymal changes than conventional radiographs and is also more sensitive in depicting the development of interstitial fibrosis (Fig. 17.15). Predominant upper lobe fibrosis and cavity or bulla formation are rare. This less common pattern of lung involvement is indistinguishable from that seen with ankylosing spondylitis and must be distinguished from postprimary fibrocavitary TB by acid-fast staining of sputum.

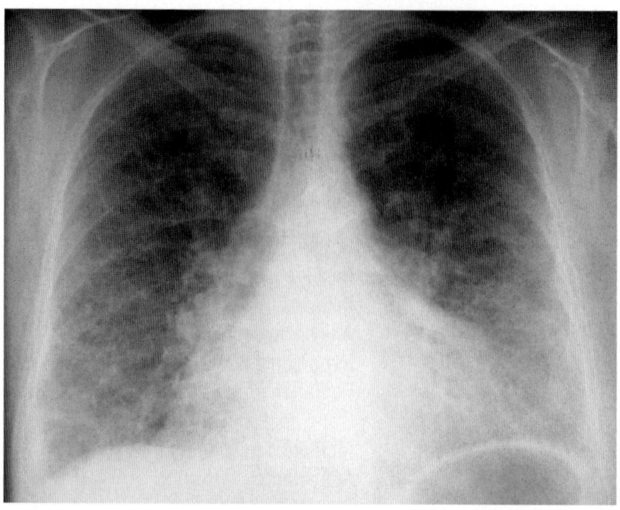

FIGURE 17.14. **Honeycombing in Rheumatoid Lung.** Posteroanterior radiograph in a patient with end-stage rheumatoid lung disease demonstrates a medium reticular process representing honeycomb lung. Note the predominant peripheral distribution of disease. Bilateral pleural effusions and cardiac enlargement caused by pericardial effusion are also evident.

TABLE 17.5 Manifestations of Rheumatoid Lung Disease

Manifestation	*Radiographic Findings*
Serositis	
Pleuritis	Pleural effusion, thickening
Pericarditis	Pericardial effusion
Interstitial pneumonitis	Pulmonary fibrosis (basilar predominance)
Necrobiotic nodules	Multiple peripheral cavitating nodules
Caplan syndrome	Multiple peripheral cavitating nodules
Bronchiolitis obliterans	Hyperinflation
Pulmonary arteritis	Pulmonary arterial hypertension and right heart enlargement
	Pulmonary hemorrhage

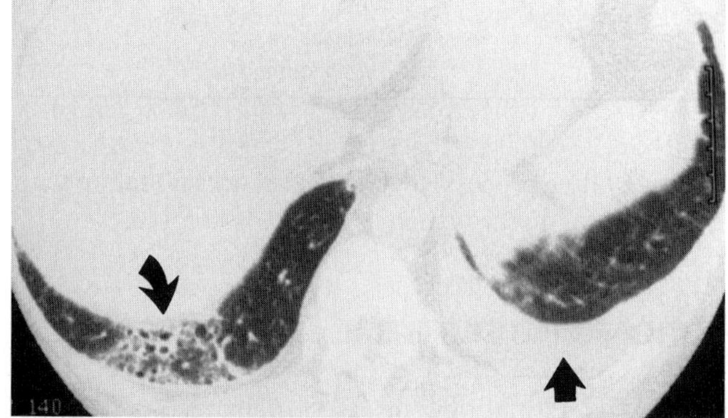

FIGURE 17.15. **Rheumatoid Lung Disease.** An HRCT through the lung bases in a patient with rheumatoid arthritis shows a focal area of honeycombing at the periphery of the right lung base (*curved arrow*). Note also the left pleural effusion (*straight arrow*), a frequent finding in rheumatoid disease.

Less common parenchymal manifestations of rheumatoid disease are lung nodules and changes attributable to COP. Necrobiotic (rheumatoid) nodules in the lung can produce peripheral well-defined nodular opacities on chest radiographs that are indistinguishable from the subcutaneous rheumatoid nodules seen on the extensor surfaces of the elbows and knees in these patients. The lung nodules commonly evolve into thick-walled cavities, which tend to wax and wane in parallel with the flares of arthritis. Similar nodules may develop in the lungs of coal miners and silica or asbestos workers with rheumatoid arthritis as a hypersensitivity response to inhaled dust particles (Caplan syndrome). Caplan syndrome is usually indistinguishable radiographically from the necrobiotic nodules of simple rheumatoid disease, although the presence of the associated characteristic small nodular or irregular parenchymal opacities of simple pneumoconiosis helps make this distinction. COP and bronchiolitis obliterans (constrictive bronchiolitis) are associated with rheumatoid disease. The clinical, functional, and radiographic findings are similar to those of COP or bronchiolitis obliterans associated with systemic lupus erythematosus (SLE), drugs, or viral infection.

Pleuritis is the most common thoracic manifestation of rheumatoid disease and is found in 20% of patients. As with pulmonary involvement, there is a male predilection for pleural disease. Unilateral or bilateral pleural effusions may be seen that are exudative and have a characteristically low glucose concentration.

Enlargement of the central pulmonary arteries and RV dilatation may be seen on chest radiographs in patients with pulmonary arterial hypertension. This is an uncommon manifestation of rheumatoid disease that usually develops secondary to diffuse interstitial fibrosis. Rarely, the pulmonary arteries are involved as a part of the systemic vasculitis seen in extra-articular rheumatoid disease. There are no parenchymal abnormalities associated with rheumatoid pulmonary arteritis.

Abnormalities that may be seen in the chest wall of individuals with rheumatoid arthritis include tapered erosion of the distal clavicles, rotator cuff atrophy with a high-riding humeral head, bilateral symmetric glenohumeral joint space narrowing with or without superimposed degenerative joint disease, and superior rib notching or erosion.

Systemic Lupus Erythematosus. This disease of young and middle-aged women typically involves inflammation of multiple organs mediated by autoantibodies and circulating immune complexes. The thorax is commonly affected and may be the initial site of involvement. The thoracic disease is often limited to the pleura and pericardium, although the lung, heart, diaphragm, and intercostal muscles are involved in as many as one third of patients. In the pleura and pericardium, a fibrinous serositis produces painful pleural and pericardial effusions that are exudative in nature. Radiographically, the pleural effusions are small or moderate in size and can be unilateral or bilateral. The effusions usually resolve with corticosteroid therapy. Pleural fibrosis, seen in a majority of patients with long-standing disease, results in diffuse pleural thickening.

Pulmonary involvement may take the form of acute lupus pneumonitis or chronic interstitial disease. Acute lupus pneumonitis is characterized by rapid onset of fever, dyspnea, and hypoxemia, which occasionally requires mechanical ventilation. These patients have pathologic changes that are indistinguishable from those seen in ARDS, with diffuse alveolar damage producing an exudative intra-alveolar edema with hyaline membrane formation. Radiographically, rapidly coalescent bilateral airspace opacities are seen, while the typical HRCT finding is one of ground-glass opacity. These findings are difficult to distinguish from those seen in diffuse alveolar hemorrhage associated with pulmonary vasculitis, severe pneumonia related to immunosuppressive therapy, or pulmonary edema secondary to renal failure. The diagnosis of acute lupus pneumonitis is made by excluding pneumonia and pulmonary edema and by noting an improvement following the initiation of immunosuppressive therapy.

Radiographic evidence of IPF is distinctly uncommon in SLE, but fibrosis is said to be present pathologically in one third of patients. When seen radiographically, the pattern is one of bibasilar reticular opacities that are indistinguishable from those seen in rheumatoid lung disease or scleroderma. Therefore, the presence of severe interstitial fibrosis in a patient with clinical features of SLE should prompt consideration of the diagnosis of an overlap syndrome (mixed connective tissue disease). As with rheumatoid lung disease and scleroderma, HRCT is the most sensitive technique for demonstrating early interstitial disease.

Additional chest radiographic findings in SLE include elevation of the hemidiaphragms with decreased lung volumes and resultant bibasilar areas of linear atelectasis. Diaphragmatic elevation is present in as many as 20% of patients and is the result of diaphragmatic weakness from a primary myopathy unrelated to corticosteroid therapy. Rarely, the central pulmonary arteries are enlarged from pulmonary arterial hypertension secondary to pulmonary vasculitis. Pulmonary embolism with or without infarction may produce peripheral parenchymal opacities and results from deep venous thrombosis that develops in the presence of a circulating lupus anticoagulant. COP has been described in patients with SLE but is indistinguishable clinically and radiographically from lupus pneumonitis, because both conditions produce parenchymal opacities that are responsive to steroids. Superior rib erosions may be seen that are indistinguishable from similar findings in rheumatoid arthritis or scleroderma.

Scleroderma produces inflammation and fibrosis of the skin, esophagus, musculoskeletal system, heart, lungs,

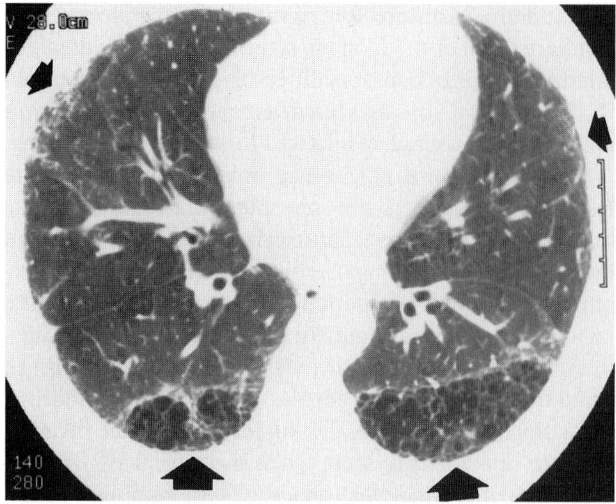

FIGURE 17.16. **Scleroderma.** An HRCT of a patient with scleroderma demonstrates minimal interstitial disease in the periphery of the middle lobe and lingula (*small arrows*), with honeycombing in the posterior subpleural portions of the lower lobes (*large arrows*).

and kidneys in young and middle-aged women. The etiology and pathogenesis are unknown. The lungs are involved pathologically in nearly 90% of patients, although only 25% of patients have respiratory symptoms or radiographic evidence of pulmonary involvement. Pulmonary function testing is more sensitive than conventional radiography in the diagnosis of lung disease and shows the typical diminished lung volumes, preserved flow rates, and low diffusing capacity of interstitial pulmonary fibrosis. Pathologically, the sequence of parenchymal and radiographic changes is indistinguishable from rheumatoid lung disease, IPF, and other forms of UIP. Severe pulmonary involvement is reflected radiographically as a coarse reticular or reticulonodular pattern involving the subpleural regions of the lower lobes. The most common HRCT findings are interlobular septal thickening, ground-glass opacities, and honeycombing (Fig. 17.16). HRCT is more sensitive than the chest radiograph in detecting early interstitial disease. Progressive loss of lung volume is seen with advancing pulmonary fibrosis. The development of large (1 to 5 cm) subpleural lower lobe cysts may lead to spontaneous pneumothorax.

Pulmonary arterial hypertension with enlarged central pulmonary arteries and RV dilatation is seen in up to 50% of patients with scleroderma and may be seen in the absence of interstitial fibrosis. In these patients, thickening and obliteration of small muscular pulmonary arteries and arterioles are responsible for the development of pulmonary arterial hypertension. Pleural effusions are significantly less common in scleroderma than in rheumatoid disease or SLE and may be a helpful distinguishing feature radiographically. Pleural thickening is more often attributable to extension of pulmonary interstitial fibrosis into the interstitial layer of the pleura than to pleuritis.

Several additional chest radiographic findings may be seen in patients with scleroderma. Eggshell calcification of mediastinal lymph nodes has been reported, although it is more common in silicosis and sarcoidosis. A dilated air-filled esophagus may be identified on the upright chest radiograph and is a manifestation of esophageal dysmotility from smooth muscle atrophy and fibrosis. An air–fluid level within a dilated esophagus suggests secondary distal esophageal stricture formation from chronic reflux esophagitis. The functional or anatomic esophageal obstruction may result in aspiration with the development of lower lobe pneumonia. Because patients with scleroderma are at a greater risk for developing lung cancer, particularly bronchioloalveolar cell carcinoma, the appearance of a mass or persistent airspace opacity should raise this possibility. Patients with the CREST syndrome (subcutaneous calcification, Raynaud phenomenon, esophageal dysmotility, sclerodactyly, and telangiectasia), a variant of scleroderma, may have radiographically visible calcifications within the subcutaneous tissues of the chest wall. Superior rib notching or erosion may be seen.

Dermatomyositis and polymyositis involve autoimmune inflammation and destruction of skeletal muscle, producing proximal muscle pain and weakness (polymyositis) and occasionally associated with a skin rash (dermatomyositis). The thoracic manifestations of these diseases include respiratory and pharyngeal muscle weakness and an associated interstitial pneumonitis. Interstitial pneumonitis, indistinguishable from that associated with rheumatoid lung disease, SLE, scleroderma, or IPF, is seen in 5% to 10% of patients. A fine reticular interstitial pattern in acute disease leads to a chronic, coarse reticular or reticulonodular process that is predominantly basilar in distribution. Most patients with polymyositis and interstitial lung disease have clinical manifestations of rheumatoid arthritis or scleroderma, and these patients tend to respond favorably to corticosteroids. As with scleroderma, the early parenchymal changes may be subradiographic but can be demonstrated on HRCT studies through the lower lobes (Fig. 17.17). Additional chest radiographic findings in polymyositis reflect the involvement of skeletal muscle. Small lung volumes with diaphragmatic elevation and basilar linear atelectasis are secondary to diaphragmatic and intercostal muscle involvement. Pharyngeal and upper esophageal muscle weakness predispose to aspiration pneumonia. The chest radiograph should be examined carefully for lung masses because bronchogenic carcinoma accounts for a significant percentage of the malignancies seen with a higher-than-normal frequency in patients with dermatomyositis or polymyositis.

Sjögren Syndrome. This autoimmune disorder of middle-aged women is characterized by the sicca syndrome of dry eyes (keratoconjunctivitis sicca), dry mouth

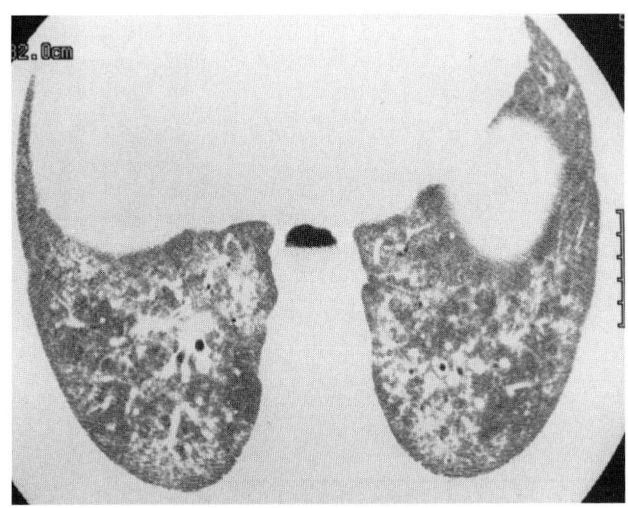

FIGURE 17.17. **Polymyositis.** An HRCT through the lung bases shows reticulation and nodules, reflecting interstitial pneumonitis in a patient with polymyositis.

(xerostomia), and dry nose (xerorhinia), which result from lymphocytic infiltration of the lacrimal, salivary, and mucous glands, respectively. Most patients with the sicca syndrome have associated manifestations of other collagen vascular diseases, such as rheumatoid arthritis, scleroderma, or SLE.

The chest is involved in approximately one third of patients with Sjögren syndrome with or without associated collagen vascular disease. The most common manifestation is interstitial fibrosis, which is indistinguishable from that seen with other collagen vascular disorders. Involvement of tracheobronchial mucous glands leads to thickened sputum with mucus plugging and recurrent bronchitis, bronchiectasis, atelectasis, and pneumonia. HRCT demonstrates both interstitial opacities and the presence of small airways involvement with bronchiolectasis and a "tree-in-bud" appearance. Pleuritis and pleural effusion are less common.

Patients with Sjögren syndrome are at increased risk for developing lymphocytic interstitial pneumonitis (LIP) and non-Hodgkin pulmonary lymphoma. The radiographic appearance of LIP is lower lobe coarse reticular or reticulonodular opacities that are indistinguishable from interstitial fibrosis. HRCT shows ground-glass opacity with scattered, thin-walled cysts. The development of lymphoma in these patients should be suspected when nodular or alveolar opacities develop in the lung in association with mediastinal lymph node enlargement.

Ankylosing Spondylitis. Approximately 1% to 2% of individuals with ankylosing spondylitis develop pulmonary disease in the form of upper lobe pulmonary fibrosis. The fibrotic changes are commonly associated with the development of bullae and cavities, which are prone to mycetoma formation with *Aspergillus*. The diagnosis should be suspected in a young to middle-aged man with characteristic spine changes (kyphosis, spinal ankylosis) seen in association with abnormally increased lung volumes and upper lobe fibrobullous disease, the latter of which simulates postprimary fibrocavitary TB.

Overlap Syndromes and Mixed Connective Tissue Disease. Some patients with collagen vascular disease have features of more than one of the recognized syndromes discussed above. These patients are classified as having an overlap syndrome with thoracic manifestations characteristic of the other disorders. Patients with a distinct form of overlap syndrome, called *mixed connective tissue disease*, have clinical features of SLE, scleroderma, and polymyositis and have serum antibodies to extractable nuclear antigen. The thoracic manifestations of mixed connective tissue disease include IPF, pulmonary arterial hypertension caused by plexogenic pulmonary arteriopathy, and pleural effusion and thickening from a fibrinous pleuritis typical of SLE.

Idiopathic Chronic Interstitial Pneumonias

The idiopathic interstitial pneumonias are characterized by an inflammatory process in the lung that can result in pulmonary fibrosis. These histologic terms provide the most precise method of classifying these disorders and include UIP, acute interstitial pneumonia (AIP), COP, respiratory bronchiolitis–associated interstitial lung disease (RB-ILD), DIP, and nonspecific interstitial pneumonia (NSIP) (2). Unfortunately, confusion arises when clinical terms are used interchangeably with the aforementioned histologic terms in describing these disorders. When possible (when the histology is known), it is most accurate to use the histologic term to describe a particular disorder, while reserving clinical terms such as *IPF* or *rheumatoid lung* for interstitial disease associated with specific clinical diseases for which histology is unavailable.

Usual Interstitial Pneumonia. UIP is the most common of the idiopathic interstitial pneumonias. It is likely the result of repetitive injury to the lung. The initial response in the lung is inflammation, which is followed by repair and eventually fibrosis. The pathologic abnormalities seen in UIP represent a spectrum of findings, characterized in the early stage of disease by marked proliferation of macrophages in the alveolar airspaces associated with a mild and uniform thickening of the interstitium by mononuclear cells. Late in the course of disease, the pathologic findings are characterized by thickening of the alveolar interstitium by mononuclear inflammatory cells and fibrous tissue. A distinguishing histologic feature of UIP is that different stages of the disease are seen simultaneously within different portions of the lung.

Patients with UIP typically present in the fifth to seventh decades, with a slight male preponderance. Presenting

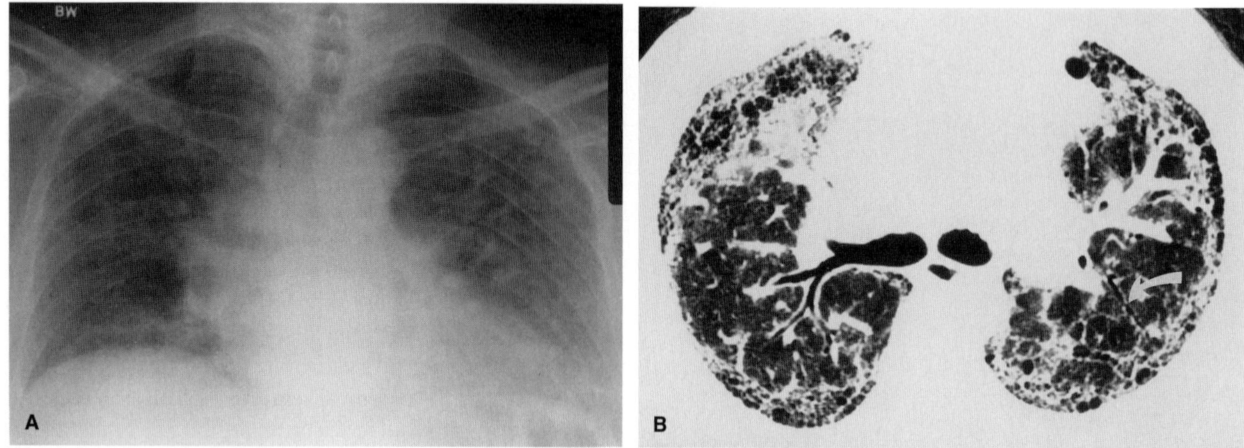

FIGURE 17.18. **Usual Interstitial Pneumonia (UIP). A.** Posteroanterior radiograph in a patient with UIP demonstrates bilateral coarse reticular opacities and diminished lung volumes. **B.** An HRCT through the mid-lungs shows honeycombing in a peripheral, subpleural distribution. Traction bronchiectasis is evident (*arrow*).

symptoms include progressive dyspnea or a nonproductive cough. Pulmonary function tests show restrictive disease and a decreased diffusing capacity for carbon monoxide (DLCO). Most cases of UIP are sporadic, but up to 30% of patients with UIP have an associated collagen vascular or immunologic disorder. This is most often rheumatoid arthritis, but it can also be SLE, scleroderma, or dermatomyositis/polymyositis.

The radiographic manifestations of UIP parallel the pathologic changes. In the early phase of disease, the chest radiograph may appear normal despite the presence of clinical symptoms and abnormalities on pulmonary function testing. The earliest radiographic changes are bibasilar fine to medium reticular opacities or ground-glass density (Fig. 17.18). As the disease progresses, a coarse reticular or reticulonodular pattern is seen, which almost invariably leads to the formation of honeycomb cysts (3 to 10 mm in diameter) and progressive loss of lung volume. Extensive pulmonary fibrosis may be associated with findings of pulmonary arterial hypertension. Upper lobe bullae may be seen and predispose to the development of spontaneous pneumothorax. Hilar lymph node enlargement and pleural effusions have been described but are rare and should suggest an alternative diagnosis.

HRCT findings in UIP differ with the stage of the disease and vary from one lung region to another. Patients with active inflammatory areas of disease, as demonstrated histologically by interstitial and intra-alveolar inflammatory changes, show areas of ground-glass density on HRCT. As fibrosis develops, findings include irregular septal or subpleural thickening (in contrast to the smooth septal thickening seen with edema or lymphangitic spread of carcinoma), intralobular lines, irregular interfaces, honeycombing, and traction bronchiectasis (Fig. 17.12). The changes are typically most severe in the peripheral and basal portions of the lungs, which can be helpful in differential diagnosis (Fig. 17.18). Mildly enlarged mediastinal lymph nodes are often seen.

In most patients, the disease progresses inexorably, with an overall mean survival of <5 years. Patients with early, active disease (positive gallium scan, ground-glass or airspace opacities radiographically) may benefit from immunosuppressive therapy with corticosteroids or cyclophosphamide, while those with end-stage fibrosis (honeycombing) will not. Most patients succumb to respiratory failure, often precipitated by infection or cardiac disease. There is an increased incidence of bronchogenic carcinoma, with adenocarcinoma the most common histologic subtype.

Acute Interstitial Pneumonia. Also known as the Hamman-Rich syndrome, AIP is an acute, aggressive form of idiopathic interstitial pneumonitis and fibrosis. Patients with AIP typically present with a brief history of cough, fever, and dyspnea that progresses rapidly to severe hypoxemia and respiratory failure requiring mechanical ventilation. The pathologic manifestations of AIP are those of ARDS, and the disease has been termed *idiopathic ARDS*. The histologic findings are those of diffuse alveolar damage with minimal mature collagen deposition. A characteristic of the process is that it is diffuse and temporally homogeneous.

Chest radiographs and HRCT scans show findings of ARDS, with diffuse ground-glass opacity and consolidation with air bronchograms (Fig. 17.19) (4). On CT, there is often a gradient of increasing density from anterior to posterior lung. Linear opacities, honeycombing, and traction bronchiectasis are uncommon. As in other forms of ARDS, mortality rates range from 60% to 90%. Fibrosis can develop but tends to stabilize and does not progress beyond the recovery phase.

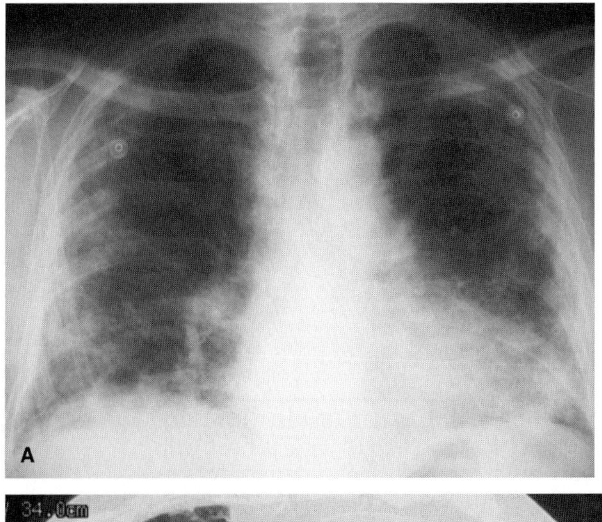

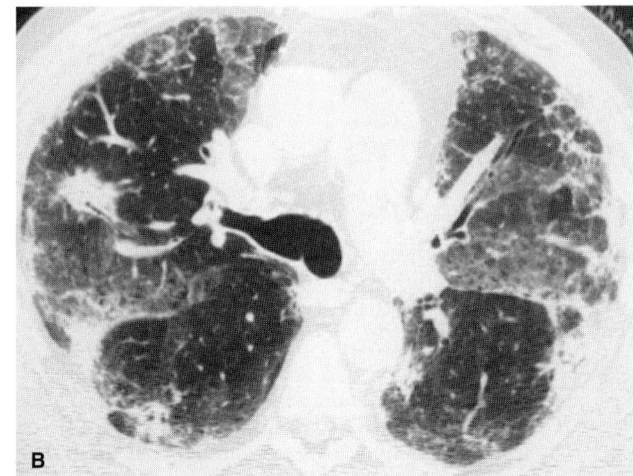

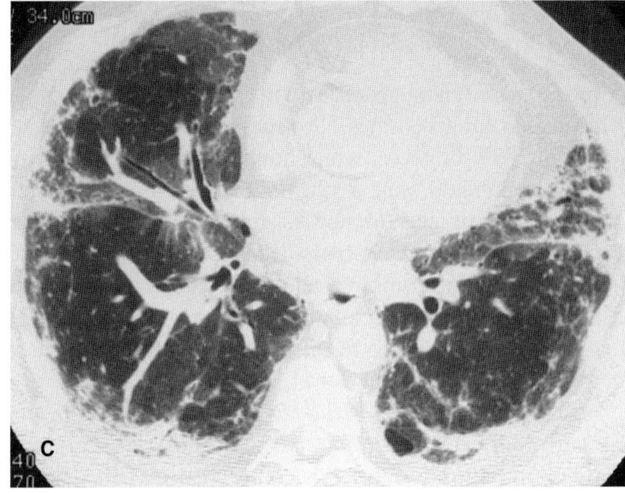

FIGURE 17.19. **Acute Interstitial Pneumonia (Hamman-Rich syndrome).** Frontal radiograph **(A)** in a patient with biopsy-proven acute interstitial pneumonia demonstrates peripheral airspace and ground-glass opacity. CT scans through the upper lobe bronchus **(B)** and lower lungs **(C)** show predominantly peripheral ground-glass and reticular opacities with scattered airspace opacities.

Cryptogenic Organizing Pneumonia. COP, also known as *idiopathic bronchiolitis obliterans with organizing pneumonia* (BOOP), is a disorder characterized by the widespread deposition of granulation tissue (fibroblasts, collagen, and capillaries) within peribronchiolar airspaces and bronchioles. Most cases of BOOP are idiopathic (i.e., COP), but a number of conditions have been associated with this disorder. These include viral infection (influenza, adenovirus, measles); toxic fume inhalation (sulfur dioxide, chlorine); collagen vascular disease (rheumatoid arthritis and SLE); organ transplantation (bone marrow, lung, and heart-lung); drug reactions; and chronic aspiration.

Patients with COP often have a subacute illness, with several months' history of nonproductive cough and dyspnea. The physical examination may reveal rales or wheezes. Pulmonary function tests usually show a restrictive pattern of disease with diminished lung volumes and normal to increased flow rates. The DLCO is significantly decreased. Pathologically, a mononuclear cell exudate in the bronchioles and surrounding alveoli organizes to form intrabronchiolar and intra-alveolar granulation tissue. A characteristic of this disease is the uniformity of the histologic changes and the absence of parenchymal distortion and fibrosis; these features help distinguish COP from UIP, which can have similar clinical, functional, and radiographic features.

Radiographs in patients with COP reveal patchy bilateral airspace or ground-glass opacities (Fig. 17.13A), with some patients showing scattered nodular opacities. The most common HRCT findings are patchy consolidation or ground-glass opacity with either a subpleural or peribronchial pattern of distribution (Fig. 17.13B). Small ill-defined peribronchial nodules are seen less commonly. Bronchiectasis and bronchial wall thickening are commonly seen in the involved areas of lung.

The diagnosis of COP can only be made by recognizing the characteristic histologic changes on open lung biopsy. The distinction of COP from IPF may be difficult but is important, because COP has a more favorable prognosis and usually responds rapidly to corticosteroid therapy. COP complicating heart-lung transplantation generally has a worse prognosis but may respond favorably to immunosuppressive therapy.

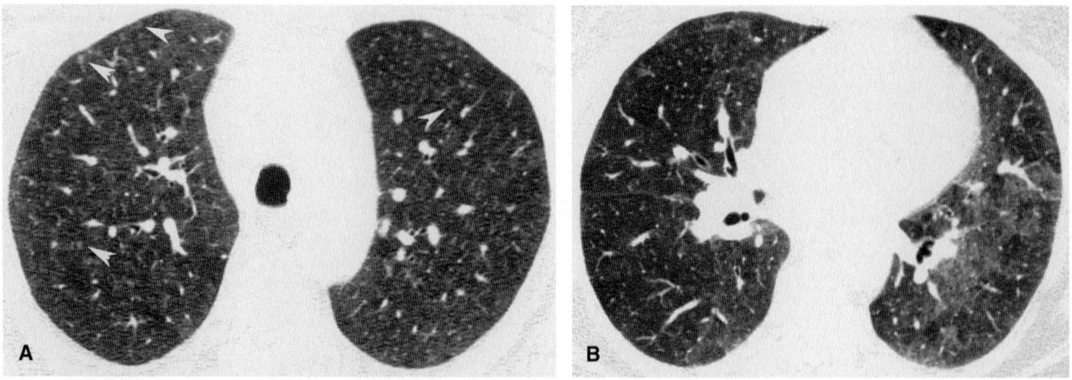

FIGURE 17.20. **Respiratory Bronchiolitis–Associated Interstitial Lung Disease (RB-ILD).** Thin-section CT scans through the upper lobes **(A)** and lower lobes **(B)** in a patient with biopsy-proven RB-ILD demonstrate bilateral centrilobular (*arrowheads*) and geographic regions of ground-glass opacity.

Respiratory Bronchiolitis–Associated Interstitial Lung Disease. Respiratory bronchiolitis is a disorder seen only in cigarette smokers and is characterized by inflammation within and around the respiratory bronchioles. The histology of RB-ILD overlaps with that of DIP, and some authors have suggested that RB-ILD is an early form of DIP. Patients with RB-ILD are typically young, heavy smokers with mild cough and dyspnea. Pulmonary function tests show restrictive or mixed restrictive-obstructive patterns. Symptoms respond to smoking cessation or steroid therapy, and there is no progression to end-stage fibrosis.

The chest radiograph is normal in up to 21% of cases of RB-ILD. Diffuse linear and nodular opacities are often seen, as is bibasilar atelectasis. The most common HRCT findings are scattered ground-glass opacities and small centrilobular nodules, often with an upper lobe–predominant distribution (Fig. 17.20). Linear opacities are rare and honeycombing is not seen. Emphysema is often a concomitant finding.

Desquamative Interstitial Pneumonia. DIP describes a histologic pattern characterized by the accumulation of macrophages within alveolar spaces. Ninety percent of patients with DIP are cigarette smokers. While focal areas of macrophage accumulation can be seen as a component of UIP, the finding in DIP is diffuse and temporally homogeneous. There are distinguishing clinical features that support the concept of two distinct entities. DIP affects younger individuals, with a mean age at diagnosis of 40 to 45, and is almost invariably associated with heavy cigarette smoking. Most importantly, DIP is more steroid-responsive than UIP and therefore carries a more favorable prognosis; the median survival for patients with DIP is 12 years, compared with 4 years for those with UIP.

DIP cannot be reliably distinguished from UIP radiographically. The typical radiographic findings in DIP are bibasilar reticular opacities with normal or minimally diminished lung volumes. Ground-glass opacities are seen in only 33% of cases, while honeycombing is rare. Up to 22% of patients have a normal chest radiograph. HRCT shows ground-glass opacities, most often within the peripheral aspects of the bases (Fig. 17.21). Irregular linear opacities, honeycombing, and traction bronchiectasis can be seen but are much less common than in UIP. Ground-glass abnormalities often improve or completely resolve with corticosteroid therapy.

Nonspecific Interstitial Pneumonia. NSIP is a recently introduced entity, used to describe interstitial pneumonias that cannot be otherwise classified as UIP, AIP, COP, RB-ILD, or DIP. Many cases of NSIP are seen in association with collagen vascular disease or as drug reactions. The pathologic changes are temporally homogeneous, as compared to UIP, which is typically heterogeneous. Pathologists generally divide NSIP into cellular and fibrotic forms of disease, with correlative findings on HRCT. Those with cellular NSIP show areas of ground-glass and consolidation on HRCT in a peripheral and lower zone distribution (Fig. 17.22). Bronchial dilatation and linear opacities are more typical of the fibrotic form of NSIP, but in distinction to UIP, honeycombing is rare. While cellular NSIP is usually responsive to steroids, fibrotic NSIP has a poor prognosis, similar to that of UIP.

Other Chronic Interstitial Lung Diseases

Neurofibromatosis (NF) is an autosomal dominant neurocutaneous syndrome, which is divided into two types: type 1, or von Recklinghausen disease, and type 2. The classic manifestations of NF 1 are cutaneous café-au-lait spots and neurofibromas of cutaneous and subcutaneous peripheral nerves and nerve roots. In addition, there is often involvement of the skeletal, vascular, and pulmonary

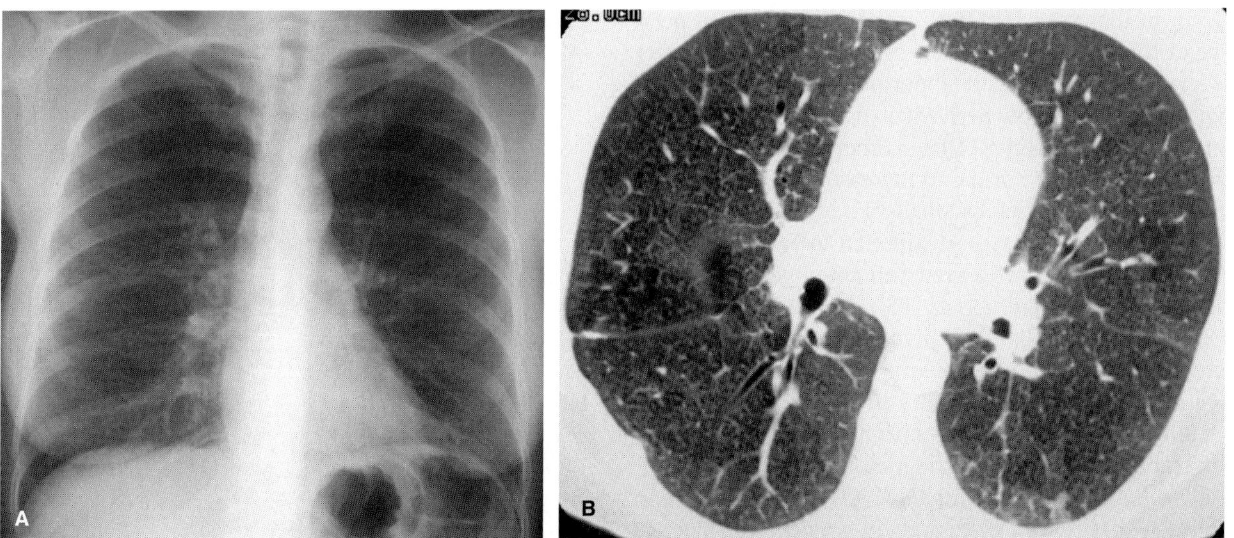

FIGURE 17.21. Desquamative Interstitial Pneumonia (DIP). Chest radiograph **(A)** and HRCT **(B)** show fine reticular or ground-glass opacities in a smoker with DIP.

systems. The condition is also associated with a variety of neoplasms, including meningiomas, optic gliomas, neurofibrosarcomas, and pheochromocytomas.

There are several thoracic manifestations of NF 1. Cutaneous and subcutaneous neurofibromas may be seen along the chest wall or projecting over the lungs. The spine may show a kyphoscoliosis, with scalloping of the posterior aspect of the vertebral bodies caused by dural ectasia. "Ribbon rib" deformities and rib notching may be seen. Mediastinal masses in patients with NF 1 include neurofibromas, lateral thoracic meningoceles, and extra-adrenal pheochromocytomas.

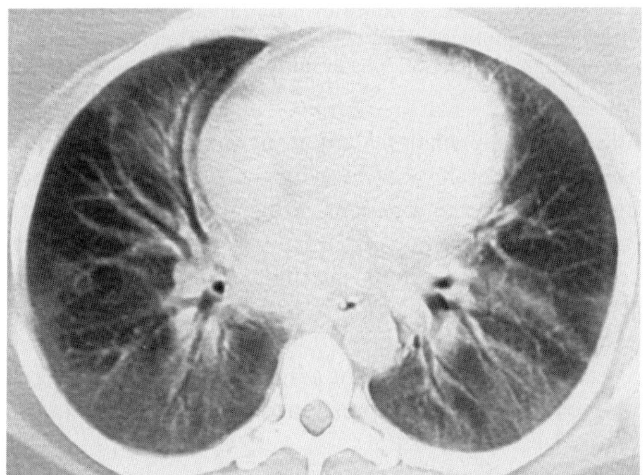

FIGURE 17.22. Nonspecific Interstitial Pneumonia (NSIP). A 10-mm axial CT scan of a 57-year-old man with cough and dyspnea shows multifocal consolidation and ground-glass opacities. Open lung biopsy demonstrated NSIP.

Parenchymal lung disease is seen in approximately 20% of patients with NF 1. The findings include diffuse interstitial fibrosis and bulla formation. The interstitial fibrosis is predominantly lower zonal and bilaterally symmetric. Bullae usually develop in the upper zones, with asymmetric involvement of the lungs. Pulmonary symptoms are usually minimal or absent, with pulmonary function tests showing a mixed obstructive/restrictive pattern. A small number of patients will develop respiratory failure caused by pulmonary fibrosis, with secondary development of pulmonary arterial hypertension and cor pulmonale.

***Tuberous Sclerosis* (TS).** TS is an autosomal dominant neurocutaneous syndrome with variable expression. The classical clinical triad of TS is seizures, mental retardation, and adenoma sebaceum. Additional manifestations include intracranial calcifications, cerebral cortical and periventricular hamartomas, renal angiomyolipomas, cardiac rhabdomyomas, retinal phakomas, and sclerotic bone lesions.

Pulmonary involvement in TS is rare and is seen in approximately 1% of cases. Patients with pulmonary TS tend to be older and have a lower incidence of seizures and mental retardation. The pulmonary involvement is indistinguishable clinically, pathologically, and radiographically from that seen in LAM. Pathologically, there is smooth muscle proliferation in the peribronchovascular and parenchymal interstitium of the lung. Small adenomatoid nodules measuring several millimeters in diameter may be seen scattered throughout the lungs.

Radiographically, there are symmetric bilateral reticular or reticulonodular opacities. In the later stages of disease, a pattern of coarse reticular or small cystic opacities may be seen. The cysts are uniform in size and

<1 cm in diameter. HRCT is best at depicting the presence of thin-walled pulmonary cysts and can help detect associated extrapulmonary abnormalities, including renal angiomyolipomas and periventricular tubera. A helpful feature in distinguishing TS from other chronic interstitial lung diseases is the normal to increased lung volumes in patients with TS caused by small airways obstruction and expiratory air trapping. In distinction to EG of lung and sarcoidosis, which have a predominant upper zone distribution of disease, pulmonary TS tends to affect the entire lung uniformly. Pneumothorax is common and results from the rupture of a subpleural cyst. Pleural effusions are uncommon. The pulmonary involvement often leads to pulmonary arterial hypertension and cor pulmonale, which are associated with a high mortality.

Lymphangioleiomyomatosis. LAM is an uncommon condition that is seen exclusively in women. The average age at diagnosis is 43 years. Although LAM shares many features with pulmonary TS, it is not an inherited condition and lacks the extrapulmonary features of TS.

On gross pathologic examination, patients with advanced LAM show replacement of the normal lung architecture by cysts. These cysts, which range from 0.2 to 2.0 cm in diameter, are separated by thickened interstitium containing numerous interlacing bundles of smooth muscle. Smooth muscle proliferation is also seen within the walls of pulmonary veins, bronchioles, and lymphatics. The smooth muscle proliferation within lymphatic channels causes lymphatic obstruction and dilatation that may lead to the development of chylothorax, chyloperitoneum, or chylopericardium. Similarly, smooth muscle proliferation within mediastinal and retroperitoneal lymph nodes may result in nodal enlargement. The perilymphatic smooth muscle proliferation and nodal enlargement help distinguish LAM pathologically from the pulmonary involvement of TS.

The patient with LAM is typically a woman of childbearing age who presents with progressive dyspnea or a spontaneous pneumothorax. Hemoptysis may be seen in some patients, presumably related to pulmonary venous obstruction by the smooth muscle proliferation.

The chest radiograph may be normal early in the disease. Eventually, symmetric bilateral fine reticular or reticulonodular opacities are seen. The late radiographic pattern is one of cysts and honeycombing; the cysts tend to have thinner walls than those seen with IPF or NF (Fig. 17.23A). As in TS, the lung volumes are typically normal or increased. Large, recurrent chylous pleural effusions may be unilateral or bilateral. Spontaneous pneumothorax is also a common finding and may be bilateral.

HRCT demonstrates thin-walled cysts distributed throughout the lungs (Fig. 17.23B). In less severely involved areas, the intervening lung is normal. Interlobular septal thickening is generally mild or absent.

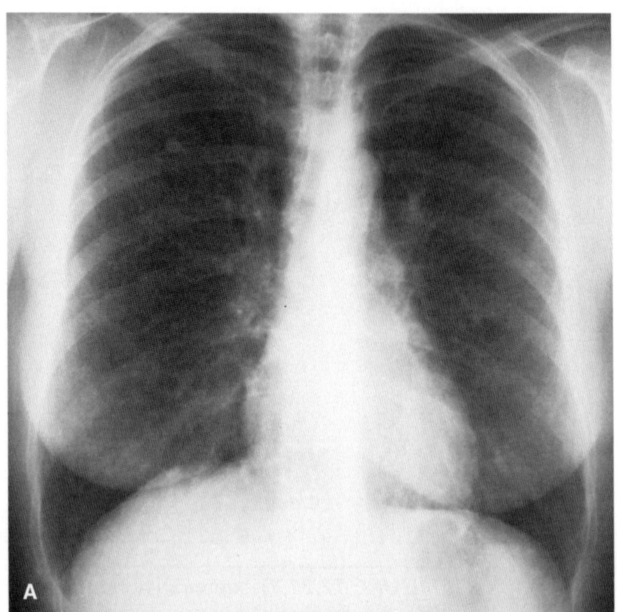

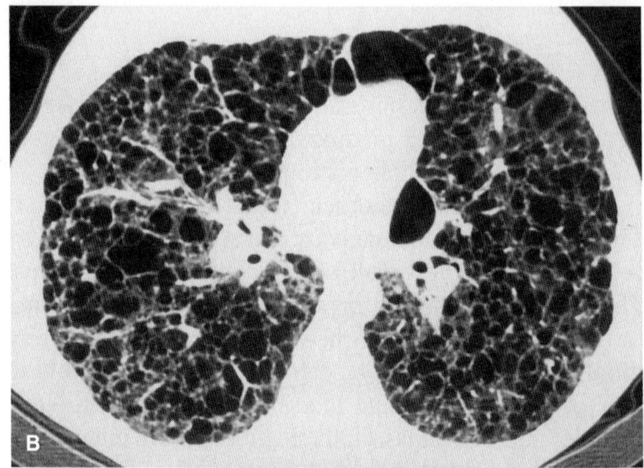

FIGURE 17.23. **Lymphangioleiomyomatosis (LAM). A.** Posteroanterior radiograph in a 36-year-old patient with LAM shows diffuse coarse reticular opacities with normal lung volumes. **B.** An HRCT in another patient with LAM shows almost complete replacement of the parenchyma by fairly uniform thin-walled cysts.

Although thin-walled cysts are seen in a variety of other diseases, most notably emphysema and EG, the HRCT findings, when seen in a patient with a characteristic history (a woman with dyspnea, spontaneous pneumothorax, and chylous pleural effusions) are diagnostic (5).

The prognosis of patients with symptomatic LAM is poor, with approximately 70% of patients dying within 5 years. In some patients, the administration of antiprogesterone agents such as tamoxifen may slow the progression of disease.

Alveolar Septal Amyloidosis. Amyloidosis encompasses a group of diseases characterized by the extracellular deposition of insoluble fibrillary proteins termed *amyloid*. Amyloid represents a number of proteins that are distinctive biochemically but similar physically in that their polypeptide chains form beta-pleated sheets. Amyloidosis has traditionally been classified into four forms: (*1*) primary, in which there is no associated chronic disease or in which there is an underlying plasma cell disorder; (*2*) secondary, in which an underlying chronic abnormality such as TB is present; (*3*) familial, which is very uncommon and usually localized to nervous tissue; and (*4*) senile, which affects many organs in patients over 70. More recently, a classification scheme has been developed that is based on the specific protein comprising amyloid. In this scheme, the most important forms are amyloid L (AL), usually seen with plasma cell dyscrasias and associated with the deposition of immunoglobulin light chains, and amyloid A (AA), which occurs in patients with chronic inflammatory diseases such as familial Mediterranean fever and certain neoplasms, including Hodgkin disease.

There are three major patterns of amyloid deposition within the lungs and airways: tracheobronchial, nodular parenchymal, and diffuse parenchymal (alveolar septal). In most cases these patterns occur independently, but there can be overlap between them.

In alveolar septal amyloidosis, the amyloid is deposited in the parenchymal interstitium and within the media of small blood vessels. Within the alveolar septa, amyloid deposits are located between the endothelial cells lining the septal capillaries and the alveolar epithelium; inflammatory cells are typically absent.

This process is usually seen in older patients who have symptoms of chronic progressive dyspnea. Recurrent hemoptysis may also be seen as a result of medial dissection of the involved pulmonary arteries. Radiographically, patients with parenchymal alveolar septal disease show evidence of interstitial disease, with fine reticular or reticulonodular opacities that may become more coarse and confluent over time. HRCT demonstrates interlobular septal thickening, reticulation, and micronodules; signs of fibrosis are uncommon, as is lymph node enlargement (4). The radiographic appearance simulates that seen in silicosis or sarcoidosis.

The diagnosis is made on lung biopsy by the identification of amorphous eosinophilic material thickening the alveolar septa that appears apple green in color when stained with Congo red and viewed under polarized light. There is no effective treatment.

Chronic Aspiration Pneumonia. Patients who repeatedly aspirate may develop chronic interstitial abnormalities on chest radiographs. With repeated episodes of aspiration over months to years, a residuum of irregular reticular interstitial opacities may persist, probably representing peribronchial scarring. A reticulonodular pattern may be seen as the result of granulomas forming around food particles. These chronic interstitial abnormalities can be observed between episodes of acute aspiration pneumonitis.

INHALATIONAL DISEASE

Pneumoconiosis

The term *pneumoconiosis* is used to describe the nonneoplastic reaction of the lungs to inhaled inorganic dust particles (6). The inorganic dust pneumoconioses result from the inhalation and retention of asbestos, silica, or coal particles within the lung. With time, the accumulation of these particles leads to two types of pathologic reaction that may be seen alone or in combination: fibrosis, which may be focal and nodular or diffuse and reticular; and the aggregation of particle-laden macrophages. Organic dust inhalational syndromes, which are discussed at the end of this section, are not associated with the retention and accumulation of particles within the lungs. Instead, the organic dusts induce a hypersensitivity reaction known as hypersensitivity pneumonitis or extrinsic allergic alveolitis.

Asbestosis. *Asbestos* is the generic term for a group of fibrous silicates that are resistant to heat and various chemical insults. Asbestos is divided into two major subgroups: the serpentines and the amphiboles. The serpentines are curly, flexible, and smooth; the only commercially important serpentine is chrysotile. The amphiboles have straight, needlelike fibers; this subgroup includes crocidolite and amosite. The different types of asbestos fibers vary in their potential to cause disease, with the amphiboles having a greater fibrogenic and carcinogenic potential than the serpentines. At present, >90% of the asbestos used in the United States is chrysotile.

Asbestos inhalation may cause disease of the pleura, parenchyma, airways, and lymph nodes. Pleural disease is the most common of these, and it usually manifests as parietal pleural plaques. Other pleural manifestations include pleural effusion, localized visceral pleural fibrosis, diffuse pleural fibrosis, and mesothelioma. The pleural manifestations of asbestos exposure are discussed in more detail in Chapter 19. The pulmonary parenchymal manifestations of asbestos inhalation include interstitial fibrosis (asbestosis), rounded atelectasis, and bronchogenic carcinoma.

Asbestosis is defined as a diffuse parenchymal interstitial fibrosis caused by the inhalation of asbestos fibers. The development of asbestosis depends on both the length and severity of exposure, and clinical manifestations are usually not apparent for 20 to 40 years following initial exposure. Pathologically, a large number of "asbestos bodies" will be seen in lung tissue. This characteristic structure consists of a core transparent asbestos fiber surrounded by a variably thick coat of iron and protein. Asbestos bodies are usually found within interstitial fibrous tissue or airspaces, and only rarely in pleural plaques. The number of asbestos bodies and fibers per gram of digested lung tissue is roughly proportional to the degree of occupational exposure and the severity of interstitial fibrosis. On gross examination of affected lungs, fibrosis is most prominent

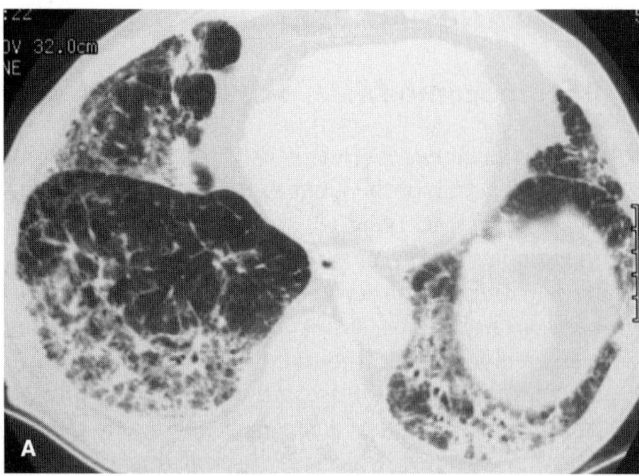

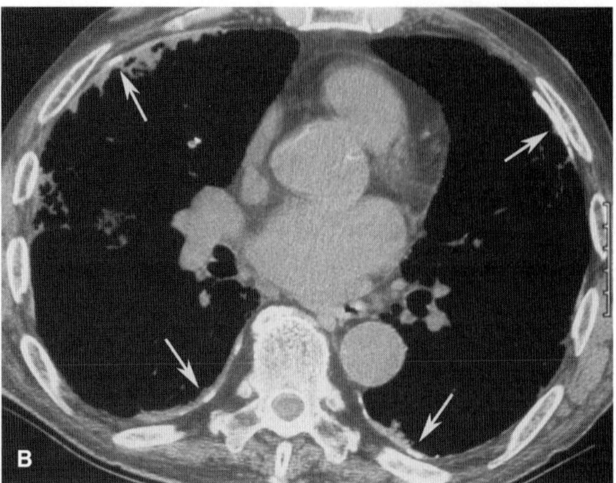

FIGURE 17.24. **Asbestosis. A.** CT through the lower lobes in a patient with asbestos exposure shows middle lobe and peripheral bilateral lower lobe reticulation and ground-glass opacity reflecting asbestosis. **B.** Scan obtained just cephalad to A at mediastinal windows shows bilateral calcified pleural plaques (*arrows*).

in the subpleural regions of the lower lobes. Microscopically, the appearance varies from a slight increase in interstitial collagen to complete obliteration of normal architecture and formation of thick fibrous (parenchymal) bands and cystic spaces (honeycombing).

The majority of patients with asbestos-related pleuropulmonary disease are asymptomatic. Patients beyond the early stages of interstitial fibrosis will often experience shortness of breath and a restrictive pattern on pulmonary function tests. These patients are also at risk of developing asbestos-associated neoplasia, particularly bronchogenic carcinoma and pleural mesothelioma, and require close clinical follow-up.

The radiographic findings in asbestosis occur in two forms: small and large opacities. Small opacities may be reticular, nodular, or a combination of the two. The changes produced on chest radiographs are divided into three stages. The earliest finding is a fine reticulation, predominantly in the lower lung zones, which is a manifestation of early interstitial pneumonitis and fibrosis. With time, the small irregular opacities become more prominent, creating a coarse reticular pattern of disease. In later stages, the reticular opacities may extend into the midlung and upper lung zones, with progressive obscuration of the cardiac and diaphragmatic margins and progressive diminution of lung volumes. Large opacities, i.e., those measuring greater than 1 cm in diameter, are invariably associated with widespread interstitial fibrosis and pleural plaques. These large opacities show lower zone predominance and may be well-defined or ill-defined and multiple.

HRCT is a sensitive indicator of both the pleural and parenchymal changes associated with clinical asbestosis. Interlobular septal thickening is the most common HRCT finding in asbestos-exposed individuals. Intralobular septal thickening and small centrilobular "dotlike" opacities, the latter caused by peribronchiolar fibrosis, are also common. Many cases will progress to honeycombing. Many of these HRCT findings overlap with those of UIP (Figs. 17.12, 17.18), but patients with asbestosis may also have pleural disease, which may help to distinguish between these two entities (Fig. 17.24). Additionally, ground-glass opacity is relatively uncommon in asbestosis compared with IPF and other forms of UIP.

Identification of intrafissural plaques, especially if they contain calcification, is also possible with HRCT. Characteristic CT features of focal lung masses in asbestos-exposed individuals may allow for conservative management of these lesions. For example, a wedge-shaped or round mass adjacent to focal pleural thickening, with evidence of lobar volume loss and a "comet tail" bronchovascular bundle coursing into it, can be confidently diagnosed as rounded atelectasis by HRCT.

Silicosis. Silica is an abundant mineral composed of regularly arranged molecules of silicon dioxide. It is ubiquitous in the earth's crust, and exposure to a high concentration may lead to pathologic and radiologic changes. Occupations associated with such levels of exposure include mining, quarrying, foundry work, ceramic work, and sandblasting.

Two distinct histopathologic reactions to inhaled silica are *silicotic nodules* and *silicoproteinosis*. Silicotic nodules measure from 1 to 10 mm in diameter and are made up of dense concentric lamellae of collagen. They are typically most numerous in the upper lobes and parahilar regions of lung; calcification or ossification of the nodules is common. Coalescence of these nodules produces areas of PMF. PMF may occupy an entire lobe, with areas of emphysema often seen adjacent to these masses. Focal necrosis is common within the central portions of these large conglomerate lesions, often the result of ischemia or superinfection by TB or anaerobic bacteria. Silicoproteinosis is a different manifestation of the disease that generally occurs in individuals exposed to very high concentrations of silica. It is characterized by filling of alveolar spaces with lipoproteinaceous material similar to that seen in idiopathic alveolar proteinosis. There is little collagen deposition associated with this reaction, and the well-defined collagenous nodule is not typically seen. Patients with both fibrotic silicosis and acute silicoproteinosis have an increased susceptibility to TB.

Exposure of 10 to 20 years is usually required for the radiographic changes of silicosis to develop. The classic radiographic appearance is multiple well-defined nodules ranging from 1 to 10 mm in diameter. These nodules, which calcify in approximately 20% of cases, are diffuse and demonstrate an upper zone predominance. A reticular pattern of disease may be seen preceding or associated with the nodular pattern and is sometimes the earliest radiographic finding. This pattern of reticulonodular opacities is often referred to as "simple" silicosis, in contrast to the large conglomerate opacities that characterize "complicated" silicosis (Fig. 17.10). These conglomerate opacities represent areas of PMF and most commonly develop in the peripheral portions of the upper and mid-lung zones. The opacities tend to migrate toward the hila, leaving areas of emphysema between the pleural surface and the areas of progressive fibrosis. These conglomerate areas may cavitate, often in association with superimposed tuberculous infection. Hilar lymph node enlargement may be seen at any stage, and these hilar nodes often demonstrate peripheral "eggshell" calcification. A variant of the classic radiographic form of the disease is seen in patients with acute heavy exposure to silica (usually sandblasters) who develop acute silicoproteinosis. This presents radiographically with diffuse airspace disease and is indistinguishable in appearance from idiopathic alveolar proteinosis. These patients are also predisposed to superinfection with *Nocardia*, which may produce masslike consolidation and chest wall involvement.

Clinically, the diagnosis of silicosis is based on identification of a diffuse reticular, nodular, or reticulonodular pattern on the chest radiograph in a patient with an appropriate exposure history. Patients may be asymptomatic for many years, but may worsen functionally in conjunction with progression of the radiographic changes. The pulmonary fibrosis and associated restrictive functional impairment of silicosis may progress even after the individual is removed from the offending environment.

Coal Worker's Pneumoconiosis. The inhalation of large amounts of carbon-containing inorganic material may lead to significant pulmonary disease. The exposure levels required to cause this disease occur almost exclusively in the workplace. Since the most common occupation producing this entity is coal mining, the resultant disease is termed coal worker's pneumoconiosis (CWP).

CWP has two characteristic pathologic findings: the coal dust macule and PMF. The coal dust macule results from the deposit of carbonaceous material within the lung. Coal dust macules are round or stellate nodules ranging in size from 1 to 5 mm. They are composed of pigment-laden macrophages with minimal or absent collagen formation. They are found within the interstitium adjacent to respiratory bronchioles, and are scattered throughout the lungs with a predilection for the apices. The coal dust macule or nodule is the hallmark of simple CWP and is generally not associated with functional impairment. In fact, radiographic abnormalities may be absent in simple CWP. Complicated CWP is characterized by the presence of PMF. PMF is defined as nodular or masslike lesions exceeding 2 to 3 cm in diameter that are composed of irregular fibrosis and pigment. PMF is most common in the posterior segments of the upper lobes and superior segments of the lower lobes. The conglomerate masses may cross interlobar fissures. Central cavitation is common and is most often a result of infarction from obliteration of pulmonary vessels by the fibrotic masses. Occasionally, superinfection of the masses by TB or fungus accounts for central necrosis and cavitation. The mass lesions of complicated CWP are similar to those seen in complicated silicosis. It should be noted that despite their name, the lesions of PMF may not progress with time and are not necessarily massive in size.

Patients with CWP usually present with respiratory difficulties only when PMF has developed, as those with simple pneumoconiosis are generally asymptomatic. In complicated CWP, there is progressive dyspnea with cor pulmonale and right heart failure. Because many coal workers also smoke cigarettes, the development of centrilobular emphysema and chronic bronchitis may complicate the clinical picture.

Radiographically, "simple" CWP presents typically as upper zone reticulonodular or small nodular opacities (6). A purely reticular pattern may also be seen, especially in the early stages of the process. The nodules range from 1 to 5 mm in diameter and correspond to conglomerates of coal dust macules seen pathologically. The lesions are indistinguishable radiographically from the nodules of simple silicosis. In as many as 10% of coal miners, some of these nodules will calcify centrally. This is in distinction to the diffuse calcification of silicotic nodules. The nodular opacities of simple CWP do not progress after coal dust exposure has ceased. The lesions of complicated pneumoconiosis (PMF) range in size from 2 cm to an entire lobe and are seen in the upper portion of the lungs. PMF usually begins peripherally as a mass with a smooth, well-defined lateral border and an ill-defined medial border. PMF gradually "migrates" toward the hilum, creating a zone of emphysema between the opacities and the chest wall. These lesions may mimic primary carcinoma, particularly if a background of nodular opacities is not appreciated. The

PMF seen with CWP may develop years after exposure to coal dust has ceased and may progress in the absence of further exposure.

Certain complicating factors may alter the radiographic appearance of CWP. TB is relatively common in patients with CWP and may produce central cavitation in some patients with PMF. Caplan syndrome or "rheumatoid pneumoconiosis," seen in coal workers with rheumatoid arthritis, is characterized radiographically by nodular opacities 0.5 to 5 cm in diameter that develop rapidly and tend to appear in crops. The nodules are more sharply defined and seen more peripherally than the masses of PMF. These lesions are not specific for CWP and may be seen in patients with silicosis or asbestosis.

Miscellaneous Pneumoconioses. A variety of inorganic dusts other than asbestos, silica, and coal dust can cause pleuropulmonary disease but are far less common. Chronic berylliosis produces a reaction that mimics sarcoidosis and is discussed in the section "Granulomatous Diseases." Aluminum workers may develop disabling pulmonary fibrosis after years of exposure to aluminum dust, usually from bauxite mining. Radiographic changes include fine to coarse reticular or reticulonodular opacities distributed throughout the lungs, along with greatly diminished lung volumes and marked pleural thickening. Apical bullae may be seen, which produce spontaneous pneumothoraces. Hard metal pneumoconiosis, formerly called giant cell interstitial pneumonitis, may result from exposure to cobalt and tungsten alloys and lead to interstitial pneumonitis with varying degrees of fibrosis. The chest radiograph demonstrates a reticulonodular pattern that may be very coarse and, if advanced, may be associated with small cystic shadows. Lymph node enlargement may be seen.

Hypersensitivity Pneumonitis

Hypersensitivity pneumonitis or *extrinsic allergic alveolitis* is an immunologic pulmonary disorder associated with the inhalation of one of the antigenic organic dusts. These dusts must be of small particle size to penetrate into the alveolar spaces and incite a host inflammatory response. A wide variety of etiologic agents have been implicated, including many thermophilic bacteria, true fungi, and various animal proteins. Some of the more common disease entities include farmer's lung, which follows exposure to moldy hay; humidifier lung, which follows exposure to water reservoirs contaminated by thermophilic bacteria; and bird-fancier's lung, which results from exposure to avian proteins in feathers and excreta.

The development of hypersensitivity pneumonitis depends upon the size, number, and immunogenicity of the inhaled organic particles and the immune response of the host. Two forms of the disease are distinguished by their clinical presentation and immunopathogenesis. Acute disease develops 4 to 6 hours following exposure to the inciting antigen and is mediated by a type 3 (immune complex) reaction. Typical symptoms include cough, dyspnea, and fever. Chronic disease is often insidious and commonly results in interstitial pulmonary fibrosis. Patients with chronic disease often have malaise, chronic cough, and progressive dyspnea. This form of disease appears to be mediated by a type 4 (cell-mediated) immune reaction.

The histopathologic features of the different types of hypersensitivity pneumonitis are usually indistinguishable, except in rare situations where antigenic material can be identified in the pathologic preparations. The pathologic features are dependent on the intensity of exposure to the allergen and on the stage of disease when tissue biopsy is obtained. Early findings include capillary congestion and inflammation within alveolar septae. In later stages of acute disease, bronchiolitis and alveolitis with granuloma formation are present. With repeated antigenic exposure, there is a progressive increase in interstitial fibrosis, which is initially patchy in distribution but may progress to diffuse interstitial fibrosis.

The radiographic changes of hypersensitivity pneumonitis parallel the pathologic findings. The chest radiograph may be normal early in the acute stage of disease. Within hours, fine nodular or ground-glass opacities develop, most often in the lower lobes; progressive airspace opacification may simulate pulmonary edema. Within hours to days, the opacities resolve and the chest radiograph becomes normal. With continued or repeated exposures, the chest radiograph will remain abnormal between acute episodes. The chronic changes appear as diffuse coarse reticular or reticulonodular opacities in the midlung and upper lung zones; a honeycomb pattern with loss of lung volume may be seen. The diagnosis of hypersensitivity pneumonitis should be considered when repeated episodes of rapidly changing ground-glass or airspace opacification are seen in a patient with underlying coarse interstitial lung disease. Hilar or mediastinal lymph node enlargement and pleural effusion are uncommon findings in patients with hypersensitivity pneumonitis.

HRCT may be very helpful in the diagnosis of hypersensitivity pneumonitis, particularly in the subacute phase, when chest radiographs may be normal or quite nonspecific. The most common findings in the acute phase of disease are airspace opacities, while the subacute phase is characterized by patchy areas of ground-glass opacity and poorly defined ("fuzzy") centrilobular nodules (Figs. 17.7, 17.11) (7). These findings may be superimposed on one another, and both show a predominance in the mid- and lower lung zones. In the chronic phase of the disease, findings are those of fibrosis: interlobular and intralobular interstitial thickening, honeycombing, and traction bronchiectasis. Distribution of disease is varied, but sometimes there is relative sparing of the costophrenic angles, which may help to distinguish hypersensitivity pneumonitis from IPF and other forms of UIP.

The diagnosis of hypersensitivity pneumonitis is made by eliciting a history that suggests a temporal relationship between the patient's symptoms and certain exposures. The intermittent exposure of susceptible persons to high concentrations of antigen leads to recurrent episodes that typically begin 4 to 6 hours following exposure. The symptoms usually persist for 12 hours and then resolve spontaneously if the exposure has been terminated. Repeated exposure to the inciting antigen will result in acute exacerbations, with typical symptoms and radiographic findings. Chronic disease is more difficult to diagnose and develops when there is a continuous low level of exposure to the antigen. The prognosis for patients whose disease is recognized at an early stage is good if the offending agent can be removed from the patient's environment. In the more insidious chronic form of disease, the diagnosis is often delayed and considerable interstitial fibrosis may be present at the time of diagnosis. These patients generally suffer from chronic respiratory insufficiency.

GRANULOMATOUS DISEASES

Sarcoidosis

Sarcoidosis is a multisystem granulomatous disease of unknown etiology characterized histologically by noncaseating granulomas that may progress to fibrosis. The disease is seen more commonly in blacks than whites and is rare in Asians. Black women are at particular risk for this disease. Most patients are 20 to 40 years of age at the time of diagnosis. However, because patients with this disease are often asymptomatic, many cases are never identified.

The etiology of sarcoidosis is unknown, although an inhaled infectious agent such as *Mycobacterium*, *Yersinia*, or a virus has been suggested. Whatever the etiologic agent, the underlying pathogenesis involves activation of pulmonary macrophages that, in turn, recruit mononuclear cells to the pulmonary interstitium, leading to the formation of granulomas. The activated macrophages also stimulate proliferation of T-helper lymphocytes in the lung, which induces an overactivity of B lymphocytes, resulting in the hypergammaglobulinemia characteristically seen in this disease. The excess number of T-helper lymphocytes in the lung may be detected in bronchoalveolar lavage fluid of patients with sarcoidosis and is helpful in the differential diagnosis of this condition.

The pathologic changes of sarcoidosis follow a fairly predictable pattern. The earliest changes involve the pulmonary interstitium, with the development of a nonspecific lymphocytic and histiocytic infiltrate. This progresses to the formation of microscopic granulomas. The granulomas contain palisading epithelioid histiocytes with intermixed multinucleated giant cells and, in contrast to tuberculous granulomas, are typically noncaseating. The giant cells in the granulomas may contain dark-staining lamellated structures within their cytoplasm called Schaumann bodies, which are characteristic of sarcoidosis. The granulomas are found most commonly within the axial (peribronchovascular) and peripheral or subpleural interstitium of the lung, but may involve the parenchymal (alveolar) interstitium and airway mucosa; the airway lesions may be visualized bronchoscopically. Involvement of the axial interstitium of the lung accounts for the high (approximately 90%) diagnostic yield of blind transbronchial biopsy in sarcoidosis, since this technique usually provides samples of the bronchial wall, the surrounding axial interstitium, and adjacent airspaces. The small granulomas usually resolve after months or years. In some patients, the microscopic granulomas coalesce to form larger nodules. Rarely, these nodules grow to form large, well-defined masses or poorly marginated opacities that contain air bronchograms and simulate an airspace-filling process. In this "alveolar" form of sarcoidosis, the airspaces are not filled with material but are compressed and obliterated by the exuberant granuloma formation within the surrounding interstitium.

In 20% of patients, fibrous tissue is deposited at the periphery of the granulomas and eventually grows inward to replace the granulomas, resulting in interstitial fibrosis. The fibrosis tends to progress over time, with the development of broad bands of fibrous tissue extending from the hilar regions toward the lung apices, producing hilar elevation and distortion of the hilar vessels and upper mediastinum. Masses of fibrous tissue may develop in the perihilar regions of the upper lobes, with peripheral areas of emphysema or cyst formation. These cysts predispose a patient to spontaneous pneumothoraces and provide a site for mycetoma formation.

Lymph node involvement in sarcoidosis is characterized by replacement of the normal nodal architecture with granulomas that are indistinguishable from those found in the pulmonary parenchyma. As with parenchymal involvement, these may regress, coalesce, or undergo fibrosis.

The clinical presentation of sarcoidosis may be dominated by pulmonary or extrapulmonary manifestations of the disease, but a considerable percentage of patients are asymptomatic and are identified by incidental findings on chest radiographs. Pulmonary symptoms are present in 25% of patients and include dyspnea and a nonproductive cough. Common extrapulmonary findings include fever, malaise, uveitis, and erythema nodosum. In a minority of patients, involvement of the liver, heart, kidneys, or CNS may dominate the clinical picture.

Common laboratory findings in sarcoidosis include hypercalcemia, hypergammaglobulinemia, and elevated serum angiotensin-converting enzyme levels. Cutaneous anergy to purified protein derivative Tubulin skin test

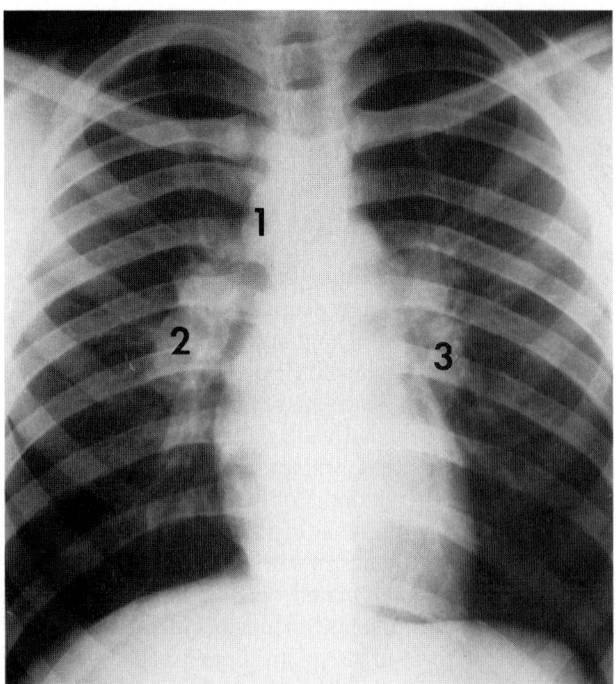

FIGURE 17.25. **Sarcoidosis.** Posteroanterior radiograph in an asymptomatic 26-year-old shows marked enlargement of right paratracheal (1), right hilar (2), and left hilar (3) lymph nodes, which is characteristic of sarcoidosis.

(PPD) reflects an abnormality of delayed hypersensitivity found in these patients. Pulmonary function tests vary from normal in those with minimal or no parenchymal disease to a severe restrictive pattern with low diffusing capacity in patients with end-stage pulmonary fibrosis.

Lymph Node Enlargement. Enlargement of mediastinal and hilar lymph nodes is found in 80% of patients with sarcoidosis and is associated with radiographically normal lungs in slightly more than half of these patients (8). The typical appearance on chest radiographs is right paratracheal and bilateral symmetric hilar lymph node enlargement (Fig. 17.25). The symmetric enlargement is a key feature that allows distinction from malignancy and TB, conditions that usually produce unilateral or asymmetric lymph node enlargement. Left paratracheal lymph node enlargement is common, as determined by CT, although enlargement of these nodes is usually not appreciated on radiographs because the region is obscured by the aorta and great vessels on frontal radiographs. The enlarged nodes tend to have a lobulated contour because the individual nodes remain discrete. Mediastinal (paratracheal) lymph node enlargement without concomitant hilar enlargement is uncommon and should suggest lymphoma or metastatic disease. Similarly, unilateral hilar nodal enlargement is unusual, seen in only 5% of individuals. Involvement of anterior mediastinal, posterior mediastinal, subcarinal, and aortopulmonary lymph nodes occurs with greater frequency than previously thought, because of the ability of CT to detect nodes in regions that are invisible on plain radiographs. Involved nodes may show contrast enhancement.

The enlarged lymph nodes regress within 2 years in 75% of affected patients. A small percentage of patients will have persistent lymph node enlargement for years. The development of parenchymal opacities concomitant with the resolution of lymph node enlargement is a helpful feature in differentiating sarcoidosis from lymphoma, in which enlarged lymph nodes do not regress when parenchymal abnormalities develop. Calcification of involved lymph nodes is seen in up to 20% of patients and may involve only the periphery of the node ("eggshell" calcification).

Lung Disease. The lung is involved radiographically in only 40% to 50% of patients with sarcoidosis, despite the nearly 90% yield from transbronchial biopsy of the lung. The earliest finding is a diffuse micronodular pattern, identical in appearance to miliary TB, which represents the superimposition of microscopic granulomas. This pattern, which is rarely identified radiographically, may precede the development of hilar lymph node enlargement. The most common parenchymal abnormality is bilateral symmetric reticulonodular opacities show a predilection for the mid- and upper lung zones (Fig. 17.26). The reticulonodular opacities represent the combination of granulomas and fibrosis. CT shows that most nodules lie predominantly in a peribronchovascular and subpleural location. The appearance of reticulonodular opacities never precedes the enlargement of hilar and mediastinal lymph nodes.

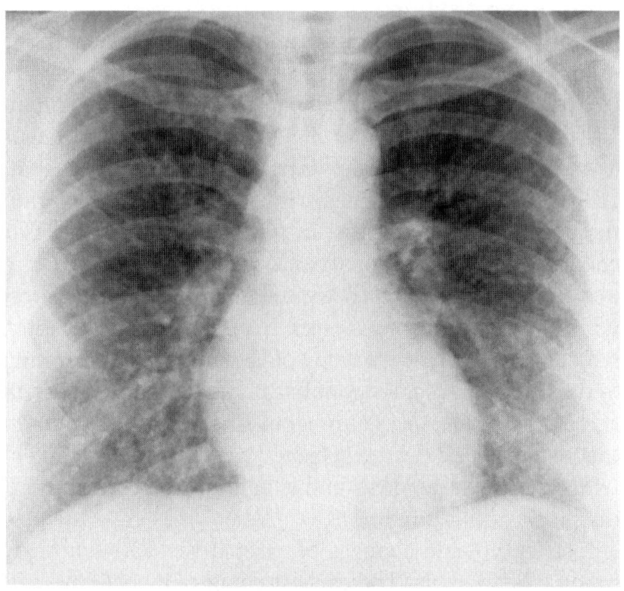

FIGURE 17.26. **Sarcoidosis.** Posteroanterior chest film in a 39-year-old black woman with mild dyspnea shows extensive bilateral reticulonodular opacities. Transbronchial biopsy showed noncaseating granulomas, which are typical of sarcoidosis.

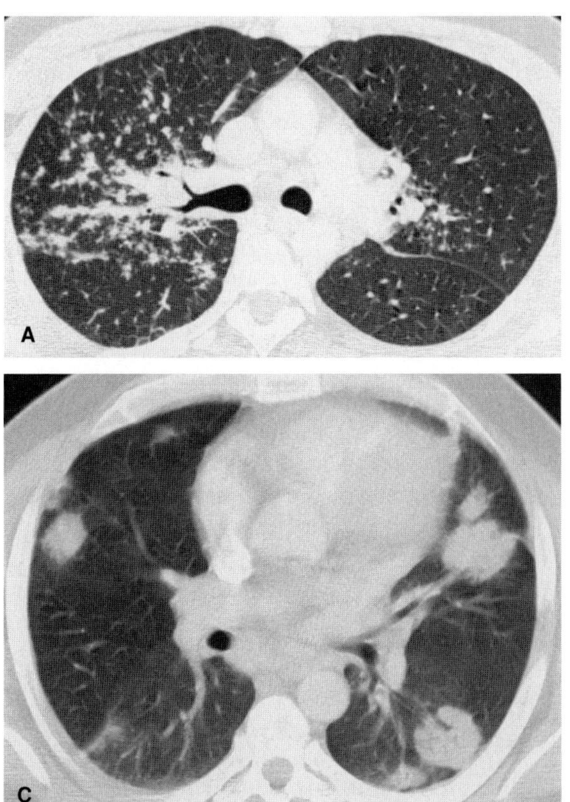
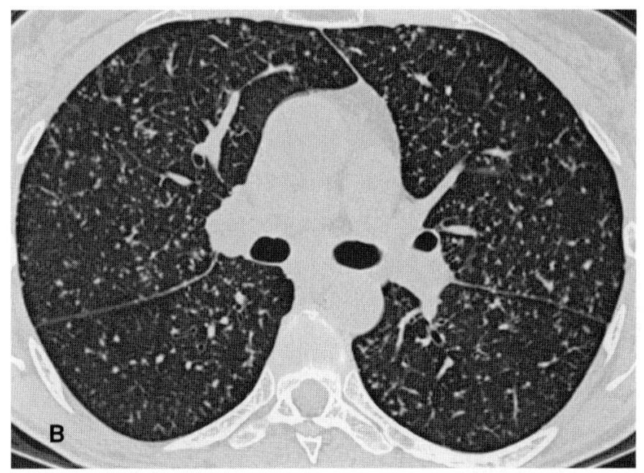

FIGURE 17.27. **CT Appearances of Sarcoidosis.** Sarcoidosis in three different patients showing typical perilymphatic nodules **(A),** miliary nodules **(B),** and masslike opacities **(C);** the latter two appearances are uncommon.

In approximately 10% of patients, the coalescence of granulomas can produce one of two unusual radiographic manifestations of parenchymal sarcoidosis. Exuberant interstitial granulomas can obliterate adjacent airspaces, producing poorly defined airspace opacities that may contain air bronchograms. In some cases, intra-alveolar inflammation and granulomas contribute to the alveolar pattern of disease. These airspace opacities are primarily seen in the peripheral portions of the midlung zone, thereby simulating eosinophilic pneumonia radiographically (Fig. 17.27). The presence of reticulonodular opacities elsewhere in the lung or concomitant symmetric hilar and mediastinal lymph node enlargement, best seen on CT and HRCT, provide important clues to the diagnosis.

Nodular or masslike sarcoidosis develops in a manner similar to alveolar disease. These masses can be quite large and typically have a sharp margin. Air bronchograms are often demonstrated on CT and HRCT; cavitation is extremely rare.

Pulmonary fibrosis develops in 20% of patients with long-standing parenchymal involvement. The chest radiograph shows coarse linear opacities extending obliquely from the hila toward the upper and mid-lung zones. There is considerable distortion and elevation of the hila, with scalloping of the lung-mediastinal interface. Occasionally, conglomerate masses of fibrosis form in the upper perihilar regions that simulate the progressive massive fibrosis of complicated silicosis. On CT, these masses contain air bronchograms with traction bronchiectasis. Distortion and obstruction of the airways from fibrosis can lead to secondary air trapping, with resultant alveolar septal disruption and bullae formation. An increase in radiographic lung volumes may accompany these cystic changes, a finding that is characteristic of bullous sarcoidosis (Fig. 17.28). Mycetomas can develop within the cysts and lead to massive hemoptysis from erosion into bronchial arteries. Cysts may also rupture into the pleural space and produce spontaneous pneumothoraces.

Pleural Changes. Pleural thickening or effusion occurs in approximately 7% of patients with sarcoidosis and is the result of granulomatous inflammation of the visceral and parietal pleura.

Miscellaneous Findings. Endobronchial granulomas can result in fibrosis of the bronchial wall and bronchostenosis. Pulmonary arterial hypertension is an uncommon finding and is usually secondary to long-standing pulmonary fibrosis.

HRCT Findings. HRCT is clearly more sensitive than chest radiographs in detecting the parenchymal abnormalities of sarcoidosis. A variety of HRCT findings have been described in this disease, which represent both the granulomatous and fibrotic response seen histologically (Fig. 17.28). The most frequent finding is the presence of interstitial nodules, 3 to 10 mm in diameter, seen as

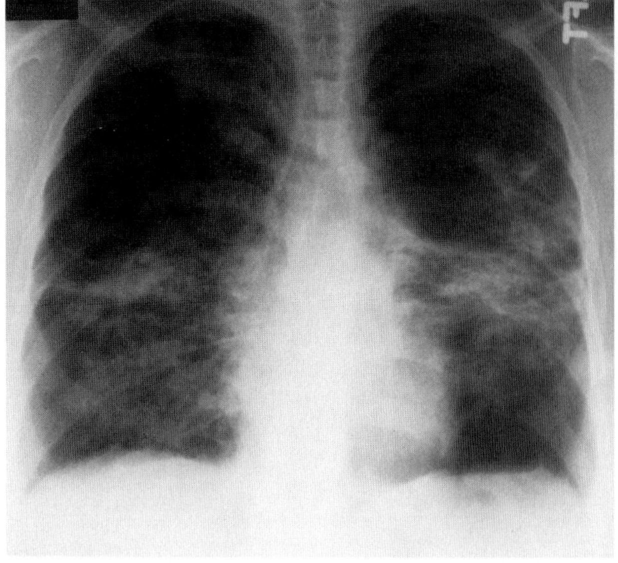

FIGURE 17.28. **Bullous Changes in Sarcoidosis.** In a 49-year-old woman with long-standing sarcoidosis, a posteroanterior chest film shows extensive middle and lower zone coarse interstitial opacities and biapical bullous disease.

nodular thickening of the peribronchoarterial (axial) interstitium and interlobular septa or as subpleural nodules. The nodules correlate closely with the coalescing noncaseating granulomas seen microscopically on tissue specimens. Septal thickening, thickening of bronchovascular bundles, architectural distortion, lung cysts, honeycombing, and central conglomerate masses with crowded, ectatic bronchi are findings indicative of fibrosis from long-standing disease. Segmental or masslike airspace opacities, termed "alveolar" sarcoid, usually indicate the presence of active disease and resolve with corticosteroid therapy. Likewise, the finding of patchy areas of ground-glass density has been shown to correlate with increased uptake on gallium scans and may be indicative of an active alveolitis. Several recent papers have showed good correlation between conventional CT and HRCT findings and pulmonary function tests.

Radiographic Staging of Sarcoidosis. The chest radiographic manifestations of sarcoidosis have been divided into five stages (Table 17.6). These stages generally parallel the course of disease and are useful for prognostic purposes. Stage 1 disease is associated with a 75% rate of resolution, whereas only 30% of patients with stage 2 and 10% of patients with stage 3 disease resolve.

The diagnosis of sarcoidosis is usually based on the histologic demonstration of noncaseating granulomas involving multiple organs. Tissue is most often obtained by bronchoscopically guided transbronchial biopsy, which provides a diagnosis in up to 90% of patients. Biopsy of organs likely to be involved in this disease, such as the liver and scalene lymph nodes, will provide a diagnosis in a majority of patients. Percutaneous needle biopsy can provide diagnostic tissue specimens in those with masslike pulmonary lesions. In certain situations, the diagnosis of sarcoidosis is made on a constellation of chest radiographic findings and characteristic eye or skin changes. In such patients, gallium scintigraphy showing a pattern of increased uptake in the hilar lymph nodes, lung, and salivary glands may be used as a confirmatory test. Gallium scanning has also been used to assess the degree of disease activity.

TABLE 17.6 Radiographic Staging of Sarcoidosis

Stage	*Radiographic Findings*
0	Normal chest radiograph
1	Bilateral hilar lymph node enlargement
2	Bilateral hilar lymph node enlargement and parenchymal disease
3	Parenchymal disease only
4	Pulmonary fibrosis

Berylliosis

Although berylliosis is actually an inhalational lung disease, it is discussed here because of the clinical, pathologic, and radiographic similarities to sarcoidosis. This uncommon disease produces noncaseating granulomas in multiple organs, with primary lung involvement. The radiographic features of berylliosis are indistinguishable from those of sarcoidosis. Hilar and mediastinal lymph node enlargement and bilateral reticulonodular opacities are the most common findings. As with sarcoidosis, progression to end-stage interstitial fibrosis with honeycombing or upper lobe bullous disease may occur, with the latter predisposing the patient to aspergilloma formation and spontaneous pneumothoraces.

Langerhans Cell Histiocytosis of Lung

The entity of LCH includes several disorders with similar pathologic features that differ in age at the time of diagnosis, mode of presentation, specific organs involved, and prognosis. The form of this disease affecting adults, also called eosinophilic granuloma (EG), presents with predominant involvement of lung and bones. The disease most commonly affects young adults and has no sex predilection. There is a very high association between pulmonary involvement and cigarette smoking.

Pathologically, LCH of lung demonstrates multiple small nodules, which are found predominantly in the axial interstitial tissues of the upper and mid-lung zones around small bronchioles. The nodules represent granulomas composed predominantly of cells with eosinophilic cytoplasm, previously called histiocytosis X cells and now known as Langerhans cells. These cells are normally found in the skin, where they act as antigen-processing cells, and appear to proliferate in the lung and other organs in response to an unidentified antigenic stimulus. In some patients, the nodular phase of disease may be preceded by an exudative phase, with filling of the alveolar spaces with a cellular exudate containing the Langerhans cells. The small peribronchiolar nodules may coalesce to form larger nodules, which may cavitate, or they may extend to infiltrate the alveolar septa and induce an interstitial inflammatory reaction. The nodules may resolve completely, but in most patients, the central portions of the nodules undergo fibrosis, producing a stellate nodular lesion that is characteristic of pulmonary LCH histologically. In the late stages, characteristic findings include fibrosis and the development of small, uniform, thin-walled cysts. Larger peripheral cysts or bullae may develop in the apical regions, presumably as a result of bronchiolar obstruction by fibrosis, with distal air trapping.

Pulmonary symptoms are present in two thirds of patients with LCH of lung at presentation. Cough and the gradual onset of dyspnea are the most common complaints. Pleuritic chest pain may indicate the development of a spontaneous pneumothorax from rupture of a subpleural cyst. The physical examination is typically unremarkable. Pulmonary function tests reflect the fibrosis and cystic changes seen in this disorder, with characteristic restrictive and obstructive patterns of disease and a diminished diffusing capacity.

The radiographic findings in LCH of the lung usually follow a predictable pattern (9). Although the earliest changes in LCH of the lung are associated with filling of alveoli, the radiographic demonstration of airspace opacities is uncommon. The earliest findings are small to medium nodular opacities that tend to have an upper and midlung zone distribution (Fig. 17.29). In some cases the nodules coalesce to form larger nodules or masses, which rarely cavitate. The nodular pattern may resolve completely or be replaced by a predominantly reticulonodular or reticular pattern that represents the fibrotic phase of the disease. Late stages of the disease are characterized by a coarse reticular pattern with intermixed thin-walled cysts. These cysts account for the relative preservation or increase in lung volumes typical of LCH, which is a distinguishing feature of this disease. Hilar or mediastinal lymph node enlargement is distinctly uncommon, a feature that helps distinguish LCH from sarcoidosis. Pneumothorax from rupture of a cyst or bulla is the presenting finding or develops during the course of disease in up to 25% of patients. Pleural effusion in the absence of a pneumothorax is rare. Extrapulmonary manifestations include well-defined lytic rib or vertebral lesions.

The parenchymal changes of LCH of the lung are best demonstrated on HRCT. HRCT in patients with a relatively short duration of symptoms (<6 months) shows well-defined interstitial nodules of varying size, sometimes with cavitation, and cyst formation in the upper lungs. More long-standing disease is characterized by larger cysts (Fig. 17.30) and honeycombing. Nodules and thick-walled cysts can transform into thin-walled cysts, suggesting that the sequence of evolution of LCH lesions is as follows: nodule right arrow cavitated nodule right arrow thick-walled cyst right arrow thin-walled cyst.

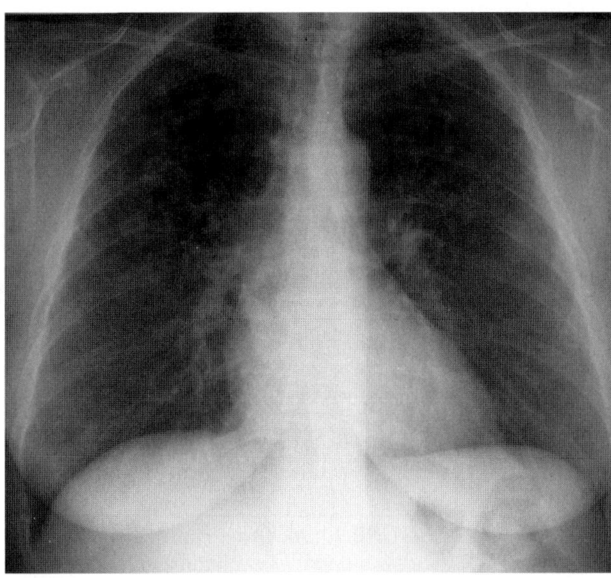

FIGURE 17.29. **Langerhans Cell Histiocytosis (LCH) of Lung.** Posteroanterior radiograph in a 52-year-old woman with LCH shows a nodular pattern with a middle and upper zone predominance.

The distinguishing features between LCH of lung and emphysema are the presence of nodules (with or without cavitation) and thin-walled cysts in LCH that lack a constant relationship to the centrilobular core structures. The HRCT distinction of LCH from LAM in a woman is more difficult; an upper zone distribution and the presence of nodules favor EG.

The diagnosis of LCH of lung is made by noting the characteristic stellate nodular lesions with Langerhans cells on open lung biopsy specimens. The treatment for symptomatic patients is corticosteroid therapy, although more than half of the patients with lung disease stabilize or improve spontaneously.

Wegener Granulomatosis

Wegener granulomatosis is a systemic autoimmune disorder characterized pathologically by a necrotizing granulomatous vasculitis involving the upper and lower respiratory tracts and kidneys. The characteristic lesions in the lungs are discrete nodules or masses of granulomatous

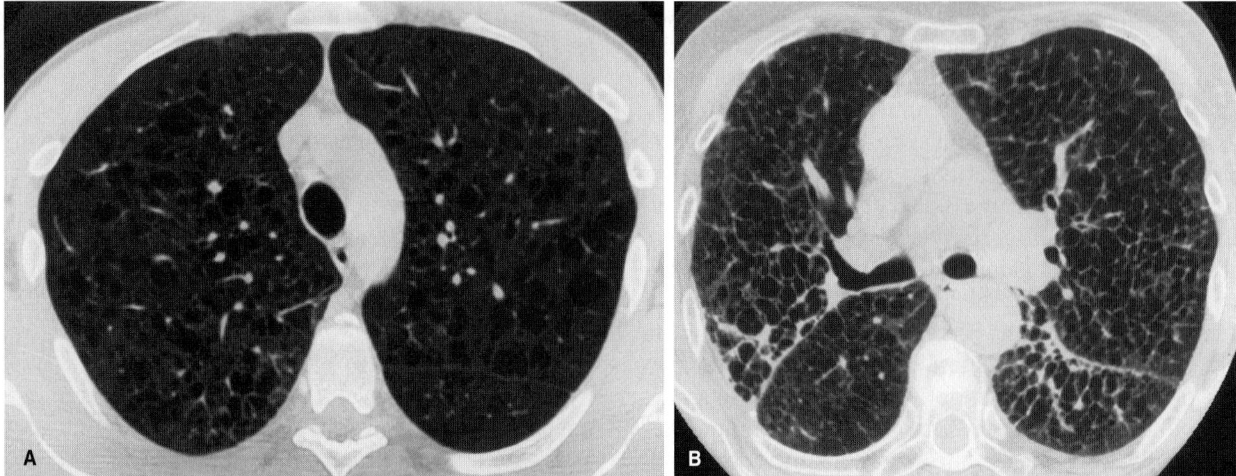

FIGURE 17.30. **Langerhans Cell Histiocytosis on HRCT. A.** An HRCT in a 39-year-old smoker with eosinophilic granuloma (EG) shows multiple cysts with thin but well-defined walls. **B.** In another patient with EG, the cysts are more extensive, with little normal intervening parenchyma. Note the irregular shape of many of these cysts.

inflammation with central necrosis and cavitation. The lesions involve pulmonary vessels, accounting for the high incidence of central necrosis and for the occasional presentation with pulmonary hemorrhage. Mucosal and submucosal lesions may be present in the tracheobronchial tree and are seen almost exclusively in women.

Most patients with Wegener granulomatosis are middle-aged, with a slight male predominance. The respiratory tract is affected in 100% of patients, with symptoms usually dominated by sinus and nasal mucosal involvement. Pulmonary involvement may be asymptomatic or manifested by cough, dyspnea, or chest pain. Presentation with pulmonary hemorrhage and hemoptysis may mimic other pulmonary-renal syndromes such as Goodpasture syndrome and idiopathic pulmonary hemorrhage. Renal involvement usually follows involvement of the respiratory tract and is seen in almost 90% of patients.

The characteristic chest radiographic features of lung involvement in Wegener granulomatosis are multiple sharply marginated nodules or masses (Fig. 17.31); solitary lesions are seen in up to one-third of patients. Irregular, thick-walled cavitary lesions are seen in 50% of patients during the course of disease (10). Localized or diffuse areas of airspace opacification may be seen, representing either hemorrhage or pneumonia, the latter often a result of complicating *Staphylococcus aureus* infection. Tracheal or bronchial lesions may be present and are usually best appreciated on CT, where they appear as calcified mucosal or submucosal deposits, producing irregular narrowing of the airway lumen. The airway lesions are usually not associated with parenchymal disease, but endobronchial lesions may produce distal atelectasis. Pleural effusion from pleural involvement is not uncommon. Pneumothorax may result from rupture of a cavitary lesion into the pleural space. Lymph node enlargement is not seen in this disease.

The diagnosis of Wegener granulomatosis should be made on biopsy of involved tissues, usually nasal mucosa or lung, that show the granulomatous inflammation and vasculitis that are characteristic of this disease. The pathologic changes in the kidneys are often nonspecific, and therefore renal biopsy is often nondiagnostic. This disease usually responds dramatically to cyclophosphamide (Cytoxan) therapy. Some patients with disease limited to the chest respond to oral co-trimoxazole (Bactrim). Untreated patients invariably die of renal failure or, less commonly, progressive respiratory disease. High serologic titers for the presence of antineutrophil cytoplasmic

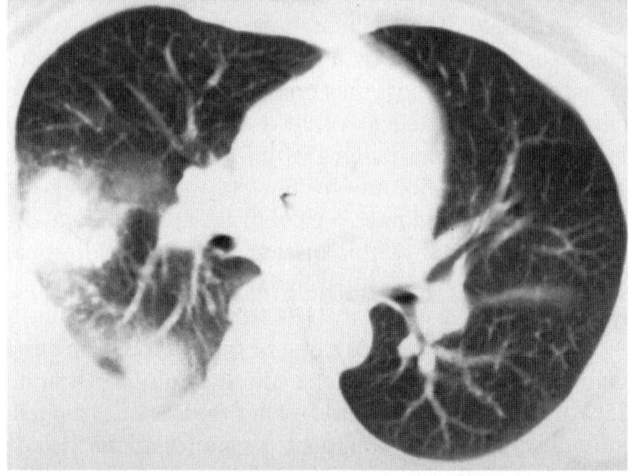

FIGURE 17.31. **Wegener Granulomatosis.** A CT examination in a patient with Wegener granulomatosis shows several large masses with indistinct margins in the right lower lobe.

antibody are specific for the diagnosis of Wegener granulomatosis, although a negative test does not exclude the diagnosis, particularly in patients with limited or inactive disease.

EOSINOPHILIC LUNG DISEASE

This term refers to a heterogeneous group of allergic diseases characterized by excess eosinophils in the lung and occasionally blood. Fraser and Pare have classified these diseases into three groups: idiopathic, those of known etiology, and autoimmune or collagen vascular disorders (Table 17.7).

Idiopathic Eosinophilic Lung Disease

The idiopathic disorders associated with eosinophilic lung disease include simple pulmonary eosinophilia, chronic eosinophilic pneumonia, and hypereosinophilic syndrome (11).

Simple pulmonary eosinophilia, also known as Löffler syndrome, is a transient pulmonary process characterized pathologically by pulmonary infiltration with an eosinophilic exudate. Most patients have a history of allergy, most commonly asthma. The characteristic radiographic findings are peripheral, homogeneous, ill-defined areas of airspace opacification that may parallel the chest wall (Fig. 17.32); this latter feature is best appreciated on CT. The opacities in Löffler syndrome have been described as fleeting, because there is a tendency for rapid clearing in one area with new involvement in other areas. A dry cough, dyspnea, and peripheral blood eosinophilia are common but are not invariably present. The diagnosis is based on the combination of pulmonary symptoms, blood eosinophilia, and characteristic radiographic findings. Most patients having a self-limiting illness that resolves spontaneously within 4 weeks.

Chronic Eosinophilic Pneumonia. Patients with symptoms and radiographic abnormalities that last longer than 1 month are considered to have chronic eosinophilic pneumonia. The clinical and radiographic features are similar to those of Löffler syndrome, although there is a distinct predilection for women. Patients are usually symptomatic with fever, malaise, and dyspnea. The pulmonary symptoms and radiographic opacities respond dramatically to corticosteroid therapy and improve within 4 to 7 days, although relapse upon discontinuation of treatment is common.

Hypereosinophilic syndrome is a systemic disorder with a male predominance that is characterized by multiple organ damage from eosinophilic infiltration of tissues. Blood eosinophilia is prolonged and marked in this condition. The major chest radiographic findings are associated with cardiac involvement and secondary congestive heart failure and include cardiomegaly, pulmonary edema, and pleural effusions. Pulmonary parenchymal infiltration with eosinophils may produce interstitial or airspace opacities.

TABLE 17.7 Eosinophilic Lung Disease

Idiopathic	Simple pulmonary eosinophilia (Löffler syndrome)
	Chronic eosinophilic pneumonia
	Hypereosinophilic syndrome
Known etiology	Drugs
	Antibiotics
	Penicillins
	Nitrofurantoin
	Nonsteroidal anti-inflammatory agents
	Aspirin
	Chemotherapeutic agents
	Bleomycin
	Methotrexate
	Parasites
	Filaria
	Strongyloides
	Ascaris
	Hookworm
Autoimmune disease	Wegener granulomatosis
	Sarcoidosis
	Rheumatoid lung disease
	Polyarteritis nodosa
	Allergic angiitis and granulomatosis (Churg-Strauss syndrome)

Müller NL, Colman N, Pare PD, Fraser RS. Fraser and Pare's Diagnosis of Diseases of the Chest (4 volume set) W.B Saunders 4th Ed Philadelphia 1999.

Eosinophilic Lung Disease of Identifiable Etiology

Pulmonary eosinophilia of known etiology includes drug and parasite-induced eosinophilic lung disease. Drugs associated with pulmonary eosinophilia include nitrofurantoin and the penicillins. The parasitic infections most commonly responsible are filaria and the roundworms *Ascaris lumbricoides* and *Strongyloides stercoralis*. These parasites may produce pulmonary eosinophilia as they migrate through the alveolar capillaries and into the alveoli during their tour of the body. These disorders are usually indistinguishable clinically and radiographically from Löffler syndrome.

Eosinophilic Lung Disease Associated With Autoimmune Diseases

A number of autoimmune disorders are associated with eosinophilic pulmonary infiltrates. These include Wegener granulomatosis, sarcoidosis, rheumatoid lung

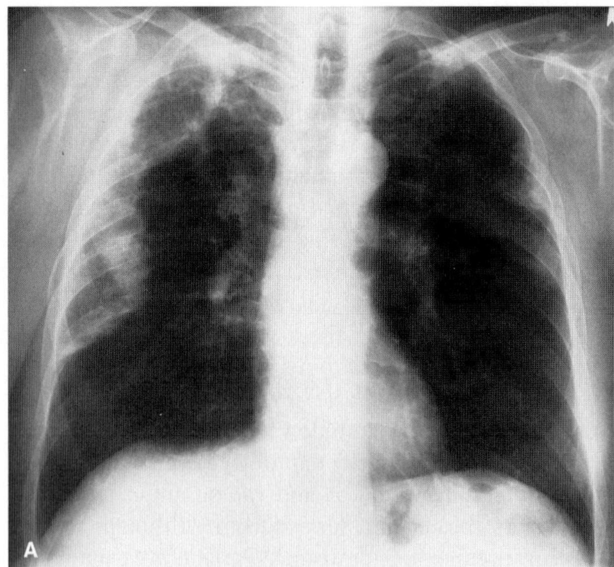

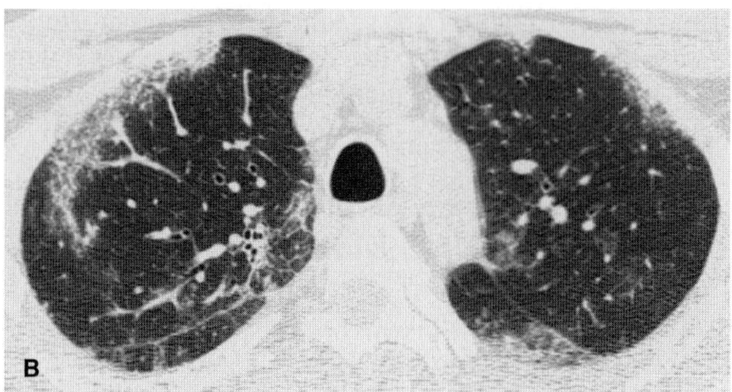

FIGURE 17.32. **Eosinophilic Pneumonia. A.** In a 38-year-old man with asthma, shortness of breath, and peripheral eosinophilia, a frontal chest film demonstrates bilateral peripheral airspace opacities. The patient's symptoms and the radiographic findings improved rapidly following initiation of corticosteroid therapy. **B.** CT scan in a different patient with eosinophilic pneumonia shows peripheral ground-glass opacity with reticulation in the upper lungs.

disease, polyarteritis nodosa, and allergic angiitis and granulomatosis. The first three disorders have a variety of thoracic manifestations and are discussed elsewhere. The predominant chest radiographic findings seen in polyarteritis nodosa represent hemorrhage caused by a vasculitis involving the bronchial arterial circulation; this condition is discussed in Chapter 14. Allergic angiitis and granulomatosis (Churg-Strauss syndrome) is a multisystem disorder in which asthma, blood eosinophilia, necrotizing vasculitis, and extravascular granulomas are invariable features. Pulmonary involvement, as seen radiographically or pathologically, is indistinguishable from chronic eosinophilic pneumonia.

MISCELLANEOUS DISORDERS

Pulmonary alveolar proteinosis (PAP) is a rare disease in which the lipoproteinaceous material surfactant deposits in abnormal amounts within the airspaces of the lung. PAP has a predilection for males in their 20s to 40s, although the disease has been reported in children. In adults, PAP has been associated with acute exposure to large amounts of silica dust (acute silicoproteinosis)—most commonly sandblasters—and immunocompromised patients with lymphoma, leukemia, or AIDS. These conditions are associated with an acquired defect of alveolar macrophages that fail to phagocytize surfactant, resulting in the accumulation of surfactant within the alveolar spaces. Pathologically, the alveoli are filled with a lipoproteinaceous material that stains deep pink with periodic acid–Schiff. The interstitium is usually not involved, but some patients may have chronic interstitial inflammation and fibrosis.

Patients with PAP are often asymptomatic, although some complain of progressive dyspnea and a nonproductive cough. The absence of orthopnea is an important clinical feature distinguishing PAP from pulmonary edema secondary to congestive heart failure.

The typical radiographic finding in alveolar proteinosis is bilateral symmetric perihilar airspace opacification, which is indistinguishable in appearance from pulmonary edema (Fig. 17.33). Airspace nodules are commonly seen at the periphery of the confluent opacities. Cardiomegaly, pleural effusions, and evidence of pulmonary venous hypertension are notably absent. CT and HRCT scans typically show geographic ground-glass opacities superimposed upon thickened interlobular and intralobular septa, a pattern that has been described as "crazy paving." While crazy paving in the proper clinical setting is characteristic of this disease, a number of conditions can produce this pattern on HRCT, including pulmonary edema (particularly permeability edema), atypical pneumonia, pulmonary hemorrhage, and rarely, bronchoalveolar cell carcinoma (12).

Patients with PAP are particularly prone to superinfection of the lung with *Nocardia, Aspergillus, Cryptococcus,* and atypical mycobacteria. The factors responsible for this propensity may include macrophage dysfunction and the favorable culture medium of intra-alveolar

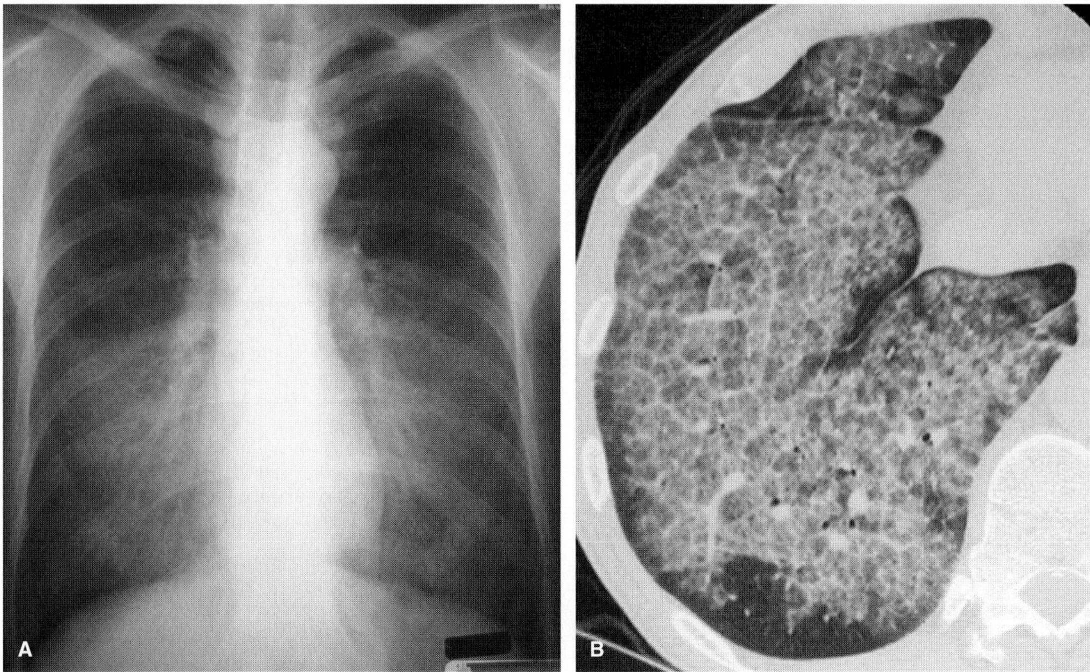

FIGURE 17.33. **Pulmonary Alveolar Proteinosis (PAP). A.** Frontal chest radiograph in a 34-year-old man with PAP demonstrates subtle bilateral ground-glass opacities. **B.** A CT scan viewed at the lung windows shows a mixed pattern of ground-glass attenuation superimposed on thickened interlobular and intralobular lines, which has been termed "crazy paving" and is characteristic of this disorder.

lipoproteinaceous material. Infection by one of these organisms should be suspected in any patient with PAP who develops symptoms of pneumonia or radiographic findings of focal parenchymal opacification or cavitation and pleural effusion. CT helps in the early detection of opportunistic infection, because pneumonia or abscess formation may be obscured by the underlying process on conventional radiographs.

Prior to the advent of bronchoalveolar lavage (BAL), one third of patients died from respiratory failure or opportunistic infections, while the remaining two thirds either stabilized or resolved spontaneously. Repeated BAL with saline has significantly reduced the mortality from this disease. The duration of treatment with BAL varies; some patients require repetitive long-term therapy, while others resolve after a single treatment. Recently, the recognition that patients with PAP have deficient levels of granulocyte macrophage–colony-stimulating factor (GM-CSF) in alveolar macrophages has led to therapy with GM-CSF, which is an alternative to lung lavage for treatment of this disease.

Alveolar microlithiasis is a rare disorder characterized by the deposition of minute calculi within the alveolar spaces. While alveolar microlithiasis can affect individuals of any age without sex predilection, there is a very high incidence of this disease in siblings. The underlying abnormality responsible for the formation of these calculi, known as calcospherites, is unknown. These are small calculi measuring less than 1 mm in diameter, which are composed of calcium phosphate. Pathologically these calculi are found within normal alveoli; interstitial fibrosis may develop in long-standing disease. The radiographic findings are specific: confluent bilateral dense micronodular opacities are seen that, because of their high intrinsic density, produce the so-called "black pleura sign" at their interface with the chest wall. Apical bullous disease is common and may lead to spontaneous pneumothorax. The diagnosis is made by a history of alveolar microlithiasis in a sibling of an affected individual and typical radiographic findings. Biopsy is usually unnecessary. The majority of patients are asymptomatic at presentation despite the marked radiographic abnormalities, a feature that is characteristic of this disorder. Most patients develop progressive respiratory insufficiency, although some remain stable for years. There is no effective treatment.

Diffuse pulmonary ossification is an uncommon condition characterized by the formation of bone within the lung parenchyma. The nodular form of this disease is seen in mitral stenosis, while more irregular ossification is seen in chronic inflammatory conditions such as amyloidosis and UIP. The condition is appreciated as nodular or linear areas of high attenuation on thin-section CT. Other conditions that can produce high-attenuation material in the lung parenchyma include pulmonary calcification in secondary hyperparathyroidism, in which there is an upper lobe predilection, and amiodarone lung toxicity, in which the deposition of an iodinated metabolite of amiodarone accumulates in the lung, liver, and thyroid.

REFERENCES

1. Kazerooni EA. High-resolution CT of the lungs. AJR Am J Roentgenol 2001;177:501–519.
2. Pandit-Bhalla M, Diethelm L, Ovella T, Sloop GD, Valentine VG. Idiopathic interstitial pneumonias: an update. J Thorac Imaging 2003;18:1–13.
3. Kim EA, Lee KS, Johkoh T, et al. Interstitial lung diseases associated with collagen vascular diseases: radiologic and histopathologic findings. Radiographics 2002;22:S151–S165.
4. Aylwin ACB, Gishen P, Copley SJ. Imaging appearance of thoracic amyloidosis. J Thorac Imaging 2005;20:41–46.
5. Pallisa E, Sanz P, Roman A, Majo J, Andreu J, Caceres J. Lymphangiomyomatosis: pulmonary and abdominal findings with pathologic correlation. Radiographics 2002;22:S185–S198.
6. Kim K-I, Kim CW, Lee MK, et al. Imaging of occupational lung disease. Radiographics 2001;21:1371–1391.
7. Lynch DA, Rose CS, Way D, King TE. Hypersensitivity pneumonitis: sensitivity of high-resolution CT in a population-based study. AJR Am J Roentgenol 1992;159:469–472.
8. Koyama T, Ueda H, Togashi K, Umeoka S, Kataoka M, Nagai S. Radiologic manifestations of sarcoidosis in various organs. Radiographics 2004;24:87–104.
9. Sundar KM, Gosselin MV, Chung H, Cahill BC. Pulmonary Langerhans cell histiocytosis: emerging concepts on pathobiology, radiology, and clinical evolution of disease. Chest 2003;123:1673–1683.
10. Mayberry JP, Primack SL, Muller NL. Thoracic manifestations of systemic autoimmune diseases: radiographic and high-resolution CT findings. Radiographics 2000;20:1623–1635.
11. Johkoh T, Muller NL, Akira M, et al. Eosinophilic lung diseases: diagnostic accuracy of thin-section CT in 111 patients. Radiographics 2000;216:773–780.
12. Holbert JM, Costello P, Li W, Hoffman RM, Rogers RM. CT features of pulmonary alveolar proteinosis. AJR Am J Roentgenol 2001;176:1287–1294.

Chapter 18

Airways Disease

Jeffrey S. Klein

Trachea and Central Bronchi
Congenital Tracheal Anomalies
Focal Tracheal Disease
Diffuse Tracheal Disease
Tracheal and Bronchial Injury
Broncholithiasis

Chronic Obstructive Pulmonary Disease
Asthma and Chronic Bronchitis
Bronchiectasis
Emphysema

Bullous Lung Disease

Small Airways Disease

TRACHEA AND CENTRAL BRONCHI

Congenital Tracheal Anomalies

Tracheal agenesis, cartilaginous abnormalities of the trachea, tracheal webs and stenosis, tracheoesophageal fistulas, and vascular rings and slings present as breathing and feeding difficulties in the neonatal and infancy period. These are uncommon congenital lesions that are discussed in Chapter 51.

Tracheoceles, also known as paratracheal air cysts, are true diverticula that represent herniation of the tracheal air column through a weakened posterior tracheal membrane. These lesions occur almost exclusively in the cervical trachea, because the pressure gradient from the extrathoracic trachea to the atmosphere with the Valsalva maneuver favors their formation in this region. Tracheoceles are usually asymptomatic and are easily recognized on fluoroscopy, CT, or contrast tracheogram.

Tracheal bronchus or bronchus suis, so-called because it is the normal pattern of tracheal branching in pigs, consists of an accessory bronchus to all or a portion of the right upper lobe that arises from the right lateral tracheal wall within 2 cm of the tracheal carina (Fig. 18.1). However, it most often supplies the apical segment of the right upper lobe. While it is usually an incidental finding on chest CT in 0.5% to 1.0% of the population, there is an association with congenital tracheal stenosis and an aberrant left pulmonary artery. Most patients are asymptomatic.

Focal Tracheal Disease

Focal disorders of the trachea may produce narrowing or dilatation of the tracheal lumen (Table 18.1) (1). Focal narrowing may be produced by extrinsic or intrinsic mass lesions, retraction, or inflammatory disorders of the tracheal wall.

Extrinsic Compression/Narrowing. The most common causes of extrinsic mass effect on the trachea are an intrathoracic goiter and a large paratracheal lymph node mass. In older individuals, a tortuous or aneurysmal transverse portion of the aortic arch may cause right lateral deviation of the distal intrathoracic trachea. Extrinsic mass effect can also be seen with congenital vascular anomalies, such as an aberrant left pulmonary artery and aortic ring, or with a large mediastinal bronchogenic cyst. Because the tracheal cartilage provides resiliency, extrinsic masses tend to displace the trachea without narrowing its lumen. Traction deformity of the trachea is generally seen in cicatrizing processes that asymmetrically affect the lung apices, most commonly chronic tuberculosis (TB) and histoplasmosis. Occasionally the distal trachea is narrowed in patients with sclerosing mediastinitis, although this disorder normally affects the central bronchi.

Focal Tracheal Stenosis. Focal tracheal or central (main and proximal lobar) bronchial narrowing may result from inflammatory disorders that affect the tracheal or central bronchial walls. Cartilaginous damage or the development of granulation tissue and fibrosis from a

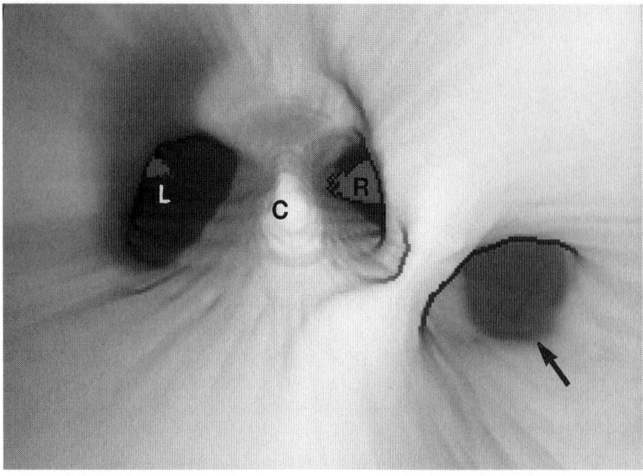

FIGURE 18.1. **Tracheal Bronchus.** Endoluminal rendering of a helical CT data set reveals an anomalous bronchus (*arrow*) arising from the right lateral tracheal wall above the tracheal carina (C). R, right main bronchus; L, left main bronchus.

TABLE 18.1 Causes of Focal Tracheal Disease

Narrowing	Extrinsic
	Thyroid goiter
	Paratracheal lymph node mass
	Asymmetric or unilateral upper lobe fibrosis
	Tuberculosis
	Histoplasmosis
	Intrinsic
	Tracheomalacia
	Endotracheal tube cuff
	Tracheostomy site
	Wegener granulomatosis
	Sarcoidosis
	Infection
	Tuberculosis
	Fungus
	Histoplasmosis
	Coccidioidomycosis
	Aspergillosis
	Scleroma
Masses	Neoplasm
	Malignant
	Primary
	Squamous cell carcinoma
	Adenoid cystic carcinoma (cylindroma)
	Metastatic
	Direct invasion
	Laryngeal carcinoma
	Thyroid carcinoma
	Esophageal carcinoma
	Bronchogenic carcinoma
	Hematogenous (endobronchial)
	Breast carcinoma
	Renal cell carcinoma
	Colon carcinoma
	Melanoma
	Benign
	Chondroma
	Fibroma
	Squamous cell papilloma
	Hemangioma
	Granular cell myoblastoma
	Nonneoplastic
	Ectopic thyroid or thymus
	Mucus
Dilatation	Tracheoceles
	Tracheomalacia
	Upper lobe fibrosis

tracheostomy or at the site of a previously inflated endotracheal tube balloon cuff can lead to focal tracheal narrowing. The tracheal stenosis has a typical hourglass deformity on frontal radiographs. Those patients with tracheomalacia from cartilage damage may only manifest narrowing during phases of the respiratory cycle when extratracheal pressure exceeds intratracheal pressure. Therefore, patients with extrathoracic tracheomalacia, most often at the site of a prior tracheostomy, demonstrate tracheal narrowing on inspiration, while patients with intrathoracic tracheomalacia, usually from prior endotracheal intubation, have tracheal narrowing on expiration. Postintubation stenosis is rare with the low-pressure, high-volume endotracheal tube cuffs in current use. Wegener granulomatosis can produce a necrotizing granulomatous inflammation of the trachea and central bronchi, leading to focal cervical tracheal narrowing or, in advanced disease, narrowing of the entire length of the trachea. The diagnosis of tracheal involvement by Wegener granulomatosis is made by the radiographic demonstration of tracheal narrowing in association with upper airway and renal involvement and characteristic findings on biopsy. Cyclophosphamide therapy administered early in the course of the disease may reduce inflammation and improve tracheal narrowing. Sarcoidosis involving the central airways may rarely cause focal tracheal or bronchial stenosis.

A number of infectious processes may result in tracheal or bronchial inflammation and stenosis. Endotracheal and endobronchial TB is usually associated with cavitary TB, where the production of large volumes of infected sputum predisposes to tracheal and central bronchial infection. Upper tracheal inflammation and stenosis may result from histoplasmosis and coccidioidomycosis. Invasive tracheobronchitis from aspergillosis, candidiasis, and mucormycosis has been described in immunodeficient patients. Scleroma is a chronic granulomatous disorder caused by infection with *Klebsiella rhinoscleromatis*. This disease is uncommon in the United States and is seen most commonly in people of lower socioeconomic standing in Central and South America and Eastern Europe. The infection begins as an inflammation of the nasal mucosa and

TABLE 18.2 Causes of Diffuse Tracheal Disease

Tracheal Narrowing	Saber-sheath trachea
	Amyloidosis
	Tracheobronchopathia osteochondroplastica
	Relapsing polychondritis
	Wegener granulomatosis
	Tracheal scleroma
Tracheal dilatation	Tracheobronchomegaly (Mounier-Kuhn syndrome)
	Tracheomalacia
	Interstitial pulmonary fibrosis

paranasal sinuses, extending inferiorly to involve the larynx, pharynx, and trachea in a minority of patients. In its chronic phase, intense granulation tissue and fibrosis lead to stenosis of the nasal cavity, pharyngeal, laryngeal, and upper trachea; the latter is seen in fewer than 10% of patients. Radiographically, the upper trachea shows irregular nodular narrowing, which may extend to involve the length of the trachea. The diagnosis is made on biopsy, which reveals granulation tissue containing large foamy histiocytes filled with the causative organism (Mikulicz cells). Antibiotic treatment is effective if administered in the early phases of infection before extensive fibrosis has developed.

Tracheal and bronchial masses are mostly neoplasms and are discussed in Chapter 15.

Focal tracheal dilatation is caused by congenital or acquired abnormalities of the elastic membrane or cartilaginous rings of the trachea. Localized tracheal dilatation may be seen with tracheoceles, with acquired tracheomalacia related to prolonged endotracheal intubation, or as a result of tracheal traction from severe unilateral upper lobe parenchymal scarring.

Diffuse Tracheal Disease

Diffuse disorders of the trachea manifest as either narrowing or dilatation of the tracheal lumen. Diffuse tracheal narrowing may be seen with saber-sheath trachea, amyloidosis, tracheobronchopathia osteochondroplastica, relapsing polychondritis, Wegener granulomatosis, or tracheal scleroma (Table 18.2) (2). The latter two conditions may cause diffuse tracheal narrowing, but more commonly the involvement is limited to the cervical trachea. These conditions are discussed in the section on focal tracheal narrowing.

Diffuse Tracheal Narrowing

Saber-sheath trachea is a fixed deformity of the intrathoracic trachea in which the coronal diameter is diminished to less than two thirds of the sagittal diameter. The tracheal wall is uniformly thickened, and calcification of the cartilaginous rings is present in most cases. This entity exclusively affects older men with functional evidence of chronic obstructive pulmonary disease (COPD). The tracheal narrowing likely reflects the chronic transmission of increased intrapleural pressure seen in obstructive lung disease and tracheal injury from chronic cough. The characteristic findings are apparent on frontal radiographs and CT (Fig. 18.2).

Amyloidosis is characterized by the deposition of a fibrillar protein-polysaccharide complex in various organs. It may involve the airways as part of localized or systemic disease. Submucosal deposits in the tracheobronchial tree are more commonly a manifestation of localized disease and may be associated with nodular or alveolar septal deposits in the lungs. Masslike circumferential deposits that irregularly narrow the tracheal lumen are best demonstrated on CT and can result in recurrent atelectasis and

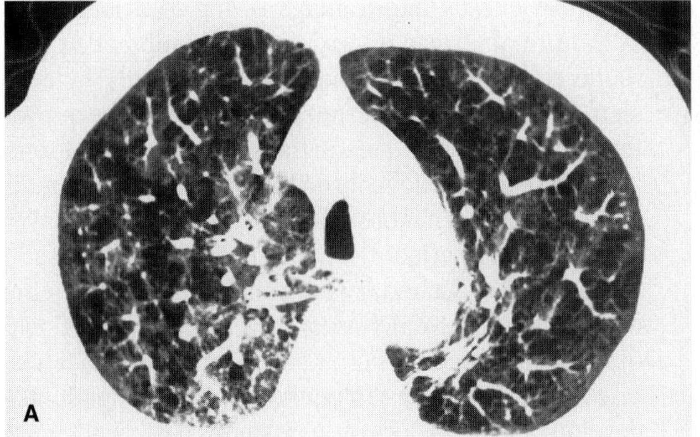

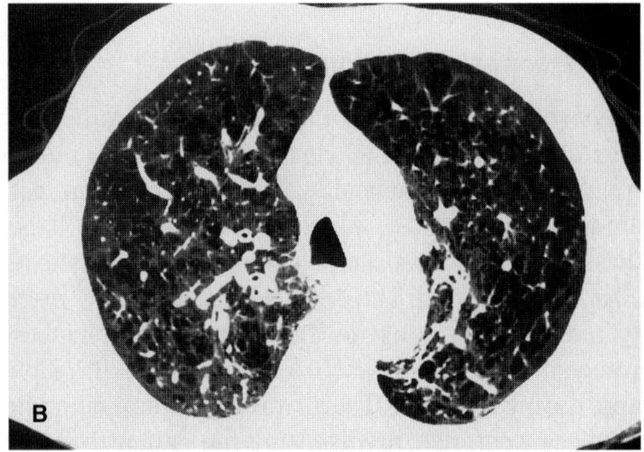

FIGURE 18.2. **Saber-Sheath Trachea in Chronic Obstructive Pulmonary Disease (COPD).** HRCT scans just above **(A)** and at the tracheal carina **(B)** in a 65-year-old man with COPD reveal coronal narrowing of the trachea, representing a saber-sheath tracheal deformity. Note additional findings associated with cigarette smoking: centrilobular emphysema and bronchial wall thickening, reflecting chronic bronchitis.

pneumonia. Calcification of these deposits occurs in only 10% of cases. The diagnosis is made by the presence of typical protein-polysaccharide deposits demonstrated on Congo red stains of tracheal or bronchial wall biopsy specimens.

Tracheobronchopathia osteochondroplastica is a rare disorder characterized by the presence of multiple submucosal osseous and cartilaginous deposits within the trachea and central bronchi of elderly men. The lesions arise as enchondromas from the tracheal and bronchial cartilage, and then project internally to produce nodular submucosal deposits that irregularly narrow the tracheal lumen and have a characteristic appearance and feel on bronchoscopy. The diagnosis is generally made on bronchoscopy and CT, where calcified plaques can be seen involving the anterior and lateral walls of the trachea. Sparing of the membranous posterior wall of the trachea, which lacks cartilage, is a helpful feature that distinguishes this entity from tracheobronchial amyloid. While usually asymptomatic, patients may have recurrent infection related to bronchial obstruction by the masses.

Relapsing polychondritis is a systemic autoimmune disorder that commonly affects the cartilage of the earlobes, nose, larynx, tracheobronchial tree, joints, and large elastic arteries. Early in the disease, tracheal wall inflammation associated with cartilage destruction leads to an abnormally compliant and dilated trachea. Later in the disease, fibrosis leads to diffuse fixed narrowing of the tracheal lumen. Respiratory complications secondary to involvement of the upper airway cartilage accounts for nearly 50% of all deaths from this condition. The diagnosis is made by noting recurrent inflammation at two or more cartilaginous sites, most commonly the pinnae of the ear (producing cauliflower ears) and the bridge of the nose (producing a saddlenose deformity). Radiographs and CT show diffuse smooth thickening of the wall of the trachea and central bronchi with narrowing of the lumen.

Diffuse Tracheal Dilatation

Tracheobronchomegaly (Mounier-Kuhn syndrome) is a congenital disorder of the elastic and smooth muscle components of the tracheal wall. An association with Ehlers-Danlos syndrome, a congenital defect in collagen synthesis, and cutis laxa, a congenital defect in elastic tissue, has been reported. The disease is found almost exclusively in men under the age of 50. Abnormal compliance of the trachea and central bronchi leads to central bronchial collapse during coughing. The airways obstruction impairs mucociliary clearance, predisposing the patient to recurrent episodes of pneumonia and bronchiectasis. Symptoms are indistinguishable from those associated with chronic bronchitis and bronchiectasis. On frontal radiographs, the trachea and central bronchi measure greater than 3.0 cm and 2.5 cm, respectively, in coronal diameter. The trachea has a corrugated appearance caused by herniation of tracheal mucosa and submucosa between the tracheal cartilages. The lungs are typically hyperinflated and may demonstrate bullae.

Tracheobronchomalacia with diffuse tracheal and central bronchial dilatation may result from a congenital or acquired defect of tracheal cartilage. The most common causes of acquired tracheomalacia are COPD, chronic bronchitis, cystic fibrosis, and relapsing polychondritis. Symptoms and radiographic findings are similar to those of tracheobronchomegaly.

In some patients with long-standing interstitial pulmonary fibrosis, diffuse tracheal dilatation may be seen. The etiology of the tracheal dilatation may relate to long-standing elevation in transpulmonary pressures caused by diminished lung compliance or to chronic coughing.

Tracheal and Bronchial Injury

Injury to the trachea or main bronchi is most often seen with blunt chest trauma from a deceleration-type injury. Concomitant aortic laceration, great vessel injury, and rib (particularly an upper anterior rib), sternum, scapula, or vertebral fracture is the rule and may dominate the clinical picture. The mechanism of injury is forceful compression of the central tracheobronchial tree against the thoracic spine during impact. The fractures generally involve the proximal main bronchi (80%) or distal trachea (15%) within 2 cm of the tracheal carina; the peripheral bronchi are involved in 5% of cases. Horizontal laceration or transection parallel to the tracheobronchial cartilage is the most common form of injury.

The diagnosis of tracheobronchial injury is often first suggested on early posttrauma chest radiographs by the presence of pneumothorax and pneumomediastinum, particularly in a patient not receiving mechanical ventilation (Fig. 18.3) (3). Typically, the pneumothorax fails to respond to chest tube drainage owing to a large air leak at the site of airway interruption. The subtended lung remains collapsed against the lateral chest wall ("fallen lung" sign) (Fig. 18.3). An aberrant endotracheal tube or overdistended balloon cuff are further clues to the presence of an unsuspected tracheobronchial disruption. As many as one third of tracheobronchial injuries have a delayed diagnosis; these patients may present with a collapsed lung or pneumonia secondary to bronchial stenosis. Definitive diagnosis is by bronchoscopy. Multidetector CT with 3-dimensional reconstruction with shaded surface display or contrast bronchography may be useful in patients who develop bronchial occlusion or stenosis because of a delay in diagnosis.

Penetrating tracheal injuries usually involve the cervical trachea and result from gunshot or stab wounds to the neck. Injury to the intrathoracic trachea is usually associated with fatal penetrating cardiovascular injury.

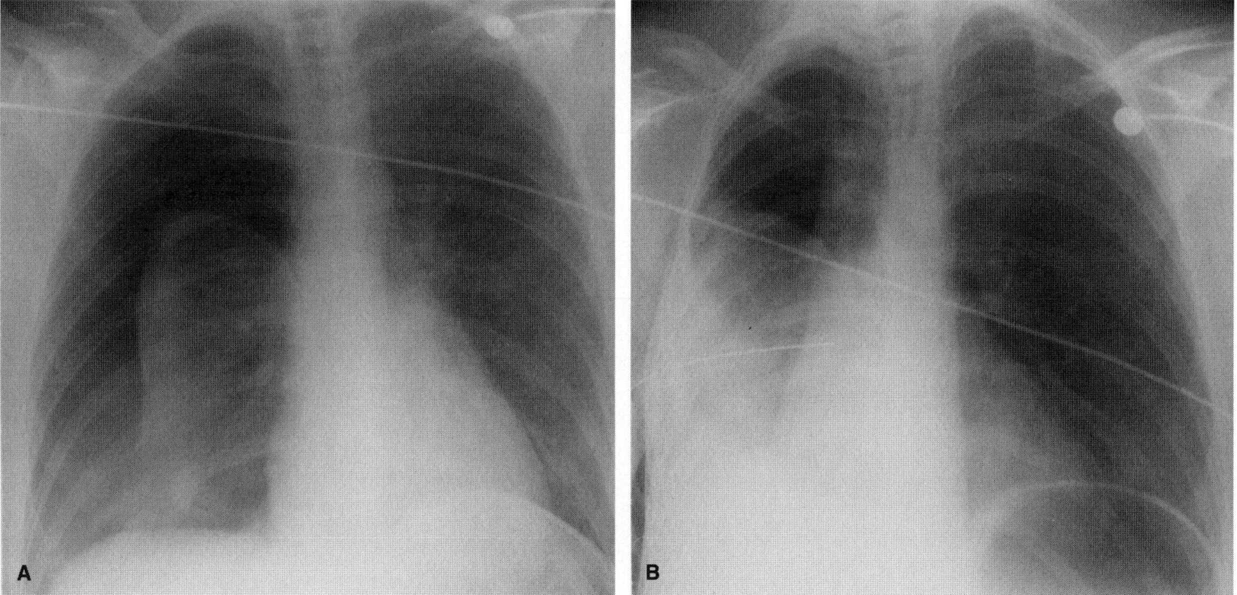

FIGURE 18.3. **Transection of the Right Main Bronchus. A.** An upright chest film shows a broken right clavicle with a large right pneumothorax and pneumomediastinum in a 24-year-old woman struck by a car. **B.** A film obtained following chest tube placement shows a persistent pneumothorax. A large air leak was noted from the tube. Bronchoscopy revealed complete disruption of the right main bronchus, which was confirmed at thoracotomy.

Broncholithiasis

Broncholithiasis, the presence of calcified material within the tracheobronchial tree, develops from erosion of a calcified peribronchial lymph node into the bronchial lumen (Fig. 18.4). Most calcified lymph nodes result from granulomatous lymph node inflammation caused by histoplasmosis or TB. Broncholiths may occlude the airway and lead to bronchiectasis, obstructive atelectasis, or pneumonia. Patients are often asymptomatic but may have cough productive of stones or calcified material (lithoptysis). Hemoptysis may develop from erosion of the broncholith into a bronchial vessel.

CHRONIC OBSTRUCTIVE PULMONARY DISEASE

The diseases known collectively as COPD include asthma, chronic bronchitis, bronchiectasis, and emphysema. The common pathophysiology in this group of diseases is obstruction to expiratory airflow.

Asthma and Chronic Bronchitis

Asthma is an airways disorder characterized by the rapid onset of bronchial narrowing with spontaneous resolution or improvement as a result of therapy. A wide variety of inciting factors and agents have been identified. Many patients have an allergic history and develop episodic bronchial constriction from excessive production of immunoglobulin E following exposure to antigenic stimuli. This results in bronchial smooth muscle contraction, bronchial wall inflammation, and excessive mucus production. These responses narrow the bronchial lumen and produce symptoms of coughing, wheezing, and dyspnea.

The radiographic findings in uncomplicated asthma are primarily the result of diffuse airways narrowing. Hyperinflation producing increased lung volume, flattening or inversion of the diaphragm, attenuation of the peripheral vascular markings, and prominence of the retrosternal airspace is the result of expiratory air trapping (4). Bronchial wall inflammation and thickening appear radiographically as peribronchial cuffing and "tram tracking." In some patients, the hila are prominent from transient pulmonary arterial hypertension caused by hypoxic vasoconstriction (Fig. 18.5).

There are several reasons to obtain a chest radiograph in patients with asthma. Tracheal and central bronchial narrowing from extrinsic or intrinsic lesions may produce dyspnea and wheezing and be mistaken for asthma. Bacterial pneumonia may induce airway hyperreactivity and present as an acute asthmatic attack. Complications of asthma may be detected on chest radiographs obtained during and following the asthmatic episode. Mucus plugs can cause bronchial obstruction and resorptive atelectasis; pneumonia can develop in these collapsed regions. Expiratory airflow obstruction with resultant alveolar rupture

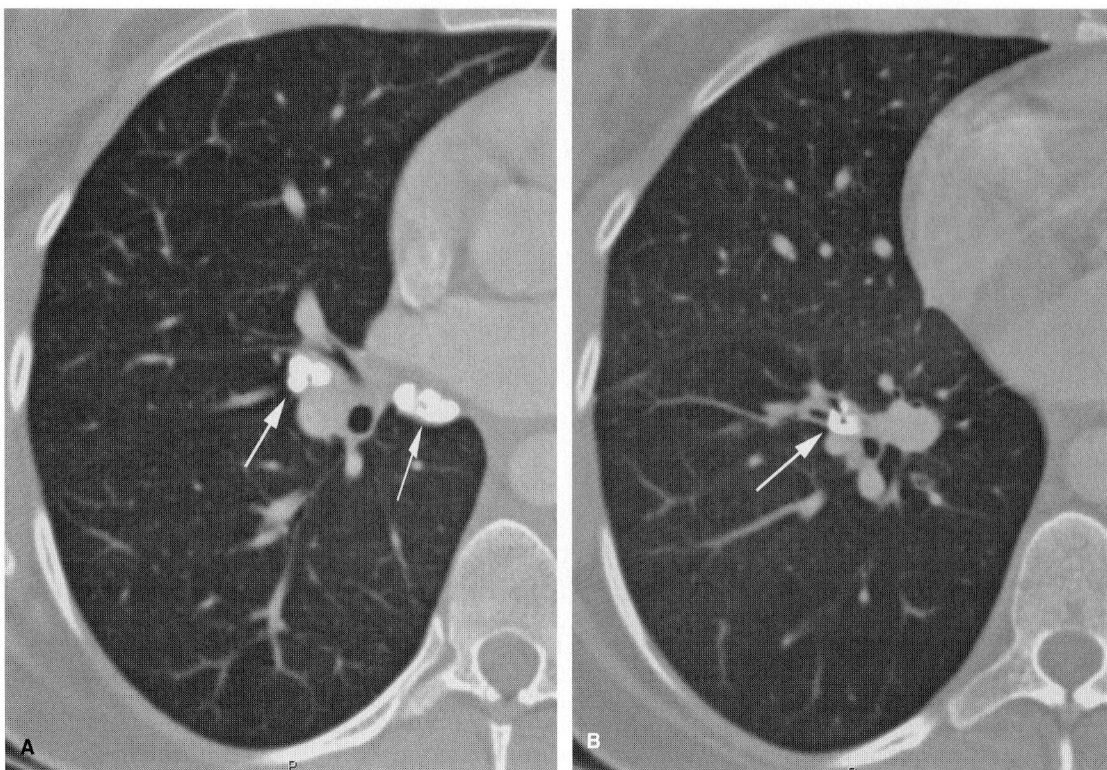

FIGURE 18.4. **Broncholithiasis.** Targeted reconstruction of the right lung from a CT in a 33-year-old woman with hemoptysis at the level of the middle lobe bronchus **(A)** and proximal basal segmental right lower lobe bronchi **(B)** show calcified lymph nodes (*arrows*) in the right hilum and azygoesophageal recess (*arrows* in A) with a calcified node within the anterior basal segmental bronchus (*arrow* in B).

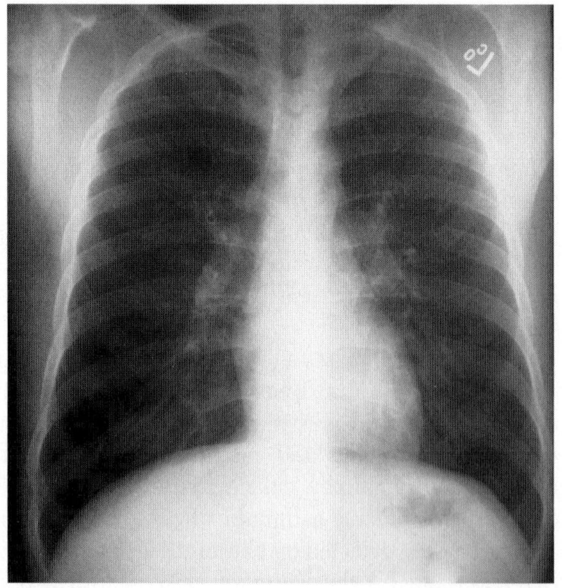

FIGURE 18.5. **Asthma.** Posteroanterior chest radiograph in a 27-year-old man suffering an acute asthma exacerbation reveals hyperinflation, bronchial wall thickening, and hilar prominence.

and dissection of air medially may produce pneumomediastinum. If the extra-alveolar air dissects peripherally to the subpleural space to form subpleural blebs, pneumothorax may result. Both pneumomediastinum and pneumothorax may be exacerbated in ventilated patients receiving high-positive-pressure ventilation.

Chronic bronchitis is a clinical and not a radiographic diagnosis. It is defined as the excess production and expectoration of sputum that occurs on most days for at least 3 consecutive months in at least 2 consecutive years. The majority of individuals with chronic bronchitis are cigarette smokers. Morphologically, the lower lobe bronchi are most often affected, with thickening of their walls from mucous gland hyperplasia. The ratio of mucous gland thickness to bronchial wall thickness is known as the Reid index; an abnormally high index (>50%) correlates strongly with symptoms of excess mucus production. Fifty percent of patients with a history of chronic bronchitis have normal chest films. Some patients show peribronchial cuffing or tram tracks when the thick-walled and mildly dilated bronchi are viewed end on or in length, respectively. Other patients have a "dirty chest," in which the peripheral lung markings are accentuated. This radiographic appearance has no definite pathologic correlate but may represent small airways disease or prominent pulmonary arteries from pulmonary arterial hypertension complicating associated centrilobular emphysema. CT in patients with chronic bronchitis may show bronchial wall thickening (Fig. 18.2B).

Bronchiectasis

Bronchiectasis is defined as an abnormal permanent dilatation of bronchi. Morphologically, bronchiectasis is divided into three groups: cylindric, varicose, and saccular (cystic). Cylindric bronchiectasis is characterized by mild diffuse dilatation of the bronchi. Varicose bronchiectasis is cystic bronchial dilatation interrupted by focal areas of narrowing, an appearance that has been likened to a string of pearls. Cystic bronchiectasis is seen as clusters of bronchi with marked localized saccular dilatation. Bronchiectasis may be localized or generalized. Localized bronchiectasis is most commonly a result of prior TB, whereas generalized bronchiectasis is seen in patients with cystic fibrosis. Patients usually have a history of chronic sputum production and recurrent lower respiratory infections. Hemoptysis associated with enlargement of bronchial arteries is common and may be massive and life threatening.

The chest radiographic findings of bronchiectasis are typically nonspecific. Scarring, volume loss, and loss of the sharp definition of the normal bronchovascular markings are present in the affected regions. Parallel linear shadows representing the walls of cylindrically dilated bronchi seen in length may be visualized. Cystic bronchiectasis has a characteristic appearance of multiple peripheral thin-walled cysts, with or without air–fluid levels, that tend to cluster together in the distribution of a bronchovascular bundle. The findings tend to be peripheral in most cases of localized bronchiectasis; central bronchiectasis is seen only in allergic bronchopulmonary aspergillosis, cystic fibrosis, bronchial atresia, or acquired central bronchial obstruction.

CT has all but eliminated the need for contrast bronchography in the evaluation of bronchiectasis. As compared to bronchography, thin-section CT scans obtained at regular intervals have an accuracy exceeding 95% in the diagnosis of bronchiectatsis (5). The CT appearance of bronchiectasis depends on the site of involvement and the type of bronchiectasis. In the upper and lower lobes, all bronchi are imaged in cross section, and their luminal diameter can be directly compared to that of the accompanying pulmonary arteries. Cylindric bronchiectasis in these regions appears as multiple dilated thick-walled circular lucencies, with the adjoining smaller artery giving each dilated bronchus the appearance of a "signet ring." In the mid-lung, where the bronchi course horizontally, the appearance is that of parallel linear opacities (tram tracks). Mucoid impaction within dilated upper or lower lobe bronchi may be mistaken for lung nodules unless one observes the vertical nature of the opacity on sequential axial images. In the mid-lung regions, impacted bronchi sectioned in length are recognized as branching, finger-like opacities. Cystic bronchiectasis in any region is easily recognized as clusters of rounded lucencies, often containing air–fluid levels; this appearance has been likened to a "cluster of grapes" (Fig. 18.6). Varicose bronchiectasis cannot be differentiated from cylindric bronchiectasis unless sectioned longitudinally in the mid-lung regions, where the pattern of dilatation simulates the contour of a caterpillar.

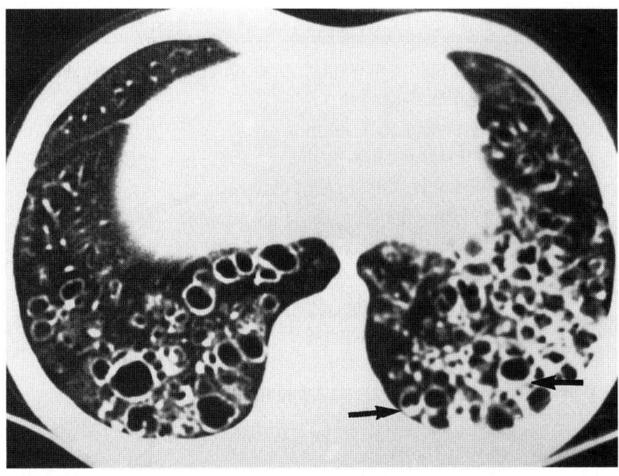

FIGURE 18.6. **Cystic Bronchiectasis.** CT scan through the lower lobes in a 12-year-old boy with severe postinfectious bronchiectasis shows clustered thin-walled cysts representing dilated bronchi in cross section. Note the presence of dependent fluid within several left lower lobe bronchi (*arrows*).

Bronchography remains the gold standard for diagnosing and evaluating the extent of bronchiectasis. However, its invasive nature and associated complications, particularly in patients with limited pulmonary reserve, preclude its routine use for the evaluation of bronchiectasis. CT has replaced bronchography for the diagnosis of bronchiectasis because it is noninvasive and highly accurate. Scans obtained at 10-mm intervals with 1.5-mm collimation and a high-spatial-resolution reconstruction algorithm are used to detect the presence and extent of disease. Currently, bronchography is limited to those patients considered for curative resection who appear to have localized disease by CT examination.

Bronchiectasis is caused by a variety of disorders, all of which predispose the bronchi to chronic inflammation, with resultant cartilage damage and dilatation (Table 18.3).

Cystic fibrosis is a hereditary disease of young Caucasians characterized in the lung by the production of abnormally thick, tenacious mucus. The thick mucus plugs the small airways and leads to bronchial obstruction and infection. A vicious cycle of recurrent infection, most often

TABLE 18.3 Specific Causes of Bronchiectasis

Localized	Tuberculous scarring, upper lobes (postprimary disease)
	Bronchial disease
	Extrinsic compression
	Enlarged hilar nodes
	Bronchial stenosis/occlusion
	Bronchial atresia
	Tuberculosis
	Sarcoidosis
	Prior bronchial injury
	Endobronchial mass
	Carcinoid tumor
	Bronchogenic carcinoma
	Foreign body
Diffuse	Cystic fibrosis
	Dysmotile cilia syndrome
	Congenital immunodeficiency
	Postinfectious
	Adenovirus (Swyer-James syndrome)
	Measles
	Pertussis
	Chronic aspiration
	Allergic bronchopulmonary aspergillosis
	Interstitial pulmonary fibrosis (traction bronchiectasis)

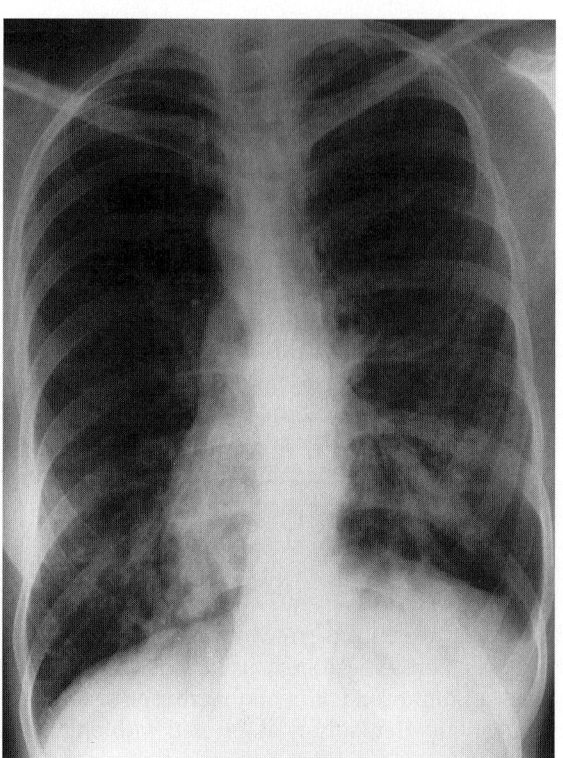

FIGURE 18.7. **Bronchiectasis in Kartagener Syndrome.** Posteroanterior chest film in a 32-year-old man with long-standing sinusitis, dextrocardia, and situs inversus reveals bilateral lower lobe bronchiectasis.

with *Pseudomonas aeruginosa* or *Staphylococcus aureus,* eventually causes severe bronchiectasis. The bronchiectasis is associated with functional airways obstruction and dyspnea. Hemoptysis, sometimes massive, may complicate the bronchiectasis and may require treatment by transcatheter bronchial artery embolization. Chest radiographs in affected adults show hyperinflation with predominantly upper lobe bronchiectasis and mucus plugging. Distal atelectasis and obstructive pneumonitis are common findings. The pulmonary hila may be prominent from enlarged lymph nodes caused by chronic infection or from vascular dilatation associated with pulmonary arterial hypertension. The diagnosis rests on a positive family history and a sweat test showing an abnormally high concentration of chloride. Improvements in antibiotic therapy and pulmonary physiotherapy have increased long-term survival, but the overall prognosis remains poor, with most patients succumbing to respiratory insufficiency in young adulthood. Recently, the use of inhaled recombinant DNAase to reduce the viscosity of tracheobronchial secretions has brought symptomatic and functional improvement to a number of patients. Lung or heart/lung transplantation is an option in selected individuals.

Dysmotile cilia syndrome is a disorder in which the epithelial cilial motion is abnormal and ineffective. A variety of structural cilial abnormalities may be found, the most common of which is an absence of the outer dynein arms of the peripheral microtubules of the cilia. The abnormality may result in rhinitis, sinusitis, bronchiectasis, dysmotile spermatozoa and sterility, situs inversus, and dextrocardia. The triad of sinusitis, situs inversus, and bronchiectasis is known as Kartagener syndrome. Chest radiographs show diffuse bronchiectasis and hyperinflation; situs inversus is seen in approximately 50% of patients (Fig. 18.7). The diagnosis is made on the basis of the clinical and radiographic findings, along with studies of cilial anatomy and motion on samples obtained from nasal biopsy.

Postinfectious Bronchiectasis. Severe childhood pneumonia, usually a sequela of infection with adenovirus, measles, or pertussis (the latter two are seen not uncommonly in nonimmunized Asian immigrants), may cause severe bronchial damage and recurrent infection with resultant bronchiectasis (Fig. 18.6). In some patients, childhood bronchitis and bronchiolitis are associated with obstructive airways disease and an underdeveloped lung, the latter known as Swyer-James syndrome (see "Small Airways Disease").

Allergic bronchopulmonary aspergillosis represents a hypersensitivity reaction to *Aspergillus* and is characterized clinically by asthma, blood eosinophilia, bronchiectasis with mucus plugging, and circulating antibodies to *Aspergillus* antigen. An immediate (type 1) hypersensitivity reaction to *Aspergillus* antigen accounts for acute episodes of wheezing and dyspnea, while an immune

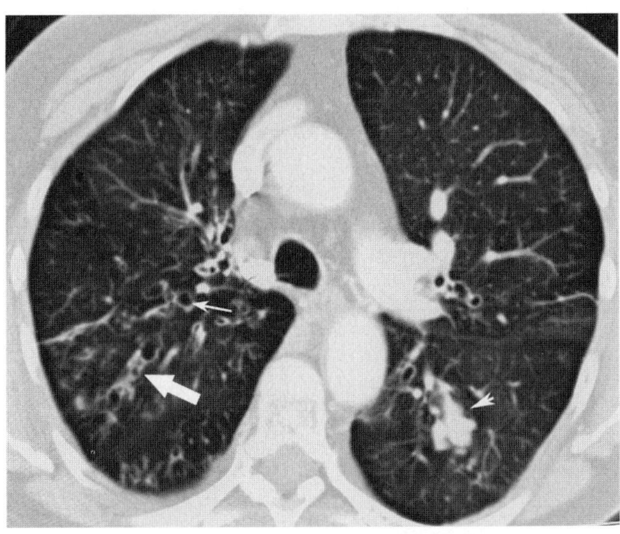

FIGURE 18.8. **Allergic Bronchopulmonary Aspergillosis (ABPA).** CT in a patient with ABPA shows mixed varicose (*large arrow*) and cystic (*small arrow*) bronchiectasis with mucus plugging evident (*arrowhead*).

complex–mediated (type 3) hypersensitivity within the lobar bronchi leads to bronchial wall inflammation and proximal bronchiectasis. Affected patients invariably have an allergic history, and it is often associated with cystic fibrosis. Patients with this disorder have recurrent episodes of cough, wheezing, and expectoration of mucus plugs. The chest radiograph is diagnostic and shows proximal, predominantly upper lobe bronchiectasis. The dilated bronchi may be seen as dilated air-filled tubules or as broadly branching opacities characteristic of mucoid impaction within the dilated bronchi. CT and HRCT are helpful in characterizing the opacities as dilated bronchi (Fig. 18.8). Corticosteroids are the treatment of choice.

Bronchial Obstruction. Bronchiectasis can develop distal to an endobronchial obstruction caused by neoplasm, atresia, or stenosis. Slow-growing central bronchogenic neoplasms that have a large endoluminal component (e.g., carcinoid tumor) may obstruct the distal bronchi and produce bronchiectasis with mucus plugging (mucoceles) (Fig. 18.9). Similarly, bronchial atresia or bronchostenosis from trauma or chronic bronchial infection (i.e., endobronchial TB) can lead to distal bronchial dilatation. The plain radiographic recognition of mucocele formation in patients with endobronchial obstruction is dependent upon adequate collateral ventilation to the lung supplied by the obstructed airway. Unfortunately, in most patients, collapse of lung around the dilated mucus-filled bronchus precludes diagnosis on plain radiographs. CT will show the central airway obstruction and dilated mucus bronchograms and can help guide bronchoscopic examination and biopsy.

Peribronchial Fibrosis. *Traction bronchiectasis* is a term used to describe the effect of severe pulmonary fibrosis on the peripheral airways. Airways that traverse regions of parenchymal fibrosis and honeycombing often become irregularly dilated as their walls are retracted by the fibrotic process. This occurs most commonly in the upper lobes in patients with long-standing TB and in the subpleural regions of the lower lobes in patients with end-stage idiopathic pulmonary fibrosis. Because the accompanying fibrosis precludes visualization of the dilated bronchi radiographically, traction bronchiectasis is best appreciated on HRCT studies of the lung.

Emphysema

Definition and Subtypes. Emphysema is a pathologic diagnosis that is defined as an abnormal, permanent enlargement of the airspaces distal to the terminal bronchiole accompanied by destruction of alveolar walls and without obvious fibrosis. The pathologic classification of emphysema is based on the portion of the secondary pulmonary lobule affected. *Centrilobular emphysema* is the most common and is characterized by airspace distention in the central portion of the lobule, with sparing of the more distal portions of the lobule. This form of emphysema affects the upper lobes to a greater extent than the lower lobes (Fig. 18.10). *Panlobular emphysema* results in uniform

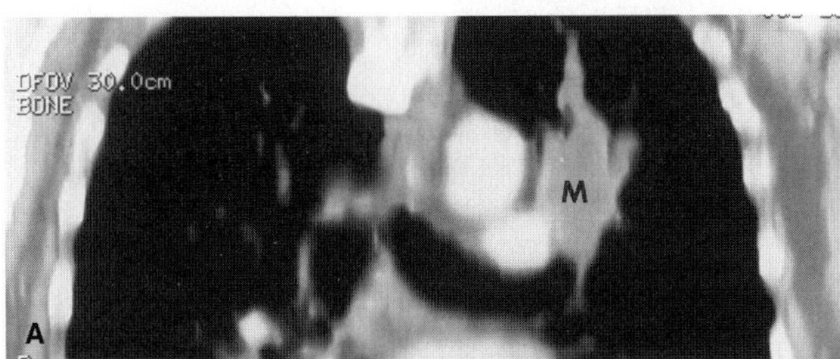

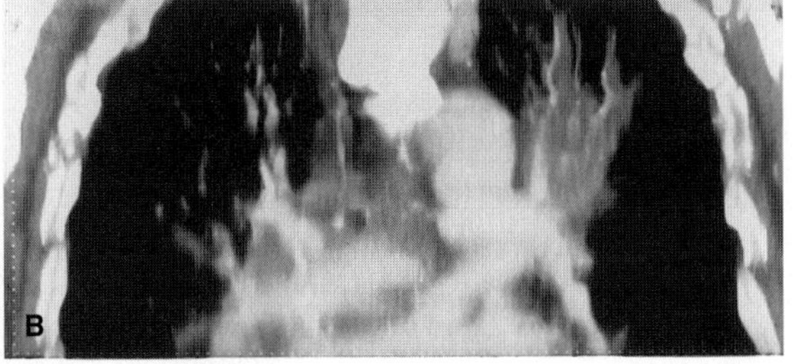

FIGURE 18.9. **Mucocele From Bronchial Carcinoid. A.** Coronal reformatted CT shows a mass (M) obstructing the left upper lobe bronchus. **B.** Coronal maximum intensity projection shows branching dilated mucus-filled bronchi paralleling arterial branches in the apicoposterior segment of the left upper lobe. Bronchoscopy revealed carcinoid tumor.

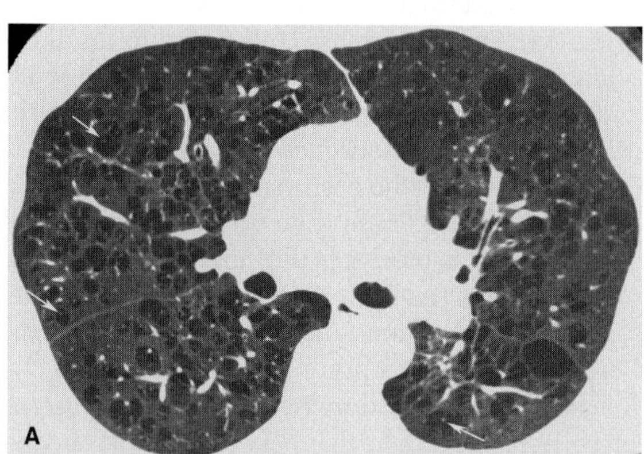

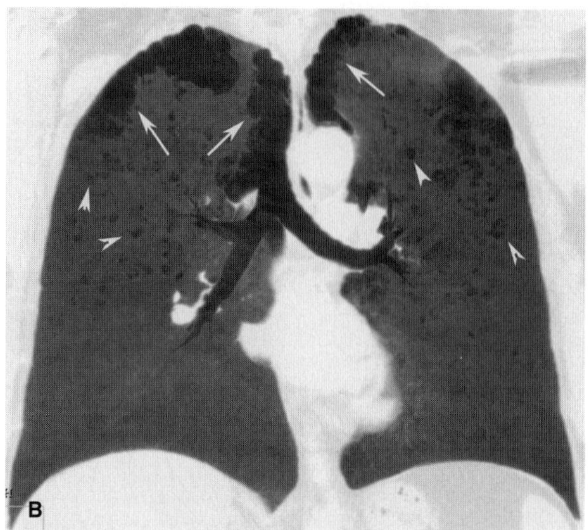

FIGURE 18.10. **Centrilobular and Paraseptal Emphysema on CT.** CT scan through the mid-lungs in a patient with centrilobular emphysema **(A)** shows discrete lucencies lacking perceptible walls and containing centrilobular artery branches (*arrows*). In another patient with both centrilobular and paraseptal emphysema **(B),** a coronal minimum intensity reconstruction shows subpleural lucencies, reflecting paraseptal emphysema (*arrows*) with associated centrilobular emphysema (*arrowheads*).

distention of the airspaces throughout the substance of the lobule, from the central respiratory bronchioles to the peripheral alveolar sacs and alveoli. In contrast to centrilobular emphysema, this form has a predilection for the lower lobes (Fig. 18.11). *Paraseptal emphysema* is seen as selective distention of peripheral airspaces adjacent to interlobular septa, with sparing of the centrilobular region. This form of emphysema is most often seen in the immediate subpleural regions of the upper lobes (Fig. 18.10). Paraseptal emphysema may coalesce to form apical bullae; rupture of these bullae into the pleural space may give rise to spontaneous pneumothoraces. *Paracicatricial* or *irregular emphysema* refers to destruction of lung tissue associated with fibrosis that bears no consistent relationship to a given portion of the lobule. It is most often seen in association with old granulomatous inflammation (Fig. 18.12).

Etiology and Pathogenesis. The most common etiologic factor for the development of emphysema is cigarette smoking. This is associated predominantly with

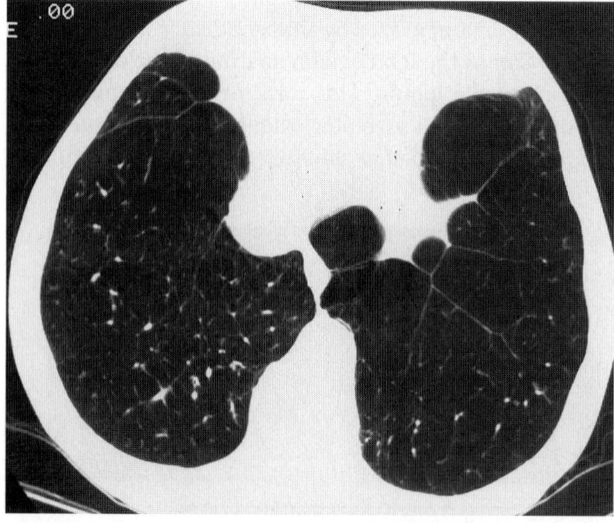

FIGURE 18.11. **Panlobular Emphysema.** HRCT through the lower lobes shows uniform destruction of secondary pulmonary lobules.

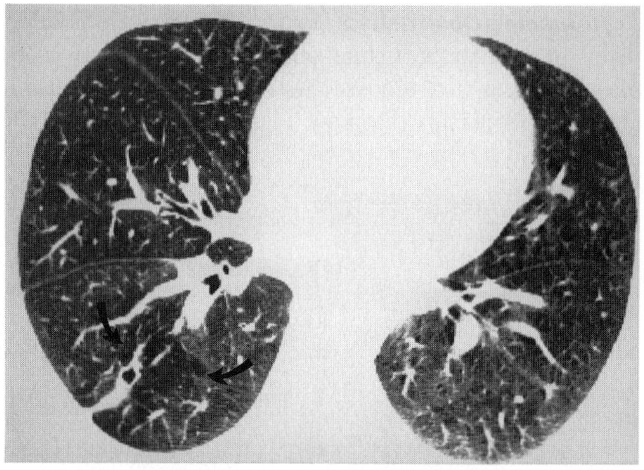

FIGURE 18.12. **Paracicatricial Emphysema.** HRCT in a patient with focal right lower lobe postinflammatory scarring and bronchiectasis shows focal hyperlucency (*arrows*) representing paracicatricial emphysema.

centrilobular emphysema but may be a contributing factor in the development of panlobular emphysema. The pathogenesis of centrilobular emphysema is complex and has not been completely elucidated. Cigarette smoke leads to excess neutrophil deposition in the lung. This results in the release of proteases (e.g., elastase) and antiprotease inhibitors, which in turn leads to destruction of alveolar septa. Inflammation and obstruction of small airways likely contributes to distal airspace distention and alveolar septal disruption. The association between deficiency of the serum protein α-1-antitrypsin (α-1-protease inhibitor) and the development of panlobular emphysema is well established. This disease is inherited as an autosomal recessive trait. Individuals who are homozygous for both recessive genes (ZZ phenotype) develop panlobular emphysema by middle age. Heterozygotes (MZ phenotype) have only a slightly increased incidence of emphysema. Cigarette smoking, by producing excess antiprotease inhibitors, can accelerate the development of emphysema in patients with the ZZ and MZ phenotypes.

Clinical Findings and Functional Abnormalities. Because a definitive diagnosis of emphysema requires tissue, the diagnosis during life is based on a combination of clinical, functional, and radiographic findings. The vast majority of patients with emphysema are long-term cigarette smokers. Symptoms associated with emphysema include dyspnea and a productive cough; the latter is attributed to chronic bronchitis, which often accompanies centrilobular emphysema. The functional hallmarks of emphysema are decreased airflow and diffusing capacity. Expiratory airflow obstruction is expressed as a decrease in the volume of air expired in the first second of a forced expiratory maneuver from total lung capacity (FEV_1) and a decrease in the ratio of FEV_1 to the total volume of air expired during a forced expiratory maneuver (FEV_1/FVC). Airflow obstruction is secondary to increased airways resistance and decreased driving pressure (i.e., elastic recoil). In patients with moderate to severe emphysema, the predominant factor limiting expiratory airflow is the decreased elastic recoil that results from parenchymal destruction. Airflow obstruction, however, is not invariably present in patients with mild emphysema. Diffusing capacity, measured by the diffusion of carbon monoxide from the alveoli into the bloodstream during a single breath hold ($DL_{CO}SB$), assesses the integrity and surface area of the alveolocapillary membrane. The diffusing capacity in emphysema is decreased because the volume of pulmonary parenchyma available for gas exchange is diminished. The severity of the emphysema correlates well with the $DL_{CO}SB$. Although an abnormal diffusing capacity is more sensitive than abnormal spirometry in diagnosing emphysema, it is nonspecific. Since $DL_{CO}SB$ depends on both the surface area available for gas diffusion and the number and hemoglobin content of red blood cells within the pulmonary capillaries, any process affecting these factors can alter the measurement of $DL_{CO}SB$. For example, a decreased $DL_{CO}SB$ can be seen in any disease that diminishes the volume of pulmonary capillaries available for gas diffusion (e.g., pulmonary embolism); interferes with gas exchange across the alveolocapillary membrane (e.g., interstitial pulmonary fibrosis); or produces airway obstruction, thereby diminishing the gas-exchanging airspaces (i.e., cystic fibrosis). Furthermore, some patients with mild to moderate morphologic emphysema can have a normal $DL_{CO}SB$.

TABLE 18.4 Radiographic Findings in Pulmonary Emphysema

Finding	*Explanation*
Diffuse hyperlucency (panlobular)	Destruction of pulmonary capillary bed and alveolar septa
Flattening and depression of the hemidiaphragms; increased retrosternal airspace (panlobular >centrilobular)	Hyperinflation caused by loss of elastic recoil of lung
Bulla	Thin-walled region of confluent (panlobular >centrilobular) emphysematous destruction
Enlarged central pulmonary arteries; right heart enlargement (centrilobular)	Loss of pulmonary capillary bed; associated chronic hypoxemia causes increased pulmonary vascular resistance
Increased peripheral vascular markings (centrilobular)	? small airways disease ? increased pulmonary vascularity

Radiologic Evaluation. Frontal and lateral chest radiographs are the initial radiographic examinations obtained in patients with suspected emphysema. The plain radiographic findings of emphysema are listed in Table 18.4 (6). Hyperinflation is the most important plain radiographic finding and reflects the loss of lung elastic recoil. It is the radiographic equivalent of an abnormally increased total lung capacity (TLC). The abnormal increase in lung volumes is best detected by noting inferior displacement and flattening of the normally convex superior hemidiaphragms, right or obtuse angles to the normally acute-angled costophrenic sulci, and an increase in anteroposterior chest diameter (best appreciated by noting an increase in the depth of the retrosternal clear space) (Fig. 18.13). Absent or attenuated peripheral vascular markings are caused by parenchymal destruction and obliteration of peripheral pulmonary arteries traversing emphysematous areas. When the characteristic thin walls of bullae are seen marginating the peripheral avascular regions, emphysema can be diagnosed with certainty. Increased radiolucency of the lungs on radiographs resulting from pulmonary hyperinflation and attenuation of peripheral vascular markings is difficult to detect because

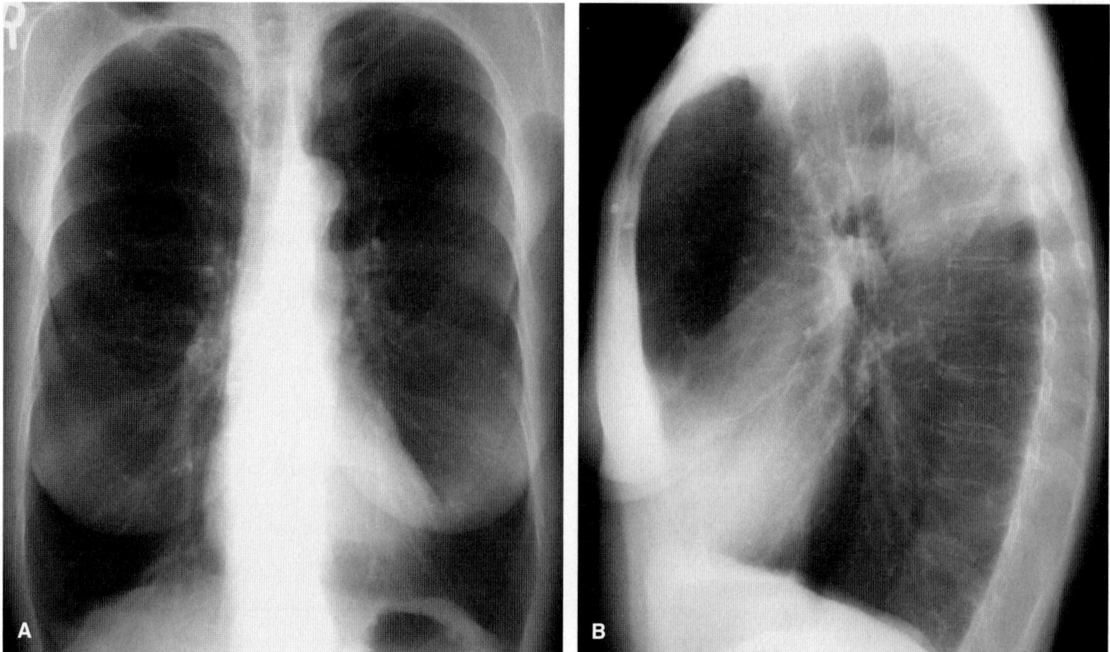

FIGURE 18.13. **Chest Radiograph of Emphysema.** Posteroanterior **(A)** and lateral **(B)** chest radiographs in a 62-year-old woman with emphysema shows hyperinflation with hyperlucency, upper lobe vascular attenuation, flattening of the diaphragms, and an increased retrosternal airspace, reflecting severe emphysema.

it is subject to various patient and technical factors and therefore is an inaccurate indicator of the presence of emphysema. The effects of emphysema and chronic hypoxemia on the right side of the heart may be appreciated as enlargement of the central pulmonary arteries and right ventricle in those with complicating pulmonary arterial hypertension and cor pulmonale. The use of the term *chronic obstructive pulmonary disease* to describe patients with the plain radiographic findings of emphysema is inaccurate and should be discouraged. COPD is a functional diagnosis, whereas the chest radiograph depicts anatomy only. In fact, patients with radiographic findings of hyperinflation and vascular attenuation, while they invariably have emphysema morphologically, may rarely lack functional evidence of airflow obstruction and therefore do not have COPD.

It is well recognized that many patients with severe centrilobular emphysema have minimal or no hyperinflation on chest radiographs, and they tend to show increased lung markings rather than peripheral vascular attenuation. These observations have led to the description of two major groups of patients with emphysema, each with distinctive radiographic patterns. Patients with predominant panlobular emphysema show hyperinflated lungs with peripheral vascular attenuation and a normal size heart and central pulmonary vessels. Bullae are common in this form of emphysema. This pattern of emphysema has been termed *arterial deficiency emphysema.* Clinically, these patients are described as "pink puffers" because of their tachypnea and normal partial pressure of oxygen. Those with centrilobular emphysema show mild hyperinflation and increased linear parenchymal markings that likely represent the small airways thickening of chronic bronchitis seen concomitantly in these patients. Bullae are uncommon in this form of emphysema. This radiographic pattern of emphysema has been termed *increased markings emphysema.* As a result of chronic hypoxemia, these individuals develop secondary polycythemia and are described as "blue bloaters." Although most patients do not fit neatly into one or the other category either clinically or radiographically, familiarity with these two patterns will allow for the correct diagnosis in the majority of patients with moderately severe or severe centrilobular or panlobular emphysema.

Widespread, extensive emphysema may be accurately diagnosed on chest radiographs, but mild disease is often not evident radiographically. The use of chest CT has allowed for the diagnosis of emphysema in the absence of chest radiographic findings of hyperinflation or parenchymal abnormalities. CT is ideally suited to the diagnosis of emphysema because of its cross-sectional nature and high contrast resolution. Early reports on the use of CT to diagnose emphysema depended on recognition of either large avascular areas or regions with abnormally low Hounsfield attenuation numbers. Thin-section CT provides better characterization of centrilobular emphysema than standard scans of 5 to 10 mm collimation.

Centrilobular emphysema on thin-section CT is seen as discrete, well-defined areas of abnormally low attenuation that lack definable walls and is situated centrally within the secondary pulmonary lobule adjacent to the bronchovascular bundle. HRCT, with its thin-collimation technique and high spatial resolution, can detect mild centrilobular emphysema that may be missed on conventional 10-mm collimated CT because of partial volume averaging of small emphysematous areas within the thickness of the scan section.

Treatment of Emphysema. Advances in operative techniques now provide two surgical options for the treatment of emphysema. Recently, a surgical technique first developed in the 1950s—lung volume reduction surgery—has been reintroduced as a method of relieving patient dyspnea by resecting severely emphysematous regions of lung and improving respiratory mechanics. This technique, which was evaluated in the National Emphysema Treatment Trial, was shown to benefit only a select group of patients with emphysema, specifically those with mostly upper lobe emphysema and low exercise capacity prior to surgery. An alternative surgical technique available to treat patients with emphysema, particularly younger patients with α-1 antitrypsin deficiency, is single or double lung transplantation. Several centers now administer intravenously pooled α-1-antitrypsin to patients with associated emphysema to prevent further damage to the lungs.

BULLOUS LUNG DISEASE

Bullae are thin-walled cystic spaces that exceed 1 cm in diameter and are found within the lung parenchyma (Fig. 18.14). Three morphologic types have been described: type 1 bullae, which are apical, subpleural rounded gas collections without septations containing a narrow neck; type 2 bullae, which are also subpleural in location but have wide necks and contain strands of residual tissue; and type 3 bullae, which are morphologically similar to type 2 bullae but are located deep within the lung substance. Bullae most often represent confluent areas of emphysematous lung and may be seen as part of generalized emphysema. However, in a minority of patients, bullae are not associated with emphysema. For example, the increased lung weight and chronically elevated transpleural pressure in patients with lower lobe interstitial pulmonary fibrosis predispose to bullae formation. Bullae may also be seen in diseases that cause chronic upper lobe fibrosis, such as sarcoidosis, pulmonary Langerhans cell histiocytosis, and ankylosing spondylitis. In these diseases, chronic bronchiolar obstruction leads to distal airspace distention, alveolar septal disruption, and the development of bullae.

Primary bullous disease (Table 18.5) is a group of disorders in which bullae are isolated lesions without intervening areas of emphysema or interstitial lung disease.

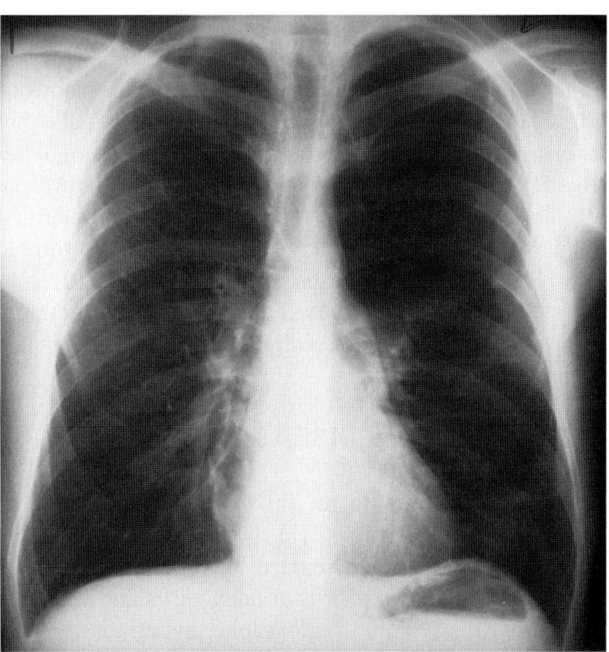

FIGURE 18.14. **Bullous Lung Disease.** Posteroanterior chest film in a 27-year-old man shows left lung and right upper lobe bullae, representing vanishing lung disease.

Primary bullous lung disease may be familial and has been found in association with Marfan or Ehlers-Danlos syndromes, intravenous drug use, HIV infection, and vanishing lung syndrome, which is an accelerated form of paraseptal emphysema seen in young adult men (Fig. 18.14). Most patients are asymptomatic unless large bullae compress normal parenchyma and cause compressive atelectasis and dyspnea. Radiographically, isolated bullae have an upper lobe distribution and appear as rounded thin-walled lucencies of varying size. These lesions can become huge as a result of air trapping and cause depression of the ipsilateral lung and hemidiaphragm and may even produce contralateral mediastinal shift. CT is useful in evaluating the extent of bullous disease and the amount of compressed pulmonary tissue.

Spontaneous pneumothorax occurs when a subpleural bulla ruptures into the pleural space. These patients may be difficult to manage; persistent air leaks lead to

TABLE 18.5 Causes of Primary Bullous Lung Disease

Familial
Vanishing lung disease
Marfan syndrome
Ehlers Danlos syndrome
Intravenous drug use
HIV infection

prolonged and often unsuccessful closed tube drainage of the pleural space and re-expansion of the lung. When a bulla becomes secondarily infected, chest radiographs or CT will demonstrate an air–fluid level within the bulla that resolves over several weeks with the administration of antibiotics. A cancer may rarely develop within the wall of a bulla. Symptomatic patients and those with enlarging bullae should be considered for bullectomy. Radioisotopic lung perfusion studies may be performed preoperatively to assess the amount of perfused and potentially functional lung parenchyma compressed by the bullae.

SMALL AIRWAYS DISEASE

Bronchiolitis refers to an inflammation of the small noncartilaginous airways (7) (Table 18.6). *Infectious bronchiolitis* is often a disease of young children caused by respiratory syncytial virus or adenovirus and produces respiratory distress and radiographic hyperinflation that are indistinguishable from asthma. However, there is an increasing recognition of infectious bronchiolitis in adults caused by a variety of microorganisms. A specific but uncommon cause of bronchiolitis is *diffuse* or *Asian panbronchiolitis*, which is associated with sinus disease and results in progressive pulmonary symptoms of airways disease, including cough and sputum production. Bronchiolar and peribronchial inflammation is commonly a result of heavy cigarette smoking. This latter disease is termed *respiratory bronchiolitis–associated interstitial lung disease* (RB-ILD), and it presents with signs and symptoms of interstitial lung disease. RB-ILD is reviewed in Chapter 17. Bronchiolitis is also a prominent feature of patients with subacute hypersensitivity pneumonitis, which is reviewed in Chapter 17. *Follicular bronchiolitis* reflects a form of diffuse lymphoid hyperplasia of peribronchiolar lymphoid follicles of unclear clinical significance seen in patients with rheumatoid arthritis or Sjögren syndrome. Thin-section CT shows ill-defined centrilobular ground-glass nodules and occasional bronchial dilatation.

Constrictive bronchiolitis, also known as *bronchiolitis obliterans,* is a subacute disease characterized pathologically by a mononuclear cell inflammatory process within the walls of respiratory bronchioles that leads to the formation of granulation tissue, which plugs small airways. This results in dyspnea and functional airways obstruction. This disorder may be idiopathic or secondary to viral infection, toxic fume inhalation, drug reaction, collagen vascular disorders (Fig. 18.15), organ transplantation, or chronic aspiration. Lung, heart-lung, and bone marrow transplant patients are particularly prone to constrictive bronchiolitis. Constrictive bronchiolitis in the adult may be the result of an early childhood lower respiratory infection with adenovirus, in which case it is known as unilateral hyperlucent lung or Swyer-James syndrome. In Swyer-James syndrome, the bronchiolitis causes diffuse small airways obliteration, air trapping, and destruction of alveolar walls and emphysema owing to overdistention of peripheral airspaces. Because postinfectious bronchiolitis obliterans affects the lungs asymmetrically and usually occurs during a period of lung growth and development, the affected lung is typically small and hyperlucent and the ipsilateral pulmonary artery is hypoplastic. Most patients with the Swyer-James syndrome are asymptomatic, while some patients complain of dyspnea or recurrent lower respiratory tract infections.

The chest radiograph in patients with pure constrictive bronchiolitis may be normal despite the presence of severe dyspnea and functional evidence of airflow obstruction. The most common radiographic abnormality in this

TABLE 18.6 Clinical and Imaging Features of Small Airways Disease

Entity	*Associated Conditions*	*CT Findings*
Infectious bronchiolitis	Viral/atypical/mycobacterial infection	Tree-in-bud opacities
Diffuse panbronchiolitis	None	Tree-in-bud opacities; bronchial dilatation/thickening
Respiratory bronchiolitis–associated interstitial lung disease	Cigarette smoking	Centrilobular and geographic ground-glass opacities
Hypersensitivity pneumonitis (subacute)	Inhaled organic antigen	Centrilobular ground-glass nodules; air trapping on expiratory scans
Follicular bronchiolitis	Rheumatoid arthritis; Sjögren syndrome	Centrilobular ground-glass nodules
Constrictive bronchiolitis	Transplant patients; drug reactions; inhalation injury	Mosaic attenuation with air trapping on expiratory scans; bronchial dilatation (late)

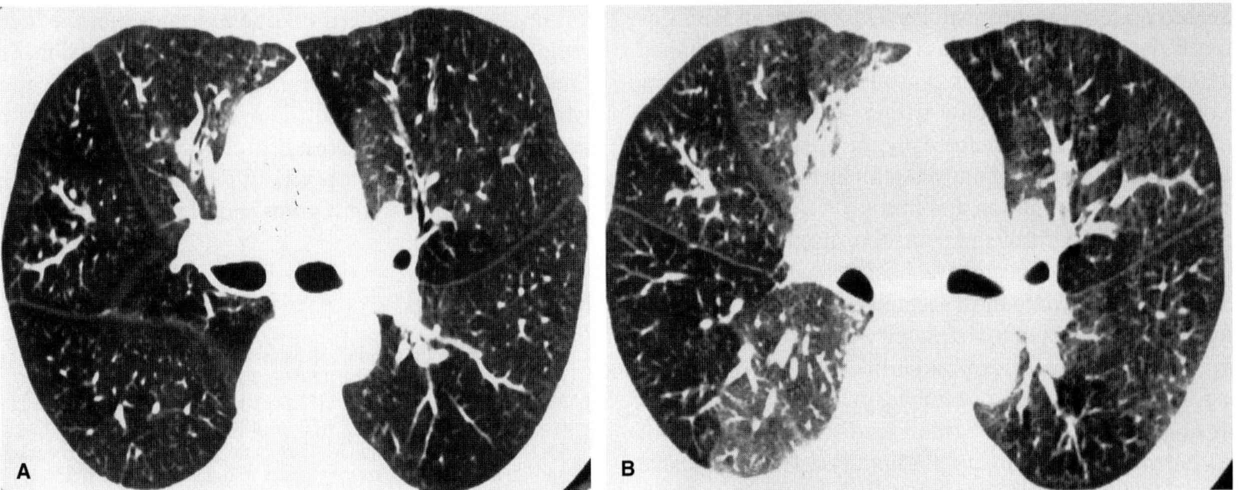

FIGURE 18.15. **Constrictive Bronchiolitis (Bronchiolitis Obliterans).** Inspiratory **(A)** and expiratory **(B)** HRCT scans in a 59-year-old woman with rheumatoid arthritis and airflow obstruction shows mosaic attenuation on the inspiratory scans with regional air trapping on expiration, representing small airways disease (bronchiolitis obliterans).

disorder is diffuse reticulonodular opacities with associated hyperinflation. Central bronchiectasis has been described, particularly in those with constrictive bronchiolitis that developed as a complication of heart-lung transplantation. In patients with Swyer-James syndrome, the affected lung is normal or small in volume, and marked unilateral air trapping is seen on fluoroscopy or expiratory films. The air trapping is caused by bronchiolar obstruction with collateral air drift to the distal airspaces on inspiration that cannot escape on expiration. The ipsilateral hilum is small and the pulmonary vasculature is reduced, accounting for the hyperlucency seen radiographically and on CT (Fig. 18.16). Perfusion lung scanning shows decreased perfusion of the affected lung, while the ventilation study shows decreased ventilation with markedly delayed radioisotope washout. This latter finding helps distinguish the Swyer-James syndrome from primary central pulmonary artery occlusion or hypoplastic lung, conditions in which ventilation is maintained.

HRCT in Small Airways Disease. HRCT is a sensitive indicator of the presence of small airways disease (7). Both direct and indirect findings may be evident on HRCT that allow detection of this process. The direct sign of small airways disease is centrilobular opacities, which represent

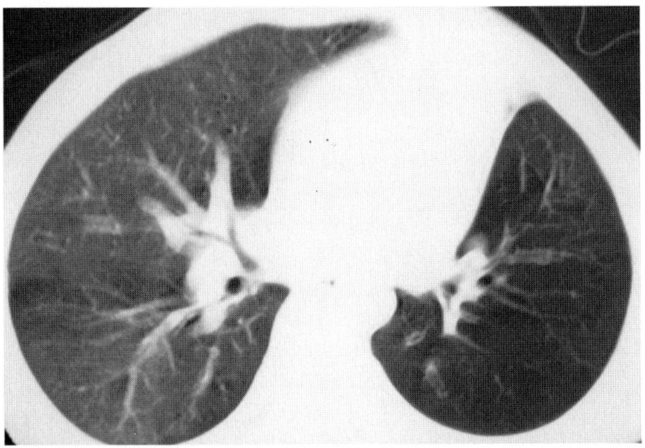

FIGURE 18.16. **Unilateral Hyperlucent Lung (Swyer-James) Syndrome.** CT scan in a 7-year-old boy with a history of neonatal pneumonia shows a small hyperlucent left lung with attenuated vascularity and central bronchiectasis.

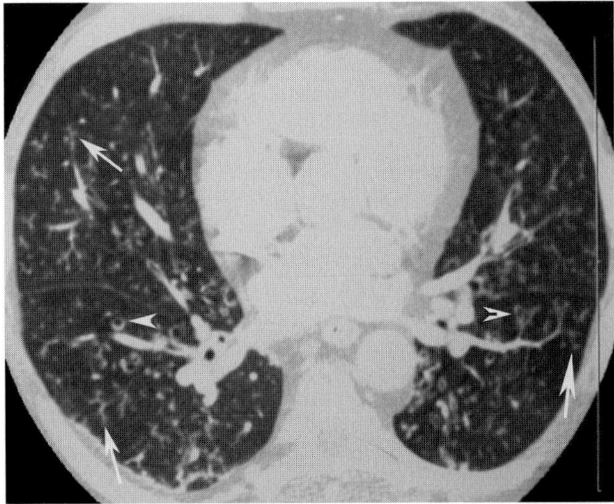

FIGURE 18.17. **Diffuse Panbronchiolitis.** CT scan through the lower lobes in a 47-year-old man with panbronchiolitis shows diffuse tree-in-bud opacities (*arrows*) with associated larger airway cylindric bronchiectasis (*arrowheads*).

diseased preterminal bronchioles. This is seen on HRCT as sharply defined or ground-glass nodules or Y- or V-shaped tubular branching opacities centrally situated within the secondary pulmonary lobule within 1 cm of the pleural surface (Fig. 18.17). Pathologically, the opacities reflect dilatation and mucus plugging of small bronchioles or peribronchiolar inflammation and fibrosis.

The indirect signs of small airways disease result from expiratory air trapping and are most easily seen on HRCT. Those portions of lung most severely affected by small airways disease are poorly ventilated and perfused and appear relatively hyperlucent adjacent to areas of normal lung. This results in an appearance on HRCT, termed "mosaic attenuation," that is virtually indistinguishable from the changes seen in primary pulmonary arterial occlusive disease. Furthermore, infiltrative processes such as *Pneumocystis jiroveci* pneumonia and desquamative interstitial pneumonitis, which produce patchy ground-glass opacification, also result in a mosaic attenuation appearance on HRCT. The use of both inspiratory and expiratory HRCT scans helps distinguish between these various disorders. In a patient with mosaic attenuation, attenuated vessels within the lucent regions of lung indicates that the lucent regions are abnormal because of decreased perfusion. This finding allows distinction from ground-glass opacification, where the caliber of vessels in normal and abnormal lung are comparable. The presence of small airways disease is confirmed on expiratory HRCT by noting air trapping within the hyperlucent regions (Fig. 18.15).

REFERENCES

1. Marom EM, Goodman PC, McAdams HP. Focal abnormalities of the trachea and main bronchi. AJR Am J Roentgenol 2001;176:707–711.
2. Marom EM, Goodman PC, McAdams HP. Diffuse abnormalities of the trachea and main bronchi. AJR Am J Roentgenol 2001;176:713–717.
3. Unger JM, Schuchmann GG, Grossman JE, et al. Tears of the trachea and main bronchi caused by blunt trauma: radiologic findings. AJR Am J Roentgenol 1989;153:1175–1180.
4. White CS, Cole RP, Lebetsky HW, et al. Acute asthma: admission chest radiography in hospitalized adult patients. Chest 1991;100:14–16.
5. Grenier P, Maurice F, Musset D, et al. Bronchiectasis: assessment by thin-section CT. Radiology 1986;161:95–99.
6. Foster WL, Gimenez EI, Roubidoux MA, et al. The emphysemas: radiologic-pathologic correlation. Radiographics 1993;13:311–328.
7. Waitches GM, Stern EJ. High-resolution CT of peripheral airways disease. Radiol Clin North Am 2002;40:21–29.

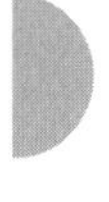

Chapter 19

Pleura, Chest Wall, Diaphragm, and Miscellaneous Chest Disorders

Jeffrey S. Klein

Pleura
Pleural Effusion
Bronchopleural Fistula
Postpneumonectomy Space
Pneumothorax
Focal Pleural Disease
Diffuse Pleural disease
Asbestos-Related Pleural Disease

Chest Wall
Soft Tissues
The Bony Thorax

Diaphragm

Congenital Lung Disease

Traumatic Lung Disease

Aspiration

Drug-Induced Chest Disease

Radiation-Induced Lung Disease

PLEURA

Pleural Effusion

Pleural Fluid Physiology and Pathophysiology. The normal volume of fluid in the pleural space is approximately 2 to 5 mL. The formation of pleural fluid follows Starling's law and depends upon hydrostatic and oncotic forces in both the systemic capillaries of the parietal pleura and the pleural space (1). Under normal conditions, pleural fluid is formed by filtration from systemic capillaries in the parietal pleura and resorbed via the parietal pleural lymphatics.

Pleural effusions may be classified by their gross appearance (bloody, chylous, purulent, serous); the causative disease (Table 19.1); or by the pathophysiology of abnormal pleural fluid formation (transudative versus exudative). This latter differentiation is made by measuring the protein, lactic acid dehydrogenase (LDH), and glucose concentration of the pleural fluid obtained by thoracentesis. Conditions associated with elevated plasma hydrostatic pressure or a decrease in plasma oncotic pressure will produce a transudative pleural effusion characterized by: (*1*) pleural/serum protein ratio <0.5, (*2*) pleural/serum LDH ratio <0.6, and (*3*) pleural LDH <200 IU/L. Left heart failure is the most common cause of pleural effusion resulting from an increase in hydrostatic pressure, which in turn is a result of pulmonary venous and capillary hypertension. Fluid overload from renal failure, pregnancy, and constrictive pericarditis are additional causes of hydrostatic pleural effusion. The hypoproteinemia associated with liver disease is the most common cause of a transudative effusion; additional causes are the nephrotic syndrome, severe malnutrition, and protein losing enteropathy. An exudative pleural effusion—characterized by: (*1*) pleural/serum protein ratio >0.5, (*2*) pleural/serum LDH ratio >0.6, and (*3*) pleural LDH >200 IU/L—is the result of increased pleural capillary permeability. Peripheral pulmonary or pleural processes that inflame the pleura (pneumonia, serositis) or directly invade the pleura (malignancy) are the most common causes of pleural exudates.

TABLE 19.1 Etiology of Pleural Effusions

Infectious	Bacterial/mycobacterial
	Viral
	Fungal
	Parasitic
Cardiovascular	Heart failure
	Pericarditis
	Superior vena cava obstruction
	Postcardiac surgery
	Myocardial infarction
	Pulmonary embolism
Neoplastic	Bronchogenic carcinoma
	Metastases
	Lymphoma
	Pleural or chest wall neoplasms (mesothelioma)
Immunologic	Systemic lupus erythematosus
	Rheumatoid arthritis
	Sarcoidosis (rare)
	Wegener granulomatosis
Inhalational	Asbestos
Trauma	Blunt or penetrating chest trauma
Abdominal disease	Cirrhosis (hepatic hydrothorax)
	Pancreatitis
	Subphrenic abscess
	Acute pyelonephritis
	Ascites (from any cause)
	Splenic vein thrombosis
Miscellaneous	Drugs
	Myxedema
	Ovarian tumor

Specific Causes of Pleural Effusion

Congestive heart failure is the condition most commonly associated with a transudative pleural effusion. The effusions are usually bilateral and larger on the right side (2). An isolated right effusion is twice as common as an isolated left effusion.

Parapneumonic Effusion and Empyema. A *parapneumonic effusion* is defined as an effusion associated with pneumonia. Peripheral parenchymal infection produces an exudative pleural effusion by causing visceral pleural inflammation that increases pleural capillary permeability. Inflammatory thickening of the pleural membranes with lymphatic obstruction may also be a contributing factor. Empyema results when the parenchymal infection extends into the pleural space. Parenchymal infections that typically result in empyema formation are bacterial pneumonia, septic emboli, and lung abscess, whereas fungal, viral, and parasitic infections are uncommon causes. Less commonly, infection may extend into the pleural space from the spine, mediastinum, and chest wall.

Forty percent of bacterial pneumonias have an associated pleural effusion. *Staphylococcus aureus* and gram-negative pneumonias are the most common cause of parapneumonic effusion and empyema. The natural history of parapneumonic effusions may be divided into three stages (3). Stage 1 is an exudative stage; visceral pleural inflammation causes increased capillary permeability and pleural fluid accumulation. Most of these sterile exudative effusions resolve with appropriate antibiotic therapy. A stage 2 parapneumonic effusion is a fibrinopurulent pleural fluid collection containing bacteria and neutrophils. Fibrin deposition on the visceral and parietal pleura impairs fluid resorption and produces loculations. If the infection is not treated, the loculations will impair attempts at closed pleural fluid drainage. A stage 3 parapneumonic effusion develops 2 to 3 weeks after initial pleural fluid formation and is characterized by the ingrowth of fibroblasts over the pleura, which produces pleural fibrosis and entraps the lung. Dystrophic calcification of the pleura may develop following resolution of the pleural infection.

Tuberculous pleural effusion or empyema resulting from the rupture of subpleural caseating granulomas may complicate pulmonary infection or occur as the primary manifestation of disease. Effusions in tuberculosis (TB) are more common in young adults with pulmonary disease and in HIV-positive individuals with severe immunodeficiency. The pleural fluid is characteristically straw colored, with greater than 70% lymphocytes and a low glucose concentration.

Radiographically, empyema most often appears as a loculated pleural fluid collection. On CT, it is elliptic in shape and is seen most often within the posterior and inferior pleural space. The collection conforms to and maintains a broad area of contact with the chest wall (Fig. 19.1). The distinction of empyema from peripheral lung abscess has important therapeutic implications; empyemas require external drainage, whereas lung abscesses usually respond to postural drainage and antibiotic therapy. Contrast-enhanced chest CT is most useful in making this distinction (Table 19.2) (4). Detection of an empyema may be difficult when there is extensive parenchymal consolidation. In these cases, CT and US are useful in detecting parapneumonic fluid collections and guiding diagnostic thoracentesis and pleural drainage. Findings on CT that are fairly specific for the presence of an exudative pleural effusion include thickening and enhancement of the parietal pleura, the presence of loculations, and the detection of discrete soft tissue lesions along the parietal pleura outlined by low-attenuation pleural fluid. Hemorrhagic effusions can occasionally be recognized on CT by their intrinsic high attenuation or the presence of a fluid–fluid level caused by dependent cellular blood elements.

Neoplasms. Pleural effusion may be seen with benign or malignant intrathoracic tumors. The tumors most commonly associated with pleural effusion are, in order of frequency, lung carcinoma, breast carcinoma, pelvic tumors, gastric carcinoma, and lymphoma. Pleural fluid may

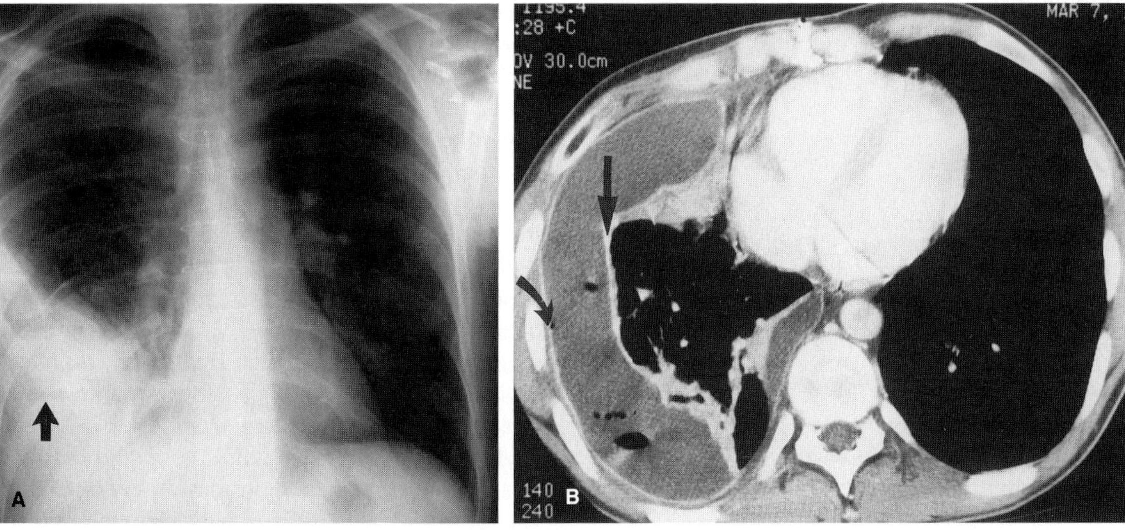

FIGURE 19.1. **Empyema on Chest Radiograph and CT. A.** Posteroanterior chest film in a patient with a recent right lower pneumonia demonstrates an oval opacity in the right lateral costophrenic sulcus containing gas (*arrow*). **B.** An enhanced CT scan shows a circumferential pleural fluid collection with enhancing visceral (*straight arrow*) and parietal (*curved arrow*) pleural layers representing an empyema. Note the contained gas pockets, indicating loculations within the collection itself.

result from pleural involvement by tumor or from lymphatic obstruction anywhere from the parietal pleura to the mediastinal nodes. The effusions are exudative and may be bloody. Demonstration of malignant cells on cytologic examination of pleural fluid obtained at thoracentesis is necessary for the diagnosis of a malignant effusion. Closed or thoracoscopic biopsy is reserved for patients with negative cytologic examination. Clues to the presence of a malignant pleural effusion include smooth or lobulated pleural thickening, mediastinal or hilar lymph node enlargement or mass, and solitary or multiple parenchymal nodules. CT is useful in demonstrating pleural masses or underlying parenchymal lesions in those with large effusions (Fig. 19.2).

Trauma. Blunt or penetrating trauma to the chest, including iatrogenic trauma from thoracotomy, thoracostomy, or placement of central venous catheters, may result in a hemothorax. Hemothorax results from laceration of vessels within the lung, mediastinum, chest wall, or diaphragm. Intrapleural blood coagulates rapidly, and septations form early. In some individuals, pleural motion causes defibrination, which lyses the clotted blood. In the acute setting, pleural fluid of high CT attenuation (>80 H) may be seen; associated rib fractures or subcutaneous emphysema should suggest the diagnosis. An acute hemothorax is treated with thoracostomy tube drainage, while thoracotomy is generally reserved for persistent bleeding or hypotension.

Esophageal perforation from prolonged vomiting (Boerhaave syndrome) or as a complication of esophageal dilatation may produce a pleural effusion, most commonly on the left side. Extravascular placement of a central line can result in a hydrothorax when intravenous solution is inadvertently infused into the pleural or extrapleural space.

Collagen Vascular and Autoimmune Disease. Systemic lupus erythematosus has a reported incidence of pleural effusions ranging from 33% to 74%. These exudative effusions are a result of pleural inflammation; patients present with pleuritic chest pain. In some cases, the nephrotic syndrome associated with systemic lupus erythematosus may produce transudative effusions.

TABLE 19.2 Empyema Versus Lung Abscess on CT

Feature	***Empyema***	***Abscess***
Shape	Oval, oriented longitudinally	Round
Margin	Thin, smooth ("split pleura" sign)	Thick, irregular
Angle with chest wall	Obtuse	Acute
Effect on lung	Compression	Consumption
Treatment	External drainage	Antibiotics, postural drainage

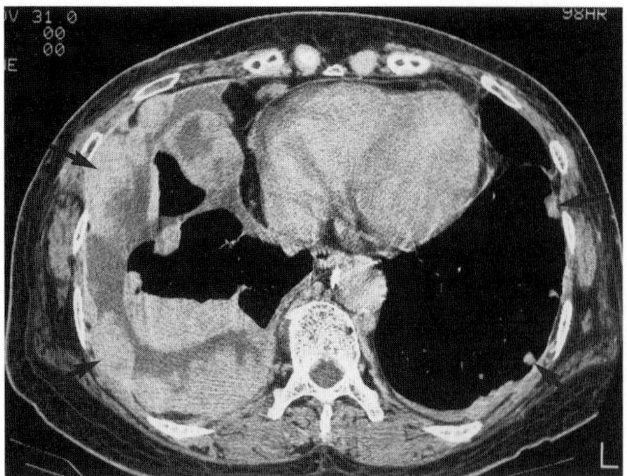

FIGURE 19.2. **Malignant Pleural Effusion: CT Diagnosis.** HRCT in a patient with breast carcinoma and a right pleural effusion on chest radiographs demonstrates multiple bilateral pleural nodules and masses (*arrows*) representing pleural metastases. The diagnosis was confirmed by US-guided right pleural biopsy.

Cardiomegaly is a common chest radiographic finding and may be caused by pericardial effusion, hypertension, renal failure, or lupus-associated endocarditis or myocarditis.

Pleural effusion is the most common intrathoracic manifestation of rheumatoid arthritis and is most frequently seen in male patients following the onset of joint disease (Fig. 19.3). The effusions occur independent of pulmonary parenchymal involvement but may develop following intrapleural rupture of peripheral rheumatoid nodules. The effusions of rheumatoid arthritis are exudative, with lymphocytosis, low glucose concentration, and low pH (<7.2). Rheumatoid effusions may persist unchanged for years.

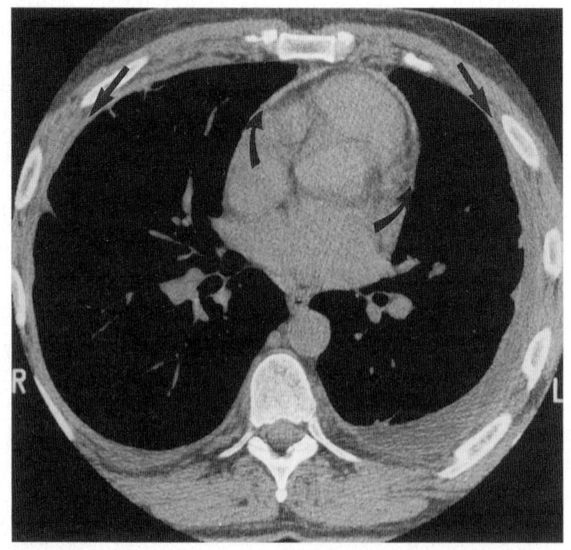

FIGURE 19.3. **Serositis in Rheumatoid Arthritis.** HRCT in a 43-year-old man with rheumatoid arthritis reveals bilateral pleural thickening (*straight arrows*) and small dependent effusions with pericardial thickening (*curved arrows*).

Autoimmune syndromes producing pleural and pericardial effusions have been described following myocardial infarction (Dressler syndrome) or cardiac surgery (postpericardiotomy syndrome). Both are characterized by fever, pleuritis, pneumonitis, and pericarditis developing within days to weeks of the precipitating event. The radiographic findings include enlargement of the cardiac silhouette, pleural effusions, and parenchymal airspace opacities. A serosanguineous exudative pleural effusion is seen in over 80% of patients. Treatment with nonsteroidal anti-inflammatory drugs usually results in symptomatic and radiographic improvement.

Abdominal Disease. Radioisotope studies have demonstrated that peritoneal fluid may enter the pleural space via transdiaphragmatic lymphatic channels or through defects in the diaphragm. The lymphatic channels are larger on the right side, accounting for the higher incidence of right-sided effusions associated with ascites or liver failure (hepatic hydrothorax).

Acute or chronic pancreatitis can cause pleural effusions that are most often left-sided because of the proximity of the pancreatic tail to the left hemidiaphragm. The effusion associated with acute pancreatitis is typically exudative and may be bloody. Pleural effusion from chronic pancreatitis may cause pleuritic chest pain and shortness of breath. Rupture of the pancreatic duct can lead to a pancreaticopleural fistula. A high amylase concentration in the pleural fluid should suggest the pancreas as the etiology of the effusion, although elevated amylase may be seen in pleural effusions caused by malignancy or esophageal perforation.

Subphrenic abscesses complicating abdominal surgery or perforation of a hollow viscus can cause diaphragmatic paresis, basilar atelectasis, and pleural effusion. Patients with a pleural effusion associated with upper abdominal pain, fever, and leukocytosis should have CT or US examination and, when feasible, percutaneous catheter drainage of the abscess.

An association between benign pleural effusions and pelvic tumors has long been recognized. First described with ovarian fibroma (Meigs syndrome), a number of pelvic and abdominal tumors, including pancreatic and ovarian malignancy, lymphoma, and uterine leiomyomas, have been found to cause pleural effusion. The effusions in Meigs syndrome are usually transudative and resolve after removal of the pelvic tumor.

Chylothorax is a pleural collection containing triglycerides in the form of chylomicrons and results from perforation of the thoracic duct that communicates with the pleural space. The thoracic duct originates from the cisterna chyli at the level of the first lumbar vertebra and ascends along the right paravertebral space, entering the thorax via the aortic hiatus. The duct crosses from right to left

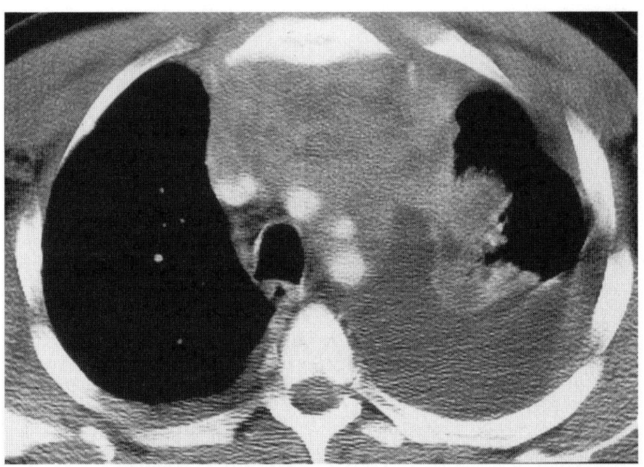

FIGURE 19.4. **Chylous Pleural Effusion Caused by Hodgkin Lymphoma.** Enhanced CT scan in a 42-year-old man with nodular sclerosing Hodgkin lymphoma shows a large anterior mediastinal mass associated with moderate left and small right pleural effusions. Chylous fluid was obtained at left-sided thoracentesis.

at the level of the sixth thoracic vertebra to lie alongside the upper esophagus. At the level of the left subclavian artery, the duct arches anteriorly to empty into the confluence of the left internal jugular and subclavian veins. Disruption of the upper duct caused by direct trauma or obstruction with rupture produces a left chylothorax, while injury to the lower intrathoracic duct produces a right chylothorax. The most common causes of chylothorax are malignancy, iatrogenic trauma, and TB (Fig. 19.4). The radiographic appearance is indistinguishable on plain radiographs and CT from other causes of free-flowing effusions. The diagnosis is confirmed by triglyceride levels exceeding 110 mg/dL in the pleural fluid.

Pulmonary Embolism. Infarction complicating pulmonary embolism is a well-recognized cause of pleural effusion. The effusion may be associated with elevation of the ipsilateral diaphragm and peripheral wedge-shaped opacities (Hampton hump). The pleural effusion is typically a small, unilateral, serosanguineous exudate.

Drugs may cause pleural effusions as a result of pleural inflammation (methysergide) or by producing a lupus-like syndrome (phenytoin, isoniazid, hydralazine, procainamide). Nitrofurantoin has been associated with an immunologic reaction that causes pleuropulmonary disease with eosinophilia.

Management of Pleural Effusion. Transudative pleural effusions are managed by treatment of the underlying disorder, because the pleura is intrinsically normal in these diseases. Management of parapneumonic effusions is best guided by evaluation of the likelihood that the effusion, if not drained, would result in prolonged hospitalization, pleural fibrosis with resultant respiratory impairment, local spread of infection, or death. This likelihood in turn is based on the anatomy, bacteriology, and chemistry (i.e., ABCs) of the fluid collection. In general, larger, loculated collections with positive gram stains or cultures and pH <7.20 are associated with a moderate to high risk for poor outcome as detailed above and should be drained if possible (5). The choice of drainage procedure depends on various factors, including patient age and underlying condition, length of illness, and access to image-guided therapy and thoracoscopy. Although intrapleural fibrinolytic therapy with streptokinase, urokinase, or tissue plasminogen activator will help a certain subset of patients with complex parapneumonic effusions (Fig. 19.5), some will require open pleural drainage by video-assisted thoracoscopic surgery (VATS) or thoracotomy with decortication.

Malignant pleural effusions most often require closed drainage and pleural sclerosis, with talc the current agent of choice. Some patients may benefit from VATS drainage and sclerosis. Select patients can be managed as outpatients with indwelling silastic catheters (e.g., Pleurx catheter), which allow intermittent patient-directed drainage of fluid. Patients with chylothorax require therapy directed at the underlying etiology (lymphoma, TB); those patients with traumatic disruption of the thoracic duct often require surgical ligation of the duct.

Patients with pleural effusions from trauma, pulmonary embolism, autoimmune disorders, and drug reactions often require no specific therapy. Exceptions include the postpericardiotomy (Dressler syndrome) patients, who are treated with nonsteroidal anti-inflammatory agents, and patients with large hemothoraces that require large bore tube drainage to prevent pleural fibrosis and lung entrapment.

Bronchopleural Fistula

A bronchopleural fistula is a communication between the lung and the pleural space that often originates from a peripheral airway. A bronchopleural fistula from a bronchus results in an empyema, while an air leak from peripheral airspaces may cause an intractable pneumothorax. Bronchopleural fistulas often develop from dehiscence of a bronchial stump following lobectomy or pneumonectomy, or as the result of a necrotizing pulmonary infection. Presenting symptoms include fever, cough, and dyspnea; large air leaks may be noted in patients with pleural drains. Radiographically, a bronchopleural fistula presents as a loculated intrapleural air and fluid collection. The development of an air–fluid level in the postpneumonectomy space or a drop in the air–fluid level during the early postoperative period, associated with shift of the mediastinum back toward the midline, should suggest the diagnosis. CT is useful in evaluating patients with suspected bronchopleural fistula and empyema (Fig. 19.6) (6). It can distinguish a hydropneumothorax from a peripheral lung abscess and occasionally demonstrates the actual fistulous communication.

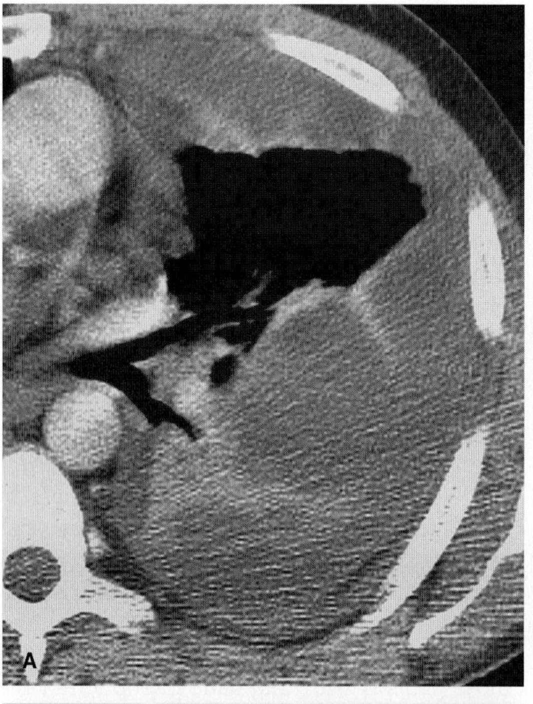

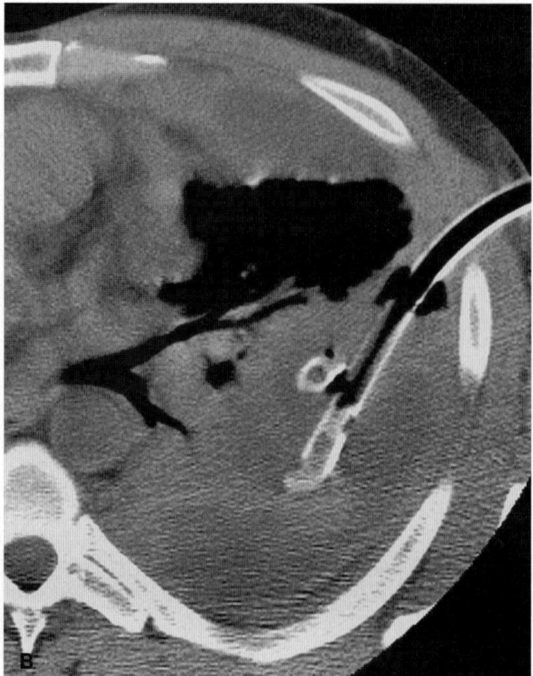

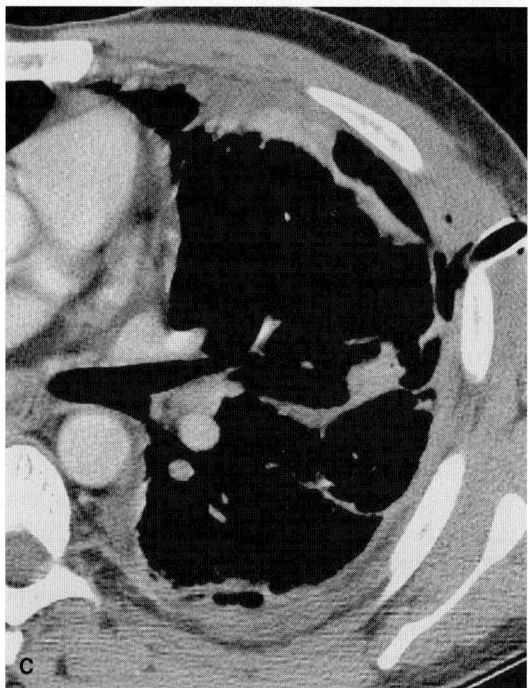

FIGURE 19.5. **CT-Guided Percutaneous Empyema Drainage Using Fibrinolytics. A.** Contrast-enhanced CT scan in a 36-year-old man with recent pneumonia and persistent fevers shows a large multiloculated left pleural effusion with underlying lingular and lower lobe atelectasis. **B.** Scan following placement of a 28-French drainage tube under CT guidance shows the tube within the parapneumonic collection. **C.** Repeat postcontrast scan after 4 days of intrapleural instillation of tissue plasminogen activator and suction drainage shows evacuation of the fluid with minimal residual consolidated lung.

Postpneumonectomy Space

Following pneumonectomy, the residual space gradually fills with fluid and appears radiographically as an opaque hemithorax with ipsilateral mediastinal shift. The radiographic findings suggesting bronchopleural fistula formation complicating pneumonectomy are described in the previous section. CT and MR are useful in evaluating the postpneumonectomy space for evidence of tumor recurrence, and may help in the diagnosis of postoperative bronchopleural fistula and empyema.

Pneumothorax

Pneumothorax results from air entering the pleural space and may be traumatic or spontaneous (Table 19.3). Spontaneous pneumothorax is further subdivided into a primary form, which has no identifiable etiology, and a secondary

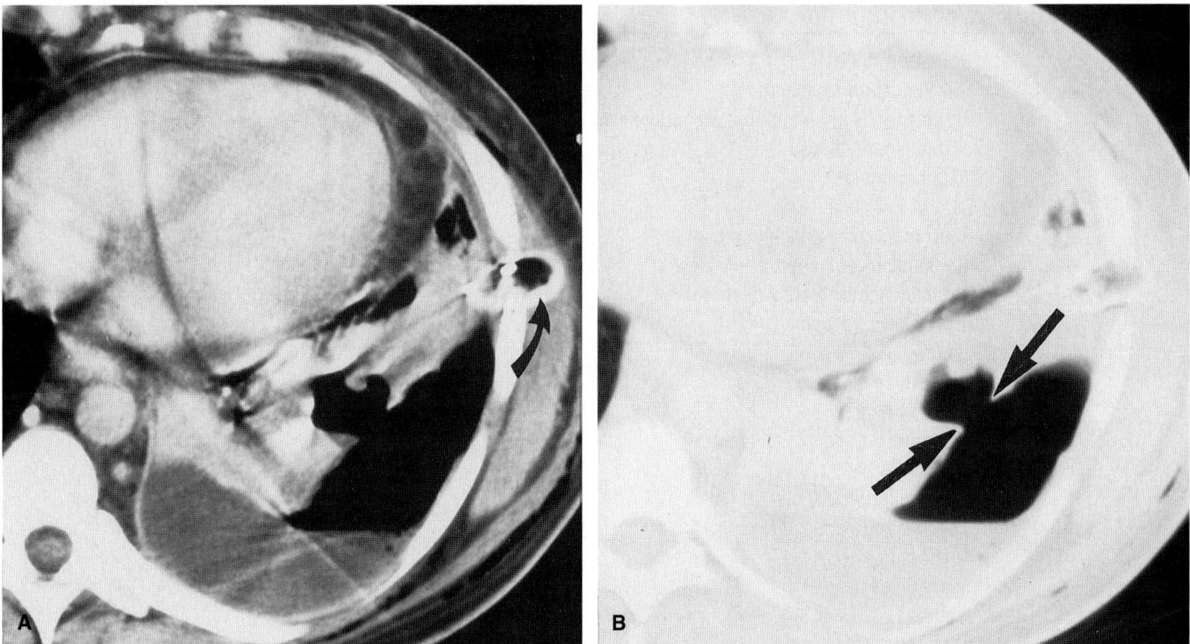

FIGURE 19.6. **Bronchopleural Fistula and Empyema Complicating Septic Emboli. A.** An enhanced CT scan in a 43-year-old woman with septic emboli complicating intravenous drug use reveals a posterior pleural air–fluid collection associated with left lower lobe consolidation. Note chest tube entering thorax laterally (*curved arrow*). **B.** The same scan at lung windows shows the left lower lobe cavity communicating with the pleural space via a breach in the visceral pleura (*straight arrows*). A properly positioned chest tube drained infected fluid and demonstrated a continuous air leak.

form, which is associated with underlying parenchymal lung disease (7). Patients with a pneumothorax typically present with the sudden onset of dyspnea and pleuritic chest pain.

Traumatic Pneumothorax. Trauma is the most common cause of pneumothorax. Penetrating injuries can produce pneumothorax by introducing air from the atmosphere into the pleural space or by laceration of the visceral pleura, resulting in an air leak from the lung. Gunshot and knife wounds to the chest and upper abdomen, central line placement, thoracentesis, transbronchial biopsy, and percutaneous needle biopsy are common penetrating injuries that cause traumatic pneumothorax. Blunt chest trauma may cause pneumothorax by two different mechanisms: (*1*) an acute increase in intrathoracic pressure results in extra-alveolar interstitial air because of alveolar disruption, which tracks peripherally and ruptures into the pleural space; and (*2*) laceration of the tracheobronchial tree can produce a pneumothorax with a large bronchopleural fistula. In patients with rib fractures, the free edge of the fractured ribs can project inward to lacerate the lung and cause pneumothorax.

Primary spontaneous pneumothorax most often occurs in young or middle-aged men. A familial incidence and a propensity for taller individuals has been noted. Affected patients often have blebs or bullae within the lung apices that are responsible for the development of recurrent pneumothoraces. Treatment of the initial episode is with closed tube drainage, with thoracoscopic bullectomy reserved for recurrent episodes or persistent air leak.

Secondary Spontaneous Pneumothorax. Multiple entities have been associated with secondary spontaneous pneumothorax. Most of these disorders have associated blebs, bullae, cysts, or cavities (Fig. 19.6), although in some patients the lungs are intrinsically normal. In the majority of the latter, there is usually a history of sudden increases in intrathoracic pressure. Chronic obstructive pulmonary disease is the most common predisposing condition. Acute obstruction to expiration from bronchoconstriction (asthma) or the performance of the Valsalva maneuver (crack cocaine or marijuana smoking, transvaginal childbirth) may cause spontaneous pneumothorax. Pneumothorax may complicate cystic lung changes in sarcoidosis, Langerhans cell histiocytosis of lung, and lymphangioleiomyomatosis. Necrotizing pneumonia or lung abscess caused by gram-negative or anaerobic bacteria, TB, or *Pneumocystis jiroveci* pneumonia can lead to pneumothorax, particularly in the mechanically ventilated patient. Metastases to the lung are an infrequent cause of pneumothorax and rarely are a presenting feature of disease. In these cases, pneumothorax develops when necrotic subpleural metastases rupture into the pleural space.

TABLE 19.3 Etiology of Pneumothorax

Trauma	Iatrogenic
	Thoracic/abdominal surgery
	Percutaneous interventional procedures
	Lung/pleural biopsy
	Thoracentesis
	Central line placement
	Aberrant feeding tube placement
	Mechanical ventilation
	Esophagoscopic biopsy/dilatation
	Bronchoscopic biopsy
	Not iatrogenic
	Penetrating injury
	Stab wound
	Gunshot wound
	Blunt injury
	Tracheobronchial disruption
	Esophageal rupture
	Rib fractures
Spontaneous	Primary (idiopathic)
	Secondary
	Obstructive airways disease
	Asthma
	Emphysema
	Infection
	Cavitating pneumonia
	Lung abscess
	Septic emboli
	Pneumatoceles
	Pulmonary infarction (rare)
	Neoplasm
	Bronchogenic carcinoma
	Pleural or chest wall neoplasm
	Metastases
	Cystic lung disease
	Sarcoidosis
	Eosinophilic granuloma
	Cystic fibrosis
	Tuberous sclerosis
	Lymphangioleiomyomatosis
	Catamenial pneumothorax
	Connective tissue disorders
	Marfan syndrome
	Ehlers-Danlos syndrome
	Cutis laxa

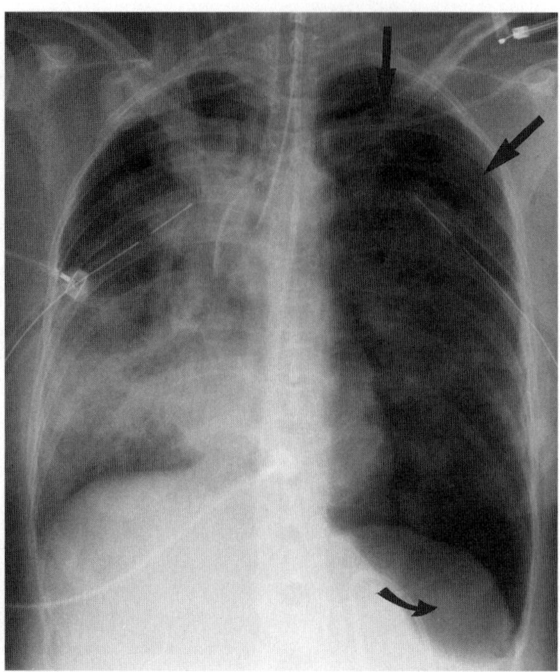

FIGURE 19.7. **Pneumothorax Complicating ARDS.** Posteroanterior chest film in a 41-year-old woman with ARDS and recurrent pneumothoraces reveals a left apical (*straight arrows*) and subpulmonic (*curved arrow*) pneumothorax despite the presence of a chest tube.

Sarcomas, particularly osteogenic sarcoma, lymphoma, and germ cell malignancies, are the most common primary malignancies to produce spontaneous pneumothorax. Marfan syndrome is the most common connective tissue disease producing pneumothorax; it usually results from the rupture of apical bullae. Other connective tissue diseases that can produce pneumothorax are Ehlers-Danlos syndrome and cutis laxa.

Mechanically ventilated patients are particularly at risk for pneumothorax because of the administration of positive pressure, emphysema, underlying or complicating necrotizing pneumonia, and frequent line placements and other invasive procedures. Not uncommonly, patients with ARDS develop small peripheral cystic airspaces, which can rupture into the pleural space (Fig. 19.7). When these are seen to develop on serial chest radiographs, impending pneumothorax can be suggested.

A particularly rare type of recurrent pneumothorax that occurs with menstruation is catamenial pneumothorax. This condition affects women in their fourth decade and is most likely caused by the cyclical necrosis of pleural endometrial implants, which creates an air leak between the lung and pleura. Rarely, air entering the peritoneal cavity during menstruation gains access to the pleural cavity via diaphragmatic defects. The predilection for right-sided pneumothoraces in this disorder indicates a key role for right-sided diaphragmatic defects. The pneumothoraces tend to be small and resolve spontaneously. Catamenial pneumothorax is managed by preventing menstruation with the administration of oral contraceptives.

Tension pneumothorax is a critical condition that most often results from iatrogenic trauma in mechanically ventilated patients. Tension pneumothorax results from a check-valve pleural defect that allows air to enter but not exit the pleural space. This leads to a pleural air collection that has a pressure exceeding atmospheric pressure during at least a portion of the respiratory cycle,

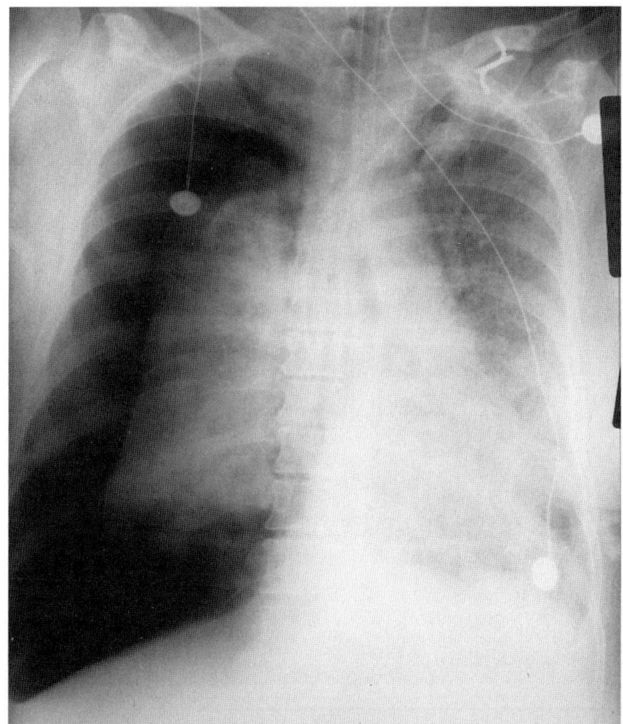

FIGURE 19.8. **Tension Pneumothorax.** Portable chest film in a 43-year-old woman with ARDS shows a large right pneumothorax with mediastinal shift and ipsilateral diaphragmatic depression, suggesting tension. Air was evacuated under pressure during emergent placement of a right chest tube.

causing complete collapse of the underlying lung and impairing venous return to the heart. Clinically, patients present with tachypnea, tachycardia, cyanosis, and hypotension. Radiographically, the involved hemithorax is expanded and hyperlucent, with a medially retracted lung, ipsilateral diaphragmatic depression or inversion, and contralateral mediastinal shift (Fig. 19.8). It is important to remember that contralateral mediastinal shift from pneumothorax does not invariably indicate tension, since a relative inequality in the degree of negative intrapleural pressure can produce shift in the absence of tension. Therefore, tension pneumothorax remains a clinical diagnosis. Immediate evacuation of the pleural space should be performed with a needle, catheter, or large-bore thoracostomy tube.

Focal Pleural Disease

Focal pleural disease may be divided into localized pleural thickening, pleural calcification, or pleural mass (Table 19.4) (8).

Localized pleural thickening from fibrosis is usually the end result of peripheral parenchymal and pleural inflammatory disease, with pneumonia the most common cause. Additional causes include pulmonary embolism

TABLE 19.4 Focal Pleural Disease

Opacities that mimic focal pleural thickening	Apical cap
	Companion shadows of first and second ribs
	Subpleural deposits of fat
Thickening	Pneumonia
	Pulmonary infarct
	Trauma
	Asbestos exposure (bilateral)
Calcification	Visceral pleura
	Hemothorax
	Empyema (tuberculosis)
	Parietal pleura
	Asbestos exposure (bilateral)
Pleural/extrapleural mass	Neoplasm
	Benign
	Fibroma
	Lipoma
	Neurofibroma
	Malignant
	Metastases (usually multiple)
	Mesothelioma (usually diffuse pleural thickening)
	Loculated pleural effusion/empyema
	Hematoma

with infarction, asbestos exposure, trauma, prior chemical pleurodesis, and drug-related pleural disease.

Pleural calcification is most often unilateral and involves the visceral pleura. It is usually the result of prior hemothorax or empyema (e.g., TB), although pleural thickening from any cause may calcify. Asbestos exposure can cause bilateral calcified parietal pleural plaques. Visceral pleural calcifications from pleural hemorrhage or infection are indistinguishable radiographically. Initially, the calcification is punctate, but it often progresses to become sheetlike. CT is particularly useful in detecting pleural calcification (Fig. 19.9). The presence of fluid within calcified pleural layers seen on CT suggests an active empyema and is most often seen in patients with prior TB. The use of CT and HRCT in the evaluation of asbestos-related focal pleural disease and calcification is discussed in a subsequent section.

Pleural Mass. Focal pleural masses are usually benign neoplasms such as lipomas; loculated pleural fluid can mimic a pleural mass radiographically. Thoracic lipomas may arise in the chest wall or subpleural fat. Subpleural lipomas produce a pleural mass and can change shape during respiration or with changes in patient positioning because of their pliable nature. Homogeneous fat attenuation on CT scan (–30 to –100 H) is diagnostic (Fig. 19.10). *Localized fibrous tumors of pleura* (LFTP) are uncommon pleural tumors (8). While most often benign, approximately 15% will recur locally after resection. These lesions appear as well-defined, spherical or oblong masses

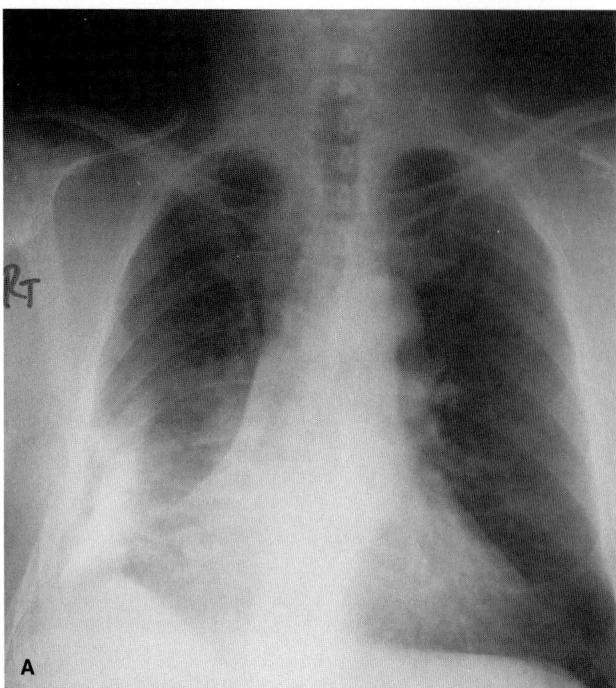

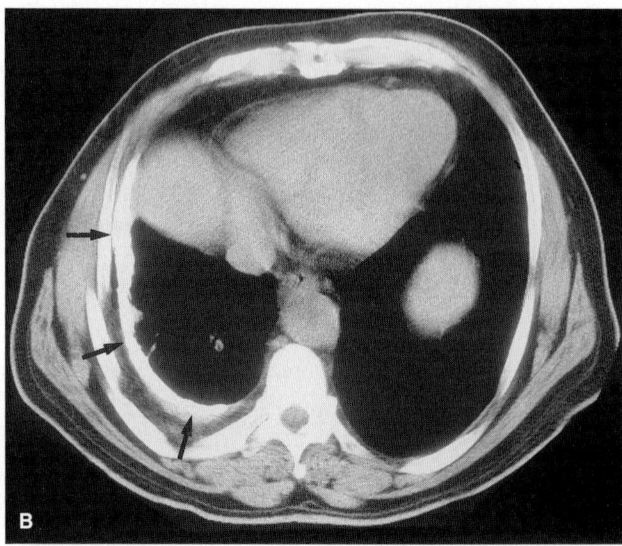

FIGURE 19.9. **Pleural Calcification Caused by Tuberculosis. A.** Posteroanterior chest radiograph in a 61-year-old man with prior TB demonstrates a small right hemithorax and a dense opacity inferolaterally. **B.** A CT scan through the lung bases shows a thick rind of pleural calcification (*arrows*) surrounding a contracted lung.

that arise from subpleural mesenchymal cells and are benign in approximately 80% of cases. These tumors are occasionally attached to the pleura by a narrow pedicle, a finding that is virtually pathognomonic and accounts for changes in intrapleural location seen with changes in patient positioning in some individuals (Fig. 19.11). CT usually shows a smoothly marginated, pleura-based soft tissue mass with either uniform soft tissue attenuation or inhomogeneous enhancement caused by areas of necrosis. An association between LFTP and hypertrophic pulmonary osteoarthropathy and hypoglycemia is recognized. Unlike malignant mesothelioma, there is no association between LFTP and asbestos exposure.

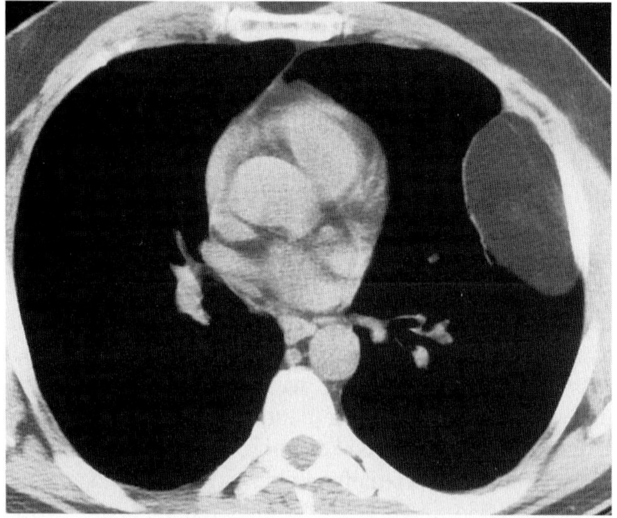

FIGURE 19.10. **Pleural Lipoma.** CT scan in a patient with an asymptomatic mass discovered as an incidental chest radiographic finding shows a left anterolateral pleura-based mass with homogeneous fatty attenuation representing a lipoma.

Diffuse Pleural Disease

Diffuse pleural disease represents diffuse pleural fibrosis (fibrothorax), pleural malignancy, or multiloculated pleural effusion (Table 19.5) (9).

Fibrothorax (diffuse pleural fibrosis) is defined as pleural thickening extending over more than one fourth of the costal pleural surface. Fibrothorax most commonly results from the resolution of an exudative pleural effusion (including asbestos-related effusions), empyema, or hemothorax. It may also be seen as a subpleural extension of diffuse interstitial fibrosis. The fibrothorax can encompass the entire lung and produce entrapment. When this causes a restrictive ventilatory defect, pleurectomy (decortication) may be necessary to restore function to the underlying lung.

Pleural Malignancy. Metastatic disease to the pleura commonly causes irregular or lobulated pleural

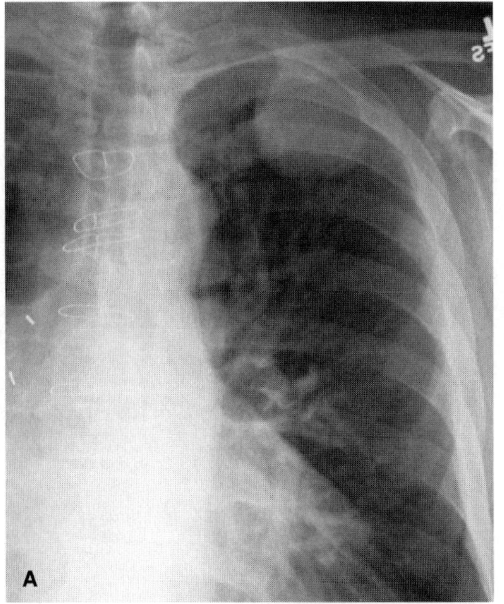

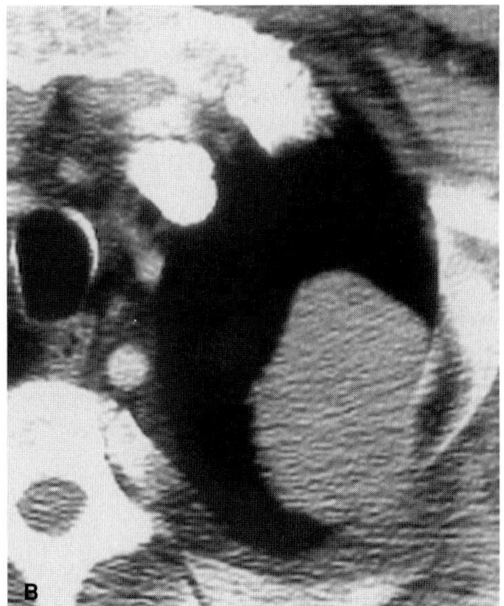

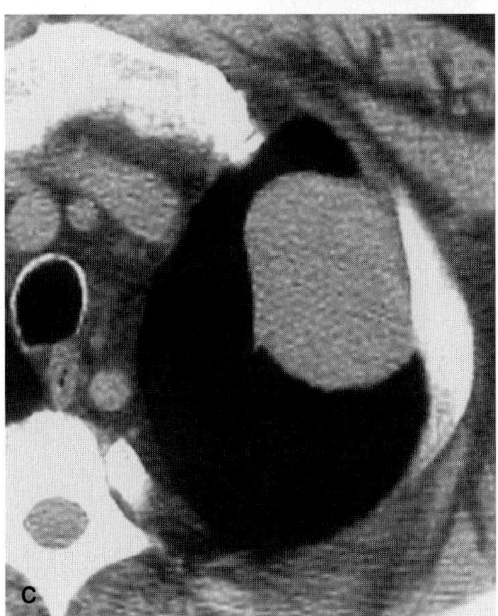

FIGURE 19.11. **Localized Fibrous Tumor of Pleura. A.** Chest radiograph in a 62-year-old man shows a smooth mass in the apex of the left lung. **B.** CT scan performed supine shows a pleural-based soft tissue mass. **C.** Prone scan, turned 180° for comparison with **B.** Shows dependent movement, suggesting that the tumor is attached by a pedicle. Biopsy proved localized fibrous tumor of pleura.

TABLE 19.5 Diffuse Pleural Disease

Smooth thickening	Pleural fibrosis
	Hemothorax
	Prior empyema or exudative effusion (including asbestos exposure)
	Interstitial pulmonary fibrosis
	Pleural effusion (particularly on supine radiographs)
Lobulated	Primary
	Mesothelioma
	Metastatic
	Adenocarcinoma of lung, breast, ovary, kidney, GI tract
	Invasive thymoma
	Lymphoma (subpleural deposits)
	Multiloculated pleural effusion/empyema

thickening, usually in association with a pleural effusion. The malignant tumors with a propensity to metastasize to the pleura include adenocarcinomas of the lung, breast, ovary, kidney, and GI tract. Malignant mesothelioma is seen almost exclusively in asbestos-exposed individuals.

Malignant pleural disease is most often caused by one of four conditions: metastatic adenocarcinoma (Fig. 19.2), invasive thymoma or thymic carcinoma, mesothelioma, and rarely non-Hodgkin lymphoma. Pleural malignancy presents radiographically as multiple discrete pleural masses or lobulated pleural thickening. The pleural lesions are often obscured by an associated malignant pleural effusion. Contrast-enhanced CT can distinguish solid pleural masses from loculated pleural fluid and can show discrete pleural masses or thickening in patients with large effusions. In contrast to benign pleural thickening, malignant pleural disease is more likely when the pleural thickening on CT is circumferential and nodular, greater than 1 cm in thickness, and/or involves the mediastinal pleura (9). Mesothelioma is radiographically indistinguishable from metastatic pleural disease and will be discussed in the next section. Chest wall invasion by pleural tumor, seen as rib destruction or soft tissue infiltration of the subcutaneous fat and musculature, is better appreciated on CT or MR than on plain films. The diagnosis of malignant pleural disease is made by cytologic examination of fluid obtained at thoracentesis, closed or thoracoscopically guided pleural biopsy, or by thoracotomy.

Asbestos-Related Pleural Disease

Prolonged exposure to the inorganic fibers generically known as asbestos can result in a variety of pleural and pulmonary disorders. Benign pleural disease is the most common thoracic manifestation of asbestos inhalation and includes pleural plaques, pleural effusions, and diffuse pleural fibrosis. Rounded atelectasis is reviewed in Chapter 12. Malignant asbestos-related pleural disease is manifested as malignant mesothelioma.

Benign Asbestos-Related Pleural Disease

Pleural plaques are the most common benign manifestation of asbestos inhalation. These plaques develop 20 to 30 years after the initial asbestos exposure and are more frequent with increasing length and severity of exposure. Asbestos plaques are found on the parietal pleura, most commonly over the diaphragm and lower posterolateral chest wall. The mediastinal pleural surface and costophrenic sulci are characteristically spared. The plaques are discrete, bilateral, slightly raised (2 to 10 mm thick) foci of pleural thickening that are pearly white and shiny in gross appearance. Histologically, the plaques are comprised of dense bands of collagen. Punctate or linear calcification within the plaques is common and is more frequent as the plaques enlarge. Asbestos bodies (short, straight asbestos fibers coated with iron and protein that microscopically look like small dumbbells) are not seen within the plaques. Visceral pleural plaques, seen as discrete flat regions of pleural thickening within the major fissures on HRCT, are most commonly associated with interstitial fibrosis. Most patients with isolated asbestos-related pleural plaques are asymptomatic.

Detection of pleural plaques on conventional radiographs is best performed with 45° oblique views that profile the anterolateral and posterolateral plaques. When viewed en face, the calcified plaques appear as geographic areas of opacity that have been likened to a holly leaf (Figs. 19.12, 19.13). CT and HRCT studies are extremely sensitive in detecting calcified and noncalcified pleural plaques in asbestos-exposed individuals and can distinguish pleural plaques and diffuse pleural fibrosis from subpleural fat deposits that may mimic pleural disease on conventional radiographs. Although plaques are invariably bilateral on gross examination of the pleural space in affected individuals, it is not unusual to see unilateral plaques (most often left-sided) on conventional radiographs or HRCT.

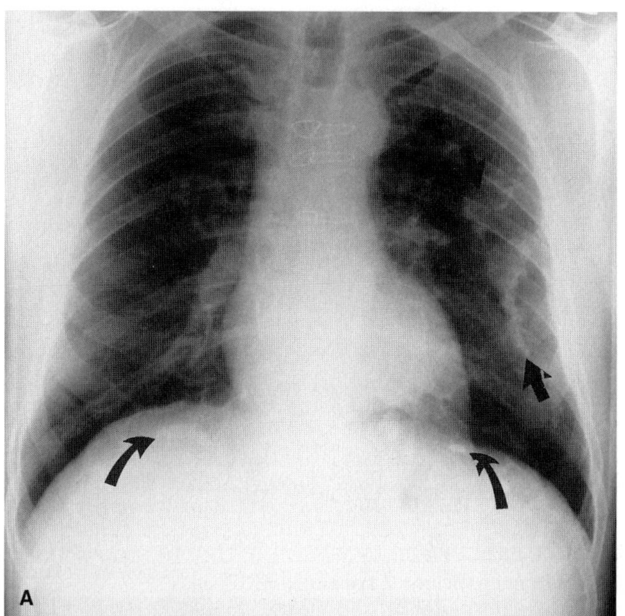

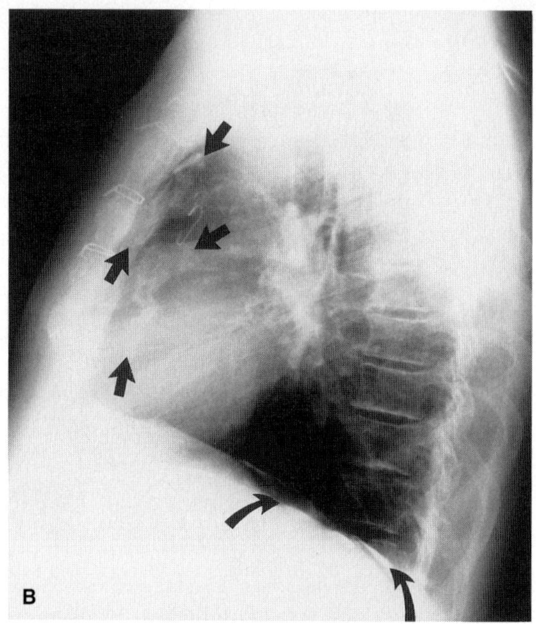

FIGURE 19.12. **Calcified Pleural Plaques.** Posteroanterior **(A)** and lateral **(B)** chest films in a 64-year-old man show bilateral diaphragmatic (*curved arrows*) and anterolateral (*straight arrows*) pleural plaques, reflecting prior asbestos exposure.

Pleural effusion occurs 10 to 20 years after the initial exposure and is the earliest manifestation of asbestos-related pleural disease. The development of asbestos-related effusions appears to be dose related. The effusions

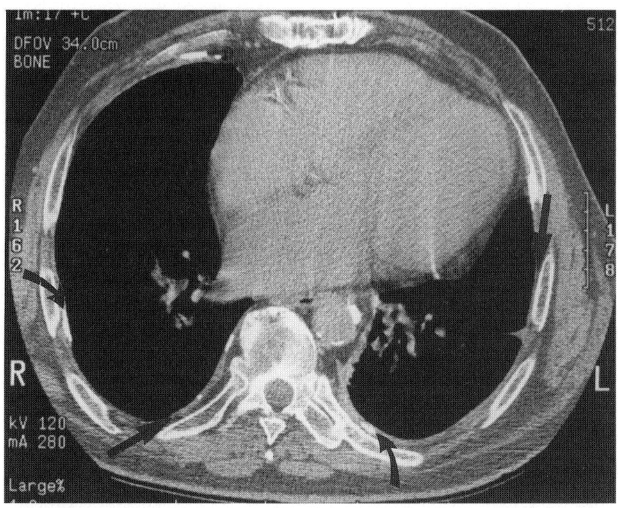

FIGURE 19.13. **Pleural Plaques and Diffuse Pleural Thickening From Asbestos Exposure.** HRCT in a 69-year-old man with benign asbestos-related pleural disease demonstrates bilateral thickening (*straight arrows*) and calcified pleural plaques (*curved arrows*).

are usually small, unilateral or bilateral, and exudative and may be bloody. The diagnosis of a benign asbestos-related pleural effusion is one of exclusion and, in addition to a history of exposure, requires the exclusion of TB or pleural malignancy (i.e., mesothelioma or metastatic adenocarcinoma). A long latency period between the initial exposure and the development of pleural effusion (>20 years) should prompt a diagnostic evaluation for malignant mesothelioma. While most asbestos-related pleural effusions resolve spontaneously, up to one third recur and some patients develop diffuse pleural fibrosis.

Diffuse pleural thickening or fibrosis may follow asbestos-related pleural effusion or result from the confluence of pleural plaques. Diffuse asbestos pleural thickening is defined as smooth, flat pleural thickening extending over one fourth of the costal pleural surface. In distinction to pleural plaques, which affect the parietal pleura alone, diffuse pleural fibrosis involves both the parietal and visceral pleura. Radiographically, diffuse pleural thickening is seen as a smooth thickening of the pleura involving the lower thorax with blunting of the costophrenic sulci. CT and HRCT are useful to determine the extent of pleural thickening, involvement of the interlobar fissures, and to detect underlying fibrotic or emphysematous lung disease (Fig. 19.13). Diffuse pleural fibrosis can result in symptomatic restrictive lung disease.

Malignant Asbestos-Related Pleural Disease

Malignant mesothelioma is a rare malignant pleural neoplasm associated with asbestos exposure. Unlike other pleural and parenchymal manifestations of asbestos, it does not appear to be dose related. Mesothelioma most often occurs 30 to 40 years after the initial exposure. Although the incidence increases with heavy exposure, malignant mesothelioma may also develop after minimal exposure and contrasts with the linear relationship between the development of benign asbestos pleural disease and the dose of asbestos exposure. Crocidolite is the fiber type most often implicated in the development of malignant mesothelioma, although chrysotile likely accounts for the majority of asbestos-related mesotheliomas, because it is the most widely used form of asbestos. Pathologically, mesothelioma is divided into epithelial, sarcomatous, and mixed types, with the epithelial form the most common and associated with a better prognosis than the sarcomatous and mixed subtypes.

Mesothelioma typically grows by contiguous spread from the pleural space into the lung, chest wall, mediastinum, and diaphragm; distant metastases are not uncommon. It most often appears radiographically as thick (>1 cm) and lobulated diffuse pleural thickening (10). Calcification or, rarely, ossification is seen in 20% of tumors, although calcified pleural plaques may be seen in uninvolved areas of the pleura. A pleural effusion is often present, which, if large, may obscure the pleural tumor. Malignant involvement of the mediastinal pleural surface may prevent contralateral mediastinal shift despite extensive pleural tumor volume and effusion, a finding that may help distinguish mesothelioma from metastatic disease. CT is the imaging modality of choice in the evaluation of malignant mesothelioma and depicts the extent of pleural involvement and invasion of the chest wall and mediastinum (Fig. 19.14). Diaphragmatic invasion by tumor, best assessed by coronal MR or reformatted multidetector CT (MDCT) scans, is important only in those patients who are considered for resection (Fig. 19.15). Adenopathy is seen in the ipsilateral hilum and mediastinum in approximately 50% of patients. While the radiologic findings may be highly suggestive of mesothelioma, metastatic pleural malignancy can have a similar appearance, so histologic confirmation is necessary.

The diagnosis of malignant mesothelioma is made histologically and often requires the use of special stains. The epithelial type of malignant mesothelioma may be indistinguishable from adenocarcinoma on light microscopy. While surgical resection by pleurectomy or extrapleural pneumonectomy may benefit selected patients with limited disease and good pulmonary reserve, the median survival from the time of diagnosis is only 6 to 12 months.

CHEST WALL

Disorders of the soft tissues or bony structures of the chest wall may come to attention because of local symptoms

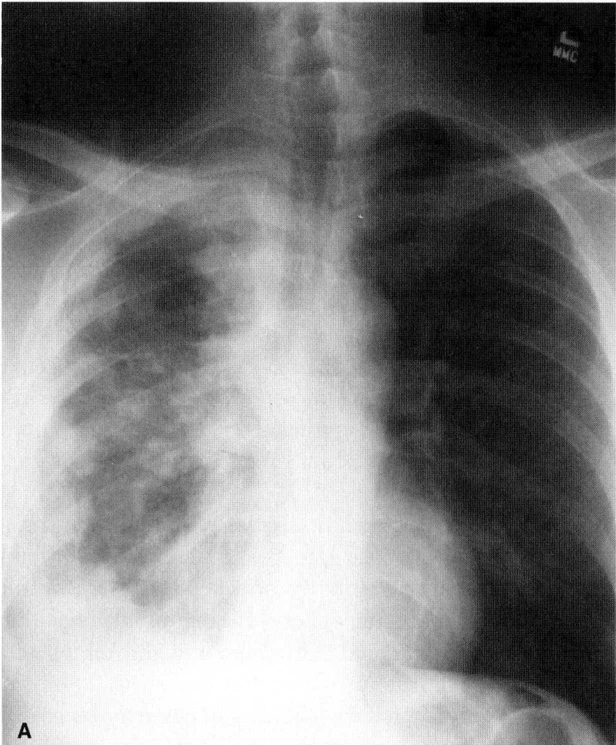

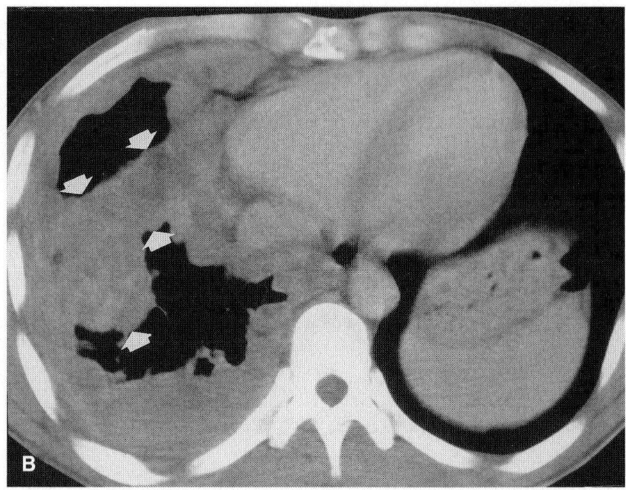

FIGURE 19.14. **Malignant Mesothelioma. A.** A posteroanterior chest radiograph in a 34-year-old man evaluated for a positive purified protein derivative tuberculin skin test (PPD) reveals lobulated right pleural thickening encompassing the right lung. **B.** A CT scan through the lung bases demonstrates a circumferential pleural soft tissue process traversing the major fissure (*arrows*). US-guided pleural biopsy revealed malignant mesothelioma.

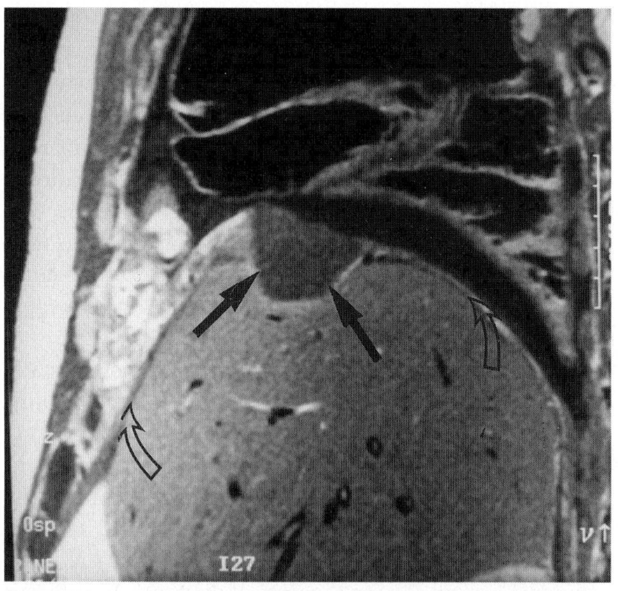

FIGURE 19.15. **Diaphragmatic Invasion of Malignant Mesothelioma on MR.** Sagittal T1WI through the dome of the right hemidiaphragm in a 53-year-old man with known pleural mesothelioma shows a basilar pleural mass (*straight arrows*) invading through the right diaphragm (*curved arrows*) into the liver. Laparoscopy confirmed the MR findings, which rendered the patient unresectable.

or physical findings, during evaluation of pulmonary or pleural disease, or as an incidental finding on radiographic studies (Table 19.6).

Soft Tissues

Congenital absence of the pectoralis muscle results in hyperlucency of the affected hemithorax on frontal

TABLE 19.6 Chest Wall Lesions

Tumors	Benign
	Mole
	Nevus
	Wart
	Neurofibroma
	Lipoma
	Hemangioma
	Desmoid
	Malignant
	Fibrosarcoma
	Liposarcoma
	Metastases
	Melanoma
	Bronchogenic carcinoma
	Askin tumor (primitive neuroectodermal tumor)
Infection (abscess)	*Staphylococcus*
	Tuberculosis
Trauma	Hematoma

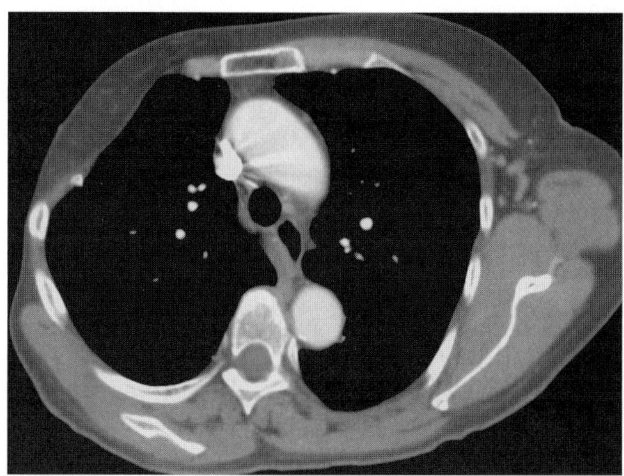

FIGURE 19.16. **Poland Syndrome.** Contrast-enhanced CT in a 62-year-old woman with Poland syndrome shows hypoplasia of right anterior ribs with absence of right pectoral muscles.

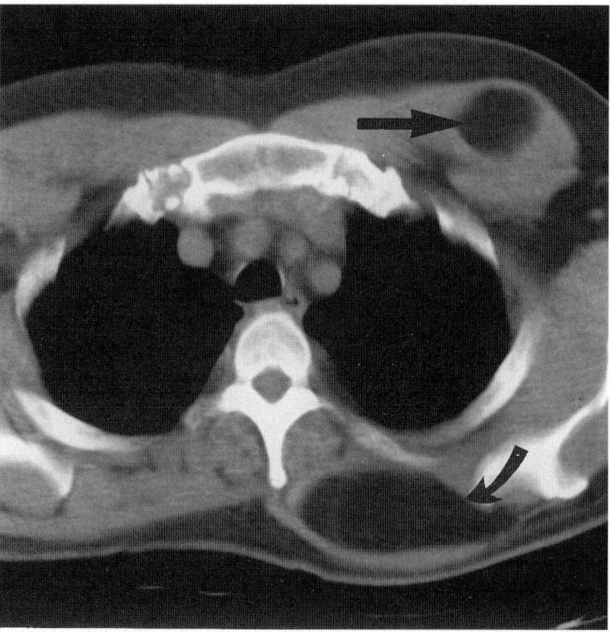

FIGURE 19.17. **Chest Wall Lipomas.** Unenhanced CT scan shows sharply circumscribed homogeneous fatty masses in the left pectoral (*straight arrows*) and rhomboid major (*curved arrows*) muscles.

radiographs. *Poland syndrome* is an autosomal recessive disorder characterized by unilateral absence of the sternocostal head of the pectoralis major, ipsilateral syndactyly, and rib anomalies. There may be associated aplasia of the ipsilateral breast (Fig. 19.16). Patients who have had a mastectomy will also show unilateral hyperlucency. In those who have undergone a modified radical mastectomy, the horizontally oriented inferior edge of the hypertrophied pectoralis minor muscle may be identified on frontal radiographs.

A variety of skin lesions such as moles, nevi, warts, neurofibromas, and accessory nipples may produce a nodular opacity on frontal radiographs that mimics a solitary pulmonary nodule. Examination of the skin surface should be performed in any patient with a new nodular opacity seen on chest radiographs, and repeat radiographs obtained with a radiopaque marker over the skin lesion will confirm the nature of the opacity and avoid unnecessary follow-up radiographs and chest CT.

Chest wall abscesses may present as localized, painful, fluctuant subcutaneous masses. *Staphylococcus* and *Mycobacterium tuberculosis* are the most common organisms responsible. The diagnosis is usually obvious clinically. Chest radiographs demonstrate a poorly defined opacity on the frontal radiograph when the abscess involves the anterior or posterior chest wall. CT shows a localized fluid collection with an enhancing wall and is used to determine the location and extent of the collection prior to open drainage.

Soft tissue neoplasms of the chest wall are rare (11). They are most often detected clinically as a mass protruding from the chest wall and appear as nonspecific extrathoracic soft tissue masses on chest radiographs. The most common benign neoplasm of the chest wall is a lipoma. Lipomas may be intrathoracic or extrathoracic, or they may project partially within and outside the thorax (dumbbell lipoma). CT shows a sharply circumscribed mass of fatty density (Fig. 19.17), while MR shows characteristic high and intermediate signal intensity on T1WIs and T2WIs, respectively. A desmoid tumor is a rare fibroblastic tumor arising within striated muscle that is histologically benign but has a tendency for local invasion. Desmoids are most common in the abdominal wall musculature of multiparous women but may arise in the chest wall musculature following local trauma. Hemangiomas are uncommon chest wall tumors. While they are often indistinguishable from other soft tissue tumors radiographically, the recognition of phleboliths, hypertrophy of involved bones, or the identification of vascular channels on contrast-enhanced CT or MR studies should suggest the diagnosis.

Fibrosarcomas and liposarcomas are the most common malignant soft tissue neoplasms of the chest wall in adults. Malignant tumors often present with symptoms of localized chest wall pain and a visible, palpable mass. Patients who have received chest wall radiation are at particular risk for developing sarcomas. Radiographically, these soft tissue masses are often associated with bony destruction. CT best depicts the bone destruction and intrathoracic component of tumor, while MR shows the extent of tumor and delineates tumor from surrounding muscle and subcutaneous fat (8). A rare malignant neoplasm arising from the chest wall of children and young adults is an Askin tumor, which arises from primitive neuroectodermal

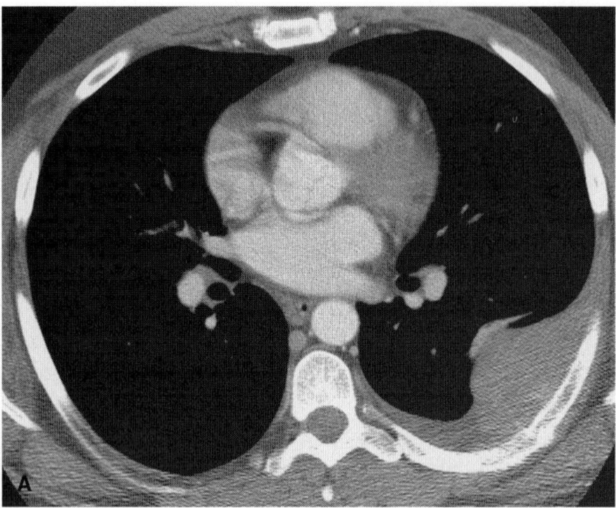

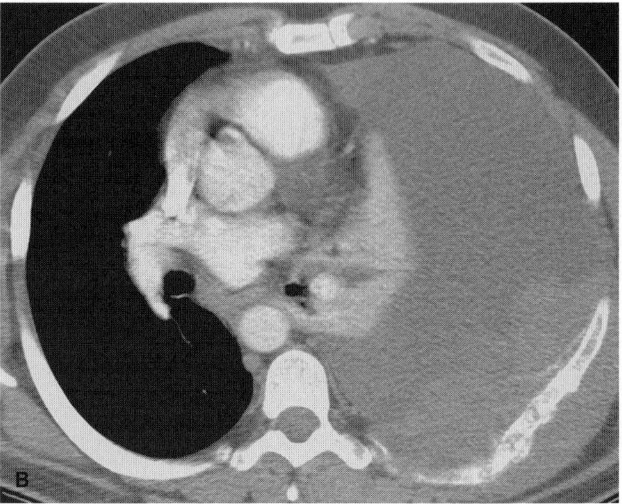

FIGURE 19.18. **Askin Tumor (Primitive Neuroectodermal Tumor) of Chest Wall. A.** Contrast-enhanced CT in a 32-year-old man demonstrates a left pleural mass with adjacent involvement of the rib and associated pleural effusion. **B.** Repeat CT obtained 1 month later shows enlargement of the mass with progressive rib involvement and a large pleural effusion with contralateral mediastinal shift. Surgical resection revealed an Askin tumor.

rests in the chest wall (Fig. 19.18). These lesions are very aggressive and associated with a high mortality rate.

The Bony Thorax

Congenital Anomalies (Table 19.7). The most common congenital anomalies of the ribs are bony fusion and bifid ribs, neither of which have clinical significance. Intrathoracic ribs are extremely rare congenital anomalies where an accessory rib arises from a vertebral body or the posterior surface of a rib and extends inferolaterally into the thorax, usually on the right side. Osteogenesis imperfecta and neurofibromatosis may be associated with thin, wavy, "ribbon" ribs. A relatively common congenital anomaly is the cervical rib, which arises from the seventh cervical vertebral body. Cervical ribs are usually asymptomatic, although in a minority of individuals with the thoracic outlet syndrome, the rib or associated fibrous bands can compress the subclavian artery, producing secondary ischemic symptoms, or compress the subclavian vein and brachial plexus, producing pain, weakness, and swelling of the upper extremity. Surgical resection of the cervical rib can relieve the symptoms in selected patients.

Rib notching is seen in a variety of pathologic conditions. Inferior rib notching is much more common than superior rib notching and is caused by enlargement of one or more of the structures that lie in the subcostal grooves (intercostal nerve, artery, or vein). The notching predominantly affects the posterior aspects of the ribs bilaterally and may be narrow, wide, deep, or shallow.

The most common cause of bilateral inferior rib notching is coarctation of the aorta distal to the origin of the left subclavian artery. In this condition, blood circumvents the aortic obstruction and reaches the descending aorta via the subclavian, internal mammary, and intercostal arteries. The increased blood flow in the intercostal arteries produces tortuosity and dilatation of these vessels, which erodes the inferior margins of the adjacent ribs. Other causes of aortic obstruction that can lead to inferior rib notching include aortic thrombosis and Takayasu aortitis. Congenital heart diseases associated with decreased pulmonary blood flow may be associated with rib notching as the intercostal arteries enlarge in an attempt to supply collateral blood flow to the oligemic lungs. Superior vena cava obstruction can cause increased flow through intercostal veins and produce rib notching.

Patients with aortic coarctation develop rib notching gradually; it is most common in adolescents and is rare in children under age 7. The first two ribs are uninvolved because the first and second intercostal arteries arise from the superior intercostal branch of the costocervical trunk of the subclavian artery and therefore do not communicate with the descending thoracic aorta. Coarctation may produce unilateral left rib notching when the aortic narrowing occurs proximal to an aberrant right subclavian artery. Unilateral right-sided notching occurs when the coarctation is proximal to the left subclavian artery. Additional causes of unilateral inferior rib notching include subclavian artery obstruction and surgical anastomosis of the proximal subclavian artery to the ipsilateral pulmonary artery (Blalock-Taussig procedure)

Multiple intercostal neurofibromas in neurofibromatosis type 1 are the most common nonvascular cause of inferior rib notching. The neurofibromas appear as multiple

TABLE 19.7 Rib Lesions

Congenital	Fusion anomalies
	Cervical rib
	Ribbon ribs
	Rib notching
	Inferior
	Coarctation of the aorta
	Tetralogy of Fallot
	Superior vena cava obstruction
	Blalock-Taussig shunt (unilateral right)
	Neurofibromatosis
	Superior
	Paralysis
	Collagen vascular disease
	Rheumatoid arthritis
	Systemic lupus erythematosus
Trauma	Healing rib fracture
Nonneoplastic tumors	Fibrous dysplasia
	Eosinophilic granuloma
	Brown tumor
Neoplasms	Benign
	Osteochondroma
	Enchondroma
	Osteoblastoma
	Malignant
	Primary
	Chondrosarcoma
	Osteogenic sarcoma
	Fibrosarcoma
	Metastatic
	Multiple myeloma
	Metastases
	Breast carcinoma
	Bronchogenic carcinoma
	Renal cell carcinoma
	Prostate carcinoma
Osteomyelitis	*Staphylococcus aureus*
	Tuberculosis
	Actinomycosis
	Nocardiosis

extrapleural soft tissue masses, most often seen in the upper paravertebral regions. Other thoracic bony manifestations of neurofibromatosis include ribbon ribs, thoracic kyphoscoliosis, and scalloping of the posterior aspect of the vertebral bodies caused by dural ectasia.

Superior rib notching is much less common than inferior rib notching. The pathogenesis of superior rib notching is unknown, although a disturbance of osteoblastic and osteoclastic activity and the stress effect of the intercostal muscles are proposed mechanisms. Paralysis is the most common condition associated with superior rib notching. Other etiologies include rheumatoid arthritis, systemic lupus erythematosus, and rarely, marked tortuosity of the intercostal arteries from severe, long-standing aortic obstruction.

Trauma. Rib and costal cartilage fractures may result from blunt or penetrating trauma to a normal ribcage or from minimal trauma to abnormal ribs, such as those affected by metastases. An acute rib fracture is seen as a thin vertical lucency; malalignment of the superior and inferior cortices of the rib may occasionally be the only radiographic finding. The tendency to affect the posterolateral aspects of the ribs explains the utility of obtaining ipsilateral posterior oblique radiographs for suspected fracture, because this projection best displays the fracture line. In any patient with an acute rib fracture, a careful search should be made for associated pneumothorax, hemothorax, and pulmonary contusion or laceration. Since the first three ribs are well protected by the clavicles, scapulae, and shoulder girdles, fracture of these ribs indicates severe trauma and should prompt a careful evaluation for associated great vessel and visceral injuries. Fracture of the tenth, eleventh, or twelfth ribs may be associated with injury to the liver or spleen. Severe blunt trauma to the ribcage, in which multiple contiguous ribs are fractured in more than one place, is termed a "flail chest." This results in a free segment of the chest wall that moves paradoxically inward on inspiration and outward on expiration. Healing rib fractures will demonstrate callus formation, which may be exuberant in patients receiving corticosteroids. Multiple contiguous healed rib fractures, particularly if bilateral, should suggest chronic alcoholism or a prior motor vehicle accident.

Nonneoplastic Lesions. The ribs are the most common site of involvement by monostotic fibrous dysplasia. The typical appearance is an expansile lesion in the posterior aspect of the rib with a lucent or ground-glass density; rarely, the lesion is sclerotic. Multiple rib involvement from polyostotic fibrous dysplasia can result in severe restrictive pulmonary disease. Eosinophilic granuloma can cause lytic lesions in patients under age 30. These are usually solitary lytic lesions, which can be expansile but do not have sclerotic margins; this latter feature helps distinguish these lesions from fibrous dysplasia (Fig. 19.19). Brown tumors from hyperparathyroidism can also produce lytic rib lesions.

Neoplasms. Primary osteochondral neoplasms or metastatic disease can involve the ribs. Osteochondromas are the most common benign neoplasm of ribs, followed in relative frequency by enchondromas and osteoblastomas (Fig. 19.20). Primary malignant neoplasms of the ribs in adults are uncommon. Chondrosarcoma is the most common primary rib malignancy, with osteogenic sarcoma and fibrosarcoma less common. Rib involvement from multiple myeloma or metastatic carcinoma can produce solitary or multiple lytic lesions and is much more common than primary tumors. Myeloma can also cause permeative bone destruction that is indistinguishable from severe osteoporosis. The diagnosis of myeloma is made by identification of a monoclonal spike on serum protein

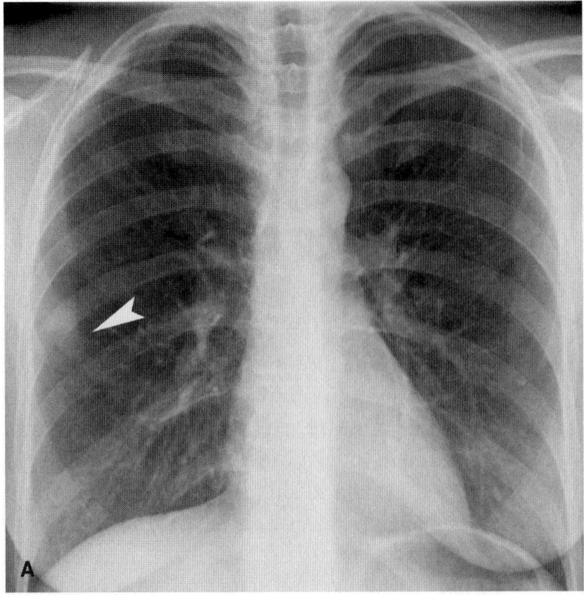

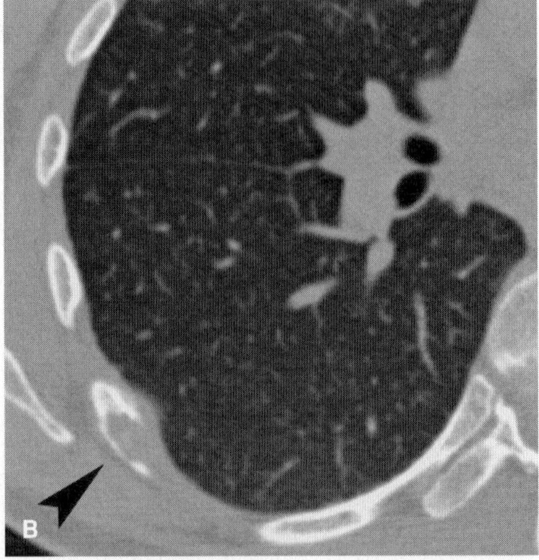

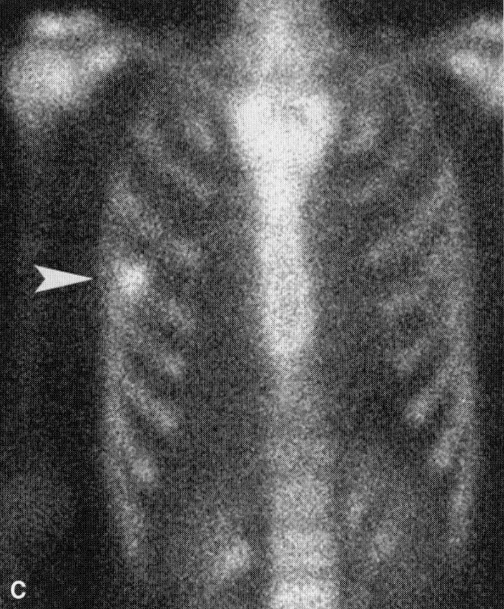

FIGURE 19.19. **Eosinophilic Granuloma of Rib.** Chest radiograph **(A)** in a 24-year-old with pleuritic chest pain shows a lytic lesion of the posterolateral right seventh rib (*arrowhead*). Thin-section CT **(B)** confirms the presence of an expansile lytic lesion (*arrowhead*), which was positive (*arrowhead*) on bone scan **(C).** Surgical resection showed eosinophilic granuloma of bone.

electrophoresis and typical findings of abnormal aggregates of plasma cells on bone marrow biopsy. The most common metastatic lesions to ribs are from bronchogenic and breast carcinoma, which produce multiple lytic lesions when dissemination is hematogenous or localized rib destruction when invasion is by direct contiguous spread. Expansile lytic rib metastases are seen most commonly from renal cell and thyroid carcinoma. Sclerotic rib metastases are most commonly seen in breast and prostate carcinoma.

Infection. Chest wall infection and osteomyelitis of the ribs usually develop from contiguous spread from the lung, pleural space, and vertebral column. Less commonly, infection complicates penetrating chest trauma or spreads to the ribs hematogenously. Pleuropulmonary infections that may traverse the pleural space and produce a chest wall infection include TB, actinomycosis, and nocardiosis. Radiographs may demonstrate bone destruction, periostitis, and subcutaneous emphysema; bone scans can detect subradiographic bone involvement. CT can demonstrate bone destruction, soft tissue swelling, and abscesses within the chest wall. Additionally, CT may show involvement of the adjacent pleural space, lung, sternum, or vertebral column.

Costal Cartilages. Ossification of the costal cartilages is a normal finding on frontal chest radiographs in adults. Female costal cartilage ossification involves the central portion of the cartilage, extending from the rib toward the sternum in the shape of a solitary finger, while male costal cartilage ossification involves the peripheral portion of the cartilage and has the appearance of two fingers ("peace" sign). These typical patterns of male and female costal cartilage ossification are seen in 70% of patients (Fig. 19.21) and do not apply to the first rib.

Scapula. Scapular abnormalities that are visible on frontal radiographs include congenital, posttraumatic, and neoplastic lesions. *Sprengel deformity* is a congenital anomaly in which the scapula is hypoplastic and elevated. The association of Sprengel deformity with an

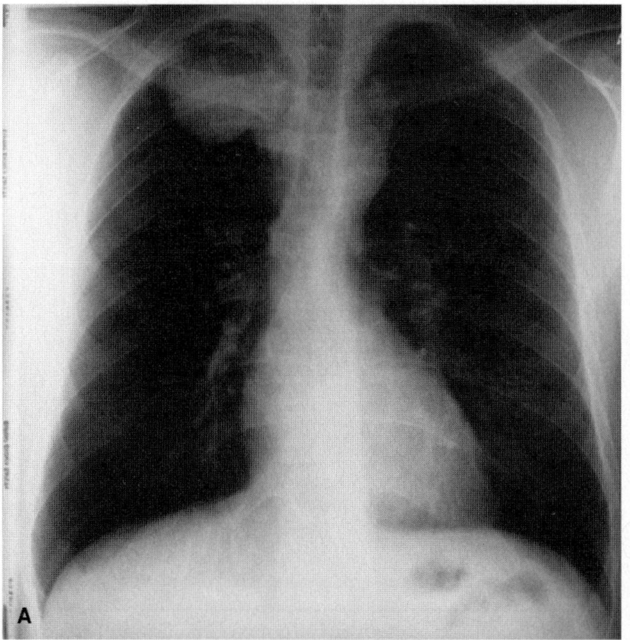

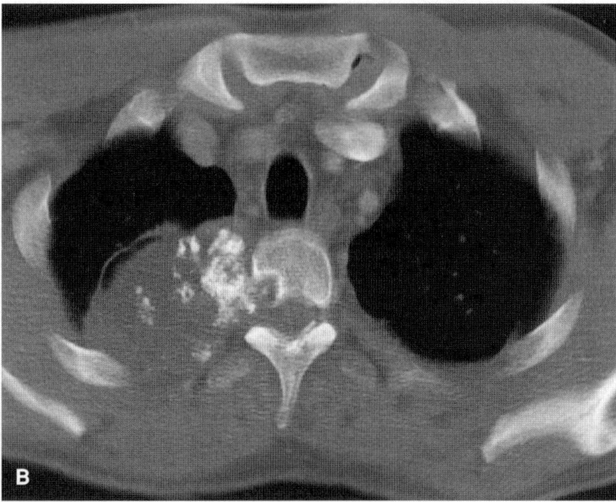

FIGURE 19.20. **Chondrosarcoma of Rib. A.** Posteroanterior chest radiograph in a 37-year-old man with a 3-month history of right shoulder pain demonstrates a right apical extrapulmonary mass. **B.** A CT scan reveals a bone-forming mass arising from the right third costotransverse junction, with erosion of the adjacent vertebral body. This chondrosarcoma was successfully resected by a combined thoracic and neurosurgical approach.

omovertebral bone, fused cervical vertebrae, hemivertebrae, kyphoscoliosis, and rib anomalies is termed the *Klippel-Feil syndrome.* Scapular fractures may result from direct trauma to the upper back and shoulder or from impaction of the humeral head into the glenoid. A winged scapula is identified when the scapula is superiorly displaced from its normal position and the inferior portion is posteriorly displaced from the chest wall, thereby foreshortening its appearance on the frontal radiograph. This deformity results from disruption in the innervation of

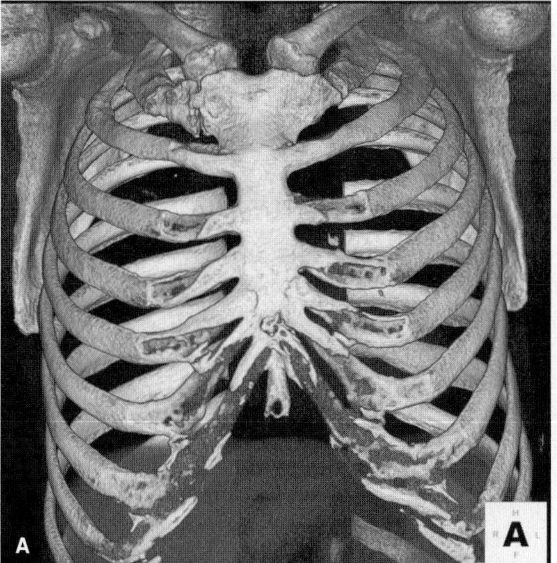

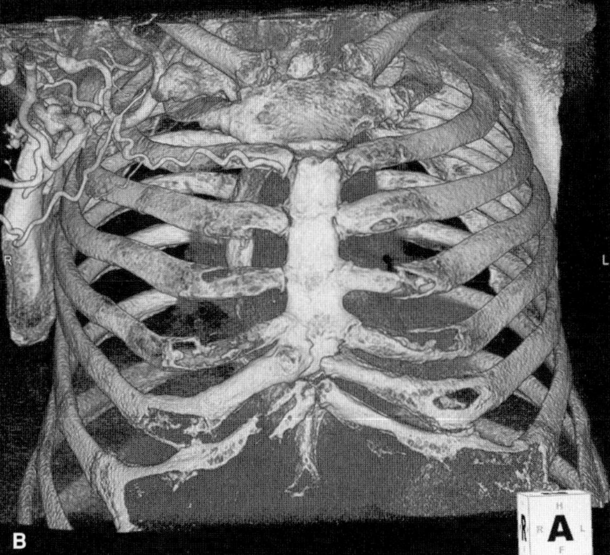

FIGURE 19.21. **Normal Ossification Patterns in Men and Women.** Shaded-surface three-dimensional reconstructions of the anterior chest wall show typical ossification patterns of costal cartilages in a woman **(A)** and a man **(B)**.

the serratus anterior muscle that maintains the scapula against the chest wall. Metastatic disease to the scapula is recognized by the presence of lytic destructive lesions; bronchogenic and breast carcinomas are the most common primary malignancies.

Clavicle. A variety of diseases can affect the clavicle. The clavicle is involved in cleidocranial dysostosis, in which there is partial or complete aplasia of the clavicle. The distal third of the clavicle is commonly fractured in blunt trauma. Rheumatoid arthritis and hyperparathyroidism are associated with erosion of the distal clavicles. The distal clavicle is sharply defined in rheumatoid arthritis and tapers to a point, whereas in hyperparathyroidism it is often widened and irregular. Additional findings in rheumatoid arthritis include narrowing of the glenohumeral joint and a high riding humeral head caused by rotator cuff atrophy. Primary malignant neoplasms of the clavicle include Ewing or osteogenic sarcoma. Metastases to the clavicle are usually associated with lesions in other portions of the bony thorax. Osteomyelitis of the clavicle is uncommon and is most often seen in intravenous drug users. Paget disease can involve the clavicle, but there is often concomitant pelvic bone and calvarial involvement.

Thoracic Spine. Numerous thoracic spine abnormalities are visible on chest radiographs. Congenital anomalies, including hemivertebrae, butterfly vertebra, spina bifida, and scoliosis, can be seen on well-penetrated frontal radiographs. Vertebral compression fractures caused by trauma, osteoporosis, or metastases are best seen on lateral radiographs and may produce an exaggerated kyphosis. Large bridging osteophytes may mimic a paraspinal mass on frontal radiographs or a pulmonary nodule on lateral films. Vertebral osteomyelitis is seen as destruction of vertebral bodies and intervertebral discs, often associated with a paraspinal abscess (Fig. 19.22). Chronic anemia in patients with thalassemia major or sickle cell disease may result in prevertebral or paravertebral masses of extramedullary hematopoiesis, which represent herniated hyperplastic bone marrow. Sickle cell anemia produces a characteristic appearance of H-shaped or "Lincoln log" vertebrae on lateral chest radiographs that is pathognomonic of this disease. Similarly, a "rugger jersey" appearance to the thoracic spine on lateral chest films suggests renal osteosclerosis.

Sternum. Developmental sternal deformities include pectus excavatum (funnel chest), pectus carinatum (pigeon breast), and abnormal segmentation. In pectus excavatum, the sternum is inwardly depressed and the ribs protrude anterior to the sternum. It often has an autosomal dominant pattern of inheritance but may occur sporadically. Pectus excavatum is commonly associated with congenital connective tissue disorders, such as Marfan syndrome, Poland syndrome, osteogenesis imperfecta, and congenital scoliosis. Most patients are asymptomatic. A clinically insignificant systolic murmur can result from compression of the right ventricular outflow tract, although some patients with pectus deformities and systolic murmurs have mitral valve prolapse. Pectus excavatum has a characteristic appearance on frontal chest radiograph. The heart is displaced to the left, and the combination of the depressed soft tissues of the anterior chest wall and the vertically oriented anterior ribs results in loss of the right heart border. The findings on frontal radiographs may be mistakenly attributed to middle lobe opacification from pneumonia or atelectasis. The typical inward depression of the midsternum and lower sternum is seen on lateral chest radiographs (Fig. 19.23). CT helps define the deformity and its effect upon the heart and mediastinal structures.

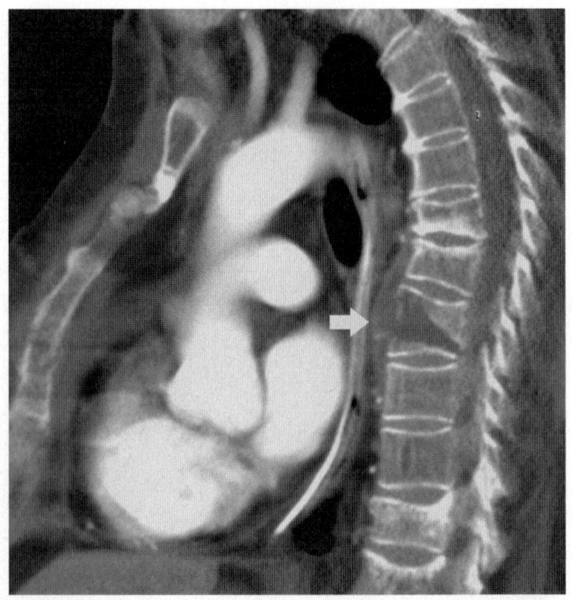

FIGURE 19.22. **Vertebral Osteomyelitis.** Sagittal maximum intensity projection reconstruction in a 72-year-old woman with back pain and staphylococcal sepsis shows an expansile lesion (*arrow*) of a midthoracic vertebral body with prevertebral soft tissue mass. CT-guided aspiration of the paravertebral mass revealed *Staphylococcus*.

Pectus carinatum is an outward bowing of the sternum that may be congenital or acquired. The congenital form is seen more commonly in boys and in families with a history of chest wall deformities or scoliosis. Congenital atrial or ventricular septal defects and severe childhood asthma account for the majority of the acquired cases of pectus carinatum. Affected patients are asymptomatic. The characteristic outward bowing of the sternum with deepening of the retrosternal airspace is seen on lateral radiographs.

Severe blunt trauma to the chest, most often associated with deceleration injury from a motor vehicle accident, can result in fracture or dislocation of the sternum. Sternal body fracture and sternomanubrial dislocation are associated with a 25% to 45% mortality rate from concomitant

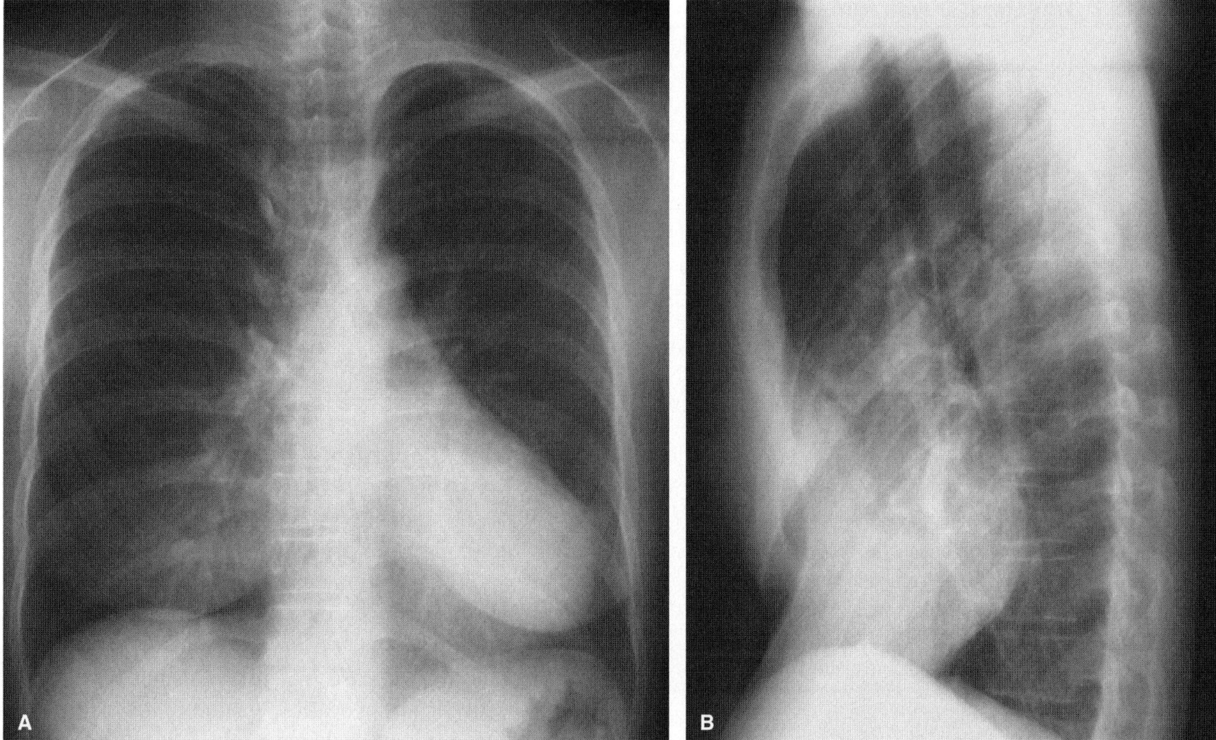

FIGURE 19.23. **Pectus Excavatum.** Posteroanterior **(A)** and lateral **(B)** chest radiographs show changes of pectus excavatum. Note the apparent middle lobe opacity that is typical of this condition.

injuries to the aorta, diaphragm, heart, tracheobronchial tree, and lung. Sternal films or lateral radiographs will show the fracture and often demonstrate a retrosternal hematoma; CT may be useful in those patients with normal plain films and a high suspicion of sternal injury.

A prior median sternotomy is the most common sternal abnormality seen on conventional radiographs and chest CT. Circular wires encompassing the sternum are seen spaced along its length within the interspaces between costal cartilages. The vertical lucency representing the sternotomy may heal, but in many patients bony union does not occur. In the early postoperative period, a retrosternal hematoma may be seen, which normally resolves within the first several weeks. The radiologist plays a key role in the evaluation of possible sternal wound infection. Plain film evidence of bony destruction and air in the sternal incision appearing days to weeks after sternotomy are specific but insensitive findings for osteomyelitis. Bone scans are not particularly useful, as there will be increased radionuclide uptake for months following sternotomy. CT is the modality of choice in the evaluation of sternal wound infection. The CT findings of sternal osteomyelitis include bone destruction, peristernal soft tissue mass, enhancing fluid collection, and gas. The extent of infection, specifically associated mediastinitis, can also be determined.

DIAPHRAGM

Unilateral Diaphragmatic Elevation. The differential diagnosis of unilateral diaphragmatic elevation is listed in Table 19.8. Eventration of the diaphragm is a result of congenital absence or underdevelopment of diaphragmatic musculature. This produces a localized elevation of the anteromedial portion of the hemidiaphragm on frontal radiographs in older individuals (Fig. 19.24), which is indistinguishable on the right from the rare foramen of Morgagni hernia. Complete diaphragmatic eventration is usually left sided and is indistinguishable radiographically from diaphragmatic paralysis.

Unilateral diaphragmatic paralysis is usually caused by surgical injury or neoplastic involvement of the phrenic nerve, which affects the right and left hemidiaphragms with equal frequency. Idiopathic phrenic nerve dysfunction resulting from a viral neuritis is a common cause of diaphragmatic paralysis in male patients and is usually right sided. A positive fluoroscopic or ultrasonographic sniff test (paradoxical superior movement of the diaphragm with sniffing, a result of the effects of negative intrathoracic pressure on a flaccid diaphragm during inspiration) is diagnostic.

Chronic loss of lung volume, particularly from collapse or resection of the lower lobe, results in diaphragmatic

TABLE 19.8 Unilateral Diaphragmatic Elevation

Eventration	
Diminished lung volume	Congenital
	Hypoplastic lung
	Acquired
	Lobar/lung atelectasis
	Pulmonary resection
Paralysis	Idiopathic
	Iatrogenic phrenic nerve injury
	Phrenic crush (tuberculosis)
	Intraoperative
	Malignant invasion of phrenic nerve
	Bronchogenic carcinoma
	Inflammation of diaphragmatic muscle
	Pleuritis
	Lower lobe pneumonia
	Subphrenic abscess
Upper abdominal mass	Hepatomegaly or liver mass
	Splenomegaly
	Gastric/colonic distention
	Ascites (usually bilateral)
	Diaphragmatic hernia*
	Subpulmonic pleural effusion*

*Apparent diaphragmatic elevation.

elevation. This is also a common sequela of chronic cicatrizing atelectasis of the upper lobe from TB.

An enlarged liver or hepatic mass can produce right hemidiaphragmatic elevation by direct pressure on the undersurface of the hemidiaphragm. Similarly, an enlarged spleen, gas-distended stomach, or enlarged splenic flexure can produce an elevated left hemidiaphragm. Irritation of the superior surface of the hemidiaphragm by a pleural or pleura-based parenchymal process (e.g., infarct, pneumonia) or of the undersurface of the diaphragm by a subphrenic abscess, hepatitis, or cholecystitis may cause the diaphragm to become flaccid, leading to elevation. A subpulmonic effusion may simulate an elevated hemidiaphragm.

Bilateral Diaphragmatic Elevation that is not effort related may be caused by a neuromuscular disturbance or intrathoracic or intra-abdominal disease. Radiographically, the diaphragms are elevated on both frontal and lateral views. Bibasilar linear atelectasis or passive lobar or segmental lower lobe atelectasis may be seen.

Bilateral phrenic nerve disruption or intrinsic diaphragmatic muscular disease will produce bilateral diaphragmatic paralysis and elevation. Common disorders include cervical cord injury, multiple sclerosis, and the myopathy

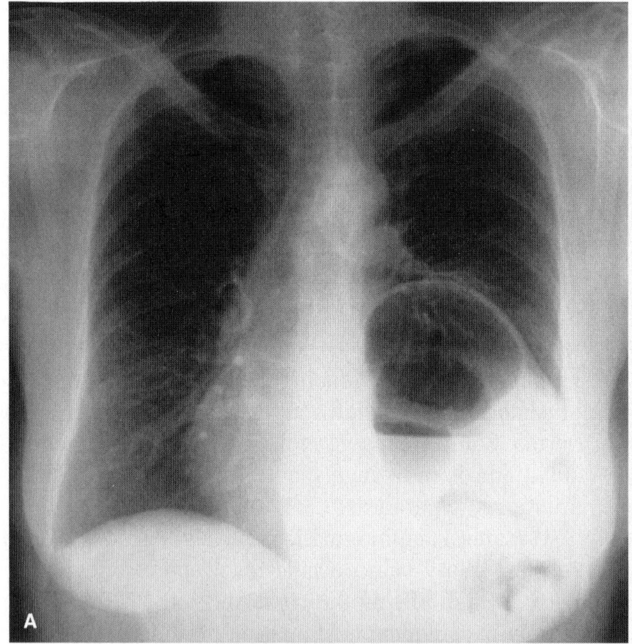

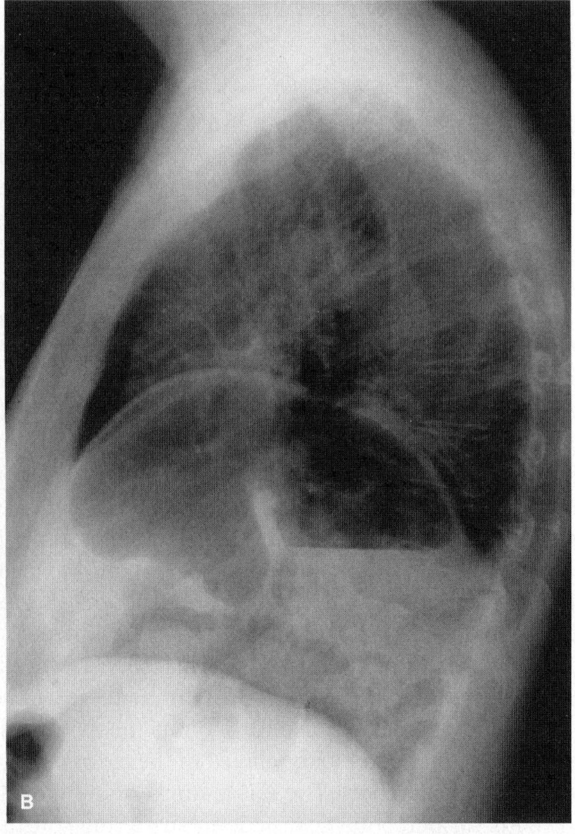

FIGURE 19.24. **Eventration of the Diaphragm.** Posteroanterior **(A)** and lateral **(B)** chest radiographs in an asymptomatic 61-year-old woman reveal marked elevation of the left hemidiaphragm representing diaphragmatic eventration.

associated with systemic lupus erythematosus. In these patients, fluoroscopic or real-time US imaging of the diaphragms demonstrates a positive sniff test.

Lung restriction caused by interstitial fibrosis, bilateral pleural fibrosis, or chest wall disease (most commonly from obesity) can produce bilateral diaphragmatic elevation. An increase in intra-abdominal volume, most often from ascites, hepatosplenomegaly, or pregnancy, can restrict diaphragmatic motion. These conditions may be distinguished from bilateral paralysis by observation of normal but diminished inferior excursion of the diaphragms on fluoroscopy, US, or inspiratory/expiratory radiographs.

Diaphragmatic Depression. Depression and flattening of one hemidiaphragm is seen with unilateral overinflation of a lung, usually as a compensatory mechanism when the contralateral lung is small or as a result of a large ipsilateral pneumothorax. Distinction between these two entities is usually possible by the clinical history and by characteristic findings in those with pneumothorax. A tension pneumothorax may cause inversion of the hemidiaphragm. Bilateral diaphragmatic depression is either a permanent finding—a result of abnormally increased lung compliance in patients with emphysema—or a transient finding in those with asthma and expiratory air trapping.

Diaphragmatic Hernias. There are three types of nontraumatic diaphragmatic hernias. The most common is the *esophageal hiatal hernia*, which represents herniation of a portion of the stomach through the esophageal hiatus. These are usually seen as incidental asymptomatic masses on chest radiographs, although some patients may have symptoms of gastroesophageal reflux or, rarely, severe pain from strangulation of the herniated stomach. Hiatal hernias are seen projecting behind the heart on frontal chest radiographs in the immediate supradiaphragmatic region of the posterior mediastinum. An air–fluid level may be seen in the hernia. An esophagram is confirmatory. CT shows widening of the esophageal hiatus and depicts the contents of the hernia sac, which often include stomach, omental fat, and, rarely, ascitic fluid (Fig. 19.25).

Bochdalek Hernia. The foramen of Bochdalek is a defect in the hemidiaphragm at the site of the embryonic pleuroperitoneal canal. Large hernias through the Bochdalek foramen present in the neonatal period with hypoplasia of the ipsilateral lung and respiratory distress. In adults, small hernias through this foramen are common and are predominantly seen on the left side, presumably because of the protective effect of the liver, which prevents herniation of right infradiaphragmatic fat through the right foramen of Bochdalek. The hernia typically appears as a

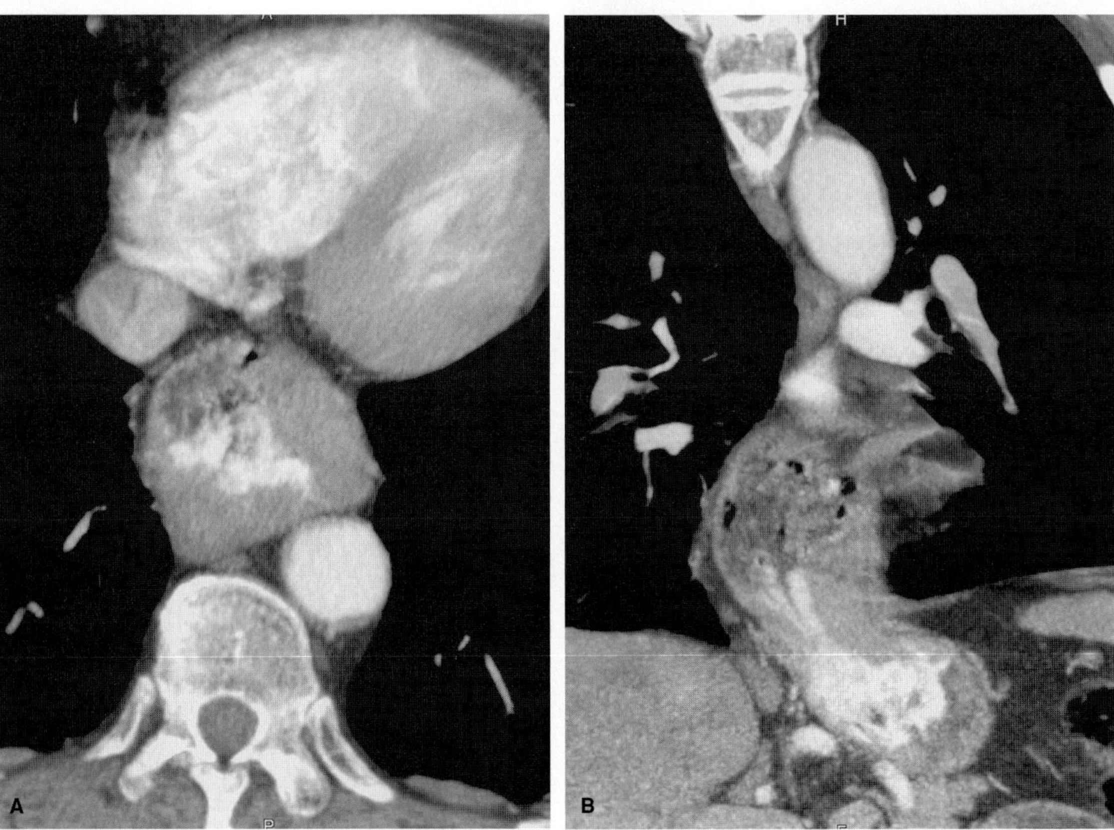

FIGURE 19.25. **Hiatal Hernia.** Axial **(A)** CT scan with coronal reconstruction **(B)** in a 73-year-old man shows a sliding hiatal hernia in the posterior mediastinum.

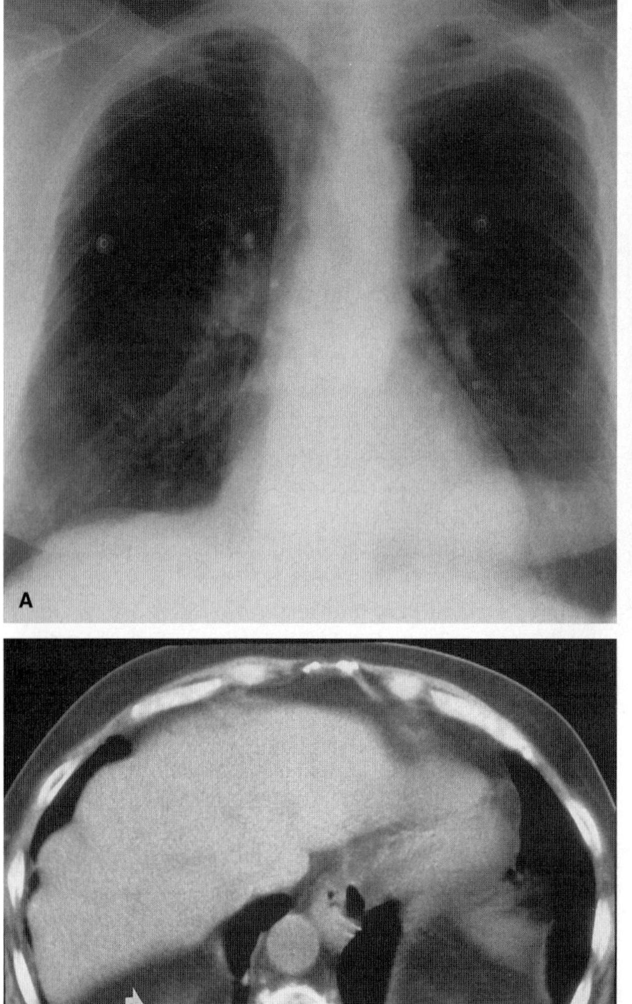

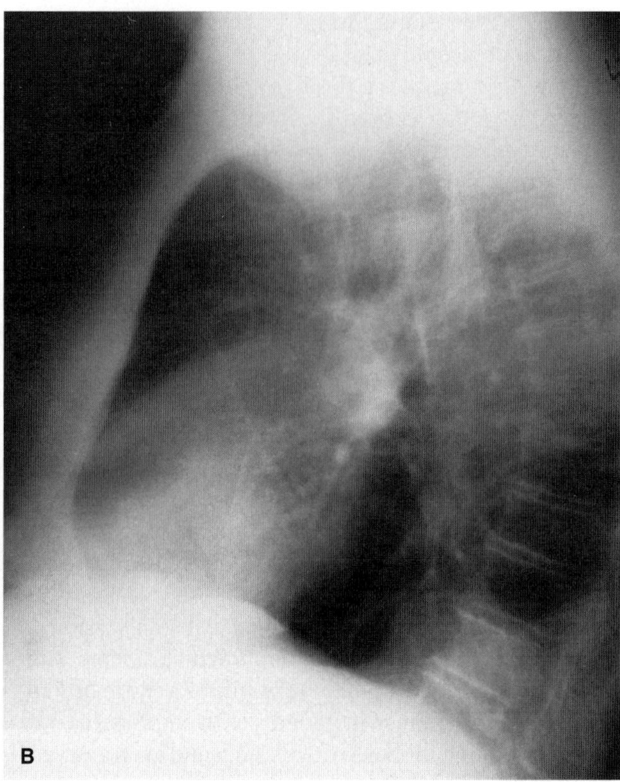

FIGURE 19.26. **Foramen of Bochdalek Hernia.** Posteroanterior **(A)** and lateral **(B)** chest radiographs in an asymptomatic 82-year-old man show a mass arising from the posterolateral aspect of the left hemidiaphragm. **C.** A CT scan through the diaphragm shows fat herniating through bilateral Bochdalek hernias. Note the top of the right kidney within the herniated fat (*arrow*).

posterolateral mass above the left hemidiaphragm, although it can occur anywhere along the posterior diaphragmatic surface (Fig. 19.26). CT shows the diaphragmatic defect with herniation of retroperitoneal fat, omentum, spleen, or kidney.

Morgagni Hernia. A defect in the parasternal portion of the diaphragm, the foramen of Morgagni, is the least common type of diaphragmatic hernia. A Morgagni hernia is invariably right sided and appears as an asymptomatic cardiophrenic angle mass. The diagnosis is made by noting herniation of omental fat, liver, or transverse colon through the paracardiac portion of the right hemidiaphragm on CT scans through the lung bases. The presence of omental vessels within a fatty paracardiac mass is diagnostic (Fig. 19.27). Coronal MR or US can demonstrate the diaphragmatic defect, distinguishing this entity from partial eventration of the hemidiaphragm.

Traumatic herniation of abdominal contents through a tear or rupture of the central or posterior aspect of the hemidiaphragm may follow blunt thoracoabdominal trauma or penetrating injury (12). The left side is affected in more than 90% of cases because the liver dissipates the traumatic forces and protects the right hemidiaphragm from injury (Fig. 19.28). Radiographically, the diagnosis should be suspected when the left hemidiaphragmatic contour is indistinct or elevated or when gas-filled loops of bowel or stomach are seen in the left lower thorax following severe trauma. Early diagnosis is often difficult because associated thoracic and abdominal injuries may obscure the clinical and radiographic findings. The diagnosis

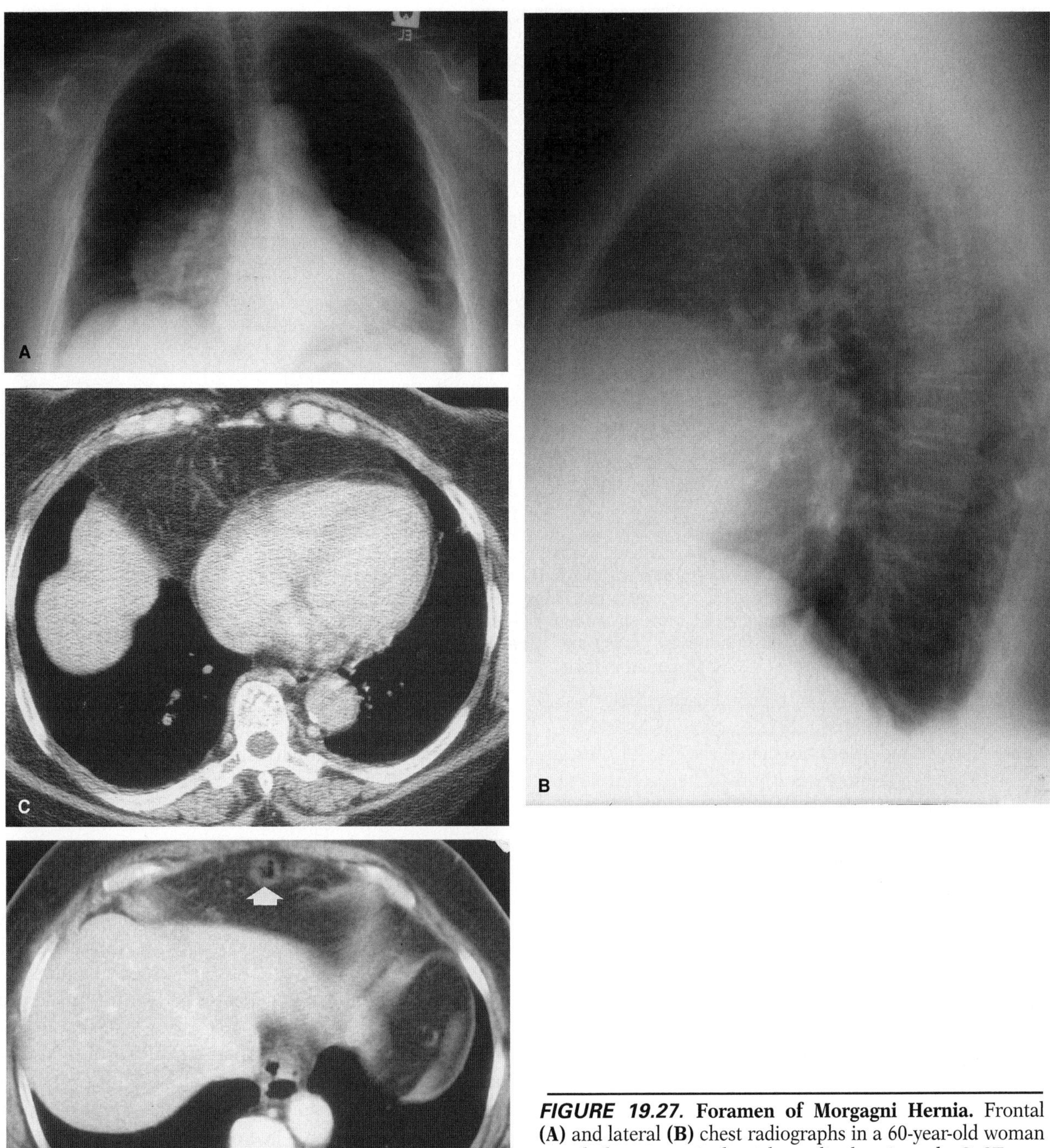

FIGURE 19.27. **Foramen of Morgagni Hernia.** Frontal **(A)** and lateral **(B)** chest radiographs in a 60-year-old woman reveal a large mass in the right cardiophrenic angle. **C.** CT scan at the level of the diaphragm shows a fatty pericardiac mass containing omental vessels. **D.** A more inferior scan demonstrates an abnormally high transverse colon (*arrow*), which is characteristic of this entity.

is often made after the traumatic episode, with symptoms caused by intestinal obstruction with strangulation (pain, vomiting, fever) or compression of the left lung (cough, dyspnea, chest pain). In addition to the stomach, the small intestine, colon, omentum, spleen, kidney, and the left lobe of the liver can also herniate through the defect. The diagnosis is usually made by upper or lower GI contrast studies demonstrating bowel herniating into the thorax through a constricting diaphragmatic defect. The resultant narrowing or "waist" of the herniated intestine as it traverses the diaphragmatic defect differentiates a hernia from simple diaphragmatic elevation. Large diaphragmatic defects may be demonstrated on MDCT scans with coronal and sagittal reconstructions, which also characterize the

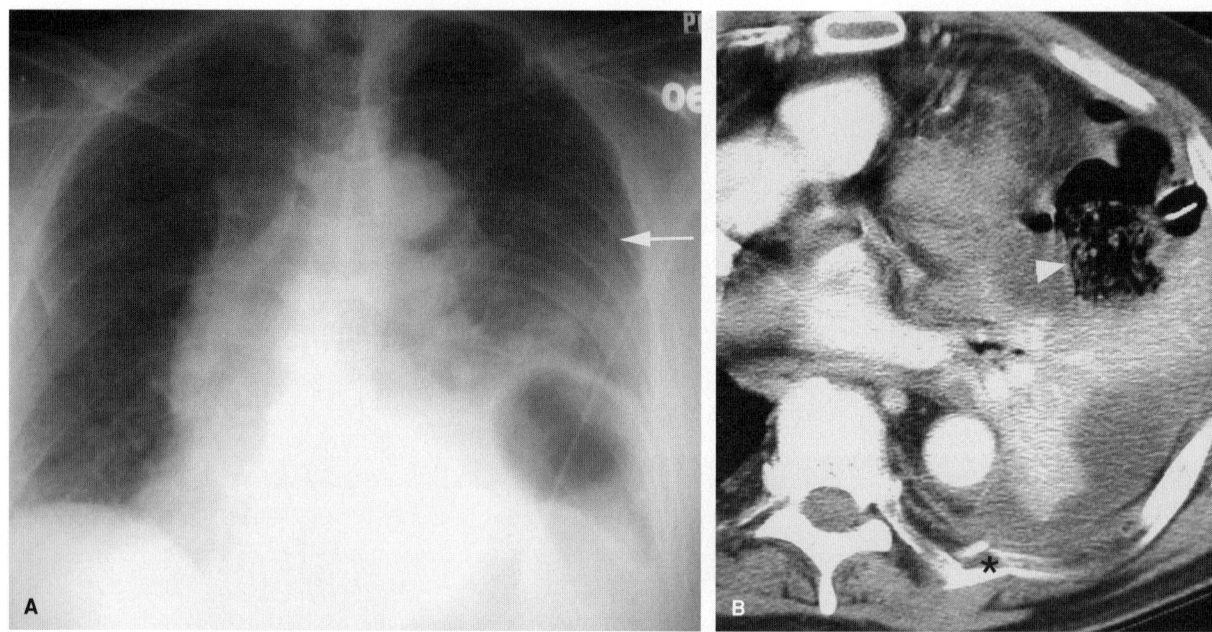

FIGURE 19.28. **Traumatic Diaphragmatic Hernia.** Frontal chest radiograph **(A)** in a 37-year-old man who sustained blunt chest trauma shows a left pneumothorax (*arrow*) and an apparently elevated left diaphragm. CT through the lower chest **(B)** shows colon (*arrowhead*) in the lower left thorax with surrounding atelectasis and effusion. Note the posterior rib fracture (*asterisk*). Surgery confirmed left diaphragmatic injury.

herniated tissues and detect associated visceral injuries. In addition to the detection of intrathoracic herniation of abdominal contents, MDCT can directly depict the diaphragmatic defect, even in the absence of visceral herniation. Other CT findings suggestive of traumatic diaphragmatic injury include thickening or retraction of the diaphragm away from the traumatic injury, a narrowing or waist of the diaphragm on the herniated viscus ("collar" or "waist" sign) and contact between the posterior ribs and the liver (right-sided injury) or stomach (left-sided injury), termed the "dependent viscera" sign. US or MR are difficult to obtain in the acute trauma setting but are occasionally useful (12).

Diaphragmatic Tumors. Primary diaphragmatic tumors are rare, with an equal incidence of benign and malignant lesions. Benign lesions include lipomas, fibromas, schwannomas, neurofibromas, and leiomyomas. Echinococcal cysts and extralobar sequestrations may be found within the diaphragm. Fibrosarcomas are the most common primary malignant diaphragmatic lesion. Radiographically, they appear as focal extrapulmonary masses obscuring all or part of the hemidiaphragm and are indistinguishable from masses arising within the diaphragmatic pleura. CT may show the origin of the mass, although the relationship of the mass to the diaphragm is best appreciated on coronal MR images or transabdominal US. Direct invasion of the diaphragm by lower lobe bronchogenic carcinoma, mesothelioma, or a subphrenic neoplasm is much more common than primary diaphragmatic malignancy.

CONGENITAL LUNG DISEASE

Bronchogenic cysts represent anomalous outpouchings of the primitive foregut that no longer communicate with the tracheobronchial tree. They are commonly present as asymptomatic mediastinal masses and are discussed in detail in Chapter 13.

Cystic adenomatoid malformation (CAM) is a lesion usually seen in newborn infants, although it occasionally presents in childhood or early adulthood. Three pathologic subtypes of CAM have been described. The most common subtype is comprised of one or several large cysts that are lined by respiratory epithelium with scattered mucous glands, smooth muscle, and elastic tissue in their walls. Multiple smaller cystic structures are present in the intervening lung between the larger cysts. Radiographically, these lesions often appear as round, air-filled masses, which exert mass effect on the adjacent lung and mediastinum (Fig. 19.29). A CAM in the left lower lobe may be difficult to distinguish from a congenital diaphragmatic hernia. Delayed clearance of fetal fluid in the newborn may give the radiographic appearance of an intrapulmonary soft tissue mass. These lesions may be identified on prenatal US examination.

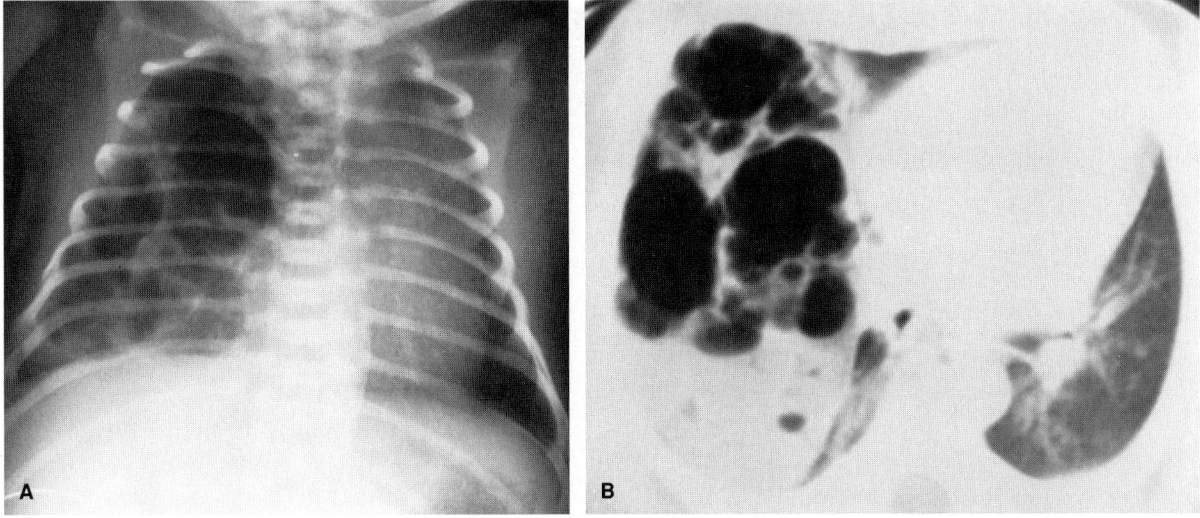

FIGURE 19.29. **Congenital Cystic Adenomatoid Malformation (CCAM). A.** Frontal chest radiograph in a newborn shows a multicystic mass in the right mid-lung and lower lung. **B.** CT scan demonstrates a complex mass occupying the middle and right lower lobes with air-filled cysts and a solid component posteriorly. Surgery revealed a CCAM of the middle lobe.

Bronchial atresia, a developmental stenosis or atresia of a lobar or segmental bronchus, produces bronchial obstruction with resultant distal bronchiectasis. Most patients are asymptomatic and are first recognized by typical findings on frontal chest radiographs, namely a rounded, oval, or branching central lung opacity representing the obstructed, mucus-filled, dilated bronchus (mucocele) with hyperlucency in that portion of lung supplied by the atretic bronchus. The overinflated lobe or segment results from air trapping in the obstructed lung as air enters by collateral air drift on inspiration but cannot empty through the proximal tracheobronchial tree on expiration. The most common site of involvement is the apicoposterior segment of the left upper lobe, followed by the segmental bronchi of the right upper and middle lobes. The combination of a central mucocele with peripheral hyperlucency in a young, asymptomatic patient is virtually diagnostic of this disorder (13).

Neonatal lobar hyperinflation (congenital lobar emphysema) may develop from a variety of disorders that produce a check-valve bronchial obstruction. These include extrinsic compression by mediastinal bronchogenic cysts, anomalous left pulmonary artery, congenital deficiency of bronchial cartilage, and congenital or acquired bronchial stenosis. The bronchial obstruction leads to air trapping on expiration, with resultant overinflation of the distal lung. In order of decreasing frequency, the left upper lobe, right middle lobe, and right upper lobe are the most common sites of involvement. Respiratory difficulties are usually evident within the first month of life, with a minority presenting later. Radiographically, hyperlucency of the affected lobe is seen with compression of adjacent lung, diaphragmatic depression, and contralateral mediastinal shift (Fig. 19.30). These findings are accentuated on expiratory films or on decubitus films obtained with the affected side down. CT, particularly when performed in expiration or with the affected side down, shows a hyperlucent, overexpanded lobe with attenuated blood vessels. Because many of these cases are not truly congenital but rather arise in the neonatal period from acquired abnormalities and because overinflation of normal alveoli without destruction of alveolar walls is seen pathologically, the term *neonatal lobar hyperinflation* has been used to more appropriately describe this syndrome. Treatment is surgical for symptomatic patients, whereas relatively asymptomatic patients are observed for spontaneous resolution. The findings in bronchial atresia and congenital lobar emphysema are reviewed in Table 19.9.

Bronchopulmonary sequestration is a congenital abnormality resulting from the independent development of a portion of the tracheobronchial tree that is isolated from the normal lung and maintains its fetal systemic arterial supply. Grossly, the sequestered lung is cystic and bronchiectatic. These patients most often present with recurrent pneumonia from recurrent infection in the sequestered lung, although some (mostly extralobar sequestrations) are discovered as asymptomatic posterior mediastinal masses on routine radiographs.

Pulmonary sequestration is divided into intralobar and extralobar forms (Table 19.10). *Intralobar sequestration* is contained within the visceral pleura of the normal lung. *Extralobar sequestration* is enclosed by its own visceral pleural envelope and may be found adjacent to the normal lung or within or below the diaphragm. Most patients

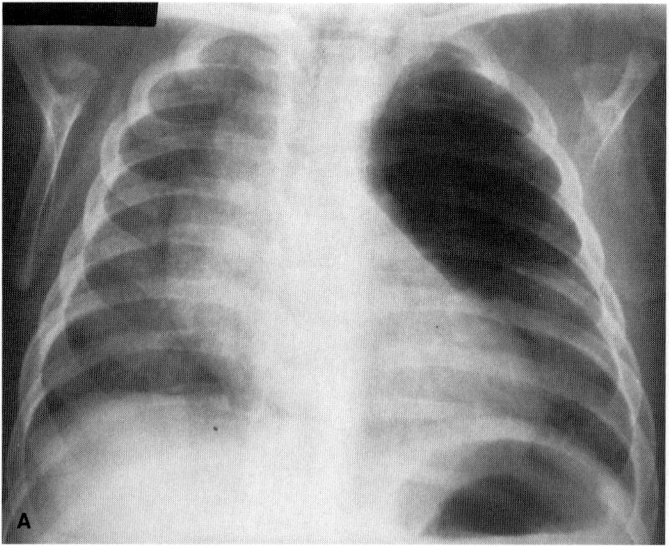

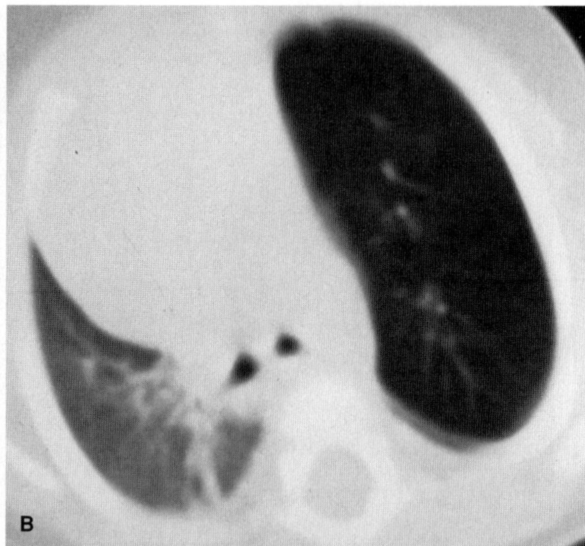

FIGURE 19.30. **Neonatal Lobar Hyperinflation. A.** Frontal chest radiograph in a 1-year-old boy shows a hyperlucent left upper lobe producing contralateral mediastinal shift. **B.** CT scan confirms the presence of an overexpanded and hyperlucent left upper lobe, representing congenital lobar emphysema.

with intralobar sequestration present with pneumonia. Extralobar sequestration is usually asymptomatic and is seen as an incidental finding in a neonate with other severe congenital anomalies. Intralobar sequestration is more common than the extralobar type, by a ratio of 3 to 1. Both forms are found in the lower lobes, but extralobar sequestration is predominantly left sided (90%), whereas one third of intralobar sequestrations are right sided. A major differentiating feature between the two types is the arterial supply to and venous drainage from the sequestered lung. An intralobar sequestration is supplied by a single large artery that arises from the infradiaphragmatic aorta and enters the sequestered lung via the pulmonary ligament. The venous drainage is via the pulmonary veins. In contrast, an extralobar sequestration receives several small branches from systemic and occasionally pulmonary arteries, with venous drainage into the systemic venous system (inferior vena cava, azygos, or hemiazygos veins).

Sequestration appears as a solid posterior mediastinal mass or as a solitary or multicystic air collection (13). Air–fluid levels are seen when infection has produced communication of the sequestered lung with the normal tracheobronchial tree. The definitive diagnosis is made by the demonstration of abnormal systemic arterial supply to the abnormal lung, which is usually accomplished by thoracic aortography, contrast-enhanced MDCT (Fig. 19.31), US, or coronal MR and MR angiography. Arteriography is usually reserved for preoperative patients in whom precise demonstration of the origin and number of the systemic feeders is necessary.

TABLE 19.9 Bronchial Atresia Versus Neonatal Lobar Hyperinflation

Diagnostic Variable	*Bronchial Atresia*	*Neonatal Lobar Hyperinflation*
Age at presentation	Teens/young adults	Neonatal period
Symptoms	Asymptomatic	Respiratory distress
Location	LUL >RUL >RML	LUL >RML >RUL
Radiographic/CT findings	Hyperlucent segment with mucocele	Hyperlucent lobe Diaphragmatic depression Mediastinal displacement
Treatment	None	Resection

LUL, left upper lobe; RUL, right upper lobe; RML, right middle lobe.

Hypoplastic lung is a developmental anomaly resulting in a small lung. It occurs secondary to congenital pulmonary arterial deficiency or following compression of the developing lung in utero from a variety of causes. Grossly, the lung is small, with a decrease in the number and size of airways, alveoli, and pulmonary arteries. Radiographically, the small lung and hemithorax are associated with ipsilateral diaphragmatic elevation and mediastinal shift, with herniation of the hyperinflated contralateral lung anteriorly toward the affected side. Hypoplastic lung can simulate total lung collapse radiographically but can usually be distinguished on clinical grounds and review of prior radiographic studies that show a small lung without evidence of pleural or parenchymal scarring.

TABLE 19.10 Pulmonary Sequestration

Diagnostic Variable	*Intralobar Sequestration*	*Extralobar Sequestration*
Frequency (of all sequestrations)	Common (75%)	Uncommon (25%)
Age at presentation	Young adult	Neonate/infant
Mode of presentation	Recurrent pneumonia	Asymptomatic
Location	Left lower lobe: 60% Right lower lobe: 40%	Left lower lobe: 90% Right lower lobe: 10%
Pleural covering	Within visceral pleura	Separate pleural layer
Associated congenital anomalies	Rare	Common (diaphragmatic eventration/hernia)
Radiographic appearance	Cystic lung mass with or without air–fluid levels	Solid peridiaphragmatic mass
Arterial supply	Single vessel from peridiaphragmatic aorta	Multiple small systemic/ pulmonary arteries
Venous drainage	Pulmonary (left-to-left shunt)	Systemic (left-to-right shunt)

Hypogenetic lung-scimitar syndrome, a variant of the hypoplastic lung, is characterized by an underdeveloped right lung with abnormal venous drainage of the lung to the inferior vena cava just above or below the right hemidiaphragm. The systemic venous drainage of the lung produces an extracardiac left-to-right shunt. The anomalous vein, which drains all or most of the right lung, may be seen as a vertically oriented curvilinear density shaped like a scimitar in the medial right lower lung, thereby giving this syndrome its common name of scimitar syndrome. The anomalies of venous drainage and lobar bronchial anatomy (usually bilateral left-sided [hyparterial] bronchial branching) have given rise to the term *congenital pulmonary venolobar syndrome*. The right pulmonary artery is invariably hypoplastic, with supply to all or part of the lung (usually the lower lobe) from the systemic circulation. Associated anomalies include eventration of the right hemidiaphragm, horseshoe lung (congenital fusion of the right and left lungs posteroinferiorly), and cardiac anomalies such as atrial septal defect (most common), coarctation of the aorta, patent ductus arteriosus, and tetralogy of Fallot. The frontal chest radiographic

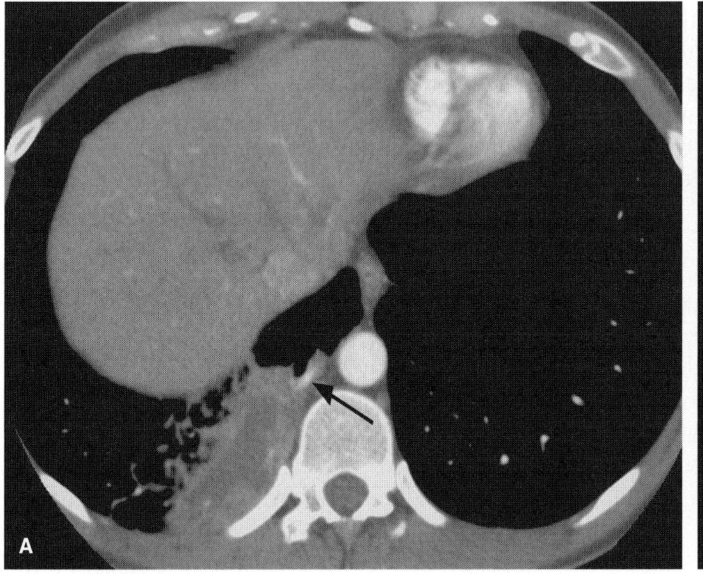

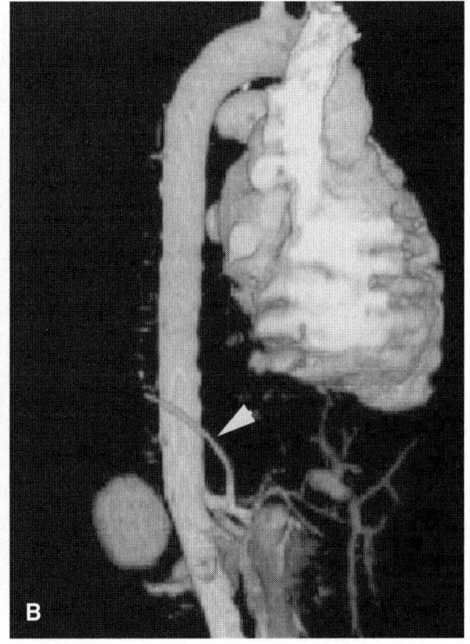

FIGURE 19.31. **Intralobar Pulmonary Sequestration.** Contrast-enhanced CT scan **(A)** in a 34-year-old pregnant woman with recurrent right lower lobe pneumonia shows focal consolidation with a feeding artery visible medially (*arrow*). Shaded-surface reconstruction **(B)** from CT angiogram shows feeding artery arising from celiac axis (*arrowhead*) to supply the right lower lobe.

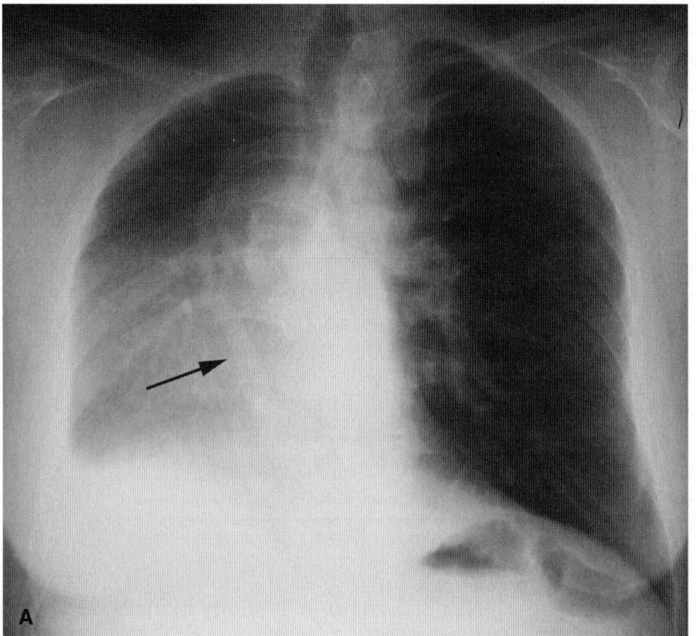

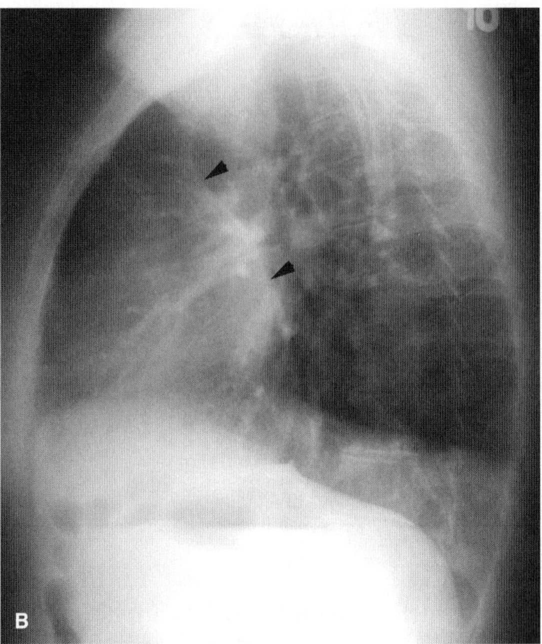

FIGURE 19.32. **Congenital Pulmonary Venolobar (Scimitar) Syndrome.** Frontal **(A)** and lateral **(B)** chest radiographs in a patient with Scimitar syndrome show a small right lung with rightward cardiomediastinal shift and a characteristic draining vein (*arrow* in **A**). The lateral film shows the interface of the hypoplastic right lung with the anteriorly situated heart and mediastinal fat (*arrowheads*) that have shifted as a result of the hypoplasia.

findings are diagnostic and include a small right hemithorax with diaphragmatic elevation or eventration, dextroposition of the heart, and herniation of left lung anteriorly into the right hemithorax (Fig. 19.32). The classic appearance of a solitary scimitar vein is seen in only one third of cases, with the remainder having multiple small draining veins. Although plain film findings are usually diagnostic, CT or MR shows the abnormal draining vein and associated abnormalities. Most patients are asymptomatic, but some may present with recurrent infection or symptoms related to a left-to-right shunt or the associated cardiac anomalies.

Arteriovenous Malformation. Pulmonary arteriovenous malformations (AVMs) are abnormal vascular masses in which a focal collection of congenitally weakened capillaries dilates to become a tortuous complex of vessels fed by a single pulmonary artery and drained by a single pulmonary vein. Most pulmonary AVMs do not come to attention until early adulthood. They are detected either incidentally, as part of a screening evaluation in patients with hereditary hemorrhagic telangiectasia (a condition that is present in approximately 80% of all patients with pulmonary AVMs), or because of a variety of symptoms. The most common pulmonary symptoms are hemoptysis and dyspnea, the latter attributable to hypoxia caused by the intrapulmonary right-to-left shunt. Nonpulmonary symptoms most often relate to CNS disease. Stroke may occur from paradoxical right-to-left cerebral emboli or from thrombosis resulting from secondary polycythemia caused by chronic hypoxemia. Brain abscess may develop from paradoxical septic emboli.

The chest radiograph of a pulmonary AVM usually shows a solitary pulmonary nodule, most often located in the subpleural portions of the lower lobes. Approximately one third of patients have multiple lesions. The lesion is often lobulated and has feeding and draining vessels emanating from the mass and extending toward the hilum. The morphology of the lesions is best demonstrated on MDCT with reconstructions. The feeding and draining vessels can be demonstrated by CT or MR. Angiography is reserved for preoperative evaluation and for patients undergoing therapeutic transcatheter embolization with spring coils or detachable occlusion balloons, which is the treatment of choice for patients with multiple AVMs.

TRAUMATIC LUNG DISEASE

Pulmonary contusion usually follows blunt chest trauma and typically develops adjacent to the site of impact. Blood and edema fluid fill the alveoli of the lung within the first 12 hours after trauma, producing scattered areas of airspace opacification that may rapidly become confluent and may be difficult to distinguish from aspiration pneumonia (Fig. 19.33). Patients may have shortness of breath and hemoptysis; blood can usually be suctioned from the

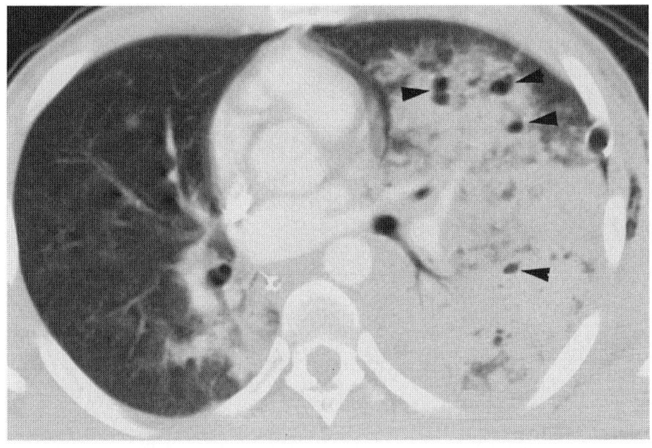

FIGURE 19.33. **Pulmonary Contusion/Traumatic Lung Cysts.** CT in a 26-year-old man who sustained severe blunt left chest trauma shows extensive contusion in the left lung, with small traumatic lung cysts (*arrowheads*) and minimal superior segment right lower lobe involvement.

endotracheal tube. The typical radiographic course is stabilization of opacities by 24 hours and improvement within 2 to 7 days. Progressive opacities seen more than 48 hours after trauma should raise the suspicion of aspiration pneumonia or developing ARDS.

Pulmonary Laceration, Traumatic Lung Cyst, and Pulmonary Hematoma. Pulmonary laceration is a common sequela of penetrating or blunt chest trauma. In the latter situation, it represents a shearing injury to the substance of the lung. The elastic properties of the lung quickly transform the linear laceration into a rounded air cyst. These cysts may be filled with varied amounts of blood as a result of laceration of pulmonary capillaries; those that are completely filled with blood are more appropriately termed *pulmonary hematomas*. On radiographs and CT, these cysts appear as rounded lucencies that may contain air or an air–fluid level (Fig. 19.33) (14). Initially, these cysts are often obscured by the adjacent contused lung, only to be recognized after resorption of the blood. The cysts tend to shrink gradually over a period of weeks to months. The term *traumatic air cysts* rather than *pneumatoceles* should be used for these lesions; the latter term is reserved for air cysts that result from a check-valve overdistention of the distal lung, as seen in staphylococcal pneumonia.

ASPIRATION

Aspiration pneumonia and *pneumonitis* are terms used to describe the different pulmonary inflammatory responses to aspirated material. As was discussed in the chapter on infection, aspiration pneumonia describes a mixed anaerobic infection resulting from the aspiration of infected oropharyngeal contents. The aspiration of oropharyngeal or gastric secretions may also occur in a "pure" form uncomplicated by anaerobic infection, producing aspiration pneumonitis.

Aspiration of oropharyngeal or gastric secretions, with or without food particles, is not an uncommon event. It is seen in debilitated patients with chronic diseases, in patients with tracheal or gastric tubes, in unconscious patients, and in those who have suffered strokes, seizures, or trauma. More chronic and less easily recognizable forms of aspiration may occur in patients with anatomic abnormalities of the upper GI tract (Zenker diverticulum, esophageal stricture) or functional disorders (gastroesophageal reflux, neuromuscular dysfunction).

Gastric fluid is highly irritating to the lungs and often stimulates explosive coughing and associated deep inspirations, leading to widespread distribution of the fluid throughout both lungs and into the peripheral airspaces. The hydrochloric acid contained in gastric fluid causes direct damage to both the bronchiolar lining and the alveolar wall. The severity of the resultant pneumonitis depends upon several factors: it is increased with a pH of the aspirated fluid <2.5, large volume of aspirated fluid, large particulate matter in the aspirated fluid, and young age. The massive aspiration of gastric contents is known as Mendelson syndrome. When the aspirate includes particulate material, the particles are distributed by gravity and may incite a granulomatous foreign body–type reaction.

Three basic radiographic patterns of aspiration pneumonitis have been observed: (*1*) extensive bilateral airspace opacification, (*2*) diffuse but discrete airspace nodular opacities, and (*3*) irregular parenchymal opacities that are not obviously airspace filling in nature (15). Parenchymal involvement is most often bilateral, with a predilection for the basal and perihilar regions. When a significant amount of admixed food is present, the opacities are usually posterior and segmental. Atelectasis is often present, presumably caused by airways obstruction by food particles. The radiographic appearance may worsen over the first few days but then demonstrates rapid improvement. A worsening of the radiographic appearance at this stage suggests development of a complicating infection, ARDS, or pulmonary embolism.

Chronic Aspiration Pneumonitis. Patients who repeatedly aspirate may develop chronic interstitial abnormalities on chest radiographs. With repeated episodes of aspiration over months to years, irregular reticular interstitial opacities may persist, probably representing peribronchial scarring. A reticulonodular pattern may be seen, caused by granulomas forming around food particles. These chronic interstitial abnormalities can be observed in between episodes of acute aspiration pneumonitis.

Exogenous lipoid pneumonia. Multifocal areas of consolidation or masses can result from the aspiration of lipid material and are classically seen in older patients with swallowing disorders or gastroesophageal reflux who ingest mineral oil as a laxative or inhale oily nose drops.

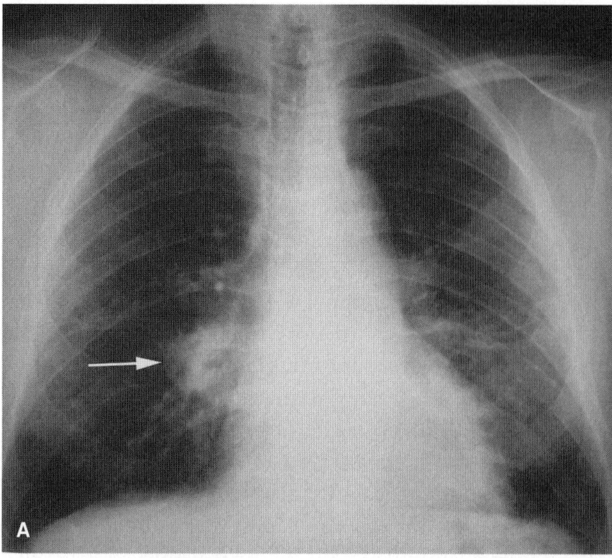

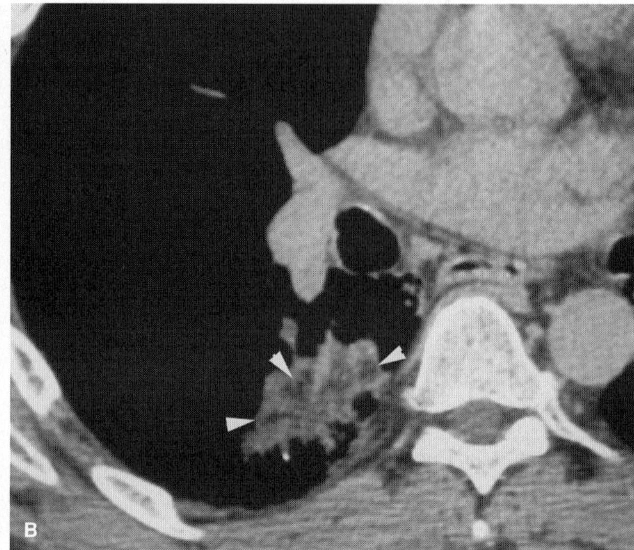

FIGURE 19.34. **Exogenous Lipoid Pneumonia.** Frontal chest radiograph **(A)** in a 77-year-old man who used mineral oil as a laxative shows a superior segment right lower lobe mass (*arrows*) with associated lower lung interstitial changes present for 3 years. Thin-section CT **(B)** at mediastinal windows shows fat attenuation within the mass (*arrowheads*), which is indicative of lipoid pneumonia.

When solitary, lesions can mimic lung cancer. CT findings of fat attenuation with a compatible clinical history are diagnostic of this entity (Fig. 19.34).

DRUG-INDUCED CHEST DISEASE

Drugs can induce a variety of adverse effects in the chest (16). The majority of cases of drug-induced chest disease are iatrogenic, though accidental or intentional drug overdoses may result in severe pulmonary disease. The changes are often difficult to distinguish from infection, pulmonary edema, or a pulmonary manifestation of the disease being treated.

Acute Reactions. There are a limited number of ways for drugs to produce acute pulmonary disease. An acute pulmonary reaction may involve a hypersensitivity response to a metabolite of the drug combined with an endogenous protein. Antibody production directed against this hapten-protein complex leads to antibody-mediated immediate or immune complex hypersensitivity reactions. In the lung, this produces bronchospasm or eosinophilic pneumonia, usually associated with fever, skin rash, and blood eosinophilia. Radiographically, fleeting peripheral patchy airspace opacities develop hours to days after the initiation of drug therapy. The opacities often respond to corticosteroid therapy. The penicillin and sulfonamide antibiotics are the drugs most often associated with hypersensitivity reactions.

The other common acute lung reaction to administered drugs is a diffuse alveolar damage that is histologically identical to the early changes of ARDS. Opiates, including heroin and crack cocaine, and chemotherapeutic agents, particularly busulfan, cytosine arabinoside, and chlorambucil, are most commonly associated with this reaction. Radiographically, the lungs show acute interstitial or airspace opacities that are indistinguishable from those of pulmonary edema, although the heart size is usually normal (Fig. 19.35). Characteristically, the edema clears as rapidly as it appeared.

Acute pulmonary hemorrhage and infarction may occur secondary to drug-induced pulmonary vasculitis, while diffuse hemorrhage may complicate anticoagulation therapy with warfarin (Coumadin) or thrombocytopenia following intensive chemotherapy administered prior to bone marrow transplantation. Penicillamine therapy has been associated with pulmonary hemorrhage in patients with rheumatoid arthritis via an unknown mechanism. Affected individuals typically have hemoptysis and a falling hematocrit that are associated with the rapid development of diffuse bilateral airspace opacities. The diagnosis is usually confirmed by noting bloody fluid return on bronchoalveolar lavage. The lavage also shows an increased percentage of alveolar macrophages containing hemosiderin deposits. The opacities of diffuse pulmonary hemorrhage resolve completely without residual scarring, while the focal opacities of pulmonary infarcts may leave pleuroparenchymal scars.

Chronic Reactions. Chronic pulmonary or pleural disease generally develops weeks to months after initial exposure to the offending drug, but can be delayed for years. The most common form of chronic lung toxicity from

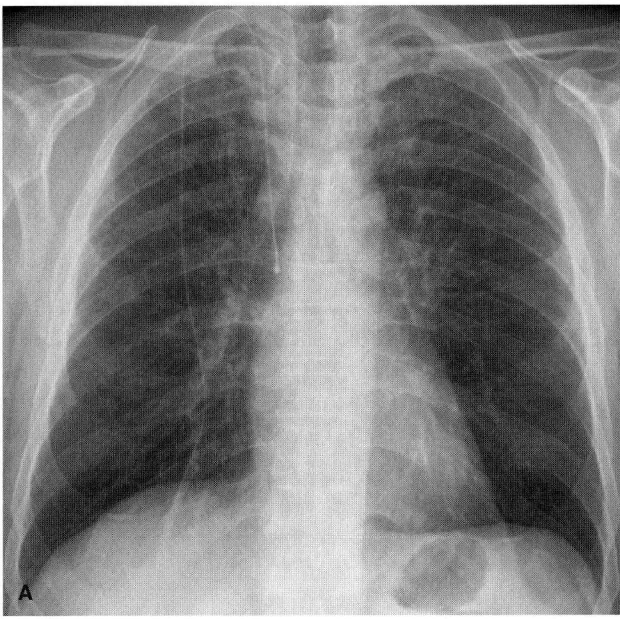

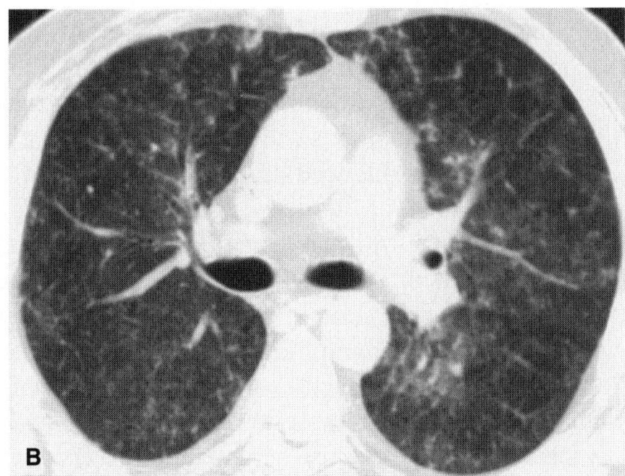

FIGURE 19.35. **Cytosine Arabinoside (Ara-C) Acute Lung Toxicity.** Chest radiograph **(A)** in a 57-year-old man with acute myelogenous leukemia and acute shortness of breath following induction chemotherapy with ara-C shows bilateral interstitial opacities. CT scan **(B)** at lung windows shows bilateral reticular opacities. Infection and edema were excluded bronchoscopically, and a diagnosis of drug toxicity was made presumptively.

drugs is that of a chronic interstitial pneumonitis, with subsequent development of pulmonary fibrosis in the healing phase of this disorder. The drugs most commonly implicated in this form of lung disease are amiodarone, nitrofurantoin, and the chemotherapeutic agents Cytoxan (cyclophosphamide), bleomycin, and methotrexate. Radiographically, there are bilateral predominantly lower lobe coarse reticular and linear opacities with diminished lung volumes. In patients undergoing chemotherapy for malignancy, the findings are difficult to distinguish from those of lymphangitic carcinomatosis, pulmonary hemorrhage, or opportunistic pneumonia, while pulmonary edema is the major differential diagnosis in patients on amiodarone therapy. The diagnosis is usually made by excluding one of these other processes. Pulmonary nodules are an uncommon manifestation of chronic lung injury from bleomycin or Cytoxan, and in this situation, they are radiographically indistinguishable from pulmonary metastases.

A number of drugs have been associated with a lupus-like syndrome that is often indistinguishable from systemic lupus erythematosus. Procainamide, hydralazine, and isoniazid are the drugs that most commonly produce a lupus-like reaction. Pleural and pericardial effusions are common. Basilar interstitial disease has been described but is uncommon.

Bronchiolitis obliterans is a small airways inflammatory process that results in granulation tissue within bronchioles. This reaction can result from a variety of insults including aspiration, organ transplantation, viral infection, collagen vascular disease, and drugs. Penicillamine administered in patients with rheumatoid arthritis is the drug most often associated with this reaction. This entity is described in more detail in Chapter 18.

A chronic granulomatous vasculitis may develop as a response to particulate substances such as talc or starch mixed with illicit intravenous drugs. This can lead to obliteration of the pulmonary vasculature, producing pulmonary hypertension and RV failure. Radiographically, the lungs may show an interstitial pattern of disease, with enlargement of the central pulmonary arteries and right heart. The radiographs may rarely show central conglomerate masses that are indistinguishable from progressive massive fibrosis of silicosis or end-stage sarcoidosis.

Enlargement of the hilar and mediastinal lymph nodes on chest radiographs is an uncommon manifestation of drug toxicity. Dilantin and methotrexate are the main drugs associated with this rare complication. The lymphadenopathy is usually part of a systemic hypersensitivity reaction and regresses with removal of the offending agent.

Nitrofurantoin is an oral antibiotic used widely in the treatment of urinary tract infections. There are two distinct patterns of nitrofurantoin-associated pulmonary reaction: acute and chronic. The acute form, seen in approximately 90% of cases, most likely represents a hypersensitivity reaction. The chest film demonstrates interstitial or mixed alveolar/interstitial infiltrates with a basal predominance, often accompanied by small pleural effusions. The chronic form occurs after weeks to years of continuous therapy and is probably caused by direct toxic damage. Interstitial pneumonitis and fibrosis indistinguishable from idiopathic pulmonary fibrosis are seen pathologically. The chest radiograph demonstrates reduced lung volumes and a diffuse reticular pattern with relative basal predominance.

Bleomycin is a cytotoxic antibiotic used in the treatment of lymphoma, squamous cell carcinoma, and testicular cancer. Bleomycin-induced lung disease is related to the cumulative dosage of the drug. Free oxygen radicals within the lung are felt to play a major role in the lung injury and account for the deleterious effects of supplemental oxygen administration in patients with bleomycin toxicity. The typical radiographic pattern is that of bilateral lower lobe reticular opacities. A minority of patients will demonstrate acute patchy or confluent airspace opacities as a result of a hypersensitivity reaction to the drug or diffuse alveolar damage. The reticular or airspace opacities tend to have a basal predominance. Solitary or multiple pulmonary nodules constitute an unusual radiographic appearance of bleomycin lung toxicity that is indistinguishable radiographically from pulmonary metastases; the lesions generally disappear following cessation of the drug.

Alkylating Agents. Drugs such as busulfan, which is used in the treatment of myeloproliferative disorders, and cyclophosphamide (Cytoxan), used widely in the treatment of malignancies and autoimmune disease, can cause clinically recognizable pulmonary toxicity in 1% to 4% of patients. Pathologic findings include organizing intra-alveolar exudate, fibrosis, and the presence of large atypical type 2 pneumocytes. Radiographically, a diffuse reticular pattern with basal predominance is seen; airspace opacities may be present and are more common with busulfan than cyclophosphamide.

Cytosine Arabinoside (Ara-C). This is an antimetabolic agent generally used to treat acute leukemia. Pulmonary toxicity develops in 15% to 30% of treated patients within 30 days of administration and is manifested as interstitial and airspace permeability pulmonary edema (Fig. 19.35).

Methotrexate is an antimetabolite used for the treatment of malignancies and autoimmune diseases such as rheumatoid arthritis and psoriasis. In contrast to bleomycin and the alkylating agents, methotrexate usually causes reversible pulmonary disease caused by a hypersensitivity reaction rather than direct toxic damage to the lung. However, diffuse alveolar damage leading to restrictive lung disease is seen in approximately 10% of cases and appears radiographically as a diffuse reticular pattern.

Amiodarone. This antiarrhythmic agent is an important cause of drug-induced pulmonary damage, affecting approximately 5% of individuals on chronic therapy. Amiodarone is concentrated in the lung and has a long tissue half-life. The exact mechanism of lung damage is unknown but relates to the accumulation of phospholipids, which disturb metabolic functions in the lung. Pathologically, there is inflammation and fibrosis of the alveolar septae, with an accumulation of lipid-laden alveolar macrophages and hyperplasia of type 2 pneumocytes.

Pulmonary toxicity begins months to years after the initiation of therapy. Patients typically present with dyspnea or a nonproductive cough, which may be difficult to distinguish from congestive heart failure or pneumonia. The chest film typically shows airspace and reticular opacities. CT findings show significant overlap with findings of pulmonary edema—which is common in these patients—with reticulation and ground-glass and airspace opacities, but findings of fibrosis and high attenuation within parenchymal abnormalities should strongly suggest amiodarone toxicity (Fig. 19.36). Amiodarone should be withdrawn or the dose diminished at the earliest sign of toxicity because the drug has an extraordinarily long half life (approximately 90 days). The cessation of amiodarone at an early stage of toxicity, with occasional use of corticosteroids, usually provides relief.

RADIATION-INDUCED LUNG DISEASE

The pulmonary effects of external irradiation, most commonly administered for palliation of unresectable bronchogenic carcinoma or metastatic disease to the chest or treatment of mediastinal Hodgkin lymphoma, depend upon several variables. The volume of lung treated will affect the incidence of radiation injury; the greater the volume irradiated, the more likely that radiation injury will occur. Most radiation treatment is limited to less than one third to one half of the lung, as an equivalent dose administered to an entire lung or both lungs would cause serious lung injury. The total dose and the method of fractionation will affect the incidence of radiation injury. Doses under 20 Gy rarely produce lung injury, while doses exceeding 30 Gy, particularly if administered to a significant portion of the lungs, have a significant incidence of radiation pneumonitis. Administration of a single large dose is more deleterious than fractionation of a similar total dose over the course of several weeks. There is variation in the susceptibility to radiation among individuals; a given dose may cause pneumonitis in one patient whereas another remains unaffected. The concomitant use of chemotherapeutic agents (particularly bleomycin) or the withdrawal of corticosteroid therapy may accentuate the deleterious effects of radiation.

The mechanism of radiation-induced lung injury is not completely understood, but the acute effects involve injury to capillary endothelial and pulmonary epithelial cells that line the alveoli. This diffuse alveolar damage produces a cellular, proteinaceous intra-alveolar exudate and hyaline

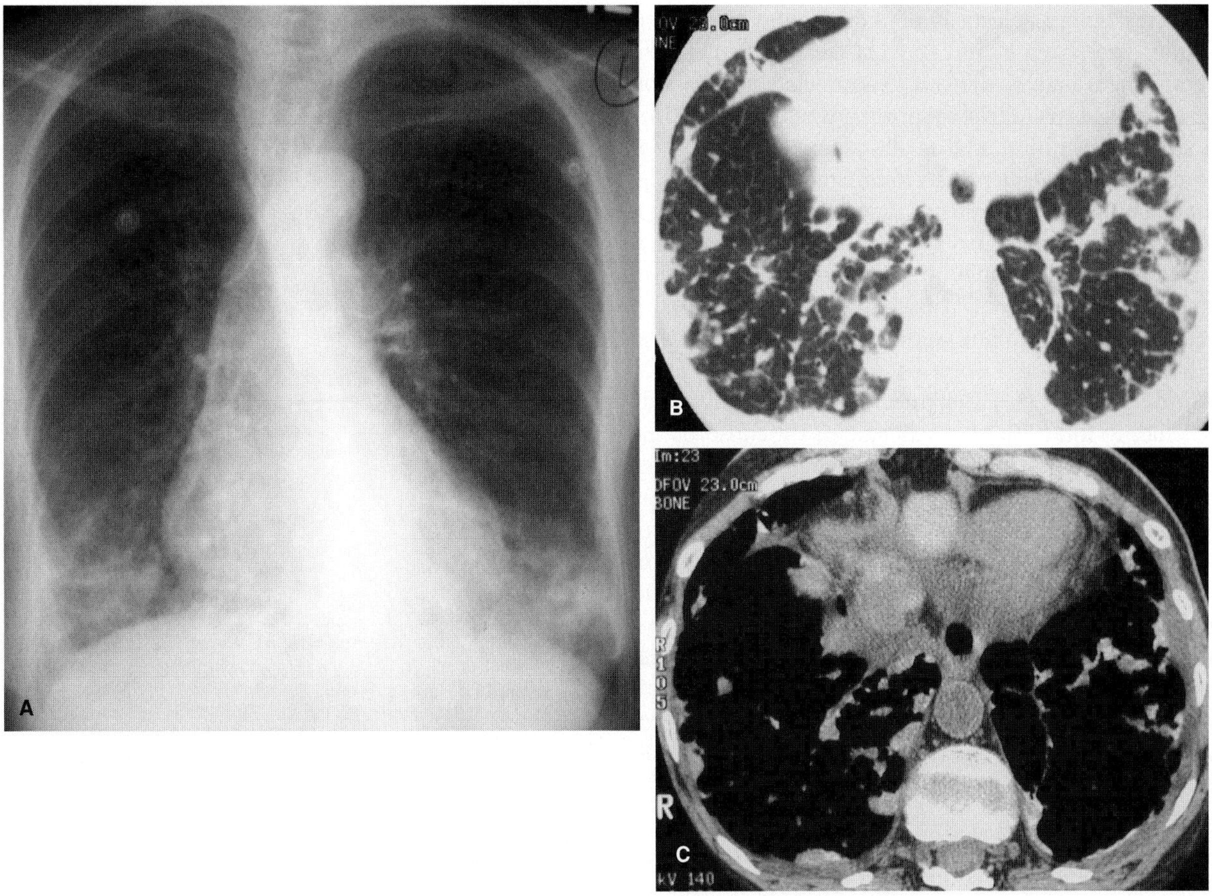

FIGURE 19.36. **Amiodarone Lung Toxicity.** Frontal chest radiograph **(A)** in a 64-year-old patient who experienced progressive shortness of breath while receiving amiodarone for ventricular tachycardia shows cardiomegaly, bibasilar coarse interstitial opacities, and small pleural effusions. Thin-section unenhanced CT scan through the lung bases at lung windows **(B)** shows coarse reticular and nodular opacities, which were high attenuation at mediastinal windows **(C),** consistent with amiodarone lung toxicity.

membranes that is indistinguishable histologically from ARDS. These changes develop 4 to 12 weeks following the completion of therapy. Whereas most patients with acute radiation pneumonitis are asymptomatic, dyspnea and a nonproductive cough may be present. Radiographically, a sharply marginated, localized area of airspace opacification is seen that does not conform to lobar or segmental anatomic boundaries and directly corresponds to the radiation port (17). Adhesive atelectasis of the involved portion of lung is common because the radiation produces a loss of surfactant by damaging type 2 pneumocytes. The pneumonitis may resolve completely with or without the administration of corticosteroids, or it may progress to pulmonary fibrosis. Pulmonary fibrosis corresponds histologically to a reparative phase, with regeneration of type 2 pneumocytes, reorganization of the parenchyma, ingrowth of granulation tissue, and eventually interstitial fibrosis. Fibrosis appears as coarse linear opacities or occasionally as a homogeneous parenchymal opacity with

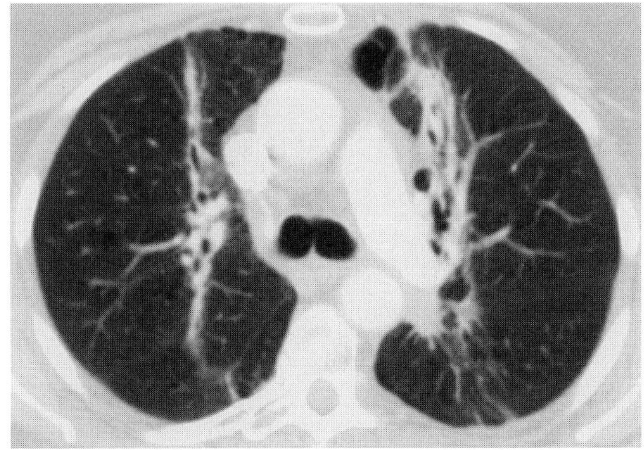

FIGURE 19.37. **Radiation Pneumonitis/Fibrosis.** CT scan at lung windows in a patient who had received radiation therapy for non–small cell lung cancer shows characteristic paramediastinal interstitial opacities sharply demarcated laterally, reflecting evolving radiation pneumonitis and fibrosis.

severe cicatrizing atelectasis of the involved portion of the lung. The sharp margination of the parenchymal fibrotic changes may be difficult to appreciate on plain radiographs but is usually obvious on cross-sectional CT or MR studies. Fibrotic tissue is characteristically low signal on T2W MR sequences, a finding that is helpful in distinguishing fibrosis from recurrent tumor, which typically produces high signal on T2WIs. The parenchymal changes are usually stable by 1 year following radiation therapy. Pleural thickening caused by fibrosis is a common finding. Small pleural and pericardial effusions are also common.

The diagnosis of radiation pneumonitis is usually made by excluding infection or malignancy as a cause of the patient's symptoms and by the presence of typical radiographic findings following a course of radiation therapy to the chest. This distinction may require bronchoalveolar lavage and transbronchial biopsy. An increased number of lymphocytes in the bronchoalveolar lavage fluid and an absence of malignant cells confirm the diagnosis. The demonstration of airspace opacification on CT that conforms to a known portal of radiation is usually sufficient for the diagnosis (Fig. 19.37). Treatment is generally supportive, with severe cases requiring corticosteroid therapy.

REFERENCES

1. Light RW. Physiology of the pleural space. In: Pleural Diseases. 4th ed. Philadelphia: Lippincott Williams & Wilkins, 2001: 8–20.
2. Peterman TA, Brothers SK. Pleural effusions in congestive heart failure and in pericardial disease. N Engl J Med 1983;309:313.
3. Light RW. Parapneumonic effusions and empyema. Clin Chest Med 1985;6:55–62.
4. Stark DD, Federle MP, Goodman PC, et al. Differentiating lung abscess and empyema: radiography and computed tomography. AJR Am J Roentgenol 1983;141:163–167.
5. Colice GL, Curtis A, Deslauriers J, et al. Medical and surgical treatment of parapneumonic effusions. An evidence-based guideline. Chest 2000;18:1158–1171.
6. Stern EJ, Sun H, Haramati LB. Peripheral bronchopleural fistulas: CT imaging features. AJR Am J Roentgenol 1996;167:117–120.
7. Baumann MH, Strange C, Heffner JE, et al. Management of spontaneous pneumothorax. An American College of Chest Physicians Delphi Consensus Statement. Chest 2001;119:590–602.
8. Muller NL. Imaging of the pleura. Radiology 1993;186:297–309.
9. Leung AN, Muller NL, Miller RR. CT in the differential diagnosis of diffuse pleural disease. AJR Am J Roentgenol 1990;154:487–492.
10. Wang ZJ, Reddy GP, Gotway MB, et al. Malignant pleural mesothelioma: evaluation with CT, MR imaging, and PET. Radiographics 2004;24:105–119.
11. Jeung M-Y, Gangi A, Gasser B, et al. Imaging of chest wall disorders. Radiographics 1999;19:617–637.
12. Iochum S, Ludig T, Walter F, Sebbag H, Grosdidier G, Blum AG. Imaging of diaphragmatic injury: a diagnostic challenge. Radiographics 2002;22:S103–S116.
13. Zylak CJ, Eyler WR, Spizarny DL, Stone CH. Developmental lung anomalies in the adult: radiologic-pathologic correlation. Radiographics 2002;22:S25–S43.
14. Wagner RB, Crawford WO Jr, Schimpf PP. Classification of parenchymal injuries of the lung. Radiology 1988;167:77–82.
15. Landay MJ, Christensen EE, Bynum LJ. Pulmonary manifestations of acute aspiration of gastric contents. AJR Am J Roentgenol 1978;131:587–592.
16. Rossi SE, Erasmus JJ, McAdams HP, Sporn TA, Goodman PC. Pulmonary drug toxicity: radiologic and pathologic manifestations. Radiographics 2000;5:1245–1259.
17. Choi YW, Munden RF, Erasmus JJ, et al. Effects of radiation therapy on the lung: radiologic appearances and differential diagnosis. Radiographics 2004;24:985–997.

SECTION IV

Breast Radiology

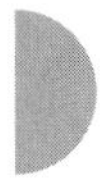

Chapter 20

Breast Imaging

Karen K. Lindfors and Huong T. Le-Petross

Screening for Breast Cancer
Screening Guidelines
Screening Outcomes
Radiation Risk
The Use of Other Imaging Modalities for Breast Cancer Screening

Evaluation of the Symptomatic Patient

Technical Considerations in Breast Imaging
Full-Field Digital Mammography
Quality Assurance
Mammographic Positioning for Screening
Interpreting the Mammogram
Diagnostic Evaluation of the Indeterminate Mammogram

Analyzing the Mammogram
Masses
Calcifications
Architectural Distortion
Increased Density of Breast Tissue
Axillary Adenopathy
The Augmented Breast
The Male Breast
Comparison With Previous Films

Magnetic Resonance Imaging

The Radiologic Report and Plan

Interventional Procedures for Nonpalpable Lesions
Percutaneous Biopsy
Localization of Occult Breast Lesions
Other Interventional Procedures

Conclusion

Breast imaging is utilized for two purposes. The first is to screen asymptomatic women for early breast cancer. The second is to evaluate breast abnormalities in symptomatic patients or patients with indeterminate screening mammograms. Screening is accomplished with standard two-view mammography, but diagnostic evaluation often requires the additional use of special mammographic views, breast US, MR, and interventional procedures.

SCREENING FOR BREAST CANCER

Breast cancer survival is influenced by the size of the tumor and the lymph node status at the time of diagnosis. Small tumors with negative axillary lymph nodes have survival rates well above 90%. Such cancers are detected far more often with screening mammography than with physical examination. It follows that screening mammography should lower mortality from breast cancer. Several randomized controlled trials have proven the efficacy of this technique.

In 1963 the Health Insurance Plan of New York (HIP) invited 31,000 women aged 40 to 64 to participate in four annual screenings for breast cancer by mammography and physical examination. This study group was compared with a control group of women who received routine medical care. Nine years after beginning the study, there was a 29% reduction in breast cancer mortality in the group receiving annual screening (1).

Other trials of mammographic screening were begun in the late 1970s and early 1980s. Four of these were carried out in Sweden and were similar in design. They were population based, meaning that all women living within a specific geographical area who were within the age range under study were included in the trial. Breast cancer mortality was compared between women invited to screening and those not invited (controls). When the data from all centers were combined, the reduction in breast cancer mortality among women age 40 to 74 was 24% in the group invited to mammographic screening (2).

The actual benefit of screening mammography for women of all ages is likely to exceed that demonstrated by the randomized clinical trials. Breast cancer mortality data on all women invited for screening, regardless of whether they actually underwent mammography, were used in calculating the reduction of mortality attributable to screening. Compliance rates for obtaining mammography among trial invitees ranged from 61% to 89%. The technology used for mammography has improved greatly since the time that the trials began, and earlier detection of breast cancer has resulted (3). Recent evaluations of the impact of mammographic screening in the community setting (service screening) have shown breast cancer mortality reductions of up to 50% among screened women; however, it is difficult to determine the contribution of screening relative to that of improvements in therapy in lowering the death rate from breast cancer (4,5).

Screening Guidelines

Updated data from the randomized, controlled trials of mammographic screening as well as information from large community-based screening programs encouraged the American Cancer Society (ACS) to update their guidelines for breast cancer screening in 2003 (6). ACS guidelines for breast cancer screening are shown in Table 20.1. Both clinical examination and mammography are essential components of a screening program, because all cancers are not seen mammographically. False-negative mammograms occur in 9% to 16% of breast cancers; these cancers are generally detected by physical examination.

The National Cancer Institute advises that women at average risk for breast cancer who are age 40 and over should undergo screening mammography every 1 to 2 years (7). The optimum interval between screens is currently the focus of considerable debate. A recent observational study showed that women aged 40 to 49 were more likely to have late-stage cancers diagnosed if they were screened at 2-year intervals versus a 1-year screening interval (8). Other studies of cancers that occur between screens have shown that a greater proportion of breast cancers grow faster in younger women than in older women (9–11). It is for this reason that the ACS has recommended *annual* mammographic screening for women at age 40 and older; yet the chance of being diagnosed with breast cancer between the ages of 40 and 49 is one in 66 women or 2%, and the chance of dying from breast cancer is 0.3 percent. Although it is clear that annual mammographic screening is more effective in reducing breast cancer deaths for women in their 40s, economic considerations may favor biennial screening.

TABLE 20.1 American Cancer Society Guidelines for Breast Cancer Screening

Age	*Clinical Examination*	*Mammography*
20–39	Every 3 years	Not recommended
40 and over	Annually	Annually

For postmenopausal women, there is some question regarding the additional benefit gained by annual screening, because studies have shown that there is no increase in late-stage cancers diagnosed if screening is done every 2 years instead of annually (8). The incidence of breast cancer does increase with age. There is no recommended age at which mammographic screening should cease. For elderly women, general health status and quality of life should be considered when deciding whether to undergo mammography.

Women at high risk for development of breast cancer should seek expert advice regarding the age at which screening should begin, the periodicity of mammography, and the possible addition of other screening modalities (such as MR). Factors known to increase a woman's risk include: (*1*) a personal history of breast cancer; (*2*) laboratory evidence that the woman is a carrier of the BRCA1 or BRCA2 genetic mutation, which confers an estimated risk of up to 80% for development of breast cancer by age 70; (*3*) having a mother, sister, or daughter with breast cancer; (*4*) atypical or precancerous lesions diagnosed on a previous breast biopsy; and (*5*) nulliparity or having a first child at age 30 or older.

When adopting a screening policy, the physician must remember that all women are at risk for developing breast cancer. The ACS estimates that one woman in every eight will develop the disease during her lifetime. The majority of women who contract breast cancer will not have histories that place them at higher risk.

Screening Outcomes

What are the expected outcomes in a group of 1,000 asymptomatic women undergoing bilateral screening mammography for the first time? Approximately 80 of these women will be recalled for additional studies. These may include magnification or other special mammographic views and US. Biopsy will be recommended in about 16 of these women, and cancer will be found in about six of them. With subsequent screenings of the same women, the number of cancers found will decrease and the positive predictive value, or percentage of women undergoing biopsy who actually have cancer, should increase.

The goal of screening asymptomatic women is to find breast cancer in its earliest stages, when survival is greatest. In a well-established screening program, more than 50% of cancers will be minimal; minimal cancers are defined as those that are noninvasive or invasive but less than 1 cm in size with negative nodes. Over 80% of breast cancer discovered by screening mammography should be node-negative (12,13).

Optimal effectiveness of a breast cancer screening program requires the use of physical examination in addition to mammographic screening. Nine percent to 16% of cancers are not visualized mammographically; such cancers are discovered on physical examination. The minimum size of breast cancers that can be felt on physical examination averages between 1.5 and 2 cm.

False-negative mammograms can occur for a variety of reasons. The palpable abnormality may not be included on a film. Dense breast parenchyma may obscure visualization of a mass. The filming technique may be suboptimal for visualization of an abnormality. The particular tumor type may not be visible mammographically, or there may be observer error in the interpretation of the mammogram. It must be emphasized that a negative mammogram should not deter further diagnostic evaluation of a clinically palpable mass.

Some breast cancers will arise in the interval between screening examinations. The number of such cancers will depend on the frequency of screening. Interval cancers tend to be more advanced at diagnosis when compared with those diagnosed at screening (10); they may be biologically more aggressive. Additionally, a previous negative mammogram or the knowledge that screening will be performed regularly may be a disincentive for patients to seek immediate medical care for a breast mass found in the interval between screens. Physicians must stress that any breast mass requires immediate attention, regardless of whether the patient has had a recent negative mammogram.

Radiation Risk

An increased susceptibility to breast cancer has been documented among women exposed to high doses of radiation (1 to 20 Gy). The survivors of the atomic bomb explosions in Japan, patients undergoing radiation therapy, and sanatoria patients undergoing multiple chest fluoroscopies for monitoring of tuberculosis therapy all have an increased incidence of breast cancer. Such data have raised questions about the risk incurred from the low doses of radiation received during screening mammography (approximately 2 mGy per view).

A controlled study of the effects of low doses of radiation, such as those received during mammography, would require large numbers of women in both the study and control groups. Close to 100 million patients in each group would be required to provide statistically significant data. Clearly, this would not be practical or possible. As such, estimates or risk have been hypothesized by extrapolation from data obtained at higher doses using a linear dose-response model.

The latest follow-up data from the Japanese atomic bomb survivors have shown progressively decreasing radiation risk with increased age at exposure. Women who were exposed in their youth and teens suffered the highest increase in risk. No increased risk was demonstrable for women aged 40 or older at exposure. Studies of the other populations sustaining significant breast radiation exposure have also supported a diminished risk with advancing age at exposure. The estimated lifetime risk of breast cancer death from a single mammogram in the age group from 40 to 49 years is approximately 2 in 1 million. In women aged 50 to 59, this risk is reduced to less than 1 in 1 million; progressive reductions in risk are seen at older ages (14).

These theoretical risks should be weighed against the risk of dying from spontaneous breast cancer, which would be approximately 700 per million in women aged 40 to 49 and 1,000 per million in women aged 50 to 59. This risk increases steadily with advancing age.

The Use of Other Imaging Modalities for Breast Cancer Screening

Mammography is the only imaging modality that has been proven to reduce breast cancer mortality when used to screen asymptomatic women. Other modalities are under investigation for their potential use in screening, particularly in high-risk women.

Several single-institution studies have shown that whole breast screening US can detect small nonpalpable invasive cancers not seen mammographically. Prevalence rates for cancers seen only on sonography are approximately 3 in 1,000, but positive predictive values for biopsies based on US alone are approximately half of those for biopsies of lesions discovered on mammography (15). US is highly dependent on the operator and on the equipment and technique used for scanning. Multi-institutional trials to assess the diagnostic yield of whole breast US with mammography compared with mammography alone for breast cancer in high-risk women are underway.

Technical advances have led to increasing interest in MR as a possible screening technique for breast cancer in certain populations. Recent data suggest that MR can reveal lesions that are missed by conventional mammography in radiographically dense breasts. The cost of MR and the necessity of contrast administration will probably prohibit its use as a general screening tool, but the technique is useful in specific cases, such as in women with a cumulative lifetime risk of breast cancer of 15% or more (16).

Other imaging technologies, such as PET, tomosynthesis, and CT, are also being explored for use in breast cancer detection and diagnosis. For the present, however, mammography remains the single best test for early detection of breast cancer; it is the "gold standard" by which all other potential screening modalities must be measured.

EVALUATION OF THE SYMPTOMATIC PATIENT

Bilateral mammography should be the first imaging study performed in patients over the age of 30 who present with breast masses that are suspicious for carcinoma. The mass should be indicated by placing a radiopaque marker over the site. This will assist the radiologist in a targeted mammographic evaluation of this area and will also ensure that the palpable abnormality corresponds to the mammographic abnormality, if one is visualized. Such correlation is important in assuring that the surgical biopsy of a palpable abnormality will encompass the mammographically suspicious area.

The primary reason for performing mammography in a patient with a suspicious palpable mass is to assess the affected breast for multifocal disease and the contralateral breast for suspicious abnormalities that should be biopsied concurrently. Mammography may also be helpful in definitively diagnosing the palpable abnormality as benign, thus avoiding biopsy.

Mammography should be performed before any intervention. A hematoma resulting from percutaneous fine-needle aspiration biopsy can look similar to a small carcinoma. When such procedures have been performed prior to mammography, it is best to perform a follow-up mammogram 4 to 6 weeks later.

If mammography is negative in a patient with a clinically evident mass and dense breasts, US is often suggested as a subsequent imaging study. US can determine whether the mass represents a simple cyst. Simple cysts are virtually never malignant and do not require aspiration unless the patient has pain related to the cyst. US cannot provide a specific diagnosis for a solid or complex mass.

Alternatively, definitive diagnosis of a palpable mass can usually be made by performing a fine-needle aspiration of the mass with a 22-gauge needle. When a simple cyst is present, the aspiration is both diagnostic and therapeutic, as all of the fluid can be withdrawn. In solid or complex masses, a cytologic examination of the cells removed at aspiration will yield the diagnosis.

In younger patients who present with breast masses, mammography must be used more judiciously. This more cautious approach is based on data from the atomic bomb survivors in Japan showing an excess risk of breast cancer in younger women exposed to high doses of radiation. These data, combined with the low incidence of breast cancer in young women (less than 1% of breast cancer occurs in women under 30), suggest that a restricted use of mammography is prudent. Some experts also believe that dense breast tissue, which is more common in younger women, limits the sensitivity of mammography, but studies have shown that mammography can demonstrate up to 90% of cancers in women under 35 (17).

Women under the age of 30 who have a focal suspicious palpable abnormality are frequently first evaluated with US. If the US is negative and the patient is over age 20, a single oblique view of the affected breast is performed to assess for suspicious microcalcifications, which would not be visualized by US. Women under age 20 should not undergo mammography.

If fine-needle aspiration is available, it may be used in lieu of imaging studies when young patients have suspicious palpable masses. In the extremely rare circumstance of a diagnosis of carcinoma, mammography can be performed subsequently. The radiologist should be aware that a previous needle aspiration may confound the mammographic assessment of the affected area, but it will not compromise assessment of surrounding or contralateral tissues.

Increased awareness of breast cancer has led many clinicians to request more imaging studies in young women. However, breast imaging cannot replace careful clinical evaluation of the breasts. If there is no suspicious focal abnormality, imaging studies will not be helpful; they may subject the patient to unnecessary risk.

TECHNICAL CONSIDERATIONS IN BREAST IMAGING

Because both high contrast and high spatial resolution are needed for optimal mammography, standard radiographic equipment cannot be utilized for this examination. Mammography must be performed on a unit dedicated to this purpose. Mammographic equipment and technique differ from standard radiography in several ways. The anode material utilized to generate the x-rays in most dedicated mammography units is molybdenum. This allows the production of lower-energy x-rays, which in turn produces greater contrast between soft tissue structures. The structures of the breast do not differ greatly in their inherent contrast, so these low-kilovolt or "softer" photons are extremely important in producing a high-contrast image. Some units also have rhodium anodes that can be used to increase the contrast in denser breasts, while keeping radiation dose and time of exposure low.

The radiologist must be able to discern tiny microcalcifications on mammograms; some of these calcifications may be 0.1 mm or less in size. The small focal spot size used in mammography units, a longer distance from the x-ray source to the image, and special high-resolution, single intensifying screens used with single-emulsion film contribute to the creation of images with high resolution.

All mammographic units are equipped with compression paddles that squeeze the breast against the film holder. Good compression of the breast is essential to high-quality mammography for several reasons. Compression spreads overlapping breast structures so that true masses can be differentiated from summation shadows that occur because of overlapping soft tissues. The breast is immobilized during compression so motion unsharpness or blurring caused by patient movement is minimized. Geometric unsharpness, caused by the finite focal spot dimension, is minimized by bringing the breast structures closer to the film. Compression renders the breast nearly uniform in thickness so the film density of tissues near the nipple will be similar to that of the tissues near the chest wall. Radiation dose can be reduced by the use of good compression; a thinner breast requires fewer photons for penetration. Beam attenuation is also reduced.

Some women find breast compression uncomfortable, but most can tolerate it once the benefits are explained. During routine mammography, the breast is compressed for a few seconds while each film is taken. Many units are equipped with automated compression devices so the technologist can release the tension immediately after the film is exposed.

Other factors are also important to consider in the production of high-quality mammograms. These include other equipment features, such as type of x-ray generator, beam filtration, and grid use, as well as film-intensifying screen combinations and the film processing system. All of these factors are interrelated and must be optimized to produce technically acceptable films of the breast.

Full-Field Digital Mammography

Full-field digital mammography (FFDM) units have been commercially available since 2000. Positioning and compression of the breast for FFDM are the same as for film screen mammography, but FFDM uses an electronic system for image capture and display. It has higher contrast resolution and equal or better dynamic range than film screen mammography. Spatial resolution is lower with FFDM, but its greater contrast resolution still makes high-quality images possible. The radiation dose from FFDM is comparable to that of film screen mammography in smaller breasts; it may be lower in larger breasts. Advantages of FFDM over film screen mammography include a higher speed of image acquisition and thus increased throughput of patients; the ability to perform image processing, which may lead to fewer repeat films because of optimization of brightness and contrast; other image-processing algorithms, which may result in increased conspicuity of certain features, including microcalcifications; integration of computer-aided detection and diagnosis software programs; electronic storage, thus eliminating lost films and the need for film storage; and the possibility of teleradiology.

Although there are technical advantages to FFDM, early clinical trials have not shown an increase in cancer detection rates with FFDM as compared to film screen mammography. FFDM technology is in its infancy; it is likely that future improvements will result in improved clinical outcomes (18).

Quality Assurance

It is the responsibility of the radiologist to assure that highest quality of breast imaging is performed at his or her facility. All standards mandated by the Mammography Quality Standards Act (MQSA) must be met. These standards apply to both film screen mammography and FFDM. MQSA was passed into law by Congress in 1992 to ensure that all women receive optimal mammography services. The law requires that every practice become accredited by the Food and Drug Administration (FDA). Specified standards for personnel (radiologists, technologists, and physicists); equipment utilized; radiation dose; and quality assurance practices are stipulated. Once FDA accreditation is granted, an annual survey by a physicist must be performed to ensure that the practice continues to meet quality control and equipment standards. All facilities performing mammography are inspected annually by an FDA inspector. Each radiologist who interprets mammograms must be fully informed of the MQSA regulations. Failure to comply with the law can result in sanctions or even closure of the mammography facility.

Mammographic Positioning for Screening

Mammography can be performed with the patient seated or standing. Most screening practices prefer the standing position because it allows faster throughput and is less cumbersome. Patients are able to lean into the unit to a greater degree when standing, thus allowing more of the posterior breast tissues to be imaged. Recumbent imaging is possible, but quite difficult; its use should be restricted to problem-solving situations.

Two views of each breast are generally utilized for screening mammography in the United States. Several European countries utilize a single mediolateral oblique (MLO) view for screening examinations, but authorities in this country have shown that one-view examinations would lead to an excessive number of patients being called back for additional views. Asking large numbers of patients to return for such views would result in unacceptable levels of patient anxiety and cost. The standard views for screening mammography are the MLO view and the craniocaudal (CC) view.

MLO View. The MLO view, when properly positioned, depicts the greatest amount of breast tissue. It is the most useful view in mammography. In those countries using single-view screening, the MLO view is preferred. To perform an MLO view, the x-ray tube and film holder, which are fixed with respect to one another, are moved to an angle that parallels the orientation of the patient's pectoralis major muscle. The technologist is given flexibility in choosing the angle so that the greatest amount of breast tissue possible can be imaged. The angle is generally between 40° and 60° from the horizontal.

The patient is asked to relax her arm and chest muscles and lean into the machine. The breast is placed on the film holder and compression is applied from the superomedial direction, the same direction from which the x-rays will be generated. The breast must be pulled anteriorly and spread in a superoinferior direction as much as possible to minimize overlapping structures and to maximize the amount of tissue imaged. The nipple should be in profile. Compression must be applied vigorously (Fig. 20.1). By convention, in the MLO view a marker indicating the side (left or right) and type of view is placed near the axillary tissues of the breast.

A properly positioned MLO mammogram should show the pectoralis major muscle down to the level of a line drawn perpendicular to the muscle through the nipple (posterior nipple line). The nipple should be in profile so that the subareolar area can be adequately evaluated. The inframammary fold should be visible to ensure that the inferior portion of the breast has been imaged (Fig. 20.2).

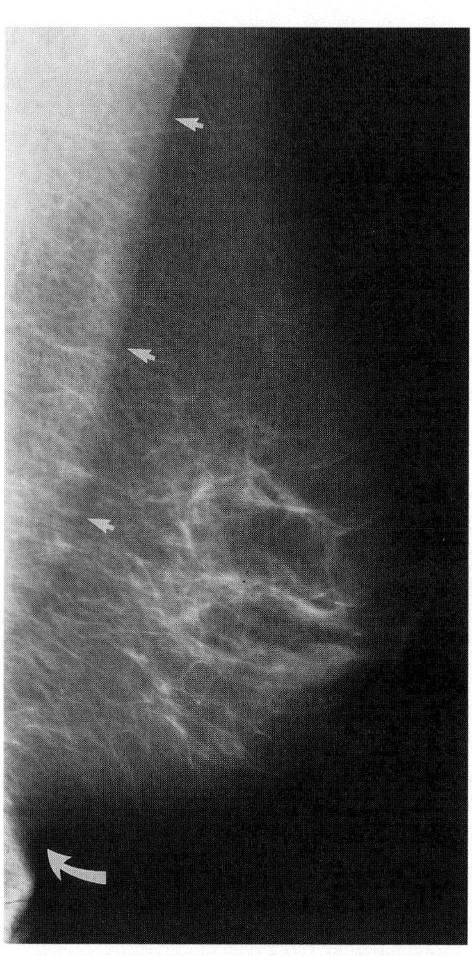

FIGURE 20.2. **Normal MLO View of Left Breast.** The pectoralis muscle (*white arrows*) is seen from the axilla to below the level of the posterior nipple line. The inframammary fold (*curved arrow*) is well seen, and the nipple is in profile.

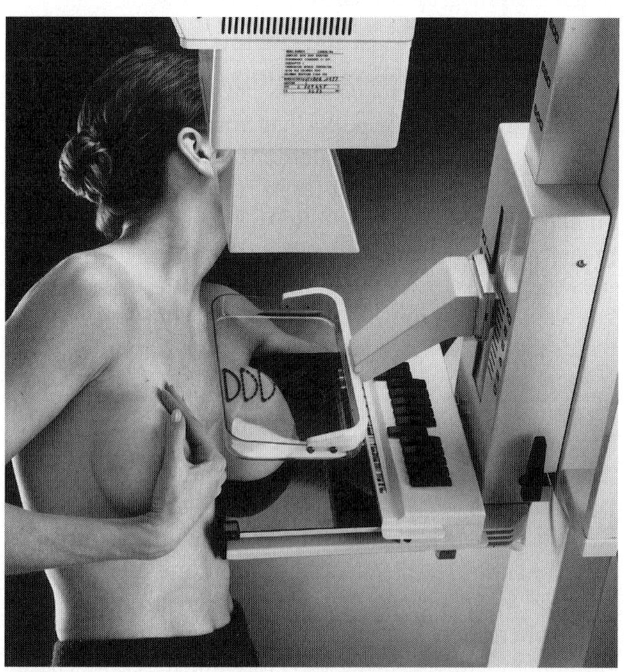

FIGURE 20.1. **Patient Positioning for an MLO View.** (Reproduced with permission from General Electric Medical Systems, Milwaukee, Wisconsin.)

CC View. For the CC view, the unit is placed in the vertical position so that the x-ray tube is perpendicular to the floor. Photons will travel from the anode, located superior to the breast, to the film underneath the breast. The breast is placed on the film holder, pulled anteriorly, and spread horizontally before the compression plate is applied to the superior skin surface (Fig. 20.3). The nipple should again be in profile. The chest wall should rest against the film holder. The markers indicating the side imaged and type of view should be placed near the skin close to the lateral aspect of the breast.

In evaluating a CC mammogram, optimal positioning can be assured when pectoralis muscle is seen centrally on the film and the nipple is in profile (Fig. 20.4). The pectoralis muscle can be visualized in about 30% of patients on the CC view. An alternative method of assuring appropriate visualization of posterior tissues is to measure the distance from the nipple to the edge of the film through the central axis of the breast; this distance should be within

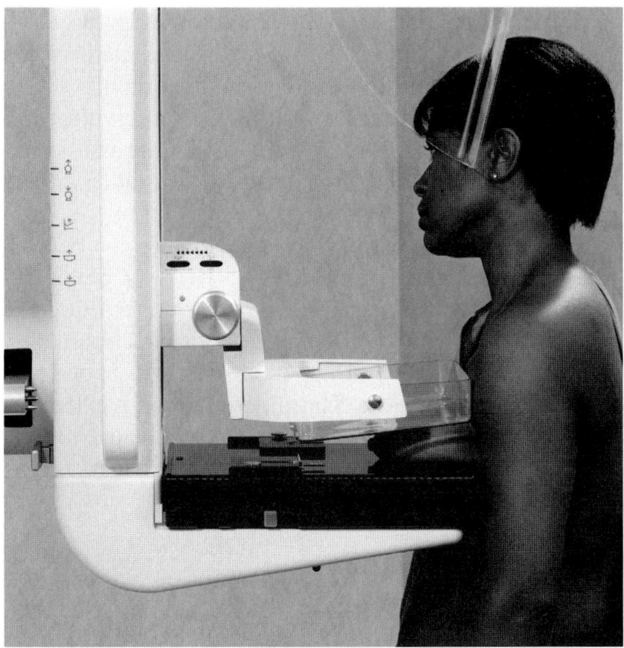

FIGURE 20.3. **Patient Positioning for the CC View.** (Reproduced with permission from Hologic Inc, Bedford, Massachusetts.)

1 cm of the length of the posterior nipple line as seen on the MLO view.

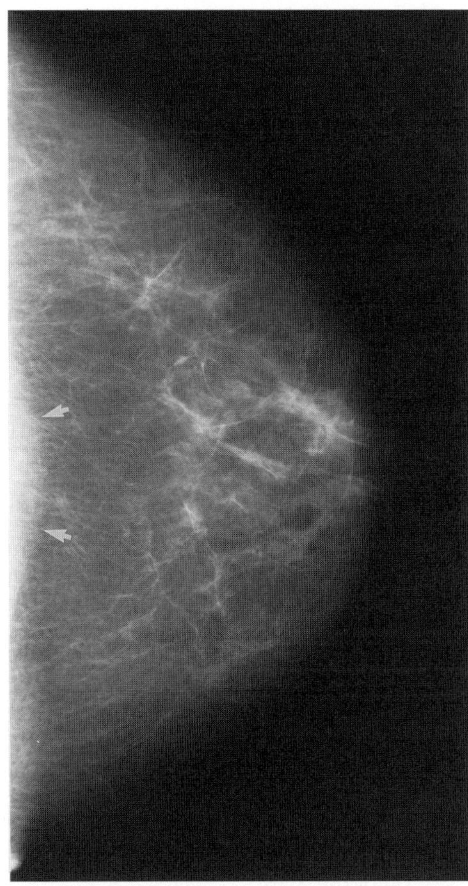

FIGURE 20.4. **Normal CC View of the Left Breast.** Note that the nipple is in profile and the pectoralis muscle (*arrows*) is seen posteriorly, indicating optimal visualization of breast tissue.

Interpreting the Mammogram

For interpretation, CC and MLO mammograms should each be viewed together in a mirror-image configuration. This will allow the radiologist to scan the breasts for symmetry. Viewing conditions are extremely important to optimal interpretation. The room must be darkened. All adjacent view box light should be blocked out. Dedicated mammography film alternators and view boxes can do this automatically. If standard view boxes or alternators are used, exposed blackened film can be cut to mask out unwanted light.

A magnifying lens should be used to examine each film thoroughly. All visible parenchyma should be scanned systematically with magnification. This will allow visualization of tiny microcalcifications and will ensure that the radiologist has examined all parts of the breast in detail.

Computer workstations should be used for interpretation of FFDM. High-resolution monitors with magnification capability are essential.

If previous mammograms are available, they should be compared to the current study so that the radiologist can evaluate the examination for any changes in the mammographic appearance of the breasts. In turn, current questionable areas can be evaluated for their stability.

In most practices, patients are asked to complete a brief history form that includes questions relevant to breast health and cancer risk. Knowledge of the patient's history will be helpful in assessing the malignant potential and likely diagnosis of a particular mammographic finding. The risk of malignancy is much greater in a 60-year-old woman than in a 30-year-old woman. A woman with a personal or close family history of breast cancer is at greater risk for development of malignancy, and the interpretation of mammographic findings should be tailored accordingly. Other information, such as previous surgical biopsies or hormone replacement intake, must also be taken into account during interpretation of the mammogram.

Correlation with the physical examination is also extremely important, so that false-negative reports can be minimized. All palpable lesions should be marked and assessed mammographically. Special views can image palpable lesions that occur in locations not included on standard mammography. The mammographer can also be certain that the mass felt corresponds to the mammographic abnormality. Areas of asymmetric tissue seen mammographically can be assessed for palpable abnormalities, which may render them more suspicious for malignancy.

Classic mammographic signs of malignancy are spiculated masses or pleomorphic clusters of microcalcifications; however, only about 40% of all occult breast carcinoma presents in these ways (19). In the remainder of cases, more subtle or indirect signs of malignancy are present. The radiologist must look at each mammogram with great care, utilizing all available diagnostic techniques so that false-negative diagnoses are minimized. This charge must be balanced against the need to minimize false-positive diagnoses. Each time a woman is subjected to a surgical biopsy, financial and emotional costs as well as risks are incurred.

Diagnostic Evaluation of the Indeterminate Mammogram

In the majority of cases, a two-view screening mammogram will provide a conclusive interpretation, but when the results of mammography are indeterminate, further evaluation is necessary; additional mammographic views (Table 20.2) (20) or US may be required for clarification. The workup must be tailored to the specific situation.

Projections other than the standard CC and MLO views may help to visualize a lesion that is seen only in one standard view or that is obscured by surrounding parenchyma. Tangential views of the skin can be used to establish a dermal location for calcifications or superficial masses. Dermal abnormalities do not represent breast cancer.

Further characterization of an abnormality can be accomplished with spot compression and magnification views. The compression plate used is much smaller than that used in standard views; therefore, greater force can be applied, which results both in further spreading of any overlying tissue and in bringing the abnormality closer to the film for increased detail. Magnification also produces finer detail, which allows more accurate assessment of the morphology of microcalcifications and the borders of masses.

Well-defined or partially obscured masses can be evaluated with US. A high-frequency (>5 MHz), handheld linear array transducer is most commonly used. A targeted evaluation of the mammographically visible abnormality is performed. Simple cysts are easily distinguishable from complex or solid masses. This differentiation is extremely important, because simple cysts are always benign and require no further workup, whereas noncystic masses may represent cancers.

ANALYZING THE MAMMOGRAM

Masses

Complete assessment of a mammographically visible, potentially malignant mass requires several steps. First, the radiologist must decide whether the mass is real. The left and right breasts must be compared in each view.

Most women have reasonably symmetric parenchyma; however, at least 3% of women have areas of asymmetric but histologically normal breast tissue. When attempting to distinguish asymmetric normal breast tissue from a true abnormality, the radiologist must look for the mammographic features of a mass. Masses have convex borders

TABLE 20.2 Diagnostic Mammographic Views

View	*Abbreviation*	*Purpose*
90° lateral	ML (mediolateral) or LM (lateral medial)	Visualize localizing lesion in one view Demonstrate milk of calcium, owing to its gravity dependency
Spot compression	—	Determine whether lesion is real or is a summation shadow
Spot compression with magnification	M	Better definition of margins of masses and morphology of calcifications
Exaggerated craniocaudal	XCCL	Show lesions in outer aspect of breast and axillary tail not seen on CC view
Cleavage view	CV	Show lesions deep in posteromedial breast not seen in CC view
Tangential	TAN	Verify skin lesions Show palpable lesions obscured by dense tissue
Roll view	RM (rolled medial) or RL (rolled lateral)	Verify true lesions Determine location of lesion seen in one view by seeing how location changes
Lateromedial oblique	LMO	Improved visualization of superomedial tissue Improved tissue visualization and comfort for women with pectus excavatum, recent sternotomy, prominent pacemaker
Implant displacement	ID	Improved visualization of native breast tissue in women with implants

and become denser toward the center. They distort the normal breast architecture. True masses are seen in multiple projections and can still be visualized when focal compression is utilized (Fig. 20.5).

Asymmetric breast parenchyma has an amorphous quality. On spot compression, the tissue spreads apart and fat can be seen interspersed with the denser breast structures in a pattern of normal architecture (Fig. 20.6). The appearance of asymmetric tissue varies significantly from one mammographic projection to another.

When evaluating the breast for a possible mass, it is important to correlate the mammographic findings with the physical examination. When a suspicious palpable abnormality corresponds to an area of asymmetry seen on mammography, a biopsy should be undertaken. In a study of 221 patients with mammographically visible asymmetries, only three patients had malignancies, and all three had suspicious, palpable abnormalities that corresponded to the visualized asymmetries (21).

Summation shadows that resemble masses on mammography can be produced by overlapping breast tissue. They are visible in only one view and usually disappear when focal compression spreads the tissues apart.

Once the radiologist has concluded that a mass is present, its margins, density, location, and size should be assessed. The number of mammographically visible masses and their similarities or differences should be analyzed. Previous films should be compared with the current study to look for new masses or an increase in the size of a mass. It is impossible to evaluate one characteristic independent of the others.

Margins

The margins of a mass are probably the most important characteristics to be assessed. Overlying breast parenchyma often obscures margin analysis, but liberal use of magnification compression views, in multiple projections, will aid the radiologist.

Spiculated Margins

Breast carcinoma classically appears as a spiculated mass on mammography (Fig. 20.7); however, fewer than 20% of nonpalpable cancers present as such (18). Most spiculated-appearing breast cancers will be infiltrating ductal carcinoma; however, tubular and lobular carcinomas can present as such. Tubular carcinomas are more well-differentiated histologically and carry a better prognosis. Lobular carcinomas comprise about 10% of all

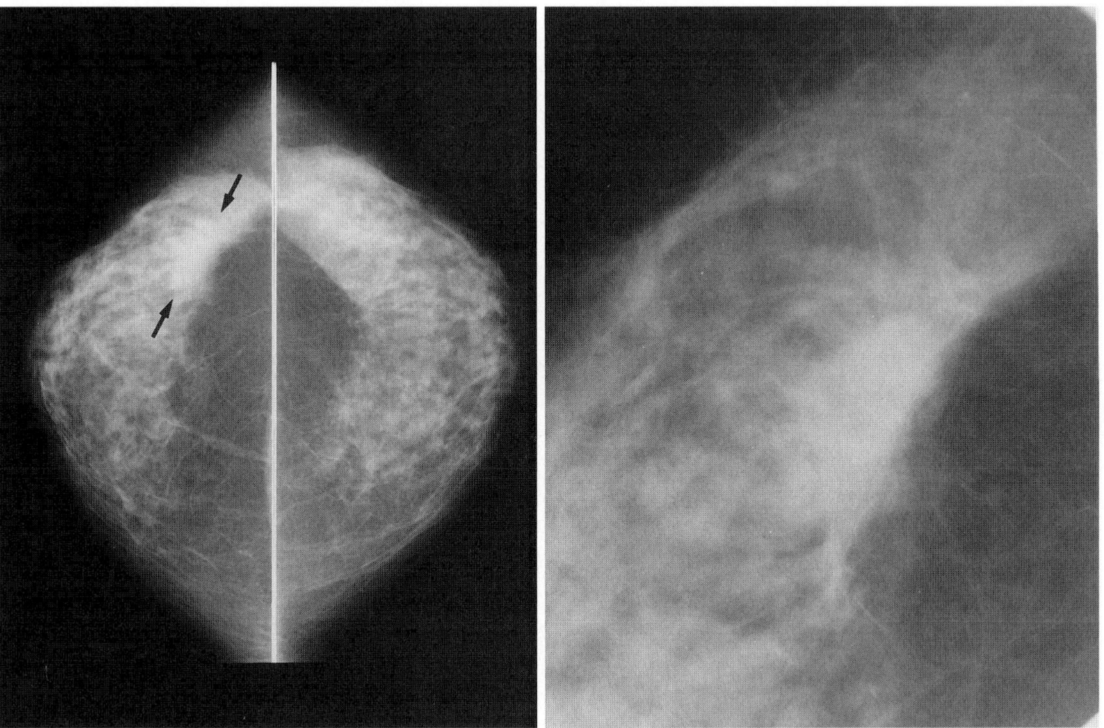

FIGURE 20.5. **Infiltrating Duct Carcinoma. A.** CC views of both breasts, showing an asymmetric area of increased density in the outer aspect of the right breast (*arrows*). **B.** Magnification compression view shows this to be a true mass with defined, convex borders and increasing density toward its center.

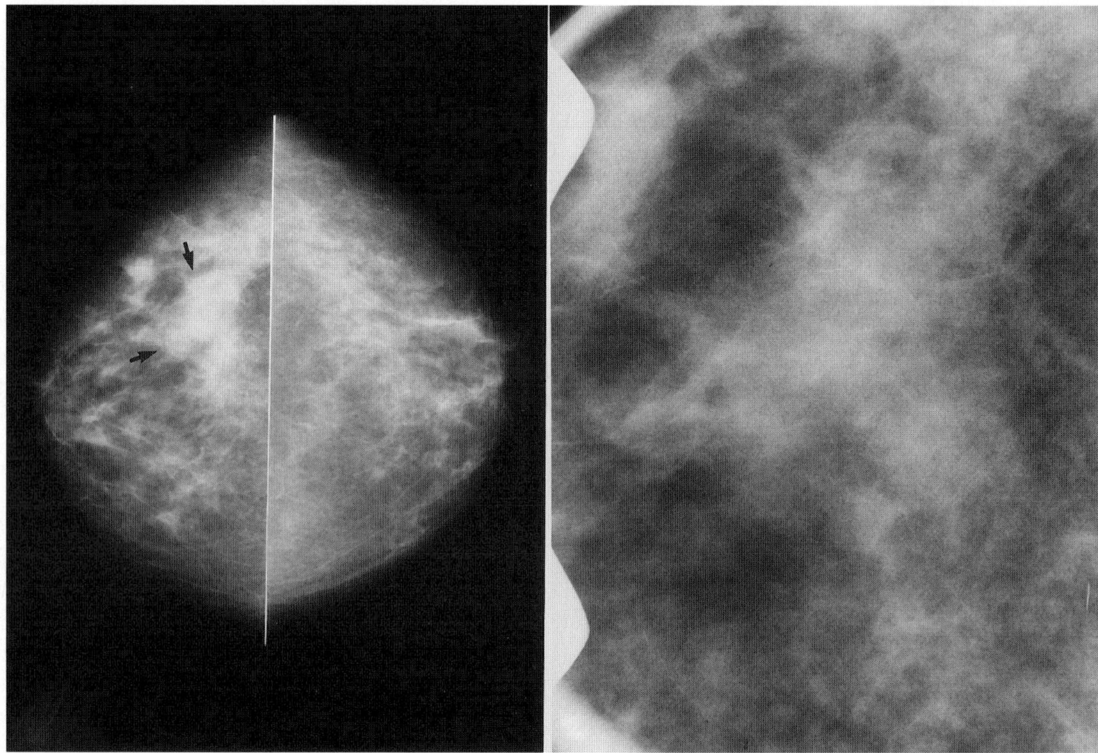

FIGURE 20.6. **Asymmetric Breast Parenchyma. A.** CC views of both breasts in an asymptomatic woman. An area of asymmetric density is seen in the outer aspect of the right breast (*arrows*). **B.** Compression magnification view demonstrates normal breast architecture in the area of increased density. These findings are consistent with histologically normal but asymmetric mammary parenchyma.

invasive carcinomas. They are not mammographically distinguishable from invasive ductal carcinomas, although they are frequently more subtle. Single rows of lobular cancer cells can infiltrate surrounding tissues, so they generally cause less tissue distortion.

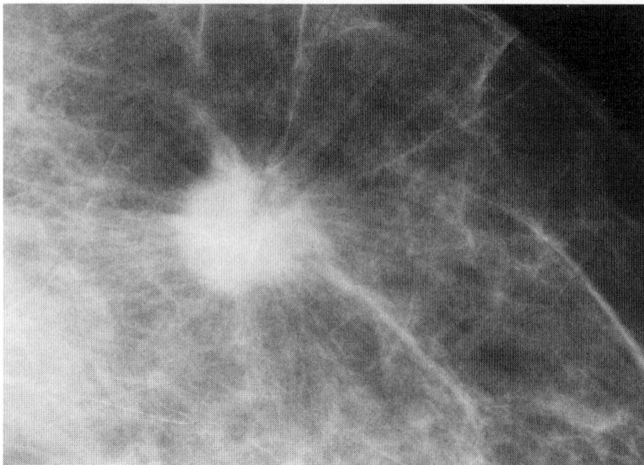

FIGURE 20.7. **Classic Breast Carcinoma.** This spiculated breast mass is an infiltrating duct carcinoma.

A very limited differential exists for a spiculated mass. ***Fat necrosis*** from a previous surgical biopsy can appear spiculated (Fig. 20.8).

Scars from previous breast surgery should be marked carefully with radiopaque wires. Comparison should be made with previous films, both to determine the location of the abnormality that underwent biopsy and to assess for any increase in size of the presumed scar. Many scars will regress with time, but others will be stable in appearance and size. Any increase in size should be viewed with suspicion and biopsy should be undertaken.

Radial scars or complex sclerosing lesions can also present as spiculated lesions. These are spontaneous lesions that are benign and consist histologically of central sclerosis and varying degrees of epithelial proliferation, represented by strands of fibrous connective tissue. Histologic differentiation of these lesions from carcinoma is mandatory.

Indistinct (Ill-Defined) Margins

Breast carcinoma can also present as a round mass with indistinct or ill-defined borders (Fig. 20.9). Benign lesions that can present as such include abscess, hematoma, and focal fibrosis.

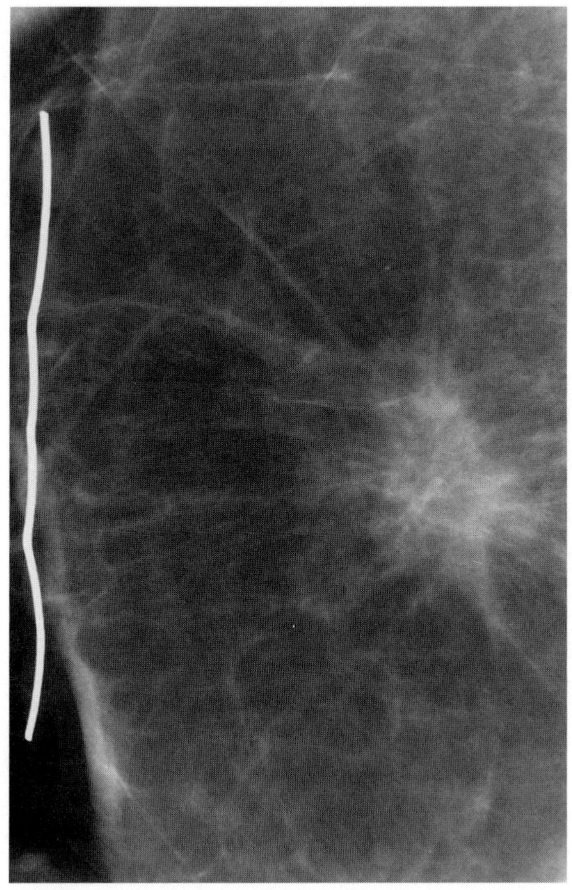

FIGURE 20.8. **Postsurgical Fat Necrosis.** This spiculated mass had been stable for 7 years. The radiopaque wire indicates the scar on the patient's skin from the previous lumpectomy.

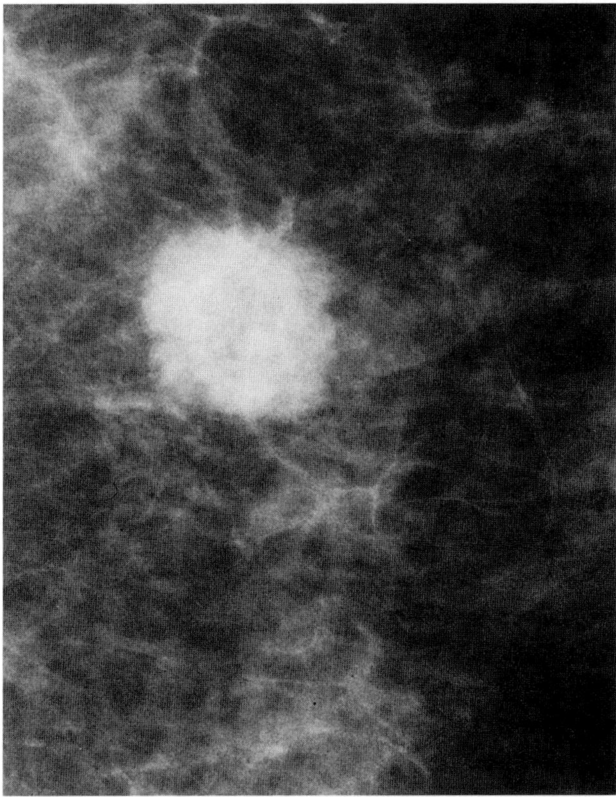

FIGURE 20.9. **Infiltrating Duct Carcinoma.** Lesion presenting as a round mass with indistinct, microlobulated borders.

Breast abscesses are most commonly seen in a subareolar location in lactating women (Fig. 20.10). Clinically, there is associated pain, swelling, and erythema.

Spontaneous hematomas are seen in women on anticoagulant therapy or in those with blood dyscrasias. They can, of course, also be secondary to trauma, needle aspiration, or surgery. Correlation with the patient's history and physical examination will be helpful in discerning whether a lesion represents a hematoma. If doubt persists as to the nature of a possible hematoma, short-interval follow-up mammograms (4 to 6 weeks later) to demonstrate resolution will be helpful (Fig. 20.11).

Circumscribed (Well-Defined) Margins

Circumscribed masses are almost always benign; however, up to 5% of masses that appear well circumscribed on conventional mammograms may represent carcinomas (22). The "halo sign," which is a partial or complete radiolucent ring surrounding a mass, is not helpful in determining benignity. Sonography should be used to assess circumscribed masses prior to any additional mammographic views; if a simple cyst is diagnosed by US, no further imaging workup is required. Magnification compression views will be of great assistance in clarifying the nature of borders of an apparently well-circumscribed solid mass. Masses that appear well circumscribed on conventional views may have indistinct or microlobulated margins on compression magnification views (23); such masses should undergo biopsy. If a solid mass appears circumscribed on magnification views and no previous mammograms are available for comparison, the mass can generally be characterized as one that has a high probability of being benign. Such masses are frequently subjected to a course of follow-up mammography. The first of these surveillance mammograms should be performed 6 months following the original study.

Cysts are the most common well-circumscribed masses seen in women between the ages of 35 and 50 (Fig. 20.12). They are rare after menopause unless hormone replacement therapy has been instituted. Cysts can be accurately diagnosed by US and are virtually never malignant. A high-frequency (generally 5 to 10 MHz) US transducer is utilized in a targeted examination of the mass in question. On sonography, cysts are round or oval, smooth-walled, anechoic, and produce enhanced through transmission of sound. They can frequently be deformed with gentle

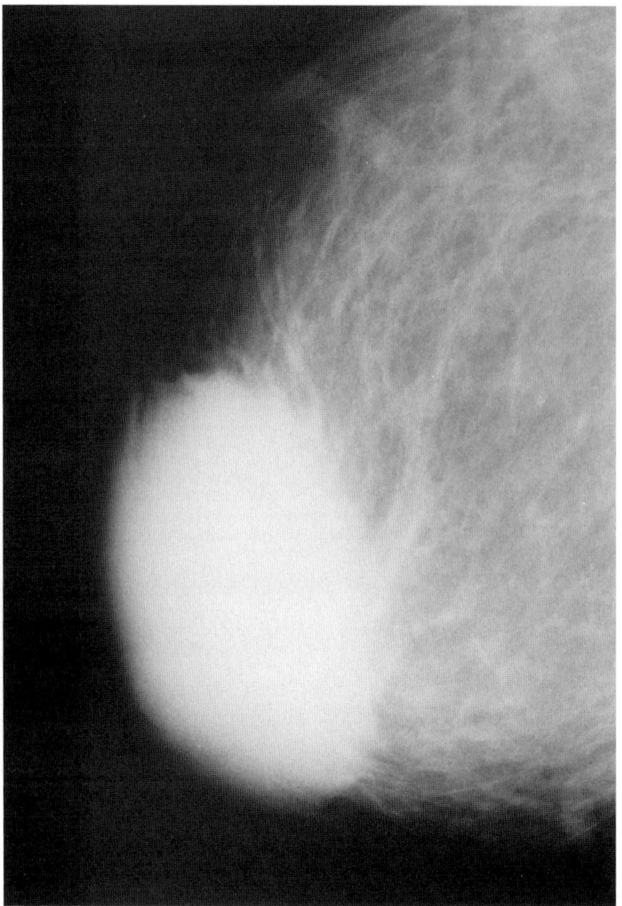

FIGURE 20.10. **Large Subareolar Abscess.** The indistinct borders of the mass are the result of surrounding inflammation.

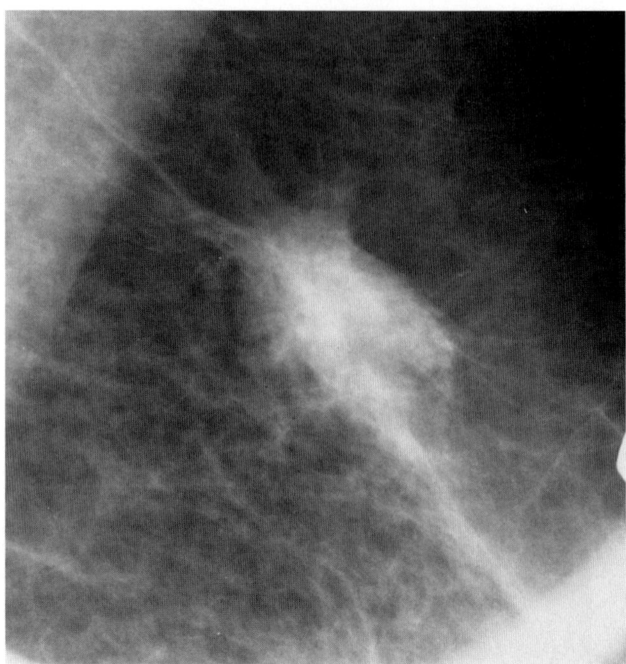

FIGURE 20.11. **Infiltrating Duct Carcinoma.** Magnification view of a palpable abnormality in the upper outer quadrant. The patient had undergone a negative fine-needle aspiration biopsy the previous day; the mammographic differential diagnosis included hematoma and carcinoma. Follow-up mammogram 6 weeks later demonstrated no resolution. Surgical biopsy showed infiltrating duct carcinoma.

pressure from the transducer. It is essential that the focal zone and gain of the US unit be optimally adjusted for the lesion so that cysts can be accurately diagnosed sonographically. The cyst must be thoroughly examined in two projections to rule out any irregularities or masses emanating from the walls.

Fibrosis is another manifestation of fibrocystic change that can be seen mammographically. It can be quite focal, giving it the appearance of a well-defined mass on the films. Such areas of focal fibrosis may also present with ill-defined borders, making them difficult to differentiate from carcinomas.

Fibroadenomas are the most common well-defined solid masses seen on mammography (Fig. 20.13). They are homogenous but frequently show large, coarse calcifications. They may have a lobulated contour, but there are usually only a few large lobulations. If a fibroadenoma is not calcified, it cannot be distinguished from a cyst by mammography. Sonography will allow characterization of fibroadenomas as solid hypoechoic masses. The peak age of patients with clinically detected fibroadenomas is 20 to 30 years; however, fibroadenomas are seen into the eighth decade. They rarely appear or grow after menopause.

Primary breast malignancies to be considered when a well-defined density is visualized on mammography are *infiltrating duct carcinoma, papillary carcinoma, mucinous carcinoma,* and *medullary carcinoma.*

Lymphoma, either primary or metastatic, may also present as a well-circumscribed mass.

Metastatic disease to the breast from other sources may present as a well-circumscribed nodule. The most common primary cancer to produce breast metastases is melanoma, but a large variety of other primary sites have also been reported to metastasize to the breast. When these malignancies are encountered, magnification compression views of the abnormality often demonstrate some irregularity to the contour of the mass (Fig. 20.14).

Density

Density is relevant to analysis of mammographically detected masses when these masses contain lucent areas indicative of fat. Breast masses that clearly contain fat are benign. The assessment of density in homogeneous nonfatty masses is not, however, useful in the prediction of benignity or malignancy.

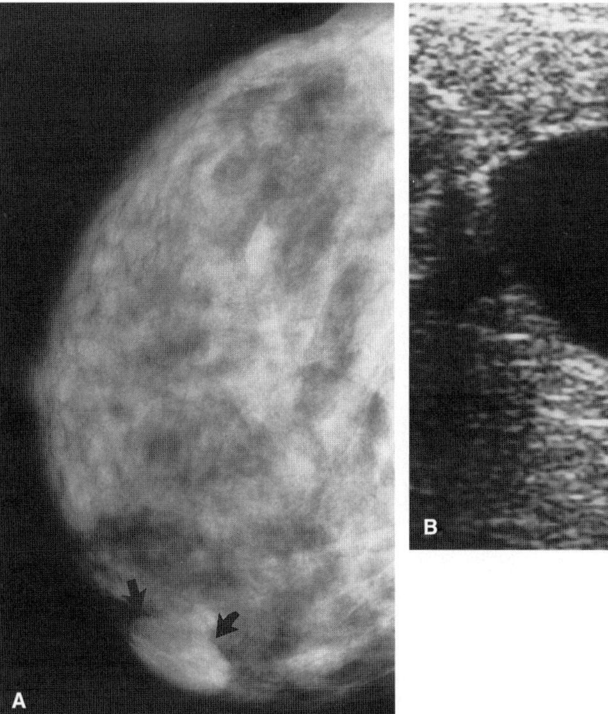

FIGURE 20.12. **Simple Breast Cyst. A.** CC mammogram demonstrates a 1.5-cm mass in a 50-year-old-woman (*arrows*). The mass is at least partially well circumscribed. **B.** US of the mass demonstrates a round, anechoic structure with well-defined margins that was enhanced through transmission of sound. These features are diagnostic of a simple cyst.

Fat Density. Benign breast lesions that are purely fat density include oil cysts from fat necrosis, lipomas, and sometimes galactoceles. *Oil cysts* are generally the result of trauma (Fig. 20.15). They are round lucent lesions surrounded by a thin capsule; often they are multiple and can demonstrate rim calcifications. *Lipomas* are similar to oil cysts in appearance; they are also lucent with a surrounding capsule. The surrounding breast architecture may be distorted because of the mass effect of the lipoma. *Galactoceles* usually occur in lactating or recently lactating women and are probably the result of an obstructed duct. If the inspissated milk is of sufficient fat quantity, these lesions will appear lucent; however, they can also be of mixed or water density.

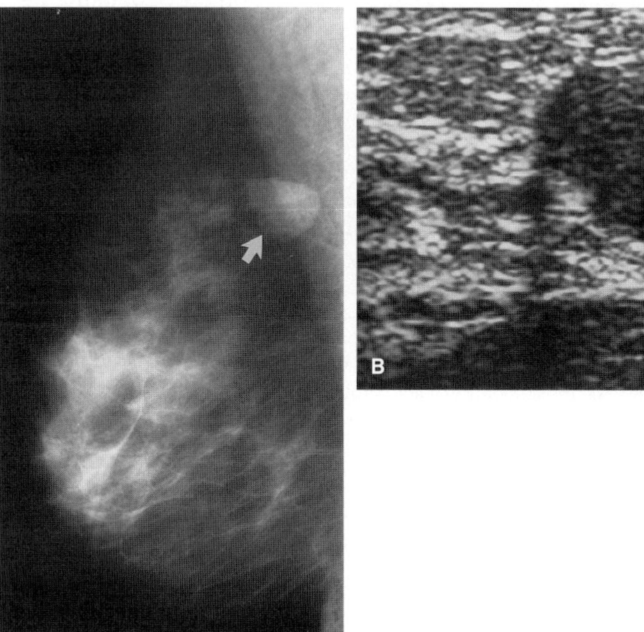

FIGURE 20.13. **Fibroadenoma. A.** MLO view of a 1.8-cm, partially well-defined mass (*arrow*). **B.** US demonstrates a solid hypoechoic mass with a macrolobulated, well-defined margin.

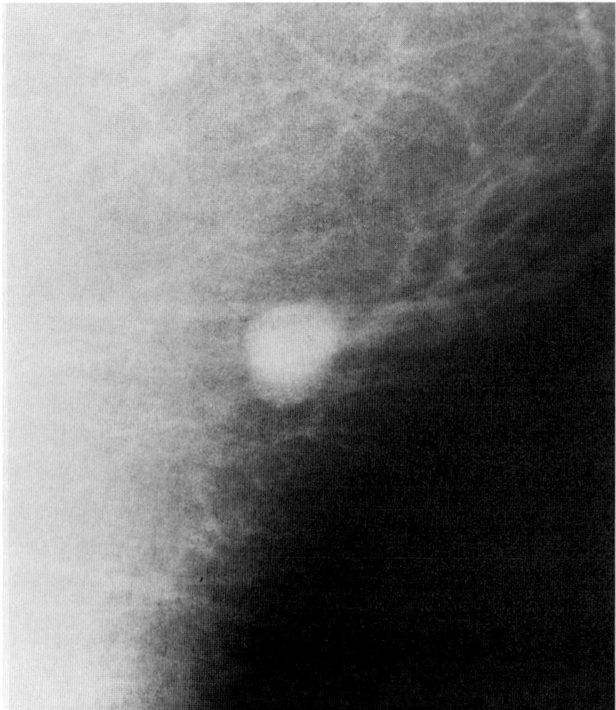

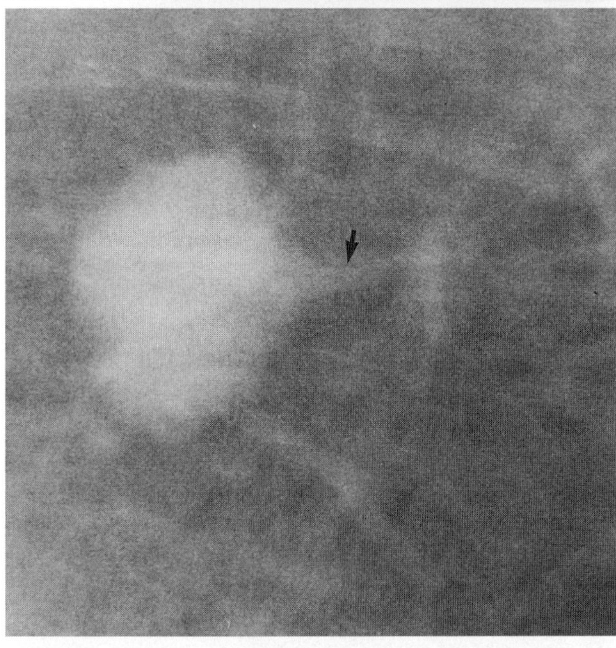

FIGURE 20.14. **Infiltrating Duct Carcinoma. A.** A well-circumscribed, 8-mm mass that had enlarged compared with a study done 1 year previously. **B.** Magnification view shows a spiculation anteriorly (*arrow*). Infiltrating duct carcinoma was proven at biopsy.

Mixed Fat and Water Density. Other benign masses that are mixed fat and water density are *hamartomas*, which are rare benign tumors, and *intramammary lymph nodes*. The latter are frequently seen on mammograms. They are generally located in the upper outer quadrant in the posterior three fourths of the breast parenchyma. They normally contain a fatty center or a lucent notch, representing fat in the hilus of the node (Fig. 20.16). Fat–fluid levels can occasionally be seen on MLO mammograms in galactoceles and postsurgical hematomas.

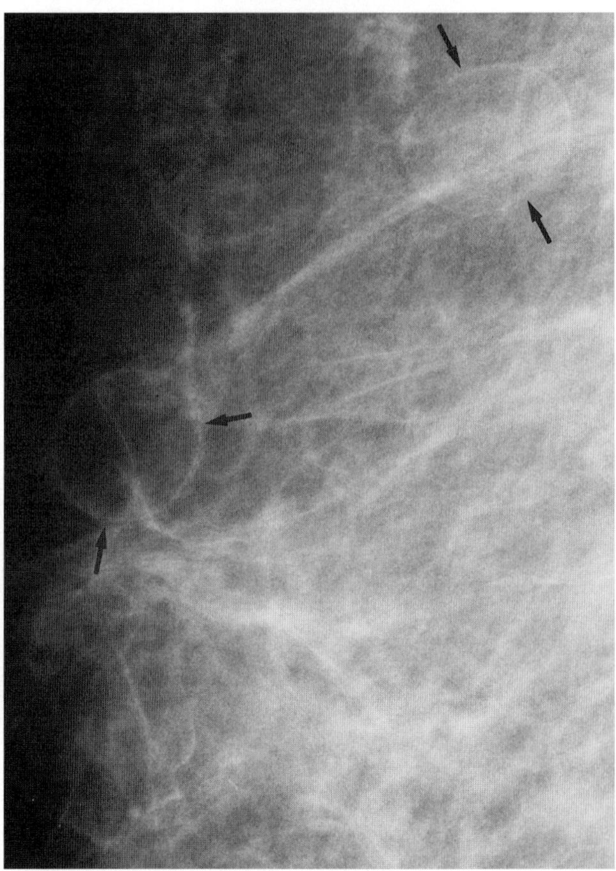

FIGURE 20.15. **Oil Cysts.** Multiple lucent masses with thin capsules (*arrows*) are characteristic of oil cysts. The patient had suffered trauma to the breast.

Location

Breast cancers can occur in any location within the breast. As such, the location of a lesion is helpful in mammographic diagnosis in only two situations. The first occurs when the mammographer is considering an intramammary lymph node in the differential. The second occurs when a lesion can be localized to the skin.

Intramammary nodes visualized on mammograms are almost always located in the upper outer quadrant of the breast. They have been noted in other locations in autopsy series, and there are rare case reports of visualization of such nodes by mammography in other locations in the breast.

Skin Lesions. If a lesion is located only on the skin, it does not represent a breast carcinoma. Frequently, however, skin lesions project over the parenchyma and can

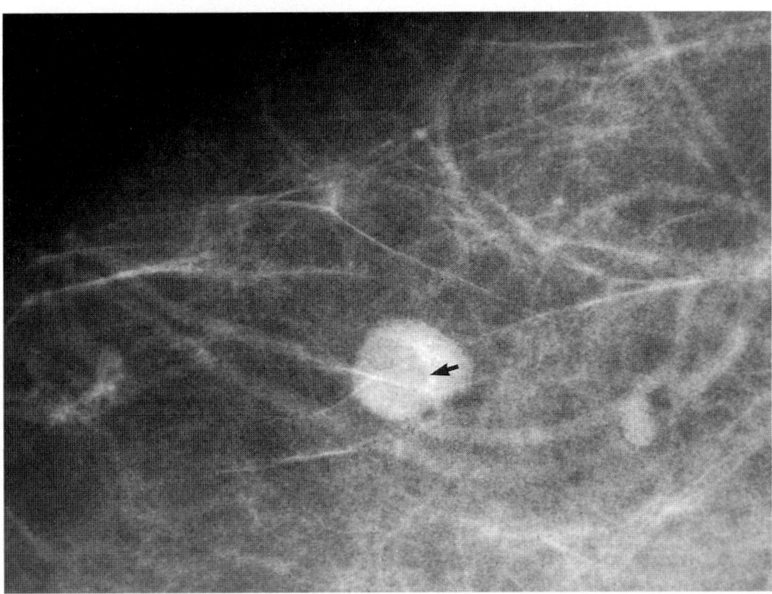

FIGURE 20.16. **Intramammary Lymph Node.** Intramammary lymph node displays a characteristic lucent center (*arrow*) and well-circumscribed margins. The node was located in the upper outer quadrant.

appear to be within the breast. Such lesions are usually recognizable by air trapping around the edges or in the interstices. This air trapping can produce a dark halo around one edge (Fig. 20.17). Air trapping will not, however, be evident with flat, pigmented skin lesions or sebaceous cysts.

It is helpful to examine the patient and place a radiopaque marker on any skin lesions or possible sebaceous cysts. The technologist can then perform a repeat film in the projection that the lesion was visualized. If necessary, this view can be followed by a tangential view to demonstrate that the lesion is located in the skin.

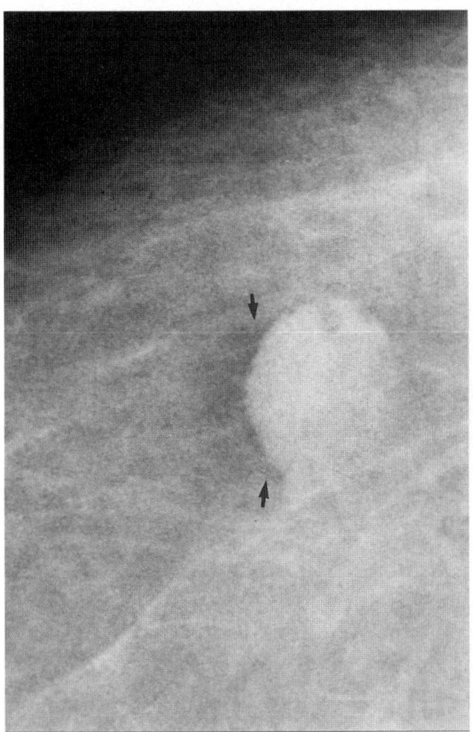

FIGURE 20.17. **Skin Nevus.** The dark halo produced around one edge is the result of air trapping (*arrows*).

Size

By itself, the size of a mammographically discovered mass is not particularly helpful in determining its etiology. A spiculated or ill-defined mass should undergo biopsy no matter what its size. However, when the mammographer is dealing with a circumscribed mass that has a much lower chance of being malignant, size may play a role in determining the next step in the workup. US is not usually helpful when lesions are less than about 3 to 5 mm in size, particularly in fatty breasts. Frequently, patients with such lesions will be asked to return in 6 months for a follow-up study to assess for interval growth. If the lesion increases in size, further investigation with US and possible biopsy can be performed. After the first 6-month follow-up, stable lesions should be followed at yearly intervals for a minimum of 3 years.

Larger, clinically occult masses require both US—to prove they are solid—and magnification views to prove they are circumscribed before surveillance mammography is suggested. Some experts advocate an upper size limit of 1 to 1.5 cm for masses that are to undergo follow-up, but recent research has shown that nonpalpable, circumscribed breast masses can be managed by periodic mammographic surveillance regardless of size (24). Generally, a 6-month follow-up of the affected breast is advocated; this is followed by a bilateral mammogram 6 months later and then annual mammography for at least 3 years to document stability.

Number Of Masses

Multiple Masses. In many cases, multiple well-defined round masses will be seen on mammography. When evident, such masses are also frequently bilateral. Multiple, bilateral round masses are usually benign. They most often represent *cysts* or *fibroadenomas*, although *multiple papillomas* can also present in this way (Fig. 20.18). In patients with a history of previous malignancy, however, *metastasis* may also be considered, although metastatic disease is much more commonly unifocal.

All lesions should be evaluated carefully. Benign and malignant lesions can coexist in the same breast. A lesion with a different, suspicious morphology should prompt a biopsy.

When evaluating the patient with similar appearing multiple, bilateral, rounded breast masses, it is not generally advisable to utilize US. US is confusing and frequently demonstrates hypoechoic areas that, although disconcerting to the radiologist, do not prove to be malignant. *Multifocal primary breast cancers* generally present as obvious ill-defined or stellate lesions that are suspicious in appearance (Fig. 20.19).

Calcifications

Clustered pleomorphic microcalcifications, with or without an associated soft tissue mass, are a primary mammographic sign of breast cancer. Such calcifications are seen in more than half of all mammographically discovered cancers; about one third of all nonpalpable cancers are manifest by calcifications alone, without an associated mass (19).

The calcifications associated with malignancy are dystrophic; they are the result of abnormalities in the tissues. Some malignant calcifications occur in necrotic tumor debris; others are the result of calcification of stagnant secretions that are trapped in the cancer (25).

Calcifications are a frequent finding on mammographic examinations. In the majority of cases, such calcifications will be benign and their origin, as such, will be easily identifiable. There is, however, a significant overlap in the appearance of benign and malignant calcifications. Only 25% to 35% of all calcifications that undergo biopsy will be malignant.

The importance of technically optimal mammography cannot be overstated when calcifications are being studied. The film exposure must be appropriate; an underexposed film can hide calcifications in a background of white breast tissue. Slight overpenetration of films is optimal for detection of calcifications. Magnification views are extremely helpful for assessing the malignant potential of a group of calcifications.

Careful analysis of the form, size, distribution, and number of calcifications, as well as any association with other soft tissue structures, will allow the radiologist to determine which calcifications are unequivocally benign and which require biopsy or follow-up studies.

Form

Benign Calcifications. Some shapes of calcifications can be easily identified as benign. Any calcification with a lucent center should not cause concern. Calcifications with lucent centers are often located in the skin. A skin marker can be placed over the calcifications and a subsequent tangential view taken to confirm their location in the skin (Fig. 20.20). Calcifications with lucent centers are also seen as a result of fat necrosis. Such calcifications can be smooth and round, or they can be eggshell-type calcifications in the walls of an oil cyst (Fig. 20.21).

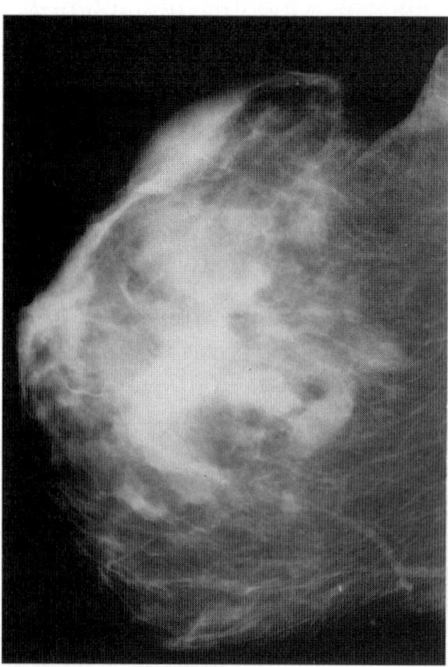
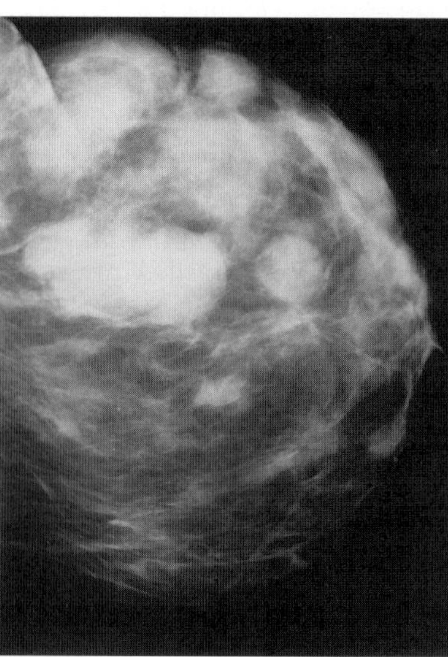

FIGURE 20.18. **Multiple Benign Masses.** Bilateral CC views show multiple large round masses in both breasts. The patient was asymptomatic. Differential diagnosis was cysts or fibroadenomas.

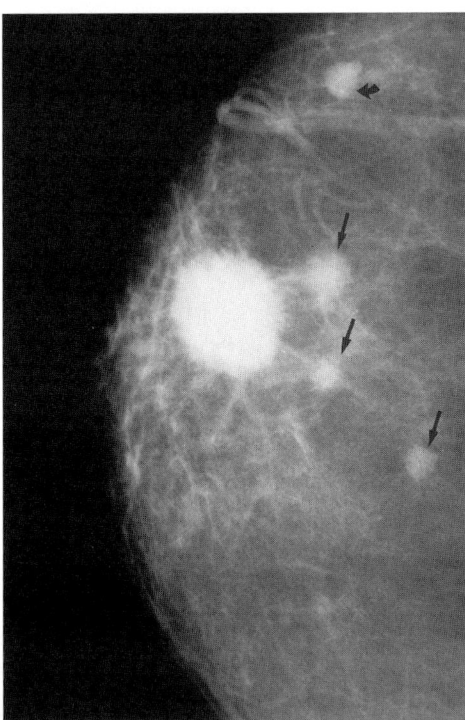

FIGURE 20.19. **Multifocal Carcinoma.** CC view. The largest mass was palpable. The others were discovered by mammography (*straight arrows*). The more well-defined nodule (*curved arrow*) probably represented an intramammary lymph node.

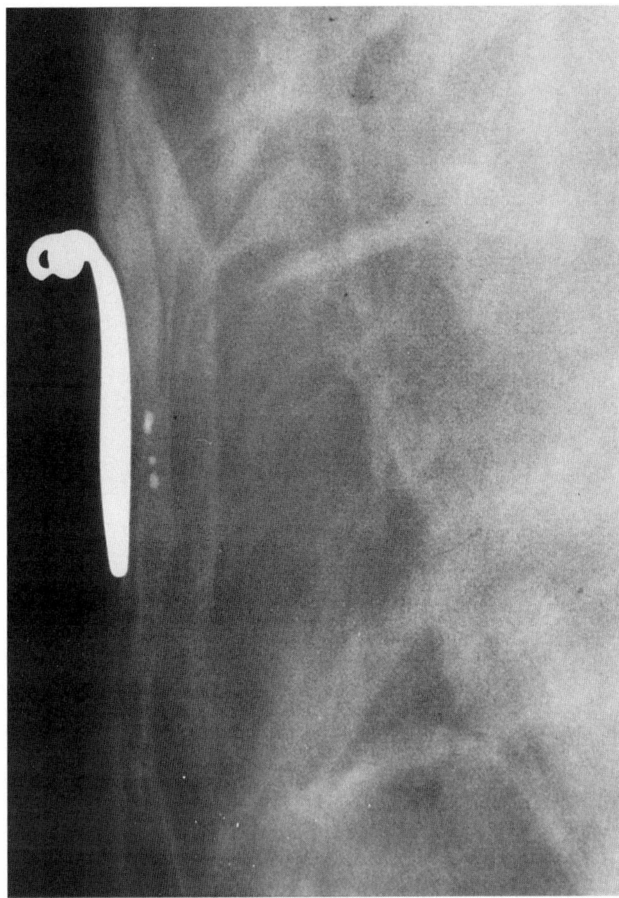

FIGURE 20.20. **Skin Calcifications.** Tangential view showing calcifications in the skin. A radiopaque marker had been placed on the skin at the site of the calcifications. This was done to facilitate positioning for the tangential view.

Calcifications that layer into a curvilinear or linear shape on 90° lateral films, yet appear as smudged clusters on CC views, are also representative of a benign process (Fig. 20.22). Such calcifications represent sedimented calcium ("milk of calcium") within the fluid of tiny breast cysts. Similar benign calcifications can also be seen within larger cysts and oil cysts. Sedimented calcium is a common finding in approximately 5% of women presenting for mammography.

Other benign calcifications that are easily recognizable by their form include arterial calcifications, the calcifications in a degenerating fibroadenoma, and calcifications associated with secretory disease. Arterial calcifications generally present as tubular parallel lines of calcium (Fig. 20.23). Occasionally, early arterial calcification can present a diagnostic problem, but this can usually be resolved by looking for soft tissue of the vessel in association with the calcification. Magnification in multiple projections can be helpful (Fig. 20.24).

Fibroadenomas can calcify in various patterns. Sometimes the calcifications are indeterminate, but the classic calcifications associated with an atrophic fibroadenoma are large, coarse, and irregular in shape (Fig. 20.25).

Secretory Disease. The calcifications associated with secretory disease are smooth, long, thick linear calcifications that radiate toward the nipple in a generally orderly pattern (Fig. 20.26). These calcifications are located in ectatic ducts. When periductal inflammation has occurred, these calcifications may appear more lucent centrally because calcium is deposited in the tissues adjacent to the ducts.

Malignant calcifications vary in shape and size (Fig. 20.27). The margins of the calcifications are jagged and irregular. Malignant calcifications are often branching. Ductal carcinoma in situ (DCIS), or noninvasive breast cancer, is most often detected mammographically as a result of such calcifications. Groups of pleomorphic calcifications that are more linear or "dot-dash" in appearance are more commonly associated with high-nuclear-grade intraductal carcinomas that have luminal necrosis (comedocarcinomas) (Fig. 20.28). The lower-grade (cribriform and micropapillary) types are often manifest by more punctate or granular appearing calcifications. The morphology of the calcification cannot, however, be used to predict the subtype of DCIS because there is

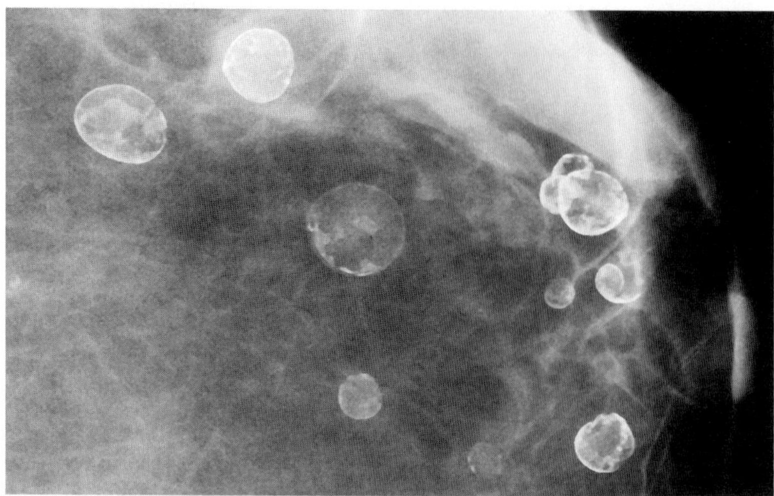

FIGURE 20.21. **Eggshell Calcifications in Oil Cysts.** These are large calcifications with lucent centers and are benign.

considerable overlap in the forms of the calcification associated with each subtype; frequently, multiple DCIS subtypes exist together in the same lesion. In the high-grade (comedo) subtype, the calcifications can be an approximate indication of the size of the tumor, although the extent of disease is often greater than mammographically predicted. In the lower-grade varieties, correlation is even poorer. The biologic behavior of these subtypes also differs; high-grade types are the most likely to recur (26).

Pleomorphic microcalcifications in association with a malignant soft tissue mass can also indicate areas of extensive intraductal component within or adjacent to the invasive tumor. It is especially important to recognize malignant calcifications that occur in tissues surrounding invasive cancers so they can be excised with the invasive tumor. Such extensive intraductal component–positive cancers also have a greater tendency to recur.

Indeterminate Calcifications. Morphologically indeterminate calcifications account for the majority of mammographically generated biopsies of calcifications (Fig. 20.29). Such calcifications are most often associated with fibrocystic change. Diagnoses included under the general category of fibrocystic disease are fibrosis, adenosis, sclerosing adenosis, epithelial hyperplasia, cysts, apocrine metaplasia, and atypical hyperplasia. Occasionally, biopsy of indeterminate calcification will yield a diagnosis of lobular carcinoma in situ (LCIS), also called lobular neoplasia. Although it is not an invasive cancer, LCIS places a woman at higher risk for development of invasive breast cancer. Mammographically, LCIS has no distinct features. If it is clinically occult, it is most often found serendipitously,

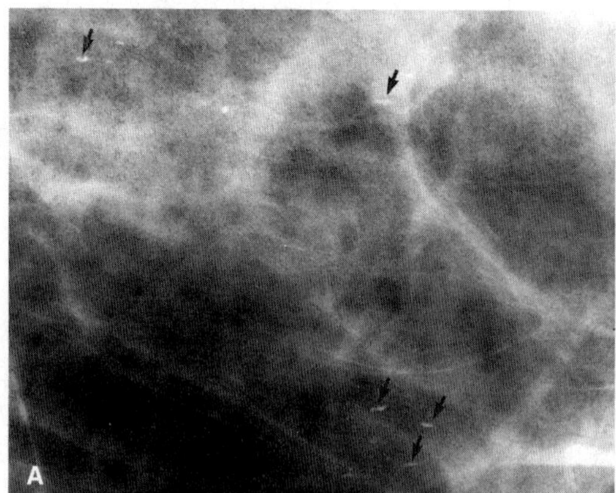

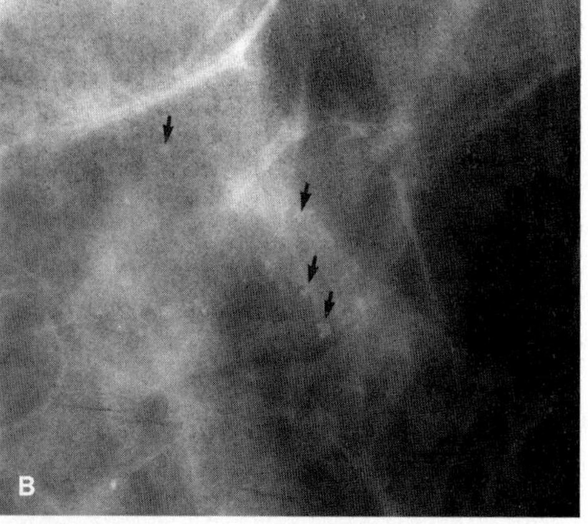

FIGURE 20.22. **Milk of Calcium in Breast Cysts. A.** Magnification of a 90° lateral mammogram showing diffuse linear calcifications (*arrows*). **B.** CC magnification view of the same area showing smudged, rounded calcifications (*arrows*). This change in configuration between views is typical of sedimented calcium. The calcium is layering in the bottom of microcysts, so it appears as a line or meniscus when viewed from the side in the lateral projection. When viewed from the top, these calcifications simply appear smudged and rounded.

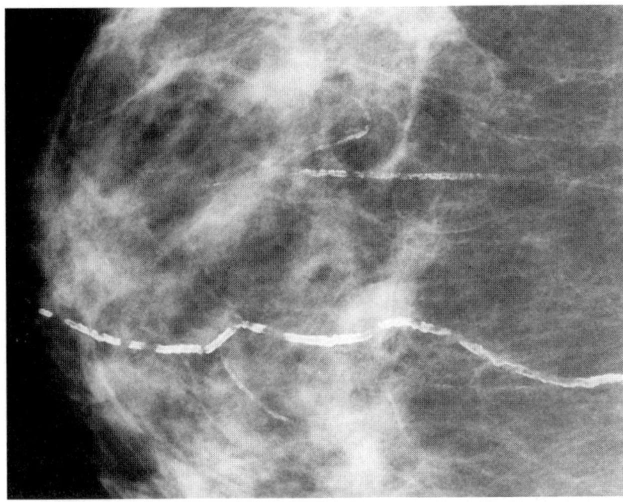

FIGURE 20.23. **Arterial Calcifications.** Arterial calcifications in the breast are identified by their location in the wall of a tortuous vessel.

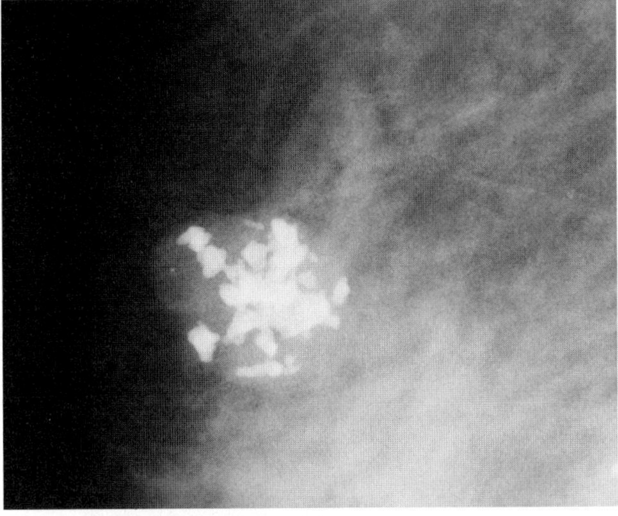

FIGURE 20.25. **Fibroadenoma.** Typical large, coarse, irregular calcifications are seen in a fibroadenoma.

adjacent to a focus of mammographically indeterminate, but histologically benign, calcifications.

Distribution

Calcifications that are widely scattered and seen bilaterally are usually indicative of a benign process, such as sclerosing adenosis or adenosis. Multiple, bilateral clusters of calcifications that appear morphologically similar are also generally benign. Careful analysis with a magnifying lens is essential in these cases so that a morphologically dissimilar cluster is not overlooked. Such calcifications should be thoroughly examined with magnification views.

Malignant calcifications usually occur in tight clusters within a small volume of tissue, but DCIS can produce calcifications that encompass large areas of the breast. Calcifications that are morphologically suspicious or indeterminate and occupy a segment of the breast should undergo biopsy.

Size

Malignant calcifications are generally smaller than 0.5 mm. Because the calcifications associated with carcinoma are so small, they are frequently referred to as *microcalcifications*. Within a cluster, there will be a variety of sizes. Benign calcifications are often larger. When benign

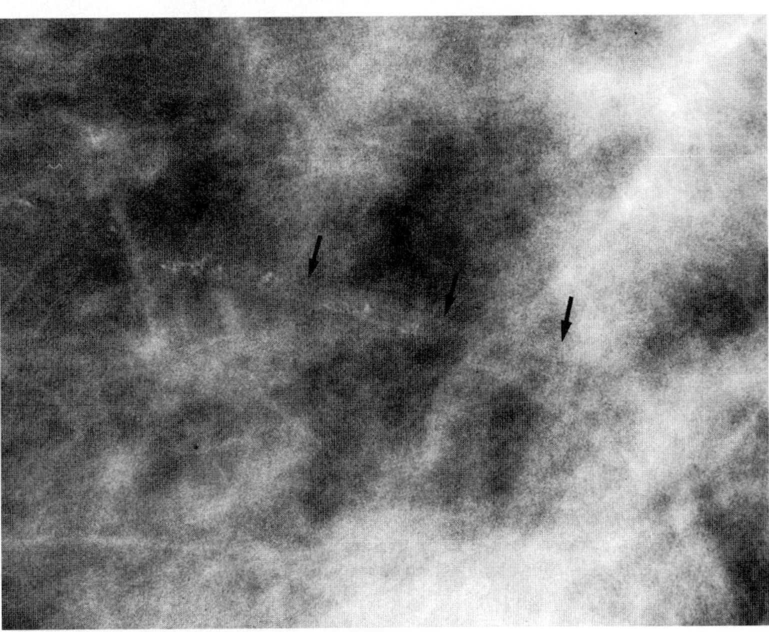

FIGURE 20.24. **Early Arterial Calcification.** Magnification view. The calcification can be seen clearly in the walls of an artery (*arrows*). The soft tissue of the artery was difficult to appreciate on the conventional views.

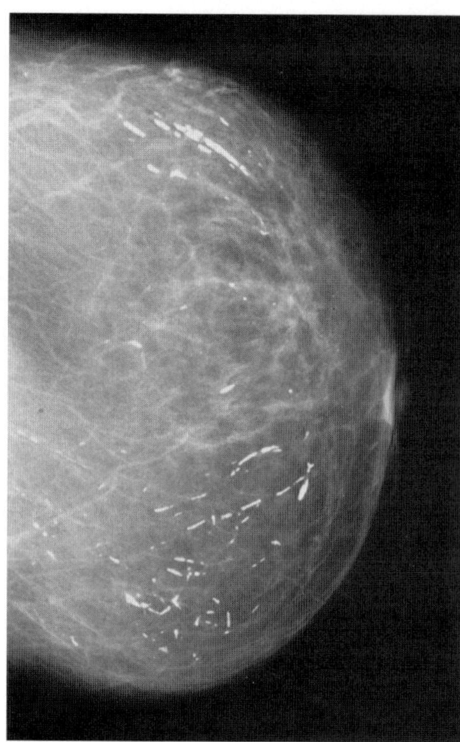

FIGURE 20.26. **Secretory Calcifications.** Craniocaudal view demonstrates long and thick calcifications in ectatic ducts that radiate toward the nipple.

disease produces clusters of calcifications, the size of these calcifications is usually similar.

Number

Calcifications associated with malignancy are generally quite numerous. The greater the number of calcifications, the more likely they are associated with malignant disease.

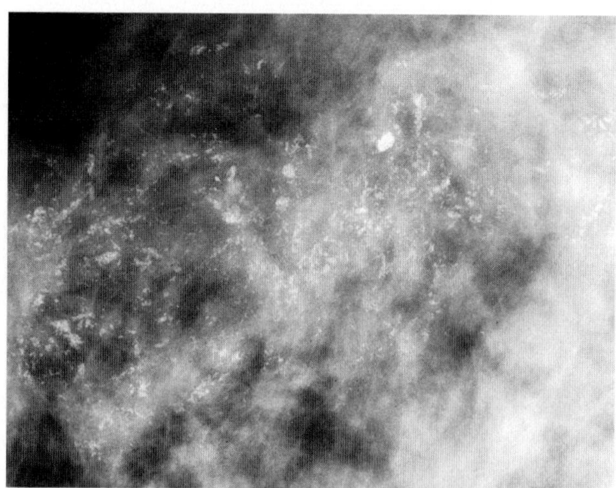

FIGURE 20.27. **Malignant Calcifications.** Magnification view of infiltrating ductal carcinoma. Note the irregular forms as well as the variety of sizes and shapes.

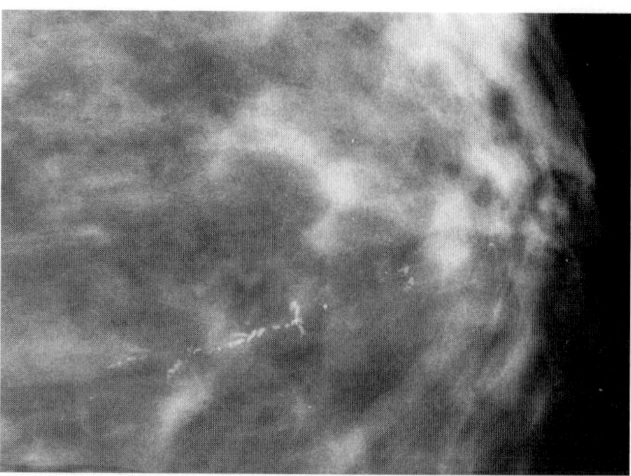

FIGURE 20.28. **Malignant Calcifications.** Dot-dash or "casting" calcifications of the comedo subtype of ductal carcinoma in situ. Note the pleomorphism in the size and shape of the calcifications. (From Kline TS, Kline IK. Breast. New York: Igaku-Shoin, 1989:201, Guides to Clinical Aspiration Biopsy Series; used with permission.)

Establishing the lower limit of the number of calcifications in a cluster that would require biopsy is extremely difficult. Assessment of the morphology of these calcifications by magnification views will influence this decision more than the actual number of calcifications.

Architectural Distortion

Breast cancer is occasionally heralded by distortion in the normal architecture of the breast (Fig. 20.30). Differential diagnosis includes fat necrosis related to scarring from previous surgery and a complex sclerosing lesion, also known as radial scar. On close inspection, fat may be seen interspersed with fibrous elements in the center of fat necrosis or complex sclerosing lesions, but this appearance is not specific for benignity. Similar findings can be seen in malignant lesions. Biopsy is necessary for differentiation.

Increased Density of Breast Tissue

Hormone Therapy. Increasing parenchymal density of breast tissue can be bilateral or unilateral. Bilateral increased density is usually the result of estrogen replacement therapy in postmenopausal women. Such hormone therapy can give the breasts a more glandular, premenopausal appearance. Intrinsic hormonal fluctuations in premenopausal, pregnant, or lactating women may cause similar changes in the density of the breasts. Hormonally related changes in breast density are not associated with skin thickening.

Inflammatory Carcinoma. A unilateral increase in breast density with associated skin thickening may be caused by several processes. The most ominous of these

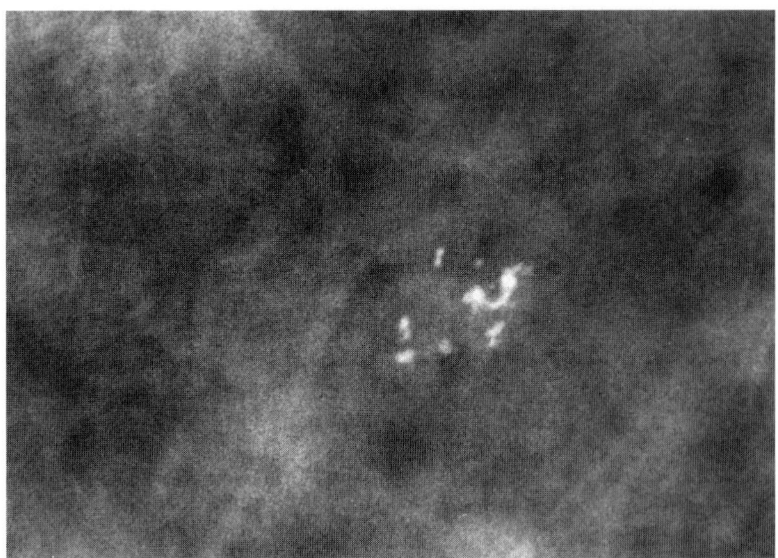

FIGURE 20.29. **Indeterminate Calcifications.** Magnification view of cluster of calcifications. There is some irregularity in shape and variation in size, but these calcifications were benign. They were associated with fibrocystic change.

is inflammatory carcinoma of the breast (Fig. 20.31). Clinically, this disease is manifest by a warm, erythematous, firm, tender breast. Histologically, the dermal lymphatics are diffusely involved. Mammographically, a focal mass may be seen within the dense tissue, but often the breast appears homogeneously dense. Inflammatory carcinoma of the breast is a locally advanced disease that carries a poor prognosis.

Radiation Therapy. A unilateral increase in parenchymal density with skin thickening can also be seen in patients who have undergone radiation therapy to the breast. Radiation changes are most pronounced during the first 6 months following therapy. They usually resolve gradually over a period of years.

Diffuse mastitis can produce a generalized skin thickening and increase in breast density. Clinical differentiation from inflammatory carcinoma is usually possible.

Obstruction to the lymphatic or venous drainage from metastatic disease, surgical removal, or thrombosis can produce a unilateral increase in breast density, with skin thickening caused by edema. The anasarca associated with congestive heart failure, renal failure, cirrhosis, or hypoalbuminemia most often presents as bilateral increased breast density with skin thickening; however, asymmetric involvement of the breasts can occur.

Correlation of physical examination findings and history will usually allow differentiation of the various causes of an increase in breast density.

Axillary Adenopathy

Axillary lymph nodes are frequently visualized on the MLO mammogram. Normally they are less than 2 cm in size and have lucent centers or notches resulting from fat in the

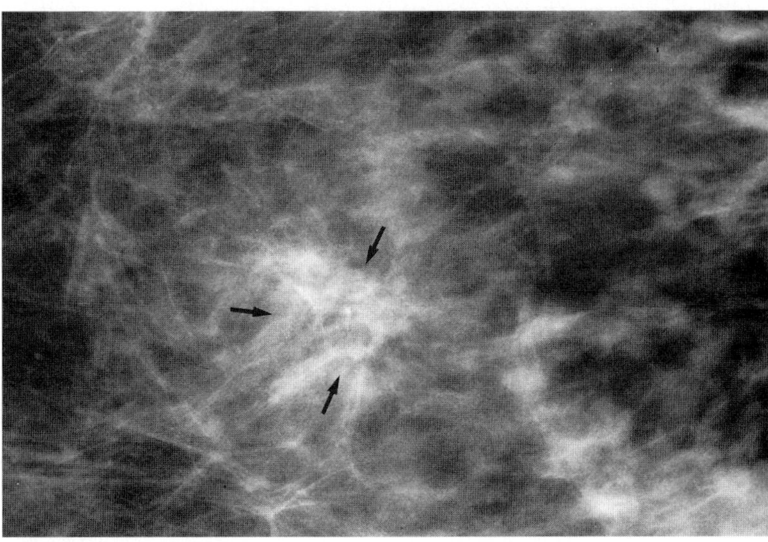

FIGURE 20.30. **Architectural Distortion Representing Breast Carcinoma.** Note how the cancer pulls the surrounding parenchyma toward it (*arrows*).

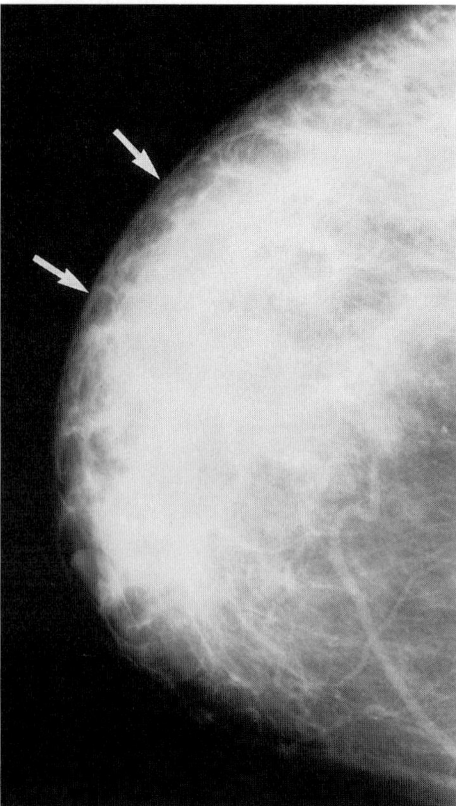

FIGURE 20.31. **Inflammatory Carcinoma.** CC view demonstrates a diffuse increase in parenchymal density, along with skin thickening laterally (*arrows*).

hilum. Fatty infiltration of the nodes themselves can cause lucent enlargement and replacement.

Pathologic axillary nodes are homogeneously dense and enlarged. A variety of processes can result in replacement of normal nodal architecture. Malignant involvement of axillary nodes can be the result of primary breast cancer, metastatic disease, lymphoma, or leukemia (Fig. 20.32). Axillary nodes can also become pathologically enlarged because of inflammation. Patients with rheumatoid arthritis, systemic lupus erythematosus, scleroderma, and psoriasis may also have axillary adenopathy.

Coarse calcifications in axillary nodes may reflect granulomatous disease. Microcalcifications are occasionally seen in nodes involved with metastatic breast cancer. Gold deposits, seen in patients being treated for rheumatoid arthritis, are occasionally seen in axillary nodes and may be confused with calcifications.

The Augmented Breast

More than 1.5 million women in the United States have undergone augmentation mammoplasty. Imaging of the augmented breast poses unique challenges. Special techniques must be employed both to screen for breast cancer and to evaluate the patient for possible complications related to the implant.

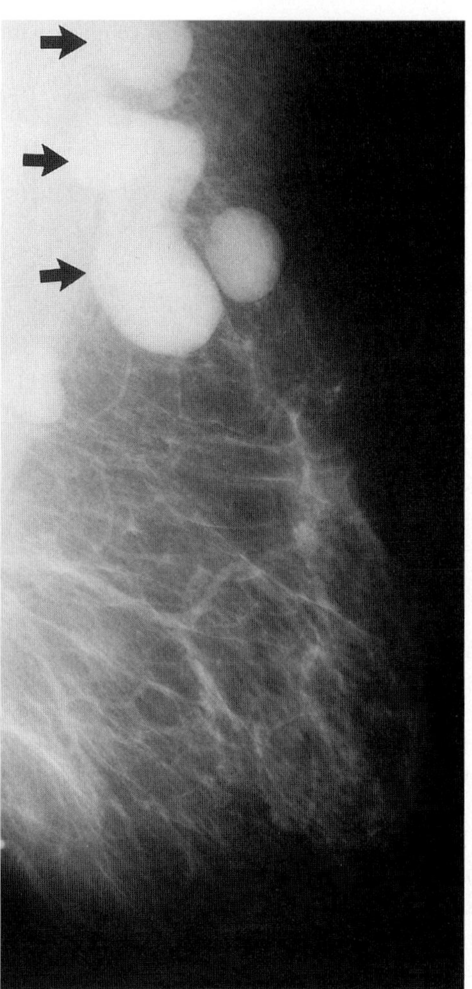

FIGURE 20.32. **Lymphoma.** Hodgkin disease involves the axillary lymph nodes. The nodes are homogeneous, dense, and enlarged (*arrows*).

Various types of implants have been used in augmentation procedures. They include silicone envelopes filled with saline or with viscous silicone gel, as well as double-lumen implants containing an inner core of silicone gel surrounded by an outer envelope filled with saline. Silicone is more radiopaque than saline, although neither allows adequate visualization of immediately surrounding tissue.

Implants can be placed either anterior (prepectoral) or posterior (subpectoral) to the pectoralis muscle. A fibrous capsule develops around the implant. Patients with prepectoral implants are subject to a greater risk of fibrous and calcific contractures around the implant. Such contractures are not only painful and deforming, but they also make mammography more difficult.

Screening mammography in the woman with implants requires the use of at least two extra views of each breast.

Standard MLO and CC views are performed with moderate compression. Then the implants are displaced posteriorly against the chest wall while the breast tissue is pulled anteriorly and compressed more vigorously (Fig. 20.33). The compression paddle keeps the implant from migrating into the field of view. Greater compression of anterior tissues allows more optimal imaging (Fig. 20.34). Both MLO and CC views are repeated using this technique. These modified views are called implant displacement views (27).

Implant displacement views are more difficult to accomplish in patients with prepectoral implants with associated capsular contractures around the implant. The implants are not easily displaced, so that less of the anterior breast tissue is depicted on the modified views. In such cases, a 90° lateral view may also be helpful in screening.

Although some breast tissue may be obscured in patients with implants, these women, when in the appropriate age groups, deserve the same careful screening examinations at the same intervals as patients without implants. The indeterminate mammogram in an implant patient should be evaluated in a manner similar to that in a patient without implants.

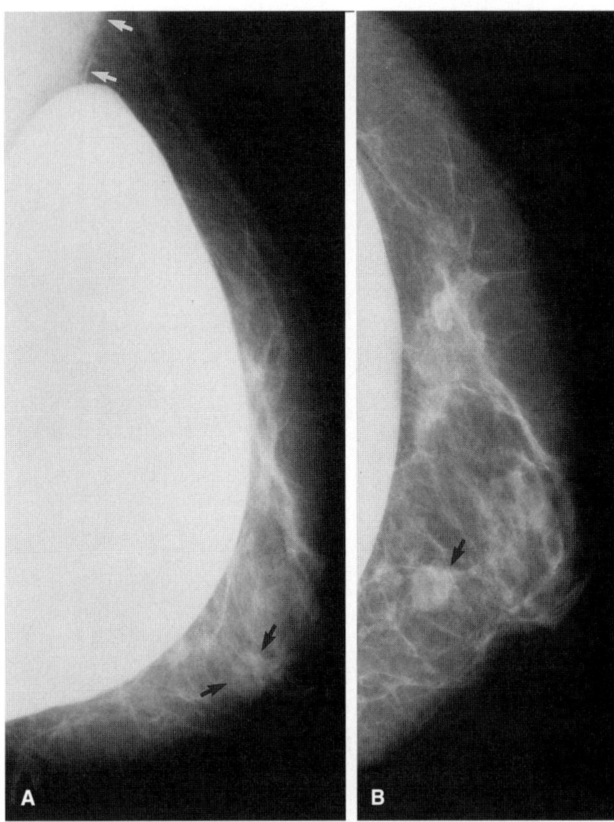

FIGURE 20.34. **Infiltrating Duct Carcinoma. A.** Standard MLO view in a patient with prepectoral silicone implants. Note the pectoralis muscle (*white arrows*) extending posterior to the implant. A poorly defined 1-cm mass (*black arrows*) was noted in the subareolar tissues. **B.** MLO implant displacement view in the same patient. The subareolar mass (*black arrow*) is more clearly defined because of greater compression of the tissues anterior to the implant. Histologic examination of the mass showed infiltrating duct carcinoma.

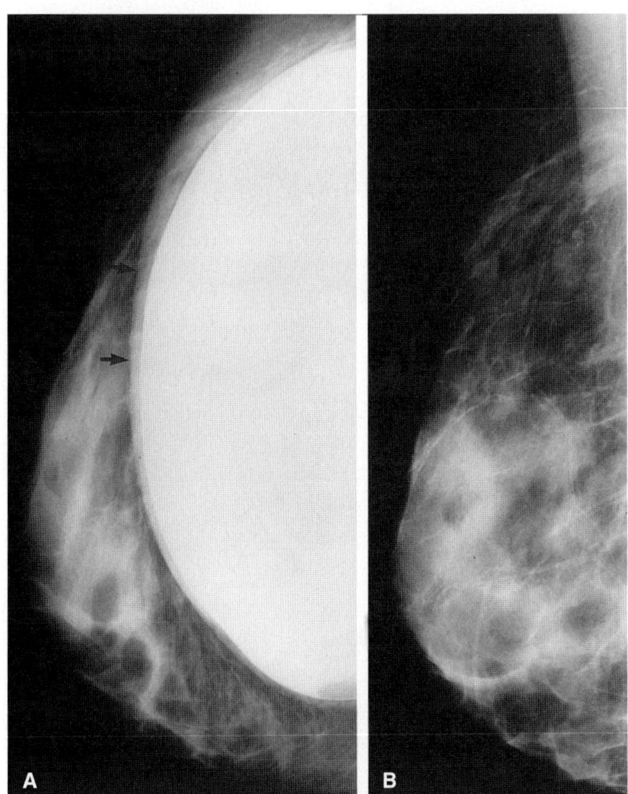

FIGURE 20.33. **Breast Implants. A.** Standard MLO view of a patient with a subpectoral silicone implant. Note the pectoralis muscle (*arrows*) anterior to the implant. **B.** MLO implant displacement view on the same patient. The implant has been displaced posteriorly, out of view, while compression has been applied anteriorly.

Women who have undergone augmentation mammoplasty may also present with abnormalities related to their implants. These include capsular contractures, herniations of the implant through rents in the capsules, implant rupture with free (extracapsular rupture) or contained (intracapsular rupture) silicone, and deflation of saline implants. Many patients will present for breast imaging subsequent to noticing a change in implant contour or size (Fig. 20.35).

Mammography is generally the first examination performed if the woman is over the age of 30; however, mammography is not useful in the detection of intracapsular silicone implant ruptures because the silicone is contained within the fibrous capsule that has developed around the implant. Extracapsular silicone implant ruptures can sometimes be detected by mammography, but often the free silicone is obscured by the overlying implant

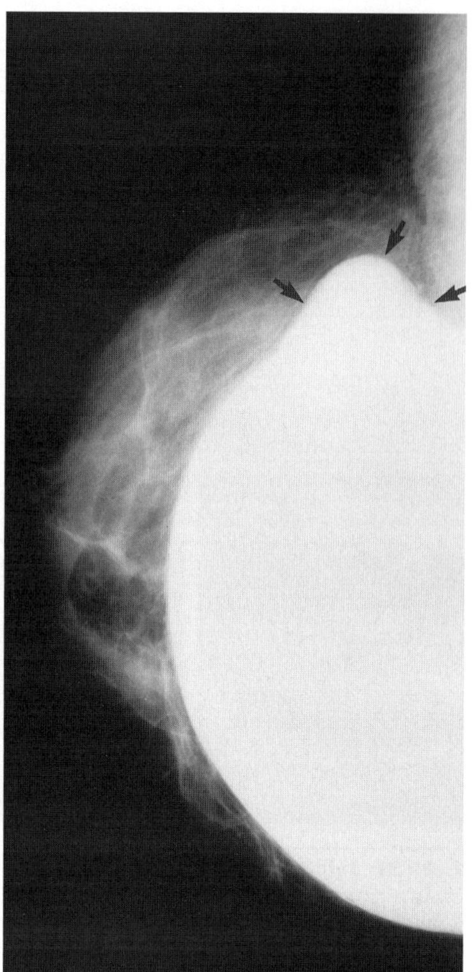

FIGURE 20.35. **Ruptured Implant.** Standard MLO view of a patient with prepectoral silicone implants. The patient had noted a new mass superolaterally in her breast. The mammogram shows an extracapsular rupture, with silicone outside the implant capsule (*arrows*) that corresponded to the palpable abnormality.

or is in an area of the breast or chest wall not imaged on the mammogram (28).

Other imaging modalities can be used for the assessment of implant complications. MR is the most accurate in identifying silicone implant rupture and in localizing free silicone (29). The protocol for breast implant evaluation consists of axial, sagittal, and/or coronal T2W sequences with and without water suppression and inversion recovery (IR) sequences with water suppression. It is essential to use several projections in implant evaluation. The most effective sequence is the IR sequence, which suppresses the fat signal. The addition of water saturation results in a silicone-only image. T2W fast spin-echo sequences, without and with water suppression, are useful for saline implants.

In intracapsular silicone implant rupture, the implant shell has ruptured but the silicone remains within the fibrous capsule. Signs of intracapsular rupture on MR can be subtle. A linguine sign indicating intracapsular rupture occurs when the collapsed implant shell floats within the silicone gel contained in the fibrous capsule (Fig. 20.36). The noose, teardrop, or keyhole signs of intracapsular rupture indicate small amounts of silicone collected in a radial fold (Fig. 20.37). Over time, microscopic silicone can leak through the intact implant shell and collect at the implant shell surface, giving a subcapsular line sign. This can be difficult to differentiate from a small intracapsular rupture. In extracapsular rupture, the envelope and fibrous capsule lose integrity, resulting in the extrusion of free silicone gel into breast tissue (Fig. 20.38). US is also used to detect implant rupture, but it has a lower sensitivity (70%) than MR (94%) (30). The specificity of both US and MR is similar (92% to 97%). The success of US in the assessment of implant integrity is highly dependent on the operator; an experienced radiologist must scan the breasts in a methodical manner.

The Male Breast

The most common indication for breast imaging in men is a palpable asymmetric thickening or mass. Gynecomastia is usually the cause. Breast cancer is rare, but can occur.

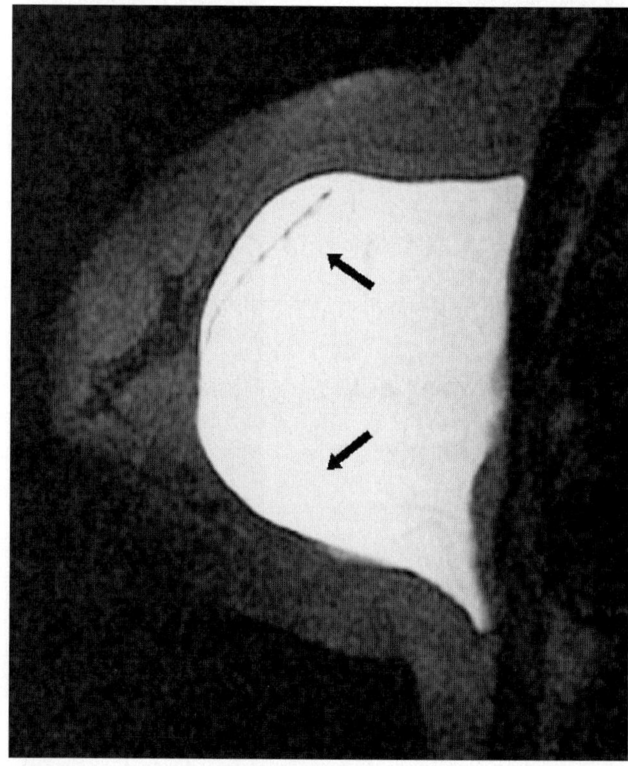

FIGURE 20.36. **MR of Intracapsular Silicone Implant Rupture.** Sagittal inversion-recovery T2WI with water suppression shows multiple low-intensity curvilinear lines (*arrows*) contained within the fibrous capsule, representing the collapsed implant shell ("linguine sign"). There is no extracapsular silicone.

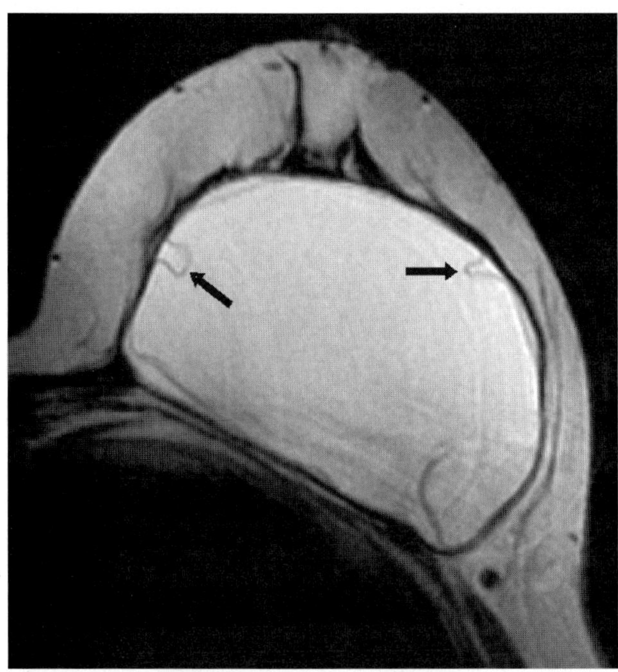

FIGURE 20.37. **MR of Subtle Intracapsular Silicone Implant Rupture.** Sagittal fast spin-echo T2WI shows a focus of silicone gel trapped within a fold of the implant shell (*arrows*), known as "noose sign," "inverted teardrop sign," or "keyhole sign."

Normal male breast appears on mammography as a mound of subcutaneous fat without glandular tissue (Fig. 20.39). The nipple is small.

Gynecomastia generally appears as a triangular or flame-shaped area of subareolar glandular tissue that points toward the nipple. Fat is interspersed with parenchymal elements. A gradual merging of the more glandular elements with the fat occurs at the deep margin (Fig. 20.40). Gynecomastia can be unilateral or bilateral. When bilateral, it is most frequently asymmetric. Many causes have been reported, including ingestion of a variety of drugs, such as reserpine, cardiac glycosides, cimetidine, and thiazides, as well as marijuana. Testicular, adrenal, and pituitary tumors are associated with gynecomastia. Chronic hepatic disease, by virtue of the body's reduced ability to clear endogenous estrogens, can also cause male breast enlargement.

Male breast cancer is mammographically similar to that found in women. It can have a variety of appearances, including an ill-defined, spiculated, or circumscribed mass (Fig. 20.41). Microcalcifications can occur.

Comparison With Previous Films

The importance of comparing current mammograms with previous films cannot be overstated. In one series, developing densities accounted for 6% of nonpalpable breast carcinomas (19). Comparison with previous films will allow detection of subtle changes, in turn suggesting the need for further evaluation of such areas at an earlier time than might be possible if no comparison had been made (Fig. 20.42). It must, of course, be remembered that benign masses may appear or enlarge over time. In fact, in the majority of cases, interval change will be benign, but such changes should be fully evaluated by correlation with the history and physical examination, as well as the use of ancillary testing methods such as US, aspiration, and biopsy.

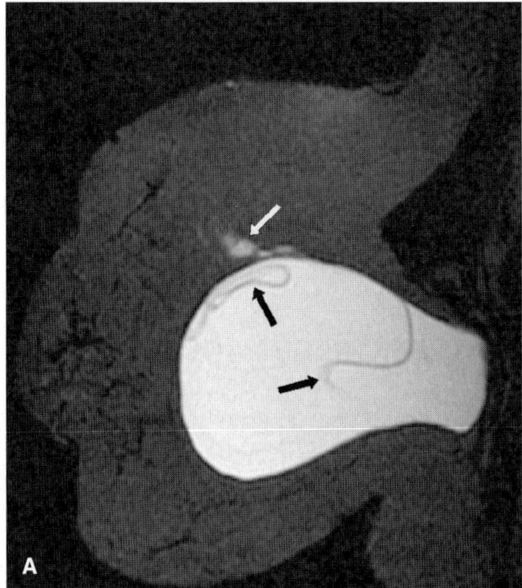

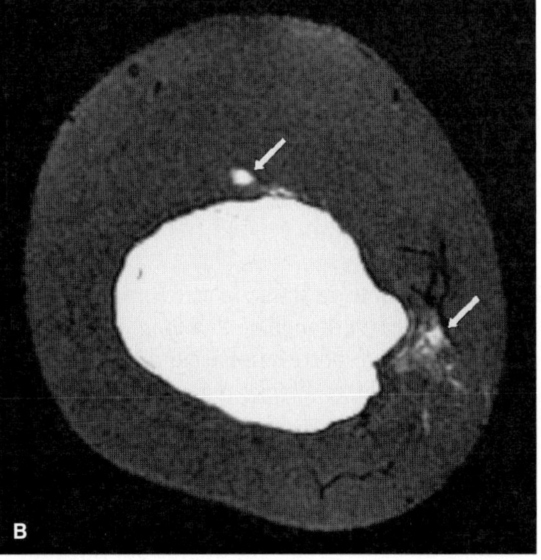

FIGURE 20.38. **MR of an Extracapsular Silicone Implant Rupture.** Sagittal **(A)** and coronal **(B)** inversion-recovery T2WIs with water suppression show extracapsular silicone (*white arrows*) in the superior and lateral left breast. The partially collapsed implant shell (*black arrow*) is seen within the silicone gel contained within the fibrous capsule that surrounds the implant.

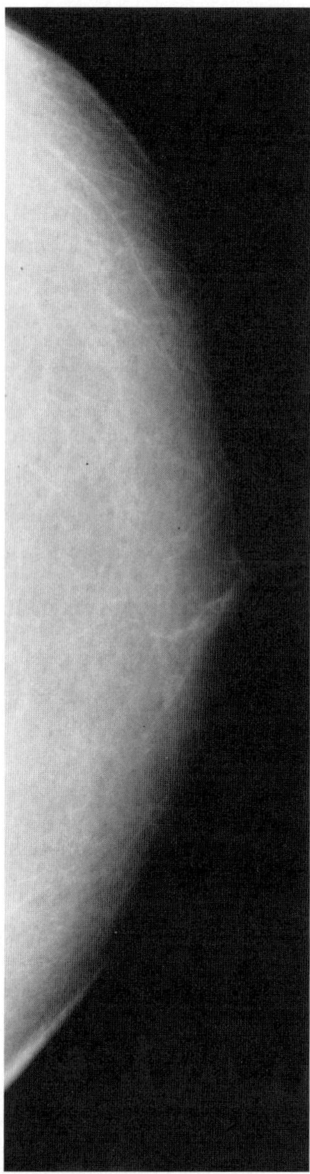

FIGURE 20.39. **Male Breast.** Relatively normal male breast, which is a mound of subcutaneous fat. Note the lack of glandular tissue.

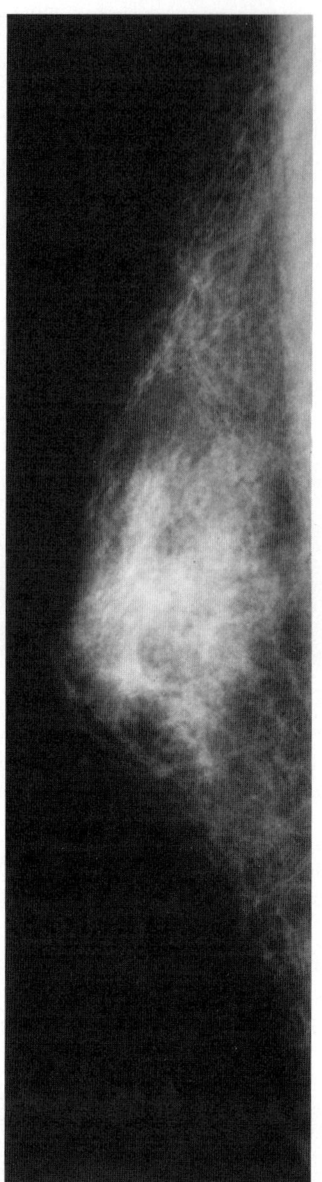

FIGURE 20.40. **Gynecomastia.** MLO view of a man with breast enlargement. Glandular tissue is seen in the subareolar area. This tissue gradually intersperses with the fat and does not appear as a mass.

Malignant masses that were stable in size for up to 4.5 years have been reported. Although such a long period of stability is unusual, these reports emphasize the need for suspicious lesions to undergo biopsy regardless of their apparent lack of change in size on serial films. Such lesions may have been overlooked or misinterpreted on a previous study.

Any new microcalcifications or increase in number of such calcifications deserve special consideration. Appropriate workup with magnification views will allow analysis of the morphology of such calcifications. Any calcifications that are not clearly benign deserve biopsy.

MAGNETIC RESONANCE IMAGING

Indications. There is growing consensus on the indications for MR of the breast. As described in the section on imaging of implants, MR is the most accurate modality for evaluating breast implant integrity. In cases of newly diagnosed invasive breast cancer, MR is superior to mammography and clinical breast examination in defining the local extent of disease (31). MR has been reported to be more sensitive than mammography in detection of multifocal or multicentric invasive tumors and in the evaluation of

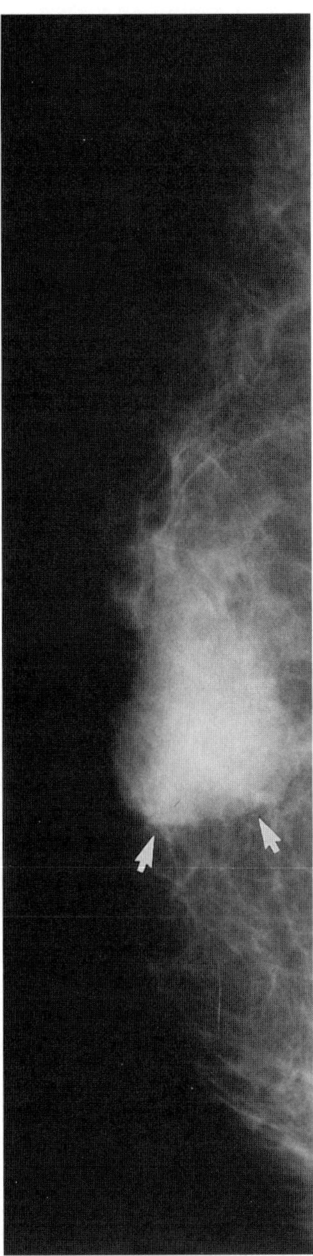

FIGURE 20.41. **Male Breast Cancer.** MLO view of the breast in a male. The mass has a defined interface with the surrounding fat (*arrows*). (Courtesy of Patricia Bell, M.D., Auburn, California.)

residual disease postlumpectomy (32–34). However, there is controversy about whether the use of MR offers meaningful clinical benefit. It is possible that women who opt for mastectomy based on MR findings may have disease that could have been controlled with radiation therapy. Further clinical trials are needed to assess the clinical utility of breast MR for determining the local extent of disease.

In patients who have undergone breast conservation therapy, differentiating lumpectomy and radiation changes from local recurrence can be difficult. MR can be helpful in these cases (35). MR is also useful in diagnosing breast cancer when the patient presents with axillary metastases and no known primary tumor (36).

The role of breast MR in screening remains controversial. MR is more costly than mammography and has high false-positive rates, making it unacceptable for the general population; however, MR does appear to have a role in screening women at high risk for development of breast cancer.

Technique. Breast MR is usually performed in a standard 1.0- to 1.5-tesla magnet. A dedicated bilateral breast surface coil should be used. The patients are imaged prone to minimize respiratory motion. Ideally, imaging should be done between days 6 and 17 of the menstrual cycle. Bilateral studies should be performed.

The breast should be imaged in axial or sagittal planes or a combination of the two. Core pulse sequences when evaluating the breast for cancer include a three-plane localizer, T1WIs, T2WIs, and two- or three-dimensional fat-suppressed gradient echo series performed before contrast administration, immediately after, and delayed. The number of postcontrast series can vary, but at least three are needed to perform kinetic enhancement curves. The T1WIs allow clear differentiation of adipose tissue from glandular tissue. T2W fat-suppressed images allow identification of fluid-filled structures such as cysts. Dynamic images obtained prior to and after IV gadolinium enhancement help to identify potential malignancies based on morphology and enhancement kinetics. The intravenous gadolinium DTPA dose ranges from 0.1 to 0.2 mmol/kg body weight.

Fat suppression can be accomplished before gadolinium administration using chemical selective fat saturation or water-only excitation techniques. After IV contrast administration, passive fat suppression can be accomplished with postprocessing image subtraction, but patient movement between precontrast and postcontrast enhanced images can degrade the images because of misregistration. Kinetic curves can be performed on enhancing lesions.

Interpretation. Each lesion should be evaluated for its shape, margin, internal architecture, precontrast T1 and T2 signal characteristic, enhancement characteristics, and change from prior studies. Predictors of benignity include smooth margins, nonenhancing internal septations, minimal or no enhancement, and diffuse patchy enhancement. Features suggestive of malignancy include spiculated or irregular borders, peripheral or rim enhancement, regional enhancement, and ductal enhancement. On the precontrast T1WI, bright T1 signal intensity is suggestive of benign etiologies such as a complicated or hemorrhagic cyst, fresh fat necrosis, or the fatty hilum of an intramammary lymph node. Simple cysts have high T2 signal intensity, whereas most invasive carcinomas have low T2 signal intensity. Medullary or mucinous carcinoma can have high T2 signal intensity and look similar to cysts on MR.

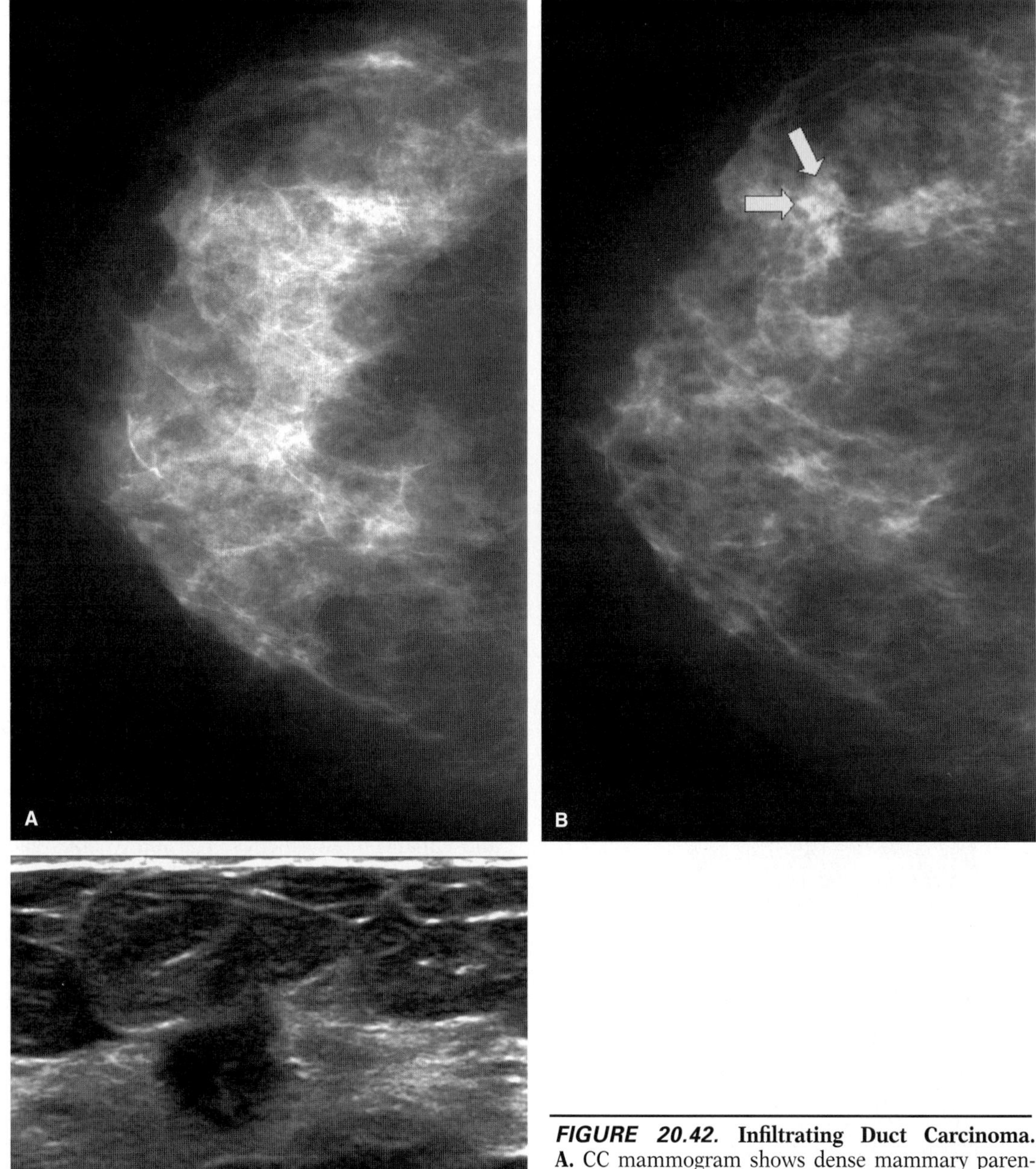

FIGURE 20.42. **Infiltrating Duct Carcinoma. A.** CC mammogram shows dense mammary parenchyma but no evidence of malignancy. **B.** Mammogram 1 year later shows development of a subtle new mass (*arrows*). **C.** US of the mass shows an irregular solid mass with indistinct margins. Biopsy demonstrated infiltrating duct carcinoma.

Kinetic curves improve the specificity of breast MR. These curves can be evaluated qualitatively according to the curve shape and classified as a persistent pattern of enhancement, a plateau of enhancement, or washout of signal intensity (37). Most invasive carcinomas demonstrate rapid initial enhancement with a plateau or washout (Figs. 20.43, 20.44). Some malignant lesions, such as DCIS, invasive lobular carcinoma, tubular carcinoma, and mucinous carcinoma, may demonstrate slow enhancement. A curve showing progressive increase in signal intensity after the first 2 minutes is more suggestive of a benign etiology. Enhancement curves are helpful for lesions that are indeterminate or benign in morphology and may influence the decision to biopsy. Any morphologically suspicious lesion, however, requires biopsy regardless of its enhancement kinetics.

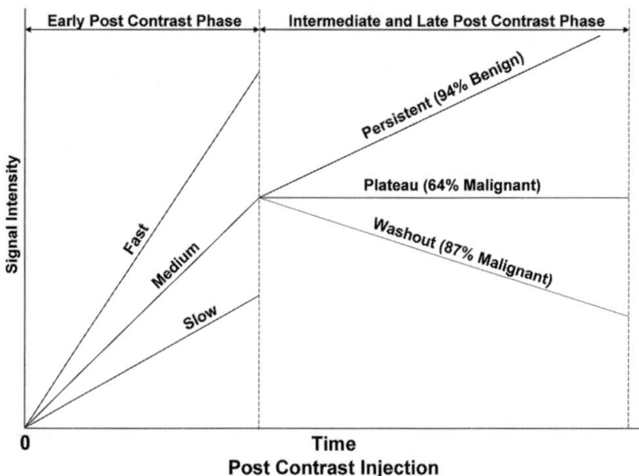

FIGURE 20.43. **Breast MR Kinetic Curves.** Schematic drawing of kinetic curves showing hypothetical signal intensities of a lesion after contrast injection. The shape of the curve aids in differentiating benign from malignant lesions. Rapid enhancement in the early postcontrast phase is more often associated with malignant lesions. Washout of contrast in the immediate and late postcontrast phases also has a higher likelihood of malignancy. Photo courtesy of Hologic, Inc, Bedford, Massachusetts.

THE RADIOLOGIC REPORT AND PLAN

The radiologic report should be clear and concise. The American College of Radiology has developed a standardized format and terminology called the Breast Imaging Reporting and Data System (BI-RADS) (38) for mammograms, breast US, and breast MR. All reports should begin with description of the overall breast composition. With mammography, this description of breast density will allow the clinician to gauge the sensitivity of the exam. The breast should be characterized as: (*1*) composed almost entirely of fat (<25% glandular); (*2*) containing scattered fibroglandular densities (25% to 50% glandular); (*3*) heterogeneously dense (51% to 75% glandular), which may obscure detection of small masses; or (*4*) extremely dense (>75% glandular), which lowers the sensitivity of mammography. A description of the significant findings on the mammogram, US or MR should follow, and there should be comparison to any previous available examinations. The most important part of the breast imaging report is the assessment category, which should fall into one of the following seven categories:

BI-RADS Category (0): **Need additional imaging evaluation and/or prior mammograms for comparison.** This category is reserved for screening exams that require further imaging workup or comparison films to fully characterize a potential abnormality. The suggested additional studies, such as US or additional mammographic views, should be specified in the report. Prior mammograms are always helpful in the interpretation of a screening study. Category 0 should, however, be used for film comparison only in cases where the radiologist feels that such films are essential to the final assessment for the patient.

BI-RADS Category (1): **Negative.** No significant findings are present on a negative mammogram. The patient should return for routine screening.

BI-RADS Category (2): **Benign finding.** There is a benign finding such as a lipoma, oil cyst, galactocele, intramammary lymph node, hamartoma, fibroadenoma, cyst, scattered round calcifications of adenosis, arterial calcifications, sedimented calcium within microcysts, secretory calcifications, duct ectasia, skin calcifications, or multiple bilateral well-circumscribed masses representing cysts or fibroadenomas. These patients should return for routine screening.

BI-RADS Category (3): **Probably benign; initial short-interval follow-up suggested.** The findings that should be included in this category are circumscribed masses, asymmetric parenchymal densities that are not associated with palpable masses and, occasionally, clusters of smooth, round, similar-appearing microcalcifications. The probability that such abnormalities represent cancer is less than 2% (39); therefore, most mammographers recommend a plan of careful follow-up. The first follow-up mammogram of the affected breast should be performed 6 months following discovery of the abnormality. If the abnormality is stable, a bilateral study should be performed 6 months later, and follow-ups should occur at yearly intervals for a period of at least 3 years. Progression of a cancerous lesion depends on tumor biology and doubling time; hence the necessity of a lengthy follow-up. Some cancers may grow slowly and others may change rapidly.

BI-RADS Category (4): **Suspicious abnormality; biopsy should be considered.** Included in this category are lesions that are not classically malignant but are suspicious enough to warrant biopsy. The probability that such a lesion will represent malignancy is approximately 25% to 35% in most practices in the United States. Category 4 lesions can be divided into three subdivisions (4A, 4B, and 4C, with 4A the lowest suspicion for malignancy and 4C the highest); this division is optional, but it may allow more meaningful correlation with biopsy results.

BI-RADS Category (5): **Highly suggestive of malignancy; appropriate action should be taken.** These are lesions that have a very high probability of being malignant and should undergo biopsy. Spiculated masses and pleomorphic clusters of calcifications are included in this category.

BI-RADS Category (6): **Known biopsy; proven malignancy; appropriate action should be taken.** These are lesions that are already known to be malignant but have not undergone definitive therapy. For example, this category should be used for proven cancers that are being

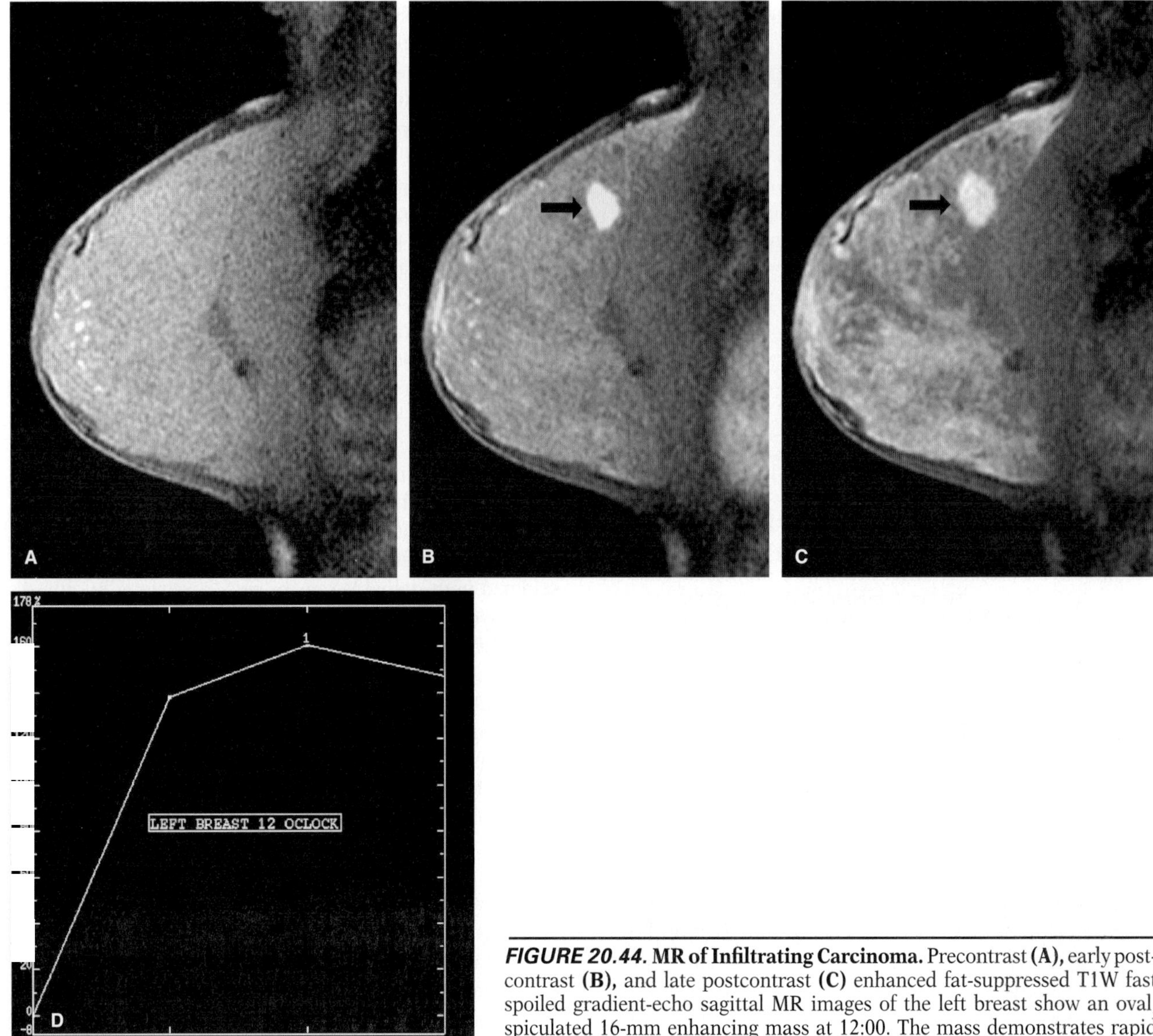

FIGURE 20.44. **MR of Infiltrating Carcinoma.** Precontrast **(A),** early postcontrast **(B),** and late postcontrast **(C)** enhanced fat-suppressed T1W fast spoiled gradient-echo sagittal MR images of the left breast show an oval, spiculated 16-mm enhancing mass at 12:00. The mass demonstrates rapid initial enhancement with washout, as shown in the kinetic curve **(D).**

imaged to assess their response to neoadjuvant chemotherapy prior to definitive surgery. Clinicians must be cautioned that mammography has a false-negative rate of 9% to 16%; therefore, a negative mammogram should not preclude biopsy of a clinically suspicious mass.

INTERVENTIONAL PROCEDURES FOR NONPALPABLE LESIONS

Mammographically suspicious abnormalities require histologic or cytologic examination for definitive diagnosis. Percutaneous, image-directed core biopsy or aspiration performed in the radiology department is the standard of care. Needle localization followed by surgical excision is reserved for cases in which the percutaneous biopsy is inconclusive or for definitive surgery after percutaneous biopsy yields a malignant diagnosis.

Percutaneous Biopsy

Increasing use of mammographic screening has led to the discovery of greater numbers of potentially malignant but clinically occult breast lesions. In the past, excisional biopsy was the only method for definitive diagnosis, but the development of imaging-guided percutaneous core biopsy of the breast now provides a more cost-effective alternative (40). Nearly all suspicious lesions are amenable to core biopsy with stereotactic, US, or MR guidance.

Core biopsy is superior to fine-needle aspiration biopsy for the following reasons:

1. Histologic evaluation of core biopsy specimens can be performed by all pathologists, whereas cytologic diagnosis of fine-needle aspirates requires that the pathologist have special expertise and training.
2. The amount of tissue obtained from core biopsies is usually sufficient for diagnosis; insufficient material for diagnosis is a frequent problem with fine-needle aspiration.
3. Differentiation of invasive from noninvasive carcinomas is usually possible with core biopsy, whereas it is not with fine-needle aspiration cytology.

Indications for core biopsy are similar to those for surgical biopsy. A full breast imaging workup must be completed before core biopsy is recommended. Core biopsy should not be substituted for short-interval follow-up of probable benign lesions, because this approach is not cost-effective and may induce increased anxiety in some women. Technical difficulties such as inadequate visualization of the lesion may occasionally preclude the use of a core biopsy.

Core biopsies can be guided by stereotactic images, US, or MR (41). Currently two types of stereotactic units are available. One can be added onto a standard mammography machine but has limited working space and requires a seated patient. The other is a prone dedicated unit that is more costly but offers the advantages of having the patient in a prone position so as to minimize movement and vasovagal reactions (Fig. 20.45). A stereotactic unit allows the x-ray tube to move independent of the compressed breast. The lesion is centered in the aperture within the compression plate, and images at negative and positive 15° are obtained. Calculation of the amount of deviation of the lesion in these two views allows the exact determination of the depth of the lesion. The needle guide is adjusted for exact positioning of the needle in three dimensions to the center of the lesion. Following the injection of local anesthetic, a small skin incision is made to permit needle entry into the breast. Positioning of the needle is verified with stereotactic views, and biopsies are taken (Fig. 20.46).

When US is used, the needle can be observed in real time as the biopsy is performed (Fig. 20.47). Adequate sonographic visualization of the lesion is essential if core biopsy is to be performed with US guidance. Most microcalcifications and some masses, particularly those in fatty-replaced breasts, cannot be visualized and hence cannot be biopsied using US. Aspiration of fluid cannot be performed through a core biopsy needle. Many lesions chosen for US-guided biopsy will be atypical cysts; in such cases it is prudent to attempt aspiration with a 22-gauge needle. If fluid is not obtained, a core biopsy can be performed.

Lesions that are seen only on MR can be biopsied in the magnet using a grid system specifically designed to fit on the breast coil. There are several MR-compatible biopsy devices that allow vacuum-assisted biopsies under MR guidance. In general, contrast enhancement is required to ensure appropriate targeting. A marking clip can be placed following an MR-guided biopsy. The clip can then be used as the target for a mammographic needle localization procedure, should that be necessary.

Either a 14-gauge automated biopsy gun or a 9- to 11-gauge vacuum-assisted needle can be used for a core biopsy. The standard 14-gauge gun works by a spring-action mechanism that fires the needle through the lesion. The inner cannula containing the tissue notch is projected through the lesion first, and the cutting cannula is then fired over it so that a small core of tissue is retained within the specimen notch. With the vacuum-assisted devices, suction is used to bring the tissue into the specimen notch of the needle, which is then cut by an inner rotating cannula. Vacuum-assisted devices generally require only a single needle pass to obtain multiple specimens, whereas standard core biopsy requires multiple passes, one for each specimen. The vacuum-assisted needle offers improved ability to adequately sample microcalcifications in comparison to the standard biopsy gun (42).

The accuracy of core biopsy in diagnosing breast carcinoma approaches that of surgical biopsy, with reported sensitivities of 85% to 100% and specificities of 96% to 100% (43). To achieve such high sensitivities and specificities, it is essential that the mammographic, sonographic, and MR appearance of the lesion be correlated with the pathologic diagnosis. If there is discordance, repeat core biopsy or excisional biopsy should be performed. In cases where atypical ductal or lobular hyperplasia is diagnosed by core biopsy, excisional biopsy should be performed,

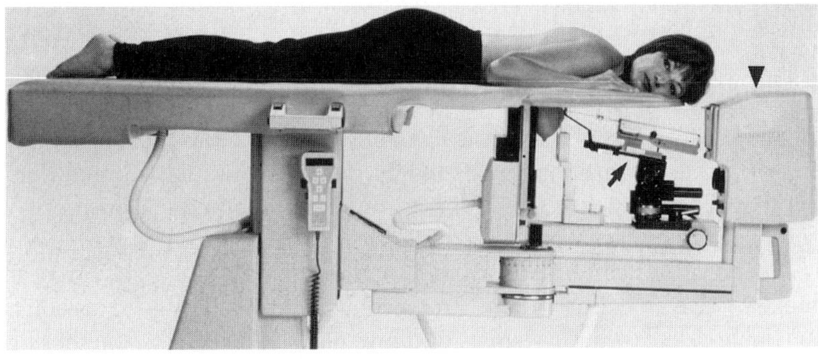

FIGURE 20.45. **Dedicated Stereotactic Biopsy Unit.** The x-ray tube (*arrowhead*) moves independent of the compressed breast so that stereotactic images can be obtained. The needle guide (*arrow*) is adjusted so that the needle will be centered in the lesion. (Reproduced with permission from Fischer Imaging Corporation, Denver, Colorado.)

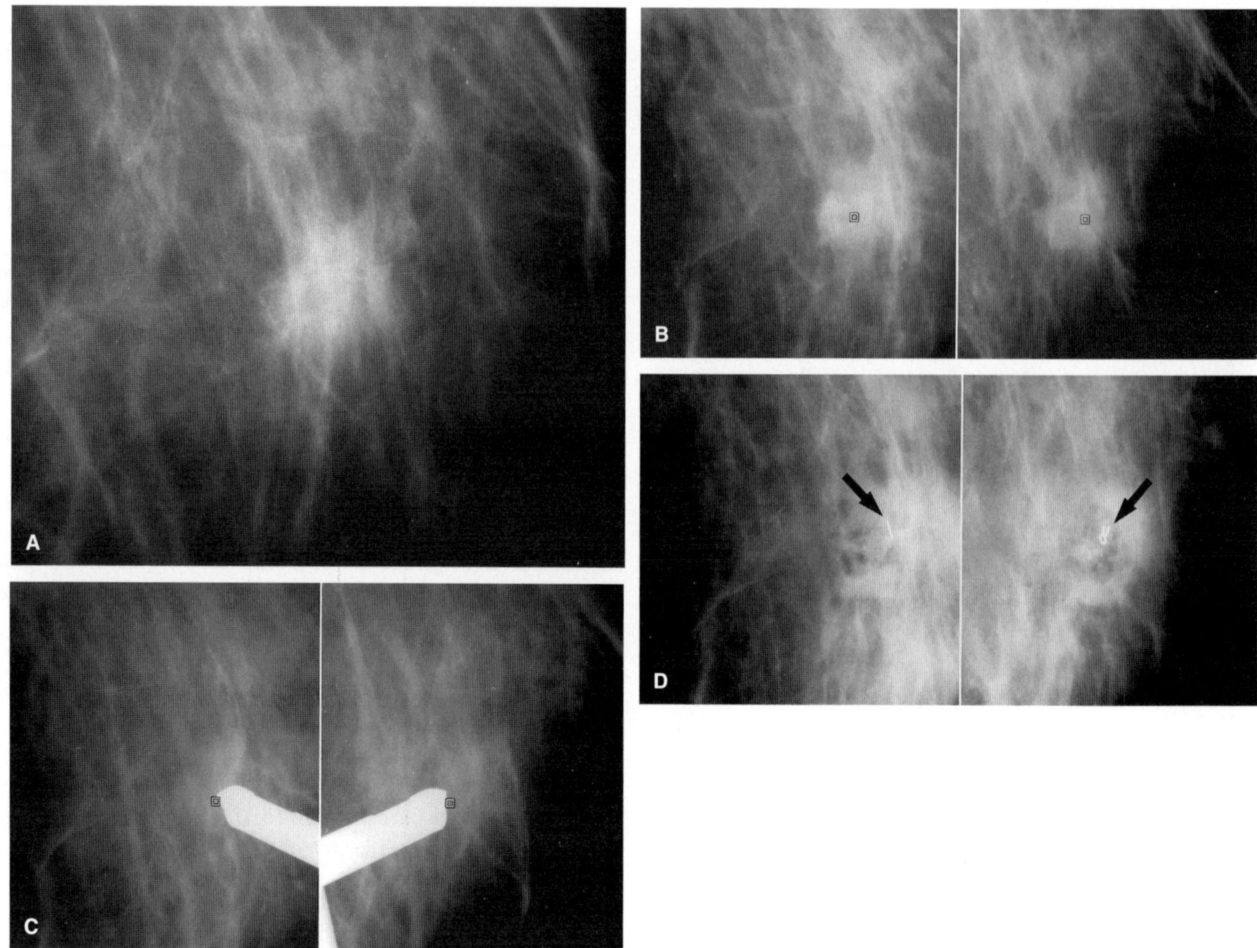

FIGURE 20.46. **Stereotactic Core Biopsy. A.** On the scout view, the lesion is centered in the aperture of the compression paddle. **B.** Stereotactic views at −15° and +15° are obtained, and the center of the lesion is marked in both views with the square target mark. **C.** After injection of local anesthetic, an 11-gauge vacuum-assisted core biopsy needle is inserted and prefire stereo images are obtained to verify appropriate positioning of the needle; the needle should be inserted to a depth that is 5 mm short of the targeted center of the lesion. The vacuum-assisted device is then fired into the lesion and multiple biopsy samples are obtained. **D.** After the biopsy is performed, a marking clip (*arrows*) is inserted and stereotactic images are obtained to verify appropriate positioning of the clip. Note air within the lesion where the biopsy specimens were obtained. In this case, the histologic diagnosis was invasive lobular carcinoma.

because 10% to 48% of these lesions will ultimately prove to be carcinoma (41). Post–core biopsy management of papillary lesions, mucin-containing lesions, LCIS, and radial scars is controversial.

Localization of Occult Breast Lesions

If surgical excision of a nonpalpable abnormality is to be performed, a localization will be required so that the surgeon is accurately directed to the lesion. Many methods for localization have been described.

Localizations can be performed using needle-wire systems or dye injection. There are several commercially available needle-wire systems. All allow placement of a wire through an introducing needle that has been positioned in the breast at the site of the abnormality. The wires differ mainly in the configuration of the anchoring end.

Injection of blue dye is a less frequently used method of localization. A needle is placed at the site of the abnormality and dye is injected. However, if there is a delay between the time of injection and surgery, diffusion of the dye through the tumors can occur, resulting in a biopsy specimen that may be larger than necessary. Methylene blue, formerly in common use for localizations, also interferes with estrogen receptor analysis.

Most mammographic units are equipped with a compression paddle that contains either one large hole marked on the edge with a grid, or a series of smaller holes marked

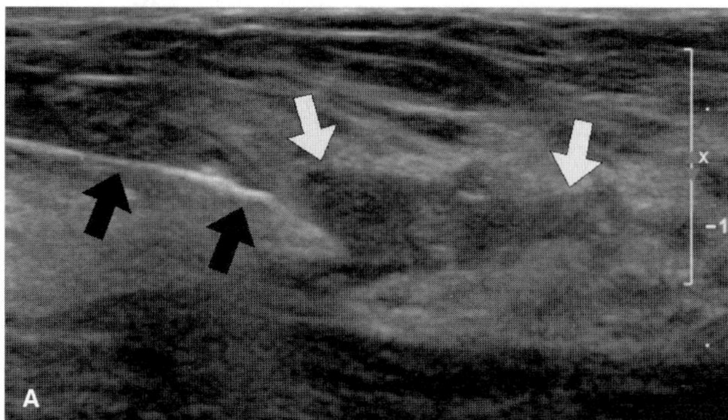

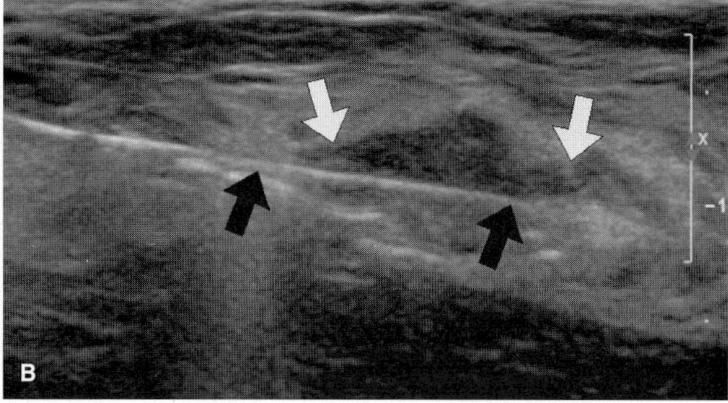

FIGURE 20.47. **US-Guided Core Biopsy.** Prefire **(A)** longitudinal US showing a 14-gauge core biopsy needle (*black arrows*) at the edge of a solid hypoechoic mass (*white arrows*). The postfire image **(B)** shows the lesion (*white arrows*) pierced by the needle (*black arrows*).

with letters or numbers. The seated patient is placed in the mammographic unit so that the lesion to be localized is located under a hole in the compression plate. The skin surface closest to the lesion should be used for needle placement. For example, if the lesion is located at 12:00, a CC approach should be used. The breast is then filmed to determine the exact location of the abnormality. A needle is inserted parallel to the x-ray beam and through the abnormal area. The position of the needle with respect to the lesion is then checked by obtaining another film. If the needle position is satisfactory, the patient, with needle in place, is carefully removed from the mammography unit so that the tube can be rotated 90°. The patient is then positioned in the unit and the affected breast compressed along an axis parallel to the needle. A film is taken to assess the depth of the needle tip with respect to the lesion. The needle must be beyond the lesion before the technician proceeds. This ensures a fixed relationship between the localizer and the lesion. Optimally, the tip of the needle for a wire localization should be 1 to 2 cm beyond the lesion. Once the depth of the needle tip is satisfactory, the wire can be inserted through the needle and the needle withdrawn, leaving the wire in place (Fig. 20.48). Alternatively, dye can be injected through the needle, which for this technique should be within the lesion or a few millimeters beyond it, and then the needle can be withdrawn. The patient is then sent to the operating room for surgical biopsy (44).

Bracketed localization is advocated for nonpalpable lesions over 2 cm in size. More than one localization wire is placed to demarcate the extent of the lesion. This technique is particularly helpful for areas of microcalcifications over 2 cm in diameter because it promotes complete removal of such lesions.

After the biopsy has been performed, the excised tissue should be sent for x-ray. This ensures that the mammographic abnormality has been removed. In a small number of cases (1% to 5%), localization will fail and the lesion will not be removed. In most of these cases, the localization will have to be repeated.

Most localizations are performed under mammographic guidance, but US and MR can also be used to guide such procedures. The technique used in US is similar to that for US-guided percutaneous biopsy. A high-frequency transducer is placed over the lesion, and the needle is introduced obliquely under real-time monitoring. When the tip is seen beyond the lesion, the wire can be inserted or the dye injected. Wire position should be confirmed by mammography.

US is most useful in guiding a localization when the abnormality is seen well in one projection but is obscured by dense tissue in the second. It may also be useful when lesions are located in areas of the breast that are difficult to position within the hole in the localized compression paddle. US can only be used when the lesion can be visualized. Microcalcifications, in general, cannot be imaged, and not all soft tissue masses are well delineated by US.

Lesions seen only on MR can be localized using the grid system that is used for MR-guided core biopsy. Freehand localizations can also be performed. Contrast enhancement is generally required to confirm the location of the lesion prior to needle placement. X-ray specimen radiography may not identify the lesion, because the contrast is no longer in the tissues. MR and pathologic correlation is, thus, extremely important. Discordant cases require postoperative MR to confirm removal of the lesion.

Other Interventional Procedures

Aspiration of sonographically atypical cysts can be performed for confirmation of the diagnosis using either US or mammographic guidance. The majority of such lesions will be smooth-walled masses that are atypical either because they lack through-transmission or because the fluid within them is not anechoic. In such cases, a 22-gauge needle can be inserted using a technique similar to that used

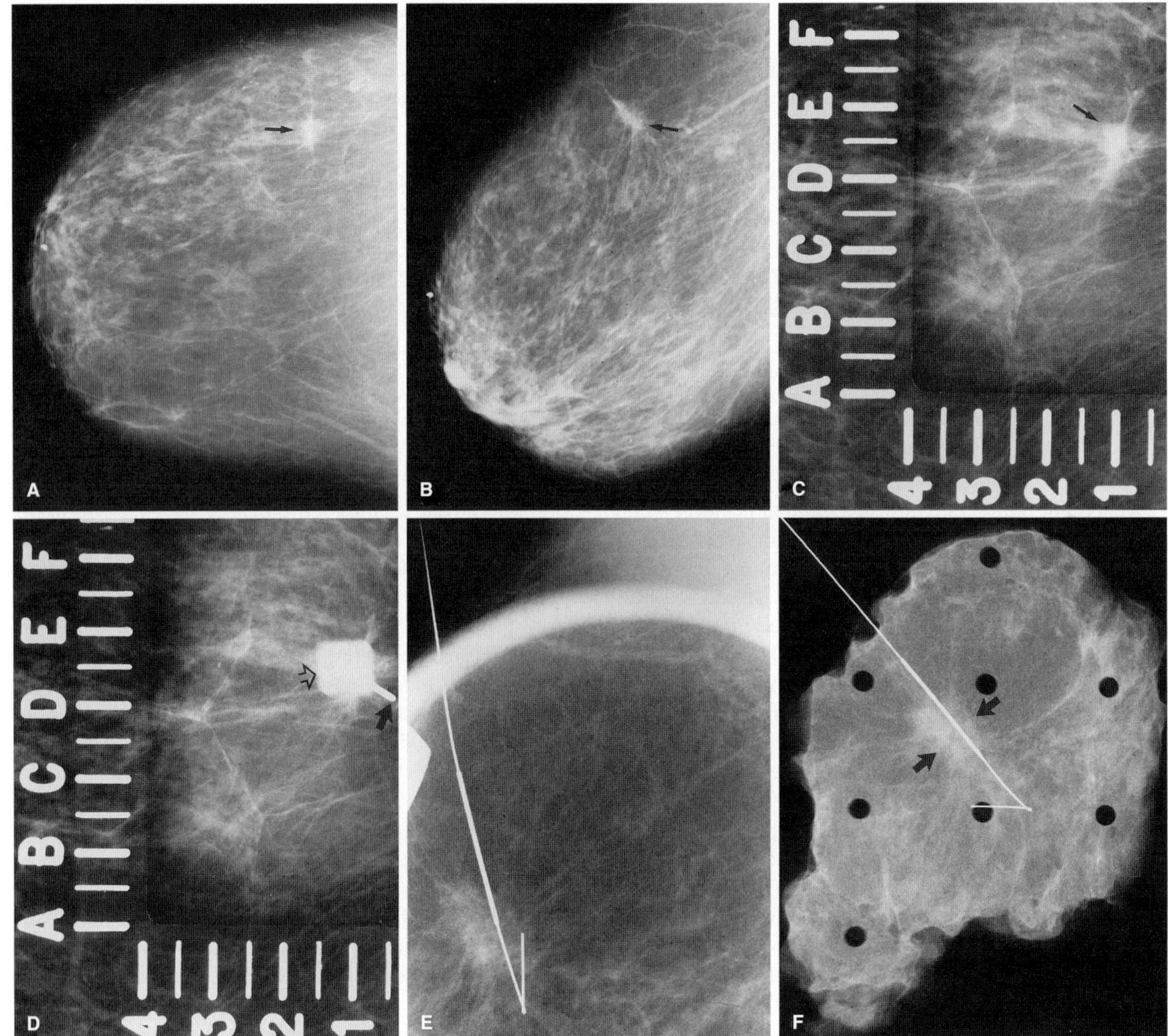

FIGURE 20.48. **Needle Localization.** CC **(A)** and MLO **(B)** mammograms show a highly suspicious spiculated mass in the upper outer quadrant (*arrows*). **C.** Localization was performed by placing the fenestrated compression plate over the lesion (*arrow*) and then placing a needle through the lesion, parallel to the x-ray beam. **D.** The hub of the needle (*open arrow*) is superimposed on the lesion; the tip (*solid arrow*) is at the posterior edge. A film is then taken in the 90° orthogonal projection and, after the depth is adjusted, the hook wire is passed through the needle. **E.** A film in the same projection demonstrates the final depth of the wire. **F.** The excised tissue is sent for specimen x-ray to confirm that the abnormality (*arrows*) has been removed. Histologic examination in this case revealed invasive lobular carcinoma.

for core biopsy. If fluid is withdrawn, the lesion should be completely aspirated. If fluid cannot be withdrawn, the lesion is presumably solid, and core biopsy can be performed.

If there is irregularity or nodularity of the cyst wall, as detected by sonography, core biopsy should be undertaken. Vacuum-assisted devices are preferable for biopsy of these types of lesions since only one needle pass is required for sampling. It is likely that the fluid surrounding such lesions will leak into the surrounding tissues at biopsy, thus rendering the lesion difficult to visualize for multiple passes. Cytologic evaluation of fluid surrounding an intracystic lesion is unreliable for diagnosis.

Ductography can be used to investigate the cause of a spontaneous nipple discharge. The procedure involves the injection of contrast material into a duct, after which films are taken to look for intraductal tumors. These are most frequently papillomas and less commonly carcinomas. The utility of this study is controversial. If the patient has a bloody discharge, some surgeons prefer to inject the discharging duct with methylene blue in the operating room before dissecting along it. Others utilize preoperative ductography to evaluate bloody discharge, reasoning that if the ductogram is negative, the patient can be observed. The use of ductography in the evaluation of a unilateral, spontaneous serous discharge is similarly controversial, since both bloody and serous fluid can be associated with small cancers that may not be visible mammographically.

CONCLUSION

Breast cancer represents a significant public health problem. More than 180,000 new cases are diagnosed and nearly 45,000 women die of the disease each year in the United States. Early detection with screening mammography is the only proven way to lower mortality from breast cancer. Diagnostic accuracy can be increased with the use of special mammographic views, US, and percutaneous biopsy techniques. Other modalities, such as MR and PET, are under study to determine their potential utility in detection and diagnosis of breast diseases. Utilization of breast imaging has increased over the last two decades, and mortality from breast cancer is declining. Our challenge, as radiologists, is to maintain the highest standards of quality in performance and interpretation of breast imaging studies; it is also to encourage all women to take regular advantage of these lifesaving techniques.

REFERENCES

1. Shapiro S. Evidence on screening for breast cancer from a randomized trial. Cancer 1977;39:2772–2782.
2. Nystrîm L, Rutqvist LE, Wall S, et al. Breast cancer screening with mammography: overview of Swedish randomized trials. The Lancet 1993;341:973–978.
3. Hendrick RE, Smith RA, Rutledge JH, et al. Benefit of screening mammography in women ages 40–49: a meta-analysis of new randomized controlled trial results. In: NIH Consensus Development Conference: Breast Cancer Screening for Women Ages 40–49, Program and Abstracts. Bethesda, MD: National Institutes of Health, 1997.
4. Paci E, Duffy SW, Giorgi D, et al. Quantification of the effect of mammographic screening on fatal breast cancers: the Florence Programme: 1990–1996. Br J Cancer 2002;87:65–69.
5. Tabar L, Vitak B, Chen HHT, Yen MF, Duffy SW, Smith RA. Beyond randomized controlled trials. Organized mammographic screening substantially reduces breast carcinoma mortality. Cancer 2001;91:1724–1731.
6. Smith RA, Saslow D, Sawyer KA, et al. American Cancer Society guidelines for breast cancer screening: update 2003. CA Cancer J Clin 2003;53:141–169.
7. von Eschenbach AC. NCI remains committed to current mammography guidelines. The Oncologist 2002;7:170–171.
8. White E, Miglioretti DL, Yankaskas BC, et al. Biennial versus annual mammography and the risk of late-stage breast cancer. J Natl Cancer Inst 2004;96(24):1832–1839.
9. Tabar L, Larsson LG, Andersson I, et al. Breast-cancer screening with mammography in women aged 40–49 years. Int J Cancer 1996;68:693–699.
10. Tabar L, Fagerberg G, Day NE, Holmberg L. What is the optimum interval between mammographic screening examinations? An analysis based on the latest results of the Swedish two-county breast cancer screening trial. Br J Cancer 1987;55:547–551.
11. Kerlikowske K, Grady D, Barclay J, et al. Effect of age, breast density, and family history on the sensitivity of first screening mammography. JAMA 1996;276:33–38.
12. Curpen BN, Sickles EA, Sollitto RA, et al. The comparative value of mammographic screening for women 40–49 years old versus women 50–64 years old. AJR Am J Roentgenol 1995;164:1099–1103.
13. Linver MN. Mammography outcomes in a practice setting by age: prognostic factors, sensitivity, and positive biopsy rate. In: National Institutes of Health Consensus Development Conference Syllabus, Breast Cancer Screening for Women Ages 40–49, January 1997, Bethesda, Maryland. Bethesda, MD: National Institutes of Health, 1997.
14. Feig SA, Ehrlich SM. Estimation of radiation risk from screening mammography: recent trends and comparison with expected benefits. Radiology 1990;174:638–647.
15. Kolb TM, Lichy J, Newhouse JH. Comparison of the performance of screening mammography, physical examination, and breast US and evaluation of factors that influence them: an analysis of 27,825 patient evaluations. Radiology 2002;225:165–175.
16. Kriege M, Brekelmans CTM, Boetes C, et al. Efficacy of MRI and mammography for breast-cancer screening in women with a familial or genetic predisposition. N Engl J Med 2004;351:427–437.
17. de Paredes ES, Marsteller LP, Eden BV. Breast cancers in women 35 years of age and younger: mammographic findings. Radiology 1990;177:117–119.
18. Lewin JM, D'Orsi CJ, Hendrick RE. Digital mammography. Radiol Clin North Am 2004;42:871–884.
19. Sickles EA. Mammographic features of 300 consecutive nonpalpable breast cancers. AJR Am J Roentgenol 1986;146:661–663.
20. Bassett LW, U.S. Agency for Health Care Policy and Research, et al. Clinical Practice Guideline no. 13: Quality Determinants of Mammography. AHCPR Publication No. 95-0632. Rockville, MD: U.S. Department of Health and Human Services, 1994:25–31.
21. Kopans DB, Swann CA, White G, et al. Asymmetric breast tissue. Radiology 1989;171:639–643.
22. Marsteller LP, de Paredes ES. Well defined masses in the breast. Radiographics 1989;9:13–37.
23. Sickles EA. Breast masses: mammographic evaluation. Radiology 1989;173:297–303.
24. Sickles EA. Nonpalpable, circumscribed, noncalcified solid breast masses: likelihood of malignancy based on lesion size and age of patient. Radiology 1994;192:439–442.
25. Bassett LW. Mammographic analysis of calcifications. Radiol Clin North Am 1992;30:93–105.
26. Harris JR, Lippman ME, Veronesi U, Willet W. Breast cancer (second of three parts). N Engl J Med 1992;327:390–398.
27. Eklund GW, Busby RC, Miller SH, Job JS. Improved imaging of the augmented breast. AJR Am J Roentgenol 1988;151:469–473.
28. Destouet JM, Monsees BS, Oser RF, et al. Screening mammography in 350 women with breast implants: prevalence and findings of implant complications. AJR Am J Roentgenol 1992;159:973–978.
29. Gorczyca DP, Schneider E, DeBruhl ND, et al. Silicone breast implant rupture: comparison between three-point Dixon and fast spin-echo MR imaging. AJR Am J Roentgenol 1994;162:305–310.
30. DeBruhl ND, Gorczyca DP, Ahn CY, et al. Silicone breast implants: US evaluation. Radiology 1993;189:95–98.
31. Morris E. Breast cancer imaging with MRI. Radiol Clin North Am 2002 May;40(3):443–466.
32. Lee SG, Orel SG, Woo IJ, et al. MR Imaging screening of the contralateral breast in patients with newly diagnosed breast cancer: preliminary results. Radiology 2003;226:773–778.
33. Liberman L, Morris EA, Kim CM, et al. MR imaging findings in the contralateral breast of women with recently diagnosed breast cancer. AJR Am J Roentgenol 2003;180:333–341.
34. Lee JM, Orel SG, Czerniecki BJ, Solin LJ, Schnall MD. MRI before reexcision surgery in patients with breast cancer. Am J Roentgenol 2004;182:473–480.

35. Lee CH, Smith RC, Levine JA, Troiano RN, Tocino I. Clinical usefulness of MR imaging of the breast in the evaluation of the problematic mammogram. AJR Am J Roentgenol 1999;173:1323–1329.
36. Orel SG, Weinstein SP, Schnall MD, et al. Breast MR imaging in patients with axillary node metastases and unknown primary malignancy. Radiology 1999;212:543–549.
37. Kuhl CK, Mielcareck P, Klaschik S, et al. Dynamic breast MR imaging: are signal intensity time course data useful for differential diagnosis of enhancing lesions? Radiology 1999;211:101–110.
38. American College of Radiology (ACR), BI-RADS Committee. ACR Breast Imaging Reporting and Data System: Breast Imaging Atlas. Reston, VA. American College of Radiology, 2003.
39. Sickles EA. Periodic mammographic follow-up of probably benign lesions: results in 3,184 consecutive cases. Radiology 1991;179:463–468.
40. Lindfors KK, Rosenquist CJ. Needle core biopsy guided with mammography: a study of cost-effectiveness. Radiology 1994;190: 217–222.
41. Berg WA. Image-guided breast biopsy and management of high-risk lesions. Radiol Clin North Am 2004;24:935–946.
42. Meyer JE, Smith DN, DiPiro PJ, et al. Stereotactic breast biopsy of clustered microcalcifications with a directional, vacuum-assisted device. Radiology 1997;204:575–576.
43. Bassett L, Winchester DP, Caplan RB, et al. Stereotactic core-needle biopsy of the breast: a report of the joint task force of the American College of Radiology, American College of Surgeons, and College of American Pathologists. Cancer 1997;47:171–190.
44. Kopans DB, Lindfors K, McCarthy KA, Meyer JE. Spring hookwire breast lesion localizer: use with rigid-compression mammographic systems. Radiology 1985;157:537–538.

SECTION V

Cardiac Radiology

Section Editor:
David K. Shelton

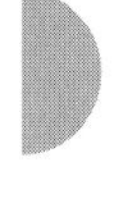

Chapter 21

Cardiac Anatomy, Physiology, and Imaging Modalities

David K. Shelton

Anatomy

Cardiac Catheterization

Chest Radiography
- Cardiac Silhouette
- Chamber Enlargement
- Abnormal Mediastinal Contours
- Cardiac Calcifications
- Pulmonary Vascularity
- The Pericardium
- Other Signs of Cardiac Disease

Nuclear Cardiology

Echocardiography

Coronary Angiography
- Coronary Anatomy
- Coronary Pathology
- Therapeutic Considerations

Cardiac Angiography

Cardiac CT

Cardiac MR

Imaging Methods. Thorough knowledge of cardiac anatomy and physiology is important as a basis for cardiac imaging. Comprehensive knowledge of cardiac imaging also requires consideration of virtually all the available imaging modalities. Chest radiography provides the initial evaluation of most cardiac patients. A barium esophagram can provide additional information because of the close relationship of the esophagus to the cardiac structures. Fluoroscopy increases the detectability of coronary and valvular calcification and provides dynamic and positional information. Transthoracic echocardiography, including pulse-wave and color-flow Doppler, and transesophageal echocardiography provide additional detailed imaging of internal cardiac anatomy and function. Nuclear cardiology, PET, and pharmacologic testing provide key functional, perfusion, and physiologic information. Cardiac and coronary angiography, although invasive, provide detailed anatomic information that can lead directly to interventional or surgical therapy. CT, multidetector CT (MDCT), CT angiography (CTA), and ultrafast CT with the use of IV iodinated contrast material are capable of providing critical information, particularly for pericardial or intracardiac disease. Recent technologic advances in the latter also allow detection of premature coronary calcification, which may have prognostic implications. MR adds three-dimensional (3D) tomographic and motion studies of the myocardium, valves, and chambers without using ionizing radiation or intravascular contrast. Cardiac imaging requires familiarity with all imaging techniques and their associated physics, 3D cardiac anatomy, cardiac physiology, and cardiac disease processes.

ANATOMY

The four-chambered heart lies primarily in the anterior left hemithorax, with the LV lying on the left hemidiaphragm (Figs. 21.1, 21.2). The RA extends to the right of midline as it receives systemic blood from the superior vena cava (SVC), inferior vena cava (IVC), and coronary sinus. The RA and RV lie primarily anterior to the planes of the LA and LV. The RV is the most anterior chamber and abuts

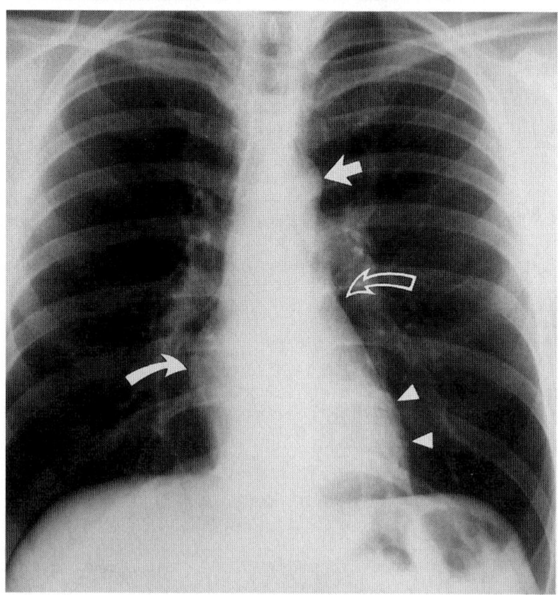

FIGURE 21.1. **Normal Posteroanterior Chest Radiograph.** Frontal view of the chest demonstrates normal heart size, contours, and chamber size. The hila and pulmonary vascularity are normal. The LV (*arrowheads*) is border-forming on the left. The RA (*curved arrow*) is border-forming on the right. The aortic knob (*arrow*) is of normal contour, and the pulmonary artery (*open arrow*) is concave.

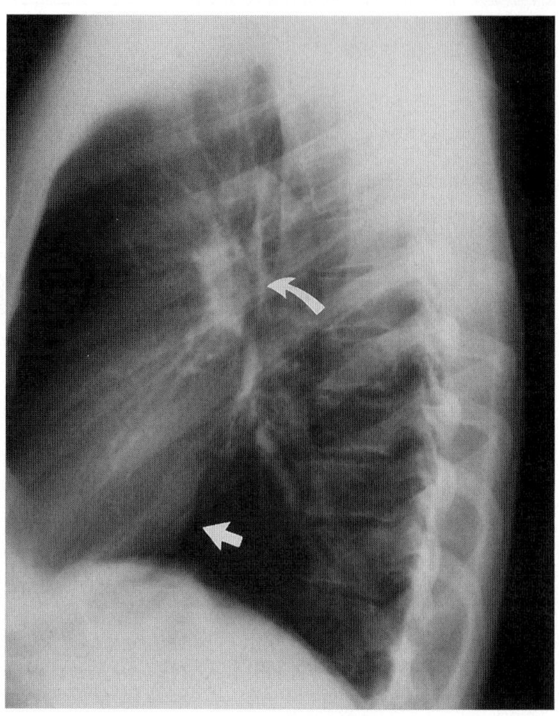

FIGURE 21.2. **Normal Lateral Chest Radiograph.** This well-positioned left lateral chest radiograph demonstrates the right ribs projected posterior to the left ribs because of divergence of the x-ray beam. The right and left bronchi are overlapped, and the sternum is seen in the lateral view. The true lateral projection allows evaluation of the inferior vena cava intersection (*arrow*) with the LV. There is no evidence of posterior displacement of the left bronchus (*curved arrow*) to indicate left atrial enlargement. There is no evidence of right ventricular encroachment into the retrosternal clear space.

the sternum (Fig. 21.3). The LA is subcarinal and midline in the thorax, being supplied by the right and left superior and inferior pulmonary veins.

Frontal Projection. The right border of the cardiac silhouette is formed primarily by the RA, with the SVC entering superiorly and the IVC often seen at its lower margin (Figs. 21.1, 21.3). The left border of the heart is created primarily by the LV and LA appendage. The pulmonary artery, aortopulmonary window, and aortic knob extend superiorly.

Lateral Projection. The RV is border-forming anteriorly adjacent to the sternum, with its outflow tract extending superiorly and posteriorly (Fig. 21.2). The LA is border-forming in the high posterior, subcarinal region. The LV is border-forming inferiorly and posteriorly.

Right Atrium. The RA is divided into two portions. The smooth posterior wall develops from the sinus venosus, with the attached SVC and IVC in continuity posteriorly (Fig. 21.4). The trabeculated anterior wall is derived from the embryonic RA. The RA appendage extends superiorly and medially from the SVC opening. The crista terminalis is a muscular ridge that runs from the mouth of the SVC and fades inferiorly to the mouth of the IVC. It divides the two portions of the atrium and corresponds to an external sulcus terminalis. The medial or posterior wall of the RA is the interatrial septum, which contains a smooth, central dimpled area called the fossa ovalis. Inflow from the SVC, IVC, and coronary sinus enters the smooth posterior portion of the RA. The SVC has a free opening, whereas the IVC is partially guarded by a thin eustachian valve, which is occasionally absent or perforated (network of Chiari). The large draining coronary vein or coronary sinus enters the RA anterior and medial to the IVC. Its opening is guarded by the thebesian valve between the orifice of the IVC and the tricuspid valve.

Right Ventricle. The RV (Figs. 21.4, 21.5) lies anterior to the left ventricular outflow tract and wraps around it and to the left. The right ventricular outflow is directed superiorly, posteriorly, and to the left. The RV is divided into a posterior or inferior portion (inflow or sinus portion), which is heavily trabeculated, and a less trabeculated anterior or superior portion (outflow tract or pulmonary conus). The two portions of the RV are divided by the crista supraventricularis, which is a muscular ridge with a septal band called the moderator band. This band is present in more than 40% of patients, connects the interventricular septum to the anterior papillary muscle, and contains the right bundle branch. The infundibulum (conus arteriosus)

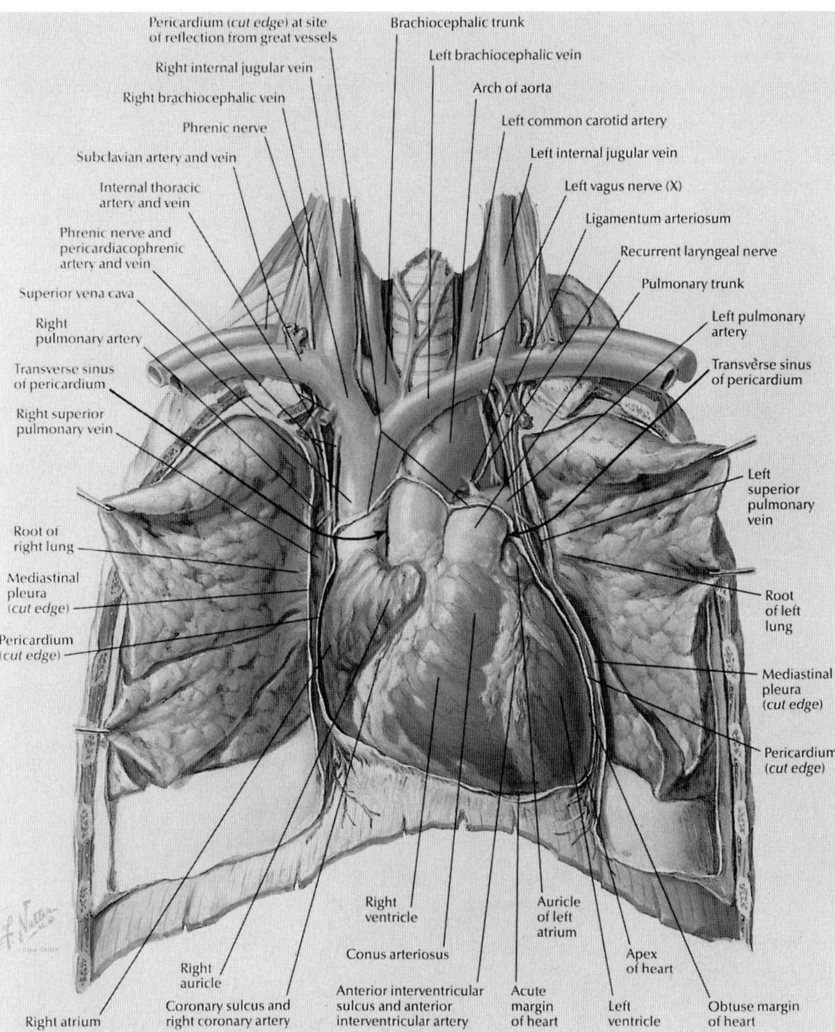

FIGURE 21.3. **Cardiothoracic Anatomy: Frontal View of the Heart After Cutaway of the Chest Wall, Pleural Surfaces, and Pericardial Surface.** Note the relationship of the RA, RV, left atrial appendage, and LV to the great vessels. (Reproduced with permission. Drawing by Frank H. Netter, MD, from Atlas of Human Anatomy. The CIBA Collection of Medical Illustrations, Clinical Symposia. West Caldwell, NJ: CIBA-Geigy Corp, 1989.)

is the smooth cephalic portion of the RV that leads to the pulmonary trunk.

Pulmonary Arteries. The muscular pulmonary conus extends to the semilunar tricuspid pulmonary valve, with the pulmonary trunk extending superiorly and to the left. The left pulmonary artery extends posteriorly as a continuation of the main pulmonary artery, coursing over the top of the left main stem bronchus and then descending posteriorly. The right pulmonary artery extends horizontally to the right, bifurcates within the pericardial sac, and exits the right hilum as the truncus anterior and interlobar arteries. The left mainstem bronchus is hyparterial, meaning that it lies below the pulmonary artery. The right bronchus is eparterial, meaning that it lies next to the right pulmonary artery.

The ligamentum arteriosum arises from the superior proximal left pulmonary artery and crosses through the aorticopulmonary window to the floor of the aorta. The ligamentum arteriosum is the remnant of the ductus arteriosus, which closes functionally in the first 24 hours and closes anatomically by 10 days following birth. Desaturated blood from the right heart circulates through the lungs and returns as oxygenated blood through the right and left superior and inferior pulmonary veins into the LA.

Left Atrium. The LA is the highest and most posterior chamber (Fig. 21.6). Its smooth walls are nestled between the right and left bronchi, and its posterior wall abuts the anterior wall of the esophagus. The left atrial appendage is a small pouch that projects superiorly and to the left and is smoother and longer than the right atrial appendage. The left atrial appendage extends anterior to the left superior pulmonary veins and is readily seen on MR and CT scans. The foramen ovale within the interatrial septum remains nominally patent in up to 25% of adults. Its inferior margin is a remnant of the septum primum and may be somewhat scalloped. The mitral valve is located anterior and inferior to the body of the LA, with the mitral valve leaflets extending into the LV.

Left Ventricle. The mitral valve is the conduit for blood flow from the LA to the LV and is in the high posterior

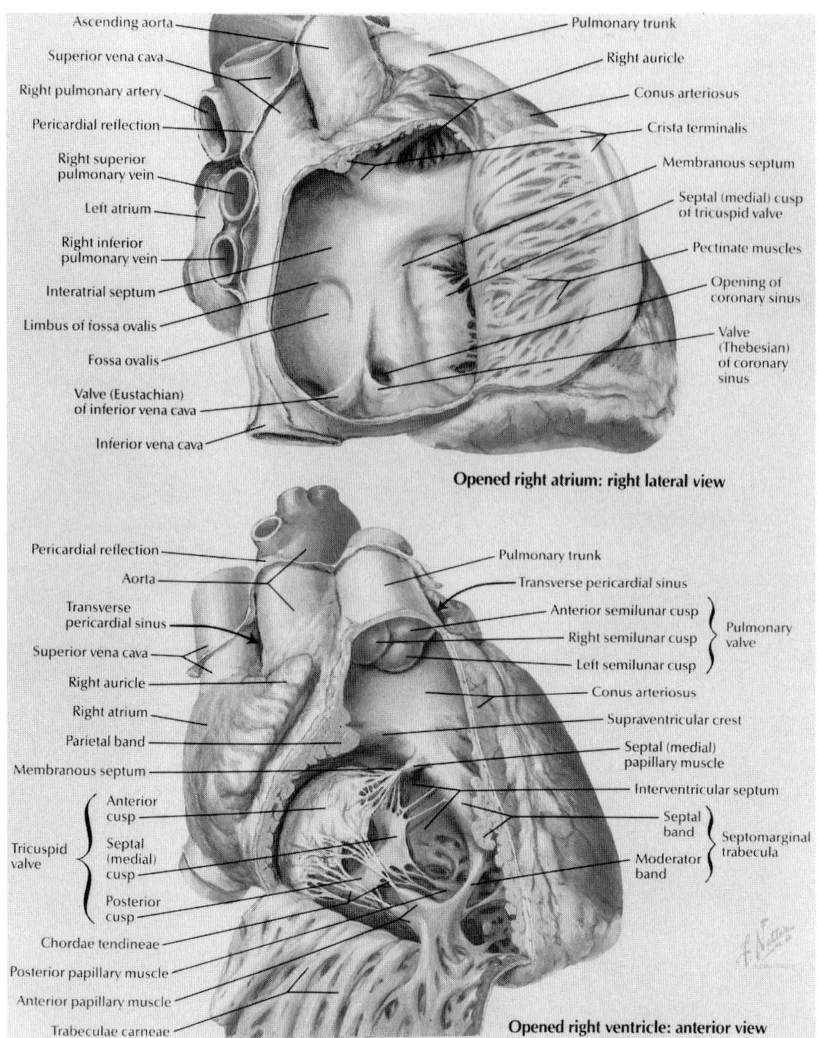

FIGURE 21.4. **Cutaway Views of the Right Atrium and Right Ventricle.** (Reproduced with permission. Drawing by Frank H. Netter, MD, from Atlas of Human Anatomy. The CIBA Collection of Medical Illustrations, Clinical Symposia. West Caldwell, NJ: CIBA-Geigy Corp, 1989.)

"valve plane" of the LV (Figs. 21.5, 21.6). The anterior or septal leaflet of the mitral valve lies near the interventricular septum and extends to the posterior (noncoronary) cusp of the aortic valve. The smaller posterior mitral leaflet lies posteriorly and to the left. The chordae tendineae are strong fibrous cords that extend from the mitral leaflets to the papillary muscles of the LV. The inflow portion of the LV is posterior to the anterior leaflet of the mitral valve. The outflow portion of the LV is anterior and superior to the anterior mitral leaflet. The interventricular septum has a high membranous portion that is contiguous with the aortic root. The more muscular inferior portion of the septum extends to the left ventricular apex. The esophagus passes immediately posterior and is in contact with the muscular wall of the LV.

Aorta. The outflow tract of the LV leads into the aortic root through the aortic valve, which is composed of right, left, and posterior (noncoronary) cusps. The sinuses of Valsalva are the reservoirs created by the closure of the aortic valve and from which the right and left coronary arteries arise. The posterior wall of the aorta is continuous with the anterior leaflet of the mitral valve and more superiorly abuts the anterior wall of the LA. The anterior wall of the aorta is continuous with the interventricular septum. After coursing superiorly and then to the left, the aorta gives off the right innominate artery, left common carotid artery, and left subclavian artery. The aortic arch is the transverse portion of the aorta that abuts the left wall of the trachea, causing a characteristic indentation.

Conduction System. The sinoatrial node consists of specialized neuromuscular tissue that measures approximately 5 to 20 mm and is located on the anterior endocardial surface of the RA, just above the SVC and right atrial appendage junction, near the crista terminalis. Electrical propagation spreads to both atria via Purkinje-like fibers and is recorded as the P wave on an electrocardiogram. The atrioventricular node is a 2- × 5-mm region of neuromuscular tissue on the endocardial surface, along the right side of the interatrial septum, just inferior to the ostium of the coronary sinus. The impulse is collected and

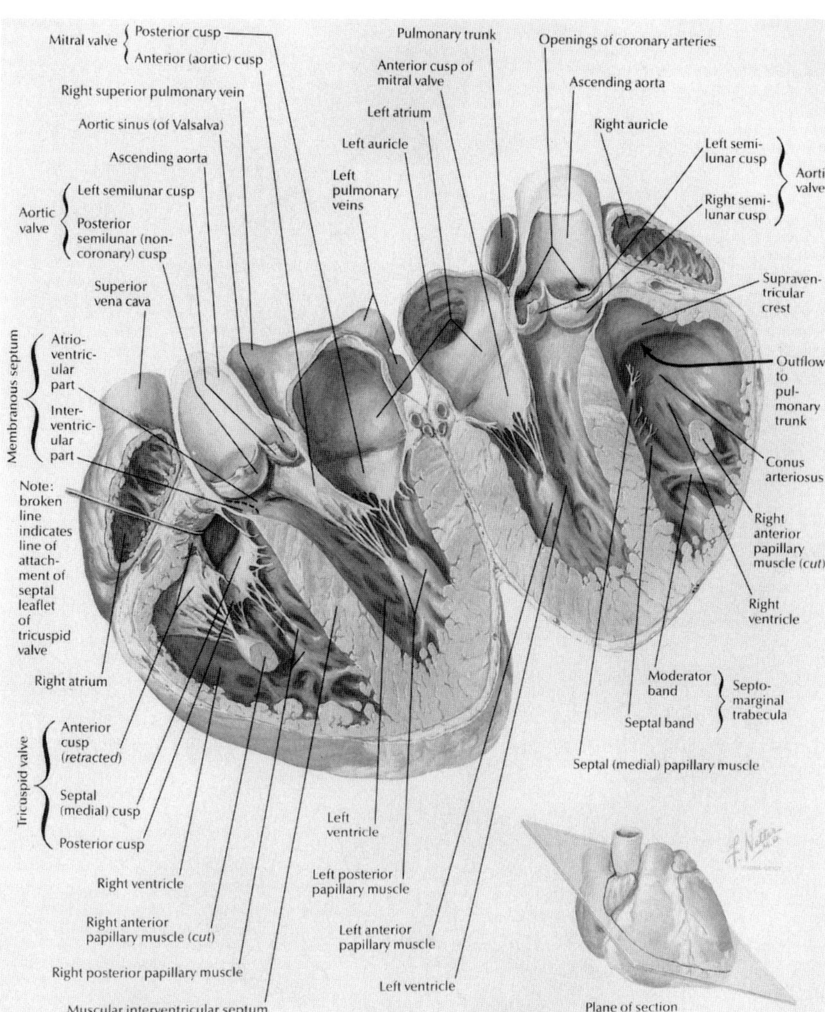

FIGURE 21.5. **Bisection Through the Heart Simulating a Four-Chamber View.** (Reproduced with permission. Drawing by Frank H. Netter, MD, from Atlas of Human Anatomy. The CIBA Collection of Medical Illustrations, Clinical Symposia. West Caldwell, NJ: CIBA-Geigy Corp, 1989.)

delayed approximately 0.7 seconds in the atrioventricular node before passing into the bundle of His. The bundle of His is a 20-mm-long tract that extends down the right side of the membranous interventricular septum. The bundle of His bifurcates into right and left bundles before arborizing through the two ventricles via the Purkinje system. The interventricular septum activates from superior to inferior, with the anterior or septal RV being the first to activate and the posterior or basal LV being the last to activate. This information is particularly useful when evaluating phase analysis or phase propagation in gated cardiac scintigraphy.

CARDIAC CATHETERIZATION

Left-sided catheterization is normally accomplished via arterial puncture in the femoral or brachial artery (Fig. 21.7). It is typically used for aortography, coronary and coronary bypass graft angiography, ventriculography, and evaluation for patent ductus arteriosus. Right-sided catheterization is typically accomplished by venous puncture in the femoral or brachiocephalic vein (Fig. 21.8). It is used for pulmonary angiography, catheterization of the RA and RV, or evaluation of shunt lesions, such as an atrial septal defect.

Important considerations include determination of the catheter course to help diagnose atrial septal defects, ventricular septal defects, patent ductus arteriosus, or persistent left SVC. During catheterization, oxygen saturation percentages are commonly determined, along with pressure measurements and pressure gradients (Table 21.1). Contrast is injected to demonstrate additional details of anatomy, as well as to evaluate for valvular lesions, chamber size, ventricular function, and wall motion.

Right atrial pressures are normally 2 to 5 mm Hg and oxygen saturation is 65% to 75%. Elevated right atrial pressures are seen with right heart failure, decreased compliance, and tricuspid valve disease. A 7% or greater increase in saturation from the IVC to the RA is considered evidence of a left-to-right shunt atrial septal defect (ASD).

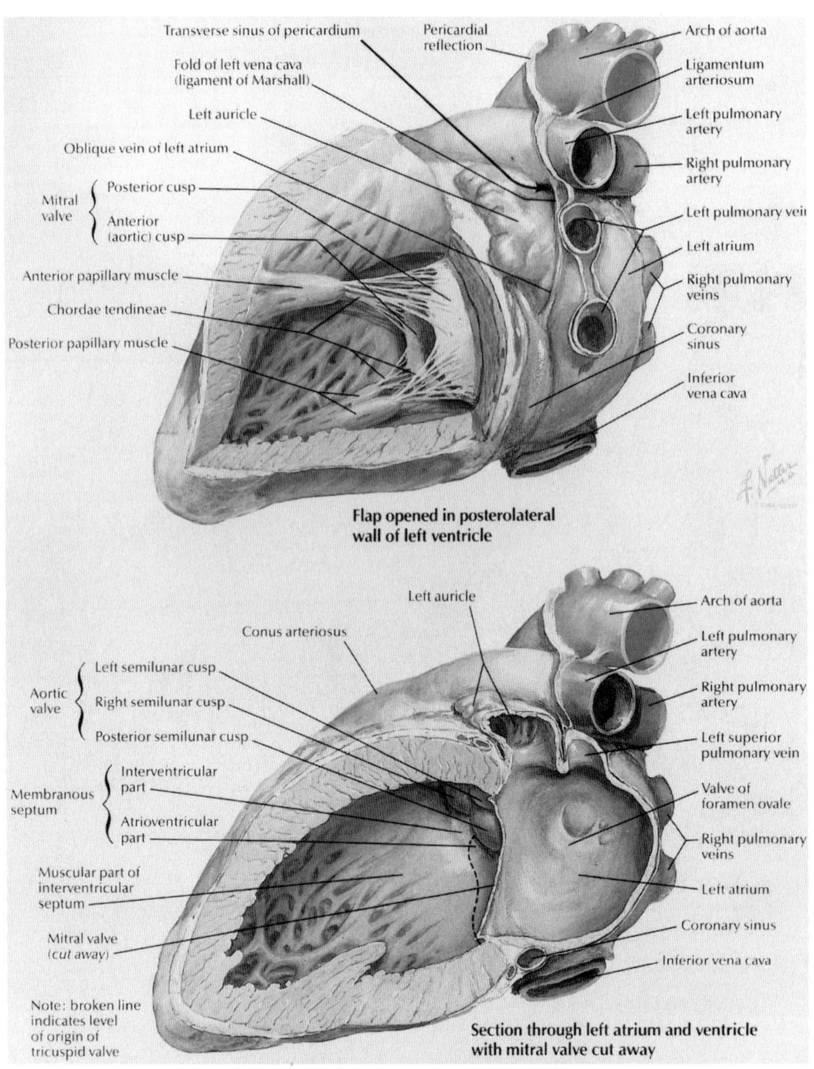

FIGURE 21.6. **Cutaway Views of the LV and LA.** (Reproduced with permission. Drawing by Frank H. Netter, MD, from Atlas of Human Anatomy. The CIBA Collection of Medical Illustrations, Clinical Symposia, 1989.)

Right ventricular pressures are typically 25 mm Hg systolic and 0 to 5 mm Hg diastolic. Elevated systolic pressures are seen with pulmonary hypertension, pulmonic valve stenosis, and congenital heart lesions such as transposition and truncus arteriosus. Diastolic pressures increase with right heart failure. Saturations should be nearly the same as right atrial saturations. A 5% increase in saturation from RA to RV suggests a ventricular septal defect.

Pulmonary arterial pressures are normally 25 mm Hg systolic and 10 mm Hg diastolic, with a mean pulmonary artery pressure of 15 mm Hg. A significant pressure gradient (>10 mm Hg) across the valve implies pulmonic valve stenosis. Increased pressures are seen with shunt lesions, pulmonary vascular disease, and pulmonary venous obstruction. Pulmonary arterial saturation should be approximately the same as right ventricular saturation, with a 3% difference considered significant for a shunt lesion.

Pulmonary capillary wedge pressure is typically 2 to 8 mm Hg and approximates the left atrial pressure unless there is evidence of pulmonary venous obstruction. Elevations in the left atrial or wedge pressure are usually seen with mitral stenosis and left-sided congestive heart failure (CHF). Normal left atrial saturation is approximately 94%, and a decrease greater than 5% implies a right-to-left shunt.

Left ventricular pressures are normally, approximately 120 mm Hg systolic and 0 to 5 mm Hg diastolic. Decreased systolic pressures are seen with shock and CHF. Elevated systolic pressures imply systemic hypertension or outlet obstruction. Increased diastolic pressure is seen with CHF. Decreased saturation at the left ventricular level would imply a right-to-left shunt. Normal aortic pressure is approximately 120 mm Hg systolic and 80 mm Hg diastolic, with a mean pressure of 70 to 100 mm Hg.

With each systolic contraction, the average stroke volume of each ventricle is 70 mL of blood (Table 21.2). End-diastolic volume is normally 125 to 150 mL for the LV and 165 mL for the RV. A normal cardiac output is 4 to 5 L/min, with a normal cardiac index of 2.8 to

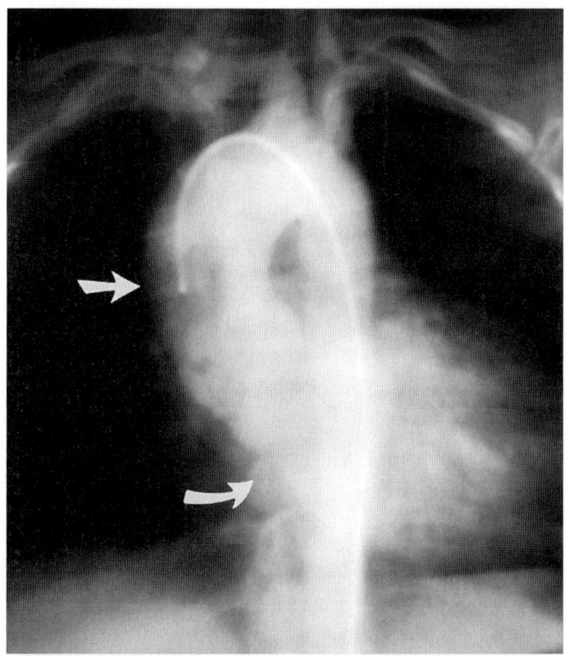

FIGURE 21.7. **Aortogram Via Transfemoral Approach.** The catheter is placed in the mildly dilated ascending aorta (*straight arrow*). Notice the reflux of contrast from the aortic valve into the LV (*curved arrow*) in this patient with aortic insufficiency.

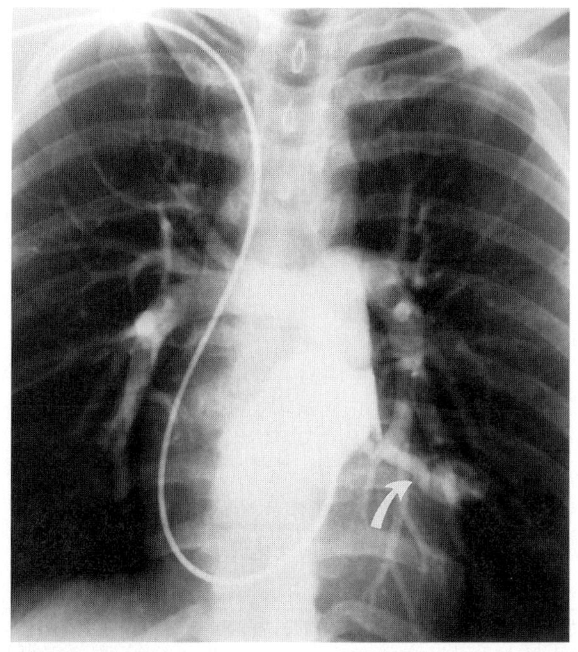

FIGURE 21.8. **Right Heart Catheterization Via the Right Subclavian Vein.** The catheter is positioned in the pulmonary conus. Contrast fills the main, right, and left pulmonary arteries. Note the arteriovenous malformation with a large feeding artery (*arrow*).

TABLE 21.1 Normal Values for Cardiac Catheterization

Site	*Pressure (mm Hg)*	*Saturation (%)*
Vena cava	5	60–65
Right atrium	2–5	65–75
Right ventricle	25/0	70
Pulmonary artery	25/10	73
Left atrium	2–8	94–98
Left ventricle	120/0–5	94–98
Aorta	120/80	94–98

4.0 L/min/m^2 of body surface area. The normal ejection fraction is 50% to 75% for the LV and 45% to 55% for the RV. Typical end-diastolic volumes are 57 mL for the RA and 50 mL for the LA. Coronary blood flow averages approximately 224 mL/min and increases by up to sixfold during exercise.

Aortic Valve. The normal aortic valve orifice is 3 cm^2. Symptoms result from aortic stenosis usually when either the orifice is less than 0.7 cm,^{2} or if aortic stenosis and insufficiency are present, when it is less than 1.5 cm^2. Mild stenosis is indicated by a pressure gradient across the aortic valve greater than 25 mm Hg, moderate stenosis by a gradient greater than 40 to 50 mm Hg, and severe stenosis by a gradient exceeding 80 mm Hg.

Mitral Valve. The mitral valve orifice usually measures 4 to 6 cm^2. Mild mitral stenosis occurs with an orifice smaller than 1.5 cm^2, moderate mitral stenosis at smaller than 1.0 cm^2, and severe mitral stenosis at smaller than 0.5 cm^2.

Pulmonic stenosis is considered significant if the right ventricular systolic pressure exceeds 70 mm Hg.

Pulmonary artery hypertension is defined as a mean pulmonary artery pressure of more than 25 mm Hg.

CHEST RADIOGRAPHY

The chest radiograph remains the mainstay for imaging of the heart and lungs. There are many approaches to

TABLE 21.2 Average Physiologic Data for Cardiac Chambers

Parameter	*Left Chambers*	*Right Chambers*
Atrial end-diastolic volume	50 mL	57 mL
Ventricular end-diastolic volume	125–150 mL	165 mL
Ejection fraction	50%–75%	45%–55%
Stroke volume	70 mL	70 mL
Cardiac output	4–5 L/min	4–5 L/min
Cardiac index	2.8–4 L/min/m^2	2.8–4 L/min/m^2

reading the radiograph. Although most radiologists initiate the process with "global perception," it is important to develop a checklist scan technique. This discussion concerns adult posteroanterior and lateral radiographs.

Cardiac Silhouette

Size. The cardiothoracic ratio should not exceed 0.5 on a 72-inch erect posteroanterior (PA) radiograph or 0.6 on a portable or anteroposterior (AP) examination. Other factors should be considered, such as fat pads and pectus deformity.

Shape. Various contour effects can offer clues to underlying disease. A "water bottle" configuration occurs with pericardial effusion or generalized cardiomyopathy. Left ventricular or "Shmoo" configuration (after Al Capp's Shmoo) describes lengthening and rounding of the left heart border, with a downward extension of the apex resulting from left ventricular enlargement. "Hypertrophy" configuration describes increased convexity of the left heart border and apex. Right ventricular hypertrophy and enlargement tend to lift the apex and create a more horizontal vector to the cardiac axis. Hypertrophy of either ventricle usually causes little enlargement of the silhouette unless dilatation is also present. Hypertrophy typically results from increased afterload, whereas dilation occurs with failure or diastolic overload. "Straightening" of the left heart border is seen with rheumatic heart disease and mitral stenosis.

"Moguls of the Heart." "Skiing the moguls of the heart" refers to the left mediastinal outline beginning at the aortic knob. A prominent knob is a clue to ectasia, aneurysm, or hypertension. Notching or a "figure 3" sign of the aorta suggests coarctation (Fig. 21.9). The second mogul is the main pulmonary artery segment. Excessive convexity is seen with poststenotic dilatation, chronic obstructive pulmonary disease, pulmonary artery hypertension, left-to-right shunts, and pericardial defects. Severe concavity suggests right-to-left shunts. The third mogul is a prominent left atrial appendage that in 90% of cases indicates prior rheumatic carditis (Fig. 21.10). It is not usually seen with other causes of left atrial enlargement. The fourth mogul is a bulge just above the cardiophrenic angle, seen with infarction or ventricular aneurysm. A fifth bulge at the cardiophrenic angle is caused by pericardial cysts, prominent fat pads, or adenopathy.

Chamber Enlargement

Left atrial enlargement is best confirmed by measuring the distance from the midinferior border of the left mainstem bronchus to the right lateral border of the left atrial density (see Fig. 21.10). This distance is less than 7 cm in 90% of normal patients and greater than 7 cm in 90% of patients with left atrial enlargement, as

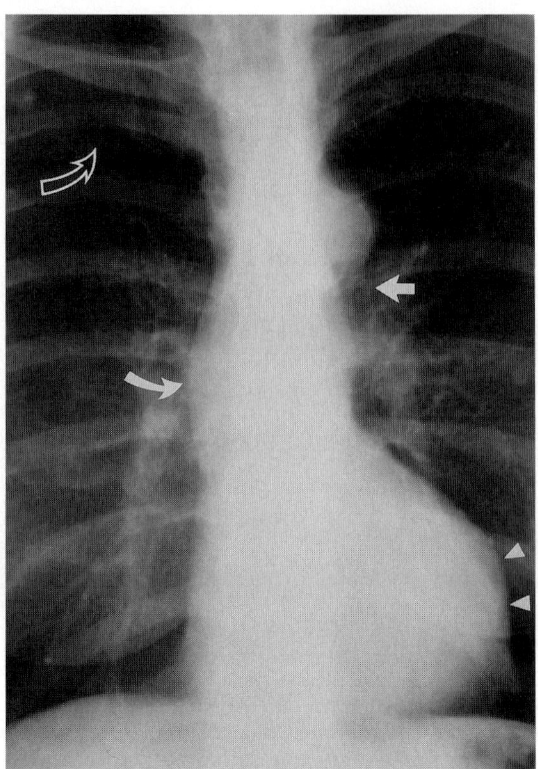

FIGURE 21.9. **Aortic Coarctation.** Notice the "figure 3 sign" or notching of the aorta near the aortic knob (*straight arrow*). The ascending aorta (*curved arrow*) is prominent, and the LV is excessively rounded (*arrowheads*). Rib notching is noted along the right fifth rib margin inferiorly (*curved open arrow*).

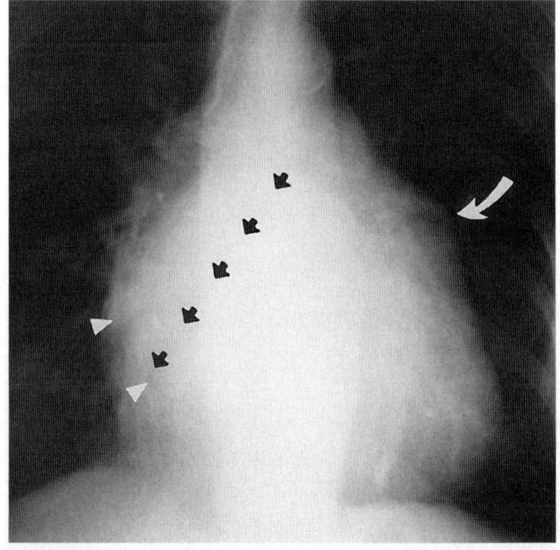

FIGURE 21.10. **Rheumatic Heart Disease.** The left atrial appendage is strikingly prominent (*curved arrow*). Splaying of the carina and a double density along the right heart border indicates left atrial enlargement (*arrowheads*). When the distance from the lateral margin of the LA to the midpoint on the undersurface of the left bronchus exceeds 7 cm, left atrial enlargement is likely (*black arrows*).

proven by echocardiography. This measurement can be approximated by placing one's right fifth finger under the left bronchus and, while keeping the fingers closed, determining whether the LA is seen beyond one's four fingertips; if so, the LA is enlarged. Less-sensitive signs of left atrial enlargement include splaying of the carinal angle, uplifting of the left mainstem bronchus, and prominence of the left atrial appendage. On occasion, the enlarged LA will displace the descending aorta to the left. Massive left atrial enlargement can result in the LA becoming border-forming on the right side, so-called "atrial escape." On lateral views, an enlarged LA will displace the left bronchus posteriorly, with the bronchi creating right and left legs for the "walking man sign." An enlarged LA also impresses against the esophagus.

Right atrial enlargement is more difficult to define on chest radiographs than left atrial enlargement, but fortunately, it is less common. Clues include a prominent atrial bulge too far to the right of the spine (more than 5.5 cm from the midline on a well-positioned PA radiograph). Another sign is elongation of the right atrial convexity to exceed 50% of the mediastinal or cardiovascular shadow. Right atrial enlargement usually accompanies right ventricular enlargement.

Left Ventricular Enlargement. On the PA view, an enlarged LV creates an elongated left heart border with the apex pointing downward. Prominent rounding of the inferior left heart border is also seen (Fig. 21.11). The lateral view shows an enlarged LV extending behind the esophagus. The Hoffman-Rigler sign for left ventricular enlargement exists when the LV extends more than 1.8 cm posterior to the posterior border of the IVC at a level 2 cm cephalad to the intersection of the LV and the IVC (Fig. 21.12). This sign requires a true lateral radiograph and can be a false-positive result if the lateral view is slightly oblique or if there is volume loss in either lower lobe. This sign can be quickly applied by using one of the "2-cm fingertips" for a quick check without a ruler.

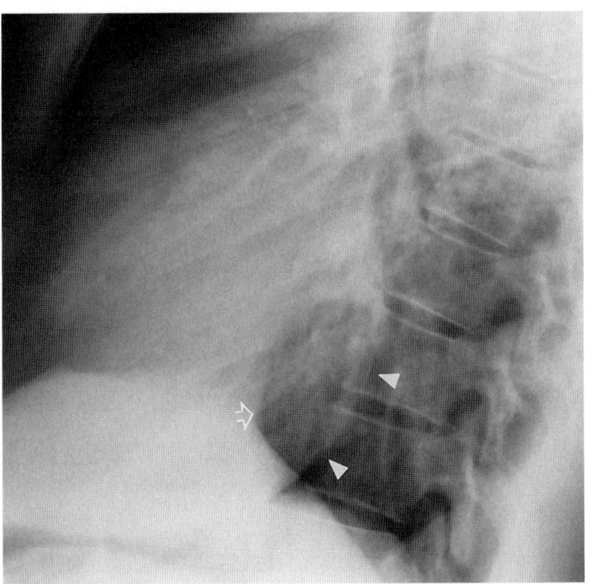

FIGURE 21.12. **Left Ventricular Enlargement on Lateral Chest Radiograph.** The posterior margin of the LV (*arrowheads*) projects prominently behind the inferior vena cava (*open arrow*) and overlaps the thoracic spine. The Hoffman-Rigler sign is positive.

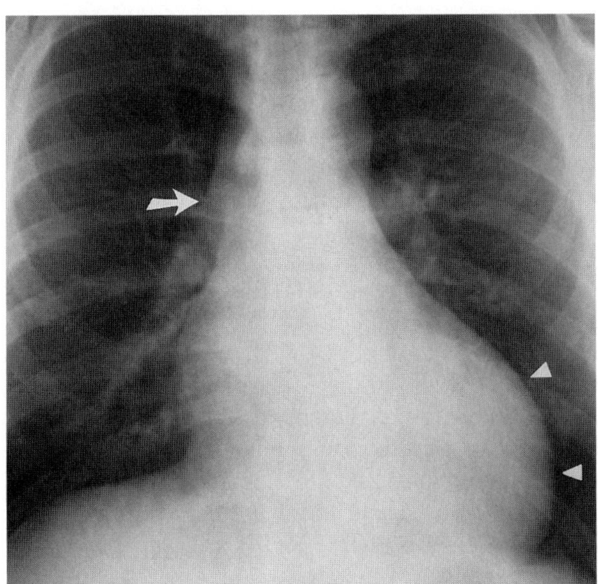

FIGURE 21.11. **Left Ventricular Enlargement on Posteroanterior Chest Radiograph.** Prominence of the LV with rounding along the inferior heart border and an apex that is pointing downward (*arrowheads*) are indicative of "left ventricular configuration." The ascending aorta (*arrow*) is dilated because of aortic stenosis and insufficiency.

Right ventricular enlargement is not as easily detected as left-sided enlargement. If the heart is enlarged and the Rigler sign does not show left ventricular enlargement, then consider right-sided enlargement. If the RV fills too much of the retrosternal clear space or "climbs" more than one third of the sternal length, then right ventricular enlargement is likely. Indirect signs such as enlargement of the pulmonary outflow tract or hilar arteries add confidence.

Abnormal Mediastinal Contours

Aorta. Dilatation of the ascending aorta as a result of poststenotic dilatation is seen in approximately 80% of patients with aortic stenosis (Fig. 21.11). It can also be seen in patients older than 50 years when there is tortuosity of the entire aorta or systemic hypertension. Ascending aortic aneurysm (calcific with syphilis, not calcified with

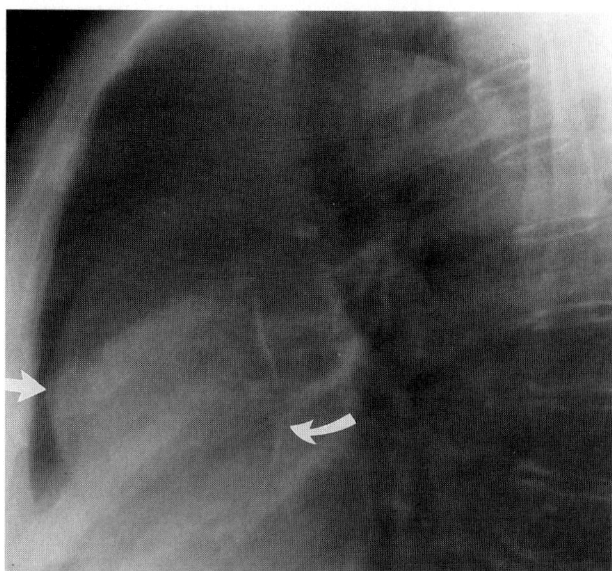

FIGURE 21.13. **Calcified Aortic Aneurysm on Lateral Chest Radiograph.** The ascending aorta is enlarged in this patient with a syphilitic calcified aortic aneurysm. The anterior margin is identified by soft tissue prominence (*straight arrow*) overlapping the retrosternal clear space. The posterior margin is identified by calcification in the wall (*curved arrow*).

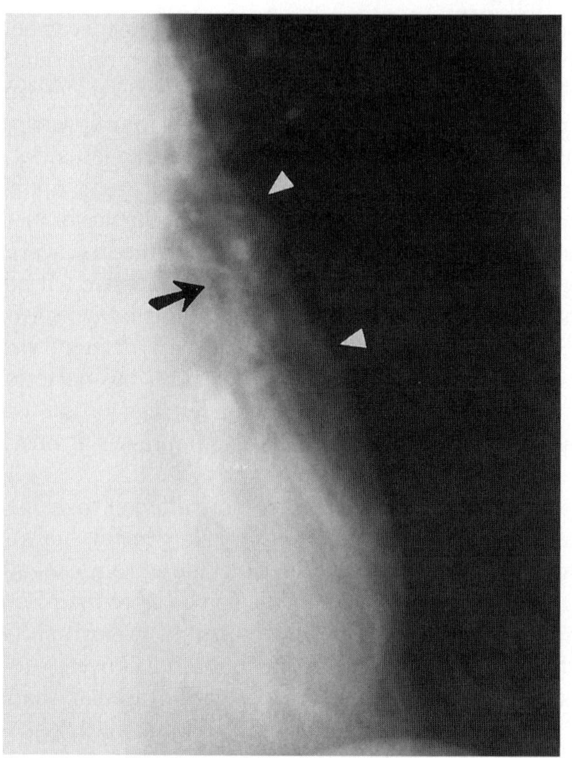

FIGURE 21.14. **Coronary Artery Calcification on Posteroanterior Chest Radiograph.** The calcification (*arrow*) is most commonly detected in the coronary artery calcification triangle along the upper left heart margin (*arrowheads*). The presence of coronary artery calcification may be indicative of coronary stenosis and ischemic heart disease.

Marfan syndrome) is another possibility (Fig. 21.13). A ductus bump adjacent to the aortic knob can be an indication of patent ductus arteriosus.

Azygos vein dilatation (>6 mm on upright PA radiograph or >1 cm on supine radiograph) is seen with intravascular volume expansion, elevated central venous pressure, and right heart failure (see Fig. 23.17). Additional causes include the Valsalva maneuver, pregnancy, renal failure, vena cava obstruction, or azygos continuation of the IVC. Dilatation of the SVC often accompanies volume expansion or elevated central venous pressure but is more difficult to detect with certainty.

Cardiac Calcifications

Coronary Calcification. Radiographs commonly demonstrate coronary artery calcification in a 3-cm triangle along the upper left heart border, called the CAC (coronary artery calcification) triangle (Figs. 21.14, 22.1). If chest pain and coronary calcification are present, there is a 94% chance the patient will show occlusive coronary artery disease at angiography. Fluoroscopic detection of coronary calcification actually has higher sensitivity and specificity in screening asymptomatic individuals than does exercise-tolerance testing. In symptomatic patients, the detection of coronary calcification approaches exercise-tolerance testing in sensitivity and exceeds exercise-tolerance testing in specificity. More than 82% of the patients with fluoroscopically demonstrated coronary artery calcification and positive exercise-tolerance testing show significant coronary artery disease at angiography. Calcifications have more significance when seen in patients under 60 years of age. Heavier and more extensive calcification correlates with more severe coronary disease. Detection of coronary calcification helps to differentiate patients with ischemic cardiomyopathy from those with nonischemic cardiomyopathy.

Valvular calcification is seen in 85% of patients with acquired valvular disease but is rarely detected in patients under 20 years of age. Aortic valve calcification is highly suggestive of valve disease. Calcific aortic stenosis is most often degenerative or atherosclerotic in origin and is usually seen in older men. Extensive aortic annulus calcification is atherosclerotic in nature and has been associated with conduction blocks.

Mitral valve calcification is highly suggestive of rheumatic valvular disease and is seen on the chest radiographs of approximately 40% of patients with mitral stenosis. It is even more common in patients with stenosis and regurgitation. Atherosclerotic calcification of the mitral annulus occurs in approximately 10% of the elderly population (Fig. 21.15). It appears as circular, ovoid, C-shaped, or J-shaped calcification in the mitral annulus and can lead to mitral valve incompetence.

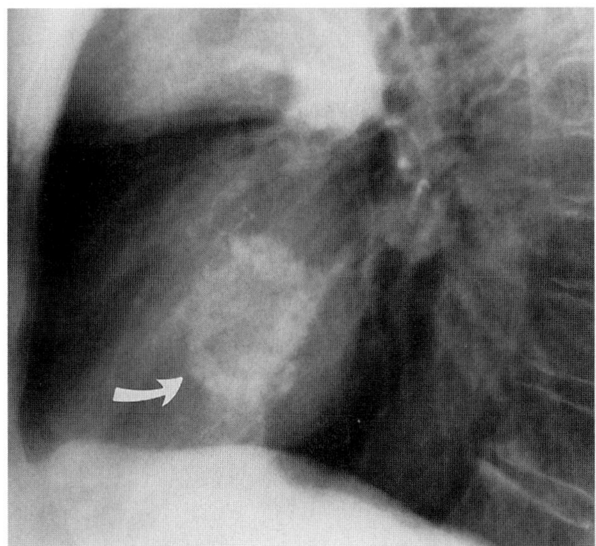

FIGURE 21.15. **Mitral Annulus Calcification on Lateral Chest Radiograph.** Ovoid calcification of the mitral annulus (*arrow*) is secondary to atherosclerosis and is commonly associated with mitral insufficiency. Mitral calcification is best seen on a lateral radiograph.

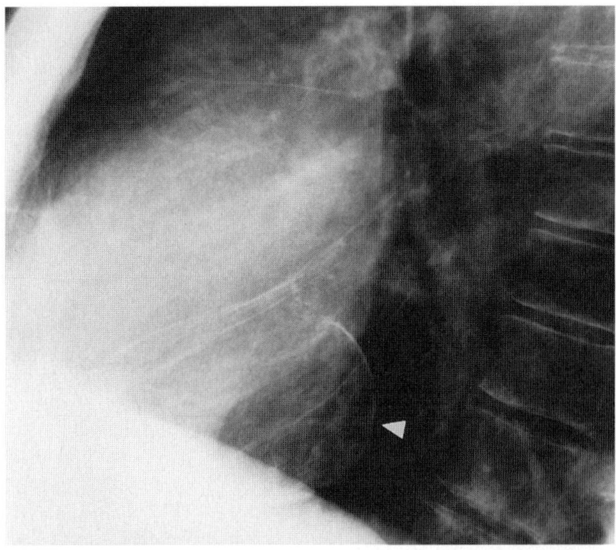

FIGURE 21.16. **Calcified Ventricular Pseudoaneurysm on Lateral Chest Radiograph.** Thin, curvilinear calcification along the posterior wall of the LV (*arrowhead*) is indicative of a ventricular pseudoaneurysm.

Sinus of Valsalva aneurysm calcification is seen as a curvilinear density anterior and lateral to the ascending aorta.

Calcified ligamentum arteriosum is seen as a linear calcification in the aortopulmonary window connecting the top of the left pulmonary artery to the floor of the aortic arch.

Calcified LA. Thin curvilinear calcification in the wall of the LA is usually associated with mitral stenosis, left atrial enlargement, atrial fibrillation, and left atrial thrombus.

Calcified pericardium is typically anterior and inferior in location. It can be single or double layered and is associated with a high incidence of constrictive pericardial hemodynamics. Causes include viral, hemorrhagic, and tuberculous pericarditis as well as postsurgical scarring.

Calcified Infarct. Dystrophic calcification may occur in the myocardial wall from prior myocardial infarction.

Calcified ventricular aneurysm. Thin curvilinear calcification anterolaterally near the apex is most often seen with true aneurysms. Posterior curvilinear calcification is usually seen in pseudoaneurysms (Fig. 21.16).

Calcified thrombus is seen as clumpy calcification in the LA or, less commonly, in the LV.

Calcified Pulmonary Arteries. Thin, eggshell-like calcification in the walls of the pulmonary arteries is virtually diagnostic of long-standing pulmonary arterial hypertension (see Figs. 22.15, 22.16).

Tumors. Rounded or stippled calcifications are seen occasionally in atrial myxomas and rarely in other cardiac neoplasms (see Fig. 22.29).

Pulmonary Vascularity

The lungs have dual blood supply, with the pulmonary arteries and the systemic bronchial arteries.

Pulmonary Arteries. Increased circulation from left-to-right shunts results in enlargement of the main and hilar pulmonary arteries with increased blood flow to the upper and lower lobes. Asymmetric blood flow can be seen with pulmonary hypoplasia, Swyer-James syndrome, and congenital lesions, such as pulmonary stenosis (increased to the left lung) or tetralogy of Fallot (increased to the right lung) (Fig. 21.17).

Bronchial arteries arise from the aorta and penetrate into the lungs, traveling with the bronchi. Tetralogy of Fallot and pseudotruncus arteriosus result in a shift to bronchial circulation. Bronchial arteries are also important in Rasmussen aneurysms from tuberculosis and systemic hypervascularity of any chronic infection.

Pulmonary arterial hypertension (Fig. 21.18) results in (*1*) dilated main pulmonary artery, (*2*) right-sided cardiac enlargement, (*3*) central enlargement of left and right pulmonary arteries, (*4*) rapid pruning of the peripheral pulmonary arteries, (*5*) decreased peripheral pulmonary circulation, (*6*) calcification of the central pulmonary arteries, and (*7*) secondary enlargement of the azygos vein.

Pulmonary aneurysms and peripheral pulmonic stenosis can also cause unusual enlargements of the pulmonary arteries and may be seen in Williams syndrome, Marfan syndrome, and collagen disorders.

Pulmonary venous hypertension (Fig. 21.19) results from mitral stenosis, mitral regurgitation, or elevated left

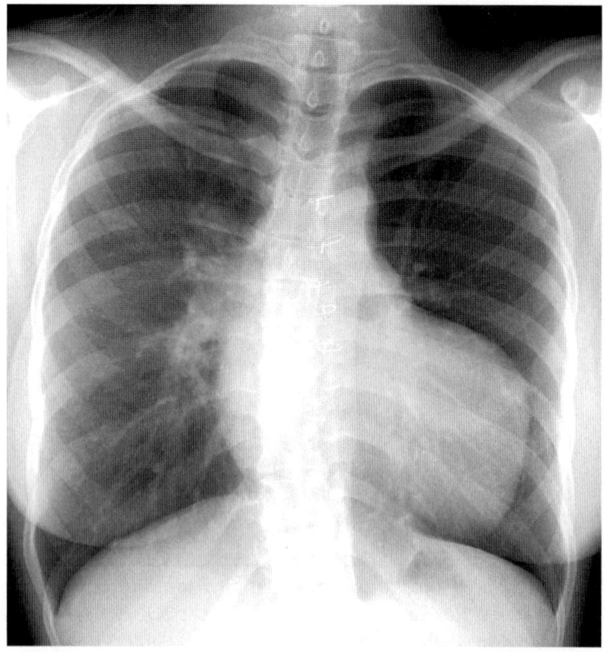

FIGURE 21.17. **Chest Radiograph on Patient With Tetralogy of Fallot.** Asymmetric blood is evident with increased flow to the right. Note also right ventricular hypertrophy configuration and concave pulmonary artery segment.

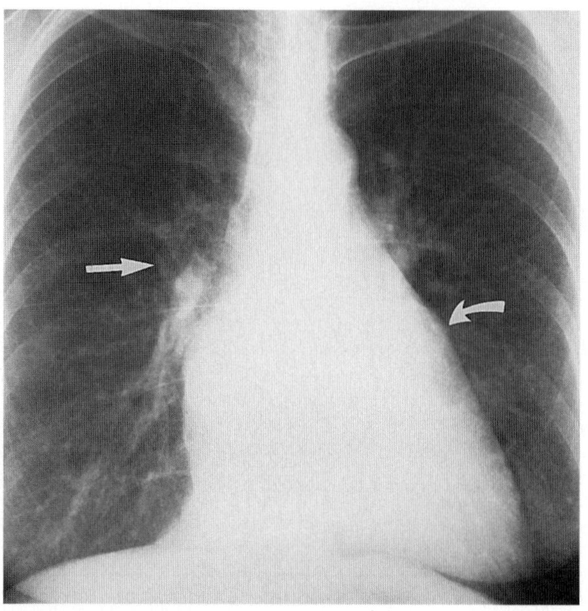

FIGURE 21.19. **Pulmonary Venous Hypertension.** Cephalization of blood flow is evident in this patient with mitral stenosis and enlarged left atrial appendage (*curved arrow*). The lower lobe vessels are constricted, and the upper lobe vessels are distended. Fullness in the hilar angle (*straight arrow*) is caused by enlargement of the superior pulmonary veins crossing between the interlobar artery and the upper lobe artery.

ventricular pressure (aortic stenosis or CHF). The normal vessel caliber in the lower lobes is greater than that in the upper lobes by a 3:2 ratio because of hydrostatic pressure and the high compliance of the venous system. Elevated venous pressure causes progressive, edematous perivascular cuffing, which occurs first in the lower vessels,

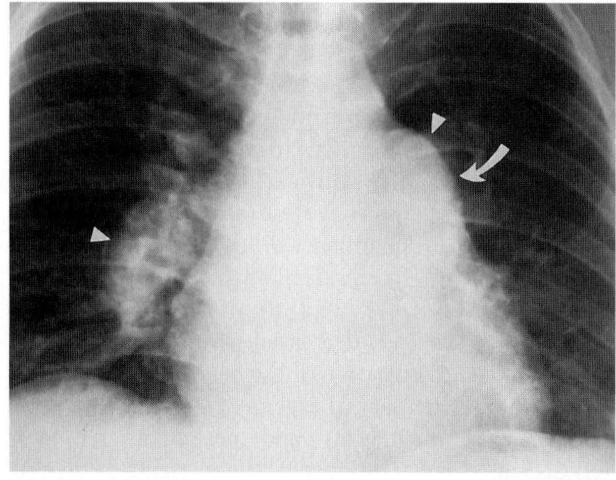

FIGURE 21.18. **Idiopathic Pulmonary Hypertension.** The main (*curved arrow*), right, and left (*arrowheads*) pulmonary arteries are dilated. The pulmonary arteries taper rapidly and peripheral pulmonary vascularity is decreased.

which have higher hydrostatic pressures. Perivascular edema in the lower lobes results in decreased compliance and progressive cephalization of blood flow. The chest radiograph will show decreased caliber of the lower lobe vessels and increased caliber of the upper lobe vessels. Cephalization of blood flow is the earliest radiographic sign of CHF and pulmonary venous hypertension. Cephalization begins at 10 to 13 mm Hg wedge pressure. Equalization of upper to lower pulmonary blood flow occurs at 14 to 16 mm Hg. Reversal of the normal distribution, with the upper lobe vessels distended and the lower lobe vessels constricted, occurs at 17 to 20 mm Hg. Hilar fullness, the "Viking helmet sign" in the hila, and filling out of the right hilar angle commonly accompany reversed flow distribution.

Pulmonary Edema. Interstitial edema with Kerley A, B, and C lines and thickened pulmonary fissures occurs at 20 to 25 mm Hg wedge pressure (Fig. 21.20). Kerley lines represent thickened interlobular septa: A lines are long, straight lines radiating toward the hila; B lines are horizontal lines connecting to the pleural surface near the costophrenic angle; and C lines are random reticular lines seen throughout the lungs. Alveolar edema begins at 25 to 30 mm Hg wedge pressure (Fig. 21.21). Chronic failure "toughens" the interstitium (often resulting in hemosiderosis and pulmonary ossification) and can add an additional protective zone of 5 mm Hg prior to the development of interstitial or alveolar edema. These

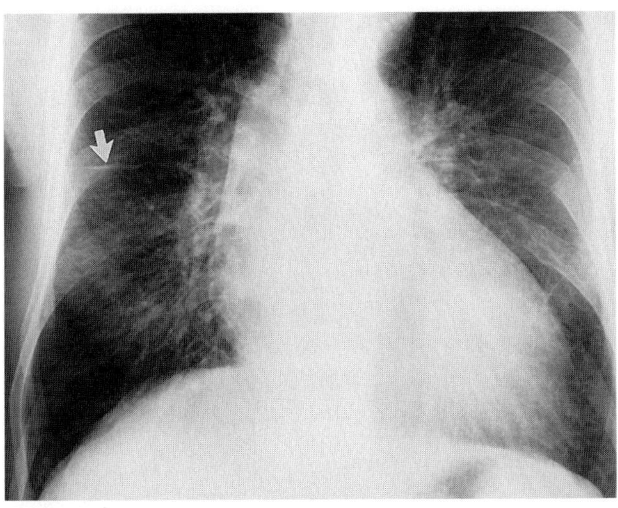

FIGURE 21.20. **Interstitial Edema.** The edema is indicated by prominent Kerley lines. Thickening of the fissures (*arrow*) is also present, along with prominence of the LV and LA and cephalization of blood flow.

progressive signs of failure have been classified as stages 1 to 4 (Table 21.3).

Congestive Heart Failure. Radiographic findings include (*1*) cardiomegaly; (*2*) left ventricular and left atrial enlargement; (*3*) cephalization of blood flow; (*4*) azygos vein and SVC distention; (*5*) perivascular cuffing with haziness and unsharpness of the pulmonary vessels; (*6*) peribronchial cuffing with thickening of the bronchial walls, seen as small "Cheerios" when viewed end on; (*7*) Kerley lines; (*8*) thickening of the pulmonary fissures; (*9*) subpleural edema; (*10*) pleural effusions, usually larger in the right hemithorax; and (*11*) alveolar edema in a "bat's wing" or "butterfly" distribution, also often more pronounced on the right.

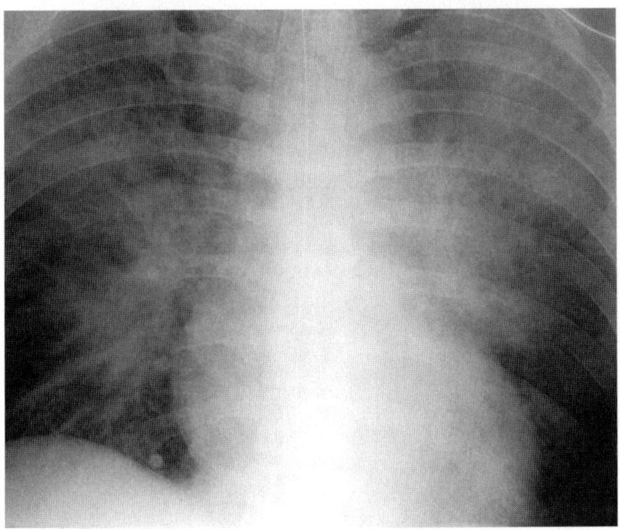

FIGURE 21.21. **Alveolar Pulmonary Edema.** Classic bat's wing or butterfly perihilar alveolar infiltrates are present in a symmetric cloudlike pattern.

TABLE 21.3 Signs of Progressive Cardiac Failure

Stage	*Sign*	*Wedge Pressure (mm Hg)*
1	Progressive cephalization	10–20
2	Interstitial edema and septal lines	20–25
3	Alveolar edema, often in bat's wing perihilar distribution	>25–30
4	Chronic or severe pulmonary venous hypertension resulting in hemosiderosis, pulmonary ossification, and chronic interstitial disease such as from long-standing mitral stenosis	>30–35

Right Heart Failure. The most common cause of right heart failure is left heart failure. Elevated left-sided pressures manifest in the pulmonary circuit and then in the right side of the heart. Long-standing venous hypertension leads to pulmonary arterial hypertension. Elevated right-sided pressures cause right ventricular hypertrophy and dilatation, as well as systemic venous dilatation involving the azygos vein, the SVC, and the jugular veins. Dilatation of the right heart can also cause tricuspid valve incompetence. Right heart failure protects the pulmonary circuit by accumulating edema and fluid outside the lungs, similar to the old therapeutic maneuver of rotating tourniquets.

Right heart failure may also occur with the dilated cardiomyopathies, including viral and alcoholic cardiomyopathy. When right heart failure is the result of pulmonary disease, such as chronic obstructive pulmonary disease, destructive lung disease, or primary pulmonary hypertension, the term *cor pulmonale* is used.

The Pericardium

The pericardium is composed of one continuous fibrous membrane that is folded back on itself, creating two layers. The inner layer of visceral pericardium, or *epicardium*, is closely attached to the myocardium and subepicardial fat. The outer layer or parietal pericardium is thicker and is often referred to simply as the pericardium.

Pericardial Effusion. Between the visceral and parietal layers is the pericardial space, which usually contains 20 mL of serous fluid. More than 50 mL of fluid is clearly abnormal, but a volume of about 200 mL is required for detection by plain film radiography. Mediastinal and epicardial fat enable the pericardium to be visualized as a thin arcuate line paralleling the anterior heart border in the retrosternal region. A pericardial stripe exceeding 2 to 3 mm is indicative of pericardial thickening or effusion. Unfortunately, the thickened pericardial stripe can be seen on the

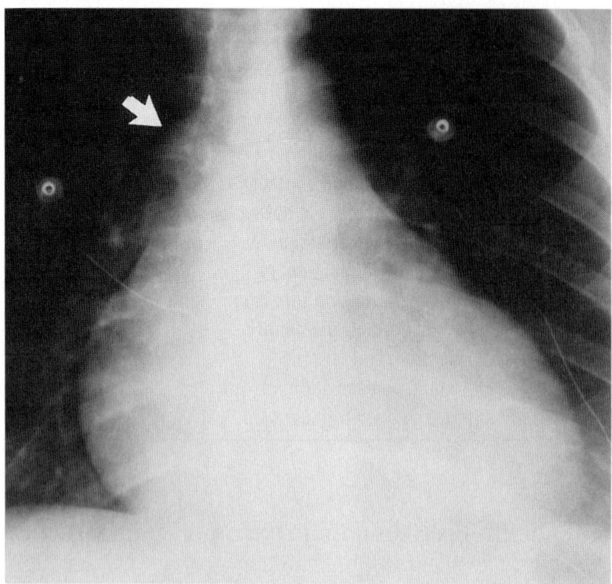

FIGURE 21.22. **Pericardial Effusion.** "Water-bottle configuration" of the cardiac silhouette is indicative of pericardial effusion or dilated cardiomyopathy. This patient with systemic lupus erythematosus has an enlarged azygos vein (*arrow*), decreased pulmonary vasculature, and clear lung parenchyma.

lateral radiograph in only about 15% of patients with pericardial effusion. The "differential density sign" refers to a lucent margin along the left heart border on the PA radiograph or along the posterior cardiac border on the lateral radiograph. It is seen in up to 63% of patients with pericardial effusion but is less specific than the thickened pericardial stripe. Large pericardial effusions cause the heart to appear on frontal radiographs in the shape of a sac of water sitting on a tabletop (Fig. 21.22).

Pneumopericardium appears on plain films as radiolucency surrounding the heart and separated from the lung by a thin white line of pericardium (Fig. 21.23). Air may also be seen outlining the pulmonary arteries or the undersurface of the heart. Pneumopericardium can be caused by trauma, infection, or pneumomediastinum. Firm attachment of the pericardium to the ascending aorta just above the main pulmonary artery acts to contain the pneumopericardium.

Other Signs of Cardiac Disease

Situs Anomalies. Careful attention should be directed at the location of the aortic arch, gastric fundus, heart, pulmonary fissures, and the branching pattern of the bronchi. Normal anatomic positioning is termed *situs solitus*. *Situs inversus* means that the patient's entire anatomic arrangement is reversed in a right-to-left direction as a "mirror image." Situs inversus is associated with a 5% to 10% incidence of congenital heart disease, compared with less than 1% incidence for situs solitus. *Dextrocardia* indicates that the heart is in the right hemithorax. The apex of the heart lies to the right, with the long axis of the heart directed from left to right. *Kartagener syndrome* is a combination of situs inversus with dextrocardia, bronchiectasis, and sinusitis (Fig. 21.24). The latter findings are caused by the abnormal mucosal cilia.

Dextroposition means the heart is shifted toward the right hemithorax. It is associated with hypoplastic right lung and an increased incidence of congenital heart

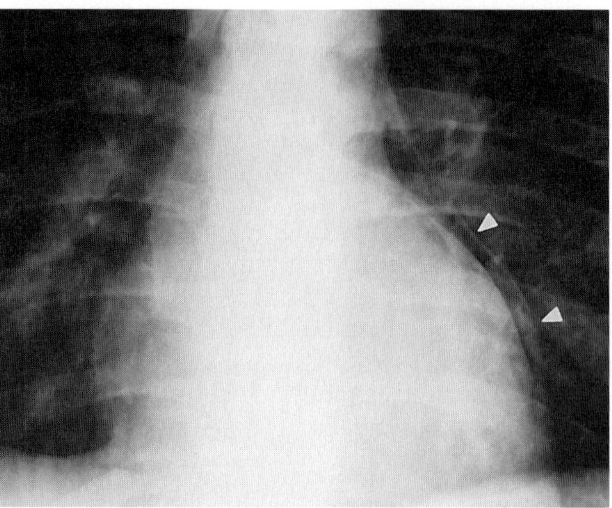

FIGURE 21.23. **Pneumopericardium.** Air within the pericardial sac enables visualization of the pericardium (*arrowheads*), seen as a thin white line paralleling the left heart border.

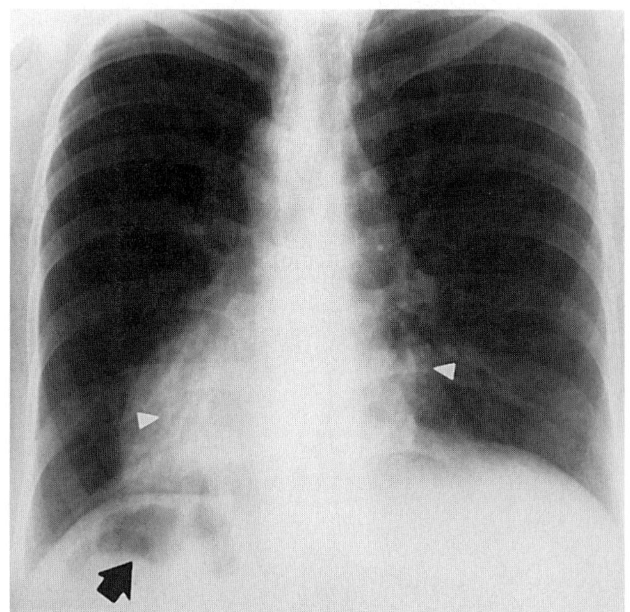

FIGURE 21.24. **Kartagener Syndrome.** Situs inversus is evident with dextrocardia and the gastric air bubble (*black arrow*) on the patient's right. Evidence of bronchiectasis is present behind the heart and in the left lower lobe (*arrowheads*).

disease, particularly left-to-right shunts. *Dextroversion* means the cardiac apex is to the right, but the stomach and aortic knob remain on the left. The LV remains on the left but lies anterior to the RV.

Dextrocardia with situs ambiguous and polysplenia is also called "bilateral left-sidedness." Each lung contains only two lobes and hyparterial bronchi. Bilateral SVCs are also common. The incidence of congenital heart disease is increased, most commonly that of atrial septal defect or anomalous pulmonary venous return. Dextrocardia with asplenia is referred to as "bilateral right-sidedness" because of bilateral minor fissures and three lobes in each lung. The cardiac anomalies are usually more complex and severe than in polysplenia.

Bony Abnormalities. Postoperative changes of sternotomy suggest prior cardiac surgery and the presence of cardiac disease. Sternal fractures from motor vehicle accidents are associated with a 50% incidence of cardiac contusion. Hypersegmentation of the sternum (more than four to five segments) is present in 90% of patients with Down syndrome and offers a clue to the presence of endocardial cushion defect or complete atrioventricular canal. Wavy retrosternal linear opacities suggest dilated internal mammary arteries associated with coarctation of the aorta. Pectus excavatum is associated with an increased incidence of mitral valve prolapse and Marfan syndrome. A barrel-shaped chest with pectus carinatum is associated with ventricular septal defects and complete atrioventricular canal. Scoliosis with a "shield chest" is seen with Marfan syndrome, aortic valve disease, coarctation, and aortic dissection.

The presence of 11 or fewer ribs is highly associated with Down syndrome and atrioventricular canal. "Ribbon ribs" or bifurcated ribs and an overcirculation pattern suggest truncus arteriosus, whereas their association with a pattern of undercirculation suggests tetralogy of Fallot. Rib notching and inferior rib sclerosis indicate collateral circulation through intercostal arteries and occur with coarctation of the aorta and Blalock-Taussig operations. The third through the eighth ribs are most commonly involved. Fractures of the first and second ribs indicate that high-velocity blunt trauma has occurred, and there is an increased risk of aortic injury.

The spine offers clues to the presence of aortic valve disease when changes of ankylosing spondylitis, neurofibromatosis, or rheumatoid arthritis are present. Scoliosis is associated with an increased incidence of congenital heart disease.

NUCLEAR CARDIOLOGY

Cardiac nuclear medicine is a central modality in cardiac imaging and is covered in detail in Chapter 57. Perfusion scans with thallium or new technetium agents are useful for diagnosing coronary ischemia and myocardial infarcts. Normal perfusion scans appear in the shape of a horseshoe in the vertical and long axes and in the shape of a doughnut in the short axis (see Fig. 57.2). The scans are accomplished during rest, with controlled exercise, or with pharmacologic stress with IV dipyridamole. The stress and redistribution or rest images appear identical in normal patients. Hypoperfused segments on stress images that fill in on rest are indicative of ischemia. Hypoperfused segments on both rest and stress images are usually infarcts or scars. Myocardial infarction scanning can be accomplished using rest perfusion agents for "cold spot" imaging or technetium pyrophosphate for "hot spot" imaging (see Figs. 22.8, 22.9). Antimyosin antibody scans have also been utilized for diagnosing and sizing myocardial infarction.

Electrocardiogram (ECG)-gated myocardial blood pool studies examine wall motion and allow calculations of left ventricular ejection fraction (see Figs. 57.10, 57.11). Ventricular function, aneurysms, and valvular disease may be studied with volume curves and functional images. Right ventricular ejection fraction calculations require first-pass examinations because of anatomic overlap of the RV with the atria in the left anterior oblique projection. First-pass cardiac studies can also diagnose SVC obstruction and left-to-right cardiac shunts. Right-to-left cardiac shunts can be evaluated and quantified with technetium macroaggregated albumin or microspheres.

SPECT imaging has greatly improved the diagnostic capabilities of myocardial perfusion imaging and infarct scans. ECG-gated SPECT is readily accomplished and adds wall motion evaluation, ventricular volumes, and ejection fraction information to the study as well. PET is a newer technology with increased resolution compared to SPECT imaging. PET can assess cardiac metabolism as well as perfusion, enhancing its ability to evaluate cardiomyopathies, ischemia, infarction, and "hibernating" or viable myocardium.

ECHOCARDIOGRAPHY

Echocardiography includes M-mode, real-time two-dimensional US, range-gated and color-flow Doppler, and transesophageal US. Transesophageal echocardiography uses a nasogastric probe with a steerable ultrasonic beam that views the heart and aorta from the close posterior position provided by the esophagus (Fig. 21.25). M-mode echocardiograms are produced by a narrow ultrasonic beam that is directed at cardiac structures and observed over time or is swept across an area of anatomy (see Figs. 21.26 to 21.28). The returning echoes produce a time–motion study of cardiac structures. With a transthoracic technique, anterior structures are usually displayed at the top of the image. The thickness and motion of the myocardium can be evaluated throughout the cardiac cycle. Pericardial effusions are shown as echo-free spaces adjacent to the myocardium (Fig. 21.26). Large pleural

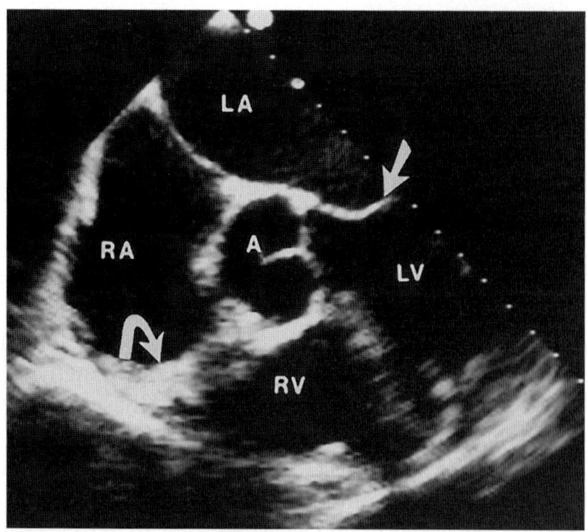

FIGURE 21.25. **Transesophageal Echocardiogram.** A five-chamber view of the heart is provided by an US probe within the esophagus. The probe is behind the LA and is depicted at the top of the image. All four chambers and the aortic valve are seen in one plane, the "five-chamber view." The LA and the RA are separated by the interatrial septum. The aortic valve (A) is readily identified in the midplane. The RV and the LV are separated by the interventricular septum. The tricuspid valve (*curved arrow*) is seen between the RA and the RV, and the mitral valve (*straight arrow*) is seen between the LA and the LV.

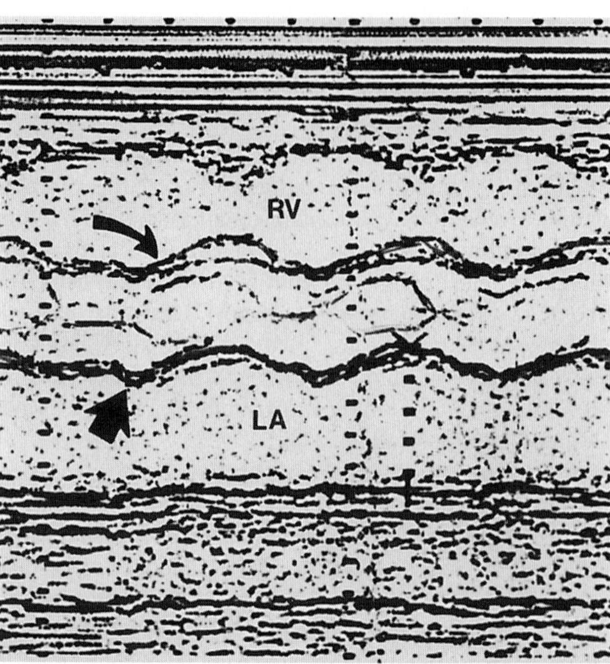

FIGURE 21.27. **Aortic Root.** An M-mode echocardiogram demonstrates anterior movement of the anterior (*curved arrow*) and posterior (*straight arrow*) walls of the aortic root during systole. The RV is seen anterior to the aortic root and the LA is seen posterior to the aortic root. Aortic valve motion can be seen within the aortic root.

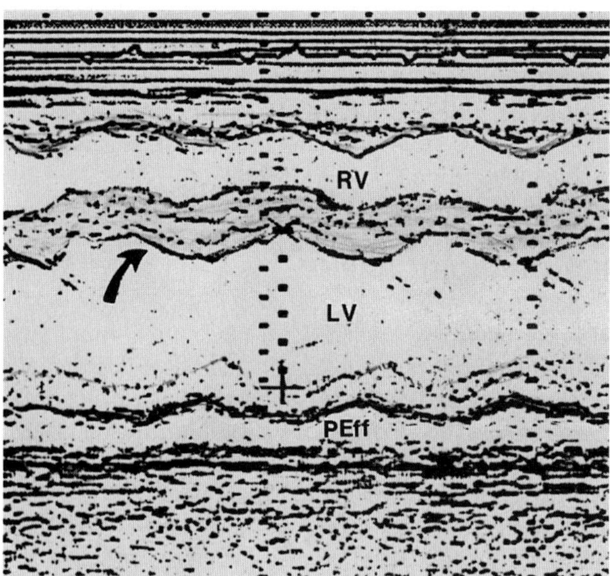

FIGURE 21.26. **Pericardial Effusion.** An M-mode echocardiogram with the ultrasonic probe at the top of the image demonstrates the RV, interventricular septum (*curved arrow*), and LV. Note the normal myocardial contractility with the interventricular septum contracting toward the posterior left ventricular wall during systole. A pericardial effusion (PEff) is seen as an echolucent space posterior to the left ventricular wall.

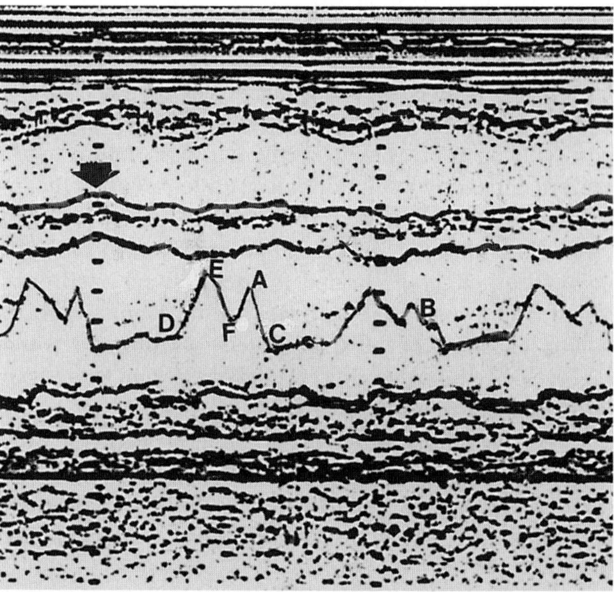

FIGURE 21.28. **Normal Mitral Valve.** An M-mode echocardiogram demonstrates the right ventricular cavity and left ventricular cavity separated by a band of echoes representing the interventricular septum (*arrow*). The moving mitral valve can be seen within the left ventricular cavity. Because of the plane of section, the full systolic motion of the myocardium is not well visualized. The points of the mitral waveform are labeled with letters.

effusions create an echolucent space posterior to the LV and pericardium.

The interventricular septum appears as a band of echoes near the midplane. It normally thickens and moves toward the posterior wall of the LV during systole (Fig. 21.26). Paradoxic septal motion may be seen in pericardial effusion, with cardiac tamponade, chronic obstructive pulmonary disease, asthma, atrial septal defects pulmonary hypertension, left bundle-branch block, and septal ischemia. The interventricular septum measures less than 10 to 11 mm at end-diastole and is compared with the thickness of the posterior wall of the LV for asymmetric or concentric hypertrophy.

The aortic root lies immediately posterior to the RV and measures 8 to 12 mm in neonates and 20 to 40 mm in adults (Fig. 21.27). The thin parallel aortic walls move anteriorly during systole. The aortic root is dilated in aortic stenosis, aortic insufficiency, tetralogy of Fallot, and aortic aneurysm. The thin aortic cusps seen within the aortic root should open widely during systole and should not reverberate.

The LA is seen posterior to the aortic root (Fig. 21.27). The normal size is no larger than 40 mm during diastole in adults. The LA is free of internal echoes and has a thin posterior wall that merges with the thicker left ventricular wall.

The LV lies inferior and lateral to the LA and is an echo-free space except for the thin chordae tendineae and the echogenic projections of the papillary muscles. The left ventricular posterior wall thickens during systole and contracts anteriorly. The transverse diameter of the LV does not normally exceed 5.7 cm during diastole. The wall measures approximately the same as the ventricular septum (10 to 11 mm).

The mitral valve produces a saw-toothed or M-shaped pattern posterior to the interventricular septum (Fig. 21.28). The anterior leaflet is the dominant echo and is continuous with the posterior wall of the aortic root. Immediately posterior to the anterior leaflet is the W-shaped pattern of the posterior leaflet. The two leaflets close during systole. The echo pattern of the anterior leaflet should be carefully scrutinized for evidence of thickening, delay in closure (seen with mitral stenosis), vegetations, prolapse, myxoma, or high-frequency vibration secondary to aortic regurgitation (Austin Flint phenomenon). The specific points of the mitral waveform are (Fig. 21.28) the following:

A point: **A**trial contraction with peak anterior opening motion

B point: notch **B**etween the A and C points representing elevated left ventricular end-diastolic pressure

C point: **C**losure of the mitral valve occurs with contraction of the LV during systole

D point: early **D**iastole when mitral valve begins to open

E point: maximal **E**xcursion of the valve opening. This is the peak of early diastolic opening and the most anterior position of the valve during diastole.

F point: most posterior point of early diastolic **F**illing prior to atrial contraction

The E–F slope is a function of the left atrial emptying rate and should be steep. With mitral stenosis, the slope will be flattened and look more squared off than M-shaped. With valve thickening and calcification, the squared-off part appears thickened.

The tricuspid valve is identified by locating the mitral valve and rotating the transducer medially. It has an M-shaped echo pattern similar to that of the mitral valve. The E–F slope is decreased with tricuspid stenosis and is increased with Ebstein anomaly, tricuspid regurgitation, and atrial septal defect.

The pulmonic valve is rather difficult to evaluate by M-mode echocardiography. The diameter of the pulmonary trunk is similar to that of the aortic root. Pulmonary valve motion is similar to aortic valve motion, except that only the posterior leaflet is well seen and there may be a small "A wave" because of atrial contraction.

CORONARY ANGIOGRAPHY

While CT coronary angiography (CTCA) is playing an increasingly important role, true coronary angiography will remain vitally important, especially in preparation for coronary intervention. Selective catheterization of the coronary arteries was first accomplished in 1959 by Sones with the use of a flexible, tapered-tip catheter using a cut-down procedure on the brachial artery. In 1966, Amplatz used J-shaped, preformed catheters with better torque control from a transfemoral approach. In 1968, Judkins used separate preformed catheters for the right and left coronary arteries. After selective catheterization of the coronary artery, hand injections of contrast verify the size and flow of the artery. The left coronary artery generally requires 7 to 9 mL of contrast at 4 to 6 mL/s, whereas 6 to 8 mL at 3 to 5 mL/s is sufficient for the smaller right coronary artery. Pressure limits for power injectors should be set at less than 150 psi. The catheter tip should not be left wedged in the coronary ostium, as this might occlude blood flow.

Complications of coronary angiography include hematoma, pseudoaneurysm, and fistula formation at the puncture site; arrhythmias, including premature ventricular contractions; heart block and asystole; myocardial infarction; stroke; emboli; and death. Indications for coronary arteriography include (*1*) confirmation of an anatomic cause for angina, (*2*) identification of high-risk lesions, (*3*) evaluation of asymptomatic patients with abnormal exercise tolerance test or occupational risk,

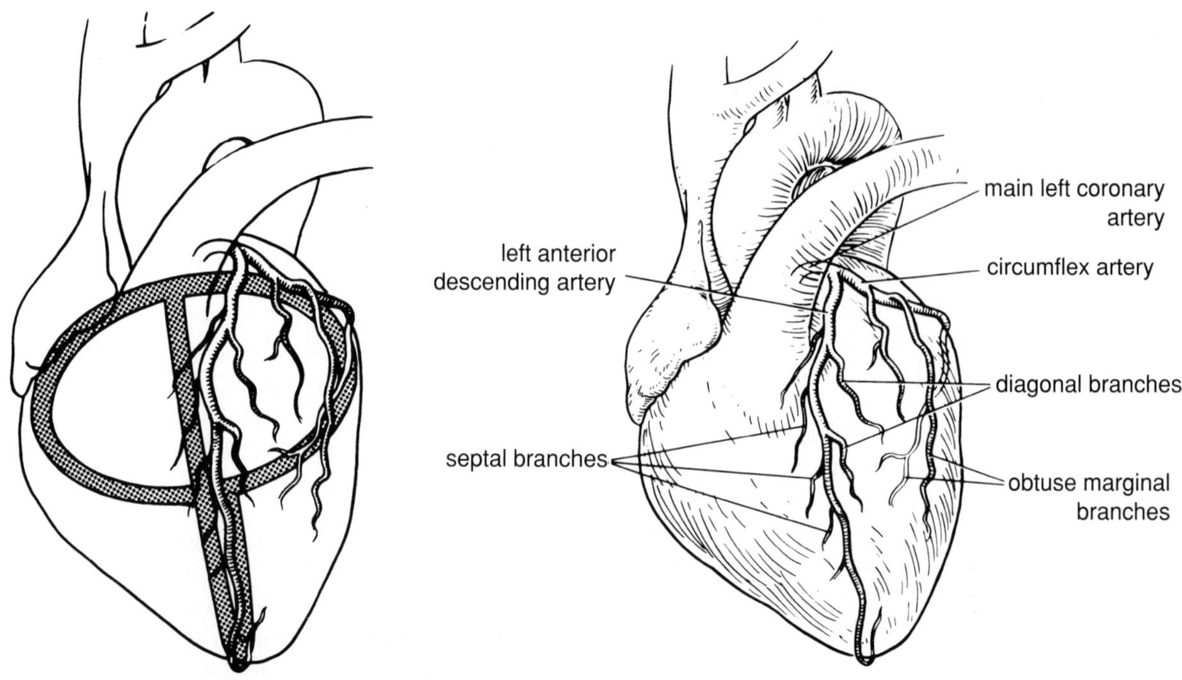

FIGURE 21.29. **Left Coronary Artery (LCA) in the Left Anterior Oblique Projection.** The LCA divides into the circumflex artery, which makes up the left side of the circle, and the left anterior descending artery, which makes up the anterior portion of the loop. Obtuse marginal branches extend from the circumflex artery; diagonal and septal branches extend from the left anterior descending artery. (Reproduced with permission from Kubicka RA, Smith C. How to interpret coronary arteriograms. Radiographics 1986;6:661–701.)

(*4*) preoperative evaluation for cardiac surgery, (*5*) evaluation of patients with coronary artery bypass grafts for stenosis or occlusion, and (*6*) evaluation of interventional therapy after myocardial infarction.

Coronary Anatomy

The right coronary artery (RCA) arises from the right coronary cusp, and the left coronary artery (LCA) arises from the left coronary cusp. Approximately 85% of patients are right dominant, meaning that the RCA supplies the posterior descending artery and the posterior and inferior surface of the myocardium. In 10% to 12% of patients, the LCA is dominant and supplies the inferior and posterior surface. Approximately 4% to 5% of patients are codominant. The LCA measures 0.5 to 1.5 cm in length before it divides beneath the left atrial appendage (Figs. 21.29, 21.30). The left anterior descending artery (LAD) extends anteriorly in the interventricular groove. The circumflex artery extends laterally and posteriorly under the left atrial appendage to the atrioventricular groove. An occasional third branch is the ramus intermedius, which extends as a first diagonal branch (d1) or a first marginal branch (m1).

The LAD gives off several septal branches that penetrate into the septum. One or more diagonal branches extend toward the anterolateral wall. Occasionally, a conus branch comes off after the first septal branch and extends to the right ventricular infundibulum. The circumflex artery gives off one or more obtuse marginal branches that supply the lateral wall of the LV.

The RCA passes anterior and to the right between the pulmonary artery and the RA (Figs. 21.31, 21.32). Its first branch is a conus branch to the pulmonary outflow tract. The second branch is the sinus node branch, with a smaller branch to the RA. Muscular branches extend into the right ventricular myocardium. At the posterior turn, a large acute marginal branch is often given off anteriorly toward the diaphragmatic surface of the RV. The RCA then extends posteriorly in the atrioventricular sulcus and makes a 90° turn toward the apex in right-dominant systems. As the posterior descending artery, it supplies branches to the diaphragmatic myocardium and the posterior one third of the interventricular septum. The distal RCA may also give off a variable number of posterolateral ventricular branches.

The coronary arteries can be visualized as a circle and loop, with the atrioventricular groove being the circle and the interventricular septum being the attached loop (Figs. 21.29 to 21.32). In the right anterior oblique projection, the circle is superimposed on itself and the loop is in profile. In the left anterior projection, the circle is more open and the loop is foreshortened. In the left anterior craniad view, there is a better, elongated view of the left main coronary artery, LAD, and ramus intermedius.

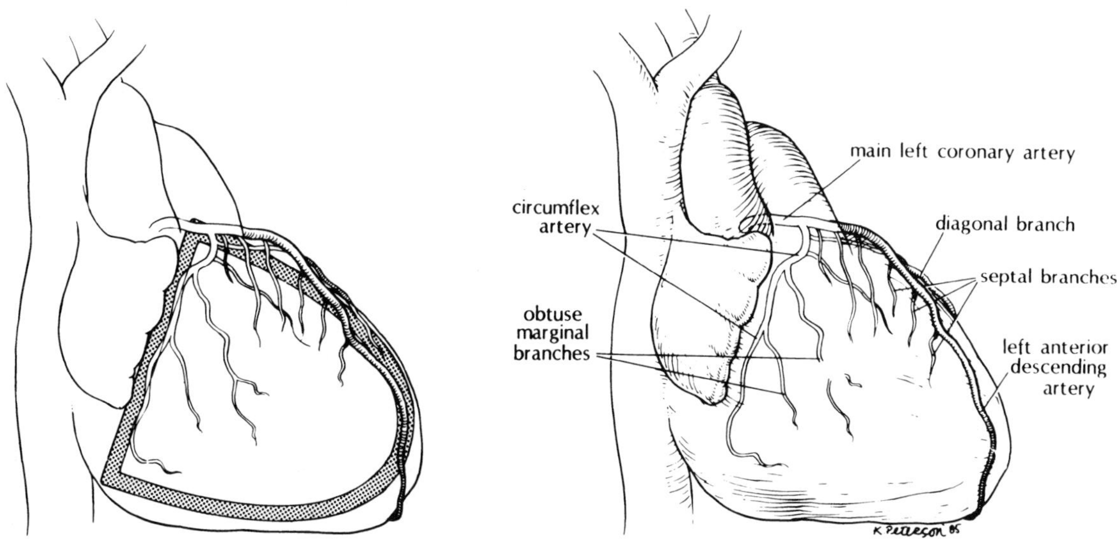

FIGURE 21.30. **Left Coronary Artery in the Right Anterior Oblique Projection.** The loop is more open in this projection, whereas the circle is superimposed. The left anterior descending artery makes up the anterior portion of the loop. The circumflex artery and its obtuse marginal branches make up the left side of the circle. (Reproduced with permission from Kubicka RA, Smith C. How to interpret coronary arteriograms. Radiographics 1986;6:661–701.)

Coronary Pathology

Fixed Coronary Stenosis. A 75% reduction in cross-sectional area is required to cause a significant reduction in blood flow (see Fig. 22.4). A 50% reduction in diameter corresponds to a 75% reduction in cross-sectional area. Other significant findings include coronary calcification, ulcerative plaques, and aneurysm formation. Collateral flow typically develops when there is greater than 85% stenosis.

Catheter spasm is most often seen in the RCA as a smooth transient narrowing 1 to 2 mm distal to

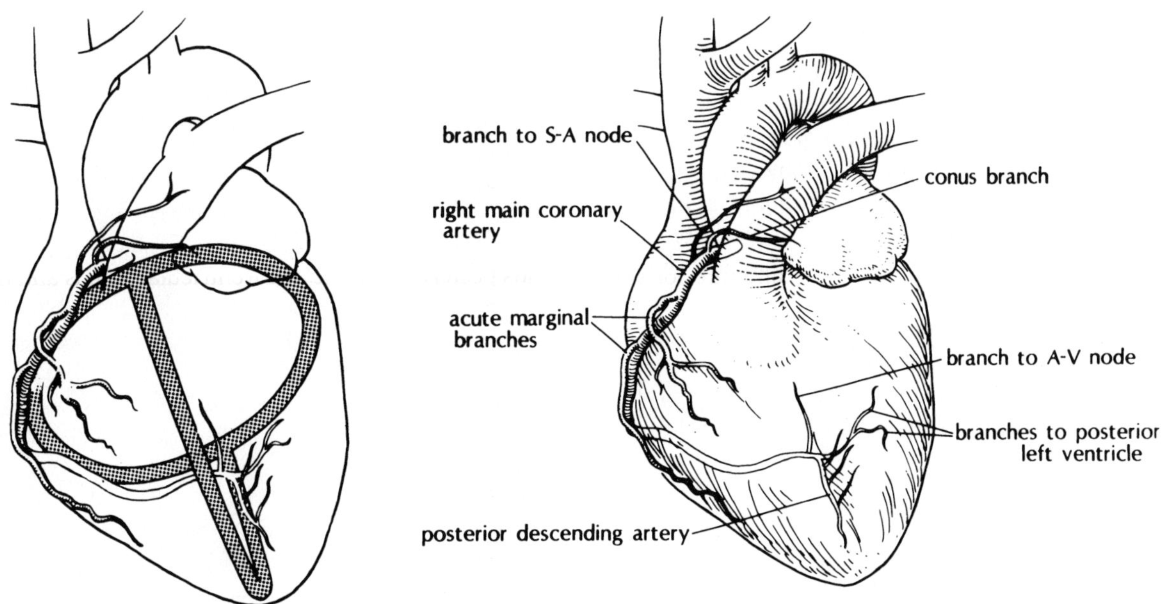

FIGURE 21.31. **Right Coronary Artery (RCA) in the Left Anterior Oblique Projection.** The right portion of the circle represents the RCA, and the posterior portion of the loop represents the posterior descending artery. S-A, sinoatrial; A-V, atrioventricular. (Reproduced with permission from Kubicka RA, Smith C. How to interpret coronary arteriograms. Radiographics 1986;6: 661–701.)

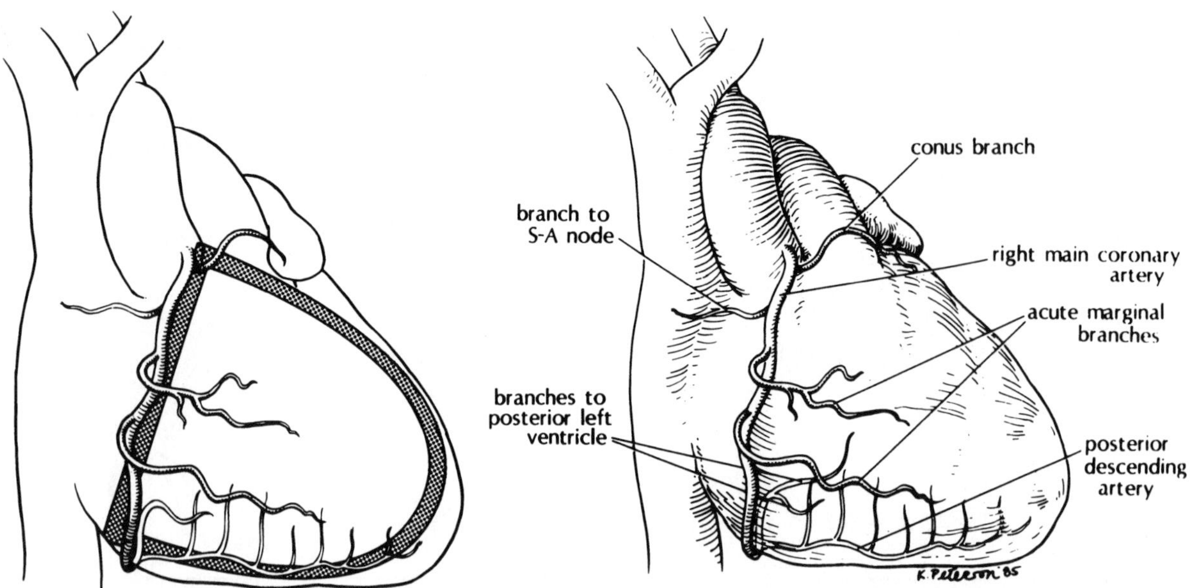

FIGURE 21.32. **Right Coronary Artery (RCA) in the Right Anterior Oblique Projection.** The RCA forms the atrioventricular circle. The loop is more opened in this projection with the posterior descending artery making up its inferior margin. S-A, sinoatrial. (Reproduced with permission from Kubicka RA, Smith C. How to interpret coronary arteriograms. Radiographics 1986;6:661–701.)

the catheter tip. The patient usually remains asymptomatic.

Prinzmetal variant angina is angina secondary to prolonged coronary spasm. IV ergonovine may be used in a provocative test to incite coronary spasm, typical symptoms, and electrocardiographic changes. Prinzmetal angina is usually treated medically.

Kawasaki syndrome is an inflammatory condition of the coronary arteries, probably attributable to a prior viral syndrome, that results in coronary stenosis and coronary aneurysms. It occasionally persists into adulthood.

Myocardial bridging describes a normal variant in which the coronary arteries penetrate and then emerge from the myocardium rather than running along the surface of the epicardium. This causes arterial constriction during systole, which reverts to normal flow during diastole.

Anomalies of the coronary arteries include multiple coronary ostia with more than one coronary artery arising directly from one coronary cusp, a single coronary artery, and origination of the LCA from the PA (Fig. 21.33).

Therapeutic Considerations

The primary modes of therapy for coronary artery disease include many efficacious medical regimens, percutaneous coronary angioplasty and stenting, and coronary artery bypass graft surgery. Coronary artery bypass grafting usually uses saphenous vein grafts or native internal mammary arteries. Surgical bypass has been shown to prolong life in left main coronary artery disease and three-vessel disease. Percutaneous coronary angioplasty (see Fig. 22.5) is considered useful for both single-vessel and multivessel disease and has an 85% to 90% initial success rate. Restenosis remains a significant problem in up to 50% of cases,

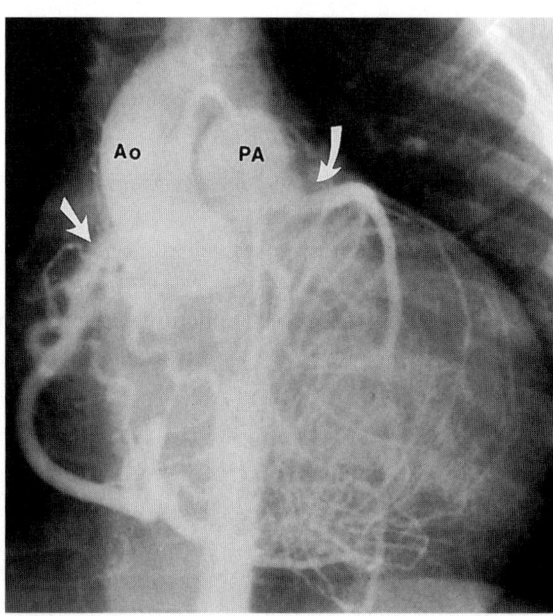

FIGURE 21.33. **Aberrant Left Coronary Artery (LCA).** The catheter in the ascending aorta (Ao) opacifies a dilated right coronary artery (RCA) (*straight arrow*). The LCA (*curved arrow*) arises from the pulmonary artery (PA) and is filled in a retrograde fashion via collateral flow from the RCA.

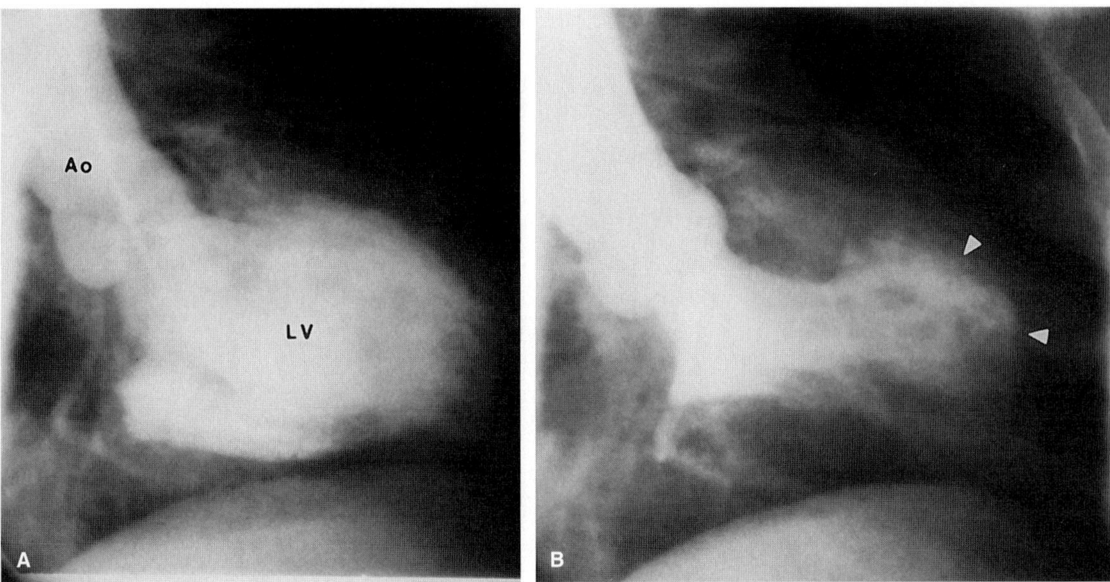

FIGURE 21.34. **Left Ventricular Aneurysm.** Diastole **(A)** and end-systole **(B)**. The left ventriculogram is accomplished with the pigtail catheter entering the LV from the aortic root (Ao). A paradoxic bulge near the apex (*arrowheads*) indicates a left ventricular aneurysm.

typically occurring within the first 6 months. Restenosis is less frequent with newer stents. Angioplasty is typically accomplished by balloon dilatation of the stenotic lesion over a guidewire. Angioplasty is considered successful when the stenosis is reduced to less than 50% of diameter narrowing, although long-term prognosis is better when there is less than a 30% residual stenosis. Directional and rotational atherectomy and atherectomy with the transluminal extraction catheter and laser angioplasty are additional percutaneous techniques that are currently used in specific situations.

CARDIAC ANGIOGRAPHY

Angiography of the heart in adults most often involves left-sided catheterization via arterial puncture with retrograde examination of the aorta, LV, and LA. Selective catheterization of the coronary arteries is also accomplished from the arterial side. Right heart angiography uses puncture of a neck or femoral vein with catheter placement in the RA, RV, pulmonary outflow tract, or pulmonary artery. Additionally, the LA or LV may be seen on delayed or "levo-phase" views from a right-sided injection. It is also possible to access the left side during right heart catheterization by puncturing the atrial septum. End-hole catheters are used for pressure measurements, and pigtail or multiple–side-hole catheters are used for intracardiac injections to avoid contrast injection into the myocardium itself. Blood flow is estimated with standard oximetry, thermodilution, and indicator dilution techniques.

Wall motion is evaluated globally and regionally. *Hypokinesia* describes diminished contractility or less systolic motion than normal. *Akinesia* denotes no systolic wall motion. *Dyskinesia* means there is paradoxic wall motion during systole. *Tardikinesia* refers to delayed contractility. *Asynchrony* refers to cardiac motion that is out of phase with the remainder of the myocardium.

Ventricular aneurysms appear as a bulge in the wall that moves paradoxically compared with other areas of the LV (Fig. 21.34). True aneurysms are lined by thinned, scarred myocardium and are typically located near the apex or anterolateral wall. Pseudoaneurysms are focal, contained ruptures that are often larger but have narrower ostia, and they are most commonly located at the inferior and posterior aspect of the LV. Intramural thrombi may be seen in up to 50% of ventricular aneurysms.

CARDIAC CT

MDCT is useful in evaluating aortic aneurysms, aortic dissections (Fig. 21.35), aortic injuries, vascular anomalies (Fig. 21.36), central pulmonary emboli (Fig. 21.37), intracardiac masses and thrombi (Fig. 21.38), pericardial thickening, fluid collections, and pericardial calcifications. Optimal contrast enhancement, ECG gating, and breath-hold technique are required for optimal studies. Ultrafast or electron beam CT (EBCT) offers the advantage of high-speed scanning to better stop action and eliminate motion artifact. Angled couch views supplement standard axial imaging. With cardiac gating, cine-CT can

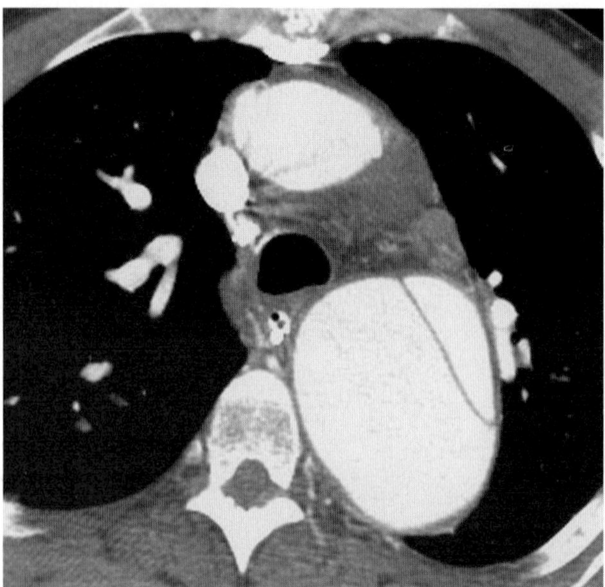

FIGURE 21.35. **Type B Aortic Dissection.** Contrast-enhanced multidetector CT scan demonstrates descending aortic aneurysm with intimal flap. The ascending aorta is normal.

provide wall motion studies, ejection fraction, and valve evaluation.

Coronary Artery Calcium Screening with CT. As previously described, coronary artery calcification has been studied extensively with chest radiography and fluoroscopy. Radiography has a sensitivity of 42% and fluoroscopy has sensitivity of 40% to 79% and specificity of 52% to 95% for detecting coronary calcification as an indicator of coronary stenosis. Coronary calcification is a significant marker for underlying atherosclerosis. EBCT has

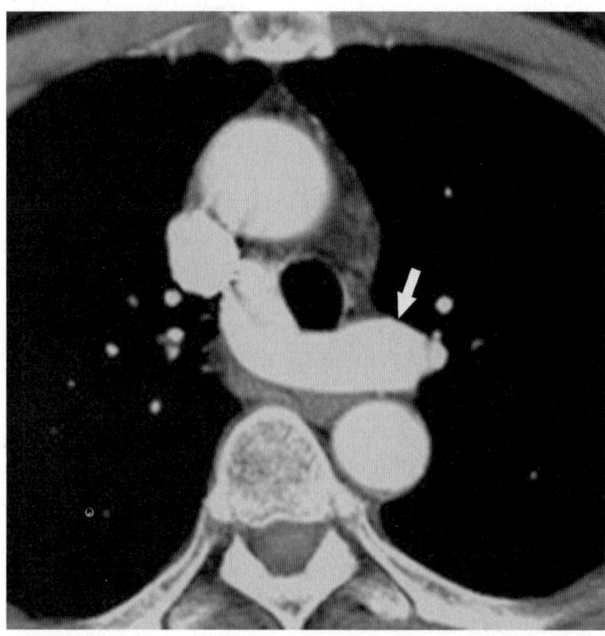

FIGURE 21.36. **Aberrant Left Pulmonary Artery.** Contrast-enhanced multidetector CT demonstrates anomalous origin of left pulmonary artery (*arrow*) from the right pulmonary artery, crossing posterior to the trachea, consistent with a pulmonary sling.

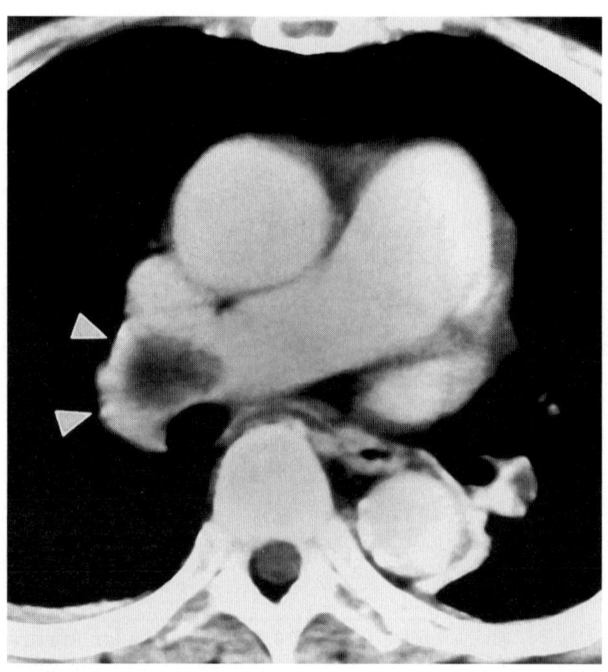

FIGURE 21.37. **Pulmonary Artery Embolus.** Contrast-enhanced CT examination shows a filling defect within the right pulmonary artery (*arrowheads*). Disappearance with time confirms an embolus. Primary neoplasms or metastatic emboli could cause a similar filling defect.

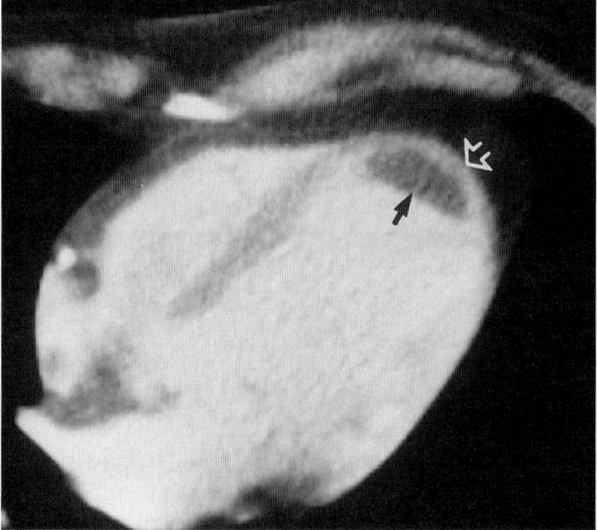

FIGURE 21.38. **Ultrafast CT (Electron Beam CT [EBCT]).** Contrast-enhanced EBCT shows intraventricular clot (*black arrow*), thinned myocardium (*white arrow*), and akinesis, secondary to anteroapical infarct. (Courtesy of William Stanford, MD.)

been studied thoroughly since the early 1990s as a coronary calcification screening modality and has a sensitivity of 70% to 74%, specificity of 70% to 91%, and negative predictive value of 97% when compared to coronary angiography (see Fig 22.2). Now multidetector CT (MDCT) has been shown to be equivalent to EBCT for coronary calcification detection and scoring.

EBCT allows 40 to 60 sections, each 1.5 to 3.0 mm, with an exposure time of 100 ms, with single breath-hold acquisition and ECG gated to end-diastole. New 16-slice, and now 64-slice MDCT equipment has taken rotation speeds down to 330 ms (0.33 sec) and resolution to 0.33 mm. MDCT coronary calcium screening is also done with ECG gating, single breath-hold, and arms up.

One method of scoring utilizes the Agatston method, in which coronary calcification is defined as an area with greater than 130 Hounsfield units (HU) and larger than 2 mm^2. A score of 1 is given for 130 to 200 HU, 2 for 201 to 299 HU, 3 for 300 to 399 HU, and 4 for 400 HU or greater. This factor is assigned and multiplied by the area of the lesion for each coronary artery territory. This score is then summed for a total coronary calcification score or Agatston score (Fig. 21.39). A score of 0 to 10 is very low to low risk, 11 to 100 is moderate risk, 101 to 400 is moderately high risk, and greater than 400 is high risk for underlying stenosis and future cardiac events. However, the specific calcified area or artery may not correlate with specific stenoses.

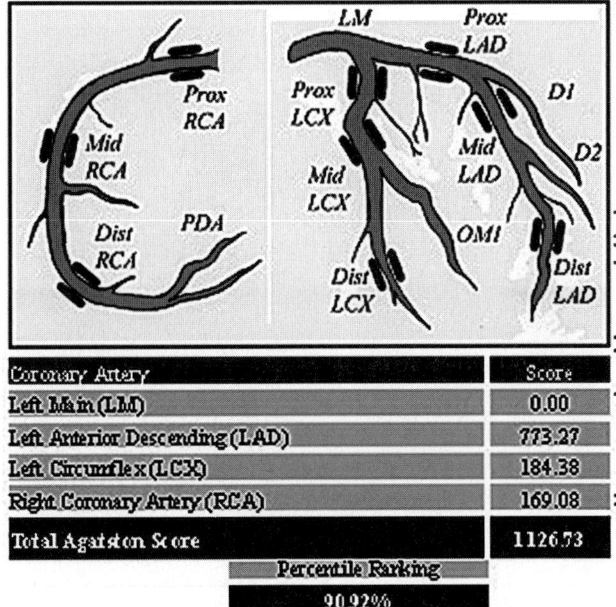

Coronary Artery	Score
Left Main (LM)	0.00
Left Anterior Descending (LAD)	773.27
Left Circumflex (LCX)	184.38
Right Coronary Artery (RCA)	169.08
Total Agatston Score	1126.73
Percentile Ranking	
90.92%	

FIGURE 21.39. **Coronary Calcification Scoring from Multidetector CT.** The report shows the score for each coronary artery and location. The summed score is over 1,100, placing the patient in the very-high-risk category.

The utility of coronary calcium screening lies in (*1*) early detection of calcium in asymptomatic patients for risk stratification and risk factor modification, (*2*) evaluation of progression or even regression of calcification as a indicator of atherosclerotic coronary disease, (*3*) its ability to demonstrate the absence of calcification, thereby essentially ruling out significant underlying coronary stenosis.

CT Coronary Angiography. EBCT and now MDCT have been also shown to be efficacious for noninvasive CTCA. Many laboratories have utilized 16-slice MDCT and more recently 64-slice MDCT for CTCA. In development are 128-slice, 256-slice, and area-detector technology. Resolution is now down to 0.33 mm with rotation speeds to 300 ms. Because faster heart rates can lead to motion artifact, slowing the heart rate to 60 or 70 bpm with oral and IV beta blockers is necessary. Contrast is delivered utilizing a peripheral or jugular vein, an 18- to 20-gauge needle, and 100 to 150 mL of isosmolar contrast at 4 mL/sec. The study is acquired with arms up, single breath-hold (10 to 30 sec) and ECG gating (prospective or retrospective). The contrast bolus is immediately followed by a saline flush of 25 to 40 mL. The scan timing can be judged with a test

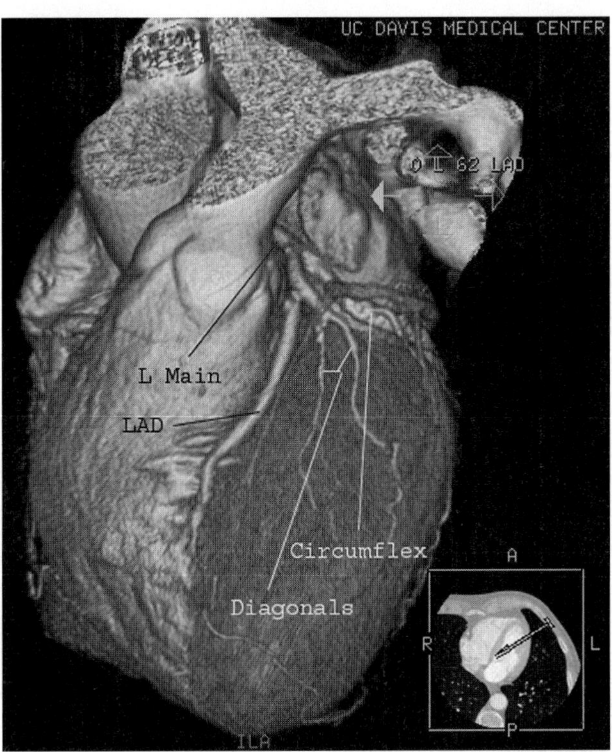

FIGURE 21.40. **Three-Dimensional Volume-Rendered CT Coronary Angiogram.** The left anterior descending (LAD), branching diagonals, and circumflex coronary arteries are well visualized in this left anterior oblique projection from 16-slice multidetector CT. The left main coronary artery is partially seen under the left atrial appendage.

bolus or begin at the end of contrast injection. Optimal image quality has peak opacification in the LV and coronary arteries, with less dense concentration in the RV and pulmonary arteries.

ECG "pulsing" can reduce tube current during systole and increase it during diastole where the target images are usually constructed. This can reduce the radiation dose by up to 50%. Reconstruction is done to 1-mm slice thickness and a medium smooth reconstruction algorithm. Past processing is very important and is often done by the radiologist, especially for 3D reconstruction.

The coronaries can be evaluated for congenital abnormalities, presurgical anatomy, coronary calcifications, and coronary plaque or stenosis utilizing volume-rendered 3D views (Fig. 21.40), 2D views, multiplanar views (Fig. 21.41), maximal intensity projections, and coronary "straightening" views (Fig. 21.42). Stenoses greater than 50% are considered hemodynamically significant and stenoses greater than 75% are considered high grade. Problems occur in grading stenoses with heavy coronary calcification and with stents. Patency, however, can be determined by evaluating coronary enhancement downstream. CTCA has also been shown to be useful and accurate for the follow-up of coronary artery bypass graft patency.

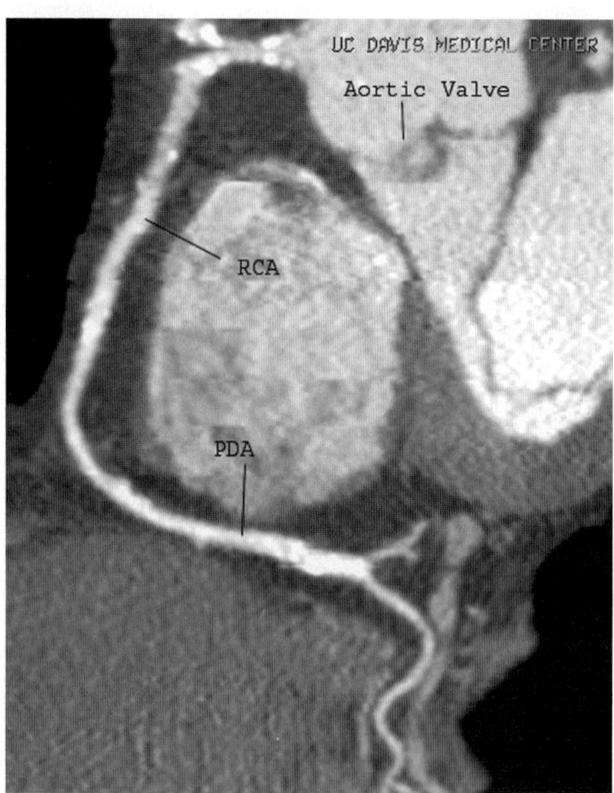

FIGURE 21.41. **Maximum Intensity Projection (MIP) CT Coronary Angiogram.** The aortic valve, right coronary artery (RCA), and posterior descending artery (PDA) are well seen in this left anterior oblique MIP from 16-slice multidetector CT.

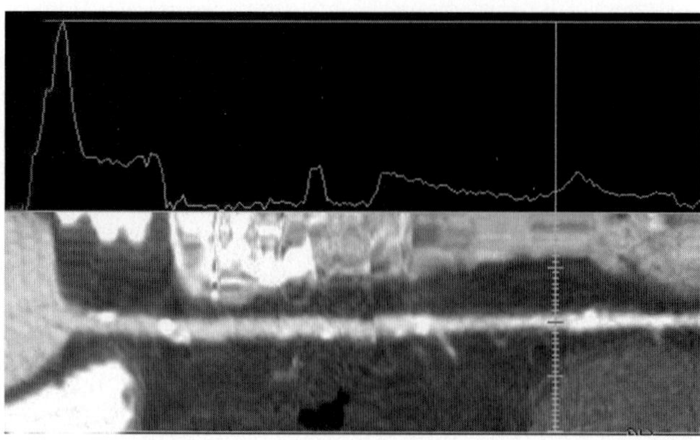

FIGURE 21.42. **Right Coronary Artery in "Straightened" Maximum Intensity Projection View.** This computer-reconstructed view effectively takes out the curves and makes it easier to see that, while there are atherosclerotic irregularities, there is no significant stenosis.

CARDIAC MR

Cardiac MR combines many of the capabilities of the other imaging modalities into one examination. These include excellent static anatomic images and dynamic motion studies for function. Cardiac MR applications include congenital heart disease, aortic and pulmonary artery disease, pericardial disease, ventricular function, valvular function, cardiomyopathies, and cardiac masses. Cardiac pacemakers are considered contraindications but most prosthetic valves can be safely studied.

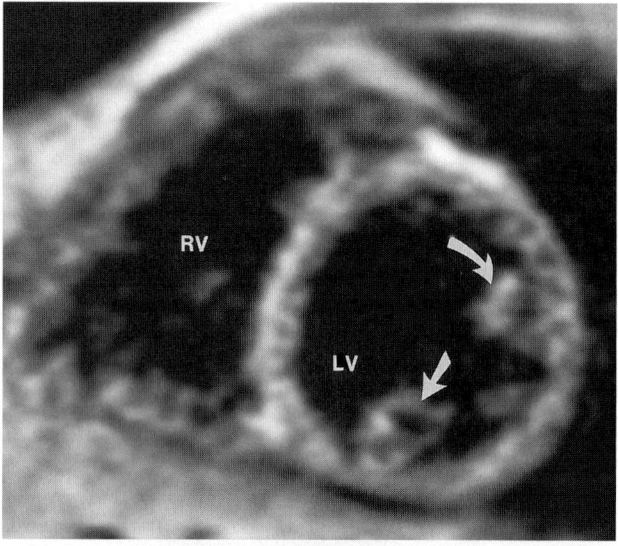

FIGURE 21.43. **Spin-Echo MR.** A tomographic slice in the short-axis projection demonstrates the RV, the interventricular septum, and the LV. The anterior (*straight arrow*) and posterior (*curved arrow*) papillary muscles are seen within the left ventricular cavity. The spin-echo technique creates a "black blood" appearance because of the signal void of moving blood.

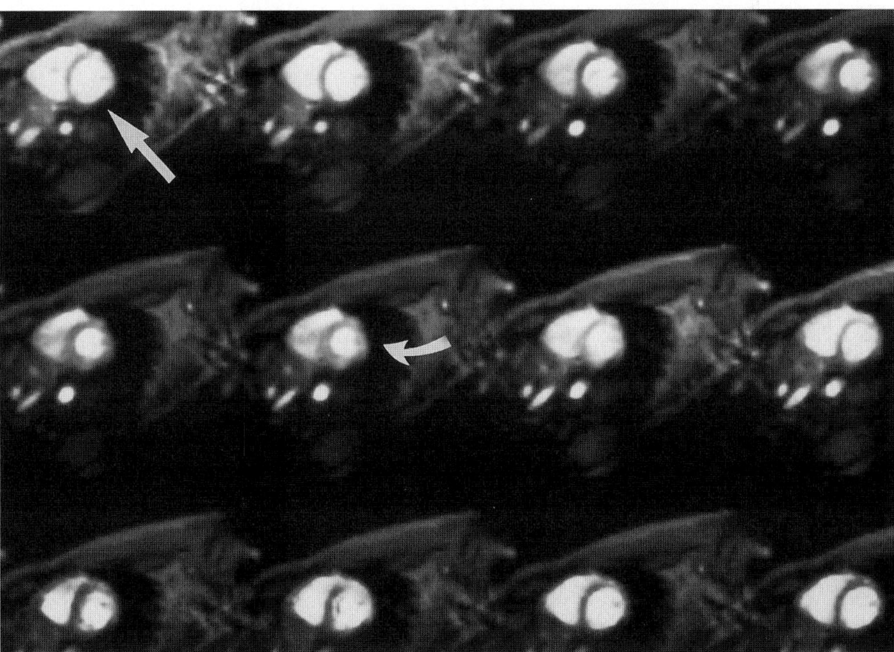

FIGURE 21.44. **Fast-Field Echo MR.** The fast-field echo technique creates a "white blood" depiction that shows flowing blood and turbulence during motion studies. The end-diastole image (*straight arrow*) has the largest ventricular size. The end-systole image (*curved arrow*) has the smallest ventricular cavity and the thickest wall.

The best anatomic depiction is accomplished on spin-echo T1WI in which the moving blood produces a signal void or "black blood" appearance (Fig. 21.43). Gradient-echo or fast-field echo images impart bright signal to coherently flowing blood, creating a "white blood" appearance that is similar to contrast studies (Fig. 21.44). Electrocardiographic gating can be used similar to gated cardiac SPECT and gated cardiac blood pool scintigraphy. Slice-specific information is acquired with reference to specific phases within the cardiac cycle. With gradient-recalled echo technique, motion studies can show flowing blood as well as myocardial contractility.

MR images are acquired as tomographic slices through any selected plane. The planes may be angled to match cardiac (e.g., short axis, four chamber) or vascular anatomy (e.g., left anterior oblique [LAO] aorta). Tissue characterization of the myocardium is accomplished using T1WI and T2WI, contrast enhancement, and spectroscopy. This may be useful for neoplastic, infiltrative, or inflammatory conditions of the myocardium.

Cardiac MR motion studies provide functional information, including wall motion analysis, systolic wall thickening, chamber volumes, stroke volumes, right and left ventricular ejection fractions, and valve evaluation (Fig. 21.45). Flowing blood becomes turbulent and loses its coherence when it passes through stenotic or regurgitant valves. The high-velocity stenotic jet or regurgitant flow is displayed as a wedge-shaped puff of dark turbulent flow, readily identified on the white blood background with the gradient-echo technique (see Figs. 22.21, 22.23). Visual and region-of-interest grading can be accomplished for stenotic or regurgitant flow based on distance, area, or regurgitant volume (see Chapter 22). The regurgitant fraction is calculated by comparing the right and left stroke volumes. Velocity-encoded cine-MR techniques using phase analysis can calculate flow velocities and flow volumes in addition to the regurgitant volumes. These techniques can be used in lieu of angiography for many cases. An understanding of MR signal characteristics and the details of 3D cardiac anatomy displayed in different tomographic planes is critical to the accurate utilization of cardiac MR.

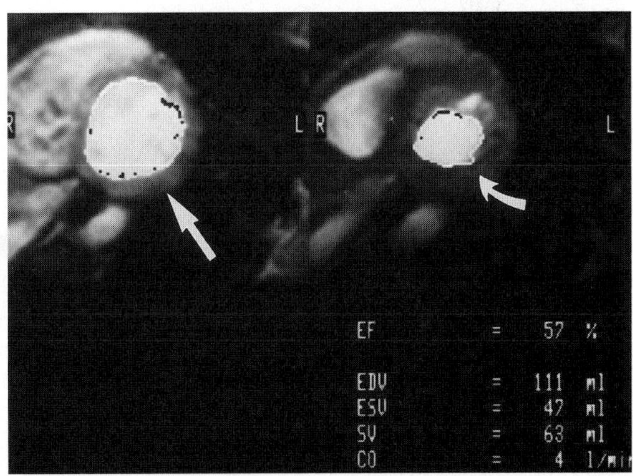

FIGURE 21.45. **MR Ejection Fraction Technique.** Regions of interest are drawn on the diastolic image (*straight arrow*) and the end-systolic image (*curved arrow*) of each slice. An area ejection fraction (EF) is then calculated for each slice. Volume ejection fraction calculations are calculated using sequential slices that include the entire ventricular volume. EDV, end-diastolic volume; ESV, end-systolic volume; SV, stroke volume; CO, cardiac output; ED, end-diastole; ES, end-systole.

SUGGESTED READINGS

Becker CR, Jakobs TF, Aydemir S, et al. Helical and single-slice conventional CT versus electron beam CT for the quantification of coronary artery calcification. AJR Am J Roentgenol 2000;174:543–547.

Bogaert J, Dymarkowski S, Taylor AM, eds. Clinical Cardiac MRI. Berlin, New York: Springer-Verlag, 2005.

Budoff MJ, Achenbach S, Duerinckx A. Clinical utility of computed tomography and magnetic resonance techniques for noninvasive coronary angiography. J Am Coll Cardiol 2003;42(11):1867–1878.

Feigenbaum H, Armstrong WF, Ryan T. Echocardiography. 6th ed. Philadelphia: Lippincott Williams & Wilkins, 2004.

Gedgaudas E, Moffer JH, Castaneda-Zuniga WR, Amplatz K. Cardiovascular Radiology. Philadelphia: WB Saunders, 1985.

Higgins CB. Essentials of Cardiac Radiology and Imaging. Philadelphia: JB Lippincott, 1992.

Kelley MJ, ed. Symposium on Chest Radiography for the Cardiologist. Philadelphia: WB Saunders, 1983. Cardiol Clin 1(4):543–750.

Kubicka RA, Smith C. How to interpret coronary arteriograms. Radiographics 1986;6:661–701.

Lardo A, Chronos NA, Fayad ZA. Cardiovascular Magnetic Resonance: Established and Emerging Applications. London: Martin Dunitz; Independence, KY: Taylor and Francis, 2003.

Lawler LP, Pannu HK, Fishman EK. MDCT evaluation of the coronary arteries, 2004: how we do it—data acquisition, postprocessing, display and interpretation. AJR Am J Roentgenol 2004;184:1402–1412.

Leschka S, Alkadhi H, Plass A, et al. Accuracy of MSCT coronary angiography with 64-slice technology: first experience. Eur Heart J 2005;26(15):1482–1487.

Lipton MJ, Boxt LM, eds. Cardiac imaging. Radiol Clin North Am 2004;42:487–697.

Marcus ML, Schelbert HR, Skorton DJ, Wolf GL. Cardiac Imaging—A Companion to Braunwald's Heart Disease. Philadelphia: WB Saunders, 1991.

Miller SW. Cardiac Imaging: The Requisites. 2nd ed. Philadelphia: Elsevier Mosby, 2005.

Netter FH. Atlas of Human Anatomy. The CIBA Collection of Medical Illustrations. West Caldwell, NJ: CIBA-Geigy, 1989.

Oudkerk M. Coronary Radiology. New York: Springer-Verlag, 2004.

Reddy GP, Higgins CB, Chao KH, Tung PP. Cardiac MR Imaging. CD-ROM. Philadelphia: Lippincott Williams & Wilkins, 2001.

Rensing BJ, Surruys PW, de Feyter PM. CT-based coronary angiography. J Invasive Cardiol 2000;12(1):23–24.

Schoepf UJ, Becker CR, Ohnesorge BM, Yucel EK. CT of coronary artery disease. Radiology 2004;232:18–37.

Schoepf UJ, Schoepf UJ. CT of the Heart: Principles and Applications. Totowa, NJ: Human Press, 2004.

Schoenhagen P, Halliburton SS, Stillman AE, et al. Noninvasive imaging of coronary arteries: current and future role of multi-detector row CT. Radiology 2004;232:7–17.

Stanford W, Thompson BH. Imaging of coronary artery calcification. Its importance in assessing atherosclerotic disease. Radiol Clin North Am 1999;37:257–272.

Stanford W, Thompson BH, Burns, TL, et al. Coronary artery calcium quantification at multi-detector row helical CT versus electron-beam CT. Radiology 2004;230:397–402.

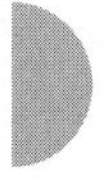

Chapter 22

Cardiac Imaging in Acquired Diseases

David K. Shelton

Ischemic Heart Disease
Coronary Artery Disease
Myocardial Infarction
Infarct Imaging

Cardiomyopathies

Pulmonary Vascular Disease

Acquired Valvular Heart Disease

Cardiac Masses

Pericardial Disease

Cardiac disease remains among the most common problems affecting patient morbidity and mortality today, despite many important dietary, pharmaceutical, interventional, and surgical advances. Most acquired cardiac diseases can be classified under six general categories: ischemic heart disease, cardiomyopathies, pulmonary vascular disease, acquired valvular disease, cardiac masses, and pericardial disease. Use of plain film radiography, fluoroscopy, US, CT, MR, nuclear imaging, and angiocardiography must be integrated with knowledge of specific disease processes.

ISCHEMIC HEART DISEASE

Coronary Artery Disease

Coronary artery disease is the most common cause of mortality in the United States, with approximately one American dying every minute. Six million to 7 million Americans have active symptoms related to ischemic heart disease. Approximately 300,000 coronary artery bypass graft (CABG) surgeries are performed per year in the United States, with a similar number of percutaneous transluminal coronary angioplasties (PTCA). There were 1.83 million cardiac catheterizations in the US in 1999 and it has been estimated to reach 3 million by 2010.

Clinical presentations include (*1*) stable angina, (*2*) unstable angina (often preinfarction), (*3*) acute myocardial infarction, (*4*) congestive heart failure secondary to chronic ischemia or prior infarction sequelae, (*5*) arrhythmias, and (*6*) sudden death. Clinical symptoms are caused by luminal abnormalities of the coronary arteries, including (*1*) atheromatous disease, (*2*) coronary thrombosis, (*3*) intraluminal ulceration and hemorrhage, (*4*) vasoconstriction, and (*5*) coronary ectasia and aneurysm. ***Vulnerable plaque*** is initiated by lipoprotein deposition into susceptible areas of the coronary walls and other arteries. Chronic inflammation elsewhere in the body, as well as in the developing plaque, is associated with cytokine and macrophage activity. A thin fibrous cap develops over the lipid core, and mechanical stress can lead to exposure to the blood products, which can then trigger the thrombotic cascade. A sequence of vulnerable plaque development, sudden rupture, and thrombosis is now known to be the leading cause of myocardial infarction.

Risk factors for development of atherosclerotic coronary artery disease include elevated serum cholesterol and C-reactive protein, tobacco smoking, diabetes, hypertension, sedentary lifestyle, obesity, age, male gender, chronic inflammation, and heredity. Aggravating conditions include aortic stenosis, ventricular hypertrophy, cardiomyopathy, coronary embolism, congenital anomalies, Kawasaki syndrome, and anemia. Noninvasive imaging is often used as a screening test. Selective coronary angiography with ventriculography and now CT coronary angiography (CTCA) can be utilized to determine coronary anatomy and to direct the specific therapy.

A typical imaging workup includes chest radiography, nuclear medicine myocardial perfusion scans, and consideration for coronary angiography. Indications for coronary

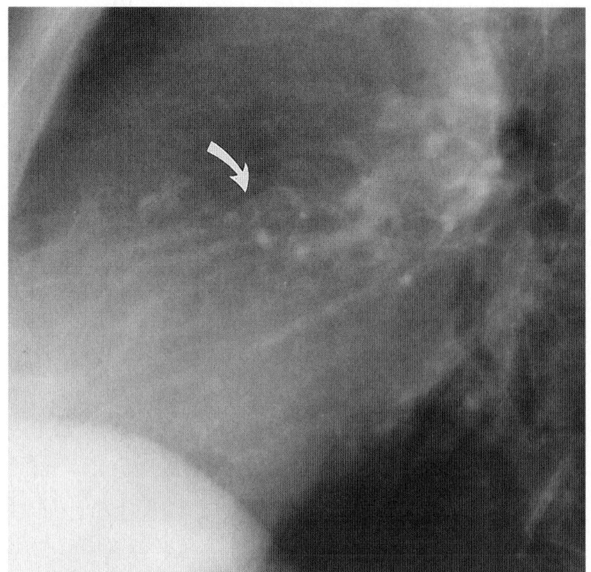

FIGURE 22.1. **Coronary Artery Calcification.** Lateral chest radiograph demonstrates coronary artery calcification (*arrow*).

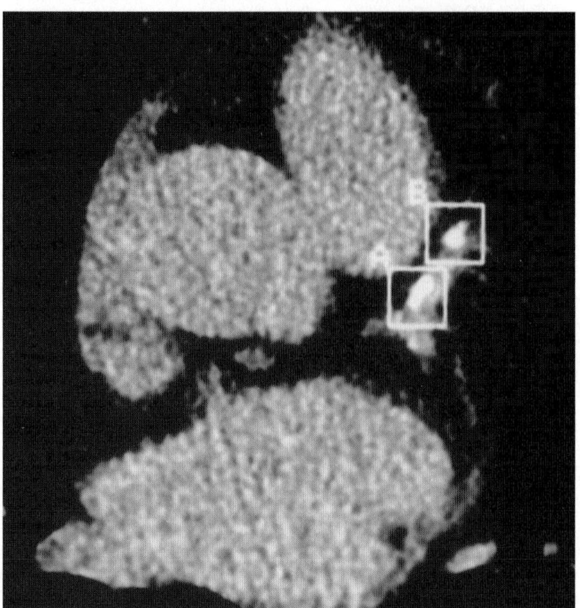

FIGURE 22.2. **CT Coronary Calcification.** Calcification is seen in the left anterior descending artery, with regions of interest (*white boxes*) placed for quantification. Electron beam CT, 100 ms, 3-mm slice, without contrast. (Courtesy of William Stanford, MD.)

angiography include angina refractory to medical therapy, unstable angina, high-risk occupation (e.g., pilot), and abnormal electrocardiograms or stress perfusion tests. Coronary angiography is considered following myocardial infarction when PTCA or intracoronary thrombolysis are being deliberated. Additional indications include development of mechanical dysfunction, progressive congestive failure, refractory ventricular arrhythmias, and follow-up after administration of IV thrombolytic agents.

Coronary artery calcification occurs in the intima and is directly related to advanced atheromatous disease and coronary narrowing (Fig. 22.1; see Fig. 21.14). Coronary calcification is detected at angiography in 75% of patients with 50% diameter stenosis. Only 11% of men without significant coronary artery disease have coronary calcification. In the asymptomatic population, the detection of coronary calcification has a predictive accuracy of 86%. In symptomatic patients, coronary calcification is seen in 50% of patients with single-vessel disease, 77% of those with two-vessel disease, and 86% of those with three-vessel disease. Fluoroscopically detected coronary calcification in the presence of angina-like chest pain is associated with coronary stenosis 94% of the time. Overall, fluoroscopic detection of coronary artery calcification has a 73% sensitivity and 84% specificity for symptomatic patients. Exercise-tolerance testing has a sensitivity of 76% to 88% and a specificity of 43% to 77%. Exercise testing with planar thallium imaging has a sensitivity and a specificity of approximately 85%.

Use of electron-beam CT (EBCT) and multidetector CT (MDCT) has improved the sensitivity for detecting coronary artery calcification to approximately 95% (Fig. 22.2). Importantly, CT also allows the grading of the severity of coronary calcification and thus can establish risk scores, which can help determine patient risk and allow follow-up after medical intervention. The absence of coronary calcification is associated with a very low risk of significant coronary disease. On the other hand, patient youth and higher calcification scores are associated with a higher risk of underlying coronary artery disease and future cardiac events. The negative predictive value of a zero calcification score is 94% to 100%. With scores greater than 400 there is a sensitivity of 82% and specificity of 62% for predicting an abnormal myocardial perfusion SPECT scan (Table 22.1).

Myocardial perfusion scanning, which uses thallium, technetium (Tc) 99m-sestamibi, Tc-99m-tetrofosmin, or Tc-99m-teboroxime, is one of the primary imaging modalities for detecting myocardial ischemia. Stress images are obtained with exercise or pharmacologic agents such as adenosine dipyridamole. SPECT has increased the sensitivity to 90% to 94% and the specificity to 90% to 95%. The hallmark for segmental ischemia is a perfusion defect on stress testing that fills in during rest (Fig. 22.3). A defect that appears stable during both stress and rest examinations is usually an infarction. "Hibernating" regions of viable myocardium associated with tight coronary stenosis may appear as fixed defects on sestamibi or tetrofosmin images or on redistribution thallium images obtained 4 hours after stress.

Stress echocardiography using either exercise or pharmacologic stress modalities has also become a widely accepted method to detect significant (>50% to 70%)

TABLE 22.1 Coronary Calcium Scoring

Calcium Score	*Interpretation*
0	No identifiable atherosclerotic plaque; very low cardiovascular disease; less than 5% chance of presence of coronary artery disease A negative examination
1–10	Minimal plaque burden Significant coronary artery disease very unlikely
11–100	Mild plaque burden Likely mild or minimal coronary stenosis
101–400	Moderate plaque burden Moderate nonobstructive coronary artery disease highly likely
Over 400	Extensive plaque burden High likelihood of at least one significant coronary stenosis (>50% diameter)

The summed coronary calcification score can be assigned a percentile ranking for sex and age as well as a risk statement. Appropriate clinical response depends on other risk factors as well.

coronary artery stenosis. With the advent of digital image acquisition and cine-loop playback, prestress echocardiographic views can be simultaneously compared with views taken either immediately postexercise or at peak pharmacologic doses. Development of new segmental wall motion abnormalities or worsening of resting abnormalities suggests stress-induced ischemia. One advantage of these techniques is that they also allow prior assessment of resting wall motion abnormalities that are consistent with either profoundly ischemic, stunned, hibernating, or infarcted myocardium.

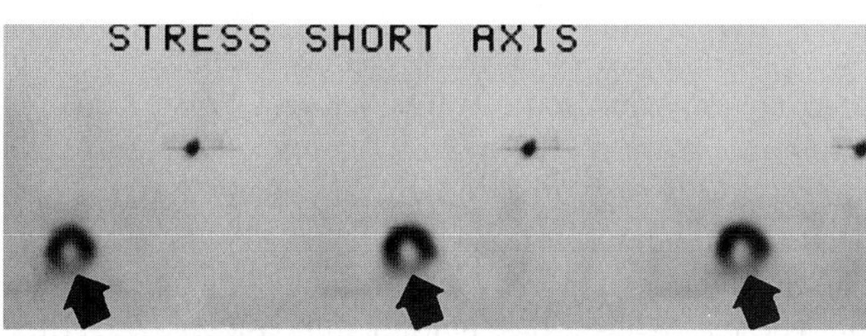

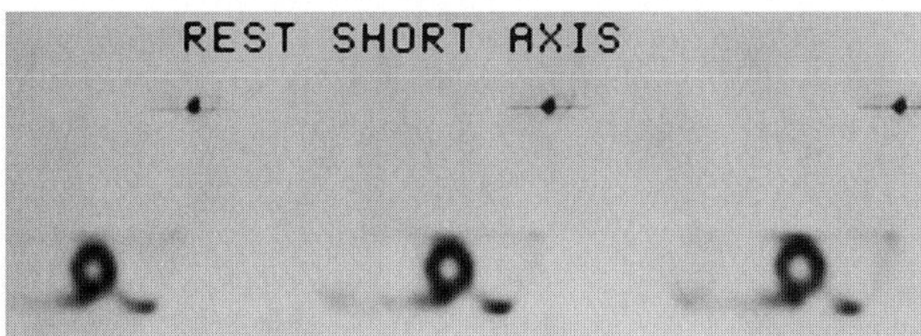

FIGURE 22.3. **Myocardial Perfusion Scan.** SPECT images of the LV in short axis projection demonstrate a defect (*arrows*) in the inferior wall of the LV during stress, which is well perfused on the rest images. This is strong evidence of ischemic heart disease when using technetium-99m-sestamibi as the radionuclide and dipyridamole for pharmacologic stress testing.

The overall sensitivity of exercise echocardiography is 76% to 97% using pharmacologic stress agents; the sensitivity is 72% to 96% with dobutamine, approximately 85% with adenosine, and 52% to 56% with a standard dose of dipyridamole. The sensitivities for these tests are lowest for single-vessel disease and improve incrementally for two- and three-vessel disease. Stress echocardiography has a specificity of 66% to 100%.

Gated blood pool scintigraphy will demonstrate exercise-induced wall motion abnormalities in 63% of patients with significant coronary artery disease. With exercise, the ejection fractions normally increase by at least 5%. Failure of ejection fraction to increase with exercise is an indication of myocardial dysfunction. Using these two findings, exercise gated blood pool scintigraphy has a sensitivity of 87% to 95% and a specificity of 92% for detection of coronary artery disease.

Coronary angiograms and CTCA (Fig. 22.4) should be evaluated for the percent of stenosis, the number of vessels

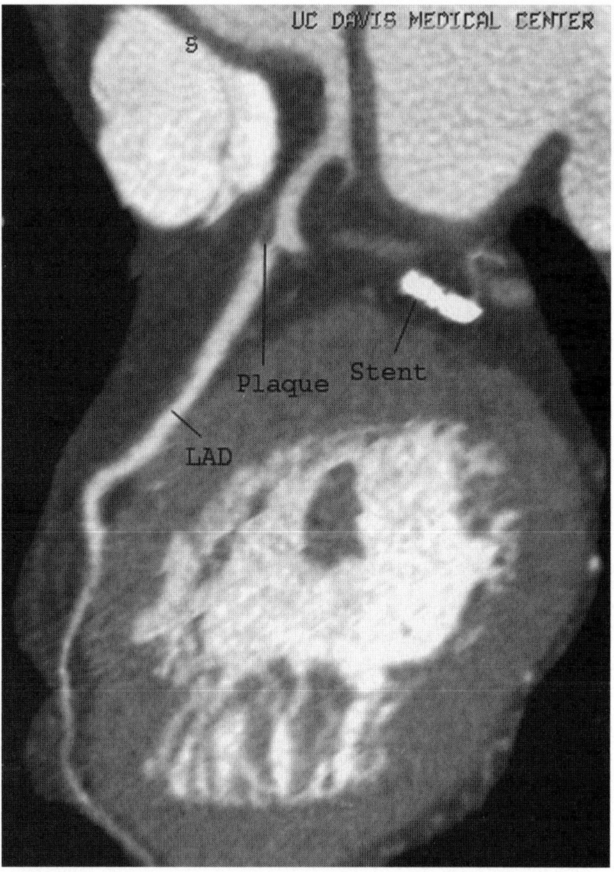

FIGURE 22.4. **CT Coronary Angiogram of Left Anterior Descending Artery (LAD).** Left anterior oblique view of maximum intensity projection from 16-slice multidetector CT, CT coronary angiogram demonstrates focal soft plaque in the proximal LAD with 70% stenosis. Percutaneous transluminal coronary angioplasty was subsequently performed.

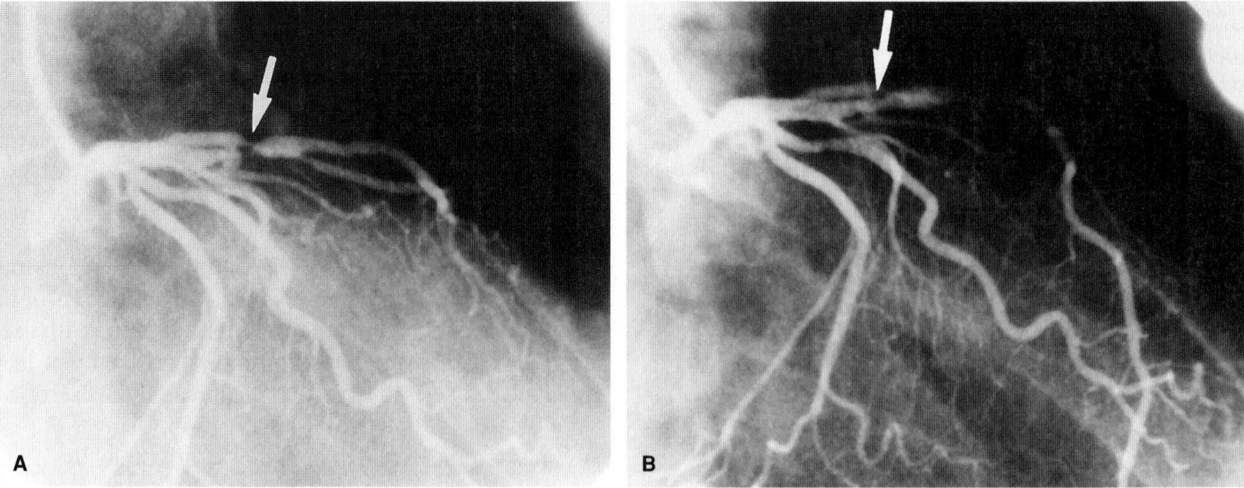

FIGURE 22.5. **Coronary Stenosis. A.** An 80% stenotic lesion (*arrow*) is identified in the left anterior descending artery (LAD) on coronary angiography. This patient was experiencing classic angina. **B.** Marked improvement in the LAD lesion (*arrow*) is evident following percutaneous transluminal coronary angioplasty. The angina symptoms resolved.

involved, focal versus diffuse disease, coronary anatomy, ectasia or aneurysm, coronary calcification, and collateral flow (Fig. 22.5). Collaterals may include epicardial, intramyocardial, atrioventricular, intercoronary, or intracoronary vessels (i.e., "bridging collateral"). The angiographer must count the number of major epicardial vessels with greater than 50% diameter narrowing. Patients are divided into one-vessel, two-vessel, or three-vessel disease on the basis of involvement of the right or left main coronary artery, left anterior descending artery and left circumflex artery. A 50% diameter narrowing roughly predicts a 75% cross-sectional area reduction, which is the physiologic point at which flow is restricted enough to result in ischemia under stress conditions. Reliability for estimating the percent diameter narrowing depends on the observer, projection, resolution, and presence of coronary calcification or ectasia. The degree of coronary disease may be assessed using percent stenosis of each individual coronary artery or of 5-mm segments of the coronary arteries. The right coronary artery is 10 cm long, the left main coronary artery is 1 cm long, the left anterior descending (LAD) is 10 cm long, and the left circumflex is 6 cm long, for a total of 27 cm. These may be divided into fifty-four 5-mm segments. This scoring system allows the interpreter to quantify the number of 5-mm segments with stenoses in the 0% to 25%, 25% to 50%, 50% to 75%, and 75% to 100% ranges. The significance of 30% to 70% lesions is often clarified by correlation with stress-induced myocardial perfusion scintigraphy.

Percutaneous transluminal angioplasty has traditionally been reserved for localized lesions in one- or two-vessel disease (Fig. 22.5), but recent published series comparing PTCA with CABG in multivessel disease revealed no difference in the endpoints of death and myocardial infarction. The PTCA group, however, required a significantly higher number of repeat procedures during follow-up, although this has improved with more frequent use of stents. CABG with the use of saphenous vein grafts or internal mammary arteries is usually reserved for more complex or longer-segment disease. CABG markers are usually placed at the anastomotic site to help the angiographer during future selective angiography. Use of the internal mammary artery has better long-term results than saphenous vein grafts and has been correlated with increased survival. Recurrence of symptoms after CABG may be because of occlusion, graft stenosis, or progression of native vessel disease. Graft stenoses and acute occlusions may be amenable to percutaneous interventional techniques. Grafts and stents can be readily evaluated with CTCA (Fig. 22.6), although the metallic stent can cause imaging problems.

Echocardiography is useful in detecting some of the long-term complications of ischemic disease, including ventricular aneurysm, thinning of myocardium, akinesia, or dyskinesia. Aneurysms are best seen at the apex and septum. Mural thrombi may also be diagnosed but are difficult to visualize at the apex. Stress echocardiography with either exercise or pharmacologic stress techniques is increasingly used to evaluate for ischemia.

CTCA is capable of establishing the patency of CABGs. Ultrafast CT (EBCT) and now MDCT have 93% sensitivity, 89% specificity, and 92% accuracy for establishing patency of CABGs. EBCT and MCDT have also shown to be extremely sensitive for detecting coronary calcification. EBCT and MDCT with contrast can also evaluate wall motion, thrombi, old infarcts, aneurysm, and pericardial abnormalities.

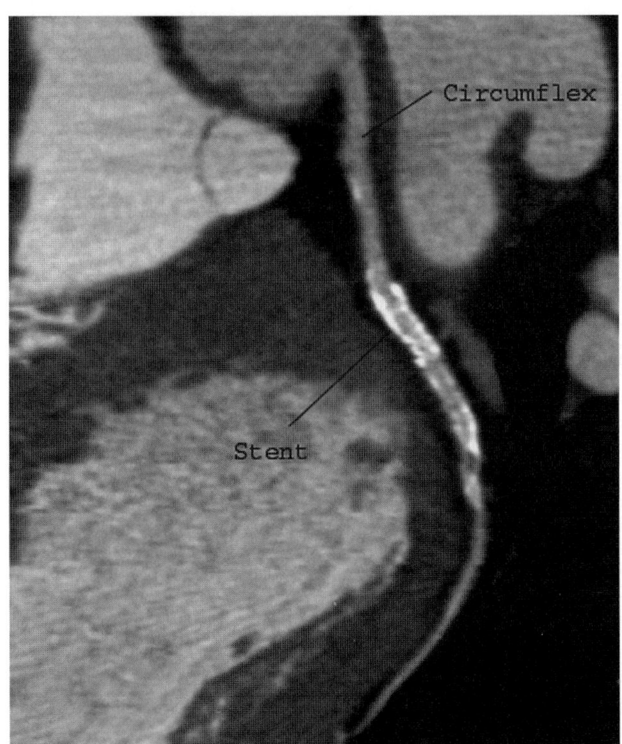

FIGURE 22.6. CT Coronary Angiogram (CTCA) of Left Circumflex. Left anterior oblique view of 16-slice multidetector CT, CTCA maximum intensity projection shows patent coronary stent with good flow and no evidence of obstruction. Coronary calcification is also evident downstream.

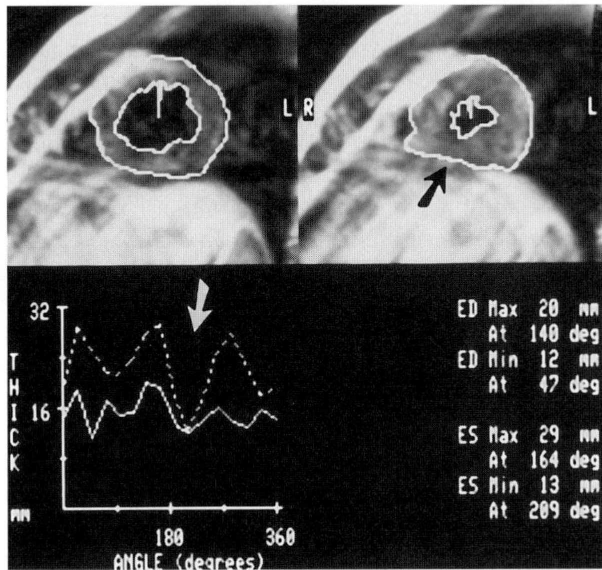

FIGURE 22.7. Wall Motion MR Evaluation. Short-axis tomographic views of the LV are used for evaluation of systolic wall thickening. Regions of interest are drawn around the myocardium in diastole (*left*) and systole (*right*). The inferior wall (*black arrow*) demonstrates hypokinesia and poor systolic wall thickening. The functional graph (*below*) confirms the findings (*white arrow*). The patient had a previous inferior wall myocardial infarction.

MR can be used (*1*) to define the location and size of previous myocardial infarctions, (*2*) to demonstrate complications of previous infarctions, (*3*) to establish the presence of viable myocardium for possible revascularization, (*4*) to differentiate acute versus chronic myocardial infarction, (*5*) to evaluate regional myocardial wall motion and systolic wall thickening (Fig. 22.7), (*6*) to demonstrate global myocardial function with right ventricular and left ventricular ejection fractions, (*7*) to demonstrate regional myocardial perfusion, and (*8*) to evaluate papillary muscle and valvular abnormalities. Gadolinium-enhanced T1WIs demonstrate areas of ischemia and reperfusion after myocardial infarction. MR with spectroscopy targeting myocardial phosphate metabolism can distinguish acute from chronic ischemia and reperfused infarcted myocardium from reperfused viable myocardium. With spin-echo imaging, MR has a 78% accuracy for establishing patency of CABGs. Cine MR with gradient echo has sensitivity of 88% to 93%, specificity of 86% to 100%, and overall accuracy of 89% to 91% for patency of CABGs.

Myocardial Infarction

After acute infarction, the chest radiograph will initially show a normal heart size in 90% of cases. Cardiomegaly and congestive failure will eventually develop in 60% to 70% of cases, more frequently with anterior wall infarction, multivessel disease, or left ventricular aneurysm. Increasing stages of pulmonary venous hypertension, particularly alveolar edema, are associated with worsened prognosis.

Complications of myocardial infarction include the following.

Cardiogenic shock implies that systolic pressure is less than 90 mm Hg and is typically associated with acute pulmonary edema and worsened prognosis.

Atrioventricular block is common, especially after inferior wall infarcts resulting from either ischemia or injury to the atrioventricular nodal branch of the right coronary artery or increased vagal tone. Complete heart block occurs with larger infarcts and has a worse prognosis.

Right ventricular infarction occurs in approximately 33% of inferior wall infarctions. Symptoms are caused by the reduction in right ventricular ejection fraction, which returns to normal within 10 days in approximately 50% of cases. The diagnosis may be established using technetium pyrophosphate (PYP) radionuclide scans. Complications include cardiogenic shock, elevated right atrial pressure, and decreased pulmonary artery pressure. Right precordial electrocardiographic leads can also assist in making the diagnosis.

Myocardial rupture (3.3% of infarcts) may occur 3 to 14 days after infarction. The mortality rate approaches

100% and accounts for 13% of myocardial infarction deaths. The chest radiograph shows acute cardiac enlargement secondary to leakage of blood into the pericardium. Rupture of the interventricular septum (1%) typically occurs between days 4 and 21, usually as a complication of anterior myocardial infarction and LAD disease. Mortality is 24% within 24 hours and 90% within 1 year. Swan-Ganz catheter measurements show an acute increase in saturation in the RV, although the wedge pressures may be normal. Chest radiographs show acute pulmonary vascular engorgement and right-sided cardiac enlargement because of left-to-right shunt. Pulmonary edema is not a typical feature. Echocardiography readily demonstrates the septal defect.

Papillary muscle rupture (1%) is suggested by abrupt onset of mitral regurgitation, with acute pulmonary edema on the radiograph. Typically, the LV is only minimally enlarged, whereas the LA enlarges quickly. Inferior infarcts are associated with posteromedial papillary rupture. Anterior infarcts less commonly affect the anterolateral papillary muscle. Mortality is 70% within 24 hours and 90% within 1 year. Echocardiography confirms the diagnosis.

Ventricular aneurysm develops in approximately 12% of survivors from myocardial infarction. Ventricular aneurysms may also be caused by Chagas disease or trauma and are rarely congenital—usually seen in young black males. Aneurysms present with congestive failure, arrhythmias, and systemic emboli. *True aneurysms* are broad-mouthed, localized outpouchings that do not contract during systole (see Fig. 22.33). They are typically anterior or apical and result from LAD disease. The chest radiograph shows a localized bulge along the left cardiac border and may show rimlike calcification in the wall (Fig. 22.8). Fluoroscopy detects up to 50% of cases, whereas 96% are detected by radionuclide ventriculography or myocardial perfusion scan. Echocardiography, contrast-enhanced CT, and MR are also accurate at detecting true aneurysms.

Pseudoaneurysms are contained myocardial ruptures consisting of a localized hematoma surrounded by adherent pericardium. Causes include infarction and trauma. Patients are at high risk for delayed rupture. Pseudoaneurysms are typically posterolateral or retrocardiac in location and have smaller mouths than true aneurysms. MR is the most accurate at detecting pseudoaneurysms, but they can also be seen with echocardiography.

Dressler syndrome (4%) is also known as the postmyocardial infarction syndrome and is similar to the postpericardiotomy syndrome complicating cardiac surgery. Onset is typically 1 week to 3 months postinjury (peak at 2 to 3 weeks), but relapses occur up to 2 years later. Presentation includes fever, chest pain, pericarditis, pericardial effusion, and pleuritis, with pleural effusion usually more prominent on the left. Dressler syndrome responds well to anti-inflammatory medications.

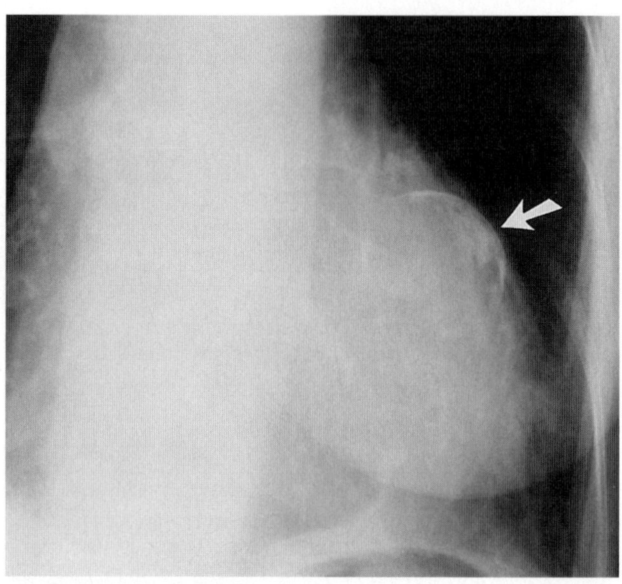

FIGURE 22.8. **Left Ventricular Aneurysm.** A localized calcified bulge (*arrow*) is seen along the left heart border, secondary to prior myocardial infarction complicated by left ventricular aneurysm.

Infarct Imaging

The indications for myocardial infarct imaging include late admission, equivocal enzymes, equivocal electrocardiogram, recent cardiac surgery or trauma, and suspicion of right ventricular infarction.

Radionuclide Imaging. "Cold spot" imaging is accomplished with thallium or technetium perfusion agents (Fig. 22.9). Sensitivity is 96% within 6 to 12 hours but is

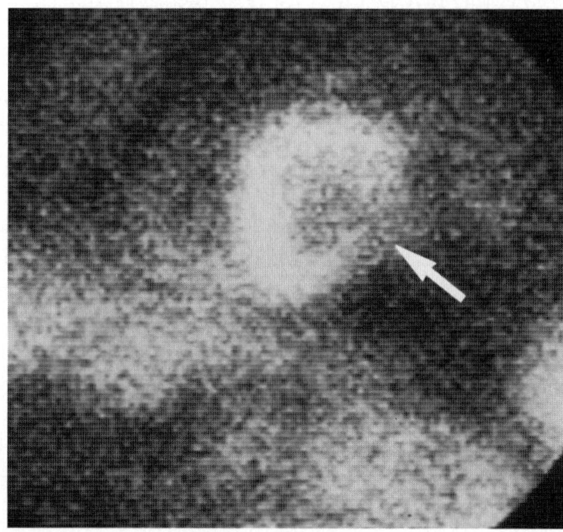

FIGURE 22.9. **Myocardial Infarction.** Resting, planar thallium image in the left anterior oblique projection demonstrates a defect in the inferoposterior wall (*arrow*), consistent with a myocardial infarction. Cold spot imaging can be accomplished almost immediately after the acute event.

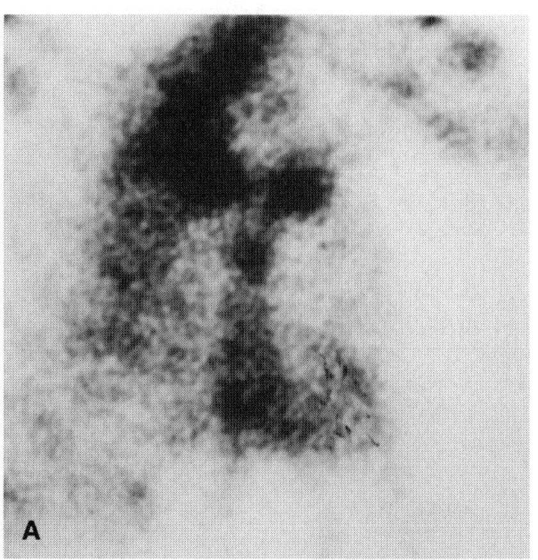

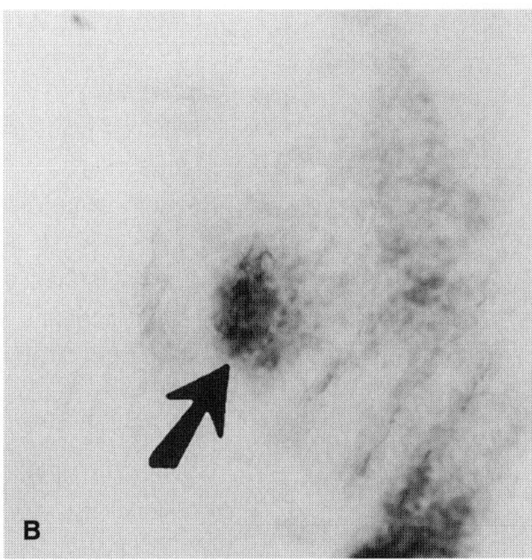

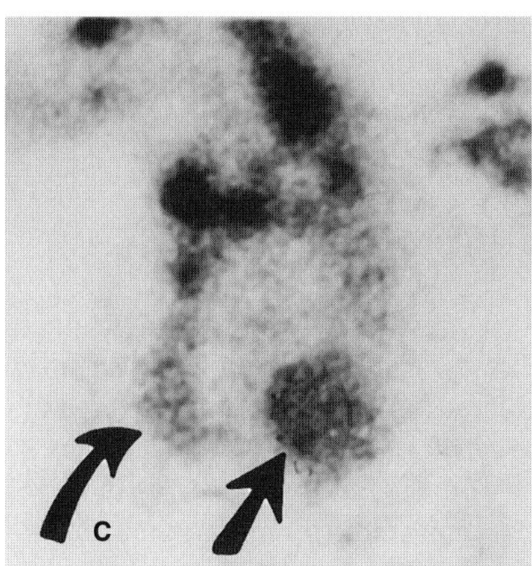

FIGURE 22.10. **Myocardial Infarct Scan.** Hot spot imaging was accomplished using pyrophosphate. Notice the uptake in the anterolateral wall of the myocardium (*arrows*), which is almost as "hot" as the sternum (*curved arrow*). Images were obtained in right anterior oblique **(A)**, left lateral **(B)**, and left anterior oblique **(C)** projections.

only 59% for remote infarction. Acute infarction cannot be distinguished from remote infarction. "Hot spot" infarct imaging uses Tc-PYP (Fig. 22.10), Tc-tetracycline, Tc-glucoheptonate, indium-111 antimyosin antibodies, or F-18 sodium fluorine. Pyrophosphate uptake occurs in myocardial necrosis as a result of PYP complexing with calcium deposits. The PYP scans turn positive at 12 hours, have peak sensitivity at 48 to 72 hours, and revert to normal by 14 days. Persistent abnormal uptake implies a poor prognosis or developing aneurysm. Cardiomyopathies and diffuse myocarditis show diffuse increased uptake. Contusions and radiation myocarditis show increased regional uptake of Tc-PYP.

EBCT and MDCT with contrast demonstrate poor perfusion of the infarcted segment immediately after administration of contrast. After a delay of 10 to 15 minutes, the normal myocardium washes out, leaving a contrast-enhanced periphery of the infarcted zone.

MR demonstrates prolongation of T1 and T2 times secondary to edema of the acutely infarcted segment. Edema occurs within 1 hour after infarct and may be associated with myocardial hemorrhage. MR has 93% sensitivity, 80% specificity, and 87% accuracy for acute myocardial infarction. The infarcted region is best delineated by high signal on T2WIs; however, surrounding edema tends to overestimate the size of the infarct. T1WIs with gadolinium demonstrate the acutely ischemic region and will help to differentiate reperfusion from occlusive myocardial infarction. Regional wall thinning and lack of systolic thickening are the best evidence of the size of the infarcted segment (Figs. 22.9, 22.11). Scar tissue will not contract, whereas viable myocardium will contract and thicken by at least 2 mm. Very high-grade stenotic lesions may result in chronically ischemic myocardium with altered metabolism. This "hibernating myocardium" may act like postinfarction scar, but it remains viable and may improve in function with revascularization. Unfortunately, it also remains at risk for acute infarction. "Stunned myocardium" describes postischemic, dysfunctional myocardium without complete necrosis, which is potentially salvageable.

Echocardiography demonstrates hypokinesis, akinesis, or dyskinesis in previously infarcted myocardial segments; however, this cannot be distinguished from stunned or hibernating myocardium. Global hypokinesis can also be seen with cardiomyopathic processes. Thinned, hyperechoic walls with resting wall motion abnormalities suggest transmural scar. Use of echocardiographic

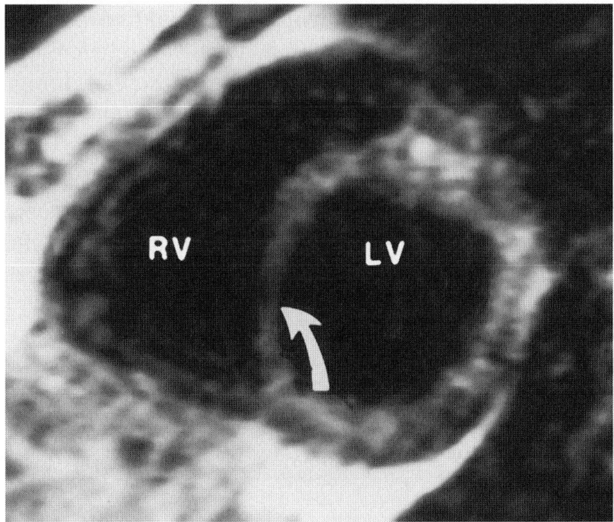

FIGURE 22.11. **Old Septal Infarction.** Spin-echo MR demonstrates fixed thinning of the myocardial wall (*arrow*) attributable to prior myocardial infarction.

microbubble contrast can enhance the infarcted region by highlighting perfused areas, resulting in a negative contrast effect at the site of the infarct.

CARDIOMYOPATHIES

The prevalence of cardiomyopathies is approximately 8 cases per 100,000 people in developed countries. One percent of cardiac deaths in the United States are attributable to cardiomyopathy. The mortality rate in men is twice that in women, and in Blacks it is twice that of Whites. In developing countries and in the tropics, the prevalence and mortality rates are much higher, probably because of nutritional deficiency, genetic factors, physical stress, untreated hypertension, and infection, especially Chagas disease.

The cardiomyopathies are a group of anomalies with three basic features: (*1*) failure of the heart to maintain its architecture, (*2*) failure of the heart to maintain normal electrical activity, and (*3*) failure of the heart to maintain cardiac output. General features of cardiomyopathies include cardiomegaly; congestive heart failure, often with relatively clear lungs; dilated LV and RV with elevated end-diastolic pressures and decreased contractility; and decreased ejection fractions. These findings are seen only in the later stages of hypertrophic and restrictive cardiomyopathies. Causes of congestive heart failure are listed in Table 22.2. The cardiomyopathies may also be divided into dilated, hypertrophic, restrictive, and right ventricular forms (Table 22.3).

TABLE 22.2 Causes of Congestive Heart Failure

- Myocardial
  - Cardiomyopathy (dilated, restrictive, hypertrophic)
  - Myocarditis
  - Postpartum cardiomyopathy
- Coronary
  - Transient ischemia
  - Chronic ischemic cardiomyopathy
  - Prior infarct or aneurysm
- Endocardial
  - Fibrosis
  - Löffler syndrome
- Valvular
  - Stenosis
  - Regurgitation
- Pericardial
  - Effusion
  - Constrictive
- Vascular
  - Hypertension
  - Pulmonary emboli
  - Arteriovenous fistula
  - Vasculitis
- Extracardiac
  - Endocrinopathy (thyroid, adrenal)
  - Toxic
  - Anemic
  - Metabolic

Dilated Cardiomyopathy. In the Western world, dilated cardiomyopathy accounts for 90% of all cardiomyopathies (Fig. 22.12). The term "congestive cardiomyopathy" should be reserved for a subgroup of the dilated cardiomyopathies for which the etiology is unknown. Specific causes for dilated cardiomyopathies should be pursued because the specific therapy may vary: (*1*) ischemic cardiomyopathy (the most common cause) because of chronic ischemia, prior infarction, or anomalous coronary arteries; (*2*) long-term sequelae of myocarditis (Coxsackie virus, most commonly); (*3*) toxins (ethanol and Adriamycin [doxorubicin]); (*4*) metabolic conditions (mucolipidosis, mucopolysaccharidosis, glycogen storage disease); (*5*) nutritional deficiencies (thiamin and selenium); (*6*) infants of diabetic mothers; and (7) muscular dystrophies.

Clinical presentation is related to congestive heart failure, although the initial presentation may include cardiac arrhythmias, conduction disturbances, thromboembolic phenomena, or sudden death. Presentation may also differ, depending on left-sided dominance, right-sided dominance, or biventricular involvement.

The chest radiograph commonly demonstrates global cardiomegaly. Larger heart sizes are associated with worse prognosis. Coronary artery calcification may be a clue to ischemic cardiomyopathy. Gated myocardial scintigraphy shows decreased left ventricular ejection fraction, prolonged pre-ejection period, shortened left ventricular ejection time, and a decreased rate of ejection. Echocardiography shows a dilated LV with global hypokinesia, thinning of the left ventricular wall and interventricular septum, decreased myocardial thickening, left atrial

TABLE 22.3 Types of Cardiomyopathies

Type	*Ventricular Wall*	*Ventricular Cavity*	*Contractility*	*Compliance*
Dilated	LV thin	LV dilated	Decreased	Normal to decreased
Hypertrophic	LV thick	LV normal to decreased	Increased	Decreased
Restrictive	Normal	Normal	Normal to decreased	Severely decreased
Uhl anomaly	RV thin	RV dilated	Decreased	Normal to decreased

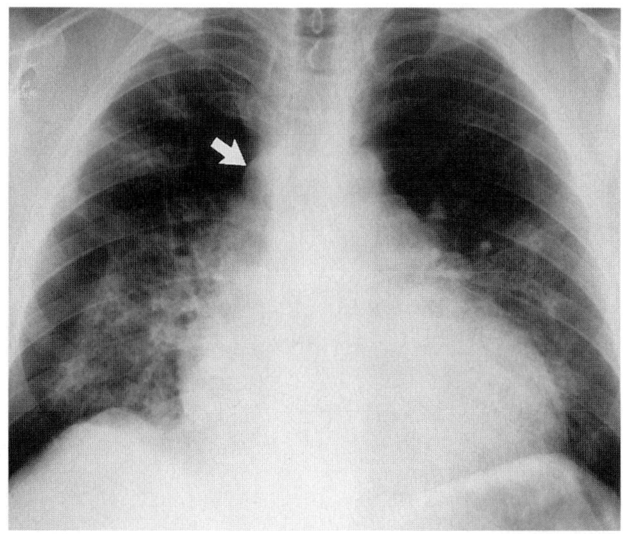

FIGURE 22.12. **Dilated Cardiomyopathy.** The typical appearance of a dilated cardiomyopathy is demonstrated with a water-bottle configuration and dilatation of the azygos vein (*arrow*). Pulmonary infiltrates are the result of pulmonary edema and capillary leak in this patient with viral myocarditis.

enlargement, and often right ventricular hypokinesia. MR shows dilatation of the specific chambers, decreased thickness of the myocardium with nonuniformity seen in prior infarctions, pericardial effusions, right and left ventricular ejection fractions, stroke volumes, wall-stress physiology, and quality of systolic wall thickening.

Hypertrophic cardiomyopathy may be familial (60%), autosomal dominant with variable penetrance, associated with neurofibromatosis and Noonan syndrome, or secondary to pressure overload. The hypertrophic cardiomyopathies are divided into two basic types: (*1*) *concentric hypertrophy,* which may be diffuse, midventricular, or apical in distribution; and (*2*) *asymmetrical septal hypertrophy* (ASH), also known as *idiopathic hypertrophic subaortic stenosis* (IHSS) (Fig. 22.13). Either form may cause some degree of muscular outflow obstruction with a systolic pressure gradient. Systemic hypertension may cause left ventricular hypertrophy followed by dilation, pulmonary venous hypertension, and increased risk of coronary artery disease.

The clinical presentation includes angina, syncope, arrhythmias, and congestive heart failure. Sudden death occurs in up to 50% of patients. The overall mortality rate is 2% to 3% per year.

On chest radiography, 50% of patients with hypertrophic cardiomyopathy will have a normal chest radiograph and 30% will have left atrial enlargement, commonly because of mitral regurgitation. Echocardiographic features of ASH include (*1*) hypertrophy of the interventricular septum (>12 to 13 mm), (*2*) abnormal ratio of thickness of the interventricular septum to the left ventricular posterior wall (>1.3:1), (*3*) systolic anterior motion of the mitral valve with mitral regurgitation, (*4*) narrowing of the left ventricular outflow tract during systole, (*5*) high velocity across the left ventricular outflow tract with delayed systolic peaks on Doppler examination, (*6*) midsystolic closure of the aortic valve, and (*7*) normal or hyperkinetic left ventricular function.

Restrictive cardiomyopathy is the least frequent form of cardiomyopathy. Etiologies include infiltrative disorders such as amyloid, glycogen storage disease, mucopolysaccharidosis, hemochromatosis, sarcoidosis, and myocardial tumor infiltration. In the tropics, endomyocardial fibrosis is highly prevalent. A rare form of endomyocardial fibrosis associated with eosinophilia is called Löffler endocardial fibrosis. Restrictive cardiomyopathy should be considered when patients present with symptoms of congestive failure without radiographic evidence of cardiomegaly or ventricular hypertrophy (Fig. 22.14). The primary differential diagnosis is constrictive pericardial disease that can be differentiated by CT or MR.

Signs and symptoms are related to congestive failure, arrhythmias, and heart block. In late stages, the electrocardiogram shows low voltage. Pathophysiology includes impaired diastolic function with decreased ventricular compliance, poor diastolic filling, and elevation of right and

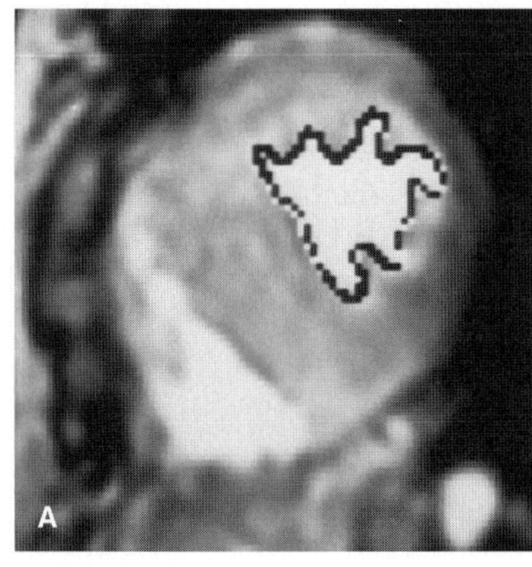

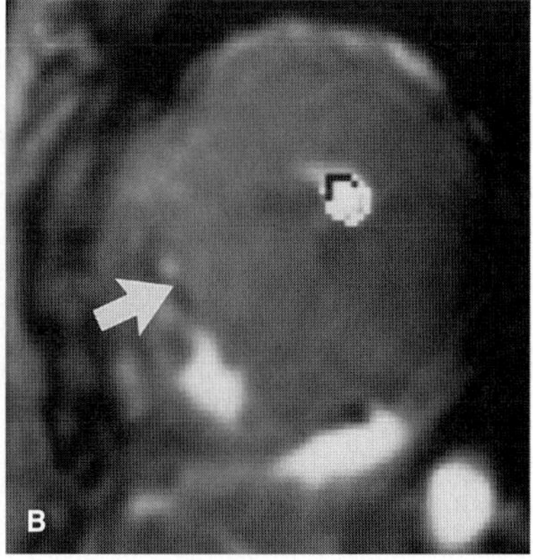

FIGURE 22.13. **Hypertrophic Cardiomyopathy.** Gradient-echo MR demonstrates marked left ventricular hypertrophy on these short-axis views of the LV obtained during diastole **(A)** and systole **(B).** Note the asymmetric thickening of the septum (*arrow*) compared with the remainder of the left ventricular myocardium. Ejection fraction is 92%.

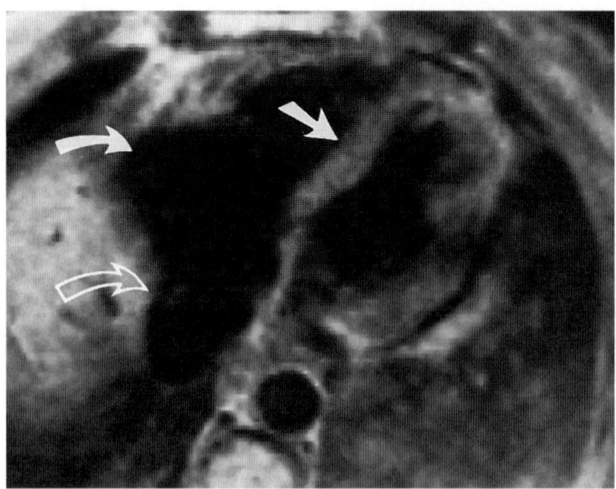

FIGURE 22.14. **Restrictive Cardiomyopathy.** Spin-echo MR demonstrates a variable high-density signal within the myocardium, a dilated RA (*closed curved arrow*), and an enlarged inferior vena cava (*open curved arrow*). The interventricular septum has an abnormal contour (*straight arrow*) because of high right ventricular pressures in this biopsy-proven case of amyloid cardiomyopathy.

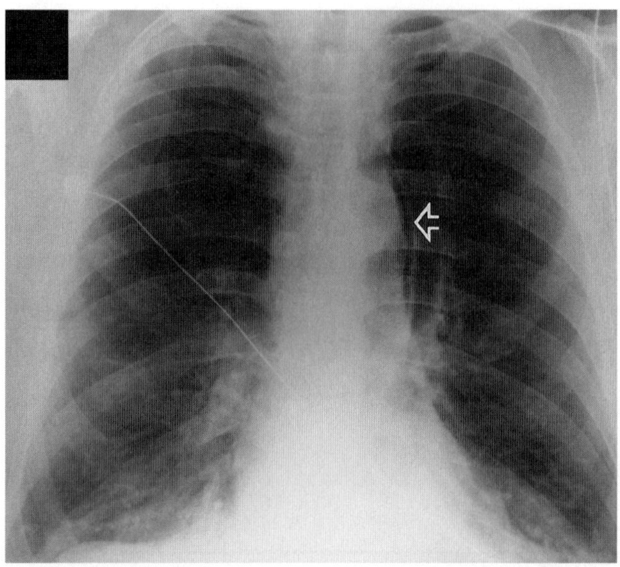

FIGURE 22.15. **Cor Pulmonale.** A posteroanterior chest radiograph demonstrates marked hyperinflation caused by chronic obstructive pulmonary disease. The anterior junction line (*arrow*) is herniated to the left of the aortic knob because of marked emphysema in the anterior segment of the right upper lobe.

left ventricular filling pressures. Early in the progression of the disease, ventricular systolic function is normal or near normal. There may be a significant decline in later stages.

The chest radiograph often shows a normal-sized heart with pulmonary congestion. Left atrial enlargement and pulmonary venous hypertension may be present. The PYP nuclear scans demonstrate hot spots in abnormal areas of myocardium in 50% to 90% of patients. Echocardiography may show decreased systolic and diastolic function, with normal to decreased ejection fractions. Mild left ventricular wall hypertrophy is often present, with a granular or "snowstorm" appearance to the myocardium, especially noted in the case of cardiac amyloidosis. MR shows high signal in the myocardium on T2WIs in patients with amyloidosis and sarcoidosis. The atria are enlarged because of elevated diastolic pressures, but ventricular volumes are often normal. Mitral regurgitation and tricuspid regurgitation are readily depicted with gradient-echo cine MR and Doppler echocardiography. The inferior vena cava and superior vena cava may be greatly dilated.

Right Ventricular Cardiomyopathies. *Cor pulmonale* is defined as right ventricular failure secondary to pulmonary parenchymal or pulmonary arterial disease. It may be considered a secondary form of right ventricular cardiomyopathy. Etiologies include (*1*) destructive pulmonary disease, such as pulmonary fibrosis and chronic obstructive pulmonary disease; (*2*) hypoxic pulmonary vasoconstriction resulting from chronic bronchitis, asthma, CNS hypoxia, or upper airway obstruction; (*3*) acute and chronic pulmonary embolism; (*4*) idiopathic pulmonary hypertension; and (*5*) extrapulmonary diseases affecting pulmonary mechanics such as chest deformities, morbid obesity (pickwickian syndrome), and neuromuscular diseases.

The end result is alveolar hypoxia leading to hypoxemia, pulmonary hypertension, elevated right ventricular pressures, right ventricular hypertrophy, right ventricular dilation, and right ventricular failure. Symptoms include marked dyspnea and decreased exercise endurance out of proportion to pulmonary function tests. Blood gases demonstrate hypoxemia and hypercapnia.

The chest radiograph shows a normal-sized heart or mild cardiomegaly (Fig. 22.15). Right ventricular and right atrial enlargement may be present. The main and central pulmonary arteries are prominent, and the periphery is oligemic. The interlobar artery typically measures more than 16 mm. The lungs show signs of chronic obstructive pulmonary disease, emphysema, or pulmonary fibrosis. Nuclear scintigraphy shows right ventricular enlargement with decrease in the right ventricular ejection fraction on first-pass examination. Echocardiography, CT, and MR show right ventricular and right atrial enlargement with thickening of the anterior right ventricular wall. M-mode echocardiography of the tricuspid valve shows a diminished A wave and a flat E–F slope. Therapy is aimed at the underlying pulmonary disorder.

Uhl anomaly was initially described as a congenital disorder with "parchment-like thinning" of the RV. More recently it has been described as an acquired disorder in infants or adults and is called "arrhythmogenic right ventricular dysplasia." This rare form of cardiomyopathy is limited to dilation of the RV, with marked thinning of the anterior right ventricular wall. MR may also show fatty infiltration of the anterior RV free wall, which is diagnostic. Clinical presentation includes syncope, recurrent ventricular tachycardia, and premature death from early congestive failure or arrhythmias. Familial occurrence has been reported, and males outnumber females by 3 to 1. Right ventricular ejection fractions are commonly reduced to less than half of normal, with mild reductions in the left ventricular ejection fraction.

PULMONARY VASCULAR DISEASE

Enlargement of the pulmonary outflow tract is seen in congenital heart disease with left-to-right shunts. Outflow tract prominence without evidence of a shunt lesion is usually the result of poststenotic dilatation secondary to pulmonary stenosis, pulmonary arterial hypertension, Marfan syndrome, Takayasu arteritis, or idiopathic dilatation of the pulmonary artery. Idiopathic dilatation of the pulmonary artery demonstrates a dilated main pulmonary artery, normal peripheral pulmonary arteries, and normal, balanced circulation. This entity is much more common in women and is often associated with a mild systolic ejection murmur, but without evidence of pulmonary stenosis.

Pulmonary arterial hypertension should be considered whenever the main pulmonary artery and left and right pulmonary arteries are enlarged (Fig. 22.16). Signs of right atrial and ventricular enlargement or hypertrophy are often present. Systolic right ventricular and pulmonary artery pressures exceed 30 mm Hg. Other findings include rapid tapering and tortuosity of the pulmonary arteries. The peripheral lung zones appear clear. Calcification within the pulmonary arterial walls is virtually diagnostic of pulmonary arterial hypertension (Fig. 22.17).

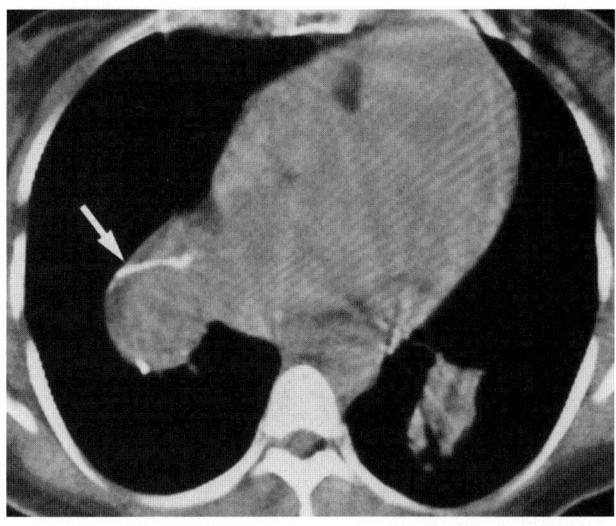

FIGURE 22.17. **Pulmonary Arterial Hypertension.** Noncontrast CT demonstrates calcification in the wall of the right pulmonary artery (*arrow*).

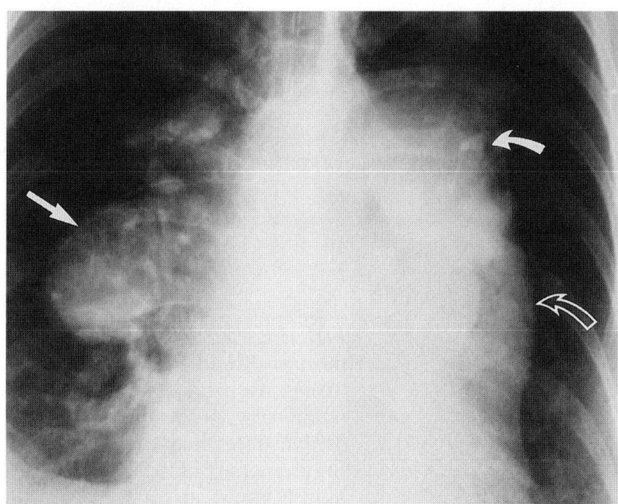

FIGURE 22.16. **Pulmonary Arterial Hypertension.** The main pulmonary artery (*curved arrow*), left pulmonary artery (*open arrow*), and right pulmonary artery (*straight arrow*) are extremely enlarged. Faint calcification is seen in the right pulmonary artery. The patient had schistosomiasis with resultant vasculitis and pulmonary arterial hypertension.

The differential diagnosis for pulmonary arterial hypertension includes long-standing pulmonary venous hypertension (e.g., mitral stenosis), Eisenmenger physiology (from long-standing left-to-right shunts), pulmonary emboli, vasculitides (such as rheumatoid arthritis or polyarteritis nodosa), and primary pulmonary hypertension. Polyarteritis nodosa is a necrotizing vasculitis involving the medium-sized pulmonary arteries. Radiographic findings include small pulmonary arterial aneurysms, focal stenoses, small infarctions, and signs of pulmonary hypertension. Primary pulmonary hypertension is most common in women in their third and fourth decades. Histologic examination reveals plexiform and angiomatoid lesions with no evidence of emboli or venous abnormalities. Symptoms include dyspnea, fatigue, hyperventilation, chest pain, and hemoptysis.

Increased pulmonary blood flow is caused by high output states and left-to-right shunts. High output states include volume loading, pregnancy, peripheral shunt lesions (arteriovenous malformations), hyperthyroidism, anemia, and leukemia (Fig. 22.18). The main and central pulmonary arteries are enlarged, with increased circulation to the lower lobes, upper lobes, and peripheral lung zones. Bronchovascular pairs show enlargement of the vascular component. The most common shunts in the adult are the acyanotic lesions, including atrial septal defect, ventricular septal defect, patent ductus arteriosus, and partial anomalous pulmonary venous return. Cyanotic lesions with

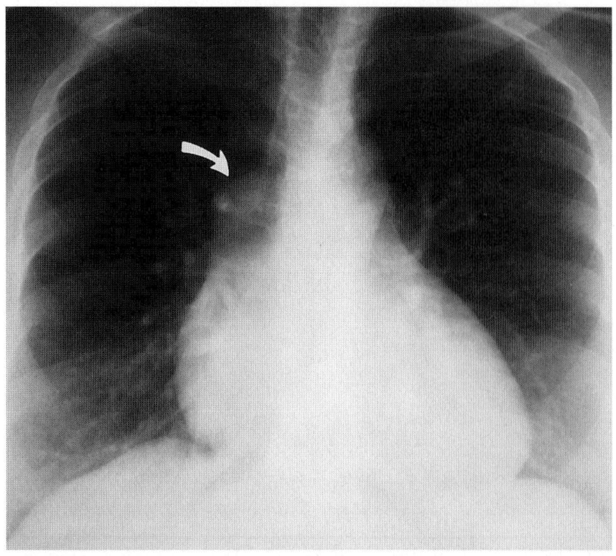

FIGURE 22.18. **High Output Failure.** Chest radiograph demonstrates cardiomegaly, vascular engorgement, and distension of the azygos vein in this pregnant patient with severe anemia. The azygos vein (*arrow*) is a good marker of intravascular volume expansion or elevated central venous pressures.

increased blood flow to the lungs include transposition of the great vessels, truncus arteriosus, total anomalous pulmonary venous return, and endocardial cushion defects. Ventricular septal defects with left-to-right shunting may occur acutely following myocardial infarction.

Decreased pulmonary blood flow with a small heart is caused by chronic obstructive pulmonary disease, hypovolemia, malnourishment, and Addison disease. When the cardiac silhouette is enlarged, the differential diagnosis includes cardiomyopathy, pericardial tamponade, Ebstein anomaly, and right-to-left shunts from congenital heart disease.

Asymmetric pulmonary blood flow may be evident on chest radiography, angiography, or nuclear medicine pulmonary perfusion scans (Fig. 22.19; see Figs. 22.15, 22.26). This may result from either decreased or increased blood flow to one lung. Pulmonary valvular stenosis often results in increased blood flow to the left lung. With resultant left pulmonary artery dilatation, tetralogy of Fallot may cause increased blood flow to the right lung (Fig. 22.15). Surgical shunts, such as the Blalock-Taussig procedure, also increase blood flow to one lung. Decreased blood flow to one lung occurs in peripheral pulmonic stenosis (see Fig. 22.26), interruption of the pulmonary artery, scimitar syndrome, pulmonary hypoplasia, Swyer-James syndrome, pulmonary emphysema, pulmonary embolism, fibrosing mediastinitis, or carcinoma affecting one artery (Fig. 22.19). When examining a chest radiograph, one must be careful to exclude technical artifacts such as lateral decentering and soft tissue asymmetry such as mastectomy. The balance of circulation and size of the central pulmonary arteries should be compared, along with the size of the bronchovascular pairs.

Pulmonary venous hypertension may be identified on radiographs, pulmonary angiograms, or nuclear medicine perfusion scans (Fig. 22.20; see Fig. 21.19). Pulmonary venous hypertension is considered mild with wedge pressures of 10 to 13 mm Hg, moderate with equalization of upper and lower lobe blood flow and wedge pressures of 14 to 16 mm Hg, or severe with the upper lobe vessels being distended more than the lower lobe vessels and wedge pressure 17 to 20 mm Hg. Progressive cephalization is accompanied by progressive secondary enlargement of the pulmonary arteries and filling out of the hilar angles. The most common cause of pulmonary venous hypertension is elevation of left atrial pressures secondary to left ventricular failure (Table 22.4).

ACQUIRED VALVULAR HEART DISEASE

Mitral stenosis in the adult is usually caused by rheumatic heart disease, with 50% of patients giving a history of

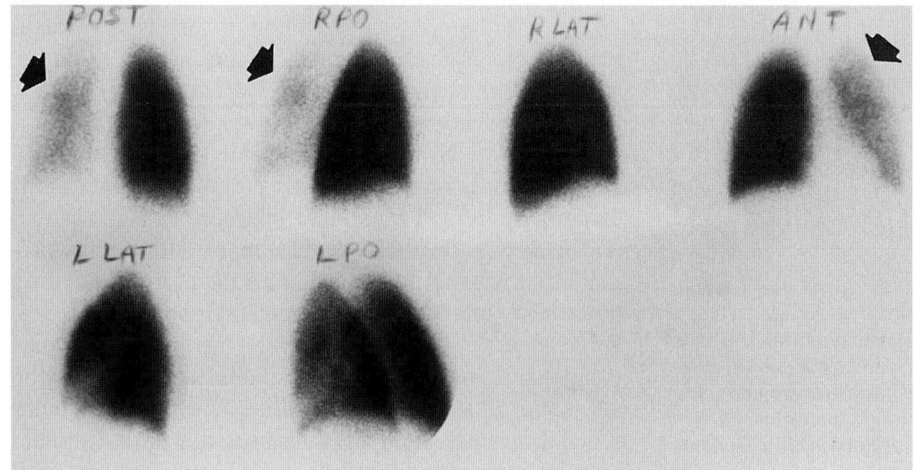

FIGURE 22.19. **Asymmetric Pulmonary Blood Flow.** Technetium-99m macroaggregated albumin pulmonary perfusion lung scan demonstrates marked reduction in the pulmonary blood flow to the left lung (*arrows*) in comparison with the right lung. A subtle left hilar mass was causing compression of the left pulmonary artery. POST, posterior; RPO, right posterior oblique; RLAT, right lateral; ANT, anterior; LLAT, left lateral; LPO, left posterior oblique.

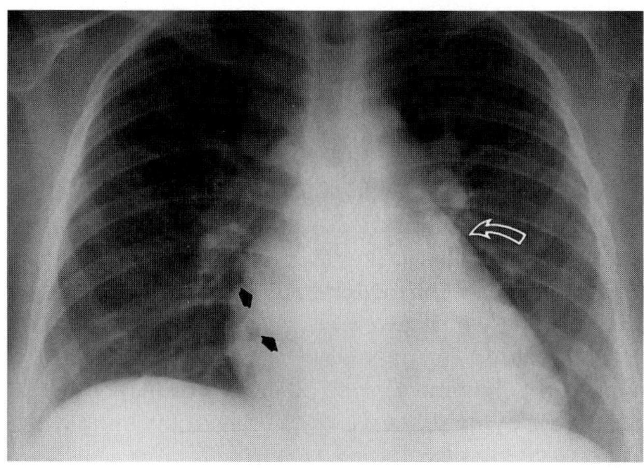

FIGURE 22.20. **Moderate Mitral Stenosis.** A chest radiograph demonstrates mild cardiomegaly with straightening of the left heart border, prominence of the left atrial appendage (*open arrow*), and evidence of left atrial enlargement (*arrows*). Cephalization of blood flow and enlargement of the pulmonary arteries indicate pulmonary venous and pulmonary arterial hypertension.

rheumatic fever. Rarely, an atrial myxoma may mimic mitral stenosis on chest radiography. The incidence of mitral stenosis is higher in women by a ratio of 8:1. *Lutembacher syndrome* is a combination of mitral stenosis with a preexisting atrial septal defect, which results in marked right-sided enlargement.

The normal mitral valve area is 4 to 6 cm^2. With mild mitral stenosis (mitral valve area <1.5 cm^2), the chest radiograph may be normal and left atrial pressures will be elevated only during exercise. Moderate mitral stenosis (valve area <1.0 cm^2) produces signs of left atrial enlargement and pulmonary venous hypertension (Fig. 22.20). Dyspnea on exertion is common. Severe mitral stenosis (valve area <0.5 cm^2) has marked left atrial enlargement, right ventricular enlargement, Kerley lines, pulmonary edema, and, occasionally, calcification in the left atrial wall. Patients are often dyspneic at rest, with resting left atrial pressure exceeding 35 mm Hg. Palpitations and atrial fibrillation with risk of atrial thrombi and systemic emboli are also common. Long-standing pulmonary venous hypertension leads to pulmonary arterial hypertension. Stages of progression of mitral stenosis are:

stage 1: pulmonary venous hypertension with hilar angle loss,
stage 2: interstitial edema with Kerley lines,
stage 3: alveolar edema, and
stage 4: chronic, recurrent congestive failure, hemosiderin deposits, and ossification or calcifications in the lung.

The chest radiograph is often characteristic, with a long, straight, left heart border; left atrial enlargement; prominence of the left atrial appendage; cephalization of blood flow, indicating pulmonary venous hypertension; pulmonary arterial hypertension; left atrial calcification; mitral valve calcification; prominent main pulmonary artery; right ventricular enlargement with filling of the retrosternal clear space; and dilatation of the inferior vena cava. Echocardiography shows a decreased E–F slope on M-mode, slow left ventricular filling, left atrial enlargement, thickened mitral valve, decreased excursion of the mitral valve with a narrow mitral orifice, parallel movement of the anterior and posterior leaflets, and atrial fibrillation. Gated nuclear angiograms are useful for following the left ventricular ejection fraction. MR grades the valvular disease and determines chamber volumes and ejection fractions. Velocity-encoded cine MR quantifies peak velocity and instantaneous blood flow. The peak gradient across the stenotic valve can be calculated when the echo times (TE) are less than 7 ms, allowing measurements of velocities up to 6 m/s. Mitral commissurotomy or balloon valvuloplasty may be performed if the leaflets are pliable and not heavily calcified. Mitral valve replacement should be considered before left ventricular failure occurs.

Mitral regurgitation associated with rheumatic heart disease used to be the most common hemodynamically significant form of mitral regurgitation in adults. Today, mitral regurgitation is more commonly the result of initial valve prolapse, followed by infarct ischemia–related papillary muscle dysfunction and rupture (Table 22.5).

The radiograph shows left atrial enlargement that is more pronounced than that seen with pure mitral stenosis (Fig. 22.21). Left ventricular enlargement is also present. Pulmonary venous hypertension is less prominent than in mitral stenosis. The radiograph is near normal with mild mitral regurgitation, shows atrial enlargement and pulmonary venous hypertension with moderate disease, and

TABLE 22.4 Causes of Pulmonary Venous Hypertension

Left ventricular failure
Mitral stenosis
Mitral regurgitation
Aortic stenosis
Aortic regurgitation
Pulmonary veno-occlusive disease
Congenital heart disease

TABLE 22.5 Causes of Mitral Regurgitation

Rheumatic heart disease
Congenital heart disease
Mitral valve prolapse
Ruptured chordae tendineae
Infectious endocarditis
Papillary muscle rupture
Mitral annulus calcification

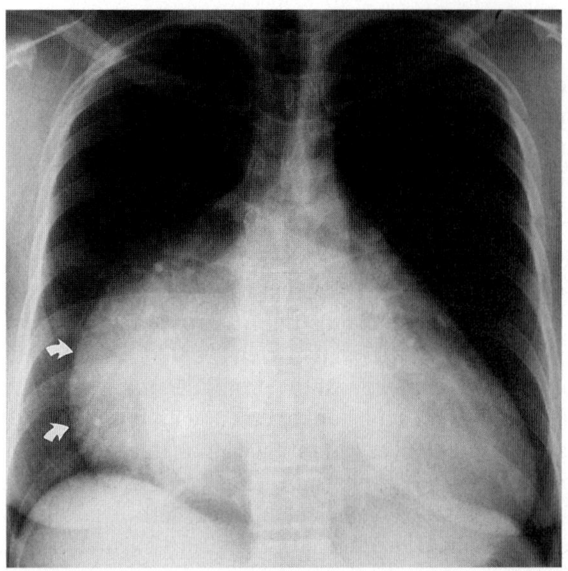

FIGURE 22.21. **Mitral Regurgitation.** A chest radiograph demonstrates marked left atrial enlargement with "atrial escape" where the LA (*arrows*) becomes border-forming along the right cardiac silhouette. Note the marked carinal splaying because of this massive left atrial enlargement.

shows progressive left atrial enlargement, left ventricular enlargement, pulmonary venous hypertension, and pulmonary edema with severe mitral regurgitation.

Echocardiography shows left atrial enlargement, left ventricular enlargement, and bulging of the atrial septum to the right. A nuclear angiogram shows a dilated LV with an elevated left ventricular ejection fraction because of the hyperdynamic status. MR using gradient echo and gated cine mode shows the regurgitant jet projecting from the LV into the LA during systole. The regurgitant jet may be graded visually as mild, moderate, or severe based on the distance it extends toward the back wall. Grade 1 regurgitation is defined as turbulent flow extending less than one third of the distance to the back wall, grade 2 is less than two thirds of the distance to the back wall, and grade 3 is more than two thirds of the distance to the back wall. The regurgitant fraction can be calculated by comparing the right and left ventricular stroke volumes, which are normally equal. The regurgitant fraction is equal to the right ventricular stroke volume minus the left ventricular stroke volume, divided by right ventricular stroke volume. Gated blood pool scintigraphy is used to follow the ejection fraction to optimize the timing of valve replacement. Echocardiography can be used to follow both the ejection fraction and left ventricular volumes.

Mitral valve prolapse is an interesting entity that has also been called "floppy mitral valve" or Barlow syndrome. It is seen in 2% to 6% of the general population and is more common in young women. It has an autosomal dominant transmission and is more common in patients with straight backs, pectus excavatum, and narrow anteroposterior diameters of the chest. Patients may be asymptomatic or have symptoms as a result of arrhythmias. A "honking" type of murmur or a murmur with midsystolic click is characteristic. The chest radiograph is usually normal, although occasionally patients will develop mitral regurgitation, left atrial enlargement, and pulmonary venous hypertension. Echocardiography demonstrates a characteristic bulging of the anterior or posterior leaflets, usually beginning during mid-systole when the valve should remain closed. This may also take the appearance of a pansystolic "hammock" type of leaflet bowing. Some patients develop myxomatous thickening of the mitral valve leaflets.

Aortic stenosis is caused by partial fusion of the commissures between the aortic valve cusps. Bicuspid aortic valve is found in 1% to 2% of the population and is present in 95% of congenital aortic stenosis. *Bicuspid aortic valve* is most common in men and is present in 25% to 50% of patients with aortic coarctation. Sixty percent of patients older than 24 years of age have calcification within the bicuspid valve. *Calcific or degenerative aortic stenosis*, on the other hand, is usually seen in older patients with systemic hypertension. It is now thought that degenerative aortic valve calcification is actually part of the atherosclerotic process and tends to progress in association with coronary calcification. Aortic valve calcification is best seen on lateral or right anterior oblique chest radiographs. Noncalcific stenosis is usually caused by rheumatic heart disease and coexists with mitral valve disease. The radiograph typically shows left ventricular hypertrophy with poststenotic dilatation of the aorta (Fig. 22.22). The ascending aorta is not normally seen on frontal chest radiographs in patients

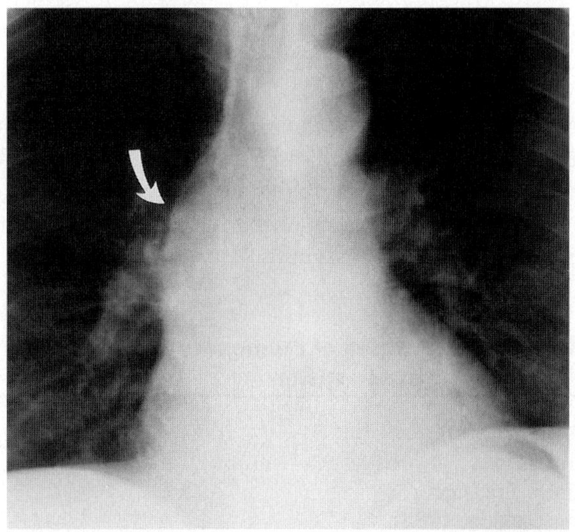

FIGURE 22.22. **Aortic Stenosis on Chest Radiograph.** Note the enlarged ascending aorta (*arrow*), highly suggestive of poststenotic dilatation in this patient with normal heart size.

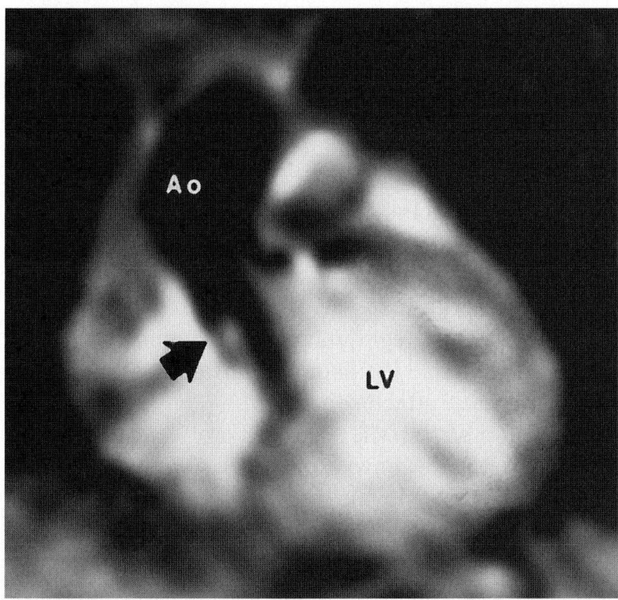

FIGURE 22.23. **Aortic Stenosis on MR.** Gradient-echo MR coronal image of the ascending aorta (Ao), aortic valve (*arrow*), and LV. Note the signal void in the entire ascending aorta as a result of marked turbulence caused by severe aortic stenosis.

who are less than 40 years of age. The echocardiogram shows dense aortic valve echoes, a dilated aortic root, hyperdynamic function, and left ventricular hypertrophy. A bicuspid valve may be directly visualized. The aortic valve area is normally 2.5 to 3.5 cm^2. Symptoms typically occur when the valve area is less than 0.7 cm^2, or less than 1.5 cm^2 if there is combined aortic stenosis and aortic insufficiency. Mild aortic stenosis is associated with a 13- to 14-mm orifice and greater than 25 mm Hg gradient. Moderate aortic stenosis has an 8- to 12-mm orifice and greater than 40 to 50 mm Hg gradient. Severe stenosis occurs at an orifice that is smaller than 8 mm with a gradient greater than 100 mm Hg. Cardiac MR and echocardiography show increased ventricular muscle mass with hypertrophy as well as turbulent flow (Fig. 22.23). MR and blood pool scintigraphy show decreased left ventricular ejection fraction, increased left ventricular emptying time, decreased rate of ejection, and a normal left ventricular filling rate.

Symptoms progress from angina to syncopal episodes to congestive failure, with the possibility of sudden death with severe stenosis. Therapy is usually valve replacement, although some cases are amenable to valvuloplasty.

Aortic insufficiency is primary when it is attributable to aortic valve disease or is secondary when it is the result of aortic root disease (Table 22.6). Physical examination reveals a water-hammer pulse, a decrescendo diastolic murmur, and, occasionally, when severe or directed toward the anterior mitral leaflet, an Austin Flint murmur caused by vibrations of the mitral valve by regurgitant flow.

TABLE 22.6 Causes of Aortic Insufficiency

Causes
Valvular
Congenital
Rheumatic
Infectious endocarditis
Trauma
Aortic root
Syphilis
Dissecting aneurysm
Marfan syndrome
Rheumatoid arthritis
Reiter syndrome
Relapsing polychondritis
Giant cell arteritis
Subvalvular
Aneurysm of sinus of Valsalva
Subaortic stenosis
High ventricular septal defect

The chest radiograph shows a dilated, calcified aortic root with a normal heart size in mild disease. With moderate disease, the LV and cardiac silhouette enlarge. With severe disease, left atrial enlargement and congestive heart failure develop. Symptoms include dyspnea on exertion, fatigue, and symptoms of congestive failure.

Echocardiography and MR show the dilated aortic root, regurgitant aortic flow, diastolic flutter of the interventricular septum or anterior mitral leaflet (Austin Flint phenomenon), left ventricular dilation, increased wall motion, increased ejection fraction, and early mitral valve closure (Fig. 22.24). The ratio of the regurgitant flow width to the

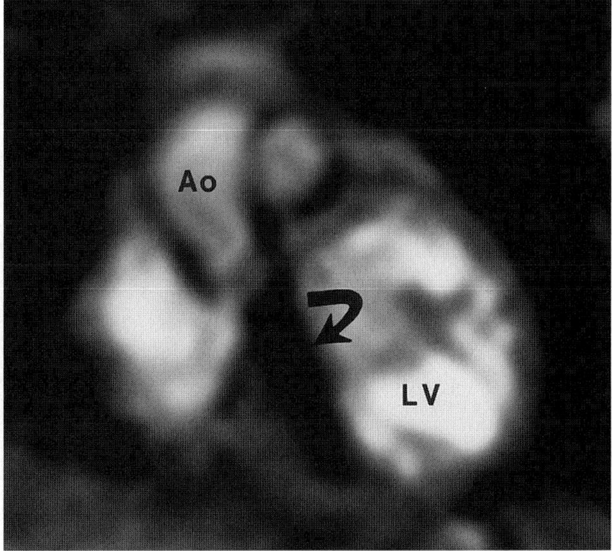

FIGURE 22.24. **Aortic Regurgitation.** Gradient-echo MR coronal image through the ascending aorta (Ao) and LV demonstrates regurgitant flow from the aortic valve into the LV (*arrow*).

aortic root is helpful for grading the severity. Ventricular function may be followed by echocardiography, nuclear scintigraphy, or MR. Once congestive failure begins to occur, the LV will dilate and the left ventricular ejection fraction will fall.

Supravalvular aortic stenosis is the result of a localized hourglass-type narrowing above the valve, a discrete fibrous-type membrane, or a diffuse hypoplastic tubular configuration of the ascending aorta. Supravalvular aortic stenosis is often associated with peripheral pulmonary stenosis and valvular or subvalvular aortic stenosis. This combination of findings is seen in Marfan syndrome or Williams syndrome. The coronary arteries are dilated because of the elevated systolic pressure and narrowing of the aortic root (<20 mm). The aortic cusps themselves are normal.

Subvalvular/subaortic stenosis may be a fixed anatomic defect or a dynamic functional obstruction. Fixed subaortic stenosis is associated with congenital heart disease, especially ventricular septal defect, in 50% of cases. Type 1 subaortic stenosis is a thin membrane located less than 2 cm below the valve. Type 2 is a thick, collar-type constriction. Type 3 subaortic stenosis is an irregular, fibromuscular type of narrowing. Type 4 is a funnel-like constriction of the left ventricular outflow tract. The mitral valve is normal.

The functional type of subaortic stenosis has also been called asymmetric septal hypertrophy, idiopathic hypertrophic subaortic stenosis, or hypertrophic obstructive cardiomyopathy. The appearances vary slightly. Findings may be evident with nuclear scintigraphy, but they are more obvious on echocardiography and MR. The interventricular septum is significantly thicker than the left ventricular free wall in 95% of patients. The left and right ventricular cavities are normal or small in 95% of patients. Systolic anterior motion of the mitral valve is best seen on echocardiography but may also be identified with MR. Asymmetric septal hypertrophy may partially obstruct outflow in systole. The aortic cusp may flutter or partially close during systole. Mitral regurgitation is a common secondary finding attributable to abnormal mitral valve position or papillary muscle attachment.

Pulmonic stenosis is seen in 8% of congenital heart disease cases and is uncommon as an acquired disease in adults. Symptoms may be secondary to cyanosis or heart failure. A systolic ejection murmur is heard over the left sternal border. The chest radiograph often shows dilatation of the main and left pulmonary arteries, with increased flow into the left lung (Fig. 22.25). Right ventricular hypertrophy or enlargement is seen on chest radiographs, MR, and echocardiography. Systolic doming of the pulmonic valve is secondary to incomplete opening and is best seen on echocardiography. Rarely, calcification may be identified in the pulmonic valve.

Valvular pulmonic stenosis is caused by partial commissural fusion in 95% of cases. Symptoms typically start during childhood and progress into adulthood. A pulmonic click is common, and the electrocardiogram often shows

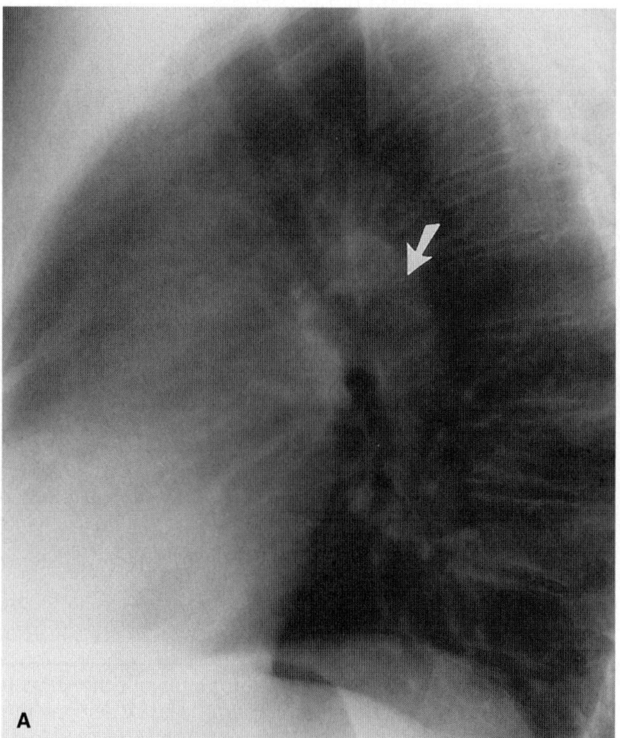

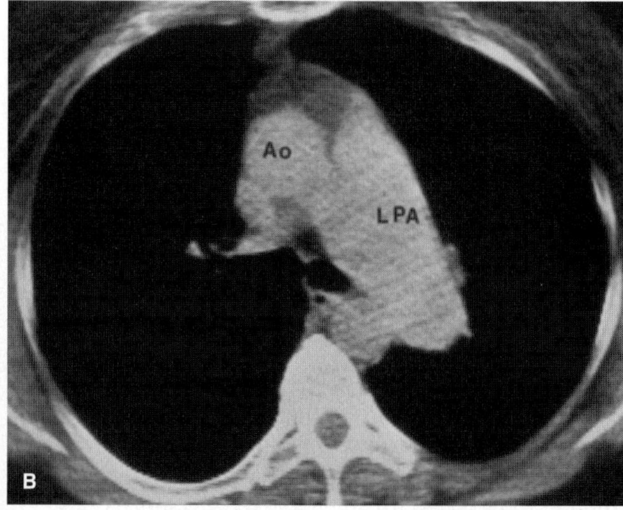

FIGURE 22.25. **Pulmonary Stenosis. A.** Lateral chest radiograph demonstrates marked poststenotic dilatation of the left pulmonary artery (*arrow*). **B.** CT through the ascending aorta (Ao) demonstrates marked dilatation of the left pulmonary artery (LPA).

right ventricular hypertrophy. On angiography, a jet of contrast may be seen extending well into the left pulmonary artery. In dysplastic pulmonic stenosis (5% of cases), the cusps are immobile, thick, and redundant. There is no click and typically no poststenotic dilatation.

Infundibular or subvalvular stenosis is common with tetralogy of Fallot and often occurs with ventricular septal defects. Because of the location of the stenosis, preferential flow goes to the right lung.

Peripheral pulmonic stenosis or supravalvular stenosis commonly (up to 60% of the time) accompanies pulmonary valvular stenosis. Sites of narrowing include the main pulmonary artery, bifurcation, lobar, and segmental arteries (Fig. 22.26). Associated syndromes include Williams syndrome, tetralogy of Fallot, Ehlers-Danlos syndrome, and postrubella syndrome. Postrubella syndrome is associated with intrauterine growth retardation, deafness, cataracts, mental retardation, and patent ductus arteriosus. Williams syndrome is associated with hypercalcemia, elfin facies, mental retardation, and supravalvular aortic stenosis. Ehlers-Danlos syndrome is a defect in collagen formation associated with joint laxity, skin stretchability, aneurysms, and mitral regurgitation.

Pulmonic insufficiency is very uncommon in adults and is usually the result of subacute bacterial endocarditis. Pulmonic insufficiency demonstrates regurgitant flow from the pulmonic valve into the RV.

Bacterial Endocarditis. Patients predisposed to subacute bacterial endocarditis (SBE) include those with rheumatic heart disease, mitral valve prolapse, aortic stenosis, aortic regurgitation, bicuspid aortic valves (50% of aortic SBE), mitral stenosis, mitral regurgitation, congenital heart disease (especially ventricular septal defect and tetralogy of Fallot), or prosthetic valves (4% of SBE), and drug addicts. IV drug abusers are particularly at risk for tricuspid valve involvement. Tricuspid valve disease is suspected when multiple septic pulmonary emboli are seen on chest radiography. *Streptococcus viridans* was previously reported as the most common bacterial etiology; however, *Staphylococcus aureus* has now become the most common bacterial agent. *Serratia* and *Pseudomonas* organisms are also common offenders, particularly in certain geographic locations. *Candida* is the most common fungal agent, followed by *Aspergillus*.

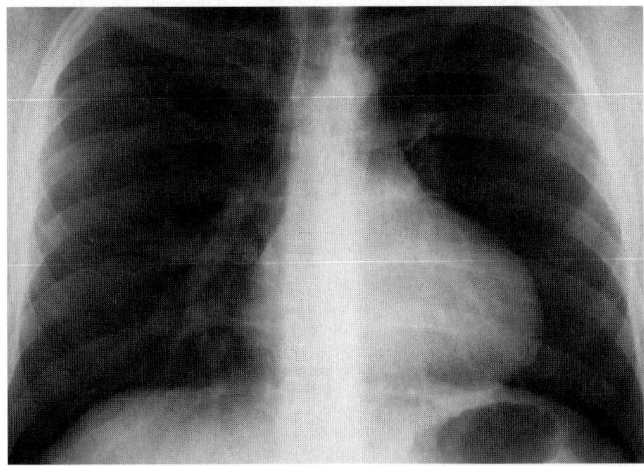

FIGURE 22.26. **Peripheral Pulmonary Stenosis.** A chest radiograph demonstrates classic right ventricular configuration indicative of right ventricular hypertrophy. Asymmetric blood flow is noted, with decreased markings in the left lung because of peripheral stenosis.

Valve vegetations, or chronic areas of thickening, can be detected in 50% to 90% of patients with known bacterial endocarditis. The vegetations cause excessive vibration of the valves during systole, and the leaflets may appear slightly thickened or fuzzy. The actual vegetations may be seen to prolapse when the valve is closed. The vegetations may cause valvular incompetence or acute valvular destruction. The vegetations may remain, even after successful antibiotic therapy. It is difficult to discern acute infective vegetations from chronic changes. Infections of prosthetic valves result in exaggerated valve motion, partial valvular obstruction, loosening of the sutures, and perivalvular leak or frank dehiscence. MR and transesophageal echocardiography are quite good at detecting perivalvular or perisutural leaks. Noninfectious vegetations and focal valve thickenings may be seen with carcinoid syndrome (right heart valves), *Libman-Sacks vegetations* of systemic lupus erythematosus, *Lambl excrescences* (focal benign thickening), and myxomatous degeneration.

Other forms of endocarditis include Chagas disease, which is common in South America and Africa. Chagas disease is a late sequelae of acute myocarditis involving the parasite *Trypanosoma cruzi*. This may result in cardiomyopathy or ventricular aneurysm. Patients with AIDS may also develop an endocarditis and cardiomyopathy, possibly because of viral infections. Indium-labeled white cell scans or gallium scans may prove useful in patients for whom echocardiography is inconclusive or in whom secondary endocardial or aortic abscess is suspected (Fig. 22.27).

CARDIAC MASSES

Cardiac masses include thrombi, primary benign tumors, primary malignant tumors, and metastatic tumors. Lipomatous hypertrophy, moderator bands, and papillary muscles may simulate cardiac masses. Because most cardiac masses do not deform the outer contours of the heart, chest radiography is typically not useful, except for the occasional calcific mass. Nuclear scintigraphy, CT, and cardiac angiography identify intracardiac masses. Echocardiography is usually the initial mode of evaluation, and MR may be helpful when there is uncertainty.

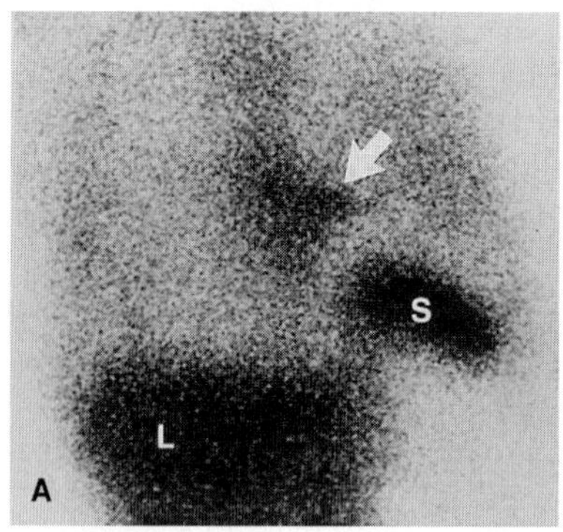

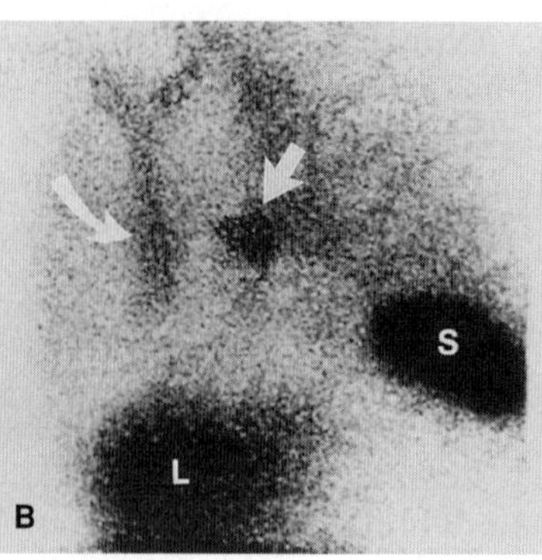

FIGURE 22.27. **Subacute Bacterial Endocarditis.** Indium-labeled white cell scan shows migration of indium-labeled white cells to the area of severe aortic endocarditis. Note the marked increased activity (*arrows*) to the left and posterior to the sternum (*curved arrow*) on these anterior **(A)** and left anterior oblique **(B)** views of the chest. L, liver. S, spleen.

Thrombi are the most frequent cause of an intracardiac mass and are most common in the LA and LV, where they present a risk of systemic emboli. Intra-atrial thrombi are usually associated with atrial fibrillation, often secondary to rheumatic heart disease. Thrombosis commonly occurs along the posterior wall of the LA. Clots within the left atrial appendage are difficult to detect on transthoracic echocardiography but are readily identified with transesophageal echo (Fig. 22.28), CT (Fig. 22.29), and MR. Left ventricular thrombi are usually secondary to recent infarction or ventricular aneurysm (Fig. 22.30). The differentiation of tumor versus clot is best done with MR using gradient-echo techniques. Clots typically have low signal, whereas tumors have intermediate signal. Clots will not enhance, whereas neoplasms will typically appear as enhancing masses on CT or MR. Cine-mode gradient-echo MR is useful for determining the morphology of a lesion. Intracardiac lipomas or lipomatous hypertrophy have characteristic bright signal on T1WIs and remain relatively bright on T2WIs. Fat-saturation sequences help to make the specific diagnosis of lipoma, which is the second most common benign tumor. MDCT can also characterize lipomas and lipomatous hypertrophy.

Benign Tumors. Atrial myxoma makes up 50% of primary cardiac tumors and is the most common primary benign tumor. It occurs most frequently in patients in the 30- to 60-year age range and is often accompanied by fever, anemia, weight loss, embolic symptoms (27%), or syncope. Most (75% to 80%) myxomas are in the LA and may mimic rheumatic valvular disease clinically (Fig. 22.31). Cardiomegaly, left atrial enlargement, pulmonary venous hypertension, and ossific pulmonary nodules may be seen. Enlargement of the left atrial appendage is uncommon. Echocardiography, CT, and MR show the atrial filling defect, which may prolapse into the LV during diastole (Fig. 22.32). Atrial myxomas may be pedunculated and are usually lobulated. On M-mode echo, the E–F slope is typically

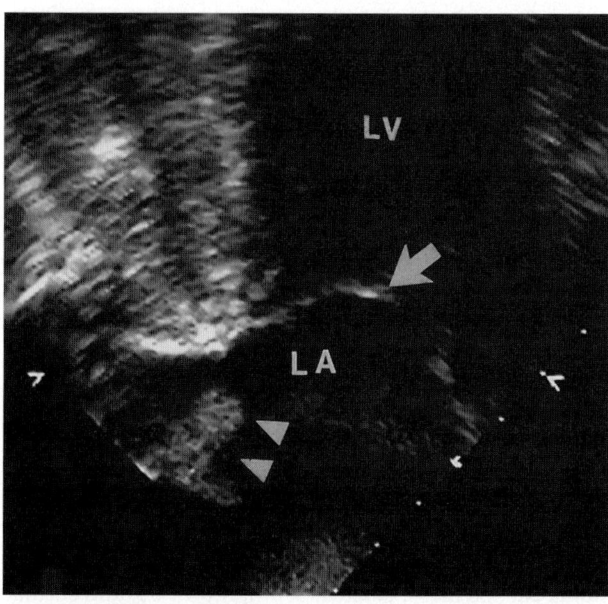

FIGURE 22.28. **Left Atrial Thrombus.** Transesophageal echo shows echogenic thrombus (*arrowheads*) in the LA. The mitral valve (*arrow*) and the LV are well seen.

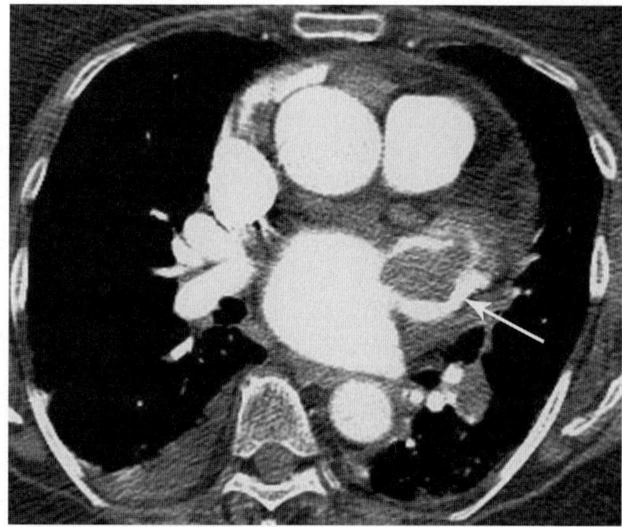

FIGURE 22.29. **CT of Left Atrial Thrombus.** Contrast-enhanced multidetector CT clearly demonstrates large thrombus (*arrow*) in the left atrial appendage.

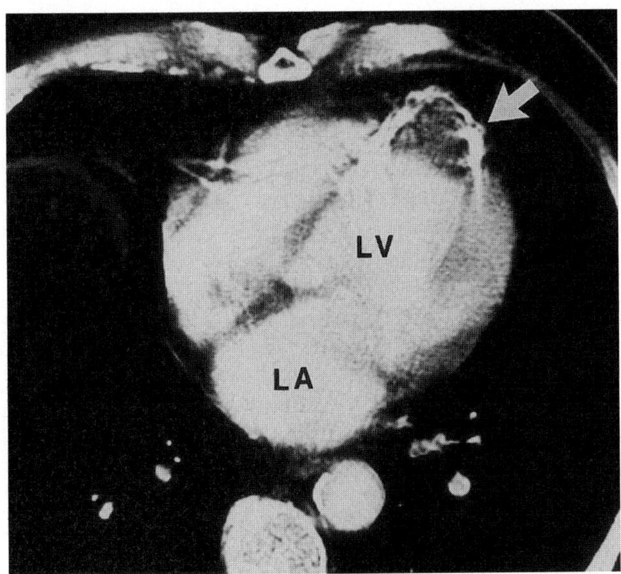

FIGURE 22.30. Left Ventricular Thrombus. Contrast-enhanced CT through the LV demonstrates calcification in an apical left ventricular aneurysm (*arrow*). Note the nonenhancing low-density thrombus within the aneurysm.

decreased, with numerous echoes seen behind the mitral valve.

Other benign tumors include lipoma, rhabdomyoma (Fig. 22.33) (found in 50% to 85% of tuberous sclerosis patients), fibromas (12% of which may calcify), and the rare teratoma. Hydatid cysts typically show a bulge along the left heart border, with associated curvilinear calcification, and are at risk for rupture into the pericardium or myocardium.

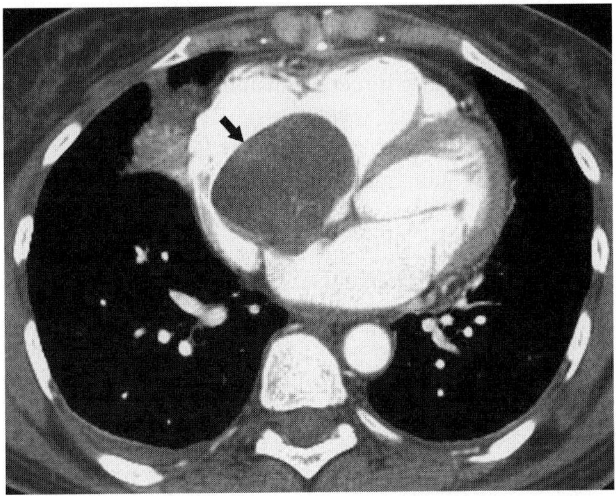

FIGURE 22.32. Multidetector CT of Right Atrial Myxoma. Contrast-enhanced multidetector CT demonstrates large right atrial myxoma (*arrow*), which was noted to prolapse through the tricuspid valve.

Malignant Tumors. Metastatic cardiac tumors are 10 to 20 times more common than primary cardiac tumors.

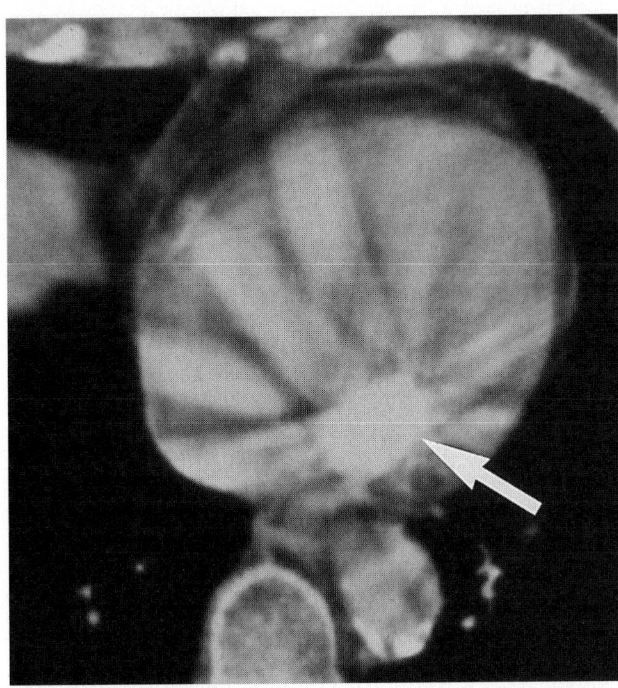

FIGURE 22.31. Left Atrial Myxoma. CT demonstrates a densely calcified mass (*arrow*) within the LA, indicative of left atrial myxoma.

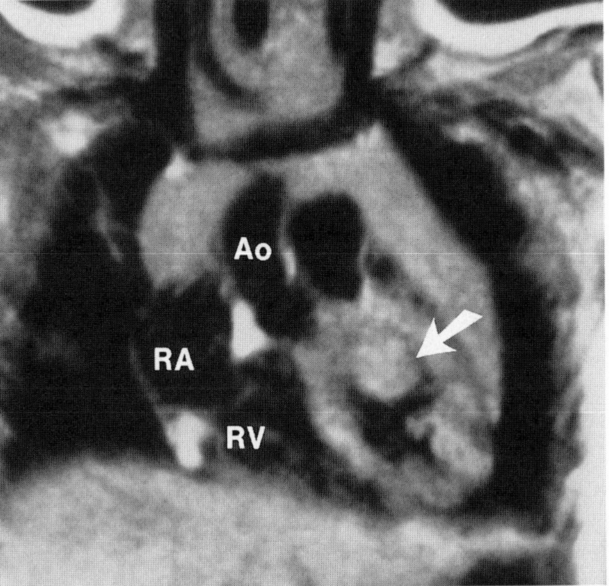

FIGURE 22.33. Left Ventricular Rhabdomyoma. Coronal spin-echo MR through the aorta (Ao) and LV demonstrates a large polypoid mass near the outflow tract of the LV (*arrow*). This patient had tuberous sclerosis, and a presumptive diagnosis of ventricular rhabdomyoma was made. Note the good delineation of the RA and RV.

Breast, lung, melanoma, and lymphoma are the most common neoplasms to metastasize to the heart. MR is excellent for detecting direct extension, intracardiac metastases, and pericardial involvement. Angiosarcoma is the most common primary malignant cardiac tumor, followed by rhabdosarcoma, liposarcoma, and other sarcomas.

PERICARDIAL DISEASE

Pericardial effusion is the most common abnormality of the pericardium. The normal pericardial stripe is 2 to 3 mm on chest radiographs and CT and less than 4 mm on MR. Plain films show thickening of the pericardial stripe or differential density sign in up to 63% of patients with pericardial effusions. The water-bottle configuration is seen in chronic effusions. Fluoroscopy shows decreased cardiac pulsations. The normal pericardium contains approximately 20 mL of fluid, whereas it takes approximately 200 mL to be detectable by plain film. Echocardiography detects very small quantities (<50 mL) of pericardial fluid, usually as a posterior sonolucent collection (Fig. 22.34). Small effusions (<100 mL) will appear as anterior and posterior sonolucent regions. Moderate-sized effusions (100 to 500 mL) demonstrate a sonolucent zone around the entire ventricle. Very large effusions (>500 mL) extend beyond the field of view and may be associated with the "swinging heart" inside the pericardium. CT is useful in detecting loculated pericardial effusions. MR may characterize the fluid. Simple serous fluid appears dark on T1WIs (probably because of fluid motion) and bright on gradient-echo images. Complicated or hemorrhagic effusions appear bright on T1WIs and dark on gradient-echo imaging (probably because of susceptibility artifact). The differential diagnosis for pericardial effusions is listed in Table 22.7.

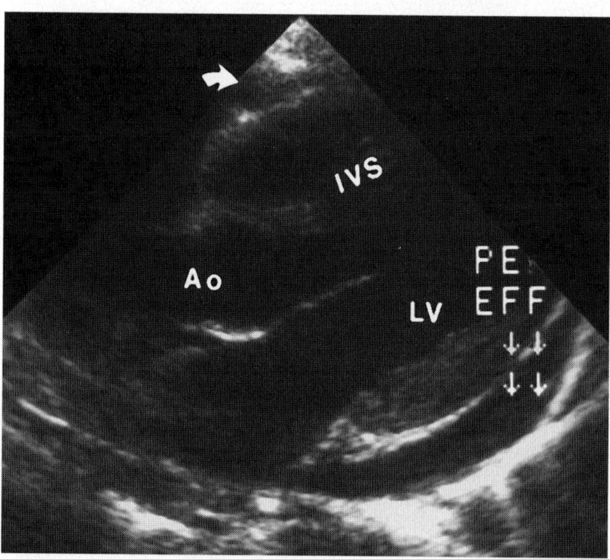

FIGURE 22.34. **Pericardial Effusion.** Longitudinal echocardiogram through the interventricular septum (IVS), aortic root (Ao), and LV demonstrates a pericardial effusion (PE EFF). A smaller anterior effusion is also noted (*arrow*).

TABLE 22.7 Causes of Pericardial Effusion

Idiopathic
Infectious
Viral (Coxsackie, echovirus, adenovirus)
Bacterial (*Staphyloccocus, Streptococcus, Haemophilus influenza*)
Fungal (*Candida, Aspergillus, Nocardia*)
Mycobacterial
Autoimmune
Systemic lupus erythematosus
Rheumatoid arthritis
Scleroderma
Dressler and postpericardiotomy syndromes
Radiation-induced
Neoplastic
Lymphoma, lung, breast metastases
Drug-induced
Procainamide, hydralazine, phenytoin
Metabolic
Uremia
Myxedema
Cholesterol
Miscellaneous
Congestive heart failure
Aortic dissection
Sarcoidosis
Pancreatitis
Trauma

Cardiac tamponade refers to cardiac chamber compression by pericardial effusion under tension, which compromises diastolic filling. *Pulsus paradoxus* describes an exaggeration of the usual drop in systolic pressure greater than 10 mm Hg during inspiration. This occurs as a result of septal shift and paradoxic septal motion during right ventricular filling. Clinical examination shows marked jugular venous distension, distant heart sounds, and a pericardial rub. The chest radiograph shows rapid enlargement of the cardiac silhouette with relatively normal-appearing vascularity. Echocardiography typically shows the septal shift, paradoxic septal motion, diastolic collapse of the RV, and cyclic collapse of the atria.

Constrictive pericardial disease is the result of fibrous or calcific thickening of the pericardium, which chronically compromises ventricular filling through restriction of cardiac motion. Age of onset is usually 30 to 50 years, and the incidence in men exceeds that in women by 3:1. The most common cause is postpericardiotomy. Other etiologies include viruses (Coxsackie B), tuberculosis, chronic renal failure, rheumatoid arthritis,

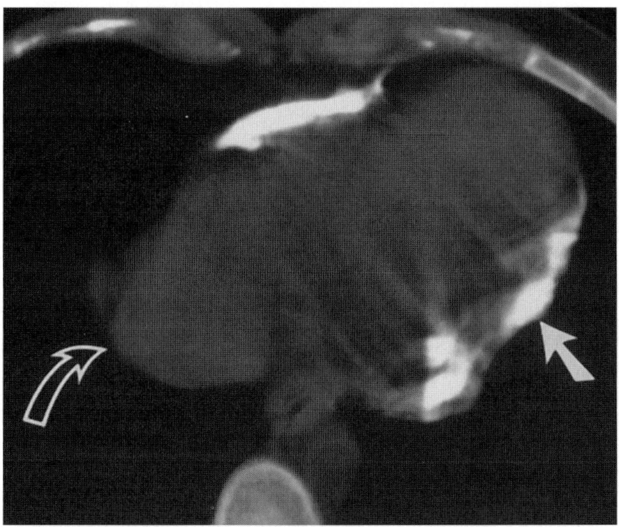

FIGURE 22.35. **Constrictive Pericarditis.** Nonenhanced CT demonstrates pericardial calcification (*closed arrow*) and a dilated inferior vena cava (*open arrow*). Note the distortion of the ventricles.

neoplastic involvement, and radiation pericarditis. Calcification is seen on radiographs in up to 50% of patients. Pleural effusions and ascites are common, and there may be an associated protein-losing enteropathy. Clinical findings include ankle edema, neck vein distension, pulsus paradoxus, pericardial diastolic knock, and ascites. Chest radiographs show normal to mildly enlarged cardiac silhouette with small atria, dilated superior and inferior vena cava and azygos vein, and a flat or straightened right heart border. Echocardiography shows thickened pericardium, abnormal septal motion, and increased left ventricular ejection fraction with small end-diastolic volume. Small effusions may be seen with "effusive constrictive pericarditis," which has both thickening and effusion.

CT is particularly good at demonstrating pericardial thickening (>3 mm) and pericardial calcification in difficult cases (Fig. 22.35). Reflux of contrast into the coronary sinus and inferior vena cava, a bowed interventricular septum, flattening of the RV, enlarged RA, ascites, and pleural effusions may also be seen. MR shows pericardial thickening (>4 mm); dilatation of the RA, inferior vena cava, and hepatic veins; sigmoid septal shift; and narrowing of the RV. Abnormal flow mechanics may also be seen in the vena cava and atria. The finding of an abnormally thick pericardium is important in differentiating constrictive pericardial disease from restrictive cardiomyopathy.

Pericardial cysts are most common in the cardiophrenic angles, with right-sided cysts more common than left-sided cysts (Fig. 22.36). They are usually asymptomatic and are more frequent in men. The cysts are attached to the parietal pericardium, are lined with epithelial or mesothelial cells, contain clear fluid, and range in size from 3 to 8 cm. They occasionally communicate with the pericardial space. CT attenuation numbers are typically 20 to 40 H and do not significantly increase with contrast enhancement. MR demonstrates characteristic low signal on T1WIs and bright signal on T2WIs. The differential diagnosis for a cardiophrenic angle mass includes pericardial cyst, fat pad, lipoma, enlarged lymph nodes, diaphragmatic hernia, and ventricular aneurysm.

Congenital absence of the pericardium (Fig. 22.37) is more common in males than females by 3:1. The age at diagnosis is infancy through age 81. Complete left-sided absence (55%) is more common than foraminal defects

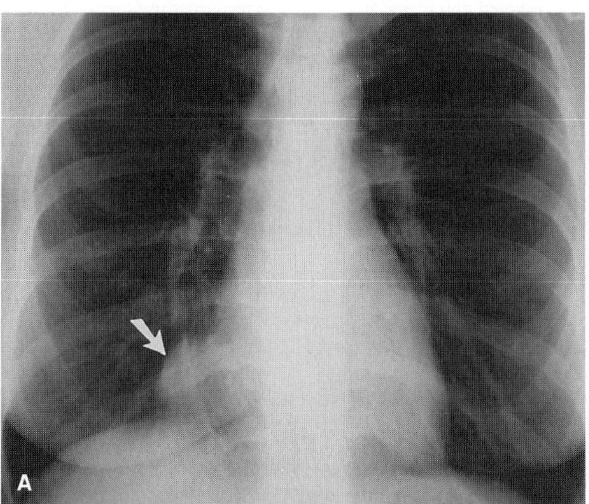

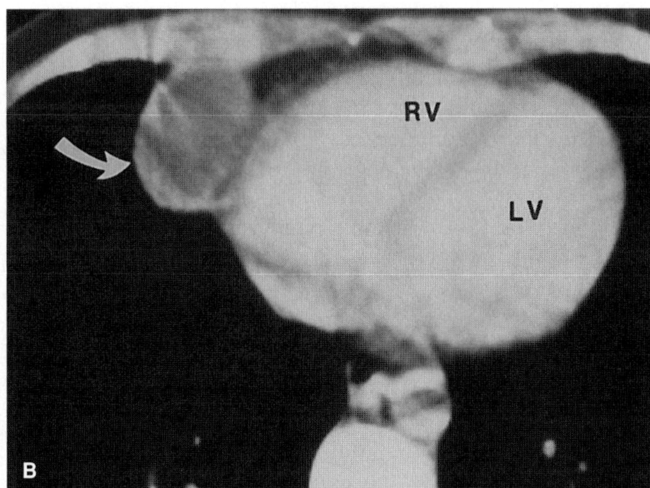

FIGURE 22.36. **Pericardial Cyst. A.** Chest radiograph demonstrates a soft tissue mass in the right cardiophrenic angle (*arrow*). **B.** Contrast-enhanced CT demonstrates near water density within the nonenhancing mass in the cardiophrenic angle, consistent with pericardial cyst.

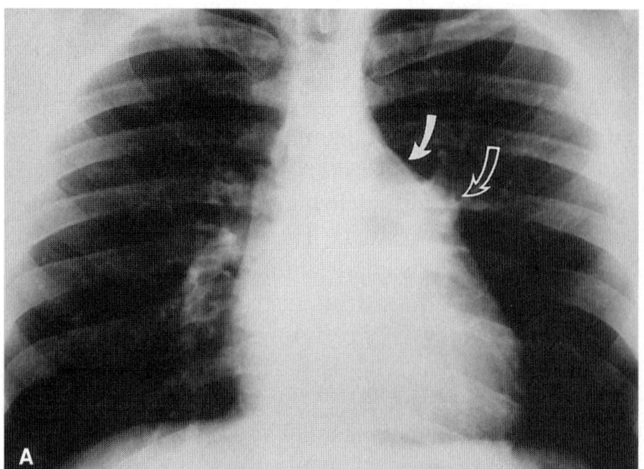

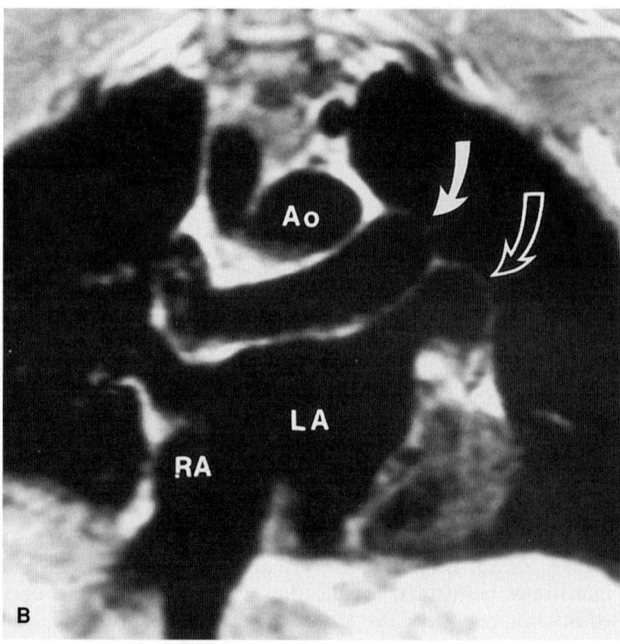

FIGURE 22.37. **Partial Absence of the Pericardium. A.** Chest radiograph demonstrates a prominence of the main pulmonary artery (*closed arrow*) and an unusual bulge along the left heart border (*open arrow*). **B.** Coronal spin-echo MR confirms enlargement of the main pulmonary artery (*closed arrow*) and shows herniation of the left atrial appendage (*open arrow*). Ao, ascending aorta.

(35%) or total absence (10%). Associated conditions include bronchogenic cysts, ventricular septal defects, diaphragmatic hernias, and sequestrations. With complete absence, the heart is shifted toward the left, with a prominent bulge of the right ventricular outflow tract, main pulmonary artery, and left atrial appendage. Insinuation of the lung into the anteroposterior window and beneath the heart is characteristic. Decubitus views show a widely swinging cardiac silhouette. Partial absence of the pericardium risks strangulation of cardiac structures, with the possibility of sudden death. Surgical closure of partial defects is usually recommended.

SUGGESTED READINGS

Becker CR, Jakobs TF, Aydemir S, et al. Helical and single-slice conventional CT versus electron beam CT for the quantification of coronary artery calcification. AJR Am J Roentgenol 2000;174:543–547.

Bogaert J, Dymarkowski S, Taylor AM, eds. Clinical Cardiac MRI. Berlin, New York: Springer-Verlag, 2005.

Budoff MJ, Achenbach S, Duerinckx A. Clinical utility of computed tomography and magnetic resonance techniques for noninvasive coronary angiography. J Am Coll Cardiol 2003;42(11):1867–1878.

DePuey EG, Berman DS, Garcia EV. Cardiac SPECT Imaging. 2nd ed. Philadelphia: Lippincott Williams & Wilkins, 2001.

Eisenberg RL. Chest and Cardiac Imaging. New York: Raven Press, 1993.

Feigenbaum H, Armstrong WF, Ryan T. Echocardiography. 6th ed. Philadelphia: Lippincott Williams & Wilkins, 2004.

Gedgaudas E, Moffer JH, Castaneda-Zuniga WR, Amplatz K. Cardiovascular Radiology. Philadelphia: WB Saunders, 1985.

Higgins CB. Essentials of Cardiac Radiology and Imaging. Philadelphia: JB Lippincott, 1992.

Kelley MJ, ed. Chest Radiography for the Cardiologist. Philadelphia: WB Saunders, 1983. Cardiol Clin 1(4):543–750.

Kubicka RA, Smith C. How to interpret coronary arteriograms. Radiographics 1986;6:661–701.

Lardo A, Chronos NA, Fayad ZA. Cardiovascular Magnetic Resonance: Established and Emerging Applications. London: Martin Dunitz; Independence, KY: Taylor and Francis, 2003.

Lawler LP, Pannu HK, Fishman EK. MDCT evaluation of the coronary arteries, 2004: how we do it—data acquisition, postprocessing, display and interpretation. AJR Am J Roentgenol 2004;184:1402–1412.

Leschka S, Alkadhi H, Plass A, et al. Accuracy of MSCT coronary angiography with 64-slice technology: first experience. Eur Heart J 2005;26(15):1482–1487.

Lipton MJ, Boxt LM, eds. Cardiac imaging. Radiol Clin North Am 2004;42:487–697.

Marcus ML, Schelbert HR, Skorton DJ, Wolf GL. Cardiac Imaging—A Companion to Braunwald's Heart Disease. Philadelphia: WB Saunders, 1991.

Miller SW. Cardiac Imaging: The Requisites. 2nd ed. Philadelphia: Elsevier Mosby, 2005.

Netter FH. Atlas of Human Anatomy. The CIBA Collection of Medical Illustrations. West Caldwell, NJ: CIBA-Geigy Corp, 1989.

Oudkerk M. Coronary Radiology. New York: Springer-Verlag, 2004.

Reddy GP, Higgins CB, Chao KH, Tung PP. Cardiac MR Imaging. CD-ROM. Philadelphia: Lippincott Williams & Wilkins, 2001.

Rensing BJ, Serruys PW, de Feyter PM. CT-based coronary angiography. J Invasive Cardiol 2000;12(1):23–24.

Schoepf UJ, Becker CR, Ohnesorge BM, Yucel EK. CT of coronary artery disease. Radiology 2004;232:18–37.

Schoepf UJ, Schoepf UJ. CT of the Heart: Principles and Applications. Totowa, NJ: Human Press, 2004.
Schoenhagen P, Halliburton SS, Stillman AE, et al. Noninvasive imaging of coronary arteries: current and future role of multi-detector row CT. Radiology 2004;232:7–17.
Stanford W, Thompson BH. Imaging of coronary artery calcification. Its importance in assessing atherosclerotic disease. Radiol Clin North Am 1999;37:257–272.
Stanford W, Thompson BH, Burns, TL, et al. Coronary artery calcium quantification at multi-detector row helical CT versus electron-beam CT. Radiology 2004;230:397–402.
Webb RB, Higgins CB. Thoracic Imaging: Pulmonary and Cardiovascular Radiology. Philadelphia: Lippincott Williams & Wilkins, 2005.
Zaret BL, Beller GA. Clinical Nuclear Cardiology. 3rd ed. Philadelphia: Elsevier Mosby, 2004.
Zipes DP, et al. eds. Braunwald's Heart Disease: A Textbook of Cardiovascular Medicine. 7th ed. Philadelphia: Elsevier Saunders, 2004.

Chapter 23

Cardiac MRI

Christopher M. Kramer

Ischemic Heart Disease

Cardiomyopathies

Pericardial Disease

Valvular Heart Disease

Congenital Heart Disease

Cardiac and Paracardiac Masses

Pulmonary Veins

Limitations/Safety

Because of advances in both technology and acquisition techniques, cardiovascular MR (CMR) has evolved rapidly, especially over the last decade. With the rising prevalence of coronary artery disease (CAD) and heart failure, the mounting enthusiasm for CMR-based cardiac assessment is readily appreciated. With one examination, LV structure, function at rest and under stress, perfusion, and viability can be evaluated with a high degree of precision while avoiding the potentially harmful effects of ionizing radiation and nephrotoxic contrast agents. Further developments are needed to bring CMR coronary arteriography into the clinical routine. Atherosclerotic plaque imaging is a growing research application that will become clinically useful with time. Other common indications for CMR will be reviewed, including imaging of cardiomyopathies, pericardial disease, valvular heart disease, congenital heart disease, cardiac masses, and pulmonary veins.

ISCHEMIC HEART DISEASE

Global Structure and Function at Rest. In patients with congestive heart failure, abnormalities in ventricular structure and function, whether characterized by visual inspection or measurement of ejection fraction, mass, or volumes, are powerful predictors of prognosis and have important therapeutic implications. Careful visual assessment of LV function by an experienced clinician is adequate in most clinical scenarios, with the caveat that great care must be taken to analyze each segment. Although a number of strategies have been devised for partitioning the myocardium, the American Heart Association currently endorses the use of a 17-sector model divided on the basis of a normal coronary distribution. For assessment of LV function with CMR, images are obtained in short-axis views covering the LV from apex to base as well as two-chamber, three-chamber, and four-chamber orientations (Fig. 23.1) to ensure visualization of all segments.

Steady-state free precession (SSFP) cine imaging is currently the optimal technique for visually assessing LV function. SSFP, in contrast to older gradient echo cine techniques, does not rely on the inflow of unsaturated spins to create contrast between the LV cavity and the endocardium. Because SSFP images are flow independent, endocardial border detection is significantly enhanced. Furthermore, SSFP provides excellent spatial and temporal resolution and a high signal-to-noise ratio, and it requires relatively short breath-holding times.

Because of its high spatial resolution, reproducibility, and 3D data that require the operator to make no geometric assumptions, CMR has evolved into the reference standard for measuring mass, chamber volumes, and ejection fraction. Because of the exceptional contrast generated between the myocardium and blood pool (Fig. 23.1), CMR enables the operator to precisely delineate both the endocardial and epicardial borders. SSFP is the favored technique for assessing ventricular dimensions. The flow-independent contrast facilitates the accurate demarcation of border contours around the papillary muscles and ventricular trabeculations, where blood pooling typically

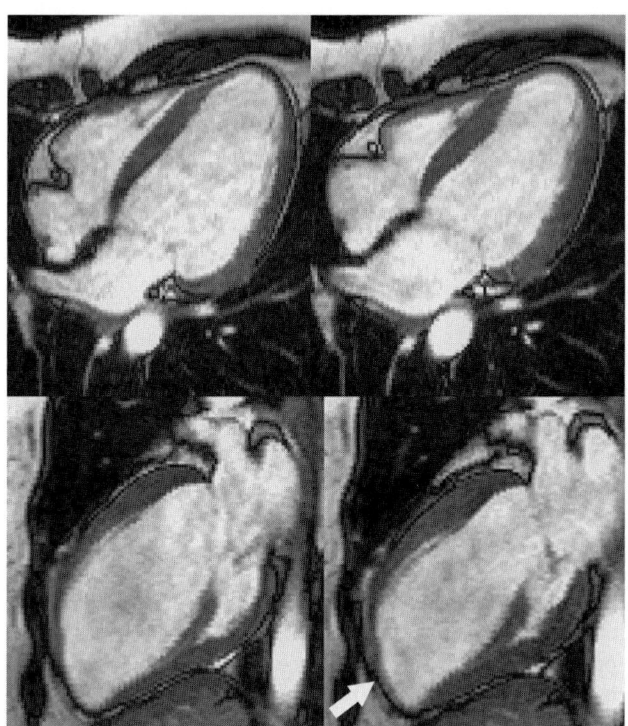

FIGURE 23.1. **LV Function.** Steady-state free precession images in two standard planes at different phases in the cardiac cycle in a patient with a prior anterior myocardial infarction (MI). The upper panels demonstrate a four-chamber long-axis image at end-diastole on the left and end-systole on the right. Note the thinned, distal anterior wall and apex (*arrow*) with reduced wall thickening during systole, which are suggestive of prior MI in that region.

occurs, particularly in patients with low-flow states such as congestive heart failure.

To calculate LV ejection fraction, mass, and volume, short-axis slices stacked from apex to base of the LV are acquired throughout the cardiac cycle, and the epicardial and endocardial contours are carefully outlined at end-diastole and end-systole. Most CMR systems have specialized software with automated border detection to assist the operator, but the technology remains limited for patients with non-geometric configurations and in those with prominent papillary muscles or heavy trabeculations. Determination of the slice area, distance between slices, slice thickness, and both end-systolic and end-diastolic volumes can then be performed using Simpson's Rule. Once these values are obtained, stroke volume (end-diastolic volume – end-systolic volume) and ejection fraction (systolic volume/end-diastolic volume × 100%) are readily measured. Myocardial mass can then be calculated by dividing the density of myocardium (1.05 g/cm^3) by the measured LV volume. The same techniques can be applied to the RV, but because of the complex 3D structure of this chamber and heavy trabeculations, the value of currently available automated border detection software is limited.

MR flow velocity mapping, a technique that can quantify flow velocity and direction on a per-pixel basis, can also be used to quantify global cardiac function. After an imaging plane is selected perpendicular to flow, velocities are acquired in the through-plane direction at multiple points in the cardiac cycle. Through summation of velocities in a selected portion of the proximal aorta, stroke volume and cardiac output can then be determined.

Regional Myocardial Function. Conventional techniques for assessing ventricular motion rely primarily on evaluating motion of the endocardial service. These methods are insensitive to the deformation within the myocardium as well as translation and torsion during contraction and relaxation. Early efforts to characterize this dynamic 3D geometry provided insight into the complexities of cardiac motion but required implantation of radiopaque markers within the myocardium. *Myocardial tagging* (Fig. 23.2) places virtual markers within the heart through the manipulation of the magnetic field to facilitate visualization and quantification of regional function, including the rotational and translational motion that has been previously difficult to analyze. CMR is currently the *only* noninvasive technique with this capability. To generate a tagged sequence, a grid consisting of nulled orthogonal lines is applied to the heart at end-diastole by altering the local magnetization with narrow and radiofrequency pulses. Because saturated rows of protons comprise this grid structure, the tagging is "embedded" in the tissue and its motion can be reliably tracked throughout the cardiac cycle. Intramural deformation can be visualized and the strain quantified at various sites within the myocardium.

Strain analysis is more accurate than planar wall thickening for detecting regional myocardial dysfunction, as this technique takes into account the motion of a selected segment in all directions simultaneously. Quantification of strain with tagged CMR can be performed with a high degree of precision, allowing for separation of the subendocardial, midmyocardial, and subepicardial layers. Although a precise assessment of 3D LV function can be achieved with this technique, the data analysis remains cumbersome and time consuming. New methods of image acquisition and postprocessing analysis are currently under investigation, such as HARP (harmonic phase) and DENSE (displacement encoding with stimulated echoes), both of which allow more rapid analysis. Although it is not ready for routine clinical application, CMR strain imaging may become the diagnostic reference standard of the future, one that will enhance our ability to identify subtle abnormalities in function during stress testing and allow for earlier detection of disease states.

Myocardial tagging techniques have already enabled researchers to achieve a better understanding of cardiac function in both normal and diseased states. Tagging has characterized regional myocardial dysfunction in acute and chronic myocardial infarction (MI), hypertrophic

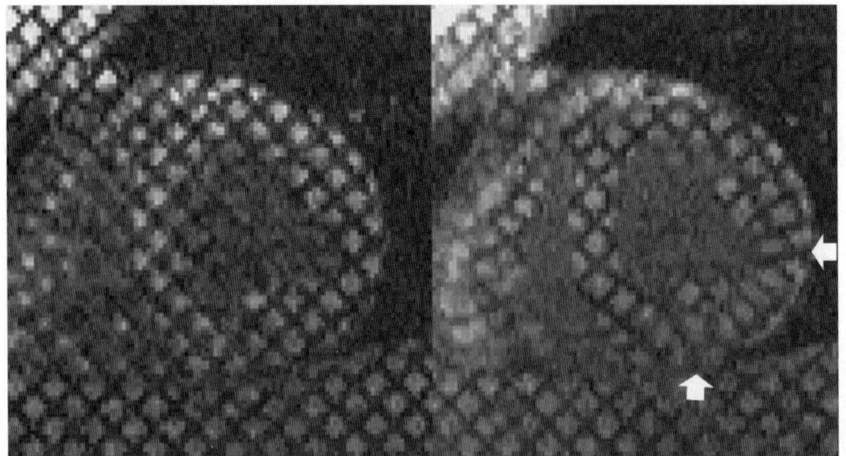

FIGURE 23.2. **Myocardial Tagging.** This technique is shown in a patient on day 3 after anterior myocardial infarction. The left panel represents a short-axis midventricular tagged image at end-diastole, while the right panel depicts the end-systolic frame at the same location. Because the tags (*dark stripes*) remain embedded within the tissue throughout the cardiac cycle, deformation can be tracked and the strain quantified. Note the normal deformation in the posterolateral wall (3:00 to 6:00 in the image) (*arrows*) and the reduced deformation in the anterior wall.

cardiomyopathy, valvular heart disease, and pulmonary hypertension. Furthermore, tagging has facilitated the detailed analysis of the local functional response of the myocardium to a number of therapies for congestive heart failure, including pharmacologic agents and surgical reduction treatments.

The role of tagging in ischemic heart disease is being established. In a recent study of 211 consecutive patients with chest pain, dobutamine CMR (DCMR) with tagging was shown to be superior to nontagged sequences for detection of significant coronary lesions with a 96% sensitivity. Among the patients with normal dobutamine CMR and no resting wall motion abnormalities, the event free survival after 17 months was 98%. Dobutamine CMR tagging has also been demonstrated to be equivalent to dobutamine stress echo in predicting functional improvement following MI with reperfusion. More recently, tagged CMR images were employed to assess timing of cardiac contraction and asynchrony in candidates for biventricular pacing.

Global Function: Stress. Dobutamine is the drug most commonly administered when performing stress CMR because of its proven efficacy in stress echocardiography (DSE). Dobutamine increases myocardial oxygen demand through its potent chronotropic and ionotropic effects. In a territory supplied by a stenotic coronary artery, inadequate blood flow is available to compensate for increased demand, resulting in ischemia. This manifests visually as a segmental wall motion abnormality, which is a reliable sign of ischemia that precedes both angina and electrocardiographic changes. Side effects of dobutamine infusion are common but typically mild, and the test is generally well tolerated, even by elderly patients. Although a number of studies have confirmed the safety and efficacy of DSE for diagnosing CAD, suboptimal image quality remains a frequently encountered drawback, occurring in up to 15% of patients studied, although problems are less common when contrast is used for LV cavity opacification (LVO).

DCMR compares favorably to DSE. DCMR requires no imaging window, which results in high-quality reproducible images, irrespective of the operator or particular patient (Fig. 23.3). Furthermore, slice position can be better reproduced during the study, ensuring that the same regions are compared both at rest and during stress.

An older study using a breath-hold gradient-echo cine technique compared high-dose DCMR and DSE in a group of 208 consecutive patients. The accuracy of DCMR in detecting ischemia was superior to that seen with second-harmonic DSE without LVO (86% versus 73%), primarily because of superior image quality. Another study enrolled 153 patients with inadequate windows by second-harmonic DSE (without LVO) and performed DCMR with both sensitivity and specificity >80%. DCMR was able to accurately diagnose ischemia in patients who were poor candidates for DSE. Subsequent follow-up demonstrated that the results could be used to predict subsequent MI and cardiovascular death.

Recently, DCMR, adenosine stress-function CMR, and adenosine first-pass perfusion were compared in 79 consecutive patients with suspected or known CAD who were scheduled for coronary angiography. Using quantitative coronary angiography as the gold standard, the sensitivity and specificity of DCMR, adenosine stress-function CMR, and adenosine magnetic resonance first-pass perfusion (MRFP) was 89% and 80%, 40% and 96%, and 91% and 62%, respectively. This study underscores the superior accuracy of dobutamine over adenosine for functional stress testing and relative advantages in specificity compared to stress-perfusion imaging.

Despite the apparent superiority of DCMR, widespread application has yet to be realized. In regard to safety, as long as online assessment of ventricular function during dobutamine infusion is used, the inability to reliably interpret electrocardiogram (ECG) recordings during testing is not a problem, since wall motion abnormalities precede ECG changes in the ischemic cascade. With respect

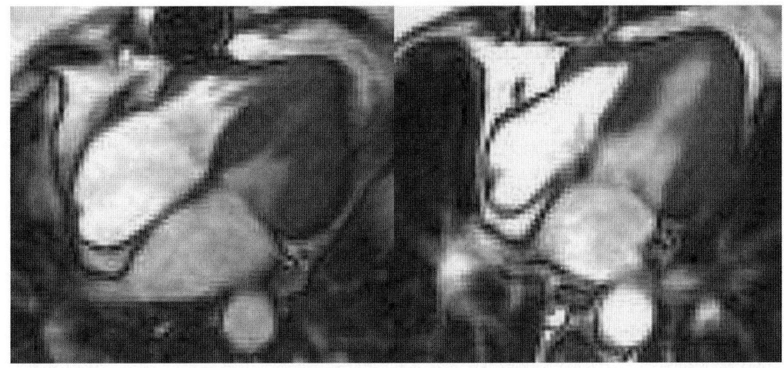

FIGURE 23.3. **Dobutamine Cardiac MR Stress Test.** Two end-systolic steady-state free precession four-chamber long-axis image frames from a dobutamine cardiac MR stress test in a patient with chest pain 10 years following left internal mammary bypass graft to the left anterior descending artery. The left frame is at a low dose of dobutamine (10 μg/kg/min) and demonstrated cavity obliteration at end-systole, implying normal systolic function. The right frame is during peak dobutamine dose (40 μg/kg/min) at a heart rate of 150 beats per minute. At peak dobutamine, note the lack of wall thickening in the apical septum consistent with disease in the bypass graft that was proven at subsequent catheterization.

to patient monitoring, all precautions observed with other modalities are mandatory with DCMR, including presence of trained clinicians and MR-compatible monitoring equipment. In case of a medical emergency, staff can provide critical life support while the patient is being moved out of the magnetic environment, a procedure that can be executed in less than 30 seconds. Significant complications from dobutamine infusion can be expected to occur in up to 0.6% of patients and include MI, sustained ventricular tachycardia, and even death. In a recent review of 1,035 consecutive patients who underwent DCMR, the only major complication consisted of one patient developing sustained ventricular tachycardia, which was successfully cardioverted.

Myocardial Perfusion. Stress-perfusion nuclear imaging is commonly performed in patients with suspected or known CAD. SPECT is the noninvasive technique most frequently employed to analyze myocardial perfusion, and on a more limited scale, PET. Although both modalities are well validated, they are hampered by limited spatial resolution, the potential risks of radiation exposure, and an inability to reliably detect subendocardial perfusion defects. First described in humans in 1992, stress magnetic resonance first-pass perfusion (MRFP) has generated a substantial amount of interest because of its favorable spatial resolution in comparison to SPECT and PET.

MRFP is performed using a T1W sequence to visualize a gadolinium-based contrast agent in transit through the heart. Following peripheral injection, the contrast is detected against the background of nulled myocardium, first in the right-sided chambers, then opacifying the left-sided cavities. The myocardium begins to enhance when the contrast reaches the ascending aorta and coronary ostia, with a peak in enhancement approximately 10 heartbeats after the LV opacifies (Fig. 23.4). Signal intensity correlates with contrast concentration. Because passage of this extracellular agent can occur in as little as 5 to 10 seconds during hyperemic conditions, rapid acquisition of images is essential, and numerous techniques to improve speed have

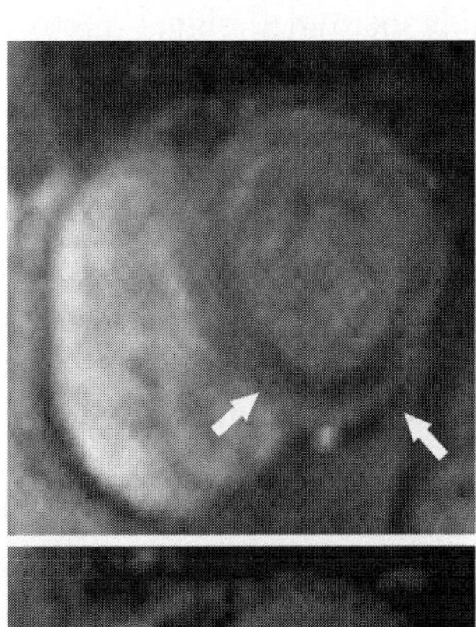

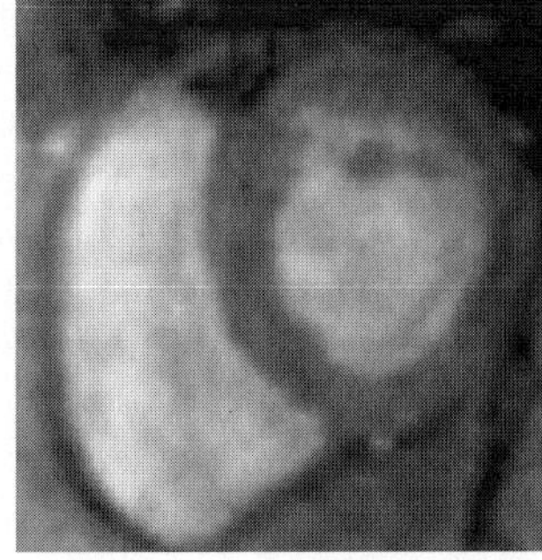

FIGURE 23.4. **MR First-Pass Perfusion.** First-pass gadolinium-enhanced hybrid gradient-echo/echo planar perfusion images in a basal short-axis plane following adenosine stress (*upper panel*) and at rest (*lower panel*) demonstrating a reversible perfusion defect in the inferior wall (5:00 to 7:00 in the image) (*arrows*). The patient was later shown to have a 99% distal right coronary artery stenosis at cardiac catheterization.

been employed. With correct patient breath-holding and proper ECG gating, a high degree of spatial resolution is preserved.

MRFP analysis relies on time-intensity curves and can be performed in a quantitative, semiquantitative, or qualitative fashion. Because the contrast agents rapidly redistribute into the extracellular space, analysis is limited to the initial upslope in the time-intensity curves, which has been shown to correlate well with measures of microsphere blood flow. In clinical practice, qualitative analysis by an experienced clinician is generally performed and relies on observer detection of regional differences in signal intensity over time. Studies evaluating the sensitivity and specificity of visual detection of perfusion defects have been encouraging.

Occlusive CAD results in a reduction in flow reserve, a characteristic feature that can be detected before either clinical symptoms or LV dysfunction are generally evident. In a viable myocardial territory supplied by a 70% stenotic coronary artery, vasodilated flow is reduced by approximately 50% when compared to flow in segments subtended by a normal coronary artery. Hence, any technique employed to detect lesions of 70% or greater must be able to differentiate at least a twofold difference in perfusion.

Validation of MRFP in humans has been performed in a series of small clinical studies employing a variety of contrast agents, analysis techniques, and reference standards. One recent study examined signal-intensity time curves in both patients and controls following dipyridamole infusion and bolus injection of gadolinium diethylenetriaminepentaacetate (Gd-DTPA). Using a linear fit to determine the upslope, the researchers defined a cutoff value between normal and ischemic myocardial segments. Diagnostic accuracy was 87% and interobserver agreement was high (0.96). In another study of 48 patients, MRFP, (13)N-ammonia PET, and quantitative coronary angiography were performed. During first pass of contrast, signal-intensity up-slopes were calculated in 32 myocardial sectors. Analysis of the subendocardial upslope data showed sensitivity and specificity of 91% and 94%, respectively, when compared to PET imaging. When compared to quantitative angiography, sensitivity and specificity were lower but were still >85%. In another study of 84 patients referred for diagnostic coronary angiography, first-pass contrast-enhanced CMR during adenosine vasodilatation was performed. Myocardial perfusion reserve index was determined from the upslope of signal intensity within the myocardium. The best results were achieved when the innermost slices were evaluated; diagnostic accuracy using this approach was 89%.

One of the more novel aspects of MRFP is that its superior spatial resolution allows for the discrimination of perfusion across layers in the same myocardial segment. Investigators have found transmural perfusion analysis useful in a number of clinical scenarios, including transplant arteriopathy, syndrome X, and transmyocardial laser revascularization. MRFP is already a powerful tool, with its capacity to detect perfusion abnormalities isolated to the endocardium, discern transmural flow gradients, and identify reductions in flow reserve that are undetectable with radionuclide imaging. With optimization of imaging sequences, development of new intravascular contrast agents, and imaging at higher field strengths, MRFP has tremendous potential for the detection of CAD.

Myocardial Viability: Contractile Reserve. Viable cardiac myocytes are alive and capable of recovery of function, while nonviability denotes cell death or irreversible myocyte damage. The identification of *viable* myocardium in patients with chronic LV dysfunction is of significant clinical relevance. With restoration of adequate blood flow, viable segments have the potential for improvement in contractile function. The prognosis of patients with viability is substantially improved with revascularization. Alternatively, patients without viability who are revascularized have higher perioperative morbidity and worse long-term outcomes. Because routine histopathologic examination of cellular elements is impractical, a number of techniques have been developed and proven useful for measuring indirect parameters of viability. Because of its ability to evaluate a number of markers proven to predict viability, CMR is rapidly becoming established as the test of choice.

The demonstration of contractile reserve is an established predictor of myocardial viability. As with echocardiography, CMR assessment of contractile reserve is performed using infusion of low dose dobutamine. Low-dose DCMR has been compared to fluorodeoxyglucose PET (FDG-PET) in 35 patients with chronic MI and segmental LV dysfunction. With end-diastolic wall thickness and improvement in systolic thickening used as markers of viability, CMR had a sensitivity, specificity, and diagnostic accuracy of 88%, 87%, and 92%, respectively, when compared to FDG-PET. When this technique was used to predict the improvement in LV function following revascularization, systolic thickening by CMR had a sensitivity and specificity of 89% and 92% for predicting recovery. Furthermore, segments that failed to improve following revascularization had a significantly lower diastolic wall thickness (6 mm versus 9.8 mm) than those that showed functional improvement. Echo-based studies have corroborated the value of end-diastolic wall thickness in predicting viability.

The utility of incorporating tagged sequences into the assessment of contractile reserve has also been demonstrated. Both DSE and low-dose DCMR with tagging were performed in a study of 22 patients with acute MI following reperfusion therapy (day 3 ± 1). At 8 weeks, both echocardiography and CMR with tagging were performed at rest to evaluate for functional recovery. Using echo as the gold standard, the overall accuracy of DSE and low-dose DCMR with tagging was similar. Recent studies of hibernating myocardium prior to and after multivessel revascularization using tagged low-dose dobutamine have demonstrated that half of dysfunctional segments recover resting function, and of the remainder, half demonstrate rest dysfunction but contractile reserve. Half of these latter segments were found to have recovered rest function when examined 3 years after revascularization.

Myocardial Viability: Infarct Imaging. Late contrast-enhanced CMR (ce-CMR) using Gd-DTPA, an extracellular/interstitial contrast agent, has proven to be a valuable tool in identifying MI and predicting the potential of infarcted myocardium to recover following revascularization (Fig. 23.5). In regions of infarction, T1 relaxation is enhanced as a consequence of increased regional uptake and retention of contrast. This phenomenon is thought to occur within infarcted zones because of increased volume of distribution as well as delayed washout of contrast. Animal studies have demonstrated that the spatial extent of late contrast enhancement on CMR very closely mirrors the distribution of myocyte necrosis early post-MI and that of collagenous scar seen at 8 weeks. Furthermore, studies have shown that in regions of the heart subjected to *reversible* injury, the retention of contrast does *not* occur. In reality, zones of ventricular dysfunction typically consist of a combination of reversibly injured (hibernating or stunned) and irreversibly injured (infarcted) myocardium.

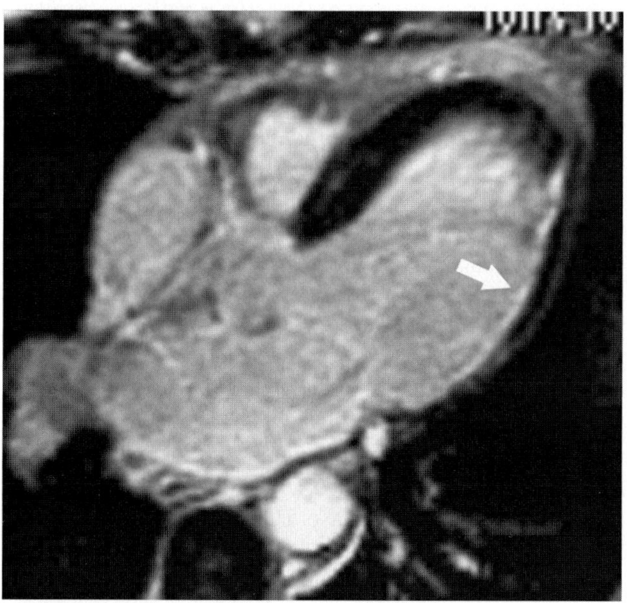

FIGURE 23.5. **Myocardial Infarction.** Contrast-enhanced inversion-recovery gradient-echo image in a four-chamber long-axis plane 10 minutes following gadolinium infusion at 0.2 mM/kg in a patient with a prior lateral wall infarction. Note the area of bright enhancement (*arrow*) in the lateral wall that subtends the inner 50% of the wall.

The power of ce-CMR is its ability to distinguish these two states within the same segment of myocardium, a feat that cannot be replicated with other techniques.

The ability of ce-CMR to identify and characterize myocardial scar has been directly compared to both SPECT and PET. In a study of 91 patients with suspected or known CAD, both ce-CMR and SPECT imaging were performed to determine the extent, location, and size of infarct scarring. Although SPECT correctly identified all patients with transmural or near-transmural scar seen on ce-CMR, SPECT failed to correctly identify nearly half of those with subendocardial infarction. Another study compared ce-CMR to PET in 31 patients with ischemic cardiomyopathy. Infarct mass correlated well between the two modalities, but ce-CMR more frequently identified scar than PET, again reflecting its superior spatial resolution.

In 2000, a landmark study was published demonstrating the utility of ce-CMR for identifying myocardial viability. Fifty patients scheduled to undergo revascularization procedures were recruited, 40 of whom had some region of hyperenhancement. Of the 2,093 myocardial segments analyzed, 804 demonstrated abnormal contractility. The likelihood of functional recovery strongly correlated with the transmural extent of scar. In patients with no hyperenhancement, 78% of segments demonstrated recovery of function. In contrast, only 1 of 58 segments with >75% transmural extent showed any improvement following revascularization, demonstrating the powerful negative predictive value of this finding. Within zones that exhibited 51% to 75% hyperenhancement, only 10% improved following revascularization. Even in regions with akinesis or dyskinesis prior to revascularization, *lack* of hyperenhancement predicted functional recovery in 100% of cases. Several subsequent studies have validated this approach for predicting recovery of function after revascularization. Some controversy persists as to which test is best for identifying viability among CMR-based techniques. A recently completed study compared the performance of low-dose DCMR with ce-CMR in predicting viability. Although no difference was appreciated in identifying viability in segments without hyperenhancement or those with scar ≥75%, DCMR was superior in predicting recovery in zones demonstrating between 1% and 74% transmural scar by late enhancement. The performance of late enhancement varied greatly depending on the cutoff values used to define viability. Ultimately, complementary use of DCMR and ce-CMR may prove to be the optimal strategy for defining viability. Although some evidence suggests that revascularization confers clinical benefits irrespective of systolic functional recovery, this hypothesis remains untested at present.

As our understanding of the nature and importance of late contrast enhancement has evolved, investigators have found that more than just the size and extent of enhanced regions have significance. Many large acute

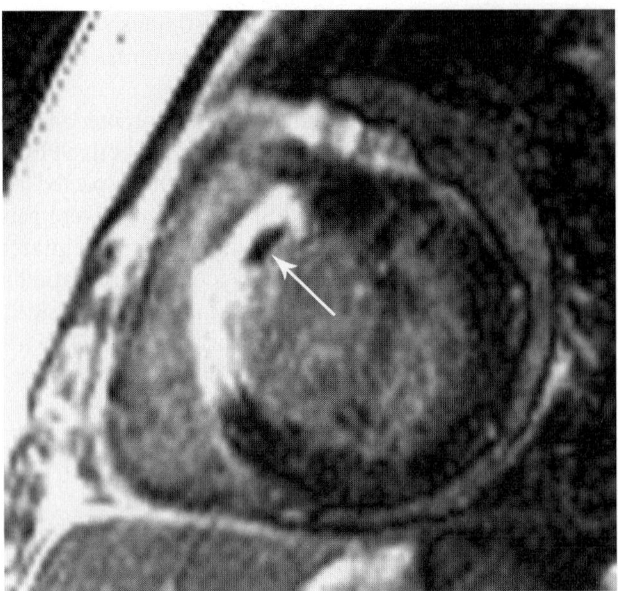

FIGURE 23.6. **Microvascular Obstruction.** Short-axis late contrast-enhanced image using an inversion-recovery gradient-echo sequence 10 minutes following gadolinium infusion at 0.2 mM/kg shows infarct scar in the septum with a small hypoenhanced zone, which is consistent with microvascular obstruction (*arrow*). This region would be deemed nonviable based on the transmural extent of hyperenhancement and presence of microvascular obstruction.

infarcts demonstrate hypoenhanced regions at the core of hyperenhanced zones, which represent areas of microvascular obstruction (Fig. 23.6). The presence of microvascular obstruction correlates strongly with infarct size and identifies regions that are truly nonviable. Moreover, microvascular obstruction has been shown to be a powerful predictor of lack of functional recovery in the infarct region and poor cardiovascular outcome in the patient post-MI. In a recent study of 110 patients post-MI, microvascular obstruction was a predictor of LV remodeling, as defined by an increase in end-diastolic volume, and was a more powerful predictor of survival than either ejection fraction or infarct size.

Coronary Arteriography. Because about 35% of patients referred for their first invasive x-ray angiogram have normal epicardial coronary arteries, an appealing role for CMR in ischemic heart disease would be the noninvasive assessment of the coronary arteries with high temporal and spatial resolution, during relatively short acquisition times. Coronary magnetic resonance angiography (CMRA) has not matured to that point yet, but substantial improvements have been achieved over the past few years. Given the small size, tortuous course, and motion of the coronary arteries, several technical challenges must be overcome to obtain images of diagnostic quality. Best in-plane resolution for CMRA is about 600 to 900 μm, which is still about twice the pixel size available in conventional angiography. Compensation for cardiac and coronary arterial motion is achieved by using short acquisition times and optimizing the timing of acquisition in middiastole, when cardiac motion is least. Respiratory motion correction can be achieved by several different techniques. The advantages of conventional breath-holding techniques are shorter acquisition times and the freedom to repeat the acquisition if the images are suboptimal, but the shorter acquisition time results in lower signal-to-noise ratio. The signal-to-noise ratio can be greatly improved upon by longer acquisition times, but this requires respiratory compensation to avoid blurring of the images. The most commonly used techniques rely on diaphragmatic navigators, in which the lung-diaphragm interface is tracked and is used to predict the motion and position of the coronary arteries. Using this method, each acquisition takes about 5 to 10 minutes, with the current navigator efficiency of 30% to 50% during free breathing.

CMRA has evolved since the early 1990s when two-dimensional fat-suppressed breath-hold techniques held early promise, with sensitivity and specificity of 90% and 92%, respectively, but fell prey to less optimal results in later studies. Several new approaches are in development in an attempt to optimize accuracy. Three-dimensional approaches are most promising; the one used most frequently is a navigator echo technique that tracks diaphragmatic motion and acquires images when the diaphragm is in a specified position. A recent multicenter study of a T_2-preparatory pulse with a gradient-echo 3D sequence and navigator echoes showed some promise, with an overall accuracy of 72%. Results in patients with left main or three-vessel CAD were quite good, with 100% sensitivity, 85% specificity, and 87% accuracy. However, the specificity on an individual vessel basis remained inadequate for screening purposes, ranging from 52% to 72% in the three major coronary vessels.

The advent of high-field (3T) coronary imaging offers enhanced image quality and resolution (Fig. 23.7) that may allow improved accuracy for detection of CAD, although large patient studies have not been performed to date using these higher field strengths.

In clinical practice, CMRA is used to assess anomalous coronary arteries, where it has been shown to be equivalent or superior to conventional coronary angiography. Other clinical applications include the evaluation of patients with Kawasaki disease. Detection of aneurysm and thrombus within aneurysms has been demonstrated with CMRA, and serial MRA avoids the risk of radiation exposure in children with Kawasaki disease.

Another clinical application of CMRA is the imaging of bypass grafts, both arterial and venous. Navigator-gated 3D CMRA has been shown to be quite accurate for identifying occlusion or stenosis. In one study of 56 vein grafts, the area under the curve by receiver-operator characteristic

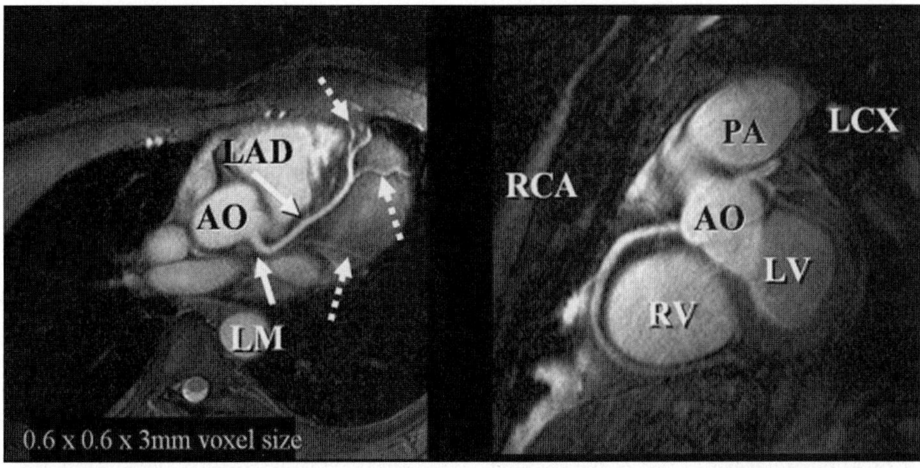

FIGURE 23.7. **Coronary MR Angiography.** Shown are curved multiplanar reformats of a three-dimensional, navigator-gated, T2-prepared gradient-echo coronary MR angiogram performed at 3.0 Tesla in a healthy volunteer. The image on the left demonstrates normal left main artery (LM, *arrow*) and left anterior descending artery (LAD, *arrow*) at high spatial resolution (0.6 × 0.6 × 3 mm voxel size) that allows visualization of diagonal and septal branches (*broken arrows*). The image on the right demonstrates the right coronary artery (RCA). AO, aorta; RV, right ventricle; LV, left ventricle; PA, pulmonary artery; LCX, left circumflex. (From Flamm SD, Muthupillai R. Coronary artery magnetic resonance angiography. J Magn Reson Imaging 2004;19:686–709; reprinted with permission.)

analysis was 0.89 and 0.89 for occlusion and 0.82 and 0.79 for stenosis >70%, with excellent interobserver agreement. A subsequent study of bypass graft patency with SSFP angiography in 25 patients showed lower specificity. Measuring flow in bypass grafts has been shown to be helpful as well. In one study of 69 patients who underwent velocity encoded flow mapping by MR at baseline and with vasodilator stress, receiver operating characteristic (ROC) analysis demonstrated sensitivity of 96% and specificity of 92% for identification of stenosis >70%, suggesting improved performance over angiography alone. However, flow scans could not be obtained in 80% of grafts.

Recent efforts have been aimed at imaging not the coronary lumen but the coronary wall itself. Black-blood MR images that null the signal from the blood are essential to visualize the coronary wall. A high-resolution black-blood CMR method without motion or blood-flow artifacts and with 0.46-mm in-plane resolution has been used to visualize the wall of major epicardial coronary arteries in a group of normal subjects and five patients with CAD. The average coronary wall thickness for each cross-sectional image in normal subjects was 0.7 mm, with a range from 0.5 to 1.0 mm. The patients with coronary disease with <40% stenosis assessed by coronary angiography showed localized wall thickness of 4.4 mm, with a range between 3.3 and 5.7 mm.

Atherosclerotic Plaque Imaging. The principle that different tissue types have different T1 and T2 appearance on CMR has been applied to characterize tissue components of atherosclerotic plaque. Bright areas on T2WIs from arterial walls correspond to regions predominantly composed of fibers, such as collagen, elastin, and proteoglycan either in media or in collagenous caps, and dark areas on T2WIs correspond to lipid-rich regions. CMR to assess atherosclerotic plaque thickness, extent, and composition in the descending aorta has been compared with trans-esophageal echocardiography (TEE), with good agreement in regards to aortic plaque type, extent, and maximum thickness. A study using multi-spectral CMR in patients prior to AAA repair demonstrated very good agreement between CMR tissue characterization and histopathology. T2WIs identified thrombus as regions of high signal and lipid core as low signal. Fibrous cap was visualized as a discrete area of uniform increased signal on T2WI. Significant enhancement of the cap was seen on T1WIs after Gd-DTPA infusion.

Because of its superficial location in the neck, minimal motion, and available tissue pathology from carotid endarterectomy, carotid artery plaque has been considered an excellent target for MR imaging of atherosclerosis (Fig. 23.8). Early on, a study demonstrated the accuracy of in vivo CMR for measuring the cross-sectional maximal wall area of atherosclerotic carotid arteries in a group of patients undergoing carotid endarterectomy. Close agreement between the in vivo and ex vivo measurements confirmed the accuracy of CMR for quantification of stenosis. Studies of plaque vulnerability have been performed, including measures of thickness of the fibrous cap, and have led to the development of a semiquantitative evaluation of fibrous cap thickness in carotid atherosclerotic plaque.

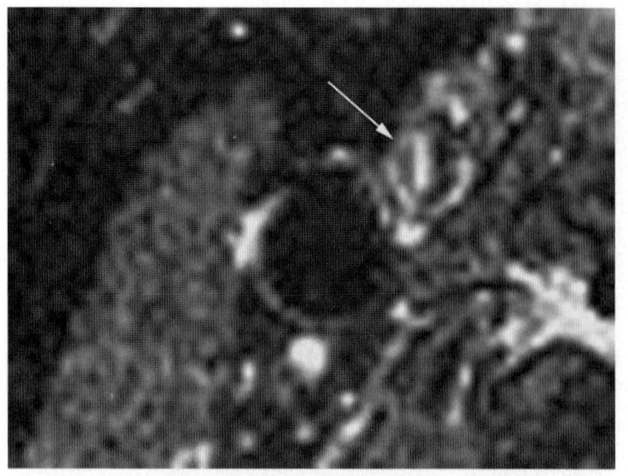

FIGURE 23.8. **MR of Atherosclerosis.** T2WI of the common carotid artery (*arrow*) in a patient with a history of a transient ischemic attack shows a significant atherosclerotic plaque burden (taking up approximately 50% of the lumen). The bright area on the luminal surface represents the fibrous cap and the darker area toward the adventitia represents the lipid core of the plaque.

This technique demonstrated its ability to differentiate among thick and thin caps and recent cap rupture. These findings are clinically relevant, as patients with rupture are likely to have symptoms such as transient ischemic attacks or stroke. The accuracy of multispectral CMR for identifying plaque components in the carotid has been carefully validated against histopathology. These techniques are currently primarily research techniques but will undoubtedly enter the clinical realm in the near future.

CARDIOMYOPATHIES

Differentiating Etiology of Cardiomyopathies. Making the etiologic diagnosis of cardiomyopathy in new-onset congestive heart failure has important therapeutic and prognostic implications, and CMR has a potentially important role to play. Prospective methods include delayed-enhancement imaging for detection of prior MI and coronary imaging for detection of obstructive CAD. Initial studies that demonstrated the utility of delayed-enhancement imaging for visualization of healed MI suggested that the presence of hyperenhancement may help to diagnose CAD. Studies of larger patient groups have shown that there are patients with nonischemic cardiomyopathy, as defined by the absence of obstructive CAD, who demonstrate delayed hyperenhancement. In the largest published study to date, a significant subset of patients (13%) had hyperenhancement that looked like prior MI, either as a result of minimal underlying CAD with thrombosis and recanalization or because of embolic infarction. Another 28% had an unusual pattern of midwall hyperenhancement that may be consistent with prior myocarditis. Thus, the presence of hyperenhancement is not necessarily diagnostic of an ischemic etiology of cardiomyopathy, although the absence of hyperenhancement is likely an excellent marker of nonischemic disease.

Myocarditis. In recent years, CMR has been added to the diagnostic armamentarium in patients with clinically suspected myocarditis as a cause of acute onset of congestive heart failure. Typically, T1W spin-echo images are obtained before and after Gd-DTPA infusion. Relative enhancement of the myocardium in patients with myocarditis is usually three to five times that of skeletal muscle. Thus, contrast enhancement may be a marker of the inflammation and edema that are the hallmarks of this disease process.

More recent studies have used the same inversion-recovery gradient-echo sequence that is used for detection of MI. Up to 88% of patients may demonstrate contrast enhancement, most frequently in the lateral free wall. In patients with biopsies taken from the area of contrast enhancement, active myocarditis is found in the majority. In biopsies from areas without contrast enhancement, active myocarditis was rarely seen. As LV function improves at follow-up, the area of contrast enhancement falls by one third. Thus, contrast enhancement appears to be a marker of active myocarditis early in the course of the disease. As it heals, a pattern of midwall hyperenhancement is often seen (Fig. 23.9). The use of CMR will continue to grow in this setting when the clinical suspicion of acute myocarditis is high.

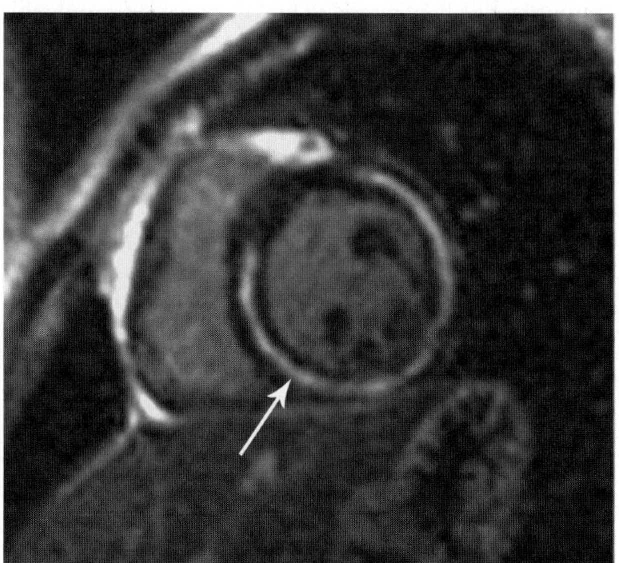

FIGURE 23.9. **Myocarditis.** Short-axis late contrast-enhanced inversion-recovery gradient-echo image obtained 10 minutes following gadolinium infusion at 0.2 mM/kg in a 10-year-old with a history of myocarditis 6 months previously. Note the band of late gadolinium enhancement in the mid-myocardium (*arrow*) that can be seen in chronic or healed myocarditis.

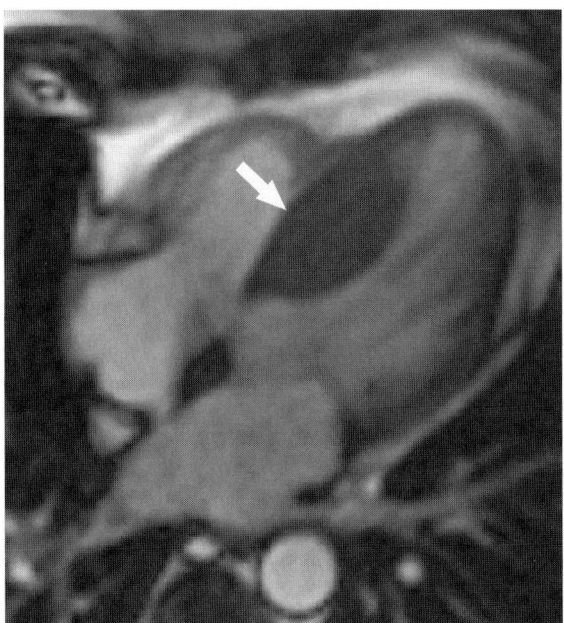

FIGURE 23.10. **Hypertrophic Cardiomyopathy.** Four-chamber long-axis steady-state free precession end-systolic image in a patient with hypertrophic cardiomyopathy and marked asymmetric septal hypertrophy (*arrow*). Note the relatively normal wall thickness in the apex and lateral walls.

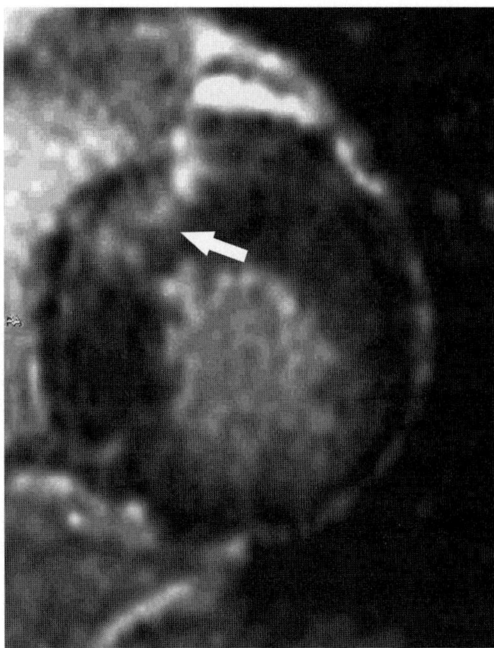

FIGURE 23.11. **Hypertrophic Cardiomyopathy.** Short-axis late contrast-enhanced inversion-recovery gradient-echo image obtained 10 minutes following gadolinium infusion at 0.2 mM/kg in the same patient as Fig. 23.10 demonstrating focal late gadolinium enhancement (*arrow*) in the septum at the anterior RV insertion site.

Hypertrophic Cardiomyopathy. The entire spectrum of the pathophysiology underlying hypertrophic cardiomyopathy (HCM) can be visualized by CMR. Cine imaging can demonstrate abnormal wall thickness (Fig. 23.10), turbulent flow in the LV outflow tract, mitral leaflet systolic anterior motion, and mitral regurgitation. Apical HCM may be more readily apparent on CMR than on echocardiography. Recent studies have shown the additive value of late Gd enhancement as a marker of fibrosis in patients with HCM. This was seen in 81% of patients with asymptomatic or minimally symptomatic HCM in regions of hypertrophy, especially at sites where the RV inserted into the ventricular septum (Fig. 23.11). The fibrosis or scar was generally patchy and its extent correlated with wall thickness and inversely with wall thickening and ejection fraction. Patients with progressive disease, defined as wall thinning, cavity dilation, or two or more risk factors for sudden death, have a greater extent of late enhancement, which is quite often diffuse as opposed to confluent. Thus, the extent of hyperenhancement likely relates to prognosis in HCM. In addition, the basal septal infarct created by ethanol septal ablation can be well visualized by ce-CMR. Despite normal to supranormal ejection fraction, intramyocardial mechanics are abnormal in HCM, as demonstrated with CMR myocardial tagging. This heterogeneity of intramural function is likely the result of the myocardial fibrosis and myofibrillar disarray that are characteristic of HCM.

Infiltrative Cardiomyopathies. Cardiac sarcoidosis is seen at autopsy in 20% to 30% of patients with systemic disease, although fewer than 25% of these patients are symptomatic. The pathophysiology involves edema, granuloma formation, and then fibrosis. Ce-CMR has proven useful for imaging these stages in the myocardium in patients with sarcoidosis. Patchy myocardial enhancement can be seen in as many as half of patients with histologically proven myocardial sarcoidosis. After 1 month of high-dose steroid therapy, the enhancement can regress.

CMR can demonstrate many of the hallmarks of amyloidosis. Deposition of amyloid fibrils can lead to concentric hypertrophy, biatrial dilatation, valvular thickening, and reduced systolic function, all of which are well demonstrated on cine imaging. One study demonstrated differentiation from HCM by the findings of atrial wall hypertrophy, RV free wall hypertrophy, and distinguishing signal characteristics on CMR. Diffuse subendocardial late enhancement using the same inversion-recovery technique used for infarct detection has been recently described as characteristic of amyloidosis, although other patterns may be seen as well (Fig. 23.12).

Typically, chronic Chagas cardiomyopathy presents with evidence of conduction system disease, congestive heart failure (often right-sided), or sudden death. In addition to the classic ECG findings of right bundle branch

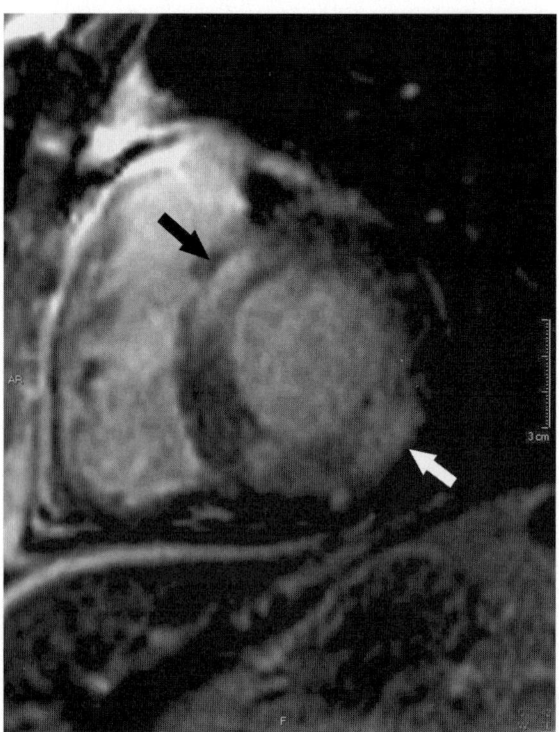

FIGURE 23.12. Infiltrative Cardiomyopathy: Amyloidosis. Short-axis late contrast-enhanced inversion-recovery gradient-echo image obtained 10 minutes following gadolinium infusion at 0.2 mM/kg in a patient with a plasma cell dyscrasia and evidence of amyloidosis on a bone marrow biopsy. There are focal regions of late gadolinium enhancement seen in the septum (*black arrow*) and inferolateral walls (*white arrow*).

block, left anterior hemiblock, atrial fibrillation, and premature ventricular complexes, cine CMR can demonstrate regional and/or global LV dysfunction with focal aneurysmal disease and RV dysfunction. Delayed enhancement on CMR can demonstrate regional LV enhancement, particularly in distributions inconsistent with CAD and more consistent with Chagas myocarditis.

Anderson-Fabry disease, an X-linked disorder of sphingolipid metabolism, can cause idiopathic myocardial hypertrophy. Approximately half of patients with this disorder demonstrate delayed contrast enhancement on CMR, especially in the basal inferolateral wall.

Arrhythmogenic RV cardiomyopathy (ARVC) is a disease of fibrofatty replacement of the RV, and occasionally of the LV as well, that presents as ventricular arrhythmias and sudden death. It is an important diagnosis to make, as it can manifest as sudden death in otherwise healthy young people and is often considered an indication for placement of an implantable cardioverter-defibrillator. The hallmark of the disease is RV dilatation and dysfunction, global and/or regional, which can be demonstrated quite readily by cine CMR (Fig. 23.13). The fatty infiltration of the RV free wall, which can be seen on T1W spin-echo imaging and with fat-suppression techniques, may be a nonspecific finding. A proportion of normal subjects and patients with other forms of arrhythmias originating in the RV, such as idiopathic RV outflow tract tachycardia, may also demonstrate focal fat infiltration in similar locations. Therefore, the RV size and functional abnormalities are more critical to making the diagnosis. Recent studies suggest that late Gd enhancement of the RV myocardium may be seen as well in this disorder.

PERICARDIAL DISEASE

CMR allows the differentiation of tissue characteristics because of differences in signal properties on T1W or T2W sequences. For example, hemorrhagic, serous, and chylous pericardial effusions can be differentiated based on their signal properties. Pericardial cysts are classically located in the right costophrenic angle and are typically high signal on T2WIs because of the proteinaceous fluid they contain (Fig. 23.14). CMR is a sensitive measure of pericardial thickness in the setting of suspected constrictive pericarditis and can make accurate measurements around both ventricles and atria, adding to other clinical and diagnostic imaging information. Physiologic parameters can also be evaluated, as CMR tissue tagging can be applied to evaluate slippage of the pericardium along the epicardium, which is often absent in pericardial constriction.

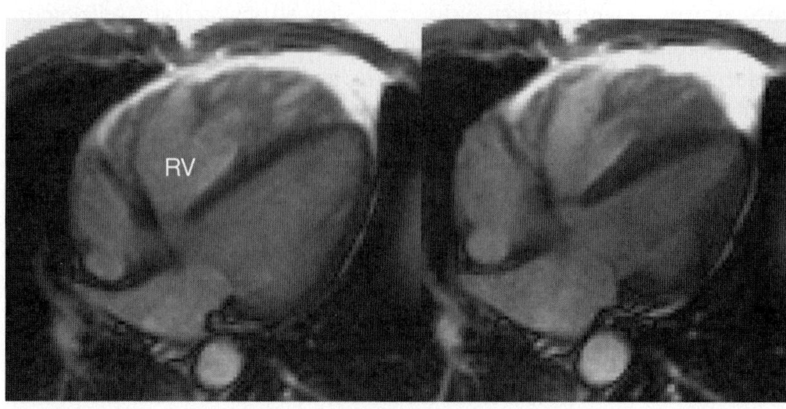

FIGURE 23.13. Arrhythmogenic RV Cardiomyopathy. End-diastolic (*left*) and end-systolic (*right*) frames from a four-chamber long-axis steady-state free precession cine acquisition in a patient with arrhythmogenic RV cardiomyopathy. The RV is dilated, with severe global systolic dysfunction consistent with that diagnosis.

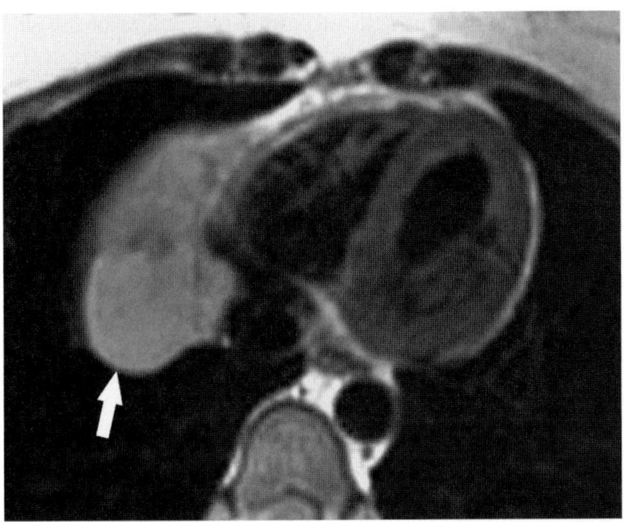

FIGURE 23.14. **Pericardial Cyst.** Axial T2W spin-echo image demonstrating a pericardial cyst (*arrow*) in the classic right costophrenic angle location and the bright signal within it noted on T2WIs.

VALVULAR HEART DISEASE

Although echocardiography is the principal imaging tool used to assess valvular disease, CMR can be used as well and is an excellent tool for quantitation. Fast spin-echo or "black blood" techniques can demonstrate excellent structural detail of valve morphology. Gradient-echo cine CMR is a "white blood" technique that has the advantage of providing multiple sequential images through the cardiac cycle in a single slice with excellent temporal resolution. Valve structure can often be well visualized (Fig. 23.15). Abnormal flow can cause dephasing of spins, which then results in a signal void and can be used for identification of regurgitant or stenotic valvular lesions (Fig. 23.16). SSFP cine CMR, the most commonly used functional sequence today, has the limitation in this setting of a short echo time (TE), which reduces spin dephasing, thereby reducing the signal void that signifies valvular disease. For this reason, gradient-echo cine CMR is often used in conjunction with SSFP when valve disease is in question.

The ability of CMR to measure the phase shifts of protons as they move through a magnetic field gradient is termed *velocity-encoded* or *phase-contrast* cine MR imaging (Fig. 23.17). The degree of phase shift can be measured to determine velocity of flow, because phase shift is proportional to motion over time. The direction of velocity encoding can be selected in any 3D orientation. The velocity map may be through-plane, with the jet perpendicular to the imaging plane, or in-plane, with the chosen plane including the jet. The Bernoulli equation ($\Delta P = 4V^2$) is used to relate velocity (V) to the pressure difference (ΔP) on either side of a stenotic orifice. Measures of velocity can be integrated over an area of interest, such as a blood vessel or cardiac chamber, and a flow volume calculated.

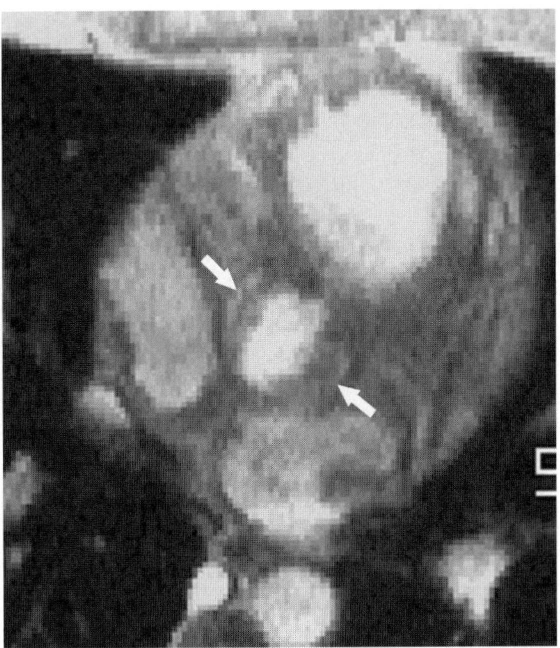

FIGURE 23.15. **Bicuspid Aortic Valve.** Shown here is a midsystolic frame of a gradient-echo image set in a double oblique orientation through the short axis of the aortic valve. Note the "fishmouth" opening of the two leaflets (*arrows*) of the aortic valve, consistent with a bicuspid valve.

Several issues must be addressed to ensure proper quantitation with the velocity-encoded CMR technique. One is the potential for malalignment of the flow

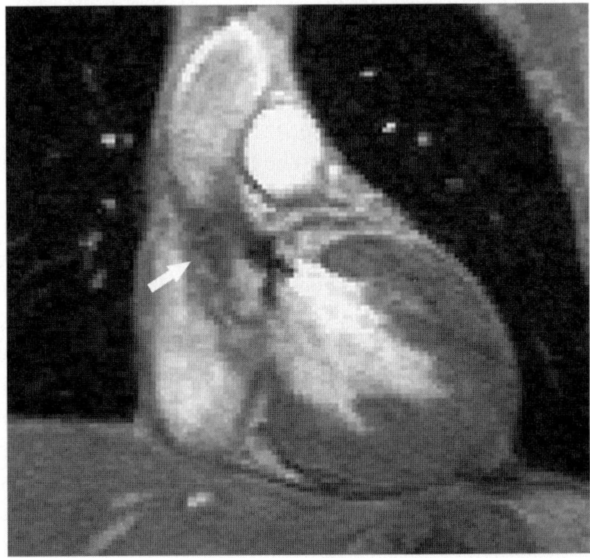

FIGURE 23.16. **Aortic Stenosis.** A midsystolic frame from a gradient-echo cine image set in a coronal view in a patient with a calcified valve (low signal in leaflets) (*arrow*) and aortic stenosis. Note the turbulence in the ascending aorta caused by dephasing of spins with high velocity flow distal to the stenotic orifice.

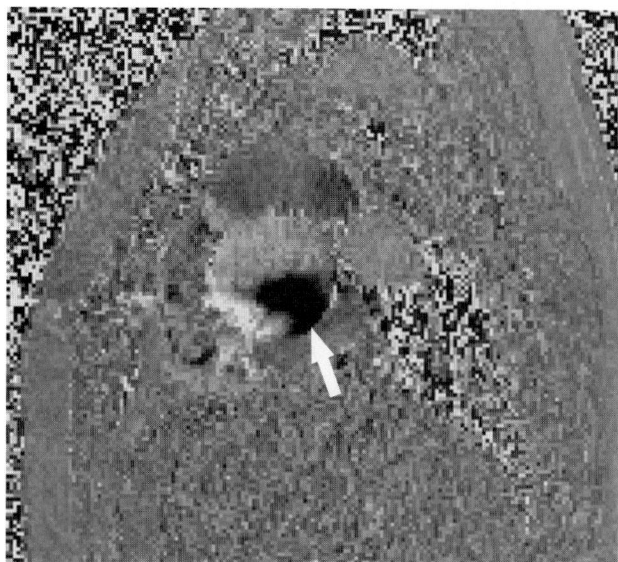

FIGURE 23.17. **Aortic Stenosis: High-Velocity Jet.** A systolic image from a phase-velocity gradient-echo image set perpendicular to the ascending aorta in a patient with aortic stenosis. The high-velocity jet in black (*arrow*) from the stenosis is seen along the wall of the ascending aorta. The direction of flow is toward the head.

direction and the direction of flow encoding. The error is proportional to the cosine of the difference between the two angles; therefore, the larger the angle, the greater the error. Thus, the imaging plane must be carefully prescribed and the decision made whether to image with through-plane or in-plane methodology. This imaging is frequently not performed with breath-holding and, therefore, respiratory motion may degrade image quality. In addition, to prevent aliasing, the operator must choose a velocity to encode prior to the acquisition that is higher than the predicted maximal velocity. The size of the region of interest used to measure velocity must be carefully chosen, depending on the need to assess the peak or mean velocity.

When using gradient-echo cine techniques, regurgitation is recognized as a signal void caused by dephasing of spins. The extent and degree of signal loss in the LA during systole correlates well with the severity of mitral regurgitation. Aortic regurgitation has likewise been measured using cine MR with evaluation of the created signal void. Many factors, however, can alter the size of signal void, reducing its effectiveness at quantitating the severity of regurgitation. These include hardware differences, complexities of regurgitant orifice size and volume, inclusion of non-regurgitant blood in jets, orientation of the imaging plane, and changes in echo time, especially with newer, faster imaging sequences. Another method to estimate severity of aortic regurgitation applies a transverse saturation band above the aorta and measures its retrograde movement in the ascending and descending aorta. The presence of marked retrograde movement of the saturation band—in principle similar to flow reversal in the descending aorta by Doppler echocardiography—is quite sensitive for severe aortic regurgitation. In patients with single isolated regurgitant lesions, the difference between RV and LV stroke volume can be calculated to estimate regurgitant volume. However, with more than one regurgitant lesion, this calculation is inaccurate.

Two different methods are used to measure regurgitant flow by velocity-encoded CMR. In one, regurgitant volume is calculated as the difference between LV and RV stroke volumes, as measured from velocities in the aorta and pulmonary artery, respectively. In isolated mitral regurgitation, this method has been shown to correlate well with color Doppler echocardiographic methods. For mitral regurgitation, aortic flow volume by velocity-encoded CMR can be subtracted from cine MR measures of LV stroke volume for accurate measures of regurgitant fraction. Velocity-encoded methods can also be applied to flow across tricuspid and pulmonic valves and are especially useful in patients with congenital heart disease, either before or after repair.

Similar to Doppler echocardiography, the examination of stenotic valvular lesions makes use of measurement of peak and mean gradients and may utilize the continuity equation to estimate functional valvular area. Velocity-encoded CMR has theoretic advantages in that there are no limitations on maximum velocity measures, it is a 3D technique, and it can examine the true direction of flow across the stenotic orifice. Potential limitations include the fact that truly perpendicular alignment of the velocity-encoded slice to the stenotic jet is problematic in eccentric jets, and its distance from the stenotic valve may cause difficulties in proper placement of the imaging plane. If it is too far removed from the valve, signal loss can occur because of turbulence. If it is too close to the valve, the leaflets may interfere with the measurement of the jet velocity. In addition, image analysis can be a prohibitively long process.

In mitral stenosis, cine gradient-echo imaging can demonstrate a signal void extending into the LV during diastole. The size of signal loss relative to LV cross-sectional area correlates quite well with catheter-measured pressure gradients. The maximum mitral leaflet separation can also be measured by cine MR, although this is a two-dimensional estimate of a 3D area. Velocity-encoded CMR with short echo times has shown excellent agreement in peak gradients in both mitral and aortic stenosis.

Both cine and velocity-encoded CMR have been used to assess the severity of aortic stenosis. The length of signal loss distal to the aortic valve has been used to grade the severity of aortic stenosis, with a good correlation with pressure gradients. Properties of cine CMR that correlate with more severe aortic stenosis include narrow high-velocity jets that extend well into the aorta distal to the valve and the presence of a prestenotic acceleration signal void proximal to the valve. Velocity-encoded techniques have also been used to estimate valve area in aortic stenosis and correlate closely with Doppler echo–derived estimates. The safety of imaging prosthetic valves of any type in high-field MR scanners has been well documented.

CONGENITAL HEART DISEASE

The versatility of CMR makes it an ideal tool for analysis of simple and complex congenital heart disease (CHD). In-depth discussion of each of the types of CHD is beyond the scope of this chapter and is covered in other chapters in this text. Structural assessment is enhanced by the ability to create 3D displays from image acquisitions. Morphologic assessment of atrial and ventricular situs and atrioventricular and ventriculoarterial connections is critical in the assessment of CHD. LV and RV volumes and mass are accurately measured in complex CHD and in the postoperative state. Valvular abnormalities can be evaluated with cine acquisitions. Shunt calculations are readily and accurately performed with phase velocity mapping of flow in the ascending aorta and main pulmonary artery. Methods for measuring intramyocardial function, such as myocardial tissue tagging, offer insight into ventricular mechanics in disease states such as single ventricles. Preoperative sizing and anatomic mapping of the central pulmonary arteries often aid with surgical planning. Assessment of congenital great vessel disease is straightforward. CMR has also become the modality of choice for postoperative assessment in this patient population.

Common congenital heart lesions include the intracardiac shunts, such as atrial septal defects (ASD) and ventricular septal defects (VSD) (Fig. 23.18). CMR is complementary to echocardiography in straightforward CHD. The exception is anomalous pulmonary venous return with the often-associated sinus venosus ASD, where CMR is more accurate than echocardiography because of its 3D coverage of the chest. In addition to cine imaging demonstrating flow, velocity-encoded imaging is useful both for sizing defects and determining shunt ratios.

Complex CHD often requires the complementary use of echocardiography. CMR has the advantage of its 3D coverage and ability to easily image the great vessels and pulmonary artery branches, a limitation of echocardiography. One example is tetralogy of Fallot, which is characterized by RV hypertrophy, membranous VSD, overriding aorta, and pulmonic or infundibular RV stenosis. CMR can easily demonstrate all aspects of this disease (Fig. 23.19), which often include systemic-to-pulmonary arterial collaterals; postoperatively, CMR can delineate residual shunting or the common finding of RV outflow tract aneurysm and pulmonic regurgitation. Other complex lesions, such as

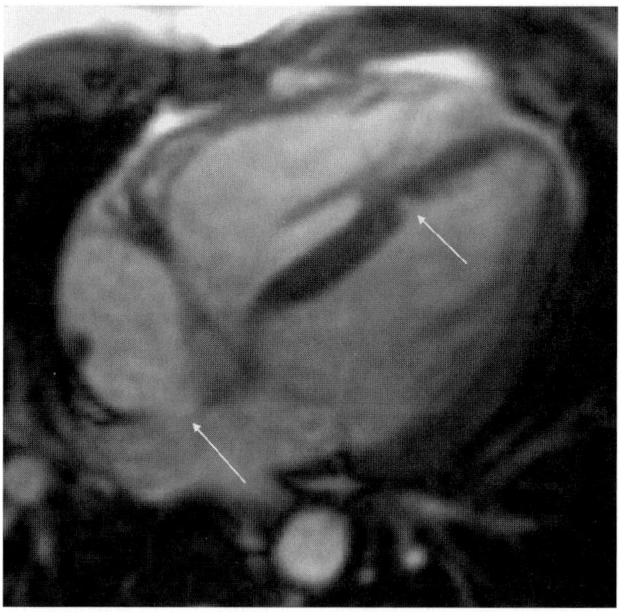

FIGURE 23.18. **Atrial and Ventricular Septal Defects.** A four-chamber long-axis steady-state free precession image in a patient with a secundum atrial septal defect (*left arrow*) as well as a muscular ventricular septal defect (*right arrow*).

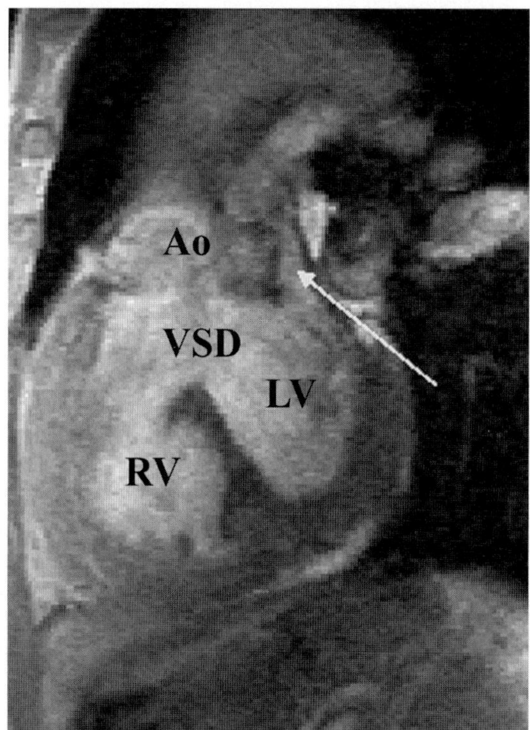

FIGURE 23.19. **Tetralogy of Fallot.** A parasagittal gradient-echo cine image in a patient with unrepaired tetralogy of Fallot. All of the findings of tetralogy are seen in this image: RV hypertrophy, a membranous ventricular septal defect (VSD), overriding aorta (Ao), and infundibular stenosis (*arrow*). LV, left ventricle.

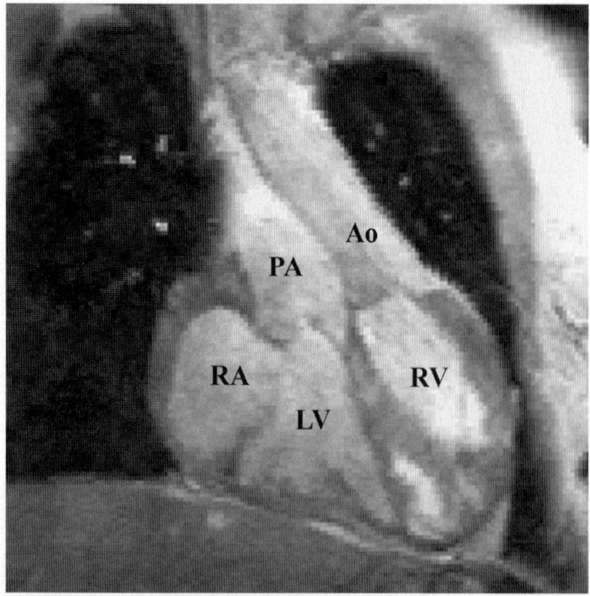

FIGURE 23.20. **D-Transposition of the Great Arteries.** Single frame from a coronal gradient-echo cine image series in a patient with D-transposition of the great arteries, also termed congenitally corrected transposition. Blood flows into the RA and then the LV, out the pulmonary artery (PA), through the lungs, into the LA (*not seen*), morphologic RV, and out the aorta (Ao). Note the abnormal positioning of the aorta to the left of the pulmonary artery.

truncus arteriosus and L-transposition of the great arteries, are diseases where CMR is well-suited to demonstrate arteriovenous connections (Fig. 23.20) and the presence and location of collateral vessels. Single ventricular hearts is another diagnosis that is well-suited to CMR, because CMR can demonstrate morphology of the single ventricle and the relationship between the aortic valve and semilunar valves, and postoperatively CMR can evaluate shunt patency and effect on underlying chambers.

CARDIAC AND PARACARDIAC MASSES

CMR provides a noninvasive, comprehensive 3D assessment of intracardiac and extracardiac structures. Although transthoracic echocardiography has traditionally been the initial test of choice for evaluating cardiac and paracardiac masses, limitations include a limited field of view and poor acoustic windows in some patients. Additionally, transthoracic echocardiography has difficulty evaluating apical, pericardial, and paracardiac masses, often making transesophageal echocardiography necessary to provide complementary information. Whereas transesophageal echocardiography has higher resolution and better acoustic windows, which aid in the detection of paracardiac, apical, and left atrial appendage masses, it has a limited field of view and is semi-invasive.

CMR is able to provide a detailed assessment of intracardiac and extracardiac masses, including their location, mobility, and relationship to other structures. Any pericardial and intramyocardial involvement and fine definition of tumor extent are easily evaluated. These features are important information for the clinician to guide therapeutic strategy. For example, extension into atrial walls generally precludes surgical removal of the entire tumor. In a study assessing the role of CMR for evaluating suspected cardiac and paracardiac masses involving the heart, CMR provided diagnostic information that affected clinical management or surgical planning in 53 of 61 patients, including showing lack of resectability or guiding the surgical approach. The advantages of CMR include its large field of view, high spatial resolution, high contrast-to-noise ratio, and multiplanar imaging capabilities. Serial CMR has also become a common modality for monitoring tumor regression after surgical, pharmacologic, and radiologic therapies.

Spin-echo CMR imaging can often suggest presence of a mass by demonstrating asymmetric thickening, cavity distortion, and intracavitary masses. Using spin echo, T1 and T2 relaxation times can be used to help differentiate tissue characteristics of different masses. While nonspecific for many primary cardiac tumors, tissue characterization by CMR can often be diagnostic for lipomas, myxomas, and lymphomas. Cysts and lipomas tend to have high signal intensity on T1W spin-echo images, similar to fat, whereas lipomas and lipomatous hypertrophy have reduced signal intensity when a fat presaturation technique is used. Conversely, tumors such as myxomas and lymphomas appear less intense on T1W spin-echo images. Myxomas often appear dark on gradient-echo cine imaging (Fig. 23.21). Relaxation times can also be used to identify acute or subacute hematomas, which appear bright on T2W spin-echo imaging.

Cine MR (either SSFP or gradient-echo) can be used to visualize valvular regurgitation or obstruction, which is important because intracavitary tumors may produce obstruction to flow into or within the heart. The dephasing of spins from turbulent blood flow provides excellent contrast in signal to help differentiate stationary from mobile objects. Cine imaging is also useful for depicting the site of attachment of tumors and prolapse of tumors through atrioventricular (AV) valves and can aid in the differentiation of certain tumors. With the exception of most atrial myxomas, tumors generally have higher signal intensities (greater than or equal to muscle) when compared to thrombus in the cardiac chambers. Myocardial tissue tagging can be applied to gradient-echo cine or multiphase T1W spin-echo imaging to help differentiate tumor from myocardium.

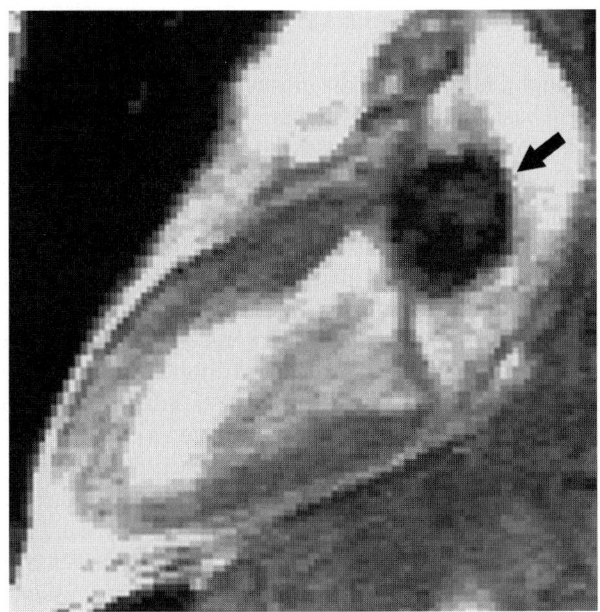

FIGURE 23.21. **Left Atrial Myxoma.** Shown here is a two-chamber long-axis gradient-echo cine image in a patient with a left atrial myxoma (*arrow*). Note the low signal of the myxoma on this gradient-echo image.

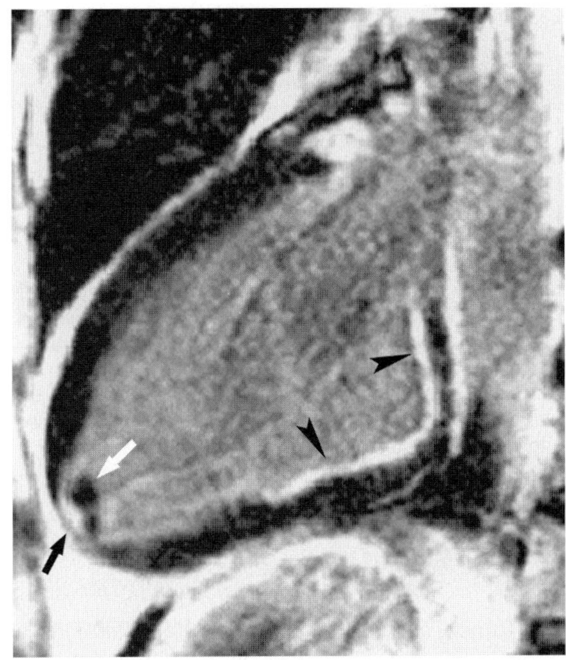

FIGURE 23.22. **Thrombus in LV.** Late contrast-enhanced image in a two-chamber orientation using an inversion-recovery gradient-echo sequence 10 minutes following gadolinium infusion at 0.2 mM/kg. Note the subendocardial hyperenhancement in the basal inferior wall (*arrowheads*) and focal transmural hyperenhancement at the apex (*black arrow*). The white arrow identifies a thrombus at the apex that fails to take up contrast.

The use of Gd-based contrast is helpful in many tumors and often shows differential contrast uptake with respect to normal myocardium. On precontrast T1W spin-echo images, cardiac tumors appear isointense in most cases and are not clearly discernible from normal myocardium based upon signal intensity. Following administration of contrast, differential uptake of contrast within the tumor compared to normal myocardium is seen as a result of the increased vascularity of the tumor. Additionally, nonvascularized, necrotic, or cystic areas inside a tumor can be differentiated because they do not accumulate contrast medium. The administration of MR contrast can also be useful to differentiate other masses from intracardiac thrombi, which generally do not take up contrast medium. Thrombi are the most frequent intracardiac mass and are most commonly located in the LA, when associated with atrial fibrillation or rheumatic heart disease, or in the LV when associated with MI or dilated cardiomyopathy. Late Gd-enhanced inversion-recovery gradient-echo CMR is best for detection of thrombus and compares favorably to cine MR and to echocardiography (Fig. 23.22).

Neoplasms of the heart may be either primary or secondary, and primary cardiac tumors may be either benign or malignant. Primary cardiac tumors are rare, with a prevalence of 0.001% to 0.3% in most autopsy series. Secondary or metastatic neoplasms of the heart are much more frequent than primary neoplasms—approximately 30 to 50 times more common (Fig. 23.23). Most primary

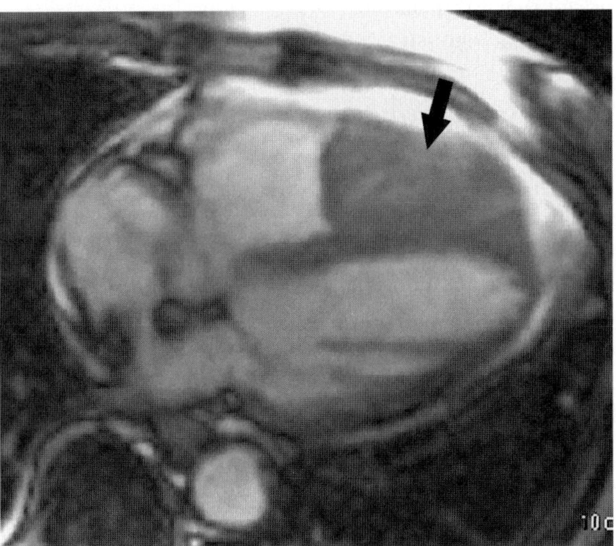

FIGURE 23.23. **Metastasis to the Heart.** Single frame from an axial steady-state free precession cine series in a patient with metastatic non–small cell lung carcinoma with tumor (*arrow*) visualized filling the RV apex.

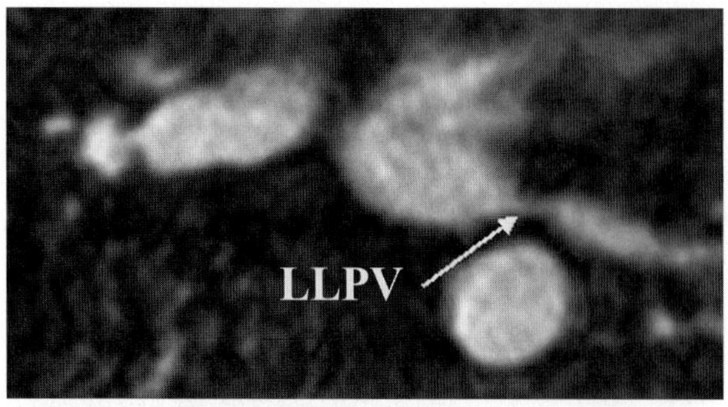

FIGURE 23.24. **Pulmonary Vein Stenosis.** Axial image taken from a maximum intensity projection (MIP) of a three-dimensional gadolinium-enhanced MR angiogram demonstrating stenosis (*arrow*) of the left lower pulmonary vein (LLPV) in an asymptomatic patient status post–radiofrequency ablation of the pulmonary veins for atrial fibrillation.

cardiac tumors are benign, are most often myxomas, and are most commonly located in the LA. Other benign tumors include lipomas, papillary fibroelastomas, fibromas, rhabdomyomas, and hemangiomas. Benign cardiac tumors are typically well circumscribed.

Malignant cardiac neoplasms are frequently invasive and may involve multiple structures. Only about 25% of primary cardiac tumors are malignant, and most of these are sarcomas. The primary malignant cardiac tumors typically involve the myocardium and the endocardial surface, while most secondary (metastatic) neoplasms to the heart involve the pericardium or epicardium, are often associated with pericardial and pleural effusions, and may cause pericardial constriction.

PULMONARY VEINS

With the recent increase in pulmonary vein mapping and isolation with radiofrequency ablation for patients with atrial fibrillation, the need for imaging techniques that demonstrate the pulmonary venous anatomy has concomitantly increased. CMR is such a technique, especially MR angiography, which allows 3D display of the pulmonary veins. The veins can be sized before and after radiofrequency ablation with CMR and can demonstrate pulmonary vein stenosis after ablation, a known complication, albeit relatively infrequent (Fig. 23.24).

LIMITATIONS/SAFETY

Although CMR provides diagnostic image quality on a consistent basis, a number of limitations remain. Patients who are morbidly obese and those who suffer significantly from claustrophobia are poor candidates. Furthermore, an inability to perform adequate breath-holding and excessive body motion can compromise image quality, although real-time imaging can overcome these potential limitations.

An ongoing concern with CMR is the interaction of the magnetic field with implanted materials or devices. While coronary stents, both uncoated and drug-eluting, and mechanical valves are safe, the presence of a cardiac defibrillator or pacemaker is currently considered a contraindication to CMR. Some of the theoretical concerns include device failure, inappropriate discharge, and lead heating resulting in thermal tissue damage. With more than 2 million devices currently implanted and that number expected to grow as the indications increase, several publications have recently surfaced that have added to our understanding of the interaction between the magnetic field and implanted cardiac devices. In a recent study, a number of cardiac devices were found to be safe when tested in a canine model at 1.5 Tesla, with smaller, more modern devices demonstrating greater MR compatibility. Although encouraging, large-scale in vivo studies are needed before CMR in this patient population can be safely recommended, and information about safety at higher field strengths is currently lacking.

SUGGESTED READINGS

Boxt LM. Magnetic resonance and computed tomographic evaluation of congenital heart disease. J Magn Reson Imag 2004;19:827–847.

Constantine G, Shan K, Flamm SD, Sivananthan MU. Role of MRI in clinical cardiology. Lancet 2004;363:2162–2171.

Dembo LG, Shifrin RY, Wolff SD. MR imaging in ischemic heart disease. Radiol Clin North Am 2004;42:651–673.

Higgins CB, de Roos A. Cardiovascular MRI and MRA. Philadelphia: Lippincott Williams & Wilkins, 2004.

Lardo AC, Fayad ZA, Chronos NAF, Fuster V, eds. Cardiovascular Magnetic Resonance: Established and Emerging Applications. London: Martin Dunitz, 2003.

Mankad S, Khalil R, Kramer CM. MRI for the diagnosis of myocardial ischemia and viability Curr Opin Cardiol 2003;18:351–356.

Manning W, Pennell D, eds. Cardiovascular Magnetic Resonance. Philadelphia: Churchill Livingstone, 2002.

Shan K, Constantine G, Sivananthan M, Flamm SD. Role of cardiac magnetic resonance imaging in the assessment of myocardial viability. Circulation 2004;109:1328–1334.

Viswamitra S, Higgins CB, Meacham DF, Mehta JL. Magnetic resonance imaging in myocardial ischemia. Curr Opin Cardiol 2004;19:510–516.

SECTION VI

Vascular and Interventional Radiology

Section Editor: Tony P. Smith

Thoracic Aorta, Pulmonary Arteries, and Peripheral Vascular Disorders

Michael J. Miller, Jr. and Tony P. Smith

Introduction to Vascular Radiology

Thoracic Aortography

Pulmonary Angiography

Bronchial Arteriography

Peripheral Arterial Disease

Uterine Artery Embolization

INTRODUCTION TO VASCULAR RADIOLOGY

The walls of both arteries and veins are made up of three layers; from the inside out, they are the *intima*, the *media*, and the *adventitia*. The intima is a single cell layer thick and has the primary function of interacting with the flowing blood—in particular, preventing thrombosis. It is by far the most chemically active layer. The media is composed for the most part of smooth muscle—more, of course, in large muscular arteries and less in smaller arteries and veins. Smooth muscle cells can contract to augment normal hemodynamic function and to respond to stress, such as with vasoconstriction (vasospasm). The adventitia is a layer of supportive connective tissue of varying thickness that surrounds and supports the media.

The anatomic structure of the vessel wall is actually simple, but its physiologic and pathologic function is very complex and for the most part poorly understood. A wide variety of disease processes can affect the vessel wall, particularly the arterial wall. These diseases include inflammation (vasculitis), fibromuscular disease, connective tissue disease, trauma, and of course degeneration (atherosclerosis), to name a few. Although we often do not understand the exact pathophysiology underlying a vessel's reaction to a particular disease process in a particular individual, the arterial wall and vessel itself have only a limited number of radiographic manifestations. When the vessel wall is "attacked," it can weaken and dilate, producing an aneurysm, or it can even rupture, causing extravasation, pseudoaneurysm formation, or arteriovenous fistulas. It can thicken either by growth of the vessel layers (intimal hyperplasia for example) or by the deposition of material, such as an atherosclerotic plaque, causing the vessel to narrow and producing stenosis or even occlusion. The vessel may lose its ability to prevent coagulation, resulting in thrombosis. As yet unknown genetic factors may induce the proliferation of vessels, resulting in arteriovenous malformations, or vessels may be induced to grow and proliferate by "acquired" factors such as within a tumor. If one keeps in mind the vessel wall, in particular the arterial wall, much of what is seen angiographically is more easily understood.

Angiographic Suite. Most angiographic suites have two major types of equipment: patient monitoring devices and radiographic equipment. Patient monitoring devices are essential to patient care during angiographic procedures, especially for conscious sedation, and there are usually one or more channels for pressure measurements. Radiographic equipment today is based on a C-arm design that allows complex angulation and is equipped for digital acquisition only. C-arm configuration allows one to set the angle for imaging; therefore the technologist no longer has to place the patient based on landmarks into the "named" positions. One is also able to acquire images at a rapid rate for long periods of time, allowing for special imaging such as bolus chasing for leg angiography and rotational angiography, which provides three-dimensional image viewing.

Tools. There are a number of *catheters* used in interventional radiology that can be loosely divided into five types: diagnostic angiographic catheters, microcatheters, drainage catheters, balloon catheters, and central venous catheters.

There are a host of properties considered in manufacturing, buying, and using *diagnostic angiographic catheters*; these include size (the smaller the better for access but size limits the lumen), shape, radiopacity, torque capacity, and softness of the distal tip. Larger-lumen diagnostic catheters are available (guiding catheters) for placement of microcatheters and angioplasty balloons in a coaxial fashion.

Microcatheters are 3 French or smaller and are designed for very distal catheterization. These catheters are placed over 0.010- to 0.018-inch guide wires. Most of their use is in the neurointerventional arena, but they are very helpful for peripheral intervention to select small vessels for embolization or infusion (e.g., chemotherapy). These catheters have a distal platinum marker but are otherwise not very radiopaque.

Drainage catheters are used frequently in interventional radiology for drainage of fluid collections, including nephrostomy, abscess, biliary gallbladder, pleural fluid, ascites, and lymphoceles. The same basic catheters are used for drainage in all such sites. Characteristics of drainage catheters include size, biocompatibility, radiopacity, and softness shape/retention property. Catheter shape is usually based on the size of the fluid collection for drainage and the retention property. The most common retention device for pigtail catheters is the retention suture. Straight catheter retention devices include the mushroom tip or inflatable balloon.

Balloon catheters can either be very soft and pliable, such as occlusion balloons or Fogarty balloons to clear thrombosis, or can be more rigid and used for dilations (angioplasty). Balloons for dilation can be divided into two main categories regarding the size of guide wire over which they are placed: 0.018 inch (or even smaller, including 0.014 inch) and 0.035 inch. The smaller guide wire lumen obviously allows the balloon to be smaller. These are the balloons used for coronary angioplasty, but they have become popular recently in peripheral and neuroradiologic interventional procedures. The smaller systems do not have the guide wire support of the larger systems, and the balloons cannot be constructed in very large diameters. Most peripheral intervention is performed with 0.035-inch wire balloon systems. There are an array of balloons in a variety of sizes. Large balloons require large access sites (introducer sheaths), especially for removal after inflation, as they do not "re-wrap" very well. An important concept to understand for the angioplasty balloon is compliance. Once the balloon reaches the manufacturer's stated size, it can be very firm (noncompliant) or it can "grow" a little with inflation (compliant). There are advantages to each. With the former, very difficult, hard lesions can be dilated. With the latter, one can "size" the balloon a little larger than its stated size by increasing the atmospheric pressure during dilation. This allows better fine-tuning of the angioplasty.

Central venous lines can be differentiated into those that have an implanted portion and those that are placed by direct puncture without implantation. The former are implanted subcutaneously and are designed for extended usage. The latter are the traditional central lines (central venous lines, Swan-Ganz catheters) that are placed for temporary care and monitoring. A special one of these is the peripherally inserted central catheter, which is placed via a peripheral arm vein coursing into the central veins for up to 6 weeks. Implanted devices can be divided into two main types: *tunneled external catheters*, placed using subcutaneous tunnels, and *implanted ports*, placed in a subcutaneous pocket. The type of device chosen depends on its clinical use and is based on a variety of factors, including number of lumens needed, frequency of use, type of use, length of use, device location, and individual patient factors. Tunneled external catheters are tunneled from the venous access site and have a retaining fabric (usually Dacron polyester) cuff to prevent dislodgment by the ingrowth of connective tissue. They are less expensive and less invasive to place than completely implanted ports but tend to have higher infection rates and are less cosmetically desirable. There are two main designs based on usage: cuffed central venous designs (e.g., Hickman) and those for hemodialysis access (e.g., PermCath). Implanted ports contain catheters that are tunneled a short distance from the venous access, where the port device is implanted in a subcutaneous pocket.

Most *guide wires* for standard angiography and interventional procedures fall into two categories based on their construction: *spring guide wires*, which are constructed of stainless steel wire tightly wound on itself to form a spring, and *nitinol guide wires*, which are constructed of a nickel-titanium alloy and an organic coating to which is bound a hydrophilic coating. This coating absorbs water and becomes very slippery. Guide wires range in size from 0.010 to 0.038 inches.

There are two types of *stents* based on mechanism of delivery: *self-expanding* and *balloon-expandable*. Self-expanding stents are composed of various metal combinations, most often either stainless steel or nitinol alloys. Balloon-expandable stents are composed for the most part of stainless steel. Self-expanding stents have the advantage of being quite flexible and can be constructed in quite large diameters but are often more difficult to place precisely because of foreshortening upon stent opening. This problem has been lessened somewhat with the nitinol varieties. Balloon-expandable stents are less flexible and are limited by balloon size but can be more precisely placed. There is much work being performed regarding drug delivery (coated stents) and covering of stents (stent grafts). Drug-coated stents are available for coronary use, but will soon be available in sizes for peripheral work as well.

A number of stents are available that are covered by fabric, producing in effect a *stent graft*. The fabric is most often polytetrafluoroethylene. Smaller varieties are used for the peripheral circulation and larger varieties are used for the aorta. In their current form, peripheral stent grafts require relatively large introducer sheaths (minimum of 7 French, up to 12 French). Those for the aorta require very large introducers (up to 30 French) and thus necessitate surgical access to the arterial entry site (usually common femoral artery).

Embolic agents can be conveniently divided into three categories, based on (*1*) location within the vascular bed where they occlude, (*2*) permanence of occlusion, and (*3*) radiopacity. Agents that occlude large vessels are considered to be proximal agents; chief among these are coils. Distal agents are smaller and flow, for example, into the nidus of an arteriovenous malformation or into a tumor bed for occlusion of small vessels. Chief among these agents are particles and liquids. A temporary agent is absorbed by the body and is principally represented by gelatin sponge. However, recanalization around an agent should also be considered temporary, as can occur with polyvinyl alcohol sponge. The major available embolic agents are outlined in Table 24.1.

Medications. A number of medications are used in the interventional suite for conscious sedation. Probably the two most common are fentanyl (Sublimaze: 25 to 100 μg bolus, 25 to 75 μg maintenance IV) and midazolam (Versed: 0.5 to 2 mg bolus, 1 mg maintenance). If these medications are administered, it is essential that the reversal agents are understood. Fentanyl is reversed with naloxone (Narcan: 0.4 to 2 mg IV). Midazolam is reversed with flumazenil (Remazicon: 0.2 mg IV over 15 seconds, with additional doses as required).

Antibiotic prophylaxis for vascular and interventional radiology is somewhat controversial. However, most clinicians suggest administration at least for contaminated (the presence of inflammation consistent with infection but no gross pus) or dirty (infected purulent site or infected GI or genitourinary (GU) site) procedures.

Intra-arterial pharmacoangiography consists of either *vasodilators* or *vasoconstrictors*. Vasodilators are used to treat vasospasm whose etiology is either iatrogenic (catheter-induced) or from other causes (trauma, medications, etc.). Two vasodilators are commonly used in vascular radiology: nitroglycerin (given intra-arterially in 100-μg doses) and papaverine (given intra-arterially in 25- to 100-mg doses). The only *vasoconstrictor* used with any frequency in vascular radiology is pitressin (Vasopressin), which was historically given intra-arterially for transcatheter therapy of lower GI bleeding, which has been mostly supplanted by embolization.

Antithrombotic agents fall into two broad categories: *anticoagulants* and *antiplatelet agents*. Anticoagulants are pharmacologic agents that inhibit thrombin generation in vivo and are usually heparin intravenously and warfarin (Coumadin) orally. These two anticoagulants have been the main stays of antithrombotic therapy for years. Newer anticoagulants such as direct thrombin inhibitors (bivalirudin, hirudin, argatroban) might offer significant advantages over heparin, but further studies are needed to demonstrate their safety and effectiveness. *Antiplatelet*

TABLE 24.1 Summary of Embolization Agents

Embolization Agent	*Constitution*	*Site of Occlusion*	*Radiopacity*	*Period of Occlusion*
Macrocoils (0.035–0.038 inch)	Stainless steel Platinum	Proximal	Excellent	Permanent
Microcoils* (0.010–0.018 inch)	Platinum	Proximal	Excellent	Permanent
Polyvinyl alcohol sponge	Denatured ethanol particles	Distal, based on size of particles, to arteriolar level	Mixed with contrast material	Temporary
Detachable balloons**	Silicone balloon	Balloon inflated to size	Inflated with isosmolar contrast	Permanent
Glue	Polymerization of cyanoacrylate	Distal based on rate of polymerization	Mixed with Ethiodol (ethiodized oil) and tantalum powder	Permanent
Alcohol	Sclerosing agent	Distal, to capillary level	Mixed with contrast powder	Permanent
Gelatin sponge	Derivative of purified pork skin	Proximal, based on size of pieces	None, except when injected with contrast	Temporary
Microspheres	Acrylic polymer	Distal, based on size of spheres, to arteriolar level	Mixed with contrast material	Unknown

*Coils are placed in the desired location by being pushed through a diagnostic angiography catheter or microcatheter. Although usually effective, the coil is not easily controlled (i.e., cannot be easily retrieved after exiting from the catheter). There are ways to control coil delivery electronically or mechanically, which are most often used in neurointerventional procedures and are not given in this table.

**Detachable balloons are currently not available in the United States.

TABLE 24.2 Commonly Used Thrombolytic Agents

Drug	Trade Name	Mechanism of Action	Dosage Via Catheter	Half-Life (minutes)
Streptokinase	Streptase	Indirect activation of plasminogen conversion	10,000-unit bolus 5,000 units/hour	18
Urokinase	Abbokinase	Tissue plasminogen activator	100,000- to 250,000-unit bolus 100,000–200,000 units/hour	15
Alteplase (rt-PA)	Activase	Tissue plasminogen activator	≤2 mg/hr infusion <40 mg total dose	5
Reteplase (r-PA)	Retevase	Tissue plasminogen activator	5- to 10-mg bolus 0.12–2 mg/hr infusion	14

rt-PA, recombinant tissue plasminogen activator; r-PA, recombinant plasminogen activator.

agents are either oral or IV. Oral antiplatelet medications include acetylsalicylic acid (either 81 mg or 325 mg) and the thienopyridines, which include ticlopidine (Ticlid: 250 mg) and clopidogrel (Plavix: 75 mg). Intravenous antiplatelet agents consist of the glycoprotein IIb/IIIa antagonists, which are the "big gun" antiplatelet agents. The best known of these is abciximab (Reopro). Antiplatelet agents have demonstrated clinical benefits in coronary interventions, particularly following stent placement. Very little data exist regarding use of these agents for peripheral interventions. However, they are used in selected situations to decrease the likelihood of thrombus formation.

Thrombolytic agents are those that actually lyse or dissolve existing thrombi, and the more commonly used agents are summarized in Table 24.2. In interventional radiology, thrombolytic agents are most often administered via a catheter directly into the thrombus located in the arterial or venous system. Catheter-directed thrombolysis is used to treat native arterial or bypass graft thrombosis, embolic occlusions, thrombosed hemodialysis access shunts, and deep venous thrombosis. The advantage of direct infusion (over empirical IV administration) is faster recanalization with a lesser dose of thrombolytic agent. Catheter-based infusion of a thrombolytic agent is an effective and well-established method of restoring blood flow in acute and subacute thrombotic occlusion. Once blood flow is reestablished, an underlying "culprit" lesion such as a stenosis is often found. The lesion that is responsible for precipitating the thrombosis must be treated. This can often be achieved with percutaneous techniques such as angioplasty or stent placement. Surgical revascularization may also be indicated, depending on the nature of the underlying problem. Occasionally, no culprit lesion is found. Thrombosis in these cases may be related to hypercoagulability, hypotension, or external compression of the graft. Remember, despite this lessened dose, these medications dissolve thromboses anywhere in the body, so the major contraindication is a known likelihood to hemorrhage (such as recent surgery, trauma, CNS lesion such as a recent stroke or tumor, etc.), and the major complication of thrombolytic therapy is likewise hemorrhage.

THORACIC AORTOGRAPHY

Anatomy. The thoracic aorta extends from the aortic valve to the diaphragm and is generally divided into three main sections: ascending aorta, arch, and descending aorta. The classic pattern of the great vessels is seen in approximately 70% of the population and consists of a right brachiocephalic, left common carotid, and left subclavian artery (Fig. 24.1). A host of variations in the origins of the great vessels from the aortic arch have been reported. The most frequent is a common origin of the right brachiocephalic and left common carotid artery (bovine anatomy), which occurs in up to 20% (see Fig. 24.4A) of the population. Other common variations include an aberrant right subclavian artery (2%) and the left vertebral artery from the arch (1%) (see Fig. 24.4C). Another important variation is the presence of an angiographically identifiable ductus diverticulum ("ductus bump"), which occurs in 9% of adults (Fig. 24.1). The ductus diverticulum appears as a fusiform dilatation along the ventromedial aspect of the proximal descending aorta adjacent to the ligamentum. In addition to the great vessels, the thoracic aorta gives rise to right and left coronary, intercostal, and bronchial arteries.

Congenital Anomalies. A number of congenital anomalies involve the arch and the branching pattern of the great vessels. The most striking is probably the *right-sided aortic arch with mirror-image branching*. There is a 98% association with congenital heart disease, the vast majority being tetralogy of Fallot. Therefore, most of these are considered congenital cardiac diseases and are often not associated with a more traditional vascular radiology practice. Two congenital anomalies are more often seen in an adult vascular radiology practice: left-sided (normal) arch with an aberrant right subclavian artery and pseudocoarctation (aortic kink) of the thoracic aorta. *Left arch with aberrant right subclavian artery* (Fig. 24.2) is the most common arch anomaly and is found in approximately 2% of individuals. It is rarely symptomatic. The right subclavian artery arises as a fourth branch of the arch and must cross the mediastinum to reach the right arm. It crosses behind

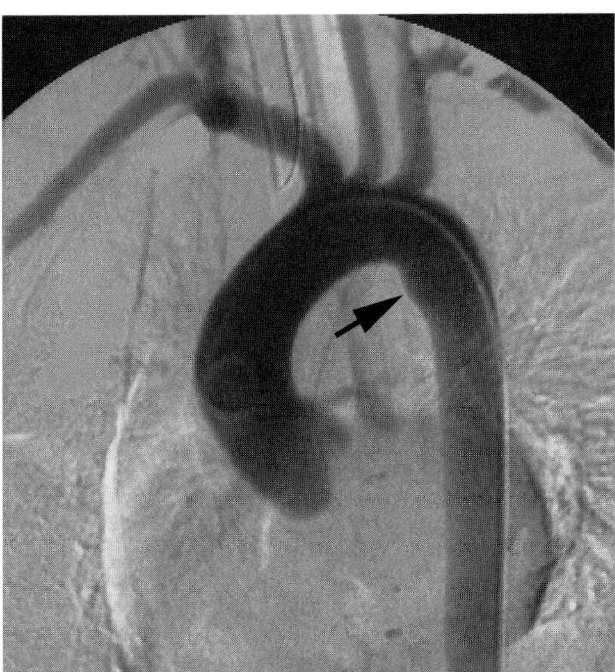

FIGURE 24.1. **Normal Aortic Arch.** Aortogram with "classic" origin pattern of the great vessels: right brachiocephalic artery, left common carotid artery, and left subclavian artery. Thoracic aortogram demonstrates a normal variant: fusiform dilatation (*arrow*) of the proximal descending aorta in the region of the ligamentum arteriosum, representing a normal ductus bump.

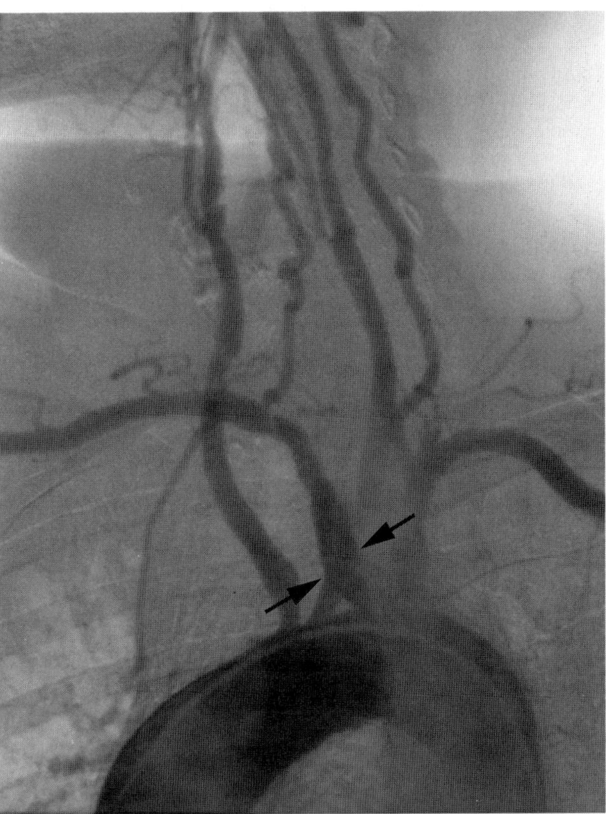

FIGURE 24.2. **Aberrant Right Subclavian Artery.** Aortogram demonstrating origin of the right subclavian artery distal to the left subclavian. Note the dilation of the origin of the right subclavian artery, representing a diverticulum of Kommerell (*arrows*).

the esophagus in 80% of cases, between the trachea and esophagus in 15%, and anterior to the trachea in 5% (Fig. 24.3A). A dilatation at the origin of the anomalous vessel is termed a *diverticulum of Kommerell* (Fig. 24.2). If large, it may cause significant posterior impression on the esophagus and result in dysphagia. The diagnosis can be confirmed with either CT or MR. Arteriography is rarely needed, but this anomaly may be encountered when angiography is performed for other reasons such as cerebral angiography. *Coarctation of the aorta* is a primary abnormality of the media with eccentric narrowing of the aortic lumen caused by infolding of the aortic wall (Fig. 24.3A). Approximately 70% of cases are associated with congenital cardiac anomalies, the most common being bicuspid aortic valve. *Pseudocoarctation* (aortic kink) (Fig. 24.3B) of the thoracic aorta is a misnomer, since it is a mild form of coarctation. The infolding occurs near the ligamentum arteriosum, similar to the localized form of coarctation. Patients are asymptomatic because of the lack of a hemodynamically significant stenosis, with a pressure gradient across the kink <10 mmHg. The ascending aorta is elongated with a high, transverse arch and redundant descending portion distal to the kink. There is a similar incidence of associated bicuspid aortic valve.

Aortic Trauma. The mechanism of thoracic aortic injury consists of either *blunt trauma* or *penetrating trauma* or, rarely, a combination of both. Although certainly less common, *penetrating trauma* to the aorta can occur, and angiographically penetrating trauma to the aorta is identical to penetrating injury to any vessel. *Blunt trauma* is far and away the most common trauma to the thoracic aorta and is most often the result of motor vehicle crashes and falls. The mechanism of blunt trauma is traditionally described as a result of sudden deceleration, with tearing of the aorta at the junction of its fixed and mobile portions: proximal ascending aorta, just beyond the left subclavian (aortic isthmus), and just above the level of the diaphragm. Another popular theory involves compression to the chest that crushes the vascular structures, while more recent data has proposed a combination of these two mechanisms.

Regardless of the mechanism of injury, aortic transaction is a clinical emergency. Classic numbers (from 1958), which combined clinical and autopsy data suggested that 85% of patients with aortic injury die at the accident scene; if untreated, most of the remaining 15% will die within 3 days. However, more recent data seem to indicate that with improvement in transport from the accident scene and prehospital treatment regimens, up to 50% of individuals with traumatic rupture of aorta reach the hospital alive.

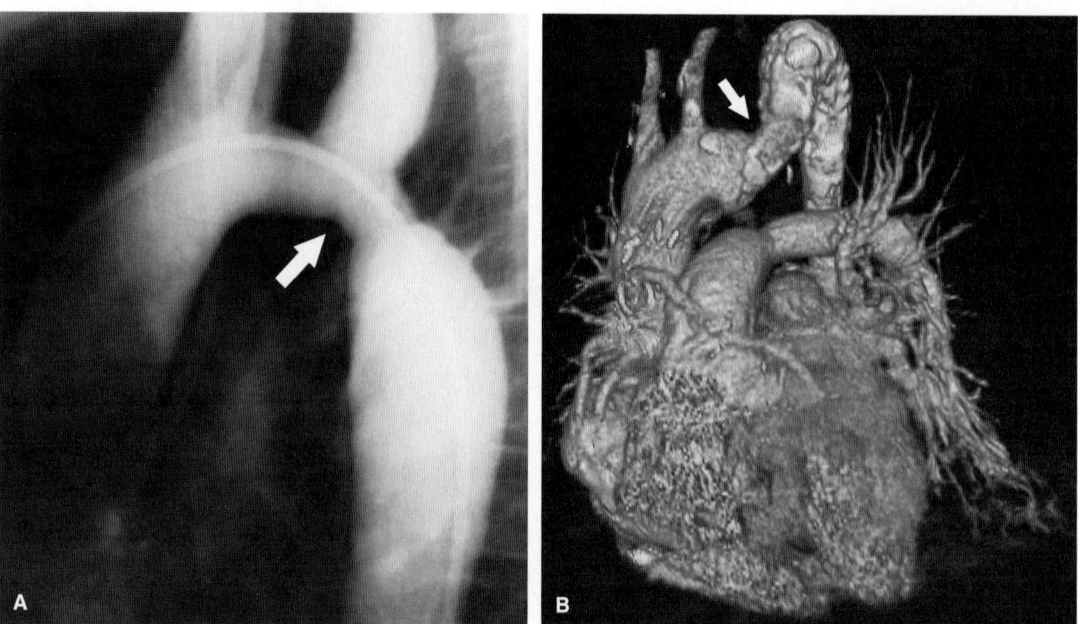

FIGURE 24.3. Coarctation of the Aorta. A. Aortic arch injection with "diffuse" type of coarctation (*arrow*), distal to the left subclavian artery. **B.** Reformatted CT angiogram of a 54-year-old man with pseudocoarctation of the aorta (*arrow*). Note smooth narrowing, which did not have a significant gradient at cardiac catheterization. (Courtesy of Dr Lynn M. Hurwitz, Durham, NC).

In addition, many of the subsequent in-hospital deaths are related to other serious concomitant injuries that inevitably occur in such serious trauma.

Aortography has been the gold standard for the diagnosis of thoracic aortic injury (Fig. 24.4A). Although relatively safe, it is time consuming, costly, invasive, and resource intensive. In near complete aortic transection, one may be unable to easily pass the catheter beyond the injury site, and a right brachial approach will be required. Because of the lack of specific clinical indicators for aortic trauma, a large number of negative aortograms have been performed. CT has replaced angiography as the initial radiographic diagnostic tool (following the chest radiograph) for blunt aortic injury. CT is widely available, and trauma patients at risk for thoracic aortic injury often require other CT examinations, e.g., head and abdomen. Findings on CT for blunt aortic trauma fall into two main categories: evidence of mediastinal hemorrhage or direct signs of aortic injury (Fig. 24.4B). Evidence of mediastinal hemorrhage includes poorly defined fat planes, mediastinal hemorrhage, perivascular hematoma, periaortic hematoma, and contrast extravasation. Direct signs of aortic injury include abnormal contour of the aorta, change in caliber of the aorta, and intraluminal irregularity (intimal flap). Using these criteria, chest CT has been shown to be extremely valuable as a screening tool, with 100% sensitivity and 100% negative predictive value for thoracic aortic injuries in some series. Because the mechanism is often difficult to determine and the physical assessment often offers little diagnostic value in these difficult patients, CT now prevents aortography in over 90% of trauma patients.

The criteria for performing aortography for suspected thoracic aortic injury are changing, and aortography is performed in most centers today based on an individual patient's needs. It is often performed to exclude aortic injury in questionable cases, particularly when determining the proximal extent of injury, when great vessel injury is suspected, or when planning endovascular rather than open surgical repair. To that end, when endovascular repair is planned, aortography is only performed during the repair process, rather than as a preliminary diagnostic study.

Angiographic findings of blunt aortic injury most often consist of an irregular outpouching just beyond the left subclavian artery, representing the aortic pseudoaneurysm, which is often bounded only by thin strands of adventitia or supported only by the adjacent mediastinum (Fig. 24.4C). Although 85% to 95% of aortic injuries found angiographically involve the aortic isthmus, one must also look for other vascular injuries in the thorax. This includes injury to the great vessels, as well as injury to the aortic valve resulting in aortic insufficiency. When performing arch aortography, the proximal great vessels must be included in the images (Fig. 24.5). A retrospective review of 89 patients with blunt chest trauma and angiographic evidence of traumatic injury to the thoracic aorta or to

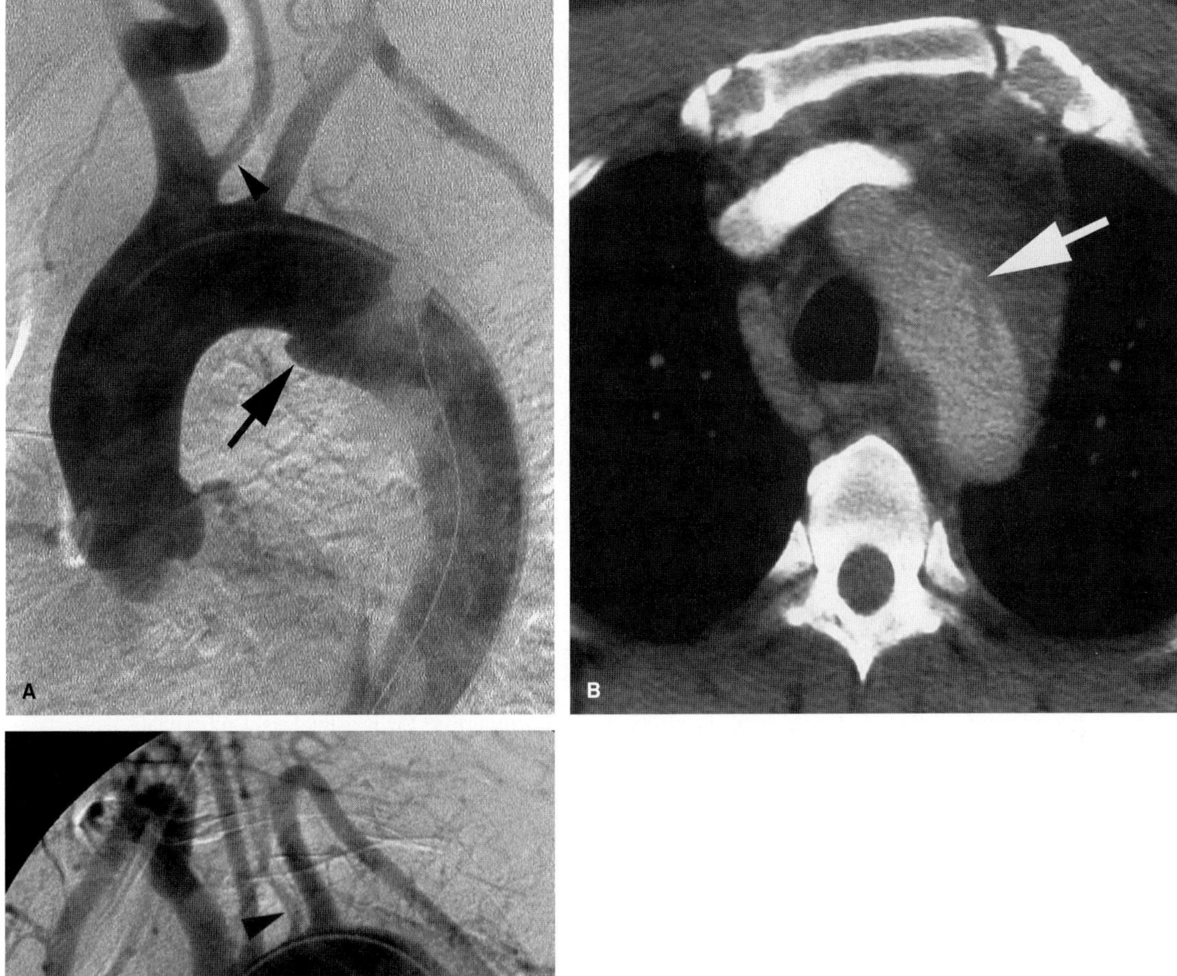

FIGURE 24.4. **Thoracic Aortic Trauma. A.** Aortogram of a 56-year-old woman following a motor vehicle crash with mediastinal hemorrhage demonstrates a nonconvex area at the aortic isthmus, suspected to be an aortic laceration (*arrow*). This was found to be a ductus bump at surgery. Normal-variant aortic arch anatomy with common origin of the right brachiocephalic artery and left common carotid artery is also present (*arrowhead*). **B.** A 37-year-old man with blunt trauma to the chest. CT demonstrates a large amount of mediastinal hemorrhage in addition to an aortic laceration (*arrow*). **C.** Aortogram of the same patient confirms the aortic laceration just distal to the left subclavian artery (*arrow*). Normal-variant aortic arch anatomy with the origin of the left vertebral artery from the aortic arch is also present (*arrowhead*).

its branches found that of the 19% of patients with ruptured aortic arch branches, 16% had an intact aorta and 3% had concomitant aortic rupture. More rarely, one may see a pseudoaneurysm of the ascending aorta just above the valve (often with aortic insufficiency) or just superior to the diaphragmatic hiatus. Frank extravasation at any of these sites is rare. A small aortic intimal tear may be the only angiographic finding, occurring in less than 10% of thoracic aortic tears.

Equivocal findings occur in <5% of aortograms, mostly because of difficulties in distinguishing the ductus bump from the contour abnormality at the isthmus (Fig. 24.4A). Keys to telling the difference are that the ductus bump is very smooth and convex without acute margins, whereas an aortic tear usually has acute margins, is irregularly shaped, and may have other associated abnormalities such as narrowing of the aorta, persistence of contrast in the outpouching, double densities, and presence of an intimal

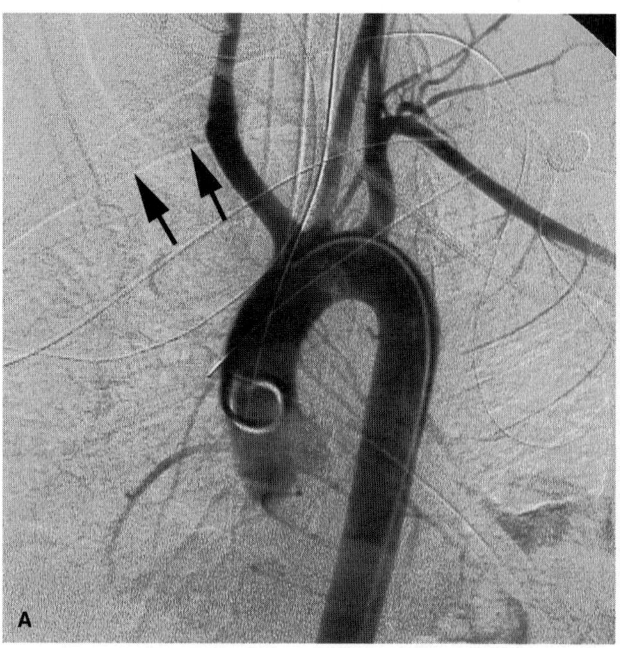

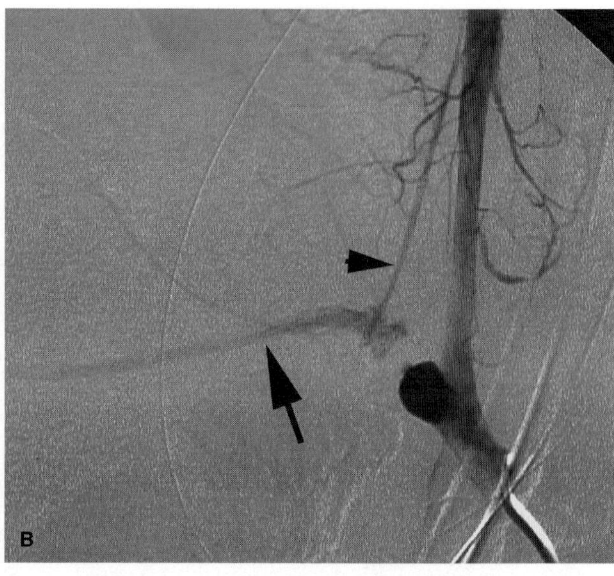

FIGURE 24.5. **Injury to Great Vessels. A.** This 23-year-old man was in a motor vehicle crash. The aortogram shows a normal arch but absence of the right subclavian (*arrows*). **B.** Selective injection of the right brachiocephalic artery shows obstruction of the proximal right subclavian artery with distal filling (*arrow*) via small collateral (*arrowhead*).

flap. It may be difficult in patients who have atherosclerosis, particularly plaque ulceration, to determine whether an angiographic abnormality is a tear or atherosclerotic disease. The presence of atherosclerotic disease elsewhere, in light of the findings on CT, helps to confirm the diagnosis.

The standard treatment for traumatic aortic injury is surgical grafting of the injured segment. This surgery is extensive, with mortality rates of 30%, often owing to other injuries related to the initial trauma. Paraplegia from open surgical repair occurs in almost 10% of patients. For these reasons, endovascular repair (stent grafting) of the injury is preferred and is becoming widely applied. Problems continue with unexpanded device size, accurate placement, and maintaining patency of the left subclavian artery. Finally, if the pseudoaneurysm of the aorta is not repaired and the tissues are strong enough to prevent rupture, a chronic saccular or fusiform pseudoaneurysm may form. Such pseudoaneurysms commonly calcify over the long term and are often diagnosed on chest radiographs.

Aneurysms of the Thoracic Aorta. Thoracic aneurysms are best classified by the portion of the aorta involved—that is, the ascending, arch, or descending thoracic aorta. This anatomic distinction is important because it allows an etiologic classification scheme. Regarding the aneurysms discussed here, those involving the ascending aorta include cystic medial necrosis, Marfan syndrome, Ehlers-Danlos syndrome, and syphilis (Figs. 24.6A, B, C). Aneurysms of the arch itself are more often atherosclerotic, as are descending thoracic aortic aneurysms. Posttraumatic thoracic aortic aneurysms most often occur at the prevalent site of injury, the aortic isthmus, while mycotic aneurysms, although more commonly associated with the ascending aorta, may occur anywhere along the course of the thoracic aorta.

Aneurysms of the ascending aorta constitute the majority of thoracic aneurysms (60%), followed by aneurysms of the descending aorta and, much more rarely, those of the arch and thoracoabdominal regions. A number of disease processes can lead to aneurysm formation in the thoracic aorta. A few of these are highlighted in this chapter because of their frequency (cystic medial degeneration, atherosclerosis, inflammation) or characteristic radiographic findings (Marfan syndrome, Ehlers-Danlos syndrome). Aneurysms of the ascending aorta most often result from cystic medial degeneration (cystic medial necrosis) (Fig. 24.6A). Cystic medial degeneration does occur in some patients with aging and appears to be accelerated by the presence of hypertension. In addition, the aortic manifestations of Marfan syndrome and Ehlers-Danlos syndrome (both described later in this chapter) result from a form of cystic medial degeneration.

Atherosclerotic disease infrequently causes aneurysms in the ascending aorta. However, aneurysms in the aortic arch are often atherosclerotic in etiology, and the most common cause of descending thoracic aortic aneurysms is certainly atherosclerotic disease. Seventy-five percent of

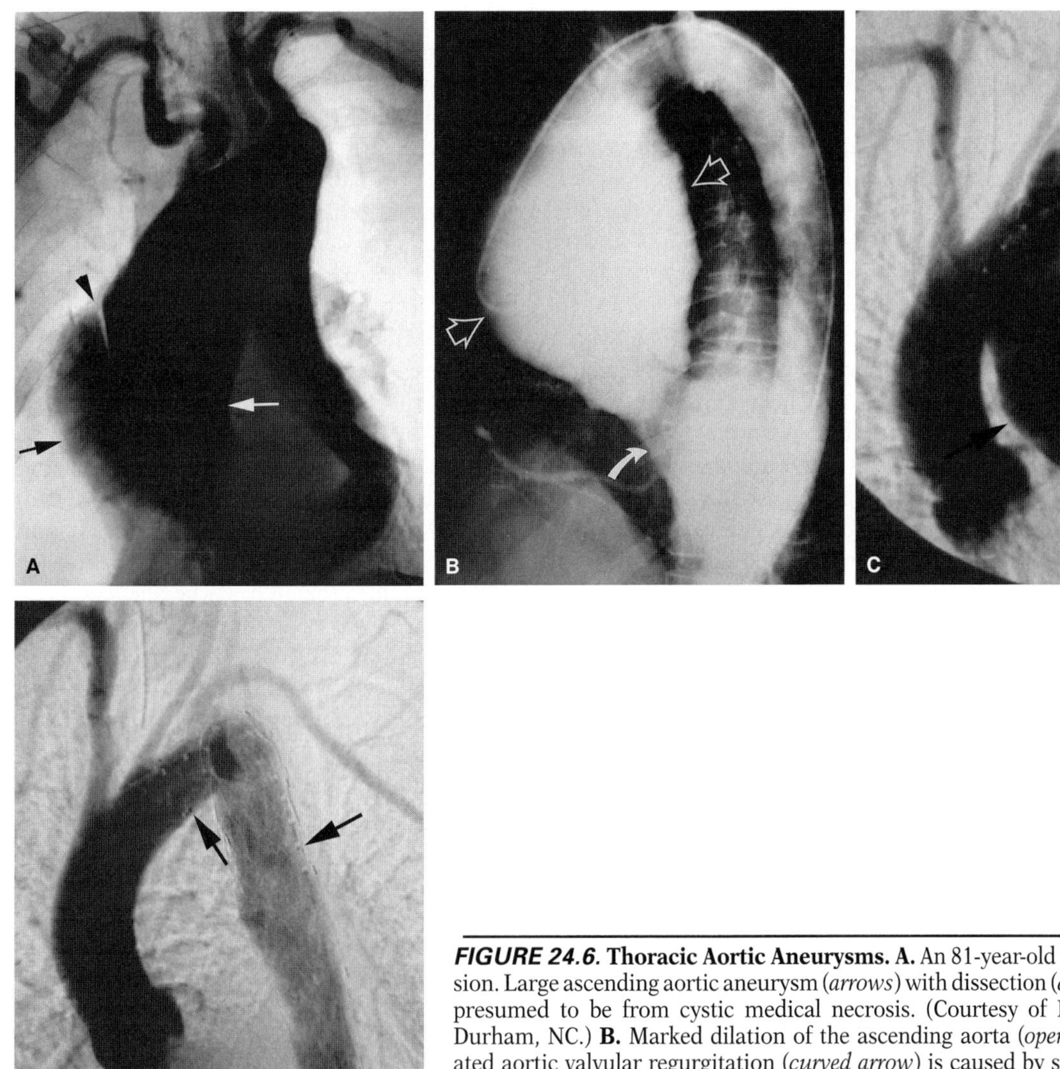

FIGURE 24.6. **Thoracic Aortic Aneurysms. A.** An 81-year-old patient with hypertension. Large ascending aortic aneurysm (*arrows*) with dissection (*arrowhead*). Aneurysm presumed to be from cystic medical necrosis. (Courtesy of Dr Joseph M. Stavas, Durham, NC.) **B.** Marked dilation of the ascending aorta (*open arrows*) with associated aortic valvular regurgitation (*curved arrow*) is caused by syphilis. **C.** Atherosclerotic aneurysm of descending aorta (*arrows*) in a 68-year-old man. **D.** Aneurysm has been successfully treated with an endograft (*arrows*). (Courtesy of Dr Richard McCann, Durham, NC.)

all thoracic aneurysms in the United States are atherosclerotic in etiology. Atherosclerosis of the thoracic aorta has the angiographic appearance of atherosclerotic disease elsewhere, including luminal irregularity by plaquing with or without calcification with degeneration of the aortic wall, resulting in thoracic aortic aneurysm formation. Atherosclerosis usually also causes stenoses/occlusions of the origins of the great vessels, particularly the left subclavian artery. Clinically, distal embolization is a feared complication, particularly stroke.

Thoracic aortic aneurysms can be diagnosed by noninvasive means, including sonography, MR, and CT, with the latter usually having the largest role. Angiography is usually obtained based on the individual needs of the patient, in particular, prior to surgical repair. Regarding the natural history of thoracic aneurysms, the best data are from the study of Davies et al, who found the growth rate for aneurysms to be greater for those of the descending aorta than for those of the ascending aorta. The mean rate of rupture or dissection was 2% per year for aneurysms under 5 cm in diameter, rose slightly to 3% per year for aneurysms 5 to 5.9 cm, and increased sharply to 7% per year for aneurysms 6.0 cm or larger. Rupture and acute dissection are the major complications of thoracic aortic aneurysms and can be fatal. Endovascular therapy using stent grafts has successfully been undertaken for descending thoracic aneurysms, and at least one device currently has Food and Drug Administration approval for this indication (Fig. 24.6D). As with thoracic aortic injury, difficulties with device size and placement continue to be problematic, but significant advances have been and will continue to be made.

Vasculitis is defined as an inflammatory process of the aorta and/or great vessels. There are a relatively large number of vasculitides, but only *Takayasu arteritis* and *infection* occur with enough frequency to deserve mention.

Although not that common in the United States, *Takayasu arteritis* presents a striking angiographic picture (Fig. 24.7). It represents a granulomatous (giant cell) inflammation of the media and adventitia of large elastic arteries. It frequently occurs in Asian women, with a female-to-male ratio of 10:1, and most often affects the thoracic aorta and its proximal branches and the pulmonary arteries. There are two relatively distinct clinical phases of the disease: an early phase and a late phase. The early phase presents with constitutional signs and symptoms and positive laboratory findings (increased erythrocyte sedimentation rate, positive C-reactive protein), but radiographic findings consist for the most part of only thickened vessel walls on CT and MR. Specifically, angiography is usually negative. The late phase has thickening of the media and adventitia, resulting in the typical angiographic findings of smooth long segment stenoses and occlusions of the proximal great vessels. Aneurysmal dilation is uncommon but can occur. Angiographic involvement has been classified into four types depending on the sites of involvement (including the great vessels, thoracic aorta, and abdominal aorta) as well as whether the disease is stenotic (as in most cases) or with dilations (rarely occurs).

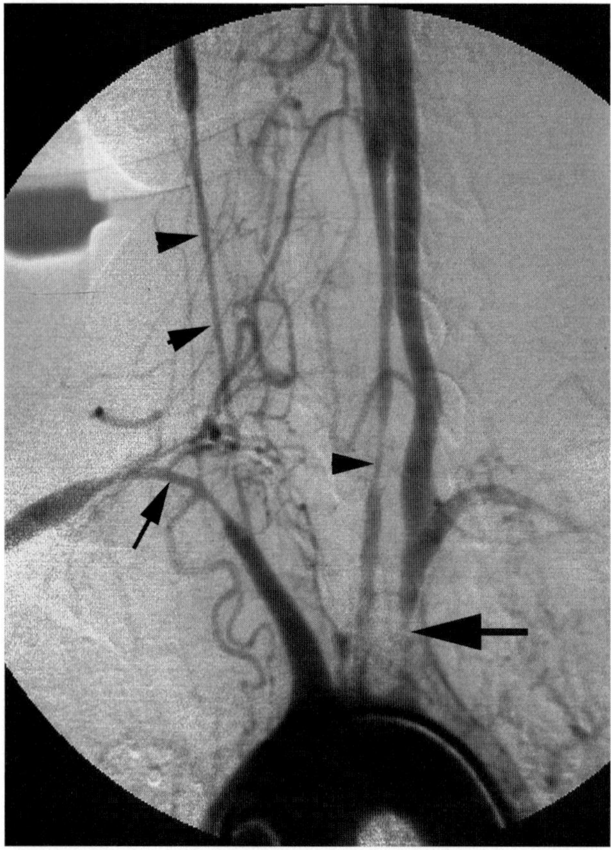

FIGURE 24.7. **Takayasu Arteritis.** A 21-year-old woman presented with seizures. Arch aortogram shows smooth narrowing of all the great vessels, including the right subclavian (*small arrow*), the right and left common carotid arteries (*arrowheads*), and the left subclavian (*large arrow*). Findings are typical of Takayasu arteritis.

Aortic infection is usually divided into two types based on the causative microorganism: syphilitic and mycotic (nonsyphilitic). *Syphilitic aortitis* occurs in approximately 12% of patients with untreated syphilis (Fig. 24.6B). It represents a direct effect of the spirochetes on the vessel wall. Syphilis was once a common cause of ascending aortic aneurysms. However, it is rarely seen today in the United States because of antibiotic therapy. There is certainly a long latency period between infection and the development of an aneurysm, most often from 10 to 25 years, and pathologically it consists of chronic inflammatory changes of the media and adventitia. The classic radiographic finding is aneurysm formation in the ascending aorta, less commonly extending into the arch. Large aneurysms are not uncommon. Fine dystrophic calcification by chest radiography, exclusively in the ascending aorta, occurs in up to 40% of cases. Aortic insufficiency is often present. There is a high likelihood of rupture if the aneurysm goes untreated.

Although the radiographic findings are not as classic as those of syphilitic aortitis, (*mycotic nonsyphilitic*) aortitis is much more common in the United States. The most common organisms are staphylococci, streptococci, and *Salmonella*, although virtually any microorganism can be the causative factor, particularly in immunocompromised patients. Although the exact mechanism of spread is unknown, bacteria destroy the aortic wall, most often resulting in irregular saccular aneurysms. Medial destruction results in aneurysm formation in 40% of patients with aortitis. When involving the aorta, it is associated with a high morbidity and mortality. Angiography demonstrates an irregular saccular aneurysm of the ascending aorta, which can also involve the arch and descending aorta, including the thoracoabdominal aorta. Any vessel can be involved, including the great vessels. Diagnosis is based on the patient's constitution, consistent with an infection.

There are two noninflammatory connective tissue diseases that bear mentioning: *Marfan syndrome* and *Ehlers-Danlos syndrome*. *Marfan syndrome* is an autosomal dominant disorder; recent studies in molecular genetics have identified the fibrillin gene product as the responsible defective connective tissue protein. Marfan syndrome affects approximately 1 per 10,000 individuals throughout the world, including both genders and all races and ethnic groups. The effects are widespread, including the eyes, skeleton, heart, and aorta, where >50% have cardiovascular complications. There is weakening of the aortic root, producing aortic ectasia and aortic insufficiency, making the patient prone to aortic dissection. Dissection or LV failure causes death in one third of patients by 32 years of

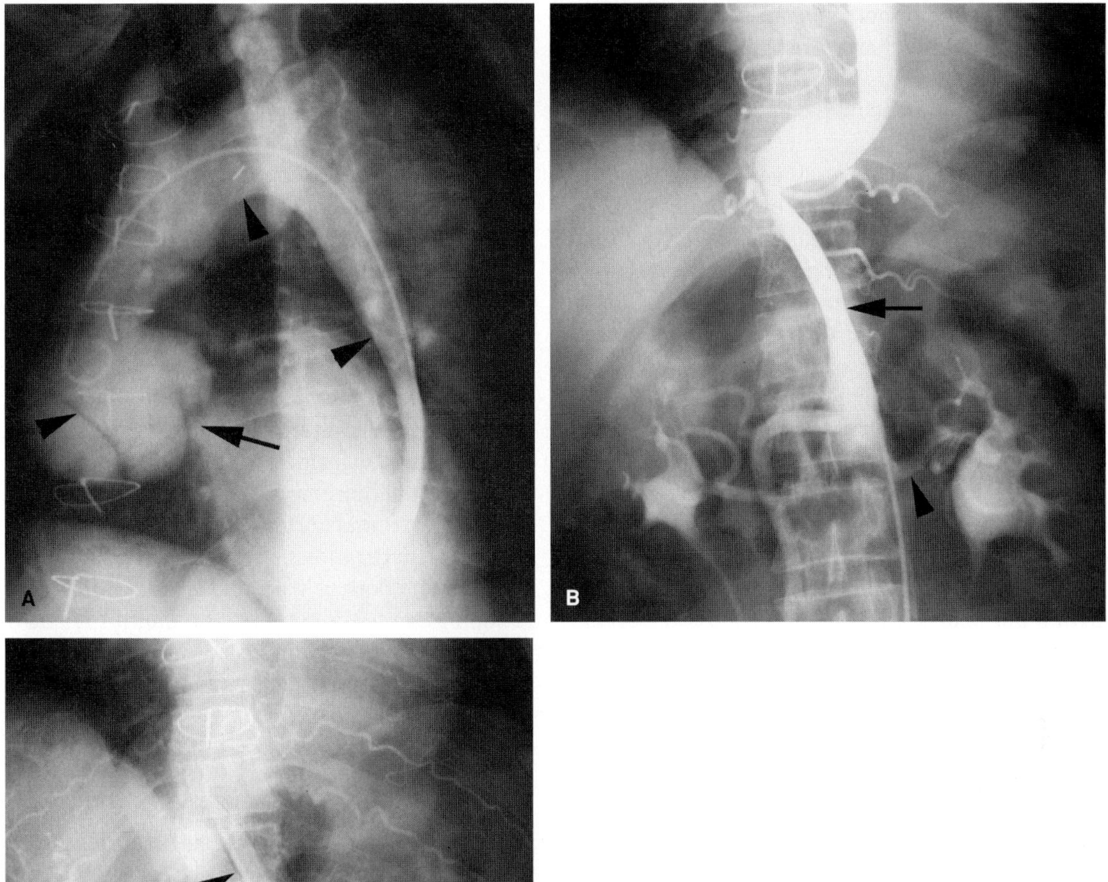

FIGURE 24.8. **Aortic Dissection. A.** Aortogram of a 47-year-old man with Marfan syndrome. Oblique arch view shows classic tulip bulb appearance of the aortic root (*arrow*). Dissection flap (*arrowheads*) is noted from the aortic root across the arch and into the descending aorta. **B.** Upper abdominal angiogram shows spiraling course of the dissection. This lumen, the true lumen, gives rise to the superior mesenteric artery (*arrow*) and the left renal artery (*arrowhead*). **C.** Later of image from abdominal aortogram shows intimal flap (*arrow*) as well as filling of the right renal artery (*arrowhead*) from the false lumen. (Courtesy Dr Joseph M. Stavas, Durham, NC.)

age and in two thirds by age 50 if untreated. The classic aortogram appearance is that of a very large aneurysmal aortic root with sinotubular ectasia (the "tulip bulb" appearance) (Fig. 24.8A). When present, aortic dissection involves the ascending aorta with or without extension into the descending (Fig. 24.8).

Ehlers-Danlos syndrome is a genetically heterogeneous group of heritable connective tissue disorders characterized by hyperextensible joints and tissue fragility. Multiple types have been described and categorized. Type IV, the type of interest here, has a defect in type III collagen presenting the characteristic vascular features, although other types have been reported to have vascular problems. Classically, type IV does not have the hyperextensibility of the large joints, although smaller joints may be minimally hypermobile. Angiographically, it tends to involve the ascending aorta, resulting in aneurysms, which are prone to dissection and rupture. Angiography should be carried out carefully as vessels are very thin and can even be perforated during catheterization.

Aortic dissection represents a laceration of the aortic intima and the inner layer of the media, resulting in a cleavage of the aortic media. Blood penetrates the aortic wall via the primary entry site and dissects the medial layers for a variable distance both upstream and particularly downstream, creating a false lumen. Blood flow may occur in both the true and false lumens, but either may be thrombosed. When blood flow exists in both lumens, there are one or more re-entry points of the false lumen into the true lumen. Aortic rupture characteristically occurs at the site of the primary entry and is the most common cause of death, with early mortality as high as 1% per hour if left untreated.

Approximately three fourths of all cases have involvement of the ascending aorta, arch, or both at autopsy. Less than 25% begin beyond the arch and 25% to 45% of dissections originate in the ascending aorta and reach the abdominal aorta. The dissection plane usually spirals as it courses downstream and may take any course. However, the typical course of an extensive dissection is usually described as the false aortic channel, expanding on the right in the arch and disrupting the right coronary artery. It then courses along the superior aspect of the arch, often involving the great vessels. If it extends distally, the false lumen most often courses to the left, involving the left renal artery. Still more distally, it tends to continue on the left side of the abdominal aorta and into the left pelvic system. Although dissection into the great vessels is quite a common finding, neurologic symptoms occur in only 20% of patients dying from dissections.

There are two basic classification systems for aortic dissection, which are based on extent of involvement. In the *DeBakey classification*, a type 1 dissection begins in the proximal aorta and courses into the descending thoracic aorta, a type 2 dissection is limited to the ascending aorta, and a type 3 dissection is limited to the descending aorta. The *Stanford classification* is based upon whether or not the ascending aorta is involved: a type A dissection involves the ascending aorta, and a type B dissection does not involve the ascending aorta. This classification scheme is based upon the need for surgical treatment of ascending aortic dissection.

There are a number of etiologic factors associated with aortic dissection. Cystic medial degeneration may be the chief predisposing factor in aortic dissection. Hypertension is present in 80% of surgical patients treated for aortic dissection and appears to be the most important predisposing factor. Atherosclerosis is present in up to two thirds of patients with an aortic dissection, although it may be coincidental rather than causative of aortic dissection. Other etiologic factors include inflammatory diseases (aortitis), blunt trauma, and iatrogenic trauma, including patients receiving catheterization, particularly patients with intra-aortic balloon counterpulsation devices. Congenital anomalies and inheritable disorders of elastic tissue (Marfan, Turner, Ehlers-Danlos syndromes) and congenitally abnormal aortic valves (particularly bicuspid aortic valve) are also associated with aortic dissection.

There are four modalities for imaging the thoracic aorta for the diagnosis of dissection: US, CT, MR, and catheter angiography. Excellent results, including sensitivities and specificities of greater than 90%, for all three noninvasive modalities have been reported. CT and MR have become the diagnostic imaging studies of choice, although transesophageal echocardiography is also applicable. However, because of its 24-hour availability and lack of invasiveness, CT is the most often employed imaging study.

Angiography was long considered the diagnostic standard for the evaluation of aortic dissection. However, prospective studies have found that for the diagnosis of aortic dissection, although the overall sensitivity of aortography is about 90%, it falls to only 77% when the definition of aortic dissection included intramural hematoma with a noncommunicating dissection. It does have advantages in that it is able to delineate the extent of the aortic dissection, including branch vessel involvement, the presence of aortic regurgitation, and patency of the coronary arteries. It is most often performed when stent grafting is being considered in the thoracic aorta or percutaneous fenestration for the abdominal aorta.

Complete diagnosis of aortic dissection requires visualization of both a true and a false lumen (Fig. 24.9). A supportive but incomplete finding for aortic dissection by angiography is compression of the true lumen by the unopacified false lumen. A number of important factors should be analyzed using angiography, including the extent of dissection, identification of the primary intimal tear (entry site), re-entry site(s), status of the aortic valve, and assessment of brachiocephalic and visceral vessels. Although a major point of aortography has been identification of the coronary vessels in relation to the exact site of intimal tear, most surgeons can visually inspect for these structures during surgery.

The classic angiographic finding of a "double barrel" aorta with an interposed intimal flap is seen in 87% of cases. The intimal flap usually begins in the right anterolateral ascending aorta and spirals to the left posterolateral aspect of the descending aorta into the abdomen (Fig. 24.8). Thus the left renal artery is frequently supplied by the false lumen, and the left iliac artery is more commonly involved when the dissection extends distally. Flow within the false lumen is slow, leading to late filling of branch vessels with their origin from this lumen. Thrombus in the false channel (25% of patients) appears as thickening of the aortic wall up to 1 cm. The true lumen is compressed and narrowed by the false channel in 85% of cases, deviating the course of a catheter.

Most diagnostic modalities for aortic dissection are aimed at the acute proximal dissection, as such a dissection requires emergency surgical intervention to prevent rupture into the pericardium. Surgery for more distal dissections (arch and beyond) in the acute setting continues to be controversial. Certainly those with perforated descending or abdominal aortas would require emergency surgery, as would those with mesenteric ischemia. However, if clinically stable, most patients are managed medically, which results in the chronic dissection often seen in imaging.

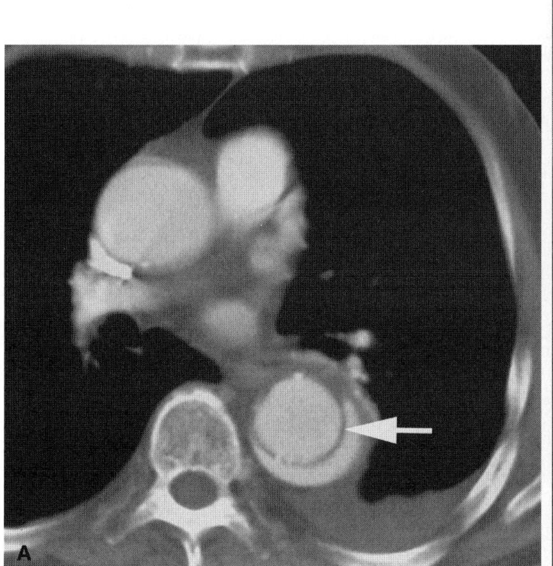

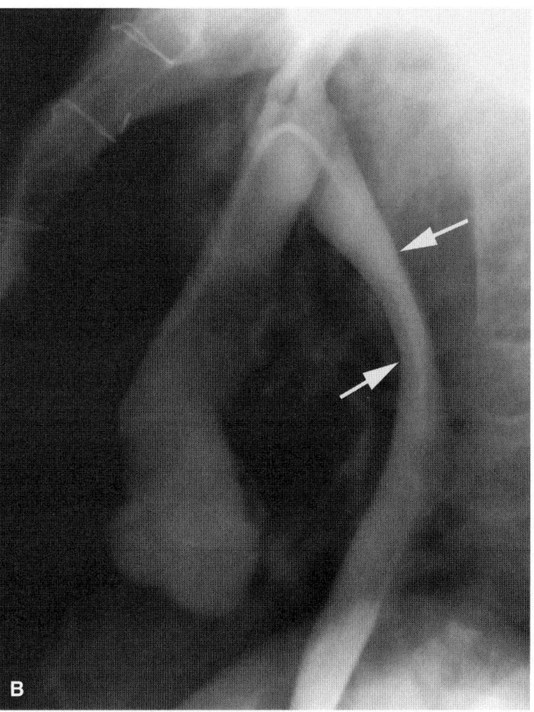

FIGURE 24.9. **Thoracic Aortic Dissection. A.** This 68-year-old man presented with chest pain. CT of thorax demonstrates the typical intimal flap of an aortic dissection (*arrow*). **B.** Lateral aortogram shows filling of the true lumen (*arrows*), which is compressed by the false lumen. The false lumen fills on later images.

The strength of angiography may be in its possibility for endovascular therapy. Although still early in the experience, promising results have been obtained and, of course, endovascular surgery avoids the risks of major thoracic surgery. However, stent grafting is limited to the descending thoracic aorta only; an ascending injury still requires open repair. Endovascular fenestration of the aorta is a method of creating an opening in the intimal flap to allow blood flow into both lumens, preserving side branch patency. Although often performed in the thoracic aorta, it is indicated for acute abdominal and distal limb ischemia and is discussed along with the abdominal aorta (see Chapter 25). Although the roles of stent grafting and fenestration are yet to be proven, they will have an impact on future therapeutic strategies.

Within the differential diagnosis of aortic dissection are the *intramural hematoma* and *penetrating aortic ulcer*. These three entities share much in common and in fact together constitute the *acute aortic syndrome*. An intramural hematoma represents a localized hematoma within the aortic wall. This usually occurs in the elder, hypertensive patient and may represent a controlled dissection, although not all experts agree on this point. It is thought to represent a localized dissection without an identifiable entry/re-entry point. It may, however, progress to dissection. Angiography plays little role in the diagnosis. CT, MR, or US are the diagnostic tests of choice and demonstrate the characteristic intramural hematoma. An atherosclerotic plaque may ulcerate into the media, resulting in a *penetrating aortic ulcer*. The presentation is usually an elderly hypertensive patient with marked atherosclerotic disease. The diagnosis is best made by CT, which demonstrates aortic ulcer, frequently associated with an intramural hematoma (Fig. 24.10A). Penetrating ulcer of the thoracic aorta is defined as an atherosclerotic lesion of the descending thoracic aorta with ulceration that penetrates the internal elastic lamina, allowing hematoma formation in the media (Fig. 24.10B). There is controversy regarding whether this lesion differs from classic acute type III aortic dissection. The plaque may precipitate localized intramedial dissection associated with a variable amount of hematoma within the aortic wall, may break through into the adventitia to form a pseudoaneurysm, or may rupture completely into the right or left hemithorax. The diagnosis is made at CT with demonstration of a contrast material–filled outpouching in the aorta in the absence of a dissection flap or false lumen and often in the presence of extensive aortic calcification. Although aortography once was the standard for the diagnosis of many aortic diseases, it has largely been replaced by CT and MR. However, angiography still plays a role when endovascular therapy with a stent graft is employed. Penetrating ulcers appear to have a greater propensity to rupture in the acute setting during conservative treatment. Thus, aggressive management is

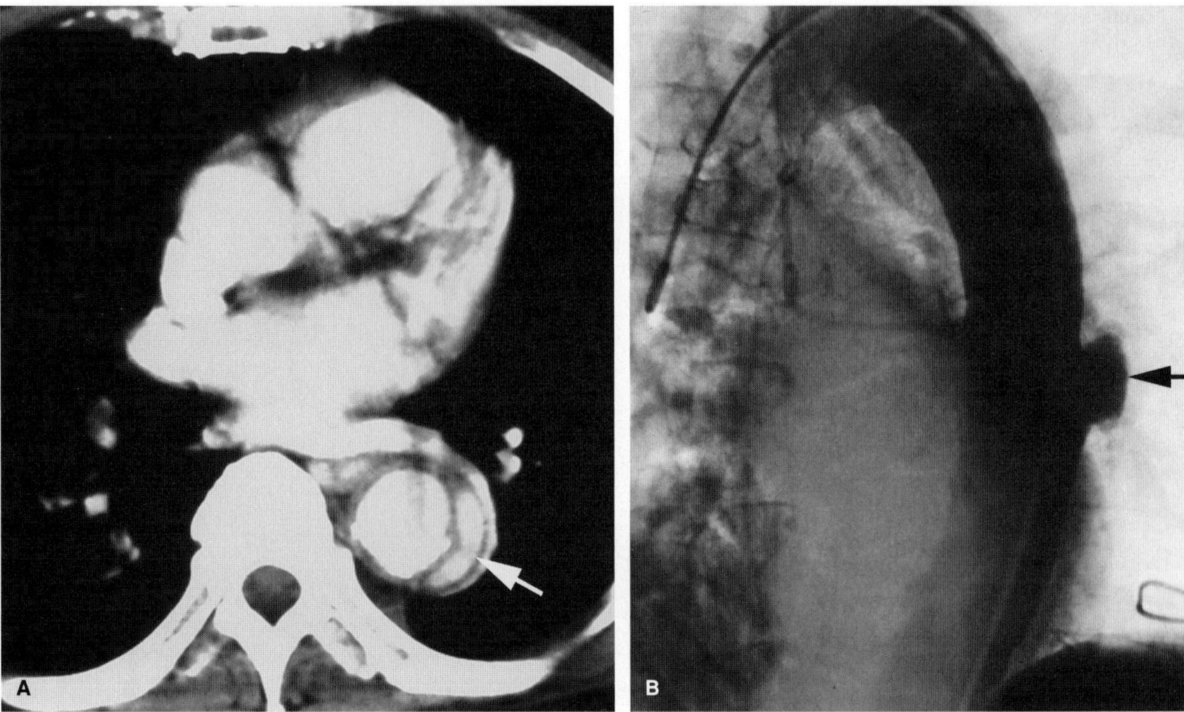

FIGURE 24.10. **Penetrating Aortic Ulcer. A.** CT of a 73-year-old man with chest pain shows an area of contrast filling with surrounding area of hemorrhage (*arrow*). Areas of calcification in the aorta signify underlying atherosclerotic disease. **B.** Oblique descending thoracic aortogram shows the ulcer crater filling with contrast material (*arrow*). Traditionally, treatment was effected by open surgery, but today this condition can be effectively treated with stent grafting.

recommended for penetrating ulcers, and a high index of suspicion must be maintained for rupture.

PULMONARY ANGIOGRAPHY

Pulmonary angiography is usually performed from the common femoral vein, but it can be performed from the internal jugular or brachial/axillary veins. Specially shaped pulmonary catheters in a 5 to 7 French multi-sidehole pigtail design with a near right-angle curve (such as the Grollman catheter) can be easily placed into the right or left pulmonary artery. Traditionally, pressures are obtained in the pulmonary artery as well as in the RA and RV. Such pressures have diagnostic value (pressures reflective of right heart function) and there has been controversy regarding perceived complications of pulmonary angiography at higher arterial pressures (discussed subsequently). Nonionic, low-osmolar contrast material is used, resulting in fewer complications and a decrease in cough reflex. Imaging is performed digitally today, with acquisition of at least 6 frames/second. The anatomy of the pulmonary arteries is variable but for the most part follows the bronchi.

Complications of pulmonary angiography have mostly been reported for the diagnosis of pulmonary embolism and are felt to be increased in the presence of pulmonary artery hypertension (usually defined as pulmonary artery systolic pressure >30 mmHg). It has been reported that pulmonary angiography is contraindicated in patients with high pulmonary artery pressures and left bundle branch block. The presence of pulmonary artery hypertension can result in right heart strain, which is exacerbated by contrast injection. However, it is not problematic with low-osmolar agents injected into the right or left pulmonary artery rather than the main pulmonary artery. The presence of an existing left bundle branch block is problematic because of its possibly inducing a right bundle block during catheterization of the right heart, resulting in total heart block. Transvenous or external pacing is recommended in this group of patients.

There may be a host of indications for pulmonary angiography in a particular patient. Such indications may include trauma, congenital anomalies (particularly with congenital heart disease), tumor encasement of vessels, pulmonary hypertension (primary), vasculitis, and stenosis. However, two overriding indications in the typical interventional radiology practice are *pulmonary embolism* (PE) and *pulmonary arteriovenous malformations* (PAVMs).

Pulmonary artery aneurysms deserve a brief discussion, even though they are rare, and even more rarely require pulmonary angiography, which is most often performed in anticipation of endovascular therapy. There are multiple etiologies for pulmonary artery aneurysms. The most striking is associated with tuberculous infection, forming the Rasmussen aneurysm. Antibiotic therapy has all but eradicated this in the United States, where the most common cause of a pulmonary artery aneurysm (pseudoaneurysm) is from iatrogenic trauma related to placement of a pulmonary artery catheter (mostly of the Swan-Ganz type).

Pulmonary Embolism. It has been estimated that PE occurs in approximately 650,000 patients annually in the United States and contributes to up to 50,000 deaths. It is said to be responsible for up to 15% of all in hospital deaths. PE disease can be divided into chronic and acute forms based on history and angiographic appearance.

Pulmonary angiography for acute PE has been all but replaced by multislice CT and is now often relegated to difficult diagnostic situations (Fig. 24.11A). There are still some advantages of pulmonary angiography. Although it is certainly less than perfect, pulmonary angiography is

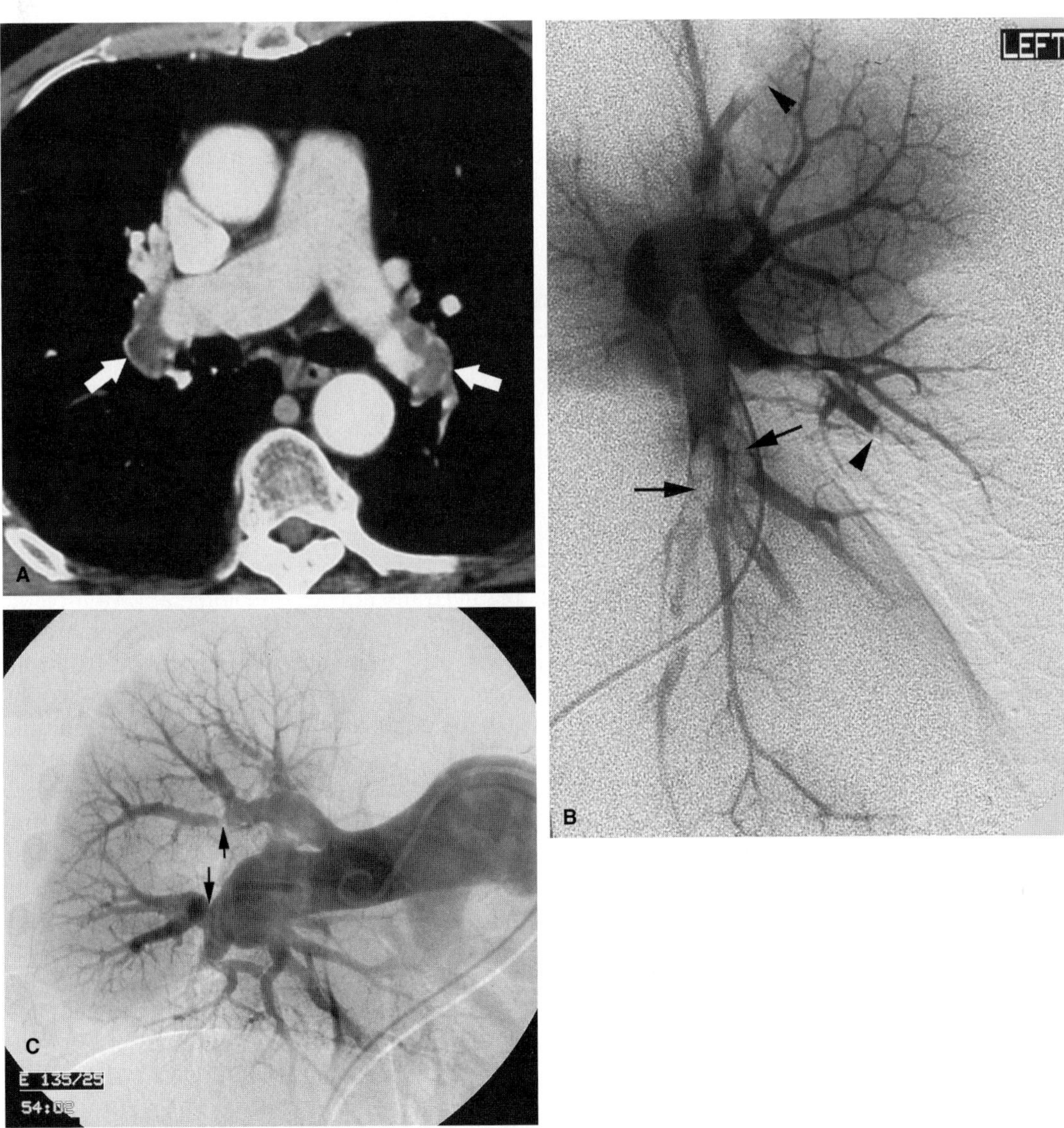

FIGURE 24.11. **Pulmonary Embolism (PE). A.** CT of a 78-year-old man with hypoxia demonstrates filling defect in the right and left pulmonary arteries, diagnostic of PE (*arrows*). **B.** Left pulmonary artery injection of a 72-year-old man who fainted demonstrates intraluminal filling defects (*arrows*) and areas of occlusion (*arrowheads*), diagnostic of acute PE. **C.** Right pulmonary angiogram of a 35-year-old woman with severe shortness of breath shows enlarged main and right proximal pulmonary arteries, with pruning of vessels distally and areas of narrowing (webbing) (*arrows*); this is diagnostic of chronic PE.

the imaging "gold standard." It allows visualization of the pelvic veins and inferior vena cava (IVC), and it provides hemodynamic parameters (pulmonary and right heart pressures) as well as an opportunity for therapy in the same sitting (filter, thrombolysis). The main disadvantage of pulmonary angiography is its invasive nature, which is not only uncomfortable for the patient but has a finite complication rate, including arrhythmias, cardiac injury (perforation), cardiac arrest, respiratory insufficiency, contrast reactions, access hematoma/thrombosis, and even death.

The diagnosis of acute PE by pulmonary angiography is only reliable when intraluminal filling defects or an occluded pulmonary artery with or without a trailing edge of clot are identified (Fig. 24.11B). Less reliable findings include area(s) of decreased flow, abnormal parenchymal stain, presence of collateral vessels, and delayed venous return. Pulmonary angiography should be performed as soon as possible, as the body tends to dissolve thrombus at a variable rate.

Approximately 0.1% to 0.2% of patients with acute PE develop chronic pulmonary hypertension. Pulmonary angiography for *chronic pulmonary embolic disease* is usually performed to confirm the diagnosis and for surgical planning for pulmonary endarterectomy. Chronic pulmonary embolic disease can be suggested from CT or MR angiography findings, but the diagnosis is confirmed by pulmonary angiography. Diagnosis of chronic PE by pulmonary angiography is based on the identification of webs, luminal irregularities, areas of abrupt vessel narrowing and/or obstruction, and dilated central pulmonary arteries consistent with arterial hypertension (Fig. 24.11C). These findings are usually bilateral. Pulmonary angiographic techniques are the same as for acute PE.

Thrombolytic therapy for acute PE has the goal of rapid clot dissolution, resulting in greater pulmonary perfusion, thus providing improved hemodynamic (right heart) status and better gas exchange. Complete clot resolution should also serve to decrease chronic vascular obstruction, hopefully preventing chronic pulmonary hypertension. All of these should reduce the morbidity and mortality of PE. Unfortunately, most of this is currently unproven. In theory, catheter-directed thrombolytic therapy should be superior to IV administration because the agent is concentrated to the region of concern and continued until thrombus has been significantly reduced. Unfortunately, the results are not clear on these points, and intra-arterial administration of thrombolytic therapy for acute PE is limited to patients who are severely ill and in need of rapid thrombus dissolution. Further studies are needed, but early data do not support the use of local thrombolytic agents over IV administration except in highly selected cases. There are currently available a number of mechanical thrombectomy devices that serve to debulk (break up) the thrombus. Small series have been published in which these instruments were applied to PE. Although the theory is very attractive, the data are scarce, very early, and completely uncontrolled.

Pulmonary arteriovenous malformations represent direct, low-pressure, artery-to-vein connections (fistulas) of the lung. Although they are associated with hereditary hemorrhagic telangiectasia (HHT) (also called Rendu-Osler-Weber syndrome) in 60% to 90% of reported cases, PAVMs may occur spontaneously (without HHT), or they may be associated with other causes such as trauma or erosion of a vessel by aneurysm, infection, or tumor.

The clinical presentation of PAVMs may be difficult to discern, because only 72% of patients have symptoms referable to the PAVM or underlying HHT. The presence of symptoms correlates best with lesion size. A single AVM <2 cm in diameter does not usually cause symptoms. The incidence of symptoms is said to be greater in patients with multiple rather than single PAVMs, and multiple PAVMs occur in approximately 35% of patients. The most common complaint in symptomatic patients with PAVM is, interestingly, epistaxis from HHT. Dyspnea is the most common complaint relative to the pulmonary system, while the most frequent serious complication is caused by paradoxical emboli to the CNS, seen in 30% of patients and consisting of strokes (18%), cerebral abscesses (9%), transient ischemic attacks (37%), and migraines (43%).

PAVMs can be diagnosed on a chest radiograph but are best diagnosed by CT, which will visualize even the small AVMs. In addition, CT is an excellent method to screen patients and for follow-up after embolotherapy. Pulmonary angiography is usually performed when contemplating transcatheter embolotherapy. Multiple views of the pulmonary vessels are necessary, and subselective injections are required to fully define the PAVM and to perform transcatheter therapy. Both lungs should be studied angiographically to look for other (multiple) PAVMs. PAVMs are categorized, based on the number and pattern of feeding arteries, as simple (one artery to one vein) or complex (multiple feeding arteries and/or draining veins). Angiographically, feeding artery(ies) and draining vein(s) are demonstrated with the malformation represented as a fistula site/aneurysmal dilation between the two (Fig. 24.12A). The angiographic picture is very characteristic and fully diagnostic.

The indications for transcatheter embolotherapy of PAVMs include exercise intolerance, prevention of neurologic complications, and prevention of lung hemorrhage (hemoptysis). Based on these indications, PAVMs are usually treated when the feeding artery is at least 3 mm in size. It is usually possible to occlude the feeding artery or arteries at the fistula site, and coils are most often used (detachable balloons are not currently available in the United States) (Fig. 24.12B). Success rates for embolotherapy are greater than 98%. Follow-up by CT to determine complete obliteration of the AVM has shown long-term success rates

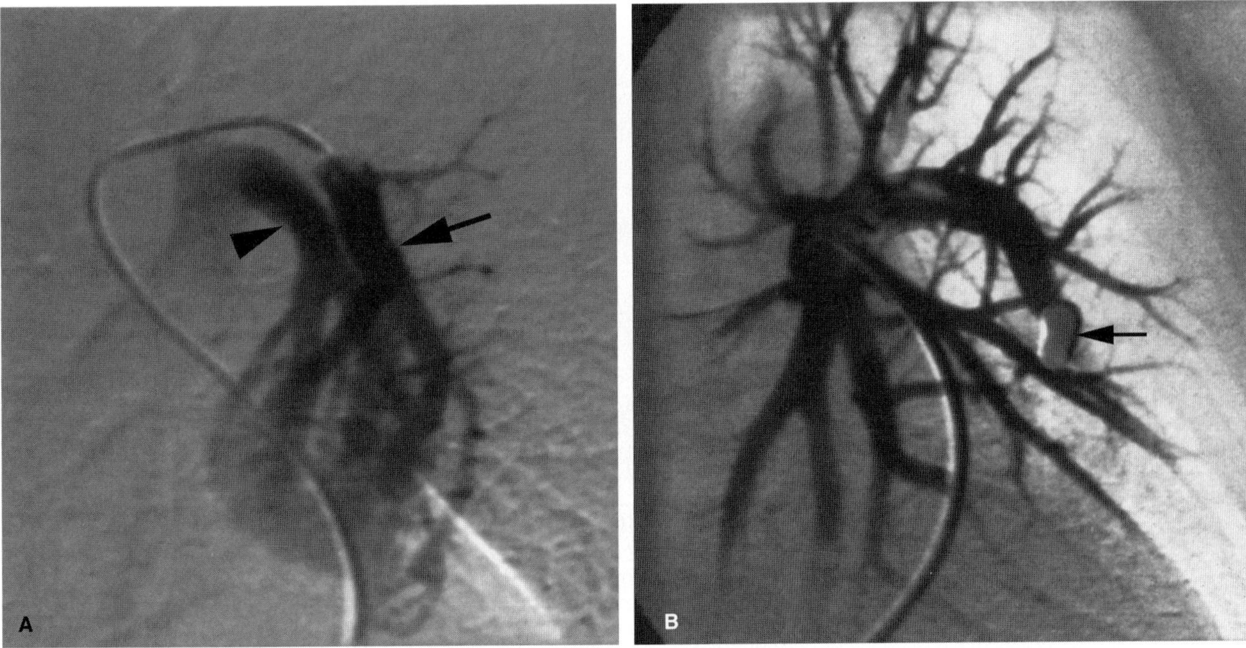

FIGURE 24.12. **Pulmonary Arteriovenous Malformation. A.** Selective angiogram of a left lower lobe pulmonary artery in a 33-year-old woman with dyspnea demonstrates a pulmonary arteriovenous malformation with a single feeding artery (*arrow*) and vein (*arrowhead*). **B.** Embolization of feeding artery with a detachable balloon (*arrow*) resulted in complete obliteration of the malformation.

of 95%. If flow is found within the AVM, additional embolotherapy is indicated.

The major complication of embolotherapy is paradoxical embolization of the coil, which is rare, occurring in <1% of all AVMs treated. Self-limiting pleurisy with minimal temperature elevation occurs in 5% to 10% of treated patients. Air embolization during treatment has been observed but has not been reported to be problematic.

BRONCHIAL ARTERIOGRAPHY

Bronchial artery anatomy is extremely variable, and the most common patterns or classification schemes vary from author to author depending on the source (autopsy, cadaveric dissections, and/or angiography). The bronchial arteries to the right and left arise from the thoracic aorta, usually from the T4 to T9 level, and 90% arise from the T5 and T6 levels. Bronchial anatomy is quite variable. The most common patterns are: three arteries (usually one right and two left) seen in 40%, single arteries bilaterally seen in 30%, and two arteries bilaterally seen in 25%. Bronchial supply may also arise in conjunction with an intercostal artery as a broncho-intercostal artery. In this situation, one must be very careful regarding supply to the spinal cord, including the anterior spinal artery (artery of Adamkiewicz).

There are a number of clinical indications for bronchial angiography, including preoperative investigation following embolic obstruction of the pulmonary arteries, congenital cardiopathy with interruption of the pulmonary artery, evaluation of the bronchial arterial system after lung transplantation, and pulmonary sequestrations. However, far and away the most common indication in an adult clinical radiology practice is for hemoptysis. Massive hemoptysis is usually defined as >600 mL/24 hours, although the numbers vary in publications from 200 to 1,000 mL/24 hours. The etiologies for hemoptysis are numerous. The most prevalent cause worldwide continues to be infection, particularly tuberculosis. In the United States, bronchogenic carcinoma, bronchitis, and bronchiectasis are the most prevalent. However, more than 20% of cases are idiopathic.

Bronchial angiography for hemoptysis is almost always performed as a precursor to planned transarterial embolotherapy of the bronchial supply. Arterial supply to the lungs can also originate as transpleural collaterals, which become enlarged because of chronic inflammation or occlusion of bronchial arteries. This is particularly true if the patient has undergone prior bronchial artery embolotherapy. Transpleural arterial collaterals originate from a number of different sites, including but not limited to the intercostal arteries; branches of the subclavian artery, including the thyrocervical and costocervical trunks as well as the internal mammary arteries; and branches of the axillary artery, particularly the thoracodorsal artery. These nonbronchial collaterals are responsible for massive

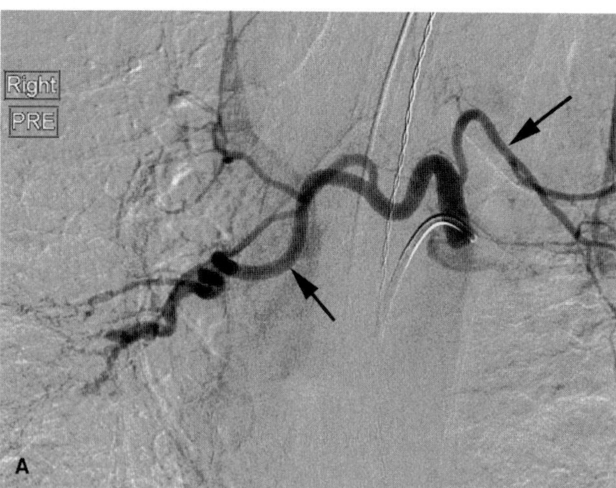

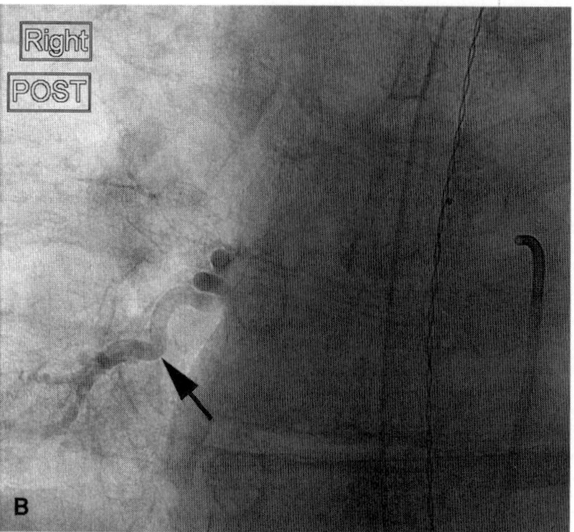

FIGURE 24.13. **Bronchial Artery Embolization. A.** Selective angiogram of 19-year-old man with hemoptysis from right upper lobe at bronchoscopy shows a common trunk for right and left bronchial arteries (*arrows*). Both sides are enlarged, with the right greater than the left. **B.** View following bronchial artery embolization with polyvinyl alcohol sponge particles shows stasis of flow in the right bronchial artery (*arrow*).

hemoptysis in up to 50% of cases. The pulmonary artery is rarely the source of hemoptysis, except with aneurysms and PAVMs.

During bronchial angiography, actual hemorrhage is very rarely seen, because such bleeding is usually intermittent and not of the degree to present as contrast extravasation angiographically. Rather, areas of hemoptysis usually originate from sites of enlarged and abnormal-appearing bronchial arteries, as seen angiographically (Fig. 24.13A). There is often hypervascularity and systemic to pulmonary arterial or venous shunting. If abnormal-appearing arteries from either the bronchial or transpleural supply are not visualized, pulmonary angiography should then be performed.

Bronchial embolotherapy is performed after selective catheterization of the bronchial arteries (Fig. 24.13B). Selective angiograms are essential to completely define the anatomy. Embolization can be performed directly through the traditional diagnostic catheter, if it can be placed well within the bronchial artery without occluding blood flow. Usually, however, embolization is performed with a coaxial system using a microcatheter. Embolization is usually performed with particles, most often polyvinyl alcohol sponge particles. The particles should be large enough to occlude at a precapillary level, thereby reducing the chances of shunting into the pulmonary venous system (effectively a right-to-left shunt). Larger particles also preserve capillary flow to critical organs supplied by the bronchial arteries, including the lungs, tracheobronchial tree, portions of the visceral pleura, esophagus, and other mediastinal tissues. Coil embolization of the proximal bronchial artery is not recommended because of collateral flow to the bronchial artery distal to the coiling.

Hemoptysis is controlled in the first 24 hours following embolotherapy in up to 98% of patients. Unfortunately, repeat hemorrhage occurs in 15% to 25% of patients within the first year. Complications from bronchial angiography and embolization are rare, consisting mostly of intimal dissections not requiring therapy (5%). Major complications are exceedingly rare, and most series report none. The most feared major complications have been for spinal cord injury. The only reported case of damage to the cord from "bronchial" embolization was in an artery arising from the seventh intercostal artery (broncho-intercostal) rather than a bronchial artery itself. There are also reports of transverse myelitis from bronchial angiography when high-osmolar contrast agents were used. It is generally believed that the risk of spinal cord damage from bronchial angiography and embolization is exceedingly low using today's techniques.

PERIPHERAL ARTERIAL DISEASE

The anatomy of the peripheral arterial system is quite straightforward. However, there are a few anatomic variants worth mentioning. Absence of the anterior or posterior tibial arteries occurs in approximately 5% of individuals. A high origin of the radial artery from either the axillary or brachial artery occurs in up to 17% of patients. A clinically confusing variant is the persistent sciatic artery, which represents a normal fetal branch of the internal iliac artery that continues into the lower extremity to provide the runoff vessels (Fig. 24.14). In the adult, it arises from the anterior division of the internal iliac artery and runs posteriorly through the sciatic notch. There is

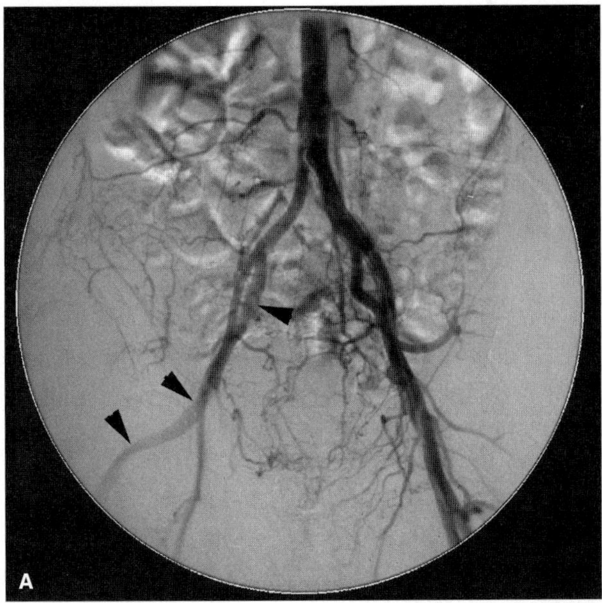

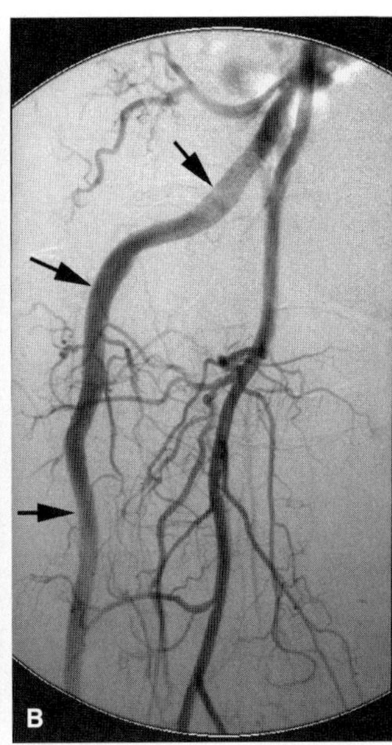

FIGURE 24.14. **Persistent Sciatic Artery. A.** Pelvic angiogram of 80-year-old man undergoing angiography for peripheral vascular disease demonstrates a large branch from the internal iliac artery (*arrowheads*) representing the persistent sciatic artery. **B.** Pelvic angiogram with imaging of the right upper leg shows enlarged branch (*arrows*) giving rise to the right superficial femoral artery, confirming the diagnosis. The left pelvic and left leg anatomy are conventional.

therefore no palpable femoral pulse, which may cause confusion on physical exam. The persistent sciatic artery is seen in <0.1% of individuals and, because of its posterior location, is subject to trauma, particularly a fall on the buttocks.

Obstructive Arterial Disease. Prior to radiographic imaging, physical examination of both the upper and lower limbs as well as laboratory assessment of the lower limbs are essential. Physical examination should include assessment of color, temperature, pulses, and evidence of tissue loss. Laboratory assessment centers around the ankle-brachial index (ABI), which is a comparison of systolic blood pressure in the arm to that in the ankle. In general, a normal ABI should be greater than 1.0. An ABI between 0.95 and 0.5 signifies intermittent to severe claudication, while one under 0.5 presents with rest pain and tissue loss. Doppler wave forms and segmental limb pressures are also useful as noninvasive means of evaluating peripheral blood flow.

Atherosclerosis is the single most common indication for peripheral angiography and intervention in the United States. Patients can present with chronic or acute symptoms (often acute on chronic). The angiographic findings are multifocal, diffuse luminal irregularities with areas of occlusion and variable calcification. The angiographic appearance of diabetic vascular disease differs from typical atherosclerosis in two main ways: dramatic vascular calcification involving arteries of all sizes, and the pattern of disease involvement is more distal, often sparring large proximal vessels. The most common locations for atherosclerotic disease of the lower limb are the superficial femoral artery (SFA) at the adductor (Hunter) canal, common iliac artery, popliteal artery, tibioperoneal trunk, and origins of the tibial arteries. Symptomatic atherosclerosis in the upper extremities is much less common. The most common site for upper-extremity atherosclerotic involvement is the proximal left subclavian artery, which can result in subclavian steal. Another prevalent site for upper-limb atherosclerotic involvement is the digital arteries of the hand.

Treatment of atherosclerotic occlusive disease is either by endovascular means or surgical bypass. The overall results of angioplasty are provided in Table 24.3 Several general principles should be kept in mind. The larger the vessel (with greater arterial blood flow), the better the results of angioplasty. Therefore, iliac artery angioplasty has traditionally been superior to angioplasty of the SFA (Fig. 24.15). Stenting has improved immediate success and long-term patency in lesions above the inguinal ligament and in the subclavian but not more distally in either limb. In general, balloon angioplasty of the iliac arteries can be performed with balloon-expandable

TABLE 24.3 Angioplasty Results of the Aorta, Pelvis, and Lower Extremity Arterial System

Location	*Technical Success (%)*	*1° Patency (%)* 1 yr	3 yr	5 yr
Aortoiliac PTA ± stent	85	88	78	75
PTA iliac stenosis	95	78	66	61
PTA iliac occlusion	83	68	60	—
Stent iliac stenosis	99	90	74	72
Stent iliac occlusion	82	75	64	—
PTA femoropopliteal	90	61	51	48
Stent femoropopliteal	98	67	—	—

PTA, percutaneous transluminal angioplasty.

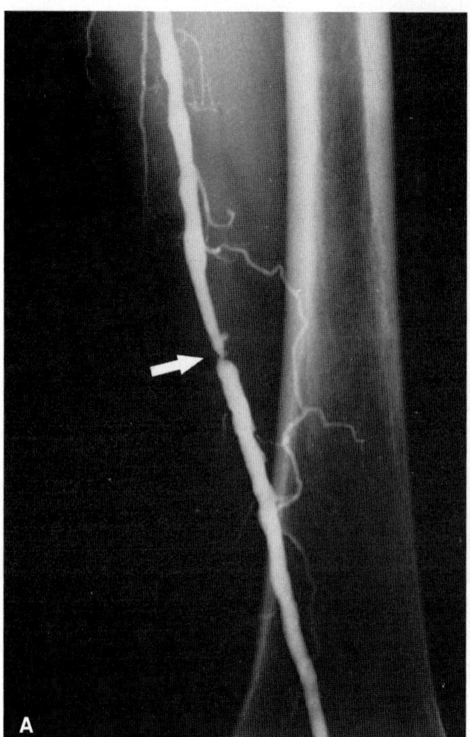

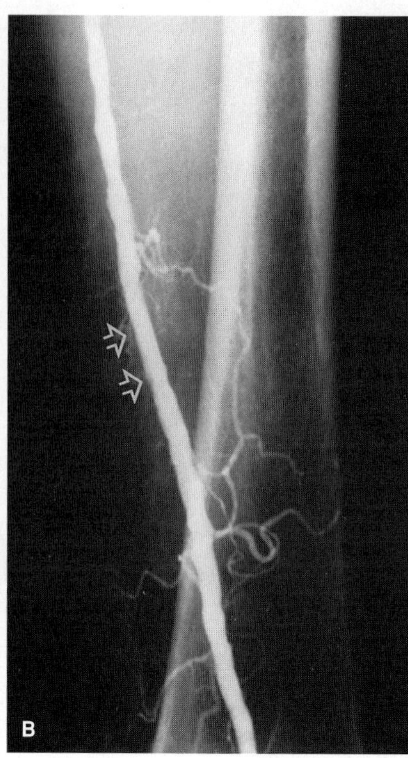

FIGURE 24.15. **Superficial Femoral Artery Atherosclerotic Stenosis. A.** Atherosclerotic changes of the superficial femoral artery are seen with a focal dominant tight stenosis (*arrow*). **B.** Following angioplasty, there is resolution of the stenosis and an excellent radiographic result (*arrows*).

or self-expanding stents, whereas stenting below the inguinal ligament is almost uniformly performed with self-expanding stents because of potential crushing of balloon-expandable stents. Concomitant medical therapy including aspirin and oral platelet inhibitors has improved outcomes, and newer devices such as drug-eluting stents, atherectomy, and brachytherapy may alter the current results. Complication rates range from approximately 3% to 6% and include minor (e.g., access hematoma) and major (e.g., vessel thrombosis, rupture) complications.

Below-knee revascularization is most often performed for limb salvage, and the results are currently imprecise at best. Wagner and Rager (1998), in a literature review of more than 1,200 patients, found the technical success for below-knee percutaneous revascularization to range from 78% to 100%, with limb salvage ranging from 52% to 88% (follow-up ranging from 8 to 24 months).

Thrombosis and Embolism. Acute ischemia of the lower extremities (in the absence of occlusion of a vascular bypass graft) is most often caused by embolism. The most common site of origin is cardiac. In situ thrombosis also occurs, typically arising from areas of severe underlying atherosclerotic disease but also in patients with coagulopathies, trauma, etc. The angiographic finding of an acute occlusion is an abrupt transition, often at bifurcation points if embolic, with poorly developed collaterals (Fig. 24.16). Blue toe syndrome represents a special embolic malady and is the clinical diagnosis of microemboli to the digital arteries of the foot. The source is distal abdominal aorta or iliac artery stenosis or aneurysm in almost 70% of cases. Stenting and recently stent grafting of lesions have been reported to be safe and effective in preventing further emboli, but long-term outcomes are still unknown. Upper-extremity embolic disease occurs with some frequency but needs to be distinguished from other entities, such as vasculitis and connective tissue diseases.

Both thrombosis and embolic disease of the limbs are amenable to treatment with transcatheter thrombolytic agents in the acute setting (Figs. 24.16, 24.17). The most important aspect when considering transcatheter treatment of arterial thrombosis is the clinical evaluation of the patient. In general, patients with pain and pallor are candidates; those with sensory and motor deficits are not and should be treated surgically. A number of catheter designs are available, including multiple-sidehole catheters, that are placed directly into the thrombus for administration of the thrombolytic agent. The patient is monitored closely in an intensive care unit during the thrombolysis process and returns to the angiography suite for follow-up angiograms and catheter manipulations and possible endovascular treatment of underlying lesions. Mechanical devices are also available for use, either instead of or in addition to intra-arterial thrombolysis.

Vasculitis is a general term for a group of diseases that involve inflammation of blood vessels. *Angiitis* and *arteritis* are both synonyms for vasculitis, literally meaning "inflammation of blood vessels" and "inflammation of arteries," respectively. Blood vessels of all sizes may be affected,

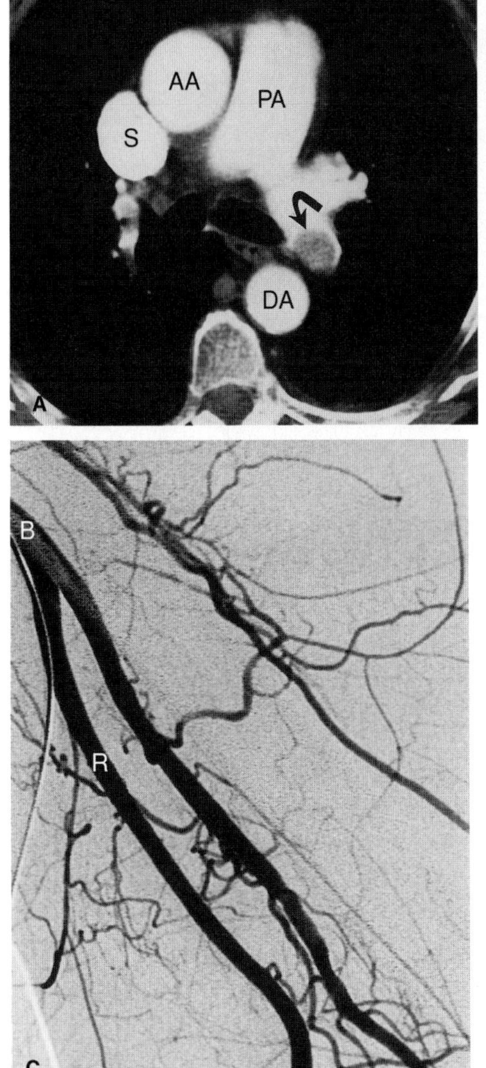

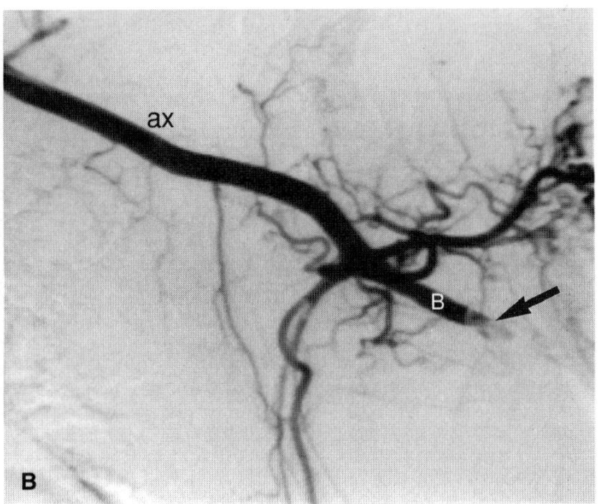

FIGURE 24.16. **Embolism Through Patent Foramen Ovale. A.** Helical CT of pulmonary arteries demonstrates pulmonary embolus (*curved arrow*). The patient presented with hypoxia and arm ischemia. PA, pulmonary artery; AA, ascending aorta; DA, descending aorta; S, superior vena cava. **B.** The proximal brachial artery (B) is occluded by an acute embolus (*arrow*). Pulmonary embolus resulted in acute elevation of pulmonary pressures, allowing systemic embolization through a patent foramen ovale. ax, axillary artery. **C.** Complete thrombolysis has been achieved. Note high origin of the radial artery (R) from the proximal brachial artery (B). (Courtesy of Pat Vogel, Sacramento, CA.)

although the size of the involved vessel varies according to the specific type of vasculitis. There are approximately 20 different disorders that are classified as vasculitis, but giant cell arteritis and Buerger disease are two main ones to remember for the peripheral arterial system, exclusive of Takayasu arteritis in the great vessels.

Giant cell arteritis typically involves the medium to large blood vessels supplying the head (temporal arteries), neck (carotid arteries), and arms (brachial arteries). It is found more frequently in women greater than 60 years of age. Angiographic findings are areas of smooth, long segment narrowing of the axillary and/or brachial arteries (Fig. 24.18). *Buerger disease* (thromboangiitis obliterans) was first reported in 1908 by Buerger, who described a disease in which the characteristic pathologic findings consisted of acute inflammation and thrombosis (clotting) of arteries and veins, primarily affecting the hands and feet. It is included here in the vasculitis section because of its inflammatory nature, but not all consider it a vasculitis. Some consider it a variation of atherosclerosis or its own pathologic entity. The typical Buerger disease patient is a young man who is a heavy cigarette smoker. More recently, however, a higher percentage of women and people over the age of 50 have been recognized to have this disease. The angiographic hallmark of Buerger disease is the "corkscrew" appearance of arteries, representing collaterals around areas of occlusion (most often at wrists and ankles), and the absence of atherosclerotic findings (Fig. 24.19). There are usually multiple segmental occlusions of the palmar and digital arteries (if there are any fingers that have yet to be amputated).

Trauma, either blunt or penetrating, can occur to any artery although it is more common to some than others. Remember that trauma includes iatrogenic injuries.

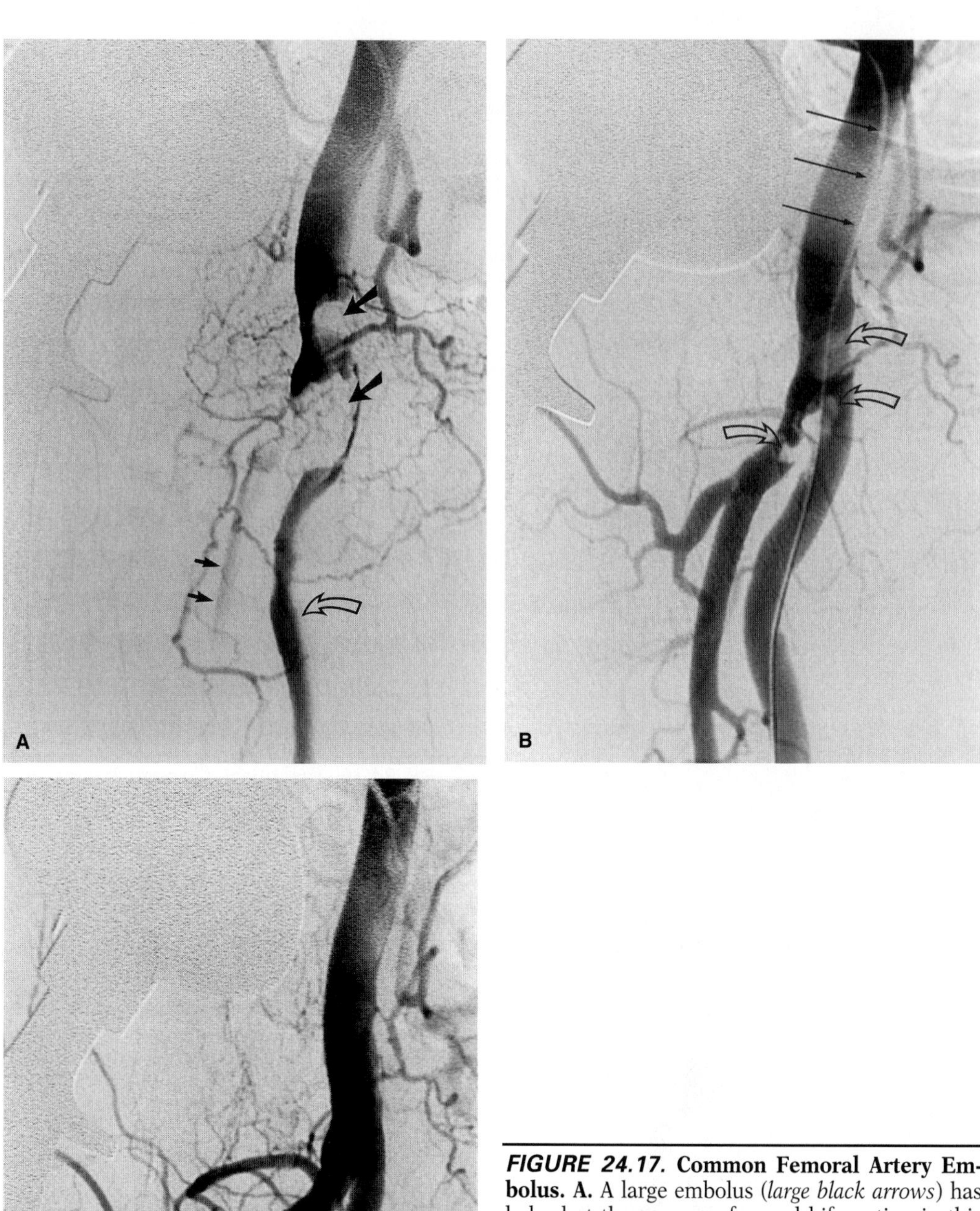

FIGURE 24.17. Common Femoral Artery Embolus. A. A large embolus (*large black arrows*) has lodged at the common femoral bifurcation in this patient with an acutely ischemic lower limb. Minimal flow is present in the profunda femoris artery (*small black arrows*) and superficial femoral artery (*curved open arrow*) distal to the embolus. **B.** After 12 hours of thrombolytic infusion, the embolus is significantly smaller (curved open arrows) and flow has improved distal to the embolus. Black arrows depict location of the guidewire. **C.** The embolus has completely resolved after 36 hours of infusion. No further intervention was necessary. p, profunda femoris artery; s, superficial femoral artery.

The angiographic findings of trauma are the same for almost any vessel injury. The range of angiographic findings of trauma include vasospasm, intimal irregularity, pseudoaneurysm, extravasation, and arteriovenous fistula (Fig. 24.20). Several special mechanisms of peripheral arterial trauma should be kept in mind, as they present a relatively characteristic angiographic picture. *Hypothenar hammer* is the consequence of repetitive palmar trauma, leading to injury of the ulnar artery as it passes adjacent to the hook of the hamate. The ulnar artery can become aneurysmal,

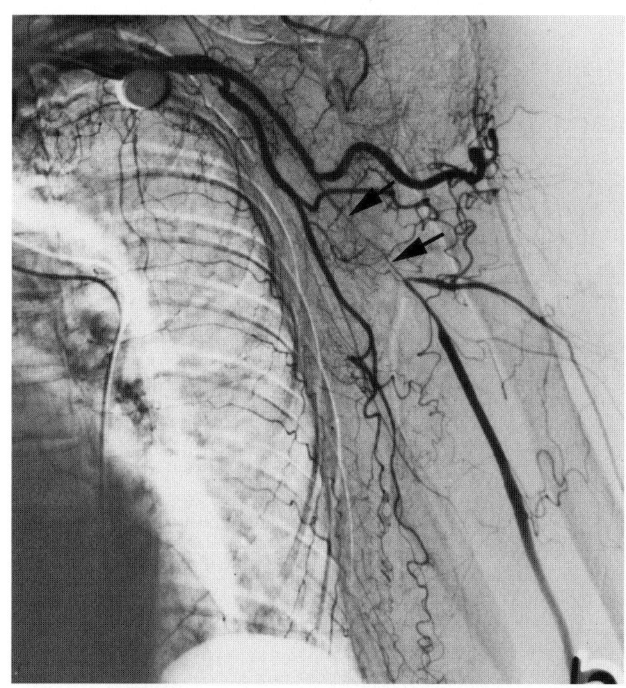

FIGURE 24.18. **Giant Cell Arteritis.** Angiogram of the left upper limb shows smooth, long segment narrowing of the brachial artery (*arrows*), classic for giant cell arteritis of the upper limb.

thrombose, or send emboli to the digital arteries. *Posterior dislocations of the knee* have the highest rates of vascular injury, although vascular injury occurs in 30% to 40% of knee dislocations overall. Angiographic findings range from small intimal tears to complete thrombosis (Fig. 24.20). *Fractures* are prone to vascular injury in a number of locations, particularly along the upper tibia/fibula and pelvic brim, where approximately 10% of patients with pelvic fractures have persistent arterial bleeding.

Endovascular treatment for trauma occupies a central position in acute therapeutic protocols. Embolotherapy consists of two main techniques: occlusion of the bleeding (parent) vessel or exclusion of the injury with preservation of the parent vessel (stent grafting). Occlusion of the bleeding vessel is usually done with coils. This of course presupposes that the bleeding vessel can be sacrificed, which is true for branches of the internal iliac, branches of the profunda femoris, geniculate branches, and the subclavian/axillary/brachial artery branches (excluding vertebral). However, the major arteries to the lower limb (common/external iliac, common/superficial femoral, popliteal) or upper limb (subclavian, axillary, brachial) cannot be sacrificed without consequence. When the vessel cannot be sacrificed, the first line of therapy is surgical. However, stent grafting offers a reasonable acute option in many of these cases. Both self-expanding and balloon-expanding stent grafts are commercially available. Placement is relatively straightforward, but most, however, require large introducer sheaths (up to 10 French). In all situations, the decision to intervene on a trauma patient must be individualized to a particular patient and the decision must be arrived upon in conjunction with the clinical trauma teams.

Fibromuscular disease (FMD) has been described in the subclavian, axillary, and brachial arteries of the upper extremities and the iliac, femoral, and popliteal arteries of the lower extremities (Fig. 24.21). The angiographic appearance is similar to that of FMD in other locations where aneurysm formation, dissection, thrombosis, and distal embolization are issues. The diagnosis is by the angiographic beaded appearance. FMD must be differentiated from standing waves, which represent a corrugated luminal contour in medium-size arteries. The etiology of the latter is unknown, but it can be diagnostically differentiated because standing waves change from one angiographic injection to the next, whereas FMD is a fixed abnormality.

Vascular Entrapment or Compression. *Thoracic outlet syndrome* corresponds to a spectrum of disorders of the upper extremities and remains a somewhat controversial subject. It represents a compression syndrome of the neurovascular bundle of an upper limb at the level of the scalene muscles and first rib. It therefore can encompass compression of the artery, vein, and/or nerve in this location. Patients can present with signs of arterial insufficiency, venous obstruction, painless wasting of intrinsic hand muscles, and pain. History and physical examination are the most important diagnostic tools, and radiographs of the chest and cervical spine and electromyography/nerve conduction studies are useful to identify other causes of pain and disability. Surgical intervention is indicated for patients failing nonoperative maneuvers and can usually yield satisfactory results.

The arterial form can be diagnosed angiographically by placing the arm into the position that most creates the symptoms and noting arterial compression compared to angiography in a neutral position (Fig. 24.22). Arterial injury, including aneurysm, stenosis, and thrombosis with or without embolic symptoms, have been found. More than 70% of patients with arterial injury have a cervical rib. However, angiography is somewhat controversial, in that arterial occlusion based on arm position can occur in normal subjects. Nerve involvement accounts for the vast majority of symptoms, whereas arterial involvement causes symptoms in less than 5% of patients.

Popliteal entrapment is a condition in which the artery and/or vein deviate around the medial head of the gastrocnemius muscle. Five variations have been described. It is usually seen in young, athletic men and should be suspected in any young patient with atraumatic leg ischemia. The diagnosis is suggested by irregularity of the popliteal artery but is confirmed by medial deviation of the popliteal artery during maneuvers of the leg and/or foot. If active

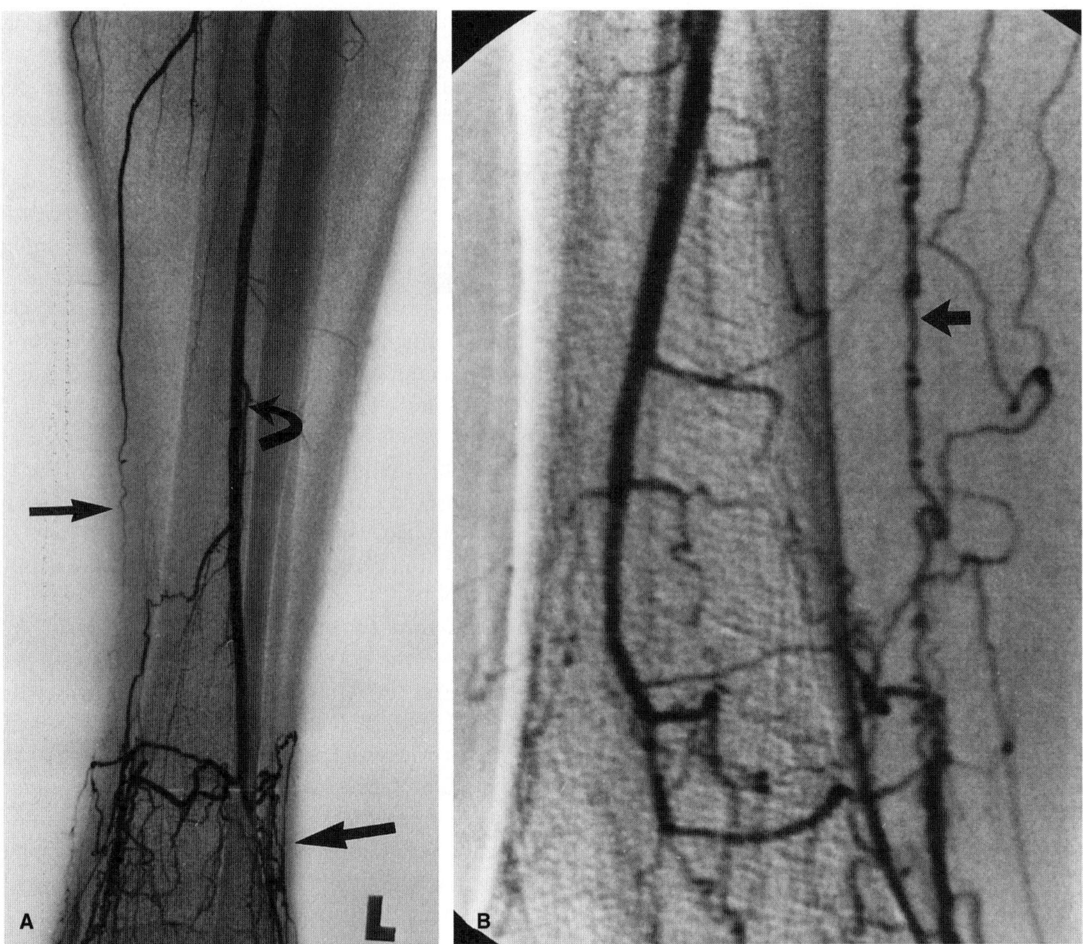

FIGURE 24.19. **Buerger Disease. A.** Arteriogram of a 37-year smoker with foot pain. Distal arterial disease with "corkscrew" vessels (*straight arrows*) are diagnostic findings specific for Buerger disease. Only the peroneal artery (*curved arrow*) is visualized. The anterior and posterior tibial arteries are occluded. **B.** An arteriogram of the opposite leg shows corkscrew vessels (*arrow*) just above the ankle.

plantar flexion and passive dorsiflexion cause the pulse to disappear or diminish by duplex Doppler, it supports the diagnosis, but 50% of normal subjects will also experience a disappearing pulse.

Angiography is the gold standard but is being supplanted by MR or CT. All studies are performed using plantar flexion and dorsiflexion. Bilateral abnormalities are found in approximately 30% of subjects, so both legs should be evaluated. Any symptomatic patient should be treated because of the natural progression to irreversible popliteal artery injury, with the potential complications of thrombosis and aneurysm formation. If the vessel is healthy, the offending muscle may be divided. Once the vessel is damaged, surgical bypass is the treatment of choice.

Adventitial Cysts and Tumors. The only role for angiography of extremity tumors is embolotherapy prior to resection of highly vascular tumors such as renal cell metastasis. *Adventitial cystic disease* is a condition in which mucin collects in the adventitial layer, most commonly in the popliteal artery, and may lead to narrowing or arterial obstruction. It is most commonly seen in young to middle-aged men, where the condition often mimics popliteal entrapment. Angiographically it is a fixed lesion, and the cystic component can be diagnosed by sonography, MR, or CT. Treatment is surgical excision of the cyst with the possible need for bypass.

Vasospasm. Spasm of the arterial system of the upper or lower extremities occurs as a response to catheter placement or trauma (including only proximity trauma). These lesions may respond to the intra-arterial administration of a vasodilator, usually 100 μg of nitroglycerin. An unusual type of systemic vasospasm is the response to the ergot alkaloids (*ergotism*). Ergotamine stimulates the contraction of smooth muscle. Angiography demonstrates long segment arterial narrowing; most often this occurs in the

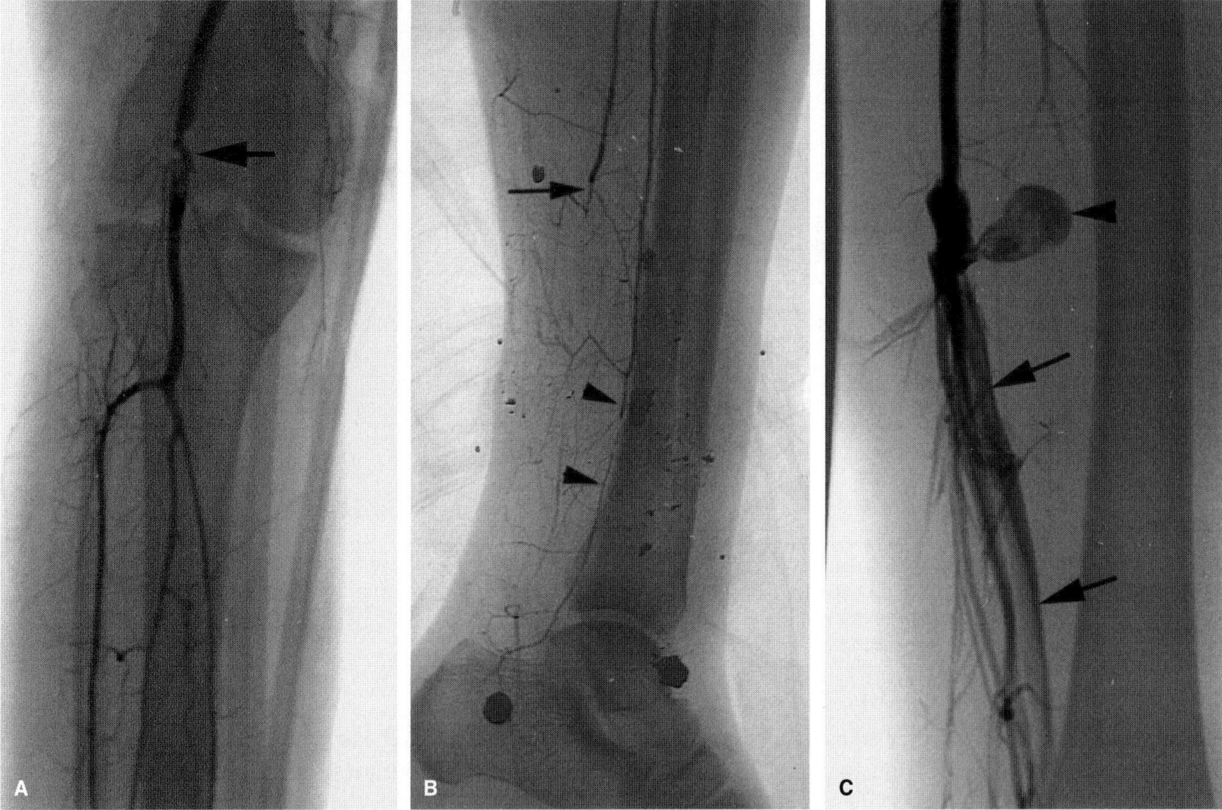

FIGURE 24.20. **Angiographic Findings of Peripheral Arterial Trauma. A.** Angiogram of the right leg of a 21-year-old man who suffered posterior knee dislocation in a motor vehicle crash demonstrates arterial injury to the popliteal artery (*arrow*). **B.** Angiogram of the left lower leg in a 21-year-old patient following gunshot wound. Vessel findings are typical of vascular trauma, including vessel occlusion (*arrow*) and vasospasm (*arrowheads*). **C.** Angiogram of a 17-year-old man obtained 3 days after gunshot wound to the thigh shows injury to superficial femoral artery with filling of the femoral vein (*arrows*), representing arteriovenous shunting and pseudoaneurysm (*arrowhead*).

lower limbs but it can occur in upper limbs as well as other arterial beds. The lesions usually reverse themselves once ergotamine use is discontinued.

Aneurysmal Disease. Aneurysms may be the result of atherosclerosis, trauma, infection, vasculitis, or connective tissue disorders. *Traumatic aneurysms* are pseudoaneurysms and are related to the site of injury. *Mycotic aneurysms* of the extremities are rare but should be considered when the location is unusual for atherosclerosis and the aneurysm architecture is quite bizarre in nature. *Atherosclerotic aneurysms* most often occur in the iliac and femoral arteries of the pelvis, the popliteal arteries of the lower limbs, and the subclavian arteries of the upper extremities. An internal iliac artery aneurysm occurs when the vessel is greater than 2 cm in diameter. Most are asymptomatic; however, the major risk is rupture. They are most often associated with abdominal aortic aneurysms. Internal iliac artery aneurysms can be effectively treated via an endovascular approach by coiling. Complications of coiling to be considered are buttock pain (claudication) and impotence in men, which are best avoided if the contralateral internal iliac artery is patent to supply collateral flow.

The exact etiology of *popliteal artery aneurysms* is unknown; however, arteriosclerosis seems to be the dominant associated factor. Approximately one third of patients are asymptomatic at the time of diagnosis. Symptomatic patients present with distal embolization or aneurysmal thrombosis that is causing claudication or popliteal occlusion. In addition, the aneurysms can rupture, causing a threat to leg viability and even becoming life threatening. This occurs much less frequently than thrombosis of the aneurysm. Diagnosis is made by physical examination and confirmed by imaging, including sonography, CT, or MR. Angiography is used to confirm the diagnosis and may be required for transcatheter thrombolytic therapy if the patient presents with thrombosis (Fig. 24.23). Thrombolysis is performed to open distal vessels, providing a target for surgical bypass. The treatment of choice is surgical ligation and bypassing the aneurysm.

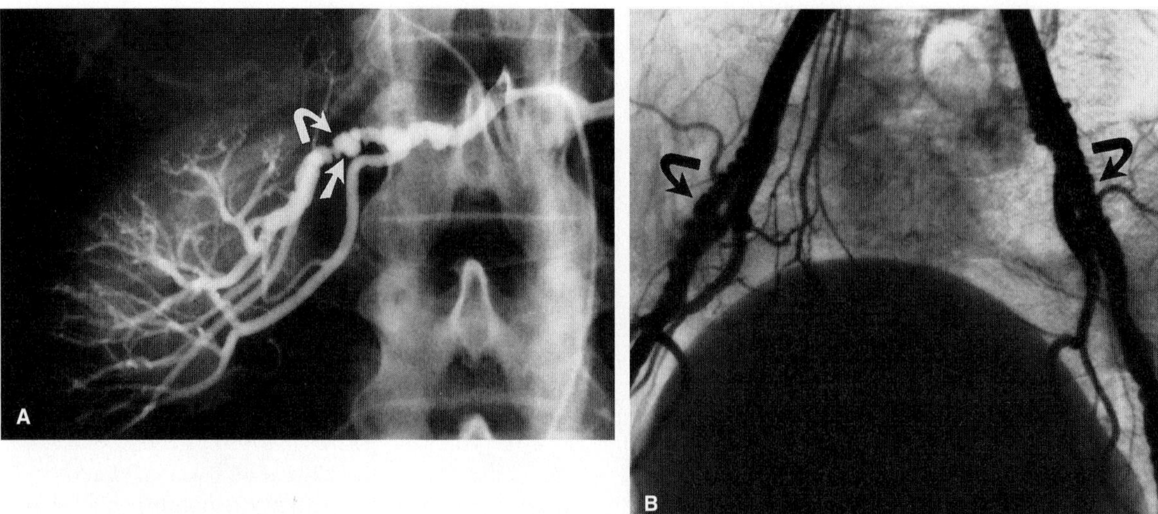

FIGURE 24.21. **Fibromuscular Dysplasia (FMD). A.** Right renal artery injection shows the beaded appearance of medial FMD (*curved arrow*) with aneurysm formation (*straight arrow*). **B.** The iliac arteries (*curved arrows*) are less commonly involved with FMD but have the same radiographic appearance.

Arteriomegaly (diffuse vascular ectasia, arteria magna, ectatic atherosclerosis) is an unusual manifestation of aneurysmal disease with diffuse, generalized dilatation of the aortoiliac and femoral vessels. It is associated with multiple aneurysms and characteristically produces severe tortuosity in the iliac arteries. Because of the capacious vascular system, increased amounts of contrast and prolonged imaging times are required.

Arteriovenous malformations (AVMs) have various classification systems but range from hemangiomatous to nidus AVMs to single-hole fistulas (or a combination of these). Sixty percent of all peripheral vascular malformations are found in the lower extremities, with another 25% in the upper extremities. The evaluation of these patients is critical to planning therapy, which includes medical, surgical, radiation, and endovascular means.

Endovascular therapy consists of transcatheter embolotherapy and/or direct percutaneous access. A wide variety of embolic agents are used and are tailored to a particular patient and their AVM, including its size, location, and architecture. Several important principles of endovascular therapy to keep in mind include: obliteration of the nidus rather than feeding arteries or draining veins, treatment of single-hole fistulas as close to the fistula site

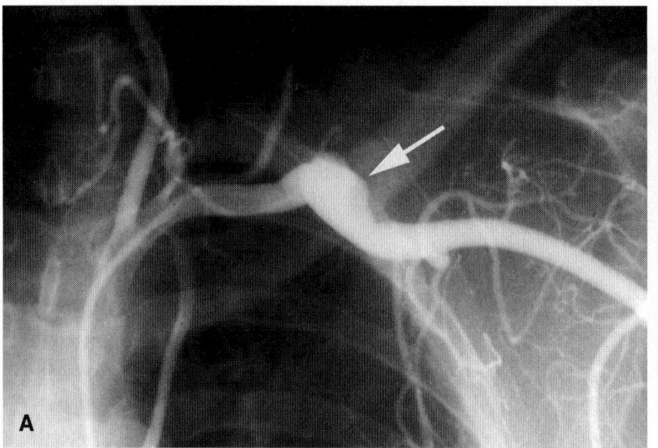

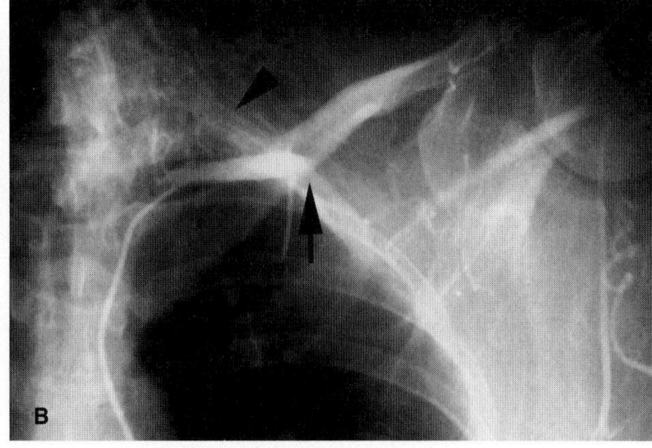

FIGURE 24.22. **Thoracic Outlet Syndrome. A.** Angiogram of left subclavian artery in a 40-year-old woman with pain upon raising arm shows filling of artery but with a fusiform aneurysm (*arrow*). **B.** When the patient elevates her arm to recreate the symptoms, the subclavian artery is completely occluded (*arrow*). Note the cervical rib (*arrowheads*).

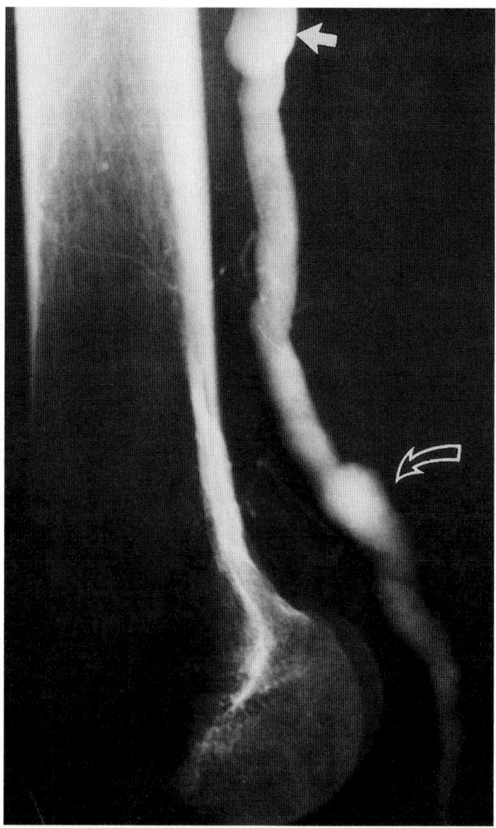

FIGURE 24.23. **Popliteal Artery Aneurysm.** Lateral view of a lower extremity arteriogram shows a distal superficial femoral artery aneurysm (*straight arrow*), a proximal popliteal artery aneurysm (*curved arrow*), and arteriomegaly.

as possible, and staged (multiple-session) embolotherapy for large extensive AVMs (remember, you can always do more but you cannot take back what is already put in). Most important, operator experience with embolic agents as well as transcatheter and percutaneous techniques is essential to ensure safety and achieve the best results.

UTERINE ARTERY EMBOLIZATION

Uterine artery embolization has been gaining favor as a treatment for symptomatic leiomyomas over the past 5 to 7 years. This offers an alternative to myomectomy or hysterectomy. Patients may present with bleeding, bulk-related symptoms, or pain. This treatment requires clinical evaluation and imaging with MR to determine the relation of the fibroid with the patient's symptoms (Fig. 24.24). MR is used to evaluate size and position of the fibroid within the uterus as well as the size of the uterus. It is also used to evaluate for other gynecologic processes, such as adenomyosis or ovarian pathology. In the setting of abnormal bleeding there is usually a submucosal component to one or more of the fibroids or adenomyosis. Pain and bulk-related symptoms may be associated with transmural or subserosal fibroids. Contrast MR is used to evaluate the vascularity of the fibroid.

Embolization is typically performed from a unilateral femoral access, with selection of both the right and left uterine arteries. Care is taken not to reflux the embolic agent into the branches of the internal iliac artery.

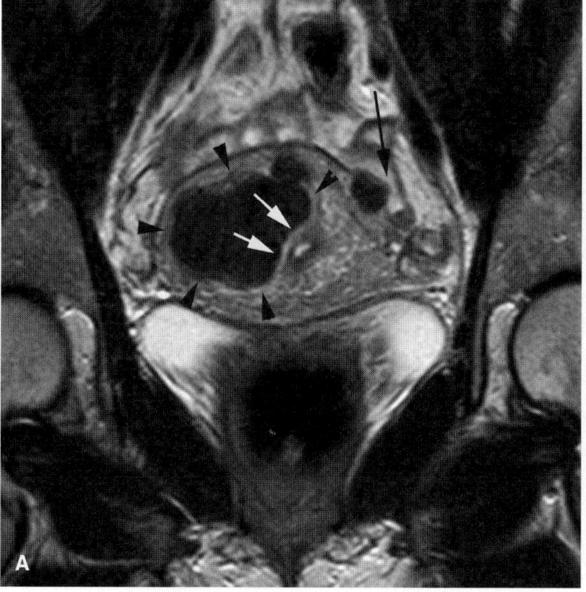

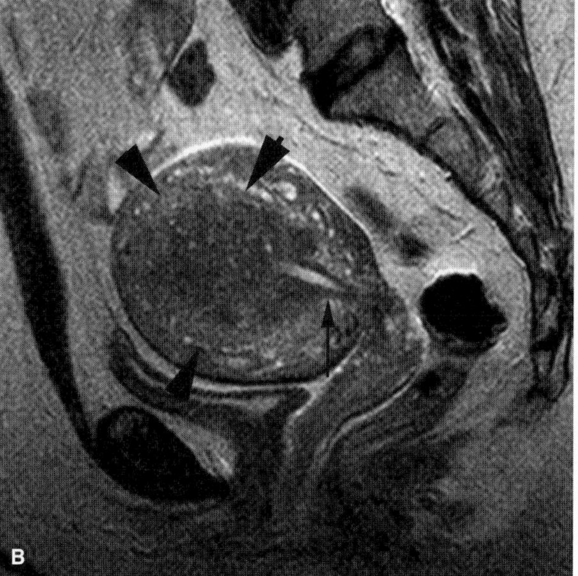

FIGURE 24.24. **Uterine Fibroids and Adenomyosis. A.** Coronal T2WI demonstrating a transmural fibroid (*black arrowheads*) with a submucosal component (*white arrows*) and a subserosal fibroid (*black arrow*). **B.** Sagittal T2WI with focal thickening of the transitional zone (*arrowheads*), compared with the normal transitional zone (*arrow*) in this patient with adenomyosis.

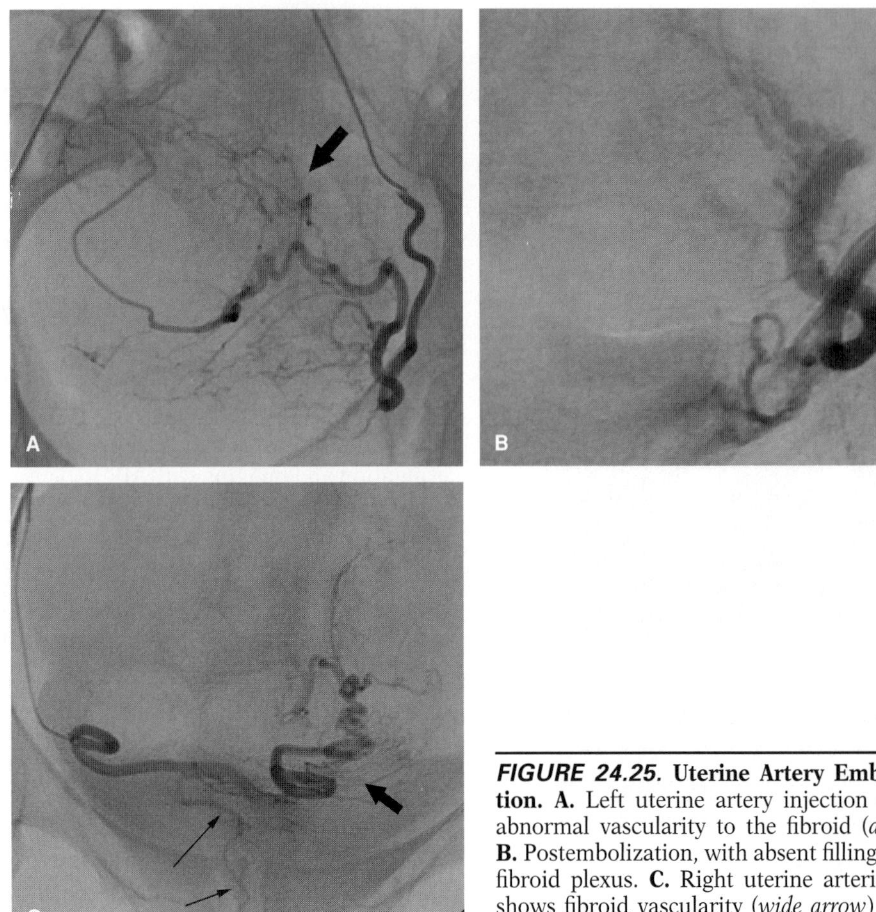

FIGURE 24.25. **Uterine Artery Embolization. A.** Left uterine artery injection shows abnormal vascularity to the fibroid (*arrow*). **B.** Postembolization, with absent filling of the fibroid plexus. **C.** Right uterine arteriogram shows fibroid vascularity (*wide arrow*) and a cervical branch (*thin arrows*).

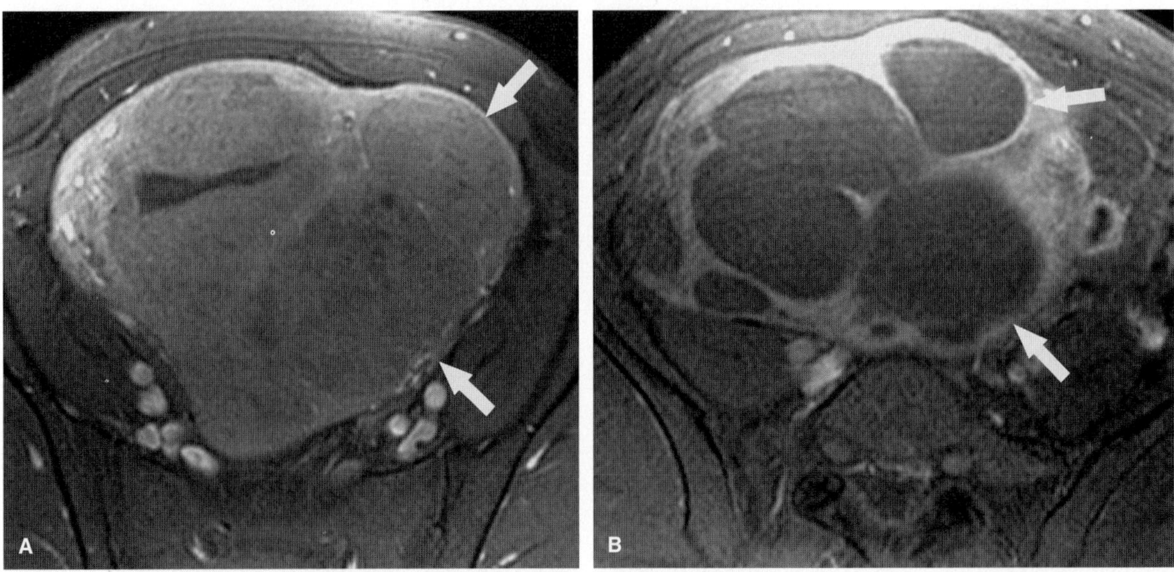

FIGURE 24.26. **Uterine Artery Embolization Follow-up. A.** Axial postcontrast MR demonstrates diffuse enhancement of multiple fibroids prior to embolization. **B.** Absence of enhancement of the fibroids 3 months following embolization is evidence of a successful procedure.

Branches of the uterine artery, such as cervical or ovarian, must be evaluated to prevent nontarget embolization. Particles ranging from 500 to 700 μm are preferred to allow for sparing of the vascular supply to the normal myometrium. The catheter should be placed in the horizontal portion of the uterine artery for injection of particles (Fig. 24.25). Devascularization of the fibroid is the targeted endpoint. Patients are kept for observation and pain control following the procedure. There is a high likelihood of postembolic syndrome with pain and fever. This is managed with anti-inflammatory agents and narcotic medication.

Follow-up MR may be used to assess the vascularity of the fibroid and determine size change, which may predict outcome as well as risk of recurrent symptoms. A reduction of 20% to 40% in the size of the fibroids and uterus is typically seen at the 3-month MR. Lack of enhancement of the fibroid is related to successful outcome and low incidence of recurrent symptoms (Fig. 24.26). The risk of delayed infection seems to be related to the presence of submucosal fibroids. Large pedunculated fibroids within the uterus carry a higher risk of infection. Other possible complications include early-onset menopause, uterine necrosis, and nontarget embolization. The impact of embolization on fertility has not yet been established.

SUGGESTED READINGS

Ahrar K, Smith DC, Bansal RC, Razzouk A, Catalano RD. Angiography in blunt thoracic aortic injury. J Trauma 1997;42:665–669.

Audet P, Therasse E, Oliva VL, et al. Infrarenal aortic stenosis: long-term clinical and hemodynamic results of percutaneous transluminal angioplasty. Radiology 1998;209:357–363.

Baum RA, Stavropoulos SW, Fairman RM, Carpenter JP. Endoleaks after endovascular repair of abdominal aortic aneurysms. J Vasc Interv Radiol 2003;14:1111–1118.

Davies RR, Goldstein LJ, Coady MA, et al. Yearly rupture or dissection rates for thoracic aortic aneurysms: simple prediction based on size. Ann Thorac Surg 2002;73:17–27.

Dormandy JA, Rutherford RB, and TASC Working Group. TransAtlantic Inter-Society Consensus (TASC), management of peripheral arterial disease (PAD). J Vasc Surg 2000;31:S1–S296.

Dyer DS, Moore EE, Ilke DN, et al. Thoracic aortic injury: how predictive is mechanism and is chest computed tomography a reliable screening tool? A prospective study of 1,561 patients. J Trauma 2000;48: 673–683.

Gossage JR, Kanj G. Pulmonary arteriovenous malformations: a state of the art review. Am J Respir Crit Care Med 1998;158:643–661.

Hovsepian DG, Siskin G, Bonn J, et al. Quality improvement guidelines for uterine artery embolization for symptomatic leiomyomata. J Vasc Interv Radiol 2004;15(6):535–541.

Leung DA, Spinosa DJ, Hagspiel KD, Angle JF, Matsumoto AH. Selection of stents for treating iliac arterial disease. J Vasc Interv Radiol 2003;14:137–152.

Parmley LF, Mattingly TW, Manion WC, et al. Nonpenetrating traumatic injury of the aorta. Circulation 1958;17:1086–1101.

Rajan D, Beecroft JT, Clark M, et al. Risk of intrauterine infectious complication after uterine artery embolization. J Vasc Interv Radiol 2004;15:1415–1421.

Shammas NW. Complications in peripheral vascular interventions: emerging role of direct thrombin inhibitors. J Vasc Interv Radiol 2005;16:165–171.

Sheth RN, Blezberg AJ. Diagnosis and treatment of thoracic outlet syndrome. Neurosurg Clin North Am 2001;12:295–309.

Townsend RN, Colella JJ, Diamond DL. Traumatic rupture of the aorta: critical decision for trauma surgeon. J Trauma 1990;30:1169–1174.

Valji K. Thoracic aorta. In Vascular and Interventional Radiology. Philadelphia: Saunders, 1999.

Valji K. Pulmonary and bronchial arteries. In Vascular and Interventional Radiology. Philadelphia: Saunders, 1999.

Wagner HJ, Rager G. Infrapopliteal angioplasty: a forgotten region? Rofo 1998;168:415–420 [German].

Chapter 25

Abdominal Arteries, Venous System, and Nonvascular Intervention

Michael J. Miller, Jr. and Tony P. Smith

Abdominal Aorta and Its Branches
Abdominal Aortography and Intervention
Renal Angiography and Intervention
Splenic Angiography and Intervention
Hepatic Angiography and Intervention
Mesenteric Angiography and Intervention

Diagnosis and Intervention of the Venous System

Nonvascular Intervention

ABDOMINAL AORTA AND ITS BRANCHES

Abdominal Aortography and Intervention

Although individualized to a particular patient and their clinical situation, angiography of the abdominal aorta is most often performed for atherosclerotic disease, both aneurismal and occlusive. Angiography is also performed for aortic dissection as well as trauma. Rarely, involvement with the vasculitides, including Takayasu arteritis, midaortic syndrome, and other etiologies, necessitates angiography.

Aneurysms. As with the thoracic aorta, there are multiple possible etiologies for abdominal aortic aneurysms, but two are of primary importance: atherosclerosis and infection. The most common etiology of abdominal aortic aneurysms (AAAs) is degenerative, which for the most part is synonymous with atherosclerotic. An *atherosclerotic AAA* is defined as enlargement of the aorta at least 1.5 times greater than the normal vessel diameter. Atherosclerotic AAAs are for the most part fusiform and often lined with mural thrombus. Although US does demonstrate the aneurysm, CT has become the diagnostic study of choice. Angiography is usually only indicated for a particular patient and their special situation. Angiography only demonstrates the true lumen, not the portion of the aneurysm, which is thrombus filled, and, of course, has a finite complication rate, as does any invasive procedure. Angiographically, an AAA is seen as an irregular, often calcified, fusiform aneurysm (Fig. 25.1A). Angiography does demonstrate the patency of the other major vessels (renals, visceral, iliacs), as well as their relationship to the AAA. Of greatest importance is the relationship of the renal arteries to the AAA, as it influences the surgical or endovascular repair.

The indication for the elective repair of an asymptomatic AAA is when the diameter exceeds 5.0 cm. It is at this diameter that the chance of rupture increases dramatically. It is common for an AAA to extend into the iliac arteries, and 99% of atherosclerotic iliac artery aneurysms are associated with an AAA. Treatment of AAAs has been traditionally by open surgical repair. However, stent graft placement has become widely used because of its minimal invasiveness (Fig. 25.1). A number of stent grafts are available; all require large (up to 30 French) access sites via the common femoral artery for placement and therefore are most often placed using surgical access to one or both groins. The grafts differ by design including segments without covering, which can be anchored above the renal arteries as well as bifurcated sections for the iliac arteries. Stent grafts can be successfully placed into AAA in over 90% of cases. However, approximately 25% will require additional endovascular procedures. To that end, one of the major concerns with the placement of grafts is the continued

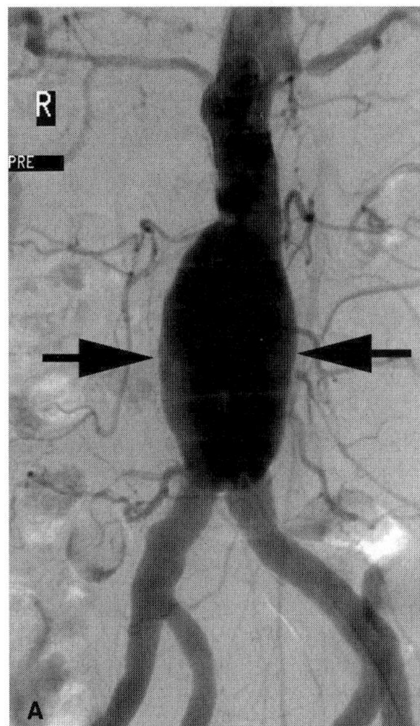

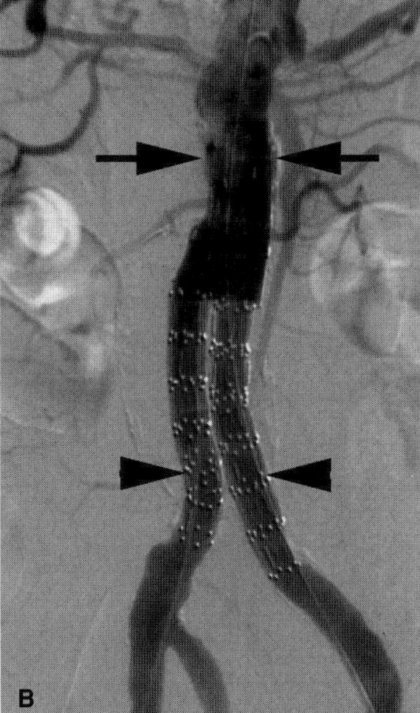

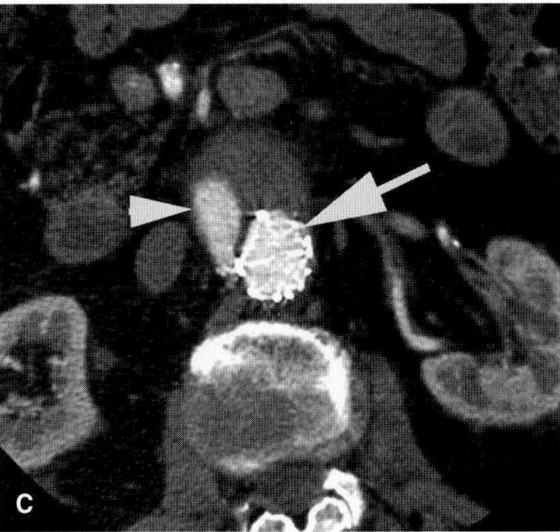

FIGURE 25.1. **Abdominal Aortic Aneurysm (AAA). A.** Aortic arteriogram in a 68-year-old man with an infrarenal demonstrates an AAA (*arrows*). **B.** The aneurysm is completely excluded by a covered stent (stent graft) (*arrows*), which was placed below the renal arteries extending into both external iliac arteries (*arrowheads*). (Courtesy Andrew H. Cragg, MD, Minneapolis, MN.) **C.** CT scan of a different patient showing a stent graft in place but with persistent filling of the aneurysm, as noted by the contrast material (*arrow*). This is a type 1 endoleak occurring at the proximal attachment site of the graft. This was repaired by placing another shorter graft (cuff) over the site.

filling (opacification) of the AAA following stent graft placement, termed *endoleaks*. Such leaks are best studied with CT (Fig. 25.1C) as well as by angiography, particularly as endovascular techniques are utilized to repair such leaks. Endoleaks are categorized into four types: type 1 is a leak at the superior or inferior attachment site, type 2 represents AAA filling via a patient arterial side branch such as a lumbar or the inferior mesenteric artery, type 3 is loss of integrity of the stent graft, and type 4 is a leak through the porous graft material. Isolated common iliac artery atherosclerotic aneurysms can be handled much like AAAs using smaller stent grafts. Internal iliac artery atherosclerotic aneurysms are probably best managed by embolizing the internal iliac aneurysm, primarily with coils.

Mycotic aneurysms or pseudoaneurysms of the abdominal aorta are a rare but life-threatening condition and are often surgical emergencies. Radiographically, they often appear saccular and very irregular. Their rate of growth and the patient's constitutional symptoms will suggest the infectious nature. The commonest pathogen is *Salmonella* species, accounting for an incidence of up to 74%.

Aortoiliac occlusive disease is most commonly caused by atherosclerosis. Patients with aortoiliac disease usually present with claudication. Bilateral buttock claudication, impotence, and absent femoral pulses are seen in the *Leriche syndrome*, although this title is often used to signify aortic occlusion by imaging rather than based on clinical symptoms. The aorta and iliac segments can be the source of distal emboli to the legs, such as the blue toe syndrome discussed later.

Radiographically, atherosclerotic involvement of the distal aorta and iliac arteries is identical to that elsewhere, with plaque formation, calcification, and vessel narrowing. Visualization of the aorta and iliac arteries as well as the entire lower extremity can be carried out with CT or MR as well as angiography. CT and MR work well for screening, but angiography remains the gold standard, and endovascular therapy can be carried out in the same sitting. Aortoiliac occlusive disease is probably best initially approached with endovascular techniques, including angioplasty with or without stent placement (Fig. 25.2). Following angiographic assessment and prior to treatment of aortoiliac lesions, pressure measurements should be obtained; a gradient of 10 mm Hg systolic is considered significant. If no gradient is noted, pressures should be augmented, with vasodilators injected intra-arterially down the leg to simulate increased blood flow to chemically mimic exercise. Another pressure gradient is then obtained, again looking for a difference of 10 mm Hg

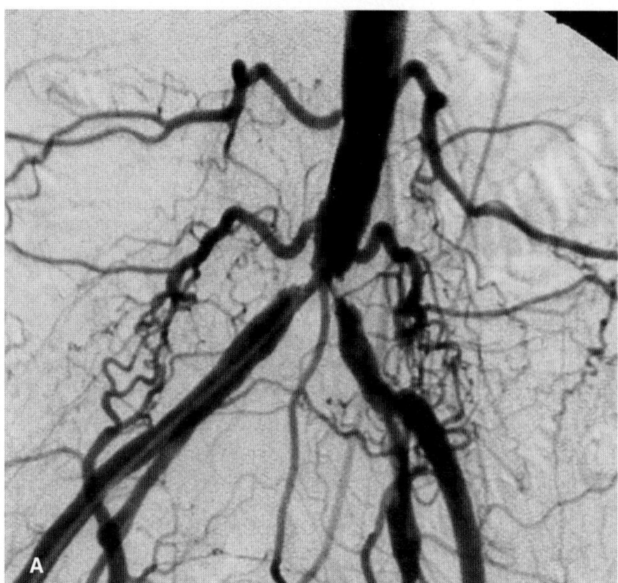

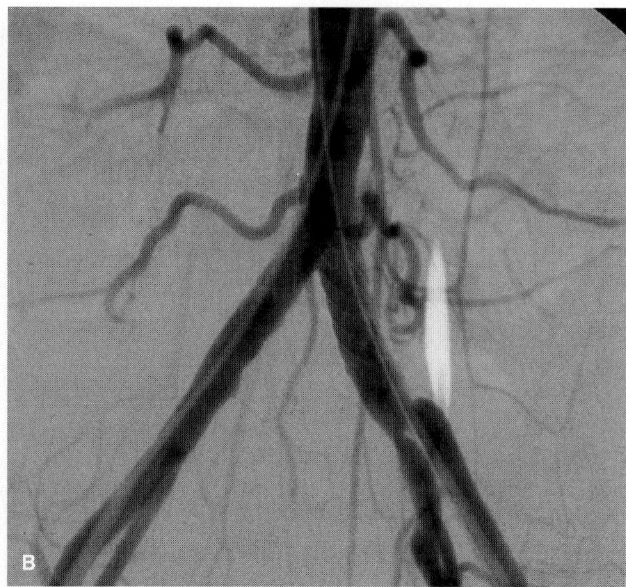

FIGURE 25.2. **Aortoiliac Stenting. A.** Pelvic angiogram in a 55-year-old woman with severe claudication demonstrates severe aortic and bilateral proximal common femoral artery atherosclerotic disease (*arrows*). **B.** Angioplasty with stents placed "kissing" in the aorta provides an excellent anatomic result.

or higher. Indications for angioplasty should take into account the patient's symptoms, appearance of the lesion, and pressure gradients.

Isolated aortic lesions are quite rare but can be effectively treated by endovascular techniques. Disease affecting both the aorta and proximal iliac arteries is usually treated with "kissing" balloons at the aortic bifurcation placed from each common femoral artery. Success can readily be achieved, even with complete occlusion of one or both iliac arteries. Stent placement for aortic or iliac disease is based on the success of angioplasty, as determined radiographically, by follow-up pressure gradients, or by intravascular sonography. Any residual gradient, vessel irregularity, or intimal flap is an indication for stent placement, although many clinicians stent these vessels primarily instead of attempting angioplasty alone. Complications of angioplasty are the same as angioplasty at other sites and include acute thrombosis, distal embolization, and vessel perforation, which occur in fewer than 5% of cases.

Aortoiliac occlusive disease can be caused by *inflammatory diseases*, in particular Takayasu arteritis, which produces a long segment, smooth narrowing of the abdominal aorta that may extend into branch vessels. *Hypoplastic aortic syndrome* is a congenital process of unknown etiology producing long segment narrowing of the aorta and is usually seen in young females. *Neurofibromatosis* may also involve the aorta, and the iliac arteries are the third most common location for *fibromuscular disease*.

Abdominal aortic dissection is almost always associated with, or is in fact an extension of, thoracic dissection. Abdominal aortic dissections are best imaged by CT, although MR does provide excellent diagnostic images. CT demonstrates both lumens, how well they fill with contrast material, the proximal and distal extent of the dissection, as well as the patency and relationship of branch vessels to the dissection. In addition to rupture, of greatest importance is how the dissection plane affects abdominal aortic branch vessels, including visceral, renal, and aortic bifurcation. Angiography is usually reserved for symptomatic patients prior to intervention. As with other imaging, it is essential that angiography demonstrate the extent of the dissection and the patency of branch vessels.

Recently, a number of newer interventional radiologic or minimally invasive techniques appear to have significantly improved the management of patients with aortic dissection. These include stent grafting for entry site closure to prevent aneurysmal widening of the false lumen, as well as percutaneous techniques, such as balloon fenestration of the intimal flap and aortic true lumen stenting to alleviate branch vessel ischemia. Aortic fenestration is a technique whereby a long needle is introduced via the groin access. Using endovascular sonography, a puncture is made from one lumen to the other. Following placement of a guide wire, a balloon is used to create an opening between the two aortic lumens to equalize the pressure between the two, which should hopefully allow reasonable flow into branch vessels from either the true or the false lumen. Aortic fenestration is a procedure reserved for emergency situations. False lumen thrombosis following entry closure with stent grafts has been observed in 86% to 100% of patients, whereas percutaneous interventions are able to effectively relieve organ ischemia in approximately 90%

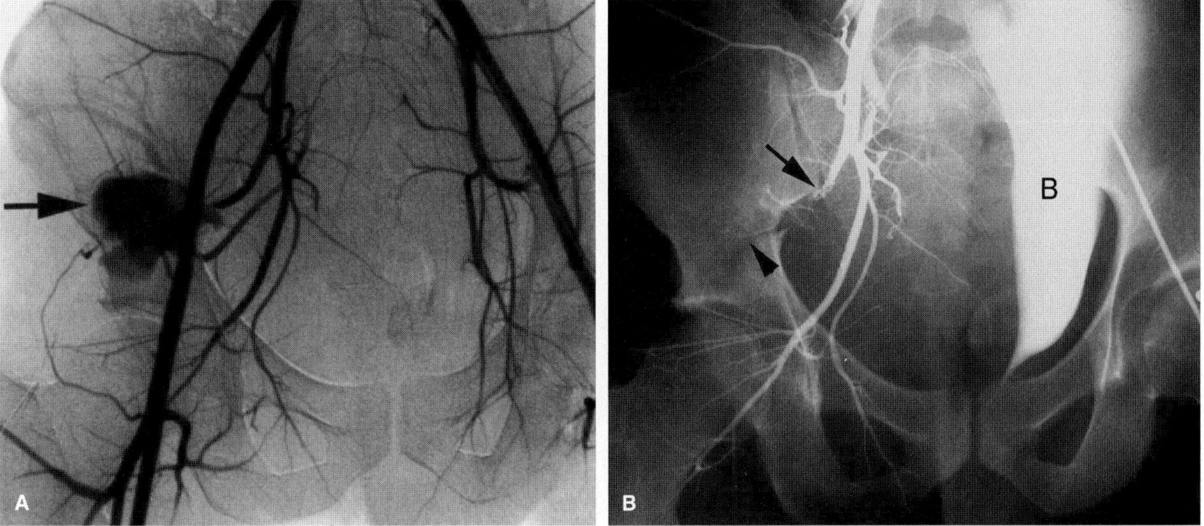

FIGURE 25.3. **Traumatic Hemorrhage in the Pelvis. A.** Pelvic angiogram in a 22-year-old man following a motor vehicle crash reveals avulsion of the superior gluteal artery with extravasation (*arrow*). **B.** Embolization of the superior gluteal was performed with coils (*arrow*), and the hemorrhage was well controlled. This unsubtracted image shows pelvic fracture (*arrowhead*) and deviation of the bladder (B) by a large pelvic hematoma.

of cases. In the years to come, it is to be expected that endoluminal techniques will become the method of choice for treating most type B dissections.

Trauma. Patients rarely survive abdominal aortic trauma, but pelvic trauma resulting in significant bleeding is more commonly seen. Most pelvic bleeding associated with pelvic fractures can be controlled by fixation devices, but those that cannot routinely turn to angiography for diagnosis and embolotherapy. Arterial bleeding is most often associated with injury to one or more branches of the internal iliac arteries. Embolization is most often performed with proximal agents—either gelatin sponge if a temporary agent is desired, or coils for more permanent occlusion. Bleeding from pelvic injury can be effectively controlled with embolotherapy, and angiographic embolization is highly effective in controlling arterial bleeding associated with pelvic fractures (Fig. 25.3). However, repeat angiography should be performed in patients with pelvic fractures and ongoing evidence of hemorrhage, demonstrated by persistent base deficit and hypotension once other potential sources of bleeding have been excluded.

Renal Angiography and Intervention

A single renal artery occurs approximately 60% of the time, with either multiple arteries or an early renal artery division in the other 40%. The most common reason to study the renal arteries in the United States is for occlusive disease and trauma; it is done less often for other abnormalities such as neoplasms.

Imaging of the renal arteries includes US, CT, and MR, with nuclear scintigraphy also playing a role in the relative perfusion of the kidney. US allows visualization of the proximal renal artery and evaluates flow, including resistance to distal flow. CT and MR provide excellent images and are useful screening tools in many centers for renal artery stenosis. However, renal angiography remains the gold standard once screening suggests an abnormality. Angiography not only provides diagnostic images, but transcatheter therapy can be applied in the same sitting and is often the primary goal for the angiographic procedure.

Renal arteries are often studied in patients with decreased renal function. In such patients, alternative imaging that does not require iodinated contrast is recommended, but when angiography is required there are several useful options. Alternative contrast agents such as carbon dioxide and gadolinium have been successfully used, particularly in conjunction with small doses of iodinated contrast. Alternatively, traditional low-molar or isosmolar iodinated contrast material may be used and kept to a minimum, especially if the patient has received preventative therapy. Chief among these is hydration, which is currently the only well proven renal protective maneuver, although agents such as fenoldopam and antioxidants (chiefly acetylcysteine) have been used.

There are a number of etiologies for *renal artery occlusive disease,* including dissection, vasospasm, vasculitis, coarctation syndromes, and neurofibromatosis, but the two most common causes by far are atherosclerosis and fibromuscular disease (FMD). These two account for 99% of the stenoses encountered in the United States, with atherosclerosis representing 65% of stenoses overall (Fig. 25.4). ***Fibromuscular disease*** is the most common cause

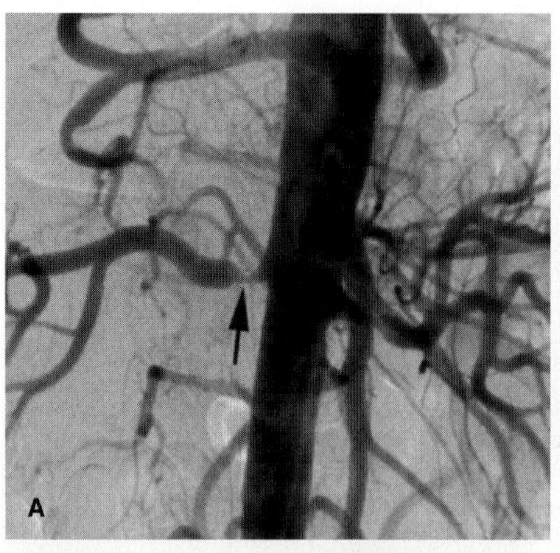

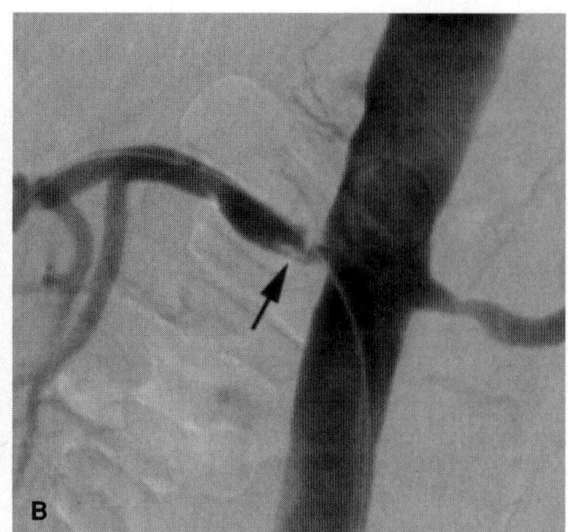

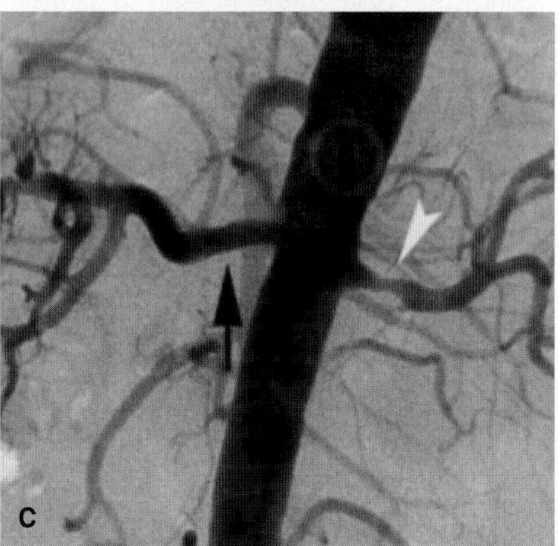

FIGURE 25.4. **Atherosclerotic Renal Artery Stenosis. A.** Aortogram in a 68-year-old woman with hypertension shows bilateral renal artery stenosis that is more pronounced on the right (*arrow*) than the left. **B.** Following angioplasty, a significant intimal dissection (flap) (*arrow*) is noted. **C.** Aortogram following placement of a balloon-expandable stent shows an excellent radiographic result (*black arrow*). Left renal artery stenosis (*white arrowhead*) is better seen here.

of renovascular hypertension in patients younger than 40 years and represents an assortment of histologic patterns, which are usually classified into three main types based on the morphologic appearance and the layer of the involved arterial wall—intimal (7% to 8%), medial (85%), and periarterial (7% to 8%)—although there are also schemes that include subclassifications of each category. Medial fibroplasia accounts for the majority of cases and has the classic "string of beads" appearance on angiography, which represents alternating weblike stenoses and aneurysms (Fig. 25.5). The middle and distal portions of the main renal artery are most frequently involved. The proximal renal artery is rarely involved alone. FMD is the most common cause of hypertension in children. It has been well shown that atherosclerotic renal disease is progressive, but it is also well documented that FMD is also progressive in nature. FMD classically responds well to angioplasty, with success rates approaching 98%. Stenting is rarely required, usually for dissections from angioplasty.

Atherosclerotic renal occlusive disease clinically presents with hypertension, renal failure, or both. Patients with atherosclerotic renal disease are usually over the age of 60 years, and the atherosclerotic lesions look like atherosclerosis elsewhere (Fig. 25.4). Atherosclerotic renal artery stenosis is amenable to angioplasty but is not as straightforward as simply dilating the lesion

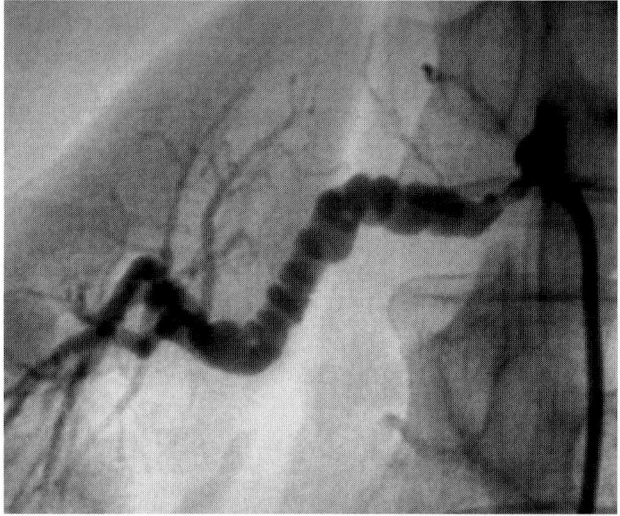

FIGURE 25.5. **Fibromuscular Disease of the Right Renal Artery.** Arteriogram in a 38-year-old with hypertension shows the typical beaded appearance of the right renal artery, diagnostic of medial fibroplasia. This is the classic "string of beads" appearance, which represents alternating weblike stenoses and aneurysms.

(Fig. 25.4). Anatomically, the atherosclerotic renal artery lesion is in both the proximal renal artery and the aorta, with the latter poorly responsive to angioplasty alone. Stenting of renal atherosclerotic lesions overcomes this problem for the most part and is now the standard, but even in light of an anatomically successful procedure, the patient may not respond very well. In fact, the vast majority of patients with hypertension (more than 95%) have essential hypertension, and etiology of renal insufficiency is often multifactorial. Whether treatment of a renal artery stenosis will actually produce a desired clinical result is difficult to predict. Renal vein renins can be measured, and elevated renin values do tend to correlate with a positive clinical result but have little predictive value when not elevated. Even pressure gradients across the stenosis are not very predictive. Therefore one can see that the results are never going to be extremely successful, as one never really knows whether the disease process (hypertension and/or renal failure) is actually caused by the renal artery stenosis until treatment is undertaken. To that end, the results of renal angioplasty are often reported as cured (off all antihypertensive medications), improved (requiring significantly less medication), or failed (no change or worsened by treatment). Based on meta-analysis data, with a mean of almost 2 years of follow-up, approximately 20% of patients are cured of hypertension with stenting, compared to only 10% following percutaneous angioplasty alone. Improvement is about the same with angioplasty alone (53%) versus stent placement (49%). Improvement in renal function is greater with angioplasty alone (38%) versus stent placement (30%). However, restenosis rates are better with stent placement (17%) when compared to angioplasty alone (26%). Angioplasty alone is usually performed for renal artery FMD, with cure rates usually in the range of 25% and improvement in the vast majority of the others.

Finally, as with any invasive procedure, there can be complications. Unfortunately, complications from renal angioplasty are not rare, with an overall complication rate of approximately 5% to 10%, most commonly worsening renal function and injury to the renal artery. In spite of the difficulties with results and the possible complications from angioplasty, endovascular therapy remains the best available treatment following medical failure. The reason to image the renal arteries in a patient with hypertension and/or renal failure is to look for a treatable cause, and a large portion of that treatment is angioplasty and stenting.

Neurofibromatosis causes renal artery stenosis by extrinsic compression of the renal artery by neurofibromata or from disorganized intimal and medial proliferation at the renal artery orifice or in the proximal renal artery. Angiography demonstrates smooth or nodular stenoses with or without associated aneurysms. Hypertension secondary to neurofibromatosis is seen mainly in children. ***Renal transplant artery narrowing*** is most often caused by surgical technical factors (acutely), intimal hyperplasia at the anastomotic site (late), or even atherosclerosis (much later), all of which may be amenable to balloon angioplasty with or without stenting.

Renal artery aneurysms, exclusive of trauma, are rare (less than 0.1%). Aneurysms are basically of two types: extrarenal, caused by atherosclerosis and FMD; and small multiple ones within the kidney, mostly indicative of ***polyarteritis nodosa*** (PAN). For unruptured hilar aneurysms, treatment is said to be indicated when the aneurysm exceeds 2 cm in size; such lesions are often amenable to endovascular therapy. PAN is a rare necrotizing vasculitis that affects the small and medium-sized arteries of multiple organs, most commonly the renal (85%) and hepatic (65%) arteries. Characteristic subcutaneous nodules are seen in 15%. The major angiographic findings are multiple, small, saccular microaneurysms; occlusions; and irregular stenoses throughout the abdominal viscera (Fig. 25.6). Microaneurysms are seen in 50% of patients, range in size from 1 to 12 mm, and are typically located at branch points. The differential diagnosis of microaneurysms includes PAN, Wegener granulomatosis, systemic lupus erythematosus, rheumatoid vasculitis, and drug abuse.

Angiography for renal neoplasms is rarely performed, most often in our experience for preoperative embolization

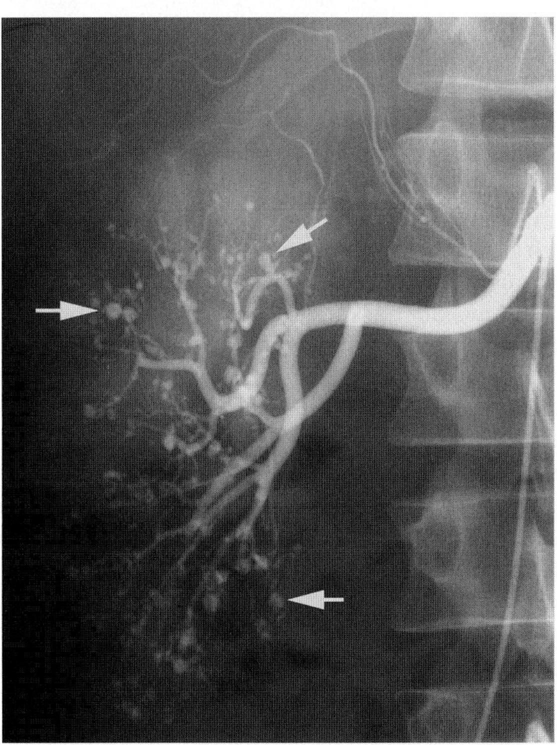

FIGURE 25.6. **Polyarteritis Nodosa.** Right renal angiogram of a 37-year-old man with a history of hypertension and IV drug abuse demonstrates multiple small renal arterial aneurysms (*arrows*). Although these findings have been reported with IV drug abuse, the most likely radiographic diagnosis is polyarteritis nodosa, which was confirmed in this patient.

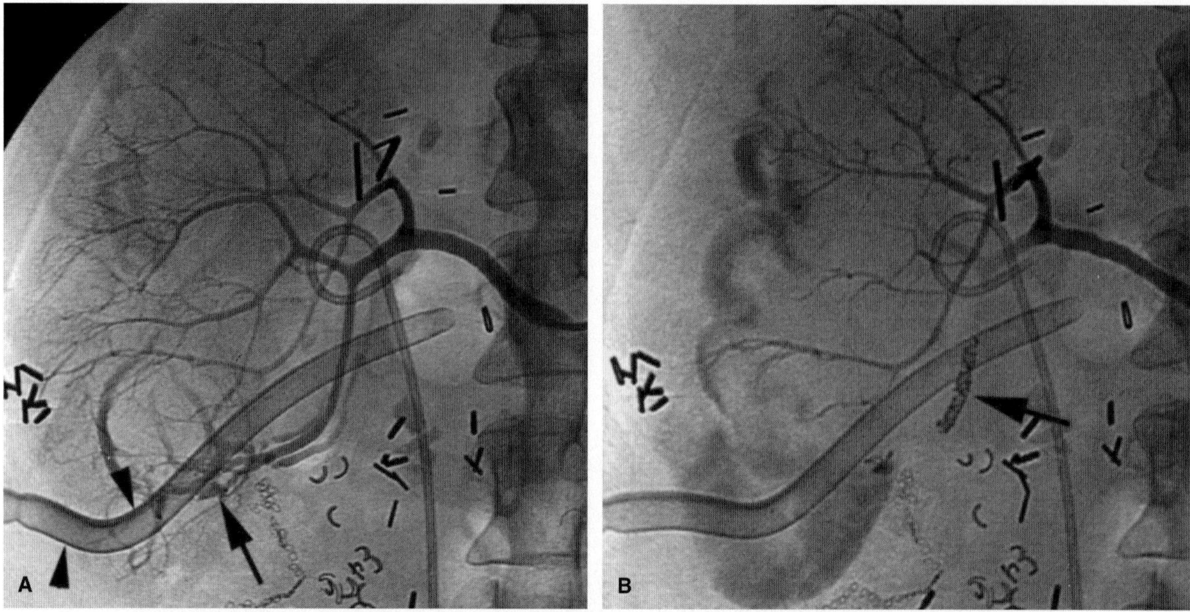

FIGURE 25.7. **Traumatic Arteriovenous Fistula. A.** Right renal angiogram in a 50-year-old man who underwent percutaneous nephrolithotomy shows a lower pole arteriovenous fistula (*arrow*) at the catheter insertion site (*arrowheads*). **B.** The vessel was occluded with microcoils (*arrows*), and the follow-up angiogram shows a good radiographic result.

prior to surgical resection or palliative for hematuria. Most hypervascular renal lesions are renal cell carcinoma, but definitive diagnosis cannot be made angiographically.

Trauma. Injury to kidney is not rare in either penetrating or major blunt trauma. A full range of vascular injuries can be seen from hematuria without visible injury (grade 1) to a shattered kidney or renal hilum avulsion (grade 5). Angiography is most often performed in these patients to determine the extent of injury and therapeutic planning, which may be surgical or via endovascular means. A special type of trauma to the kidney, of course, is iatrogenic, including biopsy or catheter placement (Fig. 25.7). This also includes the renal transplant, which might be undergoing repeated biopsies. Angiography is performed to determine the site and nature of the injury, which could be pseudoaneurysm, arteriovenous fistula, or even extravasation. Most of these injury sites are amenable to endovascular treatment, most often by subselective catheterization and coiling.

Splenic Angiography and Intervention

The splenic artery arises from the celiac artery at the hepatosplenogastric trunk. In 25% of the population, the left gastric, splenic, and hepatic arteries arise as a tripod celiac. Infrequently, the splenic may arise from the aorta or the superior mesenteric artery. The splenic artery tends to become increasingly tortuous with age. Common branches off the splenic artery include the dorsal pancreatic, arteria pancreatica magna, caudal pancreatic, left gastroepiploic, short gastric, and splenic polar branches.

There are few indications for splenic arteriogram and intervention. Prior to intervention, the patient should be informed and consent obtained. Potential complications should be discussed with the patient and the patient's family. Complications of any organ embolization also apply to the spleen, including dissection or vascular injury. Specific to the spleen are pancreatitis and splenic infarction with abscess formation. Patients should be given pneumococcal vaccine prior to the procedure, when time allows.

Trauma is a common indication for arteriographic imaging of the spleen to confirm vascular injury. The risk of delayed rupture increases with severity of splenic injury. Embolization of the splenic artery is performed as close to the injury as possible to preserve splenic tissue through collateral supply from pancreatic and short gastric collaterals (Fig. 25.8). When acute extravasation or a vascular abnormality such as pseudoaneurysm or fistula is discovered, subselective arteriography and focal occlusion of the branch of the splenic artery are performed. Coils are preferred for embolization of the main splenic artery or its branches. Delayed complications include rebleeding and abscess, which mandate splenectomy.

Hypersplenism is caused by hemolytic anemia, splenic vein thrombosis, portal venous hypertension, tumor, infiltrative diseases, myelofibrosis, and polycythemia vera. Anemia, thrombocytopenia, splenomegaly causing discomfort, and gastric varices caused by splenic vein thrombosis are indications for partial splenic infarction.

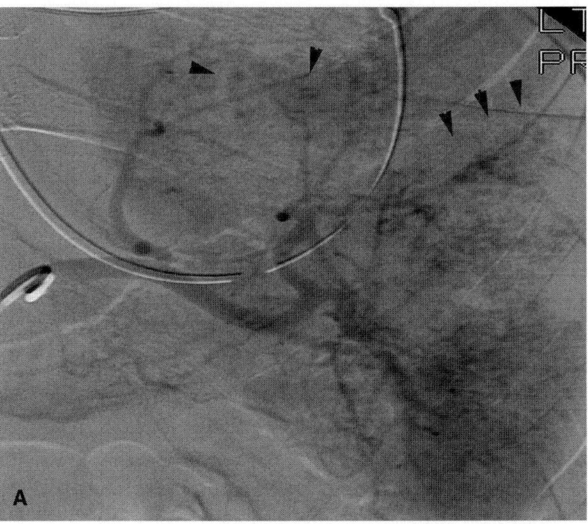

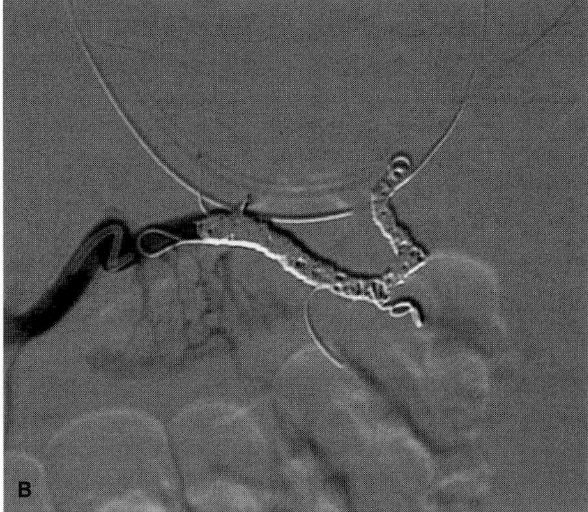

FIGURE 25.8. **Splenic Trauma. A.** Splenic arteriogram demonstrates diffuse injury of the spleen, with multiple areas of extravasation of contrast (*arrowheads*). **B.** Completion arteriogram shows occlusion of the splenic artery following coil embolization.

Embolization is performed with a distal agent, such as Gelfoam (absorbable gelatin-derived sponge), 355- to 500-μm polyvinyl alcohol particles, or 500- to 700-μm calibrated gelatin microspheres, until 60% to 70% of the splenic tissue is ablated. The catheter should be distal to the pancreatic branches prior to infusion of the embolic agent to prevent pancreatitis. Splenic abscess is a complication of splenic embolization.

Splenic artery aneurysm is the most common aneurysm outside of the aorta and iliac arteries. They are seen between the third and sixth decade of life and are more common in women. Congenital aneurysm has a higher rate of rupture. The diagnosis is made with CT or MR. Aneurysms and pseudoaneurysms are treated with coil obliteration, trapping of the arterial segment with coils, or occlusion balloons (Fig. 25.9). Blood flow to the spleen is usually preserved through short gastric collaterals. Multiple aneurysms of the main and branch vessels of the splenic artery can be seen in the setting of cirrhosis.

Hepatic Angiography and Intervention

The common hepatic artery arises from the celiac trunk. The gastroduodenal artery (GDA) is its first major branch, with the artery continuing as the proper hepatic artery. Branch arteries parallel the portal veins and supply the liver segments. In approximately 55% of people, the right, left, and middle hepatic arteries arise from the common hepatic artery. The cystic artery often arises from the right posterior branch. The middle hepatic artery may arise from either the left or right hepatic artery. It supplies liver segments IVa and IVb.

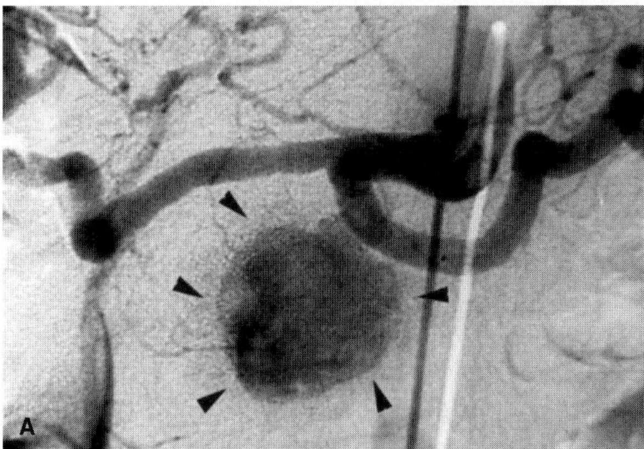

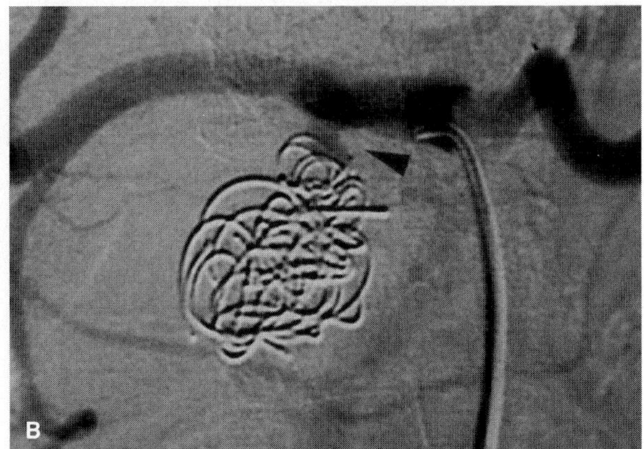

FIGURE 25.9. **Splenic Artery Pseudoaneurysm. A.** Celiac arteriogram demonstrates a large pseudoaneurysm (*arrowheads*) from the splenic artery in a patient with pancreatitis. **B.** Arteriogram following coil embolization shows a small residual neck (*arrowhead*).

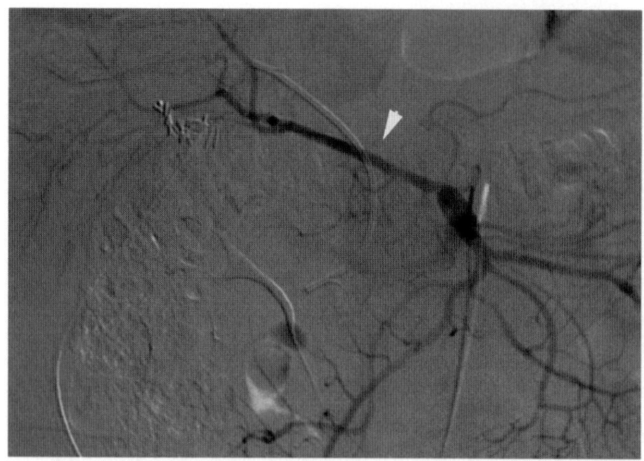

FIGURE 25.10. Replaced Right Hepatic Artery. Superior mesenteric arteriogram demonstrates a replaced right hepatic artery (*arrowhead*) arising from the superior mesenteric artery.

In approximately 2.5% of people the common hepatic artery arises from the superior mesenteric artery. An aberrant right hepatic artery exists in up to 26% of people. The most common variations are either a replaced right hepatic artery (Fig. 25.10) or an accessory artery arising from the superior mesenteric artery (SMA). An aberrant left hepatic artery exists in up to 25% of people. The left hepatic artery may arise from the left gastric artery (15%) or from the gastroduodenol artery, splenic artery, or aorta in 4% of cases. Hepatic arteriography is most commonly performed today for trauma and neoplastic disease, usually as a precursor to transcatheter intervention.

Trauma. Hepatic arteriography is used to increase the sensitivity for vascular injury, intervene upon a vascular injury demonstrated on screening CT examination, or treat a delayed complication from conservative management of a liver laceration (Fig. 25.11). Penetrating trauma is often iatrogenic, resulting from biopsies or percutaneous cholangiography with or without drainage. Indications for embolization in the acute phase include continued hemodynamic instability, arterioportal fistula, and hemobilia. In the delayed setting, pseudoaneurysm discovered on CT or US carries a 44% risk of rupture and may require emergent management.

Neoplasms are diagnosed by CT, MR, and US. Angiography is performed to determine resectability, provide an arterial roadmap, or to deliver transcatheter therapy.

Capillary hemangiomas demonstrate uniform dense staining in the late arterial phase, which persists beyond the venous phase. They usually have well-defined (but irregular) borders with a feeding artery, which is near normal in size. *Cavernous hemangiomas* have the classic appearance of contrast puddles near the periphery in well-marginated vascular spaces, while the stain persists beyond the venous phase. The lesions may be up to 15 cm in size. The feeding artery is usually normal in size. *Hemangioendotheliomas* present in infancy, either with mass effect or hepatomegaly. Most (90%) are associated with extrahepatic hemangiomas (cutaneous lesions). Lesions usually involute within 1 to 2 years. Treatment may be required if the lesions cause symptoms. Angiography shows dilated irregular vascular lakes, staining beyond the venous phase, and dilated feeding vessels. Arteriovenous

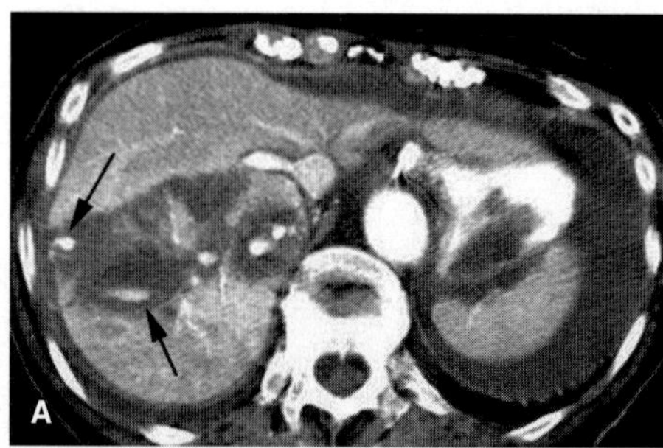

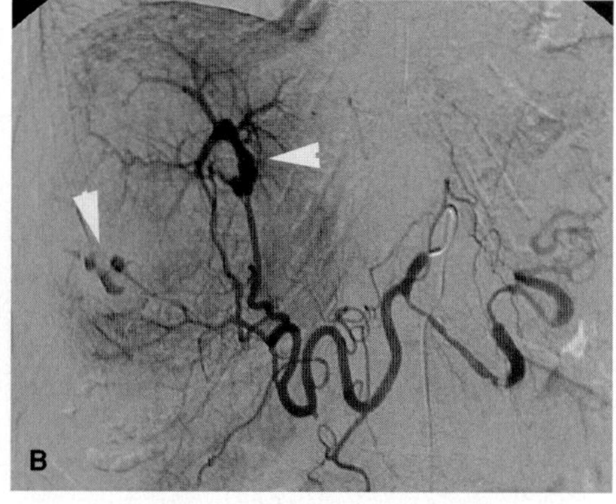

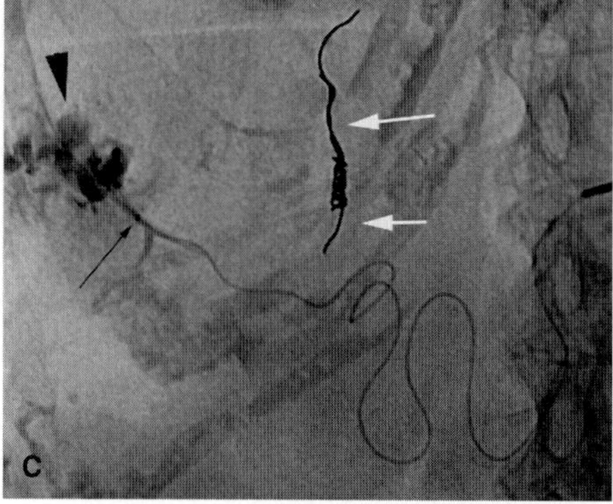

FIGURE 25.11. Active Hemorrhage: Liver Laceration. A. CT shows active hemorrhage with contrast extravasation (*arrows*) from liver lacerations caused by blunt trauma. **B.** Hepatic arteriogram demonstrates multiple arterial injuries, indicated by contrast extravasation (*arrowheads*). **C.** Arteriogram through a microcatheter (*black arrow*) shows extravasation (*black arrowhead*). Previously placed embolization coils (*white arrows*) are evident.

shunting and early opacification of hepatic veins are also described.

Angiography of *hepatoma* demonstrates a hypervascular mass with large, distorted feeding arteries. Neovascularity, intratumoral puddling of contrast, and portal vein invasion with arterioportal shunting may be demonstrated. Up to 25% of tumors are hypovascular. The combination of portal venous invasion and arterioportal shunting is pathognomonic for hepatoma. Angiography of *cholangiocarcinoma* demonstrates a hypovascular or avascular tumor without neovascularity. The most common malignant liver lesions are *metastases*. As shown on physiologic studies, the degree of vascularity and staining on angiography has little relation to tumor blood flow. Even with hypovascular metastases, the blood flow is increased relative to normal liver parenchyma. Angiography may show displacement of adjacent vessels and compressed or occluded portal veins. Arterial encasement or shunting is rare. Embolization of metastases has mixed results. Hypervascular metastases include neuroendocrine tumor, renal cell carcinoma, thyroid carcinoma, and choriocarcinoma. Hypovascular metastases include lung, esophagus, and pancreas carcinoma. Mixed vascularity is seen in breast carcinoma, ocular carcinoma, cholangiocarcinoma, and sarcoma.

Embolization. The decision to embolize a lesion involves a number of important points. First, is the portal vein patent, and in what direction is it flowing? Typically 70% of hepatic parenchymal supply is provided by the portal vein, while metastases receive blood flow primarily from the hepatic artery. Late-phase imaging of the portal vein following selective injection of the celiac, splenic, or superior mesenteric arteries can be used to confirm portal vein patency. Portal venous flow is needed to preserve functional hepatocytes in the field of planned embolization. Embolization of the hepatic artery is usually well tolerated if portal venous flow is available. Portal venous thrombosis or hepatofugal flow increases the risk of hepatic infarction. Embolization can be done in the setting of portal vein occlusion if a modified, low-dose, super-selective technique is used.

Second, are you embolizing a tumor? Tumors, which are responsive to embolization, include hepatocellular carcinoma, neuroendocrine tumors, melanoma, sarcoma, and colorectal metastases (Fig. 25.12). Tumor replacement of greater than 50% to 75% of normal liver is a contraindication to embolization. Tumors are treated with distal agents such as polyvinyl alcohol particles (100 to 300 μm or 300 to 500 μm) or calibrated gelatin microspheres (300 to 500 μm). Cytotoxic agents may improve outcomes from embolization. Most chemical embolizations are performed with a mix of Isovue (iopamidol), ethiodized oil, and cytotoxic agent in addition to the particles. Lipiodol may stay within hepatomas for up to a year while cleared from normal or cirrhotic liver within 4 weeks. Doxorubicin is used for neuroendocrine tumors, while colorectal metastases may be treated with fluorouracil and mitomycin. Attention to the cystic and gastroduodenal arteries must be taken to prevent nontarget embolization. Microcatheters facilitate subselective embolization. Patients are followed with CT or MR to detect contrast-enhancing viable tumor.

Finally, is it trauma you are treating? Proximal agents are the theme in the treatment of hepatic arterial injury. Coil embolization of the vascular injury should be performed as selectively as possible to avoid complications, including infection, ischemia, and biliary stricture. Additional complications include pseudoaneurysm, fistula, and

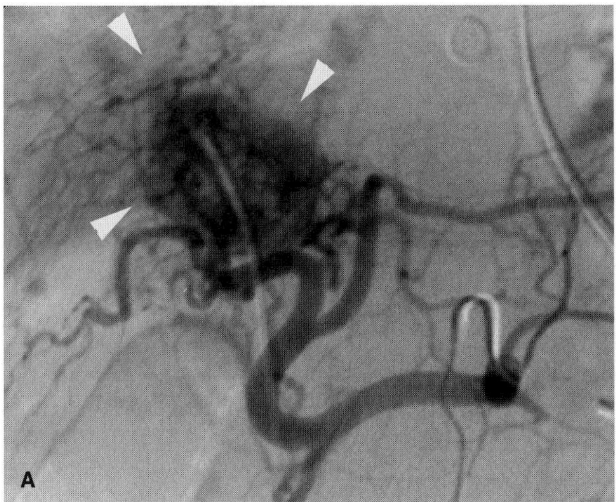

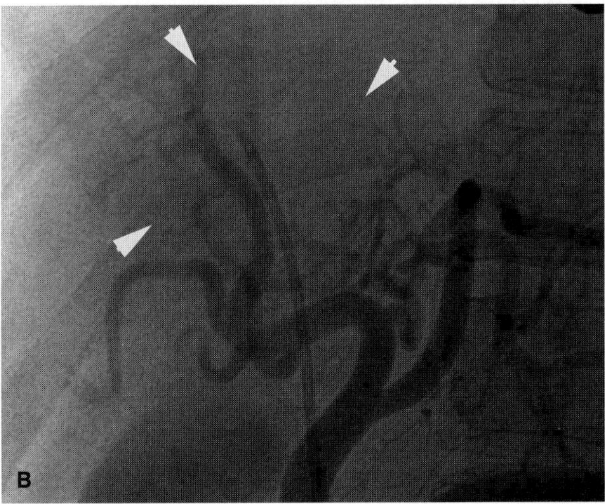

FIGURE 25.12. **Tumor Embolization. A.** Celiac arteriogram demonstrates a hypervascular mass (*arrowheads*) in the right hepatic lobe in a patient with metastatic carcinoid. **B.** Completion arteriogram following embolization with particles demonstrates absent enhancement of the mass (*arrowheads*).

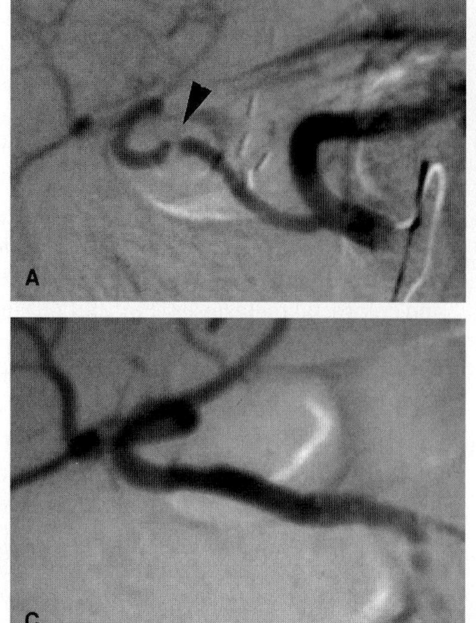

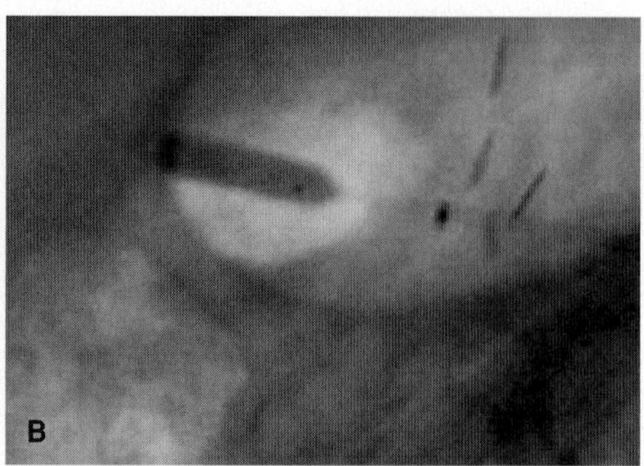

FIGURE 25.13. **Liver Transplant. A.** Celiac arteriogram reveals a high-grade anastomotic stenosis (*arrowhead*) in a patient post–liver transplant. **B.** Balloon is in place, stenting the stenosis. **C.** Completion arteriogram demonstrates resolution of the stenosis.

hemobilia. These can be treated with microcatheter subselective embolization of the source vessel. Cyanoacrylate (glue), large particles, and gelatin sponge may be used for vessels that cannot be selected primarily. Technical success is between 85% and 95 %.

Liver transplantation is now a well-accepted surgical procedure, and angiography plays a role in its planning and in the care for the patient posttransplantation. The initial planning of the transplant may be impacted by variant anatomy. Posttransplant care is usually indicated in the setting of hepatic failure or biliary strictures. Arterial anastomotic stenosis can be treated with angioplasty and stent placement (Fig. 25.13). The technique for angioplasty and stenting is covered in the aortoiliac section of this chapter. In some cases, the arteriogram precedes surgical revision. In the case of splenic arterial steal, management includes proximal embolization of the splenic artery or partial distal embolization with particles in the setting of hypersplenism.

Polyarteritis nodosa, as mentioned earlier, is a rare necrotizing vasculitis that affects the small and medium-sized arteries of multiple organs, most commonly the renal (85%) and hepatic (65%) arteries. The major angiographic findings are multiple, small saccular aneurysms, occlusions, and irregular stenoses throughout the abdominal viscera.

Mesenteric Angiography and Intervention

The celiac artery, SMA, and inferior mesenteric artery (IMA) are the main arterial supply to the gastrointestinal tract. The celiac axis originates at the T12 level, giving rise to the splenic, common hepatic, and left gastric arteries. The common hepatic artery becomes the proper hepatic artery after giving off the gastroduodenal artery, which then branches into the superior pancreaticoduodenal (anterior and posterior) and right gastroepiploic arteries. The left gastroepiploic artery and short gastric arteries are distal branches of the splenic artery. The right gastric artery is a small artery with variable origin, usually from the proper or left hepatic artery. The left gastric artery supplies the distal esophagus and the majority of the stomach while running along the lesser curvature. The gastroepiploic arteries form an anastomosing arc along the greater curvature of the stomach, supplying the bulk of the remainder of gastric flow.

The SMA originates at the T12/L1 level and supplies the entire small intestine and the proximal two thirds of the colon. The first branch is the inferior pancreaticoduodenal artery, which freely anastomoses with the superior pancreaticoduodenal artery to supply the duodenum. The remaining branches, in order of origin, are the jejunal, ileal, middle colic, right colic, and terminal ileocolic arteries. The middle colic divides into the left and right branches, which freely anastomose with the respective right and left colic (IMA) arteries. The ileocolic supplies the terminal ileum and cecum; the right colic supplies the ascending colon and hepatic flexure, and the middle colic supplies the transverse colon.

The IMA originates at the L3 level and gives rise to the left colic, sigmoid, and superior hemorrhoidal (rectal) arteries. The superior hemorrhoidal branches freely anastomose with the hemorrhoidal branches of the internal iliac system.

There are three collateral communications of the mesenteric vessels. *(1)* The marginal artery of Drummond provides anastomosis between the right colic, right and left branches of the middle colic, and the left colic arteries. It is found along the mesenteric border of the colon and is an important collateral supply in IMA occlusions. *(2)* The arc of Riolan is a variable communication between the SMA and IMA located more centrally in the mesentery than the marginal artery. *(3)* The arc of Buehler is a short, ventral artery between the main celiac and SMA and represents a persistent fetal communication.

GI hemorrhage is the most common reason to perform angiography of the mesenteric vessels. The evaluation of GI bleeding includes nasogastric tube aspirate, esophagogastric duodenoscopy, colonoscopy, radionuclide imaging (tagged red blood cells and sulfur colloid), and angiography. The application of these modalities is dependent on the likely source of bleeding and the clinical status of the patient. Hemodynamically unstable patients may require emergency angiography and/or surgery, whereas a stable patient is able to undergo a more controlled, systematic evaluation and treatment. For suspected upper GI bleeding (proximal to ligament of Treitz), the evaluation begins with gastric aspiration and endoscopy. For lower GI bleeding, evaluation by colonoscopy or radionuclide imaging localizes the site of bleeding and guides the angiographic examination to the most likely vascular territory. The most reliable angiographic sign of GI bleeding is contrast extravasation, which is seen as an amorphous contrast collection that persists through the venous phase. If the bleeding rate is rapid enough, the extravasated contrast may outline mucosal folds. The *pseudovein sign* is a linear collection of contrast between mucosal folds that simulates an enlarged vein. Bleeding must occur at a rate of at least 0.5 mL/min to be identified by angiography.

Upper GI hemorrhage is typically suspected in the setting of positive gastric aspirate and melanotic stool. First-line therapy usually consists of endoscopic evaluation and intervention. This can direct endovascular intervention when there is no angiographic evidence of bleeding. Etiologies for upper GI bleeding include Mallory-Weiss tear, hemorrhagic gastritis, gastric or duodenal ulceration, recent GI surgery, and tumor. The distribution for embolization is determined by the site of the lesion. Bleeding from the duodenum is managed with embolization of the gastroduodenal artery. Attention must be made to the retrograde filling from the pancreaticoduodenal artery. This is remedied by trapping the bleeding vessel or site. Gastric ulceration is treated with right, or more typically left, gastric arterial embolization. The technical success of embolization for upper GI bleeding is greater than 90%, while the clinical success rate ranges between 75% and 90%. Proximal agents such as coils and Gelfoam are preferred. In the setting of tumor, distal agents such as particles may be required for clinical success. In the setting of clinical failure, repeat embolization or surgical intervention may be used. Patients with prior surgical alteration require close attention if embolization is the chosen treatment, given that collateral supply to a region may be compromised, thus increasing the risk of bowel infarction.

Tumor is the most common cause for bleeding from the small bowel; it is responsible for 20% to 50% of cases. Angiography depicts tumor neovascularity (enlarged, bizarre, irregular vessels with arteriovenous shunting) with or without contrast extravasation. *Aortoenteric fistula* accounts for 10% of small bowel bleeding and is usually a complication of AAA surgery as soon as 3 weeks postoperatively. The duodenum, where it crosses over the aorta, is the source in 80% of cases. Angiography demonstrates an anterior nipplelike projection from the aortic graft anastomosis or, rarely, contrast extravasation at the fistula site. Angiography is performed using an aortic injection and treatment is urgent surgery. *Diverticula of the small bowel* are an uncommon cause of small bowel bleeding. They are located along the mesenteric border of the bowel. The jejunum is a more common bleeding source than the ileum. Bleeding is typically slow and difficult to diagnose angiographically. *Meckel diverticulum*, the omphalomesenteric duct remnant, is found along the antimesenteric border in the distal ileum. Patients present with painless bleeding caused by an ileal ulcer adjacent to the heterotopic gastric mucosa contained in the diverticulum. A radionuclide Meckel scan is more sensitive than angiography, as this demonstrates the gastric mucosa. *Inflammatory bowel disease* is identified angiographically as diffuse hyperemia, arteriovenous shunting, and oozing. *Vascular malformations* are responsible for 20% of small bowel bleeding. They may be solitary or multiple, as seen in Rendu-Osler-Weber syndrome, and usually present as chronic, recurrent bleeds.

Lower GI hemorrhage is caused most commonly by *colonic diverticula*. Although diverticula are much more common in the left colon, a bleeding diverticulum is three times more likely to be found in the right colon. *Angiodysplasia* shows the classic angiographic features of early opacification of an enlarged draining vein, persistent dense opacification of the vein, and vascular tufts along the antimesenteric border of the cecum or ascending colon. Treatment can be embolic or surgical. *Tumors* usually cause slow bleeding and anemia and are only infrequently the source of massive lower GI bleeding. When massive bleeding occurs, selective or superselective embolization with coils or particles may be performed if the patient is not a candidate for surgical resection.

Treatment of colonic bleeding has shifted toward superselective embolization with coils or particles. Despite advances in microcatheter technology, the technical success has remained constant over the years. The use of superselective embolization has increased the technical demands of the procedure (Fig. 25.14). If the catheter can

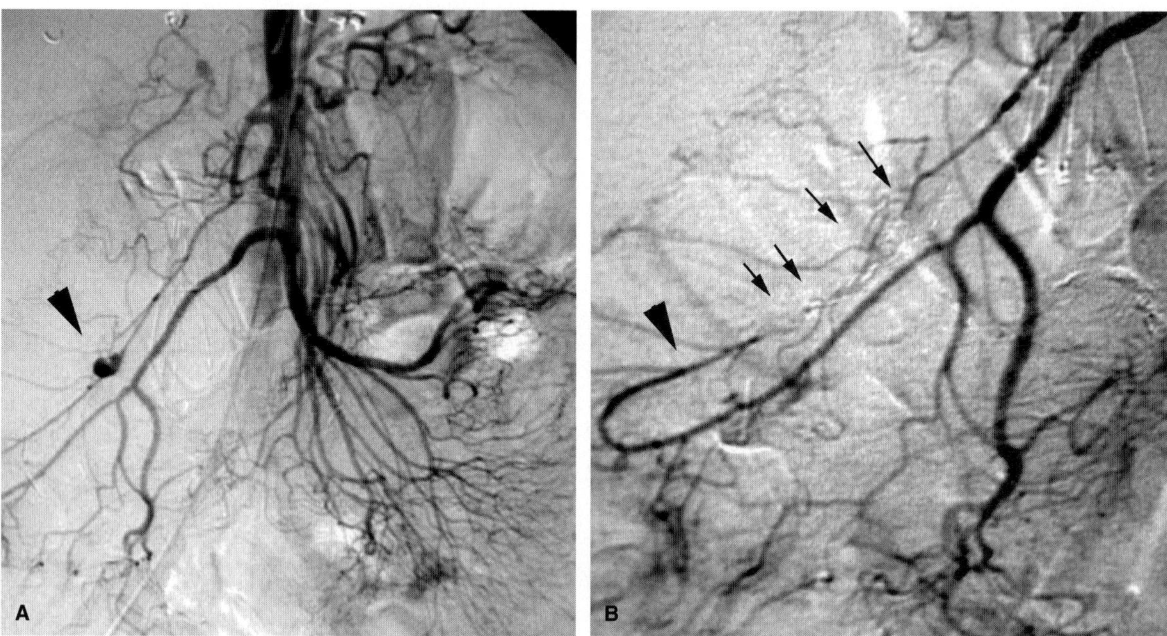

FIGURE 25.14. **Lower GI Hemorrhage. A.** Superior mesenteric artery arteriogram demonstrates extravasation (*arrowhead*) from a branch of the right colic artery. **B.** Completion arteriogram demonstrates superselective embolization of the segment (*arrows*) of the right colic artery, with preserved collateral flow (*arrowhead*) to the segment.

be advanced into the arcuate branches of the colon, collateral flow to the segment of bowel is preserved. This is thought to decrease the risk of infarction. The technical success is 70% to 100%, with a clinical success of 60% to 100%. The rate of recurrence is 19%. Coagulopathy, multiorgan failure, shock, and corticosteroids may cause clinical failure. The rate of minor complications is between 15% and 20%, while the major complication rate is 1% to 11%. In the modern series there has been no bowel infarction. This is likely related to the targeting of the vessels beyond the marginal artery. Treatment with vasopressin has been effective in lower GI bleeding but has fallen out of favor. Vasopressin administration involves placing a catheter within the source vessel and starting an initial 20-minute infusion of 0.1 IU/min, increasing up to 0.4 IU/min if necessary. Also, infusion is quite time consuming relative to embolotherapy. Complication rates have been reported as high as 20% for major and 40% for minor. Complications include myocardial infarction, bowel infarction, groin hematoma, and catheter malfunction.

Mesenteric ischemia comprises a group of disorders that have a common endpoint: bowel necrosis. The mortality rate approaches 70%. Mesenteric ischemia can be divided into acute and chronic varieties. Arterial embolism and thrombosis, nonocclusive ischemia, and mesenteric venous thrombosis are causes of *acute mesenteric ischemia*. Embolism and thrombosis account for 75% of acute ischemic episodes. Acute mesenteric ischemia may be precipitated by an embolic source, which is most commonly cardiac in origin. The angiographic appearance is of an abrupt cutoff of the SMA at the site of its most proximal branches—typically 4 to 6 cm from its origin. The abrupt cutoff has a reverse meniscus appearance because of contrast partially enveloping the embolus, which has lodged at the branch point of the SMA. Arterial thrombosis occurs on a background of preexisting severe atherosclerotic occlusive disease of the celiac artery and SMA. Symptoms of postprandial abdominal pain, weight loss, and altered bowel habits are typical. Intra-arterial infusion with thrombolytics such as tissue plasminogen activator allows for the dissolution of the clot and subsequent intervention on vascular lesions such as an ostial stenosis. Surgical intervention may be needed if bowel infarction is present.

Nonocclusive ischemia accounts for 10% of acute ischemia and is caused by conditions that produce low flow states, such as hypotension, dehydration, and low cardiac output. The bowel responds with disproportionate vasoconstriction leading to ischemia. Angiography confirms diffuse vasoconstriction without underlying structural abnormality. The classic appearance of alternating areas of vasospasm has been termed *sausage link narrowings*. Vasodilators such as papaverine can be used to improve bowel perfusion and maximize recovery. Mesenteric venous occlusion generally affects the medium-sized veins of the middle small bowel and accounts for about 10% of cases. This can be treated with catheter-directed

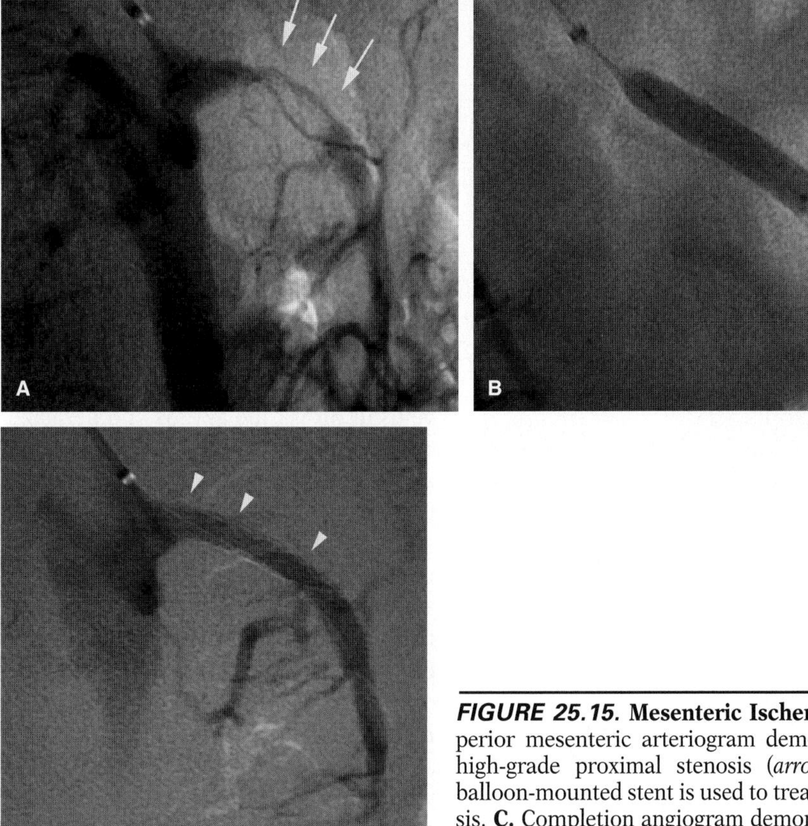

FIGURE 25.15. **Mesenteric Ischemia. A.** Superior mesenteric arteriogram demonstrates a high-grade proximal stenosis (*arrows*). **B.** A balloon-mounted stent is used to treat the stenosis. **C.** Completion angiogram demonstrates the stent (*arrowheads*) and complete resolution of the stenosis.

thrombolysis from the arterial access or via portal access from a percutaneous or transjugular route. Both mesenteric venous thrombosis and nonocclusive ischemia can present with GI bleeding.

Chronic mesenteric ischemia occurs with occlusion or high-grade stenosis of at least two of the three mesenteric arteries. Etiologies include atherosclerosis, fibromuscular dysplasia, and various vasculitides. Patients typically present with postprandial pain. The treatment is to relieve the flow-limiting lesion or occlusion with angioplasty and stenting or surgical bypass (Fig. 25.15). The vasculitides that involve the mesentery can be divided into their vascular distribution but are not very predictable for diagnosis. Treatment is specific to the etiology of the vasculitis. Drug-induced vasospasm or vasculitis must also be excluded. Stenosis of the celiac artery may be caused by extrinsic compression by the median arcuate ligament of the diaphragm. This condition has been implicated in chronic mesenteric ischemia, although this is very controversial. Angiography in the lateral projection shows a superior impression upon the proximal celiac axis that is more pronounced with expiration.

DIAGNOSIS AND INTERVENTION OF THE VENOUS SYSTEM

The superior vena cava (SVC) is formed by the junction of the short, vertically oriented right and the longer obliquely oriented left brachiocephalic veins at the level of T1. The third tributary to the SVC is the azygos vein, which enters the dorsal aspect of the SVC at its midpoint. The SVC contains no valves and is usually less than 2 cm in diameter. The inferior vena cava (IVC) is formed by the junction of the right and left common iliac veins at L5. It ascends on the right of the abdominal aorta and anterior to the spine to enter the RA at about T8. A rudimentary valve (eustachian valve) is present just prior to its entrance into the RA. The main tributaries of the IVC are the hepatic (T10), renal (L2), right adrenal, right gonadal, and lumbar veins.

The azygos venous system is an asymmetrically paired paravertebral venous complex, which provides an important collateral communication between the SVC and IVC. This system is divided into the azygos and hemiazygos veins, which lie to the right and the left of the spine,

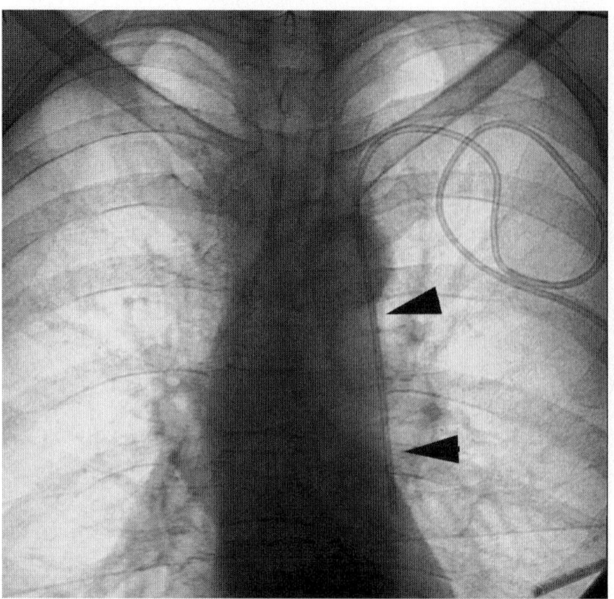

FIGURE 25.16. **Left Superior Vena Cava (SVC).** A chest radiograph demonstrates abnormal position of a central venous catheter (*arrowheads*). Blood gas analysis and contrast injection confirmed catheter position within a left-sided SVC.

respectively. Both are continuations of the ascending lumbar and subcostal veins and begin at the L1 level. The azygos follows the aorta through the diaphragm to the T6 level, where it arches anteriorly over the right mainstem bronchus to join the SVC. The hemiazygos ascends into the chest and traverses the midline to join the azygos vein at approximately T8. The azygos system serves as the most important collateral pathway when the IVC is occluded.

Central venous variants are relatively common, particularly for the IVC, and are quite important during venous intervention. A *left SVC* occurs in 0.3% of the population and descends through the left mediastinum anteriorly to join the coronary sinus, which drains into the RA (Fig. 25.16). A *double SVC* (left SVC with a normal right SVC) is the most common variation (85%). A *single left SVC* is rare and is associated with congenital heart disease. *Azygos continuation of the IVC* is caused by the absence of the intrahepatic portion of the IVC, with failure of the right subcardinal vein to anastomose with the hepatic veins. The hepatic veins drain into the RA. The renal and iliac veins drain via the azygos and hemiazygos veins into the SVC. Findings include dilatation of the azygos vein, the azygos arch, and the SVC. *Duplicated IVC* is present in 3% of the population and is a persistence of both right and left supracardinal veins (Fig. 25.17). The *left IVC* is a continuation of the left iliac vein and ascends to the left of the aorta before crossing over to join the right IVC, usually via the left renal vein. Left IVC without a right IVC occurs in 0.2% of the population and crosses the midline at the level of the renal vein. The *retroaortic left renal vein* (2%) crosses behind the aorta instead of its usual path anterior to the aorta. The presence of both retroaortic and preaortic renal veins forms the *circumaortic left renal vein* (8%), which encircles the aorta to join the IVC.

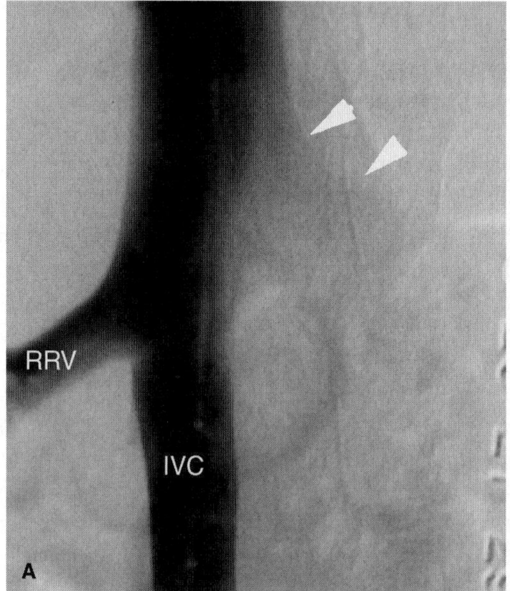

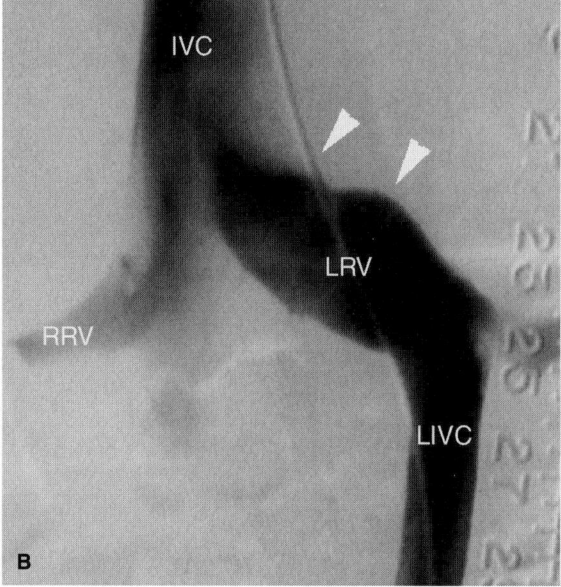

FIGURE 25.17. **Duplication Inferior Vena Cava. A.** Inferior vena cavagram demonstrates the right component of the inferior vena cava (IVC) with a large inflow from the left renal vein (*arrowheads*). The left iliac vein did not fill on this injection. **B.** Contrast injection into the left femoral vein opacifies the left IVC (LIVC), which joins the right IVC by draining through the left renal vein (LRV, *arrowheads*). RRV, right renal vein.

The deep venous drainage of the upper extremity consists of the brachial vein, which travels with its like-named artery and becomes duplicated peripheral to the elbow. The superficial venous system consists of the basilic vein, which drains into the proximal brachial vein, and the cephalic vein, which drains into the axillary vein but may drain as centrally as the subclavian or jugular veins. The axillary vein becomes the subclavian vein at the margin of the first rib.

The predominant venous system of the lower extremity is the deep system. In the calf, the deep trunks follow the named arteries. The confluence of calf veins forms the popliteal vein. The femoral vein is a continuation of the popliteal vein at the adductor hiatus. The femoral vein joins the deep femoral vein (profunda femoris) below the inguinal ligament to form the common femoral vein, which continues as the external iliac vein. The confluence of the external and internal iliac veins at the pelvic brim forms the common iliac vein. The superficial system consists of the greater and lesser saphenous veins. The greater saphenous vein courses along the medial aspect of the lower limb and enters the femoral vein below the inguinal ligament. The lesser saphenous vein commences posterior to the lateral malleolus and enters the popliteal vein above the knee joint. Both the deep and superficial venous systems contain valves.

Diagnostic evaluation of the extremity veins typically begins with US (see Chapter 40). MR, CT, and venography are useful for evaluation of both the central and peripheral venous system. Conventional venography has fallen out of favor, given the ability to evaluate for venous thrombosis on a noninvasive basis with US, CT, and MR.

Venous Access. The need for central venous access continues to increase in both hospitalized and ambulatory patients. Decisions need to be made as to which access device is most appropriate for the clinical situation. Central venous access catheters can be categorized as temporary or "permanent," tunneled or non-tunneled. The indications for placement of these catheters include access for antibiotic therapy, chemotherapy, parenteral nutrition, pain management, and hemodialysis.

Non-tunnelled, temporary catheters include triple-lumen catheters and peripherally inserted central catheters (PICCs). PICCs are inserted through a peripheral upper extremity vein. Access into the brachial, basilic, or cephalic veins allows for central placement of the catheter tip at the cavoatrial junction to reduce the risk of subclavian venous thrombosis. They can be used for access for up to 4 weeks.

Tunneled access is used to provide access for intervals of greater than 4 weeks; with proper care, these can last for longer than a year. Access via the external jugular vein is favored because its size and position lends itself for easy access and avoids some of the complications associated with subclavian access, such as pinch-off syndrome (compression between the clavicle and first rib) and subclavian stenosis. Potential complications include venous thrombosis, catheter obstruction by impingement against the vein wall, stenosis of cava, or occlusion of the catheter. A single-lumen Hickman catheter is adequate for antibiotic therapy, while hyperalimentation may require multiple-lumen access. Flow rates are the critical issue in the setting of dialysis access, so larger sized catheters are used, ranging in size from 12 French in the pediatric patient to 14 or 16 French in the adult. The catheters come premeasured and are chosen for length that will allow the catheter to bridge the cavoatrial junction into the RA. The distal catheter lumens are offset to prevent blood mixing. This is essential to prevent recirculation of the dialysate, which will prolong pump time.

Subcutaneous ports are the most cost-effective devices for venous access for more than 6 months. These are ideal for cancer patients and for patients with sickle cell disease who require pain management. The catheter is completely under the skin, which prolongs the life of the catheter and prevents infection.

Heparin solution is instilled into catheters and ports to prevent thrombosis. The access site should be kept clean, and antibiotic ointments are used at the access site to prevent catheter seeding from the skin flora. Additional complications include air embolism, access site bleeding, vessel injury, and pneumothorax.

Catheter retrieval may be required for removal of a fragment of catheter that was lost because of pinch-off syndrome, during catheter exchange, or because of placement misadventure. Retrieval is performed with a gooseneck snare, which has a snare loop at right angles to its cable. The snare comes in a variety of sizes, which are chosen to match the diameter of the vessel containing the catheter fragment (Fig. 25.18). Other foreign bodies, such as coils lost during embolotherapy, can be retrieved in a similar manner.

Inferior Vena Cava Filters. Pulmonary embolism is a major cause of morbidity and mortality, with up to 90% of pulmonary emboli originating from venous thrombosis in the lower extremity or pelvis. IVC filters are placed in patients with deep venous thrombosis (DVT) to prevent fatal pulmonary emboli. Indications for placement of IVC filters include: contraindication to anticoagulation, decreased cardiopulmonary reserve, patient noncompliance, and free-floating thrombus within the IVC. Filters may be placed prophylactically in patients with spinal injury or multiple traumatic injuries and in those undergoing pulmonary embolectomy and venous thrombolysis. The ideal filter should be efficient at trapping emboli, allow maintenance of the access site and caval patency, be easy to insert, have an indefinite life span, be potentially removable, and be MR compatible. Currently there are nine IVC filters available in the United States. These differ in

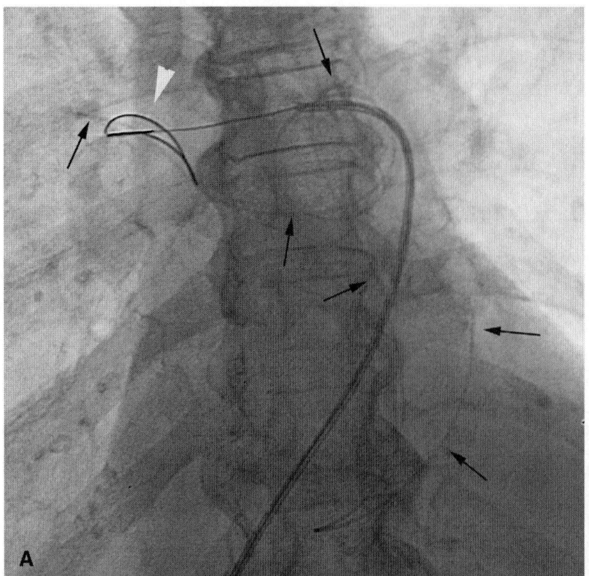

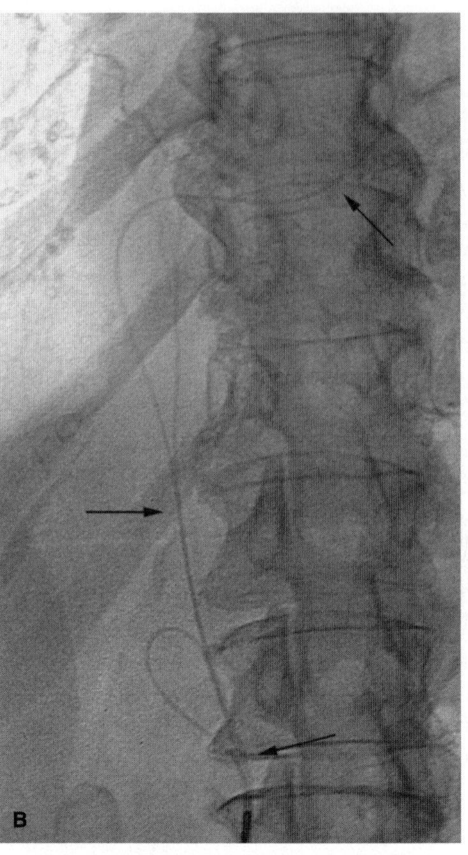

FIGURE 25.18. **Catheter Retrieval. A.** Fluoroscopic image demonstrates a peripherally inserted central catheter (PICC) line (*arrows*), which has migrated centrally through the heart and into the pulmonary artery. A gooseneck snare (*arrowhead*) has been placed in the right pulmonary artery, accessed through the IVC. The snare looped is then tightened around the wayward catheter to accomplish retrieval. **B.** The PICC line has been captured by the snare and pulled back into the IVC.

deployment, with a trend toward smaller delivery systems and the option of removal. At the time of this writing, there are three filters that have the option of removal (Günther Tulip, Cook Inc; OptEase, Cordis Corp; Recovery, C.R. Bard Inc) (see Fig. 25.21).

When placing IVC filters, access via the right femoral or right jugular vein is preferred, although the left femoral or left jugular vein may be used if other sites are occluded or otherwise unsuitable. An IVC-gram is performed to determine presence of caval thrombus, to assess the anatomy and diameter of the IVC, and to check for venous anomalies (Fig. 25.19). Reflux of contrast into, or flow of unopacified blood from, the iliac and renal veins is used to locate these vessels. Either a bony landmark or a radiopaque ruler is used as a reference marker for the renal vein level. This aids in accurate positioning of the filter just inferior to the renal veins. The filter is then deployed under fluoroscopic guidance. In patients with duplicated IVC, placement of a filter in each cava or a single suprarenal filter may be performed. Thrombus within the infrarenal cava or clot extension from a renal vein may necessitate placement in a suprarenal location. In the gravid female, placement in a suprarenal location has been recommended to avoid compression of the filter by the uterus. In addition, placement in this location should prevent embolization occurring through an enlarged ovarian vein from pelvic vein thrombosis.

Recurrence of pulmonary embolism following filter placement is in the 2.7% to 4% range. Filters vary the most in incidence of caval thrombosis, with rates in the 3% to 9% range (Fig. 25.20). Additional complications include filter migration, caval perforation, tilting of the filter, and filter fracture.

Concerns about the long-term safety of IVC filters have resulted in a trend toward retrievable filters, especially in patients with a long life expectancy or a short-term risk of thromboembolism. Indications for filter removal include migration of the filter (occasionally into the right heart) and filter infection. Retrievable filters should be removed within 10 to 14 days of placement (Fig. 25.21). Endothelialization can lead to difficulty, with explantation as soon as 12 days after placement.

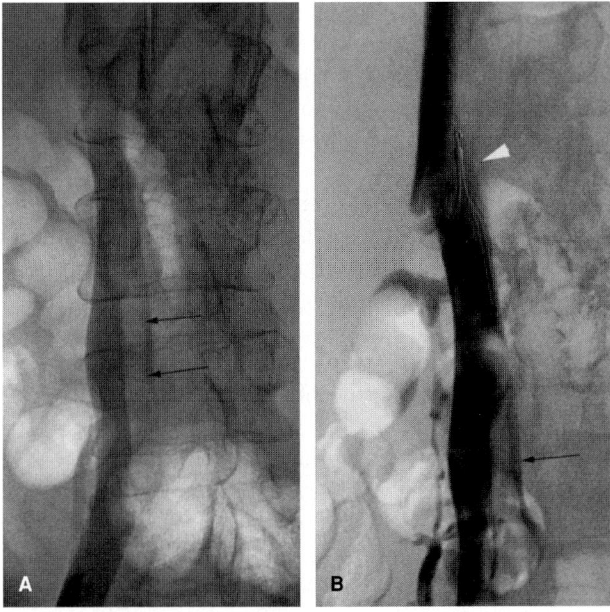

FIGURE 25.19. **Inferior Vena Cava (IVC) Filter Placement. A.** Venogram demonstrates clot (*arrows*) extending into the IVC from the left iliac vein. **B.** A filter (*arrowhead*) is demonstrated above the clot (*arrow*) within the IVC.

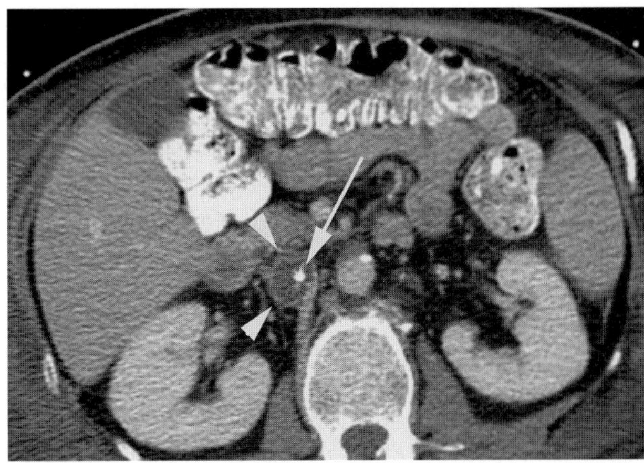

FIGURE 25.20. **Thrombus of Inferior Vena Cava (IVC) Filter.** CT of the abdomen demonstrating thrombus (*arrowheads*) surrounding the top (*arrow*) of an IVC filter. The patient had abdominal and lower extremity swelling 1 month after filter placement.

Venous Thrombolysis. Anticoagulation therapy is the standard of care for the prevention of pulmonary embolism and recurrent DVT, but it does not protect the patient from the long-term effects of DVT. Chronic venous outflow obstruction and injury to valves produce

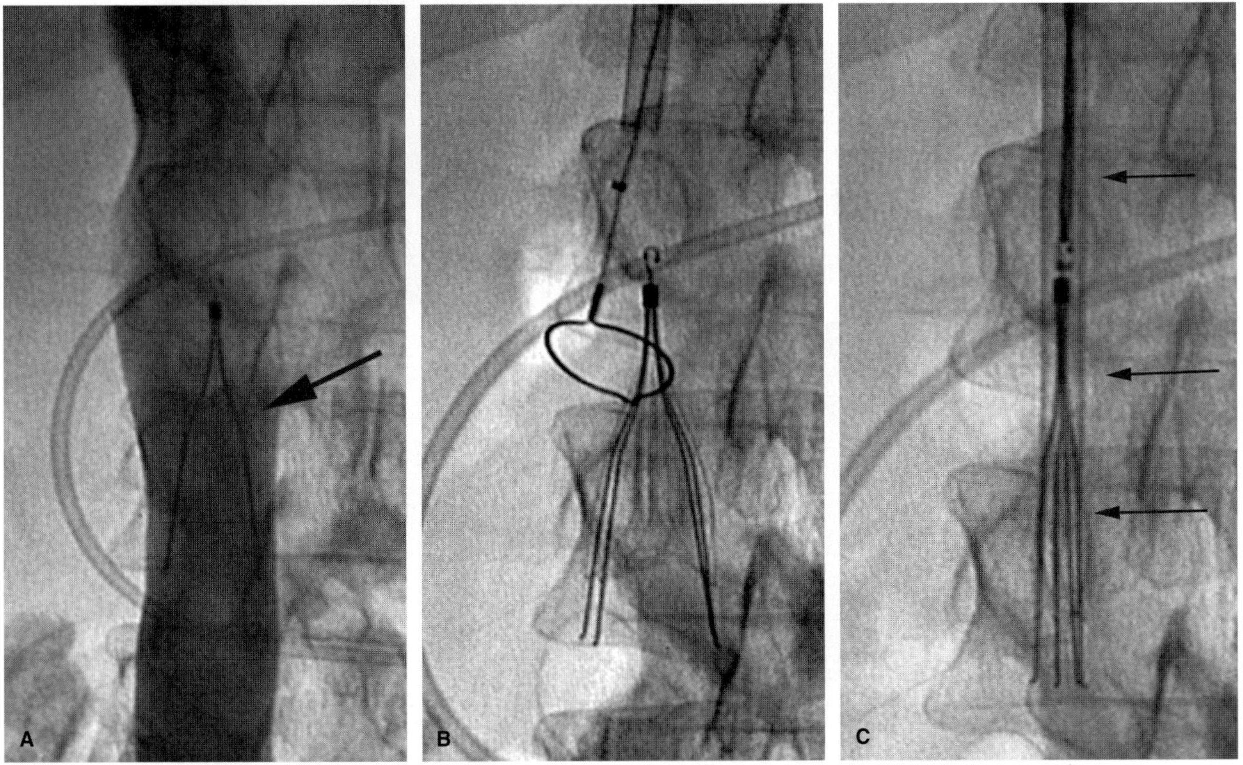

FIGURE 25.21. **Inferior Vena Cava Filter Retrieval. A.** Cavagram demonstrates a Günther Tulip filter (*arrow*) without a clot present. **B.** A gooseneck snare is used to engage the hook at the top of the filter. **C.** The filter is pulled back into and constrained by the sheath (*arrows*) and then is withdrawn through the jugular vein.

postthrombotic syndrome in 40% to 80% of patients with DVT. *Postthrombotic syndrome* refers to the chronic pain, swelling, and development of cutaneous ulcers that may follow DVT. The goal of venous thrombolysis is to remove the obstructing thrombus and to preserve venous valve function. Thrombolysis is most effective in improving vein patency and relieving symptoms when the clot extends centrally.

Patients with upper or lower extremity symptoms and documented clot may be considered for thrombolysis if they are without a contraindication for lytic therapy. Contraindications include: internal bleeding, stroke within the past 6 months, cranial or spinal surgery within the past 2 months, intracranial neoplasm, bleeding diathesis, uncontrolled hypertension, and contraindication to anticoagulation. US documents DVT in the extremity. Central extent of the clot can be evaluated with MR and CT (Fig. 25.22).

Patients with upper extremity involvement are treated with removal of the offending catheter and anticoagulation. If the patient is more symptomatic and has a documented central clot, catheter-directed thrombolysis with venous intervention may be undertaken (Fig. 25.23). For the upper extremity, the preferred access is via the brachial or basilic vein, with catheter placement into the area of thrombosis. Once lysis is complete, the offending lesion may be treated endovascularly with venoplasty or stenting. Compression syndromes may require additional surgical correction.

In the lower extremity, the popliteal vein is the preferred access to iliofemoral DVT. The popliteal vein is large enough to accommodate sheath sizes for most iliac and caval interventions (Fig. 25.24). The administration of thrombolytic agents into thrombi in the venous system is similar to the process performed in the arterial system, in that a multiple-sidehole infusion catheter is imbedded throughout the thrombus. The thrombolytic agent of choice is infused into the clot. The patient usually returns to the angiographic suite for imaging at 12 to 24 hours to assess progression of thrombolysis. Once dissolution of the thrombus has resulted in the restoration of antegrade flow, any underlying lesion can be treated with venoplasty and/or stenting. Stenting is avoided below the inguinal ligament (superficial femoral vein) because of frequent stent failure and thrombosis. For iliofemoral DVT in which symptoms have been present for less than

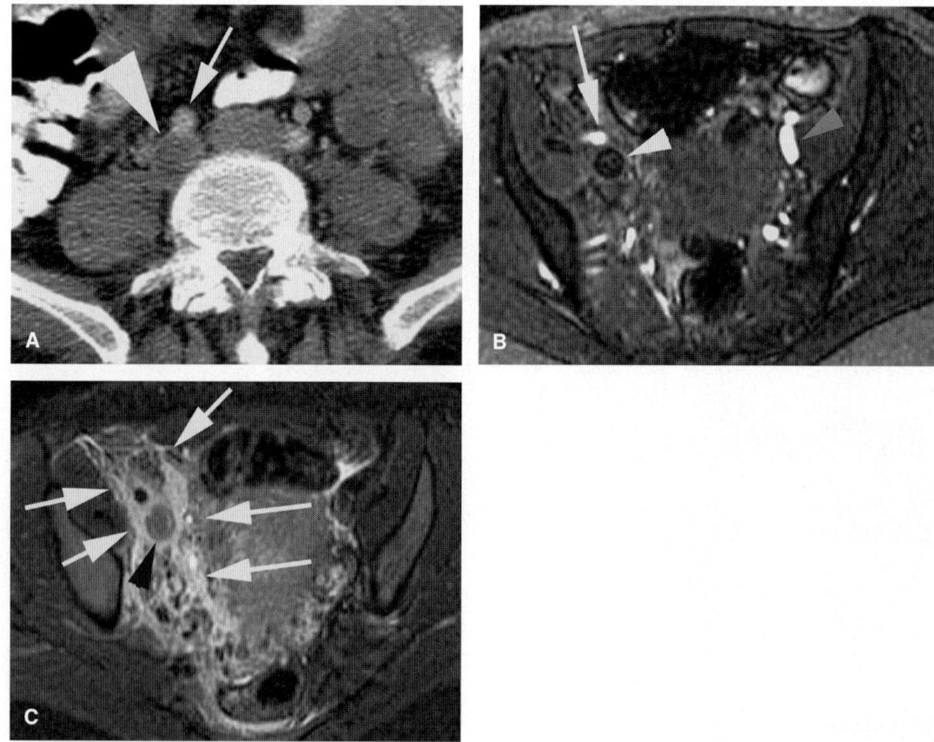

FIGURE 25.22. **Deep Venous Thrombosis: Iliac Vein. A.** Postcontrast CT shows low-attenuation clot within the right iliac vein (*arrowhead*) in comparison to the higher attenuation within the normal right iliac artery (*arrow*). **B.** Gradient MR of the pelvis shows absent flow signal (*white arrowhead*) caused by thrombus within the right iliac vein compared with the normal right iliac artery (*white arrow*) and contralateral left iliac vein (*gray arrowhead*). **C.** T2WI through the region demonstrates extensive perivascular edema (*white arrows*) and intermediate signal clot (*black arrowhead*) within the expanded right iliac vein.

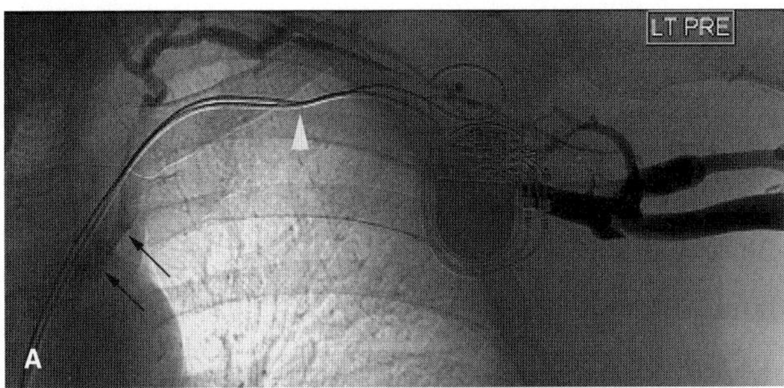

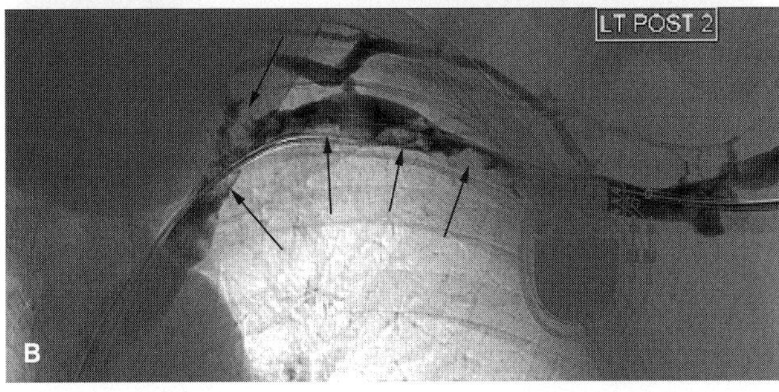

FIGURE 25.23. **Deep Venous Thrombosis: Subclavian Vein. A.** Left arm venogram in a patient with pacemaker shows lack of contrast opacification of the subclavian vein (*white arrowhead*) indicative of thrombosis along the pacemaker lead. The brachiocephalic vein (*black arrows*) fills via collaterals. **B.** Imaging following administration of thrombolytics and balloon angioplasty shows residual clots (*arrows*), which were treated with repeat angioplasty and stent placement.

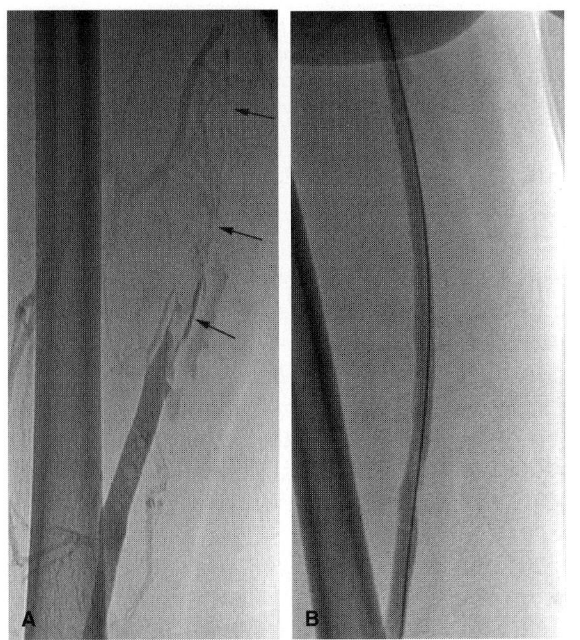

FIGURE 25.24. **Deep Venous Thrombosis: Femoral Vein. A.** Prone left leg venogram demonstrates clot (*arrows*) within the femoral vein. **B.** Venogram following 24-hour infusion of thrombolytics demonstrates complete resolution of the clot.

4 weeks, 80% to 85% of patients have completely or greatly improved partial thrombolysis. In patients in whom there is no malignancy, the 2-year iliac vein patency is as high as 75%. In well-selected patients, thrombolysis is effective and has been shown to improve quality of life with a good safety profile.

Complications of venous thrombolysis include: bleeding at the access site, hemorrhagic stroke, GI bleeding, retroperitoneal hematoma, and pulmonary embolus. Bleeding is increasingly common with higher doses of tissue plasminogen activator and anticoagulation during thrombolysis. The rate of pulmonary embolism is low. A filter may be placed if there is free-floating clot within the IVC or if clot extends above an indwelling thrombosed filter.

Phlegmasia cerulea dolens is arterial compromise of a limb caused by elevated venous pressures from massive acute venous thrombosis. In the majority of patients, DVT spares the collateral pathways. In patients with phlegmasia cerulea dolens, thrombosis involves both main and collateral venous drainage, causing swelling and severe elevations in vascular resistance and resulting in ischemia. These patients require acute treatment.

Paget-von Schrötter syndrome is compression of the subclavian vein by a cervical rib, soft tissue anomaly, or scar tissue after clavicle fracture resulting in thrombosis and arm swelling. Treatment of the offending subclavian venous stenosis becomes multidisciplinary. Stenting of these lesions should be avoided prior to surgery. Stenting often fails because of persistent extrinsic compression with stent fracture. Angioplasty may be performed to improve flow.

SVC syndrome is caused by extrinsic compression of the SVC with thrombosis. Causes include bronchogenic carcinoma (most common: up to 82%); granulomas (histoplasmosis and tuberculosis); lymphoma; intravascular foreign bodies (pacemaker leads, central venous catheters); and venous stenoses caused by chronic dialysis and venous hypertension (Fig. 25.25). In the setting of carcinoma, treatment with external beam radiation may be used initially. If symptoms persist or thrombosis has occurred, endovascular intervention can be undertaken with venoplasty and stenting.

May-Thurner syndrome involves the compression of the left iliac vein by the right iliac artery crossing over it. This is normal anatomy; however, in some patients arterial pressure on the vein results in thickening of the vein wall and narrowing of the lumen, with resulting thrombosis. In some patients, exercise alone may cause symptoms without thrombosis being present. Angioplasty and stenting may offer improvement in symptoms and long-term venous patency (Fig. 25.26).

Venous Access for Dialysis. More than 200,000 people in this country require hemodialysis. Access for hemodialysis is generally achieved through the use of arteriovenous

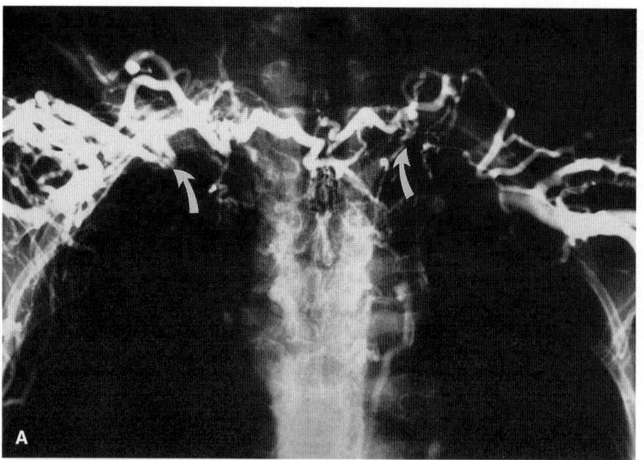

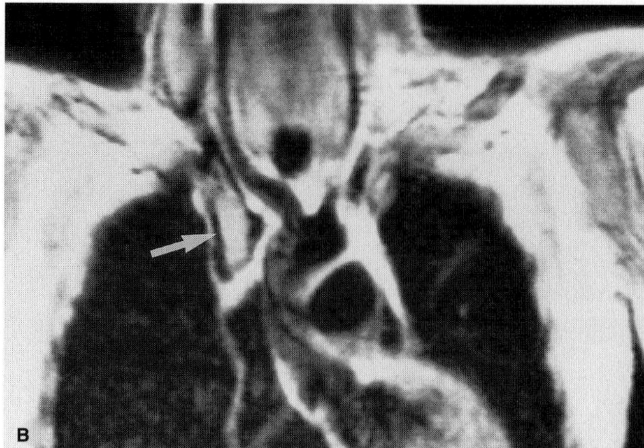

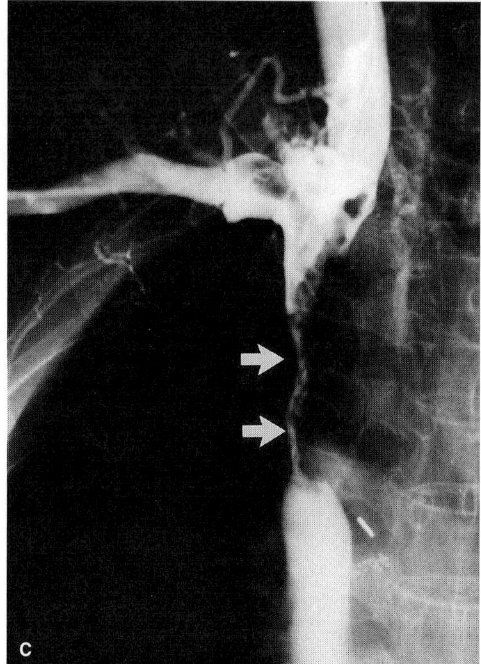

FIGURE 25.25. **Superior Vena Cava (SVC) Obstruction. A.** Dilated and tortuous collateral veins (*arrows*) carry venous return from the upper extremities. **B.** Coronal MR shows bright signal from thrombus (*arrow*) within the SVC. **C.** Contrast injection into the right subclavian vein reveals nearly complete obstruction of the SVC caused by tumor invasion (*arrows*) by bronchogenic carcinoma.

fistula (AVF) (Brescia-Cimino), bridge graft fistula, or a central venous catheter or dialysis port.

AVFs provide convenient access for hemodialysis and can last for years. In patients in whom an AVF cannot be fashioned because of inadequate native veins, a bridge graft (loop or straight) can be created between an artery and a vein using either a PTFE (polytetrafluoroethylene) material or a bovine vein. Use of the AVF is complicated by hematomas, pseudoaneurysms, stenoses, and thrombosis. Monthly monitoring of graft function is recommended. Intervention prior to graft thrombosis is preferred. High venous pressure is evidence of venous anastomotic stenosis.

Both primary fistulas and bridge grafts can be managed with percutaneous techniques in interventional radiology (Fig. 25.27). Grafts that are not amenable to percutaneous management are those that are infected, have been revised or placed within the past week, or are in patients in whom repeated graft failure has occurred within a short time of percutaneous management. Techniques for thrombectomizing dialysis grafts include mechanical thrombectomy devices, balloon thrombectomy, and thrombolytic agents. Access is gained with the puncture directed toward the venous anastomosis. The arterial end of the graft should be compressed to prevent displacement of thrombus into the parent arterial supply. The venous portion of the graft may be cleared with a balloon or mechanical device. The entire length of the graft may then be pulse-sprayed with a thrombolytic agent. A catheter is advanced through the venous anastomosis, and venography of the outflow and central veins is obtained. Any central or outflow vein stenoses and the venous anastomosis are treated with venoplasty. The graft is then accessed toward the

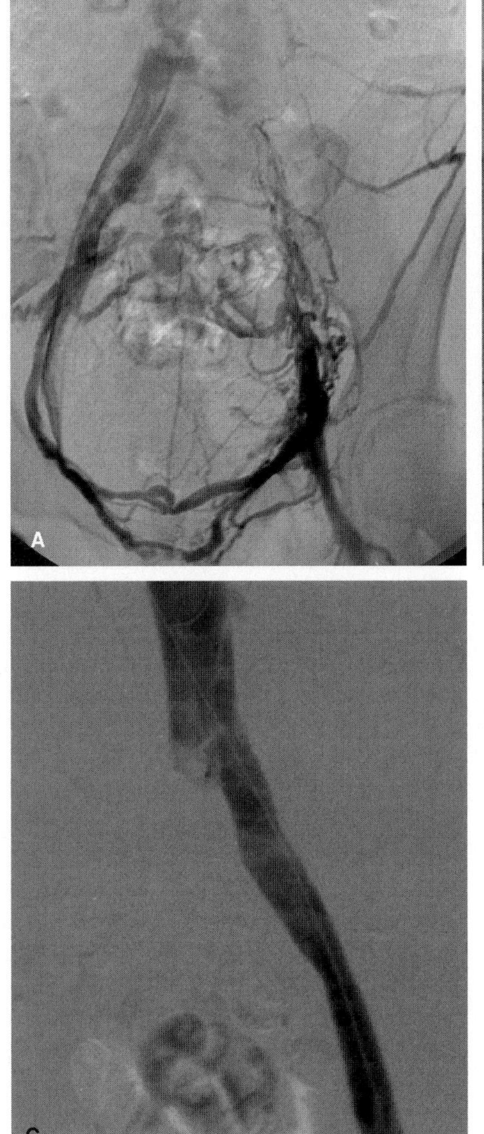

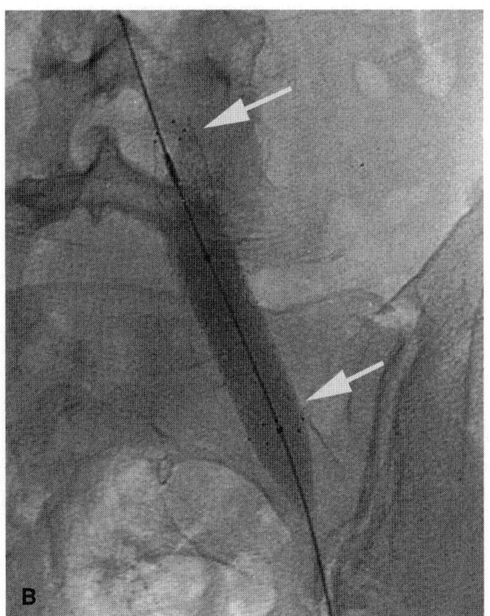

FIGURE 25.26. **May Thurner Syndrome.** **A.** Pelvic venogram demonstrates occlusion of the left common iliac vein. **B.** Following thrombolysis and angioplasty, a self-expanding stent (*arrows*) has been placed in the left iliac vein. **C.** Completion venogram demonstrating resolution of the occlusion and a patent left iliac vein.

arterial anastomosis, and a balloon thrombectomy of the arterial plug may be performed. Once function is restored, hemostasis may be achieved with manual compression or with the use of a purse-string suture. Inability to cross the venous anastomosis is a cause of technical failure. Minor complications occur in fewer than 10% of patients. Major complications occur in 1% of patients. Most of these are distal arterial emboli, which can usually be managed with catheter-directed therapy.

Budd-Chiari syndrome refers to occlusion of the hepatic veins, which occurs as result of hepatic venous or IVC outflow obstruction. Most patients have an underlying condition that predisposes to blood clotting. In up to 30% of patients, no predisposing factors are identified. Post-sinusoidal portal hypertension occurs. Patients may present with acute hepatic failure, portal hypertension, or chronic hepatic dysfunction. Angiography of the celiac and superior mesenteric artery is nonspecific. Venous studies classically show a "steeple" or "pencil point" configuration of the intrahepatic IVC (from compression by swollen liver and enlarged caudate lobe). Thrombus may be present. Hepatic vein studies show a "spiderweb" pattern of collateral veins and lymphatics (Fig. 25.28). Webs may be present but can be missed unless the catheter is directly adjacent to the web. There is usually no normal hepatic sinusoidal filling. Venoplasty of caval webs or of a segmental IVC occlusion may be used to manage these patients. The 1-year patency rate is 80% to 100%. Frequent repeat venography is needed to follow up these patients. More aggressive maneuvers such as IVC or hepatic vein stenting or placement of a transjugular intrahepatic portosystemic shunt (TIPS) may be required.

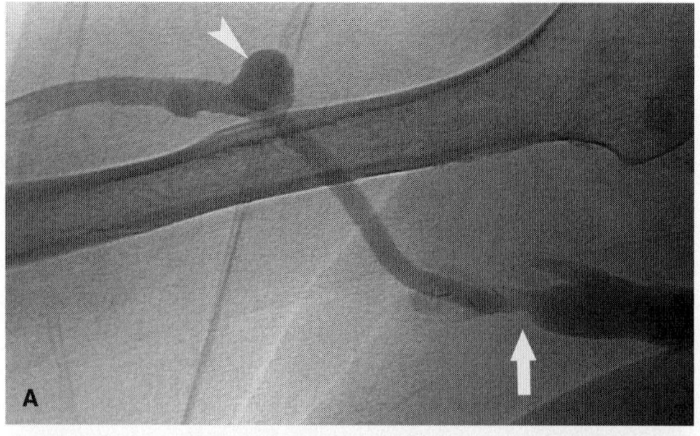

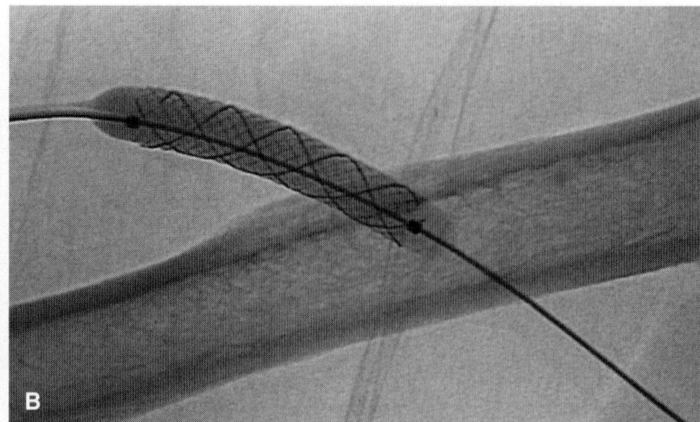

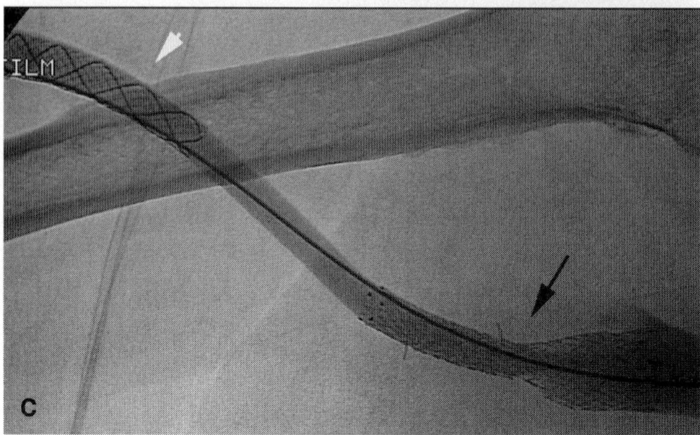

FIGURE 25.27. **Hemodialysis Fistula. A.** Fistulogram demonstrates venous anastomotic stricture (*arrow*) and a pseudoaneurysm (*arrowhead*) in a polytetrafluoroethylene graft. **B.** Balloon dilatation of a wall graft that was placed to exclude the pseudoaneurysm. **C.** Completion fistulogram demonstrates exclusion of the pseudoaneurysm (*white arrowhead*) and stenting of the venous anastomotic stricture (*black arrow*), which was resistant to balloon angioplasty.

Transjugular Intrahepatic Portosystemic Shunt. The pressure in the portal veins normally varies between 5 and 10 mm Hg. The portosystemic pressure gradient (i.e., the pressure gradient between the RA and the portal vein) normally ranges from 3 to 6 mm Hg. The definition of portal hypertension is an absolute portal pressure greater than 11 mm Hg or a portosystemic gradient above 6 mm Hg. Formation of varices (portosystemic collaterals) and subsequent bleeding occur when the portosystemic gradient is greater than 11 to 12 mm Hg. Variceal hemorrhage, ascites, spontaneous bacterial peritonitis, coagulopathy, hepatic encephalopathy, hepatorenal syndrome, and hepatopulmonary syndrome may all occur in patients with portal hypertension. Common collaterals are the coronary veins, which anastomose with the azygos system in the submucosa of the distal esophagus and gastric cardia. These abnormal vascular structures thin the overlying mucosa, project into the esophageal lumen, and are prone to erode and bleed. These are termed "uphill" varices, as opposed to the "downhill" varices seen with SVC obstruction.

The modified Child-Pugh score is a classification scheme used to assess the overall severity and prognosis of liver disease. Child class A is the mildest and Child class C

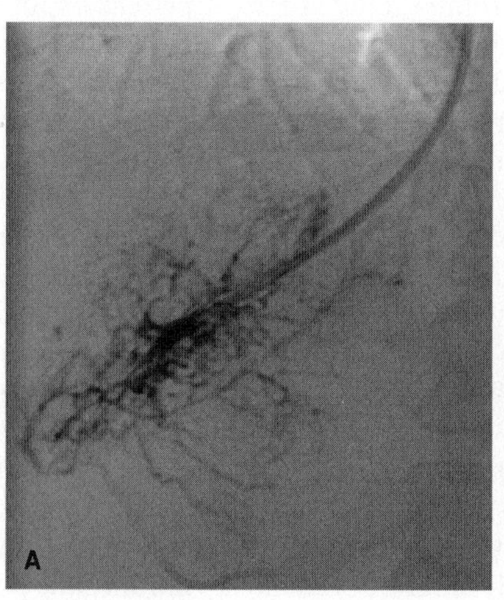

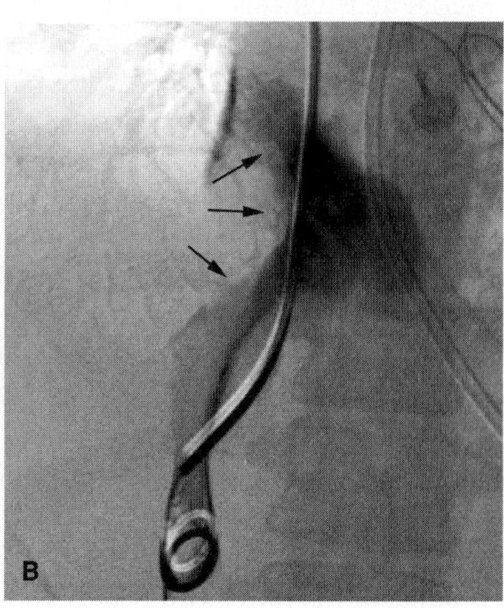

FIGURE 25.28. **Budd-Chiari Syndrome. A.** Injection of the hepatic vein shows the classic spiderweb appearance that is characteristic of Budd-Chiari Syndrome. **B.** Venogram of the intrahepatic inferior vena cava shows the mass effect (*arrows*) from the swollen liver and clot extending from the hepatic veins.

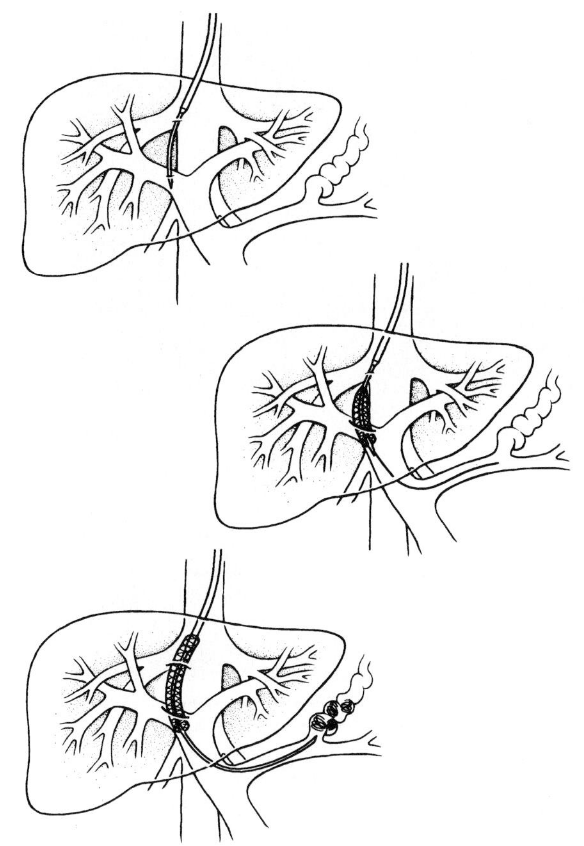

FIGURE 25.29. **Transjugular Intrahepatic Portosystemic Shunt: Step by Step. A.** The needle is shown passing from the proximal right hepatic vein into the right portal vein 2 to 3 cm from the portal vein bifurcation. Note the corkscrew appearance of the dilated coronary vein. **B.** After balloon angioplasty of the tract, a flexible wall stent is being deployed to bridge the parenchymal tract. **C.** The stent is completely deployed, creating the shunt. The coronary vein is embolized with coils in patients with ongoing or recent active bleeding. (Adapted from Zemel G, Becker GJ, Bancroft JW, et al. Technical advances in transjugular intrahepatic portosystemic shunts. Radiographics 1992;12:615–622. Used with permission.)

is the most severe. In symptomatic patients, medical management is the first line of therapy. Endoscopic management may be needed for the control of variceal bleeding from the esophagus. When medical and endoscopic management of the patient are no longer effective or fail, then decompression of the portal system should be undertaken.

TIPS is an endovascular procedure that creates a portosystemic shunt. A TIPS most closely resembles a side-to-side portocaval shunt physiologically. The shunt is typically formed between the right hepatic vein and the right portal vein (Fig. 25.29). Technical success rates for creating a TIPS are greater than 95%. Doppler US or a CT study of the liver should be obtained to confirm patency of the portal vein. Access is gained into the right internal jugular vein and a TIPS set is utilized. A number of TIPS sets are available for use by the interventionist. The right hepatic vein is accessed, and curved needle passes are made in an anterior direction to access the right portal vein. If the middle hepatic vein is used, passes are made in a posterior direction. Once the portal vein is encountered, the pressure gradient between the portal and systemic (right atrial) venous systems is measured, and portal venography is performed to determine the access point into the portal vein, length of tract, and the area to be covered by the stent. Care must be taken not to enter the extrahepatic portions of the portal vein. Following balloon dilation of the stent tract, an appropriately sized stent is deployed (Fig. 25.30). Typically a 10-mm-diameter stent will be used. The current trend is to use covered stents, as these improve patency by excluding the parenchymal tract, which promotes thrombosis and in-stent stenosis. However, covered stents are associated with trapping of portal vein branches or the IVC, so careful measurement and planning of stent placement are needed. The portosystemic pressure gradient and venography are repeated. The goal is to decrease the portosystemic gradient to less than 12 mm Hg and to see no significant filling of varices. When TIPS have been created to treat ascites, portosystemic gradients lower than 15 mm Hg are adequate.

If varices opacify following TIPS placement, embolization of the varices with coils is performed (Fig. 25.31). Proximal embolization prevents filling of the varices by its usual retrograde fashion. The coils are selected based upon the size of the vessel and should be slightly oversized to reduce the risk of distal embolization.

TIPS must be followed closely, as there is a high incidence of shunt stenosis and occlusion. Doppler US of the TIPS is required periodically for surveillance (see Chapter 40). The primary patency of TIPS at 1 year is 20% to 66%. The primary assisted patency at 1 year is 72% to 83%. Shunt dysfunction may occur early or late. Bile duct transection has been described as a potential etiology for acute shunt thrombosis. The incidence of acute thrombosis is diminished with the use of covered stents. US scans are obtained at 1, 3, and 6 months and then every 6 months thereafter.

Absolute contraindications to TIPS include severe hepatic failure and severe right heart failure. Relative contraindications include polycystic liver disease, hepatic neoplasm, hepatic encephalopathy, and portal vein thrombosis. Procedure-related complications include intraperitoneal hemorrhage (1% to 6%), hemobilia (1% to 4%), sepsis, and transient renal failure. New or worsening encephalopathy may occur in 25% of patients. In all but 4% to 7% of patients, the encephalopathy can be controlled with medical therapy. Recurrent bleeding is seen in 15% to 30% of patients. TIPS stenosis or thrombosis may be treated with balloon angioplasty with or without placement of another stent.

The population of patients receiving TIPS is often very ill. The 30-day survival of patients in whom TIPS has been

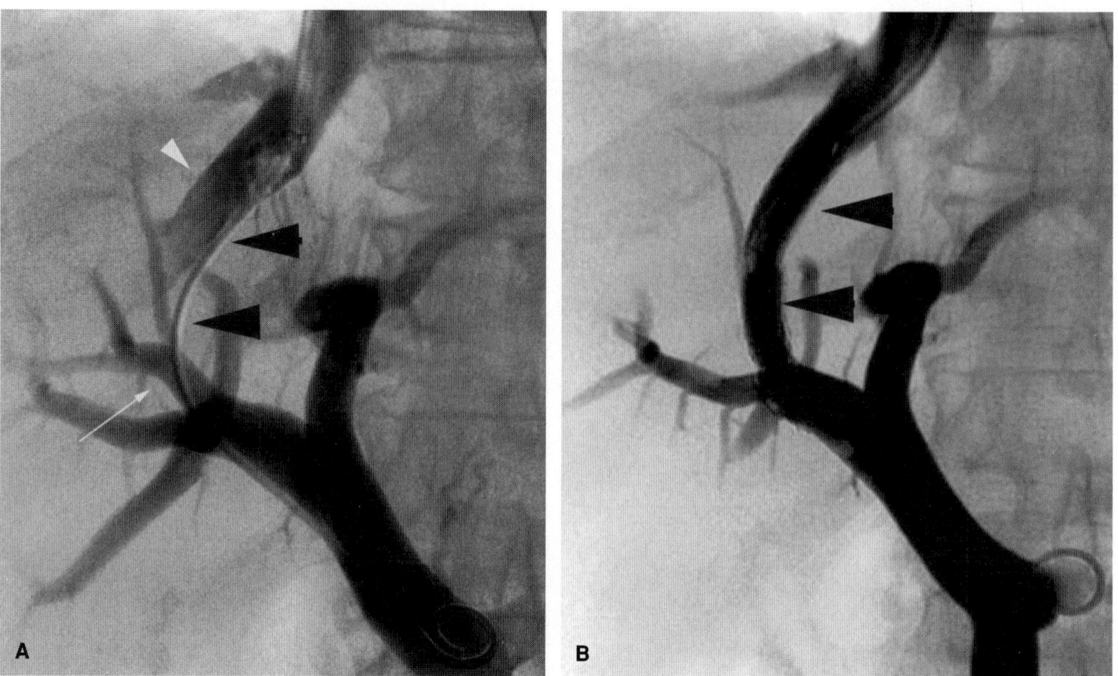

FIGURE 25.30. **Transjugular Intrahepatic Portosystemic Shunt (TIPS) Procedure. A.** Portal venogram with injection of the sheath demonstrates the hepatic vein (*white arrowhead*), right portal vein access (*white arrow*), and the parenchymal tract (*black arrowheads*). **B.** After TIPS creation, the shunt (*arrowheads*) bridges the parenchymal tract between the hepatic and portal veins.

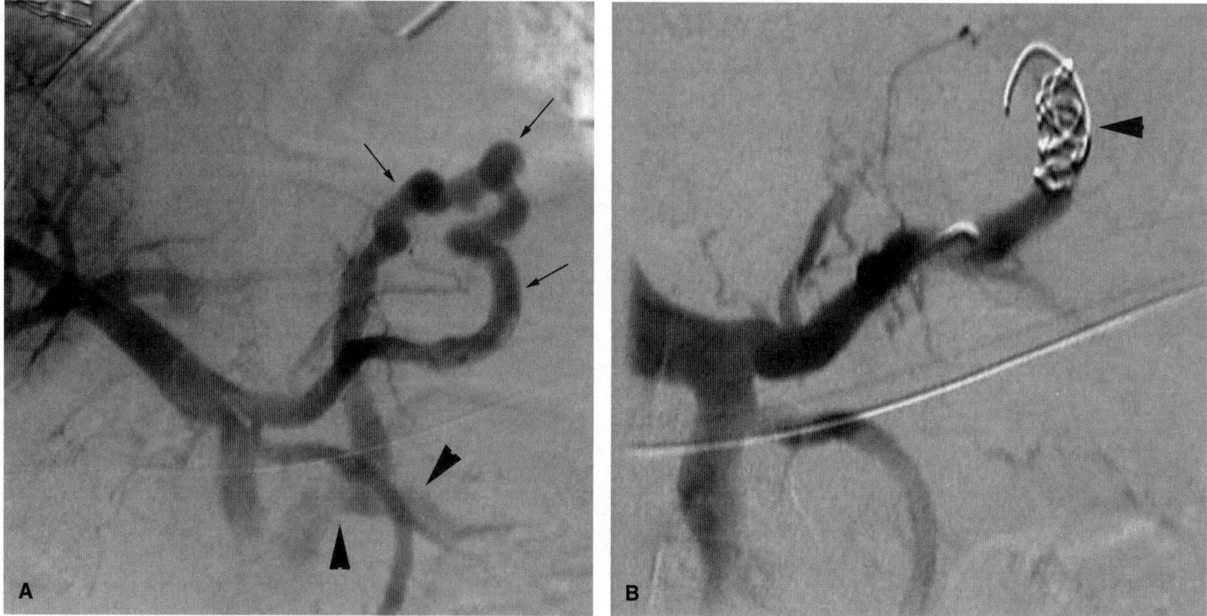

FIGURE 25.31. **Persistent Filling of Varices. A.** Portal venogram demonstrates filling of a varix (*arrows*) with a splenorenal shunt (*arrowheads*). **B.** Portal venogram shows proximal occlusion of the varix using coils (*arrowhead*).

created is 85% to 97%. A patient's status prior to the TIPS is directly related to survival post-TIPS. TIPS is best suited for Child class B and C patients, particularly those who are candidates for a liver transplant. Severe compromise of liver function and elevation of the Child score decrease survival and increase the risk of complication.

NONVASCULAR INTERVENTION

Percutaneous nephrostomy is indicated for ureteral obstruction or treatment of stones within the renal collecting system. It can also be used to access ureteral strictures for dilatation, to perform a brush biopsy of suspected tumor, or to place a ureteral stent. Urinary diversion with a nephrostomy tube is used in the setting of urine leakage including vesical-vaginal or vesical-cutaneous fistulae. Diversion of urine flow allows for closure of the fistulous tract.

The procedure may be guided by fluoroscopy using IV contrast, CT, or US. The patient is placed in a prone position. A 18- or 22-gauge needle is passed into a posterior calyx, usually at the middle or lower pole (Fig. 25.32). Ideally, the nephrostomy catheter is positioned below the 12th rib to avoid pneumothorax. However, it is often necessary to obtain access between the 11th and 12th ribs. For intercostals placement, the puncture should be made close to the top of the 12th rib to avoid the parietal pleura and the intercostal vessels. Punctures close to the neurovascular bundle may lead to increased pain.

The needle is passed through the least vascular area of the kidney, Brödel plane, by positioning the needle 30° to 45° from the vertical (Fig. 25.32). The needle is passed down the barrel of the posterior calyx, avoiding the large vascular structures in the renal pelvis. When urine is aspirated from the needle, a guidewire is advanced through the needle into the renal collecting system. The tract is dilated and the nephrostomy catheter is placed. An antegrade nephrostogram is performed to confirm catheter placement, detect urine leakage, and determine the etiology of the hydronephrosis. Patients are instructed in proper tube care. Nephrostomy catheters are typically exchanged every 3 months to prevent encrustation and occlusion.

If pyonephrosis is encountered, a urine sample is sent to microbiology, and overdistension of the collecting system is avoided to prevent bacteremia. The patient is observed carefully for septic shock. Complications of nephrostomy include hemorrhage; sepsis; pneumothorax (with an intercostal approach); urine leakage (urinoma); visceral injury (colon, liver, spleen); and catheter malfunction.

Ureteral stenting may be used for identification of the ureter during surgery or to bypass a ureteral obstruction caused by tumor, inflammation, or benign stricture. A ureteral stent catheter, usually composed of polyurethane, can be placed at the time of the initial percutaneous nephrostomy if there is no significant bleeding or edema, the ureter shows very little tortuosity, and the ureteral obstruction can be easily crossed (Fig. 25.33). If not, then a few days of drainage are recommended before stenting is undertaken. A catheter of appropriate length for the ureter is placed with the distal pigtail in the bladder and proximal pigtail in the renal pelvis. A double-J ureteral stent is a completely internal catheter that is used only if the patient can have this exchanged cystoscopically every few months.

Occasionally, a ureteral stricture will need balloon dilatation prior to stent placement. Strictures result from iatrogenic trauma, tumors of the ureter, transitional cell cancer of the bladder affecting the trigone region, and cervical cancer. Balloon dilatation with a high-pressure 5- or 6-mm balloon will suffice in most cases and allow passage of a stent. Dilatation with a cutting balloon may be necessary for difficult lesions.

Complications of ureteral stent placement include perforation of the ureter, bladder irritation with urinary frequency, catheter dislodgement, catheter encrustation resulting in occlusion, and incorrect positioning, in addition to complications of nephrostomy.

Several situations require special attention when placing nephrostomy catheters. When a nephrostomy catheter is being placed for *percutaneous stone extraction* (percutaneous nephrolithotomy), a calyx should be chosen that provides the best access to the stone. Two access sites may be needed to retrieve fragments from large staghorn calculi. Sometimes, collecting distension is needed to make room for a wire to pass into the already crowded collecting system. This can by achieved by instillation of contrast via a retrograde ureteral stent or antegrade nephrostomy. Wire access into the bladder with a second "safety wire" is recommended for the eventual dilation of the tract up to 30 French. Special attention also needs to be paid for percutaneous nephrostomy into a *horseshoe kidney*. Intervention is more complex because of altered vascular anatomy and the more anterior position of the kidney. Longer access systems are necessary, especially for stone removal cases. CT correlation is a helpful guide to anatomy and measurement. *Renal transplant* nephrostomy is usually performed with US guidance for ureteral pelvic or ureteral vesicle level obstructions. It is best in this situation to temporize with a percutaneous nephrostomy initially and then determine the best manner of treatment after discussion with transplant surgical team.

Percutaneous biliary drainage is performed most often for obstruction and less often for leakage. Biliary obstruction may be the result of extraluminal compression of the biliary tree or an intraluminal mass. Benign causes include calculi, sclerosing cholangitis, previous surgery or invasive procedure, and ischemia. Malignant obstruction

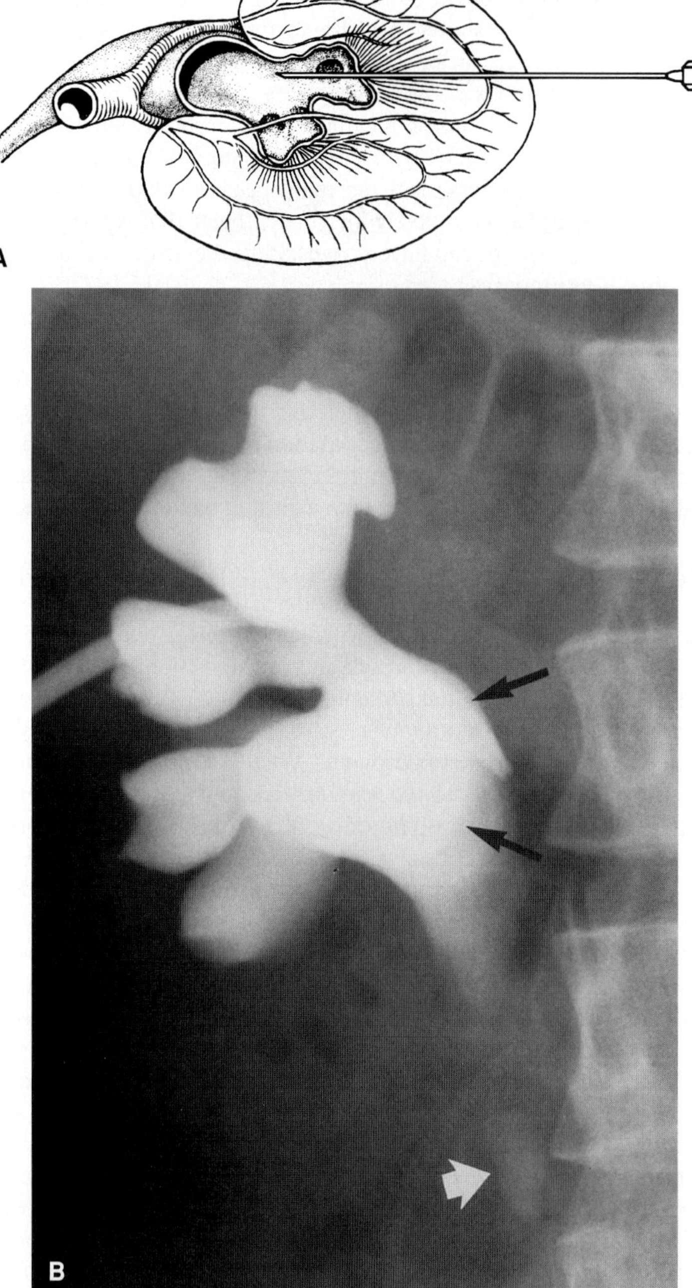

FIGURE 25.32. **Percutaneous Nephrostomy. A.** Cross section of kidney demonstrating needle path for percutaneous nephrostomy placement. Needle entry into a posterior calyx poses the least risk of hemorrhage, since it courses in the avascular plane of Brodel. (Redrawn from Kandarpa K, Aruny JE. Handbook of Interventional Radiologic Procedures. 2nd ed. Boston: Little, Brown, and Company, 1996.) **B.** Nephrostogram in a patient with obstructing stone (*white arrow*) within the proximal ureter. Note the middle-pole access of the nephrostomy with self-retaining pigtail (*black arrows*). The middle-pole access offers mechanical advantage if nephroureteral stenting is needed.

includes cholangiocarcinoma, pancreatic carcinoma, ampullary carcinoma, metastases, and lymphadenopathy. US, CT, and MR may show causes of biliary obstruction. Indications for percutaneous biliary drainage include relief of obstructive jaundice associated with pruritus, cholangitis with sepsis, brachytherapy access for malignant lesions, failed endoscopic biliary drainage, or surgically altered anatomy (Billroth II).

Patients are typically given broad-spectrum antibiotics prior to the procedure because of the high risk of bacteremia. More aggressive antibiotic therapy is needed if sepsis occurs after the procedure. Previous imaging studies are reviewed prior to the procedure for access planning. The presence of ascites is a relative contraindication. US or fluoroscopic guidance is used. From the right, the skin entry site may be up to 2 cm posterior to the midaxillary line, at about the 11th intercostal space level. Traversal of the pleural space should be avoided. From the left, access into the biliary tree may be obtained using a subxiphoid approach. Contrast injection confirms entry

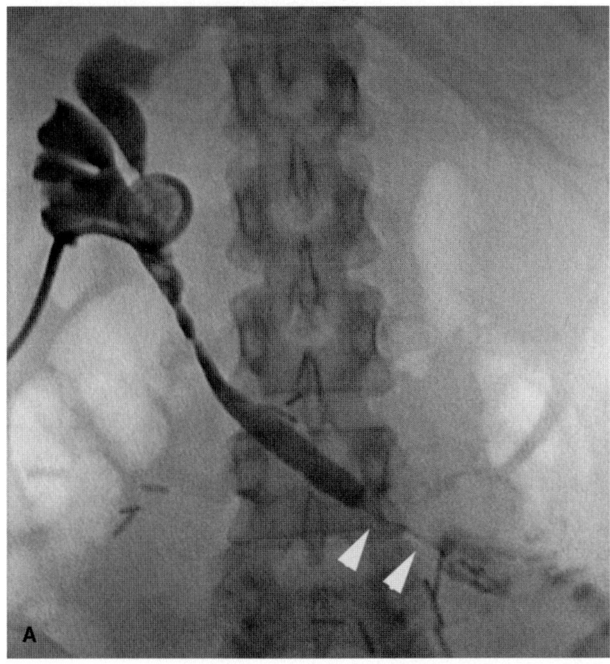

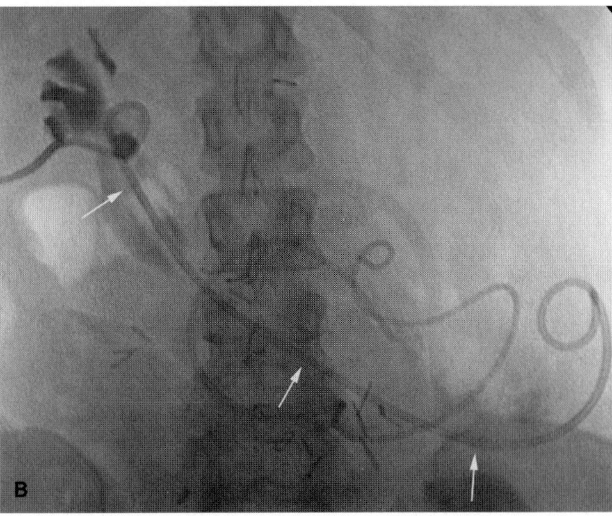

FIGURE 25.33. **Ureteral Stent Placement. A.** Nephrostogram in prone position demonstrates a stricture (*arrowheads*) at the anastomosis between the ureter and the ileal loop diversion. **B.** Postprocedure radiograph shows the nephroureteral stent (*arrows*) bridging the stenosis.

of the needle into the biliary tree (Fig. 25.34). When access into a suitable peripheral bile duct is obtained, a guidewire is inserted, and dilation of the tract is performed. Excessive manipulation within the biliary tree should be avoided. If the obstruction in the biliary tree is not traversed, a locking loop catheter may be placed above the obstruction. The biliary system should be drained for at least a day to allow for resolution of local edema and distension before making another attempt. When the obstruction is traversed, a biliary drainage catheter is inserted and the locking loop is formed within the duodenum. The catheter is placed to external gravity drainage. The catheter should be flushed with 10 mL of sterile saline two to three times daily. Routine catheter exchange is performed every three months.

Complications of biliary drainage include sepsis, hemorrhage, bile leak, cholangitis, catheter dislodgement or malfunction, fluid and electrolyte imbalance, and pneumothorax. Sepsis is caused by overdistension of an infected biliary system. Pneumothorax is a complication of

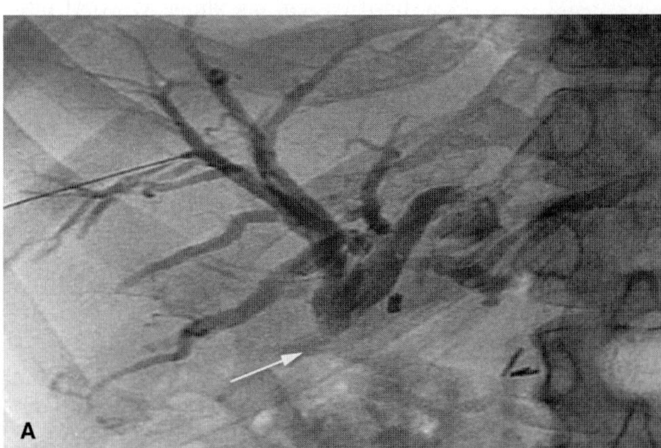

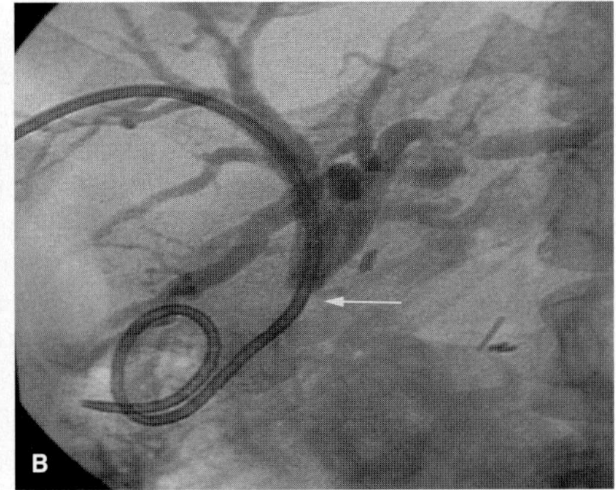

FIGURE 25.34. **Percutaneous Biliary Stent. A.** A percutaneous cholangiogram demonstrates an anastomotic stricture (*arrow*) in a patient post–biliary diversion for a laparoscopic cholecystectomy injury. **B.** A biliary drain has been placed across the anastomosis (*arrow*).

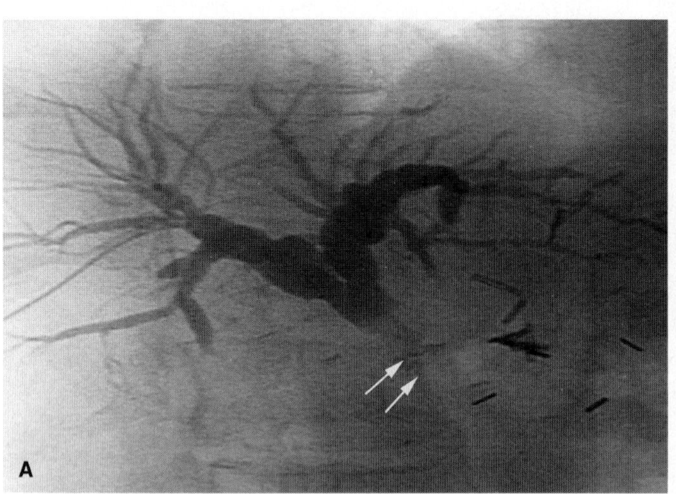

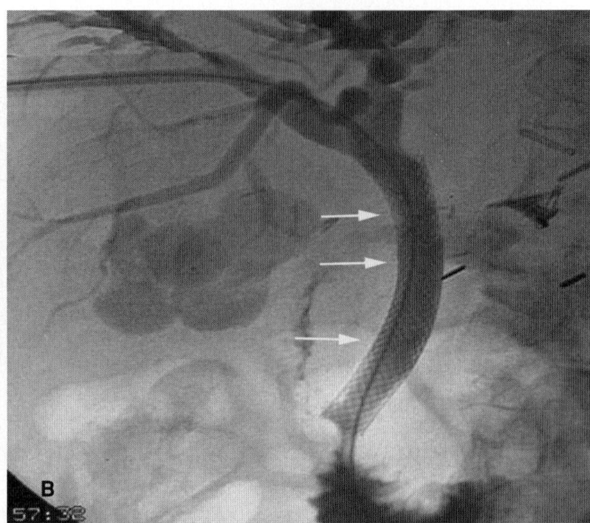

FIGURE 25.35. **Self-Expanding Biliary Stent. A.** Percutaneous cholangiogram shows common bile duct obstruction (*arrows*) in a patient with pancreatic carcinoma. **B.** Postprocedure cholangiogram shows placement of a self expanding stent (*arrows*) across the obstruction.

high access within the liver resulting in traversing of the diaphragm and lung.

In the case of malignant disease, self-expanding metallic stents can be placed within the biliary system so that patients do not have to spend the remaining few months of their lives with an external biliary drainage catheter (Fig. 25.35). Balloon dilatation of the stricture with a high-pressure or cutting balloon is performed before stent placement. Appropriate sedation must be attained, as this is very painful to the patient. The stent is placed across the obstructing biliary stricture with adequate coverage. Extension into the duodenum may be required for ampullary lesions. Tumor ingrowth through the interstices of the stent or overgrowth at the margins of the stent may lead to recurrent biliary obstruction.

Laparoscopic cholecystectomy injury to the biliary ducts deserves special attention. Biliary drainage may act as a temporizing or definitive therapy. External drainage is used to divert bile from the site of injury or from a leak from a cystic duct remnant or accessory cystic duct. When the common bile duct has been transected, access into the biliary tree may be difficult, because the biliary tree decompresses into the peritoneal cavity. An abdominal drainage catheter should be inserted into an associated biloma. Percutaneous biliary drainage may be required when endoscopic intervention fails. If possible, the site of injury is traversed with a biliary drainage catheter. This catheter may have to stay in place for weeks. If the lacerated area does not heal, then surgical repair will be needed. In cases of complete transection of the biliary tree, surgical repair is required.

Percutaneous cholecystostomy may be required in cases of calculus or acalculous cholecystitis in unstable patients. Usually, placement of a cholecystostomy tube is a temporary measure for managing a very sick patient until a cholecystectomy can be performed. The same steps apply to preparation of the patient, as described above for percutaneous biliary drainage. Antibiotic coverage is started before the procedure. US or fluoroscopic guidance is used. US guidance allows for bedside placement of the tube in very ill patients. A transhepatic approach to the gallbladder is preferred so that any leakage around the needle or catheter will be extraperitoneal. If the patient does not undergo surgery, the catheter should be left in place for approximately 6 weeks. This allows maturation of the tract and reduces the possibility of bile leakage and peritonitis. Before removal, a tube cholangiogram is performed to ensure that the cystic duct and common bile duct are patent. The catheter should not be removed if retained stones are demonstrated within the gallbladder.

SUGGESTED READINGS

Boyer H, Haskal Z. American Association for the Study of Liver Disease Practice Guidelines: the role of transjugular intrahepatic portosystemic shunt creation in the management of portal hypertension. J Vasc Interv Radiol 2005;16:615–629.

Burke D, Lewis C, Cardella J, et al. Quality improvement guidelines for percutaneous transhepatic cholangiography and biliary drainage. J Vasc Interv Radiol 2003;14:243S–246S.

Comerota AJ. Quality of life improvement using thrombolytic therapy for iliofemoral deep venous thrombosis. Rev Cardiovasc Med 2002;3(suppl 2):S61–67.

Darcy M. Treatment of lower GI bleeding: vasopressin infusion versus embolization. J Vasc Interv Radiol 2003;14:535–543.

Ferrel H, Patel N. Selection criteria for patients undergoing transjugular intrahepatic portosystemic shunt procedures: current status. J Vasc Interv Radiol 2005;16:449–455.

Goffette PP, Laterre PF. Traumatic injuries: imaging and intervention in post traumatic complications (delayed intervention). Eur Radiol 2002;12:994–1021.

Kinney TB. Update on inferior vena cava filters. J Vasc Interv Radiol 2003;14:425–440.

Leertouwer TC, Gussenhoven EJ, van Jaarsveld BC, et al. Stent placement for renal artery stenosis: where do we stand? A meta-analysis. Radiology 2000;216:78–85.

Mewissin MW, Seabrook GR, Meissner MH, et al. Catheter-directed thrombolysis for lower extremity deep venous thrombosis: report of a national multicenter registry. Radiology 1999;211:39–49.

Ramchandani P, Cardella J, Grassi CJ, et al. Quality improvement guidelines for percutaneous nephrostomy. J Vasc Interv Radiol 2003;14:277S–281S.

Shapiro M, McDonald AA, Knight D, Johannigman JA, Cuschieri J. The role of repeat angiography in the management of pelvic fractures. J Trauma 2005;58:227–231.

SECTION VII

Gastrointestinal Tract

Chapter 26

Abdomen and Pelvis

William E. Brant

Imaging Methods

Compartmental Anatomy of the Abdomen and Pelvis

Fluid in the Peritoneal Cavity

Pneumoperitoneum

Abdominal Calcifications

Acute Abdomen

Small Bowel Obstruction

Large Bowel Obstruction

Bowel Ischemia and Infarction

Abdominal Trauma

Lymphadenopathy

Abdominopelvic Tumors and Masses

Aids in the Abdomen

IMAGING METHODS

Plain film radiographs of the abdomen are important for the assessment of the acute abdomen and to serve as "scout" films prior to contrast studies. CT, US, and MR provide comprehensive evaluation of the abdomen, including the peritoneal cavity, retroperitoneal compartments, abdominal and pelvic organs, blood vessels, and lymph nodes.

COMPARTMENTAL ANATOMY OF THE ABDOMEN AND PELVIS

Knowledge of the complex compartmental anatomy of the abdomen and pelvis is fundamental to understanding the effects of pathologic processes and to correctly interpret imaging studies. An understanding of the shape and extent of anatomic compartments and their normal variations may clarify imaging findings that would otherwise be incomprehensible or lead to misdiagnosis (1). Fundamental considerations include constant anatomic landmarks, ligaments and fascia that define compartments, and normal variations in size and appearance of the various compartments and recesses. Identifying the precise compartment in which an abnormality is located determines to a great extent the origin of the abnormality.

The peritoneal cavity is divided into the greater peritoneal cavity and the lesser peritoneal cavity (the lesser sac) (Fig. 26.1). Within both portions of the peritoneal cavity are numerous recesses in which pathologic processes tend to loculate. The **right subphrenic space** communicates around the liver with the anterior subhepatic and posterior subhepatic space (Morison pouch). The Morison pouch (the right hepatorenal fossa) is the most dependent portion of the abdominal cavity in a supine patient, and it collects ascites, hemoperitoneum, metastases, and abscesses. The right subphrenic and subhepatic spaces communicate freely with the pelvic peritoneal cavity via the right paracolic gutter.

The **left subphrenic space** communicates freely with the left subhepatic space, but it is separated from the right subphrenic space by the falciform ligament and from the left paracolic gutter by the phrenicocolic ligament. The

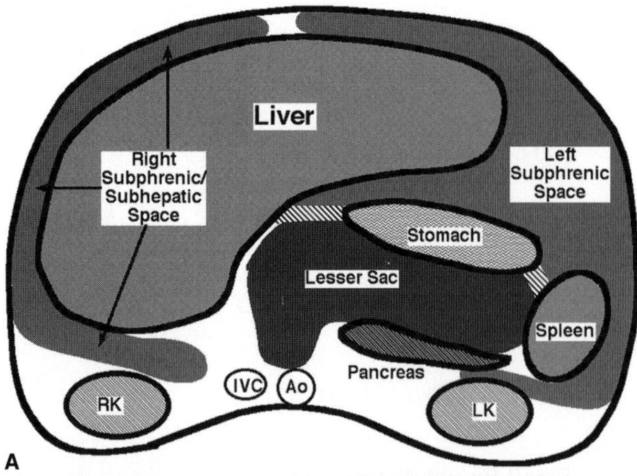

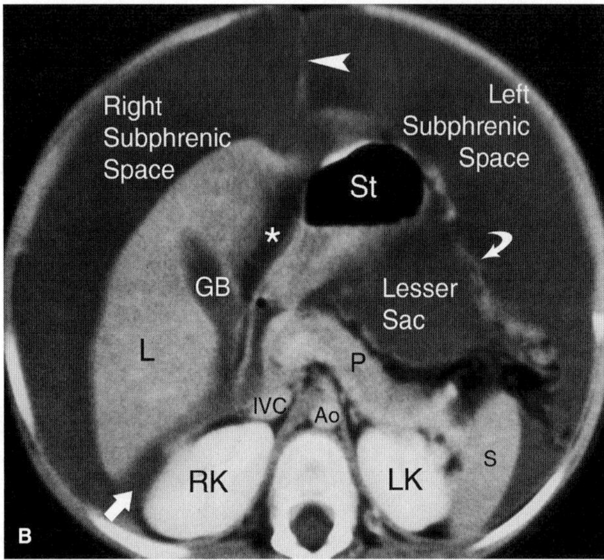

FIGURE 26.1. **Anatomy of the Peritoneal Cavity. A.** Diagram of an axial cross section of the abdomen illustrates the recesses of the greater peritoneal cavity and the lesser sac. **B.** CT scan of a patient with a large amount of ascites nicely demonstrates the recesses of the greater peritoneal cavity and the lesser sac. The lesser sac is bounded by the stomach (St) anteriorly, the pancreas (P) posteriorly, and the gastrosplenic ligament (*curved arrow*) laterally. The falciform ligament (*arrowhead*) separates the right and left subphrenic spaces. Fluid from the greater peritoneal cavity extends into the Morison pouch (*arrow*) between the liver and the right kidney. Fluid in the gastrohepatic recess (*asterisk*) separates the stomach from the liver (L). S, spleen; GB, gallbladder; RK, right kidney; IVC, inferior vena cava; Ao, aorta; LK, left kidney.

left subphrenic (perisplenic) space distends with fluid from ascites and with blood from splenic trauma. It is a common location for abscesses and for disease processes of the tail of the pancreas. The left subhepatic space (gastrohepatic recess) is affected by diseases of the duodenal bulb, lesser curve of the stomach, gallbladder, and left lobe of the liver.

Free fluid, blood, infection, and peritoneal metastases commonly settle in the pelvis because the pelvis is the most dependent portion of the peritoneal cavity (in the upright patient) and communicates with both sides of the abdomen.

The **falciform ligament** consists of two closely applied layers of peritoneum that extend from the umbilicus to the diaphragm in a parasagittal plane. The caudal free end of the falciform ligament contains the ligamentum teres, which is the remnant of the obliterated umbilical vein. Paraumbilical veins (portosystemic collateral vessels) that form in the falciform ligament are a specific sign of portal hypertension. The reflections of the falciform ligament separate over the posterior dome of the liver to form the coronary ligaments, which define the "bare area" of the liver not covered by peritoneum. The coronary ligaments reflect between the liver and diaphragm and prevent ascites and other intraperitoneal processes from covering the bare area of the liver.

The **lesser omentum,** composed of the gastrohepatic and hepatoduodenal ligaments, suspends the stomach and duodenal bulb from the inferior surface of the liver. The lesser omentum separates the gastrohepatic recess of the left subphrenic space from the lesser sac (Figs. 26.1, 26.2). The lesser omentum transmits the coronary veins (which dilate as varices) and contains lymph nodes (which enlarge with involvement by gastric carcinoma and lymphoma). The **lesser sac** is the isolated peritoneal compartment between the stomach and the pancreas. It communicates with the rest of the peritoneal cavity (the greater sac) only through the small foramen of Winslow. Pathologic processes in the lesser sac usually occur because of disease in adjacent organs (pancreas, stomach) rather than spread from elsewhere in the abdominal cavity. The lesser sac is normally collapsed but can become huge when filled with fluid.

The **greater omentum** is a double layer of peritoneum that hangs from the greater curvature of the stomach and descends in front of the abdominal viscera, separating bowel from the anterior abdominal wall (Fig. 26.2). The greater omentum encloses fat and a few blood vessels. It serves as fertile ground for implantation of peritoneal metastases and assists in loculation of inflammatory processes of the peritoneal cavity (abscesses, tuberculosis).

The retroperitoneal space between the diaphragm and the pelvic brim is divided into anterior pararenal, perirenal, and posterior pararenal compartments by the anterior and posterior renal fascia (Fig. 26.3). The **anterior pararenal space** extends between the posterior parietal peritoneum and the anterior renal fascia. It is bounded laterally by the lateral conal fascia. The pancreas, duodenal loop, and ascending and descending portions of the colon are within the anterior pararenal space. Disease in the anterior pararenal space usually originates from these organs (pancreatitis, perforating/penetrating ulcer, diverticulitis).

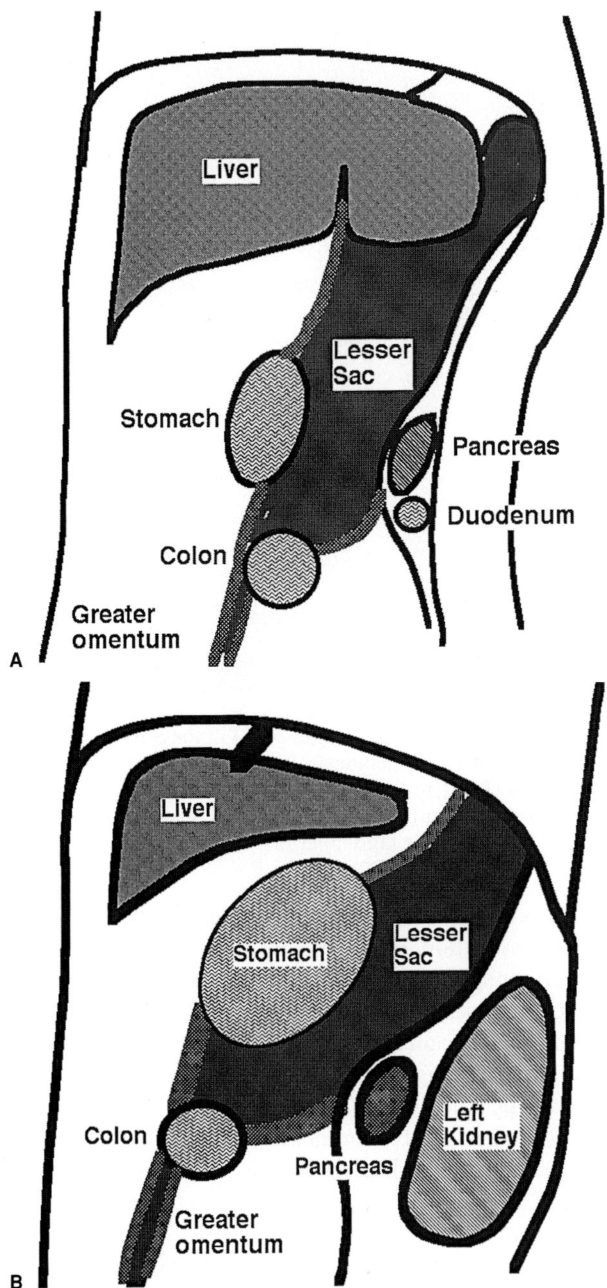

FIGURE 26.2. **The Lesser Sac.** Sagittal plane diagrams of the medial **(A)** and lateral **(B)** aspects of the lesser sac illustrate its position posterior to the stomach and anterior to the posterior parietal peritoneum covering the pancreas. Note that projections of the lesser sac extend to the diaphragm, resulting in the potential for disease processes in the lesser sac to cause pleural effusions. The coronary ligaments reflect between the liver and the diaphragm producing a bare area of liver not covered by peritoneum.

The anterior and posterior renal fascia encompass the kidney, adrenal gland, and perirenal fat within the **perirenal space.** The anterior renal fascia is thin and consists of one layer of connective tissue. The posterior renal fascia is thicker, consisting of two layers of connective tissue

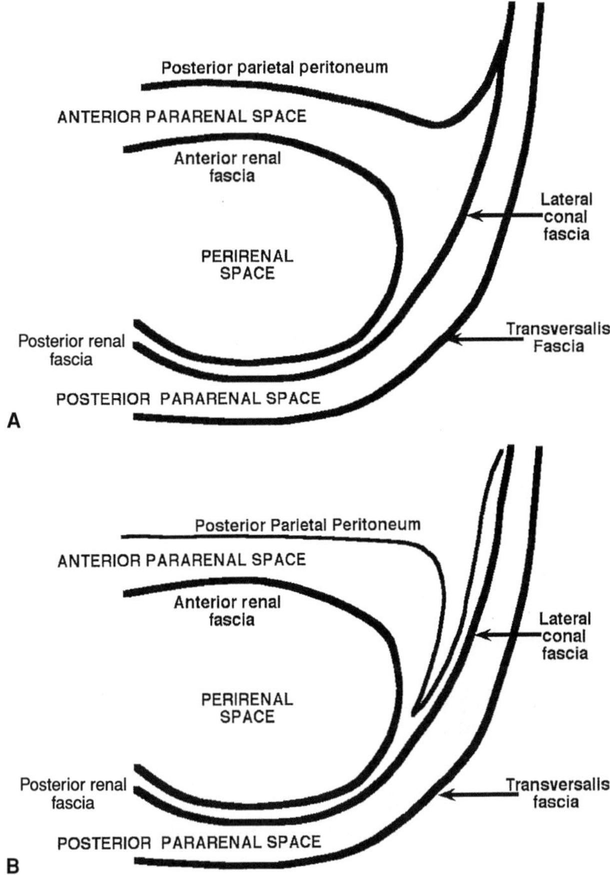

FIGURE 26.3. **Retroperitoneal Compartmental Anatomy.** Diagrams illustrate two normal variations of the reflections of the posterior parietal peritoneum around the descending colon. In **(A)** the colon is entirely retroperitoneal, and in **(B)** the peritoneum forms a deep pocket lateral to the colon, allowing intraperitoneal fluid to extend far posteriorly. Fluid or disease processes in the anterior pararenal space from the pancreas or colon may also extend posteriorly to the kidney by separating the two layers of the posterior renal fascia.

(Fig. 26.3). The anterior layer of the posterior renal fascia is continuous with the anterior renal fascia. The posterior layer of the renal fascia is continuous with the lateroconal fascia, forming the lateral boundary of the anterior pararenal space. The anterior and posterior layers of the posterior renal fascia may be separated by inflammatory processes, such as pancreatitis, extending from the anterior pararenal space. The renal fascia is bound to the fascia surrounding the aorta and vena cava; this usually prevents spread of disease to the contralateral perirenal space. However, disease processes arising from the perivascular space may extend into the perirenal space (hemorrhage from aortic aneurysm rupture, lymphoma). Fluid collections in the perirenal space are usually renal in origin (infection, urinoma, hemorrhage). Bridging septa extending between the renal fascia and the renal capsule tend to cause loculations of fluid processes in the perirenal space. The right perirenal

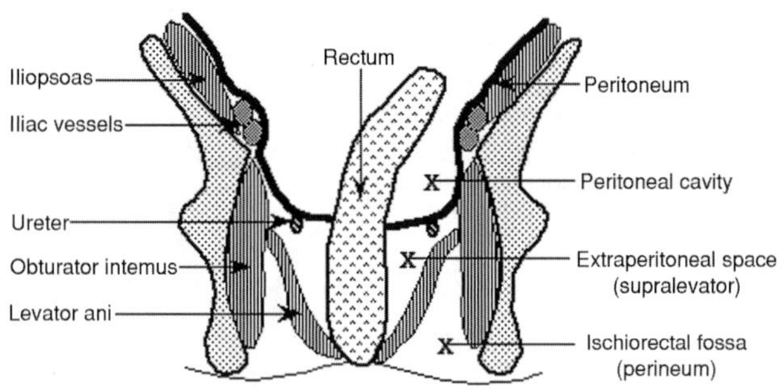

FIGURE 26.4. **Compartmental Anatomy of the Pelvis.** Diagram in the coronal plane illustrates the major anatomic compartments of the pelvis.

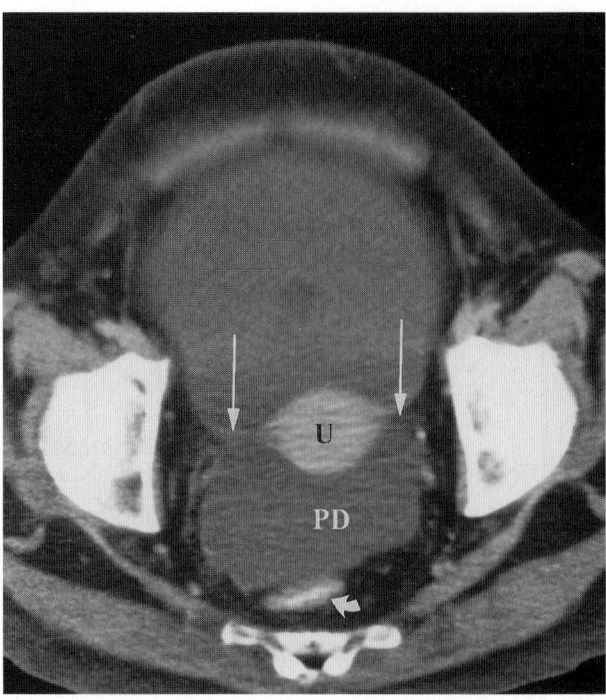

FIGURE 26.5. **Pouch of Douglas.** A CT of the pelvis in a woman with abundant ascites demonstrates fluid distension of the pouch of Douglas (PD) (cul-de-sac) posterior to the uterus (U) and anterior to the rectum (*curved arrow*). The broad ligament (*long arrows*) is outlined by fluid anteriorly and posteriorly.

space is open superiorly to the bare area of the liver, allowing spread of disease processes (infection, tumor) between the kidney and liver.

The **posterior pararenal space** is a potential space, usually filled only with fat, extending from the posterior renal fascia to the transversalis fascia. The posterior pararenal fat continues into the flank as the properitoneal fat "stripe" seen on plain films of the abdomen. The compartment is limited medially by the lateral edges of the psoas and quadratus lumborum muscles. Isolated fluid collections are rare and most commonly caused by spontaneous hemorrhage into the psoas muscle as a result of anticoagulation therapy.

The **pelvis** is divided into three major anatomic compartments (Fig. 26.4). The peritoneal cavity extends to the level of the vagina, forming the pouch of Douglas (cul-de-sac) in females (Fig. 26.5), or to the level of the seminal vesicles, forming the rectovesical pouch in males. The broad ligaments reflect over the uterus, fallopian tubes, and parametrial uterine vessels and serve as the anterior boundary of the rectouterine pouch of Douglas. The cul-de-sac is the most dependent portion of the peritoneal cavity and collects fluid, blood, abscesses, and intraperitoneal drop metastases. The **extraperitoneal space of the pelvis** is continuous with the retroperitoneal space of the abdomen, extends to the pelvic diaphragm, and includes the retropubic space (of Retzius). Pathologic processes from the pelvis spread preferentially into the retroperitoneal compartments of the abdomen. The **perineum** lies below the pelvic diaphragm. The ischiorectal fossa serves as its anatomic landmark (Fig. 26.6).

FLUID IN THE PERITONEAL CAVITY

Fluid in the peritoneal cavity originates from many different sources and varies greatly in composition. Ascites is serous fluid in the peritoneal cavity and is most commonly caused by cirrhosis, hypoproteinemia, or congestive heart failure. Exudative ascites results from inflammatory processes such as abscess, pancreatitis, peritonitis, or bowel perforation. Hemoperitoneum results from trauma, surgery, or spontaneous hemorrhage. Neoplastic ascites is associated with intraperitoneal tumors. Urine, bile, and chyle may also spread freely within the peritoneal cavity.

Plain film diagnosis of ascites requires that at least 500 mL of fluid be present. Findings are: (*1*) diffuse increase in density of the abdomen (gray abdomen); (*2*) indistinct margins of the liver, spleen, and psoas muscles; (*3*) medial displacement of gas-filled colon, liver, and spleen away from the properitoneal flank stripe; (*4*) bulging of the flanks; (*5*) increased separation of gas-filled small bowel loops; and (*6*) "dog's ears" appearance of symmetric densities in the pelvis caused by fluid spilling out of the cul-de-sac on either side of the bladder. CT demonstrates fluid density in the recesses of the peritoneal cavity (Figs. 26.1B, 26.5). The CT density of the fluid gives a clue as to its composition. Serous ascites has attenuation values near water (−10 to +10 Hounsfield units [H]). Exudative ascites is usually above +15 H, but acute bleeding into the peritoneal cavity averages +45 H. US is sensitive to small amounts of fluid in the peritoneal recesses. Care must be taken to examine the most gravity-dependent portions of the peritoneal cavity (the Morison pouch and the pelvis). Simple ascites is anechoic, and exudative, hemorrhagic, or neoplastic ascites often contains floating debris. Septations in ascites are associated with an inflammatory or

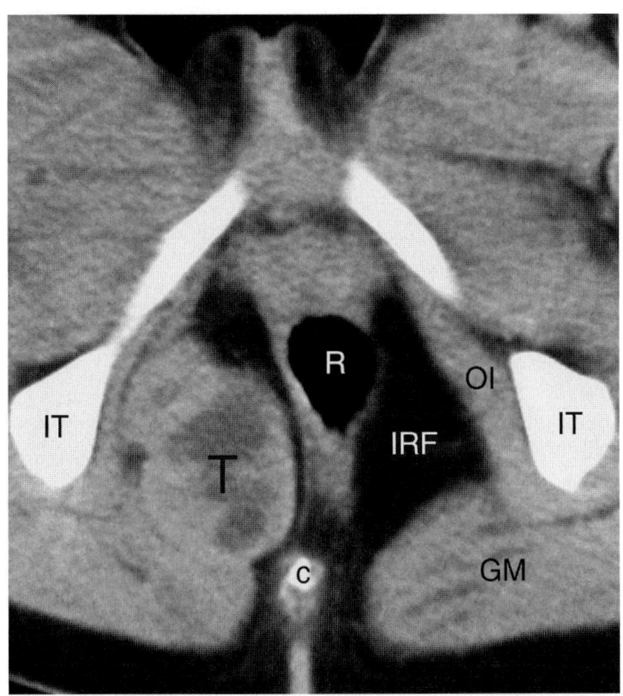

FIGURE 26.6. **Perineal Tumor.** A CT scan of a 12-year-old girl with a history of a rhabdomyosarcoma of the right leg demonstrates a tumor metastasis (T) in the right ischiorectal fossa. The left ischiorectal fossa (IRF) shows its normal appearance as a triangle of fat bordered by the rectum (R), obturator internus muscle (OI), and the gluteus muscles (GM). The ischiorectal fossa is entirely below the levator ani and is part of the perineum. c, tip of the coccyx; IT, ischial tuberosities.

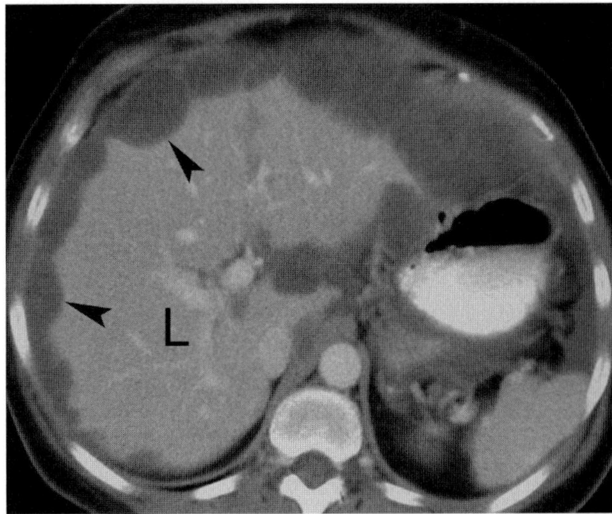

FIGURE 26.7. **Pseudomyxoma Peritonei.** CT scan of a 60-year-old man with intraperitoneal spread of mucinous adenocarcinoma of the colon shows loculations (*arrowheads*) of fluid indenting the surface of the liver (L), giving evidence of mass effect. The attenuation of the fluid measured 32 H, indicating exudative ascites.

malignant process. MR shows limited specificity for defining the type of fluid present. Serous fluid is low intensity on T1WIs and markedly increased in intensity on T2WIs. Hemorrhagic fluid shows high signal intensity on both T1WIs and T2WIs. Serous ascites is commonly bright on gradient-echo images because of fluid motion.

Pseudomyxoma peritonei refers to gelatinous ascites that occurs as a result of intraperitoneal spread of mucin-producing cells caused by rupture of appendiceal mucocele or intraperitoneal spread of mucinous adenocarcinoma of the ovary, colon, or rectum. Plain films may demonstrate punctate or ringlike calcifications scattered through the peritoneal cavity. CT demonstrates mottled densities, septations, and calcifications within the fluid. The mucinous fluid is typically loculated and causes mass effect on the liver and bowel (Fig. 26.7). US demonstrates intraperitoneal nodules that range from hypoechoic to strongly echogenic.

PNEUMOPERITONEUM

Free air within the peritoneal cavity is a valuable sign of bowel perforation, most commonly caused by duodenal or gastric ulcer perforation. However, additional causes of pneumoperitoneum include trauma, recent surgery or laparoscopy, and infection of the peritoneal cavity with gas-producing organisms. Postoperative pneumoperitoneum usually resolves in 3 to 4 days. Serial films demonstrate a progressive decrease in the amount of air present. Failure of progressive resolution or an increase in the amount of air present suggests a leak of bowel anastomosis or sepsis. Pneumoperitoneum in the absence of a ruptured viscus may occur with air introduced through the female genital tract by orogenital insufflation or in association with pulmonary emphysema, alveolar rupture, and dissection of air into the peritoneal cavity.

Plain film evidence of pneumoperitoneum is best seen on radiographs obtained with the patient in the standing or sitting position. Upright chest radiographs are the most sensitive for free air. Small amounts of air are clearly demonstrated beneath the domes of the diaphragm. Left lateral decubitus and cross-table lateral views may be used with very ill patients to demonstrate air outlining the liver. Signs of pneumoperitoneum on supine radiographs (Fig. 26.8) include the following: (*1*) gas on both sides of the bowel wall (Rigler sign), (*2*) gas outlining the falciform ligament, (*3*) gas outlining the peritoneal cavity (the "football sign"), and (*4*) triangular or linear localized extraluminal gas in the right upper quadrant. On CT, small amounts of extraluminal gas may be confused with gas within the bowel and be surprisingly difficult to recognize. Images should be examined at lung windows (window level –600 H, window width 1,000 H) to detect free

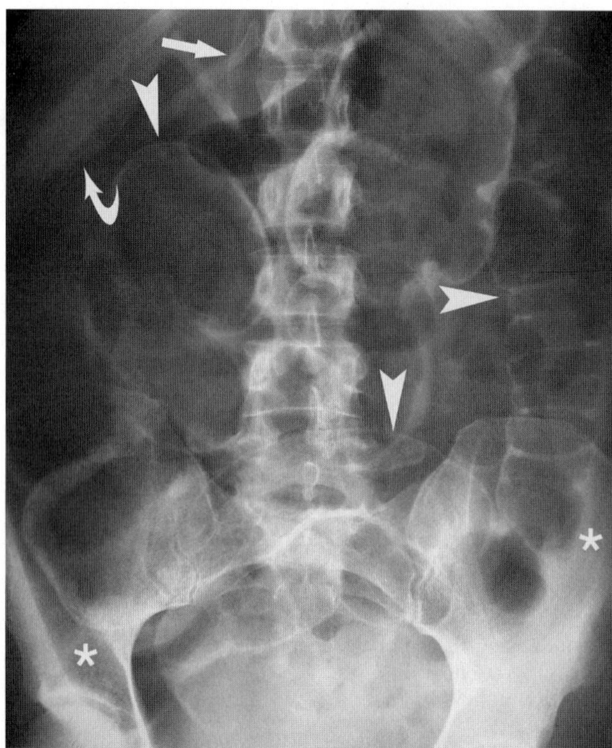

FIGURE 26.8. **Pneumoperitoneum: Radiograph.** Supine radiograph in a patient with a perforated gastric ulcer demonstrates visualization of both sides of the bowel wall (*arrowheads*), free air outlining the falciform ligament (*arrow*), free air outlining the edge of the liver (*curved arrow*), and free air outlining the pericolic gutters (*asterisk*).

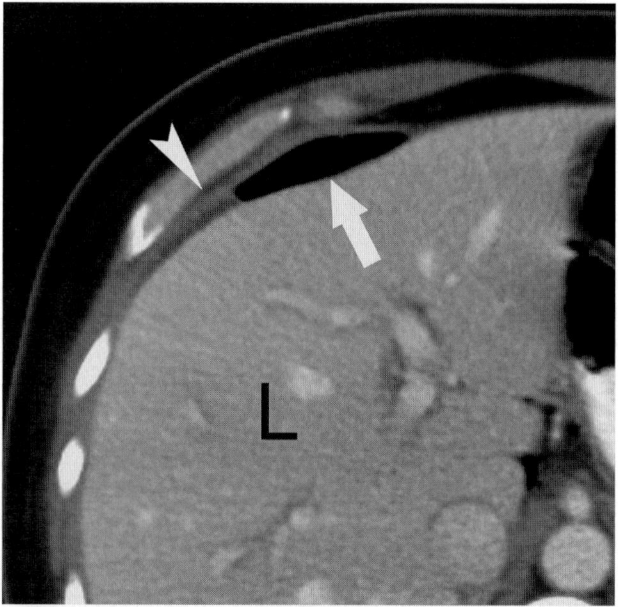

FIGURE 26.9. **Pneumoperitoneum: CT.** A collection of air (*arrow*) is seen within the peritoneal space between the liver (L) and the diaphragm (*arrowhead*). This is a prime area to search to detect small amounts of free intraperitoneal air on CT. This patient had a torn jejunum as a result of trauma from a motor vehicle collision.

intraperitoneal air. The peritoneal recess between the liver and diaphragm (Fig. 26.9) is a good place to look for pneumoperitoneum on CT.

ABDOMINAL CALCIFICATIONS

Intra-abdominal calcifications may be an important sign of intra-abdominal disease and should be searched for on every imaging study of the abdomen. CT and US are more sensitive to detection of calcifications than are plain radiographs. However, the high spatial resolution of plain film radiography commonly provides characteristic findings that allow a specific diagnosis of the nature of the calcification (2).

Vascular calcifications are common in the aorta and iliac vessels (see Fig. 26.13) of older individuals. Plaquelike vascular calcifications overlie the lumbar spine and sacrum and commonly require detailed inspection to detect. Aneurysms of the aorta are manifest by luminal diameter exceeding 3 cm, as measured between calcifications in the aortic wall (Fig. 26.10). Ringlike calcified aneurysms most commonly involve the splenic or renal arteries. *Phleboliths* are calcified thrombi in veins—most commonly visualized in the lateral aspects of the pelvis. They are round or oval calcifications up to 5 mm that commonly contain a central lucency. They may be mistaken for urinary tract calculi.

Calcified lymph nodes result most commonly from granulomatous diseases such as tuberculosis or histoplasmosis. The calcification is usually mottled and 10 to 15 mm in size. Mesenteric nodes are the most commonly calcified.

Gallstones and Gallbladder. Only about 15% of gallstones contain sufficient calcium to be identified on plain film. Most calcified gallstones contain calcium bilirubinate and have a laminated appearance, with a dense outer rim and more radiolucent center. When multiple gallstones are present, they are commonly faceted. Calcifications in the gallbladder wall (porcelain gallbladder) (Fig. 26.11) are plaquelike and oval in configuration, conforming to the size and shape of the gallbladder. Milk of calcium bile is a suspension of radiopaque crystals within gallbladder bile. Layering of the suspension can be demonstrated on erect films.

Urinary Calculi. About 85% of urinary calculi are visible on plain film. They range in size from punctate up to several centimeters. Most characteristic are the staghorn calculi, which assume the shape of the renal collecting system (Fig. 26.12). Renal calculi are differentiated from gallstones on radiographs by oblique

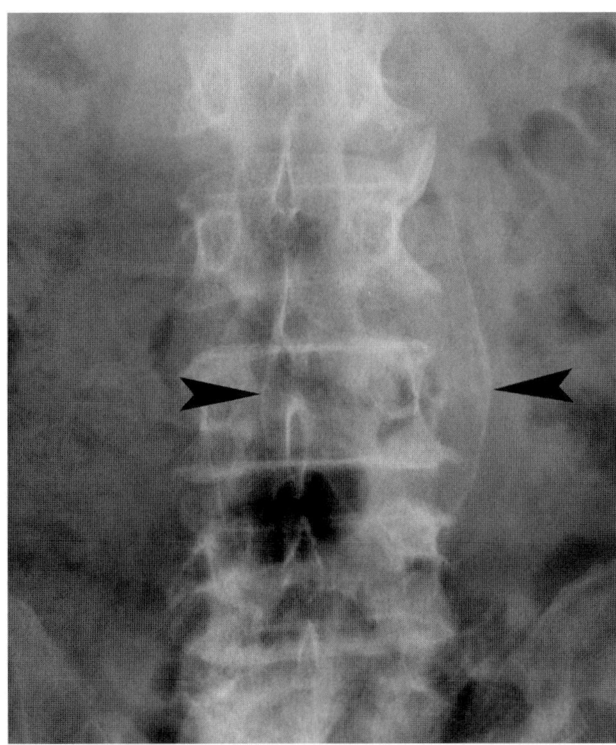

FIGURE 26.10. **Abdominal Aortic Aneurysm.** Plain radiograph demonstrates an aneurysm of the abdominal aorta, evidenced by wide separation of calcifications in the aortic wall (*arrowheads*). Calcifications in the wall overlying the spine may be difficult to visualize. A film taken with the patient in the left posterior oblique position will project the aorta away from the spine and make visualization of aortic wall calcifications easier.

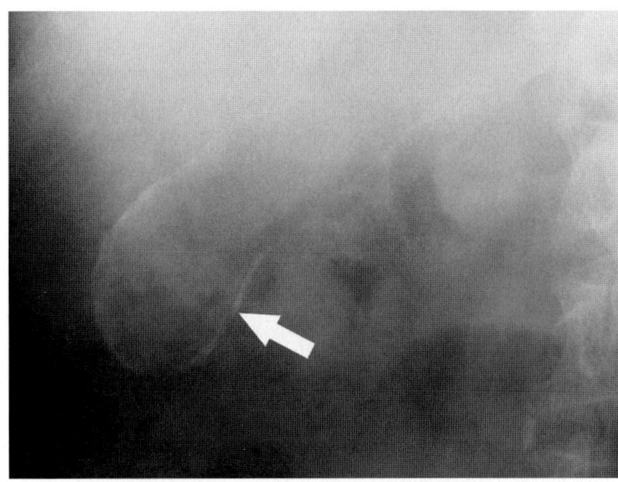

FIGURE 26.11. **Porcelain Gallbladder.** Cone-down radiograph of the right upper quadrant of the abdomen demonstrates calcification in the wall of the gallbladder (*arrow*). This finding is indicative of chronic obstruction of the cystic duct, chronic gallbladder inflammation, and an increased risk of gallbladder carcinoma.

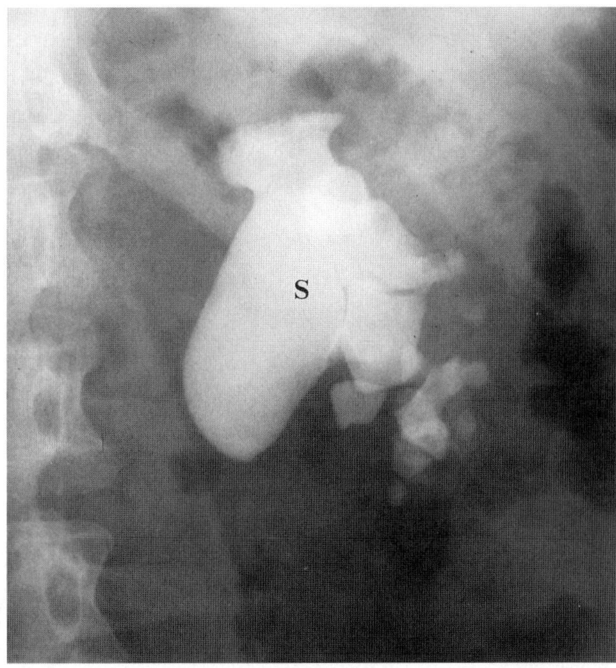

FIGURE 26.12. **Staghorn Calculus.** A plain radiograph reveals a large calculus occupying the collecting system of the left kidney and assuming its shape. Staghorn calculi (S) are usually composed of struvite and form in the presence of chronic urinary infection.

projections that confirm their posterior position, as opposed to the more anterior positions of gallstones. Ureteral calculi may be seen anywhere along the course of the ureter, but they are most common at the areas of narrowing: the ureteropelvic junction, the pelvic brim, and the vesicoureteral junction. Bladder calculi (Fig. 26.13) are single or multiple and commonly laminated, may be any size, and usually lie near the midline of the pelvis. Calculi within bladder diverticula may be eccentric to the bladder.

Liver and spleen granulomas are usually multiple, small, and dense. They are healed foci of tuberculosis, histoplasmosis, or other granulomatous disease.

Appendicoliths and enteroliths are concretions within the lumen of the bowel. Most are round or oval and have concentric laminations. Appendicoliths are strongly indicative of acute appendicitis in patients with acute abdominal pain. Enteroliths are most common in the colon and often caused by calcium deposition on an undigestible material such as a fruit pit.

Calcified adrenal glands are associated with adrenal hemorrhage in the newborn, tuberculosis, and Addison disease. The calcification is mottled and in the location of the adrenal glands on either side of the first lumbar vertebra (Fig. 26.14).

Pancreatic calcification is associated with chronic alcohol-induced pancreatitis and hereditary pancreatitis.

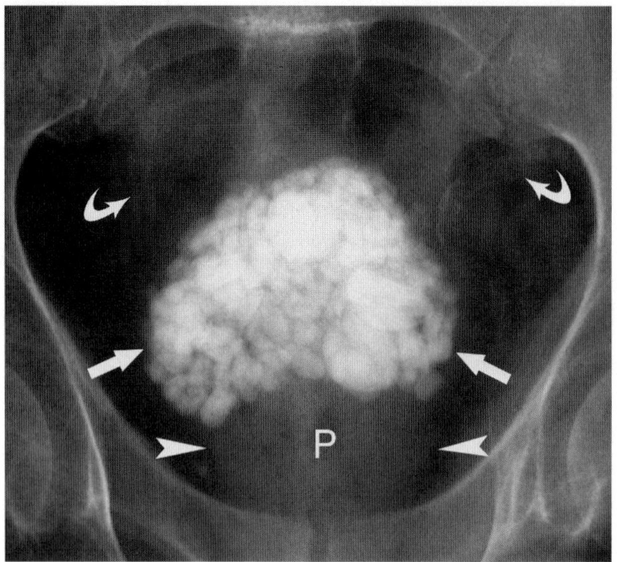

FIGURE 26.13. **Bladder Calculi.** Numerous calculi (*arrows*) in the bladder are evident on this plain radiograph of the pelvis. The large prostate (P, between *closed arrows*), responsible for urinary stasis leading to stone formation, makes a mass impression on the layering stones. Also evident are atherosclerotic calcifications in the iliac arteries (*curved arrows*).

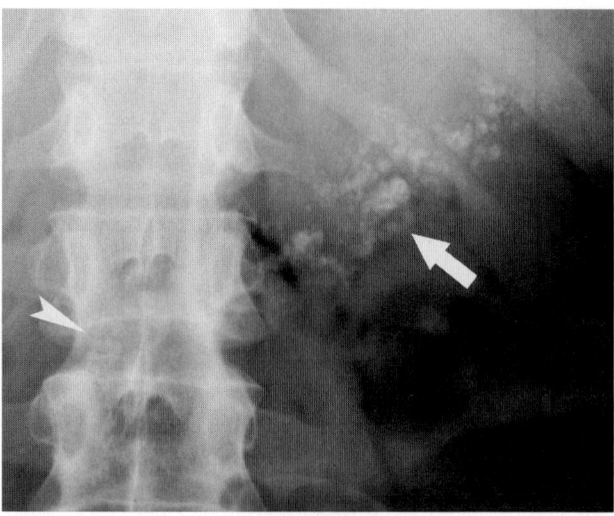

FIGURE 26.15. **Pancreatic Calcifications.** Coarse and punctate calcifications (*arrow*) extend upward across the left upper quadrant in this patient with chronic alcoholic pancreatitis. Calcifications in the pancreatic head (*arrowhead*) are obscured by the spine.

The calcifications are caused by pancreatic calculi and are usually coarse and of varying size (Fig. 26.15).

Calcified cysts may be found in the kidneys, spleen, liver, appendix, and peritoneal cavity. Calcifications in the wall of a cyst are curvilinear or ring shaped (Fig. 26.16). *Echinococcus* cysts commonly calcify and may be found in any intra-abdominal organ as well as within the peritoneal cavity.

Tumor calcification. A wide variety of different tumors of abdominal organs may contain calcifications. The coarse "popcorn" calcifications of uterine leiomyomas are most characteristic. Benign cystic teratomas may form teeth or bone. Calcified peritoneal metastases of ovarian or colon mucinous cystadenocarcinoma may outline the peritoneal cavity (Fig. 26.17). Renal cell carcinoma calcifies in up to 25% of cases.

Soft tissue calcifications may be seen with hypercalcemic states, idiopathic calcinosis, and old hematomas.

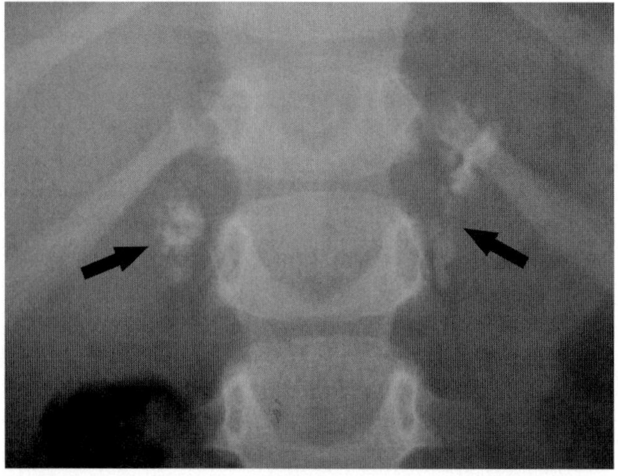

FIGURE 26.14. **Adrenal Calcifications.** Plain radiograph of the abdomen in a 4-year-old demonstrates calcification of both adrenal glands (*arrows*) resulting from bilateral adrenal hemorrhage as an infant.

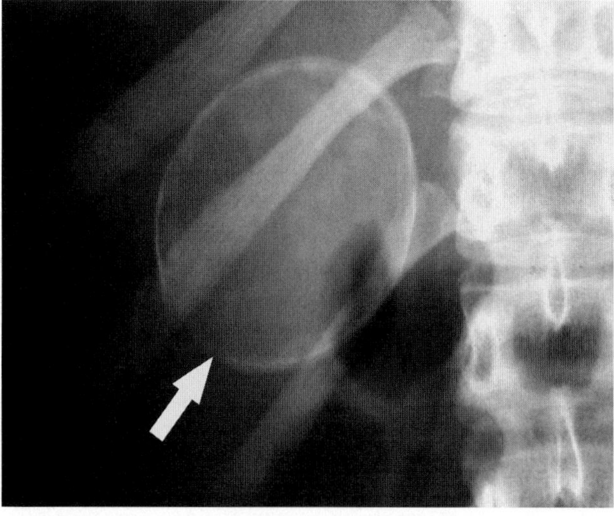

FIGURE 26.16. **Calcified Renal Cyst.** Scout radiograph for an excretory urogram shows the rim calcification (*arrow*) characteristic of wall calcification in a renal cyst.

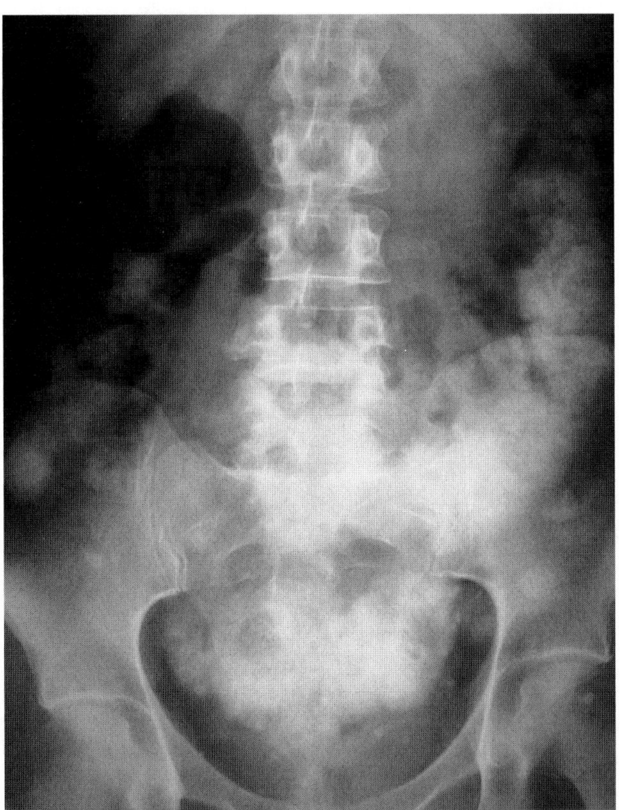

FIGURE 26.17. **Tumoral Calcifications.** Radiograph of the abdomen demonstrates cloudlike calcifications in the distribution of peritoneal recesses. These calcifications were caused by intraperitoneal spread of a papillary serous cystadenocarcinoma of the ovary.

Calcified injection granuloma from quinine, bismuth, and calcium salts of penicillin are commonly evident in the buttocks. Cysticercosis causes characteristic "rice-grain" calcifications in muscles.

Bowel contents may include bone, pits, seeds, birdshot, or medications containing iron or other heavy metals that result in abdominal opacities.

Peritoneal calcifications may be nodular or sheetlike and result most commonly from peritoneal dialysis, previous peritonitis, or peritoneal carcinomatosis (Fig. 26.17).

ACUTE ABDOMEN

The differential diagnosis of patients presenting with acute abdominal pain is extremely broad (Table 26.1). Accurate and efficient diagnosis requires cooperation between the referring physician and the radiologist to select the imaging method most likely to provide the correct diagnosis. Routine assessment of the acute abdomen commonly includes the "acute abdomen series," which consists of an erect posteroanterior chest radiograph and supine and erect or decubitus radiographs of the abdomen. The chest radiograph provides optimal detection of pneumoperitoneum and intrathoracic diseases that may present with abdominal complaints. The supine abdominal film permits diagnosis of many acute abdominal conditions, and a horizontal-beam abdominal film adds confidence to the diagnosis. CT or US are routinely obtained to provide a definitive diagnosis (3–5).

TABLE 26.1 Common Causes of Acute Abdomen

Appendicitis	Peritonitis
Acute cholecystitis	Intraperitoneal abscess
Acute pancreatitis	Retroperitoneal abscess
Acute diverticulitis	Bowel obstruction
Acute ulcerative colitis	Urinary tract infection
Pseudomembranous colitis	Urinary tract obstruction
Amebiasis	Pelvic inflammatory diseases
Acute intestinal ischemia	

Normal Abdominal Gas Pattern. Interpretation of plain abdominal radiographs routinely includes assessment of gas, fluid, soft tissue, fat, and calcium densities (Fig 26.18). Normal gas in the abdomen is predominantly swallowed air. Air–fluid levels are seen in normal patients, commonly in the stomach, often in the small bowel, but never in the colon distal to the hepatic flexure. Normal air–fluid levels in the small bowel should not exceed 2.5 cm in length. Small bowel gas usually appears as multiple small, random gas collections scattered throughout the abdomen. Small bowel gas is increased in patients who chronically swallow air or drink carbonated beverages. A normal intestinal gas pattern varies from no intestinal gas to gas within three to four variably shaped small intestinal loops measuring less than 2.5 to 3 cm in diameter. The normal colon contains some gas and fecal material and varies in diameter from 3 to 8 cm, with the cecum having the largest diameter. The term "nonspecific abdominal gas pattern" has no precise meaning and should not be used.

Dilated Bowel. The small bowel is dilated when it exceeds 2.5 to 3.0 cm in diameter. The colon is dilated when it exceeds 5 cm in diameter, and the cecum is dilated when it exceeds 8 cm in diameter. In adults, dilated small bowel can usually be differentiated from dilated large bowel by assessment of location and anatomic features. The small bowel is more central in the abdomen and is characterized by valvulae conniventes, which cross the entire diameter of the lumen. Dilated small bowel rarely exceeds 5 cm in diameter, although the large bowel is not considered dilated until it exceeds 5 cm diameter. The large bowel is more peripheral in the abdomen and is characterized by haustra that extend only part way across the lumen. The large bowel contains fecal material that has a characteristic mottled appearance. The cecum, which has the largest

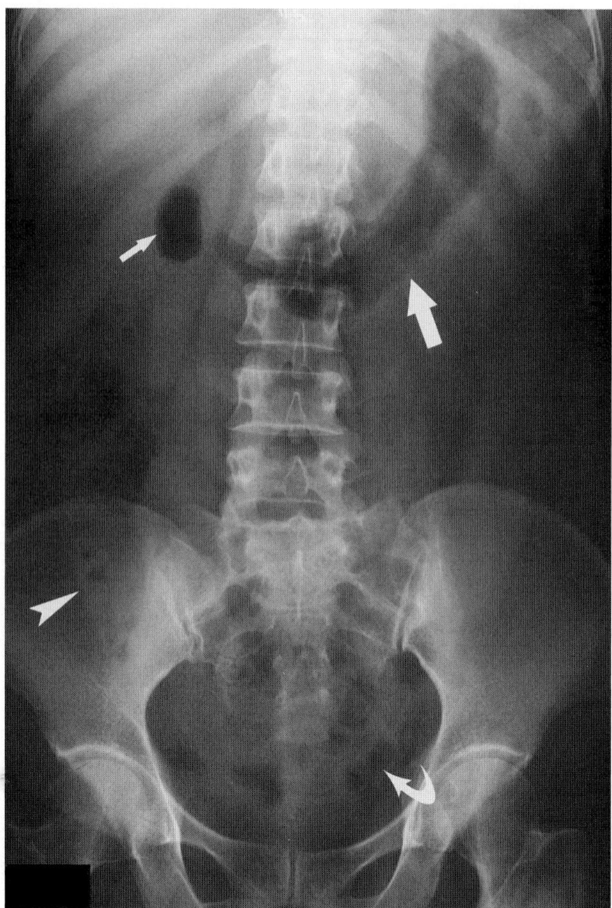

FIGURE 26.18. **Normal Bowel Gas Pattern.** Supine radiograph shows the normal distribution of gas in the stomach (*large arrow*) and duodenum (*small arrow*). The normal mottled pattern of stool is seen in the distribution of the right colon (*arrowhead*). A few gas collections within the small bowel (*curved arrow*) are seen in the pelvis.

normal diameter of the large bowel, always dilates to the greatest extent irrespective of the site of obstruction.

Adynamic Ileus. The word *ileus* means "stasis" and does not differentiate mechanical obstruction from nonmechanical stasis. The terms *adynamic ileus, paralytic ileus,* and *nonobstructive ileus* are used interchangeably and refer to stasis of bowel contents because of decreased or absent peristalsis. Common causes of adynamic ileus are listed in Table 26.2. Adynamic ileus typically demonstrates diffuse symmetric, predominantly gaseous, distension of bowel. The small bowel, stomach, and colon are proportionally dilated without an abrupt termination. More loops are dilated than with obstruction. Occasionally, adynamic ileus may result in a gasless abdomen with dilated loops of bowel that are filled only with fluid. US is useful in confirming decreased or absent peristalsis, although examination may be difficult if large amounts of gas are present.

TABLE 26.2 Common Causes of Adynamic Ileus

Drugs
Atropine, glucagon, morphine, barbiturates, phenothiazines
Metabolic causes
Diabetes mellitus, hypothyroidism, hypokalemia, hypercalcemia
Inflammation
Intestinal: gastroenteritis
Extra-intestinal: peritonitis, pancreatitis, appendicitis, cholecystitis, abscess
Postoperative: resolves in 4 to 7 days
Posttraumatic
Post–spinal injury

Sentinel loop refers to a segment of intestine that becomes paralyzed and dilated as it lies next to an inflamed intraabdominal organ. In essence, it is a short segment of adynamic ileus that appears as an isolated loop of distended intestine that remains in the same general position on serial films (Fig. 26.19). A sentinel loop should alert the clinician to the presence of an adjacent inflammatory process. A sentinel loop in the right upper quadrant suggests acute cholecystitis, hepatitis, or pyelonephritis. In the left upper quadrant, pancreatitis, pyelonephritis, or splenic injury may be suspected. In the lower quadrants, diverticulitis, appendicitis, salpingitis, cystitis, or Crohn disease are causes of a sentinel loop.

Toxic megacolon is a manifestation of fulminant colitis characterized by extreme dilation of all or a portion of the colon. In this state, peristalsis is absent and the large bowel loses all tone and contractility. The patient has progressive abdominal distension and is toxic, febrile, and

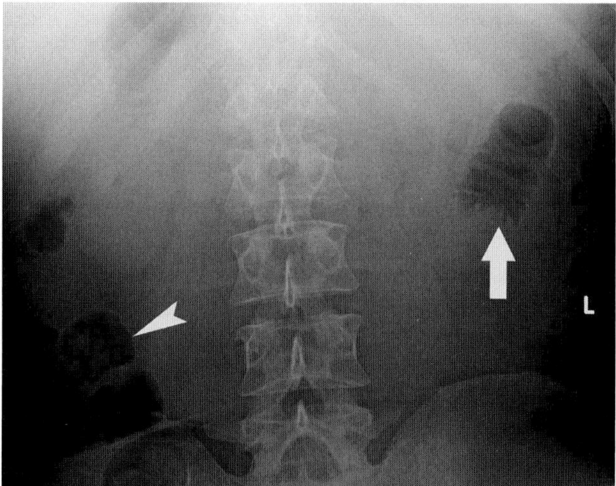

FIGURE 26.19. **Sentinel Loop.** Daily serial radiographs on this patient demonstrated a persistent loop of dilated small bowel (*arrow*) in the same location. This sentinel loop was caused by acute pancreatitis. Normal gas pattern is present in the right colon (*arrowhead*). The abdomen is otherwise devoid of intestinal gas.

TABLE 26.3 Causes of Toxic Megacolon

Ulcerative colitis: 75% of cases	Amebic colitis
Pseudomembranous colitis	Ischemic colitis
Crohn colitis	Bacterial colitis: cholera, typhoid

obtunded. Bowel sounds and bowel movements are absent. The bowel wall becomes like "wet blotting paper," and the risk of perforation is extreme. Mortality approaches 20% in toxic megacolon. Acute ulcerative colitis is the most common cause of toxic megacolon (Table 26.3). Plain films demonstrate distension of the colon with absent haustra. Dilation of the transverse colon up to 15 cm diameter is often the most striking observation. The diagnosis is suggested when the diameter of the colon exceeds 5 cm and the mucosa appears abnormal. Pseudopolyps caused by islands of edematous mucosa surrounded by extensive ulceration appear as soft tissue nodules within the air-distended colon. CT demonstrates a distended colon filled with air and fluid. The wall of the colon is thin but has an irregular nodular contour; air may be seen within the colon wall. Barium enema is absolutely contraindicated because of risk of perforation.

Mechanical bowel obstruction refers to stasis of bowel contents above a focal lesion. The obstruction may be caused by obturation (occlusion by a mass in the lumen), stenosis owing to intrinsic bowel disease, or compression of the lumen by extrinsic disease. The goal of imaging is to confirm the presence of an obstruction, identify its level, and demonstrate its cause. Radiographs can confirm the presence of bowel obstruction 6 to 12 hours before the diagnosis can usually be made clinically. When bowel obstruction occurs, the lumen of the bowel proximal to the obstruction progressively dilates because of continued secretions, swallowed fluid, air, and food, and eventual cessation of absorption. Stasis results in the overgrowth of bacteria and production of toxins that may injure the mucosa. Compromise of blood supply may occur because of distension of the bowel wall and increased intraluminal pressure. A variety of terms used clinically must be understood. **Complete obstruction** means the lumen is totally occluded, but **partial obstruction** means some bowel contents pass through. **Simple obstruction** refers to blockage of the luminal contents without interference of blood supply. **Strangulation obstruction** means that the blood supply to the bowel wall is impaired. Most strangulation obstructions are **closed-loop obstructions**— i.e., the bowel loop segment is blocked at both ends. This occurs with incarcerated hernias and volvulus.

SMALL BOWEL OBSTRUCTION

Small bowel obstruction accounts for 20% of surgical admissions for acute abdominal pain and 80% of all intestinal

TABLE 26.4 Causes of Small Bowel Obstruction

Adhesions	Volvulus
Postsurgical	Gallstone ileus
Postinflammatory	Parasites
Incarcerated hernia	Bolus of *Ascaris*
Malignancy: usually metastatic	Foreign body
Intussusception	

tract obstruction. The causes of small bowel obstruction are listed in Table 26.4. In the Western world, postsurgical adhesions account for 75% of small bowel obstructions, whereas in developing nations, 80% of small bowel obstructions are caused by incarcerated hernia but only 10% are caused by adhesions. Patients present clinically with crampy abdominal pain, abdominal distention, and vomiting. Plain films are diagnostic in only 50% to 60% of cases. Findings of small bowel obstruction are as follows: (*1*) dilated loops of small bowel (>3 cm) disproportionate to more distal small bowel or colon, (*2*) small bowel air–fluid levels that exceed 2.5 cm in length, (*3*) air–fluid levels at differing heights within the same loop (strong evidence of obstruction) (Fig. 26.20), and (*4*) small bubbles of gas trapped

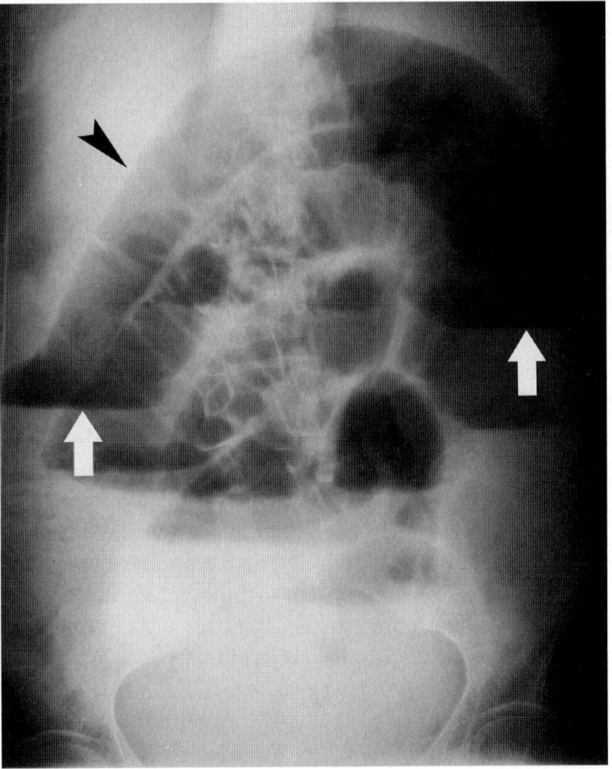

FIGURE 26.20. **Small Bowel Obstruction.** Erect radiograph of the abdomen reveals dilated air-filled loops of small bowel containing air–fluid levels at different heights within the same loop (*arrows*). Note the valvulae conniventes (*arrowhead*) that extend across the entire diameter of the bowel lumen. The small bowel obstruction was caused by adhesions.

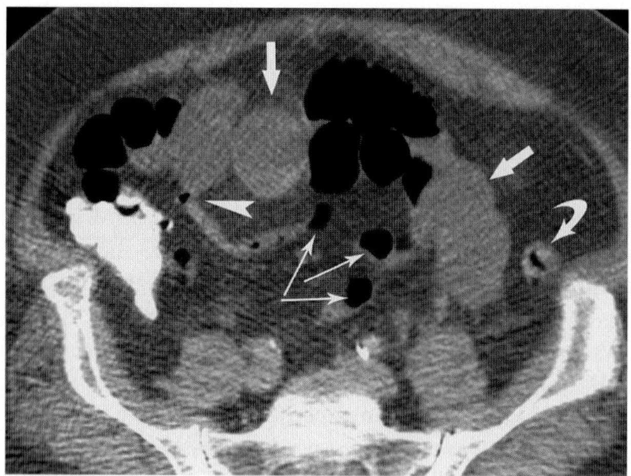

FIGURE 26.21. **Small Bowel Obstruction.** CT demonstrates dilated fluid- and air-filled loops of small intestine (*wide arrows*). A transition to nondilated bowel is evident in the distal ileum (*arrowhead*), indicating an obstructing adhesion at that point. The more distal small bowel (*thin arrows*) and the descending colon (*curved arrow*) are collapsed.

between folds in dilated, fluid-filled loops producing the "string of pearls" sign, a row of small gas bubbles oriented horizontally or obliquely across the abdomen. The level of obstruction is determined by dilated loops above the obstruction and normal or empty loops below the obstruction. Stepladder or hairpin loops of small bowel are most characteristic. Inguinal hernias, easily overlooked clinically in the obese, may be evident on radiographs. CT has become the imaging method of choice when the diagnosis is equivocal (6,7). CT offers the advantage of revealing the cause of obstruction in 70% to 90% of cases. CT diagnosis is based upon demonstration of a transition site between small bowel loops dilated with fluid or air and collapsed bowel loops distal to the obstruction (Fig. 26.21). A potential pitfall is the common finding of a collapsed descending colon, even in patients with adynamic ileus. Bowel obstruction should not be diagnosed in this setting unless an obstructing lesion is visualized at the splenic flexure. The "small-bowel feces" sign is uncommon but definitive CT evidence of bowel obstruction. Particulate feculent matter mixed with gas bubbles is seen within dilated small bowel. Abrupt beaklike narrowing, without other evidence of lesions, is indicative of adhesions as the cause of obstruction. Other causes, including tumor, abscess, inflammation, hernia, intussusception, etc., have characteristic findings.

Strangulation obstruction is associated with changes in the bowel wall and mesentery caused by impairment of blood supply. CT findings are: (*1*) circumferential wall thickening (>3 mm), (*2*) edema of the bowel wall (target or halo appearance of lucency in the bowel wall), (*3*) lack of enhancement of the bowel wall (most specific sign), (*4*) haziness or obliteration of the mesenteric vessels, and (*5*) infiltration of the mesentery with fluid or hemorrhage. Because most cases are caused by closed-loop obstruction, findings of that condition are commonly present as well.

Closed-loop obstruction is indicated by the following CT signs: (*1*) radial distribution of dilated small bowel with mesenteric vessels converging toward a focus of torsion, (*2*) U-shaped or C-shaped dilated small bowel loop, (*3*) "beak" sign at the site of torsion seen as fusiform tapering of a dilated bowel loop, (*4*) "whorl" sign of tightly twisted mesentery seen with volvulus.

Intussusception is a major cause of small bowel obstruction in children but is less common in adults (8). In adults, intussusception is often chronic, intermittent, or subacute, and it is usually caused by a polypoid tumor, such as lipoma. Additional causes are malignant tumor, Meckel diverticulum, lymphoma, mesenteric nodes, and foreign bodies. Enteroenteric intussusception occurs with small bowel tumors and sprue. Ileocolic intussusception is usually idiopathic in children but is caused by a mass in adults. Colocolic intussusception is common in adults but rare in children. Plain films in intussusception demonstrate small bowel obstruction and a soft tissue mass. Barium studies demonstrate barium trapped between the intussusceptum and the receiving bowel, forming a coiled-spring appearance. CT is usually diagnostic, demonstrating a characteristic target-like intestinal mass (Fig. 26.22). On transverse section, the inner central density is the invaginating loop, surrounded by fat-density mesentery that is enveloped by the receiving loop. US exhibits a similar "donut" configuration of alternating hyperechoic and hypoechoic rings representing alternating mucosa, muscular wall, and mesenteric fat tissues in cross section. Asymptomatic, incidental, transient intussusception without

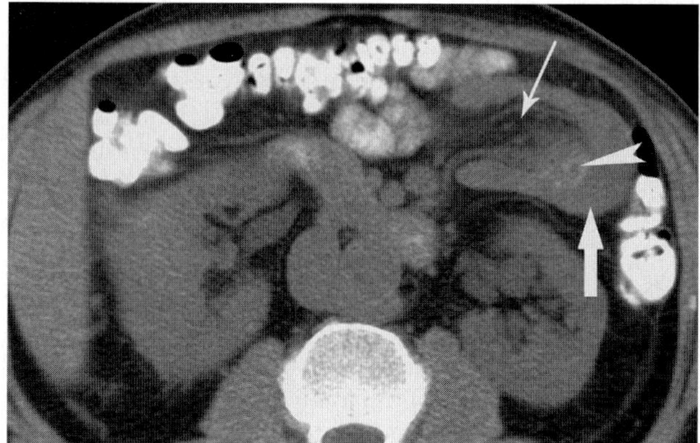

FIGURE 26.22. **Enteroenteric Intussusception.** CT performed without intravenous contrast demonstrates intussusception of small bowel, which was caused by a renal cell carcinoma metastasis to small bowel. The invaginating bowel (*arrowhead*) and its accompanying fat-containing mesentery (*thin arrow*) are seen inside of the receiving bowel (*wide arrow*).

associated small bowel infection is an increasingly common finding on CT.

Gallstone ileus is a misnomer, since it is a cause of obstruction that should be suspected in any elderly woman with small bowel obstruction. It is the cause of 24% of small bowel obstructions in patients over age 70. Because it is a disease of the elderly, insidious in onset, and difficult to diagnose, mortality is increased fivefold over mortality for small bowel obstruction caused by adhesions. Bowel obstruction is caused by a large gallstone that erodes through the gallbladder wall and passes into the intestine, usually creating a cholecystoduodenal fistula. The gallstone most commonly lodges in the distal ileum. Specific radiographic signs are present in only about half of patients. Rigler's triad consists of the following: *(1)* dilated small bowel loops (80% of cases), *(2)* air in the biliary tree or gallbladder (67%), and *(3)* calcified gallstone in an ectopic location (50%). Barium studies should include instillation of contrast into the duodenum to demonstrate passage of barium into the biliary tree. Nonopaque obstructing gallstones are demonstrated as an intraluminal mass.

LARGE BOWEL OBSTRUCTION

Large bowel obstruction is predominantly a condition of older adults and accounts for about 20% of all bowel obstructions. The cecum dilates to the greatest extent, irrespective of the site of large bowel obstruction. When the cecum exceeds 10 cm in diameter, it is at high risk for perforation, with attendant risks of peritonitis and septic shock. The common causes of large bowel obstruction are listed in Table 26.5. Most colonic obstructions occur in the sigmoid colon, where the bowel lumen is narrower and stool is more formed. Plain films are commonly diagnostic in large bowel obstruction, demonstrating dilation of the colon from the cecum to the point of obstruction. The colon distal to the obstruction is devoid of gas. When the ileocecal valve is competent, the small bowel usually contains little gas; the colon is unable to decompress into the small bowel and gaseous distension of the cecum is progressive. When the ileocecal valve is incompetent, gaseous distension of the small bowel is often present; the colon can decompress into the ileum and jejunum, and the risk of perforation of the cecum is reduced. Air–fluid levels distal to the hepatic flexure are strong evidence of obstruction unless the patient has had an enema.

Sigmoid volvulus is most common in the elderly and in individuals on high-residue diets. The sigmoid colon twists around its mesentery, resulting in a closed-loop obstruction. The proximal colon dilates while the rectum empties. Plain radiographs are usually diagnostic. The sigmoid colon appears as a large gas-filled loop without haustral markings, arising from the pelvis and extending high into the abdomen and often to the diaphragm. The three white lines formed by the lateral walls of the loop and the summation of the two opposed medial walls of the loop converge inferiorly into the left iliac fossa (Fig. 26.23). Barium enema demonstrates obstruction that tapers to a beak at the point of the twist, usually approximately 15 cm above the anal verge. Mucosal folds spiral into the beak at the point of obstruction. CT is rarely utilized. Sigmoid volvulus causes 3% to 8% of large bowel obstructions in adults and has a reported mortality of 20% to 25%.

TABLE 26.5 Causes of Large Bowel Obstruction

Colon carcinoma (50%–60%)
Metastatic disease, especially pelvic malignancies
Diverticulitis
Volvulus
Fecal impaction
Amebiasis
Ischemia
Adhesions

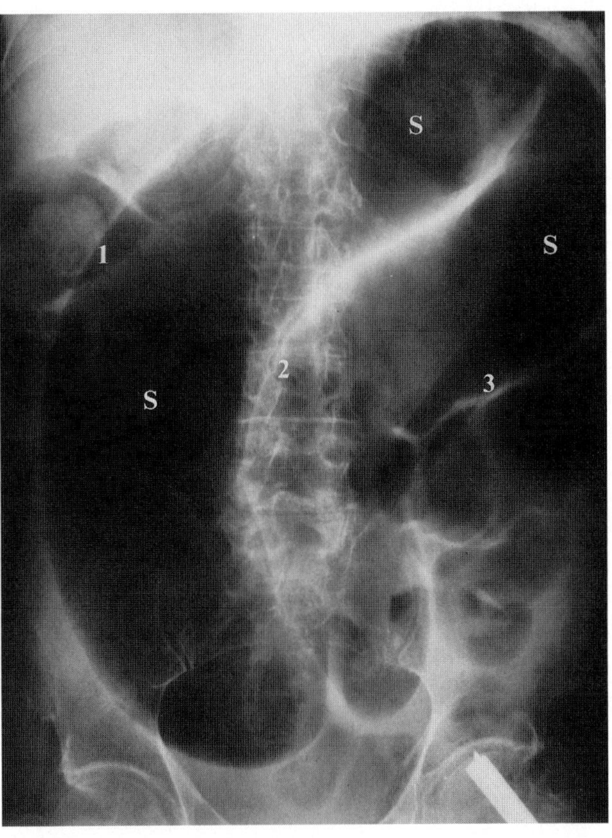

FIGURE 26.23. **Sigmoid Volvulus.** Radiograph of the abdomen demonstrates the characteristic massive dilation of the sigmoid colon (S) arising from the pelvis and extending to the left diaphragm. Three lines representing the walls of the twisted loop converging to the left lower quadrant are evident (1, 2, 3).

Cecal volvulus causes 1% to 3% of large bowel obstructions in adults and occurs most frequently in adults 30 to 60 years of age. Twisting of the cecum occurs in the ascending colon above the ileocecal valve. Two types of twisting may occur. Twisting along the long axis of the ascending colon accounts for two thirds of cases and is usually referred to as ***true cecal volvulus***. The cecum may twist and remain in the right lower quadrant of the abdomen, or it may twist and invert to occupy the left upper quadrant. ***Cecal bascule*** refers to a folding of the cecum into a position anteromedial to the ascending colon, rather like folding the toe of a sock back on itself. Bascule accounts for about one third of cases. Radiographs are usually diagnostic, showing a markedly distended loop of bowel extending from the right lower quadrant upward to the left upper quadrant or epigastrium (Fig 26.24). A single air–fluid level is often present within the dilated loop. The small bowel is distended, whereas the distal colon is decompressed. The distal ileum encircles the cecum as it rotates. CT is rarely needed but shows the dilated loop and the site of the twist or fold. Signs of small bowel obstruction may be present. Displacement of the appendix to the upper abdomen is a definitive sign. Images should be examined carefully for evidence of ischemia. A contrast enema demonstrates a beaklike or foldlike termination at the point of obstruction in the ascending colon. Mortality rates of 20% to 40% are reported because of delays in diagnosis.

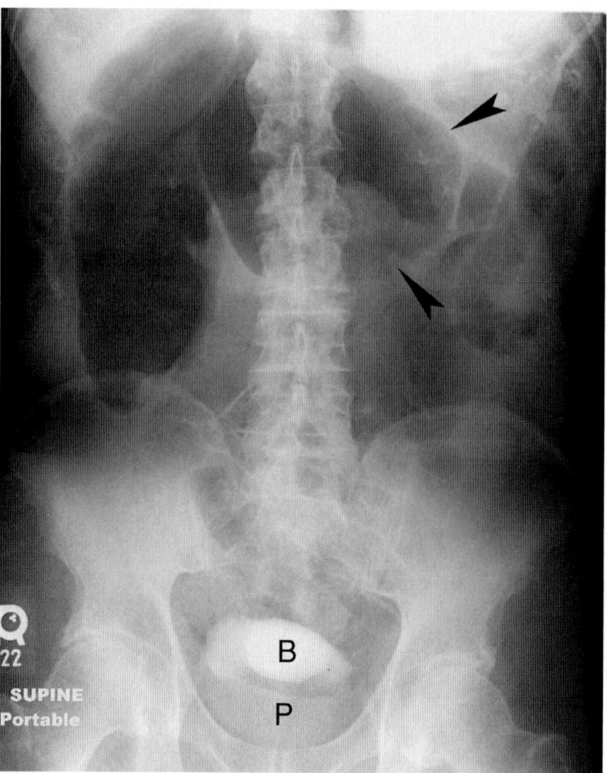

FIGURE 26.24. **Cecal Volvulus.** Supine abdominal radiograph demonstrates displacement of the dilated cecum (*arrowheads*) to the epigastrium. The more distal colon is collapsed. Previously administered IV contrast is seen in the bladder (B). The bladder base is markedly elevated by an enlarged prostrate (P).

Fecal Impaction is the most common cause of large bowel obstruction in elderly and bedridden patients. Radiographs demonstrate a large mass of stool with a characteristic mottled appearance in the distal colon. Following disimpaction, colonoscopy or barium enema should be performed to search for an obstructing carcinoma that may have caused the fecal impaction.

BOWEL ISCHEMIA AND INFARCTION

Bowel ischemia, potentially leading to infarction, is a true emergency, with high associated morbidity and mortality. Insufficient blood supply to small or large bowel may be transient and reversible or lethal (9). Causes include arterial occlusion of the mesenteric arteries by thrombus, embolus, volvulus, vasculitis, or external compression; hypotension related to congestive heart failure, sepsis, or blood loss; vasoconstrictive medications such as ergotamine, digitalis, or norepinephrine; and impaired venous drainage caused by venous thrombosis, tumor, adhesions, or volvulus. Ischemic injury starts at the mucosa and extends progressively through the bowel wall to the serosa. Contrast-enhanced multidetector CT is the imaging method of choice. Findings of bowel ischemia include: (*1*) circumferential or nodular thickening (>5 mm) of the bowel wall with infiltration of low-density edema or high-density blood, resulting from mucosal injury; (*2*) "thumbprinting" (see Fig. 32.20) resulting from this nodular infiltration of the bowel wall; (*3*) dilatation of the bowel lumen (>3 cm for small bowel; >5 cm for colon; >8 cm for cecum); (*4*) pneumatosis intestinalis (see following paragraph); (*5*) edema or hemorrhage into the mesentery; (*6*) engorged mesenteric vessels; (*7*) thrombosis of mesenteric arteries or veins; (*8*) poor enhancement of the bowel wall along its mesenteric border, which is evidence of ischemia; (*9*) poor or absent mucosal enhancement with thinning of the bowel wall, which is evidence of bowel infarction; (*10*) ascites, which is commonly present (10).

Pneumatosis intestinalis refers to the presence of gas within the bowel wall (11). It may occur as a benign entity without clinical significance, or it may be an important finding of bowel ischemia. Causes of pneumatosis intestinalis may be lumped into four categories: (*1*) bowel necrosis, usually associated with other radiographic and clinical signs of bowel ischemia; (*2*) mucosal disruption caused by ulcers, mucosal biopsies, trauma, enteric tubes, or inflammatory bowel disease; (*3*) increased mucosal permeability related to immunosuppression in AIDS, organ transplantation, or chemotherapy; and (*4*) pulmonary disease resulting in alveolar disruption and dissection of air

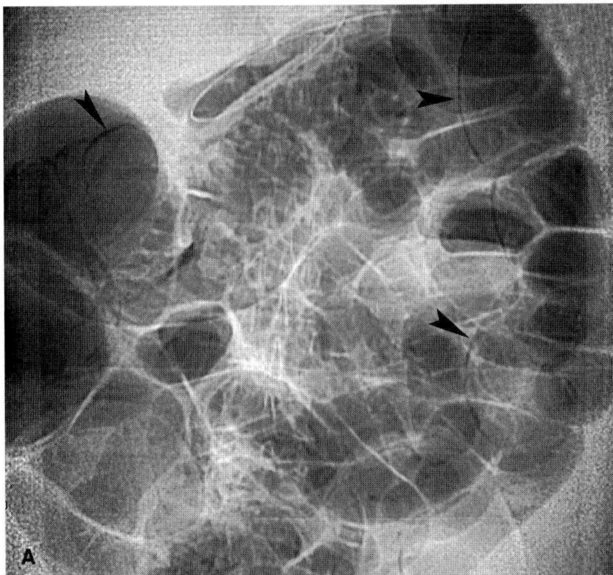

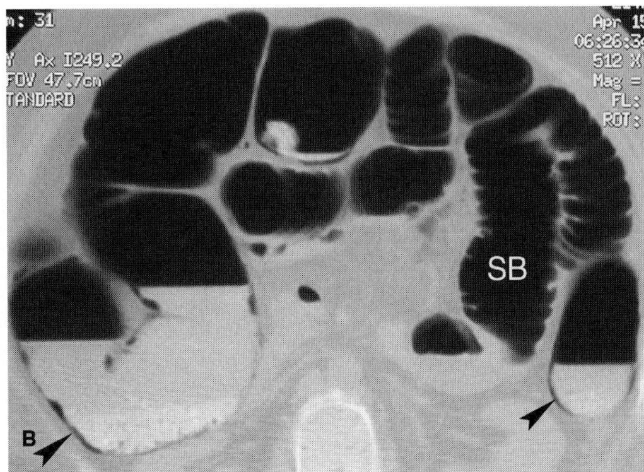

FIGURE 26.25. **Pneumatosis Intestinalis. A.** Digital radiograph scout scan from CT reveals pneumatosis of the colon as dark linear streaks of air (*arrowheads*) in the colon wall. Both small and large bowel are markedly dilated. **B.** CT image of the same patient viewed with lung windows confirms the presence of air in the colon wall (*arrowheads*). The small bowel (SB) is dilated. At surgery, both the small and large bowels were infarcted. The patient expired.

along interstitial pathways to the bowel wall. Causes of the latter include chronic obstructive pulmonary disease, asthma, cystic fibrosis, mechanical ventilation, and chest trauma. Interpretation of the imaging finding of pneumatosis must be correlated with the clinical condition of the patient. Pneumatosis in asymptomatic patients is very likely benign and incidental. Pneumatosis in seriously ill patients with abdominal pain or distension is more likely to be a sign of bowel ischemia. Pneumatosis appears on radiographs or CT as cystic air bubbles (up to several centimeters) or linear streaks of air within the bowel wall, especially in its most gravity-dependent aspect (Fig. 26.25). On CT, air bubbles within the lumen may mimic pneumatosis but should always be seen adjacent to the nondependent bowel wall. Turning the patient and rescanning may clarify the diagnosis. Air may also be evident within mesenteric vessels or within portal veins in the liver.

ABDOMINAL TRAUMA

CT of the abdomen and pelvis has become an integral part of the emergency evaluation of victims of blunt abdominal trauma (12,13). CT characterizes the precise nature of traumatic injury and is used to direct therapy, especially in patients with coexisting injuries, head trauma, or impaired consciousness caused by injury, drugs, or alcohol. Candidates for CT are patients with a history of significant blunt trauma who are hemodynamically stable. Focused abdominal sonograms for trauma (FAST scans) are often used to detect the presence of intraperitoneal fluid and triage trauma patients for CT (14). CT findings of traumatic injury include: (*1*) hemoperitoneum: acute blood within the peritoneal cavity measuring 30 to 45 H (Fig. 26.26); (*2*) sentinel clot: a focal collection of clotted blood (>60 H) that may be seen in the peritoneal cavity adjacent to an injured organ (Fig. 26.26); (*3*) active bleeding, as evidenced by hyperdense fluid (85 to 370 H) (Fig. 26.27) seen during the arterial phase of scanning with multidetector CT; (*4*) free air within the peritoneal cavity (Fig. 26.9), which is an insensitive sign of bowel injury provided that diagnostic peritoneal lavage has not been performed; (*5*) free contrast within the peritoneal cavity, which may result from oral contrast leaking from injured bowel or IV contrast leaking from a ruptured bladder; (*6*) subcapsular hematomas, which appear as crescent-shaped collections confined by the capsule of the injured organ; (*7*) intraparenchymal hematomas, which appear as irregularly shaped low-density areas within a contrast-enhanced solid organ; (*8*) lacerations, which appear as jagged linear defects (Fig. 26.27) defined by lower-density blood within a contrast-enhanced injured organ; (*9*) absence of organ enhancement, which reflects damage to the organ's arterial supply; and (*10*) infarctions, which are seen as zones of decreased contrast enhancement that extend to the capsule of a solid organ (Fig. 26.28) (15–18).

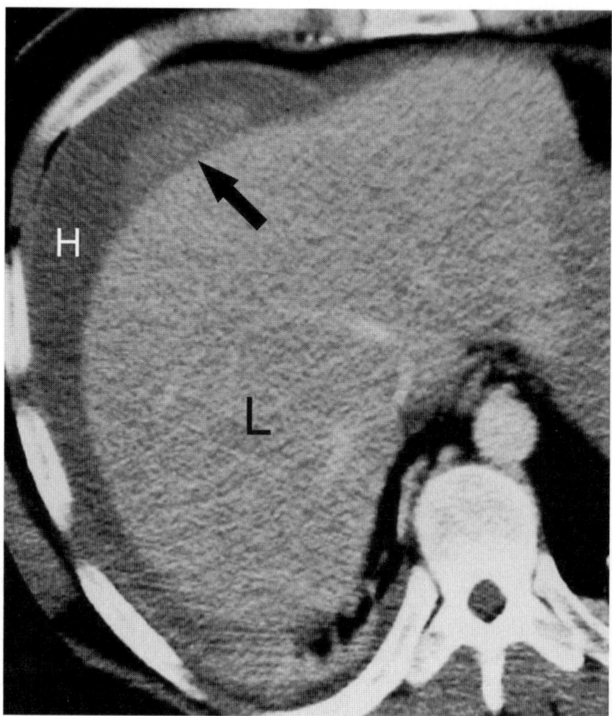

FIGURE 26.26. **Hemoperitoneum and Sentinel Clot.** CT scan shows high-attenuation fluid in the peritoneal recesses, indicating hemoperitoneum (H). A sentinel clot (*arrow*) stands out as a high-attenuation collection within the lower-attenuation liquid blood. The location of the clot suggests injury to the liver (L). A laceration of the left lobe of the liver was found at surgery.

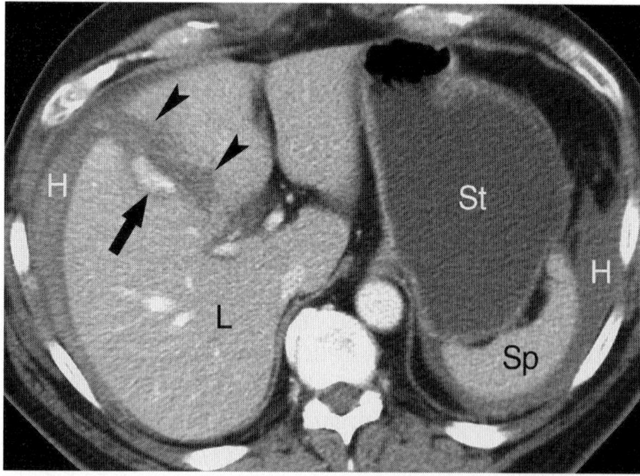

FIGURE 26.27. **Active Hemorrhage: Liver Laceration.** CT shows a jagged laceration (*arrowheads*) of the liver (L) filled with blood. A focus of continuing active hemorrhage (*arrow*) is seen as an ill-defined collection of high-attenuation contrast agent. Hemoperitoneum (H) is evident in the peritoneal recesses. Sp; spleen. St; stomach.

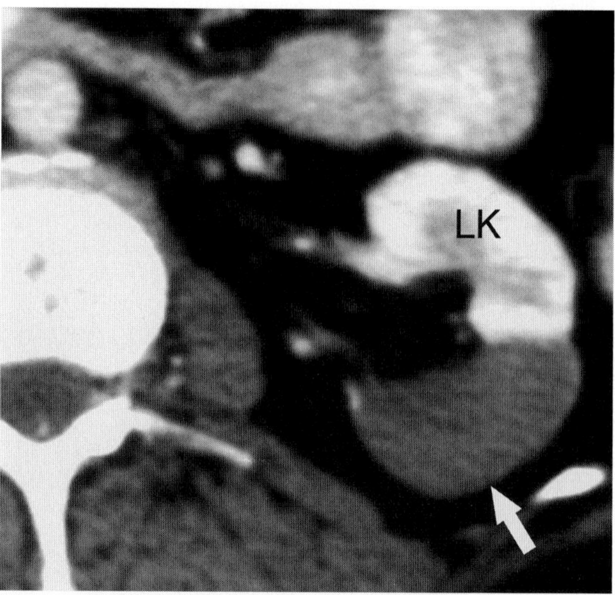

FIGURE 26.28. **Renal Infarction.** Postcontrast CT reveals a lack of enhancement (*arrow*) of the posterior portion of the left kidney (LK), which occurred as a result of an intimal tear and thrombosis of a branch renal artery occurring during a motor vehicle collision. Note that the defect in enhancement extends to the capsule of the kidney, indicating acute renal vascular injury.

LYMPHADENOPATHY

The abdomen and pelvis contain more than 230 lymph nodes that may be involved in a wide variety of neoplastic and inflammatory diseases (19). CT, US, and MR can evaluate the entire abdominopelvic lymphatic system and have replaced the older technique of lymphangiography. Unfortunately, none of the cross-sectional imaging methods can demonstrate tumor involvement of a lymph node by alteration of internal architecture. The criteria for pathologic involvement are based primarily on alterations in node size (Table 26.6). Short-axis measurements of lymph node size are preferred to determine abnormal enlargement. Morphologic patterns of pathologic lymphadenopathy include single enlarged nodes, multiple separate lobulated enlarged nodes, or bulky conglomerate masses of lymph nodes (Fig. 26.29). Calcification in enlarged nodes may be seen with inflammatory adenopathy, mucinous carcinomas, sarcomas, and treated lymphoma. CT to detect adenopathy requires optimal contrast opacification of blood vessels and the GI tract. Normal nodes are oblong in shape, homogeneous in configuration, and have short-axis diameters below the limits listed in Table 26.6. Most pathologically enlarged nodes have CT densities that are slightly lower than that of skeletal muscle. Low-density nodal metastases are commonly seen with nonseminomatous testicular carcinoma, tuberculosis, and occasionally lymphoma. US is

TABLE 26.6 Abdominal and Pelvis Lymphadenopathy: Upper Limits of Normal Node Size by Location

Node Location	*Maximum Dimension (mm)*	*Comments*
Retrocrural	6	May enlarge from disease above or below the diaphragm
Retroperitoneal	10	Multiple nodes 8 to 10 mm in size are usually abnormal
Gastrohepatic ligament	8	Must differentiate lymphadenopathy from coronary varices
Porta hepatis	6	May cause biliary obstruction
Celiac and superior mesenteric arteries	10	Also called preaortic nodes
Pancreaticoduodenal	10	Commonly involved by lymphoma and GI carcinoma
Perisplenic	10	Involved by lymphoma and GI carcinoma
Mesenteric	10	In the small bowel mesentery
Pelvic	15	Most commonly involved by pelvic tumors

almost equal to CT in accuracy for detection of lymphadenopathy; however, a skillful dedicated examination is required. Lymphoma typically produces hypoechoic or even anechoic lymphadenopathy. Masses of retroperitoneal nodes may silhouette segments of the normally echogenic wall of the aorta (the "sonographic silhouette sign"). The "sandwich sign" refers to entrapment of mesenteric vessels by masses of enlarged lymph nodes in the mesentery. MR usually provides excellent differentiation of lymph nodes from blood vessels because of flow void within vessels. However, because of the current lack of an effective GI contrast agent, loops of bowel are commonly confused with masses of nodes. On T1WIs, lymph nodes show low signal intensity compared to surrounding fat. On T2WIs, lymph nodes show high signal intensity compared to muscle. The fat-saturation technique highlights pathologic adenopathy.

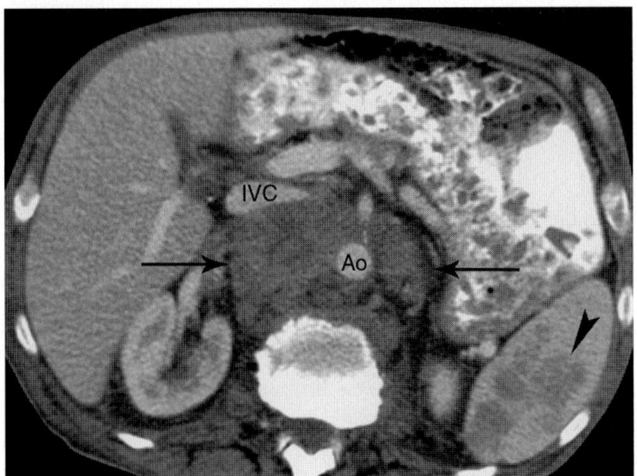

FIGURE 26.29. **Hodgkin Lymphoma.** CT shows bulky confluent adenopathy (*arrows*) in the retroperitoneum surrounding the aorta (Ao) and displacing the inferior vena cava (IVC) anteriorly. Masses of lymphoma (*arrowhead*) are also present in the spleen.

Hodgkin lymphoma is responsible for 20% to 40% of all lymphoma and is characterized histologically by the presence of the Reed-Sternberg cell. Hodgkin lymphoma has a bimodal age distribution; it most commonly affects patients aged 25 to 30 years and over 70 years. At presentation, abdominal adenopathy is present in about 25% of cases. The spleen is involved in about 40% of cases and the liver in about 8%. Involvement of the GI and urinary tracts is much less common with Hodgkin than with non-Hodgkin lymphoma.

Non-Hodgkin lymphoma is responsible for 60% to 80% of lymphomas. Non-Hodgkin lymphoma is a heterogeneous group of disorders with a confusing array of changing names and classifications. Disease severity ranges from indolent to very aggressive. Non-Hodgkin lymphomas are particularly common in patients with AIDS and other immunocompromising conditions. The non-Hodgkin lymphomas commonly involve extranodal sites, including the GI and urinary tracts. At presentation, abdominal adenopathy is present in about 50% of cases. The spleen is involved in about 40% of cases and the liver in about 14%.

Posttransplantation lymphoproliferative disorder is a spectrum of lymphoid hyperplasias and neoplasias in patients who have received solid organ transplants and immunosuppressive therapy. Up to 20% of transplant recipients may be affected. The disorder is thought to result from an Epstein-Barr virus–induced proliferation of B lymphocytes that is usually opposed by functioning T cells. However, T-cell function is limited by immunosuppressive therapy. The proliferation ranges from polyclonal, benign, and reversible to aggressive and difficult-to-treat monoclonal lymphoma. Extranodal involvement with discrete solitary, multiple, or infiltrative masses within organs is most common. Lymph node enlargement occurs near the transplanted organ but may also occur at remote sites, i.e., in the abdomen but associated with a heart or lung transplant. CT may reveal lymphadenopathy before the patient becomes symptomatic. Treatment is reduction of immunosuppressive therapy.

ABDOMINOPELVIC TUMORS AND MASSES

Peritoneal mesothelioma is an uncommon primary tumor of the peritoneal membrane. Approximately 20% to 30% of mesotheliomas arise from the peritoneum, but most of the remainder arise from the pleura. All are closely associated with asbestos exposure. CT demonstrates nodular, irregular peritoneal and omental thickening and masses, which merge to form large plaques and cakelike thickening of the omentum ("omental cake)." Adjacent bowel may be invaded and become fixed. US demonstrates the sheetlike superficial masses. Rare multilocular cystic forms of the tumor also occur. Prognosis is poor, with most patients dying within 1 year of diagnosis.

Peritoneal metastases are most commonly associated with ovarian, colon, stomach, or pancreas carcinoma. The preferential sites for tumor implantation are the pelvic cul-de-sac, right paracolic gutter, and the greater omentum. CT demonstrates tumor nodules on peritoneal surfaces ("omental cake;" Fig. 26.30), which displace bowel away from the anterior abdominal wall, tumor nodules in the mesentery, thickening and nodularity of the bowel wall owing to serosal implants, and ascites that is commonly loculated. US may directly visualize the peritoneal tumors and demonstrates secondary signs of malignant ascites, including echogenic debris in the fluid, septation, and matted bowel loops.

Lymphangiomas are benign cystic lesions that arise from lymphatic vascular channels. The cystic mass contains septations and multiple loculations containing chylous, serous, hemorrhagic, or mixed fluid. Lesions occur in the omentum, mesentery, mesocolon, and retroperitoneum. CT shows a fluid-density mass with enhancing wall and septa. US shows better the multilocular nature of the mass. The fluid contains echogenic debris. MR shows low signal on T1WIs and high signal on T2WIs for serous lymphangiomas. Those complicated by infection or hemorrhage are high signal on T1WIs.

Primary retroperitoneal neoplasms arise in the retroperitoneal tissues outside of the retroperitoneal organs. Many tumors grow quite large before discovery. Tumors displace and compress abdominal and pelvic organs. Well-defined tumors with homogeneous fat are lipomas. Heterogeneous tumors that contain areas of distinct fat density may be liposarcomas (Fig. 26.31), the most common sarcoma of the retroperitoneum, or teratomas. Other fat-containing mass lesions include adrenal myelolipoma, angiomyolipoma, omental infarction, and mesenteric panniculitis (20). Cystic tumors that enhance minimally are likely lymphangiomas. Other considerations include neurogenic tumors, such as schwannomas, neurofibromas, and ganglioneuromas; lymphoma; desmoid tumors; and malignant mesenchymomas.

Retroperitoneal fibrosis is a rare condition manifested by formation of a fibrous plaque in the lower retroperitoneum that encases and compresses the aorta, inferior

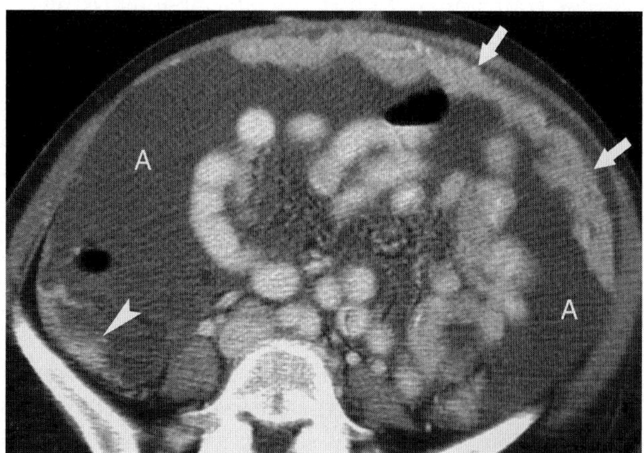

FIGURE 26.30. **Peritoneal Metastases.** A CT scan demonstrates intraperitoneal spread of ovarian carcinoma. The tumor is implanted on the omentum (*arrows*), causing the appearance of "omental cake" as the thickened omentum floats in ascites (A) between bowel loops and the abdominal wall. Nodules of tumor (*arrowhead*) are implanted on the peritoneal surface.

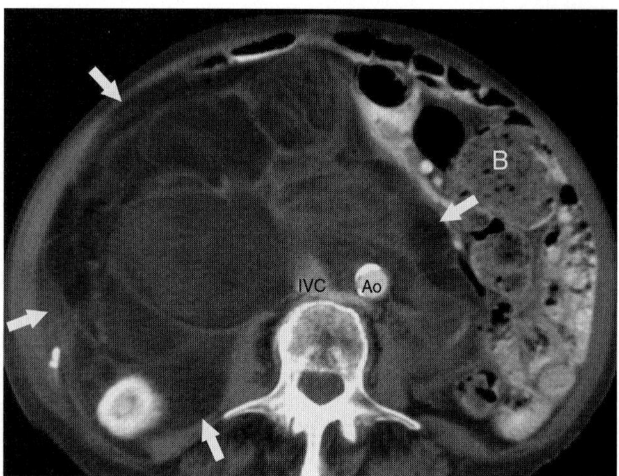

FIGURE 26.31. **Liposarcoma.** CT shows a large liposarcoma (*arrows*) that arose in the retroperitoneum as a mottled fat-density mass that distorts the inferior vena cava (IVC), surrounds the aorta (Ao), and displaces small and large bowel (B) laterally.

vena cava, and ureters. Two thirds of cases are idiopathic. Methysergide, an ergot prescribed for migraine headache, causes 12% of cases. Small foci of metastatic malignancy that elicit a fibrotic reaction in the retroperitoneum account for another 8% to 10% of cases. Inflammatory aneurysms, which induce a rind of perianeurysmal fibrosis, are responsible for 5% to 10% of cases. Other possible causes include tuberculosis, syphilis, actinomycosis, and fungi. About 15% of patients have additional fibrosing processes, including mediastinal fibrosis, Riedel fibrosing thyroiditis, sclerosing cholangitis, and fibrotic orbital pseudotumors. The fibrotic plaque is usually located over the anterior surfaces of the L4 and L5 vertebrae. In the early stages, the plaque is highly cellular and edematous; when mature, it consists of dense hyalinized collagen with few cells. Cases induced by malignancy have a few malignant cells scattered within the collagen.

The hallmark of retroperitoneal fibrosis on excretory urography is smooth extrinsic narrowing of one or both ureters in the region of L4–L5. Proximal hydronephrosis results from impairment of ureteral peristalsis. The process may extend into the pelvis and cause a teardrop configuration to the bladder and narrowing of the sigmoid colon. CT demonstrates a fibrous plaque that envelops the inferior vena cava, aorta, and often the ureters. The plaque may be midline or asymmetric, well-defined or poorly defined, localized or expansive. On MR the plaque is typically of low signal intensity on both T1WIs and T2WIs. Plaque that shows high signal intensity on T2WIs should be considered suspicious for malignancy as a cause, although early edematous plaques may have the same appearance. On US, retroperitoneal fibrosis is easily confused with lymphoma in the retroperitoneum. Both appear as confluent hypoechoic masses encasing the IVC and aorta. Typically, lymphoma extends behind the vessels and displaces them anteriorly, but retroperitoneal fibrosis does not.

Foreign bodies may be ingested or inserted, enter the abdomen or pelvis as a result of penetrating trauma, or be left behind at surgery. Recognition is important to avoid complications, which include hemorrhage, abscess formation, septicemia, bowel perforation or obstruction, or embolization. Many orally ingested foreign bodies are radiopaque, such as coins, pins, parts of toys, etc. Most will pass through the GI tract, causing only minimal mucosal damage. Large or elongated pointed objects may impinge at flexures or narrowed areas of the GI tract, such as the pylorus, duodenojejunal junction, ileocecal valve, or appendix. Button-sized batteries, such as those used in watches and hearing aids, contain highly toxic substances that can erode or perforate the bowel and can cause heavy metal poisoning if the battery ruptures. These should be followed to ensure they pass entirely through the bowel. Endoscopic or surgical removal should be considered if they fail to progress. Objects inserted into the vagina, rectum, or urethra can be removed manually or endoscopically. Retained bullets and shotgun pellets may lead to abscess formation or lead intoxication. CT is utilized to determine their exact position, complications, and the difficulty of removal. Wooden foreign bodies are usually not visualized on radiographs. CT shows high attenuation of the wooden object. US demonstrates high echogenicity with acoustic shadowing. MR shows wood to have variable intensity—usually less than that of skeletal muscle on T1WIs and T2WIs. Retained surgical sponges are a rare but dreaded complication of surgery. Retained sponges may be asymptomatic, cause an abscess, or generate a granulomatous response, inducing fibrosis and calcification. Sponges are usually detectable because of an incorporated tapelike or stringlike radiopaque marker (Fig. 26.32). CT shows a mass of soft tissue density, frequently containing air bubbles.

Radiologists should be familiar with an ever-expanding number of medical devices that appear in images of the abdomen and pelvis, including intestinal tubes, postoperative apparatus, genitourinary devices, and monitoring instruments and attachments (21).

Abscesses occur within the peritoneal cavity because of spillage of contaminated material from perforated bowel or as a complication of surgery, trauma, pancreatitis, sepsis, or AIDS. Development of an abscess is commonly insidious, and the clinical presentation is often nonspecific and confusing. The pelvis is the most common site for abscess formation. Radiograph findings include soft tissue mass, collection of extraluminal gas, viscus displacement, localized or generalized ileus, elevation of the diaphragm, pleural effusion, and pulmonary basilar changes. A focal collection of extraluminal gas is the most specific sign of abscess but is unfortunately uncommon. CT shows a loculated fluid collection, often with internal debris and fluid–fluid levels. The walls of the fluid collection are often thick and irregular. Gas within the fluid collection is strong evidence of abscess (Fig. 26.33). The fascia adjacent to the abscess is thickened, and fat surrounding the abscess may be increased in density and contain soft tissue strands because of inflammation. US demonstrates a focal fluid collection that often contains echogenic fluid, floating debris, and septations. However, completely anechoic fluid collections may also be infected. A thickened wall is usually evident. Gas within the fluid collection is evidenced by echogenic foci that produce comet-tail or reverberation artifacts. CT-directed or US-directed aspiration confirms the diagnosis, provides material for culture, and offers the opportunity for percutaneous catheter drainage.

AIDS IN THE ABDOMEN

Although advances in antiretroviral treatment have allowed many HIV-infected individuals to live productive lives, AIDS remains a worldwide epidemic, with

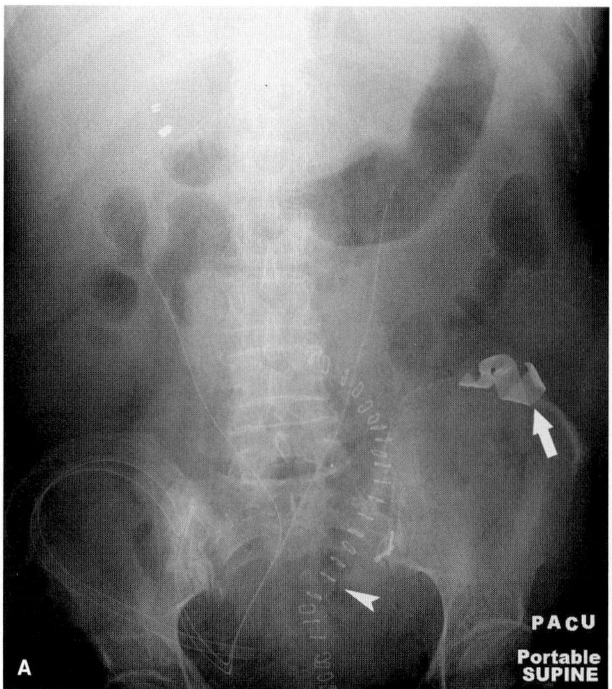

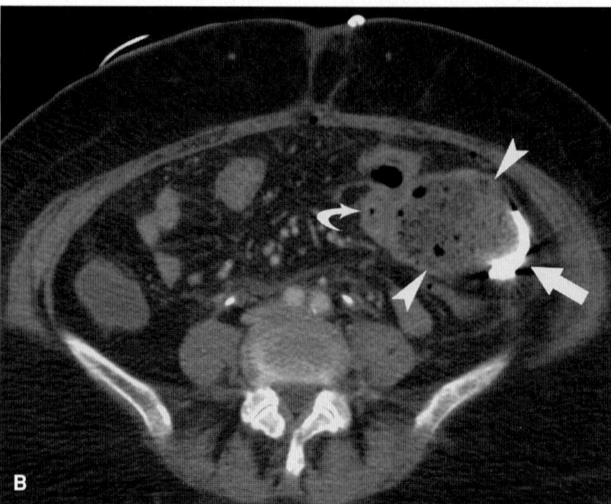

FIGURE 26.32. **Retained Surgical Sponge. A.** Digital radiograph of the abdomen taken at bedside reveals the characteristic radiopaque tape (*arrow*) that marks a surgical sponge inadvertently left within the abdominal cavity. Metallic cutaneous staples (*arrowheads*) identify the patient as having had recent surgery. **B.** CT reveals the difficulty of identifying the surgical sponge if the radiopaque marker (*straight arrow*) had not been present. The sponge (*arrowheads*) contains fluid, blood, and air bubbles, producing a pattern very similar to stool in the colon. The descending colon (*curved arrow*) is displaced medially.

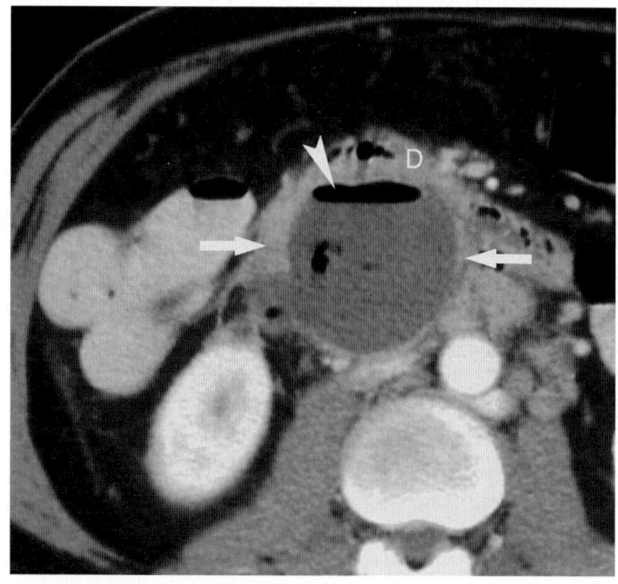

FIGURE 26.33. **Abscess.** CT reveals an abscess (*arrows*) in the retroperitoneum. The abscess contains fluid and gas (*arrowhead*). Note the discrete enhancing wall of the abscess. Duodenum (D) containing intraluminal gas is displaced anteriorly and is draped over the collection.

20 million dead and 40 million infected. Each year almost 5 million people become newly infected with HIV, and nearly 4 million die of AIDS. In the United States, approximately 40,000 people are newly infected with HIV each year and approximately 1 million people are living with HIV.

AIDS in the abdomen is characterized by multiple coexisting diseases with multicentric involvement. Up to 90% of patients with AIDS develop complaints related to the GI or hepatobiliary systems. Genitourinary tract disease affects 38% to 68% of AIDS patients. Manifestations of infectious and neoplastic processes in AIDS patients are effectively demonstrated by abdominal imaging techniques (Table 26.7).

AIDS is a disease of impaired cellular immunity caused by the retrovirus designated *human immunodeficiency virus* (HIV). The disease is characterized by multiple opportunistic infections and aggressive malignancies, most commonly Kaposi sarcoma and AIDS-related lymphoma. Infection by multiple organisms at multiple sites is the rule. Primary infection with HIV causes only minor symptoms, which may resemble infectious mononucleosis or other viral syndromes, with fevers, myalgias, transient adenopathy and skin rash. This is the stage of active viral replication and dissemination. With development of the immune response, usually within 3 months, virus

TABLE 26.7 Abdominal Imaging Findings in AIDS

Adenopathy

Persistent generalized lymphadenopathy (reactive lymphoid hyperplasia)—mild retroperitoneal adenopathy (nodes <1 cm)—precedes onset of AIDS

Lymph nodes >1.5 cm; suggests ARL, KS, MTB, MAI

Liver

Hepatitis/cirrhosis caused by HBV and HCV—especially in intravenous drug abusers

Hepatomegaly without focal lesions caused by HCV, MAI, histoplasmosis

Hepatomegaly with focal lesions caused by bacillary angiomatosis or ARL

Masses >5 cm caused by ARL, KS, or amebic abscess

Masses (2–4 cm) caused by ARL, hepatocellular carcinoma, metastatic disease

Microabscesses (<1 cm) caused by MAI, MTB, candidiasis, histoplasmosis, coccidiomycosis

Biliary tract

Acalculous cholecystitis caused by CMV, *Cryptosporidium*

AIDS-related cholangitis—resembles sclerosing cholangitis—caused by CMV, *Cryptosporidium, Microsporidium*

Papillary stenosis with dilated common bile duct

Long segment strictures of extrahepatic bile ducts

Spleen

Splenomegaly caused by OI, ARL, and portal hypertension

Focal lesions >2 cm caused by PJ, MTB, ARL

Focal lesions <1 cm caused by *Candida,* coccidiomycosis, KS, MAI, MTB, bacillary angiomatosis

GI tract

Esophagitis caused by *Candida albicans,* CMV, MTB

Gastritis/antral narrowing caused by CMV, *Cryptosporidium,* MTB, MAI, *Candida,* or toxoplasmosis

Gastric nodules/mass caused by KS or ARL

Duodenitis/small bowel thickened folds caused by *Cryptosporidium, Isospora belli, Microsporidium, Giardia lamblia,* MTB, MAI

Colitis caused by CMV, *Clostridium difficile, Salmonella, Campylobacter*

Acute proctitis/perirectal infiltrate in homosexual men caused by sexual activity and *Neisseria gonorrhea, Chlamydia,* HSV, *Treponema pallidum*

Pancreas

Acute pancreatitis caused by CMV, *Toxoplasma gondii, Cryptococcus neoformans, Candida,* and drug therapy

Irregular sclerosis with narrowing and focal dilatation of the pancreatic duct caused by CMV, *Cryptosporidium, Microsporidium*

Solitary mass—ARL or MTB more likely cause than primary pancreatic neoplasm

Kidneys

Affected by OI, KS, ARL, polypharmacy, AIDS-related renal failure

Focal pyelonephritis caused by MTB, MAI, aspergillosis, *Candida*

Parenchymal calcifications caused by PC, MAI, CMV

Multiple parenchymal masses caused by ARL

HIV nephropathy (10% of AIDS patients)—bilateral large echogenic kidneys/thick-walled collecting system owing to multiple causes—predictive of early and progressive renal failure with early mortality

Bladder

Hemorrhagic cystitis/bladder wall thickening caused by CMV, *Candida, Salmonella,* β-hemolytic streptococci

Kaposi sarcoma

Bulky adenopathy (>1.5 cm) in retroperitoneum and mesentery

GI tract wall thickening, nodules, plaques, polypoid lesions, thickened folds

Focal lesions in liver and spleen

AIDS-related lymphoma

Bulky adenopathy (>1.5 cm): mesentery, para-aortic, pelvic

Hepatosplenomegaly

Focal lesions in liver, spleen, kidney

Focal masses/wall thickening in GI tract, especially rectum and perianal area

***Mycobacterium avium-intracellulare* infection**

Bulky adenopathy (>1.5 cm): retroperitoneal + mesenteric

Hepatosplenomegaly

Rare focal lesions in liver + spleen

***Pneumocystis jiroveci* infection**

Focal lesions in liver + spleen

Diffuse or punctate calcification in liver, spleen, kidney, adrenal glands, lymph nodes

ARL, AIDS-related lymphoma; CMV, cytomegalovirus; HBV, hepatitis B virus; HCV, hepatitis C virus; HSV, herpes simplex virus; KS, Kaposi sarcoma; MAI, *Mycobacterium avium-intracellulare;* MTB, *Mycobacterium tuberculosis;* OI, opportunistic infections; PJ, *Pneumocystis jiroveci.*

levels decrease dramatically and the patient enters a clinically "silent" period, which often lasts many years. However, the CD4 receptor–coated T lymphocytes, which are primarily responsible for cell-mediated immunity, gradually but progressively decrease in number in the peripheral blood. A CD4 count below 200 cells/mm^3 (normal is 800 to 1,000 cells/mm^3) is diagnostic of AIDS.

Clinical immunodeficiency presents with signs and symptoms of impaired cellular immunity. Cellular immunity is primarily responsible for the body's defense against mycobacteria, fungi, parasites, certain viruses, and tumors. Because drug therapy has become more effective, AIDS patients live longer, develop a broader spectrum of opportunistic infections, and have a greater risk of developing AIDS-related tumors. Malignancy, rather than infection, is now a major cause of death. Although AIDS-related diseases may affect all body systems and involve every region of the body, abdominal disease is increasingly common. Abdominal imaging studies are used to document the presence and severity of complications and, in some cases, to suggest the specific cause. Patients with abdominal disease and AIDS may present with dysphagia, abdominal pain, diarrhea, fever, or progressive weight loss with muscle wasting. Barium studies are being used with declining frequency because of the lack of specificity of most findings and the expanding clinical practice of treating AIDS symptomatically without identification of a specific GI pathogen. US and CT are the most useful modalities for evaluating the solid visceral organs, adenopathy, and the peritoneal cavity. MR has made no significant contribution to evaluating the abdomen in AIDS patients. CD4 cell counts are correlated with a high risk of specific pathogens in AIDS patients. Thrush and tuberculosis are seen most commonly in patients with CD4 counts between 250 and 500 cells/mm^3. *Pneumocystis jiroveci* (formerly *P carinii*) pneumonia usually presents in patients with CD4 counts lower than 200 cells/mm^3. Kaposi sarcoma and AIDS-related lymphoma appear with counts in the range of 150 to 200 cells/mm^3. Counts of 75 to 125 cells/mm^3 are associated with esophageal candidiasis and infection with herpes simplex virus, toxoplasmosis, and cryptococcosis. Patients with CD4 counts below 50 cells/mm^3 have a median survival time of less than 1 year.

Opportunistic infections are caused by organisms that are usually effectively controlled by normal cellular immunity. *P jiroveci* causes pneumonia in nearly 80% of AIDS patients. In patients treated with prophylactic aerosolized pentamidine, extrapulmonary *P jiroveci* infection is common, affecting the liver, spleen, kidney, pancreas, and lymph nodes. *Mycobacterium avium-intracellulare* and *M tuberculosis* are also frequent infections. *M avium-intracellulare* is a cause of bulky abdominal adenopathy, hepatosplenomegaly, and focal lesions in the liver and spleen. *Candida albicans* and cytomegalovirus are common causes of esophagitis as well as gastric antritis and duodenitis. *Cryptosporidium* and *Isospora belli* are protozoans, previously found only in animals, that infect the GI tract and cause severe diarrhea. *Cryptosporidium* and cytomegalovirus are implicated as causes of AIDS-related cholangitis. Herpesvirus, *Toxoplasma gondii, Entamoeba histolytica, Giardia lamblia,* and *Cryptococcus neoformans* are additional pathogens in AIDS patients.

Kaposi sarcoma (KS) is the most common malignancy associated with AIDS and is second only to *Pneumocystis* pneumonia as the most common AIDS-defining illness. The tumor is always multicentric and arises from lymphatic epithelium found in all organs and tissues. The typical lesion is a vascular nodule on the skin or mucous membranes, in the GI tract, or in any solid visceral organ. AIDS-associated KS is divided into two clinical subtypes. *Classic KS* is a limited form of KS, with lesions mostly confined to the face, extremities, and oral mucosa; it may convert into epidemic KS at any time. *Epidemic KS* is disseminated and aggressive and requires therapy. Lesions are found in lymph nodes, visceral organs, GI tract, and bone marrow. Most patients with internal involvement have multiple lesions on the skin. KS affects the GI tract in 40% to 50% of cases, causing nodules, plaques, polypoid lesions, and thickened folds. Bulky adenopathy is sometimes present in the retroperitoneum and mesentery. Brightly enhancing lymphadenopathy is particularly suggestive of KS (79% positive predictive value). In the liver, KS lesions appear as hyperechoic nodules on US and as uniform-enhancing or ring-enhancing lesions on CT. AIDS-related KS is now believed to be caused by a herpes-type virus that is transmitted primarily by anal intercourse. KS is most common (90% to 95% of cases) in homosexual and bisexual men and is uncommon in women and heterosexual men. The diagnosis should be confirmed with biopsy to avoid misdiagnosis.

AIDS-related lymphomas are extremely aggressive neoplasms that respond poorly to therapy and commonly involve extranodal sites. Median survival is only 5 to 6 months. Extranodal involvement is found at presentation in 73% to 86% of patients, with the most common locations being the CNS (27%), bone marrow (22%), GI tract (17% to 54%), liver (12% to 29%), kidney (11%), and spleen (7%). Focal hepatic lesions are hypodense on contrast CT and vary from innumerable small lesions (<1 cm in size) to large solitary masses up to 15 cm in diameter. Hepatosplenomegaly is minimal or absent unless focal lesions are present. Spleen and renal lesions appear as hypodense nodules 1 to 3 cm in diameter. Evidence of GI tract involvement includes focal or diffuse wall thickening, which is often striking, and eccentric homogeneous masses. Rectal and perianal involvement is particularly common. Retroperitoneal or mesenteric lymph node enlargement is seen in only 64% of patients. Lymphoma may be the initial AIDS-defining illness.

REFERENCES

1. Meyers MA. Dynamic Radiology of the Abdomen: Normal and Pathological Anatomy. 5th ed. New York: Springer-Verlag, 2000.
2. Chen MYM, Bechtold RE, Bohrer SP, Dyer RB. Abdominal calcification on plain radiographs of the abdomen. Radiologist 1999;7: 65–83.
3. Gore RM, Miller FH, Pereles FS, Yaghmai V, Berlin JW. Helical CT in the evaluation of the acute abdomen. AJR Am J Roentgenol 2000;174:901–913.
4. Paulson EK, Jaffe TA, Thomas J, Harris JP, Nelson RC. MDCT of patients with acute abdominal pain: a new perspective using coronal reformations from submillimeter voxels. AJR Am J Roentgenol 2004;183:899–906.
5. Puylaert JBCM, van der Zant FM, Rijke AM. Sonography and the acute abdomen: practical considerations. AJR Am J Roentgenol 1997;168:179–186.
6. Khurana B, Ledbetter S, McTavish J, Wiesner W, Ros PR. Bowel obstruction revealed by multidetector CT. AJR Am J Roentgenol 2002;178:1139–1144.
7. Furukawa A, Yamasaki M, Furuichi K, Yokoyama K, et al. Helical CT in the diagnosis of small bowel obstruction. Radiographics 2001;21:341–355.
8. Choi SH, Han JK, Kim SH, Lee JM, et al. Intussusception in adults: from stomach to rectum. AJR Am J Roentgenol 2004;183:691–698.
9. Chou CK. CT manifestations of bowel ischemia. AJR Am J Roentgenol 2002;178:87–91.
10. Wiesner W, Khurana B, Ji H, Ros PR. CT of acute bowel ischemia. Radiology 2003;226:635–650.
11. Pear BL. Pneumatosis intestinalis: a review. Radiology 1998;207:13–19.

12. Brant WE. Abdominal trauma. In: Webb WR, Brant WE, Major N, eds. Fundamentals of Body CT. 3rd ed. Philadelphia: Elsevier/ Saunders, 2006.
13. Yoon W, Jeong YY, Kim JK, Seo JJ, et al. CT in blunt liver trauma. Radiographics 2005;25:87–104.
14. McGahan J, Richards J, Gillen M. The focused abdominal sonography for trauma scan. J Ultrasound Med 2002;2002:789–800.
15. Lane MJ, Katz DS, Shah RA, Rubin GD, Jeffrey RB. Active arterial contrast extravasation on helical CT of the abdomen, pelvis, and chest. AJR Am J Roentgenol 1998;171:679–685.
16. Brody JM, Leighton DB, Murphy BL, et al. CT of blunt trauma bowel and mesenteric injury: typical findings and pitfalls in diagnosis. Radiographics 2000;20:1525–1536.
17. Kawashima A, Sandler CM, Corl FM, et al. Imaging of renal trauma: a comprehensive review. Radiographics 2001;21:557–574.
18. Gupta A, Stuhlfaut JW, Fleming KW, Lucey BC, Soto JA. Blunt trauma of the pancreas and biliary tract: a multimodality imaging approach to diagnosis. Radiographics 2004;24:1381–1395.
19. Lucey BC, Stuhlfaut JW, Soto JA. Mesenteric lymph nodes seen at imaging: causes and significance. Radiographics 2005;25:351–365.
20. Pereira JM, Sirlin CB, Pinto PS, Casola G. CT and MR imaging of extrahepatic fatty masses of the abdomen and pelvis: techniques, diagnosis, differential diagnosis, and pitfalls. Radiographics 2005;25: 69–85.
21. Hunter TB, Taljanovic MS. Medical devices of the abdomen and pelvis. Radiographics 2005;25:503–523.

Chapter 27

Liver, Biliary Tree, and Gallbladder

William E. Brant

Liver
Anatomy
Diffuse Liver Disease
Liver Masses

Biliary Tree
Biliary Dilatation
Gas in the Biliary Tract

Gallbladder

LIVER

Imaging Methods. CT, MR, and US all produce high-quality images of the liver parenchyma. Dynamic bolus contrast–enhanced multidetector CT (MDCT) is the current method of choice for most hepatic imaging. Fast imaging techniques that control motion have increased the role of MR as a problem solver and often as the primary hepatic imaging modality. MR is preferred whenever iodinated contrast cannot be used. US is used as a screening method for patients with abdominal symptoms and suspected diffuse or focal liver disease. Color flow and spectral Doppler are used to assess hepatic vessels and tumor vascularity. Radionuclide imaging is used in the characterization of cavernous hemangiomas and focal nodular hyperplasia.

MDCT of the liver is performed using a three- or four-phase protocol of multiple scans of the entire liver. Initial noncontrast images are followed by rapid bolus IV contrast injection by a mechanical injector. Immediate images are optimally obtained during the peak arterial enhancement phase to detect hypervascular tumors and other lesions supplied primarily by the hepatic artery. Arterial-phase-enhancing lesions, like hepatocellular carcinoma (HCC), are high attenuation on a background of lower-attenuation, minimally enhanced parenchyma. Maximum enhancement of the liver is attained during the portal venous phase to demonstrate hypovascular lesions as low-attenuating masses on a background of brightly enhanced parenchyma. Delayed images are obtained several minutes after contrast injection to document late contrast fill-in of hemangioma and delayed enhancement of cholangiocarcinoma.

Hepatic MR is performed with a broad array of fast spin-echo, breath-hold gradient recall, short-time inversion-recovery, fat-suppressed, or in-phase/out-of-phase pulse sequences. The goal is to maximize lesion detection by the striking contrast resolution of MR while minimizing motion artifact by rapid-scan breath-hold sequences. Dynamic contrast enhancement is achieved with MR by repeating full liver scans multiple times in the first minutes following gadolinium injection.

US is used as a rapid screening modality to detect diseases of the gallbladder, biliary tree, and liver. Hepatic US imaging is reviewed in Chapter 36.

Radionuclide imaging of the liver is inferior to CT and MR for lesion detection but offers functional information in characterizing lesions, such as focal nodular hyperplasia. Radionuclide blood pool imaging is very useful for definitive diagnosis of cavernous hemangioma. Hepatic radionuclide imaging is reviewed in Section XII.

Fine-needle aspiration for cytology and core needle biopsy for histology, guided by US or CT, are popular and safe methods to obtain tissue diagnoses.

Anatomy

Couinaud Segments. The vascular anatomy that defines the surgical approach to lesion resection is the anatomy most relevant to liver imaging. A numbering system

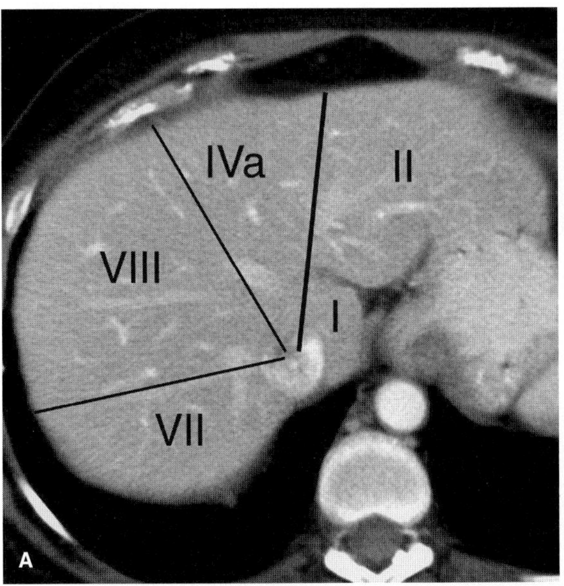

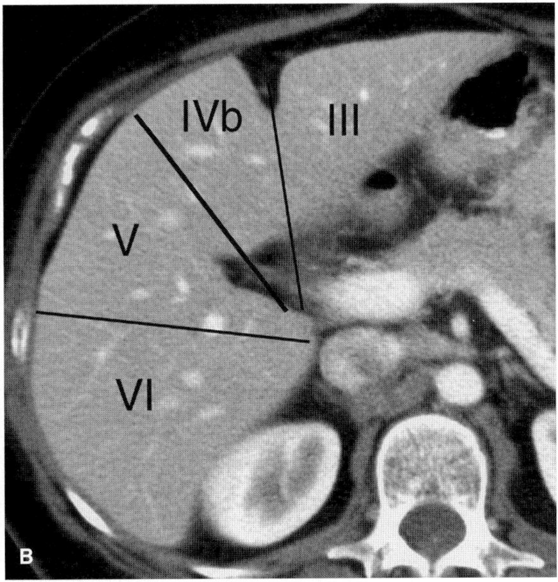

FIGURE 27.1. **Couinaud Liver Segments. A.** Superior portion of the liver. **B.** Inferior portion of the liver. CT scans illustrate the Couinaud classification of numbering of liver segments. The longitudinal plane of the right hepatic vein divides VIII from VII in the superior portion of the liver and V from VI in the inferior portion of the liver. The longitudinal plane of the middle hepatic vein through the gallbladder fossa separates IVa from VIII in the superior liver and IVb from V in the inferior liver. The longitudinal plane of the left hepatic vein and fissure of the ligamentum teres separates IVa from II in the superior liver and IVb from III in the inferior liver. The axial plane of the left portal vein separates IVa superiorly from IVb inferiorly and II superiorly from III inferiorly in the left lobe. The axial plane of the right portal vein separates VIII and VII superiorly from V and VI inferiorly in the right lobe. The caudate lobe (segment I) extends between the fissure of the ligamentum venosum anteriorly and the inferior vena cava posteriorly.

developed by Couinaud (pronounced "kwee-NO") is commonly used internationally and provides standardized identification of hepatic segments (Fig. 27.1) (Table 27.1). The eight Couinaud segments have separate vascular inflow, outflow, and biliary drainage and can each be resected without damaging the remaining segments. Division of the liver into eight segments is based on a concept of three longitudinal planes and two transverse planes. A longitudinal plane through the middle hepatic vein, inferior vena cava (IVC), and gallbladder fossa divides the liver into right and left lobes. A longitudinal plane through the right hepatic vein divides the right lobe into anterior (VIII and V) and posterior (VII and VI) segments. A longitudinal plane through the left hepatic vein divides the left lobe into medial (IVa and IVb) and lateral (II and III) segments. A transverse plane through the left portal vein divides the left lobe into superior (IVa and II) and inferior (IVb and III) segments. An oblique transverse plane through the right portal vein divides the right lobe into superior (VIII and VII) and inferior (V and VI) segments. Segment I is the caudate lobe, which extends between the fissure of the ligamentum venosum and the IVC. Hepatic venous drainage from the caudate lobe is directly into the IVC via small veins.

Blood supply to the liver is approximately two thirds via the portal vein and one third via the hepatic artery.

TABLE 27.1 American and International Nomenclature for Anatomic Segments of the Liver

American	*International*	*Number*
Caudate lobe	Caudate lobe	I
Left lobe		
Lateral segment	Left lateral superior subsegment	II
Medial segment	Left lateral inferior subsegment	III
	Left medial subsegment	IVa
Right lobe		IVb
Anterior segment	Right anterior inferior subsegment	V
Posterior segment	Right anterior superior subsegment	VIII
	Right posterior inferior subsegment	VI
	Right posterior superior subsegment	VII

Adapted from Dodd GD. An American's guide to Couinaud's numbering system. AJR Am J Roentgenol 1993;161:574-575.

When IV contrast is administered as a bolus during rapid CT scanning, the maximum liver parenchymal enhancement will be delayed 1 to 2 minutes following initiation of injection. This delay reflects the transit time of contrast agent through the GI tract and spleen before accessing the liver through the portal vein. Tumors, which are supplied primarily by the hepatic artery, will enhance maximally during the early hepatic arterial phase, while the liver parenchyma enhances maximally during the portal venous phase.

Perfusion abnormalities are seen on post–IV contrast CT and MR because of variations in hepatic arterial and portal venous blood supply to various areas of the liver (1,2). This dual blood supply has a compensatory relationship: arterial flow increases when portal venous flow decreases. Transient enhancement differences are seen during either arterial phase imaging or portal venous phase imaging on MDCT and dynamic MR. Portal venous flow may be altered by: (*1*) portal blockade by tumor or thrombus; (*2*) extrinsic compression caused by ribs or diaphragmatic slips, or by tumors on the liver capsule; or (*3*) "third inflow" from systemic veins in the pericholecystic, parabiliary, and epigastric-paraumbilical venous systems (Fig. 27.2). Hepatic arterial flow may be increased by: (*1*) focal hypervascular lesions; (*2*) inflammation of adjacent organs (cholecystitis, pancreatitis); or (*3*) aberrant hepatic arterial supply. Regional differences in blood supply related to these factors explain patterns of enhancement

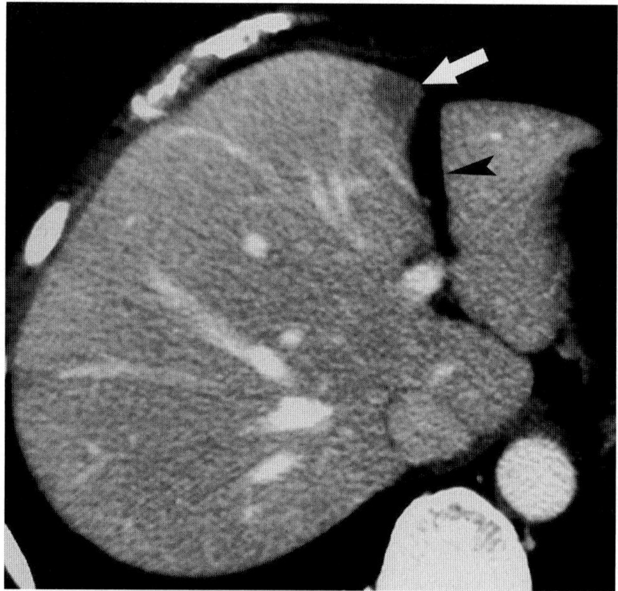

FIGURE 27.2. **Perfusion Defect.** A common perfusion defect (*white arrow*) is seen in segment IVb adjacent to the fissure of the ligamentum teres (*black arrowhead*). This perfusion defect is related to "third inflow" from paraumbilical systemic veins. Focal fatty infiltration is commonly seen in this location. Importantly, this normal variant must not be mistaken for a neoplasm.

abnormalities as well as altered patterns of diffuse liver disease, such as focal fatty deposition and focal fatty sparing in diffuse fatty infiltration.

On CT, the density of normal liver parenchyma is equal to or greater than the density of normal spleen parenchyma on unenhanced images. Following bolus IV contrast administration, the normal parenchymal enhancement is less than that of the spleen during the arterial phase and equal to or greater than that of the spleen during the portal venous phase.

On T1WI MR, the normal liver is of slightly higher signal intensity than the spleen, and most focal lesions appear as lower-intensity defects. On T2WIs, the normal liver is less than or equal to the spleen in signal strength, and most lesions appear as high-intensity foci.

Diffuse Liver Disease

Hepatomegaly. Enlargement of the liver is usually judged subjectively, based on imaging studies. Rounding of the inferior border of the liver and extension of the right lobe of the liver inferior to the lower pole of the right kidney are evidence of hepatomegaly. A liver length of greater than 15.5 cm, measured in the midclavicular line, is considered enlarged. A *Reidel lobe* is a normal variant of hepatic shape found most often in women. It refers to an elongated inferior tip of the right lobe of the liver. When a Reidel lobe is present, the left lobe of the liver is correspondingly smaller in size. The left lobe of the liver may, as a normal variant, be elongated and surround a portion of the spleen. Causes of hepatomegaly are listed in Table 27.2.

Fatty infiltration is a common and nonspecific response of hepatocytes to injury and toxins. Hepatocytes become filled with cholesterol and triglycerides. Causes include alcoholism, obesity, malnutrition, hyperalimentation, steroid therapy, diabetes mellitus, pancreatitis, glycogen storage disease, and chemotherapy. Imaging is the best diagnostic method to document the condition, since laboratory evaluation may be normal.

On CT, fat infiltration lowers the attenuation of the hepatic parenchyma and makes the liver appear less dense than the spleen (Fig. 27.3). Differences in density between liver and spleen are most reliably judged on noncontrast images. On postcontrast images, the spleen enhances maximally 1 to 2 minutes before maximal liver enhancement and is thus transiently brighter than the normal liver. Fatty-infiltrated livers enhance less than normal livers. On US, the liver parenchyma is increased in echogenicity in areas of fat infiltration. The echogenicity of the fatty liver is significantly greater than the echogenicity of the normal kidney parenchyma. This density difference (fat is bright on US and dark on CT) has been called the "flip-flop sign." Conventional spin-echo MR images show no significant abnormalities with fat infiltration. Gradient-echo imaging with fat and water molecules in-phase and out-of-phase

TABLE 27.2 Causes of Hepatomegaly

Vascular Congestion
Congestive heart failure
Hepatic vein thrombosis
Metabolic/diffuse infiltration
Fatty infiltration
Alcohol
Drugs/chemotherapy
Hepatic toxins
Gaucher disease and lipidoses
Carbohydrate
Glycogen storage diseases
Diabetes mellitus
Iron
Hemochromatosis
Amyloid
Amyloidosis
Tumor/cellular infiltrate
Diffuse metastases
Diffuse hepatocellular carcinoma
Lymphoma
Extramedullary hematopoiesis
Systemic mastocytosis
Cysts
Polycystic disease
Inflammation/infection
Hepatitis
Sarcoidosis
Tuberculosis
Malaria

is the MR method most sensitive to fatty infiltration. On in-phase images, the signal from water and fat molecules are additive. On out-of-phase images, the signals from water and fat cancel out each other. A loss of signal intensity between in-phase and out-of-phase images is indicative of fatty infiltration (Fig. 27.4). This is the same technique used to characterize benign adrenal adenomas (see Chapter 33).

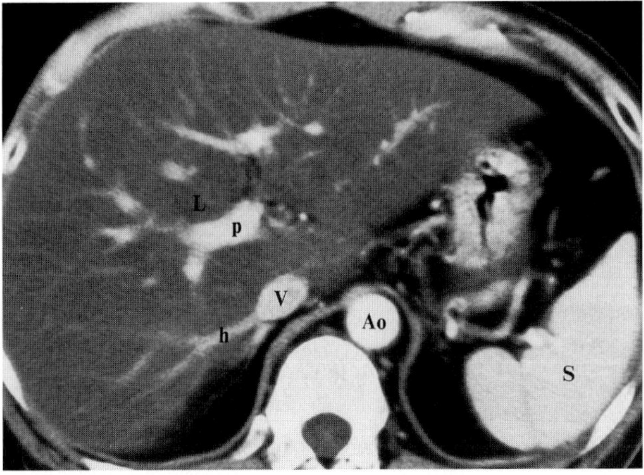

FIGURE 27.3. **Diffuse Fatty Infiltration Seen on CT.** CT reveals the density of the enhanced liver parenchyma (L) to be significantly less than the density of the enhanced splenic parenchyma (S). Portal (p) and hepatic (h) veins run their normal courses without displacement or distortion. V, inferior vena cava; Ao, aorta.

Characteristic features of fatty infiltration include lack of mass effect (no bulging of the liver contour or displacement of intrahepatic blood vessels) and angulated geometric boundaries between involved and uninvolved parenchyma. Areas of fat infiltration may be multifocal, with interdigitating fingers of normal and abnormal parenchyma. Fatty changes can develop within 3 weeks of hepatocyte insult and may resolve within 6 days of

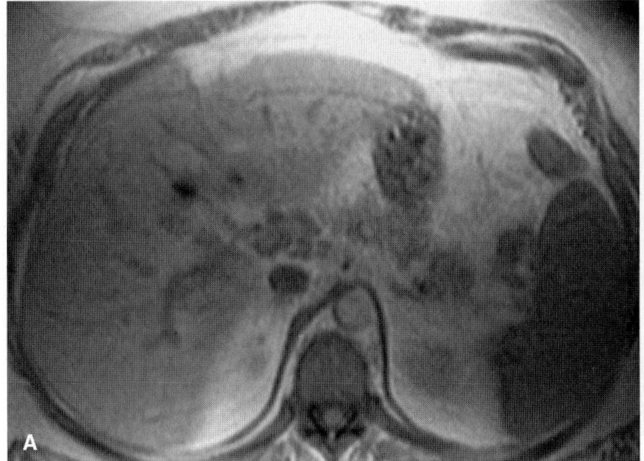

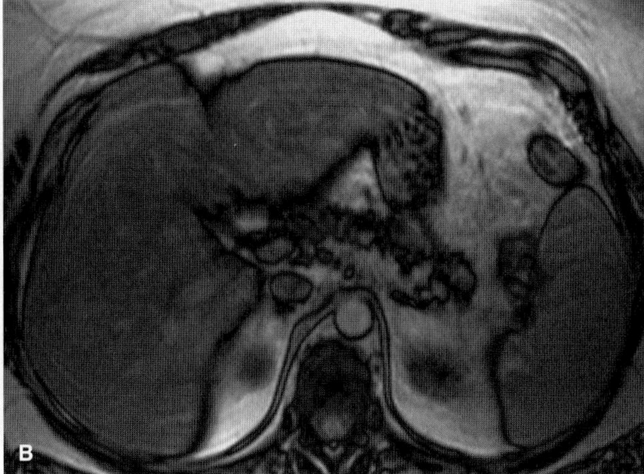

FIGURE 27.4. **Diffuse Fatty Infiltration Seen on MR. A.** In-phase gradient-recall MR. **B.** Out-of-phase gradient recall MR. The out-of-phase image shows distinct loss of signal (darkening) of the entire liver parenchyma compared to the in-phase image. The out-of-phase MR image is easily recognized by the black line surrounding soft tissue structures at the interface with abdominal fat.

removing the insult. Patterns of fatty infiltration are strongly related to hepatic blood flow.

Diffuse fatty infiltration involving the entire liver is the most common pattern. However, the degree of fat infiltration is commonly not uniform throughout the liver.

Focal fatty infiltration involves a geographic or fan-shaped portion of the liver with the same imaging features as diffuse infiltration. Vessels run their normal course through the area of involvement. Focal fatty infiltration may simulate a liver tumor; however, the area of involvement has a density characteristic of fat. Focal fatty infiltration is most common adjacent to the falciform ligament, gallbladder, and porta hepatis.

Focal sparing in a diffusely fatty-infiltrated liver may be the most confusing pattern, because spared areas of normal parenchyma may simulate a liver tumor (Fig. 27.5). The fat-spared area is most commonly located in segment IV. The fat-spared area is hypoechoic relative to the rest of the liver on US and is of higher density than the rest of the liver on CT. The remainder of the liver demonstrates features characteristic of diffuse fatty infiltration.

Nonalcoholic steatohepatitis (NASH) describes fatty liver caused by an inflammatory response that is not caused by excessive alcohol intake. NASH is related to obesity, type 2 diabetes, hyperlipidemia, and anorexia nervosa. It is a rare cause of acute fulminant hepatic failure and may progress to cirrhosis. Histology shows steatosis with parenchymal inflammation and fibrosis. Imaging features are those of diffuse fatty liver.

Acute hepatitis most commonly causes no abnormalities on hepatic imaging. In some patients, diffuse edema lowers the parenchyma echogenicity and causes the portal venules to appear unusually bright on US (3). In acute fulminant hepatitis, areas of necrosis show as ill-defined areas of low density on CT.

Chronic hepatitis is characterized pathologically by portal and perilobular inflammation and fibrosis. Imaging studies are insensitive to early pathologic changes. Fatty changes are minimal and the liver is usually not enlarged. Perihepatic lymph nodes are commonly visualized. US may show a subtle coarse increase in hepatic echogenicity. The primary role of imaging patients with chronic hepatitis is to detect hepatocellular carcinoma.

Cirrhosis is characterized pathologically by diffuse parenchymal destruction, fibrosis with alteration of hepatic architecture, and innumerable regenerative nodules that replace normal liver parenchyma. Causes of cirrhosis include hepatic toxins (alcohol, drugs); infection (viral hepatitis, especially types B and C); biliary obstruction; and heredity (Wilson disease). In the United States, 75% of patients with cirrhosis are chronic alcoholics. In Asia

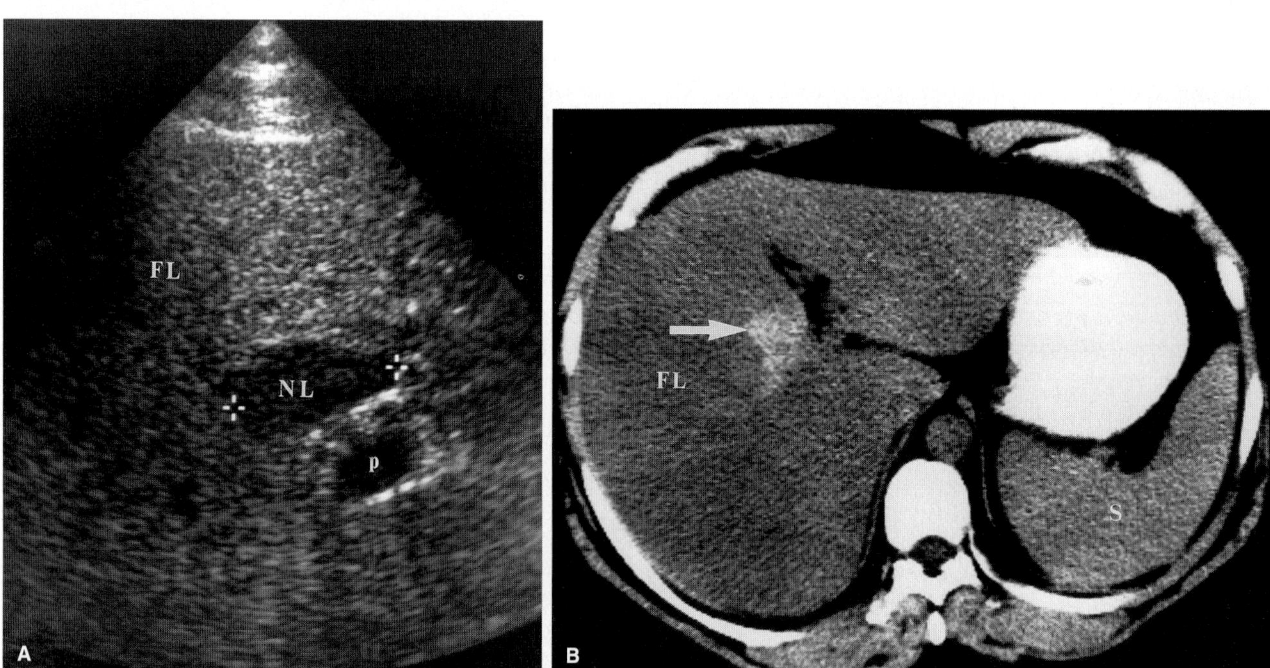

FIGURE 27.5. **Fatty Infiltration With Focal Sparing. A.** US image demonstrates a focal hypoechoic area of normal liver (NL) near the portal vein (p) in a liver (FL) that is diffusely increased in echogenicity because of fatty infiltration. **B.** CT image obtained without contrast enhancement demonstrates the spared area of normal liver (*arrow*) to be high density compared to the lower density of the fatty replaced liver (FL). Note the characteristic "flip-flop" appearance of fat density between CT and US. S, spleen.

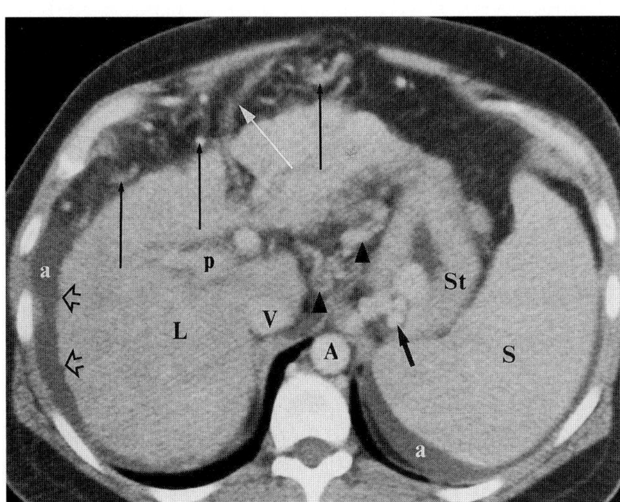

FIGURE 27.6. **Cirrhosis and Portal Hypertension.** A CT scan reveals atrophy of the liver (L) with diffuse nodularity of its surface (*open arrows*) and splenomegaly (S). Numerous enhancing portosystemic collateral vessels are evident, including perihepatic (*long black arrows*), gastrohepatic (*arrowheads*), and gastric varices (*short arrow*). A dilated periumbilical vein (*white arrow*) is seen coursing out of the fissure of the ligamentum teres into the falciform ligament. Ascites (a) is also evident. St, stomach; V, inferior vena cava; A, aorta.

and Africa, most cases of cirrhosis are caused by chronic active hepatitis. A variety of morphologic alterations are seen on imaging studies (Fig. 27.6) (4,5). These include: (*1*) hepatomegaly (early), (*2*) hepatic atrophy (late), (*3*) coarsening of hepatic parenchymal texture, (*4*) irregularity (nodularity) of the liver surface, (*5*) hypertrophy of the caudate lobe with shrinkage of the right lobe, and (*6*) regenerating nodules. Extrahepatic signs of cirrhosis include evidence of portal hypertension, splenomegaly, and ascites. The pathologic changes of cirrhosis are irreversible, but disease progression can be limited or stopped by eliminating the causative agent (stop drinking alcohol). Transjugular intrahepatic portosystemic shunts (TIPS) are effective treatment for portal hypertension and long-term control of esophageal variceal bleeding. Liver transplantation is now established as effective treatment for end-stage liver disease.

US demonstrates heterogeneous parenchyma with coarsening of the echotexture and decreased visualization of small portal triad structures. High-frequency detailed scanning of the liver surface reveals fine nodules. CT may be normal in the early stages, or it may reveal parenchymal inhomogeneity with patchy areas of increased and decreased attenuation (6). Fine or coarse nodularity of the liver surface is characteristic. Areas of fatty replacement may be evident. MR shows heterogeneous parenchymal signal on T1WIs and T2WIs. High-signal fibrosis on T2WIs is the predominant cause of the heterogeneous appearance.

TABLE 27.3 Causes of Nodules in a Cirrhotic Liver

Regenerative nodules (nodules <10 mm)
Adenomatous hyperplastic nodules (nodules >10 mm)
Hepatocellular carcinoma
Confluent fibrosis
Focal fat infiltration
Focal fat sparing
Metastases

Nodules in Cirrhosis. Nodules are a constant feature of cirrhosis (Table 27.3), and the challenge is to differentiate the ubiquitous benign nodule from HCC (7). The most common nodules are *regenerative nodules* (Fig. 27.7), which are a routine pathologic feature of cirrhosis caused by the body's attempted repair of hepatocyte injury. Regenerative nodules are composed primarily of hepatocytes that are surrounded by coarse fibrous septations. They have the same imaging characteristics as hepatic parenchyma but stand out as nodules because of their surrounding fibrous bands. Regenerative nodules are 3 to 10 mm in size. Small regenerative nodules cause the micronodular pattern of alcoholic cirrhosis. On CT, most regenerative nodules are isointense with parenchyma and are not detected. Iron deposits in regenerating nodules (siderotic nodules) will cause a slight increase in CT attenuation, causing them to appear slightly hyperintense. Regenerative nodules may be hypointense, isointense, or hyperintense on T1WIs, but they do not show the early arterial enhancement post–gadolinium administration that is typical of HCC. On T2WIs, regenerative nodules are hypointense (siderotic nodules) or isointense but are not

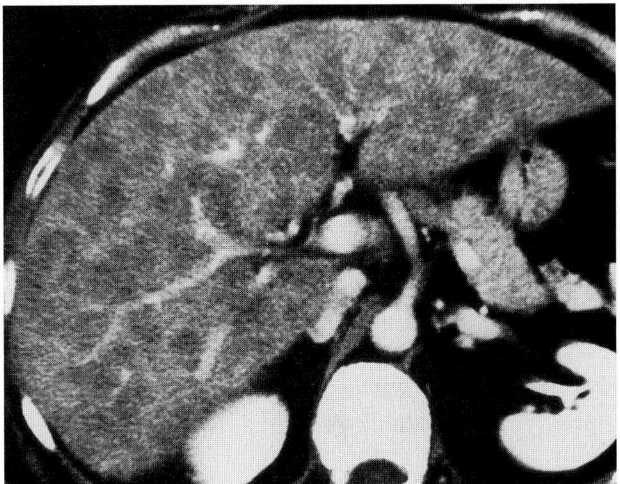

FIGURE 27.7. **Regenerative Nodules in Cirrhosis.** CT image filmed at a narrow window shows innumerable low-density small nodules evident throughout the liver in this patient with cirrhosis. Needle biopsy confirmed benign regenerative nodules.

hyperintense, providing differentiation from most liver metastases and from dysplastic nodules. *Dysplastic nodules* (adenomatous hyperplastic nodules) are proliferative precancerous lesions found in 15% to 25% of cirrhotic livers. On CT and US, adenomatous hyperplastic nodules resemble regenerative nodules but are larger than 10 mm in diameter. On MR, non–iron-containing adenomatous hyperplastic nodules are hyperintense on T1WIs and hypointense to isointense on T2WIs. High signal on a T2WI is indicative of foci of cellular atypia or malignancy. Small HCCs are variable in signal on both T1WIs and T2WIs. The most characteristic MR appearance of small HCCs is hyperintense on T1WIs and moderately hypointense on T2WIs, with homogeneous early arterial phase enhancement with rapid washout postcontrast (see Fig. 27.17). Rapid growth is characteristic. Lesions >3 cm usually have a distinct capsule. On CT, small HCCs appear as low-density, encapsulated masses that enhance rapidly and quickly become hypodense with bolus contrast dynamic scanning. Ringlike enhancement of the tumor capsule is characteristic.

Confluent fibrosis describes the masslike areas of fibrosis found in livers with advanced cirrhosis. Extensive fibrosis produces wedge-shaped or radiating bandlike masses that are hypodense on noncontrast CT and may become hyperdense post–contrast administration. Volume loss of the affected portion of the liver is a key feature. A whole hepatic segment or lobe may be replaced by fibrosis. The areas of fibrosis are hypointense to liver parenchyma on T1WIs and hyperintense on T2WIs. As mentioned previously, *focal fat infiltration* or *focal fat sparing* may also produce nodules in the cirrhotic liver. *Metastases*, especially those from breast carcinoma, may mimic the appearance of cirrhosis, with regenerative nodules. Following chemotherapy, tissue retraction of necrosing metastases with surrounding scarring may produce a condition termed *pseudocirrhosis* (6).

Portal hypertension is a pathologic increase in portal venous pressure that results in the formation of portosystemic collateral vessels that divert blood flow away from the liver and into the systemic circulation. Causes of portal hypertension include progressive vascular fibrosis associated with chronic liver disease, portal vein thrombosis or compression, and parasitic infections (schistosomiasis). Portal hypertension carries the risk of hemorrhage from varices and hepatic encephalopathy. The signs of portal hypertension include: (*1*) visualization of portosystemic collaterals (coronary, gastroesophageal, splenorenal, paraumbilical, hemorrhoidal, and retroperitoneal) (Fig. 27.6); (*2*) increased portal vein diameter (>13 mm); (*3*) increased superior mesenteric and splenic vein diameters (>10 mm); (*4*) portal vein thrombosis; (*5*) calcifications in the portal and mesenteric veins; (*6*) edema in the mesentery, omentum, and retroperitoneum; (*7*) splenomegaly owing to vascular congestion; and (*8*) ascites (8).

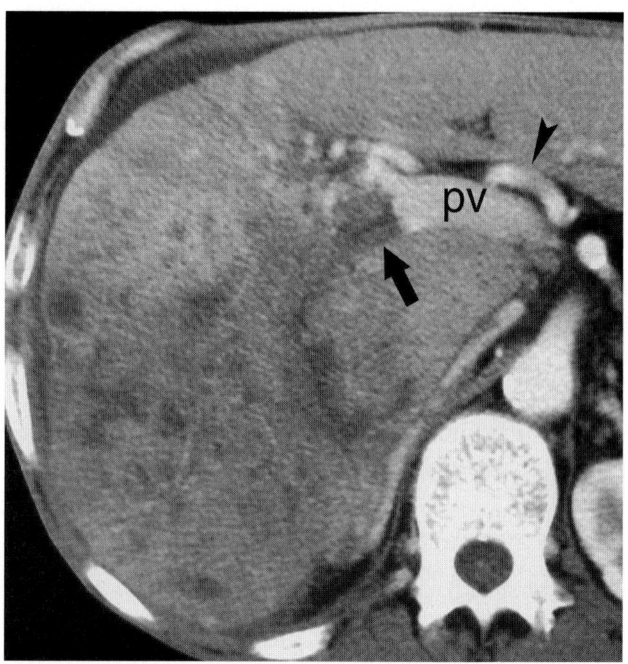

FIGURE 27.8. **Portal Vein Thrombosis: Multinodular Hepatocellular Carcinoma.** Contrast-enhanced CT demonstrates multiple hypodense nodules representing hepatocellular carcinoma that is replacing the right hepatic lobe. The portal vein (pv) is invaded by tumor (*arrow*), seen as a filling defect with the vein. The hepatic artery (*arrowhead*) is enlarged because of cirrhosis and portal hypertension.

Portal vein thrombosis may occur as a complication of cirrhosis, or it may be caused by portal vein invasion or compression by tumor (Fig. 27.8), hypercoagulable states, or inflammation (pancreatitis). The cause is unknown in 8% to 15% of patients. On CT and US, the thrombus is seen as a hypodense plug within the portal vein. On MR, the thrombus is hyperintense on T1WIs when acute and isointense when chronic. Signal in the thrombus is increased on T2WIs. Portal hypertension is exacerbated, or may be caused, by portal vein thrombosis. *Cavernous transformation* of the portal vein develops when small collateral veins adjacent to the portal vein expand and replace the obliterated portal vein. These collateral veins appear as a tangle of small vessels surrounding the thrombosed portal vein (8).

Budd-Chiari syndrome is caused by obstruction to hepatic venous outflow that may be a result of obstruction of the suprahepatic IVC by a congenital membranous web (primary type) or by thrombosis of the hepatic veins caused by tumor, hypercoagulable states, or trauma (secondary type). Blood flow to the right and left hepatic lobes is severely impaired, resulting in a characteristic "flip-flop" pattern on contrast-enhanced CT. On early images, the central liver enhances prominently, whereas the peripheral liver enhances weakly (Fig. 27.9). On delayed images, the periphery of the liver is enhanced, whereas contrast has

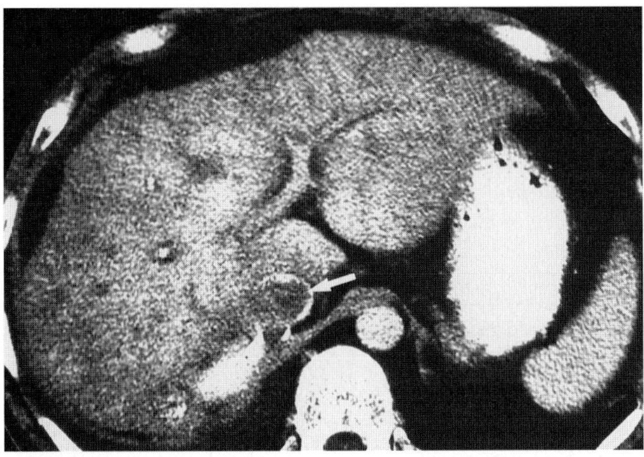

FIGURE 27.9. **Budd-Chiari Syndrome.** Early phase CT images show the markedly heterogeneous liver with prominent central and weak peripheral enhancement that is characteristic of Budd-Chiari syndrome. Tumor invasion from a right adrenal carcinoma is seen as a filling defect (*arrow*) within the inferior vena cava.

washed out of the central liver. The caudate lobe is spared because of its separate venous drainage to the IVC. The caudate lobe is characteristically enlarged and enhances normally. Thrombi may be seen in the hepatic veins, or they may be reduced in caliber and difficult to visualize. Comma-shaped intrahepatic collateral vessels may be seen on CT or MR (the "comma sign"). Multiple benign hepatic nodules up to 3 cm commonly develop. Most are detected by prominent contrast enhancement during the arterial phase or mild contrast enhancement during the portal venous phase (9).

Passive hepatic congestion is a common complication of congestive heart failure and constrictive pericarditis. Hepatic venous drainage is impaired, and the liver becomes engorged and swollen. Findings include distension of the hepatic veins and IVC, reflux of IV contrast into the hepatic veins and IVC, increased pulsatility of the portal vein, and inhomogeneous contrast enhancement of the liver. Secondary findings commonly present include hepatomegaly, cardiomegaly, pleural effusions, and ascites.

Hemochromatosis may be primary (hereditary) or secondary owing to excessive iron intake from either parenteral or dietary sources. In severe cases, CT demonstrates a diffuse increase in liver density, to 75 to 130 H. MR is more sensitive to hepatic iron overload because of the superparamagnetic effect of iron. MR demonstrates marked diffuse low signal intensity on T2WIs (Fig. 27.10) and moderate loss of signal intensity on T1WIs (10). Longstanding hemochromatosis places the patient at risk for cirrhosis and hepatocellular carcinoma.

Gas in the portal venous system is often an ominous sign associated with bowel ischemia in adults (Fig. 27.11) and necrotizing enterocolitis in infants. Additional causes include recent colonoscopy, enema administration, gastrostomy tube placement, abdominal trauma, inflammatory bowel disease, perforated gastric ulcer, necrotizing pancreatitis, diverticulitis, and abdominal abscess (8). CT reveals air in branching tubular structures that extends to the liver capsule. Air is commonly evident within

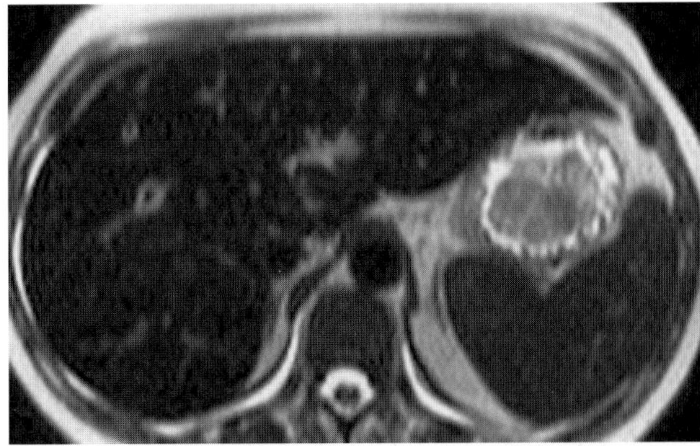

FIGURE 27.10. **Hemochromatosis.** T2W MR image demonstrates marked low signal intensity in both liver and spleen. The low signal is caused by iron deposition in the reticuloendothelial system—in this case of secondary hemochromatosis caused by multiple blood transfusions.

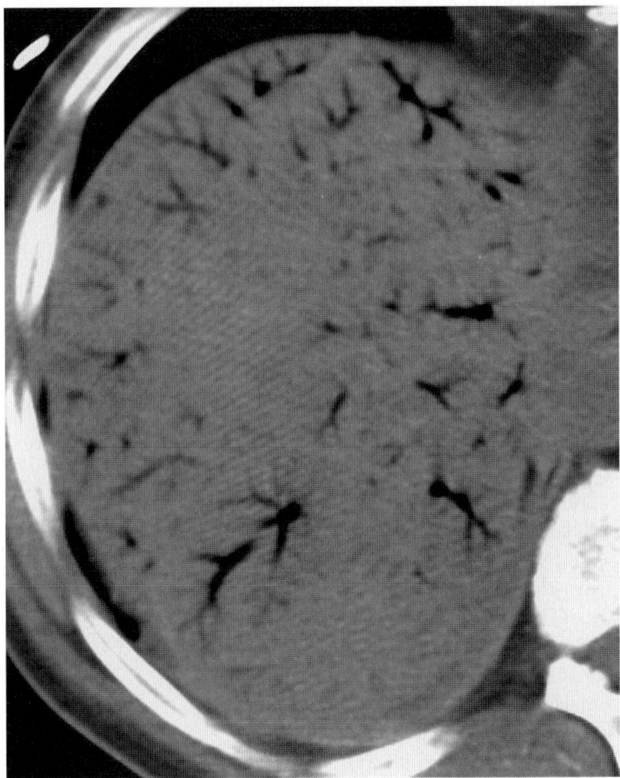

FIGURE 27.11. **Portal Venous Gas.** Noncontrast CT image reveals gas in the portal vein, seen as air-density tubular structures extending to the periphery of the liver. Gas in the biliary tree is central and does not extend into the peripheral 2 cm of the liver. In this case, portal venous gas was associated with infarction of the small bowel.

the mesenteric and portal veins. Plain radiographs show streaks of low density in the periphery of the liver. In distinction, air in the biliary tree is more central, not extending to within 2 cm of the liver capsule.

Liver Masses

A major challenge of liver imaging is to differentiate common and benign liver masses, such as cavernous hemangioma and simple hepatic cysts, from malignant masses such as metastases and hepatoma. US can definitively characterize hepatic cysts; however, benign and malignant solid masses overlap in sonographic appearance. CT can characterize most cysts and cavernous hemangiomas, but only with optimal technique and contrast administration. On MR, simple cysts and hemangiomas are hypointense on T1WIs and extremely hyperintense on T2WIs. These benign masses are typically homogeneous and have sharp outer margins. Malignant lesions on MR tend to be inhomogeneous with unsharp outer margins, peritumoral edema, and central necrosis. Most focal lesions are hypointense on T1WIs and hyperintense on T2WIs. Hyperintensity of focal lesions on T1WIs may be a result of the presence of fat, blood, proteinaceous material, or melanin in melanoma metastases (Table 27.4). Diffuse hypointensity of liver, caused by diffuse edema or iron overload, may make any lesion appear relatively hyperintense. Hypointensity on T2WIs is commonly a result of fibrosis (Table 27.5).

TABLE 27.4 Causes of Hyperintensity in Focal Liver Lesions on MR T1WIs

Fat deposits
Focal fat infiltration
Fat deposition in tumor
Hepatoma
Lipoma
Angiomyolipoma
Hepatic adenoma
Blood
Hematoma
Hemorrhage into tumor
Proteinaceous material
Proteinaceous fluid in cysts
Necrosis/hemorrhage in tumor
Abscess
Hematoma
Copper
Intratumoral copper in hepatoma
Melanin
Melanoma metastasis
Contrast enhancement
Gadolinium administration
Lipiodol administration
Ghosting artifact
Result of blood flow in adjacent vessels
Hypointensity of liver parenchyma
Edema caused by passive hepatic congestion
Iron deposition in hepatocytes

TABLE 27.5 Causes of Hypointensity in Focal Liver Lesions on MR T2WIs

Fibrous capsule
Hepatoma (24% to 42% of HCC)
Hepatic adenoma
Focal nodular hyperplasia (rare)
Fibrous central scar
Fibrolamellar HCC
Focal nodular hyperplasia

HCC, hepatocellular carcinoma.

Metastases are the most common malignant masses in the liver. Metastases are 20 times more common than primary liver malignancies. Of all patients who die of malignancy, 24% to 36% have liver involvement. Hepatic metastases most commonly originate from the GI tract, breast, and lung. A wide spectrum of appearance of metastatic disease is seen on all imaging studies (Fig. 27.12) (11). Metastases may be uniformly solid, necrotic, cystic, or calcified; they may be avascular, hypovascular, or hypervascular; they are commonly irregular and poorly marginated but may be sharp and well defined. Most characteristic is bandlike peripheral enhancement on arterial phase images, with rapid washout on delayed CT and MR images. Metastatic disease must be considered in the differential

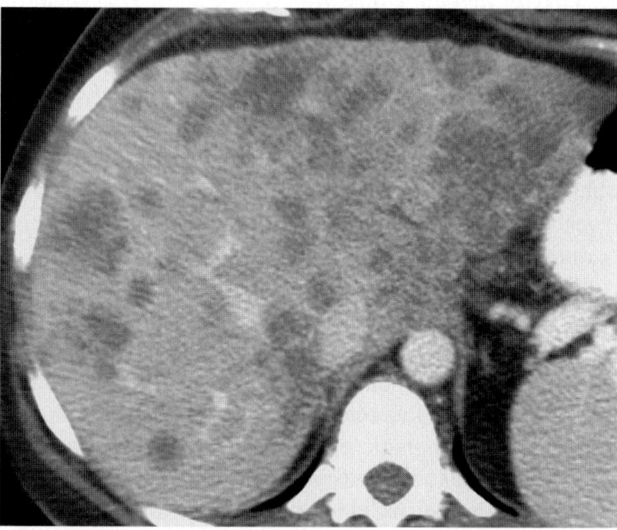

FIGURE 27.12. **Metastases.** Metastases from adenocarcinoma of the colon appear as numerous low-attenuation nodules of varying size on this portal venous phase, postcontrast CT. Note how the metastatic disease causes nodularity of the liver contour and the resemblance to regenerative nodules in cirrhosis (see Fig. 27.7).

TABLE 27.6 Causes of Multiple Small (10-mm) Lesions in the Liver

Regenerative nodules in cirrhosis
Microabscesses (immunocompromised patient)
Multiple bacterial abscesses
Histoplasmosis
Lymphoma
Kaposi sarcoma (AIDS patient)
Hepatocellular carcinoma (multinodular form)
Sarcoidosis
Gamna-Gandy bodies (portal hypertension)
Metastases
Breast carcinoma
Lung carcinoma
Ovarian carcinoma
Gastric carcinoma
Malignant melanoma
Prostate carcinoma

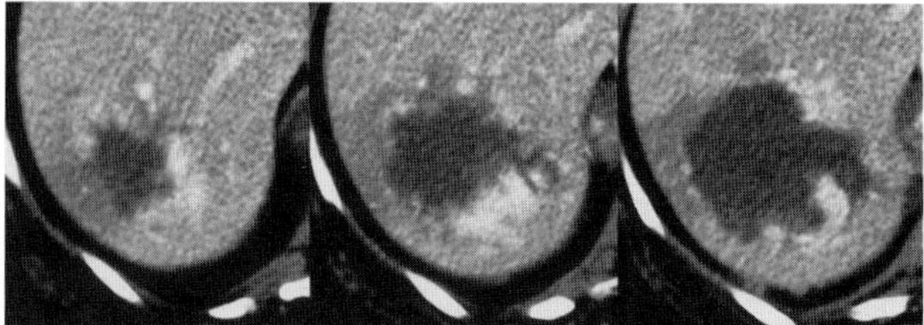
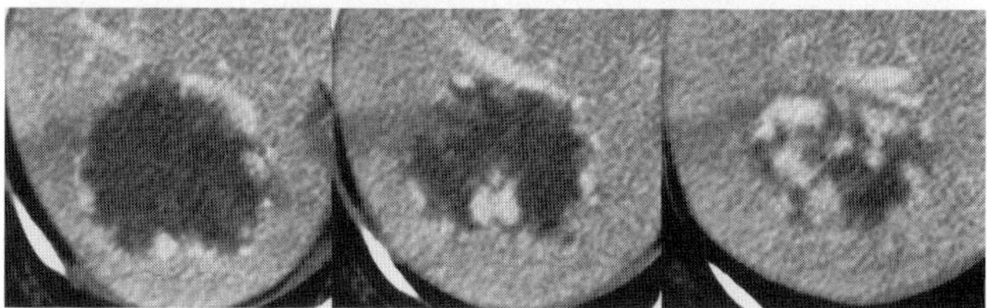

FIGURE 27.13. **Cavernous Hemangioma.** Images from a contrast-enhanced helical CT demonstrate the characteristic nodular pattern of enhancement from the periphery of the lesion.

of virtually all hepatic masses (Table 27.6). Multiplicity of lesions favors metastatic disease.

Cavernous hemangioma is second only to metastases as the most common cause of a liver mass (12). It is the most common benign liver neoplasm, found in 7% to 20% of the population and more commonly in women. Up to 10% of patients have multiple lesions, which are easily mistaken for metastases. Many hemangiomas are discovered incidentally on hepatic imaging performed for other reasons. The tumor consists of large, thin-walled, blood-filled vascular spaces separated by fibrous septa. Blood flow through the maze of vascular spaces is extremely slow, resulting in characteristic imaging findings. Thrombosis within the vascular channels may result in central fibrosis and calcification. Most lesions are smaller than 5 cm, cause no symptoms, and are considered benign incidental findings. Larger lesions (>6 cm) occasionally cause symptoms by mass effect, hemorrhage, or arteriovenous shunting. The size of most cavernous hemangiomas is stable over time. Enlargement of a lesion is cause for reassessment.

US demonstrates a well-defined, uniformly hyperechoic mass in 80% of patients. In a patient with no history of malignant disease and normal liver chemistries, follow-up only is generally recommended. No Doppler signal is obtained from most cavernous hemangiomas because the flow is too slow.

CT generally shows a well-defined, hypodense mass on unenhanced scans. Because the lesion consists mostly of blood, attenuation of the hemangioma is similar to that of blood vessels within the liver. The characteristic pattern of enhancement with bolus IV contrast is nodular enhancement from the periphery of the lesion (Fig. 27.13) that gradually becomes isodense or hyperdense compared to the liver parenchyma. The degree of contrast enhancement parallels that of hepatic blood vessels during all postcontrast phases. The contrast enhancement persists for 20 to 30 minutes following injection because of slow flow within the lesion.

Radionuclide scanning using technetium-labeled red blood cells as a blood pool agent is extremely accurate in the diagnosis of cavernous hemangioma. Hemangiomas are characterized by prolonged, intense activity within the lesion on delayed images.

MR demonstrates a well-defined homogeneous mass that is hypointense or isointense on T1WIs and brightens markedly with increasing amounts of T2 weighting. Areas of fibrosis remain dark on all image sequences. However, the MR appearance of cavernous hemangiomas overlaps that of cysts, abscesses, and hypervascular metastases. A specific diagnosis can be made by IV administration of gadolinium and observing early puddling peripheral enhancement in a pattern similar to that seen in contrast-enhanced CT.

Biopsy may be required in atypical cases. Percutaneous biopsy can be safely performed using small needles (20-gauge and smaller). The characteristic finding is blood with normal epithelial cells and no malignant cells. Biopsy with large-bore needles has been associated with hemorrhage and death.

Hepatocellular carcinoma is the most common primary malignancy of the liver. Risk factors include cirrhosis, chronic hepatitis, and a variety of carcinogens (sex hormones, aflatoxin, Thorotrast). In the United States, most HCCs are found in patients with cirrhosis (usually because of alcohol abuse). In Asia, most HCCs are found in patients with chronic active hepatitis. Hepatomas demonstrate three major growth patterns that affect their imaging appearance: diffuse infiltrative, solitary massive (Figs. 27.14, 27.15), and multinodular (Fig. 27.8). Detection of the diffuse pattern of tumor is particularly difficult,

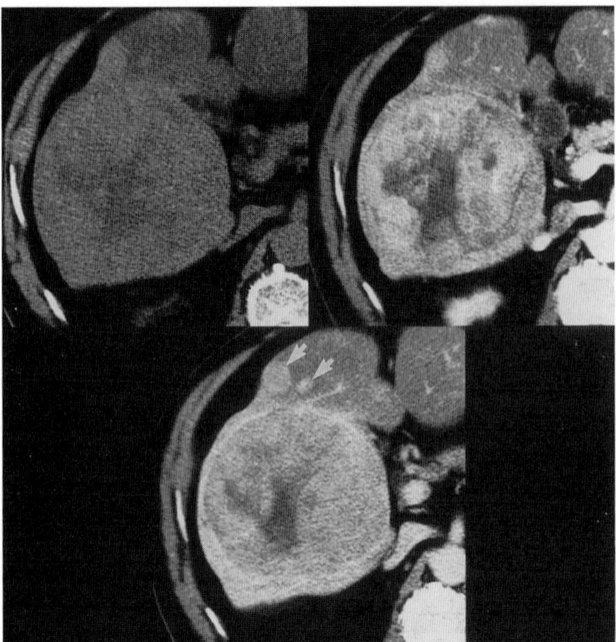

FIGURE 27.14. **Hepatocellular Carcinoma on CT.** Three-phase helical CT demonstrates the enhancement pattern of a larger hepatocellular carcinoma in the right lobe. The tumor is slightly hyperdense to parenchyma on the unenhanced scan (*upper left*) and shows intense enhancement on the early (arterial phase—*upper right*) scan and delayed (venous phase—*lower*) scan. The central low density is a result of necrosis. Note the satellite lesions (*arrows*).

especially when the liver parenchyma is already altered by diffuse hepatic disease. Approximately 24% of tumors are surrounded by a fibrous capsule. The encapsulated HCC, a variant of the solitary form, is found more frequently in Asian populations and has a better prognosis. Intratumoral hemorrhage and necrosis are common because of a

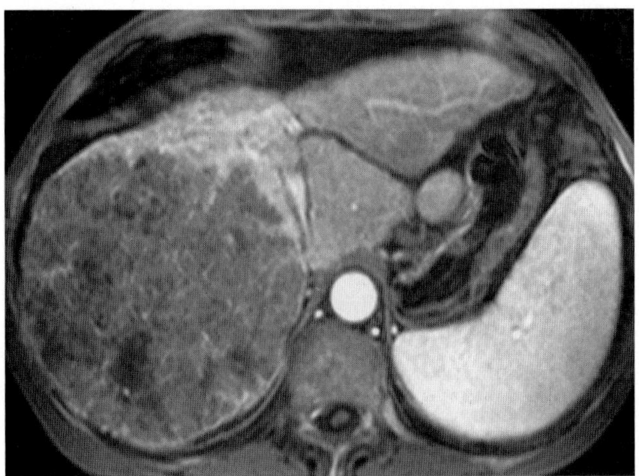

FIGURE 27.15. **Hepatocellular Carcinoma on MR.** Postcontrast T1WI shows the typical mosaic pattern of large hepatocellular carcinomas. Note the prominent enhancement in the periphery of the tumor.

TABLE 27.7 Fat-Containing Lesions in the Liver

Hepatic adenoma
Hepatocellular carcinoma
Focal fatty deposition
Lipoma
Teratoma
Liposarcoma (primary or metastatic)
Postoperative packing material (omentum)
Focal intrahepatic extramedullary hematopoiesis

lack of stroma within the tumor. Calcifications (punctate, stippled, or rimlike) occur in approximately 10% of cases. Most lesions are hypervascular and demonstrate contrast enhancement on arterial phase images, with diminishing enhancement on delayed phase images (see Fig. 27.17). Detection of hepatoma on a background of cirrhosis and regenerative nodules is a major imaging challenge. Elevation in serum α-fetoprotein is found in 90% of patients and is strongly suggestive of hepatoma in patients with cirrhosis. The tumor metastasizes to lungs, abdominal lymph nodes, adrenal glands, and bone (13).

Several imaging features are highly characteristic of HCC when present. Invasion of tumor into portal and hepatic veins occurs in up to 48% of cases (Fig. 27.8). *Tumor thrombus* is visualized as a low-density plug within an expanded vein. The intraluminal tumor enhances with contrast administration on CT and MR and may demonstrate arterial signal with Doppler US. Portal vein thrombus is more common than hepatic vein thrombus. A *tumor capsule,* when present, is visualized as a sharply marginated rim of tissue that enhances in 90% of cases. The capsule has low signal intensity on both T1WIs and T2WIs and is hypoechoic on US. *Satellite nodules* of tumor are common (Fig. 27.14). *Fatty metamorphosis* is a common histologic finding in HCC. CT may demonstrate a focal area of tumor with attenuation values of fat (Table 27.7) (14). MR confirmation of fat is performed with chemical shift imaging. A *mosaic appearance* of the tumor is considered to be characteristic but is found primarily in larger lesions (Fig. 27.15). The mosaic pattern appears as multiple nodular areas of differing CT attenuation. The pattern is more obvious with enhancement of septations on postcontrast scans. *Arterioportal shunting* is seen as early or prolonged enhancement of the portal vein or as a wedge-shaped area of parenchymal enhancement adjacent to the tumor. Abundant copper-binding protein in cancer cells may lead to *excessive copper accumulation* within the tumor. High copper concentration causes the tumor to appear hyperdense on noncontrast CT and hyperdense (because of T1 shortening effect) on T1WIs on MR.

Focal nodular hyperplasia (FNH) forms a solid mass consisting of abnormally arranged hepatocytes, bile ducts, and Kupffer cells. Most lesions are smaller than 5 cm in diameter and are hypervascular, with a central fibrous scar containing thick-walled blood vessels. Lesions are lobulated and well circumscribed but lack a capsule. These are benign lesions that do not require treatment but must be differentiated from hepatic adenoma and fibrolamellar carcinoma.

In contrast to hepatic adenoma, hemorrhage, necrosis, and infarction are extremely rare in FNH. Similar to hepatic adenoma, FNH is found most commonly in women, but it is twice as common as hepatic adenoma and is not related to oral contraceptive use. Most tumors (80% to 95%) are solitary. Because of the presence of Kupffer cells, most (50% to 70%) FNH nodules will show normal or increased radionuclide activity on technetium sulfur colloid liver-spleen scans (15). This finding is highly indicative of FNH.

On CT, MR, and US, most tumors appear homogeneous and solid. A central core scar with radiating septa is characteristic but present in only 60%. Because the cellular makeup of FNH is very similar to that of normal hepatic parenchyma, the lesion is usually isodense on noncontrast images (Fig. 27.16). The typical finding on contrast-enhanced CT and MR is intense, brief (approximately 1 minute), uniform tumor enhancement during the arterial phase. FNH is inconspicuous on US, detectable only by mass effect (bulging contour) or slight alterations in parenchymal echotexture. Some lesions have a hypoechoic halo. The central scar, if present, is often poorly visualized. Color flow imaging may show the lesion's hypervascularity. MDCT shows homogeneous hyperenhancement during the arterial phase. The lesion is often isodense during the portal phase, with enhancement of the central scar on delayed images. On MR, FNH appears homogeneous and isointense to slightly hypointense to normal parenchyma on T1WIs and isointense to slightly hyperintense on T2WIs (7). The central scar is hypointense on T1WIs and hyperintense on T2WIs. FNH shows a characteristic very intense homogeneous enhancement on arterial phase postcontrast images. The central scar and radiating septa enhance on delayed postcontrast images.

Hepatic adenomas are rare benign tumors that carry a risk of life-threatening hemorrhage and potential for malignant degeneration. Surgical removal of the tumor is advocated. They are found most commonly in women on long-term oral contraceptives. Additional risk factors include androgen steroid intake and glycogen storage disease. The tumor consists of sheets and cords of benign hepatocytes without a distinct acinar architecture. The hepatocytes occasionally contain abundant fat, detectable by imaging studies. Kupffer cells are present in some tumors but are nonfunctional; thus, hepatic adenomas appear as cold defects on technetium sulfur colloid radionuclide scans. Tumors have poor connective tissue support, making them susceptible to hemorrhage. Most tumors are solitary, smooth, and encapsulated. They do not have central scars. Tumor size is commonly 8 to 15 cm but may be up to 30 cm. Areas of necrosis, hemorrhage, and fibrosis are common (16). Liver adenomatosis is characterized by the presence of multiple adenomas in an otherwise normal liver in patients without risk factors for hepatic adenomas.

US is sensitive to high fat content or intratumoral hemorrhage, which makes the lesions appear hyperechoic. CT shows well-circumscribed tumors that are often low in attenuation because of internal fat, necrosis, or old hemorrhage. Calcifications in areas of old hemorrhage or necrosis are present in 15% of cases. Postcontrast scans show intense homogeneous enhancement during the arterial phase that becomes isodense with liver on portal venous and delayed phase scans. Tumors are hyperintense on T1WIs because of fat or hemorrhage. On T2WIs, most are hyperdense to liver and are commonly heterogeneous because of hemorrhage or necrosis. Dynamic postgadolinium scans are similar to postcontrast CT, showing intense arterial phase enhancement (Fig. 27.17), with isointensity on portal phase and delayed images.

Fibrolamellar carcinoma is a hepatocellular malignancy with clinical and pathologic features that are distinct from HCC (17). Tumors typically present as a large liver mass in a young adult (mean age, 23 years) with none of the risk factors for HCC and without elevation of α-fetoprotein levels. Cords of tumor are surrounded by prominent fibrous bands that emanate from a central fibrotic scar. The surrounding liver is usually normal, without features of cirrhosis or chronic liver disease. The characteristic appearance is a large, lobulated hepatic mass with central scar and calcifications. The central scar with radiating septa mimics the appearance of FNH. Satellite tumor nodules are occasionally present (10% to 15%). Hemorrhage and necrosis are uncommon (10%) but are occasionally massive, resulting in a multicystic appearance of the tumor. Although the tumor is less aggressive than HCC, the stage at presentation tends to be advanced, with malignant adenopathy present. Aggressive surgical management is indicated.

US shows a large, lobulated, well-defined mass with mixed echogenicity. The central scar is echogenic, if visible. On precontrast CT, the tumor is low attenuation. Calcification may be evident within the fibrous scar. The tumor enhances prominently and heterogenously on both arterial and portal venous phases (Fig. 27.18). Enhancement of the scar is most evident on delayed scans. MR shows a usually homogeneous hypointense mass (86%) or an isointense mass (14%) on T1WIs. On T2WIs the mass is usually hyperintense and much more heterogeneous. The fibrous scar is hypointense on all image sequences. Gadolinium enhancement shows the same pattern as CT.

Lymphoma involving the liver is usually diffusely infiltrative and undetectable by imaging methods. The multiple-nodule pattern found in 10% of cases resembles

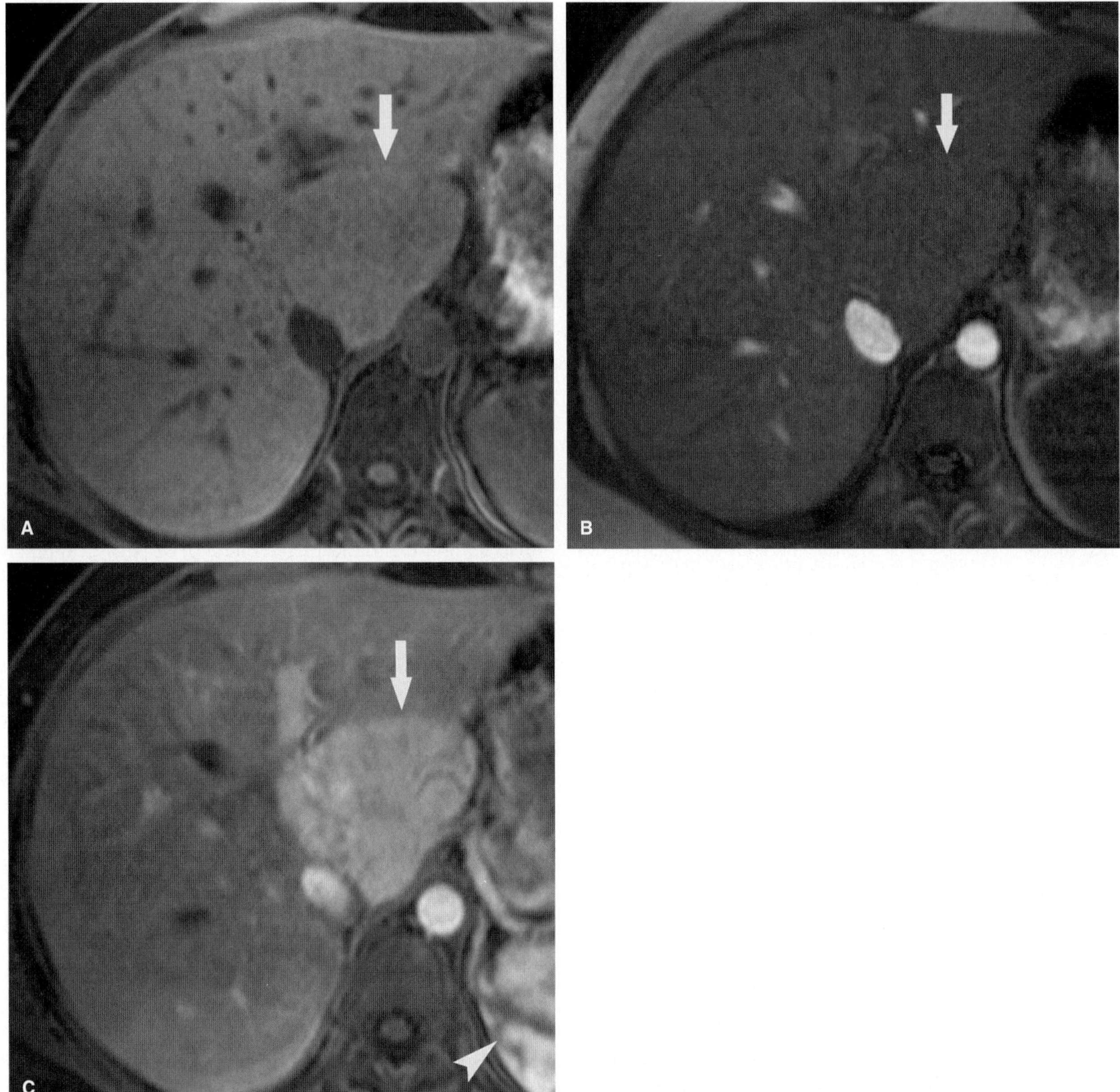

FIGURE 27.16. **Focal Nodular Hyperplasia.** The lesion (*arrows*), consisting of liver elements, is isodense with the hepatic parenchyma on a T1WI **(A)** and a gradient-recall two-dimensional time-of-flight image **(B).** The lesion is clearly depicted by intense enhancement during the arterial phase **(C),** post–gadolinium administration. This lesion lacks a central scar. Note the mottled early enhancement of the portion of the spleen (*arrowhead*) included on the image.

metastatic disease. Some cases present as a large, poorly defined, hypodense mass with or without satellite nodules. On MR, lesions are hypodense on T1WIs and hyperdense on T2WIs. Lesions enhance poorly or not at all (Fig. 27.19).

Benign hepatic cyst is the second most common benign hepatic mass, found in 5% of the population (18). Most are solitary, but they may be multiple, especially in patients with adult polycystic disease or tuberous sclerosis. Cysts range in size from microscopic to 20 cm. Hepatic cysts do not communicate with the biliary tree. Tiny cysts are responsible for many of the "hypoattenuating lesions too small to characterize" seen on MDCT. Larger cysts tend to occur in clusters with cysts of varying size, resulting in sharply defined, but lobulated, margins and septations. Hepatic polycystic disease is part of the spectrum of autosomal-dominant polycystic disease and occasionally occurs in the absence of polycystic kidneys.

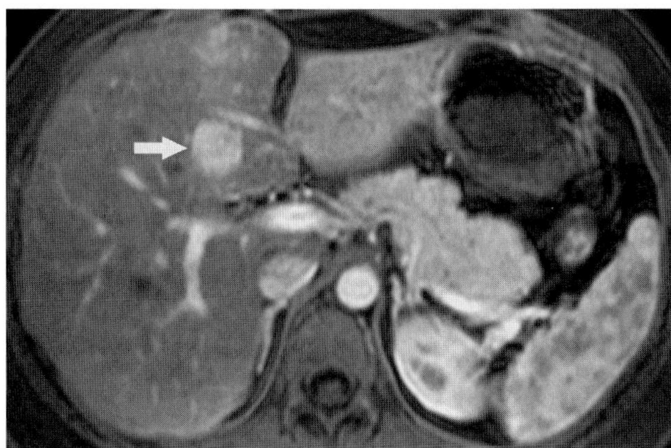

FIGURE 27.17. **Hepatic Adenoma.** Postgadolinium, T1W, fat-suppressed MR image shows intense homogeneous enhancement during arterial phase of a biopsy-proven hepatic adenoma (*arrow*). The MR appearance is indistinguishable from that of a small hepatocellular carcinoma.

US is the best imaging modality to characterize hepatic cysts. Typical cysts are anechoic with thin walls and septa and posterior acoustic enhancement. Occasionally, hepatic cysts have internal debris, especially if they have been infected. CT shows low internal attenuation near water (Fig. 27.20) (18). MR shows low internal signal on T1WIs and high internal signal on T2WIs. Cysts do not enhance following contrast administration.

Pyogenic abscess is usually caused by *Escherichia coli, Staphylococcus aureus, Streptococcus,* or anaerobic bacteria (19). Patients present with fever and pain. Destruction of liver results in a solitary cavity or a tight group of individual loculated abscesses (Fig. 27.21). A peripheral rim enhances with contrast. Gas is present within the lesion in 20% of cases (3). Diagnosis is confirmed by percutaneous aspiration. Catheter or surgical drainage is indicated.

Amebic abscess is usually solitary, with thick nodular walls (3). The lesion may be indistinguishable from pyogenic abscess (Fig. 27.22); however, the patient is often

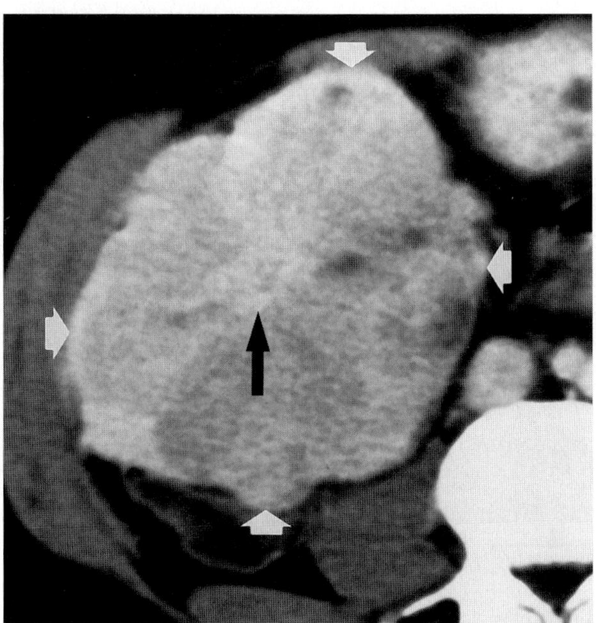

FIGURE 27.18. **Fibrolamellar Hepatocellular Carcinoma.** CT scan demonstrates a large tumor (between *white arrows*) extending caudally from the right lobe of the liver. A characteristic stellate central scar (*black arrow*) is present.

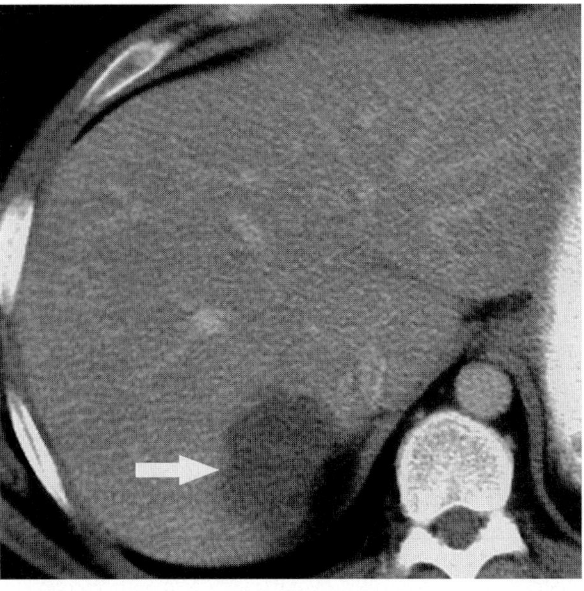

FIGURE 27.19. **Hepatic Lymphoma.** CT shows a poorly marginated, hypodense, nonenhancing nodule (*arrow*) that proved on biopsy to be non-Hodgkin lymphoma.

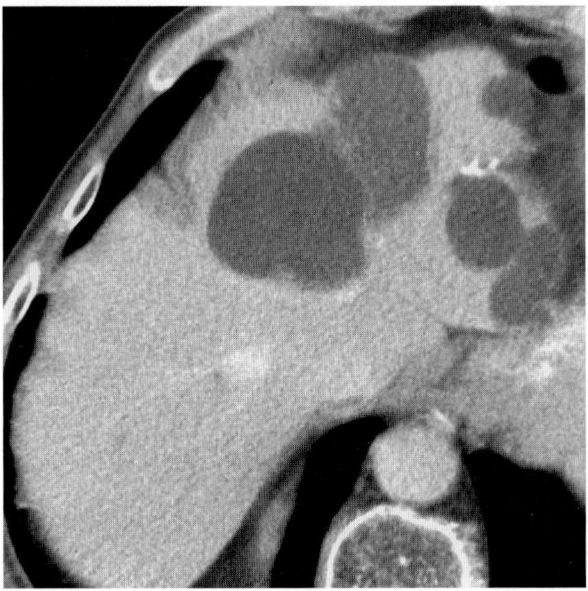

FIGURE 27.20. **Hepatic Cysts.** Multiple hepatic cysts are an incidental finding on this postcontrast CT in a 78-year-old patient.

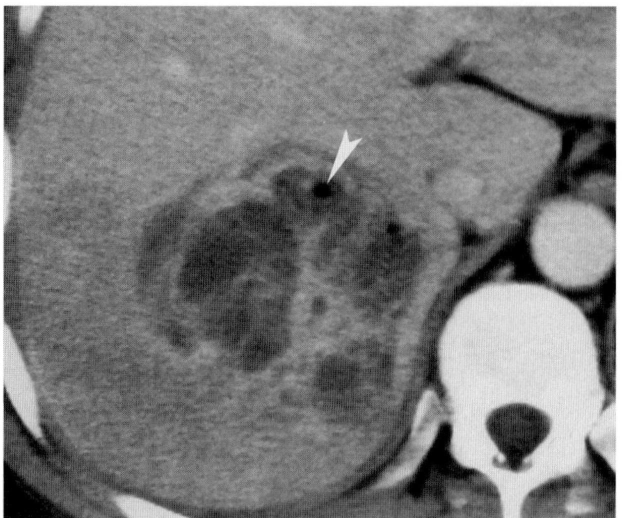

FIGURE 27.21. **Pyogenic Abscess.** CT scan shows multiple low-density areas separated by enhancing septa and representing abscess locules. Several air bubbles (*arrowhead*) are evident within the lesion.

more acutely ill and has a history of travel to endemic areas (India, Africa, East Asia, Central and South America). Amebic abscesses commonly occur in the right lobe of the liver, often cause elevation of the right hemidiaphragm, and may rupture through the diaphragm into the pleural space. In the United States, the diagnosis is typically confirmed by serology and the patient is treated with metronidazole. In endemic areas, the diagnosis is confirmed by aspiration of "anchovy paste" material, and the patient is treated by repeated aspiration or catheter drainage.

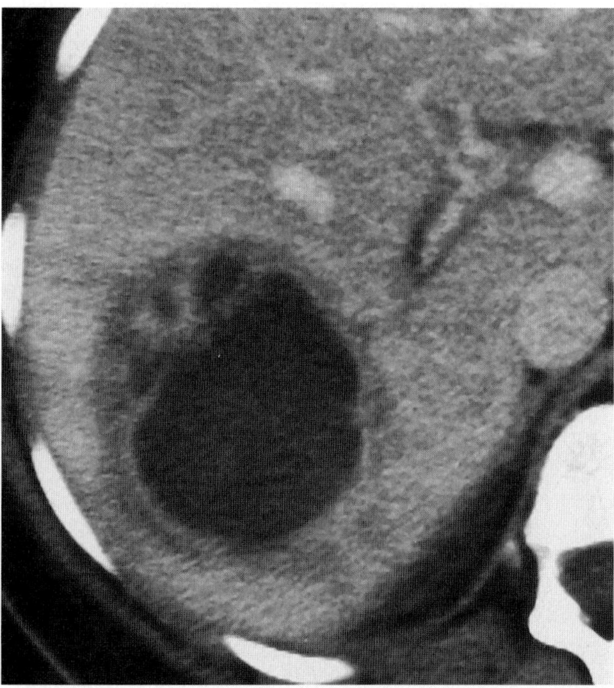

FIGURE 27.22. **Amebic Abscess.** Postcontrast CT image reveals a thick-walled fluid collection in the right hepatic lobe. Differentiation of amebic from pyogenic liver abscess is made by history, serology, or image-guided aspiration.

Echinococcus cyst is caused by infestation with *Echinococcus granulosus* or *E multilocularis* tapeworm (19). The parasite is endemic in central and northern Europe, the Mediterranean, northern Asia, China, Japan, Turkey, and parts of North America. The liver is the most common organ affected (95%). Single or multiple cystic masses usually have well-defined walls that commonly calcify (50%). The cyst wall and septations usually enhance. Daughter cysts may be visualized within the parent cyst (75%). Diagnostic aspiration carries a risk of anaphylactic reaction. Treatment is mebendazole or surgical excision.

Cystic/necrotic tumor must always be considered for atypical cystic masses. Metastases may be necrotic or predominantly cystic. Biliary cystadenoma and cystadenocarcinomas are rare primary tumors that resemble mucinous cystic tumors of the pancreas. Undifferentiated embryonal sarcomas are seen in older children, adolescents, and young adults (18).

Small hypoattenuating lesions are detected with increased frequency on MDCT because of thinner collimation, improved resolution, and rapid, multiphase, postcontrast scanning (Fig. 27.23). Lesions smaller than 1 cm

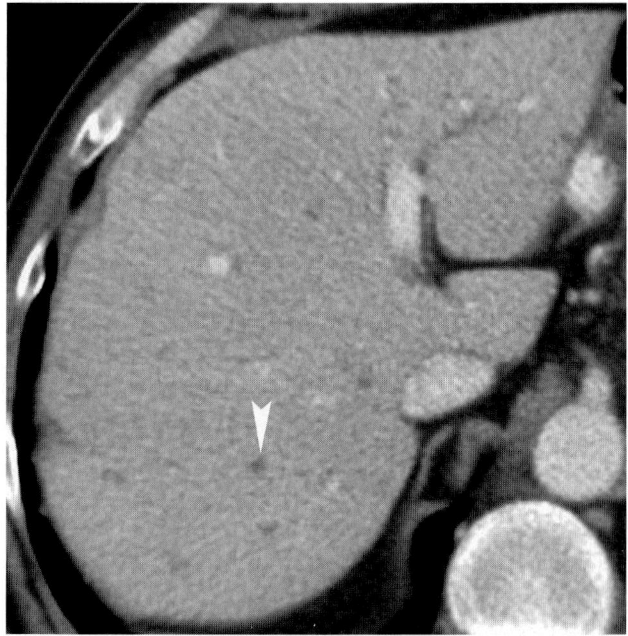

FIGURE 27.23. **Too Small to Characterize.** Multidetector CT shows multiple, tiny, low-attenuation lesions (*arrowhead*) that are too small to definitively characterize. Even in patients with known malignancy, these lesions are usually benign. However, on follow-up in some patients, they will prove to be early metastatic lesions. They are usually identified only on high-quality postcontrast CT. Image-guided biopsy cannot usually be performed because the lesions cannot be identified on US or noncontrast CT.

are difficult to characterize and often too small to biopsy. Differential diagnoses include cysts, hemangiomas, and metastases. Statistically, most of these tiny lesions are benign. In a patient with known malignancy, follow-up scans are needed to exclude metastatic disease. In a series of patients with known malignancy, lesions were metastases in 12% of cases (20).

BILIARY TREE

Imaging Methods. Imaging of the biliary tree uses assorted techniques that differ in degrees of invasiveness. US and CT are highly sensitive in the detection of dilation of the bile ducts, though they are somewhat less effective in identifying its cause. US is the preferred screening method for biliary obstruction because of its low cost and convenience. Unenhanced helical CT has a reported sensitivity of 88% in detection of stones in the common bile duct. MR can also demonstrate biliary dilation and may be more effective than CT or US in demonstrating associated tumors.

MR cholangiopancreatography (MRCP), performed using extreme T2W sequences, offers a noninvasive method of high-resolution imaging of the biliary tree (21). MRCP takes advantage of the long T2 characteristic of bile. Extreme T2 weighting demonstrates bright bile ducts with dark surrounding soft tissues (Fig. 27.24). However, any static fluid will also be bright on MRCP images, so ascites, hepatic and renal cysts, and fluid in the bowel may obscure the biliary tree. Similar to contrast cholangiography, stones are seen as hypodense filling defects (Table 27.8).

Endoscopic retrograde cholangiography and percutaneous transhepatic cholangiography supplement cross-sectional imaging methods by providing access to the biliary tree for contrast injection and subsequent catheter drainage or biliary stent placement. Operative cholangiography is used to visualize nonpalpable bile duct stones at surgery, and T-tube cholangiography is used to visualize common duct stones following surgery. Radionuclide imaging utilizing technetium-99m-iminodiacetic acid is useful for showing the patency of biliary-enteric anastomoses and for demonstrating bile leaks and fistulae. Scintigraphy has the greatest sensitivity for early obstruction. IV cholangiography involves the use of highly toxic contrast agents and has been abandoned in favor of other techniques. Functional CT and MR cholangiography using oral cholangiographic agents, iopanoic acid (Telepaque) for CT, and mangafodipir trisodium for MR are under investigation.

TABLE 27.8 Causes of Filling Defects in the Bile Ducts

Biliary stones
Air bubbles
Blood clots
Neoplasms
Cholangiocarcinoma
Ampullary carcinoma
Granular cell myoblastoma
Mesenchymal tumor
Parasites
Ascaris lumbricoides
Liver fluke

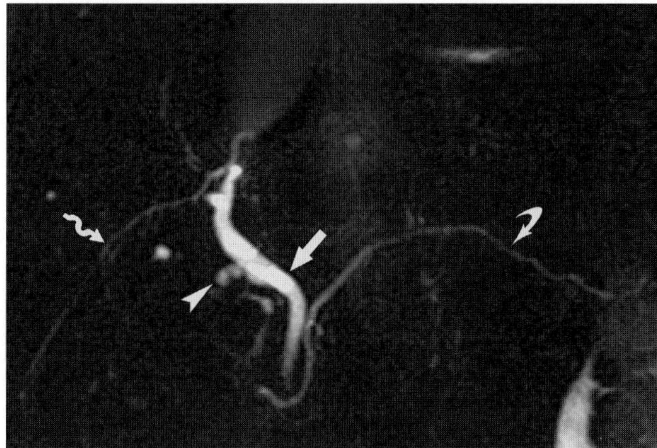

FIGURE 27.24. **Normal MR Cholangiopancreatography (MRCP).** Image from a MRCP in a patient who has had a cholecystectomy shows the cystic duct remnant (*arrowhead*), normal common bile duct (*straight arrow*), normal pancreatic duct (*curved arrow*), and normal major intrahepatic bile ducts (*squiggly arrow*).

Anatomy of the Biliary Tract. The bile ducts arise as bile capillaries between hepatocytes and join progressively larger branches until two main trunks are formed, draining the right and left lobes of the liver. The ducts of the left hepatic lobe are more anterior than those of the right hepatic lobe. This relationship must be kept in mind when contrast cholangiography is performed. Contrast agents flow to the most dependent portions of the biliary tree and may not opacify nondependent ducts. Failure to fill ducts before gravitational repositioning must not be interpreted as evidence of obstruction.

The right and left hepatic ducts combine to form the *common hepatic duct* (CHD), which courses with the portal vein and hepatic artery in the porta hepatis. The *cystic duct* courses posteriorly and inferiorly from the gallbladder to join the CHD and form the *common bile duct* (CBD). The CBD runs ventral to the portal vein and to the right of the hepatic artery, descending from the porta hepatis along the free right margin of the hepatoduodenal ligament to the duodenal bulb. The distal third of the CBD turns caudally and descends in the groove between the descending duodenum and the head of the pancreas, just anterior to the IVC. The CBD tapers distally as it ends in the *sphincter of Oddi*, which protrudes into the duodenum as the *ampulla of Vater*. The CBD and the pancreatic duct share a common orifice in 60% of individuals and have separate orifices in the remainder. However, because of their close proximity, tumors of the ampulla region generally obstruct both ducts. The CHD and CBD are considered to be extrahepatic bile ducts (EHBDs).

Normal intrahepatic bile ducts (IHBDs) are occasionally seen on US and on postcontrast helical CT with thin (5-mm) collimation. Normal IHBDs do not exceed 40% of the diameter of the adjacent portal vein, or 2 mm in diameter in the central liver or 1.8 mm in diameter in the peripheral liver. The extrahepatic CBD is routinely visualized and does not exceed 6 to 7 mm in internal diameter. Normal ducts appear larger on contrast cholangiography studies because of distention and magnification. Slightly larger common ducts are also normal in elderly patients because of elastic tissue degeneration with aging. Cholecystectomy is not proven to alter normal common duct size. Care must be taken to differentiate an enlarged common duct from an enlarged hepatic artery. Color Doppler is useful to make this differentiation on US. Contrast enhancement of blood vessels makes differentiation easy on CT.

MRCP and cholangiographic studies demonstrate IHBD branches that parallel the portal veins and correspond to the Couinaud segments of the liver (22). The right hepatic duct drains segments V to VIII and is formed by the junction of the more horizontal coursing right posterior duct draining VI and VII and the more vertically coursing right anterior duct draining V and VIII. The left hepatic duct is formed by segmental ducts draining segments II, III, and IV. The duct of the caudate lobe (I) joins either the right or left hepatic duct. Variations include drainage of the right posterior duct into the left hepatic duct (13% to 19%); triple confluence, with the right posterior, right anterior, and left hepatic ducts uniting at a single position (11%); and anomalies of the cystic duct, including low insertion on the CBD, long parallel course with the CHD, and insertion on the medial rather than the lateral side of the CBD. These anomalies have significant importance to the biliary surgeon.

Biliary Dilatation

CT, US, and MR are highly effective at demonstrating the anatomic finding of biliary dilatation, which is usually equated with biliary obstruction. However, biliary obstruction may be present intermittently or in the early stage without biliary dilation being present. Alternatively, biliary dilatation may be present without obstruction, such as after surgical decompression or bypass. Patients with clinical evidence of biliary obstruction (i.e., elevated alkaline phosphatase and direct hyperbilirubinemia) may not have biliary dilation. Hepatitis causes swelling of hepatocytes, which blocks biliary capillaries and causes intrahepatic cholestasis without surgical obstruction.

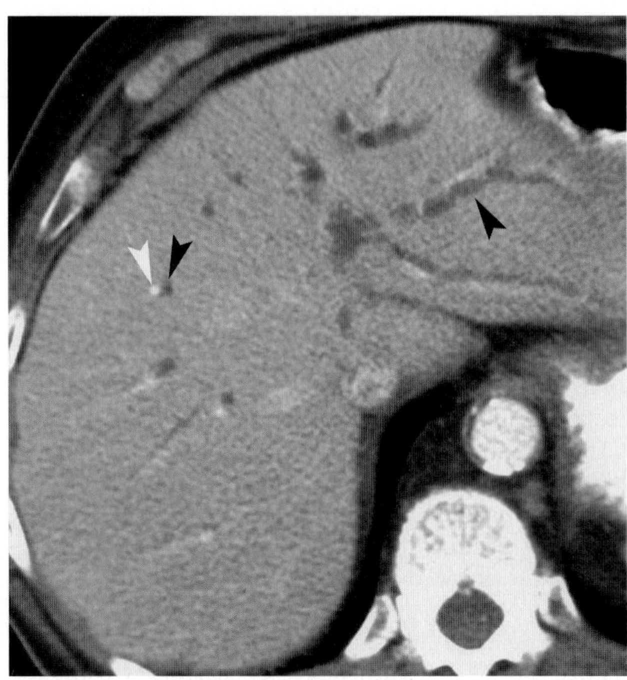

FIGURE 27.25. **Biliary Dilation.** A CT scan demonstrates dilated intrahepatic ducts (*black arrowheads*), which are easily differentiated from portal veins (*white arrowhead*) and hepatic veins by contrast enhancement of the blood vessels. Note that the diameter of the bile ducts clearly exceeds 40% of the diameter of the adjacent portal vein. Biliary dilatation in this patient was caused by adenocarcinoma of the head of the pancreas.

Signs of biliary dilation include the following: (*1*) multiple branching tubular, round, or oval structures that course toward the porta hepatis; (*2*) diameter of intrahepatic bile ducts larger than 40% of the diameter of the adjacent portal vein (Fig. 27.25); (*3*) dilation of the common duct greater than 6 mm; and (*4*) gallbladder diameter greater than 5 cm, when obstruction is distal to the cystic duct. Benign disease is responsible for approximately 75% of cases of obstructive jaundice in the adult, while malignant disease causes the remainder. Gradual tapering of a dilated common duct suggests benign stricture. Gallstones may be identified in the bile duct surrounded by a crescent of bile. Abrupt termination of a dilated common duct is characteristic of a malignant process (23).

Infected bile is present in up to 10% of cases of complete biliary obstruction and 60% of cases of partial or intermittent biliary obstruction. IV antibiotic therapy is warranted prior to biliary interventional procedures in the obstructed patient.

Causes of biliary dilation and obstruction (Table 27.9) include the following.

Choledocholithiasis is responsible for approximately 20% of cases of obstructive jaundice in the adult (Fig. 27.26). Gallstones are present in the gallbladder in

TABLE 27.9 Causes of Biliary Tract Obstruction

BENIGN (75% of cases)
- Benign stricture
  - Surgery/instrumentation
  - Trauma
  - Stone passage
  - Pancreatitis
  - Cholangitis
  - Choledochal cyst
- Stone impacted in duct
- Parasite (*Ascariasis*)
- Liver cyst

MALIGNANT (25% of cases)
- Pancreatic carcinoma
- Ampullary/duodenal carcinoma
- Cholangiocarcinoma
- Metastasis

10% of the population, but the presence of stones in the gallbladder does not necessarily mean that stones are the cause of ductal obstruction. In addition, 1% to 3% of patients with choledocholithiasis will have no stones in the gallbladder.

The sensitivity of US for stones in the bile ducts ranges from 20% to 80%. Stone detection by US is much improved when the CBD is dilated and the pancreatic head is well visualized. CT sensitivity is 70% to 80%, with stones appearing as intraluminal masses of varying attenuation. The "target sign" or "crescent sign" describes the appearance

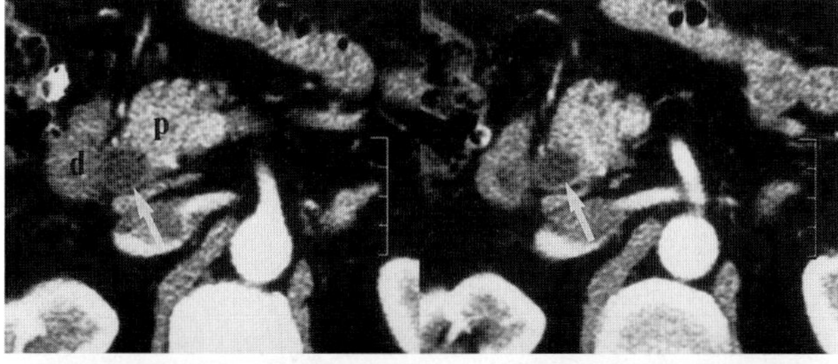

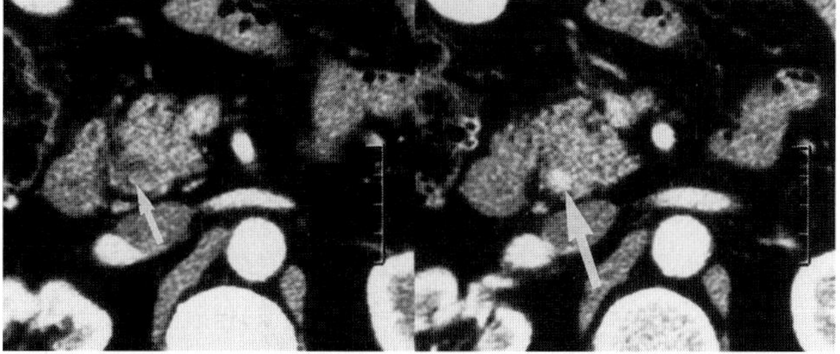

FIGURE 27.26. **Obstructing Stone in Common Bile Duct.** Serial CT images obtained from a jaundiced patient demonstrate dilatation of the common bile duct (*small arrows*) caused by an obstructing high-density gallstone (*large arrow*) impacted in the distal common bile duct. Note the course of the common bile duct in relationship to the head of the pancreas (p) and descending duodenum (d).

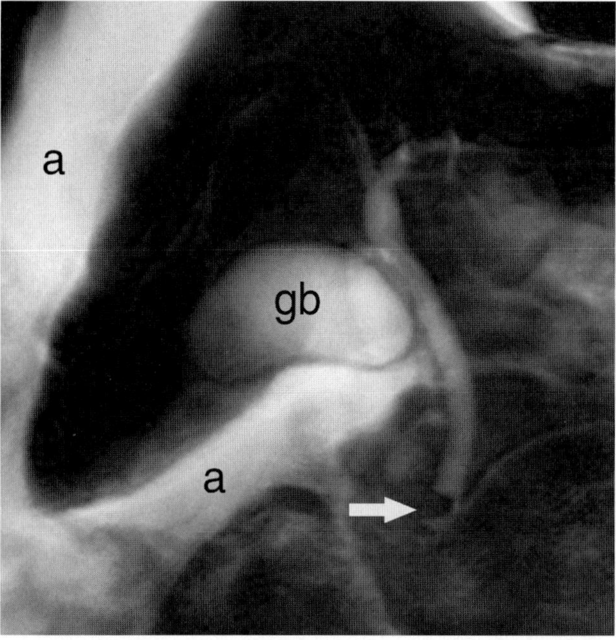

FIGURE 27.27. **Choledocholithiasis.** MR cholangiopancreatography image demonstrates two stones (*arrow*) seen as filling defects in the distal common bile duct. Ascites (a) outlines the liver. A normal gallbladder (gb) is evident.

of an intraluminal stone that is partially surrounded by a crescent of low-attenuation bile (24). Contrast studies and MRCP have the highest sensitivity for stone detection (95% to 99%) and demonstrate stones as dark filling defects within bright bile (Fig. 27.27).

Benign stricture is the cause of 40% to 45% of obstructive jaundice in the adult. Causes of benign stricture include trauma, surgery, prior biliary interventional procedures, recurrent cholangitis, previous passage of stones through the bile ducts, radiation therapy, and perforated duodenal ulcer. The wall of the involved CBD enhances minimally with benign strictures, while hyperenhancement of the CBD during the portal venous phase is evidence of malignant stricture (25).

Pancreatitis is responsible for approximately 8% of cases of biliary obstruction. Inflammation, fibrosis, and inflammatory masses narrow the bile ducts.

Primary sclerosing cholangitis (PSC) is associated with a history of ulcerative colitis in 50% to 70% of cases (26). PSC is characterized by insidious onset of jaundice, with progressive disease affecting both IHBDs and EHBDs. Alternating dilation and stenosis (Fig. 27.28) produces a characteristic beaded pattern of the IHBDs. Small saccular outpouchings (duct diverticula), demonstrated on cholangiography, are considered to be pathognomonic. Complications include biliary cirrhosis (50%) and cholangiocarcinoma.

AIDS-associated cholangitis is characterized by thickening of the walls of the bile ducts and the gallbladder

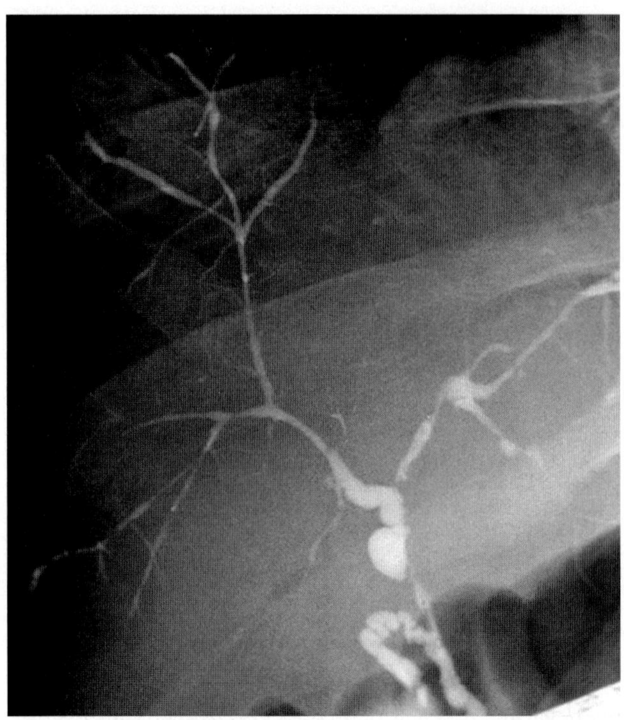

FIGURE 27.28. **Primary Sclerosing Cholangitis.** Radiograph from an endoscopic retrograde cholangiography demonstrates the focal irregular strictures and focal mild dilatation of intrahepatic bile ducts that are typical of early stage sclerosing cholangitis.

because of inflammation and edema. Infection by opportunistic organisms, most commonly cytomegalovirus and *Cryptosporidium*, as well as reaction to HIV itself, are implicated as the causes of observed disease. Bile ducts are commonly dilated in association with stenosis at the ampulla. Ulcers in the common duct, inflammatory changes in the duodenum, and additional evidence of infection with opportunistic organisms are commonly associated.

Recurrent pyogenic cholangitis has been called *Oriental cholangiohepatitis* because it is an endemic disease in Southeast Asia (27). It is characterized by recurrent attacks of jaundice, abdominal pain, fever, and chills. Intrahepatic and extrahepatic bile ducts are dilated and filled with soft pigmented stones and pus. The disease is associated with parasitic infestation (clonorchiasis, ascariasis) and nutritional deficiency. Findings include intraductal stones, severe extrahepatic biliary dilation, focal strictures, and straightening and rigidity of intrahepatic ducts. Complications include liver abscess, biloma, pancreatitis, and cholangiocarcinoma.

Caroli disease is an uncommon congenital anomaly of the biliary tract characterized by saccular ectasia of the IHBDs without biliary obstruction (28). Only one hepatic lobe or segment may be affected. The EHBDs are spared in 50% of cases. Findings include: (*1*) saccular dilatation of IHBDs, giving the appearance on cross-sectional imaging of scattered intrahepatic cysts that communicate with the biliary tree; (*2*) enhancing fibrovascular bundles seen centrally within many of the dilated ducts, producing the characteristic "central dot sign;" (*3*) segmental distribution of the bile duct abnormality, with normal appearance of unaffected liver segments; (*4*) cholangiography showing a characteristic pattern of focal biliary narrowing and saccular dilatation; and (*5*) dilatation of the CBD (10 to 30 mm) in half of cases. The disease is associated with medullary sponge kidney and autosomal-recessive polycystic kidney disease. Complications include pyogenic cholangitis, liver abscess, and biliary stones. Cholangiocarcinoma develops in 7% of cases. Most cases present in childhood. Autosomal-recessive inheritance is evident in many cases.

Choledochal cysts are uncommon congenital anomalies of the biliary tree characterized by cystic dilation of the bile ducts (29). Many (60%) present in infancy or childhood, while others present in adulthood. Some are discovered by fetal US. The condition is much more common in females (70% to 84% of cases). Patients present with abdominal pain, mass, and jaundice. The Todani classification (1977) is typically used to describe choledochal cysts (Fig. 27.29). Type 1 lesions are most common (80% to 90%) and appear as fusiform or saccular dilatations (Fig. 27.30) of the CHD, CBD, or segments of each. Type 2 lesions are diverticula of the CBD attached by a narrow

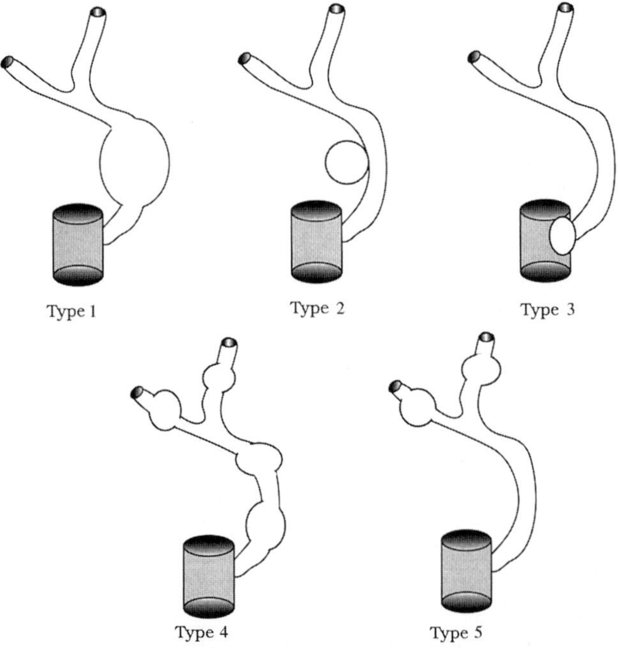

FIGURE 27.29. **Classification of Congenital Biliary Cysts.** Type 1 choledochal cysts (80% to 90% of cases) are focal, saccular or fusiform, dilatations of the common bile duct. Type 2 cysts (2%) are true diverticula of the common bile duct. Type 3 cysts (1.4% to 5%) are termed choledochoceles and are dilatations of the terminal intraduodenal portion of the common bile duct. A type 4 classification (19%) refers to multiple intrahepatic and extrahepatic bile duct cysts. Caroli disease is classified as type 5.

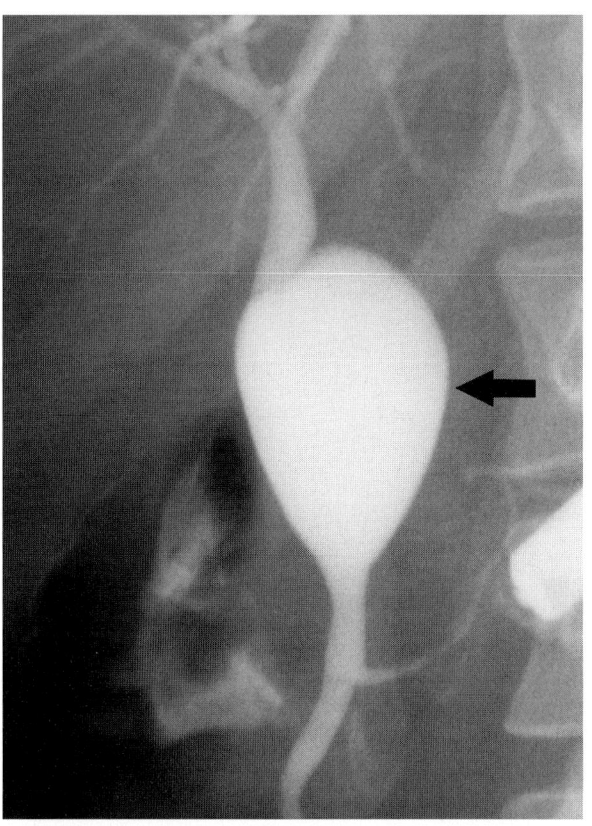

FIGURE 27.30. **Type 1 Choledochal Cyst.** Radiograph from endoscopic retrograde cholangiography demonstrates saccular dilation (*arrow*) of the common bile duct, which is typical of the most common form of choledochal cyst: type 1.

stalk. Type 3 lesions are termed *choledochoceles* and are focal dilatations of the intraduodenal portion of the CBD, closely resembling ureteroceles. Type IV lesions are defined as multiple focal dilatations of the IHBDs and EHBDs usually with a focal large cystic dilatation of the CBD. Type 5 lesions are referred to as Caroli disease, which is more properly classified as a disease separate from choledochal cyst.

Pancreatic and ampullary carcinomas are the cause of 20% to 25% of cases of biliary obstruction in the adult. Metastatic disease from lung, breast, GI tumors, and lymphoma accounts for 2% of cases.

Cholangiocarcinoma is the second most common malignant primary hepatic tumor (30). Tumors arise from the epithelium of bile ducts and are usually adenocarcinomas (90%). Growth patterns include mass forming, periductal infiltrating, and intraductal polypoid. *Peripheral cholangiocarcinoma* (10%) presents as an intrahepatic hypodense mass, with adjacent biliary dilatation present in only 25% of cases (Fig. 27.31). MDCT demonstrates delayed, mild, thin, incomplete, rimlike enhancement with low tumoral attenuation in most cases. *Hilar cholangiocarcinoma* (Klatskin tumor) (25%) occurs near the junction of the right and left bile ducts (Fig. 27.32). The tumor is usually small, poorly differentiated, and aggressive and causes

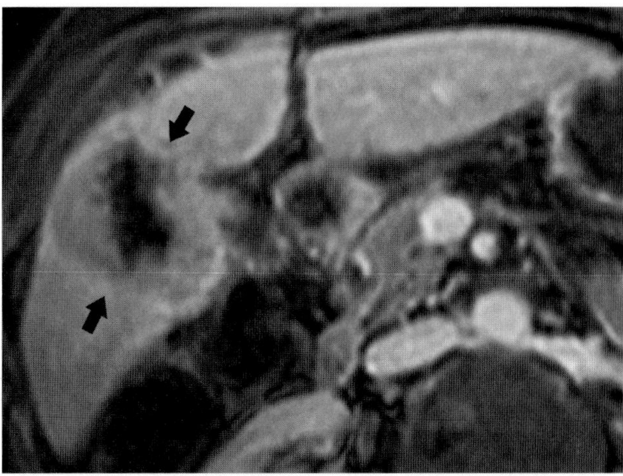

FIGURE 27.31. **Cholangiocarcinoma: Peripheral.** Postcontrast, T1W, fat-suppressed MR shows a heterogeneous mass (*between arrows*) within the liver. Biopsy confirmed cholangiocarcinoma. No dilated bile ducts were evident.

obstruction of both ductal systems. *Extrahepatic cholangiocarcinoma* (65%) causes stenosis or obstruction of the CBD in most cases (95%) and presents as an intraductal polypoid mass in 5%. Infiltrating cholangiocarcinoma shows thickening of the wall of the involved bile duct, with

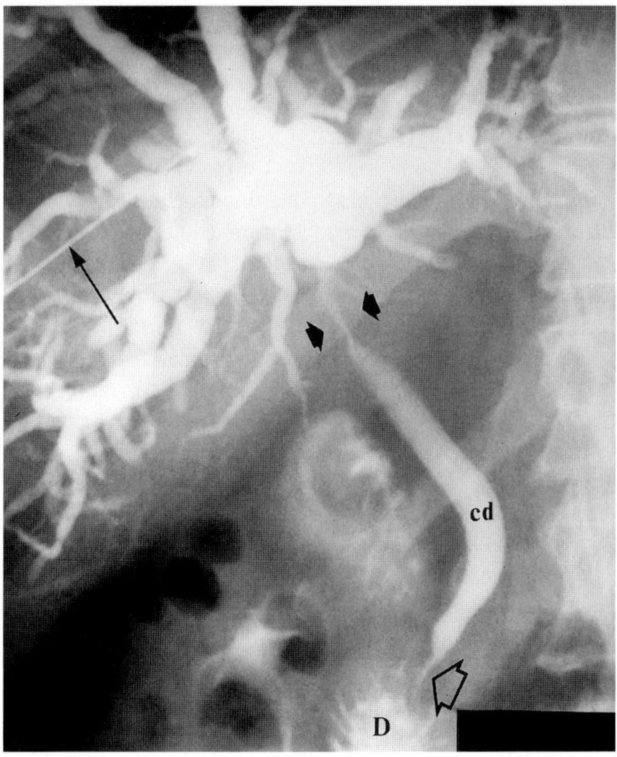

FIGURE 27.32. **Cholangiocarcinoma: Hilar.** Percutaneous transhepatic cholangiogram (PTC) demonstrates abrupt focal narrowing (*short arrows*) of the proximal common bile duct (cd) near the bifurcation. The intrahepatic bile ducts are diffusely dilated. The common bile duct shows normal narrowing at the ampulla of Vater (*open arrow*). The PTC needle (*long arrow*) is evident. D, duodenum.

hyperenhancement during the arterial phase (25). Predisposing conditions include choledochal cyst, ulcerative colitis, Caroli disease, *Clonorchis sinensis* infection, and PSC. The tumor may be infiltrative, desmoplastic, and small, making imaging detection as well as needle biopsy difficult. Abrupt stricture and thickening of the duct wall may be the only findings. Cross-sectional imaging is used to detect adenopathy and hepatic metastases. Prognosis is poor, with fewer than 20% of tumors being resectable.

Gas in the Biliary Tract

Gas in the biliary tract is most commonly encountered in the patient with a surgically created biliary-enteric anastomosis or who has received a sphincterotomy to facilitate stone passage (Table 27.10).

Cholecystoduodenal fistula is most commonly caused by erosion of a gallstone through the gallbladder and into the duodenum. When the gallstone is large, it may cause small bowel obstruction, i.e., "gallstone ileus." The gallstone may also erode into the colon and pass spontaneously in the feces. Cholecystoduodenal fistula is most common in women because of the higher incidence of gallstones.

Choledochoduodenal fistula is caused by a penetrating peptic ulcer eroding into the common bile duct (Fig. 27.33).

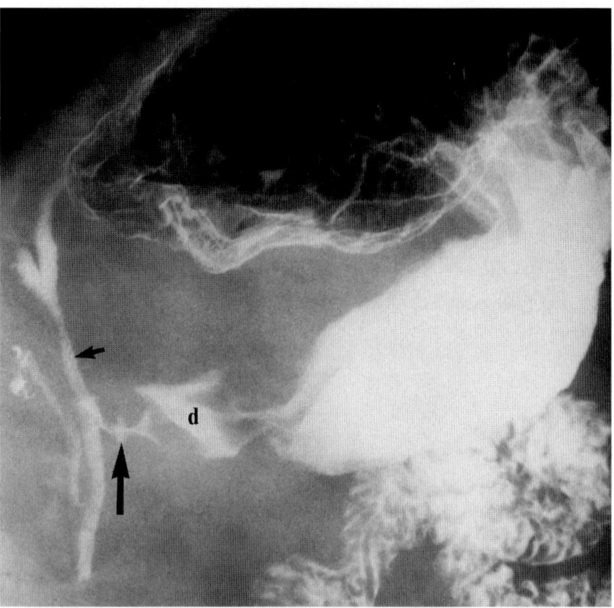

FIGURE 27.33. **Choledochoduodenal Fistula.** An upper GI series demonstrates filling of the bile ducts because of a penetrating duodenal ulcer that created a fistula (*large arrow*) between the duodenum (d) and the bile ducts (*small arrow*).

GALLBLADDER

Imaging Methods. US is the imaging method of choice for the gallbladder. It offers high anatomic detail, convenience, and cost efficiency. Gallbladder US is reviewed in detail in Chapter 36. Cholescintigraphy utilizing technetium-99m-iminodiacetic acid has sensitivity and specificity comparable to US for the diagnosis of acute cholecystitis. Oral cholecystograms have been abandoned in favor of other imaging methods. However, oral biliary contrast agents, previously used for oral cholecystograms, are currently utilized for CT cholangiography. Plain radiographs demonstrate calcified gallstones, porcelain gallbladder, and emphysematous cholecystitis. CT, as the imaging method of choice for the acute abdomen, frequently provides imaging diagnosis of gallbladder disease (31).

TABLE 27.10 Causes of Gas in the Biliary Tract

Postsurgical
Sphincterotomy
Choledochoduodenostomy
Choledochojejunostomy
Biliary-enteric fistula
Cholecystoduodenal fistula (gallstone erodes into CBD)
Choledochoduodenal fistula (ulcer penetrates CBD)
Surgery/trauma
Tumor erosion with fistula
Infection
Emphysematous cholecystitis
Pyogenic cholangitis

CBD, common bile duct.

Anatomy. The gallbladder lies on the underside of the liver, in the fossa formed by the junction of the left and right lobes. While the position of the fundus is inconsistent, the neck of the gallbladder is invariably positioned in the porta hepatis and major interlobar fissure. The gallbladder fundus frequently causes a mass impression on the top of the duodenal bulb. Kinking and folding of the gallbladder is common and generally easily recognized by careful image analysis. The so-called phrygian cap, which is descriptive of folding of the gallbladder fundus, is a common normal variant. Septa within the gallbladder may be partial or complete. The spiral valves of Heister are small folds in the cystic duct.

The normal gallbladder is well distended with bile following a 4-hour fast and is easily visualized. A gallbladder larger than 5 cm in diameter is considered enlarged (hydropic), while a gallbladder smaller than 2 cm in diameter is considered contracted. The normal gallbladder wall does not exceed 3 mm in thickness—measured from gallbladder lumen to liver parenchyma—when the gallbladder is distended. The normal gallbladder lumen is free of particulate debris and is fluid density on imaging studies.

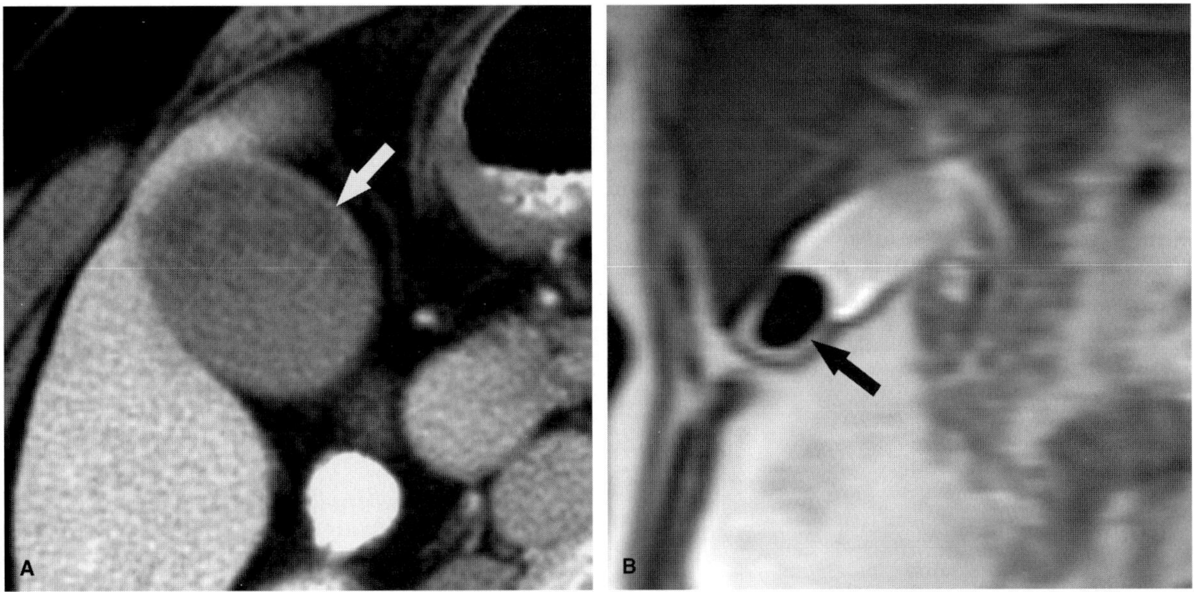

FIGURE 27.34. **Cholelithiasis. A.** CT reveals numerous subtle low-attenuation floating gallstones (*arrow*) within the gallbladder. The stones are nearly isodense with bile. Stones may be overlooked on CT because they are isodense with bile or because of their small size. **B.** Coronal T2WI shows a large gallstone (*arrow*) as a filling defect within high-signal bile.

Gallstones are present in 8% of the general population and 15% of the population aged 40 to 60 years. Approximately 85% of gallstones are predominantly cholesterol, while 15% are predominantly bilirubin (pigment stones) related to hemolytic anemia. Approximately 10% of stones are sufficiently radiopaque to be detected by conventional radiographs as laminated or faceted calcifications. Fissures within gallstones may contain nitrogen gas that appears on plain film as branching linear lucencies resembling a "crow's foot." Gallstones are most common in women (female:male = 4:1) and in patients with hemolytic anemia, diseases of the ileum, cirrhosis, and diabetes mellitus (32).

US detects 95% of all gallstones, whereas CT detects only 80% to 85%. Gallstones vary in CT attenuation, from fat density to calcium density (Fig. 27.34). Up to 20% of gallstones are isodense with bile and not detected by CT, while some gallstones are missed because of their small size. Care must be taken to avoid interpreting contrast in adjacent bowel as cholelithiasis.

Contrast studies, MRCP, and T2WIs demonstrate gallstones as "filling defects"—rounded or faceted dark objects within high-density bile.

Differential considerations for lesions in the gallbladder that may be mistaken for gallstones include the following.

Sludge balls or tumefactive biliary sludge result from biliary stasis. The bile thickens and forms mobile masses that move with changes in patient position.

Cholesterol polyps are common benign, polypoid masses that result from accumulation of triglycerides and cholesterol in macrophages in the gallbladder wall. They are of no clinical significance. All are 10 mm or smaller.

Adenomyomatosis may be focal and present as a polypoid mass fixed to the gallbladder wall.

Adenomatous polyps are small, usually flat masses fixed to the gallbladder wall.

Gallbladder carcinoma may present as a polypoid mass. Most are 1 cm or larger. Gallstones are usually present.

Acute Cholecystitis. Acute inflammation of the gallbladder is caused by gallstones obstructing the cystic duct in 90% of cases. *Acalculous cholecystitis* occurs nearly always in patients with predisposing conditions (listed subsequently). Cholescintigraphy and US have comparable sensitivities and specificities in the diagnosis of acute cholecystitis.

Scintigraphic diagnosis of acute cholecystitis is based on obstruction of the cystic duct with nonvisualization of the gallbladder. The normal gallbladder demonstrates progressive accumulation of radionuclide activity over 30 minutes to 1 hour following injection of technetium-99m-iminodiacetic acid. Delayed visualization of the gallbladder may be seen in patients with biliary stasis caused by fasting or hyperalimentation. Delayed images taken at 4 hours post-radionuclide injection are needed to assess for this possibility. The test is considered positive if there is prompt tracer accumulation in the liver with excretion of tracer into the bowel and without gallbladder visualization at 4 hours. The test may be considered positive at 1 hour post-radionuclide injection if the gallbladder does not visualize within 20 minutes of IV injection of morphine.

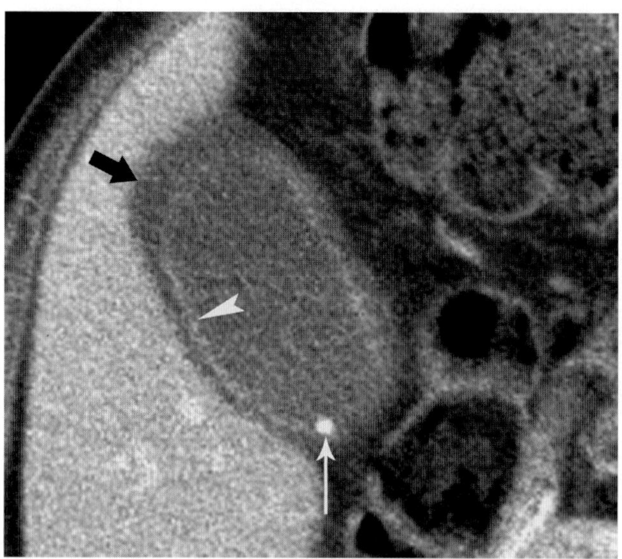

FIGURE 27.35. **Acute Cholecystitis.** Postcontrast CT demonstrates fluid (*black arrow*) around the enhancing mucosa (*white arrowhead*) of the gallbladder and a small, high-attenuation gallstone (*thin arrow*) within the gallbladder lumen in a patient with acute, severe right upper quadrant pain. Surgery confirmed acute cholecystitis.

Confident US diagnosis of acute cholecystitis requires the presence of three findings: cholelithiasis; edema of the gallbladder wall, seen as a band of echolucency in the wall; and a positive sonographic Murphy sign.

CT demonstrates the following (Fig. 27.35): gallstones, distended gallbladder, thickened gallbladder wall, subserosal edema, high-density bile, intraluminal sloughed membranes, inflammatory stranding in pericholecystic fat, pericholecystic fluid, blurring of the interface between gallbladder and liver, and prominent arterial phase enhancement of the liver adjacent to the gallbladder (31).

Acalculous cholecystitis causes special problems in diagnosis because the cystic duct is often not obstructed. Inflammation may be the result of gallbladder wall ischemia or direct bacterial infection. Patients at risk for acalculous cholecystitis include those with biliary stasis caused by lack of oral intake, posttrauma, postburn, postsurgery, or on total parenteral nutrition. Scintigraphy usually demonstrates lack of gallbladder visualization. Although this finding is 90% to 95% sensitive for acalculous cholecystitis, it is only 38% specific. False-positive conditions for nonvisualization include hyperalimentation and prolonged severe illness, which are predisposing conditions for acalculous cholecystitis. US demonstrates a distended tender gallbladder with thickened wall but without stones. Many patients are too ill to elicit a reliable sonographic Murphy sign.

Sludge is a term used to describe the presence of thick particulate matter in highly concentrated bile. Calcium bilirubinate and cholesterol crystals precipitate in the bile when biliary stasis is prolonged because of a lack of oral intake, hyperalimentation, or biliary obstruction. Sludge appears as echodense bile on US and as high-attenuation bile on CT. Because sludge may be found in a fasting but otherwise normal patient, its presence is not definitive evidence of gallbladder disease. Pus, blood, and milk of calcium are additional causes of dense bile.

Complications of acute cholecystitis include the following.

Gangrenous cholecystitis indicates the presence of necrosis of the gallbladder wall. The patient is at risk for gallbladder perforation. Findings include mucosal irregularity and asymmetric thickening of the gallbladder wall with multiple lucent layers, indicating mucosal ulceration and reactive edema.

Perforation of the gallbladder is a life-threatening complication seen in 5% to 10% of cases. Perforation may occur adjacent to the liver, resulting in pericholecystic abscess; into the peritoneal cavity, resulting in generalized peritonitis; or into adjacent bowel, resulting in biliary-enteric fistula. Overall mortality is as high as 24%. A focal pericholecystic fluid collection suggests pericholecystic abscess.

Emphysematous cholecystitis results from infection of the gallbladder with gas-forming organisms, usually *E coli* or *Clostridium perfringens*. Approximately 40% of patients are diabetic. Gallstones may or may not be present. Gas is demonstrated within the wall or within the lumen of the gallbladder by plain film or CT. On US, intramural gas has an arc-like configuration that is difficult to differentiate from calcification and porcelain gallbladder.

Mirizzi syndrome refers to the condition of biliary obstruction resulting from a gallstone in the cystic duct eroding into the adjacent common duct and causing an inflammatory mass that obstructs the common duct. Visualization of a stone at the junction of the cystic duct and the common hepatic duct in a patient with biliary obstruction and gallbladder inflammation suggests the diagnosis.

Chronic cholecystitis includes a spectrum of pathology that shares the presence of gallstones and chronic gallbladder inflammation. Patients with chronic cholecystitis complain of recurrent attacks of right upper quadrant pain and biliary colic. Imaging findings include gallstones, thickening of the gallbladder wall, contraction of the gallbladder lumen, delayed visualization of the gallbladder on cholescintigraphy, and poor contractility. Variants of chronic cholecystitis include the following.

Porcelain gallbladder describes the presence of dystrophic calcification in the wall of an obstructed and chronically inflamed gallbladder (Fig. 27.36). The condition is associated with gallstones in 90% of cases. Porcelain gallbladder carries a 10% to 20% risk of gallbladder carcinoma. Cholecystectomy is usually indicated.

Milk of calcium bile, also called limy bile, is associated with an obstructed cystic duct, chronic cholecystitis, and gallstones. Particulate matter with a high concentration of

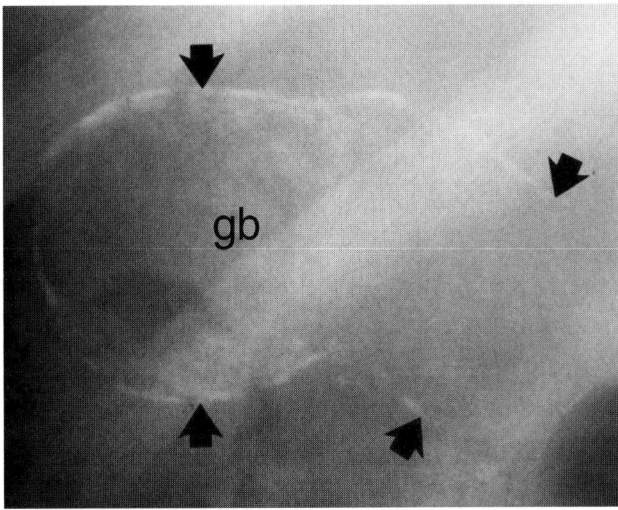

FIGURE 27.36. **Porcelain Gallbladder.** Conventional radiograph of the right upper quadrant of the abdomen shows calcification (*arrows*) in the wall of the gallbladder (gb). This finding is indicative of chronic obstruction of the cystic duct with chronic cholecystitis. The risk of gallbladder carcinoma is increased.

calcium compounds is precipitated in the bile, making the bile radiopaque on plain films or CT. Dependent layering of bile can be demonstrated on plain film radiographs. The bile is extremely echogenic on US, and gallstones may be visualized within it.

Xanthogranulomatous cholecystitis is an uncommon variant of chronic cholecystitis characterized by nodular deposits of lipid-laden macrophages in the gallbladder wall and proliferative fibrosis. Imaging findings include marked wall thickening (2 cm), fat-density nodules in the wall, and narrowing of the lumen. Cholelithiasis is frequently present. The condition is difficult to differentiate from gallbladder carcinoma.

Thickening of the gallbladder wall is present when the wall thickness at the hepatic aspect of the gallbladder exceeds 3 mm in patients who have fasted at least 8 hours. Conditions associated with wall thickening include the following.

Acute and Chronic Cholecystitis. Wall thickening is a usual feature of acute cholecystitis and is present in 50% of cases of chronic cholecystitis.

Hepatitis causes reduction in bile flow, which results in reduced gallbladder volume and thickening of the gallbladder wall in approximately half of patients.

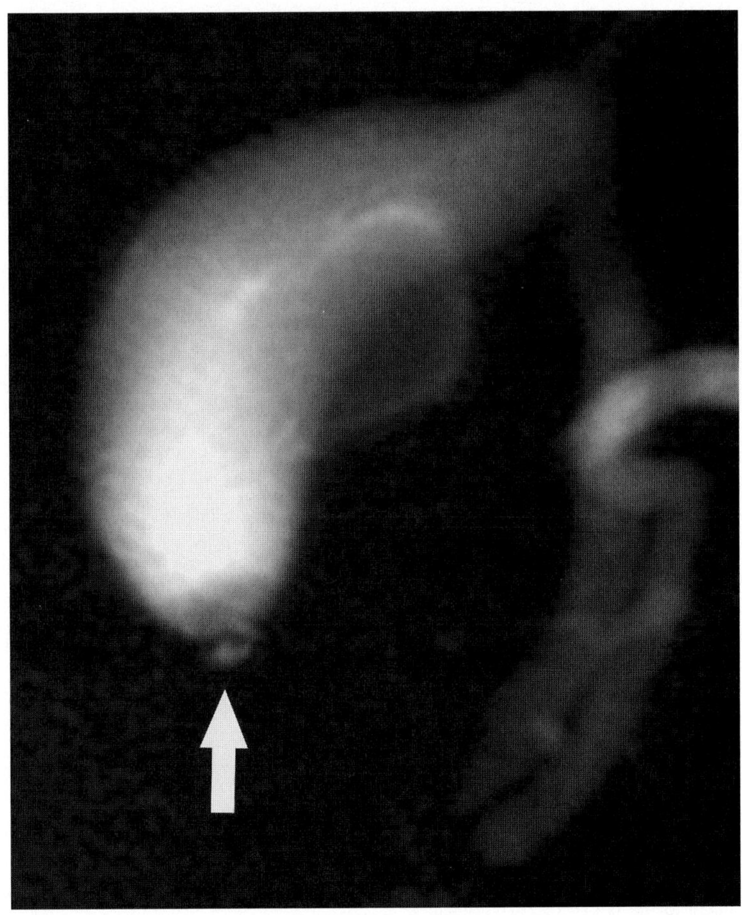

FIGURE 27.37. **Adenomyomatosis of the Gallbladder.** An MR cholangiopancreatography image shows focal thickening of the wall of gallbladder fundus with a Rokitansky-Aschoff sinus (*arrow*) extending into the thickened wall.

Portal venous hypertension and *congestive heart failure* may cause wall thickening by passive venous congestion.

AIDS is associated with thickening of the gallbladder wall and the walls of the bile ducts. Opportunistic organisms are sometimes present.

Hypoalbuminemia is associated with thickened gallbladder wall in 60% of patients.

Gallbladder carcinoma usually presents as a focal mass but may cause only focal wall thickening.

Adenomyomatosis is the most frequent benign condition of the gallbladder and is characterized by hyperplasia of the mucosa and smooth muscle. It is usually focal and in the fundus, but may be diffuse, involving the entire gallbladder. Outpouchings of mucosa into or through the muscularis form characteristic Rokitansky-Aschoff sinuses (Fig. 27.37). The condition has no malignant potential. Coexisting gallstones are commonly present (33).

Gallbladder Carcinoma. Adenocarcinoma of the gallbladder is commonly overlooked or misdiagnosed preoperatively. The presence of gallstones in 70% to 80% of cases masks the findings of cancer, especially with US examination. Gallbladder carcinoma is most often a tumor of elderly women (>60 years, female:male = 4:1). Patients present with pain, anorexia, weight loss, and jaundice. Calcification of the gallbladder wall (porcelain gallbladder) is a risk factor. Imaging findings include the following: (*1*) intraluminal soft tissue mass (Fig. 27.38); (*2*) focal or diffuse thickening of the gallbladder wall; (*3*) soft tissue mass replacing the gallbladder; (*4*) gallstones; (*5*) extension of tumor into the liver, bile ducts, and adjacent bowel; (*6*) dilated bile ducts; and (*7*) metastases to periportal and peripancreatic lymph nodes and liver. Most tumors are unresectable at discovery (34).

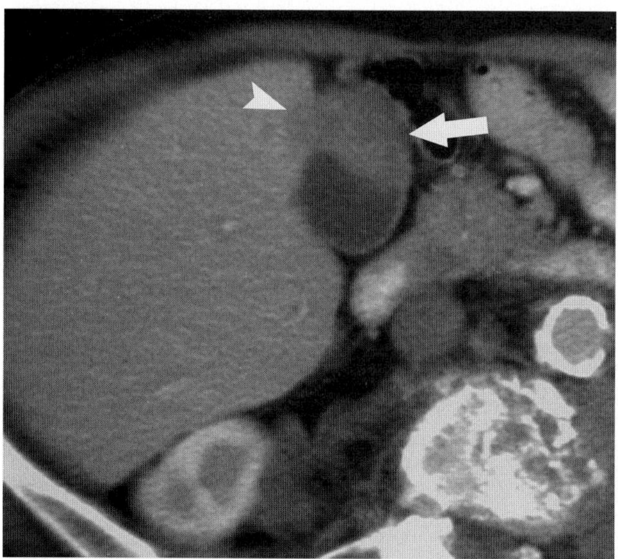

FIGURE 27.38. **Gallbladder Carcinoma.** Postcontrast CT shows an enhancing soft tissue mass (*arrow*) within the lumen of the gallbladder. Direct invasion of tumor into the adjacent liver parenchyma is evident (*arrowhead*).

REFERENCES

1. Colagrande S, Centi N, La Villa G, Villari N. Transient hepatic attenuation differences. AJR Am J Roentgenol 2004;183:459–464.
2. Yoshimitsu K, Honda H, Kuroiwa T, Irie H, et al. Unusual hemodynamics and pseudolesions of the noncirrhotic liver at CT. Radiographics 2001;21:S81-S96.
3. Mortele KJ, Segatto E, Ros PR. The infected liver: radiologic-pathologic correlation. Radiographics 2004;24:937–955.
4. Dodd GDI, Baron RL, Oliver JHI, Federle MP. Spectrum of imaging findings of the liver in end-stage cirrhosis: part II, focal abnormalities. AJR Am J Roentgenol 1999;173:1185–1192.
5. Dodd GDI, Baron RL, Oliver JHI, Federle MP. Spectrum of imaging findings of the liver in end-stage cirrhosis: part I, gross morphology and diffuse abnormalities. AJR Am J Roentgenol 1999;173:1031–1036.
6. Gupta AA, Kim DC, Krinsky GA, Lee VS. CT and MRI of cirrhosis and its mimics. AJR Am J Roentgenol 2004;183:1595–1601.
7. Hussain SM, Zondervan PE, Ijzermans JNM, Schalm SW, et al. Benign versus malignant hepatic nodules: MR imaging findings with pathologic correlation. Radiographics 2002;22:1023–1039.
8. Gallego C, Velasco M, Marcuello P, Tejedor D, De Campo L, Friera A. Congenital and acquired anomalies of the portal venous system. Radiographics 2003;22:141–159.
9. Brancatelli G, Federle MP, Graziola L, Golfieri R, Lencioni R. Benign regenerative nodules in Budd-Chiari syndrome and other vascular disorders of the liver: radiologic-pathologic and clinical correlation. Radiographics 2002;22:847–862.
10. Tani I, Kurihara Y, Kawaguchi A, et al. MR imaging of diffuse liver disease. AJR Am J Roentgenol 2000;174:965–971.
11. Sica GT, Ji H, Ros PR. CT and MR imaging of hepatic metastases. AJR Am J Roentgenol 2000;174:691–698.
12. Vilgrain M, Boulos L, Vullierme M-P, Denys A, Terris B, Menu Y. Imaging of atypical hemangiomas of the liver with pathologic correlation. Radiographics 2000;20:379–397.
13. Lee KHY, O'Malley MEO, Kachura JR, Haider M, Hanbidge A. Hepatocellular carcinoma: imaging and imaging-guided intervention. AJR Am J Roentgenol 2003;180:1015–1022.
14. Prasad SR, Wang H, Rosas H, et al. Fat-containing lesions of the liver: radiologic-pathologic correlation. Radiographics 2005;25:321–331.
15. Hussain SM, Terkivatan T, Zondervan PE, et al. Focal nodular hyperplasia: findings at state-of-the-art MR imaging, US, CT, and pathologic analysis. Radiographics 2004;24:3–19.
16. Graziola L, Federle MP, Brancatelli G, et al. Hepatic adenomas: imaging and pathologic findings. Radiographics 2001;21:877–894.
17. McLarney JK, Rucker PT, Bender GN, et al. Fibrolamellar carcinoma of the liver: radiologic-pathologic correlation. Radiographics 1999;19:453–471.
18. Mortele KJ, Ros PR. Cystic focal liver lesions in the adult: differential CT and MR imaging features. Radiographics 2001;21:895–910.
19. Kawamoto S, Soyer PA, Fishman EK, Bluemke DA. Nonneoplastic liver disease: evaluation with CT and MR imaging. Radiographics 1998;18:827–848.
20. Schwartz LH, Gandras EJ, Colangelo SM, Ercolani MC, Panicek DM. Prevalence and importance of small hepatic lesions found at CT in patients with cancer. Radiology 1999;210:71–74.
21. Jara H, Barish MA. MR cholangiopancreatography techniques. Semin Ultrasound CT MRI 1999;20:281–293.
22. Mortele KJ, Ros PR. Anatomic variants of the biliary tree: MR cholangiographic findings and clinical applications. AJR Am J Roentgenol 2001;177:389–394.
23. Soto JA, Alvarez O, Lopera JE, et al. Biliary obstruction: findings at MR cholangiography and cross-sectional MR imaging. Radiographics 2000;20:353–366.
24. Miller FH, Hwang CM, Gabriel H, Goodhartz LA, Omar AJ, Parsons WG III. Contrast-enhanced helical CT of choledocholithiasis. AJR Am J Roentgenol 2003;181:125–130.

25. Choi SH, Han JK, Lee JM, et al. Differentiating malignant from benign common bile duct stricture with multiphasic helical CT. Radiology 2005;236:178–183.
26. Vitellas KM, Keogan MT, Freed KS, et al. Radiologic manifestations of sclerosing cholangitis with emphasis on MR cholangiopancreatography. Radiographics 2000;20:959–975.
27. Lim JH. Oriental cholangiohepatitis: pathologic, clinical, and radiologic features. AJR Am J Roentgenol 1991;157:1–8.
28. Levy AD, Rohrmann CA Jr, Murakata LA, Lonergan GJ. Caroli's disease: radiologic spectrum with pathologic correlation. AJR Am J Roentgenol 2002;179:1053–1057.
29. Kim OH, Chung HJ, Choi BG. Imaging of the choledochal cyst. Radiographics 1995;15:69–88.
30. Lim JH. Cholangiocarcinoma: morphologic classification according to growth pattern and imaging findings. AJR Am J Roentgenol 2003;181:819–827.
31. Grand D, Horton KM, Fishman EK. CT of the gallbladder: spectrum of disease. AJR Am J Roentgenol 2004;183:163–170.
32. Bortoff GA, Chen MYM, Ott DJ, Wolfman NT, Routh WD. Gallbladder stones: imaging and intervention. Radiographics 2000;20:751–766.
33. Levy AD, Murakata LA, Abbott RM, Rohrmann CA Jr. Benign tumors and tumorlike lesions of the gallbladder and extrahepatic bile ducts: radiologic-pathologic correlation. Radiographics 2002;22:387–413.
34. Levy AD, Murkata LA, Rohrmann CA Jr. Gallbladder carcinoma: radiologic-pathologic correlation. Radiographics 2001;21:295–314.

Chapter 28

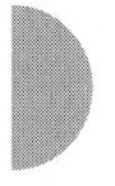

Pancreas and Spleen

William E. Brant

Pancreas
Imaging Techniques
Anatomy
Pancreatitis
Solid Lesions of the Pancreas
Cystic Lesions of the Pancreas

Spleen
Imaging Techniques
Anatomy
Splenomegaly
Cystic Lesions of the Spleen
Solid Lesions of the Spleen
AIDS

PANCREAS

Imaging Techniques

CT, US, and MR provide high-quality images of the pancreatic parenchyma and are used as the primary imaging modalities for the pancreas (Fig. 28.1). Multidetector CT (MDCT) optimizes contrast enhancement for detection of small tumors and provides the capability of CT angiography to detect vascular involvement by pancreatic tumor. Improved techniques and the use of gadolinium enhancement have increased the capability of MR to detect and characterize pancreatic lesions. Endoscopic retrograde cholangiopancreatography (ERCP) provides excellent visualization of the lumen of the pancreatic duct (Fig. 28.2), which is usually affected by any mass lesion of the pancreas. This procedure is performed by endoscopic cannulization of the bile and pancreatic ducts, followed by injection of a contrast agent and filming. MR cholangiopancreatography (MRCP) offers a noninvasive method of imaging the pancreatic duct as well as the biliary system (1). Secretin administration during MRCP increases pancreatic secretions and improves visualization of the pancreatic duct. Arteriography is now routinely performed using CT and MR angiographic techniques (CTA, MRA). US- and CT-guided biopsy and drainage procedures play a major role in the diagnosis and treatment of pancreatic diseases.

Anatomy

The pancreas is a tongue-shaped organ, approximately 12 to 15 cm in length, that lies within the anterior pararenal compartment of the retroperitoneum (Fig. 28.1). The pancreas is posterior to the left lobe of the liver, the stomach, and the lesser sac. It is anterior to the spine, the inferior vena cava, and the aorta. Pancreatic tissue is best recognized by identification of the vessels around it. The neck, body, and tail of the pancreas lie ventral to the splenic vein, with the tail extending into the hilum of the spleen. The splenic vein and pancreas are located anterior to the superior mesenteric artery. The head of the pancreas wraps around the junction of the superior mesenteric vein and the splenic vein, with the uncinate process of the pancreatic head extending under the superior mesenteric vein just anterior to the inferior vena cava. The splenic artery courses through the pancreatic bed in a tortuous course. Atherosclerotic splenic artery calcifications are easily mistaken for pancreatic calcifications. The lumen of the splenic artery may be mistaken for pancreatic cysts or a dilated pancreatic duct on CT without contrast or on US.

Maximum dimensions for pancreatic size are a 3.0-cm diameter for the head, 2.5-cm diameter for the body, and 2.0-cm diameter for the tail. The gland is somewhat larger in young patients and progressively decreases in size with age. Because the gland is not encapsulated, fatty

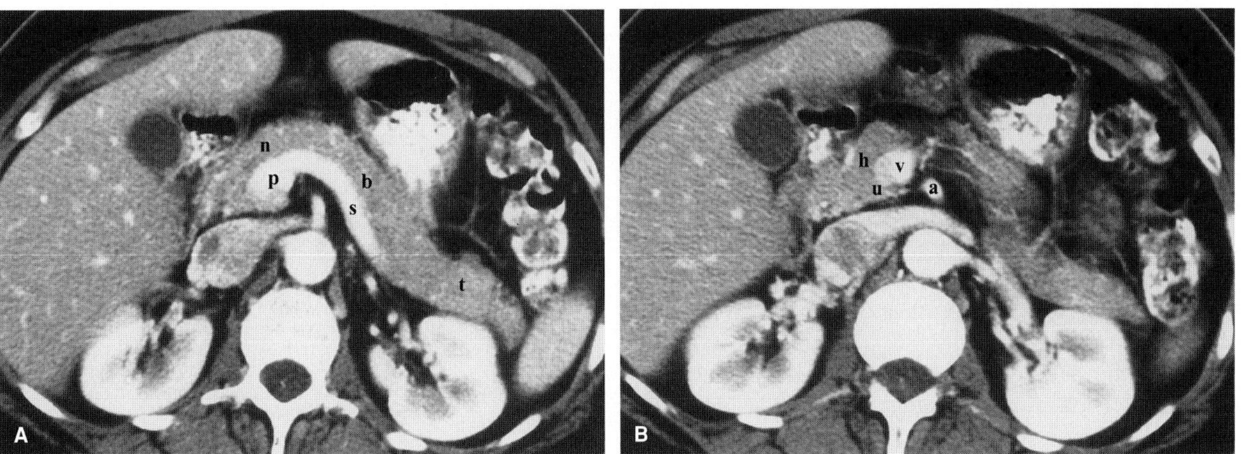

FIGURE 28.1. **Normal Pancreas as Seen on CT. A.** Image through neck (n), body (b) and tail (t) of the pancreas. **B.** Image through head (h) and uncinate process (u) of the pancreas. The majority of the pancreas lies anterior to the splenic vein (s) and its junction with the superior mesenteric vein (v), which forms the portal vein (p). The head and uncinate process lie caudal to the majority of the pancreas. The superior mesenteric artery (a) arises from the aorta posterior to the splenic vein and courses caudally, just to the left of the superior mesenteric vein. The superior mesenteric artery is normally surrounded by a collar of clear fat.

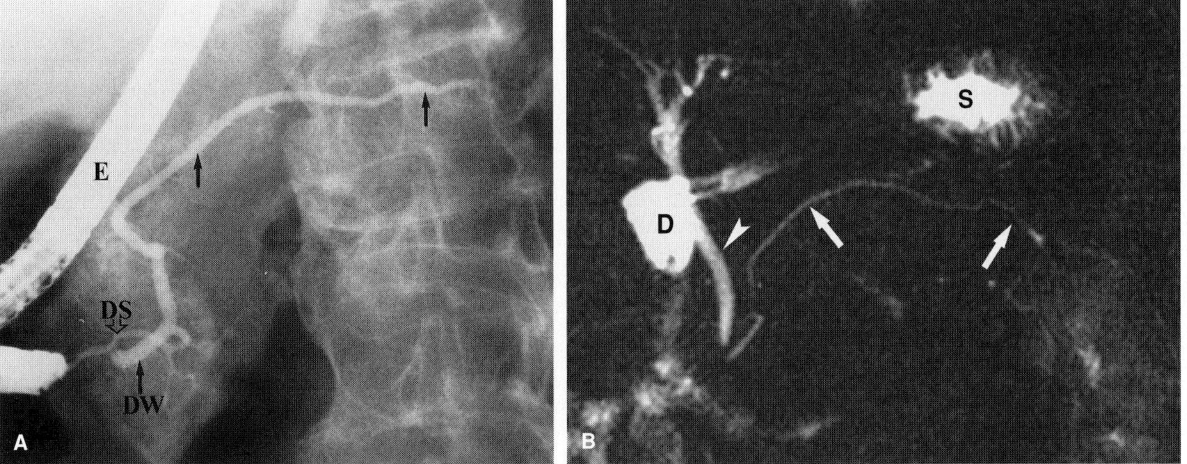

FIGURE 28.2. **Normal Pancreatic Ducts. A.** Radiograph from endoscopic retrograde cholangiopancreatogram demonstrates the main duct of Wirsung (*DW, black arrows*) and the accessory duct of Santorini (*DS, open arrow*). In this patient, the main duct drained separately into the major papilla (of Vater), with a different orifice for the common bile duct. The accessory duct drained into the minor papilla. Both ampullae were cannulated endoscopically and injected before this radiograph. A number of different variants of pancreatic duct anatomy exist. This variant is found in about 35% of individuals. Embryologically, the main duct is formed by the entire duct of the ventral pancreatic bud and the distal portion of the duct of the dorsal pancreatic bud. The main duct may join the common bile duct or it may have a separate orifice in the major papilla. The proximal portion of the duct of the dorsal pancreatic bud may be obliterated or persist as the accessory duct. E, endoscope. **B.** Image from an MR cholangiopancreatogram (MRCP) in a different patient. The pancreatic duct and the common bile duct are well visualized. This patient has had a cholecystectomy. MRCP offers the obvious advantage of being noninvasive. S, stomach. D, duodenal bulb.

infiltration between the lobules in older patients gives the pancreas a delicate, feathery appearance on CT. The pancreatic duct is visualized with thin-slice CT and with US. It normally measures 3 to 4 mm in diameter in the head and tapers smoothly to the tail. Films from ERCP show that the normal duct is a bit larger owing to magnification effect and distension resulting from contrast injection (Fig. 28.2). The duodenum cradles the pancreatic head in the C-loop. Many pancreatic abnormalities show secondary effects on the duodenum, and occasionally on the stomach and colon.

On MR, the pancreas is best seen on fat-suppressed T1WIs (2,3). High protein content in the exocrine pancreas results in high signal of the pancreatic parenchyma, which is difficult to differentiate from fat on non–fat-suppressed T1WIs. Tumors are typically of lower signal than pancreatic parenchyma on T1WIs. On T2WIs, pancreatic tissue is variable in signal intensity, from as low as the liver to as high as fat. Cystic lesions are bright and easily seen on T2WIs. Gadolinium will enhance the parenchyma, whereas adenocarcinoma enhances poorly and remains low signal on postcontrast T1WIs.

Pancreatitis

Acute pancreatitis is generally diagnosed clinically. The role of imaging is to clarify the diagnosis when the clinical picture is confusing, to assess severity, to determine prognosis, and to detect complications (4). Inflammation of the pancreatic tissue leads to disruption of small pancreatic ducts, resulting in leakage of pancreatic secretions. Because the pancreas lacks a capsule, the pancreatic juices have ready access to surrounding tissues. Pancreatic enzymes digest fascial layers, spreading the inflammatory process to multiple anatomic compartments. Causes of acute pancreatitis are listed in Table 28.1. Imaging studies of acute pancreatitis may be normal in mild cases. Contrast-enhanced MDCT provides the most comprehensive initial assessment (5,6); however, US is useful for follow-up of specific abnormalities, such as fluid collections. Abnormalities that may be seen in the pancreas include: (*1*) focal or diffuse parenchymal enlargement, (*2*) changes in density because of edema, and (*3*) indistinctness of the margins of the gland owing to inflammation. Abnormalities in the peripancreatic tissues include stranding densities in the fat with indistinctness of the fat planes and thickening of affected fascial planes. Complications demonstrated by imaging are listed in Table 28.2, and a few are shown in Figs 28.3, 28.4, and 28.5. US- or CT-directed aspiration biopsy may be needed to confirm the presence of pancreatic abscess. Image-directed catheter placement is an alternative to surgical drainage of pancreatic fluid collections (7). Contrast-enhanced MR is equivalent to CT in the assessment of pancreatitis (2).

TABLE 28.1 Causes of Acute Pancreatitis

Alcohol abuse—most common cause of chronic pancreatitis
Gallstone passage/impaction—most common cause of acute pancreatitis
Metabolic disorders
- Hereditary pancreatitis—autosomal dominant
- Hypercalcemia
- Hyperlipidemia—types 1 and 5
- Malnutrition

Trauma
- Blunt abdominal trauma
- Surgery
- Endoscopic retrograde cholangiopancreatography

Penetrating ulcer
Malignancy
- Pancreatic adenocarcinoma
- Lymphoma

Drugs—steroids, tetracycline, furosemide, many others
Infection
- Viral—mumps, hepatitis, infectious mononucleosis, AIDS
- Parasites—*Ascariasis, Clonorchis*

Structural
- Choledochocele
- Pancreas divisum

Idiopathic—20% of cases of acute pancreatitis

TABLE 28.2 Complications of Acute Pancreatitis

Pancreatic fluid collections (collections of enzyme-rich pancreatic juice)
- Acute: resolve spontaneously in 50% of cases; may be intrapancreatic, anterior pararenal space, lesser sac, or extend anywhere in the abdomen, into solid organs, or even into the chest
- Pseudocyst: round or oval, encapsulated pancreatic fluid collection encased by a distinct fibrous capsule; require at least 4 weeks to develop; about 50% will spontaneously resolve, whereas the remainder will require catheter or surgical drainage

Liquefactive necrosis of pancreatic parenchyma—seen as lack of parenchymal enhancement during bolus contrast administration on CT, often multifocal. Morbidity and mortality increase dramatically when necrosis is present.

Infected necrosis—bacterial infection in necrotic tissue. Seen as an area of nonenhancing pancreatic tissue containing gas. Confirmed with needle aspiration. Infected necrosis generally requires surgical drainage.

Abscess—circumscribed collection of pus in area with little or no necrosis tissues. Seen as a fluid collection with a thick wall. Effectively treated with catheter drainage.

Hemorrhage—resulting from erosion of blood vessels and tissue necrosis. CT shows high-attenuation blood in the retroperitoneum.

Pancreatic ascites—leakage of pancreatic secretions into peritoneal cavity.

Pseudoaneurysm—autodigestion of arterial walls by pancreatic enzymes results in pulsatile mass that is lined by fibrous tissue and maintains communication with parent artery.

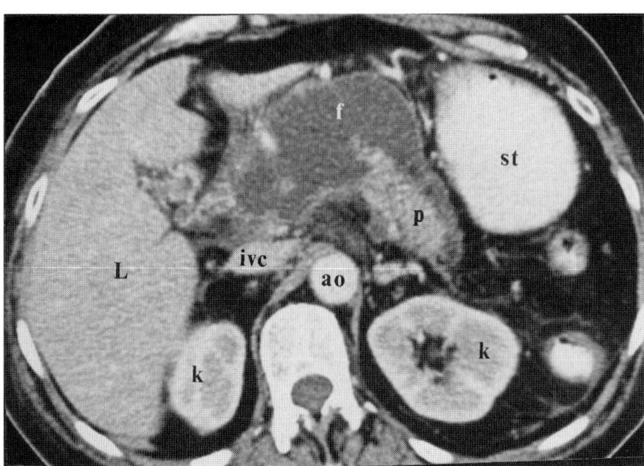

FIGURE 28.3. Acute Necrotizing Pancreatitis. CT scan performed with rapid bolus administration of IV contrast demonstrates enhancement of only the distal body of the pancreas (p). The pancreatic head and neck did not enhance and are lost in the fluid (f) extending from the pancreatic bed. This CT finding is indicative of pancreatic necrosis. st, stomach; L, liver; ivc, inferior vena cava; ao, aorta; k, kidney.

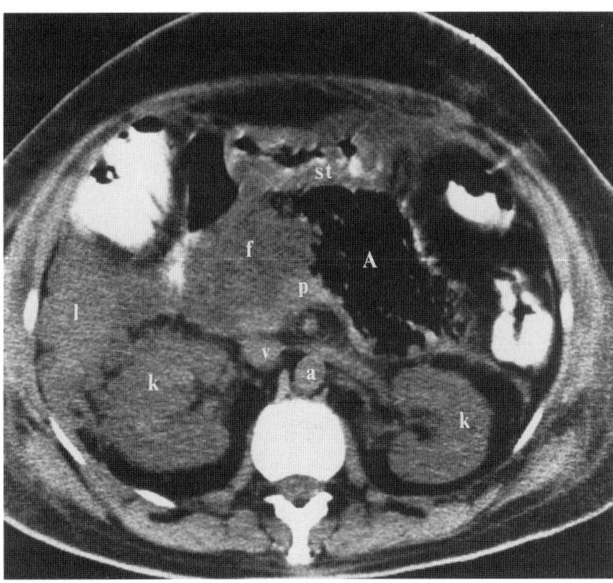

FIGURE 28.5. Pancreatic Abscess. Air (A) and fluid (f) extend from the bed of the pancreas (p) on this CT scan performed without IV contrast. Air in the pancreatic bed is indicative of abscess and/or fistulous communication with bowel. st, stomach; l, liver; v, inferior vena cava; a, aorta; k, kidney.

Chronic pancreatitis is caused by recurrent and prolonged bouts of acute pancreatitis, which cause parenchymal atrophy and progressive fibrosis. Both the exocrine and endocrine functions of the pancreas may be impaired. The most common causes are alcohol abuse (70%) and biliary stone disease (20%). Many of the remaining patients may have autoimmune pancreatitis that responds to steroid therapy. The clinical diagnosis is often vague, so imaging is used both to confirm the diagnosis and to detect complications. The morphologic changes of chronic pancreatitis include (*1*) dilation of the pancreatic duct (70% to 90% of cases), usually in a beaded pattern of alternating areas of dilation and constriction (Fig. 28.6); (*2*) decrease in visible pancreatic tissue because of atrophy; (*3*) calcifications (40% to 50% of cases) in the pancreatic parenchyma that vary from finely stippled to coarse, usually associated with alcoholic pancreatitis (Fig. 28.7); (*4*) fluid collections that are both intrapancreatic and extrapancreatic;

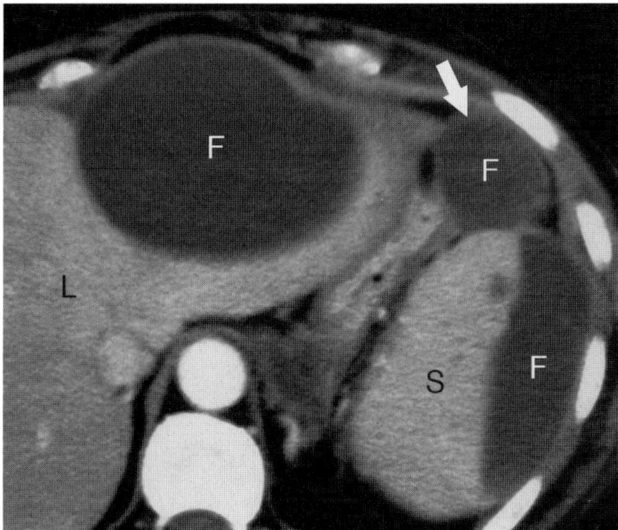

FIGURE 28.4. Pancreatic Fluid Collections. Three fluid collections (F) occurred as complications of acute pancreatitis. Pancreatic fluid dissected to subcapsular locations in the liver (L) and spleen (S), and one collection (*arrow*) developed within the peritoneal cavity.

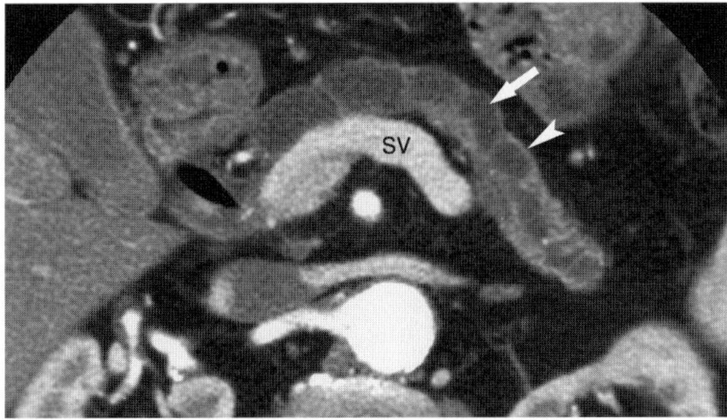

FIGURE 28.6. Chronic Pancreatitis. CT demonstrates marked beaded dilatation of the pancreatic duct (*arrow*) associated with atrophy (*arrowhead*) of the pancreatic parenchyma. These are characteristic findings of chronic pancreatitis.

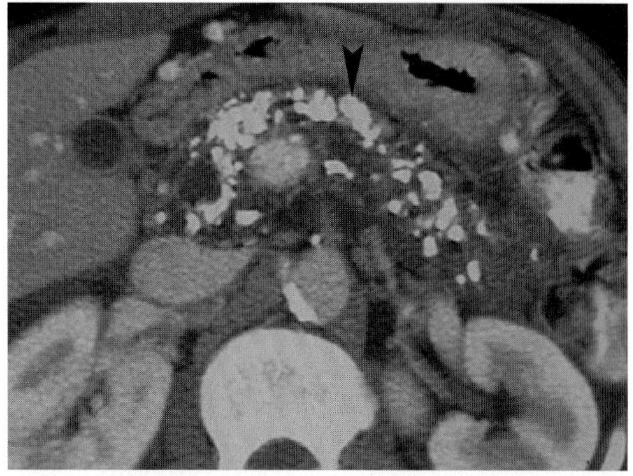

FIGURE 28.7. **Chronic Pancreatitis.** CT in a patient with a history of chronic alcohol abuse reveals innumerable coarse calcifications (*arrowhead*) throughout the pancreas. This finding is most common in chronic pancreatitis caused by alcoholism.

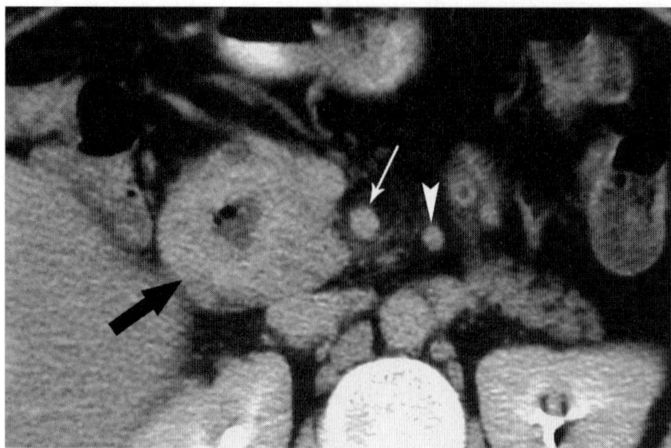

FIGURE 28.8. **Pancreatic Carcinoma: Resectable.** This adenocarcinoma (*black arrow*) of the pancreatic head proved to be surgically resectable. Central necrosis produced low density and air bubbles in the middle of the lesion. The superior mesenteric artery (*white arrowhead*) and vein (*white arrow*) are spared of involvement.

(*5*) focal enlargement of the pancreas owing to benign inflammation and fibrosis; (*6*) dilation of the biliary duct because of fibrosis or mass in the pancreatic head; and (*7*) fascial thickening and chronic inflammatory changes in surrounding tissues. Differentiation between an inflammatory mass resulting from chronic pancreatitis and that of pancreatic carcinoma frequently requires image-directed biopsy. MR reveals the fibrosis and parenchymal atrophy as a loss of the bright signal of pancreas parenchyma normally seen on T1W fat-suppressed images (3). Parenchymal enhancement on MR is heterogeneous early and increases on delayed images. MRCP and ERCP demonstrate the characteristic changes in the pancreatic duct (3). Calcifications are demonstrated by CT, US, and plain radiographs but are easily overlooked on MR. Autoimmune pancreatitis is characterized by diffuse narrowing of the pancreatic duct and a well-defined capsule that surrounds the pancreas and shows delayed contrast enhancement (8).

Solid Lesions of the Pancreas

Pancreatic carcinoma (ductal adenocarcinoma) is a highly lethal tumor that is usually unresectable at presentation. The average survival time of a patient with this disease is only 5 to 8 months. It accounts for 3% of all cancers and is second only to colorectal cancer as the most common digestive tract malignancy. Radiographic assessment of resectability is critical, because surgical resection offers the only hope of cure, yet the surgery itself carries a high morbidity. Scanning by CT should include rapid bolus contrast injection and thin slices (9). Adenocarcinoma appears as a hypodense mass that distorts the contour of the gland. Associated findings include obstruction of the common bile duct and pancreatic duct and atrophy of pancreatic tissue beyond the tumor. Metastases commonly go to regional nodes, liver, and the peritoneal cavity. Signs of potential resectability (Fig. 28.8) include isolated pancreatic mass with or without dilation of the bile or pancreatic ducts, or combined dilation of both the bile and pancreatic ducts without an identifiable pancreatic head mass. Signs of unresectability include: (*1*) extension of the tumor beyond the margins of the pancreas, (*2*) tumor involvement of adjacent organs, (*3*) enlarged regional lymph nodes (>15 mm), (*4*) encasement or obstruction of peripancreatic arteries or veins (Fig. 28.9) (10),

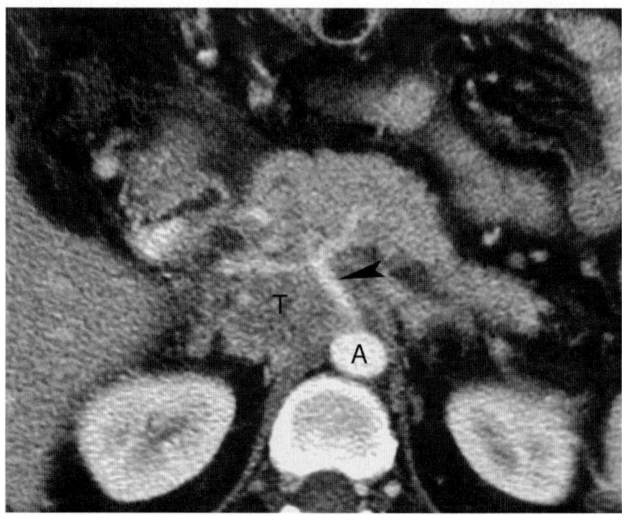

FIGURE 28.9. **Pancreatic Carcinoma: Nonresectable.** Pancreas tumor (T) encases and narrows the celiac axis (*arrowhead*) and its branches, and partially envelopes the aorta (A). This cancer is not resectable by CT criteria.

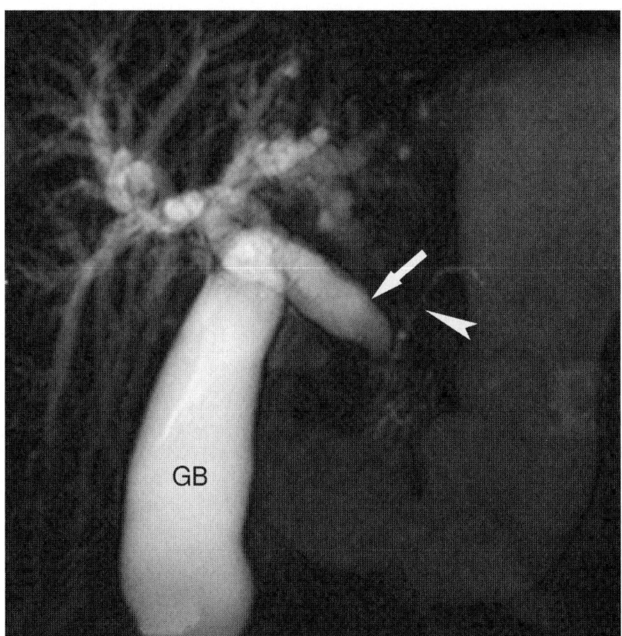

FIGURE 28.10. **Pancreatic Carcinoma.** Coronal plane image from an MR cholangiopancreatogram demonstrates a dilated gallbladder (GB), diffuse dilatation of the intrahepatic biliary tree, and marked dilatation of the common bile duct (*arrow*) that ends abruptly at the tumor (not visualized on this image). The pancreatic duct (*arrowhead*) was not obstructed by the tumor and is normal in caliber.

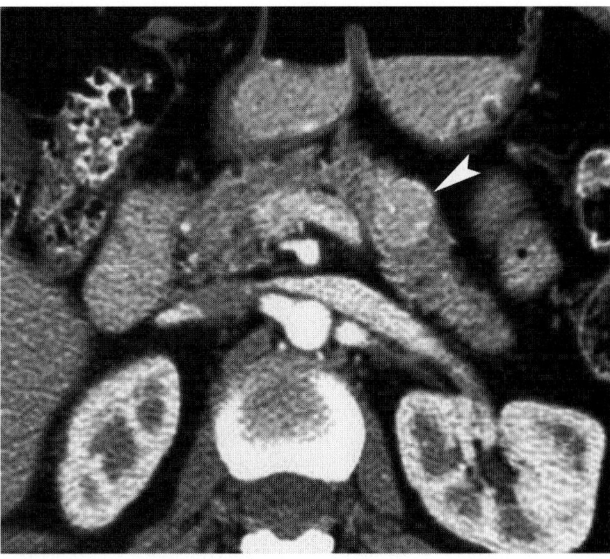

FIGURE 28.11. **Insulinoma.** A small insulin-secreting islet cell tumor (*arrow*) is identified by bright enhancement during arterial phase of contrast injection by multidetector CT.

(*5*) metastases in the liver, and (*6*) peritoneal carcinomatosis. Only 10% to 15% of patients have tumors that are potentially resectable using these criteria. Image-guided biopsy can confirm the diagnosis in patients whose tumors are deemed unresectable. Tumor recurrence following the Whipple procedure is best detected with MDCT (11). MR shows low-signal infiltrative tumor surrounded by high-signal enhanced parenchyma on a postcontrast T1WI. MRCP defines ductal anatomy with dilatation proximal to the stricturing tumor (Fig. 28.10). MRA and MR venography are excellent in identifying vascular involvement by tumor.

Chronic pancreatitis may produce a mass that mimics pancreas carcinoma. Beaded dilatation of the pancreatic duct is characteristic of chronic pancreatitis, whereas smooth ductal dilatation is most frequent with carcinoma. Calcifications within the mass are common with chronic pancreatitis and are very rare with adenocarcinoma. Islet cell tumors more commonly contain calcifications. As many as 14% of patients with pancreas adenocarcinoma also have chronic pancreatitis. Image-guided biopsy is usually needed to provide a definitive diagnosis, but a negative biopsy is not always definitive because of sampling errors.

Islet Cell Tumors. Functioning islet cell tumors produce distinct clinical syndromes and usually present while the tumors are small (12). Insulinomas present with hypoglycemia, and gastrinomas present with peptic ulcers, diarrhea caused by gastric hypersecretion, or Zollinger-Ellison syndrome. Other islet cell tumors include glucagonoma (diabetes mellitus and painful glossitis), somatostatinoma (diabetes and steatorrhea), and VIPoma (massive watery diarrhea). Nonfunctioning islet cell tumors are clinically silent until they present with symptoms of a growing, usually large, mass. Functioning tumors vary in malignant potential, from 10% for insulinoma to 60% for gastrinoma and 80% for glucagonoma. Up to 80% of nonfunctioning tumors are malignant. Functioning islet cell tumors vary in size from 0.4 to 4.0 cm and require strict attention to technique for accurate preoperative identification (13). Most small islet cell tumors cannot be identified on precontrast CT. Because the lesions tend to be hypervascular, bolus contrast administration during rapid, thin-slice, MDCT scanning through the pancreatic bed offers the best chance of lesion visualization. The tumor stands out as an enhancing nodule within the pancreas (Fig. 28.11). Sonography has proved extremely valuable for tumor localization during surgery. Islet cell tumors appear as hypoechoic masses within the pancreas. Octreotide is a somatostatin analogue that is used for scintigraphic detection of islet cell tumors. Nonfunctioning islet cell tumors tend to be much larger—6 to 20 cm diameter (Fig. 28.12). Imaging findings include coarse calcifications, cystic degeneration, necrosis, local and vascular invasion, and metastases. On MR, most islet cell tumors are hypointense on T1WIs and hyperintense on T2WIs and demonstrate bright arterial enhancement on dynamic postcontrast T1WIs (Fig. 28.13).

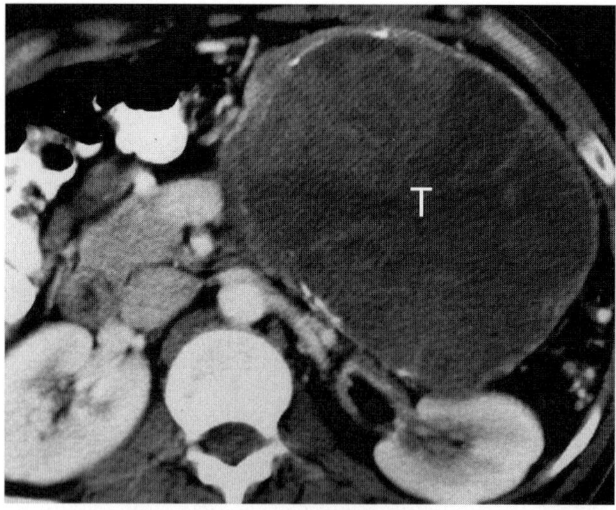

FIGURE 28.12. **Nonfunctioning Malignant Islet Cell Tumor.** A huge tumor mass (T) arises from the tail of the pancreas. This tumor grew to a large size before producing symptoms. Note the heterogeneous attenuation, which is characteristic of large islet cell malignancies.

Metastases to the pancreas are most frequent with renal cell carcinoma and bronchogenic carcinoma (14). Lesions may appear as a solitary, well-defined, heterogenously enhancing mass, as diffuse heterogeneous enlargement of the pancreas, or as multiple nodules. Tumors have no predilection for any particular portion of the pancreas. On MR, most lesions are low signal on T1WIs and high signal on T2WIs. Melanoma metastases are characteristically hyperintense on T1WIs because of the paramagnetic properties of melanin.

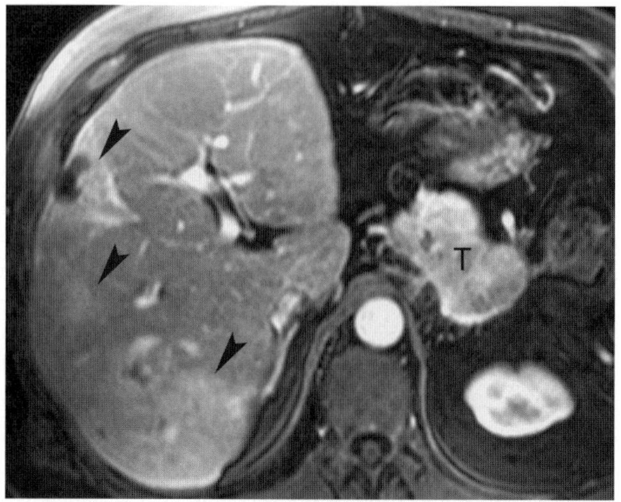

FIGURE 28.13. **Malignant Islet Cell Tumor.** Fat-suppressed T1W early phase postcontrast MR demonstrates bright enhancement of the primary tumor (T) as well as its metastases (*arrowheads*) in the liver.

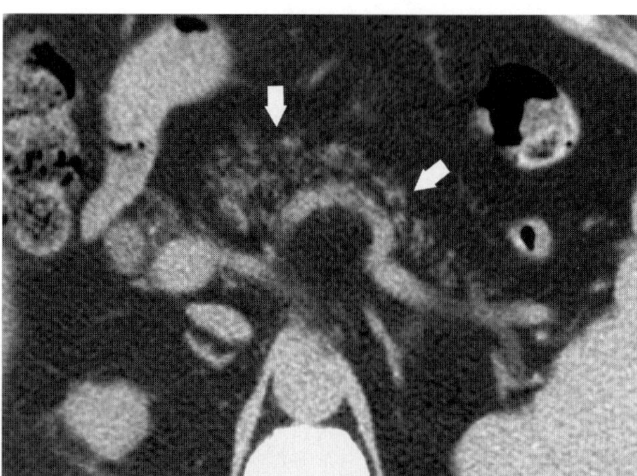

FIGURE 28.14. **Diffuse Fatty Infiltration of the Pancreas.** CT shows diffuse fatty infiltration between the lobules of the pancreas (*arrows*) in a 70-year-old obese patient.

Lymphoma may involve the pancreas as a primary site (rare) or by direct extension from disease in the retroperitoneum (15). On CT, most lesions are homogeneous and of lower attenuation than muscle, and they show limited enhancement. Lesions may be a localized, well-defined mass, or they may be infiltrating diffusely enlarging or replacing the gland. Attenuation may be so low as to appear cystic.

Fatty lesions of the pancreas, similar to those of the liver, include diffuse fatty infiltration, focal fatty infiltration, focal fatty sparing, and lipoma (16). Diffuse infiltration is associated with aging and obesity and is seen with pancreatic atrophy. Fat infiltrates between the lobules of pancreatic parenchyma (Fig. 28.14). In patients with cystic fibrosis, pancreatic parenchyma is eventually completely replaced by fat. Focal fatty sparing in diffuse infiltration may simulate a pancreatic mass, especially when it involves the head or uncinate process. Focal fatty infiltration may involve any portion of the pancreas. Lipomas are rare, usually solitary, fat-density masses that are usually incidental findings but may occasionally obstruct the pancreatic or bile ducts.

Cystic Lesions of the Pancreas

Pseudocysts resulting from pancreatitis are the most common pancreatic cystic lesions (17). They are of fluid density and have a definable fibrous wall that may be calcified. Internal septations and multiple loculations are common (18).

Abscess must be considered in any patient with a cystic pancreatic lesion and a fever. Most abscesses have indistinct walls and contain fluid and debris. The presence of gas bubbles within the cystic mass is good evidence for abscess. Image-directed aspiration confirms the diagnosis and may be followed by percutaneous catheter placement for treatment. Abscesses usually occur as a complication of pancreatitis.

True pancreatic cysts, with epithelial lining, are found in 10% of patients with autosomal-dominant polycystic disease, 30% of patients with von Hippel-Lindau syndrome, and some patients with cystic fibrosis. They appear as well-defined, fluid-filled masses with walls of variable thickness. Patients with von Hippel-Lindau syndrome are prone to islet cell tumors and microcystic adenomas, in addition to multiple pancreatic cysts.

Cystic tumors of the pancreas are uncommon (5% to 15% of pancreatic cysts) (18,19). Islet cell tumors may appear cystic because of extensive necrosis (13). Cystic teratomas rarely arise in the pancreas and usually have characteristic hair, fat, calcifications, and cystic and solid components.

Microcystic adenoma (serous cystadenoma) is a benign pancreatic tumor composed of innumerable small cysts 1 mm to 2 cm in size. The lining epithelial cells are rich in glycogen, resulting in the alternate name of *glycogen-rich cystadenoma*. The cysts may be so small that the tumor appears as a solid lesion on imaging studies. A characteristic feature is a central stellate fibrous scar, which may be calcified. Approximately 80% of patients with this disease are age 60 or older. This tumor is common in patients with von Hippel-Lindau syndrome. Noncontrast CT shows a well-defined mass with low attenuation near water density. Contrast enhancement is usually marked, with demonstration of multiple internal septations in a honeycomb appearance (Fig. 28.15). US commonly shows an echogenic mass, with only a few of the larger cysts visible.

Macrocystic serous cystadenoma, consisting of a unilocular or bilocular cyst larger than 2 cm, accounts for approximately 10% of serous cystadenomas (20). Most are smaller than 5 cm. These benign tumors are indistinguishable from potentially malignant mucinous cystic tumors (Fig. 28.16) (21).

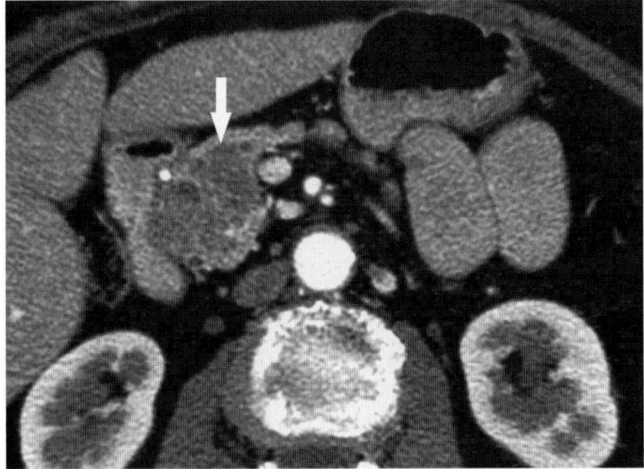

FIGURE 28.15. **Microcystic Serous Cystadenoma.** Enhanced CT shows a mass (*arrow*) in the pancreatic head consisting of innumerable cysts that are so small the low-attenuation mass appears almost solid.

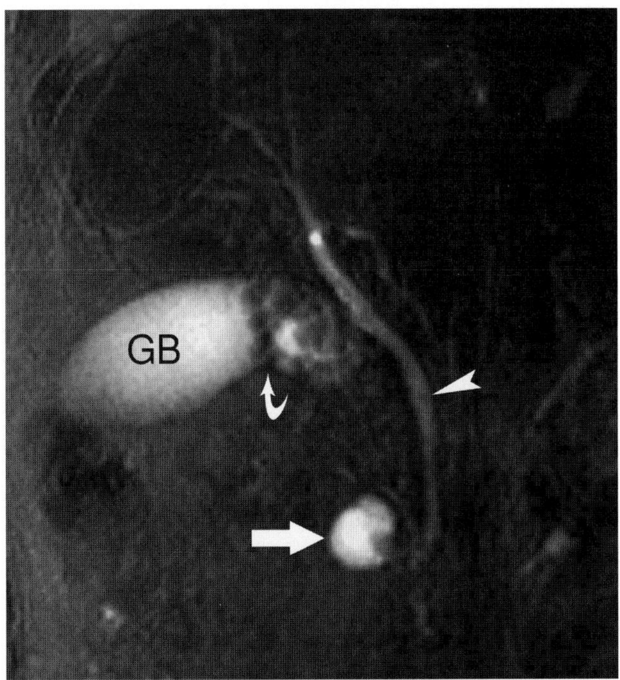

FIGURE 28.16. **Macrocystic Serous Cystadenoma.** MR cholangiopancreatography image in sagittal plane shows a 3-cm cystic mass (*straight arrow*) in the head of the pancreas. A single fine septation is present within the cyst. The appearance suggests mucinous cystic neoplasm, but pathology confirmed a benign macrocystic serous cystadenoma. The common bile duct (*arrowhead*) and intrahepatic bile ducts are normal. The gallbladder (GB) shows a layer of gallstones (*curved arrow*). The patient is supine.

Mucinous cystic neoplasm has previously been known as *macrocystic adenoma* or *mucinous cystadenoma/cystadenocarcinoma* (Fig. 28.17) (20). Lesions are 2 to 30 cm in size and consist of a mucin-filled cyst, which is bounded by a thick fibrous capsule lined by mucin-producing cells. CT shows a multilocular or unilocular cyst in the body or tail of the pancreas. Individual cysts are generally larger than 2 cm and six or fewer in number. Thin sections and contrast enhancement best demonstrate the tumor detail. MR with contrast enhancement provides optimal detail of the structure inside the cyst. Because all mucinous tumors carry a risk of malignancy, surgical resection is the treatment of choice (19). Metastases to the liver tend to be cystic.

Intraductal papillary mucinous neoplasm (IPMN) is the recently adopted preferred term for pancreatic tumors that produce an excessive amount of mucin, resulting in marked dilatation of the pancreatic duct and cystic enlargement of the branch ducts (22,23). IPMN of the main

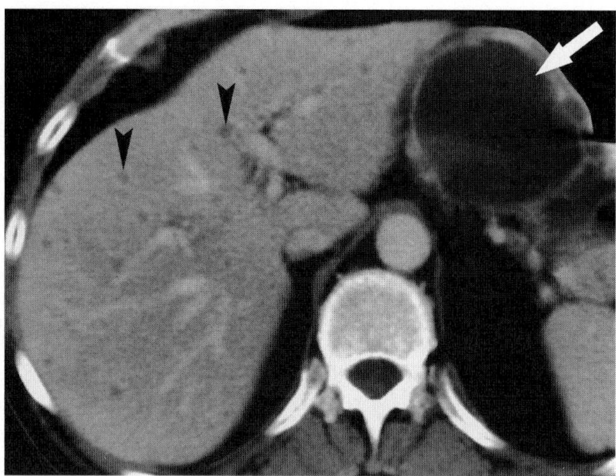

FIGURE 28.17. **Mucinous Cystic Neoplasm (Cystadenocarcinoma).** CT demonstrates a 5-cm unilocular cystic tumor (*arrow*) (*arrowheads*) within the liver proved to be metastases.

duct type is associated with dilatation of the entire main pancreatic duct (Fig. 28.18). Papillary solid tumor excrescences may be seen within the dilated duct. Only a thin rim of atrophic pancreatic parenchyma is present. ERCP demonstrates a bulging papilla with mucin protruding from the orifice. IPMN of the branch duct–type appears as a focal group of small cysts (1 to 2 cm in diameter) that intercommunicate through dilated branch ducts (Fig. 28.19). These lesions are most common in the uncinate process. Some lesions consist of a single unilocular cyst. Pancreatic parenchyma adjacent to the lesions atrophies and becomes the capsule of the cystic mass (20).

Duodenal diverticula filled only with fluid may mimic a cystic pancreatic lesion (24).

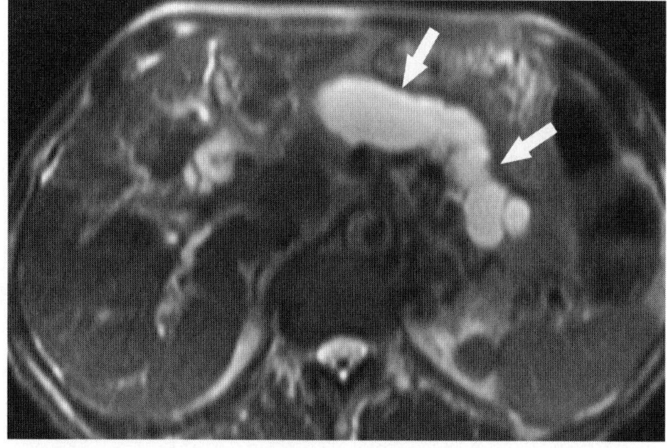

FIGURE 28.18. **Intraductal Papillary Mucinous Neoplasm, Main Duct Type.** Axial T2WI shows massive dilatation of the main pancreatic duct (*arrows*). No discernible pancreatic parenchyma is evident.

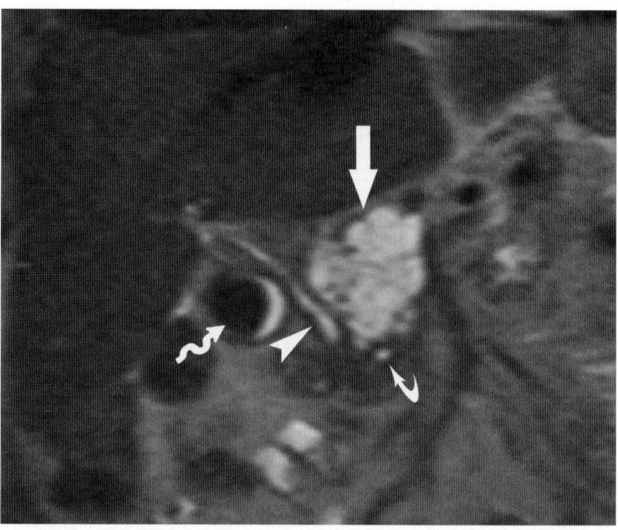

FIGURE 28.19. **Intraductal Papillary Mucinous Neoplasm (IPMN), Branch Duct Type.** Coronal T2WI shows a multilobulated cystic mass (*straight arrow*) occupying the neck and head of the pancreas. Pathology after surgical removal confirmed IPMT. The common bile duct (*arrowhead*) is normal. A portion of the normal main pancreatic duct (*curved arrow*) is also evident on this image. A large gallstone (*squiggly arrow*) is present in the gallbladder.

SPLEEN

Imaging Techniques

CT and US remain the major techniques for imaging the splenic parenchyma (25). Technetium sulfur colloid radionuclide scanning images both the liver and the spleen and can be used to confirm the presence of functioning splenic tissue. MR is somewhat disappointing in its ability to demonstrate splenic abnormalities, because the signal intensity of the splenic parenchyma tends to parallel the signal intensity of pathologic lesions and shows insufficient contrast differentiation to identify the lesions. With the use of gadolinium enhancement, MR imaging of the spleen is improved.

Anatomy

The spleen is the body's largest lymphoid organ. Although it serves as a site of blood formation in the fetus, there is no hematopoietic activity in the normal adult spleen. The spleen sequesters abnormal and aged red and white blood cells and platelets and serves as a reservoir for red blood cells. The spleen occupies the left upper quadrant of the abdomen, just below the diaphragm and posterior and lateral to the stomach. Its diaphragmatic surface is smooth and convex, conforming to the shape of the diaphragm, whereas its visceral surface has concavities for the stomach, kidney, colon, and pancreas. Spleen size varies with age, nutrition, and hydration. The spleen is relatively large in children, reaching adult size by age 15. The average spleen dimensions in adults are 12 cm in length, 7 cm in width, and 3 to 4 cm in thickness. The spleen progressively decreases in size with age. The splenic artery and vein course through the pancreas to the splenic hilum, where they divide into multiple branches. Splenic arteries are end arteries without anastomoses or collateral supply. Occlusion of the splenic artery or its branches produces infarction. On all imaging studies, the spleen has a homogeneous appearance. On both CT and MR, lesions are best demonstrated on contrast-enhanced images. On noncontrast CT, the normal spleen density is less than or equal to the density of normal liver. On MR, the spleen signal intensity is lower than hepatic parenchyma on T1WIs and higher than liver parenchyma on T2WIs (26). US demonstrates a midlevel, even echo pattern for the splenic parenchyma.

Transient pseudomasses are formed during rapid IV bolus administration of both CT and MR contrast agents because of variable rates of blood flow through the splenic parenchyma (Fig. 28.20). Images obtained during the arterial phase demonstrate irregular defects in parenchymal enhancement (27). One or 2 minutes later, the entire spleen is homogeneously enhanced on both CT and MR. Diffuse liver disease is associated with more prominent splenic pseudomasses during early enhancement.

Lobulations and clefts in the splenic contour are common and must not be mistaken for masses or splenic fractures.

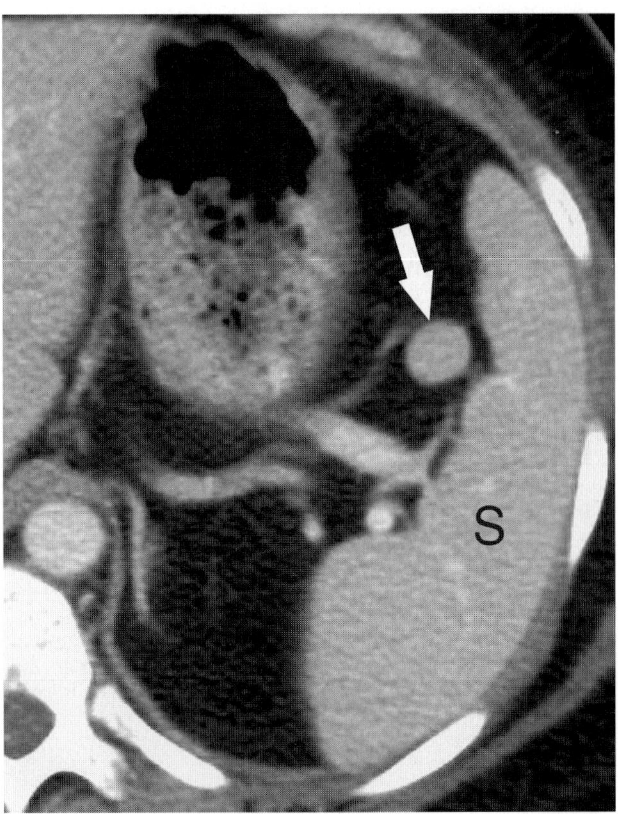

FIGURE 28.21. **Accessory Spleen.** An accessory spleen (*arrow*) is seen in the splenic hilum. Accessory spleens have the same imaging characteristics as the parent spleen (S).

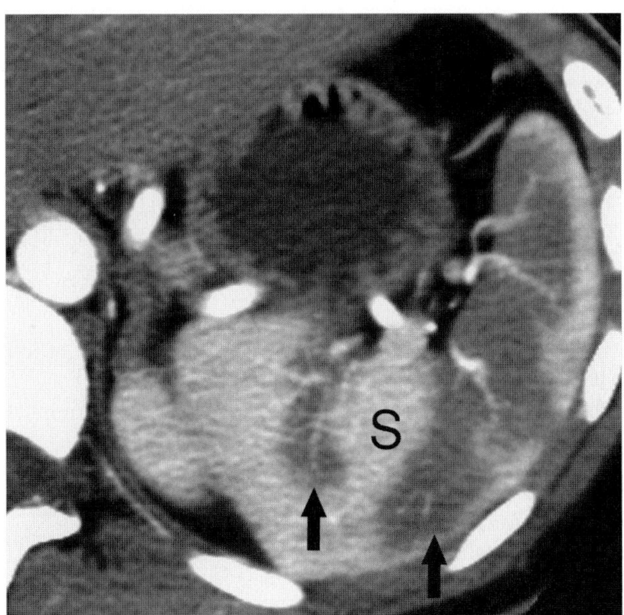

FIGURE 28.20. **Transient Pseudomasses in Spleen.** Multidetector CT image obtained during the arterial enhancement phase of IV contrast injection shows normal early flow enhancement defects (*arrows*) in the spleen (S).

Accessory spleens are found in 10% to 16% of normal individuals (28). These appear as round masses, 1 to 3 cm in size, and of the same texture as normal splenic parenchyma (Fig. 28.21). They may be single or multiple and are usually located near the splenic hilum. Technetium sulfur colloid radionuclide scans can be used to confirm suspected accessory spleens as functioning splenic tissue.

Wandering spleen is the term applied to a normal spleen that is positioned out of its normal location in the left upper quadrant. Laxity of the splenic ligaments, commonly found in association with abnormalities of intestinal rotation, allows the spleen to be positioned anywhere in the abdominal cavity. A wandering spleen may present as a palpable abdominal mass, although most cause no symptoms. The diagnosis is made by recognizing the normal shape and tissue texture of the spleen and the absence of normal spleen in the left upper abdomen and by identifying the blood supply from splenic vessels. Radionuclide scans can confirm functioning splenic tissue.

Splenosis refers to multiple implants of ectopic splenic tissue that may occur after traumatic splenic rupture. Splenic tissue can implant anywhere in the abdominal cavity, or even in the thorax if the diaphragm has been ruptured. Splenosis complicates 40% to 60% of splenic

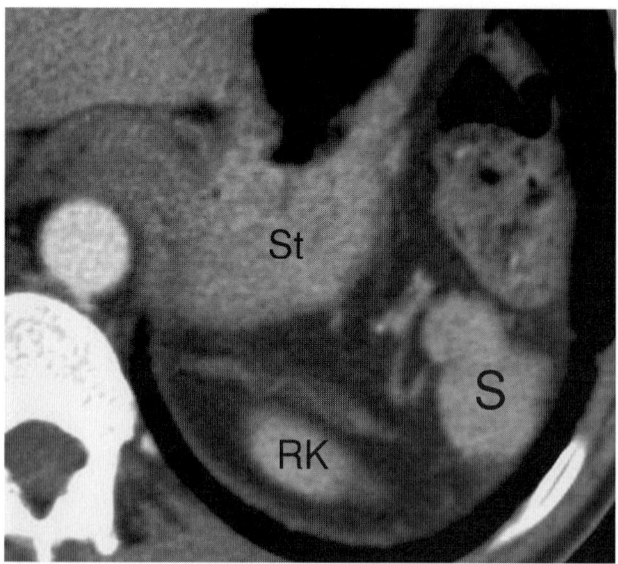

FIGURE 28.22. **Splenic Regeneration.** Hypertrophy of remnants of splenic tissue deposited on the diaphragm after traumatic splenic rupture has created a homogeneously enhancing mass of functioning splenic tissue (S). This patient has a history of splenectomy. LK, left kidney; St, stomach.

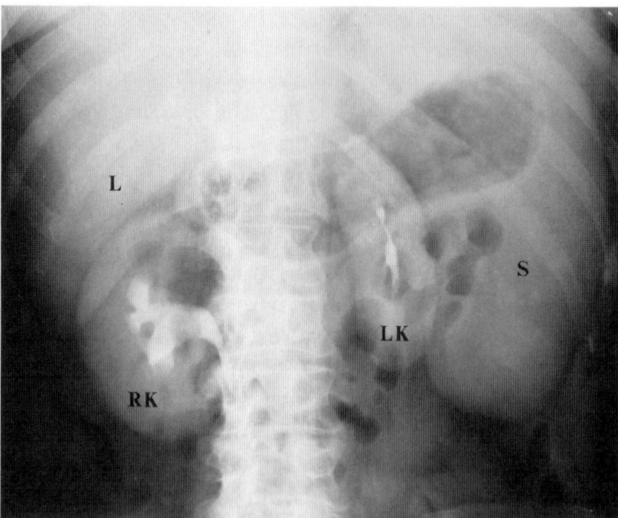

FIGURE 28.23. **Splenomegaly.** Radiograph from an excretory urogram demonstrates a massively enlarged spleen (S) in a patient with rheumatoid arthritis and Felty syndrome. The left kidney (LK) is compressed and rotated by the large spleen. The inferior margin of the spleen extends well below the inferior margin of the liver (L). RK, right kidney.

injuries. The splenic implants are usually multiple and vary in size and shape. The tissue fragments enlarge over time and may simulate peritoneal metastases. Functioning splenic tissue is confirmed by radionuclide scanning.

Splenic Regeneration. After splenectomy, remaining accessory spleens or splenules resulting from traumatic peritoneal seeding of splenic tissue may enlarge and resume the function of the resected spleen. When the spleen is removed, bits of nuclear material, called Howell-Jolly bodies, are routinely seen in red cells on peripheral blood smears. Disappearance of these Howell-Jolly bodies from peripheral blood is a clinical sign of splenic regeneration. Imaging studies demonstrate single or multiple spleen-like masses (Fig. 28.22) in the abdominal cavity in patients with a history of splenectomy.

Polysplenia is a rare congenital anomaly that features multiple small spleens, usually located in the right abdomen and associated with situs ambiguous. Both spleens are two-lobed. Most patients also have cardiovascular anomalies.

Asplenia (Ivemark syndrome) is the congenital absence of the spleen, found in association with bilateral right-sidedness, midline liver, and bilateral three-lobed lungs. Major cardiac anomalies are present in 50% of cases. Most patients die before 1 year of age.

Splenomegaly

The diagnosis of splenic enlargement on imaging studies is usually made subjectively. Although quantitative methods have been attempted, none have proved popular. Findings that suggest splenomegaly are (*1*) any spleen dimension greater than 14 cm, (*2*) projection of the spleen ventral to the anterior axillary line, (*3*) inferior spleen tip extending more caudally than the inferior liver tip, or (*4*) inferior spleen tip extending below the lower pole of the left

TABLE 28.3 Causes of Splenomegaly

Congestive
Portal hypertension (50% of cases)
Portal vein thrombosis
Myeloproliferative disorders
Leukemia
Lymphoma (30% of cases)
Polycythemia vera
Idiopathic thrombocytopenia purpura
Sickle cell disease (in infants)
Thalassemia major
Hereditary spherocytosis
Myelofibrosis
Infection
Malaria (universal in endemic areas)
Schistosomiasis (endemic areas)
Infectious mononucleosis
Subacute bacterial endocarditis
AIDS
IV drug abuse
Infiltrative
Systemic lupus erythematosus
Amyloidosis
Gaucher disease

kidney. Enlarged spleens frequently compress and displace adjacent organs, especially the left kidney (Fig. 28.23). The causes of splenomegaly are exhaustive (Table 28.3). Most do not produce a change in spleen density, so differentiation is based upon associated imaging findings or on clinical evaluation. MR offers no significant benefit in the differential diagnosis of splenomegaly. Mild to moderate splenomegaly is seen with portal hypertension, AIDS, storage diseases, collagen vascular disorders, and infection. More marked splenomegaly is usually associated with lymphoma, leukemia, infectious mononucleosis, hemolytic anemia, and myelofibrosis.

Cystic Lesions of the Spleen

Posttraumatic cysts are false cysts that lack an epithelial lining (29). They generally have thick walls and septations that commonly become calcified (30% to 40%) (Fig. 28.24). The internal fluid may be complex owing to blood products, cholesterol crystals, or cellular debris. Posttraumatic cysts result from previous hemorrhage, infarction, or infection. They account for 80% of all splenic cysts.

Epidermoid cysts are true epithelial-lined cysts that are probably developmental in origin. They have the same appearance as posttraumatic cysts but less frequently have calcification in their walls (5%).

Pancreatic pseudocysts extend beneath the splenic capsule by tracking along the pancreatic tail to the splenic hilum. Splenic subcapsular pancreatic fluid collections develop in 1% to 5% of patients with pancreatitis (Fig. 28.4).

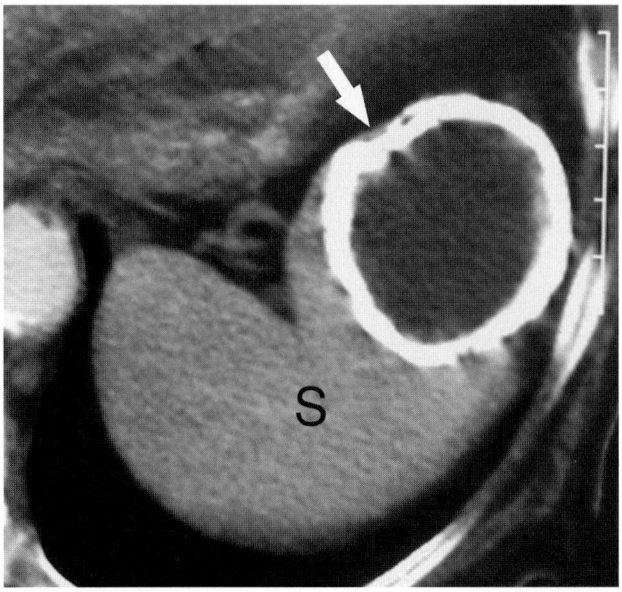

FIGURE 28.24. **Posttraumatic Splenic Cyst.** The well-defined cyst with thick, densely calcified walls (*arrow*) seen in the spleen (S) on this CT scan is the result of an old intrasplenic hemorrhage.

Internal debris and hemorrhage are commonly present. Imaging studies demonstrate associated findings of pancreatitis.

Bacterial abscesses occur most commonly in spleens that are already diseased. They present with vague symptoms but have a high mortality when left untreated. They result from hematogenous spread of infection (75%), trauma (15%), or infarction (10%). Abscesses appear as single or multiple low-density masses with ill-defined thick walls. US commonly demonstrates internal echoes caused by inflammatory debris. Abscesses are low intensity on T1WIs and high intensity on T2WIs. They may contain gas or demonstrate air–fluid levels. Perisplenic fluid collections and left pleural effusions are common. Image-guided aspiration confirms the diagnosis. Treatment is by catheter drainage or splenectomy.

Microabscesses are found in patients with immune systems compromised by AIDS, organ transplantation, lymphoma, or leukemia. The causes of microabscesses include fungi, tuberculosis, *Pneumocystis jiroveci* (Fig. 28.25),

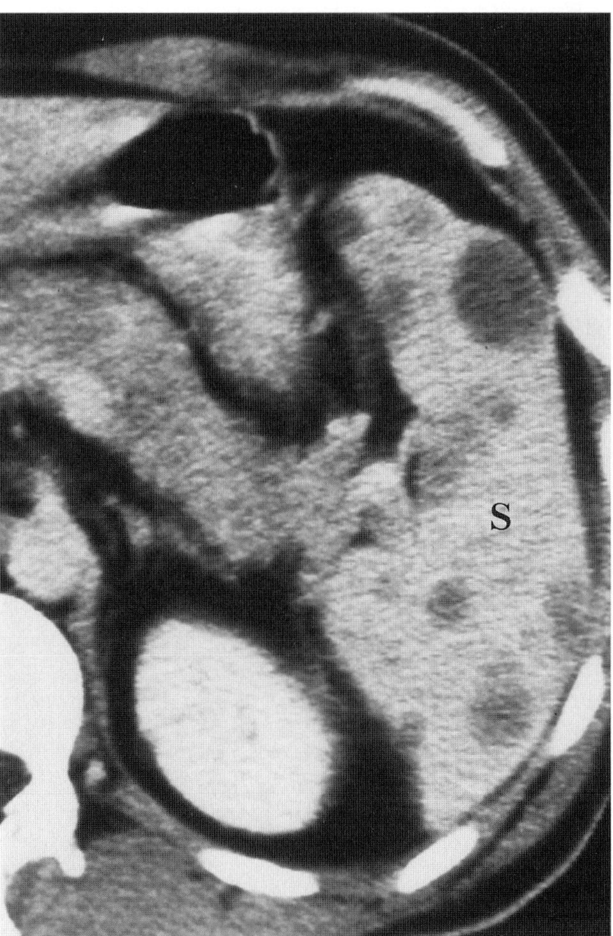

FIGURE 28.25. **Microabscesses in the Spleen.** Multiple lucent defects of varying size in the spleen (S) of this patient with AIDS are attributable to *Pneumocystis jiroveci* infection.

TABLE 28.4 Causes of Multiple Small (10-mm) Lesions in the Spleen

Microabscesses (immunocompromised patients)
Multiple bacterial abscesses
Histoplasmosis
Lymphoma
Kaposi sarcoma (AIDS patients)
Sarcoidosis
Gamna-Gandy bodies (portal hypertension)
Metastases
Breast carcinoma
Lung carcinoma
Ovarian carcinoma
Gastric carcinoma
Malignant melanoma
Prostate carcinoma

histoplasmosis, and cytomegalovirus. Imaging studies demonstrate multiple small defects in the spleen, usually 5 to 10 mm but up to 20 mm, in size. The differential diagnosis of multiple small low-density splenic defects is listed in Table 28.4.

Hydatid cysts in the spleen are found in only 2% of patients with hydatid disease. Hydatid cysts are usually also present in the liver or lung. The lesions consist of spherical mother cysts that contain smaller daughter cysts and have internal septations and debris representing hydatid sand. Ringlike calcifications in the wall are usually prominent in the chronic stage.

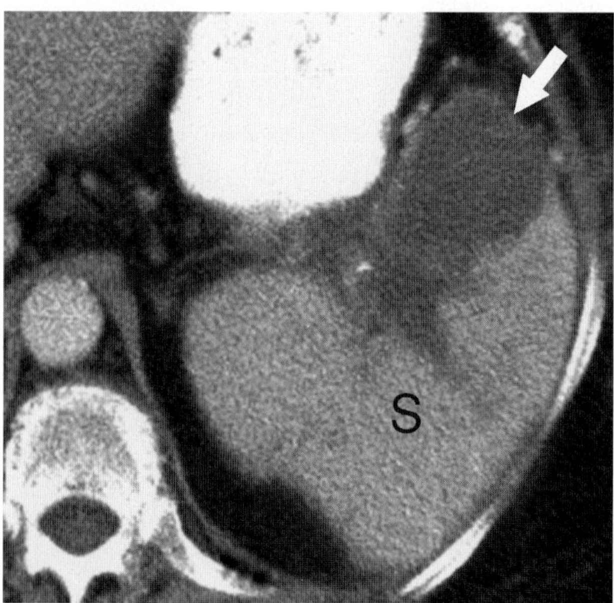

FIGURE 28.26. **Lymphoma.** Contrast-enhanced CT demonstrates a lobulated low-attenuation mass (*arrow*) within the parenchyma of the spleen (S). Note the resemblance to the splenic flow defect illustrated in Fig. 28.20.

Solid Lesions of the Spleen

Lymphoma is the most common malignant tumor involving the spleen. Commonly, a spleen involved with lymphoma appears normal on all imaging studies. CT is only 65% sensitive in demonstrating splenic involvement with lymphoma. Patterns of involvement that are visible on imaging studies include diffuse splenomegaly, multiple masses of varying size, miliary nodules resembling microabscesses, large solitary mass (Fig. 28.26), and direct invasion from adjacent lymphomatous nodes. Adenopathy is frequently evident elsewhere in the abdomen when the spleen is involved with lymphoma. Lymphoma is a common predisposing condition for splenic infarction.

Metastases are found in the spleen on autopsy series in up to 7% of patients who die of cancer. Most splenic metastases are microscopic and are not detected by imaging studies. The most common tumors to metastasize to the spleen are malignant melanoma and lung, breast, ovary, prostate, and stomach carcinoma. Metastases appear as single or multiple low-density masses. On MR, metastases are low intensity on T1WIs and high intensity on T2WIs. The increased signal intensity of the lesions parallels the increased signal intensity of the normal splenic parenchyma on T2WIs, and the lesions may not be evident. Contrast enhancement is recommended for both CT and MR demonstration of metastases. Calcification is rare. Melanoma metastases commonly appear cystic.

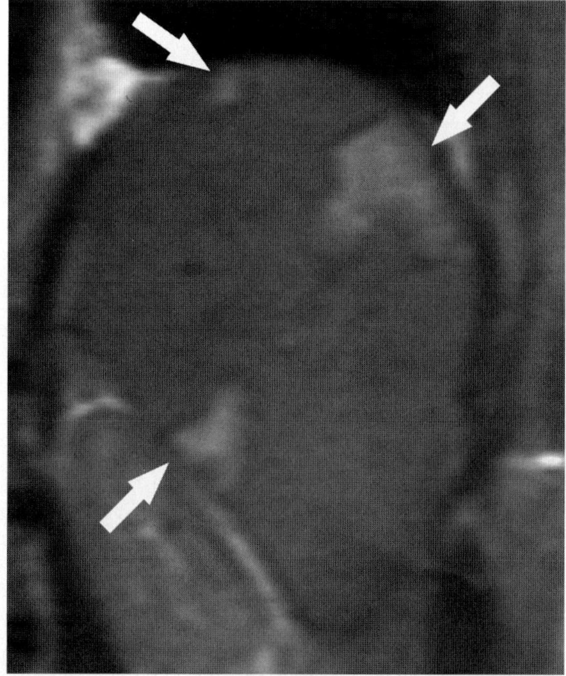

FIGURE 28.27. **Splenic Infarction.** Coronal plane MR with T2 weighting demonstrates three splenic infarcts (*arrows*) as high-signal areas of parenchyma that extend characteristically to the splenic capsule.

Infarction is produced by occlusion of the main or branch splenic arteries. Causes of infarction include emboli (owing to endocarditis, atherosclerotic plaques, or cardiac valve thrombi); sickle cell disease; pancreatitis; pancreatic tumors; and arteritis. Additional predisposing conditions include myeloproliferative disorders, hemolytic anemias, and sepsis. Infarcts classically appear as wedge-shaped defects in the splenic parenchyma. However, multiple infarcts may fuse, and the wedge shape may be lost. The key finding is extension of the abnormal parenchymal zone to an intact splenic capsule (Fig. 28.27). Splenomegaly, especially when caused by lymphoma, is a predisposing condition. Complications of splenic infarctions include subcapsular hematomas, infection, and splenic rupture with hemoperitoneum.

Gamna-Gandy bodies (also called *siderotic nodules*) are small hemorrhages in the spleen caused by portal hypertension (26). They are seen best on MR as multiple small low-intensity nodules on T1WIs (Fig. 28.28) and T2*WIs. Signal intensity is low because of hemosiderin content. They do not enhance.

Hemangioma is the most common primary neoplasm of the spleen, found in 14% of patients on autopsy

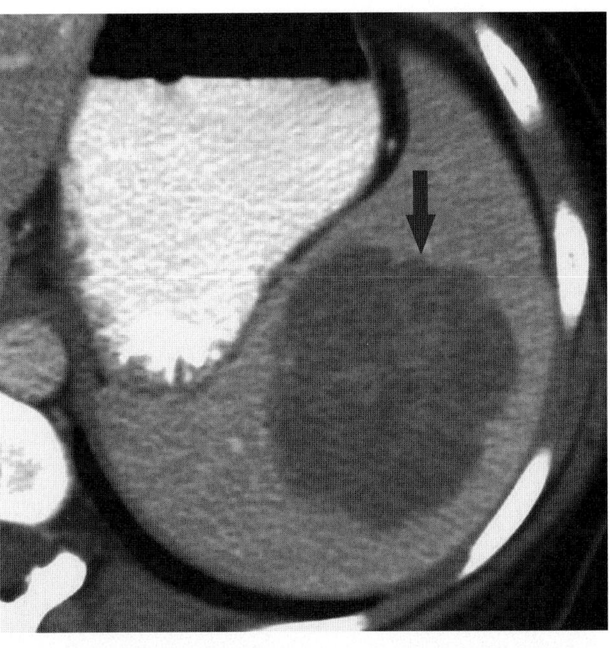

FIGURE 28.29. **Hemangioma Spleen.** Postcontrast CT shows this splenic hemangioma (*arrow*) to be an inhomogeneous, minimally enhancing, lobulated, low-attenuation mass.

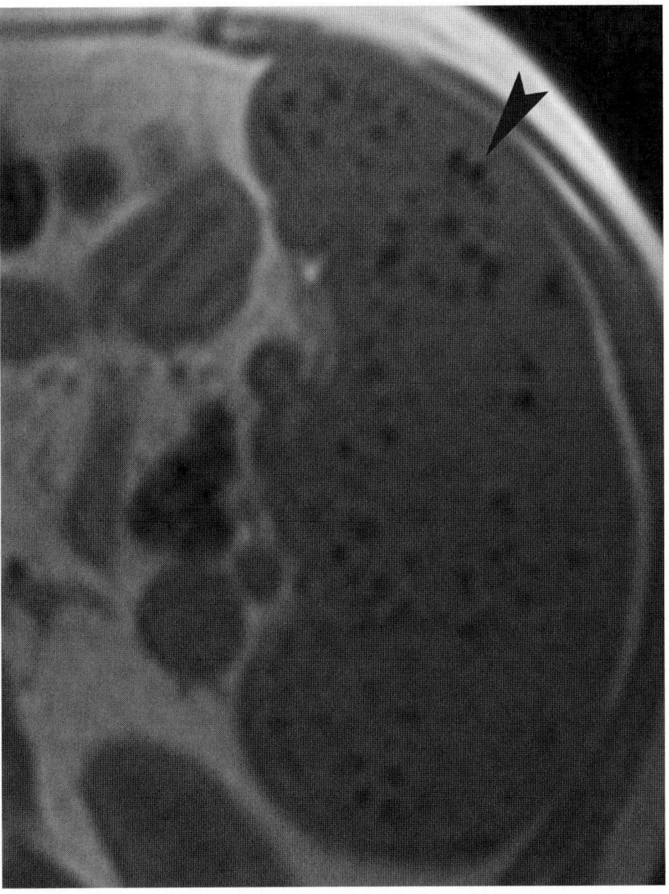

FIGURE 28.28. **Gamna-Gandy Bodies.** Axial T1WI shows numerous low-signal nodules (*arrowhead*) throughout the splenic parenchyma in a patient with splenomegaly and portal hypertension. These represent hemosiderin deposits from previous tiny intraparenchymal hemorrhages.

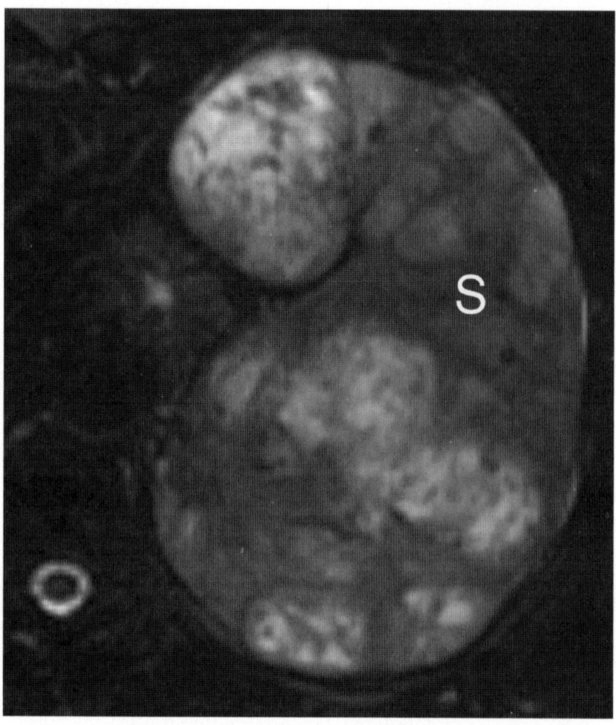

FIGURE 28.30. **Angiosarcoma Spleen.** Axial T2WI shows nearly complete replacement of the parenchyma of the spleen (S) with numerous heterogeneous high-signal nodules of various sizes. Pathology confirmed nearly complete involvement of the spleen with angiosarcoma.

series (30). The tumor consists of vascular channels of varying size lined by a single layer of endothelium. Imaging studies demonstrate an appearance similar to that of hemangiomas in the liver. US shows a well-defined hyperechoic mass. On CT, the lesion may appear solid and may have central punctate or peripheral curvilinear calcification. On MR, the lesion is low in signal intensity on T1WIs and high in signal intensity on T2WIs. The contrast enhancement pattern is variable (Fig. 28.29). The nodular enhancement from the periphery described for liver hemangiomas is not often seen with splenic hemangiomas.

Angiosarcoma is very rare but is still the most common malignancy arising in the spleen (31). The tumor is aggressive, usually presenting with widespread metastases, especially to the liver. Imaging studies demonstrate multiple well-defined enhancing nodules or diffuse spleen abnormality (Fig. 28.30). Patients with Thorotrast exposure are at increased risk.

AIDS

Splenomegaly associated with generalized lymphoid hyperplasia is the most common finding in patients with AIDS. Focal lesions in the spleen are usually caused by opportunistic infections such as pneumocytes, *Pneumocystis jiroveci,* atypical mycobacterium, or *Candida. Pneumocystis jiroveci* infection may cause multiple splenic calcifications (Table 28.5). AIDS-associated lymphoma and Kaposi sarcoma may also cause single or multiple solid-appearing lesions in the spleen.

TABLE 28.5 Causes of Multiple Splenic Calcifications

Histoplasmosis
Tuberculosis
Healed *Pneumocystis jiroveci* (AIDS patient)
Phleboliths
Hemangiomas

REFERENCES

1. Reuther G, Kiefer B, Tuchmann A, Pesendorfer FX. Imaging findings of pancreaticobiliary duct diseases with single-shot MR cholangiopancreatography. AJR Am J Roentgenol 1997;168:453–459.
2. Miller FH, Keppke AL, Dalal K, et al. MRI of pancreatitis and its complications: part 1, acute pancreatitis. AJR Am J Roentgenol 2004;183:1637–1644.
3. Miller FH, Keppke AL, Wadhwa A, et al. MRI of pancreatitis and its complications: part 2, chronic pancreatitis. AJR Am J Roentgenol 2004;183:1645–1652.
4. Balthazar EJ. Acute pancreatitis: assessment of severity with clinical and CT evaluation. Radiology 2002;223:603–613.
5. Mortele KJ, Wiesner W, Intriere L, et al. A modified CT severity index for evaluating acute pancreatitis: improved correlation with patient outcome. AJR Am J Roentgenol 2004;183:1261–1265.
6. Paulson EK, Vitellas KM, Keogan MT, et al. Acute pancreatitis complicated by gland necrosis: spectrum of findings on contrast-enhanced CT. AJR Am J Roentgenol 1999;172:609–613.
7. Lee MJ, Wittich GR, Mueller PR. Percutaneous intervention in acute pancreatitis. Radiographics 1998;18:711–724.
8. Irie H, Honda H, Baba S, et al. Autoimmune pancreatitis: CT and MR characteristics. AJR Am J Roentgenol 1998;170:1323–1327.
9. Tamm EP, Silverman PM, Charnsangavej C, Evans DB. Diagnosis, staging, and surveillance of pancreatic cancer. AJR Am J Roentgenol 2003;180:1311–1323.
10. Novick SL, Fishman EK. Three-dimensional CT angiography of pancreatic carcinoma: role in staging extent of disease. AJR Am J Roentgenol 1998;170:139–143.
11. Bluemke DA, Abrams RA, Yeo CJ, Cameron JL, Fishman EK. Recurrent pancreatic adenocarcinoma: spiral CT evaluation following the Whipple procedure. Radiographics 1997;17:303–313.
12. Buetow PC, Miller DL, Parrino TV, Buck JL. Islet cell tumors of the pancreas: clinical, radiologic, and pathologic correlation in diagnosis and localization. Radiographics 1997;17:453–472.
13. Sheth S, Hruban RK, Fishman EJ. Helical CT of islet cell tumors of the pancreas: typical and atypical manifestations. AJR Am J Roentgenol 2002;179:725–730.
14. Scatarige JC, Horton KM, Sheth S, Fishman EK. Pancreatic parenchymal metastases: observations on helical CT. AJR Am J Roentgenol 2001;176:695–699.
15. Merkle EM, Bender GN, Brambs H-J. Imaging findings in pancreatic lymphoma: differential aspects. AJR Am J Roentgenol 2000;174:671–675.
16. Katz DS, Hines J, Math KR, et al. Using CT to reveal fat-containing abnormalities of the pancreas. AJR Am J Roentgenol 1999;172:393–396.

17. Demos TC, Posniak HV, Harmath C, Olson MC, Aranha G. Cystic lesions of the pancreas. AJR Am J Roentgenol 2002;179:1375–1388.
18. Kim YH, Saini S, Sahani D, Hahn PF, et al. Imaging diagnosis of cystic pancreatic lesions: pseudocyst versus nonpseudocyst. Radiographics 2005;25:671–685.
19. Spinelli KS, Fromwiller TE, Daniel RA, et al. Cystic pancreatic neoplasms: observe or operate. Ann Surg 2004;239:651–657.
20. Grogan JR, Saeian K, Taylor AJ, et al. Making sense of mucin-producing pancreatic tumors. AJR Am J Roentgenol 2001;176:921–929.
21. Khurana B, Mortele KJ, Glickman J, Silverman SG, Ros PR. Macrocystic serous adenoma of the pancreas: radiologic-pathologic correlation. AJR Am J Roentgenol 2003;181:119–123.
22. Lim JH, Lee G, Oh YL. Radiologic spectrum of intraductal papillary mucinous tumor of the pancreas. Radiographics 2001;21:323–340.
23. Sohn TA, Yeo CJ, Cameron JL, et al. Intraductal papillary mucinous neoplasms of the pancreas: an updated experience. Ann Surg 2004;239:788–797.
24. Stone EE, Brant WE, Smith GB. Computed tomography of duodenal diverticula. J Comput Assist Tomogr 1989;13:61–63.
25. Brant WE, Jain KA. Current imaging of the spleen. Radiologist 1996;3:185–192.
26. Ito K, Mitchell DG, Honjo K, et al. MR imaging of acquired abnormalities of the spleen. AJR Am J Roentgenol 1997;168:697–702.
27. Urban BA, Fishman EK. Helical CT of the spleen. AJR Am J Roentgenol 1998;170:997–1003.
28. Mortele KJ, Mortele B, Silverman SG. CT features of accessory spleen. AJR Am J Roentgenol 2004;183:1653–1657.
29. Urritia M, Mergo PJ, Ros LH, Torres GM, Ros PR. Cystic lesions of the spleen: radiologic-pathologic correlation. Radiographics 1996;16:107–129.
30. Abbott RM, Levy AD, Aguilera NS, Gorospe L, Thompson WM. Primary vascular neoplasms of the spleen: radiologic-pathologic correlation. Radiographics 2004;24:1137–1163.
31. Thompson WM, Levy AD, Aguilera NS, Gorospe L, Abbott RM. Angiosarcoma of the spleen: imaging characteristics in 12 patients. Radiology 2005;235:106–115.

Chapter 29

Pharynx and Esophagus

William E. Brant

Imaging Methods

Anatomy

Normal Swallowing and Motility

Motility Disorders

Outpouchings

Esophagitis

Esophageal Stricture

Enlarged Esophageal Folds

Mass Lesions/Filling Defects

Esophageal Perforation and Trauma

IMAGING METHODS

The upper GI series (UGI), also called a barium meal, is a barium examination of the alimentary tract from the pharynx to the ligament of Treitz. A barium swallow or esophagram is a study more dedicated to evaluation of swallowing disorders and suspected lesions of the pharynx and esophagus. Barium sulfate preparations are ingested orally, and filming is performed during fluoroscopy. The fluoroscopic examination is commonly videotaped or digitally stored to allow for more detailed review of swallowing dynamics and motility. Double-contrast techniques, using mucosal coating with barium combined with luminal distension, are preferred for mucosal detail. Distension of the pharynx is provided by having the patient phonate. Distension of the esophagus is attained by having the patient ingest gas-producing crystals. The full-column, or single-contrast, technique uses barium suspension alone to fill and distend the esophagus. Mucosal relief views are collapsed views of the barium-coated esophagus.

Cross-sectional imaging techniques are used to stage malignancies of the pharynx and esophagus and to clarify findings seen with other imaging methods. CT complements barium studies and endoscopy of the esophagus by demonstrating the esophageal wall and adjacent structures to determine the extent of disease (1). CT is poor at evaluating the mucosa and generally cannot differentiate inflammatory and neoplastic conditions. MR is preferred over CT for evaluation of the nasopharynx and is an alternative to CT for demonstrating the extent of esophageal disease. The clear depiction of blood vessels by MR is useful in confirming the presence of varices and in evaluating mediastinal vascular anatomy. Endoscopic sonography is useful for demonstration of tumor penetration of the esophageal wall (2).

This chapter reviews the pharynx, studied as part of a barium examination and for assessment of swallowing disorders. Cross-sectional imaging of the neck and pharynx is reviewed in Chapter 9.

ANATOMY

The pharynx extends from the nasal cavity to the larynx and is arbitrarily divided into three compartments (Fig. 29.1). The *nasopharynx* extends from the skull base to the soft palate. Its function is entirely respiratory, and the nasopharynx is not considered further in this chapter. The *oropharynx* is posterior to the oral cavity and extends from the soft palate to the hyoid bone. The *hypopharynx* (laryngopharynx) extends from the hyoid bone to the cricopharyngeus muscle. The base of the tongue forms the anterior boundary of the oropharynx. The outline of the surface of the tongue is nodular because of the presence of lymphoid tissue forming the lingual tonsils and the circumvallate papillae, which contain taste buds. The lingual tonsils may hypertrophy and mimic a neoplasm. The epiglottis and aryepiglottic folds separate the larynx

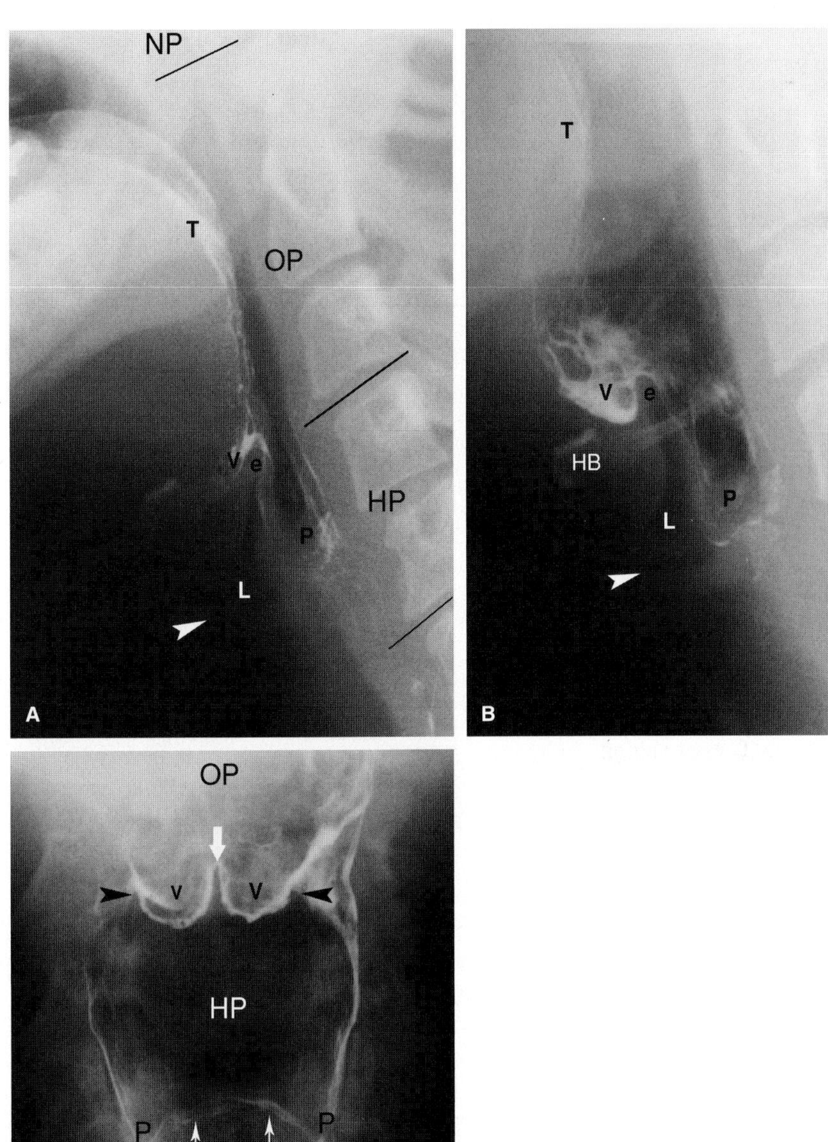

FIGURE 29.1. **Double-Contrast Pharyngogram.** Three radiographs of the pharynx coated with barium demonstrate normal anatomic structures: **(A)** nondistended lateral view; **(B)** distended lateral view, obtained by having the patient phonate "eee..."; and **(C)** frontal (anteroposterior) view. The nasopharynx (NP) extends from the skull base to the soft palate. The oropharynx (OP) spans from the soft palate to the hyoid bone (HB). The hypopharynx (HP) extends from the hyoid bone to the cricopharyngeus muscle (C5–C6), which demarcates the pharynx and esophagus. The epiglottis (e) closes during swallowing to protect the larynx (L) from aspiration. The cricoid cartilage makes a prominent impression on the hypopharynx (*long white arrows*). The base of the tongue (T) has a normal lobulated appearance owing to nodular lymphoid tissue. The valleculae (V) are recesses between the tongue and epiglottis, bordered by the median glossoepiglottic fold (*thick white arrow*) and the lateral glossoepiglottic folds (*black arrowheads*). The pyriform recesses (P) extend laterally and posterior to the larynx. The pyriform recesses are commonly slightly asymmetric in size. The laryngeal ventricle (*white arrowhead*) is faintly visualized, outlined by air between the false vocal cords above and the true vocal cords below.

from the oropharynx and hypopharynx. The *valleculae* are two symmetric pouches formed in the recess between the base of the tongue and the epiglottis. They are divided medially by the median glossoepiglottic fold and bounded laterally by the lateral glossoepiglottic folds. The *piriform sinuses* are deep, symmetric, lateral recesses formed by the protrusion of the larynx into the hypopharynx.

The esophagus extends from the cricopharyngeus muscle at the level of C5–C6 to the gastroesophageal junction (GEJ). The esophagus is a muscular tube formed by an outer longitudinal muscle layer and an inner circular muscle layer lined by stratified squamous epithelium. The esophagus lacks a serosal layer, which allows for rapid spread of tumor into adjacent tissues. The proximal third of the esophagus is predominantly striated muscle, whereas the distal two thirds, below the level of the aortic arch, is predominantly smooth muscle. Normal extrinsic impressions on the esophagus are made by the aortic arch, the left mainstem bronchus, and the LA. The normal esophageal mucosa is smooth and featureless when fully distended on air-contrast barium studies (3). With partial collapse, multiple longitudinal folds, 1 to 2 mm in thickness, become evident. Multiple regular, transverse folds, 1 mm thick, result from contraction of the longitudinal fibers in the muscularis mucosa (see Fig. 29.17). This pattern is called *feline esophagus* because it is typical of a

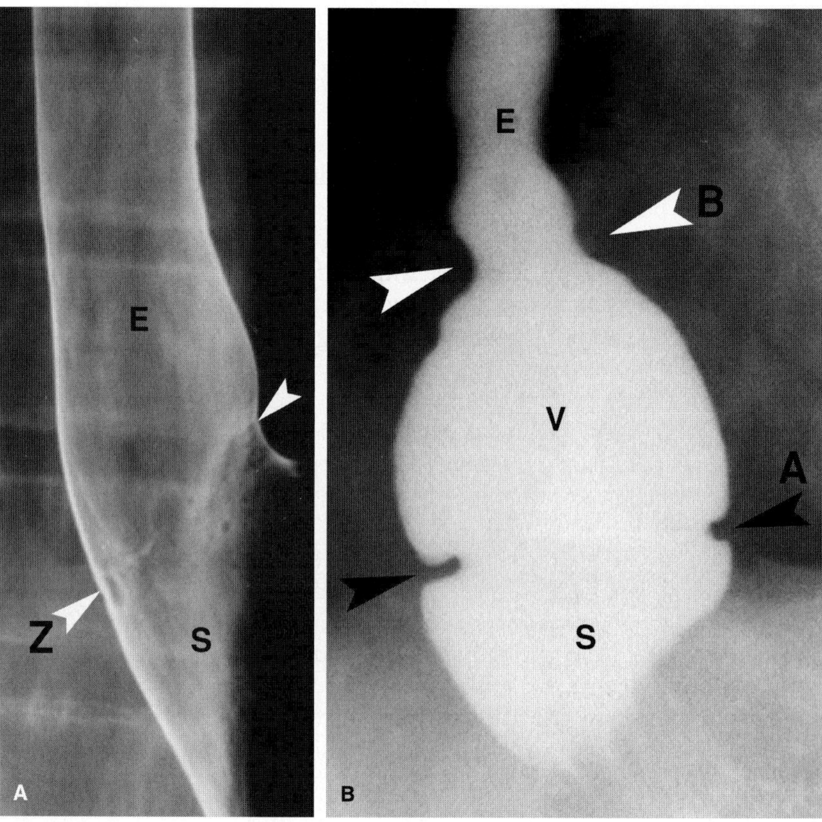

FIGURE 29.2. **Anatomy of the Gastroesophageal Junction (GEJ).** Radiographs from a double-contrast barium study **(A)** and a single-contrast barium study **(B)** demonstrate the physiologic and anatomic landmarks of the GEJ. The Z line (Z, *white arrowheads*), seen best on the double-contrast study, marks the junction of the squamous epithelium of the esophagus (E) and the columnar epithelium of the stomach (S). The single-contrast study demonstrates the esophageal vestibule (V) demarcated by the muscular A ring (A, *white arrowheads*) and the mucosal fold of the B ring (B, *black arrowheads*). The vestibule marks the location of the lower esophageal sphincter. The Z line and the B ring are markers of the GEJ. Their location relative to the esophageal hiatus in the diaphragm varies with swallowing and other physiologic motions. The double-contrast study shows the featureless mucosal pattern of the well-distended normal esophagus.

normal esophagus in cats. In humans, it may be an early sign of dysmotility or esophagitis.

On cross-sectional imaging, the esophagus appears as an oval of soft tissue density usually surrounded by fat. The esophagus may contain air or contrast located centrally within its lumen. Eccentric contrast or air should be considered abnormal. The wall of the distended esophagus should not exceed 3 mm in thickness.

The anatomy of the esophagogastric region is complex (Fig. 29.2). The length of the esophagus is tubular, and its termination is saccular. The saccular termination is called the *esophageal vestibule.* The tubulovestibular junction is formed by a symmetric muscular ring called the *A ring.* The *B ring* is an asymmetric mucosal ring or notch that occurs at the junction of esophageal squamous epithelium with gastric columnar epithelium. This squamocolumnar junction is also marked by the *Z line,* a thin ragged line of demarcation seen on double-contrast views of the lower esophagus. The B ring and the Z line are considered to be radiographic markers of the GEJ.

The esophageal hiatus is an angled opening in the diaphragm formed by the edges of the diaphragmatic crura. On CT and MR, the crura appear, often prominently, as teardrop-shaped structures of muscle density. With normal breathing, the proximal vestibule and A ring lie in the thorax. The midvestibule is in the esophageal hiatus, and the distal vestibule and B ring are in the abdomen. With swallowing, the vestibule opens and moves upward and the B ring may be seen 1 cm above the diaphragm.

NORMAL SWALLOWING AND MOTILITY

The normal process of swallowing can be divided into oral, pharyngeal, and esophageal phases. The oral stage involves the voluntary transport of a bolus from the oral cavity into the pharynx. The soft palate elevates and the tongue depresses to accommodate the bolus and channel it into the oropharynx. The oropharynx and hypopharynx receive the bolus and conduct it to the esophagus. Breathing is halted while the larynx elevates, the laryngeal vestibule closes, and the epiglottis and aryepiglottic folds close over the opening into the larynx and deflect the bolus through the lateral piriform recesses.

The functional upper esophageal sphincter (UES), formed by the cricopharyngeus and other pharyngeal muscles, opens to receive the bolus. Peristalsis conveys ingested material through the tubular esophagus to the stomach. *Primary* peristalsis consists of a rapid wave of inhibition that opens the sphincters, followed by a slow wave of contraction that moves the bolus. Normal peristalsis will clear the esophagus completely with each swallow. Radiographically, primary peristalsis appears as a stripping wave that traverses the entire esophagus from top to bottom. *Secondary* peristalsis is initiated by distension of the esophageal lumen. The peristaltic wave starts in the midesophagus and spreads simultaneously up and down the esophagus to clear reflux or any part of a bolus left behind. Secondary waves have the same radiographic appearance as primary waves, except that they start at the point of the retained barium bolus. *Tertiary* waves are nonproductive contractions associated with motility disorders. Irregular contractions follow one another at close intervals from the top to the bottom of the esophagus. These nonperistaltic contractions cause a corkscrew or beaded appearance of the esophageal barium column. The functional lower esophageal sphincter (LES) at the level of the esophageal vestibule relaxes and opens in response to swallowing, primary peristalsis, and proximal esophageal dilation.

Oral and pharyngeal swallowing are evaluated fluoroscopically with the patient in an upright position simulating normal eating. The lateral projection is most useful. Studies are videotaped or digitally stored for subsequent detailed study. Esophageal motility is evaluated by observing fluoroscopically at least five separate swallows of barium with the patient in a prone oblique position. The patient must be instructed to swallow only once, as continuous swallowing distends the esophagus and makes impossible the evaluation of primary peristalsis.

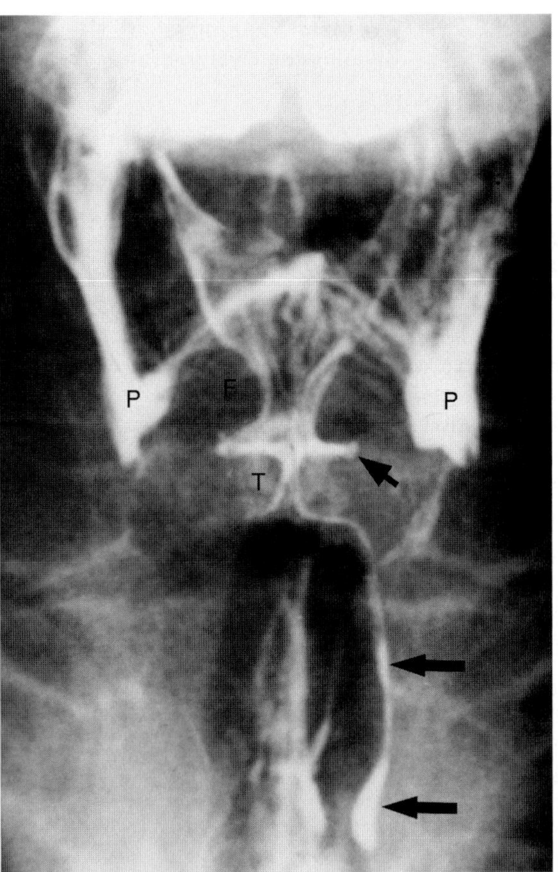

FIGURE 29.3. **Aspiration on a Barium Swallow.** Frontal radiograph taken during a barium swallow examination demonstrates the appearance of aspiration. Barium coats the surface of the false cords (F), the intervening laryngeal ventricle (*arrowhead*), and the true vocal cords (T). Barium coating to this level would be diagnostic of laryngeal penetration. However, barium coating is seen in the proximal trachea (*arrows*) indicating that aspiration has occurred. Barium is also seen pooling in the piriform recesses (P). This is a normal finding.

MOTILITY DISORDERS

Difficulty with swallowing has an increasingly high prevalence with age. Symptoms of abnormal oral or pharyngeal swallowing include difficulty initiating swallowing, globus sensation (lump in throat), cervical dysphagia, nasal regurgitation, hoarseness, coughing, or choking. Symptoms suggesting esophageal dysfunction include heartburn, dysphagia, "indigestion," and chest pain. *Dysphagia* is defined as the awareness of swallowing difficulty during the passage of solids or liquids from mouth to stomach. Patients complain of food "sticking in the throat" and of painful swallowing (odynophagia). These symptoms may be caused by anatomic abnormalities, tumors, or motility disorders. The patient's subjective assessment of the location of the abnormality is not reliable. Detailed dynamic barium studies of the entire oropharyngeal-esophageal pathway with videofluoroscopy are needed for complete evaluation. Motility disorders that may cause dysphagia or aspiration are reviewed in this section. Radiographic findings of functional abnormalities of the pharynx and esophagus increase in prevalence with age, may not correlate with specific symptoms, and must be interpreted with caution.

Signs of Pharyngeal Dysfunction. *Pharyngeal stasis*, indicative of impaired pharyngeal transport, is seen as increased residual volume of swallowed material filling the valleculae and piriform sinuses (4). *Laryngeal penetration* is defined as entry of barium into the laryngeal vestibule without passage below the vocal cords. *Aspiration* implies barium passage below the vocal cords (Fig. 29.3). Any of these findings may precipitate a cough. Laryngeal penetration and tracheobronchial aspiration are associated with an increased risk of pneumonia, especially in hospitalized patients. *Nasal regurgitation* occurs when the soft palate does not make a good seal against the posterior pharyngeal wall. Causes include neurologic impairment, muscular dystrophies, and structural defects in the palate. The major causes of pharyngeal dysfunction are listed in Table 29.1.

Cricopharyngeal achalasia is attributable to failure of complete relaxation of the UES, commonly resulting in dysphagia and aspiration. Barium swallow demonstrates

TABLE 29.1 Causes of Pharyngeal Swallowing Dysfunction

Aging (primary presbyphagia)
Neurologic disease
Cerebrovascular accident
Multiple sclerosis
Movement disorders
Neurodegenerative diseases
CNS infections
Muscle disease
Muscular dystrophies
Myasthenia gravis
Structural abnormalities
Pharyngeal webs
Zenker diverticulum
Tumors
Medications
Radiation
Gastroesophageal reflux
Zenker diverticulum
Trauma
Postsurgical changes
Malignancy
Oral cavity
Pharynx
Larynx

a shelflike impression (*cricopharyngeal bar*) on the barium column at the pharyngoesophageal junction at the level of C5–C6. The pharynx is distended, and barium may overflow into the larynx and trachea. Because some normal individuals have a prominent cricopharyngeal impression, controversy exists as to how prominent the impression must be to be considered significant. Narrowing of the lumen by more than 50% of its usual diameter is generally accepted as a definite cause of dysphagia. Cricopharyngeal dysfunction is commonly associated with neuromuscular disorders of the pharynx.

Esophageal achalasia is a disease of unknown etiology characterized by (*1*) absence of peristalsis in the body of the esophagus, (*2*) marked increase in resting pressure of the LES, and (*3*) failure of the LES to relax with swallowing. The abnormal peristalsis and LES spasm result in a failure of the esophagus to empty. Pathologically, cases show a deficiency of ganglion cells in the myenteric plexus (Auerbach plexus) throughout the esophagus. The clinical presentation is insidious, usually at age 30 to 50 years, with dysphagia, regurgitation, foul breath, and aspiration. Radiographic signs include (*1*) uniform dilatation of the esophagus, usually with an air–fluid level present; (*2*) absence of peristalsis, with tertiary waves common in the early stages of the disease; (*3*) tapered "beak" deformity at the LES because of failure of relaxation (Fig. 29.4); and (*4*) increased incidence of epiphrenic diverticula and esophageal carcinoma. Achalasia is treated with balloon dilation or Heller myotomy. Diseases that may mimic esophageal achalasia include the following.

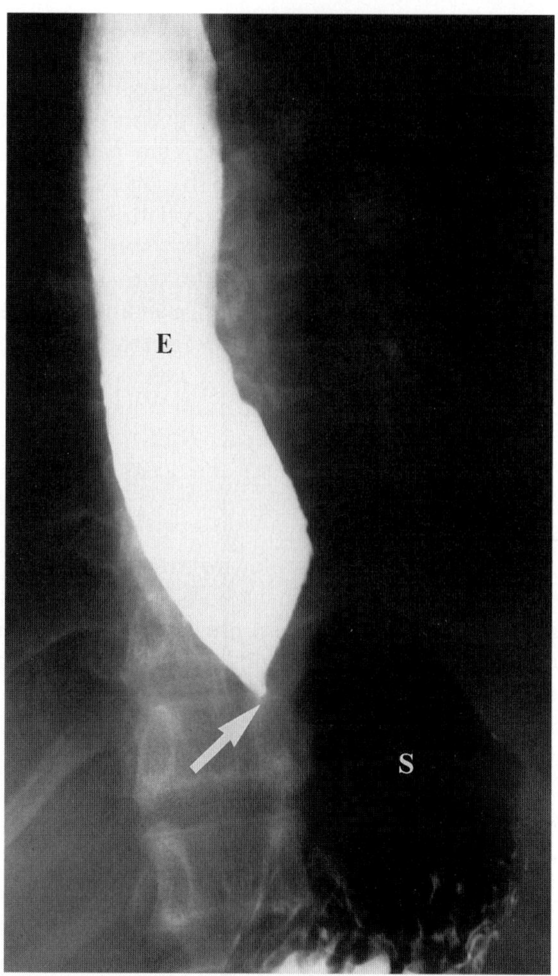

FIGURE 29.4. **Esophageal Achalasia.** Radiograph from an upper GI series reveals uniform dilatation of the esophagus (E) to the level of the gastroesophageal junction, where a beak (*arrow*) is formed by the barium column. Repeated observation by fluoroscopy confirmed failure of relaxation of the lower esophageal sphincter and prolonged retention of barium in the esophagus, even in the upright position. The differential diagnosis for narrowing of the distal esophagus includes tumor, strictures (most often caused by gastroesophageal reflux disease), Chagas disease, and post-vagotomy effect. S, stomach.

Chagas disease is caused by the destruction of ganglion cells of the esophagus as the result of a neurotoxin released by the protozoa *Trypanosoma cruzi,* which is endemic to South America, especially eastern Brazil. The radiographic appearance of the esophagus is identical to that seen in achalasia. Associated abnormalities include cardiomyopathy, megaduodenum, megaureter, and megacolon.

Carcinoma of the GEJ may mimic achalasia, but it tends to involve a longer (>3.5-cm) segment of the distal esophagus, is rigid, and tends to show more irregular tapering of the distal esophagus and mass effect.

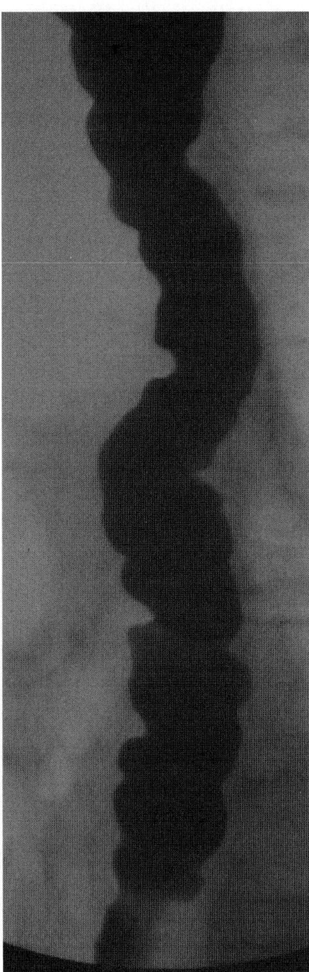

FIGURE 29.5. **Diffuse Esophageal Spasm.** Image from a barium esophagram demonstrates numerous ineffective tertiary contractions throughout the esophagus. The lower esophageal sphincter was dysfunctional, not opening appropriately on fluoroscopic examination.

Peptic strictures are usually associated with normal primary peristalsis.

Diffuse esophageal spasm is a syndrome of unknown cause characterized by multiple tertiary esophageal contractions (Fig. 29.5), thickened esophageal wall, and intermittent dysphagia and chest pain. Primary peristalsis is usually present, but the contractions are infrequent. Most patients are middle-aged. The LES is frequently dysfunctional, and the condition commonly improves with balloon dilatation of the LES.

Neuromuscular disorders are a common cause of abnormalities of the oral, pharyngeal, or esophageal phases of swallowing. The most common causes of neurologic dysfunction are cerebrovascular disease and stroke. Additional causes include parkinsonism, Alzheimer disease, multiple sclerosis, neoplasms of the CNS, and posttraumatic CNS injury. Diseases of striated muscle, such as muscular dystrophy, myasthenia gravis, and dermatomyositis, predominantly affect the pharynx and proximal third (striated muscle portion) of the esophagus.

Scleroderma is a systemic disease of unknown cause characterized by progressive atrophy of smooth muscle and progressive fibrosis of affected tissues. Women are most commonly affected and are usually age 20 to 40 years at the onset of disease. The esophagus is affected in 75% to 80% of patients. Radiographic findings (Fig. 29.6) include (*1*) weak to absent peristalsis in the distal two thirds (smooth muscle portion) of the esophagus, (*2*) delayed esophageal emptying, (*3*) a stiff dilated esophagus that does not collapse with emptying, and (*4*) wide gaping LES with free gastroesophageal reflux. Despite free reflux, tight strictures of the distal esophagus are uncommon.

Postoperative states, including surgery for malignancy of the tongue, larynx, and pharynx, commonly impair swallowing function as well as alter the morphology. Surgical resection is aimed at providing at least a 1-cm

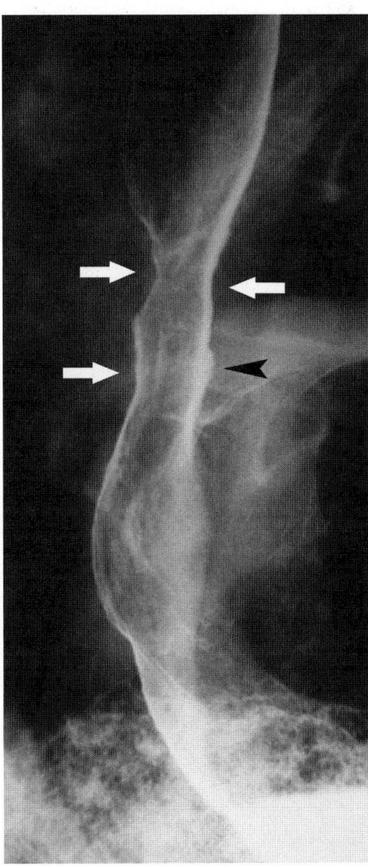

FIGURE 29.6. **Scleroderma.** Double-contrast esophagram in a patient with scleroderma demonstrates a stiff esophagus with peristalsis. The gastroesophageal junction is gaping, and free gastroesophageal reflux was observed. Reflux esophagitis has resulted in mild stricturing (*white arrows*) of the esophagus and focal ulcers (*black arrowhead*).

margin free of tumor and often results in the removal of large blocks of tissue and functional alteration of the structures that remain.

Esophagitis frequently results in abnormal esophageal motility and visualization of tertiary esophageal contractions.

Gastroesophageal reflux disease (GERD) occurs as a result of incompetence of the LES. The resting pressure of the LES is abnormally decreased and fails to increase with raised intra-abdominal pressure. As a result, increases in intra-abdominal pressure exceed LES pressure, and gastric contents are allowed to reflux into the esophagus. Symptoms of GERD include substernal burning pain ("heartburn"), postural regurgitation (in the supine position), and development of reflux esophagitis, dysphagia, and odynophagia. Complications of GERD include reflux esophagitis (RE), stricture, and development of Barrett esophagus. The radiographic diagnosis of GERD may be difficult, because 20% of normal individuals show spontaneous reflux on UGI examination, and patients with pathologic GERD may not demonstrate reflux without provocative tests. Monitoring of esophageal pH for 24 hours in an ambulatory patient is the most sensitive means of diagnosing abnormal gastroesophageal reflux.

Hiatus hernia is often considered synonymous with GERD. There is, however, a poor correlation between the presence of hiatus hernia and GERD or reflux esophagitis. One area of controversy is the definition of hiatus hernia and the criteria used for diagnosis. The simplest definition is protrusion of any portion of the stomach into the thorax. Three types of hiatal hernia are described (5). The most common (95%) is the *sliding hiatus hernia,* with the GEJ displaced more than 1 cm above the hiatus. The esophageal hiatus is often abnormally widened to 3 to 4 cm (Fig. 29.7). The upper limit of normal hiatal width is 15 mm, and this is most easily measured by CT. The gastric fundus may be displaced above the diaphragm and present as a retrocardiac mass on chest radiographs. The presence of an air–fluid level in the mass suggests the diagnosis. Small, sliding hiatus hernias commonly reduce in the upright position. The mere presence of a sliding hiatus hernia is of limited clinical significance in most cases. The function of the LES and the presence of pathologic gastroesophageal reflux are the crucial factors in producing symptoms and causing complications. Much less common is the *paraesophageal hiatus hernia,* in which the GEJ remains in its

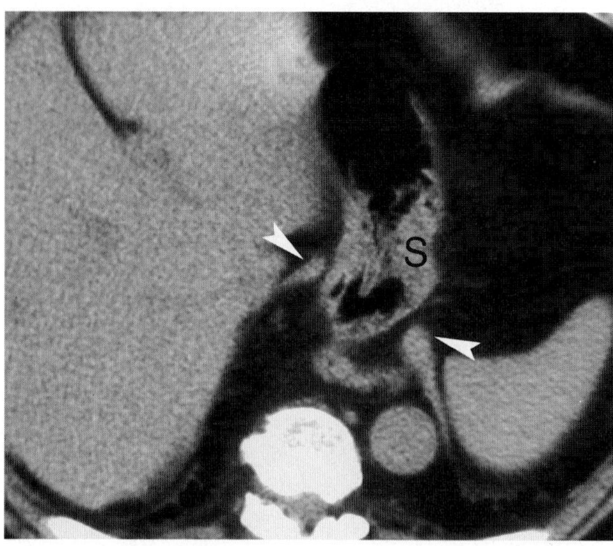

FIGURE 29.7. **Sliding Hiatus Hernia.** CT demonstrates a 26-mm gap between the crura (*arrowheads*) of the diaphragm. The normal esophageal hiatus should not exceed 15 mm. The stomach (S) extends through the hiatus and is positioned both above and below the diaphragm. The gastroesophageal junction was seen at a higher level in the thorax.

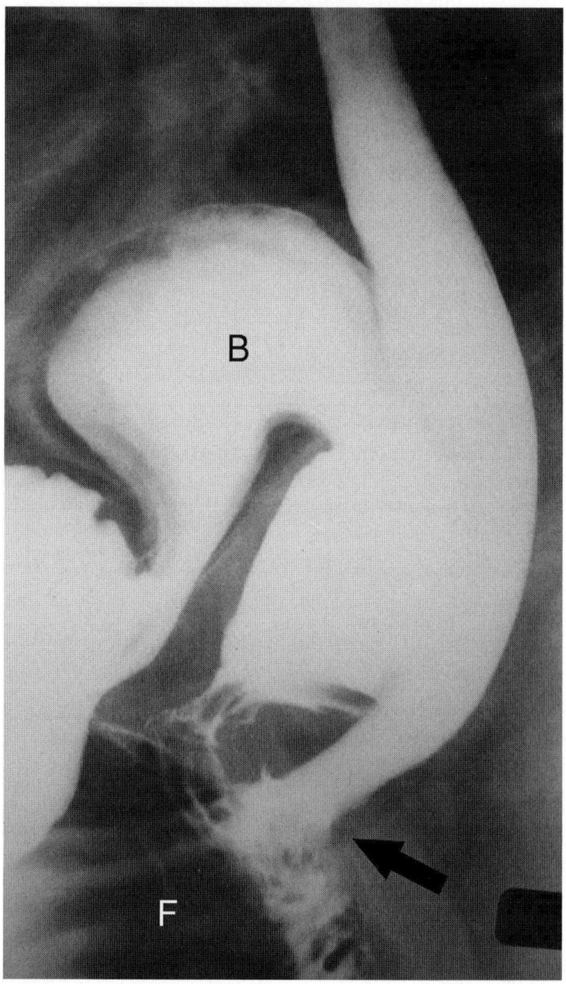

FIGURE 29.8. **Paraesophageal Hiatal Hernia.** Radiograph from an upper GI series shows the characteristic findings of paraesophageal hiatal hernia. The gastroesophageal junction (*arrow*) and fundus (F) of the stomach are below the diaphragm, while a portion of the body (B) of the stomach herniates through the hiatus into the chest and then doubles back into the abdomen.

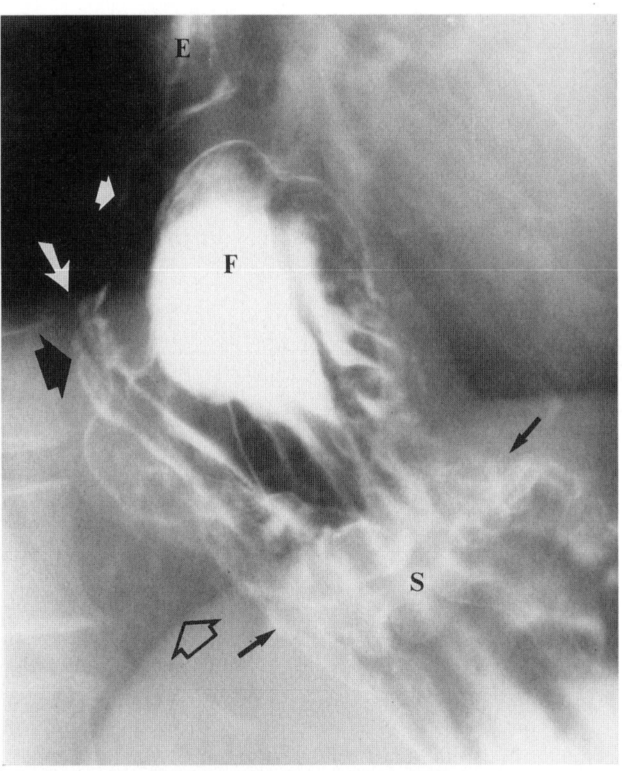

FIGURE 29.9. **Compound Hiatus Hernia.** Left posterior oblique view from an upper GI series demonstrates a large hiatus hernia. The fundus (F) of the stomach (S) extends well above the level of the left hemidiaphragm (*open arrow*). The widened (6-cm) esophageal hiatus makes an impression (*small black arrows*) on the body of the stomach. The gastroesophageal junction (*wide black arrow*) is 5 cm above the left hemidiaphragm. The distal esophagus (*wide white arrow*) is bowed around the herniated stomach. The right hemidiaphragm (*white arrow*) projects well above the left hemidiaphragm on this view.

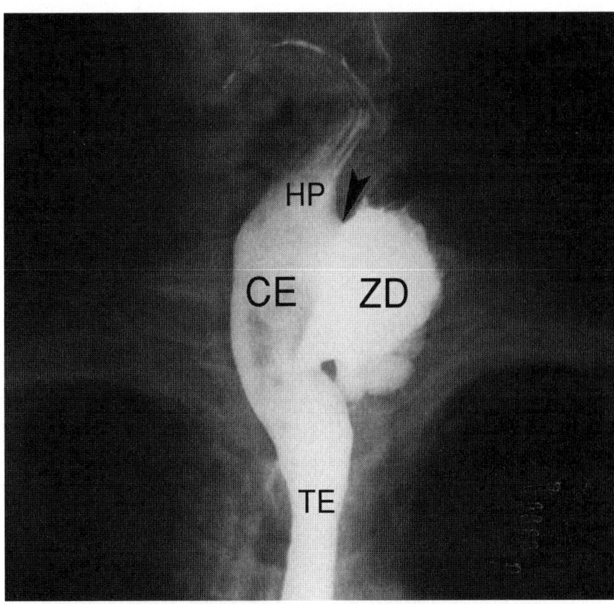

FIGURE 29.10. **Zenker Diverticulum.** Barium swallow examination demonstrates the characteristic barium-filled outpouching, indicating a Zenker diverticulum (ZD) at the junction of the hypopharynx (HP) and cervical esophagus (CE). Note that the neck of the diverticulum (*arrowhead*) is at a more cephalad location than its base, encouraging the trapping of food and liquid. TE, thoracic esophagus.

normal location while a portion of the stomach herniates above the diaphragm (Fig. 29.8). The *mixed or compound hiatal hernia* is the most common type of paraesophageal hernia (Fig. 29.9). The GEJ is displaced into the thorax with a large portion of the stomach, which is usually abnormally rotated. Paraesophageal hernias, especially when large with most of the stomach in the thorax, are at risk for volvulus, obstruction, and ischemia.

OUTPOUCHINGS

Lateral pharyngeal diverticula are protrusions of pharyngeal mucosa through areas of weakness of the lateral pharyngeal wall and are most common in the region of the tonsillar fossa and thyrohyoid membrane. They reflect increased intrapharyngeal pressure and are seen most commonly in wind instrument players.

Zenker diverticulum arises in the hypopharynx just proximal to the UES. It is located in the posterior midline at the cleavage plane (known as Killian dehiscence) between the circular and oblique fibers of the cricopharyngeus muscle. The diverticulum has a small neck that is higher than the sac, resulting in the trapping of food and liquid within the sac (Fig. 29.10). The distended sac may compress the cervical esophagus. Symptoms include dysphagia, halitosis, and regurgitation of food.

Midesophageal diverticula may be pulsion or traction diverticula. Pulsion diverticula occur as a result of disordered esophageal peristalsis (Fig. 29.11). Traction diverticula occur because of fibrous inflammatory reactions of adjacent lymph nodes. Most midesophageal diverticula have large mouths and empty well, so they are usually asymptomatic.

Epiphrenic diverticula occur just above the LES, usually on the right side. They are rare and usually found in patients with esophageal motility disorders (Fig. 29.12). Because they have a small neck that is higher than the sac, they may trap food and liquids and cause symptoms.

Sacculations are small outpouchings of the esophagus that usually occur as a sequela of severe esophagitis (Fig. 29.13). They are thought to result from the healing and scarring of ulcerations. Sacculations tend to change in size and shape during fluoroscopic observation. Smooth contours help to differentiate sacculations from ulcerations.

Intramural pseudodiverticula are the dilated excretory ducts of deep mucous glands of the esophagus (6). They appear as flask-shaped barium collections that

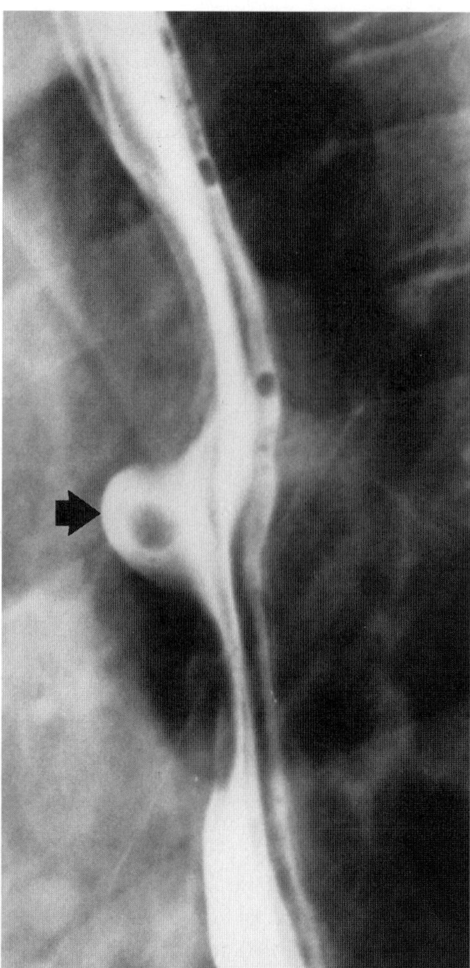

FIGURE 29.11. **Pulsion Diverticulum.** A barium swallow examination demonstrates a persistent mucosal outpouching (*arrow*) in the midesophagus. The patient was asymptomatic. Pulsion diverticula are formed when the mucosa and submucosa herniate through the muscularis.

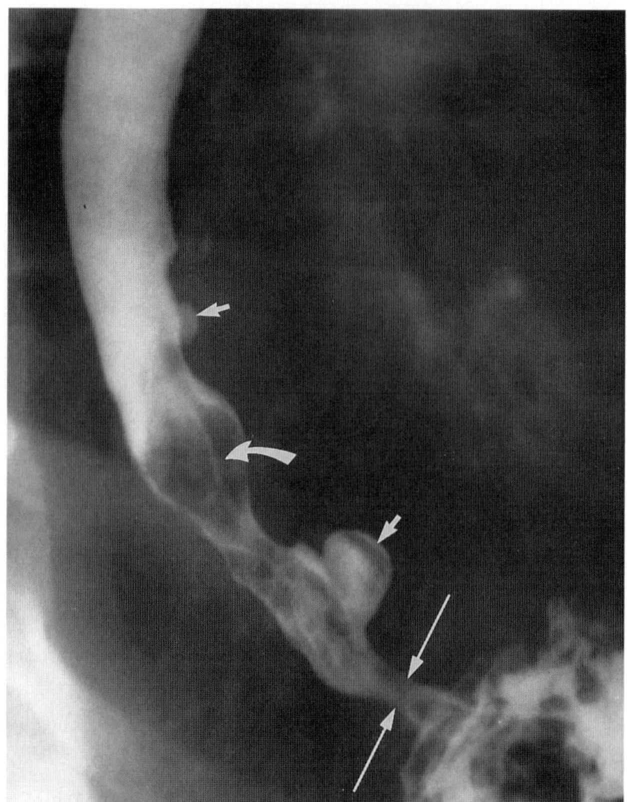

FIGURE 29.12. **Epiphrenic Diverticula.** A stricture (*long arrows*) of the distal esophagus has resulted in the formation of pulsion diverticula (*short arrows*). The filling defects (*curved arrow*) in the barium column are caused by retained boluses of meat proximal to the stricture.

extend from the lumen or as lines and flecks of barium outside the esophageal wall. They tend to occur in clusters and in association with strictures. Liner tracks of barium ("intramural tracking") commonly bridge adjacent pseudodiverticula.

ESOPHAGITIS

Esophagitis is a common disease with many causes. Radiologic evaluation will detect most cases of moderate to severe esophagitis but will demonstrate fewer than half the cases of mild esophagitis. Attention to excellent technique and use of double-contrast studies are essential. Radiographic signs of esophagitis include (*1*) thickened esophageal folds (>3 mm), (*2*) limited esophageal distensibility (asymmetric flattening), (*3*) abnormal motility, (*4*) mucosal plaques and nodules, (*5*) erosions and ulcerations, (*6*) localized stricture, and (*7*) intramural pseudodiverticulosis (barium filling of dilated 1- to 3-mm submucosal glands). Ulcers are a hallmark finding of esophagitis. Small ulcers (<1 cm) are found with RE, herpes, acute radiation, drug-induced esophagitis, and benign mucous membrane pemphigoid. Larger ulcers (>1 cm) are characteristic of cytomegalovirus, HIV, Barrett esophagus, and carcinoma. CT usually reveals nonspecific findings of thickening of the wall (>5 mm) and target sign with hypoattenuating thickened wall and high-attenuation enhancing mucosa (7).

Reflux esophagitis is the result of esophageal mucosal injury caused by exposure to gastroduodenal secretions. The severity depends on the concentration of caustic agents, including acid, pepsin, bile salts, caffeine, alcohol, and aspirin, as well as the duration of contact with the esophageal mucosa. The findings of RE are always most prominent in the distal esophagus and GEJ (Fig. 29.13). Early changes of RE include mucosal edema, which is manifested as a granular or nodular pattern of the distal esophagus. In contrast to the distinct borders of *Candida* plaques and nodules, RE nodules have poorly defined borders. Inflammatory exudates and pseudomembrane formation may mimic fulminant *Candida* esophagitis;

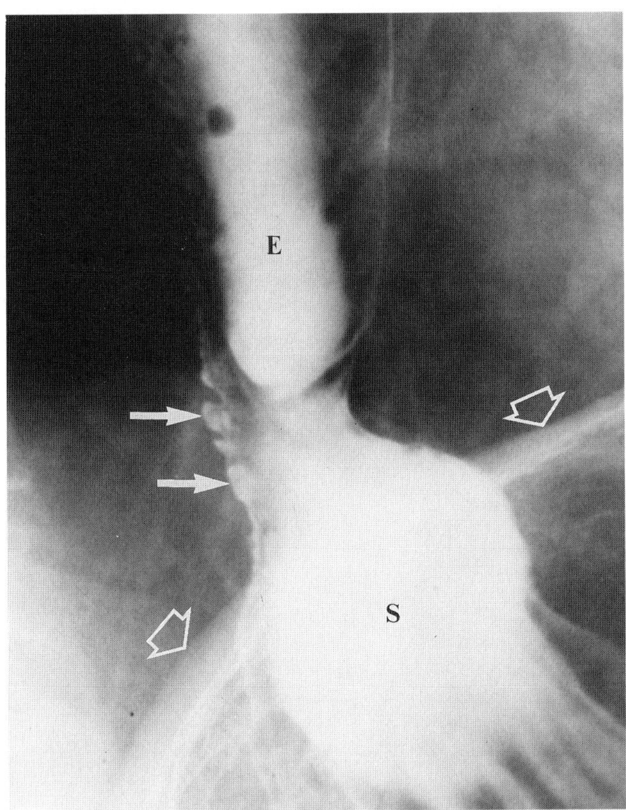

FIGURE 29.13. **Reflux Esophagitis.** A barium esophagram demonstrates stiffness and narrowing of the distal esophagus just above the level of the diaphragm (*open arrows*). Several prominent sacculations (*arrows*) are present, indicating long-standing and severe esophagitis. E, esophagus; S, stomach.

however, the patient has symptoms of reflux rather than severe odynophagia. RE is the most common cause of esophageal ulcerations. The ulcers appear as discrete linear, punctate, or irregular collections of barium, usually surrounded by a radiolucent mound of edema. Prominence of the ulcerations in the distal rather than proximal or midesophagus is the key to differentiating RE ulcers from those of herpes or drug-induced esophagitis. Complications of RE include ulceration, bleeding, stricture, and Barrett esophagus.

Barrett esophagus is an acquired condition of progressive columnar metaplasia of the distal esophagus caused by chronic GERD. Columnar rather than squamous epithelium lines the distal esophagus. The prevalence of Barrett esophagus in patients with reflux esophagitis is about 10%, but increases to 37% in patients with scleroderma. It is premalignant, with a 30- to 40-fold increased risk of developing adenocarcinoma, resulting in a 15% prevalence of adenocarcinoma in patients with Barrett esophagus. Clinical presentation is usually indistinguishable from that of RE. Adenocarcinoma may develop at any age. The characteristic radiographic appearance of Barrett esophagus is a high (midesophageal) stricture or deep ulcer in a patient with GERD. A reticular mucosal pattern of the esophageal mucosa, resembling areae gastricae of the stomach, is also suggestive. The diagnosis is confirmed by endoscopy and biopsy.

Infectious esophagitis is found most commonly in patients with compromised immune systems. It is increasingly common because of the use of steroids and cytotoxic drugs and because of the increasing prevalence of AIDS.

Candida albicans is by far the most common cause of infectious esophagitis and is highly prevalent in patients with AIDS. Additional risk factors include malignancy, radiation, chemotherapy, and steroid treatments. *Candida* of the oropharynx (thrush) is commonly present and is usually evident on physical examination. Odynophagia is a prominent symptom. Discrete plaquelike lesions demonstrated by double-contrast esophagrams are most characteristic (Fig. 29.14). The plaques appear as longitudinally

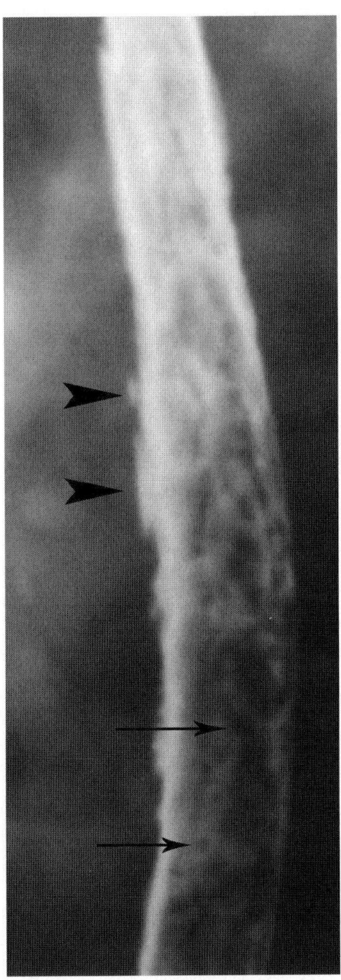

FIGURE 29.14. **Candida Esophagitis.** Barium esophagram in an immunocompromised patient on chemotherapy demonstrates "shaggy" esophageal mucosa caused by multiple confluent plaques (*arrows*) and shallow ulcers (*arrowheads*) produced by *Candida albicans* esophagitis.

oriented linear or irregular discrete filling defects etched in white with intervening normal-appearing mucosa. The lesions may be tiny and nodular, or they may be giant and coalescent with pseudomembranes. Ulcers tend to be small (<1 cm) and may be punctate, round, oval, or linear. Fulminant disease produces a "foamy esophagus," with a pattern of tiny bubbles at the top of the barium column.

Herpes simplex esophagitis begins as discrete vesicles that rupture to form discrete mucosal ulcers. The ulcers may be linear, punctate, or ringlike and have a characteristic radiolucent halo. Discrete ulcers on a background of normal mucosa involving the midesophagus are most characteristic of herpes. Nodules and plaques are usually absent.

Cytomegalovirus is a cause of fulminant esophagitis in patients with AIDS. Cytomegalovirus esophagitis is characteristically manifest as one or more large, flat mucosal ulcers (Fig. 29.15). Endoscopic biopsy or culture confirms the diagnosis.

HIV esophagitis causes giant ulcers and severe odynophagia. Electron microscopy reveals HIV particles in the ulcers. The ulcers are large, flat, and usually in the midesophagus.

Tuberculosis. The esophagus is the least common portion of the GI tract to be involved by tuberculosis. Manifestations include ulceration, stricture, sinus tracts, and abscess formation (Fig. 29.16).

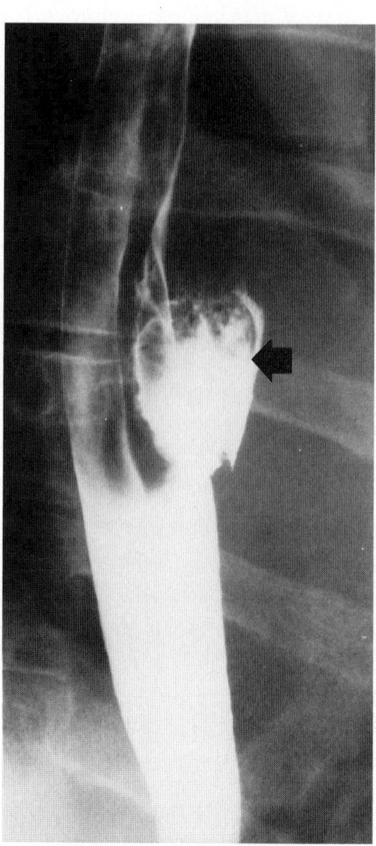

FIGURE 29.16. **Tuberculous Esophagitis.** Tuberculosis in an immunocompromised patient has ulcerated the esophagus and causes a periesophageal abscess (*arrow*).

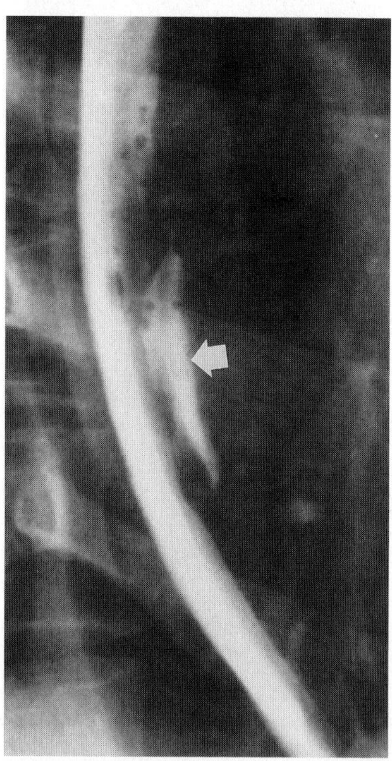

FIGURE 29.15. **Cytomegalovirus Esophagitis.** A large flat mucosal ulcer (*arrow*) in the distal esophagus is characteristic of Cytomegalovirus esophagitis in a patient with AIDS.

Drug-induced esophagitis is the result of intake of oral medications that produce a focal inflammation in areas of contact with the mucosa. Drugs that cause this condition include tetracycline, doxycycline, quinidine, aspirin, indomethacin, ascorbic acid, potassium chloride, and theophylline. The radiographic appearance may be identical to that of herpes esophagitis, with discrete ulcers separated by normal mucosa in the midesophagus (Fig. 29.17). The diagnosis is suggested by a history of recent drug ingestion. Healing usually occurs within 7 to 10 days of discontinuing the offending medication.

Corrosive ingestion usually occurs as an accident in children or a suicide attempt in adults. Alkaline agents (e.g., liquid lye) produce deep (full-thickness) coagulation necrosis. Acid agents tend to produce more superficial injury. Ulceration, esophageal perforation, and mediastinitis may complicate the acute injury. Late complications are fibrosis and long or multiple strictures.

Crohn disease may rarely manifest as discrete aphthous ulcers in the esophagus. Involvement of the small or large bowel by Crohn disease is virtually always present. Crohn disease of the esophagus should not be considered unless Crohn disease of the bowel is already evident.

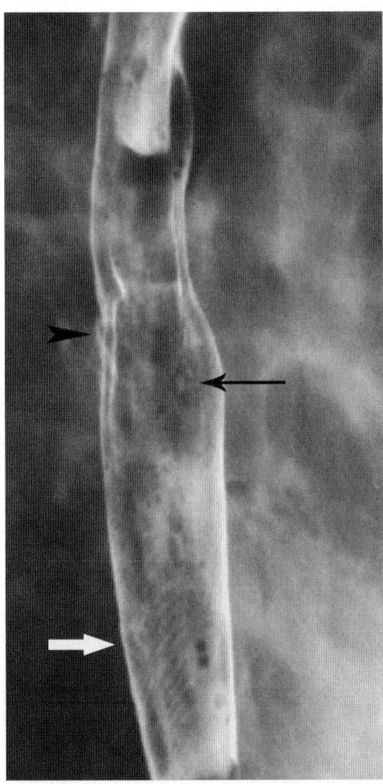

FIGURE 29.17. **Drug-Induced Esophagitis.** Air-contrast esophagram demonstrates discrete shallow ulcers en face (*black arrow*) and in profile (*arrowhead*). The ulcers were caused by stasis of tetracycline capsules in the esophagus. Multiple regular, thin, transverse folds (*white arrow*) in the distal esophagus are typical of feline esophagus, a finding suggestive of esophagitis.

Radiation esophagitis occurs in patients with a history of thoracic radiation therapy for malignant disease. Acute radiation may cause shallow or deep ulcers in the area of involvement. With the development of fibrosis, the peristaltic wave is interrupted, and a long smooth stricture may develop within the radiotherapy field. Higher radiation doses, in the range of 45 to 60 Gy, are associated with development of strictures. Simultaneous radiotherapy and doxorubicin hydrochloride (Adriamycin) chemotherapy greatly accentuates esophageal inflammation. UGI will show a variable-length segment of esophageal narrowing, multiple discrete ulcers, or a granular mucosal pattern within the radiation field.

ESOPHAGEAL STRICTURE

Strictures are defined as any persistent intrinsic narrowing of the esophagus (6). The most common causes are fibrosis induced by inflammation and neoplasm. Because radiographic findings are not reliable in differentiating benign from malignant strictures, all should be evaluated endoscopically (8). Distal esophageal strictures are caused by GERD, scleroderma, and prolonged nasogastric intubation. Upper and middle esophageal strictures most commonly result from Barrett esophagus, mediastinal radiation, caustic ingestion, and skin diseases associated with mucosal ulceration, such as pemphigoid, erythema multiforme, and epidermolysis bullosa dystrophica. Benign strictures typically show smoothly tapering, concentric narrowing (Fig. 29.18). Malignant strictures are characteristically abrupt, asymmetric, eccentric narrowings with irregular, nodular, mucosa (Fig. 29.19). Tapered margins may occur with malignant lesions because of the ease of submucosal spread of tumor (9).

Esophagitis. Chronic inflammation induces progressive fibrosis that eventually narrows the esophageal lumen. Acute and chronic findings of esophagitis commonly overlap.

Reflux esophagitis (GERD) is the most common cause of esophageal stricture. Reflux strictures are usually confined to the distal esophagus and may be tapered, smooth, and circumferential (the classic appearance) (Fig. 29.18) or asymmetric and irregular. Small smooth sacculations and fixed transverse folds are characteristic and caused

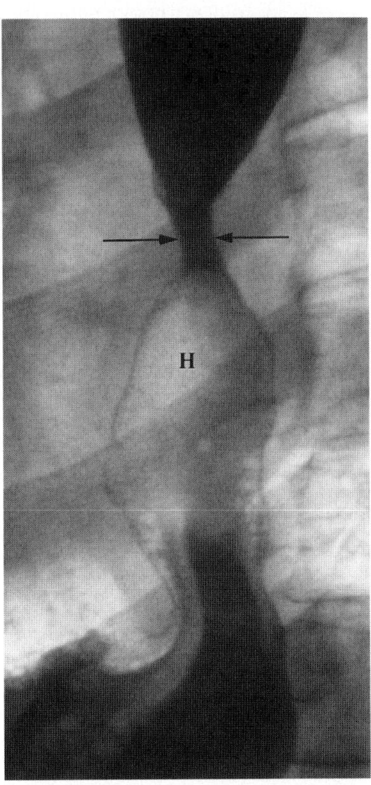

FIGURE 29.18. **Benign Stricture Resulting from Reflux Esophagitis.** A short, narrowed area (*arrows*) of the distal esophagus extends to the top of a hiatus hernia (H) in this patient with chronic gastroesophageal reflux. Note the tapered margins and concentric shape of the stricture, which are typical for a benign stricture.

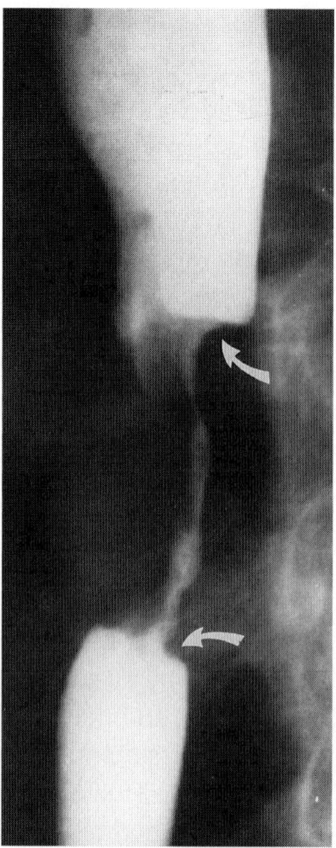

FIGURE 29.19. **Malignant Stricture.** A squamous cell carcinoma of the midesophagus causes an abrupt narrowing with irregular mucosa. The prominent shoulders (*arrows*) are characteristic of tumor. Differential diagnosis of strictures of the upper and midesophagus includes Barrett esophagus, mediastinal irradiation, caustic ingestion, and drug-induced esophagitis.

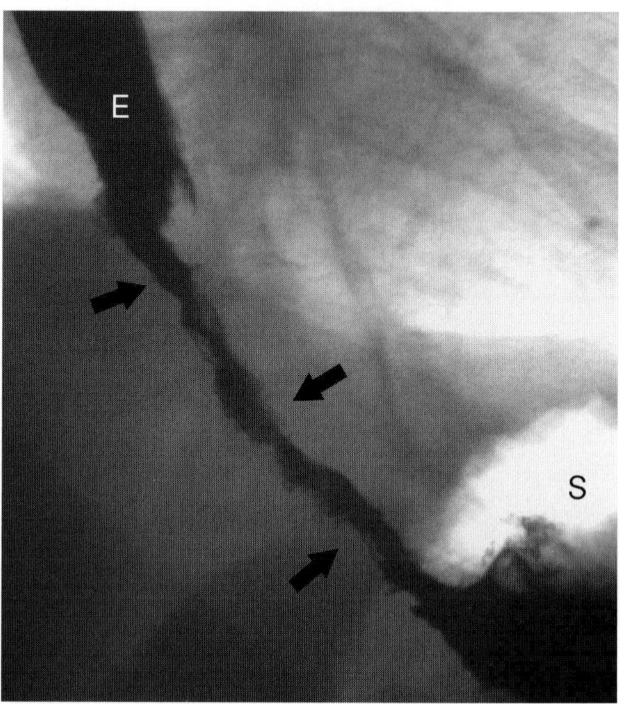

FIGURE 29.20. **Long Stricture Resulting from Esophageal Carcinoma.** A long-segment stricture (*arrows*) of the distal esophagus (E) is apparent on this barium esophagram. The column of barium is abruptly narrowed to a thin, markedly irregular channel. Differential diagnosis of long-segment strictures of the esophagus include reflux esophagitis, caustic ingestion, complicated scleroderma, and radiation esophagitis. S, stomach.

by scarring. Long-segment stricture may be induced by long-term nasogastric intubation. Zollinger-Ellison syndrome can lead to severe RE because of the high acid content of refluxed gastric contents. A *Schatzki ring* is a pathologic ringlike stricture at the level of the B ring caused by RE.

Barrett esophagus strictures tend to be high in the midesophagus and may be smooth and tapered or ringlike narrowings. The high position is caused by a tendency for strictures to occur at the squamocolumnar junction, which has been displaced to a position well above the GEJ.

Corrosives strictures are long and symmetric. They commonly develop years after the initial injury.

Radiation strictures are confined to the radiotherapy field. They are smooth and tapered and usually in the upper or midesophagus.

Neoplasm. An irregular, ulcerated, circumferential narrowing is most typical of a malignant stricture (Fig. 29.19). Infiltrative tumors may cause smooth, rigid narrowing of the esophagus without a clear zone of transition. The mucosa may not be altered until tumor spread is substantial. Because longitudinal spread of tumor along the length of the esophagus is typical, long-segment strictures caused by carcinoma are common (Fig. 29.20).

Webs are thin (1 to 2 mm), delicate membranes that sweep partially across the lumen (Fig. 29.21). They occur in both the pharynx and esophagus and are commonly multiple. Pharyngeal webs arise most commonly from the anterior wall of the hypopharynx. Esophageal webs may occur anywhere, but they are most common in the cervical esophagus just distal to the cricopharyngeus impression. Most are incidental findings; however, they occasionally cause sufficient obstruction to result in dysphagia.

Extrinsic Compression. Malignancy or inflammation in the mediastinum may encase the esophagus and narrow its lumen. Causes include lung carcinoma, lymphoma, metastasis to mediastinal nodes, tuberculosis, and histoplasmosis.

ENLARGED ESOPHAGEAL FOLDS

Esophagitis. Thick folds occur most commonly with RE. Additional findings associated with esophagitis, such as ulcerations and nodules, are commonly present.

Varices appear as serpiginous filling defects (Fig. 29.22) that change in size with changes in intrathoracic

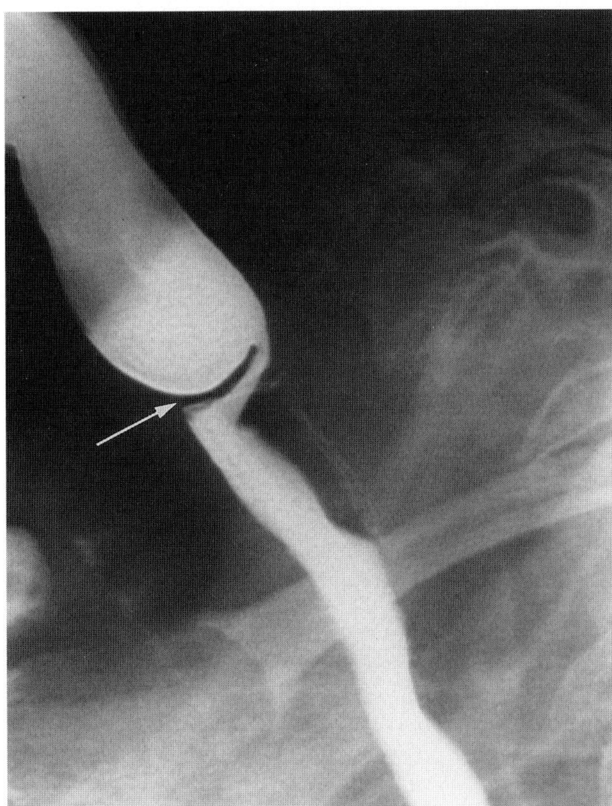

FIGURE 29.21. **Esophageal Web.** Lateral oblique view from a barium esophagram reveals a thin membrane (*arrow*) that extends across the lumen of the proximal esophagus, leaving only a narrow lumen for passage of food. The esophagus is dilated proximal to the web.

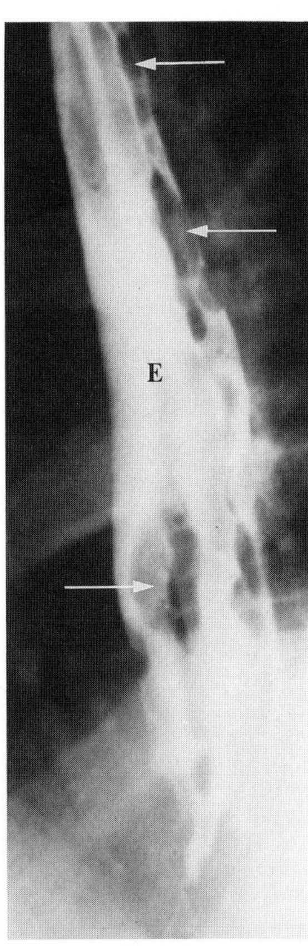

FIGURE 29.22. **Varices.** A single-contrast barium esophagram demonstrates sinuous tubular and nodular filling defects (*arrows*) in the esophagus (E). This patient has cirrhosis, portal hypertension, and a history of upper GI bleeding.

pressure and that collapse with esophageal peristalsis and distension. They are best demonstrated on UGI with mucosal relief views. Spiral CT with bolus contrast enhancement demonstrates varices as enhancing vascular structures within and adjacent to the esophageal wall near the GEJ. MR is also effective in demonstrating varices as vascular spaces, with signal void because of flowing blood.

Uphill varices refer to the portosystemic collateral veins that enlarge because of portal hypertension. Coronary vein collaterals connect with gastroesophageal varices that drain into the inferior vena cava via the azygos system. Uphill varices are usually only present in the distal esophagus. *Downhill varices* are formed as a result of obstruction of the superior vena cava with drainage from the azygos system through esophageal varices to the portal vein. Downhill varices usually predominate in the proximal esophagus.

Lymphoma may infiltrate the submucosa and thicken the folds. Lymphoma rarely involves the esophagus directly and is virtually never primary in the esophagus.

Varicoid carcinoma causes thick, tortuous, longitudinal folds that resemble varices but are rigid and persistent.

MASS LESIONS/FILLING DEFECTS

Pharyngeal carcinomas are well demonstrated by double-contrast pharyngography. Barium studies may detect tumors that are difficult to visualize endoscopically. Radiographic signs include (*1*) intraluminal mass, seen as a filling defect, abnormal luminal contour, or focal increased density; (*2*) mucosal irregularity owing to ulceration or mucosal elevations; and (*3*) asymmetric distensibility caused by infiltrating tumor or extrinsic nodal mass. Most pharyngeal tumors are squamous cell carcinomas, which may arise on the base of the tongue, palatine tonsil, posterior pharyngeal wall, or the piriform sinus (Fig. 29.23). Laryngeal tumors may impress on the pharynx or extend into it. Staging is best performed by CT or MR.

Lymphoma of the pharynx is usually manifested as a large, bulky tumor of the lingual or palatine tonsils. Lymphoma constitutes 15% of oropharyngeal tumors.

Esophageal carcinoma is squamous cell carcinoma in 85% to 90% of cases; the remainder are adenocarcinoma arising in Barrett esophagus (Fig. 29.24), undifferentiated, or miscellaneous cell types. Because of rapid spread to

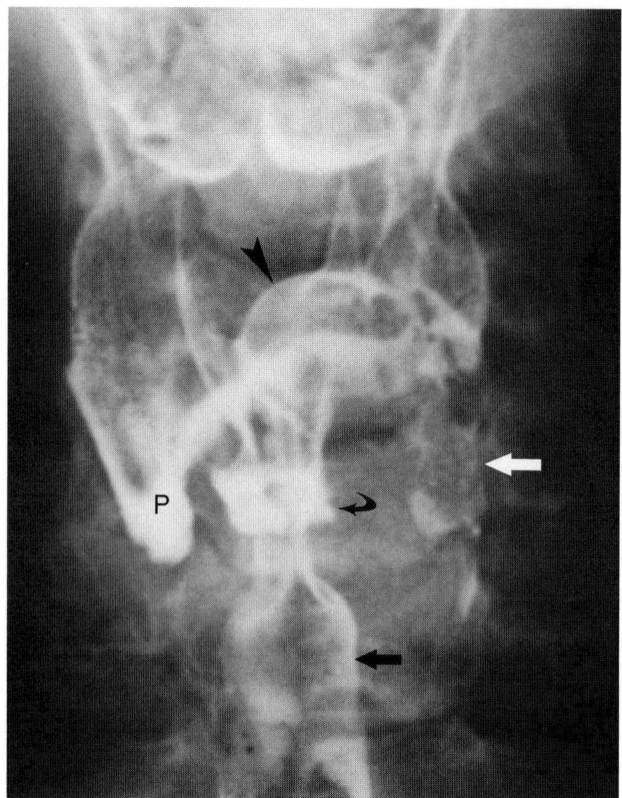

FIGURE 29.23. **Carcinoma in the Piriform Recess.** Frontal view from a barium swallow examination demonstrates a mass mostly filling the left piriform recess (*white arrow*) and bulging into the hypopharynx (*black arrowhead*). The right piriform recess (P) has a normal appearance. The presence of the mass has caused aspiration. Barium is seen filling the larynx (*black curved arrow*) and extending into the trachea (*black arrow*).

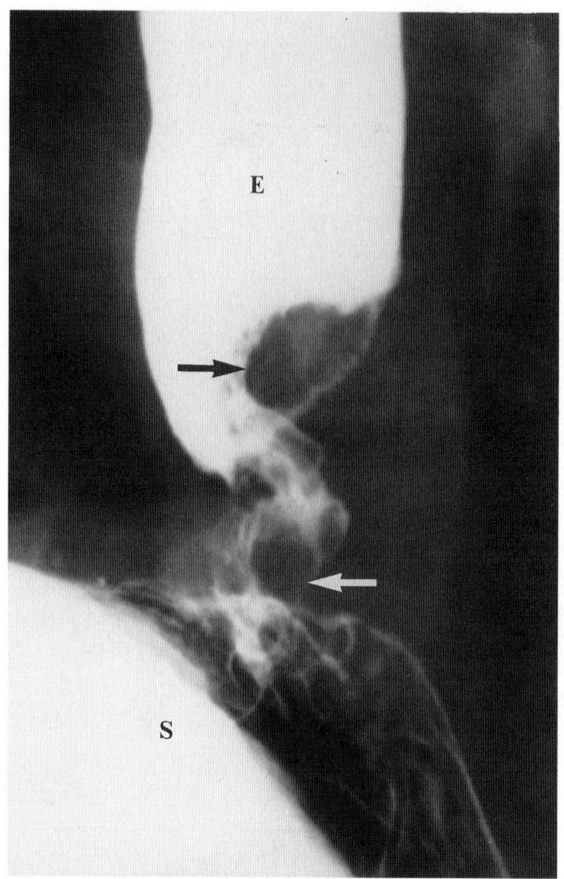

FIGURE 29.24. **Adenocarcinoma in Barrett Esophagus.** A tumor in the distal esophagus (E) forms nodular (*arrows*) narrowing of the barium column. Endoscopy confirmed adenocarcinoma arising in Barrett esophagus. S, stomach.

adjacent structures, esophageal carcinoma is deadly, with a 5-year survival of only 5%. The tumor assumes four basic radiographic patterns. An annular constricting lesion, appearing as an irregular ulcerated stricture, is most common (Figs. 29.19, 29.20). The polypoid pattern causes an intraluminal filling defect (Fig. 29.25). The infiltrative variety grows predominantly in the submucosa and may simulate a benign stricture. The least common pattern is that of an ulcerated mass. Risk factors include cigarette and alcohol abuse, corrosive ingestion, and carcinoma of the head and neck. The typical patient is a 65-year-old man.

The tumor spreads quickly by direct invasion into adjacent tissues because of the lack of a serosal covering on the esophagus. Lymphatic spread may go to nodes in the neck or mediastinum or below the diaphragm, depending on the location of the primary tumor in the esophagus. Hematogenous spread is to lung, liver, and adrenal glands.

CT, MR, or endoscopic US are used to define the extent of disease and determine surgical resectability (Fig. 29.26) (2). Findings include irregular thickening of the esophageal wall, eccentric narrowing of the lumen, dilation of the esophagus above the area of narrowing, invasion of periesophageal tissues, and metastases to mediastinal lymph nodes and the liver. Obliteration of the fat space between the aorta, esophagus, and vertebral body is highly predictive of invasion of the aorta.

Gastric adenocarcinoma spreads from the fundus and GEJ into the distal esophagus. Adenocarcinoma of the distal esophagus may be either primary gastric or primary esophageal, arising in Barrett esophagus (Fig. 29.24).

Leiomyoma, while rare, is still the most common benign neoplasm of the esophagus, accounting for 50% of all benign esophageal neoplasms. Gastrointestinal stromal tumors are rare in the esophagus. The tumor is firm and well-encapsulated and arises in the wall. Ulceration is rare. Most are asymptomatic and discovered incidentally. Men aged 25 to 35 years are affected most commonly (male-to-female ratio = 2:1). On UGI, most appear as smooth, well-defined wall lesions, although rarely they may be pedunculated or polypoid. Coarse calcifications are occasionally present and strongly indicative of leiomyoma. CT demonstrates a smooth, well-defined mass of uniform

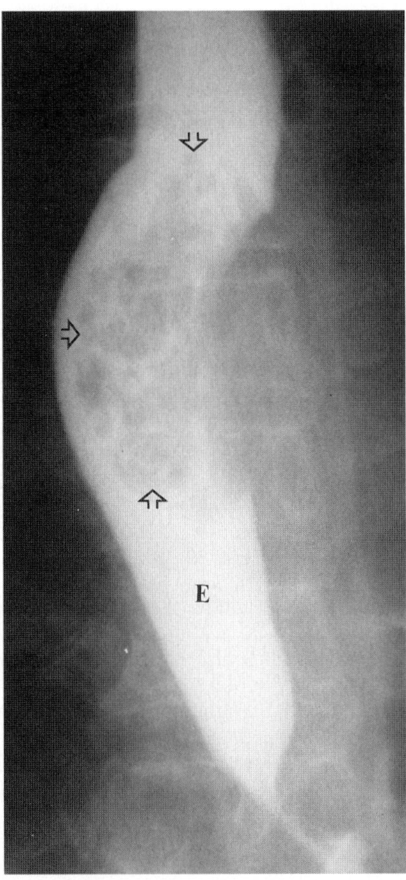

FIGURE 29.25. **Polypoid Squamous Cell Carcinoma.** This esophageal carcinoma appears as a polypoid mass (*arrows*) in the midesophagus (E) on this barium esophagram. Barium outlines the lobulations in the tumor.

soft tissue density (1). The esophageal wall is eccentrically thickened. Leiomyosarcoma of the esophagus is exceedingly rare, accounting for fewer than 1% of esophageal malignancies. Malignant lesions are typically heterogeneous with a large exophytic component.

Polyp. Fibroepithelial or fibrovascular polyps are a rare cause of esophageal filling defects. They appear as large ovoid or elongated intraluminal masses in the upper esophagus.

Esophageal duplication cysts are congenital abnormalities that are usually incidental findings presenting without symptoms. Most (60%) occur in the lower esophagus. CT shows a well-defined cystic mass. Differential diagnosis includes bronchogenic and neurenteric cyst.

Extrinsic lesions may invade the esophagus or simulate an esophageal mass or filling defect. Causes include mediastinal adenopathy, lung carcinoma, and vascular structures.

Aberrant right subclavian artery arises from the aorta distal to the left subclavian artery. To reach its destination, it must cross the mediastinum behind the esophagus. It causes a characteristic upward-slanting linear filling defect on the posterior aspect of the esophagus (Fig. 29.27).

ESOPHAGEAL PERFORATION AND TRAUMA

Esophageal perforation is a life-threatening event requiring prompt diagnosis and treatment. More than half of cases are related to esophageal instrumentation.

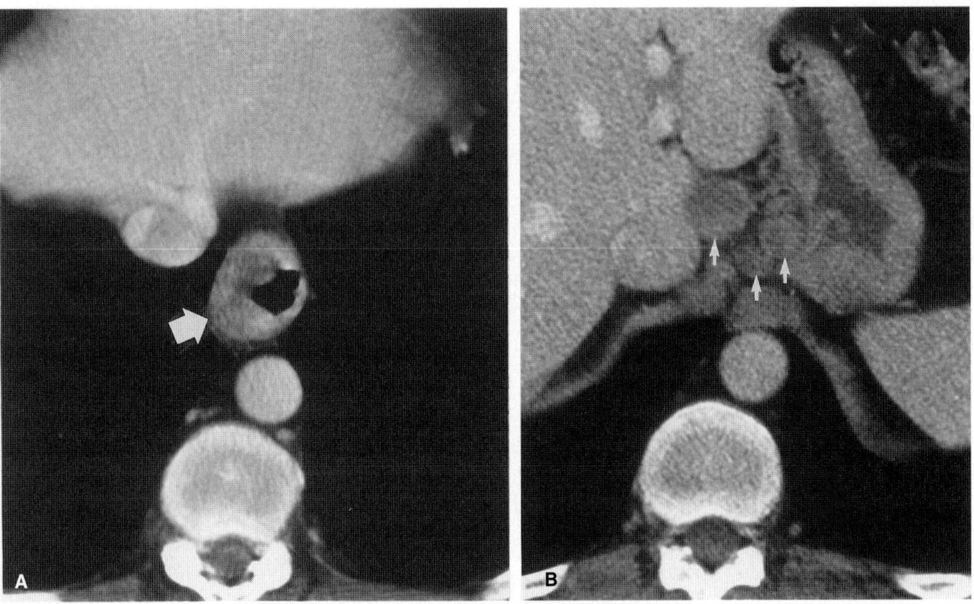

FIGURE 29.26. **Esophageal Carcinoma. A.** CT image of the distal esophagus demonstrates eccentric thickening of the wall (*arrow*) as a result of tumor. **B.** CT image just below the level of the gastroesophageal junction in the same patient reveals enlarged lymph nodes (*arrows*) in the gastrohepatic ligament because of metastases.

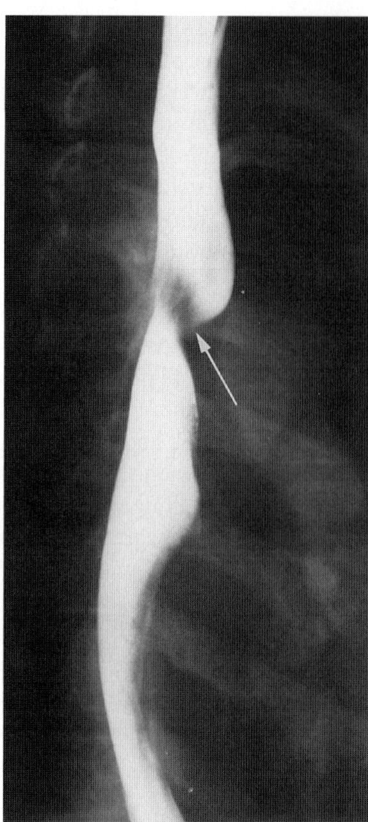

FIGURE 29.27. **Aberrant Right Subclavian Artery.** Frontal view from a barium esophagram reveals an aberrant right subclavian artery that arises from the aortic arch distal to the left subclavian artery and crosses behind the esophagus, causing a tubular extrinsic impression (*arrow*) on the esophagus slanting upward and to the patient's right.

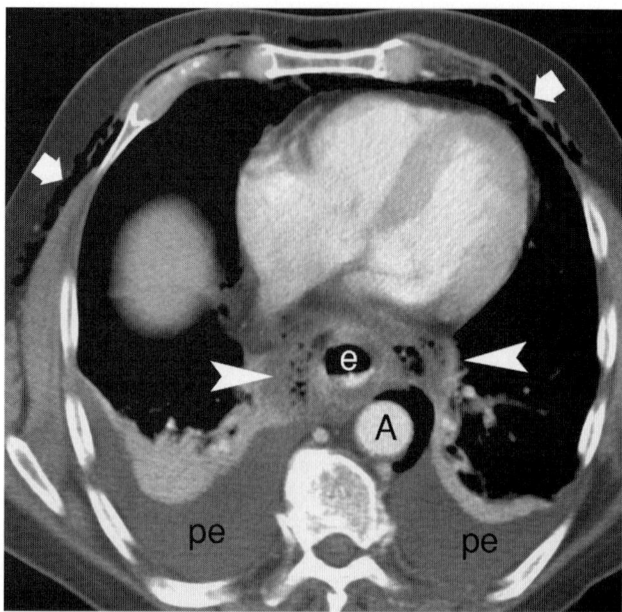

FIGURE 29.28. **Esophageal Perforation.** CT scan through the lower thorax shows bubbles of air and fluid in the mediastinum (*arrowheads*) and around the thoracic aorta (A). Air and contrast distend the esophagus (e). Air has dissected into the subcutaneous tissues (*arrows*). Bilateral pleural effusions (pe) are also evident. Esophageal perforation occurred during endoscopic esophageal stenting.

Bleeding can be profuse, and infection is a great risk. Plain films demonstrate subcutaneous, cervical, or mediastinal emphysema within 1 hour of perforation. Chest radiographs may show a widened mediastinum and pleural effusion or hydropneumothorax. Contrast studies should be performed initially with low-osmolar water-soluble agents and, if negative, followed by repeating the study with barium (10). The key finding is focal or diffuse extravasation of contrast outside the esophagus. CT demonstrates fluid collections, extraluminal contrast, and air in the mediastinum (Fig. 29.28).

Trauma. Endoscopy, esophageal dilation procedures, or any type of instrumentation may perforate the esophageal wall. Knife and bullet wounds may perforate the esophagus. Blunt trauma may tear the esophagus by an explosive increase in intraesophageal pressure.

Boerhaave syndrome refers to rupture of the esophageal wall as a result of forceful vomiting. The tear is virtually always in the left posterior wall, near the left crus of the diaphragm. Esophageal contents usually escape into the left pleural space or into the potential space between the parietal pleura and left crus.

Mallory-Weiss tear involves only the mucosa and not the full thickness of the esophagus. The tears are usually caused by violent retching. Although endoscopy usually identifies the lesion, it is commonly missed on UGI. When seen, the tear appears as a longitudinally oriented barium collection, 1 to 4 cm in length, in the distal esophagus. It may be a cause of copious hematemesis.

Foreign body impaction in adults is usually attributable to bones or boluses of meat. Children may ingest any foreign object, including toys, coins, and jewelry. Bones usually lodge in the pharynx, most often near the cricopharyngeus muscle. Meat impacts in the distal or midesophagus. Perforation occurs in only 1% of cases, but the risk increases if impaction persists more than 24 hours. Bones in the pharynx are difficult to differentiate from calcification of the thyroid and cricoid cartilages. Contrast studies show nonopaque foreign bodies as filling defects. Impacted foreign bodies may be removed by use of a Foley balloon catheter or wire basket or by gaseous distension of the esophagus with gas-producing crystals.

REFERENCES

1. Noh HM, Fishman EK, Forastiere AA, Bliss DF, Calhoun PS. CT of the esophagus: spectrum of disease with emphasis on esophageal carcinoma. Radiographics 1995;15:1113–1134.
2. Iyer RB, Silverman PM, DuBrow RA, Charnsangave C. Imaging in the diagnosis, staging, and follow-up of colorectal cancer. AJR Am J Roentgenol 2002;179:3–13.

3. Gore RM, Ghahremani GG, Miller FH. Mucosal features of the alimentary tract on double contrast barium studies. Radiologist 1995;2:283–295.
4. Dodds WJ, Logemann JA, Stewart ET. Radiologic assessment of abnormal oral and pharyngeal phases of swallowing. AJR Am J Roentgenol 1990;154:965–974.
5. Abbara S, Kalan MMH, Lewicki AM. Intrathoracic stomach revisited. AJR Am J Roentgenol 2003;181:403–414.
6. Luedtke P, Levine MS, Rubesin SE, Weinstein DS, Laufer I. Radiologic diagnosis of benign esophageal strictures: a pattern approach. Radiographics 2003;23:897–909.
7. Berkovich GY, Levine MS, Miller WT Jr. CT findings in patients with esophagitis. AJR Am J Roentgenol 2000;175:1431–1434.
8. Karasick S, Lev-Toaff AS. Esophageal strictures: findings on barium radiographs. AJR Am J Roentgenol 1995;165:561–565.
9. Gupta S, Levine MS, Rubesin SE, Katzka DA, Laufer I. Usefulness of barium studies for differentiating benign and malignant strictures of the esophagus. AJR Am J Roentgenol 2003;180:737–744.
10. Swanson JO, Levine MS, Redfern RO, Rubesin SE. Usefulness of high-density barium for detection of leaks after esophagogastrectomy, total gastrectomy, and total laryngectomy. AJR Am J Roentgenol 2003;181:415–420.

Chapter 30

Stomach and Duodenum

William E. Brant

Imaging Methods
Anatomy

Stomach
Helicobacter pylori Infection
Gastric Filling Defects/Mass Lesions
Thickened Gastric Folds/Thickened Wall
Gastric Ulcers

Duodenum
Duodenal Filling Defects/Mass Lesions
Thickened Duodenal Folds
Duodenal Ulcers and Diverticula
Duodenal Narrowing
Upper GI Hemorrhage

Imaging Methods

As endoscopy has become more commonplace, the utilization of fluoroscopy to study the upper GI tract has continued to diminish. CT competes with endoscopic US to evaluate the extraluminal component of disease (1). Nonetheless, a high-quality upper GI (UGI) series provides excellent evaluation of the stomach and duodenum and remains part of the radiologic armamentarium (2). To attain a high sensitivity for the examination and to avoid missing significant pathology, multiple techniques must be used for the UGI series. The single-contrast technique of filling and distending the stomach and duodenum with barium suspension is one such technique. It is usually supplemented by compression procedures, which are effective in demonstrating abnormalities of the distal stomach and duodenum. The mucosal relief technique, which entails using small amounts of barium to coat the mucosa without distending the bowel, is useful in demonstrating abnormalities such as varices. The double-contrast technique, which uses high-density barium suspensions to coat the mucosa, and ingestible effervescent granules to distend the organ, is optimal for demonstration of subtle features of the mucosal surface. As with any radiographic examination, attention to detail and tailoring the examination for the clinical problem are essential in producing good results.

CT, with use of air-contrast distension techniques, is a valuable adjunct to barium studies and endoscopy to document abnormalities of the wall of the stomach wall and duodenum and to determine the extent of extraluminal disease (3). Optimal distension of the stomach and duodenum is mandatory for accurate CT interpretation (1). Gastric and duodenal distension may be attained by filling the organs with water or positive contrast agents, or by using effervescent granules to cause gaseous distension (4). The patient should be positioned to optimize distension of the GI tract portion of greatest interest. MR and US have limited roles in the evaluation of the luminal GI tract.

Anatomy

The GI tract is essentially a hollow tube consisting of four concentric layers of tissue. The innermost layer exposed to the lumen is the *mucosa*. The mucosa consists of epithelium supported by loose connective tissue of the lamina propria and a thin band of smooth muscle called the muscularis mucosae. The *submucosa* provides connective tissue support for the mucosa. The submucosa contains the primary vascular and lymphatic channels, lymphoid follicles, and autonomic nerve plexuses. The major muscular structure of the bowel wall is the *muscularis propria*, which comprises inner circular and outer longitudinal layers. The *serosa* or adventitia is the outer covering of the bowel. Lymphoid tissue in the GI tract is located in the mucosa (epithelium and lamina propria), the submucosa, and the mesenteric lymph nodes. As the major component of the mucosa-associated lymphoid tissue (MALT), lymphoid tissue plays a major role in host immune defenses and is a site of significant disease (5).

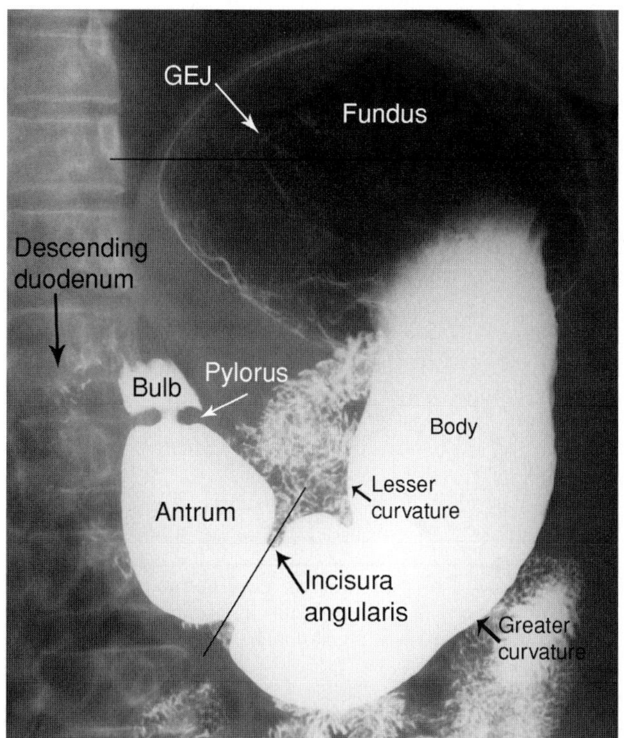

FIGURE 30.1. **Anatomy of the Upper GI Tract.** A prone right anterior oblique image of the stomach taken during an upper GI series demonstrates normal radiographic anatomy. The fundus is that portion of the stomach above the level of the gastroesophageal junction (GEJ). The incisura angularis is the angular notch on the lesser curvature that serves as a landmark dividing the body and antrum of the stomach. The greater curvature serves as the attachment for the greater omentum. The partially contracted pylorus is the valve between the stomach and the duodenum. The bulb is the pyramid-shaped first portion of the duodenum. The descending duodenum is faintly outlined by barium on this image.

The appearance and position of the stomach and duodenum vary considerably from one individual to another. The terms used to describe the anatomic divisions of the stomach and duodenum are illustrated in Fig. 30.1. *Cardia* refers to the region of the gastroesophageal junction (GEJ). The *fundus* is that portion of the stomach above the level of the GEJ. The *body* of the stomach is the central two thirds, from the cardia to the *incisura angularis*. The incisura angularis is an acute angle formed on the lesser curvature that marks the boundary between the body and the antrum. The parietal cells, which produce hydrochloric acid, and the chief cells, which produce pepsin precursors, are located in the fundus and body. The *antrum* is the distal third of the stomach and contains gastrin-producing cells but no acid-secreting cells.

The *pylorus* is the junction of the stomach with the duodenum, and the *pyloric canal* is the channel through the pylorus. The *duodenal bulb*, or cap, is the pyramidal first portion of the duodenum. The gallbladder frequently makes a prominent impression on the top of the bulb. The duodenal bulb, like the stomach, is covered on all surfaces by visceral peritoneum. The remainder of the duodenum is retroperitoneal and within the anterior pararenal compartment.

The second or descending portion of the duodenum is lateral to the head of the pancreas. The common bile duct and pancreatic duct pierce the medial aspect of the descending duodenum at the ampulla of Vater. The third or horizontal portion of the duodenum passes to the left between the superior mesenteric vessels and the inferior vena cava and aorta. The fourth or ascending portion of the duodenum ascends on the left side of the aorta to the level of L2 and the ligament of Treitz, where it turns abruptly ventrally to form the duodenal-jejunal flexure.

The term *areae gastricae* refers to the detailed pattern of the gastric mucosa as demonstrated by double-contrast technique (Fig. 30.2). Normal areae gastricae varies from a fine reticular pattern to a course nodular pattern. The hallmark of normal is the regularity of the pattern in all areas in which it is visualized. The term *rugae* refers to the gastric mucosal folds that produce distinct radiolucent ridges when the stomach is partially distended. Rugae are composed of mucosa, the lamina propria, the muscularis mucosae, and portions of the submucosa. Disease in any of these structures may cause thickening of the gastric folds.

The *lesser curvature* of the stomach is attached to the liver by the lesser omentum. The greater omentum attaches to the *greater curvature* of the stomach. The lesser sac is the intraperitoneal space posterior to the stomach and anterior to the pancreas.

On CT the normal gastric wall is 7 to 10 mm thick (6), and the normal duodenal wall is less than 3 mm thick. Both organs must be fully distended to accurately assess wall thickness (4). A prominent pseudotumor, caused

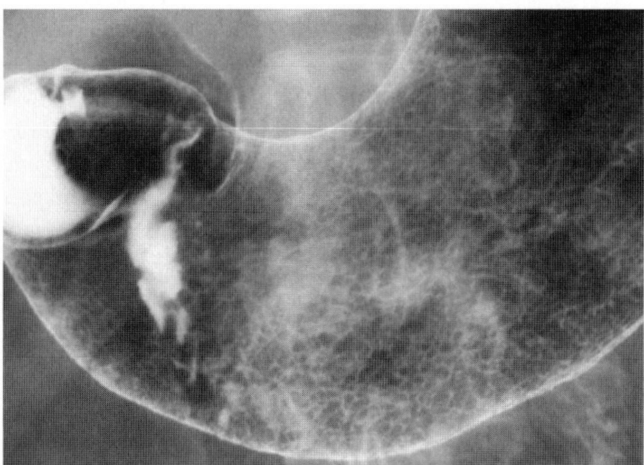

FIGURE 30.2. **Normal Areae Gastricae.** Double-contrast technique provides distension of the stomach with coating of its mucosa to demonstrate the normal pattern of areae gastricae produced by small polygonal mounds of normal gastric mucosa.

by inadequate distension, is often seen on CT near the GEJ.

STOMACH

Helicobacter pylori Infection

H. pylori infection has been identified as the major cause of chronic gastritis, duodenitis, benign gastric and duodenal ulcers, gastric adenocarcinoma, and MALT lymphoma (7). *H. pylori* is a gram-negative spiral bacillus that colonizes the stomachs of as much as 80% of some populations. It will infect only gastric-like epithelium and is usually localized to the gastric antrum, living on surface epithelial cells beneath the mucous coat. It survives in gastric acid by using a powerful urease enzyme to break down urea into ammonia and bicarbonate, creating a more alkaline environment for itself. The prevalence of infection increases with age (>50% of Americans over age 60), in lower socioeconomic populations, and in developing countries. Infection is chronic and causes a superficial gastritis, which is most commonly asymptomatic. Approximately 70% of peptic gastric ulcers, 95% of duodenal ulcers, and 50% of gastric adenocarcinomas are caused by this infection. Diagnosis of *H. pylori* infection is made by serology, urease breath tests, and endoscopic biopsy. Treatment is usually a combination of two to four drugs, including one or more antibiotics, histamine-2 receptor blockers (H_2 blockers) to decrease acid secretion, and occasionally a bismuth compound. Cure rates of 90% are reported, although antibiotic resistance is emerging. Although spontaneous elimination of infection is rare, treatment of asymptomatic infected individuals is not currently recommended.

Gastric Filling Defects/Mass Lesions

Gastric carcinoma is the third most common GI malignancy, following colon and pancreatic carcinoma. Most (95%) are adenocarcinomas; the remainder are diffuse anaplastic (signet-ring) carcinoma, squamous cell carcinoma, or rare cell types. Predisposing factors include smoking, pernicious anemia, atrophic gastritis, and gastrojejunostomy. *H. pylori* infection increases the risk of gastric carcinoma sixfold and is the cause of approximately half of gastric adenocarcinoma cases. Peak age is from 50 to 70 years, with men predominating (2:1). The incidence of gastric carcinoma is as much as five times higher in Japan, Finland, Chile, and Iceland than in the United States. Mortality is high, with a 5-year survival rate of 10% to 20%.

The tumor assumes four common morphologic growth patterns. One third are polypoid masses that present as filling defects within the gastric lumen (Fig. 30.3). Many of these are broad-based and papillary in configuration. Another third are ulcerative masses presenting as malignant gastric ulcers. The remainder are infiltrating, presenting as scirrhous carcinomas (15%), or superficial spreading, producing plaquelike tumors or bizarre thickened folds. Scirrhous carcinoma is characterized by diffuse infiltration of the gastric wall by poorly differentiated or undifferentiated carcinomatous cells (Fig. 30.4). The wall of the stomach is thickened and rigid. The terms "linitis plastica" and "water-bottle stomach" may be applied to describe the resulting stiff, narrowed stomach (Fig. 30.5). Additional causes of narrowed stomach are listed in Table 30.1.

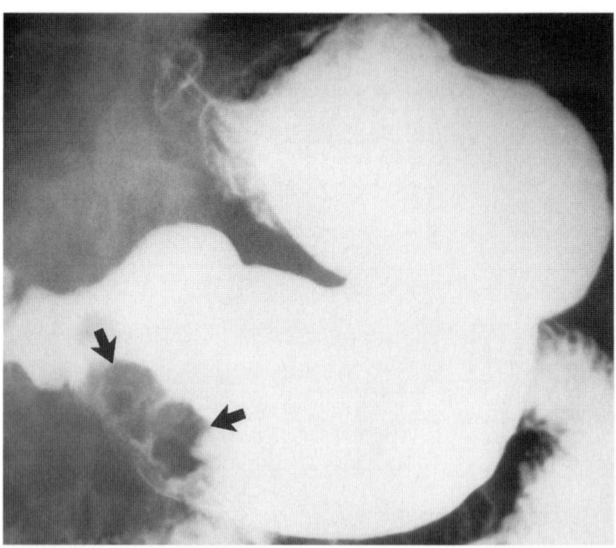

FIGURE 30.3. **Polypoid Gastric Carcinoma.** Single-contrast technique upper GI series reveals a lobulated filling defect (*arrows*) in the antrum of the stomach.

Superficial spreading carcinoma spreads through the mucosa and submucosa, producing nodular thickening or superficial mucosal ulceration. Intraluminal mass effect

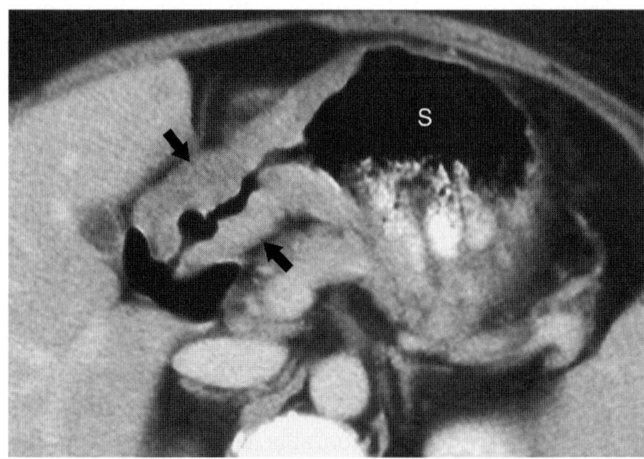

FIGURE 30.4. **Scirrhous Carcinoma.** CT demonstrates nodular thickening (*arrows*) of the antrum of the stomach (S) caused by poorly differentiated gastric adenocarcinoma. The outer margin of the stomach is well defined, giving evidence against extension of tumor through the wall. Note the fixed narrowing of the gastric lumen.

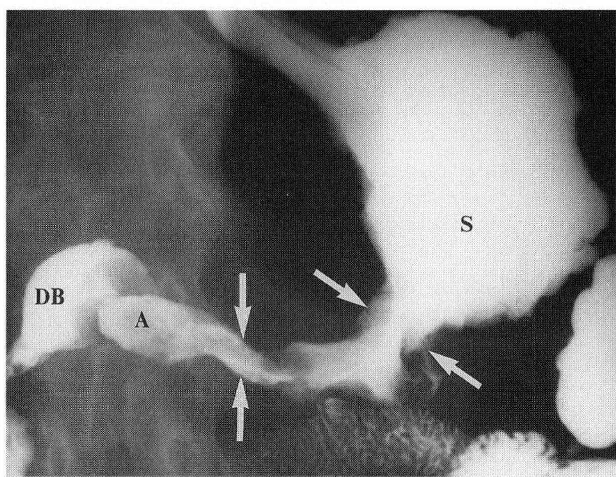

FIGURE 30.5. **Linitis Plastica.** Scirrhous gastric carcinoma causes fixed nodular narrowing (*arrows*) of the body and antrum (A) of the stomach (S). No peristalsis through this portion of the stomach was observed at fluoroscopy. Biopsy yielded undifferentiated adenocarcinoma. DB, duodenal bulb.

is minimal; however, the involved areas are thickened and rigid, and involved rugae are thickened and distorted. Cancers are most common near the cardia (44%), in the antrum, and along the lesser curvature. The tumor spreads by direct invasion through the gastric wall to involve perigastric fat and adjacent organs, or it may seed the peritoneal cavity. Lymphatic spread is to regional lymph nodes, including perigastric nodes along the lesser curvature, celiac axis, and hepatoduodenal, retropancreatic, mesenteric, and paraaortic nodes. Hematogenous metastases involve the liver, adrenal glands, ovaries, and, rarely, bone and lung. Intraperitoneal seeding presents as carcinomatosis or Krukenberg ovarian tumors.

TABLE 30.1 Possible Causes of Narrowed Stomach

Neoplastic
- Gastric adenocarcinoma (linitis plastica)
- Lymphoma (antral narrowing + extension into duodenum)
- Metastases (linitis plastica resulting from breast carcinoma)
- Kaposi sarcoma (AIDS)

Inflammatory
- *Helicobacter pylori* gastritis (usually antral narrowing)
- Corrosive ingestion (usually acid)
- Radiotherapy (after 4.5 Gy)
- AIDS (*Cryptosporidium* infection) (narrowed antrum + small bowel involvement)
- Eosinophilic gastroenteritis (narrowing + wall thickening)
- Infection (tuberculosis + syphilis [both rare])
- Crohn disease (rare)
- Sarcoidosis (usually asymptomatic)

Extrinsic compression
- Pancreatitis
- Pancreatic carcinoma
- Omental cake

Early gastric cancers appear on barium studies as: (*1*) gastric polyps, with risk of malignancy increased for lesions larger than 1 cm; (*2*) superficial plaquelike lesions or nodular mucosa; and (*3*) shallow, irregular ulcers with nodular adjacent mucosa. These lesions are most sensitively detected on double contrast studies.

CT and MR are used to determine the extent of tumor to facilitate preoperative planning (3). Transmural extension, intraperitoneal spread, or distant metastases limit treatment to palliative surgery or chemotherapy. Findings include (*1*) focal, often irregular, wall thickening (>1 cm) (8); (*2*) diffuse wall thickening as the result of tumor infiltration (linitis plastica) (contrast enhancement is common); (*3*) intraluminal soft tissue mass; (*4*) bulky mass with ulceration; (*5*) rare, large, exophytic tumor resembling leiomyosarcoma; (*6*) extension of tumor into perigastric fat; (*7*) regional lymphadenopathy; and (*8*) metastases in the liver, adrenal, and peritoneal cavity. Mucinous adenocarcinomas frequently contain stippled calcifications. Findings used to differentiate gastric malignancies are listed in Table 30.2.

TABLE 30.2 Gastric Malignancies

Tumor	*Imaging Features*
Gastric adenocarcinoma	Focal wall thickening (>1 cm suggests malignancy)
	Diffuse wall thickening (linitis plastica)
	Large mass
	Ulcerated mass that is predominantly intraluminal
	Soft tissue stranding from mass into perigastric fat
	Adenopathy, peritoneal implants, distant metastases
Gastric lymphoma	Marked wall thickening (4–5 cm)
	Circumferential wall thickening without luminal narrowing
	Homogeneous attenuation of tumor
	Multiple polyps with ulceration
	Extensive adenopathy, especially if below the renal hila
	Transpyloric tumor spread to the duodenum
Malignant GI stromal tumors	Large, heterogeneous exophytic mass (>5 cm)
	Extensive ulceration of the mass
	Prominent necrosis, hemorrhage, liquefaction
	Calcification within the tumor
Metastases to stomach	Wall thickening similar to primary carcinoma
	Focal intramural mass
	Ulcerated mural nodule
	Direct invasion of the stomach from adjacent tumor

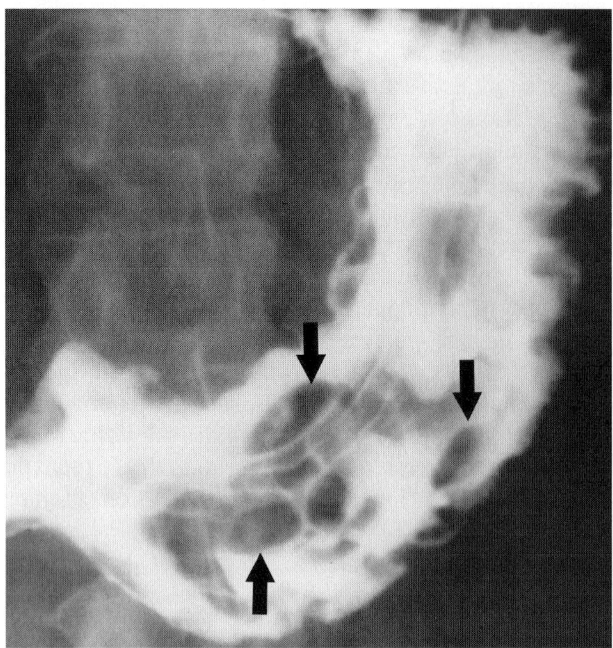

FIGURE 30.6. **Mucosa-Associated Lymphoid Tissue (MALT) Lymphoma.** Upper GI series shows multiple smoothly marginated polypoid nodules of varying size and shape in the stomach (*arrows*). Multiple polypoid nodules may also be seen with gastric carcinoma.

Lymphoma accounts for 2% of gastric neoplasms. The stomach is the most common site of involvement of primary GI lymphoma, accounting for approximately 50% of cases (9). Most (80%) gastric lymphomas are non-Hodgkin, B-cell type (3). Chronic infection of the gastric epithelium with *H. pylori* is associated with a risk of developing MALT gastric lymphomas, which are more indolent and have a better prognosis than B-cell lymphomas (10). Because lymphoma remains confined to the bowel wall for prolonged periods of time, it has a better prognosis than carcinoma, with 5-year survival rates in the 62% to 90% range. Lymphoma demonstrates four morphologic patterns: polypoid solitary mass, ulcerative mass, multiple submucosal nodules (Fig. 30.6), and diffuse infiltration. UGI series findings include the following: (*1*) polypoid lesions, (*2*) irregular ulcers with nodular thickened folds, (*3*) bulky tumors with large cavities, (*4*) multiple submucosal nodules that commonly ulcerate and create a target or "bull's-eye" appearance, (*5*) diffuse but pliable wall and fold thickening, and (*6*) rarely, linitis plastica appearance of diffuse, stiff narrowing (Fig. 30.7) (5). Multiplicity of lesions favors MALT lymphoma as the diagnosis.

CT is the primary imaging modality used to stage lymphoma. CT findings that are helpful in differentiating gastric lymphoma from carcinoma include (*1*) more marked thickening of the wall (may exceed 3 cm) (Fig. 30.8), (*2*) involvement of additional areas of the GI tract (transpyloric spread of lymphoma to the duodenum in 30%), (*3*) absence of invasion of the perigastric fat, (*4*) absence of luminal narrowing despite extensive involvement, and (EMPHASIS EMPH-TYPE="italic">5) more widespread and bulkier adenopathy.

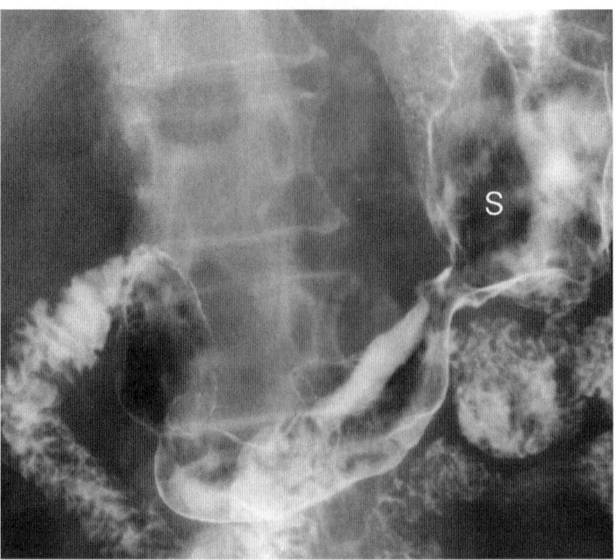

FIGURE 30.7. **Gastric Lymphoma.** Upper GI series reveals striking narrowing of the body and antrum of the stomach (S). Note the abnormal folds in the fundus, indicating diffuse involvement of the stomach. This linitis plastica appearance is much less common with lymphoma than with adenocarcinoma.

GI stromal tumors (GISTs) are the most common mesenchymal tumor to arise from the GI tract (11). Most, but not all, tumors previously classified as leiomyomas, leiomyosarcomas, and leiomyoblastomas are now classified as GISTs. Approximately 60% to 70% of GISTs arise in the stomach, and 10% to 30% of these are malignant. True leiomyomas and leiomyosarcomas are very rare in the stomach.

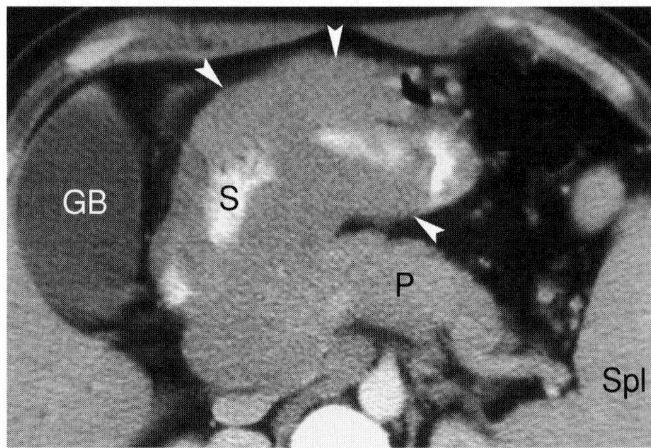

FIGURE 30.8. **Gastric Lymphoma.** CT demonstrates marked thickening (*arrowheads*) of the gastric wall with a homogeneous tumor. The gastric tumor blends into and involves the pancreas (P). The lumen of the stomach (S) is irregularly narrowed. GB, gallbladder; Spl, spleen.

Long-term silent growth to a large size is characteristic. The overlying mucosa is commonly ulcerated. Dystrophic calcification is relatively common in both benign and malignant tumors and helps differentiate these lesions from other gastric tumors. Histologic differentiation of benign from malignant tumors is difficult; the differentiation is based upon size, gross appearance, and behavior of the tumor. On UGI series, GISTs appear as submucosal nodules and masses (Fig. 30.9). Ulceration causes a bull's-eye appearance and may be responsible for significant bleeding (Fig. 30.10).

CT is useful in characterizing the tumors because they are predominantly extraluminal. Benign tumors are smaller (average of 4 to 5 cm), are homogeneous in density, and show uniform diffuse enhancement. Malignant tumors tend to be larger (>10 cm) with central zones of low density caused by hemorrhage and necrosis and show irregular patterns of enhancement (Fig. 30.10) (12).

Metastases may present as submucosal nodules or ulcerated masses (Fig. 30.11). Most are hematogenous metastases. Common primary tumors are melanoma and breast and lung carcinoma. Breast cancer metastases cause linitis plastica.

Kaposi sarcoma, usually found in patients with AIDS, demonstrates a wide spectrum of appearances, including

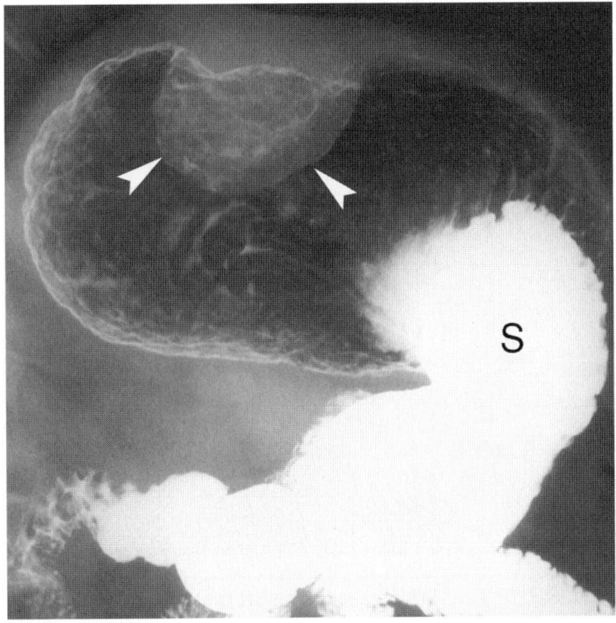

FIGURE 30.9. **Gastrointestinal Stromal Tumor (GIST).** A benign GIST (*arrowheads*) demonstrates the characteristic findings of a submucosal mass on an upper GI series. The mass protrudes into the lumen of the stomach (S). The surface of the mass is coated with barium and outlined by air in the fundus. The margin of the lesion is very well defined.

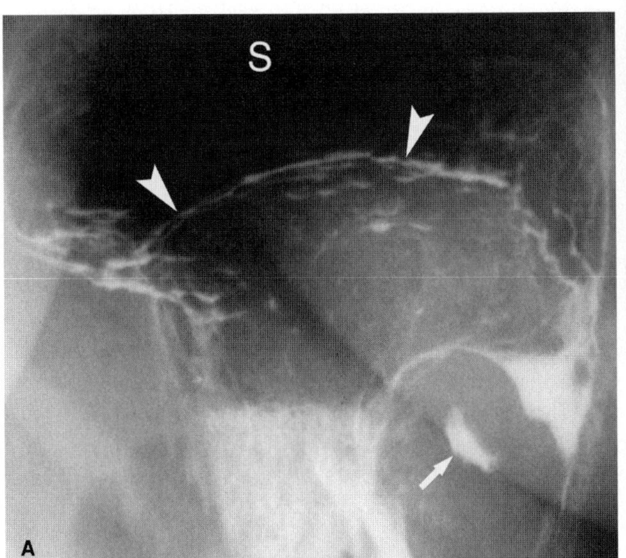

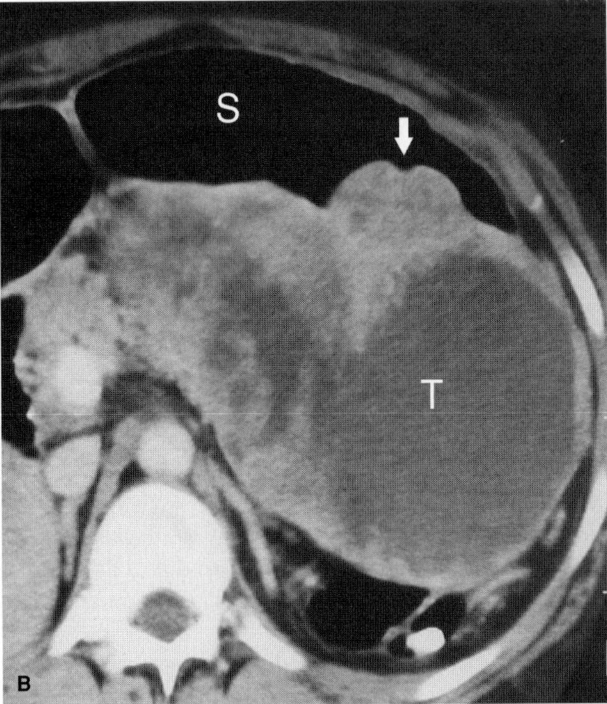

FIGURE 30.10. **Malignant Gastrointestinal Stromal Tumor (GIST). A.** Radiograph in lateral upright position from an upper GI series demonstrates a huge mass (*arrowheads*) impressing into the lumen of the stomach (S). A mound of tumor contains an irregular ulcer (*arrow*) that collects barium within its crater. **B.** CT of the same patient reveals the tumor (T) to be heterogeneous, with large low-attenuation areas representing necrosis. The ulcer (*arrow*) and tumor mound protruding into the lumen of the stomach (S) are evident.

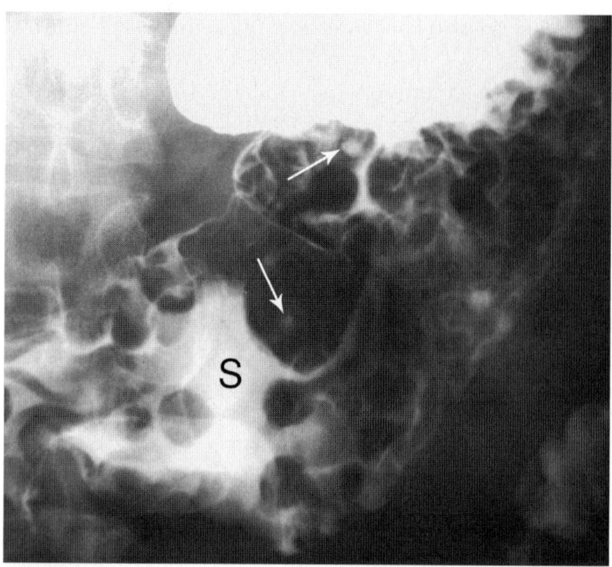

***FIGURE 30.11.* Metastases to the Stomach.** Metastases from malignant melanoma produce innumerable polypoid nodules protruding into the stomach (S). Some are ulcerated (*arrows*), producing a target appearance.

polypoid mass, thickened folds, multiple submucosal masses, and linitis plastica.

Villous tumors are adenomatous polypoid masses that produce multiple frondlike projections. Most are solitary and 3 to 9 cm in size, although giant tumors may be as large as 15 cm. Malignant potential is high and varies with size of the lesion (50% for lesions of 2 to 4 cm, 80% for lesions >4 cm). Barium trapped in the clefts between fronds produces a characteristic "soap-bubble" appearance. The tumors are mobile and deform with compression. All should be treated as malignant lesions.

Polyps are lesions that protrude into the lumen. Their appearance on double-contrast UGI series depends on whether they are on the dependent or nondependent surface. A polyp on the dependent surface appears as a radiolucent filling defect in the barium pool; a polyp on the nondependent surface is covered with a thin coat of barium. The x-ray beam catches its margin in tangent, resulting in a lesion whose margins are etched in white. The *bowler hat sign* is produced by the acute angle of attachment of the polyp to the mucosa. The *Mexican hat sign* consists of two concentric rings and is produced by visualizing a pedunculated polyp end-on. Polyps are commonly multiple (Table 30.3).

Hyperplastic polyps account for 80% of gastric polyps. Most are less than 15 mm in diameter. They are not neoplasms but rather hyperplastic responses to mucosal injury, especially gastritis. They may be located anywhere in the stomach and are frequently multiple but have no malignant potential. *Adenomatous polyps* account for 15% of gastric polyps and are true neoplasms with malignant potential. Most are solitary, located in the antrum, and larger than 2 cm in diameter. Polyps that are larger than 1 cm, lobulated, or pedunculated should have biopsies taken of them because of the risk of malignancy. *Hamartomatous polyps* occur in Peutz-Jeghers syndrome. They have no malignant potential.

TABLE 30.3 Multiple Gastric Filling Defects

Hyperplastic polyps
Adenomatous polyps (especially with polyposis syndromes)
Metastases
Lymphoma
Varices

Lipomas are submucosal neoplasms composed of mature benign fatty material (13). The UGI series reveals a smooth well-defined submucosal lesion that occasionally ulcerates. CT provides a definitive diagnosis by demonstration of a sharply circumscribed wall mass with uniform fat attenuation (14).

Ectopic pancreas is a common intramural lesion, usually found in the antrum. Lobules of heterotopic pancreatic tissue, up to 5 cm in size, are covered by gastric mucosa. Most are nipple-shaped or cone-shaped with small central orifices.

Bezoar/Foreign Body. The term *bezoar* refers to an intraluminal gastric mass consisting of accumulated ingested material. Bezoars may be composed of a wide variety of substances: trichobezoars are composed of hair, whereas phytobezoars are composed of fruit or vegetable products. Any ingested foreign body may produce an intraluminal filling defect.

Extrinsic Impression. Masses adjacent to the stomach may produce filling defects. Extrinsic masses on the dependent surface produce ill-defined radiolucencies. The mucosa may be impressed upon by an extrinsic mass and be seen in profile as a white line. Pancreatic, splenic, hepatic, and retroperitoneal masses may impress upon the stomach. CT is excellent for demonstrating the nature of an extrinsic mass impression.

Thickened Gastric Folds/ Thickened Wall

Gastric folds are usually considered to be thickened if they exceed 1 cm in the fundus and 5 mm in the antrum.

Normal Variant. Gastric folds are normally most prominent in the fundus and upper third of the greater curvature. Thickened folds—even larger than 1 cm—in this region are often normal, but they require evaluation to exclude pathology.

Gastritis is a convenient label used to describe a wide variety of diseases affecting the gastric mucosa (15). Most of these diseases are inflammatory. Gastritis is much more common than gastric ulcers (16). The hallmarks of gastritis are thickened folds and superficial mucosal ulcerations (erosions). The thickened folds are usually caused by mucosal edema and superficial inflammatory infiltrate. *Erosions* are defined as defects in the mucosa that do not penetrate beyond the muscularis mucosae. *Aphthous ulcers* (also called *varioliform erosions*) are complete erosions that appear as tiny central flecks of barium surrounded by a radiolucent halo of edema (Fig. 30.12). Incomplete erosions appear as linear streaks and dots of barium. Erosions heal without scarring. Barium precipitates may mimic erosions, appearing as distinct punctate barium spots but without the distinctive radiolucent halo of a true erosion.

H. pylori gastritis is the most common form of gastritis. Although most people who are infected with *H. pylori* are asymptomatic, most have gastritis endoscopically and pathologically. Almost all patients with benign gastric and duodenal ulcers have *H. pylori* gastritis. UGI findings of *H. pylori* gastritis include: (*1*) thickening (<5 mm) of gastric folds, (*2*) nodular folds, (*3*) erosions, (*4*) antral narrowing, (*5*) inflammatory polyps, (*6*) antral narrowing, and (*7*) enlarged areae gastricae.

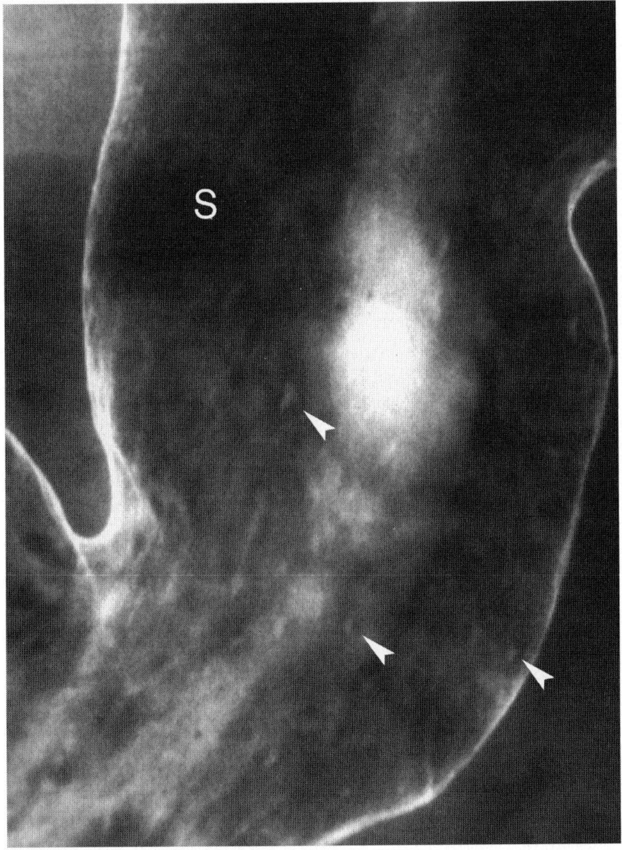

FIGURE 30.12. **Erosive Gastritis.** Double-contrast upper GI series demonstrates numerous aphthous ulcers (*arrowheads*) throughout the stomach (S). The characteristic appearance of aphthous ulcers is a persistent small collection of barium surrounded by a tiny lucent mound of edema. This patient had a recent heavy intake of alcohol.

Erosive gastritis is most often caused by alcohol, aspirin and other nonsteroidal anti-inflammatory agents, or steroids. Double-contrast UGI findings include: (*1*) erosions (aphthous ulcers) (Fig. 30.12); (*2*) thickened, nodular folds in the antrum; (*3*) limited distensibility of the antrum; and (*4*) wall stiffness and limited peristalsis.

Crohn gastritis characteristically involves the gastric antrum and proximal duodenum. Early stage disease manifests as aphthous ulcers identical to those seen with erosive gastritis. More advanced disease shows antral narrowing, wall thickening, and fistulas.

Atrophic gastritis is a chronic autoimmune disease that destroys the fundic mucosa but spares the antral mucosa. Destruction of parietal cells results in decreased acid and intrinsic factor production, which leads to vitamin B_{12} deficiency and pernicious anemia. Antibodies to parietal cells and intrinsic factors are found in peripheral blood samples. Characteristic UGI findings are: (*1*) decreased or absent folds in the fundus and body ("bald fundus"); (*2*) narrowed, tube-shaped stomach (fundal diameter <8 cm); and (*3*) small (1 to 2 mm) or absent areae gastricae.

Phlegmonous gastritis is an acute, often fatal, bacterial infection of the stomach. Streptococci are the most common cause, but a variety of other bacteria have also been identified. It may arise as a complication of septicemia, gastric surgery, or gastric ulcers. Multiple abscesses are formed in the gastric wall, which is markedly thickened. The rugae are swollen. Barium may penetrate into abscess crypts in the gastric wall. Peritonitis develops in 70% of cases. Healing usually results in a severely contracted stomach.

Emphysematous gastritis is a form of phlegmonous gastritis caused by gas-producing organisms, usually *Escherichia coli* or *Clostridium welchii*. Most cases are caused by caustic ingestion, surgery, trauma, or ischemia. Multiple gas bubbles are apparent within the wall of the stomach.

Eosinophilic gastroenteritis is a diffuse infiltration of the wall of the stomach and small bowel by eosinophils. Any or all layers of the wall may be involved. The condition is associated with a peripheral eosinophilia as high as 60%. Initially, the folds are markedly thickened and nodular, especially in the antrum. When chronic, the antrum is narrowed with a nodular "cobblestone" mucosal pattern.

Ménétrier disease, also called giant hypertrophic gastritis, is a rare condition characterized by excessive mucus production, giant mucosal hypertrophy, hypoproteinemia, and hypochlorhydria. UGI findings include: (*1*) markedly enlarged (>5 mm) and tortuous but pliable folds in the fundus and body, especially along the greater curvature, with sparing of the antrum (Fig. 30.13); and (*2*) hypersecretion

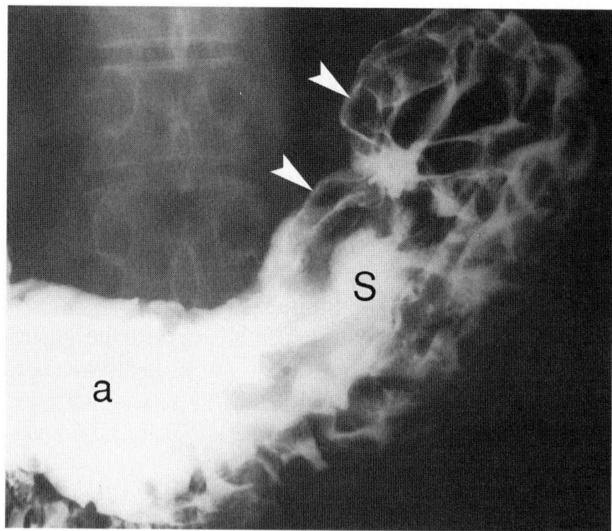

FIGURE 30.13. **Ménétrier Disease.** Upper GI series reveals marked thickening of the mucosal folds (*arrowheads*) in the fundus and proximal body of the stomach (S). The gastric antrum (a) is not involved.

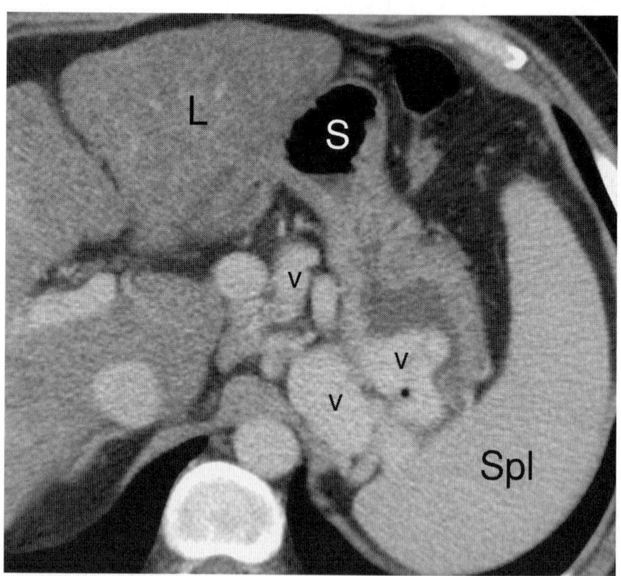

FIGURE 30.14. **Gastric Varices.** Helical CT with bolus IV contrast reveals enhancing varices (v) outside the stomach (S) in the gastrohepatic ligament and protruding into the gastric lumen. The liver (L) is nodular in contour, indicating the presence of cirrhosis. The spleen (Spl) is enlarged, providing further evidence of portal hypertension.

that has diluted the barium and impaired mucosal coating. CT demonstrates thick, nodular folds with smooth serosal surface and normal gastric wall thickness between folds.

Varices appear as smooth, lobulated filling defects resembling thickened folds. They are most common in the fundus and usually accompany esophageal varices. Isolated gastric varices may occur with splenic vein occlusion. CT with bolus contrast enhancement is an excellent method for confirming the presence of gastric varices as well as demonstrating their cause (Fig. 30.14). CT shows well-defined clusters of rounded and tubular enhancing vessels. Additional findings of portal hypertension may be evident.

Neoplasm. Lymphoma and superficial spreading gastric carcinoma may produce distorted rigid gastric folds that are commonly ulcerated and appear nodular. The distal stomach is the most common location for neoplasms.

Gastric Ulcers

An ulcer is defined as a full-thickness defect in the mucosa. It frequently extends to the deeper layers of the stomach, including the submucosa and muscularis propria. About 95% of ulcerating gastric lesions are benign. All gastric ulcers should be examined endoscopically or be followed to complete radiographic healing.

Signs of an ulcer as demonstrated by double-contrast UGI series include (*1*) a barium-filled crater on the dependent wall (Fig. 30.15), (*2*) a ring shadow caused by barium coating the edge of the crater on the nondependent wall, (*3*) a double ring shadow if the base of the ulcer is broader than the neck, and (*4*) a crescentic or semilunar line when the ulcer is seen on tangent oblique view. Some ulcers may be linear or rod-shaped. Ulcers are multiple in about 20% of patients.

Peptic Ulcer Disease. Benign gastric ulcers are caused by *H. pylori* infection (70%) and by nonsteroidal anti-inflammatory medications (30%). Duodenal ulcers are usually associated with increased production of acid. Gastric ulcers occur with normal or even decreased acid levels (17). However, hydrochloric acid must be present for peptic ulceration to occur. Patients usually present with aching or burning pain within several hours after eating. Some patients with ulcers may be asymptomatic. The major complications of peptic ulcer disease are bleeding, obstruction, and perforation. Bleeding occurs in 15% to 20% of patients and is manifest by melena, hematemesis, or hematochezia. Gastric outlet obstruction complicates approximately 5% of cases. Ulcers may perforate into the free abdominal cavity or penetrate into adjacent organs. Free perforations usually present with an acute abdomen. Ulcer penetration into an adjacent organ is usually heralded by a marked increase in abdominal pain.

Benign Ulcers. Most (95%) gastric ulcers currently diagnosed in the United States are benign (17). The hallmark of benign ulcers—and the basis for most radiographic signs of benignancy—is mucosa that is intact to the very edge of an undermining ulcer crater. However, it should be recognized that even if the ulcers are radiographically

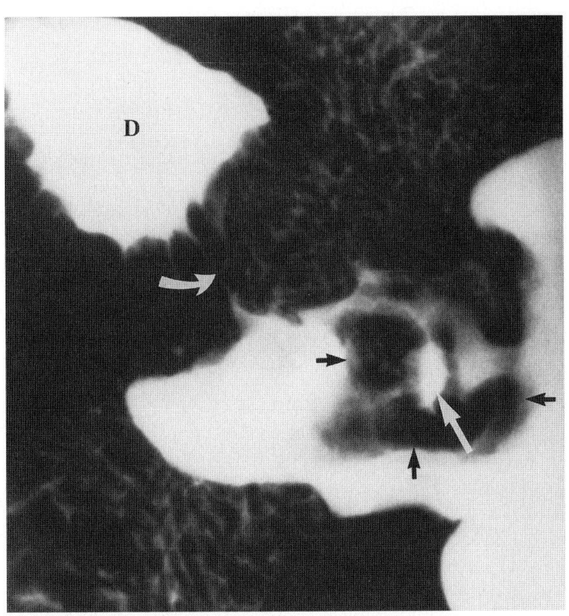

FIGURE 30.15. **Benign Gastric Ulcer.** Spot film from an upper GI series demonstrates a benign gastric ulcer (*straight white arrow*) in the antrum. Prominent nodular folds (*black arrows*) surround the ulcer crater. The normal contracted pyloric channel (*curved white arrow*) is seen as a thin line of barium. D, normal distended duodenal bulb.

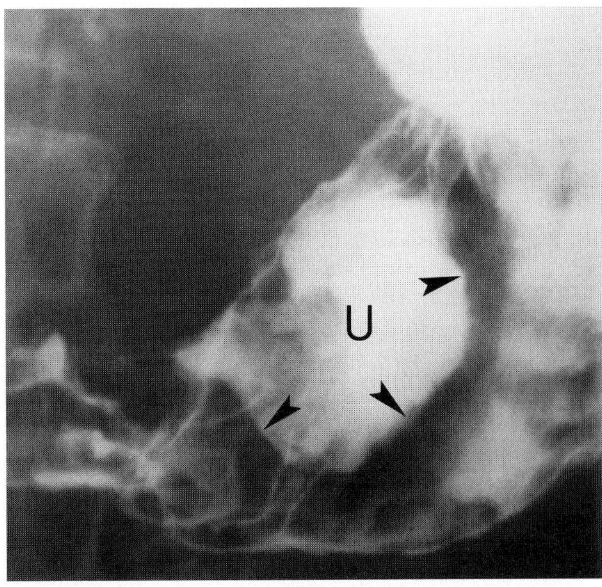

FIGURE 30.16. **Carmen Meniscus Sign.** A large, flat, malignant ulcer (U) traps barium within its rounded edges, seen as a band of lucency (*arrowheads*) surrounding the barium collection. The barium collection is convex toward the gastric lumen.

"benign," as many as 3% will actually be malignant. Demonstration of complete and sustained healing is considered the only reliable radiographic evidence of benign ulcer. Signs of benignancy include (*1*) a smooth ulcer mound with tapering edges, (*2*) an edematous ulcer collar with overhanging mucosal edge, (*3*) an ulcer projecting beyond the expected lumen, (*4*) radiating folds extending into the crater, (*5*) depth of ulcer greater than width, (*6*) sharply marginated contour, and (*7*) Hampton line (a thin, sharp, lucent line that traverses the orifice of the ulcer). A Hampton line, best demonstrated on spot films obtained with compression, is caused by an overhanging gastric mucosa in an undermined ulcer.

The size, depth, and location of the ulcer, along with the contour of the ulcer base, are of no diagnostic value in differentiating benign from malignant ulcers. The differential diagnosis of "benign ulcer" includes *H. pylori* peptic disease, gastritis, hyperparathyroidism, radiotherapy, and Zollinger-Ellison syndrome.

Malignant ulcers demonstrate signs that are the antithesis of benign ulcers. Evidence of irregular tumor mass or infiltration of the surrounding mucosa is evidence of malignancy. Signs of malignancy include (*1*) location within the lumen of the stomach; (*2*) eccentric location within the tumor mound; (*3*) width greater than depth; (*4*) nodular, rolled, irregular, or shouldered edges; and (*5*) Carmen meniscus sign (describes a large flat-based ulcer with heaped-up edges that fold inward to trap a lens-shaped barium collection that is convex toward the lumen) (Fig. 30.16). The differential diagnosis of "malignant ulcer" includes gastric adenocarcinoma, lymphoma, leiomyoma, and leiomyosarcoma.

CT is useful in demonstrating the extent of the tumor mass and the degree of involvement of the gastric wall.

DUODENUM

Duodenal Filling Defects/Mass Lesions

In the duodenal bulb, 90% of tumors are benign. In the second and third portions of the duodenum, tumors are 50% benign and 50% malignant. In the fourth portion of the duodenum, most tumors are malignant. Small, benign tumors of the duodenum usually present as smooth, polypoid filling defects. CT is helpful, but not specific, in predicting malignancy. Biopsy is usually required. Signs of malignancy include the following: (*1*) central necrosis, (*2*) ulceration or excavation, (*3*) exophytic or intramural mass, and (*4*) evidence of tumor beyond the duodenum.

Duodenal adenocarcinoma, although it is the most frequent malignant tumor of the duodenum, is a rare lesion (18). Malignant tumors are most common in the periampullary region and are rare in the bulb. Morphologic patterns include polypoid mass, ulcerative mass, and annular constricting lesion. Metastases to regional lymph nodes are present in two thirds of patients at presentation. CT demonstrates the local extent of the tumor, as well as nodal and liver metastases.

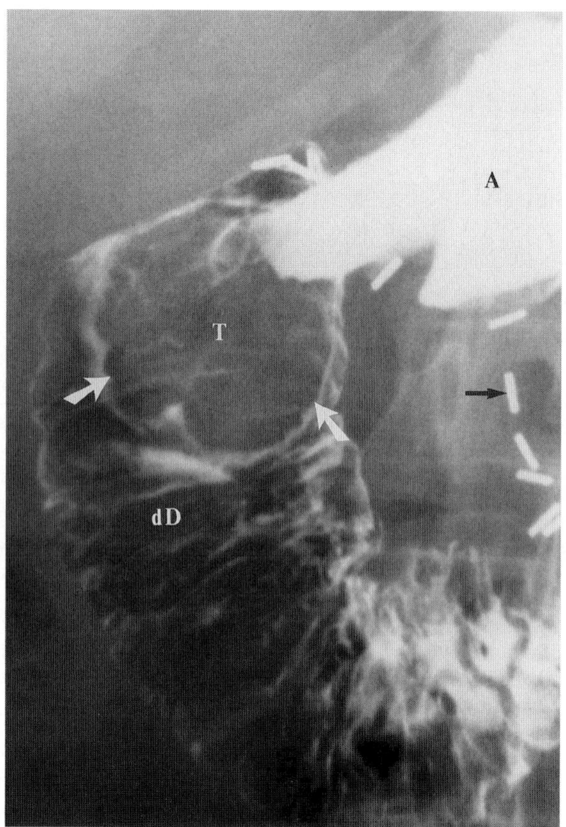

FIGURE 30.17. **Metastasis to Duodenum.** Double-contrast upper GI image demonstrates a lobulated tumor (T, *white arrows*) within the lumen of the descending duodenum (dD). Surgical biopsy revealed renal cell carcinoma metastatic to the duodenum. The surgical clips (*black arrow*) are from a radical left nephrectomy. A, antrum of the stomach.

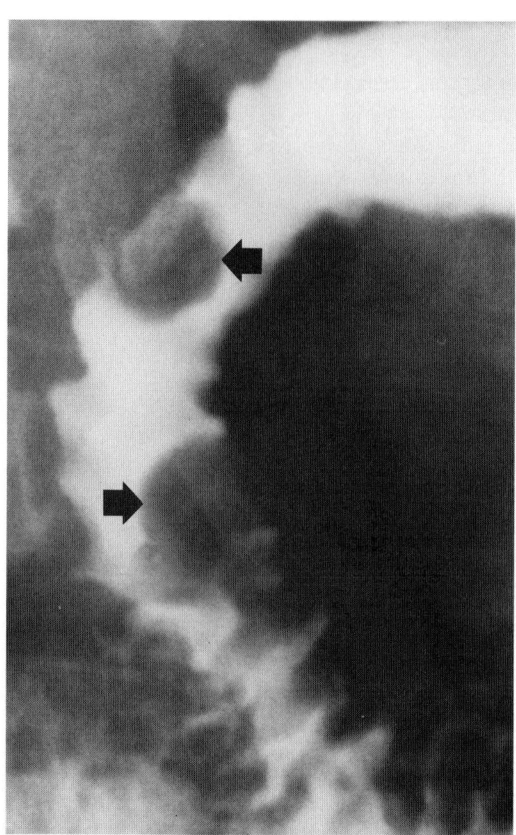

FIGURE 30.18. **Benign Gastrointestinal Stromal Tumor in Duodenum.** Spot view from an upper GI (UGI) series shows two round, smooth filling defects (*arrows*) in the descending duodenum. Endoscopic biopsy confirmed two leiomyomas. The UGI appearance is nonspecific.

Metastases to the duodenum may occur in the wall or subserosa of the duodenum. As the tumor grows, it may extend into the lumen and present as an intraluminal mass (Fig. 30.17) that may ulcerate. The most common primaries are breast, lung, and other GI malignancies. The duodenum may be invaded by tumors of adjacent organs, including the pancreas and kidney.

Lymphoma in the duodenum usually presents as nodules with thickened folds. The nodules associated with lymphoma are distinctly larger than those seen with benign lymphoid hyperplasia.

Duodenal adenoma presents as a polypoid lesion that may be pedunculated or sessile. Multiple adenomatous polyps are associated with polyposis syndromes. Villous adenomas have a high incidence of malignant degeneration and a characteristic "cauliflower" appearance on double-contrast UGI series.

GISTs of the duodenum present as an intramural, endoluminal, or exophytic mass, most commonly in the second or third portion of the duodenum (Fig. 30.18) (11). Ulceration is common. Malignant tumors range up to 20 cm in size and are most common in the more distal duodenum. Malignant GISTs are the second most common primary malignant tumor of the duodenum.

Lipoma of the duodenum is a soft tumor that may grow to a large size (14). Definitive diagnosis can be made by CT demonstration of a uniform, fat-density mass.

Lymphoid hyperplasia presents as small (1 to 3 mm) polypoid nodules located diffusely throughout the duodenum. The condition is usually benign, especially in children. It is associated with immunodeficiency in some adults. No evidence supports the concept that lymphoid hyperplasia is a precursor to lymphoma.

Gastric Mucosal Prolapse/Heterotopic Gastric Mucosa. Gastric mucosa may prolapse through the pylorus during peristalsis and cause a lobulated filling defect at the base of the duodenal bulb. The diagnosis is suggested by the characteristic location and change in configuration with peristalsis.

Heterotopic gastric mucosa in the duodenal bulb is common on endoscopy (12%) but less frequently evident radiographically. The lesion has the appearance of areae gastricae in the duodenal bulb or as clusters of 1- to 3-mm plaques on the smooth duodenal bulb mucosa. It may also appear as a solitary polyp that is indistinguishable from other polypoid lesions of the duodenum.

Brunner Gland Hyperplasia/Adenoma. The Brunner glands are located in the submucosa of the proximal two-thirds of the duodenum and secrete an alkaline substance that buffers gastric acid. Diffuse nodular gland hyperplasia is a common cause of multiple filling defects and is associated with hyperacidity. Brunner gland adenoma presents as a solitary filling defect and is identical in appearance to other benign duodenal nodules.

Ectopic pancreas may also occur in the duodenum, most commonly in the proximal descending portion. A solitary mass with a central dimple is most characteristic.

Extrinsic mass impressions on the duodenum may be made by the gallbladder; masses in the liver, pancreas, adrenal gland, kidney, or colon; pancreatic fluid collections; adenopathy; or aneurysms.

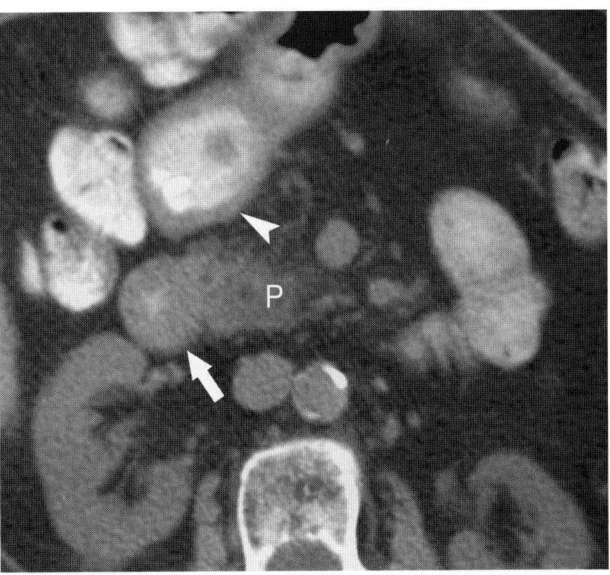

FIGURE 30.19. **Duodenitis.** CT scan performed with oral but without IV contrast shows diffuse circumferential thickening of the wall of the duodenum (*arrow*). Slight thickening of the wall of the gastric antrum (*arrowhead*) is also present. The inflammatory changes were confirmed by endoscopy and were believed to be caused by anti-inflammatory medications. P, head of the pancreas.

Thickened Duodenal Folds

The valvulae conniventes, or Kerckring folds, of the small bowel begin in the second portion of the duodenum and continue throughout the remainder of the small bowel. The valvulae conniventes are permanent circular folds of mucosa supported by a core of fibrovascular submucosa. They are normally several millimeters wide and remain visible even with full distension of the duodenum. Folds wider than 2 to 3 mm are usually considered thickened.

Normal Variant. Thickened folds are a nonspecific radiographic finding that may be found in normal individuals. The radiographic diagnosis of a pathologic condition is more confident when there are additional findings.

Duodenitis refers to inflammation of the duodenum without discrete ulcer formation (16). The major cause of duodenitis is *H. pylori* infection. Alcohol and anti-inflammatory medications cause a few cases. UGI findings include (*1*) thickening (>4 mm) of the proximal duodenal folds, (*2*) nodules or nodular folds (enlarged Brunner glands), (*3*) deformity of the duodenal bulb, and (*4*) erosions. CT shows nonspecific wall thickening (Fig. 30.19).

Pancreatitis and cholecystitis thicken the duodenal folds by paraduodenal inflammation. Both may also cause mass impressions on the duodenal lumen. CT or US demonstrate the extent and nature of the paraduodenal process.

Crohn disease of the duodenum usually involves the first and second portions and is almost always associated with contiguous involvement of the stomach. Duodenal involvement is apparent by thickened folds, aphthous ulcers, erosions, and single or multiple strictures.

Parasites. Giardiasis is caused by an overgrowth of the parasite *Giardia lamblia* in the duodenum and jejunum. Many patients are asymptomatic carriers, but patients with invasion of the gut wall have abdominal pain, diarrhea, and malabsorption. Giardiasis is a frequent cause of travelers' diarrhea. Radiographic findings include (*1*) distorted, thickened folds in the duodenum and jejunum; (*2*) hypermotility and spasm; and (*3*) increased secretions.

Strongyloidiasis is caused by infection with the nematode *Strongyloides stercoralis*, which is found in all areas of the world but is most common in the warm, moist regions of the tropics. As with giardiasis, many patients are asymptomatic carriers. Invasion of the intestinal wall causes vomiting and malabsorption. UGI findings include edematous folds, spasm, dilation of the proximal duodenum, and diffuse mucosal ulceration.

Lymphoma presents with nodular thickened folds.

Intramural hemorrhage is caused by trauma, anticoagulation, and bleeding disorders (1). The regular pattern of thickened folds resembles a stack of coins. Partial or complete duodenal obstruction is usually present. The fixed retroperitoneal position of the third portion of the duodenum makes it susceptible to blunt abdominal trauma and compression against the lumbar spine.

Duodenal Ulcers and Diverticula

Duodenal ulcers are caused by *H. pylori* infection in 95% of cases. Addition causes include anti-inflammatory medications, Crohn disease, Zollinger-Ellison syndrome, viral infections, or penetrating pancreatic cancer. Duodenal

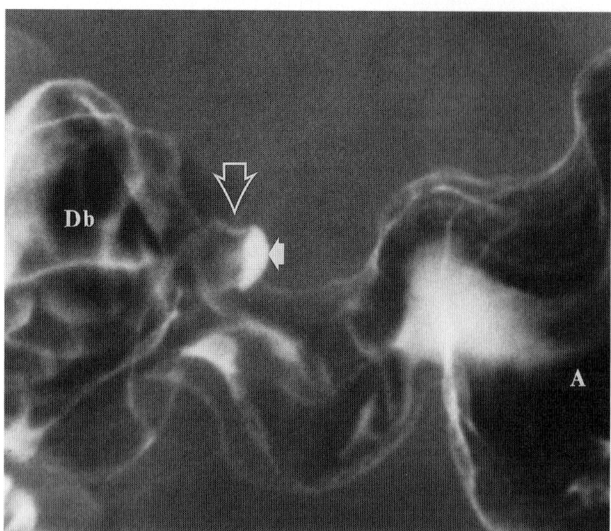

FIGURE 30.20. **Peptic Ulcer.** An upper GI series demonstrates a persistent barium collection (*closed arrow*) that projects beyond the lumen of the base of the duodenal bulb (Db). A well-defined ulcer collar (*open arrow*) is present. A, gastric antrum.

ulcers are associated with acid hypersecretion. Most (95%) are in the duodenal bulb, with the anterior wall most often involved (17). Radiographic diagnosis of a duodenal ulcer depends upon demonstration of the ulcer crater or niche (Fig. 30.20). En face, the crater appears as a persistent collection of barium or air. In profile, ulcers project beyond the normal lumen. Thickened folds often radiate toward the ulcer crater, which may be surrounded by a mound of edema. Although duodenal ulcers are usually round or oval, linear ulcers also occur. Most duodenal ulcers are smaller than 1 cm in diameter. Giant ulcers larger than 2 cm resemble diverticula or a deformed bulb. Ulcer craters have no mucosal lining and therefore no mucosal relief pattern, and they do not contract with peristalsis. Ulcer scarring may cause a pattern of radiating folds with a central barium collection that is indistinguishable from that of an acute ulcer. Endoscopy may be required to make the differentiation. Postbulbar ulcers represent about 5% of the total but are more commonly associated with serious upper GI hemorrhage (19). Most involve the second and third portions of the duodenum, which are frequently narrowed.

Complications of duodenal ulcer disease include obstruction, bleeding, and perforation. Bleeding from a duodenal ulcer is most efficiently diagnosed endoscopically. Perforation may be manifest by pneumoperitoneum or a localized abnormal gas collection. Peptic duodenal ulcer is not a premalignant condition.

Zollinger-Ellison syndrome is caused by a gastrin-secreting islet cell tumor (gastrinoma). Gastrinomas are found in the pancreas (75%), duodenum (15%), and in 10% in extraintestinal sites (liver, lymph nodes, and ovary). The islet cell tumor is malignant in 60% of cases. Gastrinomas also occur as part of the hereditary syndrome of multiple endocrine neoplasia, type 1 (MEN-1). Continuous gastrin secretion results in marked hyperacidity and multiple peptic ulcers in the duodenum, stomach, and jejunum. UGI studies show pathognomic findings of (*1*) multiple peptic ulcers in the stomach, duodenal bulb, and, most characteristically, in the postbulbar duodenum; (*2*) hypersecretion with high volumes of gastric fluid diluting the barium and impairing mucosal coating; and (*3*) thick edematous folds in the stomach, duodenum, and proximal jejunum.

Flexural pseudotumors are a common cause of a duodenal filling defect with a central barium collection, mimicking an ulcerated lesion. Appearing as rounded, swirled mucosal folds on the inner aspect of the flexure at the apex of the bulb, these tumors are redundant mucosa and have a variable appearance on different projections.

Duodenal diverticula are common (5% of UGI series) and usually incidental findings. They may be multiple and may form in any portion of the duodenum but are most common along the inner aspect of the descending duodenum (Fig. 30.21). Diverticula are differentiated from ulcers on a UGI series by demonstration of mucosal folds entering the neck of the diverticulum and change in appearance with peristalsis. On plain abdominal radiographs, duodenal diverticula may be seen as abnormal air collections. On CT they may be filled with fluid and mimic a pancreatic pseudocyst, or they may contain air and fluid and mimic

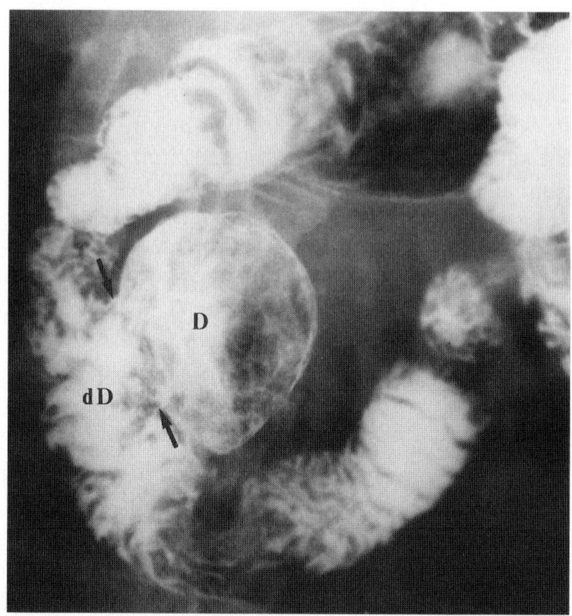

FIGURE 30.21. **Duodenal Diverticulum.** Radiograph from an upper GI series demonstrates contrast and air filling a duodenal diverticulum (D) that originates from the medial aspect of the descending duodenum (dD). The neck of the duodenum is indicated by arrows.

a pancreatic abscess (20). Rare complications include perforation and hemorrhage. Diverticula adjacent to the ampulla of Vater may rarely obstruct the common bile duct or pancreatic duct.

Intraluminal diverticula are caused by a thin, incomplete, congenital diaphragm that is stretched by the intraluminal contents to form a "windsock" configuration within the duodenum (Fig. 30.22).

Duodenal Narrowing

Annular pancreas is the most common congenital anomaly of the pancreas. Pancreatic tissue encircles the descending duodenum and narrows its lumen. The abnormality occurs when the bilobed ventral component of the pancreas fuses with the dorsal pancreas on both sides of the duodenum. Although it often presents in childhood, especially in children with Down syndrome, about half of cases do not present until adulthood. Symptomatic adults present with nausea, vomiting, abdominal pain, and occasionally jaundice. The UGI series typically demonstrates eccentric or concentric narrowing of the descending duodenum (Fig. 30.23). Annular

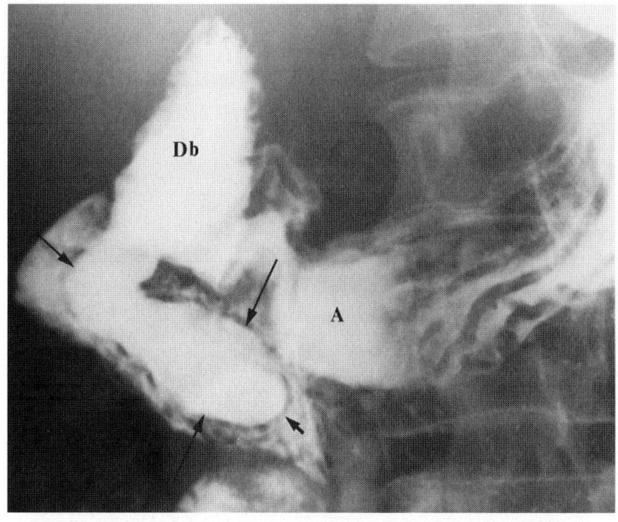

FIGURE 30.22. **Intraluminal Duodenal Diverticulum.** A upper GI series demonstrates a barium-filled "sock" (*long arrows*) within the lumen of the descending duodenum. The radiolucent wall of the diverticulum (*short arrow*) is outlined by barium, both within the diverticulum and within the lumen of the duodenum. Db, duodenal bulb; A, gastric antrum.

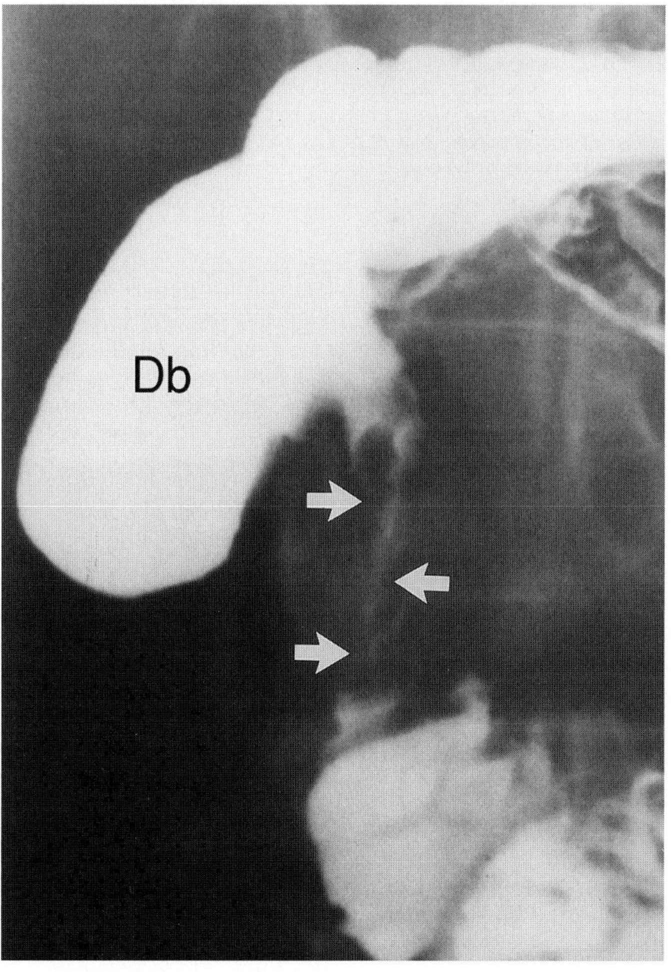

FIGURE 30.23. **Annular Pancreas.** Upper GI series demonstrates a 3-cm long circumferentially narrowed segment (*arrows*) of the descending duodenum. No ulceration was evident. CT confirmed an annular pancreas. Db, duodenal bulb.

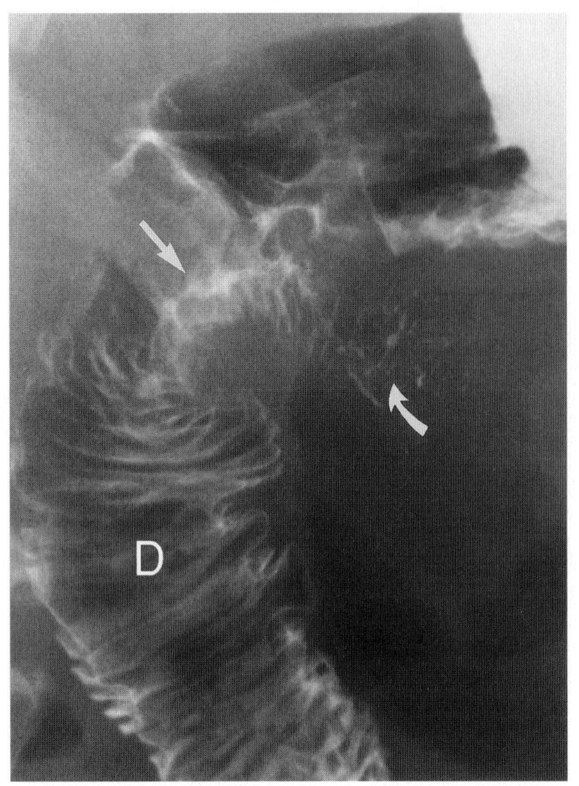

FIGURE 30.24. **Pancreatic Carcinoma.** Double-contrast upper GI series reveals narrowing (*straight arrow*) of the proximal descending duodenum, with ulceration that allowed tracking of barium (*curved arrow*) into the pancreas. The cause was carcinoma of the pancreas. Normal folds and mucosal pattern are seen in the more distal descending duodenum (D).

pancreas is associated with a high incidence of postbulbar peptic ulceration in adults. CT confirms the diagnosis by demonstration of pancreatic tissue encircling the duodenum. Endoscopic retrograde cholangiopancreatography demonstrates an annular pancreatic duct encircling the duodenum.

Duodenal adenocarcinoma can present as a circumferential constricting lesion with tumor shoulders, giving evidence of mass effect. Ulceration is common. CT demonstrates the extent of the lesion.

Pancreatic carcinoma may also encircle (Fig. 30.24) and obstruct the pancreas. Jaundice with dilatation of the bile and pancreatic ducts are usually present.

Lymphoma causes marked wall thickening and bulky paraduodenal lymphadenopathy that may narrow the lumen.

Postbulbar ulcer is commonly associated with narrowing of the lumen of the second and third portions of the duodenum.

Extrinsic compression caused by inflammation or tumor in adjacent organs, especially the pancreas, may constrict the duodenal lumen.

Upper GI Hemorrhage

UGI hemorrhage refers to bleeding with the site of origin proximal to the ligament of Treitz. This hemorrhage has an average mortality of 8% to 10%. Causes in an approximate order of frequency are (*1*) duodenal ulcer, (*2*) esophageal varices, (*3*) gastric ulcer, (*4*) acute hemorrhagic gastritis, (*5*) esophagitis, (*6*) Mallory-Weiss tear, (*7*) neoplasm, (*8*) vascular malformation, and (*9*) vascular enteric fistula.

Barium studies should be avoided in patients in the acute stages of UGI hemorrhage. Endoscopy is much more accurate than a UGI series in demonstrating the bleeding site (95% versus 45%). The UGI series may identify a lesion but will not indicate whether that lesion is responsible for the bleeding. Also, retained barium in the GI tract following a UGI series will usually make performance of angiography impossible. Helical CT angiography shows promise in identifying the bleeding site. Conventional angiography is used to localize active bleeding sites and provide therapy by infusion of vasoconstrictors or performance of transcatheter embolization.

REFERENCES

1. Jayaraman MV, Mayo-Smith WW, Movson JS, Dupuy DE, Wallach MT. CT of the duodenum: an overlooked segment gets its due. Radiographics 2001;21(special issue):147–160.
2. Goldberg HI, Margulis AR. Gastrointestinal radiology in the United States: an overview of the past 50 years. Radiology 2000;216:1–7.
3. Ba-Ssalamah A, Prokop M, Uffman M, Pokieser P, Teleky B, Lechner G. Dedicated multidetector CT of the stomach: spectrum of diseases. Radiographics 2003;23:625–644.
4. Horton KM, Fishman EK. Current role of CT in imaging of the stomach. Radiographics 2003;23:75–87.
5. An SK, Han JK, Kim YH, et al. Gastric mucosa-associated lymphoid tissue lymphoma: spectrum of findings at double-contrast gastrointestinal examination with pathologic correlation. Radiographics 2001;21:1491–1504.
6. Fishman EK, Urban BA, Hruban RH. CT of the stomach: spectrum of disease. Radiographics 1996;16:1035–1054.
7. Pattison CP, Combs MJ, Marshall BJ. Helicobacter pylori and peptic ulcer disease: evolution to revolution to resolution. AJR Am J Roentgenol 1997;168:1415–1420.
8. Insko EK, Levine MS, Birnbaum BA, Jacobs JE. Benign and malignant lesions of the stomach: evaluation of CT criteria for differentiation. Radiology 2003;228:166–171.
9. Levine MS, Rubesin SE, Pantongrag-Brown L, et al. Non-Hodgkin's lymphoma of the gastrointestinal tract: radiographic findings. AJR Am J Roentgenol 1997;168:165–172.
10. Park M-S, Kim KW, Yu J-S, et al. Radiographic findings of primary B-cell lymphoma of the stomach: low-grade versus high-grade malignancy in relation to the mucosa-associated lymphoid tissue concept. AJR Am J Roentgenol 2002;179:1297–1304.
11. Sandrasegaran K, Rajesh A, Rydberg J, Rushing DA, et al. Gastrointestinal stromal tumors: clinical, radiologic, and pathologic features. AJR Am J Roentgenol 2005;184:803–811.
12. Kim H-C, Lee JM, Kim WK, et al. Gastrointestinal stromal tumors of the stomach: CT findings and prediction of malignancy. AJR Am J Roentgenol 2004;183:893–898.
13. Park SH, Han JK, Kim TK, et al. Unusual gastric tumors: radiologic-pathologic correlation. Radiographics 1999;19:1435–1446.
14. Thompson WM. Imaging and findings of lipomas of the gastrointestinal tract. AJR Am J Roentgenol 2005;184:1163–1171.

15. Furth EE, Rubesin SE, Levine MS. Pathologic primer on gastritis: an illustrated sum and substance. Radiology 1995;197:693–698.
16. Gelfand DW, Ott DJ, Chen MYM. Radiologic evaluation of gastritis and duodenitis. AJR Am J Roentgenol 1999;173:357–361.
17. Dickerson BA, Ott DJ, Chen MYM, Gelfand DW. Peptic ulcer disease: pathogenesis, radiologic features, and complications. Acad Radiol 2000;7:355–364.
18. Ott DJ, D'Alessio TL, Chen MYM. Duodenal neoplasms: pathology and radiologic imaging. Radiologist 2001;8:203–212.
19. Carucci LR, Levine MS, Rubesin SE, Laufer I. Upper gastrointestinal tract barium examinations of postbulbar duodenal ulcers. AJR Am J Roentgenol 2004;182:927–930.
20. Stone EE, Brant WE, Smith G. Computed tomography of duodenal diverticula. Comput Assist Tomogr 1989;13:61–64.

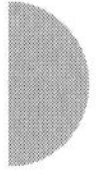

Chapter 31

Mesenteric Small Bowel

William E. Brant

Imaging Methods
Anatomy
Small Bowel Filling Defects/Mass Lesions
Mesenteric Masses
Diffuse Small Bowel Disease
Small Bowel Erosions and Ulcerations
Small Bowel Diverticula

Imaging Methods

Disease of the mesenteric small intestine is relatively rare (1). Detailed radiographic study of the small bowel is justified only when clinical suspicion of small bowel disease is high. Small bowel disease is usually manifest by four major symptoms: colic, diarrhea, malabsorption, and bleeding. Colic is defined as recurrent and spasmodic abdominal pain, with periods of relief every 2 to 3 minutes. Diarrhea caused by small bowel disease is less urgent than that caused by colon disease. Malabsorption is manifest by steatorrhea, foul-smelling stools, and weight loss. Bleeding from small bowel disease is usually occult and manifest by anemia. Because the majority of the mesenteric small intestine is out of reach of the endoscopist, diagnostic radiology has the primary responsibility for its evaluation.

The traditional method for radiographic examination of the small bowel is the small bowel follow-through examination (SBFT) (Fig. 31.1) tacked onto a standard upper GI series. The patient is asked to continue drinking barium while a series of supine abdominal films are obtained until the terminal ileum and cecum are filled with barium. Fluoroscopic examination of the small bowel is then attempted. This study is notoriously insensitive. It is limited by overlap of bowel loops, poor distension, flocculation of barium, intermittent barium filling, and unpredictable transit time. Visualization of the distal ileum may be improved with double-contrast technique by insufflating the colon with air (SBFT with peroral pneumocolon).

Enteroclysis, or the small bowel enema, is the preferred method for detailed radiographic examination (Fig. 31.2). This study provides more uniform distension of the bowel, even distribution of barium, superior anatomic detail, and shorter overall examination time (1). The study is performed by passing a specially designed enteroclysis catheter (12 to 14 French) through the mouth or nose and into the distal duodenum or proximal jejunum. A guidewire is used for directional control of the catheter during manipulation under fluoroscopy. The study may be performed single contrast (with approximately 600 mL of barium) or double contrast (with 200 mL of barium followed by 1,000 mL of methylcellulose to advance the barium and distend the bowel). The small bowel lumen and mucosal surface are best demonstrated by barium studies. CT complements the barium examination by demonstrating the extraluminal component of bowel disease. In addition, CT evaluates the mesentery, adjacent solid organs, the peritoneal cavity, and the retroperitoneum. CT signs that aid in the differentiation of benign and malignant disease are listed in Table 31.1 (2,3). CT enteroclysis combines the total opacification of the small bowel achieved by contrast infusion through a nasoenteric tube with thin-section multidetector CT imaging (4). MR enteroclysis is an emerging technique utilizing fast thin-section MR imaging of the small bowel after it has been well distended by nasojejunal catheter infusion of isosmotic water solution.

Anatomy

The mesenteric small intestine is a tube approximately 7 m long that lies totally within the greater peritoneal cavity. The jejunum is arbitrarily defined as the proximal

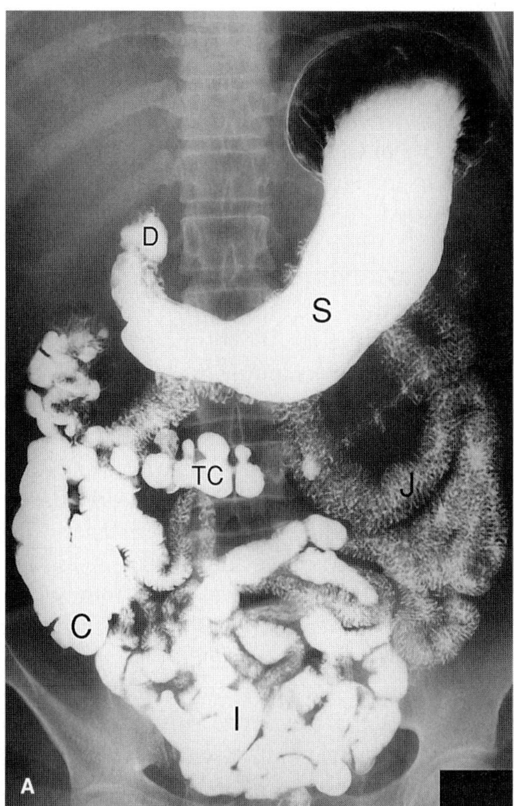

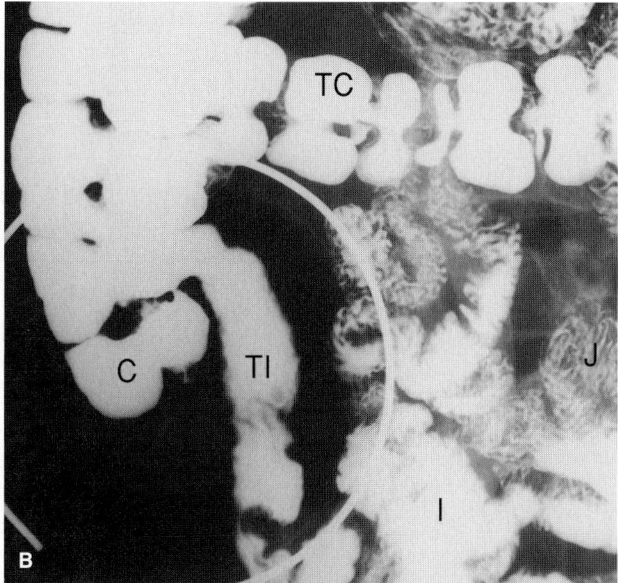

FIGURE 31.1. **Normal Small Bowel Follow-Through. A.** Prone abdominal radiograph. **B.** Spot-compression view of the terminal ileum. The small bowel is demonstrated on an upper GI series by having the patient ingest additional barium and by obtaining additional radiographs to document passage of barium through the small bowel into the colon. The loops of jejunum (J) have a delicate feathery appearance in the left upper abdomen, whereas the loops of ileum (I) are coarse and featureless in the right lower abdomen. Barium has filled portions of the cecum (C) and ascending and transverse colon (TC), the latter identified by its haustral folds. Colonic haustral folds extend only partway across the bowel lumen, and small bowel folds extend completely across the bowel lumen. The spot compression provides separation of bowel loops in the right lower quadrant to optimally demonstrate the terminal ileum (TI). S, stomach; D, duodenum.

two fifths of the mesenteric intestine, while the ileum is the distal three fifths. The jejunum and ileum are suspended from the posterior abdominal wall by the small bowel mesentery. The small bowel mesentery is composed of connective tissue, blood vessels, and lymphatic vessels, and it is covered by peritoneum, which reflects from the posterior parietal peritoneum (5). The root of the small bowel mesentery extends obliquely from the ligament of Treitz, just left of the L2 vertebra, to the cecum, near the right sacroiliac joint. On CT the mesentery is defined by its normal vascular structures, which are outlined by fat between loops of bowel. Normal mesenteric lymph nodes may be seen as soft tissue–density nodules that are 5 mm or smaller. The concave border of the small bowel loops is the *mesenteric border,* where the mesentery attaches. The convex border, facing away from the mesentery, is called the *antimesenteric border.* Identification of the border involved by disease can be of diagnostic value.

On CT and barium studies, the jejunum has a feathery mucosal pattern, more prominent valvulae conniventes, a wider lumen, and a thicker wall. The ileum has a less featured mucosal pattern; thinner, less frequent folds; a narrower lumen; and a thinner wall. The transition between jejunum and ileum is gradual, and all loops are freely mobile. The ileum has larger and more numerous lymphoid follicles in the submucosa. The villi are fingerlike projections that extend from the entire mucosal surface of the small bowel. They are composed of loose connective tissue of the lamina propria. Tiny capillaries and lymphatic vessels (lacteals) extend to the submucosal vessels. The combination of valvulae conniventes and villi greatly expands the absorptive surface area of the small intestine. The caliber of the normal small bowel lumen is less than 3 cm, with normal fold thickness of less than 2 mm and normal wall thickness of 3 mm. Normal lymph nodes seen in the mesentery are smaller than 4 mm in diameter.

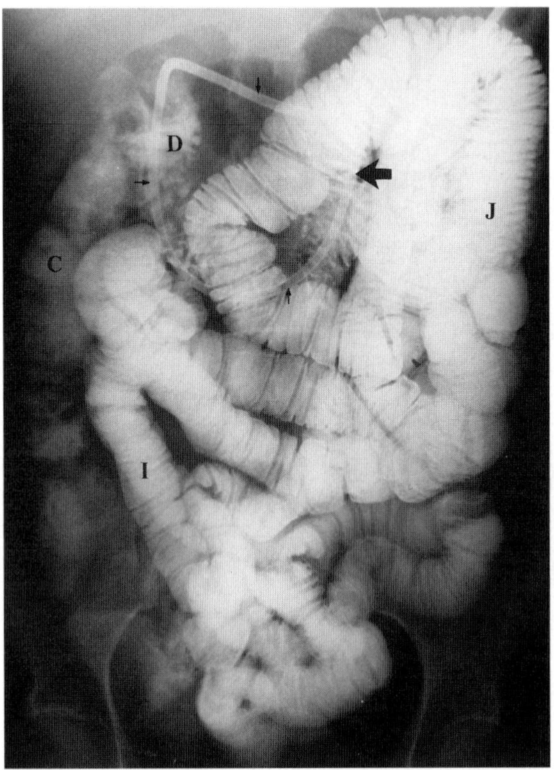

FIGURE 31.2. **Normal Enteroclysis.** The enteroclysis catheter (*small arrows*) has been passed through the C-loop of the duodenum to the location of the ligament of Treitz (*large arrow*) with fluoroscopy used to guide catheter manipulation. The enteroclysis technique provides uniform distension of the jejunum (J) and ileum (I). Barium fills portions of the ascending colon (C). Note the small bowel folds crossing the entire diameter of the small bowel lumen. D, duodenum.

TABLE 31.1 Diagnostic Findings of CT of the Gastrointestinal Tract

Benign Lesion	Neoplastic Lesion
Circumferential thickening	Eccentric thickening
Symmetric thickening	Asymmetric thickening
Thickening <1 cm	Thickening >2 cm
Segmental or diffuse involvement	Focal soft tissue mass
Thickened mesenteric fat	Abrupt transition
Wall is homogeneous soft tissue density	Lobulated contour
"Double halo sign": dark inner ring/bright outer ring	Spiculated outer contour
"Target sign": bright inner, dark middle, bright outer	Luminal narrowing
	Regional adenopathy
	Liver metastases

Small Bowel Filling Defects/ Mass Lesions

Neoplasms of the small intestine are rare, accounting for only 2% to 3% of GI tumors. Benign neoplasms are about equivalent to malignant neoplasms in overall frequency. However, when the patient presents with symptoms, malignancy is three times more common. Presenting afflictions include obstruction, pain, weight loss, bleeding, and palpable mass.

Carcinoid tumors are the most common neoplasm of the small intestine, accounting for about one third of all small bowel tumors (6). They are considered a low-grade malignancy that may recur locally or metastasize to the lymph nodes, liver, or lung. They arise from endocrine cells (enterochromaffin or Kulchitsky cells) deep in the mucosa. These cells produce vasoactive substances, including serotonin and bradykinins. About 20% of all carcinoid tumors arise in the small bowel, most commonly in the ileum, where 30% are multiple. Only 7%—those with liver metastases—present with carcinoid syndrome (cutaneous flushing, abdominal cramps, and diarrhea) because the liver inactivates the vasoactive substances. The tumors grow slowly but cause a marked fibrotic response of the bowel wall and mesentery, because the serotonin produced by the tumor induces an intense local desmoplastic reaction. Complications include stricture, obstruction, and bowel infarction induced by fibrosis of the mesenteric vessels. The tumors may be pedunculated and cause intussusception. Radiographic signs of fibrosis and metastases resemble the findings of Crohn disease and overshadow demonstration of the primary tumor. Barium studies show: (*1*) luminal narrowing, (*2*) thickened and spiculated folds, (*3*) separation of bowel loops by mesenteric mass or (*4*) bowel loops drawn together by fibrosis, and (*5*) primary lesion appearing as a small (<1.5-cm) mural nodule or intraluminal polyp. CT findings that are pathognomonic of carcinoid tumor are (Fig. 31.3): (*1*) sunburst pattern of radiating soft tissue density in the mesenteric fat because of mesenteric fibrosis; (*2*) bowel wall thickening; (*3*) primary lesion appearing as a small, lobulated soft tissue mass, occasionally with central calcification, usually in the distal ileum; and (*4*) enlarged mesenteric nodes and liver masses caused by metastatic disease.

Adenocarcinoma of the small bowel is about half as common as carcinoid tumor. It is most frequent in the duodenum (50%) and proximal jejunum and is uncommon in the distal ileum, where carcinoid is most common. Most patients are symptomatic at presentation, and 30% have a palpable mass. Patients with adult celiac disease, Crohn disease, and Peutz-Jeghers syndrome are at increased risk for small bowel carcinoma. Complications include bleeding, obstruction, and intussusception. Prognosis is poor, with a 5-year survival rate of 20%. Metastatic spread is by intraperitoneal seeding, lymphatic channels to regional

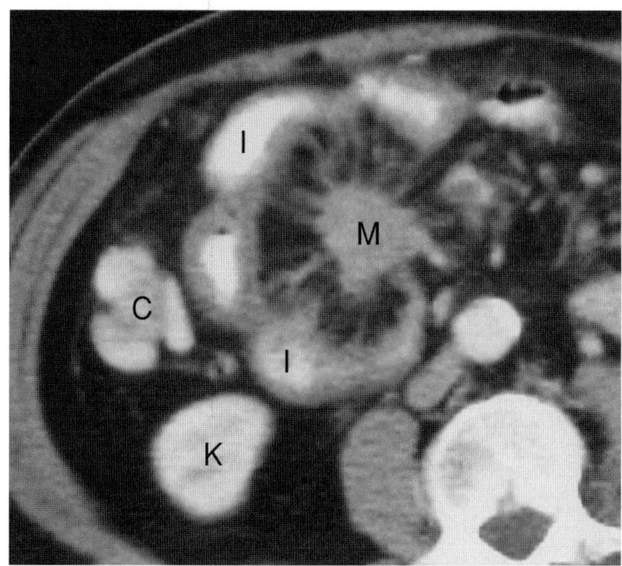

FIGURE 31.3. **Carcinoid Tumor.** CT scan shows classic "sunburst" appearance of radiating strands and mesenteric mass (M) caused by carcinoid tumor arising in the ileum (I). C, ascending colon; K, kidney.

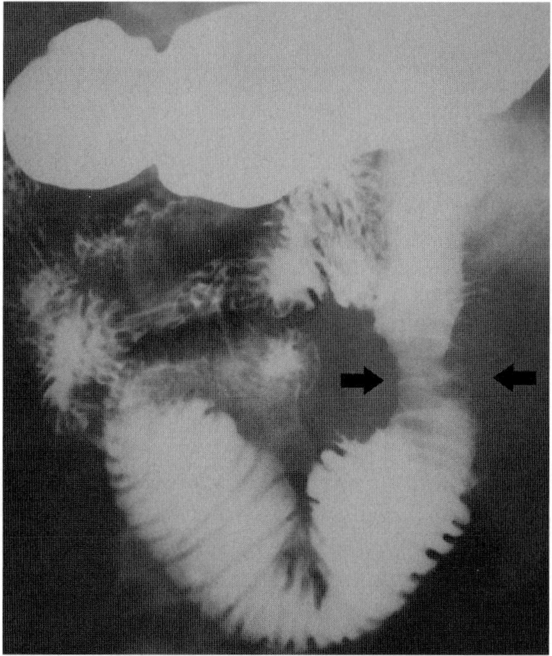

FIGURE 31.4. **Adenocarcinoma of the Jejunum.** Small bowel follow-through study demonstrates fixed constricting lesion (*arrows*) of the jejunum. The folds in the involved area are thickened and effaced.

nodes, and portal veins to the liver. Morphologically the tumor may be infiltrating, producing strictures; polypoid, producing filling defects; or ulcerating. Barium studies typically show a characteristic "apple core" stricture of the small bowel (Fig. 31.4). CT (Fig. 31.5) demonstrates (*1*) a solitary mass in the duodenum or jejunum (up to 8 cm diameter), (*2*) an ulcerated lesion, or (*3*) abrupt irregular circumferential narrowing of the bowel lumen, with abrupt edges to the thickened wall.

Lymphoma is responsible for about 20% of all small bowel malignant tumors. The GI tract is the most common site for an extranodal origin of lymphoma, and the small bowel is most commonly involved (7). Most cases are non-Hodgkin lymphoma of the B-cell type. Non-Hodgkin lymphoma clinically involves the GI tract in 30% of cases overall. Lymphoma is most frequent in the distal ileum, where the concentration of lymphoid tissue is the greatest. Morphologic patterns of involvement include diffuse infiltration, exophytic mass, polypoid mass, and multiple nodules. Multiple sites of involvement are seen in 10% to 25% of cases. Aneurysmal dilation of the lumen is a feature of lymphoma caused by replacement of the muscularis and destruction of the autonomic plexus by tumor without inducing fibrosis. As a result, obstruction is uncommon. Barium studies most commonly reveal: (*1*) wall thickening with irregular, distorted folds caused by submucosal infiltration of cells (Fig. 31.6); (*2*) fold thickening that may be smooth and regular in early stages because of lymphatic blockage in the mesentery; (*3*) effacement of folds in later stages with greater cell infiltration into the bowel wall; (*4*) narrowed, widened, or normal lumen;

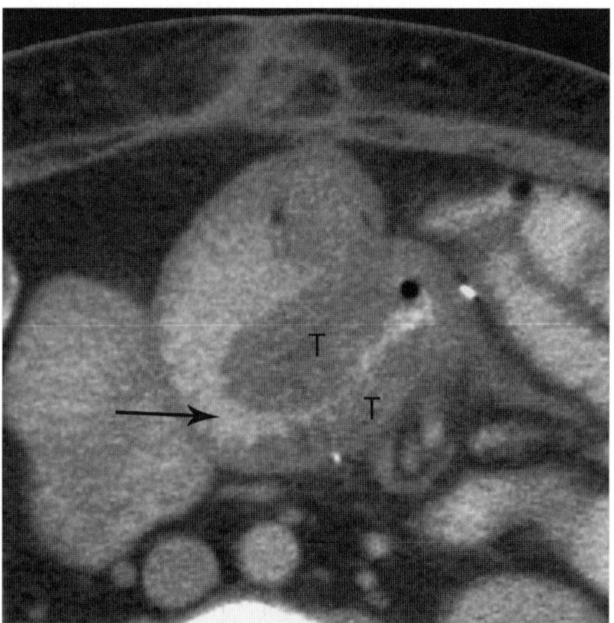

FIGURE 31.5. **Adenocarcinoma of the Jejunum.** CT image from another patient demonstrates tumor infiltration (T) of the wall of the jejunum resulting in constriction of the lumen (*arrow*). The complete examination revealed additional signs of small bowel obstruction.

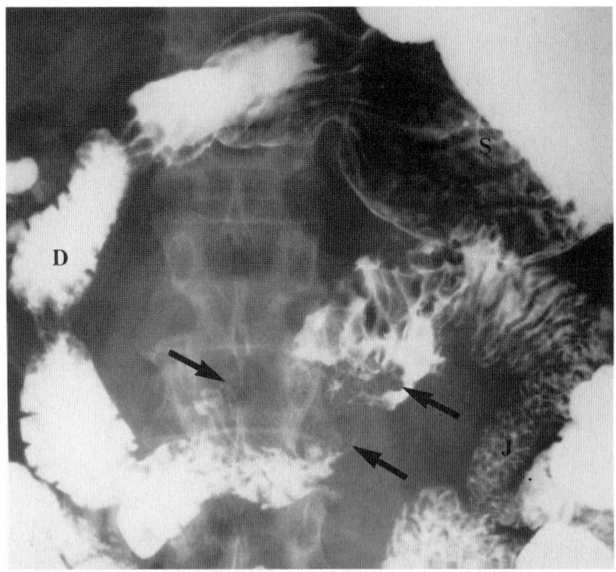

FIGURE 31.6. **Non-Hodgkin Lymphoma.** An upper GI series demonstrates polypoid filling defects (*arrows*) in the third portion of the duodenum (D) caused by masses of lymphoma in the bowel wall. The duodenal C-loop is widened and the jejunum (J) is displaced laterally. S, stomach.

(*5*) cavitary lesions containing fluid and debris; (*6*) polypoid masses that may cause intussusception; (*7*) rare multiple filling defects that are larger than 4 mm, variable in size, and nonuniform in distribution. Shallow ulceration is common. CT demonstrates: (*1*) circumferential wall thickening involving a long segment of small bowel, (*2*) effacement of folds, (*3*) mucosal nodularity, and (*4*) eccentric wall thickening (Fig. 31.7). Exophytic lymphoma is generally of uniform soft tissue density and enhances little, if any, with IV contrast administration. This is a differentiating finding in comparison with GI stromal tumors (GISTs) and adenocarcinoma, which usually enhance prominently. CT readily demonstrates associated findings of lymphoma, including mesenteric and retroperitoneal adenopathy and hepatosplenomegaly. The mesentery may show a large confluent mass encasing multiple bowel loops or enlarged individual nodes (Fig. 31.8). The "sandwich sign" refers to the sparing of rind of fat surrounding mesenteric vessels that are encased by lymphomatous nodes.

Burkitt lymphoma in North America usually presents with intestinal involvement, especially of the ileocecal area in children and young adults. The malignancy is aggressive, with rapid doubling time and poor prognosis. Imaging studies show bulky tumors.

AIDS-related lymphoma is an aggressive high-grade non-Hodgkin lymphoma with poor prognosis. Extranodal involvement, including small bowel lymphoma, is common. Adenopathy may be caused by lymphoma, Kaposi sarcoma, or *Mycobacterium avium-intracellulare* infection.

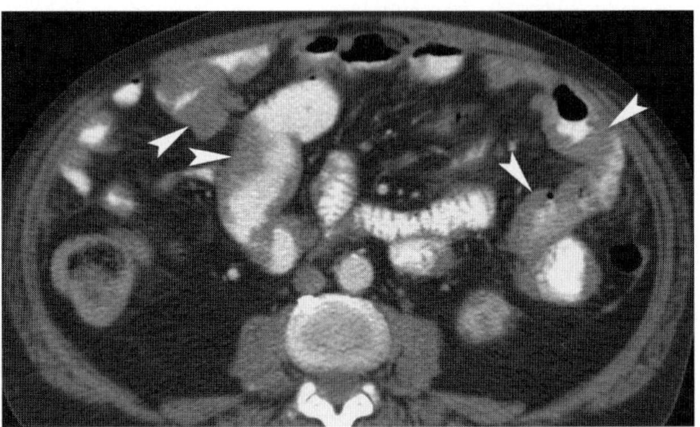

FIGURE 31.7. **Non-Hodgkin Lymphoma.** CT image shows eccentric wall thickening (*arrowheads*) of multiple loops of the small bowel.

Radiographic findings are identical to those seen in immunocompetent patients.

Nodular lymphoid hyperplasia may involve the entire small bowel. The condition is differentiated from lymphoma by the uniform small size of the nodules (2 to 4 mm) and their even distribution throughout the area of involvement (Fig. 31.9). Lymphoid hyperplasia confined to the terminal ileum and proximal colon is usually considered incidental and may be related to recent viral infection. Diffuse lymphoid hyperplasia is associated with hypogammaglobulinemia, especially low IgA.

Metastases to the small bowel are common. The two most frequent routes are by peritoneal seeding, usually involving the mesenteric border, and by hematogenous spread, which usually implants on the antimesenteric border. Intraperitoneal implantation on the small bowel serosa is most commonly the result of ovarian carcinoma in women and colon, gastric, and pancreatic carcinoma in men. The mesenteric border of the small bowel is

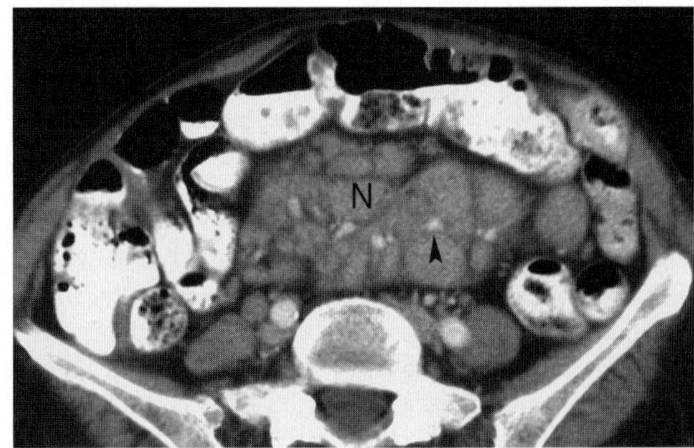

FIGURE 31.8. **Sandwich Sign: Mesenteric Lymphoma.** CT demonstrates confluent masses of enlarged lymph nodes (N) in the small mesentery producing the "sandwich sign" by engulfing mesenteric blood vessels (*arrowhead*).

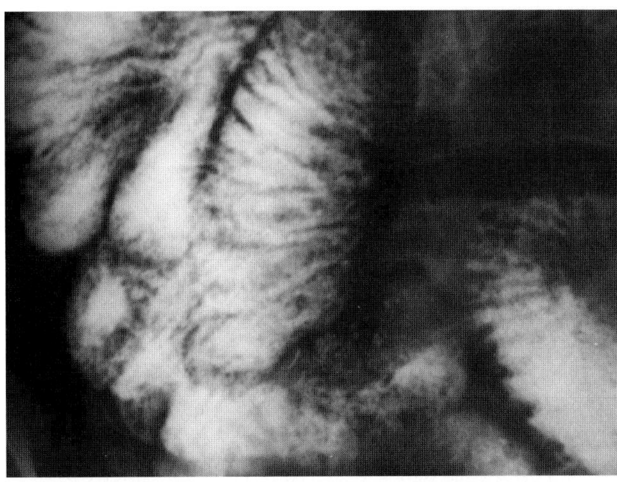

FIGURE 31.9. **Nodular Lymphoid Hyperplasia.** Numerous tiny nodules cause tiny filling defects that distort the regular fold pattern of the small bowel on this radiograph from a small bowel follow-through examination.

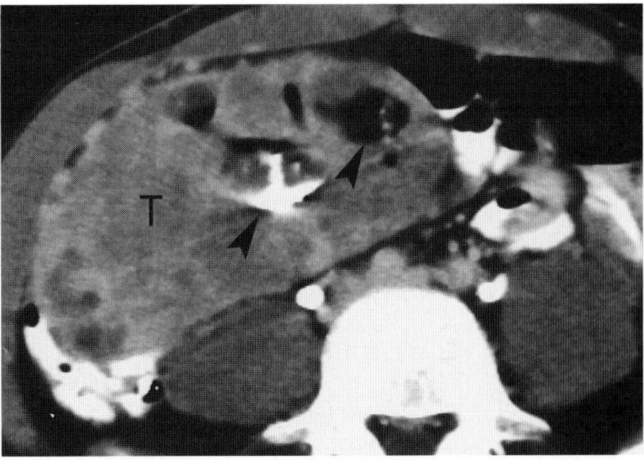

FIGURE 31.10. **Malignant GI Stromal Tumor of the Ileum.** Contrast-enhanced CT reveals a large heterogeneous tumor (T) that envelops loops of ileum (*arrowheads*). Areas of low attenuation within the tumor represent hemorrhage, necrosis, and cystic change.

favored by the flow of fluid along the small bowel mesentery, from the left upper to the right lower abdomen. Implantation is most common along the terminal ileum, cecum, and ascending colon. Peritoneal implants on the parietal peritoneum and omentum (omental cake), as well as in the pouch of Douglas, are demonstrated by CT. Barium studies demonstrate nodules and tethering of folds caused by mesenteric fibrosis. Hematogenous metastases are deposited along the antimesenteric border where the submucosal blood vessels arborize. Common primary malignancies are melanoma; lung, breast, and colon carcinoma; and embryonal cell carcinoma of the testes. Barium studies demonstrate mural nodules of uniform or varying size anywhere in the small bowel. They may appear as target lesions, or they may ulcerate or cavitate. Direct extension to involve the small bowel is seen with malignancies of the pancreas and colon.

Kaposi sarcoma in AIDS patients commonly involves the small intestine. About half of patients with skin lesions have intestinal lesions as well. Barium studies demonstrate multiple mural nodules, which are often centrally umbilicated. CT demonstrates mesenteric, retroperitoneal, and pelvic adenopathy.

Gastrointestinal Stromal Tumors. As in the stomach, most tumors that were previously classified as leiomyomas and leiomyosarcomas are now classified as GISTs (8). Approximately 20% to 30% of GISTs arise throughout the small intestine, and they tend to be more aggressive than gastric tumors of the same size (9). Tumors present with obstruction or intestinal bleeding. Barium studies show a well-defined submucosal mass with smooth mucosa. Tumors that exceed 2 cm tend to ulcerate whether they are benign or malignant. On CT, benign GISTs are homogeneous, with attenuation similar to muscle. Malignant GISTs tend to be larger (>5 cm) and heterogeneous, with prominent areas of low-attenuation necrosis and hemorrhage (Fig. 31.10). Nodal metastases are uncommon. Calcifications are infrequent. MR shows the solid portions of the lesions to be low signal on T1WIs and high signal on T2WIs. Solid areas show distinct contrast enhancement. Hemorrhage shows characteristic MR signal dependent on its age.

Adenoma accounts for about 20% of benign small bowel neoplasms. It is more common in the duodenum than in the mesenteric small intestine. The tumor is a benign proliferation of glandular epithelium and has the potential for malignant degeneration. Barium studies demonstrate an intraluminal polyp with a finely lobulated surface.

Lipoma is most common in the ileum (10). The tumor arises from the fat of the submucosa. Lipomas account for about 17% of benign small bowel tumors. Most are asymptomatic incidental findings, although some may cause bleeding or intussusception. CT demonstration of a fat-density (-50 to -100 H) tumor is diagnostic (Fig. 31.11).

Hemangioma is usually solitary and submucosal, projecting into the lumen as a polyp. These tumors are located predominantly in the jejunum. About two thirds present with bleeding. Barium studies demonstrate a small polyp. The occasional presence of a calcified phlebolith suggests the diagnosis. They account for fewer than 10% of benign small bowel tumors.

Polyposis syndromes cause multiple polypoid lesions of the small bowel. The differential diagnosis includes metastases, lymphoma, nodular lymphoid hyperplasia, Kaposi sarcoma, and carcinoid tumors.

Peutz-Jeghers syndrome is an autosomal-dominant inherited condition consisting of multiple hamartomatous

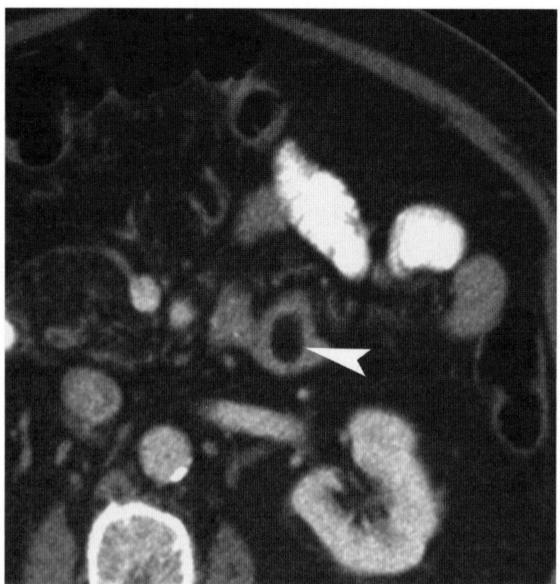

FIGURE 31.11. **Small Bowel Lipoma.** A fat-density mass (*arrowhead*) within a loop of proximal ileum was the cause of partial small bowel obstruction. CT demonstration of a mass of pure fat density is diagnostic of lipoma.

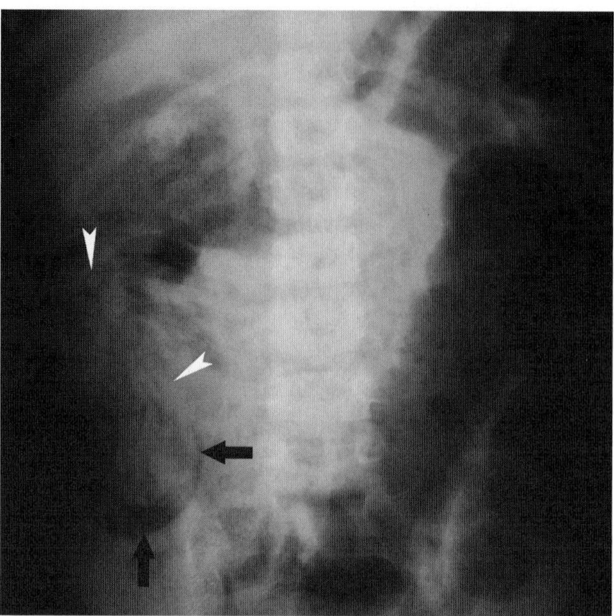

FIGURE 31.12. **Ascaris Infestation.** Plain radiograph demonstrates diffuse intestinal dilation. Roundworms in the ileum are seen as round and tubular soft tissue densities outlined by intestinal gas (*white arrowheads*). A large bolus of entangled worms (*black arrows*) plugged the distal ileum, causing small bowel obstruction.

polyps in the small intestine (most common), colon, and stomach associated with melanin freckles on the facial skin, palmar aspects of the fingers and toes, and mucous membranes (11). Hamartomatous polyps are a nonneoplastic, abnormal proliferation of all three layers of the mucosa, epithelium, lamina propria, and muscularis mucosae. The polyps are most common in the jejunum, are usually pedunculated, and are variable in size up to 4 cm. Patients are at increased risk for intussusception, GI tract adenocarcinoma, and extraintestinal malignancy (breast, pancreas, ovary). Barium studies demonstrate myriad polyps in involved areas of small intestine, separated by normal bowel segments.

Cronkhite-Canada syndrome involves the small bowel in about half of cases with multiple inflammatory polyps. The colon and stomach are always involved.

Gardner syndrome of inherited adenomatous polyposis coil usually includes a few adenomatous polyps in the small bowel.

Juvenile GI polyposis is most common in the colon but occasionally involves the small bowel. Inflammatory polyps containing cysts filled with mucin develop secondary to chronic irritation. Most are round, smooth, and pedunculated.

Ascariasis is caused by infestation with the roundworm *Ascaris lumbricoides.* Ascariasis is found worldwide but is most common in Asia and Africa. Endemic areas in the United States include rural southern Appalachia and the Gulf Coast states. Infestation is acquired by ingesting food or water contaminated with *Ascaris* eggs. The eggs hatch in the small bowel. Larvae penetrate the wall and migrate through the vascular system to the lungs, where they molt and grow before migrating up the bronchi and trachea to the larynx, where they are again swallowed. Worms mature in the small bowel, especially in the jejunum, and may reach 15 to 35 cm in size. New generations of infective ova are excreted in feces. A large bolus of worms may obstruct the small bowel, especially in children, or cause intussusception. Worms can be identified on plain abdominal radiographs in 70% of cases (Fig. 31.12). Barium studies demonstrate worms as long linear filling defects. Barium ingested by the worms may be seen in their intestinal tracts as long, stringlike white lines.

Mesenteric Masses

Masses arising in the small bowel mesentery frequently present as a palpable abdominal mass (12). The mesenteric fat may be infiltrated by edema, hemorrhage, or inflammatory cells. The disorders may be diseases of the small intestine or be primary to the mesentery itself. CT, US, and MR provide the most diagnostic information.

Lymphoma causing bulky adenopathy is the most common solid mesenteric mass. Confluent adenopathy surrounds mesenteric vessels and fat, producing the "sandwich sign" (Fig. 31.8). Adenopathy is commonly present in the retroperitoneum and elsewhere.

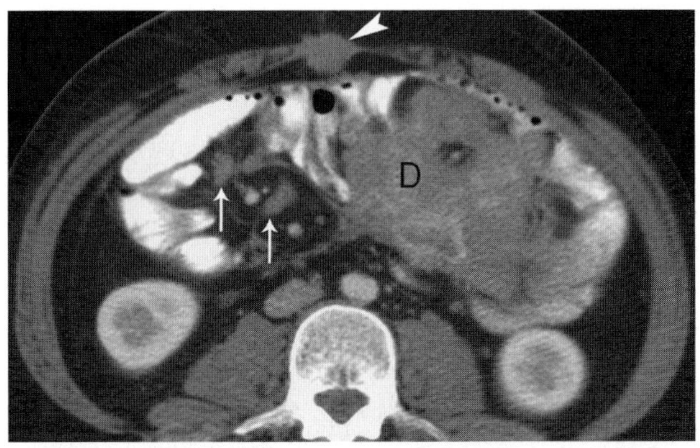

FIGURE 31.13. **Mesenteric Desmoid.** Multiple desmoid tumors are evident on this CT image. A large desmoid (D) infiltrates the mesentery, displacing bowel loops. Two smaller desmoid tumors (*arrows*) appear as soft tissue nodules within the mesentery. Another desmoid tumor (*arrowhead*) expands the linea alba in the midline of the anterior abdominal wall.

Metastases may implant in the mesentery and produce a large mesenteric mass without impingement of the bowel lumen, or they may implant adjacent to bowel, narrowing the bowel lumen. Carcinoid and small bowel adenocarcinoma metastases produce a prominent desmoplastic reaction in the mesentery, whereas melanoma produces no mesenteric retraction.

Mesenteric desmoid tumors are benign but locally aggressive, solid, fibrous, mesenteric tumors (13). They may be solitary (28%) or multiple (72%) and associated with Gardner syndrome. These tumors commonly recur after surgical resection. US and CT demonstrate a homogeneous solid mass with well-defined (68%) or infiltrative borders (Fig. 31.13). Attenuation is similar to that of muscle. Tumors commonly also occur within the muscles of the anterior abdominal wall or in the psoas muscles.

GISTs may arise primarily in the mesentery or omentum or may be found as metastases from tumors arising elsewhere. On CT, tumors appear as large, well-defined masses with prominent areas of low density representing hemorrhage and necrosis (14).

Mesenteric cysts are lymphangiomas that arise in the root of the small bowel mesentery. Most are thin walled and multiloculated with internal fluid that may be chylous, serous, or bloody. US demonstrates a well-defined cyst with internal debris, along with fluid–debris or fluid–fat levels. CT shows a cystic mass displacing loops of small bowel anteriorly and laterally. On MR, cyst contents are hyperintense on T2WIs and hypointense on T1WIs when serous, or hyperintense on T1WIs when chylous or hemorrhagic.

GI duplication cyst is a congenital, either partial or complete, replica of the small bowel. Most arise from the distal small bowel and may communicate with the normal intestinal lumen at one or both ends, or not at all. They are lined by intestinal epithelium. US, CT, and MR reveal a thick-walled cyst, usually with serous contents. Malignancies (adenocarcinoma) may arise within duplication cysts.

Mesenteric teratoma is heterogeneous with cystic and solid components. Demonstration of calcium or fat is a clue to radiographic diagnosis.

Sclerosing mesenteritis is an uncommon inflammatory condition affecting the root of the mesentery, with variable inflammation, fat necrosis, and fibrosis. CT shows soft tissue infiltration of the mesentery, so-called "misty mesentery." The cause is unknown. Patients commonly present with abdominal pain.

Diffuse Small Bowel Disease

Students of radiology dread learning about diseases of the small bowel, because they are numerous, obscure, and confusing and lead to long lists of differential diagnoses (see Tables 31.3 to 31.5). A few common diseases cause the majority of small bowel abnormalities that most radiologists will encounter in routine practice (1). The rest of the list must be known to pass board examinations. Five rules, learned well, help to simplify the problem:

Rule #1. Dilatation of the small bowel lumen indicates small bowel obstruction or dysfunction of small bowel muscle.

Rule #2. Thickening of small bowel folds indicates infiltration of the submucosa.

Rule #3. Uniform, regular, straight thickening indicates infiltration by fluid (edema or blood).

Rule #4. Irregular, distorted, nodular thickening indicates infiltration by cells or other nonfluid material.

Rule #5. The specific diagnosis requires matching the small bowel pattern with the clinical data.

The normal values for small bowel luminal diameter and fold anatomy are given in Table 31.2.

Dilated Small Bowel Lumen (Table 31.3). The hallmark of mechanical bowel obstruction is a point of transition between dilated bowel and nondilated bowel at the site

TABLE 31.2 Normal Small Bowel Measurements

	Normal Values	
Feature	***Jejunum***	***Ileum***
Diameter of lumen	3.0 cm	2.5 cm
Diameter of lumen during enteroclysis	4.5 cm	3.5 cm
Thickness of folds	2 mm	2 mm
No. of folds	4 to 7 per inch	2 to 4 per inch
Depth of folds	8 mm	8 mm
Thickness of bowel wall	3 mm	3 mm

TABLE 31.3 Causes of Dilated Small Bowel (>3 cm)

Obstruction (transition zone between dilated and nondilated bowel)
- Adhesions (75% of small bowel obstruction)
  - Postsurgical
  - Postperitonitis
- Incarcerated hernia
- Volvulus
- Extrinsic tumor
- Congenital stenosis
- Intraluminal lesion
  - Tumor: usually malignant
  - Intussusception
  - Foreign body
  - Gallstone ileus
  - Bezoar
  - Ascaris (bolus of worms)
  - Meconium

Muscle dysfunction (no transition zone)
- Adynamic ileus
  - Surgery
  - Trauma
  - Peritoneal inflammation
  - Ischemia
  - Drugs
    - Opiates
    - Barbiturates
    - Anticholinergics
  - Vagotomy
  - Diabetic neuropathy
  - Metabolic disorders
    - Electrolyte imbalance
- Collagen diseases
  - Scleroderma
  - Dermatomyositis
- Malabsorption syndromes
  - Celiac disease
- Chronic idiopathic pseudoobstruction

of obstruction. With muscle dysfunction, the small bowel dilatation is diffuse, with no transition point. If no coexisting mucosal disease is present, the small bowel folds are straight and regular (Fig. 31.14). See Chapter 26 for an expanded discussion of this topic.

Thickened Folds: Straight and Regular (Table 31.4). Infiltration of edema fluid or hemorrhage into the submucosa results in uniform, straight thickening of the folds (Fig. 31.15). Hemorrhage usually causes thicker folds than edema and may result in scalloping or "thumbprinting" of some folds.

Thickened Folds: Irregular and Distorted (Table 31.5). This is the most difficult category of abnormality because many conditions are unusual. The distribution of fold abnormality helps to limit the differential diagnosis (Fig. 31.16).

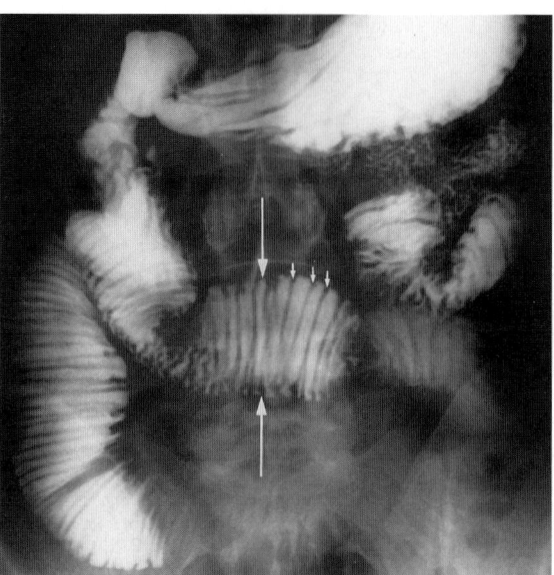

FIGURE 31.14. **Dilated Small Bowel, Normal Folds.** Small bowel follow-through examination reveals dilation of the small bowel lumen (>5 cm between *large arrows*) with normal thickness of well-defined folds (*small arrows*). The reason was small bowel obstruction caused by adhesions.

Some conditions are included in several categories. Early Crohn disease is characterized by edema and regular folds. More advanced Crohn disease has inflammatory cell infiltrate and irregular folds. Lymphoma in the mesentery obstructs lymphatics and causes edema, and lymphoma in the bowel wall causes nodular, irregular folds. Lymphoma and Crohn disease are the two most commonly encountered small bowel diseases.

Scleroderma produces atrophy of the muscularis of the small bowel by the process of progressive collagen deposition, resulting in flaccid, atonic, dilated bowel. The valvulae conniventes are normal or thinned (Fig. 31.17). A "hide-bound" appearance of thinned folds tethered together is produced by contraction of the longitudinal muscle layer to a greater extent than the circular muscle layer. Excessive contraction of the mesenteric border of the small bowel results in formation of mucosal sacculations along the antimesenteric border. The jejunum and duodenum are more severely involved than the ileum. The diagnosis is confirmed by skin changes and characteristic involvement of the esophagus. Malabsorption eventually occurs.

Adult celiac disease (nontropical sprue) presents with malabsorption, steatorrhea, and weight loss. Gluten, an insoluble protein found in wheat, rye, oats, and barley, acts as a toxic agent to the small bowel mucosa. The mucosa becomes flattened and absorptive cells decrease in number; villi disappear. The submucosa, muscularis, and serosa remain normal. Patients with long-term sprue have an increased risk of lymphoma and GI carcinoma. The

TABLE 31.4 Thickened Small Bowel Folds: Straight and Regular

Intestinal edema (diffuse)
- Hypoproteinemia
- Congestive heart failure
- Portal hypertension
- Lymphatic obstruction
  - Tumor infiltration (lymphoma)
  - Radiation
  - Fibrosis of the mesentery
  - Lymphangiectasis
- Zollinger-Ellison syndrome
- Lactase deficiency

Intestinal edema (short segment)
- Crohn disease
- Eosinophilic gastroenteritis

Hemorrhage into bowel wall (long segment)
- Trauma
- Ischemia
- Anticoagulant therapy
- Bleeding disorders
- Vasculitis
  - Henoch-Schönlein syndrome
  - Connective tissue disease
  - Radiation
  - Thromboangiitis obliterans

Stomach and small bowel involved
- Ménétrier disease
- Zollinger-Ellison syndrome
- Crohn disease
- Lymphoma
- Eosinophilic gastroenteritis

Implies submucosal infiltration by fluid.

classic radiographic findings are as follows: (*1*) dilated small bowel (Fig. 31.18), (*2*) normal or thinned folds, (*3*) a decreased number of folds per inch in the jejunum, and (*4*) an increased number of folds per inch in the ileum ($\geq$5). Findings are best demonstrated by enteroclysis. Detection of five or more folds per inch in the jejunum makes the diagnosis unlikely. Fluid excess is often evident in the ileum. Transient intussusceptions may be observed. Typical CT findings are distal small bowel dilatation, dilution of intraluminal contrast by high intraluminal fluid content, and enlarged lymph nodes in the mesentery (15).

Tropical sprue has similar clinical and radiographic findings as nontropical sprue but is confined to East Asia and Puerto Rico. The disease responds to administration of folate and antibiotics.

Lactase Deficiency. Lactase is required within the absorptive cells of the jejunum to properly digest disaccharides. Several population groups, including Chinese, Arabs, Bantu, and Eskimos, may become totally deficient in lactase during adult life. Secondary lactase deficiency may develop with alcoholism, Crohn disease, and use of drugs such as neomycin. The nondigested lactose in the

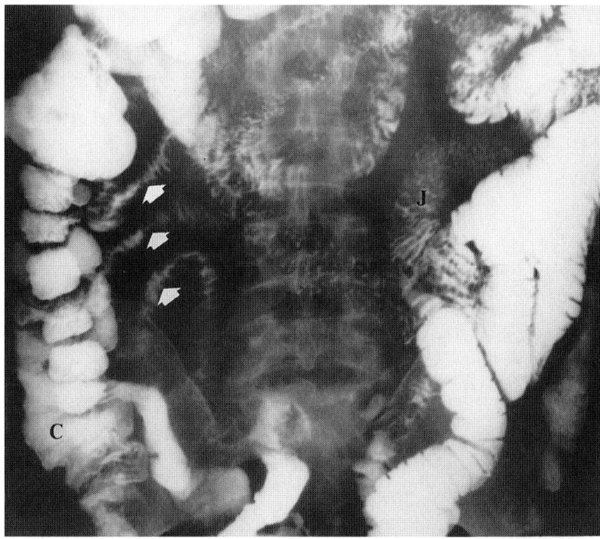

FIGURE 31.15. **Thickened Folds, Regular: Intestinal Ischemia.** Barium examination demonstrates a striking separation of multiple loops of ileum (*arrows*), indicating thickening of the bowel walls. The folds in involved loops are thickened and nodular because of edema and hemorrhage resulting from ischemia. A repeat study 1 month later documented complete resolution of all findings. C, colon; J, jejunum.

TABLE 31.5 Thickened Small Bowel Folds: Irregular and Distorted

Proximal (predominantly duodenum + jejunum)
- Giardiasis
- Strongyloides
- Whipple disease
- Eosinophilic gastroenteritis
- Zollinger-Ellison syndrome

Distal (predominantly ileum)
- Lymphoma
- Crohn disease
- *Yersinia/Campylobacter*
- *Salmonella*
- Tuberculosis
- Behçet disease
- Cystic fibrosis
- AIDS-related infections

Diffuse
- Lymphoma
- Polyposis syndromes
- Amyloidosis
- Histoplasmosis
- Systemic mastocytosis
- Waldenström macroglobulinemia
- Lymphoma

Stomach and small bowel involved
- Lymphoma
- Crohn disease
- Eosinophilic gastroenteritis
- Whipple disease
- Tuberculosis
- Mastocytosis

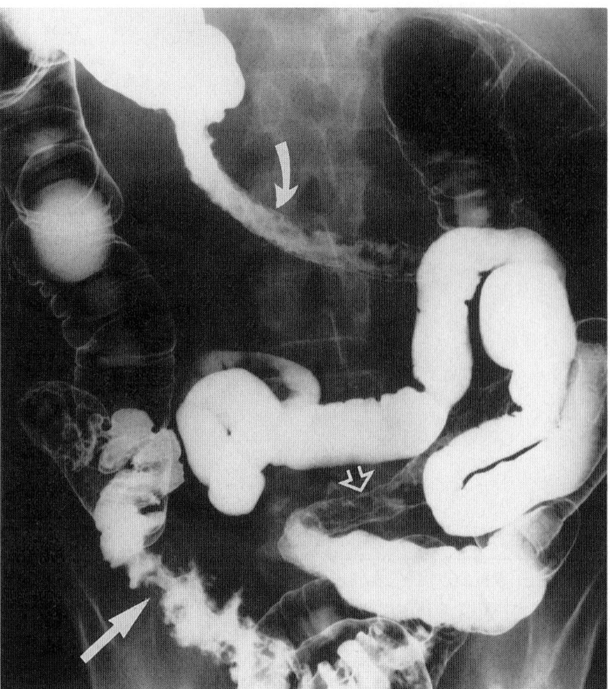

FIGURE 31.16. **Thickened Folds, Irregular: Crohn Disease.** Crohn disease of the ileum causes thickened folds (*straight arrow*) that are irregular and distorted. A more proximal segment of jejunum (*open arrow*) is effaced and narrowed. The transverse colon (*curved arrow*) is narrowed and stiffened and has multiple inflammatory polyps producing filling defects. This is an excellent example of the "skip lesions" that are characteristic of Crohn disease.

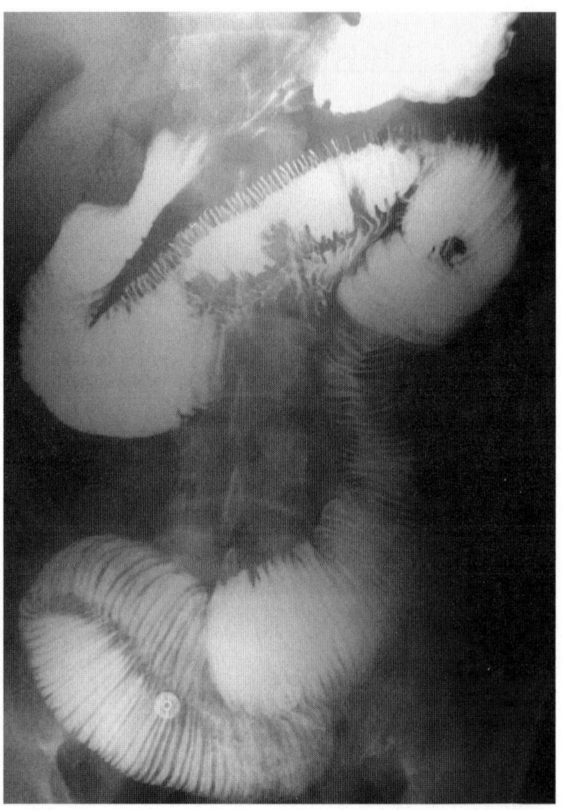

FIGURE 31.17. **Scleroderma.** Radiograph from a small bowel follow-through examination demonstrates dilatation of the jejunum with thin normal folds, an appearance commonly seen with scleroderma. Luminal dilatation is caused by smooth muscle dysfunction in the bowel wall.

small bowel causes increased intraluminal fluid and dilated small bowel with normal folds.

Intestinal ischemia may result from embolism or thrombosis of the superior mesenteric artery or vein (16). Patients may present with acute abdomen or vague symptoms. Arterial occlusion may be caused by embolus, vasculitis, trauma, or adhesions. Venous thrombosis results from hypercoagulability states (neoplasms, oral contraceptives); inflammation (pancreatitis, peritonitis, abscess); or stasis (portal hypertension, congestive heart failure). Plain films demonstrate gaseous distention, thickened mucosal folds ("thumbprinting") (Fig. 31.15), and, in some cases, intramural or portal venous gas. CT is preferred to barium studies to demonstrate characteristic abnormalities: dilated lumen, thickened bowel wall (Fig. 31.19), absent or poor enhancement of the bowel wall, engorged mesenteric vessels, thrombus in the mesenteric arteries or veins, and intramural or venous gas (17).

Radiation enteritis occurs when large doses of radiation are given to adjacent organs. The small bowel is the most radiosensitive organ in the abdomen. Long segments of bowel may be involved, with thickening of folds and bowel wall. Peristalsis is impaired. Progressive fibrosis leads to tapered strictures, commonly involving long segments. The bowel may be kinked and obstructed by adhesions. Fistulas to the vagina or other organs may also result. CT demonstrates wall thickening and increased density of the mesentery, along with fixation of bowel loops (Fig. 31.20).

Lymphangiectasia refers to gross dilation of the lymphatic vessels in the small bowel mucosa and submucosa. The primary form is a congenital lymphatic blockage, which is often associated with asymmetric edema of the extremities. Despite being congenital, symptoms often do not occur until young adulthood. Patients present with protein-losing enteropathy, diarrhea, steatorrhea, and recurrent infection. Secondary lymphangiectasia refers to lymphatic obstruction caused by radiation, congestive heart failure, or mesenteric node involvement by malignancy or inflammation. The diagnosis is confirmed by jejunal biopsy. Barium study findings include diffuse fold thickening that is most pronounced in the jejunum, increased intraluminal fluid, and groups of tiny (1-mm) nodules owing to distended villi. The pattern closely resembles Whipple disease. CT helps the differentiation by revealing thickening of the bowel wall and mesenteric adenopathy in secondary lymphangiectasia.

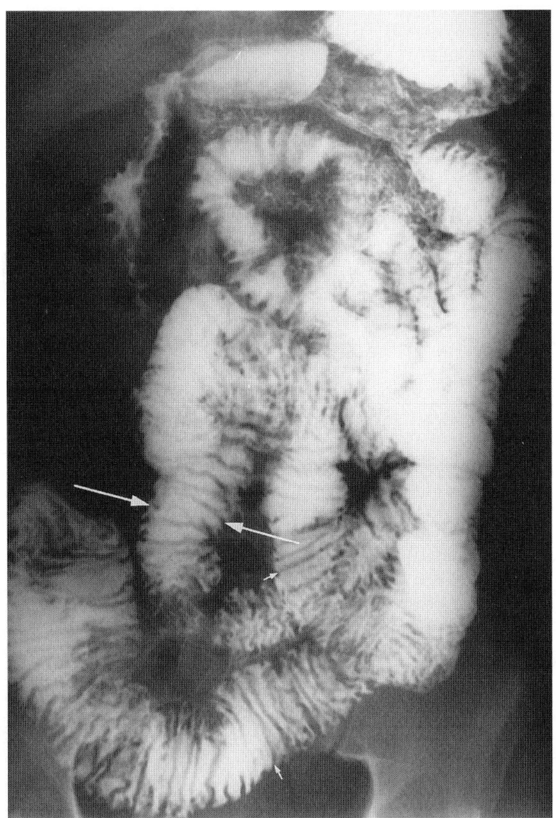

FIGURE 31.18. **Adult Celiac Disease.** Small bowel follow-through examination demonstrates dilation of the lumen of the small bowel (4 cm between *long arrows*). The folds are of normal thickness (*small arrows*), ie, less than 3 mm. This patient with malabsorption became asymptomatic on a gluten-free diet.

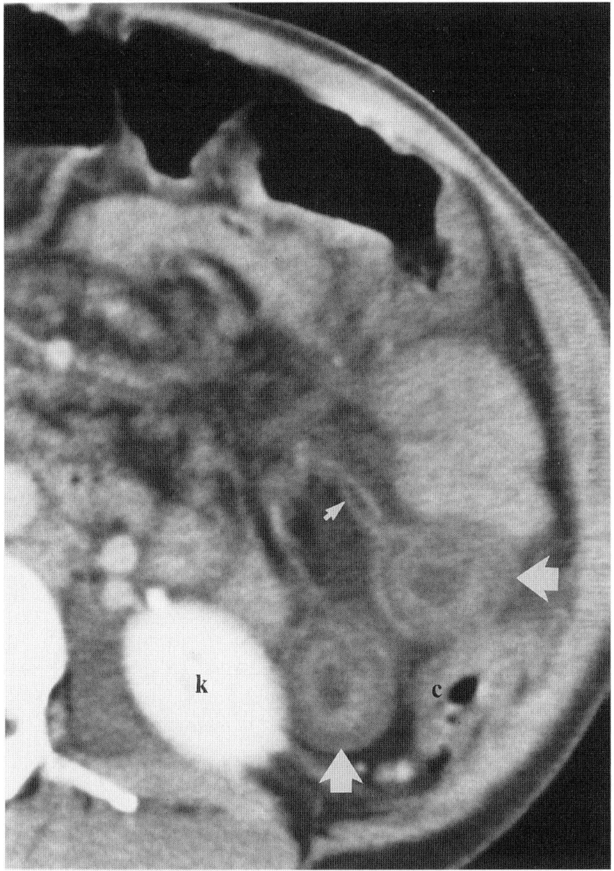

FIGURE 31.19. **Intestinal Ischemia.** CT demonstrates circumferential thickening of small bowel loops (*large arrows*) caused by intestinal ischemia owing to portal vein thrombosis. A characteristic, benign, "target" appearance of bowel wall thickening is evident. The mesentery is edematous and congested (*small arrow*). c, descending colon; k, kidney.

Eosinophilic gastroenteritis virtually always affects the gastric antrum as well as all or part of the small bowel. Intense infiltration of eosinophils in the lamina propria causes thickening of the bowel wall and mucosal folds, often with luminal narrowing. Barium studies show thickened and straightened folds. Thickening of the bowel wall is evidenced by wide separation between bowel loops. CT shows thickened distorted folds in the distal stomach and proximal small bowel (15). Most patients have a history of allergic disorders. The disease is self-limited, but recurrences are frequent.

Amyloidosis is a disease complex associated with extracellular infiltration of an amorphous protein material in body tissues. The disease may be primary or associated with multiple myeloma (10% to 15%), rheumatoid arthritis (20% to 25%), or tuberculosis (50%). Most cases are systemic, but 10% to 20% are localized. The small bowel is the most common site of GI involvement. Amyloid deposits are seen throughout the wall of the small bowel, especially within the walls of small blood vessels, resulting in ischemia and infarction. Deposits in the muscularis impair motility. Diffuse, irregular thickened folds may be seen throughout the small bowel. Nodules are sometimes present. CT demonstrates symmetric wall thickening of affected bowel without luminal dilatation or hypersecretion (15). Small mesenteric lymph nodes may be evident. Diagnosis is confirmed by biopsy.

Systemic mastocytosis is a proliferation of mast cells in the skin, bones, lymph nodes, and GI tract. Urticaria pigmentosa is the characteristic skin manifestation. Osteoblastic bone changes are found in 70% of cases. Lymphadenopathy and hepatosplenomegaly are often present. The bowel wall and mucosal folds are thickened, and mucosal nodules up to 5 mm are often evident (Table 31.6).

Whipple disease is an uncommon systemic disorder affecting the GI tract, joints, CNS, and lymph nodes. The disease is caused by Whipple bacilli—gram-positive, rod-shaped bacteria that are found within macrophages in many organs and tissues. Patients may present with arthritis, neurologic symptoms, or steatorrhea. Generalized lymphadenopathy is usually present. Enteroclysis

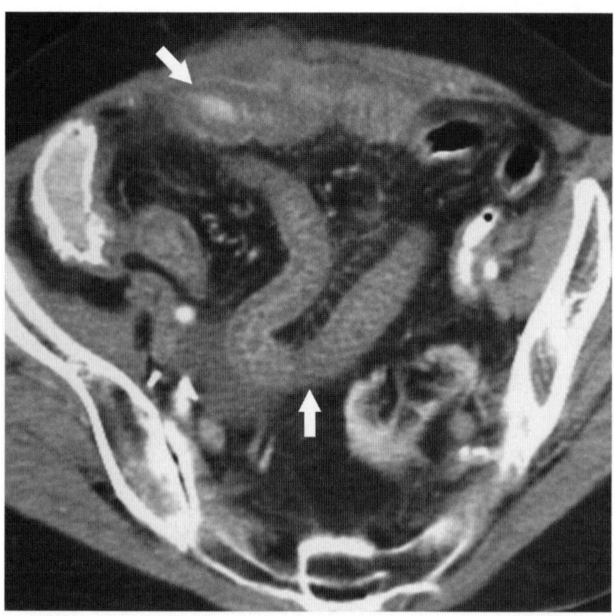

FIGURE 31.20. **Radiation Enteritis.** CT image through the pelvis in a patient with cervical carcinoma treated with radiation reveals long segments of small bowel (*arrows*) with wall thickening and infiltrated mesentery.

demonstrates irregularly thickened folds that are most prominent in the jejunum. Demonstration of tiny (1-mm) sandlike nodules spread diffusely over the mucosa or in small groups is strong evidence of the disease. Increased luminal fluid is usual. CT reveals thick folds, especially in the jejunum, without significant dilatation. Low-density or fat-density nodes in the mesentery are characteristic (15).

AIDS Enteritis. In addition to lymphoma and Kaposi sarcoma, AIDS patients are predisposed to multiple opportunistic infections of the GI tract. Infective agents usually occur in combination and in multiple GI sites.

Cryptosporidium and *Isospora belli* are protozoans that may infest the proximal intestine and cause a cholera-like diarrhea, with life-threatening fluid loss. Barium studies show thickened folds and marked increased fluid.

Cytomegalovirus causes disease in the small bowel and colon as well as the lungs, liver, and spleen. Mucosal ulceration with bleeding and perforation are the major intestinal manifestations. Barium studies show thickened folds, loop separation, ulcers, and fistulae.

Mycobacterium avium-intracellulare is a common systemic infection in AIDS involving lung, liver, spleen, bone marrow, lymph nodes, and the intestinal tract. Barium studies show thickened, nodular folds with a sandlike mucosal pattern. CT demonstrates retroperitoneal and mesenteric adenopathy and focal lesions in the liver and spleen.

Candida, Amoeba histolytica, Giardia, Strongyloides, herpes simplex, and *Campylobacter* may also occur in AIDS patients.

TABLE 31.6 Tiny Small Bowel Nodules

Nodular lymphoid hyperplasia (2–4 mm)
Lymphoma (>4 mm)
Amyloidosis
Whipple disease (1–2 mm)
Mycobacterium avium-intracellulare
Lymphangiectasia
Systemic mastocytosis (<5 mm)

Small Bowel Erosions and Ulcerations

Crohn disease is an inflammatory disease of uncertain etiology that may involve the GI tract from the esophagus to the anus. The disease is characterized by erosions, ulcerations, full-thickness bowel wall inflammation, and formation of noncaseating granulomas. Patients present, usually in their 20s and 30s, with diarrhea, abdominal pain, weight loss, and often fever. The typical course is one of remissions, relapse, and progression of disease. Patterns of GI involvement include colon and terminal ileum (55%), small bowel alone (30%), colon alone (15%), and proximal small bowel without terminal ileum (3%). Radiographic hallmarks of Crohn disease are: (*1*) aphthous erosions (see Fig. 30.12); (*2*) confluent deep ulcerations; (*3*) thickened and distorted folds (Fig. 31.16); (*4*) fibrosis with thickened walls, contractures, and stenosis; (*5*) involvement of the mesentery; (*6*) asymmetric involvement, both longitudinally and around the lumen; (*7*) skip areas of normal intervening bowel between diseased segments (Fig. 31.16); and (*8*) fistula and sinus tract formation. Aphthous ulcers are shallow, 1- to 2-mm depressions usually surrounded by a well-defined halo. Deep ulcerations are larger and often linear, forming fissures between nodules of elevated edematous mucosa ("cobblestone pattern") (Fig. 31.21). Fibrosis and progressive thickening of the bowel wall narrows the lumen, particularly of the terminal ileum, producing the "string sign" (Figs. 31.22, 31.23). Mesenteric involvement is best demonstrated by CT. Ulceration along the mesenteric border may extend between the leaves of the mesentery. The mesenteric fat is infiltrated; the mesentery is thickened and retracted.

Complications of Crohn disease are common and well shown by CT and MR (18). Obstruction is usually partial and caused by strictures or areas of severe ulceration and spasm. Fistulae are formed in 19% of patients with small bowel disease. Fistulae are abnormal communications between two epithelial-lined organs. Most frequent are ileocolonic and ileocecal, but enterocutaneous, enterovesical, and colovesical fistulae are also common. Sinus tracts extend into inflammatory extraluminal masses from the bowel lumen (Fig. 31.22). Abscess and phlegmon formation in the mesentery, peritoneal cavity,

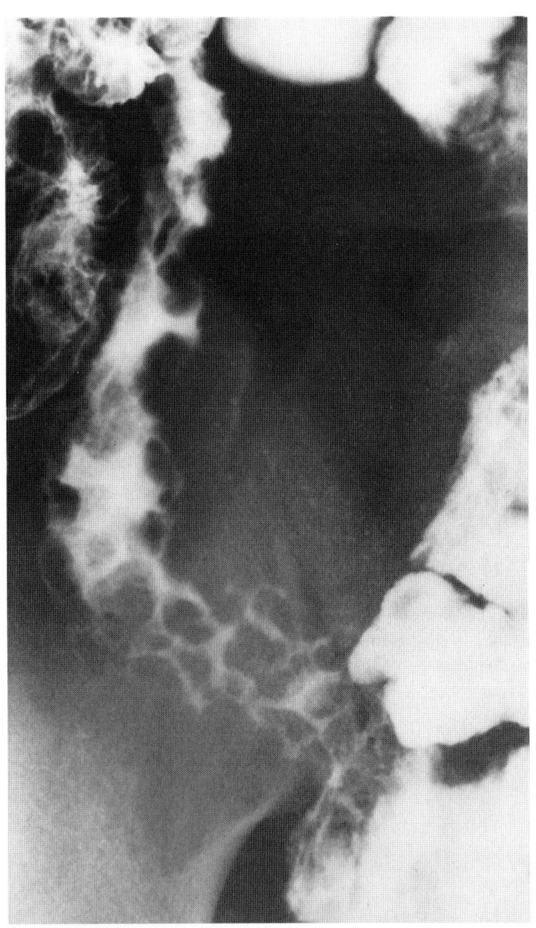

FIGURE 31.21. **Crohn Disease: Cobblestone Pattern.** Cone-down view of the terminal ileum reveals a cobblestone pattern of ulcerations and fissures between mounds of unaffected mucosa.

retroperitoneum, and abdominal wall are common. Free perforation occurs in 3% of cases. Most perforations are confined and form sinus tracts or fistulae. Carcinomas of the small and large bowel are increased in frequency, with a prevalence of about 0.5% in Crohn disease patients. Derangements of intestinal absorption cause megaloblastic anemia (vitamin B_{12} deficiency) and an increased incidence of gallstones and renal stones. Up to 20% of patients have arthritis or spondylitis that mimics ankylosing spondylitis.

Yersinia enterocolitis is caused by infection with the gram-positive bacilli *Yersinia enterocolitica* or *Y pseudotuberculosis*. Infection causes an acute enteritis with abdominal pain, fever, and often bloody diarrhea that mimics acute appendicitis or acute Crohn disease. Children and young adults are most often affected. The infection runs a self-limited course of 8 to 12 weeks. Diagnosis is confirmed by stool culture. Radiographic findings are most pronounced in the last 20 cm of the ileum. They include aphthous ulcers, nodules up to 1 cm, wall thickening, and thickened folds that become effaced with increasing edema. Nodular lymphoid hyperplasia may appear during the resolution stage.

Campylobacter fetus jejuni infection is clinically and radiographically similar to *Yersinia* enterocolitis. The disease usually lasts 1 to 2 weeks, but relapses are common. Diagnosis is by stool culture.

Behçet disease is a multisystem disease caused by a small vessel vasculitis that affects eyes, joints, skin, CNS, and the intestinal tract (19). Prominent clinical features include relapsing iridocyclitis, mucocutaneous ulcerations, vesicles, pustules, and mild arthritis. Intestinal disease most commonly involves the ileocecal region, where Crohn

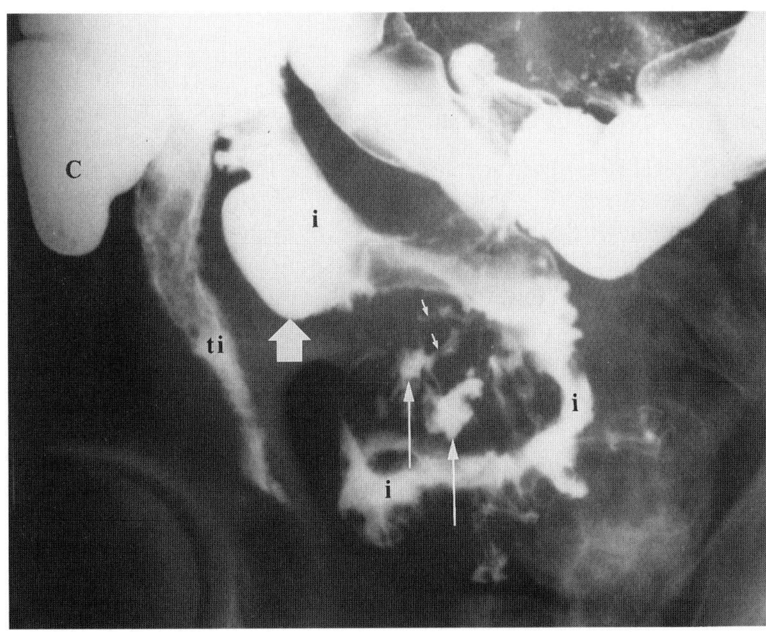

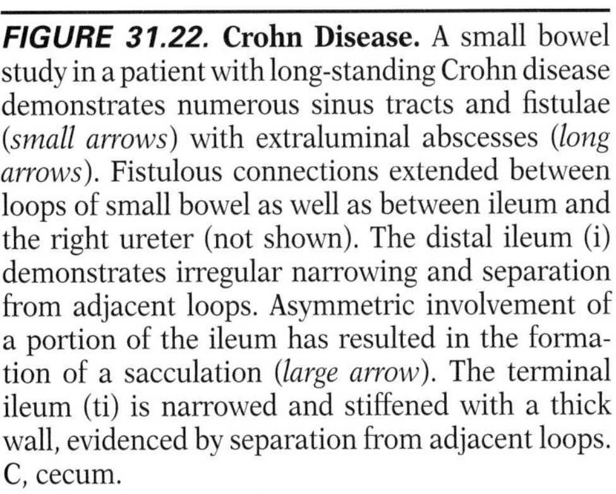
FIGURE 31.22. **Crohn Disease.** A small bowel study in a patient with long-standing Crohn disease demonstrates numerous sinus tracts and fistulae (*small arrows*) with extraluminal abscesses (*long arrows*). Fistulous connections extended between loops of small bowel as well as between ileum and the right ureter (not shown). The distal ileum (i) demonstrates irregular narrowing and separation from adjacent loops. Asymmetric involvement of a portion of the ileum has resulted in the formation of a sacculation (*large arrow*). The terminal ileum (ti) is narrowed and stiffened with a thick wall, evidenced by separation from adjacent loops. C, cecum.

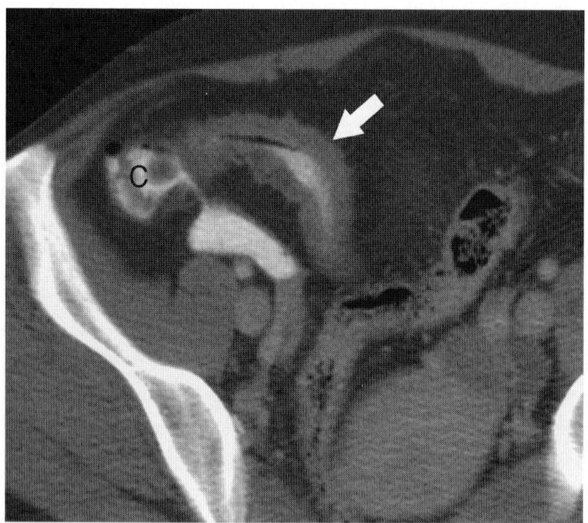

FIGURE 31.23. Crohn Disease: Terminal Ileitis. CT of the right lower quadrant shows the circumferential wall thickening of the terminal ileum (*arrow*) that narrows the lumen, producing the "string sign" seen on barium studies. C, cecum.

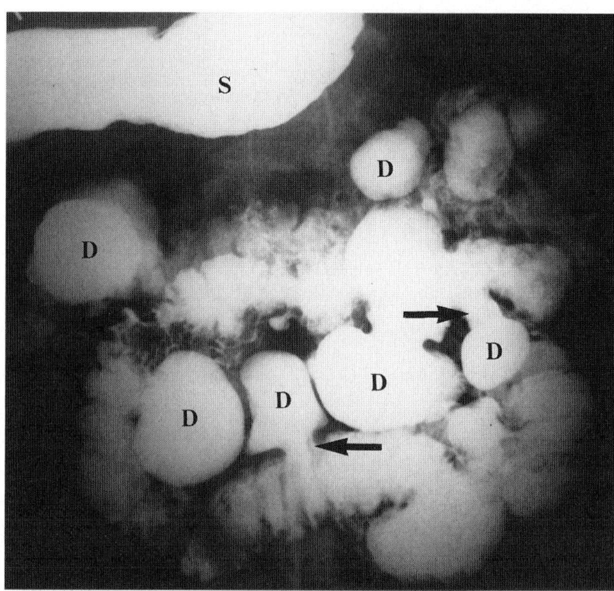

FIGURE 31.24. Small Bowel Diverticula. A small bowel series demonstrates numerous diverticula (D) extending from the duodenum and jejunum. The necks (*arrows*) of several diverticula are shown particularly well. S, stomach.

disease is closely mimicked with aphthous erosions, deep ulceration, stenosis, and fistula formation. Complications include bowel perforation and peritonitis.

Tuberculosis presents as peritonitis or focal infection of the gut, most commonly involving the ileocecal area, closely mimicking Crohn disease. Fewer than half of patients have concurrent evidence of pulmonary tuberculosis. Barium studies demonstrate inflamed mucosa with transverse and stellate ulcers. The affected bowel becomes rigid and narrowed, with nodular mucosa. The ileocecal valve is stiff and gaping with narrowed terminal ileum and cecum. CT shows characteristic findings of mesenteric adenopathy, high-density ascites, and peritoneal thickening accompanying the bowel wall thickening.

Small Bowel Diverticula

Small bowel diverticula are most common in the jejunum along the mesenteric border. They are outpouchings of mucosa through the bowel wall and between the leaves of the mesentery. They are commonly multiple and often asymptomatic. However, because of stasis of bowel contents within them, bacterial overgrowth may occur, resulting in deconjugation of bile salts and malabsorption. Vitamin B_{12} absorption may also be impaired, resulting in megaloblastic anemia. Additional complications include obstruction, acute diverticulitis, hemorrhage, and volvulus. Plain films may reveal featureless ovoid collections of air. Barium studies show the outpouchings; most have a neck smaller in diameter than the outpouching itself (Fig. 31.24). The diverticulum lacks mucosal folds and does not contract because of the lack of muscle within its wall. Diverticula are difficult to recognize on CT.

Meckel diverticulum is the most common congenital anomaly of the GI tract, present in 2% to 3% of the population (20). The diverticulum varies from 2 to 8 cm in length and is located on the antimesenteric border of the ileum, up to 2 m from the ileocecal valve. The tip of the diverticulum may be attached to the umbilicus by a remnant of the vitelline duct. Ectopic gastric mucosa is present in up to 62% of cases. Peptic secretions may cause ulceration and bleeding. Other complications are intussusception, volvulus, and perforation. Radionuclide (technetium-99m-pertechnetate) scanning for ectopic gastric mucosa is the test of choice but is less reliable in adults than in children, and gives negative results when the diverticulum does not contain gastric mucosa. Enteroclysis is then the best method to demonstrate the diverticulum, which appears as a blind sac attached to the antimesenteric border of the ileum. On CT, Meckel diverticulitis appears as a blind-ending pouch of variable size and wall thickness, with inflammatory changes in an adjacent mesentery (21).

Pseudodiverticula or sacculations are outpouchings along the antimesenteric border of the small bowel caused by disease of the small bowel. They occur most commonly in association with Crohn disease or scleroderma. With fibrosis and contraction of the mesenteric border of the bowel, the unsupported antimesenteric border becomes pleated and forms sacculations.

REFERENCES

1. Hara AK, Leighton JA, Sharma VK, Heigh RI, Fleischer DE. Imaging of small bowel disease: comparison of capsule endoscopy, standard endoscopy, barium examination, and CT. Radiographics 2005;25:697–718.
2. Wittenberg J, Harisinghani MG, Jhaveri K, Varghese J, Mueller PR. Algorithmic approach to CT diagnosis of the abnormal bowel wall. Radiographics 2002;22:1093–1109.
3. Balthazar EJ. CT of the gastrointestinal tract: principles and interpretation. AJR Am J Roentgenol 1991;156:23–32.
4. Bender GN, Maglinte DDT, Klopper VR, Timmons JH. CT enteroclysis: a superfluous diagnostic procedure or valuable when investigating small-bowel disease. AJR Am J Roentgenol 1999;172: 373–378.
5. Okino Y, Kiyosue H, Mori H, et al. Root of the small-bowel mesentery: correlative anatomy and CT features of pathologic conditions. Radiographics 2001;21:1475–1490.
6. Horton KM, Kamel I, Hofmann L, Fishman EK. Carcinoid tumors of the small bowel: a multitechnique imaging approach. AJR Am J Roentgenol 2004;182:559–567.
7. Levine MS, Rubesin SE, Pantongrag-Brown L, et al. Non-Hodgkin's lymphoma of the gastrointestinal tract: radiographic findings. AJR Am J Roentgenol 1997;168:165–172.
8. Levy AD, Remotti HE, Thompson WM, Sobin LH, Mietten M. Gastrointestinal stromal tumors: radiologic features with pathologic correlation. Radiographics 2003;23:283–304.
9. Sandrasegaran K, Rajesh A, Rydberg J, et al. Gastrointestinal stromal tumors: clinical, radiologic, and pathologic features. AJR Am J Roentgenol 2005;184:803–811.
10. Thompson WM. Imaging and findings of lipomas of the gastrointestinal tract. AJR Am J Roentgenol 2005;184:1163–1171.
11. Cho GJ, Bergquist K, Schwartz AM. Peutz-Jeghers syndrome and the hamartomatous polyposis syndromes: radiologic-pathologic correlation. Radiographics 1997;17:785–791.
12. Sheth S, Horton KM, Garland MR, Fishman EK. Mesenteric neoplasms: CT appearances of primary and secondary tumors and differential diagnosis. Radiographics 2003;23:457–473.
13. Azizi L, Balu M, Belkacem A, Lewin M, et al. MRI features of mesenteric desmoid tumors in familial adenomatous polyposis. AJR Am J Roentgenol 2005;184:1128–1135.
14. Kim H-C, Lee JM, Kim SH, et al. Primary gastrointestinal stromal tumors in the omentum and mesentery: CT findings and pathologic correlations. AJR Am J Roentgenol 2004;182:1463–1467.
15. Horton KM, Fishman EK. Uncommon inflammatory diseases of the small bowel. AJR Am J Roentgenol 1998;170:385–388.
16. Bradbury MS, Kavanagh PV, Bechtold R, et al. Mesenteric venous thrombosis: diagnosis and noninvasive imaging. Radiographics 2002;22:527–541.
17. Wiesner W, Khurana B, Ji H, Ros PR. CT of acute bowel ischemia. Radiology 2003;226:635–650.
18. Furukawa A, Saotome T, Yamasaki M, Maeda K, et al. Cross-sectional imaging in Crohn disease. Radiographics 2004;24:689–702.
19. Ha HK, Lee HJ, Yang S-K, Ki WW, et al. Intestinal Behçet syndrome: CT features of patients with and patients without complications. Radiology 1998;209:449–454.
20. Levy AD, Hobbs CM. Meckel diverticulum: radiologic features with pathologic correlation. Radiographics 2004;24:565–587.
21. Bennett GL, Birnbaum BA, Bathazar EJ. CT of Meckel's diverticulitis in 11 patients. AJR Am J Roentgenol 2004;182:625–629.

Chapter 32

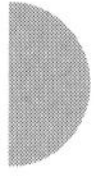

Colon and Appendix

William E. Brant

Colon
Imaging Methods
Anatomy
Colon Filling Defects/Mass Lesions
Colon Inflammatory Disease
Diverticular Disease
Lower GI Hemorrhage

Appendix
Imaging Methods
Anatomy
Acute Appendicitis
Mucocele of the Appendix
Appendiceal Tumors

COLON

Imaging Methods

The primary imaging methods for detection and characterization of colon abnormalities have continued to evolve over time. The persistently expanding availability of colonoscopy has continued to reduce the role of barium enema in imaging the colon. On the other hand, the use of CT to image the abdomen and pelvis continues to increase, making CT often the preferred method for initial detection of colon disease. CT (virtual) colonography challenges the role of traditional colonoscopy for polyp and cancer detection. Once a possible neoplastic lesion is discovered, however, colonoscopy or proctoscopy is usually used for biopsy. The single-contrast barium enema is still occasionally used for the evaluation of colonic obstruction and fistulas and in old, seriously ill, or debilitated patients. The double-contrast (air-contrast) barium enema (Fig. 32.1) is favored for detection of small lesions (<1 cm), for documentation of inflammatory bowel disease, and for detailed imaging evaluation of the rectum (1). Colonoscopy is sporadically limited by occasional failure to reach the right colon. In such cases, barium enema or virtual colonoscopy is utilized to complete the examination. As elsewhere in the GI tract, CT complements colonoscopy and barium examinations by demonstrating intramural and extracolonic components of disease. It is excellent for demonstrating extrinsic inflammatory and neoplastic processes that affect the colon: abscesses, sinuses, and fistulas.

CT and MR imaging have been utilized for initial staging of colorectal carcinoma. However, both methods are limited in their ability to determine the extent of bowel wall tumor infiltration and involvement of regional lymph nodes. Transrectal US is more accurate than CT or MR in determining local tumor extent of rectal carcinomas, and it is used in the evaluation of other rectal and perirectal disease (2). For the initial staging of colorectal carcinoma, CT and MR should be reserved for patients with suspected widespread local or disseminated disease. CT is useful in screening for recurrence of colorectal carcinoma because it can provide a comprehensive examination of the liver, abdominal cavity, and entire colon. MR is sensitive but nonspecific for the detection of local recurrence of rectal carcinoma.

CT colonography (Fig. 32.2) is becoming a viable alternative to invasive colonoscopy to screen for colorectal cancer (3). The procedure begins with diligent bowel preparation, identical to that used for invasive colonoscopy. A rectal tube is inserted and the colon is insufflated with carbon dioxide or room air. Multidetector CT of the entire extent of the colon with the patient in supine position is obtained in a single breath-hold utilizing 1.25- to 2.5-mm collimation and a reconstruction interval of 1 mm. The scan is repeated with the patient in prone position. Commercially available software programs that provide endoluminal display and "fly-through" capabilities provide three-dimensional volume-rendering image processing. Image viewing and interpretation are usually performed using

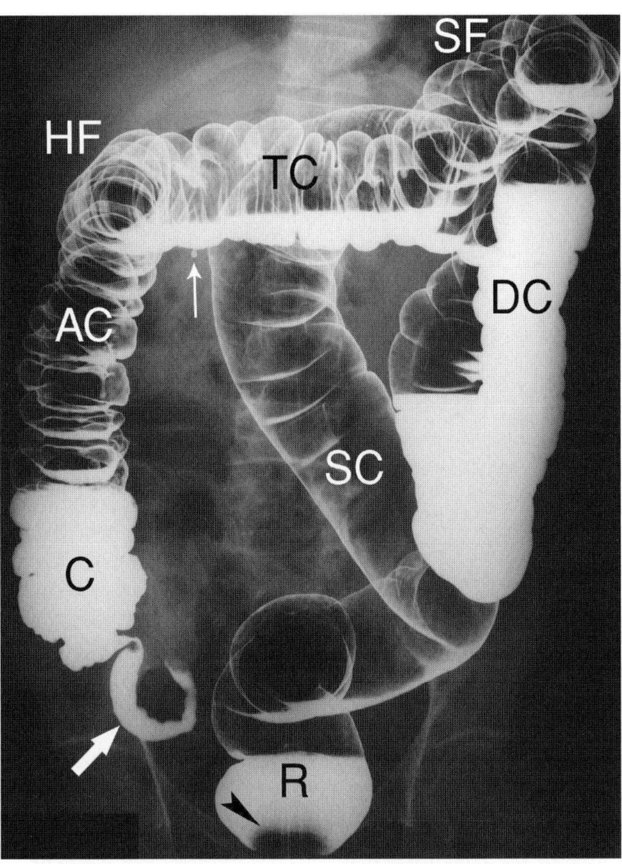

FIGURE 32.1. Double-Contrast Barium Enema. An upright radiograph from a double-contrast barium enema demonstrates normal colon anatomy. The appendix (*larger white arrow*) extends from the cecum (C). The ascending colon (AC) extends to the hepatic flexure (HF), the coils of which must be examined by multiple oblique views. The transverse colon (TC) extends to the splenic flexure (SF), which continues as the descending colon (DC). This patient has a long sigmoid colon (SC) that extends high into the abdomen. The transverse colon is relatively short. Patients with a short sigmoid colon usually have a long, redundant transverse colon. The distended balloon at the tip of the enema catheter causes a lucent filling defect (*black arrowhead*) in the rectum (R). A tiny intramural diverticulum (*smaller white arrow*) is seen in the proximal transverse colon.

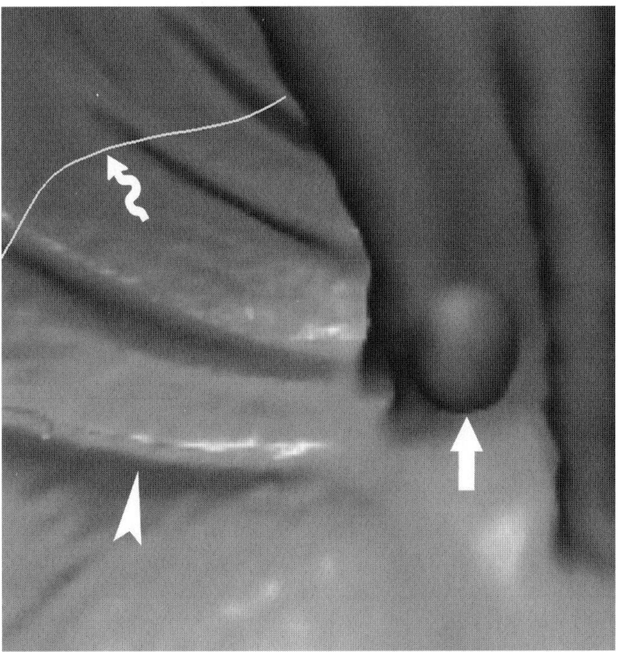

FIGURE 32.2. Polyp on Virtual Colonography. Three-dimensional reconstructed image shows a 7-mm polyp (*straight arrow*) extending into the lumen of the colon. Multiple normal-appearing folds (*arrowhead*) are evident. The white line (*curvy arrow*) shows the colon "fly-through" path. Images are usually reviewed in color on a computer workstation.

both standard two-dimensional axial CT reconstructions and three-dimensional volume-rendered images on a computer workstation. The role of virtual colonoscopy in imaging the colon and screening for colorectal cancer is still being debated.

Anatomy

The large intestine consists of the cecum and appendix, colon, rectum, and anal canal. It is approximately 1.5 m in length from the ileum to the anus. The large intestine is characterized by the *taenia coli,* three longitudinal bands of muscle that traverse the colon and shorten it to form *haustra,* the sacculations created by puckering of the bowel wall. The major functions of the large intestine are the formation, transport, and evacuation of feces. These functions require mobility, absorption of water, and secretion of mucus. Infrequent peristalsis transports feces from the ascending and transverse colon to the sigmoid colon, where fecal material is stored until defecation. The cecum and ascending colon absorb water from the highly liquid material received from the ileum. Mucus secreted by mucosal goblet cells protects the mucosa from injury and is secreted in profuse amounts when the mucosa is irritated or injured.

The cecum is the large blind pouch that extends below the level of the ileocecal valve. The cecum generally lies in the right iliac fossa but may be quite mobile. It is usually covered on all sides by peritoneum (intraperitoneal), but it may be fixed extraperitoneally and covered by peritoneum on its ventral surface only. The appendix is a long wormlike tube that hangs from near the apex of the cecum. The ileocecal valve consists of two lips that project into the cecum, forming a sometimes prominent mass.

The ascending colon is extraperitoneal, lying in the anterior pararenal space and covered by peritoneum on its ventral surface only. The hepatic flexure forms two curves. The proximal, more posterior curve is closely related to the descending duodenum and right kidney. The more distal anterior curve is closely related to the gallbladder.

The transverse colon is intraperitoneal and suspended from the transverse mesocolon, which arises from the peritoneum to cover the pancreas and sweep transversely across the upper abdomen. The transverse mesocolon limits the superior extent of the small bowel loops. The splenic flexure is closely related to the tail of the pancreas and the caudal aspect of the spleen. The splenic flexure is anchored to the diaphragm by the phrenicocolic ligament, which serves as a boundary between disease processes of the left subphrenic space and the left paracolic gutter.

The descending colon, like the ascending colon, is extraperitoneal within the anterior pararenal space and is covered by peritoneum only on its ventral surface. The sigmoid colon forms a redundant loop of variable length from the distal descending colon in the left iliac fossa to the rectum. The sigmoid colon is completely intraperitoneal and is suspended by the sigmoid mesocolon, which allows considerable mobility. The sigmoid colon penetrates the peritoneum at the level of vertebrae S2 to S4 to continue as the extraperitoneal rectum. The rectum extends for approximately 12 cm, in close relationship with the sacrum. Peritoneum forming the pouch of Douglas covers the ventral and lateral aspects of the rectum. The anal canal is 3 to 4 cm long and is invested by the sphincter ani and levator ani muscles. A series of vertical folds forms the rectal columns of Morgagni, beneath which are the veins that, when dilated, are hemorrhoids. The colon is recognized on imaging studies by its course, haustral markings, and fecal content. The thickness of the wall of the normal colon does not exceed 5 mm.

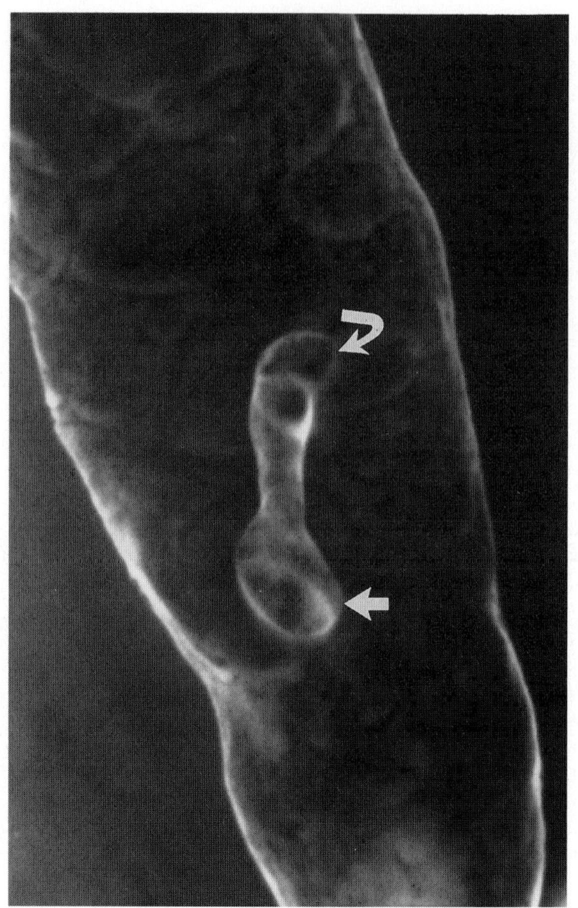

FIGURE 32.3. **Pedunculated Polyp.** Double-contrast barium enema demonstrates a long-stalked pedunculated polyp with a bulbous tip (*straight arrow*) arising (*curved arrow*) from the mucosa of the descending colon.

Colon Filling Defects/Mass Lesions

Filling defect refers to a radiolucency in a barium pool caused by a protruding mass lesion. On barium enema examinations, filling defects may be polyps, tumors, plaques, air bubbles, feces, mucus, or foreign objects. Polyps are protrusions from the mucosa that produce filling defects in pools of barium or are etched in white when coated by barium and outlined by air on double-contrast studies. Polyps may be pedunculated on a stalk (Fig. 32.3) or sessile. They may appear as "bowler hats" (Fig. 32.4) when viewed obliquely. The term *polyp* is generic for a protruding lesion and does not imply a histologic diagnosis. Air bubbles rise to the highest point of a contrast column (the "carpenter's level" sign), but fecal material usually remains dependent. Plaques are flat lesions that barely rise above the mucosal surface.

Colorectal adenocarcinoma is the most common malignancy of the GI tract and the second most common malignant tumor in the United States. Approximately 50% arise in the rectum and rectosigmoid area. Another 25% occur in the sigmoid colon, and the remaining 25% are evenly distributed throughout the remainder of the colon. Nearly all cancers of the colon are adenocarcinomas arising from preexisting adenomas. Most tumors are annular constricting lesions, 2 to 6 cm in diameter, with raised everted edges and ulcerated mucosa (Fig. 32.5). Polypoid tumors are less common, with some having the frond-like appearance of villous carcinoma. Infiltrating scirrhous tumors—common in gastric carcinoma—are rare in the large intestine, unless the patient has ulcerative colitis. The tumor spreads by direct invasion through the bowel wall into pericolonic fat (Fig. 32.6) and adjacent organs, through lymphatic channels to regional nodes, and hematogenously through the portal veins to the liver and systemic circulation. Intraperitoneal seeding from a tumor that penetrates the colon wall may also occur. Obstruction is the most frequent complication. Other complications are uncommon but include perforation (Fig. 32.7), intussusception, abscess, and fistula formation. Up to 20% of patients have a second tumor of the large bowel at diagnosis, usually an adenoma or another carcinoma. Approximately 5% of patients will have a second colorectal carcinoma,

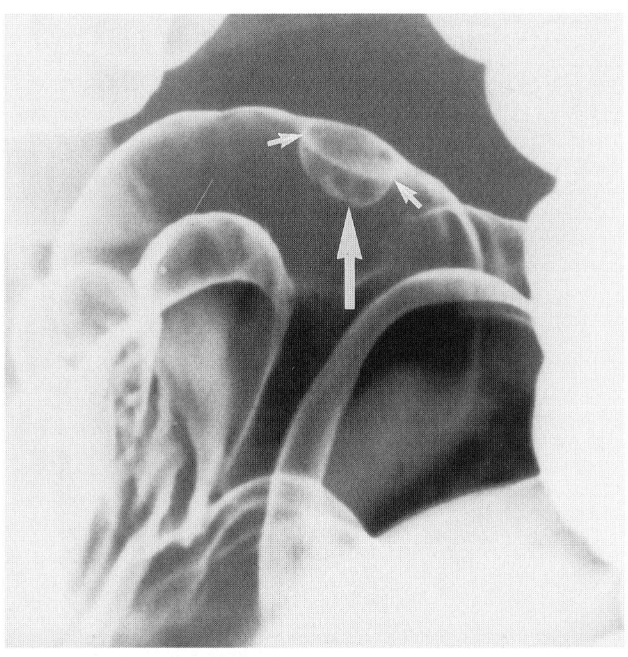

FIGURE 32.4. **Bowler Hat Sign.** The "bowler hat" sign is produced by barium coating both the body of the polyp (*large arrow*) and the recesses (*small arrows*) between the base of the lesion and the normal colonic mucosa.

either simultaneously or diagnosed subsequently. Patients with ulcerative colitis, Crohn disease, familial adenomatous polyposis syndrome, and Peutz-Jeghers syndrome are at increased risk of colon carcinoma.

Local disease staging is best evaluated with transrectal or colonoscopic US. CT and MR are used for more advanced disease and to detect recurrence (4). Microscopic invasion through the bowel wall and tumor involvement of normal-size lymph nodes are not detected by CT or MR. Cross-sectional imaging findings include: (*1*) polypoid primary tumor (usually >1 cm); (*2*) "apple-core" lesions, with bulky, irregular thickening of the colon wall and irregular narrowing of the lumen; (*3*) cystic, necrotic, and hemorrhagic areas within the tumor mass, especially when the tumor is large; (*4*) linear soft tissue stranding into the pericolonic fat, which is often indicative of tumor extension through the bowel wall; (*5*) enlarged regional lymph nodes (>1 cm) representing lymphatic spread of tumor; (*6*) distant metastases, especially in the liver (5). When tumors cause colonic obstruction, edema and/or ischemia may thicken the wall of the uninvolved colon proximal to the tumor.

Tumor recurrences are most common (*1*) at the operative site, near the bowel anastomosis; (*2*) in lymph nodes that drain the operative site; (*3*) in the peritoneal cavity; and (*4*) in the liver and distant organs. Because the entire abdominal cavity must be surveyed to detect tumor recurrence, CT is the current method of choice.

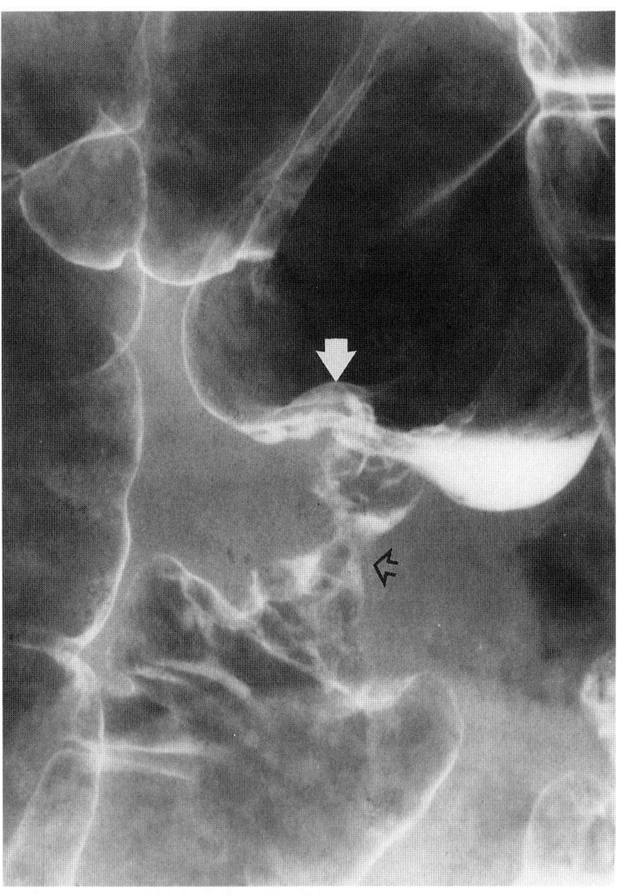

FIGURE 32.5. **Colon Carcinoma.** Radiograph of the sigmoid colon from a double-contrast barium enema demonstrates a characteristic "apple core" constricting lesion of colon carcinoma. The lumen is markedly narrowed (*open arrow*), and the shoulders of the tumor cause a mass impression on the adjacent distended lumen (*solid arrow*).

Polyps. A polyp is defined as a localized mass that projects from the mucosa into the lumen. Because the majority of colorectal cancers are believed to arise from preexisting adenomatous polyps, the detection of colon polyps is a major indication for barium studies of the colon. The following "rules of thumb" can be applied. Polyps smaller than 5 mm are almost all hyperplastic, with a risk of malignancy less than 0.5%. Polyps between 5 and 10 mm are 90% adenomas, with a risk of malignancy of 1%. Polyps between 10 and 20 mm are usually adenomas, with a risk of malignancy of 10%. Polyps larger than 20 mm are 50% malignant.

Hyperplastic polyps are nonneoplastic mucosal proliferations. They are round and sessile. Nearly all are smaller than 5 mm.

Adenomatous polyps are distinctly premalignant and a major risk for development of colorectal carcinoma. Adenomatous polyps are neoplasms with a core of connective tissue. Approximately 5% to 10% of the population older than 40 years have adenomatous polyps.

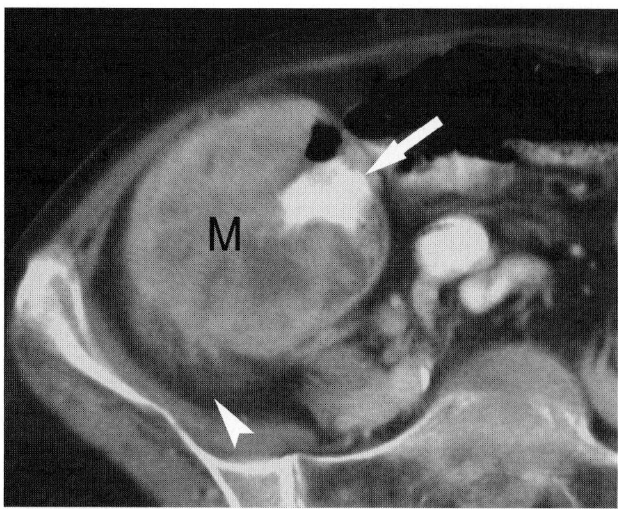

FIGURE 32.6. **Cecal Carcinoma.** CT reveals a large mass (M) representing adenocarcinoma of the cecum. Note the asymmetric, irregular narrowing of the cecal lumen (*arrow*). Soft tissue stranding (*arrowhead*) extending well into the pericecal fat is indicative of tumor extension through the wall of the colon.

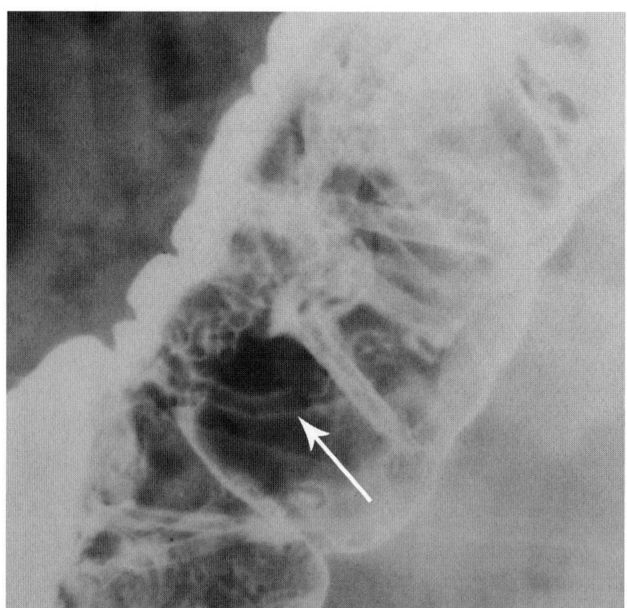

FIGURE 32.8. **Postinflammatory Filiform Polyps.** Detail view from an air-contrast barium enema in a patient with ulcerative colitis shows the characteristic wormlike appearance of postinflammatory filiform polyps (*arrow*). Numerous polyps are present.

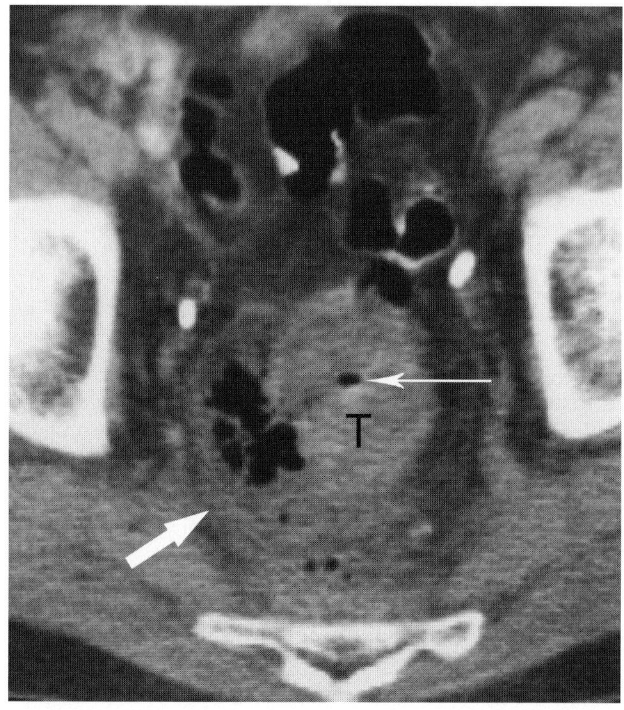

FIGURE 32.7. **Rectal Carcinoma With Perforation.** An aggressive rectal carcinoma (T) markedly thickens the wall of the rectum and narrows its lumen to a tiny channel (*thin arrow*). The tumor has perforated the wall of the rectum, resulting in a perirectal abscess (*wide arrow*); this is shown on CT as soft tissue and fluid density with air bubbles replacing the perirectal fat.

Hamartomatous polyps (juvenile polyps) represent approximately 1% of colon polyps. They are a common cause of rectal bleeding in children. The Peutz-Jeghers polyp is a type of hamartomatous polyp.

Inflammatory polyps are usually multiple and associated with inflammatory bowel disease (Fig. 32.8). They account for less than 0.5% of colorectal polyps.

Familial adenomatous polyposis syndrome is approximately two thirds inherited and one third spontaneous. The inheritance pattern is autosomal dominant with high penetrance. The polyps are tubulovillous adenomas, which usually are evident by age 20. Colorectal cancer will eventually develop in nearly all patients, so total colectomy with rectal mucosectomy and ileoanal pouch construction is the current recommended therapy. Polyps typically carpet the entire colon (Fig. 32.9). Patients are at risk for numerous extracolonic manifestations, including carcinomas of the small bowel, thyroid carcinoma, and mesenteric fibromatosis. Patients with associated bone and skin abnormalities, including cortical thickening of the ribs and long bones, osteomas of the skull, supernumerary teeth, exostoses of the mandible, dermal fibromas, desmoids, and epidermal inclusion cysts, have been diagnosed as *Gardner syndrome.* Those with associated tumors of the CNS have been grouped as *Turcot syndrome.* These are variations of the same disease.

Hamartomatous Polyposis Syndromes. Hamartomatous polyps are nonneoplastic growths with a smooth

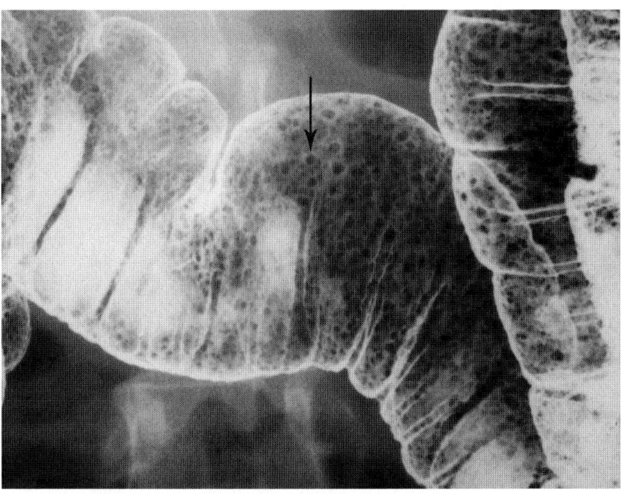

FIGURE 32.9. **Familial Adenomatous Polyposis Syndrome.** Cone-down image from a double-contrast barium enema reveals the colonic mucosa to be carpeted with innumerable small polyps, seen as tiny filling defects (*arrow*).

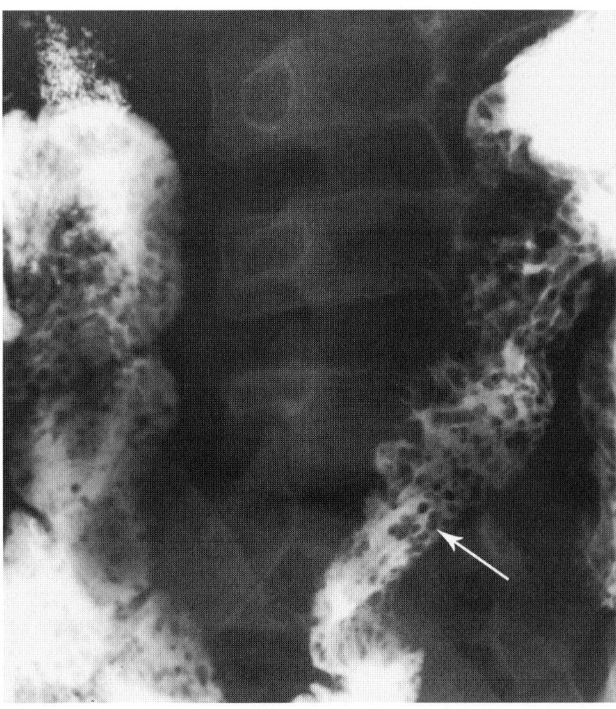

FIGURE 32.10. **Nodular Lymphoid Hyperplasia.** Single-contrast barium enema in a young patient with hypogammaglobulinemia shows numerous small nodules (*arrow*) throughout the colon.

muscle core covered by mature glandular epithelium (6). The hamartomatous polyps associated with various syndromes have minor histologic differences. These lesions carry no risk of malignant transformation. However, patients with hamartomatous polyposis syndromes may also develop adenomatous polyps, which do carry a risk of malignancy.

Peutz-Jeghers syndrome predominantly involves the small bowel, but most cases have gastric and colon polyps as well. The condition is autosomal dominant with incomplete penetrance. Dark pigmented spots on the skin and mucous membranes are characteristic. Risk of carcinoma arising from coexisting adenomatous polyps is 2% to 20%. Patients are at risk for breast, uterine, and ovarian cancer and early age cancer of the pancreas.

Cowden disease is a syndrome of multiple hamartomas, including hamartomatous polyposis of the GI tract, with goiter and thyroid adenomas and increased risk of breast cancer and transitional cell carcinoma of the urinary tract. The syndrome is autosomal dominant and affects mainly Caucasians. All patients have mucocutaneous lesions with facial papules, oral papillomas, and palmoplantar keratoses.

Cronkhite-Canada syndrome is a disease of older patients with a mean age of onset of 60 years. Polyps are distributed throughout the stomach, small bowel, and colon. Associated skin findings include nail atrophy, brownish skin pigmentation, and alopecia. Patients present with watery diarrhea and protein-losing enteropathy.

Lymphoid hyperplasia may involve the colon. The normal lymphoid follicular pattern of diffuse tiny nodules 1 to 3 mm in diameter (Fig. 32.10) with characteristic umbilication is most common in the terminal ileum and cecum but may involve any portion of the colon. The nodular lymphoid hyperplasia pattern of diffuse nodules larger than 4 mm is associated with allergic, infectious, and inflammatory disorders.

Lymphoma. The colon is less commonly involved with lymphoma than the stomach or small bowel. Involvement of the cecum or rectum is most common with anal and rectal lymphoma, which is increasingly frequent in AIDS patients. Morphologic patterns include small to large nodules, which may ulcerate, excavitate, and perforate, and diffuse infiltration of the bowel wall, resulting in bulbous folds and thickened bowel wall (Fig. 32.11). As in the small intestine, marked narrowing of the lumen is uncommon, and aneurysmal dilation occurs when transmural disease destroys innervation. The diffuse multinodular form may be difficult to differentiate from nodular lymphoid hyperplasia. Lymphoma nodules vary in size, although lymphoid hyperplasia nodules are uniform in size. Non-Hodgkin lymphoma is most common.

GI stromal tumors (GISTs) account for nearly all mesenchymal tumors of the colon. True colonic leiomyomas and leiomyosarcomas are very rare (7). GISTs are much less common in the colon than in the stomach and small bowel, accounting for only 7% of the total. As in the remainder of the GI tract, they may appear as exophytic, mural, or intraluminal masses. Ulceration is relatively

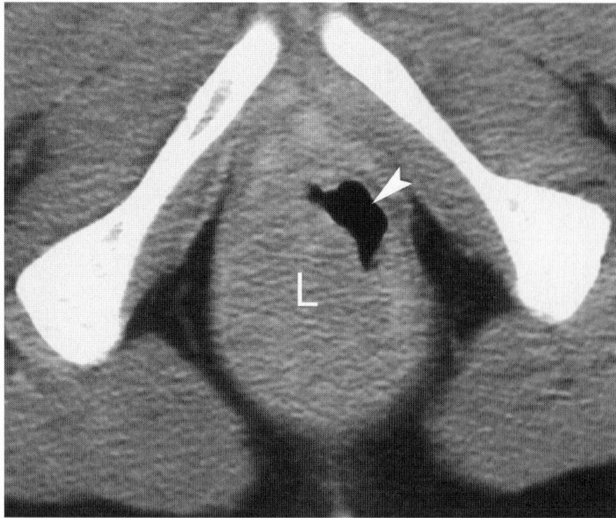

FIGURE 32.11. **Rectal Lymphoma.** CT demonstrates a prominent mass of lymphoma (L) that causes irregular narrowing of the lumen (*arrowhead*) of the rectum. Note the homogeneous attenuation of the lymphomatous mass. The CT appearance is indistinguishable from adenocarcinoma of the rectum.

frequent. Hemorrhage, cystic change, necrosis, and calcification are more common in larger tumors (Fig. 32.12).

Lipoma is the most common submucosal tumor of the colon. It is most frequent in the cecum and ascending colon. Nearly 40% present with intussusception. Barium studies demonstrate a smooth, well-defined, elliptic filling defect, usually 1 to 3 cm in diameter. The tumors are soft and change shape with compression. CT demonstration of a fat-density tumor is definitive.

Extrinsic masses commonly cause mass effect on the colon that may simulate intrinsic disease (Fig. 32.13).

Endometriosis commonly implants on the sigmoid colon and rectum (8). Defects are frequently multiple and of variable size. Lesions are commonly within the cul-de-sac. Barium studies demonstrate sharply defined defects that compress but do not usually encircle the lumen. CT demonstrates complex cystic pelvic masses with high-density fluid components. Multiple pelvic organs may be incorporated into the mass. MR demonstrates masses with signal characteristics of hemorrhage.

Benign pelvic masses such as ovarian cysts, cystadenomas, teratomas, and uterine fibroids produce smooth extrinsic mass impressions on the colonic wall. The colon is displaced but not invaded.

Malignant pelvic tumors and metastases may involve the colon by contiguous spread, by spreading along mesenteric fascial planes, by intraperitoneal seeding, through lymphatic channels, or by embolus through blood vessels. The involved colon demonstrates thickening of the wall, separation of folds, spiculation, angulations, narrowing, and serosal plaques. Metastases often cannot be differentiated

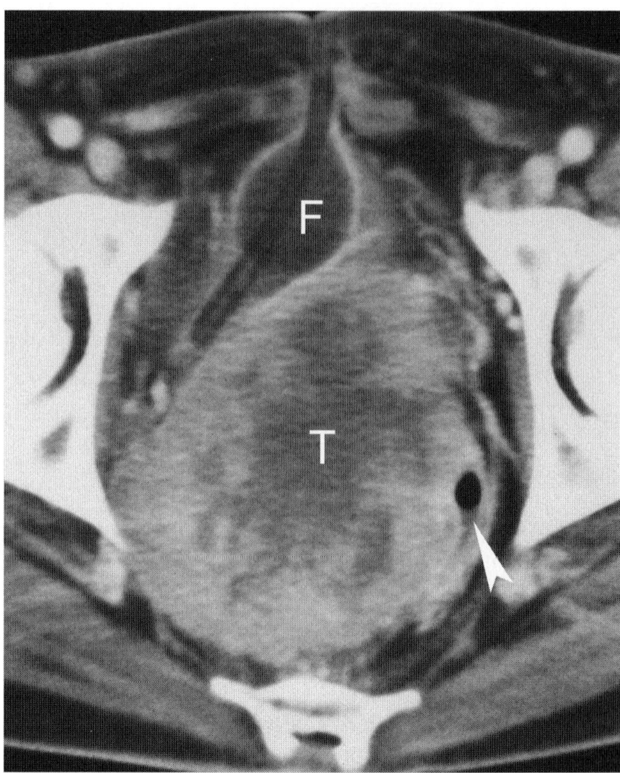

FIGURE 32.12. **Malignant GI Stromal Tumor of the Rectum.** A CT scan shows a large tumor (T) with an irregular low-density area of central necrosis arising exophytically from the wall of the rectum (*arrowhead*), which is displaced laterally and anteriorly. The tumor obstructed the bladder outlet, necessitating placement of a suprapubic Foley catheter (F).

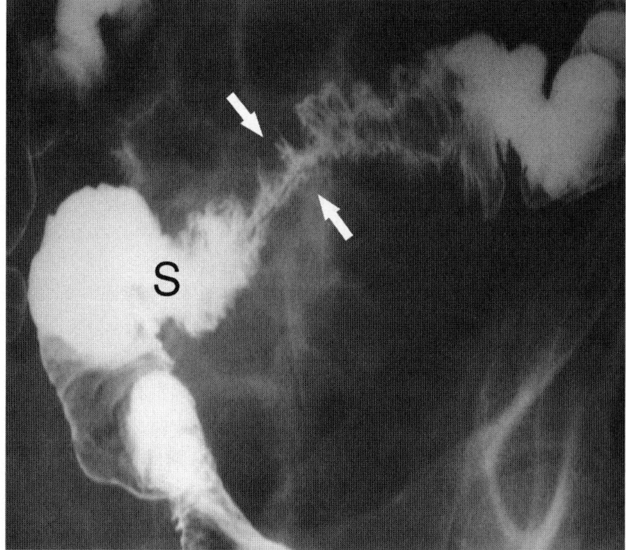

FIGURE 32.13. **Serosal Metastases Involving the Colon.** Metastases from carcinosarcoma of the uterus implanted on the serosal surface of the sigmoid colon (S) cause narrowing and spiculation (*arrows*) of the lumen.

from primary tumors by imaging methods. Crohn disease and metastatic disease may also look exactly alike radiographically. CT and MR demonstrate contiguous involvement of the colon and rectum by pelvic tumors.

Extrinsic inflammatory processes, such as appendicitis, pelvic abscess, diverticular abscess, and pelvic inflammatory disease, cause mass effect, asymmetric tethering, and spiculation.

Colon Inflammatory Disease

Ulcerative colitis is an uncommon idiopathic inflammatory disease involving primarily the mucosa and submucosa of the colon (9). The peak age for its appearance is 20 to 40 years, but onset of disease after age 50 is common. The disease consists of superficial ulcerations, edema, and hyperemia. The radiographic hallmarks of ulcerative colitis are granular mucosa, confluent shallow ulcerations, symmetry of disease around the lumen, and continuous confluent diffuse involvement (Table 32.1). An early fine granular pattern is produced by mucosal hyperemia and edema that precede ulceration. Superficial ulcers spread to cover the entire mucosal surface. The mucosa is stippled, with barium adhering to the superficial ulcers. *Collar button ulcers* (Fig. 32.14) are deeper ulcerations of thickened edematous mucosa with crypt abscesses extending in the submucosa. A coarse granular pattern is produced later by the replacement of diffusely ulcerated mucosa with granulation tissue. Late changes include a variety of polypoid lesions. *Pseudopolyps* are mucosal remnants in areas of extensive ulceration. *Inflammatory polyps* are small islands of inflamed mucosa. *Postinflammatory polyps* are mucosal tags that are seen in quiescent phases of the disease. *Filiform polyps* are postinflammatory polyps with a characteristic wormlike appearance (Fig. 32.8). They are typically seen in an otherwise normal-appearing colon. *Hyperplastic polyps* may occur during healing after mucosal injury. Involvement typically extends from the rectum proximally in a symmetric and continuous pattern. The terminal ileum is nearly always normal. Rare *backwash ileitis* may produce an ulcerated but patulous terminal ileum. CT findings include: (*1*) wall thickening, often with a "halo sign" of low-density submucosal edema; (*2*) narrowing of the lumen of the colon; (*3*) pseudopolyps; and (*4*) pneumatosis coli with megacolon. Complications of ulcerative colitis include: (*1*) strictures (Fig. 32.15), usually 2 to 3 cm or longer and commonly involving the transverse colon and rectum; (*2*) colorectal adenocarcinoma, with an approximate risk of 1% per year of disease; (*3*) toxic megacolon (2% to 5% of cases) as the initial manifestation; and (*4*) massive hemorrhage. Associated extraintestinal diseases include sacroiliitis mimicking ankylosing spondylitis (20% of cases), eye lesions including uveitis and iritis (10% of cases), cholangitis, and an increased incidence of thromboembolic disease.

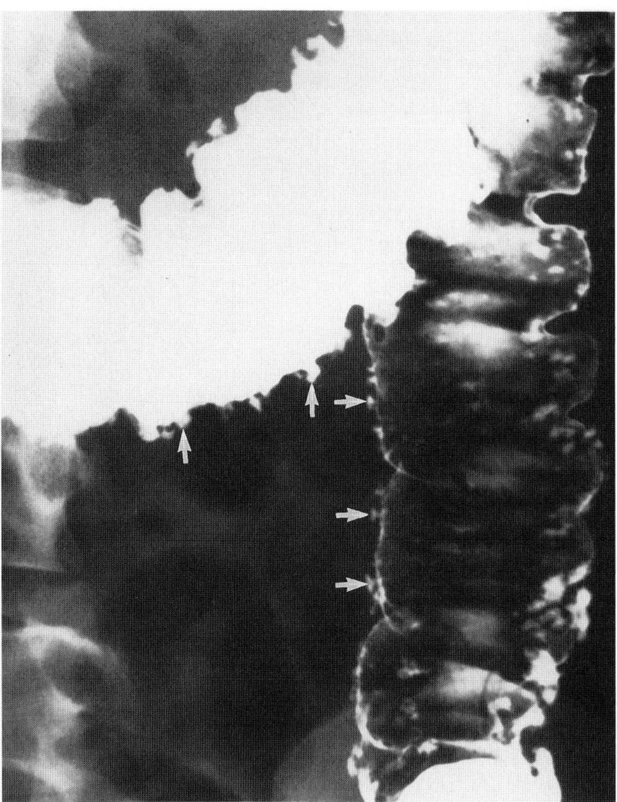

FIGURE 32.14. **Ulcerative Colitis.** Double-contrast barium enema shows a pattern of continuous involvement of the colon with innumerable submucosal collar button ulcers (*arrows*).

TABLE 32.1 Ulcerative Colitis Versus Crohn Colitis

Ulcerative Colitis	*Crohn Colitis*
Circumferential disease	Eccentric disease
Regional (continuous disease)	Skip lesions (discontinuous disease)
Predominantly left-sided	Predominantly right-sided
Rectum usually involved	Rectum normal in 50% of cases
Confluent shallow ulcers	Confluent deep ulcers
No aphthous ulcers	Aphthous ulcers early
Collar button ulcers	Transverse and longitudinal ulcers
Terminal ileum usually normal	Terminal ileum usually diseased
Terminal ileum patulous	Terminal ileum narrowed
No pseudodiverticula	Pseudodiverticula
No fistulas	Fistulas common
High risk of cancer	Low risk of cancer
Risk of toxic megacolon	No toxic megacolon

Crohn disease involves the colon in two thirds of cases and is isolated to the colon in approximately one third of all cases. Hallmarks of Crohn colitis include early aphthous ulcers, later confluent deep ulcerations, predominant right colon disease, discontinuous involvement with intervening regions of normal bowel, asymmetric

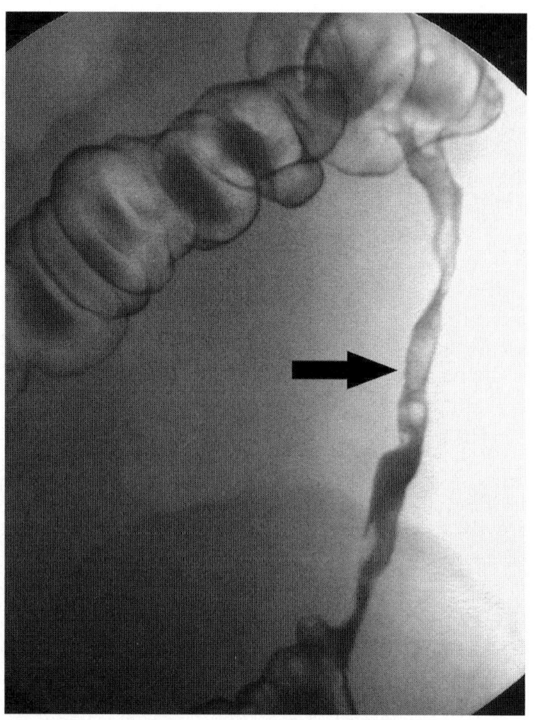

FIGURE 32.15. **Ulcerative Colitis Stricture.** A long-segment stricture (*arrow*) is typical of inflammatory bowel disease rather than malignancy. Air-contrast barium enema shows irregular narrowing of the lumen of the descending colon.

involvement of the bowel wall, strictures, fistulas, and sinus formation (Fig. 32.16) (Table 32.1). Pseudodiverticula of the colon are formed by asymmetric fibrosis on one side of the lumen, causing saccular outpouches on the other side. Involvement of the rectum is characterized by deep rectal ulcers and multiple fistulous tracts to the skin.

Infectious colitis may be caused by a variety of bacteria (*Salmonella, Shigella, Escherichia coli*); parasites; viruses (cytomegalovirus, herpes); and fungi (histoplasmosis, mucormycosis). Most cause a pancolitis with edema and inflammatory wall thickening with infiltration of pericolonic fat. Pericolonic fluid and intraperitoneal fluid may be present (Fig. 32.17).

Toxic megacolon is a potentially fatal condition characterized by marked colonic distension and risk of perforation. It occurs as a complication of fulminant colitis, often caused by ulcerative colitis, Crohn disease, pseudomembranous colitis, use of antidiarrheal drugs, and hypokalemia. Transmural inflammation causes deep ulcers that may extend to the serosa surface, large areas of denuded mucosa, and loss of muscle tone. Radiographic findings include: (*1*) marked dilatation of the colon (transverse colon >6 cm) with absence of haustral markings, (*2*) edema and thickening of the colon wall, (*3*) pneumatosis coli, and (*4*) evidence of perforation. Barium studies should be avoided because of risk of perforation.

Pseudomembranous colitis is an inflammatory disease of the colon (and occasionally the small bowel) characterized by the presence of a pseudomembrane of necrotic

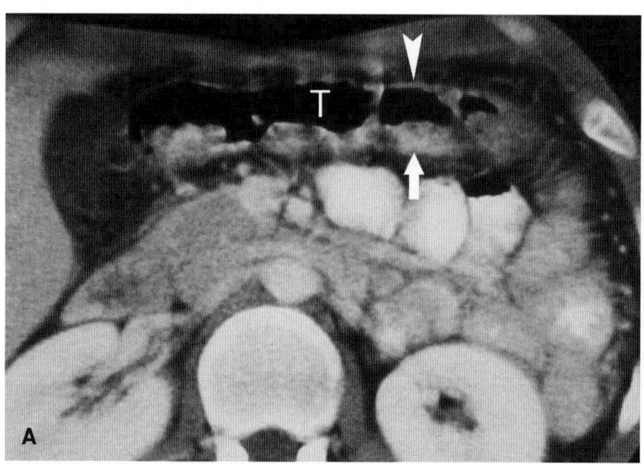

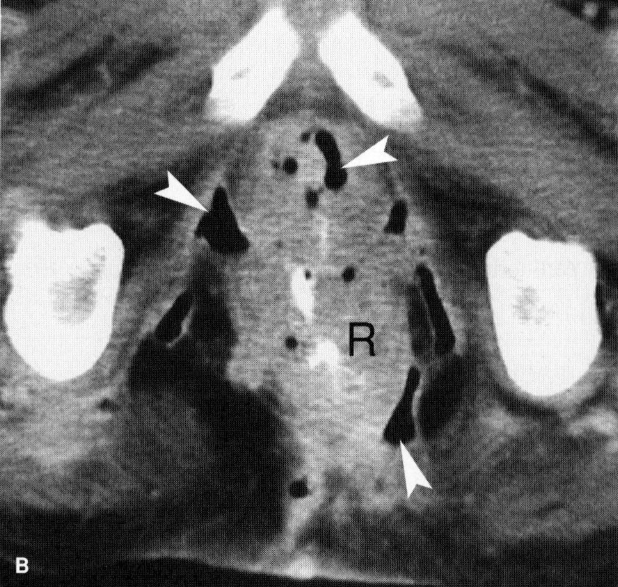

FIGURE 32.16. **Crohn Colitis. A.** CT scan through the transverse colon (T) demonstrates the asymmetric thickening of the colon wall characteristic of Crohn colitis. The anterior wall (*arrowhead*) is normal, and the posterior wall (*arrow*) is thickened and nodular. **B.** A more caudal CT scan in the same patient demonstrates numerous air-containing perineal cutaneous fistulas (*arrowheads*) surrounding the rectum (R).

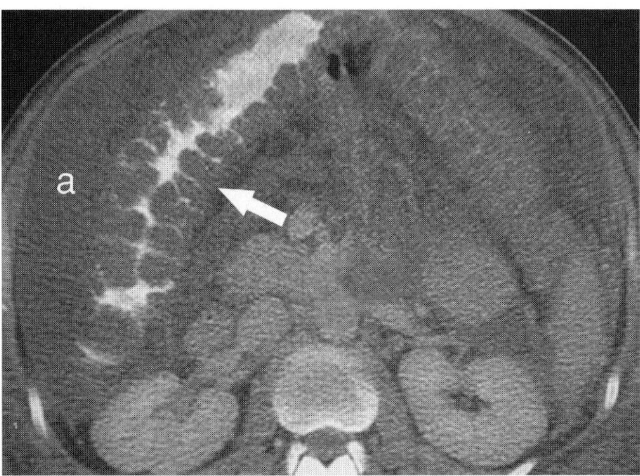

FIGURE 32.17. **Infectious Colitis.** CT demonstrates marked thickening of the wall (*arrow*) of the transverse colon. Pericolonic fat is diffusely infiltrated, and ascites (a) is present. This patient was proven to have colitis caused by Cytomegalovirus.

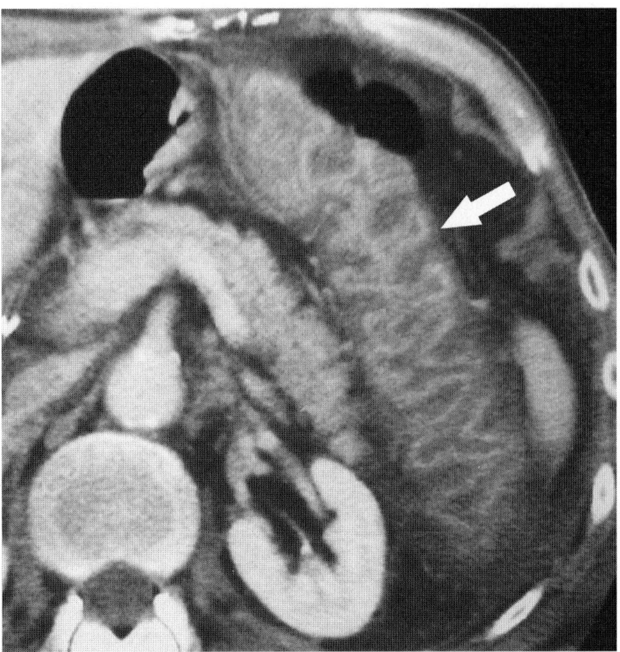

FIGURE 32.18. **Pseudomembranous Colitis.** The wall of the transverse colon (*arrow*) is markedly and diffusely thickened, trapping intraluminal contrast between the folds and producing the "accordion sign" on this CT scan. This patient developed *Clostridium difficile* colitis caused by broad-spectrum antibiotic therapy.

debris and overgrowth of *Clostridium difficile* (10). There are many contributing causes, including antibiotics (any that change bowel flora), intestinal ischemia (especially following surgery), irradiation, long-term steroids, shock, and colonic obstruction. The disease presents as fulminant inflammatory bowel disease with diarrhea and foul stools. Plain radiographs may reveal: (*1*) dilated colon, (*2*) nodular thickening of the haustra, and (*3*) ascites. The colon may be greatly dilated, and toxic megacolon has been reported. Barium enema demonstrates an irregular lumen with thumbprint indentations similar to ischemic colitis. Superficial ulcers are common. Plaquelike defects on the mucosal surface are caused by the pseudomembranes. The colitis is frequently patchy in distribution, with sparing of the rectum. The condition is commonly first detected on CT, which shows: (*1*) marked wall thickening up to 30 mm (average 15 mm) with halo or target appearance, (*2*) characteristic stripes of intraluminal contrast media trapped between nodular areas of wall thickening (the "accordion sign") (Fig. 32.18), (*3*) mild pericolonic fat inflammation disproportionate with the marked colonic wall inflammation, and (*4*) ascites (35%).

Amebiasis is an infection by the protozoan parasite *Entamoeba histolytica*. The disease exists worldwide but is particularly common in South Africa, Central and South America, and Asia. At least 5% of the population of the United States harbor amebae. Encysted amebae are ingested with contaminated food and water. The cyst capsule is dissolved in the small bowel, releasing trophozoites that migrate to the colon and burrow into the mucosa, forming small abscesses. The infection can spread throughout the body by hematogenous embolization or direct invasion. Amebic colitis produces dysentery with frequent bloody mucoid stools. Barium studies demonstrate a disease that closely mimics Crohn colitis, with aphthous ulcers, deep ulcers, asymmetric disease, and skip areas. The cecum and rectum are the primary sites of colonic disease. The terminal ileum is characteristically not involved. Complications include strictures, amebomas consisting of a hard fixed mass of granulation tissue that may simulate carcinoma, toxic megacolon, and fistulas, particularly following surgical intervention. Amebic liver abscess results from the spread of infection through the portal system and may be complicated by diaphragm perforation, pleural effusion, and thoracic disease.

Typhilitis is a potentially fatal infection of the cecum and ascending colon usually seen in patients who are neutropenic and immunocompromised by chemotherapy. Concentric, often marked, thickenings of the wall of the cecum and ascending colon with prominent pericolonic inflammatory changes are characteristic (Fig. 32.19). Patients are at risk for colon ischemia.

Ischemic colitis mimics ulcerative colitis and Crohn colitis, both clinically and radiographically (11). The causes of ischemic colitis include arterial occlusion caused by arteriosclerosis, vasculitis, or arterial emboli; venous thrombosis owing to neoplasm, oral contraceptives, and other hypercoagulation conditions; and low-flow states such as hypotension, congestive heart failure, and cardiac arrhythmias. The pattern of involvement generally follows the distribution of a major artery and is the clue to

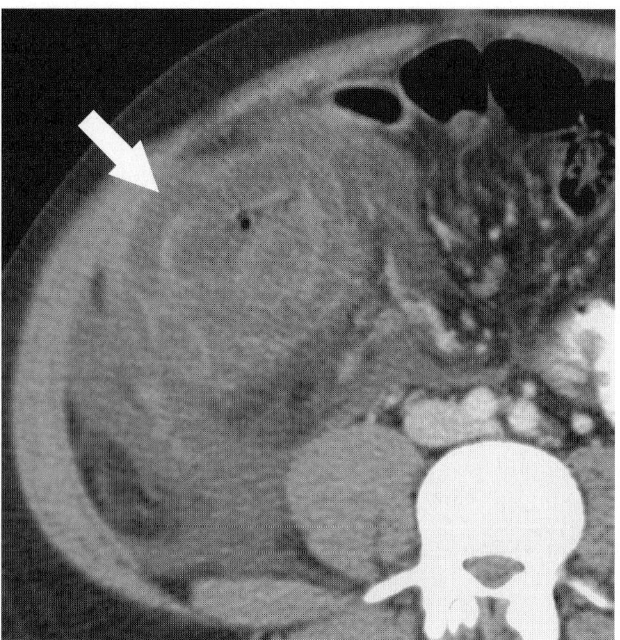

FIGURE 32.19. **Typhilitis.** The wall of the cecum (*arrow*) is markedly thickened and edematous, demonstrating the target sign. The pericecal fat is infiltrated with fluid. The mucosa enhances weakly, indicating ischemia. This patient was neutropenic because of chemotherapy.

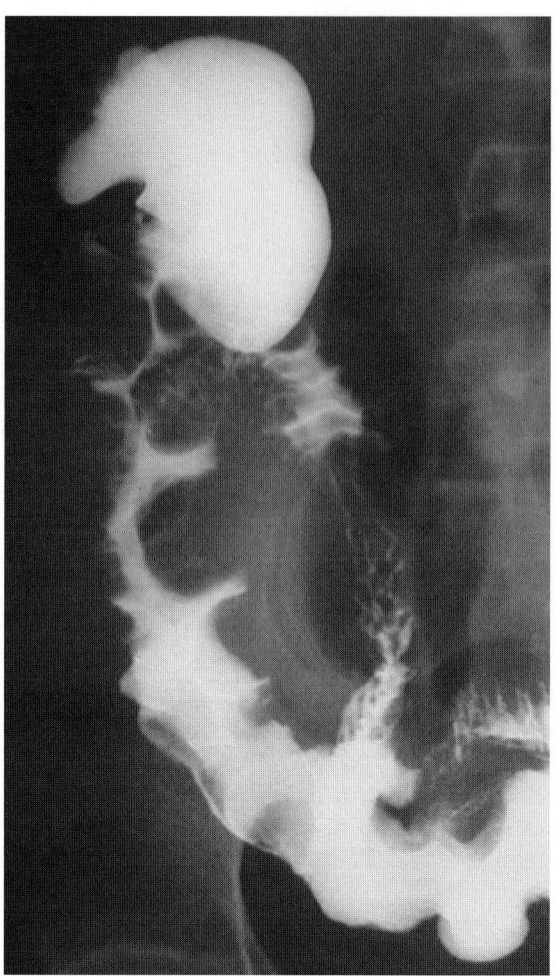

FIGURE 32.20. **Ischemic Colitis.** Double-contrast barium enema shows thumbprinting pattern (*arrows*) involving the proximal portion of a redundant transverse colon (T). H, hepatic flexure.

diagnosis. The superior mesenteric artery supplies the right colon from the cecum to the splenic flexure. The inferior mesenteric artery supplies the left colon from the splenic flexure to the rectum. The splenic flexure region and descending colon are watershed areas and most susceptible to ischemic colitis. Early changes include thickening of the colon wall, spasm, and spiculation. As blood and edema accumulate within the bowel wall, multiple nodular defects are produced in a pattern called "thumbprinting" (Fig. 32.20). Progression of the disease results in ulcerations, perforation, scarring, and strictures. CT demonstrates symmetric or lobulated thickening of the bowel wall, with an irregularly narrowed lumen. Submucosal edema may produce a low-density ring bordering on the lumen (target sign). Air in the abnormal bowel wall (pneumatosis) is highly suggestive of ischemia. Thrombus may occasionally be demonstrated within the superior mesenteric artery or vein.

AIDS-associated colitis occurs most commonly in AIDS patients with CD4 lymphocyte counts below 200. Causative organisms are most commonly Cytomegalovirus or *Cryptosporidium,* although HIV itself may cause ulceration and colitis. Right colon disease is most common, with wall thickening and ulceration.

Radiation colitis may be indistinguishable radiographically from early ulcerative colitis. The diagnosis is made by confirmation that the involved colon is within an irradiation field. The rectosigmoid region is most commonly involved, owing to radiation of pelvic malignancy. Colitis is produced by a slowly progressive endarteritis that causes ischemia and fibrosis. Radiographic findings include thickened folds, spiculation, ulceration, stricture, and occasionally fistula formation. Fibrosis results in a rigid, featureless bowel. Healing may include formation of pseudopolyps and postinflammatory polyps.

Cathartic colon is caused by chronic irritation of the mucosa by laxatives, including castor oil, bisacodyl, and senna. The involved colon may be dilated and without haustra, or narrowed. The right colon is most commonly affected. Bizarre contractions are often observed. The diagnosis is made by clinical history.

Diverticular Disease

Colon diverticulosis is an acquired condition in which the mucosa and muscularis mucosae herniate through the muscularis propria of the colon wall, producing a saccular outpouching. Colon diverticula are classified as false diverticula because the sacs lack all of the elements of the normal colon wall. The condition is rare in those younger than 25 but becomes more common with age thereafter to affect 50% of the population over age 75. The major risk factor for diverticulosis is a low-residue diet. The condition is very uncommon in cultures where a high-residue diet is the norm, such as African native populations. The formation of diverticular sacs is usually associated with thickening of the muscularis propria, including both the circular muscle and the taenia coli. Severely affected portions of bowel are usually shortened in length, resulting in crowding of the thickened circular muscle bundles. Muscle dysfunction associated with diverticulosis may result in pain and tenderness without evidence of inflammation. Diverticulosis without diverticulitis is a cause of painless colonic bleeding that may be brisk and life threatening. Plain abdominal radiographs demonstrate diverticula as gas-filled sacs parallel to the lumen of the colon. Barium studies show diverticula as barium or gas-filled sacs outside the colon lumen. Sacs vary in size from tiny spikes to 2 cm in diameter. Most are 5 to 10 mm in diameter. They may occur anywhere in the colon but are most common and usually most numerous in the sigmoid colon. Some sacs are reducible and may disappear with complete filling of the lumen. Others may contain fecal residue. The associated muscle abnormality is seen as thickening and crowding of the circular muscle bands with spasm and spiked irregular outline of the lumen. CT demonstrates the muscle hypertrophy as a thickened colon wall and distorted luminal contour. The diverticula are shown as well-defined gas-, fluid-, or contrast-filled sacs outside the lumen (Fig. 32.21).

Diverticulitis is inflammation of diverticula, usually with perforation and intramural or localized pericolic abscess (12). Diverticulitis eventually complicates approximately 20% of the cases of diverticulosis. Clinical signs include painful mass, localized peritoneal inflammation, fever, and leukocytosis. Complications of diverticulitis include bowel obstruction, bleeding, peritonitis, and sinus tract and fistula formation. Diverticulitis is a less common cause of colon obstruction than is colon carcinoma. Obstruction caused by diverticulitis is often temporarily relieved by smooth muscle relaxants such as glucagon. Colon bleeding is more often associated with diverticulosis than diverticulitis. Most diverticular abscesses are quickly walled off and confined, but free perforation with pus and air in the peritoneal cavity and diffuse peritonitis may occur. Sinus tracts may lead to larger abscess cavities in the peritoneal or retroperitoneal compartments. Fistulas are most common to the bladder (Fig. 32.22), vagina, or skin, but they may develop to any lower abdominal organ, including fallopian tubes, small bowel, and other parts of the colon. Diverticulitis of the right colon may

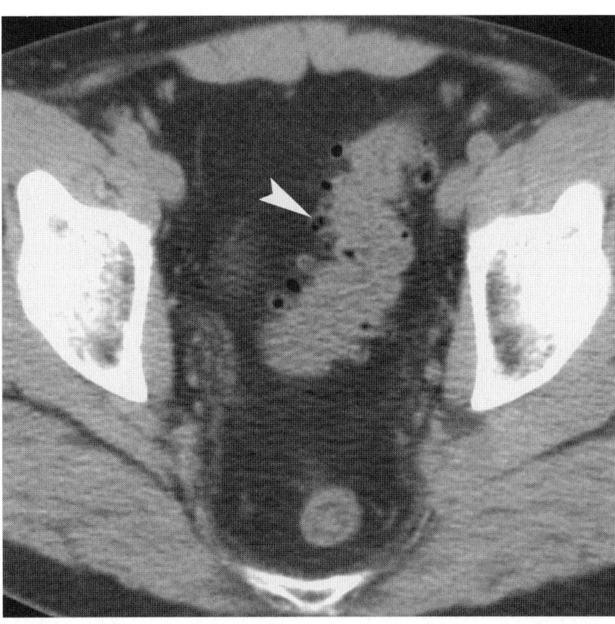

FIGURE 32.21. **Diverticulosis.** A noncontrast CT scan demonstrates air-filled outpouchings (*arrowhead*), representing diverticula in the sigmoid colon. Note the absence of soft tissue stranding or fluid in the adjacent fat, indicating that no inflammation is present.

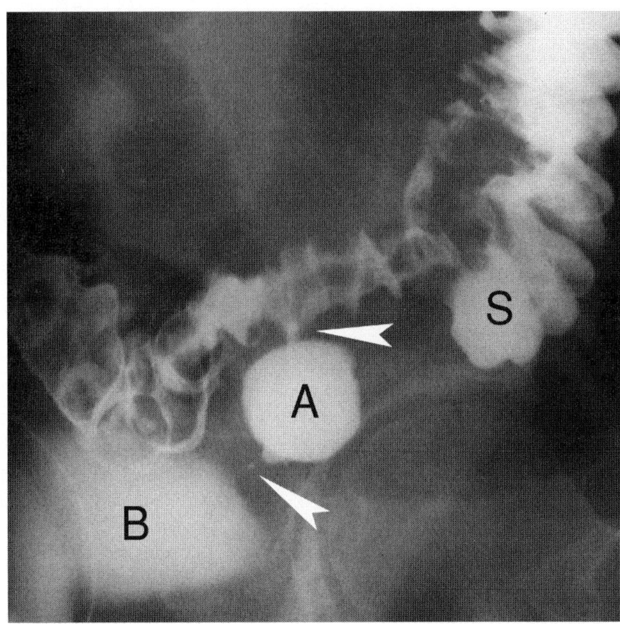

FIGURE 32.22. **Diverticular Abscess and Colovesical Fistula.** Single-contrast barium enema demonstrates barium filling a diverticular abscess (A) and opacifying the bladder (B). Thin columns of barium (*arrowheads*) outline fistulous tracts extending from the bowel lumen to abscess and from abscess to the bladder. The lumen of the sigmoid colon (S) is irregularly narrowed by the inflammatory process.

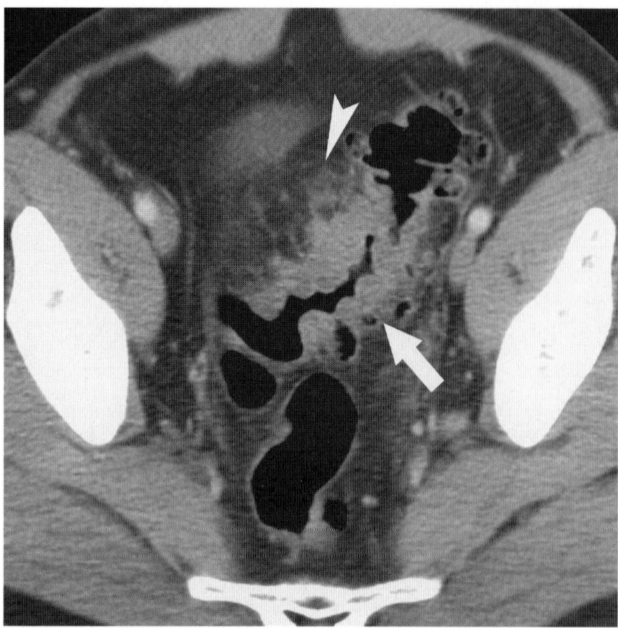

FIGURE 32.23. **Diverticulitis.** A CT scan demonstrates focal, marked thickening of the wall (*arrow*) of the sigmoid colon. Stranding into the adjacent fat (*arrowhead*) is indicative of inflammation. Because of the close resemblance of diverticulitis to colon carcinoma on CT, this patient must be followed to confirm complete resolution.

be mistaken clinically for acute appendicitis. Diverticulitis is efficiently diagnosed radiographically by barium enema or CT. Barium enema examination is considered safe, except when signs of free intraperitoneal perforation or sepsis are present. Hallmarks of diverticulitis on barium enema include deformed diverticular sacs, demonstration of abscess, and extravasation of barium outside the colon lumen. The smooth outlines of the involved sacs are deformed by inflammation and perforation. The resulting abscess causes extrinsic mass effect on the adjacent colon. The colon lumen is narrowed but tapers at the margins of narrowing, in contrast to the abrupt narrowing of carcinoma. Barium leaks into the abscess cavities or it may form tracks paralleling the colon lumen and often connecting multiple perforated sacs (the "double track" sign). CT excels at demonstrating the paracolic inflammation and abscess associated with diverticulitis, as well as complications such as colovesical fistula. CT findings are: (*1*) localized wall thickening (Fig. 32.23), (*2*) inflammation of pericolonic fat, (*3*) pericolonic abscess, and (*4*) diverticula at or near the site of inflammation.

Lower GI Hemorrhage

Although upper GI hemorrhage is usually readily diagnosed by gastric aspirate and endoscopy, lower GI hemorrhage is difficult to localize, even during surgery. The common causes of lower GI hemorrhage are listed in Table 32.2. Radionuclide imaging studies are often selected as the screening examination of choice for confirming the presence of, and often localizing, lower GI bleeding. Technetium-99m-sulfur colloid or technetium-99m-red blood cell studies are capable of detecting bleeding at rates below 0.1 mL/min. A negative scintigraphic study usually precludes the need for urgent angiography. Angiography requires bleeding rates of 0.5 mL/min or greater; however, angiography is more specific than scintigraphy in demonstrating the anatomic cause of bleeding and offers the possibility of nonoperative treatment by embolization. Colonoscopy is usually unrewarding because of the large quantities of sticky, melanotic stool. Barium enema is not used to evaluate acute hemorrhage, because it usually cannot locate the source of bleeding and will interfere with any subsequently needed angiographic procedure. Multidetector CT performed without intraluminal contrast shows promise in the detection of hemorrhage by documenting intraluminal extravasation of intravenously administered contrast (13).

TABLE 32.2 Causes of Lower GI Hemorrhage

Cause	*Percentage of Cases*
Colon diverticula	40
Angiodysplasia	17–30
Colon carcinoma	7–16
Polyps	8
Rectal trauma/fissure/hemorrhoids	7
Duodenal ulcer	Rare
Meckel diverticulum	Rare
Bowel ischemia	Rare

Angiodysplasia refers to ectasia and kinking of mucosal and submucosal veins of the colon wall. The condition results from a chronic, intermittent obstruction of the veins where they penetrate the circular muscle layer. A maze of distorted, dilated vascular channels replaces the normal mucosal structures and is separated from the bowel lumen only by a layer of epithelium. Angiodysplasia is acquired and probably related to aging. The average age of affected patients is 65 years. Bleeding is usually chronic, resulting in anemia, but may be acute and massive. Angiography demonstrates a tangle of ectatic vessels without an associated mass.

APPENDIX

Imaging Methods

Filling of the appendix is attained most reliably by single-contrast barium enema examination. The appendix is also frequently visualized on abdominal films obtained 6 to

48 hours following oral administration of barium. Failure to fill the appendix with barium on barium enema examination is not definitive evidence of appendiceal disease. Both CT and US have proven extremely useful in the diagnosis of appendiceal disease, especially acute appendicitis (14).

Anatomy

The appendix arises from the posteromedial aspect of the cecum at the junction of the taenia coli, approximately 1 to 2 cm below the ileocecal valve. The appendix is a blind-ended tube that is 5 to 10 mm in diameter (on barium studies) and approximately 8 cm in length, although it may be up to 30 cm long. Its mucosa is heavily infiltrated with lymphoid tissue. The appendix is quite variable in position: it may be pelvic, retrocecal, or retrocolic, and it can be intraperitoneal or extraperitoneal in location. The appendix always arises from the cecum on the same side as the ileocecal valve. A posterior position of the ileocecal valve indicates a posterior position of the appendix. On CT and US, the normal appendix appears as a thin-walled tube less than 6 mm in diameter (Fig. 32.24).

Acute Appendicitis

Acute appendicitis is the most common cause of acute abdomen. Frequently the clinical diagnosis is straightforward. However, patients with atypical presentations cause diagnostic problems. The most difficult patients are women of childbearing age, in whom ruptured ovarian cysts and pelvic inflammatory disease may mimic acute appendicitis. Acute appendicitis results from obstruction of the appendiceal lumen. Continued mucosal secretions cause dilation and increased intraluminal pressure that impairs venous drainage and results in mucosal ulceration. Bacterial infection causes gangrene and perforation with abscess. Most periappendiceal abscesses are walled off, but free perforation and pneumoperitoneum occasionally occur.

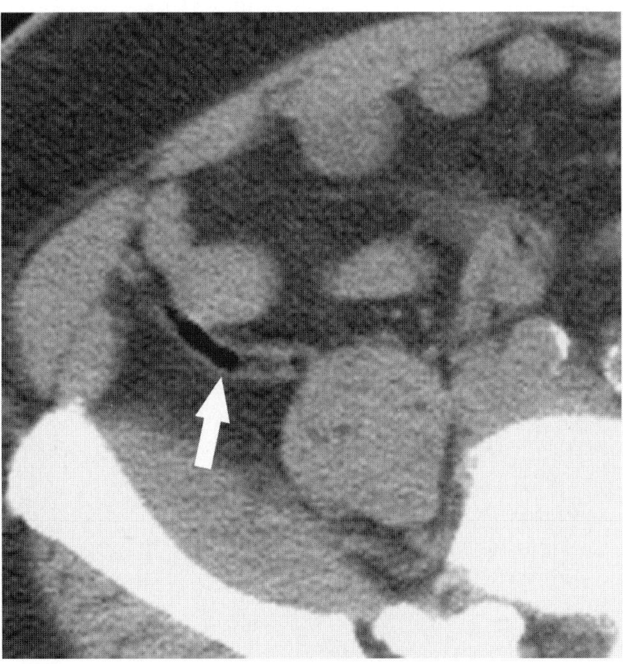

FIGURE 32.24. **Normal Appendix.** A noncontrast CT image shows a normal appendix (*arrow*) as a small gas-filled tubular structure with a blind end.

Plain films will demonstrate an appendiceal calculus (appendicolith or fecalith) in approximately 14% of patients with acute appendicitis. An appendicolith is formed by calcium deposition around a nidus of inspissated feces. The resultant calcification is usually laminated, with a radiolucent center. Appendiceal abscess or periappendiceal inflammation may result in a visible soft tissue mass in the right lower quadrant. The lumen of the cecum, as outlined by gas, will be deformed; localized ileus may be evident. Barium enema examination is frequently nonspecific. Complete filling of the appendix to its bulbous tip is strong evidence against appendicitis. However, nonfilling of the appendix, as would be expected with luminal obstruction, has no diagnostic value of its own. Mass impression on the cecum has many causes besides appendicitis.

US, using the graded compression technique, is quite accurate in providing a definitive diagnosis and is commonly the imaging technique of choice in women of childbearing age and in children. Slow graded compression is applied with a near-focus transducer to the area of maximum tenderness (14). The normal appendix has a diameter of less than 6 mm when compressed. US signs of acute appendicitis are: (*1*) a noncompressible appendix larger than 6 mm in diameter, measured outer wall to outer wall (Fig. 32.25), and (*2*) visualization of a shadowing appendicolith. With perforation, sonography demonstrates a loculated pericecal fluid collection, a discontinuous wall of the appendix, and prominent pericecal fat. When the US examination is negative for appendicitis, an alternate diagnosis can frequently be suggested based on visualized abnormalities.

CT is the imaging method of choice in men, in older patients, and when periappendiceal abscess is suspected (15). Definitive CT diagnosis of acute appendicitis is based on finding: (*1*) an abnormally dilated (>6 mm), enhancing appendix (Fig. 32.26); (*2*) enhancing appendix surrounded by inflammatory stranding or abscess; or (*3*) pericecal abscess or inflammatory mass with a calcified appendicolith (16,17). A inflammatory mass is seen as indurated soft tissue with a CT density greater than 20 H. A liquified mass less than 20 H in CT density is evidence of abscess (Fig. 32.27). Abscesses larger than 3 cm generally require

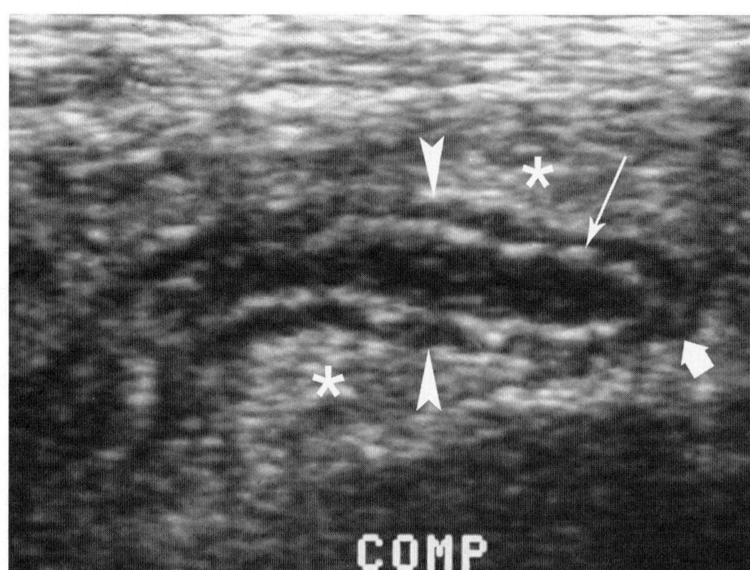

FIGURE 32.25. **Acute Appendicitis: US.** Graded compression US demonstrates a distended appendix with a diameter (between *arrowheads*) of 10 mm. The mucosal interface produces a bright echogenic line (*thin arrow*). The blunt tip (*wide arrow*) confirms identification of this tubular structure as the appendix. Inflammation of the periappendiceal fat (*asterisk*) increases its echogenicity. Surgery confirmed an acutely inflamed and focally necrotic appendix.

surgical or catheter drainage. Smaller abscesses commonly resolve on antibiotic treatment alone.

Mucocele of the Appendix

Mucocele refers to distension of all or a portion of the appendix with sterile mucus (18). The lumen is obstructed by appendicolith, foreign body, adhesions, or tumor. Some cases are caused by mucinous cystadenomas or cystadenocarcinomas of the appendix. Continued secretion of mucus produces a large (up to 15 cm), well-defined, cystic mass in the right lower quadrant (Fig. 32.28). Peripheral calcification may be present. Rupture of the mucocele may result in pseudomyxoma peritonei. Gelatinous implants spread throughout the peritoneal cavity, causing adhesions and mucinous ascites.

Appendiceal Tumors

Carcinoid is the most common tumor of the appendix, accounting for 85% of all tumors (18). The appendix is the most common location for carcinoid tumor, accounting for 60% of all carcinoids. Most occur near the tip and are round, nodular tumors up to 2.5 cm. Most are solitary

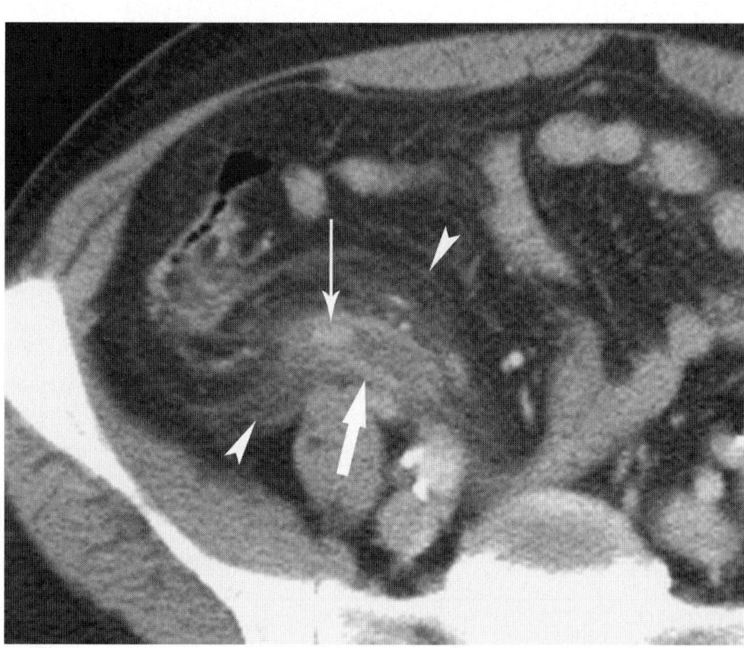

FIGURE 32.26. **Acute Appendicitis: CT.** CT image shows a dilated appendix (*wide arrow*) measuring 8 mm in diameter with irregularly thickened and indistinct walls. Marked stranding (*arrowheads*) in the periappendiceal fat is indicative of inflammation. An appendicolith (*thin arrow*) is seen in the lumen of the appendix.

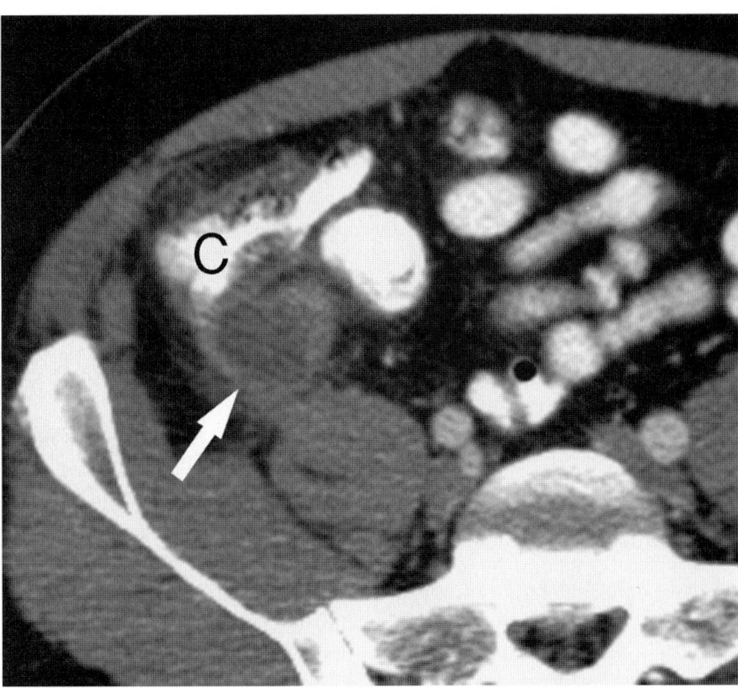

FIGURE 32.27. **Appendiceal Abscess.** CT demonstrates a thick-walled fluid collection (*arrow*) adjacent to the cecum (C). Inflammatory stranding is seen in the nearby fat. The appendix was not visualized. Surgery revealed a ruptured appendix with a focal abscess.

and have fewer tendencies to metastasize than carcinoids elsewhere in the GI tract. Carcinoid syndrome is rare, and the mesenteric reaction seen with small bowel carcinoid is usually absent.

Adenomas occur in the appendix, usually in association with familial multiple polyposis. Isolated adenomas are usually mucinous cystadenomas associated with mucocele of the appendix.

Adenocarcinoma of the appendix is rare and is usually discovered in the clinical setting of suspected appendicitis in an older adult. Imaging demonstrates a soft tissues mass within or replacing the appendix (18).

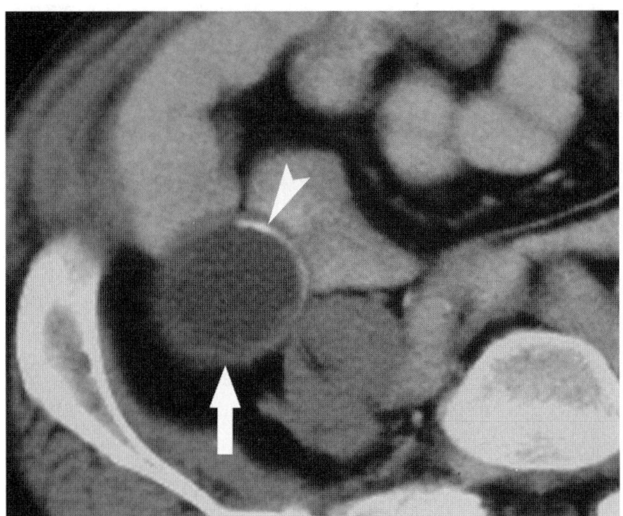

FIGURE 32.28. **Appendiceal Mucocele.** CT reveals a tubular cystic mass (*arrow*) with calcification in its wall (*arrowhead*) in the right lower quadrant of the abdomen.

REFERENCES

1. Levine MS, Rubesin SE, Laufer I, Hermlinger H. Diagnosis of colorectal neoplasms at double-contrast barium enema examinations. Radiology 2000;216:11–18.
2. Bipat S, Glas AS, Slors FJM, et al. Rectal cancer: local staging and assessment of lymph node involvement with endoluminal US, CT and MR imaging–a meta-analysis. Radiology 2004;232:773–783.
3. Macari M, Bini EJ, Jacobs SL, Lange N, Lui YW. Filling defects at CT colonography: pseudo- and diminutive lesions (the good), polyps (the bad), flat lesions, masses, and carcinomas (the ugly). Radiographics 2003;23:1073–1091.
4. Iyer RB, Silverman PM, DuBrow RA, Charnsangave C. Imaging in the diagnosis, staging, and follow-up of colorectal cancer. AJR Am J Roentgenol 2002;179:3–13.
5. Horton KM, Abrams RA, Fishman EK. Spiral CT of colon cancer: imaging features and role in management. Radiographics 2000;20:419–430.
6. Harned RK, Buck JL, Sobin LH. The hamartomatous polyposis syndromes: clinical and radiologic features. AJR Am J Roentgenol 1995;164:565–571.
7. Levy AD, Remotti HE, Thompson WM, Sobin LH, Mietten M. Gastrointestinal stromal tumors: radiologic features with pathologic correlation. Radiographics 2003;23:283–304.
8. Szucs RA, Turner MA. Gastrointestinal tract involvement by gynecologic diseases. Radiographics 1996;16:1251–1270.
9. Chen MYM, Anthony EY, Ott DJ, Scharling ES, Gelfand DW. Colitis: causes, pathology, and imaging. Radiologist 2001;8:119–128.
10. Kawamoto S, Horton KM, Fishman EK. Pseudomembranous colitis: spectrum of imaging findings with clinical and pathologic correlation. Radiographics 1999;19:887–897.
11. Balthazar EJ, Yen BC, Gordon RB. Ischemic colitis: CT evaluation of 54 cases. Radiology 1999;211:381–388.

12. Horton KM, Corl FM, Fishman EK. CT evaluation of the colon: inflammatory disease. Radiographics 2000;20:399–418.
13. Tew K, Davies RP, Jadun CK, Kew J. MDCT of acute lower gastrointestinal bleeding. AJR Am J Roentgenol 2004;182:427–430.
14. Abu-Yousef MM. Ultrasonography of the right lower quadrant. Ultrasound Q 2001;17:211–225.
15. Levine CD, Aizenstein O, Lehavi O, Blachar A. Why we miss the diagnosis of appendicitis on abdominal CT: evaluation of imaging features of appendicitis incorrectly diagnosed by CT. AJR Am J Roentgenol 2005;184:855–859.
16. Vaswani KK, Seth SK, Vitellas KM, Reader DW, et al. Normal appendix, appendicitis, and complications: CT evaluation—a practical approach and challenges for diagnostic radiologists. Radiologist 2002;9:31–45.
17. Rao PM. Technical and interpretative pitfalls of appendiceal CT imaging. AJR Am J Roentgenol 1998;171:419–425.
18. Pickhardt PJ, Levy AD, Rohrmann CA Jr, Kende AI. Primary neoplasms of the appendix: radiologic spectrum of disease with pathologic correlation. Radiographics 2003;23:645–662.

SECTION VIII

Genitourinary Tract

Chapter 33

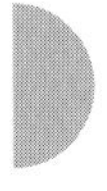

Adrenal Glands and Kidneys

William E. Brant

Adrenal Glands
Imaging Methods
Anatomy
Endocrine Syndromes
Benign Adrenal Lesions
Malignant Adrenal Lesions
Problematic Adrenal Lesions

Kidneys
Imaging Methods
Anatomy
Congenital Renal Anomalies
Solid Renal Masses
Cystic Renal Masses
Renal Cystic Disease
Renal Infections
Renal Parenchymal Disease
Nephrocalcinosis

ADRENAL GLANDS

Imaging Methods

Challenges in adrenal imaging occur in three major clinical settings. First, a patient is referred for adrenal imaging because a hormonally active adrenal tumor is suspected on a clinical basis. The role of imaging is to locate and characterize the lesion. Second, adrenal imaging is requested to evaluate for metastatic disease. Third, an adrenal mass may be incidentally detected on imaging studies performed for other indications. The significance of the finding must be assessed both radiographically and clinically. CT is usually the adrenal imaging modality of choice in adults (1). MR provides high-quality images of adrenal lesions, and chemical-shift imaging characterizes benign adrenal adenomas (2). US is excellent for screening the adrenal glands in infants and children, especially for detection of adrenal hemorrhage. Arteriography, venography, venous sampling, radionuclide imaging, and percutaneous biopsy are reserved for selected problem cases.

Anatomy

The adrenal glands are composed of an outer cortex and an inner medulla that are functionally independent and distinct. The cortex secretes steroid hormones, including cortisol, aldosterone, androgens, and estrogens. The medulla produces catecholamines.

The adrenal glands lie within the perirenal space and are surrounded by fat. The right adrenal gland is located posterior to the inferior vena cava (IVC) at the level where the IVC enters the liver. The right adrenal gland is between the right lobe of the liver and the right crus of the diaphragm, just above the upper pole of the right kidney. The left adrenal gland lies just medial and anterior to the upper pole of the left kidney, posterior to the pancreas and splenic vessels, and lateral to the left crus of the diaphragm. On cross-sectional imaging, the adrenal glands appear triangular, linear, or inverted V- or Y-shaped. Each limb is smooth in outline and uniform in thickness, with straight or concave borders. The limbs are 4 to 5 cm in length and 5 to 7 mm in thickness. The adrenal glands are of uniform soft tissue density on CT and US. On MR, the normal adrenal is hypointense, about equal to striated muscle, on T1WIs. On T2WIs, the adrenals are isointense or slightly hypointense compared with the liver and hypointense compared with the spleen. Chemical-shift MR imaging is used to demonstrate intracellular fat in benign adrenal adenomas by utilizing in-phase (IP) and out-of-phase (OP) gradient-recalled sequences (2). Intracellular fat demonstrates a loss of signal on OP images compared to IP images. Fat-saturation MR is used to demonstrate macroscopic fat seen in adrenal myelolipomas. Macroscopic fat shows a loss of signal intensity on fat-saturation images compared to pulse sequences of the same technique without fat saturation.

Adjacent structures may cause problems in adrenal imaging by mimicking adrenal masses. Tortuous splenic vessels, splenic lobulations, pancreatic projections, exophytic upper pole renal masses, portosystemic venous collaterals, retroperitoneal adenopathy, gastric diverticula, and portions of the stomach may all cause adrenal pseudotumors. Judicious use of oral and IV contrast on CT, or supplemental US or MR studies, will reveal the true nature of these conditions.

Endocrine Syndromes

Cushing syndrome is caused by excessive amounts of hydrocortisone and corticosterone released by the adrenal cortex. Clinical signs include truncal obesity, easy bruisability, generalized weakness, diabetes mellitus, and oligomenorrhea. Adrenal hyperplasia causes 70% of cases of noniatrogenic Cushing syndrome. The hyperplasia is stimulated in 90% of cases by a pituitary microadenoma that produces adrenocorticotropic hormone (ACTH). MR of the sella is recommended for suspected pituitary adenomas. In 10% of cases, the source of ACTH is ectopic, usually from lung malignancies. Benign adrenal adenomas cause 20% of cases of Cushing syndrome, and adrenal carcinoma causes the remaining 10%.

Conn syndrome, produced by elevated levels of aldosterone, causes 1% to 2% of systemic hypertension. The clinical diagnosis is made by findings of persistent hypokalemia, increased serum and urine aldosterone, and decreased renin activity in the plasma. A solitary, benign, hyperfunctioning adrenal adenoma is the cause of 80% of cases, and adrenal hyperplasia is the cause of the remaining 20%. Adenomas are treated with surgical resection, whereas hyperplasia is treated medically. Adenomas that produce Conn syndrome tend to be small (<2 cm); therefore, strict attention to excellent CT technique using thin slices is necessary for accurate localization. Adrenal venous sampling is used to confirm the site of excess aldosterone secretion and to differentiate adenoma from hyperplasia in problem cases.

Adrenogenital syndrome usually occurs in newborns and infants who have an enzyme deficiency (11β- or 22-hydroxylase), leading to deficient production of cortisol and aldosterone, and an excess of precursors, especially androgens. These infants have adrenal hyperplasia, which is usually well demonstrated by US. Both adrenal adenomas and carcinomas may be a cause of masculinizing or feminizing syndromes in older patients.

Addison disease refers to primary adrenal insufficiency, which occurs only after 90% of the adrenal cortex is destroyed. The most common cause (60% to 70%) in the United States is idiopathic atrophy, which is probably an autoimmune disorder. The adrenal glands shrink and may not be detectable with imaging methods. Additional causes include tuberculosis, histoplasmosis, infarction, disseminated fungal infection, lymphoma, and metastatic tumor. Adrenal calcification suggests prior tuberculosis or histoplasmosis. Bilateral enlargement is seen with active infection. Lymphoma and metastases replace the glands with tumor.

Pheochromocytoma is a rare tumor that causes hypertension, headaches, and tremors. Paroxysmal attacks are characteristic but not always present. Symptoms are produced by excessive secretion of catecholamines by the tumor. Pheochromocytoma is said to follow the "rule of tens": 10% are bilateral, 10% are extra-adrenal, 10% are malignant, and 10% are familial. Pheochromocytoma is associated with multiple endocrine neoplasia (MEN II), von Hippel-Lindau syndrome, and neurofibromatosis. Because 90% of pheochromocytomas arise in the adrenal medulla, the adrenal glands are usually scanned first. CT is the usual imaging method of choice. The literature has traditionally advised against the use of IV contrast media in patients with pheochromocytoma because of a presumed risk of precipitating adrenergic crisis. More recent experience indicates a high level of safety with nonionic contrast media. Most tumors are larger than 2 cm in diameter. Tumors vary from purely solid to complex to predominantly cystic (Fig. 33.1). Calcification is rare but is usually "eggshell" in configuration when present. Pheochromocytomas show poor contrast washout, similar to adrenal metastases on delayed postcontrast CT scans (3). If no lesion is found and clinical suspicion remains high, then scanning must be expanded to include the chest and remainder of the abdomen and pelvis. Extra-adrenal sites for pheochromocytoma include the organ of Zuckerkandl near the bifurcation of the

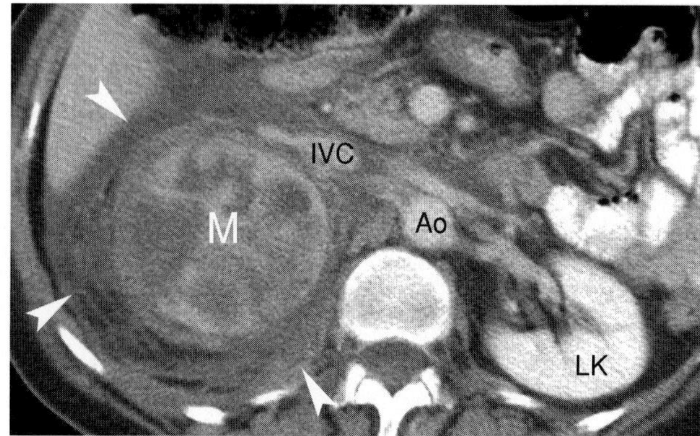

FIGURE 33.1. **Pheochromocytoma With Spontaneous Hemorrhage.** Postcontrast CT shows a heterogeneous adrenal mass (M) with hemorrhage (*arrowheads*) into the perinephric space. The inferior vena cava (IVC) is displaced anteriorly by the mass. Ao, aorta; LK, left kidney.

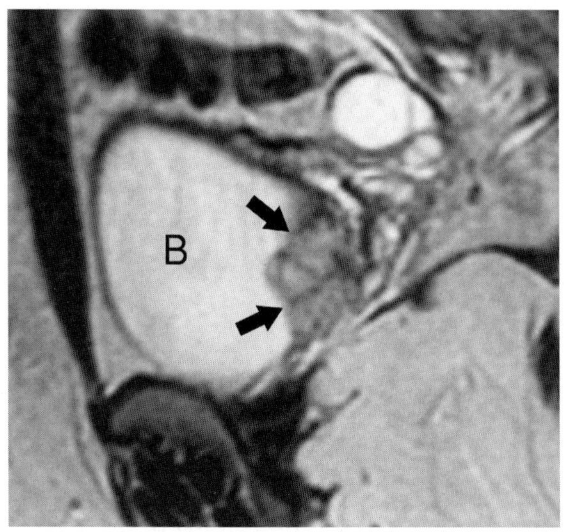

FIGURE 33.2. **Pheochromocytoma in Bladder Wall.** T2W sagittal MR image demonstrates a lobulated mass (*arrows*) in the posterior wall of the bladder (B). Surgical excision confirmed a pheochromocytoma.

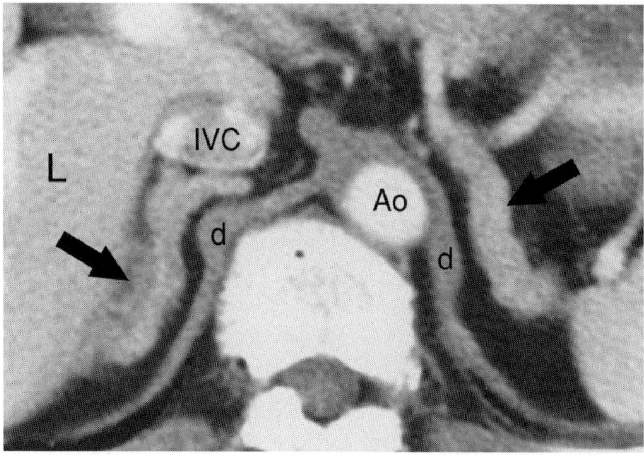

FIGURE 33.3. **Adrenal Hyperplasia.** The limbs of both adrenal glands (*arrows*) are thickened and somewhat nodular. Differential considerations include hyperplasia, metastases, and granulomatous disease. Note the anatomic landmarks for the adrenal glands: d, crura of the diaphragm; L, right lobe of the liver; IVC, inferior vena cava; Ao, aorta.

aorta, the bladder (Fig. 33.2), and the para-aortic sympathetic chain. MR may be the modality of choice to search for extra-adrenal pheochromocytoma (4). The tumor demonstrates very bright signal intensity on T2WIs that makes it stand out from surrounding structures. Tumors enhance moderately with IV contrast administration. Chemical shift MR shows no change in signal intensity between IP and OP images. Radionuclide scans using ^{131}iodine- or ^{123}iodine-metaiodobenzylquanidine (MIBG) are also effective in localizing pheochromocytoma. Atypical appearance of the tumor is relatively common on all imaging modalities (5). Pheochromocytoma is the most common adrenal tumor to hemorrhage spontaneously (Fig. 33.1).

Benign Adrenal Lesions

Adrenal hyperplasia is the cause of 70% of cases of Cushing syndrome and 20% of cases of Conn syndrome. Adrenal hyperplasia is important to differentiate from adrenal adenoma as a cause of endocrine syndromes. The syndrome is usually treated medically when hyperplasia is causative, whereas surgical removal of hyperfunctioning adrenal adenomas is usually curative. Half of the cases of biochemically hyperplastic glands will appear anatomically normal on CT and MR. In the remainder of cases, both glands will be diffusely enlarged but maintain their normal adrenal shape (Fig. 33.3). Uncommonly, hyperplasia may appear nodular and mimic solitary or multiple adenomas. In diffuse hyperplasia, the limbs of the adrenal glands are longer than 5 cm and exceed 10 mm in thickness. Chemical-shift MR occasionally shows a loss of signal on OP images. Metastatic disease, tuberculosis, and histoplasmosis may also cause diffuse adrenal enlargement and mimic the appearance of adrenal hyperplasia.

Adrenal adenomas may secrete excessive hormone and cause one of the endocrine syndromes, or they may be nonhyperfunctional and present as an unsuspected adrenal mass. Nonhyperfunctional adrenal adenomas are incidental findings in as much as 3% to 5% of the population. The function of an adenoma cannot be determined by imaging appearance but is assessed clinically or, in problem cases, by venous sampling. Patients with hyperfunctioning adenomas are cured by surgical excision. The most likely cause of an incidentally discovered adrenal mass is a benign nonhyperfunctioning adenoma. These must be differentiated from an unsuspected metastasis or a rare, small, adrenal carcinoma. Incidental discovery of an adrenal metastasis as the first manifestation of an occult primary tumor is a rare event. On CT, benign adenomas are typically small (<4 cm), well-defined, smooth, round, and homogeneous (Fig. 33.4). Because benign adenomas are rich in lipids, they tend to be low in CT density. On a nonenhanced CT scan, a measured CT density of less than 10 H is strongly predictive of benign adenoma and virtually excludes a metastatic lesion. Benign adenomas enhance homogeneously but to a variable amount with IV contrast administration. Adrenal masses cannot be adequately characterized as benign by CT attenuation values on immediate postcontrast CT. On MR, T1WIs show adenomas to be homogeneous and hypointense or isointense relative to the liver. On T2WIs, benign adenomas are usually isointense or slightly hyperintense to liver. Some adenomas are substantially hyperintense to liver on T2WIs and overlap with the appearance of adrenal metastases. Malignant

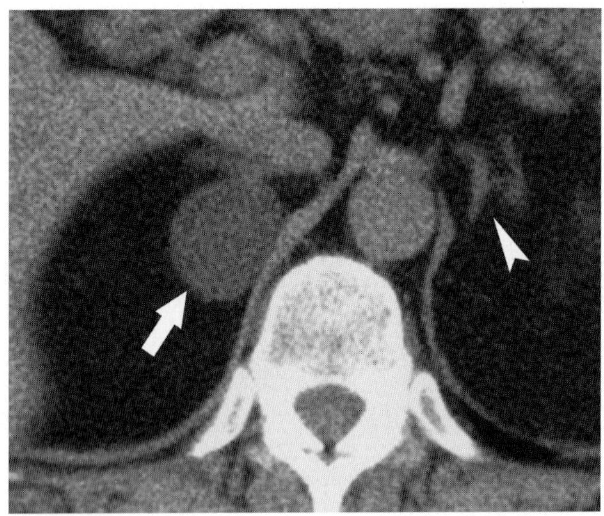

FIGURE 33.4. **Benign Adrenal Adenoma.** Noncontrast CT reveals a small homogeneous well-defined right adrenal mass (*arrow*). The attenuation of -2H is indicative of benign lipid-rich adrenal adenoma. The left adrenal gland (*arrowhead*) is normal in appearance.

lesions and pheochromocytoma tend to be very hyperintense to liver. Use of chemical-shift MR can identify the high intracellular fat content that is characteristic of benign functional adenomas (2). The US appearance parallels that of CT, with benign adenomas being small (<4 cm), well-defined, and homogeneous in echogenicity. Larger masses with heterogeneous echogenicity tend to be malignant.

Adrenal myelolipomas are rare, nonfunctioning benign tumors arising from bone marrow elements in the adrenal gland (6). The tumors have no malignant potential. They range in size up to 30 cm and are frequently inhomogeneous because of their mixed components of marrow fat and hemopoietic tissue. Calcifications are present in 20%. Identification of regions of macroscopic fat within the tumor by CT or MR is definitive in making the diagnosis (Fig. 33.5). CT attenuation under −30 H is definitive. Fat-saturation pulse sequences showing decreased signal confirm the diagnosis on MR. On US, they may be extremely echogenic and blend in with retroperitoneal fat.

Adrenal hemorrhage is most common in newborn infants, usually induced by episodes of hypoxia, birth trauma, or septicemia (7). Most cases are bilateral. In children, adrenal hemorrhage may be associated with child abuse. In adults, trauma and infection are the most common causes of adrenal hemorrhage. Unilateral hemorrhage is most common in adults, with the right adrenal most frequently affected. Bilateral hemorrhage may cause adrenal insufficiency. Hemorrhage on CT is hypodense compared with the liver and spleen on contrast-enhanced studies (Fig. 33.6). Stranding in the periadrenal fat and thickening of the adjacent fascia are additional findings.

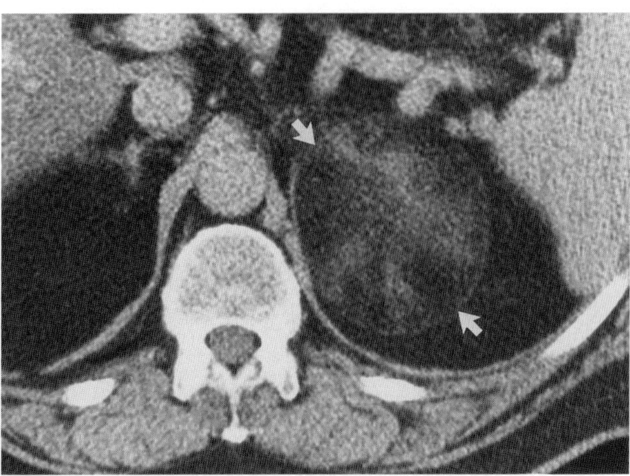

FIGURE 33.5. **Adrenal Myelolipoma.** Lesion (*between arrows*) of the left adrenal gland has large internal areas of fat density that are identical to surrounding retroperitoneal fat. Inhomogeneous attenuation is common and results from the mixture of bone marrow hemopoietic tissue with bone marrow fat.

MR is highly sensitive and specific for adrenal hemorrhage, with imaging features dependent on the age of the hemorrhage. Acute hemorrhage is isointense on T1WIs and low intensity on T2WIs. Subacute hemorrhage is bright on T1WIs and either dark or bright on T2WIs. Old hemorrhage with hemosiderin content is low signal on both T1WIs and T2WIs. US demonstrates a hypoechoic mass that shrinks and becomes less echogenic over time.

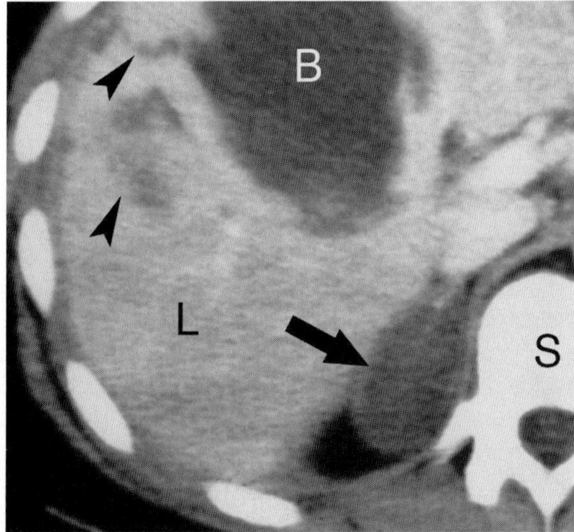

FIGURE 33.6. **Adrenal Hemorrhage.** Postcontrast CT shows posttraumatic hemorrhage (*arrow*) into the right adrenal gland. Blunt trauma to the abdomen compresses the right adrenal gland between the liver (L) and the spine (S), resulting in adrenal hemorrhage. This patient also has areas of fracture and hemorrhage (*arrowheads*) within the liver, as well as a biloma (B).

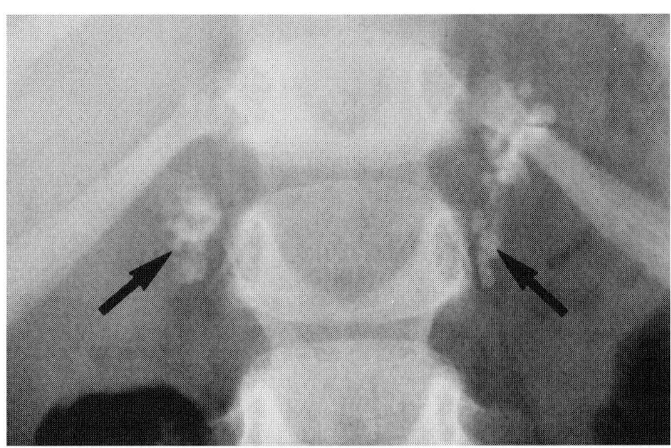

FIGURE 33.7. **Adrenal Calcification.** Plain radiograph of the abdomen in a 4-year-old child demonstrates calcification of both adrenal glands (*arrows*) resulting from bilateral adrenal hemorrhage as an infant.

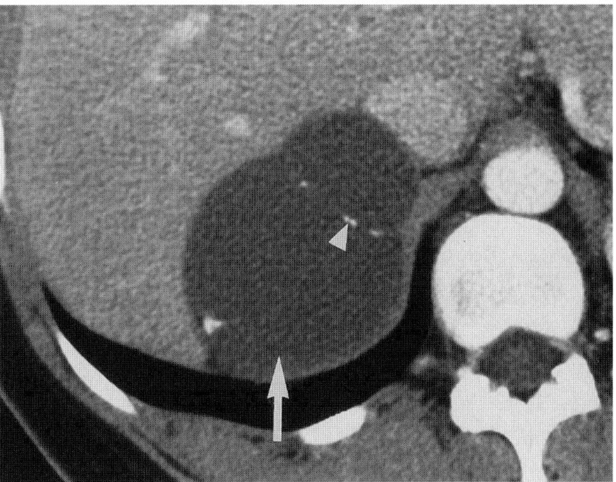

FIGURE 33.8. **Posthemorrhagic Adrenal Cyst.** CT shows a well-defined, fluid-density lesion (*arrow*) of the right adrenal gland. Calcification (*arrowhead*) is evident in the wall and in the septation.

Adrenal calcifications, in both children and adults, most commonly result from adrenal hemorrhage (Fig. 33.7). Tuberculosis and histoplasmosis may cause diffuse adrenal calcification associated with Addison disease. Adrenal tumors that calcify include neuroblastoma and ganglioneuroma in children and adrenal carcinoma, pheochromocytoma, and ganglioneuroma in adults. Adrenal pseudocysts attributable to previous hemorrhage are the most common calcified adrenal masses in adults. Wolman disease is a rare, autosomal recessive lipid disorder associated with enlarged calcified adrenal glands, hepatomegaly, and splenomegaly.

Adrenal cysts are rare lesions that usually produce no symptoms and are discovered incidentally. True cysts are lined with endothelium or epithelium. Pseudocysts have a fibrous wall without lining cells and usually result from adrenal hemorrhage or infarction. Parasitic cysts are usually echinococcal in origin. Adrenal cysts are more common in women and may be found at any age. Cysts can be classified as uncomplicated and benign when they have thin walls ($\geq$3 mm) with or without calcification, internal water density, do not exceed 5 to 6 cm, and show no internal enhancement on CT. Calcification in cyst walls and septa is a common finding in all types of cysts (Fig. 33.8). Endothelial cysts tend to be multilocular with septal calcification. Hemorrhagic pseudocysts are usually unilocular with calcification in the wall. US demonstrates thin-walled, anechoic cysts that may be septated. Uncomplicated cysts have uniform low-intensity contents on T1WIs and uniform high-intensity contents on T2WIs; they show no internal enhancement with gadolinium. Cysts that are larger than 6 cm, have thick walls or solid components, show internal contrast enhancement on CT or MR, are inhomogeneous on MR, have echogenic fluid or internal debris on US, or produce symptoms should be considered for surgical removal. These lesions may be cysts complicated by hemorrhage or may be tumors with cystic degeneration, including metastases and pheochromocytoma. Percutaneous biopsy of the cyst wall is difficult, and percutaneous aspiration of cyst fluid may not be reliable to exclude malignancy.

Malignant Adrenal Lesions

Adrenal metastases are exceedingly common, found in 27% of patients with malignant disease on autopsy series. The most common primary tumors are lung, breast, melanoma, GI, and renal. Small lesions (<3 to 4 cm) tend to be homogeneous, well-defined, and difficult to distinguish from benign, nonhyperfunctioning adenomas. To complicate the issue, even in patients with known primary malignancy, up to 50% of small adrenal masses are benign adenomas and not metastases. On CT and MR, larger lesions (>4 cm) generally show features characteristic of malignancy, including inhomogeneous density, inhomogeneous but progressive enhancement (Fig. 33.9), irregular outline, thick irregular rim, and invasion of adjacent structures.

Adrenal carcinoma is an uncommon but lethal tumor. Most are large and invasive at presentation. About half the carcinomas are hyperfunctioning and cause endocrine syndromes, most commonly Cushing syndrome, virilization, or feminization. The typical CT appearance is a large mass (4 to 20 cm) with areas of central necrosis and hemorrhage and a pattern of irregular enhancement. On delayed postcontrast CT scans, enhancement washout is significantly less than with benign adrenal adenomas and is similar to the poor washout of adrenal metastases (3). Adrenal tumors larger than 4 to 5 cm should be removed because of the significant risk of carcinoma. Calcification is present

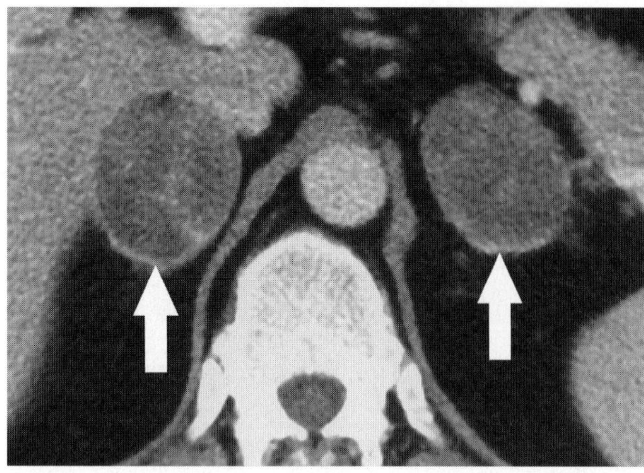

FIGURE 33.9. **Adrenal Metastases.** Contrast-enhanced CT demonstrates bilateral inhomogeneous adrenal masses. Adrenal protocol CT with delayed images showed minimal contrast washout at 15 minutes, indicating a high likelihood of malignancy. The lesions are metastases from lung carcinoma.

in 30% of the tumors. Hepatic and lymph node metastases are common. Tumor thrombus in the renal vein or IVC may be evident. Large tumors may be difficult to differentiate from hepatic masses. On MR, T1WIs demonstrate an inhomogeneous large mass that is predominantly hypointense compared with liver. Signal intensity is increased on T2WIs, especially in areas of necrosis (Fig. 33.10). Gadolinium enhancement or gradient-echo imaging is useful to detect tumor thrombus. US with Doppler is also excellent for the evaluation of tumor thrombosis.

Problematic Adrenal Lesions

Small (<4 cm), well-defined, homogeneous, uniformly enhancing adrenal masses are usually benign nonhyperfunctioning adrenal adenomas (1,8). However, small metastases to the adrenal gland may have an identical appearance. Both lesions are relatively common in patients with known malignant disease (9). Benign adenomas are common incidental imaging findings on patients studied for other reasons. Lesions with this appearance are therefore problematic.

Fortunately, both CT and MR can definitively characterize these lesions in the majority of cases. Functioning adrenal tissue concentrates cholesterol as a precursor of adrenal hormones. Approximately 70% of benign adenomas are lipid rich and contain detectable amounts of intracellular cholesterol and other lipids. These lesions are characterized as benign by CT demonstration of uniform low attenuation (<+10 H) on nonenhanced scans, or by chemical-shift MR demonstrating a distinct visual loss of signal on OP images compared to IP images (Fig. 33.11).

The remaining 30% of benign adrenal adenomas are lipid poor and do not meet these criteria. These can usually characterized by adrenal protocol contrast-enhanced CT imaging of the adrenal glands immediately following bolus IV contrast injection and at 10 to 15 minutes postinjection to demonstrate characteristic rapid washout of contrast agent (Fig. 33.12). Attenuation of the adrenal mass is measured on the immediate postcontrast images. Attenuation of the mass is then measured on the delayed postcontrast images. A relative percentage washout of >50% indicates a benign adenoma. Metastases show slow contrast washout or even an increase in attenuation on delayed images. Pheochromocytomas and adrenocortical carcinomas show enhancement loss similar to that of adrenal metastases (3). Masses that fail to meet these criteria for a benign adenoma remain indeterminate and generally undergo follow-up or biopsy, depending on the clinical circumstances. To date, contrast washout studies have only been effective utilizing CT and iodinated contrast. Washout studies using MR and gadolinium have not been proven reliable. Chemical-shift MR may characterize as benign some of the lesions that do not meet criteria for benignancy on noncontrast CT (10). Smooth enlargement or slight nodularity of the adrenal gland is not indicative of the presence of metastatic disease.

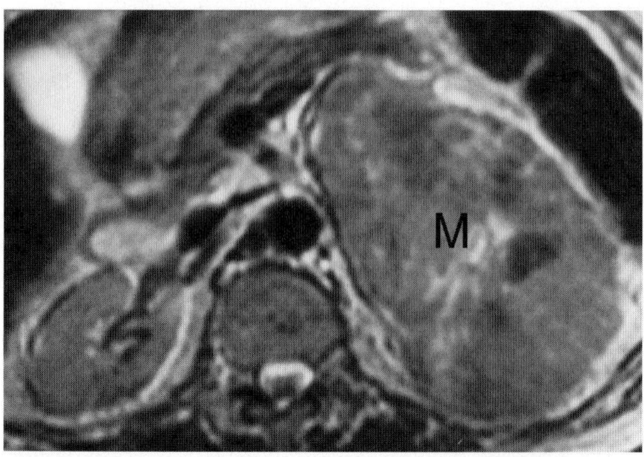

FIGURE 33.10. **Adrenal Carcinoma.** T2WI shows a huge inhomogeneous left adrenal mass (M). Areas of high and low signal intensity represent necrosis and hemorrhage.

KIDNEYS

Imaging Methods

Excretory urography (XU), also called IV pyelography (IVP), has been the traditional method of imaging the kidneys (Fig. 33.13); however, US, CT, and MR all provide better images of the renal parenchyma and have, in most practices, largely replaced XU. Multidetector CT (MDCT) with IV contrast administration is currently the best imaging study to detect and evaluate suspected

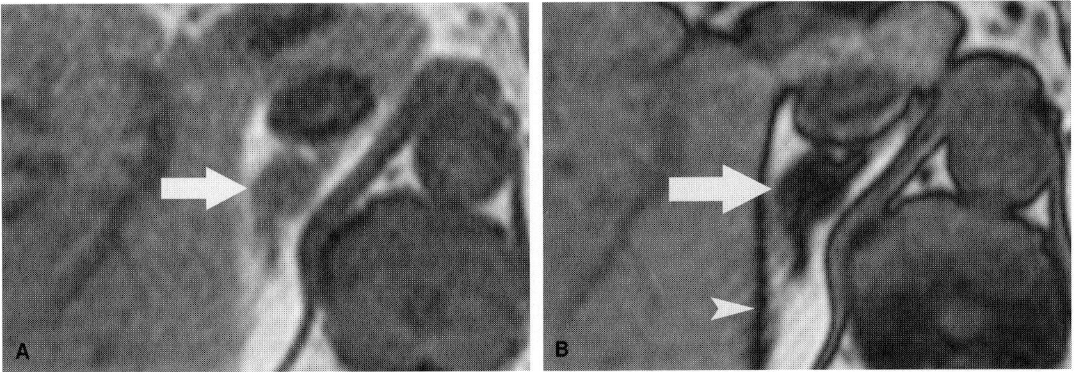

FIGURE 33.11. **Benign Lipid-Rich Adrenal Adenoma on MR.** Chemical-shift imaging is used to characterize a lipid-rich adenoma in a patient with a history of renal cell carcinoma. **A.** In-phase MR image shows a small right adrenal mass (*arrow*) with signal intensity slightly less than that of the liver. **B.** Out-of-phase MR image shows the distinct loss of signal intensity caused by intracellular fat that characterizes lipid-rich adrenal adenomas. Note the black band (*arrowhead*) at interfaces between soft tissue and fat produced by chemical-shift artifact. This finding allows immediate recognition of the out-of-phase MR image.

renal tumors. MDCT is usually performed as a multistage study using thin slices. Precontrast scans are obtained from the kidneys through the bladder to detect urinary stones and calcifications. Arterial-phase scans through the kidneys show early enhancement of renal tumors. The renal cortex enhances before the renal medulla, resulting in the characteristic *corticomedullary phase* appearance. Because the medulla is unenhanced, small medullary lesions may be missed during this phase. At approximately 120 seconds following onset of contrast injection, the renal parenchyma is normally uniformly enhanced (the *nephrogram phase* scan). A *pyelogram phase* scan at 3 to 5 minutes shows contrast filling of the collecting system and ureters. MDCT allows acquisition of thin slices that may be reformatted into three-dimensional images of the collecting systems and ureters (Fig. 33.14) mimicking an IVP but with the improved contrast resolution of CT (11). This type of study has been called a CT-IVP.

MR is a substitute for CT for patients in whom the use of IV iodinated contrast agents is contraindicated or whenever the CT study is equivocal. Multiphase post-gadolinium administration acquisitions provide images very similar to multiphase postcontrast MDCT. MR urography provides effective evaluation of the uroepithelial tissue (12). US is used primarily as a screening study to detect hydronephrosis and demonstrate kidney size. Color Doppler US is valuable in the assessment of venous involvement by renal tumors.

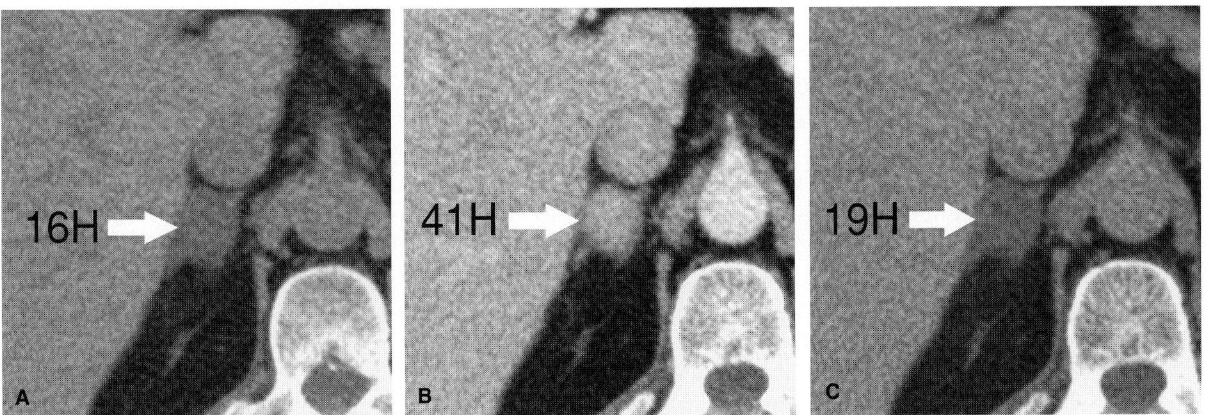

FIGURE 33.12. **Benign Lipid-Poor Adrenal Adenoma on CT. A.** Precontrast scan shows a small right adrenal mass (*arrow*) with attenuation of 16 H—too high to characterize as a lipid-rich adrenal adenoma. **B.** Image at 1 minute post-IV contrast administration shows enhancement of the lesion to 41 H. **C.** Delayed image obtained at 15 minutes postcontrast administration shows >50% enhancement loss, to 19 H. This characterizes this lesion as a lipid-poor adrenal adenoma.

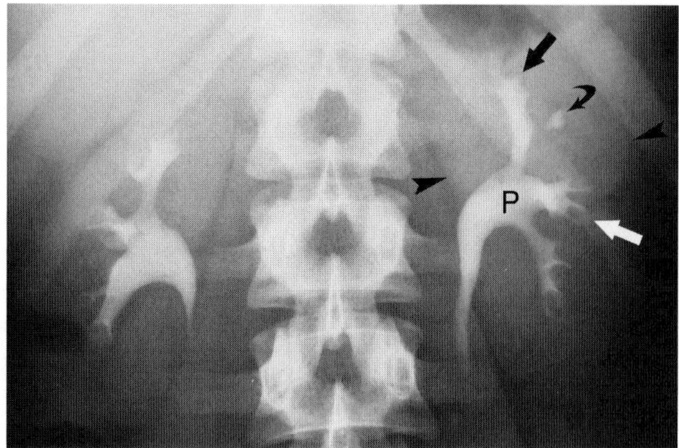

FIGURE 33.13. **Normal Excretory Urogram (IV Pyelography).** A radiograph of the kidneys taken 5 minutes after IV contrast injection demonstrates the enhanced renal parenchyma (*between arrowheads*) and the filled collecting system (P). The calyces (*white arrow*) are sharp and cup-shaped to accept the apex of the medullary pyramids. Upper-pole calyces (*black arrow*) are usually compound because of drainage of multiple pyramids. Oblique views may be needed to confirm the normal appearance of calyces oriented anteriorly or posteriorly (*curved arrow*). The normal kidney is equal in length to between three and four vertebral bodies.

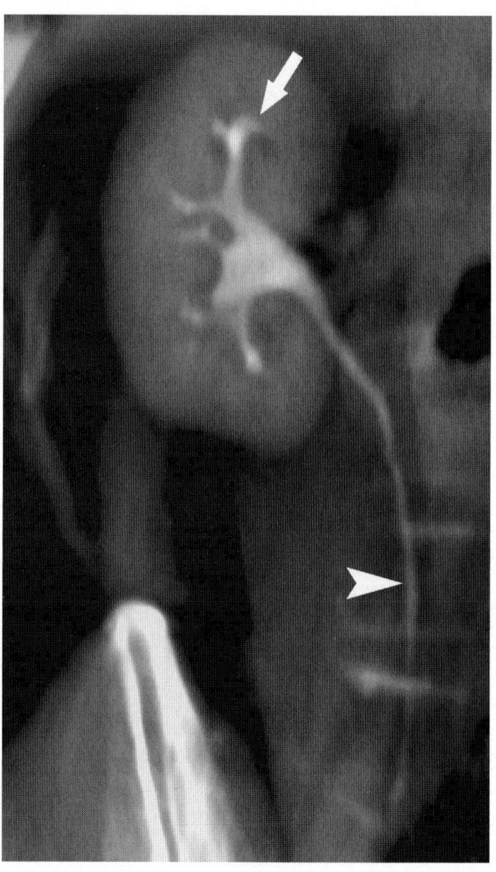

FIGURE 33.14. **CT-IVP.** Oblique coronal image reconstructed from thin axial slices obtained by multidetector CT nicely demonstrates the renal parenchyma and the ureter (*arrowhead*). The detail of the calyces (*arrow*) is not as well shown as on a traditional IV pyelogram.

Anatomy

The kidneys are located within the cone of renal fascia (Gerota fascia), surrounded by the fat of the perirenal space. The kidney is made up of lobes that consist of a pyramid-shaped medulla surrounded by cortex, except at the apex of the pyramid. The cortex consists of all the glomeruli, proximal and distal convoluted tubules, and accompanying blood vessels. The *peripheral cortex* is immediately beneath the renal capsule, and the *septal cortex* extends down between the pyramids as the columns of Bertin. A prominent intrarenal septal cortex may simulate a renal mass. The medullary pyramids consist of the collecting tubules and the long, straight portions of the loops of Henle, as well as accompanying blood vessels. The apex of each pyramid is directed at the renal sinus and projects into a calyx. The term *papilla* refers to the innermost zone of the medulla, closest to the draining calyx. The kidneys gradually increase in size from birth to age 20. Renal length is relatively stable at 9 to 13 cm from ages 20 to 50 and gradually decreases thereafter.

Simple calyces are cup-shaped structures that drain one renal lobe. Compound calyces drain several renal lobes and are more complex in shape. Compound calyces are more common at the poles of the kidney and are more prone to intrarenal reflux. The shape of each calyx is determined by the shape of the papilla. Disease of the papilla is reflected in the appearance of the calyx. The minor calyces join to form major calyces (infundibula), which drain into the renal pelvis. The appearance of the calyces and pelvis varies widely from patient to patient and often from one kidney to another, even in the same patient. About 10% of the renal collecting systems are bifid or completely duplicated.

The main renal arteries originate laterally from the aorta, just below the origin of the superior mesenteric artery. The right renal artery courses posterior to the IVC, whereas the left renal artery courses posterior to the left renal vein. The main renal artery divides into ventral and dorsal branches as it enters the renal hilum. These branches divide into segmental arteries that supply separate portions of the kidney. Each is an end artery without anastomoses. Supplied segments of the kidney are therefore highly subject to infarction caused by emboli or occlusion. Interlobar arteries arise from segmental arteries and course in the columns of Bertin. Arcuate arteries are continuations of the interlobar arteries and course parallel to the renal capsule at the corticomedullary junction. Arcuate arteries give rise to intralobular arteries. Arterial divisions down to the level of the arcuate artery are demonstrable by color Doppler US.

The tight fibrous capsule that covers the kidney produces a sharp renal margin on CT. Perirenal fat continues into the renal sinus, outlining blood vessels and the collecting system. The renal fascia is commonly visualized on CT, especially when the fascia is thickened. Connective tissue septa extending between the renal capsule and the renal fascia subdivide the perirenal space into compartments and may be seen as linear strands in the perirenal fat.

On MR, T1WIs demonstrate a high-density cortex and a lower-density medulla. With T2WIs, both the cortex and medulla brighten, but corticomedullary differentiation is often lost. The collecting systems may be difficult to visualize unless filled with urine or contrast agent.

XU will demonstrate corticomedullary differentiation when bolus contrast administration and rapid sequence filming are used. Because contrast agents are excreted by glomerular filtration, the cortex is opacified first, and then the medulla is opacified as contrast passes into the collecting tubules. A tomogram late in the nephrogram phase will demonstrate uniform enhancement of the renal parenchyma. By 5 minutes postinjection, the collecting structures and ureters should be opacified.

Because the kidneys actively concentrate contrast in the collecting tubules, renal masses seen on CT and XU will be hypodense compared with the enhanced renal parenchyma.

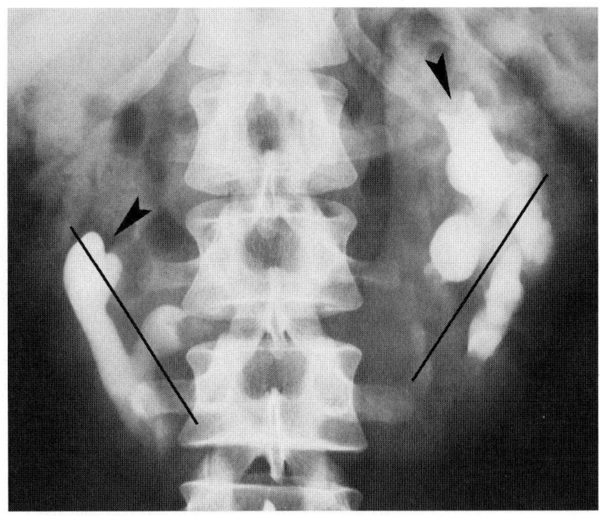

FIGURE 33.15. **Horseshoe Kidney.** Radiograph from an excretory urogram demonstrates the two kidneys extending across the spine and joined at their lower poles. Note the reversal of the long axis of each kidney (*black lines*), with the lower poles converging instead of diverging. The calyces (*arrows*) are blunted, reflecting urinary stasis created by the ureters having to cross anteriorly over the joined parenchyma.

Congenital Renal Anomalies

Renal agenesis is associated with genital tract anomalies in the female. Ipsilateral adrenal agenesis is found in 10% of cases. In the remainder, the adrenal gland may appear enlarged. Compensatory hypertrophy of the opposite kidney is usually evident.

Horseshoe kidney is the most common renal fusion anomaly. The lower poles of the kidneys are joined across the midline by a fibrous or parenchymal band. As a result of fusion, the kidneys are malrotated, with the renal pelvises directed more anteriorly and the lower pole calyces directed medially (Fig. 33.15). The fused kidney is low in position in the abdomen because normal ascent is prevented by renal tissue encountering the inferior mesenteric artery in the midline. Renal arteries are frequently multiple and ectopic in origin. Complications include increased susceptibility to trauma and urinary stasis, leading to stones and infection. The midline isthmus of the kidney is identified by cross-sectional imaging.

Crossed-fused renal ectopia may present as an abdominal mass, because both kidneys are on the same side of the abdomen (Fig. 33.16). Renal arteries are invariably aberrant. The ureters insert in their normal locations in the bladder trigone.

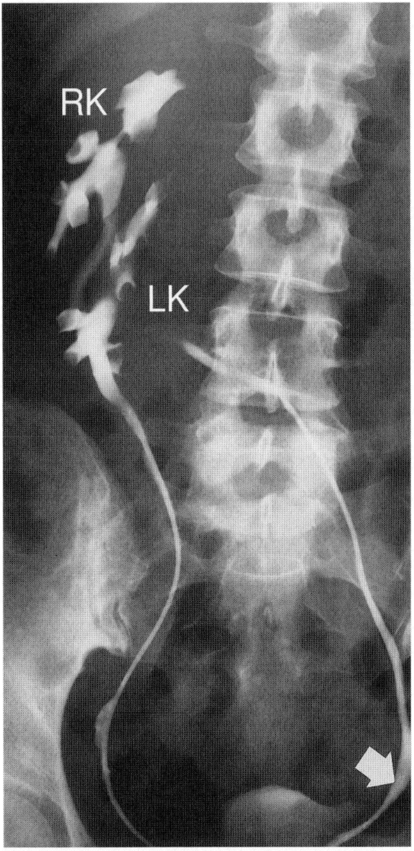

FIGURE 33.16. **Crossed-Fused Renal Ectopia.** The left kidney (LK) is ectopic on the right side of the abdomen, and its parenchyma is fused to the parenchyma of the right kidney (RK). Note that the left ureter (*arrow*) inserts normally into the bladder.

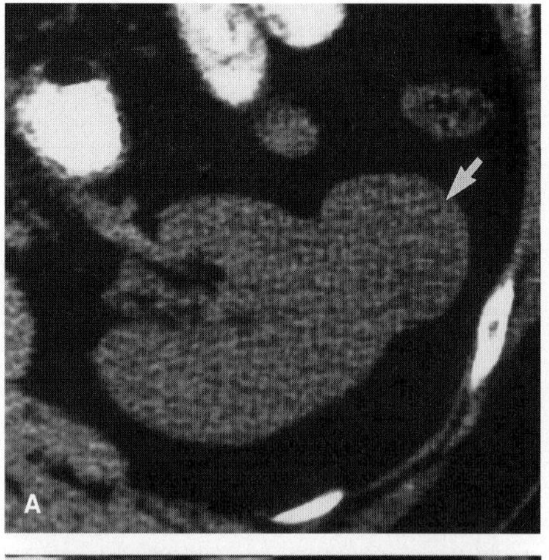

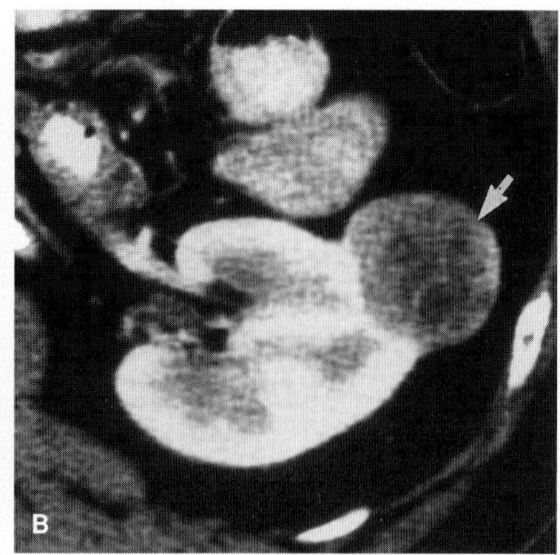

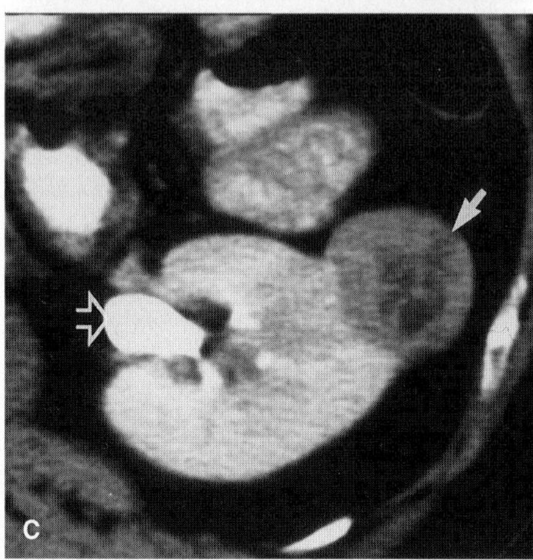

FIGURE 33.17. **Renal Cell Carcinoma.** Three-phase helical CT demonstrates a solid mass (*arrows*) with internal necrosis arising from the left kidney. **A.** Precontrast scan shows that the mass is isodense with unenhanced renal parenchyma. **B.** Cortical nephrogram phase shows early enhancement of the mass. The renal cortex is enhanced, whereas the medullary pyramids have not yet received the contrast agent. **C.** Pyelogram phase (delayed) scan shows that the mass remains hypodense to the enhanced renal parenchyma. Contrast has now opacified the collecting system (*open arrow*).

Solid Renal Masses

Renal cell carcinoma (RCC) accounts for 85% of all renal neoplasms. It is more common in men (male-to-female ratio = 3:1) aged 50 to 70 years and is bilateral in 2% of cases. Because surgical resection provides the only chance for cure, early detection and accurate staging are critically important. Treatment is radical nephrectomy with removal of the renal fascia and its contents including the kidney, adrenal gland, perinephric fat, and hilar lymph nodes. Small RCCs (<3 cm) have been treated with partial nephrectomy with good results. Any solid renal mass should be considered suspect for RCC (Fig. 33.17). Hemorrhage and necrosis are common, and cystic and multicystic forms (Fig. 33.18) are also seen (5% to 10% of cases). Stippled central or peripheral calcifications are present in 10% of cases. The tumors are commonly hypervascular, with numerous abnormal feeding vessels visualized. Tumor growth into the renal vein occurs in 30% of cases and extends into the IVC in 5% to 10% of cases (Fig. 33.19). Detection of venous invasion is critical to surgical planning. Metastases are present at diagnosis in 40% of cases. The tumor metastasizes most commonly to lung, local lymph nodes, liver, bone, adrenal glands, and the opposite kidney. Chest CT and radionuclide bone scans are effective in demonstrating distant metastases. Prognosis is directly related to the stage of the tumor at the time of diagnosis.

Contrast-enhanced CT is usually the tumor evaluation and staging method of choice (Table 33.1) (13). The tumor appears as a heterogeneously enhancing mass that is less dense than enhanced renal parenchyma. Low-density areas within the tumor reflect hemorrhage and necrosis. CT is not accurate in the differentiation of stage I and stage II tumors, but this is of limited treatment significance. Stranding densities in the perirenal fat are usually attributable to edema or fibrosis from previous inflammation and are not a reliable sign of tumor spread. Discrete soft tissue nodules in the perirenal fat are highly predictive of tumor spread into the fat. Preoperative percutaneous biopsy is indicated only when the tumor is believed to be metastatic on imaging studies. In this case, percutaneous biopsy of a metastatic lesion is usually more fruitful than biopsy of the renal tumor itself, because well-differentiated RCC may be difficult to differentiate cytologically from normal renal cells. Venous tumor thrombus is seen as a low-density filling defect within a contrast-enhanced vein that is usually enlarged.

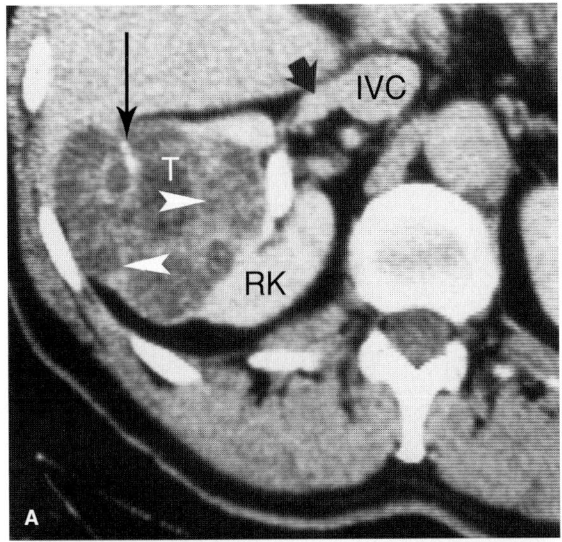

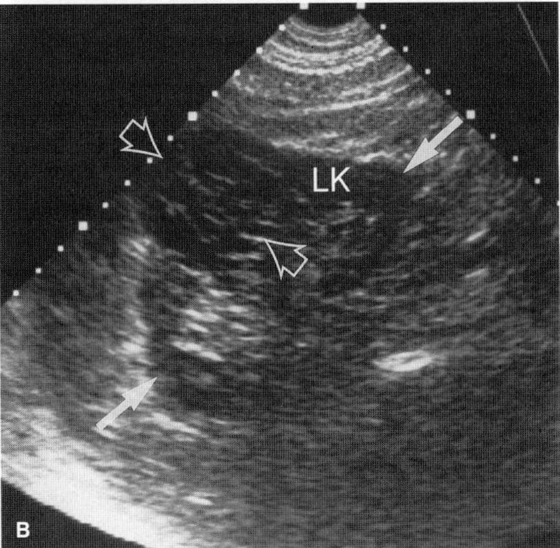

FIGURE 33.18. **Renal Cell Carcinoma: Multicystic Appearance. A.** Contrast-enhanced CT scan reveals a lobulated tumor (T) in the right kidney (RK). Septations (*arrowheads*) are evident between low-attenuation cystic areas. A focal calcification (*long black arrow*) is also present. The right renal vein (*black arrow*) and the inferior vena cava (IVC) are free of tumor thrombus. **B.** An US image in a different patient shows a multicystic mass (*between open arrows*) arising from the lateral aspect of the left kidney (LK; *between closed arrows*). The thin septations were lined by clear cells, which is typical of renal cell carcinoma.

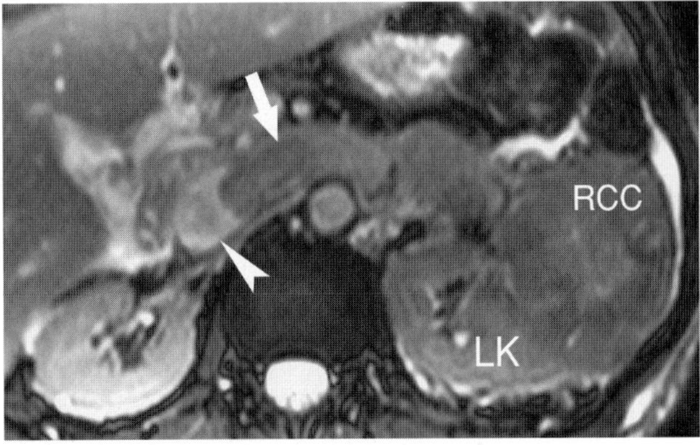

FIGURE 33.19. **Renal Cell Carcinoma: Venous Involvement.** T2WI demonstrates inhomogeneous renal cell carcinoma (RCC) in the left kidney (LK). Tumor extends through the left renal vein (*arrow*) and into the inferior vena cava (*arrowhead*).

On MR, RCC is isointense or hyperintense compared with renal parenchyma on T1WIs and shows distinct enhancement with gadolinium administration. Hyperintensity on T1WIs usually reflects tumoral hemorrhage, but fat-suppression sequences should be used to ensure the high signal is not because of fat. Most RCCs are heterogeneous on T2WIs, reflecting areas of tumor, necrosis, hemorrhage, and hemosiderin (Fig. 33.19). The staging accuracy of MR and CT is about equal. US demonstrates solid RCCs as a heterogeneous, hypoechoic or mildly hyperechoic mass. Areas of hemorrhage and necrosis appear cystic. Doppler US of the renal vein and IVC shows tumor thrombus by demonstration of echogenic material in the vein associated with partial or complete absence of blood flow. XU is insensitive to small tumors, demonstrating only about half of the 2- to 3-cm tumors that are shown by CT. Larger tumors appear as contour bulges on the renal outline, defects in the nephrogram, or areas of mottled enhancement or by the presence of calcification.

Angiomyolipoma (AML) is an uncommon (1% to 3% of renal neoplasms) benign mesenchymal tumor composed of varying amounts of fat, smooth muscle, and abnormal blood vessels lacking elastic tissue. Most (80%) are solitary unilateral tumors; they are discovered most commonly in middle-aged women. The remaining 20% are found in patients with tuberous sclerosis. These tumors are commonly multicentric and bilateral. Because of the abnormally thin-walled vessels, the tumors are prone to hemorrhage, which may be massive. Large solitary lesions are usually surgically removed. Follow-up of small lesions reveals slow growth. Imaging studies reflect the tissue composition of the tumor and can range from almost purely fat density to nearly homogeneously solid muscle density. Tumors may be as large as 20 cm and may be predominantly exophytic, mimicking nonrenal tumors. CT demonstration of even small quantities of fat density within the tumor is considered diagnostic of AML (Fig. 33.20). Thin-section MDCT is the preferred method to demonstrate fat in problem cases. Smooth muscle and vascular components of the tumor are seen as nodules and strands of soft tissue density. Vascular areas of the tumor may show striking contrast enhancement. In a few reported cases, fat has been detected in association with calcification in an RCC. In these cases, the calcification was shown histologically to be ossification with associated marrow fat. Fat density

TABLE 33.1 Staging of Renal Cell Carcinoma

Robson Stage	TNM Stage	Description	Imaging Findings
I		Confined within renal capsule	Sharp renal margin
	T1	Tumor <2.5 cm	
	T2	Tumor >2.5 cm	
II	T3a	Spread to perinephric fat but confined within the renal fascia	Poorly defined margin Discrete soft tissue nodules in perirenal fat
III-A		Tumor thrombus in veins	Enlarged vessels + intraluminal mass
	T3b	Tumor in renal vein only	
	T3c	Tumor in IVC below diaphragm	
	T4b	Tumor in IVC above diaphragm	
III-B	N1–N3	Spread to local lymph nodes	Local lymph nodes >15 mm diameter
III-C		Tumor thrombus in vein and tumor spread to local lymph nodes	Enlarged vessels + intraluminal mass Local lymph nodes 15 mm diameter
IV-A	T4a	Direct invasion of adjacent organs	Tumor invasion of adjacent organs
IV-B	M1a–M1d N4	Distant metastases	Distant metastases

Adapted from Robson CJ, Churchill BM, Anderson W. The results of radical nephrectomy for renal cell carcinoma. J Urol 1969;101:297; and American Joint Committee on Cancer. Beahrs O, ed. Manual for Staging of Cancer. 3rd ed. Philadelphia: Lippincott, 1988.

in a solid renal tumor without calcification is diagnostic of AML. US characteristically demonstrates a strikingly hyperechoic solid mass. Echogenicity of the tumor often exceeds that of renal sinus fat. Small tumors (<2 cm) are common incidental findings. On MR, T1WIs demonstrate the high signal intensity of fat, which should be confirmed by fat-suppression technique. Coronal and sagittal MR is useful in confirming the renal origin of large masses.

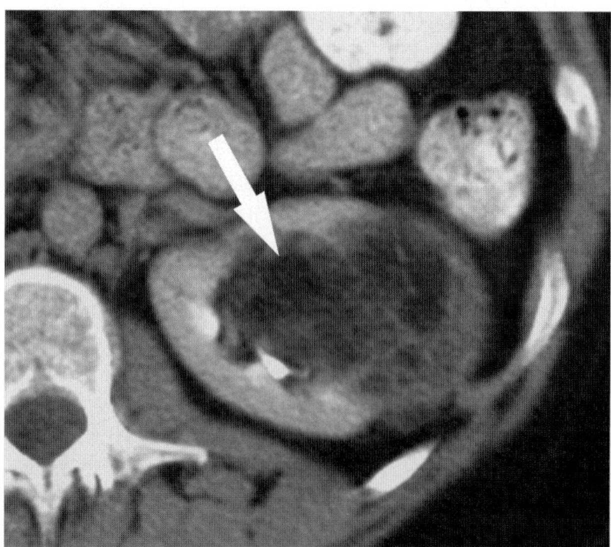

FIGURE 33.20. **Angiomyolipoma.** Postcontrast CT demonstrates a tumor infiltrating the left kidney. Areas of fat density (*arrow*) are mixed with strands and foci of soft tissue density. The appearance is characteristic of angiomyolipoma. Compare the fat-density regions within the tumor with subcutaneous and retroperitoneal fat.

Oncocytoma is a rare (3% to 6% of renal neoplasms), well-encapsulated, benign tumor composed of eosinophilic cells called oncocytes. Tumors can be large (up to 25 cm), but they average 5 to 8 cm. Hemorrhage and necrosis are rare. Most are solitary, but 6% are multiple or bilateral. Large tumors demonstrate a stellate central scar that is suggestive of the diagnosis. Angiography classically demonstrates a "spoke-wheel" configuration of radiating vessels. Most oncocytomas are indistinguishable from RCC by all imaging methods and must be surgically removed to confirm the diagnosis.

Lymphoma. Although primary renal lymphoma is rare, the kidney is commonly involved by metastatic lymphoma or by direct invasion. Most cases are non-Hodgkin lymphoma (Fig. 33.21). Patterns of renal involvement include

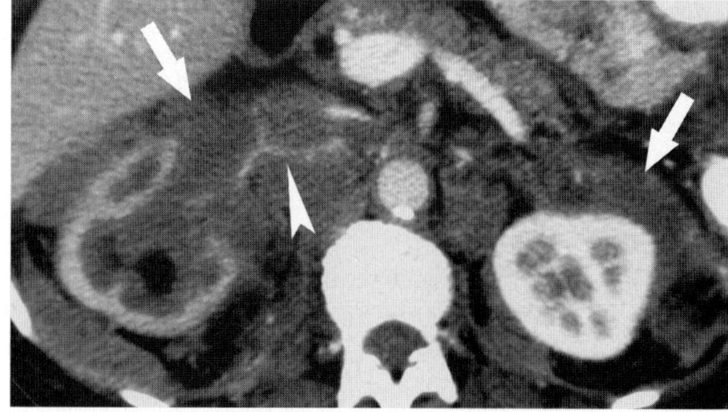

FIGURE 33.21. **Renal Lymphoma.** Non-Hodgkin lymphoma (*arrows*) infiltrates the perirenal space partially surrounding both kidneys. Note the impaired contrast enhancement of the right kidney, which is caused by lymphomatous involvement of the right renal blood vessels (*arrowheads*). The tumor infiltrates the sinus and parenchyma of the right kidney.

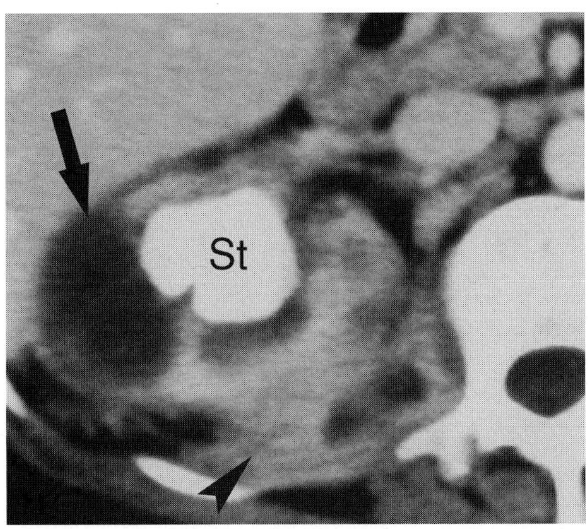

FIGURE 33.22. **Xanthogranulomatous Pyelonephritis.** Post-contrast CT shows a poorly functioning right kidney with a large obstructing stone (St) occupying the renal pelvis. A low-attenuation mass (*arrow*) replaces renal parenchyma. Inflammatory change (*arrowhead*) extends into the perirenal space.

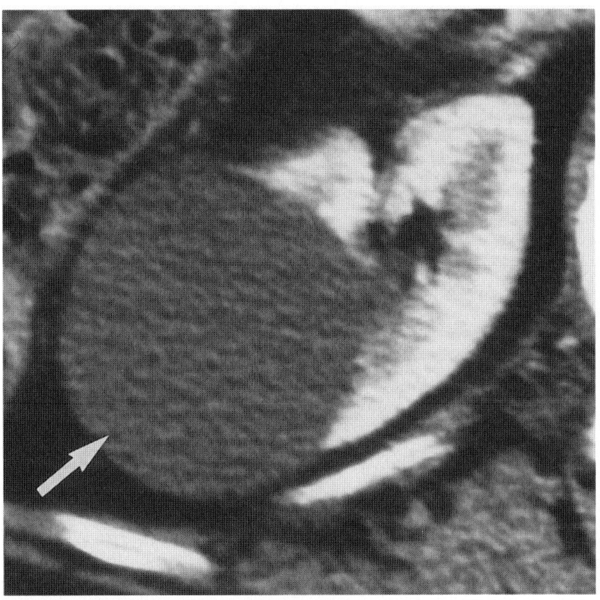

FIGURE 33.23. **Simple Renal Cyst.** A large cyst (*arrow*) arising from the right kidney shows characteristic CT features. The cyst is of uniform low density and has a sharp margin with the renal parenchyma, and its wall is imperceptible.

diffuse disease enlarging the kidney, multiple bilateral solid renal masses, solitary bulky tumor, tumor invasion into the renal sinus, and perirenal tumor surrounding the kidneys (14). CT shows lymphoma as a homogenous, round, poorly enhancing mass. Extensive retroperitoneal adenopathy favors the diagnosis.

Metastases. The kidneys are a frequent site of hematogenous metastases; however, most are detected late in the course of malignancy. Most metastases appear as multiple, bilateral, small, irregular renal masses. Some are large, solitary, and indistinguishable from RCC. Common primary tumors include lung, breast, and colon carcinoma and melanoma.

Xanthogranulomatous pyelonephritis is a rare inflammatory lesion that may diffusely involve an obstructed kidney or present as a focal renal mass. An obstructing stone, often a staghorn calculus, is usually present (Fig. 33.22). The kidney is chronically infected, most commonly with *Proteus mirabilis*, and does not function in the affected areas. The renal parenchyma is destroyed and replaced by xanthoma cells, which are lipid-laden macrophages. CT and US demonstrate focal or diffuse hydronephrosis and a complex mass with areas of high and low density.

Cystic Renal Masses

Simple renal cysts are the most common type renal mass. They are found in half the population older than age 55. Small cysts are asymptomatic. Large cysts (>4 cm) occasionally cause obstruction, pain, hematuria, or hypertension. Cysts are commonly multiple and bilateral. US, CT, and MR can each make a definitive diagnosis. US criteria for simple renal cyst are: (*1*) round or oval anechoic mass, (*2*) increased through transmission, (*3*) sharply defined far wall, and (*4*) thin or imperceptible cyst wall. CT signs include: (*1*) sharp margination with the renal parenchyma, (*2*) no perceptible wall, (*3*) homogeneous attenuation near water density (−10 to +10 H), and (*4*) absence of contrast enhancement (Fig. 33.23). MR criteria include: (*1*) homogeneous, sharply defined, round or oval mass; (*2*) homogeneous low signal intensity on T1WIs; and (*3*) homogeneous high signal intensity similar to that of urine on T2WIs. No enhancement should be seen after gadolinium administration. XU shows cysts as lucent defects in the nephrogram, with sharp round borders with the renal parenchyma. A beak or claw sign may be produced by the enhancing renal parenchyma. Findings on XU are not sufficiently specific to characterize renal masses as cysts. Sonography is the most cost-effective method to evaluate renal masses detected by XU.

Complicated Cyst. Simple renal cysts may be complicated by hemorrhage or infection. The resulting change in imaging characteristics may make differentiation from cystic renal tumors difficult (15). Bosniak developed a classification system for cystic masses that helps to categorize these problematic lesions (16).

Category I lesions are simple cysts with the imaging findings just listed. US and CT are definitive when all characteristic findings are present.

Category II lesions are benign, with no further imaging or follow-up needed. Three types of cysts are in this

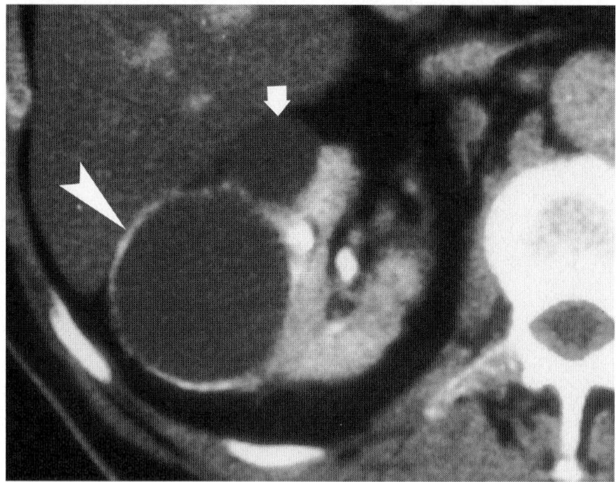

FIGURE 33.24. **Complicated Renal Cyst.** CT demonstrates a small simple renal cyst (*arrow*) and a larger renal cyst complicated by a thin rim of calcification in its wall (*arrowhead*). This larger cyst would be classified as a benign renal cyst, Bosniak category II.

category: (*1*) cysts with delicate thin septations no more than 1 to 2 mm thick, (*2*) cysts with delicate thin calcification in the wall or septum (Fig. 33.24), and (*3*) cysts that are hyperdense (60 to 100 H) on CT because of high concentration of protein or blood breakdown products and smaller than 3 cm. Larger lesions thought to be benign but with less characteristic findings are classified as category IIF lesions. Bosniak recommends imaging follow-up of IIF lesions at 3, 6, and 12 months.

Category III lesions are indeterminate lesions that may be malignant. Most should be treated surgically. Findings include thick irregular calcification, irregular margins, thick or enhancing septa, areas of nodularity, thick walls, and multilocular appearance. Lesions in this category include hemorrhagic or infected simple cysts, multilocular cystic nephroma, multiloculated cysts, and cystic forms of RCC.

Category IV lesions are necrotic cystic neoplasms or tumors that arise in the wall of a cyst. Findings include irregular solid nodules, irregular thick shaggy walls, and septa with contrast enhancement of solid areas.

Small renal lesions may be particularly difficult to classify. Thin-section CT with bolus contrast enhancement and great attention to detail will assist in correct classification of lesions. MR signal intensity depends on the amount of blood or proteinaceous material present within the cyst. Cyst fluid with signal characteristics similar to those of urine suggests a simple cyst. Higher signal intensity on T1WIs suggests a complicated cyst, which may be indistinguishable from a solid mass.

Renal abscess usually results from pyelonephritis complicated by liquefactive necrosis. A focal renal mass with a thick wall is the most common appearance. Associated inflammatory changes include stranding densities in the perirenal space and thickening of the renal fascia (Fig. 33.25). Renal abscesses may extend into the perirenal space and demonstrate an associated perirenal fluid collection.

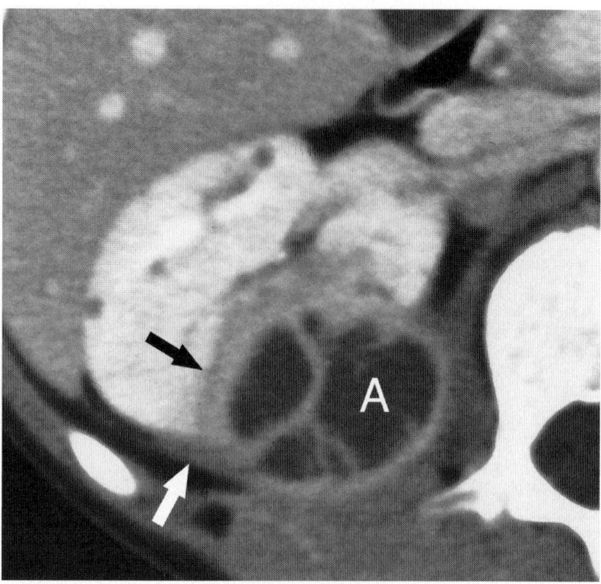

FIGURE 33.25. **Renal Abscess.** The right renal abscess (A) has characteristic thick walls and septations and internal fluid density. Edema reduces the CT density of the renal parenchyma adjacent to the mass (*black arrow*) and infiltrates the perirenal space (*white arrow*). This patient also has multiple small renal cysts caused by autosomal dominant polycystic disease.

Renal cell carcinoma may appear as a predominantly cystic or multiloculated cystic mass. Malignant tumor cells line the walls and septa. Thick walls, thick septations, and contrast enhancement are usually evident.

Multilocular cystic nephroma is an uncommon benign neoplasm consisting of a cluster of noncommunicating cysts of varying size, separated by connective tissue septations. The tumor has a thick capsule with thin septations. They are discovered most commonly in male infants and children (<4 years) and middle-aged women (40 to 60 years). Surgical excision is usually recommended in adults to exclude RCC.

Renal Cystic Disease

Autosomal dominant polycystic disease is transmitted by autosomal dominant inheritance but usually manifests clinically later in life. Renal parenchyma is progressively replaced by multiple noncommunicating cysts of varying size (Fig. 33.26). Renal volume increases with the number and size of the renal cysts. The cysts are commonly complicated by internal hemorrhage. The condition can

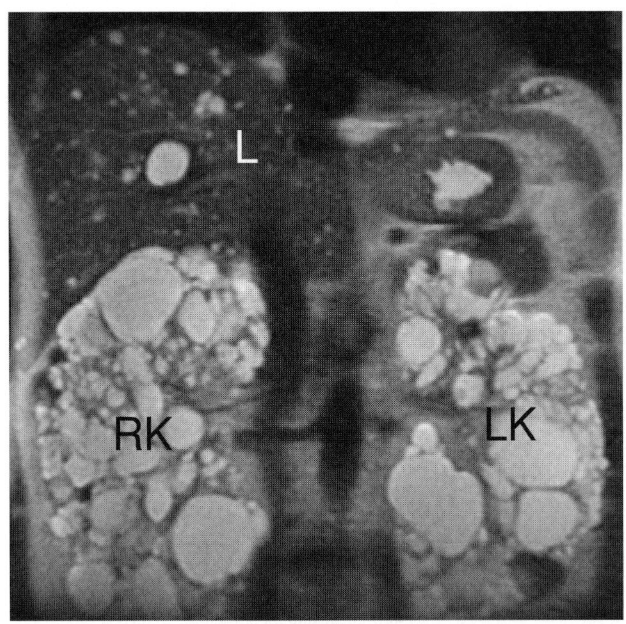

FIGURE 33.26. **Autosomal Dominant Polycystic Disease.** Coronal T2WI shows extensive replacement of the renal parenchyma with innumerable cysts of various sizes. Cysts are also seen in the liver (L). Both kidneys (RK, LK) are massively enlarged.

be detected in neonates and children, but most patients present clinically between ages 30 and 50 years with hypertension and renal failure. Imaging diagnosis is confirmed by demonstration of cysts in the liver (60% of patients), pancreas (10% of patients), and often other organs. Extrarenal cysts seldom cause clinical problems. Associated cardiovascular abnormalities include intracranial aneurysms (20% of patients), mitral valve prolapse, bicuspid aortic valve, aortic aneurysms, and aortic dissections.

Multiple simple cysts must be differentiated from adult polycystic disease. Patients with multiple simple cysts are usually older and have fewer cysts, usually no renal failure, and no family history of renal cystic disease. Cysts are not found in other organs.

Von Hippel-Lindau disease is associated with multiple renal and pancreatic cysts, pheochromocytomas, and frequently multiple and bilateral RCCs (24% to 45% of patients). Associated lesions include retinal angiomas and cerebellar hemangioblastomas. The disease is inherited with an autosomal dominant pattern that is not expressed in every individual with the gene (17).

Tuberous sclerosis combines multiple renal cysts and multiple AMLs. Cutaneous, retinal, and cerebral hamartomas are associated. This condition also has an autosomal dominant inheritance pattern.

Acquired uremic cystic kidney disease is the term applied to the development of multiple cysts in the native kidneys of patients on long-term hemodialysis. Affected

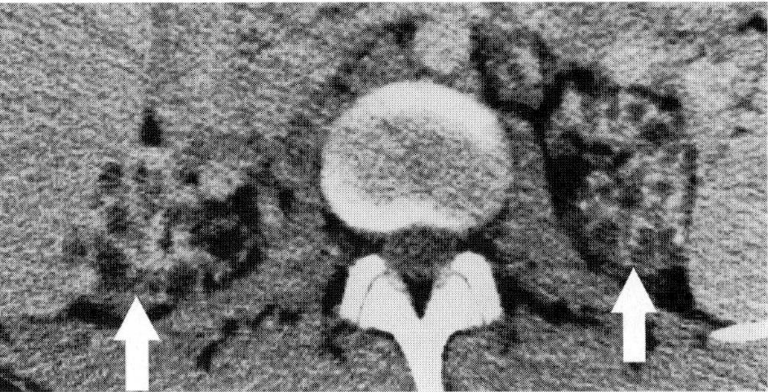

FIGURE 33.27. **Acquired Uremic Cystic Kidney Disease.** Noncontrast CT reveals that both kidneys (*arrows*) are small and contain numerous small cysts. The patient has been on hemodialysis for 8 years.

kidneys are usually small, reflecting the chronic renal disease. Cysts are predominantly cortical and rarely exceed 2 cm (Fig. 33.27). Solid renal adenomas and RCCs (7%) also develop and are prone to spontaneous hemorrhage.

Autosomal recessive polycystic kidney disease usually presents in the neonate and is detectable in the fetus. The condition is bilateral, relatively symmetric, and characterized by marked enlargement of the kidneys and occasionally the liver. Affected patients have a combination of cystic renal disease and hepatic fibrosis. The disease runs a spectrum from severe renal disease at birth (infantile polycystic disease) to relatively mild renal disease with development of hepatic fibrosis and liver failure in childhood (juvenile polycystic disease). The primary defect in the kidneys is diffuse dilatation of the collecting tubules (Fig. 33.28). Early prognosis depends on the number of abnormal nephrons. Most infants who present

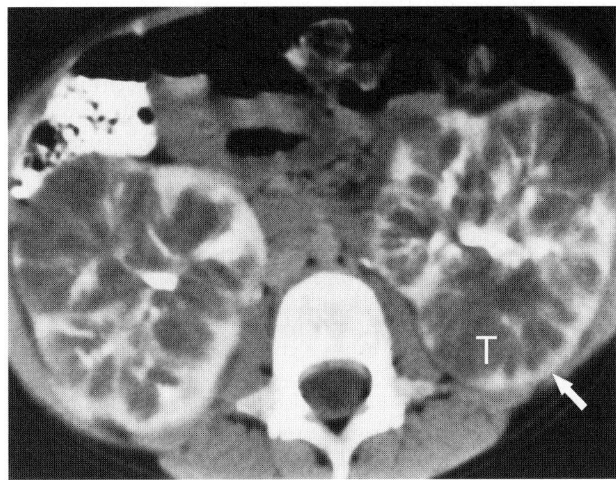

FIGURE 33.28. **Autosomal Recessive Polycystic Disease.** Contrast-enhanced CT in a 5-year-old child shows massive kidneys. The enhanced cortex (*arrow*) is thinned, and nonenhanced collecting tubules (T) in the medulla are enlarged. No discrete cysts are evident.

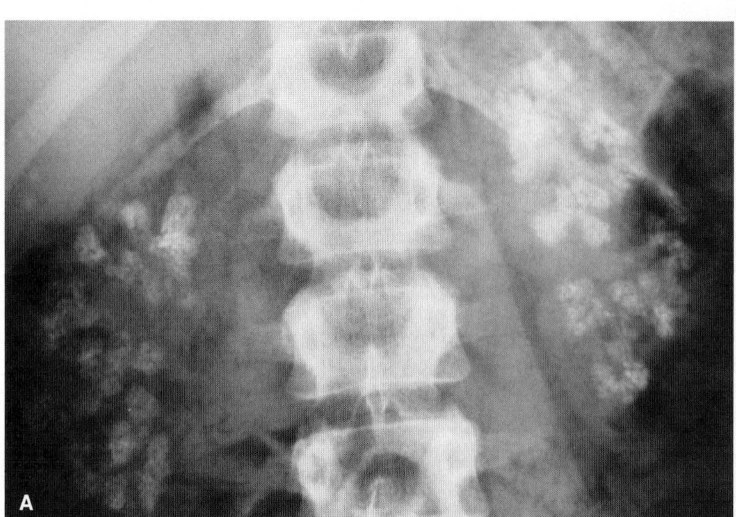

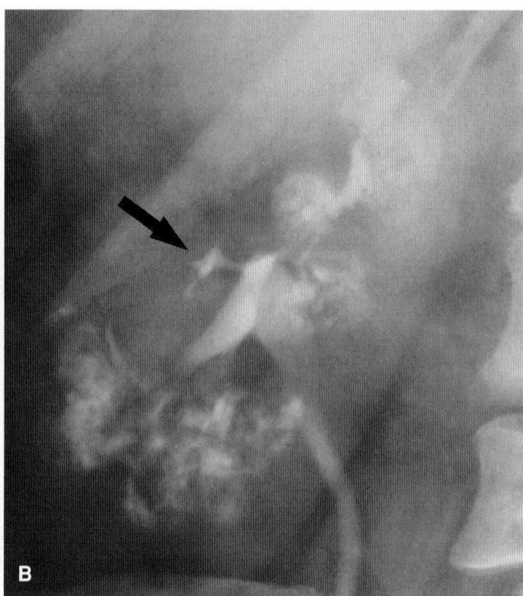

FIGURE 33.29. **Nephrocalcinosis and Medullary Sponge Kidney. A.** Plain radiograph demonstrates innumerable calcifications in the medullary regions of both kidneys. The stones form in the dilated collecting tubules in the medullary pyramids. **B.** Image from an excretory urogram in another patient shows the cystic and tubular dilatation of the collecting tubules that is characteristic of medullary sponge kidney. Stasis within the abnormal tubules leads to stone formation and predisposition to infection. Note that not all medullary pyramids (*arrow*) are affected—another characteristic feature of medullary sponge kidney.

in renal failure die in the neonatal period. Infants with a larger number of normal nephrons have mild renal impairment and present at age 3 to 5 years with progressive liver failure and portal hypertension. US is used to make the diagnosis in most cases. Both kidneys are large and echogenic centrally, with a sonolucent rim of compressed cortex. Visualized cysts are generally small (<5 mm). Children with less severe renal disease develop larger cysts. US shows an enlarged, echogenic liver with splenomegaly, dilated portal vein, and enlarged portosystemic collateral vessels in the older children who develop liver disease.

Medullary sponge kidney refers to dysplastic dilatation of the collecting tubules in the papilla (Fig. 33.29). The dilatation is cylindric or saccular in configuration. The condition causes urinary stasis in the papilla, which results in stone formation and occasionally infection. Most patients are asymptomatic. There is no genetic predisposition and no risk of renal failure. The kidneys remain normal in size. The condition is usually bilateral and symmetric but may be focal, unilateral, or asymmetric. Striations or saccular contrast collections in the papilla on excretory urography are most characteristic. Stones in the papilla cause increased echogenicity in the medulla on US.

Uremic medullary cystic disease presents with renal failure, anemia, and salt wasting. The basic defect is progressive tubular atrophy with glomerular sclerosis and formation of medullary cysts. The medullary cysts are generally too small to be visualized by current imaging methods. Kidney size is normal or small. Renal parenchymal echogenicity is usually increased.

Multicystic dysplastic kidney is usually diagnosed in utero or at birth. The classic multicystic dysplastic kidney appears as a mass of noncommunicating cysts of varying size. With time, the kidney progressively atrophies, so in the adult a nubbin of tissue, which is often calcified, is all that remains. The ureter is commonly atretic.

Renal Infections

Acute pyelonephritis is usually the result of ascending urinary tract infection caused by gram-negative organisms, especially *Escherichia coli*. Uncomplicated infection requires no imaging and often shows no imaging abnormalities. Imaging evaluation is indicated in patients who fail to respond to treatment or are severely ill. CT is more sensitive than US in demonstrating subtle changes in the renal parenchyma associated with uncomplicated pyelonephritis. Complications such as renal or perirenal abscess are well demonstrated by CT or US. Predisposing factors include diabetes, obstruction, immune system compromise, drug abuse, chronic debilitating disease, and incomplete antibiotic treatment. CT is normal in some patients with mild uncomplicated pyelonephritis. In most patients, edema causes diffuse or focal swelling. Areas of high attenuation on precontrast scans suggest hemorrhagic inflammation. Contrast enhancement reveals

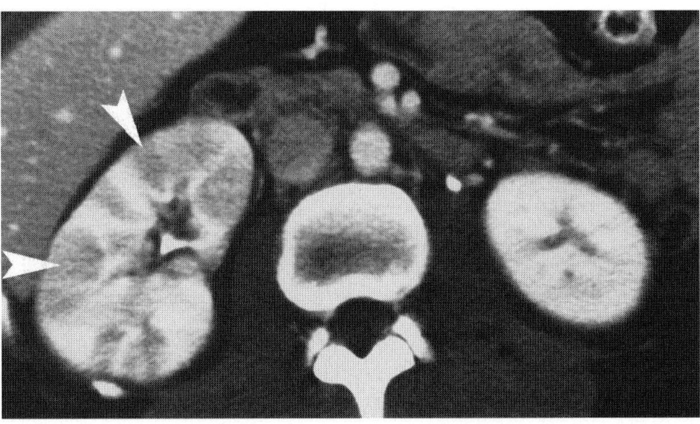

FIGURE 33.30. **Acute Pyelonephritis.** Edema and swelling associated with acute renal infection cause wedge-shaped defects (*arrowheads*) in the enhanced parenchyma of the right kidney. The left kidney is normal.

streaks and wedges of low attenuation extending to the renal capsule (Fig. 33.30), often associated with thickened septa in perinephric fat and thickening of the Gerota fascia. Inflammatory low-density masses may form in the renal parenchyma. A variety of confusing terms, including "lobar nephronia" and "focal bacterial nephritis," have been applied to these masses. The Society of Uroradiology recommends abandoning these terms and using only the terms "acute pyelonephritis" with or without "focal, multifocal, or diffuse swelling." Complications of acute pyelonephritis include intrarenal (Fig. 33.25) and perirenal abscess (Fig. 33.31).

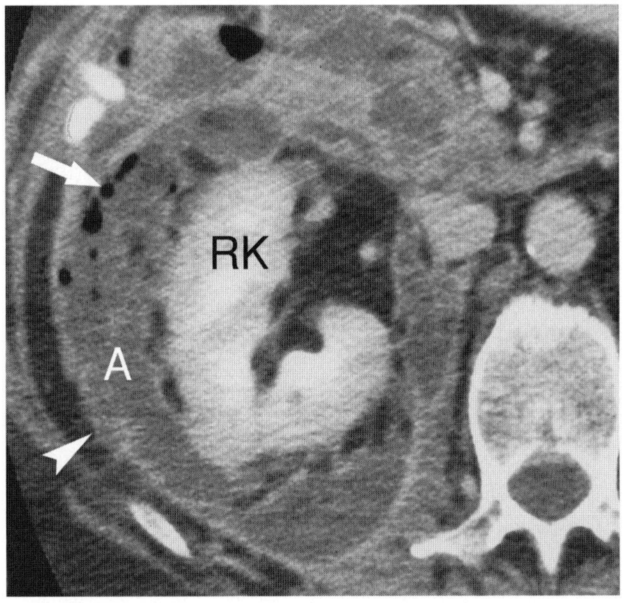

FIGURE 33.31. **Perirenal Abscess.** Contrast-enhanced CT scan discloses a low-density fluid collection (A) in the perirenal space between the right kidney (RK) and the thickened renal fascia (*arrowhead*). Gas bubbles (*arrow*) are seen within the perirenal abscess.

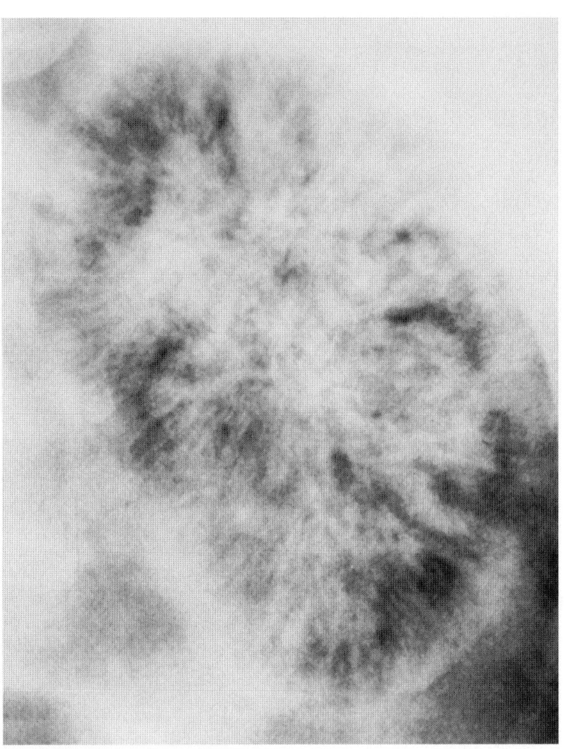

FIGURE 33.32. **Emphysematous Pyelonephritis.** Plain radiograph of the left kidney shows striations in the renal parenchyma caused by interstitial gas. This finding is indicative of life-threatening infection.

Emphysematous pyelonephritis is a form of acute pyelonephritis with air in the renal parenchyma. Most cases occur in patients with diabetes, obstruction, or immune system compromise. The condition is rapidly progressive and often life threatening. Mixed flora infection with gram-negative organisms is most common. Plain films and CT demonstrate streaks and collections of gas within the renal parenchyma (Fig. 33.32).

Chronic Pyelonephritis and Reflux Nephropathy. Chronic pyelonephritis refers to chronic interstitial nephritis caused by infection. In children, vesicoureteral reflux of infected urine is the most common cause of chronic pyelonephritis. Intrarenal reflux, usually most prominent at the upper pole, damages the papilla, resulting in calyceal blunting with overlying cortical scarring. This process of progressive renal injury associated with reflux is referred to as *reflux nephropathy*. Adults may show stable residual findings of this childhood disease. Chronic pyelonephritis in adults is most commonly associated with calculi and chronic obstruction. Neurogenic bladder, ileal conduits, and other causes of urinary stasis are predisposing conditions. Both reflux nephropathy of childhood and chronic pyelonephritis in adults show similar imaging findings. The hallmark is a focal cortical scar that overlies a blunted calyx (Fig. 33.33). The disease is classically lobar,

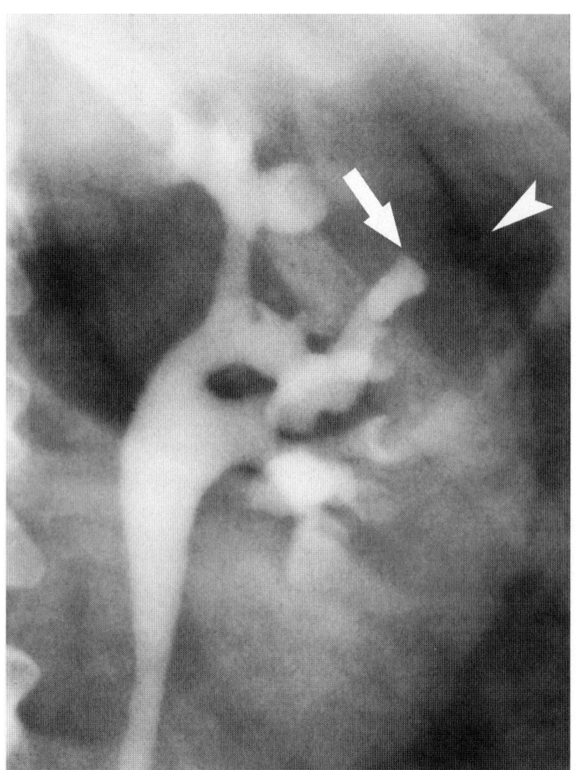

FIGURE 33.33. **Reflux Nephropathy.** Radiograph of the left kidney obtained as part of an excretory urogram demonstrates a blunted calyx (*arrow*) with an overlying cortical scar (*arrowhead*). These findings are indicative of reflux nephropathy.

with normal lobes with normal calyces interposed between diseased lobes. These findings are best demonstrated on excretory urography but may also be evident on US and CT.

Renal tuberculosis may follow primary pulmonary tuberculosis by as much as 10 to 15 years. Active pulmonary tuberculosis is present in only 10% of cases of renal tuberculosis. Only 30% of cases show any chest radiograph evidence of prior tuberculosis. Patients present with asymptomatic hematuria or sterile pyuria. Imaging studies often initially suggest the diagnosis when it is unsuspected clinically. The hallmarks of renal tuberculosis include (*1*) parenchymal destruction and cavity formation eventually leading to parenchymal scarring, (*2*) parenchymal masses owing to granuloma formation, (*3*) fibrosis leading to strictures of the collecting system and ureters, and (*4*) a wide variety of patterns of calcification (18). End-stage nonfunctional tuberculous kidneys may be hydronephrotic sacs or appear as atrophic and calcified masses in the renal bed (Fig. 33.34).

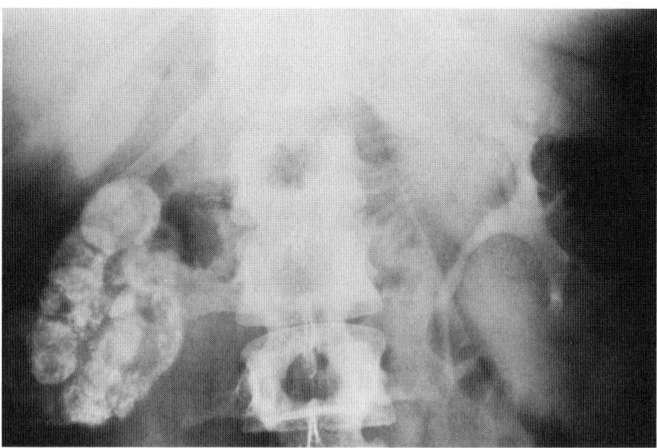

FIGURE 33.34. **End-Stage Renal Tuberculosis.** The right kidney is small, nonfunctioning, and completely calcified because of chronic tuberculous infection. The left kidney is enlarged owing to compensatory hypertrophy resulting from long-standing reduced right renal function.

Renal Parenchymal Disease

Renal Failure. In patients with renal failure, US is usually requested to exclude hydronephrosis, assess renal size, and identify renal parenchymal disease. Bilateral hydronephrosis is a rare, but potentially reversible, cause of renal failure. Patients with acute renal failure and large or normal-size kidneys often require biopsy for definitive diagnosis of renal parenchymal disease. Patients with small (<9 cm) kidneys usually have irreversible end-stage renal disease and do not benefit from biopsy. Measurements of renal cortical thickness are unreliable in assessing residual renal function. Sonographic signs of renal parenchymal disease include a diffuse increase in parenchymal echogenicity, often associated with loss of corticomedullary differentiation. Sonographic characterization of renal parenchymal changes correlated with renal size shortens the differential diagnosis of "medical renal disease" to a limited degree (see Table 36.3).

Acquired Immunodeficiency Syndrome. Renal disease in AIDS encompasses a broad spectrum of abnormalities. AIDS-related nephropathy refers to focal and segmental glomerulosclerosis with associated tubular abnormalities. Diffuse renal infection with associated calcification resulting from *Pneumocystis jiroveci* (formerly *P carinii*), *Mycobacterium avium intracellulare,* and *M tuberculosis* has been reported. Patients with AIDS are exposed to many nephrotoxic drugs. Associated diseases such as lymphoma and dehydration caused by diarrhea and vomiting may contribute to renal injury. More than 50% of patients with AIDS demonstrate increased renal parenchymal echogenicity.

Bilateral small kidneys (<9 cm) imply a systemic disease process that injures both kidneys and usually reduces their function (Table 33.2). The conditions listed are generally indistinguishable by imaging methods.

Bilateral large kidneys (>13 cm) imply a systemic process that adds to renal size by deposition of protein, cells,

TABLE 33.2 Causes of Bilateral Small Kidneys

Arterial hypotension (acute contrast reaction)
Generalized arteriosclerosis
Nephrosclerosis because of systemic hypertension
Chronic glomerulonephritis
Uremic medullary cystic disease

Adapted from Davidson AJ. Radiology of the Kidney. Philadelphia: WB Saunders, 1985:179.

or fluid (Table 33.3). Acute tubular necrosis is the most common cause of acute renal failure. Acute tubular necrosis is most commonly precipitated by renal ischemia or exposure to nephrotoxic substances, including radiographic contrast agents.

Unilateral small kidney suggests global injury to the renal parenchyma as a result of a local unilateral process rather than a systemic process (Table 33.4). Renal artery stenosis causes chronic renal ischemia and is a cause of systemic hypertension. The involved kidney is small and demonstrates a delayed nephrogram and a delay in the collecting system opacification on XU. Global renal infarction occurs as a result of sudden occlusion of a main renal artery because of embolus, thrombus, or trauma. Radiation nephritis results from inclusion of the kidney in a field of therapeutic radiation. Postobstructive atrophy may follow relief of chronic obstruction. Postinflammatory atrophy follows chronic infection. Congenital hypoplasia is an underdeveloped kidney with a reduced number of lobes (<5 lobes); the opposite kidney usually shows compensatory hypertrophy.

TABLE 33.3 Causes of Bilateral Large Kidneys

Proliferative disorders
Acute glomerulonephritis
Lupus nephritis
Diabetic glomerulosclerosis
Parenchymal edema
Acute tubular necrosis
Acute cortical necrosis
Acute bilateral pyelonephritis
Cell infiltration
Lymphoma
Leukemia
Protein deposition
Multiple myeloma
Amyloidosis
Urate deposition
Urate nephropathy

Adapted from Davidson AJ. Radiology of the Kidney. Philadelphia: WB Saunders, 1985:221.

TABLE 33.4 Causes of Unilateral Small Kidney

Renal artery stenosis
Global renal infarction
Radiation nephritis
Postobstructive atrophy
Postinflammatory atrophy
Congenital hypoplasia

Adapted from Davidson AJ. Radiology of the Kidney. Philadelphia: WB Saunders, 1985:151.

Unilateral Large Kidney. With the exception of a duplicated collecting system and compensatory hypertrophy, unilateral large kidneys are the result of acute local insults that affect only one kidney (Table 33.5). Renal vein thrombosis and renal artery infarction result in enlarged swollen kidneys in the acute state and small kidneys in the chronic state. Acute obstruction and acute pyelonephritis cause edematous, swollen kidneys. Compensatory hypertrophy is usually associated with a small or poorly functioning opposite kidney. Duplication of the collecting system is proved by excretory urography.

Nephrocalcinosis

Nephrocalcinosis is a broad term that refers to pathologic deposition of calcium in the renal parenchyma. Nephrocalcinosis is usually bilateral and the result of systemic disorders.

Cortical nephrocalcinosis is unusual, representing fewer than 5% of nephrocalcinoses. Causes include acute cortical necrosis precipitated by severe ischemia, chronic glomerulonephritis, and primary hyperoxaluria.

Medullary nephrocalcinosis is far more common and is usually related to hypercalcemic or hypercalciuric states (Table 33.6). Note that echogenic renal pyramids may result from medullary nephrocalcinosis, as well as other causes (Fig. 33.29).

TABLE 33.5 Causes of Unilateral Large Kidney

Acute renal vein thrombosis
Acute arterial infarction
Obstructive uropathy
Acute pyelonephritis
Duplicated collecting system
Compensatory hypertrophy

Adapted from Davidson AJ. Radiology of the Kidney. Philadelphia, WB Saunders, 1985:255.

TABLE 33.6 Causes of Medullary Nephrocalcinosis

Hyperparathyroidism
Medullary sponge kidney
Renal tubular acidosis (distal form)
Milk-alkali syndrome
Hypervitaminosis D
Hypercalcemic/hypercalciuric states

REFERENCES

1. Mayo-Smith WW, Boland GW, Noto RB, Lee MJ. State-of-the-art adrenal imaging. Radiographics 2001;21:995–1012.
2. Elsayes KM, Mukundan G, Narra VR, et al. Adrenal masses: MR imaging features with pathologic correlation. Radiographics 2004;24:S73–S86.
3. Szolar DH, Korokin M, Reittner P, et al. Adrenocortical carcinomas and adrenal pheochromocytomas: mass and enhancement loss evaluation at delayed contrast-enhanced CT. Radiology 2005;234:479–485.
4. Elsayes KM, Narra VR, Leyendecker JR, et al. MRI of adrenal and extraadrenal pheochromocytoma. AJR Am J Roentgenol 2005;184: 860–867.
5. Blake MA, Kalra MK, Maher MM, et al. Pheochromocytoma: an imaging chameleon. Radiographics 2004;24:S87–S99.
6. Kenney PJ, Wagner BJ, Rao P, Heffess CS. Myelolipoma: CT and pathologic features. Radiology 1998;208:87–95.
7. Kawashima A, Sandler CM, Ernst RD, et al. Imaging of nontraumatic hemorrhage of the adrenal gland. Radiographics 1999;19:949–963.
8. Caoilli EM, Korobkin M, Francis IR, et al. Adrenal masses: characterization with combined unenhanced and delayed enhanced CT. Radiology 2002;222:629–633.
9. Dunnick NR, Korobkin M. Imaging of adrenal incidentalomas: current status. AJR Am J Roentgenol 2002;179:559–568.
10. Haider MA, Ghai S, Jhaveri K, Lockwood G. Chemical shift MR imaging of hyperattenuating (>10 HU) adrenal masses: does it still have a role? Radiology 2004;231:711–716.
11. Joffe SA, Servaes S, Okon S, Horowitz M. Multi-detector row CT urography in the evaluation of hematuria. Radiographics 2003;23: 1441–1456.
12. Blandino A, Gaeta M, Minutoli F, Salamone I, et al. MR urography of the ureter. AJR Am J Roentgenol 2002;179:1307–1314.
13. Sheth S, Scatarige JC, Horton KM, Corl FM, Fishman EK. Current concepts in the diagnosis and management of renal cell carcinoma: role of multidetector CT and three dimensional CT. Radiographics 2001;21:S237–S254.
14. Sheeran SR, Sussman SK. Renal lymphoma: spectrum of CT findings and potential mimics. AJR Am J Roentgenol 1998;171:1067–1072.
15. Hartman DS, Choyke PL, Hartman MS. A practical approach to the cystic renal mass. Radiographics 2004;24:S101–S115.
16. Bosniak MA. The current radiological approach to renal cysts. Radiology 1986;158:1–10.
17. Taouli B, Ghouadni M, Correas J, et al. Spectrum of abdominal imaging findings in von Hippel-Lindau disease. AJR Am J Roentgenol 2003;181:1049–1054.
18. Jung YY, Kim JK, Cho K-S. Genitourinary tuberculosis: comprehensive cross-sectional imaging. AJR Am J Roentgenol 2005;184: 143–150.

Chapter 34

Pelvicaliceal System, Ureters, Bladder, and Urethra

William E. Brant

Pelvicalliceal System and Ureter
- Imaging Methods
- Anatomy
- Congenital Anomalies
- Renal Stone Disease
- Hydronephrosis
- Filling Defects/Masses in Pelvicaliceal System or Ureter
- Stricture of Pelvicaliceal System or Ureter
- Papillary Cavities

Bladder
- Imaging Methods
- Anatomy
- Thickened Bladder Wall/Small Bladder Capacity
- Calcified Bladder Wall
- Bladder Wall Masses/Filling Defects
- Pear-Shaped Bladder/Extrinsic Masses
- Bladder Outpouchings/Fistulas
- Bladder Trauma

Urethra
- Imaging Methods
- Anatomy
- Pathology

PELVICALICEAL SYSTEM AND URETER

Imaging Methods

The choices for imaging of the pelvicaliceal system and ureters have expanded. An excretory urogram (XU), also called an intravenous pyelogram (IVP), has been the traditional choice. This study is performed by obtaining a series of radiographs at various times and in various projections following IV administration of contrast agent. The images of the collecting system are routinely of high quality and remain the gold standard. However, detection of lesions in the renal parenchyma is limited. With the development of multidetector CT (MDCT) and continued improvement in MR, we now have available the CT-IVP and the MR-IVP, which combine optimal imaging of the renal parenchyma with satisfactory images of the collecting system and ureters. Thin-slice MDCT can be reformatted in longitudinal planes to provide visualization of the collecting system (see Fig. 34.14) comparable to that obtained with the XU (1). MR urography can be performed without the use of IV contrast utilizing T2 weighting to provide visualization of urine-filled structures (2). Poor renal function or high-grade obstruction limits the use of IV contrast agents because of poor concentration of contrast within the collecting system. Retrograde pyelography, performed by cystoscopic catheterization of the ureteral orifice followed by injection of contrast, is independent of renal function, provides high-quality images of the ureter and the collecting system, and is another alternative commonly utilized by urologists. When a percutaneous nephrostomy catheter has been placed in the collecting system, antegrade pyelography is an additional choice. US is the imaging method of choice for screening for hydronephrosis but is limited in its ability to demonstrate small uroepithelial tumors. CT, routinely performed without IV or oral contrast agents, has supplanted plain radiographs and IVP in the diagnosis of renal stones in the kidneys and ureters.

Anatomy

The collecting tubules of the medullary pyramid coalesce into a variable number of papillary ducts that pierce the tip of the papilla and drain into the receptacle of the collecting

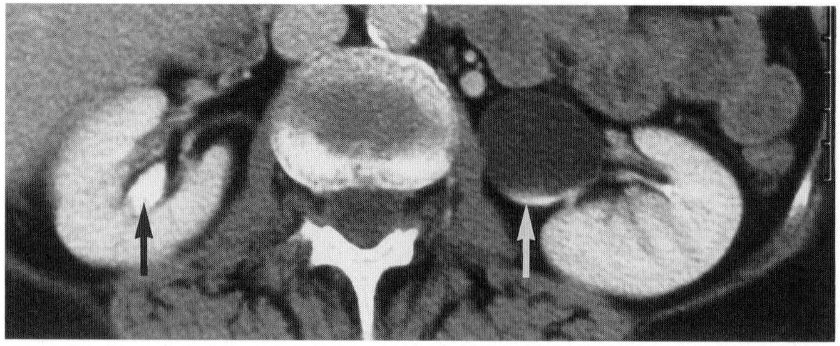

FIGURE 34.1. **Extrarenal Pelvis.** The position of the left renal pelvis (*white arrow*) outside of the renal sinus enables the pelvis to distend with urine and to be larger than the normal right renal pelvis (*black arrow*). The extrarenal pelvis is a normal variant, not to be mistaken for hydronephrosis.

system, called a *minor calix*. The projection of the papilla into the calix produces a cup shape. The sharp-edged portion of the minor calix that projects around the sides of a papilla is called the *fornix* of the calix. Compound calices, usually found at the poles of the kidney, are formed by the projection of two or more papillae into the calix. *Infundibula* extend between minor calices and the renal pelvis. The renal pelvis is triangular, with its base within the renal sinus. The apex of the pelvis extends outward and downward to join the ureter. A so-called *extrarenal pelvis* is predominantly outside the renal sinus and is larger and more distensible than an intrarenal pelvis surrounded by renal sinus fat (Fig. 34.1). An extrarenal pelvis is a normal variant that should not be confused with hydronephrosis. There is endless variety in the size and arrangement of calices and in the shape and appearance of the renal pelvis.

The ureters have an outer fibrous adventitia that is continuous with the renal capsule and with the adventitia of the bladder. The muscularis, responsible for ureteral peristalsis, consists of outer circular and inner longitudinal muscle bundles. The mucosa lining the entire pelvicaliceal system, ureters, and bladder is *transitional epithelium*. The ureters enter the bladder at an oblique angle. When the bladder wall contracts, the ureteral orifices are closed. The ureters propel urine by active peristalsis, which can be visualized fluoroscopically and by US. Jets of urine opacified by contrast are frequently seen within the bladder on XU and CT. Because of peristalsis, the diameter of the ureter at any particular instant is highly variable. Three main points of ureteral narrowing, where calculi are likely to become impacted, are (*1*) the ureteropelvic junction (UPJ), (*2*) the site at which the ureter crosses the pelvic brim, and (*3*) the ureterovesical junction (UVJ).

Congenital Anomalies

Ureteral duplication occurs in 1% to 2% of the population (Fig. 34.2). Unilateral duplication is six times more common than bilateral duplication (3). The *Weigert-Meyer rule* states that with complete ureteral duplication, the ureter draining the upper pole passes through the bladder wall to insert inferior and medial to the normally placed ureter that drains the lower pole (see Fig. 34.22). The upper pole ureter often ends as an ectopic ureterocele that is obstructed because of its ectopic insertion. The lower pole ureter inserts in or near the normal location in the bladder trigone and is subject to vesicoureteral reflux because of distortion of its passage through the bladder wall by the ectopic ureterocele. Complications of complete

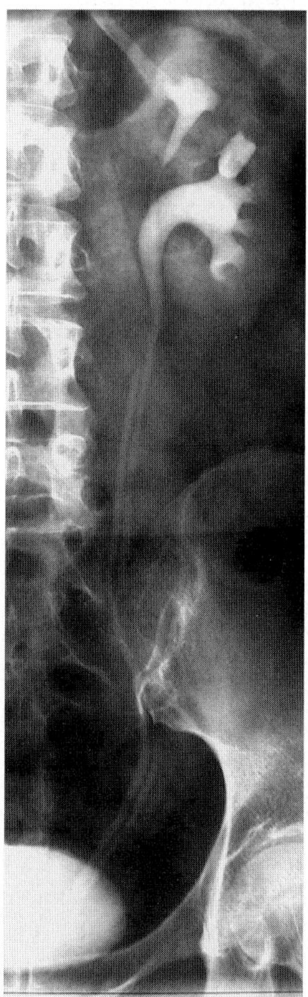

FIGURE 34.2. **Ureteral Duplication.** The left collecting system and ureter are completely duplicated. The ureter draining the upper pole of the left kidney inserts into the bladder inferior and medial to the insertion of the ureter draining the lower pole collecting system.

duplication include urinary tract infection, vesicoureteral reflux, and ureteropelvic junction obstruction of the lower pole system. Reflux into the lower pole collecting system in childhood may produce scarring and deformity of the lower pole of the kidney.

XU commonly demonstrates poor function or nonfunction of the obstructed upper pole system. The lower pole system is displaced inferiorly and commonly shows a "drooping lily" appearance. Reflux nephropathy of the lower pole system may be evident. US, CT, or MR demonstrates cystic dilatation of the upper pole system, usually with marked parenchymal thinning. The upper pole ureter is commonly tortuous and dilated. The ectopic ureterocele and its associated dilated ureter may simulate a multiseptated cystic mass in the pelvis.

Bifid renal pelvis occurs in 10% of the population. Separate pelvises draining the upper and lower poles join at the ureteropelvic junction. This anomaly has no pathologic consequences.

Ureteropelvic junction obstruction is a common congenital anomaly that may go undiagnosed until adulthood (4). The amount of hydronephrosis and parenchymal atrophy present depends on the severity of obstruction. The condition is bilateral in 30% of cases but is often not symmetric. XU and US demonstrate pelvicaliectasis, with sharply defined narrowing at the ureteropelvic junction (Fig. 34.3). The ureter is not dilated. In 15% to 20% of cases, an aberrant renal vessel causes the obstruction. MDCT is effective in demonstrating the crossing vessel. In the majority of cases, the precise cause is unknown.

Retrocaval ureter is a developmental variant in which the right ureter passes behind the inferior vena cava at the level of the L3 or L4 vertebra (Fig. 34.4). The ureter exits anteriorly between the cava and the aorta to return to its normal position. The condition is associated with varying degrees of urinary stasis and proximal pyeloureterectasis. The anomaly is caused by faulty embryogenesis of the inferior vena cava, with abnormal persistence of the right subcardinal vein anterior to the ureter instead of the right supracardinal vein posterior to the ureter.

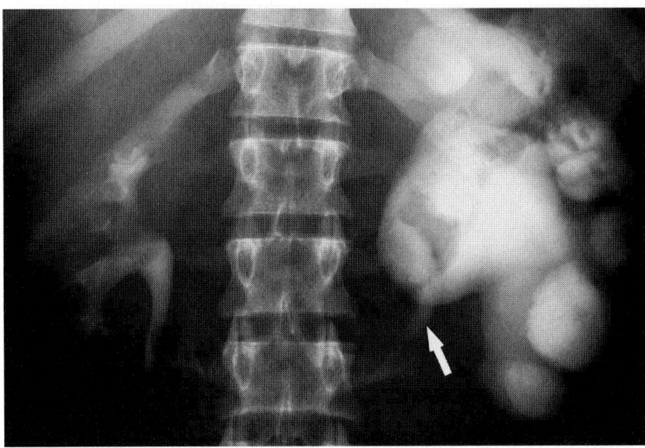

FIGURE 34.3. **Ureteropelvic Junction (UPJ) Obstruction.** An excretory urogram demonstrates marked dilatation of the left renal collecting system. The degree of dilatation indicates a chronic, likely congenital, process. The proximal ureter (*arrow*) is normal in caliber, indicating obstruction at the level of the UPJ. The right renal collecting system is normal in appearance.

Renal Stone Disease

Routine use of noncontrast CT has revolutionized the imaging evaluation of renal stone disease, nearly completely replacing plain radiographs and XU for the diagnosis of acute ureteral obstruction by renal stones (5). *Nephrolithiasis* refers to the presence of calculi in the renal collecting system. Nearly 10% of the population will form a renal stone in their lifetime. Sufficient calcium oxalate or calcium phosphate is present in 80% of renal calculi for them to be radiopaque on plain radiographs. Struvite (magnesium ammonium phosphate) stones, formed in the presence of alkaline urine and infection, make up another 15% of renal calculi and are also radiopaque on radiographs. Struvite is the most common component of staghorn calculi (Fig. 34.5). Cystine stones comprise 1% to 2% of renal stones, are mildly radiopaque, and are found only in patients with congenital cystinuria. The remaining 3% to 4% of renal stones are composed of urate or xanthines and are radiolucent on radiographs. A major advantage of noncontrast CT is that (nearly) all stones are opaque on CT. The primary limitation of CT is the small size of the stone rather than its attenuation. On soft tissue windows, urinary calculi appear as high-attenuation objects. The single uncommon exception is crystalline stones associated with the use of protease inhibitors (indinavir) in the treatment of HIV infection. These stones are low attenuation on CT but may cause ureteral obstruction. On CT, calcium oxalate and calcium phosphate stones are 800 to 1,000 H, struvite stones are 330 to 900 H, cystine stones are 200 to 880 H depending on calcium content, and uric acid stones are 150 to 500 H. High CT attenuation makes calculi easy to differentiate from other collecting system lesions, such as tumors, hematoma, fungus balls, or sloughed papilla, which are all usually <50 H.

Complications of renal calculi include obstruction, ureteral stricture, chronic renal infection, and loss of renal function. Acute flank pain is a common complaint of patients seeking emergency medical treatment. Renal colic, caused by a calculus obstructing the ureter, is the most common cause of acute flank pain and is the usual major consideration for diagnostic imaging. Although most calculi can be detected on plain radiographs, difficulties in localization to the ureter and differentiation from other calcifications limits the sensitivity of plain radiography for ureteral stones to as low as 45% with a specificity of only 77% (6). Noncontrast CT has a sensitivity of 97% and

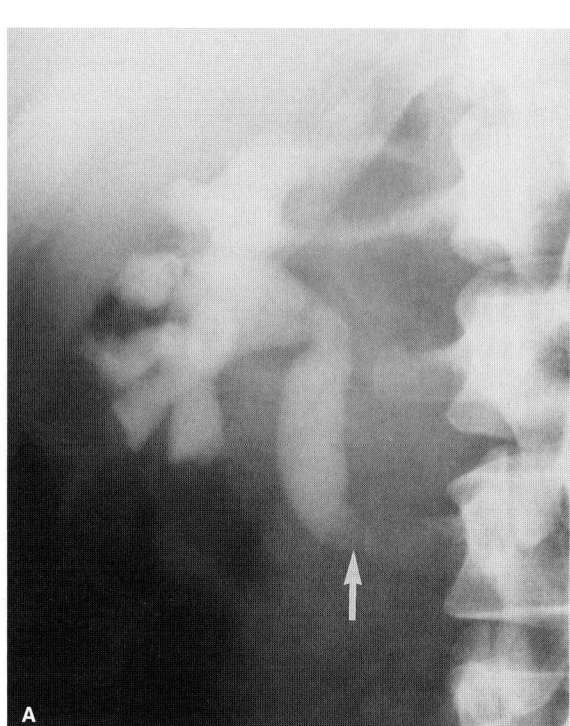

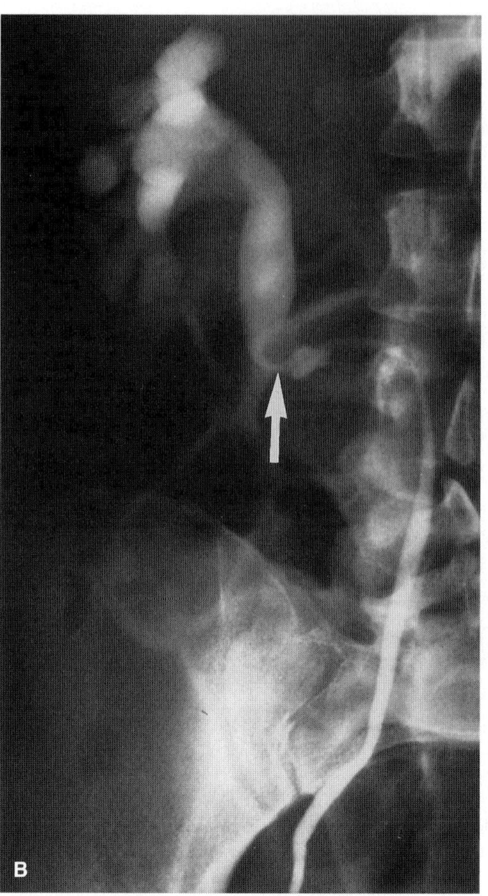

FIGURE 34.4. **Retrocaval Ureter. A.** The right renal collecting system and proximal right ureter are dilated. At the level of the transverse process of the L3 vertebra (*arrow*), the ureter makes an abrupt turn to the left. The more distal ureter was poorly visualized but did not appear dilated on this excretory urogram. **B.** Retrograde ureterogram documents the characteristic appearance of the ureter (*arrow*), which courses behind the inferior vena cava at the level of the sharp bend.

specificity of 96% for ureteral calculi (7). US has a sensitivity for stone detection of only 24% compared to unenhanced CT (8). An additional advantage of noncontrast CT in the diagnosis of acute flank pain is demonstration of pathology other than a ureteral stone. Among the numerous possibilities are acute appendicitis, incarcerated hernia, ovarian cyst, diverticulitis, and pyelonephritis (9).

Noncontrast renal stone CT is a helical or multidetector CT of the urinary tract performed without oral or IV contrast (Fig. 34.6). The thin slice (1.3 mm) capability of MDCT is optimal for this indication. Stones appear as geometric or oval, high-attenuation foci (5,10). Stone location within the ureter is confirmed by location along the course of the ureter and the presence of a halo of soft tissue surrounding the calculus ("tissue rim sign"). Findings of obstruction include: (*1*) mild dilatation of the pelvicaliceal system and ureter (>3 mm) proximal to the stone; (*2*) slight decrease in attenuation of the affected kidney caused by edema; and (*3*) perinephric soft tissue stranding, representing edema in the perinephric fat. Focal perinephric fluid collections represent forniceal rupture caused by high-grade obstruction coupled with high urine output. Pitfalls in diagnosis include: (*1*) peripelvic cysts or extrarenal pelvis simulating hydronephrosis; (*2*) preexisting stranding in the perinephric fat caused by previous inflammation, especially in older patients; (*3*) atherosclerotic calcifications; (*4*) recent stone passage without a stone currently present; and (*5*) phleboliths. Phleboliths are calcifications within thrombosed veins and are particularly common in the pelvis. Differentiation from stones is made by: (*1*) location not along the course of the ureter; (*2*) absence of a tissue rim sign; (*3*) presence of a "tail sign," a tubular "tail" extending from the calcification, representing a thrombosed vein; and (*4*) relatively low attenuation of phleboliths (mean value of 160 H). The probability that a calcification represents a phlebolith is less than 3% when the attenuation is >300 H.

Stones smaller than 6 mm are likely to pass spontaneously through the ureter within 6 weeks. Stones larger than 6 mm are more likely to remain lodged in the ureter

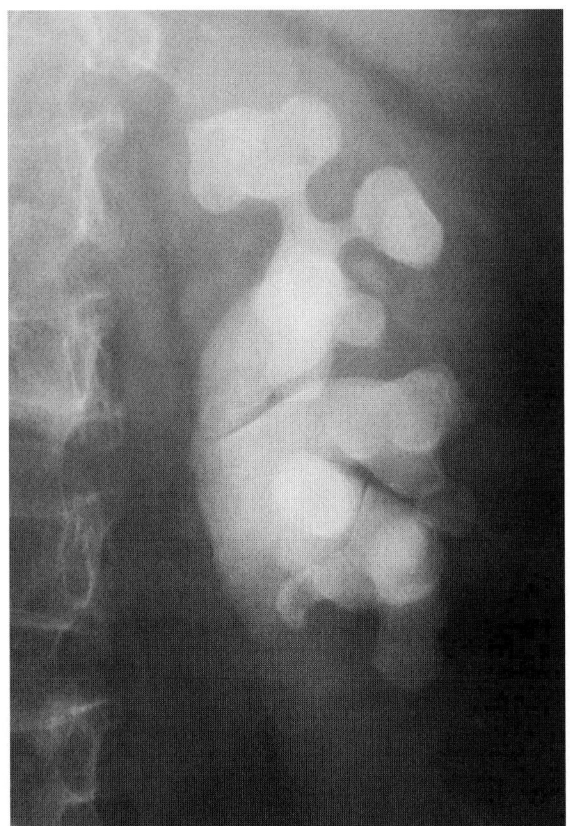

FIGURE 34.5. **Staghorn Calculus.** A plain radiograph (without radiographic contrast agent) demonstrates a complex calculus creating a cast of the collecting system of the left kidney. This staghorn calculus, named (imprecisely) for its resemblance to the antlers of a male deer, is formed in the presence of obstruction with chronic infection and is composed of struvite.

and require intervention for removal. Calculi are most likely to be found at the three points of ureteral narrowing previously described.

Hydronephrosis

Hydronephrosis is defined as dilatation of the upper urinary tract. Hydronephrosis is not synonymous with obstruction but has a number of causes, which are described in this section. The terms *caliectasis, pyelectasis,* and *ureterectasis* are more precise in describing dilatation of portions of the urinary tract. US is an excellent screening modality for determining the presence of urinary tract dilation.

Obstruction. The causes of obstruction include stone, stricture, tumor, and extrinsic compression. The degree of dilatation produced by obstruction varies. In general, the more proximal and the more chronic the obstruction, the greater the degree of dilatation. Acute obstruction produced by an impacted stone often produces minimal dilatation. US demonstrates hydronephrosis as separation of normal sinus echogenicity by anechoic urine in the collecting system. The calices become enlarged and blunted and are seen to connect with the dilated renal pelvis. Medullary pyramids may be hypoechoic, especially in children, and must be differentiated from dilated calices. Pyramids are more peripheral, are surrounded by more echogenic cortex, and do not connect with the renal pelvis. A peripelvic cyst can easily be mistaken for hydronephrosis on US. XU signs of obstruction (Fig. 34.7) include (*1*) increasingly dense nephrogram with time, (*2*) delay in appearance of

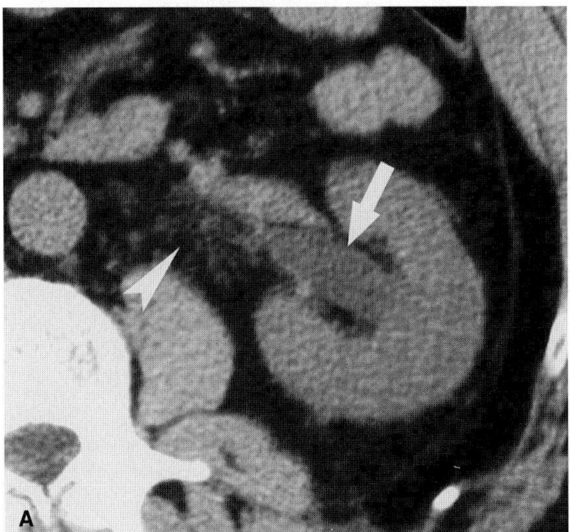

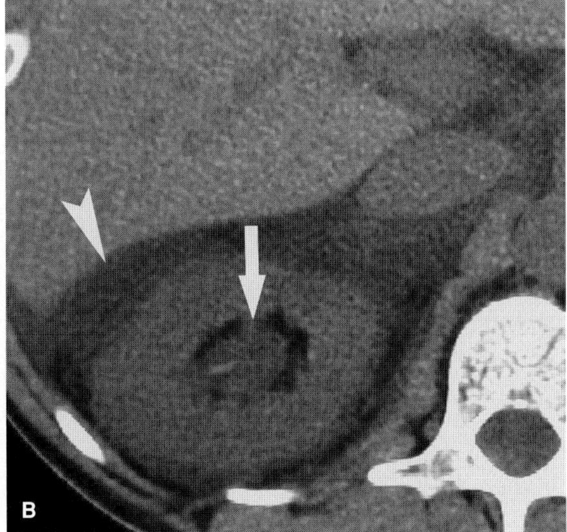

FIGURE 34.6. **Noncontrast Renal Stone CT. A.** CT image through the kidneys in a patient with left flank pain demonstrates mild enlargement of the left renal pelvis (*arrow*). Streaks and strands of edema (*arrowhead*) are seen in the fat adjacent to the renal pelvis. **B.** CT in a different patient with a stone in the distal ureter shows mild hydronephrosis (*arrow*) associated with fluid in the perinephric space (*arrowhead*). These findings indicate rupture of the collecting system at a fornix resulting from high-grade obstruction and high urine output. (*continued*)

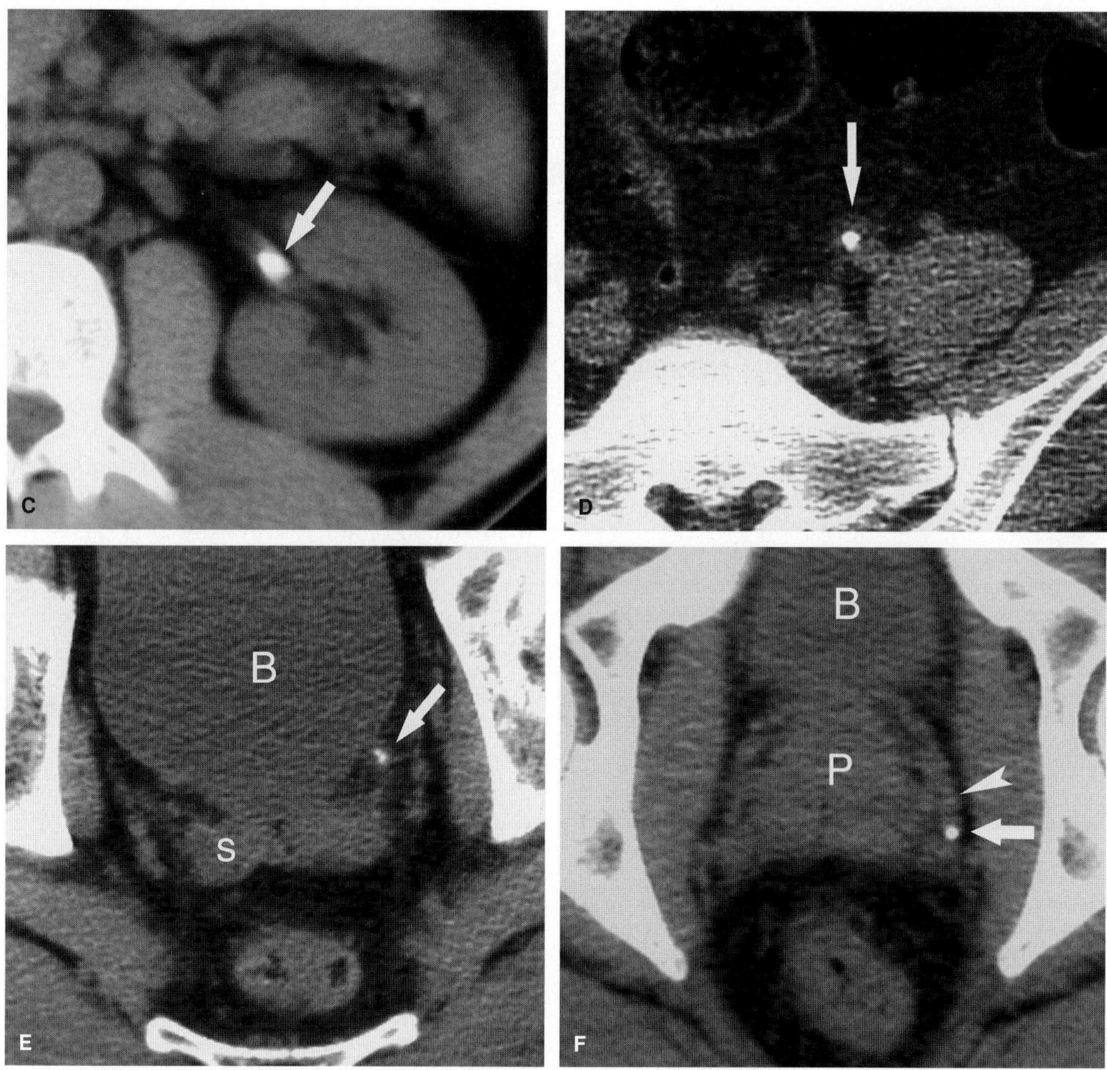

FIGURE 34.6. *(Continued)* **C.** A stone (*arrow*) at the ureteropelvic junction is apparent in this patient. Absence of hydronephrosis or edema in the perinephric fat indicates that obstruction is very low grade. Note that the rim of tissue around the stone is somewhat obscured by bloom artifact from the marked high attenuation of the stone. **D.** A stone in the left ureter (*arrow*) has impacted at the level of the pelvic brim. Note the irregular shape; this is characteristic of renal stones. The rim of soft tissue density surrounding the stone represents the swollen wall of the ureter ("tissue rim sign"). **E.** CT at the level of the seminal vesicles (s) shows a high-density stone (*arrow*) in the distal left ureter. The "tissue rim sign" is evident. "Nearly all" urinary tract stones appear white on CT viewed at soft tissue windows. **F.** A more caudal image at the level of the base of the prostate (P) shows a phlebolith (*arrow*), not to be mistaken for a ureteral stone. The location is below the level of the distal ureter, and the calcification lacks a tissue rim sign. The tubular structure (*arrowhead*) extending from the calcification represents the thrombosed vein (the tail sign). B, bladder.

contrast in the collecting system, and (*3*) dilated pelvicaliceal system and ureter to the point of obstruction. *Pyelosinus reflux* may result from rupture of a fornix precipitated by contrast-induced diuresis superimposed on the increased hydrostatic pressure of an obstructed pelvicaliceal system. Urine and contrast extravasate into the renal sinus and perirenal space. CT demonstrates dilatation of the collecting system, either with or without use of IV contrast. Delay in opacification of the obstructed kidney and dependent layering of unopacified urine over heavier contrast media may also be evident. The location and cause of obstruction can usually be identified.

Pyonephrosis refers to infection in an obstructed kidney. Pyonephrosis can result in rapid destruction of the renal parenchyma and must be treated promptly by relief of obstruction by ureteral stent or nephrostomy tube

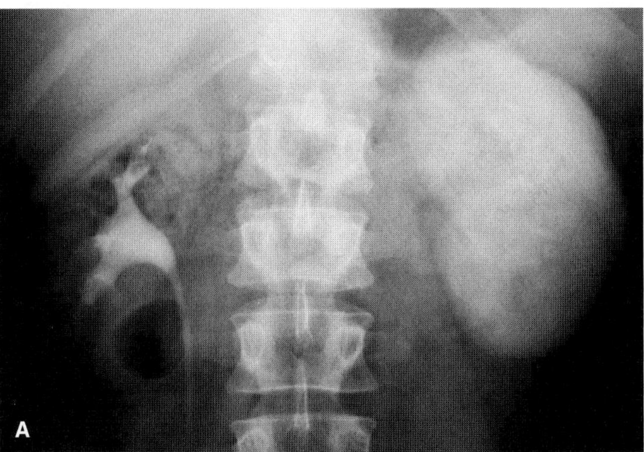

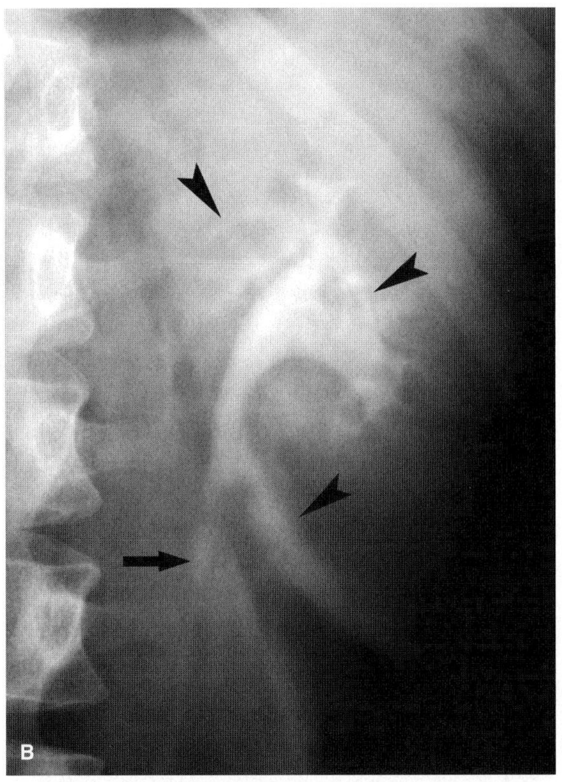

FIGURE 34.7. **Obstruction With Pyelosinus Reflux. A.** Radiograph obtained 10 minutes after IV injection of contrast demonstrates a persisting dense nephrogram in the left kidney with delay of contrast excretion into the collecting system. The patient had an obstructing stone at the ureterovesical junction. The right kidney is normal. **B.** Radiograph obtained 2 hours after contrast injection reveals leakage of contrast (*arrowheads*) out of the left collecting system and into the renal sinus and the perirenal and periureteric spaces. Overdistension of the obstructed collecting system because of the diuretic effect of the contrast agent resulted in rupture of a caliceal fornix. The left ureter (*arrow*) is filled with contrast.

placement and antibiotics. US classically demonstrates a dilated collecting system filled with layering echogenic pus and debris. Shadowing calculi may also be evident. CT is better than US in demonstrating the site and cause of obstruction. XU is usually not useful, because the affected kidney functions poorly or not at all.

Vesicoureteral reflux is a common cause of hydronephrosis in children. The basic defect is an abnormal ureteral tunnel at the ureterovesical junction and associated urinary tract infection. In adults, vesicoureteral reflux is usually associated with neurogenic bladder or bladder outlet obstruction. Chronic vesicoureteral reflux of infected urine causes reflux nephropathy. Vesicoureteral reflux is confirmed by demonstrating retrograde filling of the ureters on voiding cystourography or radionuclide cystography.

Congenital megaureter is the result of an aperistaltic segment of the lower ureter causing a functional obstruction and resulting in dilatation of the proximal ureter. The aperistaltic segment of the ureter demonstrates smoothly tapered narrowing without evidence of mechanical obstruction.

Prune belly syndrome, also called Eagle-Barrett syndrome, is a congenital disorder manifested by absence of the abdominal wall musculature, urinary tract anomalies, and cryptorchidism. The ureters are markedly dilated and tortuous, the bladder is large and distended, and the posterior urethra is dilated.

Polyuria, associated with acute diuresis and diabetes insipidus, may cause mild to severe hydronephrosis.

Filling Defects/Masses in Pelvicaliceal System or Ureter

Calculi are the most common cause of filling defects in the contrast-filled collecting system (Fig. 34.8) or ureter. Most calculi (>85%) are radiopaque on plain radiographs. Noncontrast CT demonstrates all calculi as high-density objects with a CT density of >100 H. The presence of contrast agent in the collecting system commonly obscures detection of calculi on CT. On MR, stones are seen as foci of absent signal within the collecting system.

Blood clots cause radiolucent filling defects that can be differentiated from soft tissue tumors by their change in appearance over time. Attenuation values on CT are usually <50 H.

Transitional cell carcinoma (TCC) accounts for 85% to 90% of all uroepithelial tumors (11). Most (85%) have a papillary growth pattern that is exophytic, polypoid, and attached to the mucosa by a stalk. These lesions cause a distinct filling defect in the collecting system (Fig. 34.9) or ureter. A stippled pattern of contrast material within the interstices of the papillary lesion is characteristic. Tumors in the ureter may demonstrate a "champagne glass" sign (Fig. 34.10) of ureteral dilatation distal to a filling defect. This sign distinguishes tumor from a calculus that

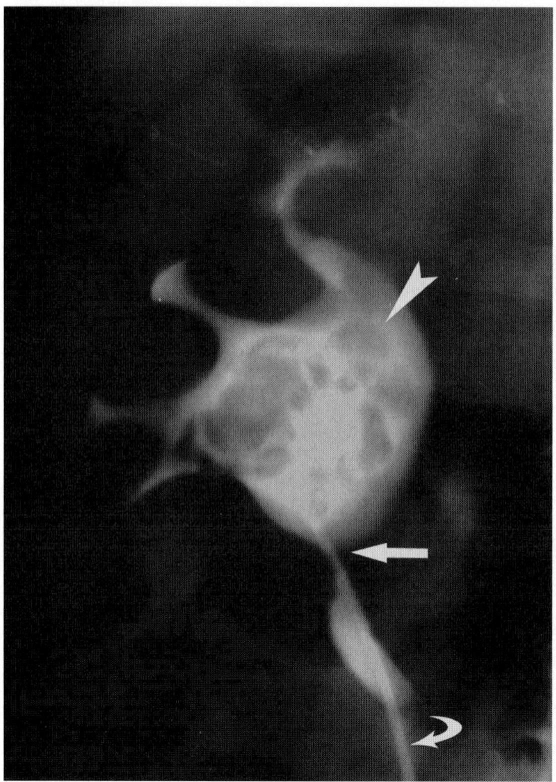

FIGURE 34.8. **Multiple Calculi in the Renal Pelvis.** A retrograde pyelogram demonstrates multiple filling defects (*arrowhead*) in the right renal pelvis that proved to be radiolucent calculi. Contrast was injected into the renal pelvis via a catheter (*curved arrow*) in the right ureter that was inserted at cystoscopy. A stricture at the ureteropelvic junction (*straight arrow*) caused stasis in the renal pelvis, promoting stone formation.

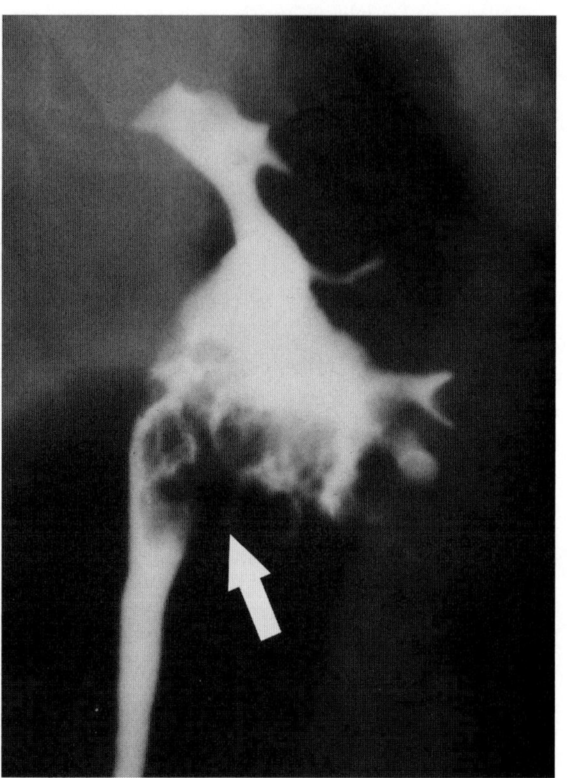

FIGURE 34.9. **Transitional Cell Carcinoma of the Renal Pelvis.** Radiograph from a retrograde pyelogram of the left kidney reveals a multilobulated filling defect (*arrow*) in the left renal pelvis. Biopsy confirmed transitional cell carcinoma.

impacts in the ureter and causes distal spasm and narrowing. Nonpapillary tumors are nodular or flat and tend to be infiltrating and aggressive. They cause strictures of the collecting system or ureter, rather than filling defects. Most TCCs occur in men (male-to-female ratio = 4:1) aged 60 and older. A variety of chemical agents used in the textile and plastic industries, drugs (including cyclophosphamide and phenacetin), chronic urinary stasis (horseshoe kidney), and smoking play a role in the etiology of these tumors. The tumor metastasizes most commonly to regional lymph nodes, liver, lung, and bone. TCC exhibits a strong tendency toward multiplicity. Patients with upper tract TCC have multicentric tumors in 20% to 44% of cases, and those with TCC of the ureter develop bladder TCC in 20% to 37% of cases. Careful evaluation of the entire urinary tract is warranted, both at initial diagnosis and for follow-up. Standard treatment of TCC is total nephroureterectomy and excision of a cuff of the bladder surrounding the ureteral orifice.

CT demonstrates a mass within the collecting system (Fig. 34.11). Densities range from 8 to 30 H unenhanced and 18 to 55 H after contrast administration, enabling clear differentiation from calculi. CT demonstrates the extent of the tumor, including invasion of the kidney or surrounding structures, lymphadenopathy, and distant metastases (Table 34.1). US demonstrates renal TCC as a discrete hypoechoic mass within the renal sinus. Small lesions may be subtle and easily missed. The absence of acoustic shadowing usually provides differentiation from calculi, although a few high-grade tumors may cast acoustic shadows.

Squamous cell carcinoma accounts for 10% of uroepithelial tumors. Chronic infection, calculi, and phenacetin abuse are major predisposing factors. Most tumors are infiltrating and superficially spreading, producing strictures or subtle filling defects. Imaging appearance is indistinguishable from that of TCC.

Metastases are a rare cause of filling defects. Common primary tumor sites are the breast, skin (melanoma), lung, stomach, and cervix.

Papillary necrosis is ischemic necrosis of the tips of the medullary pyramids. Causes include infection, tuberculosis, sickle cell trait and disease, diabetes, and analgesic nephropathy. Necrotic papilla may remain in situ, slough into the collecting system causing a mobile filling defect, or disappear, resulting in a contrast collection in the papilla or

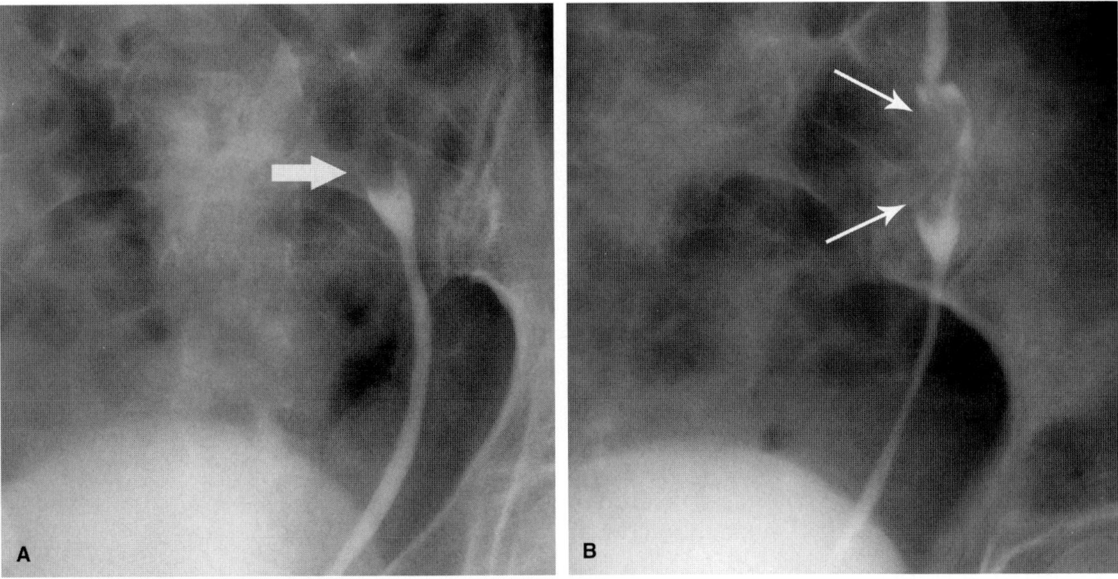

FIGURE 34.10. Transitional Cell Carcinoma of the Ureter. A. A retrograde ureterogram demonstrates widening of the ureter (*arrow*) distal to an obstructing tumor. The distal ureter assumes a champagne glass configuration because of the slow growth of the tumor. **B.** Additional contrast administration demonstrates the full extent of the tumor (*between arrows*).

a blunted calix. Sloughed papilla may obstruct the ureter and cause renal colic.

Fibroepithelial polyp is a benign fibrous polyp covered by transitional epithelium. It is most common in young adult men. The polyp is mobile and hangs from the mucosa by a long, thin stalk (Fig. 34.12).

Pyeloureteritis cystica is a benign process of submucosal cyst formation associated with chronic urinary tract infection. Multiple, small (2 to 3 mm), smooth, round filling defects in the ureter are characteristic (Fig. 34.13). Cysts in the renal pelvis tend to be larger (up to 2 cm).

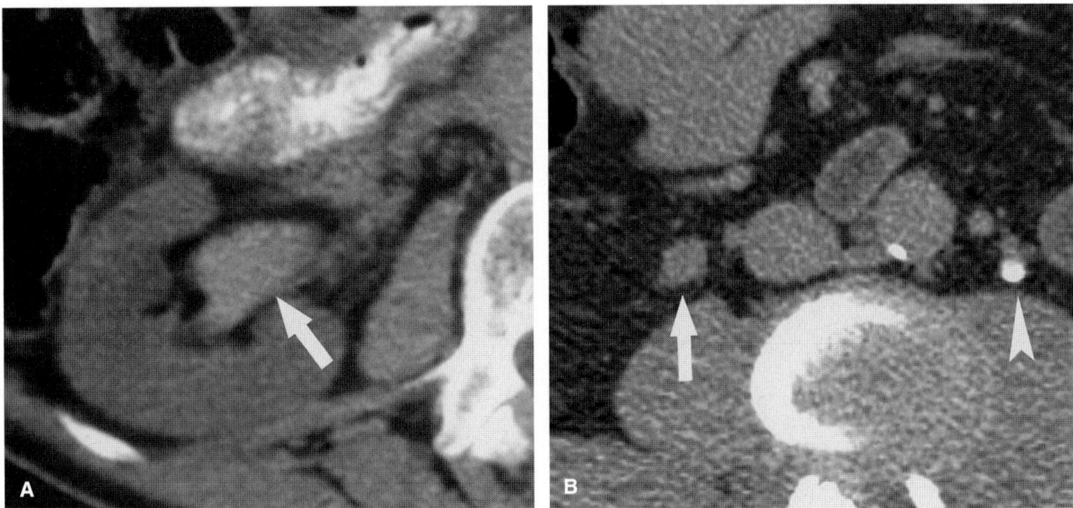

FIGURE 34.11. Transitional Cell Carcinoma (TCC) on CT. A. Image from a noncontrast renal stone CT shows an intermediate-attenuation mass (*arrow*) distending the right renal pelvis. Differential diagnosis would include blood clot versus tumor. Biopsy reveals transitional cell carcinoma. **B.** Postcontrast CT demonstrates an enlarged right ureter (*arrow*) with ill-defined margins. This image was obtained at the level of a ureteral stricture. The ureter above this level was distended and filled with contrast. Surgery confirmed TCC. The left ureter (*arrowhead*) is filled with contrast and is normal in appearance.

TABLE 34.1 Staging of TCC in the Renal Pelvis and Ureter

Stage	Description
I	Tumor limited to uroepithelial mucosa and lamina propria
II	Tumor invades into, but not beyond, muscularis
III	Tumor invades beyond muscularis into periureteric or peripelvic fat or renal parenchyma
IV	Tumor invades adjacent organs or spreads through the kidney into perinephric fat

Adapted from American Joint Committee on Cancer. Manual for Staging of Cancer. 4th ed. Philadelphia: Lippincott, 1992:205–207.

Leukoplakia is a rare inflammatory condition of the uroepithelium related to chronic urinary tract infection and calculi. Squamous metaplasia with keratinization and desquamation results in irregular plaques in the renal pelvis, proximal ureter, and bladder. A key clinical feature is passage of flakes of desquamated epithelium in the urine. Leukoplakia is considered a premalignant condition in the bladder but not in the ureter.

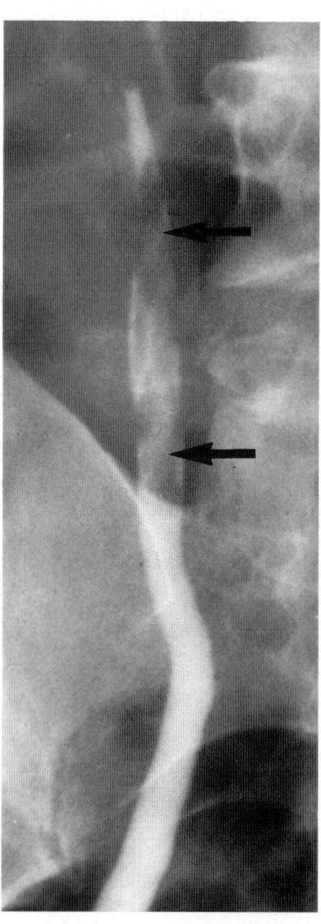

FIGURE 34.12. **Fibroepithelial Polyp.** The long, sinuous filling defect (*arrows*) in the ureter is characteristic of fibroepithelial polyp.

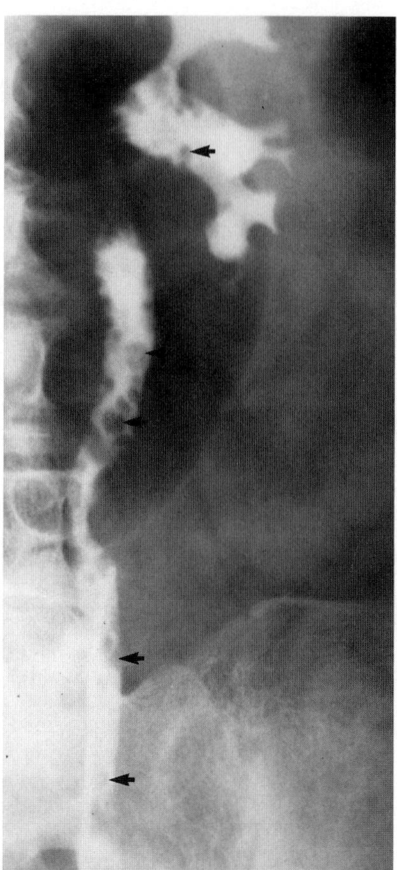

FIGURE 34.13. **Pyeloureteritis Cystica.** Retrograde pyeloureterogram demonstrates numerous well-defined, rounded filling defects (*arrows*) representing submucosal cysts in the left renal pelvis and ureter. The patient had a history of recurrent urinary tract infection.

Malacoplakia is another rare inflammatory condition of the uroepithelium caused by chronic infection, especially by *Escherichia coli.* Smooth submucosal nodules composed of histiocytes produce multiple smooth filling defects in the distal ureter and bladder. This condition is not premalignant.

Stricture of Pelvicaliceal System or Ureter

A stricture is a fixed narrowing of the pelvicaliceal system or ureter. Strictures should be confirmed with multiple views taken in different projections. A diagnosis of ureteral stricture should never be made unless dilatation of the ureter or pelvis above the point of narrowing is present. Active peristalsis and the numerous normal kinks and bends in the ureter mimic strictures but lack the combination of fixed narrowing with proximal dilatation.

Inflammation From Stone. An impacted calculus may cause inflammation, which results in scarring and fibrosis and produces a stricture.

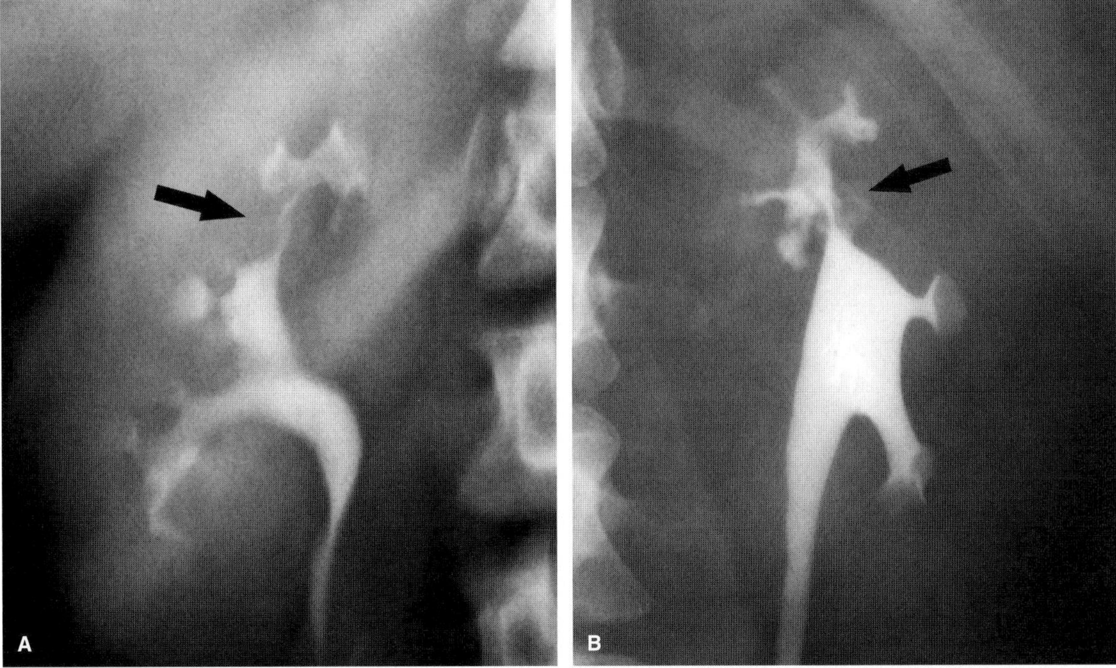

FIGURE 34.14. **Infundibular Strictures. A.** Radiograph from an excretory urogram demonstrates fixed narrowing (*arrow*) of the upper pole infundibulum. The stricture was caused by infiltrating transitional cell carcinoma. **B.** Radiograph from a retrograde ureterogram shows narrowing of the upper pole infundibulum (*arrow*). Active renal tuberculosis with fibrosis was the cause of infundibular stricture in this patient. Note the additional areas of narrowing and irregularity affecting upper pole collecting structures.

Posttraumatic strictures result from surgery and instrumentation.

Uroepithelial Tumor. The infiltrating growth pattern of TCC characteristically causes strictures of the collecting system or ureters (Fig. 34.14). These account for 15% of TCCs. Squamous cell carcinoma is usually manifest as a stricture of the pelvis or ureter.

Tuberculosis and schistosomiasis are two chronic inflammatory processes that are characterized by fibrosis and strictures (Fig. 34.14). Differentiation from TCC may be difficult by imaging studies but may be suggested by history.

Extrinsic encasement by tumor or inflammatory processes is a common cause of stricture. Causes include lymphoma, cervical carcinoma, colon carcinoma, endometriosis, Crohn disease, diverticulitis, and pelvic inflammatory disease.

Papillary Cavities

Caliceal diverticula are uroepithelium-lined cavities in the renal parenchyma that communicate via a narrow channel with the fornix of a nearby calix (Fig. 34.15). They may be congenital, developing from a ureteral bud remnant, or acquired because of infection, reflux, or rupture of a cyst.

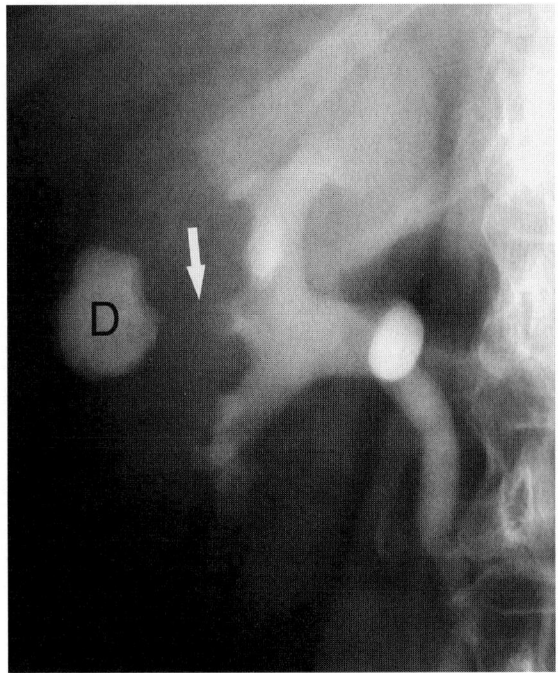

FIGURE 34.15. **Caliceal Diverticulum.** An excretory urogram reveals a contrast-filled diverticulum (D) in the renal parenchyma. A tiny stream of contrast (*arrow*) fills the tract, providing communication between the diverticulum and the caliceal fornix.

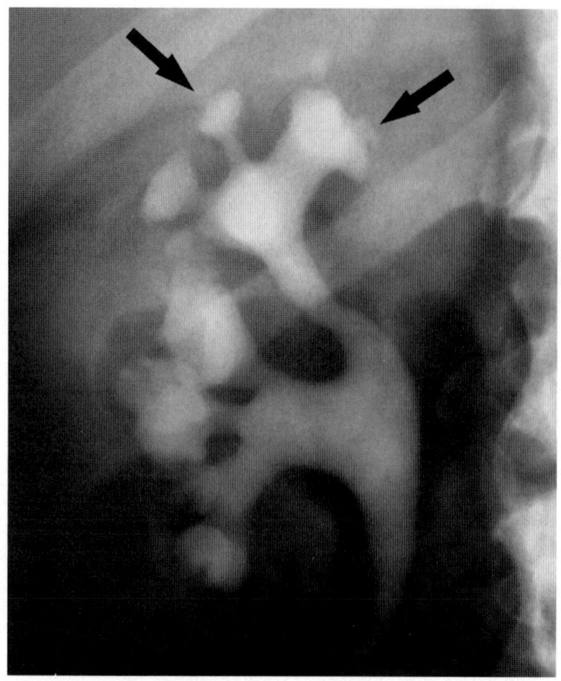

FIGURE 34.16. **Papillary Necrosis.** Multiple cavities (*arrows*) in the papilla filled with contrast during this excretory urogram in a patient with sickle cell trait. Most calices are blunted. Low oxygen tension and high blood osmolality in the papillary tips predispose to sickling and ischemic injury.

Papillary necrosis may result in cavities at the papillary tips that fill with contrast on both antegrade and retrograde studies (Fig. 34.16). Larger cavities cause blunting of the calices.

BLADDER

Imaging Methods

Evaluation of the bladder by standard XU is usually sufficient to exclude most radiographically detectable bladder lesions. A cystogram, performed by instilling contrast agents directly into the bladder, provides a more detailed examination. Fluoroscopic examination is performed during bladder filling to detect reflux. Films are obtained in frontal, lateral, and oblique positions. Films obtained during voiding demonstrate the bladder outlet and urethra. Postvoid films document residual urine. Diagnosis of bladder lesions is made by cystoscopy and biopsy. This procedure is commonly performed prior to any imaging because the patient has hematuria. CT and MR are used primarily to stage known bladder neoplasms. The urine-filled bladder is routinely used as a sonographic window to the pelvis. Intraluminal masses, calculi, bladder wall thickness, and bladder emptying can be reliably assessed by US (see Chapter 37).

Anatomy

The normal filled urinary bladder is oval, with the floor parallel to and 5 to 10 mm above the superior aspect of the symphysis pubis. The size and shape of the bladder vary with the degree of bladder filling. The superior surface is covered by peritoneum, which extends to the side walls of the pelvis. The sigmoid colon and loops of small bowel, as well as the uterus in females, lie on top of the bladder and may cause mass impressions on the bladder dome. The inferior surface is extraperitoneal. Anteriorly, the bladder is separated from the symphysis pubis by fat in the extraperitoneal space of Retzius. Posteriorly, the bladder is separated from the uterus by the uterovesical peritoneal recess in females and from the rectum by the rectovesical peritoneal recess in males.

The lining mucosa of the bladder is loosely attached to the muscular coat, so when the bladder is contracted, the mucosa appears wrinkled. The bladder wall has four layers: (*1*) an outer connective tissue adventitia, (*2*) smooth muscle consisting of circular muscle fibers sandwiched between inner and outer layers of longitudinal fibers, (*3*) submucosal connective tissue (the lamina propria), and (*4*) the mucosa of transitional epithelium. The *trigone* is a triangle at the bladder floor formed by the two ureteral orifices and the internal urethral orifice. With voiding, the trigone descends 1 to 2 cm and transforms from a flat surface into a cone with the urethra at the apex.

On MR, the bladder wall is often indistinguishable from low-intensity urine on T1WIs. On T2WIs, the low-intensity bladder wall is well outlined by high-intensity urine and perivesical fat. Chemical-shift artifact at water–fat interfaces may interfere with assessment of tumor invasion of the bladder wall.

Bladder exstrophy results from a congenital deficiency in development of the lower anterior abdominal wall. The bladder is open, and its mucosa is continuous with the skin. Epispadias and wide diastasis of the symphysis pubis are associated. Ureteral obstruction and umbilical and inguinal hernias are common. Management includes urinary diversion, bladder augmentation, and skin grafting.

Urachal remnant diseases may be discovered in asymptomatic adult patients on CT or US examinations performed for other reasons (12). The urachus is the vestigial remnant of the urogenital sinus and allantois. It is a tubular structure that extends from the bladder dome to the umbilicus along the anterior abdominal wall. The median umbilical ligament is its obliterated residual.

Patent urachus accounts for 50% of cases. The persistent communication between the bladder and umbilicus causes a urine leak, usually resulting in discovery during the neonatal period. Some patients are asymptomatic until an obstructive lesion of the lower urinary tract opens the un-obliterated urachus, resulting in an umbilical-urinary fistula.

Umbilical-urachal sinus (15% of cases) is a blind-ended dilatation of urachus at the umbilical end that may cause a persistent umbilical discharge. Imaging shows a tubular structure in the midline abdominal wall extending caudally from the umbilicus.

Vesical-urachal diverticulum (5%) is an outpouching of the bladder in the anterior midline location of the urachus. This is seen in adults with bladder outlet obstruction as a fluid-filled sac extending cranially from the bladder in midline abdominal wall. Stasis of urine in the diverticulum causes infection, stone formation, and a risk of carcinoma developing within the diverticulum.

Urachal cyst (30%) develops if the urachus is closed at both ends but remains patent in the middle. Imaging shows a fluid-filled cyst in the midline abdominal wall, usually in the lower third of the urachus. Infection may complicate the usually simple nature of the fluid and may result in calcification of the cyst wall.

Urachal carcinoma is usually an adenocarcinoma (90%) and represents 0.5% of bladder carcinomas. Tumors are seen most commonly between ages 40 and 70. They are asymptomatic until they present with local invasion or metastatic disease.

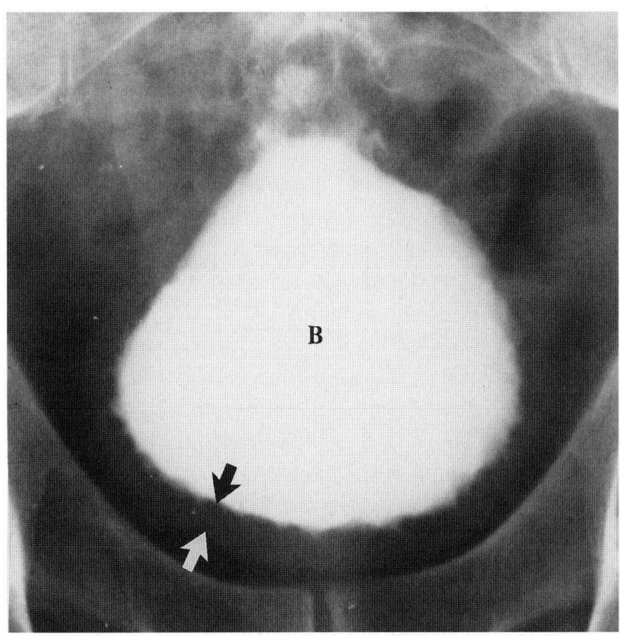

FIGURE 34.17. **Bladder Wall Thickening.** Radiograph from a cystogram in a patient with a neurogenic bladder and chronic urinary tract infections demonstrates a thickened bladder wall (*between arrows*) outlined by the contrast agent inside the bladder (B) and pelvic fat outside the bladder. Note the irregular contour of the bladder lumen, which is caused by trabeculation of the muscle of the bladder wall.

Thickened Bladder Wall/ Small Bladder Capacity

The normal wall of a well-distended bladder should not exceed 5 to 6 mm in thickness (Fig. 34.17). The following conditions are associated with abnormal thickening of the bladder wall and, often, reduced bladder capacity.

Benign prostatic hypertrophy affects 50% to 75% of men over age 50. The enlarged prostate projects into the base of the bladder, uplifting the bladder trigone and causing "J-hooking" of the distal ureters (Fig. 34.18). Chronic bladder outlet obstruction results in thickening and trabeculation of the bladder wall. Prostate calcifications and bladder stones may be present. Prostate carcinoma must also be considered as a cause of prostate enlargement, although imaging methods cannot reliably differentiate benign enlargement from malignancy.

Urethral stricture and posterior urethral valves cause chronic obstruction to the outflow of urine from the bladder. The bladder wall thickens, reflecting muscle hypertrophy in an attempt to overcome the obstruction. Voiding or retrograde urethrography demonstrates the urethral abnormality.

Neurogenic bladder may be spastic or atonic. Causes include meningomyelocele, spinal trauma, diabetes mellitus, poliomyelitis, CNS tumor, and multiple sclerosis. Neurogenic bladders are prone to urinary stasis, chronic infection, and stone formation. Most neurogenic bladders eventually become trabeculated, thick walled, and reduced in capacity.

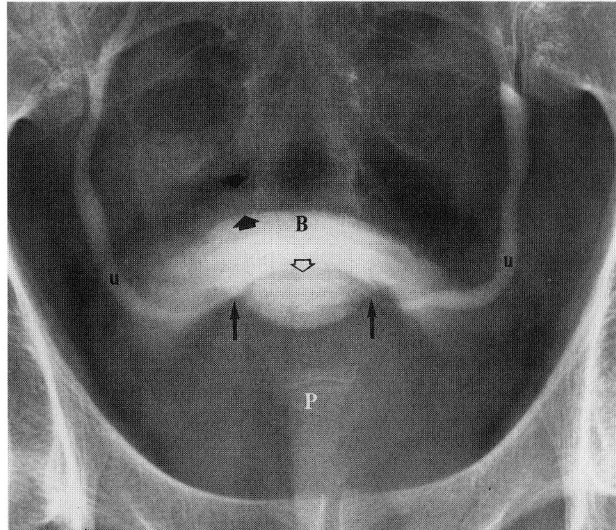

FIGURE 34.18. **Benign Prostatic Hypertrophy.** A radiograph from an excretory urogram shows marked uplifting of the bladder base because of massive enlargement of the prostate (P). The trigone (*open arrow*) and ureteral orifices (*black arrows*) are markedly elevated, resulting in a J-shaped appearance to the distal ureters (u). The bladder wall is thickened (between *black arrowheads*), and the bladder (B) mucosal pattern is prominent.

Cystitis. Inflammation of the bladder has many causes, including infection (bacteria, adenovirus, tuberculosis, schistosomiasis); drugs (cyclophosphamide); radiation; and autoimmune reactions. MR demonstrates mucosal edema and inflammation as high signal intensity on T2WIs, which are easily differentiated from the normal low-signal bladder wall.

Cystitis cystica is characterized by multiple fluid-filled submucosal cysts. Most cases are associated with bladder infection.

Cystitis glandularis is a further progression of cystitis cystica with proliferation of mucous-secreting glands in the lamina propria. The cysts vary in size and may obstruct the ureteral orifice. Cystitis glandularis may be a precursor of adenocarcinoma of the bladder.

Bullous edema of the bladder wall is usually associated with chronic irritation from indwelling catheters. Grape-like cysts elevate the mucosa.

Interstitial cystitis is a chronic, idiopathic inflammation of the bladder found most often in women. Bladder capacity is progressively diminished, and the bladder wall thickens and becomes trabeculated and fibrotic.

Hemorrhagic cystitis is characterized by hemorrhage into the mucosa and submucosa. It is caused by bacterial or adenovirus infection.

Eosinophilic cystitis is an infiltration of the bladder wall by eosinophils. The cause is uncertain. The bladder wall is greatly thickened and frequently nodular.

Emphysematous cystitis is a form of bladder inflammation with gas within the bladder wall (Fig. 34.19). It is associated with poorly controlled diabetes mellitus, bladder outlet obstruction, and infection with *E coli,* which ferment sugar in the urine to release carbon dioxide and hydrogen gasses. Gas within the bladder lumen is seen with emphysematous cystitis, instrumentation, and vesicocolic fistula.

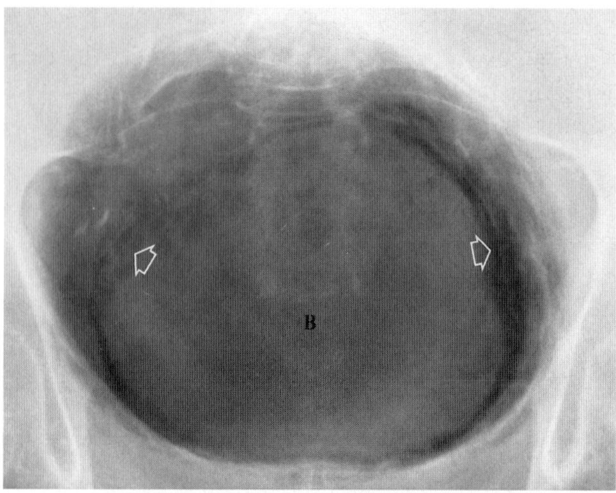

FIGURE 34.19. **Emphysematous Cystitis.** Air in the bladder wall is seen as a pattern of layering linear lucencies (*open arrows*) outlining the bladder (B) on this plain radiograph in a 67-year-old man with cystitis caused by Escherichia coll.

Calcified Bladder Wall

Schistosomiasis of the urinary tract is caused by infestation with *Schistosoma haematobium.* The disease is most prevalent in North Africa, the Nile Valley, and Egypt. The larval cercariae of the blood fluke penetrate the skin of humans in infected water, enter the lymphatic vessels, and eventually circulate to the portal venous system, where the organism matures into adulthood. Adult females migrate to the vesical venous plexus and lay their eggs in the wall of the urinary bladder and ureter. The eggs incite a fibrosing granulomatous reaction that results in beaded stenosis and irregular dilatation of the ureters, along with calcification of the walls of the distal ureters and bladder. The calcification is entirely the result of calcification of the eggs embedded within the wall (Fig. 34.20). The ureters become aperistaltic, resulting in vesicoureteral reflux. Eventually, the bladder may become shrunken, fibrotic, and contracted. Fistulas may develop in the perineum and scrotum. Renal disease develops slowly as the result of functional obstruction and reflux.

Tuberculosis affects the kidneys primarily and the ureters and bladder secondarily. Calcification affects the ureters proximally and may eventually extend into

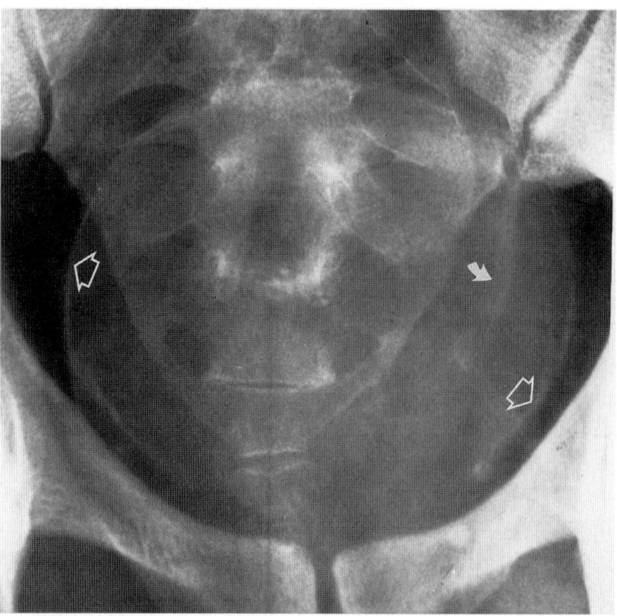

FIGURE 34.20. **Infestation With Schistosoma haematobium.** Plain radiograph demonstrates calcification in the wall of the bladder (*open arrows*) and in the wall of the left ureter (*curved arrow*). The bladder is filled with urine. The patient is a 25-year-old Egyptian man.

the distal ureters and bladder. Tuberculous infection of the bladder causes wall thickening and reduced capacity. Calcification of the bladder wall is uncommon and patchy.

Cystitis. Postirradiation cystitis, chronic infection, and cyclophosphamide-induced cystitis cause curvilinear or flocculent bladder wall calcification.

Neoplasm. Transitional cell and squamous cell carcinomas of the bladder may rarely calcify (1% to 7% incidence). Tumor calcification may be punctate or curvilinear and is best demonstrated by CT.

Bladder Wall Masses/Filling Defects

Simple ureterocele is a congenital prolapse of the dilated distal ureter and orifice into the bladder lumen at the normal insertion site of the ureter into the trigone. It is usually an incidental finding in adults, although larger, simple ureteroceles may be associated with ureter obstruction, infection, and stone formation. XU demonstrates a rounded filling defect in the bladder at the ureteral insertion (Fig. 34.21). A "cobra head" or "spring onion" appearance is characteristic. A radiolucent halo is produced by the wall of the ureter, which is outlined both inside and outside by contrast. US demonstrates a cystic mass at the ureteral orifice. Peristalsis of the ureter causes alternate filling and emptying of the ureterocele, as seen on real-time US.

Ectopic ureterocele is usually associated with ureteral duplication. Females with ectopic ureters are prone to urinary incontinence because the ureter may insert distal to the external sphincter into the vestibule, uterus, or vagina. In males, the ectopic ureter usually inserts proximal to the external sphincter; no incontinence results. Insertion sites include the lower bladder, posterior urethra, seminal vesicles, vas deferens, and ejaculatory duct. Large ectopic ureteroceles may obstruct the opposite ureter or cause bladder outlet obstruction because of their mass effect. The ectopic ureterocele appears as a cystic mass at the ectopic site of ureter insertion. The ureter is dilated and tortuous (Fig. 34.22).

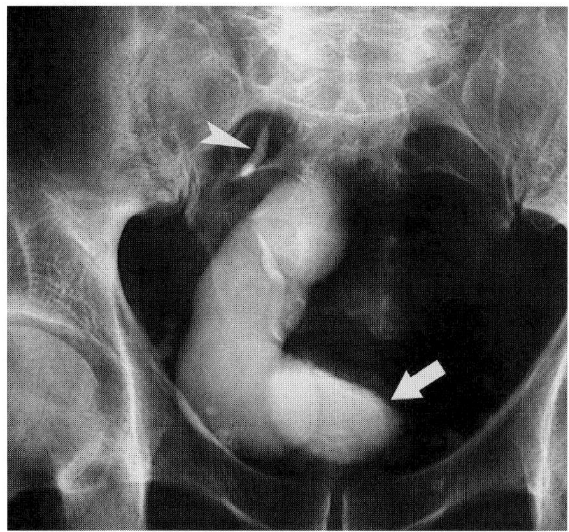

FIGURE 34.22. **Obstructed Duplication: Ectopic Ureterocele.** Radiograph from an excretory urogram shows a normal ureter (*arrowhead*) from the normal lower pole of the kidney and a dilated ureter with ectopic ureterocele (*arrow*) from the obstructed upper pole of the kidney. The ectopic ureter inserts medial and caudal to the normal insertion of the upper pole ureter.

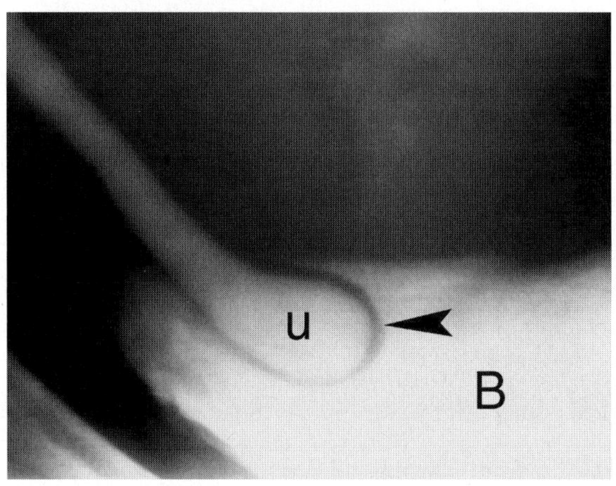

FIGURE 34.21. **Simple Ureterocele.** Radiograph from an excretory urogram demonstrates mild dilation of the right ureter associated with a simple ureterocele (u) that protrudes into the lumen of the bladder (B). The radiolucent wall of the ureterocele (*arrowhead*) is outlined by contrast within the ureterocele and contrast within the bladder lumen. The wall of the ureterocele is made up of the wall of the ureter and the bladder mucosa.

Transitional cell carcinoma of the bladder is the most common urinary tract neoplasm. TCC of the bladder is 50 times more common than TCC of the ureter. Although bladder tumors commonly develop in patients with primary TCC of the renal pelvis or ureter, only 2% to 4% of patients with bladder carcinoma have TCC of the ureter. Nonetheless, all patients with TCC deserve detailed screening of the entire uroepithelium. Bladder cancers are classified as superficial (papillary tumors confined to the mucosa and associated with a high likelihood of multiplicity and recurrence following resection) or invasive (penetrating into and through the bladder wall, resulting in local extension and metastases). Cross-sectional imaging is used to stage known bladder carcinoma (Table 34.2). TNM staging is favored over the older, but still used, Jewett-Marshall-Strong staging system (13). Bladder carcinoma spreads by direct invasion through the bladder wall, by lymphatic spread to regional lymph nodes, or by hematogenous spread, most commonly to bones, liver, and lung (13). Approximately 5% of patients have distant metastases at initial diagnosis.

XU has played a major role in screening the uroepithelium. Most bladder tumors appear as irregular filling

TABLE 34.2 Staging of TCC in the Bladder

Jewett-Strong-Marshall System	TNM System	Description	CT and MR Findings
0	T1s	Carcinoma in situ	Flat tumor too small to be detected
0	Ta	Papillary tumor, confined to epithelium	Tumor confined to bladder wall; outer bladder wall is intact
A	T1	Tumor invades lamina propria	Tumor confined to bladder wall; outer bladder wall is intact
B1	T2	Tumor invades inner half of muscle layer	Tumor confined to bladder wall; outer bladder wall is intact
B2	T3a	Tumor invades outer half of muscle layer	Tumor extends through the bladder wall but not into perivesical fat
C	T3b	Tumor invades perivesical fat	Tumor extends into perivesical fat
D1	T4a	Tumor invades surrounding organs	Tumor invades other pelvic organs
D1	T4b	Tumor invades pelvic or abdominal wall	Tumor invades pelvic side wall
D1	N1–N3	Pelvic lymph node metastases	Pelvic nodes >1.0 cm

Adapted from Kundra V, Silverman PM. Imaging in the diagnosis, staging, and follow-up of cancer of the urinary bladder. AJR Am J Roentgenol 2003;180:1045–1054.

defects (Fig. 34.23). Tumors larger than 1.5 cm are reliably detected by XU with inclusion of a postvoid film. The tumor may obstruct a ureteral orifice. Cystoscopic biopsy confirms the diagnosis. CT and MR are approximately equally useful in staging bladder cancer (14). CT demonstrates TCC as a soft tissue mass projecting into the bladder lumen or as a focal thickening of the bladder wall. Enhancing tumor is best seen against a background of low-attenuation urine distending the bladder (Fig 34.24). Tumor enhancement peaks during the first 60 seconds following contrast injection, allowing the optimal identification of tumor invasion. When contrast has filled the bladder, tumor is seen as low-attenuation polypoid or plaquelike

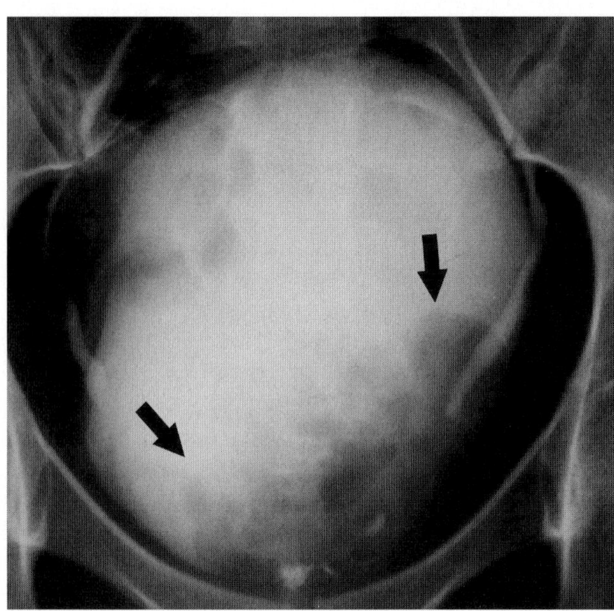

FIGURE 34.23. **Transitional Cell Carcinoma.** Radiograph from an excretory urogram reveals a lobulated mass (*arrows*) causing a large filling defect in the base of the bladder (B). Both ureters are visualized.

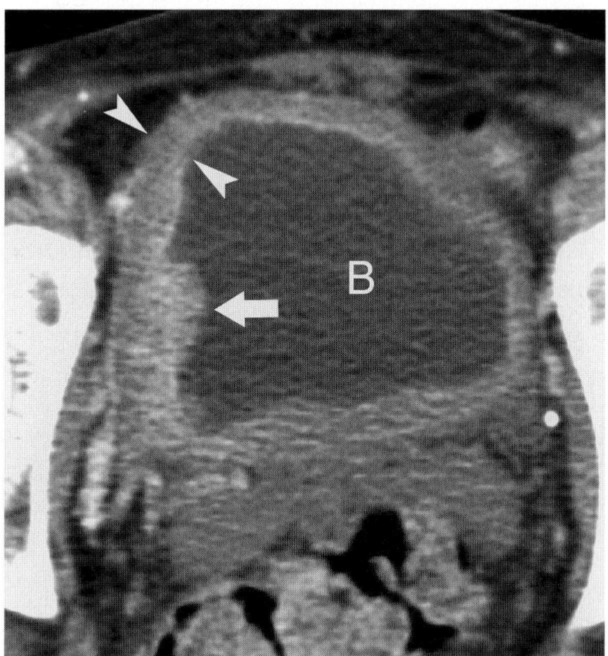

FIGURE 34.24. **Transitional Cell Carcinoma on CT.** CT image demonstrates a flat mucosal lesion (*arrow*) arising from the right lateral wall of the bladder (B). Contrast enhancement of the lesion is slightly greater than that of the bladder wall, revealing the extent of the tumor. This is a T1 lesion (i.e., confined to the bladder wall). The bladder wall is thickened (between *arrowheads*) and irregular because of muscle hypertrophy induced by the chronic obstruction of an enlarged prostate. On this early phase CT image, the bladder is distended with low-attenuation urine.

mural nodule against a background of high-attenuation, contrast-opacified urine. Calcifications are seen in 5% of tumors. Perivesical spread is seen as soft tissue–density tumor in the perivesical fat. Previous biopsy, inflammation, and postradiation changes make image interpretation more difficult.

On MR, TCC is intermediate signal, equal to muscle, on T1WIs (15). Invasion of perivesical fat and involvement of lymph nodes are best determined on T1WIs. Depth of bladder wall invasion is determined on T2WIs. Tumor is slightly higher in signal than bladder wall muscle but lower in signal than urine. Bladder wall invasion is suggested by disruption of the low-signal muscle layer. Postcontrast images are routinely T1WIs with fat suppression to aid in detection of enhancing tumor in perivesical fat. TCC enhances earlier than bladder muscle, so dynamic imaging should be performed following gadolinium injection. Lesions with shaggy irregular outer borders with streaky areas or high signal in perivesical fat are classified as T3b. Tumor extension to the pelvic sidewall, abdominal wall, or adjacent organ is classified as T4a or T4b. Coronal and sagittal plane images improve the accuracy of staging on MR (13,15).

US demonstrates exophytic tumors as polypoid masses extending from the bladder wall. Infiltrating tumors may show as focal thickening of the bladder wall. Tumors may be difficult to recognize in the presence of diffuse bladder wall thickening and trabeculation.

Squamous cell carcinoma accounts for 4% of bladder malignancy. It tends to develop in bladders that have been chronically irritated by stones and infection and is highly associated with bladder schistosomiasis. Most tumors have invaded the bladder wall and many have metastasized to distant sites at the time of diagnosis (16).

Adenocarcinoma is rare, accounting for fewer than 1% of bladder malignancies. Most cases are associated with bladder exstrophy or urachal remnants.

Benign bladder tumors include leiomyoma, hemangioma, pheochromocytoma, and neurofibroma. They produce smooth filling defects.

Blood clots in the bladder are usually irregular in shape, move with changes in patient position, and change in size and appearance over time.

Bladder stones may migrate from the kidney or form primarily within the bladder (Fig. 34.25) because of urinary stasis or a foreign body. Solitary stones are most common. Stones must be removed to cure chronic bladder infection. Chronic bladder stones increase the risk of developing bladder carcinoma.

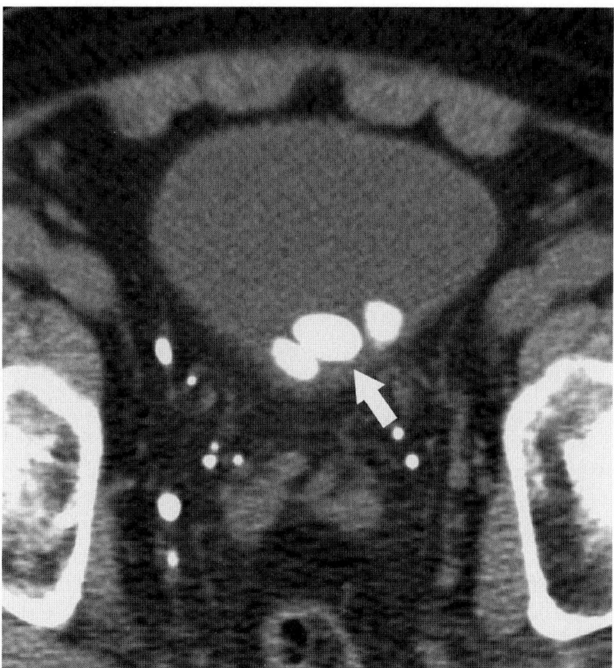

FIGURE 34.25. **Bladder Stones.** Multiple high-attenuation stones (*arrow*) are seen within the lumen of the bladder on this noncontrast CT. Contrast opacification of the bladder may obscure the presence of bladder stones. This patient has a neurogenic bladder, which has resulted in chronic urine stasis within the bladder.

Pear-Shaped Bladder/Extrinsic Mass

Lymphadenopathy is a common cause of extrinsic mass impression on the bladder. Lymphoma and metastases from malignancies of the pelvic organs are common causes.

Pelvic hemorrhage indents the bladder and displaces it to the opposite side. CT and MR confirm the presence of hematoma.

Pelvic lipomatosis refers to a condition of excessive perirectal and perivesical fat in the pelvis. The bladder is elongated and lifted up and out of the pelvis. Fat density is evident on CT and MR.

Iliac artery aneurysms tend to be clinically silent, but rupture is common and associated with high mortality. Calcification in the aneurysm may be apparent. Most iliac artery aneurysms are associated with aortic aneurysms.

Pelvic tumors may be manifest on plain film or excretory urography by mass impression on the bladder.

Psoas muscle hypertrophy may also cause a pear-shaped bladder.

Bladder Outpouchings/Fistulas

Bladder diverticula are herniations of the bladder mucosa between interlacing muscle bundles. Most are located posterolaterally, near the ureterovesical junction (Fig. 34.26). Diverticula may contain stones or tumor and occasionally do not fill on cystograms. Complications of bladder

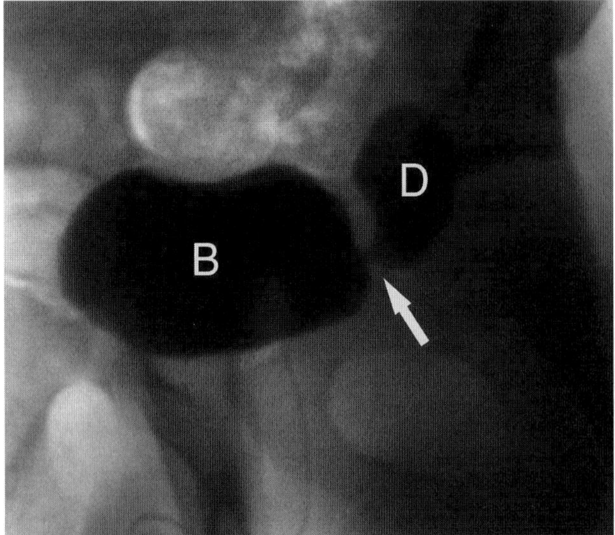

FIGURE 34.26. **Bladder Diverticulum.** Oblique digital radiograph obtained during a cystogram reveals a congenital bladder diverticulum (D) in a child. The diverticulum connects to the bladder (B) via a narrow channel (*arrow*) through the bladder wall. Diverticula that originate near the ureterovesical junction may induce vesicoureteral reflux.

diverticula include urinary stasis, infection, stone formation, vesicoureteral reflux, and bladder outlet obstruction.

Vesicocolonic fistula most commonly occurs as a complication of diverticulitis. Additional causes include colon or bladder carcinoma, ulcerative colitis, and Crohn disease. The bladder is chronically infected, and the patient may complain of pneumaturia and fecaluria. The diagnosis is often made clinically. Barium enema and cystography detect only 35% of vesicocolonic fistulas. The fistulous tract is occasionally demonstrated by CT.

Vesicovaginal fistula is usually a complication of gynecologic surgery, especially for cervical carcinoma. Obstetric injury is an occasional cause.

Vesicoenteric fistulas are almost always attributable to Crohn disease.

Bladder Trauma

Susceptibility of the bladder to traumatic injury depends largely on the degree of bladder filling at the time of injury. A distended bladder is more prone to injury than a collapsed bladder.

Extraperitoneal bladder rupture (80% of bladder ruptures) results from puncture of the bladder by a spicule of bone from a pelvic fracture. Contrast extravasates into the extraperitoneal compartments, most commonly the retropubic space of Retzius (Fig. 34.27). Contrast extravasation may extend into the anterior abdominal wall, thigh, and scrotum. XU is not an adequate screening method.

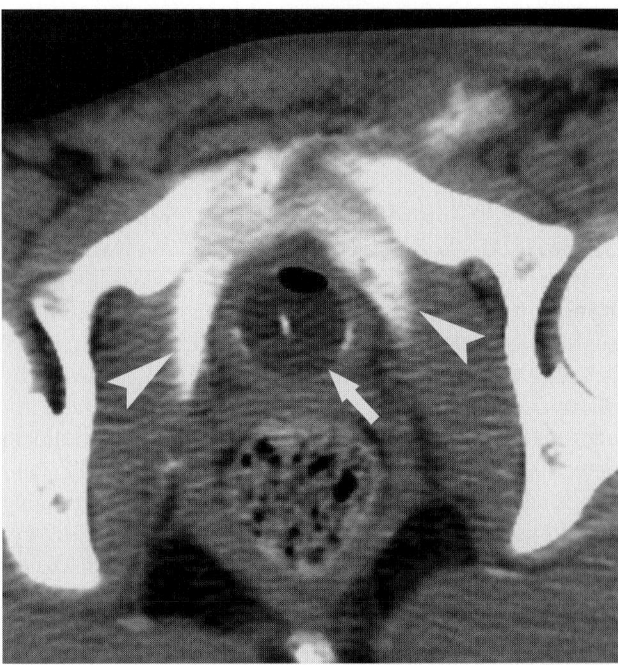

FIGURE 34.27. **Extraperitoneal Bladder Rupture.** Image from a CT cystogram performed in a patient with a pelvic fracture reveals contrast extravasation (*arrowheads*) from the bladder into the retropubic space of Retzius, indicating bladder rupture into the extraperitoneal compartment. Contrast was instilled into the bladder via a Foley catheter (*arrow*).

Cystography or CT with distension of the bladder to at least 250 mL is required to exclude bladder rupture.

Intraperitoneal bladder rupture (20% of bladder ruptures) results from application of blunt trauma to a distended bladder. The sudden rise in intravesical pressure results in rupture of the bladder dome and extravasation into the peritoneal space. Contrast material flows into

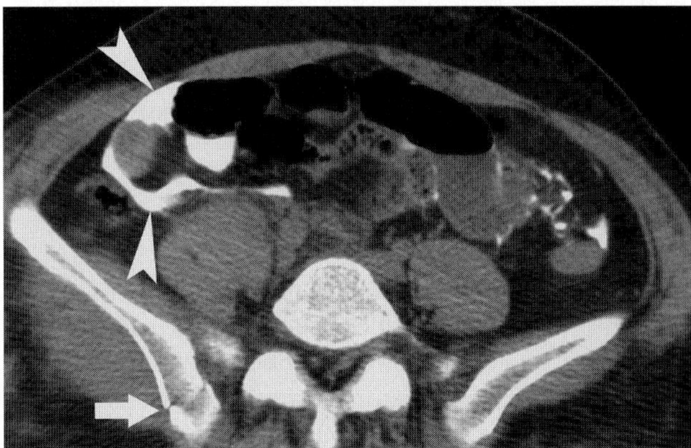

FIGURE 34.28. **Intraperitoneal Bladder Rupture.** Image from a CT cystogram demonstrates extravasation of contrast from the bladder into the intraperitoneal space. Contrast (*arrowheads*) enveloping loops of bowel confirms its intraperitoneal location. This finding on a CT cystogram is diagnostic of intraperitoneal bladder rupture. A fracture (*arrow*) of the ilium is evident.

the paracolic gutters and outlines the loops of the bowel (Fig. 34.28). Intraperitoneal bladder rupture may clinically mimic acute renal failure. Urine output is decreased or absent, and serum creatinine is increased because of absorption of urine by the peritoneal surface.

URETHRA

Imaging Methods

The urethra is studied by retrograde and voiding urethrography (Fig. 34.29) (17). The retrograde urethrogram is a simple study of the anterior male urethra. Contrast medium is injected into the anterior urethra by means of a syringe or catheter that occludes the meatal orifice. Films are exposed in the right posterior oblique projection. The anterior urethra normally distends fully because of resistance of the external sphincter at the level of the urogenital diaphragm. Complete filling of the posterior urethra is not possible because contrast runs freely into the bladder. Voiding cystourethrography is performed by filling the bladder with contrast via a catheter. The catheter is removed, and films are obtained while the patient urinates into a basin on the fluoroscopy table. The voiding urethrogram demonstrates distension of both the posterior and anterior urethra. Radiographic study of the female urethra may be conducted by voiding cystourethrogram or by retrograde urethrogram with a specially designed double-balloon catheter. The female urethra is also well studied by transrectal or perineal US and by CT and MR (18,19).

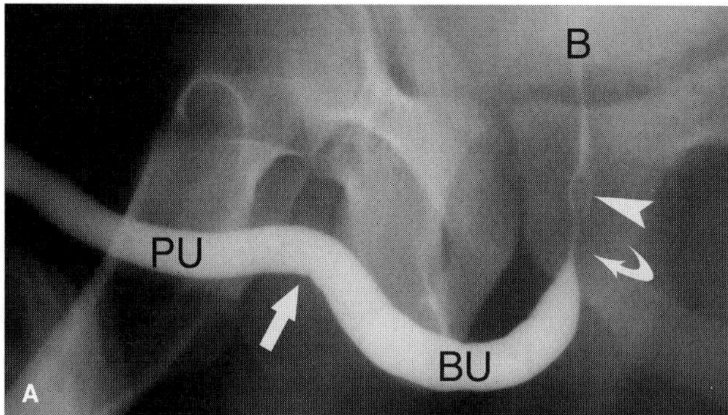

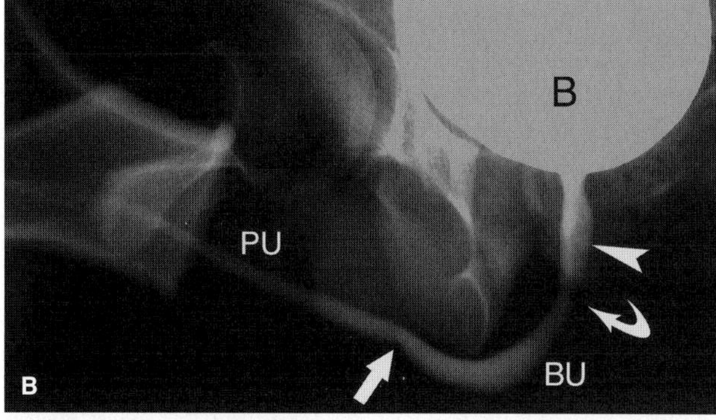

FIGURE 34.29. **Normal Male Urethra. A.** Retrograde urethrogram (RUG). **B.** Voiding cystourethrogram (VCUG). The anterior urethra consists of the penile and bulbous urethra. The penile urethra (PU) extends from the urethral meatus to the suspensory ligament of the penis (*straight arrows*) at the penoscrotal junction. The bulbous urethra (BU) extends from the penoscrotal junction to the urogenital diaphragm (*curved arrows*), marked by the tip of the cone on the RUG and the slight narrowing of urethral caliber on the VCUG. The posterior urethra consists of the membranous urethra and the prostatic urethra. The membranous urethra (*curved arrows*) is only 1 cm in length and is entirely within the muscle of the urogenital diaphragm. On a RUG, the membranous urethra extends between the tip of the cone and the verumontanum. The verumontanum (*arrowheads*) is a nodular structure that produces a filling defect on the urethrograms by bulging into the prostatic urethra. The prostatic urethra extends from the inferior aspect of the verumontanum to the base of the bladder (B).

Anatomy

The male urethra is divided into posterior and anterior portions by the inferior aspect of the urogenital diaphragm (Fig. 34.29). The posterior urethra consists of the *prostatic urethra* within the prostate gland, from the bladder neck to urogenital diaphragm, and the short *membranous urethra,* which is totally contained within the 1-cm thick urogenital diaphragm. The anterior urethra extends from the urogenital diaphragm to the external urethral meatus. It consists of the *bulbous urethra,* which extends from the urogenital diaphragm to the penoscrotal junction, and the *penile urethra,* which extends to the urethral meatus. The anterior urethra is entirely contained within the corpus spongiosum penis, except for the proximal 2 cm of the bulbous urethra, called the *pars nuda.* The prostatic urethra runs vertically through the prostate over a length of 3 to 4 cm. An oval filling defect in the midportion of the posterior wall is the *verumontanum.* The ejaculatory ducts open into the urethra on either side of the verumontanum, and the prostatic glands empty into the urethra by multiple small openings that surround the verumontanum. The *utricle,* a müllerian remnant, is a small, saccular depression in the middle of the verumontanum. The distal end of the verumontanum marks the beginning of the membranous urethra, which extends to the apex of the cone of the bulbous urethra. The voluntary external urethral sphincter within the urogenital diaphragm entirely surrounds the membranous urethra. The *Cowper glands* are pea-sized accessory sex glands within the urogenital diaphragm on either side of the membranous urethra. Their ducts empty into the bulbous urethra 2 cm distally (Fig. 34.30).

On retrograde urethrography, the bulbous urethra tapers to a cone shape as the urethra enters the external sphincter. The apex of the cone marks the division between the membranous and bulbous urethra. The penoscrotal junction, which divides the bulbous and penile

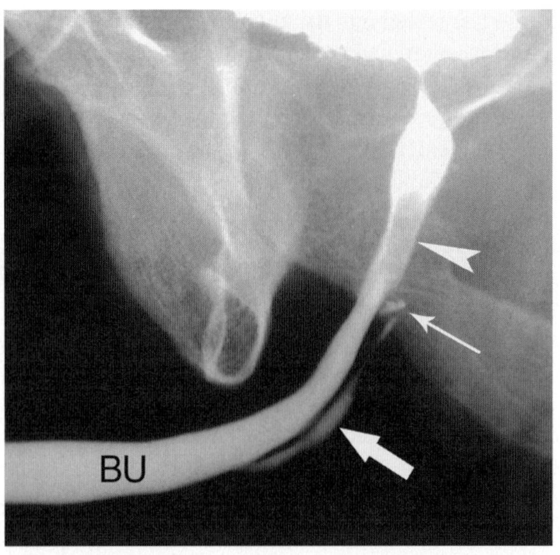

FIGURE 34.30. **Cowper Glands.** Radiograph from a voiding cystourethrogram shows filling of the ducts to Cowper glands. The glands (*thin arrow*) are in the urogenital diaphragm, and their ducts (*wide arrow*) drain into the bulbous urethra (BU). The verumontanum (*arrowhead*) produces its usual filling defect in the contrast column.

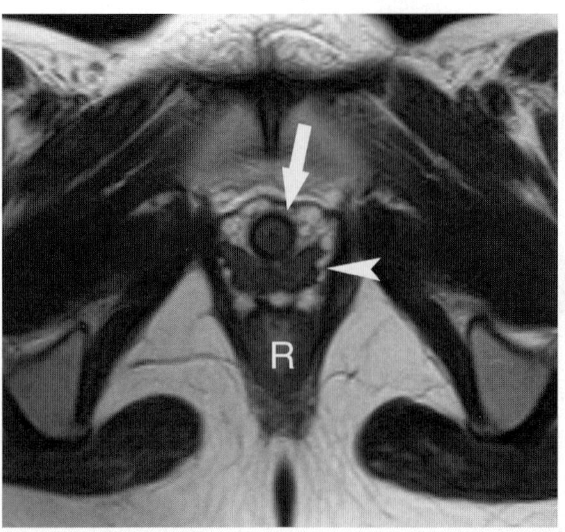

FIGURE 34.31. **Normal Female Urethra.** T2WI demonstrates the zonal anatomy of the female urethra (*arrow*) in the anterior wall of the vagina (*arrowhead*). The outer smooth layer is low signal (*dark*), the submucosal layer is moderately bright, and the central mucosa is dark. The rectum (R) is seen posteriorly.

urethra, is marked by the suspensory ligament of the penis, which causes a normal bend in the urethra. The entire anterior urethra is lined by the *glands of Littre* (see Fig. 34.32), whose secretions lubricate the urethra. Cowper ducts and the utricle occasionally fill with contrast during urethrography in a normal patient; however, the filling of these structures with contrast occurs much more commonly in the presence of urethral strictures. Visualization of the glands of Littre is always abnormal and is associated with chronic inflammation and urethral stricture. Reflux of contrast into the prostatic ducts is also abnormal and is associated with prostatitis and distal urethral stricture.

The female urethra varies in length from 2.5 to 4 cm. The urethra is embedded in the anterior wall of the vagina and is lined throughout by periurethral glands. On MR, the urethra is isointense with the vaginal muscle on T1WIs. On T2WIs, the normal urethra demonstrates a characteristic target appearance (Fig. 34.31), with dark inner and outer rings and a middle zone of high signal intensity. The middle zone corresponds to highly vascular submucosa and enhances markedly with gadopentetate administration. The dark inner zone is mucosa, and the dark outer zone is urethral smooth muscle.

Pathology

Urethral strictures are abnormal narrowings of the urethra caused by fibrous scar tissue. They may involve the entire urethra or only a small portion. Abrupt, short-segment strictures are usually traumatic. Long-segment strictures may be either traumatic or inflammatory (Fig. 34.32). Causes of traumatic urethral strictures include instrumentation, indwelling catheters, prostatectomy procedures, chemical injury (podophyllin), straddle injuries (usually of the bulbous urethra), and pelvic fractures. Most inflammatory strictures are attributable to gonorrhea. Bacteria become sequestered in the glands of Littre and incite the formation of granulation tissue and fibrosis. Additional etiologies include chlamydia, mycoplasma, tuberculosis, and schistosomiasis. Complications of urethral strictures include the following:

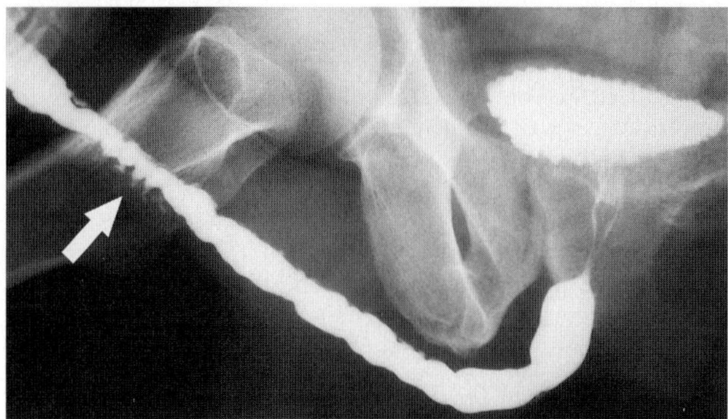

FIGURE 34.32. **Urethral Strictures, Glands of Littre.** Retrograde urethrogram demonstrates multiple strictures in the penile and bulbous urethra. Filling of the glands of Littre (*arrow*) is evidence of urethritis. This patient had a history of multiple episodes of gonorrhea.

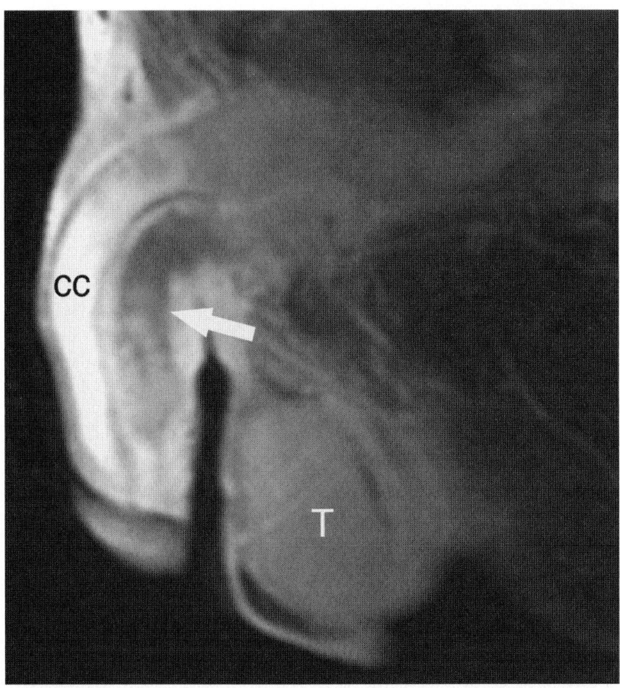

FIGURE 34.33. **Carcinoma of the Penile Urethra.** Sagittal MR image shows recurrent squamous cell carcinoma as abnormal low signal (*arrow*) filling and distending the penile urethra within the corpus spongiosum. This patient has already experienced partial resection of the tip of his penis for carcinoma. One of the corpora cavernosa (cc) is seen anteriorly. A normal testis (T) is also shown.

- *Periurethral abscess* usually develops on the ventral surface and may drain into the lumen or onto the skin, creating a periurethral fistula.
- *False passage* is the most common complication of urethral stricture. It is usually iatrogenic because of attempted passage of catheters or instruments past the obstruction.
- *Stasis and infection* may cause disease of the more proximal urinary tracts, including hydronephrosis, bladder hypertrophy, calculi, and chronic inflammation.
- *Carcinoma of the urethra* occurs as a complication of chronic urethritis and stricture. Carcinomas may appear as filling defects in the urethra or as changes in appearance of the stricture. Most are squamous cell carcinomas and most involve the anterior urethra. MR is the imaging method of choice for showing extent of tumor (Fig. 34.33). Rare tumors of the posterior urethra are usually TCCs that occur as part of multiple uroepithelial neoplasia.

Urethral diverticula are smooth, saclike outpouchings of the urethra. They may be congenital or the result of infection or trauma. Because they serve as a site of urinary stasis, stone formation and recurrent infection are common complications. A diverticulum of the female urethra

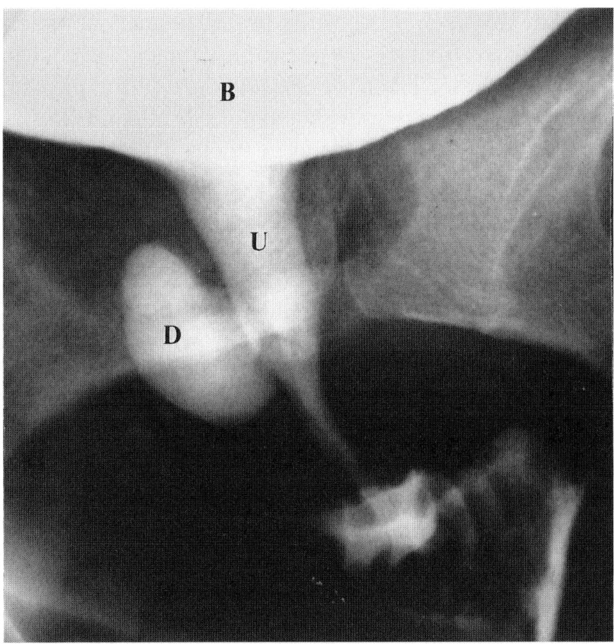

FIGURE 34.34. **Urethral Diverticulum.** Voiding cystourethrogram in a woman with recurrent urinary tract infections fills a urethral diverticulum (D). B, bladder; U, urethra.

is an uncommon cause of recurrent urinary tract infection. It may be demonstrated by a postvoid film of an excretory urogram, voiding cystourethrogram (Fig. 34.34), transrectal or transperineal US, or MR (19).

Traumatic injury to the posterior urethra occurs in about 10% of pelvic fractures. The junction between the

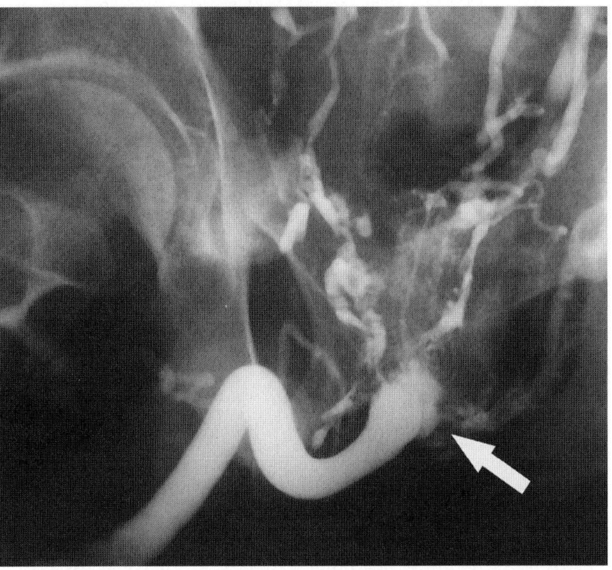

FIGURE 34.35. **Traumatic Urethral Transection.** Radiograph from a retrograde urethrogram shows transection of the urethra at the level of the urogenital diaphragm (*arrow*). Contrast extravasates into adjacent tissues and intravasates into pelvic veins.

prostatic and membranous urethra is the most common site of injury. Injury is suspected in patients with pelvic fractures or when blood is present at the urethral meatus. Retrograde urethrography should precede attempts at urethral catheterization. If a bladder catheter has already been inserted, the urethra can be studied by inserting a small (8 French) pediatric feeding tube adjacent to the catheter and injecting contrast. The classification of posterior urethral injury is as follows: *Type 1* is a stretch injury caused by pelvic hematoma; *Type 2* is a rupture of the membranous urethra at the apex of the prostate, with extravasation above the urogenital diaphragm; *Type 3* is a rupture of both the membranous and bulbous urethra, with disruption of the urogenital diaphragm and contrast extravasation both above and below the diaphragm (Fig. 34.35) (17).

A "straddle injury"—ie, falling astride a fixed object—commonly injures the bulbous urethra. Instrumentation, foreign body insertion, or direct trauma to the penis may injure the penile urethra. Long-term bladder catheterization may injure any portion of the urethra. Autodigestion of the urethra because of drainage of pancreatic exocrine enzymes has been reported as a complication of pancreatic transplantation, with pancreatic drainage into the bladder. Complications of urethral injury are common and include stricture, incontinence, impotence, and pelvic and perineal sinus tracts and fistulas.

REFERENCES

1. Kawashima A, Vrtiska TJ, LeRoy AJ, et al. CT urography. Radiographics 2004;24:S35–S58.
2. Blandino A, Gaeta M, Minutoli F, et al. MR urography of the ureter. AJR Am J Roentgenol 2002;179:1307–1314.
3. Fernbach SK, Feinstein KA, Spencer K, Lindstrom CA. Ureteral duplication and its complications. Radiographics 1997;17:109–127.
4. Lawler LP, Jarret TW, Corl FM, Fishman EK. Adult ureteropelvic junction obstruction: insights with three-dimensional multidetector row CT. Radiographics 2005;25:121–134.
5. Brant WE. Spiral CT replaces IVP and KUB for renal stone disease. Diag Imag 2001;Jun:51–57.
6. Levine JA, Neitlich J, Verga M, Dalrymple NC, Smith RC. Ureteral calculi in patients with flank pain: correlation of plain radiography with unenhanced helical CT. Radiology 1997;204:27–31.
7. Chen MYM, Scharling ES, Zagoria RJ, et al. CT diagnosis of acute flank pain from urolithiasis. Semin Ultrasound CT MRI 2000;21:2–19.
8. Fowler KAB, Lochem JA, Duchesne JH, Williamson MR. US for detecting renal calculi with nonenhanced CT as a reference standard. Radiology 2002;222:109–113.
9. Rucker CM, Menias CO, Bhalla S. Mimics of renal colic: alternative diagnoses at unenhanced helical CT. Radiographics 2004;24:S11–S33.
10. Katz DS, Hines J, Rausch DR, et al. Unenhanced helical CT for suspected renal colic. AJR Am J Roentgenol 1999;173:425–430.
11. Wong-You-Cheong JJ, Wagner BJ, Davis CJ Jr. Transitional cell carcinoma of the urinary tract: radiologic-pathologic correlation. Radiographics 1998;18:123–142.
12. Yu J-S, Kim KW, Lee H-J, et al. Urachal remnant diseases: spectrum of CT and US findings. Radiographics 2001;21:451–461.
13. Kundra V, Silverman PM. Imaging in the diagnosis, staging, and follow-up of cancer of the urinary bladder. AJR Am J Roentgenol 2003;180:1045–1054.
14. Kim JK, Park SY, Ahn HJ, Kim CS, Cho K-S. Bladder cancer: analysis of multi-detector row helical CT enhancement pattern and accuracy in tumor detection and perivesical staging. Radiology 2004;231:725–731.
15. Tekes A, Kamel IR, Imam K, et al. MR imaging features of transitional cell carcinoma of the urinary bladder. AJR Am J Roentgenol 2003;180:771–777.
16. Tekes A, Kamel IR, Chan TY, Schoenberg MP, Bluemke DA. MR imaging features of non-transitional cell carcinoma of the urinary bladder with pathological correlation. AJR Am J Roentgenol 2003;180:779–784.
17. Kawashima A, Sandler CM, Wasserman NF, et al. Imaging of urethral disease: a pictorial review. Radiographics 2004;24:S195–S216.
18. Prasad SR, Menias CO, Narra VR, et al. Cross-sectional imaging of the female urethra: technique and results. Radiographics 2005;25:749–761.
19. Hahn WY, Israel GM, Lee VS. MR of female urethral and periurethral disorders. AJR Am J Roentgenol 2004;182:677–682.

Chapter 35

Genital Tract: Radiographic Imaging and MR

William E. Brant

Female Genital Tract
Anatomy
Congenital Anomalies
Gynecologic Malignancy
Benign Conditions

Male Genital Tract
Testes and Scrotum
Prostate and Seminal Vesicles

FEMALE GENITAL TRACT

The primary modality for imaging of the female genital tract is US using transabdominal and transvaginal techniques (1). MR and CT are used to stage and follow up pelvic malignancies and to supplement US by providing additional characterization of lesions. MR, because of its excellent capacity to differentiate tissue types, is particularly useful in making an imaging diagnosis of pelvic disease (see Chapter 1) (2). In addition, many uterine and adnexal lesions may be discovered incidentally by pelvic CT or MR performed for other reasons (3). Hysterosalpingography (HSG) is combined with US, CT, and MR to diagnose congenital anomalies of the female genital tract and mechanical causes of infertility. The HSG is performed by cannulating the cervix and injecting a contrast agent into the lumina of the uterus and fallopian tubes. Free communication of these lumina with the peritoneal cavity should be evident. Sonohysterography is an alternative to HSG. Isotonic saline is injected into the uterine cavity while the uterus is examined sonographically (4). Sonography of the genital tract is reviewed in Chapter 37.

Anatomy

The uterus is a pear-shaped muscular organ located between the bladder and rectum. The anterior and posterior surfaces of the uterus are covered by peritoneum, the folds of which extend laterally to the pelvic sidewalls, forming the *broad ligament*. Peritoneum reflecting off the uterus and the bladder forms a shallow anterior vesicouterine pouch. Posteriorly, the peritoneum reflects onto the rectum and forms a deep rectouterine pouch or cul-de-sac. Anteriorly, a "bare area" of extraperitoneal space is present between the lower uterus and bladder. Posteriorly, the peritoneum completely covers the uterus and the posterior vaginal fornix. Only the thin wall of the vagina separates the vaginal cavity from the cul-de-sac, allowing potential transvaginal access to the intraperitoneal space by ultrasound-guided culdocentesis or biopsy. The uterus, cervix, and upper one-third of the vagina are derived from the Müllerian ducts, while the lower two-thirds of the vagina arise from the urogenital sinus. *Parametrium* refers to the connective tissue adjacent to the uterus between the folds of the broad ligament and adjacent to the vagina. Uterine vessels and lymphatics pass through the parametrium. The fundus of the uterus is that portion that extends cephalad from the origin of the fallopian tubes. The body extends from the fallopian tubes to the isthmus, a slight constriction that marks the location of the internal cervical os. The cervix is cylindric in shape and 3 to 4 cm in length. Its lower portion, including the external os, protrudes into the vagina and is surrounded by the vaginal fornices. The ureters pass 2 cm lateral to the supravaginal portion of the cervix. The ***vagina*** is a muscular tube that is a flattened oval shape on cross-sectional images.

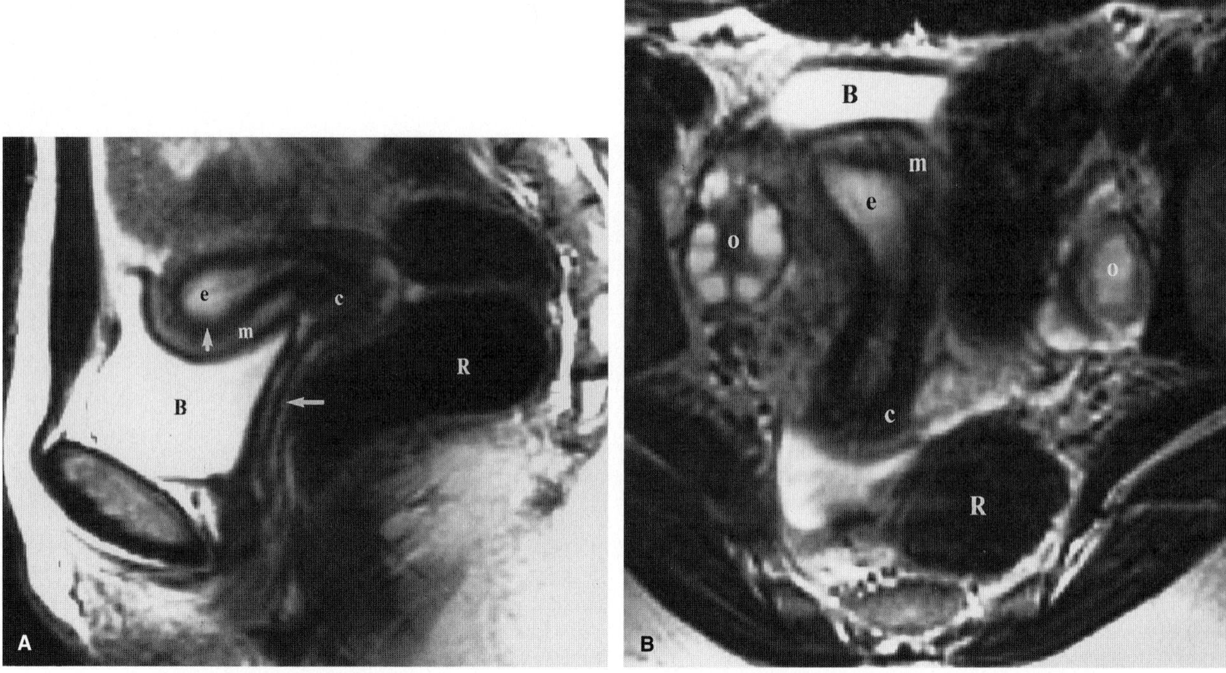

FIGURE 35.1. **Normal MR Anatomy: Female. A.** Sagittal midline T2WI. **B.** Axial T2WI. The uterus is in a normal anteverted position impressing on the bladder (B). The high-signal-intensity endometrium (e) is surrounded by the low-signal-intensity junctional zone (*arrowhead*) and the intermediate-signal-intensity myometrium (m). The cervix (c) is lower in signal intensity than the myometrium. Multiple follicles are seen on both ovaries (o). The vagina (*arrow*) has high-intensity epithelium and low-intensity muscular walls. R, rectum.

Ovaries vary in size and appearance depending on the woman's age, hormonal status, and stage of the menstrual cycle (5). The adult ovary is oval, with maximal dimensions of 5 × 3 × 2 cm. Abnormalities of size are best determined by calculating ovarian volume using the formula length × width × thickness × 0.523. Maximum ovarian volume is 9 mL before menarche, 22 mL in menstruating women, and 6 mL in postmenopausal women. The location of the ovaries is variable in different patients and even in the same patient at different times, depending on degree of bladder filling and the presence and size of other structures in the pelvis. The typical location is lateral, superior, or posterior to the uterine fundus or in the cul-de-sac. When the uterus is retroverted, the ovaries are anterior or lateral to the uterus. The pelvic ureters form an important anatomic landmark that assist in the recognition of the origin of pelvic masses (5). The ovaries are anterior to the ureters, so an ovarian mass will displace the ureter posteriorly or posterolaterally. Iliac lymph nodes are lateral to ureters, so adenopathy will displace the ureters medially or anteromedially.

Normal MR Anatomy. The internal anatomy of the uterus is depicted best on T2WIs (6). On T2WIs, the *endometrium* appears as a high-signal-intensity central stripe surrounded by the low-signal-intensity *junctional zone* (Fig. 35.1). The bulk of the *myometrium* is intermediate signal intensity. The low signal intensity of the inner junctional zone of the myometrium is caused by its lower water content. On T1WIs, the entire uterus is low in signal intensity and the internal anatomy of the uterus is poorly demonstrated. With gadolinium enhancement, uterine zonal anatomy is shown on T1WIs. The cervix is largely composed of collagenous tissues that are low in signal intensity on both T1WIs and T2WIs, providing a dark background for visualization of hyperintense cervical carcinomas. The endocervical epithelium and mucus are homogeneous high signal on T2WIs. High-resolution MR using surface or intravaginal coils shows two zones in the cervical fibromuscular stroma: a darker inner zone that is contiguous with the uterine junctional zone and an intermediate signal outer zone that is distinctly darker than the myometrium. Vaginal anatomy is also best seen on T2WIs, which shows the muscular vaginal wall as low in signal and the epithelium and mucus as high in signal. The normal ovaries of fertile women are easily identified by the bright signal of the follicles on T2WIs. The follicles are low or intermediate in signal on T1WIs. The cortex of the ovary in the premenopausal

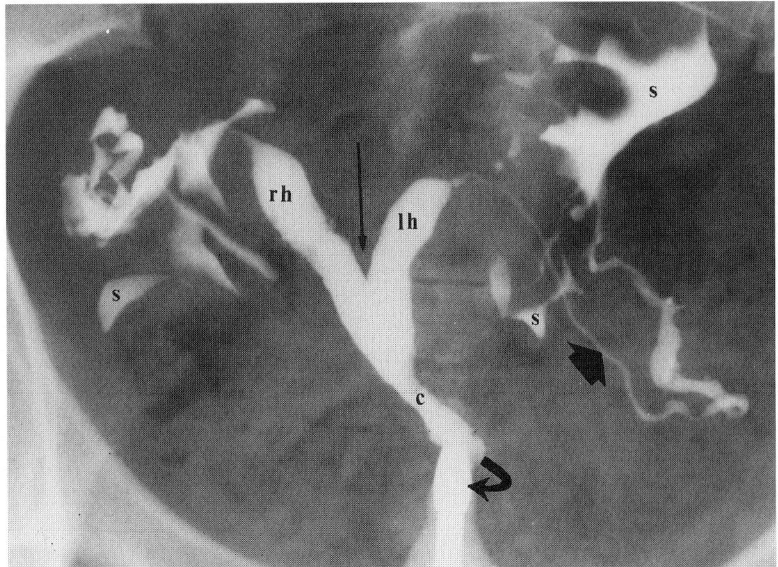

FIGURE 35.2. **Septate Uterus.** Hysterosalpingogram demonstrates two horns of the uterine cavity (rh, lh) separated by a muscular septum (*long arrow*). The lumen of the left fallopian tube is well demonstrated (*arrowhead*), while the lumen of the right fallopian tube is obscured by the superimposed contrast. Free spill of contrast into the peritoneal cavity is evident (s), confirming the patency of the fallopian tubes. A contrast agent was injected into the uterus after placing a cannula (*curved arrow*) into the cervix (c).

woman is darker in the signal than the medulla on T2WIs. The postmenopausal ovary is more difficult to identify because of the absence of follicles and the nearly equal signal intensity of the cortex and medulla on both T1WIs and T2WIs.

Normal CT Anatomy. Because the position of the uterus is so variable and CT is limited to axial slices, the outline of the uterus may appear lobulated or bulbous solely because of position. The uterus is uniform in soft tissue density, and its internal anatomy is not well demonstrated by CT. Because the myometrium is highly vascular, the uterus enhances more than most other pelvic organs. Fluid in the uterine cavity is usually low density. The ovaries are easily mistaken for unopacified bowel loops in the pelvis. Ovarian follicles are recognized by their fluid attenuation (7). The vagina is seen in cross section as a flattened ellipse of soft tissue density between the bladder and rectum. Normal fallopian tubes are not demonstrated by CT.

Hysterosalpingography is primarily used for the evaluation of infertility to demonstrate the morphology and patency of the uterine canal and fallopian tubes (Fig. 35.2). Contrast injected into the uterine cavity outlines the endocervical canal, uterine cavity, and lumen of the fallopian tubes, with free spill of contrast into the peritoneal cavity in the normal patient. The uterine cavity is sharply defined and triangular in shape, with normal mild concavity in the fundal region. The size of the cavity varies with parity. The endocervical canal is cylindric in shape, 3 to 4 cm in length, and 1 to 3 cm in width. Folds in the endocervical mucosa form a normal serrated appearance. The normal fallopian tubes are 10 to 12 cm long, extending from the cornua of the uterus. The lumen is threadlike (1 to 2 mm) until it reaches the ampulla, where it expands to 5 to 10 mm and rugal folds become visible. Patency of the tubes is confirmed by dispersal of contrast within the peritoneal cavity with outlining of bowel loops.

Congenital Anomalies

Congenital anomalies of the female genital tract are a common cause of infertility, seen in up to 9% of women evaluated for infertility or recurrent abortion. In addition, unrecognized anomalies may be mistaken for other types of pathology, such as leiomyoma. Most anomalies result from arrested development or incomplete fusion of the paired müllerian duct that forms the uterus, cervix, and fallopian tubes (8). Urinary tract abnormalities are found in 20% to 50% of patients with uterine anomalies. Arrested müllerian duct development may result in uterine aplasia or unicornuate uterus with a single fallopian tube. Ipsilateral renal agenesis is found in 5% to 20% of patients with these anomalies. Failure of complete fusion of the müllerian duct results in varying degrees of duplication: *uterus didelphys*, with two uteri, two cervices, and two vaginas; *bicornuate uterus* with two uterine horns, one (*unicollis*) or two (*bicollis*) cervices, and one vagina; or an *arcuate* (septate) uterus with a midline septum that divides the uterus into two cavities (Figs. 35.2, 35.3). Uterine anomalies should be suspected when the uterus appears abnormal in size, contour, or position. The classification of the anomaly is made by a combination of physical examination and MR examination. HSG is used to demonstrate the uterine cavity and fallopian tubes.

Gynecologic Malignancy

Ovarian cancer represents 3% of all malignancy in women but accounts for 15% of all cancer deaths. There are more than 20 histologic types of ovarian malignancy; however,

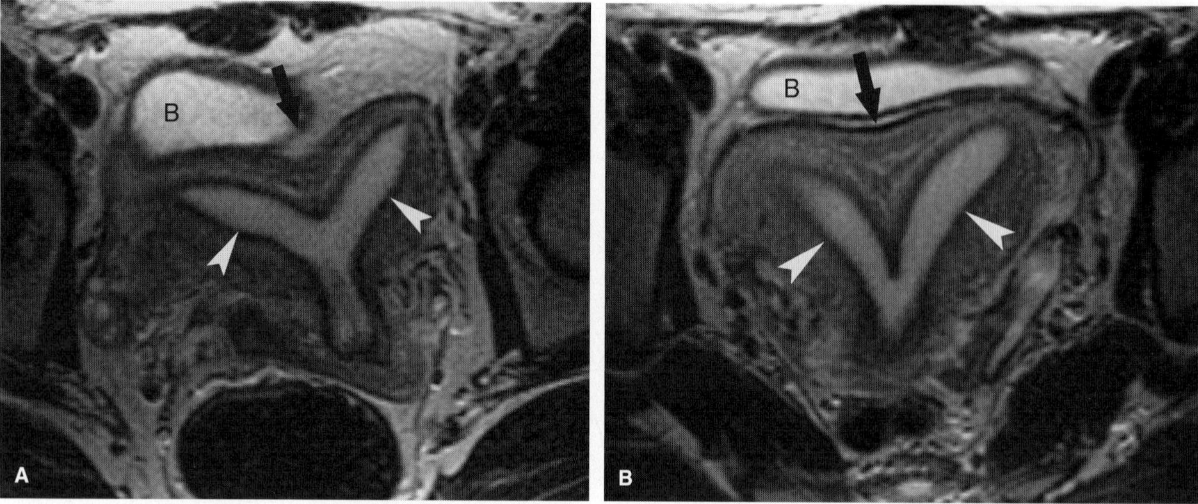

FIGURE 35.3. **Uterine Anomalies. A.** Bicornuate uterus. **B.** Septate uterus. Axial T2WIs of the uterus in two patients demonstrate the characteristic difference between a bicornuate uterus **(A),** with a surface indentation at the fundus (*arrow*) that divides the uterus into two separate horns (*arrowheads*) and a septate uterus **(B),** showing a thick muscular septum and only a slight surface indentation at the fundus (*arrow*). Two uterine cavities (*arrowhead*) are present in both cases. Uterine anomalies represent a continuous spectrum of abnormality. B, bladder.

epithelial (70%) and germ cell (15%) tumors account for the majority. Approximately 40% of ovarian tumors are malignant, two thirds are cystic, and 25% are bilateral. The peak age of onset of ovarian cancer is 55 to 59. Ovarian malignancy has an insidious onset and a silent growth pattern that results in advanced disease at presentation in 70% of cases. CA-125 is a serologic marker for ovarian cancer that is found to be elevated in 80% of women with ovarian cancer. Unfortunately, it is more likely to be abnormal in advanced cancers and is elevated in only 25% to 50% of stage 1 ovarian cancers. Survival correlates directly with the stage of disease, which also determines treatment (Table 35.1).

MR and CT signs of ovarian malignancy are similar to those listed for US in Chapter 37 (7). Wall thickness greater than 3 mm, nodularity, vegetations, solid components, evidence of invasion of adjacent structures, ascites, contrast enhancement of the peritoneum, and adenopathy are evidence of malignancy (Fig. 35.4). Ovarian carcinoma spreads primarily by peritoneal seeding, with small tumor nodules implanting on the peritoneum, mesentery, and omentum, and malignant ascites (Figs. 35.5, 35.6). Secondary patterns of spread include direct extension to adjacent structures, lymphatic metastases to pelvic and retroperitoneal nodes, and late hematogenous spread to lung, liver, and bones. CT is used primarily for follow-up of known ovarian cancer. Because ovarian cancer is usually staged with surgical laparotomy, initial radiographic tumor staging is indicated only for clearly advanced cases (9). Initial treatment is total abdominal hysterectomy, bilateral salpingo-oophorectomy, omentectomy, and tumor debulking. Both CT and MR are poor at detecting peritoneal metastases. The presence of ascites is highly predictive of the presence of peritoneal metastases. A careful search for focal peritoneal thickening and tiny nodules should be conducted. Thickening of the bowel wall and distortion of bowel loops suggests intestinal involvement. No imaging method can reliably differentiate benign from

TABLE 35.1 Ovarian Cancer Staging (FIGO)

Stage	Description
I	**Tumor limited to ovaries**
Ia	Growth limited to one ovary
Ib	Growth limited to both ovaries
Ic	With malignant ascites or malignant peritoneal washings
II	**Tumor involves one or both ovaries with pelvic extension**
IIa	Extension to uterus and/or fallopian tubes
IIb	Extension to other pelvic tissues
IIc	With malignant ascites or malignant peritoneal washings
III	**Tumor involves one or both ovaries with peritoneal extension outside the pelvis and/or regional lymph node metastasis**
IIIa	Microscopic peritoneal metastasis beyond pelvis
IIIb	Macroscopic peritoneal metastasis beyond pelvis, 2 cm or smaller in greatest dimension; nodes are negative
IIIc	Peritoneal metastasis beyond pelvis more than 2 cm in greatest dimension and/or regional lymph node metastasis
IV	**Distant metastases**

FIGO, International Federation of Gynecology and Obstetrics.

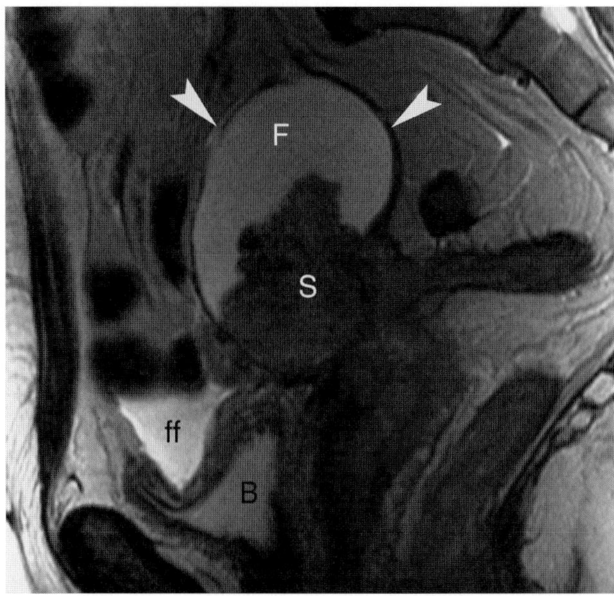

FIGURE 35.4. **Cystadenocarcinoma of Ovary.** Sagittal plane T2WI in a 63-year-old woman demonstrates a cystic adnexal mass (*arrowheads*) with a prominent solid component (S), highly indicative of malignancy. The fluid content (F) of the mass was high signal on both T1WIs and T2WIs, indicating internal hemorrhage or high protein content. Free intraperitoneal fluid (ff) is also present, indicating a high likelihood of intraperitoneal metastases. B, bladder.

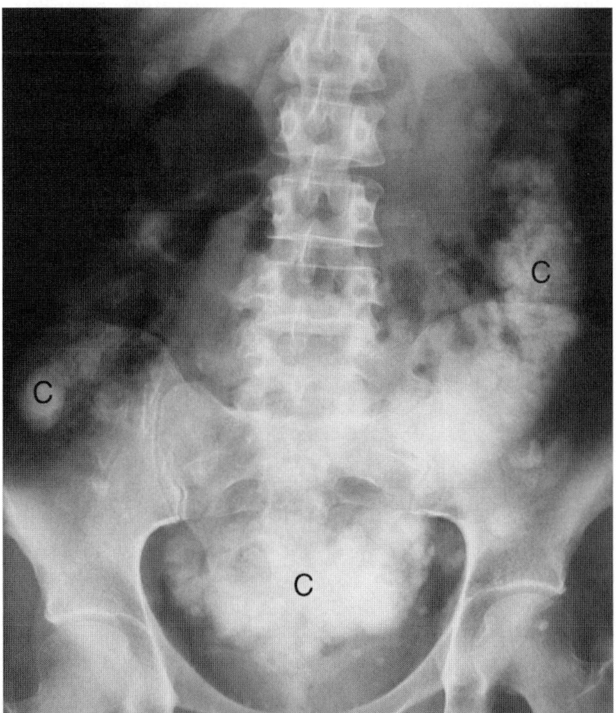

FIGURE 35.5. **Metastatic Ovarian Carcinoma.** A plain radiograph of the abdomen demonstrates calcified implants of ovarian carcinoma (C) throughout the peritoneal cavity. The pathologic diagnosis was metastatic papillary serous cystadenocarcinoma of the ovary.

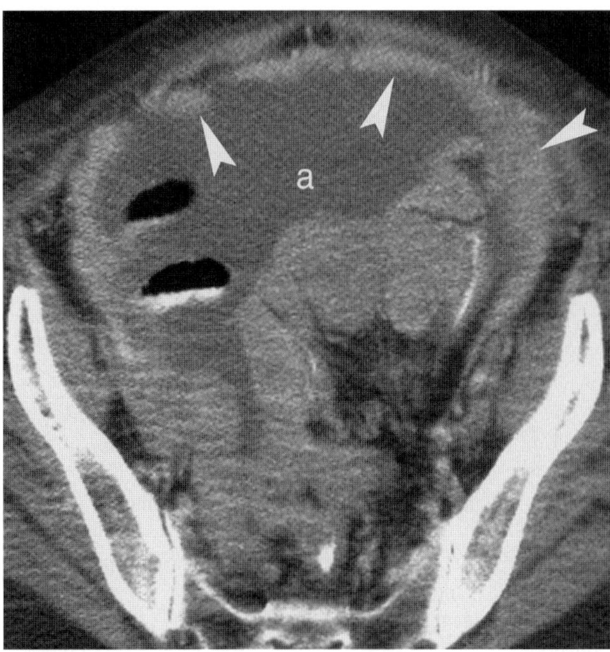

FIGURE 35.6. **Peritoneal Metastases of Ovarian Carcinoma.** CT image demonstrates nodular tumor implants (*arrowheads*) on the parietal peritoneum, well outlined by ascites (a).

malignant ovarian masses. This is not surprising because many cases are borderline malignant, even histologically.

Cervical cancer is the most common gynecologic malignancy. Squamous carcinoma accounts for 95% and adenocarcinoma for 5% of these cases. The peak age of onset is 45 to 55 years, but it is the second most common malignancy in women aged 15 to 34. Cervical cancer spreads predominantly by direct extension to involve the vagina, paracervical and parametrial tissues, and the bladder and rectum. Obstruction of the ureters is particularly common because of their proximity to the cervix. Lymphatic metastases to the pelvic, inguinal, and retroperitoneal nodes are common. Hematogenous metastases to the lung, bone, and brain occur only late in the course of the disease.

MR is usually preferred to CT for staging of proven disease (Table 35.2) (10,11). On T1WIs, cervical carcinoma is isointense with the myometrium. On T2WIs, the tumor is higher in signal compared with the lower signal of normal cervical tissue (12). A continuous rind of low-signal cervical stroma surrounding the tumor is reliable evidence of the absence of parametrial invasion (Fig. 35.7). Signs of side wall invasion include tumor abutting or extending to within 3 mm of pelvic musculature. High-intensity signal in the parametrium on T2WIs is evidence of parametrial invasion. Vaginal involvement is evidenced by loss of the normal thin rind of vaginal muscle on T2WIs.

Local staging by CT is limited by the fact that up to 50% of tumors are isodense to cervical tissue on both contrast and noncontrast scans (Fig. 35.8). Visible tumor is

TABLE 35.2 Cervical Cancer Staging (FIGO)

Stage	Description
0	**Carcinoma *in situ***
I	**Tumor confined to cervix**
Ia	Preclinical invasive carcinoma diagnosed by microscopy only; invasion no deeper than 5 mm and no wider than 7 mm
Ib	Clinical lesions confined to cervix
II	**Tumor invades beyond cervix but not to pelvic wall or lower third of vagina**
IIa	Without parametrial invasion
IIb	With parametrial invasion
III	**Tumor extends to pelvic wall and/or involves lower third of vagina and/or causes hydronephrosis**
IIIa	No extension to pelvic side wall
IIIb	Extension to pelvic sidewall or hydronephrosis
IV	
IVa	Tumor invades mucosa of bladder or rectum and/or extends to pelvic side walls
IVb	Distant metastases

FIGO, International Federation of Gynecology and Obstetrics 1995. Montreal.

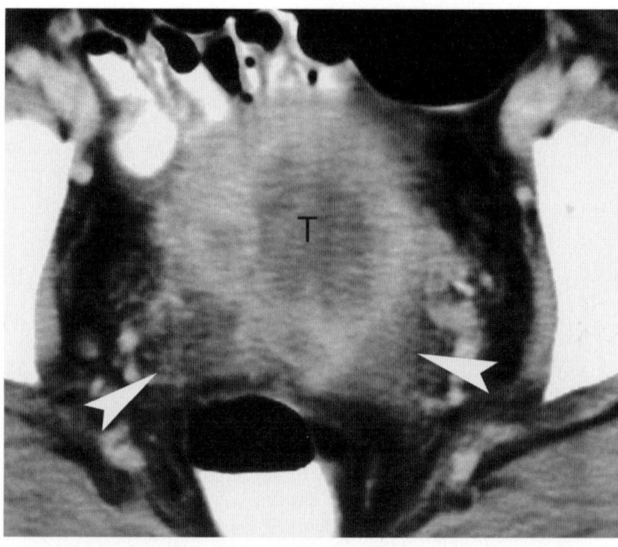

FIGURE 35.8. **Cervical Carcinoma, Stage IIb, on CT.** Heterogeneous tumor (T) has completely replaced the cervix on this CT scan. Stranding densities (*arrowheads*) into the paracervical fat indicate parametrial invasion by tumor.

heterogeneously hypodense on postcontrast scans. Both MR and CT use node enlargement (>10 mm in short axis) as the primary criterion for involvement. This is inherently inaccurate, because cervical cancer is known to involve nodes without enlarging them. Central necrosis within a lymph node is highly predictive of tumor involvement, regardless of node size. Lymphatic spread involves internal and external iliac, presacral, and paraaortic nodes. Distant metastases most commonly involve liver, lung, and bone. Imaging studies should include the kidneys to assess for obstruction.

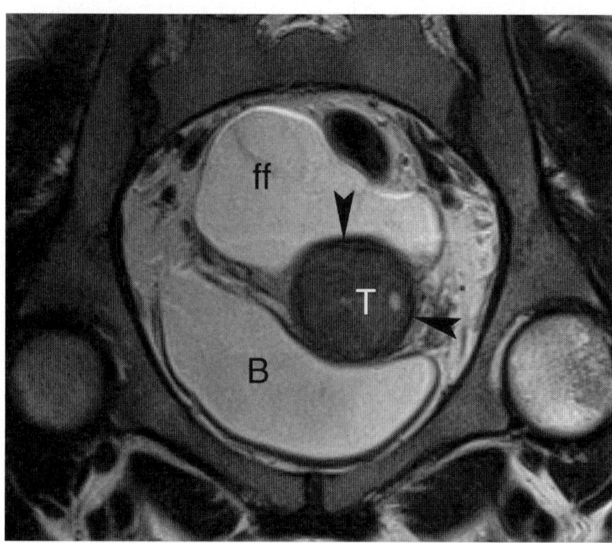

FIGURE 35.7. **Cervical Carcinoma, Stage IA, on MR.** This T2WI was obtained in an oblique coronal plane to the patient to image the cervix in transverse orientation. The tumor (T), appearing dark gray, has nearly completely replaced the normal cervix, seen only as a black rim (*arrowheads*). No parametrial invasion is evident. Free intraperitoneal fluid (ff) is seen in the cul-de-sac. B, bladder.

Endometrial carcinoma is now the most common invasive gynecologic malignancy. Histologically, it is 95% adenocarcinoma and 5% sarcoma. The peak age at onset is 55 to 62 years, with postmenopausal vaginal bleeding as the key symptom. The tumor spreads initially by invasion into the myometrium and cervix, followed by lymphatic spread to the pelvic and retroperitoneal nodes, then continued direct spread into the broad ligaments, parametrium, and ovaries. Peritoneal seeding will occur with penetration of the uterine serosa. Hematogenous spread to the lung, bone, liver, and brain occurs late in the course of the disease.

Prognosis and treatment depend on stage of the disease (Table 35.3), with the most critical factors being the depth of myometrial invasion and the involvement of lymph nodes. Lymph node metastases are unlikely if myometrial invasion is less than 50%. MR staging is more accurate than CT staging (13). On MR, the signal from tumor is similar to that of endometrium (14). Tumor is isointense to myometrium on T1WIs and hyperintense to myometrium on T2WIs (Fig. 35.9). Evidence of tumor includes thickening and poor definition of the endometrium. Large tumors appear as a polypoid mass that expands the uterine cavity. Tumor enhancement with gadolinium is variable and may be less than or greater than enhancement of

TABLE 35.3 Endometrial Cancer Staging (FIGO)

Stage	Description
0	Carcinoma *in situ*
I	
Ia	Tumor limited to endometrium
Ib	Tumor invasion of <50% thickness of myometrium
Ic	Tumor invasion of >50% thickness of myometrium
II	
IIa	Tumor invades cervical mucosa
IIb	Tumor invades cervical mucosa and stroma
III	
IIIa	Tumor invades uterine serosa and/or adnexa, and/or positive peritoneal cytology
IIIb	Metastases to vagina
IIIc	Metastases to pelvic and/or paraaortic lymph nodes
IV	
IVa	Tumor invades bladder and/or bowel mucosa
IVb	Distant metastases, including intra-abdominal and/or inguinal lymph nodes

FIGO, International Federation of Gynecology and Obstetrics.

myometrium and endometrium. Invasion of myometrium is determined on postcontrast T2WIs. An intact junctional zone myometrium is evidence of the absence of myometrial invasion (stage Ia). Pitfalls for myometrial invasion include thinning of the myometrium by rapidly expanding tumors. Cervical invasion is determined on sagittal T2WIs and postcontrast sequences, with enhancing tumor seen within the dark tissue of the cervix. T1WIs show parametrial invasion into fat. Invasion of the bladder and rectum is evidenced by disrupted tissue planes and tumor signal with bladder or rectal wall on T2WIs. On CT, the depth of myometrial invasion is determined on postcontrast images. The tumor enhances less than myometrium. Obstruction of the cervix results in filling of the uterine cavity with fluid of variable density (Fig. 35.10). Cervical involvement (stage II disease) appears as heterogeneous enlargement of the cervix. Parametrial invasion appears as irregular margins of the uterus, parametrial soft tissue stranding, or parametrial mass. CT and MR evidence of nodal metastases are lymph nodes larger than 10 mm in short axis.

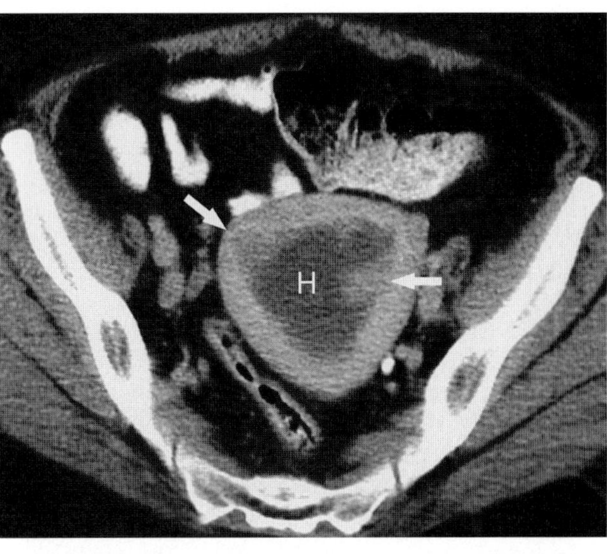

FIGURE 35.10. **Endometrial Carcinoma, Stage Ib, on CT.** Postcontrast CT image shows enhancing tumor nodules (*arrows*) outlined by low-attenuation hemorrhagic fluid (H) within the uterine cavity. Tumor invasion is difficult to assess because the tumor is nearly isointense with enhanced myometrium. The stage was proven to be Ib at surgery.

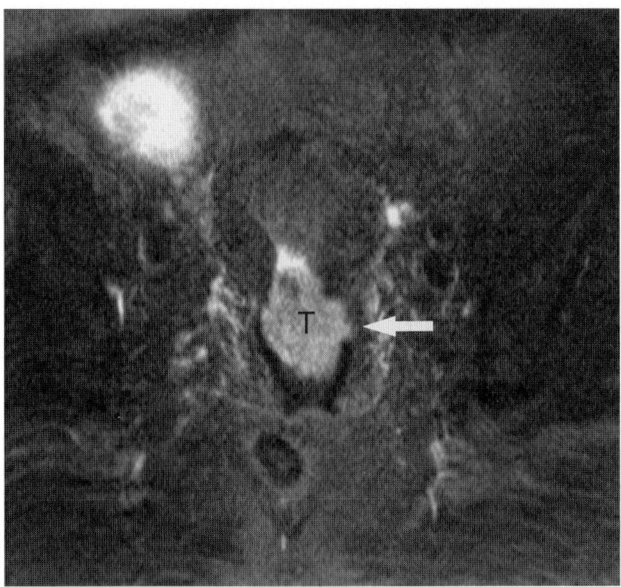

FIGURE 35.9. **Endometrial Carcinoma, Stage Ic, on MR.** Axial-plane T2WI with fat saturation shows endometrial carcinoma (T) invading more than 50% of the thickness of the myometrium (*arrow*). This tumor is distinctly high signal compared to myometrium.

Uterine sarcomas are the most aggressive of the uterine tumors (15). Sarcomas may be suspected when uterine masses are large and heterogeneous. Malignant *mixed müllerian tumors* are large solid tumors with prominent necrosis and hemorrhage that expand the uterine cavity and invade the myometrium. Lymphatic and peritoneal spread are common. *Leiomyosarcomas* usually present as a rapidly growing pelvic mass. The uterus is enlarged with a markedly heterogeneous mass with extensive necrosis, hemorrhage, and frequently calcifications (Fig. 35.11). Imaging differentiation from a degenerated benign leiomyoma is not possible unless signs of malignant spread of tumor are evident. Endometrial stromal sarcomas appear as polypoid endometrial masses that invade the myometrium.

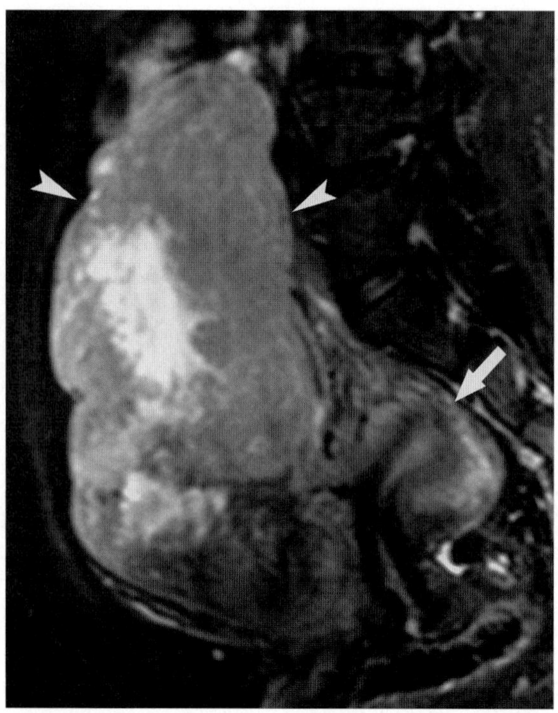

FIGURE 35.11. **Leiomyosarcoma.** T2WI shows a huge heterogeneous tumor mass (*arrowheads*) arising from the anterior wall of the retroflexed uterus (*arrow*). Note that the uterine cavity is intact. The exophytic myometrial origin and heterogeneity of the mass are indicative of either a degenerated leiomyoma or a leiomyosarcoma. The latter diagnosis was confirmed at surgery.

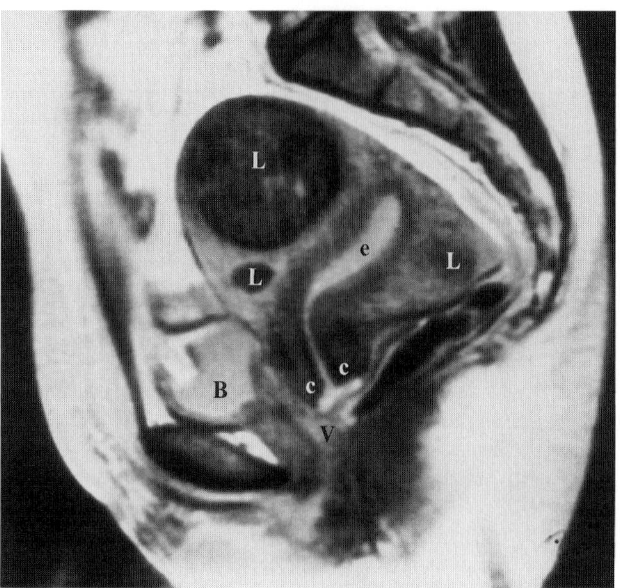

FIGURE 35.12. **Multiple Leiomyomas.** A midsagittal T2WI of the pelvis demonstrates multiple leiomyomas (L), which greatly enlarge and distort the uterus. The endometrial cavity (e) of the uterus and the cervix (c) are clearly demonstrated. B, bladder; V, vagina.

Benign Conditions

Leiomyomas are the most common uterine tumor, affecting 50% of women of reproductive age. Most women are asymptomatic, but the tumors may cause excessive bleeding, pelvic pain, mass symptoms, and infertility. Tumors are benign and made up of smooth muscle and a variable amount of fibrous tissue. Tumors with scant fibrous tissue enhance brightly, while those with abundant fibrous tissue enhance poorly. Most tumors are intramural (within the myometrial wall), while others are submucosal (beneath the endometrium) or subserosal (beneath the serosa). Subserosal or submucosal tumors may be pedunculated on long stalks. Submucosal tumors are prone to ulcerate, resulting in severe menorrhagia.

MR provides the best characterization of size, number, and location (16). Leiomyomas are usually low signal compared to myometrium on both T1WIs and T2WIs, although visualization is best on T2WIs (Fig. 35.12). Areas of degeneration and cystic change cause inhomogeneous high internal signal. The tumors are well demarcated from adjacent myometrium by a discrete rim of low signal. Contrast enhancement does not improve leiomyoma detection or characterization. On CT, leiomyomas appear as homogeneous or heterogeneous masses that may be hypodense, isodense, or hyperdense relative to enhanced myometrium. Coarse calcifications within the mass are common and characteristic (Fig. 35.13). Cystic degeneration produces interior low density. Diffuse enlargement of the uterus and lobulation of its contour are common. Pedunculated leiomyomas may appear as adnexal rather than uterine masses.

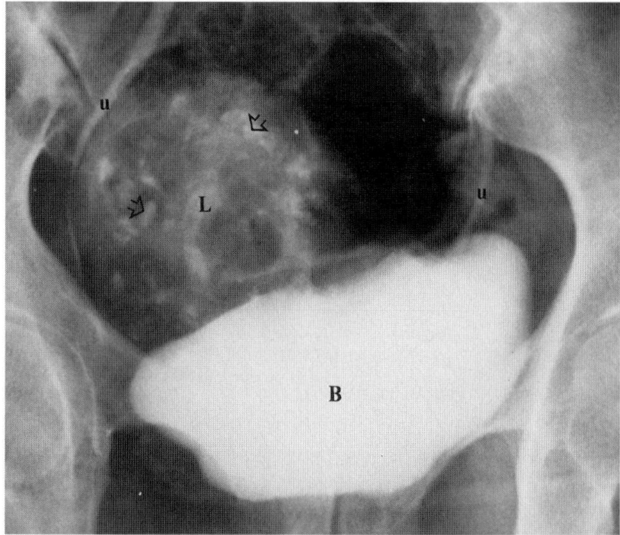

FIGURE 35.13. **Leiomyoma Calcifications.** A radiograph of the pelvis obtained as part of an excretory urogram demonstrates a leiomyoma (L) causing a mass impression on the bladder (B). Multiple characteristic "popcorn" calcifications (*open arrows*) are evident. u, ureters.

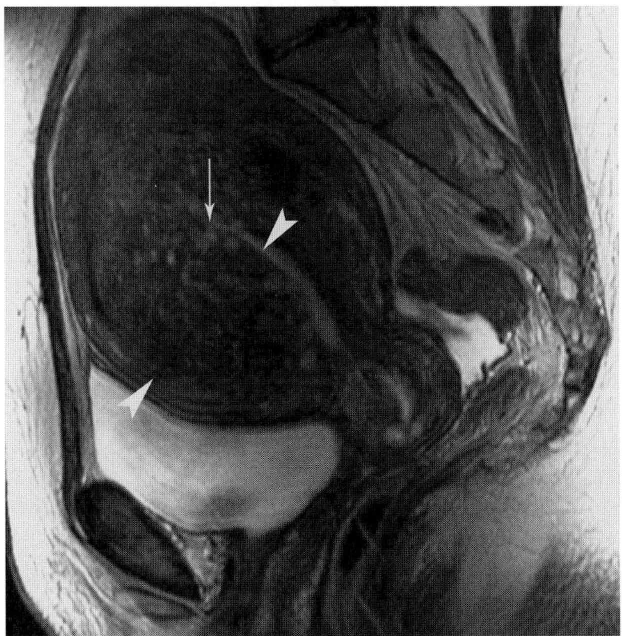

FIGURE 35.14. **Adenomyosis.** Sagittal T2WI shows marked widening of the junctional zone myometrium (*between arrowheads*), a key finding of adenomyosis. Small cysts seen as bright round foci (*long arrow*) are also characteristic.

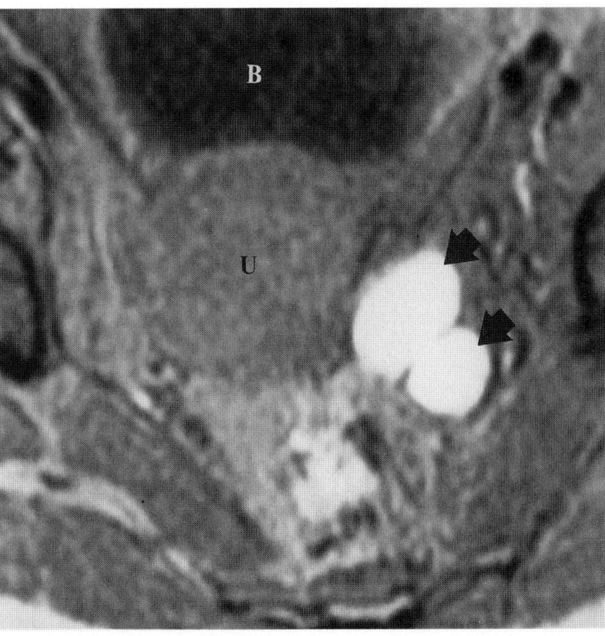

FIGURE 35.15. **Hemorrhagic Follicular Cysts.** Fat-suppressed T1WI shows high signal in two left ovarian cysts (*arrows*), indicating internal hemorrhage. The cysts are well-defined, homogeneous, and lack any solid component. U, uterus; B, bladder.

Adenomyosis is a benign disease of the uterus characterized by the presence of ectopic endometrial glands and stroma within the myometrium, eliciting surrounding myometrial hypertrophy (17). Patients present with dysmenorrhea or menorrhagia. The disease may be focal or diffuse. MR provides the best detection of the disease (18). *Diffuse disease* is indicated by regular or irregular thickening of the junctional zone myometrium >12 mm. The low signal abnormality corresponds to myometrial hypertrophy. Half of patients also demonstrate high-signal foci within the myometrium corresponding to islands of endometrial glands with cystic change or hemorrhage (Fig. 35.14). *Focal disease* is evidenced by low-signal masses within the myometrium on T2WIs. These masses are isointense to myometrium on T1WIs. High-signal foci, occasionally seen on T1WIs, represent hemorrhage. Differentiation from leiomyomas is difficult. Leiomyomas are characteristically well circumscribed, while adenomyomas are poorly defined with vague margination. Adenomyosis is not routinely evident on CT. US findings are commonly subtle and nonspecific.

Nabothian cysts are retention cysts of the mucous-secreting glands of the cervical epithelium. They are common and are seen on MR as bright, round, well-defined structures in the cervix on T2WIs. On T1WIs, they are isointense to urine or muscle.

Physiologic ovarian cysts contain simple fluid that is low signal on T1WIs and high signal on T2WIs. A uniform, thin, dark wall is evident on T2WIs. Gadolinium enhancement of the cyst wall is common but not constant. On CT they are well defined, thin walled, and have homogeneous internal density near water. Size under 2.5 cm is indicative of physiologic ovarian follicle.

Hemorrhagic functional ovarian cysts appear high signal on T1WIs if a large amount of methemoglobin is present (Fig. 35.15). If predominantly intact red blood cells are present, the cyst appears low signal on T2WIs. Thus, hemorrhagic cysts may be low signal on both T1WIs and T2WIs, high signal on T1WIs and low signal on T2WIs, or low signal on T1WIs and high signal on T2WIs. Layering of blood products may be present. The absence of gadolinium enhancement differentiates blood clot that is adherent to the cyst wall from clot that has formed a solid nodule. On CT, hemorrhagic cysts appear as thin-walled cysts with internal density near water or higher, depending on the physical state of the blood products. Atypical cysts can be followed with US to determine if they resolve after one or two menstrual cycles.

Endometriosis is the presence of endometrial tissue outside of the uterus (19). The endometrial implants respond to hormonal stimulation, resulting in recurrent bleeding, inflammation, and fibrosis. Hallmarks of disease include numerous tiny implantations of endometrial tissue on peritoneal surfaces, development of endometriomas (endometrial cysts filled with hemorrhage), and formation of adhesions between surrounding tissues. The most

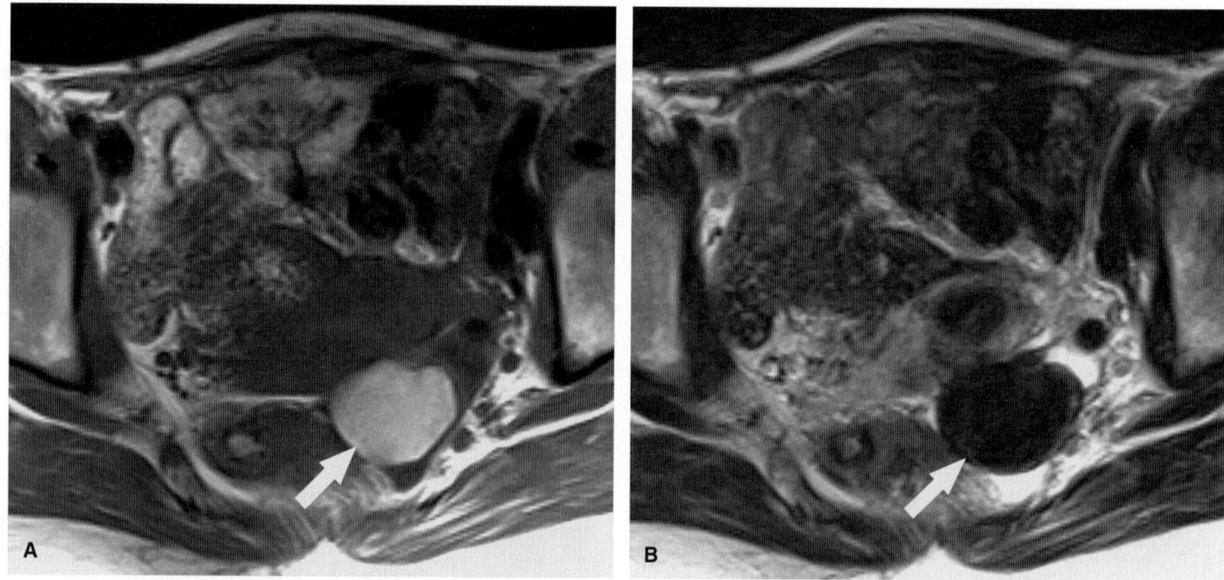

FIGURE 35.16. **Endometrioma on MR. A.** T1WI. **B.** T2WI. A cystic mass (*arrows*) in the cul-de-sac is high signal on the TIWI and shows characteristic loss of signal on the T2WI (T2 shading). The loss of signal is caused by the presence of methemoglobin within the cyst resulting from multiple episodes of internal hemorrhage.

common sites of involvement are the ovaries, the cul-de-sac, and peritoneal reflections over the uterus, fallopian tubes, bladder, and rectosigmoid colon.

All imaging modalities have high sensitivity for detection of endometriomas, but they all lack the ability to reliably detect tiny endometrial implants, which are commonly smaller than 3 mm. Endometriomas ("chocolate cysts") contain blood products of various ages, reflecting recurrent episodes of bleeding and corresponding to the menstrual cycle. They are characteristically multiple and bilateral. MR shows the cysts to be homogeneous high intensity on T1WIs and characteristically low signal on T2WIs, a finding termed "T2 shading" (Fig. 35.16). Loss of signal on T2WIs is caused by the presence of methemoglobin within the cysts (20). Iron concentration and viscosity increase within the cysts as water is resorbed. Cysts may appear heterogeneous because of the varying age of contained blood products. The cyst wall is usually low in signal, representing fibrous tissue or hemosiderin. Fat-saturation T1WIs improve visualization of small implants on peritoneal surfaces. On CT, endometriomas appear as complex cystic pelvic masses, frequently with relatively high-density fluid components. Inflammation and fibrosis are prominent. Multiple pelvic organs may be incorporated into a mass. Hydrosalpinx is a common associated finding (30%).

Hydrosalpinx is a common finding on HSG performed for infertility (Fig. 35.17). Occlusion of the fallopian tube, caused by infection, surgery, or endometriosis, results in fluid accumulation and dilatation of the tube. The most common cause is pelvic infection. CT and MR demonstrate hydrosalpinx as a sausage-, C-, or S-shaped adnexal structure distended with fluid of variable character.

Pelvic inflammatory disease is a common affliction of women of reproductive age. Endometritis and myometritis are treated medically. Imaging is performed to detect *tubo-ovarian abscess* and *pyosalpinx,* complications that are treated surgically. Early findings include pelvic edema

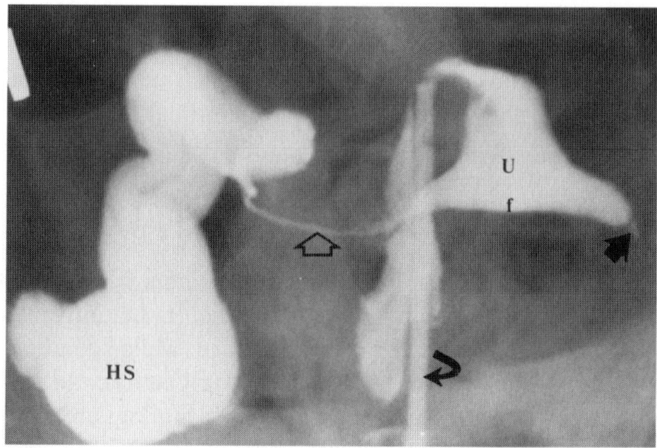

FIGURE 35.17. **Hydrosalpinx.** Hysterosalpingography demonstrates a retroflexed uterus (U), with the fundus (f) directed posteriorly and inferiorly. The left fallopian tube is occluded at the isthmus (*black arrow*). The right fallopian tube (*open arrow*) is massively dilated at its distal end, forming a hydrosalpinx (HS). Occlusion of the right fallopian tube is confirmed by the absence of peritoneal spill. The curved arrow indicates the cervical cannula.

and stranding in the parametrium and paraovarian tissues. Pyosalpinx appears as a thick-walled hydrosalpinx that contains complex fluid. Tubo-ovarian abscess appears as a thick-walled, fluid-filled adnexal mass that incorporates the ovary and commonly a dilated fallopian tube (21). Gas bubbles are occasionally present within the collection and are highly indicative of abscess.

Benign cystic teratoma, or dermoid cyst, is the most common germ cell neoplasm of the ovary (22). Lesions contain mature elements derived from ectoderm, mesoderm, or endoderm, resulting in a broad range of appearances. Mean patient age at discovery is 30 years. Most lesions are discovered incidentally while the patients are asymptomatic. The cysts are filled with liquid sebaceous material that is fat density on MR and CT. Internal contents include the Rokitansky nodule, which commonly includes hair, teeth, bone, or cartilage. US features are usually characteristic, but lesions may be discovered or further characterized by MR or CT. MR shows the sebaceous material as very high intensity on T1WIs. Signal is usually decreased on T2WIs, approximating fat signal. Fat content is confirmed by in-phase and out-of-phase gradient recall images or frequency-selective fat-saturation images. CT demonstration of fat density within a cystic adnexal mass is definitive (Fig. 35.18). CT and plain radiographs show bone and tooth formation within the mass (Fig. 35.19).

Fibrotic neoplasms account for 4% of ovarian tumors (1). Because they are solid masses and are commonly (40% of cases) associated with ascites, they may mimic ovarian cancers. Tissue types include fibromas, thecomas, and fibrothecomas arising from ovarian stroma. MR shows a well-defined ovarian mass that is predominantly low signal on both T1WIs and T2WIs. Scattered high-signal areas within the mass on T2WIs represent focal edema or cystic change.

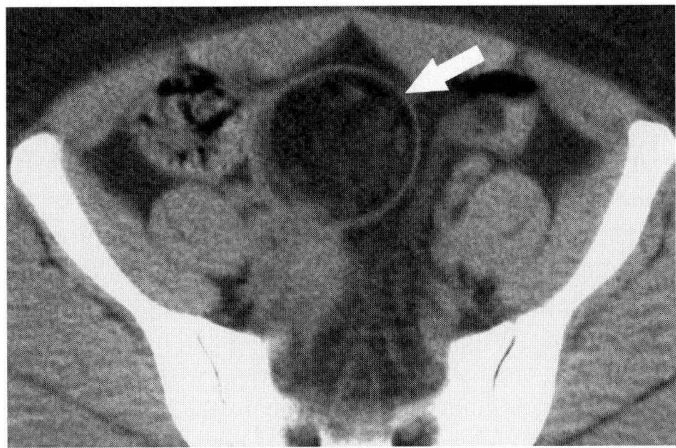

FIGURE 35.18. **Benign Cystic Teratoma.** CT performed without contrast reveals a fat-density mass (*arrow*) in the pelvis of a 28-year-old woman. The appearance is diagnostic of a benign cystic teratoma.

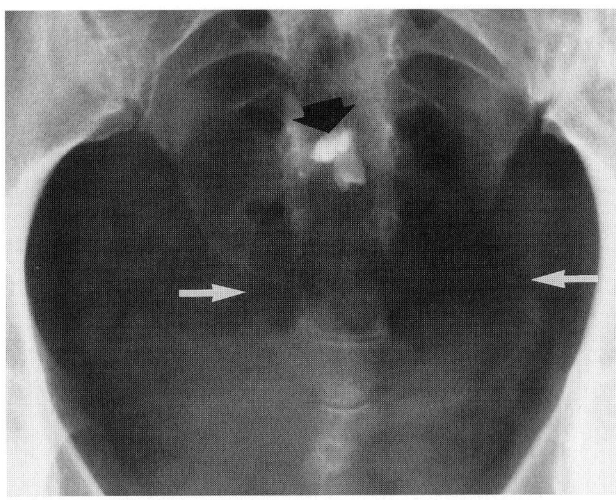

FIGURE 35.19. **Benign Cystic Teratoma.** A plain radiograph of the pelvis in a young woman demonstrates several well-formed teeth (*black arrow*). A subtle, well-defined mass of fat density is also present (*white arrows*). These findings are diagnostic of benign cystic teratoma.

Adnexal torsion may be initially diagnosed, or confirmed, by CT or MR examination (23). Key findings include a smooth-walled adnexal mass, which serves as a nidus for twisting. The torsed mass demonstrates concentric wall thickening. The ipsilateral fallopian tube appears as an amorphous mass or tube with thickened walls. The uterus is deviated toward the torsed adnexa. Signs of hemorrhagic infarction of the torsed adnexa include marked thickening of the wall of the adnexal mass (>10 mm), hemorrhage within the mass and within the twisted tube, and hemoperitoneum.

MALE GENITAL TRACT

Testes and Scrotum

US, supplemented by color Doppler, is the imaging method of choice to evaluate the testes and scrotal contents. MR using surface coils offers excellent spatial resolution, greater tissue contrast, and wider field of view but has the disadvantages of greater cost and lesser availability. Radionuclide imaging provides useful information about perfusion but with limited anatomic detail. CT is useful in the staging of testicular tumors and in locating undescended testes that are not found by US. This chapter reviews MR and CT imaging. US imaging of scrotal contents is reviewed in Chapter 37.

Normal MR Anatomy. Because of its high fluid content, the testes are of uniform intermediate signal on T1WIs and uniform high signal—slightly less than water—on T2WIs (Fig. 35.20). The tunica albuginea forms a well-defined

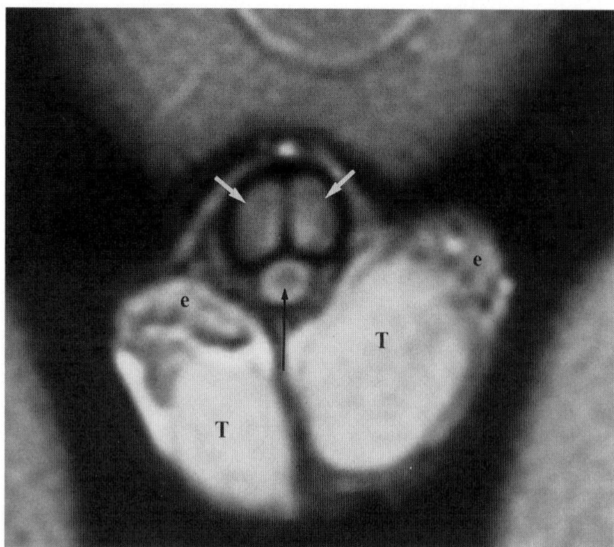

FIGURE 35.20. **Normal MR Anatomy: Male.** Coronal T2WI shows both testes (T) and the penis in cross section. The testes are high in signal because of their high fluid content. The epididymis (e) is also high signal on T2WIs but less than that of the testes. The paired corpora cavernosa (*white arrows*) are well demonstrated. The corpus spongiosum contains the urethra (*black arrow*).

1-mm-thick rim. Septations are often visualized radiating from the mediastinum to the tunica albuginea. A small amount of fluid is normally present in the scrotum between the layers of the tunica vaginalis. The epididymis is isointense to the testes on T1WIs and brightens on T2WIs, though to a lesser extent than the testis. The scrotum is intermediate signal, reflecting the dartos muscle. The spermatic cord appears as numerous tubular structures, representing the arteries and veins, with MR signal determined by blood flow.

Undescended Testis. CT and MR are used to localize undescended testes not demonstrated by US to be within the inguinal canal. The testis, if present, will be seen between the lower pole of the kidney and the internal inguinal ring. In 3% to 5% of cases, the testis is congenitally absent. The undescended testis appears as an oval soft tissue mass up to 4 cm in size. Because the undescended testis is usually atrophic, MR may show low or intermediate signal instead of high signal on T2WIs.

Neoplasms. Germ cell tumors, stromal tumors, lymphoma, and leukemia all appear on T2WIs as low-signal areas of tumor within the high-signal normal testicular parenchyma (24). Normal parenchymal septations are disrupted by the tumor. High-signal areas within tumors correspond to areas of hemorrhage. MR cannot reliably differentiate benign from malignant tumors. CT and MR are used for staging of tumors. Lymphatic spread of tumor is most common, with a usual pattern of orderly ascending nodal involvement. Initial spread is along gonadal lymphatic vessels, following the testicular veins to the renal hilar nodes. Lymphatic metastases may also follow the external iliac chain to the paraaortic nodes. The internal iliac and inguinal nodes are rarely involved. Extensive metastatic involvement of the lymph nodes mimics lymphoma in young males. A primary tumor in the testis may be clinically occult, yet is effectively demonstrated by US. Hematogenous spread to the lungs usually follows lymphatic spread, except in choriocarcinoma, which spreads hematogenously early.

Scrotal Fluid Collections. Simple hydroceles show signal characteristics of water: low signal on T1WIs and high signal on T2WIs (25). Hematoceles and pyoceles show high signal on T1WIs, reflecting complex fluid or high protein content. Epididymal cysts show the signal of simple fluid. Spermatoceles commonly contain fat and protein, causing high signal on T1WIs, and layering debris may be evident. Varicoceles appear as serpiginous tubular structures in the spermatic cord. Signal intensity corresponds to slow blood flow.

Epididymitis/Orchitis. Orchitis causes inhomogeneous signal on both T1WIs and T2WIs, indistinguishable from tumor. With epididymitis, the epididymis is enlarged, but signal intensity on T2WIs is unpredictable and may be increased, decreased, or normal. Dilated vessels in the spermatic cord reflect hypervascularity. Hydrocele is usually present.

Testicular torsion is best evaluated with Doppler US or scintigraphy. With acute torsion, MR may demonstrate a characteristic twisted pattern of torsion of the spermatic cord, with impaired blood flow evident. The testis appears heterogeneous on all image sequences.

Prostate and Seminal Vesicles

No imaging modality can reliably demonstrate the presence or absence of cancer in the prostate. That diagnosis relies on biopsy, which is best performed using transrectal US for guidance. MR with endorectal coils and transrectal US offer the best promise for staging of local disease. Either CT or MR may be used to demonstrate evidence of nodal and distant tumor spread.

Normal MR Anatomy. The prostate is divided into three glandular zones surrounding the urethra (Fig. 35.21). The *peripheral zone* contains approximately 70% of the prostate tissue and is draped around the remainder of the gland like a glove holding a baseball. Most prostate cancers (70%) arise in the peripheral zone. The *transitional zone* consists of two small areas of periurethral glandular tissue. Although it contains only 5% of the prostatic tissue in the normal young man, it is the site of benign prostatic hypertrophy and may enlarge greatly in the older man. The *central zone* consists of the glandular tissue at the base of the prostate, through which course the ducts of the vas deferens and seminal vesicles and the ejaculatory ducts.

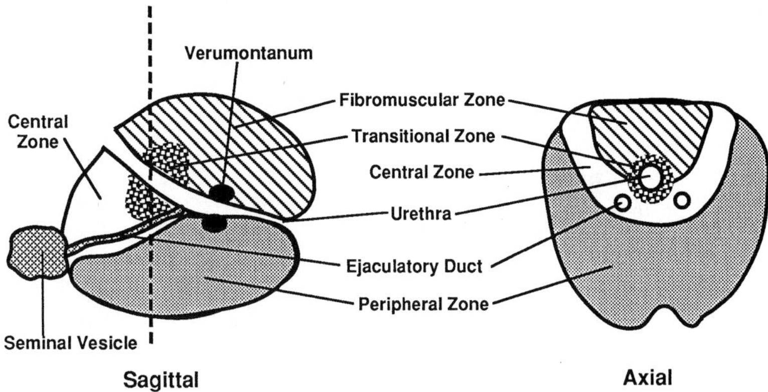

FIGURE 35.21. **Zonal Anatomy of the Prostate.** The anatomy is illustrated in the midsagittal plane (*left*) and the axial plane (*right*) at the level of the vertical dashed line on the left.

Although the central zone makes up 25% of prostate glandular tissue, only 10% of cancers arise there. The anterior portion of the prostate is occupied by nonglandular tissue called the anterior *fibromuscular stroma.* The *base* of the prostate is that portion adjacent to the base of the bladder and the seminal vesicles. The *apex* of the prostate rests on the urogenital diaphragm.

The seminal vesicles are symmetrically sized, lobulated, teardrop-shaped, coiled ducts that occupy the groove between the base of the bladder and the base of the prostate posteriorly. Prominent veins are frequently visualized in the periprostatic tissues. Lymphatic drainage of the prostate goes to regional pelvic lymph nodes, with channels to paraaortic and inguinal nodes. Periprostatic venous connections to vertebral veins offer a route for the hematogenous spread of tumor to the axial skeleton.

On T1WIs, the prostate gland is uniform intermediate to low signal, similar to skeletal muscle. The high-signal periprostatic fat defines the margin of the prostate. Periprostatic veins and neurovascular bundles are low signal. T2WIs demonstrate the internal structure (zonal anatomy) of the prostate (Fig. 35.22). The peripheral zone is high in signal because of its higher water content and looser acinar structure. The central zone is lower in signal because of its more compact muscle fibers and acinar structure. The central and transitional zones become heterogeneous with age and the development of benign prostatic hyperplasia. The anterior fibromuscular stroma is low in signal and has poorly defined margins. The seminal vesicles are low to intermediate signal on T1WIs and brighten greatly on T2WIs because of fluid within the tubules. The normal size of the seminal vesicles varies widely, and slight asymmetry is common (26).

Normal CT Anatomy. The prostate gland is seen at the base of the bladder, just posterior to the symphysis pubis, as a homogeneous rounded soft tissue organ up to 4 cm in maximal diameter. Prostate zonal anatomy is not demonstrated by CT. A well-defined plane of fat separates the prostate from the obturator internus. The paired seminal vesicles produce a characteristic "bowtie"-shaped soft tissue structure in the groove between the bladder base and the prostate.

Prostate carcinoma is the third leading cause of cancer death in men. Approximately 10% of men over age 50 will develop clinical prostate carcinoma in their lifetime. Despite the high prevalence and importance of prostate disease, treatment remains extremely controversial. One of the difficulties of dealing with prostate cancer is differentiating tumors with biologic aggressiveness from those that are incidental findings. Nearly 50% of men older than 75 years of age will have prostate carcinoma on biopsy or autopsy. However, many of these cancers will not affect the patient's lifespan. The tumor is uncommon before

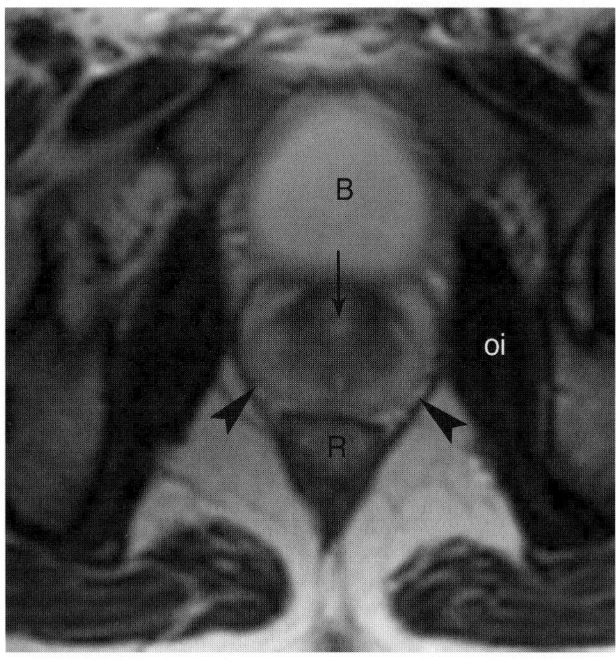

FIGURE 35.22. **Normal Prostate on MR.** Axial plane T2WI of a normal prostate in a 40-year-old man demonstrates the high-intensity peripheral zone (*arrowheads*), the urethra (*long arrow*), and the surrounding lower-intensity transitional zone. B, bladder; r, rectum; oi, obturator internus muscle.

TABLE 35.4 Prostate Cancer Staging: 1992 Revision of TNM Classification

Stage	Description
Primary tumor	
TX	**Not assessable**
T0	**Not evident**
T1	**Clinically apparent, not palpable or visible by imaging**
T1a	Found incidentally in 5% or less of tissue resected
T1b	Found incidentally in more than 5% of tissue resected
T1c	Identified by needle biopsy because of elevated PSA
T2	**Palpable or visible by imaging**
T2a	Involves half of one lobe or less
T2b	Involves more than half of one lobe, but not both lobes
T2c	Involves both lobes
T3	**Extends through prostate capsule**
T3a	Found unilaterally
T3b	Found bilaterally
T3c	Invades seminal vesicles
T4	**Fixed, or invades other structures**
T4a	Invades bladder neck, external sphincter, or rectum
T4b	Invades levator muscles or is fixed to pelvic wall
Regional lymph nodes	
NX	Regional lymph nodes cannot be assessed
N0	No regional lymph nodes metastases
N1	Metastases to single lymph node 2 cm or smaller in greatest dimension
N2	Metastases to single lymph node 2 to 5 cm in greatest dimension, or to multiple lymph nodes all <5 cm in greatest dimension
N3	Metastases to regional lymph node >5 cm in greatest dimension
Distant metastases	
MX	Metastases cannot be assessed
M0	No distant metastases
M1	Distant metastases present

Adapted from Schroeder FH, Hermanek P, Denis L, et al. The TNM classification of prostate cancer. Prostate 1992;4(suppl):129–138.

age 50 and increases in incidence thereafter. The Gleason histologic grading system is used to assess the degree of differentiation of the tumor. A grade 1 is well differentiated, and a grade 5 is anaplastic. The Gleason score varies from 2 to 10 and adds the Gleason grade for the predominant and the secondary portions of the tumors. Tumor staging is by the American Urological Association system (Table 35.4).

Most tumors are adenocarcinoma (95%). Prostate cancer spreads by local extension, from lymphatic vessels to regional nodes, and by hematogenous dissemination. Penetration of tumor through the capsule or into the seminal vesicles greatly worsens the prognosis. Involvement of the axial skeleton by hematogenous metastases is common. Metastases to the lungs, liver, and kidneys occur in the terminal phases of the disease.

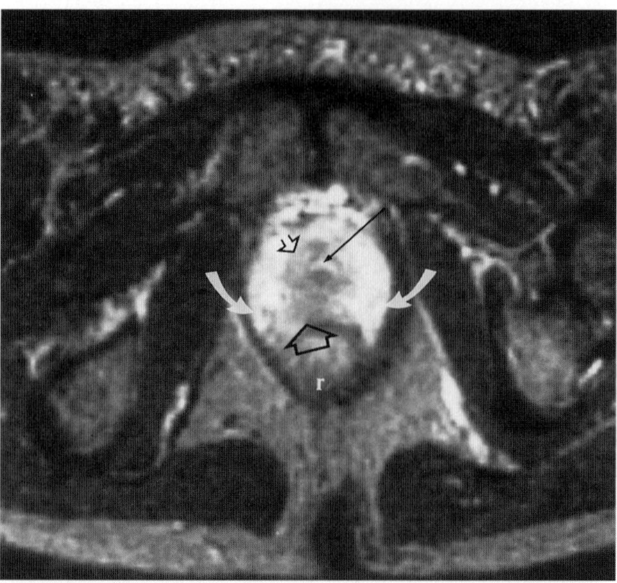

FIGURE 35.23. **Prostate Carcinoma.** Proton density–weighted axial plane MR image demonstrates a low-intensity prostate carcinoma (*large open arrow*) in the peripheral zone (*curved arrows*). The tumor is confined to the prostate gland and measures approximately 2 cm. The urethra (*long arrow*) and dark transitional zone (*small open arrow*) are evident. r, rectum.

On MR T2WIs, cancers appear as areas of low signal within the high-signal peripheral zone (Fig. 35.23). Cancer is isointense with prostate tissue on T1WIs, which are best used for assessing invasion of periprostatic fat and for detecting nodal involvement. Recent biopsy limits the specificity of MR because areas of hemorrhage may mimic tumor. Criteria for extracapsular extension of tumor include: (*1*) asymmetry of neurovascular bundles, (*2*) tumor envelopment of neurovascular bundle, (*3*) angulated contour of the prostate gland, (*4*) irregular, spiculated margins of the prostate gland, and (*5*) obliteration of the retroprostatic angle (26). CT is limited to the demonstration of adenopathy and distant spread of tumor, because it cannot differentiate tumor from benign hyperplasia within the gland. Some (~50%) cancers are detectable as a focus of contrast enhancement in the peripheral zone on multidetector CT.

Benign prostatic hyperplasia begins at approximately age 40 and eventually occurs in all men. Hypertrophy and hyperplasia occur in glandular tissue in the transitional and periurethral zones, accompanied by proliferation of supporting smooth muscle and stromal cells. The end result is focal or diffuse enlargement of the prostate. Pressure on the urethra obstructs bladder outflow and results in symptoms of hesitancy, decreased force and caliber of the urine stream, dribbling, frequency, nocturia, and postvoid residual. This progressive process is combatted by hypertrophy of the bladder wall musculature. Advanced symptoms require medical therapy balloon

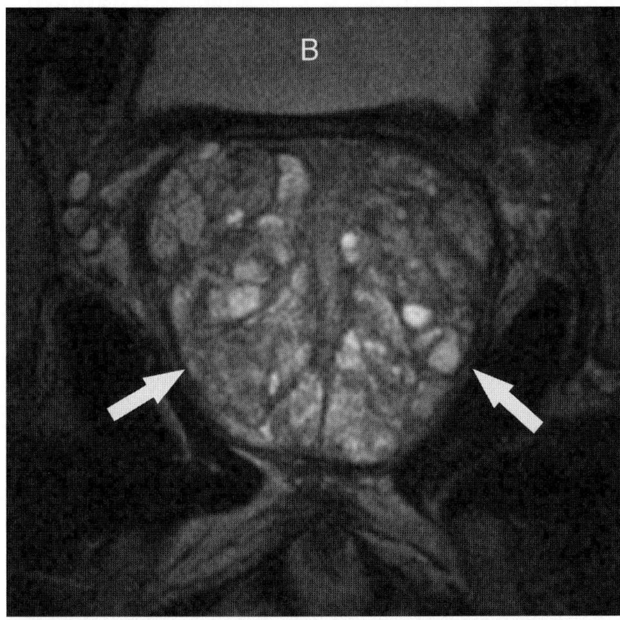

FIGURE 35.24. **Benign Prostatic Hypertrophy.** T2WI in the axial plane shows marked diffuse enlargement of the prostate gland (*arrows*) with heterogeneous signal and cystic change. The normal zonal anatomy of the prostate is not evident. B, bladder.

dilatation, stents, or transurethral resection. CT findings include: (*1*) enlargement of the prostate, commonly with lobulated contour and visible high- and low-density nodules; (*2*) coarse calcifications; (*3*) cystic degeneration; and (*4*) bladder wall thickening and trabeculation. MR shows prostate enlargement with heterogeneous central gland on T2WIs (Fig. 35.24). Areas of cystic degeneration are low signal on T1WIs and high signal on T2WIs.

REFERENCES

1. Jeong YY, Outwater EK, Kang HK. Imaging evaluation of ovarian masses. Radiographics 2000;20:1445–1470.
2. Siegelman ES, Outwater EK. Tissue characterization in the female pelvis by means of MR imaging. Radiology 1999;212:5–18.
3. Saini A, Dina R, McIndoe GA, et al. Characterization of adnexal masses with MRI. AJR Am J Roentgenol 2005;184:1004–1009.
4. Berridge DL, Winter TC. Saline infusion sonohysterography: technique, indications, and imaging findings. J Ultrasound Med 2004; 23:97–112.
5. Saksouk FA, Johnson SC. Recognition of the ovaries and ovarian origin of pelvic masses with CT. Radiographics 2004;24:S133–S146.
6. Outwater EK, Talerman A, Dunton C. Normal adnexa uteri specimens: anatomic basis of MR imaging features. Radiology 1996; 201:751–755.
7. Jung SE, Lee JM, Rha SE, et al. CT and MR imaging of ovarian tumors with emphasis on differential diagnosis. Radiographics 2002;22:1305–1325.
8. Troiano RN, McCarthy SM. Müllerian duct anomalies: imaging and clinical issues. Radiology 2004;233:19–34.
9. Woodward PJ, Hosseinzadeh K, Saenger JS. Radiologic staging of ovarian carcinoma with pathologic correlation. Radiographics 2004;24:225–246.
10. Pannu HK, Corl FM, Fishman EK. CT evaluation of cervical cancer: spectrum of disease. Radiographics 2001;21:1155–1168.
11. Kaur H, Silverman PM, Iyer RB, et al. Diagnosis, staging, and surveillance of cervical carcinoma. AJR Am J Roentgenol 2003;180:1621–1632.
12. Okamoto Y, Tanaka YO, Nishida M, et al. MR imaging of the uterine cervix: imaging-pathologic correlation. Radiographics 2003;23:425–445.
13. Kinkel K, Kaji Y, Yu KK, Segal MR. Radiologic staging in patients with endometrial cancer: a meta-analysis. Radiology 1999;212:711–718.
14. Lee EJ, Byun JY, Kim B, et al. Staging of early endometrial carcinoma: assessment with T2-weighted and gadolinium-enhanced T1-weighted MR imaging. Radiographics 1999;19:937–945.
15. Rha SE, Byun JY, Jung SE, et al. CT and MRI of uterine sarcomas and their mimickers. AJR Am J Roentgenol 2003;181:1369–1374.
16. Murase E, Siegelman ES, Outwater EK, et al. Uterine leiomyomas: histopathologic features, differential diagnosis, and treatment. Radiographics 1999;19:1179–1197.
17. Tamai K, Togashi K, Ito T, et al. MR imaging findings of adenomyosis: correlation with histopathologic features and diagnostic pitfalls. Radiographics 2005;25:21–40.
18. Byun JY, Kim SE, Choi BG, et al. Diffuse and focal adenomyosis: MR imaging findings. Radiographics 1999;19:S161–S170.
19. Woodward PJ, Sohaey R, Mezzetti TP, Jr. Endometriosis: radiologic-pathologic correlation. Radiographics 2001;21:193–216.
20. Gougoutas CA, Sigelman ES, Hunt J, Outwater EK. Pelvic endometriosis: various manifestations and MR imaging findings. AJR Am J Roentgenol 2000;175:353–358.
21. Sam JW, Jacobs JE, Birnbaum BA. Spectrum of CT findings in acute pyogenic pelvic inflammatory disease. Radiographics 2002;22:1327–1334.
22. Outwater EK, Siegelman ES, Hunt JL. Ovarian teratomas: tumor types and imaging characteristics. Radiographics 2001;21:475–490.
23. Rha SE, Byun JY, Jung SE, et al. CT and MR imaging features of adnexal torsion. Radiographics 2002;22:283–294.
24. Woodward PJ, Sohaey R, O'Donoghue MJ, Green DE. Tumors and tumorlike lesions of the testes: radiologic-pathologic correlation. Radiographics 2002;22:189–216.
25. Woodward PJ, Schwab C, Sesterhenn IA. Extratesticular scrotal masses: radiologic-pathologic correlation. Radiographics 2003;23: 215–240.
26. Claus FG, Hricak H, Hattery RR. Pretreatment evaluation of prostate cancer: role of MR imaging and 1H MR spectroscopy. Radiographics 2004;24:S167–S180.

SECTION IX

Ultrasonography

Chapter 36

Abdomen Ultrasound

William E. Brant

Peritoneal Cavity
Retroperitoneum
Liver
Bile Ducts
Gallbladder
Spleen
Pancreas
Adrenal Glands
Kidneys

Ultrasound (US) is firmly established as a primary imaging modality for comprehensive evaluation of the abdomen, including the abdominal organs, the peritoneal cavity, and the retroperitoneum (1). Its role includes screening for disease, evaluation and follow-up of known abnormalities, and guidance of biopsy, aspiration, and catheter drainage procedures. Comprehensive examination commonly includes the use of Doppler and color flow imaging, as well as specialized techniques of transvaginal or transrectal US to demonstrate pelvic extension of disease. This chapter provides the basic information needed to understand the effective use of US in examining the abdomen.

PERITONEAL CAVITY

Normal US Anatomy. The normal peritoneal cavity is a potential space best appreciated when fluid is present (2). The peritoneal membrane lines the abdominal cavity and covers—in whole or in part—the intra-abdominal organs. Numerous peritoneal ligaments, folds, and recesses are visualized when outlined by fluid within the peritoneal cavity. US examination for the presence of fluid includes inspection of the subdiaphragmatic and subhepatic regions, the pericolic gutters, and the pelvic cul-de-sac. Tiny volumes of intraperitoneal fluid are best detected by transvaginal US examination of the cul-de-sac. Firm transducer pressure and changes in patient position are needed to inspect between bowel loops for fluid collections. Solid organs and fluid serve as sonographic windows to the abdomen, whereas gas in the bowel and the ribs, spine, and bony pelvis serve as obstacles.

Intraperitoneal Fluid. Fluid within the peritoneal cavity flows, under the effect of gravity, along peritoneal reflections to peritoneal recesses (Fig. 36.1) (2). The hepatorenal recess (Morison pouch) and the pelvic cul-de-sac are the two most dependent recesses in the supine patient. They connect via the paracolic gutters. Fluid outlining the intraperitoneal organs provides an opportunity to evaluate organ surface abnormalities, such as the fine nodularity of cirrhosis. Transudative ascites, urine, and bile are anechoic. Fluid with echogenic particles, layering debris, or septations may be hemorrhage, pus, malignant ascites, or spilled GI contents.

Free intraperitoneal fluid outlines recesses and compartments that retain their normal shape. Loops of bowel float and sway freely within free fluid. Loculated fluid collections, abscesses, and cystic masses create their own space, displace bowel and adjacent organs, and are usually more round and tense.

Intraperitoneal Abscess. Although CT is commonly preferred for detection of small intraperitoneal abscesses, US readily demonstrates most abscesses and is effectively used to guide aspiration and catheter drainage (Fig. 36.2). Because abscesses most commonly form in the dependent recesses, the pelvis must be included in every examination. Abscesses appear as loculated collections of fluid that may be anechoic to densely echogenic. Fluid levels, internal debris, septations, thick walls, and gas within the abscess are common. Gas is brightly echogenic and associated with reverberation artifact and acoustic shadowing. An abscess containing extensive gas may be mistaken for gas-filled bowel and overlooked. Some abscesses appear solid. Changes in patient position show shifting of the particle pattern when liquid. Doppler and color flow US

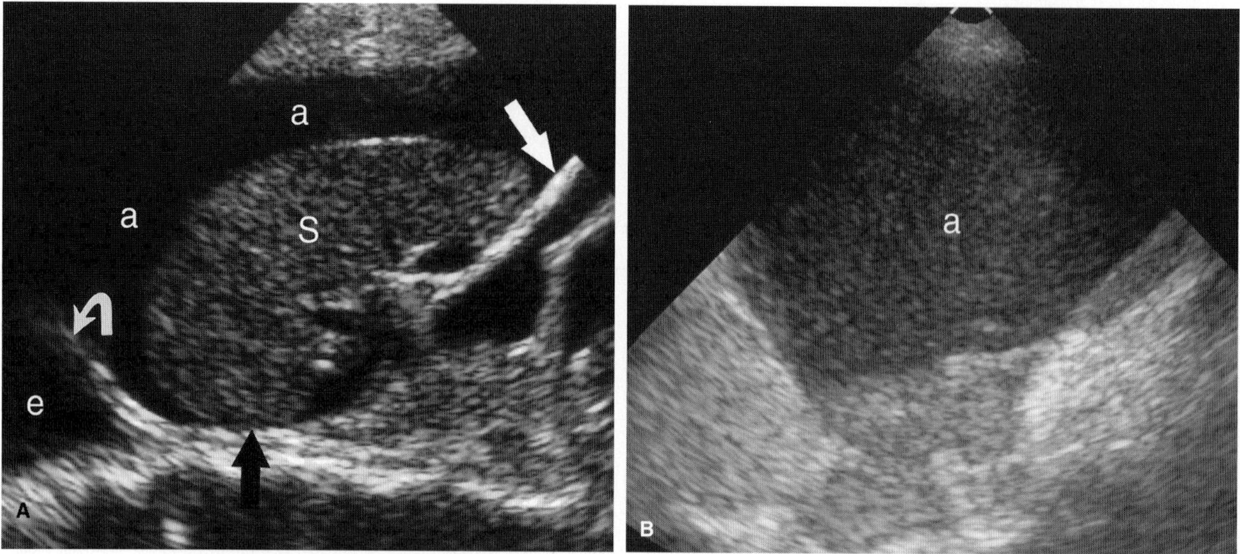

FIGURE 36.1. **Ascites. A.** Longitudinal US image shows anechoic ascites (a) surrounding the spleen (S). Fluid outlines the gastrosplenic ligament (*white arrow*). Note the small bare area of the spleen (*black arrow*), where reflections of the peritoneum from the spleen to the diaphragm prevent access of intraperitoneal fluid. A left pleural effusion (e) is seen above the diaphragm (*curved arrow*). **B.** US image of the right lower quadrant of the abdomen reveals ascites (a) containing echogenic particulate matter. This exudative ascites resulted from a bowel perforation.

show the absence of internal blood vessels within echogenic fluid collections or the presence of blood vessels within solid tissue. Abscesses have mass effect and displace adjacent structures.

Intraperitoneal Tumor. Metastases are the most common tumor of the peritoneal surface. Fluid and gravity distribute malignant cells throughout the peritoneal cavity, where they implant upon visceral or parietal peritoneal surfaces. The greater omentum is fertile ground and thickens with tumor implantation to form "omental cake," a layer of solid tissue separating bowel from contact with the anterior abdominal wall (Fig. 36.3). Metastatic implants

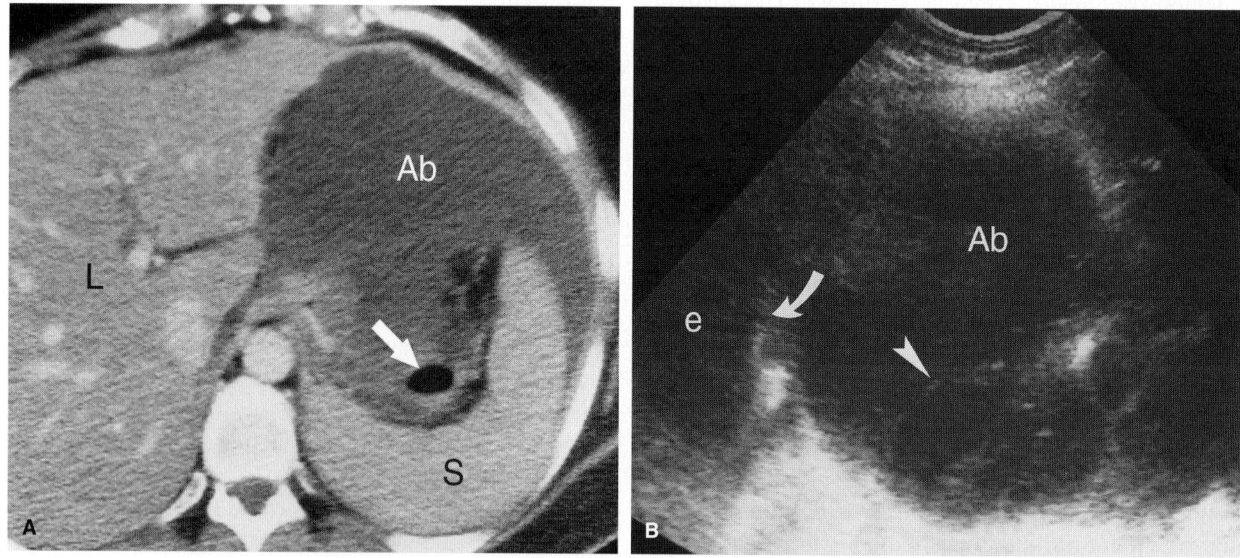

FIGURE 36.2. **Left Subphrenic Abscess. A.** CT scan demonstrates a loculated fluid collection (Ab) in the left subphrenic space following gastric bypass surgery. The stomach (*arrow*) is displaced posteriorly. L, liver; S, spleen. **B.** US in the same patient demonstrates internal septations (*arrowhead*) within the fluid collection (Ab) that are not apparent on the CT study. A pleural effusion (e) is seen above the diaphragm (*curved arrow*). The abscess contained gram-negative organisms.

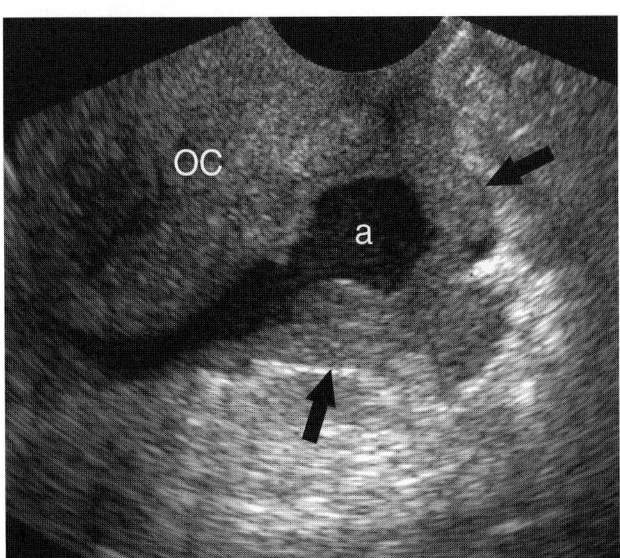

FIGURE 36.3. **Peritoneal Metastases.** US image shows solid tumor implanted on the omentum creating "omental cake" (OC). Solid tumor causes lumpy thickening of the peritoneal surfaces (*arrows*). Malignant ascites (a) contains floating echogenic debris. The primary tumor was ovarian carcinoma.

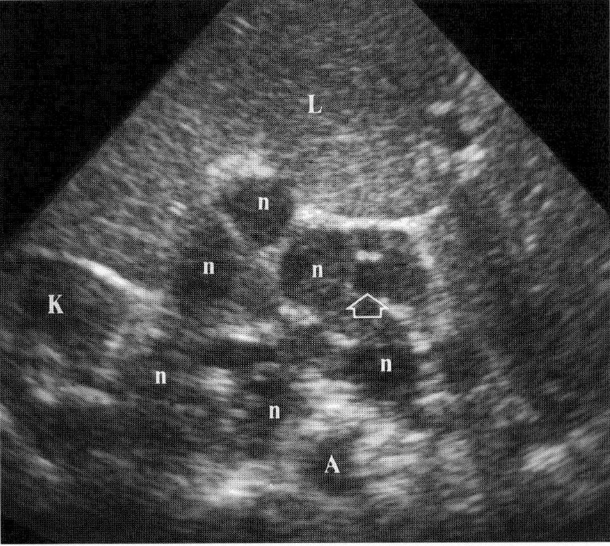

FIGURE 36.4. **Adenopathy Caused by Lymphoma.** An axial-plane US demonstrates multiple enlarged hypoechoic lymph nodes (n) surrounding and displacing the aorta (A) and celiac axis (*open arrow*). The adenopathy extends into the hilum of the right kidney (K). L, liver.

appear as hypoechoic solid masses of varying size on peritoneal surfaces. Ascites is usually present, with echogenic debris and septations common. The most common tumors of origin are ovarian, colon, pancreas, and gastric carcinoma.

Primary peritoneal tumors include mesothelioma, desmoids, carcinoids, primary peritoneal serous papillary carcinoma, and lymphoma. These appear as predominantly hypoechoic solid masses. Acoustic shadows may arise from dense fibrous tissue or calcifications.

RETROPERITONEUM

Normal US Anatomy. The retroperitoneum is that portion of the abdomen behind the posterior parietal peritoneum. The anatomy of its three compartments is described in Chapter 26. US of the abdominal aorta and inferior vena cava (IVC) is discussed in Chapter 40. The crura of the diaphragm must not be mistaken for retroperitoneal adenopathy. Both are hypoechoic linear bands of muscle. The right crus is larger, more lobular, and inserts lower, extending to the L3 vertebral body. The left crus is more uniform in thickness, inserting on the L1 and L2 vertebral bodies. The crura serve as landmarks for identification of the adrenal gland. The psoas and quadratus lumborum muscles show the typical hypoechoic pattern of muscle, with longitudinally oriented echogenic fibrous strands dividing muscle bundles. Echogenic retroperitoneal fat surrounds and defines organs, vessels, and other structures.

Retroperitoneal Adenopathy. Enlarged individual lymph nodes are homogeneous, hypoechoic, and round or oval (Fig. 36.4). Accentuated sound transmission may be present, and some enlarged solid nodes are so hypoechoic they appear cystic. A solitary node larger than 1.5 cm in short axis diameter, or multiple nodes larger than 1.0 cm each, are considered to be pathologically enlarged. Lymphoma is characterized by confluence of enlarged nodes to form a solid mass that surrounds vessels and organs. Causes of retroperitoneal adenopathy are lymphoma (most common); tumor metastases (testicular, renal, pelvic, GI malignancies, and melanoma); and infection, especially in AIDS patients.

Retroperitoneal tumors are most commonly of mesenchymal origin and include liposarcoma, leiomyosarcoma, and malignant fibrous histiocytoma. These are aggressive tumors that invade organs and muscles and are difficult to remove surgically. Most are large, heterogenous, and partially cystic. Germ cell tumors in the retroperitoneum may be primary or secondary and either benign or malignant. The sonographic features of the various tumors overlap, and US examination does not yield a specific diagnosis. Benign lipoma may be suggested when the tumor is isoechoic to retroperitoneal fat.

Retroperitoneal fluid collections include hemorrhage, infection, urinoma, pancreatic fluid collections, and cystic masses (lymphoceles, lymphangiomas, renal cysts, and teratomas). Portosystemic collaterals and other enlarged blood vessels are differentiated by Doppler US. As within the peritoneal cavity, retroperitoneal fluid may be anechoic or echogenic, with particulate cellular debris and layering fluid levels. Echogenic clotted blood may appear as a solid mass. Absence of internal vascularity on Doppler examination and change in appearance with time are distinguishing features.

LIVER

US is an efficient imaging method to screen patients for diffuse and focal hepatic disease (3–5). For focal liver metastases, its sensitivity approaches that of CT and MR; however, its images are more difficult to reproduce for follow-up comparisons, and benign and malignant nodules cannot usually be distinguished. Color Doppler US is valuable for the assessment of liver vasculature, for the diagnosis of portal and hepatic vein thrombosis and portal hypertension, and in evaluating the vascularity of liver tumors.

Normal US Anatomy. The echogenicity of the liver parenchyma is homogeneous and equal to or slightly greater than that of the kidney (Fig. 36.5A). The surface of the liver is normally smooth, and the inferior margin of the liver is sharp-edged. The lobar and segmental anatomy of the liver is described and illustrated in Chapter 27. The hepatic veins are seen as echolucent tubes with thin walls that converge into the IVC. The portal veins, hepatic arteries, and bile ducts, encompassed by fibrofatty tissue, form the portal triads, which are normally visualized as echogenic foci throughout the liver. Doppler US is used to differentiate blood vessels from bile ducts and small hepatic cysts and to confirm blood flow.

Fatty infiltration causes an increase in echogenicity of the liver, making affected areas distinctly more echogenic than normal renal parenchyma (4). Fatty infiltration also increases the attenuation of the US beam, diminishing visualization of the diaphragm and commonly requiring a lower-frequency transducer to examine deep portions of the liver (Fig. 36.5B). The hepatic echotexture appears coarsened, and visualization of the portal triads is decreased. The various patterns of fatty infiltration are reviewed in Chapter 27. The "flip-flop" pattern of fatty infiltration as seen on US compared with CT is useful in confirming a diagnosis of focal fatty infiltration and focal fat sparing. Fat-infiltrated areas are bright on US and dark on CT. Focally sparred areas within diffuse fatty infiltration are dark on US and bright on CT.

Acute hepatitis results in diffuse hepatic edema, which reduces the echogenicity of the liver, resulting in a "starry sky" appearance. The portal triads appear unusually bright on the darkened background of edematous parenchyma. The starry sky appearance has also been described with diffuse leukemic or lymphomatous infiltrate, toxic shock syndrome, and diffuse decrease in glycogen stores in the liver.

Passive hepatic congestion refers to stasis of blood in the liver owing to congestive heart failure. US findings

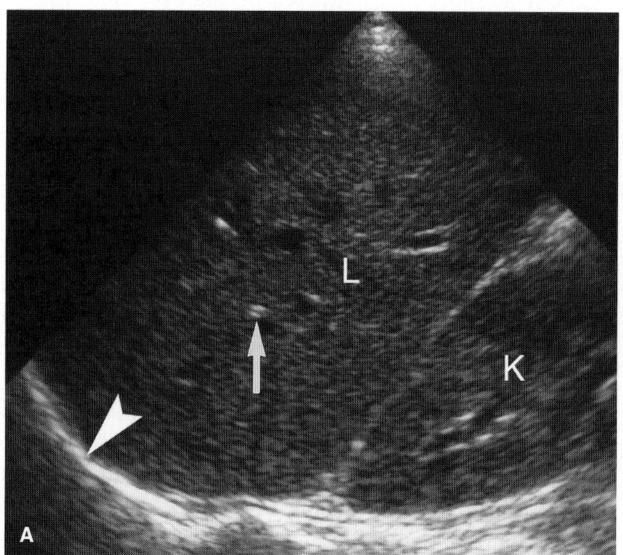

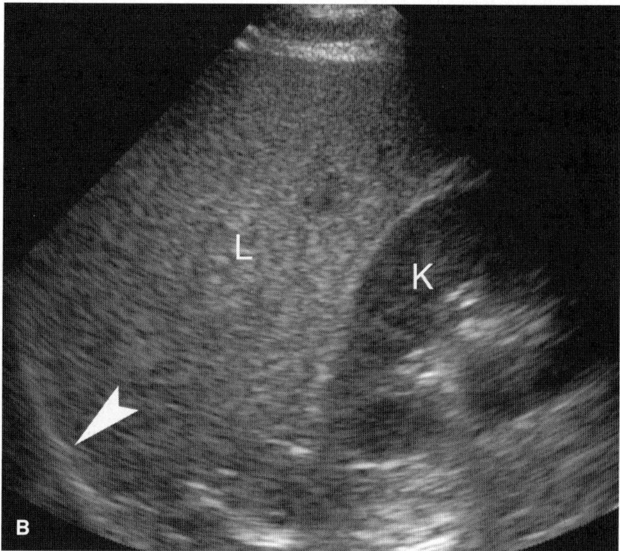

FIGURE 36.5. **Normal and Diffuse Fatty Liver. A.** Longitudinal US image demonstrates normal liver (L) and right kidney (K). The liver parenchyma is of uniform echogenicity, approximately equal to the parenchymal echogenicity of the kidney. The liver is well visualized to the level of the diaphragm (*arrowhead*). Small portal triad structures (*arrow*) are seen throughout the liver parenchyma. **B.** Diffuse fatty infiltration of the liver (L) markedly increases liver parenchymal echogenicity compared to that of the kidney (K). No portal triads are seen, and the diaphragm (*arrowhead*) is less well visualized.

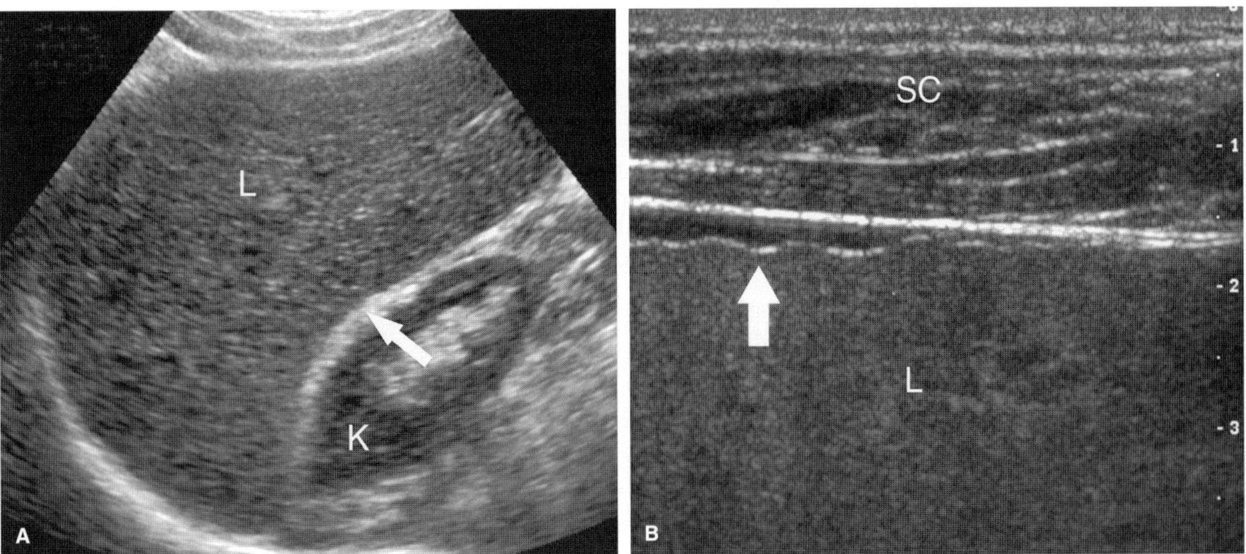

***FIGURE 36.6.* Cirrhosis. A.** Longitudinal US image of the liver (L) shows coarsening of the echotexture, loss of visualization of portal triads, and nodularity characteristic of cirrhosis. The deep surface of the liver (*arrow*) shows the fine nodular contour typical of alcoholic cirrhosis. Note that the echogenicity of the cirrhotic liver is close to the echogenicity of the normal kidney (K). Cirrhosis coarsens hepatic echotexture. Fatty infiltration increases hepatic echogenicity. **B.** A linear array transducer produces a detailed image of the liver (L) surface showing the nodular contour (*arrow*) of cirrhosis. SC, subcutaneous tissues. This technique is helpful in revealing the morphologic changes of cirrhosis.

include hepatomegaly, distention of the IVC and hepatic veins, and pulsatile portal vein flow seen on Doppler caused by transmission of right atrial activity through congested sinusoids. Ascites, pleural effusion, and pericardial effusion are often present.

Cirrhosis. US reflects the morphologic changes in the liver associated with cirrhosis (4). Hepatic echotexture is usually coarsened and heterogeneous, with numerous vague nodules commonly evident (Fig. 36.6). When examined with high-frequency transducers, the surface of the liver shows fine or coarse nodularity. Echogenicity is increased in proportion to the degree of fatty infiltration. With alcoholic cirrhosis, the right lobe is shrunken, and the left lobe and caudate lobe are enlarged. Advanced cirrhosis results in a small liver with nodular contour. The normal triphasic Doppler waveform of the hepatic veins is flattened in cirrhosis, with loss of the reverse-flow component caused by atrial systole. US is insensitive (<45%) to detection of malignancy in cirrhotic livers; however, US demonstration of a discrete focal mass is highly predictive of malignancy.

Portal Hypertension. US evidence of portal hypertension includes demonstration of portosystemic collateral vessels, dilatation of the portal vein (>13 mm), dilatation of the splenic and superior mesenteric veins (>10 mm), splenomegaly, and ascites. The hepatic artery may be enlarged and tortuous. Doppler demonstration of reversed (hepatofugal) flow in the portal vein is diagnostic of portal hypertension (Fig. 36.7). Flow in a dilated paraumbilical vein traversing the falciform ligament and anterior abdominal wall is also highly specific for portal hypertension. Color Doppler US is very useful in the detection of splenorenal, retroperitoneal, and coronary vein collaterals.

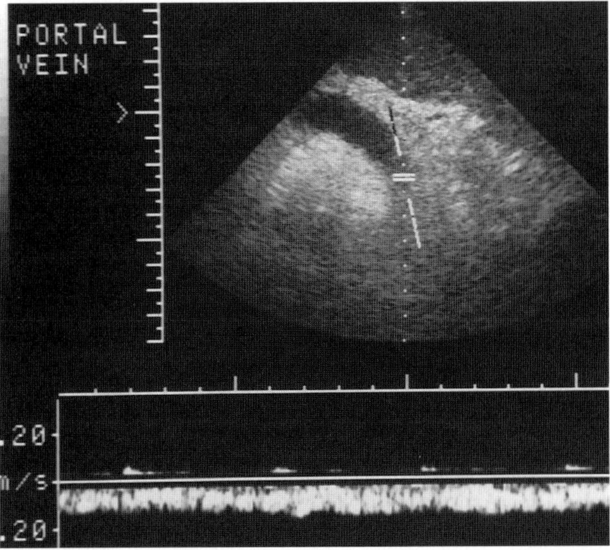

***FIGURE 36.7.* Reversed Flow in the Portal Vein.** The spectral waveform below the baseline indicates venous flow away from the transducer. The anatomic image confirms that the flow direction is out of, instead of into, the liver, indicating advanced portal hypertension.

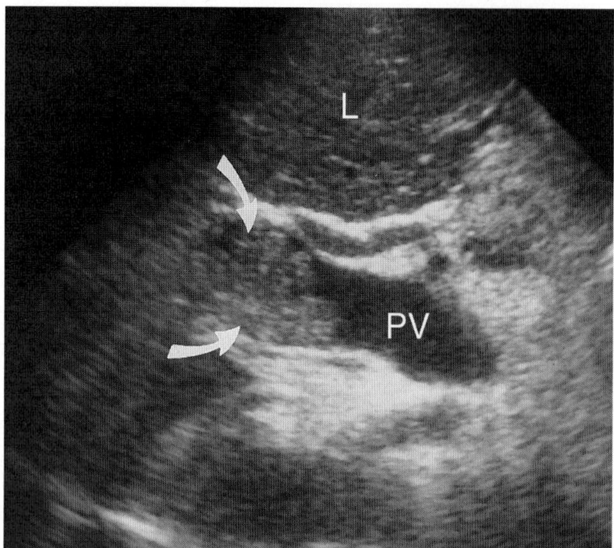

FIGURE 36.8. **Portal Vein Thrombosis.** The portal vein (PV) is enlarged and partially filled with tumor thrombus (*arrows*) from hepatocellular carcinoma. L, liver.

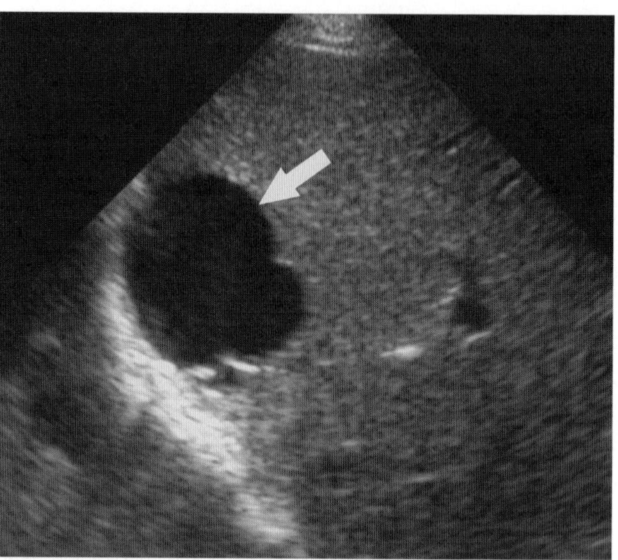

FIGURE 36.9. **Benign Hepatic Cyst.** A hepatic cyst (*arrow*) has sharply defined walls and anechoic contents. Benign hepatic cysts are rarely simple. They tend to occur in clusters, have thin septations, and lobulated contours. No solid nodular component is evident.

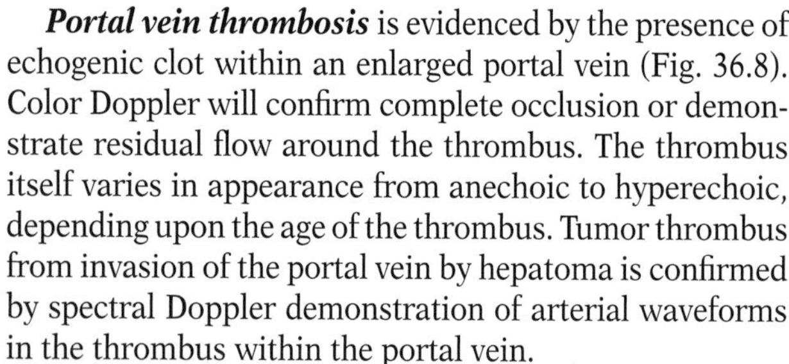

Portal vein thrombosis is evidenced by the presence of echogenic clot within an enlarged portal vein (Fig. 36.8). Color Doppler will confirm complete occlusion or demonstrate residual flow around the thrombus. The thrombus itself varies in appearance from anechoic to hyperechoic, depending upon the age of the thrombus. Tumor thrombus from invasion of the portal vein by hepatoma is confirmed by spectral Doppler demonstration of arterial waveforms in the thrombus within the portal vein.

Cysts are common and easily identified and characterized by US (Fig. 36.9). Benign hepatic cysts contain anechoic fluid, have thin walls, and demonstrate posterior acoustic enhancement. Most are septated and have a lobulated, rather than spherical, contour. They vary in size from tiny to huge and are commonly multiple, producing a "bunch of grapes" appearance. Small cysts may mimic vessels on quick inspection. Doppler is useful to confirm their avascular nature.

Cavernous hemangiomas are commonly identified on hepatic sonograms. The classic US appearance is a well-defined, homogeneous, hyperechoic mass (Fig. 36.10). Doppler usually shows no internal blood flow, although on occasion with slow-flow, high-sensitivity settings, very low-velocity flow is detected. Large lesions may contain hypoechoic thrombosis, fibrosis, and calcification. Most lesions remain stable in size over time, but about 2% show enlargement. Classic-appearing lesions in patients with normal liver function tests usually require no follow-up. Atypical lesions should have a 6-month follow-up US or be confirmed with other imaging modalities, as discussed in Chapter 27.

Metastases vary greatly in appearance from hypoechoic to hyperechoic and from homogeneous to heterogeneous to calcified (Fig. 36.11). Metastatic disease must be considered in the differential diagnosis of all solid and atypical cystic lesions in the liver. In 90% of cases, metastatic disease is multifocal in the liver.

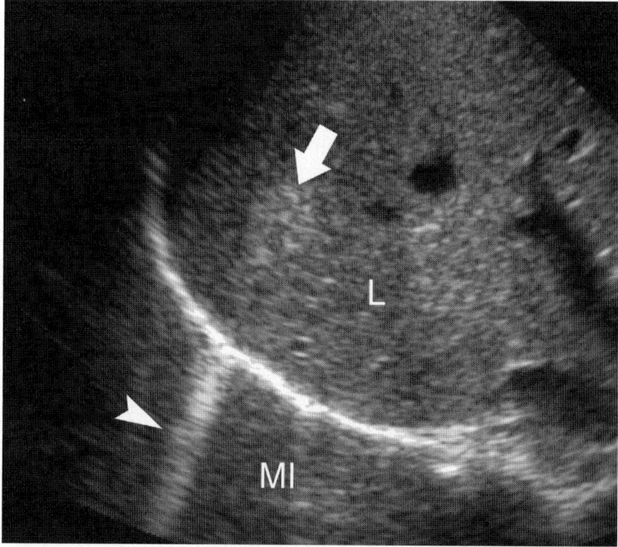

FIGURE 36.10. **Cavernous Hemangioma.** A small, incidentally discovered, cavernous hemangioma is seen as a well-defined echogenic mass in the liver (L). Acoustic enhancement, caused by the mostly fluid (blood) content of the lesion, is best appreciated in the mirror image (MI) of the liver projected above the diaphragm.

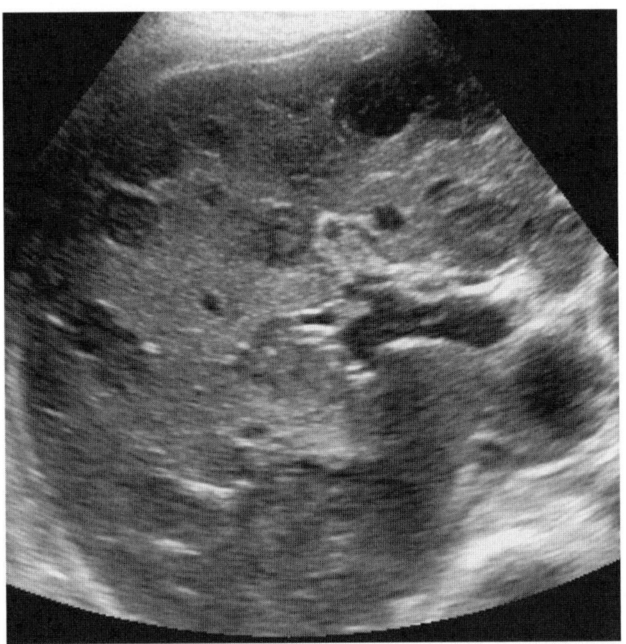

FIGURE 36.11. **Metastases.** Metastases from a retroperitoneal sarcoma are seen as innumerable heterogeneous hypoechoic solid masses in the liver.

Hepatocellular carcinoma may be solitary, multifocal, or diffuse (Fig. 36.12). Detection in the diseased liver is commonly difficult with US. Most are hypervascular, with prominent vascularity shown by color Doppler. Tumor invasion of the portal and hepatic veins is common. Tumors may be hyperechoic with internal fat to hypoechoic and heterogeneous because of nonliquefactive necrosis. Any solid mass detected by US in a diseased liver is suspicious for hepatocellular carcinoma.

Abscesses usually appear as complex fluid collections containing echogenic fluid, fluid–fluid layers, or gas (Fig. 36.13). Healed abscesses commonly calcify.

Microabscesses occur most commonly in immunocompromised patients with fungal or parasitic septicemia. Target lesions with central echogenic spot and peripheral hypoechoic halo are common. The differential diagnosis of multiple small (<10-mm) lesions in the liver is given in Table 27.6.

Other masses, including hepatic adenoma, focal nodular hyperplasia, sarcoma, and peripheral cholangiocarcinoma, have a varied and nonspecific sonographic appearance. They range from hypoechoic to hyperechoic and may contain areas of internal hemorrhage, necrosis, fibrosis, or calcification. Characterization of these nonspecific masses is often best performed with three-phase contrast-enhanced multidetector CT. The final diagnosis often depends on percutaneous biopsy.

Transjugular intrahepatic portosystemic shunt (TIPS) function is routinely monitored by Doppler US examination (6). TIPS are used to treat complications of portal hypertension, including intractable ascites and bleeding from varices. Stenosis and occlusion rates for TIPS approach 50% at 6 months and can reach up to 87% by 1 year. Evidence of stent stenosis include a maximum intrastent velocity of <90 cm/s or a focal jet

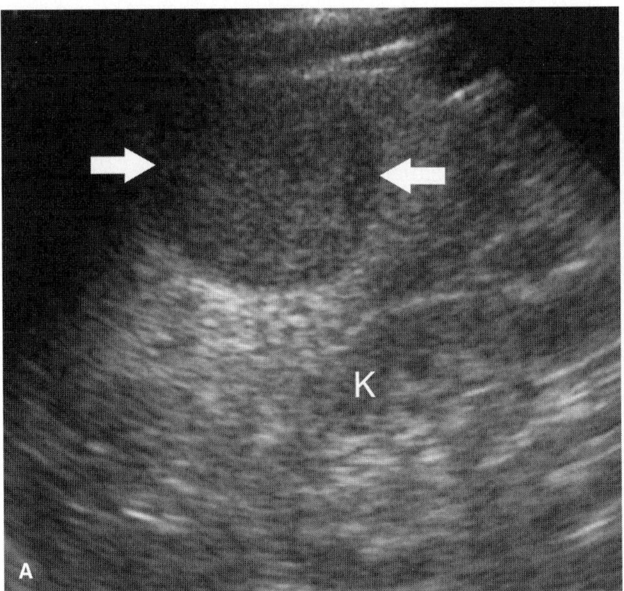

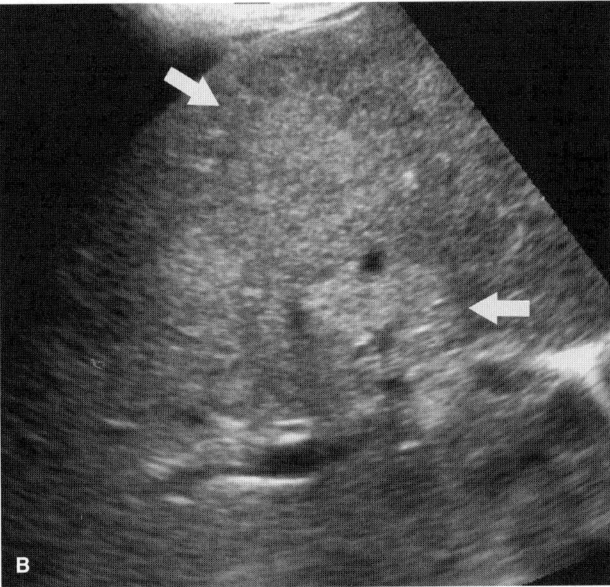

FIGURE 36.12. **Hepatocellular Carcinoma. A.** A well-differentiated hepatocellular carcinoma appears as a well-defined mass (*arrows*) within an echogenic cirrhotic liver. K, Kidney. **B.** A poorly differentiated hepatocellular carcinoma appears as multiple poorly defined echogenic masses (*arrows*) within a cirrhotic liver.

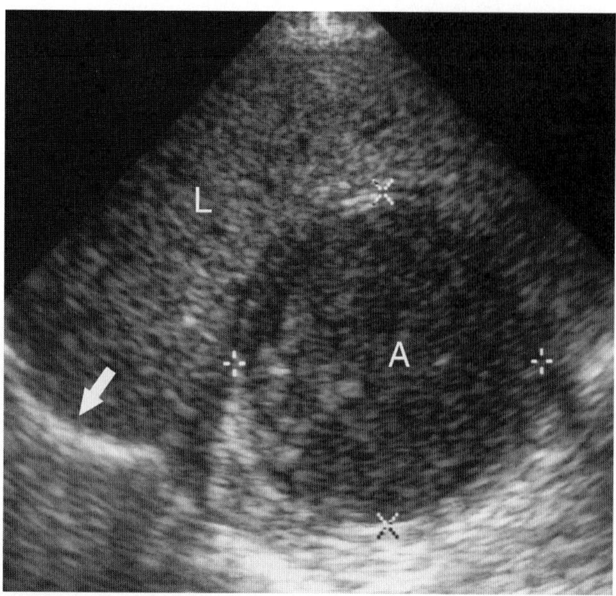

FIGURE 36.13. **Amebic Abscess.** A well-defined hypodense mass (A, between calipers) is seen in the right lobe of the liver (L). Note the proximity to the right hemidiaphragm (*arrow*). Amebic abscesses in the liver may rupture through the diaphragm into the right pleural space.

with increase in flow velocity >60 cm/s. Blood flow in the portal veins in a patient with normal shunt function is usually hepatofugal (into the stent). Relapse of portal venous flow back into the liver parenchyma (hepatopetal) may be a sign of shunt malfunction.

Liver Transplants. US with Doppler is the imaging method of choice for evaluation of liver transplants (7). Peritransplant fluid collections are common in the immediate posttransplant period. Simple anechoic fluid collections include ascites, bile, and lymph. Fluid with particulate matter is usually pus or blood. Hepatic artery complications account for 60% of vascular complications and include thrombosis, stenosis, and pseudoaneurysms. Thrombosis and stenosis of the portal vein or IVC are uncommon. Bile leaks, bile duct anastomotic strictures, necrosis of bile ducts, and stones in the bile ducts account for 25% of complications. Posttransplantation lymphoproliferative disorder occurs 4 to 12 months after transplantation. Focal solid hypoechoic masses may be seen within or adjacent to the transplanted liver. Hepatocellular carcinoma is a risk for the immunocompromised posttransplant patient.

BILE DUCTS

Normal US Anatomy. Intrahepatic bile ducts run in the portal triads in the company of the portal veins and hepatic arteries. Normal intrahepatic ducts may be visualized with high-resolution US. Intrahepatic ducts normally do not exceed 2 mm in diameter in the central liver or 40% of the diameter of the adjacent portal vein. The junction of the right and left lobe bile ducts to form the common hepatic duct marks the division between the intrahepatic and extrahepatic portions of the biliary tree. The junction of the cystic duct with the common hepatic duct marks the commencement of the common bile duct. Because this junction is seldom visualized with US, the generic term "common duct" is used to identify the duct in the porta hepatis. The common duct courses anterior to the main portal vein, the right portal vein, and the right hepatic artery in the portal region. The hepatic artery is commonly tortuous in the porta hepatis, but the common duct runs a straight course parallel to the portal vein. This straight portion of the common duct is routinely measured, with normal values for the diameter (from inner wall to inner wall) of 4 to 6 mm in adults. After age 60, an additional millimeter per decade is added to the normal range, so a 70-year-old patient may have a normal common duct as large as 7 mm (8).

As the portal triad structures course through the free edge of the hepatoduodenal ligament, a "Mickey Mouse" configuration is formed, with the common duct forming Mickey's right ear (Fig. 36.14). The normal common bile duct can be traced as it descends adjacent to the pancreatic head to its insertion at the ampulla of Vater. Normal variants that may cause confusion include a "replaced" right hepatic artery arising from the superior mesenteric artery and coursing between the portal vein and IVC to the porta hepatis. An elongated gallbladder neck may be mistaken for a dilated common duct. Low insertion of the cystic duct causes the appearance of two common ducts. Doppler identification of vascular structures is helpful in confusing cases.

Dilatation of the Biliary Tree. Dilated intrahepatic ducts are tortuous like the branches of an oak tree, exceed 40% of the diameter of the adjacent portal vein, and are visualized in the periphery of the liver (8). US shows "too many tubes" in the liver, and color Doppler US offers rapid differentiation of patent blood vessels and dilated bile ducts (Fig. 36.15). Dilated extrahepatic ducts exceed 6 to 7 mm in diameter and appear as enlargements of Mickey's right ear in the hepatoduodenal ligament. The dilated duct should be followed to the level of obstruction, where careful evaluation will demonstrate the cause of obstruction in 80% of patients.

Choledocholithiasis. Stones in the bile ducts appear as echogenic objects within the lumen of the duct (Fig. 36.16). Unfortunately, not all intraluminal stones will cast a distinct acoustic shadow; therefore, technique must be optimized to demonstrate shadowing. Nonetheless, US detection of obstructing common duct stones is only about 75% sensitive. Abrupt termination of a dilated common duct is an indication for MR cholangiography.

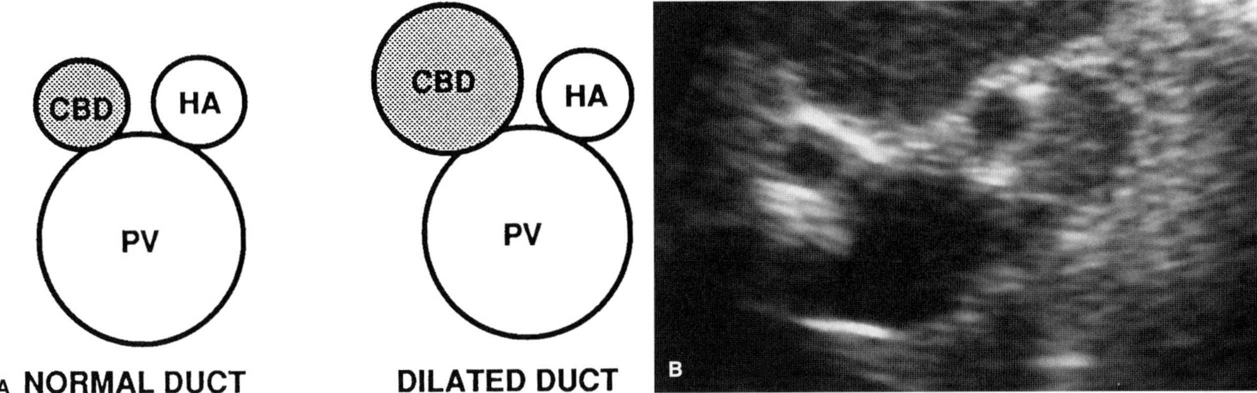

FIGURE 36.14. **"Mickey Mouse" Configuration of the Portal Triad. A.** Anatomic drawing demonstrates the anatomic relationships of the common bile duct (CBD), hepatic artery (HA), and portal vein (PV). Dilation of the common bile duct enlarges Mickey's right ear. **B.** US image of Mickey Mouse.

Calcification in the hepatic artery may mimic the appearance of stones in the biliary tree.

Gas in the biliary tree is most commonly the result of surgical procedures, such as sphincterotomy or choledochoenterostomy (see Table 27.10). Additional causes include gas-producing infection; fistulous connection with the intestinal tract (gallstone ileus, perforating duodenal ulcer); and trauma. Air in bile ducts causes bright linear or globular reflections with shadowing and ring-down artifacts. Air will move in the biliary tree with changes in patient positioning. Ducts are usually dilated when air is present.

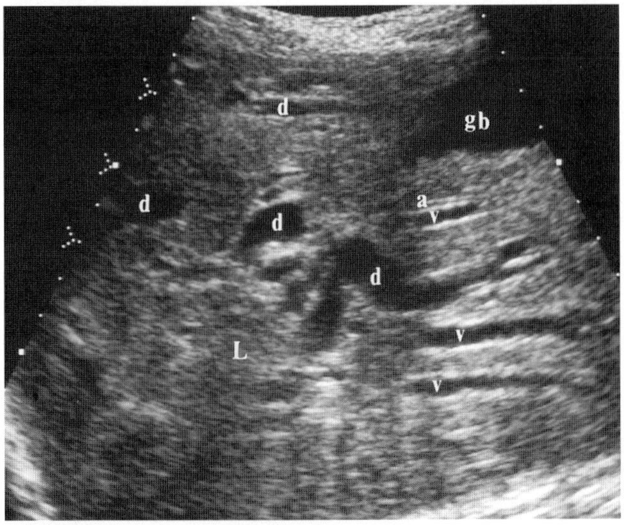

FIGURE 36.15. **Bile Duct Dilation.** Longitudinal US image demonstrates "too many tubes" in the liver (L). Dilated bile ducts (d), veins (v), and arteries (a) are most easily distinguished by use of spectral or color Doppler. Dilated bile ducts tend to be more tortuous and less uniform in diameter than arteries or veins. gb, gallbladder.

Cholangiocarcinoma. Hilar cholangiocarcinoma (Klatskin tumor) and extrahepatic cholangiocarcinoma tend to be small (<3 cm) when they present with biliary obstruction. US demonstrates the tumor as a focal mass at the point of obstruction (Fig. 36.17), nodular thickening of the bile duct wall, or polypoid intraluminal mass. The visualized mass is most commonly isoechoic with the

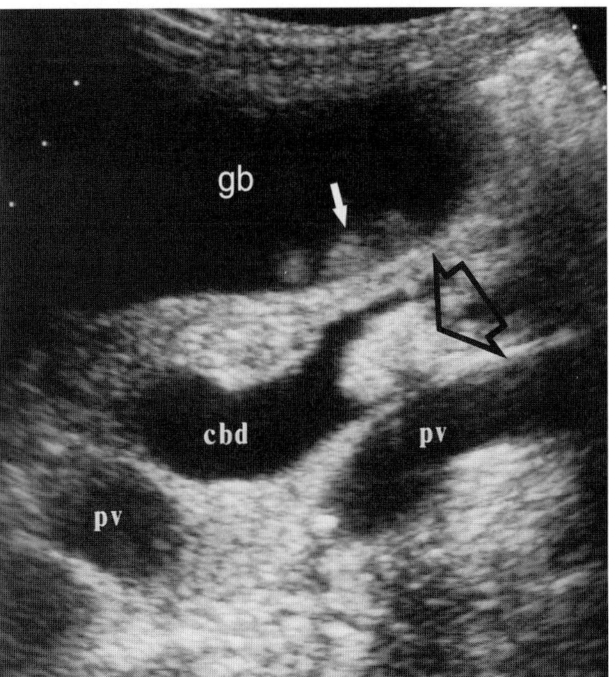

FIGURE 36.16. **Choledocholithiasis.** US image of the porta hepatis demonstrates a large stone (*open arrow*) obstructing the common bile duct (cbd) and resulting in its dilation (13 mm diameter). The gallbladder (gb) is dilated and contains several non-shadowing sludge balls (*white arrow*) formed as a result of biliary stasis. pv, portal vein.

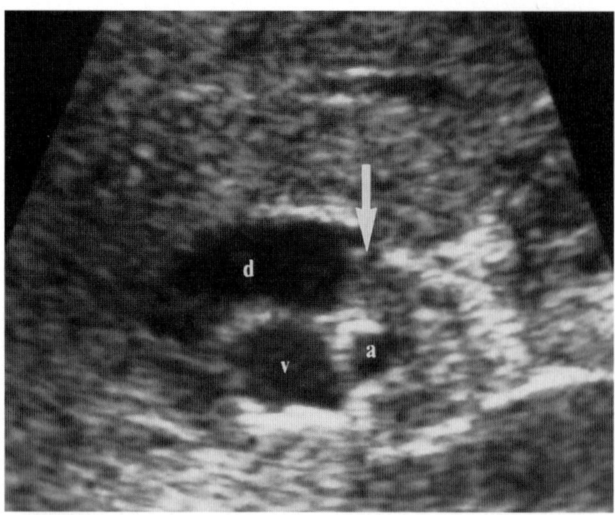

FIGURE 36.17. **Cholangiocarcinoma.** Tumor (*arrow*) obstructs and dilates the common bile duct (d) in the porta hepatis. v, portal vein; a, hepatic artery.

liver parenchyma but may be hypoechoic or hyperechoic. Abrupt termination of a dilated duct without visualization of a mass may be the only finding. Adjacent portal veins may be invaded and obstructed by tumor.

Oriental Cholangiohepatitis (Recurrent Pyogenic Cholangitis). US reveals bile ducts that are focally dilated or stenotic. Multiple stones with and without shadowing are evident in the bile ducts. Debris ("biliary mud") may fill and layer within dilated ducts. Most patients originate from Southeast Asian countries, where the disease is endemic.

AIDS-related cholangitis features dilated intrahepatic and extrahepatic bile ducts with thickening of the walls of the bile ducts and gallbladder. Sludge is commonly seen, but stones are usually not present. A unique finding is an echogenic nodule, representing edema of the papilla of Vater at the termination of the dilated common bile duct.

Biliary Ascariasis. Worms that colonize the intestinal tract may find their way into the biliary tree and gallbladder. Living worms may obstruct the biliary tree and gallbladder and cause cholangitis, cholecystitis, and pancreatitis, with a high associated mortality. Worms are seen by US as moving tubular echogenic structures with an echolucent core.

Congenital Biliary Cysts. The classification of congenital biliary cysts is illustrated in Chapter 27. US is excellent in demonstrating the morphology of cystic masses and their relationship to the biliary tree.

GALLBLADDER

Normal US Anatomy. The gallbladder is found on the undersurface of the liver, with the gallbladder neck positioned in the interlobar fissure. Normal bile is anechoic. The normal wall does not exceed 3 mm in thickness. The mucosa is echogenic and the smooth muscle layer of the wall is hypoechoic. The diameter of the gallbladder is less than 4 cm in 96% of normal individuals. The length of the gallbladder is highly variable, and measurement is not diagnostically useful. Most patients are examined after an overnight fast, although a 4-hour fast is usually sufficient to ensure gallbladder distension. Patients are examined in multiple positions to displace gallstones and demonstrate their mobility. The neck region should be carefully examined to avoid overlooking impacted stones. Normal folds in the gallbladder neck and cystic duct may cause acoustic shadows and mimic gallstones (9).

Echogenic Bile. Bile becomes echogenic when it is highly concentrated and cholesterol crystals and calcium bilirubinate granules precipitate as *sludge*. Sludge commonly layers in the gallbladder (Fig. 36.18) and may become quite viscous and form "sludge balls" or tumefactive sludge. Sludge balls usually move within the gallbladder but do not cast acoustic shadows. Floating cholesterol crystals are seen as bright reflectors with short "comet-tail" artifacts. Air in bile has a similar appearance. Sludge is not definitive evidence of gallbladder disease but is indicative of prolonged lack of bile turnover in the gallbladder. Prolonged fasting is the most common cause, but sludge is usually present with gallbladder and biliary obstruction. Sludge is not produced by the routine overnight fast advised in preparation for gallbladder examination. Additional causes of echogenic bile are blood, pus, and parasites.

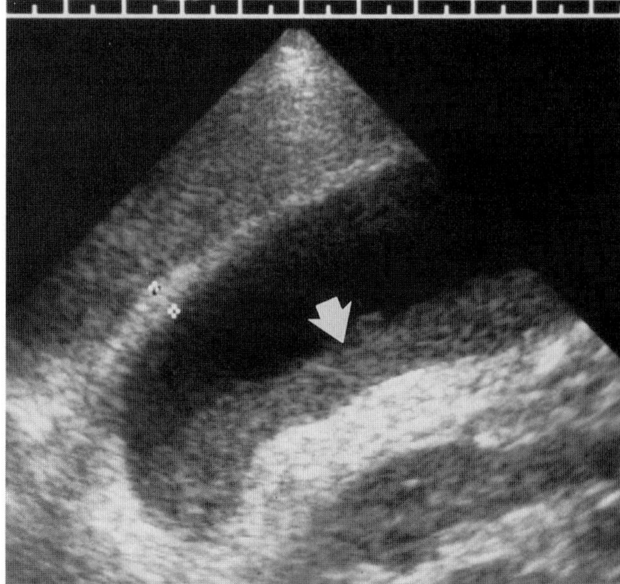

FIGURE 36.18. **Echogenic Bile.** Highly concentrated echogenic bile (*arrow*) layers dependently within the gallbladder. The gallbladder wall is thickened (between cursors) to 6 mm in this patient with acute cholecystitis.

TABLE 36.1 Causes of Gallbladder Wall Thickening

Contracted gallbladder after eating
Gallbladder disease
Acute cholecystitis
Chronic cholecystitis
Adenomyomatosis
Gallbladder carcinoma
AIDS cholangiopathy
Sclerosing cholangitis
Nonbiliary disease
Hypoproteinemia
Ascites
Edema caused by congestive heart failure
Hepatitis
Portal hypertension
Portal lymph node obstruction
Cirrhosis

Thickened Gallbladder Wall. The gallbladder wall is considered thickened when it exceeds 3 mm, as measured between the gallbladder lumen and the liver parenchyma. Causes of thickening include gallbladder disease and nonbiliary processes (Table 36.1). The most common causes are ascites, hypoproteinemia, and cholecystitis.

Gallstones. US is the imaging method of choice for detection of gallstones with its sensitivity of greater than 90%. Gallstones appear within the gallbladder lumen as echogenic objects that cast acoustic shadows and move with changes in patient position (Fig. 36.19). When these findings are present, specificity for gallstones is 100%. However, the demonstration of acoustic shadowing is strongly dependent on technique. When shadows are not evident with a suspected gallstone, a switch to a higher-frequency transducer with the focal zone adjusted at the depth of the stone will commonly demonstrate the elusive shadow.

Gallstones may be nonmobile because of adhesion to the gallbladder wall, but acoustic shadowing should be demonstrable. Cholesterol polyps and adenomatous polyps are nonmobile, nonshadowing soft tissue nodules attached to the gallbladder wall. Sludge balls appear as echogenic foci that move or are adherent to the wall but do not shadow.

Wall-Echo-Shadow (WES) Sign. When the gallbladder is completely filled with gallstones, a confident diagnosis becomes more difficult because the gallbladder resembles an air-filled loop of bowel. The WES sign is definitive evidence of a stone-filled gallbladder (Fig. 36.20). Gallstones produce a "clean" dark shadow, and air in the bowel produces a "dirty" brighter shadow.

Polyps appear as echogenic nonshadowing nodules that extend from the gallbladder wall (Fig. 36.21). Most are cholesterol polyps, which are smaller than 1 cm and are

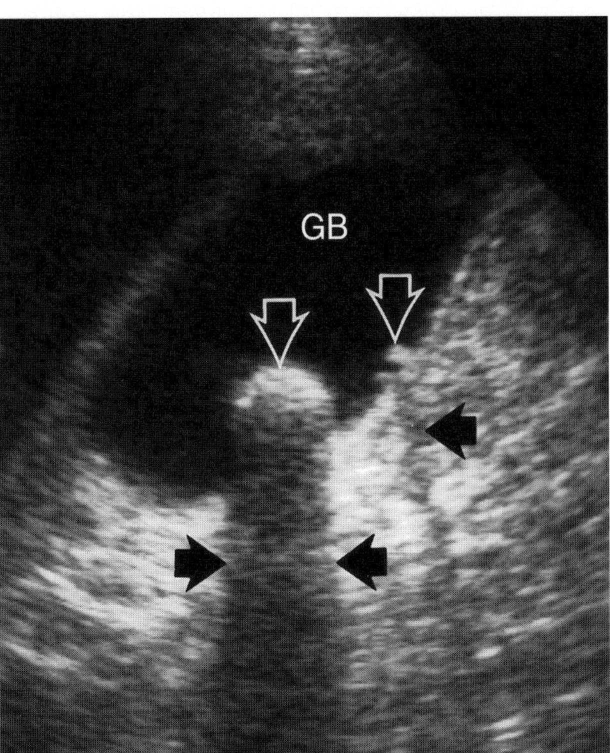

FIGURE 36.19. **Gallstones.** US demonstrates focal echodensities of varying size (*open arrows*) within the gallbladder lumen (GB). Acoustic shadows (*closed arrows*) extend from the echodensities. Moving the patient into the upright position resulted in a change in position of the gallstones.

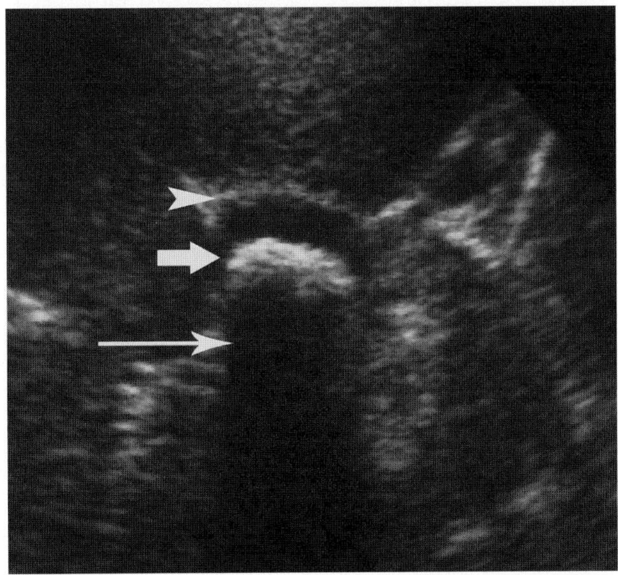

FIGURE 36.20. **Wall-Echo-Shadow Sign.** A thin layer of bile separates the gallbladder wall (*arrowhead*) from the bright echo (*short arrow*) of gallstones, which cast a dense acoustic shadow (*long arrow*). This appearance has also been called the "double arc shadow sign."

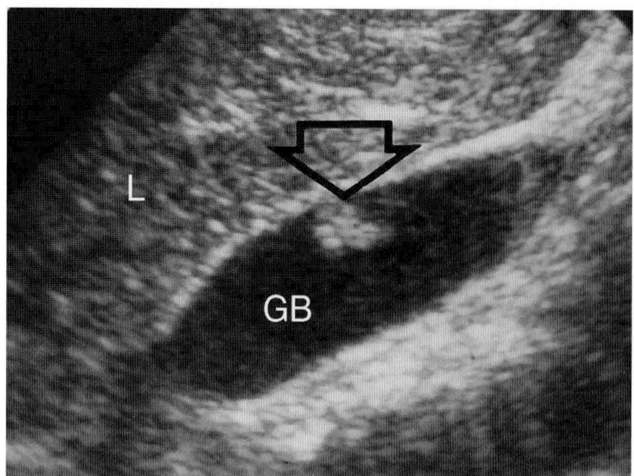

FIGURE 36.21. **Cholesterol Polyp.** An echogenic nodule (*arrow*) extends from the nondependent wall of the gallbladder into the lumen (gb). The lesion does not cause acoustic shadowing. L, liver.

commonly multiple. Adenomatous polyps are rare and indistinguishable from cholesterol polyps. Polyps larger than 1 cm may be malignant.

Acute Cholecystitis. US is commonly performed in patients who present with acute right upper quadrant pain. US evidence of acute cholecystitis includes (Fig. 36.22): (*1*) gallstones, (*2*) thickened gallbladder wall, (*3*) focal gallbladder tenderness elicited by transducer pressure directly over the gallbladder (positive sonographic Murphy sign), (*4*) pericholecystic fluid, (*5*) dilated gallbladder, and (*6*) power Doppler evidence of wall hyperemia. A positive Murphy sign is highly predictive of acute cholecystitis (92%). A negative or equivocal Murphy sign is evidence against acute cholecystitis. A striated appearance of a thickened gallbladder wall is evidence of gangrenous cholecystitis. Pericholecystic fluid collections larger than 1 cm are evidence of gallbladder perforation. The absence of gallstones is not evidence against cholecystitis in patients who are at risk for acalculous cholecystitis (Fig. 36.23). These patients usually have a prolonged illness associated with major surgery, trauma, burns, prolonged hospitalization, parenteral nutrition, and sepsis.

Emphysematous cholecystitis is usually caused by ischemia in elderly patients with diabetes. Gas develops in the gallbladder wall and lumen in association with gas-producing bacterial infection of the gallbladder. Perforation occurs commonly, and mortality is high. The diagnosis is suggested on US by bright reflections in the gallbladder wall associated with ring-down artifact. Gas bubbles in the lumen move and produce comet-tail artifacts. Air may be present in the bile ducts. The diagnosis is confirmed by CT or radiograph confirmation of air in the gallbladder. Immediate surgery is indicated.

Gallbladder Carcinoma. Because gallstones are usually present, the signs of gallbladder carcinoma may be overlooked during US examination. Three major patterns

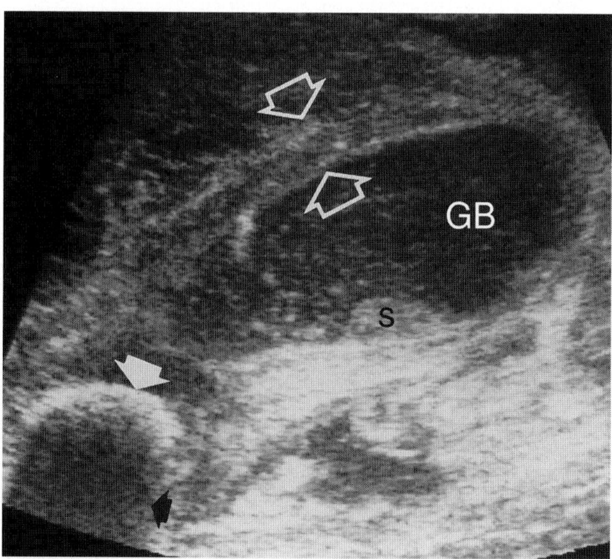

FIGURE 36.22. **Acute Cholecystitis.** US image through the long axis of the gallbladder (GB) demonstrates a large gallstone (*solid white arrow*) impacted in the neck of the gallbladder and casting an acoustic shadow (*black arrow*). The gallbladder wall is thickened (*open arrows*) and edematous. Echogenic sludge (s) is seen within the gallbladder lumen, giving evidence of bile stasis. A sonographic Murphy sign was present.

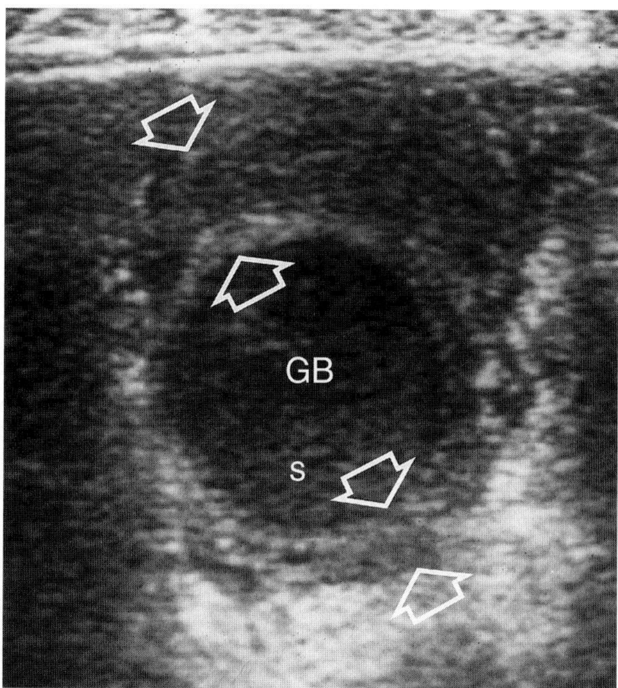

FIGURE 36.23. **Acalculous Cholecystitis.** Transverse image of the gallbladder (GB) demonstrates marked thickening and edema of the wall (*arrows*) and echogenic sludge (s) in the lumen. A sonographic Murphy sign was elicited. No gallstones were present.

of disease have been described. A mass replacing the gallbladder is the most common appearance (40% to 65% of cases). A normal gallbladder is not evident. The mass is strikingly heterogeneous because of enveloped gallstones, tumor, and necrotic debris. Diffuse or focal thickening of the gallbladder wall is the second pattern, seen in 20% to 30% of cases. The wall is thicker and more irregular than walls thickened by other causes. The least common pattern (5% to 10% of cases) is a soft tissue mass within the gallbladder lumen (Fig. 36.24). An intraluminal mass larger than 10 mm is suspicious for cancer. Cholesterol polyps are usually smaller than 5 mm, and benign adenomatous polyps uncommonly exceed 10 mm in diameter. Additional findings associated with gallbladder cancer include biliary obstruction, adenopathy, liver metastases, and invasion of adjacent structures (10).

Porcelain gallbladder refers to calcification of the gallbladder wall complicating chronic cholecystitis. US demonstrates a highly echogenic wall with acoustic shadowing. Porcelain gallbladder is a predisposing condition to gallbladder carcinoma.

Adenomyomatosis appears on US as focal or diffuse thickening of the gallbladder wall (11). The gallbladder fundus is nearly always involved. Rokitansky-Aschoff sinuses are a characteristic morphologic feature (Fig. 36.25). These are pockets of mucosa within the hypertrophied smooth muscle wall. These pockets commonly contain precipitated cholesterol crystals, which are very echogenic and produce comet-tail artifacts. This benign condition has no malignant potential but may mimic gallbladder carcinoma on US studies.

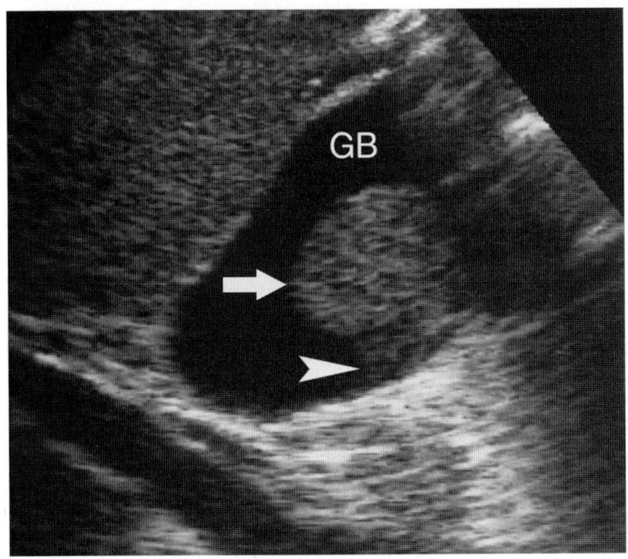

FIGURE 36.24. **Gallbladder Carcinoma.** A soft tissue mass (*arrow*) extends into the gallbladder lumen (GB) from an area of focally thickened gallbladder wall (*arrowhead*).

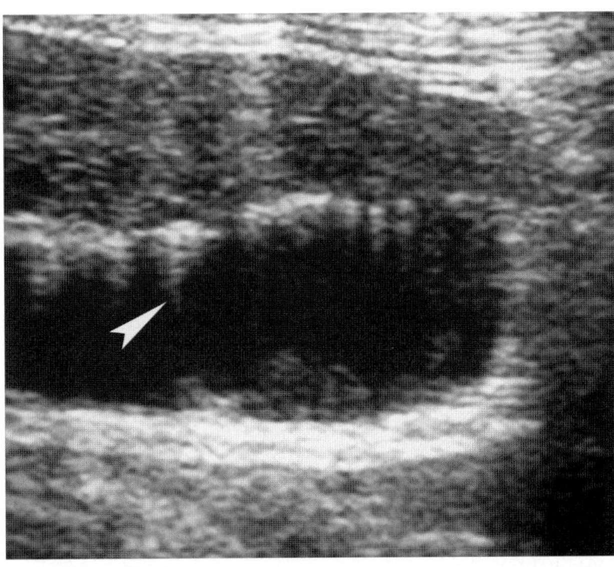

FIGURE 36.25. **Adenomyomatosis.** V-shaped comet-tail artifacts (*arrowhead*) extend from the gallbladder wall thickened because of adenomyomatosis. The comet-tail reverberation artifacts are caused by precipitation of cholesterol crystals within Rokitansky-Aschoff sinuses.

SPLEEN

Normal US Anatomy. The spleen is best visualized with US with a posterolateral intercostal approach and the patient supine (12). If the patient is in a right lateral decubitus position, the spleen may be difficult to visualize because of expansion of the left lung. When the spleen is large, an anterior subcostal approach with the patient in deep inspiration is also useful. The splenic parenchyma is homogeneous and normally more echogenic than the liver (Fig. 36.26). Its borders are smooth, sharply defined, and commonly lobulated. Doppler US demonstrates the splenic artery and vein in the splenic hilum and their branches within the spleen.

Accessory spleens (splenules) appear as rounded, well-defined masses in or near the splenic hilum (Fig. 36.26). They are homogeneous and isoechoic with spleen parenchyma. Blood supply by branches of the splenic artery or vein is diagnostic.

Splenomegaly is evidenced by splenic length >14 cm or thickness >6 cm. The parenchyma usually remains homogeneous and normal in appearance, regardless of the cause of splenic enlargement (see Table 28.3).

Posttraumatic cysts account for 80% of cystic lesions of the spleen. Most are well defined and anechoic, with accentuated through-transmission. Thick walls with ringlike calcification are common.

True epithelial cysts are indistinguishable from posttraumatic cysts, although calcification in the wall is less common.

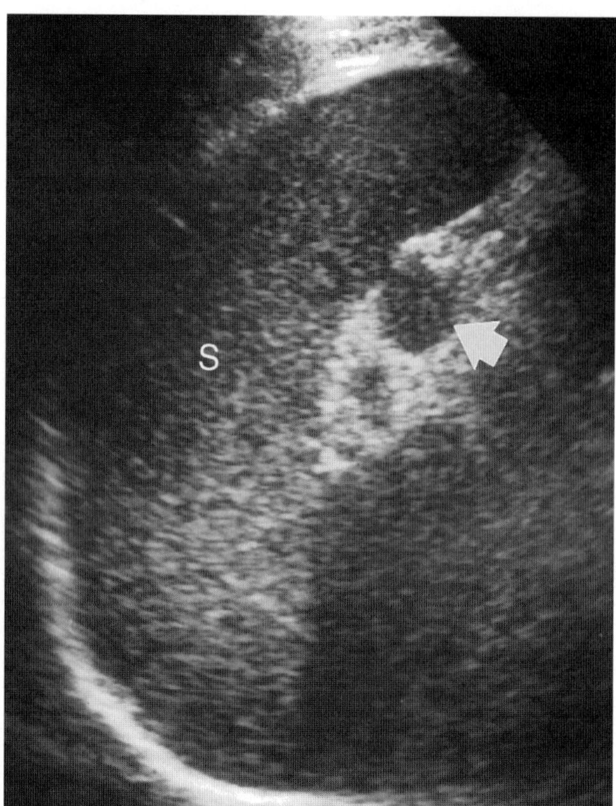

FIGURE 36.26. **Normal Spleen With Splenule.** A well-defined nodule (*arrow*) with the same echotexture as the splenic parenchyma is seen in the splenic hilum. The spleen (s) has a normal US appearance.

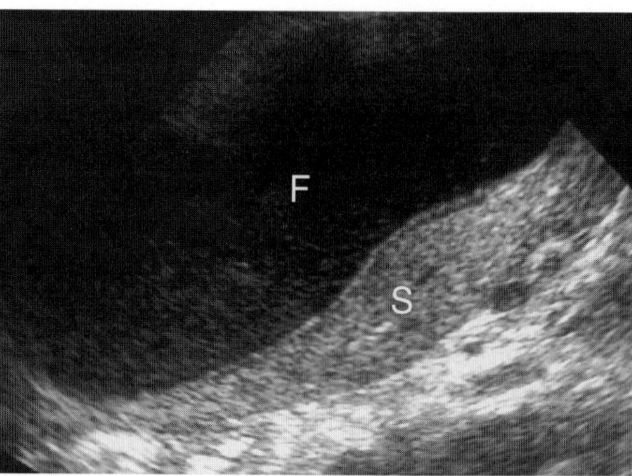

FIGURE 36.27. **Subcapsular Pancreatic Fluid Collection in the Spleen.** Pancreatic fluid (F) owing to acute pancreatitis has tracked beneath the splenic capsule and compressed the splenic parenchyma (S).

Pancreatic fluid collections are nearly always subcapsular in location (Fig. 36.27). Fluid flows from the pancreas to the spleen along the course of the splenic artery and vein. Associated findings of pancreatitis confirm the diagnosis.

Aneurysms of the splenic artery are common and present as a hypoechoic mass in the region of the splenic hilum. Atherosclerotic calcification in the aneurysm wall is usually present. Doppler US reveals arterial blood flow. Rupture causes a high mortality. Pseudoaneurysms of the splenic artery are usually caused by pancreatitis. Real-time scanning reveals a fluid collection with thin, noncalcified walls. Doppler US demonstrates internal arterial flow and communication with the splenic artery.

Abscesses usually demonstrate echogenic fluid, layering debris, and air, although some contain anechoic fluid (Fig. 36.28). US-guided percutaneous aspiration for diagnosis and catheter placement for treatment are safe procedures.

Microabscesses are most common in immunocompromised patients. High-frequency transducers reveal multiple tiny hypoechoic lesions. Common causes are *Mycobacterium tuberculosis*, *M avium intracellulare*, *Candida*, and

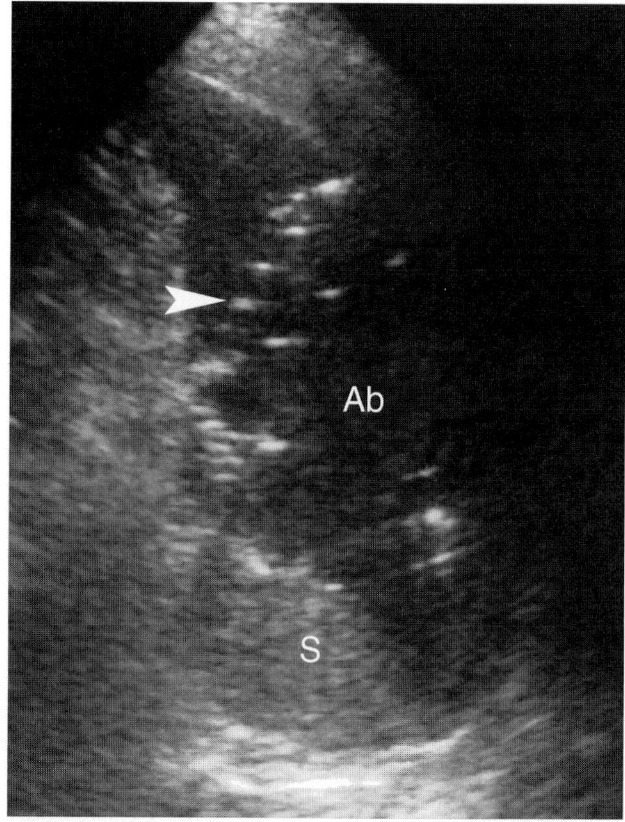

FIGURE 36.28. **Splenic Abscess.** Coronal plane US image demonstrates extensive destruction of the splenic parenchyma by a large abscess (Ab) containing air bubbles seen as mobile echogenic foci distributed through the fluid of the abscess (*arrowhead*). Only a small remnant of normal splenic parenchyma (S) remains.

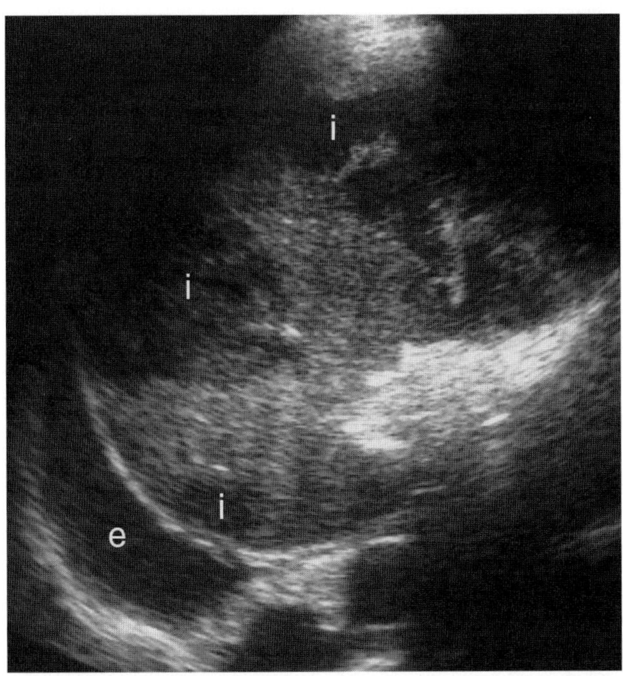

FIGURE 36.29. **Splenic Infarctions.** Acute splenic infarctions (i) appear as irregular and wedge-shaped, peripheral hypoechoic regions in the spleen. An associated pleural effusion (e) is also evident.

Pneumocystis jiroveci (formerly *P carinii*). The differential diagnosis is listed in Table 28.4.

Lymphoma. Hypoechoic lesions in the spleen in patients with lymphoma are very likely to be foci of lymphoma. Lesions range from numerous and small to solitary and large. However, the spleen may be enlarged without lymphoma involvement or appear normal and still be diffusely infiltrated.

Infarctions appear hypoechoic or anechoic and are usually wedge-shaped and characteristically extend to the splenic capsule (Fig. 36.29). Parenchymal borders may be sharply defined or irregular. Hemorrhage associated with infarction may dissect beneath the capsule, or the capsule may rupture, resulting in hemoperitoneum. Most patients with infarction have a predisposing cause, such as splenomegaly or lymphoma involving the spleen.

Hemangiomas are usually homogeneous and hyperechoic, but they have a much more variable appearance than in the liver. A complex mass appearance with multiple cystic areas has been described. Calcifications occur in areas of fibrosis.

Metastases are nonspecific in appearance; they are usually hypoechoic and multiple.

Hematoma. Sonography is now commonly used to screen for free intraperitoneal blood in patients who have suffered blunt abdominal trauma. Splenic lacerations and subcapsular and intraparenchymal hematomas are commonly demonstrated. The US appearance of the hematoma varies with age and composition. Most are well defined and hypoechoic.

PANCREAS

Normal US Anatomy. The pancreas can be a difficult organ to image with US. Vascular landmarks are the key to its identification (Fig. 36.30). The body and tail of the pancreas are immediately anterior to the splenic vein as it courses from the splenic hilum toward the liver. The neck of the pancreas is anterior to the junction of the splenic vein with the superior mesenteric vein, which marks the commencement of the portal vein. The head of the pancreas envelops this confluence and lies anterior to the IVC. It is important to remember that a portion of the pancreatic head—the uncinate process—lies caudal to level of the splenic vein, between the superior mesenteric vein and the IVC.

The echogenicity of the pancreas depends upon the amount of fatty infiltration. In children and young adults, the pancreas is about equal in echogenicity to the liver. In older adults, the pancreas becomes more echogenic with progressive fat infiltration between lobules of pancreatic parenchyma. The pancreatic duct is commonly seen in normal individuals. The normal duct does not exceed 3 mm in diameter and tapers progressively toward the tail.

The left lobe of the liver serves as the best sonographic window to the pancreas. The distal stomach lies between the liver and the pancreas. The hypoechoic muscular wall of the stomach should not be mistaken for the pancreatic duct. Gas in the stomach—or more often in the transverse colon—often prevents visualization of the pancreas, especially if the left lobe of the liver is small. Progressive transducer pressure is most effective in displacing gas to visualize the pancreas. The tail of the pancreas can be visualized through the spleen by concentrating on the region of the splenic hilum.

Acute Pancreatitis. US findings include: diffuse glandular enlargement, decrease in echogenicity because of edema, and poorly defined gland margins (Fig. 36.31). In mild cases, the US examination may be normal. Focal pancreatitis most commonly involves the pancreatic head. US examination should include documentation of the presence of gallstones and dilatation of the biliary tree. The ampullary region should be carefully examined for an impacted gallstone. US is excellent for detection and follow-up of fluid collections (Fig. 36.32). Fluid accumulates most commonly around the pancreas, in the lesser sac, and in the splenic hilum. Examination should be extended into the pelvis, especially if fluid is seen tracking caudal to the pancreas. Discrete cystic collections should be examined with Doppler US to detect pseudoaneurysms.

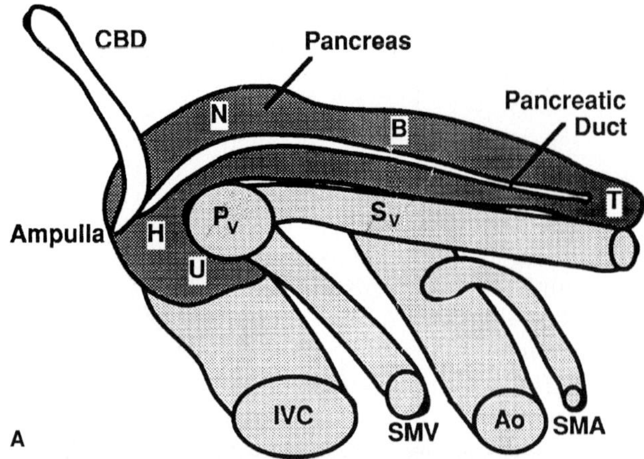

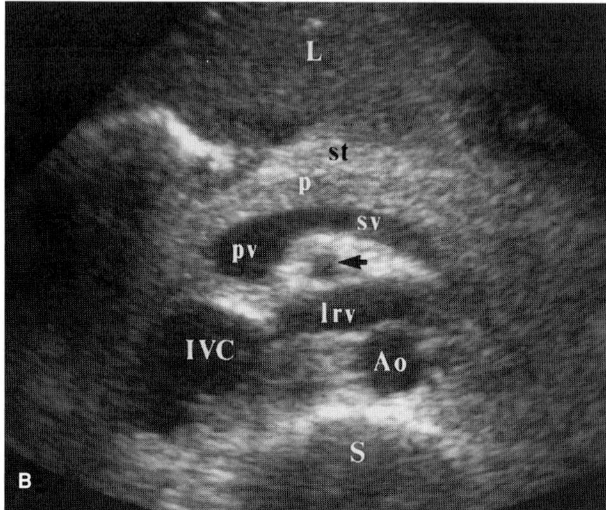

FIGURE 36.30. **Normal Pancreas Anatomy.** A diagram **(A)** and an US in transverse plane **(B)** demonstrate the normal US anatomy of the pancreas. The majority of the pancreas lies anterior to the splenic vein (sv) and its junction with the superior mesenteric vein (SMV), which forms the portal vein (pv). The head (H) and uncinate process (U) of the pancreas cradle the origin of the portal vein. The pancreatic neck (N) is anterior to the sv-SMV confluence, and the uncinate process and inferior vena cava (IVC) are posterior to the confluence. The superior mesenteric artery (SMA, *arrow*) arises from the aorta (Ao) dorsal to the splenic vein. The left renal vein (lrv) passes between the SMA and aorta to the IVC. The left lobe of the liver (L) offers a good sonographic window to the pancreas. The stomach (st) and lesser sac (collapsed) are anterior to the pancreas. CBD, common bile duct; S, spine; B, body of the pancreas; T, tail of the pancreas; p, pancreas.

The splenic, portal, and superior mesenteric veins should be examined for evidence of thrombosis.

Chronic Pancreatitis. Because of fibrosis and diffuse glandular atrophy, the pancreas is reduced in size and increased in echogenicity, making its identification with US more difficult. Calcifications produce focal echodensities and, often, acoustic shadowing. The pancreatic duct shows a pattern of alternating dilatation and constriction. Calcifications are commonly seen within the duct (Fig. 36.33). Signs of acute pancreatitis are commonly superimposed on chronic pancreatitis.

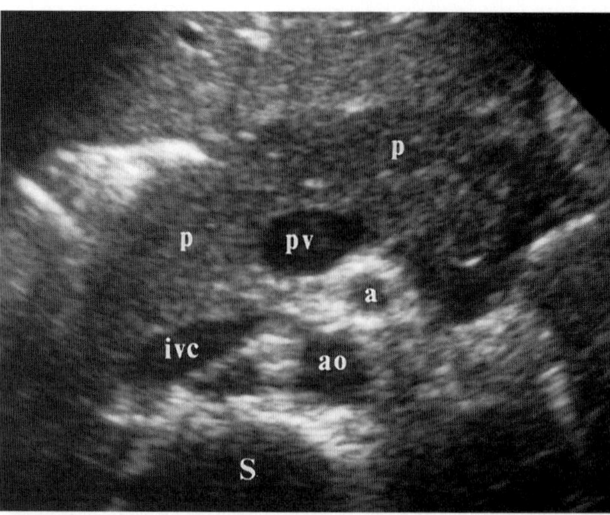

FIGURE 36.31. **Acute Pancreatitis.** Axial-plane US image reveals a diffuse decrease in the echogenicity of the pancreatic parenchyma (p) compared to the liver (L) because of diffuse edema of acute inflammation. The normal pancreas is more echogenic than normal liver (Fig. 36.30B). No discrete fluid collections were evident. pv, portal vein; a, superior mesenteric artery; ivc, inferior vena cava; ao, aorta; S, spine.

A mass of solid fibrinous tissue caused by chronic pancreatitis may be indistinguishable from adenocarcinoma. Ductal dilatation may be present. A major use of US is to guide percutaneous biopsy to provide pathologic differentiation of this common clinical problem.

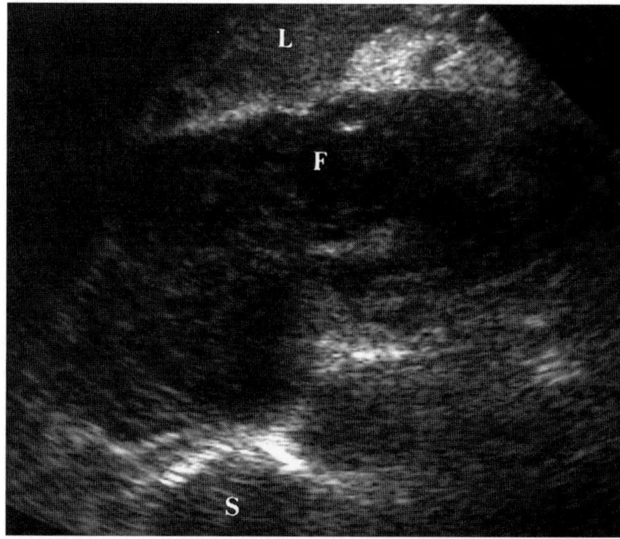

FIGURE 36.32. **Necrotizing Pancreatitis.** The anatomic landmarks for the pancreas are obliterated and replaced by heterogeneous fluid (F) in this patient with acute severe necrotizing pancreatitis. S, spine; L, liver.

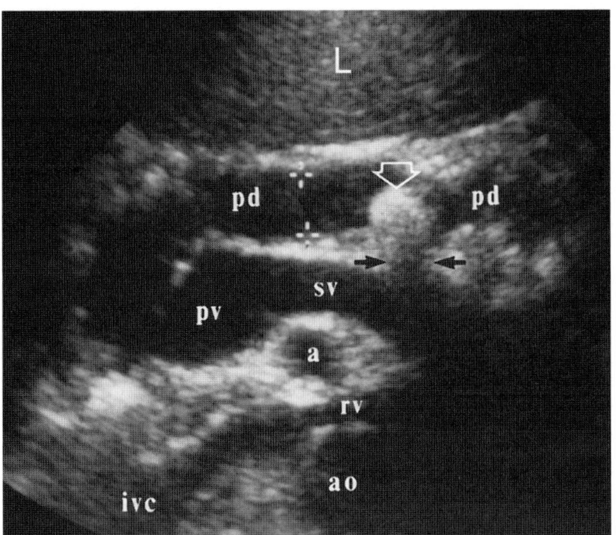

FIGURE 36.33. **Chronic Pancreatitis.** US in axial plane demonstrates a calculus (*open arrow*) in the markedly dilated pancreatic duct (pd). The calculus is seen as an echogenic focus with acoustic shadowing (*black arrows*). The pancreatic parenchyma is atrophic, consistent with chronic pancreatitis. The pancreatic duct measures 8.7 mm in diameter (*calipers*). A detailed knowledge of anatomy is needed to correctly identify all structures visualized. Doppler US is helpful in confirming vascular structures. ao, aorta; a, superior mesenteric artery; ivc, inferior vena cava; rv, left renal vein; sv, splenic vein; pv, portal vein; L, liver.

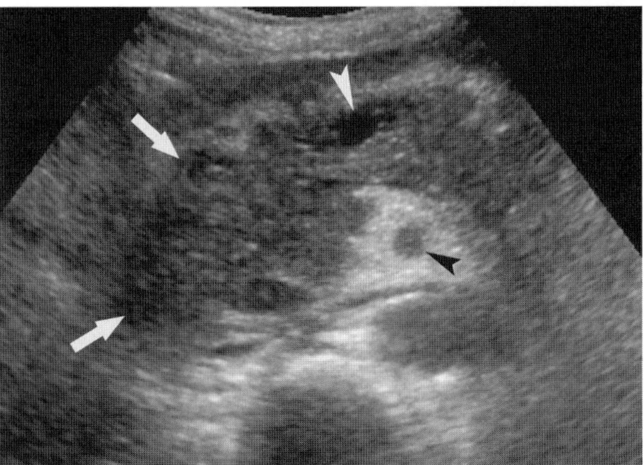

FIGURE 36.34. **Adenocarcinoma of the Pancreas.** The tumor is seen as a subtle hypoechoic mass (*arrows*) enlarging the head of the pancreas. The tumor margins are poorly defined. The pancreatic duct (*white arrowhead*) is dilated and terminates abruptly as it encounters the tumor. The superior mesenteric artery (*black arrowhead*) and its surrounding collar of echogenic fat are preserved.

Adenocarcinoma appears as a hypoechoic mass or as a subtle alteration of acoustic texture in the pancreas (Fig. 36.34). Biliary and pancreatic ductal obstruction is easily identified. Sudden termination of dilated ducts in a hypoechoic mass is characteristic. Doppler US is used to detect any vascular encasement or invasion, which commonly makes the tumor nonresectable. The liver and retroperitoneum should be carefully examined for metastatic nodules and adenopathy.

Islet cell tumors are predominantly hypoechoic compared to pancreatic parenchyma. Cystic degeneration, hemorrhage, fibrosis, and calcification cause wide variations in appearance. Transabdominal US detects 20% to 75% of insulinomas and only 20% to 30% of gastrinomas. Endoscopic US improves detection to the 77% to 94% range. Intraoperative US demonstrates 75% to 100% of small tumors and serves as a major aid to the surgeon having difficulty identifying the tumor.

Metastases, especially from colon carcinoma, may mimic pancreatic adenocarcinoma.

Lymphoma commonly involves the peripancreatic lymph nodes, causing multiple or confluent hypoechoic masses.

Pseudocysts appear as well-defined, smooth-walled, anechoic masses. Multiple loculations and internal septations are common. Internal debris and fluid–fluid levels are indicative of hemorrhage or infection. US is an excellent way to provide imaging follow-up of pseudocysts to confirm resolution or determine the need for drainage.

Abscess. US demonstrates a fluid collection that is usually ill defined and contains echogenic fluid. Gas bubbles that move, shadow, and cause comet-tail artifacts are strong evidence of infection. US is used to guide aspiration and catheter drainage.

Multiple pancreatic cysts are seen in patients with autosomal dominant polycystic disease and those with von Hippel-Lindau syndrome. Solitary true epithelial-lined cysts are rare.

Pseudoaneurysms develop in the peripancreatic region most commonly as a complication of pancreatitis with enzyme erosion of arterial walls. US demonstrates a discrete cystic mass in close proximity to an artery. Doppler US confirms arterial flow within the lumen of the pseudoaneurysm. A small neck of connection with the parent artery can be identified by flow jets.

Microcystic adenoma (serous cystadenoma), although composed of innumerable small cysts, commonly appears as a solid lesion on US (13). A few larger cysts may be demonstrated (Fig. 36.35). An echogenic central stellate scar with calcification is characteristic. CT should be performed to demonstrate distinctive enhancement of honeycomb septations.

Mucinous cystic neoplasms demonstrate cysts 2 cm or larger in size. Internal septations and papillary projections from walls that are 1 to 2 mm thick are demonstrated (13). Doppler commonly demonstrates flow within septa and solid components. All mucinous tumors are potentially malignant.

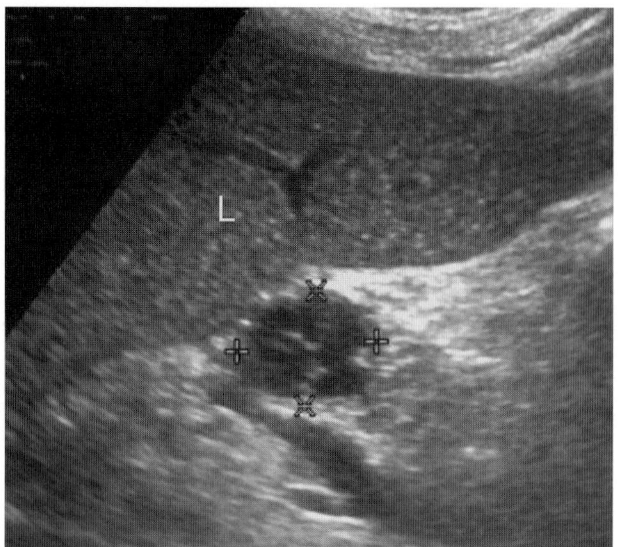

FIGURE 36.35. **Microcystic Adenoma of the Pancreas.** Sagittal-plane US image through the left lobe of the liver (L) reveals a small tumor (between *calipers*) of the pancreatic body consisting of multiple small cysts.

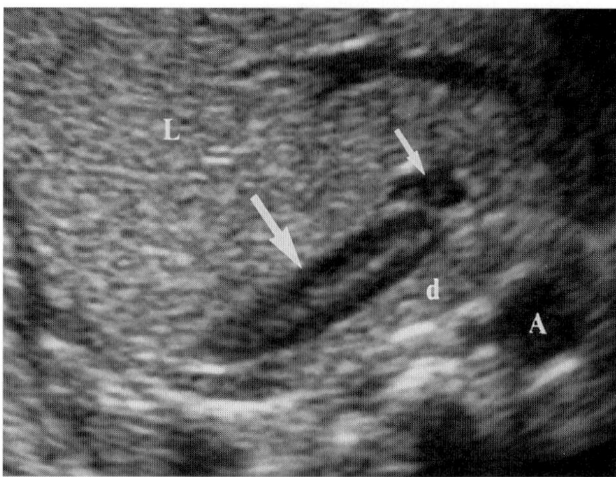

FIGURE 36.36. **Normal Adrenal Gland.** Transverse US image in an infant demonstrates the normal anatomic landmarks for identification of the right adrenal gland (*large arrow*), which are found posterior to the inferior vena cava (*small arrow*), between the right lobe of the liver (L) and the right crus (d) of the diaphragm. A, aorta.

Intraductal papillary mucinous tumors produce focal multicystic masses (branch duct type) or marked diffuse dilation of the pancreatic duct (main duct type) (13). Ductal dilatation is produced by secretion of large volumes of mucin.

ADRENAL GLANDS

Normal US Anatomy. The normal adrenal glands may be difficult to visualize sonographically in the adult but are usually quite prominent in the newborn (Fig. 36.36). The right adrenal gland is best seen on a transverse image just above the upper pole of the right kidney. The Y- or V-shaped adrenal gland is seen just posterior to the IVC as the IVC enters the liver. The right adrenal is visualized between the right lobe of the liver and the right crus of the diaphragm. The left adrenal is best seen between the upper pole of the left kidney and the aorta on an angled coronal plane. The adrenals are hypoechoic compared to retroperitoneal fat and isoechoic compared to the crura of the diaphragm. The medulla is seen as a thin echogenic line surrounded by the hypoechoic cortex. The limbs of the normal adult adrenal gland are 4 to 5 cm long and 5 to 7 mm wide. In infants, the adrenal glands normally appear large because of persistence of the "fetal" portion of the gland. The fetal cortex rapidly involutes in the first 3 weeks of life.

Although CT is more sensitive than US for detection of small adrenal masses, US is useful for characterizing adrenal masses as cystic, follow-up of presumed benign adrenal masses, and confirming the origin of large retroperitoneal masses (14).

Adrenal hyperplasia appears as bilateral diffuse enlargement or as multiple bilateral small nodules. Hyperplastic glands are seen with adrenal endocrine syndromes. The differential diagnosis of bilateral enlarged adrenal glands includes infection (especially tuberculosis, histoplasmosis, and Cytomegalovirus); metastatic disease; and lymphoma. Patients with AIDS may have adrenal enlargement caused by mycobacterial, fungal, or viral infection.

Adrenal adenomas appear as solid, homogeneous, adrenal masses with echogenicity similar to that of the renal parenchyma (Fig. 36.37). US offers no specific findings that differentiate benign from malignant masses. Masses larger than 4 cm should be considered suspicious for malignancy.

Adrenal carcinomas are indistinguishable from adenomas when the tumor is small (<4 cm). Larger carcinomas are inhomogeneous with areas of necrosis, hemorrhage, and calcification. Real-time imaging and Doppler are useful to detect tumor invasion of adrenal or renal veins and the IVC.

Pheochromocytoma arising in the adrenal gland can usually be demonstrated by US, because most are large (5 to 6 cm). Most are sharply marginated and predominantly solid; cystic areas of necrosis and hemorrhage are commonly present (Fig. 36.38). Predominantly cystic pheochromocytomas are less common.

Adrenal myelolipoma appears as a highly echogenic mass in the adrenal bed. They may be easily overlooked. Mixed hyperechoic and hypoechoic areas correspond to fatty and myeloid elements within the tumor. The diagnosis is confirmed by demonstration of internal fat density by

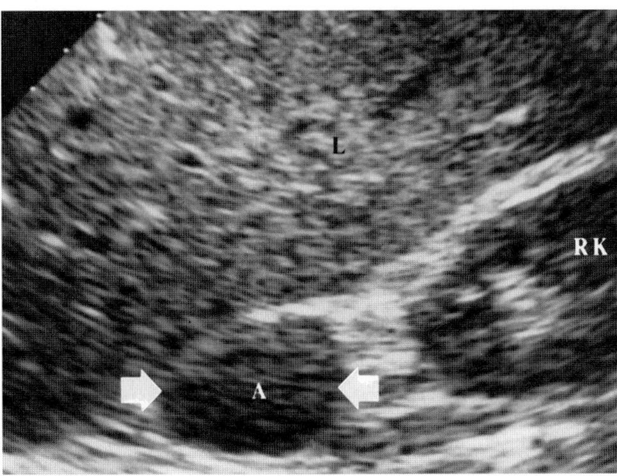

FIGURE 36.37. **Benign Adrenal Adenoma.** Longitudinal US demonstrates a homogeneous 3.5-cm mass (A, between *arrows*) arising from the right adrenal gland. The mass is outlined by echogenic fat. This is a nonhyperfunctioning adrenal adenoma that was discovered incidentally. L, liver; RK, right kidney.

CT or MR. Other echogenic masses in the adrenal region include renal angiomyolipoma, teratoma, lipoma, and liposarcoma.

Adrenal Cysts. US may be utilized to differentiate benign cysts from cystic tumors. Uncomplicated benign cysts have thin walls and septa (<3 mm), anechoic internal fluid, and demonstrate accentuated through-transmission. Calcification in walls and septa is common in all types of benign cysts. Echogenic internal fluid or debris, thick walls, solid components, and large size (>6 cm) suggest malignancy.

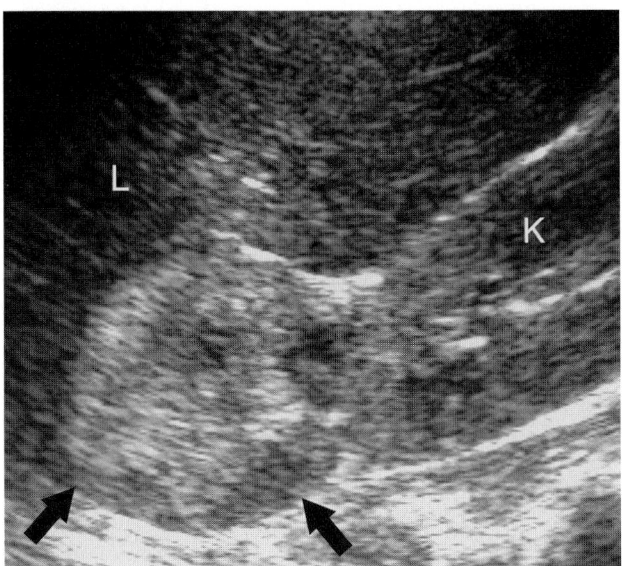

FIGURE 36.38. **Pheochromocytoma.** Longitudinal-plane US demonstrates an adrenal tumor (*arrows*) posterior to the liver (L) and superior to the right kidney (K). The tumor is heterogeneous in echogenicity, with highly echogenic areas that correspond to foci of internal hemorrhage.

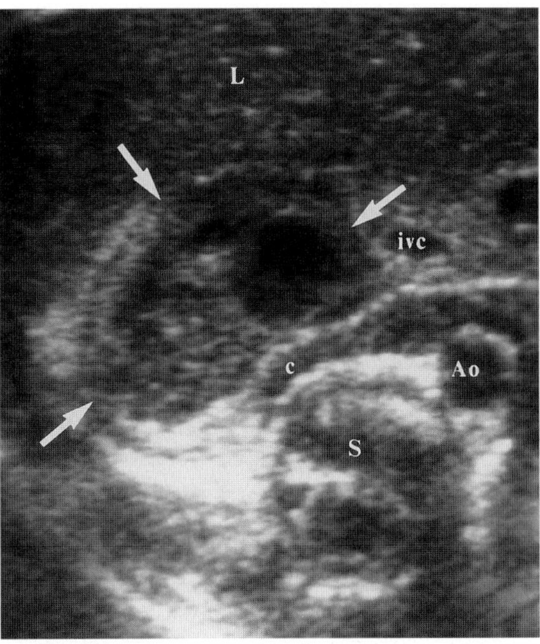

FIGURE 36.39. **Adrenal Hemorrhage.** The adrenal gland in a 2-week-old infant is identified by its location between the liver (L), the inferior vena cava (ivc), and the right crus of the diaphragm (c). Ao, aorta; S, spine.

Adrenal Hemorrhage. US initially demonstrates hyperechoic, masslike enlargement of the adrenal gland (Fig. 36.39). With time, the adrenal mass rapidly becomes hypoechoic and progressively decreases in size. The gland may return entirely to normal, or it may evolve into a pseudocyst that commonly develops calcifications in its walls within 2 to 4 weeks of the hemorrhage. Eventual collapse of the pseudocyst results in coarsely calcified adrenal glands. In the neonate, adrenal hemorrhage is usually bilateral and caused by hypoxic stress. In the adult, adrenal hemorrhage is usually unilateral and right sided (85%). Most adult cases of adrenal hemorrhage are associated with blunt abdominal trauma.

KIDNEYS

Normal US Anatomy. On US examination, the renal cortex is isoechoic or slightly hypoechoic compared to the liver and distinctly hypoechoic compared to the spleen (Fig. 36.40) (14). The medullary pyramids are visualized as hypoechoic, cone-shaped structures surrounded by the more echogenic cortex. This corticomedullary differentiation is striking in the newborn and becomes less noticeable with age. Lucent pyramids should not be mistaken for

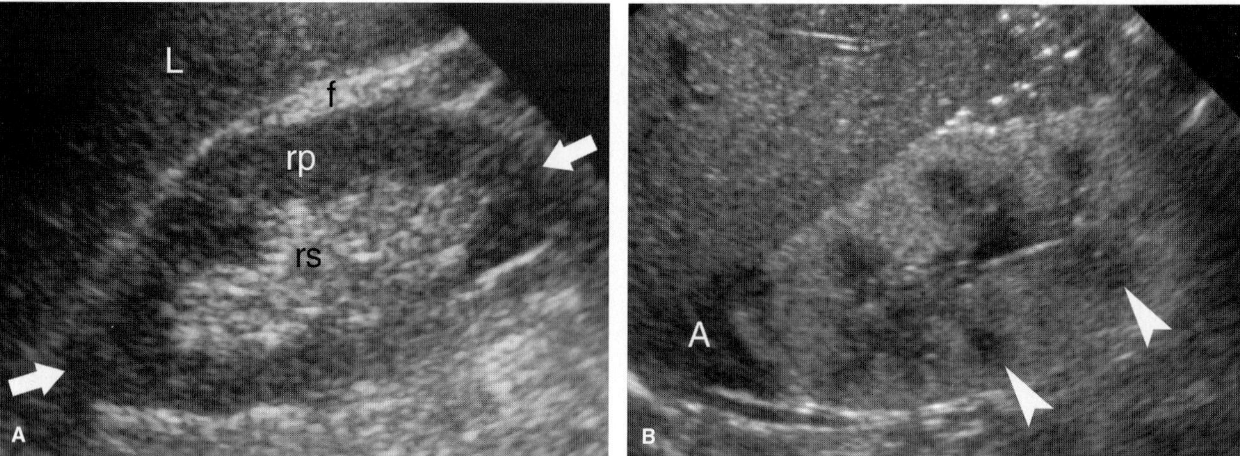

FIGURE 36.40. **Normal Kidneys. A.** Adult kidney. A long-axis US view of the right kidney (between *arrows*) obtained through the liver (L) demonstrates echogenicity of the normal renal parenchyma, which is approximately equal to the echogenicity of the normal liver. The renal sinus (rs), which contains vessels, the collecting system, and fat, is hyperechoic compared to the renal parenchyma (rp). The margins of the kidney are outlined by echogenic perirenal fat (f). Morison pouch is a recess of the peritoneal cavity between the kidney and the liver that usually fills with fluid when ascites is present. **B.** Newborn kidney. In newborns and infants, the renal cortex is more echogenic than in older children and adults, causing the medullary pyramids (*arrowheads*) to appear more lucent and resemble hydronephrosis. Note that the lucent pyramids correspond anatomically to the location of the renal medulla, that the pyramids do not interconnect, and that the renal pelvis is not dilated. The adrenal gland (A) is normally prominent in size in the newborn.

hydronephrosis. The central sinus contains fat, blood vessels, the collecting system, and lymphatic vessels. Central sinus echogenicity is the same as that of perirenal fat. Blood vessels appear as lucent tubular structures, with flow demonstrated by Doppler. In well-hydrated patients, minimally dilated collecting structures may be normally visualized. The contour of the kidney is smooth and may be lobulated by the normal renal lobes. Adult kidneys range from 9 to 13 cm in length. The *junctional parenchymal defect* is a normal anatomic variant caused by incomplete fusion of the upper and lower poles of the kidney. Sonography demonstrates a wedge-shaped echogenic defect in the renal parenchyma at the junction of the upper and middle thirds of the kidney.

Obstruction. US is commonly the imaging method of first choice for the diagnosis of urinary obstruction, but there are numerous pitfalls in using US to make this diagnosis. The key US finding in obstruction is hydronephrosis. Hydronephrosis is recognized as fluid distension of the collecting system, with communication between round, fluid-filled calices and the dilated renal pelvis (Fig. 36.41). A dilated ureter appears as a fluid-filled tube extending from the renal pelvis. However, in acute obstruction, such as from a stone impacted in the ureter, the degree of collecting system dilatation may be slight, even though the obstruction is severe. Moreover, the presence of hydronephrosis does not always mean obstruction. Additional causes of pelvocaliectasis are listed in Table 36.2. Structures that may mimic hydronephrosis include peripelvic cysts (Fig. 36.42), multiple simple cysts in the renal sinus, and an extrarenal pelvis. An *extrarenal pelvis* is one that extends outside the renal sinus. This type of pelvis is commonly filled with fluid but is a normal variant not associated with

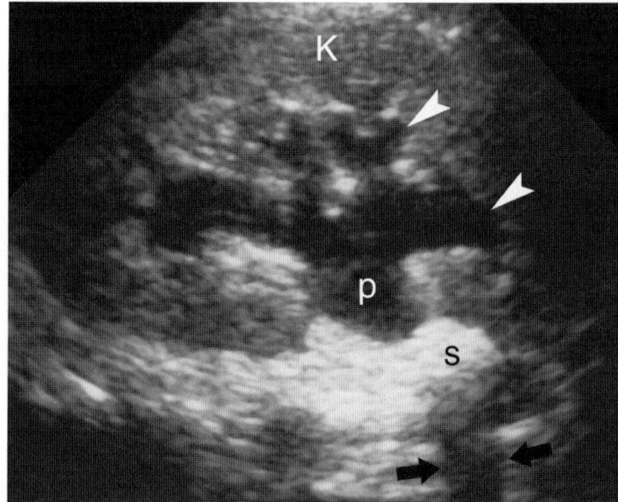

FIGURE 36.41. **Hydronephrosis Caused by Ureteropelvic Junction Calculus.** Coronal-plane US of the right kidney (K) reveals mild dilation of the calices (*arrowheads*) and renal pelvis (p) owing to an impacted stone (s) at the ureteropelvic junction. Note the dark acoustic shadow (between *arrows*) cast by the calculus.

TABLE 36.2 Causes of Hydronephrosis

Obstruction
Vesicoureteral reflux
Distended bladder
Relieved obstruction with persistent dilatation
Pregnancy
Diabetes insipidus
Active diuresis

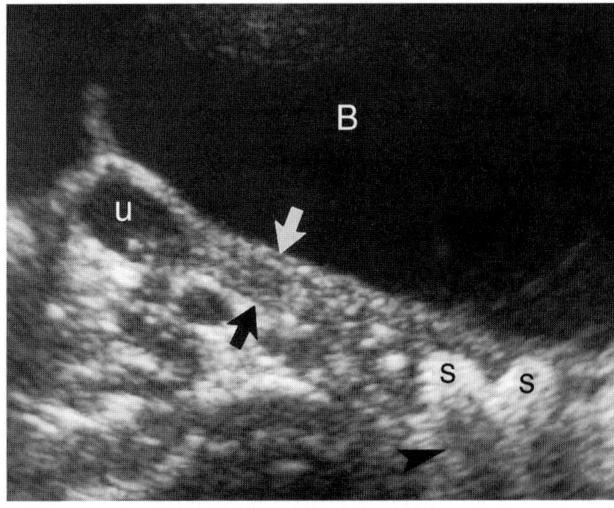

FIGURE 36.43. **Calculi in Distal Ureter.** Sagittal-plane US image of the distal right ureter (u) through the bladder (B) demonstrates two stones (s) impacted at the ureterovesical junction. Faint acoustic shadows (*arrowhead*) are cast by the stones. Just proximal to the stones, the ureter is filled with echogenic debris (*arrows*) owing to infection developing as a result of urinary stasis.

dilated calices or ureter. Comparison with previous studies may help in making the correct diagnosis. The ureterovesical junction should be examined with color Doppler to detect the presence or absence of a ureteral jet. Doppler evaluation of the renal arteries may also be helpful. A resistance index greater than 0.70 in the arcuate artery suggests obstruction.

Stones. All renal stones, regardless of composition, appear on US as bright, echogenic foci (Fig. 36.43) (15). Stones as small as 5 mm may be identified if they cast an acoustic shadow. However, when acoustic shadowing is not evident, often because of technical factors, small stones may be overlooked because they blend in with echogenic renal sinus fat. Technical factors that improve the capability to demonstrate shadowing include: imaging the stone in the focal zone of the transducer, centering the stone within the US beam, and using high-frequency transducers.

Nephrocalcinosis refers to calcification in the renal medullary pyramids, which appear echogenic rather than echolucent (Fig. 36.44). US is highly sensitive to even faint calcification that may not be visible on plain radiographs. Acoustic shadowing is present only when calcification is dense. Common causes include furosemide therapy in the newborn, hypercalciuric states such as hyperparathyroidism, medullary sponge kidney, and renal tubular acidosis.

Diffuse Renal Parenchymal Disease. US is commonly used to evaluate patients with acute and chronic renal failure. Rarely (<5% of cases), bilateral renal obstruction will be a cause of acute renal failure. Causes of bilateral obstruction include leaking abdominal aortic aneurysm, tumor (especially cervical carcinoma), and retroperitoneal

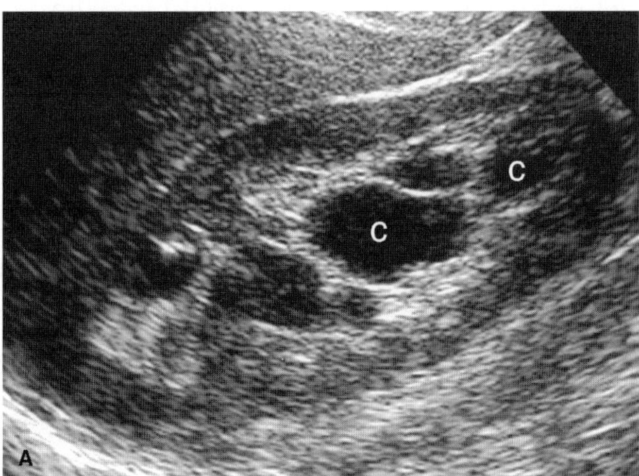

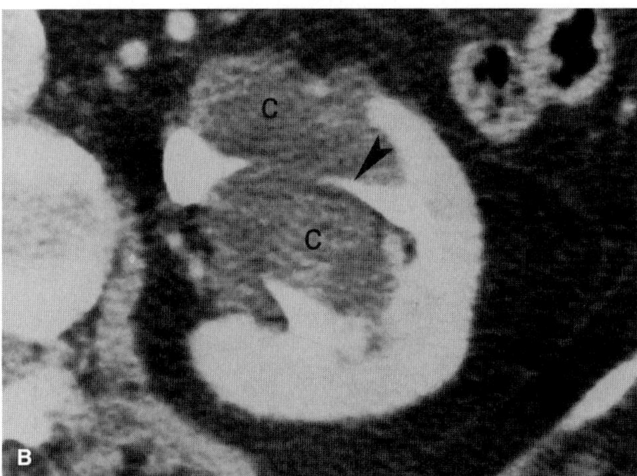

FIGURE 36.42. **Peripelvic Cyst. A.** Long-axis US image of the left kidney reveals fluid-filled structures (c) in the renal sinus. Lobulations of the cystic mass resemble dilated calices. **B.** A CT image of the left kidney reveals that the calices and pelvis (*arrowhead*) are stretched around the peripelvic cysts (c). Cysts that arise in the renal sinus assume the shape of the sinus as they slowly enlarge, mimicking hydronephrosis.

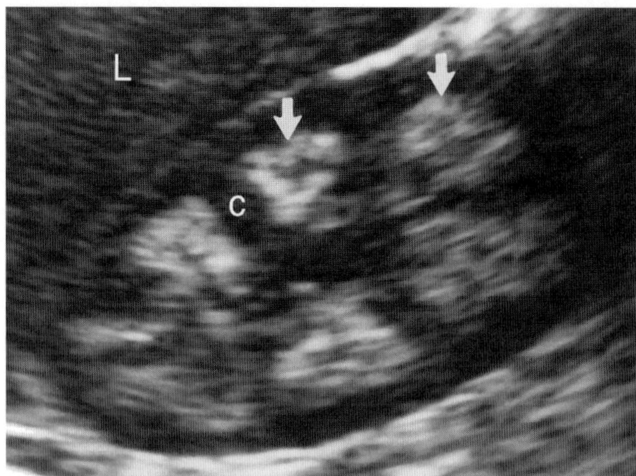

FIGURE 36.44. **Medullary Nephrocalcinosis.** Longitudinal US of the right kidney imaged through the liver (L) demonstrates abnormal increased echogenicity of the medullary pyramids (*arrows*). Compare to Fig. 36.40. The echogenicity of the intrarenal cortex (c) (columns of Bertin) is normal.

fibrosis. These rare cases will benefit from relief of obstruction. In the remainder of patients, US reveals the size and morphology of the kidneys. End-stage renal disease is associated with small, echogenic, often difficult-to-visualize kidneys (Fig. 36.45) (Table 36.3). When the kidneys are smaller than 9 cm in adults, reversible renal disease is unlikely and renal biopsy is seldom justified. Diffuse and focal renal parenchymal thinning and scarring provide rough estimates of renal parenchymal loss. Enlarged kidneys (>12 cm) suggest an infiltrative process such as acute glomerulonephritis, leukemia, lymphoma, or renal vein thrombosis (edema). AIDS nephropathy is characterized by an enlarged, diffusely echogenic kidney (Fig. 36.46). Enlarged kidneys are an indication for Doppler examination of the renal veins and may warrant a renal biopsy to detect

TABLE 36.3 Medical Renal Diseases With Echogenic Renal Parenchyma in Adults

Acute glomerulonephritis
Chronic glomerulonephritis
Hypertensive nephrosclerosis
Diabetic glomerulosclerosis
Lupus nephritis
Lymphoma
AIDS
Amyloidosis

a treatable condition. US may demonstrate an unsuspected condition, such as a form of renal cystic disease.

Renal Masses. Sonography plays a significant role in both the detection and characterization of renal masses. Real-time grayscale US is used to determine whether a mass is a simple cyst, a complicated cyst, a complex mass, or an entirely solid mass. Doppler is used to demonstrate the internal vascularity to characterize a neoplasm.

Simple cysts are diagnosed accurately and easily by US (Fig. 36.47). Characteristic findings are: (*1*) anechoic contents, (*2*) well-defined far wall, (*3*) acoustic enhancement deep to the lesion, and (*4*) imperceptibly thin walls. Small cysts may have artifactual internal echoes owing to slice thickness limitations. Acoustic enhancement may depend upon optimizing technique. All cysts should have a sharply defined back wall. Cysts with thin septations or thin peripheral curvilinear calcifications still qualify as benign cysts.

Complicated cysts have any of the following findings, which disqualify their characterization as a simple cyst: internal debris, echogenic clot, fluid–debris levels, thick septations, thick walls, blood vessels in septations, thick or coarse calcification. Differential diagnosis of a

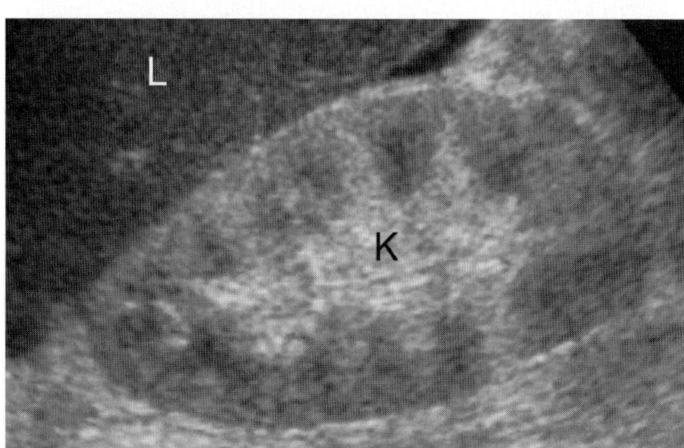

FIGURE 36.45. **End-Stage Kidney Failure.** In this patient with advanced renal failure, both kidneys (K) are small (<9 cm in length) and diffusely echogenic. The echogenicity of the renal parenchyma exceeds that of the liver parenchyma (L).

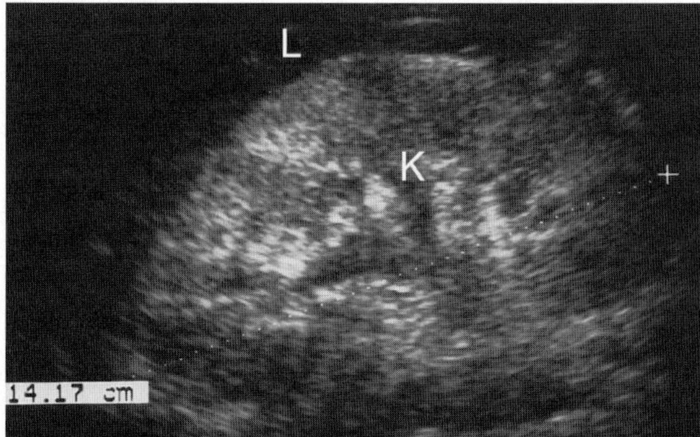

FIGURE 36.46. **AIDS Nephropathy.** Both kidneys in this patients with AIDS and impaired renal function were diffusely enlarged (>14 cm) and diffusely increased in echogenicity. Compare the right kidney parenchyma (K) to the liver parenchyma (L).

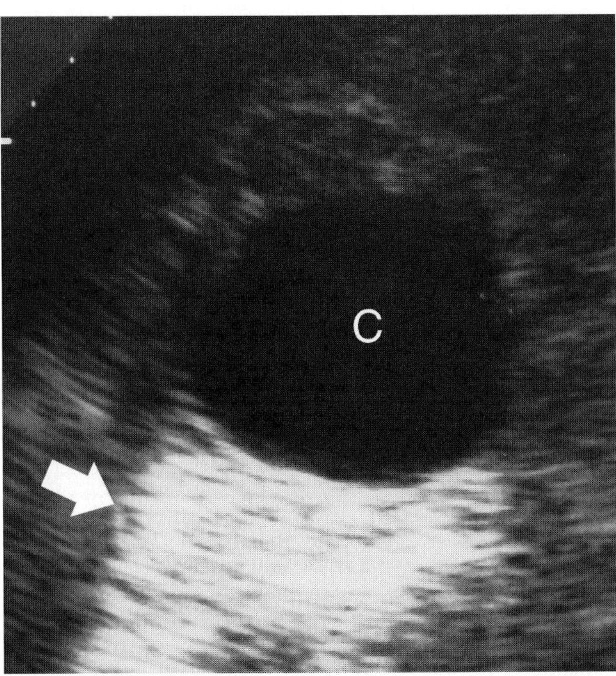

FIGURE 36.47. **Simple Renal Cyst.** Transverse image of the kidney shows a simple renal cyst (C) with imperceptibly thin walls, anechoic internal fluid, and accentuated sound transmission (*arrow*).

complicated cystic mass includes: hemorrhage or infection in simple cyst, cystic tumor, abscess, obstructed upper pole duplication, caliceal diverticulum, lymphoma, aneurysm, and pseudoaneurysm.

Peripelvic cysts form in the renal sinus, are multilobed, and may closely resemble hydronephrosis. Peripelvic cysts are differentiated from hydronephrosis by demonstration of lack of communication with each other or dilated renal pelvis, echogenic fat between the tip of the medullary pyramid and the cyst, and lack of a dilated ureter. Problem cases require excretory urography or CT.

Renal cystic disease is discussed in detail in Chapter 33. US is a reliable, safe, and accurate method to demonstrate the size, number, and character of cysts in the kidney as well as other organs (Figs. 36.48 to 36.50).

Renal cell carcinoma (RCC) is by far the most common solid renal mass in adults (Fig. 36.51). On US, 50% are hyperechoic compared to renal parenchyma, 30% are isoechoic, 10% are hypoechoic, 5% to 10% are predominantly cystic, and 20% to 30% have coarse, punctate, central calcification. Highly echogenic RCC may be confused with angiomyolipoma (AML), although RCC tends to be more heterogeneous and may have cystic components. CT or MR may be needed to demonstrate fat in the tumor. Isoechoic tumors are detected when they distort the renal contour. Tumors become cystic because of necrosis and internal hemorrhage. Doppler demonstration of internal vascularity is strong evidence of RCC.

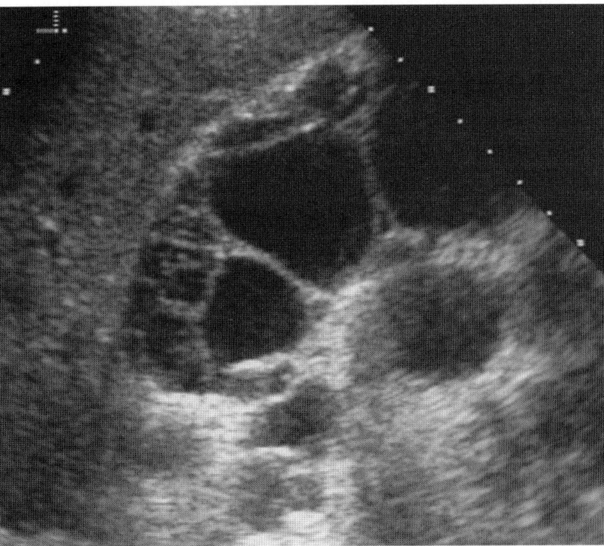

FIGURE 36.48. **Autosomal Dominant Polycystic Disease.** The kidney of a 57-year-old patient with a family history of cystic renal disease shows replacement of the renal parenchyma with innumerable cysts of varying size. Both kidneys were greatly enlarged.

With detection of a solid renal mass, the US examination should be extended to detect tumor invasion of the renal vein and IVC (Fig. 36.52). Signs of tumor thrombus include: echogenic mass in vein, enlarged vein, enlarged collateral vein, lack of or displacement of venous flow on color Doppler, and arterial Doppler signal within the vein caused by tumor neovascularity.

Angiomyolipoma. The classic US appearance of AML, seen in 80% of cases, is a uniformly hyperechoic renal mass with sharp borders (Fig. 36.53). The echogenicity of the mass is at least equal to that of renal sinus fat. Tumors

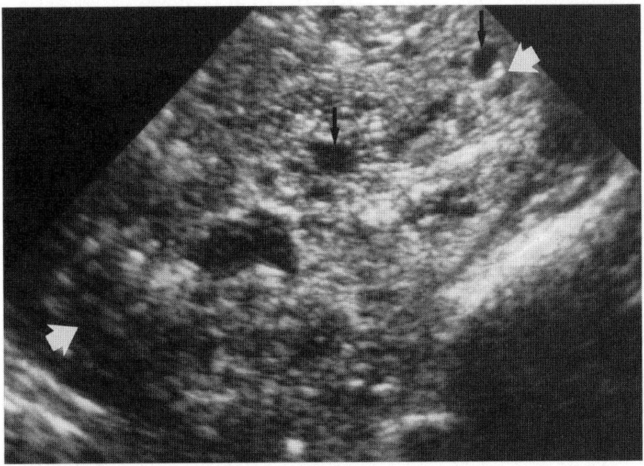

FIGURE 36.49. **Autosomal Recessive Polycystic Disease.** The kidney (between *white arrows*) of a 5-year-old with impaired renal and hepatic function shows mottled increased echogenicity and several small parenchymal cysts (*black arrows*).

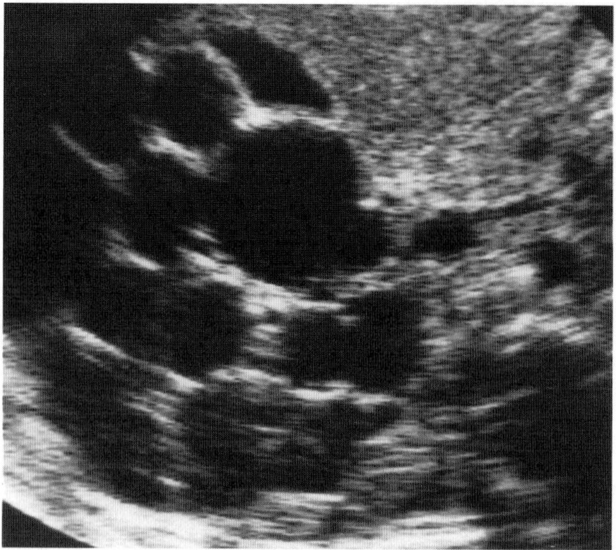

FIGURE 36.50. **Multicystic Dysplastic Kidney.** The right kidney is totally replaced by cysts of varying size, in a classic appearance of multicystic dysplastic kidney. The left kidney appeared normal. A radionuclide scan demonstrated absent function on the right and normal function on the left.

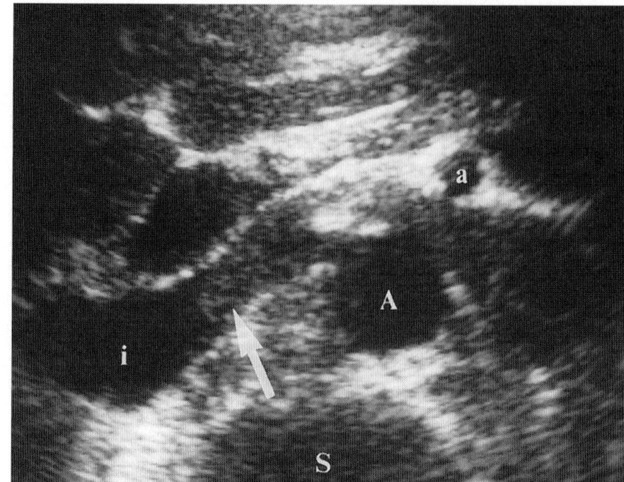

FIGURE 36.52. **Extension of Renal Cell Carcinoma into Renal Vein.** Transverse image reveals an enlarged left renal vein, with intraluminal soft tissue (*arrow*) extending to its junction with the inferior vena cava (i) in patient with renal cell carcinoma in the left kidney. A, aorta; a, superior mesenteric artery; S, spine.

that lack substantial fat are often indistinguishable from other renal tumors. Weak acoustic shadowing in the absence of calcification is seen with AML but not with RCC. AML is typically hypervascular but rarely has any cystic components. Definitive diagnosis is made by CT or MR demonstration of fat within the tumor. Calcification in the tumor is extremely rare.

Transitional cell carcinoma (TCC) is easy to overlook on US examination. Tumors may be small, infiltrative, or stenosing. A solid mass within or arising from the central renal sinus is suspicious (Fig. 36.54). US is best used to differentiate a solid mass in the renal sinus from a peripelvic cyst. Focal hydronephrosis may be caused by a small TCC, or TCC may appear as a soft tissue nodule within a dilated pelvis.

Lymphoma typically produces multiple hypoechoic masses, each of which has a uniform pattern of fine, low-level echoes that reflect the homogeneous cellular structure. Doppler demonstration of internal vessels differentiates lymphoma from cysts containing echogenic fluid.

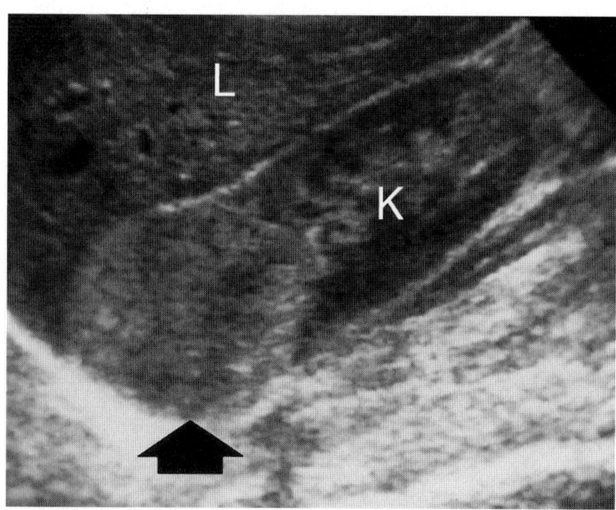

FIGURE 36.51. **Renal Cell Carcinoma.** An US image in the long axis of the right kidney (K) reveals a solid, hyperechoic mass (*arrow*) at the upper pole. L, liver.

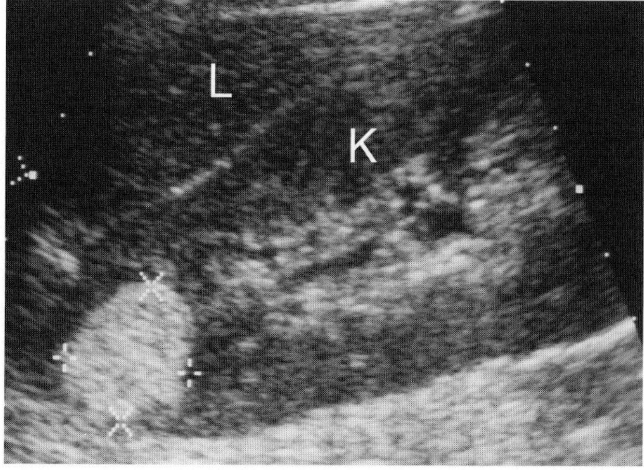

FIGURE 36.53. **Angiomyolipoma.** An US image through the long axis of the right kidney (K) demonstrates a well-defined, uniformly hyperechoic tumor (between *calipers*) in the upper pole. This appearance is strongly suggestive of angiomyolipoma. L, liver.

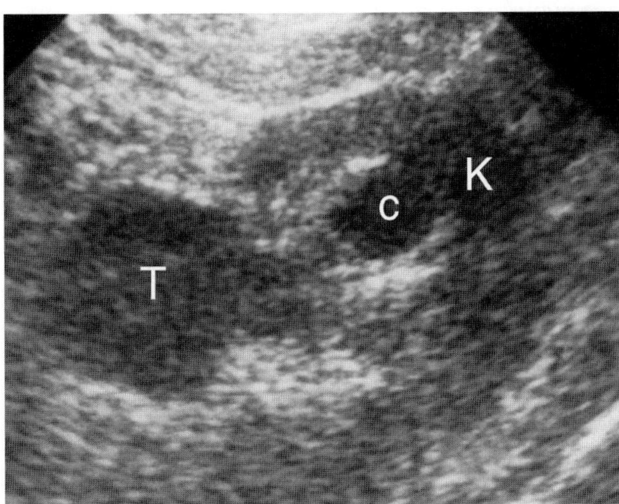

FIGURE 36.54. **Transitional Cell Carcinoma.** An US image of the left kidney (K) in the transverse plane shows the tumor (T) as a hypoechoic mass. The echogenicity of the mass is only slightly greater than that of a dilated calix (c).

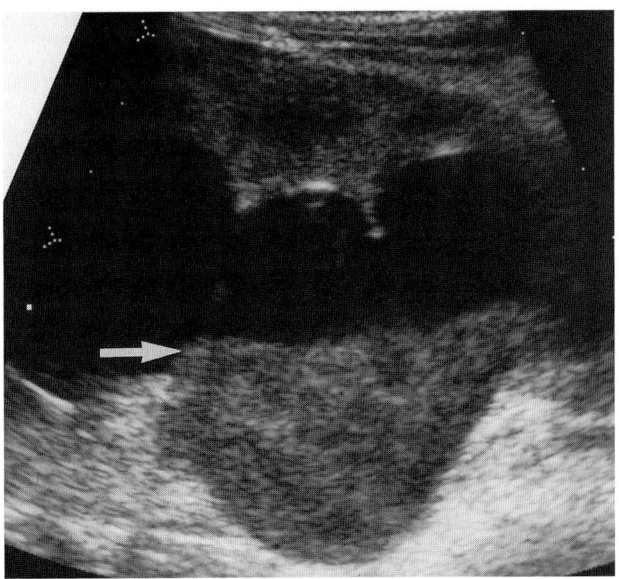

FIGURE 36.56. **Pyonephrosis.** US view of the left kidney with the patient in the right lateral decubitus position reveals layering pus (*arrow*) in a dilated, obstructed collecting system.

Growth patterns include single dominant mass, multiple masses, diffuse infiltration causing renal enlargement, and invasion of the renal sinus from confluent retroperitoneal adenopathy.

Acute pyelonephritis frequently produces no US abnormalities. Severe cases alter the echogenicity of the renal parenchyma owing to edema, local inflammation, and focal bleeding (Fig. 36.55). Masslike areas of focal inflammation have been called "lobar nephronia," "focal nephritis," and a variety of other names that mostly cause confusion. These findings should be viewed as US evidence of severe pyelonephritis and probably nothing more. US is performed in patients with urinary tract infection to detect hydronephrosis, renal abscess, or perirenal abscess. Color flow Doppler increases the sensitivity of US examination by demonstrating edematous areas of pyelonephritis as foci of decreased parenchymal blood flow. This finding correlates with the foci of decreased enhancement that are characteristic of pyelonephritis on CT.

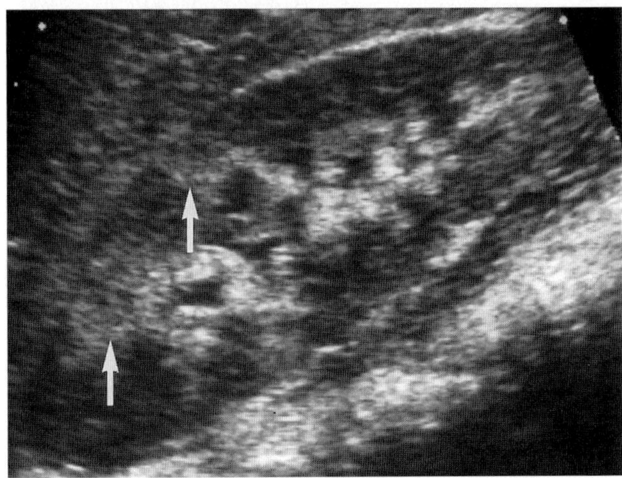

FIGURE 36.55. **Acute Pyelonephritis.** Focal areas of increased echogenicity (*arrows*) indicate inflammation and hemorrhage caused by acute bacterial infection.

Pyonephrosis refers to infection within a dilated and obstructed renal collecting system. Echogenic debris, often with a shifting urine–debris level (Fig. 36.56), is seen within a dilated pelvicaliceal system in an infected patient. Gas in the collecting system produces shifting echogenic foci with shadowing and reverberation artifact. About 10% of cases of pyonephrosis are indistinguishable from uncomplicated hydronephrosis, so guided aspiration for diagnosis is indicated in clinically suspicious cases. Pyonephrosis is an indication for urgent percutaneous or surgical drainage.

Renal abscess appears as a poorly marginated intrarenal cystic mass containing echogenic fluid (Fig. 36.57). The appearance may change rapidly over a few days with extension of infection into and beyond the perirenal space. Small abscesses may be effectively treated with antibiotics, but larger abscesses (>2 cm) may require percutaneous drainage. Extensive perirenal abscess usually requires surgical drainage.

Renal tuberculosis is characterized by the multiplicity of findings present, including parenchymal scarring, calcification, intraparenchymal cavities with echogenic contents, and dilated calices without accompanying dilatation of the renal pelvis. US findings are seldom specific.

Xanthogranulomatous pyelonephritis is suggested by US demonstration of a shadowing stone in the renal

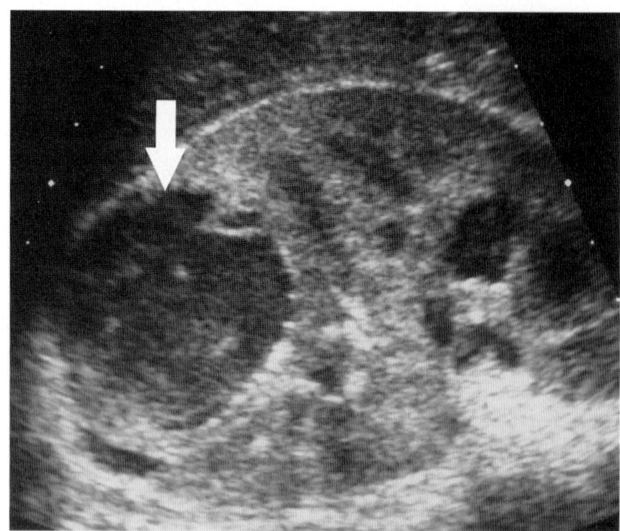

FIGURE 36.57. **Renal Abscess.** A cystic mass (*arrow*) in the upper pole of the kidney contains heterogeneous echogenic fluid. US-guided aspiration yielded coliform bacteria.

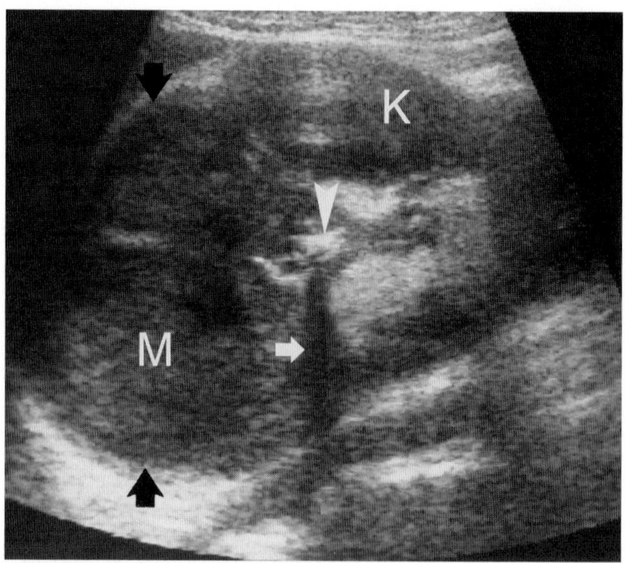

FIGURE 36.58. **Xanthogranulomatous Pyelonephritis.** Long-axis US of the right kidney (K) reveals a hypoechoic mass (M, between *black arrows*) enlarging the upper pole. An obstructing stone (*arrowhead*) casting an acoustic shadow (*white arrow*) is seen in the renal sinus. The kidney was chronically infected and was surgically removed, confirming xanthogranulomatous pyelonephritis.

pelvis, dilated collecting structures commonly filled with echogenic debris, masslike distortion and enlargement of the kidney, and extension of disease into the perirenal space (Fig. 36.58). The renal parenchyma is frequency hypoechoic, reflecting edema and inflammation.

Reflux nephropathy is suggested by US findings of focal renal parenchyma thinning with an underlying echogenic scar extending from the renal sinus toward the periphery, or a dilated calix beneath the parenchymal thinning. The process is distinctly focal, with the remainder of the kidney usually appearing normal.

Renal artery stenosis may be a difficult US diagnosis to make because of limited visualization of the renal arteries in large patients and the frequency of accessory renal arteries that may be stenosed and cause hypertension but are not detected with US (16). Significant renal artery stenosis is evidenced by parvus-tardus spectral waveforms in intrarenal arteries (Fig. 36.59) (see Chapter 40). Normal intrarenal artery spectral waveforms demonstrate a nearly vertical early systolic upstroke. Parvus-tardus waveforms show a diminished peak systolic velocity (parvus) and a delayed time to peak systole (tardus). Systolic acceleration values under 300 cm/s^2 are abnormal. Additional signs of renal artery stenosis are main renal artery peak systolic velocity greater than 100 cm/s and renal artery to aortic peak systolic velocity ratio of greater than 3.5.

Renal vein thrombosis occurs in clinical settings of nephrotic syndrome, dehydration, trauma, coagulopathy, or thrombosis of the IVC. Acute complete thrombosis causes an enlarged, hypoechoic, edematous kidney without detectable blood flow in the renal vein by spectral or color Doppler. Waveforms in the renal artery are diminished in velocity and show a high resistance pattern, with diminished diastolic forward flow. Incomplete venous thrombosis usually does not enlarge the kidney. Clot may be seen in the renal vein, with flow on color Doppler diverted around the thrombus. Enlarged venous collateral vessels may be visualized.

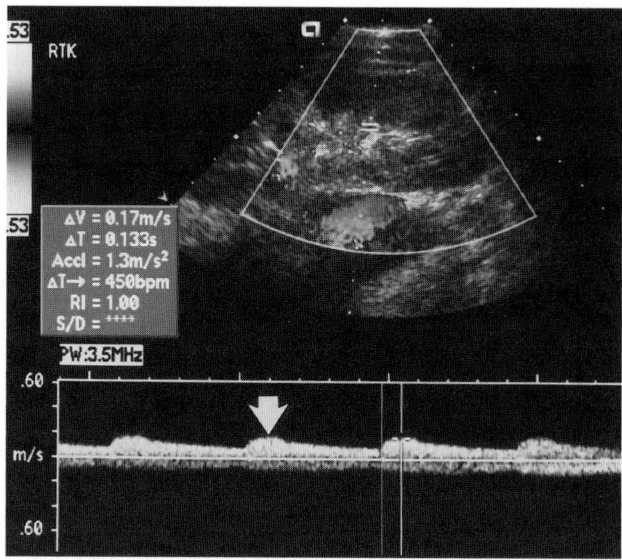

FIGURE 36.59. **Renal Artery Stenosis.** Doppler spectrum obtained from an intrarenal artery reveals tardus-parvus waveform with delayed and stunted peak systolic velocities (*arrow*).

Renal transplant evaluation includes detailed US imaging and Doppler examination (17). Visualization of small fluid-filled collecting structures is common and normal. Serial US examinations, or radionuclide renograms, are often needed to confirm that hydronephrosis is caused by obstruction. Perirenal fluid collections are common and include: hematoma, seroma, urinoma, lymphocele, and abscess. US-guided aspiration is used to obtain fluid for laboratory differentiation. Doppler US is used to visualize and confirm patency of the entire length of the renal artery and vein. Doppler waveforms and resistive indices are not useful in differentiating acute rejection from acute tubular necrosis from acute drug reaction in the setting of acute transplant dysfunction. US-guided parenchymal biopsy is commonly used to make the diagnosis histologically.

REFERENCES

1. Brant WE. Ultrasound. Philadelphia: Lippincott Williams & Wilkins, 2001.
2. Hanbidge AE, Lynch D, Wilson SR. Ultrasound of the peritoneum. Radiographics 2003;23:663–684.
3. Brant WE. Liver. In: Brant WE, ed. The Core Curriculum: Ultrasound. Philadelphia: Lippincott Williams & Wilkins, 2001:35–54.
4. Tchelepi H, Ralls P, Radin R, Grant E. Sonography of diffuse liver disease. J Ultrasound Med 2002;21:1023–1032.
5. Tchelepi H, Ralls P. Ultrasound of focal liver masses. Ultrasound Q 2004;20:155–169.
6. Wachsberg RH. Doppler ultrasound evaluation of transjugular intrahepatic portosystemic shunt function: pitfalls and artifacts. Ultrasound Q 2003;19:139–148.
7. Crossin JD, Muraldi D, Wilson SR. US of liver transplants: normal and abnormal. Radiographics 2003;23:1093–1114.
8. Parulekar SG. Transabdominal sonography of bile ducts. Ultrasound Q 2002;18:187–202.
9. Gore RM, Yaghmai V, Newmark GM, et al. Imaging benign and malignant disease of the gallbladder. Radiol Clin North Am 2002;40:1307–1323.
10. Levy AD, Murkata LA, Rohrmann CA Jr. Gallbladder carcinoma: radiologic-pathologic correlation. Radiographics 2001;21:295–314.
11. Levy AD, Murakata LA, Abbott RM, Rohrmann CA Jr. Benign tumors and tumorlike lesions of the gallbladder and extrahepatic bile ducts: radiologic-pathologic correlation. Radiographics 2002;22: 387–413.
12. Brant WE, Jain KA. Current imaging of the spleen. Radiologist 1996;3:185–192.
13. Demos TC, Posniak HV, Harmath C, Olson MC, Aranha G. Cystic lesions of the pancreas. AJR Am J Roentgenol 2002;179:1375–1388.
14. Brant WE. Renal, bladder, and adrenal ultrasound. In: Brant WE, ed. The Core Curriculum: Ultrasound. Philadelphia: Lippincott Williams & Wilkins, 2001:103–151.
15. Durr-e-Sabih, Khan AN, Craig M, Worrall JA. Sonographic mimics of renal calculi. J Ultrasound Med 2004;23:1361–1367.
16. Lavoipierre AM, Dowling RJ, Little AF. Ultrasound of the renal vasculature. Ultrasound Q 2000;16:123–132.
17. Baxter GM. Imaging in renal transplantation. Ultrasound Q 2003; 19:123–138.

Chapter 37

Genital Tract and Bladder Ultrasound

William E. Brant

Female Genital Tract
Uterus
Ovaries and Adnexa

Male Genital Tract
Testes and Scrotum
Prostate

Bladder

FEMALE GENITAL TRACT

US is the primary imaging modality for evaluation of the female genital tract and pelvis (1). US is used as an adjunct to physical examination to confirm the presence of a pelvic mass and to evaluate its size, contour, and character; determine the organ of origin; evaluate for involvement of other organs; and detect the presence of ascites, hydronephrosis, and metastases. The US examination is initiated transabdominally using the distended urinary bladder as a window to the pelvis. The transvaginal approach is used to improve visualization of all lesions and to overcome the limitations of limited bladder filling and obesity. Color flow US is used to identify pelvic blood vessels, identify vascular lesions of the pelvis, and detect neovascularity of tumors. Saline infusion sonohysterography (SHG) utilizes real-time US imaging of the uterus during injection of the uterine cavity with sterile saline to detect and characterize abnormalities of the uterus and endometrium (2).

Uterus

Normal US Anatomy. The uterus in the postpubertal woman is smoothly contoured and pear-shaped (Fig. 37.1). The myometrium is uniformly midlevel in echogenicity, with the endometrium distinctly more echogenic. The thickness of the endometrial echo varies with menstrual state. The innermost myometrium, called the *junctional zone,* may appear as a thin hypoechoic layer adjacent to the echogenic endometrial stripe. Maximum normal uterine dimensions in the adult woman are 9 cm in length, 6 cm in width, and 4 cm in anteroposterior diameter. Following menopause, the uterus atrophies to approximately $6 \times 2 \times 2$ cm. The prepubertal infantile uterus is cigar-shaped. The cervix makes up about one third the length of the uterus in the adult woman and about two thirds of the length of the uterus in the prepubertal girl. Normal uterine positions in the pelvis include tilted forward (anteverted; this is the most common), tilted backward toward the sacrum (retroverted), or folded anteriorly (anteflexed) or posteriorly (retroflexed) (Fig. 37.2). The normal uterus may also be tilted right or left toward the pelvic side walls. The position of the uterus is altered by the degree of bladder filling and the presence of pelvic masses. The retroverted or retroflexed uterus appears more globular on transabdominal scanning. The normal vagina appears as a flattened muscular tube with echogenic mucosa.

The US examination must always be correlated with the stage of the menstrual cycle, which affects the normal brightness and thickness of the endometrium (Fig. 37.1). At the end of menstruation, the endometrium is discrete and thin (2 to 3 mm). During the *proliferative phase,* the endometrium assumes a three-layer appearance. The basal endometrium, adjacent to the junctional zone myometrium, remains echogenic, whereas the functional endometrium, which will thicken and eventually slough with menstruation, is relatively hypoechoic during the first half of the menstrual cycle. The three layers are formed by the anterior and posterior basal endometrium and the echogenic stripe that marks the uterine cavity. Measurement of endometrial thickness is defined by the added thickness of the anterior and posterior endometrium. Any fluid or blood within the uterine cavity is excluded. At midcycle, the endometrium normally measures 8 to 10 mm in double-layer thickness. From ovulation to menstruation, through the *secretory phase,* the endometrium

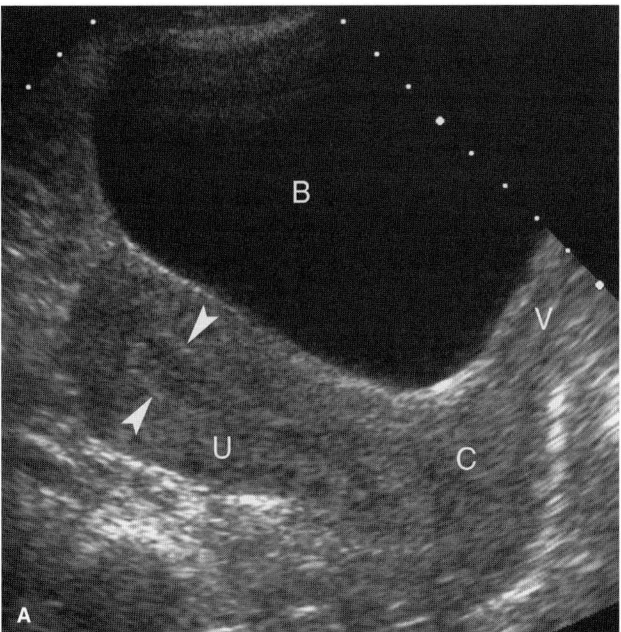

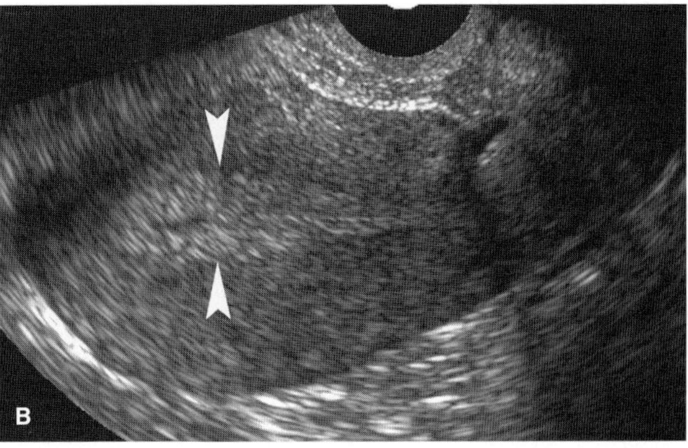

FIGURE 37.1. **Normal Uterus. A.** Transabdominal sagittal plane image through the urine-filled bladder (B) demonstrates the smooth contour and pear shape of the normal uterus (U). The endometrium (between *arrowheads*) is more echogenic than the surrounding myometrium. This image demonstrates the typical three-layer appearance of proliferative phase endometrium. The cervix (C) protrudes into the upper vagina (V) at the intersection between the long axis of the uterus and the axis of the vagina. **B.** Transvaginal sagittal-plane image of the uterus demonstrates the improved resolution of this technique. The endometrium (between *arrowheads*) is more sharply defined and the myometrium is more clearly evaluated. This image demonstrates the typical uniformly echogenic appearance of secretory phase endometrium.

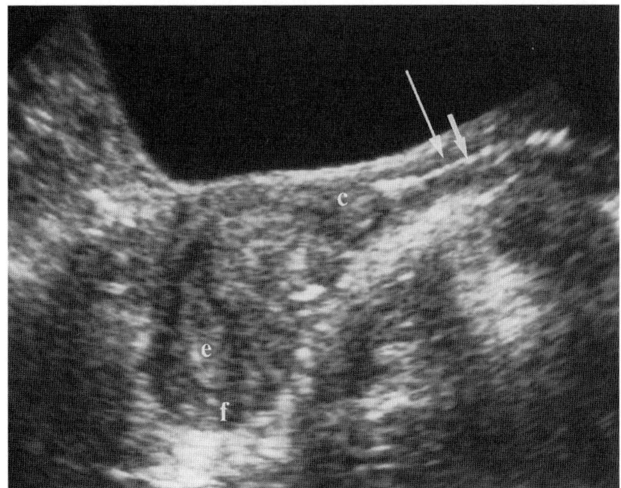

FIGURE 37.2. **Retroflexed Uterus.** The uterus is flexed with the fundus (f) directed posteriorly toward the sacrum on this sagittal midline transbladder image. A retroflexed or retroverted uterus may be mistaken for a pelvic mass on both physical examination and US. The vagina is well seen with its hypoechoic muscular walls (*long arrow*) and echogenic mucosa (*short arrow*). c, cervix; e, endometrium.

progressively thickens up to 14 mm and becomes more uniformly echogenic. The junctional zone myometrium appears as a hypoechoic halo surrounding the bright endometrium. In the normal postmenopausal woman, the echogenic endometrium does not exceed 5 to 7 mm in thickness. During the normal fertile years, pregnancy must always be considered in evaluation of the female genital tract. Abnormalities of the first trimester of pregnancy are reviewed in Chapter 38.

Congenital anomalies are best defined by correlation of physical examination, US or MR imaging, and hysterosalpingography. US may define two uterine horns, two distinct endometrial cavities, and an abnormal shape of the uterus. The kidneys should be examined for associated anomalies, such as renal agenesis.

Leiomyomas (fibroids) are exceedingly common benign smooth muscle tumors of the myometrium that develop in women of all ages. They are suspected when the uterus is enlarged or altered in contour. Leiomyomas are virtually always multiple. They may be completely within the myometrium, subserosal, or submucosal. Leiomyomas may also be pedunculated and predominantly extrauterine, simulating an adnexal mass. Color flow US demonstration of vascular supply contiguous with the myometrium

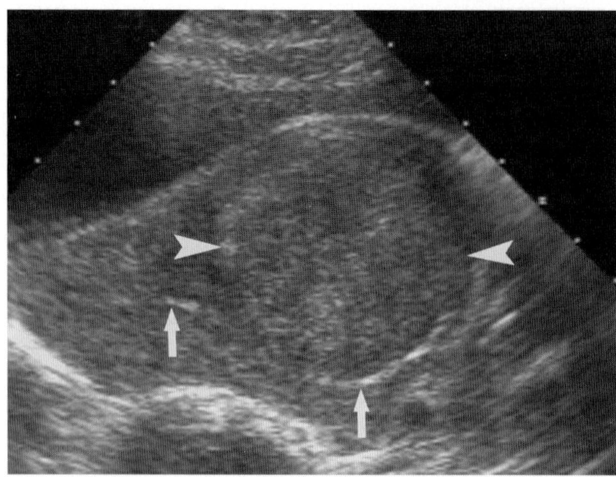

FIGURE 37.3. **Leiomyoma.** Transvaginal image of the uterus shows a hypoechoic leiomyoma (between *arrowheads*) displacing the endometrium (*arrows*) and impinging on the uterine cavity.

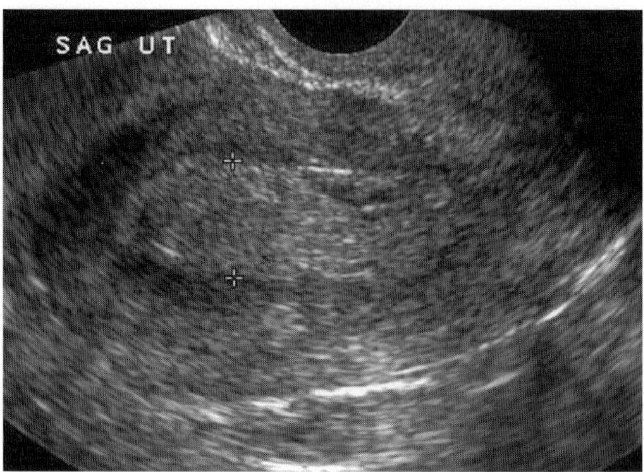

FIGURE 37.4. **Endometrial Carcinoma.** Transvaginal US reveals a thickened endometrium measured at 14 mm between calipers in a postmenopausal woman with vaginal bleeding. Biopsy confirmed endometrial carcinoma.

is definitive in confirming the uterine origin of these exophytic leiomyomas. Uncomplicated leiomyomas may be isoechoic, hypoechoic, or hyperechoic compared to normal myometrium. Leiomyomas may undergo atrophy, internal hemorrhage, cystic degeneration, fibrosis, and calcification. A "popcorn" pattern of calcification is characteristic and definitive on plain film radiographs. On US they are typically heterogeneous and vary from hypoechoic (Fig. 37.3) to hyperechoic, sometimes causing acoustic shadowing. No imaging modality can reliably differentiate a benign leiomyoma from the rare leiomyosarcoma. Retroposition of the uterus and uterine anomalies, such as a bicornuate uterus, must be differentiated from leiomyoma. Leiomyomas may cause menorrhagia or vaginal bleeding unrelated to menstrual cycles. Exophytic tumors may torse and may be a cause of acute pelvic pain. The tumors are responsive to female hormones and commonly accelerate in growth during pregnancy. Correspondingly, they involute with menopause.

Arcuate artery calcifications are seen as discrete echogenic foci in the outer third of the myometrium of postmenopausal women. They are seen more commonly in women who are diabetic or hypertensive.

Thickened Endometrium. The thickness of the endometrium must always be correlated with age, menstrual history, and stage of the menstrual cycle (3). The full thickness of the echogenic endometrium, including both anterior and posterior endometrium, is measured perpendicular to the long axis of the uterus. In women with active menstrual cycles, the endometrial stripe may measure up to 14 mm during the secretory phase. However, in postmenopausal women the endometrium normally does not exceed 5 mm in thickness. Hormone replacement therapy thickens the endometrium in postmenopausal women by 1 to 2 mm. In women with abnormal vaginal bleeding, US demonstration of abnormal endometrial thickness is an indication for endometrial biopsy. A normal endometrial thickness measurement averts the need for biopsy. In a postmenopausal woman, endometrial thickness <5 mm is indicative of endometrial atrophy. The causes of thickening of the endometrium include the following:

1. *Endometrial carcinoma.* Thickness of the stripe may be uneven, with an ill-defined irregular contour. Less commonly, the cancer appears as a heterogeneous focal mass. This cancer is most common in women over age 50. Postmenopausal vaginal bleeding is a common presentation (Fig. 37.4).
2. *Endometrial hyperplasia* is caused by unopposed or prolonged estrogen stimulation and is most common in perimenopausal and postmenopausal women. The endometrium is thickened and inhomogeneous, with small cysts commonly present. Only biopsy can differentiate endometrial hyperplasia from endometrial cancer.
3. *Endometrial polyps* result from focal hyperplasia or adenomatous neoplasia of the endometrium. They are most common between ages 30 and 60. Malignant transformation is reported in 1% to 4% of cases. About 20% are multiple. US demonstrates a focal echogenic polypoid mass in the endometrium or diffuse endometrial thickening. SHG is helpful in demonstrating the polypoid nature of the endometrial mass (Fig. 37.5).
4. *Other* less common causes include endometritis, tamoxifen therapy, incomplete abortion, metastatic carcinoma, and submucosal leiomyoma. The precise diagnosis is determined by endometrial biopsy. Pregnancy must never be forgotten as a possibility.

Endometrial atrophy is a normal finding in a postmenopausal women. However, it is also the most common

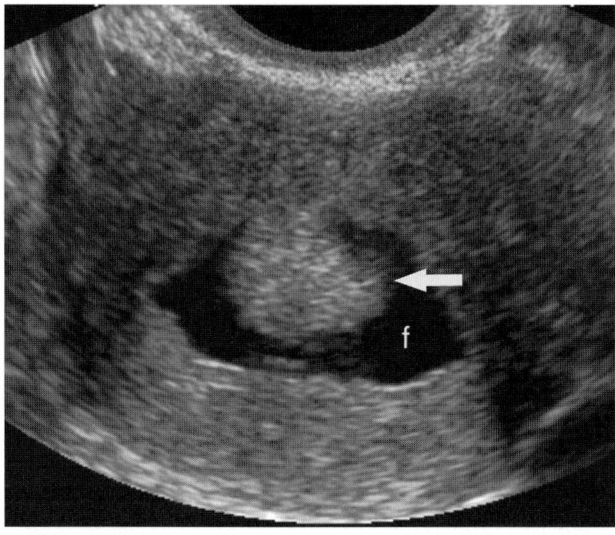

FIGURE 37.5. **Endometrial Polyp.** Transvaginal image in transverse plane taken during a sonohysterography clearly reveals the polypoid nature of the endometrial mass (*arrow*). Injected sterile saline fluid (f) distends the uterine cavity.

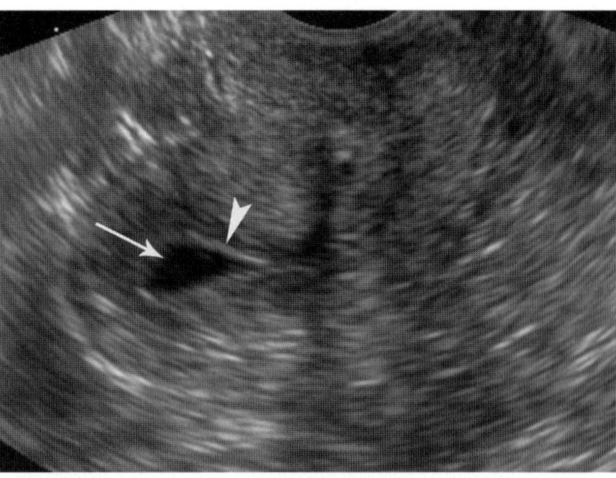

FIGURE 37.7. **Fluid in the Endometrial Cavity.** Anechoic fluid (*arrow*) is evident within the uterine cavity on this transvaginal US image of the uterus of a 75-year-old woman. The endometrium (*arrowhead*) is thin and normal. This patient has atrophic cervical stenosis.

cause of postmenopausal bleeding. US demonstrates a uniformly thin endometrium, with double-layer thickness less than 5 mm (Fig. 37.6).

Fluid in the endometrial cavity may be blood, mucus, or purulent material. *Hematometra* refers to blood in the endometrial cavity and *hematocolpos* describes blood filling the vagina. In postmenopausal women, causes of fluid in the uterine cavity include cervical stenosis (Fig. 37.7), cervical carcinoma, endometrial carcinoma, endometrial polyps, and pyometrium. In premenopausal women, causes include congenital obstruction caused by an imperforate hymen, vaginal septum, vaginal or cervical atresia; acquired cervical obstruction caused by instrumentation, radiation, or carcinoma; menorrhagia; and pregnancy.

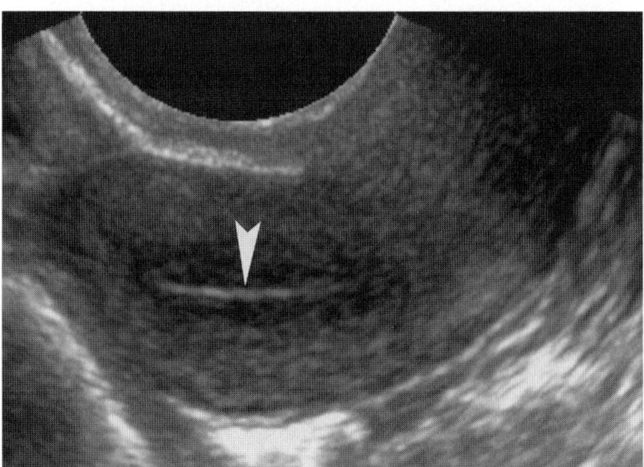

FIGURE 37.6. **Endometrial Atrophy.** Transvaginal sonogram in longitudinal plane reveals a very thin endometrium (*arrowhead*) measuring only 2 mm in a postmenopausal woman with vaginal bleeding. This is diagnostic of endometrial atrophy as the source of her bleeding. No biopsy is necessary.

Adenomyosis is the condition of diffuse or focal invasion of the myometrium by benign endometrium ("internal endometriosis"). It is found commonly in multiparous women over age 30. The diffuse form is most common, with islands of endometrium scattered throughout the myometrium. The localized form results in a mass—an adenomyoma—within the myometrium. A broad spectrum of sonographic appearance is related to the distribution of ectopic endometrium, the presence and number of cysts within the ectopic endometrium, and the amount of associated myometrial hypertrophy (4). The most common US findings are: (*1*) diffuse abnormal hypoechoic or heterogeneous echotexture of the myometrium (Fig. 37.8), (*2*) poor definition or nodularity of the junction between endometrium and myometrium, (*3*) subendometrial echogenic nodules, (*4*) subendometrial myometrial cysts (1 to 5 mm), and (*5*) subendometrial hypoechoic linear striations (4). The uterus is usually enlarged (5). Leiomyomas are commonly present as well, frequently masking the coexistence of adenomyosis. MR provides the best detection and characterization of adenomyosis.

Nabothian cysts result from obstruction of the ducts of the mucus-secreting glands of the epithelial lining of the cervix and are commonly visualized on transvaginal US. They are anechoic and frequently multiple and vary in size, from 2 to 3 mm up to 4 cm.

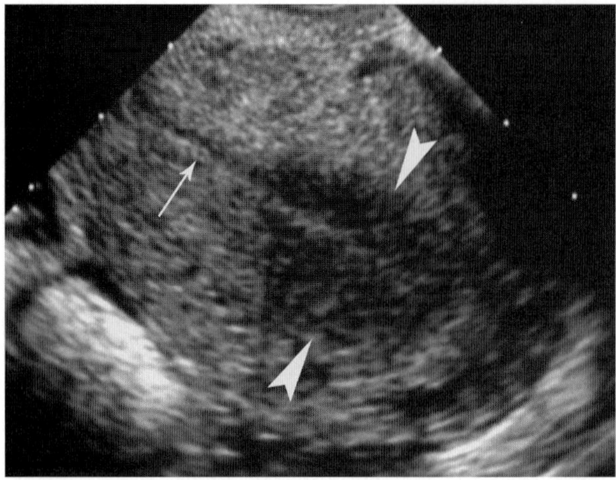

FIGURE 37.8. **Adenomyosis.** The junctional zone myometrium is irregularly thickened (*arrowheads*), poorly marginated, and markedly hypoechoic on this transvaginal US image in a woman with abnormal vaginal bleeding and pelvic pain. MR and pathology at hysterectomy confirmed adenomyosis.

Ovaries and Adnexa

Normal US Anatomy. The term *adnexa* refers to the ovaries, fallopian tubes, broad ligament, and ovarian and uterine vessels, all of which may be involved in pathologic conditions. US demonstrates the ovaries as oval soft tissue structures with multiple small cystic follicles. The ovaries average 4 × 3 × 2 cm in size, with a maximum of 5 cm in any one dimension. The maximum ovarian volume for an adult woman, calculated by the standard formula (length × width × height × 0.523), is 22 mL. The ovaries show characteristic morphologic changes with the menstrual cycle (Fig. 37.9). Following menstruation, the ovaries are at their smallest, with the follicles measuring less than 5 mm. During the estrogen phase, follicles enlarge to 10 to 15 mm, with one dominant follicle attaining 20 to 25 mm by midcycle. Rupture of the dominant follicle releases the ovum, and the *corpus luteum* forms at the site of the dominant follicle. Ovulation releases fluid, which pools in the cul-de-sac. All remaining follicles normally involute following ovulation. Hemorrhage into the corpus luteum or any follicle produces a *hemorrhagic functional cyst.* The ovaries vary widely in location but usually lie in a shallow ovarian fossa in the angle between the external iliac vessels anteriorly and the ureter posteriorly with the fallopian tubes draped over and around them. The fallopian tubes are not visualized unless enlarged; however, the broad ligament is clearly seen when it is outlined by fluid in the pelvis. Transvaginal US is the most effective way to evaluate the ovaries. *Postmenopausal ovaries* are atrophic, lack follicles, and are often difficult to visualize. Mean ovarian volume decreases from 8 mL at age 40 to 44 to less than 1.0 mL at age 70. Maximum ovarian volume in a postmenopausal woman is 6 mL. Focal *calcifications* in otherwise normal-appearing ovaries are a common and benign finding (6).

Functional ovarian cysts are the most common ovarian masses (7). Small cysts, up to 2.5 cm, should generally be considered to be normal follicles. Pathologic *follicular cysts* up to 20 cm result from excessive accumulation of fluid or internal hemorrhage. They basically represent follicles that fail to regress. *Corpus luteal cysts* result from hemorrhage into a physiologic corpus luteum. Functional cysts may rupture or undergo torsion. Diagnosis is made by the demonstration of a round, smooth, usually unilocular

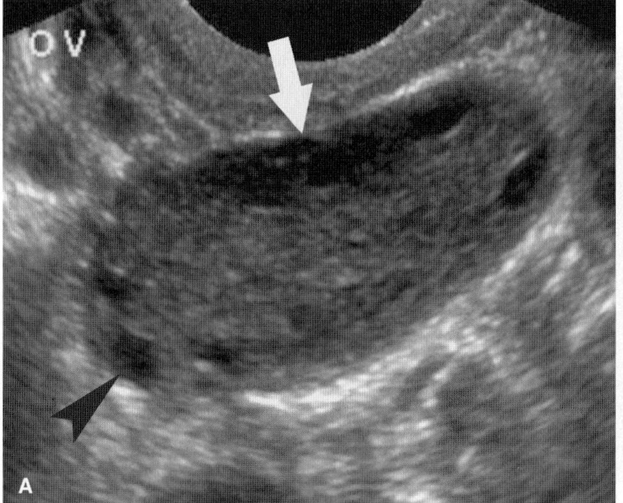

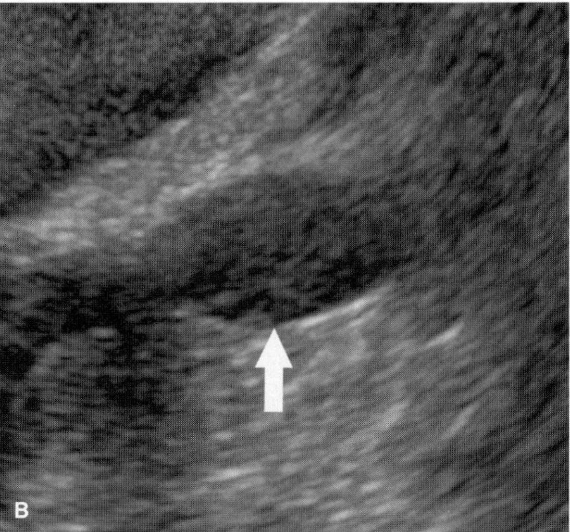

FIGURE 37.9. **Normal Ovaries.** Transvaginal US shows normal ovaries (*arrows*) in a woman of childbearing age **(A)** and in a postmenopausal woman **(B).** Ovaries in the premenopausal woman are larger and demonstrate follicles (*arrows*), which are landmarks for identification of the ovary. Ovaries in postmenopausal women are smaller and lack follicles.

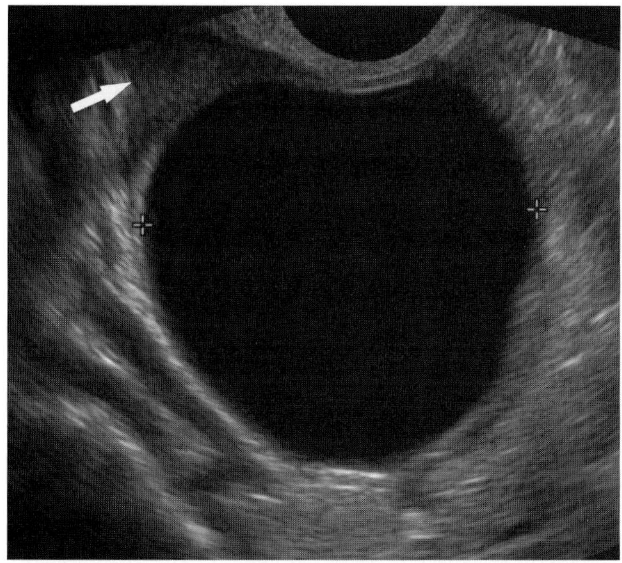

FIGURE 37.10. **Functional Ovarian Cyst.** Transvaginal US demonstrates a well-defined, thin-walled, anechoic ovarian cyst (between *calipers*) in a 36-year-old woman. A small portion of the ovary (*arrow*) is visible on this image. The appearance is typical of functional ovarian cyst. On follow-up US examination 10 weeks later, the cyst had resolved.

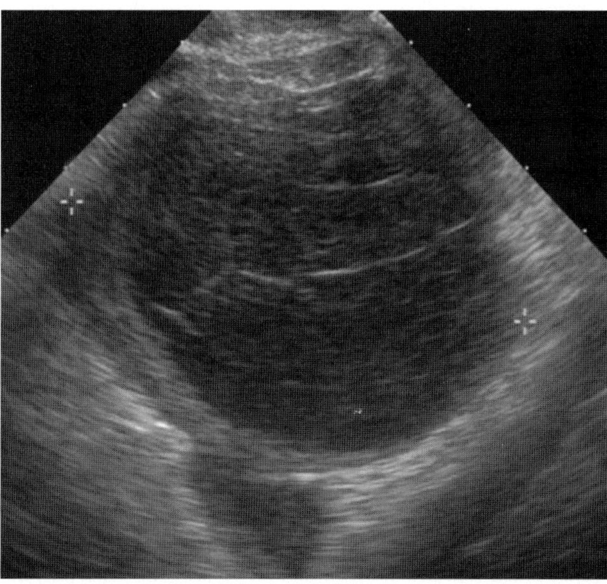

FIGURE 37.11. **Hemorrhagic Functional Cyst.** Transvaginal US shows the complex internal echogenicity of a hemorrhagic functional cyst (between *calipers*), which resolved on follow-up US examination 2 months later. The lacy internal appearance is characteristic of evolving hemorrhage.

ovarian cyst that resolves on follow-up examination after one or two menstrual cycles (Fig. 37.10).

Hemorrhagic ovarian cysts result from hemorrhage into a functional cyst. US shows a broad spectrum of findings (8): (*1*) the key finding is a cystic mass with internal echoes; (*2*) accentuated through-transmission reflects its cystic nature; (*3*) wall thickness is variable (between 2 and 20 mm); (*4*) blood flow in the wall is commonly prominent and does not differentiate hemorrhagic cyst from tumor; (*5*) internal echogenicity depends upon the physical state of the hemorrhage; (*6*) the cyst may appear solid, but color flow US shows no internal blood vessels; (7) clots adherent to the wall mimic neoplastic papillary projections but lack blood flow; (*8*) a weblike pattern of lacy internal echoes is characteristic (Fig. 37.11). Follow-up US usually shows complete resolution within two menstrual cycles.

Postmenopausal ovarian cysts are benign serous inclusion cysts found in 15% of asymptomatic postmenopausal women. US features are: (*1*) small size (<5 cm); (*2*) smooth, thin walls of uniform thickness (<3 mm); (*3*) anechoic fluid contents; and (*4*) absence of septations, nodules, or any soft tissue component. Over time, these cysts commonly change their size or disappear. Cysts with these characteristics are extremely unlikely to be malignant.

Pelvic inflammatory disease and endometriosis have a very similar appearance on all imaging studies and are considered together. Both cause masses that are predominantly cystic with complex internal fluid and adhesions that may encompass adjacent structures such as the ovary or bowel into a complex mass (9). Differentiation is made primarily by clinical history. *Pelvic inflammatory disease* refers to acute or chronic inflammation of the tubes, ovaries, and pelvic peritoneum (10). Patients are usually in their teens and 20s and present with pain, fever, and vaginal discharge. Causes of the disease include gonococcus, chlamydia, anaerobic bacteria, and tuberculosis. The disease runs a spectrum from endometritis to salpingitis to hydrosalpinx and tubo-ovarian abscess. US demonstrates a complex, ill-defined adnexal mass that often includes a dilated, pus-filled fallopian tube, swollen ovary, and adhesions to adjacent structures (Fig. 37.12). Fluid is usually present in the cul-de-sac. *Endometriosis* is the occurrence of aberrant endometrial tissue outside the uterus. Patients are commonly in their 20s and 30s and present with infertility, dysmenorrhea, and dyspareunia. Many cases involve tiny (1- to 2-mm) implants on the peritoneum that are not visualized by US. Transvaginal US distinctly improves detection. Larger deposits may form cystic masses filled with old, echogenic blood, a condition termed a "chocolate cyst" or endometrioma. *Endometriomas* appear as single or (characteristically) multiple adnexal masses with diffuse low-level internal echoes (Fig. 37.13). Hyperechoic foci in the wall of an internally echogenic cyst are characteristic (11).

Ovarian tumors, whether benign or malignant, are predominantly cystic. The tumors most commonly encountered are the epithelial tumors, serous and mucinous

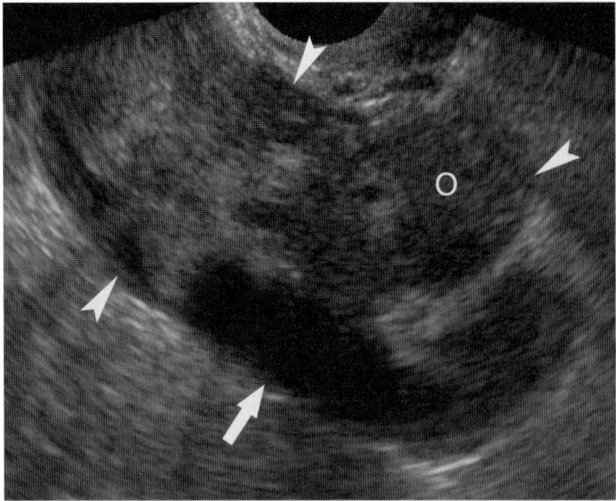

FIGURE 37.12. **Tubo-ovarian Abscess.** US of the adnexa reveals a complex mass (*arrowheads*) enveloping the ovary (O) and tube (*arrow*). Physical examination revealed marked pelvic tenderness with fixation of the pelvic organs.

cystadenoma and cystadenocarcinoma, and benign cystic teratoma. US is used to differentiate functional ovarian cysts from ovarian tumors and to provide findings used to assess the risk of malignancy.

Benign cystic teratomas, also called *dermoid cysts*, are benign germ cell tumors usually discovered in patients aged 10 to 30 years (12). They are the most common ovarian neoplasm and are bilateral in 15% to 25% of cases. Although predominantly cystic, the presence of mature ectodermal elements such as bone, teeth, and hair give them a complex and varied appearance. Most tumors can be diagnosed by US. Three appearances are most common. The most characteristic appearance is a cystic mass with complex fluid and a mural nodule (the "dermoid plug"). Fluid–fluid levels, representing fatty sebum floating on aqueous liquid, are common (Fig. 37.14). Another classic finding is the "tip of the iceberg" appearance of an echogenic mass that fades into acoustic shadowing because of sound absorption. The third common pattern appears as multiple fine echogenic strands representing hair within the cyst cavity. The diagnosis can often be confirmed by a plain radiograph that demonstrates teeth or bone. CT or MR confirmation of fat content is also definitive.

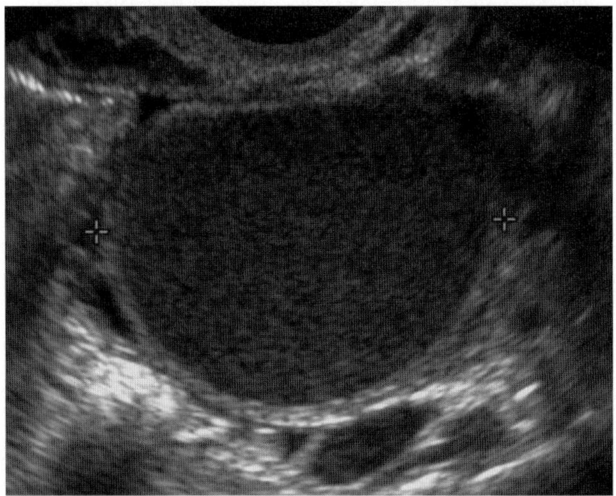

FIGURE 37.13. **Endometrioma.** Transvaginal sonogram shows an adnexal cyst (between *calipers*) with uniform thin wall and homogeneous fine internal echoes. This appearance may be seen with either a hemorrhagic ovarian cyst or an endometrioma. Endometrioma should be suspected if the cyst fails to resolve within 2 months.

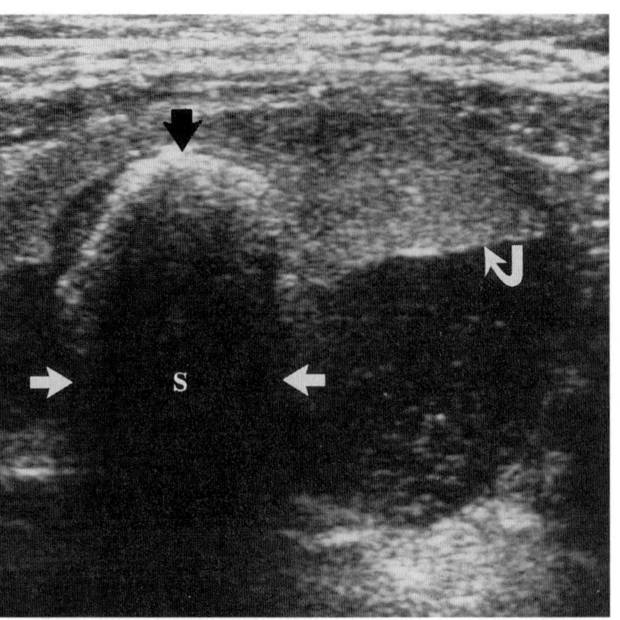

FIGURE 37.14. **Benign Cystic Teratoma.** US of a pelvic mass demonstrates a fluid–fluid layer (*curved arrow*) and a large area of calcification (*black arrow*) with acoustic shadowing (S, between *white arrows*). Surgery confirmed a benign cystic teratoma containing teeth (the calcified portion) along with fat and hair (the fluid–fluid layer).

Epithelial tumors arise from the epithelial covering of the ovary. As a group, they account for 65% to 75% of all ovarian neoplasms. Most present as predominantly cystic masses. Pathologic differentiation of benign and malignant forms is sometimes difficult, resulting in some being classified as "borderline" malignant or tumor of "low malignant potential." Bilateral tumors are common and more frequent with malignant types.

Serous cystadenoma and cystadenocarcinoma comprise 30% of all ovarian neoplasms and 40% of all ovarian malignancies. Serous cystadenomas are thin-walled, usually unilocular, cysts with anechoic fluid. Serous cystadenocarcinomas are multiloculated, with thick walls, thick septa, and papillary projections into fluid that may be echogenic.

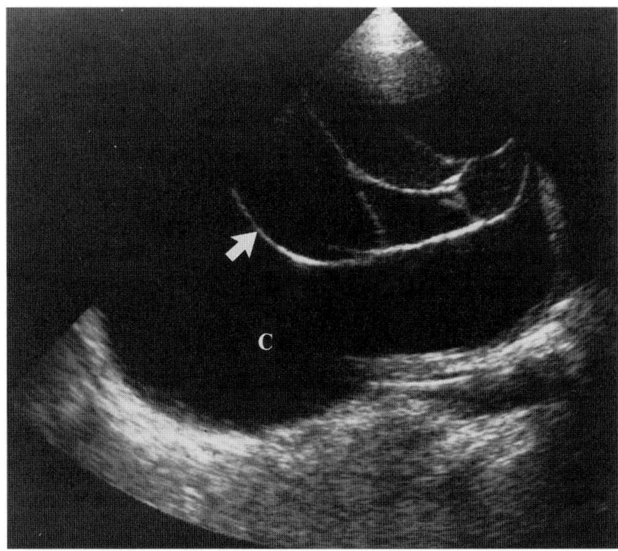

FIGURE 37.15. **Benign Mucinous Cystadenoma.** This ovarian tumor caused a huge mass, filling the pelvis and lower abdomen. US examination confirmed a cystic mass (C) with a network of fine septations (*arrow*). The absence of detectable solid components suggests a benign tumor.

Blood flow is usually documented within septa and papillary projections.

Mucinous cystadenoma and cystadenocarcinoma comprise 20% of ovarian neoplasms. About 85% are benign. Mucinous tumors may be huge, filling the pelvis and extending high into the abdomen. Most have multiple septations (Fig. 37.15) and contain fluid that is echogenic because of the presence of mucin. Rupture spreads mucin-secreting cells throughout the peritoneal cavity and may result in pseudomyxoma peritonei.

Endometrioid tumors are nearly always malignant. Most are cystic masses with papillary projections.

Other epithelial cell tumor types include clear cell carcinoma (unilocular cyst with a mural nodule); Brenner tumor (solid, benign); and undifferentiated epithelial tumor (aggressive, ill-defined, cystic or solid).

Germ cell tumors include the benign cystic teratoma previously described; struma ovarii, in which thyroid tissue predominates; dysgerminomas, which consist of undifferentiated germ cells; yolk sac (endodermal sinus) tumor; and immature teratoma. The latter tumors are malignant and predominantly solid with small areas of hemorrhage or necrosis.

Stromal tumors include Sertoli-Leydig cell tumors (which may cause masculinization and are malignant in 10% to 20% of cases), thecoma (which produces estrogen), and fibromas (which are associated with ascites and pleural effusions, i.e., Meigs syndrome). US reveals a solid hypoechoic mass that often causes striking sound attenuation. Pedunculated leiomyomas have a similar appearance. Physical connection to and vascular supply from the uterus differentiates leiomyomas from solid stromal tumors.

Metastases to the ovary occur most commonly with GI and breast carcinomas. A *Krukenberg* tumor is a metastasis to the ovary from a mucin-producing tumor of the GI tract. Most metastases to the ovary are bilateral and solid. Cystic metastases may be indistinguishable from a primary ovarian tumor.

Signs of Malignancy. Because most pelvic masses are discovered, or initially evaluated, by US, every effort should be made to assess the risk of malignancy (13,14). Transvaginal US aids substantially in the evaluation. The following signs correlate with an increased risk of malignancy (15):

1. Solid consistency: the more solid tissue present, the greater the risk of malignancy. Solid tissue includes thick walls, thick septations, papillary projections, and solid tumor mass (Fig. 37.16). Unilocular cysts or cysts with thin septations are likely to be benign. Thick-walled, multilocular masses with solid nodules are likely to be malignant. Echogenic solid masses, or portions of masses, that transmit sound poorly are likely to be malignant.
2. Size greater than 10 cm correlates with a 64% risk of malignancy in postmenopausal women. Masses under 5 cm are more likely to be benign.
3. Color flow US demonstration of blood vessels within papillary projections is evidence of neoplasm and provides differentiation from avascular blood clots adherent to the cyst wall. Vascularized papillary projections are more common with malignant neoplasms.
4. Color flow US demonstration of blood vessels within septations is strong evidence of neoplasm. Hemorrhagic functional cysts may be complex in appearance

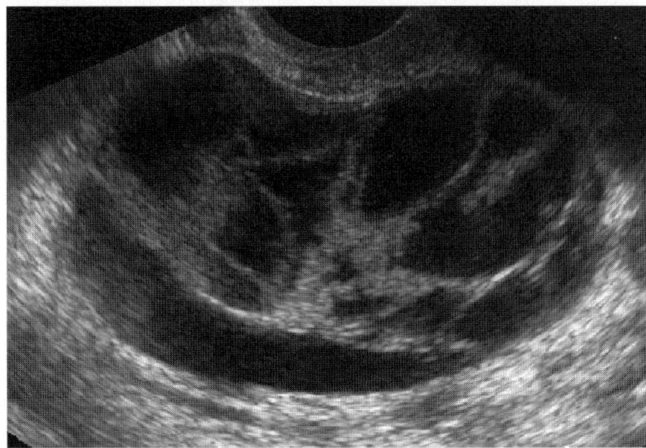

FIGURE 37.16. **Ovarian Carcinoma.** Transvaginal sonogram of an adnexal mass shows it to be predominantly cystic but with prominent septations of irregular thickness and nodularity. Color Doppler US showed blood vessels coursing through the nodules and septa, confirming neoplastic tissue. Pathologic diagnosis was clear cell carcinoma of the ovary.

but lack internal vascularity. Blood flow in the wall of cystic masses is commonly seen with both benign and malignant lesions.

5. Age: The risk of malignancy of an ovarian mass increases with the patient's age, from 24% between ages 50 and 60 years to 60% above age 80.
6. Extension of tumor outside the ovary to the uterus, broad ligament, or other pelvic organs is strong evidence of malignancy. However, inflammatory processes, such as tubo-ovarian abscess and endometriosis, may produce similar extension of disease.
7. Ascites, even in the absence of visualized tumor implants, is an ominous finding in the presence of an adnexal mass. Peritoneal implants from ovarian carcinoma are commonly minute and may not be detected by US or other imaging methods.
8. Evidence of metastatic spread, including tumor implants on peritoneal surfaces, omental cake, and enlarged lymph nodes, is a clear sign of malignancy (Fig. 37.17).

Adnexal torsion is a result of axial rotation of the ovary and/or tube about its vascular pedicle and causes acute severe pelvic pain because of arterial occlusion and venous stasis. The torsed ovary becomes swollen, hemorrhagic, and often necrotic, depending on the severity of torsion. An ovarian cyst or mass usually serves as the lead point. The fallopian tube is commonly torsed as well, adding to the complexity of the adnexal mass. US reveals an enlarged ovary, which appears as a swollen hemorrhagic edematous mass with peripheral follicles. Free fluid is frequently present in the cul-de-sac. Differentiation from other complex masses is often not possible. Doppler evaluation is not always reliable because of normal variations in adnexal flow and the common occurrence of intermittent torsion (16). Reduced or absent arterial flow to the involved ovary suggests the diagnosis. The presence of central venous flow is indicative of ovarian viability.

Polycystic ovary syndrome is a clinical and biochemical diagnosis based on findings of hirsutism, amenorrhea, infertility, and obesity. US only defines the morphology of the ovaries. In 70% of cases, both ovaries are enlarged and contain multiple follicles (usually >10 to 12 follicles per ovary). In 30% of cases, the ovaries are completely normal in size and appearance. Patients with anovulatory menstrual cycles, especially young female athletes, may have ovaries with multiple follicles but lack the clinical features of polycystic ovary syndrome.

Nonovarian cysts in the pelvis include abscess from appendicitis or diverticulitis, urachal cysts in the midline

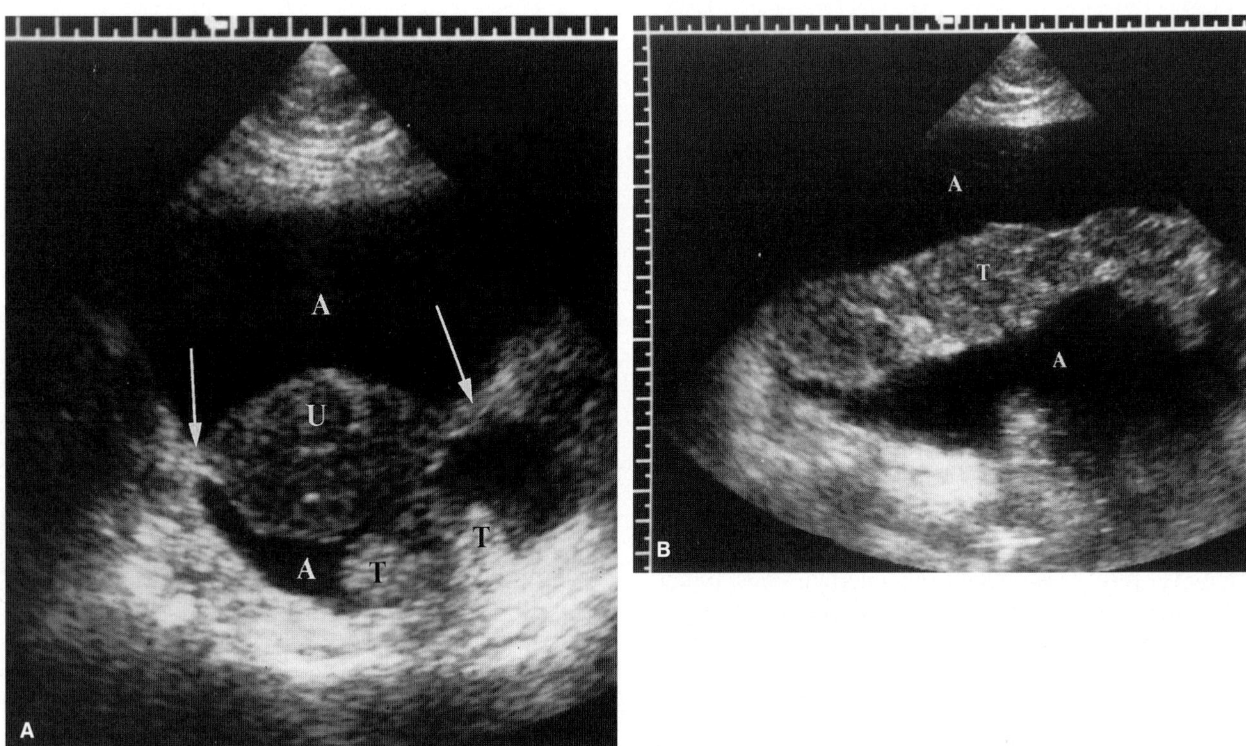

FIGURE 37.17. **Metastatic Ovarian Carcinoma. A.** US image of the pelvis in a 68-year-old woman presenting with sudden onset of ascites confirmed ascites (A) with tumor implants (T) on the peritoneal surfaces. The uterus (U) is seen in transverse section, with the broad ligaments (*arrows*) outlined by fluid. **B.** Sagittal US image from the upper abdomen demonstrates tumor implantation (T) on the greater omentum outlined by fluid (A). This appearance has been called "omental cake."

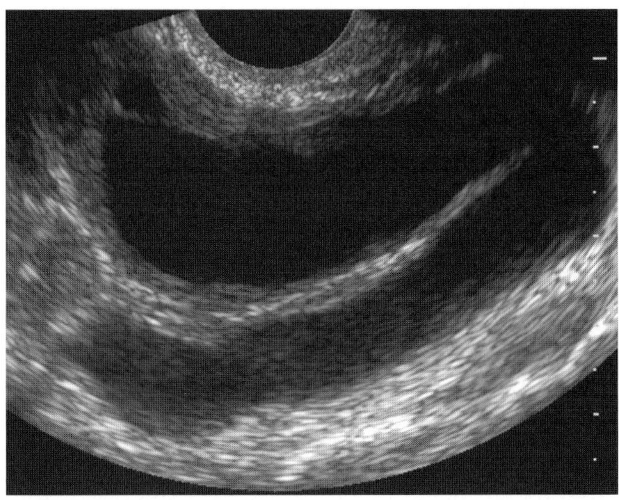

FIGURE 37.18. **Hydrosalpinx.** Transvaginal US demonstrates the tubular nature of an adnexal mass, confirming hydrosalpinx.

above the bladder, lymphocele in patients with prior pelvic node dissection, and *paraovarian cysts* in the mesosalpinx arising from wolffian duct remnants. Sonographic demonstration of a separate ovary on the same side as the adnexal mass suggests the diagnosis of nonovarian mass.

Hydrosalpinx can produce a large complex cystic mass. US shows a thin-walled or thick-walled tubular mass that is commonly elongated and folded on itself (Fig. 37.18) (17). Folds in the dilated fallopian tube may simulate septa in an ovarian tumor. Fluid within the mass is commonly echogenic. Transvaginal US is best for demonstrating the tubular nature of the mass. Other findings of pelvic inflammatory disease may be present. *Carcinoma of the fallopian tube* is rare. US shows features of a malignant adnexal mass.

Peritoneal inclusion cysts are relatively common inflammatory cysts of the peritoneal cavity that result from adhesions that envelop an ovary (18). The diseased peritoneum loses its ability to absorb fluid. Secretions from an active ovary confined by adhesions produces an expanding pelvic mass. Patients present with pain or a pelvic mass. Most have a history of previous pelvic surgery, infection, trauma, or endometriosis. US demonstrates a complex fluid collection occupying pelvic recesses and containing the ovary (Fig. 37.19). Septations, loculations, and particulate matter within the contained fluid are common.

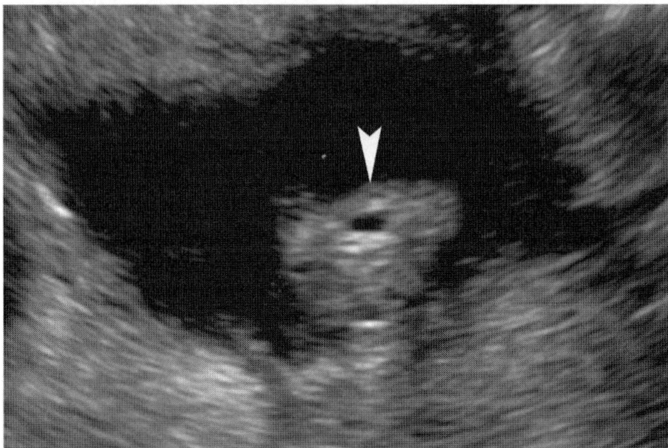

FIGURE 37.19. **Peritoneal Inclusion Cyst.** Sonogram reveals a fixed pelvic fluid collection with angulated boundaries and fluid occupying the peritoneal recesses. The collection encloses the ovary (*arrowhead*), which is identified by the presence of follicles.

MALE GENITAL TRACT

Testes and Scrotum

Normal US Anatomy. The normal testis is ovoid and smooth, measuring approximately 3.5 cm in length and 2.0 to 3.0 cm in diameter (Figs. 37.20, 37.21). It is covered by a dense, fibrous capsule called the *tunica albuginea.* The testis consists of 250 lobules made up of seminiferous tubules, which are the site of spermatozoa development. The seminiferous tubules unite to form the tubuli recti, rete testes, and finally efferent ductules, which exit the testis at the mediastinum. The mediastinum is an invagination of the tunica albuginea on the posterior surface of the testes that provides access for the testicular vessels

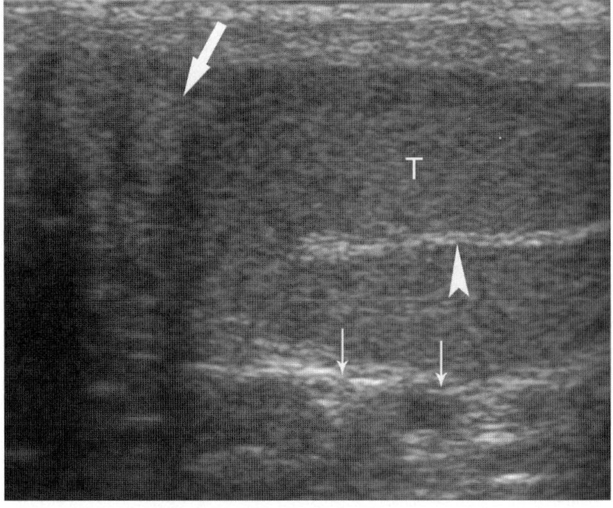

FIGURE 37.20. **Normal Testis.** US image demonstrates normal scrotal anatomy. The parenchyma of the testis (T) is of uniform midlevel echogenicity. The mediastinum of the testis (*arrowhead*) forms a bright, echogenic line caused by the infolding of the tough fibrous capsule, the tunica albuginea. The epididymis exits the testis through the mediastinum, forming the nodular head (<1 cm diameter) of the epididymis (*large arrow*) at the upper pole of the testis. The epididymis (*small arrows*) continues as a convoluted tube along the posterior aspect of the testis to its lower pole, where it reverses course and straightens out to become the vas deferens, which continues past the upper pole of the testis into the spermatic cord.

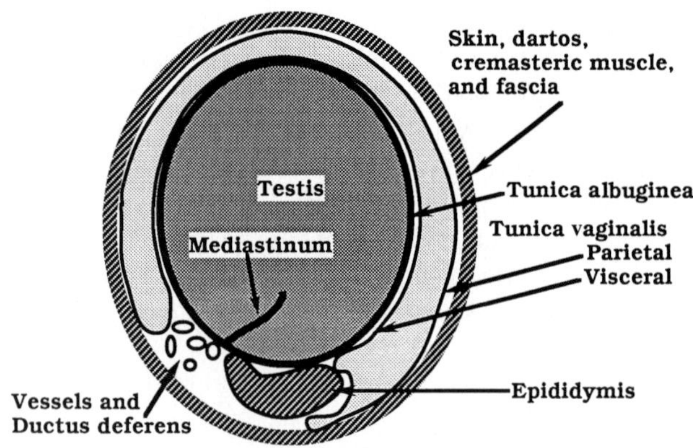

FIGURE 37.21. **Normal Scrotal Anatomy.** Drawing of a cross section of the scrotum demonstrates the testis, encapsulated by the tunica albuginea and largely surrounded by the potential space lined by the tunica vaginalis. The testis is attached to the scrotal wall posteriorly, where the testicular blood vessels, ductus deferens, and epididymis reside.

and exit for efferent ductules. The efferent ductules carry seminal fluid to the epididymis.

The epididymis is a highly convoluted tubule that is tightly applied to the posterior aspect of the testis. The *head of the epididymis* (globus major) is the enlarged (7- to 8-mm-diameter) superior portion of the epididymis adjacent to the superior pole of the testes. The body of the epididymis is 1 to 2 mm in diameter and courses caudally along the posterolateral testis. The tail (globus minor) is the pointed lower extremity of the epididymis at the lower pole of the testis. The ductus deferens is the continuation of the epididymis that ascends along the posteromedial aspect of the testis to become a component of the spermatic cord and traverse the inguinal canal. The *appendix testis* is a müllerian duct remnant seen as a small, oval structure just beneath the head of the epididymis. The *appendix epididymis* is a small, stalked appendage of the epididymal head. Torsion of the appendix testis or appendix epididymis may clinically mimic testicular torsion.

The scrotum consists of many layers of different tissue. The thickness of the scrotal skin is usually 3 to 6 mm, with a maximum of 8 mm. The *tunica vaginalis* is a peritoneal membrane that forms a closed serous sac that covers the medial, anterior, and lateral aspects of the testis and the lateral aspect of the epididymis. This space normally contains 1 to 2 mL of fluid. Excessive fluid in this space is termed a *hydrocele.* The tunica vaginalis leaves a bare area posteriorly that anchors the testis to the scrotal wall. A midline septum divides the scrotum into two separate compartments.

The spermatic cord is formed at the internal inguinal ring, courses through the inguinal canal and abdominal wall, and suspends the testes in the scrotum. The spermatic cord consists of the ductus deferens; the testicular, deferential, and external spermatic arteries; the pampiniform plexus of veins; lymphatic vessels; and the covering cremaster muscle. Enlargement of the pampiniform plexus of veins is termed a *varicocele*. Color flow and power Doppler US evaluate arterial flow in the spermatic cord and testes. After entering the testis, the testicular artery forms the capsular arteries, which course just beneath the tunica albuginea. The capsular arteries give rise to the centripetal branches, which flow toward the mediastinum through the testicular parenchyma. Because vascularity of the testes is quite variable, color flow images of one testis should always be compared to color flow images of the opposite testis.

US demonstrates the testes to be homogeneous in echogenicity, with an echotexture similar to the thyroid. The mediastinum is seen as a prominent echogenic line along the posterior aspect of the testis. Fluid in the space formed by the tunica vaginalis provides the best visualization of the components of the epididymis. The epididymis has a coarser, more heterogeneous appearance than the testis (19,20).

Undescended testis. About 3% of full-term newborns have an undescended testis. Most of these testes will spontaneously descend by 1 year of age, leaving 1% with cryptorchidism. Spontaneous descent after 1 year of age is unlikely. To preserve fertility, orchiopexy is recommended by 2 years of age. Long-term retention of an undescended testis is associated with a dramatically increased risk of testicular neoplasm, especially seminoma. The undescended testis may be located anywhere along the course of descent, from the lower pole of the kidney to the superficial inguinal ring. Most are identified by US and are within the inguinal canal (70% to 80%). The remainder, located in the abdomen, are best demonstrated by CT or MR. The inguinal canal runs an oblique, medially directed course through the flat muscles of the abdominal wall between the deep and superficial inguinal rings. The deep inguinal ring is located midway between the anterior superior iliac spine and the symphysis pubis. The superficial inguinal ring is located just above the pubic crest. Most undescended testes are atrophic, as small as 1 cm in size, and appear hypoechoic compared to normal testis. The bulbous termination of the gubernaculum, called the pars infravaginalis gubernaculi, must not be mistaken for the undescended testis. The gubernaculum is a cordlike structure that guides the testes into the scrotum during descent. The gubernaculum atrophies after normal testicular descent, but when descent is incomplete, the pars infravaginalis gubernaculi persists as a fibrous or gelatinous mass. Correct identification of the testis is assured by demonstration of the testicular mediastinum.

Acute scrotal pain is a common indication for US examination (Table 37.1). Doppler US has largely replaced radionuclide studies as the imaging method of first choice.

Testicular torsion results from anomalous suspension of the testis by a long spermatic cord with associated

TABLE 37.1 Causes of Acute Painful Scrotum

Common
Acute epididymitis/orchitis
Acute testicular torsion
Uncommon
Torsion of appendix epididymis
Torsion of appendix testis
Incarcerated inguinal hernia
Hemorrhage into a testicular tumor

complete investment of the testis and epididymis by the tunica vaginalis, resulting in the testis being not securely anchored to the scrotum. This anatomic variant is usually bilateral and has been termed the "bell-clapper" deformity. Surgical correction within 6 hours of torsion will usually preserve testicular function. Delay of surgery for 12 hours or more results in a salvage rate under 20%. The peak ages for testis torsion are the newborn period and ages 13 to 16 years. US findings of acute torsion include enlargement of the testis and epididymis, with a diffuse but sometimes heterogeneous decrease in echogenicity because of edema. The spermatic cord is enlarged and the Doppler signal from the spermatic cord is decreased or lost (21). Demonstration of normal flow on one side and absent or decreased flow on the symptomatic side provides the most reliable evidence of torsion and testicular ischemia (Fig. 37.22). Spontaneous detorsion may result in reactive hyperemia which mimics epididymo-orchitis.

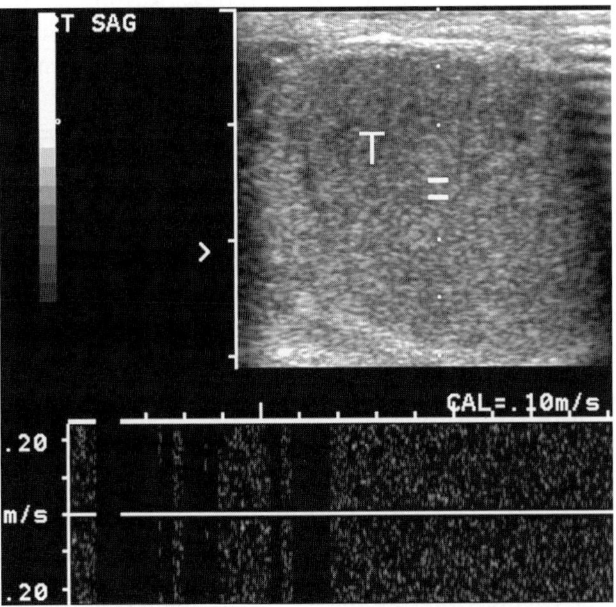

FIGURE 37.22. **Testicular Torsion.** Spectral Doppler shows no evidence of blood flow within the testis (T). Careful examination with color flow US confirmed this finding.

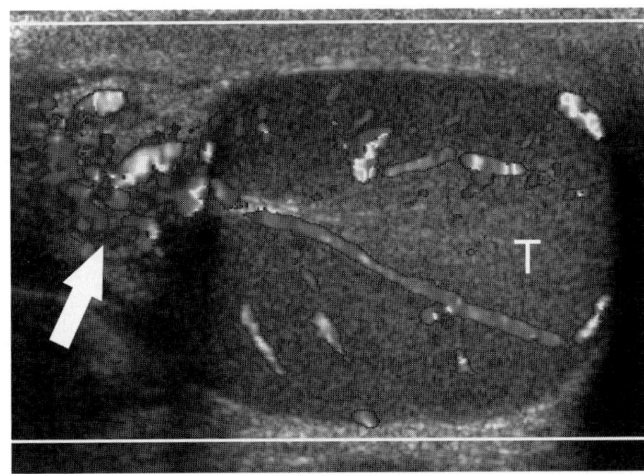

FIGURE 37.23. **Acute Epididymo-orchitis.** Color flow US image (shown in grayscale) demonstrates enlargement and marked hypervascularity of the epididymis (*arrow*). The testis (T) is mildly increased in vascularity as well.

A clinical history of decreasing pain prior to sonography suggests the possibility of detorsion.

Acute Epididymo-orchitis. Although testicular torsion is most common in patients under 20 years, acute epididymitis is more common after age 20. The onset of pain and swelling is more gradual with epididymitis. Pyuria is commonly present. *Escherichia coli, Staphylococcus aureus*, gonococcus, and tuberculosis are the most common causative organisms. US demonstrates thickening and enlargement of the epididymis associated with decreased echogenicity and indicating edema. Color Doppler demonstrates diffuse increased blood flow on the affected side as compared to the opposite side (Fig. 37.23). Hypervascularity may be confined to the epididymis or the testis, or it may involve both. Hydrocele is common. Inflammatory changes in the testis occur in 20% of cases. The inflamed testis is hypoechoic because of edema (Fig. 37.24).

Torsion of the appendix testis or appendix epididymis is a common cause of acute scrotal pain in children (22). Presentation mimics testicular torsion. US demonstrates an enlarged hypoechoic mass medial or posterior to the epididymal head and associated with hydrocele, thickening of the scrotal wall, and normal testes. Treatment is symptomatic, with spontaneous resolution expected.

Scrotal masses. US is 80% to 95% accurate in differentiating intratesticular from extratesticular masses. The majority of intratesticular masses are malignant (Table 37.2). Every intratesticular lesion should be considered to be potentially malignant until it is proven to be benign. Most extratesticular lesions are benign and are caused by inflammation or trauma (Table 37.3).

Primary testicular neoplasms constitute 4% to 6% of all male genitourinary tumors and 1% of all male malignancies. Most (95%) are germ cell tumors. These occur

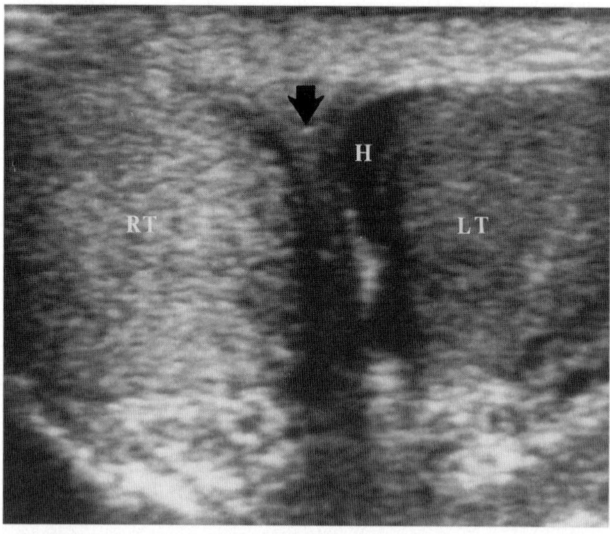

FIGURE 37.24. **Acute Orchitis.** Transverse US view of the scrotum demonstrates the left testis (LT) to be diffusely hypoechoic compared to the right testis (RT). A small hydrocele (H) is seen in the left hemiscrotum. The midline septum (*arrow*) dividing the scrotum into two separate compartments is evident.

most commonly in the 25- to 35-year-old age group and present as a unilateral painless mass.

Seminomas constitute 50% of germ cell tumors. They are less aggressive and are sensitive to radiation therapy. Seminomas are histologically monotonous, consisting of sheets of uniform cells intermixed with fibrous strands. Reflecting the histology, US demonstrates the tumor to be homogeneous and hypoechoic (Fig. 37.25).

TABLE 37.2 Differential Diagnosis of Intratesticular Lesions

Malignant
Primary germ cell tumor
  Seminoma
  Nonseminoma
  Embryonal cell carcinoma
  Teratoma
  Choriocarcinoma
  Mixed cell tumor
Secondary malignancy
  Leukemia and lymphoma
  Metastasis

Benign
Inflammatory
  Orchitis
  Epididymo-orchitis
  Mumps
  Abscess
Torsion/infarction
Gonadal stromal tumor
  Leydig cell tumor
  Sertoli cell tumor
Cysts
  Cyst of the tunica albuginea
  Benign testicular cyst
Trauma/hemorrhage

TABLE 37.3 Differential Diagnosis of Extratesticular Lesions

Extrinsic to epididymis
Scrotal fluid collections
  Hydrocele
  Hematocele
  Pyocele
Varicocele
Scrotal hernia

Epididymal lesions
Cystic
  Spermatocele
  Epididymal cyst
  Abscess
Solid
  Sperm granuloma
  Epididymitis
  Sarcoidosis
  Adenomatoid tumor

Nonseminomatous tumors. The remainder of germ cell malignancies can be grouped as nonseminomatous tumors. As a group they are more aggressive and are resistant to radiation therapy. Cell types include embryonal cell carcinoma (20% to 25%), teratoma (5% to 10%), and choriocarcinoma (1% to 3%). The remainder are of mixed cell type. All tend to appear as heterogeneous masses because of mixed cellularity as well as the presence of hemorrhage and necrosis. US shows irregular areas of high and low density, cystic areas, and calcification (Fig. 37.26). A hydrocele is present in 15% of patients with germ cell tumors. Both CT and MR are excellent methods for initial tumor staging and follow-up.

Lymphoma, leukemia, and metastases from other primary tumors are more common than germ cell tumors in patients over age 50. The testis serves as a sanctuary for disease because of ineffective access of chemotherapy. Involvement of the testis may be diffuse or focal. Tumors are usually of lower echogenicity than normal parenchyma (Fig. 37.27). Careful comparison with the opposite testis may be necessary for detection of lesions. Renal cell and prostate carcinoma are the most common tumors to metastasize to the testis.

Gonadal Stromal Tumors. Leydig and Sertoli cell tumors account for 3% to 6% of all testicular tumors; 3% are bilateral; up to 15% are malignant. They appear as small, solid masses.

Testicular microlithiasis appears on US as diffuse, punctate, nonshadowing, hyperechoic foci throughout the testicular parenchyma (Fig. 37.28). It is a benign condition of microcalcifications within the seminiferous

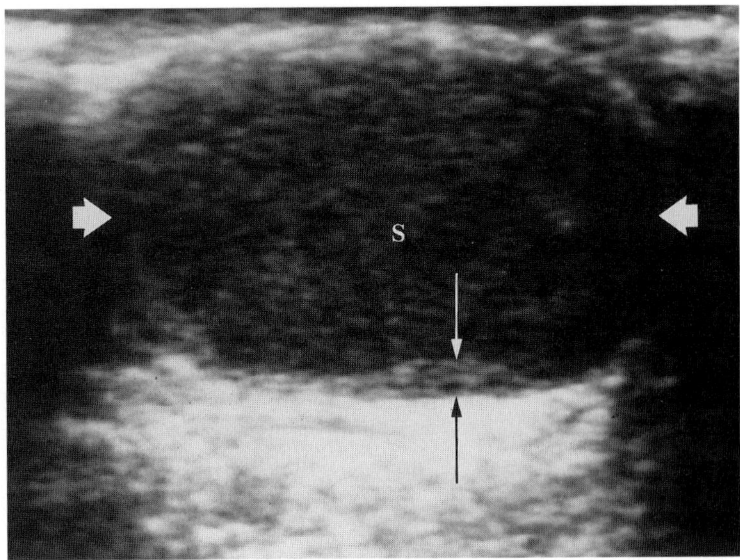

FIGURE 37.25. **Seminoma.** Longitudinal US demonstrates near-complete replacement of the testes (between *wide arrows*) by a homogeneous hypoechoic mass (S) that proved to be seminoma. Only a thin rim of normal testicular parenchyma remains (between *thin arrows*).

tubules, but it is associated with an incidence of testicular carcinoma as high as 40%. Nearly all cases are bilateral. Additional associations include cryptorchidism and infertility.

Cysts. Benign testicular cysts are incidental findings in 8% to 10% of males (23). Cysts of the tunica albuginea are well defined, small (2 to 5 mm in diameter), and peripheral. Both types are filled with serous fluid (Fig. 37.29).

Dilated rete testis may mimic a complex intratesticular mass. US demonstrates multiple small spherical or tubular cystic structures in the region of the mediastinum of the testis (Fig. 37.30). Nearly all cases are associated with abnormalities of the epididymis, including spermatocele, epididymal cysts, or history of epididymitis or vasectomy.

Orchitis and Abscess. Most inflammations of the testis are associated with epididymitis. Mumps is an additional cause of orchitis. The testis with orchitis is enlarged with edematous areas that may be irregular in outline (Fig. 37.24). A fluid-filled mass suggests abscess formation. Testicular abscess may rupture through the tunica albuginea and result in a pyocele.

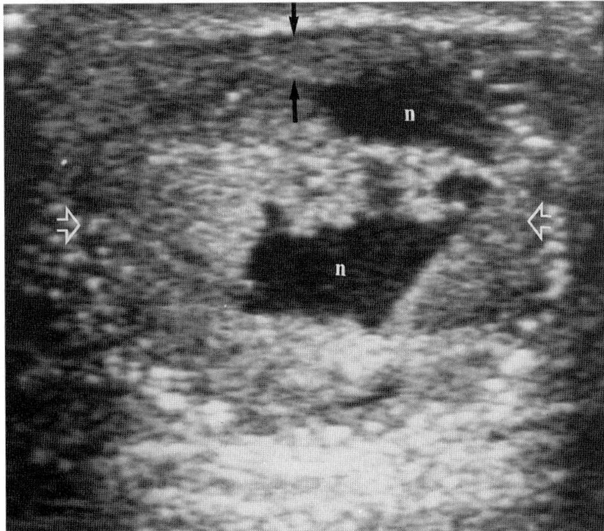

FIGURE 37.26. **Choriocarcinoma.** An US view of a testis in long axis demonstrates a large tumor (between *open arrows*) replacing the testicular parenchyma. Note the marked inhomogeneity of the tumor with large areas of necrosis (n). The residual testicular parenchyma is indicated by the black arrows.

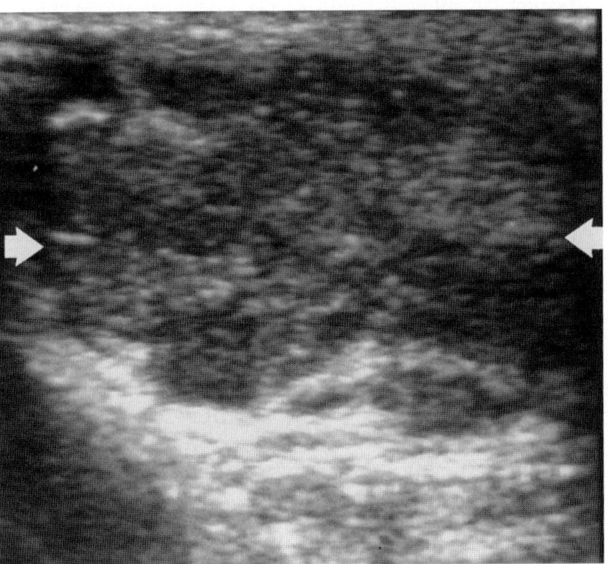

FIGURE 37.27. **Malignant Melanoma Metastasis.** Long-axis view of the testis reveals complete replacement of parenchyma by an inhomogeneous, predominantly hypoechoic tumor (between *arrows*). No recognizable normal parenchyma remains.

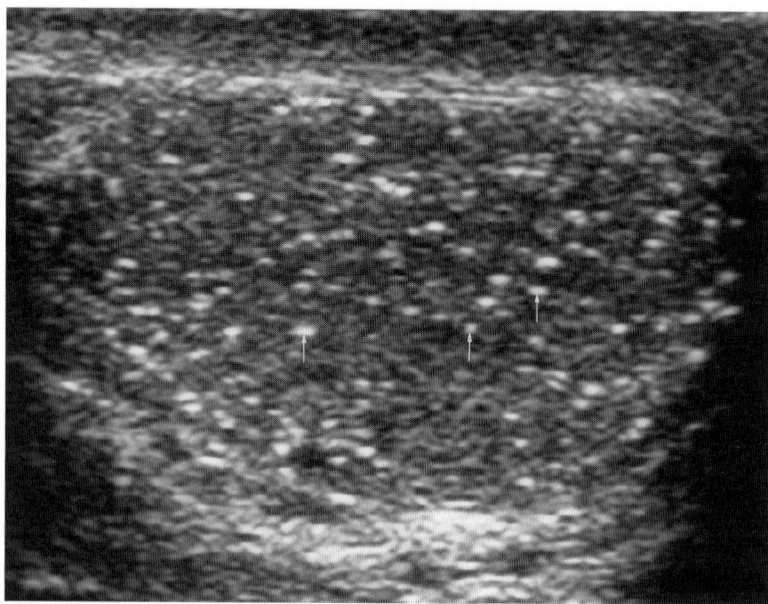

FIGURE 37.28. **Testicular Microlithiasis.** Innumerable tiny echogenic spots (*arrows*) are evident throughout the testicular parenchyma. This benign condition is associated with a significant risk of testicular carcinoma.

Infarction. Testis infarction may result from torsion or trauma. The infarct may appear as a focal low-density area or as diffuse low density of the entire testis. With time, the testis shrinks and becomes fibrotic.

Trauma/Hemorrhage. In the setting of trauma, the role of imaging is to detect a ruptured testis. Most (90%) ruptured testes can be salvaged by surgery performed in the first 72 hours following trauma. Intratesticular hematoma and hematocele are the major indicators of testis rupture. The normal shape and clear definition of the testis are lost (Fig. 37.31). Discrete fractures are identified in a minority of cases. Color Doppler US is useful in detecting intratesticular vascular disruption and in avoiding mistaking a normal vascular cleft for a fracture.

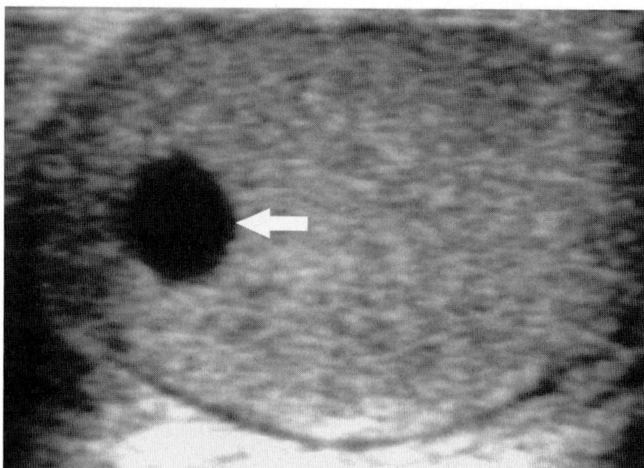

FIGURE 37.29. **Testicular Cyst.** A benign testicular cyst is viewed as a well-defined, spherical, uniformly anechoic mass (*arrow*) within the testis. Care must be taken to differentiate simple testicular cysts from cystic necrosis within testicular tumors.

Scrotal Fluid Collections. A *hydrocele* is the accumulation of serous fluid between the visceral and parietal layers of the tunica vaginalis (Fig. 37.32). It is the most common cause of painless scrotal swelling. Although many cases are idiopathic, hydrocele may accompany malignant

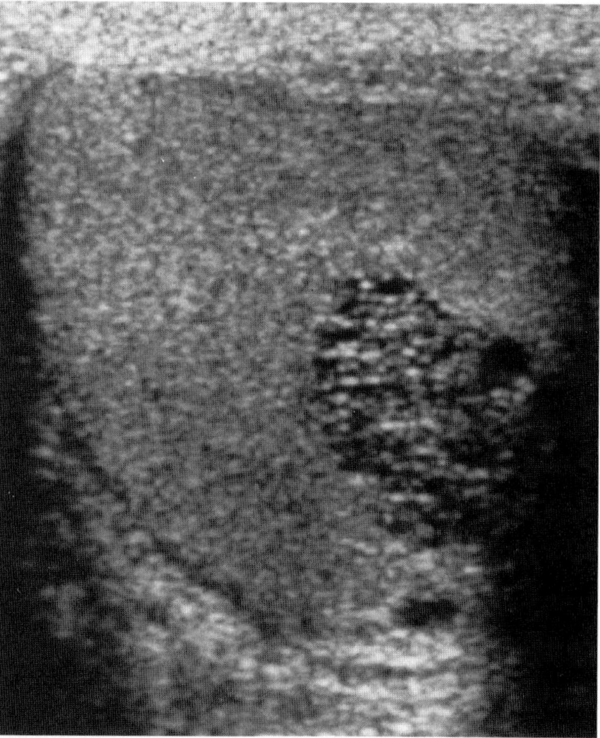

FIGURE 37.30. **Dilated Rete Testis.** A complex-appearing mass is made up of numerous tiny cystic tubular structures and is located in the mediastinum of the testis.

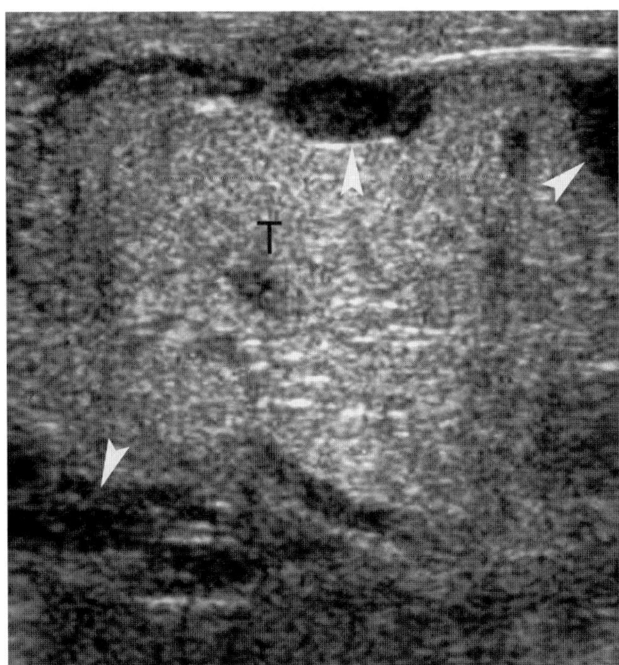

FIGURE 37.31. **Fractured Testis.** The testis (T) is heterogeneous and its normal shape is disrupted. Multiple areas of hemorrhage (*arrowheads*) are evident. This man had been injured in a motorcycle accident.

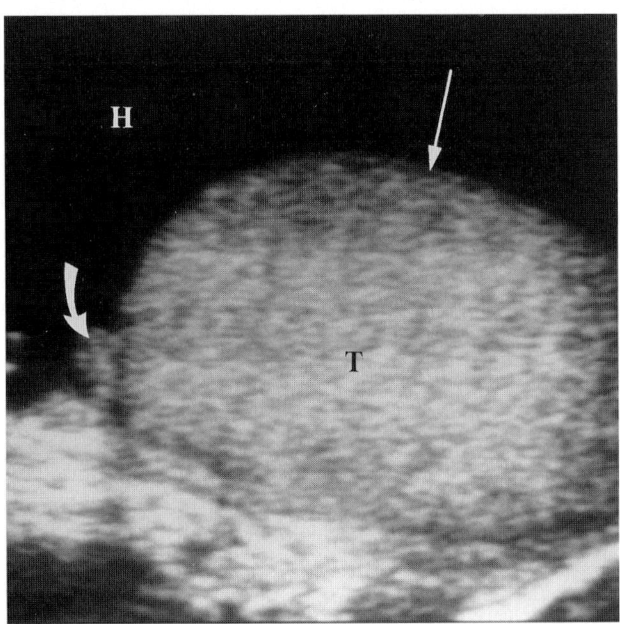

FIGURE 37.32. **Large Hydrocele.** An US image through the long axis of the testis (T) demonstrates its homogeneous midlevel echogenicity. The head of the epididymis is seen as a small nodular structure (*curved arrow*) at the superior aspect of the testis. The tunica albuginea (*straight arrow*) is the tough fibrous capsule that covers the testis. The hydrocele (H) surrounds all portions of the testis except its posterior portion, where the testis is attached to the scrotal wall.

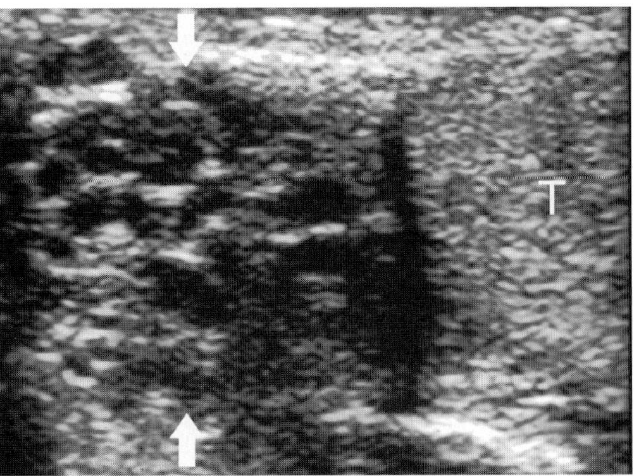

FIGURE 37.33. **Varicocele.** Sagittal view of the scrotum demonstrates a network of curving tubular structures (between *arrows*) at the superior pole of the testis (T). Color Doppler US confirmed slow venous flow within these dilated vessels.

tumors, torsion, and inflammation. *Hematoceles* result from trauma or surgery. *Pyoceles* usually result from rupture of an abscess into the space between the layers of the tunica vaginalis. Internal septations and loculations are common with hematoceles and pyoceles.

Varicoceles are dilated serpiginous veins of the pampiniform plexus (Fig. 37.33). They occur in 15% to 20% of males and are the most common correctable cause of male infertility. Acute onset of a varicocele in an adult male aged 40 or older may be a sign of neoplastic obstruction of the ipsilateral gonadal or renal vein.

Scrotal hernias may contain omentum, small bowel, or colon. The herniated mass extends through the inguinal canal to the scrotum (Fig. 37.34).

Cystic Epididymal Lesions. *Spermatoceles* are cysts of the epididymal head that contain sperm and cellular debris. *Epididymal cysts* contain clear serous fluid and may occur anywhere along the course of the epididymis. Loculations and septations within the cysts are common (Fig. 37.35). Spermatoceles range in size up to several centimeters.

Solid Epididymal Lesions. *Sperm granuloma* form when sperm extravasate into the soft tissues surrounding the epididymis. *Chronic epididymitis,* which results from incompletely resolved acute epididymitis, causes an irregular, hard, tender mass (Fig. 37.36). *Sarcoidosis* may cause a painless, solid epididymal mass and involve the testis. *Adenomatoid tumors* are benign, slow-growing epididymal neoplasms.

Prostate

The major indication for transrectal US of the prostate gland is to guide needle biopsy for diagnosis of prostate cancer (24). Early enthusiasm for use of transrectal US

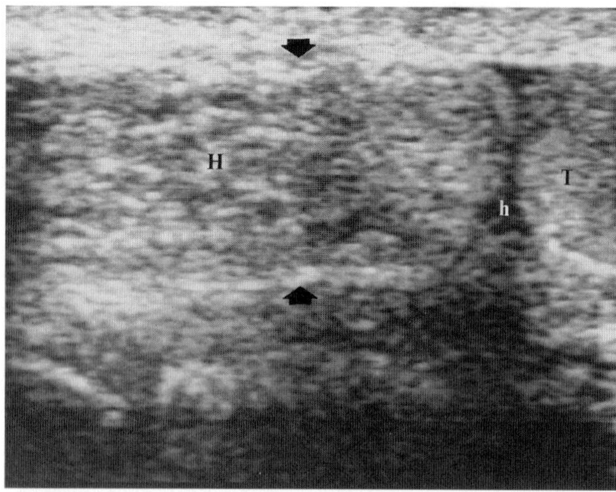

FIGURE 37.34. **Inguinal Hernia.** Sagittal plane image reveals a moderately echogenic mass in the inguinal canal (H, between *arrows*). With straining, the mass approached the superior pole of the testis (T). With relaxation in the supine position, the hernia was reduced. A small hydrocele (h) was also present. Surgery confirmed a small inguinal hernia, with omentum extending through the inguinal canal into the superior aspect of the scrotum.

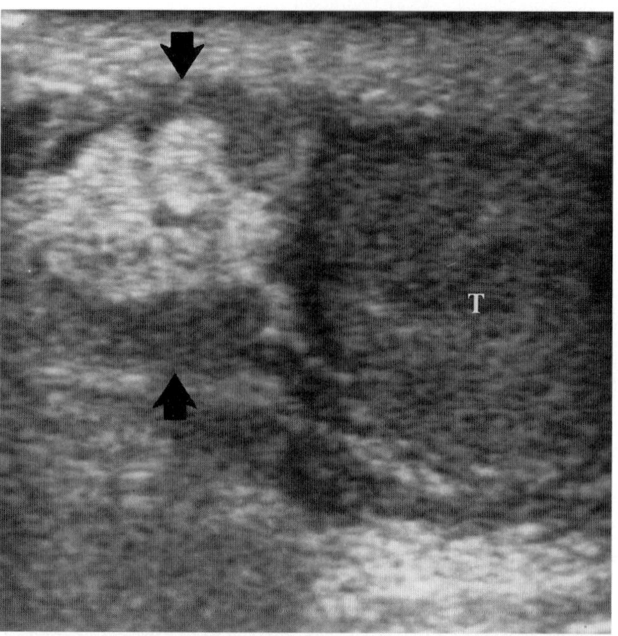

FIGURE 37.36. **Chronic Epididymitis.** The epididymis (*arrows*) is grossly enlarged and has a large central echogenic area, representing fibrosis and chronic inflammation. The testis (T) is diffusely hypoechoic because of diffuse orchitis.

as a screening examination for prostate cancer has been dampened by well-documented sensitivity of only 60% for US examination alone. Additional indications for US include detection of abscess or infertility with suspicion of obstruction of the ejaculatory ducts or atresia of the seminal vesicles and for examination of the posterior urethra (25).

Normal US Anatomy. On transabdominal US, the prostate is seen as a rounded organ at the base of the bladder (see Fig. 37.42). Enlargement of the prostate elevates the base of the bladder. The urethral orifice can usually be identified as a V-shaped indentation in the prostate. The zonal anatomy of the prostate is described in Chapter 35. On transrectal US, the central and peripheral zones are nearly equal in echogenicity and are usually distinguished mainly by position. It is useful to describe the gland on US as having a *peripheral zone* and an *inner gland* composed of the central and transitional zones and their pathologic alterations (Fig. 37.37). The anterior fibromuscular stroma is seen as a hypoechoic area at the anterior superior aspect of the gland. US can be used to calculate the volume of the prostate gland using the formula width × height × length × 0.52. A prostate that is larger than 30 mL (or 30 g) is considered enlarged. The seminal vesicles are seen as hypoechoic, lobulated, tubular structures in the groove between the base of the bladder and the base of the prostate (Fig. 37.38).

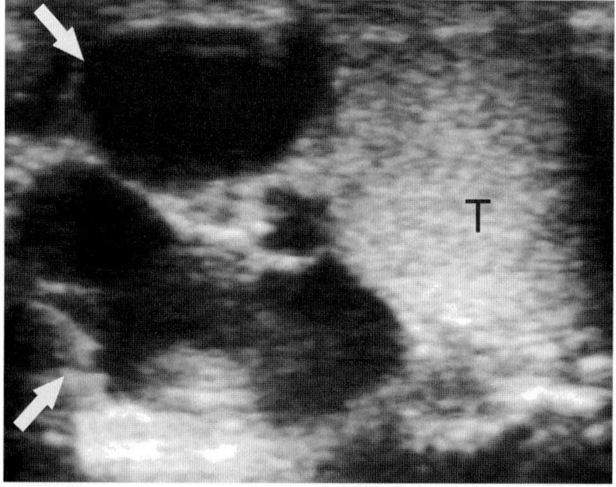

FIGURE 37.35. **Spermatocele.** US image displays a complex, septated extratesticular cyst (*arrows*) at the superior pole of the testicle (T). Debris within the spermatocele produces floating particles within the fluid.

Prostate carcinoma screening currently includes digital rectal examination and serum prostate-specific antigen (PSA) testing. PSA is a glycoprotein produced only by the prostate gland. Elevated PSA levels suggest the presence of cancer with the risk of malignancy increasing with the PSA value. The normal serum PSA level is 0 to 4 ng/mL. False-positive elevation of PSA levels is generally caused by benign prostate hyperplasia (BPH). For this reason, some centers use a PSA-density calculation, i.e., PSA value divided by size of the prostate estimated clinically or measured by transabdominal or transrectal US. US signs of

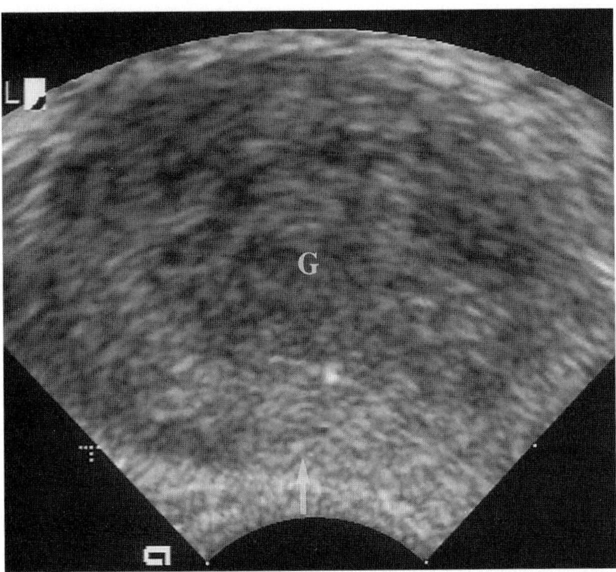

FIGURE 37.37. **Prostate Anatomy.** Transrectal US images of the prostate are routinely viewed inverted. The transducer is at the bottom rather than the top of the image. This sagittal image shows the normal peripheral zone (*arrow*) to be slightly echogenic compared to the hypoechoic, more heterogeneous central gland (G).

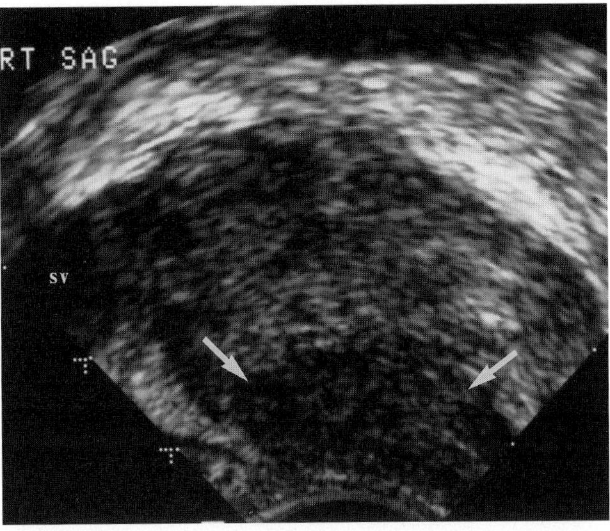

FIGURE 37.39. **Prostate Cancer.** Right sagittal transrectal US image shows a distinct hypoechoic nodule (*arrows*) in the peripheral zone. US-guided transrectal needle biopsy confirmed prostate carcinoma. sv, seminal vesicle.

prostate cancer are: (*1*) presence of a distinct hypoechoic nodule (Fig. 37.39), (*2*) poorly marginated hypoechoic area in the peripheral zone, (*3*) mass effect on surrounding tissues, (*4*) asymmetric enlargement of the prostate, (*5*) deformation of prostatic contour, (*6*) heterogeneous area in the homogeneous gland, and (*7*) focal increased vascularity in the peripheral zone with color flow US (26). All findings are nonspecific (Table 37.4), and random biopsies of the prostate yield carcinoma as commonly as 20% of the time.

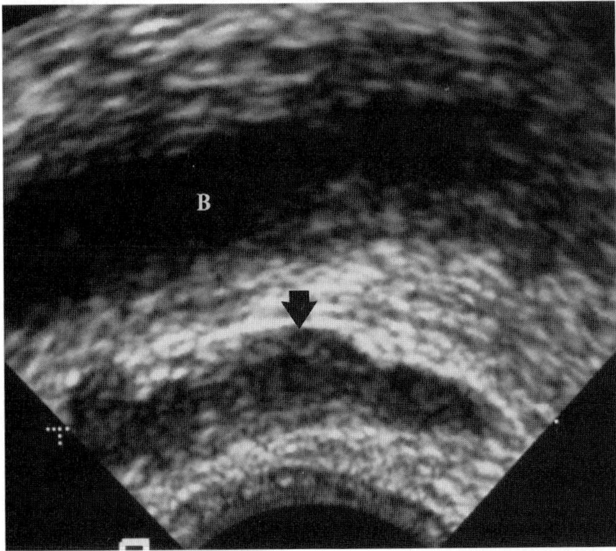

FIGURE 37.38. **Normal Seminal Vesicles.** Transrectal US image shows the normal hypoechoic convoluted tubular appearance of the seminal vesicle (*arrow*). B, bladder.

Sonographic guidance provides a safe and accurate method to obtain tissue from specific areas of the prostate gland. Indications for US-guided needle biopsy include: suspicious palpable nodule, suspicious nodule visualized by US, or elevated PSA. Both transrectal and transperineal routes are used for prostate biopsy. The transperineal route is more painful, and the transrectal route requires preprocedure antibiotics. Our practice had been to routinely obtain a total of six to ten 18-gauge core biopsy specimens from different areas of the gland, always including all four quadrants.

Benign prostatic hyperplasia is a nodular hypertrophy of the glandular tissue of the transitional zone, usually beginning in the fifth decade of life. The transitional zone becomes enlarged and heterogeneous and compresses the urethra and the central zone (Fig. 37.40). Discrete nodules, some with cystic changes, may be visualized. The enlargement is often marginated circumferentially by a

TABLE 37.4 Causes of Peripheral Hypoechoic Nodule in the Prostate

Carcinoma
Benign prostatic hypertrophy
Prostatitis
Infarction
Fibromuscular hyperplasia

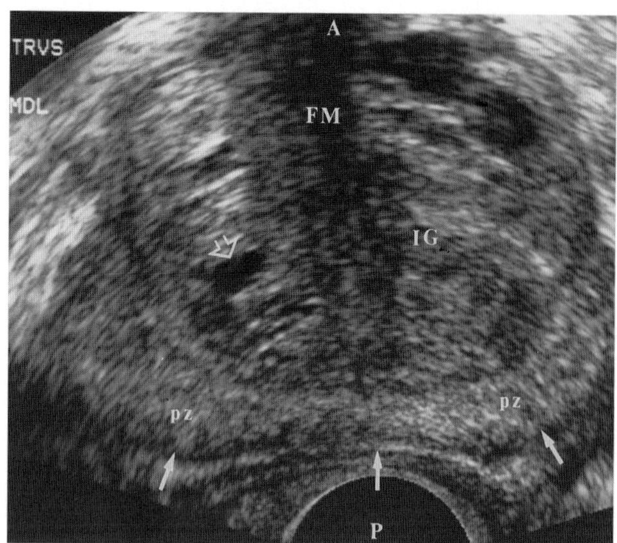

FIGURE 37.40. **Benign Prostatic Hypertrophy.** Transrectal axial US view through the midprostate demonstrates excellent differentiation of a normal peripheral zone (pz, *solid arrows*). The inner gland (IG) demonstrates mild enlargement and heterogeneity that is characteristic of benign prostatic hypertrophy. A small prostatic cyst is evident (*open arrow*). The hypoechoic fibromuscular zone (FM) is anterior. A, anterior; P, posterior.

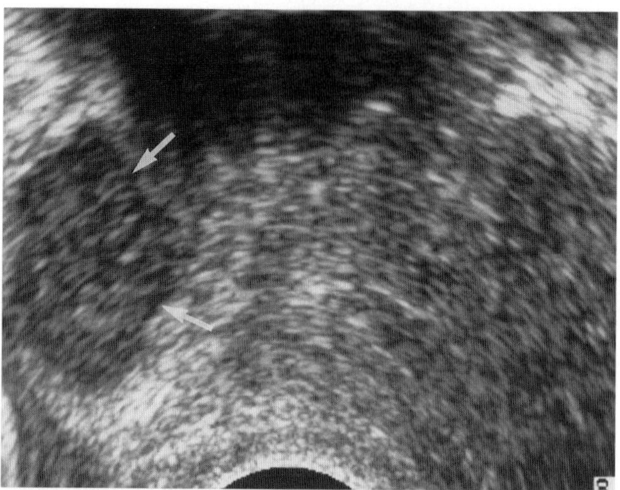

FIGURE 37.41. **Prostate Abscess.** Transverse transrectal US reveals an abscess (*arrows*) in the right side of the prostate gland in a patient with fever, pelvic pain, and pyuria. The abscess contained purulent debris, which was seen on US as floating particulate matter.

pseudocapsule. The size of the prostate exceeds 30 g (mL). The prostatic urethra becomes elongated, tortuous, and compressed, causing bladder outlet obstruction. Stasis of urine may lead to the formation of bladder stones. The bladder base is commonly elevated, and the bladder wall may be thickened.

Acute prostatitis is usually caused by *E coli* infection. The gland is swollen and edematous. Prostatic abscess is demonstrated by US as a focal collection of echogenic fluid within the gland (Fig. 37.41). Septations may be present. Transrectal US may be used to direct needle aspiration of a suspected abscess.

Chronic prostatitis results from incompletely resolved acute prostatitis. Large prostatic calculi are common and serve as a reservoir for persistent and relapsing infection.

Prostatic calculi form spontaneously or result from chronic inflammation. Most calculi are periurethral and develop from the corpora amylacea, a proteinaceous material formed in the prostate gland. On US, calculi are brightly echogenic and commonly produce acoustic shadows. Although they may be found in areas of cancer, they are not a sign of cancer and do not develop from the malignant process.

Prostatic cysts are relatively common findings on prostate imaging examinations. Cystic lesions of the prostate are listed in Table 37.5.

Ejaculatory duct obstruction is an uncommon but treatable cause of male infertility. Causes include congenital obstruction, urethritis, and instrumentation. The normal ejaculatory ducts are not commonly visible on transrectal US. Obstruction of the ducts is suggested by presence of a cyst posterior to the prostatic urethra, commonly associated with dilatation of the seminal vesicles. Needle aspiration or surgical resection of the obstructing cyst is frequently curative.

BLADDER

The full bladder is used as an acoustic window to the pelvis for evaluation of the genital tract (Fig. 37.42). Abnormalities of the bladder may be mistaken for abnormalities of other organs of the pelvis. Alternatively, large cystic masses may be mistaken for the bladder. US is valuable for evaluation of bladder wall, distal ureters, and intravesical and extravesical masses (19).

Normal US Anatomy. The urine-filled bladder is thin walled and contains anechoic urine. The normal wall measures 3 mm when the bladder is distended and 5 mm when collapsed. The volume of bladder contents may be calculated by the standard formula for volume of a prolate

TABLE 37.5 Cystic Lesions in the Prostate

Müllerian duct cyst (midline)
Utricle cyst (midline)
Prostate retention cyst (associated with benign prostate hyperplasia)
Seminal vesicle cyst
Ejaculatory duct cyst

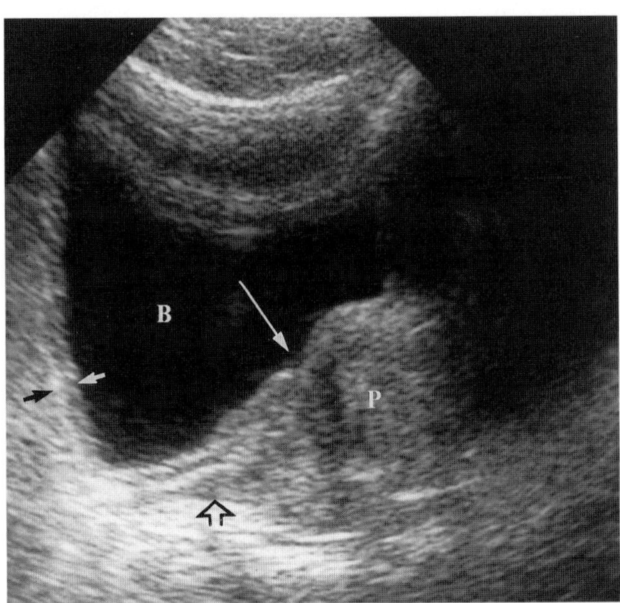

FIGURE 37.42. **Enlarged Prostate.** Midline sagittal US image shows an enlarged prostate (P) protruding into and elevating the base of the bladder (B). The urethral orifice (*long arrow*) forms a V-shaped depression in the prostate. The seminal vesicles (*open arrow*) are also seen. The bladder wall is mildly thickened (between *short arrows*).

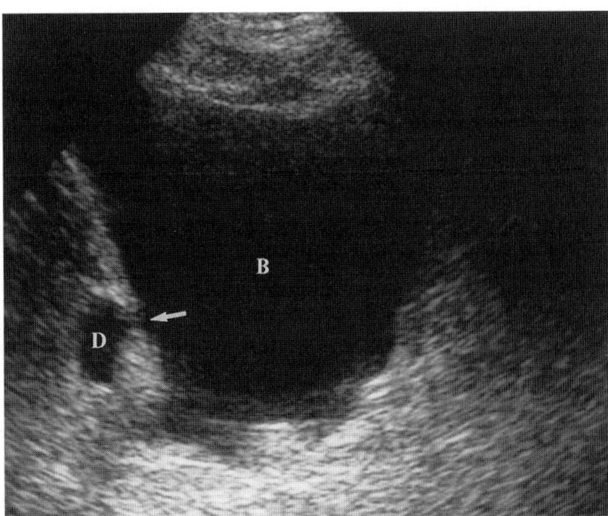

FIGURE 37.43. **Bladder Diverticulum.** Axial-plane image shows a urine-filled diverticulum (D) projecting through a defect (*arrow*) in the bladder wall. B, bladder.

ellipse (length × width × height × 0.52). US measurements may be used to calculate postvoid urine residual and overdistended bladder volumes when the bladder is neurogenic. Ureteral jets are spurts of urine into the bladder caused by ureteral peristalsis. They are best visualized by color Doppler but are occasionally seen on grayscale US as swirling microbubbles. Visualization of ureteral jets confirms patency of the ureter.

Bladder diverticula appear as fluid-filled sacs that project from the bladder wall. Bladder mucosa herniates through a defect in the bladder wall, producing a fluid-filled mass that communicates with the main bladder lumen through a small orifice (Fig. 37.43). The wall of the diverticulum lacks a muscle layer and is thinner than the bladder wall. The orifice may be inconspicuous and require a diligent search to detect. Color Doppler may be used to detect a jet of urine flow through the diverticular orifice when pressure is applied to the lower abdomen. Diverticula may not empty completely with voiding and serve as a site of urine stasis, predisposing to infection and stone formation. US may demonstrate floating and layering debris in the urine, with infection and shadowing stones within the diverticulum or bladder. The presence of a soft tissue mass within the diverticulum suggests a complicating carcinoma.

Simple ureteroceles produce small, oval, fluid-filled masses projecting into the bladder lumen. The size of the ureterocele changes as it fills and empties with ureteral peristalsis. The location at the ureterovesical junction may be confirmed by observing ureteral jets that originate from the ureterocele.

Ectopic ureteroceles are found with ureteral duplication and produce fluid-filled masses of variable size in the bladder lumen. The ureterocele commonly remains unchanged in size after voiding. The distal ureter is dilated and tortuous (Fig. 37.44).

Bladder carcinoma may appear as a polypoid mass or as focal, multifocal, or diffuse thickening of the bladder wall. An irregular papillary surface of the tumor may be evident. Tumors may be single or multiple, and they occur with increased incidence within diverticula. Tumor can be differentiated from blood clot by Doppler demonstration of blood vessels within the mass. Bladder carcinoma is difficult to differentiate from benign bladder wall thickening unless a polypoid mass is present. Early stage tumors are usually not demonstrated with US.

Bladder stones appear as brightly echogenic objects that cast acoustic shadows. Most stones will move with changes in patient position, but some are adherent to the bladder wall. Stones may also be seen in the distal ureter, in ureteroceles, and in diverticula.

Foreign bodies are usually echogenic and linear, angulated, or geographic in appearance, rather than round or oval like stones. Many will cast acoustic shadows and move within the bladder.

Blood clots may produce layering fluid–debris levels when small or heterogeneous masses when large. Doppler shows no internal vascularity. Clots change in appearance and size with time.

Bladder outlet obstruction causes muscle hypertrophy and trabeculation of the bladder wall. US demonstrates

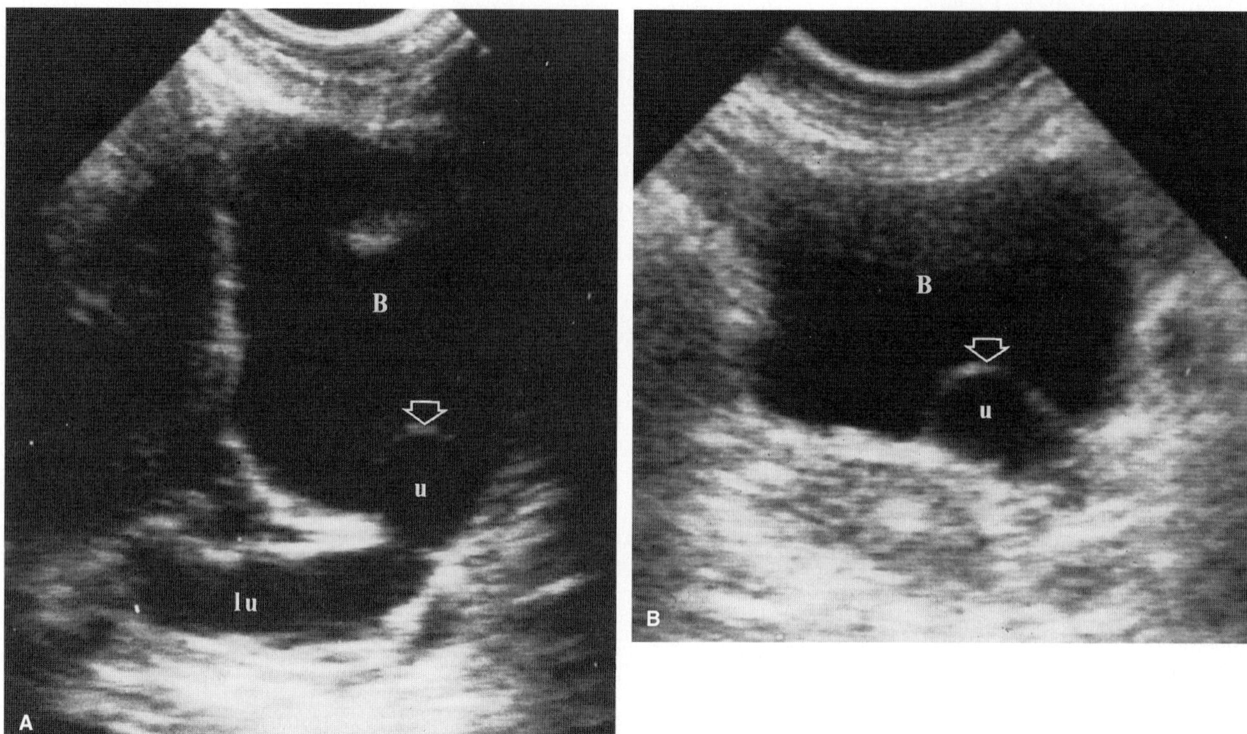

FIGURE 37.44. **Ectopic Ureterocele.** US images in left sagittal **(A)** and transverse **(B)** planes demonstrate an ectopic ureterocele (u) of the left upper pole ureter (lu) protruding into the lumen of the bladder base. The upper pole collecting system was hydronephrotic, but the lower pole collecting system was normal. The wall of the ureterocele (*arrows*) is clearly seen. A ureterocele changes in size with peristalsis of the ureter. B, bladder.

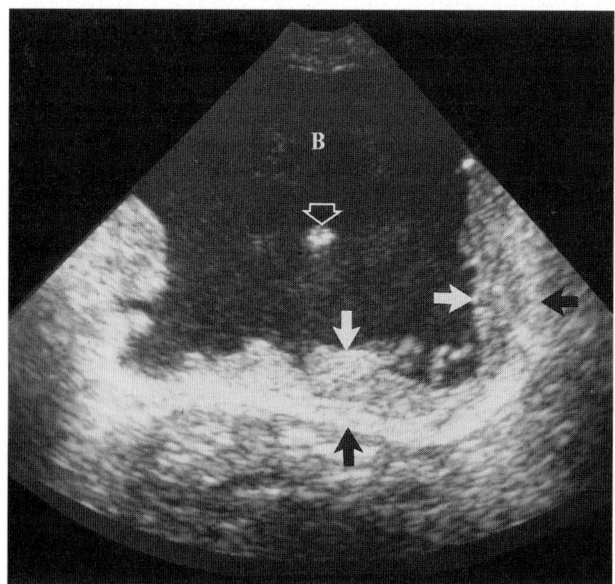

FIGURE 37.45. **Thickened Bladder Wall.** Axial US of a neurogenic bladder (B) demonstrates marked thickening (*arrows*) of the bladder wall with trabeculation. The patient had an indwelling Foley catheter, the tip of which is evident (*open arrow*).

thickening of the wall and marked irregularity of its luminal surface (Fig. 37.45). Causes include prostate enlargement, neurogenic bladder, urethral stricture, ectopic ureterocele, tumors, and blood clots.

Cystitis resulting from any cause may produce focal or diffuse thickening of the bladder wall, often associated with layering or masslike echogenic debris within the urine. The mucosa may be raised and echolucent because of edema. Air within the bladder wall or lumen produces bright echoes with acoustic shadowing or ring-down artifact.

REFERENCES

1. Brant WE. Female pelvis ultrasound. In: Brant WE, ed. The Core Curriculum: Ultrasound. Philadelphia: Lippincott Williams & Wilkins, 2001:179–224.
2. Berridge DL, Winter TC. Saline infusion sonohysterography: technique, indications, and imaging findings. J Ultrasound Med 2004; 23:97–112.
3. Nalaboff KM, Pellerito JS, Ben-Levi E. Imaging of the endometrium: disease and normal variants. Radiographics 2001;21:1409–1424.
4. Atri M, Reinhold C, Mehio AR, Chapman WB, Bret PM. Adenomyosis: US features with histologic correlation in an in vitro study. Radiology 2000;215:783–790.

5. Reinhold C, Tafazoli F, Mehio A, et al. Uterine adenomyosis: endovaginal US and MR imaging features with histopathologic correlation. Radiographics 1999;19:S147–S160.
6. Brown DL, Frates MC, Muto MG, Welch WR. Small echogenic foci in the ovaries: correlation with histologic findings. J Ultrasound Med 2004;23:307–313.
7. Jeong YY, Outwater EK, Kang HK. Imaging evaluation of ovarian masses. Radiographics 2000;20:1445–1470.
8. Swire MN, Castro-Aragon I, Levine D. Various sonographic appearances of the hemorrhagic corpus luteum cyst. Ultrasound Q 2004; 20:45–58.
9. Woodward PJ, Sohaey R, Mezzetti TP Jr. Endometriosis: radiologic-pathologic correlation. Radiographics 2001;21:193–216.
10. Horrow MM. Ultrasound of pelvic inflammatory disease. Ultrasound Q 2004;20:171–179.
11. Patel MD, Feldstein VA, Chen DC, et al. Endometriomas: diagnostic performance of US. Radiology 1999;210:739–745.
12. Outwater EK, Siegelman ES, Hunt JL. Ovarian teratomas: tumor types and imaging characteristics. Radiographics 2001;21:475–490.
13. Brown DL, Doubilet PM, Miller GH, et al. Benign and malignant ovarian masses: selection of the most discriminating gray-scale and Doppler sonographic features. Radiology 1998;208:103–110.
14. Buy J-N, Ghossain MA, Hugol D, et al. Characterization of adnexal masses: combination of color Doppler and conventional sonography compared with spectral Doppler analysis alone and conventional sonography alone. AJR Am J Roentgenol 1996;166:385–393.
15. Fleischer AC. Sonographic assessment of the morphology and vascularity of ovarian masses. Ultrasound Q 2002;18:81–88.
16. Albayram F, Hamper UM. Ovarian and adnexal torsion: spectrum of sonographic findings with pathologic correlation. J Ultrasound Med 2001;20:1083–1089.
17. Benjaminov O, Atri M. Sonography of the abnormal fallopian tube. AJR Am J Roentgenol 2004;183:737–742.
18. Jain KA. Imaging of peritoneal inclusion cysts. AJR Am J Roentgenol 2000;174:1559–1563.
19. Brant WE. Scrotal ultrasound. In: Brant WE, ed. The Core Curriculum: Ultrasound. Philadelphia: Lippincott Williams & Wilkins, 2001: 331–348.
20. Akin EA, Khati NJ, Hill MC. Ultrasound of the scrotum. Ultrasound Q 2004;20:181–200.
21. Dogra VS, Rubens DJ, Gottlieb RH, Bhatt S. Torsion and beyond: new twists in spectral Doppler evaluation of the scrotum. J Ultrasound Med 2004;23:1077–1085.
22. Baldisserotto M, Ketzer de Souza JC, Pertence AP, Dora MD. Color Doppler sonography of normal and torsed testicular appendages in children. AJR Am J Roentgenol 2005;184:1287–1292.
23. Dogra VS, Gottlieb RH, Rubens DJ, Liao L. Benign intratesticular cystic lesions: US features. Radiographics 2001;21:S273–S281.
24. Altman AL, Resnick MI. Ultrasonographically guided biopsy of the prostate gland. J Ultrasound Med 2001;20:159–167.
25. Brant WE. Prostate and seminal vesicle ultrasound. In: Brant WE, ed. The Core Curriculum: Ultrasound. Philadelphia: Lippincott Williams & Wilkins, 2001: 499–509.
26. Frauscher F, Klauser A, Halpern EJ. Advances in ultrasound for detection of prostate cancer. Ultrasound Q 2002;18:135–142.

Chapter 38

Obstetric Ultrasound

William E. Brant

First Trimester
Normal Gestation
Abnormal Pregnancy
Gestational Trophoblastic Disease

Fetal Measurements and Growth

The Fetal Environment
Uterus and Adnexa in Pregnancy
Placenta and Membranes
Amniotic Fluid
Multiple Pregnancy

Fetal Anomalies
General
Central Nervous System, Face, and Neck
Chest and Heart
Abdomen
Skeleton

Imaging Methods. US is the imaging method of choice for dating the pregnancy, monitoring fetal growth, assessing fetal well-being, and evaluating fetal anatomy and maternal pelvic organs (1,2). Transvaginal sonography is particularly useful in the assessment of first-trimester pregnancy and in the demonstration of fetal anatomic structures deep in the pelvis. Modern US offers superb anatomic detail in real time, keeping up with the frequently vigorous motion of the fetus. MR is used occasionally as a supplement to US imaging when the US examination is equivocal. MR offers excellent detail of maternal pelvic organs, unobscured by bone, gas, or fat (3). Demonstration of fetal anatomy is limited by fetal motion but may be overcome by fetal sedation and fast scanning techniques. CT is the method of choice for pelvimetry, now a rarely used technique.

The obstetric US examination consists of a survey of the uterus and maternal pelvic organs, measurements of the fetus to date the pregnancy and assess fetal growth, and a survey of fetal anatomy. Standards for the performance of obstetric US examinations have been published by the American Institute of Ultrasound in Medicine (AIUM) and endorsed by the American College of Radiology (ACR) and the American College of Obstetricians and Gynecologists (ACOG) (4). In the first trimester, the location and appearance of the gestational sac are documented. The presence or absence of a yolk sac and embryo is confirmed. If an embryo is present, the crown-rump length (CRL) is measured, and fetal cardiac activity is documented. Fetal number is determined and the uterus and adnexa are examined. Second- and third-trimester sonography includes assessment of fetal life and number; fetal position; amount of amniotic fluid; placental location and appearance; fetal measurements (biparietal diameter, head circumference, abdominal circumference, femur length); and evaluation of the uterus and adnexa. Assessment of fetal anatomy includes the cerebellum, cisterna magna, lateral cerebral ventricles, choroid plexus, midline falx, cavum septi pellucidi, a four-chamber view of the heart and ventricular outflow tracts, and images of the entire spine, stomach, kidneys, bladder, umbilical cord insertion site, umbilical cord vessel number, and arms and legs. The literature refers to "level 1" obstetric US as routine or standard examinations and "level 2" (specialized or detailed) examinations as targeted to scrutinize fetal anatomy and detect anomalies.

FIRST TRIMESTER

The first trimester covers the period from conception to the end of the 13th menstrual week. This includes the entire embryonic period (0 to 10 weeks) and is a time of dynamic growth and the differentiation and development of most organ systems. The embryo and fetus have the greatest risk of maldevelopment, injury, and death during this period because of external factors (infection, drugs, radiation, etc.) or chromosome abnormalities. About 40% of implanted zygotes are menstrually aborted, and another 25% to 35% of surviving embryos will threaten to abort during the first trimester.

Normal Gestation

The presence of a pregnancy is confirmed by a positive serum β-human chorionic gonadotropin (β-hCG) test or by a positive enzyme-linked immunoassay (ELISA) urinary pregnancy test. Radioimmunoassay for serum β-hCG allows pregnancy to be detected within 2 weeks of conception (as early as 23 menstrual days) and before a normal gestational sac can be detected by either transabdominal or transvaginal US. The early gestational sac can be seen by transvaginal sonography at 3.5 to 4.5 menstrual weeks as a tiny cystic structure implanted within the echogenic decidua: the ***intradecidual sign*** (Fig. 38.1). This sign is not specific for early intrauterine pregnancy and may be mimicked by fluid collections or decidual cysts in the presence of ectopic pregnancy. A normal gestational sac is visualized by the transabdominal approach by 5 menstrual weeks. The normal gestational sac appears on US as a smoothly contoured, round or oval, fluid-containing structure positioned in the endometrial cavity near the fundus of the uterus (Table 38.1). The normal sac has an echogenic border greater than 2 mm thick, which represents the choriodecidual reaction. A ***double decidual sac sign*** is evident in about 85% of normal pregnancies. The double sac sign is produced by visualization of three layers of decidual reaction early in pregnancy (Fig. 38.2). The term *decidua* refers to the endometrium of the pregnant uterus. The *decidua vera* lines the endometrial cavity, and the *decidua capsularis* covers the gestational sac. The *decidua basalis* contributes to the formation of the

TABLE 38.1 US Characteristics of a Normal Gestational Sac[a]

Intradecidual sign—before 5 weeks' GA
Double decidual sac sign—after 5 weeks' GA (>98% of IUP)
Well-defined round/or oval anechoic sac
Echogenic decidua >2 mm thick
Position in upper uterine body midway between uterine walls
Growth in MSD >1.2 mm/day
Yolk sac 2 to 6 mm in diameter:
Always present when MSD ≥20 mm on transabdominal US
Always present when MSD ≥8 mm on transvaginal US
Embryo:
Always present when MSD ≥25 mm on transabdominal US
Always present when MSD ≥16 mm on transvaginal US

[a]The gestational sac diameter is measured in three orthogonal planes, and the measurements are averaged to calculate MSD.
IUP, intrauterine pregnancy; MSD, mean sac diameter.
Adapted from Nyberg DA, Laing FC, Filly RA, et al. Ultrasonographic differentiation of the gestational sac of early intrauterine pregnancy from the pseudogestational sac of ectopic pregnancy. Radiology 1983;146:755–759; and from Levi CS, Lyons EA, Lindsay DJ. Early diagnosis of nonviable pregnancy with endovaginal US. Radiology 1988;167:383–385.

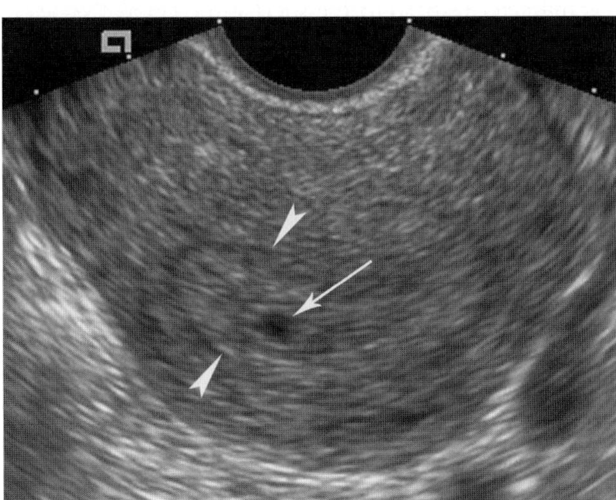

FIGURE 38.1. **Intradecidual Sign.** Transvaginal US image of the uterus in a transverse plane demonstrates a tiny gestational sac (*arrow*) implanted within the thickened decidual (between *arrowheads*). The size of the sac corresponds to a pregnancy of approximately 4 weeks' menstrual age.

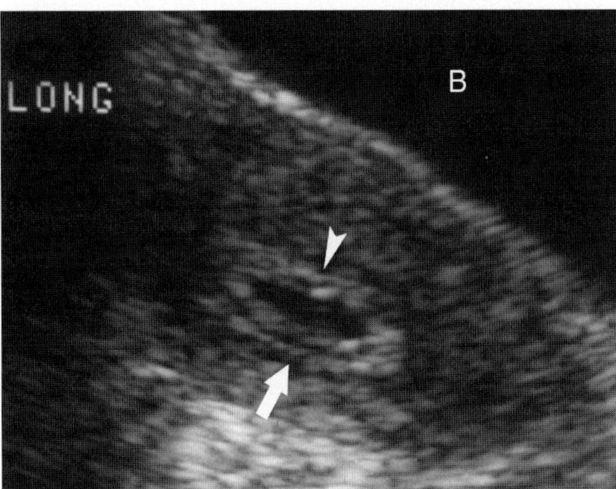

FIGURE 38.2. **Double Decidual Sac Sign.** A longitudinal image of the uterus obtained transabdominally through a filled bladder (B) demonstrates a gestational sac with two decidual layers in the uterine cavity. The two echogenic lines (*arrow*) are formed by the decidua vera lining the endometrial cavity and the decidua capsularis covering the gestational sac. The placental implantation site on the anterior aspect of the uterus (*arrowhead*) has a single echogenic stripe owing to the decidua basalis.

placenta at the site of implantation. A small amount of fluid in the endometrial cavity separates the decidua vera from the decidua capsularis, enabling visualization of the "double sac." The free margin of the gestational sac consists of chorion and decidua capsularis and is normally at least 2 mm thick. The double sac is not complete because of placental attachment to the uterine wall. A well-visualized double sac is excellent evidence of intrauterine pregnancy. An absent double sac sign is evidence of an abnormal intrauterine pregnancy or an ectopic pregnancy.

The ***yolk sac*** is a 2- to 6-mm-diameter, spherical, cystic structure (Fig. 38.3) that is connected to the midgut of the embryo by a thin stalk, the *vitelline duct*. A Meckel diverticulum is a remnant of the connection of the vitelline duct (also called the *omphalomesenteric duct*) to the distal ileum. The yolk sac is the earliest site of blood cell formation in the embryo. It floats freely in fluid between the amniotic and chorionic membranes. It is generally the earliest structure visualized within the gestational sac and serves as definitive evidence of early pregnancy. The yolk sac should always be visualized in normal pregnancy in gestational sacs of 20-mm mean sac diameter by transabdominal US or 8-mm mean sac diameter by transvaginal US.

The earliest demonstration of the embryo is the ***double bleb sign***, which is produced by the amniotic sac and the yolk sac with the embryonic disc between them (Fig. 38.4). Embryos as small as 2 mm can be detected by transvaginal US. The earliest embryonic cardiac activity can be detected by careful inspection of the embryonic disc by real-time US. Transvaginal sonography may demonstrate tiny normal embryos (<5 mm) in which cardiac activity cannot be confirmed. Cardiac activity should always be seen transvaginally in embryos that can be visualized by transabdominal US.

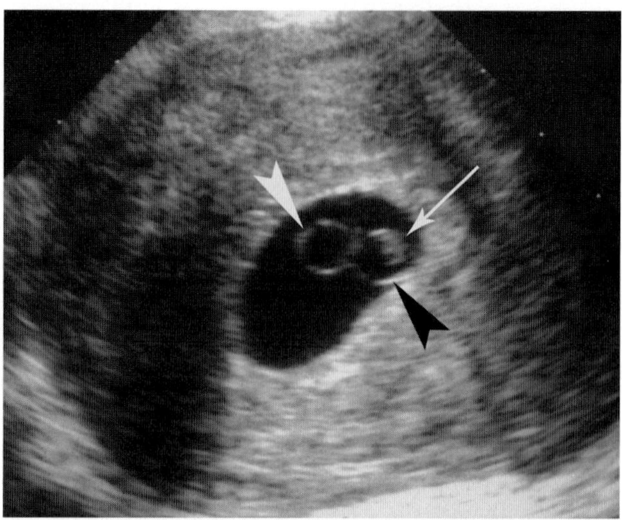

FIGURE 38.4. **Double Bleb Sign.** The double bleb is formed by the yolk sac (*white arrowhead*) and the amniotic sac (*black arrowhead*) suspended in the fluid of the early chorionic sac. The embryo is seen as a tiny disclike structure (*arrow*) within the amniotic sac. Early cardiac activity can frequently be observed in the tiny embryo.

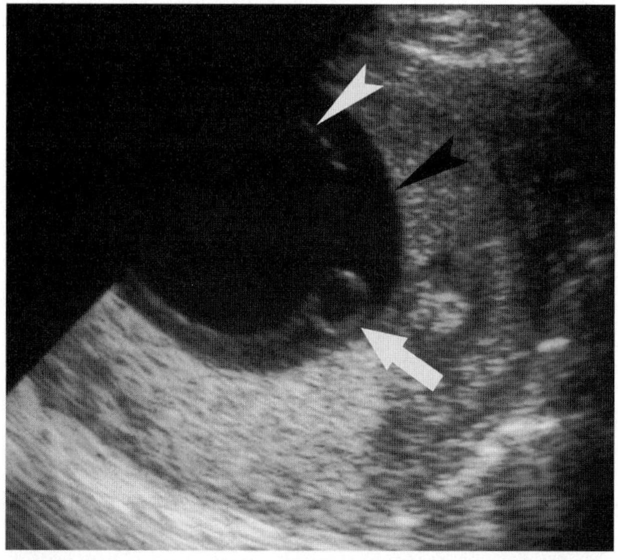

FIGURE 38.3. **Yolk Sac.** The yolk sac (*arrow*) is seen within the gestational sac by transvaginal US. The normal yolk sac is less than 6 mm in diameter, spherical, and fluid filled with a thin wall. The yolk sac is in the fluid space between the thin membrane of the amnion (*white arrowhead*) and the chorion (*black arrowhead*), which defines the limit of fluid within the gestational sac.

Gestational age in the first trimester is estimated by measuring the mean diameter of the gestational sac (mean sac diameter [MSD]) or the CRL of the embryo or fetus. A normal gestational sac grows at a rate of approximately 1.2 mm/day MSD.

Patients who present with vaginal bleeding and pelvic pain during the first trimester are commonly referred for US examination. The differential diagnosis is listed in Table 38.2.

TABLE 38.2 Differential Diagnosis of Vaginal Bleeding in the First Trimester

Spontaneous abortion
Anembryonic pregnancy
Embryonic demise
Demise of a twin
Ectopic pregnancy
Subchorionic hemorrhage
Implantation bleeding
Gestational trophoblastic disease

Abnormal Pregnancy

Abortion is the termination of pregnancy before 20 weeks' gestational age. *Spontaneous abortion* is the termination of pregnancy by natural causes. Approximately 10% to 15% of all known pregnancies end in spontaneous abortion. Up to 60% of spontaneous abortions have chromosomal abnormalities. A number of clinical terms are used to describe abortion. *Threatened abortion* refers to the occurrence of vaginal bleeding and uterine cramping with a closed cervical os in early pregnancy. Threatened abortion complicates roughly 25% of all pregnancies. *Inevitable abortion* presents with cervical dilation and fetal or placental tissues within the cervical os. With *complete abortion,* all uterine contents have been expelled. *Incomplete abortion* refers to the presence of residual products of conception within the uterus. In *missed abortion,* the fetus has died but remains within the uterus. *Habitual abortion* is defined as three or more successive spontaneous abortions. *Anembryonic pregnancy* or *blighted ovum* is a pregnancy in which the embryo has died and is no longer visible or never developed.

"Empty" Gestational Sac. A gestational sac without an embryo demonstrated by US is compatible with a very early intrauterine pregnancy or a nonviable intrauterine pregnancy (anembryonic pregnancy) (Fig. 38.5). An empty gestational sac must be differentiated from a pseudogestational sac associated with ectopic pregnancy (Fig. 38.6). A gestational sac is considered to be abnormal if it demonstrates the following features (Table 38.3): large size without an embryo or yolk sac, distorted shape, irregular contour, thin or weak choriodecidual reaction, absence of a double decidual sac, or abnormal position. Any one of the major criteria or three of the minor criteria are considered diagnostic. Large sac size without visualized yolk sac

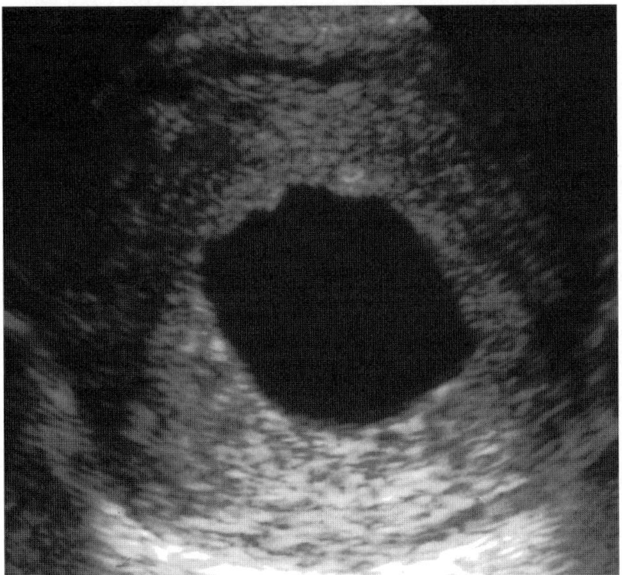

FIGURE 38.5. **Anembryonic Pregnancy.** An empty gestational sac measuring 31 mm in mean sac diameter (MSD) is demonstrated within the uterus by transvaginal US. The margin of the sac is irregular in contour and the decidual reaction is poorly defined. In a normal intrauterine pregnancy, a yolk sac should always be demonstrable by transvaginal US when the MSD exceeds 8 mm and an embryo should be seen when the MSD exceeds 16 mm.

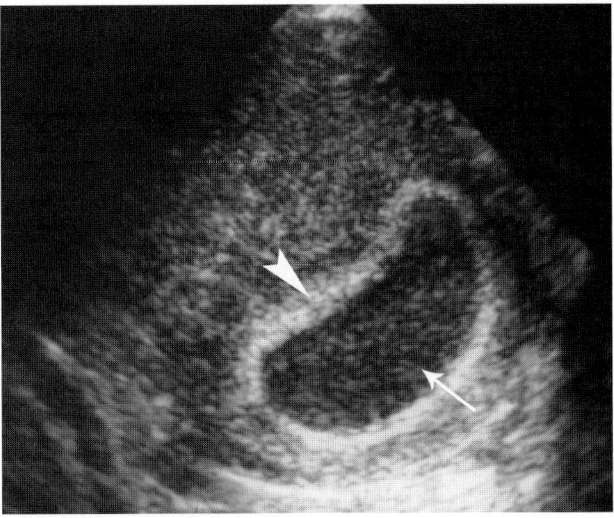

FIGURE 38.6. **Pseudogestational Sac.** Fluid within the endometrial cavity (*arrow*) in a patient with an ectopic pregnancy mimics an intrauterine gestational sac. The intrauterine fluid is echogenic, indicative of blood. The decidual reaction (*arrowhead*) will be present whether the pregnancy is intrauterine or ectopic.

TABLE 38.3 US Characteristics of an Abnormal Gestational Sac[a]

Major criteria
Absence of yolk sac when:
MSD $\geq$20 mm on transabdominal US
MSD $\geq$8 mm on transvaginal US
Absence of embryo when:
MSD $\geq$25 mm on transabdominal US
MSD $\geq$16 mm on transvaginal US
Distorted sac shape
Growth <1 mm MSD/day
Minor criteria
Irregular sac contour
Thin decidual reaction <2 mm
Weak decidual echo amplitude
Absent double decidual sac sign
Sac positioned low in the uterus

[a]The gestational sac diameter is measured in three orthogonal planes, and the measurements are averaged to calculate the mean sac diameter (MSD).

Adapted from Nyberg DA, Laing FC, Filly RA, et al. Ultrasonographic differentiation of the gestational sac of early intrauterine pregnancy from the pseudogestational sac of ectopic pregnancy. Radiology 1983;146: 755–759; and from Levi CS, Lyons EA, Lindsay DJ. Early diagnosis of nonviable pregnancy with endovaginal US. Radiology 1988;167:383–385.

or embryo and a distorted sac contour have a reported 100% specificity and positive predictive value for identification of nonviable pregnancy. The original criteria described for transabdominal US have been refined by the use of transvaginal transducers, which improve visualization of anatomic detail. Most authors recommend allowing a 1- to 2-mm margin of error and repeating any equivocal scans in several days. Growth of the gestational sac of less than 1 mm/day MSD is strong evidence of abnormal sac development.

Embryonic or fetal demise is diagnosed by US confirmation of the absence of cardiac activity. Absence of cardiac activity in a fetus or an embryo large enough to be visualized by transabdominal US is definitive evidence of death. Because of the increased sensitivity of transvaginal US in demonstrating cardiac activity, all cases of suspected demise of small embryos should be confirmed by transvaginal US, which may demonstrate cardiac activity, even in embryos as small as 1.5 mm CRL. Transvaginal US may also visualize small, normal, living embryos (<5 mm CRL) without demonstrating cardiac activity. Absence of cardiac activity in embryos larger than 5 mm on transvaginal US is considered diagnostic of embryonic demise (missed abortion). Embryos smaller than 5 mm without cardiac activity should be rescanned in a few days to confirm viability. M-mode US is used to document visualized cardiac activity.

Quantitative serum β-hCG levels have been correlated with US findings to assist in the identification of abnormal pregnancies. Great caution is advised, however, because of differences in the way that individual laboratories report serum β-hCG results and in the wide variation in values obtained by different laboratories. Discriminatory levels will vary with the resolution of the US scanner used and with the laboratory reporting the hormonal assay.

Ectopic pregnancy occurs in only 1.4% of all pregnancies, but it is the major cause of pregnancy-related maternal deaths (5). Misdiagnosis of ectopic pregnancy remains one of the most common areas for medical malpractice litigation. Patients at high risk for ectopic pregnancy include those with a history of pelvic inflammatory disease, tubal surgery, endometriosis, ovulation induction, previous ectopic pregnancy, or use of intrauterine device for contraception. Most (95%) ectopic pregnancies occur in the fallopian tube, most commonly in the isthmic portion. Interstitial ectopic pregnancies, which develop in the portion of the tube passing through the uterine wall, may grow to large size before rupture, resulting in catastrophic hemorrhage. Additional sites for ectopic implantation include the abdominal cavity, ovary, and cervix. All patients with a positive pregnancy test (serum β-hCG) and vaginal bleeding, pelvic pain, or adnexal mass must be considered at risk for ectopic pregnancy (6).

A completely confident diagnosis of ectopic pregnancy can be made sonographically only when a living embryo or

TABLE 38.4 Risk of Ectopic Pregnancy as Determined by US Findings

Finding	*Approximate Risk*
IUP confirmed	
General population	1 in 30,000
Patient taking ovulation-inducing drugs	1 in 6,000–7,000
IUP not confirmed	43%
Living ectopic fetus	100%
Adnexal mass	83%
Moderate/large fluid	83%
Adnexal mass + pelvic fluid	94%
Normal pelvic sonogram	8%

IUP, intrauterine pregnancy.
Adapted from Mahony BS, Filly RA, Nyberg, DA, Callen PW. Sonographic evaluation of ectopic pregnancy. J Ultrasound Med 1985;4:221–228.

a gestational sac containing a yolk sac is positively demonstrated to be in a position outside of the uterus (18% to 26% of ectopic pregnancies) (7). Transvaginal US increases the possibility of demonstrating a live ectopic pregnancy. In any other circumstance, we are dealing with a situation of relative risk (Table 38.4). When an intrauterine pregnancy is documented by US, the risk of coexisting ectopic pregnancy is extremely low, estimated at 1 in 30,000. Concurrent intrauterine and extrauterine pregnancies do occur, however, especially in patients taking ovulation-inducing drugs, in whom the risk of ectopic pregnancy is increased to 1 in 6,000 to 7,000. When an adnexal mass other than a corpus luteal cyst is demonstrated, or when a moderate or large amount of fluid is present in the pelvis, the risk of ectopic pregnancy is high. Even when the US examination is entirely normal but without definitive evidence of intrauterine pregnancy, a patient with a positive pregnancy test remains at risk for ectopic pregnancy. The role of US, then, is to demonstrate findings that determine relative risk. This assessment, in conjunction with clinical history and physical examination, determines the next step in the patient's evaluation.

US findings in ectopic pregnancy include demonstration of an extrauterine gestational sac appearing as a fluid-containing structure with an echogenic ring, the ***tubal ring sign*** (40% to 68% of ectopic pregnancies) (Fig. 38.7) (7). A living or dead embryo might or might not be evident. The ectopic gestational sac must be differentiated from a corpus luteal cyst, which develops on the ovary at the site of ovulation. The corpus luteal cyst appears as a thin-walled cyst projecting eccentrically from the ovary. Clotted blood from hemorrhage within a corpus luteal cyst may simulate an embryo. A key differentiating finding is whether the cystic mass arises from the ovary. Most ectopic pregnancies occur within the fallopian tube and are separate from the ovary. Implantation of ectopic pregnancy on the ovary is a rare event. Corpus luteal cysts always arise from the

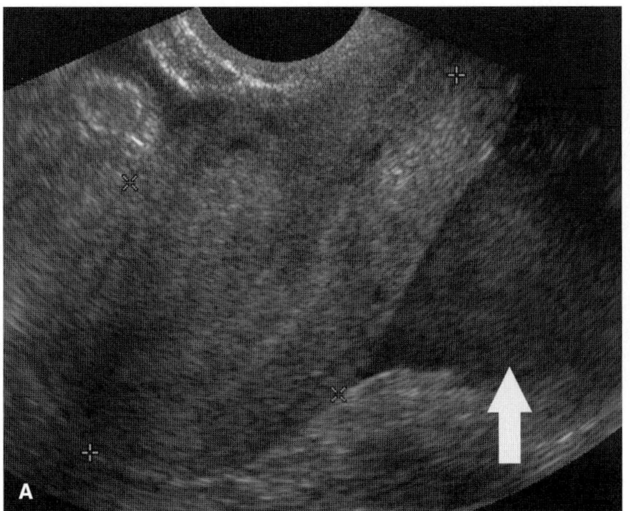

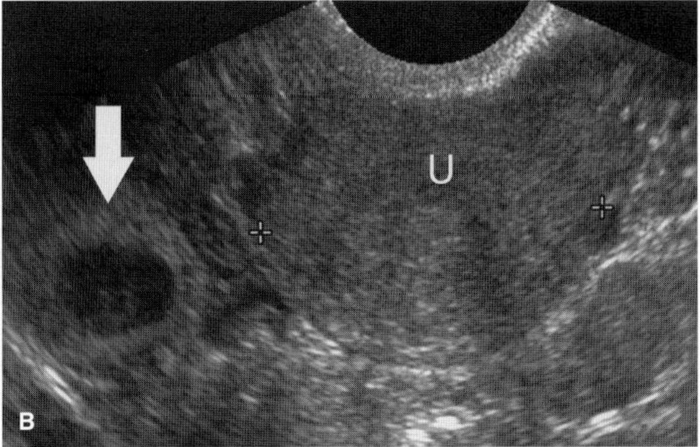

FIGURE 38.7. **Ectopic Pregnancy. A.** Transvaginal US in a longitudinal plane demonstrates an empty uterus (between *calipers*) in a pregnant patient. Echogenic blood (*arrow*) distends the cul-de-sac. **B.** Transverse transvaginal image reveals a tubal ring sign (*arrow*) in the right adnexa, which is highly indicative of ectopic pregnancy. u, uterus (between *calipers*).

ovary. Hematosalpinx or ruptured ectopic pregnancy may appear as an amorphous solid or complex adnexal mass lacking an embryo or sac. Blood in the cul-de-sac usually appears as echogenic fluid, but it may be entirely echolucent if liquid, or echogenic and solid-appearing if clotted. Stimulation of the endometrium by the hormones associated with the ectopic pregnancy causes thickening and increased echogenicity of the endometrium, termed the "decidual reaction." Blood in the uterine cavity produces a ***pseudogestational sac*** in up to 20% of ectopic pregnancies (Fig. 38.6). A true gestational sac is differentiated from a "pseudosac" by the presence of a yolk sac or embryo. A double decidual sac sign suggests a true gestational sac, but is not totally reliable because some pseudosacs may also show a double decidual sac sign. Doppler studies demonstrate absent or minimal peritrophoblastic flow with pseudosacs and high-velocity, low-impedance flow with true gestational sacs.

Subchorionic hemorrhage is a common finding in the bleeding pregnant patient before 20 weeks' gestational age (5). All cases are believed to develop because of venous bleeding from separation of the margin of the placenta. The hematoma collects preferentially beneath the chorion because the chorion is more easily separated from the myometrium than is the placenta. Patients may be asymptomatic if the hematoma remains confined, or they may present with vaginal bleeding if the hematoma leaks through the cervix. In most patients, a subchorionic hematoma is an innocent finding; however, an increased rate of spontaneous abortion has been reported in some series associated with large hematomas (>60 mL), advanced maternal age (>35 years), and early gestational age (<8 weeks). The US appearance of the hemorrhage varies with age (Fig. 38.8). Acute bleeding is anechoic to hypoechoic. With clotting, it becomes hyperechoic and heterogeneous. With lysis, the hematoma reverts to being hypoechoic to anechoic.

Implantation bleeding is a nonspecific term that refers to small collections of blood at the site of attachment of the chorion to the endometrium. These are in essence small areas of subchorionic hemorrhage that occur early

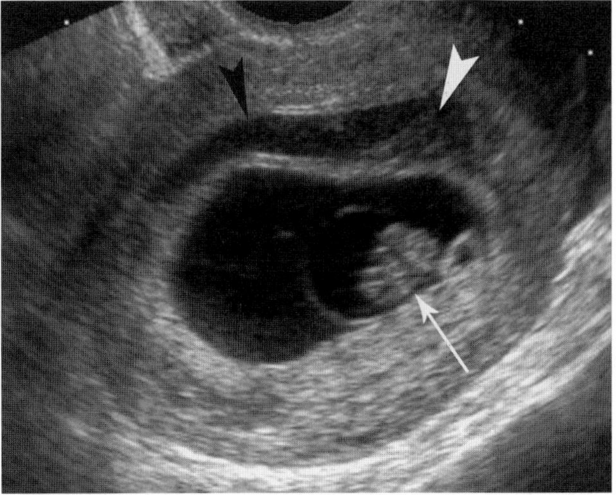

FIGURE 38.8. **Subchorionic Hemorrhage.** Hemorrhage (*black arrowhead*) is seen in the uterine cavity between the decidua capsularis and the decidua vera. Some of the blood is clotted and appears more echogenic (*white arrowhead*) than the liquid blood. A live embryo (*arrow*) was present within its amniotic sac.

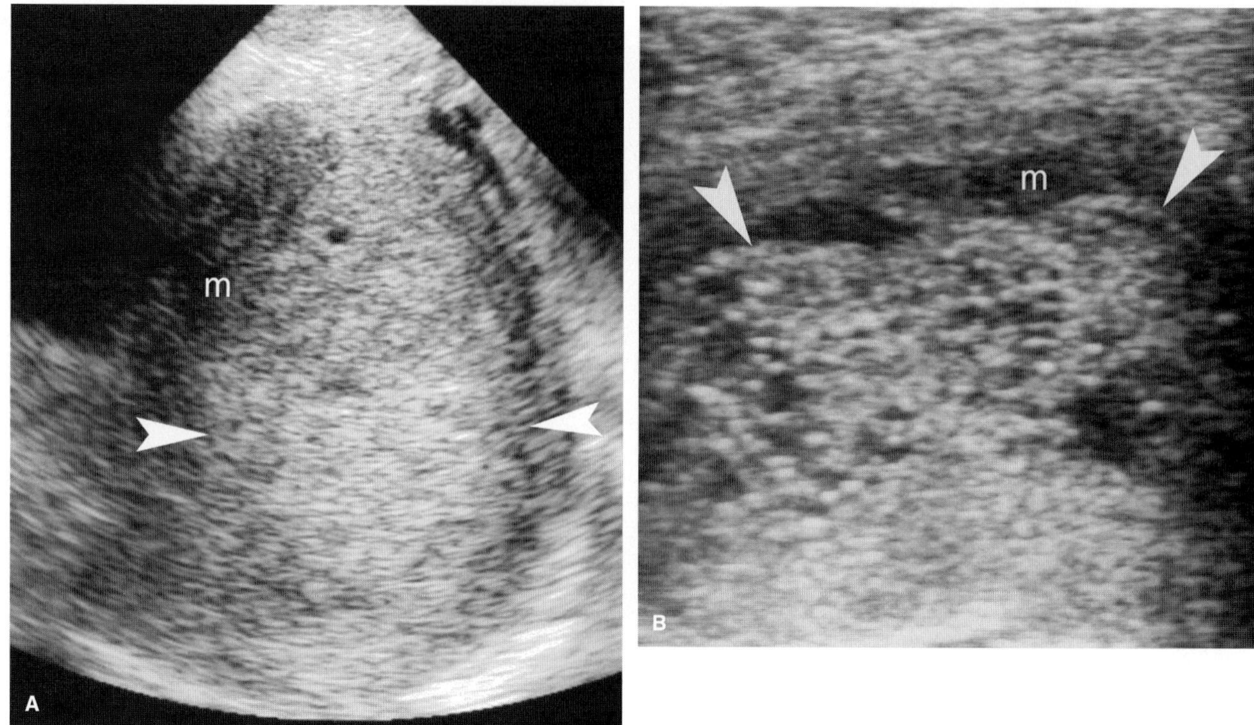

FIGURE 38.9. **Hydatidiform Mole. A.** Transvaginal US shows the "snowstorm" appearance of a molar pregnancy (between *arrowheads*) filling the uterine cavity in the first trimester. **B.** In another patient examined early in the second trimester, more discrete cysts are seen within the molar tissue (*arrowheads*). m, myometrium.

in pregnancy. US follow-up is warranted to assess for progression.

Gestational Trophoblastic Disease

Gestational trophoblastic disease is a group of neoplasms that range from benign to highly malignant. All are derived from abnormal placental tissues and occur as sequelae to pregnancy. Both benign and malignant tumors produce β-hCG. Marked elevation of β-hCG levels is characteristic, and serial measurement is a sensitive and reliable indicator of tumor activity. Gestational trophoblastic disease complicates about 1 in 1,000 to 2,000 pregnancies in the United States but has a much higher incidence in East Asia and in Latin America (8).

Hydatidiform mole is the most common (80%) and most benign form of the disease but maintains a potential for malignant sequelae. The placenta demonstrates edema and proliferation of trophoblasts. The villi become swollen and vesicular, resembling a bunch of grapes. Patients present with hyperemesis, pregnancy-induced hypertension, and vaginal bleeding. The uterus may be enlarged (50%), normal (35%), or small (15%) for dates. Two types of hydatidiform mole exist. *Complete mole* (classic mole) (70%) involves the entire placenta, lacks a fetus, and is diploid in karyotype. *Partial mole* (30%) involves only a portion of the placenta, is associated with an abnormal fetus, and is triploid in karyotype (owing to fertilization of an ovum by two sperm). This condition is lethal to the fetus. Rarely, a normal fetus may coexist with a complete mole in a twin pregnancy. Prognosis for the normal fetus in these cases is grim because of maternal complications of the mole.

US in complete mole classically demonstrates the uterus to be filled with innumerable tiny cysts, often described as a "snowstorm" appearance in the first trimester because of the multiple echogenic foci (Fig. 38.9) (8). Discrete vesicles 2 to 30 mm in size are more commonly seen in the second trimester. Partial mole demonstrates vesicular changes in only a portion of the placenta. The associated triploid fetus has multiple anomalies. Early in the first trimester, the classic appearance may not be evident. Molar pregnancy may appear as an anechoic fluid collection that mimics anembryonic pregnancy, or it may appear echogenic and solid. Transvaginal US helps to demonstrate the characteristic vesicles. *Theca lutein cysts* are seen as large, septated, bilateral cysts that massively enlarge the ovaries in up to 50% of cases (Fig. 38.10). Theca lutein cysts are caused by ovarian hyperstimulation resulting from high circulating levels of β-hCG.

Invasive mole (chorioadenoma destruens) refers to invasion of molar tissue into, but usually not beyond, the

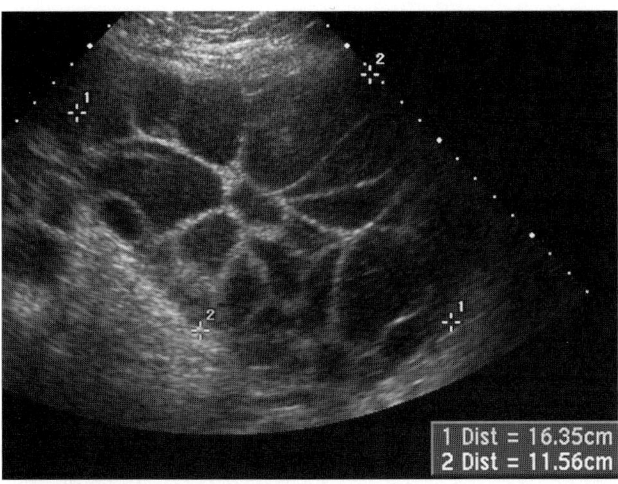

FIGURE 38.10. **Theca Lutein Cysts.** Transabdominal image demonstrates the ovary (between *calipers*) to be greatly enlarged by numerous cysts in this patient with a twin pregnancy following infertility therapy. The β-hCG level was greatly elevated.

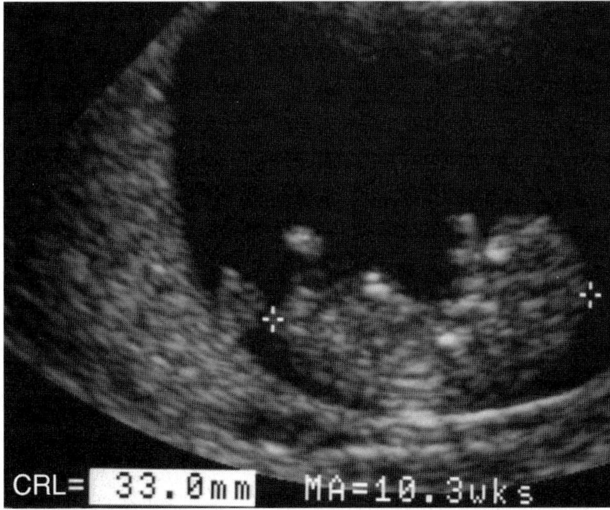

FIGURE 38.11. **Crown-Rump Length (CRL).** The CRL is measured from the top of the head to the bottom of the torso (between *cursors*).

myometrium. It is seen in about 10% of patients and is usually evident after treatment for hydatidiform mole.

Choriocarcinoma is a highly aggressive malignancy that forms only trophoblasts without any villous structure. Choriocarcinoma is locally invasive, spreads into the myometrium and parametrium, and hematogenously metastasizes to any site in the body. β-hCG levels that rise or plateau in the 8 to 10 weeks following evacuation of molar pregnancy should suggest invasive or metastatic gestational trophoblastic disease.

US is relatively insensitive in demonstrating a locally invasive mole. Nodules in the myometrium are suggestive, but the sonographic appearance overlaps that of degenerating fibroids and ovarian dysgerminomas. CT and MR demonstrate uterine enlargement, focal myometrial masses, dilated vessels, and areas of hemorrhage and necrosis within highly vascular tumor. Metastases may be found in any organ.

FETAL MEASUREMENTS AND GROWTH

Dating the pregnancy and determining the appropriateness of fetal growth are essential to obstetric care. Clinical dating is based on history of the mother's last menstrual period (LMP) and bimanual assessment of uterine size. Sonographic dating is based on measurements of the gestational sac and the embryo or fetus. Serial measurements of fetal parameters are used to document growth. By convention, pregnancies are dated from the first day of the LMP. The terms *gestational age* (GA), which is the clinical standard, and *menstrual age* are usually considered to be synonymous terms and are based on the average 28-day menstrual cycle. Conception is assumed to occur 14 days following the LMP. Term is 40 weeks, with an acceptable range of 37 to 42 weeks.

Gestational sac size is used in the first trimester to estimate GA when no embryo is visualized. The gestational sac diameter is measured in three orthogonal planes, and the results are averaged. The MSD is accurate to within approximately 1 week's menstrual age.

Crown-rump length is measured from the top of the head to the bottom of the torso of the visualized embryo or fetus (Fig. 38.11). The CRL is useful until about 10 to 12 weeks' GA, when other fetal measurements become more accurate. Charts provide GA estimations accurate to approximately 0.5 week's menstrual age.

Biparietal diameter (BPD) is measured on an axial image of the fetal head at the level of the third ventricle and thalamus (Fig. 38.12). By convention, the measurement is made from the outer table of the near cranium to the inner table of the far cranium. The measurement is affected by head shape and provides an inaccurate estimate of GA if significant *dolichocephaly* (elongated skull) or *brachycephaly* (round skull) is present.

Head circumference (HC) is the outer perimeter of the fetal cranium, measured in the same plane as the BPD (Fig. 38.12). The HC measurement is relatively independent of head shape.

Abdominal circumference (AC) is the outer perimeter of the fetal abdomen, measured on an axial plane image at the level of the intrahepatic portion of the umbilical vein (Fig. 38.13).

Femur length (FL) is the measurement of the ossified portion of the femoral diaphysis (Fig. 38.14). The entire femur must be imaged, and the femoral shaft must be centered in the beam so that it casts an acoustic shadow.

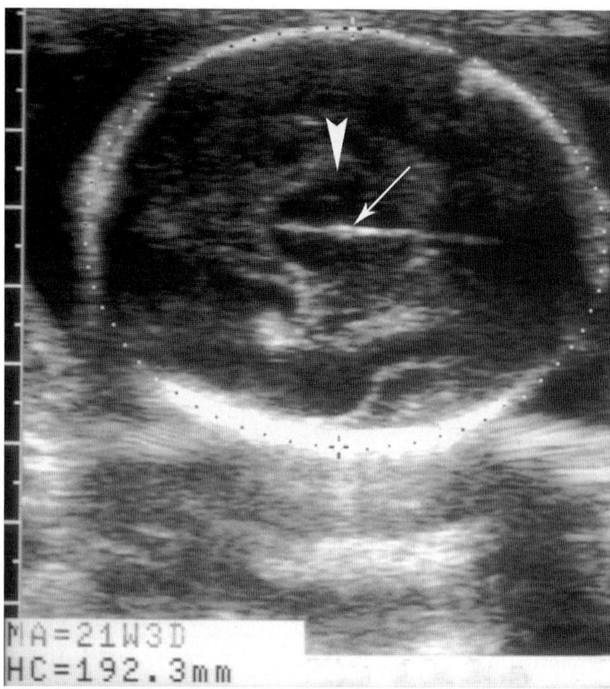

FIGURE 38.12. **Transthalamic (Biparietal Diameter/Head Circumference) Plane.** Axial image of the fetal cranium demonstrates the paired thalami (*arrowhead*) on either side of the midline third ventricle (*long arrow*). The biparietal diameter is measured in this plane from the outer surface of the near cranium to the inner surface of the far cranium. The head circumference is measured in this same plane as shown.

GA estimates are most accurate in early pregnancy and become progressively less accurate as the pregnancy advances. The composite age, calculated by averaging the GA estimates of multiple parameters, is more accurate

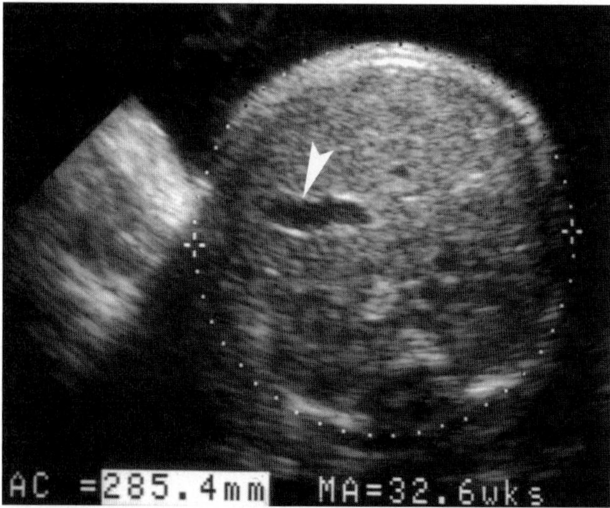

FIGURE 38.13. **Abdominal Circumference.** The correct plane of measurement of the abdominal circumference is an axial plane showing a round abdomen at the level of the umbilical vein (*arrowhead*) junction with the left portal vein.

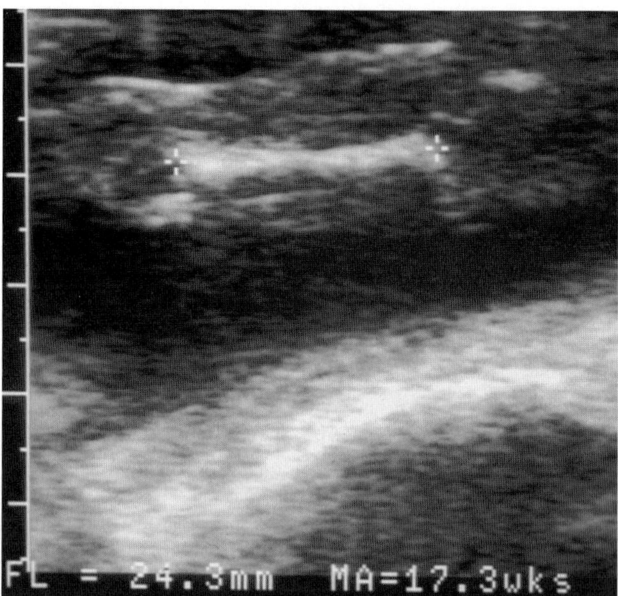

FIGURE 38.14. **Femur Length.** The femur length is the measurement of the ossified portion of the femoral diaphysis (between *calipers*).

than any single parameter because fetal anomalies may make individual parameters inaccurate for estimation of GA. Body parts with structural anomalies should be excluded from the composite GA estimation. The composite of BPD, HC, AC, and FL measurements predicts GA, which is accurate to about 1.2 weeks at 12 to 18 weeks, but the composite age is accurate to only about 3.1 weeks at 36 to 42 weeks. GA is assigned at the time of the first US and is not changed thereafter. All subsequent US examinations are compared with the first examination to assess fetal growth.

Intrauterine Growth Retardation (IUGR). Fetuses with impaired intrauterine growth have an increased risk of intrauterine demise and a perinatal mortality rate four to eight times greater than normal-sized fetuses (9). Half the survivors have significant morbidity, including intrapartum fetal distress, hypoglycemia, hypocalcemia, meconium aspiration pneumonia, impaired immune function, retarded neurologic development, and learning disabilities. A fetus or newborn is considered small for gestational age (SGA) if its weight is below the 10th percentile for GA. This definition will encompass normal infants who are constitutionally small as well as infants with IUGR who are pathologically small. The challenge is to separate the growth-restricted fetuses from those who are normal. Impaired growth may be caused by factors that are intrinsic to the fetus or related to a hostile fetal environment (Table 38.5). Fetuses with intrinsic insults have fixed defects and will not benefit from early delivery. The pattern of growth impairment occurs early in the second trimester and tends to be symmetric, in that the head, abdomen,

TABLE 38.5 Causes of Intrauterine Growth Retardation

Intrinsic causes
- Chromosome abnormalities (trisomy, triploidy)
- Intrauterine infection (rubella, CMV, toxoplasmosis)
- Structural abnormalities (congenital heart disease)
- Teratogen exposure

Extrinsic causes
- Primary placental insufficiency
- Maternal hypertension
- Chronic maternal diseases (anemia, renal failure)
- Maternal malnutrition
- Maternal smoking, alcohol, and drug abuse
- Multiple gestation

CMV, Cytomegalovirus.

and femur are all proportionally small. Fetuses exposed to an extrinsically impaired growth environment will usually benefit from therapy that commonly includes early delivery. Growth impairment occurs in the late second and third trimesters and tends to be asymmetric, in that the fetal abdomen is disproportionally small relative to the head and femur. The AC is small because of diminished glycogen stores in the fetal liver and decreased subcutaneous fat.

Many US criteria have been proposed to diagnose IUGR, but none individually are highly accurate. A multiparameter approach using estimated fetal weight (EFW), amniotic fluid volume, and the presence or absence of maternal hypertension has the greatest accuracy for diagnosis (9). The first step in diagnosis is to establish an accurate GA. An early US provides assignment of GA, which should not be changed on subsequent examinations. When the initial US is not obtained until the third trimester, GA is assigned on the basis of BPD, HC, and FL measurements, recognizing the imprecision of GA estimations in the third trimester. EFW is determined from established charts by measurement of AC and BPD, or AC and FL. The error range of these weight predictions is large: 15% to 18% for 95% of cases and even greater for 5% of cases. IUGR is diagnosed confidently when the EFW is below the sixth percentile for GA and is excluded when the EFW is above the 20th percentile for GA. When the EFW is between the sixth and 20th percentiles, IUGR is diagnosed if oligohydramnios or maternal hypertension is present, and it is likely not present if the amniotic fluid volume is normal or elevated and the mother is normotensive. US follow-up of fetuses with IUGR should be performed weekly or biweekly and include measurement of growth parameters, assessment of amniotic fluid volume, biophysical profile score, and umbilical cord Doppler. Normal fetal weight gain in the third trimester is 100 to 200 g/week. An amniotic fluid index of 5 cm or less (oligohydramnios) is strongly predictive of poor outcome.

Biophysical profile is a test to identify compromised fetuses. Four parameters assess for acute hypoxia: reactive fetal heart rate (nonstress test), respiratory activity, gross motor movements, and fetal tone. One parameter, the amniotic fluid volume, evaluates for chronic hypoxia. A variety of different techniques is used for assessment and scoring. A score of 2 is given for a normal response, and 0 is given for an abnormal response. The fetus is at extreme risk for fetal demise within 1 week with a total score of 0 or 2, and it is at no immediate risk with a total score of 8 or 10.

Umbilical cord Doppler US is not accurate in the diagnosis of IUGR, but it is valuable for monitoring the pregnancy and detecting fetal compromise. Spectral Doppler tracings are obtained from the umbilical artery in a free-floating loop of umbilical cord. Evidence of high vascular resistance in the placenta, manifest by a systolic-to-diastolic ratio (see Chapter 40) of 4.0 or greater, or the absence of forward flow in diastole, is strongly predictive of severe fetal compromise. Reversal of flow in diastole is a particularly ominous finding, indicative of high risk for fetal demise within 1 to 7 days if the fetus is left in utero (Fig. 38.15).

Fetal macrosomia is defined as estimated fetal weight above the 90th percentile for GA or a fetal weight above 4,000 g. Risk factors include maternal diabetes, maternal obesity, previous history of macrosomic infant, and

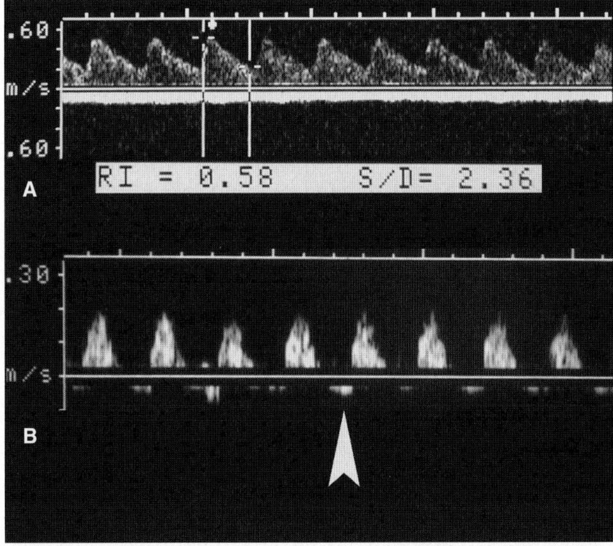

FIGURE 38.15. **Umbilical Artery Doppler. A.** Spectral Doppler tracing from an umbilical artery shows a normal pattern with forward flow maintained throughout diastole and a low vascular resistance with resistive index (RI) = 0.58. **B.** Spectral Doppler in a severely growth-retarded fetus shows a high vascular resistance pattern with flow toward the placenta during systole and reversal of blood flow direction during diastole (*arrowhead*). This finding is highly indicative of severe fetal distress. This fetus died 4 days after this examination.

excessive weight gain during pregnancy. Complications of macrosomia are manifest at delivery and include shoulder dystocia, traumatic delivery, fractures, brachial plexus injury, perinatal asphyxia, neonatal hypoglycemia, and meconium aspiration.

THE FETAL ENVIRONMENT

Uterus and Adnexa in Pregnancy

Uterine leiomyomas (fibroids) are the most common solid pelvic masses encountered during pregnancy (10). Fibroids commonly enlarge and undergo cystic degeneration induced by hormonal stimulation as the pregnancy advances. They are associated with bleeding, premature uterine contractions, malpresentation, and mechanical obstruction during labor. Leiomyomas must be differentiated from uterine contractions. Contractions are transient, although they may persist up to an hour. Contractions typically appear homogeneous and isoechoic with the myometrium. They bulge the inner, but generally not the outer, margin of the uterine wall. Leiomyomas are persistent, are more heterogeneous, may have calcifications, and typically bulge the outer margin of the uterine wall. Doppler US demonstrates splaying of myometrial vessels around leiomyomas but no vessel displacement in areas of myometrial contraction.

Corpus luteal cysts are the most common cystic pelvic masses found in pregnancy. Internal hemorrhage causes enlargement up to 10 to 15 cm, internal echoes, and septations. Most of these cysts regress by 16 to 18 weeks' GA. Differential diagnosis includes benign cystic teratoma, cystadenoma, hydrosalpinx, and paraovarian cyst (10).

Theca lutein cysts form because of an exaggerated corpus luteum response to high levels of β-hCG. They appear as bilateral multicystic enlargement of the ovaries. They occur with gestational trophoblastic disease, pregnancy with more than one fetus, or in association with the use of ovulation-inducing drugs (Fig. 38.10).

Cervical incompetence may be congenital or may result from cervical lacerations, excessive cervical dilation, or therapeutic abortion. The incompetent cervix is incapable of retaining a pregnancy to term. Preterm delivery is the single most common cause of a poor neonatal outcome. An obstetric history of recurrent loss of pregnancy in the second trimester establishes the diagnosis. US is used to measure and follow cervical length and appearance. Scans are best performed transvaginally or translabially from the introitus with the bladder empty. A full urinary bladder compresses the lower uterus and falsely elongates the length of the cervix. The normal cervical length is 26 to 50 mm throughout gestation. Cervical length is measured in the sagittal plane between the internal os (marked by a V-shaped notch) and the external os (marked by a triangular echodensity) (Fig. 38.16). The endocervical canal is seen as a thin hypoechoic or hyperechoic line. The relative risk of preterm delivery increases as cervical length decreases, with the greatest risk for cervical lengths under 3.0 cm. Cervical dilation is measured between the anterior and posterior surface of the cervical canal. Dilation of the cervical canal >8 mm is indicative of cervical incompetence. Membranes may be seen bulging into the cervical canal. Sutures associated with cervical cerclage used to treat cervical incompetence are seen on US as echogenic linear structures with acoustic shadowing.

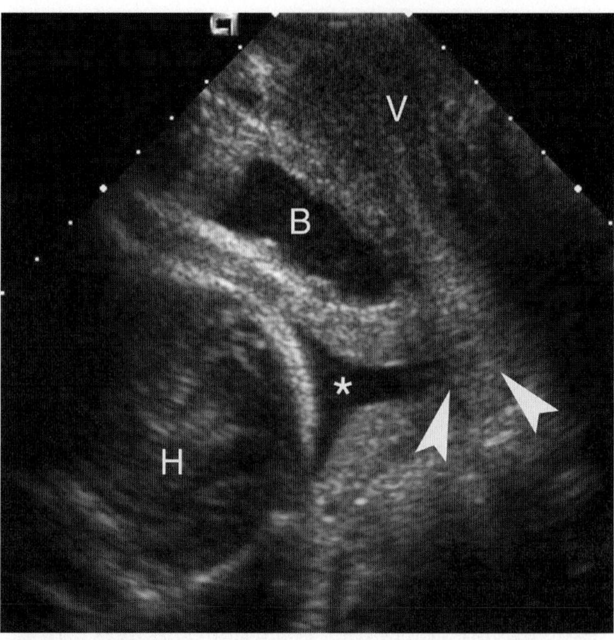

FIGURE 38.16. **Cervical Incompetence.** The cervix is best evaluated with a translabial view with the bladder (B) empty. The transducer is aimed down the long axis of the vagina (V). The cervix, measured between the internal os and the external os (*arrowheads*), is shortened to 9 mm in this patient with a history of multiple spontaneous abortions in the second trimester. The cervix is also dilated, allowing amniotic fluid (*asterisk*) to enter the endocervical canal. The fetal head (H) is presenting at the internal cervical os.

Placenta and Membranes

Normal placenta is first apparent on US at about 8 weeks as a focal thickening at the periphery of the gestational sac (2). The disclike shape of the placenta becomes evident by 12 weeks, and by 18 weeks the placenta is finely granular and homogeneous, with a smooth covering chorionic membrane along its fetal surface. The *retroplacental complex* of decidual and myometrial veins forms a prominent sonographic landmark (Fig. 38.17). As the gestation advances, the placenta becomes more heterogeneous, with focal echolucencies owing to venous lakes and areas of fibrin deposition. Septations become prominent

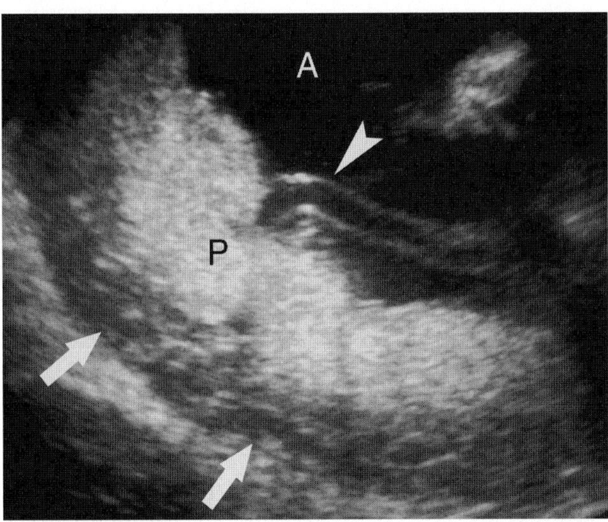

FIGURE 38.17. **Normal Placenta.** A transabdominal scan demonstrates a normal placenta (P) and the insertion site of the cord onto the placenta (*arrowhead*). The retroplacental complex of veins (*arrows*) appears as a network of tubular lucencies beneath the placenta. A, amniotic cavity.

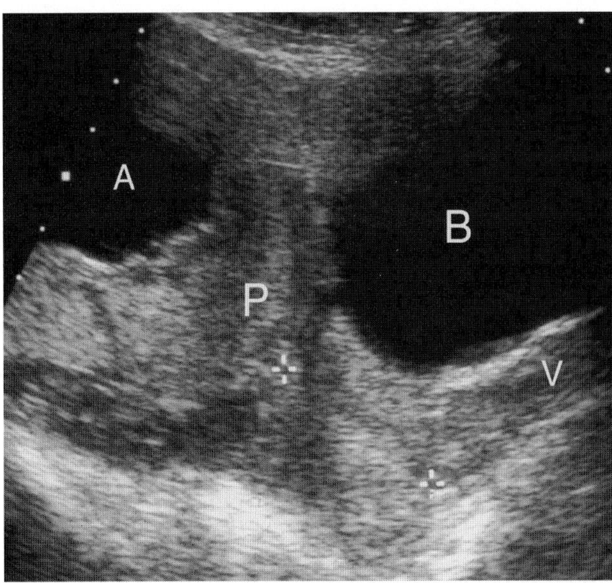

FIGURE 38.18. **Placenta Previa.** Transabdominal US shows a normal cervix (between *cursors*) measuring 34 mm. The placenta (P) covers the internal os. A, amniotic cavity; B, bladder; V, vagina.

US features throughout the placenta and cause undulations of the placental surface. Calcifications occur along the septations and are dispersed randomly throughout the placenta. These are normal changes of placental aging and should not be interpreted as indicators of disease. The normal placenta has a maximum thickness of 4 cm and a minimal thickness of 1 cm. Thick placentas are associated with maternal diabetes, maternal anemia, hydrops from immune and nonimmune causes, and chronic uterine infections. Thin placentas are associated with preeclampsia, placental insufficiency, IUGR, and trisomies 13 and 18.

Placenta previa is present when part or all of the placenta covers the internal cervical os. Placenta previa is present at term in 0.3% to 0.6% of live births. Placenta previa is suggested by US in as many as 45% of pregnancies examined in the first and second trimesters. These cases are the result of low implantation of the placenta and filling of the bladder, which distorts the lower uterine segment and cervix. As the pregnancy progresses, the muscular portion of the cervix elongates and increases the distance from the margin of the placenta to the cervical os. Risk factors for placenta previa include scarring of the lower uterine segment associated with previous cesarean section, previous placenta previa, surgical scars, and multiple previous pregnancies. Patients usually present with painless vaginal bleeding in the third trimester. Bleeding is initiated by the effacement of the cervix and dilation of the cervical os, which disrupts the vascular bed of the placenta. US confirmation of placenta previa is performed transperineally, with the bladder empty to allow optimal identification of both the edge of the placenta and the internal os of the cervix. When the placenta covers the entire cervical os, the previa is complete (Fig. 38.18). When an edge of the placenta covers a portion of the cervical os, the previa is partial or marginal.

Vasa previa is present when placental blood vessels, or the umbilical cord, are adherent to the membranes that cover the cervix. The vessels tear as the cervix dilates, resulting in fetal hemorrhage and death. Color Doppler is used to identify blood vessels fixed in place over the internal cervical os.

Placental abruption is defined as the premature separation of a normally positioned placenta from the myometrium. Separation is associated with hemorrhage from the maternal vessels at the base of the placenta. Abruption complicates 0.5% to 1.3% of pregnancies and is implicated in 15% to 25% of perinatal deaths. Risk factors include maternal hypertension, smoking, cocaine abuse, and previous history of abruption. *Subchorionic hemorrhage* (marginal abruption) occurs because of a separation at the edge of the placenta. Bleeding is usually venous and preferentially accumulates beneath the chorionic membrane adjacent to the placenta. *Retroplacental hemorrhage* occurs with more central abruption. Bleeding is usually arterial and accumulates beneath the placenta as an anechoic or mixed hypoechoic mass (Fig. 38.19). The hemorrhage may be isoechoic and difficult to differentiate from the placental tissue. The diagnosis is suggested by demonstrating disruption of the retroplacental complex of veins and thickening of the placenta (>4 cm).

Placenta accreta is an abnormal adherence of the placenta to the uterine wall. Invasion of the uterine wall by the placenta is referred to as *placenta increta,* and penetration of the uterine wall is *placenta percreta.* The decidua basalis

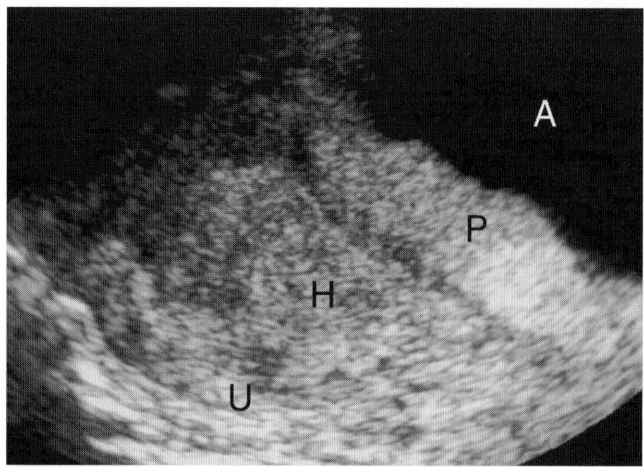

FIGURE 38.19. **Placental Abruption.** The placenta (P) is displaced away from the wall of the uterus (U) by an echogenic hematoma (H). Note the absence of visualization of the retroplacental complex of veins. A, amniotic cavity.

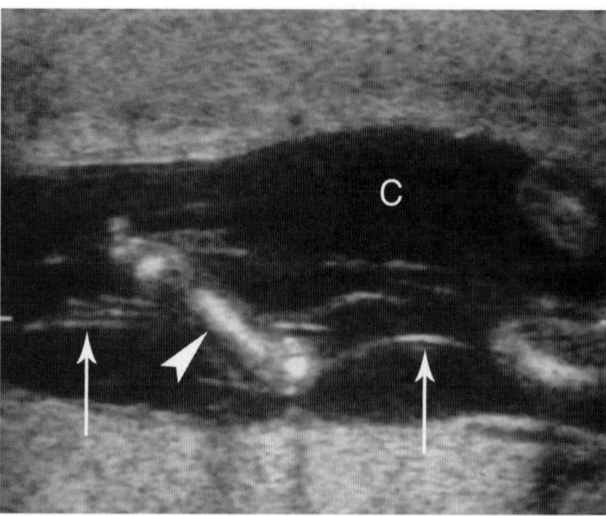

FIGURE 38.20. **Amniotic Band Syndrome.** The forearm (*arrowhead*) of a fetus at 15 weeks' GA is entangled within fibrous bands (*arrows*) that extend across the chorionic cavity (C).

and retroplacental complex of veins are completely or partially absent. Failure of the abnormally adherent placenta to separate completely from the myometrium after delivery results in copious hemorrhage. Risk factors include prior cesarean section, prior placenta accreta, and prior placenta previa. Scarring of the uterus results in the defective formation of decidua. US findings include absence of normal vascular channels in the retroplacental region, increased echogenicity of tissues deep to the placenta, and visualization of retroplacental vessels within the bladder lumen. Placenta previa is usually also present.

Chorioangioma is a benign vascular placental mass supplied by the fetal circulation. It appears on US as a solid hypoechoic, sometimes septated, mass in the placenta, usually close to the chorionic surface. Doppler demonstration of arterial waveforms at the fetal heart rate in vessels supplying the tumor is diagnostic. Vascular shunting may cause fetal high-output cardiac failure and fetal hydrops.

Umbilical Cord. The normal umbilical cord consists of two arteries and one vein surrounded by Wharton jelly. It has a normal diameter of 1 to 2 cm. A single-artery umbilical cord is found in about 1% of pregnancies and has a 10% to 20% association with congenital malformations. Associated anomalies include cardiac, urinary tract, and CNS malformations, omphalocele, trisomy 13, and trisomy 18. Masses in the umbilical cord include allantoic cysts, hematomas, hemangiomas, and teratomas.

Placental membranes consist of an outer layer *(chorion)* and an inner layer *(amnion)*. These membranes commonly remain separated by a layer of fluid until 14 to 16 weeks' GA, when the two membranes fuse. The amnion is visualized on US as a thin membrane floating in fluid. The chorion is identified as the membrane that confines fluid within the gestational sac. Occasional persistence of chorioamnionic separation into the third trimester is believed to be of no clinical significance.

Amniotic band syndrome is caused by the early (before 10 weeks' GA) disruption of the amnion, which enables the fetus to enter the chorionic cavity (Fig. 38.20). The fetus becomes entangled in fibrous bands that cross the chorionic cavity. Entrapment of fetal parts results in amputation deformities that range from mild to incompatible with life. Typical abnormalities include asymmetric absence of the cranium resembling anencephaly, encephaloceles, gastroschisis and truncal defects, spinal deformities, and extremity amputations. The amniotic bands trapping the fetus may be visualized.

Amniotic sheets (uterine synechia) are membranous structures that project into the uterine cavity. They demonstrate a characteristic appearance with a bulbous-free edge, thinner midportion, and a thickened base (Fig. 38.21). The fetus is able to move freely about the sheet of tissue. No fetal deformities are associated with this condition, which makes it distinct from the amniotic band syndrome. The amniotic sheets arise from folding of the chorioamnionic membranes over an intrauterine adhesion. Patients at increased risk for amniotic sheets include those with prior history of dilation and curettage, therapeutic abortion, or endometritis. An increased rate of cesarean section because of fetal malpresentation has been reported.

Amniotic Fluid

Normal amniotic fluid is essentially a dialysate of maternal serum in early pregnancy. As the pregnancy advances, fetal urine becomes the major source of amniotic fluid. The

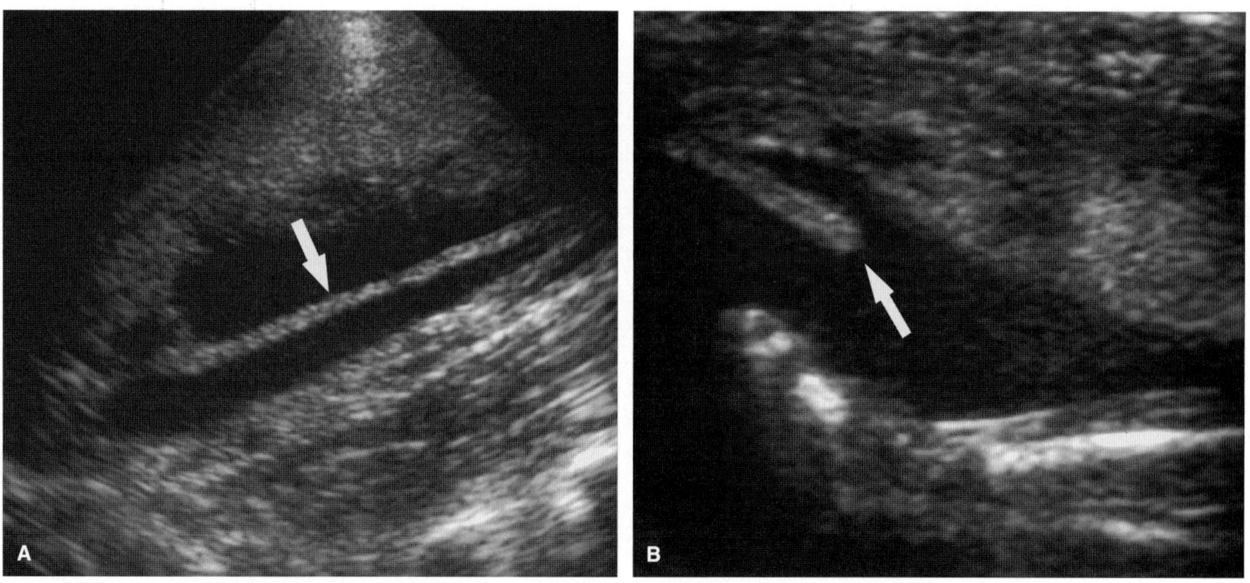

FIGURE 38.21. **Amniotic Sheet. A.** A fibrous band covered by chorioamnionic membranes (*arrow*) extends across the amniotic cavity. The uterine synechia forms a shelflike structure that partially compartmentalizes the uterine cavity. The fetus has free access to both compartments. **B.** The characteristic free edge (*arrow*) of the amniotic sheet is demonstrated.

composition of amniotic fluid is dynamic, with turnover of the entire volume every 3 hours. The fetus swallows amniotic fluid at a rate up to 450 mL per 24 hours. Transudate from the fetal lungs contributes a small volume. Water crosses placental membranes in response to osmotic gradients. Amniotic fluid is essential in promoting normal development and maturation of the fetal lungs. Suspended particles in amniotic fluid visualized by US are attributable to normal vernix (desquamated fetal skin), blood, or meconium.

Amniotic fluid index is a rough US measurement of amniotic fluid volume obtained by measuring the vertical diameter of the deepest pockets of fluid in the four quadrants of the uterus and adding these values together. Pockets are selected that do not include fetal parts or umbilical cord. Normal values are 5 to 20 cm.

Polyhydramnios is an excessive amount of amniotic fluid, traditionally defined as greater than 2 L of fluid at delivery. US is used to confirm excessive fluid any time in pregnancy. Because amniotic fluid volume is difficult to measure accurately, the diagnosis is usually made subjectively by visual inspection. The visual proportion of fluid relative to the size of the fetus is greatest early in the second trimester and decreases progressively to term. Polyhydramnios is suggested by large pockets of fluid relative to the size of the fetus and the age of the pregnancy. An amniotic fluid index greater than 20 cm or a single fluid pocket greater than 8 cm deep is strongly suggestive of polyhydramnios. Another clue is failure of the fetal abdomen to be in contact with both anterior and posterior uterine walls after 24 weeks' GA. Excessive fluid is associated with preterm labor, premature rupture of membranes, and substantial maternal discomfort. About 60% of cases are idiopathic; 15% to 20% are related to maternal disease (diabetes mellitus, preeclampsia, anemia, obesity); and 20% to 25% are associated with fetal anomalies. About half of all fetuses with anomalies will have polyhydramnios. Gross polyhydramnios has a higher association with fetal anomalies than mild polyhydramnios. Associated anomalies include anencephaly, encephalocele, GI obstructions, abdominal wall defects, achondroplasia, and hydrops (isoimmunization).

Oligohydramnios refers to an abnormally low amniotic fluid volume. Fluid pockets are small or absent, fetal parts are crowded, fetal surface features such as the face are difficult to visualize, and the amniotic fluid index measures less than 5 cm. Measurement of the largest fluid pocket in the vertical direction of less than 1 cm is indicative of severe oligohydramnios. Causes of oligohydramnios include premature rupture of membranes, IUGR, renal anomalies (lack of urine output), fetal death, eclampsia, and postdate pregnancies. A major complication of severe oligohydramnios is fetal lung immaturity.

Multiple Pregnancy

Twins occur in 1 of every 90 births. Morbidity and mortality are significantly increased in twin pregnancy compared with singleton pregnancy. Twins account for 12% to 13% of all neonatal deaths. Morbidity associated with multiple pregnancy includes prematurity, polyhydramnios, increased incidence of congenital anomalies, discordant growth, and cord accidents. Relative risk is increased if the fetuses share a placenta (monochorionic twins, 20%) as opposed to each fetus having its own placenta (dichorionic twins, 80%). Twins that share a single amniotic cavity (monoamniotic twins) have the highest risk for morbidity, including conjoined twinning and intertwining of the umbilical cords. Visualization of two separate placentas, or determination that the twins are of different sex, is definitive proof of lower-risk dichorionic twinning. Unfortunately, about half of dichorionic twins will have a fused placenta. Visualization of a membrane separating the twins confirms diamniotic twins. Monochorionic twins usually have vascular anastomoses at the placental level, making them at risk for twin transfusion syndrome and twin embolization syndrome.

Twin transfusion syndrome results from shunting of blood from one twin to the other through vascular connections in the placenta. The abnormality ranges in severity from minor discordance in growth to severe IUGR in one twin, with hydropic fluid overload in the other twin. Severe disparity in amniotic fluid volume may be present, with one twin experiencing polyhydramnios while the other twin is virtually anhydramniotic ("a stuck twin" compressed against the uterine wall by the amnion). The mortality rate is as high as 70%.

Twin embolization syndrome is an uncommon complication of the death of one twin in utero. Blood products from the dead twin are shunted through placental interconnections to the live twin, resulting in disseminated intravascular coagulopathy and multifocal tissue infarction.

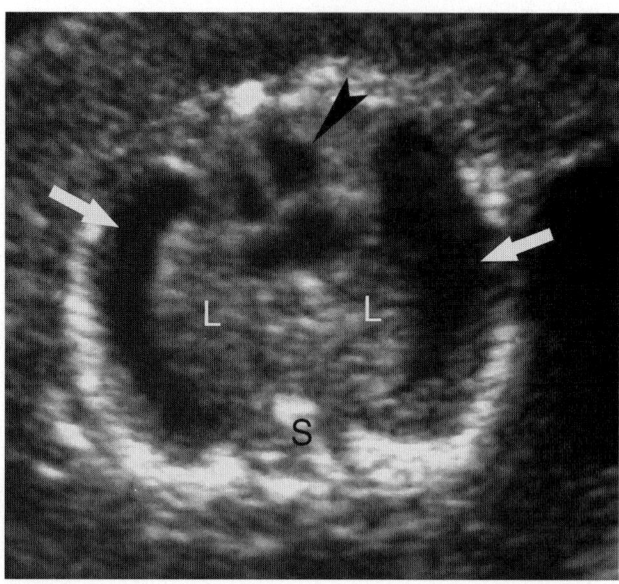

FIGURE 38.22. **Fetal Hydrops.** A transverse image through the fetal thorax at the level of a four-chamber view of the heart (*black arrowhead*) demonstrates bilateral pleural effusions (*white arrows*) outlining the lungs (L). The fetal chest is viewed from above, with the spine (S) posterior. This fetus also had ascites.

FETAL ANOMALIES

General

Fetal hydrops refers to the pathologic accumulation of fluid in body cavities and tissues. US demonstrates ascites, pleural and pericardial effusions, and subcutaneous edema (Fig. 38.22). *Immune hydrops* is caused by blood group incompatibility between mother and fetus. Current treatment, including fetal transfusion, is highly successful. *Nonimmune hydrops* is caused by a host of conditions, including cardiac disorders, infections, chromosomal anomalies, twin pregnancy, urinary obstruction, and umbilical cord complications. The cause of many cases is not identified. The prognosis for nonimmune hydrops remains poor.

Alpha-Fetoprotein (AFP) and Triple Marker Screening. AFP is a protein produced by the fetal liver. Concentrations of AFP are highest in the fetal serum, with small amounts present in the amniotic fluid (AF-AFP) and minute amounts detectable in maternal serum (MS-AFP). Open neural tube and other skin defects in the fetus allow AFP to leak into the amniotic fluid and maternal serum in abnormally large quantities. Routine MS-AFP screening is performed to aid in detection of neural tube defects and other fetal anomalies. *Triple marker screening* refers to expanded maternal serum screening programs that have added β-hCG and unconjugated estriol (uE3) determinations to MS-AFP screening (11). Results are reported as multiples of the median (MOM) values. AFP is considered elevated when it is *greater than* 2.50 MOM. Low values for the triple marker screen are correlated with maternal age to yield a risk for chromosome abnormalities, especially trisomy 21 and trisomy 18. The MS-AFP or triple marker screening blood tests are performed at 16 to 18 weeks' GA as determined by menstrual history. The normal values for MS-AFP vary with GA, reaching maximum values at 30 to 32 weeks' gestation. Patients with abnormal MS-AFP or triple marker screening are routinely referred for US dating, detailed fetal examination, and consideration of amniocentesis for karyotyping. The differential diagnosis for elevated AFP is listed in Table 38.6.

Chromosome abnormalities are suspected when multiple or major fetal anomalies are detected by US. Advanced maternal age (>35 years at delivery) or a parent or previous child with aneuploidy or chromosomal translocation anomalies are risk factors for fetal chromosome abnormalities. Fetuses with structural anomalies detected on US have an 11% to 35% risk of associated chromosome abnormality. Fetal conditions with significant high risk of associated chromosome abnormality include holoprosencephaly, Dandy-Walker syndrome, cystic hygroma,

TABLE 38.6 Causes of Elevated MS-AFP

Erroneous gestational dating
Multiple pregnancy
Fetal demise
Neural tube defects:
  Anencephaly
  Spina bifida
  Encephaloceles
Abdominal wall defects:
  Gastroschisis
  Omphalocele
Amniotic band syndrome
Cystic hygroma
Placental abnormalities:
  Subchorionic hemorrhage
  Chorioangioma
Unexplained—fetus is at high risk for:
  IUGR
  Fetal death
  Preterm delivery
  Preeclampsia
  Oligohydramnios

MS-AFP, maternal serum level of alpha-fetoprotein; IUGR, intrauterine growth retardation.

cardiac malformations, omphalocele, duodenal atresia, facial anomalies, and early symmetric IUGR. Chromosome analysis is performed on samples obtained by amniocentesis or chorionic villous sampling.

Trisomy 21, Down syndrome, is the most common chromosome abnormality, occurring in 1 of 660 births. Although women older than age 35 have a 1 in 250 risk of carrying a fetus with trisomy 21, 80% of fetuses with Down syndrome are born to younger women (11). Triple marker serum screening will detect about 60% of affected fetuses. A variety of US findings serve as markers for the condition (12). Major structural defects found in Down fetuses include congenital heart disease (endocardial cushion defect), duodenal atresia, and hydrocephalus. *Nuchal fold thickening* greater than 3 mm in the first trimester or greater than 6 mm in the second trimester is strongly associated. The skinfold is measured from the occipital bone to the external skin surface on the transcerebellar plane view. If two or more of the following findings are present, trisomy 21 is likely: short femur, short humerus, echogenic bowel, mild fetal renal pyelectasis, intracardiac echogenic focus, hypoplastic middle phalanx of fifth finger.

Trisomy 18 is the second most common chromosome anomaly, occurring in 1 of 3,000 births. A large number of structural abnormalities may occur, but the most common identified by US are IUGR (74%), complex congenital heart disease (52%), choroid plexus cysts (47%), congenital diaphragmatic hernia, omphalocele, neural tube defects, Dandy-Walker syndrome, clenched hands, and single umbilical artery (12).

Central Nervous System, Face, and Neck

Anomalies of the CNS occur in 1 of 1,000 live births (2). Survivors are often severely disabled and require long-term care. Effective US screening for CNS anomalies can be performed by examination of three crucial axial planes through the fetal brain. The *transthalamic plane* is used to measure the BPD and HC (Fig. 38.12). Abnormalities of head shape, microcephaly, macrocephaly, and major structural abnormalities are evident in this plane. The third ventricle varies in appearance from a single echogenic line to a slitlike structure narrower than 3.5 mm. The *transventricular plane* is an axial plane at the level of the ventricular atria (Fig. 38.23). The dominant landmark is the echogenic choroid plexus, which normally fills the atrium nearly completely. Measurements of atrial diameter made perpendicular to the walls do not normally exceed 10 mm. The *transcerebellar plane* is an axial scan at approximately 10° to 15° of inclination from the canthomeatal line. The anatomic landmarks include the inferior portion of the third ventricle and the cerebellar hemispheres, which are outlined by fluid in the cisterna magna (Fig. 38.24). The normal cisterna magna measures 2 to 11 mm in width. A small cisterna magna (<2 mm) suggests a Chiari II

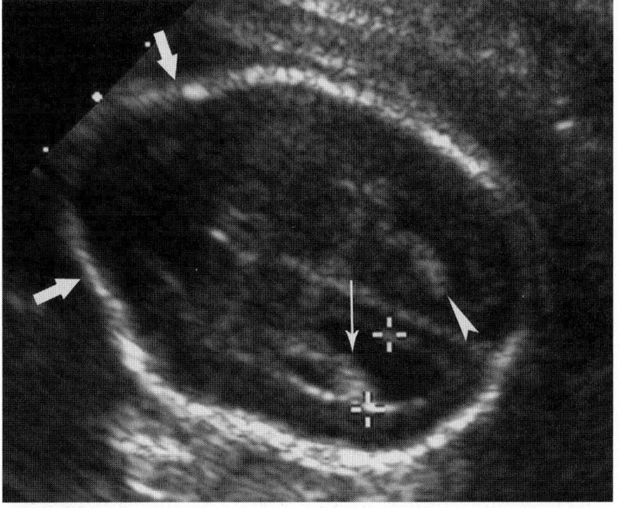

FIGURE 38.23. **Transventricular Plane: Early Ventriculomegaly.** The choroid plexus (*thin arrow*) hangs dependently in the atria of the lateral ventricle (between *cursors*). The choroid plexus (*arrowhead*) in the near ventricle also hangs dependently. The ventricular atrium is measured from its medial wall to its lateral wall (between *cursors*). The normal ventricular atrium does not exceed 10 mm in width at any time during pregnancy. The diameter of the atrium in this case measures 12 mm, indicating ventriculomegaly. This fetus has a spina bifida defect with associated Arnold-Chiari II malformation as the cause of ventriculomegaly. Note the bossing of the frontal bones (*thick arrows*), which gives the outline of the cranium an appearance similar in shape to a lemon (lemon head).

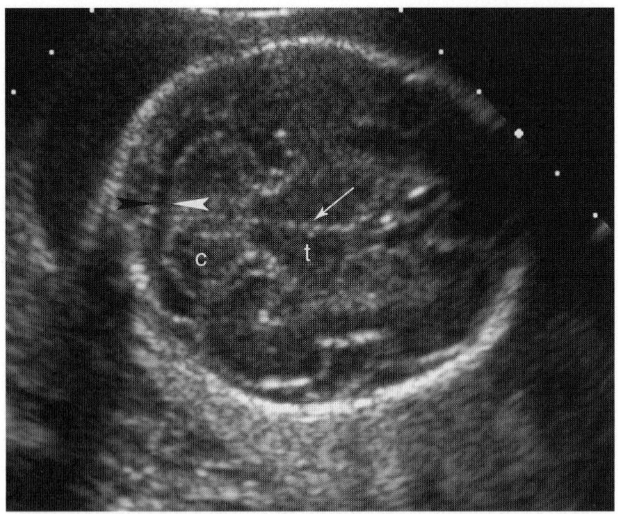

FIGURE 38.24. **Transcerebellar Plane.** Landmarks for the transcerebellar plane are the thalami (t), third ventricle (*arrow*), and cerebellar hemispheres (c). The cisterna magna (between *arrowheads*) is measured from the vermis (*white arrowhead*) to the occiput (*black arrowhead*). The normal cisterna magna measures 2 to 11 mm throughout pregnancy.

malformation but may also be seen with massive ventriculomegaly. A large cisterna magna (>11 mm) may be a normal variant (mega–cisterna magna) or indicate Dandy-Walker malformation, arachnoid cyst, or cerebellar hypoplasia. When these three planes are anatomically normal, the risk of CNS anomaly is minute (0.005%). An algorithm for sorting out fetal CNS anomalies is given in Table 38.7.

Ventriculomegaly is an anatomic finding with many causes that can be grouped into the categories of obstructive hydrocephalus (obstruction to flow of CSF), cerebral atrophy (ex vacuo), and maldevelopment (such as agenesis of the corpus callosum). Ventriculomegaly detected in utero carries a poor prognosis. Up to 80% of fetuses with ventriculomegaly have associated anomalies. The US signs of ventriculomegaly include diameter of the ventricular atrium >10 mm, separation of choroid plexus from the ventricular wall by >3 mm, and a "dangling choroid." The choroid plexus hangs dependently in the ventricle and marks the position of the lateral ventricular wall. The most common causes of ventriculomegaly in the fetus are Chiari II malformation and aqueductal stenosis (Fig. 38.25).

TABLE 38.7 Algorithm for Diagnosis of Congenital Brain Abnormalities[a]

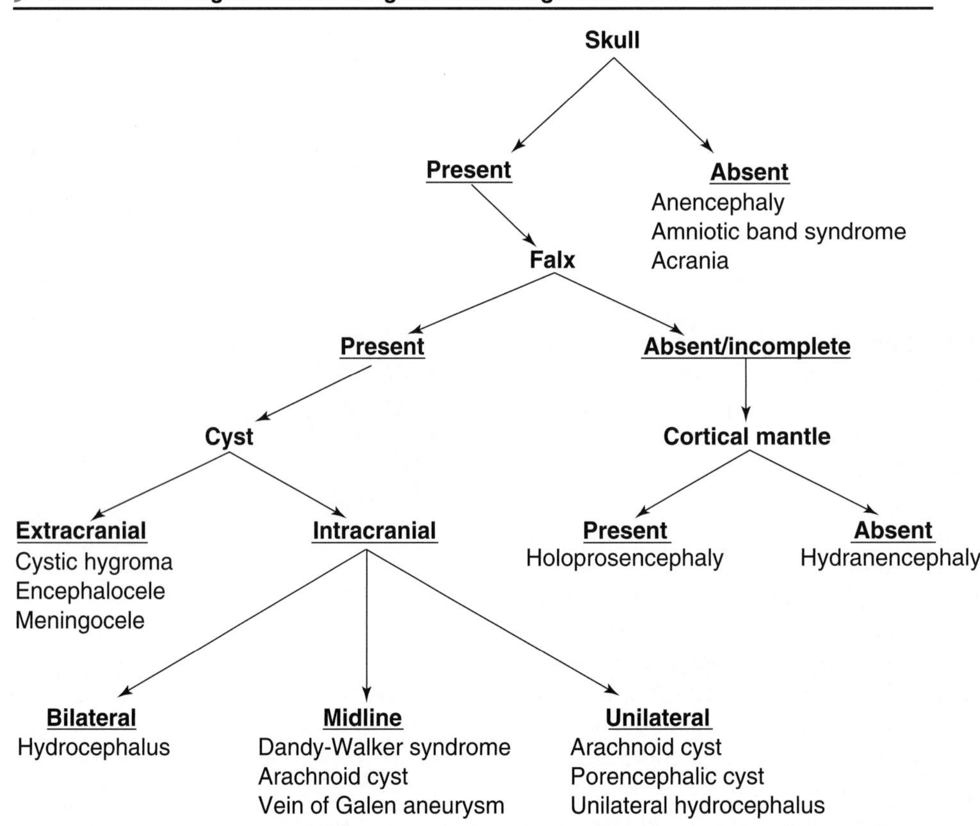

[a]From Carrasco CR, Stierman ED, Hornsberger HR, Lee TG. An algorithm for prenatal ultrasound diagnosis of congenital CNS abnormalities. J Ultrasound Med 1985;4:163–168.

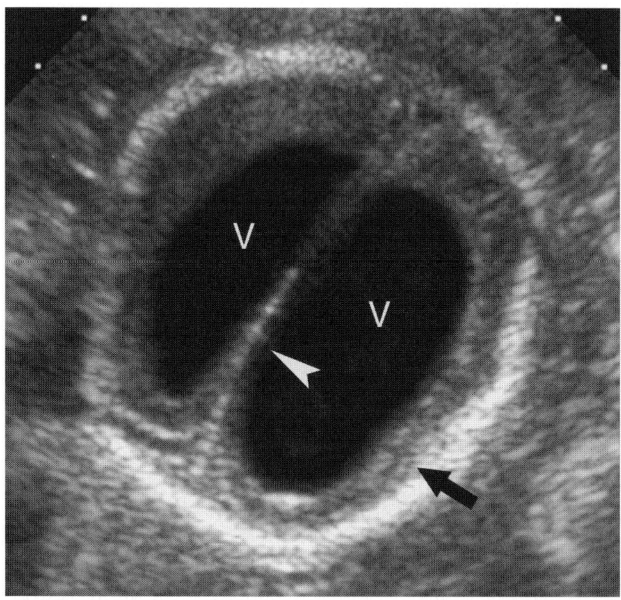

FIGURE 38.25. **Ventriculomegaly.** An axial image of the fetal brain in fetus with aqueduct stenosis demonstrates marked enlargement of the lateral ventricles (V). The falx (*arrowhead*) is seen as an echogenic stripe in the midline. A rind of cortex (*arrow*) is present. These latter two findings differentiate ventriculomegaly from hydranencephaly and holoprosencephaly.

Anencephaly is the most common neural tube defect. US findings include absence of the cranial vault and cerebral hemispheres above the level of the orbits (Fig. 38.26). The cerebral hemispheres may be replaced by an amorphous neurovascular mass (area cerebrovasculosa). The condition is inevitably fatal.

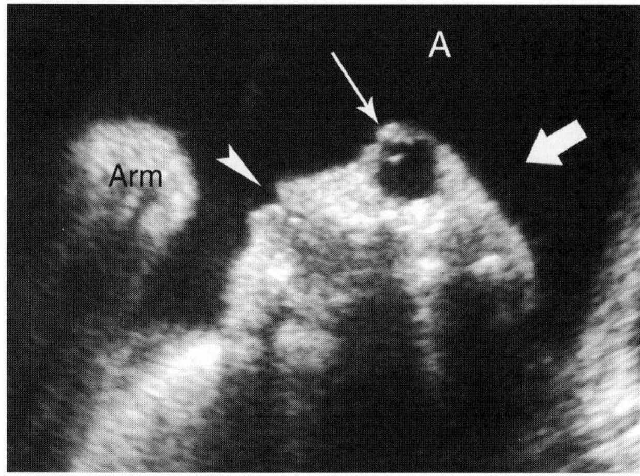

FIGURE 38.26. **Anencephaly.** A sagittal image through the head of a fetus demonstrates absence of the cranial vault (*thick arrow*) above the level of the eye (*thin arrow*). The mouth and lips are evident (*arrowhead*). The volume of amniotic fluid is increased. Polyhydramnios is common in the presence of anencephaly. Arm, fetal arm.

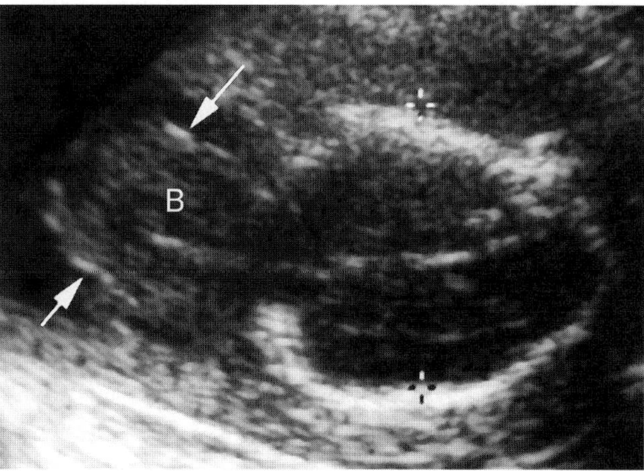

FIGURE 38.27. **Encephalocele.** Axial US image through the fetal skull demonstrates herniation of brain tissue (B) through a large defect in the skull, forming an occipital encephalocele (between *arrows*). The intracranial contents are reduced and the biparietal diameter (between *cursors*) is less than expected for gestational age because of the encephalocele.

Cephaloceles are fluid-filled and/or brain tissue–filled sacs that protrude through a defect in the bony calvaria. They are found in the occipital (75%), frontoethmoid (13%), and parietal (12%) regions. Meningoceles contain only CSF, whereas encephaloceles contain brain tissue (Fig. 38.27).

Spina bifida refers to a spectrum of spinal abnormalities resulting from failure of the complete closure of the neural tube. The condition ranges from simple nonfusion of the vertebral arches with intact skin (spina bifida occulta); to protruding sacs containing CSF, spinal cord, or nerve roots (myelomeningocele); to a totally open spinal defect (myeloschisis). Spina bifida may occur anywhere in the spine but most often occurs in the lumbosacral region. US findings (Fig. 38.28) include: outward splaying, rather than inward convergence, of the laminae; defect in the soft tissues overlying the bony abnormality; and a protruding sac containing fluid and often neural tissues. The associated functional neuromuscular defect often results in club foot deformities and dislocated hips. Associated cranial abnormalities of the Chiari II malformation provide clues to the presence of the spinal defect. Ventriculomegaly is present in 75% of cases. The "lemon sign" refers to bossing of the frontal bones, causing a lemon-shaped appearance to the head in the axial plane (Fig. 38.23). The "banana sign" is produced by compression of the cerebellar hemispheres into a banana shape. The cisterna magna is small or obliterated.

Chiari II malformation is associated with 95% of myelomeningoceles. The cranial abnormality consists of caudal displacement of the cerebellar tonsils, pons, and medulla. The fourth ventricle is elongated, the posterior fossa is small, and the cisterna magna is obliterated.

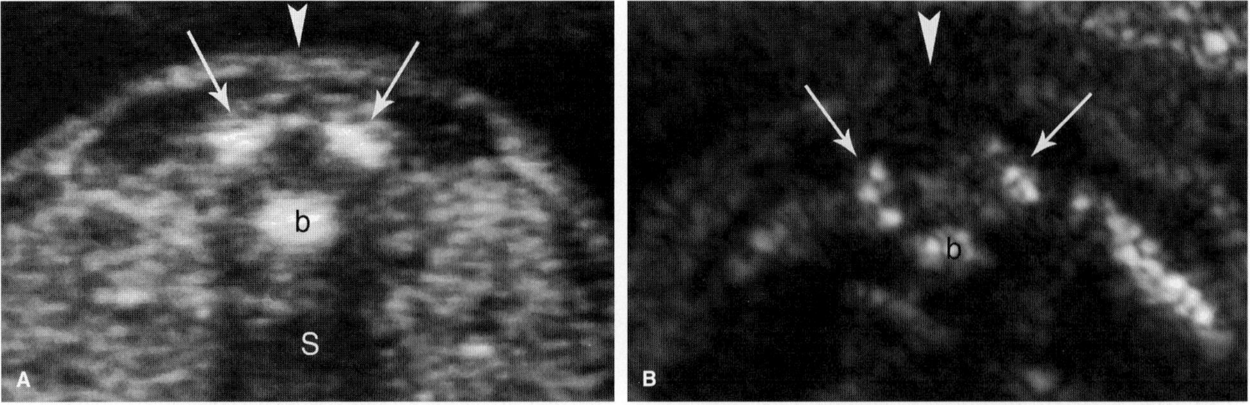

FIGURE 38.28. **Normal Spine and Spina Bifida. A.** Normal spine. Posterior transverse image through a normal fetal spine at the L4-L5 level demonstrates the ossified portion of the vertebral body (b) anteriorly and the converging ossified portions of the lamina (*arrows*) posteriorly. The skin overlying the posterior aspect of the vertebra is intact (*arrowhead*). The spine normally casts an acoustic shadow (S). **B.** Spina bifida. Posterior transverse image through a spina bifida defect demonstrates the ossified portion of the vertebral body (b) anteriorly and the diverging ossified portions of the lamina (*arrows*) posteriorly. A defect is evident in the overlying skin (*arrowhead*).

Holoprosencephaly refers to a spectrum of disorders characterized by a failure of the prosencephalon to divide and form separate right and left hemispheres and thalami. Associated facial anomalies including hypotelorism, cyclopia, and proboscis are common. *Alobar* holoprosencephaly is the most severe form and demonstrates absence of the falx and interhemispheric fissure with a single midline ventricle (Fig. 38.29). The *semilobar* and *lobar* forms demonstrate greater degrees of midline separation.

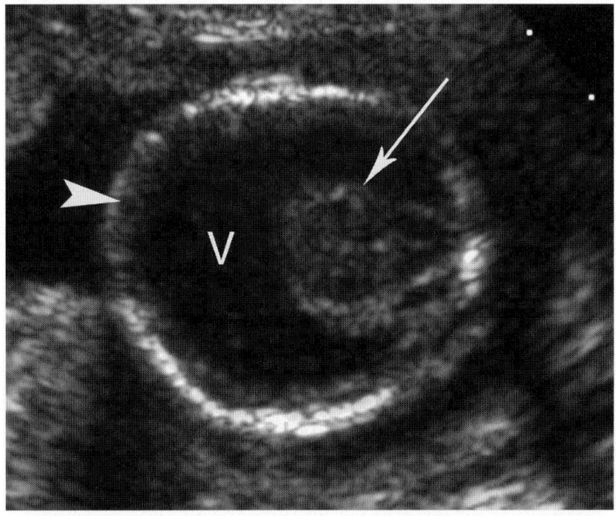

FIGURE 38.29. **Holoprosencephaly.** Image through the cranium of a fetus reveals a single large midline ventricle (V) and fused thalami (*arrow*). A thin rim of cortex (*arrowhead*) is present. These findings are characteristic of alobar holoprosencephaly. The fetal face should be examined for associated defects such as midline cleft and proboscis.

Hydranencephaly refers to total destruction of the cerebral cortex, believed to be caused by the occlusion of the internal carotid arteries. The cranial vault contains fluid, but no cortical mantle of brain tissue is visible (Fig. 38.30). The falx may be present but is usually incomplete. The brainstem and structures supplied by the vertebral arteries appear normal.

Dandy-Walker malformation results from the maldevelopment of the roof of the fourth ventricle. The cisterna magna is enlarged and communicates directly with the fourth ventricle through its absent roof. The posterior fossa is enlarged, and the tentorium is elevated. The cerebellar hemispheres are usually hypoplastic (Fig. 38.31). Hydrocephalus is usually present. The condition varies in severity across a broad spectrum. Less severe abnormalities are usually called Dandy-Walker variants. Arachnoid cysts and large cisterna magna are differentiated by their lack of communication with the fourth ventricle.

Choroid plexus cysts are found in 1% to 3% of normal fetuses during the second trimester. The cysts themselves cause no clinical problem and nearly always resolve. Because they are present in up to 47% of fetuses with trisomy 18, their discovery causes concern for the presence of chromosome abnormality. In nearly all cases, detailed US examination, which should include echocardiography and examination of the fetal hands, will demonstrate additional structural abnormalities that justify amniocentesis for karyotyping. Trisomy 18 is unlikely and amniocentesis is not indicated if detailed US examination of the fetus is normal.

Cleft lip and cleft palate account for 13% of all congenital anomalies found in the United States. *Lateral cleft* is most common and involves both lip and palate in 50% of

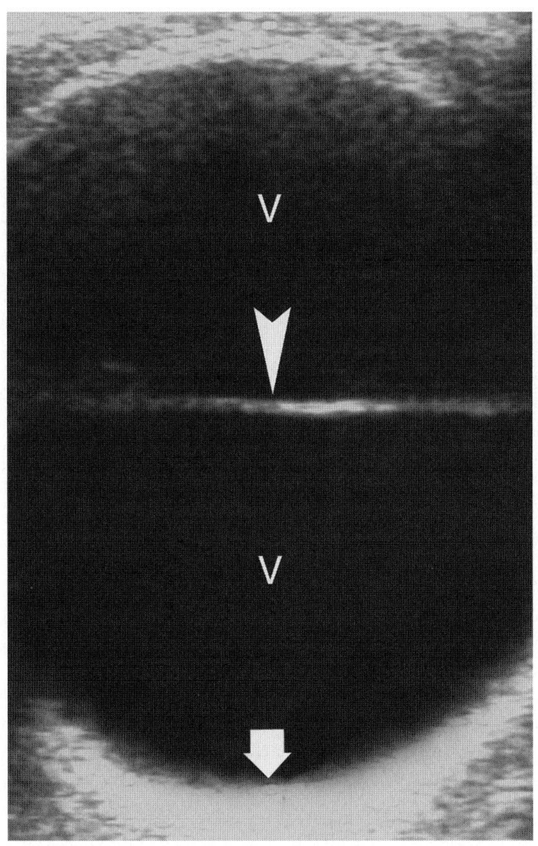

FIGURE 38.30. **Hydranencephaly.** Axial sonogram through the brain of a near-term fetus demonstrates two massive ventricles (V), a well-defined midline falx (*arrowhead*) and total absence of detectable cortical tissue (*arrow*). These findings are characteristic of hydranencephaly.

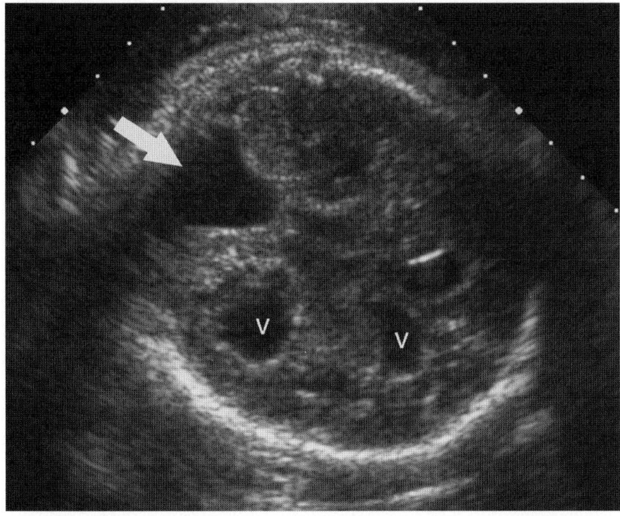

FIGURE 38.31. **Dandy-Walker Malformation.** Coronal plane image demonstrates cystic enlargement of the posterior fossa (*arrow*). The lateral ventricles (V) are enlarged, indicating associated hydrocephalus.

cases, the lip alone in 25%, and the palate alone in 25%. The condition is bilateral in 20% to 25% of cases. Up to 60% of affected fetuses have additional anomalies, including polydactyly, congenital heart disease, and trisomy 21. US diagnosis is made on demonstration of a groove extending from one of the nostrils through the lip (Fig. 38.32) (13). *Median cleft* is a completely different entity associated with holoprosencephaly and accounting for fewer than 0.7% of all cases of cleft lip. A coronal plane sonogram of the face demonstrates a wide central defect in the upper lip and palate.

Cystic hygroma is a fluid collection in the fetal neck caused by failure of the lymphatic system to develop normal connections with the venous system in the neck. US demonstrates a bilateral nuchal cystic mass with a prominent midline septum that represents the nuchal ligament (Fig. 38.33). Up to 70% have abnormal karyotypes, usually Turner syndrome or Down syndrome. Generalized lymphangiectasia and fetal hydrops may occur and are always fatal when they do.

Chest and Heart

Congenital diaphragmatic hernia is a disorder in which abdominal contents protrude into the thorax through defects in the diaphragm. The most common type involves the foramen of Bochdalek at the posterolateral aspect of the diaphragm. The majority (75%) occur on the left side (Fig. 38.34). Anteromedial defects at the foramen of Morgagni also occur. US findings include: fluid-filled, solid, or multicystic mass in the chest; displacement of the heart and mediastinum; absence of the stomach in the abdomen; and polyhydramnios. Associated defects, especially cardiac and CNS, are common. Mortality is high (50% to 80%) because of pulmonary hypoplasia.

Cystic adenomatoid malformation is a congenital hamartomatous lesion of the lung that usually affects one lobe. The lesion consists of single or multiple cysts that vary in size from microscopic to larger than 2 cm. Type 1 lesions appear on US as single or multiple cysts larger than 2 cm. Type 2 lesions consist of multiple smaller cysts of uniform size (<2 cm). Type 3 lesions appear as echogenic solid masses because the cysts are microscopic (Fig. 38.35). Polyhydramnios and fetal hydrops may occur. Some of these lesions resolve spontaneously in utero.

Pulmonary sequestration is a mass of lung tissue supplied by systemic arteries and separated from its normal bronchial and pulmonary vascular connections (14). *Intralobar sequestrations* (75% to 85%) are contained within the pleural covering of an otherwise normal lobe of the lung. Pulmonary venous drainage is maintained. US detection in the fetus is rare. *Extralobar sequestrations,* although less common (15% to 25%), are much more frequently evident on fetal US. These are accessory lobes contained within their own pleura and supplied by both

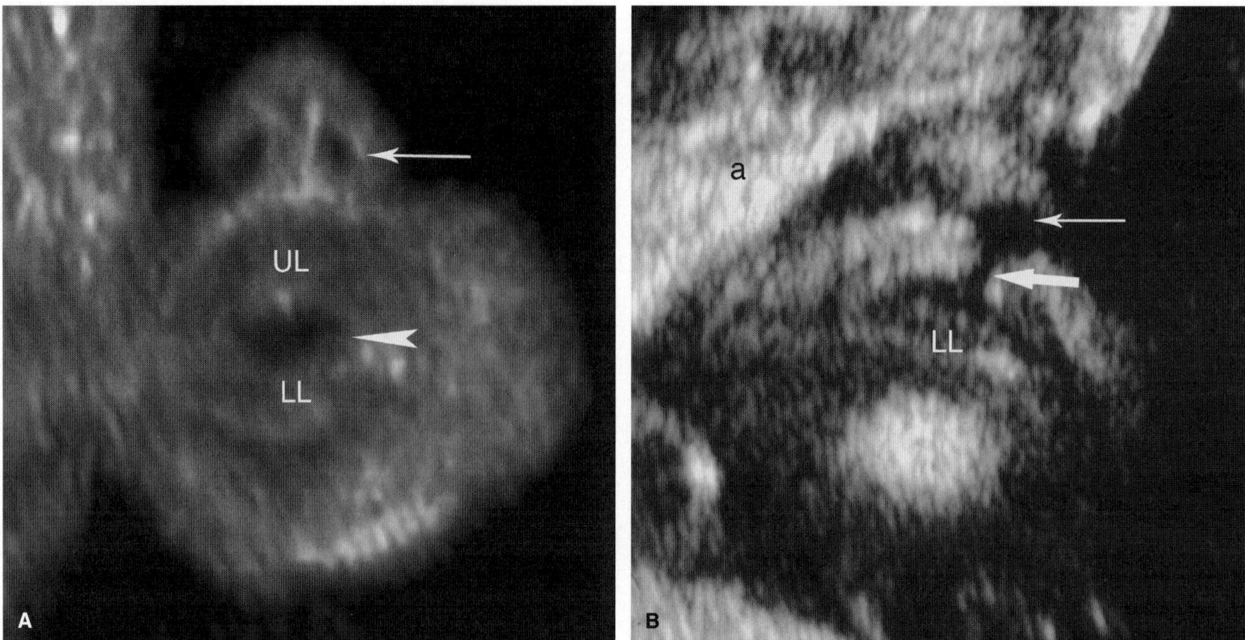

FIGURE 38.32. **Cleft Lip. A.** Coronal view of a normal fetal face ("up your nose" view) shows both nares (*arrow*), an open mouth (*arrowhead*), and the muscles of the upper (UL) and lower (LL) lips. **B.** Matching coronal view of another fetus reveals a cleft (*thick arrow*) in the left upper lip extending into the left nares (*thin arrow*). The mouth is slightly open. The lower lip (LL) is apparent. An arm (a) extends across the face.

systemic arteries and veins. US demonstrates a homogeneous, echogenic, solid lung mass that displaces the mediastinum. Color Doppler is used to demonstrate the systemic supplying artery arising from the thoracic aorta. Hydrops may occur.

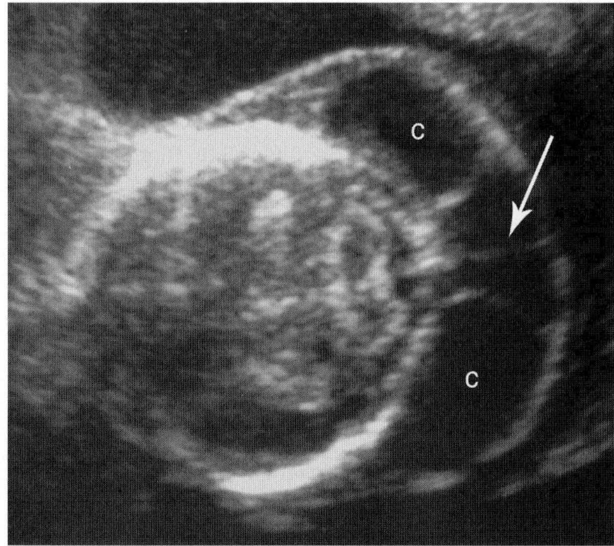

FIGURE 38.33. **Cystic Hygroma.** A multiseptated cystic mass (c) extends over the occipital region of the fetal skull. Cystic hygroma is differentiated from occipital cephalocele by demonstration of the midline septum (*arrow*) owing to the nuchal ligament and by absence of a bony defect in the skull.

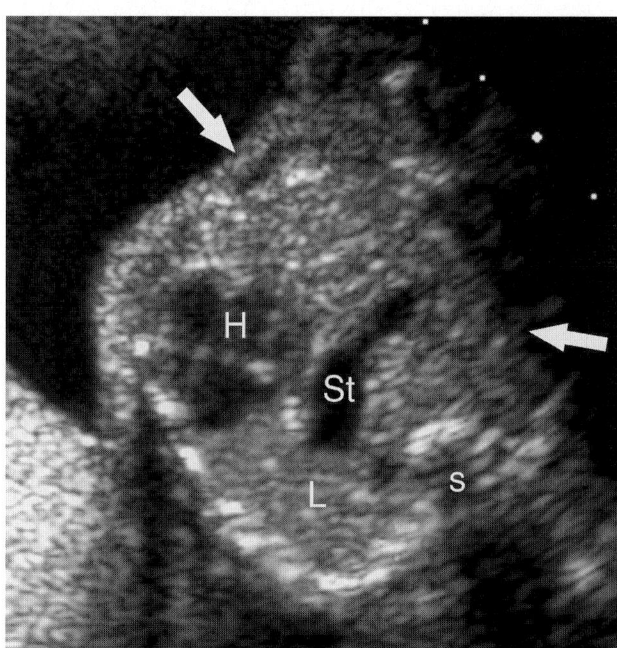

FIGURE 38.34. **Congenital Diaphragmatic Hernia.** Axial plane image of the fetal thorax stomach (St) and small bowel (between *arrows*) herniated into the left thorax. The heart (H) is shifted markedly into the right thorax and is abnormally rotated. Only a small volume of compressed right lung (L) is present. Severe pulmonary hypoplasia is likely, and the prognosis for this fetus is grim. The spine (s) is seen posteriorly.

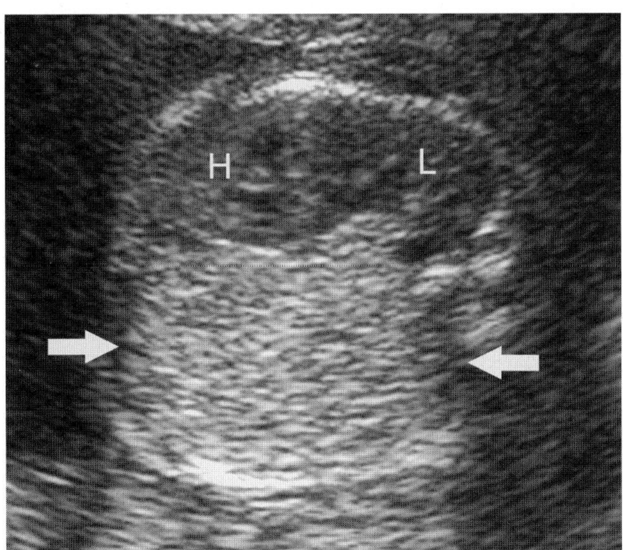

FIGURE 38.35. **Cystic Adenomatoid Malformation.** An echogenic solid-appearing mass (between *arrows*) is seen in the right thorax, displacing and compressing the heart (H). A small portion of the compressed left lung (L) is evident. The appearance is characteristic of type 3 cystic adenomatoid malformation.

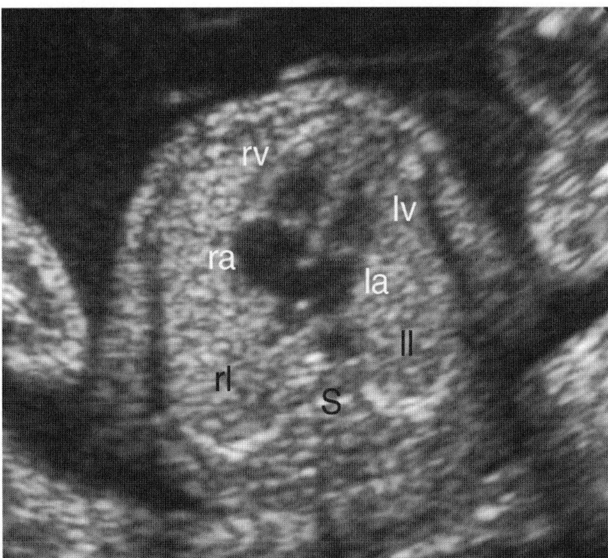

FIGURE 38.36. **Normal Four-Chamber Heart View.** Axial sonogram through the fetal chest demonstrates the normal heart and fluid-filled lungs in an 18-week fetus. The right ventricle (rv) and left ventricle (lv) are approximately equal in size, as are the right atrium (ra) and left atrium (la). The heart normally occupies about one-third of the cross-sectional area of the thorax. The developing lungs are echogenic. The spine (S) is seen posteriorly. rl, right lung; ll, left lung.

Fetal Heart Anomalies. Congenital heart disease is a major cause of neonatal morbidity and mortality (15). Precise US diagnosis of fetal heart abnormalities often requires specialized equipment and a high level of expertise. The presence of many major structural abnormalities of the fetal heart can be recognized on the four-chamber heart view (Fig. 38.36). The four-chamber view is obtained on an axial scan through the fetal chest, just above the diaphragm. The apex of the heart is directed at the left anterior chest wall at a 45° angle on the same side as the fetal stomach. Deviation from this position suggests a cardiac malformation or a thoracic mass. Pericardial effusions appear as an anechoic band surrounding the myocardium. The ventricles are approximately equal in size and slightly smaller than their corresponding atria. Motion of the atrioventricular valves is observed in this plane. Papillary muscles in the ventricles may be echogenic and prominent. Discrepancies in chamber size or valve motion suggest cardiac malformations, and detailed fetal echocardiography is necessary.

Abdomen

Normal Fetal Abdomen. The abdomen of the fetus is significantly different from the abdomen of the older child or adult (16). The abdomen of the fetus is large relative to its body length compared with the adult. The liver is large, and the left lobe is larger than the right lobe. The umbilical vein is an important US landmark. Half the blood it carries goes directly to the inferior vena cava via the ductus venosus. The remainder perfuses the liver via the left portal vein. The adrenal glands are up to 20 times larger in relative size because of the presence of the "fetal zone." The pelvis is relatively small, and the pelvic organs extend into the lower abdomen. Swallowing begins at 11 to 12 weeks' GA. The fetal stomach should be filled with swallowed fluid by 18 weeks' GA. The small bowel is moderately echogenic, centrally located, and blends with the liver. By the third trimester, peristalsis in small bowel loops can be observed. The visualized small bowel loops are normally less than 6 mm in diameter and less than 15 mm in length. The colon is visualized after 20 weeks as a tubular structure around the periphery of the abdomen. The colon progressively fills with meconium but does not exceed 23 mm in diameter. Normal fetal kidneys are seen as paired, slightly hypoechoic structures adjacent to the spine. The renal sinus appears as an echogenic stripe. Fetal lobulation causes an undulating contour of the kidneys. The length of normal fetal kidneys in millimeters is approximately equal to GA in weeks. The bladder should be observed to fill and empty. Because amniotic fluid is predominantly urine, a normal amniotic fluid volume implies at least one functioning kidney.

Absent Stomach. Failure to visualize the fetal stomach by 18 weeks' GA is a significant abnormality in about half of cases. Causes include obstruction (esophageal atresia, chest mass); impaired swallowing (facial clefts

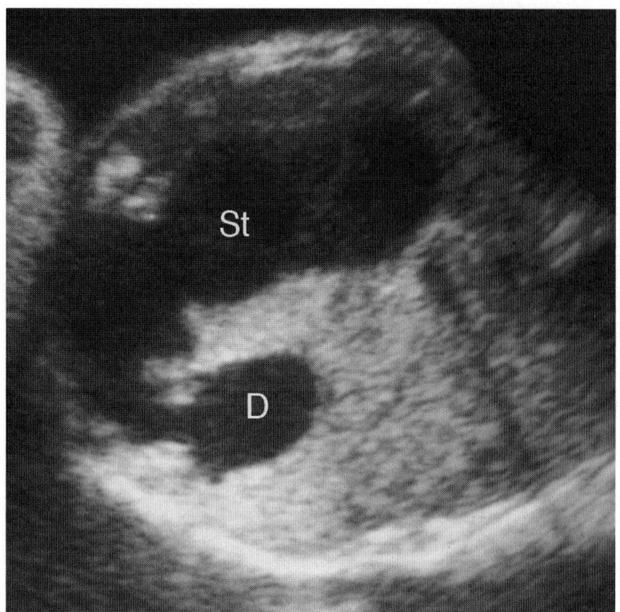

FIGURE 38.37. **"Double Bubble."** Fluid distension of the stomach (St) and the duodenal bulb (D) is caused by obstruction at the level of the descending duodenum.

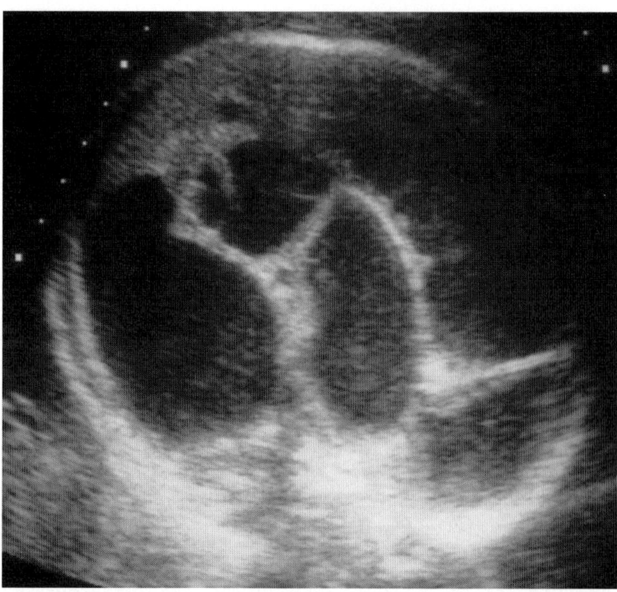

FIGURE 38.38. **Small Bowel Obstruction.** Ileal atresia was the cause of markedly dilated loops of small bowel seen throughout the abdomen.

and neuromuscular disorders); low amniotic fluid volume; and ectopic stomach (diaphragmatic hernia). In the remaining cases, absence of fluid in the stomach is a normal variant, probably representing recent gastric emptying. Follow-up US is warranted to detect delayed filling.

Double bubble is descriptive of fluid distension of the stomach and proximal duodenum (Fig. 38.37). Fluid dilatation of the duodenum is abnormal and indicative of duodenal atresia or stenosis, annular pancreas, or volvulus. Down syndrome should be considered. Half of cases have additional anomalies.

Bowel obstruction is suggested by dilation of the small bowel to larger than 6 mm (Fig. 38.38). Causes include jejunal or ileal atresia or stenosis, volvulus, meconium ileus, and enteric duplication. A dilated and tortuous ureter should not be misinterpreted as dilated bowel.

Meconium ileus causes small bowel obstruction by impaction of abnormally thick meconium in the distal ileum. Meconium ileus is nearly always associated with cystic fibrosis. The combination of dilated bowel with echogenic meconium suggests the diagnosis.

Meconium peritonitis results from perforation of a bowel segment. Spillage of meconium into the peritoneal cavity causes a sterile peritonitis that results in calcifications in the peritoneal cavity, meconium pseudocysts, ascites, bowel dilatation, and polyhydramnios. The cause is commonly not identified but may be caused by vascular insult to small bowel. Identified causes include meconium ileus (cystic fibrosis), bowel atresia, and volvulus.

Echogenic Bowel. Meconium, which consists of desquamated cells, proteins, and bile pigments, fills the distal small bowel by 15 to 16 weeks. Its US appearance ranges from echolucent to moderately echogenic. Small bowel is considered abnormally echogenic when its echogenicity is equal to or greater than that of adjacent bone. This finding is normal in half of cases but serves as a marker of significant abnormality in the other half. Associations include cystic fibrosis, chromosome abnormalities (trisomy 21, trisomy 18), small bowel atresia, volvulus, and fetal viral infection (Cytomegalovirus).

Urinary Obstruction. The most common causes of hydronephrosis in the fetus are ureteropelvic junction obstruction, ectopic ureterocele, and posterior urethral valves (Fig. 38.39). Dilation of the renal pelvis to greater than 10 mm in anteroposterior diameter or greater than 50% of the anteroposterior diameter of the kidney in axial section, or unequivocal caliectasis, are definitive evidence of significant hydronephrosis. Assessment of bladder filling and amniotic fluid volume is necessary to determine the severity of obstruction.

Minimal dilatation of the renal pelvis presents a frequent clinical problem. Up to 20% of fetuses show a slightly large renal pelvis (greater than or equal to 3 mm), and another 40% show detectable (1- to 2-mm) fluid distension of the pelvis. This mild dilatation is most often caused by physiologic vesicoureteral reflux, which is normal during the second and third trimesters. Because some significant obstructions may show only mild dilatation in the second trimester, follow-up US in the third trimester is warranted

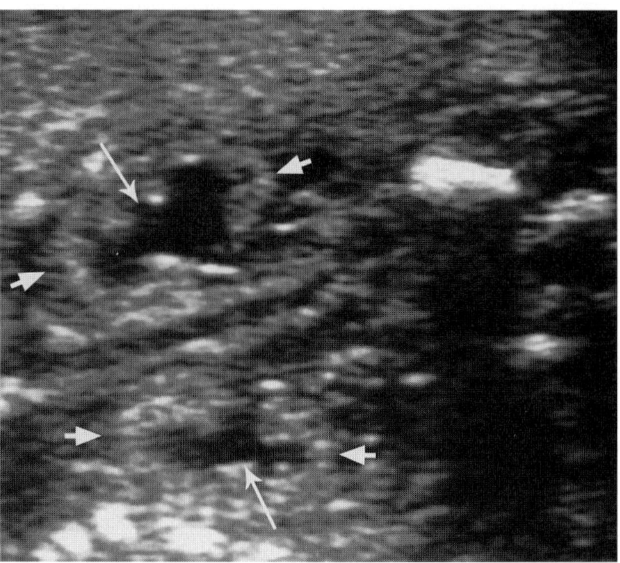

FIGURE 38.39. **Hydronephrosis.** Coronal plane image through the fetal abdomen reveals bilateral hydronephrosis (*thin arrows*) resulting from posterior urethral valves. Calices and the renal pelvis are dilated. Both kidneys (between *short arrows*) are normal in size.

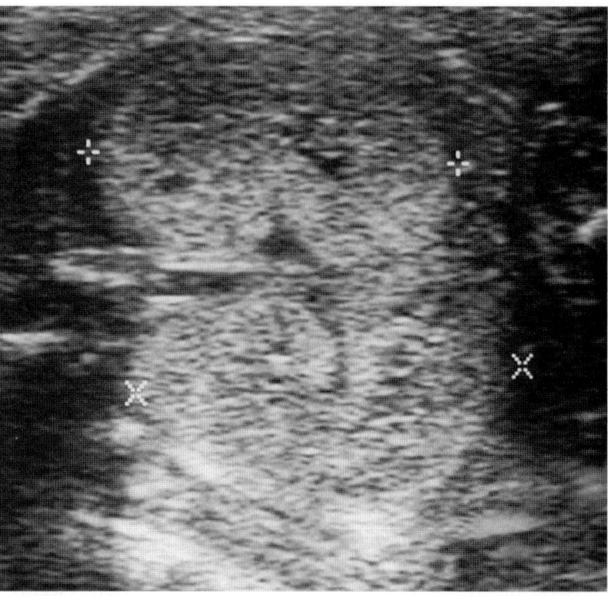

FIGURE 38.40. **Autosomal Recessive Polycystic Kidney Disease.** Coronal-plane image in a 22-week fetus shows two markedly enlarged, highly echogenic kidneys (between *cursors*) filling and distending the abdomen. Each kidney exceeded 5 cm in length. Severe oligohydramnios was present. This appearance is characteristic of the infantile form of autosomal recessive polycystic disease.

to detect development of caliectasis or progression of pyelectasis. Elective postnatal US examinations of equivocal cases should be performed at 1 to 2 weeks of age to avoid underestimation of hydronephrosis because of the normal oliguria that occurs during the early postnatal period.

Renal cystic disease is commonly detected in utero. *Multicystic dysplastic kidney* appears as multiple noncommunicating cysts of varying size. Because the affected kidneys do not function, bilateral multicystic dysplastic kidney is associated with severe oligohydramnios and is not compatible with life. Massive enlargement of both kidneys in association with oligohydramnios suggests *autosomal recessive polycystic kidney disease*. The kidneys are predominantly echogenic, with a sonolucent rim. Discrete cysts are usually not evident. *Autosomal dominant polycystic kidney disease* is occasionally detected in utero (Fig. 38.40). The kidneys are enlarged but lack the sonolucent rim of autosomal recessive polycystic kidney disease. Occasionally, discrete cysts are visualized. *Obstructive uropathy* such as posterior urethral valves may result in cystic renal dysplasia. Affected kidneys are hydronephrotic, with increased parenchymal echogenicity and cysts of varying size. The kidneys may be dysplastic without cysts being visualized by US.

Gastroschisis results from a defect in the anterior abdominal wall on the right side of the umbilicus (17). The defect is usually 2 to 5 cm in size. Bowel herniates through the defect and floats freely in the amniotic fluid, with no covering membrane (Fig. 38.41). Small defects may be associated with bowel ischemia, which results in thickening of the wall of the herniated bowel. The cord insertion site is normal. Gastroschisis is most commonly an isolated defect without chromosomal anomaly or recurrence risk. Postnatal repair is usually successful, so the prognosis is excellent when no other anomalies are present.

Omphalocele is a more serious abdominal wall defect that is about equal in frequency to gastroschisis (17). The defect is midline at the umbilicus with herniation of

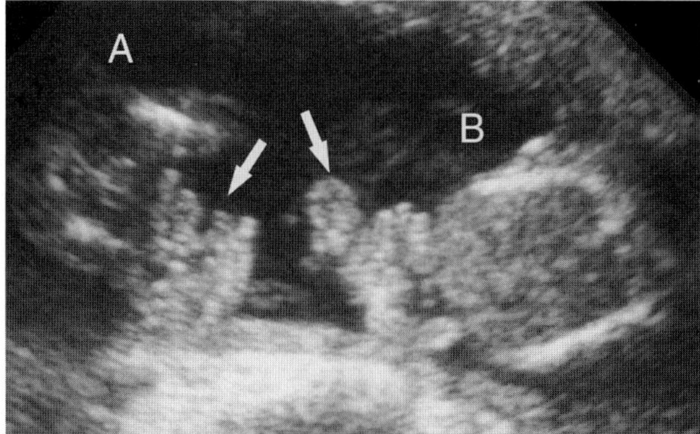

FIGURE 38.41. **Gastroschisis.** Image of a twin pregnancy, with the twins labelled A and B, shows that each fetus has gastroschisis. Multiple herniated bowel loops (*arrows*) float freely in amniotic fluid. No covering membrane is present. The cord insertion site of each twin fetus was normal.

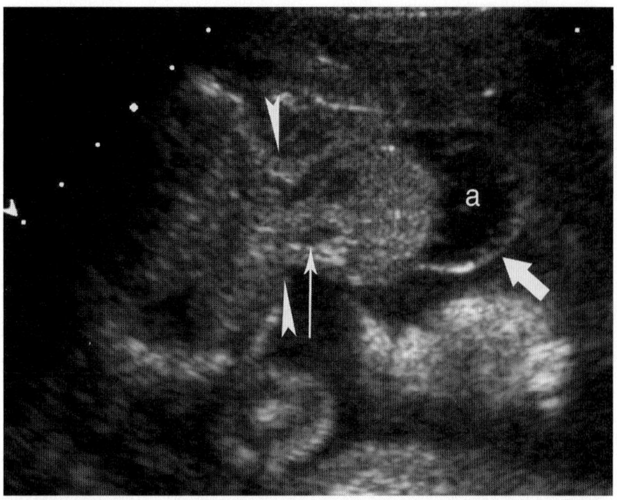

FIGURE 38.42. **Omphalocele.** Transverse image of the fetal abdomen at the level of the umbilicus shows liver herniating through a defect (between *arrowheads*) in the anterior abdominal wall. The defect involves the umbilical cord (*thin arrow*). A covering membrane (*wide arrow*) is easily seen because it is outlined by ascites (a) within the omphalocele and amniotic fluid.

abdominal contents into the base of the umbilical cord (Fig. 38.42). Both liver and bowel are commonly present in the herniation. A membrane consisting of peritoneum and amnion covers the omphalocele. The umbilical cord inserts through the membrane. Associated anomalies are common (67% to 88% of cases) and include cardiac, CNS, urinary tract, and GI malformations. Chromosome anomalies are found in up to 40% of cases. The ventral wall defect may include the heart (ectopia cordis).

Skeleton

Skeletal dysplasias are a heterogeneous group of disorders of skeletal growth that result in bones of abnormal size and shape (18). US findings that are highly associated with the presence of a generalized skeletal dysplasia include shortening of extremity bones, fractures, bowing of long bones, demineralization, and a small thorax (Fig. 38.43). A finding of short femur length mandates detailed bone examination, with measurement of additional long bones. A ratio of femur length to foot length of less than 0.9 suggests a skeletal dysplasia, whereas a ratio greater than 0.9 is usually associated with a constitutionally small or growth-retarded fetus. Additional findings that help categorize the skeletal dysplasia include polydactyly, abnormal head shape, spine anomalies, midface hypoplasia, abnormal bone configuration, ventriculomegaly, polyhydramnios, and hydrops. Precise diagnosis of a skeletal dysplasia may be difficult unless there is a family history. An algorithmic approach is recommended.

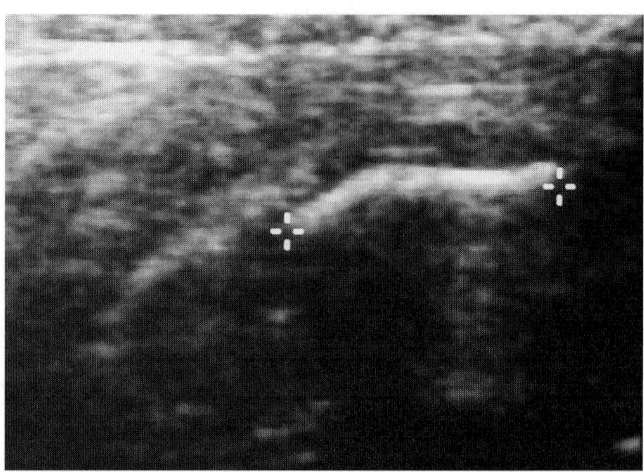

FIGURE 38.43. **Micromelic Dwarf.** A longitudinal image of the femur demonstrates poor mineralization, central bowing, and length that is markedly short for gestational age.

Thanatophoric dwarfism is the most common lethal skeletal dysplasia. Distinguishing features include small thorax, cloverleaf skull, large head, hydrocephalus, and polyhydramnios. *Achondroplastic dysplasia* is an autosomal dominant trait that is lethal in homozygous form and nonlethal in heterozygous form. Because at least one parent must have the condition, the US diagnosis is made on the basis of proximal limb shortening. *Osteogenesis imperfecta* is a heterogenous group of disorders with both autosomal dominant and recessive inheritance patterns. The hallmark of the disease is osteoporosis, which may manifest on US as diminished bone echogenicity. Additional features include bone thickening with fractures and callus formation, bone bowing, a small chest, and protuberant abdomen.

Examination of the fetal hands and feet may yield characteristic findings that suggest a variety of syndromes and chromosome abnormalities. Clenched hands with overlapping index fingers suggests trisomy 18. Polydactyly with polycystic kidneys suggests Meckel-Gruber syndrome. Hypoplasia of the middle phalanx of the fifth digit in association with femur and humerus shortening suggests Down syndrome.

REFERENCES

1. Brant WE. Obstetric ultrasound: first trimester. In: Brant WE, ed. The Core Curriculum: Ultrasound. Philadelphia: Lippincott Williams & Wilkins, 2001:225–256.
2. Brant WE. Obstetric ultrasound: second and third trimesters. In: Brant WE, ed. The Core Curriculum: Ultrasound. Philadelphia: Lippincott Williams & Wilkins, 2001:257–329.
3. Coakley FV, Glenn OA, Qayyun A, Barkovich AJ, Goldstein R, Filly RA. Fetal MRI: a developing technique for the developing patient. AJR Am J Roentgenol 2004;182:243–252.
4. American Institute of Ultrasound in Medicine. AIUM Practice Guidelines for the Performance of an Antepartum Obstetric Ultrasound Examination. Rockville: American Institute of Ultrasound in Medicine, 2003.

5. Dogra V, Paspulati RM, Bhatt S. First trimester bleeding evaluation. Ultrasound Q 2005;21:29–85.
6. Dialani V, Levine D. Ectopic pregnancy: a review. Ultrasound Q 2004;20:105–117.
7. Ignacio EA, Hill MC. Ultrasound of the acute female pelvis. Ultrasound Q 2003;19:86–98.
8. Zhou Q, Lei X-Y, Xie Q, Cardoza JD. Sonographic and Doppler imaging in the diagnosis and treatment of gestational trophoblastic disease. J Ultrasound Med 2005;24:15–24.
9. Smith-Bindman R, Chu PW, Ecker JL, et al. US evaluation of fetal growth: prediction of neonatal outcomes. Radiology 2002;223: 153–161.
10. Di Salvo DN. Sonographic imaging of maternal complications of pregnancy. J Ultrasound Med 2003;22:69–89.
11. DeVore GR, Romero R. Combined use of genetic sonography and maternal serum triple-marker screening: an effective method for increasing the detection of Trisomy 21 in women younger than 35 years. J Ultrasound Med 2001;20:645–654.
12. Nyberg DA, Souter VL. Sonographic markers of fetal trisomies. J Ultrasound Med 2001;20:655–674.
13. Mulliken JB, Benacerraf BA. Prenatal diagnosis of cleft lip: what the sonologist needs to tell the surgeon. J Ultrasound Med 2001;20:1159–1164.
14. Dhingsa R, Coakley FV, Albanese CT, Filly R, Goldstein R. Prenatal sonography and MR imaging of pulmonary sequestration. AJR Am J Roentgenol 2003;180:433–437.
15. Barboza JM, Dajani NK, Glenn LG, Angtuaco TL. Prenatal diagnosis of congenital cardiac anomalies: a practical approach using two basic views. Radiographics 2002;22:1125–1138.
16. Hertzberg BS, Kliewer MA. Ultrasound of the fetal gastrointestinal tract. Radiologist 1996;3:123–129.
17. Brant WE. Sonographic evaluation of the fetal abdominal wall. Radiologist 1995;2:149–161.
18. Parilla BV, Leeth EA, Kambick MP, Chilis P, MacGregor SN. Antenatal detection of skeletal dysplasias. J Ultrasound Med 2003;22:255–258.

Chapter 39

Chest, Thyroid, Parathyroid, and Neonatal Brain Ultrasound

William E. Brant

Chest
Pleural Space
Lung Parenchyma
Mediastinum

Thyroid
Thyroid Nodules
Diffuse Thyroid Disease

Parathyroid
Hyperparathyroidism

Neonatal Brain
Congenital Brain Abnormalities
Infection
Ischemic Brain Injury

CHEST

US is an excellent supplement to plain film radiography and CT for the problem-solving evaluation of the chest and to guide interventional procedures in the thorax (1–6). US can image into and through pleural effusions and lung consolidation to evaluate the thorax that is opacified on plain radiographs. Its portability allows evaluation of critically ill patients who are impractical to move for a CT. US examination of the chest must always be correlated with available chest radiography.

Pleural Space

Normal US Anatomy. Air in the lungs completely reflects the US beam and prohibits examination deeper into the chest. However, when pleural fluid displaces air-filled lungs away from the chest wall, disease in the pleural space can be optimally evaluated with US. The pleural space is examined by a direct intercostal approach, with the US transducer applied directly to the chest, or by an abdominal approach, imaging through the diaphragm from the abdomen. The ribs are used as sonographic landmarks for direct chest imaging (Fig. 39.1). A linear array transducer applied to the chest wall shows the ribs as curving echoes that cast acoustic shadows. The visceral pleura/air-filled lung interface is seen within 1 cm of the rib echo as a bright echogenic surface that moves with respiration (the "gliding sign"). The moving lung surface is well visualized when the transducer is turned to parallel the intercostal space. The tiny normal amount of fluid in the pleural space is seen just superficial to the gliding pleura. From the abdomen, the diaphragm is seen as a bright curving interface because of complete sound reflection from the air-filled lung above it (Fig. 39.2). Organs beneath the diaphragm (liver, spleen) are artifactually reproduced above the diaphragm because of multipath sound reflection (the "mirror image" artifact).

Pleural fluid displaces the lung away from the chest wall, allowing visualization of the pleural space (Figs 39.1C, 39.2B). Most pleural fluid is anechoic, or hypoechoic with floating particulate matter (7). The fluid separates the visceral and parietal pleural surfaces. From an abdominal approach, hypoechoic fluid is seen above the diaphragm, the inside of the thorax is visualized, and the mirror-image artifact is not present. Septations not evident on CT are commonly visualized by US. Collapsed or consolidated lung moves with respiration within the fluid in the pleural space. Fluid that is echogenic, contains floating particles or layering debris, or is septated is an exudate (Fig. 39.3). Fluid that is anechoic may be a transudate,

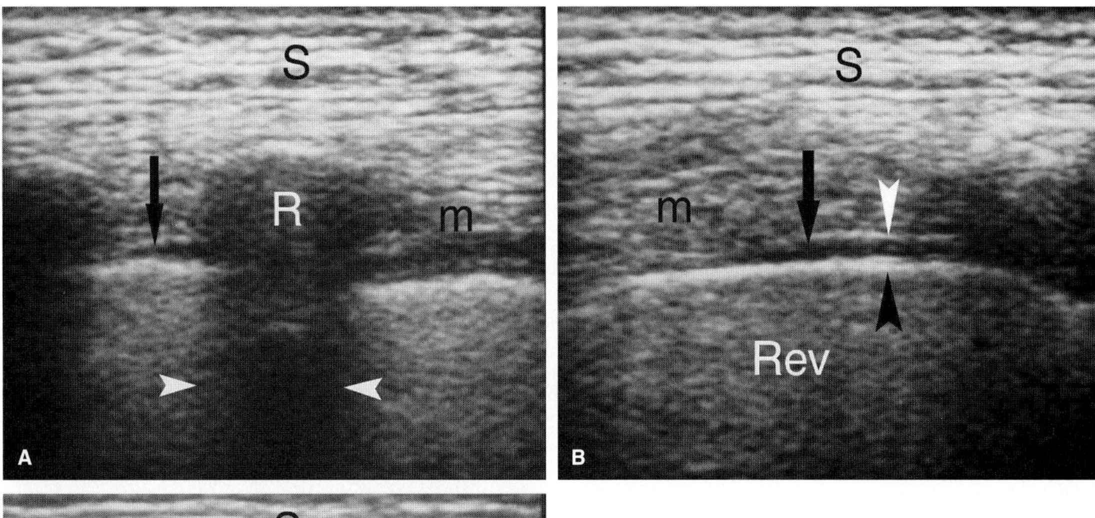

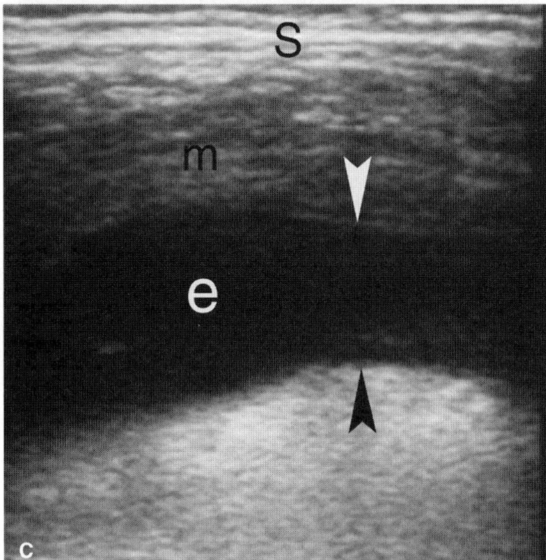

FIGURE 39.1. **Pleural Space: Intercostal Scan. A.** Longitudinal US image of the chest shows a rib (R) and its acoustic shadow (between *arrowheads*). The pleural space is approximately 1 cm deep to the surface of the rib (*arrow*). Intercostal muscle (m) is seen between the ribs. **B.** Aligning the transducer parallel to the ribs in the intercostal space enables improved visualization of the pleural space (*arrow*). The visceral pleura/air-filled lung interface (*black arrowhead*) is identified by its movement with respiration: the "gliding sign." The visceral pleura is separated from the parietal pleura (*white arrowhead*) by a thin layer of pleural fluid in the pleural space (*arrow*). The air-filled lung is obscured by reverberation artifact (Rev). **C.** A pleural effusion (e) separates the visceral pleura (*black arrowhead*) from the parietal pleura (*white arrowhead*). m, intercostal muscle; S, subcutaneous fatty tissue.

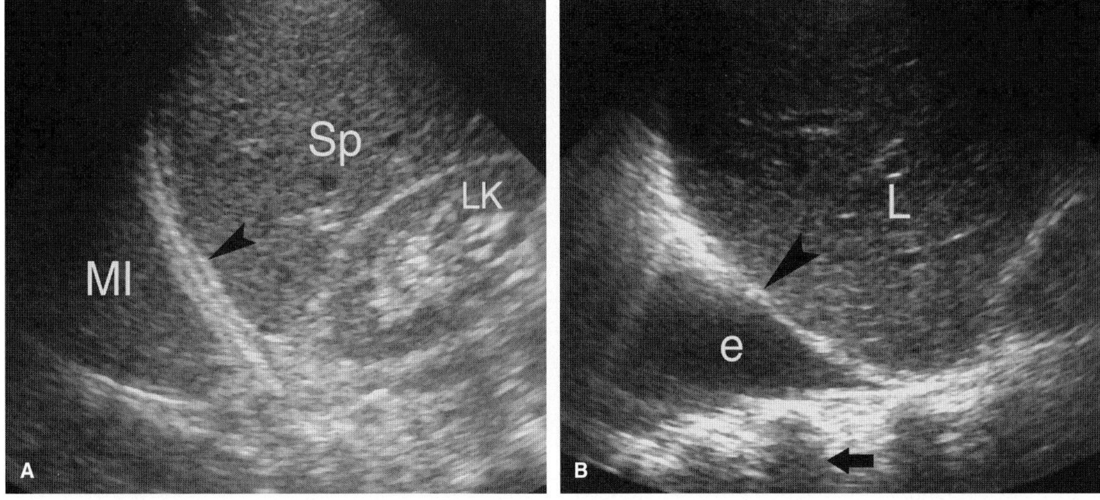

FIGURE 39.2. **Pleural Space: Abdominal Scan. A.** Examination of the chest can be performed from an abdominal approach, using the liver or spleen (Sp) as a sonographic window. The diaphragm is seen as a bright curving line (*arrowhead*). Normal air-filled lung causes the spleen to be reproduced as a mirror-image artifact (MI) above the diaphragm. LK, left kidney. **B.** A pleural effusion (e) eliminates the mirror-image artifact and allows visualization of the chest, wall characterized by ribs and rib shadows (*arrow*) through the diaphragm (*arrowhead*) and pleural space. L, Liver.

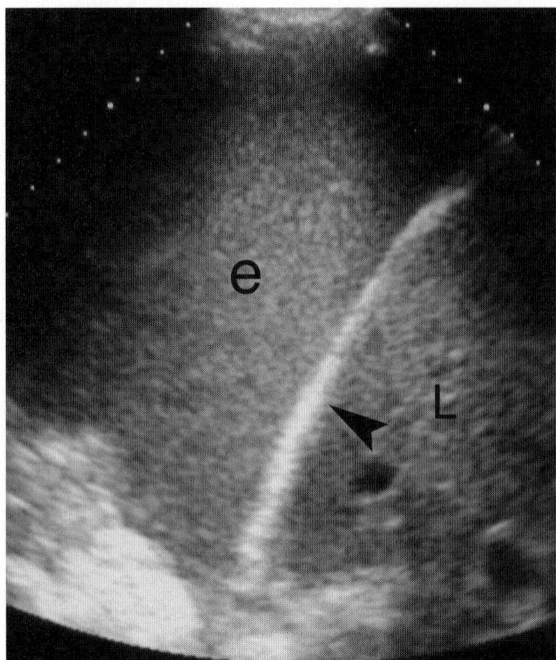

FIGURE 39.3. **Echogenic Pleural Effusion.** An empyema associated with a right lower lobe pneumonia appears on US as an echogenic effusion (e). Innumerable moving floating particles were observed within the fluid on real-time US examination. The liver (L) is very similar in echogenicity. The diaphragm (*arrowhead*) is seen as a curving, brightly echogenic line.

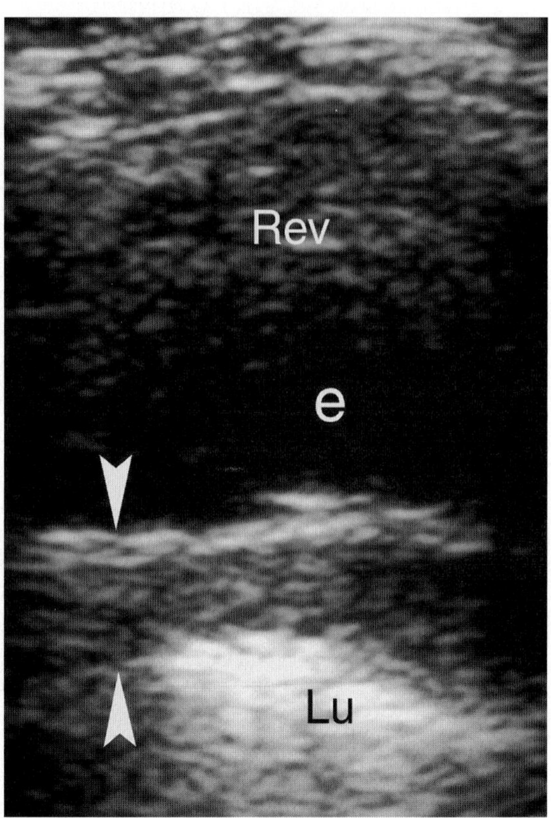

FIGURE 39.4. **Pleural Thickening.** Intercostal US image demonstrates a moderate volume pleural effusion (e). The visceral pleura (between *arrowheads*) is thickened because of chronic inflammation. The parietal pleura is obscured in the near field by reverberation artifact (Rev). The air-filled lung (Lu) is brightly echogenic.

exudate, or even empyema. Loculations of pleural fluid and suspected empyemas can be localized and evaluated, with US visualization used to guide needle aspiration and drainage catheter placement.

Pleural thickening complicates inflammatory and malignant disease of the thorax. US demonstrates uniform, undulating, or plaquelike thickening of the pleura (Fig. 39.4). The visceral pleura is easily evaluated. The parietal pleura is partially obscured by reverberation artifact in the near field.

Pleural Masses. Pleural metastases or tumors such as mesotheliomas are seen as nodular pleural thickening or hypoechoic soft tissue masses in the pleural space projecting from the pleural surface.

Pneumothorax can be diagnosed by US. Pneumothorax produces a highly echogenic reflective line very similar to that of air-filled lung but lacking the "gliding sign" associated with respiratory movement. Pneumothorax is also indicated by loss of visualization of a previously visualized lung lesion that occurs during an invasive procedure.

Lung Parenchyma

Normal US Anatomy. The normal air-filled lung with its covering visceral pleura completely blocks transmission of US into the thorax. The gliding visceral surface of the lung is easily seen, but reverberation artifact is displayed deep to that surface. However, consolidation, atelectasis, or tumor that extends to the visceral pleural surface produces a window for US examination. When scanning the thorax from the abdomen, the normal air-filled lung produces a mirror-image artifact.

Consolidation refers to filling of the air spaces of the lung with fluid and inflammatory cells. This process "solidifies" the lung and provides a medium for sound transmission (Fig. 39.5). The consolidated lung appears solid and hypoechoic, with echogenicity similar to that of liver tissue. *Sonographic air bronchograms* and *sonographic air alveolograms* may be seen within the consolidated lung. Air-filled bronchi produce bright branching linear reflections. Air trapped in alveoli surrounded by consolidated lung produces globular bright echoes with comet-tail artifacts. *Sonographic fluid bronchograms* appear as anechoic fluid-filled tubes extending from the hilum of the lung. Color flow US demonstrates pulmonary vessels extending through the consolidated lung.

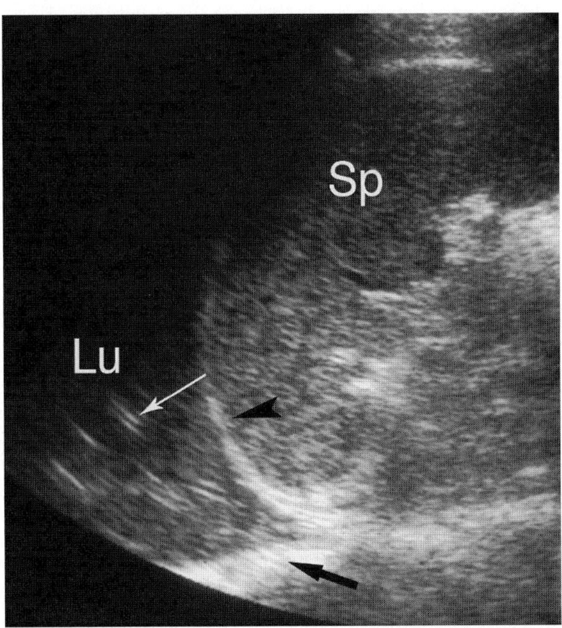

FIGURE 39.5. **Lung Consolidation.** US image obtained using the spleen (Sp) as a sonographic window in a patient with left upper quadrant pain reveals an unsuspected pneumonia in the left lower lobe of the lung (Lu). Inflammatory fluid and cells solidify the lung, replacing air and allowing visualization of the chest wall (*black arrow*) through the airless lung. Sonographic fluid bronchograms (*white arrow*) are seen within the pneumonia. The diaphragm (*arrowhead*) produces a bright, curving echo.

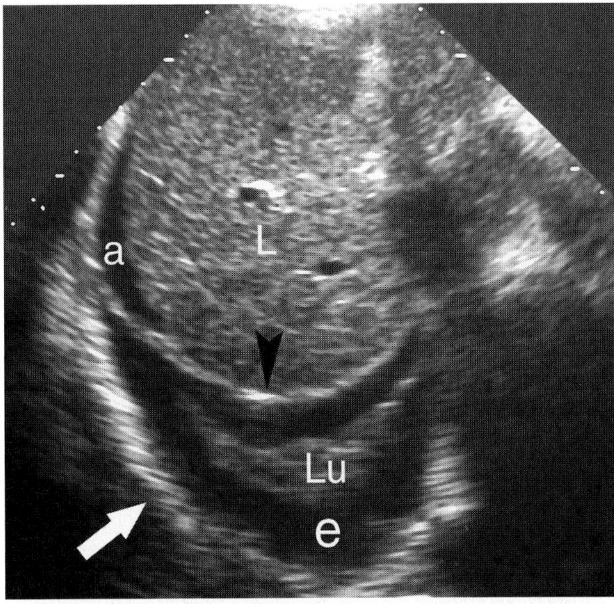

FIGURE 39.6. **Atelectasis.** A transverse image through the liver (L) reveals a pleural effusion (e) surrounding a tongue of collapsed lung (Lu). The patient also has ascites (a). The diaphragm (*arrowhead*) produces a thin, curving, bright echo. The chest wall (*arrow*) produces a thick, curving, bright echo.

Atelectasis. Collapse of the airspaces with absorption of air also results in solidification of the lung. With atelectasis, the lung volume is decreased and bronchi and pulmonary blood vessels are crowded together. Collapsed lung always accompanies large pleural effusions (Fig. 39.6). The atelectatic lung is wedge-shaped and sharply defined by its covering pleura.

Lung masses surrounded by air-filled lung are not visualized by US, but those that extend to the visceral pleura or are accompanied by peripheral consolidation or atelectasis may be seen and evaluated (Fig. 39.7). US guidance may be effectively used to aspirate or biopsy lung masses in areas that are difficult to access with CT or fluoroscopy. Central tumor necrosis, hemorrhage within tumors, and lung abscesses are effectively evaluated.

Pulmonary sequestration is a congenital partition of lung tissue that does not communicate with the bronchial tree. Most occur at the lung base. Intralobar sequestrations are within the visceral pleura. Extralobar sequestrations are invested by their own separate pleura. US is used to confirm the diagnosis by demonstration of a feeding artery arising from the aorta. Extralobar sequestrations drain via a systemic vein, whereas intralobar sequestrations connect to the pulmonary veins.

Mediastinum

Normal US Anatomy. The superior and anterior mediastinum are effectively evaluated with US using a parasternal or supramanubrial approach. The posterior mediastinum is less accessible because of spine and lung. Large lesions create sonographic windows to the mediastinum. Imaging downward into the superior mediastinum from just above the sternal manubrium demonstrates the innominate veins and the arteries arising from the aortic arch. Doppler US assists in the identification of vessels.

Vascular Lesions. Elongation and tortuosity of the brachiocephalic artery are common causes of mediastinal widening in older adults. This diagnosis is easily confirmed by US, which can also exclude other masses of the superior mediastinum.

Mediastinal Masses. Thymic masses, substernal extension of thyroid enlargement, adenopathy, and other mediastinal masses are effectively demonstrated by US, which can confirm their cystic or solid nature and vascularity. Lesions that can be visualized by US can usually be biopsied using US guidance to avoid critical structures (Fig. 39.8). Continuation of thyroid tissue into the mediastinum is a straightforward diagnosis. Enlarged lymph nodes are usually homogeneous and hypoechoic. Confluent adenopathy caused by lymphoma produces a solid, homogeneous, hypoechoic mass that encompasses and displaces blood vessels.

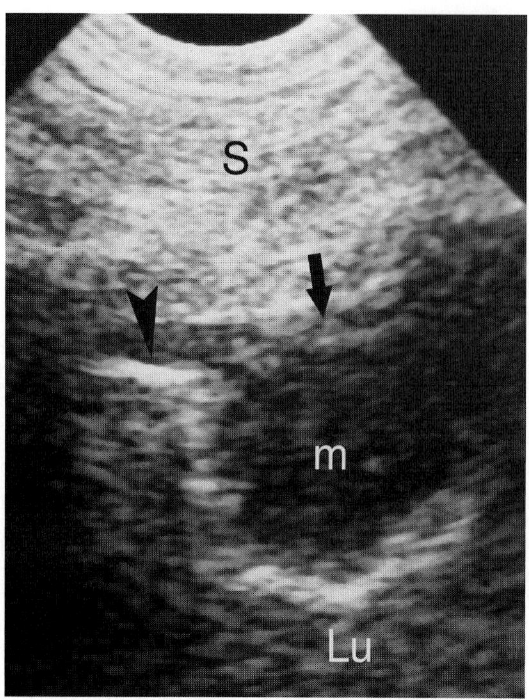

FIGURE 39.7. **Peripheral Lung Mass.** Intercostal US scan shows a 3-cm lung mass (m) abutting the pleural surface. Note how the bright echo from the visceral pleura/air-filled-lung interface (*arrowhead*) is obliterated over the mass (*arrow*). The hypoechoic mass stands out because it is surrounded by echogenic, air-filled lung (Lu). Fine-needle biopsy, which was precisely guided by US visualization into the mass without transgressing air-filled lung, confirmed squamous cell carcinoma. This patient has abundant subcutaneous fatty tissue (S).

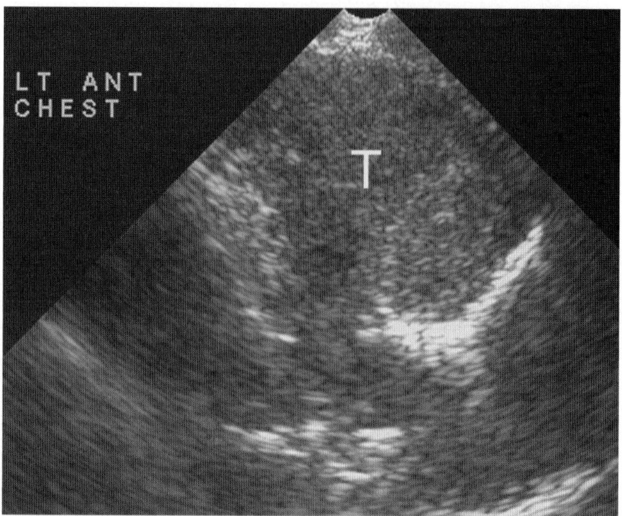

FIGURE 39.8. **Mediastinal Mass.** A left parasternal US image shows a large solid mediastinal mass (T). US-guided fine-needle and core biopsies were easily performed and confirmed a malignant thymoma.

THYROID

Imaging of the thyroid gland is a controversial topic (8,9). Thyroid nodules are exceedingly common, although thyroid cancer is uncommon and death from thyroid malignancy is rare. High-resolution US is extremely sensitive in detecting thyroid nodules; however, imaging signs to differentiate benign from malignant lesions are nonspecific and unreliable (10). This creates a recurring clinical problem of what to do with the many nodules detected sonographically. Because of this difficulty, the indications for US of the thyroid are debated. US is used to precisely guide percutaneous biopsy of thyroid nodules, to screen patients at high risk for thyroid cancer, to identify recurrent disease in patients with known thyroid cancer, and to determine whether palpable nodules arise from the thyroid gland. CT and MR supplement US by staging of invasive thyroid cancers, evaluating for postoperative recurrence of thyroid cancer, and demonstrating extension of goiter into the thorax. Radionuclide imaging, discussed in a subsequent chapter, evaluates the physiologic function of the gland and determines the activity of nodules.

Normal US Anatomy. The thyroid gland consists of paired lobes of nearly equal size ($5 \times 2 \times 2$ cm) connected across the trachea by a thin thyroid isthmus (Fig. 39.9). The thyroid parenchyma is homogeneous, with fine medium-level echogenicity greater than muscle. Anatomic landmarks include the midline air-filled trachea, which casts an air shadow; the common carotid artery and internal jugular vein, which parallel the lateral edge of the thyroid lobes; the longus colli muscles posteriorly; and the sternohyoid, sternothyroid, and sternocleidomastoid muscles anteriorly. Small pools of colloid (colloid cysts) are routinely visualized within the normal gland. The thyroid

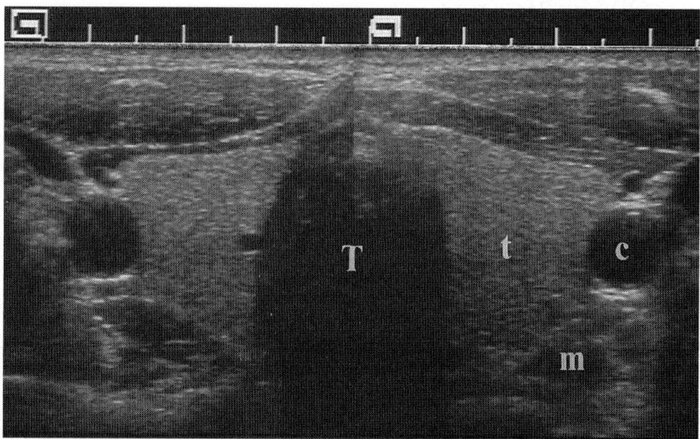

FIGURE 39.9. **Normal Thyroid.** Symmetric lobes of homogeneous thyroid tissue (t) are seen on either side of the trachea (T) on this transverse image. Anatomic landmarks include the carotid arteries (c) and longus colli muscle (m).

TABLE 39.1 Differentiation of Benign and Malignant Thyroid Nodules

Evidence Favoring Benign Nodule	*Evidence Favoring Malignant Nodule*	*Indeterminate Evidence Found With Both Benign and Malignant Nodules*
Extensive cystic component Sharply defined margin Peripheral calcification Homogeneously hyperechoic Comet tail artifacts	Irregular contour Poor margination Microcalcifications Size >4 to 5 cm Single cold nodule on radionuclide scan (15% malignant)	Hypoechoic nodule Isoechoic nodule Solid nodule Amorphous dense calcification Echolucent halo
Multiple nodules on radionuclide scan	Age <20 years History of neck irradiation, especially in childhood	Multiple nodules on US Increased flow on color Doppler US
Hot on radionuclide scan	Family history of thyroid malignancy, especially medullary carcinoma Male	

lobes are often mildly asymmetric in size. The esophagus may protrude from behind the trachea on the left side and must not be mistaken for a thyroid or parathyroid mass or lymph node (see Fig. 39.15). The superior thyroid artery and vein are imaged between the upper pole of the thyroid and the longus colli. The recurrent laryngeal nerve and inferior thyroid artery and vein are seen posterior to the lower poles. The thyroid is easily imaged with the patient in a supine position, with the neck extended by placement of a pillow beneath the shoulders.

Thyroid Nodules

The Problem. Thyroid nodules can be palpated in 4% to 7% of the general population and are found at autopsy in 50% of thyroid glands that are normal to palpation. High-resolution US demonstrates thyroid nodules in 35% to 45% of asymptomatic adults, with a higher incidence of nodules in women. Thyroid cancer, on the other hand, affects only 0.1% of the population. Thyroid cancer accounts for less than 1% of all cancers and is the cause of less than 0.5% of all cancer deaths. The ratio of benign thyroid nodules to thyroid cancer can be estimated at 500:1. The challenge of imaging studies and clinical evaluation is to establish the likelihood of malignancy and to select out for surgery only those patients with thyroid malignancy.

US is highly sensitive for the detection of thyroid nodules; however, its specificity for determining malignancy is low. Neither MR nor CT can improve that specificity. This is not surprising, because the histologic differentiation of benign follicular adenoma from well-differentiated follicular carcinoma is based solely on identification of vascular invasion. Radionuclide imaging is far less sensitive than US in the demonstration of thyroid nodules. Although no signs are specific, multiple parameters can be used together to make a clinical judgement regarding the risk of thyroid malignancy (Table 39.1). Nodules considered suspicious for malignancy should undergo fine-needle aspiration biopsy (FNA) for diagnosis. US is a precise imaging method to guide FNA.

Although true thyroid cysts are extremely rare, many benign nodules demonstrate cystic degeneration. An extensive cystic component is strong evidence of benignancy. Most of these benign cystic lesions demonstrate internal debris and some degree of wall irregularity and solid components. This finding is not specific, however. Although most thyroid cancers are solid masses, some have cystic areas within them. Radionuclide scans classify nodules as hypofunctioning ("cold"), hyperfunctioning ("hot"), or indeterminate. Single cold nodules have a 15% incidence of malignancy, and malignancy is exceedingly rare in hot nodules. If a radionuclide scan demonstrates multiple nodules, the risk of malignancy is about 1%. However, demonstration of multiple nodules by US is *not* a sign of benignancy (Table 39.2). Papillary thyroid cancer is multicentric in 20% of cases, and benign nodules are found to coexist with thyroid cancer in 33% of cases undergoing surgery. Most benign nodules and most thyroid cancers are hypoechoic relative to normal thyroid parenchyma. However, a nodule that is predominantly hyperechoic is very likely to be benign. Benign nodules tend to be well marginated and smooth in contour. Malignancies are usually poorly marginated and irregular in contour (11). However, many thyroid nodules violate these trends. An echolucent rim is a sign of a slow-growing nodule but may be found with both benign and malignant nodules. Up to 20% of malignant nodules have a sonolucent peripheral halo. Calcifications are common in all thyroid nodules. Peripheral or eggshell calcification is highly

TABLE 39.2 Causes of Multiple Thyroid Nodules on US

Common
Multinodular goiter
Multiple benign adenomas
Hashimoto thyroiditis (micronodules)
Subacute thyroiditis
Chronic thyroiditis
Uncommon
Carcinoma + benign adenomas
Anaplastic carcinoma
Lymphoma
Acute thyroiditis

characteristic of benign lesions, whereas microcalcifications (small echodense particles, usually without acoustic shadows) are strongly indicative of malignancy. Amorphous dense calcifications are found with both benign and malignant nodules. Comet-tail artifacts, which arise from inspissated colloid, are a strong sign of a benign nodule (12). A history of neck irradiation, particularly in childhood, increases the risk of malignancy by fivefold to 10-fold. Regression of nodule size following thyroid hormone therapy is a sign of a benign nodule. Color flow US is not helpful in the differentiation of benign versus malignant thyroid nodules. Biopsy is indicated for all nodules with malignant features and for nodules larger than 15 mm with indeterminate features. Nodules smaller than 15 mm can be followed by physical examination for evidence of enlargement.

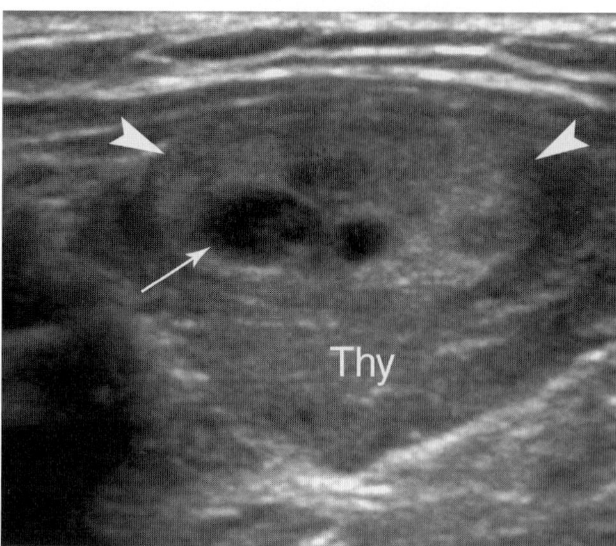

FIGURE 39.10. **Adenomatous Nodule.** Longitudinal image of the thyroid gland reveals a dominant nodule (between *arrowheads*) with cystic change (*arrow*). US-guided fine-needle aspiration biopsy yielded a cytologic diagnosis of "colloid nodule," indicating visualization of benign thyroid cells and thyroid colloid. "Colloid nodules" is the usual cytologic term for adenomatous nodules. Note the homogeneous pattern of the visualized normal thyroid parenchyma (Thy).

Benign Thyroid Nodules

Adenomatous nodules, also called *colloid nodules*, are the most common thyroid nodule. They are not neoplasms but benign growths resulting from cycles of hyperplasia and involution of thyroid tissue. They are usually multiple and associated with diffuse enlargement of the thyroid gland. Individual nodules are isoechoic or hypoechoic to thyroid parenchyma, and they commonly show degenerative changes, with prominent cystic components, necrosis, hemorrhage, and calcification (Fig. 39.10).

Follicular adenoma is the most common benign neoplasm. Autonomous hyperfunctioning adenomas are a cause of hyperthyroidism, but most adenomas cause no alteration of overall thyroid function. Most are solitary, solid, and well encapsulated. They may be hypoechoic, hyperechoic, or isoechoic to thyroid parenchyma (Fig. 39.11). Hyperfunctioning adenomas are commonly strikingly hypervascular on color flow US. Degenerative changes include focal necrosis, hemorrhage, edema, infarction, fibrosis, and calcification. Differentiation from follicular carcinoma is difficult; therefore, an FNA cytologic diagnosis of follicular neoplasm is commonly considered an indication for surgical removal.

Thyroid cysts are extremely rare, epithelial-lined, simple cysts. Most cystic nodules found in the thyroid are actually cystic degeneration of an adenomatous nodule ("colloid cyst") or a follicular adenoma.

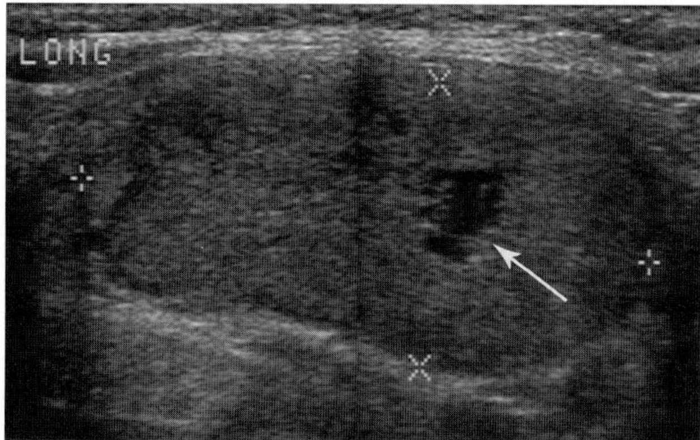

FIGURE 39.11. **Follicular Neoplasm.** US-guided fine-needle aspiration yielded abundant follicular cells from this dominant thyroid nodule (between *cursors*). An irregular area of cystic change is evident (*arrow*). Because a diagnosis of follicular carcinoma could not be excluded, this lesion was surgically removed. No histologic evidence of malignancy was present. Follow up showed no recurrence and no evidence of metastatic disease.

Hemorrhage may occur into an adenomatous nodule or a follicular adenoma, or spontaneously into normal parenchyma. Patients present with sudden neck pain and subsequent swelling. US reveals a hypoechoic nodule with internal debris.

Malignant Thyroid Nodules

Papillary thyroid carcinoma (75% of thyroid cancers) is one of the least aggressive cancers in humans. Most patients are female (4:1). Nodules are hypoechoic and commonly multiple. Punctate internal calcification (Fig. 39.12), representing psammoma bodies, is common (42%) and highly indicative of malignancy. Involved cervical nodes may contain similar calcifications. The tumor spreads commonly to regional nodes, but rarely (2% to 3% of cases) to lung and bone. The 5-year survival rate is 95% to 99% (13).

Follicular thyroid carcinoma (10% to 15%) is also a slow-growing malignancy, but invasion of blood vessels is characteristic, with hematogenous spread to lung and bone common. Lymphatic spread to cervical nodes is uncommon. Most tumors are solitary, isoechoic, and ill defined. Cystic areas, hemorrhage, and necrosis are common. The 5-year survival rate is about 65%.

Medullary thyroid carcinoma (5%) is a neuroendocrine malignancy that arises from parafollicular C cells that secrete calcitonin, which serves as a tumor marker. About 20% of cases are familial and associated with multiple endocrine neoplasia (MEN 2). US appearance is similar to that of papillary carcinoma, with coarse internal calcifications common (80%). The 5-year survival rate is 65%.

Anaplastic thyroid carcinoma (<5%) is a lethal malignancy of the elderly. The tumor grows rapidly and metastasizes widely. US shows a ill-defined, inhomogeneous, hypoechoic, solid mass. Nodal metastases are commonly present. The 5-year survival rate is under 4%.

Thyroid Cancer Staging. When US, CT, or MR is used for initial staging of thyroid malignancy or follow-up for recurrence, one must consider the common routes of spread of the specific type of malignancy to optimally plan the imaging study. The impressive contrast resolution of MR makes it excellent for determining involvement of muscles, larynx, esophagus, and other cervical structures by large, invasive tumors. Recurrence of tumor may be demonstrated by MR. On T2WIs, tumor has high signal intensity, brighter than muscle, and fibrosis in the thyroid bed has low signal intensity that is less than or equal to that of muscle. Lymph node involvement is determined primarily by size criteria. Normal lymph nodes in the neck are less than 10 mm in diameter.

Lymphoma accounts for 4% of thyroid malignancies and is most common in elderly women. Most is of the non-Hodgkin type. A solitary, strikingly hypoechoic mass is most common, although some cases demonstrate multiple nodules. Associated enlarged cervical nodes are common. Nearly all patients with primary thyroid lymphoma also have Hashimoto thyroiditis.

Metastasis. Metastatic disease to the thyroid gland is rare. The most common primary tumors to metastasize to the thyroid are breast, lung, kidney, and malignant melanoma.

Diffuse Thyroid Disease

The diagnosis of most diffuse diseases of the thyroid is made clinically, and US is seldom indicated. US can be helpful when thyroid enlargement is asymmetric and a neoplasm is suspected.

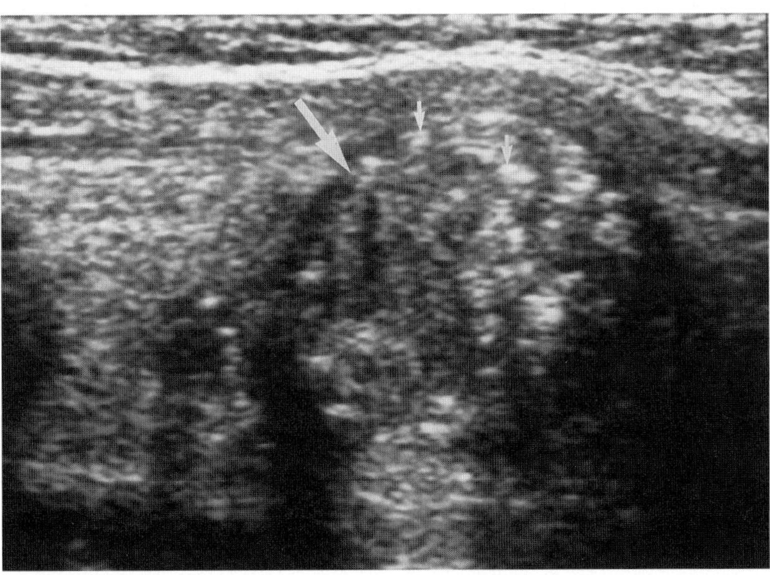

FIGURE 39.12. **Papillary Carcinoma of the Thyroid.** Longitudinal image reveals a solid nodule (*large arrow*) containing numerous microcalcifications (*small arrows*). The presence of microcalcifications in a thyroid nodule is highly indicative of malignancy. Biopsy proved papillary carcinoma.

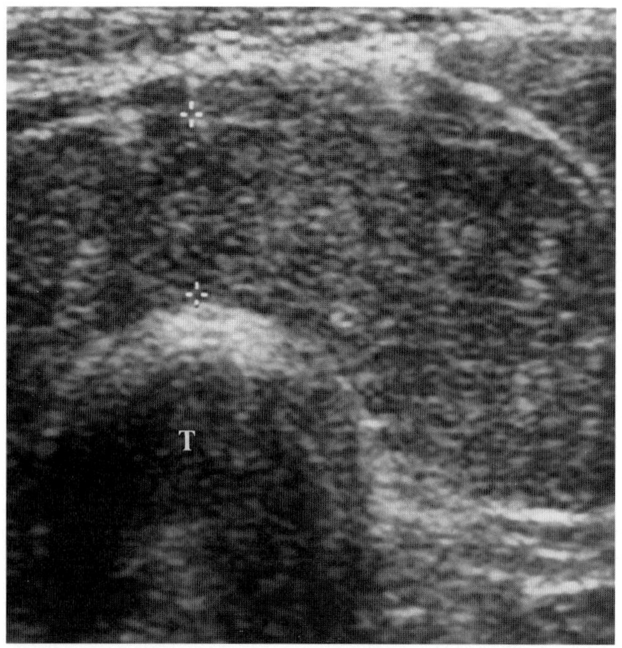

FIGURE 39.13. **Goiter.** Transverse image shows thickening of the thyroid isthmus to 12 mm (between *cursors*). T, trachea.

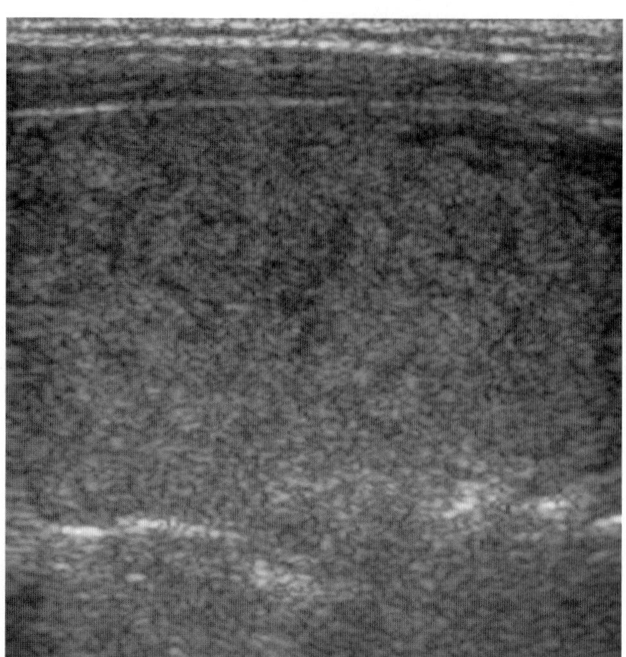

FIGURE 39.14. **Hashimoto Thyroiditis.** Longitudinal image through one lobe of the thyroid shows heterogeneous parenchyma, with a myriad of indistinct tiny nodules.

Goiter is a general term indicating diffuse thyroid enlargement. Goiter may be associated with increased, decreased, or normal thyroid function. The range of normal thyroid size is great. Thyroid enlargement is best judged subjectively. Helpful US signs of thyroid enlargement are thickening of the isthmus greater than 3 mm and outward bulge of the anterior surface of the gland (Fig. 39.13). US measurement is useful in assessing and following thyroid gland size in determining response to therapy.

Nontoxic goiter is caused by iodine deficiency, goitrogens in the diet, or deficiency of thyroid enzymes. US shows an enlarged gland with homogeneous parenchyma.

Adenomatous goiter, also called multinodular goiter, affects about 5% of the population of the United States. Adenomatous hyperplasia is the cause of 80% of thyroid nodules. Adenomatous goiter refers to the generalized enlargement of the thyroid that occurs when multiple hyperplastic nodules are present. US shows coarsening and heterogeneity of the thyroid parenchyma (see Fig. 39.15), with coarse calcifications commonly present. Each nodule must be individually evaluated for signs of malignancy.

Hashimoto thyroiditis (chronic lymphocytic thyroiditis) is an autoimmune disease that affects primarily women. About 10% to 15% of patients are clinically hypothyroid. It is the most common cause of hypothyroidism and goiter in adults in the United States. Circulating antithyroid antibody is associated with diffuse lymphomatous infiltration of the gland. US demonstrates diffuse thyroid enlargement with inhomogeneous low-density parenchyma. No normal parenchyma is present. A pattern of multiple, tiny nodules, 1 to 6 mm in size, is highly indicative of the disease (Fig. 39.14). Patients are at risk for development of lymphoma. Large, hypoechoic nodules should be considered for biopsy.

Graves disease is the most common cause of hyperthyroidism. The gland is usually enlarged twofold to threefold, homogeneous, and without nodules. Color Doppler US demonstrates striking, diffuse, increased vascularity with multiple small areas of intrathyroid flow (the "thyroid inferno").

Subacute (viral) thyroiditis, also called De Quervain or granulomatous thyroiditis, presents with thyroid pain and hyperthyroidism following an upper respiratory infection. Iodine uptake is usually decreased or absent in the acute stages. The disease runs a subacute course of a few weeks to a few months. Affected portions of the gland are swollen, edematous, and hypoechoic on US.

Acute suppurative thyroiditis is a rare bacterial infection of the thyroid gland. Often only a portion of the gland is involved. US is helpful in the detection and aspiration of abscesses.

Riedel thyroiditis is a rare inflammatory disease of progressive fibrosis that eventually destroys the thyroid gland and commonly extends into the neck. The gland is diffusely enlarged and inhomogeneous. US is used to show extension into the neck with encasement of cervical blood vessels.

PARATHYROID

Imaging of the parathyroid glands is another controversial topic. The primary indication is preoperative localization of parathyroid adenomas or hyperplastic parathyroid glands in the setting of clinically diagnosed hyperparathyroidism (10). Preoperative localization makes resection easier and reduces surgical morbidity. Preoperative imaging is particularly useful in patients with previous neck surgery. US, CT, MR, and radionuclide imaging have all been used in this setting. Of these, radionuclide imaging is the most sensitive and accurate. However, because 80% to 85% of abnormal parathyroid glands are located in the neck, US is able to demonstrate the majority. Imaging has no role in hypoparathyroidism.

Normal US Anatomy. Normal parathyroid glands measure only 5 × 3 × 1 mm in size and are not usually demonstrated by any imaging method. Most enlarged glands are found beneath the thyroid lobes, between the trachea and carotid sheath. The esophagus commonly protrudes out from behind the trachea, particularly on the left side. This normal structure should not be mistaken for a thyroid or parathyroid lesion (Fig. 39.15). Ectopic glands may be found between the upper pole of the thyroid and the thymus.

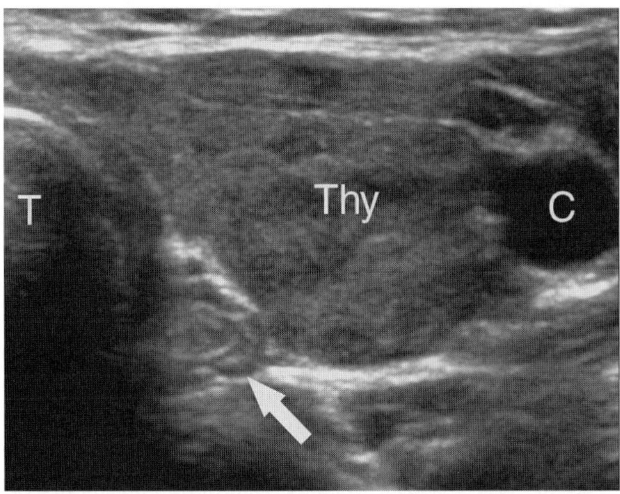

FIGURE 39.15. **Normal Esophagus.** Transverse US image of the thyroid gland (Thy) reveals an apparent nodule (*arrow*) deep to the thyroid and extending laterally from the acoustic shadow of the trachea (T). Having the patient swallow confirms that this structure is the normal esophagus. Note the multilayered echo pattern characteristic of the GI tract. The esophagus should not be mistaken for a thyroid or parathyroid lesion. This patient's thyroid gland is diffusely heterogeneous, characteristic of adenomatous goiter. C, common carotid artery.

Hyperparathyroidism

Primary hyperparathyroidism is a common disease that affects women two to three times more commonly than men. More than half the patients are above age 50. A single, benign, hyperfunctioning adenoma is the cause in 85% of cases (14). Multiple gland enlargement is responsible for 14% of cases and parathyroid carcinoma is the cause of 1% of cases. Most cases of hyperplasia involve all glands, although usually asymmetrically. The diagnosis is suspected on the basis of unexplained hypercalcemia and is confirmed by an elevated serum parathyroid hormone level. In secondary and tertiary hyperparathyroidism, elevated parathormone levels are caused by diffuse or nodular glandular hyperplasia. Secondary hyperparathyroidism occurs as a result of chronic hypocalcemia in patients with chronic renal failure. The parathyroid glands are overstimulated and become hyperplastic. When the chronically overstimulated glands become autonomous, the term *tertiary hyperparathyroidism* is used. Parathormone may also be produced by nonendocrine tumors, such as renal cell and bronchogenic carcinoma.

Parathyroid adenomas appear on US as homogeneous, hypoechoic, solid, oval, and well-defined masses (Fig. 39.16) between 8 and 15 mm in size (15). Color Doppler demonstrates hypervascularity. On T1WIs, adenomas show low intensity, similar to muscle. On T2WIs, the adenomas showed high intensity, similar to or greater than fat. Because adenomas may be isointense with fat, T2WIs alone provide an incomplete examination. CT is best performed with IV contrast to demonstrate the contrast-enhancing parathyroid nodules. Rarely, parathyroid adenomas may show cystic degeneration or calcification. Thyroid nodules may appear similar to parathyroid adenomas on US, although degenerated parathyroid adenomas may mimic cystic thyroid masses. US may be used to guide needle biopsy. Cells of parathyroid origin can be readily differentiated from thyroid cells cytologically, although fluid aspirated from degenerated parathyroid nodules has high parathyroid hormone levels.

Parathyroid hyperplasia affects all the parathyroid glands, but the degree of enlargement is frequently asymmetric. Hyperplastic glands have the same imaging characteristics as parathyroid adenomas.

Parathyroid carcinoma is distinguished by larger size (>20 mm) versus parathyroid adenomas. Tumors are usually more heterogeneous, with cystic degeneration and occasional calcification. The contour is lobulated or ill-defined. Color flow US is useful to demonstrate invasion

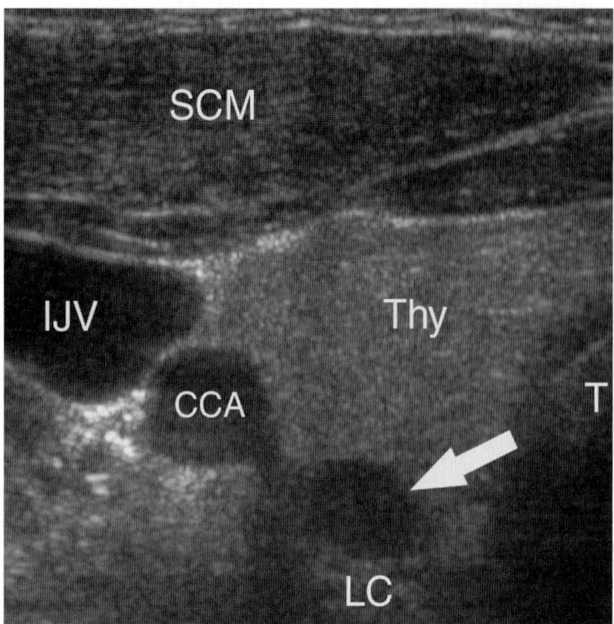

FIGURE 39.16. **Parathyroid Adenoma.** Transverse US image shows the characteristic appearance and location of a parathyroid adenoma (*arrow*), deep to the thyroid gland (Thy), superficial to the longus colli muscle (LC), medial to the common carotid artery (CCA), and lateral to the acoustic shadow of the trachea (T). IJV, internal jugular vein; SCM, sternocleidomastoid muscle.

of adjacent vessels or muscle. The diagnosis is most commonly confirmed at surgical resection.

Ectopic parathyroids are best localized by radionuclide imaging. CT or MR is usually needed to show the anatomic relationships when they are located in the mediastinum (Fig. 39.17).

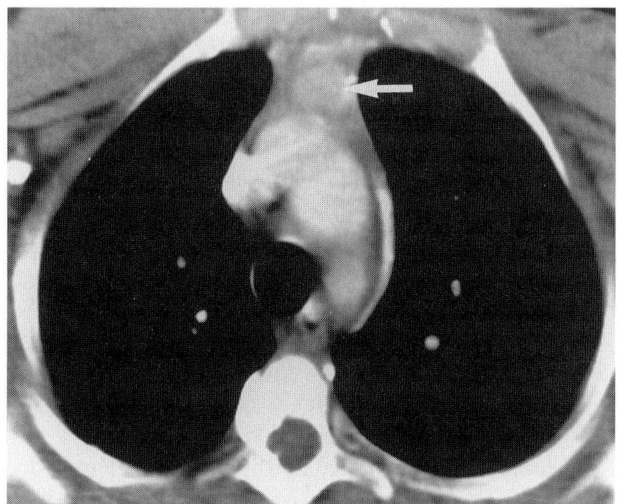

FIGURE 39.17. **Ectopic Parathyroid Adenoma.** Contrast-enhanced CT of the chest confirms the presence of an ectopic parathyroid adenoma (*arrow*) in the mediastinum just anterior to the top of the aortic arch.

NEONATAL BRAIN

Sonography of the neonatal brain has become an integral part of the care of the neonate, allowing detailed evaluation of intracranial structures to be performed at the infant's bedside. The standard examination is relatively simple to perform, takes only a few minutes, and requires no sedation. The fact that the examination can be performed portably in the nursery, where the infant can be kept warm and well monitored, offers great advantage over CT and MR brain imaging. Indications for neonatal head US include: detection and confirmation of congenital brain abnormalities, detection and follow-up of hydrocephalus and other sequelae of infection, and evaluation for brain injury caused by hypoxia (16,17).

Normal US Anatomy. Routine cranial sonograms are performed through the anterior fontanel. The anterior fontanel remains open until about 2 years of age, but examinations may be difficult after 12 to 14 months of age because of its smaller size. Standard views are taken in coronal and sagittal planes and are frequently supplemented by views in the axial plane, or through the posterior fontanel, open sutures, or the foramen magnum. Examinations are performed at bedside while the infant is kept warm, covered, and monitored in the isolette. The infant is positioned to optimize access to the anterior fontanel. High-frequency 5- and 7.5-MHz sector transducers with a wide angle of view are preferred. The transducer is thoroughly cleansed with alcohol between each patient. In the coronal plane (Fig. 39.18), the brain is examined from anterior to the frontal horns to the occipital cortex. Standard views are recorded through the frontal horns, third ventricle, and trigone. Sagittal views (Fig. 39.19) include midline and parasagittal scans obtained 10° laterally through the frontal horns and bodies of the lateral ventricles and 20° laterally through the temporal horns. Axial views (Fig. 39.20) through the thin squama of the temporal bone provide excellent demonstration of the third ventricle, the cortex abutting the inside of the cranium, and the circle of Willis for Doppler studies. Key anatomic landmarks to be identified on every cranial US include: the lateral, third, and fourth ventricles; cavum septum pellucidum/cavum vergae; corpus callosum; choroid plexus in the temporal horn, atrium, and body of the lateral ventricles and in the roof of the third ventricle; cerebellar vermis; caudate nucleus, thalamus and caudothalamic groove. The posterior fontanel and foramen magnum can be effectively used as windows to the posterior fossa.

Congenital Brain Abnormalities

Congenital brain abnormalities are among the most common human malformations. With obstetric US becoming routine, most brain abnormalities are detected or

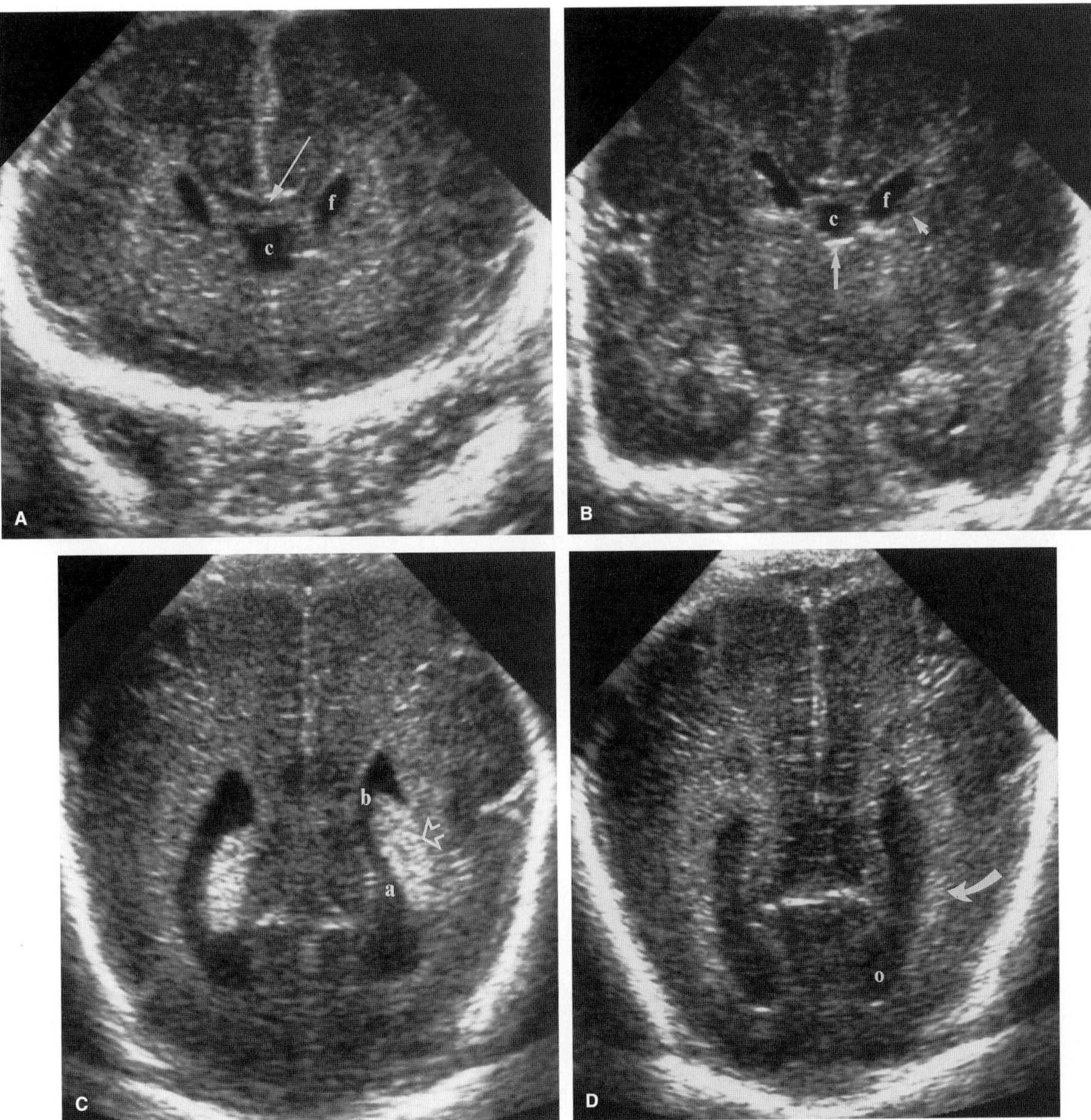

FIGURE 39.18. **Normal Cranial US: Coronal Plane.** The normal brain of a 29-week premature infant is imaged through the anterior fontanel. **A.** Anterior image shows frontal horns of the lateral ventricles (f), cavum septum pellucidum (c), and corpus callosum (*long arrow*). **B.** Midline image shows choroid plexus in the roof of the third ventricle (*longer arrow*), cavum septum pellucidum (c), frontal horns of the lateral ventricle (f), and caudate nucleus (*shorter arrow*). **C.** Posterior image through the body (b) and atria (a) (trigone) of the lateral ventricles demonstrates the choroid plexus (*open arrow*), which lies dependently against the down (left) side of the ventricles. **D.** More posteriorly angled image shows the occipital horns (o) of the lateral ventricles and the moderately echogenic normal periventricular white matter (*curved arrow*).

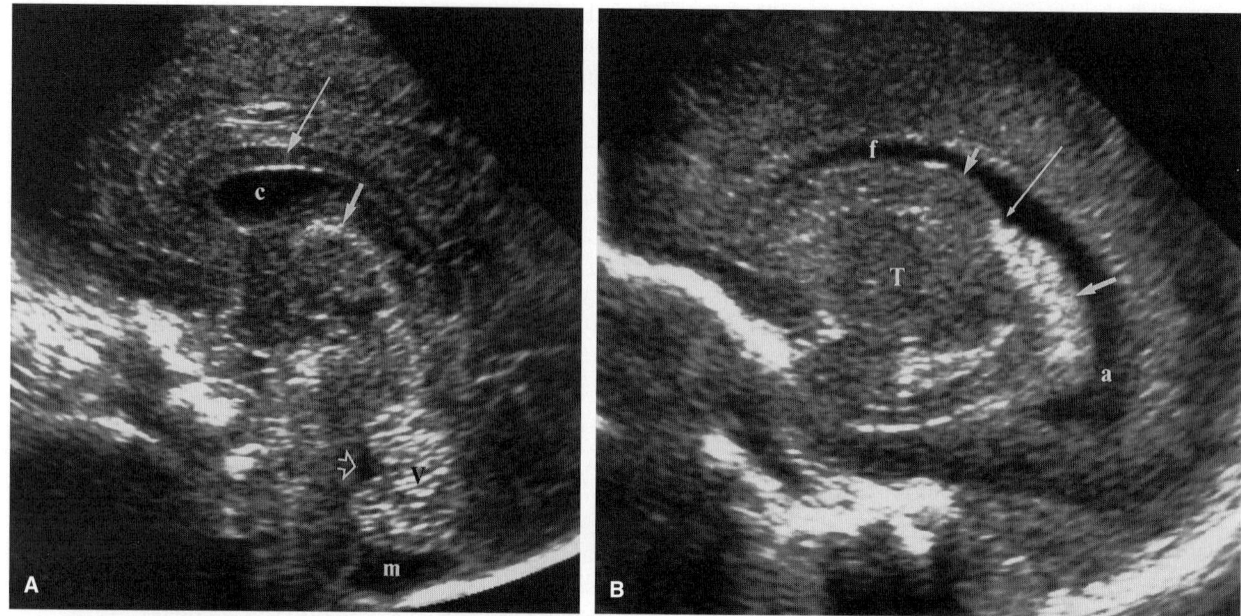

FIGURE 39.19. **Normal Cranial US: Sagittal Plane. A.** Midline image shows the corpus callosum (*long arrow*), cavum septum pellucidum (c), echogenic choroid plexus in the roof of the 3rd ventricle (*short arrow*), echogenic cerebellar vermis (V), the fourth ventricle (*open arrow*), and the cisterna magna (m). **B.** Laterally angled image shows the frontal horn (f) and atrium (a) of the lateral ventricle, the caudate nucleus (*short arrow*), caudothalamic groove (*long arrow*), choroid plexus (*medium arrow*), and thalamus (T).

suspected in utero. Anomalies of the face, head, or other organ systems in the newborn suggest possible brain anomalies. Cranial US in the neonate can be used in these settings to confirm suspected abnormalities. Discussions of the classifications and findings of various brain malformations are provided in other chapters.

Infection

Meningitis occurs as a result of hematogenous spread of bacteria from respiratory infections, or direct spread from ear or sinus infections. *Haemophilus influenza, Escherichia coli,* and group B streptococci are the most common

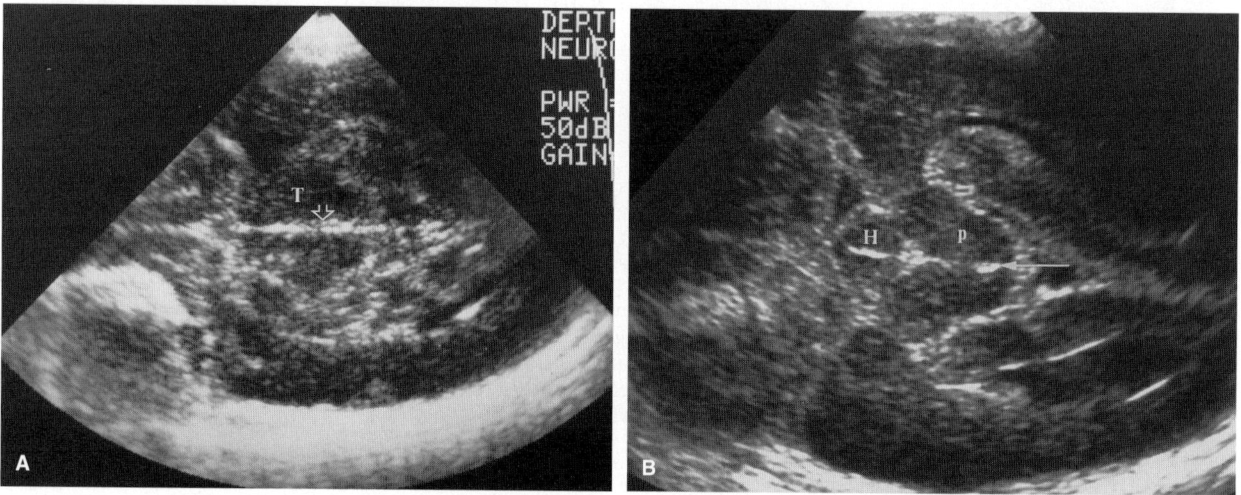

FIGURE 39.20. **Normal Cranial US: Axial Plane. A.** Image shows the walnut-shaped thalamus (T), which contains the third ventricle (*open arrow*). **B.** Image at a slightly lower level shows the hypothalamus (H) and heart-shaped cerebral peduncles (p). The aqueduct of Sylvius is seen as an echogenic dot (*arrow*) posteriorly. The circle of Willis surrounds the hypothalamus in the suprasellar cistern.

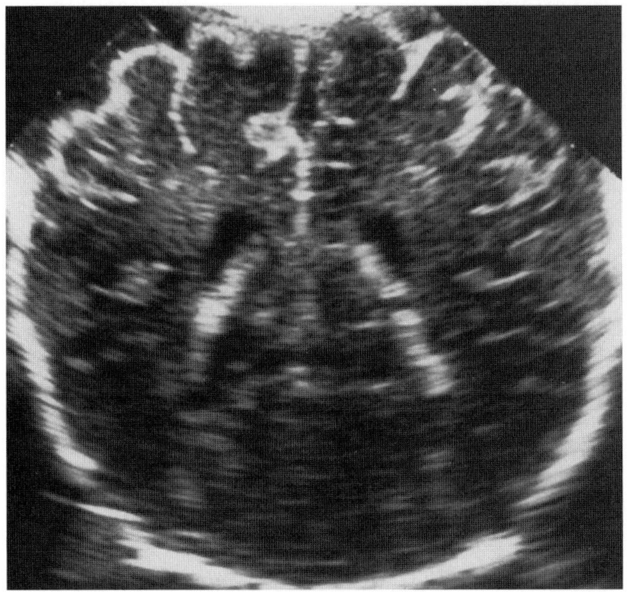

FIGURE 39.21. **Meningitis.** Coronal-plane US shows marked increased echogenicity of the gyri and sulci associated with diffuse brain atrophy and causing increased extraaxial fluid spaces.

causative organisms. Bacteria in the subarachnoid space cause inflammation of the pia and arachnoid. US findings (Fig. 39.21) in meningitis include: (*1*) echogenic sulci; (*2*) echogenic debris in the ventricles; (*3*) enlarged ventricles, often caused by obstruction by inflammatory exudate; (*4*) increased echogenicity and shaggy thickening of the ependyma; and (*5*) transient extra-axial fluid collections. US may be used to detect complications, including persistent hydrocephalus, abnormal parenchymal echogenicity representing infarction or cerebritis, and brain abscess.

TORCH organisms can cause congenital infections affecting the CNS. TORCH refers to ***T****oxoplasma gondii,* **o**ther conditions including syphilis, **r**ubella, **C**ytomegalovirus (CMV), and **h**erpes simplex type 2. Congenital CMV infection is the most common and may cause severe brain destruction. Necrotizing periventricular infection causes periventricular calcification, subependymal cysts, and microcephaly. Toxoplasmosis causes scattered brain calcifications especially in the basal ganglia, multicystic encephalopathy, and porencephaly. Herpes causes cystic periventricular encephalomalacia, hemorrhagic infarction, and scattered brain calcifications, as well as retinal dysplasia. Rubella uncommonly causes recognizable brain injury, but microcephaly, vasculopathy, and massive calcification have been reported.

Ischemic Brain Injury

Premature infants born at less than 34 weeks' gestational age or with birth weight less than 1,500 g are extremely susceptible to ischemic brain injury. Subependymal hemorrhage in the residual germinal matrix and periventricular leukomalacia are the two most common forms of hypoxic brain injury in premature infants. They are responsible for a 5% to 15% incidence of cerebral palsy (spastic motor deficits) and a 25% to 50% incidence of cognitive disabilities in surviving premature infants. Cranial sonograms are routinely performed on premature infants to

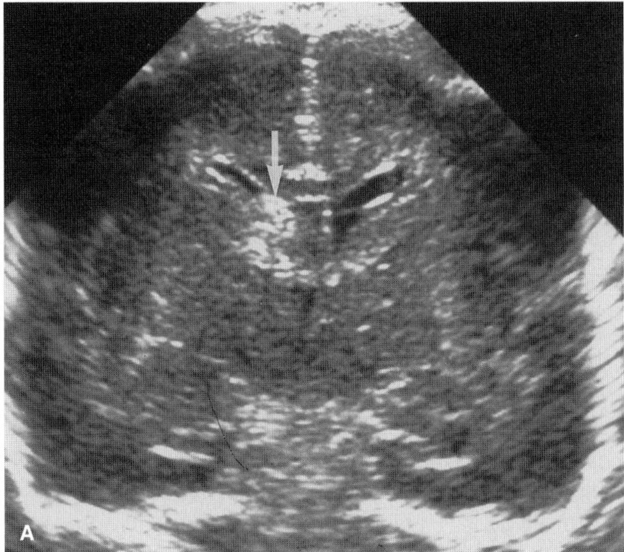

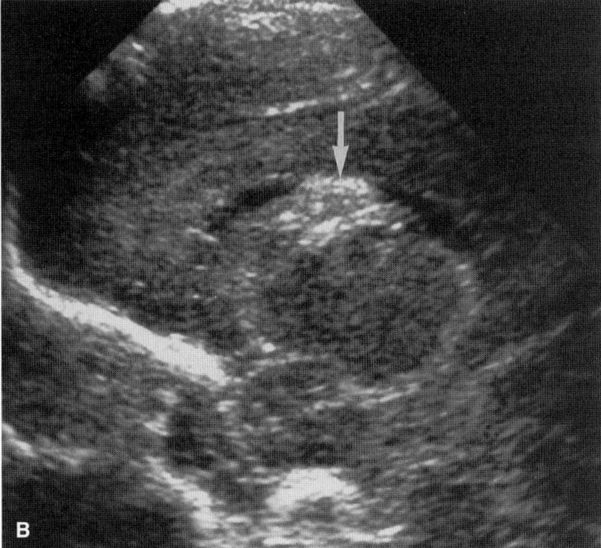

FIGURE 39.22. **Grade 1 Germinal Matrix Hemorrhage.** Coronal **(A)** and angled sagittal **(B)** images show abnormal echogenicity (*arrows*) overlying the caudate nucleus, indicating germinal matrix hemorrhage.

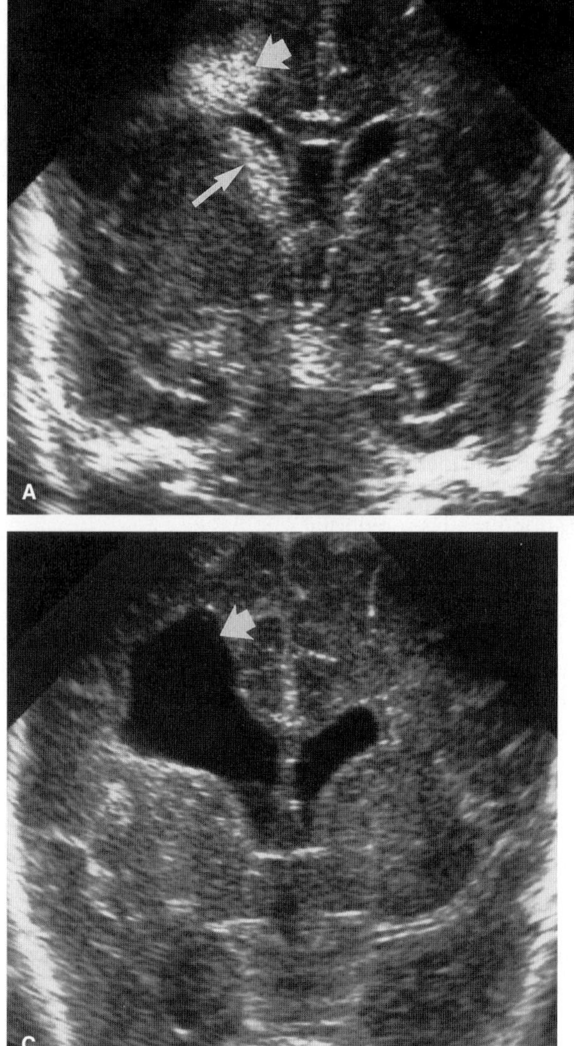
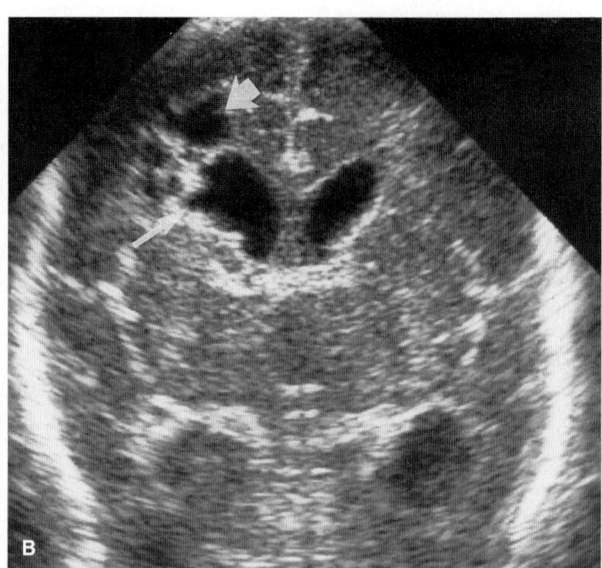

FIGURE 39.23. **Grade 4 Germinal Matrix Hemorrhage Resulting in Porencephaly. A.** Coronal brain image on the second day of life for a premature infant shows hemorrhage in the caudate nucleus (*long arrow*) and in the periventricular brain parenchyma (*short arrow*). **B.** Image obtained 1 month later shows small area of porencephaly extending into the caudate nucleus (*long arrow*) and focus of cystic encephalomalacia in the brain parenchyma (*short arrow*). The ventricles are enlarged. **C.** Follow-up image obtained at 15 weeks of age shows large area of brain destruction, resulting in porencephaly (*short arrow*).

detect these brain injuries and to monitor for treatable complications.

Germinal matrix is a fragile gelatinous mass of tissue found in the fetal brain between the ependyma lining the ventricles and the caudate nucleus. The germinal matrix is highly vascular and is a major source of hemorrhage when it becomes ischemic. The germinal matrix is the source of neuroblasts and spongioblasts, which migrate to the brain surface to form the glial cells of the cortex. The germinal matrix involutes by 32 weeks of gestational age, so only premature infants are susceptible to germinal matrix hemorrhage (GMH).

Germinal matrix hemorrhage, also called subependymal or intraventricular hemorrhage, occurs in the residual germinal matrix overlying the frontal horn and body of the lateral ventricles. The incidence is reported at 30% to 55% in infants born at 24 to 32 weeks' gestation. Most hemorrhages originate in the region of the *caudothalamic groove* (Fig. 39.22), where the germinal matrix is most prominent in the premature infant. The hemorrhage may remain confined but commonly ruptures into the ventricle, resulting in intraventricular hemorrhage, ependymitis, and hydrocephalus. Most (97%) GMH occurs in the first week after birth. Ventriculomegaly develops in the first 2 weeks after hemorrhage and may persist for 3 to 6 months.

US demonstrates confined subependymal hemorrhage as a focus of bright echogenicity anterior to the caudothalamic groove (Fig. 39.22). On coronal views, the echogenic clot is at the floor of the frontal horn, obscuring the caudate nucleus. Hemorrhage into the ventricle is seen as echogenic clots in an enlarging ventricle. Hemorrhage frequently has the same echogenicity as the choroid plexus and can be differentiated from the choroid plexus by location and appearance. Because no choroid plexus is

TABLE 39.3 Classification of Germinal Matrix Hemorrhage

Grade	Description
1	Small hemorrhage confined to germinal matrix
2	Small hemorrhage with extension into lateral ventricles; ventricles may dilate transiently but are not filled with blood
3	Large hemorrhage that fills and dilates the ventricles with blood
4	Intraparenchymal hemorrhagic venous infarction caused by obstruction of the medullary veins draining the periventricular white matter

present in the frontal and occipital horns of the lateral ventricles, any echogenic foci in these locations likely represent hemorrhage. Asymmetric enlargement of the choroid plexus is suspicious for hemorrhage. Parenchymal hematomas (Fig. 39.23) result from hemorrhagic infarction caused by obstruction of the medullary veins by the GMH. A commonly used grading system for classifying the severity of hemorrhage is described in Table 39.3. The sonographic appearance of hematomas follows a predictable evolution. The hematoma is initially densely echogenic and becomes progressively echolucent centrally as it shrinks. Clots in the ventricles characteristically maintain an echogenic rim. Eventually the clots resolve completely. Cellular debris from the hemorrhage is seen as echogenic material floating within the intraventricular CSF. Hydrocephalus is a common sequela of GMH. Hydrocephalus may result from obstruction of CSF pathways by clot, organizing ependymitis, or arachnoid granulation obstruction. Spastic paralysis results from injury to the corticospinal tracts as they course in close proximity to the site of hemorrhage. Cognitive defects and learning disorders may also result from the brain injury.

Periventricular leukomalacia refers to lesions caused by hypoxic injury in the periventricular white matter. The periventricular white matter, at the angles of the lateral ventricles, is in a watershed zone between the arterial blood supply of the basal ganglia and the immature arterial supply to the cerebral cortex. After 34 weeks' gestational age, maturation of the cerebral arterial supply moves the watershed zones from the periventricular area to the cortex between cerebral artery territories. Hypoxia in the premature infant may cause infarction of the periventricular white matter, followed by necrosis, cyst formation, and gliosis. This injury results from arterial infarction, whereas the parenchymal injury from GMH results from venous infarction. The initial injury is usually not detected by US unless the damaged area of the brain becomes echogenic because of hemorrhage. In this case, US demonstrates foci of increased echogenicity in the periventricular white matter at the lateral angles of the lateral ventricles. This finding resolves in 2 to 4 weeks, when periventricular cysts may be visualized (Fig. 39.24). Within 2 to 4 months, these

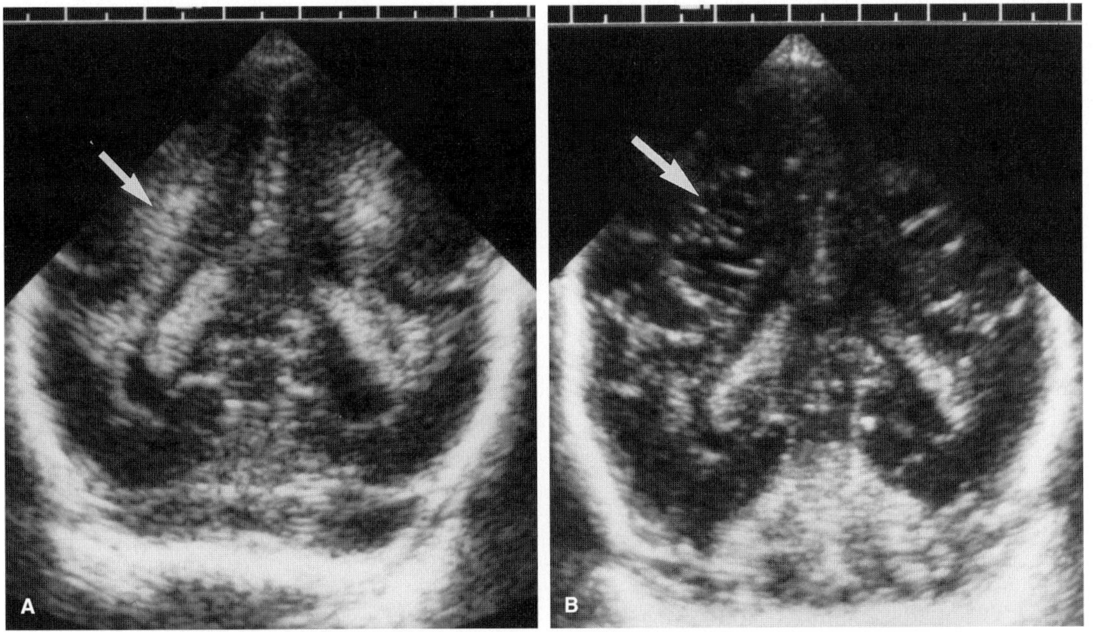

FIGURE 39.24. **Periventricular Leukomalacia. A.** US obtained a few hours after an episode of severe hypoxia in a premature infant shows increased echogenicity (*arrow*) in the periventricular white matter bilaterally. **B.** Follow-up US 1 month later shows the characteristic periventricular cysts (*arrow*) resulting from white matter necrosis.

cysts may enlarge, coalesce and form porencephalic cysts, resolve completely, or result in ventriculomegaly owing to brain atrophy.

Diffuse cerebral edema may result from profound cerebral ischemia in premature or full-term infants. US signs of diffuse cerebral edema include decreased visibility of the sulci and gyri, slitlike ventricles, and diffuse increased parenchymal echogenicity. Severe hypoxia may cause cystic areas of brain destruction and diffuse brain atrophy, resulting in microcephaly, and severe motor and mental impairment. Slitlike lateral ventricles as an isolated finding is a common normal variant in premature infants. Other, often subtle, signs of cerebral edema must be present before the diagnosis can be made sonographically. CT and MR are more sensitive than US for evidence of diffuse hypoxic injury in infants.

Neurodevelopmental deficits are caused by injury to the brain parenchyma on account of GMH, periventricular leukomalacia, or diffuse hypoxia. Spastic diplegia or quadriplegia is caused by injury to the corticospinal tracts. Developmental delay, learning disabilities, and mild mental retardation also occur. Severe mental retardation is uncommon. More severe long-term prognosis is associated with grade 3 and grade 4 GMH, persistence of ventriculomegaly, large parenchymal cysts, and brain atrophy.

REFERENCES

1. Brant WE. Interventional procedures in the thorax. In: McGahan J, ed. Interventional Ultrasound. Baltimore: Williams & Wilkins,1990: 85–100.
2. Brant WE. Diagnostic and interventional ultrasonography of the thorax. Perspect Radiol 1990;3:95–109.
3. Brant WE. Chest. In: McGahan JP, Goldberg BB, eds. Diagnostic Ultrasound: A Logical Approach. Philadelphia: Lippincott-Raven, 1998:1063–1086.
4. Brant WE. Chest ultrasound. In: Brant WE, ed. The Core Curriculum: Ultrasound. Philadelphia: Lippincott Williams & Wilkins,2001: 433–456.
5. Brant WE. The thorax. In: Rumack CM, Wilson SR, Charboneau JW, eds. Diagnostic Ultrasound. St. Louis: Mosby, 2004:603–623.
6. Gupta S, Seaberg K, Wallace MJ, et al. Imaging-guided percutaneous biopsy of mediastinal lesions: different approaches and anatomic considerations. Radiographics 2005;25:763–788.
7. Wernecke K. Sonographic features of pleural disease. AJR Am J Roentgenol 1997;168:1061–1066.
8. Brant WE. Thyroid, parathyroid, and neck ultrasound. In: Brant WE, ed. The Core Curriculum: Ultrasound. Philadelphia: Lippincott Williams & Wilkins, 2001:349–364.
9. Ahuja A, Metreweli C. Ultrasound of thyroid nodules. Ultrasound Q 2000;16:111–121.
10. Khati N, Adamson T, Johnson KS, Hill MC. Ultrasound of the thyroid and parathyroid glands. Ultrasound Q 2003;19:162–176.
11. Iannuccilli JD, Cronan JJ, Monchik JM. Risk for malignancy of thyroid nodules assessed by sonographic criteria. J Ultrasound Med 2004;23:1455–1464.
12. Ahuja A, King W, Metreweli C. Clinical significance of the comet-tail artifact in thyroid ultrasound. J Clin Ultrasound 1996;24:129–133.
13. Jun P, Chow LC, Jeffrey RB. The sonographic features of papillary thyroid carcinomas. Ultrasound Q 2005;21:39–45.
14. McDonald DK, Parman L, Speights VO. Primary hyperparathyroidism due to parathyroid adenoma. Radiographics 2005;25: 829–834.
15. Gotway MB, Leung JW, Gooding GA, et al. Hyperfunctioning parathyroid tissue: spectrum of appearances on noninvasive imaging. AJR Am J Roentgenol 2002;179:495–502.
16. Brant WE. Neonatal neurosonography. In: Brant WE, ed. The Core Curriculum: Ultrasound. Philadelphia: Lippincott Williams & Wilkins, 2001:365–388.
17. Benson JE, Bishop MR, Cohen HL. Intracranial neonatal ultrasonography: an update. Ultrasound Q 2002;18:89–114.

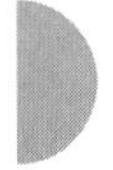

Chapter 40

Vascular Ultrasound

Raymond S. Dougherty and William E. Brant

Doppler Basics

Carotid Ultrasound
Plaque Evaluation
Stenosis
Occlusion
Common Pitfalls

Abdominal Vessels
Anatomy
Aneurysm
Thrombosis

Tips Evaluation

Peripheral Arteries
Arterial Puncture Complications
Aneurysm
Stenosis and Occlusion
Graft Surveillance

Venous Ultrasound
Lower Extremity
Upper Extremity

Spectral Doppler US and color flow vascular imaging supplement grayscale US by identifying blood vessels, confirming the presence of blood flow and its direction, detecting vessel stenosis and occlusion, assessing the perfusion of organs and tumors, and characterizing blood flow dynamics to detect physiologic abnormalities (1–5). This chapter reviews the basics of vascular US examination and Doppler interpretation.

DOPPLER BASICS

Doppler effect refers to the change in the frequency of sound waves that occurs on account of the motion of a sound source, a sound reflector, or a sound receiver. Johann Doppler of Salzburg, Austria, described this phenomenon in 1842. In medical diagnosis, the Doppler effect is used to confirm blood flow by detecting the change in frequency of US waves that occurs when sound is reflected from moving clumps of red blood cells (RBCs). The echoes reflected from RBCs are very weak, with a signal intensity up to 10,000 times less than that of contiguous soft tissue; thus, Doppler US instruments require a high sensitivity to weak signals, and instrument settings must be routinely optimized.

Doppler shift is the change in frequency between the US waves emitted by the transducer and the US waves returning to the transducer after reflection from moving RBCs (Fig. 40.1). This shift in sound frequency results from the Doppler effect. The reflected sound frequency increases when blood flow direction is toward the Doppler signal and decreases when the direction is away from the Doppler signal. An increase in frequency is termed a *positive Doppler shift;* the sound waves are compressed by encountering RBCs moving toward the sound source. A decrease in frequency is termed a *negative Doppler shift,* because the reflected sound waves are stretched by RBCs moving away from the sound source. The presence of a Doppler shift within a blood vessel confirms the presence of blood flow. The direction of the Doppler shift toward higher or lower frequency indicates the direction of blood flow. Doppler shift frequencies are within the range of human hearing and produce distinctive audible sound patterns that characterize normal and abnormal arterial and venous blood flow.

Doppler Equation. The Doppler equation describes, in mathematical form, the relationship between the Doppler

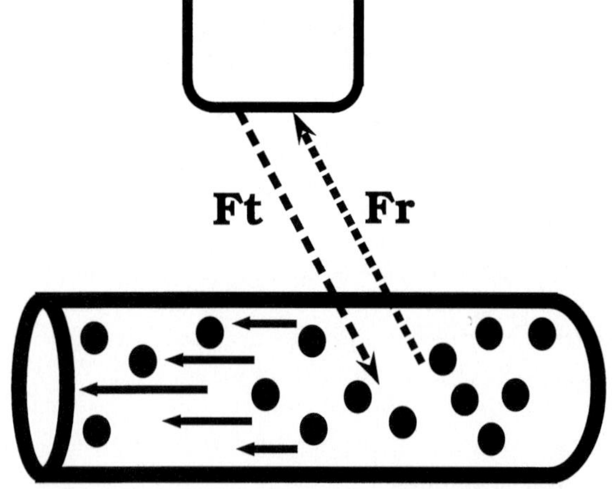

FIGURE 40.1. **Doppler Frequency Shift.** The transmitted Doppler US beam (Ft) encounters red blood cells moving toward it within a visualized blood vessel. The red blood cell motion causes an increase in frequency of the returning echo (Fr) because of the Doppler effect. The US instrument detects and measures the frequency of the returning Doppler signal, confirming the presence of blood flow and its direction by the presence and direction of the Doppler frequency shift.

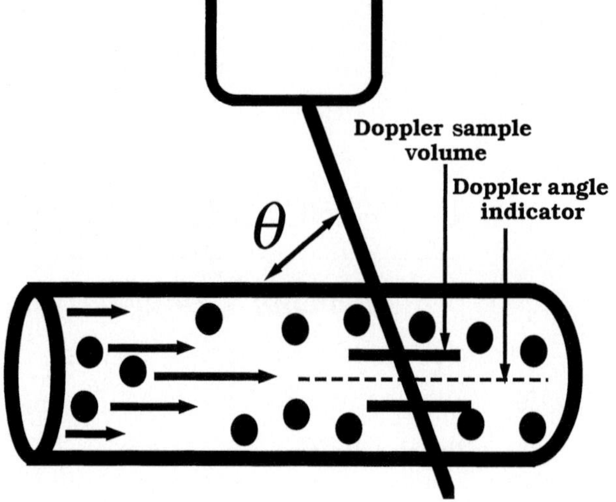

FIGURE 40.2. **Doppler Angle.** The Doppler angle (θ) is defined as the angle between the Doppler US beam and the direction of blood flow, which is assumed to be parallel to the walls of the blood vessel. The Doppler sample volume is indicated by two parallel lines. The Doppler angle indicator is displayed as a dashed line within the sample volume. The US unit has a control knob that is used to align the Doppler angle indicator with the blood vessel walls.

frequency shift (ΔF) and the velocity (V) of the moving RBCs that produce the shift.

$$\Delta F = (Fr - Ft) = \frac{2(V)(Ft)(\cos\theta)}{C}$$

ΔF = (Fr − Ft) = the Doppler frequency shift

Ft = frequency of the transmitted Doppler US beam (the transducer frequency)

Fr = frequency of the reflected US beam (shifted by RBC motion)

V = RBC velocity (blood flow velocity)

θ = the Doppler angle = the angle between the direction of blood flow and the direction of the Doppler US beam

C = speed of sound in tissue (assumed to be constant at 1,540 m/s)

The frequency shift (ΔF) is proportional to the following: (*1*) the velocity (V) of the moving RBCs; (*2*) the frequency of the transmitted Doppler US beam (Ft); and (*3*) the cosine of the angle between the incident Doppler US beam and the direction of blood flow. This angle is called the *Doppler angle* and is symbolized by the Greek letter theta (θ). The direction of blood flow is assumed to be parallel to the walls of the visualized blood vessel being interrogated (Fig. 40.2). The Doppler US beam can be steered by controls on the US unit. The direction of the Doppler beam is indicated on the US image by a dotted or dashed line.

The fact that the Doppler frequency shift is directly proportional to the *cosine* of the Doppler angle has important implications (Table 40.1). First, the largest frequency shift—that is, the largest Doppler signal—will be obtained when the Doppler US beam is directed straight down the barrel of the vessel ($\theta = 0°$, cosine $0° = 1$). Second, no Doppler shift will occur when the Doppler US beam is directly perpendicular to blood flow ($\theta = 90°$, cosine $90° = 0$). Small errors in Doppler angle estimation cause only small errors in velocity calculations at small Doppler angles, but small errors in Doppler angle estimation cause large errors in velocity calculations at angles close to 90°. *As a general rule, Doppler scanning should be performed to keep Doppler angles at 60° or less.*

By algebraic manipulation we can rewrite the Doppler equation as follows:

$$V = \frac{(\Delta F)(C)}{2(Ft)(\cos\theta)}$$

TABLE 40.1 Cosine Values

Angle	*Cosine*
0°	1
10°	0.98
20°	0.93
30°	0.87
40°	0.77
50°	0.64
60°	0.50
70°	0.34
80°	0.17
90°	0

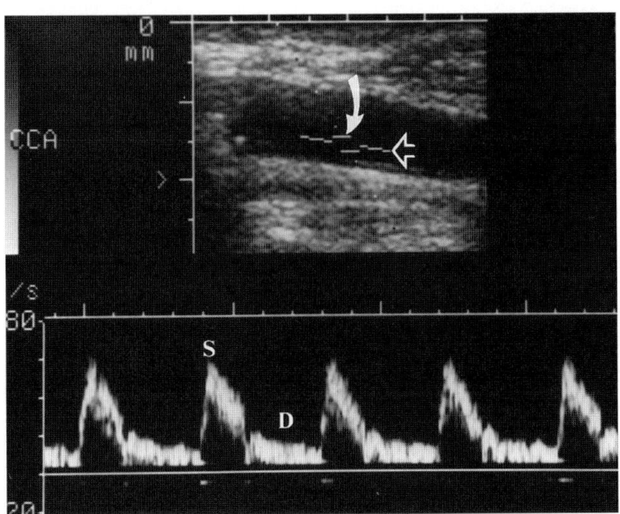

FIGURE 40.3. **Duplex Doppler US.** US image shows the Doppler spectrum of the common carotid artery. The vertical scale shows blood flow velocity in meters per second. The horizontal scale shows time in seconds. The Doppler trace demonstrates peak velocities in systole (S) and low flow velocities in diastole (D). A 2-mm Doppler sample volume (*curved arrow*) is placed by the sonographer in the midportion of the artery visualized by real-time US. Only Doppler shifts originating from this sample volume are analyzed for display. An estimated Doppler angle of 50° is communicated to the US unit computer by aligning the angle indicator (*open arrow*) parallel to the vessel walls.

The US unit detects and measures the frequency of the Doppler beam reflected from moving RBCs (Fr) and calculates the Doppler frequency shift ($\Delta F = Ft - Fr$). The transmission frequency (Ft) is determined by the transducer chosen to perform the examination. The speed of sound in human tissue is assumed to be constant (C). The operator communicates the Doppler angle to the US unit by aligning the Doppler angle "wings" to be parallel with the walls of the vessels examined (Figs. 40.2, 40.3).

Because the depth of a structure in an US image is measured by the time delay between transmission of the US into tissue and the return of the echo from the structure, Doppler information can be limited to a selected Doppler "sample volume" by use of a "time window." The length of the time window determines the size of the sample volume, and the time delay of the time window determines its depth. Thus, we can restrict Doppler information to a small portion of a single visualized vessel. On most Doppler US units, the size and location of the Doppler sample volume is indicated by two short parallel lines along the Doppler beam indicator line (Figs. 40.2, 40.3). Simultaneous grayscale imaging plus Doppler scanning is called *duplex US*. Both spectral and color Doppler imaging are examples of duplex imaging.

Doppler Spectral Display. Returning Doppler signals are processed using a fast Fourier transform spectrum analyzer that sorts the range and mixture of Doppler frequency shifts into individual components and displays them as a function of time on a velocity (or frequency shift) scale (Fig. 40.3). Analysis is performed rapidly enough to be displayed in real time. The horizontal scale (x axis) of the Doppler spectrum represents time in seconds. The vertical scale (y axis) represents blood flow velocity in m/s or cm/s. Because velocity and Doppler frequency shift are directly related mathematically, Doppler frequency shift may alternatively be used on the vertical scale without changing the appearance of the Doppler spectrum. Since blood flow velocity provides the most diagnostically useful information, velocity is the usual choice for the vertical axis. Each pixel (dot) in the spectral display represents a group of RBCs moving at a specific velocity at a given moment in time. The more RBCs that are moving at that specific velocity and time, the brighter the pixel. Flow toward the Doppler beam (positive frequency shift) is displayed above the zero baseline, and flow away from the Doppler beam (negative frequency shift) is displayed below the zero baseline. Peaks of higher velocity occur during ventricular systole, and periods of lower velocity represent ventricular diastole.

Spectral Waveforms. Different blood vessels have unique flow characteristics that can be recognized by the Doppler spectral waveform (Doppler "signature") that they produce (6,7). Factors that affect the appearance of the spectral waveform include cardiac contraction, vessel compliance, and downstream vascular resistance. Cardiac arrhythmias are reflected in the periodicity of the systolic peaks and the velocities reached during each cardiac contraction. A major determinant of the spectral waveform's appearance is the resistance to blood flow offered by the vascular bed supplied by the artery being studied. Arteries can be categorized as high resistance or low resistance, based upon their Doppler spectral waveform. *High-resistance* spectral waveforms are characterized by velocities that increase sharply with systole, decrease rapidly with cessation of ventricular contraction, and show little or no forward flow during diastole (Fig. 40.4). Blood flow direction may reverse briefly during early diastole,

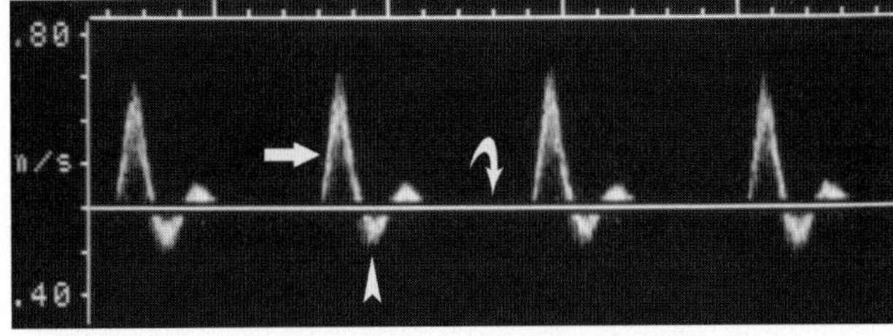

FIGURE 40.4. **High-Resistance Doppler Spectrum.** A high-resistance waveform is characterized by rapid systolic upstroke (*straight arrow*), low flow velocities during diastole (*curved arrow*), and, commonly, reversal of flow direction (*arrowhead*) in early diastole. This Doppler spectrum was obtained from the common femoral artery.

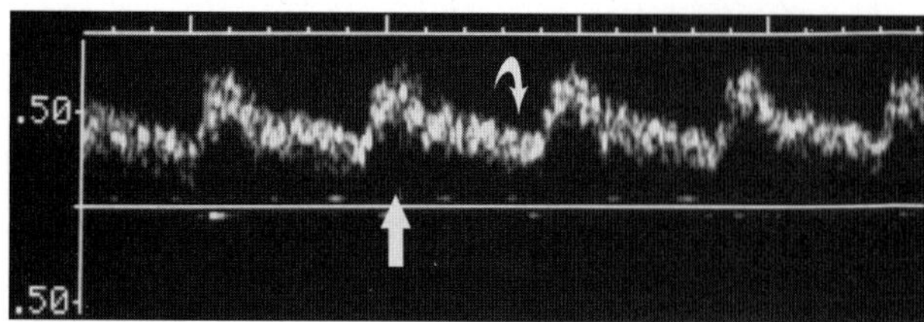

FIGURE 40.5. **Low-Resistance Doppler Spectrum.** A low-resistance waveform is characterized by relatively high flow velocities throughout diastole (*curved arrow*). The narrow spectrum and clean systolic window (*straight arrow*) are characteristic of laminar blood flow. This Doppler spectrum was obtained from the internal carotid artery.

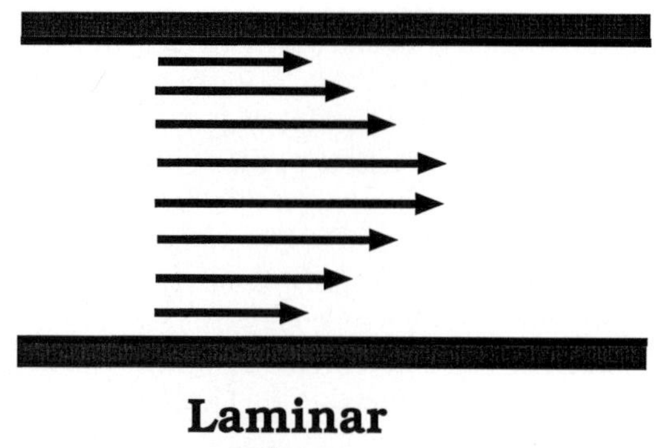

FIGURE 40.6. **Laminar Blood Flow.** Blood flow in most normal arteries is arranged in an orderly layering pattern, with the highest velocity at midstream and the lowest velocity near the vessel wall.

producing a triphasic waveform. Blood flow in high-resistance arteries is always under considerable pressure and encounters constricted arterioles that impede forward blood flow. Pulse pressures traveling down the arterial tree are highly reflected, which results in minimal flow to the capillary bed during diastole. Diastolic flow velocity is low, absent, or reversed, and pulse pressure is high. The ratio of systolic velocity to diastolic velocity (pulsatility) is high. Arteries that normally show a high-resistance Doppler waveform include arteries that supply primarily skeletal muscle at rest, including the iliac, femoral, popliteal, subclavian, and brachial arteries. The external carotid artery waveform is relatively high resistance in appearance.

Low-resistance spectral waveforms are characterized by a slower increase in flow velocity with onset of systole and a gradual decrease in velocity during diastole, with continued forward flow throughout the cardiac cycle (Fig. 40.5). Arteries that supply vital organs characteristically have a low-resistance waveform. These include the internal carotid, hepatic, and renal arteries. The superior mesenteric artery waveform has a high-resistance pattern during fasting and a low-resistance pattern after eating, reflecting the opening of intestinal tract arterioles and increased intestinal blood flow induced by food in the gut. The common carotid artery, with 70% of its blood flow going to the internal carotid artery, has a low-resistance spectral waveform.

Laminar Blood Flow. Most normal arteries and large veins have a laminar pattern of blood flow. Blood flow velocity is highest at the center of the vessel and progressively diminishes closer to the vessel wall (Fig. 40.6). The Doppler waveform of laminar flow is characterized by a "narrow spectrum"—a narrow band of blood flow velocities throughout the cardiac cycle with a "window" beneath the spectral trace in systole (Fig. 40.4). Large arteries such as the aorta have "plug" flow characterized by a uniform flow velocity extending from the center to near the vessel wall. At vessel bifurcations, the division of blood flow results in a small area of normal reversed blood flow near the vessel wall, opposite the flow divider (Fig. 40.7).

Tortuous blood vessels demonstrate normal slowing of blood flow on the inner aspect of the curve, with acceleration of blood flow on the outer aspect of the curve. The highest velocities are seen at the outer aspect of the curving vessel, rather than at midlumen. Blood flow velocity returns to a laminar distribution a short distance downstream from the curve.

Disturbed Blood Flow. Turbulent and disturbed spectral waveforms are usually, but not always, indicative of pathologic changes in blood flow. Disturbed blood flow is a loss of the normal orderly laminar flow pattern. Characteristic spectral Doppler signs of disturbed blood flow are: increased velocity, spectral broadening, simultaneous

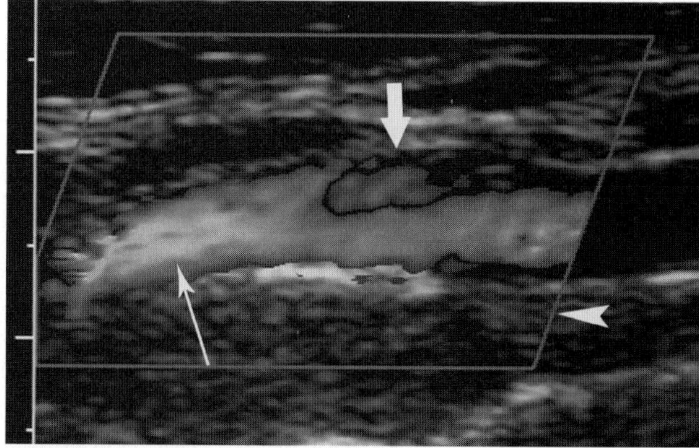

FIGURE 40.7. **(Color Plates) Normal Flow Reversal at Bifurcation.** Flow in the internal carotid artery is shown in red, with areas of higher flow velocity shown in yellow. A normal area of blood flow reversal (*short arrow*) is seen in the carotid bulb. Note how the true color change is outlined in black. The color Doppler interrogation area is marked on the image by the box outlined in white (*arrowhead*). Higher velocity in the middle of the vessel, shown in yellow (*long arrow*), is indicative of laminar blood flow in the artery.

forward and reverse flow, and fluctuations of flow velocity with time (5). Peak systolic velocity increases with severity of vessel stenosis. *Spectral broadening* is widening of the spectral waveform that reflects a broader range of flow velocities within the Doppler sample volume. Spectral broadening increases with the severity of flow disturbance. However, normal spectral broadening occurs when the size of the Doppler sample volume is large compared to the size of the vessel, or when the sample volume is placed near the vessel wall instead of midlumen. Flow velocity fluctuation and simultaneous forward and reverse flow characterize turbulence. Turbulence is most pronounced just downstream from a severe vessel stenosis, where eddy currents are produced as the high-velocity flow slows and occupies a larger vessel area.

Velocity Ratios. Blood flow velocity calculations are dependent upon accurate estimation of the Doppler angle. When the Doppler angle cannot be determined because of poor visualization of the interrogated blood vessel or the vessel's tortuosity (as with the umbilical artery in the cord), velocity cannot be accurately calculated. When the Doppler angle indicator is not displayed, the US instrument calculates Doppler velocities using Doppler equation by assuming that the Doppler angle is 0° (cosine 0° = 1). Velocity ratios can be calculated from the spectral waveform and can be used to estimate vascular resistance and hemodynamics. The ratios are independent of absolute velocity measurements. The velocity ratios in common use are listed in Table 40.2.

Assessing Arterial Stenosis. Acute narrowing of the blood vessel lumen disturbs laminar flow. Doppler characterization of vessel stenosis is based upon changes in blood flow pattern and velocity. To assess the degree of stenosis, Doppler spectra are routinely obtained in three areas of the vessel lumen (Fig. 40.8): (*1*) proximal to stenosis, (*2*) at the point of maximal stenosis, and (*3*) 1 to 2 cm downstream from the stenosis. Laminar flow is generally present proximal to the stenosis. Within the stenotic zone, velocity is increased but usually remains laminar. The severity of stenosis correlates best with the highest blood flow velocity during peak systole. The highest velocity may be in a very small region, and a careful search of the vessel is necessary. In the poststenotic zone, flow spreads out, causing turbulence and eddy currents to occur and produce broadening of the Doppler spectrum. Downstream from severe stenosis (>50%) the Doppler signals are dampened, producing the *parvus-tardus waveform*. Flow velocities are low (parvus) with a slow systolic upstroke (tardus) (see Fig. 40.22) (8,9).

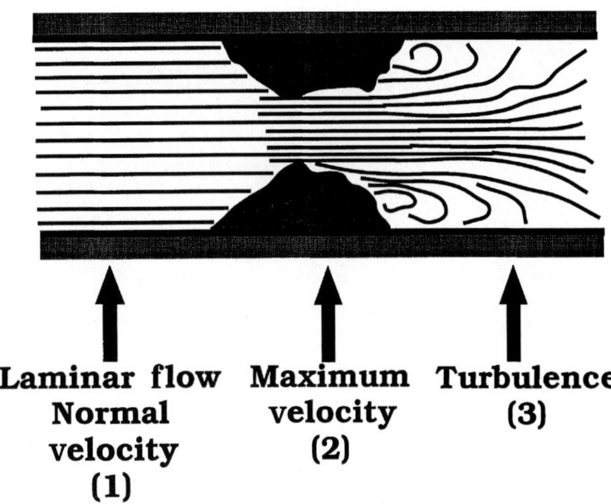

FIGURE 40.8. **Assessment of Arterial Stenosis.** To assess a vessel plaque for stenosis, Doppler spectra are obtained: (*1*) proximal to the plaque, where blood flow velocity is normal and flow is laminar; (*2*) in the area of the plaque where flow usually remains laminar but where flow velocity is at maximum; and (*3*) downstream from the plaque, where turbulence and eddy currents are detected.

Color Flow US. Currently, three different techniques are used to produce color flow US images.

1. *Color Doppler imaging* (CDI) superimposes Doppler flow information on a standard grayscale B-mode real-time US image (10,11). The B-mode image is displayed in shades of gray, and the Doppler flow information is displayed on the same image in color (Fig. 40.9). Most of the same principles and limitations of spectral Doppler apply to color Doppler imaging.
2. *Color Doppler energy* (CDE), also termed *power Doppler*, displays color flow information obtained from integration of the power of the Doppler signal rather the Doppler frequency shift itself (1,12–14). Power Doppler displays information more directly related to the number of moving RBCs than to their velocity (Fig. 40.10). CDE is relatively angle independent and is more sensitive to slow flow than CDI.
3. The third method of color flow imaging is called *color velocity imaging* (CVI) (15). Color velocity imaging is not a Doppler technique; instead, CVI tracks the movement of structure in the US image from one moment to the next. In effect, CVI images blood like a soft tissue and stores a unique texture pattern for comparison with a subsequent image. Movement of the blood flow speckle pattern is displayed as a color flow image.

TABLE 40.2 Doppler Velocity Ratios

A/B ratio (systolic/diastolic ratio)	$= \frac{\text{Peak systolic velocity}}{\text{End-diastolic velocity}}$
Resistance Index (RI) (Pourcelot Index [PoI])	$= \frac{\text{Peak systolic velocity} - \text{end-diastolic} - \text{velocity}}{\text{Peak systolic velocity}}$
Pulsatility Index (PI)	$= \frac{\text{Peak systolic velocity} - \text{end-diastolic} - \text{velocity}}{\text{Temporal mean velocity}}$

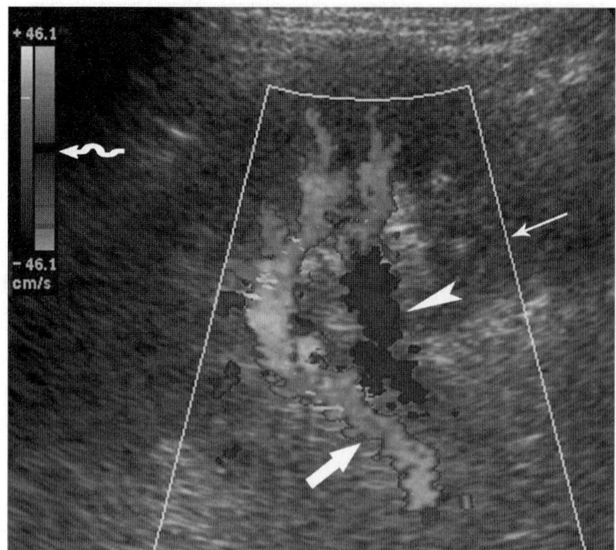

FIGURE 40.9. **(Color Plates) Color Doppler Image.** This color Doppler image of blood flow in the kidney displays arteries entering the kidney in red (*wide arrow*) and the veins leaving the kidney in blue (*arrowhead*). The color Doppler area of interrogation (sample volume) is etched by thin green lines (*thin arrow*). Any detected Doppler shift within this area is displayed in color. The kidney and surrounding tissue are displayed in grayscale. The color Doppler map on the left is set to show blood flow toward the Doppler beam in red/yellow at the top of the scale and blood flow away from the Doppler beam in blue/green at the bottom of the scale. The zero flow baseline is represented by the black bar (*squiggly arrow*) in the center of the color map.

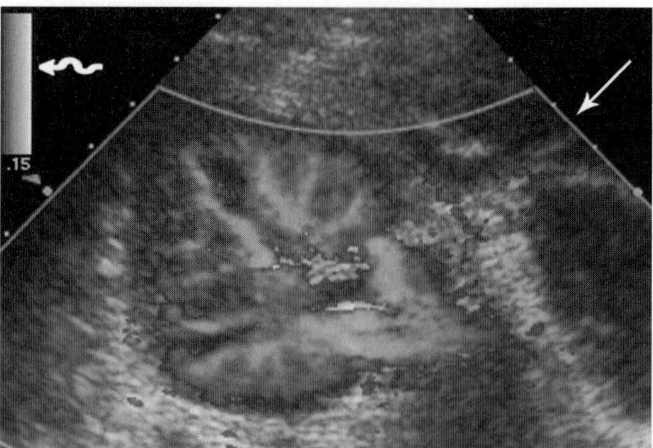

FIGURE 40.10. **(Color Plates) Power Doppler (Color Doppler Energy [CDE]) Image.** Power Doppler image of a transplant kidney in the transverse plane shows the increased sensitivity of CDE. Blood vessels are detected more peripherally in the kidney. However, power Doppler lacks the capability to show blood flow direction. Arteries and veins are displayed in the same color shades. The CDE area of interrogation is indicated by the white box (*thin arrow*). The CDE color map is shown at the left (*squiggly arrow*).

On the color Doppler, image flow directed toward the transducer is usually colored red, whereas flow away from the transducer is usually colored blue. The operator may arbitrarily change the coloring of the Doppler information. The color map used is displayed as part of the color US image. Faster blood flow velocities are colored in lighter shades, whereas slower blood flow is colored in darker shades. Color shading is dependent on mean velocities, not peak velocities. Thus, peak velocities cannot be estimated from the color image alone and must be determined from spectral Doppler. A normal laminar flow pattern will demonstrate lighter shades in the midstream and darker shades near the vessel walls, reflecting rapid flow in the middle of the vessel and slower flow near its walls. Disturbed flow, such as turbulence, is indicated by a wide range of colors in a scrambled pattern.

Changes in color within a blood vessel on a color flow US image may be caused by: (*1*) change in the Doppler angle, (*2*) change in blood flow velocity, (*3*) aliasing, or (*4*) artifact. A change in Doppler angle causes a change in Doppler frequency shift, which, on a color flow image, produces a change in the color displayed. Variations in the Doppler angle may be caused by divergence of US beams emanating from sector or curved array transducers, a blood vessel curving through the color image, or a combination of both. Color flow images are used to detect changes in blood flow velocity for further analysis by spectral Doppler. To interpret a color flow image, inspect the color map for color display orientation, then analyze the image for variations in Doppler angle and blood flow velocity.

Doppler Artifacts. A variety of artifacts distort Doppler information and limit the information provided.

Aliasing is a limitation of pulsed Doppler US that occurs with both spectral and color flow Doppler (11,16). Aliasing happens with high-velocity blood flow and improper velocity scale and baseline settings. Aliasing on spectral displays is seen as a "wraparound" of peak velocities to the opposite end of the scale (Fig. 40.11). The highest velocities are cut off one side of the scale and artifactually displayed on the opposite side of the scale. Aliasing on color Doppler "wraps around" high velocities onto the opposite color scale (Fig. 40.12). For example, velocities too high for the red-scale setting are artifactually displayed as shades of blue. Color aliasing must be distinguished from true color changes caused by flow reversal or changes in the Doppler angle. True color changes are always surrounded by a black border, whereas color shifts related to aliasing lack this black border.

Aliasing occurs when the pulse Doppler sampling rate is too low for a given Doppler signal frequency, thus resulting in an inaccurate frequency measurement. The US instrument measures the frequency of returning Doppler signal, piece by piece, by a series of pulses. The rate at which pulses can be transmitted (the *pulse repetition frequency*

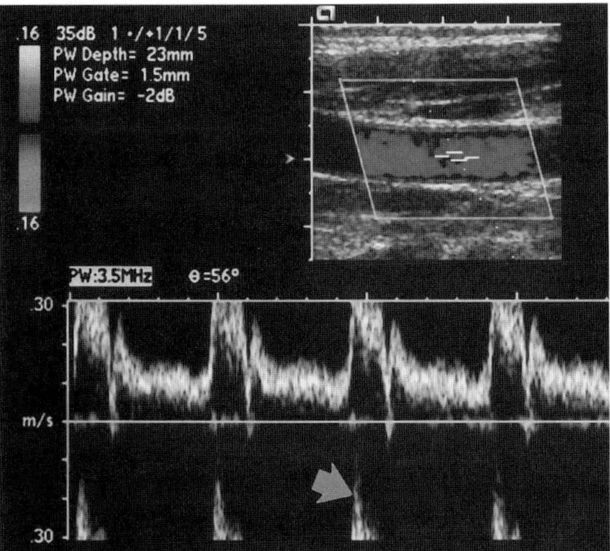

FIGURE 40.11. **(Color Plates) Aliasing on Spectral Doppler.** The high-velocity peaks (*arrow*) of the spectral Doppler display are cut off at the top, "wrapped around," and displayed at the bottom of the spectral display. The spectral Doppler scale on the left is set with a Nyquist limit of 0.30 m/s, too low for the peak velocities encountered within the interrogated blood vessel.

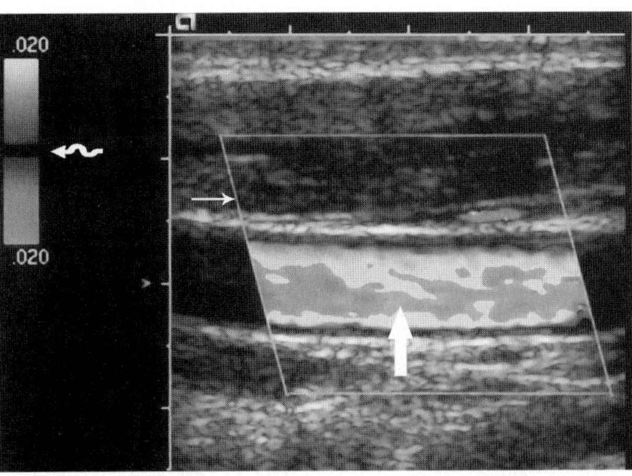

FIGURE 40.12. **(Color Plates) Aliasing on Color Doppler Imaging.** The color map (*squiggly arrow*) is set for red/yellow color at the top of the scale to indicate flow toward the Doppler beam and for blue/green color at the bottom of the scale to indicate flow away from the Doppler beam. The direction of the Doppler beam is indicated by the parallel sides (*thin arrow*) of the color Doppler sample volume box, shown in white. The dominant color within the visualized blood vessel is red/yellow, indicating that the direction of blood flow is from right to left. The higher velocity of blood flow in the center of the blood vessel (*wide arrow*) exceeds the low-velocity scale setting (Nyquist limit = 0.020 m/s) and is displayed in green, the high-velocity color on the opposite end of the color scale. The lack of a black border around the color shift is a sign of aliasing.

[PRF]) is limited by the depth of the vessel interrogated. Deeper vessels require more time for the US beam to travel to the vessel and for the echo to return. To avoid aliasing, the PRF must be at least twice the frequency of the signal to be detected. The maximum frequency that can be accurately detected without aliasing is called the *Nyquist limit* and is equal to half the PRF. The Nyquist limit is displayed at the top and bottom of the spectral Doppler scale and the color map. On color Doppler images, aliasing may be helpful and serve as a tag for high velocities associated with significant stenosis. Aliasing may be eliminated by proper adjustment of the Doppler scale and baseline settings, by using a lower Doppler transmission frequency, or by increasing the Doppler angle.

Incorrect Doppler Gain. When the Doppler gain is set too low, Doppler information may be lost and blood flow may not be demonstrated. The color Doppler image with gain that is too high demonstrates color in non-flow areas and random color noise. Correct gain settings are attained by turning up the gain setting until noise appears on the image and then slightly lowering the setting.

Velocity Scale Errors. Velocity range settings that are too high may obscure low-velocity flow, which is lost in noise and the wall filter near the baseline. Vessels that are patent but with very slow flow may be considered thrombosed. When velocity scale settings are too low, aliasing occurs. Such aliasing is corrected by adjusting scale and baseline settings.

Color Flash. Any motion of a reflector relative to the transducer produces a Doppler shift. Rapid movement of the transducer itself may produce a Doppler shift and a flash of color projected over the grayscale image. Most instruments incorporate motion discriminators that suppress color flash in hyperechoic but not in hypoechoic areas. Color flash is accentuated in cysts, the gallbladder, and other hypoechoic nonvascular structures. High color sensitivity settings accentuate color flash.

Tissue Vibration Artifact. Tissue vibration may produce color display in perivascular tissues, indicating flow where none is present. Tissue vibration artifact is produced in non-flow areas by bruits, arteriovenous fistulas, and shunts.

Fluid Motion. Color signal can be produced during CDI by motion of fluids other than blood. Motion of fluid within cysts and bowel may be misinterpreted as blood flow. Ureteral peristalsis produces a jet of color in the bladder that confirms patency of the ureter.

CAROTID ULTRASOUND

Stroke. Approximately 700,000 strokes occurred in the United States in 2002, resulting in 163,000 deaths. It is projected that the direct and indirect public healthcare cost of

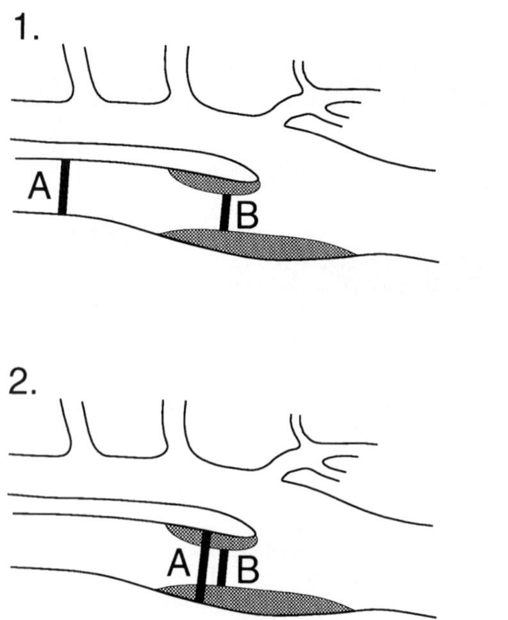

FIGURE 40.13. **Percent Carotid Stenosis.** Carotid percent stenosis: (A − B)/A × 100% **1.** North American Symptomatic Carotid Endarterectomy Trial classification. **2.** European Carotid Stenosis Trial (traditional) classification. See text for further explanation.

stroke in 2005 will approach $56 billion. Atherosclerotic lesions of the extracranial vessels are estimated to cause 75% of strokes that have either a thrombotic or embolic cause (17).

During the last 15 years, the management of atherosclerotic carotid disease has changed significantly. In 1991, two randomized prospective multicenter studies, the North American Symptomatic Carotid Endarterectomy Trial (NASCET) (18) and the European Carotid Stenosis Trial (ECST) (19), demonstrated a clear benefit of carotid endarterectomy in patients with an internal carotid artery (ICA) stenosis ≥70% of the diameter, as defined by conventional angiography. An important difference between the NASCET and ECST studies is the method of measuring the stenosis (Fig. 40.13). NASCET measured the degree of narrowing as the ratio of the diameter of the stenosis to the diameter of the normal ICA distal to the stenosis on catheter angiography. The ECST measured carotid stenosis in the more traditional fashion, by comparing the residual lumen diameter to an approximation of the original vessel diameter. A 70% ECST stenosis is approximately equal to a 50% NASCET stenosis.

NASCET found an unequivocal difference between the risk of stroke in patients receiving the best medical care alone and those undergoing endarterectomy. The risk of ipsilateral stroke at 2 years is 26% for those treated medically and 9% for those treated surgically. Additional data from NASCET published in 1998 showed modest benefits of endarterectomy for stenoses measuring 50% to 69% as long as the rate of the institution's serious surgical complication rate was <2% (20). Similarly, the ECST found a sixfold decrease in stroke in endarterectomy patients. If the stenoses had been measured as in the NASCET study, this decrease may have been more significant. Most investigators regard the NASCET study as the gold standard that makes carotid endarterectomy the standard of care for symptomatic carotid stenosis ≥70% and, in selected cases, ≥50%. No patients benefit with a stenosis <50%. The ECST found that patients with stenoses <30% diameter are best managed medically.

The Asymptomatic Carotid Atherosclerosis Study (ACAS) (21) demonstrated a 53% aggregate risk reduction with carotid endarterectomy for stenosis ≥60% of the diameter in asymptomatic individuals. In men, the risk reduction is 66%; in women, 17%. Three other studies (22–24) do not corroborate the ACAS study and suggest there may be no benefit of endarterectomy over medical therapy in asymptomatic patients with a stenosis ≥60%. These studies are not perfect and have been criticized. The management of the asymptomatic stenosis remains controversial.

Carotid angioplasty and stenting (CAS) has emerged as an alternative to endarterectomy. Its relative risk and efficacy are currently being evaluated. Some investigators believe the indications for CAS should be the same as for endarterectomy. Because of the lack of consensus, the Collaborative Panel of the American Society of Interventional and Therapeutic Neuroradiology (ASTIN), the American Society of Neuroradiology (ASNR), and the Society of Interventional Radiology (SIR) published guidelines that recommend CAS only for patients with severe symptomatic stenosis who are not medically fit for endarterectomy or in whom the surgery would be technically difficult (25).

Carotid Anatomy. The right common carotid artery (CCA) arises from the bifurcation of the innominate artery. The left CCA arises from the aortic arch. The CCAs ascend anterolaterally up the neck, medial to the jugular vein, and lateral to the thyroid. Each artery measures 6 to 8 mm in diameter. US evaluation of the CCA often demonstrates the three layers of the normal vessel wall: the echogenic intima, hypoechoic media, and echogenic adventitia. The distance between these two echogenic lines (intima-media complex) is normally less than 1.1 mm. The CCA dilates in the common carotid bulb and bifurcates into the internal (ICA) and external (ECA) carotid arteries at the C3–C4 level. The bifurcation may occur anywhere from the C1 level to the T2 level. The ECA assumes an *anteromedial* course off the carotid bulb 70% of the time. It is intermediate (overlaps the ICA) in 20% of patients and reversed (lateral) in 10% of patients. The ECA has branch vessels that supply the head and face. It measures 3 to 4 mm in diameter. The ICA assumes a *posterolateral* course off the carotid bulb, supplies the brain, and measures 5 to 6 mm in diameter. The portion of the arterial wall between the

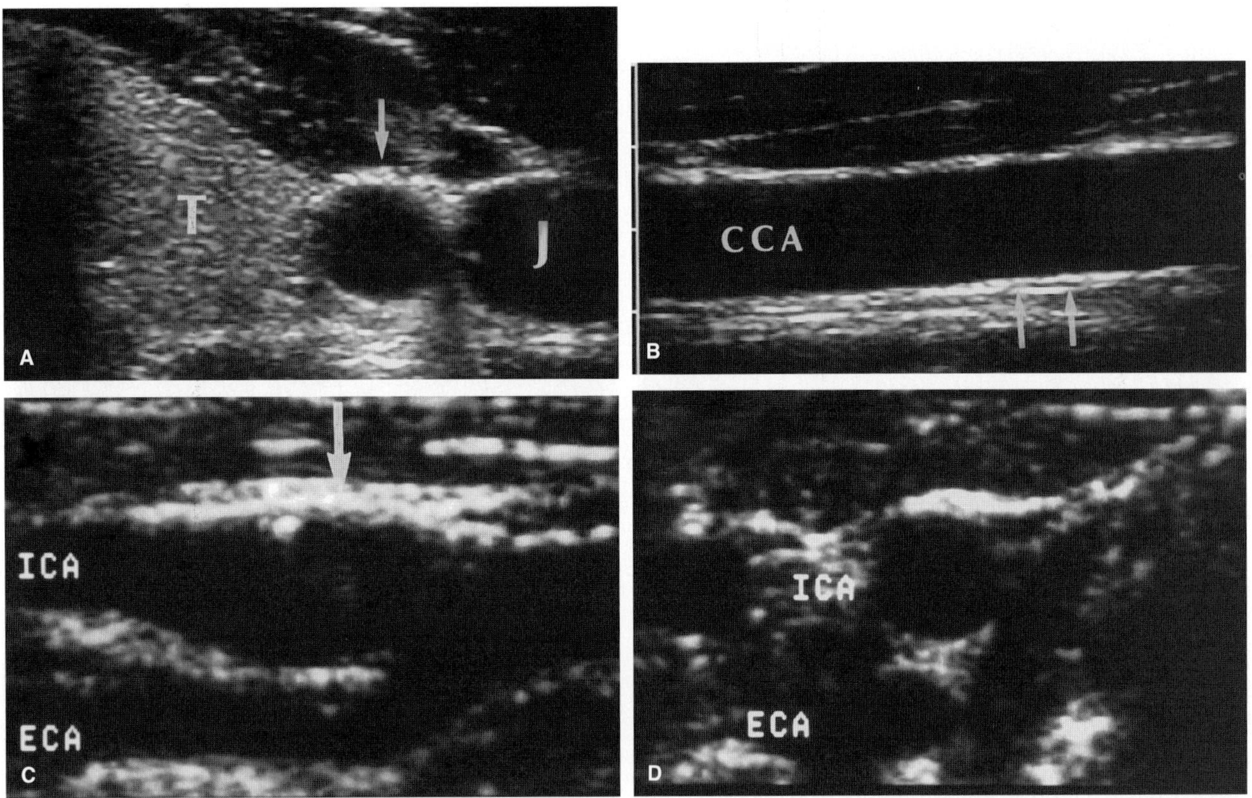

FIGURE 40.14. **Carotid Anatomy. A.** Transverse grayscale US image of the left CCA (*arrow*) at the level of the thyroid (T). The CCA is positioned medial to the jugular vein (J) and lateral to the thyroid. **B.** Longitudinal image of the right CCA. Normal intima-media complex (*arrows*). **C.** Longitudinal image of the carotid bifurcation and carotid bulb (*arrow*). **D.** Transverse image of the carotid bifurcation. CCA, Common carotid artery; ICA, internal carotid artery; ECA, external carotid artery.

ICA and ECA at their origin is called the *flow divider.* The vertebral arteries are the first branches of the subclavian arteries, with the left the same size or larger than the right in 75% of cases. They ascend in the transverse foramen of C2 to C6. Normal carotid anatomy is illustrated in Figure 40.14. Sonographic characteristics that aid in the differentiation of the ICA and ECA are shown in Figs. 40.15 and 40.16 and in Table 40.3.

Technique. Duplex US of the carotid arteries is performed with the patient in the supine position using a linear 5- to 10-MHz transducer. The patient's head is rotated away from the side being examined. The cervical carotid arteries are evaluated in the longitudinal plane using grayscale, color flow, and spectral Doppler imaging. Findings are confirmed in the transverse plane.

Plaque Evaluation

Intimal Hyperplasia. Diffuse thickening of the intima-media complex of the CCA has been linked to an increased risk of atherosclerotic vascular disease, including transient ischemic attack (TIA), stroke, and coronary artery disease. The normal intima-media thickness (IMT) is dependent upon age and gender. In general, the normal IMT is <0.8 mm and abnormal is >1.1 mm. Indeterminate values range between 0.8 and 1.1 mm. Serial wall thickness measurements have been used to monitor the clinical response to specific treatments for atherosclerosis (26–29).

Plaque Formation. Carotid plaques are most commonly found within 2 cm of the bifurcation. Injury to the vascular endothelium results in the deposition of a fatty streak in the wall of the artery. Plaque growth results from progressive deposition of lipids, proliferation of smooth muscle cells, and migration of fibrocytes. The "vulnerable" plaque contains a lipid core with a variable fibrous cap. As the plaque increases in size, the shearing forces of blood flow cause repeated episodes of fissuring and intraplaque hemorrhage with interval healing. During this process, the plaque can rupture, causing cerebral emboli (30).

Plaque Characterization. No universal system exists to characterize plaque. Plaque is usually described by surface characteristics, density, and texture (Figs. 40.17, 40.18) (26,30–32).

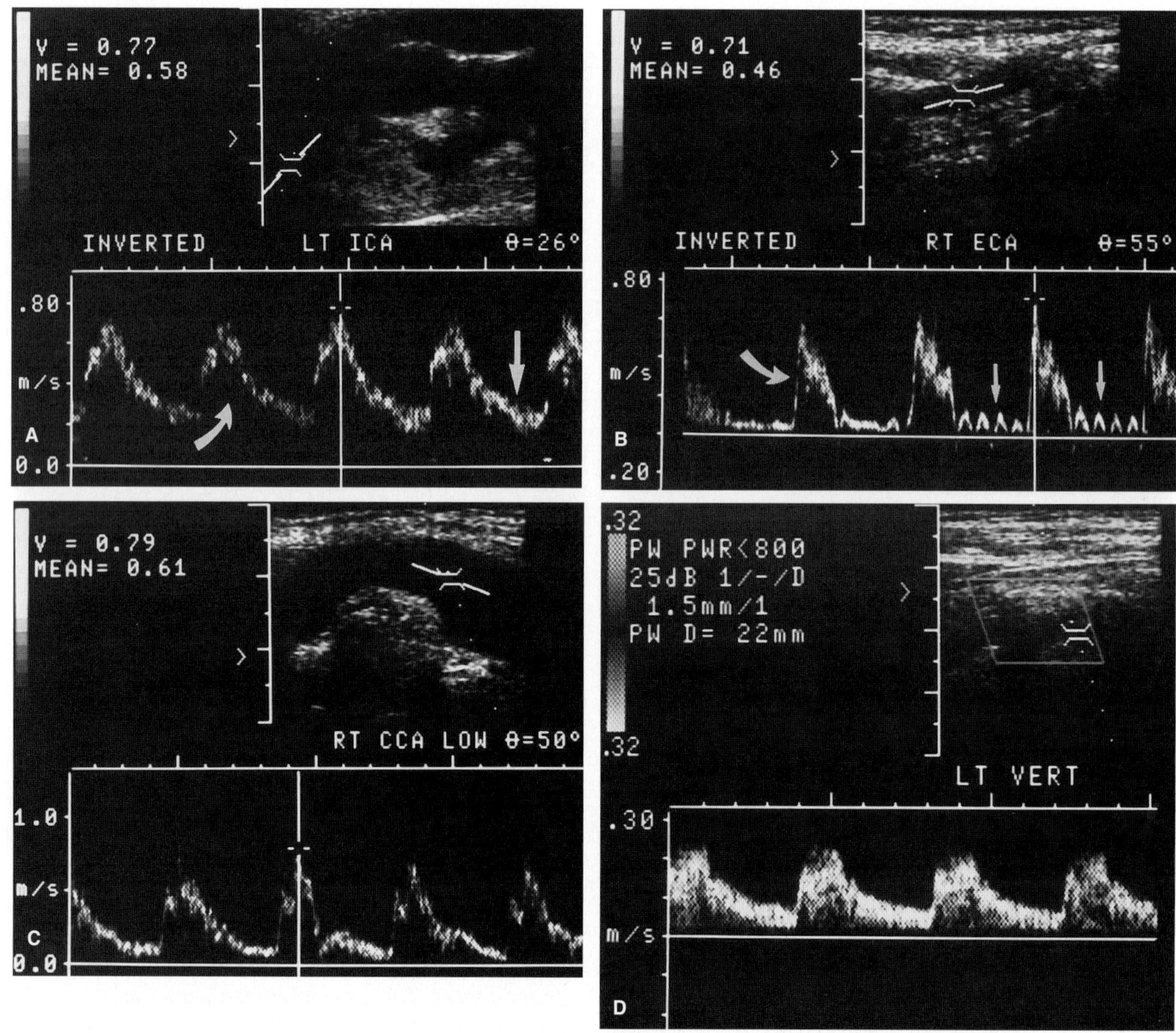

FIGURE 40.15. **Normal Carotid Spectral Waveforms. A.** Internal carotid artery (ICA): low-resistance waveform. Note the prominent diastolic flow (*arrow*) and clean systolic window (*curved arrow*). **B.** External carotid artery (ECA): high-resistance waveform. The rapid systolic upstroke is characteristic (*curved arrow*). The "sawtooth" pattern (*arrows*) is the result of the temporal tap. The sonographer palpates the pulse and then digitally taps either the superficial temporal or preauricular branch of the ECA. The tapping is transmitted back to the ECA as the "sawtooth" pattern on the spectral display. This maneuver helps distinguish the ECA from the ICA (no "sawtooth") in difficult cases. **C.** Common carotid artery (CCA): hybrid waveform. The CCA typically is more ICA-like, because 70% of its blood flows into the ICA. **D.** Vertebral artery (VA): low-resistance waveform. The VA often demonstrates spectral broadening because of its small size and location (poor visualization). Note the filling in of the systolic window with spectral broadening (*curved arrow*).

Surface characteristics are smooth, irregular, and ulcerated. With sensitivity and specificity of approximately 60%, US is unreliable in the diagnosis of plaque ulceration. Grayscale US findings suggestive of ulceration include undercutting of the plaque margin, a sonolucent area that extends to the surface of the plaque, and a divot or crater on the surface of the plaque. Color Doppler may demonstrate flow into the crater with flow reversal.

Hypoechoic, isoechoic, and *hyperechoic* are the terms used to describe plaque density. The more hypoechoic (or anechoic) the plaque, the higher its lipid content. Isoechoic plaques contain more smooth muscle, and hyperechoic plaques contain a large amount of fibrous tissue. Color Doppler is useful to help identify areas of anechoic plaque not seen in the vessel lumen because they are isoechoic with blood.

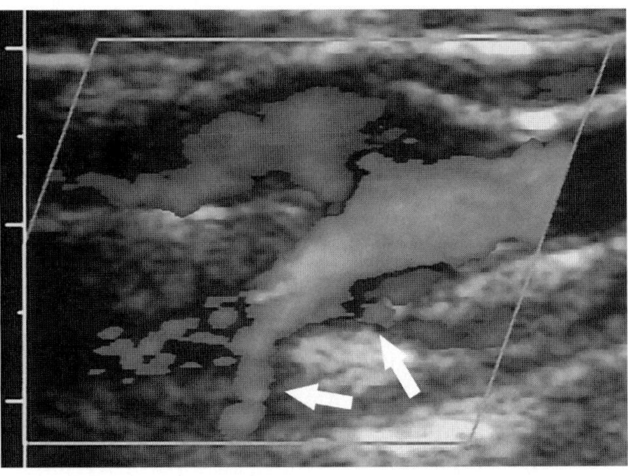

FIGURE 40.16. **(Color Plates) External Carotid Artery.** Note vessel branches (*arrows*).

TABLE 40.3 Internal Carotid Artery Versus External Carotid Artery

Internal Carotid Artery	*External Carotid Artery*
Larger (6 mm)	Smaller (3 to 4 mm)
No branches	Branch vessels
Usually posterolateral	Usually anteromedial
Courses posteriorly to mastoid	Courses anteriorly to face
Low-resistance flow pattern	High-resistance flow pattern
Carotid bulb at origin	"Temporal tap" maneuver

Plaque texture is either homogeneous or heterogeneous. Because of its high content of fibrous tissue, homogeneous plaque is smooth and similar in echotexture to the surrounding soft tissues. Heterogeneous plaque is complex, with at least one focal area of sonolucency representing intraplaque hemorrhage. Intraplaque hemorrhage is identified on sonography with approximately a 90% sensitivity and 85% specificity. Heterogeneous plaque can have

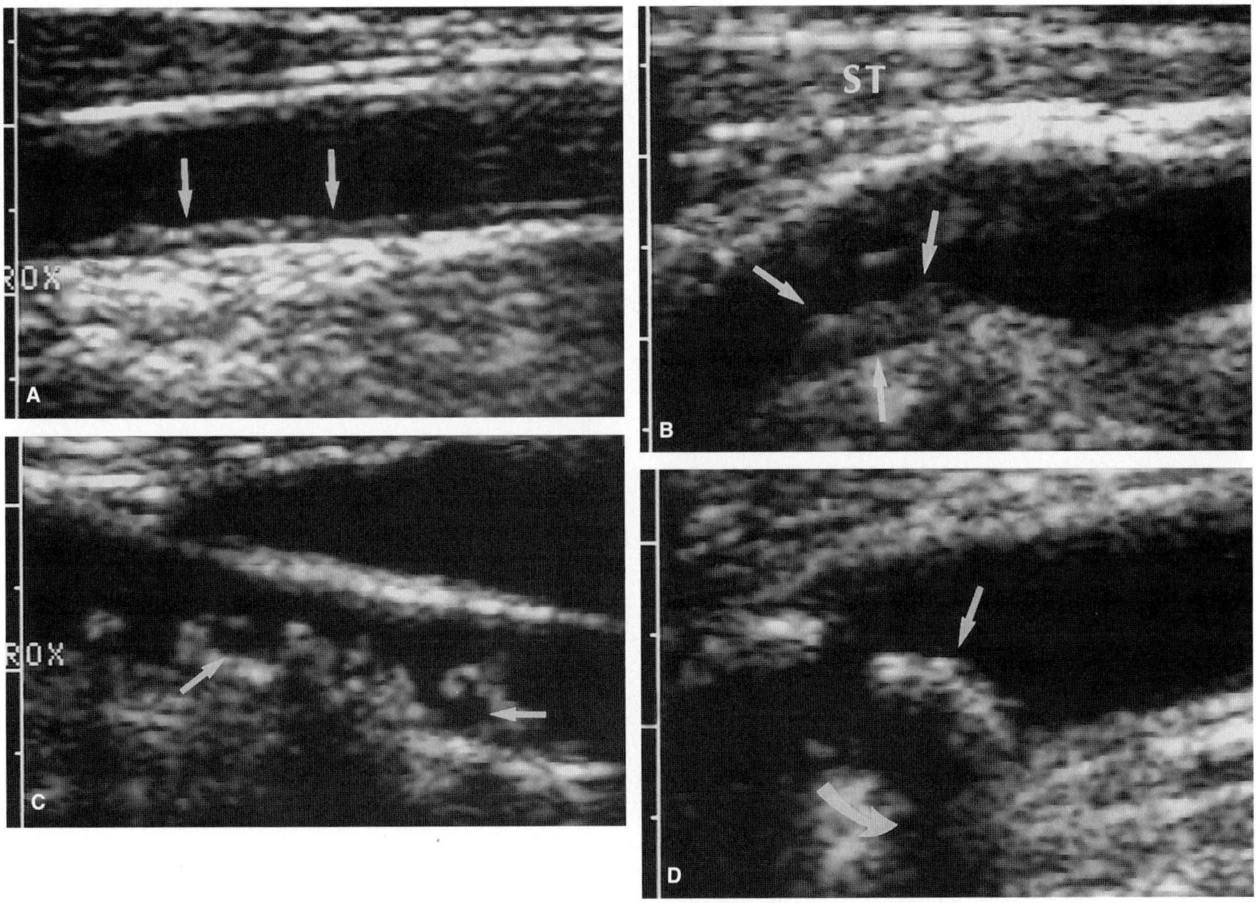

FIGURE 40.17. **Plaque. A.** Intimal hyperplasia (*arrows*). **B.** Predominantly homogeneous plaque (*arrows*) demonstrates echotexture similar to that of the surrounding soft tissue (ST). **C.** Heterogeneous plaque with sonolucent areas representing intraplaque hemorrhage (*arrows*). **D.** Calcified plaque (*arrow*) with distal acoustic shadowing (*curved arrow*).

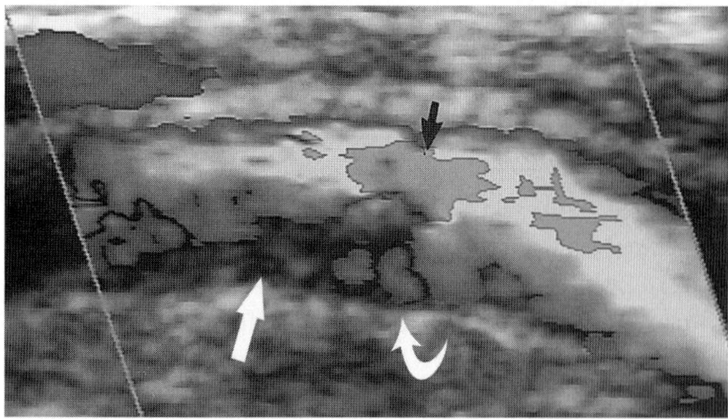

FIGURE 40.18. **(Color Plates) Ulcerated Plaque.** Color Doppler demonstrates a heterogeneous plaque (*white arrow*) with a vortex of color (flow reversal) extending into the plaque. This represents an angiographically proven ulcer crater (*curved arrow*). An area of green color shift (*black arrow*) represents aliasing owing to increased flow velocity caused by stenosis.

either a smooth or irregular surface. All ulcerated plaques are heterogeneous, but not all heterogeneous plaques ulcerate. Plaque calcification is a nonspecific finding and is seen in both homogeneous and heterogeneous plaque.

Plaque Significance. Heterogeneous plaque is a risk factor for a subsequent neurologic event. However, many asymptomatic individuals have heterogeneous plaque. How many of these individuals have a subsequent TIA or stroke remains controversial. No study to date demonstrates a definite stroke reduction from endarterectomy or medical management based on the US characteristics of plaque. Polak et al (33) found that the severity of ICA stenosis more closely predicts stroke or TIA than plaque characterization. In the authors' opinion, until conclusive evidence exists that plaque morphology can predict stroke, spectral Doppler (velocity parameters) and diameter stenosis (residual vessel lumen) remain the most important factors in carotid duplex interpretation.

Stenosis

Duplex US is well established in screening for carotid stenosis. *Properly performed*, duplex US has sensitivity and specificity exceeding 90%. However, many studies, including NASCET, have shown only marginal diagnostic accuracy (sensitivity, 67%; specificity, 78%). Most investigators believe the poor statistics are caused by suboptimal quality control and no standardization of the duplex scans by the institutions involved in the study. The cost-effectiveness of duplex sonography is well recognized when symptomatic individuals are screened. The rate of positive angiograms (>50% stenosis) increases from 30% to more than 70%, thus decreasing the number of unnecessary angiograms and their associated risk (34).

ICA Stenosis. Numerous velocity criteria exist for grading ICA stenosis. The most common velocity parameters include peak systolic velocity (PSV), end-diastolic velocity (EDV), and peak systolic velocity ICA to CCA ratio. Color Doppler and grayscale images are used to aid interpretation, particularly when the velocity parameters are discordant. Color Doppler mapping of the ICA also aids in identifying areas of suspected high flow (aliasing), significantly shortening the examination time (Fig. 40.19).

PSV is the most accurate parameter for a stenosis greater than 50% and less than 90%. A stenosis of less than 50% is more accurately graded with grayscale and color flow imaging in the transverse plane. At approximately 50% stenosis, spectral broadening of the ICA waveform and a mild increase in PSV are noted. Above 90% to 95% stenosis, the PSV falls as stenosis approaches occlusion.

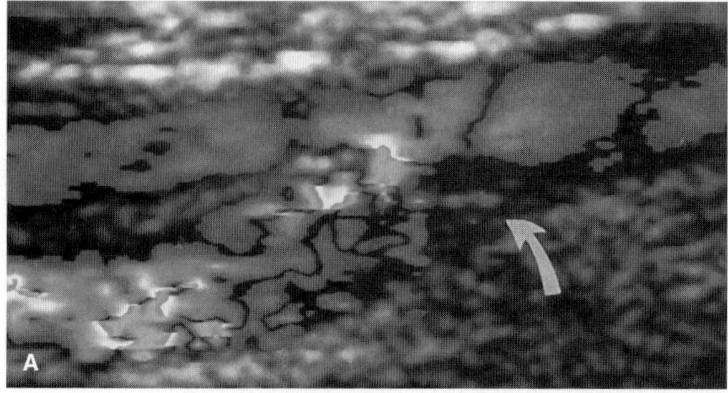

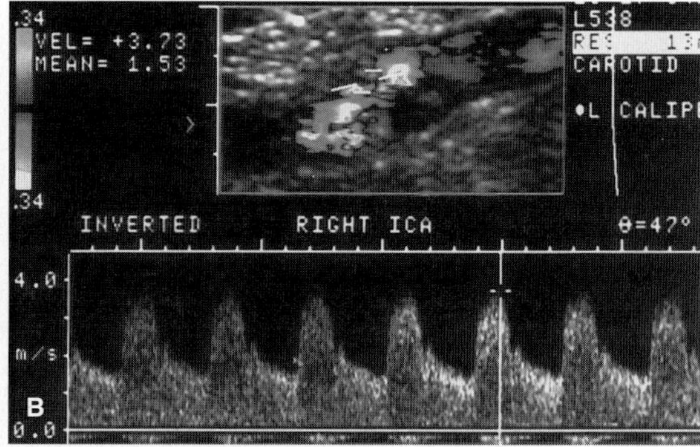

FIGURE 40.19. **(Color Plates) Internal Carotid Artery (ICA) Stenosis. A.** Longitudinal color Doppler image of the carotid bifurcation demonstrates an eccentric atherosclerotic plaque (*arrow*) at the origin of the ICA. The markedly heterogeneous color display distal to the plaque is indicative of severe turbulence caused by significant stenosis. The color Doppler image is used to direct placement of the spectral Doppler sample volume in the area of maximum flow velocity. **B.** Spectral Doppler waveform shows measurement of peak systolic flow velocity at 3.73 m/s (*upper left*), indicating critical stenosis. Note "filling in" of the Doppler waveform, known as spectral broadening, indicative of turbulence.

TABLE 40.4 Abnormal Common Carotid Artery (CCA) Velocities

Symmetric CCA Velocities	
Bilateral Low <50 cm/s	**Bilateral High >100 cm/s**
Low cardiac output	High cardiac output
Congestive heart failure	Hypertension
Cardiomyopathy	Hyperthyroid
Pericardial effusion	Bradycardia
Wide-diameter arteries	Narrow-diameter arteries
Asymmetric CCA Velocities	
Unilateral Low <50 cm/s	**Unilateral High >100 cm/s**
Severe proximal stenosis	Technical (i.e., tortuous)
Severe distal stenosis or occlusion	CCA stenosis
Wide-diameter CCA	Narrow-diameter CCA
Long-segment stenosis	Contralateral severe stenosis

The ICA/CCA ratio is most helpful when the CCA velocities are abnormal (Table 40.4). The EDV (>100 cm/s) helps to distinguish high-grade stenoses from lesser degrees of stenosis.

Since the NASCET study, many investigators have published revised criteria for grading ICA stenosis (Table 40.5) (35–46). These studies demonstrate the wide variability between vascular laboratories. Most vascular labs in North America have adopted the NASCET criteria (percent stenosis) for grading carotid disease. Because the distal lumen diameter of the ICA varies among normal individuals and is affected by perfusion pressure, some investigators believe residual lumen diameter is more accurate and a better predictor of stroke. A residual lumen diameter of <1.5 mm suggests a hemodynamically significant stenosis in most patients. For example, a 1.5-mm residual lumen diameter represents a 75% NASCET stenosis if the distal lumen measures 6 mm but only a 62% stenosis if the distal

TABLE 40.5 Doppler Criteria Based on NASCET

Author	*Cutoff (% Stenosis)*	*Parameter*	*Value*
Hunink et al. (1993) (35)	70	PSV	>230 cm/s
Moneta et al. (1993) (36)	70	SVR	>4.0
Neale et al. (1994) (37)	70	PSV	>270 cm/s
		EDV	>110 cm/s
Faught et al. (1994) (38), Hood et al. (1996) (41)	70	PSV	>130 cm/s
		EDV	>100 cm/s
Carpenter et al. (1995) (39)	60	PSV	>170 cm/s
		EDV	>40 cm/s
		SVR	>2.0
		DVR	>2.4
Moneta et al. (1995) (40)	60	PSV	>290 cm/s
		EDV	>80 cm/s
Browman et al. (1995) (43)	70	PSV	>175 cm/s
		PSV	<40 cm/s
Carpenter et al. (1996) (42)	70	PSV	>210 cm/s
		EDV	>70 cm/s
		SVR	>3.0
		DVR	>3.3
AbuRahma et al. (1998) (44)	50	PSV	>140 cm/s
	60	PSV	>150 cm/s
	70	EDV	>65 cm/s
		PSV	>150 cm/s
		EDV	>90 cm/s
Grant et al. (1999) (45)	60	PSV	>175 cm/s
	70	SVR	>2.5
		PSV	>200 cm/s
		SVR	>3.0
Huston et al. (2000) (46)	50	PSV	>130 cm/s
	70	SVR	>1.6
		PSV	>230 cm/s
		EDV	>70 cm/s
		SVR	>3.2

NASCET, North American Symptomatic Carotid Endarterectomy Trial; PSV, peak systolic velocity; EDV, end-diastolic velocity; SVR, peak systolic velocity ratio (ICA/CCA); DVR, end-diastolic velocity ratio (ICA/CCA).

TABLE 40.6 Society of Radiologists in Ultrasound Consensus Panel for Grayscale and Doppler US Criteria[a]

Degree Stenosis (%)	*ICA PSV (cm/s)*	*Plaque Estimate (%)*	*ICA/CCA (PSV Ratio)*	*ICA EDV (cm/s)*
Normal	<125	None	<2.0	<40
<50	<125	<50	<2.0	<40
50–69	125–230	≥50	2.0–4.0	40–100
≥70 but <near occlusion	>230	≥50	>4.0	>100
Near occlusion	High, low, or undetectable	Visible	Variable	Variable
Total occlusion	Undetectable	Visible, no detectable lumen	Not applicable	Not applicable

[a]From Grant et al. (49).
ICA, internal carotid artery; CCA, common carotid artery; PSV, peak systolic velocity; EDV, end-diastolic velocity.

lumen measures 4 mm (47,48). Each vascular US laboratory must develop its own criteria that correlate with conventional angiography, MR angiography (MRA), CT angiography (CTA), clinical outcomes data, and the desired sensitivity and specificity at their institution. Because of the lack of standardization of performance of carotid duplex examinations, the Society of Radiologists in Ultrasound has developed a consensus statement, which serves as a useful guide (49). Their conclusions are shown in Table 40.6.

CCA Stenosis. The normal velocity in the CCA is 50 to 100 cm/s in the population over age 50. No velocity tables exist for grading CCA stenosis. However, some vascular labs use ICA parameters. Along with grayscale and color flow imaging, a PSV ratio can be used to estimate the percent stenosis. The velocity at the stenosis is divided by the velocity proximal to the stenosis (Table 40.7, Fig. 40.20). If a significant stenosis exists in the extreme proximal portion of the CCA or at its origin, the CCA may have a parvus-tardus waveform (Fig. 40.21).

ECA Stenosis. Because the ECA predominantly supplies the face, the degree of stenosis (or occlusion) does not affect clinical management or stroke reduction. However, a significant ECA stenosis can alter the waveform of the CCA and cause elevated flow velocities in the ICA. A high-grade ECA stenosis may cause a neck bruit.

Vertebral Artery Stenosis. No well-established velocity parameters exist for determination of vertebral artery stenosis. Because treatment is limited and the vertebral artery origin and size are so variable, the detection of stenosis and occlusion is not clinically useful. Analysis is usually limited to confirming the presence and normal direction of blood flow.

TABLE 40.7 Peak Systolic Velocity Ratio (SVR) and % Stenosis

Velocity Ratio	*Diameter Stenosis*
2:1	50%
3.5:1	75%
7:1	90%

Occlusion

CCA occlusion is easily identified on duplex scanning. No spectral waveform or color flow can be elicited. Echogenic clot can often be seen filling the CCA lumen. Antegrade flow is usually present in the ipsilateral ICA, secondary to retrograde flow through the ECA to the carotid bifurcation and into the ICA. Spectral analysis in this situation demonstrates reversed flow in the ECA (Fig. 40.22).

ICA occlusion is suggested when no flow is identified in the vessel with spectral analysis and color flow imaging. On grayscale, the ICA diameter may be small and filled with echogenic thrombus. A brief systolic pulse (followed by a flow reversal) is usually present at the proximal end of the obstruction owing to the "thumping" of blood against the occlusion. The CCA waveform has a high-resistance flow pattern, with decreased diastolic flow velocity more characteristic of the ECA. This pattern is often called "externalization of the CCA" (Fig. 40.23). If the patient has well-developed ipsilateral ECA-to-ICA collateral flow intracranially, the CCA may not be externalized. In this circumstance, the ECA waveform becomes more low resistance or ICA-like, often called "internalization of the ECA" because it then supplies brain parenchyma (Fig. 40.24).

The distinction between total occlusion of the ICA and trickle flow is of critical importance. Patients with trickle flow are candidates for carotid endarterectomy, and those with total occlusions are not (Fig. 40.25). Despite advances in duplex US, 5% to 7% of trickle flow is not detected on grayscale, spectral Doppler, or color Doppler imaging. Power Doppler may improve the detection rate. MRA has an accuracy similar to that of duplex US. Therefore, catheter angiography is still recommended to exclude a "string sign" when the Doppler suggests occlusion. CTA is performed in lieu of catheter angiography in some settings.

Innominate or subclavian artery occlusion proximal to the origin of the vertebral artery results in the

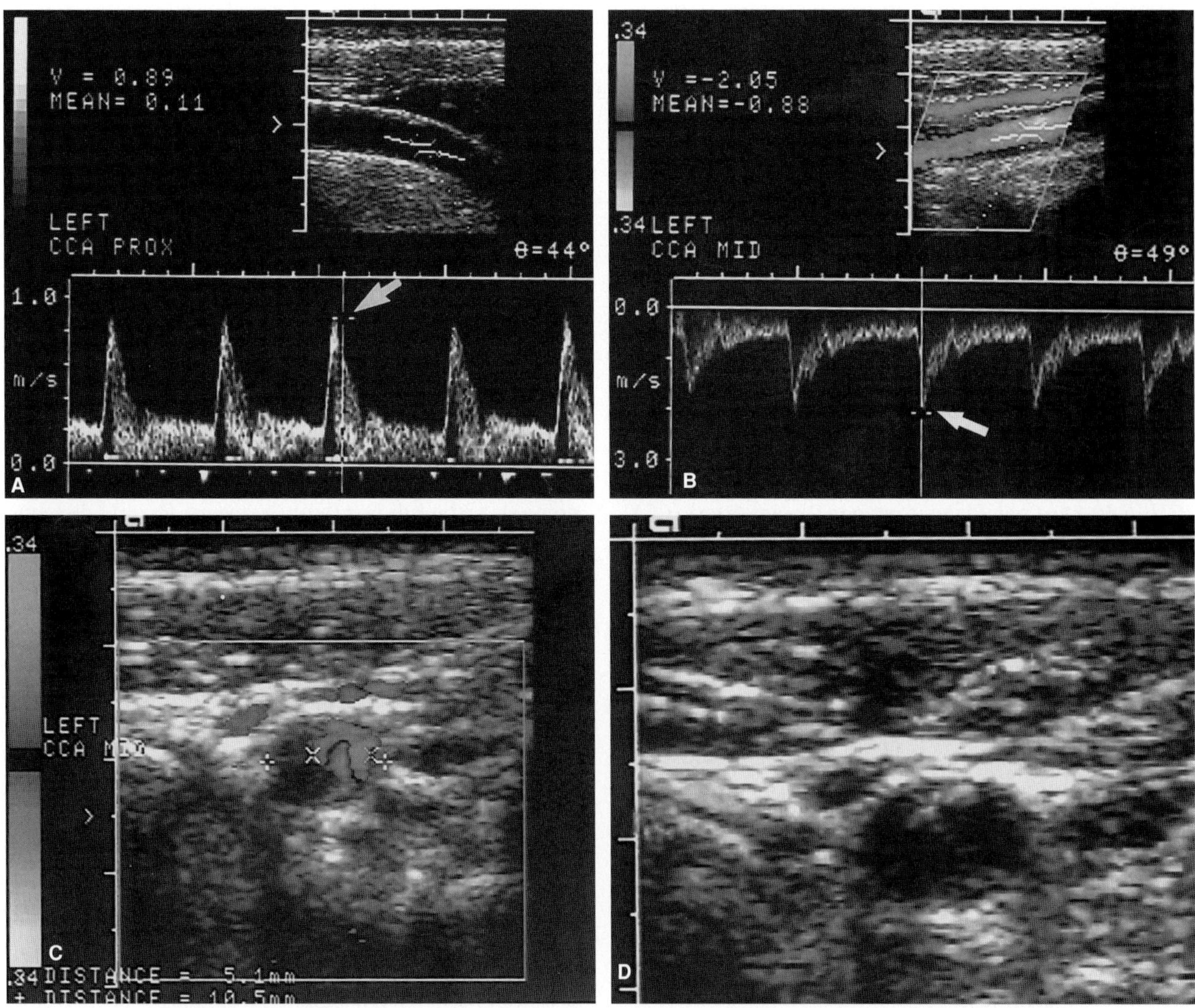

FIGURE 40.20. **(Color Plates) Common Carotid Artery (CCA) Stenosis. A.** Proximal left CCA peak systolic velocity is 0.89 m/s (*arrow*). **B.** Mid-left CCA peak systolic velocity is 2.05 m/s (*arrow*). The velocity ratio (mid/proximal) is 2.3, indicating a ≥50% diameter left CCA stenosis (see Table 40.7). Transverse color Doppler **(C)** and grayscale **(D)** images confirm the degree of stenosis secondary to mildly heterogeneous plaque. MR angiography graded the stenosis at 60% diameter.

subclavian steal syndrome. In this circumstance, the upper extremities receive blood from the CCA through the circle of Willis and down the vertebral artery. Spectral Doppler demonstrates reversed flow in the vertebral artery. Partial subclavian steal results in reversed flow during systole and antegrade flow during diastole in the vertebral artery because of severe stenosis of the innominate or left subclavian artery (Fig. 40.26).

Common Pitfalls

Angle of Insonation. The technician must ensure that the angle of insonation is between 30° and 60°. Spectral analysis with angles of interrogation >60° may cause large errors in velocity calculation.

Tortuous and Narrow Vessels. The laminar flow pattern is disrupted as blood flows through a sharp bend. Reporting of the higher velocity at the outer bend in a tortuous vessel may overestimate the degree of stenosis or falsely suggest a stenosis when none is present (Fig. 40.27).

Carotid Bulb. Normal flow reversal is usually noted in the carotid bulb opposite the flow divider (Fig. 40.7) and should not be mistaken for pathologic flow.

Calcified Plaque. Dense calcification can make it impossible to obtain velocities in portions of the ICA because of acoustic shadowing. As a result, a significant stenosis may not be detected. Color flow imaging is helpful in this situation. If the color flow into and out from behind the plaque is homogeneous, the presence of a significant stenosis is unlikely. However, if flow proximal to the plaque is

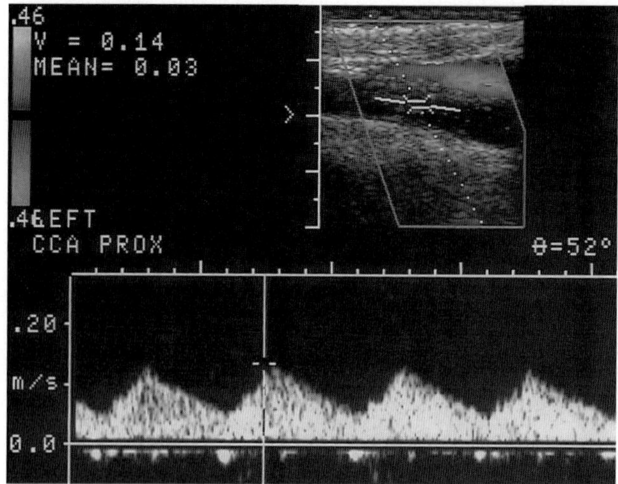

FIGURE 40.21. **(Color Plates) Common Carotid Artery (CCA) Origin Stenosis.** A parvus-tardus waveform is shown in the left proximal CCA, with a low peak systolic velocity of 0.14 m/s (*upper left*) corresponding to an angiographically proven severe origin stenosis of the left CCA.

homogeneous and flow distal to the plaque is heterogeneous, a significant stenosis should be suspected (Fig. 40.28).

Contralateral High-Grade Carotid Stenosis. With unilateral ICA occlusion or high-grade stenosis, flow velocity in the contralateral CCA and ICA may be elevated to maintain cerebral perfusion pressure.

Bilateral ICA disease causes physiologic flow alterations that complicate determining which side represents the more significant disease.

Tandem Lesions. The presence of more than one high-grade stenotic lesion can lead to interpretation errors. A significant intracranial ICA lesion causes a reduction in PSV, with absence of diastolic flow in the cervical portion of the ICA. Alternatively, a significant proximal CCA lesion lowers the PSV and increases the diastolic flow. In either circumstance, a stenosis in the cervical ICA may be underestimated.

Mistaking ECA for ICA When ICA Is Occluded. Remember that the ECA waveform may be internalized because of collateral flow. Use the temporal tap and look for branch vessels to identify the ECA (Figs. 40.16, 40.24).

Near Occlusion of the ICA. As the ICA approaches occlusion, the PSV and EDV may approach normal. The severity of the stenosis can be grossly underestimated if grayscale and color flow imaging are not performed.

Postendarterectomy. Following endarterectomy, the vein or polytetrafluoroethylene (PFTE) patch sutures may remain visible along the arterial wall (Fig. 40.29). A patulous carotid artery at the operative site is common. Complications include restenosis (~10% to 15% within the first year because of intimal hyperplasia), intimal flaps, and clamp strictures. Intraoperative US can be used to assess surgical result prior to closure. The postendarterectomy waveform often has a high-resistance flow pattern like that of the ECA. Turbulent flow is often noted because of the absence of the smooth endothelial lining.

Duplex US following carotid stent placement requires further study. No criteria have been established. It is recommended that carotid US be performed immediately after stent placement to establish a baseline. Serial color Doppler and spectral analysis may be useful in predicting stent stenosis if there is a change from baseline.

Nonatherosclerotic Carotid Disease. Remember that not all carotid disease is atherosclerotic. Takayasu arteritis and radiation fibrosis cause diffuse concentric wall thickening and narrowing of the lumen. Fibromuscular dysplasia in the cervical CCA produces irregular intimal thickening over the full length of the artery. Carotid dissection can be traumatic, inflammatory, degenerative, or spontaneous. Systolic flow reversal and intimal flaps can be seen. Carotid body tumors or vascular invasion from metastases can be visualized with duplex scanning.

Valvular Heart Disease. Significant aortic stenosis produces a bilateral parvus-tardus waveform, and aortic insufficiency demonstrates a bisferious pulse, with the second systolic peak higher than the first.

A simplified approach to carotid duplex interpretation is provided in Table 40.8. The ideal carotid imaging algorithm remains controversial, and a detailed discussion is beyond the scope of this chapter. For both medical and economic reasons, a combination of noninvasive studies—MRA and duplex US—has replaced catheter angiography in most patients. In our institutions, duplex US is used to screen patients. If a significant stenosis is suspected, an MRA is performed for confirmation. Catheter angiography is reserved for difficult cases and to confirm carotid occlusion. CTA is becoming more accepted in this role and may replace catheter angiography.

The reader is referred to the excellent pictorial essay of Romero et al on the interpretative pitfalls of carotid duplex US (50).

ABDOMINAL VESSELS

Anatomy

Abdominal Aorta. The abdominal aorta enters the abdomen through the aortic hiatus of the diaphragm and descends just to the left of midline and anterior to the spine. It bifurcates into the bilateral common iliac arteries at approximately the level of L4. The aorta has five main branches. Three originate from the ventral aorta: the celiac axis, the superior mesenteric artery, and the inferior mesenteric artery. The left and right renal arteries originate from the aorta laterally. The proximal aorta measures 2.5 cm and tapers distally to measure about 1.5 to 2.0 cm

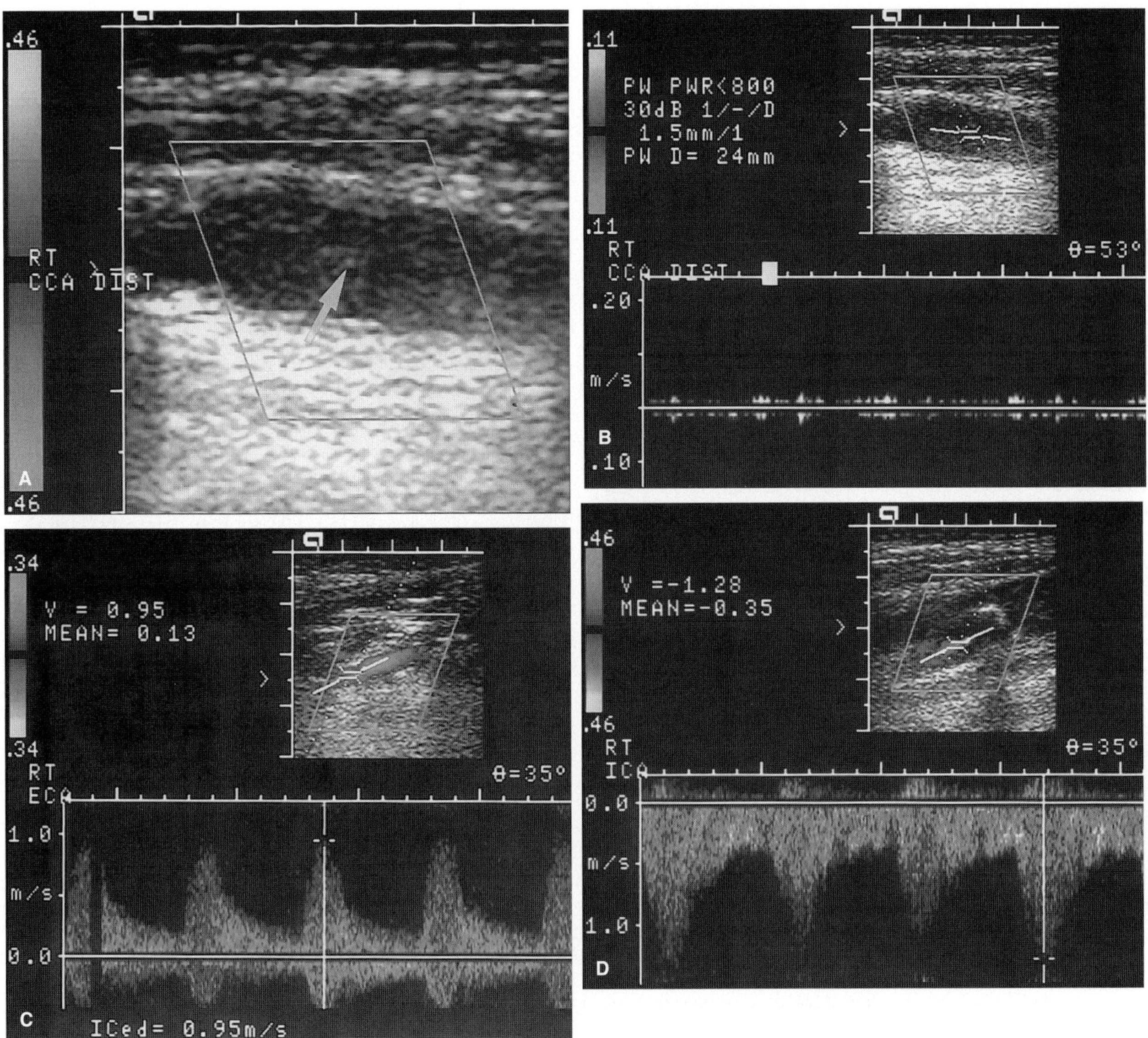

FIGURE 40.22. **(Color Plates) Common Carotid Artery (CCA) Occlusion. A.** Longitudinal color Doppler image of the right CCA showing echogenic thrombus (*arrow*) with absence of color, indicating no blood flow. **B.** Spectral Doppler confirms no CCA flow. The irregular signal near the baseline is due to noise. **C.** Spectral Doppler of the right external carotid artery demonstrates retrograde flow (toward the heart). **D.** Spectral Doppler of the right internal carotid artery shows antegrade flow (toward the head). See text for explanation.

at the bifurcation (Fig. 40.30). Spectral analysis demonstrates a triphasic waveform. Color Doppler is useful to identify thrombus.

Inferior Vena Cava. The inferior vena cava (IVC) courses toward the heart just to the right of midline and to the right of the aorta. As it reaches the liver, the IVC is contained in a deep groove on its posterior surface. It traverses the diaphragm and empties into the RA. Sonographically detectable branches include the hepatic and renal veins. The renal veins are anterior to their corresponding arteries and enter the IVC at right angles. The left renal vein is three times longer than the right. The hepatic veins enter the IVC from the posterior surface of the liver. Many embryologic variations of the IVC exist, including an interrupted IVC that does not extend above the renal arteries, a left-sided IVC, and a duplicated IVC. The left renal vein can be retroaortic or circumaortic. Spectral analysis of the IVC demonstrates the classic "sawtooth" pattern from cardiac and respiratory pulsations similar to the hepatic veins. Distally near the common iliac veins, there is a more phasic pattern similar to that seen in the proximal extremities.

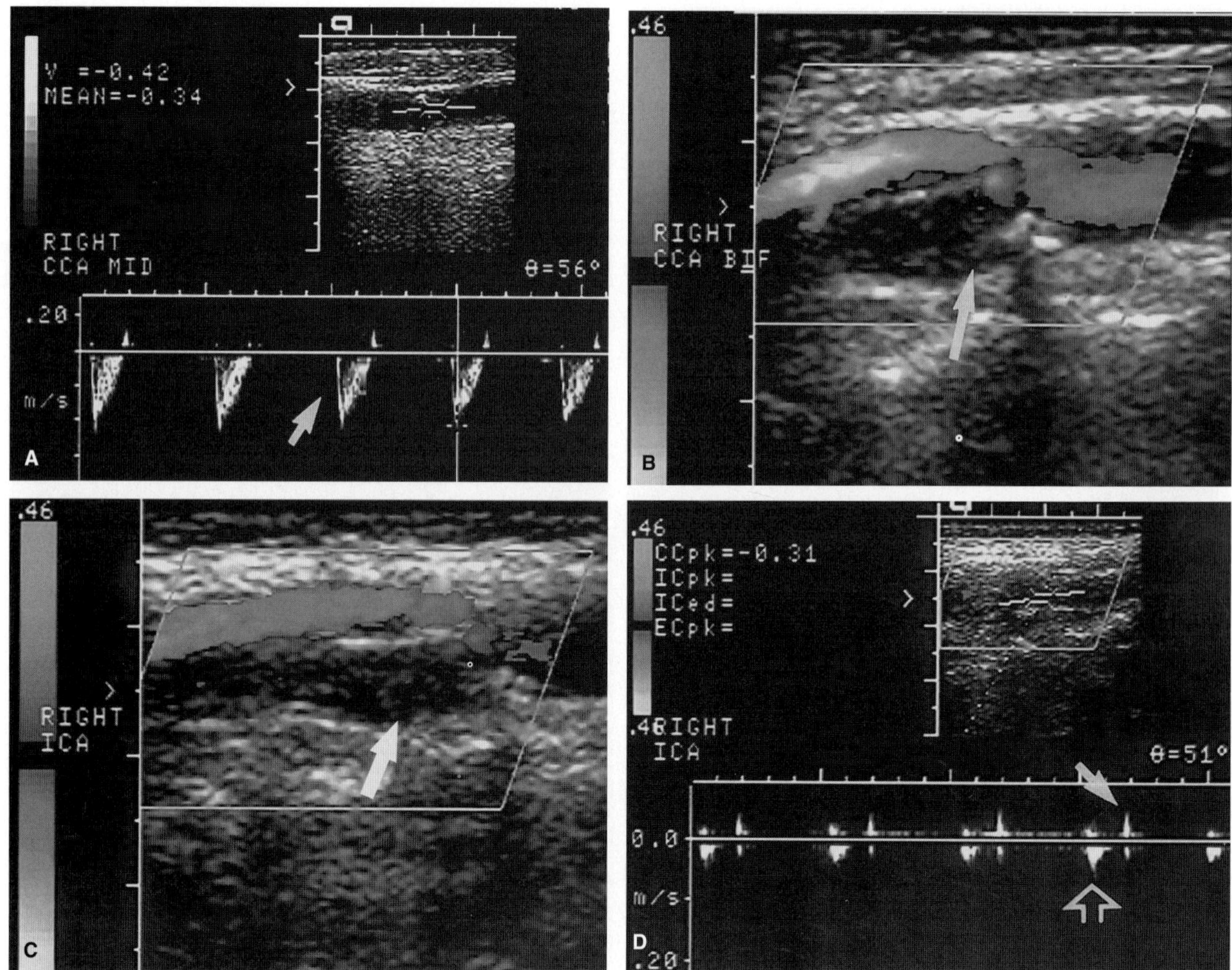

FIGURE 40.23. **(Color Plates) Internal Carotid Artery (ICA) Occlusion. A.** Spectral Doppler waveform in the right mid–common carotid artery (CCA) illustrates "externalization" of the CCA (*arrow*). The CCA waveform resembles the high-resistance external carotid artery (ECA) waveform. Longitudinal color Doppler images of the right carotid bifurcation **(B)** and right ICA **(C)** demonstrate echogenic thrombus and the absence of color flow (*arrow*) in the ICA. Color Doppler flow (*red*) is present in the ECA. **D.** Spectral Doppler interrogation of the ICA at the proximal end of the occlusion shows the typical bidirectional flow. Antegrade flow (*open arrow*) slams into the occlusion, resulting in flow reversal (*arrow*). During scanning, an audible carotid "thump" can be heard.

Aneurysm

Abdominal Aorta Aneurysm (AAA). More than 90% of AAAs involve the infrarenal aorta. Most are fusiform and enlarge at the rate of 2 to 4 mm per year. Surgery is recommended for aneurysms >5 cm. This recommendation stems from the autopsy data of Darling et al of aneurysm rupture rates, shown in Table 40.9 (51). The rupture rate for an aneurysm >5 cm is currently estimated at about 8% per year, with lifetime risks of 25% to 49% (52); thus, surgery is reasonable but not universally accepted. Some surgeons operate on smaller aneurysms (52,53). Some use rapid expansion rates (>1 cm per year) as an additional criteria for elective surgery for aneurysms <6 cm (54). Currently, no definitive patient selection process exists for elective aneurysm repair. Aneurysm size, clinical risk factors, and operative mortality (1% to 3% in experienced centers) are important factors. The development of endovascular aortic stent graft techniques for the treatment of AAAs has significantly reduced the major morbidity associated with standard surgical repair. However, agreement on the indications and limitations of their use has not been reached.

Duplex US has a diagnostic accuracy approaching 100% and is readily available and cost effective. Therefore, it has become the imaging modality of choice for diagnosing and following asymptomatic AAAs. The aorta is imaged from the diaphragm to the iliac bifurcation using a 3.5- to

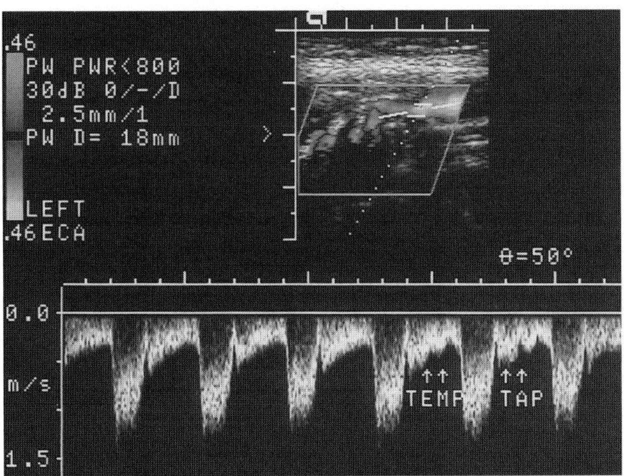

FIGURE 40.24. **(Color Plates) Internal Carotid Artery (ICA) Occlusion.** Color image and spectral Doppler demonstrate "internalization" of the external carotid artery (ECA) waveform because of ICA occlusion, with intracranial ECA collateral flow to the ICA system. The temporal tap (*arrows*) confirms that the artery visualized is the ECA.

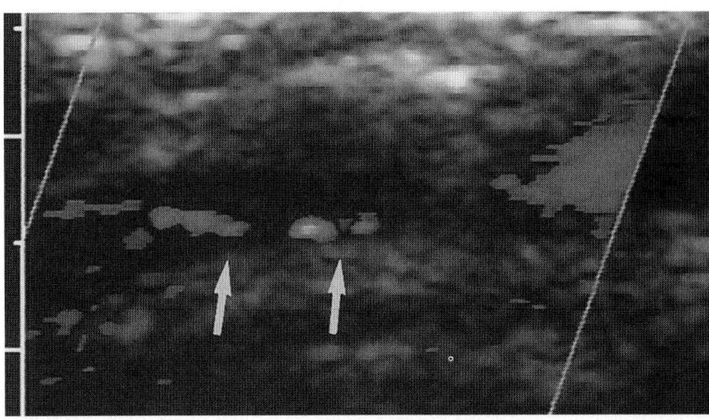

FIGURE 40.25. **(Color Plates) String Sign.** Near occlusion of the right internal carotid artery demonstrates "trickle flow" (*arrows*).

5.0-MHz transducer in both the longitudinal and transverse planes. Limitations include patient obesity, bowel gas, and difficulty identifying the origins of the renal arteries. An AAA is defined as a focal enlargement of the aorta greater than 3 cm in the anteroposterior (AP) diameter. The AP dimension of the aorta should be measured in both the transverse and longitudinal planes to assure accuracy. Many atherosclerotic aortas are tortuous and if measured obliquely, measurement errors occur. The AP dimension can be overestimated in the transverse plane and underestimated in the longitudinal plane. The authors report the longitudinal measurement, provided it is concordant with the transverse measurement. The length and width of the aneurysm are also reported. The aorta normally tapers from proximal to distal. If it enlarges distally, it is technically considered aneurysmal regardless of the absolute measurement (Fig. 40.31).

In addition to sizing the aneurysm, US can identify intraluminal thrombus, which generally appears hypoechoic. Thrombus can be isoechoic to blood within the aorta, making it invisible on grayscale imaging; therefore, color Doppler is useful in this situation. Inflammatory aneurysms have a hypoechoic ring surrounding the aorta that corresponds to the perianeurysmal fibrosis. Aortic rupture can be diagnosed with US if a retroperitoneal hematoma is present. CT is the diagnostic modality of choice for suspected leaking aneurysm, rupture, and inflammatory aneurysm and for defining the

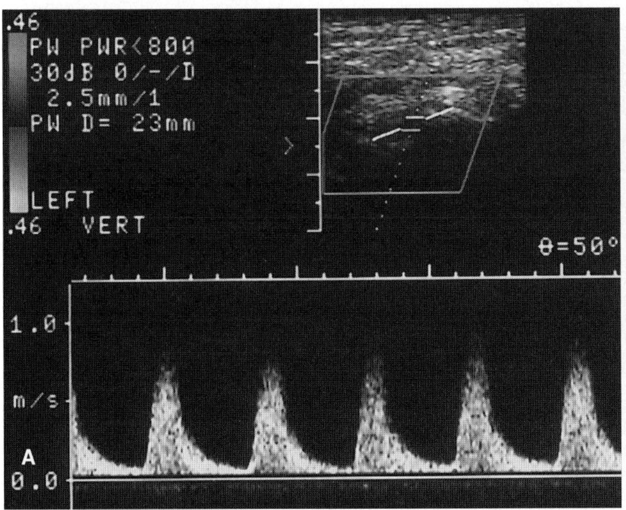

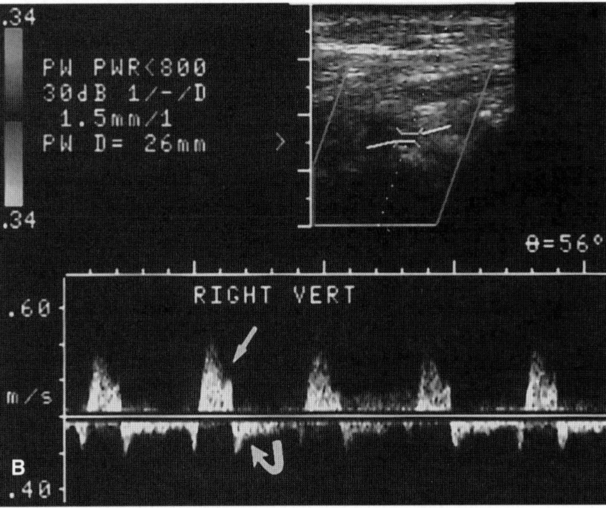

FIGURE 40.26. **Subclavian Steal. A.** Flow is reversed in the left vertebral artery (flow is away from the brain). **B.** Partial subclavian steal in another patient results in reversed flow during systole (*arrow*) and antegrade flow during diastole (*curved arrow*).

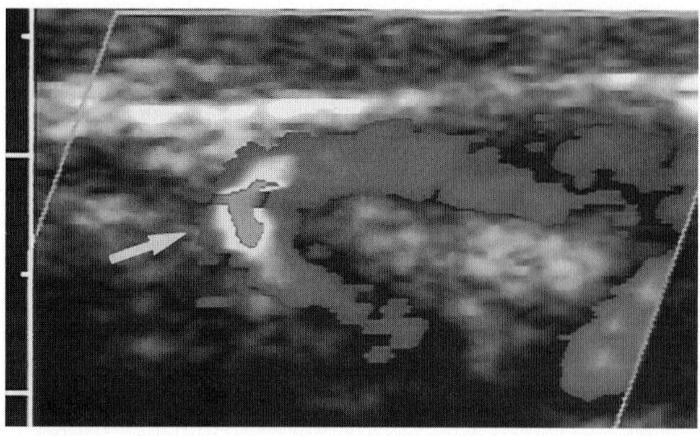

FIGURE 40.27. **(Color Plates) Tortuous Vessel.** Color Doppler image of the internal carotid artery shows a sharp turn. Aliasing and turbulence (*arrow*) indicate the disruption in laminar flow as blood flows around a bend.

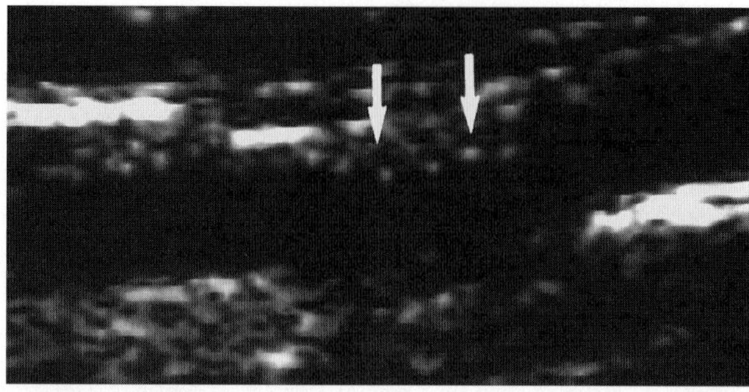

FIGURE 40.29. **Postendarterectomy.** Note the typical "dot-dash" pattern of the synthetic polytetrafluoroethylene sutures (*arrows*).

relationship of the aneurysm to the surrounding retroperitoneal structures.

Following AAA repair, the aortic graft demonstrates discrete echogenic walls. US is used to confirm patency of the graft, assess for perigraft fluid collections, and evaluate for anastomotic stenosis or aneurysm. Perigraft fluid collections seen more than 3 months after surgery may indicate hemorrhage or infection. Anastomotic aneurysms typically occur at the iliac anastomosis. They appear as focal circumscribed bulges off the distal end of the graft.

Abdominal aortic dissection can be diagnosed with US when an intimal flap is identified or color flow US identifies flow in the false lumen (Fig. 40.32). Chronic dissection is difficult to identify, because the false lumen is often filled with clot. CT and MR remain the preferred diagnostic modalities.

Iliac Artery Aneurysm. Approximately two thirds of AAAs extend into the common iliac arteries; however, extension into the external iliac artery is uncommon. The normal common iliac arteries measure <15 mm in the AP dimension. Isolated iliac artery aneurysms are rare. Common iliac artery aneurysms can rupture or erode into the adjacent iliac vein, colon, or ureter.

Thrombosis

IVC Thrombosis. The IVC is examined in sagittal, coronal, and transverse planes using a 3.5- to 5.0-MHz transducer. The renal and hepatic vein communications with the IVC are usually seen. The characteristic waveform in the IVC results from transmission of right atrial pulsations. The

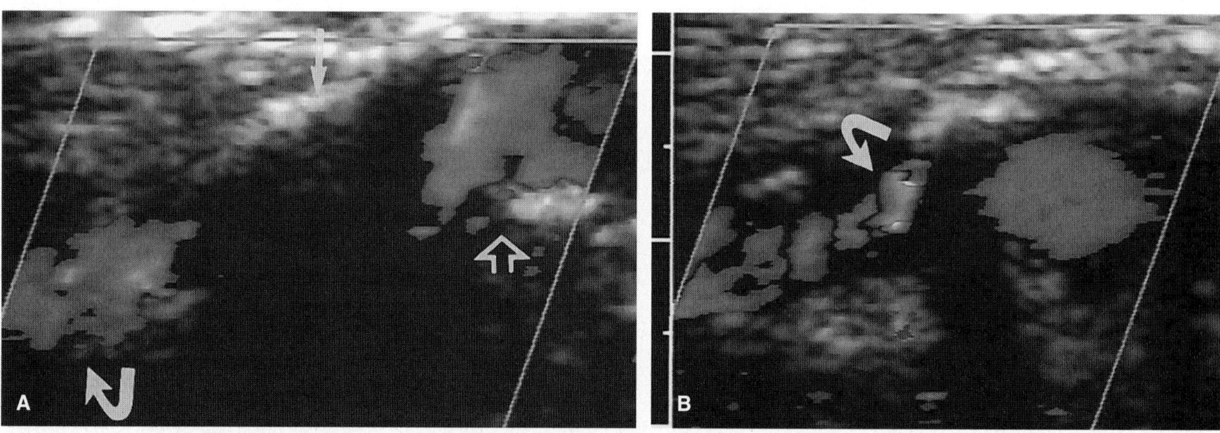

FIGURE 40.28. **(Color Plates) Calcified Plaques. A.** Longitudinal color Doppler image of a right internal carotid artery. Visualization of the lumen is limited behind a calcified plaque (*arrow*) because of sound absorption/shadowing. However, the flow is homogeneous (*red*) both entering (*open arrow*) and exiting (*curved arrow*) from behind the plaque. The absence of turbulent flow after the plaque bodes against a significant stenosis. **B.** In contrast, this longitudinal color Doppler image demonstrates heterogeneous or turbulent flow (aliasing) exiting from behind the calcified plaque (*curved arrow*). This patient had a severe stenosis at angiography despite only mild to moderate elevation of velocity.

TABLE 40.8 Carotid Duplex Interpretation: Checklist

1. Keep angle of insonation <60°.
2. Is the CCA flow normal (50 to 100 cm/s)?
3. If CCA velocities are normal and symmetric, use the PSV to grade stenosis.
4. If CCA velocities abnormal or asymmetric, use ICA/CCA ratio and search for cause.
5. Use the EDV to help identify very high-grade stenosis; >100 cm/s suggests >80% diameter stenosis
6. Confirm all findings on grayscale and color Doppler; measure diameter stenosis/residual lumen
7. Assess direction of flow in vertebral arteries.

CCA, common carotid artery; PSV, peak systolic velocity; EDV, end-diastolic velocity; ICA/CCA, ICA peak systolic velocity/CCA peak systolic velocity.

tracing is similar to that of the hepatic veins. Patency is confirmed by color flow and a normal spectral tracing.

IVC thrombosis usually extends from the peripheral veins. Bilateral lower extremity edema is present, and if acute, patients typically experience severe pain. Other clinical symptoms and signs are related to organ involvement (e.g., renal failure, bowel ischemia). Grayscale imaging demonstrates intraluminal clot (Fig. 40.33) that often expands the IVC. Remember that congestive heart failure also distends the hepatic veins and the IVC. With the current high-resolution transducers, slow-flowing blood can be mistaken for clot. Doppler demonstrates the absence of flow in complete occlusion and diverted flow with partial obstruction. In partial thrombosis, the spectral waveform is usually blunted, with loss of the transmitted cardiac pulsation and respiratory phasicity.

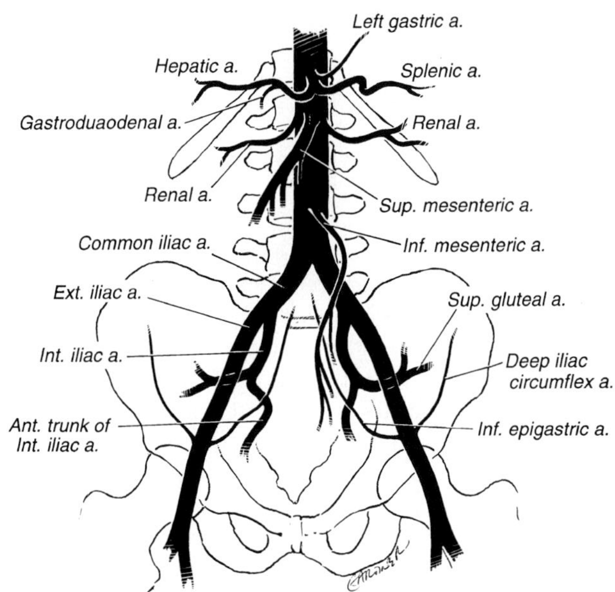

FIGURE 40.30. **Normal Abdominal Aorta and Major Arterial Branch Anatomy.**

TABLE 40.9 Aortic Aneurysm Rupture

Size	***Rupture Rate***
<4 cm	10%
4 to 7 cm	25%
7 to 10 cm	45%
>10 cm	60%

Tumor extension into the IVC causes a tumor thrombosis (Fig. 40.33), which appears similar to bland thrombus. If arterial flow is identified in the IVC lumen within the mass, the diagnosis of tumor thrombus can be made confidently. The most common tumor to extend into the IVC is renal cell carcinoma. Less common tumors include hepatoma, adrenal cell carcinoma, pheochromocytoma, and lymphoma. Benign tumors that rarely invade the IVC include angiomyolipoma and atrial myxoma. Leiomyosarcoma is the most common primary tumor of the IVC. Extrinsic compression from any intraperitoneal or retroperitoneal process such as lymphadenopathy, hepatomegaly, retroperitoneal fibrosis, or hematoma can cause obstruction and thrombosis of the IVC.

Budd-Chiari syndrome (segmental obstruction of the hepatic veins) can involve the IVC. Causes include hypercoagulable states, posttraumatic causes, tumor invasion, and membranous obstruction of the suprahepatic IVC (web or diaphragm). US demonstrates echogenic thrombus within, reduced caliber of, or nonvisualization of the hepatic veins. The spectral waveform is often monophasic.

Aortic Thrombosis. Grayscale imaging of the abdominal aorta may be normal with aortic thrombosis, because aortic thrombosis can occur in the absence of an aneurysm and the clot can be echolucent. Spectral and color Doppler imaging confirm the presence of a thrombosis.

TIPS EVALUATION

Transjugular intrahepatic portosystemic shunt (TIPS) has become commonplace in the treatment of life-threatening portal venous hypertension with variceal bleeding refractory to sclerotherapy and intractable ascites. It is also indicated for hepatic hydrothorax, hepatorenal syndrome, and Budd-Chiari Syndrome. The TIPS procedure involves creating a tract between a hepatic vein and a portal vein, most commonly the right hepatic vein and the right portal vein. Shunt stenosis occurs in approximately 60% of cases within the first 12 months. Because early shunt malfunction is often asymptomatic, the ability to predict shunt failure is of prime importance. If diagnosed, reintervention can be performed in a timely fashion to prevent a catastrophic complication (e.g., variceal bleed) and to increase the longevity of the stent. TIPS patency rates of >90% at

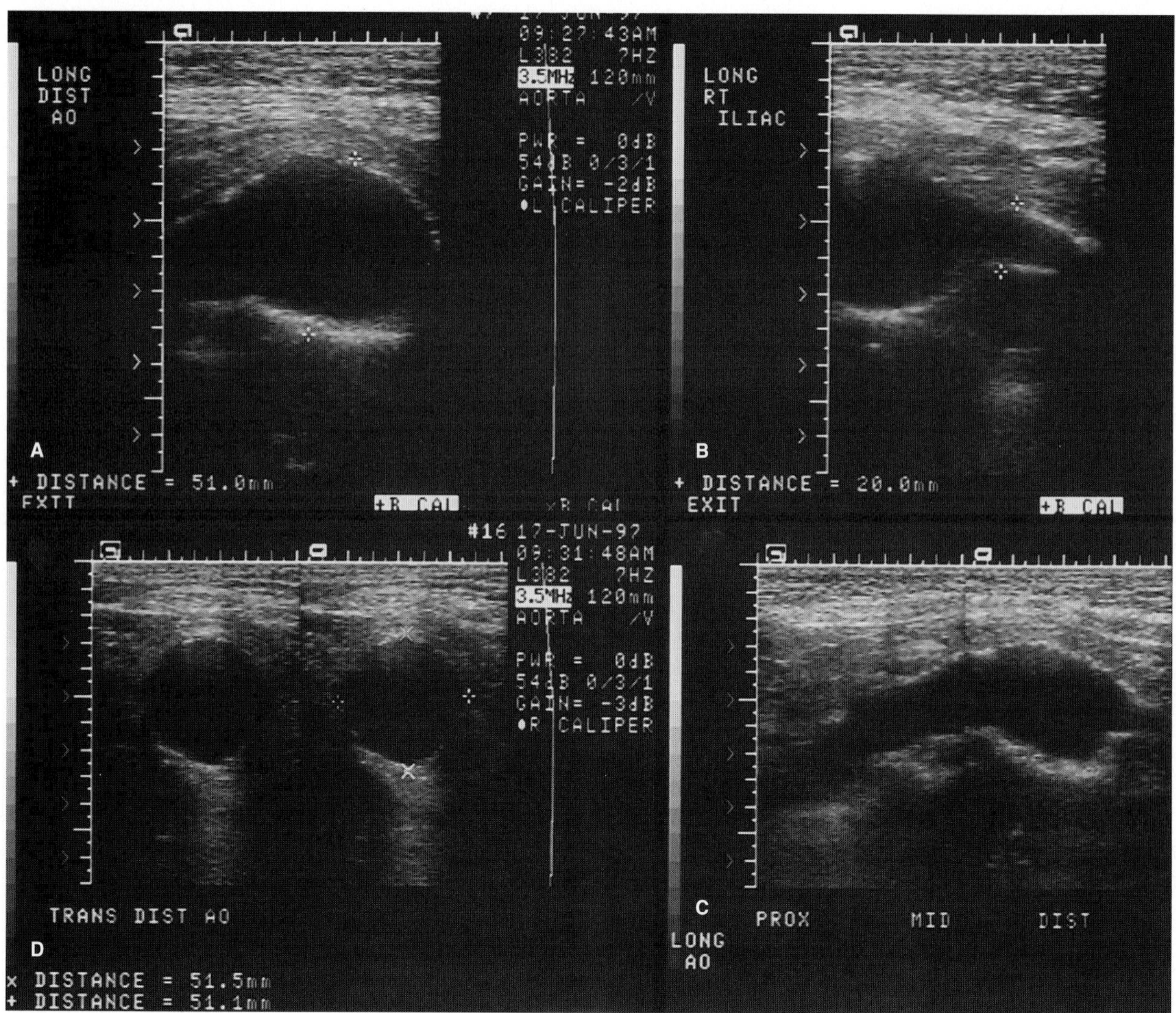

FIGURE 40.31. **Abdominal Aortic Aneurysm (AAA). A.** Longitudinal image of a distal AAA measuring 5.1 cm in the anteroposterior dimension (*cursors*). **B.** Longitudinal image shows extension of the aneurysm into the right common iliac artery, which measures 20 mm in diameter (*cursors*). **C.** The maximum dimension of the aneurysm is confirmed in the transverse plane. **D.** Longitudinal image showing the fusiform nature of the AAA.

4 years have been obtained with rigorous shunt surveillance (55,56).

Technique. The patient is imaged using a 2.5- to 3.5-MHz curvilinear or sector transducer. A common US protocol for monitoring a TIPS calls for a pre-TIPS US, an US within 24 hours following the procedure, another US at 3 months after TIPS, and then US examinations at 6-month intervals. Additional interval US is performed if the clinical situation suggests shunt malfunction (e.g., recurrent bleeding or ascites). Transjugular portal venograms are routinely performed at 6 months and 1 year following the procedure and then annually (57).

The pre-TIPS US defines the anatomy and establishes the patient's baseline hemodynamics prior to the procedure. Grayscale US evaluates the size and echotexture of the hepatic and splenic parenchyma. Spectral and color Doppler examinations establish the patency and direction of flow in the main, right, and left portal veins; the hepatic veins; and the IVC. Velocity measurements are obtained in the main portal vein and hepatic arteries. Enlarged collateral vessels (patent umbilical vein, etc.) are documented, and the amount of ascites is noted. The right internal jugular vein is assessed for patency.

After the TIPS procedure, the shunt is easily visualized on US as an echogenic tubular structure coursing from a portal vein to hepatic vein. The anatomic survey is repeated, as per the pre-TIPS protocol. In addition, duplex interrogation of the stent is performed. The

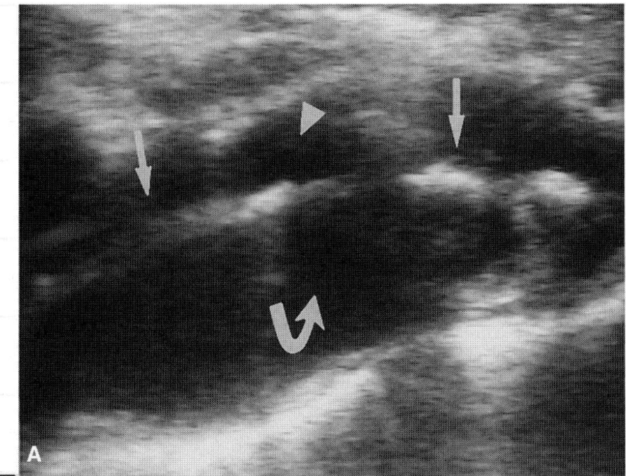

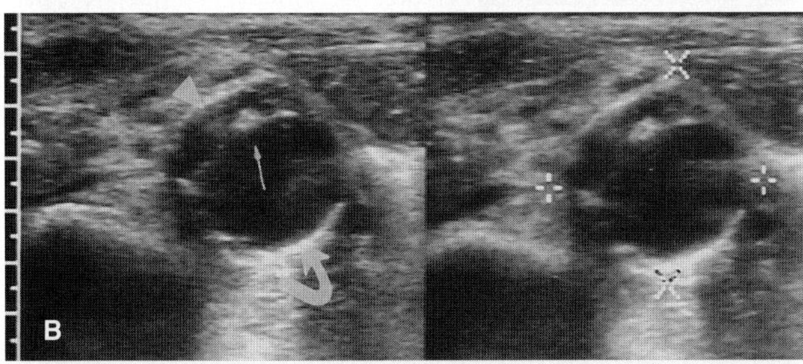

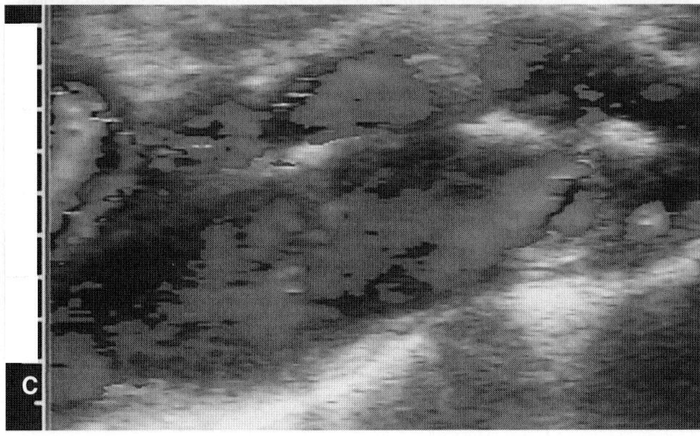

FIGURE 40.32. **(Color Plates) Aortic Dissection.** Longitudinal **(A)** and transverse **(B)** images of a 4.2-cm aortic aneurysm with dissection. An echogenic intimal flap is identified (*arrows*), separating the true lumen (*arrowhead*) from the false (*curved arrow*) lumen. **C.** Longitudinal color Doppler image demonstrates antegrade flow in the smaller true lumen (*red*) and retrograde flow in the larger false lumen (*blue*).

angle-corrected PSVs at the portal vein end of the stent, mid-stent, and hepatic vein end of the stent are obtained. Normal postshunt velocities range from ~100 to 200 cm/s. Following shunting, the collateral vessels disappear and ascites resolves in many patients. In two thirds of patients, blood flow in the right and left portal vein reverses (becomes hepatofugal) secondary to diversion through the stent. The immediate post-TIPS US establishes a new baseline and looks for immediate thrombosis of the stent and hemorrhagic complications (Fig. 40.34) (57–59).

Shunt malfunction usually results from thrombosis or pseudointimal hyperplasia of the stent. The latter can occur within a few weeks after TIPS, and significant stenoses are often detected within 6 months. Stenosis is usually focal and can occur anywhere in the stent but is more common in the hepatic vein end. Diffuse pseudointimal hyperplasia occurs less commonly.

Nearly all shunt stenoses manifest as decreased velocity within the stent because of preferential shunting through the lower-resistance collateral venous pathways present in portal hypertension. However, several researchers have shown high-velocity stenosis within the TIPS stent (59). Duplex US is nearly 100% accurate in detecting shunt occlusion. No spectral waveform or color flow is identified within the shunt (Fig. 40.35).

The methodology, parameters, location of velocity measurements within the stent, small patient numbers, and individual patient manifestations of portal hypertension have made establishing universally accepted criteria for shunt malfunction difficult.

US is a screening test used to decide when transjugular portography should be performed. The absolute or temporal change in PSV within the shunt is an indicator of shunt malfunction. Measuring the PSV in more than one region within the stent increases the chance of finding an early focal stenosis. A peak shunt velocity of <50 cm/s portends a bad prognosis. This velocity has been used as a threshold value to predict shunt malfunction. Although 90% specific, it lacks the sensitivity (25% to 57%) needed for a screening test (57,60,61). This low sensitivity casts doubt on the utility of Doppler US as a screening test (56,62). However, increasing the peak velocity threshold to <90 cm/s improves the sensitivity to ~90% (59). A temporal stent velocity decrease of more than 50 cm/s from baseline indicates a potential shunt malfunction, and portography is warranted. Shunt velocities >200 cm/s suggest shunt stenosis, particularly if the velocity has increased >50 cm/s above the established baseline (63). Because velocity in the main portal vein increases after shunting, a decrease in the main portal vein velocity below 30 cm/s indicates possible shunt stenosis (59). Recurrence of ascites, recanalization of collateral pathways, and return of hepatopetal flow in the right and left portal veins are other indicators of shunt malfunction. Parameters for the early detection of shunt malfunction are shown in Table 40.10. If any of these changes occur, the patient is referred for transjugular portography and potential shunt revision (Fig. 40.36).

PERIPHERAL ARTERIES

In the lower extremity, duplex US is the diagnostic modality of choice for evaluating the complications of arterial puncture and monitoring arterial bypass grafts. This noninvasive technique is also evolving as an important adjunct

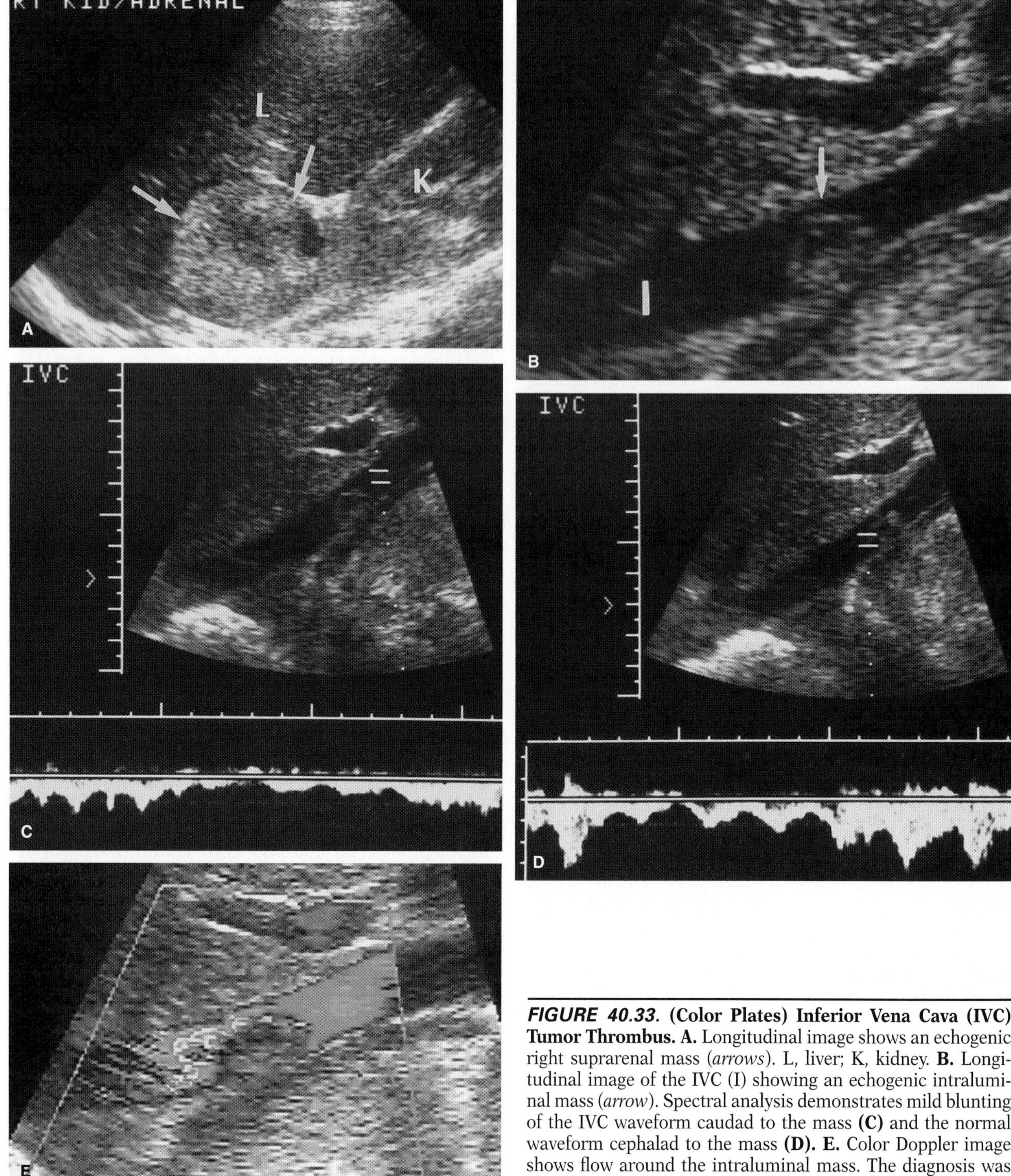

FIGURE 40.33. **(Color Plates) Inferior Vena Cava (IVC) Tumor Thrombus. A.** Longitudinal image shows an echogenic right suprarenal mass (*arrows*). L, liver; K, kidney. **B.** Longitudinal image of the IVC (I) showing an echogenic intraluminal mass (*arrow*). Spectral analysis demonstrates mild blunting of the IVC waveform caudad to the mass **(C)** and the normal waveform cephalad to the mass **(D). E.** Color Doppler image shows flow around the intraluminal mass. The diagnosis was pheochromocytoma with tumor extension into the IVC.

in the evaluation of atherosclerotic peripheral vascular disease (ASPVD). In the upper extremity, ASPVD is uncommon distal to the subclavian arteries. Therefore, US is limited to evaluation of thoracic outlet syndrome (discussed in the section "Venous Ultrasound") and dialysis grafts.

Anatomy. In the lower extremity (Fig. 40.37), the femoral and popliteal arteries travel with an accompanying vein. The patient is imaged supine using a 5- to 10-MHz linear transducer. The common femoral artery arises at the inguinal ligament and quickly bifurcates into the

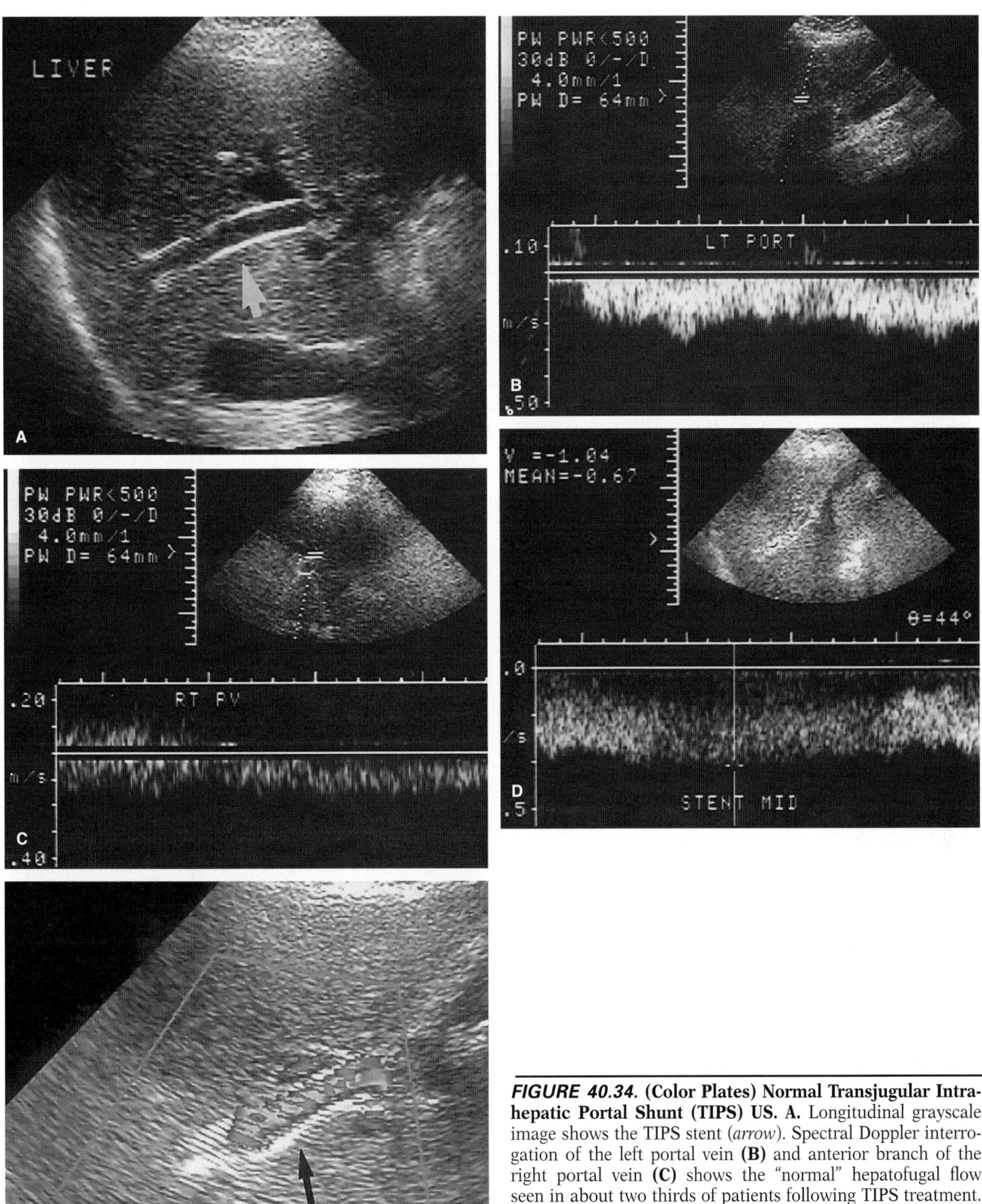

FIGURE 40.34. **(Color Plates) Normal Transjugular Intrahepatic Portal Shunt (TIPS) US. A.** Longitudinal grayscale image shows the TIPS stent (*arrow*). Spectral Doppler interrogation of the left portal vein **(B)** and anterior branch of the right portal vein **(C)** shows the "normal" hepatofugal flow seen in about two thirds of patients following TIPS treatment. The Doppler tracings are below the baseline, indicating flow away from the transducer. **D.** Normal midstent velocity of 1.04 m/s. **E.** Color Doppler image demonstrates a patent TIPS stent (*arrow*).

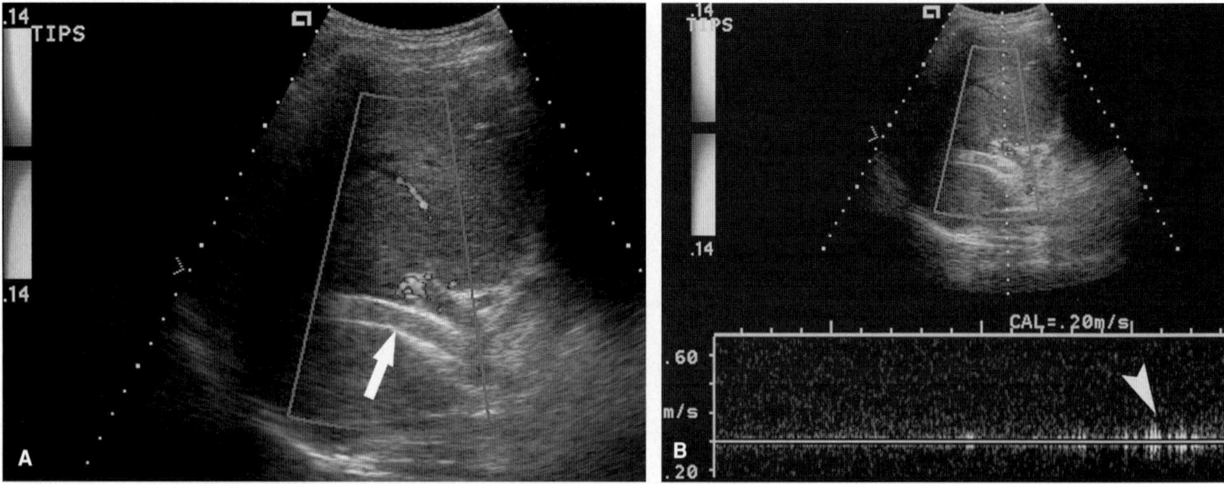

FIGURE 40.35. **(Color Plates) Transjugular Intrahepatic Portal Shunt (TIPS) Occlusion.** Color Doppler **(A)** and spectral Doppler **(B)** show an occluded TIPS shunt. Echogenic thrombus (*arrow*) is seen in the stent, with the absence of flow on color flow imaging. The pulsed wave Doppler shows artifact (*arrowhead*) but no flow.

profunda femoris and superficial femoral artery (SFA). The SFA travels along the anteromedial thigh, through the adductor (Hunter) canal, and becomes the popliteal artery. Below the knee, the popliteal artery branches into the anterior tibial artery and a short tibioperoneal trunk that quickly bifurcates into the peroneal and posterior tibial arteries. The anterior tibial artery descends anteriorly and terminates in the dorsalis pedis artery. The peroneal artery terminates above the ankle; the posterior tibial artery continues behind the medial malleolus, supplying the plantar surface of the foot. The normal Doppler waveform is a high-resistance, triphasic pattern. The first phase is the high velocity component during ventricular systole. PSV decreases from proximal to distal, averaging about 110 cm/s in the femoral artery and 70 cm/s in the popliteal artery. The second phase is postsystolic reversal of flow because of the increased resistance in the small distal vessels and capillary bed. The third phase is a small amount of forward flow in late diastole caused by elastic recoil of the vessel wall.

In the upper extremity, the right subclavian artery arises from the innominate artery, and the left subclavian artery originates from the aortic arch. Their origins can usually be identified from a supraclavicular approach. The subclavian arteries lie superficial to the veins. The distal subclavian artery is difficult to visualize because of the clavicle and is generally better imaged from an infraclavicular approach. The subclavian artery continues as the axillary artery, and the axillary artery becomes the brachial artery, which courses along the medial aspect of the arm. At the elbow, the brachial artery branches into the ulnar and radial arteries, which continue into the hand, forming the palmar arches. As in the leg, the Doppler waveforms are high resistance and triphasic. Peak systolic velocity is 110 cm/s in the proximal subclavian artery and decreases to about 85 cm/s in the axillary artery.

TABLE 40.10 Doppler Indicators of TIPS Malfunction (59,63)

Criteria	*Shunt Abnormal If:*
Shunt velocity	Peak <90 or ≥190 cm/s
Temporal shunt velocity change	Decrease or increase >50 cm/s
	Decrease >40 cm/s
	Increase >60 cm/s
Main portal vein velocity	Peak <30 cm/s
Collaterals	Recurrent, new, or increased
Ascites	Recurrent, new, or increased
Right/left portal vein flow	Hepatofugal to hepatopetal

TIPS, transjugular intrahepatic portosystemic shunt.

Arterial Puncture Complications

Pseudoaneurysm is a contained rupture of an artery wall with a persistent connection (neck) to the artery, resulting in a pulsatile mass (64–67). Most are seen in the common femoral artery as a complication of arterial catheterization. Other etiologies are surgery or trauma. The increased number of percutaneous interventions, use of large-bore catheters, longer indwelling catheter time, and routine postprocedure anticoagulation have increased the incidence of pseudoaneurysm to as high as 6%.

US reliably differentiates pseudoaneurysms from other groin masses. Grayscale imaging demonstrates a predominantly echolucent mass, sometimes multilocular, that may

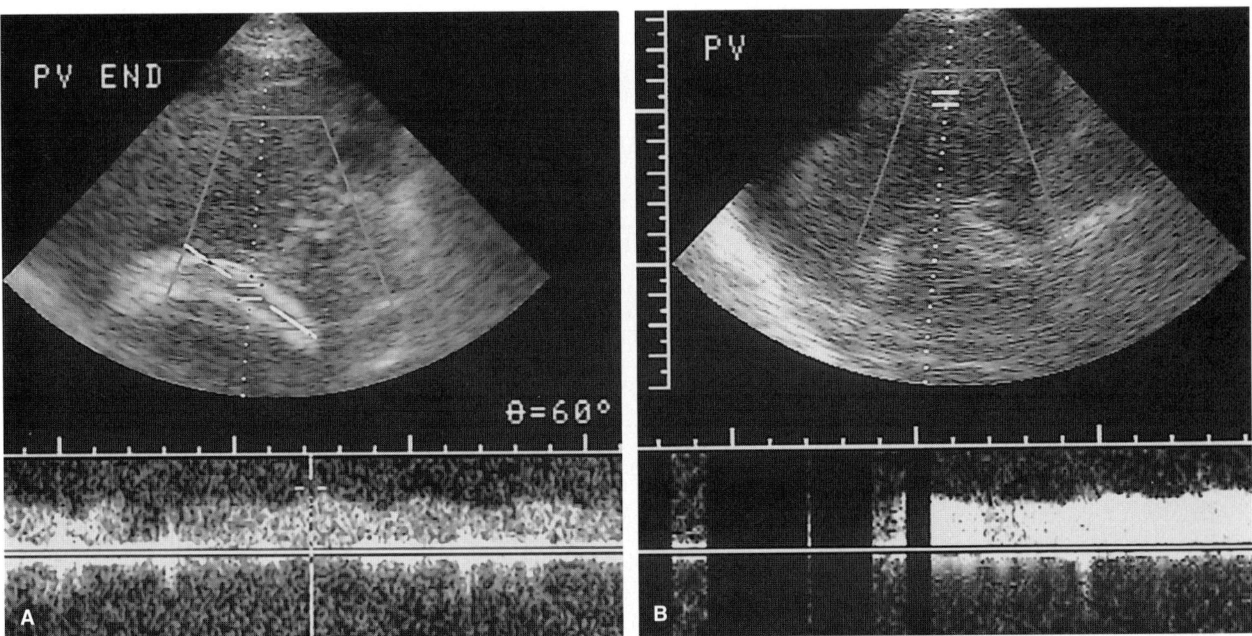

FIGURE 40.36. **Transjugular Intrahepatic Portal Shunt (TIPS) Malfunction.** On follow-up US, the same patient as seen in Fig. 40.34 shows a decreased velocity within the stent of 0.33 m/s **(A)** and hepatopetal flow (above the baseline) in the right portal vein **(B),** indicating shunt stenosis. The patient underwent successful shunt revision.

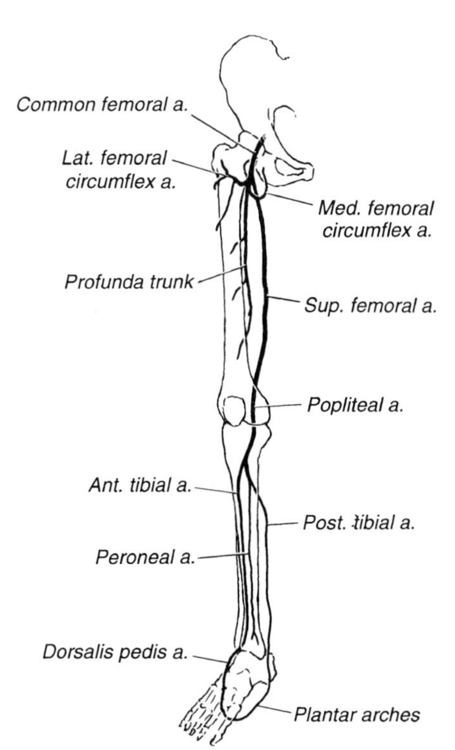

FIGURE 40.37. **Normal Lower Extremity Arterial Anatomy.**

contain internal echoes or mural thrombus. The mass is located immediately adjacent to the artery. Color Doppler demonstrates the connection to the artery and documents flow within the mass in the typical "yin-yang" pattern. Interrogation over the neck shows the characteristic "to and fro" spectral waveform (Figs. 40.38, 40.39).

US-guided compression is a safe, successful, and cost effective method of treating postcatheterization pseudoaneurysms. Pain, distal embolization, rupture and thrombosis of the femoral artery, deep venous thrombosis (DVT), and technical failures are potential complications. Pain medications and local anesthesia are given at the patient's request. Contraindications include infection, high puncture above the inguinal ligament, and large hematomas. A contraindication or technically inadequate compression occurs in about 10% to 15% of patients.

The neck of the pseudoaneurysm is compressed using direct pressure from the US transducer during color flow imaging. Enough pressure is applied to obliterate flow in the pseudoaneurysm while maintaining flow in the common femoral artery. Distal pulses are monitored. Compression is held for 20 to 30 minutes and then slowly released. If flow into the pseudoaneurysm is detected, compression is immediately resumed. This cycle is continued until no extraluminal flow is seen and the pseudoaneurysm is completely thrombosed (Fig. 40.38D). If operator or patient fatigue occurs (usually after 1 to 2 hours) before complete thrombosis is achieved, the process can be repeated the following day. The authors have had several cases of apparent

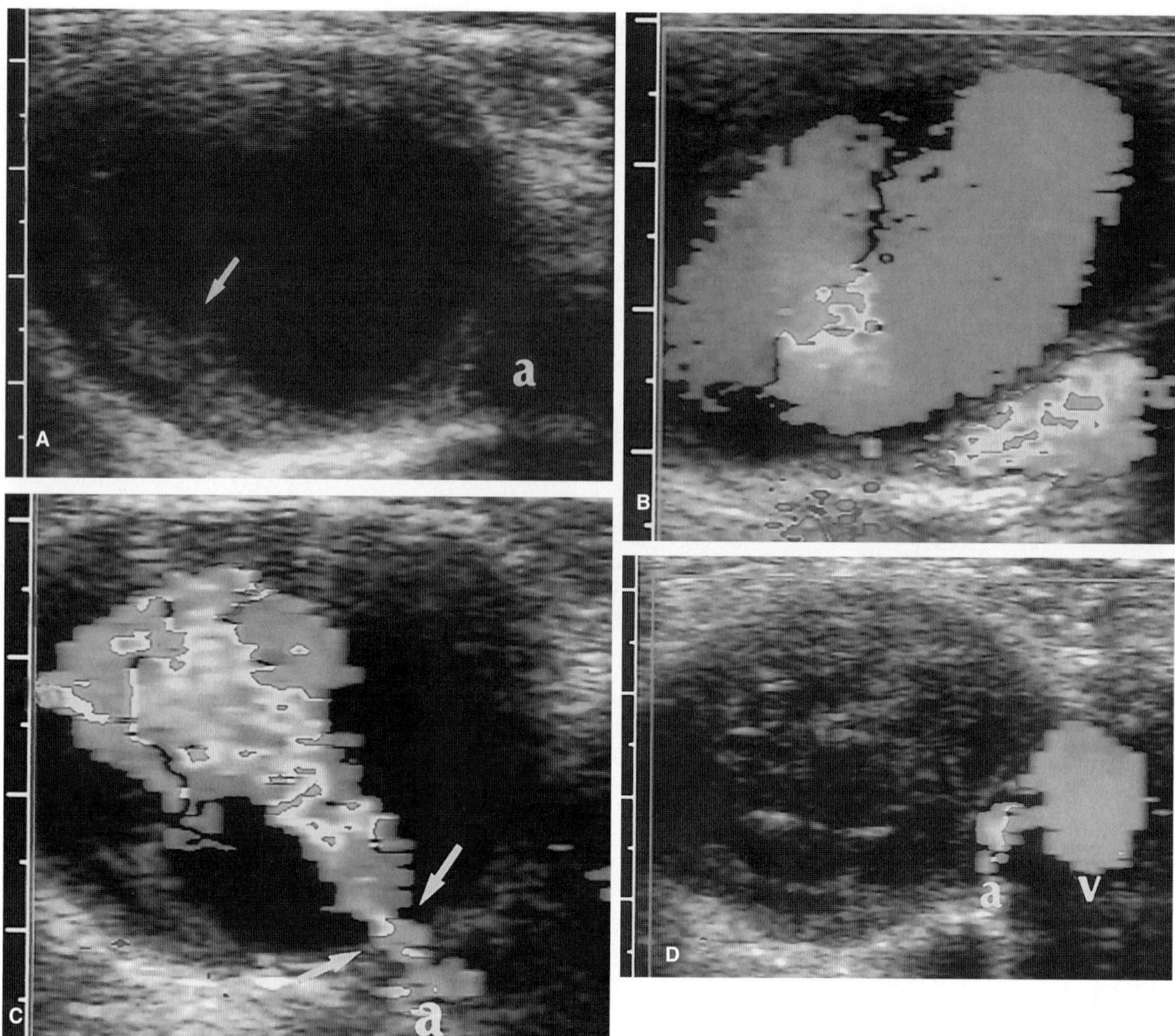

FIGURE 40.38. **(Color Plates) Pseudoaneurysm. A.** An echolucent mass with thrombus (*arrow*) is seen adjacent to the common femoral artery (a). **B.** Color Doppler image demonstrates the characteristic swirling or "yin-yang" flow. **C.** Transverse color Doppler image demonstrates the neck of the pseudoaneurysm with a "jet" (*arrows*) of blood flow into the mass. **D.** Following successful compression, no flow is seen within the thrombosed pseudoaneurysm. a, Common femoral artery; v, common femoral vein.

failure that on 24-hour follow-up reexamination had spontaneously thrombosed. In the rare circumstance of a recurrent pseudoaneurysm, recompression is almost always successful. Although the compression technique is usually performed in the groin, it can be successfully performed for pseudoaneurysms that have resulted from brachial or axillary artery procedures.

US-guided thrombin injection into the pseudoaneurysm has supplanted US compression as the treatment of choice in most institutions. It is much less time consuming and better tolerated by the patient. Color Doppler is used to guide the injection of 0.5 to 1.0 mL of thrombin (1,000 IU/mL) directly into the pseudoaneurysm cavity. Care is taken to avoid direct injection of the femoral artery or the neck of the pseudoaneurysm. Usually, complete thrombosis of the pseudoaneurysm occurs in 20 to 30 seconds. Occasionally, delayed thrombosis spontaneously occurs or a second injection is required.

Properly performed, technical success of those pseudoaneurysms that are amenable to compression approaches 80% to 90%. These figures exclude those that are not compressible for technical reasons or patient discomfort. Anticoagulation decreases the success rate, but compression is still successful in about two thirds of patients. Success rates for thrombin injection range from 92% to 100%, including those on anticoagulation therapy. The complication rate for thrombin injection is remarkably low. A 2% reperfusion of the pseudoaneurysm occurs,

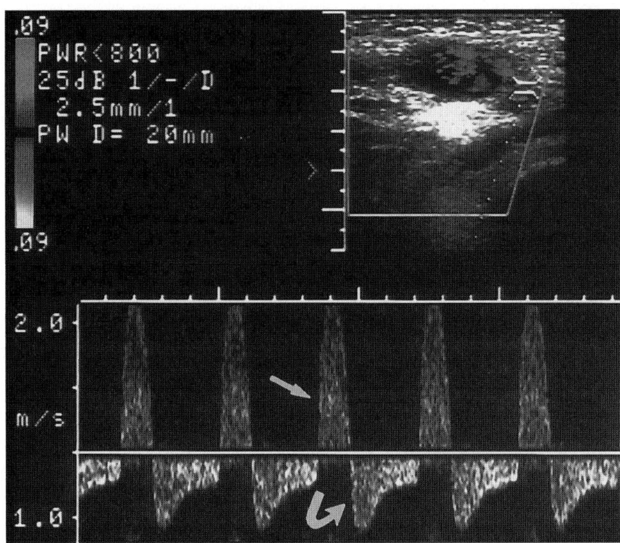

FIGURE 40.39. **(Color Plates) Pseudoaneurysm.** Spectral Doppler tracing over the neck of a pseudoaneurysm showing the characteristic "to and fro" waveform. During systole, blood flows into the pseudoaneurysm (*arrow*), and during diastole (*curved arrow*), blood flows out of the pseudoaneurysm.

but nearly all recurrences respond to a reinjection. Thromboembolic events are reported in 0.8% of cases. Fever, presumably brought on by allergic reaction, occasionally occurs. Some patients (41%) report groin pain following the procedure, ranging from slight to severe, at 1 week postprocedure.

The relative ease of performance, short procedure time, success rate in patients on anticoagulation therapy, and low complication rate have made thrombin injection the procedure of choice for the treatment of femoral artery and amenable brachial artery pseudoaneurysms.

Arteriovenous fistulas (AVFs) generally result from simultaneous puncture of the artery and vein. Less common than pseudoaneurysms, AVFs are often small and resolve spontaneously. In a large AVF, the feeding artery has a low-resistance waveform with increased diastolic flow, which is atypical for an extremity artery. The draining vein is distended and demonstrates high-velocity pulsatile flow. These characteristic findings are usually only present within several centimeters of the fistula (Fig. 40.40). Spectral Doppler waveforms are obtained in the artery and vein just above and just below the suspected site of the fistula. With a small AVF, duplex imaging may be normal. Color flow imaging guides the placement of the Doppler gate. Color Doppler shows a heterogeneous and markedly disorganized color pattern overlying the fistula caused by soft tissue vibration. This appearance is sometimes called a *color Doppler bruit.* With appropriate technical adjustments, the fistulous tract can often be seen (64,65).

Hematoma. Perivascular masses immediately following arterial puncture are most commonly hematomas. Sonographically, hematomas range from anechoic to hypoechoic with a complex echo pattern. No internal flow can be demonstrated. Hematomas cannot be distinguished from thrombosed pseudoaneurysms, seromas, or abscesses.

Aneurysm

The popliteal arteries are the most common site of aneurysm in the peripheral vascular system. The popliteal artery is considered aneurysmal when it measures >2 cm. Unlike aneurysms in the abdominal aorta, popliteal aneurysms are unlikely to rupture. Mural thrombus within the aneurysms may cause distal embolization and potential limb loss. No good surgical size criteria exist for aneurysms in the peripheral arterial system. Surgery is performed on any aneurysm that is the source of distal embolization and is considered for aneurysms >2 cm.

Stenosis and Occlusion

In most circumstances, the diagnosis of significant peripheral arterial occlusive disease is made on clinical grounds based on the symptom of claudication and findings of a physical exam. Noninvasive testing is used primarily to confirm the clinical suspicion prior to angiography. The primary noninvasive techniques include continuous wave Doppler, plethysmography, the ankle-brachial index (ABI), segmental pressure measurements, and pulse volume recordings. Discussion of these modalities is beyond the scope of this chapter. Evaluation with duplex US (65,68,69) continues to evolve for the diagnosis of peripheral vascular stenosis in the native arterial system. It remains complementary to the clinical evaluation but may have a role in selecting patients for percutaneous intervention rather than surgery. Vascular surgeons typically require either catheter, CT, or MR angiography for an arterial road map preoperatively. In addition, definitive treatments—angioplasty or stent placement—can often be performed at the time of the diagnostic study.

Peripheral arterial mapping is performed with a linear 5- to 7.5-MHz transducer. Grayscale imaging locates the vessels and evaluates plaque. Color Doppler mapping decreases the imaging time by identifying areas of narrowing and turbulent flow, where spectral tracings are then obtained.

The previously described waveform changes that occur before, at, and after a stenosis apply in the peripheral arterial system. Proximal to a significant stenosis, the waveform may be normal or demonstrate a monophasic waveform, decreased PSV, and no diastolic flow. A high-velocity jet is usually at (or just after) the stenosis. Distal to a significant stenosis, the parvus-tardus waveform may be seen. The waveforms can be markedly different for the same

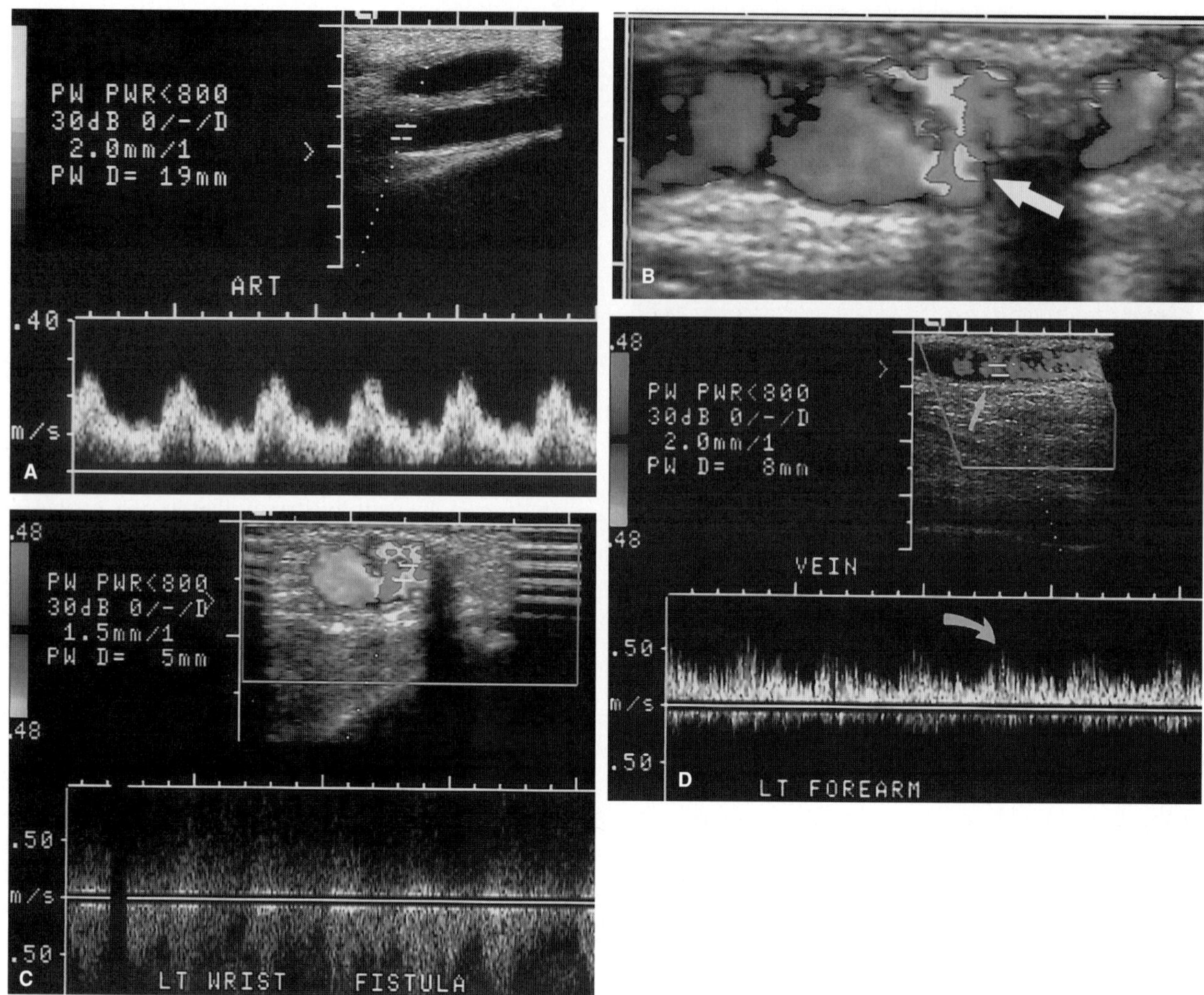

FIGURE 40.40. **(Color Plates) Arteriovenous Fistula in the Left Wrist. A.** The feeding artery demonstrates a low-resistance waveform, which is uncharacteristic of an extremity artery. **B.** Color Doppler image demonstrates the typical heterogeneous, turbulent flow pattern (*arrow*) at the level of the fistula. **C.** Pulsed wave Doppler tracing showing a pulsatile, turbulent (spectral broadening) waveform with bidirectional flow at the level of the fistula. **D.** The draining vein is dilated (*arrow*) and exhibits a pulsatile (arterialized) waveform (*curved arrow*).

degree of stenosis in different individuals. This difference is influenced by blood inflow, runoff, collateral flow, and medications.

Because of the wide range of normal velocities, the PSV has not been reliable in grading stenosis. Instead, *velocity ratios* are more predictive. The high velocity in the stenosis is divided by the "normal" velocity proximal to the stenosis. Although the numbers vary among investigators, the percent stenosis using velocity ratios can be estimated using the values shown in Table 40.7. A severe or hemodynamically significant stenosis (decreased blood pressure and blood flow across the lesion) in the peripheral system represents a >50% diameter stenosis. The PSV is doubled and the waveform is monophasic. Properly performed, sensitivities for detecting stenoses in the femoral-popliteal arteries are 85% to 90%.

Duplex US has a sensitivity above 90% in diagnosing occlusion in the lower extremity. Most errors in diagnosis are technical; most commonly, "trickle" flow is overlooked.

Graft Surveillance

In contrast to native vessels, sonography has established itself as the noninvasive modality of choice in monitoring peripheral bypass grafts (65,68,70).

Synthetic Grafts. Dacron (polyester fiber) grafts typically give a corrugated appearance, whereas PTFE grafts

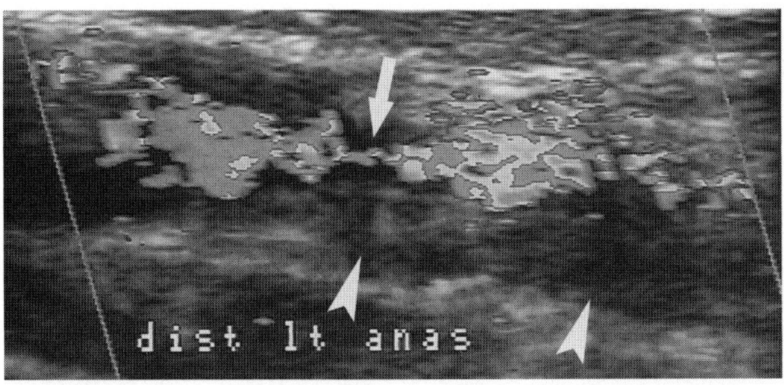

FIGURE 40.41. **(Color Plates) Synthetic Graft Anastomotic Stenosis.** Longitudinal color Doppler image at the left distal anastomosis of an aorto-bi-iliac graft. Predominantly homogeneous fibrointimal hyperplasia (*arrowheads*) and a significant stenosis (*arrow*) are evident. The velocity proximal to the graft is ~0.53 m/s and at the anastomosis it is 1.80 m/s. According to Table 40.7, this represents about a 75% diameter stenosis (confirmed angiographically).

typically show two parallel echogenic lines. Synthetic grafts are rarely used for grafting below the knee. Graft failure is usually a result of a complication at the anastomotic connections to the native artery (Fig. 40.41), such as stenosis or pseudoaneurysm. Anastomotic pseudoaneurysms may not have the typical appearance described previously in this chapter, because the communication between the pseudoaneurysm and the bypass graft anastomosis is almost always larger than those acquired following arterial puncture. Occasionally, a patulous anastomosis can mimic a pseudoaneurysm (Fig. 40.42). Such complications typically occur within the first 2 years following surgery. Progressive disease in the native arteries causes failure because of poor inflow or outflow. Fibrointimal hyperplasia within the graft lumen is a late complication, usually occurring 5 to 10 years after surgery. No good data exist using velocity criteria for evaluation of synthetic graft failure, but velocity ratios are commonly used.

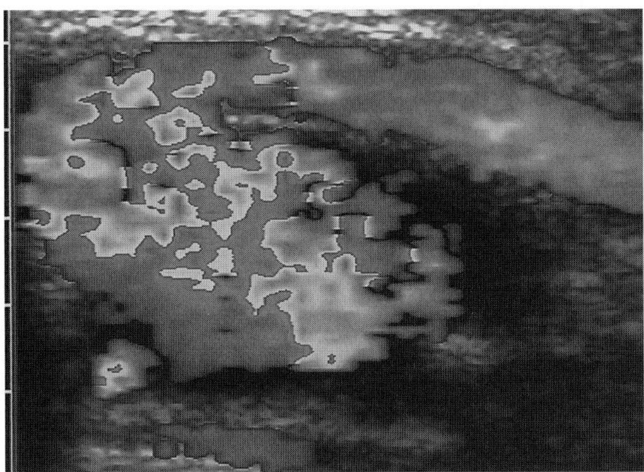

FIGURE 40.42. **(Color Plates) Graft Anastomosis.** Color Doppler image shows heterogeneous flow pattern at a patulous proximal femoral-popliteal graft anastomosis. A graft anastomotic pseudoaneurysm has a similar appearance.

Autologous Vein Grafts. Two techniques are typically performed. The most common is the reversed saphenous vein graft; the second is the in situ graft. In the former, the vein is removed from its normal location, reversed, and anastomosed to the proximal and distal artery. For the in situ graft, only the proximal and distal ends of the saphenous vein are mobilized and anastomosed to the proximal and distal artery. In this type of graft, the venous valves are lysed to allow flow down the extremity. Duplex graft surveillance and early intervention result in a 5-year graft patency rate of 82% to 93%. Without surveillance, only a 60% to 85% patency rate is expected. Graft surveillance is recommended every 2 to 3 months during the first postoperative year and every 6 to 12 months in subsequent years.

During the first month following surgery, Doppler is used to assess the technical success of the operation. Perivascular fluid collections, anastomotic failure, poor vein selection, AVF, and residual valves are detected. Most important, Doppler confirms patency of the graft.

Between 1 month and 2 years following surgery, intimal hyperplasia causes a focal stenosis in about 20% of patients. The hyperplasia usually occurs at the site of venous valves. Grayscale and color flow are used to identify areas of potential stenosis. The velocity obtained at the suspected stenosis is divided by the velocity in the graft 2 to 4 cm more proximal. A doubling of velocity at the stenosis is considered to be a 50% diameter or significant stenosis. This roughly corresponds to a PSV of 180 cm/s. The protocol is slightly modified at the anastomoses: the velocity at the proximal anastomosis is divided by the velocity 4 to 6 cm distally into the graft. At the distal anastomosis, the velocity is divided by the velocity in the native artery in a "normal" segment distal to the graft. It is not uncommon for the velocity ratio at the distal anastomosis to be 2, because the distal native arteries are usually smaller than the graft. A velocity in the graft <45 cm/s usually indicates impending graft failure. This protocol has proven more sensitive to early graft abnormalities than clinical symptoms or ABI measurements. The reported accuracy approaches 95%, but Doppler tends to overestimate the stenosis. Intervention is generally considered for a stenotic lesion when the velocity triples (Figs. 40.43, 40.44 and Table 40.11).

Graft failures later than 2 years after surgery are usually caused by progression of native atherosclerotic vascular disease.

Dialysis Grafts. Dialysis grafts are typically inserted into the forearm with a side-to-side, end-to-side, or loop anastomosis. They can be either synthetic or autologous vein. The primary indication for Doppler evaluation is patency. Complications include anastomotic pseudoaneurysms, aneurysms, or stenoses. Accuracy of Doppler US for the detection of stenosis approaches 90%.

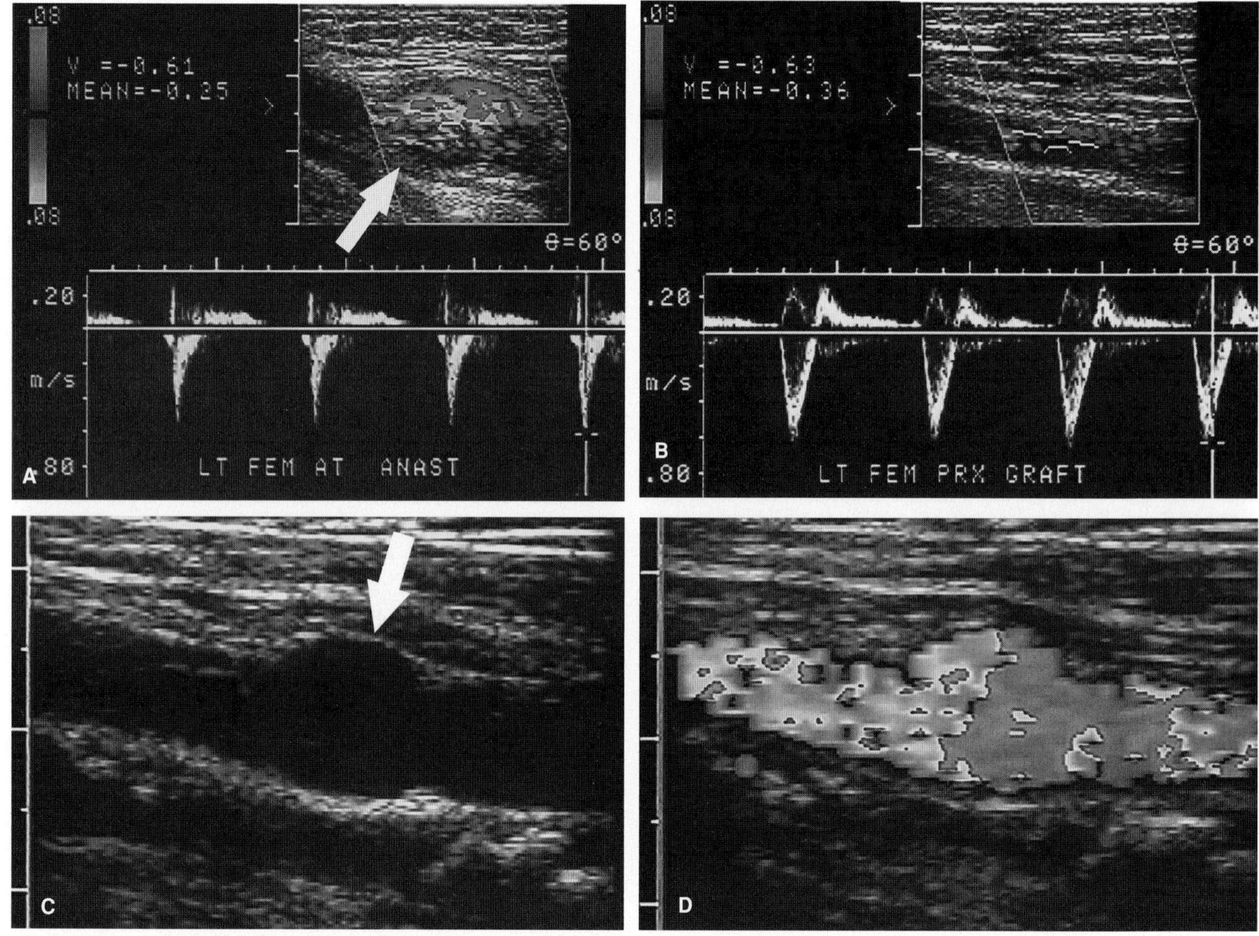

FIGURE 40.43. **(Color Plates) Reversed Saphenous Vein Graft. A.** Spectral Doppler tracing at the proximal anastomosis of a left femoral-popliteal vein graft has a velocity of 0.61 m/s. Mild aneurysmal dilatation and heterogeneous flow (*arrow*) are not uncommon. **B.** Velocity obtained 4 to 6 cm into the graft is nearly identical (0.63 m/s), indicating no significant anastomotic stenosis. **C.** Mild saccular dilatation within the graft (*arrow*) corresponds to the location of a saphenous vein valve. **D.** Longitudinal color Doppler image confirms patency at the valve. Stenoses most commonly occur at the location of the valves.

VENOUS ULTRASOUND

Lower Extremity

Duplex US is clearly recognized as the diagnostic modality of choice for the evaluation of lower extremity swelling for DVT (71–73). Cronan et al pooled data from multiple studies and demonstrated a sensitivity of 95% and a specificity of 98%. Other modalities, such as MR venography and contrast venography, are reserved for instances when duplex is nondiagnostic, pelvic or IVC clot is suspected, or if calf clot will be treated. CT venography is performed in conjunction with CT pulmonary angiography in some institutions.

Anatomy. The deep venous system of the lower extremity consists of veins that parallel the arteries both anatomically and in name (Fig. 40.45). In the calf, the anterior tibial, posterior tibial, and peroneal veins converge just below the knee to form the popliteal vein. The popliteal vein continues into the thigh through the adductor canal as the superficial femoral vein (SFV). Near the groin, the profunda femoris vein joins the SFV to form the common femoral vein (CFV). The popliteal vein and SFV are partially or completely duplicated about 25% of the time. The calf veins have many normal variations. We tend to use the term *femoral vein* in lieu of *superficial femoral vein* to avoid confusion with the superficial venous system. Thrombus within the SFV is considered DVT and is a risk factor for pulmonary embolus.

The greater and lesser saphenous veins comprise the superficial venous system of the lower extremity (Fig. 40.45). The greater saphenous vein (GSV) originates on the medial side of the ankle, ascends anteromedially along the thigh, and empties into the CFV at the inguinal ligament.

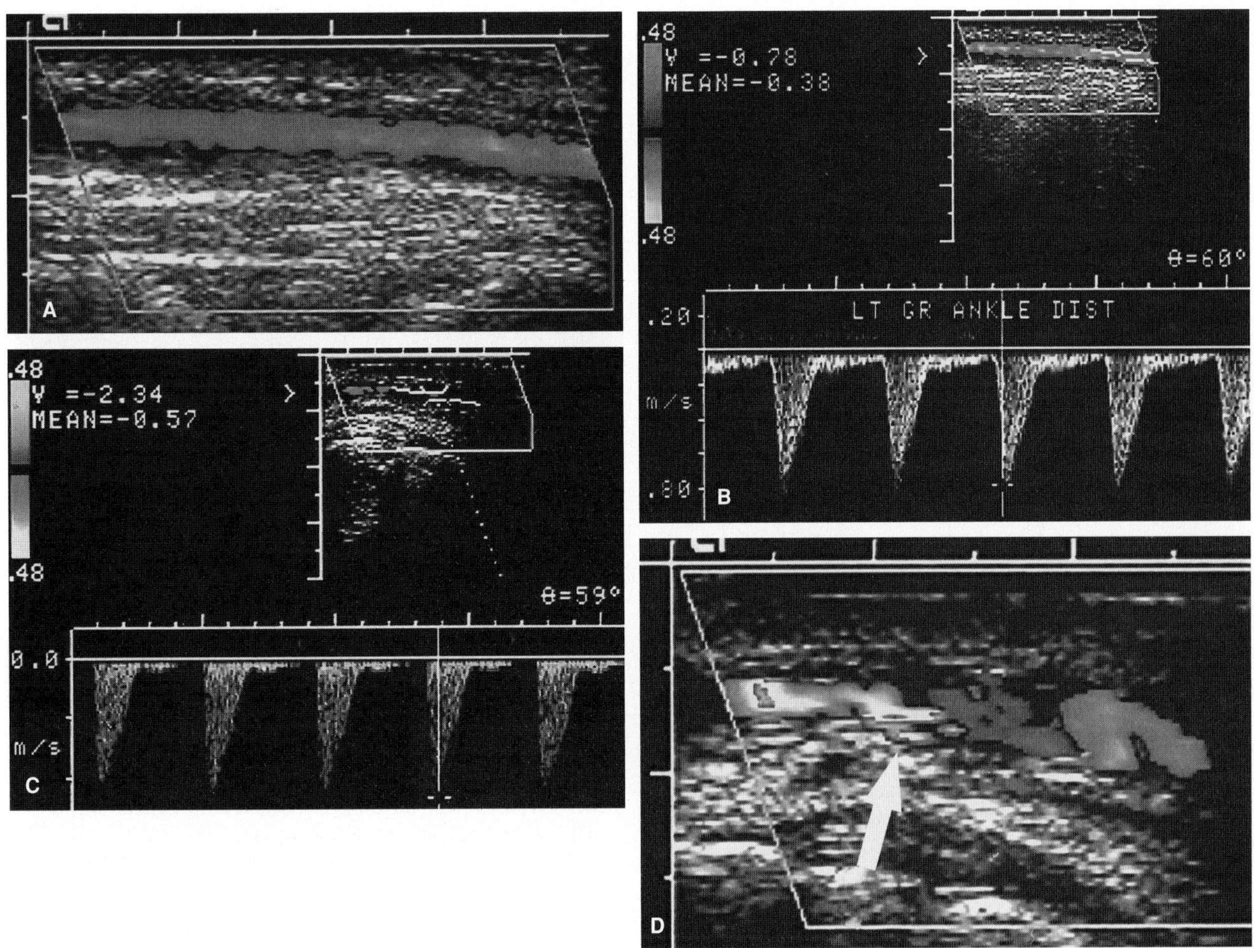

FIGURE 40.44. **(Color Plates) Popliteal to Plantar Artery Vein Graft Stenosis.** Color Doppler US **(A)** and spectral tracing **(B)** within the vein graft demonstrate homogenous color flow (*red*) and a velocity of 0.78 m/s. More distally within the graft the velocity has increased to 2.34 m/sec **(C)** and heterogeneous, turbulent flow (*arrow*) is noted on color Doppler **(D).** According to Table 40.7, this tripling of the velocity corresponds to approximately a 75% stenosis. This patient had a nonhealing foot ulcer that responded to surgical revascularization.

The lesser saphenous vein (LSV) originates laterally at the ankle and ascends posteriorly along the calf. It usually empties into the popliteal vein or, rarely, into the profunda femoris or GSV. Small perforating veins containing valves connect the superficial to the deep system in the calf and lower thigh. Flow is directed from the superficial system to the deep system.

TABLE 40.11 Principles of Vein Graft Surveillance

Color Doppler entire graft to identify significant flow abnormalities
Interrogate suspicious areas with pulsed Doppler

- PSV >180 cm/s indicates ~50% stenosis
- Velocity ratio >2 indicates ~50% stenosis

Flow rate <45 cm/s suggests impending graft failure
Marked velocity changes on serial examinations suggest stenosis
Waveform change from triphasic to monophasic is consistent with either proximal or distal stenosis

PSV, peak systolic velocity.

The CFV ascends medial to the artery into the pelvis and becomes the external iliac vein. The internal iliac vein joins the external iliac vein to become the common iliac vein over the sacrum. The common iliac veins join to form the IVC.

Technique. The deep veins of the lower extremity are examined from the inguinal ligament (junction of the GSV with the CFV) through the popliteal fossa. Examination of the CFV/SFV is performed in the supine position with a linear 5- to 7.5-MHz transducer in a slight reverse Trendelenburg position. In the transverse plane, compression and release of the veins are performed every 1 cm to the popliteal fossa. Behind the knee, the popliteal vein is examined in a similar fashion, with the patient prone and knee flexed 15°. If a thrombus is present, longitudinal views are

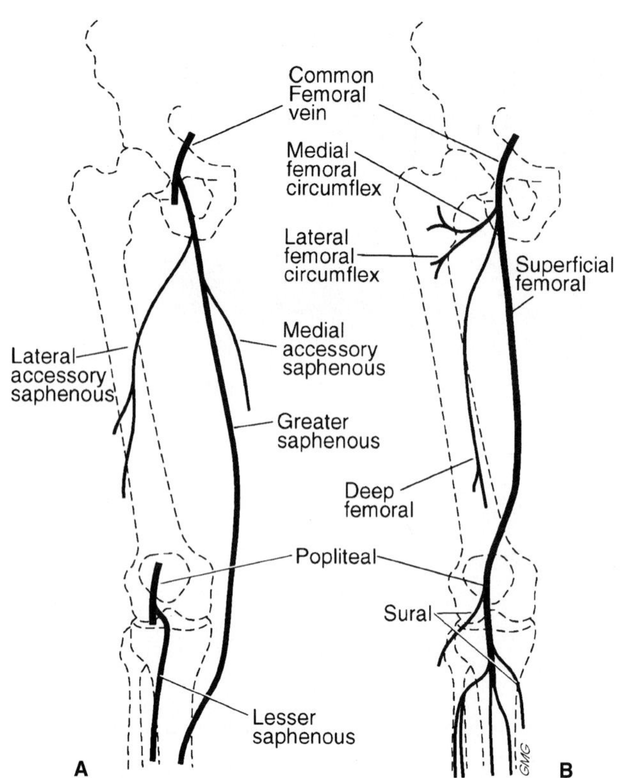

FIGURE 40.45. **Lower Extremity Venous Anatomy. A.** Superficial system. **B.** Deep system.

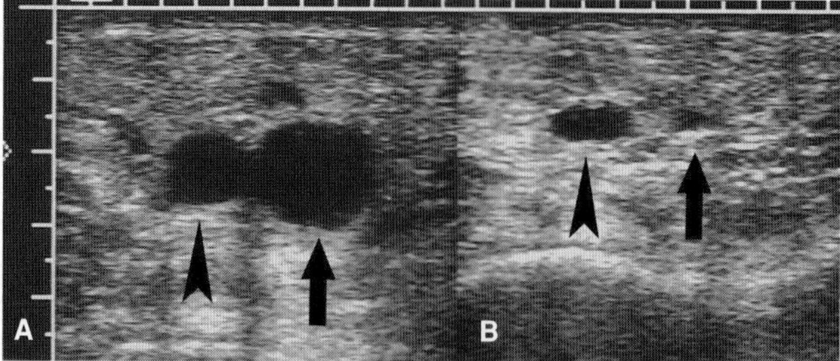

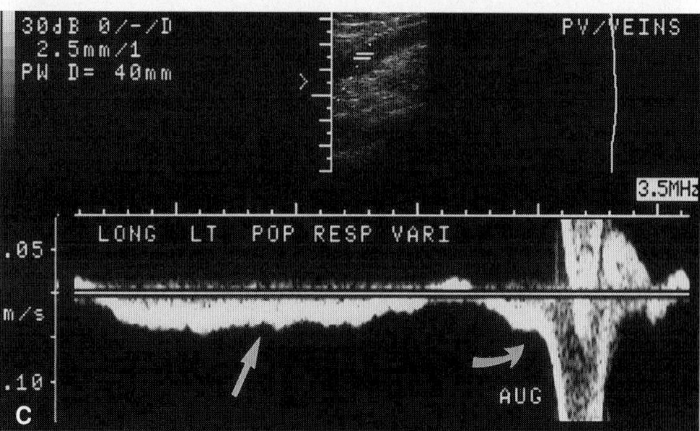

FIGURE 40.46. **Normal Venous Compressibility, Respiratory Phasicity, and Augmentation. A.** Transverse grayscale imaging demonstrates the normal common femoral artery (*arrowhead*) and vein (*arrow*). **B.** With compression, the normal vein (*arrow*) is obliterated and the arterial lumen (*arrowhead*) persists. Enough compression has been applied to deform the arterial lumen (making it more oval) but not obliterate it. **C.** Spectral Doppler shows the normal respiratory phasicity (*arrow*) and augmentation from squeezing the calf (*curved arrow*) in the normal popliteal vein.

performed to determine its extent. Doppler interrogation demonstrates respiratory phasicity, and augmentation of flow is created by squeezing the calf or having the patient plantar flex the foot (Fig. 40.46). Color Doppler evaluation confirms vein patency and unidirectional flow and is particularly useful in challenging areas or in patients who are difficult to examine (e.g., the adductor canal and obese patents). The increased sensitivity of power Doppler occasionally augments the color Doppler examination.

Because of the many anatomic variations and duplications of the calf veins, duplex US is time consuming and probably does not have the diagnostic accuracy needed to exclude a small thrombus. Most clinicians do not anticoagulate an isolated calf DVT because they are not a cause of pulmonary emboli and often spontaneously resolve. For these reasons, we do not routinely perform duplex US of the calf veins. Up to 20% of calf vein DVTs propagate to the popliteal or SFV. Serial evaluation every 3 to 5 days is therefore important in patients who remain symptomatic with conservative therapy to diagnose clot propagation and prevent pulmonary embolus.

Deep Venous Thrombosis. Risk factors for developing DVT include prolonged immobilization, age, pregnancy, oral contraceptives, surgery, trauma, myocardial infarction, congestive heart failure, malignancy, polycythemia, prior DVT, or any other hypercoagulable state. The clinical presentation and physical exam findings are unreliable in making the diagnosis. Differential diagnoses include Baker cyst; cellulitis; popliteal artery aneurysm; edema from multiple causes (congestive heart failure, lymphatic, renal failure, etc.); chronic venous insufficiency; extrinsic venous compression; superficial thrombophlebitis; and hematomas. The importance of making the diagnosis cannot be underestimated, since 90% of pulmonary emboli arise in the lower extremities and untreated DVT results in pulmonary embolus in up to 50% of cases.

The most accurate US criterion for the diagnosis of DVT is loss of compressibility of the vein. The veins of the deep venous system are generally easily compressible with light pressure. The maximum pressure required to obliterate a normal vein in any patient is less than that required to deform the shape of the adjacent artery. Other findings include distension of the vein and visualization of intraluminal thrombus (Fig. 40.47). Because a significant number of clots are isoechoic to flowing blood, the latter

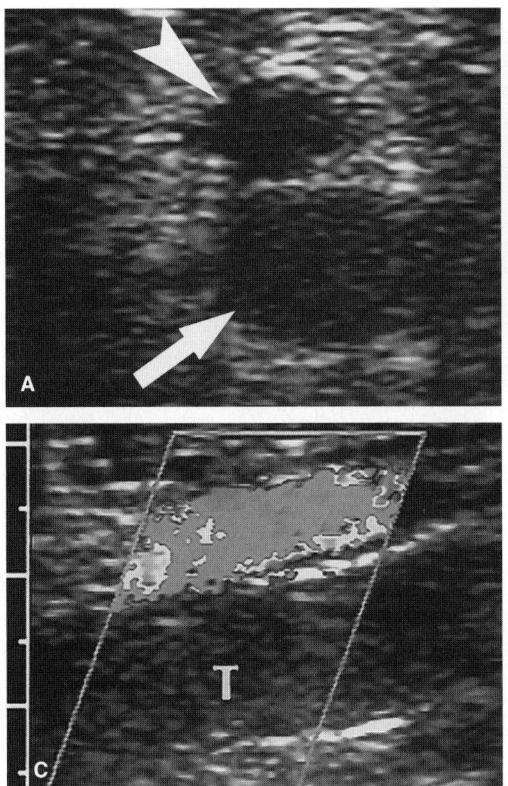

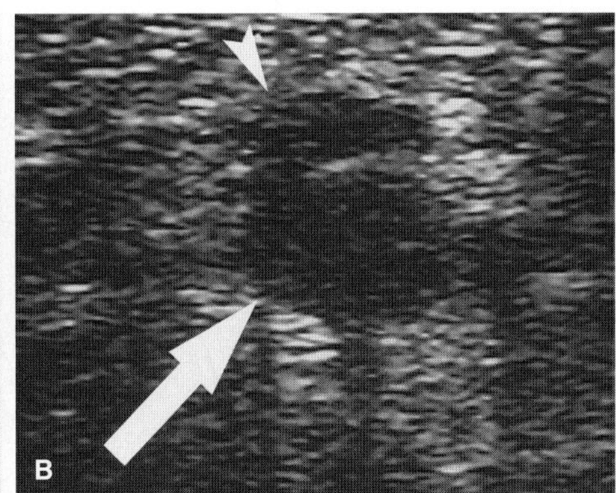

FIGURE 40.47. **(Color Plates) Deep Venous Thrombosis.** Transverse images without **(A)** and with **(B)** compression demonstrate a noncompressible, distended superficial femoral vein (*arrow*) diagnostic of a DVT. Note that enough pressure has been applied to deform the artery (*arrowhead*) when compared to the adjacent image without compression. **C.** Longitudinal color Doppler image of the superficial femoral vein demonstrates echogenic thrombus (T) and no color flow. Flow is present in the superficial femoral artery anteriorly.

finding is less reliable. Color Doppler demonstrates an intraluminal defect or color void. Several studies have shown that color Doppler imaging may be as accurate as compression US. Spectral Doppler exhibits a lack of augmentation of signal when the clot is between the point of interrogation and the foot. Doppler may also show a loss of respiratory phasicity caudad to the clot. If the respiratory phasicity is lost in the CFV, an iliac vein or IVC clot should be suspected. Loss of augmentation of signal in the CFV with release of Valsalva is also suggestive of a more cephalad obstruction. A complete evaluation utilizes all the above techniques.

It is important to realize the limitations of US diagnosis. The iliac and pelvic veins are not adequately evaluated in most patients. Obesity and severe edema can cause technically inadequate examinations. The adductor canal can be difficult to visualize, even in thin patients. The saphenous vein or collaterals can be mistaken for the SFV. Duplications of the deep venous system can lead to diagnostic error, particularly if one system is clotted and the other is patent. Extrinsic venous compression by nodes or tumor can cause loss of respiratory phasicity and augmentation.

The distinction between ***acute*** and ***chronic*** DVT is difficult on all imaging modalities, including contrast venography. Six months following a DVT, 50% of patients have persistent abnormalities on US. Typically, chronic clot does not expand the lumen of the vein and appears more echogenic than an acute clot. Echogenic strands are often noted in the lumen. The walls of the vein also appear thickened, irregular, and echogenic, and the vein is incompletely compressible (Fig. 40.48). Color Doppler often demonstrates collateral vessels. The authors obtain a baseline duplex US just prior to discontinuing anticoagulation therapy to help distinguish acute versus chronic changes in the future. Otherwise, with recurrent symptoms, a chronic DVT may be inadvertently diagnosed as an acute or recurrent DVT, subjecting the patient to lifelong anticoagulation therapy. If a clot appears chronic and unchanged from baseline, an interval follow-up US in 2 to 3 days is performed to assess for change. Superimposition of acute clot on chronic changes remains a difficult US diagnosis. Venography may be required.

Chronic venous insufficiency occurs in approximately 40% of individuals following an episode of acute DVT (74). However, the majority of patients with venous insufficiency have incompetent valves, unrelated to DVT. Venous insufficiency results when the lower-extremity venous valves are destroyed or become incompetent. It is very common and is estimated to affect 25% of women and 15% of men. Color Doppler or spectral Doppler detects valvular insufficiency by demonstrating flow reversal from the deep venous system to the superficial venous system for >1

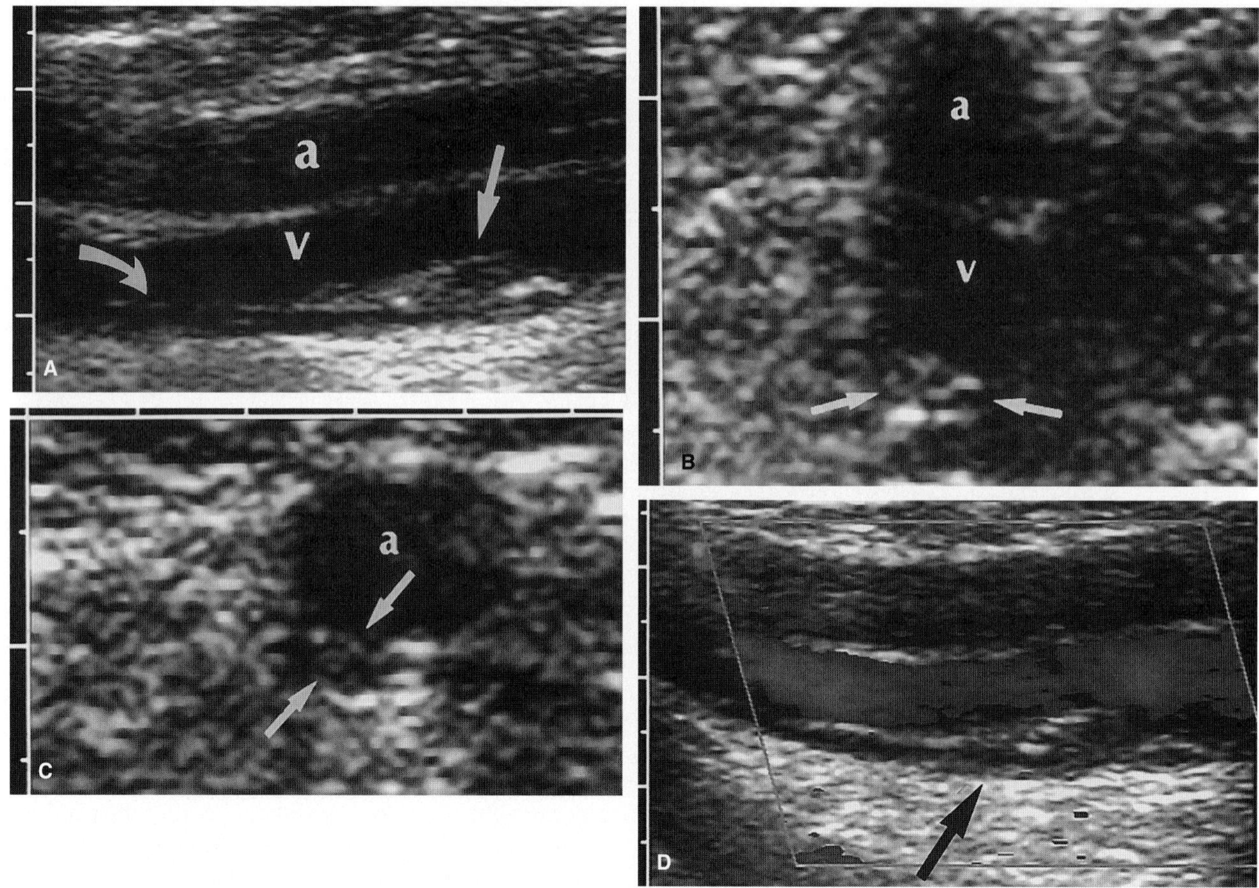

FIGURE 40.48. (Color Plates) Chronic Deep Venous Thrombosis. A. Longitudinal image of the right superficial femoral vein (SFV) (v) and the superficial femoral artery (SFA) (a) in a patient with a prior DVT. The wall of the vein appears thickened and irregular, with areas of increased echogenicity (*arrow*). An echogenic strand is seen within the lumen (*curved arrow*). **B.** Transverse image through the SFV without compression shows the thickened, irregular wall inferiorly (*arrow*). The vein is not distended. **C.** Transverse image shows complete compression except for the thickened wall (*arrows*). **D.** Longitudinal color Doppler image confirms the grayscale findings (*arrow*), showing patency of the residual lumen (*blue*). Serial examinations were unchanged.

second during Valsalva or augmentation. This technique is easily performed in both the supine and upright positions. Interrogation is performed in the GSV just before it enters the CFV and in the LSV just prior to joining the popliteal vein (Fig. 40.49). Compression of the thigh muscle while interrogating the venous system more distally demonstrates reversed flow or augmentation (valvular incompetence). Both the deep system cephalad to the popliteal vein and the saphenous system can be evaluated with this technique. Reversal of flow from the deep to the superficial system through the perforating veins can often be documented. Many variations of thigh and calf compression techniques are reported in the literature.

Vein mapping using duplex US is a valuable adjunct to the vascular surgeon in preoperative evaluation for autologous vein grafts. The GSV is most commonly used for vein grafts, but any vein can be used as long as the diameter is >3 mm without varicosities. The course of the vein is marked with a permanent marker, and all branch points are labeled. The exam is time consuming, and it is important to communicate with the vascular surgeon to make certain the desired veins are mapped and adequate for the procedure planned.

Upper Extremity

Although not as well studied, duplex US has become a useful screening modality for the venous evaluation of the upper extremity, particularly for DVT and symptoms suggestive of thoracic outlet syndrome (75,76).

Anatomy. The superficial venous system is the primary drainage pathway for the upper extremity. The basilic vein courses along the ulnar side of the forearm and medial upper arm and continues as the axillary vein. The cephalic

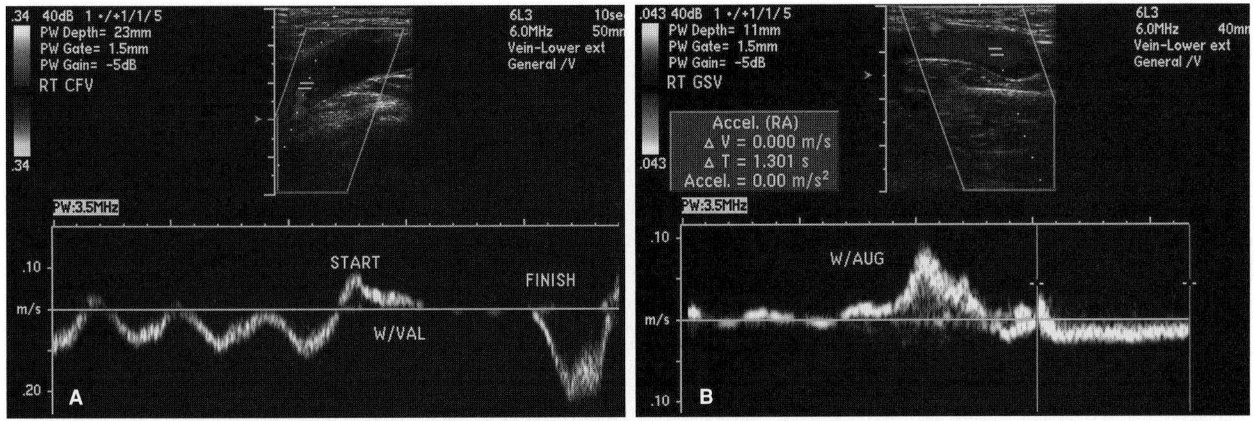

FIGURE 40.49. **(Color Plates) Venous Insufficiency. A.** Normal. Duplex imaging in the common femoral vein (CFV) near its junction with the greater saphenous vein (GSV). The patient performs a Valsalva maneuver (start). No flow is noted during Valsalva. The patient breathes (finish), and "augmented" flow is noted toward the heart (normal). No reversed flow (reflux) is noted. **B.** Reflux. Duplex interrogation in the GSV just prior to joining the CFV. Calf augmentation is performed. Note the flow toward the feet (reversed) in the GSV for >1 second following augmentation (flow below baseline between cursors). Courtesy of Robert A. Jesinger, M.D., and David Grant United States Air Force Medical Center, Travis Air Force Base, California.

vein ascends on the radial aspect of the forearm and continues laterally to the shoulder. The cephalic vein joins the axillary vein just below the clavicle. The axillary vein continues as the subclavian vein at the lateral border of the first rib (Fig. 40.50). After it receives the internal jugular vein, it continues as the brachiocephalic vein to the superior vena cava. The deep system consists of small, paired brachial veins that course with the artery and empty into the basilic vein.

Technique. A complete evaluation of the upper extremity includes the bilateral evaluation of the axillary, subclavian, and internal jugular veins. The same technique used

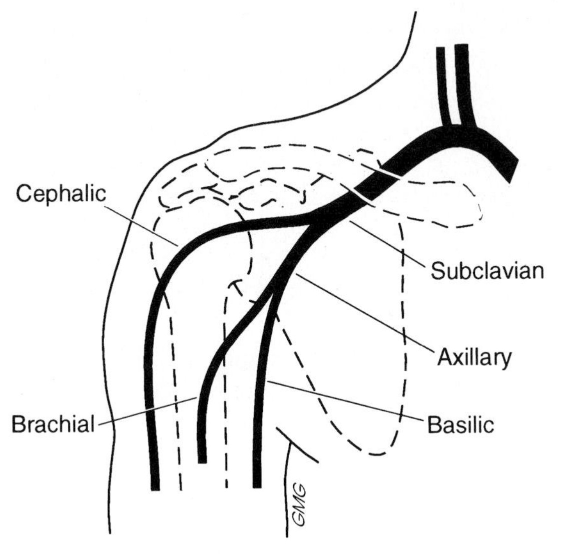

FIGURE 40.50. **Upper Extremity Venous Anatomy.**

for the lower extremity can be applied in the upper extremity above the elbow. Evaluation of the central veins, especially the subclavian, is limited because the overlying clavicle restricts visualization; thus the compression technique cannot be used. Color Doppler is the mainstay of evaluation of the central veins.

In lieu of compression, the "sniff" test is useful in the subclavian vein. With sniffing, the diameter of the subclavian vein will decrease and often completely collapse. With Valsalva, the vein will increase in diameter. These maneuvers are performed bilaterally and the response compared.

Duplex evaluation of venous waveforms reveals normal respiratory phasicity and transmitted cardiac pulsations (Fig. 40.51) in the central veins. The greater the distance from the thoracic inlet, the more monophasic the waveform will be. Loss of the normal pulsatility (monophasic waveform) centrally when compared to the contralateral side suggests a proximal central obstruction (Fig. 40.50).

Deep Venous Thrombosis. Upper-extremity DVT is usually the result of a current or previous indwelling catheter. A coexistent ipsilateral internal jugular vein clot is often present (Fig. 40.52). Venous stasis in the upper extremity caused by extrinsic compression or thoracic outlet syndrome is less common. In contrast to the lower extremity, upper extremity DVT is associated with pulmonary embolism in only 12% of cases. The diagnosis of DVT employs the same principles as for the lower extremity, in addition to the techniques described in the previous paragraphs (Fig. 40.53). Although no large studies have compared duplex US to contrast venography, most consider US as the initial imaging modality. Contrast venography, CT venography, and MR venography are reserved for patients

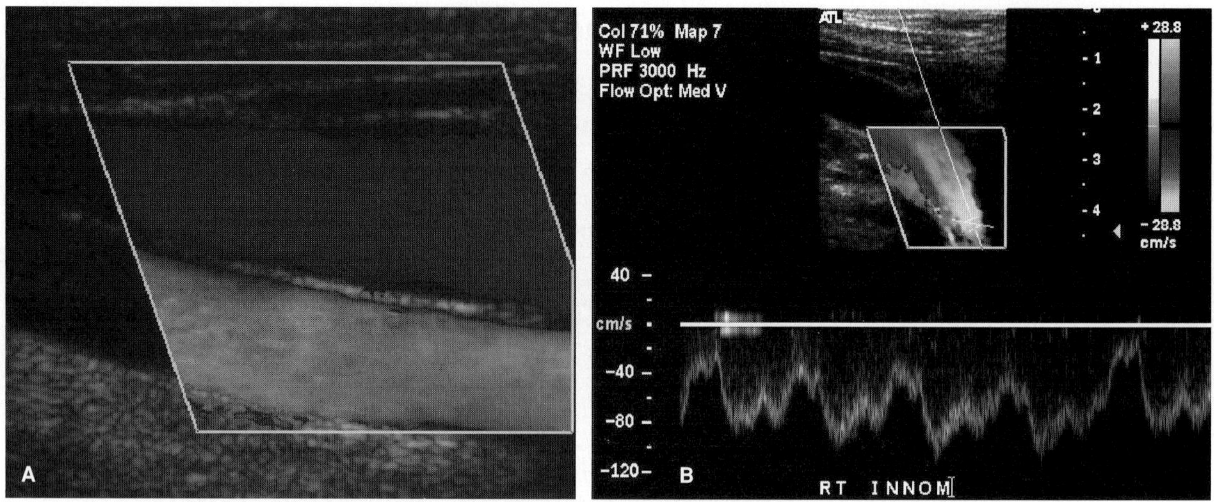

FIGURE 40.51. **(Color Plates) Normal Upper Extremity Venous US. A.** Color Doppler image shows normal wall-to-wall color flow in the jugular vein in blue and in the carotid artery in red. **B.** Normal venous waveform in the innominate vein demonstrates respiratory phasicity and transmitted cardiac pulsations.

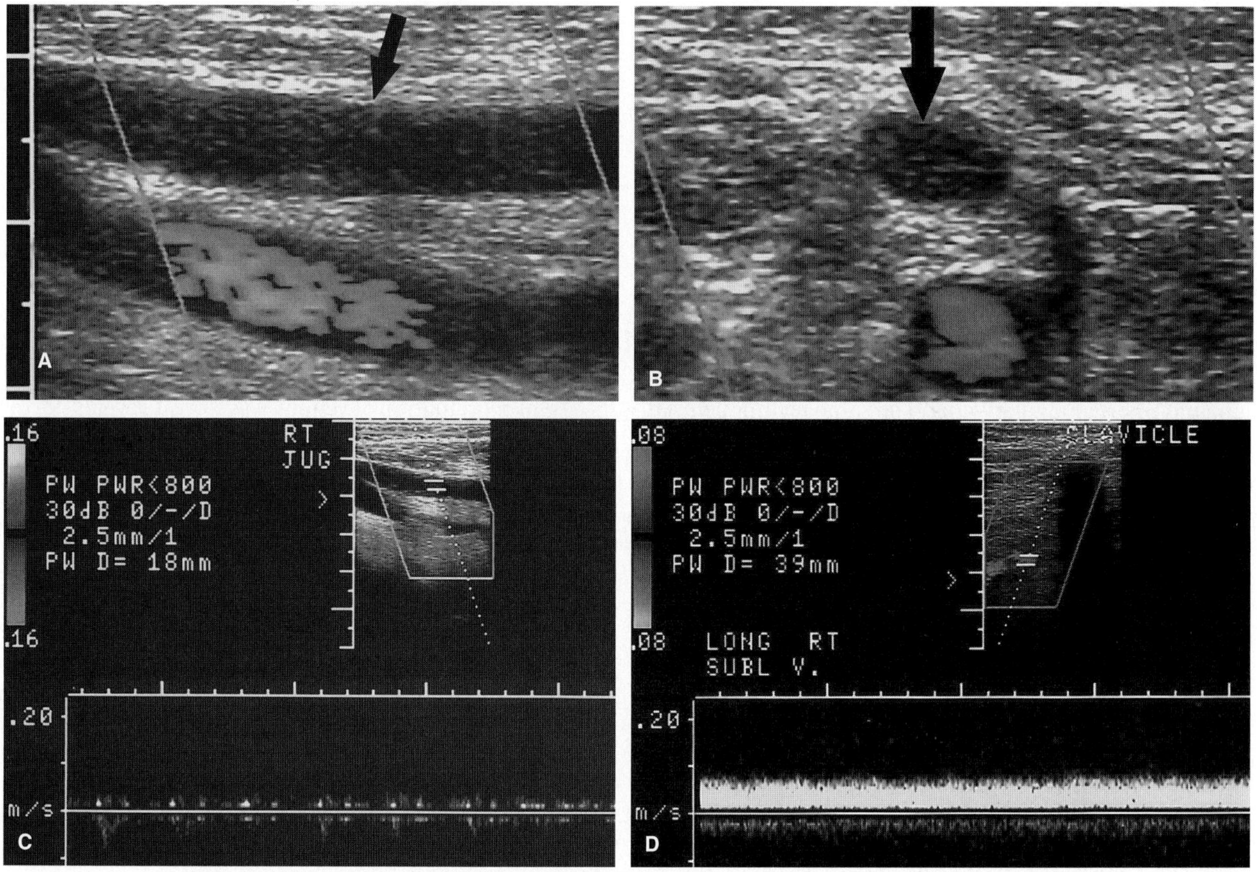

FIGURE 40.52. **(Color Plates) Internal Jugular Vein Thrombosis.** Longitudinal **(A)** and transverse **(B)** color Doppler images of the right internal jugular (IJ) vein show noncompressible echogenic thrombus (*arrows*). Color flow (*red*) is seen in the right common carotid artery and no flow is seen in the IJ vein. **C.** Spectral Doppler confirms no flow in the right IJ vein. **D.** The proximal right subclavian vein has a blunted, monophasic waveform, suggesting a central obstruction. CT revealed a left brachiocephalic vein thrombosis.

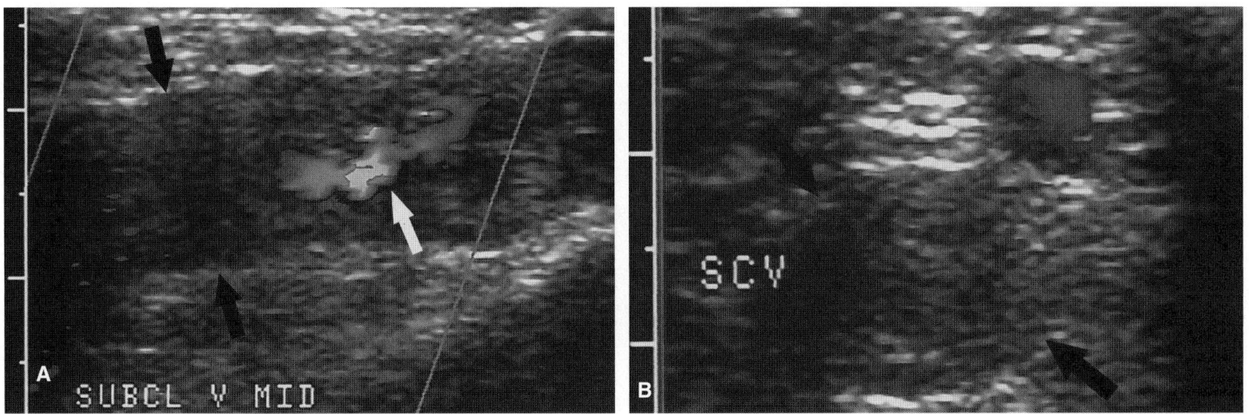

FIGURE 40.53. **(Color Plates) Subclavian Vein Thrombosis.** Longitudinal **(A)** and transverse **(B)** color Doppler images of the right subclavian vein (SCV). The distended vein is filled with echogenic thrombus (*black arrows*). The longitudinal image demonstrates some residual patent lumen (*white arrow*).

with a high clinical suspicion despite a negative duplex examination.

Thoracic Outlet Syndrome. The most common presentation for a patient with thoracic outlet syndrome is pain caused by compression of the brachial plexus. Venous obstruction resulting in arm swelling is more common than arterial obstruction. Venous compression occurs on the subclavian vein as it passes between the first rib and scalene muscles at the thoracic inlet. Intermittent arm swelling, effort thrombosis, and pain are the usual symptoms. If frank clot is not identified, the patient should be examined with the arm at the side and at various degrees of abduction. When pulse wave and color Doppler imaging are used, compression is likely if flow ceases or a dampening of the waveform occurs. No dampening is seen on the unaffected side. Similarly, a blunted arterial waveform or absent flow is seen if the subclavian artery is affected (Figs. 40.54, 40.55).

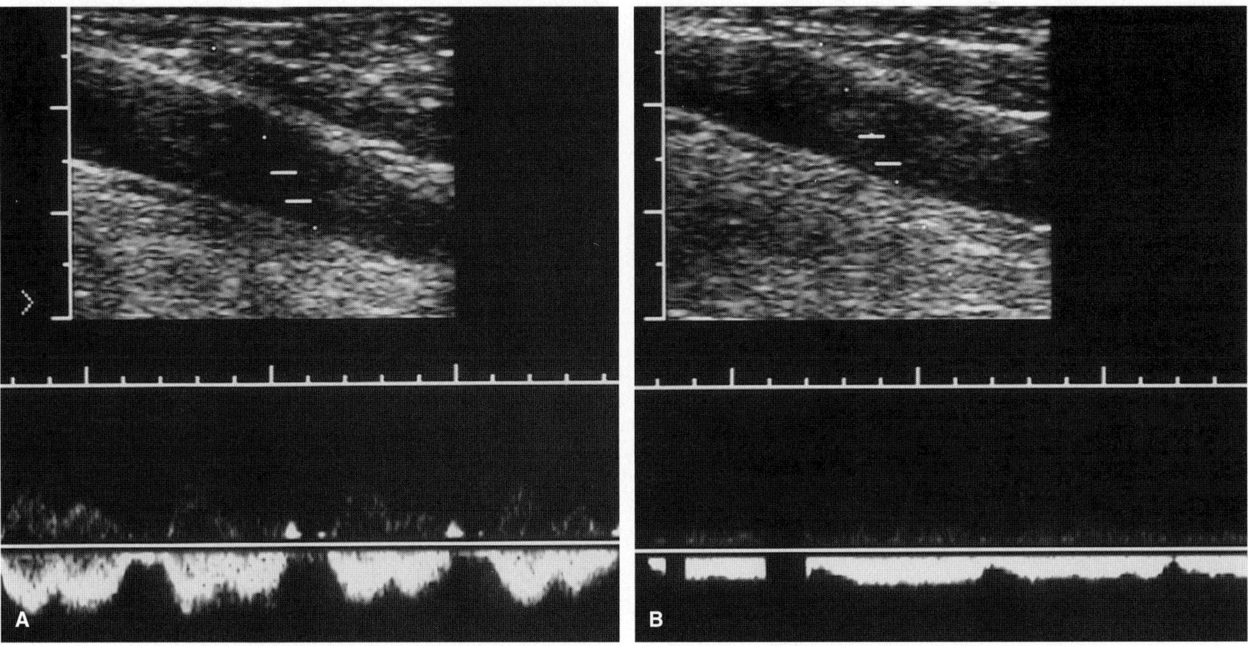

FIGURE 40.54. **Thoracic Outlet Syndrome: Venous. A.** Normal subclavian vein waveform with the arm at the patient's side. **B.** With the arm abducted, the Doppler tracing is blunted (more monophasic). The contralateral side demonstrated no blunting of the waveform with abduction.

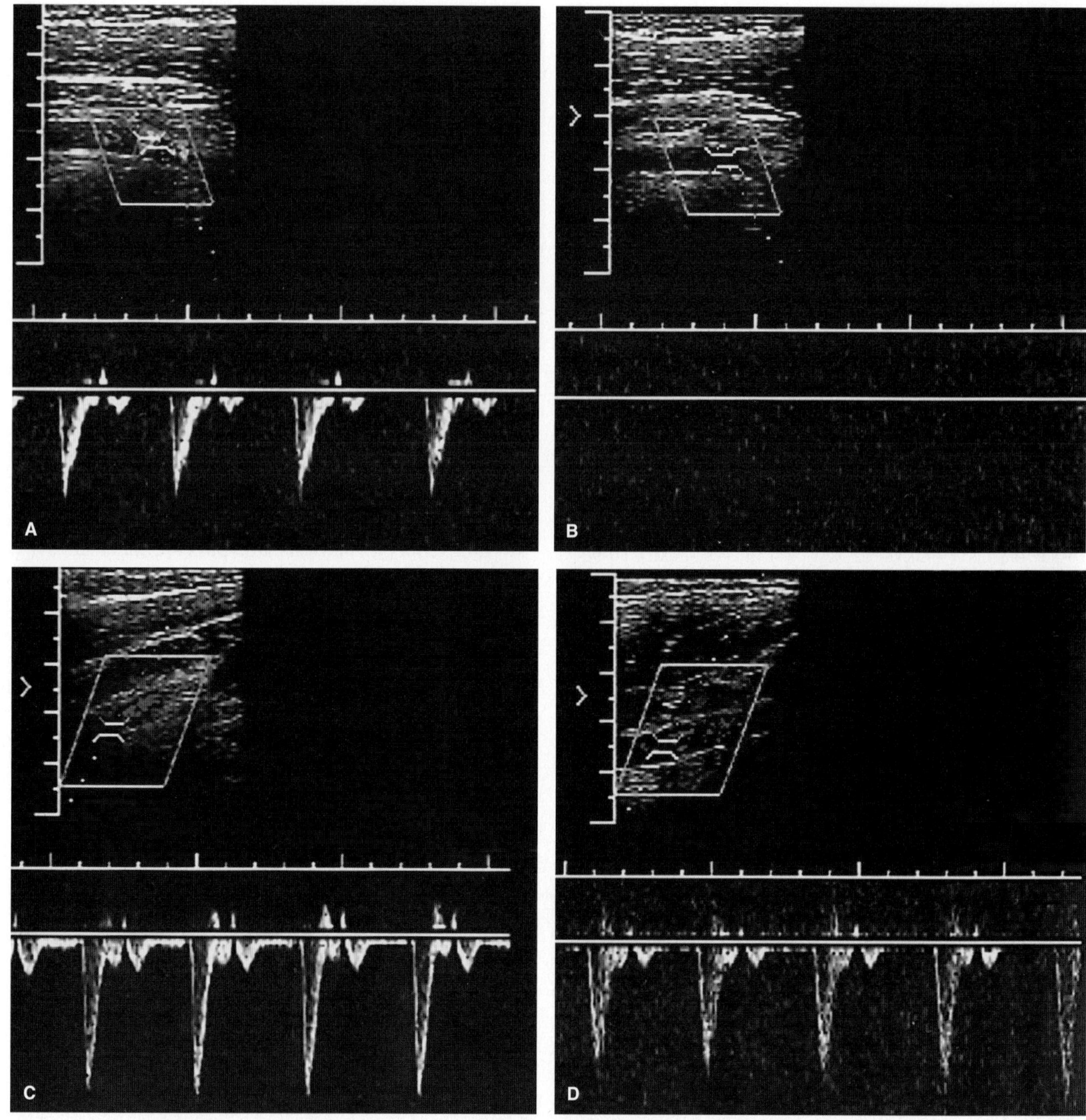

FIGURE 40.55. **Thoracic Outlet Syndrome: Arterial. A.** Normal triphasic, high-resistance waveform in the left subclavian artery with the arm at the patient's side. **B.** Abduction of the left arm causes obliteration of the left radial pulse on physical exam. The Doppler tracing confirms the clinical finding, demonstrating complete occlusion of the left subclavian artery. **C.** and **D.** The right subclavian artery has normal triphasic, high-resistance flow with the arm at the patient's side and in abduction (no thoracic outlet syndrome).

REFERENCES

1. Newman JS, Adler RS, Bude RO, Rubin JM. Detection of soft-tissue hyperemia: value of power Doppler sonography. AJR Am J Roentgenol 1994;163:385–389.
2. Nelson TR, Pretorius DH. The Doppler signal: where does it come from and what does it mean? AJR Am J Roentgenol 1988;151: 439–447.
3. Boote EJ. Doppler US techniques: concepts of blood flow detection and flow dynamics. Radiographics 2003;23:1315–1327.
4. Campbell SC, Cullinan JA, Rubens DJ. Slow flow or no flow? Color and power Doppler US pitfalls in the abdomen and pelvis. Radiographics 2004;24:497–506.
5. Kruskal JB, Newman PA, Sammons LG, Kane RA. Optimizing Doppler and color flow US: application to hepatic sonography. Radiographics 2004;24:657–675.

6. Zwiebel WJ, Fruechte D. Basics of abdominal and pelvic duplex: instrumentation, anatomy, and vascular Doppler signatures. Semin Ultrasound CT MRI 1992;13:3–21.
7. Maulik D. Hemodynamic interpretation of the arterial Doppler waveform. Ultrasound Obstet Gynecol 1993;3:219–227.
8. Kotval PS. Doppler waveform parvus and tardus: a sign of proximal flow obstruction. J Ultrasound Med 1989;8:435–440.
9. Bude RO, Rubin JM, Platt JF, et al. Pulsus tardus: its cause and potential limitations in detection of arterial stenosis. Radiology 1994;190:779–784.
10. Powis RL. Color flow imaging. Radiographics 1994;14:415–428.
11. Mitchell DG. Color Doppler imaging: principles, limitations, artifacts. Radiology 1990;177:1–10.
12. Weskott HP. Amplitude Doppler US: slow blood flow detection tested with a flow phantom. Radiology 1997;202:125–130.
13. Bude RO, Rubin JM. Power Doppler sonography. Radiology 1996;200:21–23.
14. Rubin JM, Bude RO, Carson PL, et al. Power Doppler US: a potentially useful alternative to mean frequency-based color Doppler US. Radiology 1994;190:853–856.
15. Bohs LN, Friemel BH, McDermott BA, Trahey GE. Real-time system for angle-independent US of blood flow in two dimensions: initial results. Radiology 1993;186:259–261.
16. Pellerito JS, Troiano RN, Quedens-Case C, Taylor KJW. Common pitfalls of endovaginal color Doppler flow imaging. Radiographics 1995;15:37–47.
17. American Heart Association. Heart Disease and Stroke Statistics, 2005;16–20, 53.
18. North American Symptomatic Carotid Endarterectomy Trial Collaborators. Beneficial effect of carotid endarterectomy in symptomatic patients with high-grade carotid stenosis. N Engl J Med 1991;325:445–453.
19. European Carotid Surgery Trialist's Collaborative Group. MRC European carotid surgery trial: interim results for symptomatic patients with severe (70–99%) or with mild (0–29%) carotid stenosis. Lancet 1991;337:1235–1243.
20. Barnett HJM, Taylor DW, Eliasziw M, et al. Benefit of Carotid endarterectomy in symptomatic moderate or severe stenosis. N Engl J Med 1998;339:1415–1425.
21. Executive Committee for the Asymptomatic Carotid Atherosclerosis Study. Endarterectomy for asymptomatic carotid artery stenosis. JAMA 1995;273:1421–1428.
22. Hobson RW, Weiss DG, Fields WS, et al. Efficacy of carotid endarterectomy for asymptomatic carotid stenosis. N Engl J Med 1993;328:221–227.
23. Mayo Asymptomatic Carotid Endarterectomy Study Group. Results of a randomized controlled trial of carotid endarterectomy for asymptomatic carotid stenosis. Mayo Clin Proc 1992;67: 513–518.
24. The CASANOVA Group. Carotid surgery versus medical therapy in asymptomatic carotid stenosis. Stroke 1991;22:1229–1235.
25. Barr JD, Connors JJ III, Sacks D, et al. Quality improvement guidelines for the performance of cervical carotid angioplasty and stent placement. Am J Neuroradiol 2003;24:2020–2034.
26. Carroll BA. Carotid sonography. Radiology 1991;178:303–313.
27. O'Leary DH, Polak JF. Intima-media thickness: a tool for atherosclerosis imaging and event prediction. Am J Cardiol 2002;90(suppl): 18L–21L.
28. Burke GL, Evans GW, Riley WA, et al. Arterial wall thickness is associated with prevalent cardiovascular disease in middle-aged adults. The atherosclerosis risk in communities (ARIC) study. Stroke 1995;26:386–391.
29. Gaitini D, Soudack M. Diagnosing carotid stenosis by Doppler sonography: State of the art. J Ultrasound Med 2005;24:1127–1136.
30. Polak JF. Carotid ultrasound. Radiol Clin North Am 2001;39(3): 569–589.
31. Bluth EI, Stavros AT, Marich KW, et al. Carotid duplex sonography: a multicenter recommendation for standardized imaging and Doppler criteria. Radiographics 1988;8:487–506.
32. Polak JF. Sonographic evaluation of the carotid arteries in patients with transient ischemic attacks, strokes, or carotid bruits. In: Bluth EI, ed. Syllabus: A Special Course in Ultrasound: Presented at the 82nd Scientific Assembly and Annual Meeting of the Radiological Society of North America, December 1–6, 1996. Oak Brook, IL: Radiological Society of North America, 1996:91–97.
33. Polak JF, O'Leary DH, Kronmal RA, et al. Sonographic evaluation of carotid artery atherosclerosis the elderly: relationship of disease severity to stroke and transient ischemic attack. Radiology 1993;188:363–370.
34. O'Leary DH, Clouse ME, Potter JE, et al. The influence of noninvasive tests on the selection of patients for carotid angiography. Stroke 1995;16:264–267.
35. Hunink MG, Polak JF, Barlan MM, et al. Detection and quantification of carotid artery stenosis: efficacy of various Doppler velocity parameters. AJR Am J Roentgenol 1993;160:619–625.
36. Moneta GL, Edwards JM, Chitwood RW, et al. Correlation with North American Symptomatic Carotid Endarterectomy Trial (NASCET) angiographic definition of 70% to 99% internal carotid artery stenosis with duplex scanning. J Vasc Surg 1993;17:152–157.
37. Neale ML, Chambers JL, Kelly AT et al. Reappraisal of duplex criteria to assess significant carotid stenosis with special reference to reports from the North American Symptomatic Carotid Endarterectomy Trial and the European Carotid Surgery Trial. Stroke 1994;20: 642–649.
38. Faught WE, Mattos MA, van Bemmelen PS, et al. Color-flow duplex scanning of carotid arteries: new velocity criteria based on receiver operator characteristic analysis for threshold stenoses used in the symptomatic and asymptomatic carotid trials. J Vasc Surg 1994;19:818–828.
39. Carpenter JP, Lexa FJ, Davis JT. Determination of sixty percent or greater carotid artery stenosis by duplex Doppler ultrasonography. J Vasc Surg 1995;22:697–705.
40. Moneta JL, Edwards JM, Papanicolaou G, et al. Screening for asymptomatic internal carotid artery stenosis: duplex criteria for discriminating 60% to 99% stenosis. J Vasc Surg 1995;21:989–994.
41. Hood DB, Mattos MA, Mansour A, et al. Prospective evaluation of new duplex criteria to identify 70% internal carotid artery stenosis. J Vasc Surg 1996;23:254–261.
42. Carpenter JP, Lexa FJ, Davis JT. Determination of duplex Doppler US criteria appropriate to the North American Symptomatic Carotid Endarterectomy Trial. Stroke 1996;27:695–699.
43. Browman MW, Cooperberg PL, Harrison PB, et al. Duplex ultrasonography criteria for internal carotid stenosis of more than 70% diameter: angiographic correlation and receiver operating characteristic curve analysis. Can Assoc Radiol J 1995;46:291–295.
44. AbuRahma AF, Robinson PA, Strickler DL, et al. Proposed new duplex classification for threshold stenose used in various symptomatic and asymptomatic carotid endarterectomy trials. Ann Vasc Surg 1998;12:349–358.
45. Grant EG, Duerinckx AJ, El Saden S, et al. Doppler sonographic parameters for detection of carotid stenosis: Is there an optimum method for their selection? Am J Roentgenol 1999;172:1123–1129.
46. Huston J III, James EM, Brown RD Jr., et al. Redefined duplex ultrasonographic criteria for diagnosis of carotid artery stenosis. Mayo Clin Proc 2000;75:1133–1140.
47. Suwanwela N, Can U, Furie KL, et al. Carotid Doppler ultrasound criteria for internal carotid artery stenosis based on residual lumen diameter calculated from en bloc carotid endarterectomy specimens. Stroke 1996;27:1965–1969.
48. Ackerman RH, Candia MR. Identifying clinically relevant carotid disease. Stroke 1994;25:1–3.
49. Grant EG, Benson CB, Moneta GL, et al. Carotid artery stenosis: gray-scale and Doppler US diagnosis—Society of Radiologists in Ultrasound Consensus Conference. Radiology 2003;229(2):340–346.
50. Romero JM, Lev MH, Chan S, et al. US of neurovascular occlusive disease: interpretive pearls and pitfalls. Radiographics 2002;22: 1165–1176.
51. Darling RC, Messina CR, Brewster DC, et al. Autopsy study of unoperated abdominal aortic aneurysms. Circulation 1977;56:161–164.
52. Geroulakis G, Nicolaides A. Infrarenal abdominal aortic aneurysms. Eur J Vasc Surg 1992;6:616–622.
53. Ernst CB. Abdominal aortic aneurysm. N Engl J Med 1993;16: 1167–1172.
54. Scott RAP, Wilson NM, Ashton HA, et al. Is surgery necessary for abdominal aortic aneurysm less than 6 cm in diameter? Lancet 1993;342:1395–1396.

55. Wachsberg RH. Doppler ultrasound evaluation of transjugular intrahepatic portosystemic shunt function. Ultrasound Q 2003;19(3): 139–148.
56. Jalan R, Lui HF, Redhead DN, Hayes PC. TIPSS 10 years on. Gut 2000;46:578–581.
57. Feldstein VA, Patel MD, LaBerge JM. Transjugular intrahepatic portosystemic shunts: accuracy of Doppler US in determination of patency and detection of stenosis. Radiology 1996;201:141–147.
58. Foshager MC, Ferral H, Finlay DE, et al. Color Doppler sonography of transjugular intrahepatic portosystemic shunts (TIPS). AJR Am J Roentgenol 1994;163:105–111.
59. Kanterman RY, Darcy MD, Middleton WD, Sterling KM, Teefey SA, Pilgram TK. Doppler sonography findings associated with transjugular intrahepatic portosystemic shunt malfunction. AJR Am J Roentgenol 1997;168:467–472.
60. Murphy TP, Beecham RP, Kim HM, et al. Long-term follow-up after TIPS: use of Doppler velocity criteria for detecting elevation of the portosystemic gradient. J Vasc Interv Radiol 1998;9:275–281.
61. Haskal ZJ, Carroll JW, Jacobs JE, et al. Sonography of transjugular intrahepatic portosystemic shunts: detection of elevated portosystemic gradients and loss of shunt function. J Vasc Interv Radiol 1997;8:549–556.
62. Owens CA, Bartolone C, Warner DL, et al. The inaccuracy duplex ultrasonography in predicting patency of transjugular intrahepatic portosystemic shunts. Gastroenterology 1998;114:975–980.
63. Dodd GD, Zajko AB, Orons PD, et al. Detection of transjugular intrahepatic portosystemic shunt dysfunction: value of duplex Doppler sonography. AJR Am J Roentgenol 1995;164:1119–1124.
64. Carroll BA. Pulsatile groin mass in the post-catheterization patient. In: Bluth EI, ed. Syllabus: A Special Course in Ultrasound: Presented at the 82nd Scientific Assembly and Annual Meeting of the Radiological Society of North America, December 1–6, 1996. Oak Brook, IL: Radiological Society of North America, 1996:107–115.
65. Pellerito JS. Current approach to peripheral arterial sonography. Radiol Clin North Am 2001;39(3):553–567.
66. Foshager MC, Finlay DE, Longley DG, et al. Duplex and color Doppler sonography of complications after percutaneous interventional vascular procedures. Radiographics 1994;14:239–253.
67. Krueger K, Zaehringer M, Strohe D, et al. Postcatheterization pseudoaneurysm: results of US-guided percutaneous thrombin injection in 240 patients. Radiology 2005;236:1104–1110.
68. Zwiebel WJ. Painful legs after walking. In: Bluth EI, ed. Syllabus: A Special Course in Ultrasound: Presented at the 82nd Scientific Assembly and Annual Meeting of the Radiological Society of North America, December 1–6, 1996. Oak Brook, IL: Radiological Society of North America, 1996:133–141.
69. Polak JF. Arterial sonography: efficacy for the diagnosis of arterial disease of the lower extremity. AJR Am J Roentgenol 1993;161: 235–243.
70. Beidle TR, Brom-Ferral R, Letourneau JG. Surveillance of infrainguinal vein grafts with duplex sonography. AJR Am J Roentgenol 1994;162:443–448.
71. Dorfman GS, Cronan JJ. Venous ultrasonography. Radiol Clin North Am 1992;30:879–893.
72. Cronan JJ. Venous thromboembolic disease: the role of US. Radiology 1993;186:619–630.
73. Bluth EI. Leg swelling with pain or edema. In: Bluth EI, ed. Syllabus: A Special Course in Ultrasound: Presented at the 82nd Scientific Assembly and Annual Meeting of the Radiological Society of North America, December 1–6, 1996. Oak Brook, IL: Radiological Society of North America, 1996:99–105.
74. Min RJ, Khilnani NM, Golia P. Duplex ultrasound evaluation of lower extremity venous insufficiency. J Vasc Interv Radiol 2003;14: 1233–1241.
75. Beidle TR, Letourneau JG. Arm swelling. In: Bluth EI, ed. Syllabus: A Special Course in Ultrasound: Presented at the 82nd Scientific Assembly and Annual Meeting of the Radiological Society of North America, December 1–6, 1996. Oak Brook, IL: Radiological Society of North America, 1996:125–132.
76. Wadhwani R, Chaubal N, Sukthankar R, et al. Color Doppler and duplex sonography in 5 patients with thoracic outlet syndrome. J Ultrasound Med 2001;20:795–801.

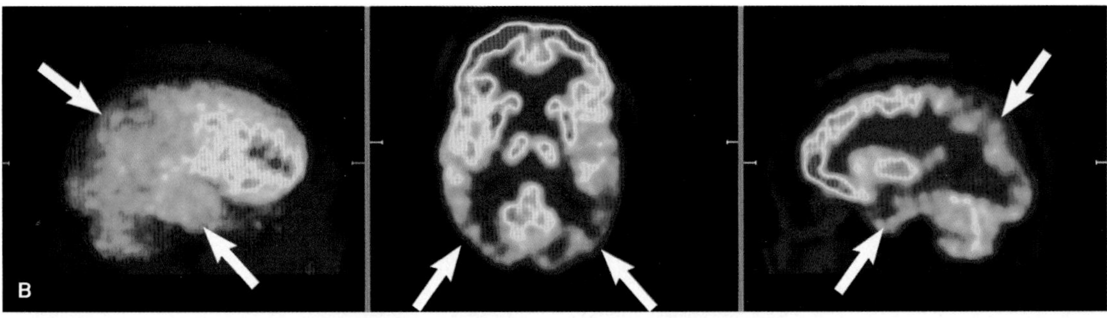

FIGURE 7.26B. **Alzheimer Disease (AD).**

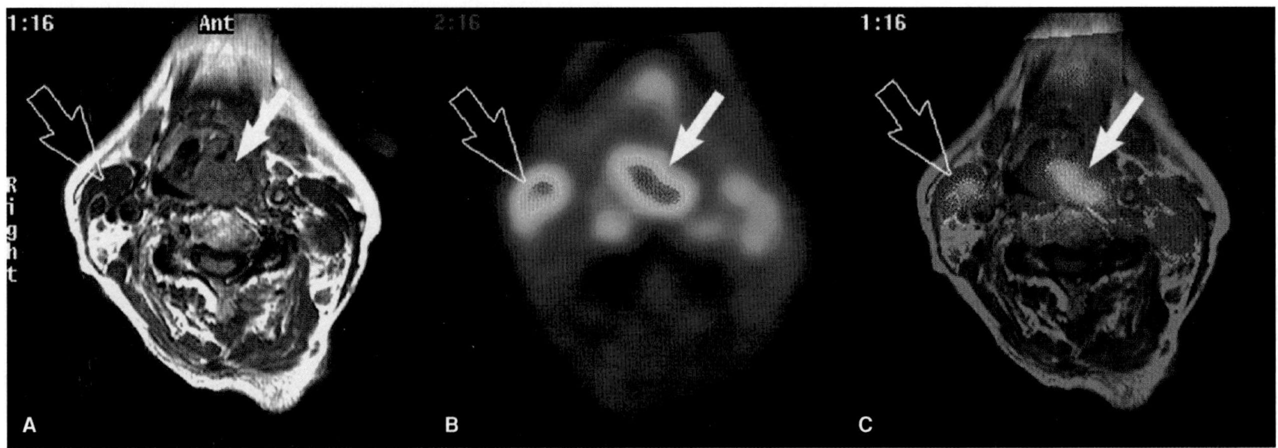

FIGURE 9.1. **Positron Emission Tomography (PET).**

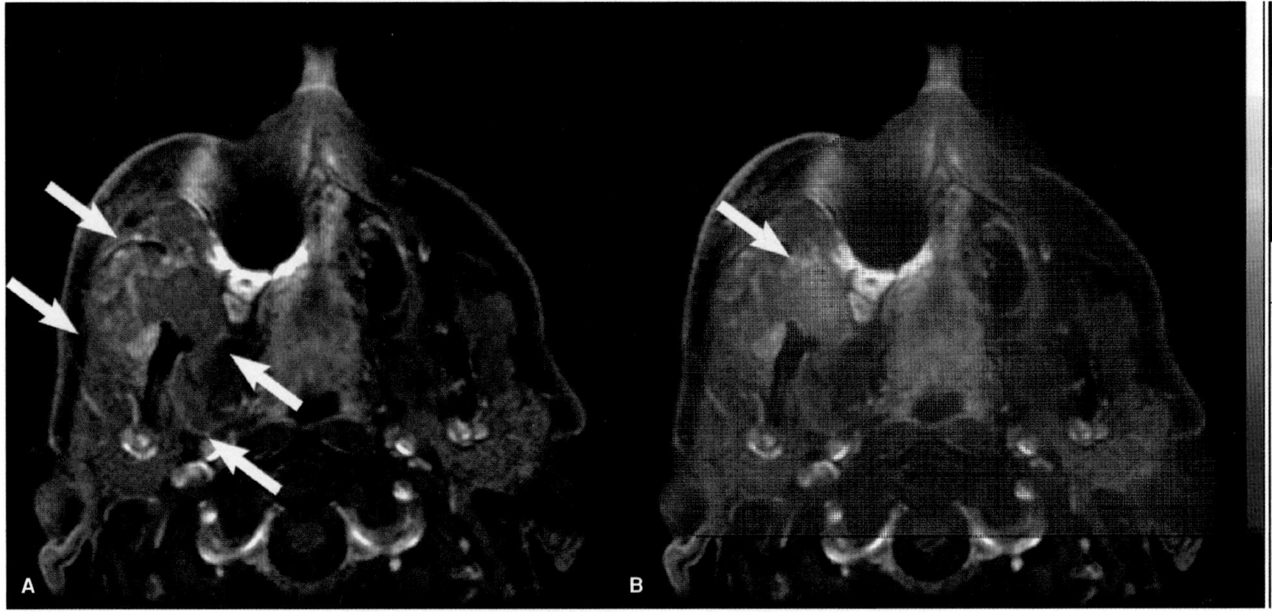

FIGURE 9.7. **Non-Hodgkin Lymphoma of the Masticator Space.**

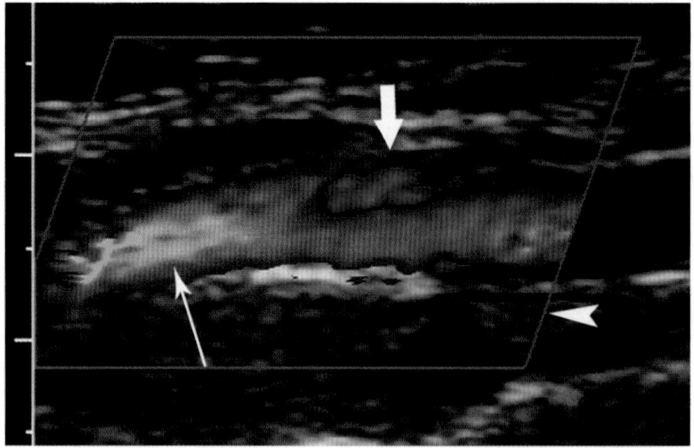

FIGURE 40.7. Normal Flow Reversal at Bifurcation.

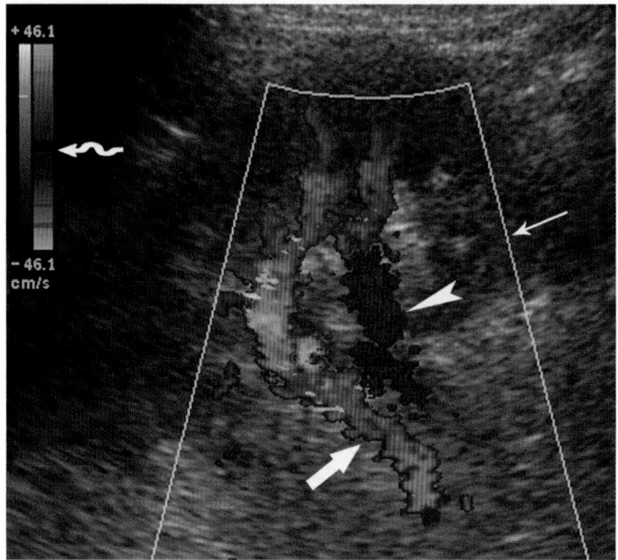

FIGURE 40.9. Color Doppler Image.

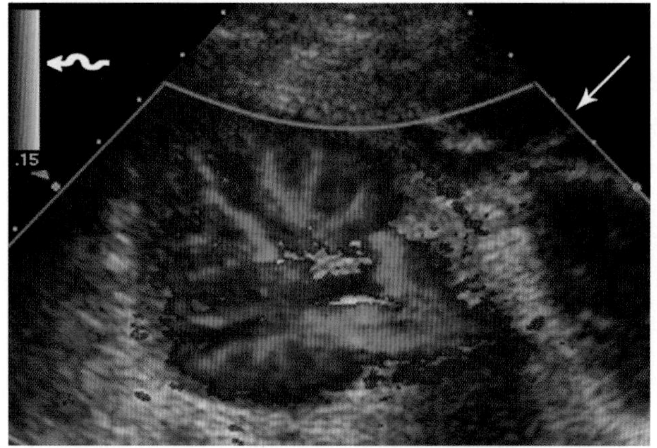

FIGURE 40.10. Power Doppler (Color Doppler Energy [CDE]) Image.

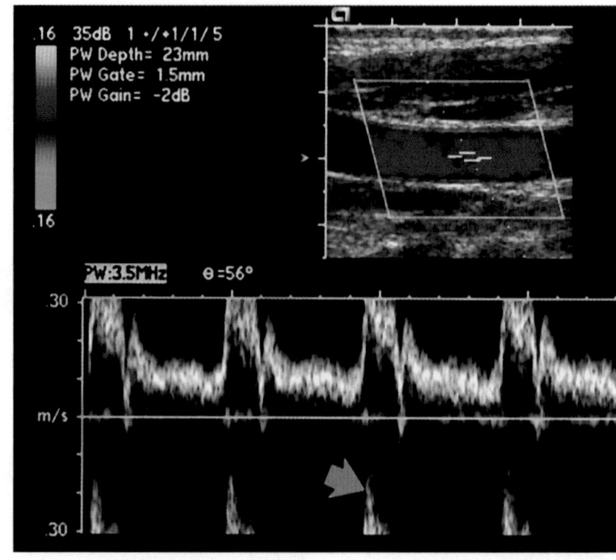

FIGURE 40.11. Aliasing on Spectral Doppler.

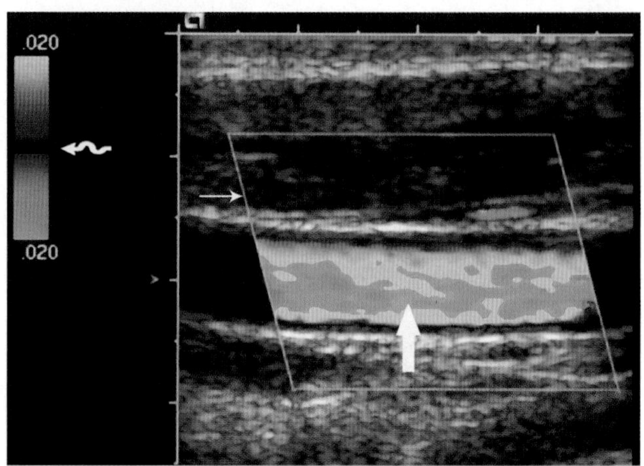

FIGURE 40.12. Aliasing on Color Doppler Imaging.

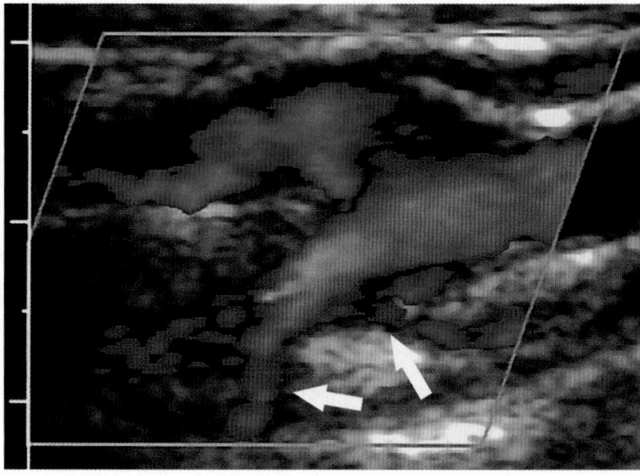

FIGURE 40.16. External Carotid Artery.

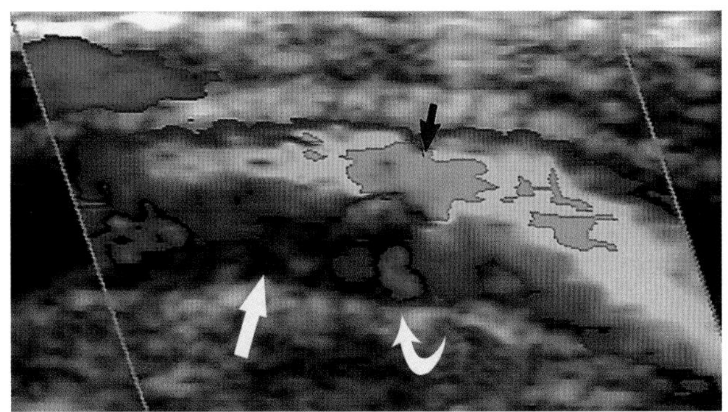

FIGURE 40.18. **Ulcerated Plaque.**

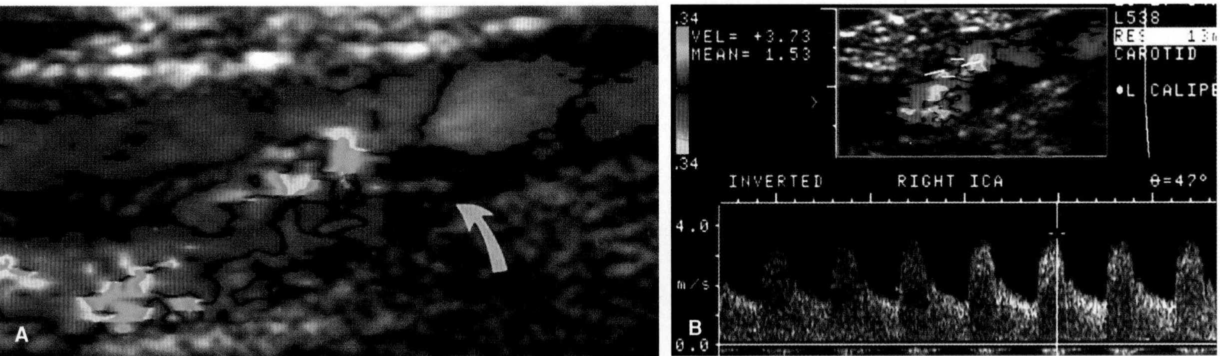

FIGURE 40.19. **Internal Carotid Artery (ICA) Stenosis.**

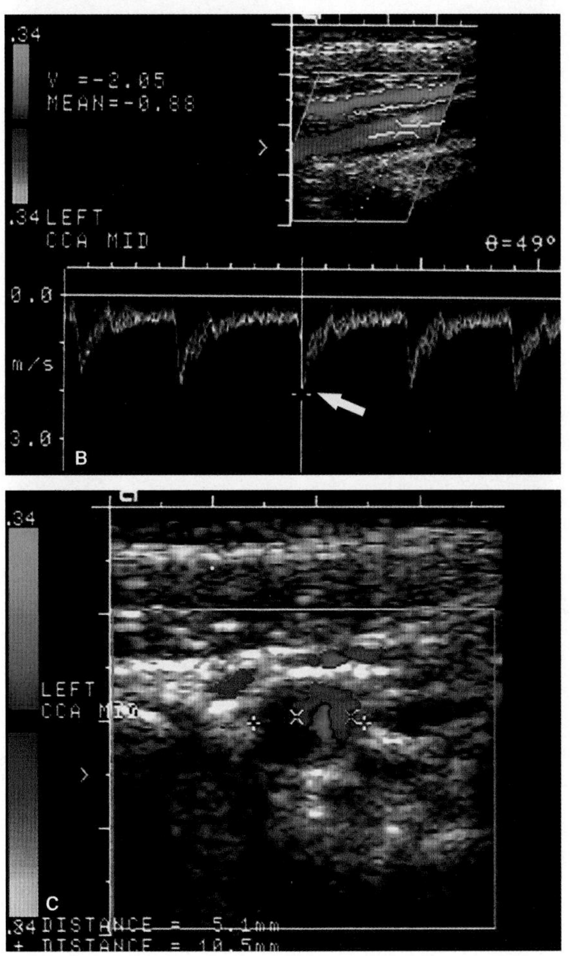

FIGURE 40.20B, C. **Common Carotid Artery (CCA) Stenosis.**

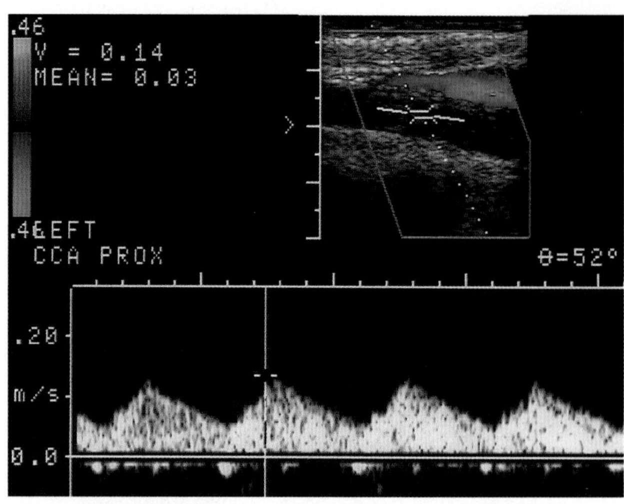

FIGURE 40.21. **Common Carotid Artery (CCA) Origin Stenosis.**

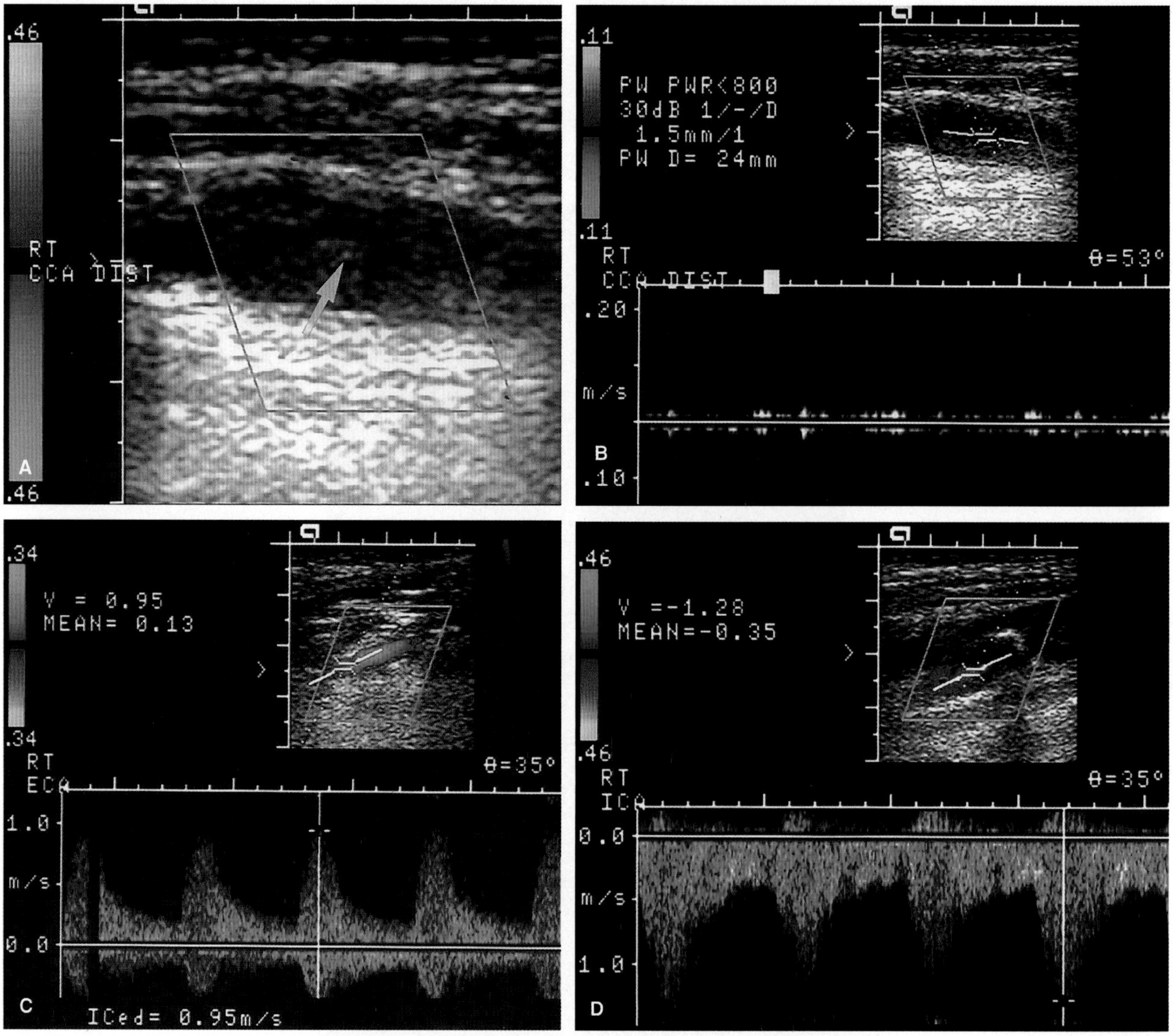

FIGURE 40.22. **Common Carotid Artery (CCA) Occlusion.**

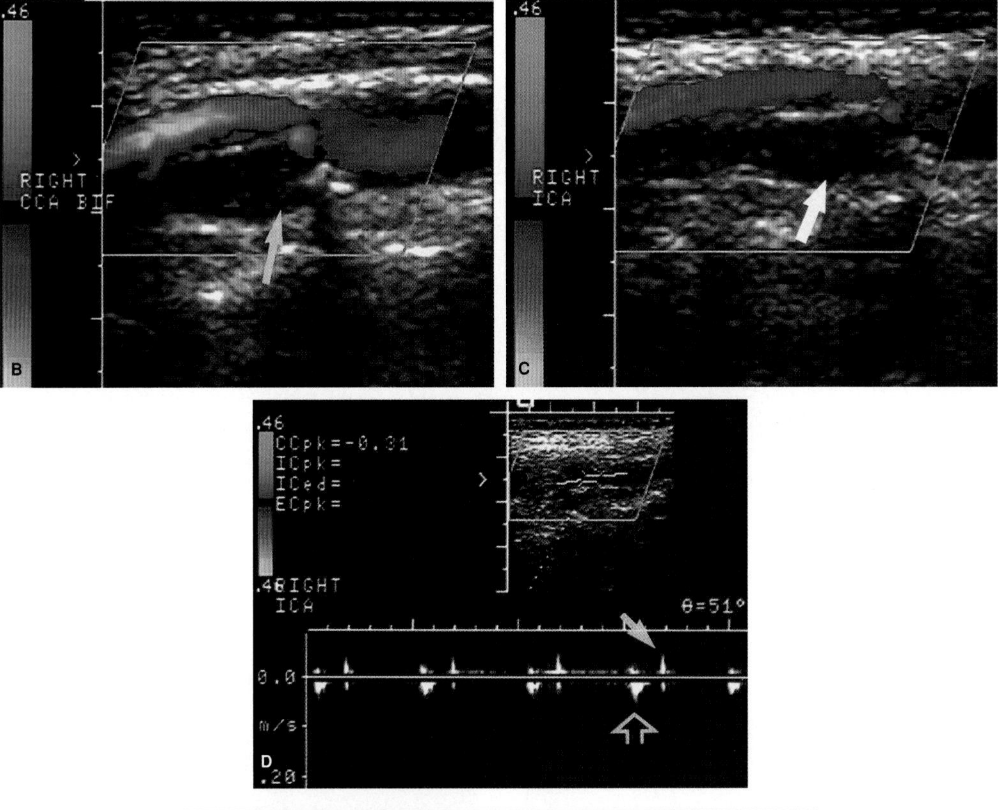

FIGURE 40.23B–D. **Internal Carotid Artery (ICA) Occlusion.**

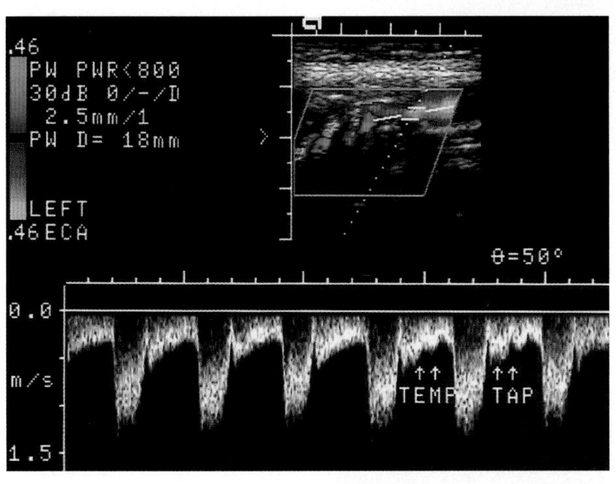

FIGURE 40.24. **Internal Carotid Artery (ICA) Occlusion.**

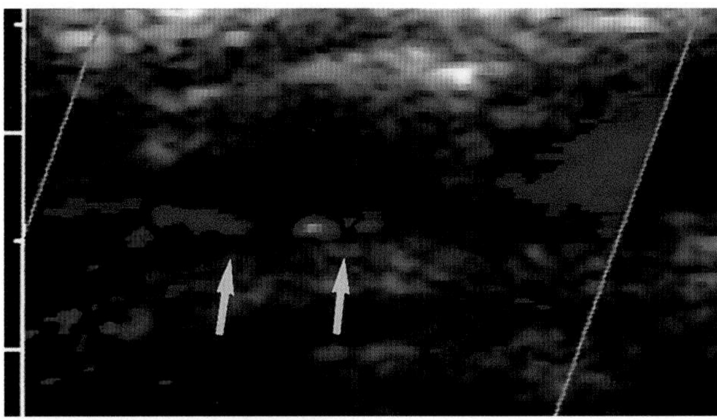

FIGURE 40.25. **String Sign.**

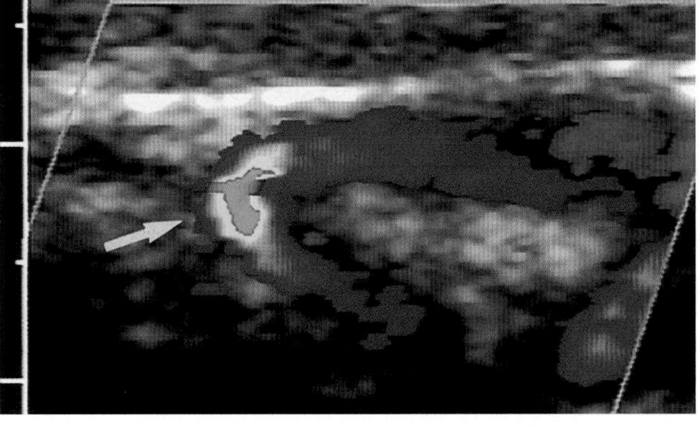

FIGURE 40.27. **Tortuous Vessel.**

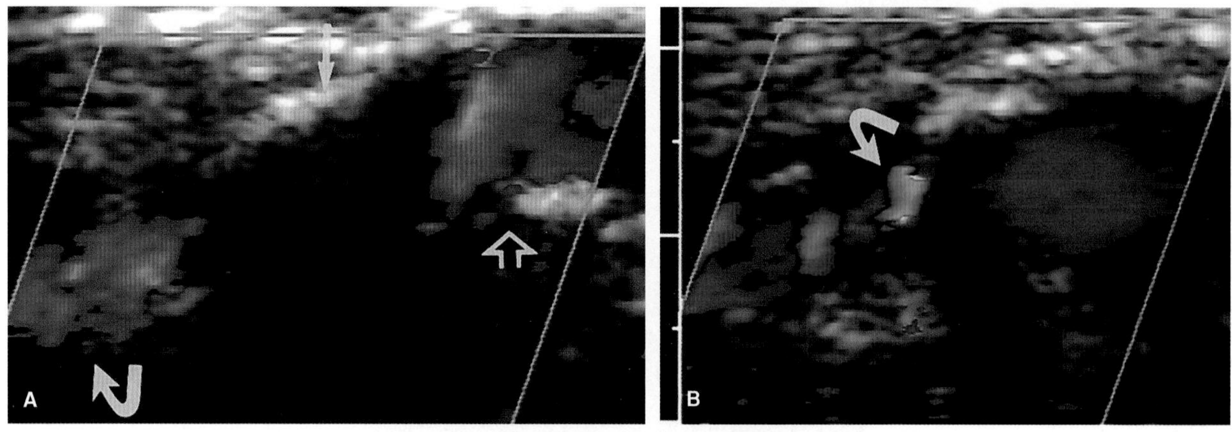

FIGURE 40.28. Calcified Plaques.

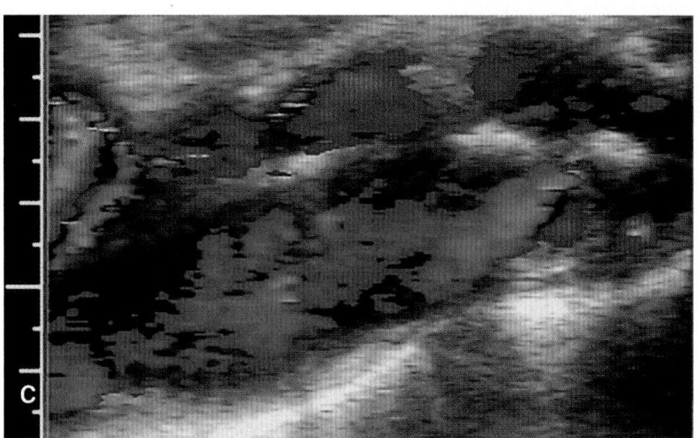

FIGURE 40.32C. Aortic Dissection.

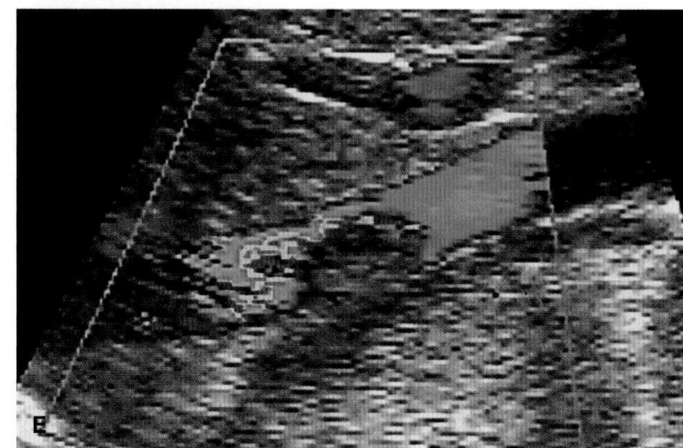

FIGURE 40.33E. Inferior Vena Cava (IVC) Tumor Thrombus.

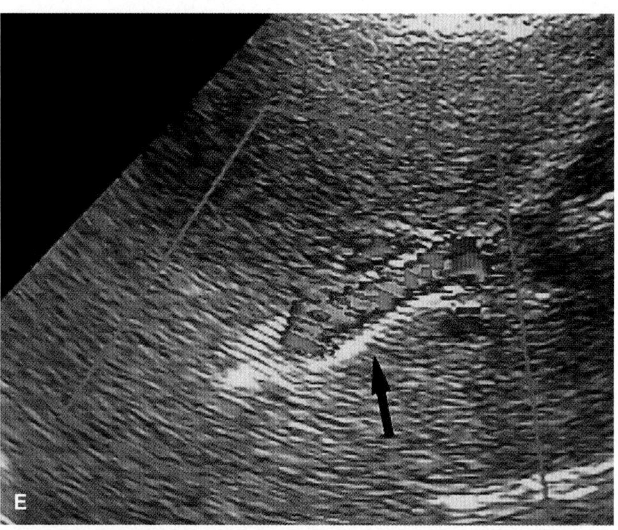

FIGURE 40.34E. Normal Transjugular Intrahepatic Portal Shunt (TIPS) US.

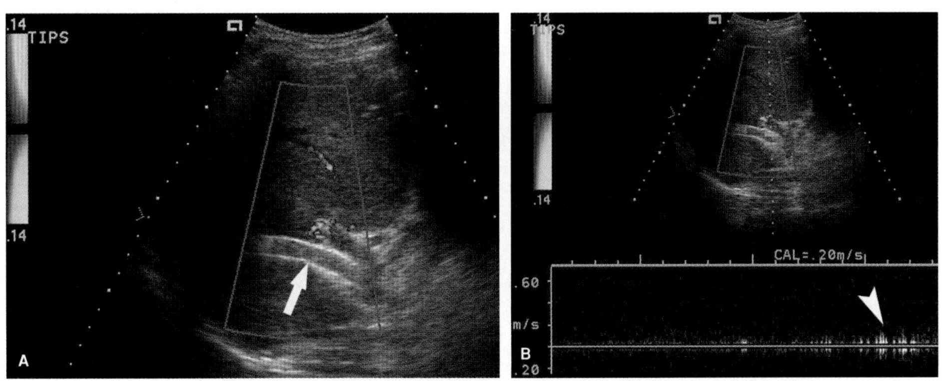

FIGURE 40.32. **Transjugular Intrahepatic Portal Shunt (TIPS) Occlusion.**

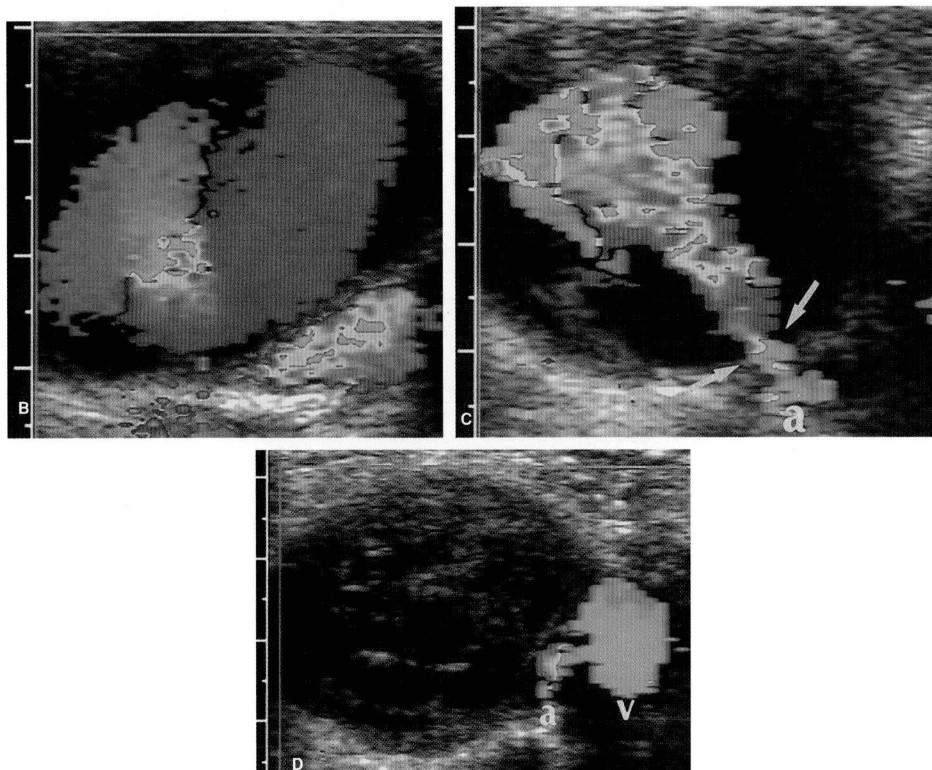

FIGURE 40.38B–D. **Pseudoaneurysm.**

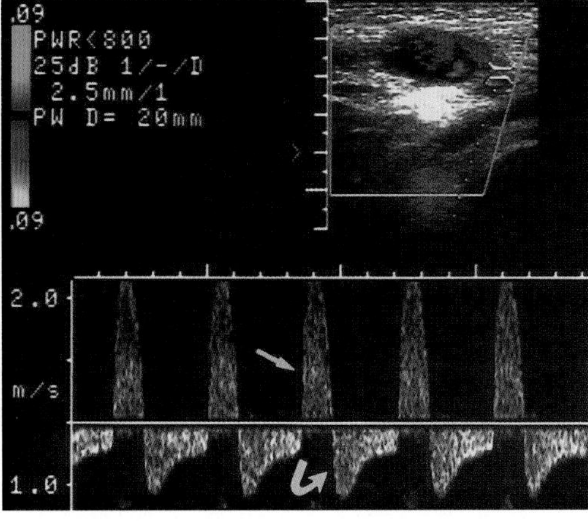

FIGURE 40.39. **Pseudoaneurysm.**

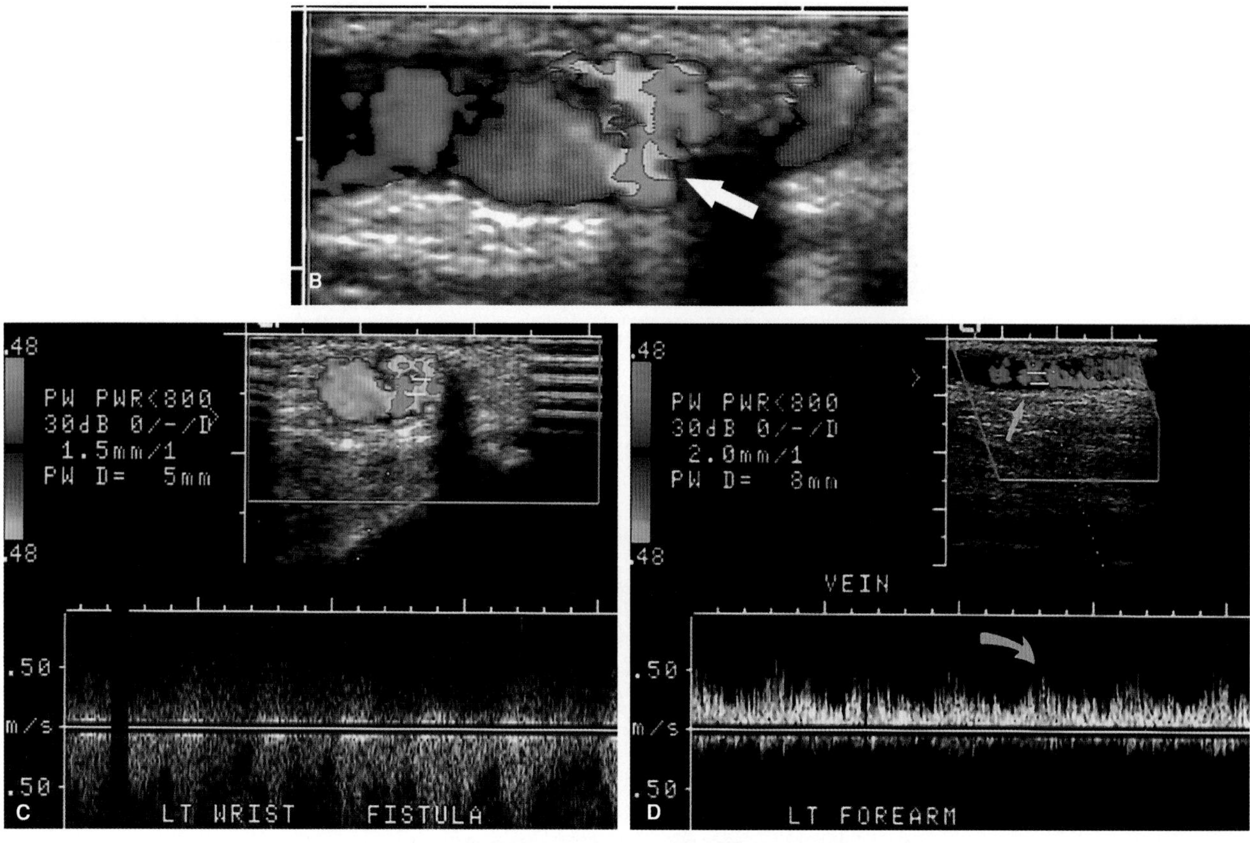

FIGURE 40.40B–D. **Arteriovenous Fistula in the Left Wrist.**

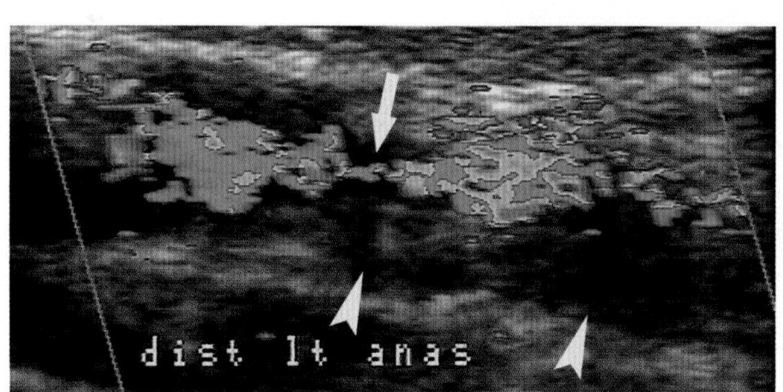

FIGURE 40.41. **Synthetic Graft Anastomotic Stenosis.**

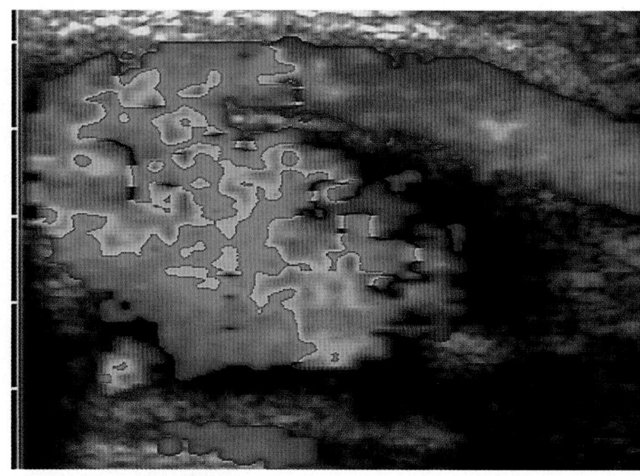

FIGURE 40.42. **Graft Anastomosis.**

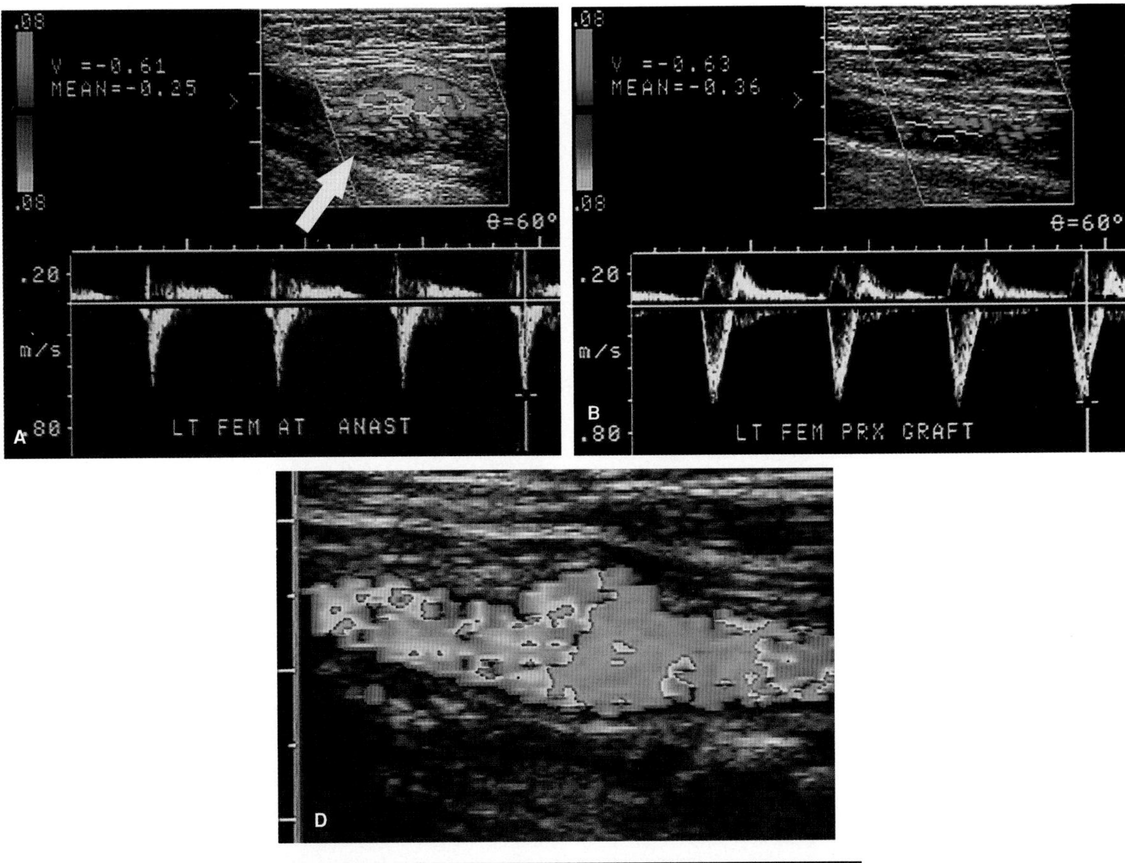

FIGURE 40.43A, B, D. Reversed Saphenous Vein Graft.

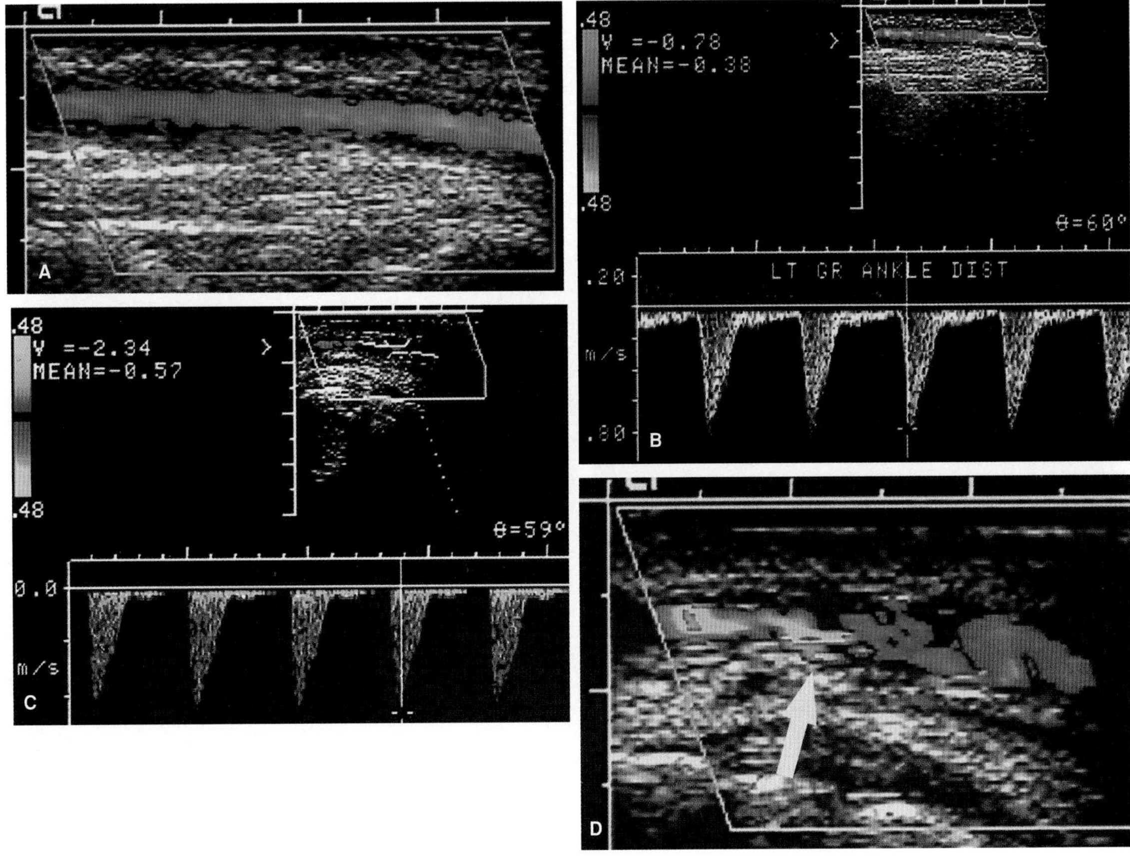

FIGURE 40.44. Popliteal to Plantar Artery Vein Graft Stenosis.

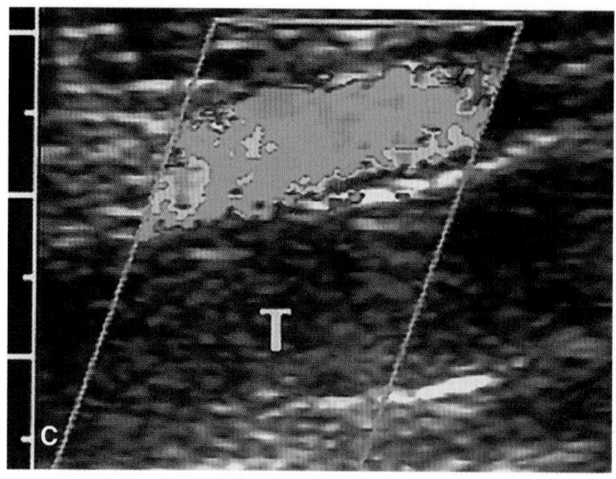

FIGURE 40.47C. **Deep Venous Thrombosis.**

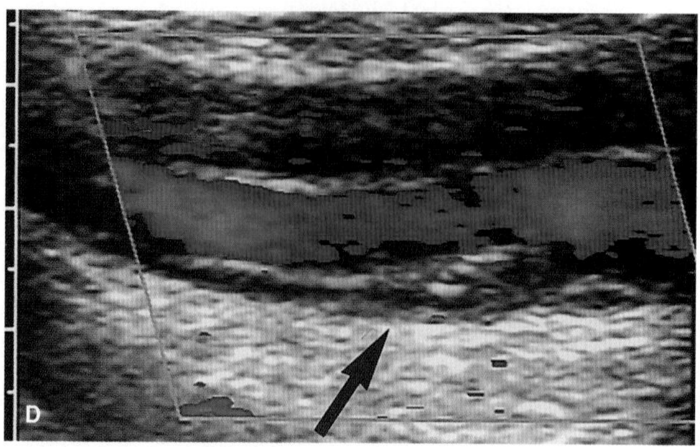

FIGURE 40.48D. **Chronic Deep Venous Thrombosis.**

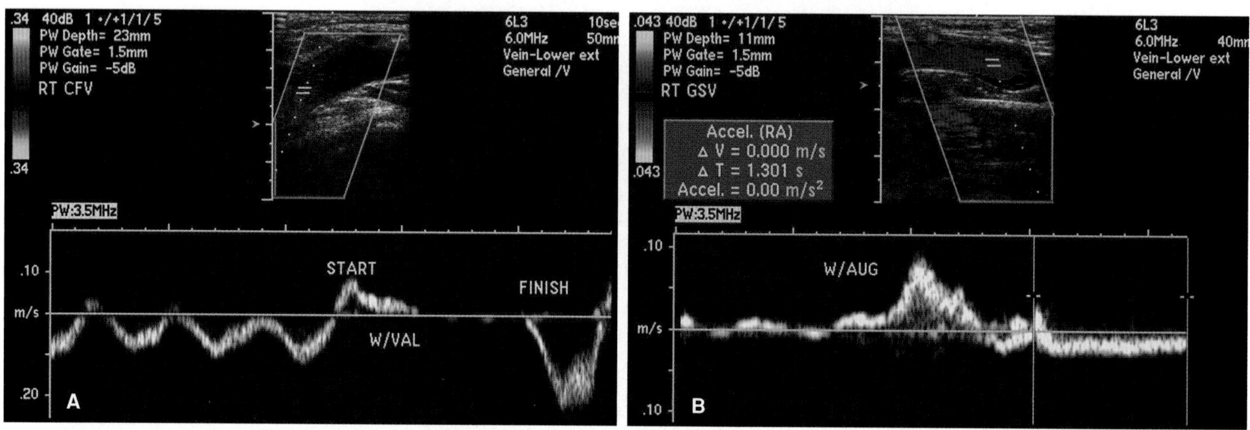

FIGURE 40.49. **Venous Insufficiency.**

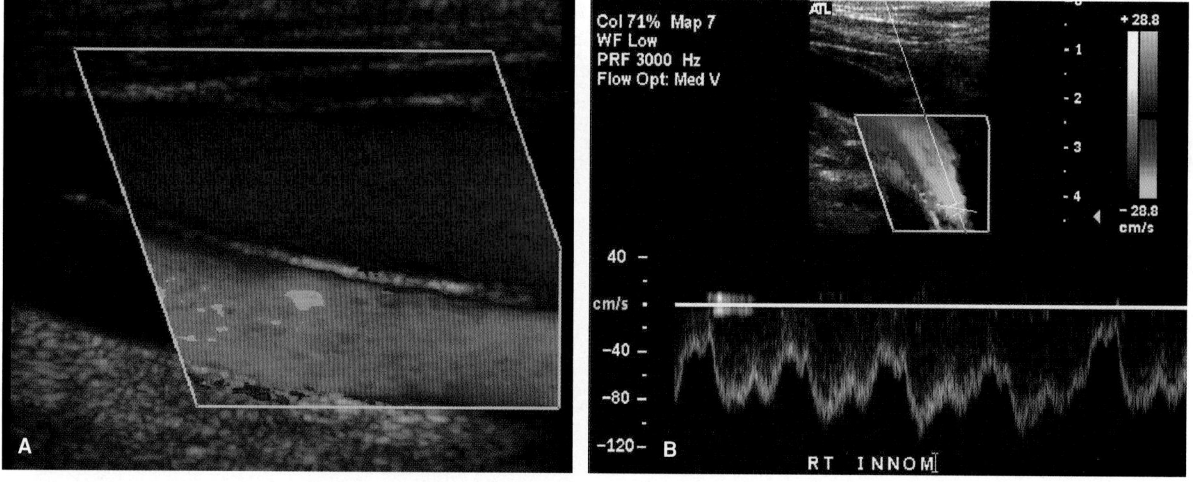

FIGURE 40.51. **Normal Upper Extremity Venous US.**

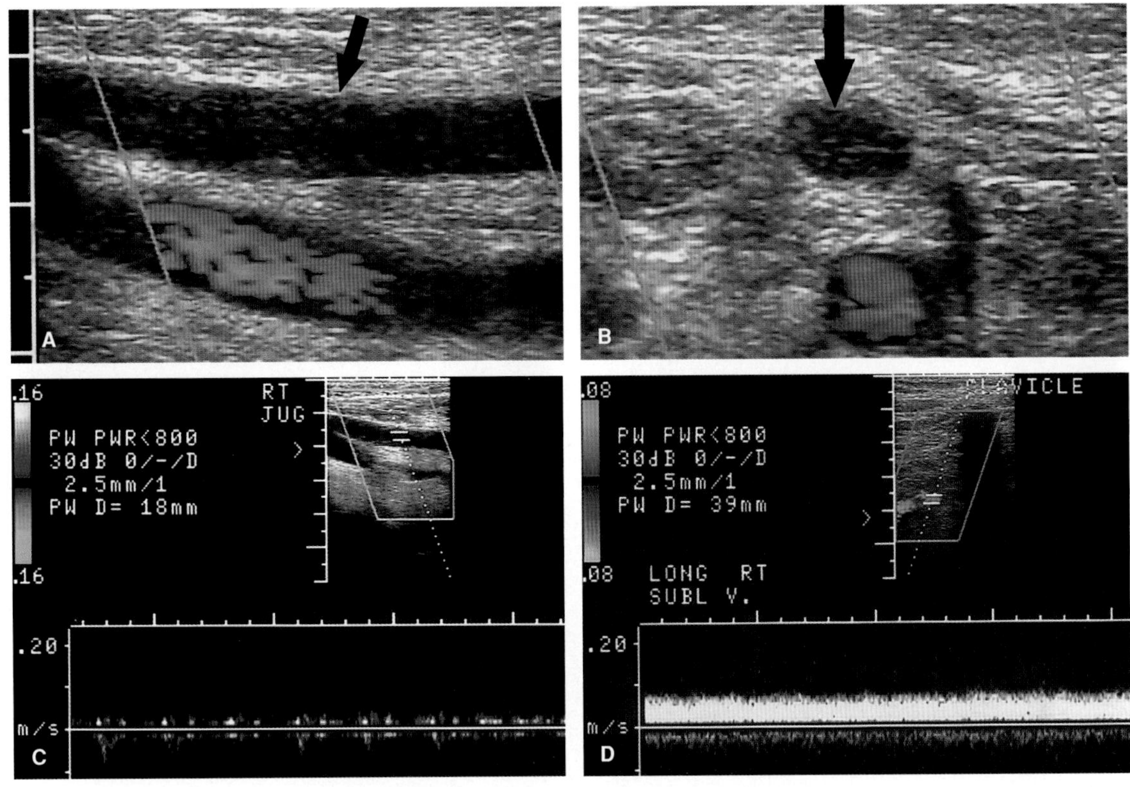

FIGURE 40.52. **Internal Jugular Vein Thrombosis.**

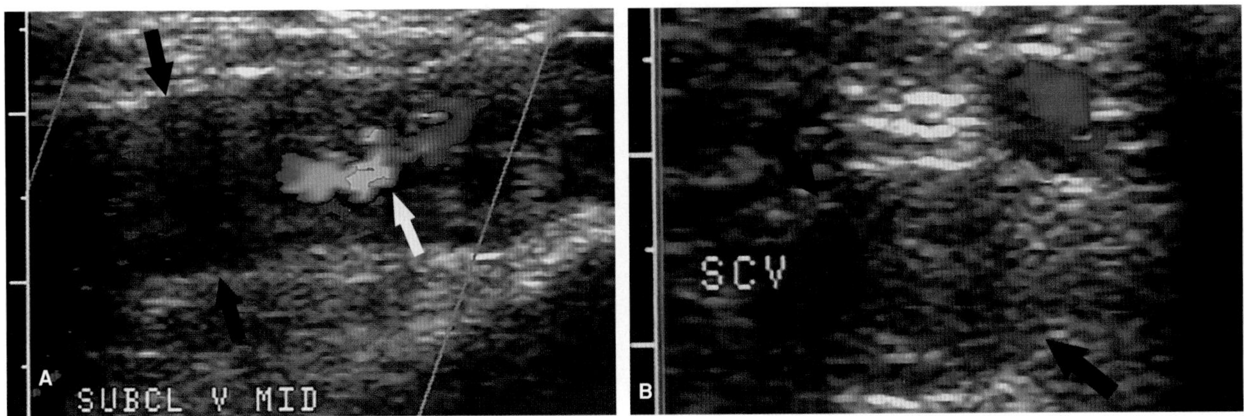

FIGURE 40.53. **Subclavian Vein Thrombosis.**

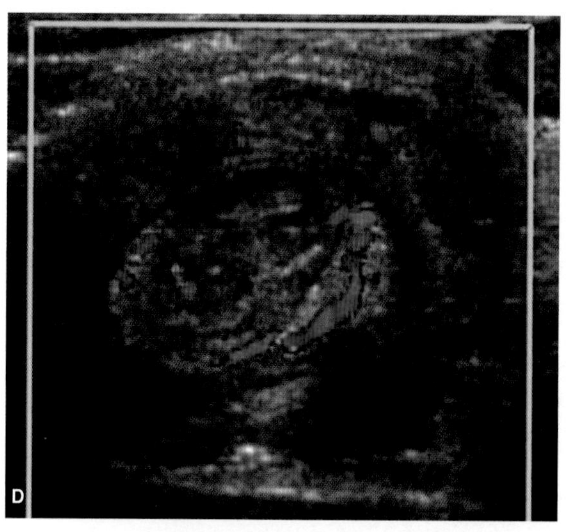

FIGURE 52.19D. Intussusception.

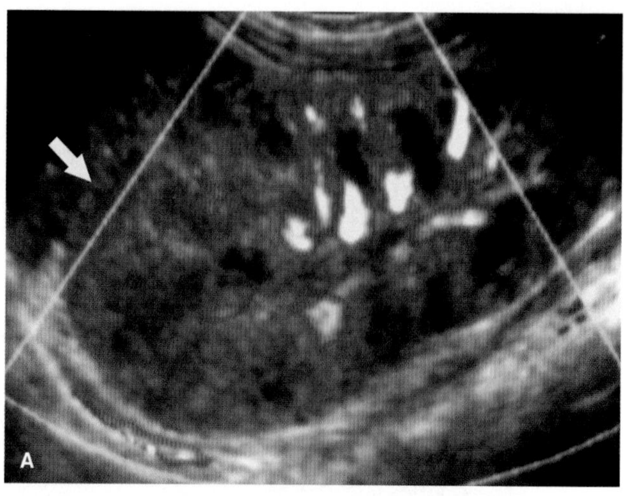

FIGURE 52.40A. Renal Abscess.

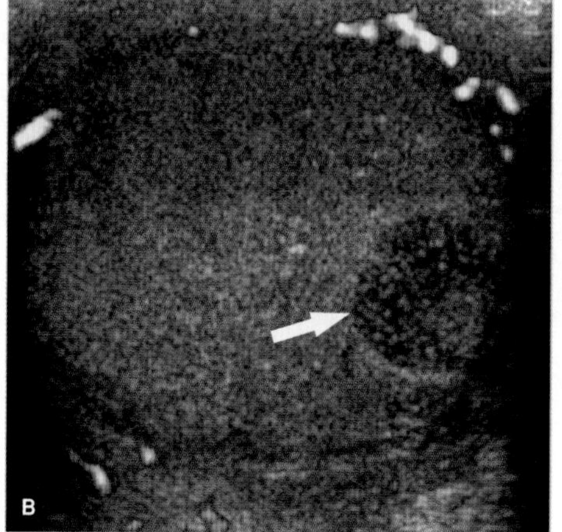

FIGURE 52.54B, C. Testicular Torsion.

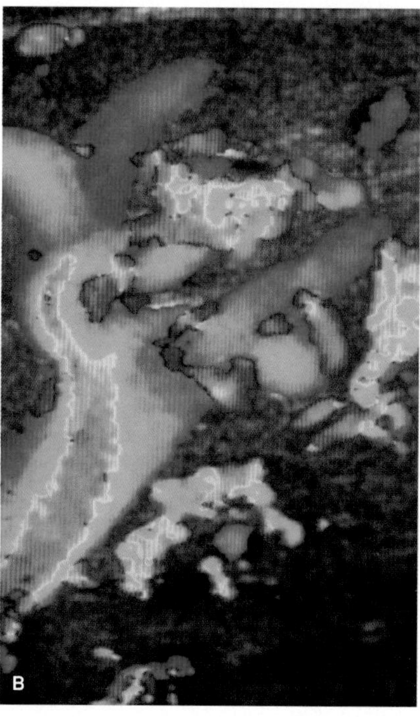

FIGURE 52.64B. Vascular Neoplasms of the Liver.

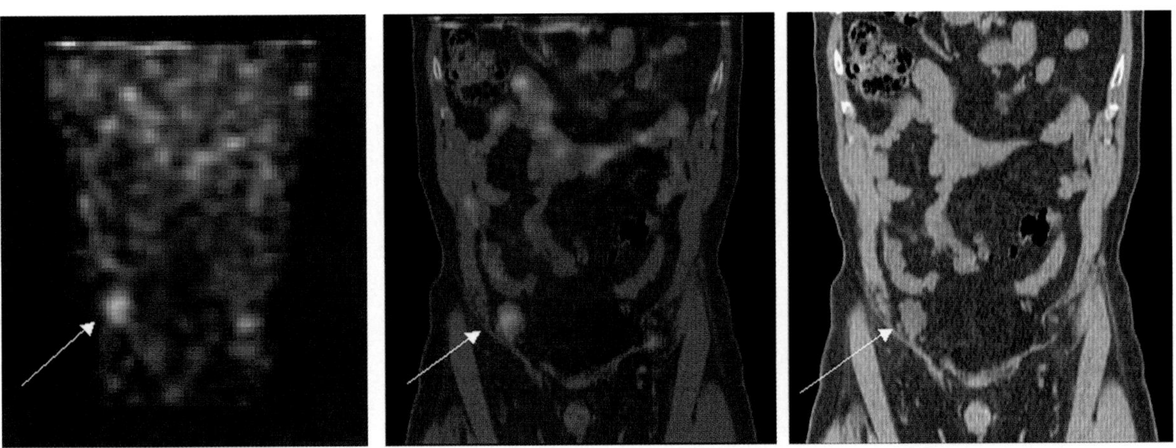

FIGURE 62.11. **SPECT-CT of Metastatic Prostate Carcinoma With ProstaScint.**

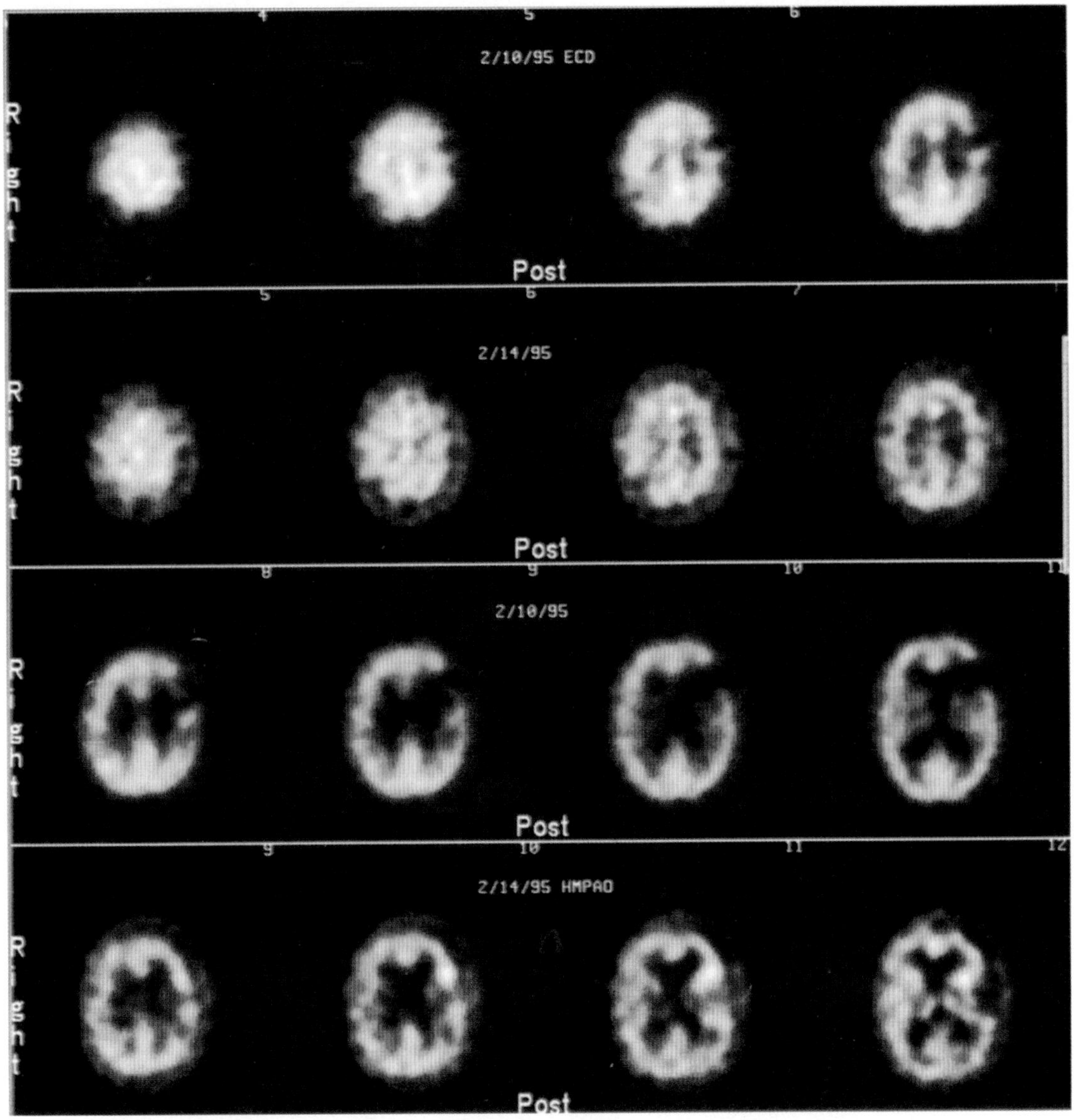

FIGURE 63.2. **Ethyl Cysteinate Dimer (ECD) Versus Hexamethylpropyleneamine Oxime (HMPAO) in Luxury Perfusion.**

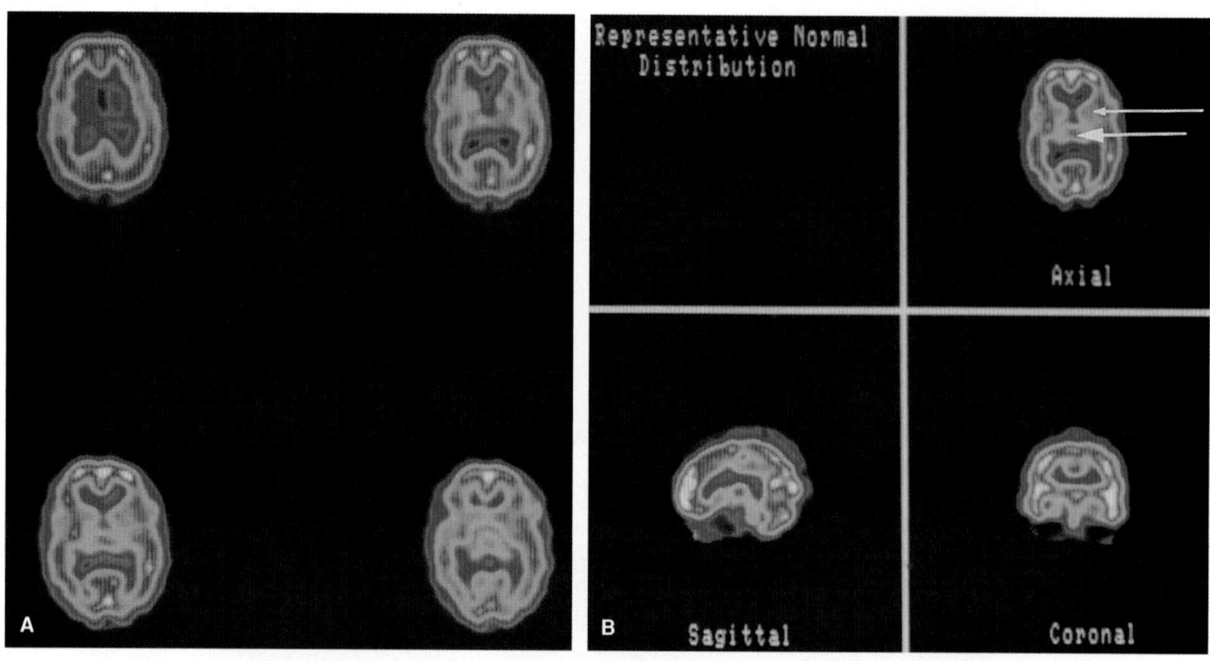

FIGURE 63.3. **Normal Hexamethylpropyleneamine Oxime (HMPAO) Study.**

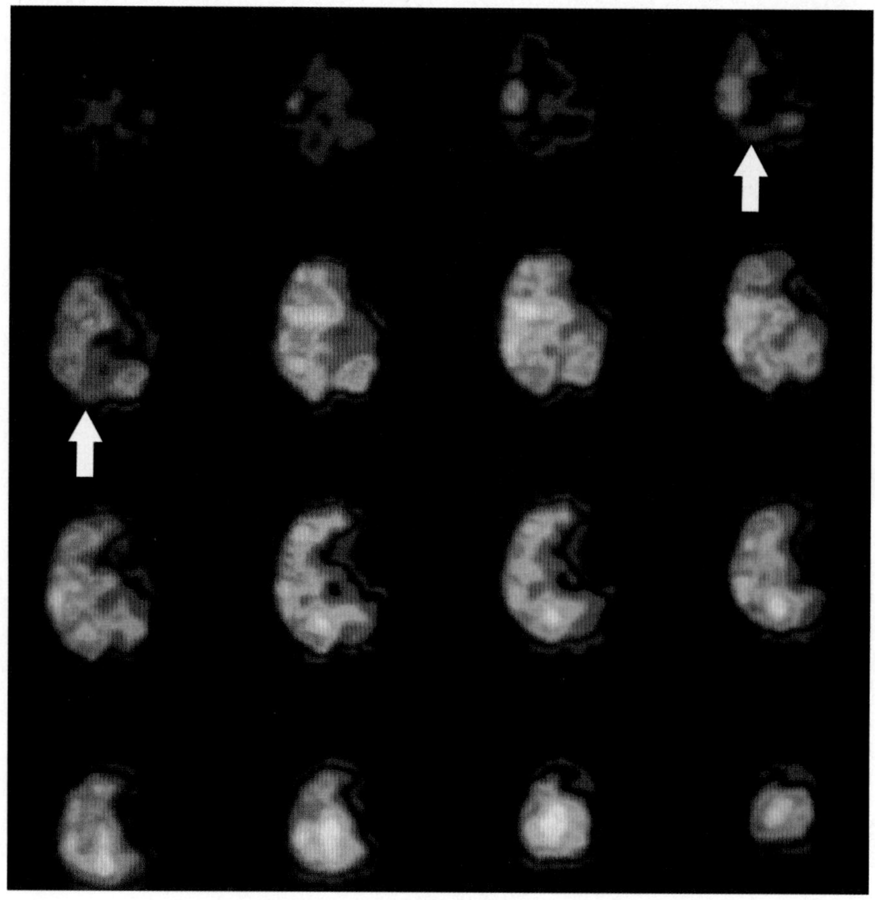

FIGURE 63.4. **Cerebral Infarction.**

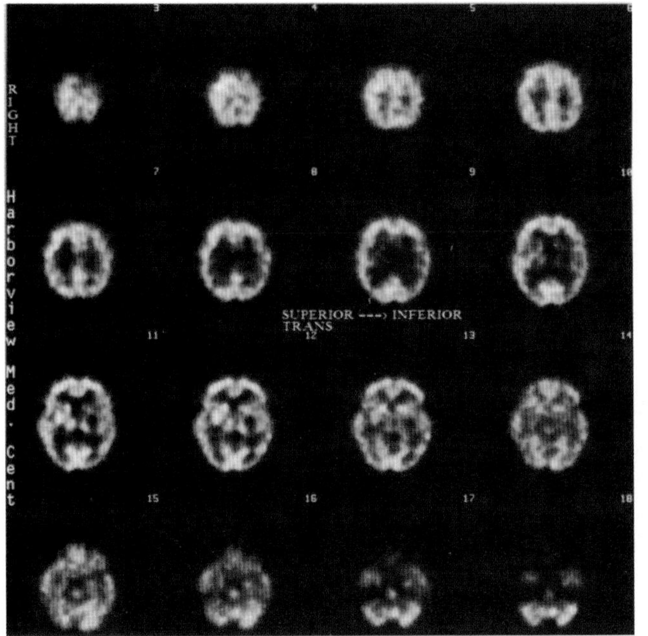

FIGURE 63.5. Subcortical Cerebral Infarct.

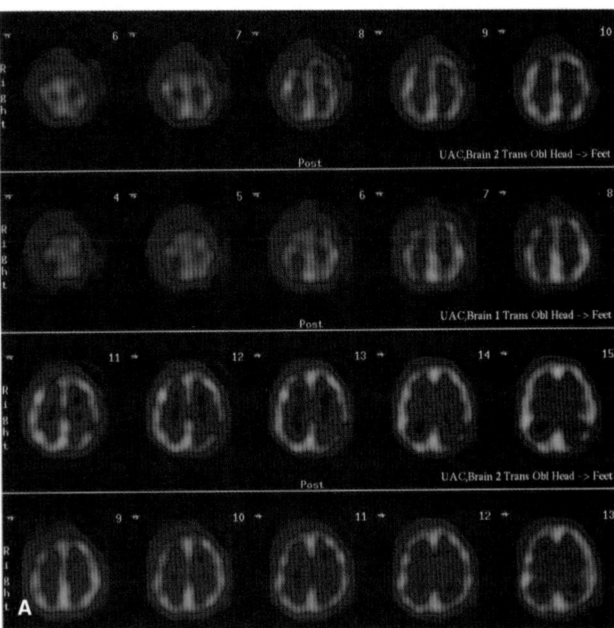

FIGURE 63.6A. Subarachnoid Hemorrhage and Cerebral Vasospasm.

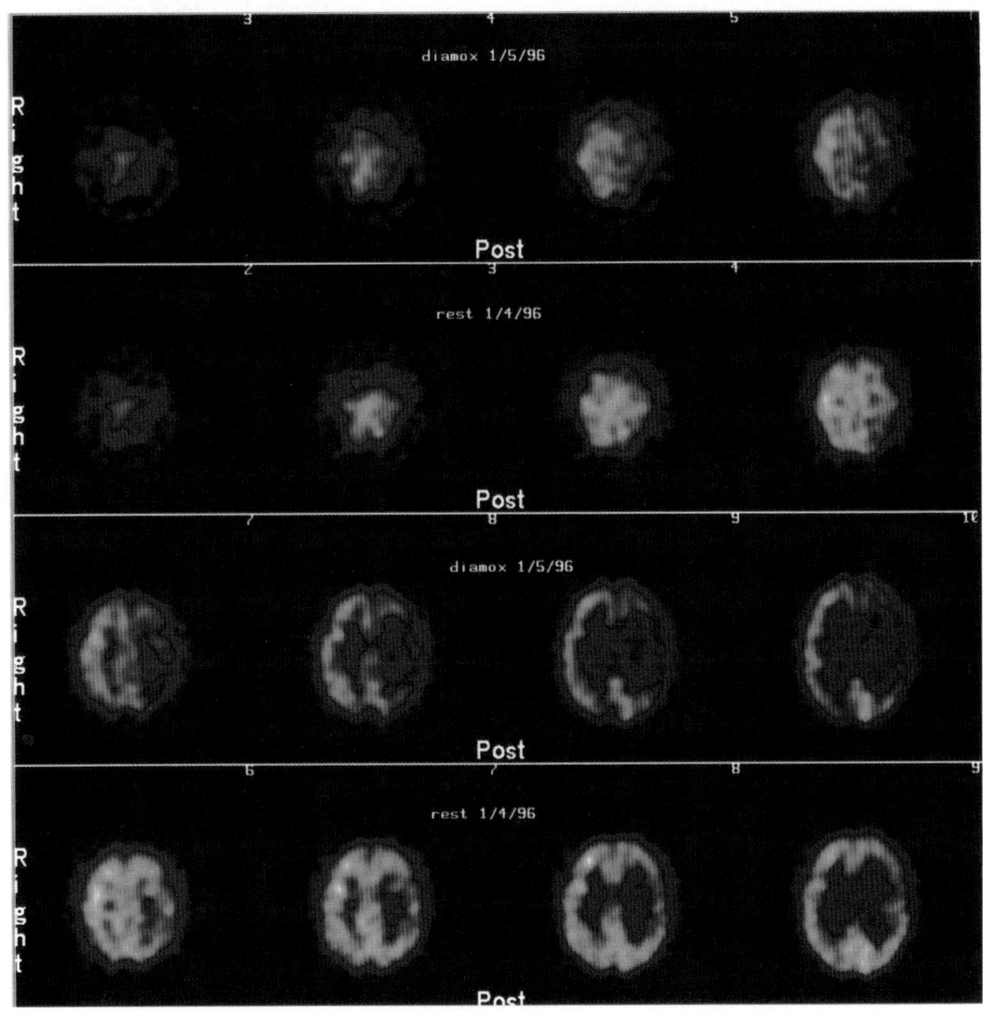

FIGURE 63.7. Acetazolamide Vascular Reserve Testing in Occlusive Carotid Disease.

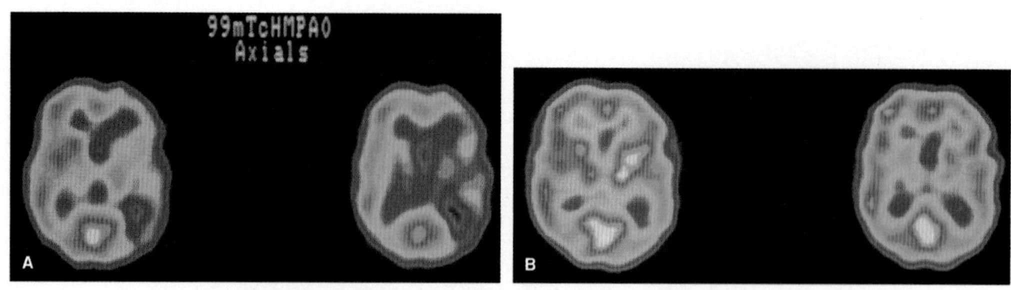

FIGURE 63.8. Positive Balloon Occlusion Study.

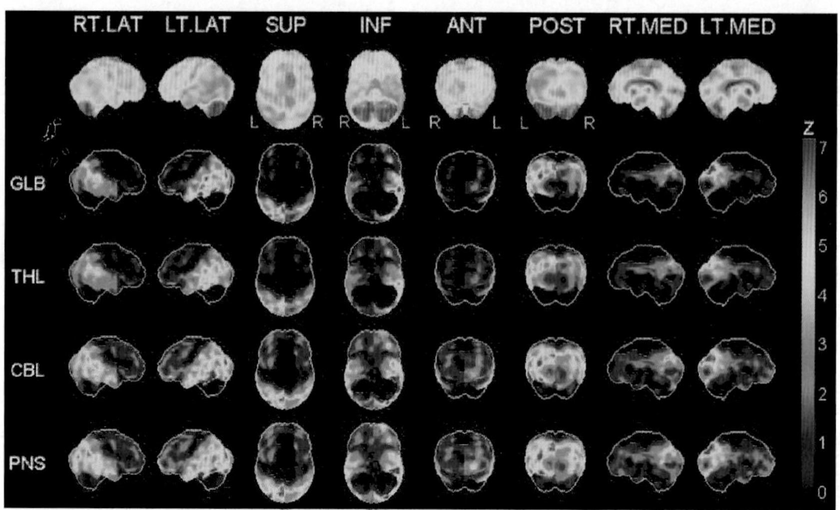

FIGURE 63.10. Three-dimensional SSP Display of SPECT in Alzheimer Disease.

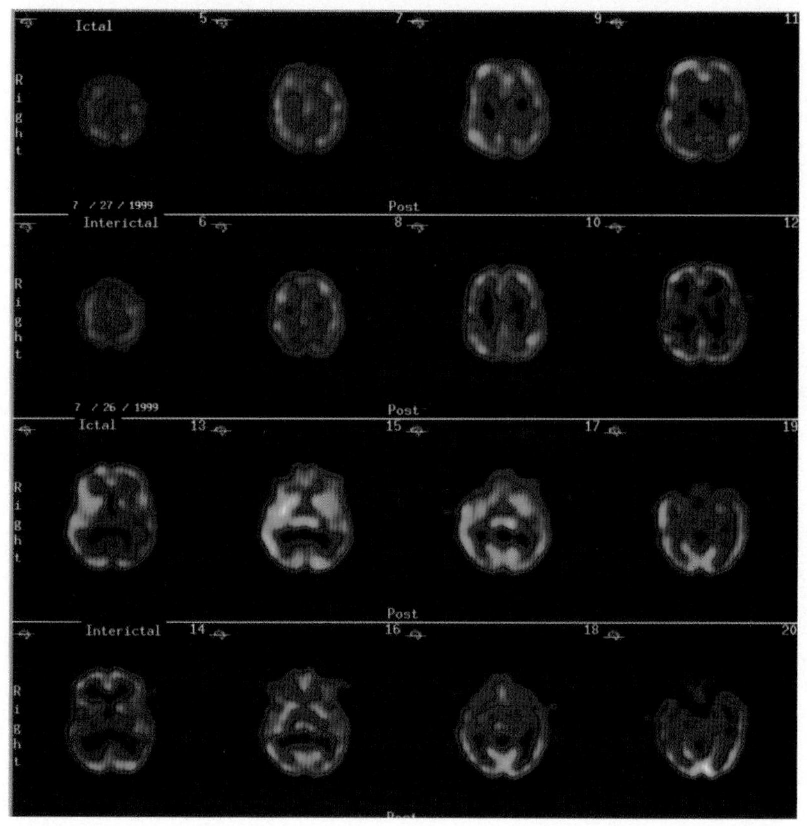

FIGURE 63.11. Ictal and Interictal SPECT Scans in Complex Partial Epilepsy.

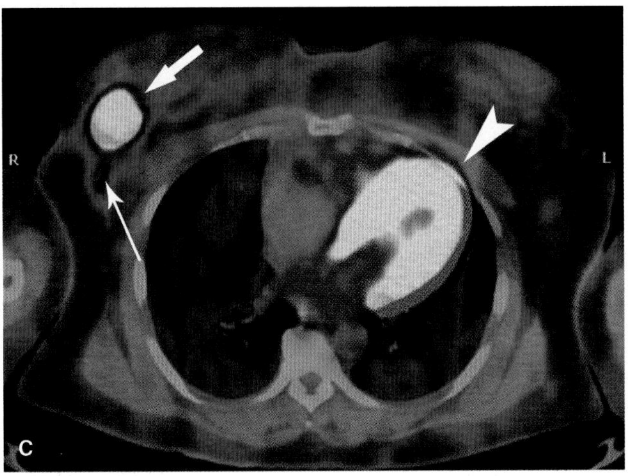

FIGURE 64.1C. **Breast Cancer PET-CT.**

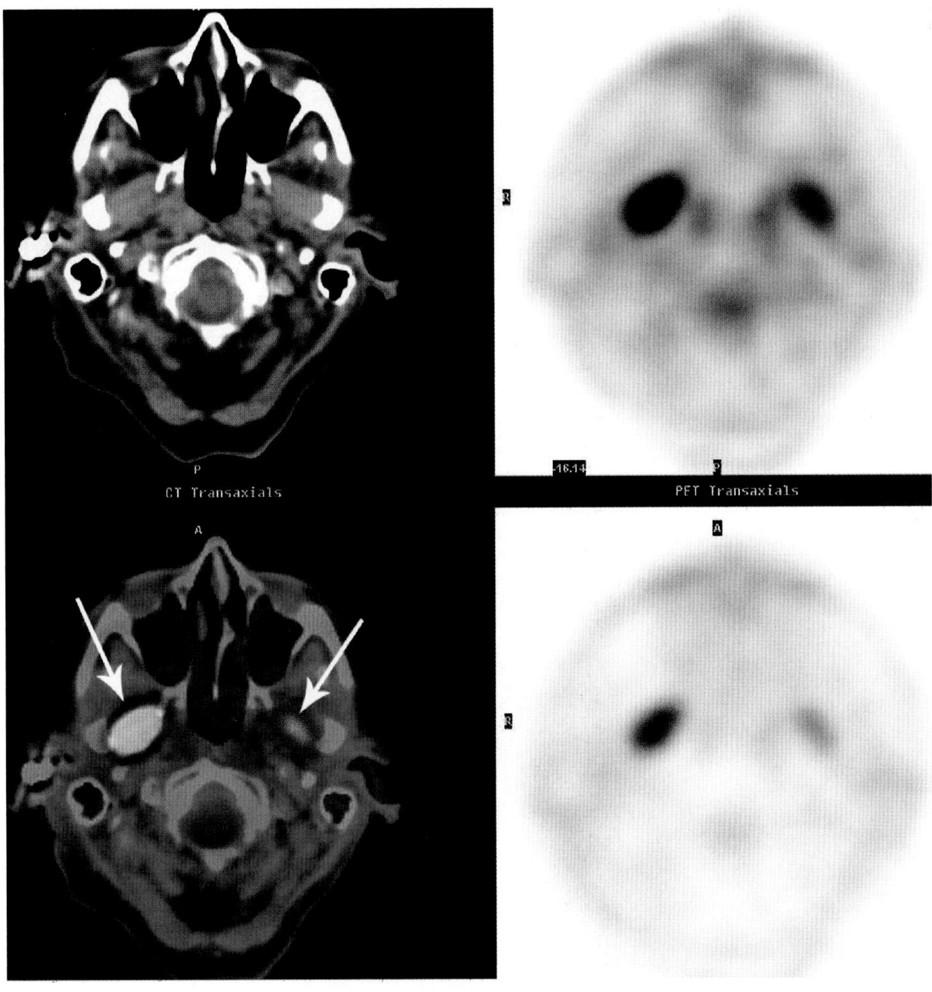

FIGURE 64.2. **Physiologic Fluorodeoxyglucose (FDG) Activity in Muscle.**

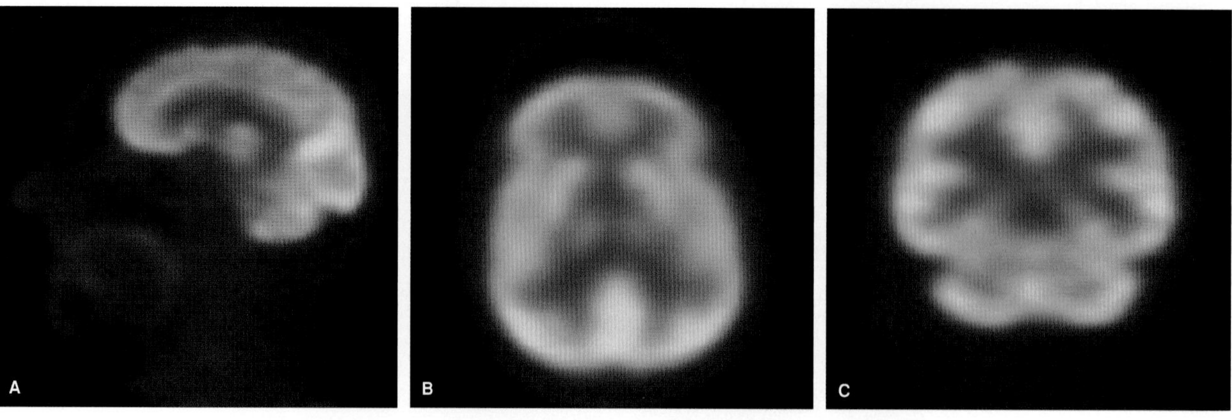

FIGURE 64.3. **Physiologic Fluorodeoxyglucose (FDG) Activity in the Brain.**

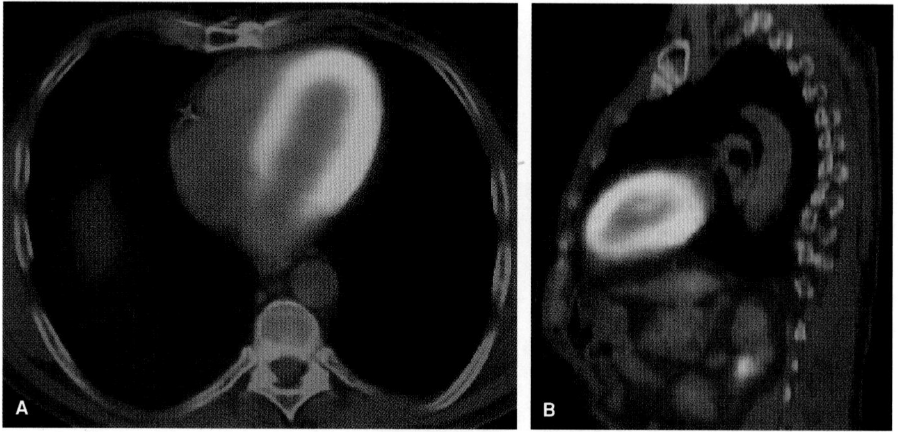

FIGURE 64.4. **Physiologic Fluorodeoxyglucose (FDG) Activity in the Heart.**

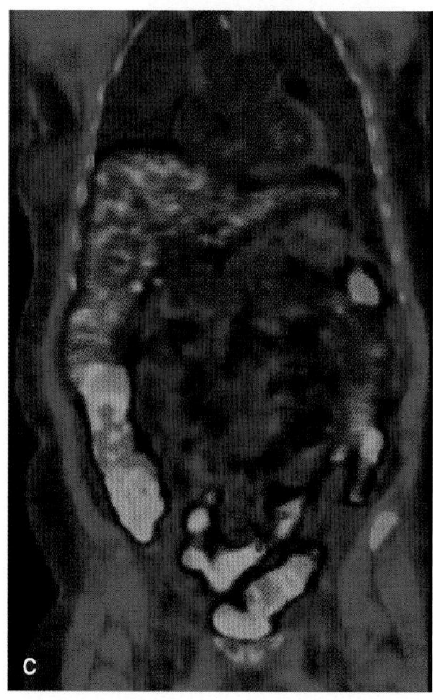

FIGURE 64.6C. **Massive Physiologic Colon Activity.**

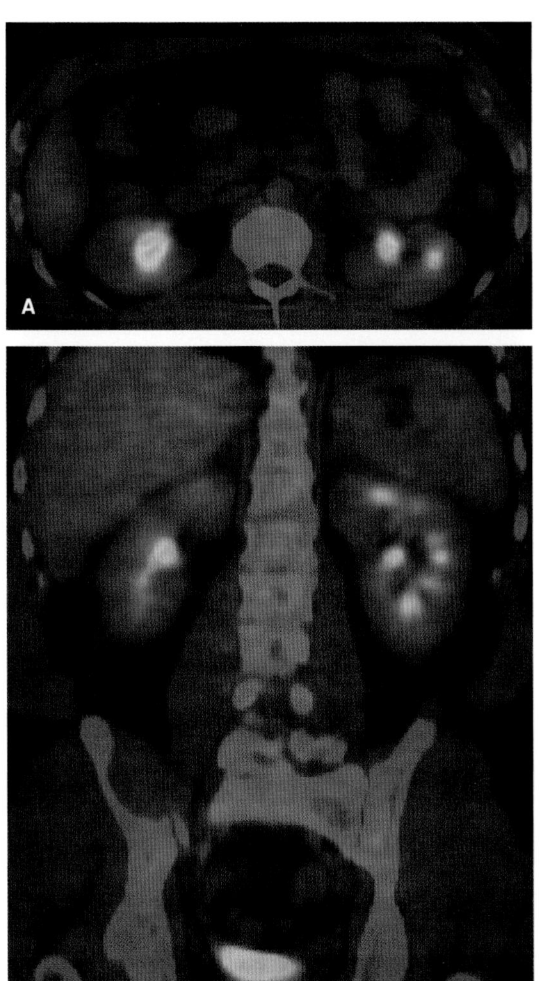

FIGURE 64.7. **Normal Physiologic Activity in the Urinary Tract.**

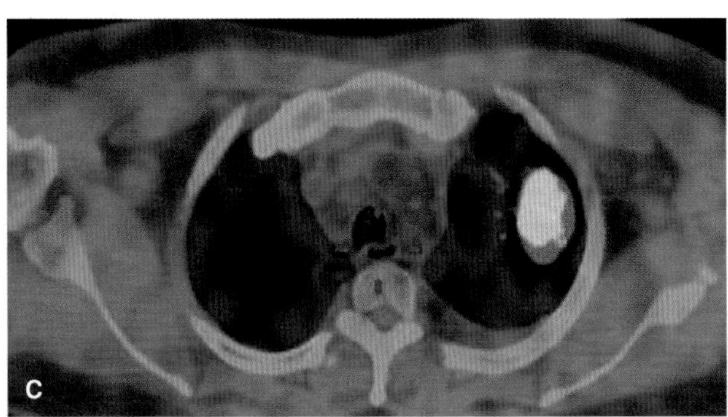

FIGURE 64.8C. **Hot Pulmonary Nodule: Bronchogenic Carcinoma.**

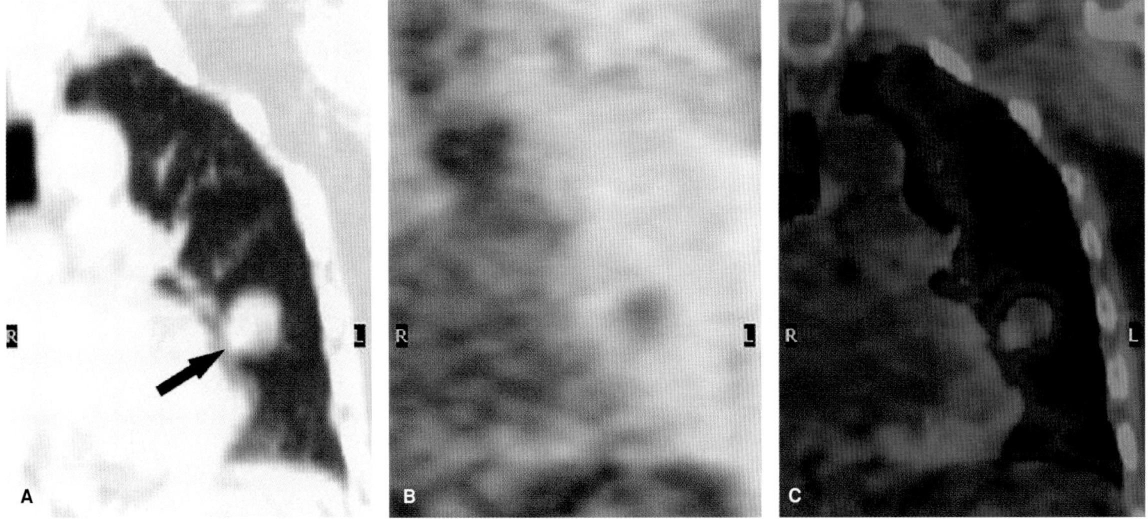

FIGURE 64.9. **Warm Pulmonary Nodule: Bronchoalveolar Carcinoma.**

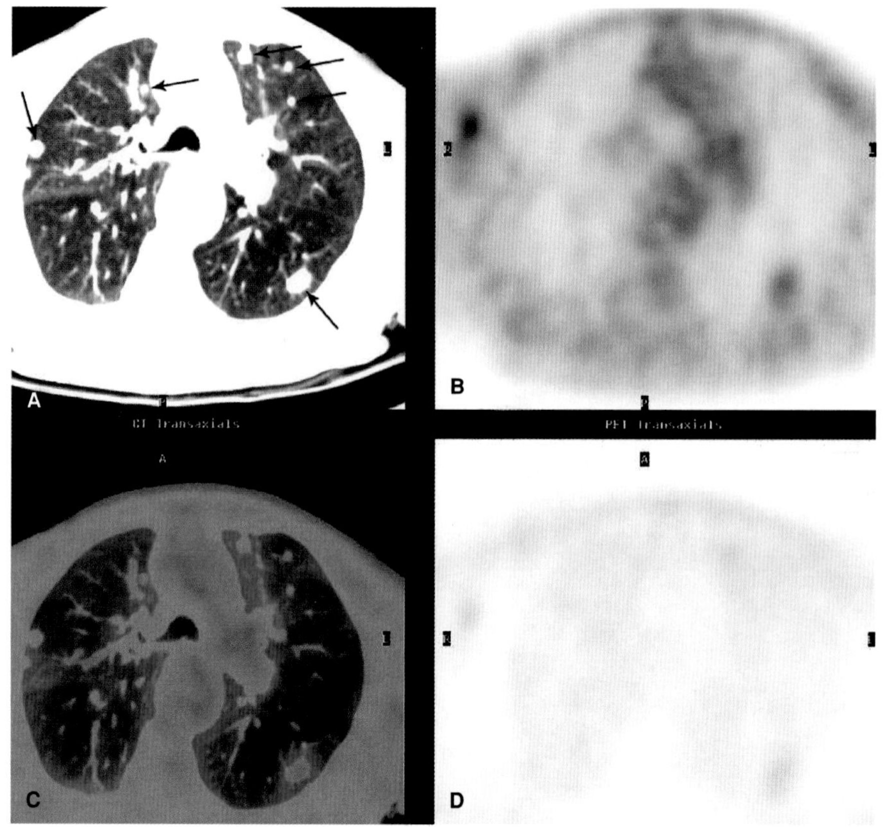

FIGURE 64.10. **Multiple Pulmonary Nodules.**

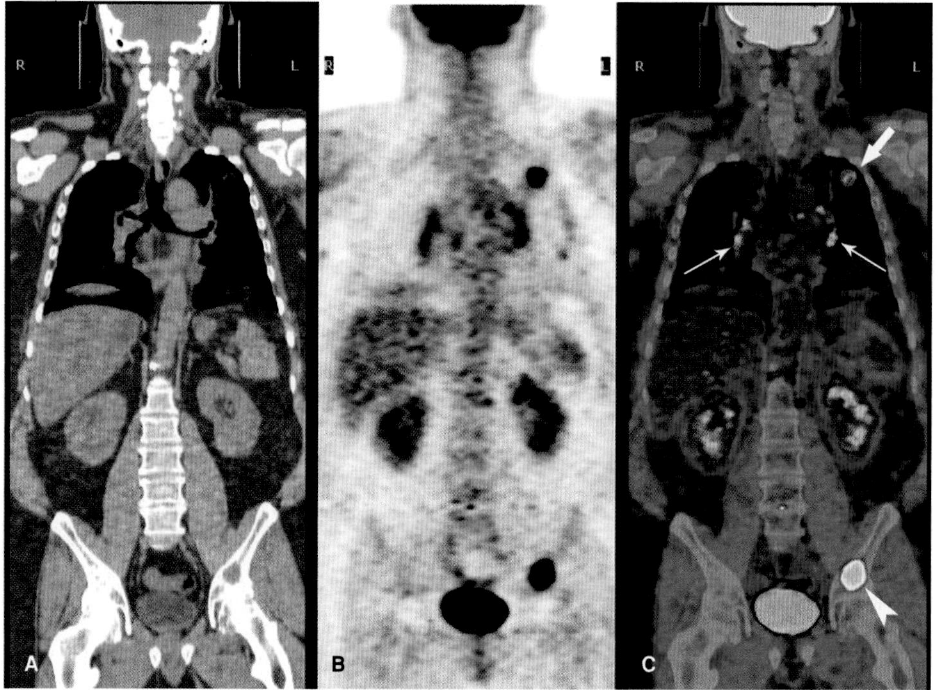

FIGURE 64.11. **Lung Cancer Staging.**

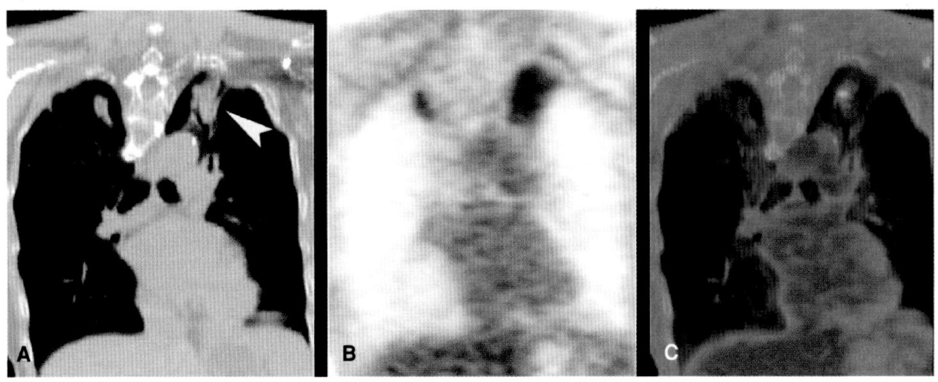

FIGURE 64.12. Postradiation Pneumonitis.

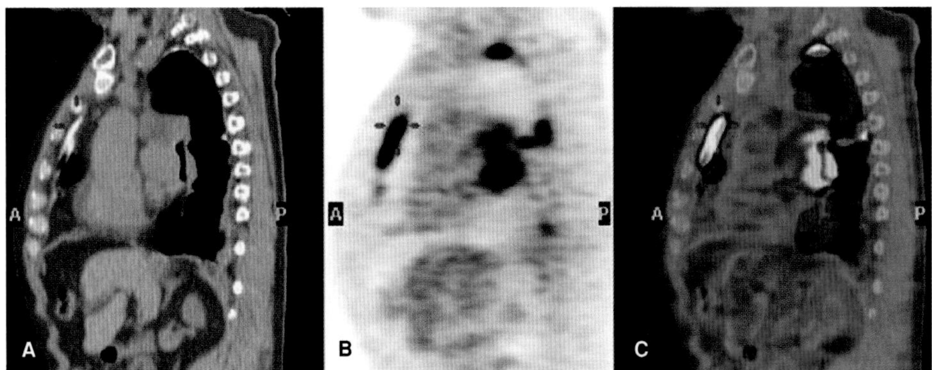

FIGURE 64.13. Lymphoma Staging.

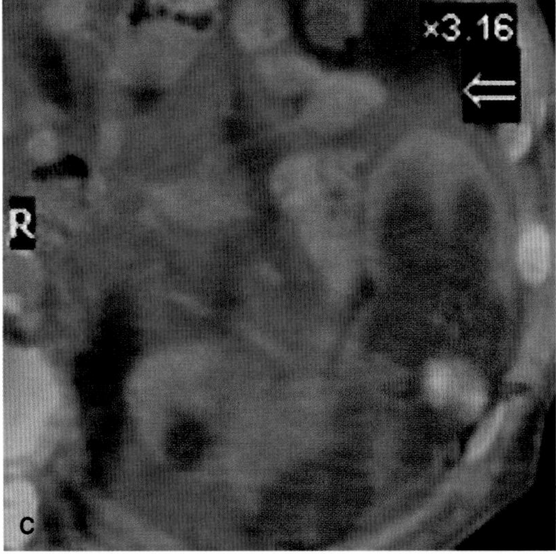

FIGURE 64.14C. Spleen Lymphoma.

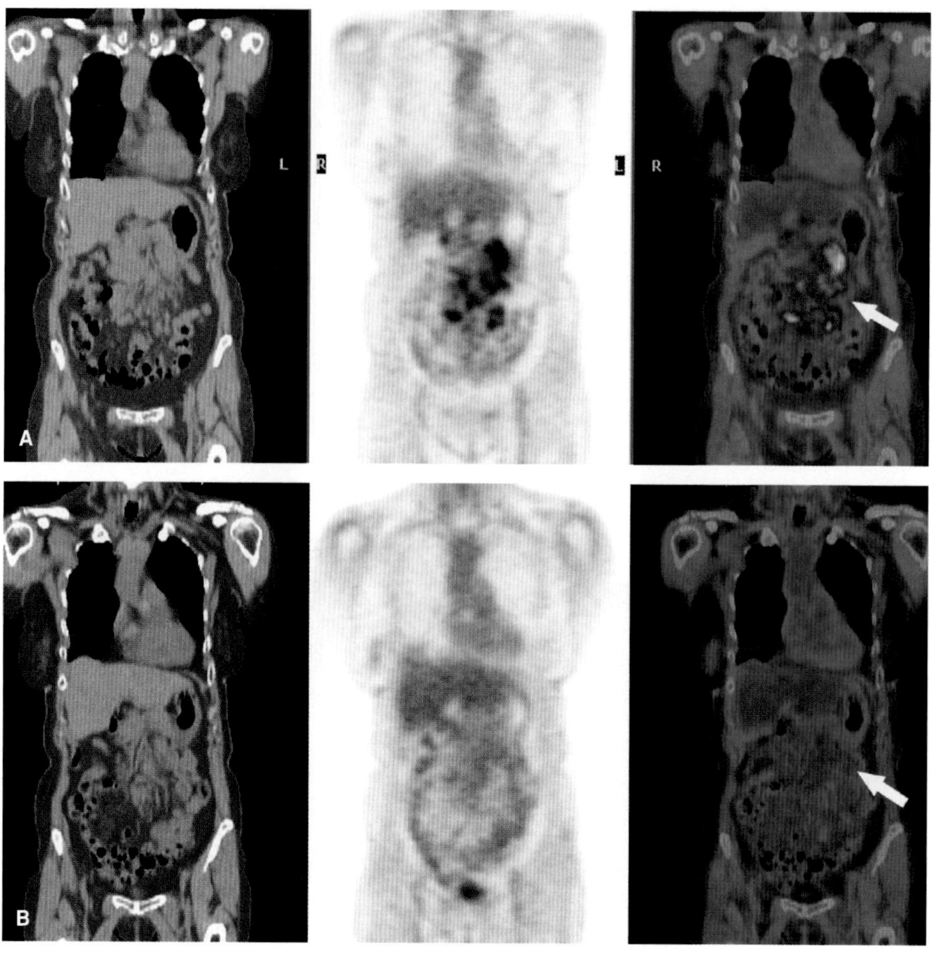

FIGURE 64.15. Lymphoma: Early Response to Therapy.

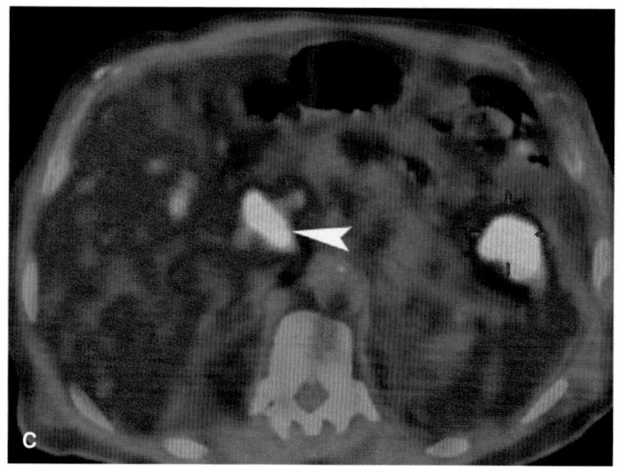

FIGURE 64.16C. Colon Cancer Staging.

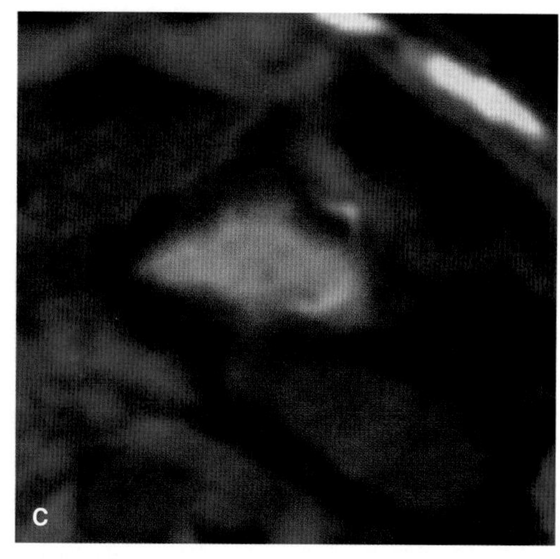

FIGURE 64.17C. Colon Cancer: Anastomosis Activity.

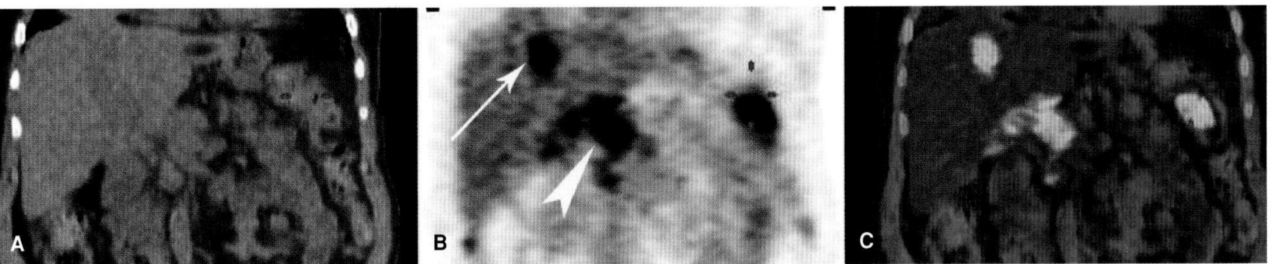

FIGURE 64.18. **Hepatic Metastasis: Colon Cancer.**

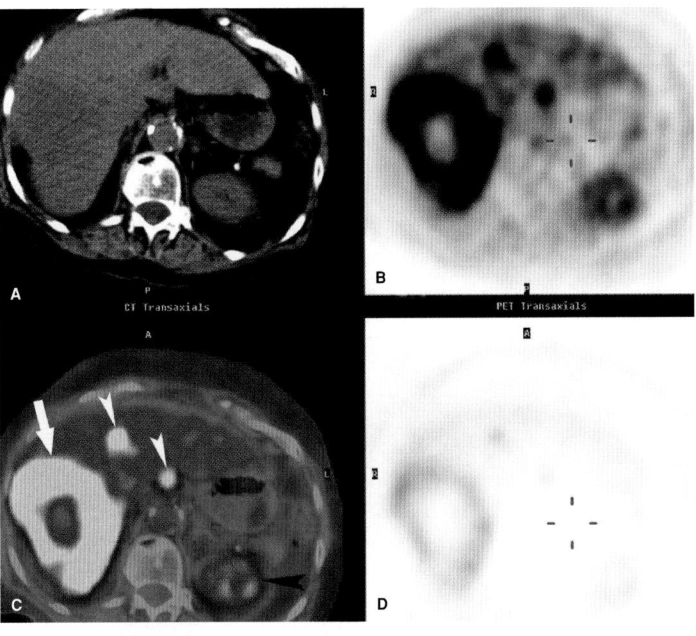

FIGURE 64.19. **Necrotic Hepatic Metastasis.**

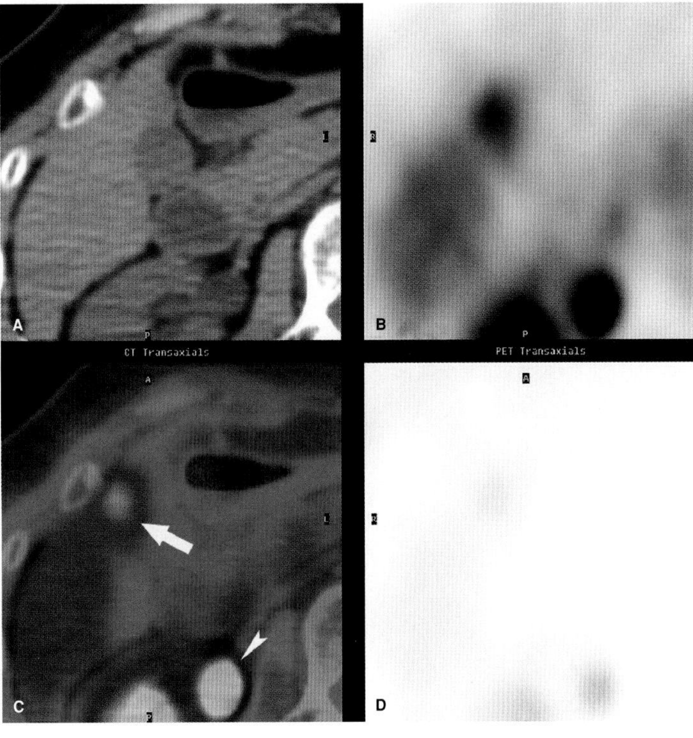

FIGURE 64.20. **Chronic Cholecystitis.**

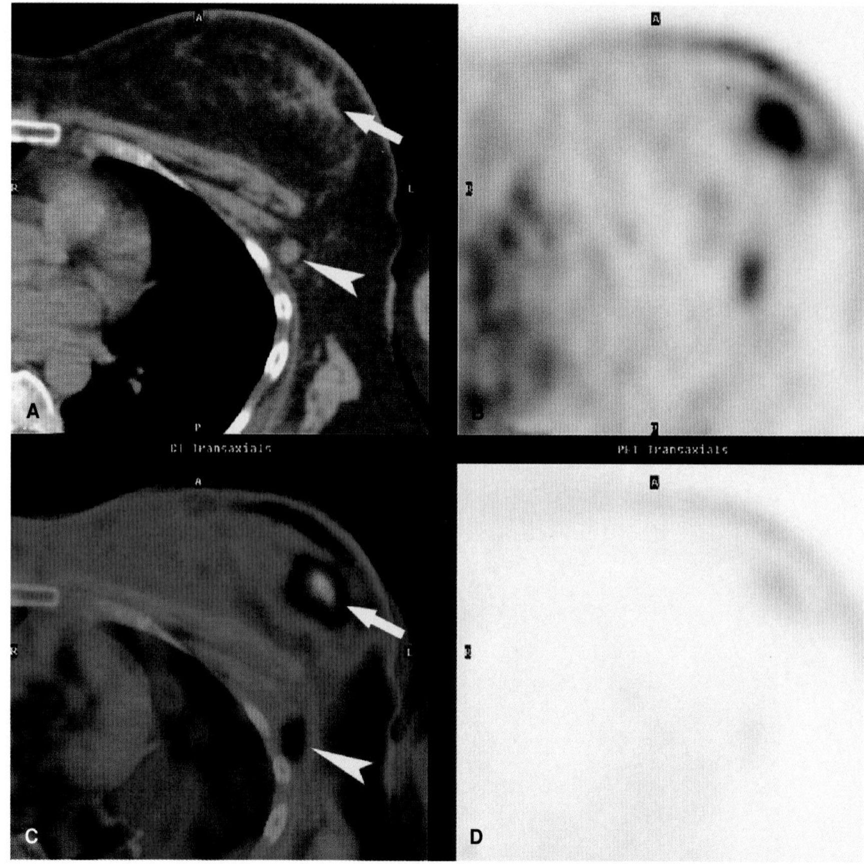

FIGURE 64.21. **Breast Cancer: Axillary Node Metastasis.**

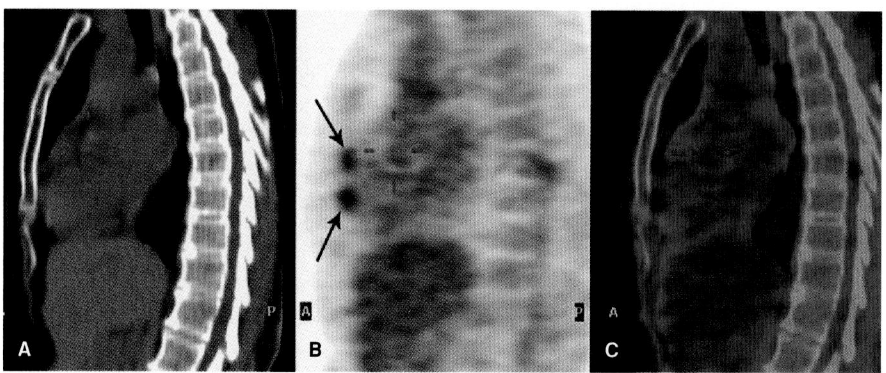

FIGURE 64.22. **Breast Cancer: Internal Mammary Node Metastases.**

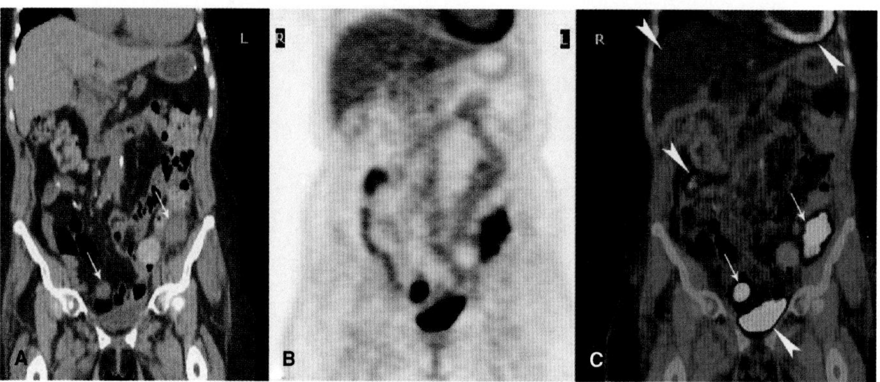

FIGURE 64.23. **Uterine Cancer Recurrence.**

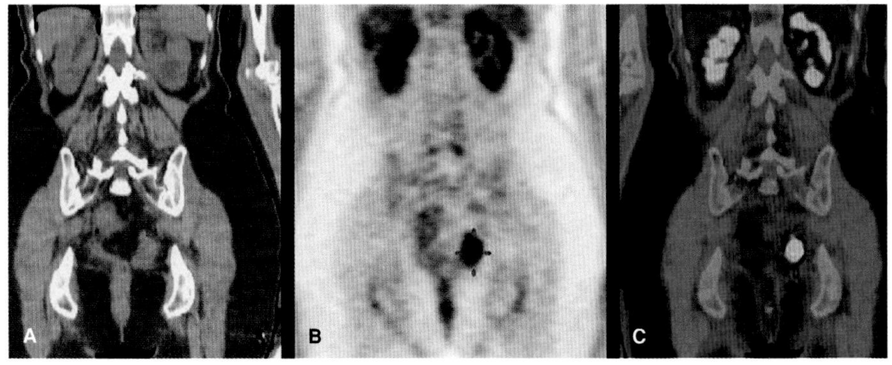

FIGURE 64.24. **Ovarian Cancer, Stage 1.**

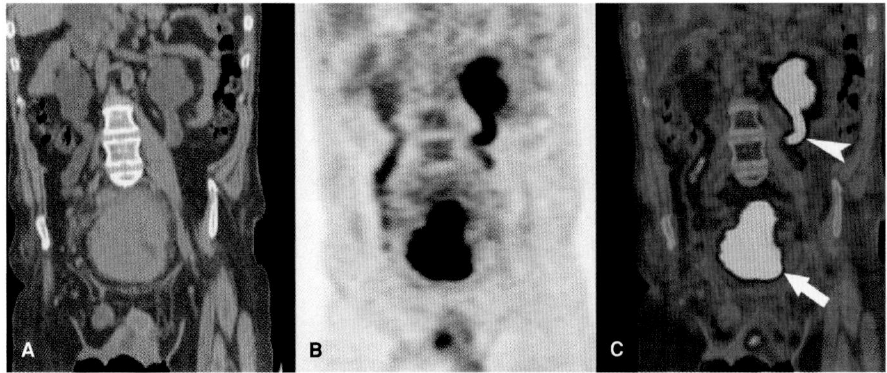

FIGURE 64.25. **Transitional Cell Carcinoma of the Bladder.**

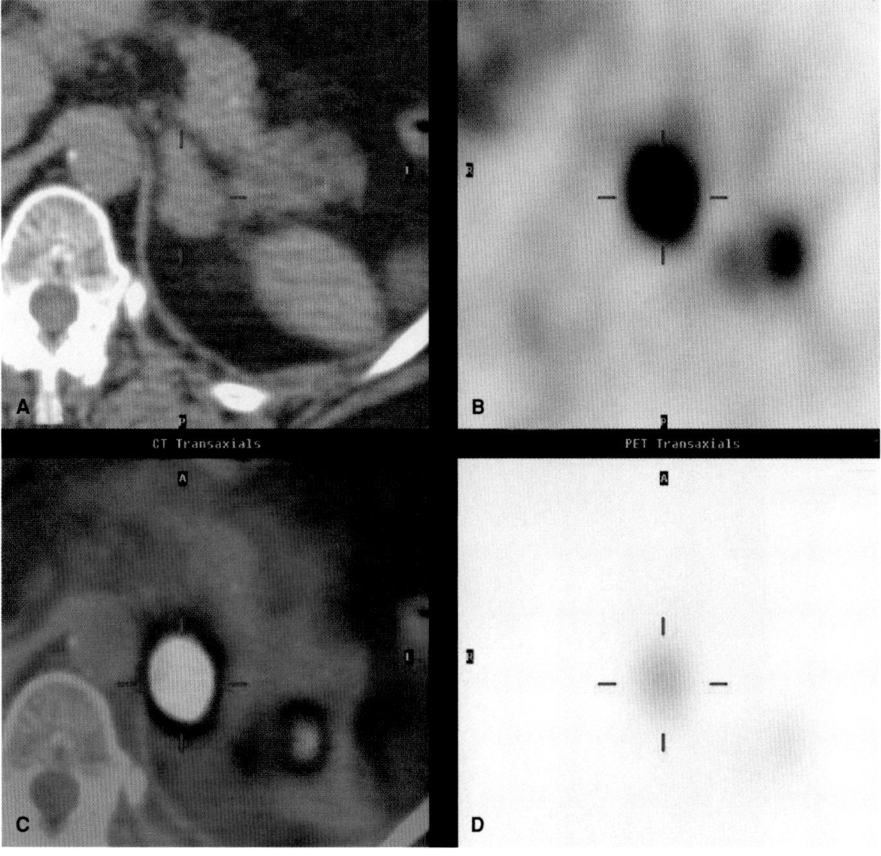

FIGURE 64.26. **Adrenal Metastasis.**

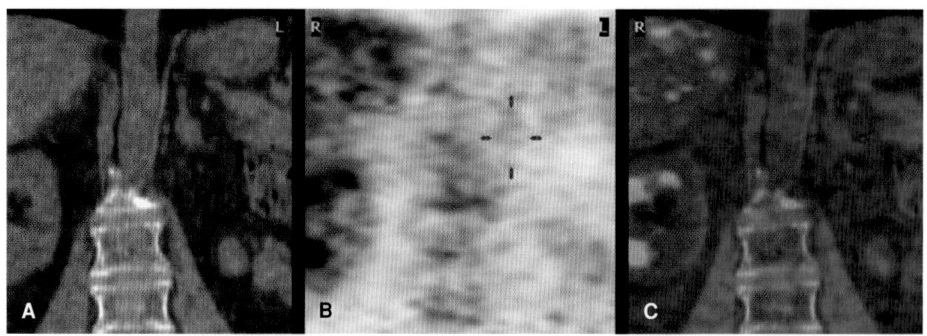

FIGURE 64.27. **Benign Adrenal Adenoma.**

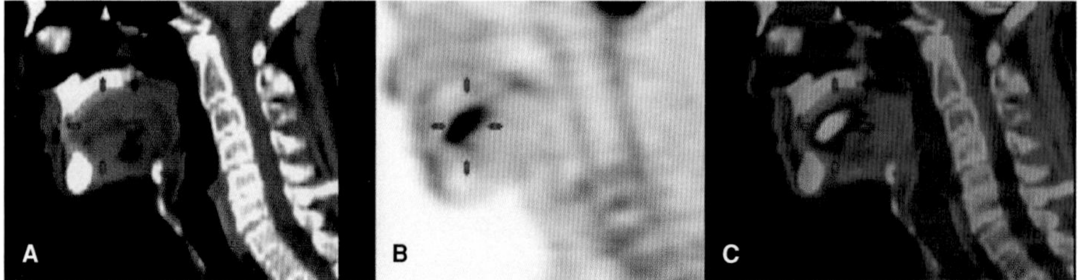

FIGURE 64.28. **Squamous Cell Carcinoma of the Tongue.**

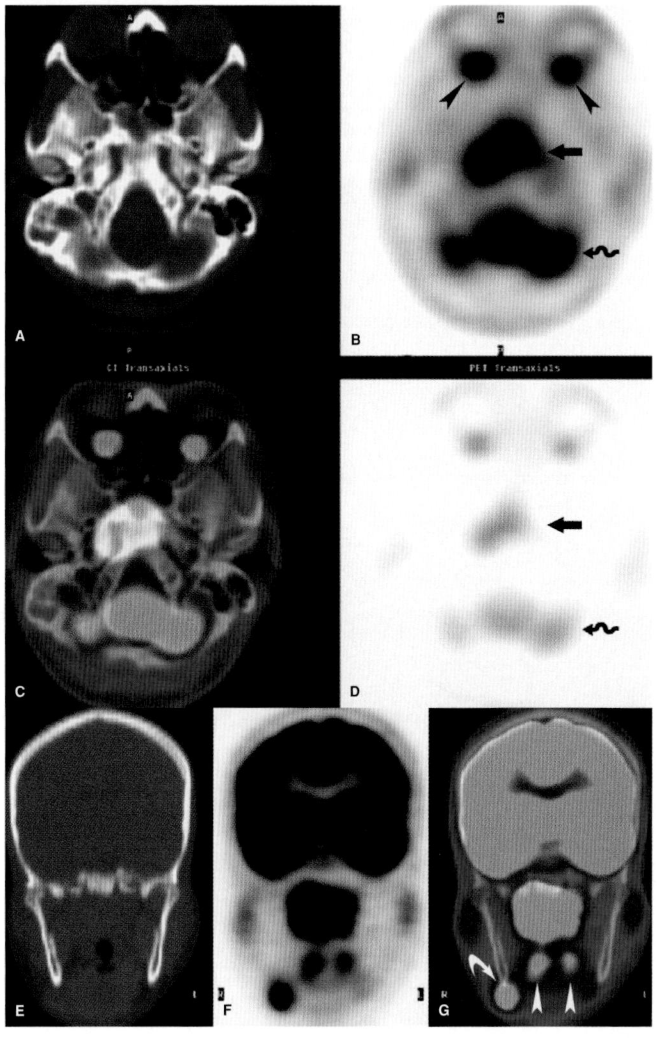

FIGURE 64.29. **Metastatic Squamous Cell Carcinoma of the Nasopharynx.**

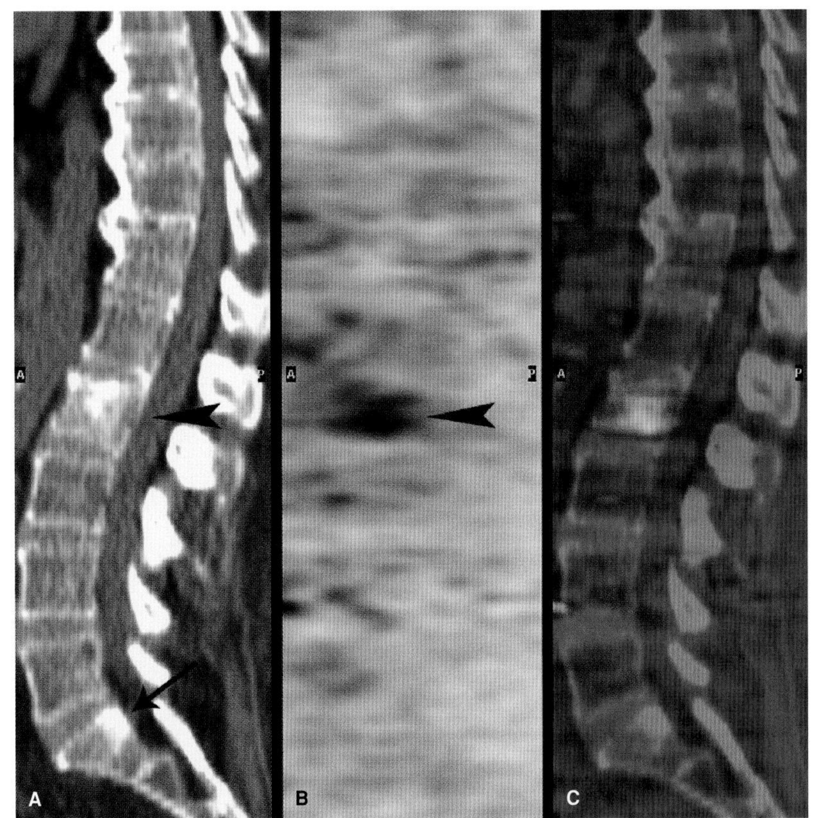

FIGURE 64.30. **Metastasis to Spine.**

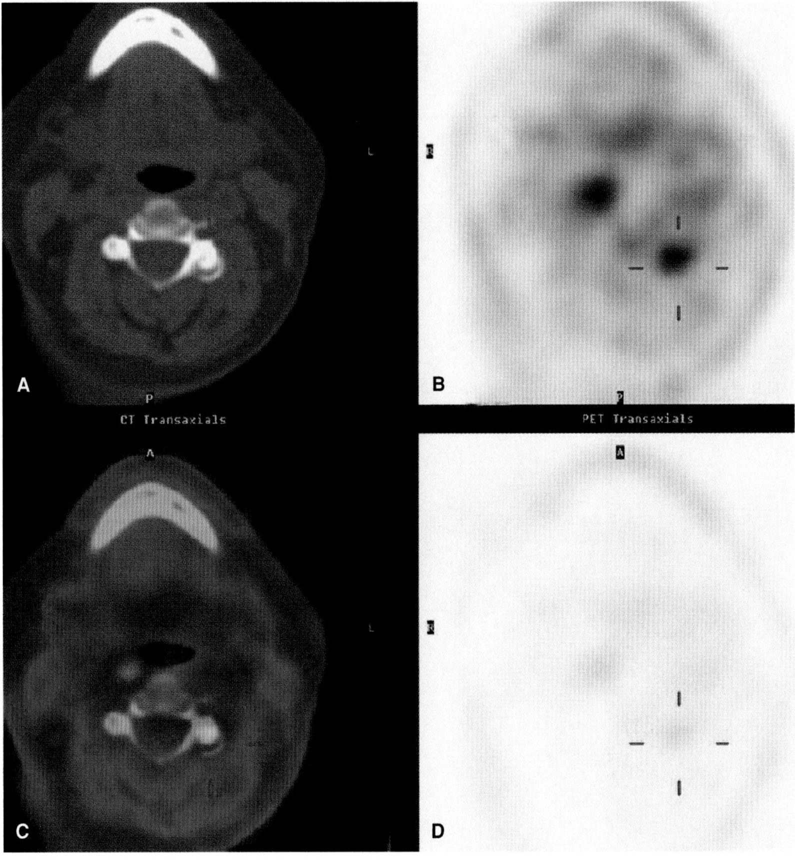

FIGURE 64.31. **Facet Hypertrophy, Not Metastasis.**

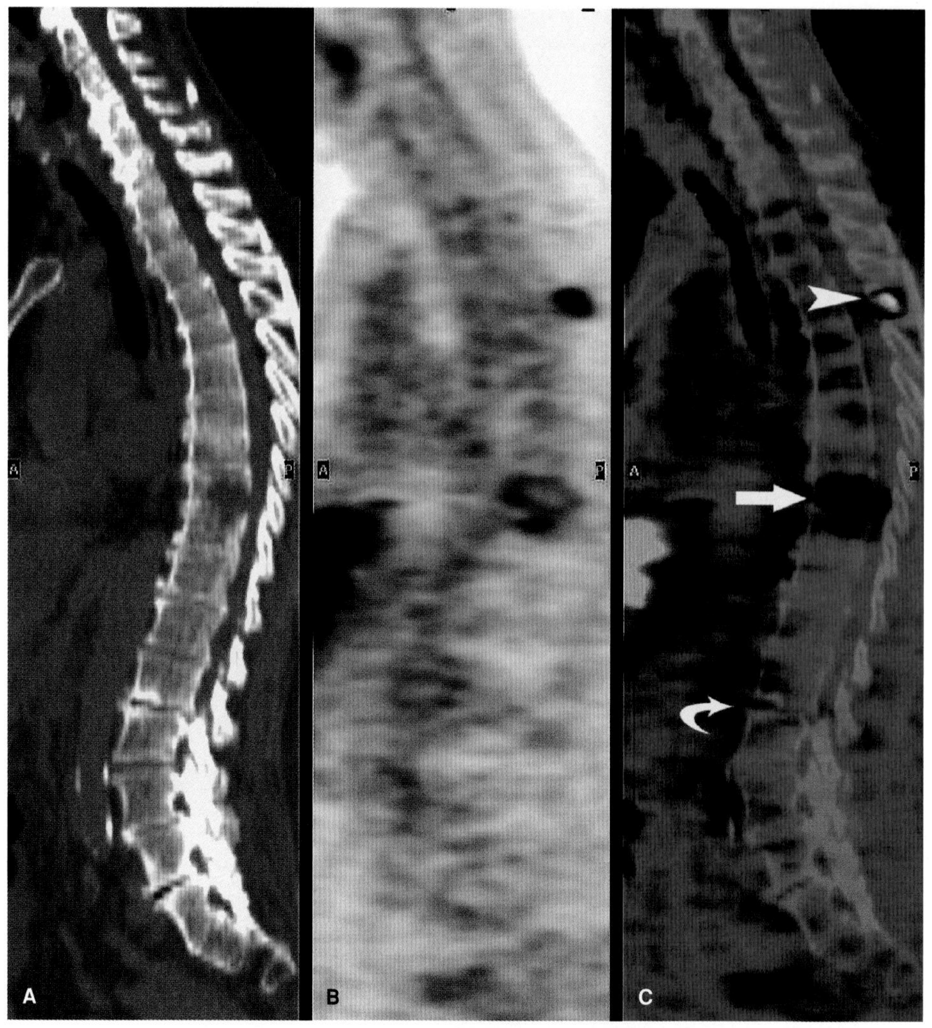

FIGURE 64.32. **"Hot" and "Cold" Osseous Metastases.**

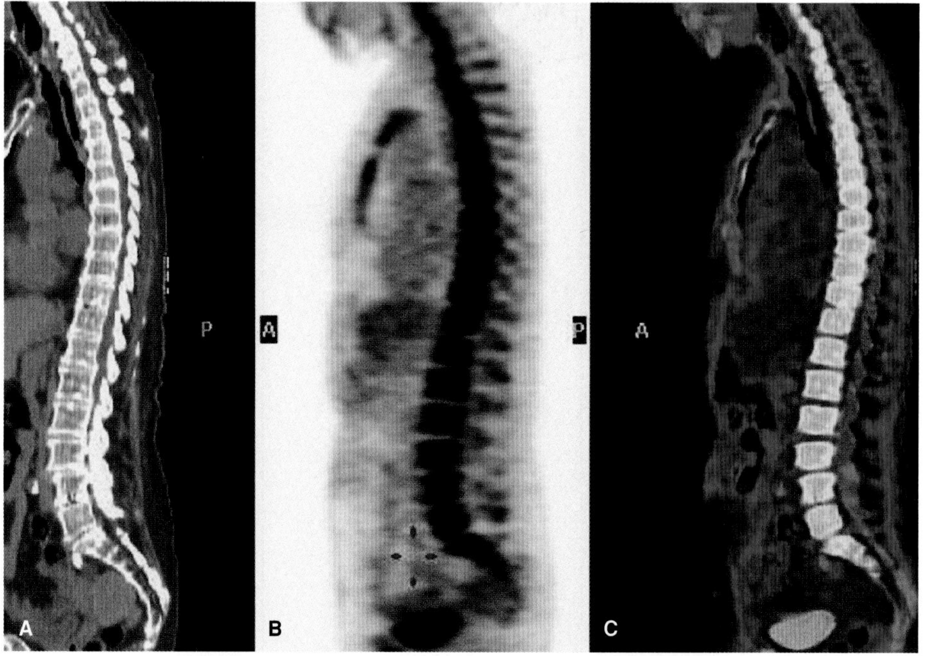

FIGURE 64.33. **Benign Hypermetabolic Bone Marrow.**

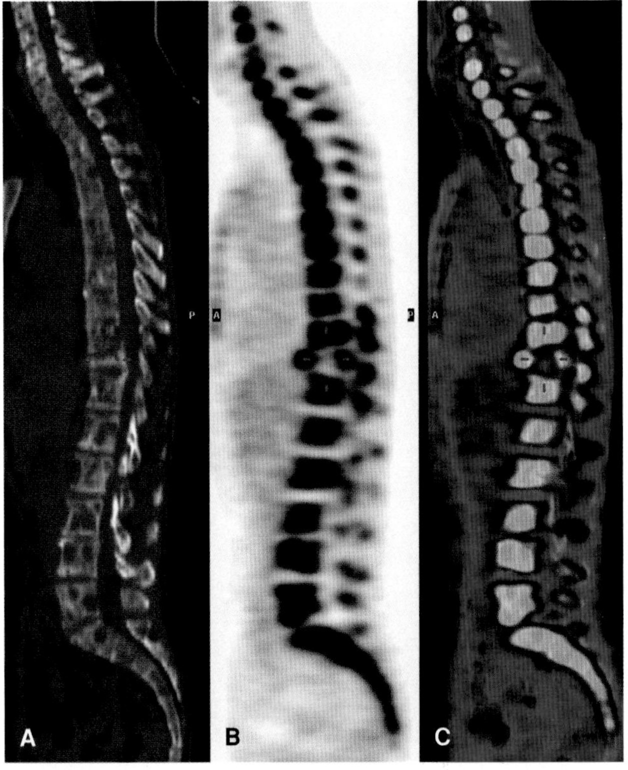

FIGURE 64.34. Diffuse Metastatic Disease With Hypermetabolic Bone Marrow.

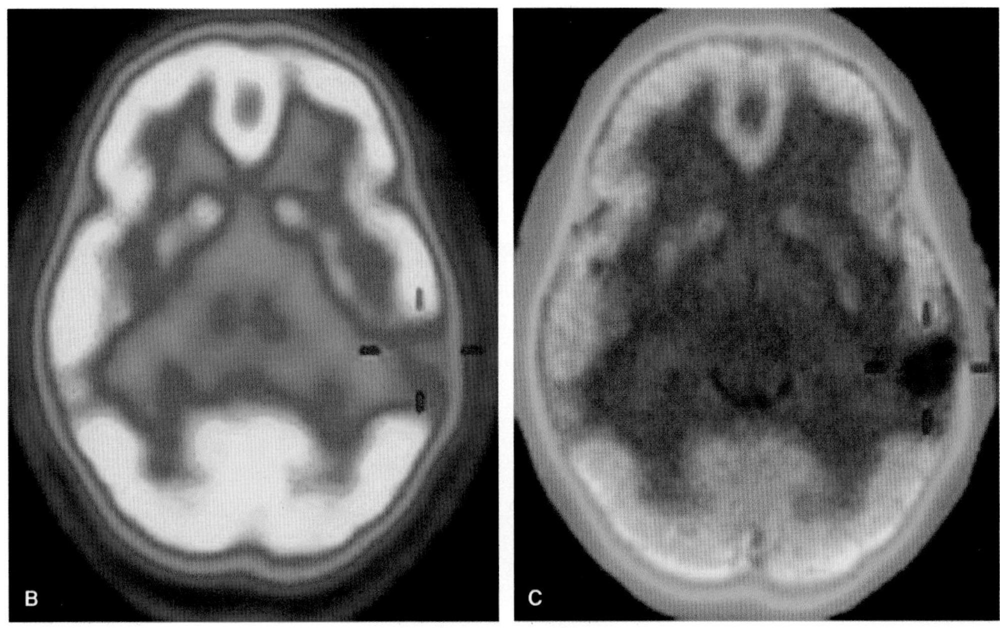

FIGURE 64.35B, C. Benign Intra-axial Brain Cyst.

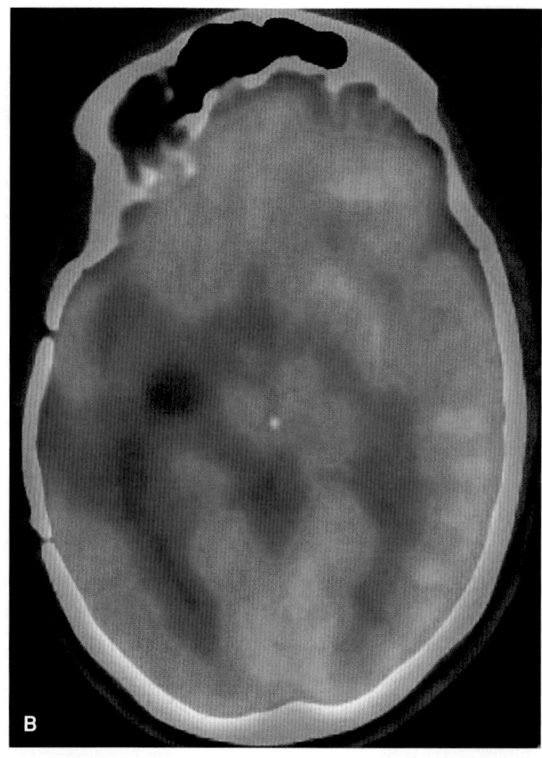

FIGURE 64.36B. Absence of Residual Brain Tumor.

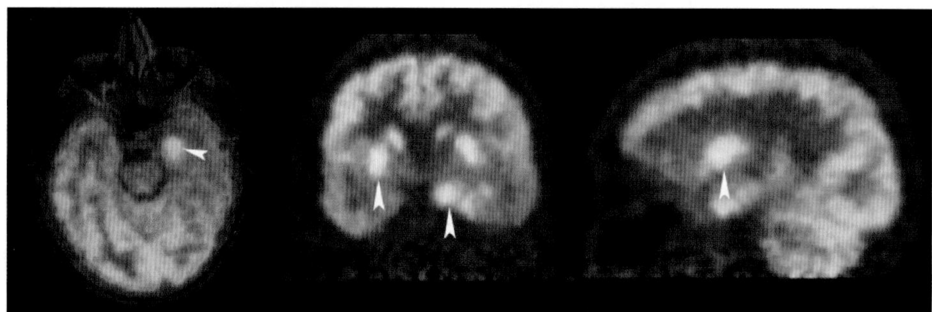

FIGURE 64.37. Brain Metastases.

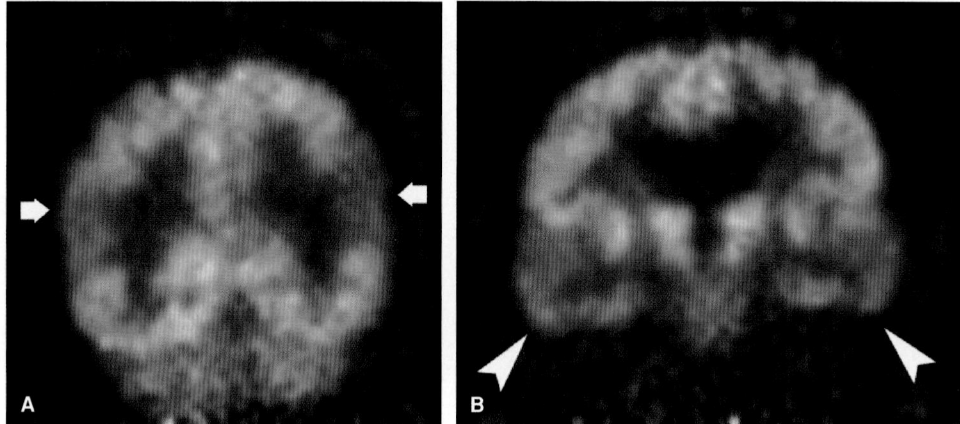

FIGURE 64.38. Alzheimer Dementia.

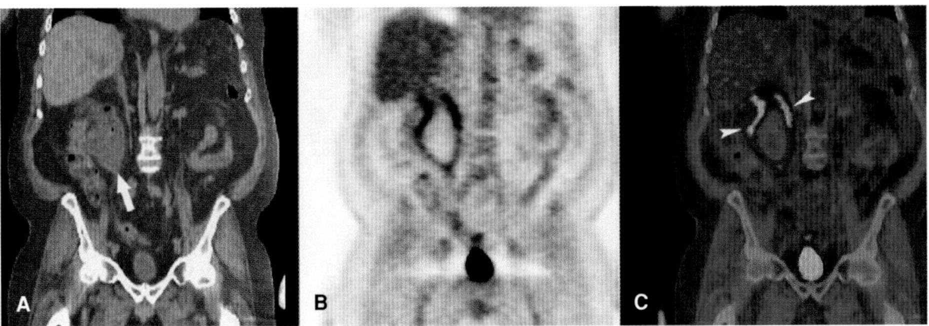

FIGURE 64.40. Abdominal Abscess.

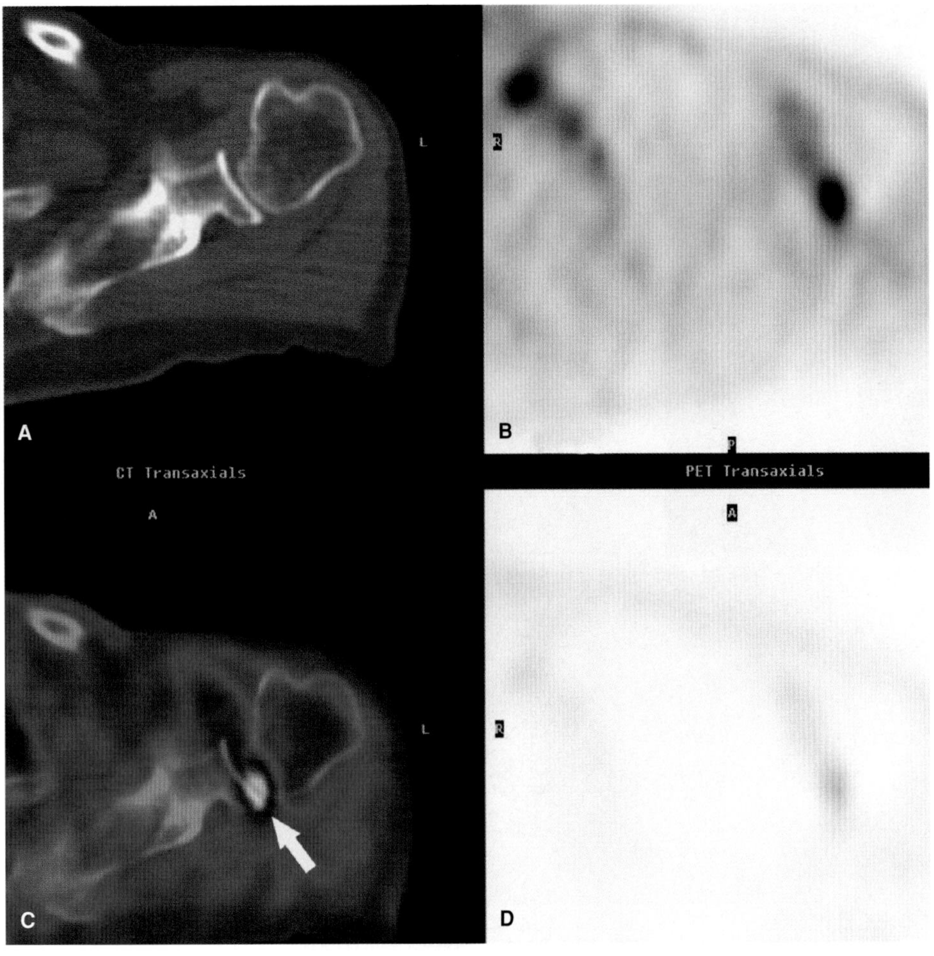

FIGURE 64.41. Shoulder Arthritis.

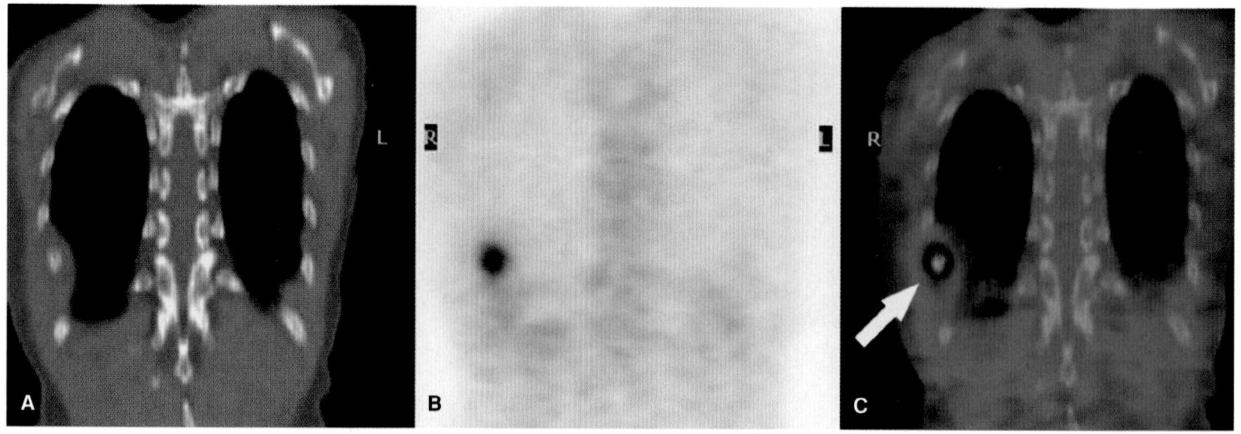

FIGURE 64.42. **Rib Fracture.**

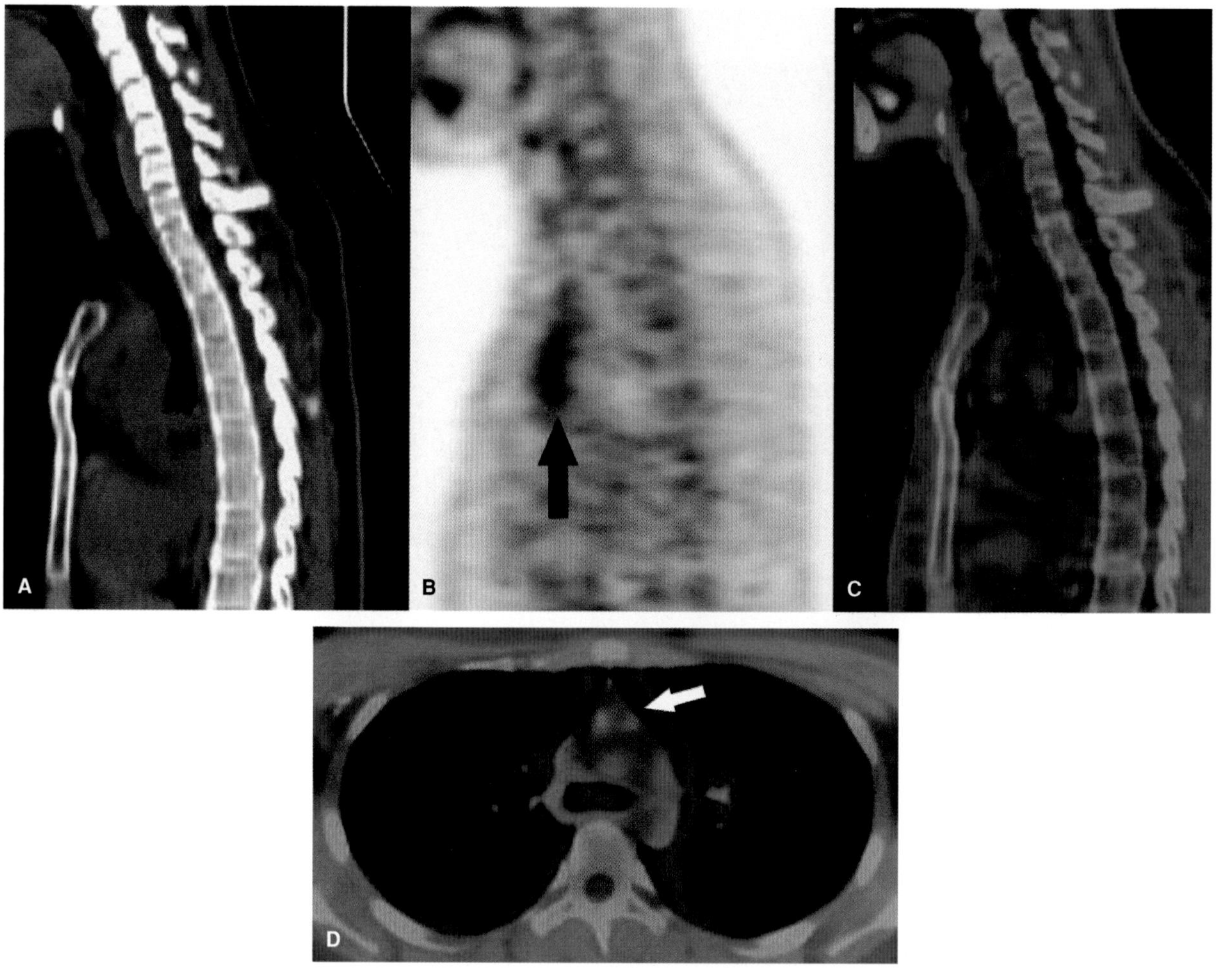

FIGURE 64.43. **Thymic Rebound.**

SECTION X

Musculoskeletal Radiology

Chapter 41

Benign Cystic Bone Lesions

Clyde A. Helms

Fegnomashic
- Fibrous Dysplasia
- Enchondroma and Eosinophilic Granuloma
- Giant Cell Tumor
- Nonossifying Fibroma
- Osteoblastoma
- Metastatic Disease and Myeloma
- Aneurysmal Bone Cyst
- Solitary Bone Cyst
- Hyperparathyroidism (Brown Tumors)
- Infection
- Chondroblastoma
- Chondromyxoid Fibroma

Summary

Differential Diagnosis of a Sclerotic Lesion

A benign, bubbly, cystic lesion of bone is one of the more common skeletal lesions that a radiologist encounters. The differential diagnosis can be quite lengthy and is usually structured on how the lesion looks to the radiologist, using his or her experience as a guide. This method, called *pattern identification,* certainly has merit, but it can lead to a very long differential diagnosis and many erroneous conclusions if not tempered with some logic.

In general, if a differential diagnosis will yield the correct diagnosis 95% of the time, most would consider it a useful differential list; however, it would not be appropriate to accept a 1-in-20 miss rate for fractures and dislocations. In general, the shorter the differential diagnosis list, the more helpful it is to clinicians and the easier it is to remember. A shorter differential list will usually have a lower accuracy rate than a long list; however, many times the longer lists contain such rare entities that the accuracy does not really increase substantially. For most of the entities in bone radiology, a 95% accurate differential is acceptable. If one wants to be more accurate than that, more diagnoses can simply be added to the list of differential possibilities.

When the differential diagnosis is long, as in the differential for bubbly, cystic lesions of bone, it can be difficult to recall all of the entities that should be mentioned. A mnemonic can be helpful in recalling long lists of information and is recommended.

FEGNOMASHIC

FEGNOMASHIC is a mnemonic that serves as a nice starting point for discussing possibilities that appear as benign, cystic lesions in bone. This mnemonic has been in general use for many years. By itself, it is merely a long list—14 entities—and it needs to be coupled with other criteria to shorten the list into a manageable form for each particular case. For instance, the age of the patient will help add or eliminate many of the possibilities. If multiple lesions are present, only half a dozen entities need to be discussed. Methods of narrowing the differential are discussed later in this chapter.

The first step in approaching a benign, cystic bone lesion is to be certain it is really benign. The criteria for differentiating benign lesions from malignant lesions are covered in Chapter 42. Once it is established that the lesion is truly a benign, cystic lesion, FEGNOMASHIC will enable a differential diagnosis that is at least 95% accurate. Memorization of the 14 entities in this differential is easily done (Table 41.1).

The next step after learning the names of all of the lesions is getting some idea of each lesion's radiographic appearance. This is when experience becomes a factor. For the medical student or first-year resident, it is difficult to go beyond saying that they all look cystic, bubbly, and benign. The fourth-year resident should have no trouble

TABLE 41.1 Discriminators for Benign Lytic Bone Lesions—Mnemonic: FEGNOMASHIC

Letter	*Represents*	*Characteristics*
F	Fibrous dysplasia	No periosteal reaction
E	Enchondroma	1. Calcification present (except in phalanges) 2. Painless (no periostitis)
	Eosinophilic granuloma	Younger than age 30
G	Giant cell tumor	1. Epiphyses closed 2. Abuts the articular surface (in long bones) 3. Well defined with a nonsclerotic margin (in long bones) 4. Eccentric
N	Nonossifying fibroma	1. Younger than age 30 2. Painless (no periostitis) 3. Cortically based
O	Osteoblastoma	Mentioned when aneurysmal bone cyst (ABC) is mentioned (especially in the posterior elements of the spine)
M	Metastatic diseases and myeloma	Older than age 40
A	Aneurysmal bone cyst	1. Expansile 2. Younger than age 30
S	Solitary bone cyst	1. Central 2. Younger than age 30
H	Hyperparathyroidism (brown tumor)	Must have other evidence of hyperparathyroidism
I	Infection	Always mention
C	Chondroblastoma	1. Younger than age 30 2. Epiphyseal
	Chondromyxoid	No calcified matrix

differentiating between a unicameral bone cyst and a giant cell tumor because he or she has seen examples of each many times before and knows their appearance.

After getting a feel for what each lesion looks like radiographically and overcoming the frustration that builds when one realizes that many of them look alike, one should try to learn ways to differentiate each lesion from the others. I have developed a number of keys that I call *discriminators,* which help to differentiate each lesion. These discriminators are 90% to 95% useful (I will mention when they are more or less accurate, in my experience) and are by no means intended to be absolutes or dogma. They are guidelines but have a high accuracy rate.

Textbooks rarely state that a finding "always" or "never" occurs. They temper descriptions with "virtually always," "invariably," "usually," or "characteristically." I have tried to pick out findings that come as close to "always" as I can, realizing that I will only be approximately 95% accurate. That is good enough for most radiologists.

The following is only a brief description of each entity; more complete descriptions are readily available in any skeletal radiology text. What is emphasized here are the points that are unique for each entity, thereby enabling differentiation from the others. Table 41.1 is a synopsis of these discriminators.

Fibrous Dysplasia

Fibrous dysplasia is a benign congenital process that can be seen in a patient of any age and can look like almost any pathologic process radiographically. It can be wild looking, discretely lucent, patchy, sclerotic, expansile, multiple, and many other descriptions. It is, therefore, difficult to look at a bubbly lytic lesion and unequivocally say it is or is not fibrous dysplasia. It would be better if the FEGNOMASHIC differential started on a positive note, say, with giant cell tumor or chondroblastoma, for which there are some definite criteria. However, because fibrous dysplasia is first on the list, we might as well deal with it.

How do you know whether to include or exclude fibrous dysplasia if it can look like almost anything? Experience is the best guideline. In other words, look in a few texts and find as many different examples as possible; get a feeling for what fibrous dysplasia looks like.

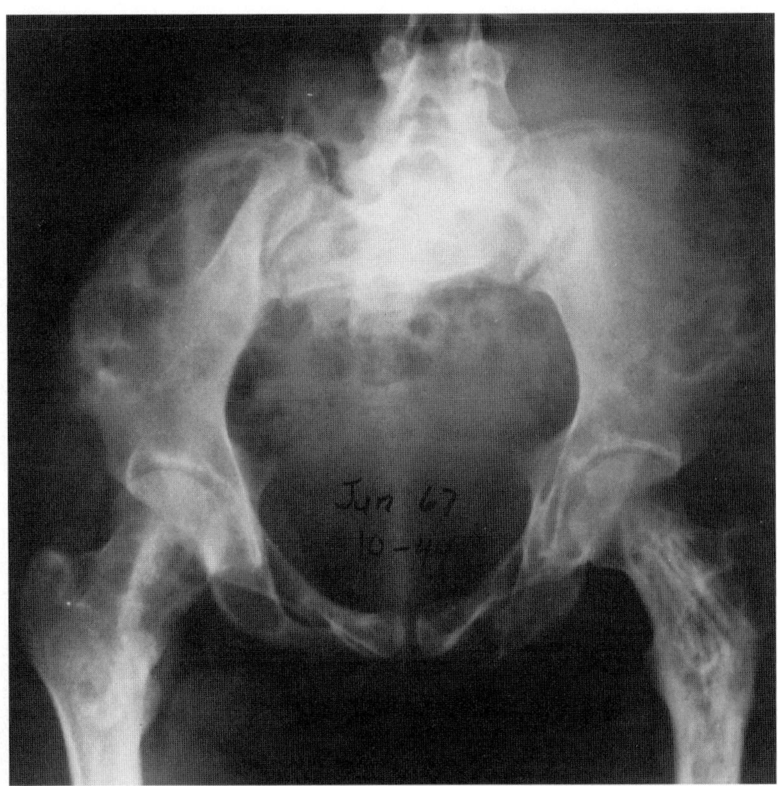

FIGURE 41.1. Fibrous Dysplasia. This patient has polyostotic fibrous dysplasia with diffuse involvement of the pelvis as well as the proximal femurs.

Fibrous dysplasia will not have periostitis associated with it; therefore, if periostitis is present, one may safely exclude fibrous dysplasia. Fibrous dysplasia virtually never undergoes malignant degeneration and should not be a painful lesion unless there is a fracture. An occult fracture often occurs in long bones with fibrous dysplasia; therefore, it is not unusual to have it present with pain and no obvious fracture seen in a long bone. Pain in a flat bone, such as the ribs or pelvis (non–weight-bearing bones), should not occur with fibrous dysplasia.

Fibrous dysplasia can be either monostotic (most commonly) or polyostotic and has a predilection for the pelvis, proximal femur, ribs, and skull. When it is present in the pelvis, it is invariably present in the ipsilateral proximal femur (Figs. 41.1, 41.2). I have seen only one case in which the pelvis was involved with fibrous dysplasia, and the proximal femur was spared. The proximal femur, however, may be affected alone, without involvement in the pelvis (Fig. 41.3).

Fibrous dysplasia often involves the ribs. It typically has an expansile, lytic appearance in the posterior ribs (Fig. 41.4) and a sclerotic appearance in the anterior ribs.

The classic description of fibrous dysplasia is that it has a ground-glass or smoky matrix. This description confuses people as often as it helps them, and I do not recommend using "ground-glass appearance" as a buzz word for fibrous dysplasia. Fibrous dysplasia is often purely lytic and becomes hazy or takes on a ground-glass look as the matrix

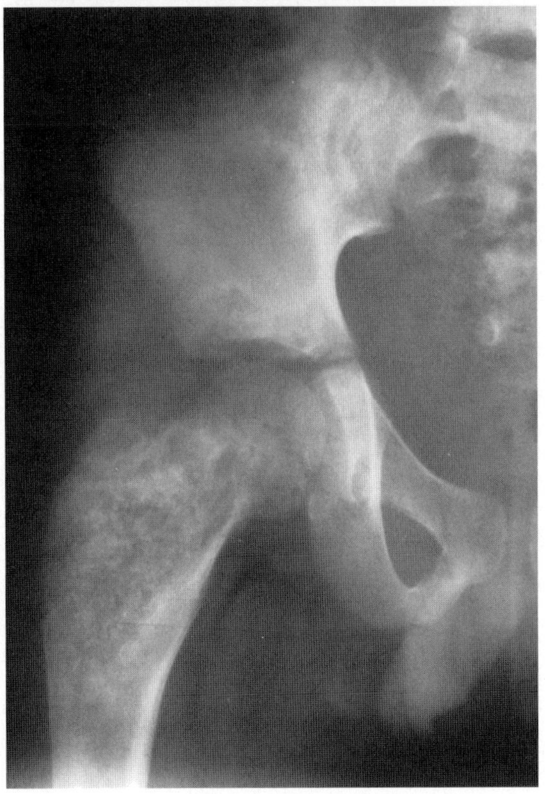

FIGURE 41.2. Fibrous Dysplasia. This patient has polyostotic fibrous dysplasia with involvement of the right femur as well as the supraacetabular portion of the ilium. When the pelvis is involved with fibrous dysplasia, the ipsilateral femur on the affected side is invariably also involved.

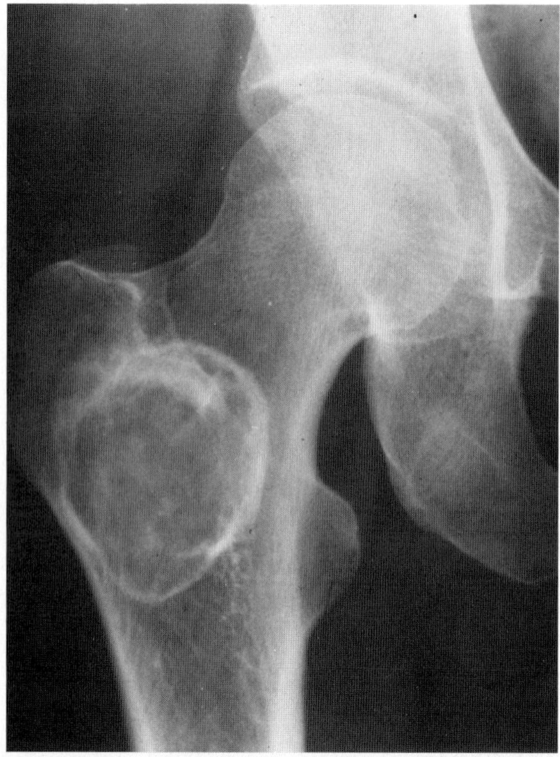

FIGURE 41.3. **Fibrous Dysplasia.** This patient has a well-defined lytic lesion with a hazy, ground-glass appearance in the neck of the right femur. The pelvis was uninvolved. It is not unusual for monostotic fibrous dysplasia to involve the proximal femur and spare the pelvis.

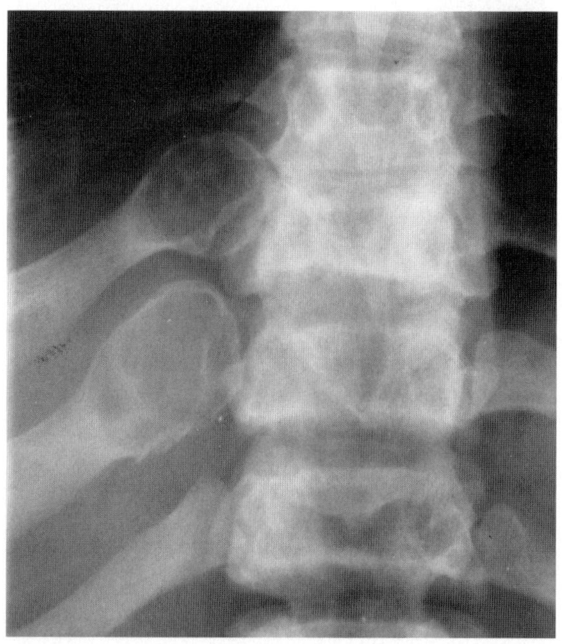

FIGURE 41.4. **Fibrous Dysplasia.** When fibrous dysplasia affects the ribs, the posterior ribs often demonstrate a lytic expansile appearance, as in this example. When the anterior ribs are involved, they are most often sclerotic in appearance. Note also the involvement of the thoracic spine.

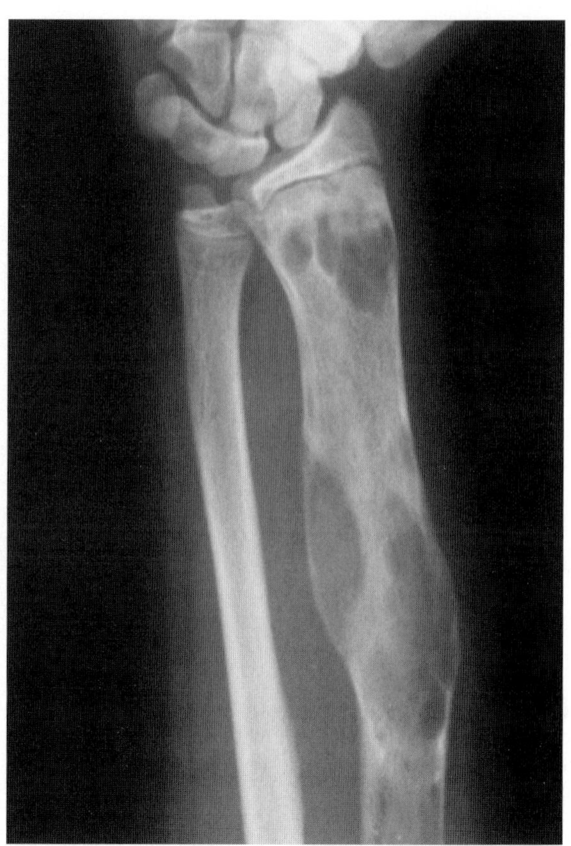

FIGURE 41.5. **Fibrous Dysplasia.** Polyostotic fibrous dysplasia is seen in the radius in this child. Parts of this lesion have a hazy, ground-glass appearance, whereas others are more lytic appearing. A hazy, ground-glass appearance is often present in fibrous dysplasia, but just as often, the appearance can be purely lytic or even sclerotic.

calcifies (Fig. 41.5). It can go on to calcify significantly, and then it presents as a sclerotic lesion. Also, I often see lytic lesions with a pathologic diagnosis other than fibrous dysplasia that have a distinct ground-glass appearance; therefore, the "ground-glass" qualifier can be misleading.

Adamantinoma. When a lesion is encountered in the tibia that resembles fibrous dysplasia, an adamantinoma should also be considered. An adamantinoma is a malignant tumor that radiographically and histologically resembles fibrous dysplasia (Fig. 41.6). It occurs almost exclusively in the tibia and the jaw (for unknown reasons) and is rare. Because it is rare, one may choose not to include it in the differential—a misdiagnosis will not occur more than once or twice in a lifetime.

McCune-Albright Syndrome. Polyostotic fibrous dysplasia occasionally occurs in association with café-au-lait spots on the skin (dark-pigmented, frecklelike lesions) and precocious puberty. This complex is called McCune-Albright syndrome. The bony lesions in this syndrome, and even in the simple polyostotic form, often occur unilaterally—that is, throughout one half of the body. This

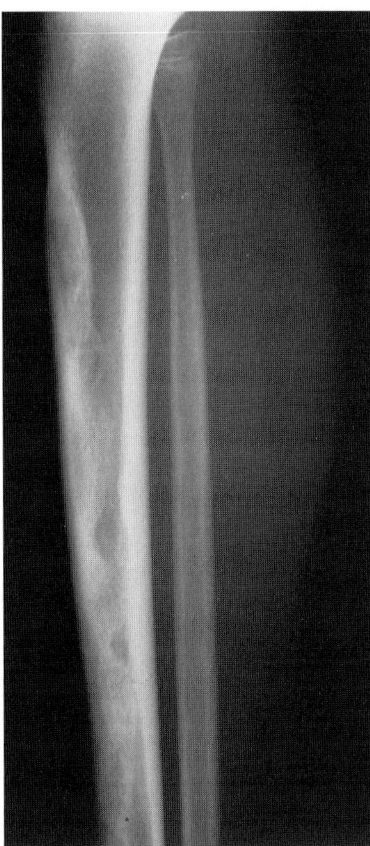

FIGURE 41.6. **Adamantinoma.** This mixed lytic and sclerotic process in the midshaft of the tibia is characteristic for fibrous dysplasia. An adamantinoma has an identical appearance and should be considered in any tibial lesion that resembles fibrous dysplasia. Biopsy showed this to be an adamantinoma.

does not happen often enough to be of any diagnostic use in differentiating fibrous dysplasia from other lesions.

The presence of multiple lesions of fibrous dysplasia in the jaw has been termed *cherubism*. This is from the physical appearance of the child with puffed-out cheeks having an angelic look. The jaw lesions of cherubism regress in adulthood.

Discriminator. No periosteal reaction.

Enchondroma and Eosinophilic Granuloma

Enchondromas occur in any bone formed from cartilage and may be central, eccentric, expansile, or nonexpansile. They invariably contain calcified chondroid matrix, except when in the phalanges. An enchondroma is the most common benign cystic lesion in the phalanges (Fig. 41.7). If a cystic lesion is present without calcified chondroid matrix anywhere except in the phalanges, I do not include enchondroma in my differential.

Often it is difficult to differentiate between an enchondroma and a bone infarct. An infarct usually has a well-defined, densely sclerotic, serpiginous border (Fig. 41.8), whereas an enchondroma does not (Fig. 41.9). An enchondroma often causes endosteal scalloping, whereas a bone infarct will not. Although these criteria are helpful in separating an infarct from an enchondroma, they are not foolproof.

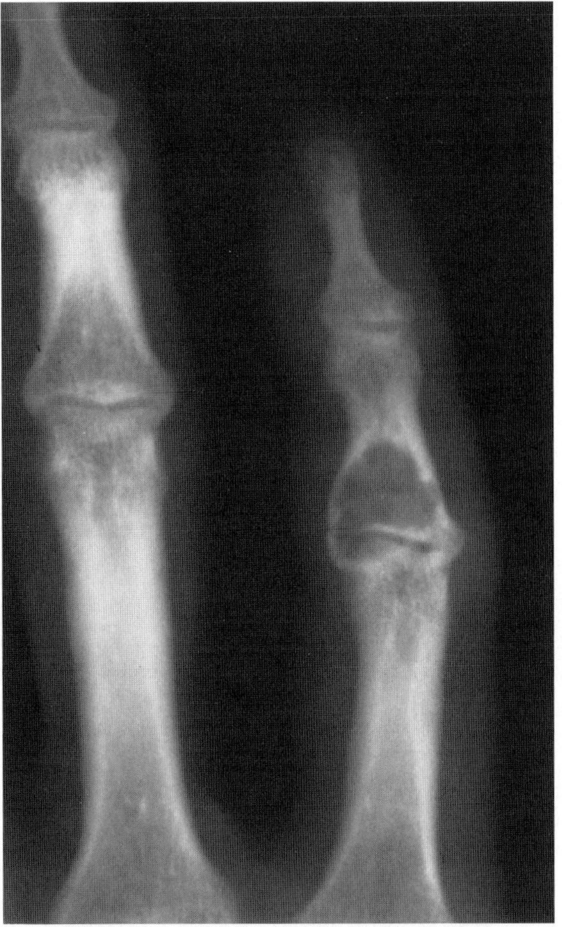

FIGURE 41.7. **Enchondroma.** A lytic lesion in the phalanges is most commonly an enchondroma. This is the only location in the skeleton where an enchondroma does not contain calcified chondroid matrix. These most often present with pathologic fractures, as in this example.

It is difficult, if not impossible, to differentiate an enchondroma from a chondrosarcoma. Clinical findings (primarily pain) serve as a better indicator than radiographic findings, and indeed pain in an apparent enchondroma should warrant surgical investigation. Periostitis should not be seen in an enchondroma either. Trying to differentiate histologically an enchondroma from a chondrosarcoma is also difficult, if not impossible, at times. Biopsy of an apparent enchondroma should not be performed routinely for histologic differentiation.

Multiple enchondromas occur on occasion; this condition has been termed Ollier disease (Fig. 41.10). It is not

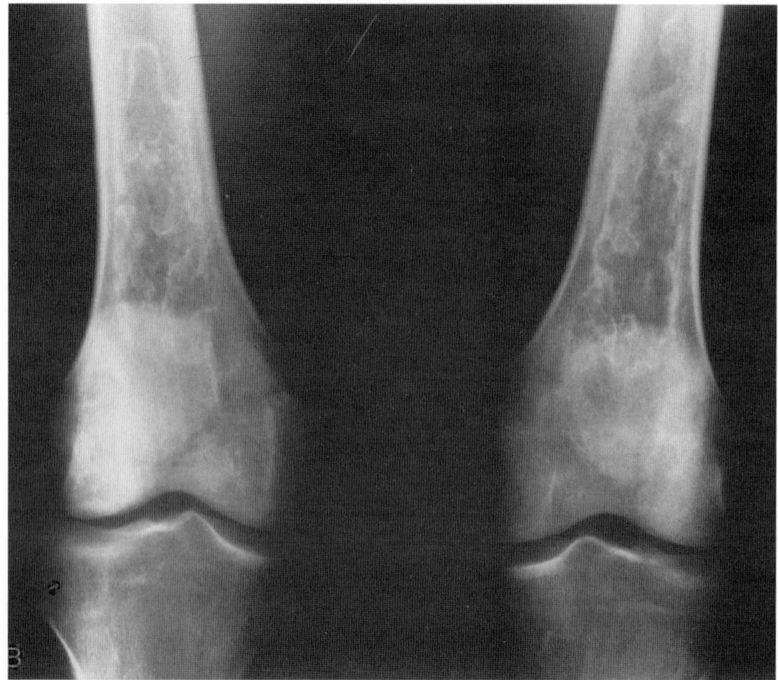

FIGURE 41.8. **Bone Infarct.** These lytic lesions in the distal femurs with calcified, serpiginous borders are typical for bone infarcts. Occasionally, the differential between a bone infarct and an enchondroma can be difficult on plain films; however, in this example, infarcts are easily diagnosed.

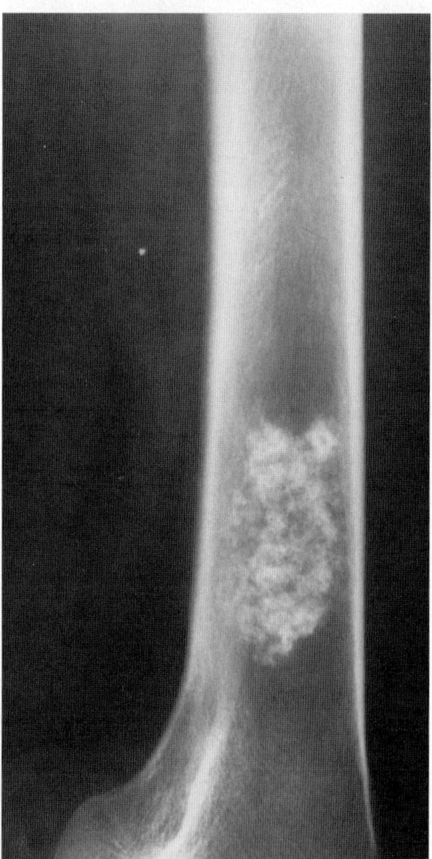

FIGURE 41.9. **Enchondroma.** This lesion in the distal right femur shows the stippled, punctate calcification typical for chondroid matrix seen in an enchondroma.

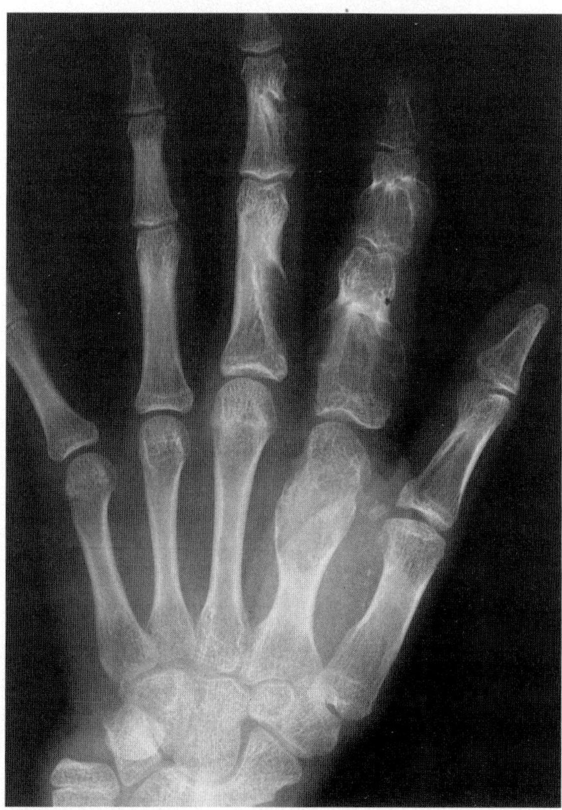

FIGURE 41.10. **Ollier Disease.** Multiple enchondromas are present throughout the hand. This is a typical example of Ollier disease.

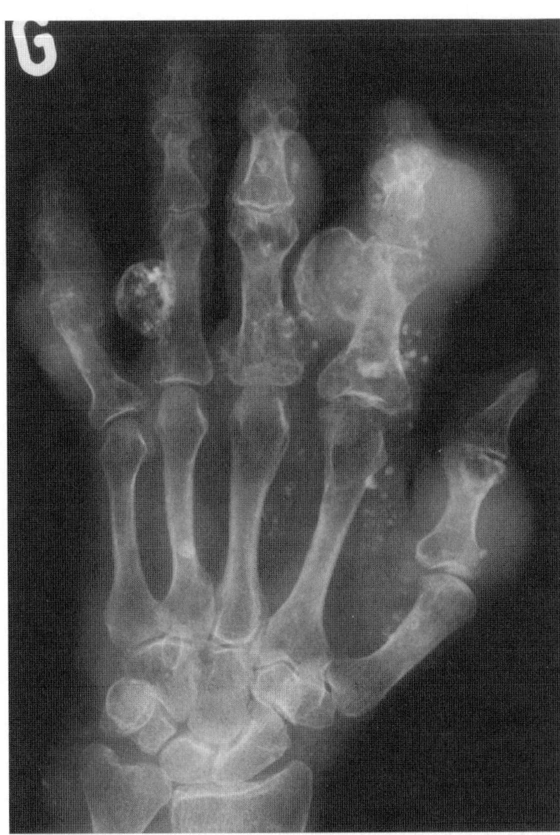

FIGURE 41.11. **Maffucci Syndrome.** Multiple enchondromas associated with phleboliths are present in the phalanges. This combination of findings invariably represents hemangiomas and enchondromas in Maffucci syndrome.

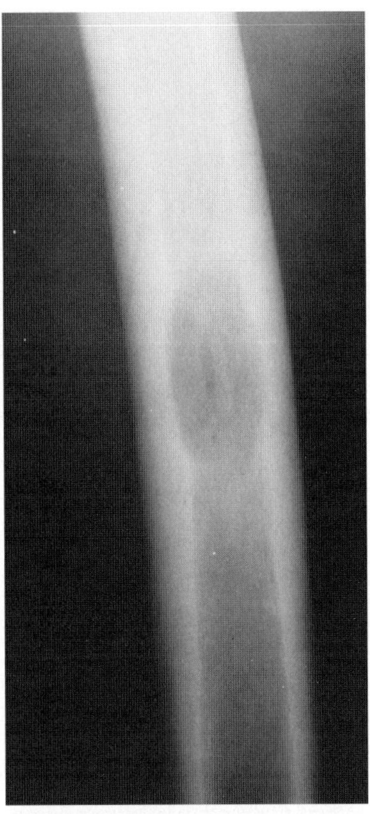

FIGURE 41.12. **Eosinophilic Granuloma (EG).** A well-defined lytic lesion is seen involving the midfemur in this 20-year-old patient. Biopsy showed this to be EG.

hereditary and does not have an increased rate of malignant degeneration. The presence of multiple enchondromas associated with soft tissue hemangiomas is known as Maffucci syndrome (Fig. 41.11). This syndrome also is not hereditary; however, it does have an increased incidence of malignant degeneration of the enchondromas.

Discriminators. 1. Must have calcification (except in phalanges). 2. No periostitis or pain.

Eosinophilic granuloma (EG) is a form of histiocytosis X, the other forms being Letterer-Siwe disease and Hand-Schüller-Christian disease. Although these forms may be merely different phases of the same disease, most investigators categorize them separately. The bony manifestations of all three disorders are similar and are discussed in this review simply as EG.

Unfortunately for radiologists, EG has many appearances (1). It can be lytic or sclerotic, it may be well defined or ill defined, it might or might not have a sclerotic border, and it might or might not elicit a periosteal response. The periostitis, when present, is typically benign in appearance (thick, uniform, wavy) but can be lamellated or amorphous. EG can mimic Ewing sarcoma and present as a permeative (multiple small holes) lesion.

How, then, can one distinguish EG from any of the other lytic lesions in this differential? Remember that it is difficult to exclude EG from almost any differential of a bony lesion, be it benign or malignant. EG occurs almost exclusively in patients under 30 years (usually <20 years); therefore, the patient's age is the best criterion. I recommend mentioning EG as a differential possibility for any lesion in a patient less than the age of 30. Because EG can look like anything, so long as the radiograph is not of an arthritide or trauma, EG can be mentioned without even looking at the film!

EG is most often monostotic (Fig. 41.12), but it can be polyostotic (Fig. 41.13) and, thus, has to be included whenever multiple lesions are present in a patient younger than the age of 30 years.

EG might or might not have a soft tissue mass associated, so the presence or absence of a soft tissue mass will not help in the differential diagnosis. I know of no entity in which the presence or absence of an associated soft tissue mass will warrant inclusion or exclusion of the process from a differential. It is important to note the presence of a soft tissue mass (or its absence), but this will do little to narrow the differential diagnosis.

Most radiologists are inept at evaluating the soft tissues because they are difficult to see, and CT and MR have made

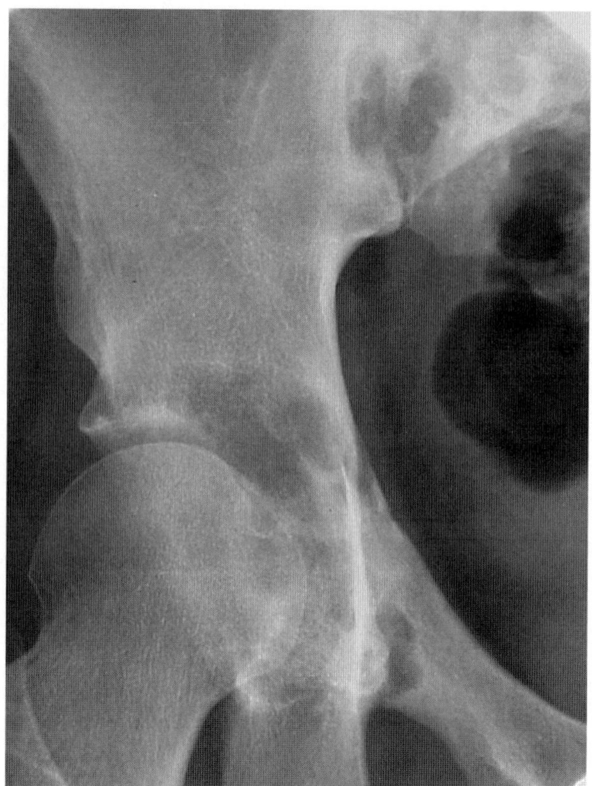

FIGURE 41.13. **Eosinophilic Granuloma (EG).** Well-defined lytic lesions are present throughout the pelvis in this 24-year-old patient. In addition to the lesion around the right hip, a lesion is seen at the right sacroiliac joint. Biopsy showed this to be EG.

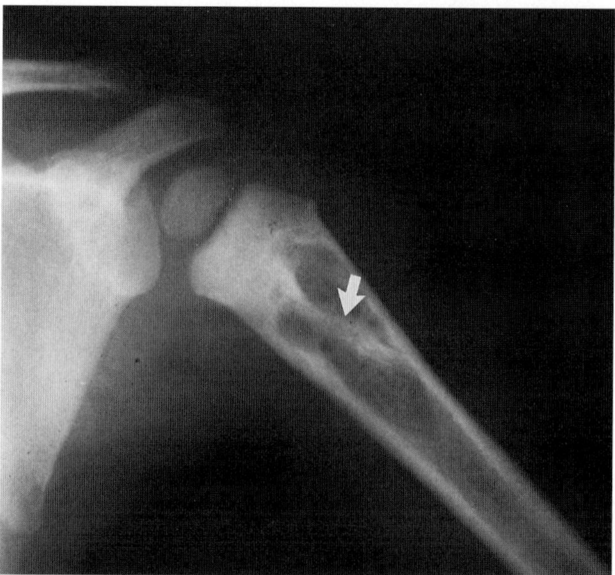

FIGURE 41.14. **Eosinophilic Granuloma (EG).** This well-defined lytic lesion contains a bony sequestrum (*arrow*), which is typical for osteomyelitis or EG. Biopsy revealed this to be EG.

it unnecessary in most cases to rely on plain films alone for the soft tissues. Fortunately, in most cases, the presence or absence of a soft tissue mass will not alter the differential diagnosis. The treating physician will undoubtedly want to know whether the soft tissues are involved and to what extent; this can be satisfactorily demonstrated with MR.

EG occasionally has a bony sequestrum (Fig. 41.14). Only a few other entities have been described that on occasion have bony sequestra: osteomyelitis, lymphoma, and fibrosarcoma; therefore, when a sequestrum is identified, EG, osteomyelitis, lymphoma, and fibrosarcoma should be considered. As discussed in Chapter 47, an osteoid osteoma will often give an appearance of a sequestration when the nidus is partially calcified. Clinically, EG might or might not be associated with pain; therefore, clinical history is noncontributory for the most part.

Discriminator. Must be under age 30 years.

Giant Cell Tumor

Giant cell tumor is an uncommon, somewhat controversial lesion with several schools of thought as to its radiographic appearance. I subscribe to the most widely used approach, as do the majority of radiologists and pathologists (2).

First, it is important to realize that one is unable to tell whether a giant cell tumor is benign or malignant, regardless of its radiographic appearance. Histologically, a giant cell tumor cannot be divided into either a benign or a malignant category. Most surgeons curettage and pack the lesions and consider them benign unless they recur. Even then, they can still be benign and recur a second or third time. About 15% of giant cell tumors are thought to be malignant on the basis of their recurrence rate. When malignant, they can metastasize to the lungs, but they do so infrequently.

Four classic radiographic criteria for diagnosing giant cell tumors exist. If any of these criteria are not met when looking at a lesion, giant cell tumor can be eliminated from the differential diagnosis.

1. Giant cell tumor occurs only in patients with closed epiphyses; this is valid at least 98% to 99% of the time and is extremely useful. I do not entertain the diagnosis of giant cell tumor in a patient with open epiphyses.
2. The lesion must be epiphyseal and abut the articular surface (Fig. 41.15). There is disagreement as to whether giant cell tumors begin in the epiphyses or metaphyses or from the physeal plate itself; however, except for rare cases, when radiologists see the lesions, they are epiphyseal and are flush against the articular surface. The metaphysis also has some of the tumor in it because the lesions are generally very large. When one sees a giant cell tumor, it will be epiphyseal. Perhaps more importantly, it should be flush against the articular surface of the joint. This occurs in 98% to 99% of giant cell tumors; therefore, if I have a lesion that is

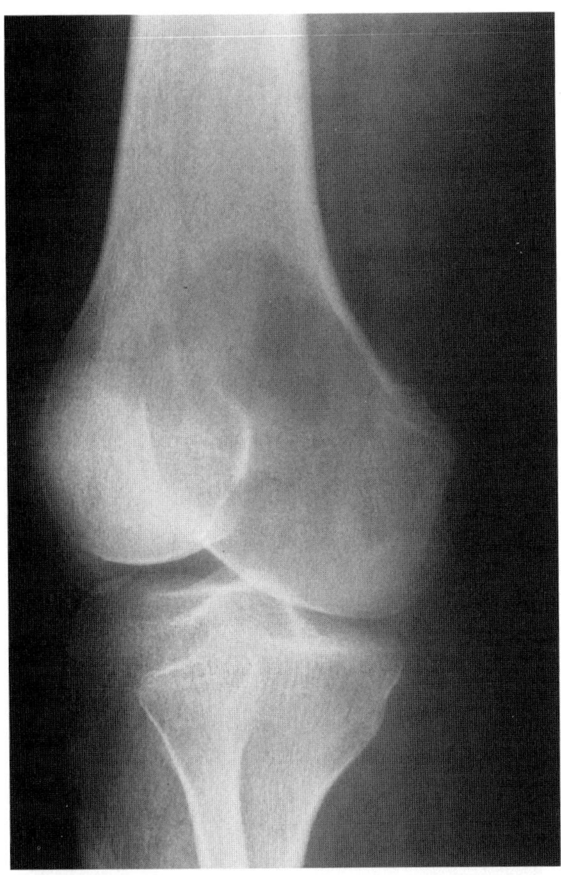

FIGURE 41.15. **Giant Cell Tumor.** A well-defined lytic lesion without a sclerotic margin is seen abutting the articular surface of the distal femur in a patient who has closed epiphyses. These are all characteristics of a giant cell tumor.

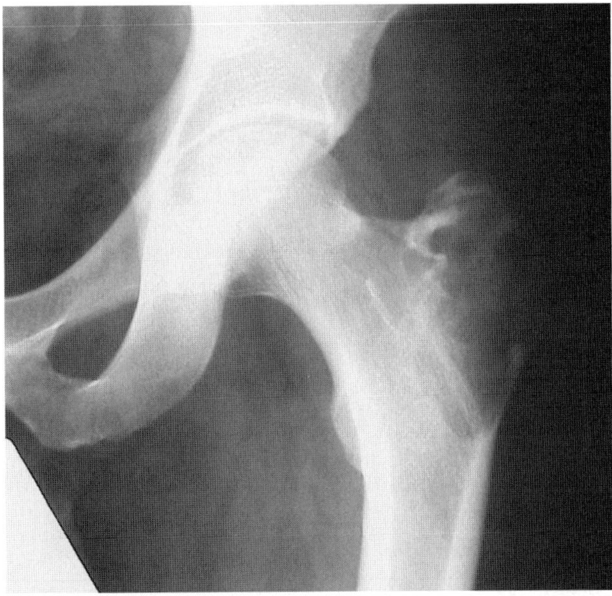

FIGURE 41.16. **Giant Cell Tumor.** This well-defined lytic lesion that does not have a sclerotic margin completely involves the greater trochanter. The apophyses have the same differential diagnosis as lesions in the epiphyses, which makes giant cell tumor a strong possibility in this example. Biopsy showed this to be a giant cell tumor.

separated from the articular surface by a definite margin of normal bone, I will not include giant cell tumor in the diagnosis. This rule does not apply in flat bones, such as in the pelvis or in the apophyses (Fig. 41.16), which have no articular surfaces.

3. Giant cell tumors are said to be eccentrically located in the bone, as opposed to being centrally placed in the medullary cavity. When a bony lesion is quite large, it can be difficult to tell whether it is central or eccentric. I do not find this to be a terribly useful description, but it is one of the classic "rules" of a giant cell tumor.
4. The lesion must have a sharply defined zone of transition (border) that is not sclerotic. This is a very helpful finding in giant cell tumor. The only places this does not apply is in flat bones, such as the pelvis (Fig. 41.17) and the calcaneus.

It is important to realize that the four criteria for a giant cell tumor apply only to giant cell tumors and not to any other lesion. For instance, I know of no other lesion that depends on whether the epiphyses are open or closed. No other lesion in any of my lists uses as a diagnostic factor whether the zone of transition is sclerotic or not (many lesions, such as nonossifying fibromas, will usually have a sclerotic margin, but it does not occur often enough to include as a discriminator). No other lesion must always abut the articular surface, and no other lesion has the classic

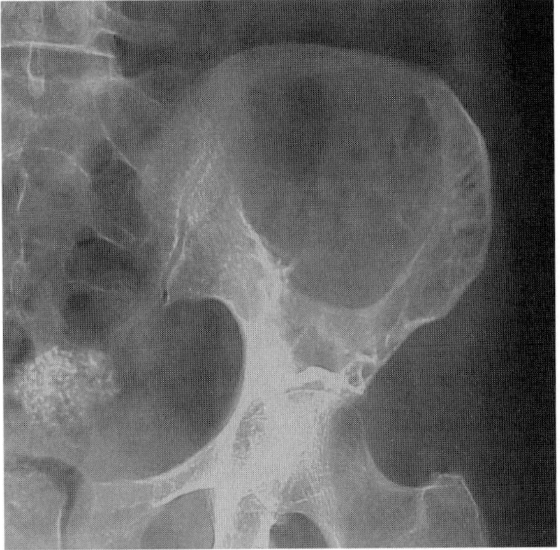

FIGURE 41.17. **Giant Cell Tumor.** A large, well-defined lytic lesion in the iliac wing is seen, which does contain a sclerotic margin and does not appear to abut any articular surface. The pelvis is a good location for giant cell tumor, which this proved to be at biopsy. The usual rules for giant cell tumors such as presence of a nonsclerotic margin do not apply in flat bones.

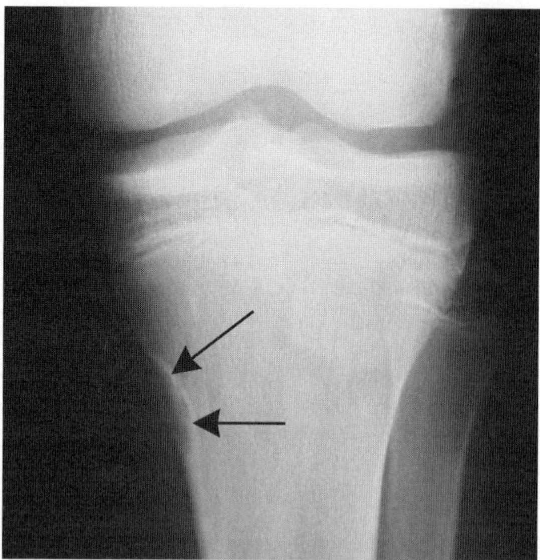

FIGURE 41.18. **Fibrous Cortical Defect.** A well-defined lytic lesion is seen in the medial metaphysis of this tibia (*arrows*), which is typical for a fibrous cortical defect.

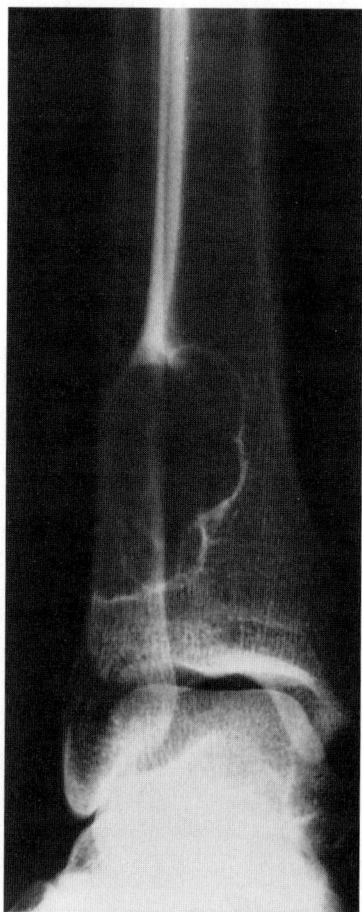

FIGURE 41.19. **Nonossifying Fibroma.** A large, well-defined lytic lesion, which is slightly expansile with scalloped sclerotic margins, is seen in the distal tibia in this young patient. This is a characteristic appearance of a nonossifying fibroma. The examination was obtained for a sprained ankle and not for this asymptomatic lesion.

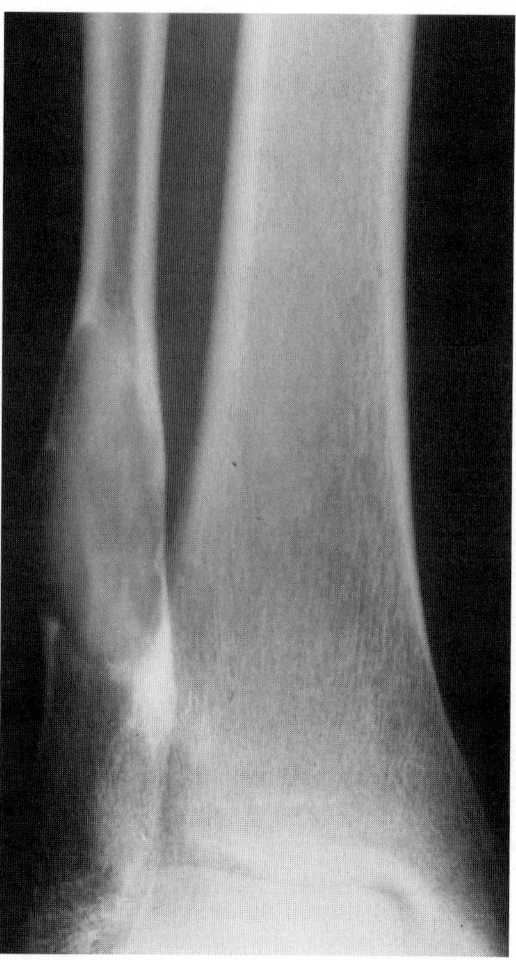

FIGURE 41.20. **Nonossifying Fibroma.** A well-defined, expansile lytic lesion in the distal fibula is noted in this asymptomatic patient, which is characteristic for a nonossifying fibroma.

description of being eccentrically placed (although several lesions, including nonossifying fibroma and chondromyxoid fibroma, are eccentric most of the time).

Although these four criteria apply well for giant cell tumor, they do not apply at all for any other lesions. Residents have a tendency to apply these criteria to every lytic lesion encountered for the simple reason that they have learned the four criteria.

Once one of the criteria is violated, the remainder do not even have to be used to eliminate a giant cell tumor. For instance, if a lytic lesion is found in the mid-diaphysis of a bone, giant cell tumor can be excluded. There is no need to check further to see whether it is eccentric, whether it has a nonsclerotic margin, or whether the epiphyses are closed.

Again, these rules will be greater than 95% effective and, in my experience, close to 99% effective. It should be noted that these criteria only apply to giant cell tumors of long bones. They would not work, for instance, in the pelvis or the calcaneus, two locations where giant cell tumors often occur. If one or two cases are found that do not fit the criteria, another pathologist should review the slides.

Many pathologists refer to aneurysmal bone cysts as giant cell tumors; hence, they have giant cell tumors that do not obey any of the criteria. These pathologists may be correct, but they are not in the mainstream of what most people use for giant cell tumor criteria, both radiographically and histologically.

Discriminators. 1. Epiphyses must be closed. 2. Must abut the articular surface. 3. Must be well defined with a nonsclerotic margin. 4. Must be eccentric.

Nonossifying Fibroma

Nonossifying fibroma (NOF) is probably the most common bone lesion encountered by radiologists. It reportedly occurs in up to 20% of children and usually spontaneously regresses, so as to be seen only rarely after the age of 30. "Fibrous cortical defect" is a common synonym, although some people differentiate the two lesions on the basis of size, with a fibrous cortical defect being smaller than 2 cm in length (Fig. 41.18) and an NOF being larger than 2 cm (Fig. 41.19). Histologically, these lesions are identical; therefore, it seems appropriate to refer to them all as NOFs rather than to subdivide them by their size.

NOFs are benign, asymptomatic lesions that typically occur in the metaphysis of a long bone, emanating from the cortex. They classically have a thin, sclerotic border that is scalloped and slightly expansile (Fig. 41.20); however, this is a general description that probably applies to only 75% of the lesions and could equally apply to most of the lesions in FEGNOMASHIC. They do not have to have expansion or a scalloped or sclerotic border and are not limited to the metaphyses. Then how are they best recognized? The best way is to familiarize oneself with their general appearance by looking at examples in textbooks. That can be done in 15 minutes. It is important to recognize these lesions because they are what I call "don't touch" lesions (see Chapter 46); that is, the radiologist's diagnosis should be the final word and thereby supplant a biopsy. These lesions are so characteristic that no differential diagnosis should be entertained, although a few entities can indeed occasionally simulate them.

If a CT or MR is obtained of an NOF, there will often appear to be interruption of the cortex, which can be misinterpreted as cortical destruction (Fig. 41.21). This merely represents cortical replacement by benign fibrous tissue and should not warrant further investigation.

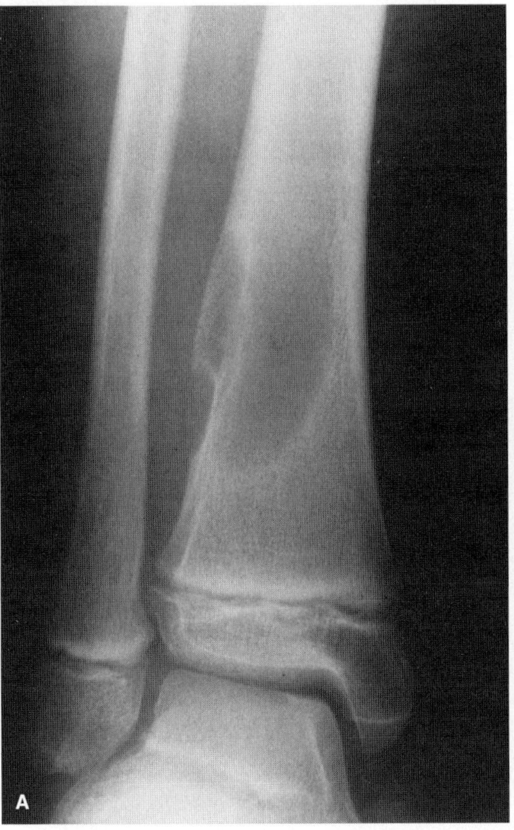

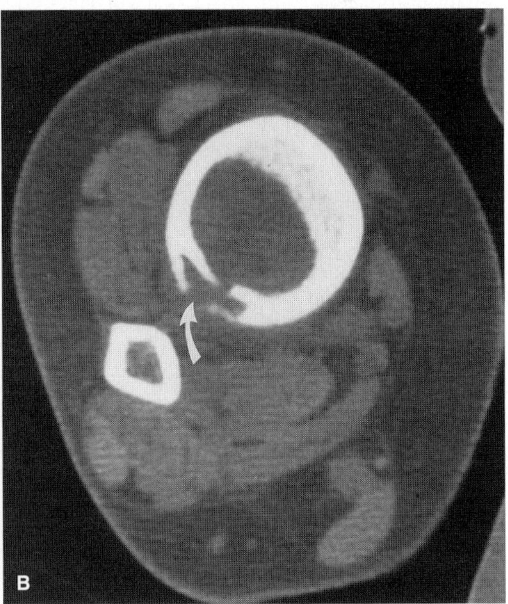

FIGURE 41.21. **Nonossifying Fibroma. A.** A well-defined, lytic lesion that is minimally expansile is seen in the distal tibia in this child who was examined for a sprained ankle. **B.** A CT examination showed apparent cortical destruction (*arrow*), which was believed to be suggestive of an aggressive lesion. Biopsy showed this to be a nonossifying fibroma. Both CT and MR will often show apparent cortical destruction, which is merely cortical replacement by benign fibrous tissue.

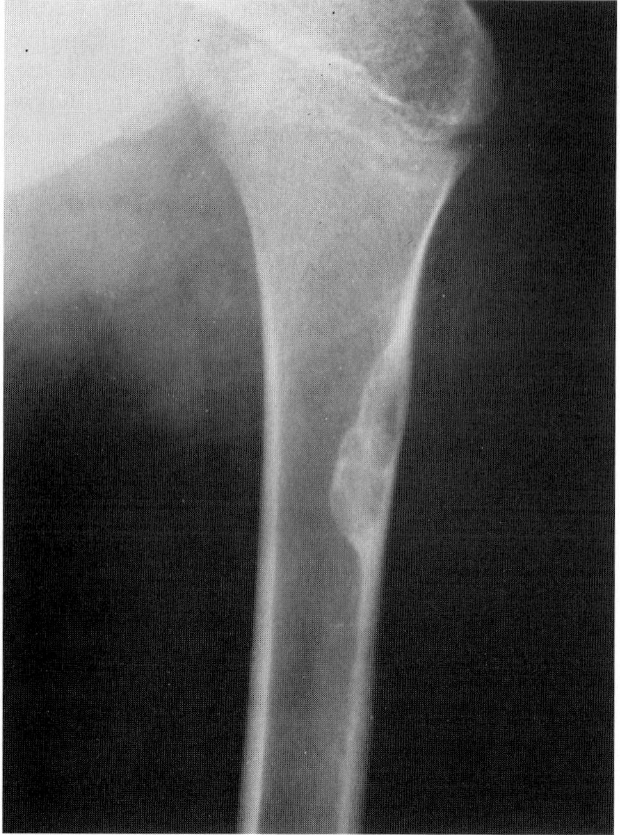

FIGURE 41.22. **Healing Nonossifying Fibroma.** A predominantly sclerotic lesion, which is minimally expansile and well defined, is seen in the proximal humerus in this child who is asymptomatic. This is a typical appearance of a disappearing or healing nonossifying fibroma. With time, this lesion will melt into the normal bone and essentially disappear.

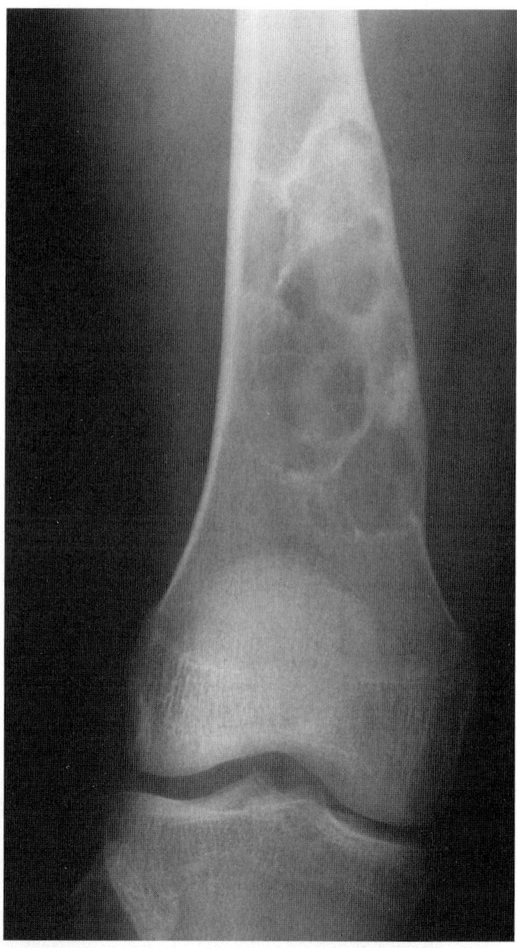

FIGURE 41.23. **Nonossifying Fibroma.** This large, well-defined lytic lesion with faint sclerotic margins is seen in the distal femur. It has a very typical appearance for a giant cell tumor; however, it has sclerotic margins and does not abut the articular surface. The lesion underwent biopsy and was found to be a nonossifying fibroma.

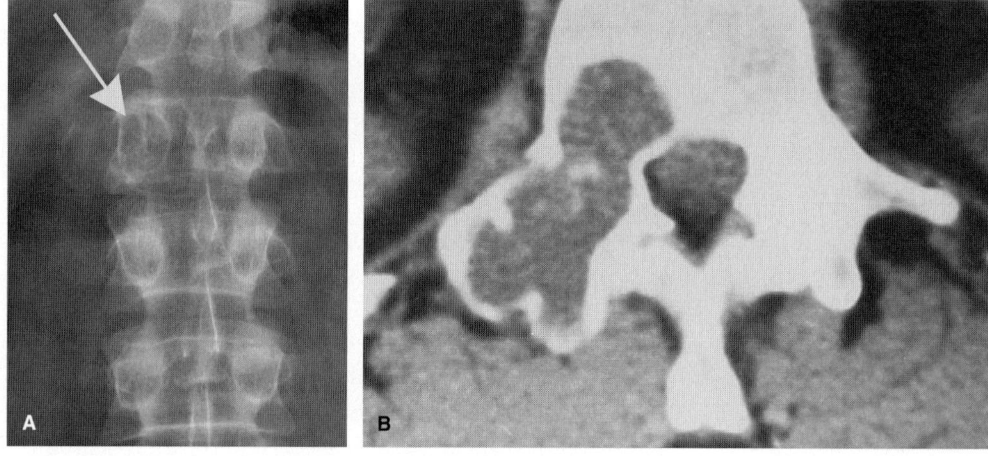

FIGURE 41.24. **Osteoblastoma. A.** A lytic expansile lesion involving the right T12 pedicle (*arrow*) and transverse process is seen on this anteroposterior plain film. **B.** The lesion is seen on CT to extend into the vertebral body. It has intact cortices and contains some calcified matrix. This is a classic example of an osteoblastoma of the spine.

If the patient is older than 30 years of age, NOF should not be included in the differential diagnosis. NOFs must be asymptomatic and exhibit no periostitis, unless there is an antecedent history of trauma. They routinely "heal" with sclerosis and eventually disappear (Fig. 41.22), usually around the ages of 20 to 30 years. During this healing period, they can appear hot on a radionuclide bone scan because there is osteoblastic activity. These lesions can occasionally get quite large (Fig. 41.23); therefore, growth or change in size should not alter the diagnosis. They are most commonly seen about the knee but can occur in any long bone. Occasionally, multiple NOFs are seen about the knee, each of which is characteristic in appearance.

Discriminators. 1. Must be younger than age 30 years. 2. No periostitis or pain. 3. Cortically based.

Osteoblastoma

Osteoblastomas are rare lesions that could justifiably be excluded from this differential without the fear of missing a diagnosis more than once in a lifetime. Why, then, include them? The mnemonic FEGNOMASHIC would not have nearly the same ring without the extra vowel, so osteoblastoma remains.

Osteoblastomas have two appearances: (*1*) They look like large osteoid osteomas and are often called *giant osteoid osteomas*. Because osteoid osteomas are sclerotic lesions and do not resemble bubbly lytic lesions, this is not the type of osteoblastoma we are concerned with in this differential. (*2*) They simulate aneurysmal bone cysts (ABCs). They are expansile, often having a "soap-bubble" appearance. If an ABC is being considered, so should an osteoblastoma. Osteoblastomas commonly occur in the posterior elements of the vertebral bodies, and about half of the cases demonstrate speckled calcifications (Fig. 41.24). A classic radiology differential is that of an expansile lytic lesion of the posterior elements of the spine, which includes osteoblastoma, ABC, and tuberculosis.

Discriminator. Mentioned when ABC is mentioned (especially in the posterior elements of the spine).

Metastatic Disease and Myeloma

Metastatic disease should be considered for any lytic lesion—benign or aggressive in appearance—in a patient over 40 years of age. Metastatic disease can appear perfectly benign radiographically (Fig. 41.25), so it is not valid to say, "Because this lesion looks benign, it should not be a metastasis." Most metastatic disease has an aggressive appearance and will not be in the FEGNOMASHIC differential, but a significant number of metastases appear benign. In fact, metastases can have any radiographic appearance; therefore, any bone lesion in a patient older than the age of 40 should have metastatic disease as a consideration, unless trauma or arthritis is the primary concern.

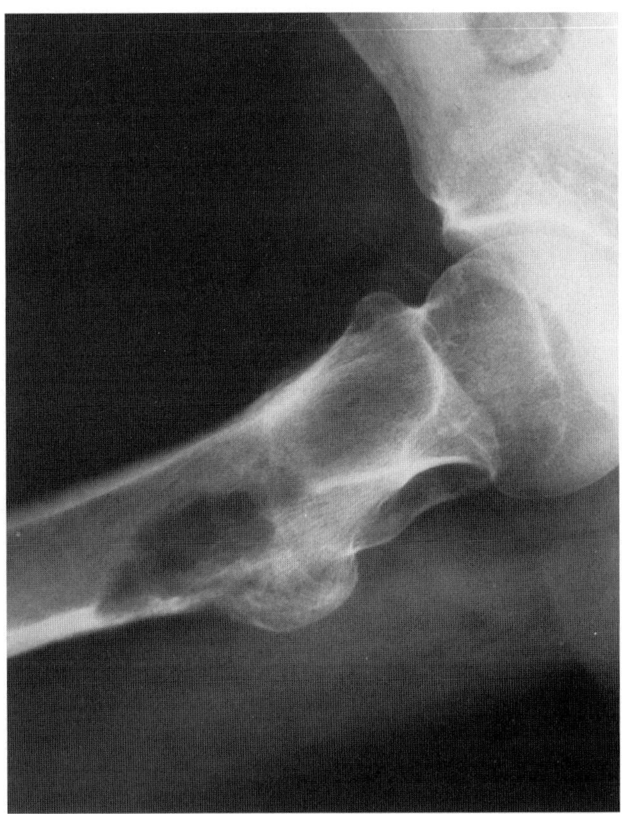

FIGURE 41.25. **Metastatic Disease.** A well-defined lytic lesion is seen in the proximal femur in this 50-year-old patient who had pain associated with this lesion. Biopsy showed this to be a renal metastasis. A significant number of metastatic lesions can have a completely benign appearance, as in this example.

For statistical purposes, I do not mention metastatic disease in a patient younger than age 40. I will be correct more than 99% of the time using 40 as a cutoff age. Otherwise, metastatic diseases would have to be mentioned in every single case of a lytic lesion, and I prefer to limit the list of differential possibilities. I am not claiming that metastatic disease does not occur in patients younger than age 40—only that I consider it acceptable to miss it (unless given a history of a known primary neoplasm).

Myeloma. Although myeloma most commonly presents as a diffuse permeative process in the skeleton (Fig. 41.26), it can present as either a solitary lesion (Fig. 41.27) or as multiple lytic lesions. Bubbly, lytic bone lesions of myeloma are more correctly called *plasmacytomas*. I mention plasmacytoma separately from metastatic disease because it can occur in a slightly younger population (age greater than 35 years is my cutoff) and can precede clinical or hematologic evidence of myeloma by 3 to 5 years. In general, there is no harm in lumping all metastatic disease, including myeloma, into one group and using greater than age 40 as the limiting factor.

Virtually any metastatic process can present as a lytic, benign-appearing lesion; therefore, it serves no purpose to

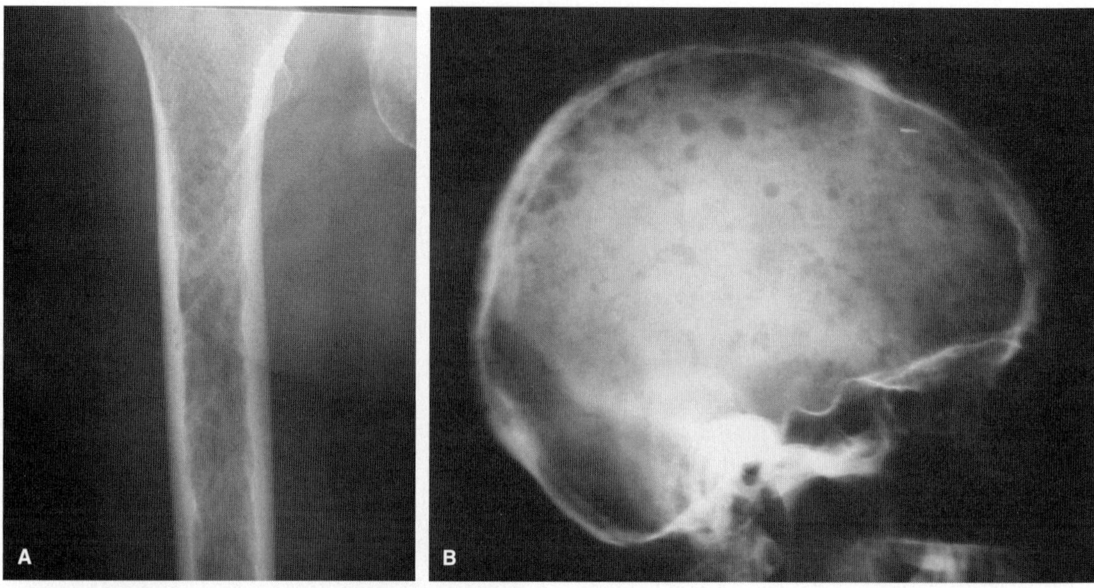

FIGURE 41.26. **Multiple Myeloma. A.** A diffuse permeative pattern is present throughout the femur in this patient with multiple myeloma. **B.** A lateral skull film shows a typical presentation of multiple myeloma in the skull with multiple small holes throughout the calvaria, which are well defined.

try to guess the source of the metastatic disease from its appearance. In general, lytic expansile metastatic diseases tend to come from thyroid and renal tumors (Fig. 41.28). The only metastatic lesion that is said to always be lytic is renal cell carcinoma.

Discriminator: Must be older than age 40 years.

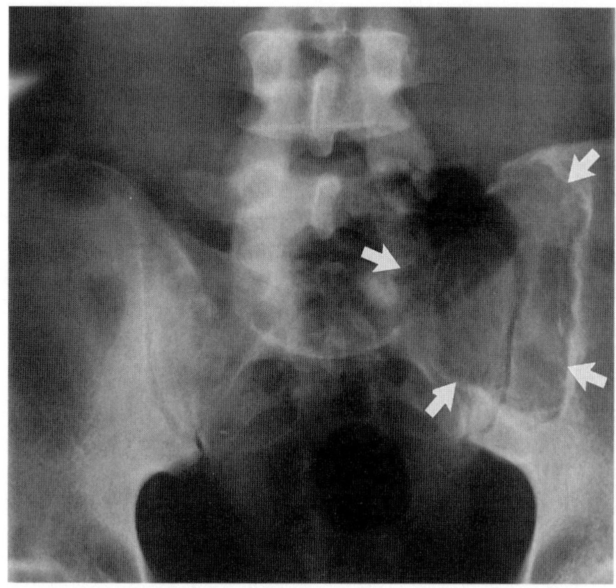

FIGURE 41.27. **Plasmacytoma.** A large, well-defined lytic lesion is seen in the left ilium (*arrows*) in this patient with multiple myeloma. This is a common location for a plasmacytoma. Like metastases, plasmacytomas often have a completely benign appearance.

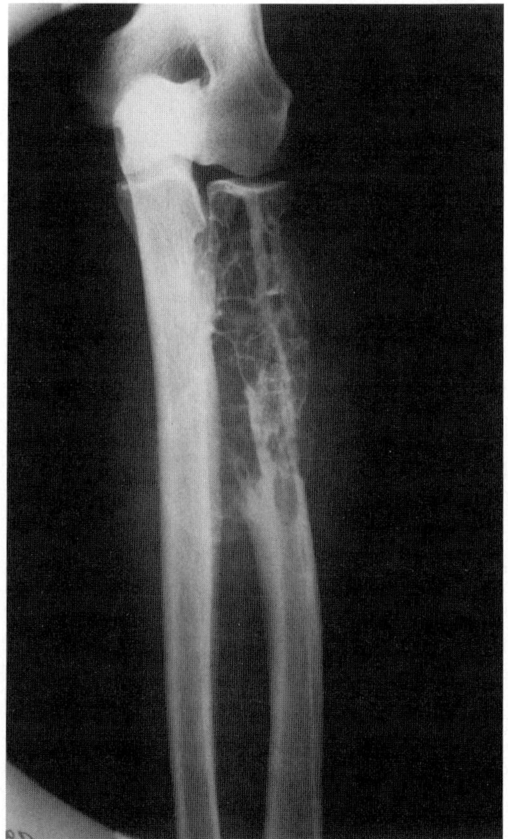

FIGURE 41.28. **Metastatic Disease.** An expansile lesion with a soap-bubble appearance is present in the proximal radius in a patient with renal cell carcinoma. An expansile lytic lesion is a common finding with renal or thyroid metastatic disease.

Aneurysmal Bone Cyst

Aneurysmal bone cysts (ABCs) are the only lesions I know of that are named for their radiographic appearance. They are virtually always aneurysmal or expansile (Figs. 41.29, 41.30). Rarely, an ABC will present before it is expansile, but that is unusual enough not to worry about. Aneurysmal bone cysts occur primarily in patients who are younger than age 30, although occasionally one will be encountered in older patients. I use bony expansion and age of less than 30 years as fairly rigid guidelines and seldom miss the diagnosis of ABC. They often have fluid–fluid levels on CT or MR (Fig. 41.31), although this is a nonspecific finding, as many other lesions can have fluid–fluid levels.

ABCs are, like giant cell tumors, somewhat controversial. There are apparently two types of ABCs: a primary type and a secondary type. The secondary type occurs in conjunction with another lesion or from trauma, whereas a primary ABC has no known cause or association with other lesions. Secondary ABCs have been said to occur with giant cell tumors, osteosarcomas, and almost any other lesion. I have seen dozens of ABCs and have seen only a few in association with another lesion. As to occurring after trauma, I do not understand why they would be age-limited if trauma were causative. Also, malignant tumors

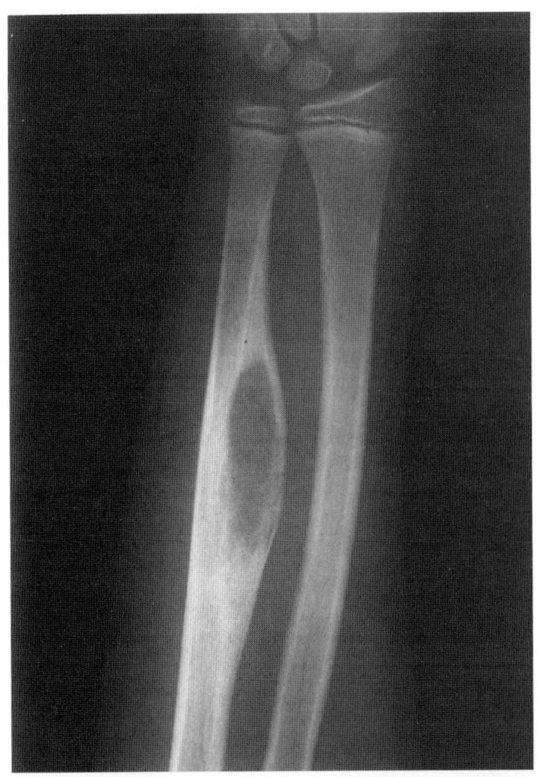

FIGURE 41.30. **Aneurysmal Bone Cyst.** A well-defined expansile lesion is seen in the midshaft of the ulna in a child who presented with pain in this region. This is a characteristic appearance for an aneurysmal bone cyst.

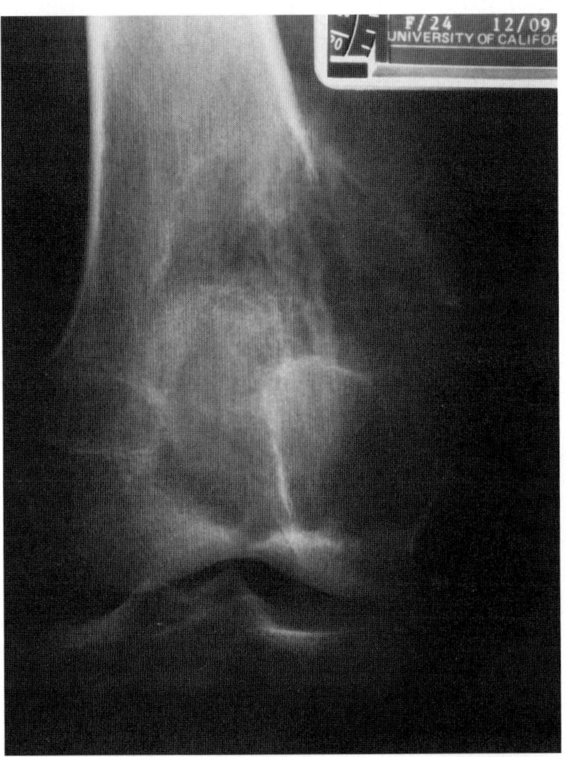

FIGURE 41.29. **Aneurysmal Bone Cyst.** An expansile lytic lesion is present in the distal femur in this 24-year-old patient who presents with pain. This is a fairly typical appearance for an aneurysmal bone cyst.

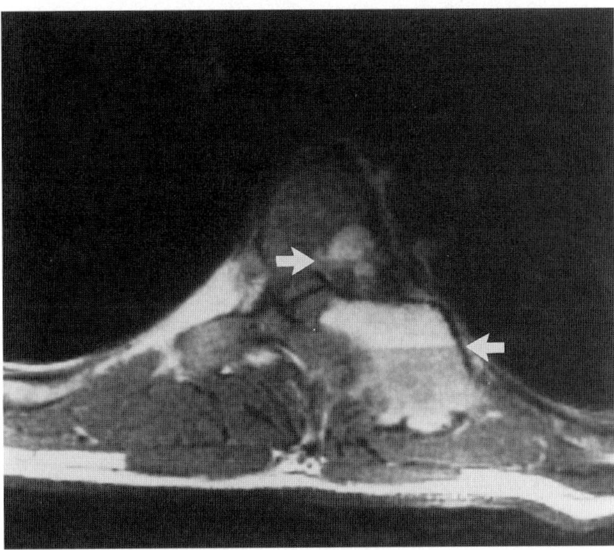

FIGURE 41.31. **Aneurysmal Bone Cyst.** An axial T2WI through a thoracic vertebral body shows an expansile lesion involving the posterior elements that has several fluid–fluid levels (*arrows*). This is a typical appearance for an aneurysmal bone cyst.

were once thought to occur after trauma because of the frequent association of a history of antecedent trauma with malignant bone tumors. This is not seriously considered today and is thought to be coincidental. I suspect that ABCs and trauma are also coincidental, but this is mere speculation.

ABCs typically present because of pain. They can occur anywhere in the skeleton, and there is no location that would make them more highly ranked in the differential diagnosis. As with osteoblastoma, they often occur in the posterior elements of the spine.

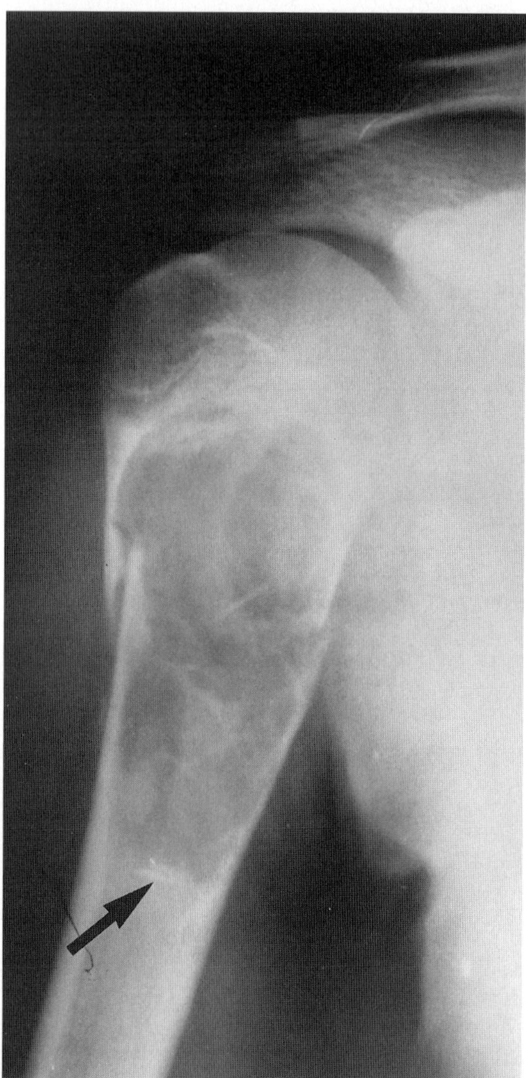

FIGURE 41.32. **Solitary Bone Cyst.** A well-defined lytic lesion is present in the proximal humerus in this child who suffered a fracture through the lesion. The location and central appearance, as well as the age of the patient, are characteristic for a solitary bone cyst. A piece of cortical bone has broken off and descended through the serous fluid contained within the lesion and can be seen in the dependent portion of the lesion (*arrow*) as a fallen fragment sign. A fallen fragment sign is said to be pathognomonic for a unicameral bone cyst.

Discriminators. 1. Must be expansile. 2. Must be younger than age 30 years.

Solitary Bone Cyst

Solitary bone cysts are also called *simple bone cysts* or *unicameral bone cysts*. They are not necessarily unicameral (one compartment), however. This is the only lesion in FEGNOMASHIC that is always central in location. Many of the other lesions may be central, but a solitary bone cyst can be excluded if it is not. It is one of the few lesions that does not occur most commonly around the knees. Two thirds to three fourths of these lesions occur in the proximal humerus (Fig. 41.32) and proximal femur (Fig. 41.33). Application of this rule alone is not that helpful, or one third to one fourth of lesions would be missed.

Solitary bone cysts are usually asymptomatic unless fractured, which is a common occurrence. Even when pathologic fractures occur, they rarely form periostitis. A classic radiographic finding for a solitary bone cyst is the fallen fragment sign (see Fig. 41.32). This occurs when a piece of cortex breaks off after a fracture in a solitary bone cyst, and the piece of cortical bone sinks to the gravity-dependent portion of the lesion. This has not been

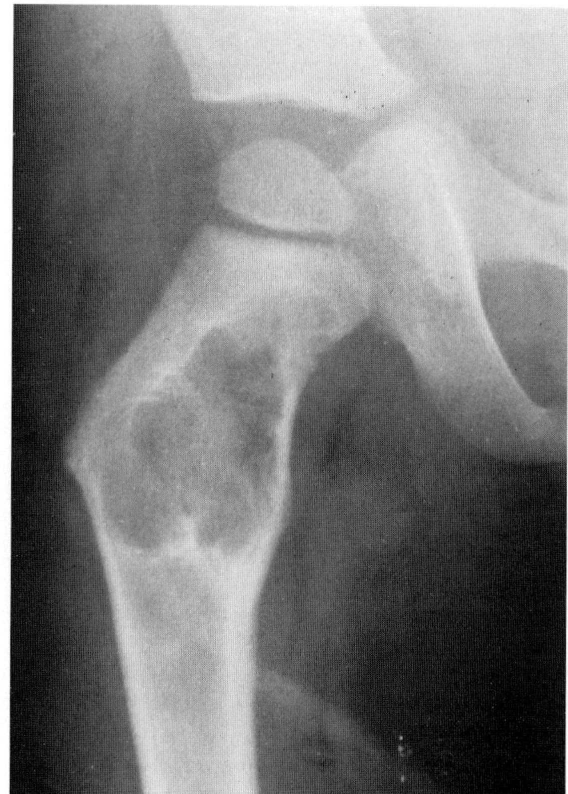

FIGURE 41.33. **Solitary Bone Cyst.** A well-defined lytic lesion, which is central in location, is seen in the proximal femur in this child. This is characteristic for a solitary bone cyst.

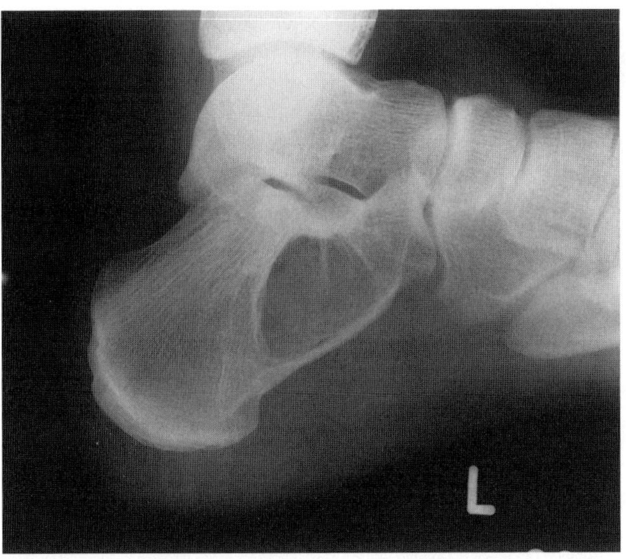

FIGURE 41.34. **Solitary Bone Cyst.** A well-defined lytic lesion is seen in the calcaneus abutting the inferior surface, which is typical in location and appearance for a solitary bone cyst. A solitary bone cyst in the calcaneus occurs almost exclusively in this location and is not subject to pathologic fracture as readily as when one occurs in the proximal femur and humerus.

described in any other lesion and indicates a fluid-filled cystic lesion, rather than a lesion filled with matrix.

Solitary bone cysts occur almost exclusively in young patients (under age 30). Although long bones are most commonly involved, solitary bone cysts have been described in almost every bone in the body. They begin at the physeal plate in long bones and grow into the shaft of the bone; therefore, they are not epiphyseal lesions. They can, however, extend up into an epiphysis after the plate closes, but this is unusual. A fairly common location is in the calcaneus, where they have a characteristic location adjacent to the inferior surface of the calcaneus (Fig. 41.34).

Discriminators. 1. Must be central. 2. Must be younger than age 30 years. 3. No periostitis.

Hyperparathyroidism (Brown Tumors)

Brown tumors of hyperparathyroidism (HPT) can have almost any appearance, from a purely lytic lesion (Fig. 41.35) to a sclerotic process. Generally, when the patient's HPT is treated, the brown tumor undergoes sclerosis and will eventually disappear. If a brown tumor is going to be considered in the differential diagnosis, additional radiographic findings of HPT should be seen. Subperiosteal bone resorption is pathognomonic for HPT and should be

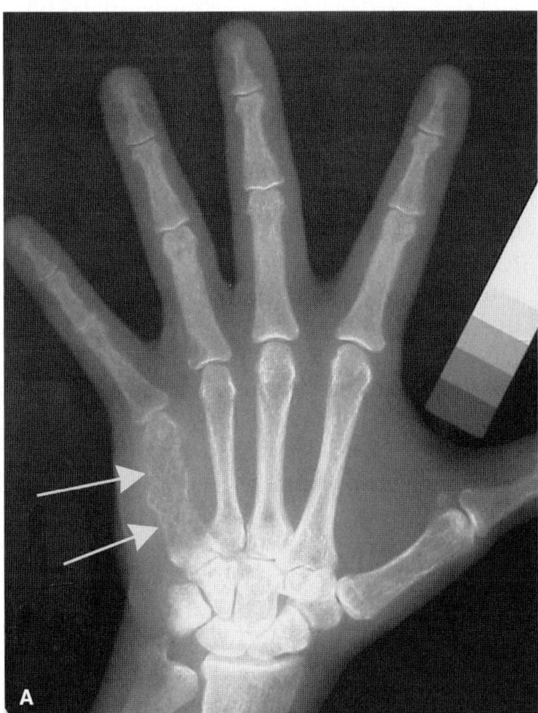

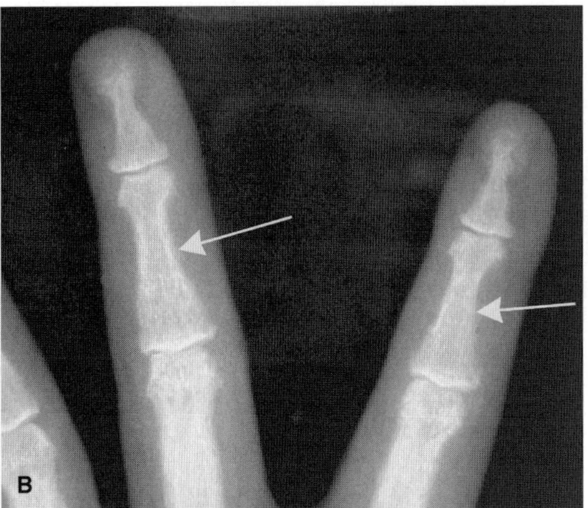

FIGURE 41.35. **Brown Tumor. A.** An expansile lytic lesion is seen in the fifth metacarpal (*arrows*), and a second, smaller lytic lesion is seen in the proximal portion of the fourth proximal phalanx. **B.** This patient is noted to have subperiosteal bone resorption, best seen in the radial aspect of the middle phalanges (*arrows*) as indistinct, interrupted cortex. This makes the diagnosis of hyperparathyroidism with multiple brown tumors most likely.

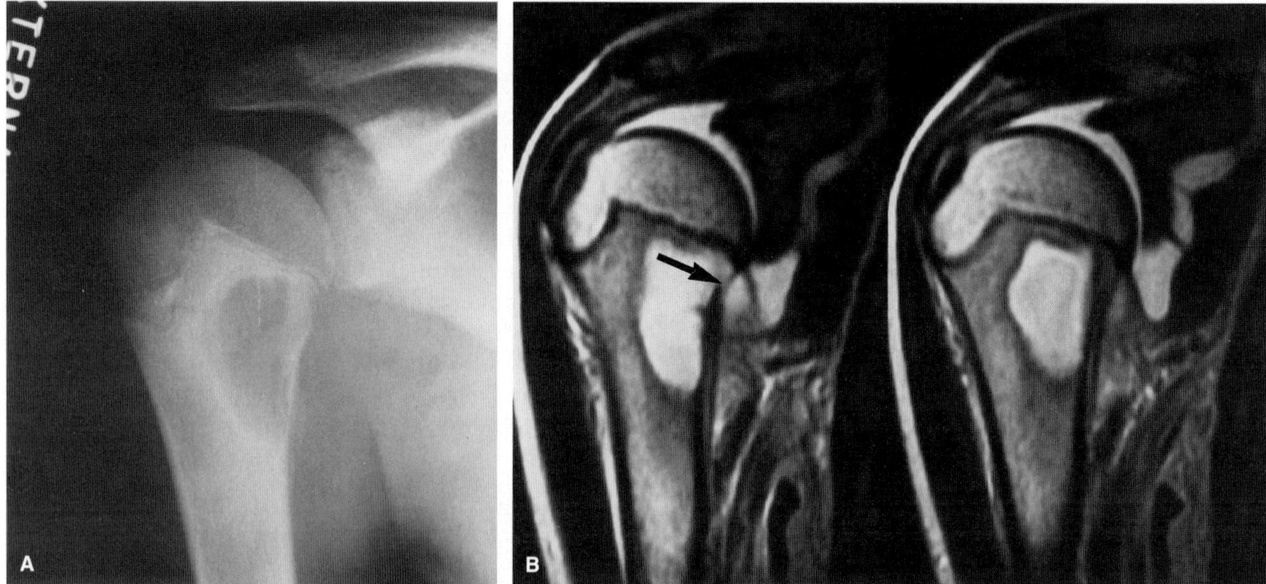

FIGURE 41.36. **Osteomyelitis. A.** A plain film of the proximal humerus in this child with shoulder pain reveals a well-defined lytic lesion in the medial metaphysis. **B.** T2WI of the humerus shows the lesion to have high signal and an associated joint effusion. The probable site of connection to the joint can be seen (*arrow*), which likely represents a draining abscess. Aspiration of the joint fluid revealed pus. This is a large focus of osteomyelitis or Brodie abscess.

searched for in the phalanges (particularly in the radial aspect of the middle phalanges) (Fig. 41.35), distal clavicles (resorption), medial aspect of the proximal tibias, and sacroiliac joints. If the physes are open, they should have a frayed, ragged appearance, as in rickets, owing to the effect of parathormone. Osteoporosis or osteosclerosis might suggest that renal osteodystrophy with secondary HPT is present, but subperiosteal resorption must be present, or brown tumor can be safely excluded from the differential.

Most authorities believe that brown tumors occur most commonly in primary HPT; however, because we see so many more patients with secondary HPT, more brown tumors are seen in patients with secondary rather than primary HPT.

Discriminator. Must have other evidence of HPT.

Infection

Infection. Unfortunately, there is no reliable way radiographically to exclude a focus of osteomyelitis. It has a protean radiographic appearance and can occur at any location and in a patient of any age. It might or might not be expansile, have a sclerotic or nonsclerotic border, or have associated periostitis (3). Therefore, infection will be in almost every differential diagnosis of a lytic lesion, which is acceptable, as it is one of the most common lesions encountered. Soft tissue findings such as obliteration of adjacent fat planes are notoriously unreliable and even misleading, because tumors and EG can do the same thing.

When osteomyelitis occurs near a joint, if the articular surface is abutted, invariably the joint will be involved and show cartilage loss, an effusion (Fig. 41.36), or both. This finding is not particularly helpful, as any lesion can cause an effusion, but it is occasionally useful in ruling out osteomyelitis when no effusion is present and the lesion abuts the articular surface.

If a bony sequestrum is present, osteomyelitis should be strongly considered (Fig. 41.37). As mentioned previously, the only lesions described that demonstrate sequestra are infection, EG, lymphoma, and fibrosarcoma, with osteoid osteoma sometimes mimicking a sequestrum. The finding of a sequestrum in osteomyelitis can be significant for treatment in that it usually requires surgical removal rather than antibiotics alone because a sequestrum is a focus of devitalized bone that does not have a blood supply and will not be effectively treated with parenteral medication. For this reason, CT is routinely recommended when osteomyelitis is considered.

Discriminator. None.

Chondroblastoma

Chondroblastomas are rare lesions but are among the easiest lesions for radiologists to deal with because they occur only in the epiphyses (Fig. 41.38) (a handful of cases have been reported in the metaphyses, but this is rare) and they occur almost exclusively in patients younger than the age of 30 years. Between 40% and 60% demonstrate calcification, so the absence of calcification is not helpful. Presence

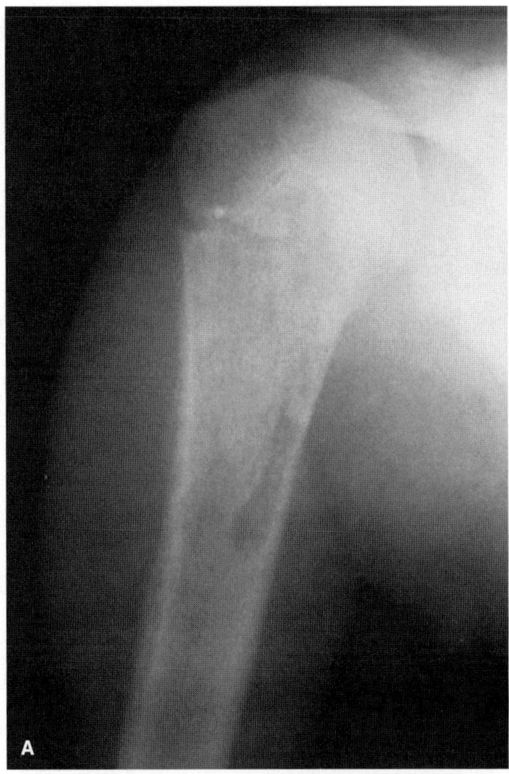

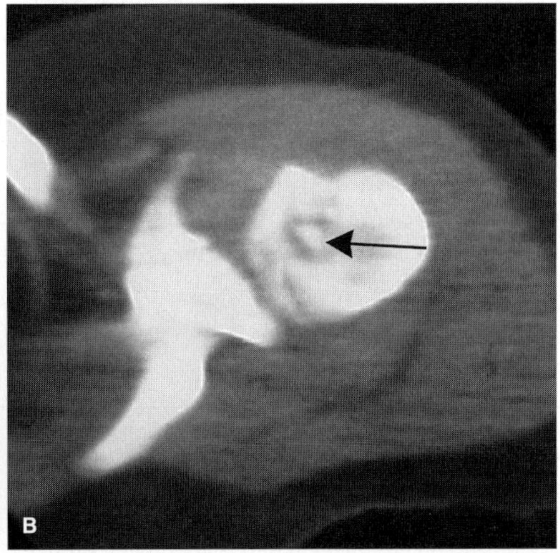

FIGURE 41.37. **Osteomyelitis. A.** A lytic lesion is present in the proximal humerus, which has some associated periostitis laterally. **B.** CT scan through this area reveals a lytic lesion that contains a calcific density within (*arrow*), which is a bony sequestrum. This is an area of osteomyelitis with a bony sequestration.

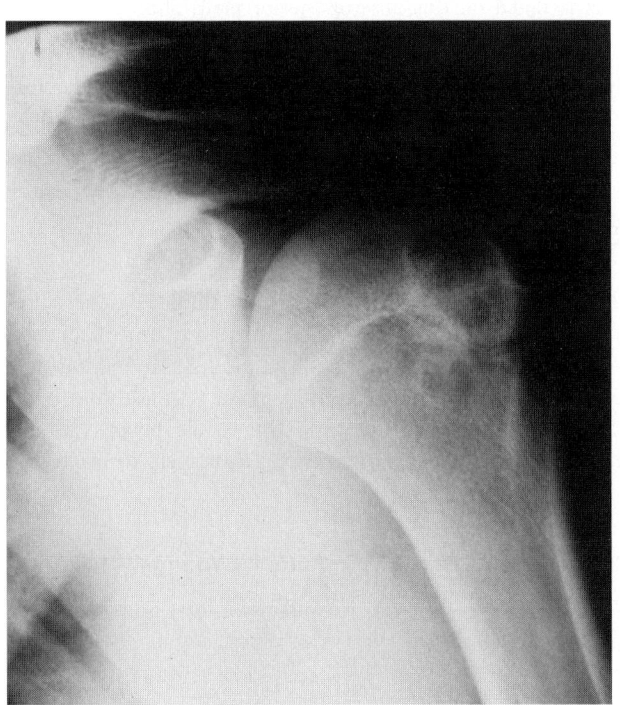

FIGURE 41.38. **Chondroblastoma.** A plain film in this young patient shows a well-defined lytic lesion in the greater tuberosity of the humerus. Biopsy showed this to be a chondroblastoma.

of calcification is helpful, as long as one is certain that it is not detritus or sequestra from infection or EG, both of which can occur in the epiphyses.

The differential diagnosis of a lytic lesion in the epiphysis of a patient under 30 years of age is simple: (*1*) infection (most common), (*2*) chondroblastoma, and (*3*) giant cell tumor (which has its own diagnostic criteria, so it can usually be definitely ruled out or in). This is an old, classic differential and probably encompasses 98% of epiphyseal lesions.

A caveat on epiphyseal lesions is to always consider the possibility of a subchondral cyst or geode (Fig. 41.39), which has been described in four disease processes: (*1*) degenerative joint disease (must have joint space narrowing, sclerosis, and osteophytes); (*2*) rheumatoid arthritis; (*3*) calcium pyrophosphate dihydrate crystal disposition disease or pseudogout; and (*4*) avascular necrosis. The clinician must be certain no joint pathology that might indicate one of these processes is present, or an unnecessary biopsy of a geode might be performed on the basis of the differential of an epiphyseal lesion.

Apophyses are identical to epiphyses as far as the differential diagnosis of lytic lesions, with the exception of geodes, which only occur adjacent to articular surfaces. The carpal bones, the tarsal bones, and the patella have

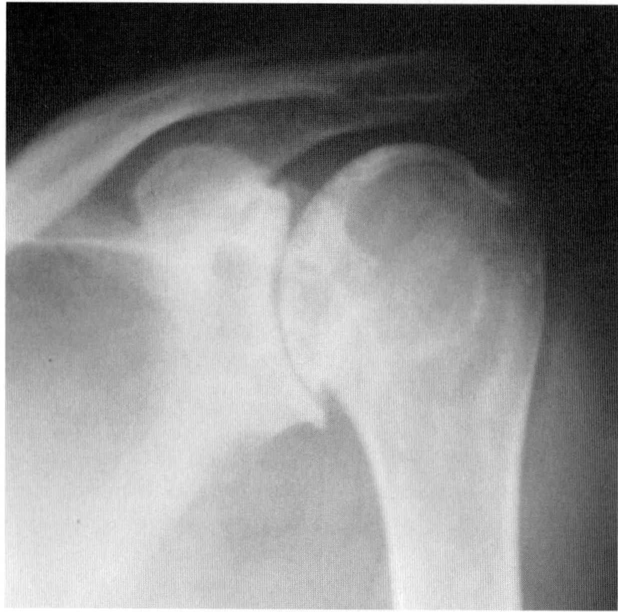

FIGURE 41.39. **Geode.** A large, well-defined lytic lesion in the proximal humerus is present, which is associated with marked degenerative disease of the glenohumeral joint. When definite degenerative joint disease is present and associated with a lytic lesion, the lytic lesion should be considered to be a geode. A biopsy was performed, which confirmed this to be a geode, or subchondral cyst; however, the biopsy could have been avoided.

a tendency to behave like epiphyses in their differential diagnosis of lesions. Therefore, a lytic lesion in these areas has a similar differential diagnosis as an epiphyseal lesion.

Discriminator. 1. Must be younger than age 30. 2. Must be epiphyseal.

Chondromyxoid Fibroma

Chondromyxoid fibroma, like osteoblastoma, is such a rare lesion that failure to mention it is probably not going to result in missing more than one in a lifetime. Why include it, then? I recommend not including it, but it is part of the classic FEGNOMASHIC differential. If it is mentioned, at least know what it looks like. Basically, chondromyxoid fibromas resemble NOFs. Unlike NOFs, however, they can be seen in a patient of any age. Chondromyxoid fibromas often extend into the epiphyses (Fig. 41.40), whereas NOFs rarely do. Also, they can present with pain, which will not occur with an NOF. They have been reported to progress from a benign process to an aggressive and even malignant lesion, but this is extremely rare. Although chondromyxoid fibromas are cartilaginous lesions, calcified cartilage matrix is virtually never seen radiographically.

Discriminator. 1. Mention when an NOF is mentioned. 2. No calcified matrix.

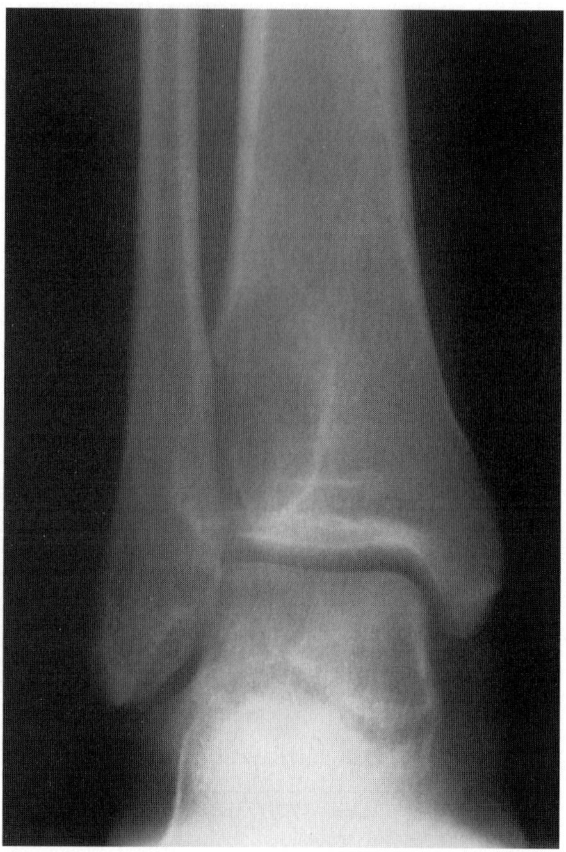

FIGURE 41.40. **Chondromyxoid Fibroma.** A well-defined lytic lesion in the distal tibia that extends slightly into the epiphysis is noted on this anteroposterior plain film. A nonossifying fibroma could certainly have this appearance; however, this underwent biopsy and was found to be a chondromyxoid fibroma. Chondromyxoid fibromas often extend into the epiphysis, as in this example, whereas nonossifying fibromas usually do not.

SUMMARY

That, in essence, is the differential diagnosis for a benign cystic lesion of bone. It is probably 98% accurate, which is good enough for most radiologists. To increase the accuracy to 99%, it would be necessary to add many uncommon or rare lesions, and the whole process would become too confusing for most radiologists to learn and

TABLE 41.2 Lesions in Patients Younger Than 30 Years of Age

Eosinophilic granuloma
Aneurysmal bone cyst
Nonossifying fibroma
Chondroblastoma
Solitary bone cyst

TABLE 41.3 "Automatics"

Younger than age 30
Infection
Eosinophilic granuloma
Older than age 40
Infection
Metastatic disease and myeloma

TABLE 41.5 Epiphyseal Lesions

Infection
Giant cell tumor
Chondroblastoma
Geode

apply. If there is a favorite lesion that is not on this list, by all means add it. Likewise, if the list is already too cumbersome, forget about osteoblastoma and chondromyxoid fibroma. I am unable to make it much simpler than that and still be reasonably accurate.

Some of the lesions I have purposefully omitted are intraosseous ganglion, pseudotumor of hemophilia, hemangioendothelioma, ossifying fibroma, intraosseous lipoma, glomus tumor, neurofibroma, plasma cell granuloma, and schwannoma. Others could be added to this list, of course, but are best left to the pathologist—not the radiologist—for the diagnosis.

There are several features that are somewhat useful in separating the various lesions in FEGNOMASHIC. For instance, if the patient is younger than the age of 30 years, be sure to consider *EG, chondroblastoma, NOF, solitary bone cyst,* and *ABC* (Table 41.2). If the patient is over 30 years of age, those five lesions can be excluded. Note that this is not a differential diagnosis for lesions in patients under age 30; it simply means these entities should not be mentioned in older patients. For those younger than age 30, other lesions such as fibrous dysplasia and infection must also be mentioned.

There are a few lytic lesions that have no good discriminators other than age and, therefore, must be mentioned routinely. I call these lesions "automatics" because one should automatically mention them regardless of the location or appearance of the lesion. *Infection* and *EG* must be mentioned for those younger than age 30, whereas *metastatic disease* and *infection* must be included in any differential in a patient older than age 40 (Table 41.3). These lesions have a protean radiographic appearance and should be mentioned not only in the benign cystic differential but also for an aggressive lesion.

If periostitis or pain is present (assuming no trauma, which can be a foolhardy assumption), you can exclude *fibrous dysplasia, solitary bone cyst, NOF,* and *enchondroma* (Table 41.4). If the lesion is epiphyseal, the differential is *infection, giant cell tumor, chondroblastoma* (and do not forget *geodes*) (Table 41.5). If the patient is over 40 years of age, add *metastatic disease* and *myeloma* and remove *chondroblastoma* from the epiphyseal list.

The epiphyseal differential tends to apply also to the tarsal bones (especially the calcaneus), the carpal bones, and the patella. In the calcaneus, a unicameral bone cyst should also be considered and has a characteristic appearance and location (see Fig. 41.34). Apophyses are "epiphyseal equivalents" and have the same differential as epiphyses. The difference between an epiphysis and an apophysis is that epiphyses contribute to the length of a bone, whereas apophyses serve as ligamentous attachments.

A classic differential for benign, cystic rib lesions is the mnemonic FAME, in which F = *fibrous dysplasia,* A = *ABC,* M = *metastatic diseases* and *myeloma,* and E = *enchondroma* and *EG* (Table 41.6). If multiple lytic lesions are present, FEEMHI is a useful mnemonic of the lesions in FEGNOMASHIC that can be multiple: F = *fibrous dysplasia,* E = *enchondroma,* E = *EG,* M = *metastatic disease* and *myeloma,* H = *hyperparathyroidism* (brown tumor), and I = *infection* (Table 41.7).

A few findings that just do not seem to narrow the differential diagnosis are presence or absence of a soft tissue mass, expansion of the bone (except it must be present in an ABC), sclerotic or nonsclerotic border (except it must be nonsclerotic in giant cell tumor), presence or absence of bony struts or compartments in the lesion, and size of the lesion.

If calcified matrix is identified in a lesion, it is tempting to narrow the differential to either the osteoid series

TABLE 41.4 Lesions That Have No Pain or Periostitis

Fibrous dysplasia
Enchondroma
Nonossifying fibroma
Solitary bone cyst

TABLE 41.6 Differential for Rib Lesions

Fibrous dysplasia
Aneurysmal bone cyst
Metastatic disease and myeloma
Enchondroma and eosinophilic granuloma

TABLE 41.7 Multiple Lesions (FEEMHI)

Fibrous dysplasia
Eosinophilic granuloma
Enchondroma
Metastatic disease and myeloma
Hyperparathyroidism (brown tumors)
Infection

or the chondroid series of lesions, depending on the character of the matrix. Be careful of this. Very few radiologists can reliably differentiate chondroid from osteoid matrix. Routine calcification of a lesion or debris, detritus, or sequestrations in osteomyelitis can mimic chondroid or osteoid calcification and be misleading. The only lesion that must exhibit calcified matrix is the enchondroma (except in the phalanges). Chondroblastomas and osteoblastomas demonstrate calcified matrix about half the time, and chondromyxoid fibromas never have radiographically demonstrable calcified matrix.

DIFFERENTIAL DIAGNOSIS OF A SCLEROTIC LESION

Many lytic lesions spontaneously regress and are not usually seen in patients over 30 years of age. When these lesions regress, they often fill in with new bone and have a sclerotic or blastic appearance. Therefore, when a sclerotic focus is identified in a 20- to 40-year-old patient, especially if it is an asymptomatic, incidental finding, the

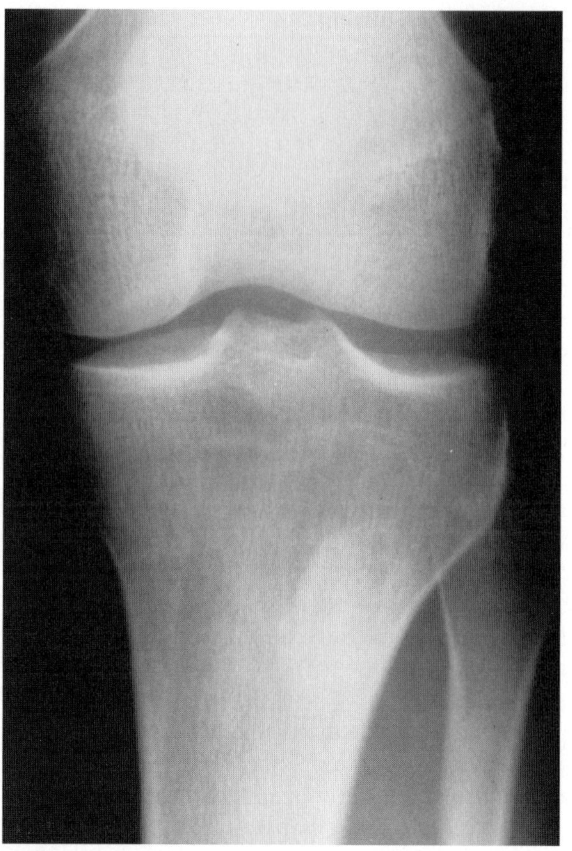

FIGURE 41.41. **Healing Nonossifying Fibroma.** A plain film of the knee in this 25-year-old patient reveals a sclerotic lesion in the proximal tibia, which is a healing or resolving nonossifying fibroma.

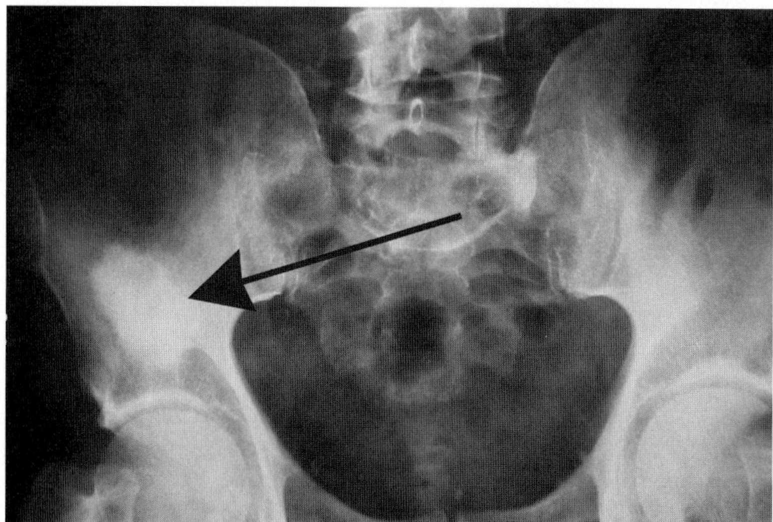

FIGURE 41.42. **Giant Bone Island.** A large sclerotic lesion is present in the right supraacetabular region of the ilium (*arrow*), which represents a giant bone island. The slightly feathered margins of the trabeculae, which blend in with the normal bone, and the long axis of the lesion being in the direction of primary weight bearing are characteristic for a bone island.

following lesions should be considered: NOF (Fig. 41.41), EG, aneurysmal bone cyst, solitary bone cyst, and chondroblastoma. Several other lesions should be included that can also appear sclerotic: fibrous dysplasia, osteoid osteoma, infection, brown tumor (healing), and perhaps a giant bone island (Fig. 41.42). In any patient older than the age of 40 years, the number one possibility should be metastatic disease.

REFERENCES

1. David R, Oria R, Kumar R, et al. Radiologic features of eosinophilic granuloma of bone. Pictorial essay. AJR Am J Roentgenol 1989;153: 1021–1026.
2. Dahlin D. Giant cell tumor of bone: highlights of 407 cases. AJR Am J Roentgenol 1985;144:955–960.
3. Gold R, Hawkins R, Katz R. Pictorial essay. Bacterial osteomyelitis: findings on plain radiography, CT, MR, and scintigraphy. AJR Am J Roentgenol 1991;157:365–370.

Chapter 42

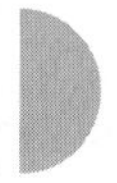

Malignant Bone and Soft Tissue Tumors

Clyde A. Helms

Radiographic Findings

Tumors

RADIOGRAPHIC FINDINGS

Malignant bone tumors, thankfully, are not very common. Nevertheless, every radiologist should be able to recognize them and give a useful differential diagnosis. First, how does one recognize a malignant tumor and differentiate it from a benign process? This can be difficult and is often impossible. Recognizing that it is *aggressive* is usually easy, but stating that it is *malignant* is another matter altogether. Processes such as infection and eosinophilic granuloma (EG) can mimic malignant tumors and are, of course, benign. They will often be included in the differential diagnosis of an aggressive lesion, along with malignant tumors. What radiologic plain film criteria are useful for determining malignant versus benign? Standard textbooks give four aspects of a lesion to be examined: (*1*) cortical destruction, (*2*) periostitis, (*3*) orientation or axis of the lesion, and (*4*) zone of transition. Let me discuss each of these criteria and show why only the last one—the zone of transition—is accurate to a 90% plus rate. It is important to recognize that these are plain film criteria and do not apply to CT or MR imaging in many instances.

Cortical Destruction. Benign fibro-osseous lesions and cartilaginous lesions often have part of their noncalcified matrix (fibrous matrix or chondroid matrix, both of which are radiolucent on plain films) replacing cortical bone, which can give the false impression of cortical destruction on plain films (Fig. 42.1) or CT. Also, benign processes such as infection and EG can cause extensive cortical destruction and mimic a malignant tumor. It is well known that aneurysmal bone cysts cause such thinning of the cortex as to make the cortex radiographically undetectable (Fig. 42.2). For these reasons, cortical destruction can occasionally be misleading. Cortical destruction always makes one think of a malignant lesion when using the "gestalt approach," but the lesion must also have other criteria for a malignant process, such as a wide zone of transition.

Periostitis. Periosteal reaction occurs in a nonspecific manner whenever the periosteum is irritated, whether by a malignant tumor, a benign tumor, infection, or trauma. Callus formation in a fracture is actually just periosteal reaction of the most benign type. Periosteal reaction occurs in two types: benign or aggressive, based more on the timing of the irritation than on whether it is a malignant or benign process causing the periostitis. For example, a slow-growing benign tumor will cause thick, wavy, uniform, or dense periostitis (Fig. 42.3A) because it is a low-grade chronic irritation that gives the periosteum time to lay down thick new bone and remodel into more normal cortex. A malignant tumor causes a periosteal reaction that is high grade and more acute; hence, the periosteum does not have time to consolidate. It appears lamellated (onion-skinned) (Fig. 42.3B) or amorphous or even sunburst-like. If the irritation stops or diminishes, the aggressive periostitis will solidify and appear benign. Therefore, when periostitis is seen, the radiologist should try to characterize it into either a benign (thick, dense, wavy) type or an aggressive (lamellated, amorphous, sunburst) type.

Unfortunately, judging a lesion by its periostitis can be very misleading. First, it takes considerable experience to characterize periostitis accurately, because many times the reaction is not clearly benign or aggressive. Second, many benign lesions cause aggressive periostitis, such as infection, EG, aneurysmal bone cysts, osteoid osteomas, and even trauma. Detection of *benign* periostitis, however, can be very helpful because malignant lesions will not cause benign periostitis. Some investigators with great experience in dealing with malignant bone tumors state that the only

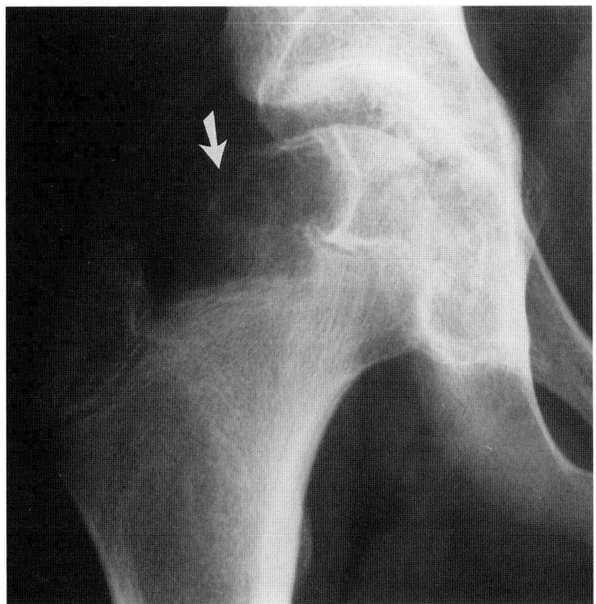

FIGURE 42.1. **Apparent Cortical Destruction.** This benign chondroblastoma has noncalcified chondroid tissue replacing cortical bone in the proximal femur (*arrow*), which gives this lesion a destructive appearance. This is an example of cortical replacement, rather than cortical destruction, which can be very confusing if one uses cortical destruction as a criterion for aggression or malignancy. Note in this example that the zone of transition is narrow, as one would expect in a benign lesion such as this.

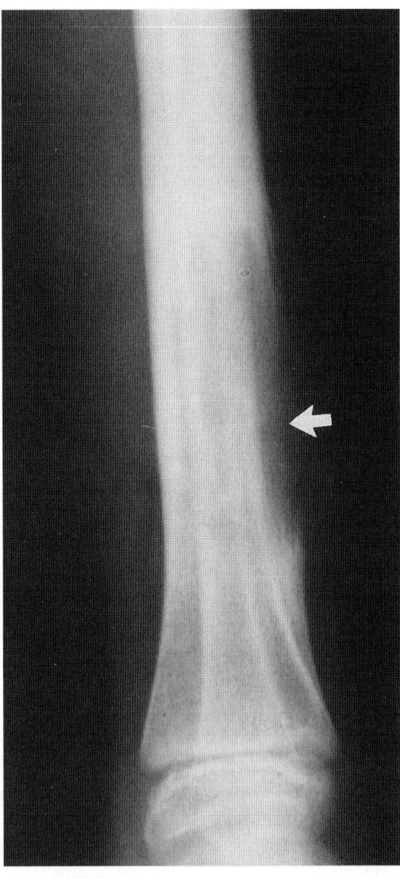

FIGURE 42.2. **Aneurysmal Bone Cyst.** This benign lesion has thinned the cortex to such a degree as to make it imperceptible (*arrow*). As in Fig. 42.1, this could be misconstrued as cortical destruction, giving the false impression of a malignant or very aggressive lesion.

way benign periostitis can occur in a malignant lesion is if there is a concomitant fracture or infection. Exceptions to this are extremely uncommon.

Orientation or axis of the lesion is a very poor determinant of benign versus aggressive lesions and rarely helps determine into which category the lesion should be placed. It has been said that if a lesion grows in the long axis of a long bone, rather than being circular, it is benign. However, there are simply too many exceptions to this rule for it to be helpful. For example, Ewing sarcoma, an extremely malignant lesion, usually has its axis along the shaft of a long bone. Conversely, many fibrous cortical defects are circular yet totally benign. Thus, the axis of the lesion is not helpful in assessing benignity versus malignancy.

Zone of transition is without question the most reliable plain film indicator for benign versus malignant lesions. Unfortunately, it also has some drawbacks. The zone of transition is the border of the lesion with the normal bone. It is said to be "narrow" if it is so well defined that it can be drawn with a fine-point pen (Fig. 42.4). If it is imperceptible and cannot be clearly drawn at all, it is said to be "wide" (Fig. 42.5). Obviously, all shades of gray lie in between, but most lesions can be characterized as having either a narrow or a wide zone of transition. If the lesion has a sclerotic border, it, of course, has a narrow zone of transition. If a lesion has a narrow zone of transition, a benign process should be considered as the most likely possibility.

The exceptions to this are rare. If a lesion has a wide zone of transition, it is aggressive, although not necessarily malignant. As with aggressive periostitis, many benign lesions as well as malignant lesions can cause a wide zone of transition. A few of the same processes that can cause aggressive periostitis and thereby mimic a malignant tumor can have a wide zone of transition (i.e., infection and EG). They are aggressive in their radiographic appearance because they are usually fast-acting, aggressive lesions. The zone of transition is usually easier to characterize than the periostitis; in addition, it is always present to evaluate, whereas many lesions (whether benign or malignant) have no periostitis. For these reasons, the zone of transition is the most useful indicator of whether a lesion is benign or malignant.

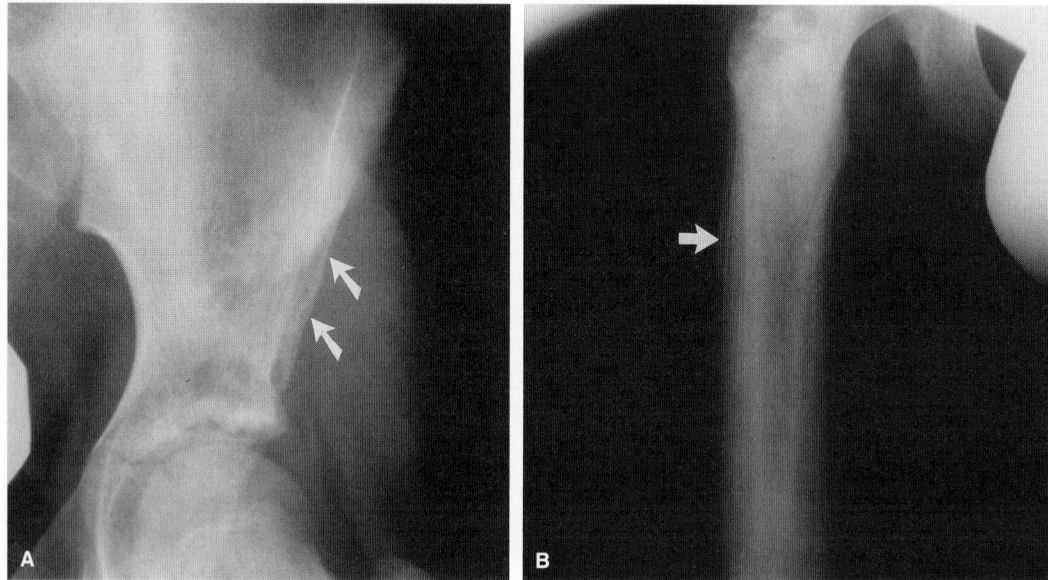

FIGURE 42.3. **Periostitis. A.** Benign periostitis. Thick, wavy periostitis (*arrows*) along the ilium in a child with a permeative lesion in the pelvis is characteristic for infection or eosinophilic granuloma. Ewing sarcoma was initially considered in the differential; however, the benign periostitis would make a malignant lesion very unlikely. Biopsy showed this lesion to be eosinophilic granuloma. **B.** Aggressive periostitis. Lamellated or onion-skin periostitis (*arrow*) is characteristic of an aggressive process, such as in this patient with Ewing sarcoma of the femur. Again, this aggressive type of periostitis could conceivably occur in a benign process such as infection or eosinophilic granuloma.

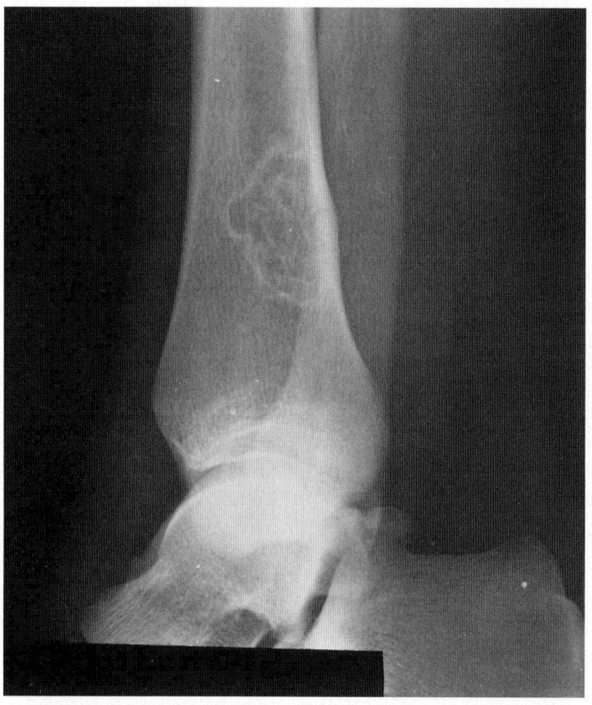

FIGURE 42.4. **Narrow Zone of Transition.** When the margins of a lesion can be drawn with a fine-point pen, as in this example, it is said to be a narrow zone of transition, which is characteristic of a benign lesion. A narrow zone of transition might or might not have a sclerotic border. This is a nonossifying fibroma.

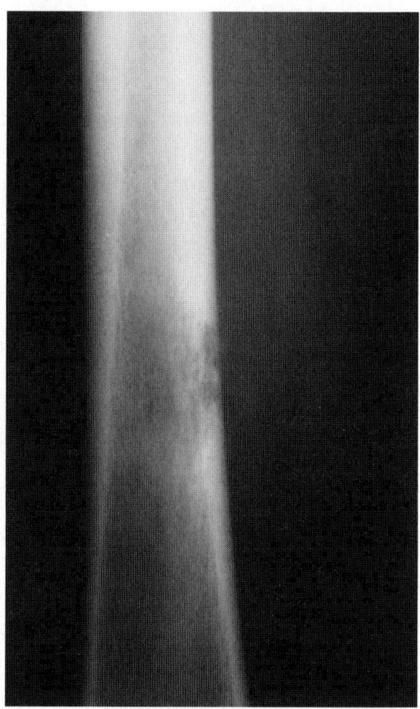

FIGURE 42.5. **Wide Zone of Transition.** A lytic, permeative process is seen in the midshaft of the femur in this patient that on biopsy was found to be a malignant fibrous histiocytoma. The zone of transition in this lesion is said to be wide, as it cannot be easily drawn with a fine-point pen. A permeative lesion such as this, by definition, has a wide zone of transition.

TABLE 42.1 Ages of Patients With Malignant Tumors

Age (y)	*Possible Diagnoses*
1–30	Ewing sarcoma, osteogenic sarcoma
30–40	Giant cell tumor, parosteal sarcoma, fibrosarcoma, malignant fibrous histiocytoma, 1° lymphoma of bone
Over 40	Chondrosarcoma, metastatic disease, myeloma

A lesion consisting of multiple small holes is said to be *permeative* (see Chapter 45 for discussion of the difference between a permeative and a pseudopermeative lesion). It has no perceptible border and therefore has a wide zone of transition. Round cell tumors such as multiple myeloma, reticulum cell sarcoma (primary lymphoma of bone), and Ewing sarcoma are typical of this type of lesion. Infection and EG also can have this same appearance.

Once it is decided that a particular lesion is most likely malignant, the differential is fairly straightforward. First, the list of malignant tumors is relatively short; and second, most tumors follow somewhat strict age groupings. Jack Edeiken, one of the preeminent bone radiologists of our era, evaluated 4,000 malignant bone tumors and found that they could be diagnosed correctly 80% of the time just by using the patient's age. He basically divides the tumors into decades of when they usually affect a patient. For example, osteosarcoma and Ewing sarcoma are the only childhood primary malignant tumors of bone, and after the age of 40, only metastatic disease, myeloma, and chondrosarcoma are common (Table 42.1). Although there are certainly outliers that are uncommon, these age guidelines are extremely useful. It is inappropriate to mention Ewing

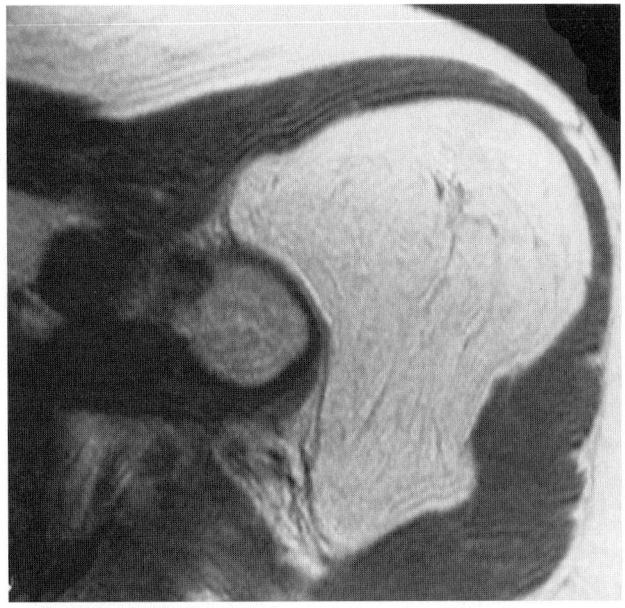

FIGURE 42.6. **Lipoma.** This axial proton-density image (time of repetition 2,000; time of echo 20) through the pelvis shows a large mass lateral to the femur, which has sharp margins and signal characteristics similar to the subcutaneous fat. This is a lipoma. Lipomas will usually contain a small amount of low-signal linear tissue, as in this example, which should not be cause to consider this lesion malignant.

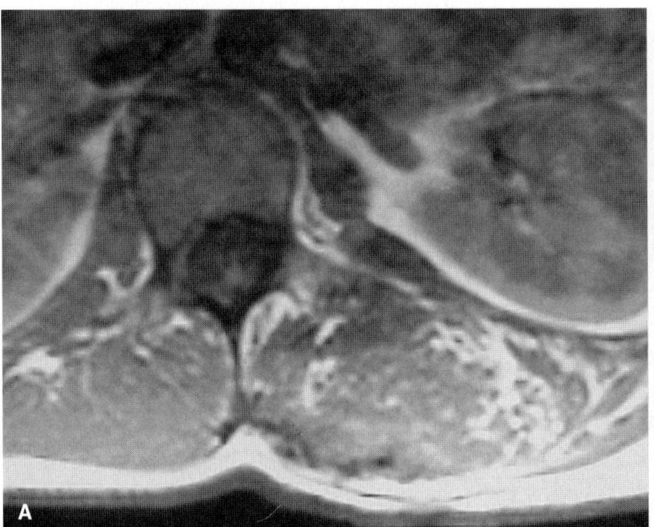

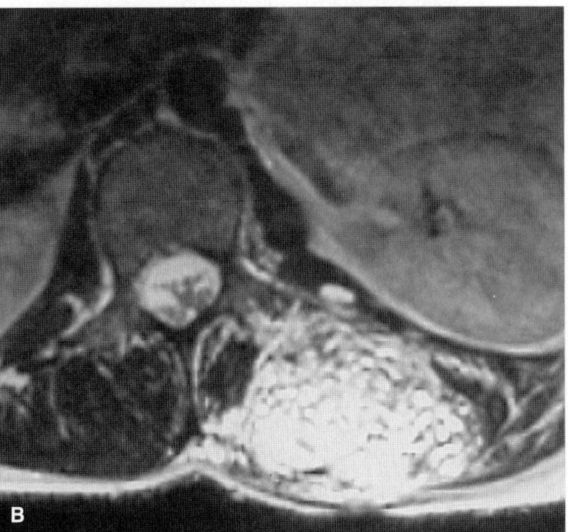

FIGURE 42.7. **Hemangioma. A.** A T1W axial image (time of repetition [TR] 600; time of echo [TE] 11) through the midback in a 30-year-old patient with a mass shows a predominantly low-signal mass with stippled areas of high signal representing fat around numerous vessels. **B.** A fast spin-echo T2W axial image (TR 3,700; TE 102) reveals inhomogeneous high signal with punctate areas of very bright signal representing vessels. Hemangiomas typically have mixed fatty and vascular tissue, which gives high signal on both T1 and T2 sequences.

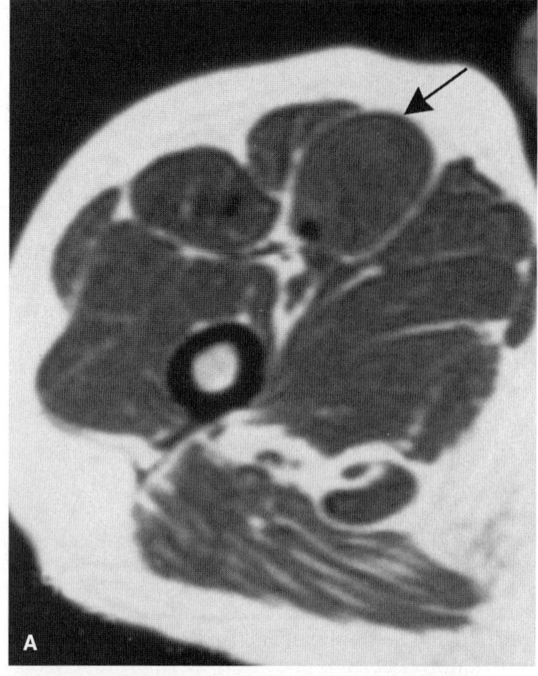

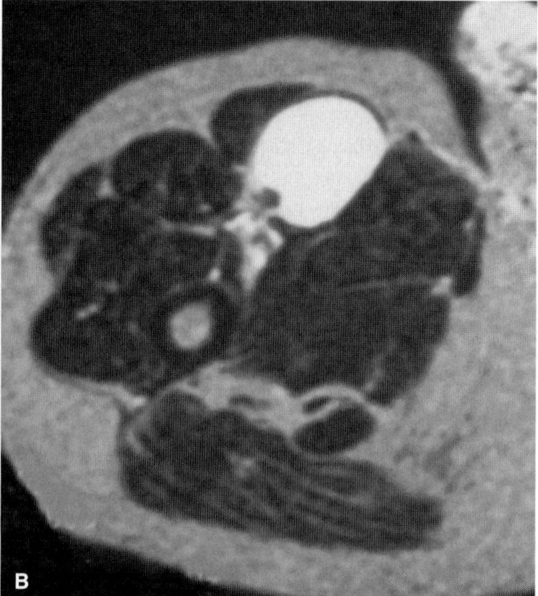

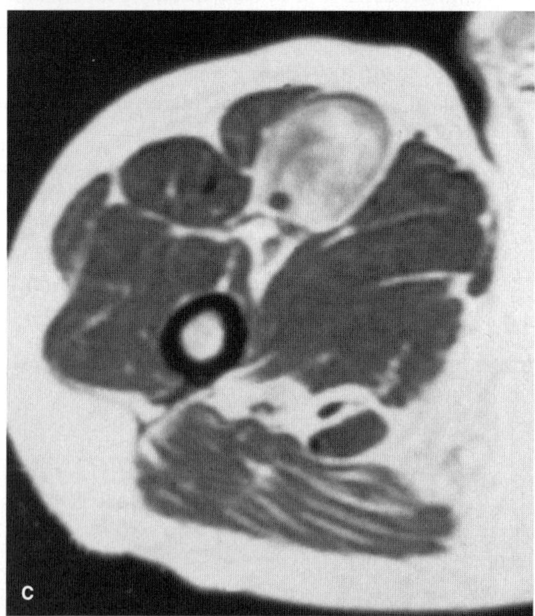

FIGURE 42.8. **Schwannoma. A.** A T1W axial image (time of repetition 600; time of echo 11) shows a mass (*arrow*) in the anterior thigh. **B.** A T2WI shows homogeneous high signal identical to that seen in a fluid collection. **C.** A T1WI taken after administration of gadolinium shows diffuse enhancement of the mass, indicating that this is a solid tumor. Biopsy revealed this to be a schwannoma.

sarcoma in a 40-year-old patient or metastatic disease in a 15-year-old patient, unless there is a known primary tumor. In fact, any bone lesion, regardless of its appearance, could be a metastatic lesion and would be suspicious in a patient with a known primary tumor.

Magnetic Resonance Imaging. Although plain films are the best modality for characterizing a bony lesion—that is, the ability to distinguish benign from malignant and generating a differential diagnosis—MR is without question the imaging procedure of choice for determining the extent of a lesion, both in the skeleton and in the soft tissues. For this reason, if resection of a tumor is contemplated, MR should be performed.

In assessing benignity versus malignancy, MR is somewhat controversial (1). Benign lesions tend to be well marginated, to have uniform and homogeneous signal, not to encase neurovascular structures, and not to invade bone. Malignant lesions tend to have irregular margins and inhomogeneous signal, and they may encase neurovascular structures or invade bone.

Although almost all tumors will have low signal on T1WI, which become very high in signal intensity with

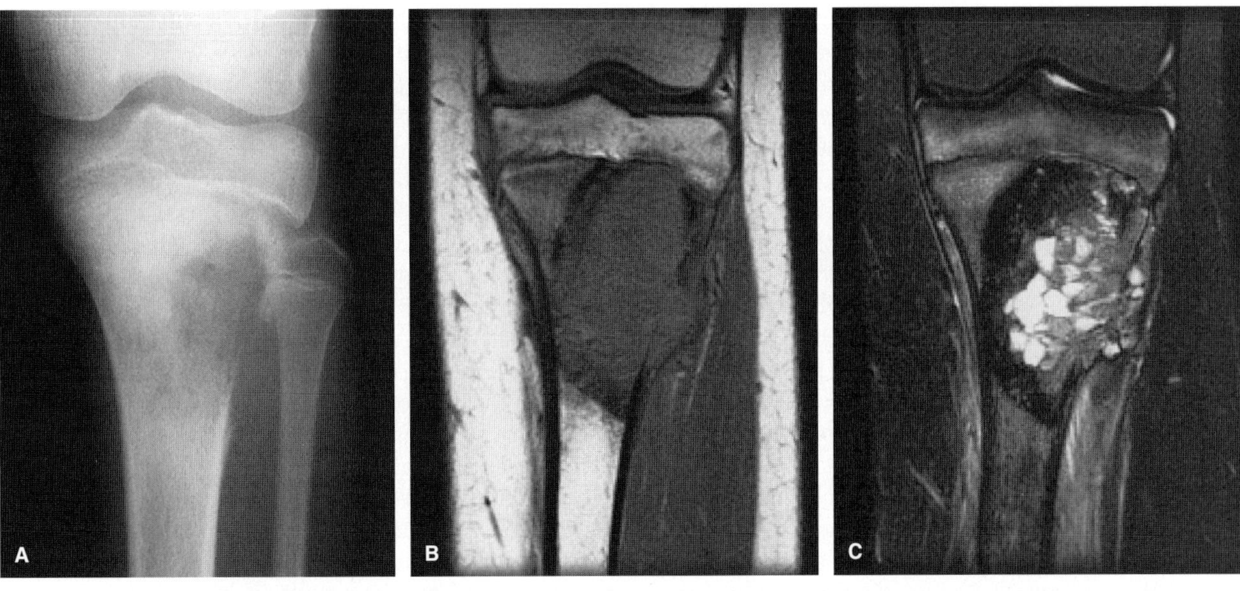

FIGURE 42.9. **Osteosarcoma. A.** A mixed lytic and sclerotic lesion in the proximal tibia of a child is noted, which is characteristic for an osteogenic sarcoma. **B.** A coronal T1WI shows the full extent of the lesion with some soft tissue extension. **C.** These findings are also observed on the T2WI.

T2 weighting (as will fluid collections), there are a few exceptions. Fibrosarcomas, malignant fibrous histiocytomas, and desmoid tumors can occasionally demonstrate low signal on both T1W and T2W sequences. Any tumor with calcification will be low in signal on both T1 and T2 sequences.

In some instances, MR will characterize the lesion better than plain films and enable a specific diagnosis to be made. Lipomas are easily diagnosed with MR by their homogeneous high signal on T1WIs and sharp margins, whether they are intraosseous or in the soft tissues (Fig. 42.6). Hemangiomas and arteriovenous malformations most commonly have mixed high and low signal on both sequences because of the combination of fatty elements and blood (Fig. 42.7). They characteristically have low-signal serpiginous vessels visible.

The finding of a low-signal mass on a T1WI that is high in signal on a T2WI is suspicious for a tumor, but this is a very nonspecific finding and needs to be correlated clinically. Intramuscular injection sites can mimic soft tissue tumors, as can any area of soft tissue trauma. Many malignant tumors exhibit high signal radiating from involved bone, which is soft tissue edema and virtually indistinguishable from tumor spread.

Gadolinium should be routinely given when a presumed fluid collection is found that is not an obvious ganglion or bursa to differentiate a solid mass (which will diffusely enhance with contrast) from a fluid collection (which will have rim enhancement) (Fig. 42.8).

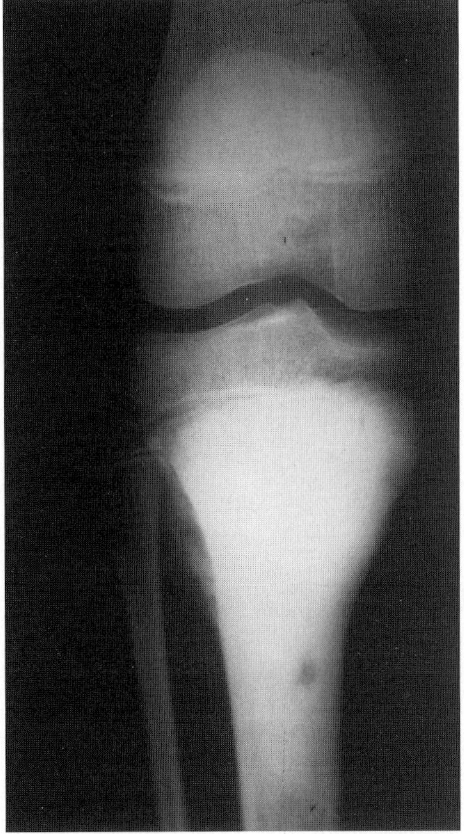

FIGURE 42.10. **Osteosarcoma.** A densely sclerotic lesion in the proximal tibia of a child is seen, which is characteristic for an osteosarcoma.

TUMORS

Osteosarcoma is the most common malignant primary bone tumor. These occur almost exclusively in children and young adults (<30 years old). Some texts describe a second peak of osteosarcoma around the sixth decade, but this is probably because of secondary osteosarcoma in Paget disease and because of prior radiation. Although osteosarcoma typically occurs toward the end of a long bone, it may occur anywhere in the skeleton with enough frequency that location is not a helpful discriminator. These lesions are usually destructive, with obvious sclerosis present from either tumor new bone formation or reactive sclerosis (Figs. 42.9, 42.10); however, on occasion an osteosarcoma can be entirely lytic. These are usually telangiectatic osteosarcomas. There are many different types and classifications of osteosarcomas, but it serves little purpose for the radiologist to try to distinguish between most of them. MR of an osteosarcoma generally reveals a large soft tissue component with heterogeneous high and low signal on both T1WIs and T2WIs (Fig. 42.9).

Parosteal osteosarcoma should be distinguished from central osteosarcoma. A parosteal osteosarcoma originates from the periosteum of the bone and grows outside the bone (Fig. 42.11). It often wraps around the diaphysis without breaking through the cortex at all. It occurs in an older age group than the central osteosarcomas and is not as aggressive or as deadly as long as it has not extended into the medullary portion of the bone. Treatment used to consist of merely shaving the tumor off the bone from which it was arising; however, recurrence rates were so high that now wide, en bloc excisions are performed. Once a parosteal osteosarcoma violates the cortex of the adjacent bone, it is considered to be as aggressive as a central osteosarcoma and is treated in a similar fashion—that is, by amputation or radical excision. The radiologist needs to evaluate the lesion for invasion of the adjacent cortex to help determine treatment and prognosis. This is best done with CT or MR (Fig. 42.12). A common location from which parosteal osteosarcomas arise is the posterior femur, near the knee.

A lesion that can mimic an early parosteal osteosarcoma in this location is a *cortical desmoid tumor.* A cortical desmoid tumor is an avulsion injury that is totally benign but can appear somewhat aggressive. Unfortunately, it can appear malignant histologically, so biopsy can lead to disastrous consequences. Amputations for benign cortical desmoid tumors that were confused with malignancies have occurred.

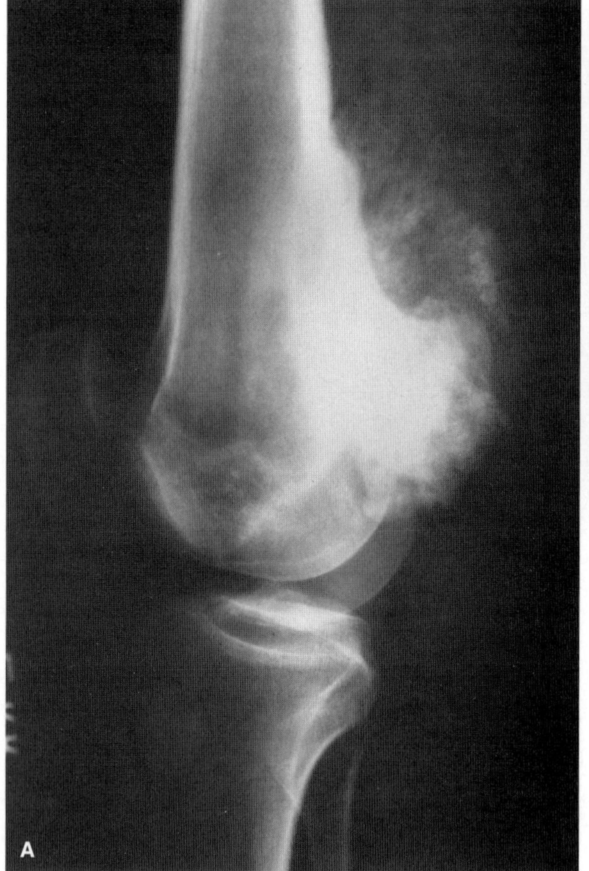

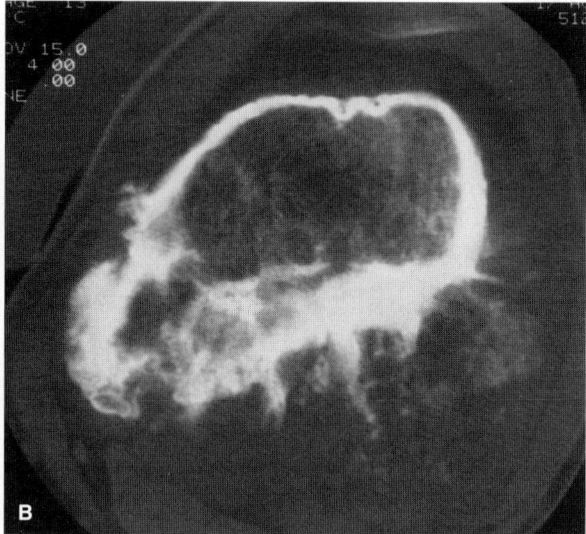

FIGURE 42.11. **Parosteal Osteosarcoma. A.** A lateral plain film of the knee shows a bony lesion emanating from the posterior cortex of the distal femur with a large, calcified soft tissue mass. Note that the densest calcification is central and the periphery is only faintly calcified; these characteristics are typical for a parosteal osteosarcoma. **B.** CT through the lesion reveals the tumor to be invading the medullary portion of the bone. This is a poor prognostic sign and is essential information to the surgeon.

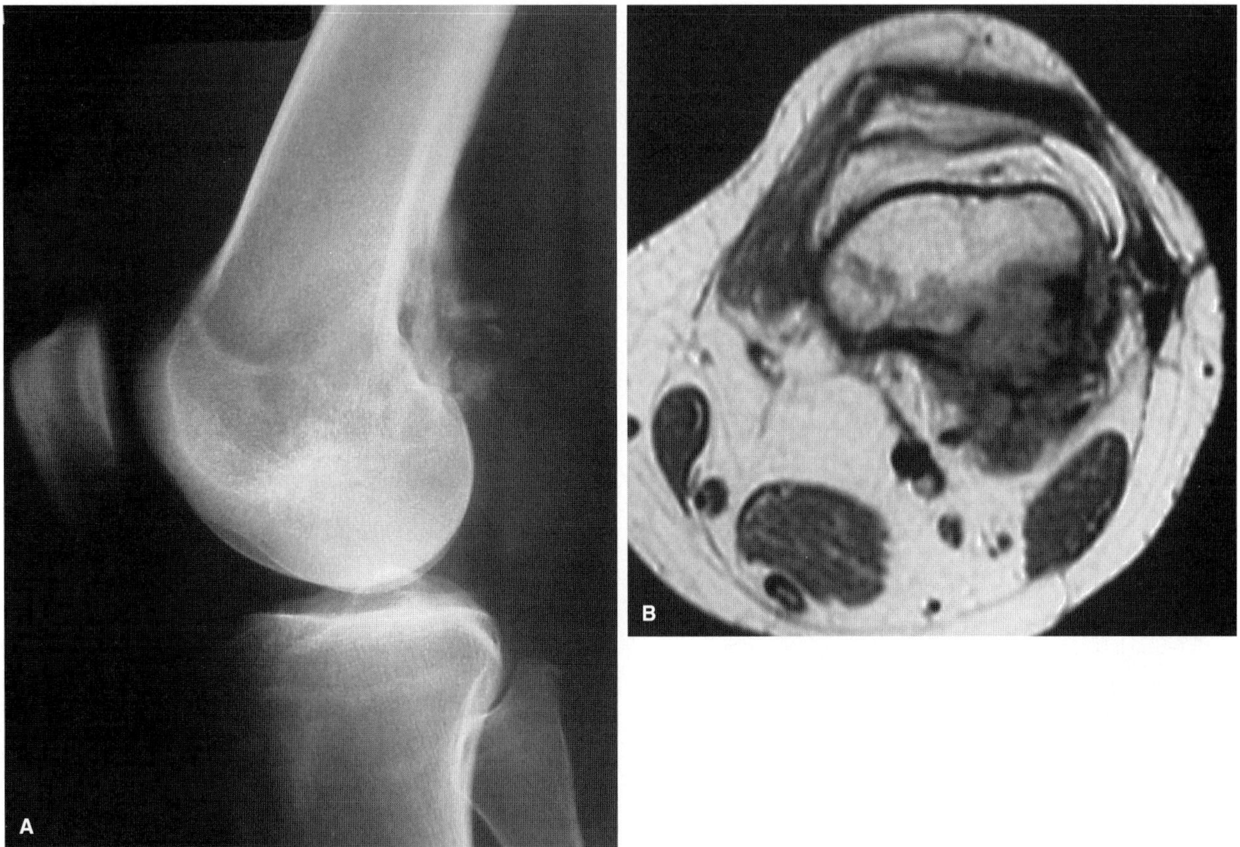

FIGURE 42.12. **Parosteal Osteosarcoma. A.** A lateral plain film in a different patient with a parosteal osteosarcoma shows soft tissue calcification extending from the posterior femur. **B.** A proton-density axial image reveals considerable bony involvement. It also shows that the vascular structures are uninvolved with the soft tissue component.

Another lesion that can be confused with a parosteal osteosarcoma is an area of *myositis ossificans.* Like cortical desmoid tumors, areas of myositis ossificans can be histologically confused for malignancies, with disastrous consequences. Differentiation is, of course, vital. Fortunately, differentiation between parosteal osteosarcoma and myositis ossificans is usually easily done radiographically. (See Chapter 46 for discussion of differential points between parosteal osteosarcoma, myositis ossificans, and cortical desmoid tumors.)

Ewing sarcoma is classically a permeative (multiple small holes) lesion in the diaphysis of a long bone in a child (see Fig. 42.3B). Only about 40% of these tumors occur in the diaphysis, however, with the remainder being metaphyseal and diametaphyseal and in flat bones. They tend to occur primarily in children and adolescents, although a significant number occur in patients in their 20s, especially in flat bones. Although they are most often permeative in appearance, they can elicit reactive new bone that can give the lesion a partially sclerotic or "patchy" appearance. Ewing sarcomas often have an onion-skin type of periostitis, but they can also have periostitis that is sunburst-like or amorphous in character (Fig. 42.13). Rarely, if ever, will a Ewing sarcoma have benign-appearing periostitis (thick, uniform, or wavy).

If benign periostitis is present, other lesions should be considered instead, such as infection and EG. The classic differential diagnosis for a permeative lesion in a child is Ewing sarcoma, infection, and EG. These three entities can appear radiologically identical. Ewing sarcoma should be removed from the differential diagnosis if definite benign periostitis or a sequestration is present. The presence or absence of a soft tissue mass is not helpful in distinguishing between these three lesions. The presence of symptoms is not helpful, because all three entities can be symptomatic.

Chondrosarcomas have a protean appearance that makes it difficult, at times, to make the diagnosis with any assurance. They most commonly occur in patients older than age 40. Chondrosarcoma rarely occurs in children, although occasionally one will be encountered from malignant degeneration of an osteochondroma. It can be

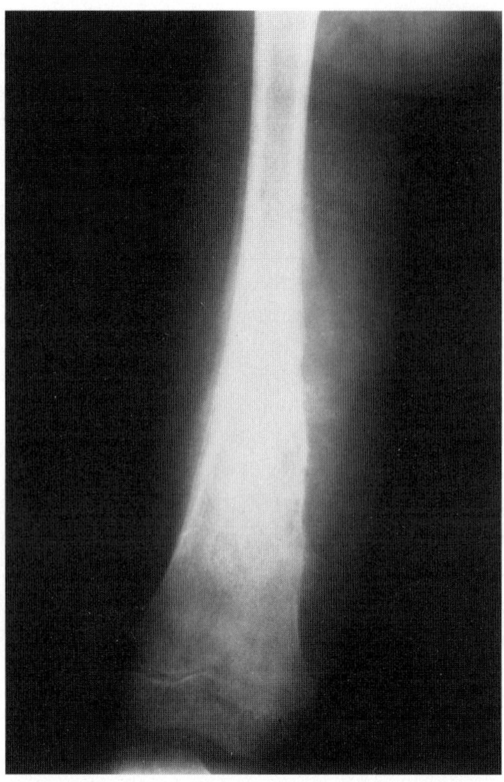

FIGURE 42.13. **Ewing Sarcoma.** An anteroposterior plain film of the femur of a child shows a predominantly sclerotic process with large amounts of sunburst periostitis in the diaphysis, which on biopsy was found to be Ewing sarcoma.

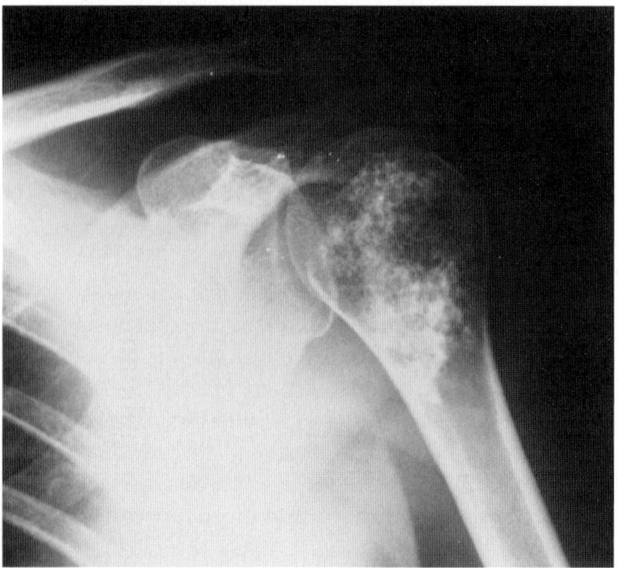

FIGURE 42.14. **Chondrosarcoma.** Typical snowflake or popcornlike amorphous calcification in the proximal humerus is seen, which is typical of an enchondroma. However, this patient had pain associated with this lesion, and on biopsy, this was found to be a chondrosarcoma.

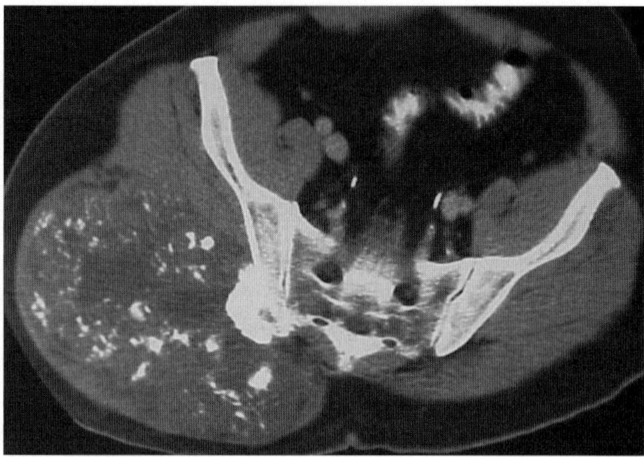

FIGURE 42.15. **Chondrosarcoma.** A large soft tissue mass with amorphous, irregular calcification is seen in a lesion arising from the ilium on this CT of the pelvis. This is typical for a chondrosarcoma.

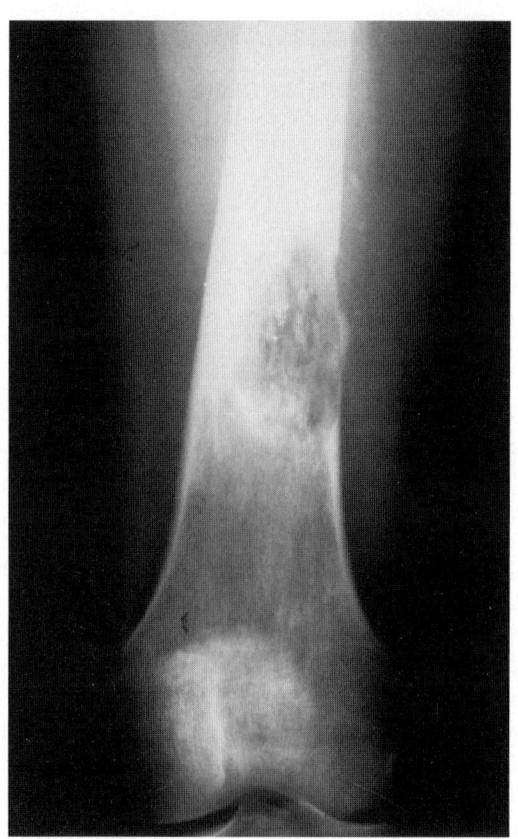

FIGURE 42.16. **Fibrosarcoma.** An ill-defined lytic lesion that is permeative or moth-eaten in appearance is seen in the diaphysis of the femur that on biopsy was shown to be a fibrosarcoma.

extremely difficult to differentiate histologically a low-grade chondrosarcoma from an enchondroma (2). The diagnosis of chondrosarcoma usually initiates radical excision and therapy, although it is debatable (and somewhat controversial) whether a low-grade chondrosarcoma is even a malignant tumor. For these reasons, the diagnosis of "possible chondrosarcoma" should be reserved for those lesions that are painful (Fig. 42.14) or that show definite aggressive characteristics, such as periostitis and destruction. The truth of the matter is neither radiologists nor pathologists can reliably distinguish between enchondromas and low-grade chondrosarcomas. MR can be very useful in distinguishing a benign enchondroma from a chondrosarcoma. If a soft tissue mass or edema is present, it is unlikely to be an enchondroma.

Chondrosarcoma should be considered in the diagnosis any time there is a bony or soft tissue mass with amorphous, snowflake calcification in an older patient (>40 years) (Fig. 42.15). Without the presence of calcified chondroid matrix, the lesion is indistinguishable from any other aggressive lytic lesion, such as metastatic disease, plasmacytoma, fibrosarcoma, malignant fibrous histiocytoma, or infection. Usually the radiologist can only give a long differential diagnosis such as this, which is entirely acceptable. The lesion will have to undergo biopsy at any rate, so it is not necessary for the radiologist to make the diagnosis. This is the case for most malignant tumors.

Malignant Giant Cell Tumor. It is said that approximately 15% of giant cell tumors are malignant; however, this statement is based on their rate of recurrence rather than on the presence of metastatic disease, which is rare. Unfortunately, there does not seem to be any way to predict which giant cell tumors will become malignant. Radiologically, benign and malignant giant cell tumors appear identical. Histologically, benign and malignant giant cell tumors appear the same. If metastases (usually to the lung) occur, the tumor is considered by most oncologists to be malignant. This is quite rare. Malignant giant cell tumors tend to occur primarily in the fourth decade of life.

Fibrosarcomas are lytic malignant tumors that do not produce osteoid or chondroid matrix. True fibrosarcomas are today considered to be very uncommon lesions, with most of what were once called fibrosarcomas actually being malignant fibrous histiocytomas (MFHs). They usually do not cause reactive new bone and, therefore, are almost always lytic in appearance. This lytic appearance may take any form, from permeative (Fig. 42.16) to moth-eaten to a fairly well-defined area of lysis (Fig. 42.17). The age range for fibrosarcoma is quite broad, but they tend to predominate in the fourth decade. This is one of the few malignant tumors that can, on occasion, have a bony sequestrum.

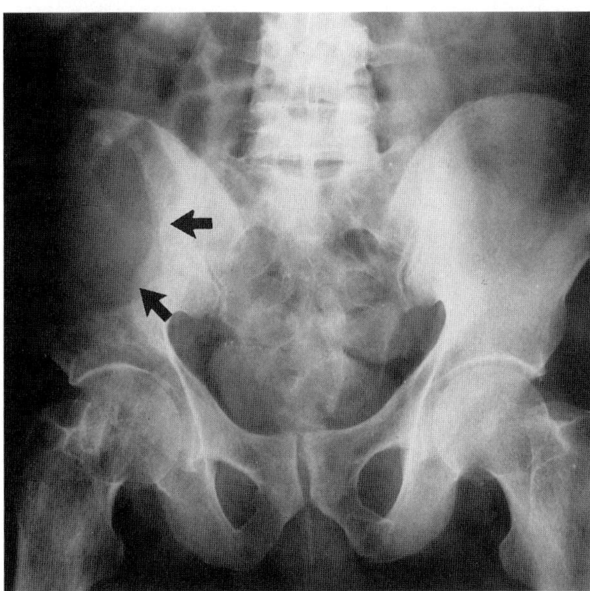

FIGURE 42.17. **Fibrosarcoma.** A large, lytic, destructive process of the entire right iliac wing (*arrows*) is noted, which is fairly well defined. On biopsy, this was shown to be a fibrosarcoma. Fibrosarcomas can be very slow growing and will occasionally have a narrow zone of transition such as this.

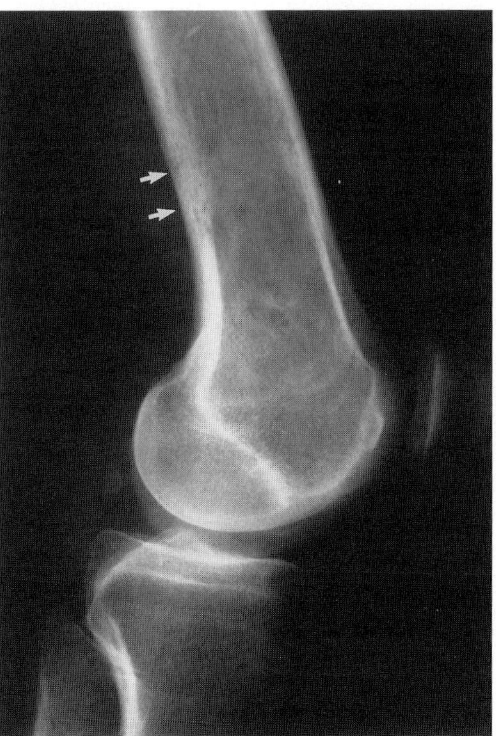

FIGURE 42.18. **Malignant Fibrous Histiocytoma.** A moth-eaten or permeative process in the distal femur, with some involvement of the posterior cortex (*arrows*), is seen on this lateral radiograph. In a patient younger than the age of 30 years, Ewing sarcoma, eosinophilic granuloma, or infection would be the differential diagnosis. In a patient older than age 30, infection and malignant fibrous histiocytoma would be more common. A 1° lymphoma of bone could have a similar appearance.

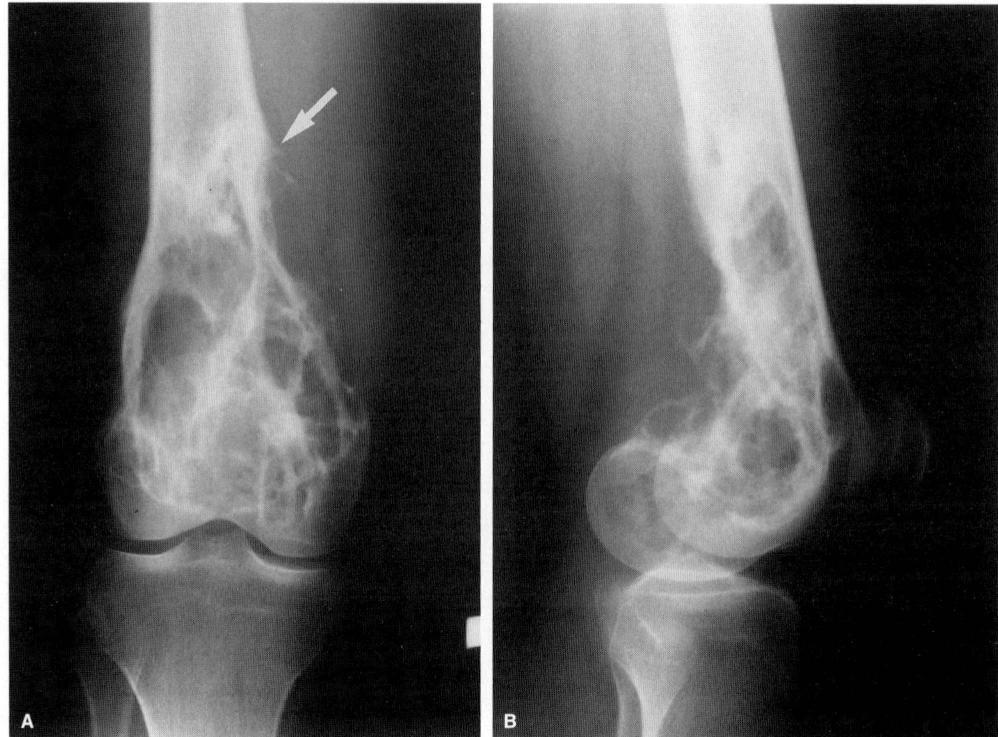

FIGURE 42.19. **Desmoid Tumor.** A multilocular, heavily septated, destructive, lytic lesion of the distal femur is noted in these anteroposterior **(A)** and lateral **(B)** plain films of the femur, which is fairly characteristic for a desmoid tumor. The thick septa and narrow zone of transition are characteristic of a benign process, whereas the Codman triangle (*arrow*) and large amount of bony destruction indicate an aggressive process.

Malignant fibrous histiocytoma was originally classified as a fibrosarcoma by most pathologists but has come into its own grouping in the past few decades. MFH is one of the most common soft tissue tumors, with true fibrosarcomas, as mentioned earlier, being uncommon. Radiologically, when they arise in bone, they appear identical to fibrosarcomas: lytic lesions with variations extending from permeative (Fig. 42.18) to fairly well defined. Like fibrosarcomas, they may, on occasion, have a bony sequestrum.

Desmoid tumor (not to be confused with a cortical desmoid; see Chapter 46) is a half-grade fibrosarcoma. It has also been called a *desmoplastic fibroma* or *aggressive fibromatosis*. They most commonly arise in the soft tissues and are uncommon in the bony skeleton. These lesions, like fibrosarcoma, are lytic when in bone but are usually fairly well defined because of their slow growth. They often have benign periostitis present that has thick spicules or "spikes." They usually have a multilocular appearance with thick bony septa (Fig. 42.19). They are slow growing and do not metastasize, but they can exhibit inexorable tumor extension into surrounding soft tissues, with devastating results. Like fibrosarcoma and malignant fibrous histiocytomas, these lesions can exhibit a bony sequestrum.

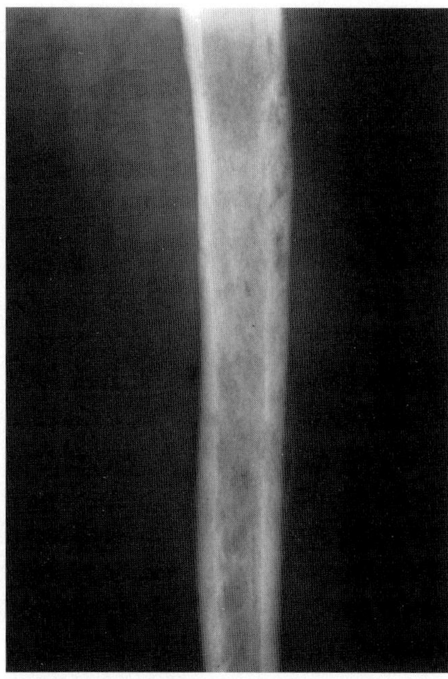

FIGURE 42.20. **Primary Lymphoma of Bone.** A diffuse permeative pattern is seen throughout the humerus in this 35-year-old patient, which is characteristic of primary lymphoma of bone.

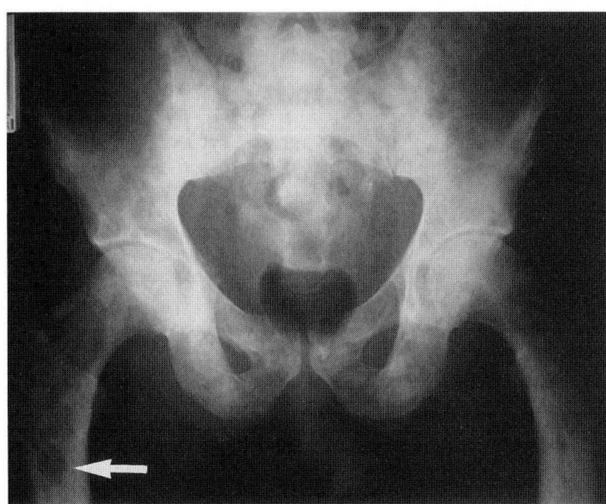

FIGURE 42.21. **Metastatic Prostate Carcinoma.** Diffuse blastic metastases are seen throughout the pelvis and proximal femurs with a lytic, destructive lesion seen in the right proximal femur (*arrow*). Prostate metastases tend to be blastic but can occasionally be lytic.

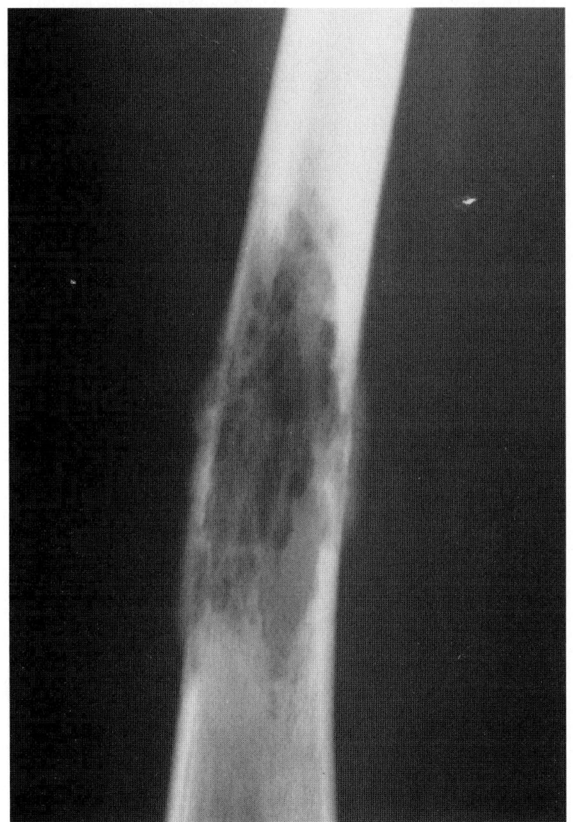

FIGURE 42.22. **Metastatic Renal Cell Carcinoma.** A lytic lesion in the diaphysis of the femur is noted, which is typical for renal cell carcinoma. As many as one third of renal cell carcinomas present initially with a bony metastasis. Renal cell carcinoma virtually never presents with a blastic metastatic focus.

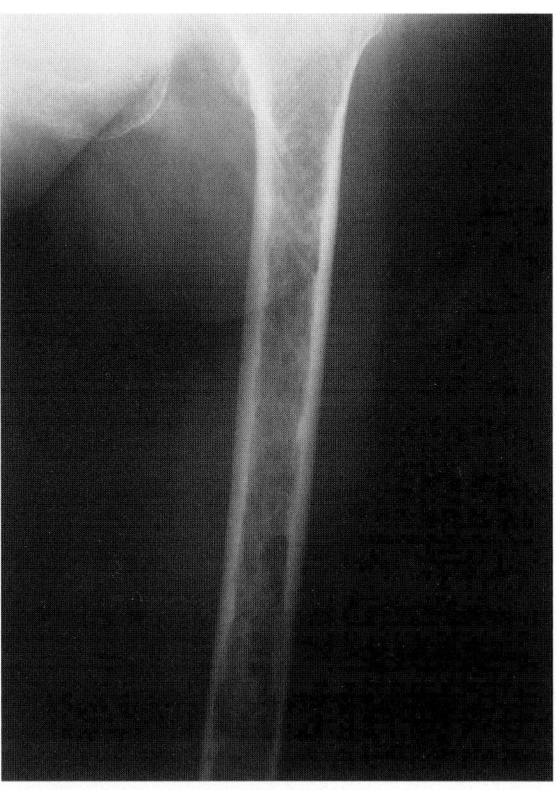

FIGURE 42.23. **Multiple Myeloma.** A diffuse, moth-eaten pattern is seen throughout the diaphysis of the femur in this 45-year-old patient, which is characteristic for myeloma. Primary lymphoma of bone could have a similar appearance.

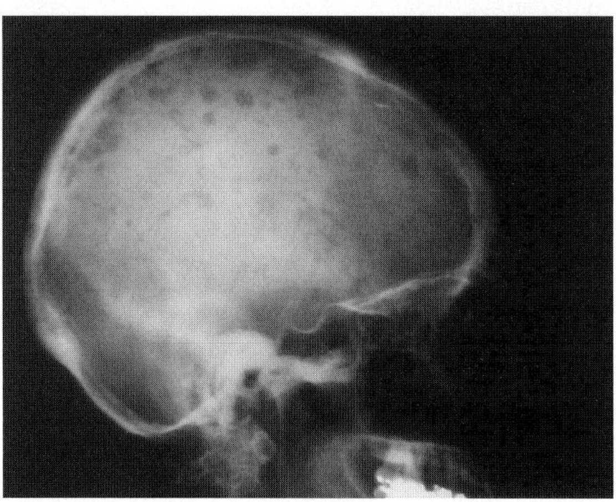

FIGURE 42.24. **Multiple Myeloma.** A lateral view of the skull shows multiple lytic lesions in the calvaria, which is a characteristic appearance of multiple myeloma.

Primary lymphoma of bone (reticulum cell sarcoma) is a neoplasm with a radiologic appearance identical to that of Ewing sarcoma—that is, a permeative or moth-eaten pattern (Fig. 42.20). Primary lymphoma of bone tends to occur in an older age group than Ewing sarcoma, and, whereas Ewing sarcomas are typically systemically symptomatic, patients with primary lymphoma of bone are often asymptomatic. It is said to be the only malignant tumor that can involve a large amount of bone while the patient is asymptomatic.

Metastatic disease must be included in any differential diagnosis of a bone lesion in a patient older than age 40. Metastatic lesions can have virtually any appearance. They can mimic a benign lesion or an aggressive primary bone tumor. It can be difficult, if not impossible, to judge the origin of the tumor from the appearance of the metastatic focus, although some appearances are fairly characteristic. For instance, multiple sclerotic foci in a man are most likely prostatic metastases (Fig. 42.21), although lung, bowel, or almost any other metastatic tumor could present like this. In a woman, the same picture would most likely be caused by breast metastases. Although nearly every metastatic bone lesion can be either lytic or blastic, the only primary tumor that virtually never presents with blastic metastatic disease is renal cell carcinoma. The classic differential diagnosis for an expansile, lytic metastasis is renal cell or thyroid carcinoma (Fig. 42.22).

Myeloma. Like metastases, myeloma should only be considered in a patient older than the age of 40 years, although some radiologists use age 35 for the lower limits of myeloma. Myeloma typically has a diffuse permeative appearance (Fig. 42.23) that can mimic a Ewing sarcoma or primary lymphoma of bone. Because of the age criteria, Ewing sarcoma and myeloma are not in the same differential, however. Myeloma frequently involves the calvaria (Fig. 42.24). Rarely, myeloma can present with multiple sclerotic foci, thus resembling diffuse metastatic disease. Myeloma is one of the only lesions that is not characteristically hot on a radionuclide bone scan; therefore, radiologic "bone surveys" are performed in place of radionuclide bone scans when evidence of myeloma is found clinically. Occasionally, myeloma will present with a lytic bone lesion called a *plasmacytoma.* This lesion can mimic any lytic bone lesion, benign or aggressive, in its appearance; it can precede other evidence of myeloma by up to 3 years.

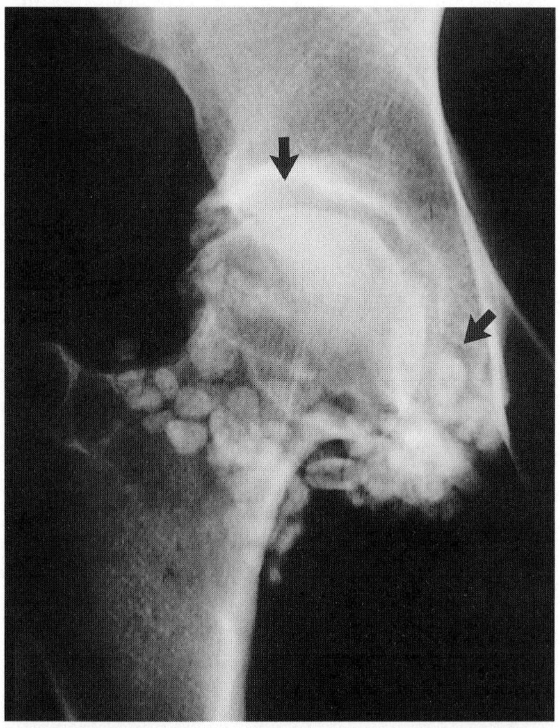

FIGURE 42.25. **Synovial Osteochondromatosis.** Multiple calcific loose bodies in a hip joint, as in this example, are virtually pathognomonic for synovial osteochondromatosis. Notice the erosions in the acetabulum (*arrows*). In up to 20% of cases, the loose bodies are not ossified; in such cases, this process is indistinguishable from pigmented villonodular synovitis.

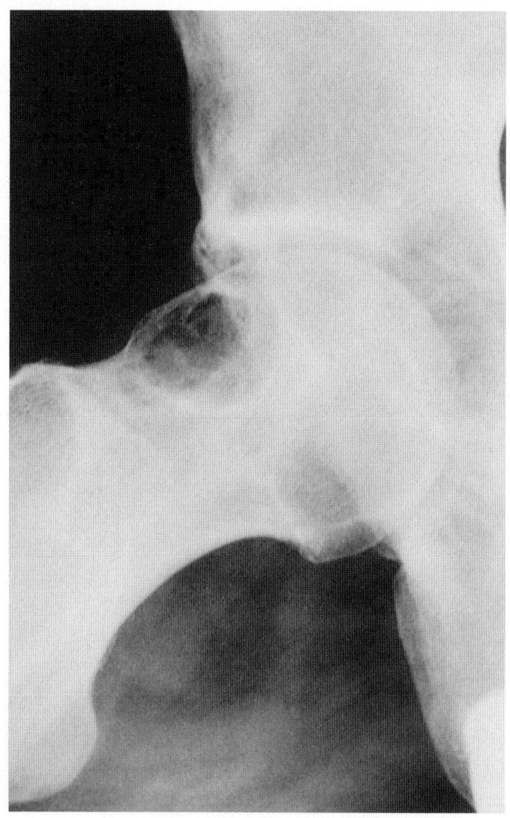

FIGURE 42.26. **Pigmented Villonodular Synovitis (PVNS).** Large erosions in the femoral head and acetabulum are characteristic for PVNS; however, nonossified synovial osteochondromatosis could present similarly.

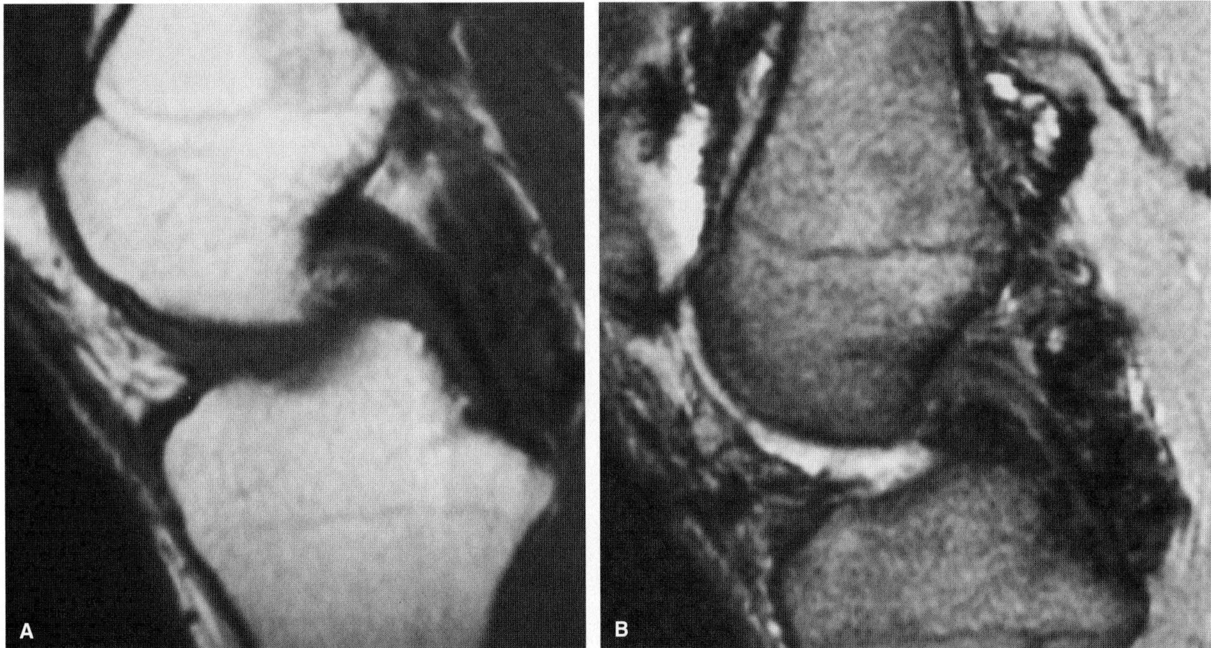

FIGURE 42.27. **Pigmented Villonodular Synovitis (PVNS).** Proton-density **(A)** (time of repetition [TR] 1,500; time of echo [TE] 20) and T2W **(B)** (TR 3000; TE 60) sagittal images of the knee in this patient with painful swelling show diffuse low signal throughout the synovium. The low signal on both T1WIs and T2WIs is typical for hemosiderin deposits in PVNS.

Soft Tissue Tumors. There is no concise, useful differential diagnosis for soft tissue tumors, whether or not there is calcification, bony destruction, fat plane involvement, and so forth. The two most common soft tissue tumors, *malignant fibrous histiocytoma* and *liposarcoma,* should be mentioned as the most likely possibilities for any soft tissue tumor, but any cell type can produce a benign or malignant tumor and mimic any other soft tissue tumor. A lipoma, obviously, can be distinguished by the appearance of fat, but a liposarcoma might or might not have fat present. There are at least three subtypes of liposarcomas, two of which have only small amounts of fat present. Therefore, the radiologist is generally left to giving descriptions of size and extent of the tumor and letting the pathologist determine the diagnosis.

Synovial sarcomas or synoviomas, only rarely originate in a joint. They are often adjacent to joints. There are no malignant tumors that routinely need to be considered in the differential diagnosis of joint lesions. Synovial sarcomas are one of two types of tumors (along with neural tumors) that are typically homogeneously bright on T2WIs—to the extent that they can be mistaken for a fluid collection. As mentioned previously, whenever a mass is found on MR that resembles a fluid collection in a location that is atypical for a ganglion or bursa, gadolinium must be given to determine whether it is indeed fluid or a solid mass.

Synovial osteochondromatosis is a benign joint lesion that probably occurs from metaplasia of the synovium and

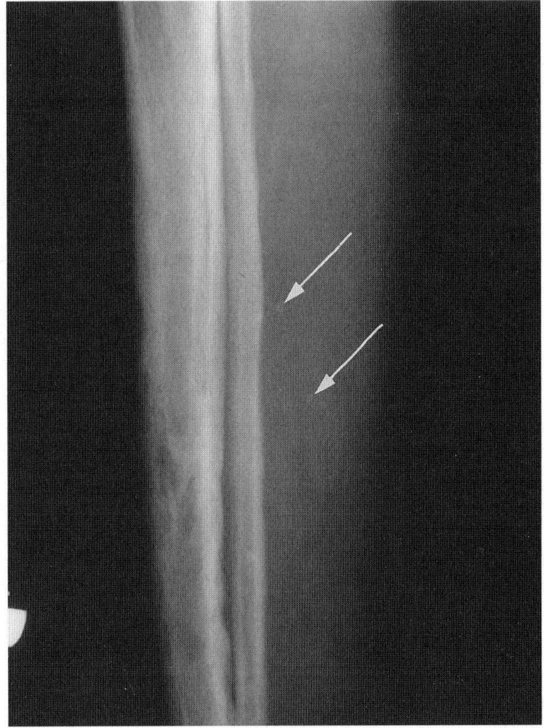

FIGURE 42.28. **Hemangioma.** Multiple, irregular, lytic lesions, predominantly cortical in nature, are seen in the tibia in this patient with a soft tissue mass. Cortical holes such as this occur almost exclusively in radiation and soft tissue hemangioma. Note the phleboliths in the posterior soft tissues (*arrows*), which are often seen in hemangioma and make this an easy diagnosis.

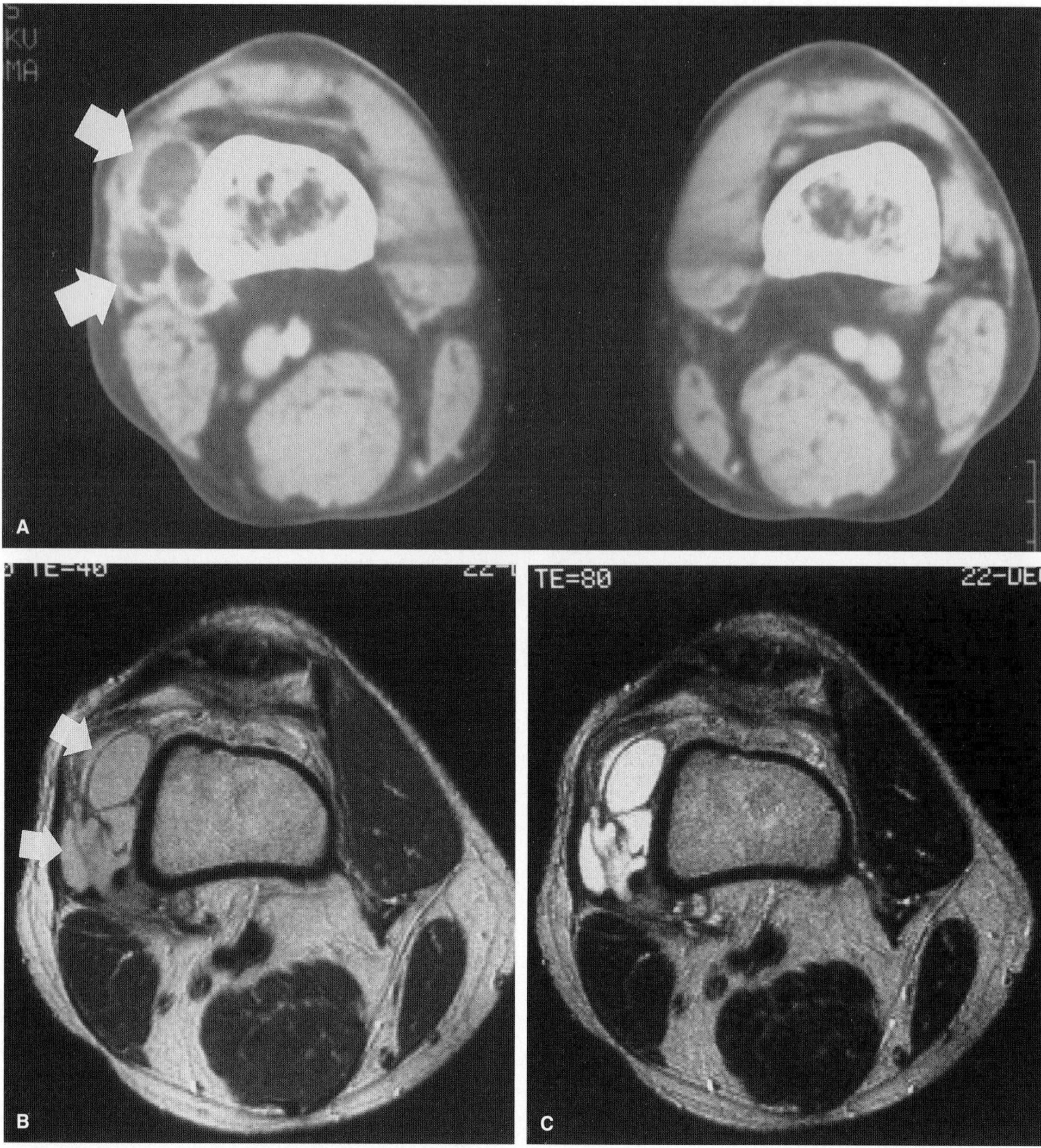

FIGURE 42.29. **Atypical Synovial Cyst. A.** CT scan through the distal femurs in a patient with a soft tissue mass around the right knee shows a multilocular soft tissue mass adjacent to the distal right femur (*arrows*). **B.** A proton-density MR (time of repetition [TR] 2,000; time of echo [TE] 40) through the same area shows intermediate-intensity signal in a homogeneous multilocular soft tissue mass (*arrows*). **C.** A T2WI (TR 2,000; TE 80) shows high-intensity signal in the lesion, which is typical for fluid, although a tumor could have these signal characteristics. This was an atypical synovial cyst arising from the knee joint.

leads to multiple calcific loose bodies in a joint. This can histologically mimic a chondrosarcoma and therefore is best diagnosed radiographically, as it has a pathognomonic radiographic appearance (Fig. 42.25). Up to 20% of the time, the loose bodies do not calcify, however, and the osteochondromatosis then can mimic pigmented villonodular synovitis.

Pigmented villonodular synovitis is a benign synovial soft tissue process that causes joint swelling and pain and, occasionally, joint erosions (Fig. 42.26). It virtually never has calcifications associated with it. The MR appearance of pigmented villonodular synovitis is characteristic. Marked low signal lining the synovium is seen on T1WIs and T2WIs because of the hemosiderin deposits (Fig. 42.27). Chronic bleeding into a joint, so-called hemosiderotic arthritis, can have a similar appearance but is encountered uncommonly.

Hemangiomas will often have phleboliths associated with them and often cause cortical holes in adjacent bone that can mimic a permeative or moth-eaten pattern (Fig. 42.28) in a pseudopermeative pattern. The true permeative pattern of round cell lesions occurs in the intramedullary or endosteal part of the bone and can be differentiated from a pseudopermeative pattern by the intact cortex.

Atypical synovial cysts, such as Baker cysts around the knee, can present as soft tissue masses and result in an unnecessary biopsy. On CT, these lesions may not be appreciated as fluid-filled lesions, and their association with a joint can be easily overlooked. MR will demonstrate a very high signal intensity with T2 weighting that is very homogeneous and often septated (Fig. 42.29). Gadolinium should be given to determine whether it is truly a fluid collection or a solid mass. As mentioned previously, synovial sarcomas and neural tumors often mimic fluid collections on T2WIs.

REFERENCES

1. Berquist T, Ehman R, King B, Hodgman C, et al. Value of MR imaging in differentiating benign from malignant soft-tissue masses: study of 95 lesions. AJR Am J Roentgenol 1990;155:1251–1255.
2. Brien EW, Mirra JM, Kerr R. Benign and malignant cartilage tumors of bone and joint: their anatomic and theoretical basis with an emphasis on radiology, pathology and clinical biology. 1. The intramedullary cartilage tumors [review]. Skeletal Radiol 1997;26(6):325–353.

Chapter 43

Skeletal Trauma

Clyde A. Helms

Spine

Hand and Wrist

Arm

Pelvis

Leg

Most of the differential diagnoses in skeletal radiology that I use are geared to be 95% inclusive; that is, the correct diagnosis will be mentioned 95% of the time. The yield can be increased by lengthening the list, but if the list gets too long, it will become unwieldy and less useful for the clinician. In trauma cases, however, being right 95% of the time is not good enough. Missing the correct diagnosis 5% of the time is unacceptable. Fractures simply should not be missed.

Before reviewing specific examples, the reader should keep a few key points in mind concerning radiology of trauma. First, have a high index of suspicion. Every radiologist in the world has missed fractures on radiographs because he or she was not sufficiently attuned to the possible presence of a fracture. Often, the history is either nonexistent or misleading, so that the anatomic area of concern is overlooked. When in doubt, examine the patient. Orthopaedic surgeons rarely miss seeing fractures on radiographs because they have examined the patient, they know where the patient hurts, and they have a high index of suspicion. Second, always get two radiographs at 90° to each other in every trauma case. A high percentage of fractures are seen only on one view (the anteroposterior [AP] or the lateral) and will therefore be missed unless two views are routinely obtained. Third, once a fracture is identified, do not forget to look at the rest of the film. About 10% of all cases have a second finding that often is as significant or even more so than the initial finding. Many fractures have associated dislocation, foreign bodies, or additional fractures, so be sure to examine the entire film.

Finally, do not hesitate to obtain a CT scan or an MR study if the plain films fail to confirm what is believed to be present clinically. MR imaging is being used more frequently as a primary imaging tool for trauma, replacing CT or radionuclide studies in cases in which the plain films are negative or equivocal. Make sure that an expensive examination such as CT or MR is truly going to affect patient care rather than just show an abnormality and then result in the same treatment whether positive or negative. For example, there is no reason to perform a CT scan or an MR study to find a subtle or occult fracture of the radial head in the elbow, because the patient is going to have a posterior splint regardless of the results of the advanced study (assuming the patient had trauma to the elbow, has pain, and the plain film shows a displaced fat-pad, indicative of fluid in the joint). On the other hand, an elderly patient who has hip pain after a fall and has a negative plain film would benefit from an MR study because his treatment will vary based on whether an occult fracture is present.

SPINE

The cervical spine (C-spine) is one of the most commonly filmed parts of the body in a busy emergency department and can be one of the most difficult examinations to interpret. One of the most important pieces of information for the radiologist to have is the clinical history. If the patient has been involved in an automobile accident and has no neck pain, it is extremely unlikely that a fracture is present (1). So-called precautionary radiographs are not justified. On the other hand, if the plain films are negative in a trauma victim who has neck pain or neurologic deficits, a CT scan should be obtained.

Usually, a cross-table lateral view of the C-spine is obtained first to avoid unduly moving the patient who might

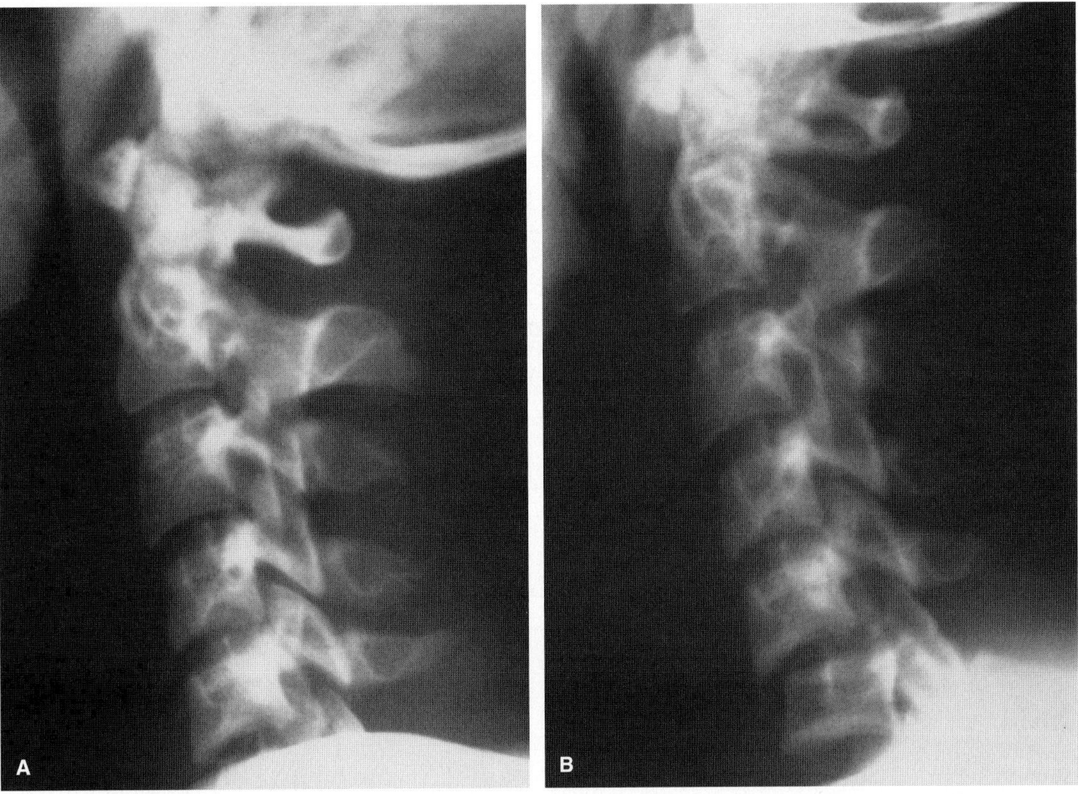

FIGURE 43.1. **Shoulders Obscuring C5–C6 Dislocation.** This patient presented to the emergency department after an injury suffered while diving into a shallow swimming pool. He had neck pain but no neurologic deficits. **A.** The initial radiograph obtained of the cervical spine was interpreted as within normal limits. Only five cervical vertebrae are visible, however, because of high-riding shoulders. **B.** A repeat examination with the shoulders lowered reveals a dislocation of C5 on C6. To visualize C7, the shoulders were lowered even further. The C7 vertebral body must be visualized on every lateral cervical spine examination in a trauma setting.

have a cervical fracture. If the lateral C-spine appears normal, the remainder of the C-spine series, including flexion and extension views (if the patient can cooperate) is obtained.

What does one look for on the lateral C-spine? First, make certain that all seven cervical vertebral bodies can be visualized. A large number of fractures are missed because the shoulders obscure the lower C-spine levels (Fig. 43.1). If the entire cervical spine is not visualized, repeat the film with the shoulders lowered.

Next, evaluate five parallel (more or less) lines for step-offs or discontinuity as follows (Fig. 43.2):

Line 1 is the prevertebral soft tissue and extends down the posterior aspect of the airway; it should be several millimeters from the first three or four vertebral bodies and then moves further away at the laryngeal cartilage. Line 1 should be less than one vertebral body width from the anterior vertebral bodies from C3 or C4 to C7, and it should be smooth in its contour.

Line 2 follows the anterior vertebral bodies and should be smooth and uninterrupted. Anterior osteophytes can encroach on this line and extend beyond it and should therefore be ignored in drawing this line. Interruption of the anterior vertebral body line is a sign of a serious injury (Fig. 43.1B).

Line 3 is similar to the anterior vertebral body line (line 2) except that it connects the posterior vertebral bodies. Like line 2, it should be smooth and uninterrupted, and any disruption signifies a serious injury.

Line 4 connects the posterior junction of the lamina with the spinous processes and is called the spinolaminal line. The spinal cord lies between lines 3 and 4; therefore, any offset of either of these lines could mean a bony structure is impinging on the cord. It takes very little force against the cord to cause severe neurologic deficits, and any bony structure lying on the cord must be recognized as soon as possible.

Line 5 is not really a line so much as a collection of points—the tips of the spinous processes. They are quite variable in their size and appearance, although C7 is consistently the largest. A fracture of one of the spinous processes by itself is not a serious injury, but it occasionally heralds other, more serious injuries.

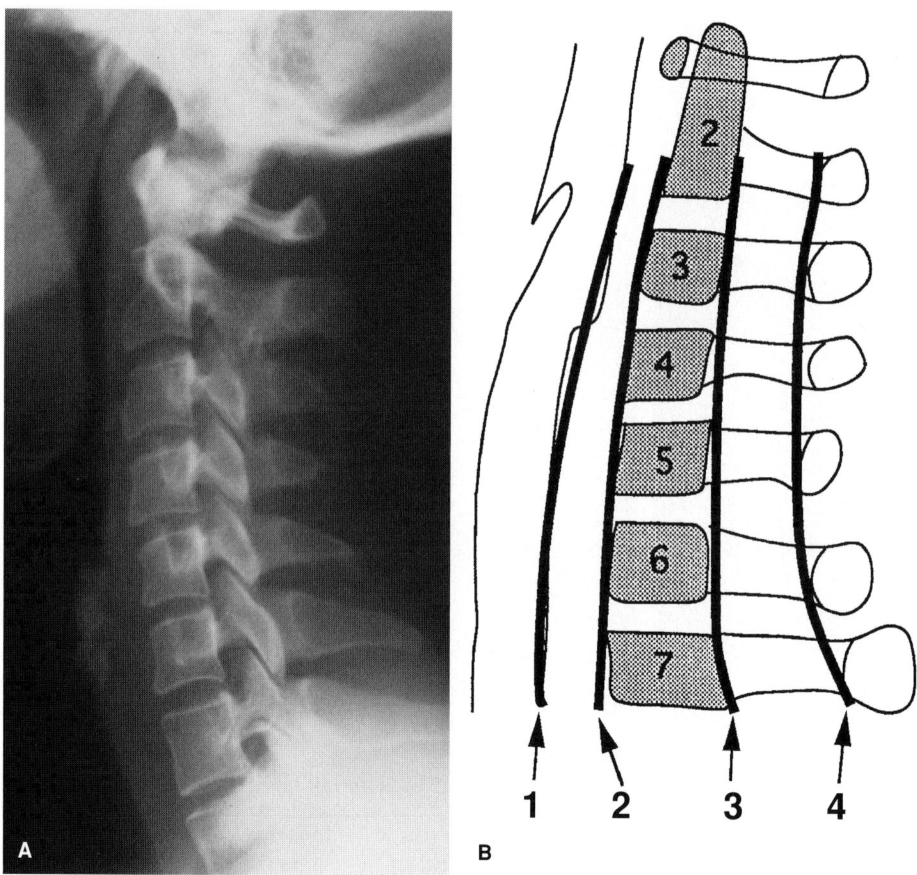

FIGURE 43.2. **Normal Lateral Cervical Spine (C-spine). A.** Lateral radiograph of a normal cervical spine. **B.** Diagrammatic representation of a lateral C-spine showing four parallel lines that should be observed in every lateral C-spine examination. Line 1 is the soft tissue line that is closely applied to the posterior border of the airway through the first four or five vertebral body segments; it then widens around the laryngeal cartilage and runs parallel to the remainder of the cervical vertebrae. Line 2 demarcates the anterior border of the cervical vertebral bodies. Line 3 is the posterior border of the cervical vertebral bodies. Line 4 is drawn by connecting the junction of the lamina at the spinous process, which is called the spinolaminal line. It represents the posterior extent of the central canal that contains the spinal cord itself. These lines should be generally smooth and parallel, with no abrupt step-offs.

After visually inspecting these five lines on the lateral C-spine film, then inspect the C1–C2 area a little more closely. Make certain that the anterior arch of C1 is no more than 2.5 mm from the dens (Fig. 43.3). Any greater separation than this (except in children, for whom up to 5.0 mm can be normal) is suspicious for disruption of the transverse ligament between C1 and C2 (Fig. 43.4).

The disk spaces are examined next to see that there is no inordinate widening or narrowing, either of which could indicate an acute traumatic injury. If a disk space is

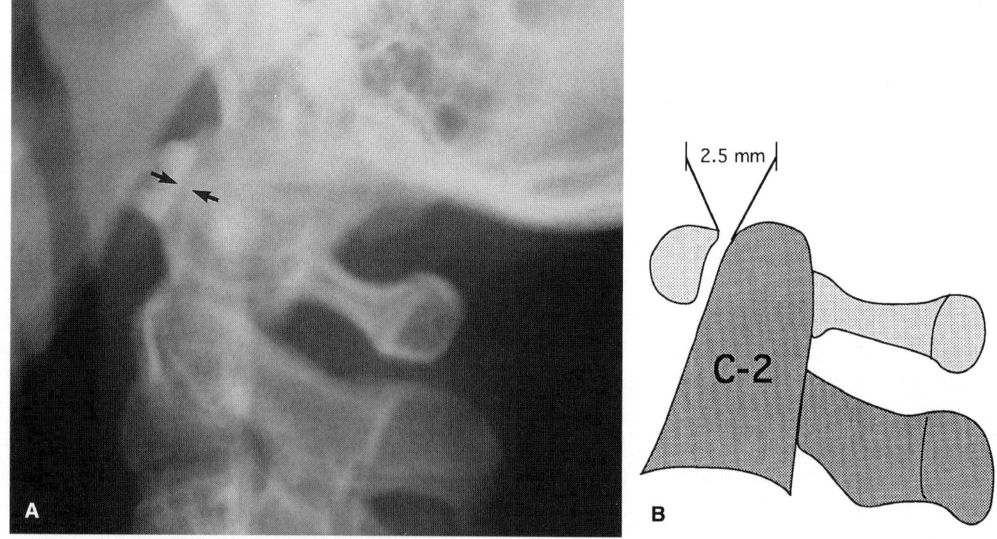

FIGURE 43.3. **Normal C1 and C2.** A lateral radiograph **(A)** and drawing **(B)** of the upper cervical spine showing the normal distance of less than 2.5 mm from the anterior arch of C1 to the odontoid process (dens) of C2 (*arrows*).

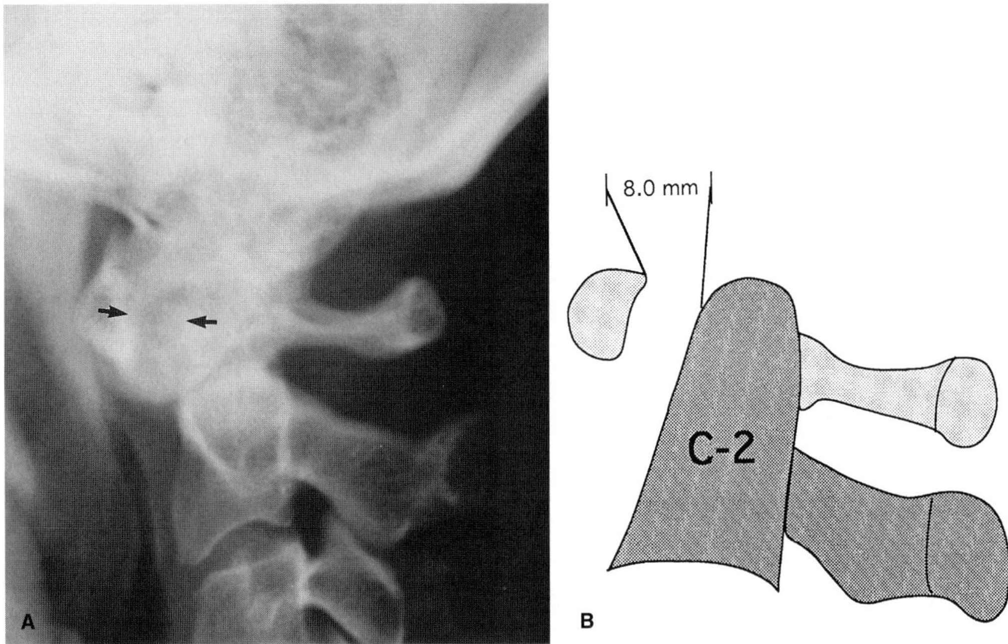

FIGURE 43.4. **C1–C2 Dislocation.** A lateral radiograph **(A)** and drawing **(B)** of the upper cervical spine in a patient who suffered trauma to the neck shows that the anterior arch of C1 is 9 mm anterior to the odontoid process of C2 (*arrows*). This is diagnostic of a dislocation of C1 on C2 and indicates rupture of the transverse ligaments that normally hold these vertebral segments together.

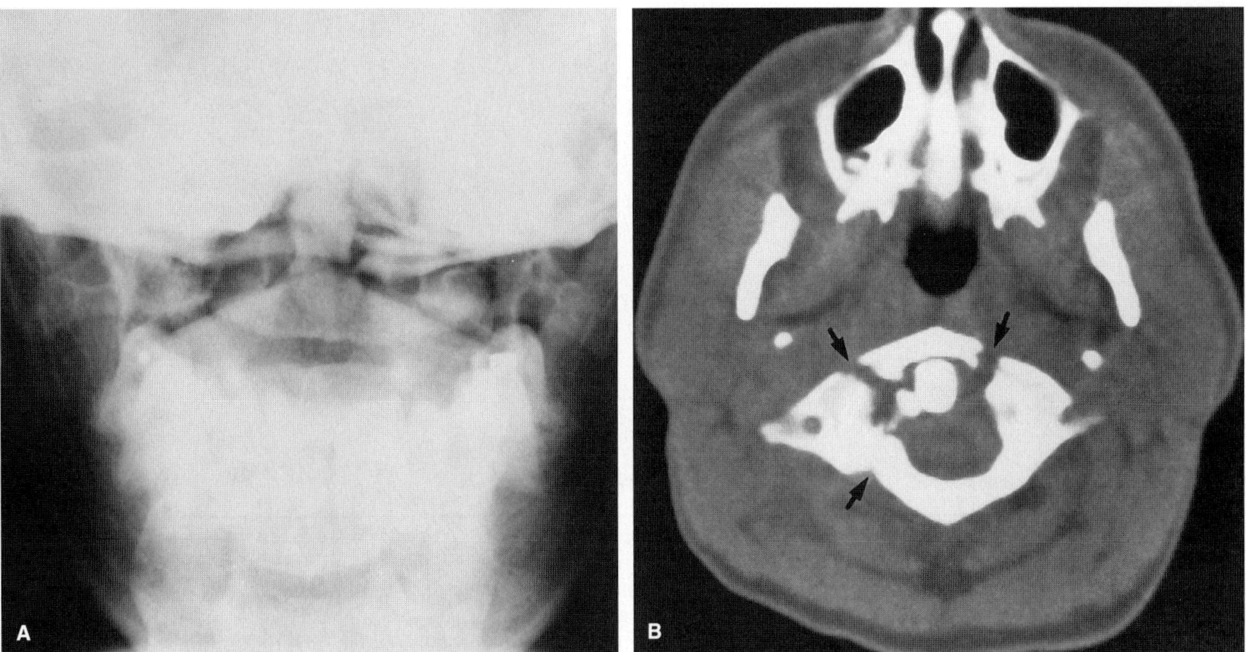

FIGURE 43.5. **Jefferson Fracture. A.** An anteroposterior open-mouth odontoid view is suspicious for the lateral masses of C1 being laterally displaced on the body of C2. Because of overlying structures, however, this is difficult to appreciate. **B.** A CT examination was obtained and shows multiple fracture sites in the C1 ring (*arrows*). This is called a Jefferson fracture. CT should be routinely used in spinal trauma because of frequent shortcomings of plain films.

narrowed, it will usually be secondary to degenerative disease, but the clinician must make certain that associated osteophytosis and sclerosis are present before diagnosing degenerative disease.

The examination of the lateral C-spine as described here can be done in less than 1 minute. If it is normal, then the remainder of the examination can be completed, including flexion and extension views. It is imperative that the patient initiate the flexion and extension without help from the technician or anyone else. A patient, if conscious and alert, will not injure himself or herself with voluntary flexion and extension and will have muscle guarding preventing

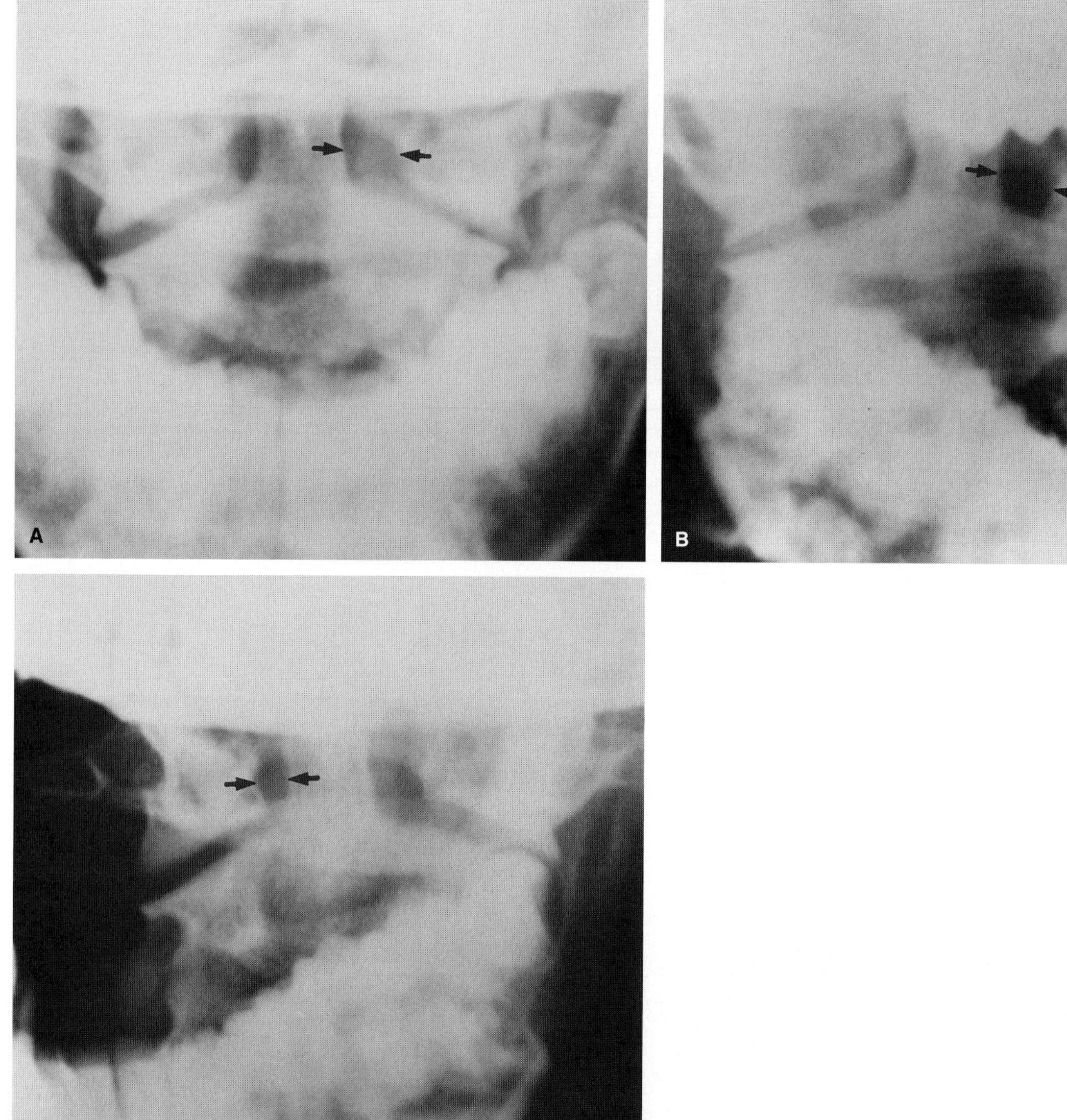

FIGURE 43.6. **Rotatory Fixation of the Atlantoaxial Joint.** This patient presented to the emergency department with pain and decreased motion in the cervical spine. **A.** An anteroposterior open-mouth odontoid view shows that the space on the left side of the odontoid between the odontoid and the lateral mass of C1 (*arrows*) is wider than the corresponding space on the right side. This is often the result of rotation. Therefore, open-mouth odontoid views with right and left obliquities were obtained. **B.** This view shows rotation of the patient's head to the left, which causes the space on the left side of the odontoid process (*arrows*) to be wider than that on the right, which is appropriate. **C.** This view, however, shows that when the patient turns the head to the right, the space on the right (*arrows*) does not get wider than the space on the left. This is diagnostic of rotatory fixation of the atlantoaxial joint.

motion if there is an injury present. Even gentle pressure to aid in flexion or extension can cause severe injury if a fracture or dislocation is present.

A few examples of fractures, dislocations, and other abnormalities are illustrated in the following paragraphs.

Jefferson Fracture. A blow to the top of the head, such as when an object falls directly on the apex of the skull, can cause the lateral masses of C1 to slide apart, splitting the bony ring of C1. This is called a Jefferson fracture (Fig. 43.5). It nicely illustrates how a bony ring will not break in just one place, but must break in several places. This is a rule that is seldom violated. All the vertebral rings, when fractured, must fracture in two or more places. The bony rings of the pelvis behave similarly.

CT is excellent at demonstrating the complete bony ring of C1 and shows the fractures, as well as any associated soft tissue mass, much better than plain films do. For correct diagnosis of a Jefferson fracture on plain film, the lateral masses of C1 must extend beyond the margins of the C2 body (Fig. 43.5A). The presence of asymmetry of the spaces on either side of the dens is not enough to make the diagnosis, as this can be normally asymmetric with rotation or with rotatory fixation of the atlantoaxial joint.

Rotatory fixation of the atlantoaxial joint is a somewhat controversial, little-understood process in which the atlantoaxial joint becomes fixed and the C1–C2 bodies move en mass instead of rotating on one another. It is easily diagnosed with open-mouth odontoid views. In the normal odontoid view, the spaces lateral to the dens (odontoid) are equal. With rotation of the head to the left, the space on the left widens, and with rotation to the right the space on the right widens. With rotatory fixation, one of the spaces is wider than the other and stays wider, even with rotation of the head to the opposite side (Fig. 43.6). This is a

FIGURE 43.7. **Clay Shoveler's Fracture.** A nondisplaced fracture of the C7 spinous process (*arrow*) is noted that is diagnostic of a clay shoveler's fracture.

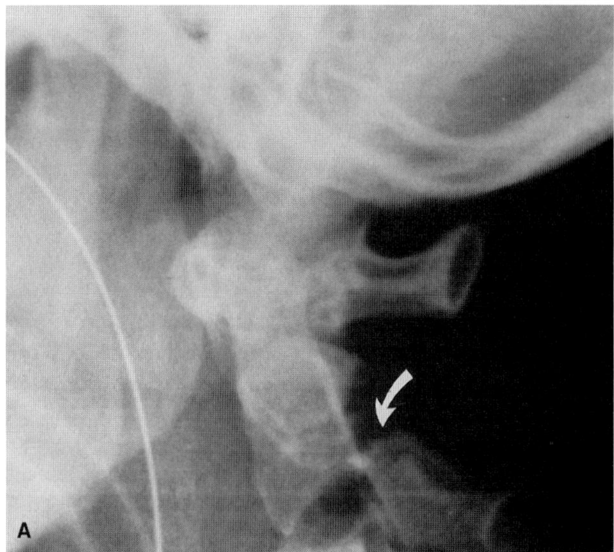

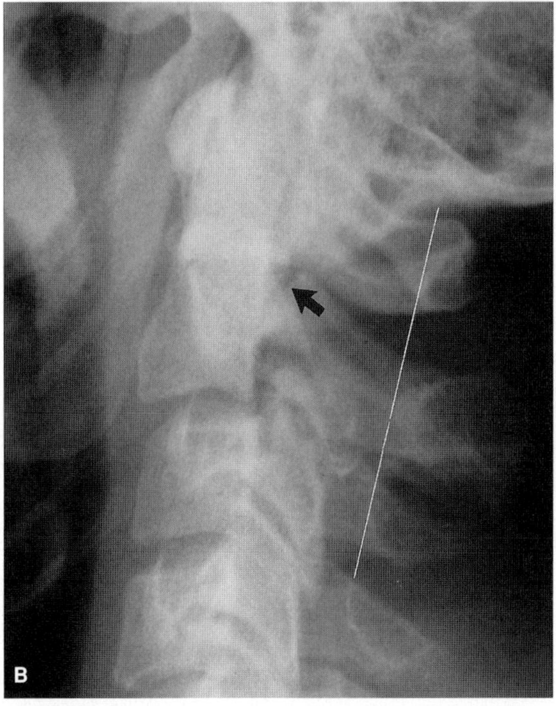

FIGURE 43.8. **Hangman's Fracture. A.** Lateral films of a patient with a hangman's fracture shows an obvious example of the posterior elements of the C2 vertebral body fractured and displaced inferiorly (*arrow*). **B.** This view shows a very subtle fracture through the posterior elements of C2 (*arrow*) in another patient. A line drawn through the spinolaminal lines of the posterior elements shows that the C2 spinolaminal line is offset posteriorly in this example.

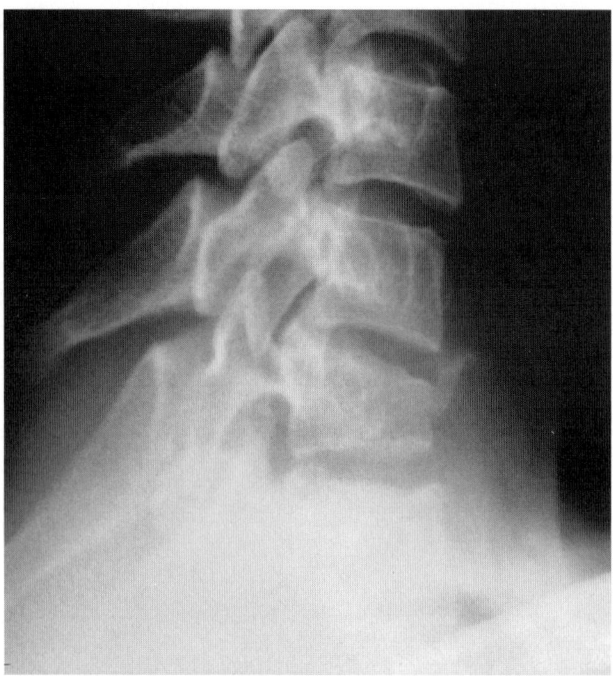

FIGURE 43.9. **Flexion Teardrop Fracture.** This patient suffered a hyperflexion injury in an automobile accident and presented to the emergency department with severe neurologic deficits. A lateral radiograph of the lower cervical spine shows wedging anteriorly of the C7 vertebral body, with some displacement of the posterior vertebral line at C7 into the central canal. A small avulsion fracture off the anterior body is also noted.

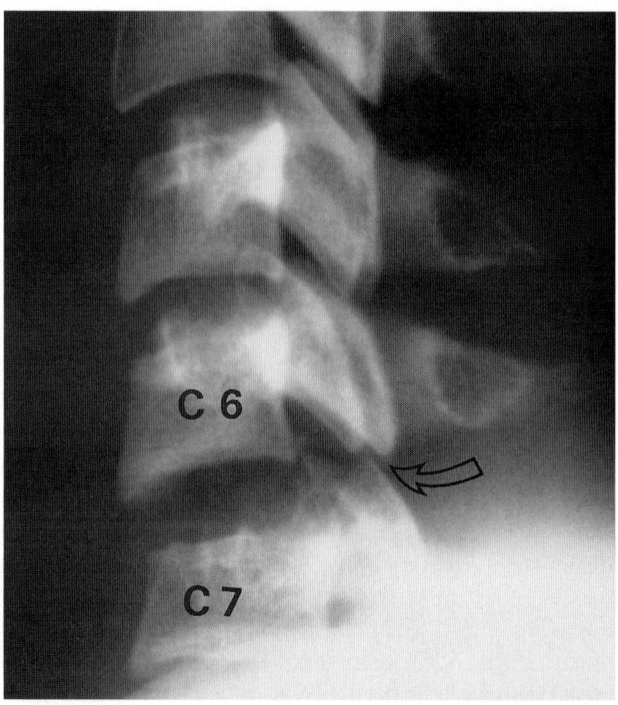

FIGURE 43.10. **Unilateral Locked Facets.** The C6-C7 disk space is abnormally widened, and the C7 vertebra is posteriorly located in relation to C6. Also note the C7 facets, which are dislocated and locked on the C6 facets (*arrow*). When the facets are perched in this manner, it is termed *locked facets*, which are unilateral in this example.

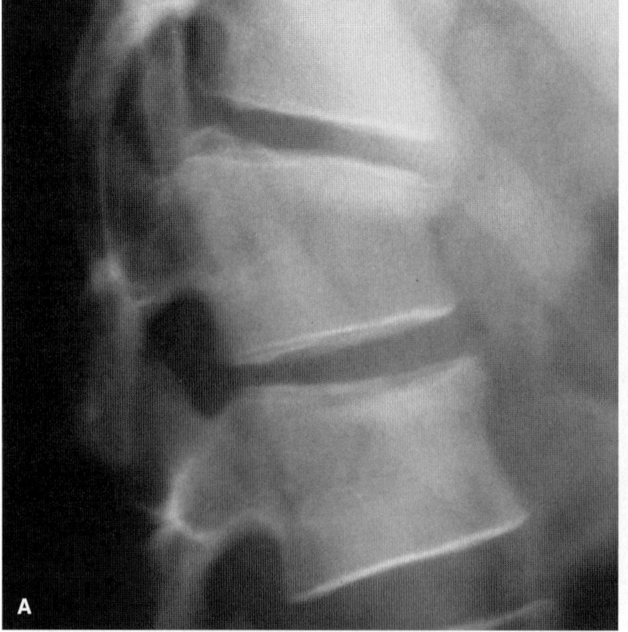

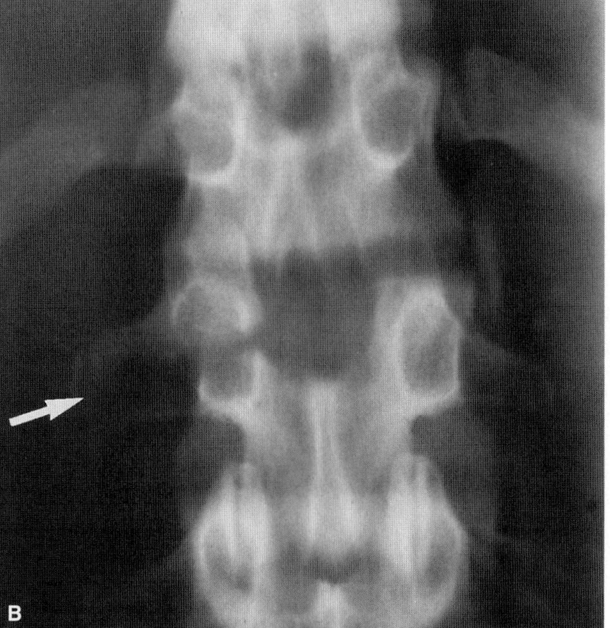

FIGURE 43.11. **Seatbelt Fracture.** Hyperflexion at the waist can cause anterior wedging of the vertebral body in the lower thoracic or upper lumbar region as shown in **(A).** By itself, although painful, it is somewhat innocuous; however, **(B)** shows a horizontal fracture through the right transverse process and pedicle (*arrow*) caused by extreme traction during the flexion injury. When fracture of the posterior elements occurs, this injury is considered to be unstable and potentially debilitating. Any anterior wedging injury to a vertebral body should have the posterior elements of that level closely inspected.

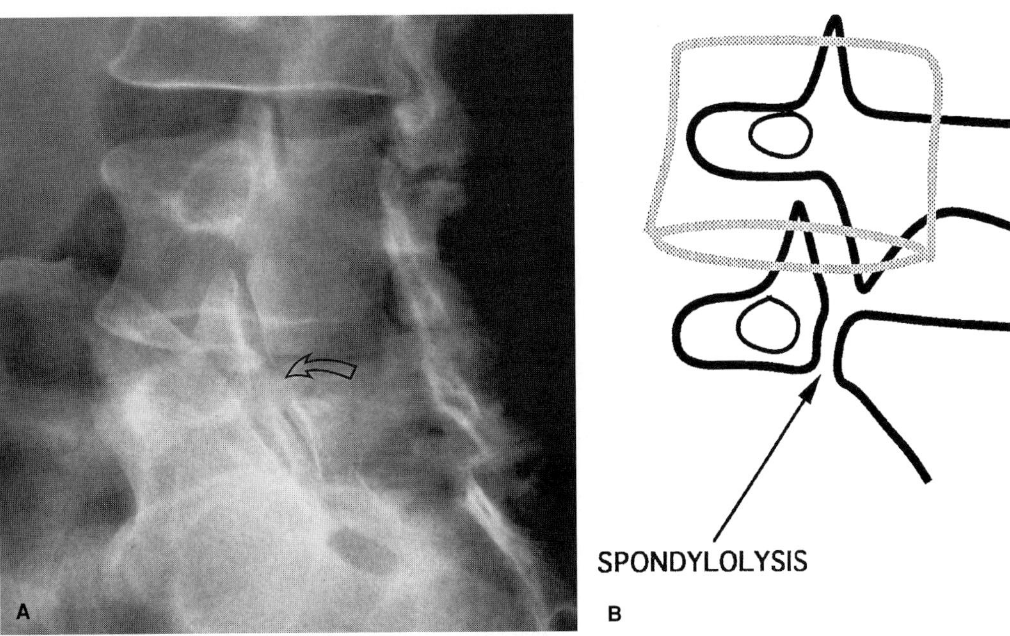

FIGURE 43.12. **Spondylolysis. A.** An oblique plain film of the lumbar spine shows a defect in the neck of the "Scottie dog" at L5 (*arrow*), which is diagnostic of a spondylolysis. **B.** A drawing of an oblique view of the lumbar spine shows how a spondylolysis appears as a "collar" around the Scottie dog's neck.

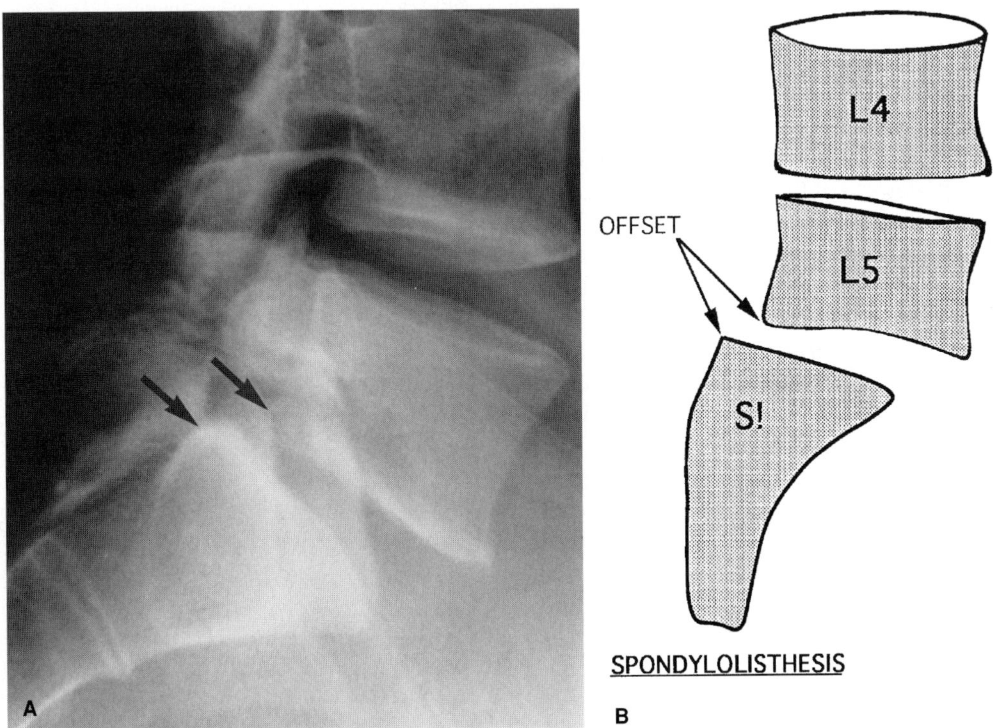

FIGURE 43.13. **Spondylolisthesis. A.** A lateral plain film of the lumbar spine shows that the L5 vertebral body is slightly anteriorly offset on the S1 body, as noted by the posterior margins (*arrows*). **B.** The drawing illustrates this more clearly. Because this offset is less than 25%, as measured by the length of the S1 endplate, it is termed a grade 1 spondylolisthesis. A grade 2 offset is more than 25% but less than 50% of the length of the S1 endplate.

relatively innocuous malady that by itself is usually treated with a soft cervical collar, gentle traction, or both. However, on rare occasions it is associated with disruption of the transverse ligaments at C1–C2 (diagnosed by an increase of more than 2.5 mm in the space between the anterior arch of C1 and the dens), and when it is, it is then a serious problem. It usually presents spontaneously or after very mild trauma such as an unusual sleeping position.

"Clay-Shoveler's" Fracture. Another relatively innocuous injury is a fracture of the C6 or C7 spinous process, which is called a "clay-shoveler's" fracture. Supposedly, workers shoveling sticky clay would toss shovels full of clay over their shoulders; once in a while, the clay would stick to the shovel, causing the ligaments attached to the spinous processes (supraspinous ligaments) to undergo tremendous force, pulling on the spinous process and avulsing it. This can occur at any of the lower cervical spinous processes (Fig. 43.7).

"Hangman's" Fracture. A "hangman's" fracture is an unstable, serious fracture of the upper C-spine that is caused by hyperextension and distraction (such as hitting one's head on a dashboard). This is a fracture of the posterior elements of C2 and, usually, displacement of the C2 body anterior to C3 (Fig. 43.8). These patients actually do better than one might think. They often escape neurologic impairment because the fractured posterior elements of C2, in effect, cause decompression and take pressure off the injured area.

Flexion-Teardrop Fracture. Severe flexion of the C-spine can cause a disruption of the posterior ligaments with anterior compression of a vertebral body. This is called a flexion "teardrop" fracture (Fig. 43.9). A teardrop fracture is usually associated with spinal cord injury, often a result of displacement of the posterior portion of the vertebral body into the central canal.

Unilateral Locked Facets. Severe flexion associated with some rotation can result in rupture of the apophyseal joint ligaments and facet joint dislocation. This can result in locking of the facets in an overriding position that, in effect, causes some stabilization to protect against further injury. This is called unilateral locked facets (Fig. 43.10). It occasionally occurs bilaterally.

"Seatbelt Injury." "Seatbelt injury" is seen secondary to hyperflexion at the waist (as occurs in an automobile accident while restrained by a lap belt). This causes distraction of the posterior elements and ligaments and anterior compression of the vertebral body. It usually involves the T12, L1, or L2 level. Several variations of this injury can occur: a fracture of the posterior body is called a Smith fracture, and a fracture through the spinous process is called a Chance fracture. Horizontal fractures of the pedicles, laminae, and transverse processes can also occur (Fig. 43.11).

Spondylolysis. A somewhat controversial spinal abnormality that may or may not be caused by trauma is spondylolysis. Spondylolysis is a break or defect in the pars interarticularis portion of the lamina (Fig. 43.12). On oblique views, the posterior elements form the figure of a "Scottie dog," with the transverse process being the nose, the pedicle forming the eye, the inferior articular facet being the front leg, the superior articular facet representing the ear, and the pars interarticularis (the portion of the lamina that lies between the facets) equivalent to the neck of the dog. If a spondylolysis is present, the pars interarticularis, or the neck of the dog, will have a defect or break. It often looks as if the dog has a collar around the neck.

The cause of spondylolysis is controversial but is thought to be congenital and/or posttraumatic. Many believe this is a stress-related injury from infancy that develops when toddlers try to walk and repeatedly fall on their buttocks, sending stress to their lower lumbar spine. The significance of spondylolysis is just as controversial as its etiology. More and more clinicians are coming to the viewpoint that a spondylolysis is an incidental finding with no

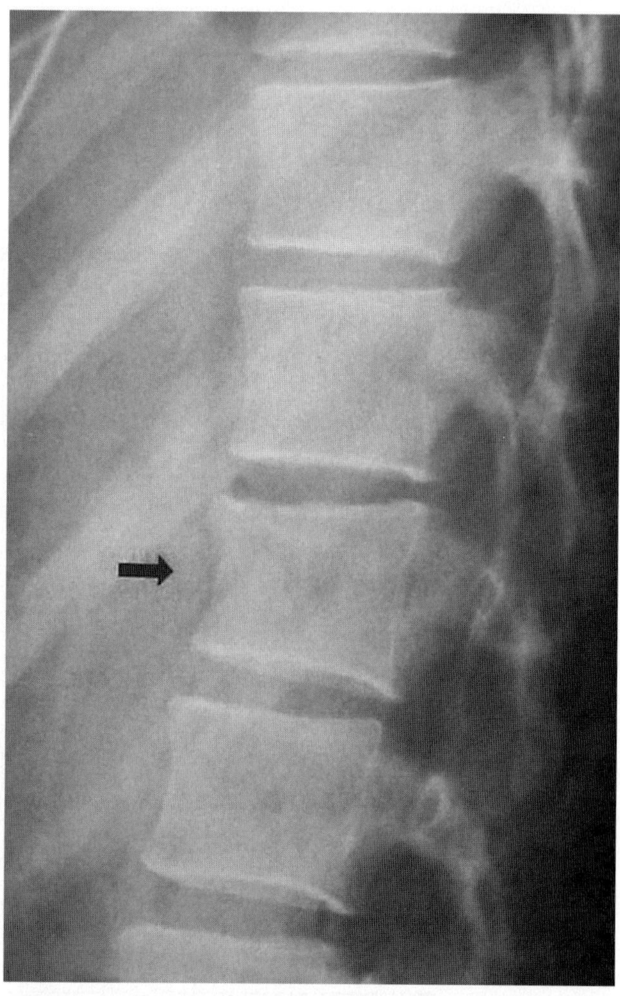

FIGURE 43.14. **Anterior Wedge Compression Fracture.** Anterior compression of this lower thoracic spine vertebral body (*arrow*) is present, which may or may not be acute. If the patient has pain in this area, it is most likely acute and must be protected with a back brace until the symptoms abate.

clinical significance in most cases. It has been reported in up to 10% of the asymptomatic population. Certainly some patients have pain related to a spondylolysis and get relief after rest or immobilization, and some require surgical stabilization. It is important to identify spondylolysis preoperatively in patients undergoing lumbar discectomy, so that the possibility of clinical symptoms from the spondylolysis that can mimic disk symptoms can be evaluated. Although plain films can usually show spondylolysis, CT will show it to better advantage and will demonstrate any associated disk disease. MR will show spondylolysis, but it can be difficult to see and is easily overlooked with this method.

If spondylolysis is bilateral and the vertebral body in the more cephalad position slips forward on the more caudal body, *spondylolisthesis* is said to be present (Fig. 43.13). Spondylolisthesis may or may not be symptomatic and by itself has no clinical significance. If severe, it can cause neuroforaminal stenosis and can impinge on the nerve roots in the central spinal canal. If it is symptomatic, it can be stabilized surgically.

Other Abnormalities. Anterior wedge compression fractures of the spine are commonly seen (Fig. 43.14), especially at the thoracolumbar junction, because of an old injury; they are passed off by the radiologist, if they are mentioned at all, as incidental findings. The problem with this assumption is that you cannot tell from a plain film if the fracture is old or new, even if degenerative changes are present (which are often not related to the fracture). If acute and left unprotected, a wedge compression fracture can proceed to delayed further collapse, with resulting severe neurologic deficits (Fig. 43.15). This is called Kümmel disease and typically occurs 1 to 2 weeks after the initial trauma. Multiple lawsuits have been filed against radiologists who failed to mention minor anterior wedging of a vertebral body that went on to further collapse, with associated paraplegia. All that needs to be mentioned is that a fracture is present that is of indeterminate age and requires clinical correlation. If the patient has pain in that location, a back brace must be worn until they are pain free. Old films can help determine whether it is an old fracture. If no pain is present on physical exam, it can be safely assumed to be an old fracture. It is not necessary to obtain a CT or MR even if pain is present, because the treatment will be the same regardless of what the CT or MR reveals. No spine surgeon will operate on a stable spine fracture without kyphosis or neurologic deficits, so the CT or MR adds nothing but time and expense.

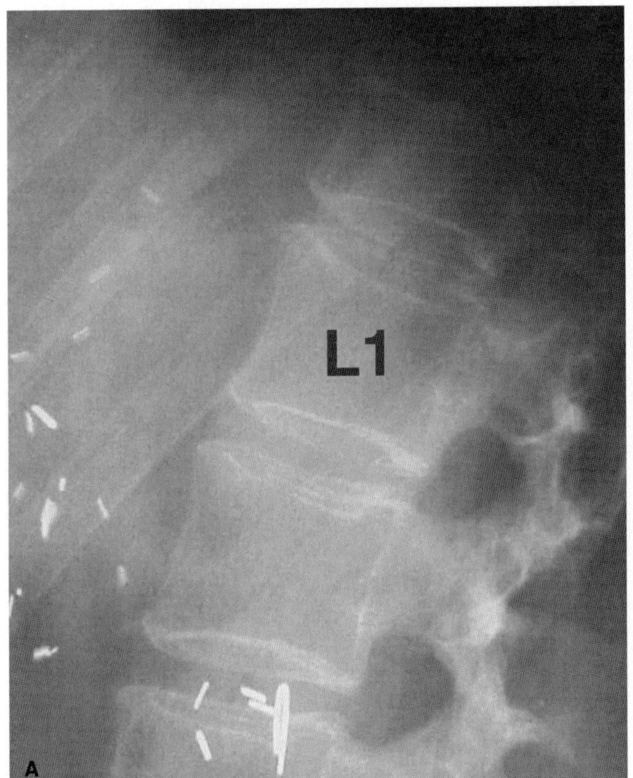

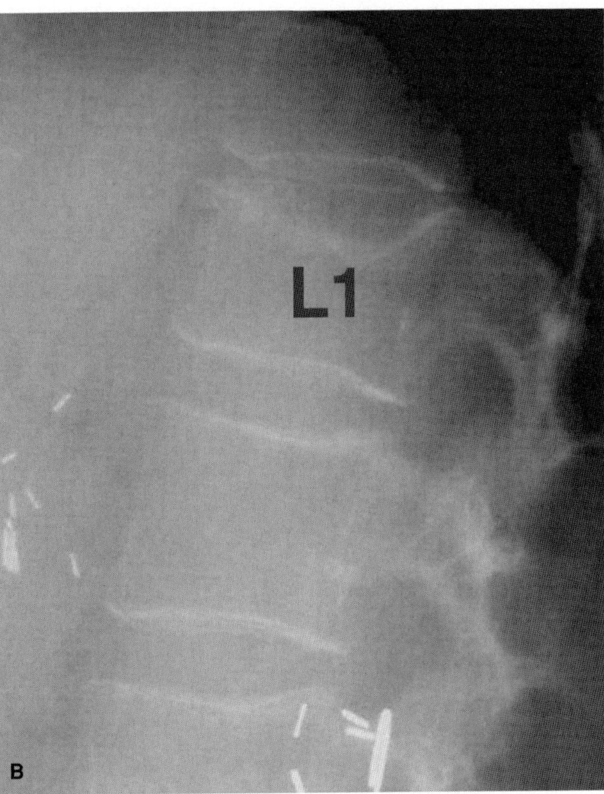

FIGURE 43.15. **Kümmel Disease. A.** Very minimal anterior wedging of the L1 vertebral body is noted by comparing the height of the anterior body versus the posterior height. This patient had been in an automobile accident and complained of back pain. No treatment for his back was given. **B.** After several weeks of continuing pain, he presented with leg weakness, which proceeded to paraplegia. A spine film showed progression of the vertebral body collapse of L1. This almost certainly could have been avoided with simple bracing of the spine after the initial injury.

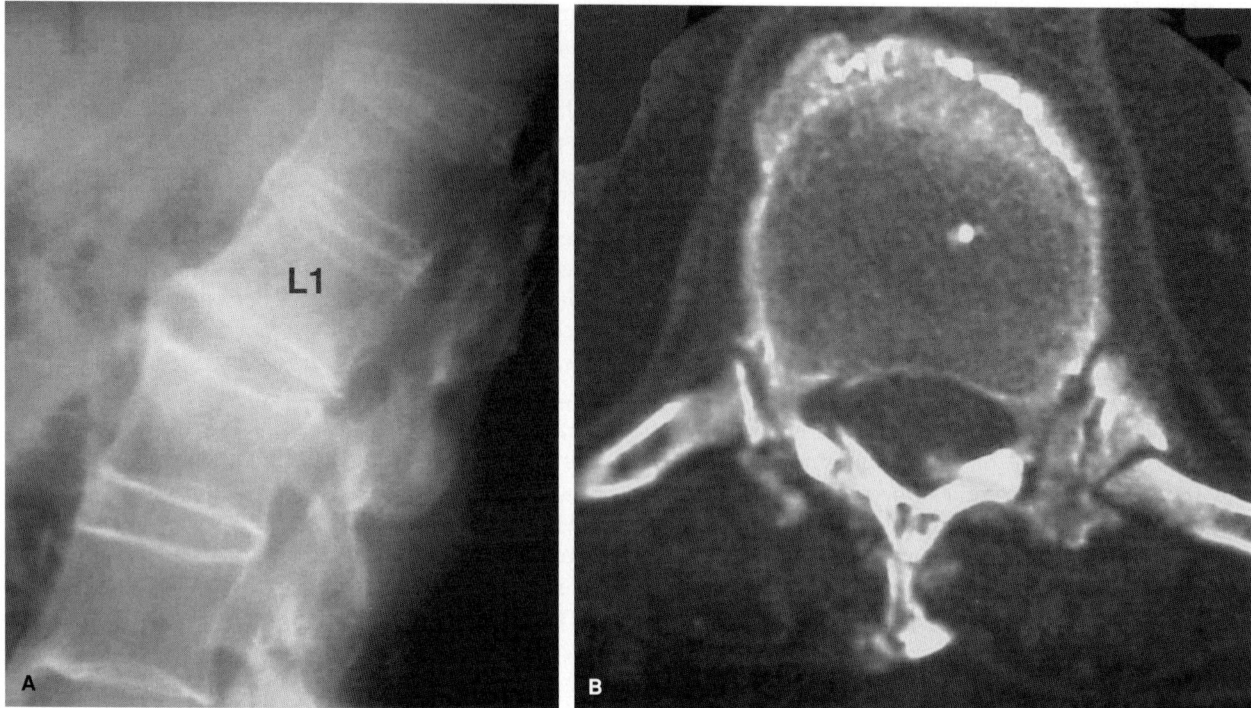

FIGURE 43.16. **Spine Fracture in Ankylosing Spondylitis. A.** A lateral plain film of the spine following trauma shows fusion anteriorly, which was secondary to ankylosing spondylitis. Minimal anterior wedging of the L1 vertebral body is present, which was overlooked. **B.** Two weeks later, a CT of the spine was performed because of the sudden onset of paralysis. This axial image through L1 shows a fracture of the posterior elements, which was undoubtedly present on the initial visit to the emergency room. Patients with ankylosing spondylitis need to be examined closely for any back pain following trauma and imaged with CT or MR if any pain is present.

Patients who have fusion of their spine from ankylosing spondylitis, and, to a lesser extent, from diffuse idiopathic skeletal hyperostosis, are at a very high risk of spinal fractures from even relatively minor trauma. Patients with ankylosing spondylitis typically have marked osteoporosis, which further magnifies their risk of fracture. A fused spine is more likely to fracture than a normal spine in a manner similar to a long glass pipette breaking more easily than a short one because it has a long lever arm. A small force at one end is greatly magnified further down the lever arm. For that reason, a patient with ankylosing spondylitis should be treated as though a spinal fracture is present if they have back pain following trauma. CT and/or MR are mandatory if plain films are negative (Fig. 43.16).

HAND AND WRIST

Several seemingly innocuous fractures in the hand require surgical fixation rather than just casting and should therefore be recognized by the radiologist as serious injuries.

Bennett Fracture. One such fracture is a fracture at the base of the thumb into the carpometacarpal joint—a Bennett fracture (Fig. 43.17). Because of the insertion of the strong thumb adductors at the base of the thumb, it is almost impossible to keep the metacarpal from sliding off its proper alignment. It almost always requires internal fixation. The radiologist occasionally has to remind a nonorthopaedic practitioner of this, as well as closely examine the alignment of a Bennett fracture in plaster that has not been internally fixed with wires.

A comminuted fracture of the base of the thumb that extends into the joint has been termed a *Rolando fracture* (Fig. 43.18), and a fracture of the base of the thumb that does not involve the joint has been called a *pseudo-Bennett fracture*.

Mallet finger or baseball finger is an avulsion injury at the base of the distal phalanx (Fig. 43.19) where the extensor digitorum tendon inserts. With the extensor tendon inoperative, the distal phalanx flexes without opposition, which can result in a flexion deformity and inability to extend the distal phalanx if not properly treated.

Volar Plate Fracture. A fracture at the volar aspect of the base of the interphalangeal and metacarpophalangeal joints from an avulsion of the volar plate can appear innocent but often requires surgical intervention. The volar plate is a dense fibrocartilaginous band that covers the joint on the volar aspect and can get interposed in the joint once it is torn, often requiring surgical removal.

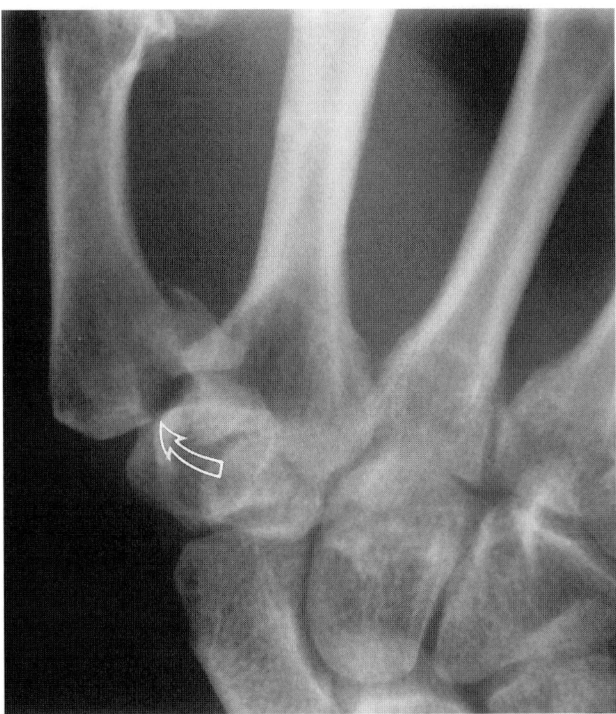

FIGURE 43.17. **Bennett Fracture.** A small corner fracture of the base of the thumb is noted that involves the articular surface of the base of the thumb (*arrow*); this is a serious injury that almost always requires internal fixation.

"Gamekeeper's Thumb." Another innocent-appearing fracture that often requires internal fixation is an avulsion on the ulnar aspect of the first metacarpophalangeal joint (Fig. 43.20); this is where the ulnar collateral ligament of the thumb inserts. If the ulnar collateral ligament is torn, normal function of the thumb can be impaired, and this can have a serious result if not properly treated. This injury is called a "gamekeeper's thumb" because of the propensity of English game wardens to acquire it from breaking rabbits' necks between their thumb and forefinger. A more current scenario is falling on a ski pole and having the pole jam into the webbing between the thumb and index finger. This avulsion injury usually requires pinning to fix the ligament securely.

Lunate/Perilunate Dislocation. A fall on the outstretched arm can result in any number of wrist fractures and dislocations. One serious such injury is the lunate/perilunate dislocation. This occurs when the ligaments between the capitate and the lunate are disrupted, allowing the capitate to dislocate from the cup-shaped articulation of the lunate. This is best seen on lateral views. Ordinarily, on the lateral view the capitate should be seen seated in the cup-shaped lunate (Figs. 43.21, 43.22A). In a dorsal dislocation (the capitate occasionally dislocates volarly, but this is uncommon), the capitate and all of its surrounding bones, including the metacarpals, come to lie dorsal to a line drawn through the radius and the lunate (Figs. 43.22B, 43.23). If the capitate then pushes the lunate volarly and tips it over, a line drawn up through the radius shows that the lunate is volarly displaced, and the line goes through the capitate. This has been termed a lunate dislocation (Figs. 43.22C, 43.24). Failure to diagnose and treat this disorder can result in permanent median nerve impairment, as the nerve can get impinged by the volarly displaced lunate.

A lunate or perilunate dislocation can be diagnosed on an AP view of the wrist by noting a triangular or pie-shaped lunate (Fig. 43.24B). Ordinarily, the lunate has a rhomboid

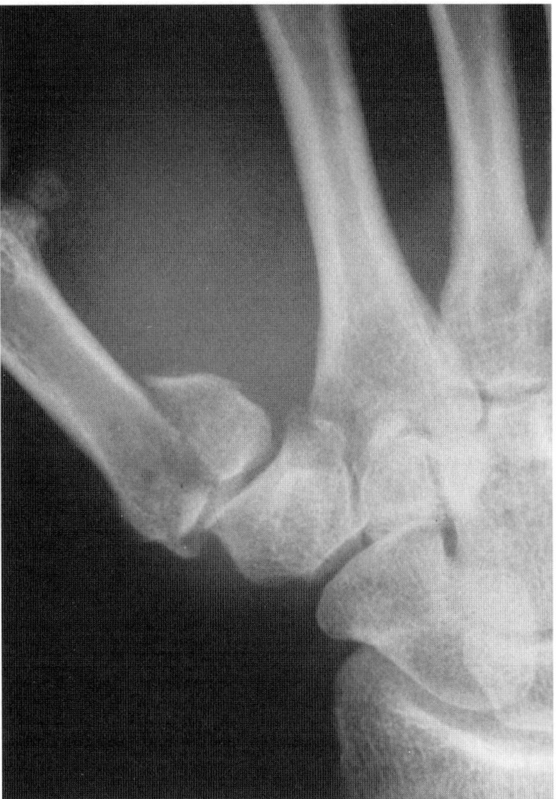

FIGURE 43.18. **Rolando Fracture.** A comminuted fracture of the base of the thumb that extends into the articular surface is a more serious type of Bennett fracture, which has been termed a Rolando fracture.

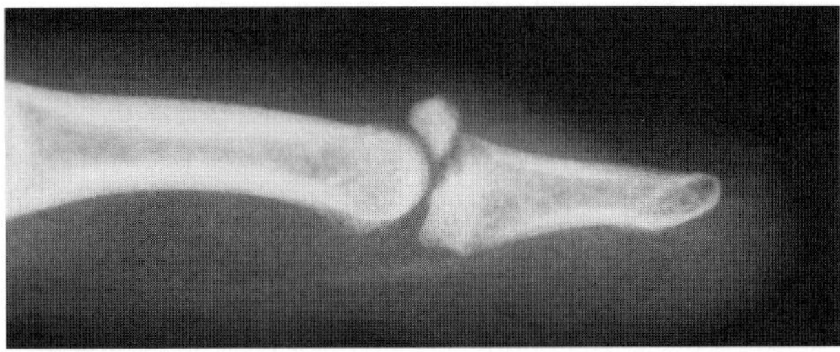

FIGURE 43.19. **Mallet Finger.** A small avulsion injury is noted at the base of the distal phalanx, which is where the extensor digitorum tendon inserts. This is termed a mallet finger or baseball finger because it is often caused by a baseball striking the distal phalanx and causing the avulsion.

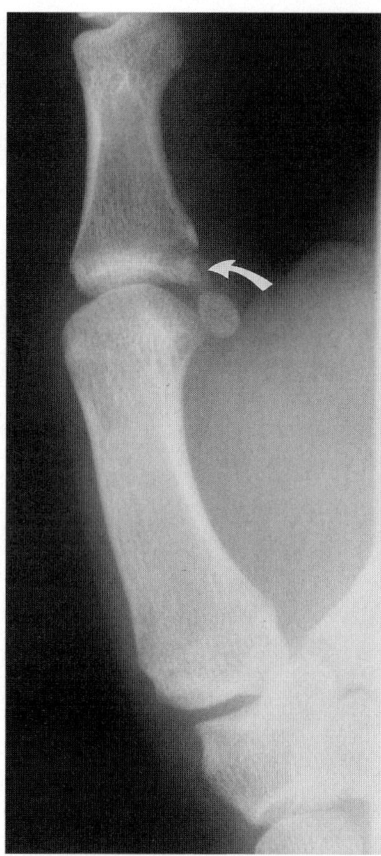

FIGURE 43.20. **Gamekeeper's Thumb.** A small avulsion injury on the ulnar aspect of the first metacarpophalangeal joint (*arrow*) is diagnostic of a gamekeeper's thumb. This is the insertion site for the ulnar collateral ligament and usually requires internal fixation.

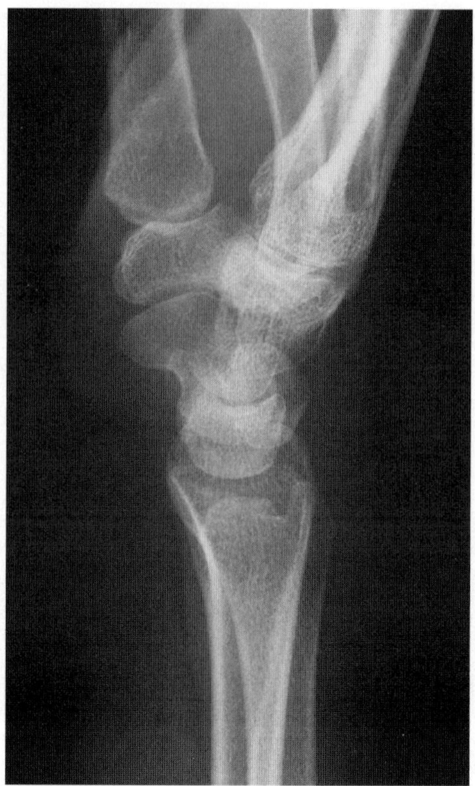

FIGURE 43.21. **Normal Lateral Radiograph of the Wrist.** The normal lateral view should show the lunate seated in the distal radius and the capitate seated in the lunate. A line drawn up through the radius should connect all three structures. Compare this radiograph with the drawing in Fig. 43.22A.

shape on the AP view, with the upper and lower borders parallel.

Several fractures are known to be associated with a perilunate dislocation, the most common of which is a transscaphoid fracture. The capitate, radial styloid, and triquetrum are also known to fracture frequently when a perilunate dislocation occurs.

Hook of the Hamate Fracture. One of the most difficult wrist fractures to identify radiologically is a fracture of the hook of the hamate. A special view, the carpal tunnel view, should be obtained when trying to see the hook of the hamate. This view is obtained with the wrist (palm down) flat on an x-ray plate and the fingers pulled dorsally. The x-ray beam is angled about 45°—parallel to the palm of the hand so that the carpal tunnel is in profile. The hook of the hamate is seen as a bony protuberance off the hamate on the ulnar aspect of the carpal tunnel. A fractured hook of the hamate is often identified with the carpal tunnel view (Fig. 43.25) but occasionally can be very difficult to visualize. A CT scan will often show an obvious fracture that the plain film does not (Fig. 43.26) and should be considered

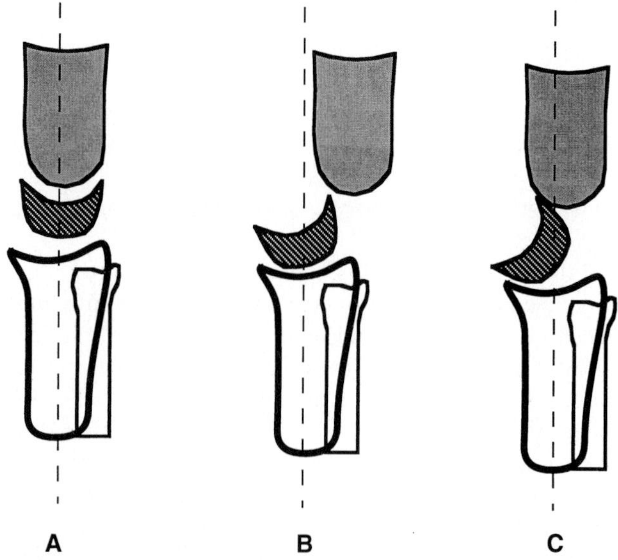

FIGURE 43.22. **Perilunate and Lunate Dislocations.** Schematic depiction of normal lateral wrist **(A),** perilunate dislocation **(B),** and lunate dislocation **(C).** (Dorsal is to the right.)

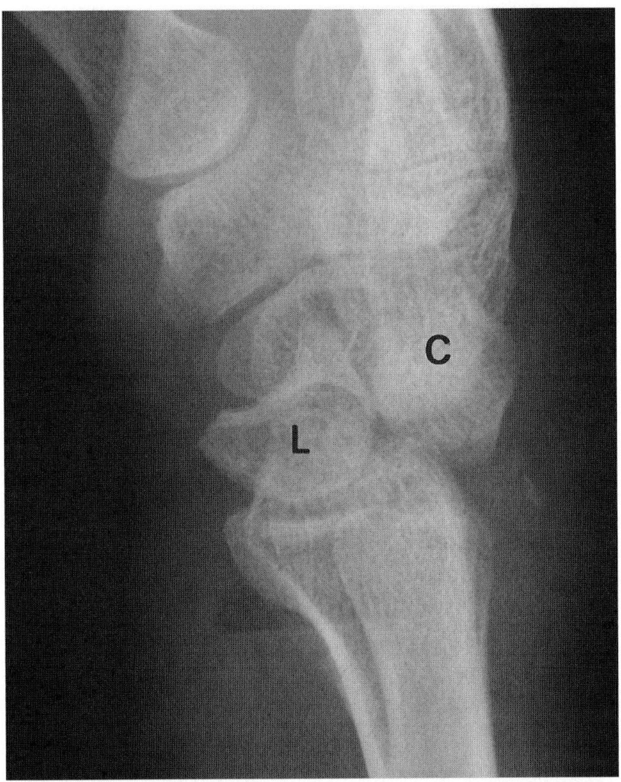

FIGURE 43.23. Perilunate Dislocation. Although the lunate (L) is in a normal relationship to the distal radius, the capitate (C) and the remainder of the wrist are dorsally displaced in relation to the lunate. Compare this radiograph with the drawing in Fig. 43.22B.

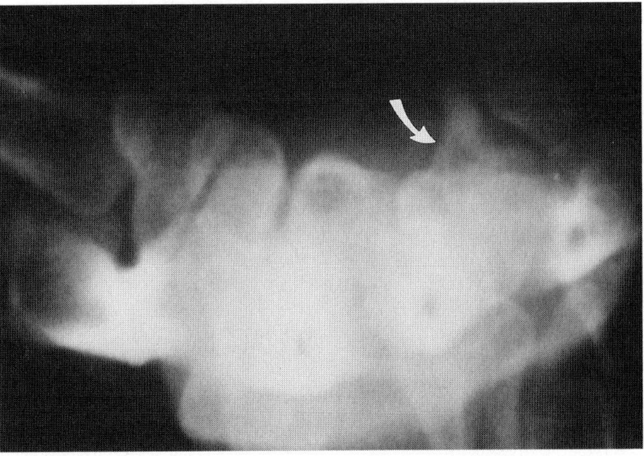

FIGURE 43.25. Fracture of the Hook of the Hamate. The hook of the hamate is seen on a carpal tunnel view in this patient and has an area of sclerosis with a faint cortical break (*arrow*). This represents a fracture at the base of the hook of the hamate.

in any possible carpal fracture when plain films are not diagnostic.

A fracture of the hook of the hamate most commonly occurs from a fall on the outstretched hand. A clinical setting that has gained attention in sports medicine circles is that of a professional athlete who participates in an activity in which the butt of a club, bat, or racket is held in the palm of the hand. Overswinging can result in the butt of the club levering off the hook of the hamate. This has been seen in professional baseball players, tennis players, and golfers. It is not seen as often in amateurs because they usually are not strong enough to exert enough force to lever the hook off and, if they do, will usually terminate that activity, allowing healing, whereas a professional will continue participation, which can lead to a nonunion of the fracture.

Rotary subluxation of the navicular is another wrist injury seen after a fall onto the outstretched hand. This results from rupture of the scapholunate ligament, which allows the scaphoid (navicular) to rotate dorsally. On an

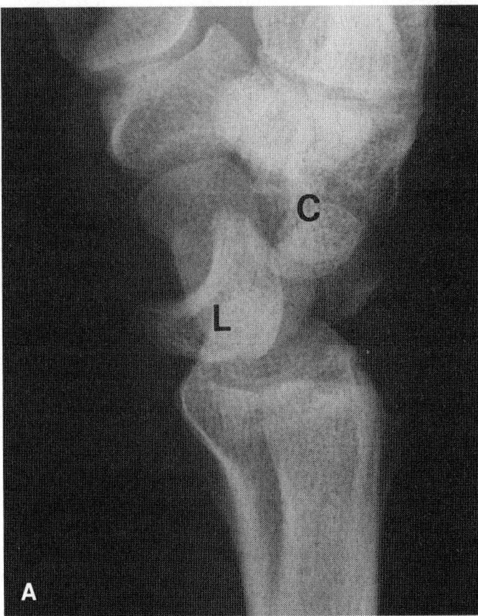

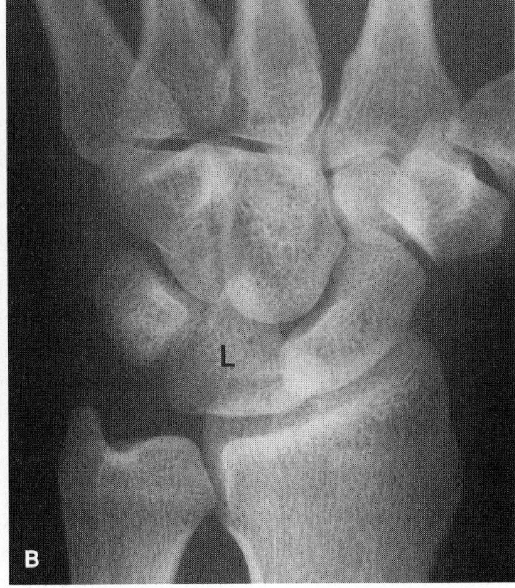

FIGURE 43.24. Lunate Dislocation. A. The lateral radiograph of the wrist shows the lunate (L) tipped off of the distal radius, whereas the capitate (C) seems to be normally aligned in relation to the radius yet is dislocated from the lunate. Compare this with the drawing in Fig. 43.22C. **B.** Anteroposterior view shows a pie-shaped lunate (L) rather than a lunate with a more rhomboid shape. A pie-shaped lunate on an anteroposterior view is diagnostic of a perilunate or lunate dislocation.

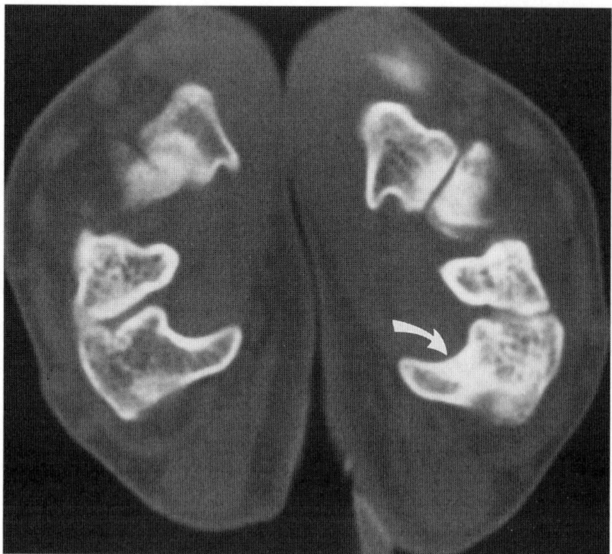

FIGURE 43.26. **Fractured Hamate.** A CT scan through the wrist in this patient shows a faint lucency surrounded by sclerosis in the left hamate (*arrow*), which represents a fracture through the base of the hook of the hamate with moderate reactive sclerosis. This could not be seen in the plain films, even in retrospect.

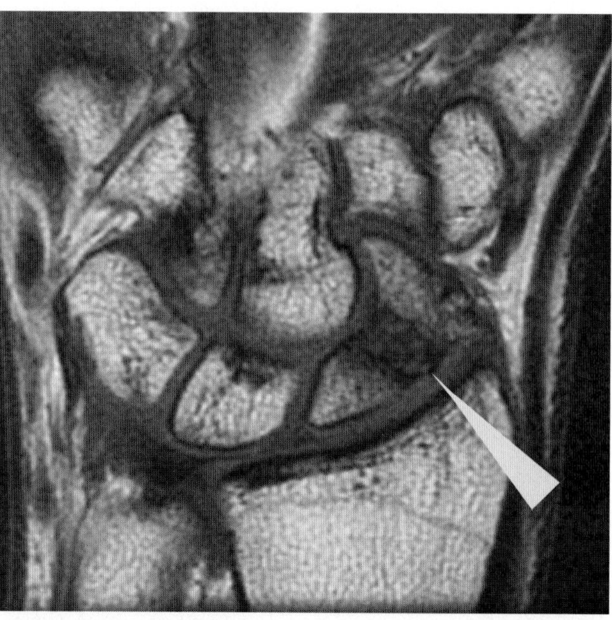

FIGURE 43.28. **Scaphoid Fracture.** A coronal T1WI of the wrist in a patient with snuffbox tenderness and a normal plain film shows a fracture of the mid-waist of the scaphoid (*arrow*).

AP wrist plain film, a space is seen between the navicular and the lunate (Fig. 43.27), where ordinarily they are closely apposed. This has been called the "Terry Thomas" sign after a famous British actor (circa 1950s) who had a gap between his two front teeth.

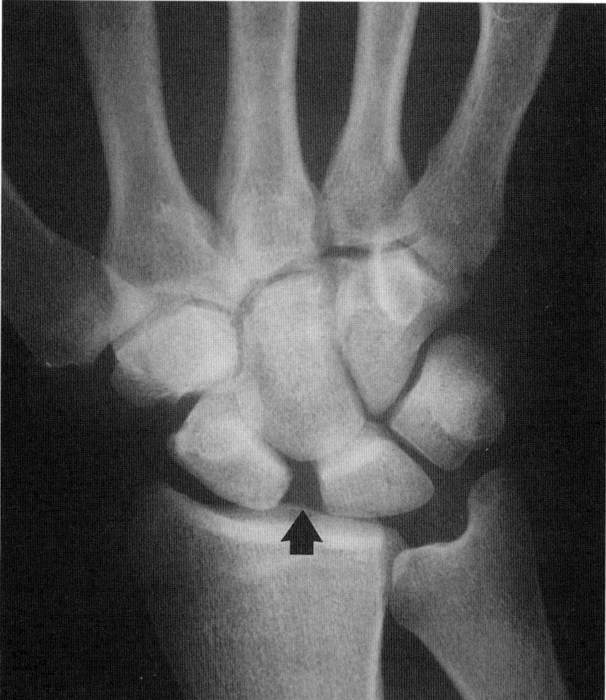

FIGURE 43.27. **Rotatory Subluxation of the Navicular.** An anteroposterior view of the wrist shows a gap or space between the navicular and the lunate (*arrow*). This is abnormal and represents the "Terry Thomas" sign, which means that the scapholunate ligament is ruptured. This is diagnostic of a rotatory subluxation of the navicular.

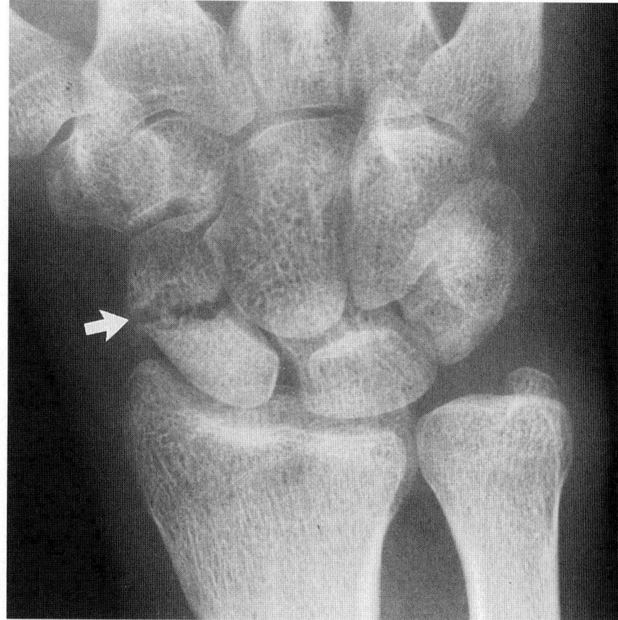

FIGURE 43.29. **Avascular Necrosis of the Navicular.** An anteroposterior view of the wrist shows a fracture through the waist of the navicular (*arrow*). The proximal half of the navicular is slightly sclerotic in relation to the remainder of the carpal bones, which indicates avascular necrosis of the proximal half.

Navicular Fracture. A fracture of the navicular is a potentially serious injury because of the high rate of avascular necrosis (AVN) that occurs with this injury. When AVN occurs, it usually requires surgical intervention with a metallic screw and bone grafting to obtain healing. This fracture can be very difficult to detect initially; therefore, whenever a fracture of the navicular is clinically suspect (trauma with pain over the snuffbox of the wrist), the wrist should be casted and repeat radiographs obtained in 1 week. Often, the fracture is then visualized because of the disuse osteoporosis and hyperemia around the fracture site. Thus, in the acute setting, a negative film does not exclude a fractured scaphoid. Instead of casting the wrist and repeating the films in a week, many patients now get immediate MR to determine whether a fracture is present (Fig. 43.28). This has been shown to be less expensive overall than having the patient casted and reexamined in a week (2).

If AVN of the navicular develops, it is the proximal fragment that undergoes necrosis because the blood supply to the navicular begins distally and runs proximally. A fracture with disruption of the blood supply thus leaves the proximal pole without a vascular supply; hence, it dies. AVN is diagnosed by noting increased density of the proximal pole of the navicular compared with the remainder of the carpal bones (Fig. 43.29).

AVN can occur in other carpal bones, most commonly the lunate. This is called *Kienböck malacia* and is most often caused by trauma; however, it is also thought to be idiopathic. It is diagnosed by noting the increased density in the lunate, which may or may not go on to collapse and fragmentation (Fig. 43.30). It often requires surgical bone grafting and, occasionally, removal or proximal carpal row fusion. It has a high association with a discrepancy between the length of the radius and the ulna as seen at the radiocarpal joint. If the ulna is shorter than the radius, it is termed *negative ulnar variance* and there is an increased incidence of Kienböck malacia (Fig. 43.30). If the ulna is longer than the radius, it is termed *positive ulnar variance* and there is an increased incidence of triangular fibrocartilage tears.

A common avulsion fracture in the wrist is a triquetral fracture. It is best seen on a lateral film, which shows a small chip of bone off the dorsum of the wrist (Fig. 43.31). This is virtually pathognomonic of an avulsion from the triquetrum.

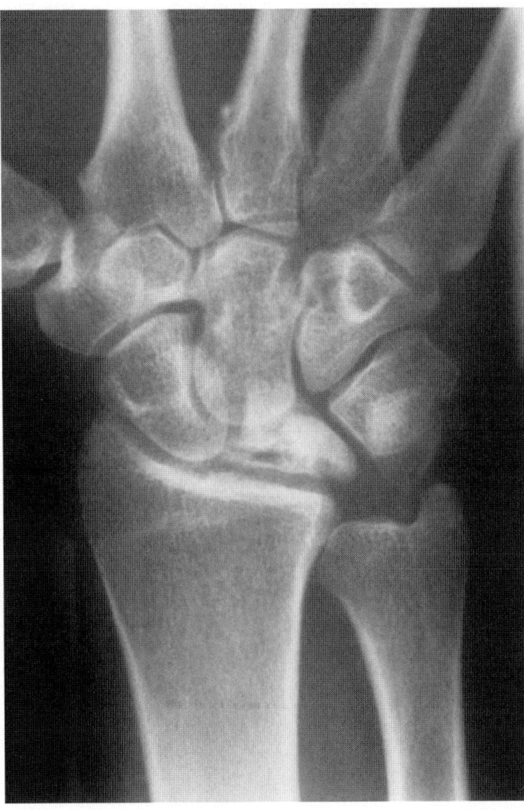

FIGURE 43.30. **Kienböck Malacia.** An anteroposterior view of the wrist reveals the lunate to be sclerotic and abnormal in shape. The lunate has collapsed because of aseptic necrosis. This is known as Kienböck malacia. Note that the ulna is shorter than the radius; this is termed negative ulnar variance, which is often associated with Kienböck malacia.

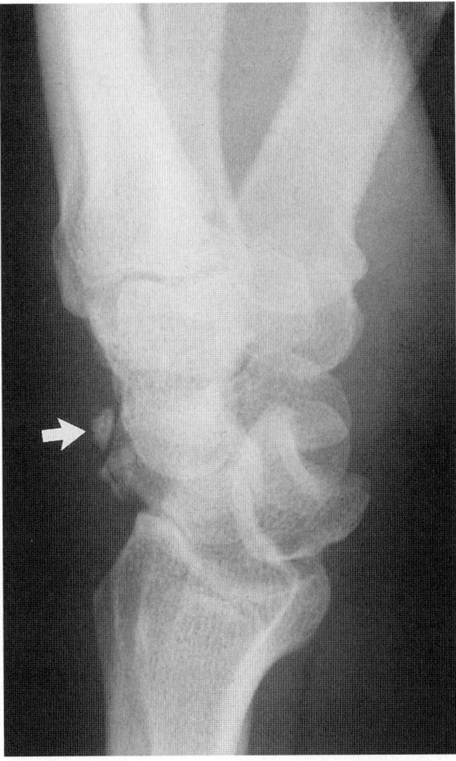

FIGURE 43.31. **Triquetral Fracture and Perilunate Dislocation.** A perilunate or lunate dislocation is present (it is difficult to classify exactly which has occurred, because both the lunate and the capitate are out of their normal position). A small avulsion is seen on the dorsum of the wrist (*arrow*), which is virtually diagnostic of an avulsion off the triquetrum. It is often associated with a lunate or perilunate dislocation.

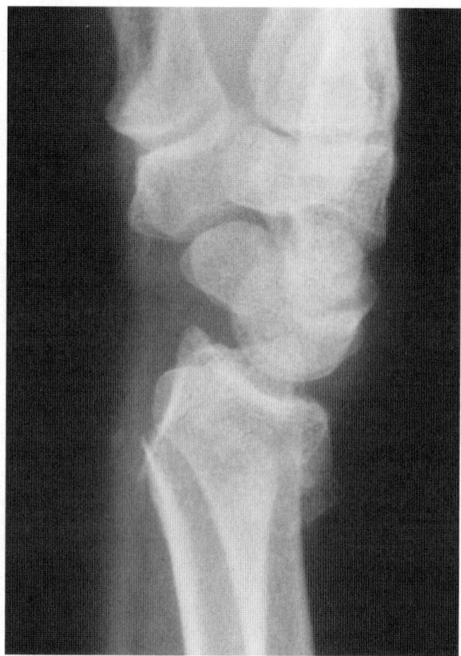

FIGURE 43.32. **Colles Fracture.** A fracture of the distal radius with dorsal angulation is noted, which has been termed a Colles fracture.

ARM

Colles Fracture. One of the most common fractures of the forearm is a fracture of the distal radius and ulna after a fall on an outstretched arm. This results in a dorsal angulation of the distal forearm and wrist and is called a Colles fracture (Fig. 43.32). When the fracture angulates volarly, it is called a *Smith fracture* (Fig. 43.33). A Smith fracture is much less common than a Colles fracture. Sometimes the radius and ulna suffer a traumatic insult, and the force on the bones causes bending instead of a frank fracture. This has been termed a *plastic bowing deformity* of the forearm (Fig. 43.34) and is often treated by breaking the bones while the patient has undergone anesthesia and resetting them. Left untreated, a plastic bowing deformity can result in reduced supination and pronation.

Monteggia Fracture. The forearm is a two-bone system that has some of the same properties as a ring bone. As mentioned previously, a solid ring cannot break in only a single place; it must break in at least two places. In the forearm, a fracture of one bone should be accompanied by a fracture of the other. If the second fracture is not present,

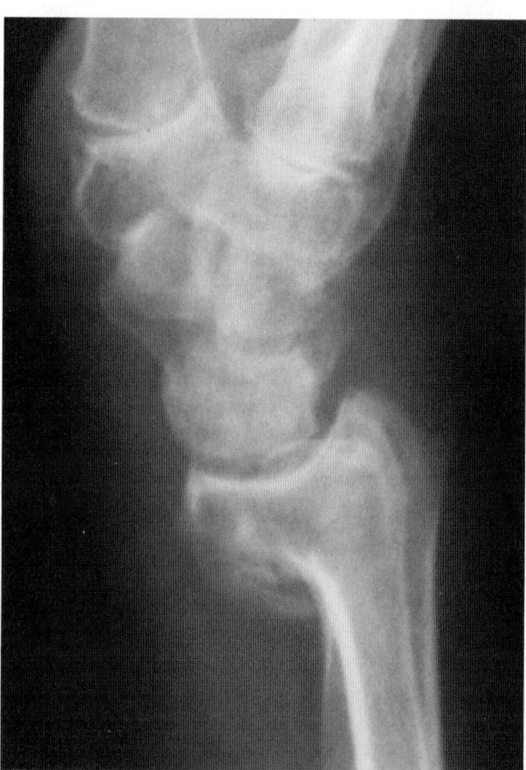

FIGURE 43.33. **Smith Fracture.** A fracture of the distal radius with volar angulation such as this is called a Smith fracture. This is a much less common injury than the Colles fracture, shown in Fig. 43.32.

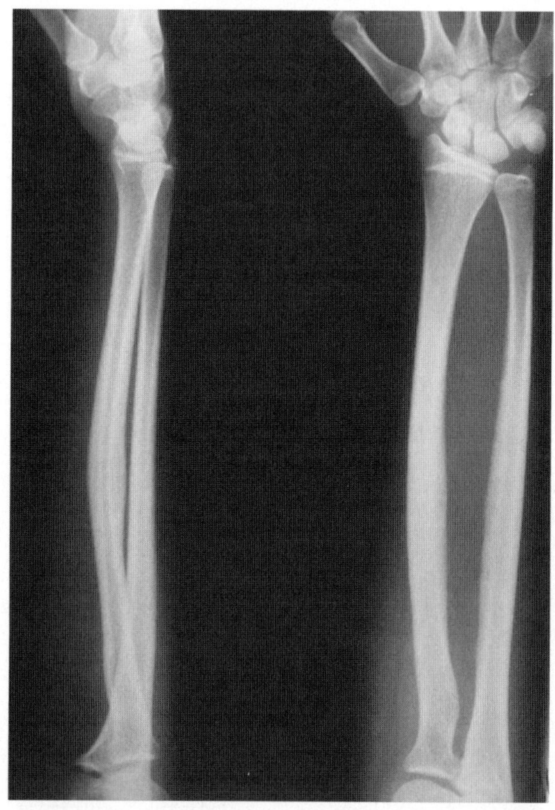

FIGURE 43.34. **Plastic Bowing Deformity of the Forearm.** These anteroposterior and lateral views of the forearm of a child show the radius to be abnormally bowed anteriorly. This has been termed a plastic bowing deformity of the forearm and occurs only in children.

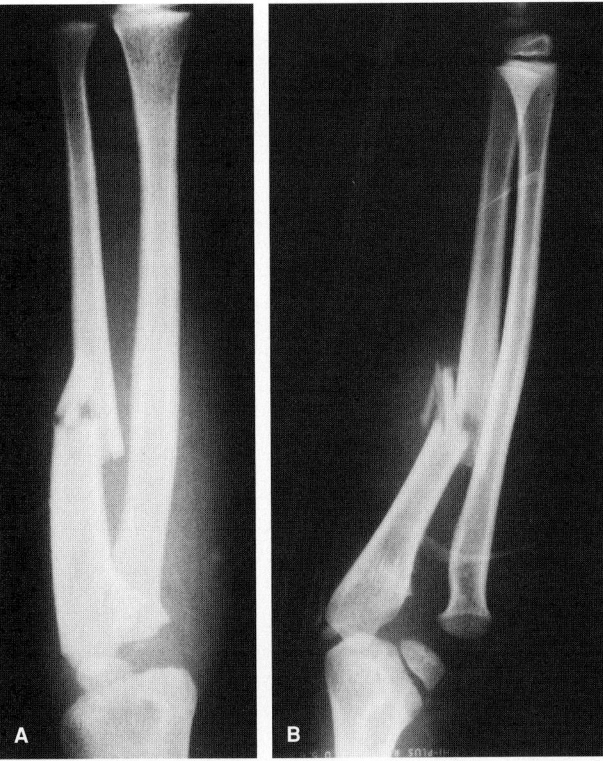

FIGURE 43.35. **Monteggia Fracture.** A blow to the forearm such as with a police officer's nightstick can result in a fracture of the ulna. Although the head of the radius appears normally placed in an anteroposterior view **(A),** the lateral examination **(B)** reveals that the head of the radius is displaced. Failure to recognize this abnormality can result in death of the radial head, with subsequent elbow dysfunction. This illustrates the importance of always obtaining two views of a bone after trauma.

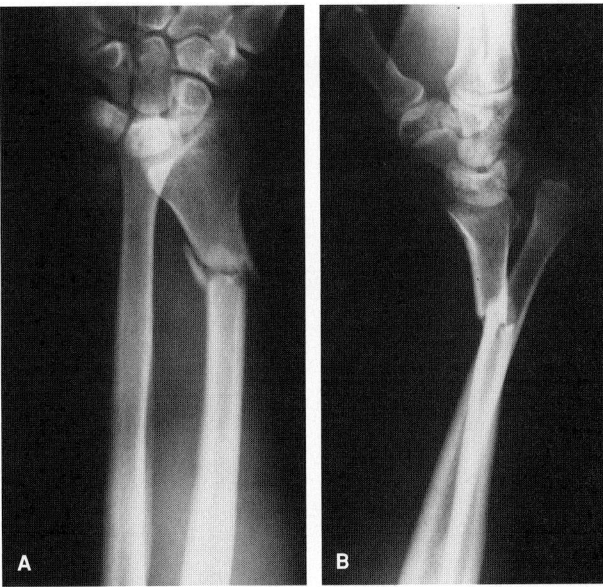

FIGURE 43.36. **Galeazzi Fracture. A.** A fracture of the distal radius in this patient is seen on the anteroposterior view without a definite fracture of the ulna. **B.** This view shows an obvious dislocation of the distal ulna, which would almost certainly not be missed clinically. This has been termed a Galeazzi fracture and is much less common than the Monteggia fractures.

a dislocation of the nonfractured bone usually occurs. The most common example of this is a fracture of the ulna with a dislocation of the proximal radius (Fig. 43.35). This is called a Monteggia fracture. The dislocated radial head can be missed clinically and develop into AVN, with subsequent elbow dysfunction. Whenever the forearm is fractured, the elbow must be examined to exclude a dislocation.

Galeazzi Fracture. A fracture of the radius with dislocation of the distal ulna is called a Galeazzi fracture (Fig. 43.36). This is less common than a Monteggia fracture.

A helpful indicator of a fracture about the elbow is a displaced posterior fat-pad. Ordinarily, the posterior fat-pad is not visible on a lateral view of the elbow because it is tucked away in the olecranon fossa of the distal humerus. When the joint becomes distended with blood secondary to a fracture, the posterior fat-pad is displaced out of the olecranon fossa and is visible on the lateral view (Fig. 43.37A). Therefore, in the setting of trauma, a visible posterior fat-pad indicates a fracture. In an adult (epiphyses closed), the fracture site is almost always the radial head (Fig. 43.37B). In a child (epiphyses open), it is usually indicative of a supracondylar fracture (Fig. 43.38).

Often, the fracture itself is not visualized, and extraordinary steps are taken by clinicians and radiologists alike to demonstrate the fracture. These steps include oblique views, special radial head views, tomograms, and even CT or MR. These are absurd attempts to document pathology that will be treated identically whether or not it is radiographically recorded. As long as there is no obvious deformity or loose body, it does not matter whether the fracture is definitely identified or not in a patient with a posttraumatic painful elbow and a visible posterior fat-pad. An infection, an arthritide, or any elbow effusion could cause a joint effusion and a displaced posterior fat-pad, but the clinical setting would not be to rule out a fracture.

The anterior fat-pad also gets displaced with a joint effusion. Ordinarily it is visible as a small triangle just anterior to the distal humeral diaphysis on a lateral film (Fig. 43.39). With an effusion, it gets displaced superiorly and outward from the humerus and has been called a "sail sign" because it resembles a spinnaker sail (see Figs. 43.37, 43.38).

Shoulder dislocations are generally easily diagnosed, both clinically and radiographically. The most common shoulder dislocation is the anterior dislocation. It is at least 10 times more common than a posterior dislocation. For all practical purposes, anterior and posterior dislocations are the only two types of shoulder dislocations about which to be concerned.

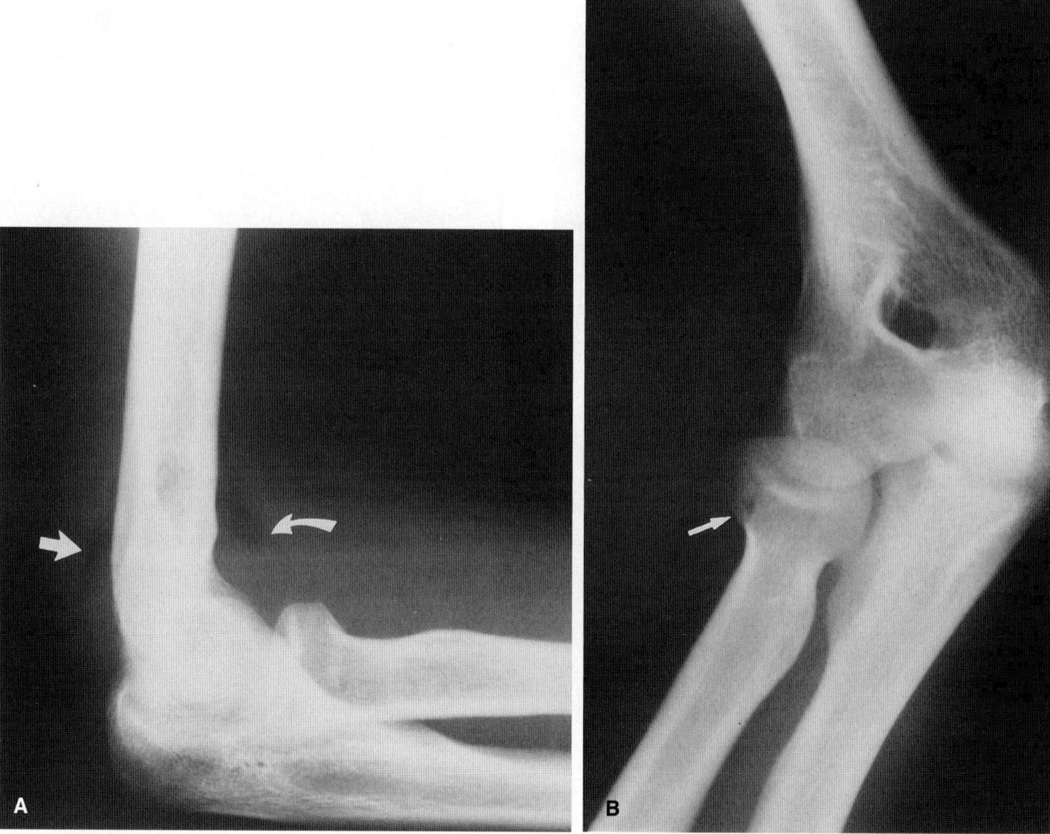

FIGURE 43.37. **Displaced Elbow Fat-Pads. A.** On the lateral view of this elbow, the posterior fat-pad is faintly visible (*arrow*) and the anterior fat-pad is elevated and anteriorly displaced (*curved arrow*). These findings indicate a fracture about the elbow that in an adult should be in the radial head. **B.** An oblique view shows the fracture of the radial head (*arrow*). Even without seeing the fracture on the radiographs, it should be surmised to be present when the posterior fat-pad is visualized in the setting of trauma. The elevated and displaced anterior fat-pad has been termed a sail sign.

An *anterior dislocation* occurs when the arm is forcibly externally rotated and abducted. This is commonly seen when football players "arm tackle," when kayakers "brace" with the paddle above their heads and allow their arms to get too far posterior, when skiers plant their uphill pole and get it stuck, and from other similar athletic positions. Radiographically, the diagnosis is easily made on an AP shoulder film: the humeral head is seen to lie inferiorly and medial to the glenoid (Fig. 43.40). The humeral head often impacts on the inferior lip of the glenoid, causing an indentation on the posterosuperior portion of the humeral head; this is called a *Hill-Sachs deformity.* The presence of a Hill-Sachs deformity is said to indicate a greater likelihood of recurrent dislocation, and some surgeons use it as an indicator to intervene surgically to prevent a recurrence. A bony irregularity or fragment off the inferior glenoid, which occurs from the same mechanism as the Hill-Sachs deformity, is called a *Bankart deformity.* It is not seen radiographically as often as the Hill-Sachs deformity.

A *posterior dislocation* can be a difficult diagnosis to make, both clinically and radiographically. An AP view may look completely normal, or nearly so. On the AP view of a normal shoulder, the humeral head should slightly overlap the glenoid (Fig. 43.41), forming what has been called the "crescent sign." In a patient with a posterior dislocation, this crescent of bony overlap is usually absent and a small space is seen between the glenoid and the humeral head (Fig. 43.42).

The best way to unequivocally diagnose a dislocated shoulder is to obtain a transscapular view. An axillary view will show basically the same thing but requires the patient to move the arm and shoulder, which can be painful and may even re-dislocate the shoulder if it has spontaneously reduced itself. The transscapular view is obtained by angling the x-ray beam across the shoulder in the same plane as the blade of the scapula. This gives an en face view of the glenoid, and the humeral head can easily be related to it as either normal, anterior (Fig. 43.43), or posterior.

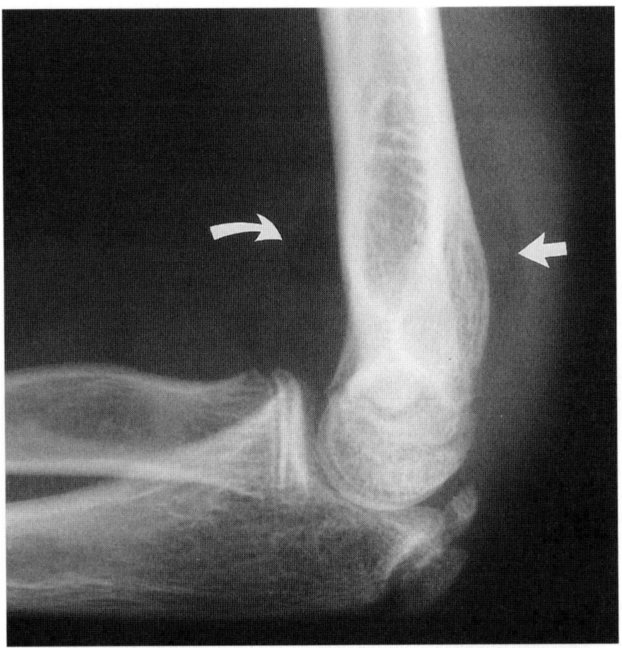

FIGURE 43.38. **Displaced Elbow Fat-Pads.** A lateral view of the elbow in this child shows a posterior fat-pad (*arrow*) and a sail sign anteriorly (*curved arrow*). This is indicative of a fracture about the elbow, which in a child (epiphyses are open) usually means a supracondylar fracture.

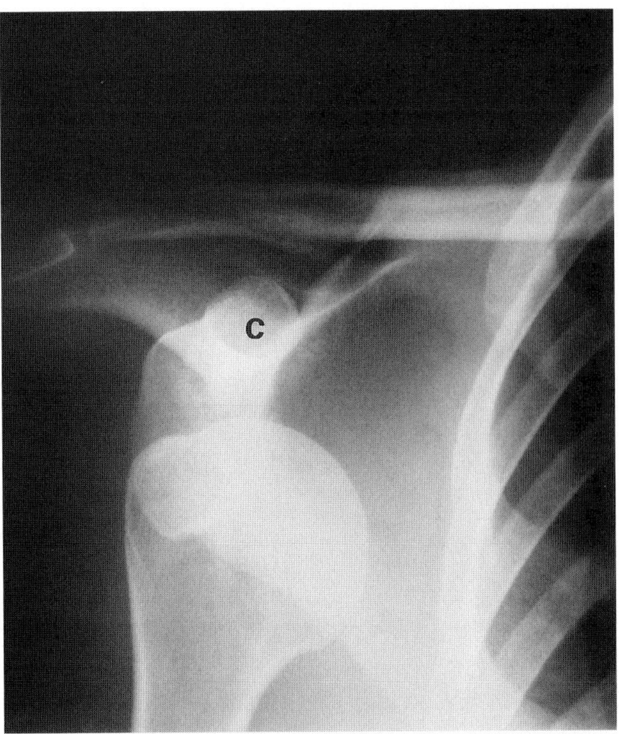

FIGURE 43.40. **Anterior Shoulder Dislocation.** An anteroposterior view of the right shoulder shows the humeral head to lie medial to the glenoid and inferior to the coracoid process (C). This is diagnostic of an anterior dislocation of the shoulder.

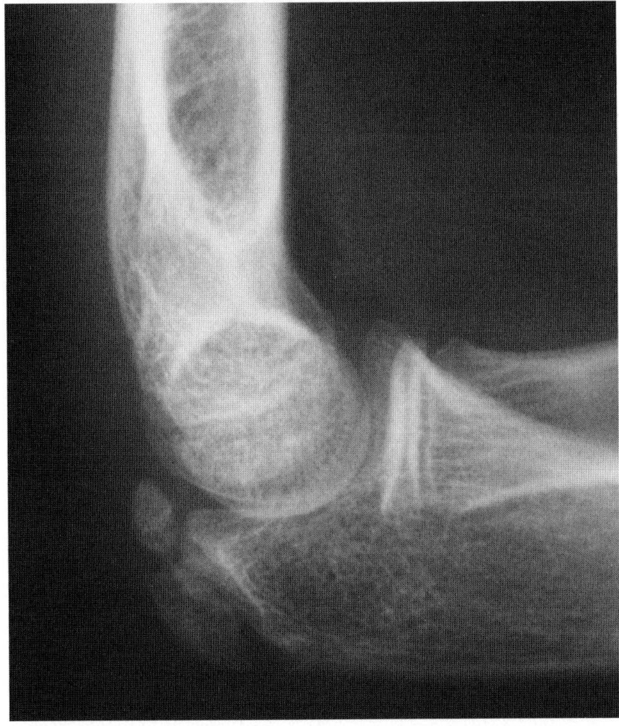

FIGURE 43.39. **Normal Anterior Fat-Pad of the Elbow.** Note the lucency just anterior to the humerus of this normal elbow and compare this with the sail sign of the anterior fat-pads in Figs. 43.37 and 43.38.

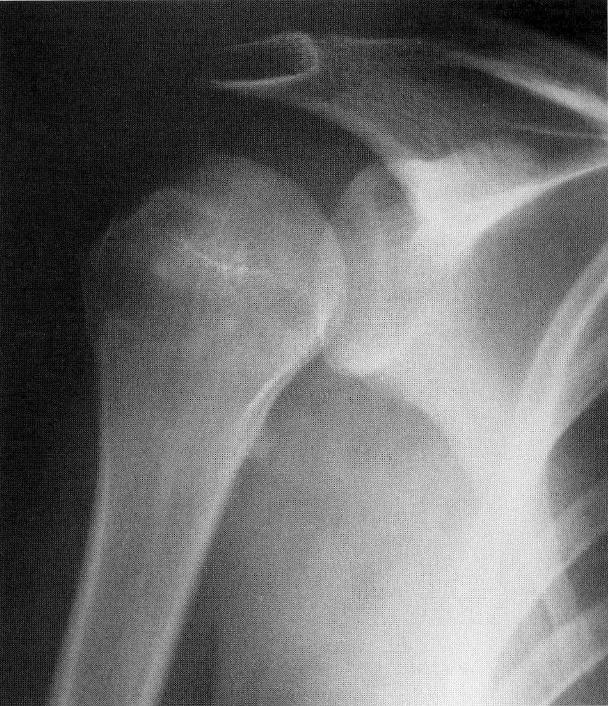

FIGURE 43.41. **Normal Anteroposterior View of the Shoulder.** Note in this example of a normal shoulder that the humeral head slightly overlaps the glenoid, which has been termed the crescent sign.

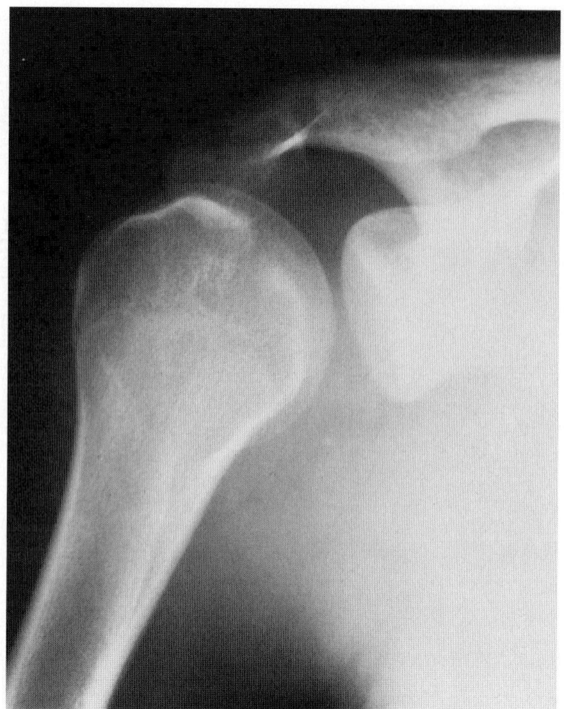

FIGURE 43.42. **Posterior Shoulder Dislocation.** Note that the humeral head in this patient is slightly displaced from the glenoid on the anteroposterior view. This is termed absence of the crescent sign and is often seen with a posterior dislocation. Compare this with the normal shoulder in Fig. 43.41.

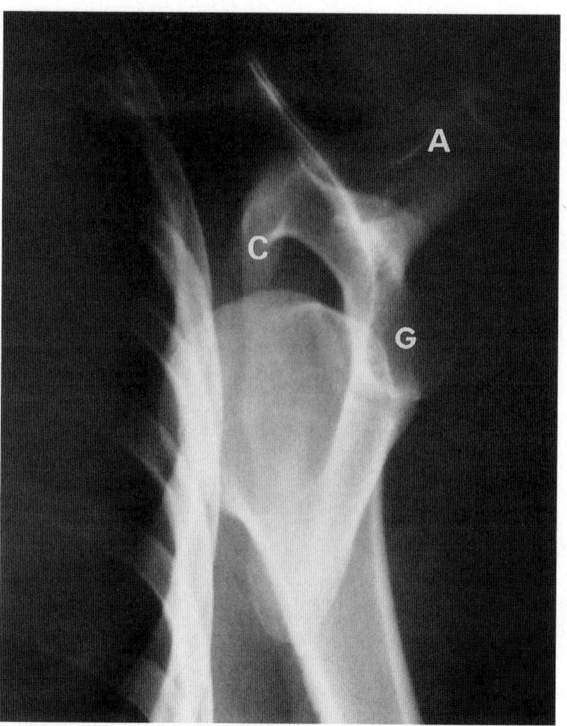

FIGURE 43.43. **Transscapular View of an Anterior Dislocation.** This transscapular view of the shoulder is obtained by aiming the x-ray beam parallel to the shoulder blade. The coracoid process (C) can be seen anteriorly, and the spine of the acromion (A) can be seen posteriorly. Both of these structures extend inwardly and meet at the glenoid (G). The humeral head is seen in this example to lie anterior to the glenoid.

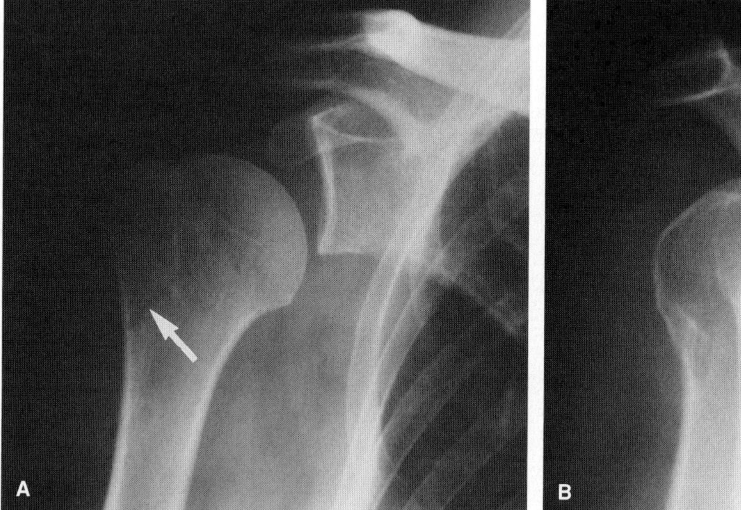

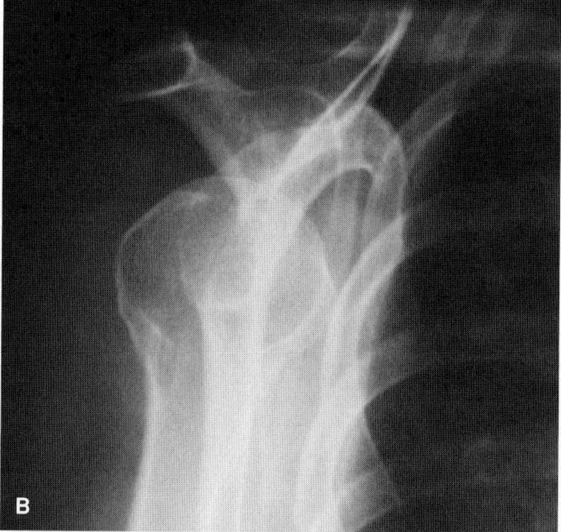

FIGURE 43.44. **Pseudodislocation of the Shoulder. A.** An anteroposterior view of the shoulder in this patient who had trauma to the shoulder shows the humeral head to be inferiorly placed in relation to the glenoid with absence of the normal crescent sign. A dislocation was suspected. **B.** The transscapular lateral film, however, reveals that the humeral head is normally placed over the glenoid. This is a pseudodislocation owing to a hemarthrosis. A search for an occult fracture should be made. In this case, a fracture can be seen in **(A)** (*arrow*), which caused bleeding into the joint.

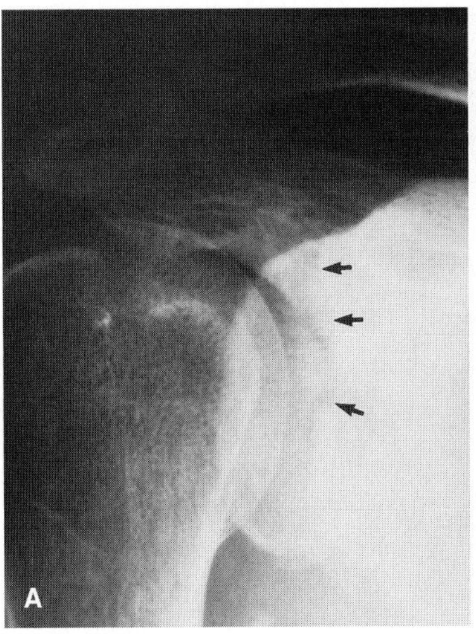

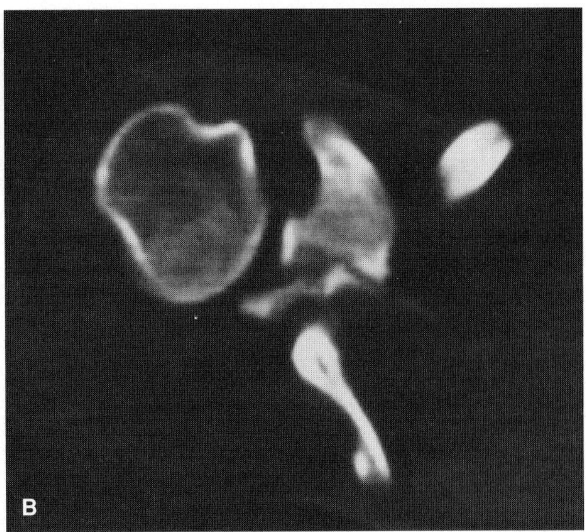

FIGURE 43.45. **Fracture of the Glenoid. A.** An anteroposterior view of the shoulder demonstrates a faint lucency, indicative of a fracture of the glenoid (*arrows*), with a fragment of bone seen inferior to the joint. **B.** The full extent of the fracture cannot be appreciated until the CT is examined. On the CT scan, the fracture can be seen to extend fully through the scapula and is seen to be slightly displaced in the articular portion.

Because of frequently overlapping ribs and clavicles, the exact anatomy is often difficult to discern on the transscapular view. To find the glenoid, one has to find the coracoid, the spine of the acromion, and the blade of the scapula. These three structures all lead to the glenoid and form a "Y" around it. All that is necessary to find the center of the glenoid is to find two of those bony landmarks, usually the coracoid and the blade of the scapula. The humeral head can then be found and its position determined.

An entity that can be mistaken for a dislocated shoulder is a traumatic hemarthrosis, which displaces the humeral head inferolaterally on the AP film (Fig. 43.44). Because the anterior dislocation displaces inferomedially, it should not be confused with this. The posterior dislocation will easily be excluded by looking at a transscapular view. This has been termed a pseudodislocation. It should be recognized so that attempts to "reduce" the "dislocation" are not made. Also, it can suggest a subtle or occult humeral head fracture.

If a fracture is suspected about the shoulder and the plain films are negative or equivocal, a CT scan should be performed. A complex joint such as the shoulder or hip is best examined with CT scanning when the full extent of the fracture needs to be identified (Fig. 43.45).

PELVIS

Fractures of the pelvis, especially those involving the acetabulum, can be difficult to evaluate completely with plain films alone. CT scanning should be considered in almost all acetabular fractures because of the possibility of free fragments and subtle fractures that do not show on plain films (Fig. 43.46).

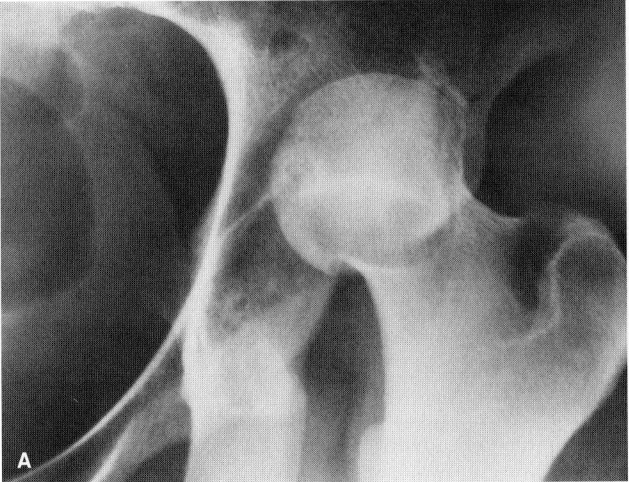

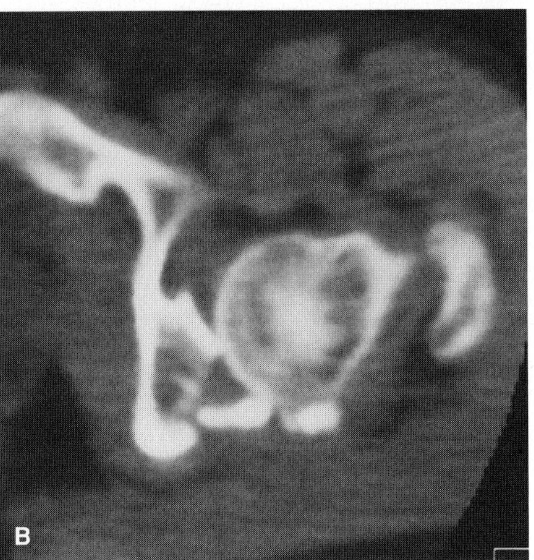

FIGURE 43.46. **Dislocation of the Hip. A.** An anteroposterior plain film of the left hip shows dislocation of the femoral head, which lies slightly superior to the acetabulum. **B.** Fractures are easily identified on CT. A cortical break through the articular surface of the posterior acetabulum, as well as the dislocation, is identified.

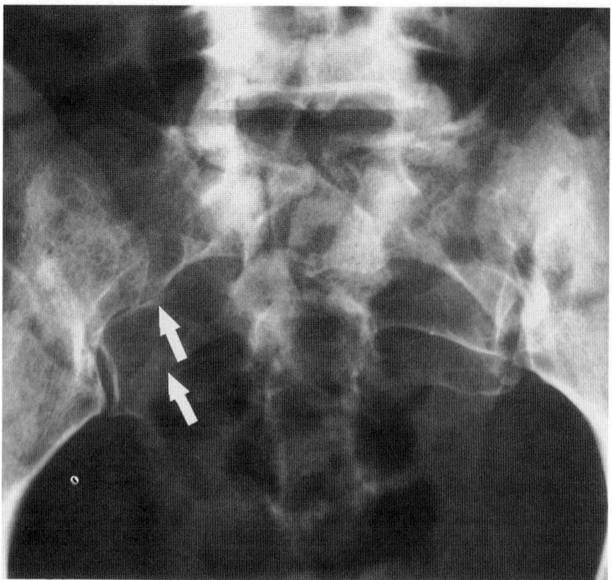

FIGURE 43.47. **Fracture of the Sacrum.** An anteroposterior view of the sacrum in this patient shows normal arcuate lines on the left side of the sacrum that are interrupted on the right side (*arrows*). Interruption of these lines indicates a fracture through this portion of the sacrum.

Sacral fractures are said to occur in half of the cases of pelvic fractures. They can be difficult to see on even the best of films because the sacrum is often hidden by bowel gas. In looking for sacral fractures, one should examine the arcuate lines of the sacrum bilaterally to see whether they are intact. Fractures often interrupt these lines and, because of the side-to-side asymmetry, can therefore be easily identified (Fig. 43.47).

Sacral stress fractures in patients who are osteoporotic or who have undergone radiation therapy can present as patchy or linear sclerosis on the sacral alae that may or may not show cortical disruption on plain films (Fig. 43.48A). These should be differentiated from metastatic disease because of their characteristic location, appearance, and history of prior radiation and by visualization of a cortical break. CT will usually, but not always, demonstrate cortical disruption (Fig. 43.48B). These fractures have a characteristic appearance on radionuclide bone scans (Fig. 43.49A), which is termed the "Honda sign" because of its appearance to the logo of the car. The Honda sign is seen only with bilateral stress fractures; unilateral fractures will have increased radionuclide uptake throughout one sacral ala. MR will demonstrate an area of diffuse low signal on T1WIs corresponding to the area of involvement (Fig. 43.49B). Sacral stress fractures have also been termed *insufficiency fractures,* indicating that the underlying bone is abnormal, similar to a pathologic fracture.

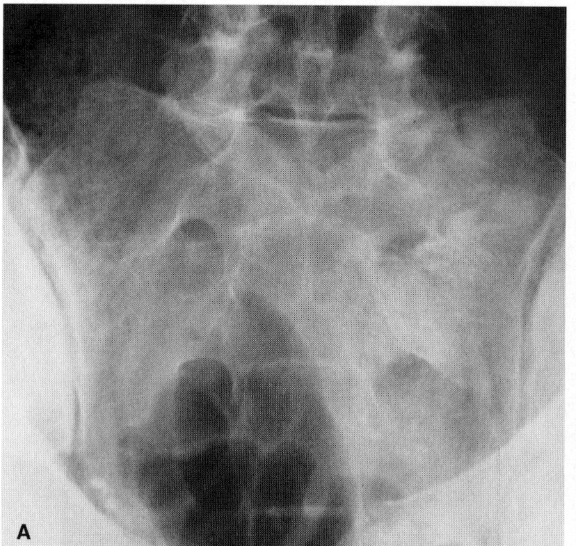

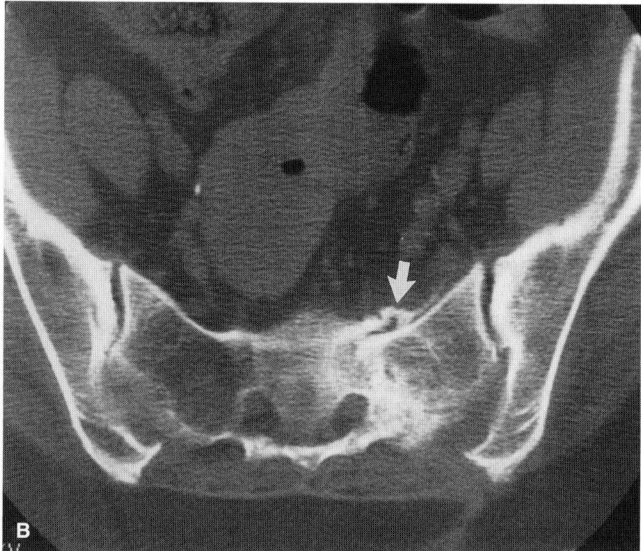

FIGURE 43.48. **Sacral Stress Fracture. A.** Faint sclerosis is noted in the left part of the sacrum as compared with the right in this patient complaining of pelvic pain. A radionuclide bone scan showed increased isotope uptake on the left half of the sacrum, and metastatic disease was postulated. **B.** A CT scan through this region demonstrates a cortical disruption (*arrow*), indicative of a fracture. These are characteristic plain film and CT appearances of a stress fracture of the sacrum.

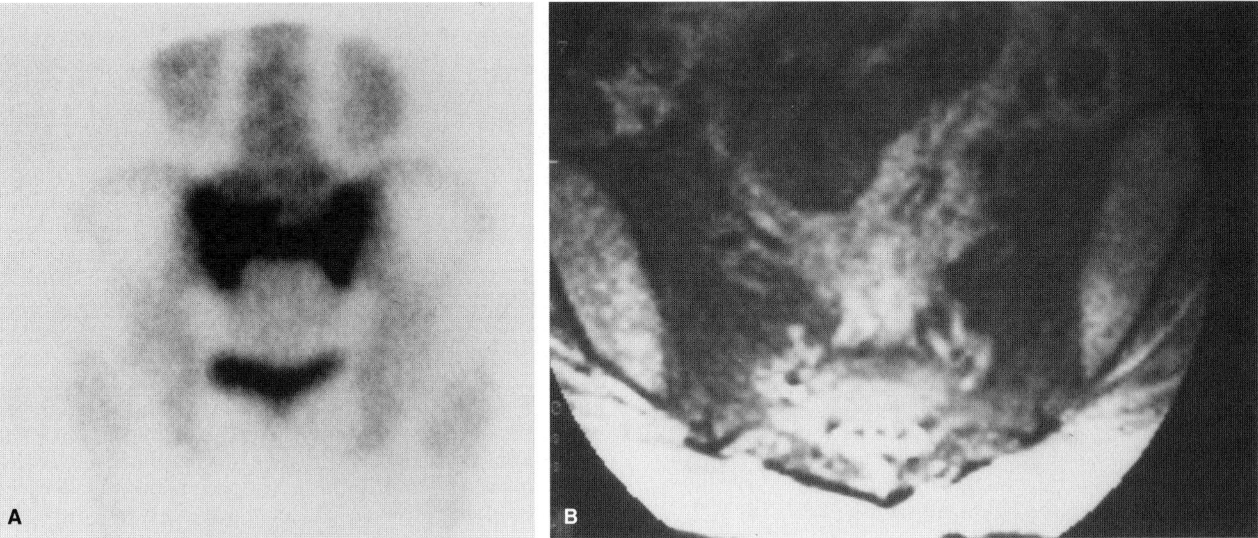

FIGURE 43.49. **Sacral Stress Fracture. A.** A radionuclide bone scan in an osteoporotic patient with pelvic pain shows a classic "Honda sign" seen with bilateral sacral stress fractures. **B.** A T1W coronal MR in this patient shows diffuse low signal throughout the sacrum adjacent to the sacroiliac joints bilaterally. This represents edema and hemorrhage in the fractures and corresponds to the bone scan Honda sign.

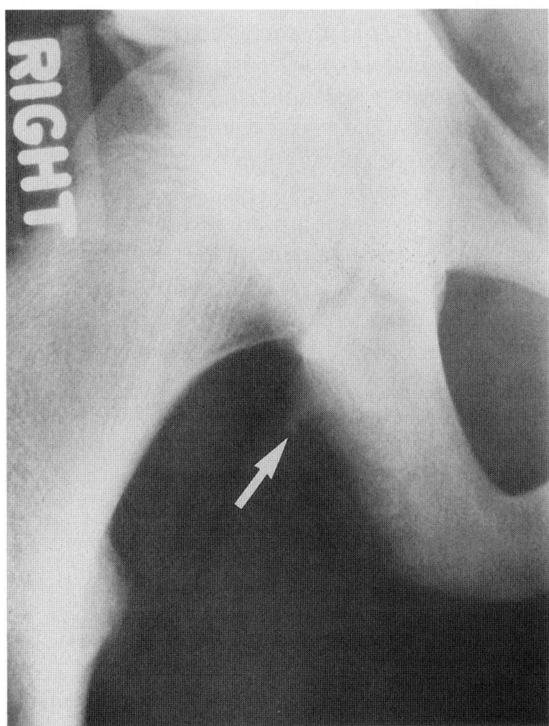

FIGURE 43.50. **Avulsion Off the Ischium.** An anteroposterior view of the pelvis shows an area of cortical disruption and periostitis at the right ischium (*arrow*) in a patient complaining of pain at this site. These findings are characteristic for an ischial avulsion and should not undergo biopsy.

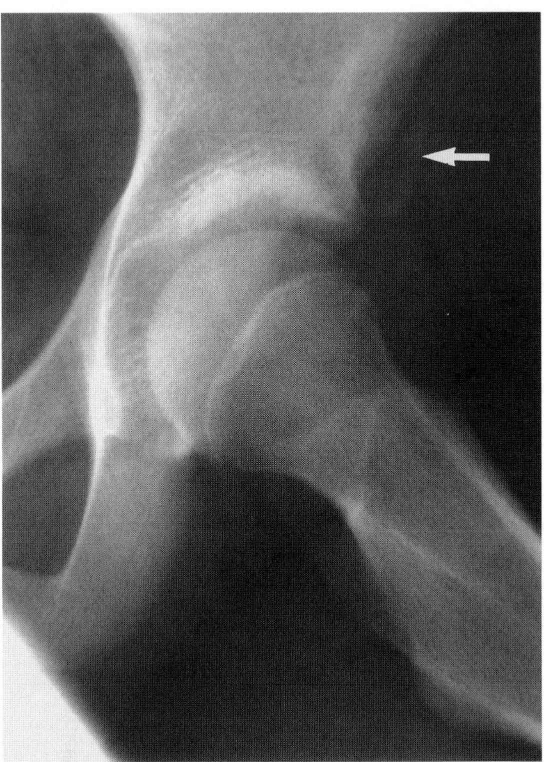

FIGURE 43.51. **Rectus Femoris Avulsion.** An anteroposterior plain film of the left hip shows a faint calcific density superior to the acetabulum (*arrow*), which is characteristic for an avulsion of the rectus femoris muscle from the anterior inferior iliac spine.

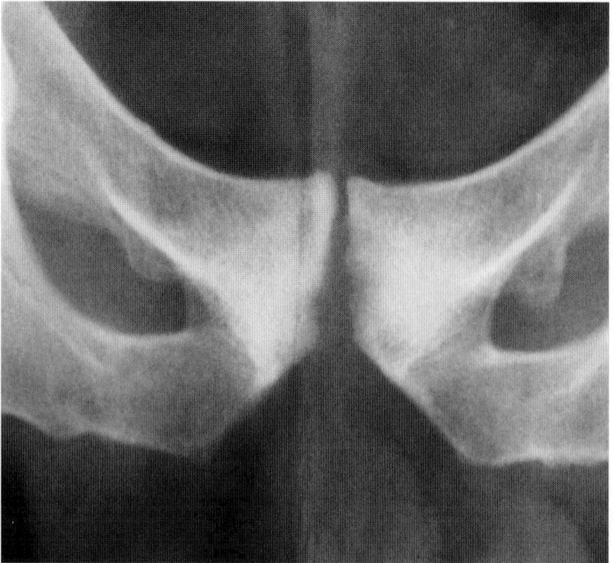

FIGURE 43.52. **Osteoarthritis of the Symphysis Pubis.** Sclerosis with erosion is noted at the symphysis in this ultramarathoner complaining of severe pubic pain. This is characteristic of degenerative joint disease (DJD) or osteoarthritis at this site in such an overuse setting. Erosions are ordinarily not seen in DJD, except in certain joints such as the symphysis pubis, sacroiliac, and the acromioclavicular.

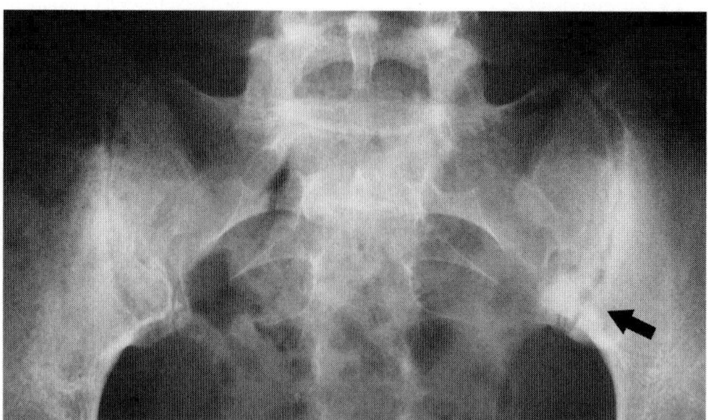

FIGURE 43.53. **Osteoarthritis of the Sacroiliac Joint.** Sclerosis and erosions (*arrow*) are seen in the left sacroiliac joint in this young professional dancer. Although this has the appearance of an inflammatory arthritis, this is also seen in degenerative joint disease or osteoarthritis secondary to overuse.

Avulsion injuries affect the pelvis quite often and should be easily recognized by radiologists. On occasion, an avulsion injury can have an aggressive appearance and, if not diagnosed radiographically, a biopsy might be performed. This can be calamitous, as avulsion injuries have been known to mimic malignant lesions histologically, with a misdiagnosis leading to radical treatment (Fig. 43.50). Therefore, when an avulsion injury is a consideration, it becomes a "do not touch" lesion (see Chapter 46). Common sites for pelvic avulsions include the ischium, the superior and inferior anterior iliac spines (Fig. 43.51), and the iliac crest. These injuries are said to be fairly common in long jumpers, sprinters, hurdlers, gymnasts, and cheerleaders.

Another area in the pelvis that can demonstrate radiologic findings as a result of stress is the symphysis pubis. In ultramarathoners, cross-country skiers, soccer players, and other athletes, the symphysis can be affected by degenerative joint disease (DJD) or osteoarthritis (Fig. 43.52). The hallmarks of DJD are sclerosis, joint space narrowing, and osteophytosis (see Chapter 44). In certain joints, however, erosions can occur as a result of DJD. These joints include the temporomandibular joint, the acromioclavicular joint, the symphysis pubis, and the sacroiliac joint.

When the sacroiliac joints are involved with DJD, this can closely resemble a human leukocyte antigen–B27 spondyloarthropathy (Fig. 43.53) and lead to erroneous diagnosis and treatment. Large osteophytes can develop across the sacroiliac joints and mimic sclerosis or even a tumor (Fig. 43.54).

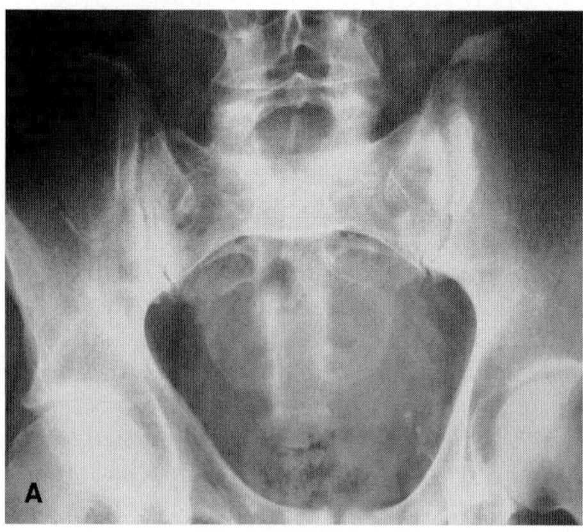

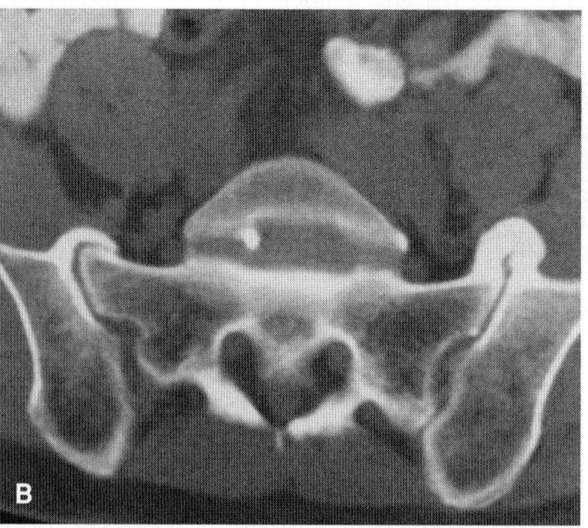

FIGURE 43.54. **Sacroiliac Osteophytes. A.** An anteroposterior view of the pelvis in this marathoner shows dense sclerosis over both sacroiliac joints. **B.** A CT through this area demonstrates dense, bridging osteophytes, characteristic of degenerative joint disease.

LEG

Overt fractures in the femur and lower leg are, for the most part, straightforward and deserve no special radiologic treatment for fear of missing subtle abnormalities.

Stress fractures, however, need to be considered in anyone with hip or leg pain, because overlooking the diagnosis can lead to a complete fracture. The most serious stress fracture, and fortunately, one of the rarest, is the femoral neck stress fracture (Fig. 43.55). Many of these progress to complete fractures (Fig. 43.56) that, with continued weight bearing, can displace; these are very serious lesions.

Stress fractures also occur in the distal diaphysis of the femur and in the proximal, middle, and distal thirds of the tibia. All of these stress fractures need to be treated with the utmost caution, because complete fractures are not uncommon with continued stress (Fig. 43.57). Sclerosis in a weight-bearing bone that has a horizontal or oblique linear pattern should be considered a stress fracture until proved otherwise. A history of repetitive stress is not always associated, so the diagnosis should not depend solely on the history.

A stress fracture occasionally will appear somewhat aggressive, with aggressive periostitis and no definite linearity to the sclerosis (Fig. 43.58A). If this is mistaken for a tumor and undergoes biopsy, it can be confused with a malignancy, with subsequent radical therapy. Therefore, these should not undergo biopsy under any circumstance. If the clinical presentation is unusual for a stress fracture and the plain films are not diagnostic, additional films should be obtained 1 or 2 weeks later. CT and MR sometimes will better delineate the lesion (Fig. 43.58B). Stress fractures can be difficult to diagnose radiologically early on but should be straightforward after several weeks.

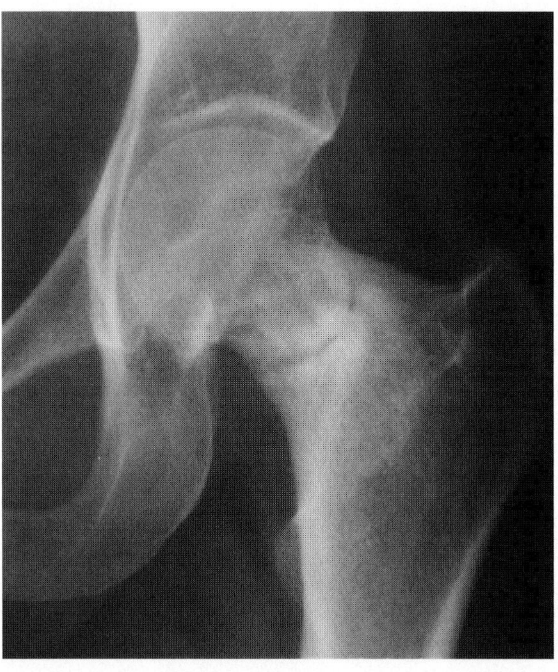

FIGURE 43.56. **Stress Fracture of the Femoral Neck.** A linear lucency with surrounding sclerosis is seen in the femoral neck in this jogger with hip pain. This is a severe femoral neck stress fracture.

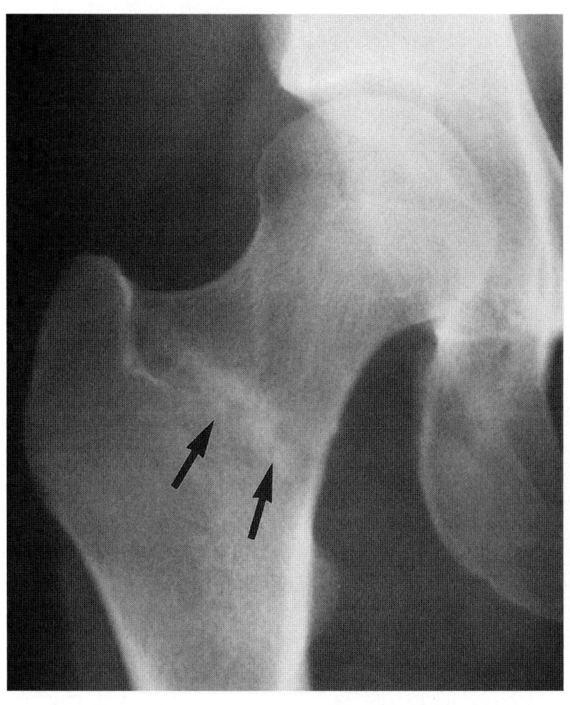

FIGURE 43.55. **Femoral Stress Fracture.** An area of linear sclerosis (*arrows*) is seen at the base of the femoral neck in a runner with hip pain. This is diagnostic of a stress fracture of the femur.

One final stress fracture that deserves mention because it is frequently misdiagnosed clinically and overlooked radiographically is the calcaneal stress fracture (Fig. 43.59). It is often clinically misdiagnosed as a "heel spur" or plantar fasciitis and can be a somewhat subtle radiographic finding.

Hip Fracture. Overt fractures in the lower extremity are uncommonly missed on radiographs; however, a few exceptions should be noted. Hip fractures in the elderly population can be very difficult to detect (Fig. 43.60), and a high index of suspicion should be maintained. A negative plain film in an elderly patient with hip pain after trauma (even relatively mild trauma) does not exclude a femoral neck fracture. MR has been shown to be very useful in demonstrating femoral neck fractures that are occult (Fig. 43.61).

Tibial Plateau Fracture. Another fracture that can be difficult to exclude on routine plain films is a tibial plateau

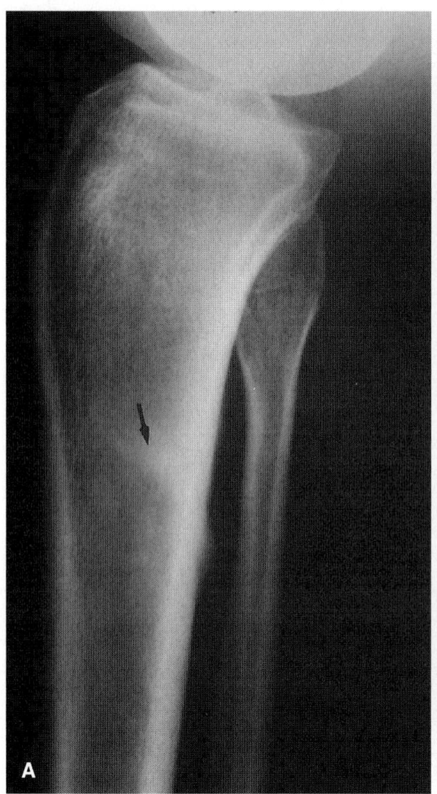

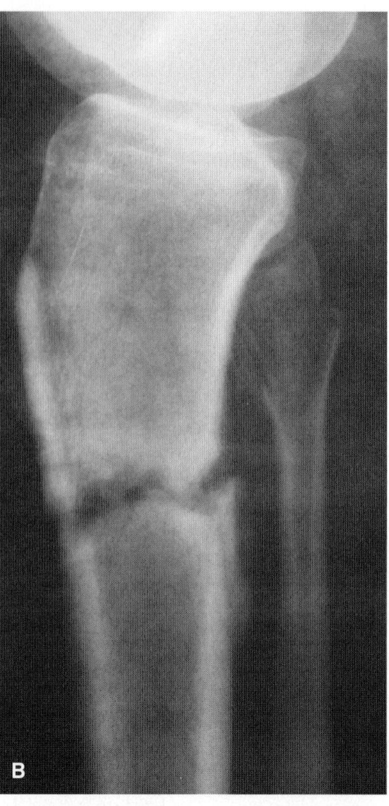

FIGURE 43.57. **Stress Fracture of the Proximal Tibia. A.** A faint linear sclerotic area (*arrow*) is seen, which is characteristic for a stress fracture of the proximal tibia. **B.** This view shows the result of continued exercise in this patient: a complete fracture of the tibia and of the proximal fibula.

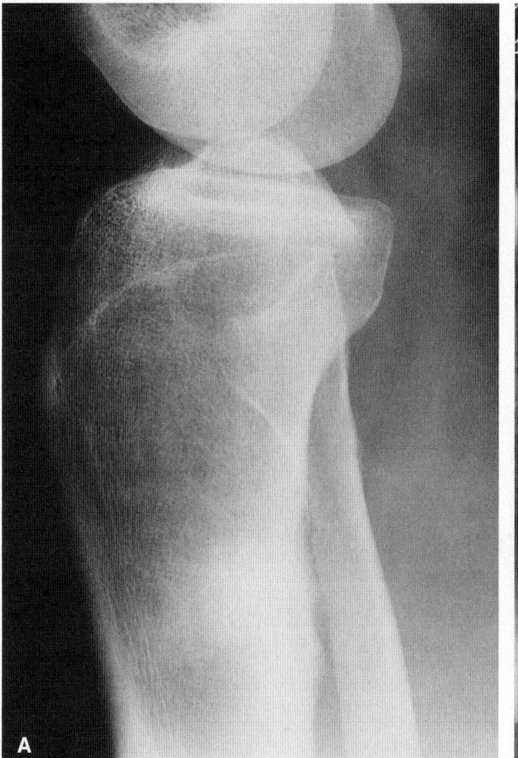

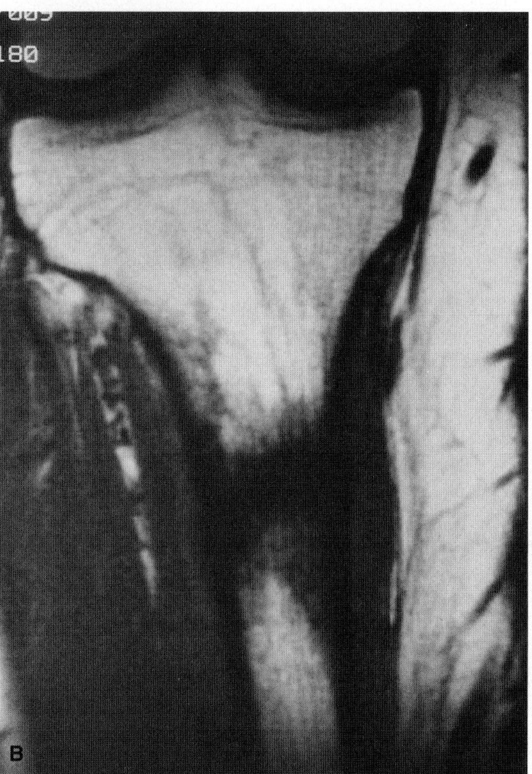

FIGURE 43.58. **Stress Fracture of the Tibia. A.** An irregular focus of sclerosis is seen in the posterior proximal tibia with adjacent periostitis. There was concern that this might represent a primary bone tumor, and the surgeons recommended a biopsy. **B.** An MR scan was performed, however, which shows a linear low signal area running obliquely across the tibia on this T1W coronal image, which is characteristic for a stress fracture. No significant soft tissue mass was found. The patient's recent history included an increase in his jogging. A stress fracture was diagnosed on the basis of these images.

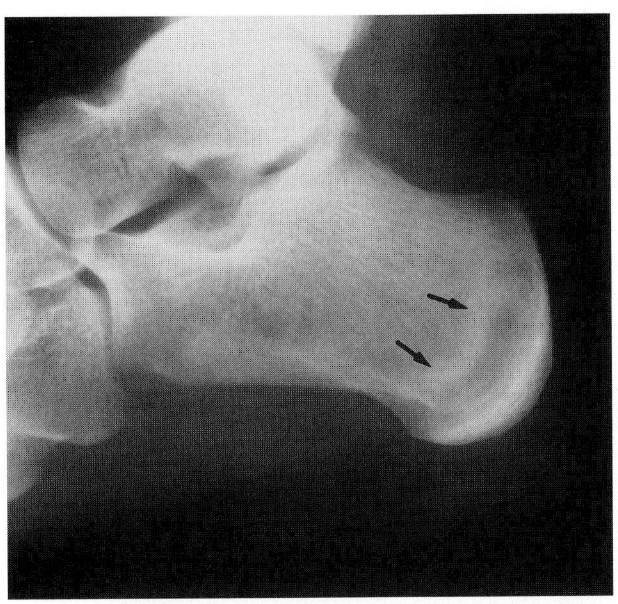

FIGURE 43.59. **Calcaneal Stress Fracture.** A linear band of sclerosis is seen in the posterior calcaneus (*arrows*), which is diagnostic for a stress fracture of the calcaneus.

fracture. A cross-table lateral plain film should be obtained in cases of knee trauma to look for a fat–fluid level (Fig. 43.62); this indicates a fracture that allows fatty marrow to leak into the knee joint. In the appropriate clinical setting, MR or CT may be necessary to make the diagnosis.

Lisfranc Fracture. A serious fracture in the foot that can be missed radiographically when little or no displacement occurs is the so-called Lisfranc fracture (Fig. 43.63). It is named after a surgeon in Napoleon's army who would perform forefoot amputations in patients with gangrenous toes caused by frostbite. The Lisfranc fracture is a fracture-dislocation of the tarsometatarsals. If the dislocation is slight, it can be easily overlooked. A key to normal alignment is that the medial border of the second metatarsal should always line up with the medial border of the second cuneiform. If it does not, a Lisfranc fracture-dislocation should be suspected. This fracture is seen most commonly in patients who catch the forefoot in something such as a hole in the ground, or a horseback rider who falls and hangs by the forefoot in the stirrups. It is commonly seen as a neurotrophic or Charcot joint in diabetics.

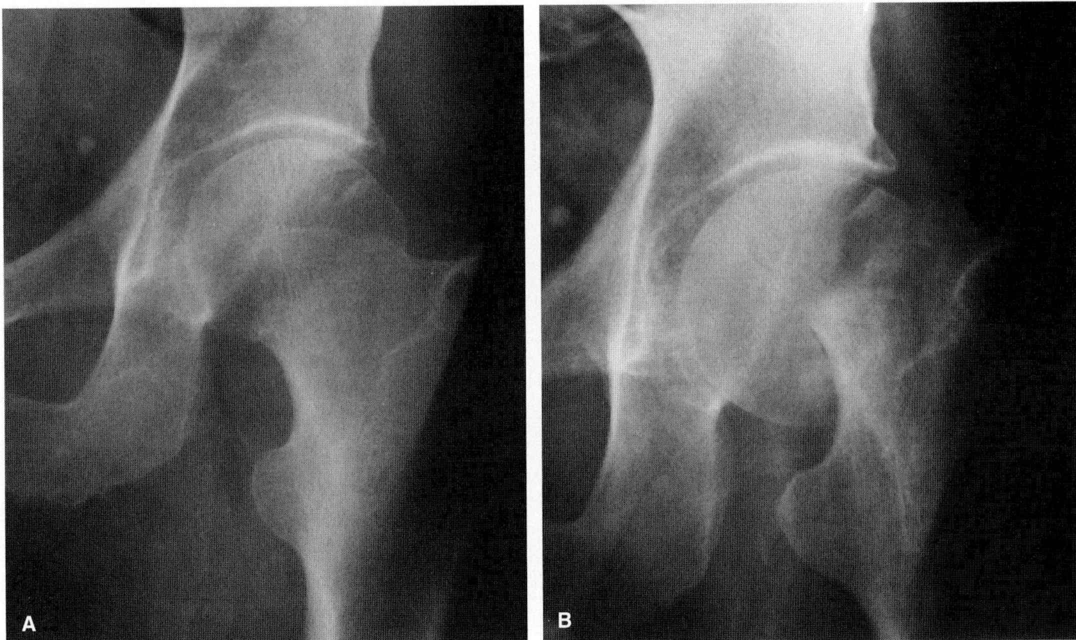

FIGURE 43.60. **Fracture of the Hip. A.** An anteroposterior view of the hip of an elderly man was obtained following a fall. It was interpreted as normal, and the patient was dismissed from the emergency department. Two weeks later, the patient returned to the emergency department unable to walk, and another radiograph **(B)** was obtained. It shows a complete fracture through the femoral neck. In retrospect, the fracture can be faintly seen in **(A)** and should have been picked up initially. Fractures of the hip in the elderly can be very difficult to see and should be diligently searched for with additional views when the clinical setting is appropriate.

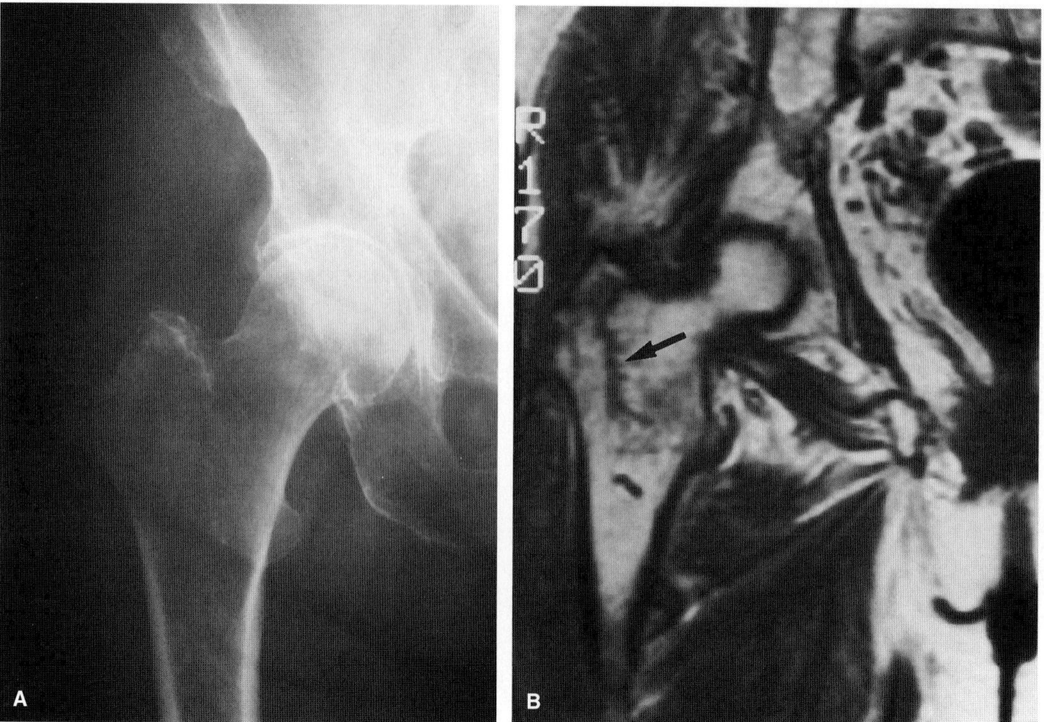

FIGURE 43.61. **Occult Fracture of the Hip. A.** An anteroposterior plain film in an elderly patient with hip pain after a fall appears normal. **B.** A coronal T1WI was obtained because of the clinical suspicion of a fracture and shows linear low signal in the intertrochanteric region (*arrow*), confirming the fracture.

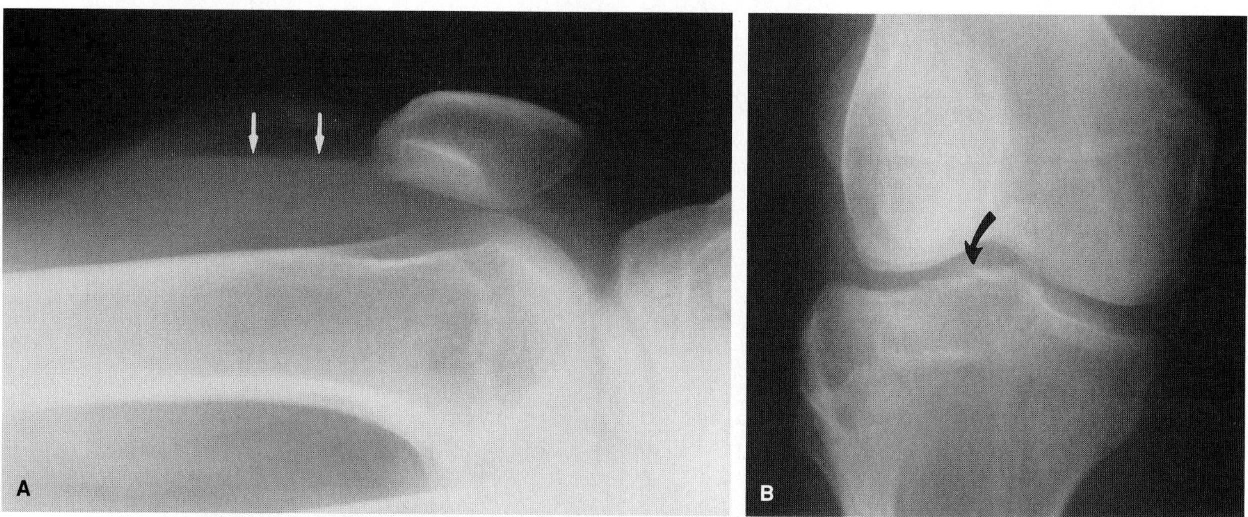

FIGURE 43.62. **Tibial Plateau Fracture. A.** A cross-table lateral plain film of the knee reveals a fat–fluid level (*arrows*), which indicates a fracture with fatty marrow leaking into the joint. **B.** An anteroposterior view shows a barely discernible fracture (*arrow*) near the tibial spines, indicative of a tibial plateau fracture.

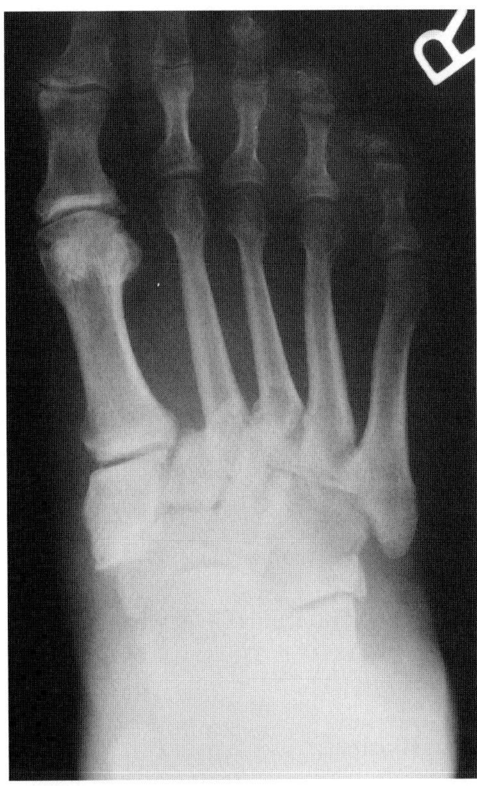

FIGURE 43.63. **Lisfranc Fracture.** An anteroposterior view of the foot in this patient shows a space between the first and second metatarsals with the base of the second metatarsal displaced off the second cuneiform. This is indicative of a Lisfranc fracture dislocation.

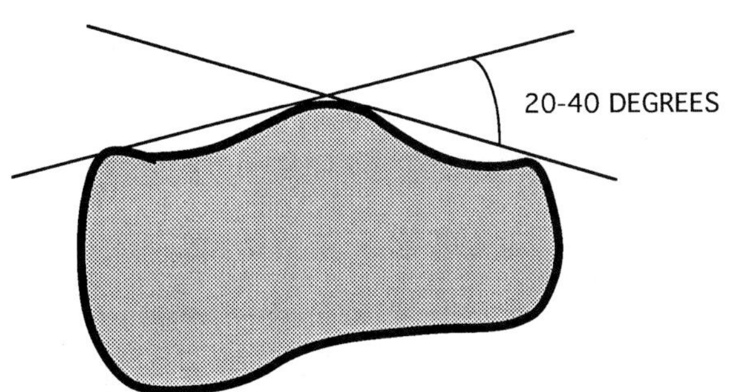

FIGURE 43.64. **Böhler Angle in a Normal Calcaneus.** This drawing depicts the normal calcaneus with a line across the anterior process extending to the apex of the calcaneus intersecting with a line from the posterior portion of the calcaneus to the apex. This is termed the Böhler angle, and when it becomes flattened or smaller than 20°, a calcaneal fracture should be diagnosed.

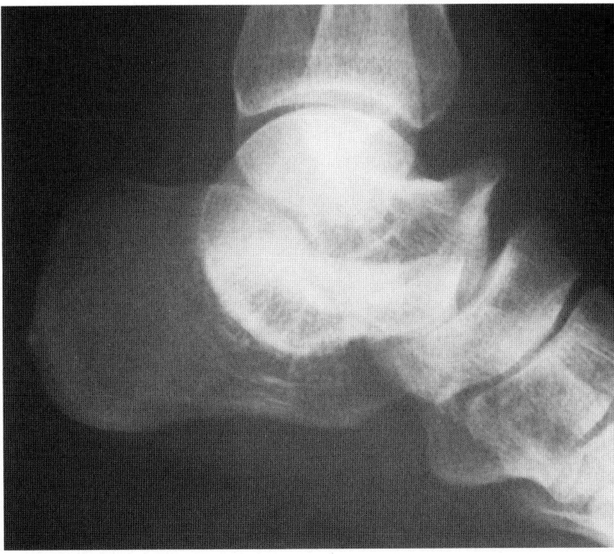

FIGURE 43.65. **Calcaneal Fracture.** The Böhler angle in this calcaneus is smaller than 20°, which is indicative of a fracture of the calcaneus.

Fracture of the calcaneus can be difficult to appreciate on routine radiographs. The Böhler angle is a normal anatomic landmark that should be looked for in every foot film when trauma has occurred (Fig. 43.64). An angle narrower than 20° indicates a compression of the calcaneus, as seen in jumping injuries (Fig. 43.65).

This is a fairly simplified overview of some commonly overlooked fractures and dislocations and should not be interpreted as a substitute for the more complete texts listed in the references (3–5).

REFERENCES

1. Mirvis S, Diaconis J, Chirico P, Reiner B, Joslyn J, Militello P. Protocol-driven radiologic evaluation of suspected cervical spine injury: efficacy study. Radiology 1989;170:831–834.
2. Dorsay TA, Major NM, Helms CA. Cost-effectiveness of immediate MR imaging versus traditional follow-up for revealing radiographically occult scaphoid fractures." AJR Am J Roentgenol 2001;177(6): 1257–1263.
3. Rogers LF. Radiology of Skeletal Trauma. 3rd ed. New York: Churchill Livingstone, 2002.
4. Rockwood CA Jr, Green DP. Fractures in Adults. 5th ed. Philadelphia: Lippincott Williams & Wilkins, 2001.
5. Harris JH Jr, Harris WH. The Radiology of Emergency Medicine. 4th ed. Baltimore: Lippincott Williams & Wilkins, 2000.

Chapter 44

Arthritis

Clyde A. Helms

Osteoarthritis

Rheumatoid Arthritis

HLA-B27 Spondyloarthropathies

Crystal-Induced Arthritis

Collagen-Vascular Diseases

Sarcoid

Hemochromatosis

Neuropathic or Charcot Joint

Hemophilia, Juvenile Rheumatoid Arthritis, and Paralysis

Synovial Osteochondromatosis

Pigmented Villonodular Synovitis

Sudeck Atrophy

Joint Effusions

Avascular Necrosis

OSTEOARTHRITIS

Osteoarthritis, or degenerative joint disease (DJD), is the most common arthritide. It is believed to be caused by trauma—either overt or as an accumulation of microtrauma over years, although there is also a hereditary form called primary osteoarthritis that occurs primarily in middle-aged women. The hallmarks of DJD are *joint space narrowing, sclerosis,* and *osteophytosis* (Table 44.1 and Fig. 44.1). If all three of these findings are not present on a radiograph, another diagnosis should be considered. Joint space narrowing is the least specific finding of the three, yet it is virtually always present in DJD. Unfortunately, it is also seen in almost every other joint abnormality.

Sclerosis should be present in varying amounts in all cases of DJD unless severe osteoporosis is present. Osteoporosis will cause the sclerosis to be diminished. For instance, in long-standing rheumatoid arthritis in which the cartilage has been destroyed, DJD often occurs with very little sclerosis. Osteophytosis will also be diminished in the setting of osteoporosis. Otherwise, sclerosis and osteophytosis should be prominent in DJD.

The only disorder that will cause osteophytes without sclerosis or joint space narrowing is diffuse idiopathic skeletal hyperostosis (1). This is a common bone-forming disorder that at first glance resembles DJD, except that there is no joint space narrowing (or disk space narrowing in the spine) and there is no sclerosis (Fig. 44.2). Diffuse idiopathic skeletal hyperostosis (DISH) is not believed to be caused by trauma or stress, as is DJD, and is not painful or disabling, as DJD can be. Millions of dollars per year are awarded to federal employees upon retirement, representing disability payments for supposed DJD acquired during their employment, when in fact, these retirees have diffuse idiopathic skeletal hyperostosis and have been misdiagnosed. Osteoarthritis is divided into two types: primary and secondary. Secondary osteoarthritis is what radiologists refer to when speaking of DJD. It is, as mentioned, secondary to trauma of some sort. It can occur in any joint

TABLE 44.1 Hallmarks of Degenerative Joint Disease

Joint space narrowing
Sclerosis
Osteophytes

in the body but is particularly common in the hands, knees, hips, and spine.

Primary osteoarthritis is a familial arthritis that affects middle-aged women almost exclusively and is seen only in the hands. It affects the distal interphalangeal joints, the proximal interphalangeal joints, and the base of the thumb in a bilaterally symmetric fashion (Fig. 44.3). If it is not bilaterally symmetric, the diagnosis of primary osteoarthritis should be questioned.

A type of primary osteoarthritis that can be very painful and debilitating is ***erosive osteoarthritis.*** It has the identical distribution mentioned for primary osteoarthritis but

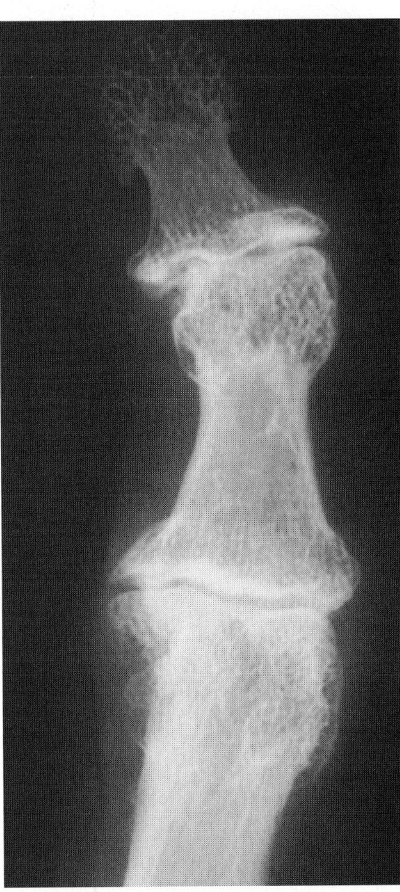

FIGURE 44.1. **Osteoarthritis (DJD).** Plain film of a finger with osteoarthritis (DJD) of the distal and proximal interphalangeal joints. Both joints demonstrate joint space narrowing, subchondral sclerosis, and osteophytosis, which are hallmarks of DJD.

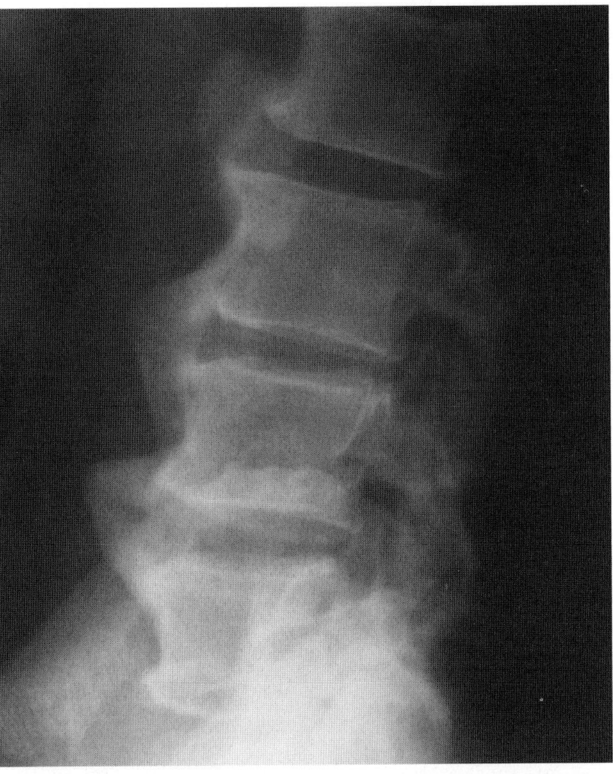

FIGURE 44.2. **Diffuse Idiopathic Skeletal Hyperostosis (DISH).** A lateral view of the lumbar spine shows extensive osteophytosis without significant disk space narrowing or sclerosis. This is a classic picture for diffuse idiopathic skeletal hyperostosis.

is associated with severe osteoporosis of the hands, as well as erosions. It is uncommon, and radiologists generally see little of this disorder. It is also called Kellgren arthritis.

There are a few exceptions to the classic triad of findings seen in DJD (sclerosis, joint space narrowing, and osteophytes). Several joints also exhibit erosions as a manifestation of DJD: the *temporomandibular joint,* the *acromioclavicular joint,* the *sacroiliac joints,* and the *symphysis pubis* (Table 44.2). When erosions are seen in one of these joints, DJD must be considered, or inappropriate treatment may be instituted (Fig. 44.4).

A subchondral cyst, or *geode* (taken from the geologic term used when a volcanic rock has a gas pocket that leaves a large cavity in the rock), is often found in joints

TABLE 44.2 Joints That Have Erosions as a Feature of Degenerative Joint Disease

Sacroiliac
Acromioclavicular
Temporomandibular
Symphysis pubis

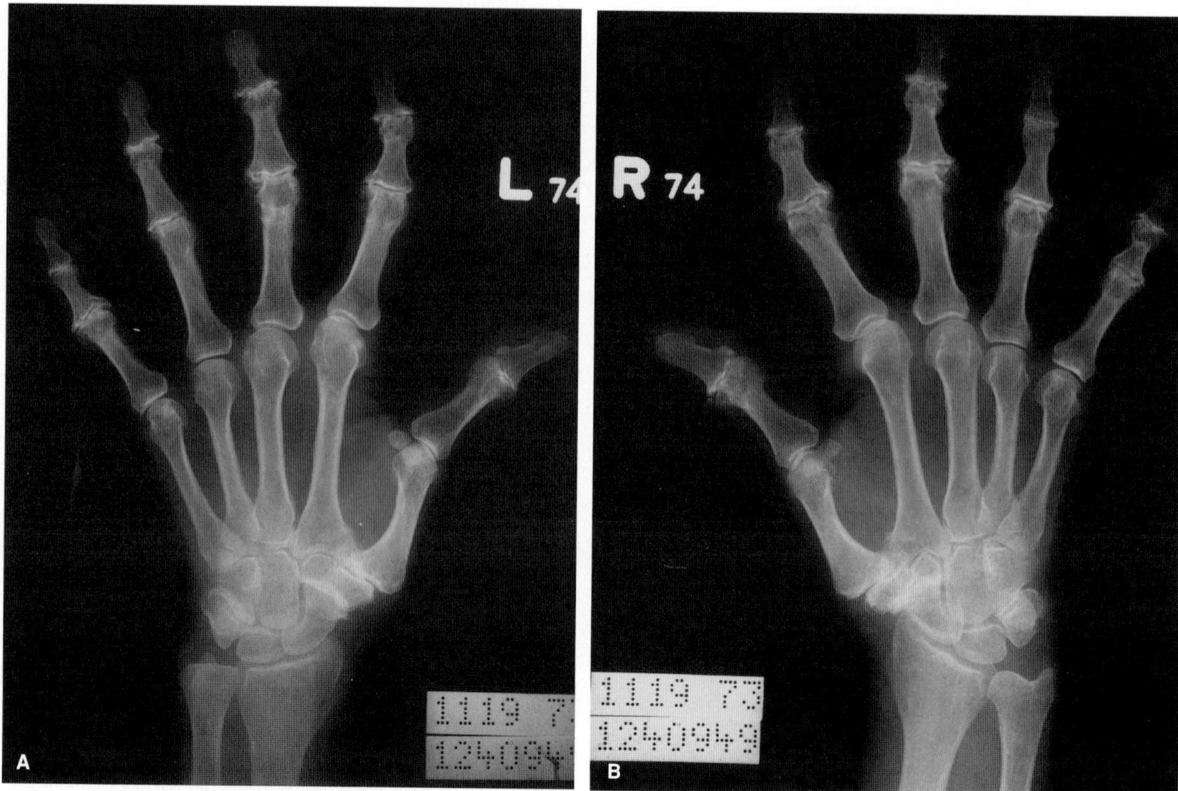

FIGURE 44.3. **Primary Osteoarthritis.** Bilateral hand films in a patient with primary osteoarthritis. Present are classic findings of osteophytosis, joint space narrowing, and sclerosis at the distal interphalangeal joints, the proximal interphalangeal joints, and at the base of the thumb. This is bilaterally symmetric, which is typical for primary osteoarthritis.

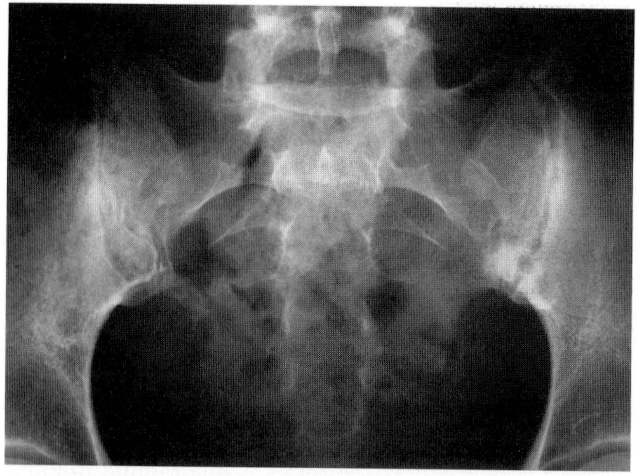

FIGURE 44.4. **Osteoarthritis of the Sacroiliac (SI) Joint.** A young woman who is a professional dancer complained of left-sided hip pain. An anteroposterior film of the pelvis demonstrated left SI joint sclerosis, joint irregularity, and erosions. A complete workup to rule out a human leukocyte antigen (HLA) –B27 spondyloarthropathy was negative, and no laboratory or clinical evidence for infection was found. Her clinical history pointed to this being completely occupation-related, and an aspiration biopsy to rule out infection was therefore not performed. This is not an unusual appearance for degenerative joint disease of the SI joint.

affected with DJD. Geodes are cystic formations that occur around joints in a variety of disorders (including, in addition to DJD, *rheumatoid arthritis, calcium pyrophosphate dihydrate crystal deposition disease* (CPPD) and *avascular necrosis*) (Table 44.3) (2). Presumably, one method of geode formation takes place when synovial fluid is forced into the subchondral bone, causing a cystic collection of joint fluid. Another etiology is following a bone contusion, in which the contused bone forms a cyst. They rarely cause problems by themselves but are often misdiagnosed as something more sinister (Fig. 44.5).

RHEUMATOID ARTHRITIS

Rheumatoid arthritis is a connective tissue disorder of unknown etiology that can affect any synovial joint in the body. The radiographic hallmarks are *soft tissue swelling,*

TABLE 44.3 Diseases in Which Geodes Are Found

Degenerative joint disease
Rheumatoid arthritis
Calcium pyrophosphate dihydrate deposition disease (CPPD)
Avascular necrosis

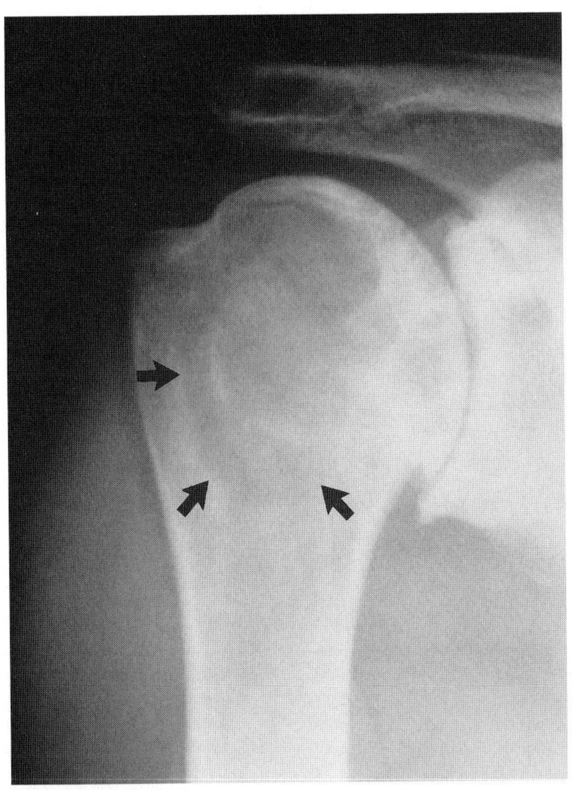

FIGURE 44.5. **Subchondral Cyst or Geode of the Shoulder.** This patient has marked degenerative joint disease (DJD) of the shoulder, with joint space narrowing, sclerosis, and osteophytosis. A large lytic process (*arrows*) is seen in the humeral head, which is a subchondral cyst or geode often seen in association with DJD. Because of the DJD in the shoulder, a biopsy to rule out a more sinister lesion in the humeral head should be avoided.

osteoporosis, joint space narrowing, and *marginal erosions.* In the hands, it is classically a *proximal* process that is *bilaterally symmetric* (Table 44.4 and Fig. 44.6). There are so many exceptions to these rules, however, that I have come to regard them as no better than 80% accurate. Rheumatoid arthritis has a large variety of appearances, and from its radiographic appearance alone, it can be very difficult to diagnose with any degree of assurance.

Rheumatoid arthritis in large joints is fairly characteristic in that it causes marked joint space narrowing and is associated with osteoporosis. Erosions might or might not

TABLE 44.4 Hallmarks of Rheumatoid Arthritis

Soft tissue swelling
Osteoporosis
Joint space narrowing
Marginal erosions
Proximal distribution (hands)
Bilateral symmetry

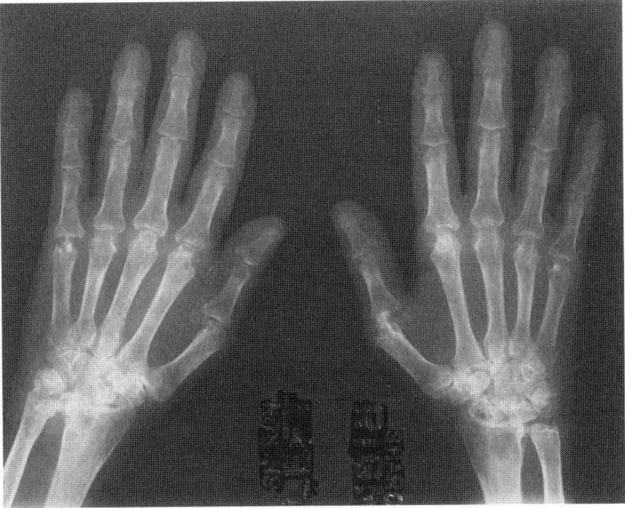

FIGURE 44.6. **Rheumatoid Arthritis.** An erosive arthritis affecting primarily the carpal bones and the metacarpophalangeal joints is seen that has associated osteoporosis and soft tissue swelling (note the soft tissue over the ulnar styloid processes). It is a bilaterally symmetric process in this patient, which is classic.

be present and tend to be marginal—that is, away from the weight-bearing portion of the joint. In the hip, the femoral head tends to migrate axially, whereas in osteoarthritis, it tends to migrate superolaterally (Figs. 44.7, 44.8). In the shoulder, the humeral head tends to be "high-riding" (Fig. 44.9). Other things to think of when confronted with a high-riding shoulder are a torn rotator cuff and calcium pyrophosphate dihydrate deposition disease (CPPD) (Table 44.5).

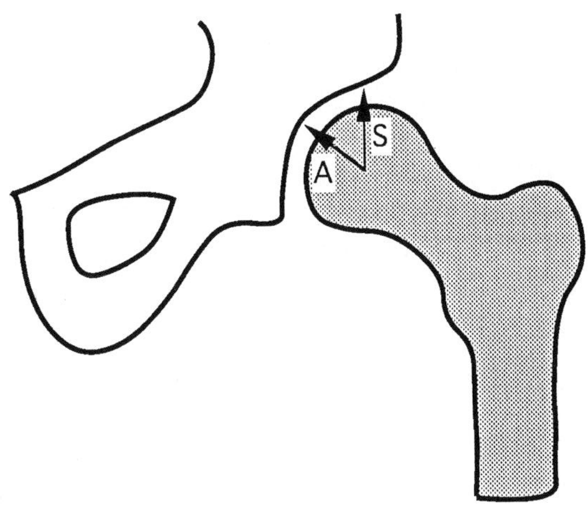

FIGURE 44.7. **Migration of the Femoral Head.** A drawing of the hip showing routes of migration of the femoral head. Osteoarthritis of the hip tends to cause superior (S) migration of the femoral head in relation to the acetabulum, whereas rheumatoid arthritis tends to cause axial (A) migration of the femoral head in relation to the acetabulum.

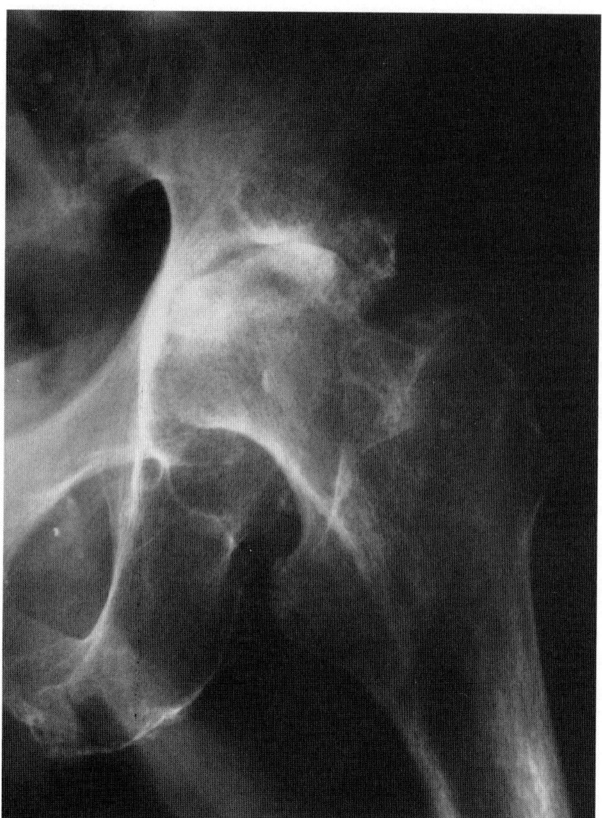

FIGURE 44.8. **Rheumatoid Arthritis of the Hip.** Note the severe joint space narrowing in this patient with rheumatoid arthritis. The femoral head has migrated in an axial direction, with fairly concentric joint space narrowing. Minimal secondary degenerative changes have occurred, as noted by the sclerosis in the superior portion of the joint; however, these have been diminished somewhat by the osteoporosis that usually accompanies rheumatoid arthritis.

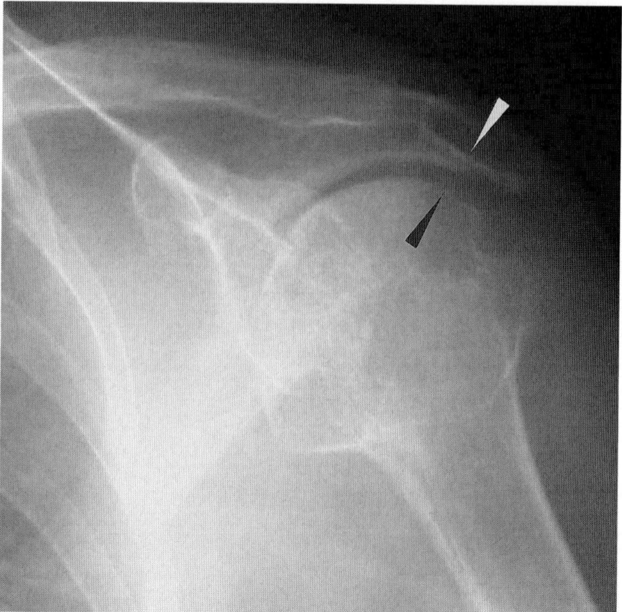

FIGURE 44.9. **Rheumatoid Arthritis in the Shoulder.** An anteroposterior view of the shoulder in this patient with rheumatoid arthritis shows that the distance between the acromion and the humeral head is diminished (*arrowheads*). Ordinarily, this space is about 1 cm in width to allow the rotator cuff to pass freely beneath the acromion. This is a common finding in rheumatoid arthritis as well as in calcium pyrophosphate dihydrate deposition disease.

When rheumatoid arthritis is long-standing, it is not unusual for secondary DJD to superimpose itself on the findings one would expect with rheumatoid arthritis. This picture of DJD differs somewhat from that usually seen, in that the sclerosis and osteophytes are considerably diminished in severity as compared with the joint space narrowing (Fig. 44.10).

HLA-B27 SPONDYLOARTHROPATHIES

A group of diseases that was formerly known as rheumatoid variants is now known as the seronegative, HLA-B27–positive spondyloarthropathies. These disorders are all linked to the human leukocyte antigen (HLA)-B27 histocompatibility antigen. Included in this group of diseases are ankylosing spondylitis, inflammatory bowel disease, psoriatic arthritis, and Reiter syndrome (also called reactive arthritis). They are characterized by bony ankylosis, proliferative formation of new bone, and predominantly axial (spinal) involvement.

One of the more characteristic findings in these disorders is that of *syndesmophytes* in the spine. A syndesmophyte is a paravertebral ossification that resembles an osteophyte, except that it runs vertically, whereas an osteophyte has its orientation in a horizontal axis. Sometimes it can be difficult to decide whether a particular paravertebral ossification is an osteophyte or a syndesmophyte based on its orientation alone (Fig. 44.11). Bridging osteophytes and large syndesmophytes can have a similar appearance, with an orientation halfway between vertical and horizontal. To evaluate those cases, one must look at the other vertebral bodies and use the ossifications on them to determine whether they are osteophytes or syndesmophytes. If no other level is involved, the two might not be distinguishable.

Syndesmophytes are classified as to whether they are marginal and symmetric or nonmarginal and asymmetric. A marginal syndesmophyte has its origin at the edge

TABLE 44.5 Causes of High-Riding Shoulder

Rheumatoid arthritis
Calcium pyrophosphate dihydrate deposition disease (CPPD)
Torn rotator cuff

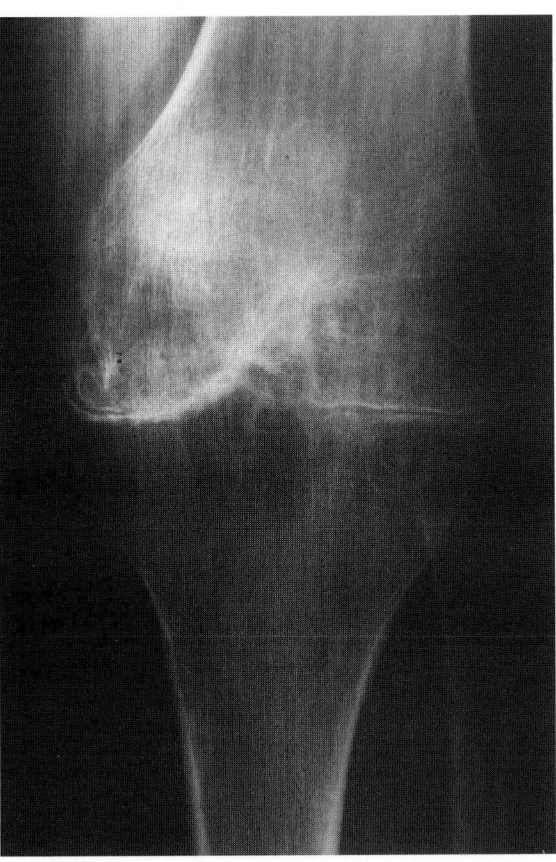

FIGURE 44.10. Secondary Degenerative Joint Disease (DJD) in the Knee in a Patient With Rheumatoid Arthritis. This patient has a history of long-standing rheumatoid arthritis. An anteroposterior view of the knee shows severe osteoporosis and joint space narrowing. Secondary DJD is occurring, as evidenced by the sclerosis and osteophytosis; however, these findings are out of proportion to the severe joint space narrowing. When DJD narrows a joint to this extent, the osteophytosis and sclerosis are invariably much more pronounced.

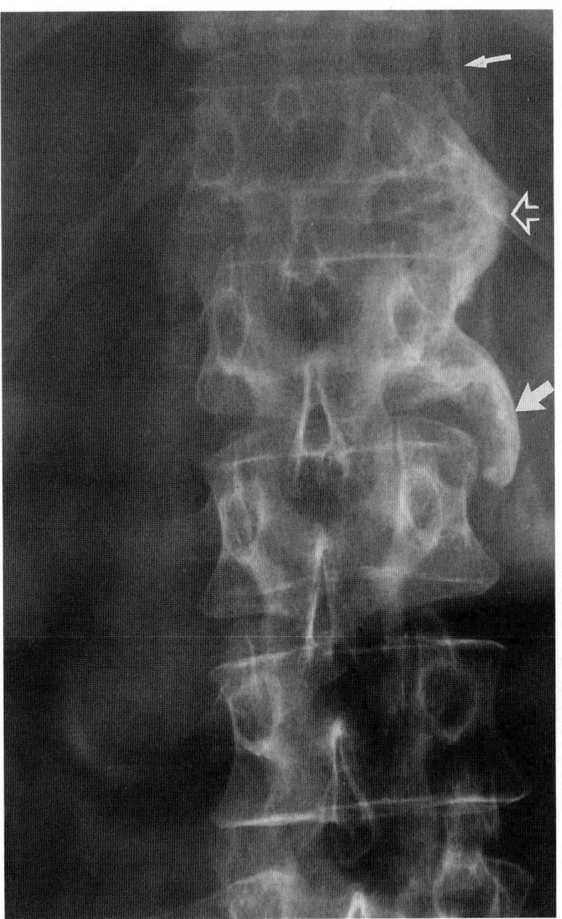

FIGURE 44.11. Psoriasis With Syndesmophytes. The large paravertebral ossification on the left side of the T12-L1 disk space (*open arrow*) is difficult to differentiate between an osteophyte and a syndesmophyte. Either could have this appearance. The paravertebral ossification at the left L1-L2 disk space (*large solid arrow*) definitely has a vertical rather than a horizontal orientation, however, as does the faint ossification seen at the T11-T12 disk space (*small solid arrow*). These definitely represent syndesmophytes. It makes sense, therefore, to assume that the ossification at the T12-L1 disk space is almost certainly a syndesmophyte as well. This patient has large nonmarginal, asymmetric syndesmophytes, which are typical of psoriatic arthritis or Reiter disease. This patient has psoriatic arthritis.

or margin of a vertebral body and extends to the margin of the adjacent vertebral body. They are invariably bilaterally symmetric, as viewed on an anteroposterior (AP) spine film. Ankylosing spondylitis classically has marginal, symmetric syndesmophytes (Fig. 44.12). Inflammatory bowel disease has an identical appearance when the spine is involved. Nonmarginal, asymmetric syndesmophytes are generally large and bulky. They emanate from the vertebral body, away from the endplate or margin, and are unilateral or asymmetric as viewed on an AP spine film (Figs. 44.11, 44.13). Psoriatic arthritis and Reiter syndrome classically have this type of syndesmophyte.

Involvement of the sacroiliac (SI) joints is common in the HLA-B27 spondyloarthropathies. The patterns of involvement, like the patterns of involvement of the spine, are somewhat typical for each disorder. Ankylosing spondylitis and inflammatory bowel disease typically cause bilaterally symmetric SI joint disease, which is initially erosive in nature and progresses to sclerosis and fusion (Figs. 44.14, 44.15). It is extremely unusual to have asymmetric or unilateral SI joint disease in these two disorders.

Reiter syndrome and psoriatic arthritis can exhibit unilateral or bilateral SI joint involvement. It seems that it is bilateral about 50% of the time. It is often asymmetric when it is bilateral, but exact symmetry can be difficult to assess; therefore, when involvement is definitely bilateral and not clearly asymmetric, consider the SI joints to be in the bilateral symmetric category. This means that if there is bilateral, symmetric SI joint disease, it could be caused by any of the four HLA-B27 spondyloarthropathies. If there

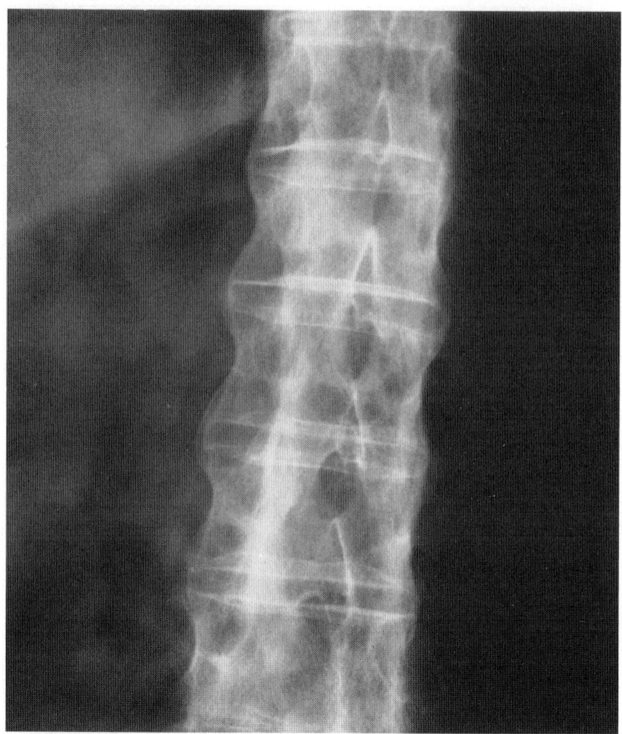

FIGURE 44.12. **Marginal, Symmetric Syndesmophytes in Ankylosing Spondylitis.** Bilateral marginal syndesmophytes are seen bridging the disk spaces throughout the lumbar spine in this patient. This is a so-called bamboo spine and is classic for ankylosing spondylitis and inflammatory bowel disease.

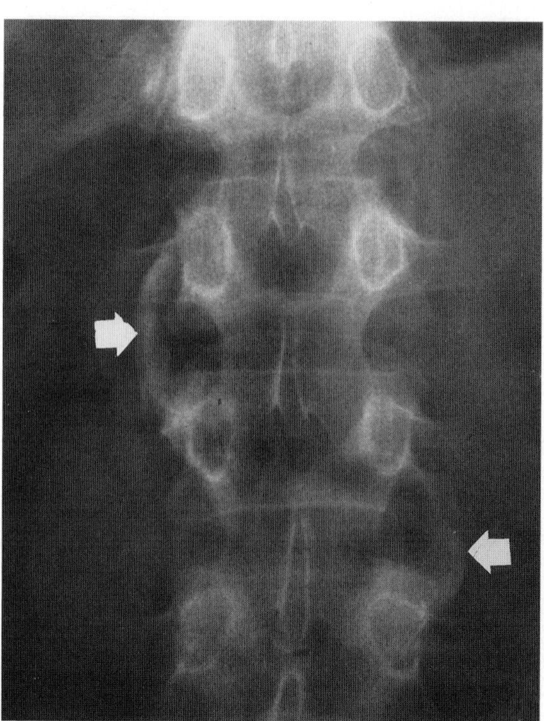

FIGURE 44.13. **Syndesmophytes in Psoriatic Arthritis.** Large, bulky, nonmarginal, asymmetric syndesmophytes (*arrows*) are seen in this patient with psoriatic arthritis.

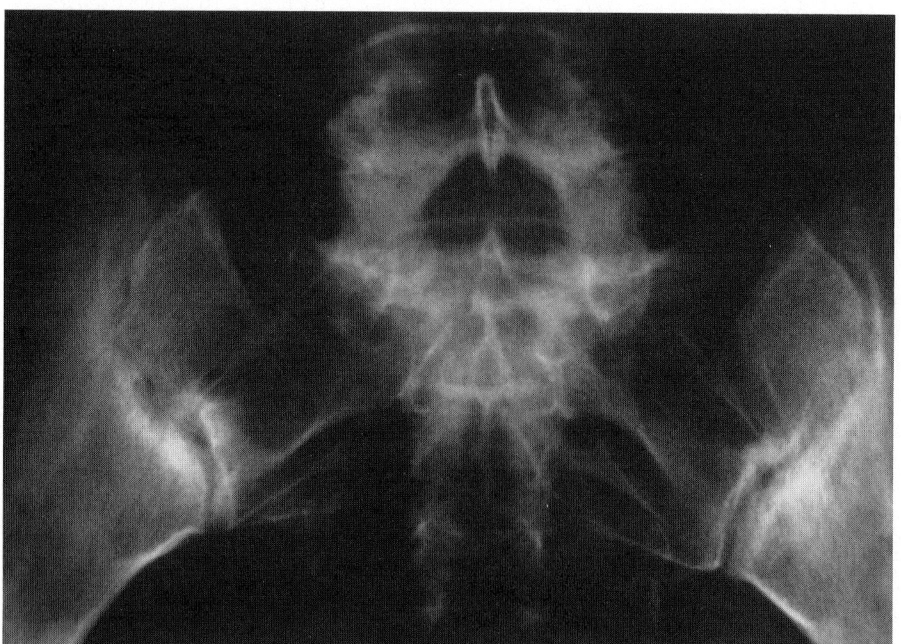

FIGURE 44.14. **Ankylosing Spondylitis.** Bilateral symmetric sacroiliac joint sclerosis and erosions are seen in this patient with ankylosing spondylitis. Inflammatory bowel disease could have a similar appearance. Although this is classic for these two disorders, it would not be that unusual for psoriatic disease or Reiter syndrome to have this same appearance. Although less likely, it would be possible for infection and even degenerative joint disease to be bilateral in this fashion.

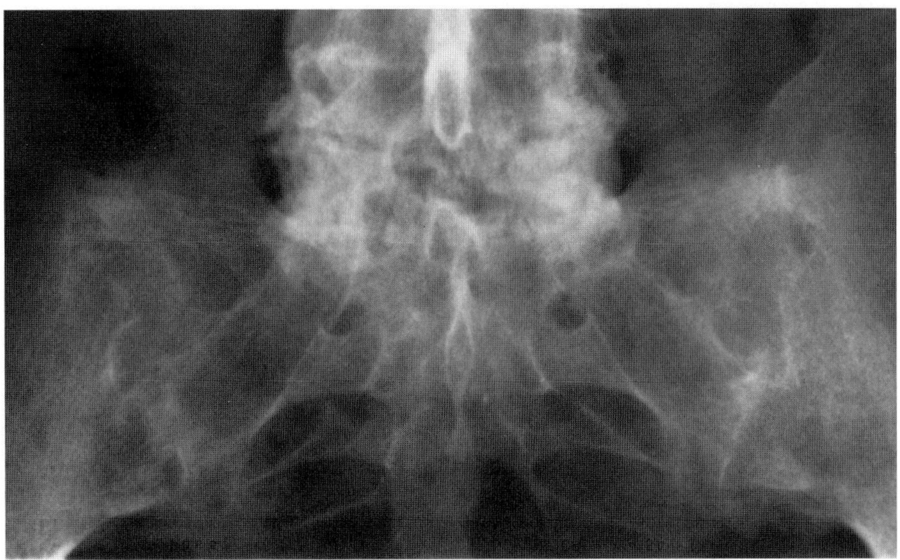

FIGURE 44.15. **Fusion of the Sacroiliac (SI) Joints in Ankylosing Spondylitis.** Bilateral complete fusion of the SI joints in this patient with ankylosing spondylitis makes the SI joints totally indistinguishable. Inflammatory bowel disease could have a similar appearance.

is unilateral (or clearly asymmetric) SI joint involvement, one can exclude ankylosing spondylitis and inflammatory bowel disease and consider Reiter syndrome or psoriatic disease. In this latter example, one would also have to consider infection and DJD (remember that DJD can cause erosions in the SI joints). Although it is seen less commonly, gout can also affect the SI joints unilaterally (Table 44.6 and Figs. 44.4, 44.16).

CT can be very helpful in examining the SI joints and is considered by many to be the diagnostic procedure of choice because of the unobstructed view of the entire joint (Fig. 44.17).

Large joint involvement with the HLA-B27 spondyloarthropathies is uncommon (except for ankylosing spondylitis), but when it does occur, the arthropathy will resemble rheumatoid arthritis (Fig. 44.18). The hips are involved in up to 50% of patients with ankylosing spondylitis.

Small joint involvement, specifically in the hands and feet, is not common in ankylosing spondylitis and inflammatory bowel disease. Psoriatic arthritis causes a distinctive arthropathy that is characterized by its distal predominance, proliferative erosions, soft tissue swelling, and periostitis. Proliferative erosions are different from the clean-cut, sharply marginated erosions seen in all other erosive arthritides, in that they have fuzzy margins with wisps of periostitis emanating from them (Fig. 44.19A). The severe forms are often associated with bony ankylosis across joints (Fig. 44.19B) and arthritis mutilans deformities. A fairly common finding is a calcaneal heel spur that has fuzzy margins, as opposed to the well-corticated heel spur seen in DJD or posttraumatically (Fig. 44.20).

Reiter syndrome causes identical changes in every respect to psoriatic arthritis, with the exception that the hands are not as commonly involved as the feet. The

TABLE 44.6 Causes of Sacroiliac Joint Disease

Ankylosing spondylitis
Inflammatory bowel disease
Psoriatic arthritis
Reiter syndrome
Infection
Degenerative joint disease
Gout

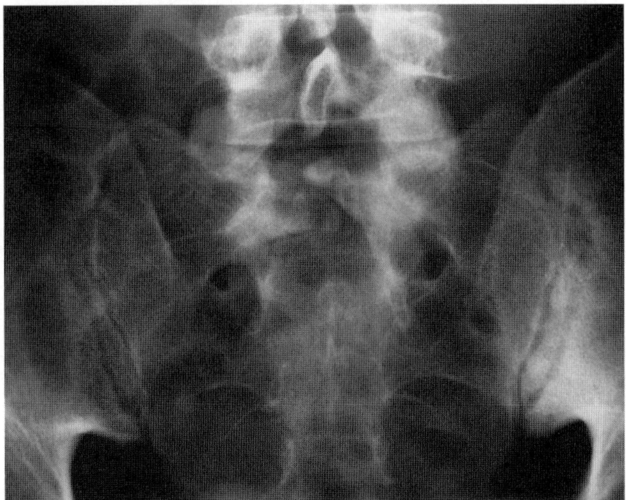

FIGURE 44.16. **Psoriatic Arthritis With Sacroiliac (SI) Joint Disease.** Unilateral SI sclerosis and erosions are seen in this patient with psoriatic arthritis. Ankylosing spondylitis and inflammatory bowel disease virtually never have this appearance.

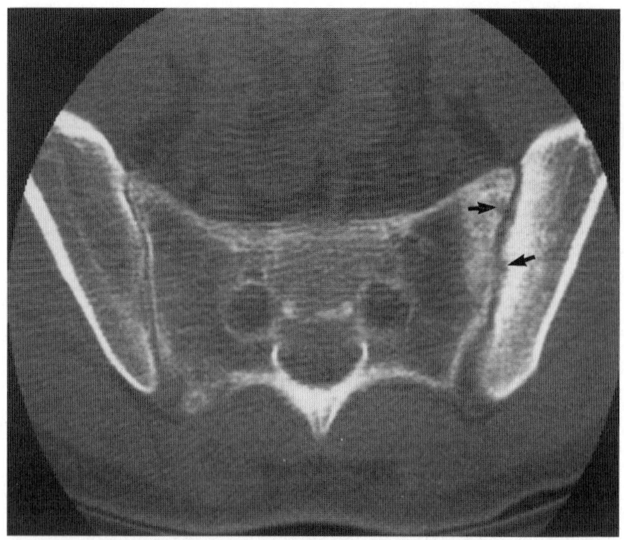

FIGURE 44.17. **CT of the Sacroiliac (SI) Joints in Psoriasis.** A CT scan through the SI joints in this patient with psoriatic arthritis shows unilateral SI joint sclerosis and erosions (*arrows*), typical for psoriatic arthritis or Reiter disease.

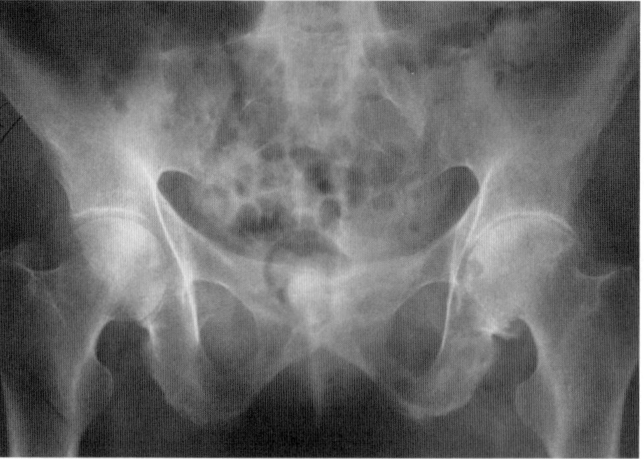

FIGURE 44.18. **Ankylosing Spondylitis With Hip Disease.** Anteroposterior view of the pelvis in this patient with ankylosing spondylitis shows bilateral complete fusion of the sacroiliac joints. Concentric left hip joint narrowing is present with axial migration of the femoral head. This would be a typical finding in rheumatoid arthritis or, as in this example, in ankylosing spondylitis. Note the secondary degenerative joint disease changes in the left hip as well.

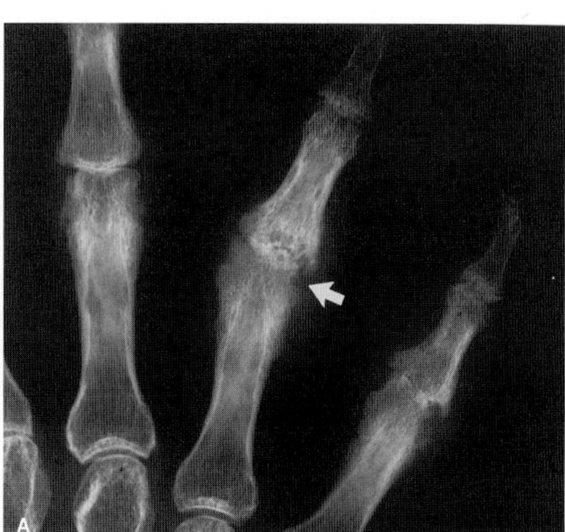

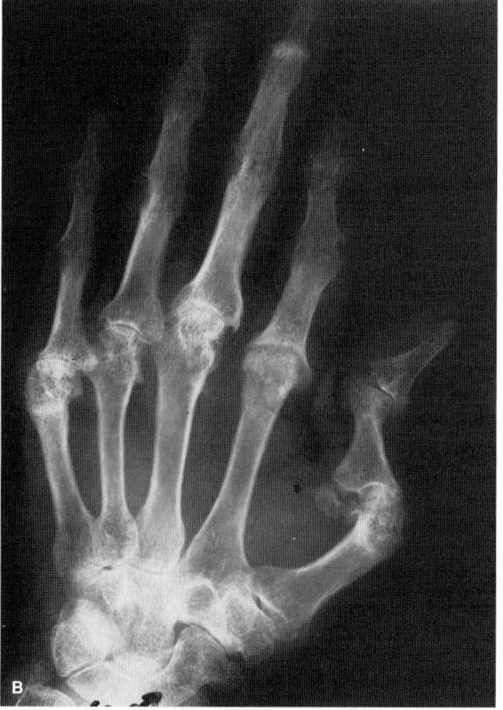

FIGURE 44.19. **Psoriatic Arthritis. A.** Cartilage loss at the proximal interphalangeal joints of the third, fourth, and fifth digits in this hand is apparent, with erosions noted most prominently in the fourth digit (*arrow*). These erosions are not sharply demarcated but are covered with fluffy new bone. These are termed proliferative erosions. Note also the periostitis along the shafts of each of the proximal phalanges. **B.** Advanced psoriatic arthritis. Fusion or ankylosis is apparent across the proximal interphalangeal joints of the second through the fifth digits. Several of the distal interphalangeal joints are also ankylosed. Severe joint space narrowing at the metacarpophalangeal joints is noted. This distal distribution is typical for psoriatic arthritis in advanced stages.

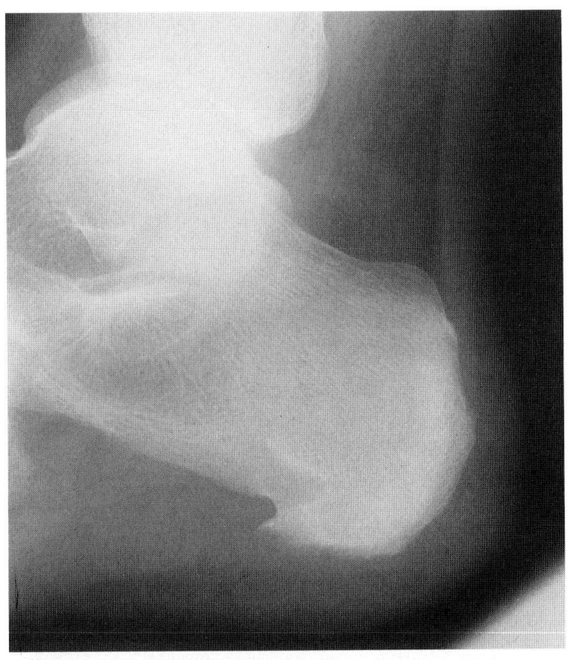

FIGURE 44.20. **Reiter Syndrome.** Lateral view of a calcaneus in a patient with Reiter syndrome shows poorly defined new bone on the posteroinferior margin of the calcaneus with a calcaneal spur which is also poorly defined. This is typical of psoriatic or Reiter disease, as opposed to the well-formed calcaneal spur in degenerative joint disease.

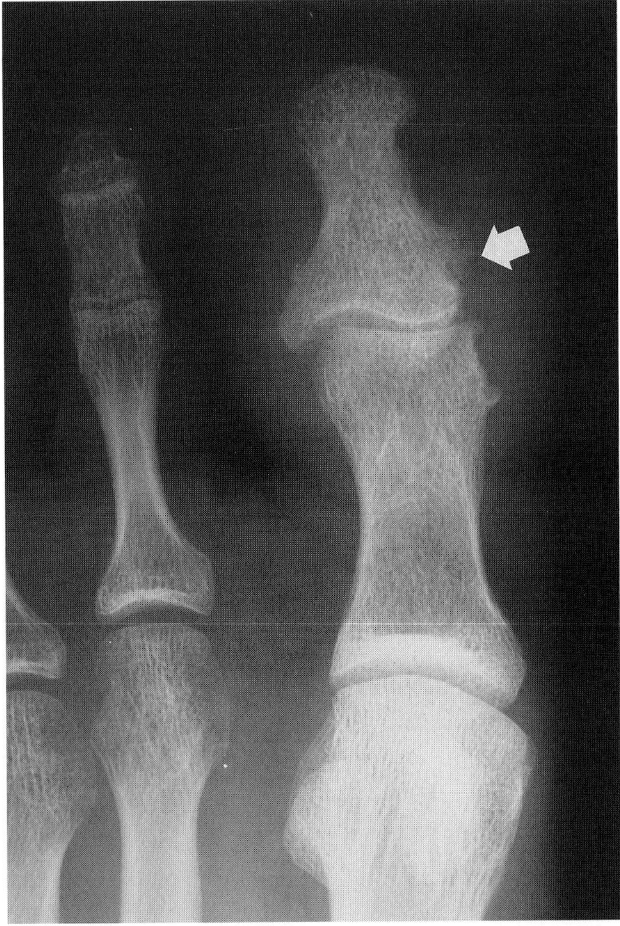

FIGURE 44.21. **Reiter Syndrome.** Anteroposterior view of the large toe in a patient with Reiter disease shows fluffy periostitis (*arrow*) in the erosions adjacent to the interphalangeal joint of the great toe. Marked soft tissue swelling is also present throughout the great toe. These changes are typical in appearance and location for Reiter disease or psoriatic arthritis.

interphalangeal joint of the great toe is a commonly affected location in Reiter disease (Fig. 44.21).

CRYSTAL-INDUCED ARTHRITIS

The crystal-induced arthritides include, primarily, gout and pseudogout (CPPD). Ochronosis and Wilson disease are so rare that they are not discussed in this chapter.

Gout is a metabolic disorder that results in hyperuricemia and leads to deposition of monosodium urate crystals in various sites in the body, especially in the joint cartilage. The actual causes of the hyperuricemia are myriad and include heredity.

The arthropathy caused by gout is very characteristic radiographically. It takes 4 to 6 years for gout to cause radiographically evident disease, and most patients are treated successfully long before the destructive arthropathy occurs; therefore, gouty arthritis is not commonly encountered. The classic radiographic findings in gout are *well-defined erosions,* often with sclerotic borders or overhanging edges; *soft tissue nodules* that calcify in the presence of renal failure; and a *random distribution* in the hands *without marked osteoporosis* (Table 44.7 and Fig. 44.22). Even though erosions with overhanging edges occur with gout, they can occur in other disorders as well and are by no means pathognomonic. The sclerotic margins of the erosions are rarely seen in any other arthritide; therefore, this is a very useful differential point. Gout typically affects the metatarsophalangeal joint of the great toe (Fig. 44.23). In the advanced stages, it can be very deforming (Fig. 44.24). Patients with gout often have chondrocalcinosis because they have a predisposition for pseudogout (CPPD). As many as 40% of patients with gout concomitantly have CPPD.

TABLE 44.7 Hallmarks of Gout

Well-defined erosions (sclerotic margins)
Soft tissue nodules
Random distribution
No osteoporosis

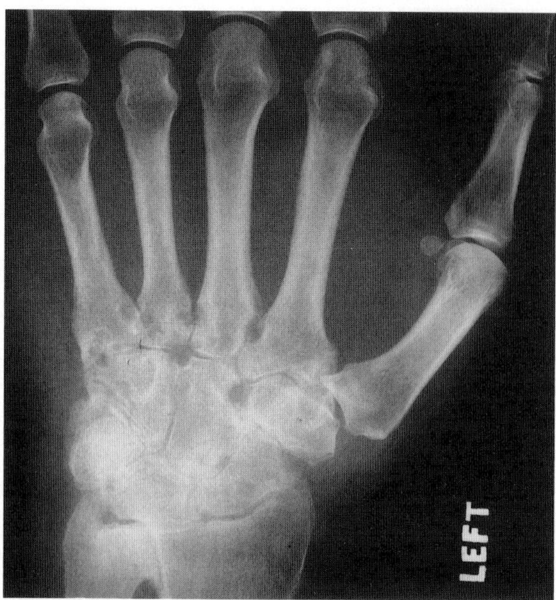

FIGURE 44.22. **Gout.** Sharply marginated erosions, some with a sclerotic margin, are noted throughout the carpus and proximal metacarpals. These erosions are classic in gout. Note the absence of marked demineralization.

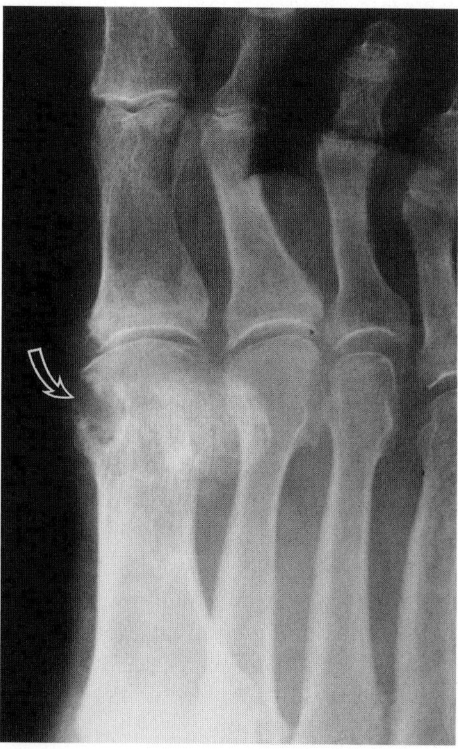

FIGURE 44.23. **Gout.** A sharply marginated erosion with an overhanging edge (*arrow*) and a sclerotic margin is seen in the metatarsophalangeal in the great toe in this patient with gout. This appearance and location are classic for gout, whereas psoriatic arthritis and Reiter disease usually involve the interphalangeal joint and do not have erosions that are this sharply marginated.

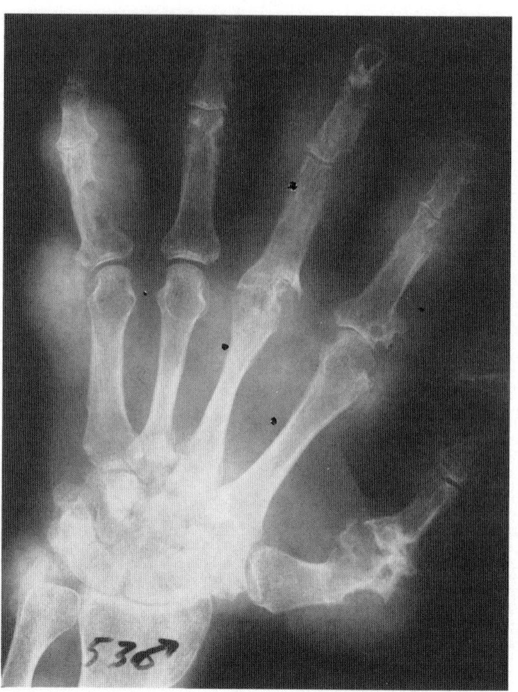

FIGURE 44.24. **Advanced Gout.** Marked diffuse and focal soft tissue swelling is present throughout the hand and wrist in this patient with long-standing gout. Destructive, large, well-marginated erosions, some with overhanging edges, are noted near multiple joints. The focal areas of soft tissue swelling are called tophi, some of which are calcified. These only calcify with coexistent renal disease.

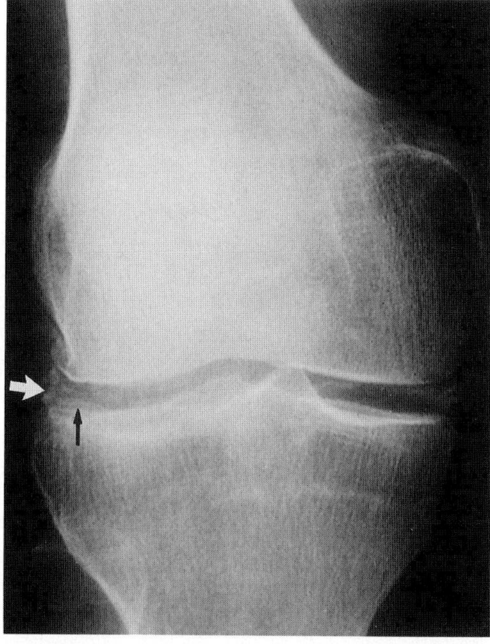

FIGURE 44.25. **Chondrocalcinosis in the Knee.** Cartilage calcification known as chondrocalcinosis is seen in the fibrocartilage (*white arrow*) and in the hyaline articular cartilage (*black arrow*) in this patient with calcium pyrophosphate dihydrate deposition disease.

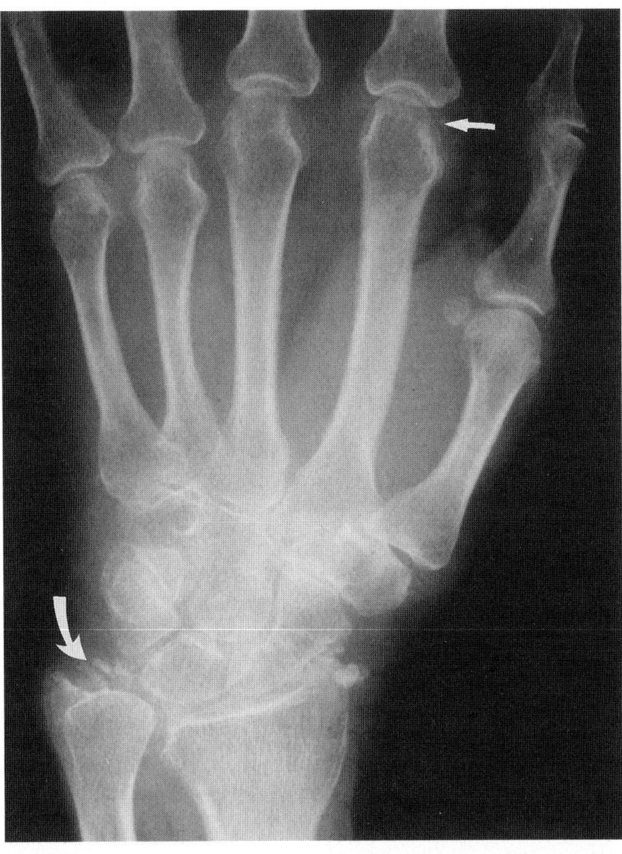

FIGURE 44.26. **Chondrocalcinosis in the Wrist.** This patient with calcium pyrophosphate dihydrate deposition disease exhibits chondrocalcinosis in the triangular fibrocartilage of the wrist (*curved arrow*). A small amount of chondrocalcinosis is also seen in the second metacarpophalangeal (*small arrow*). Triangular ligament calcification is one of the more common locations for chondrocalcinosis to occur.

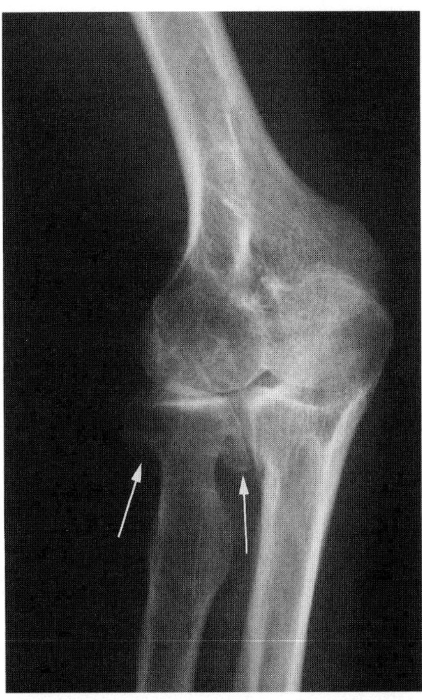

FIGURE 44.27. **Calcium Pyrophosphate Dihydrate Crystal Deposition Disease (CPPD) Arthropathy.** Degenerative joint disease (DJD) of the elbow is seen in this patient with CPPD. Note the joint space narrowing, with minimal sclerosis and large osteophytes (*arrows*). Osteophytes of this nature are termed drooping osteophytes and are often seen in CPPD. The elbow is an unusual place for DJD to occur except in the setting of CPPD or trauma.

Pseudogout has a classic triad: pain, cartilage calcification, and joint destruction. The patient may have any combination of one or more of this triad at any one time. Each of these is addressed individually in some detail in this chapter, but note that two of the three are radiographic findings. This is a disorder that is best diagnosed radiographically.

The pain of CPPD is nonspecific. It can mimic that of gout (hence the term "pseudogout"), infection, or just about any arthritis. It typically is intermittent for a large number of years until DJD occurs and becomes the main cause of pain.

TABLE 44.8 Most Common Location of Chondrocalcinosis in Calcium Pyrophosphate Dihydrate Deposition Disease

Knee
Triangular fibrocartilage of wrist
Symphysis pubis

Cartilage calcification, known as chondrocalcinosis, can occur in any joint but tends to affect a few select sites in most patients. These are the medial and lateral compartments of the *knee* (Fig. 44.25), the *triangular fibrocartilage of the wrist* (Fig. 44.26), and the *symphysis pubis* (Table 44.8). Chondrocalcinosis in these areas is virtually diagnostic of CPPD (3). When CPPD crystals are deposited in the soft tissues, such as in the rotator cuff of the shoulder, a radiograph cannot differentiate between CPPD and calcium hydroxyapatite, which occurs in calcific tendinitis. Calcium hydroxyapatite does not occur in the joint cartilage except in extremely unusual cases; therefore, all chondrocalcinosis can be considered to be secondary to CPPD.

The joint destruction or arthropathy of CPPD is virtually indistinguishable from that of DJD. In fact, it is DJD. It is caused by CPPD crystals eroding the cartilage. There are a few features of the DJD caused by CPPD that will help distinguish it from DJD caused by trauma or overuse, however. The main difference is location. The DJD of CPPD has a proclivity for the *shoulder*, the *elbow* (Fig. 44.27), the *radiocarpal joint* in the wrist (Fig. 44.28), the *patellofemoral joint* of the knee, and the metacarpophalangeal joints in the hand (Table 44.9). These are areas of wear and tear not normally involved by DJD (such as in the distal

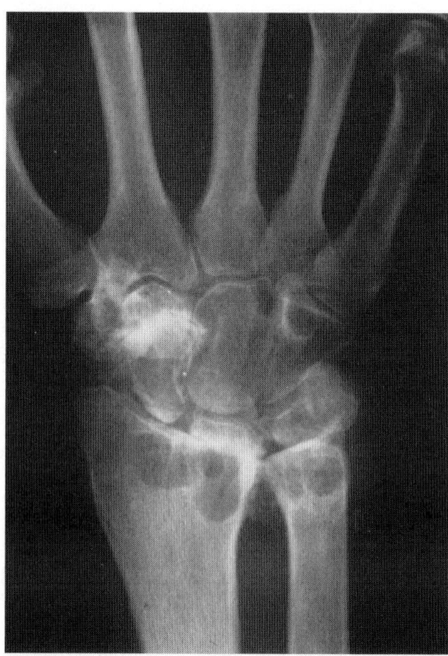

FIGURE 44.28. **Calcium Pyrophosphate Dihydrate Crystal Deposition Disease (CPPD) Arthropathy.** Marked degenerative joint disease (DJD) at the radiocarpal joint is seen in this patient with CPPD. Severe joint space narrowing and sclerosis with large subchondral cysts or geodes are all hallmarks of DJD. This is an unusual location for DJD except in the setting of CPPD or trauma.

interphalangeal joints of the hand, the hip, and the medial compartment of the knee). When DJD is seen in the joints that CPPD tends to involve, a search for chondrocalcinosis should be made. If necessary, a joint aspiration for CPPD crystals may be required to confirm the diagnosis.

Occasionally, the arthropathy of CPPD causes such severe destruction that a neuropathic or Charcot joint is mimicked on the radiograph. This has been termed a *pseudo-Charcot joint*. It is not a true Charcot joint because of the presence of sensation (4).

There are three diseases that have a high degree of association with CPPD. These are *primary hyperparathyroidism, gout,* and *hemochromatosis* (Table 44.10). This is not a differential diagnosis for chondrocalcinosis; rather, these are diseases that tend to occur at the same time as CPPD. If the patient has one of these three disorders, he or she is more likely to have CPPD than is an unaffected person. There is probably no good reason to work up every patient with chondrocalcinosis for one of the three associated diseases because they are so uncommon and CPPD is extremely common.

TABLE 44.9 Most Common Location of Arthropathy in Calcium Pyrophosphate Dihydrate Deposition Disease

Shoulder
Radiocarpal joint
Patellofemoral joint
Elbow
Metacarpophalangeal joints in hand

TABLE 44.10 Diseases With High Association With Calcium Pyrophosphate Dihydrate Deposition Disease

Primary hyperparathyroidism
Gout
Hemochromatosis

COLLAGEN-VASCULAR DISEASES

Scleroderma, systemic lupus erythematosus, dermatomyositis, and mixed connective tissue disease are all grouped together as collagen-vascular diseases. The striking abnormality in the hands in each of these disorders is osteoporosis and soft tissue wasting. Systemic lupus erythematosus characteristically has severe ulnar deviation of the phalanges (Fig. 44.29). Erosions are generally not a feature of these disorders. Soft tissue calcifications are typically present in scleroderma (Fig. 44.30) and dermatomyositis. The calcifications in scleroderma are typically subcutaneous, whereas in dermatomyositis they are intramuscular in location. Mixed connective tissue disease is an overlap of scleroderma, systemic lupus erythematosus, polymyositis, and rheumatoid arthritis. It has a myriad of radiographic findings.

SARCOID

Sarcoidosis is a disease that causes deposition of granulomatous tissue in the body—primarily in the lungs, but also in the bones. In the skeletal system, it has a predilection for the hands, where it causes lytic destructive lesions in the cortex. These often have a so-called lacelike appearance, which is characteristic (Fig. 44.31). Sarcoidosis can have associated skin nodules inthe hands.

HEMOCHROMATOSIS

Hemochromatosis is a disease of excess iron deposition in tissues throughout the body that leads to fibrosis and eventual organ failure. Twenty percent to 50% of patients with hemochromatosis have a characteristic arthropathy in the hands that should suggest the diagnosis. The classic radiographic changes are essentially DJD that involves the second through the fourth metacarpophalangeal joints (Fig. 44.32). Up to 50% of patients with hemochromatosis also have CPPD; therefore, a search should be made for chondrocalcinosis. Another finding that is often seen in hemochromatosis is called "squaring" of the metacarpal heads, which appear enlarged and blocklike as a result of the large osteophytes commonly seen in this

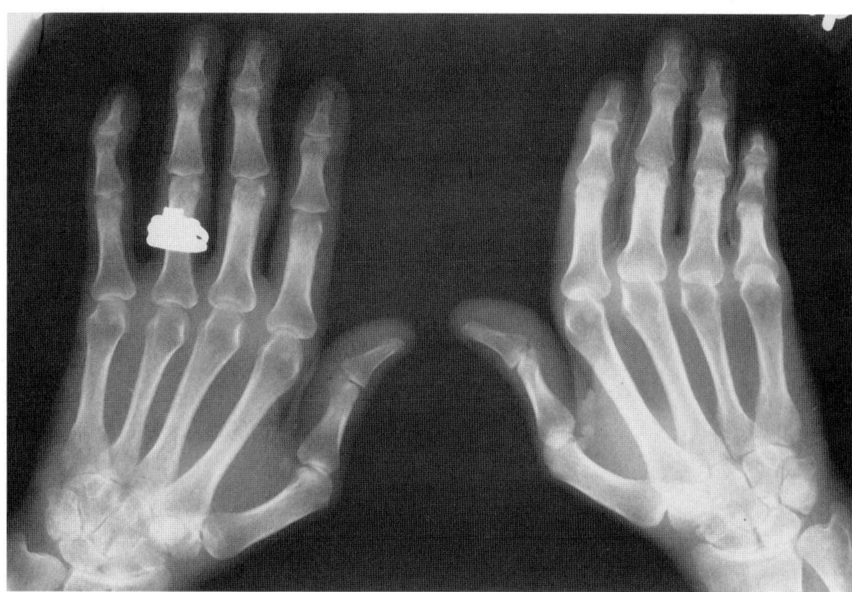

FIGURE 44.29. **Systemic Lupus Erythematosus.** Marked soft tissue wasting, as noted by the concavity in the hypothenar eminence, and ulnar deviation of the phalanges, seen primarily in the right hand, are hallmarks of systemic lupus erythematosus.

disorder. The osteophytes are often said to be "drooping" because of the unusual way they hang off the joint margin.

NEUROPATHIC OR CHARCOT JOINT

The radiographic findings for a Charcot joint are characteristic and almost pathognomonic. A classic triad has been described that consists of *destruction, dislocation,* and *heterotopic new bone* (Table 44.11 and Fig. 44.33).

Joint destruction is seen in every type of arthritis and therefore seems very nonspecific; however, nothing causes such severe destruction in a joint as a Charcot joint. Progressive joint destruction occurs in a neuropathic joint because the joint is rendered unstable by inaccurate muscle action and is unprotected by intact nerve reflexes. Early in the development of a Charcot joint, the joint destruction may appear to be merely joint space narrowing. It is extremely difficult to make the diagnosis this early. In the spine, instead of joint space destruction, there is disk space destruction (Fig. 44.34).

Dislocation, like joint destruction, can be present in varying degrees. Early on, the joint may have subluxation instead of dislocation.

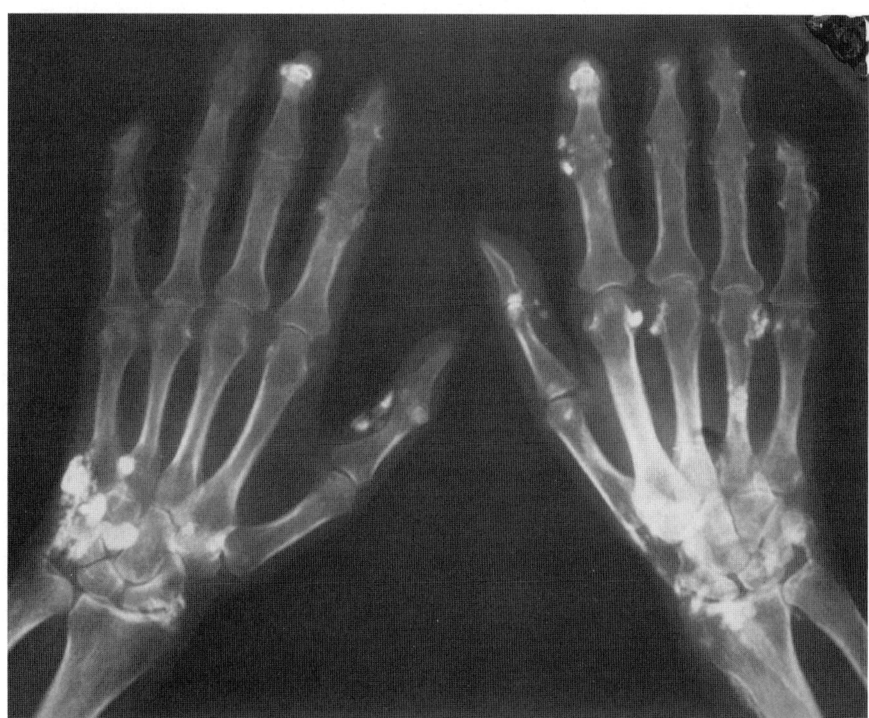

FIGURE 44.30. **Scleroderma.** Diffuse subcutaneous soft tissue calcification is seen throughout the hands and wrists in this patient with scleroderma. Soft tissue wasting and osteoporosis are also present, as well as bone loss in multiple distal phalanges secondary to the vascular abnormalities often present in this disease.

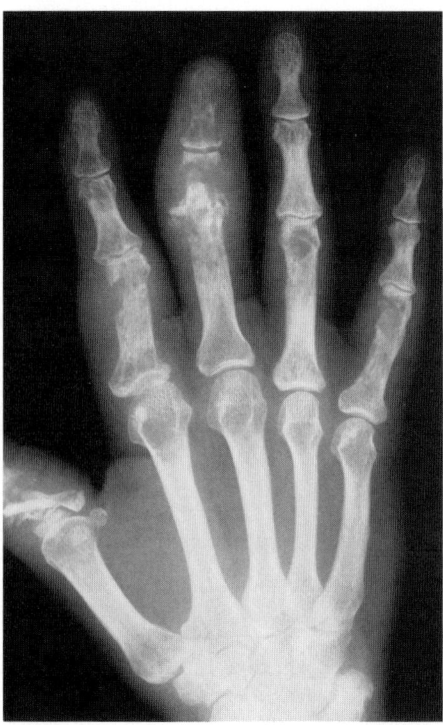

FIGURE 44.31. **Sarcoid.** Anteroposterior view of the hand in this patient with sarcoid demonstrates classic changes of bony involvement with this granulomatous process. Note the lacelike pattern of destruction, which is seen most prominently in the proximal phalanges and in the distal third phalanx. Soft tissue swelling and some areas of severe bony dissolution are also noted, which occur in more advanced patterns of sarcoid. These changes are typically limited to the hands but can rarely occur in other parts of the skeleton.

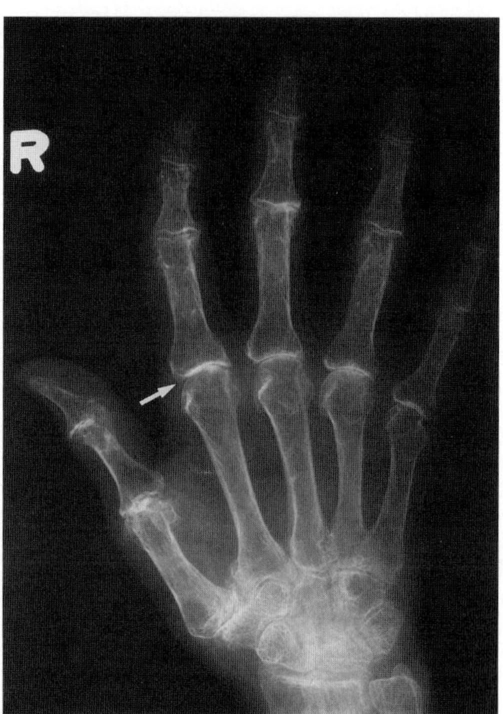

FIGURE 44.32. **Hemochromatosis.** Anteroposterior view of the hand in this patient with hemochromatosis shows severe joint space narrowing throughout the hand, which is most marked at the metacarpophalangeal joints. Associated sclerosis at the metacarpophalangeal joints with large osteophytes seen off the metacarpal heads suggests degenerative joint disease (DJD). These are very unusual joints for DJD to occur in, yet this is the classic appearance of hemochromatosis. No chondrocalcinosis is seen in the triangular cartilage in this patient; however, a small amount of chondrocalcinosis can be seen at the second metacarpophalangeal joint (*arrow*). Fifty percent of patients with hemochromatosis also have calcium pyrophosphate dihydrate deposition disease.

Heterotopic new bone has also been termed debris or detritus and consists of soft tissue calcification or clumps of ossification adjacent to the joint. It, too, can be present in varying amounts.

The most commonly seen Charcot joint today is in the foot of a diabetic. The disease typically affects the first and second tarsometatarsal joints in a fashion similar to a Lisfranc fracture (Fig. 44.35).

Tabes dorsalis from syphilis is rarely seen today. More commonly seen is a Charcot joint in a patient with paralysis who continues to use the affected limb for support. A Charcot joint that is also seen on occasion is the so-called pseudo-Charcot joint in CPPD.

HEMOPHILIA, JUVENILE RHEUMATOID ARTHRITIS, AND PARALYSIS

Why would clinically disparate entities like paralysis, juvenile rheumatoid arthritis (JRA), and hemophilia be covered in the same section? Because they are usually radiographically indistinguishable.

The classic findings for JRA and hemophilia are *overgrowth of the ends of the bones* (epiphyseal enlargement) associated with *gracile diaphyses* (Fig. 44.36). Joint destruction might or might not be present. A finding that is purported to be classic for JRA and hemophilia is widening of the intercondylar notch of the knee. This sign can be quite variable and difficult to apply. It is rarely present when the other classic signs are not also present and obvious.

Another process that can mimic the findings of JRA and hemophilia is a joint that has undergone disuse from para- lysis (Fig. 44.37). It has always been said that the reason the epiphyses are overgrown in JRA and hemophilia is

TABLE 44.11 Hallmarks of a Neuropathic Joint

Joint destruction
Dislocation
Heterotopic new bone formation

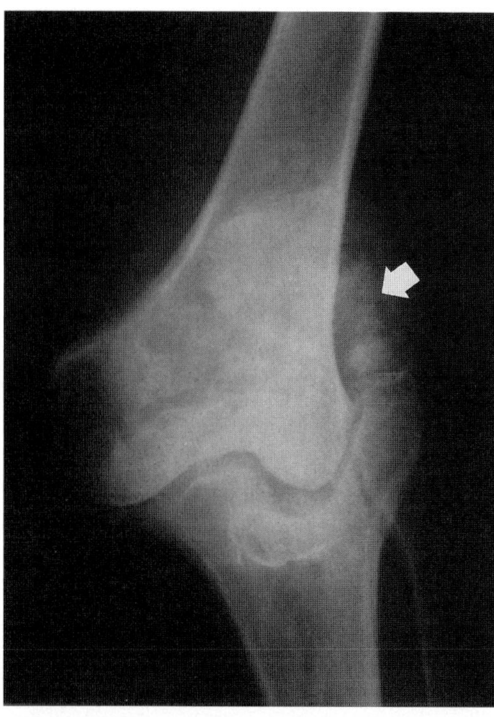

FIGURE 44.33. **Charcot Joint.** Anteroposterior view of the knee in this patient with tabes dorsalis shows the classic changes of a neuropathic or Charcot joint. Note the severe joint destruction, the subluxation, and the heterotopic new bone (*arrow*).

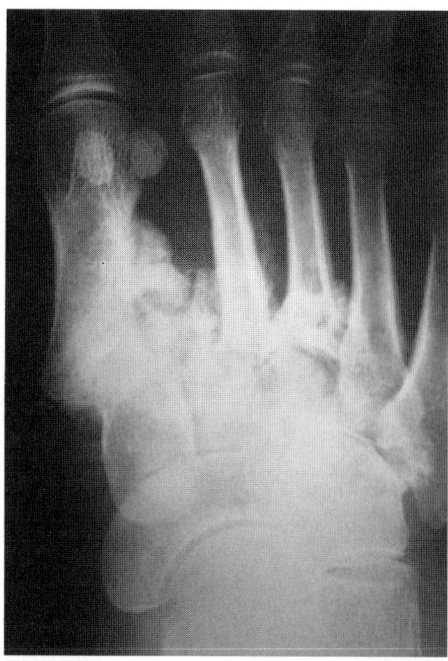

FIGURE 44.35. **Lisfranc Charcot Joint.** Dislocation of the second and third metatarsals along with joint destruction and large amounts of heterotopic new bone are present in the foot of this diabetic patient. These findings are classic for a Charcot joint, which has been termed a Lisfranc fracture-dislocation. It is most commonly seen secondary to trauma rather than as a Charcot joint but is the most common neuropathic joint seen today.

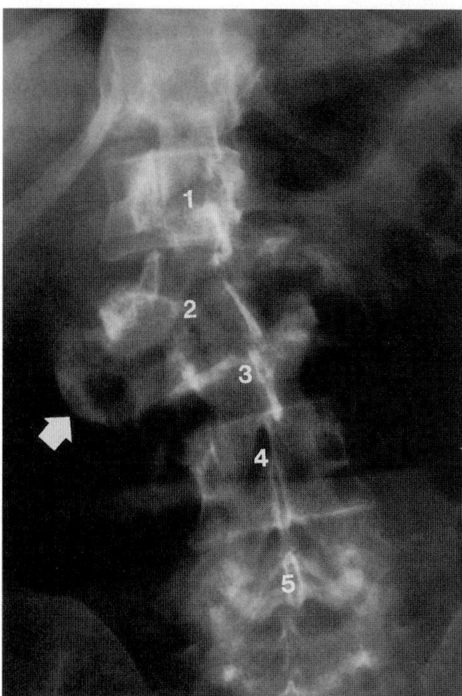

FIGURE 44.34. **Charcot Spine.** Anteroposterior view of the spine in this paraplegic patient shows severe destruction of the L2 and L3 vertebral bodies and the intervening disk space, heterotopic new bone (*arrow*), and malalignment or dislocation. Numbers indicate lumbar vertebrae.

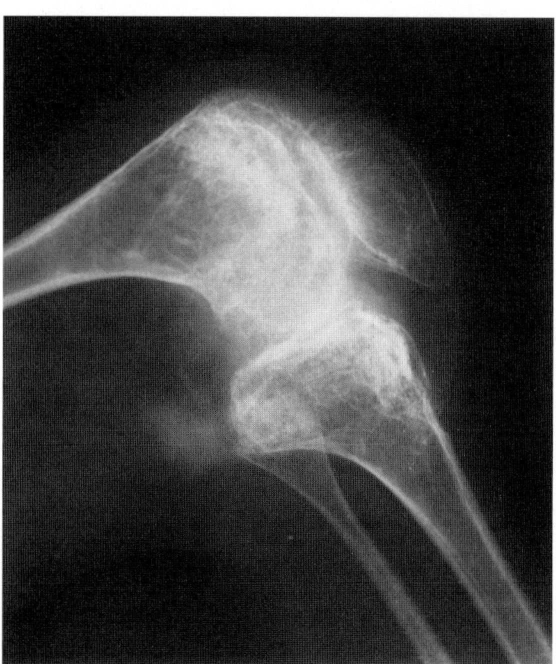

FIGURE 44.36. **Juvenile Rheumatoid Arthritis (JRA).** A lateral view of the knee in this patient with JRA shows the classic findings of overgrowth of the ends of the bones and associated gracile diaphyses. These changes can also be seen in patients with hemophilia or paralysis.

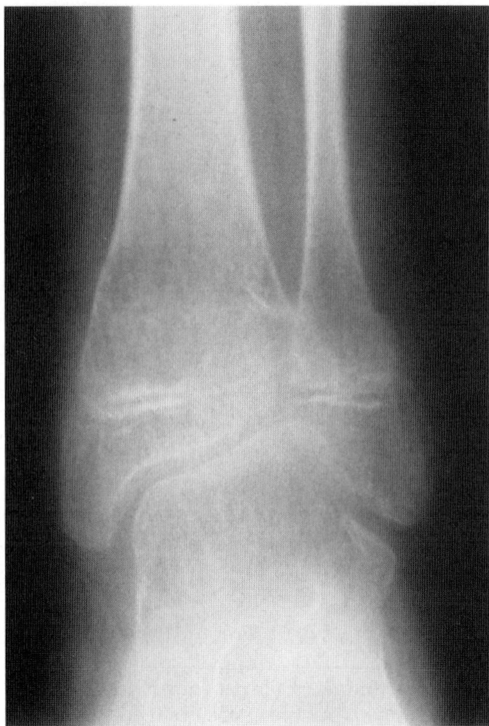

FIGURE 44.37. **Muscular Dystrophy Simulating Juvenile Rheumatoid Arthritis (JRA) or Hemophilia.** Anteroposterior view of the ankle in this patient with muscular dystrophy shows subtle changes of overgrowth of the distal tibia and fibular epiphyses. Marked tibiotalar slant, which can also be present in JRA or hemophilia, is also present.

because of the hyperemia; however, many other things cause hyperemia without affecting the size of the epiphyses (such as rheumatoid arthritis and infection). The common denominator shared by JRA, hemophilia, and paralysis is disuse. This is most likely what causes the overgrowth of the ends of the bones that is seen in all three of these disorders.

SYNOVIAL OSTEOCHONDROMATOSIS

Synovial osteochondromatosis is a relatively common disorder caused by a metaplasia of the synovium that results in deposition of foci of cartilage in the joint. Most of the time, these cartilaginous deposits calcify and are readily seen on a radiograph (Fig. 44.38). It is most commonly seen in the knee, hip, and elbow. Up to 30% of the time, the cartilaginous deposits do not calcify. In these cases, all that is seen on the radiograph is a joint effusion, unless erosions or joint destruction occur (Fig. 44.39).

The calcifications begin in the synovium and then tend to shed into the joint, where they can cause symptoms of free fragments, or "joint mice." They then embed into the synovium and tend not to be free in the joint after a while. It is usually necessary to perform a complete synovectomy to relieve the symptoms.

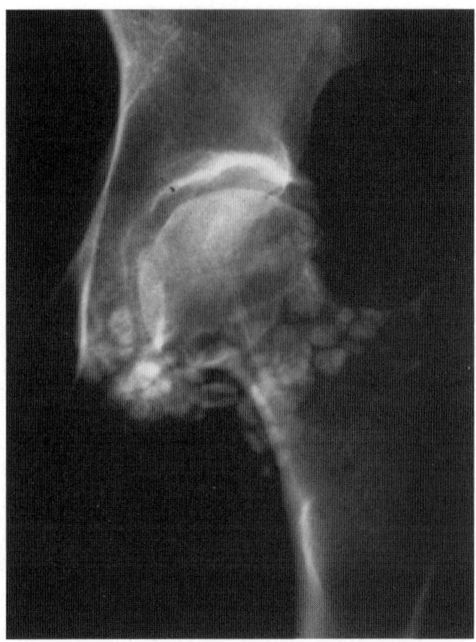

FIGURE 44.38. **Synovial Osteochondromatosis.** Anteroposterior view of the hip in this patient with left hip pain shows multiple calcified loose bodies in the hip joint, which is virtually diagnostic of synovial osteochondromatosis.

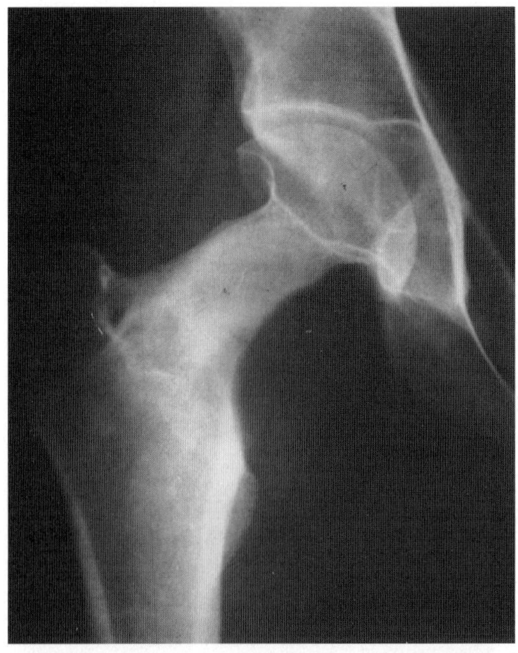

FIGURE 44.39. **Synovial Osteochondromatosis Without Calcification.** Anteroposterior view of the hip in this patient shows that the femoral neck is eroded, with the femoral head having an "apple core" appearance. This has occurred from the pressure erosion of multiple nonossified loose bodies in the joint. This is nonossified synovial osteochondromatosis (probably more properly termed synovial chondromatosis). It usually does not cause this degree of bony erosion and is indistinguishable from pigmented villonodular synovitis.

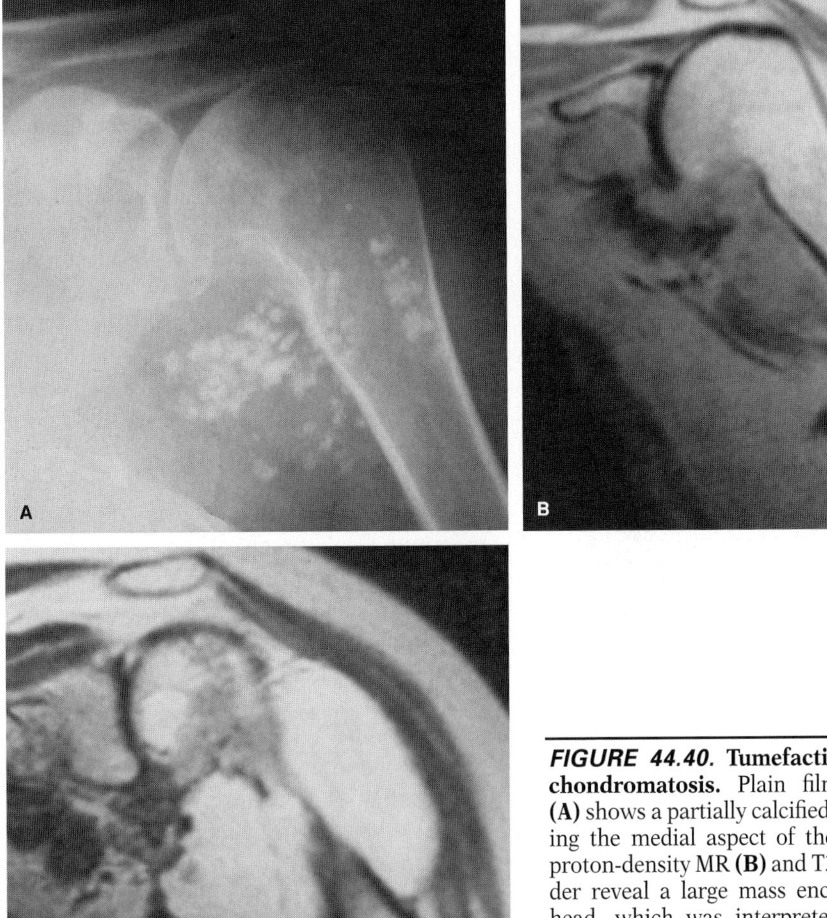

FIGURE 44.40. **Tumefactive Synovial Osteochondromatosis.** Plain film of the shoulder **(A)** shows a partially calcified mass which is eroding the medial aspect of the humerus. Coronal proton-density MR **(B)** and T2WI **(C)** of the shoulder reveal a large mass encircling the humeral head, which was interpreted as a sarcoma. A biopsy was performed and called "chondrosarcoma," which resulted in a forequarter amputation. The intra-articular nature of the mass was not appreciated until after the radical surgery, when it was correctly recognized as synovial chondromatosis.

An uncommon presentation that can lead to diagnostic confusion is when the loose bodies are tightly packed in a joint, giving it the appearance of a tumor on MR (Fig. 44.40). This has been termed *tumefactive synovial chondromatosis*. If a biopsy is performed, it can get interpreted as a chondrosarcoma and treated with resultant radical surgery. Because no malignant tumors arise in joints, this should not present a problem in diagnosis.

PIGMENTED VILLONODULAR SYNOVITIS

Pigmented villonodular synovitis (PVNS) is a rare chronic inflammatory process of the synovium that causes synovial proliferation. A swollen joint with lobular masses of synovium occurs and causes pain and joint destruction (Fig. 44.41). It rarely, if ever, calcifies. It has been termed *giant cell tumor of tendon sheath* and *tendon sheath xanthoma* when it occurs in a tendon sheath, which is not unusual. Joints with PVNS look radiographically identical to noncalcified synovial osteochondromatosis, yet they are much less common. Therefore, whenever PVNS is a consideration, synovial chondromatosis should be mentioned. PVNS has a characteristic appearance on MR, with low-signal hemosiderin seen lining the synovium on both T1WIs and T2WIs (Fig. 44.42).

SUDECK ATROPHY

Also known as shoulder-hand syndrome and reflex sympathetic dystrophy, Sudeck atrophy is a poorly understood joint affliction that typically occurs after minor trauma to an extremity, resulting in pain, swelling, and dysfunction. Severe, patchy osteoporosis and soft tissue swelling are seen radiographically (Fig. 44.43). It typically affects the distal part of an extremity, such as a hand or foot, yet intermediate joints such as the knee and hip are believed by some to be occasionally involved. The pain usually

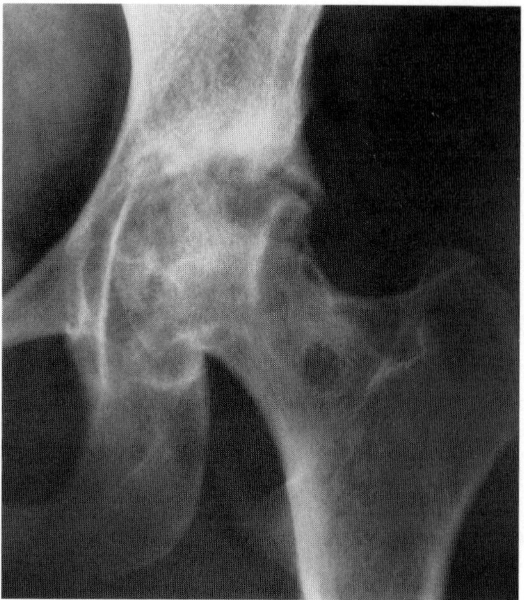

FIGURE 44.41. **Pigmented Villonodular Synovitis.** Anteroposterior view of the hip in this patient shows joint space destruction and bony erosions throughout the femoral head and neck. Pigmented villonodular synovitis or synovial chondromatosis could have this appearance.

subsides, but the osteoporosis may persist. With time, the swelling will subside and the skin may become atrophic. It is important for the radiologist to recognize the aggressive osteoporosis in this disorder and differentiate it from disuse osteoporosis so that the treating physician can begin aggressive physical therapy.

JOINT EFFUSIONS

Most joint effusions are clinically obvious and do not require radiographic validation. The elbow is an exception. In the setting of trauma to the elbow, an effusion indicates a fracture. The radiographic signs of an elbow effusion are generally clearly seen (displaced fat-pads, as described in Chapter 43) and have been proven valid. Clinical determination of an elbow effusion can be difficult; therefore, the radiologist can be very helpful in this area.

Clinical determination of a hip effusion is also very difficult. The presence of a hip effusion can be valuable in certain clinical settings. For instance, a patient with pain in the hip and an effusion should have the joint aspirated to rule out an infection. If only pain is present, an aspiration would probably not be performed. The radiology literature mentions displacement of the fat stripes about the hip as an indicator for an effusion, but this has been proved to be unfounded. The only fat-pad around the hip that gets displaced with an effusion is the obturator internus, and it is seen uncommonly.

The radiographic sign for a knee effusion that seems to be the most reliable is the measurement of the distance between the suprapatellar fat-pad and the anterior femoral fat-pad (Fig. 44.44). A distance between these two fat-pads of more than 10 mm is definite evidence for an effusion. A distance of less than 5 mm is normal. A distance of 5 to 10 mm is equivocal. It does not make any difference if there is an effusion in the knee—treatment is the same, regardless. If it were vital to the patient, one could aspirate the joint or perform an MR study to find out. I should

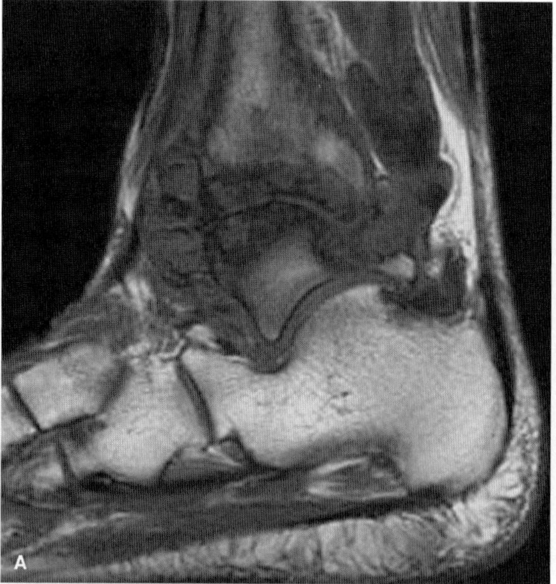

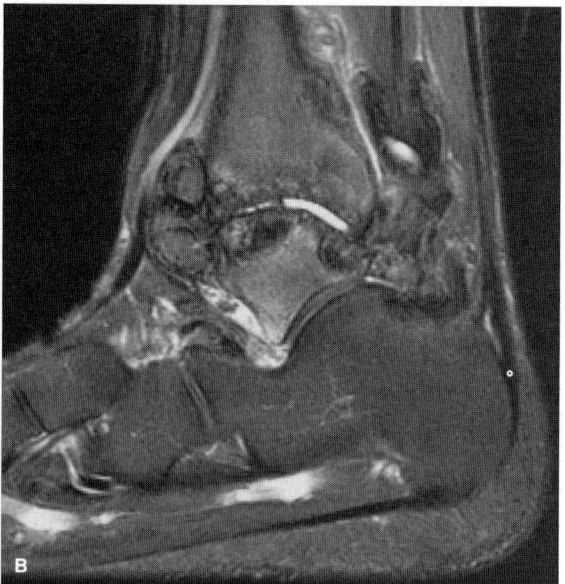

FIGURE 44.42. **Pigmented Villonodular Synovitis (PVNS).** Sagittal T1W **(A)** and fast spin-echo T2W **(B)** images of an ankle with PVNS show a soft tissue mass emanating from the ankle joint, which is low signal on both sequences and has very low signal hemosiderin lining parts of the synovium, which is characteristic for PVNS.

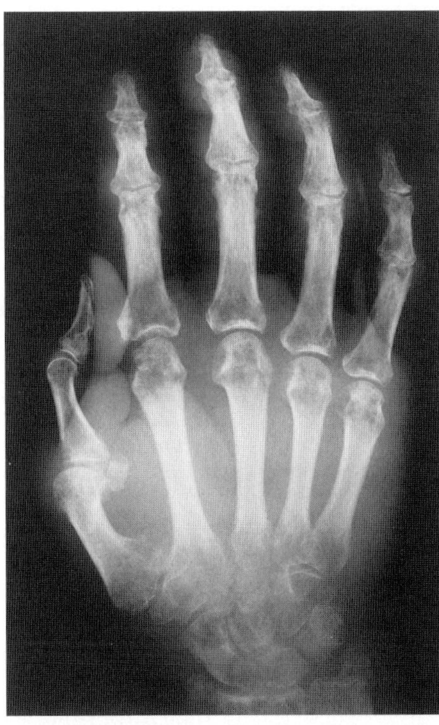

FIGURE 44.43. **Sudeck Atrophy.** Diffuse soft tissue swelling and marked osteoporosis that is so aggressive it has a spotty or permeative appearance is noted around all of the joints in the hand. This patient experienced severe hand pain and dysfunction following minor trauma. This is characteristic of Sudeck atrophy.

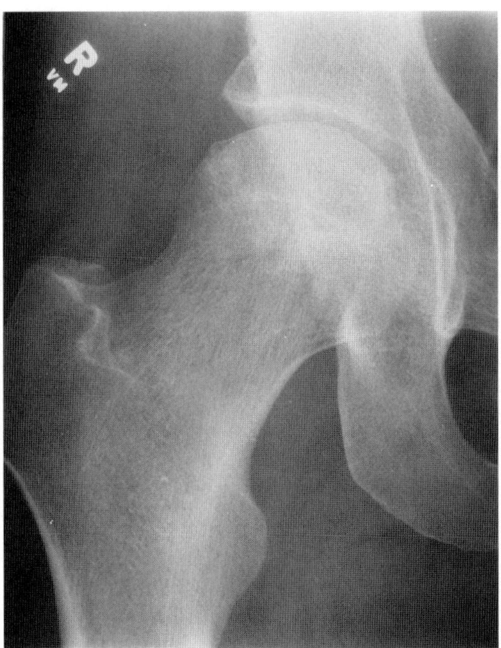

FIGURE 44.45. **Early Avascular Necrosis of the Hip.** Patchy sclerosis is present in the femoral head in this patient with a renal transplant and avascular necrosis of the right hip. No subchondral lucency or articular surface irregularity in the weight-bearing region is yet present, with the exception of a small cortical irregularity seen laterally.

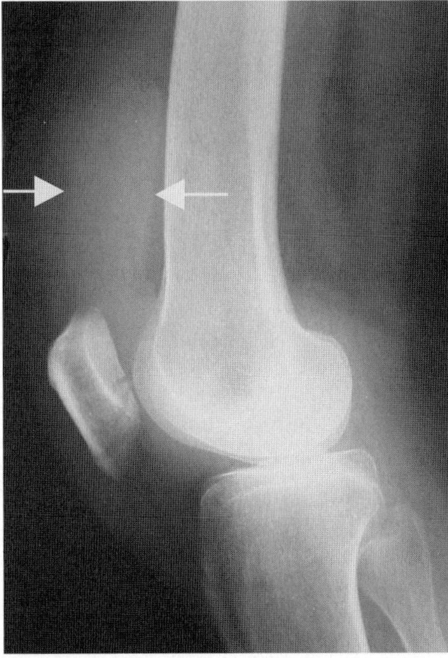

FIGURE 44.44. **Knee Joint Effusion.** This patient has joint fluid in the knee, with widely displaced fat-pads. The suprapatellar fat-pad (*left arrow*) is more than 5 mm from the anterior suprafemoral fat-pad (*right arrow*), which indicates a joint effusion. The patella is fractured.

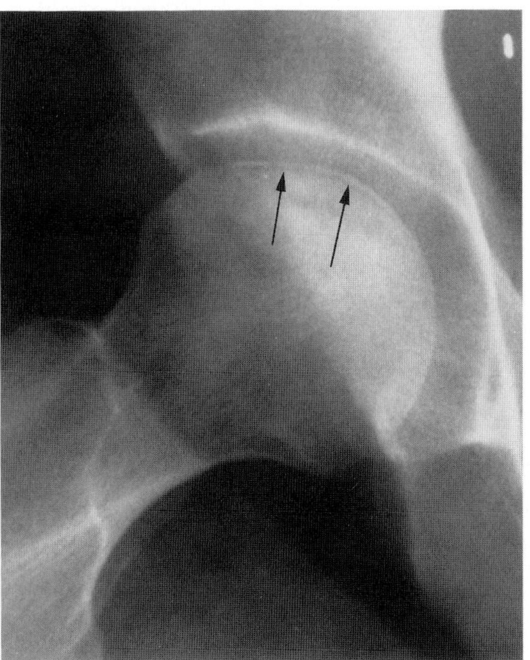

FIGURE 44.46. **Avascular Necrosis (AVN) of the Hip.** Subchondral lucency (*arrows*) is seen in the weight-bearing portion of this hip with AVN. Patchy sclerosis throughout the femoral head is also noted.

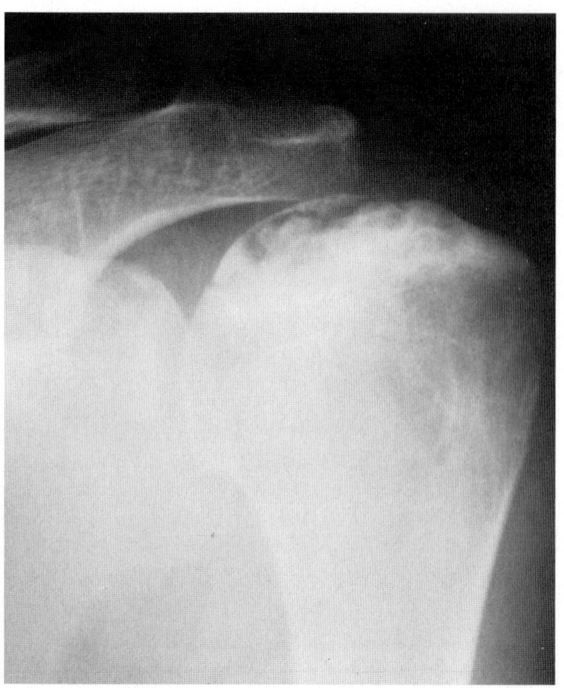

FIGURE 44.47. **Avascular Necrosis (AVN) of the Shoulder.** Articular surface collapse is present in this shoulder with longstanding AVN. Dense bony sclerosis is also present.

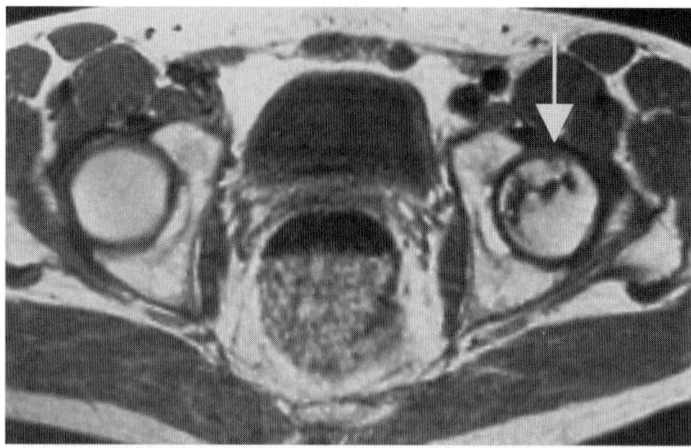

FIGURE 44.48. **Avascular Necrosis of the Hip.** An axial T1WI (time of repetition 600; time of echo 20) of the hips shows a focal area of abnormality in the left femoral head (*arrow*), which is characteristic for AVN. The low-signal, serpiginous border is a typical finding, as is the anterior location.

point out that an MR should never be performed just to see whether there is fluid in the joint.

Shoulder effusions are very difficult to detect unless they are massive enough to displace the humeral head inferiorly, as with a fracture and hemarthrosis (see Chapter 43). Fortunately, as with most other joints, treatment is not based solely on the presence or absence of an effusion, so it hardly matters. The same is true in the ankle, wrist, and smaller joints.

AVASCULAR NECROSIS

Avascular necrosis (AVN), or osteonecrosis, can occur around almost any joint for a host of reasons, including steroid use, trauma, a variety of underlying disease states, and even idiopathically. It is often seen in renal transplant patients.

The hallmark of AVN is increased bone density at an otherwise normal joint. Increased density at a narrowed joint usually indicates DJD; however, if either osteophytes or joint space narrowing are absent, another disorder should be considered.

The earliest sign of AVN is a joint effusion. This often is not visible radiographically or is so nonspecific that it does not help with the diagnosis unless the clinical setting had already raised suspicion for AVN. The next sign for AVN is a patchy or mottled density (Fig. 44.45). In the

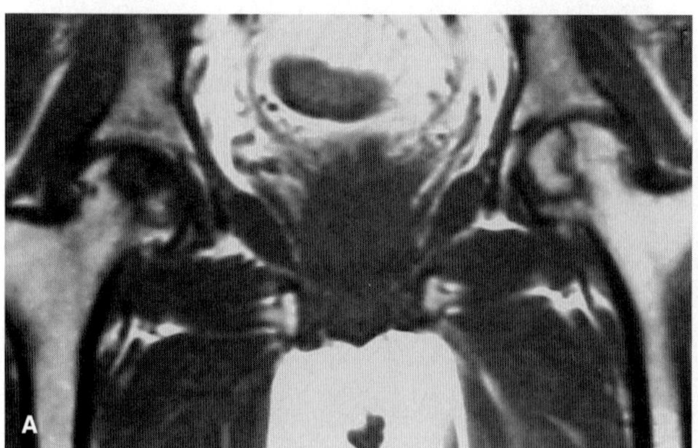

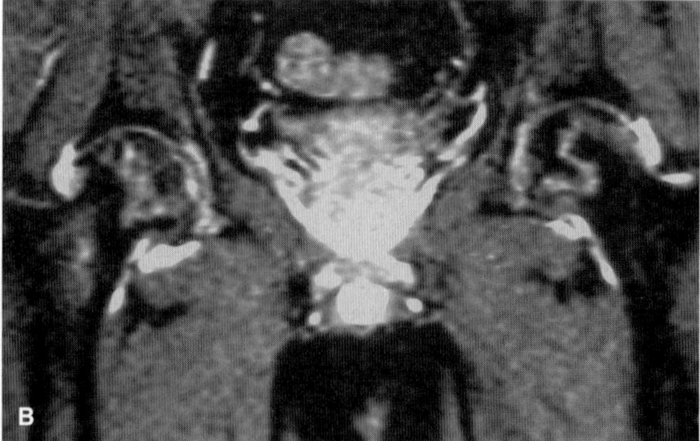

FIGURE 44.49. **Avascular Necrosis (AVN) of the Hip.** Coronal T1WI **(A)** (time of repetition 600; time of echo 20) and coronal STIR **(B)** images show bilateral AVN.

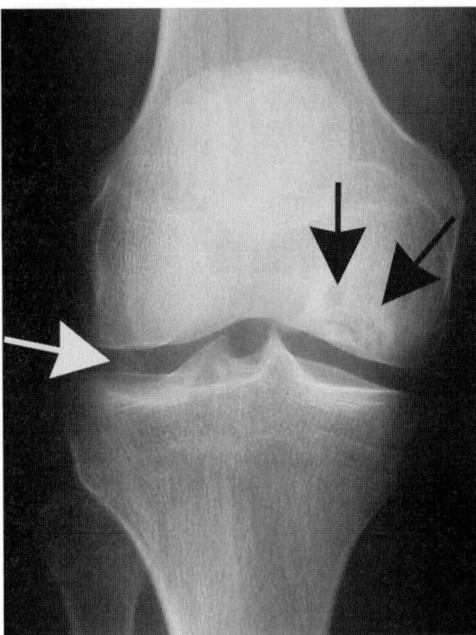

FIGURE 44.50. **Osteochondritis Dissecans.** A small focal area of avascular necrosis (AVN) in the medial epicondyle of the femur (*black arrows*) is present, which is an area of osteochondritis dissecans. Part of the area of AVN has shed a bony fragment (*white arrow*) that is loose in the joint, which is known as a loose body or "joint mouse."

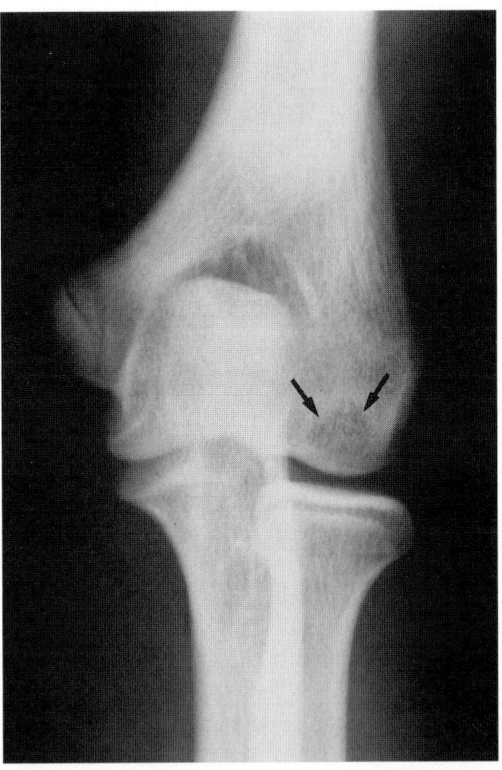

FIGURE 44.52. **Osteochondritis Dissecans of the Elbow.** The third most common site for osteochondritis dissecans is in the capitellum of the elbow. The faint lucency seen in this capitellum (*arrows*) was at first believed to be a chondroblastoma or an area of infection.

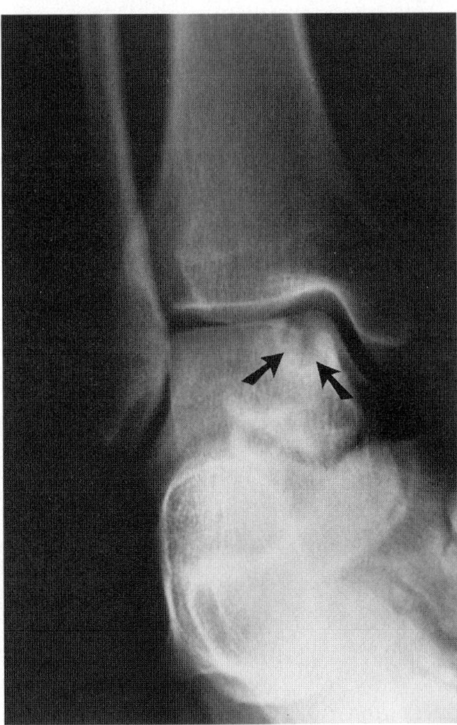

FIGURE 44.51. **Osteochondritis Dissecans of the Talus.** A focal area of avascular necrosis in the talus, as seen here (*arrows*), is called osteochondritis dissecans. The talus is the second most common site after the knee and, as in the knee, can cause a joint mouse, or loose body in the joint.

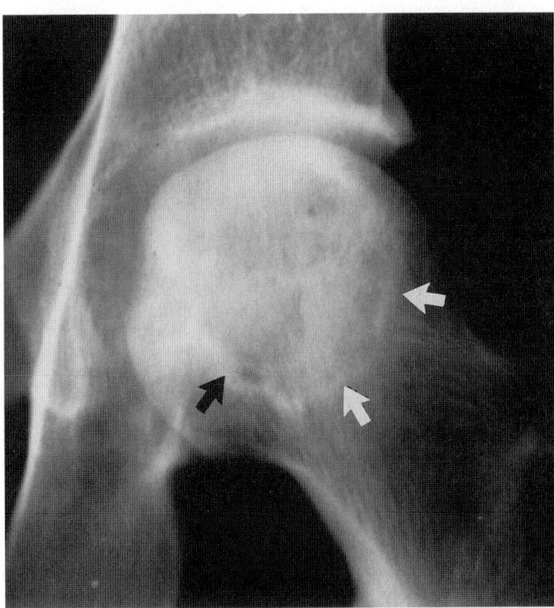

FIGURE 44.53. **Geode in the Hip.** A large cystic lesion (*arrows*) is seen in this patient with avascular necrosis (AVN) of the hip. Note the adjacent patchy sclerosis, indicative of AVN. A subchondral cyst or geode should be considered any time a lytic lesion is found around a joint.

knee, this density increase can occur throughout an entire condyle, whereas in the hip, it often involves the entire femoral head. Next, a subchondral lucency often develops that forms a thin line along the articular surface (Fig. 44.46). This lucent line has been described as being an early indicator for AVN, whereas, in fact, it is a late finding. Also, the lucent line stage is often not present in the evolution of AVN. Therefore, use of the lucent line as one of the main criteria for AVN can lead to missing early findings in some cases and missing the diagnosis completely in others.

The final sign in AVN is collapse of the articular surface and joint fragmentation (Fig. 44.47). I must stress that these changes all occur on only one side of a joint, which makes for an easy diagnosis because almost everything else around joints involves both sides of the joint.

MR is extremely useful in evaluating AVN. It is the most sensitive imaging study available, often showing AVN when plain films or radionuclide scans are normal (5). In the hip, AVN typically has an area of low or mixed signal on T1WIs that is located in the anterosuperior portion of the femoral head (Figs. 44.48, 44.49). If the anterior portion of the femoral head is not involved, the diagnosis of

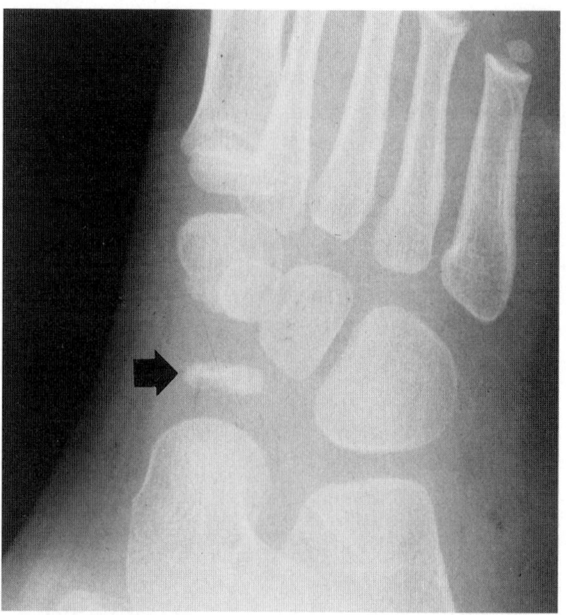

FIGURE 44.55. **Köhler Disease.** Flattening and sclerosis of the tarsal navicular (*arrow*) in children is thought by many to be avascular necrosis and is called Köhler disease. Others have found this to be an asymptomatic normal variant and believe that it is an incidental finding.

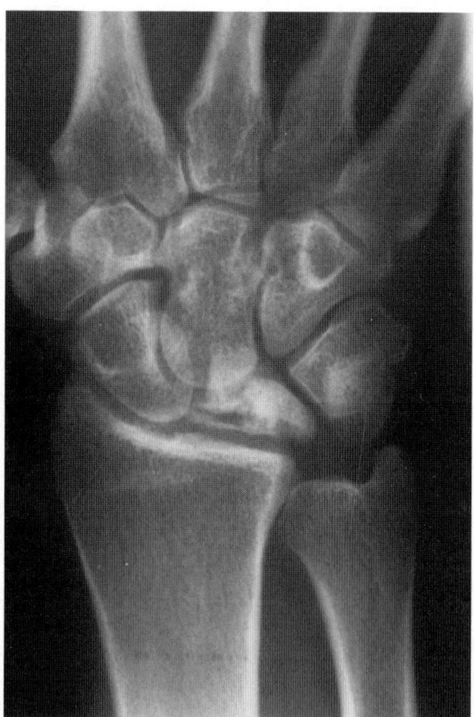

FIGURE 44.54. **Kienböck Malacia.** Avascular necrosis (AVN) of the lunate, or Kienböck malacia, is demonstrated in this patient's wrist. The increased density and partial fragmentation of the lunate are characteristic for AVN. Also, note the slightly shortened ulna (in comparison with the radius), which is called negative ulnar variance. Negative ulnar variance is said to have a high association with Kienböck malacia.

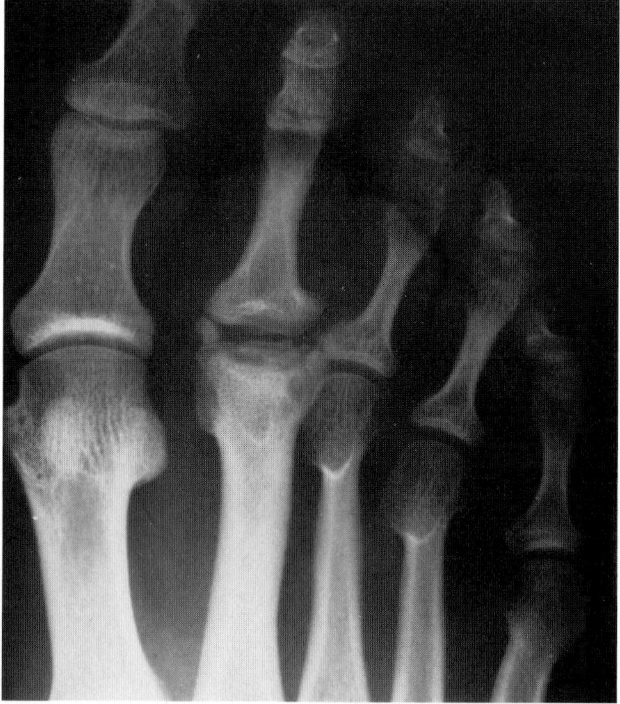

FIGURE 44.56. **Freiberg Infraction.** Flattening, collapse, and sclerosis of the second metatarsal head, as seen in this patient, is typical of avascular necrosis or Freiberg infraction. It can also involve the second, third, or fourth metatarsal heads. Note the compensatory hypertrophy of the cortex of the second metatarsal, which is invariably found with this disorder.

AVN should be questioned, as it is uncommon for this condition to present otherwise. Posterior femoral head AVN can occasionally be found after posterior dislocation of the hip because of impaction of the femoral head on the posterior column of the acetabulum.

A form of AVN that is smaller and more focal than that just described is osteochondritis dissecans. It is most likely caused by trauma; however, this is controversial, with one school of thought believing the cause is idiopathic. It occurs most often in the knee at the medial epicondyle (Fig. 44.50). It also is frequently seen in the dome of the talus (Fig. 44.51) and occasionally in the capitellum (Fig. 44.52). Osteochondritis dissecans frequently leads to a small fragment of bone being sloughed off and becoming a free fragment in the joint, i.e., a "joint mouse" (see Fig. 44.50).

AVN is one of the disorders around joints in which subchondral cysts or geodes can occur. It is the only one of the four disorders (rheumatoid arthritis, DJD, and CPPD being the others) that can have an essentially normal joint and have a geode (Fig. 44.53). The other abnormalities will have any or a combination of joint space narrowing, osteophytes, osteoporosis, chondrocalcinosis, or other findings.

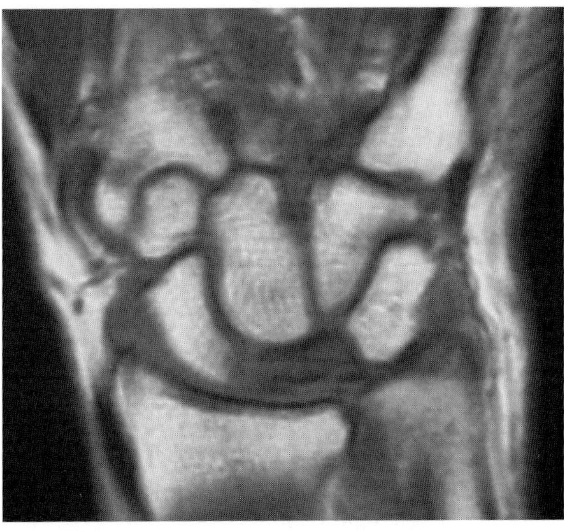

FIGURE 44.58. **Kienböck Malacia.** A coronal T1WI (time of repetition 600; time of echo 20) of the wrist shows low signal throughout the lunate, which is characteristic for avascular necrosis of the lunate, or Kienböck malacia.

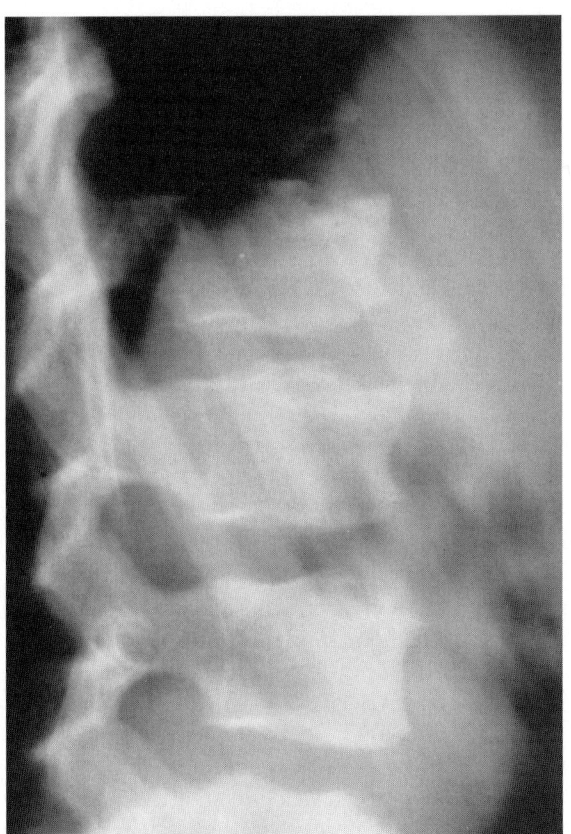

FIGURE 44.57. **Scheuermann Disease.** Avascular necrosis of the apophyseal rings of the vertebral bodies is called Scheuermann disease. He originally described a painful kyphosis with multiple vertebral bodies involved. It is most commonly seen without kyphosis or pain and with only a few vertebral bodies involved.

A host of names have been ascribed to certain bones with AVN, usually with the eponym being the first person to describe the disorder. These have been called osteochondroses. They are believed to be idiopathic for the most part but can also occur secondary to trauma. A few of the more common bones involved are the following: the carpal lunate in Kienböck malacia (Fig. 44.54); the tarsal navicular in Köhler disease (Fig. 44.55); the metatarsal heads in Freiberg infraction (Fig. 44.56); the femoral head in Legg-Perthes disease; the ring epiphyses of the spine in Scheuermann disease (Fig. 44.57); and the tibial tubercle in Osgood-Schlatter disease, also called surfer's knees. MR can be very useful in identifying AVN in these sites. It shows diffuse low signal on T1WIs that involves the entire area of AVN (Fig. 44.58).

REFERENCES

1. Resnick D, Shaul S, Robins J. Diffuse idiopathic skeletal hyperostosis with extraspinal manifestations. Radiology 1975;115:513–524.
2. Resnick D, Niwayama G, Coutts R. Subchondral cysts (geodes) in arthritic disorders: pathologic and radiographic appearance of the hip joint. AJR Am J Roentgenol 1977;128:799–806.
3. Resnick D, Niwayama G, Goergen T, et al. Clinical, radiographic and pathologic abnormalities in calcium pyrophosphate dihydrate deposition disease (CPPD): pseudogout. Radiology 1977;122:1–15.
4. Helms CA, Chapman GS, Wild JH. Charcot-like joints in calcium pyrophosphate dihydrate deposition disease. Skeletal Radiol 1981;7:55–58.
5. Mitchell D, Kressel H, Arger P, et al. Avascular necrosis of the femoral head: morphologic assessment by MR imaging, with CT correlation. Radiology 1986;161:739–742.

Chapter 45

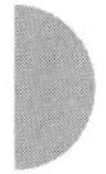

Metabolic Bone Disease

Clyde A. Helms

Osteoporosis

Osteomalacia

Hyperparathyroidism

Hypoparathyroidism

Pseudohypoparathyroidism and Pseudopseudohypoparathyroidism

Pituitary Gland Hyperfunction

Thyroid Gland Hyperfunction

Thyroid Gland Hypofunction

Osteosclerosis

OSTEOPOROSIS

Osteoporosis is defined as diminished bone *quantity* in which the bone is otherwise normal. This contrasts to osteomalacia, in which the bone quantity is normal but the *quality* of the bone is abnormal in that it is not normally mineralized. Osteomalacia results in excess nonmineralized osteoid. It is not possible in most cases to distinguish between osteoporosis and osteomalacia on plain films; hence, many prefer the term "osteopenia" for the plain film finding of diminished mineralization.

There are myriad causes of osteoporosis, the most common of which is primary osteoporosis (so-called senile osteoporosis or osteoporosis of aging). This is seen most commonly in postmenopausal women and is a major health concern because of the increase in vertebral body and hip fractures in this patient population.

Secondary osteoporosis implies that an underlying disorder, such as thyrotoxicosis or renal disease, has caused the osteoporosis. Only about 5% of osteoporosis cases are of the secondary type. The differential diagnosis for secondary osteoporosis is quite long and probably should not be memorized. One cannot even be sure whether it is osteoporosis or osteomalacia on the basis of plain films; therefore, the differential for presumed osteoporosis would have to include the causes of osteomalacia.

The main radiographic finding in osteoporosis is thinning of the cortex. Although this can be seen in any bone, it is most reliably demonstrated in the second metacarpal at the middiaphysis. Normal metacarpal cortical thickening should be approximately one fourth to one third the thickness of the metacarpal (Fig. 45.1). In osteoporosis, this cortical thickness is decreased (Fig. 45.2). The metacarpal cortex (and all bony cortices, for that matter) decreases in thickness normally with age and is thinner in women than in men of the same age. Several tables have been published that give normal metacarpal cortical measurements, with age and sex adjustments to assist in the determination of normal. Unfortunately, these only determine the mineralization of the peripheral skeleton and do not seem to relate to whether vertebral body or hip fractures will occur.

Measurement of the bone mineral content in the axial skeleton can be done by one of several methods that use CT to assess bone quantity in the spine. There is much debate about which method is superior and even about whether knowledge of the bone mineral content is clinically more helpful than just knowing the age and sex of the patient, which is fairly accurate for predicting the bone mass quantity.

Exercise and proper diet seem to help delay the onset of primary osteoporosis. Calcium additives have not been shown to reverse the process of primary osteoporosis. Estrogen clearly plays a role in alleviating postmenopausal osteoporosis, yet its use in a widespread manner is somewhat controversial.

A type of osteoporosis that can be seen in a patient of any age is ***disuse osteoporosis***. It results from immobilization from any cause, most commonly following treatment

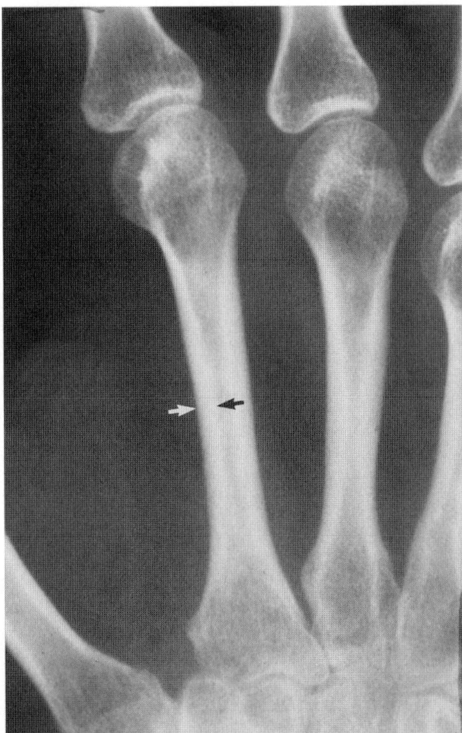

FIGURE 45.1. **Normal Mineralization.** The cortical width (*arrows*) at the mid–second metacarpal in this patient with normal mineralization is greater than one third of the total width of the metacarpal.

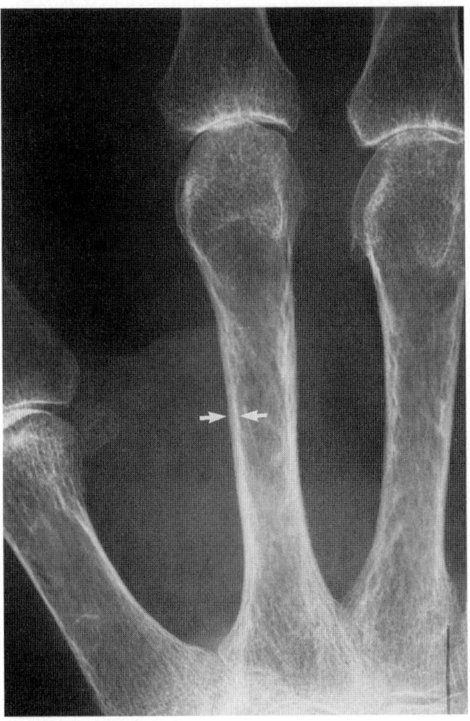

FIGURE 45.2. **Osteoporosis.** Severe cortical narrowing (*arrows*) at the midsecond metacarpal cortex is seen in this patient with severe osteoporosis. Note the intracortical tunneling, which occurs in more aggressive forms of osteoporosis.

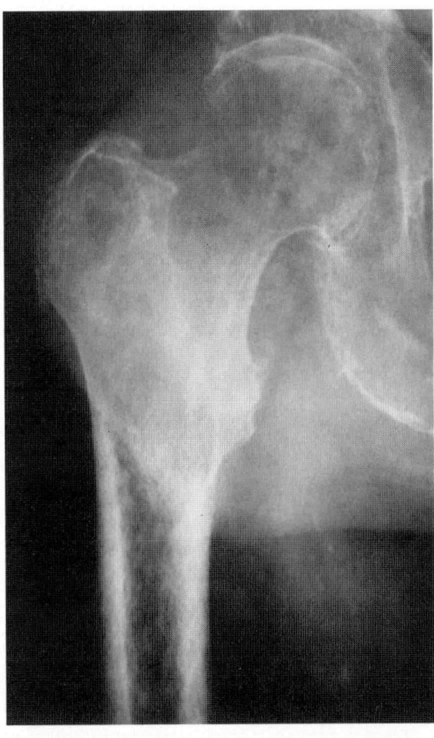

FIGURE 45.3. **Disuse Osteoporosis.** A mottled, patchy appearance is present in the proximal right femur in this patient with aggressive disuse osteoporosis secondary to an amputation. Note the mottled, irregular cortex seen in the femoral shaft, which is representative of cortical holes that can be seen in aggressive osteoporosis.

of a fracture. The radiographic appearance of disuse osteoporosis differs from that of primary osteoporosis in that it occurs somewhat more rapidly and gives the bone a patchy appearance (Fig. 45.3). This is from osteoclastic resorption in the cortex, which causes intracortical holes. If the disuse were to continue, the bone would resemble any bone with marked osteoporosis, that is, severe cortical thinning.

Occasionally, aggressive osteoporosis from disuse can mimic a permeative lesion, such as a Ewing sarcoma or multiple myeloma, because of the multiple cortical holes that project over the medullary space, thus resembling a medullary permeative process (Fig. 45.4). The way to differentiate a true intramedullary permeative process from an intracortical process such as osteoporosis is to observe the cortex and see whether it is solid or riddled with holes (Fig. 45.5). If the cortex is solid, one can assume the permeative process is emanating from the medullary space (Fig. 45.6); if the cortex has multiple small holes, the clinician can assume the permeative pattern is from the cortical process. I call a permeative appearance that is secondary to cortical holes a "pseudopermeative" process to distinguish it from a true permeative process (1).

Other causes for a pseudopermeative process include hemangioma and radiation. A hemangioma can cause cortical holes in two ways: from focal hyperemia causing

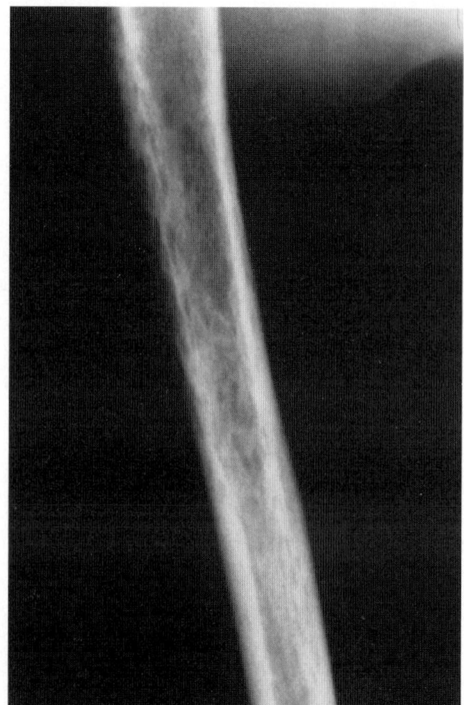

FIGURE 45.4. **Aggressive Osteoporosis.** Multiple small holes are seen in the cortex and overlying the medullary space in the proximal humerus of this patient who has suffered a stroke. This represents aggressive osteoporosis from disuse and is mimicking an aggressive permeative process. These holes are, however, almost entirely within the cortex of the bone.

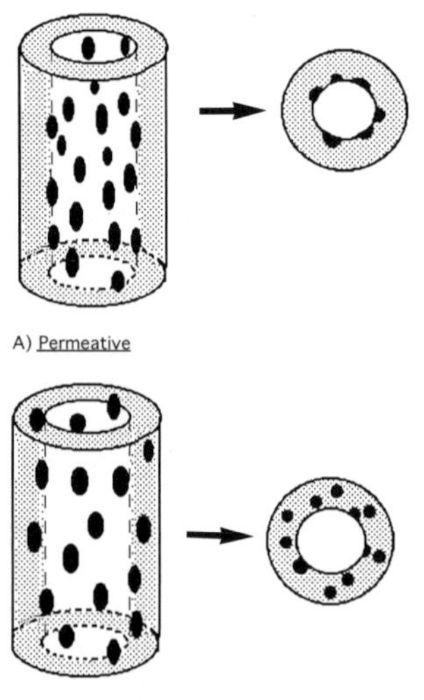

FIGURE 45.5. **Differentiation of Permeative Process. A.** Schematic of a permeative lesion. A true permeative process has multiple small holes secondary to endosteal involvement, with sparing of the cortex. This represents a marrow process. **B.** Schematic of a pseudopermeative process. A pseudopermeative process such as osteoporosis has multiple small cortical holes that are then superimposed over the marrow, giving an appearance similar to that of a permeative process.

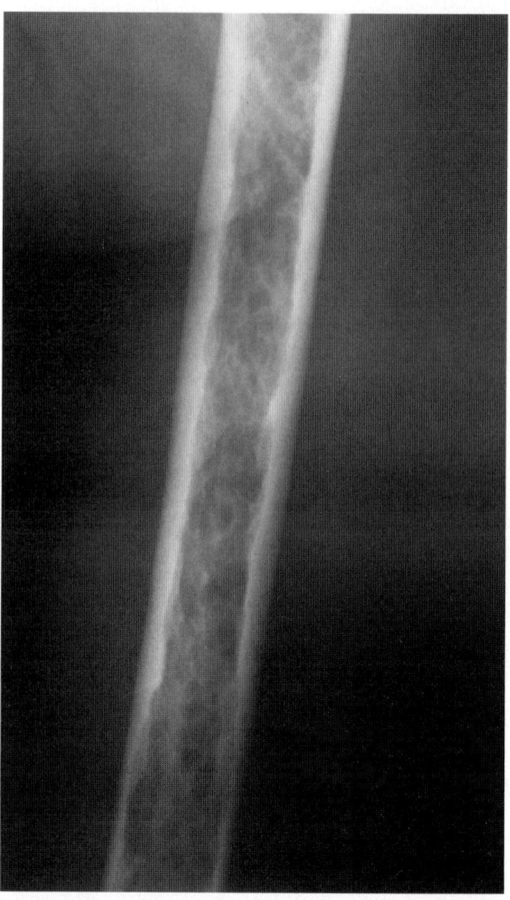

FIGURE 45.6. **Myeloma Causing a Permeative Process.** A diffuse permeative process throughout the femur is seen in this patient with myeloma. Note that the cortex is solid, although the endosteum has some scalloping. This is a true permeative process.

focal osteoporosis, or by the blood vessels themselves tunneling through the cortex (Fig. 45.7). Radiation can cause cortical holes in bone and mimic a permeative pattern because of the death of cortical osteocytes, which can result in large lacunae in the cortex (Fig. 45.8). The cortical holes from radiation can be large, in which case they would not be confused with a true permeative process, but they can also be small and resemble an aggressive lesion.

If a permeative lesion is found, the differential diagnosis is usually an aggressive process such as Ewing sarcoma, infection, or eosinophilic granuloma in a young person (<30 years of age) or multiple myeloma, metastatic carcinomatosis, or primary lymphoma of bone in an older patient. If, however, the permeative pattern is a result of cortical holes—that is, a pseudopermeative pattern—the differential diagnosis is considerably less sinister: *aggressive osteoporosis, hemangioma,* or *radiation changes.* This differential diagnosis does not arise often but is very useful when it does (Table 45.1).

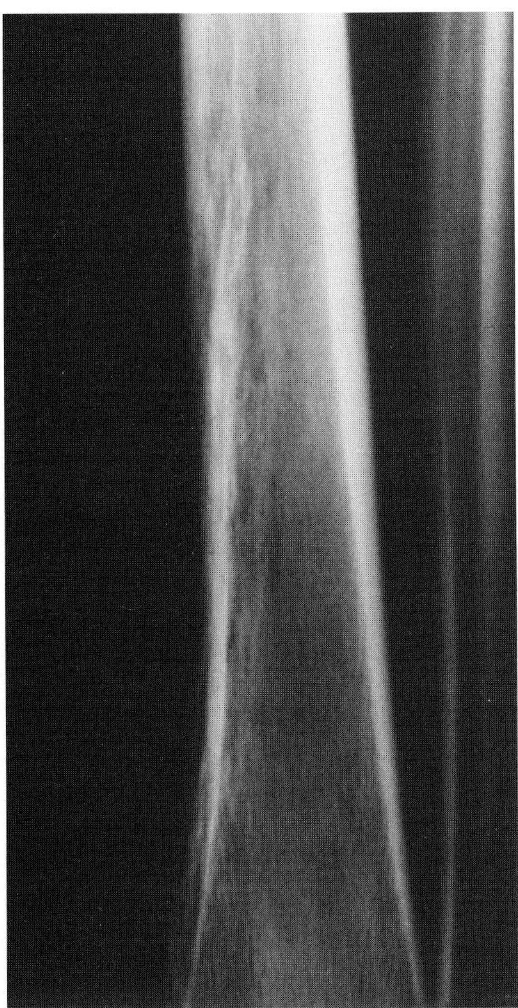

FIGURE 45.7. **Pseudopermeative Process Secondary to Hemangioma.** A permeative pattern is seen in the distal tibia in this patient with pain and swelling. It was thought to represent a Ewing sarcoma, and a biopsy was performed, with subsequent heavy loss of blood. This was found to be a hemangioma. An examination of the cortex demonstrates that the medial aspect is diffusely riddled with cortical holes, compared with the lateral aspect. The endosteum laterally also is completely spared, making a marrow process very unlikely. Hemangioma, radiation, and osteoporosis can cause a pseudopermeative process, although in this example, osteoporosis and radiation would be unlikely because of its focal nature.

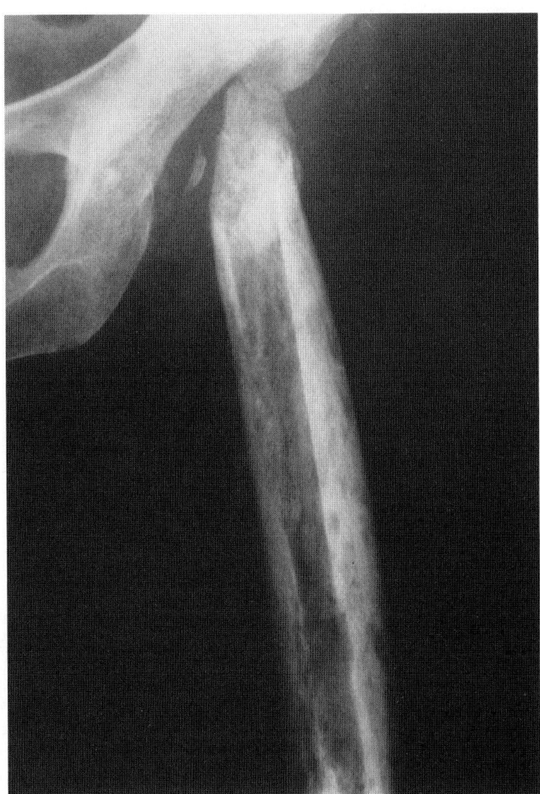

FIGURE 45.8. **Pseudopermeative Pattern Secondary to Radiation.** This patient had a fibrosarcoma treated with excision of the femoral head and subsequent radiation. A follow-up film shows a diffuse permeative pattern throughout the proximal femur. Because the cortex is riddled with holes, it was thought that this was secondary to radiation rather than tumor recurrence. This is a pseudopermeative appearance secondary to radiation.

OSTEOMALACIA

Osteomalacia, as mentioned earlier, is the result of too much nonmineralized osteoid. The most common cause is renal osteodystrophy. The plain radiographic findings are almost identical to those of osteoporosis, and, for the most part, the two disorders are indistinguishable. The only finding that is pathognomonic for osteomalacia is a Looser fracture, which is a fracture through large osteoid seams (Fig. 45.9). They are extremely uncommon but tend to occur in the femur, pelvis, and scapula.

In children, osteomalacia is called ***rickets***. It causes the epiphyses to become flared and irregular and the long bones to undergo bending from the bone softening (Fig. 45.10). As in adults, the most common cause is renal disease, although other causes such as biliary disease and dietary insufficiencies are occasionally seen.

HYPERPARATHYROIDISM

Hyperparathyroidism (HPT) occurs from excess parathyroid hormone. Parathyroid hormone (PTH) causes osteoclastic resorption in bone, which leads to osteoporosis and

TABLE 45.1 Differential Diagnosis of Pseudopermeative Pattern

Aggressive osteoporosis
Hemangioma
Radiation

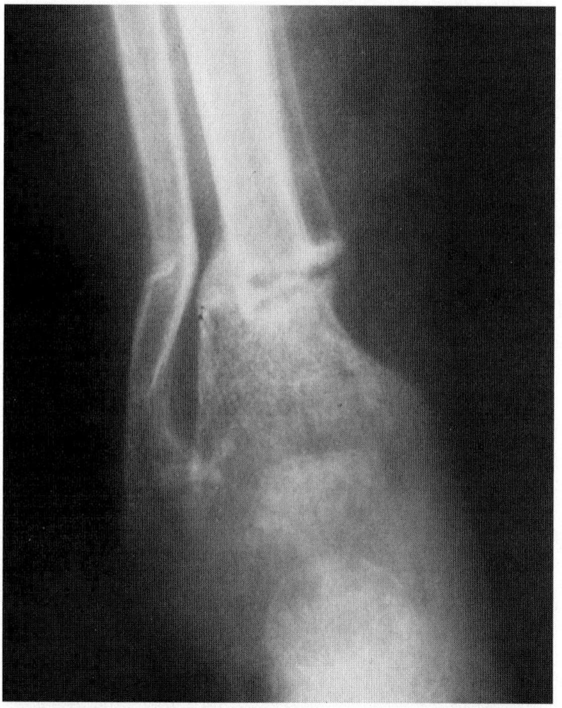

FIGURE 45.9. **Looser Fractures in Osteomalacia.** Horizontal fractures of the tibia and the fibula are present in this child with osteomalacia (rickets). Fractures of this type are called Looser fractures and are virtually pathognomonic for osteomalacia; however, they are rarely seen.

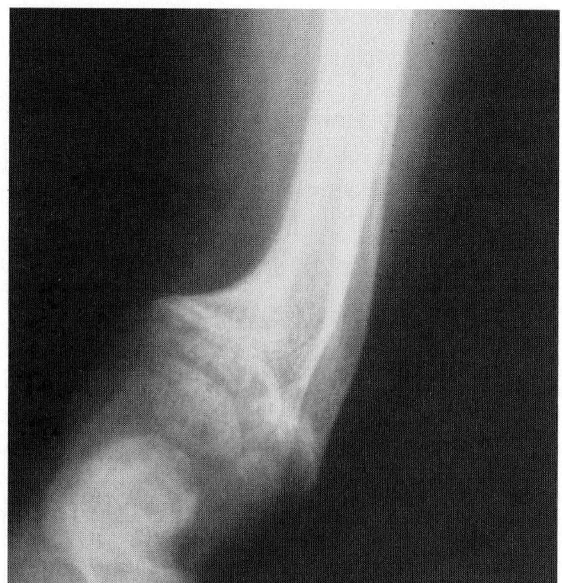

FIGURE 45.10. **Rickets.** Osteomalacia in children is called rickets and is identified by fraying and splaying of the epiphyses, as well as bending of the bone secondary to softening. This patient had renal osteodystrophy.

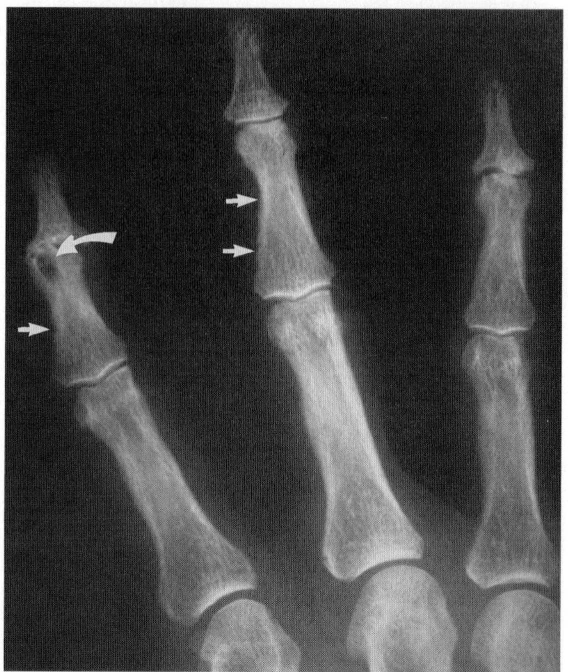

FIGURE 45.11. **Hyperparathyroidism (HPT).** Subperiosteal bone resorption can be seen at the radial aspect of the middle phalanges (*straight arrows*), which is pathognomonic for HPT. The lytic lesion seen in the distal middle phalanx (*curved arrow*) may be a small brown tumor.

osteomalacia. Primary HPT is caused by parathyroid adenomas and hyperplasia. Up to 40% of patients with primary HPT will demonstrate skeletal abnormalities radiographically. The most common cause of HPT is from renal disease, which leads to secondary HPT. Secondary HPT is the result of the parathyroids secreting excess PTH in response to the hypocalcemia that occurs.

The radiographic sign that is pathognomonic for HPT is subperiosteal bone resorption. It is seen most commonly on the radial aspect of the middle phalanges of the hand (Fig. 45.11), but it can be seen in any long bone in the body. It is commonly seen on the medial aspect of the proximal tibia, at the sacroiliac joints (Fig. 45.12), and in the distal clavicle.

Other radiographic findings include osteosclerosis, which is usually diffuse but often involves the spine in a manner resembling the stripes on rugby jerseys, hence the name "rugger jersey spine" (Fig. 45.13). Brown tumors are cystic lesions that are often expansile and aggressive in appearance (Fig. 45.14). They were once said to be more common in primary HPT but today are seen more commonly in association with secondary HPT because of the overwhelming preponderance of patients with secondary disease compared with primary disease. A brown tumor can have a variety of appearances, so its only unique characteristic is its association with subperiosteal bone

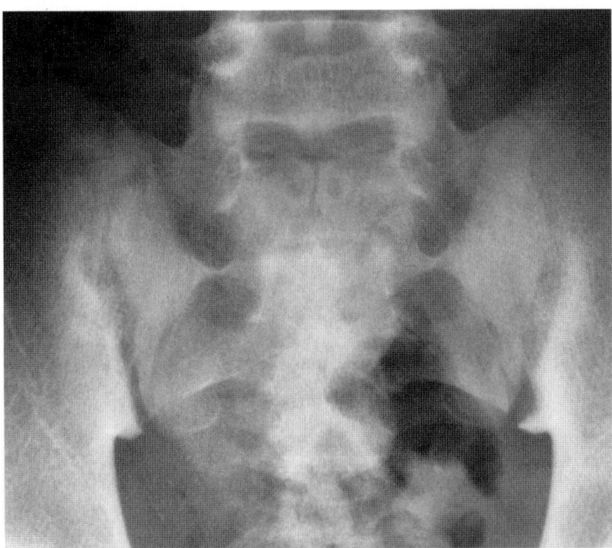

FIGURE 45.12. **Hyperparathyroidism (HPT).** Bilateral sacroiliac joint erosive changes with sclerosis are present in this patient with renal osteodystrophy and secondary HPT. Bilateral sacroiliac joint changes such as this are often seen with HPT.

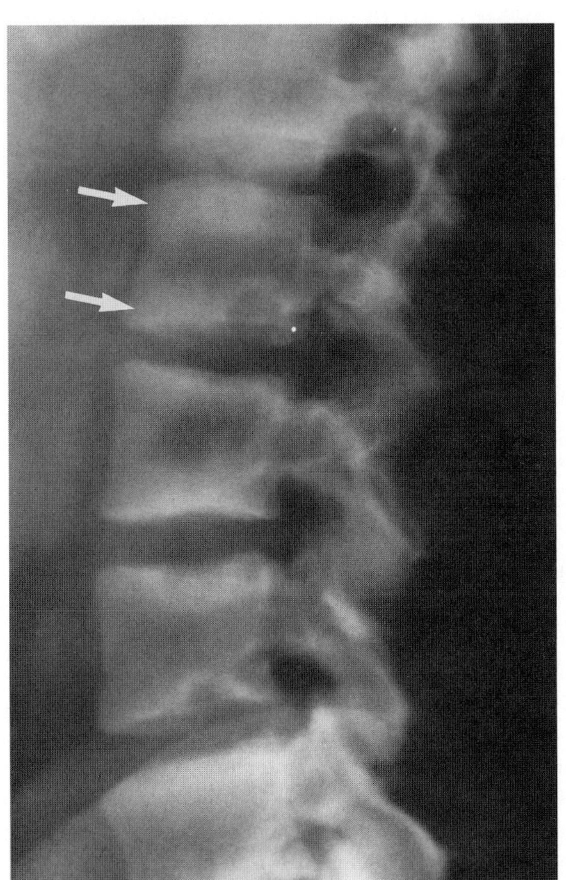

FIGURE 45.13. **Hyperparathyroidism (HPT).** Sclerotic bands present at the vertebral body endplates (*arrows*) are characteristic of a rugger jersey spine. This is seen in HPT.

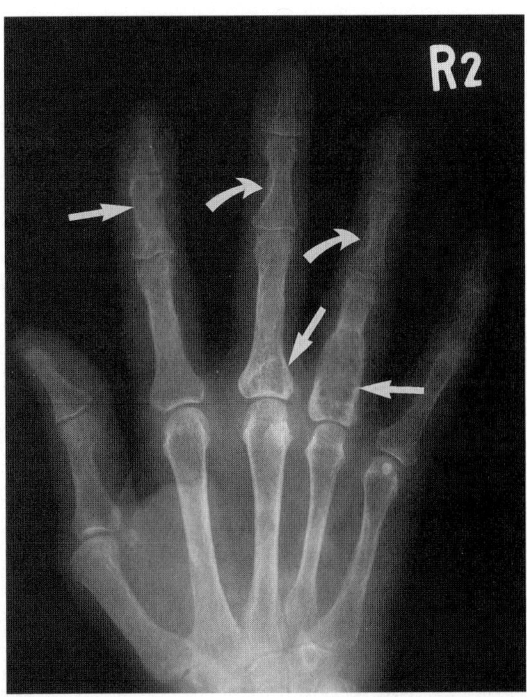

FIGURE 45.14. **Brown Tumors in Hyperparathyroidism (HPT).** Several lytic lesions are present in the phalanges (*straight arrows*) in this patient with HPT; these are brown tumors. Note the subperiosteal bone resorption in the radial aspect of the middle phalanges (*curved arrows*), which is pathognomonic for HPT.

resorption. If the underlying HPT is treated, the subperiosteal resorption may disappear before the brown tumor does. This is not commonly seen, however.

Metabolic bone surveys (plain films of the hands, spine, and long bones) were once routinely obtained in patients to look for subperiosteal bone resorption, brown tumors, osteosclerosis, calcifications, and Looser fractures. They are no longer recommended, however, as the yield of positive findings is extremely low and a positive finding will rarely affect treatment. In place of the metabolic bone survey, it is now recommended that plain films of the hands be obtained to look for subperiosteal resorption (2). A radionuclide bone scan can be obtained in selected cases, which will show increased radionuclide uptake by brown tumors and Looser fractures. Also, investigation of causes of hypercalcemia, which can be caused by metastatic disease or metabolic bone disease, should include a bone scan (3).

HYPOPARATHYROIDISM

Hypoparathyroidism occurs because of a deficiency of the parathyroid glands, which secrete abnormally low amounts of PTH. Few skeletal changes occur in hypoparathyroidism. The calvaria on occasion will show thickening, and calcification in the basal ganglia of the brain has been described.

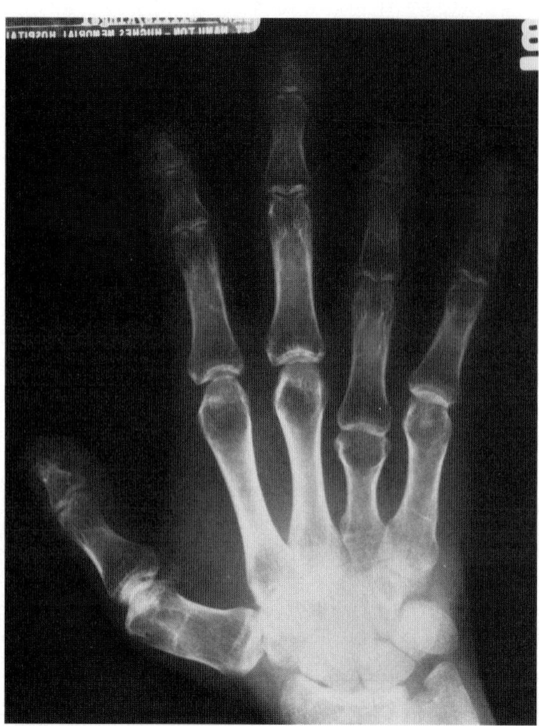

FIGURE 45.15. **Pseudohypoparathyroidism.** Brachydactyly is present in several of the metacarpals in this patient with pseudohypoparathyroidism. A short fourth metacarpal, as seen here, is a frequent finding in this entity.

PSEUDOHYPOPARATHYROIDISM AND PSEUDOPSEUDOHYPOPARATHYROIDISM

Pseudohypoparathyroidism is caused by a congenital failure of tissues to respond to PTH. The parathyroid glands are normal in these cases. Treatment of these patients with PTH is of no help because the problem lies in the end organs, not in the parathyroid glands. A characteristic appearance is seen in these patients: obesity, round facies, short stature, and brachydactyly (Fig. 45.15). The tubular bones of the hands and feet are often all short. In pseudopseudohypoparathyroidism, there is no parathyroid abnormality and no end-organ problem; these patients merely resemble patients with pseudohypoparathyroidism. In summary, hypoparathyroidism is a parathyroid gland problem, pseudohypoparathyroidism is an end-organ problem, and pseudopseudohypoparathyroidism mimics pseudohypoparathyroidism morphologically.

PITUITARY GLAND HYPERFUNCTION

A secreting adenoma or hyperplasia of the anterior lobe of the pituitary gland will result in accelerated bone growth. If it occurs before the epiphyses close, it causes giantism.

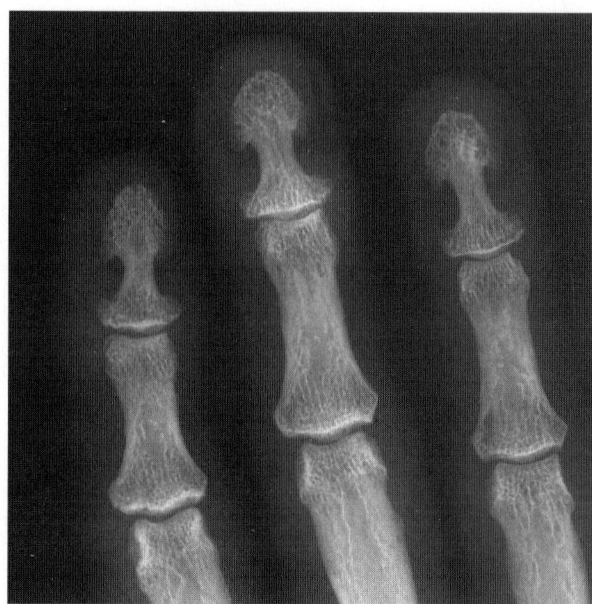

FIGURE 45.16. **Acromegaly.** Enlargement of the distal tufts in the phalanges (so-called spade tufts) is characteristic in acromegaly.

If it occurs after the epiphyses are closed, the result is acromegaly.

Acromegaly has several characteristic radiographic features in the skeletal system. The skull film invariably shows calvarial thickening, enlarged sinuses, and an enlarged sella turcica. The jaw is prognathic. The terminal tufts of the distal phalanges become hypertrophied and have a so-called spade appearance (an appearance not unlike a spade or shovel) (Fig. 45.16). The joint spaces are occasionally minimally enlarged because of hypertrophy of the hyaline articular cartilage. Early DJD ensues because the cartilage itself is abnormal. The soft tissues also hypertrophy, with various measurements of soft tissue thickening used by some as an indicator for acromegaly. For instance, thickening of the heel pad adjacent to the calcaneus has been used as a sign of acromegaly.

THYROID GLAND HYPERFUNCTION

In children, hyperthyroidism can result in increased skeletal maturation; however, this is seldom marked. A rare manifestation of hyperthyroidism in adults is thyroid acropachy. This occurs only after prior thyroidectomy, and the cause is unknown. A characteristic-appearing periostitis occurs in the metacarpals and phalanges of the hands and feet (Fig. 45.17). It invariably involves the ulnar aspect of the fifth metacarpal, a useful differential point that can be used to tell thyroid acropachy from other causes of diffuse periostitis, such as hypertrophic pulmonary osteoarthropathy and pachydermoperiostitis, a rare form of idiopathic periostitis and skin thickening.

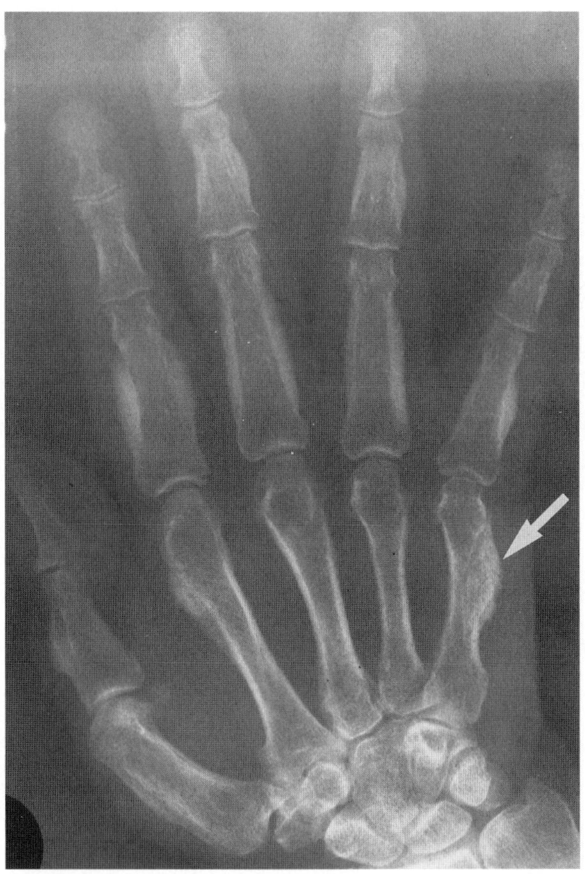

FIGURE 45.17. **Thyroid Acropachy.** Extensive periostitis is noted in the metacarpals and phalanges in this patient with thyroid acropachy. It is characteristic to have marked involvement of the ulnar aspect of the fifth metacarpal (*arrow*) in this entity.

THYROID GLAND HYPOFUNCTION

Decreased thyroid secretion, or cretinism, results in delayed skeletal maturation in children. Delay in ossification of epiphyseal centers with occasional appearance of "stippled" epiphyses is seen. A delay in epiphyseal closure also occurs, in some instances with failure of epiphyseal closure noted in the third and fourth decade.

OSTEOSCLEROSIS

The radiographic finding of diffuse increased bone density, osteosclerosis, is somewhat uncommon, yet every radiologist must have a differential diagnosis for this process. Fortunately, it is a rather short differential, and there are criteria to narrow down the list of possibilities.

The list of diseases that can cause diffuse osteosclerosis is quite long, but a list that includes 95% to 98% of the pathologic processes is all that is really necessary. The entities I include in the differential diagnosis of diffuse osteosclerosis are listed in Table 45.2.

TABLE 45.2 Differential Diagnosis of Diffuse Bony Sclerosis (Dense Bones)

Renal osteodystrophy
Sickle cell disease
Myelofibrosis
Osteopetrosis
Pyknodysostosis
Metastatic carcinoma
Mastocytosis
Paget disease
Athletes
Fluorosis

The mnemonic I use to remember them is "*R*egular *S*ex *M*akes *O*ccasional *P*erversions *M*uch *M*ore *P*leasurable *A*nd *F*antastic." I will cover each of these topics in generalities, trying to point out the features of each that should be looked for to allow inclusion or exclusion from the differential.

Renal Osteodystrophy. Anything that causes HPT can cause osteosclerosis, but renal disease is by far the most common disease in which osteosclerosis is seen. Although the most common presentation of renal osteodystrophy is osteopenia, about 10% to 20% of patients with renal osteodystrophy will exhibit osteosclerosis, and the reasons for it are unknown. As mentioned previously, the sine qua non of renal osteodystrophy is subperiosteal bone resorption, seen earliest and most reliably at the radial aspect of the middle phalanges of the hands. Without this finding, osteosclerosis caused by renal disease should not be entertained.

Sickle Cell Disease. As in renal osteodystrophy, the underlying cause of dense bones in sickle cell disease is unknown. It occurs in a small percentage of patients. Additional signs to look for are bone infarcts and step-off deformities of the vertebral body endplates (Fig. 45.18). These are also called "fish" vertebrae because they resemble the vertebrae found in fish. Avascular necrosis of the hip is frequently an accompanying finding.

Myelofibrosis. Also called *agnogenic myeloid metaplasia,* myelofibrosis is a disease caused by progressive fibrosis of the marrow in patients older than 50 years of age. It leads to anemia, with marked splenomegaly and extramedullary hematopoiesis. Whenever osteosclerosis is seen in a patient older than 50 years of age, a search should be made for a large spleen and extramedullary hematopoiesis (Fig. 45.19).

Osteopetrosis is a hereditary abnormality that results in extremely dense bones throughout the skeleton (Fig. 45.20). There are congenital and tarda forms, with different degrees of severity in each. The congenital form occurs at birth and can be lethal. Anemia, jaundice, hepatosplenomegaly, and infections are often present in this form. The tarda form is seen in older children and adults

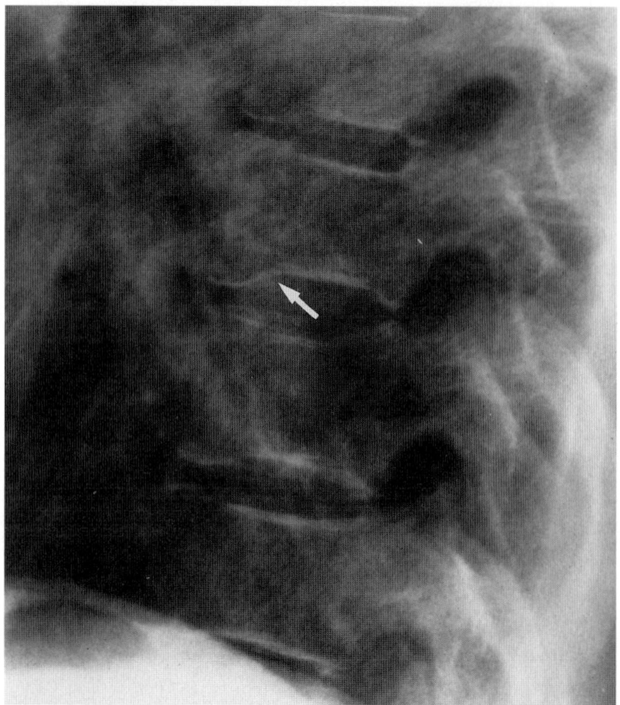

FIGURE 45.18. Sickle Cell Disease. Step-off deformities (*arrow*) are seen in the endplates of several vertebral bodies in this patient with sickle cell disease. They are also nicknamed "fish vertebrae."

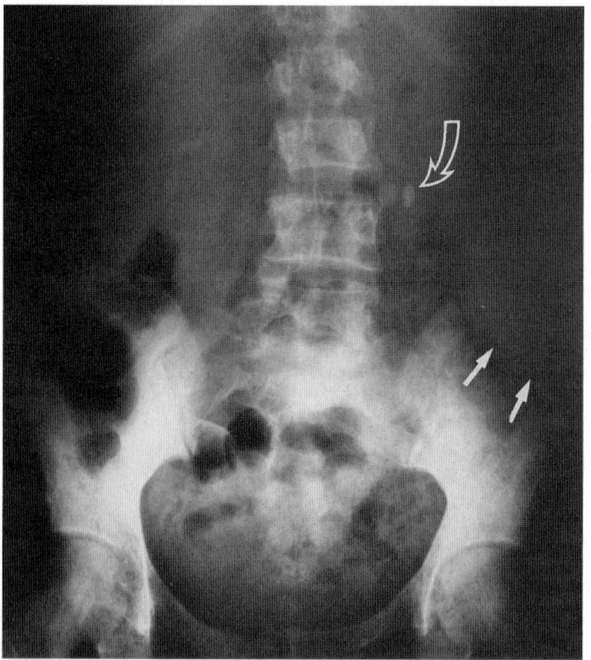

FIGURE 45.19. Myelofibrosis. Diffusely increased bone density is seen throughout the pelvis and spine in this patient with myelofibrosis. The spleen is markedly enlarged (*straight arrows*), and opaque iron tablets (*curved arrow*) can be seen, which were taken for the anemia that is often found in this disorder.

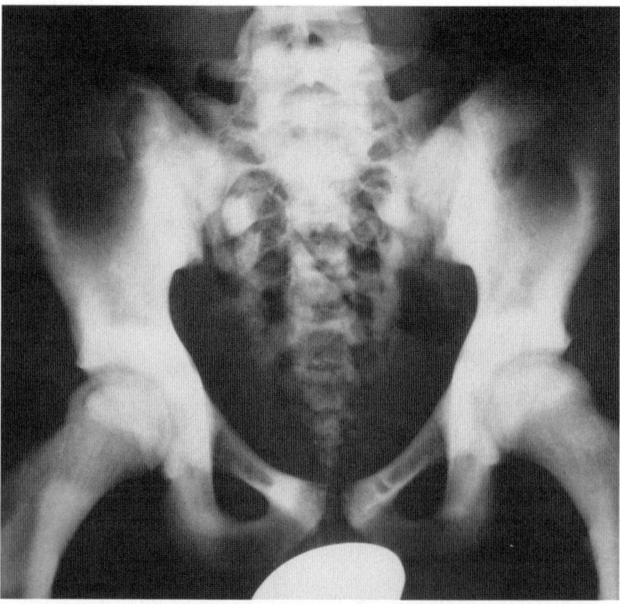

FIGURE 45.20. Osteopetrosis. Marked, diffuse bony sclerosis is seen throughout the skeleton in this patient with osteopetrosis.

and has milder clinical problems—in fact, it may be so mild that it has no clinical findings. Although uncommon, it is not so rare that one will never see a case; therefore, it should be included in this differential diagnosis. A characteristic finding is the so-called bone-in-bone appearance often seen in the vertebral bodies, in which the vertebrae have a small replica of the vertebral body inside the normal one. Also characteristic are "sandwich vertebrae," in which the endplates are densely sclerotic, giving the appearance of a sandwich (Fig. 45.21). The sandwich vertebrae appearance resembles a rugger jersey spine but the pattern is much denser and more sharply defined.

Pyknodysostosis is the other congenital abnormality with dense bones that should be considered in the differential diagnosis of osteosclerosis. It is seen less commonly than osteopetrosis. These patients are typically short and have hypoplastic mandibles. The distinguishing radiographic finding that is essentially pathognomonic is acroosteolysis with sclerosis. The distal phalanges often have the appearance of chalk that has been put into a pencil sharpener: they are pointed and dense (Fig. 45.22). No other disease process has this appearance. Another name for this disorder is Toulouse-Lautrec syndrome, named for the famous artist who was afflicted with pyknodysostosis.

Metastatic Carcinoma. Only rarely will diffuse metastatic carcinoma cause a problem in diagnosis. I have seen only a handful of cases in which diffuse metastatic carcinoma mimicked diffuse osteosclerosis, and in every case, the primary tumor was either prostate or breast

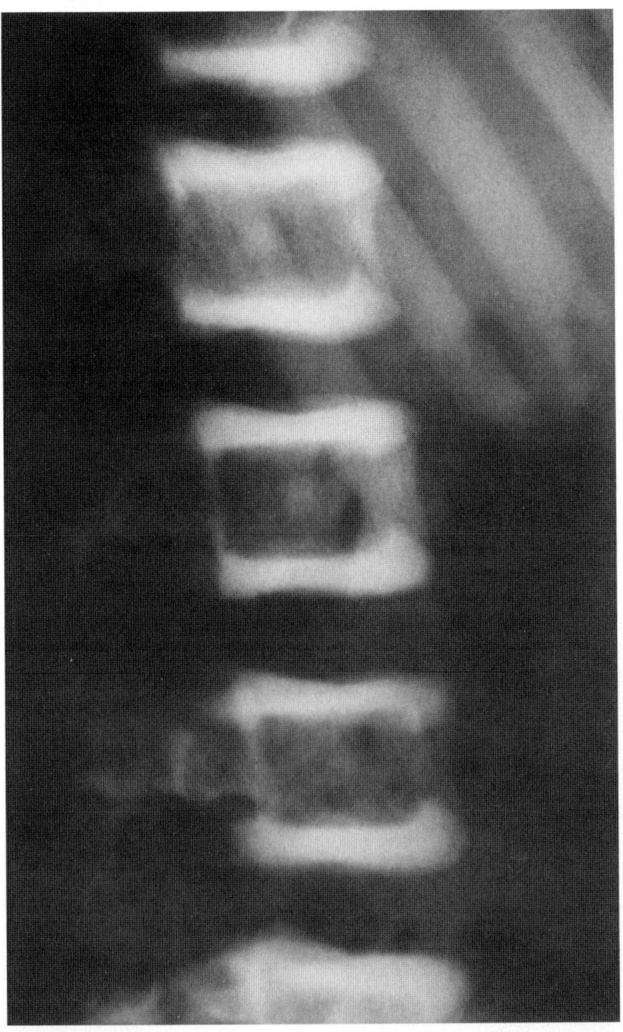

FIGURE 45.21. **Sandwich Vertebrae.** Dense bands of sclerosis parallel to the endplates are seen in this patient with osteopetrosis. These are called sandwich vertebrae, which are much more distinct than the dense bands of sclerosis seen in a rugger jersey spine (see Fig. 45.13).

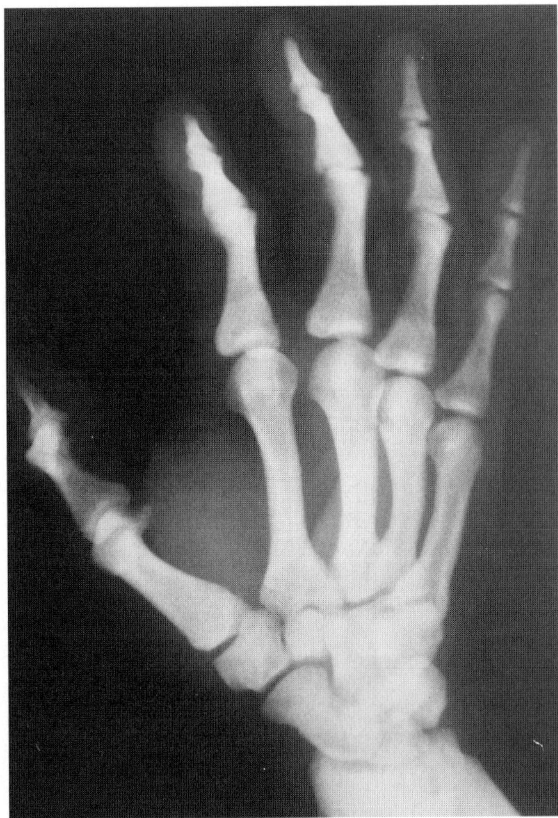

FIGURE 45.22. **Pyknodysostosis.** Diffuse, dense sclerosis is seen throughout the hand and wrist in this patient with pyknodysostosis. Note the absent distal phalangeal tufts, which appear pointed and sclerotic; this appearance is virtually pathognomonic for pyknodysostosis.

carcinoma. If cortical destruction or a lytic component is present, it simplifies the differential diagnosis, so a search should be made for these.

Mastocytosis is another rare disorder that can cause uniformly increased bone density. Unfortunately, there are no other plain film findings that might help with the diagnosis. Patients with this disease have thickened small bowel folds with nodules, but, of course, to see these, an upper GI contrast study must be performed (Fig. 45.23). Urticaria pigmentosa is a characteristic skin lesion found in these patients.

Paget Disease. Diffuse Paget disease that could be confused with one of the other diseases in the differential diagnosis of generalized osteosclerosis is very rare. Paget disease classically causes bony enlargement (Fig. 45.24),

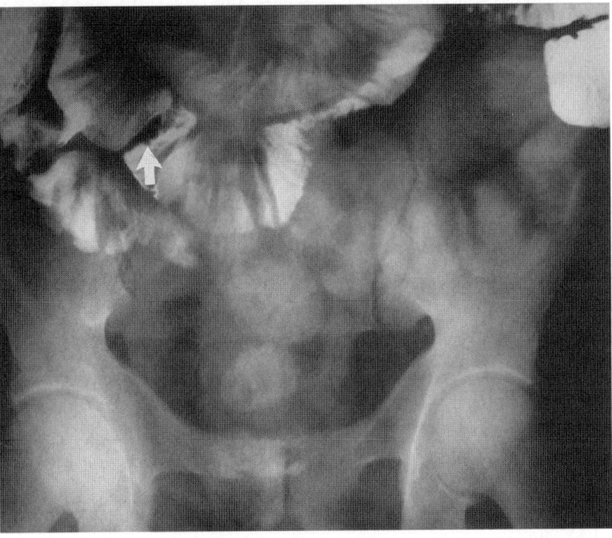

FIGURE 45.23. **Mastocytosis.** Uniformly increased bone density is seen throughout the pelvis in this patient with mastocytosis. In the small bowel, thickened folds with nodules (*arrow*) can be seen in this barium study; these are often found in mastocytosis.

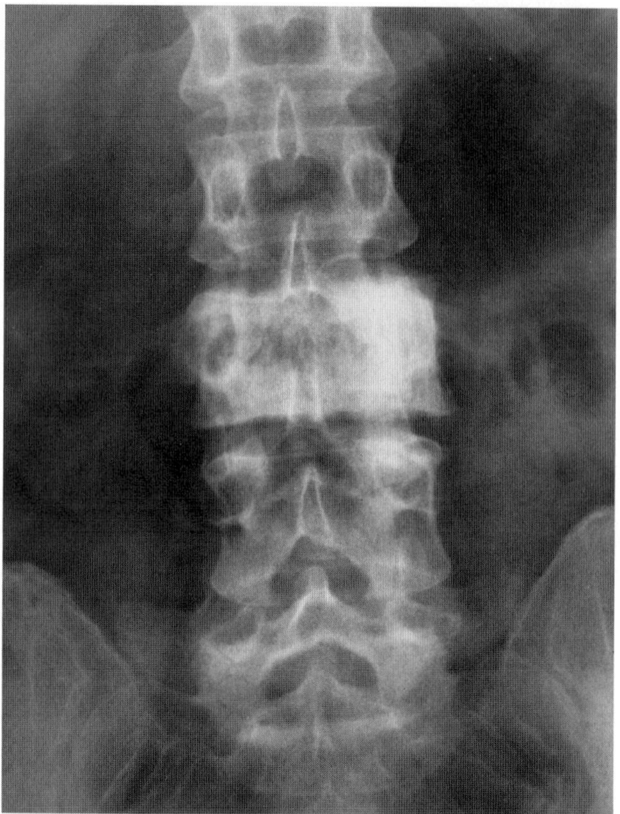

FIGURE 45.24. **Paget Disease.** Dense, bony sclerosis with overgrowth of the vertebral body is seen at the L3 vertebra in this patient with Paget disease. The left L3 pedicle is markedly dense and enlarged.

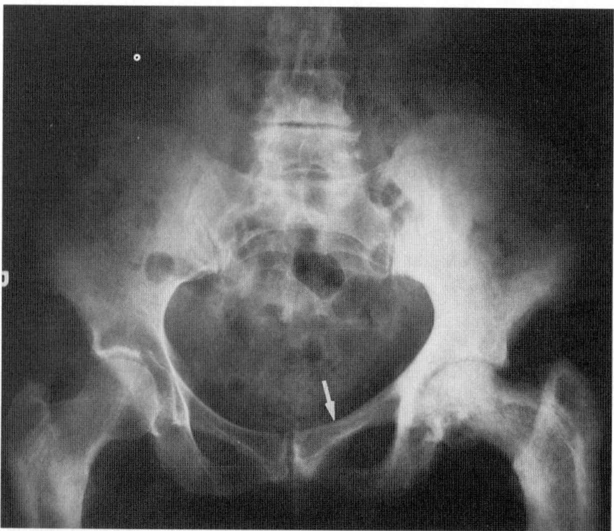

FIGURE 45.25. **Paget Disease.** Bony sclerosis with some bony enlargement is seen in the left pelvis and proximal femur of this patient and is characteristic of Paget disease. Note the cortical thickening of the left superior pubic ramus (*arrow*), which is called thickening of the iliopectineal line and is commonly seen in Paget disease.

but this is not always present. It occurs most commonly in the pelvis (Fig. 45.25), where it has been said that the iliopectineal line on the pelvic brim must be thickened if Paget disease is present. In fact, the iliopectineal line is usually, but not always, thickened. Paget disease can occur in any bone in the body, including the smaller bones of the hands and feet.

Paget disease has three distinct phases that are visible radiographically: a lytic phase, a sclerotic phase, and

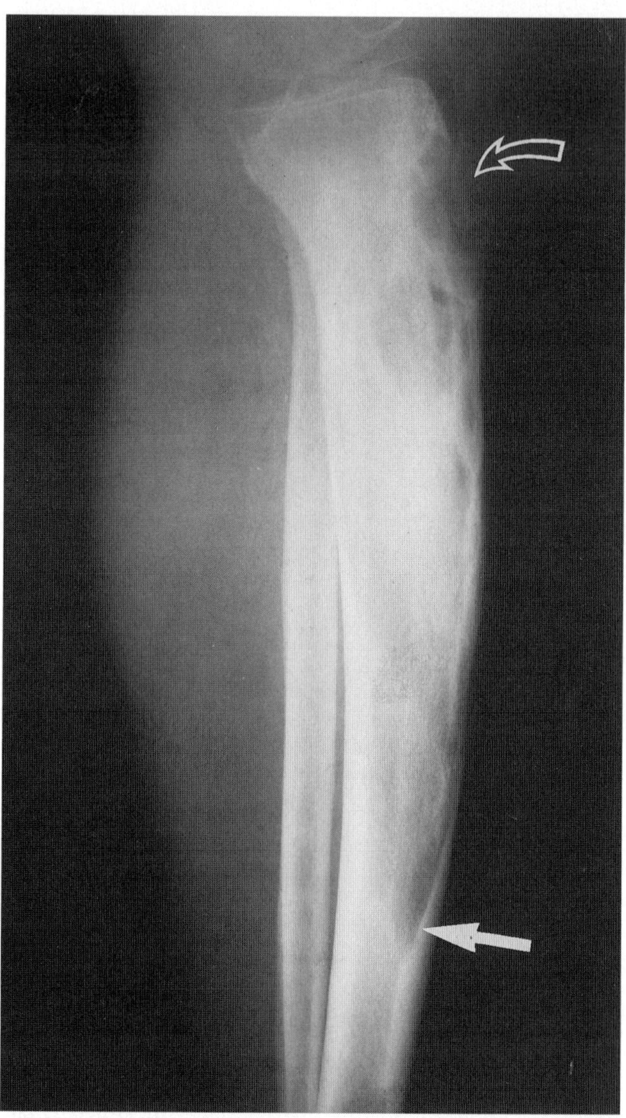

FIGURE 45.26. **Paget Disease.** A lytic process involving the proximal two thirds of the tibia is noted and has a blade-of-grass or flame-shaped leading edge (*straight arrow*), which is characteristic for Paget disease. This represents the lytic phase of Paget disease. The sclerotic phase of Paget disease can be seen in the midportion of this lesion, and an area of probable sarcomatous degeneration can be seen in the proximal tibia (*curved arrow*), where apparent cortical destruction is noted. This represents all three phases or stages of Paget disease.

a mixed lytic-sclerotic phase. The lytic phase often has a sharp leading edge, called a flame-shaped or blade-of-grass leading edge (Fig. 45.26). In a long bone, with the sole exception being the tibia, Paget disease always starts at the end of the bone; therefore, if a lesion is present in the middle of a long bone and does not extend to either end, one can safely exclude Paget disease.

Athletes. Conventional radiographs of professional athletes quite often demonstrate increased cortical thickness and apparent diffuse osteosclerosis, to the point of appearing pathologic. Undoubtedly, increased stress causes hypertrophy of bone as well as muscle. The increased density in these otherwise normal subjects is occasionally misinterpreted as abnormal, with extensive workups and even bone biopsy resulting.

Fluorosis is a rare disorder that is usually a result of chronic intake of fluoride in certain geographic areas where large amounts of fluoride are present in the drinking water. It can also be a result of long-term therapy with sodium fluoride for osteoporosis. A radiographic finding that patients with fluorosis often have is ligamentous calcification. Calcification of the sacrotuberous ligament is said to be characteristic for fluorosis.

There are other categories of disease that could be covered in a chapter on metabolic bone disease, but most of the remaining disorders are exceedingly rare and not likely to be seen by most radiologists on a routine basis.

REFERENCES

1. Helms C, Munk P. Pseudopermeative skeletal lesions. Br J Radiol 1990;63:461–467.
2. Cooper KL. Radiology of metabolic bone disease. Endocrinol Metab Clin North Am 1989;18:955–976.
3. McAfee JG. Radionuclide imaging in metabolic and systemic skeletal diseases. Semin Nucl Med 1987;17:334–349.

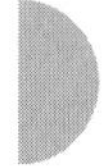

Chapter 46

Skeletal "Don't Touch" Lesions

Clyde A. Helms

Posttraumatic Lesions

Normal Variants

Obviously Benign Lesions

Skeletal "don't touch" lesions are those processes that are so radiographically characteristic that a biopsy or additional diagnostic tests are unnecessary. Not only does the biopsy result in unnecessary morbidity and cost, but in some instances, as discussed in this chapter, a biopsy can also be frankly misleading and lead to additional unnecessary surgery.

Most radiology training stresses giving a differential diagnosis of a lesion, leaving it up to the clinician to decide between the various entities. For the "don't touch" lesions, however, a differential list is inappropriate, as that often makes the next step in the decision-making process a biopsy. Because these lesions do not need to undergo biopsy for a final diagnosis, a radiologic diagnosis should be made without a list of differential possibilities. These lesions can be classified into three categories: (*1*) posttraumatic lesions, (*2*) normal variants, and (*3*) lesions that are real but obviously benign.

POSTTRAUMATIC LESIONS

Myositis ossificans is an example of a lesion that should not undergo biopsy because its aggressive histologic appearance can often mimic a sarcoma (1). Unfortunately, radical surgery has been performed based on the histologic appearance of myositis ossificans when the radiologic appearance was diagnostic. The typical radiologic appearance of myositis ossificans is circumferential calcification with a lucent center (Fig. 46.1). This is often best appreciated on a CT scan (Fig. 46.2). A malignant tumor that mimics myositis ossificans has an ill-defined periphery and a calcified or ossific center (Fig. 46.3). Periosteal reaction can be seen with myositis ossificans or with a tumor. Occasionally, the peripheral calcification of myositis ossificans can be too faint to appreciate; in these cases, a CT scan should help, or delayed films 1 or 2 weeks later are recommended. Biopsy should be avoided when myositis ossificans is a clinical consideration. MR can be misleading because the peripheral calcification is not as well seen, and edema in the soft tissues can extend beyond the calcific rim (Fig. 46.4).

Avulsion Injury. Another posttraumatic entity in which a biopsy can be misleading is any avulsion injury (2,3). These injuries can have an aggressive radiographic appearance, but because of their characteristic location at ligament and tendon insertion sites (e.g., anteroinferior iliac spine or ischial tuberosity), they should be recognized as benign. (Figs. 46.5, 46.6). As with myositis ossificans, delayed films of several weeks will usually allow the problem case to become more radiographically clear. Biopsy can lead to the mistaken diagnosis of a sarcoma and should therefore be avoided. Any area undergoing healing can have a high nuclear-to-chromatin ratio and a high mitotic figure count, thereby occasionally simulating a malignancy histologically.

Cortical desmoid is a process on the medial supracondylar ridge of the distal femur that is considered by many to be the result of an avulsion of the adductor magnus muscle. It occasionally simulates an aggressive lesion radiographically, and histologically, it can look malignant (4). In many instances, biopsy has led to amputation for this benign, radiographically characteristic lesion (Figs. 46.7, 46.8). Cortical desmoids occur only on the posteromedial epicondyle of the femur. They might or might not be associated with pain and can have increased radionuclide uptake on a bone scan. They might or might not exhibit periosteal new bone and usually occur in young people. Biopsy should be avoided in all cases. Painful cortical

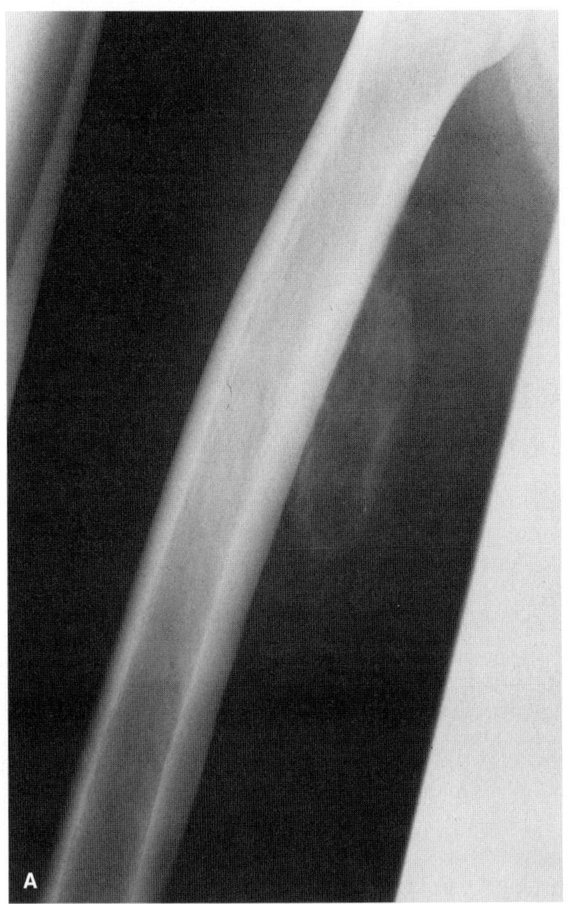

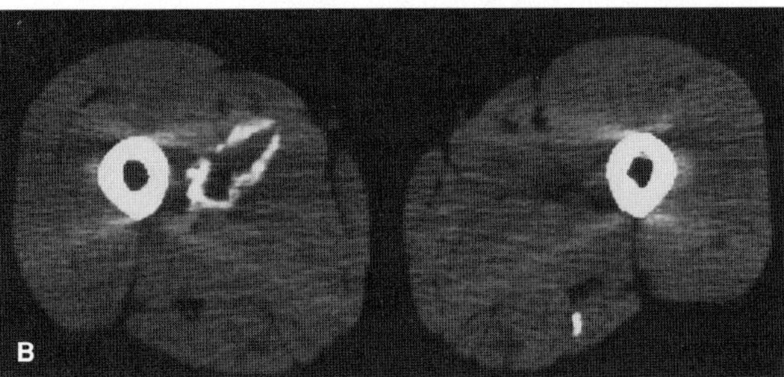

FIGURE 46.1. **Myositis Ossificans.** A plain film of the femur **(A)** in this patient who presented with a soft tissue mass shows a calcific density adjacent to the posterior cortex of the femur, which is calcified primarily in its periphery. If it is difficult to determine from the plain film alone that this is definitely peripheral, circumferential calcification, a CT scan **(B)** can be helpful in showing that the calcification is unequivocally peripheral in nature. This is virtually diagnostic of myositis ossificans.

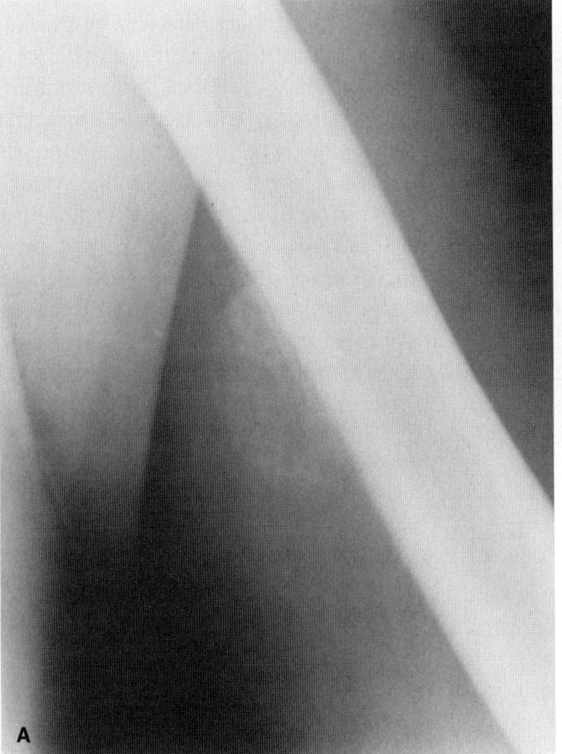

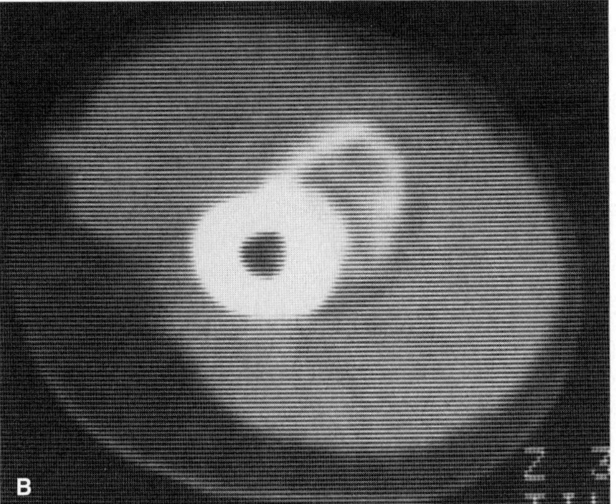

FIGURE 46.2. **Myositis Ossificans. A.** Hazy calcification is seen adjacent to the humeral shaft, with underlying periosteal reaction noted. It is difficult to ascertain whether the calcification is circumferential. **B.** A CT scan through this mass shows that the calcification is unequivocally circumferential in nature, making the diagnosis of myositis ossificans a certainty.

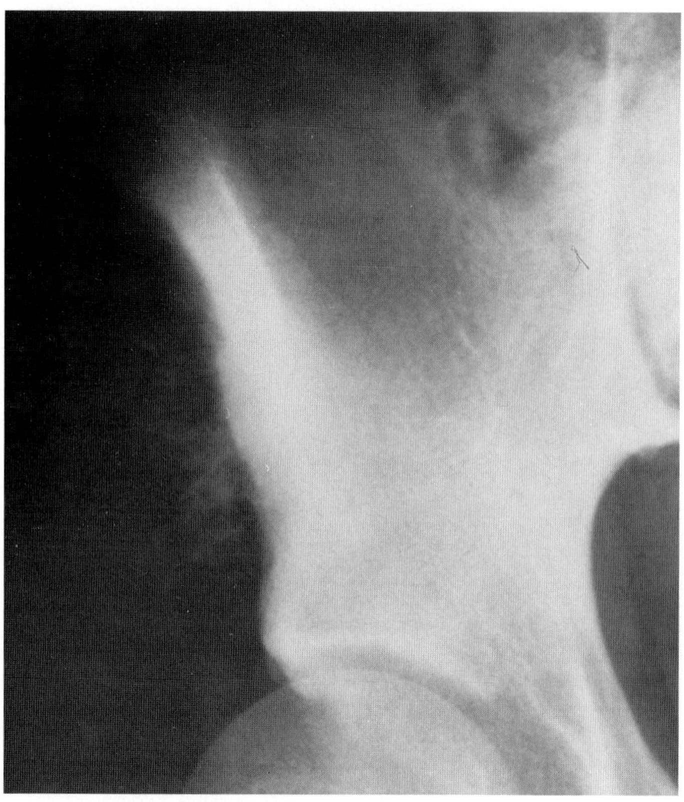

FIGURE 46.3. **Osteogenic Sarcoma.** Hazy, ill-defined calcification is seen adjacent to the iliac wing in this patient, which can be ascertained from the plain film as definitely not circumferential in nature. Although a prior history of trauma was obtained in this case, myositis ossificans is not a consideration with this appearance of calcification. Biopsy showed this to be an osteogenic sarcoma.

desmoids should become asymptomatic with rest. They are often seen as an incidental finding on MR of the knee and have a characteristic appearance (Fig. 46.9).

Trauma can lead to large, cystic geodes or subchondral cysts near joints and can be mistaken for other lesions, resulting in a biopsy being ordered. Although the biopsy specimen is not likely to mimic a malignant process, it is nevertheless avoidable. Because geodes from degenerative joint disease are almost always associated with additional findings such as joint space narrowing, sclerosis, and osteophytes, a diagnosis should be made radiographically (Fig. 46.10). On occasion, however, the additional findings are subtle and can be missed (Fig. 46.11). Geodes can also occur in the setting of calcium pyrophosphate dihydrate crystal disease, rheumatoid arthritis, and avascular necrosis (5,6).

Discogenic Vertebral Sclerosis. An entity that is often confused for metastatic disease to the spine is discogenic vertebral disease. It can mimic metastatic disease very closely, and unless the radiologist is familiar with this process, it can lead to an unnecessary biopsy (7). Discogenic vertebral disease most often is sclerotic and focal (Fig. 46.12). It is always adjacent to the endplate, and the associated disk space should be narrow. Osteophytosis is invariably present. It really is a variant of a Schmorl node and should not be confused with a metastatic focus. On occasion it can be lytic or even mixed lytic-sclerotic. The typical clinical setting is a middle-aged woman with chronic low back pain. Old films often confirm the benign nature of this process. In the setting of disk space narrowing and osteophytosis, focal sclerosis adjacent to an endplate should not undergo biopsy (8).

Fracture. Occasionally, a fracture will be the cause of extensive osteosclerosis and periostitis, which can mimic a primary bone tumor (Fig. 46.13). Lack of immobilization can result in exuberant callus, which can be misinterpreted as aggressive periostitis or even new tumor bone. Results of a biopsy in such a case might resemble a malignant lesion; therefore, any case associated with trauma should be carefully reviewed for a fracture.

Pseudodislocation of the Humerus. Another traumatic process that can be misdiagnosed radiologically, leading to inappropriate treatment and morbidity, is a pseudodislocation of the humerus (Fig. 46.14). This results from a fracture with hemarthrosis, which causes distension of the joint and migration of the humeral head inferiorly (9). An axial or transscapular view shows it is not anteriorly or posteriorly dislocated (the usual forms of shoulder dislocation) but merely inferiorly subluxated. On an anteroposterior view, it can mimic a posterior dislocation in that the normal superimposition of the humeral head and the glenoid is missing. Often, attempts are made to "relocate" the humeral head, which, of course, are both fruitless (because it is not dislocated) and painful. A fracture is invariably present, and if not seen on the initial films, it should be sought with additional views. The

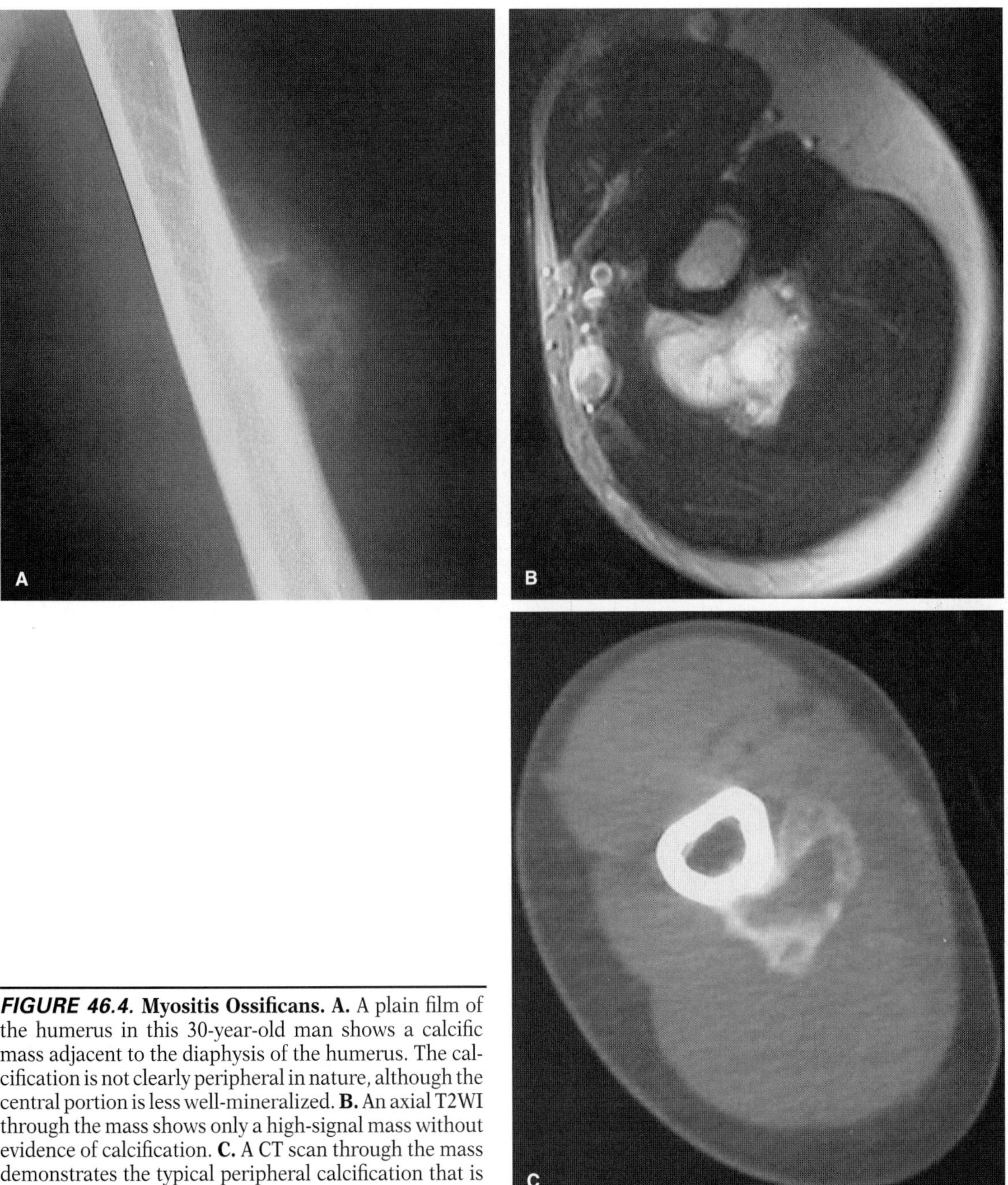

FIGURE 46.4. Myositis Ossificans. A. A plain film of the humerus in this 30-year-old man shows a calcific mass adjacent to the diaphysis of the humerus. The calcification is not clearly peripheral in nature, although the central portion is less well-mineralized. **B.** An axial T2WI through the mass shows only a high-signal mass without evidence of calcification. **C.** A CT scan through the mass demonstrates the typical peripheral calcification that is virtually pathognomonic for myositis ossificans.

transscapular or the axial view is the key to making the diagnosis of a pseudodislocation. If necessary, the joint can be aspirated to confirm the presence of a bloody effusion and to show the normal position of the humeral head when fluid has been removed from the joint.

NORMAL VARIANTS

Dorsal Defect of the Patella. A normal variant that has been described in the patella that can be mistaken for a pathologic process is a lytic defect in the upper outer quadrant called a dorsal defect of the patella (Fig. 46.15) (10). It can mimic a focus of infection, osteochondritis dissecans, or a chondroblastoma. It is a normal developmental anomaly, however, and because of its characteristic location, it should not undergo biopsy. On MR, it will have an appearance similar to that of many other bony lesions—that is, low signal on T1WIs and high signal on T2WIs (Fig. 46.16).

Pseudocyst of the humerus is another entity that is often mistaken for a lytic pathologic lesion (Fig. 46.17). This is merely an anatomic variant caused by increased

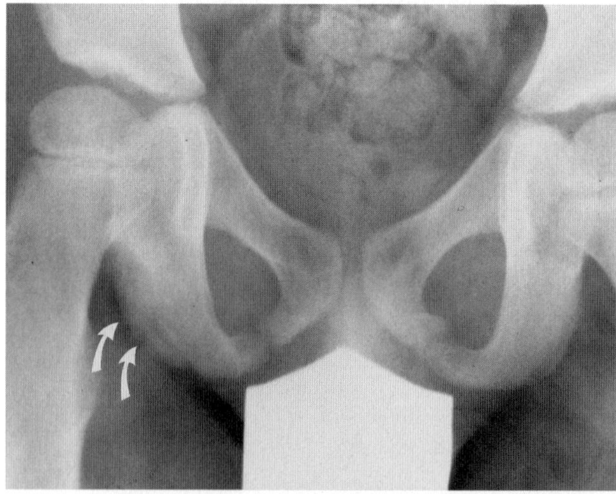

FIGURE 46.5. **Avulsion Injury.** Cortical irregularity (*arrows*) at the ischial tuberosity in this patient with pain over this region raises the question of possible tumor. This is a classic appearance, however, for an avulsion injury from this region, and a biopsy should be avoided.

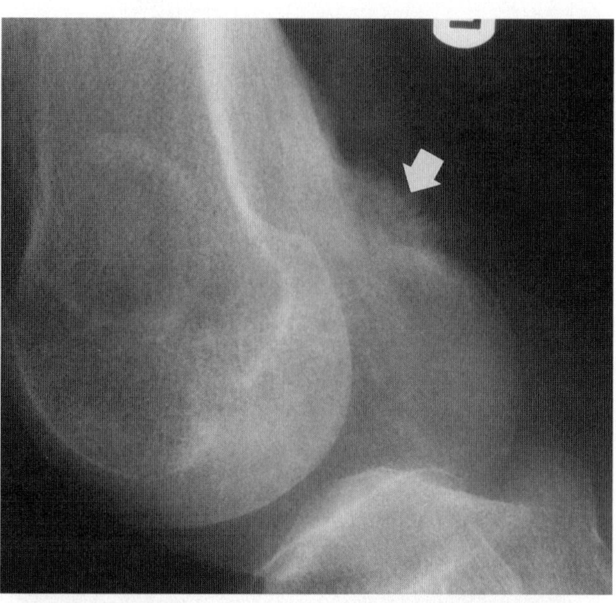

FIGURE 46.7. **Cortical Desmoid.** A focal cortical irregularity in this patient is seen in the posterior aspect of the femur (*arrow*), with adjacent periostitis noted. Although a tumor such as an early parosteal osteosarcoma could perhaps have this appearance, this is a characteristic location and appearance for a cortical desmoid and should not undergo biopsy. Pain will disappear with rest.

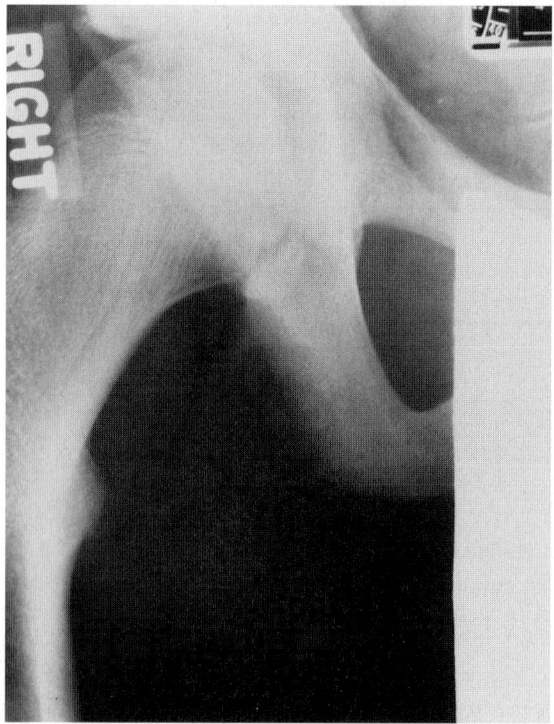

FIGURE 46.6. **Avulsion Injury.** Cortical irregularity with a Codman triangle of periostitis is seen along the ischial tuberosity, which was at first believed to represent a malignancy. However, because of the characteristic location, an avulsion injury was considered and the lesion was observed. It healed without sequelae.

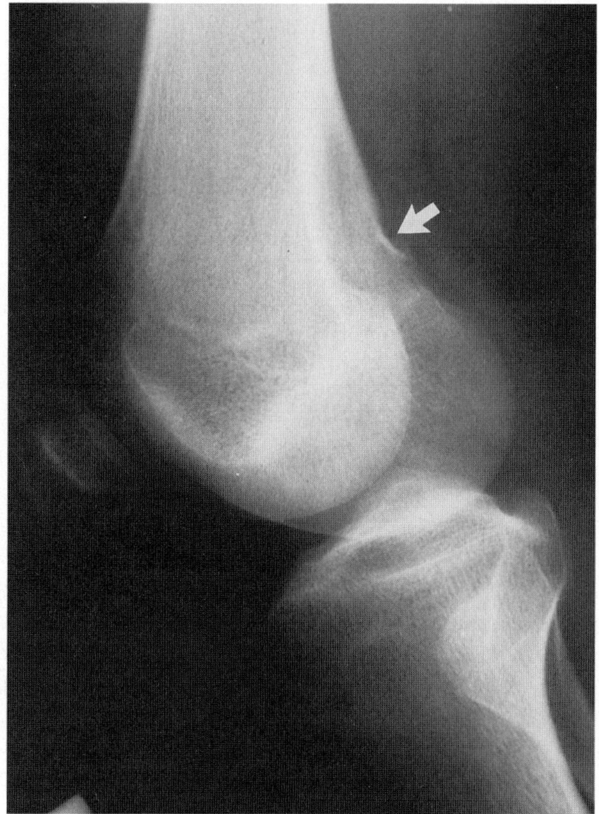

FIGURE 46.8. **Cortical Desmoid.** A well-defined cortical defect is seen in the posterior distal femur (*arrow*), which is a common appearance for a fairly well-healed cortical desmoid.

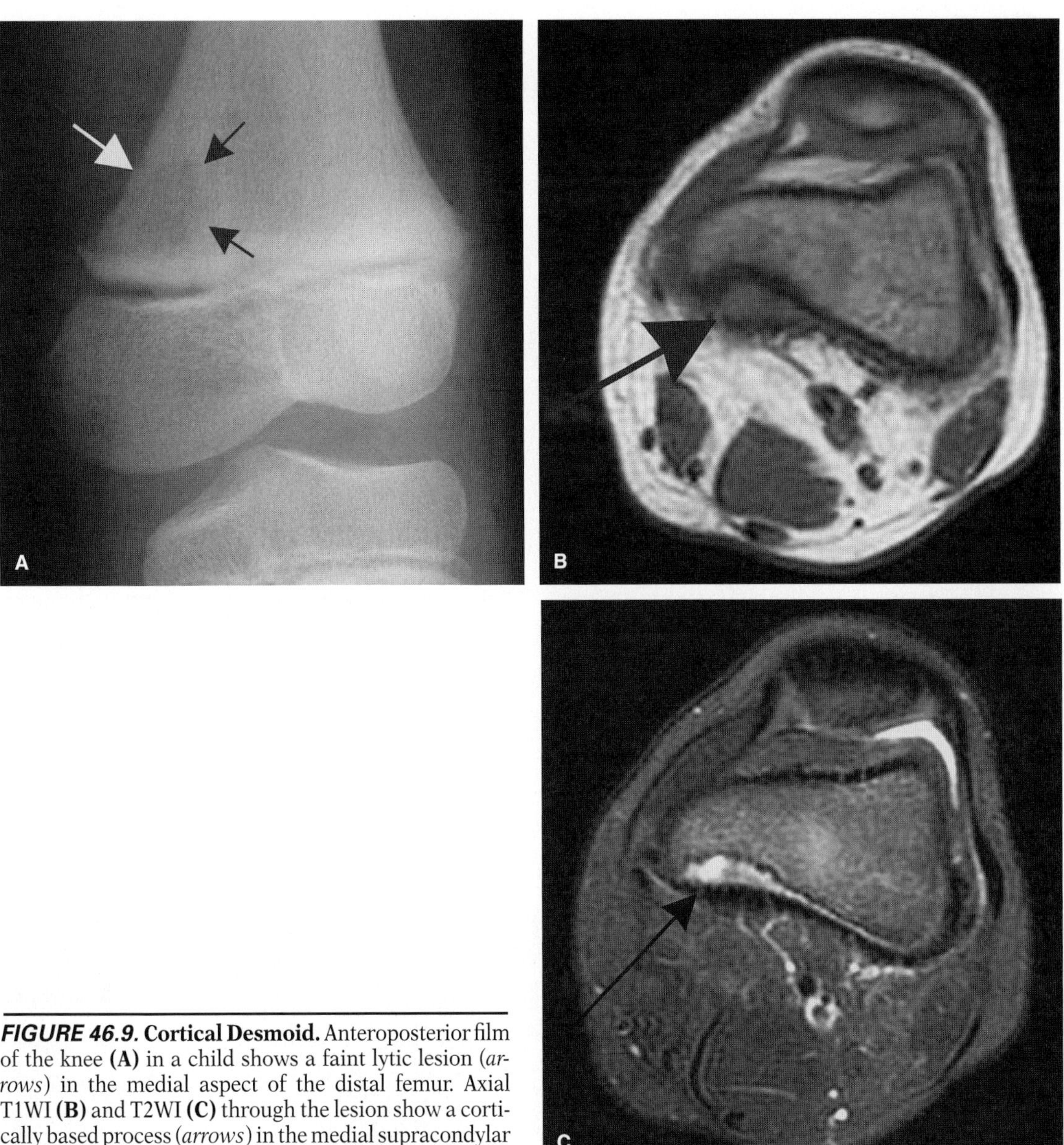

FIGURE 46.9. **Cortical Desmoid.** Anteroposterior film of the knee **(A)** in a child shows a faint lytic lesion (*arrows*) in the medial aspect of the distal femur. Axial T1WI **(B)** and T2WI **(C)** through the lesion show a cortically based process (*arrows*) in the medial supracondylar ridge, which is characteristic for a cortical desmoid.

cancellous bone in the region of the greater tuberosity of the humerus, giving this region a more lucent appearance on radiographs (11,12). With hyperemia and disuse caused by rotator cuff problems or any other shoulder disorder, this area of lucency may appear strikingly more lucent and mimic a lytic lesion. Many of these have mistakenly undergone biopsy, and several have even had repeat biopsies after the initial pathology report stated "normal bone, no lesion in specimen." Because of the associated hyperemia from the shoulder disorder (be it rotator cuff injury or another condition), a bone scan can show increased radionuclide uptake and thus sway the surgeon to perform a biopsy of this normal variant. It is radiographically characteristic in its location and appearance and should not undergo biopsy. Although other lesions, such as a chondroblastoma, an infection, or even a metastatic focus, could occur in a similar location, they do not have quite the same appearance as a pseudocyst of the humerus.

Os odontoideum is a normal variant of the cervical spine that may, in fact, be posttraumatic (13). It is an unfused dens that may move anterior to the C2 body with flexion and can mimic a fractured dens (Fig. 46.18). Many of these require surgical fixation; some surgeons fuse every case, believing that they are all unstable. Radiologists should recognize that this process is not acute, thus, saving the patient from halo fixation and possible immediate surgical intervention. Most of these cases are seen after trauma, and if no neurologic deficits are present, these patients can be seen electively and spared the morbidity

(*text continues on p. 1179*)

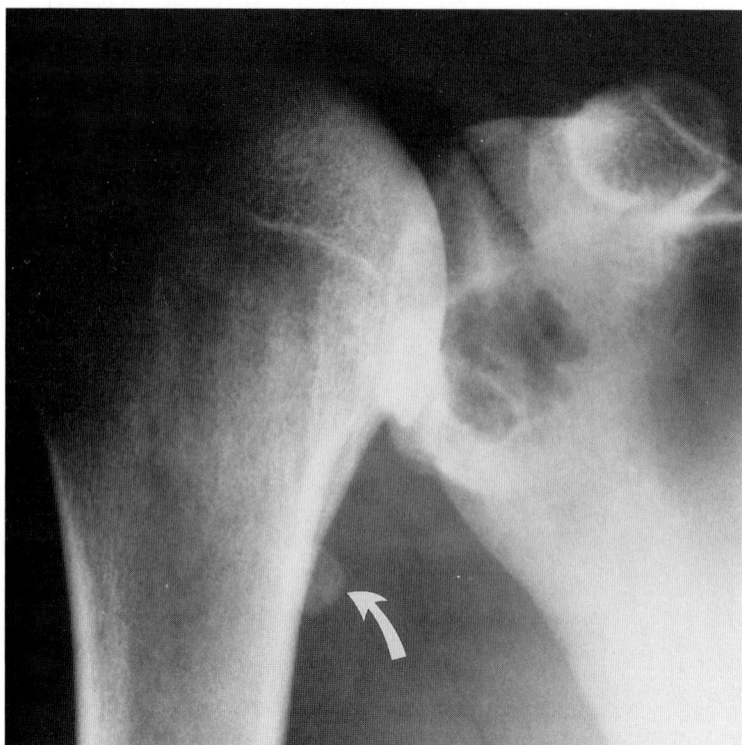

FIGURE 46.10. **Geode.** A large cystic lesion was found in the shoulder in this middle-aged weightlifter, and the possibility of a metastatic process was considered. Because the humeral head has sclerosis and osteophytosis as well as a loose body in the joint (*arrow*), degenerative disease of the shoulder was diagnosed; this makes the cystic lesion almost certainly a geode or subchondral cyst.

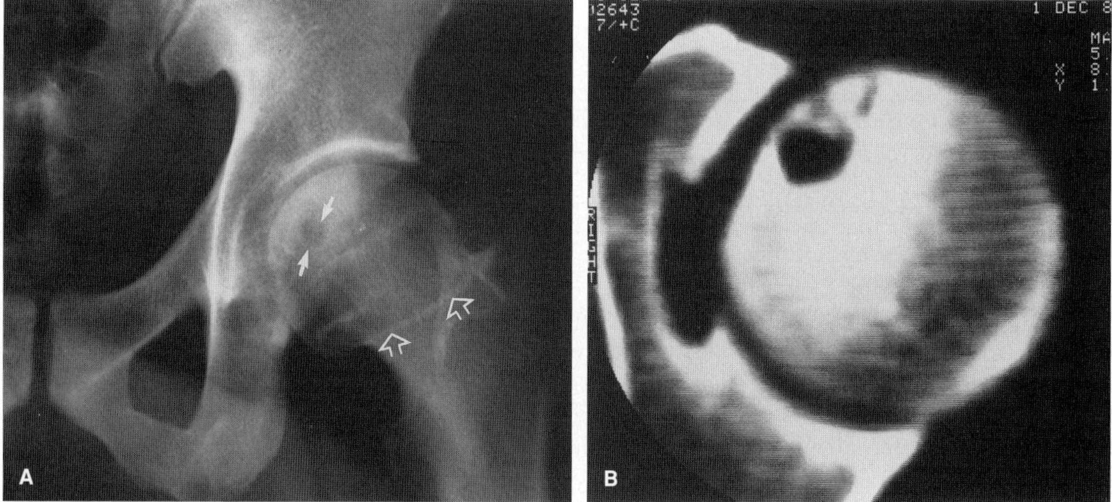

FIGURE 46.11. **Geode. A.** A cystic lesion was noted in the femoral head (*solid arrows*) of a young man with a painful hip. **B.** A CT scan through this area shows the subarticular nature and adjacent sclerosis. The differential diagnosis of infection, eosinophilic granuloma, and chondroblastoma was given. A ring of osteophytes (*open arrowheads*) was noted in retrospect on the plain film **(A)** in the subcapital region, which indicates degenerative disease of the hip. Degenerative joint disease is extremely unusual in a 20-year-old healthy man; however, it makes the lytic lesion in the femoral head almost certainly a subchondral cyst or geode. This was an active soccer player who had been playing with pain in his hip for several years following an injury that had caused the degenerative disease. Unfortunately, a biopsy was performed anyway and a subchondral cyst or geode was confirmed.

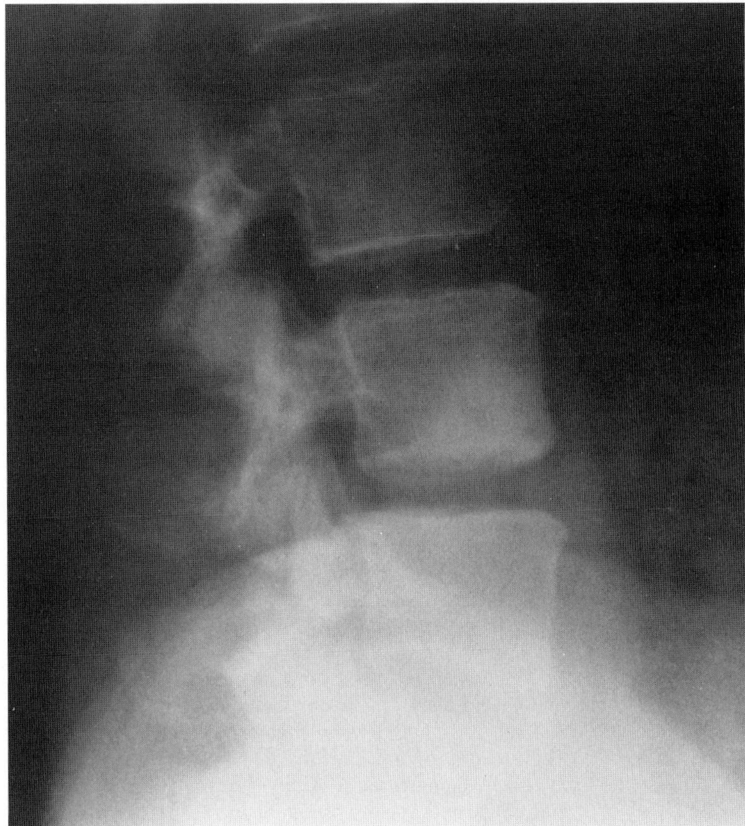

FIGURE 46.12. **Discogenic Vertebral Sclerosis.** This patient has sclerosis on the inferior portion of the L4 vertebral body associated with minimal osteophytosis and joint space narrowing at the adjacent disk space. This is the classic appearance for discogenic vertebral sclerosis, and a biopsy to rule out metastatic disease should not be performed.

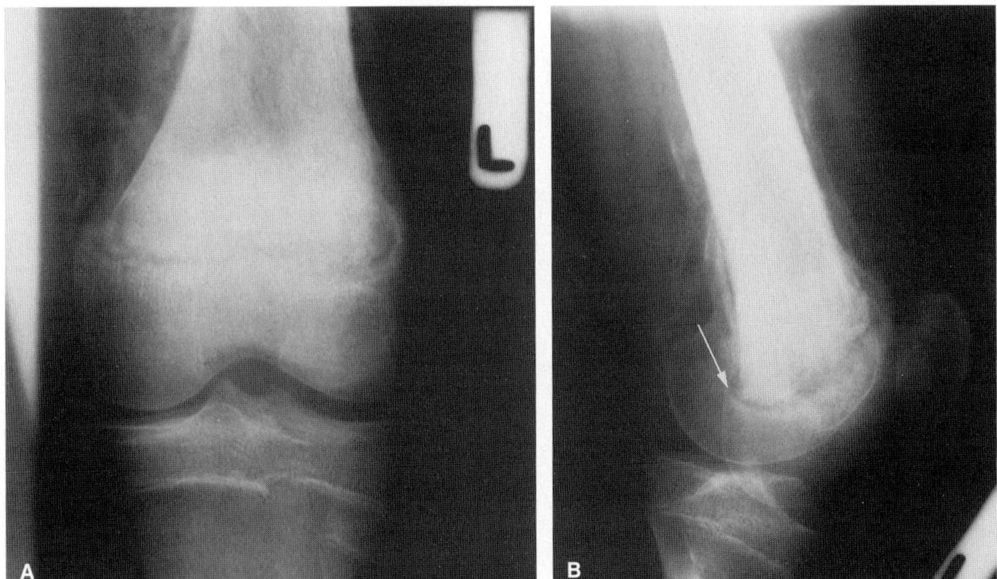

FIGURE 46.13. **Fracture Mimicking Osteosarcoma. A.** This 16-year-old patient had experienced pain around the knee for 2 weeks before these radiographs. The knee films showed diffuse sclerosis and extensive periostitis about the distal femur, which is thought to be characteristic for an osteogenic sarcoma. The periosteal reaction, however, was thought to be much too thick, dense, and wavy to represent a malignant type of periostitis. **B.** A small offset of the epiphysis can be seen (*arrow*), which indicates an epiphyseal slippage consistent with a Salter epiphyseal fracture. This teenager had fallen off a bicycle and fractured the femur, yet continued to be active. The lack of immobility caused exuberant periostitis or callus with a large amount of reactive sclerosis, all of which mimicked an osteogenic sarcoma.

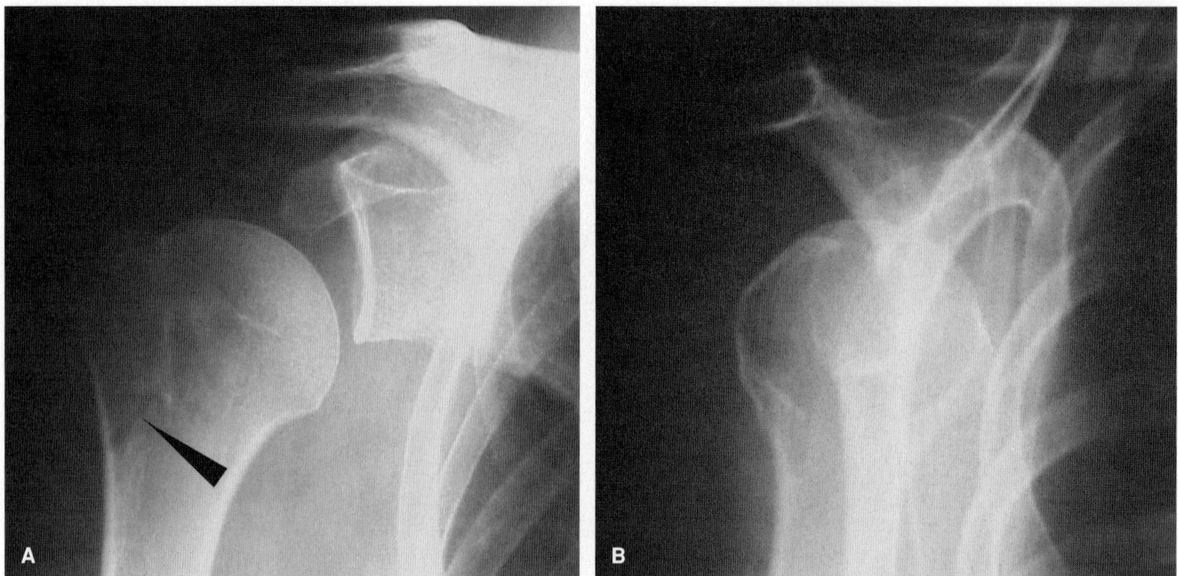

FIGURE 46.14. **Pseudodislocation of the Shoulder. A.** This patient experienced trauma to the shoulder, with resultant pain and immobility, and was thought to have a dislocation of the shoulder after the anteroposterior film was seen. The humeral head is inferiorly placed in relation to the glenoid; however, this is not the characteristic location of an anterior or posterior dislocation. **B.** The transscapular view shows that the humeral head is situated normally over the glenoid, without anterior or posterior dislocation. These findings are characteristic for a pseudodislocation caused by hemarthrosis, or blood in the joint, which allows the shoulder to be subluxed rather than dislocated. When a pseudodislocation is seen, as in this example, search for an occult fracture should ensue. In this case, as seen on **(A),** a fracture (*arrowhead*) was initially missed.

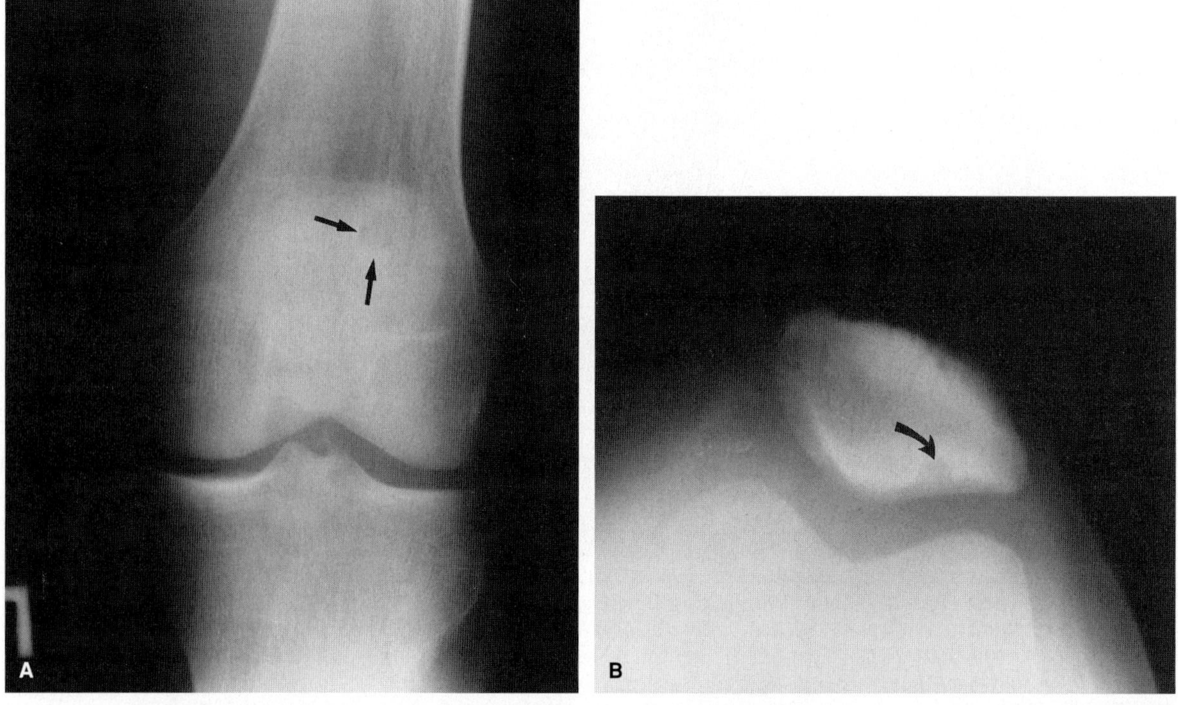

FIGURE 46.15. **Dorsal Defect of the Patella.** A lytic defect in the upper outer quadrant of the patella was seen in this patient on the anteroposterior film **(A)** and the axial or sunrise view **(B)** (*arrows*), which is characteristic for a normal variant called dorsal defect of the patella. It occurs only in the upper outer quadrant and should be asymptomatic.

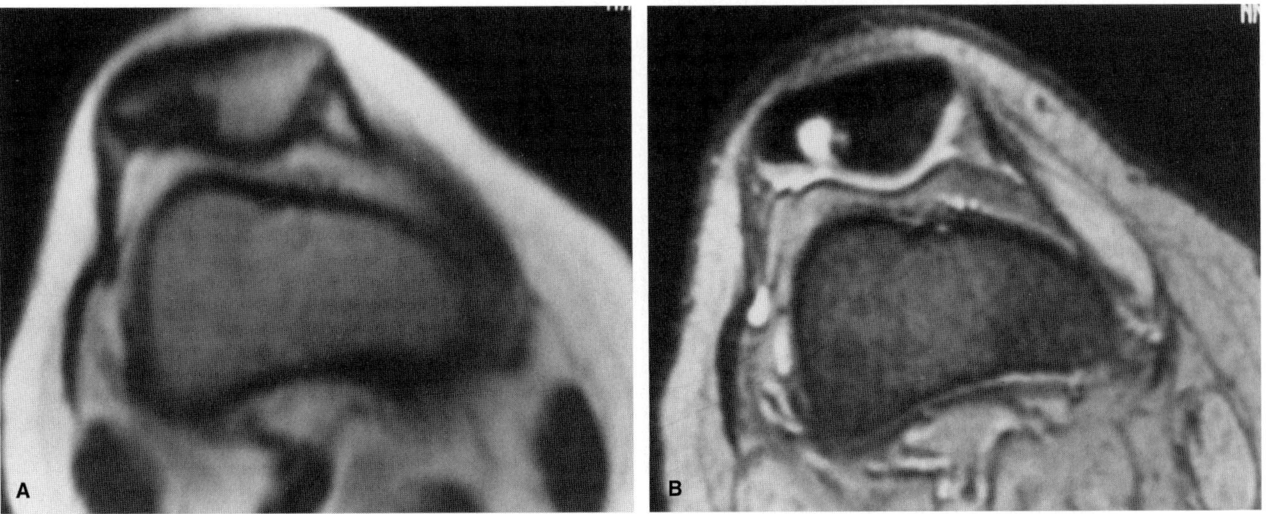

FIGURE 46.16. **Dorsal Defect of the Patella. A.** Axial T1WI shows a focal area of low signal in the patella in a subarticular location in the lateral facet of the patella. **B.** The axial T2WI shows high signal in the lesion. This is typical in location and appearance for a dorsal defect of the patella.

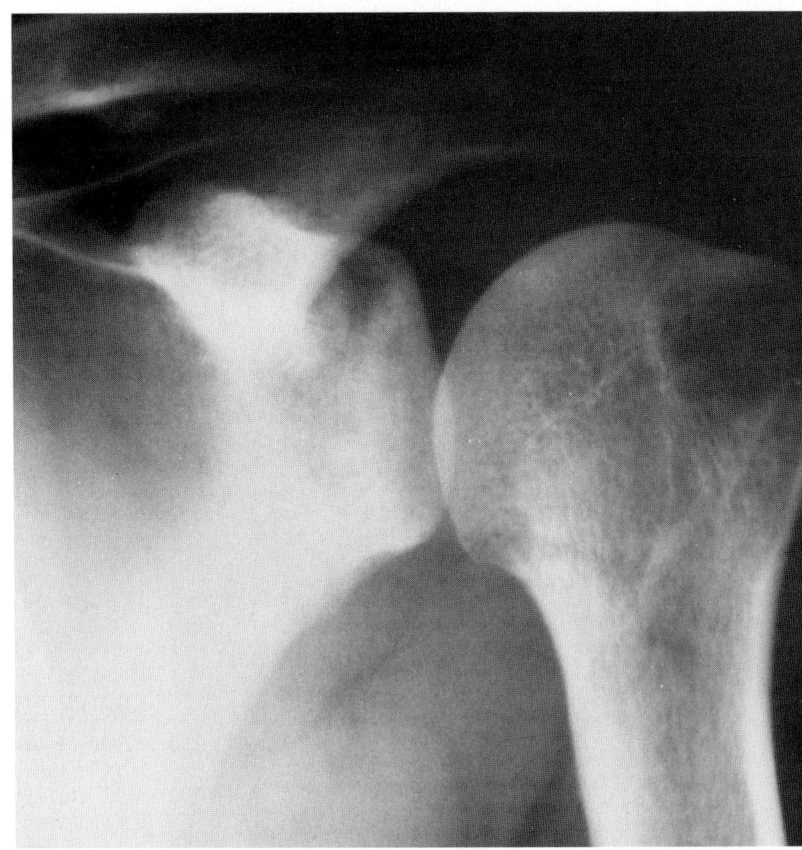

FIGURE 46.17. **Pseudocyst of the Humerus.** A well-defined lytic process is seen in the greater tuberosity, which was thought to represent a lytic lesion. This patient was symptomatic and had increased radionuclide uptake on an isotope bone scan. However, this is a characteristic location and appearance for a pseudocyst of the humerus, which merely represents decreased cortical bone in this region. This becomes more pronounced when pain in the shoulder is present and hyperemia or disuse osteoporosis occurs.

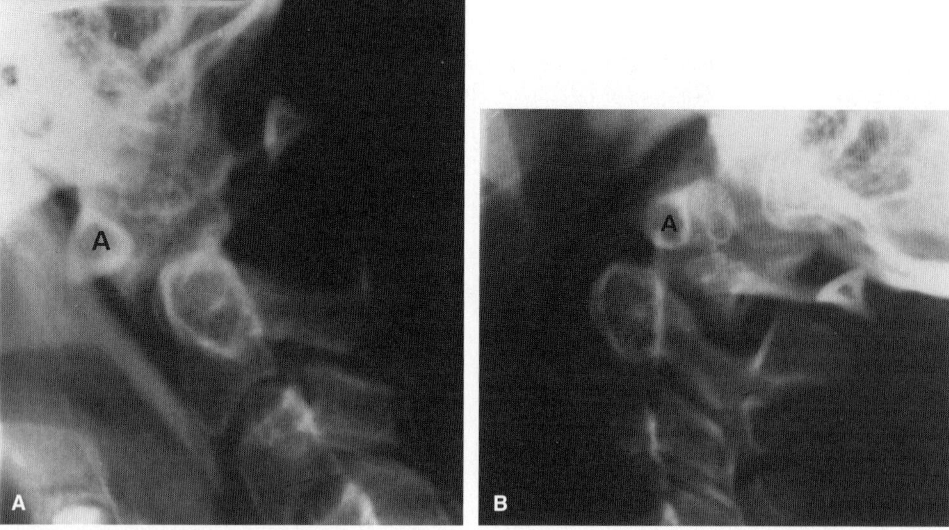

FIGURE 46.18. **Os Odontoideum.** Flexion **(A)** and extension **(B)** views show the anterior arch (A) of the C1 vertebrae has moved markedly anterior in relation to the body of C2 in flexion. The odontoid or dens is difficult to see but appears to be separated from the body of C2. Because of the smooth borders of the separated dens and because of the cortical hypertrophy of the anterior arch of C1, this can safely be called an os odontoideum, which is a congenital or long-standing posttraumatic abnormality rather than an acute fracture. Obviously, patients with this condition should have no neurologic problems, yet in many instances are still believed to be unstable and undergo surgically fusion. This, however, can be done on an elective basis.

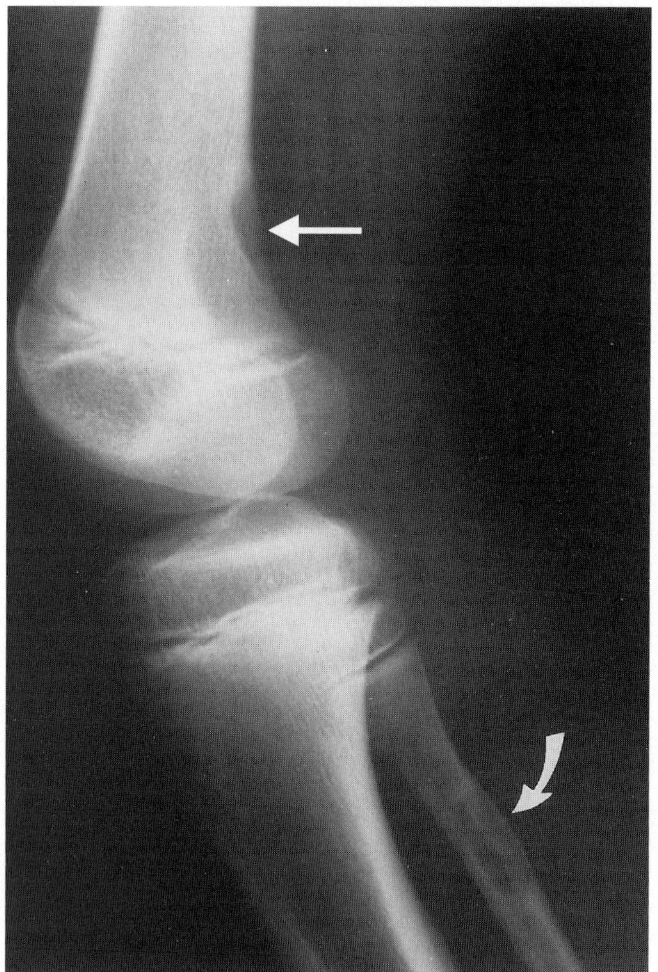

FIGURE 46.19. **Nonossifying Fibroma.** A well-defined, slightly expansile, lytic lesion is seen in the fibula (*lower curved arrow*); this is characteristic for a nonossifying fibroma. A second lytic lesion is seen in the posterior distal femur (*upper curved arrow*), which is also typical in appearance for a nonossifying fibroma.

associated with treatment of the acutely fractured cervical spine. The radiologic signs of an os odontoideum are the smooth, often well-corticated, inferior border of the dens and the hypertrophied, densely corticated anterior arch of C1 (14). This latter finding presumably represents compensatory hypertrophy and indicates a long-standing condition.

OBVIOUSLY BENIGN LESIONS

Multiple real lesions exist that should be recognized radiographically as benign and left alone. These are lesions that should be diagnosed by the radiologist, not the pathologist. Listing a differential in these cases often spurs the surgeon to a biopsy, when, in fact, no biopsy should be necessary.

Nonossifying fibroma (NOF) is perhaps the most often encountered lesion in this category. NOF is identical to a fibrous cortical defect, but the term is usually reserved for defects larger than 2 cm. They are, classically, lytic lesions located in the cortex of the metaphysis of a long bone and have a well-defined, often sclerotic, scalloped border with slight cortical expansion (Fig. 46.19). They are found almost exclusively in patients younger than the age of 30 years; hence, the natural history of the lesion is involution. As they involute, they fill in with new bone, giving it a sclerotic appearance (Fig. 46.20) thus, they can have some increased radionuclide activity on bone scans. They are most often mistaken for an area of infection, eosinophilic granuloma, fibrous dysplasia, or aneurysmal bone cyst. They are asymptomatic and have never been reported to

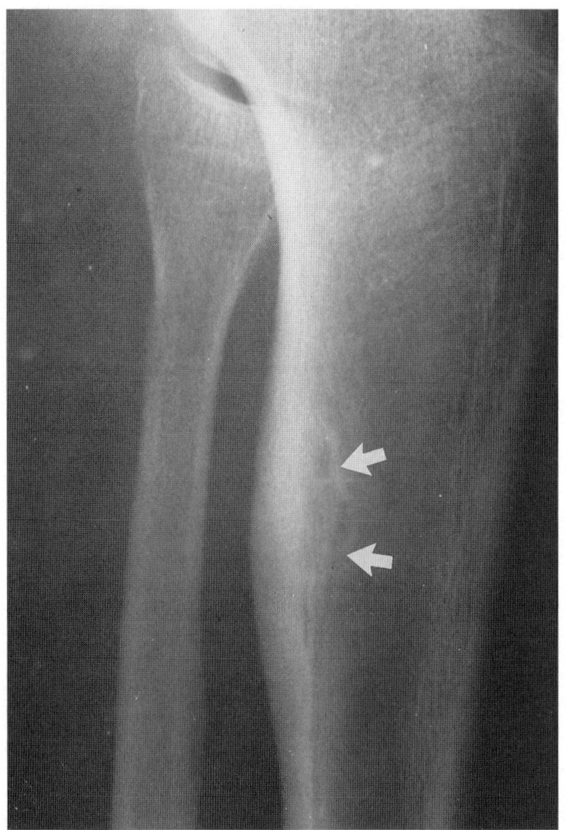

FIGURE 46.20. **Healing Nonossifying Fibroma.** A minimally sclerotic process is seen in the proximal tibia (*arrows*), which was thought by the surgeons to represent a focus of infection or an osteoid osteoma, even though the patient was asymptomatic. This is a characteristic appearance for a disappearing or healing nonossifying fibroma and should not undergo biopsy.

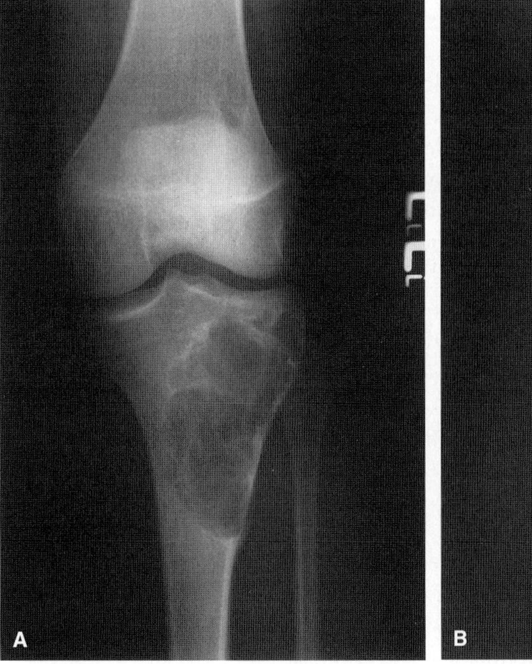

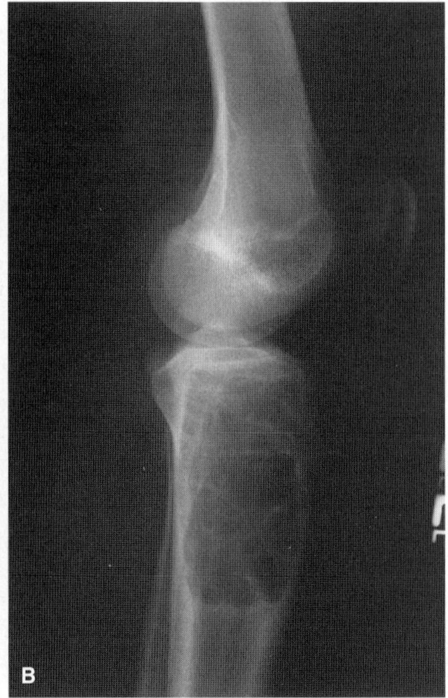

FIGURE 46.21. **Nonossifying Fibroma.** Anteroposterior **(A)** and lateral **(B)** films of the tibia show a large, well-defined, minimally expansile lytic lesion of the proximal tibia, which is characteristic for a nonossifying fibroma. Even though the patient was asymptomatic, biopsy was performed and the diagnosis confirmed.

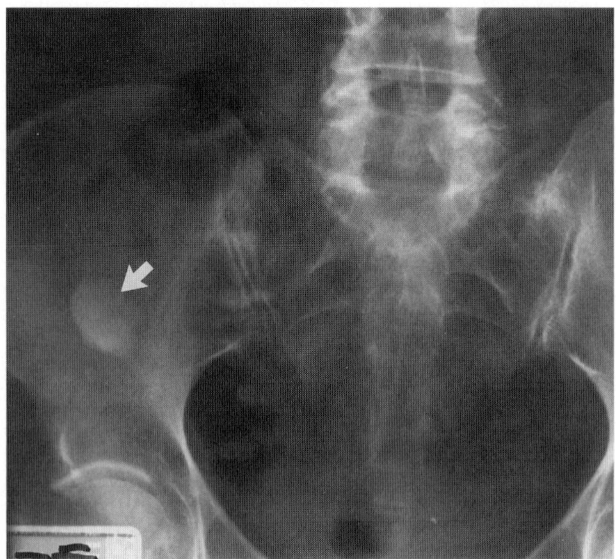

FIGURE 46.22. **Giant Bone Island.** A large sclerotic focus is seen in the right iliac wing (*arrow*). Note how the lesion is somewhat spherical or oblong and in the lines of trabecular stress, which is characteristic for a bone island. This patient was asymptomatic and had no evidence of a primary carcinoma.

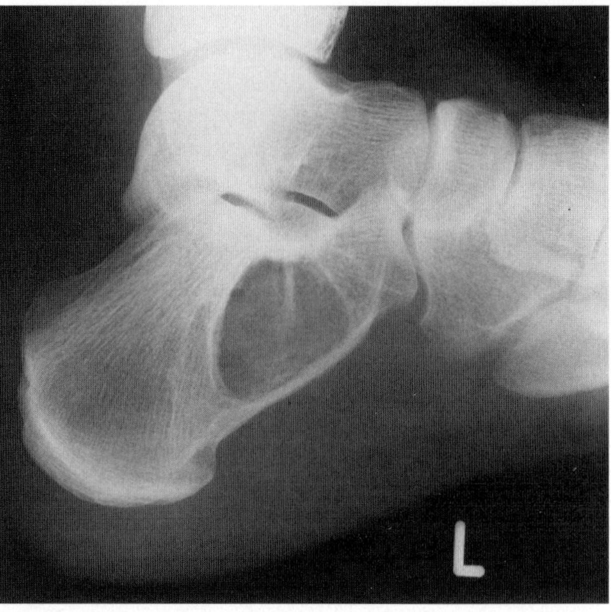

FIGURE 46.23. **Unicameral Bone Cyst.** A well-defined lytic lesion on the anteroinferior portion of the calcaneus, as in this example, is virtually pathognomonic for a unicameral bone cyst or simple bone cyst. Because this is an area of diminished stress, it is thought to be unnecessary to curettage and pack this lesion prophylactically in an effort to avoid a pathologic bone fracture, which is often done in the femur and humerus with unicameral bone cysts.

be associated with malignant degeneration. On occasion, a pathologic fracture can occur through these lesions, but most surgeons do not advocate prophylactic curettage to prevent fracture, as with unicameral bone cysts. NOFs can be quite large but invariably have a benign appearance (Fig. 46.21), and biopsy should be avoided. Their asymptomatic nature should help differentiate them from most of the other lesions in the differential diagnosis and thereby preclude even giving a differential diagnosis. On occasion, they are found to be multiple, yet each lesion is so characteristic as to be easily diagnosed.

Bone islands are not a radiographic dilemma when they are 1 cm or smaller. Occasionally, however, they grow to golf ball size or larger and mimic sclerotic metastases (Fig. 46.22). They are always asymptomatic. Radiographically, two signs can be found to help distinguish giant bone islands from metastases. First, bone islands usually are oblong, with their long axis in the axis of stress on the bone: for example, in a long bone they align themselves along the axis of the diaphysis. Second, the margins of a bone island, when examined closely, will show bony trabeculae extending from the lesion into the normal bone in a spiculated fashion (15). This is characteristic of a bone island and helpful in differentiating it from a more aggressive process.

Unicameral bone cysts are often prophylactically curettaged and packed so as to prevent fracture with subsequent deformity. When these cysts occur in the calcaneus, however, they should be left alone. They always occur in the anteroinferior portion of the calcaneus (Fig. 46.23), an

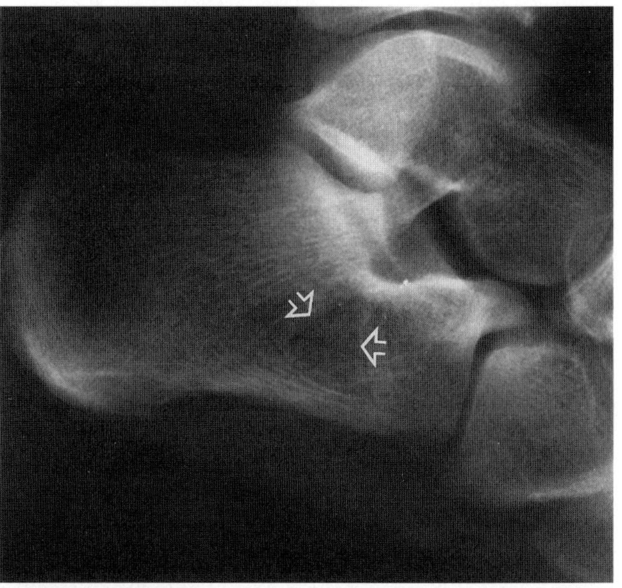

FIGURE 46.24. **Pseudocyst of the Calcaneus.** An area of radiolucency is seen on the anteroinferior portion of the calcaneus (*arrows*) similar to the example in Fig. 46.23, but it is not as well defined. This is a pseudocyst similar to the pseudocyst of the humerus that results from diminished stress through this region.

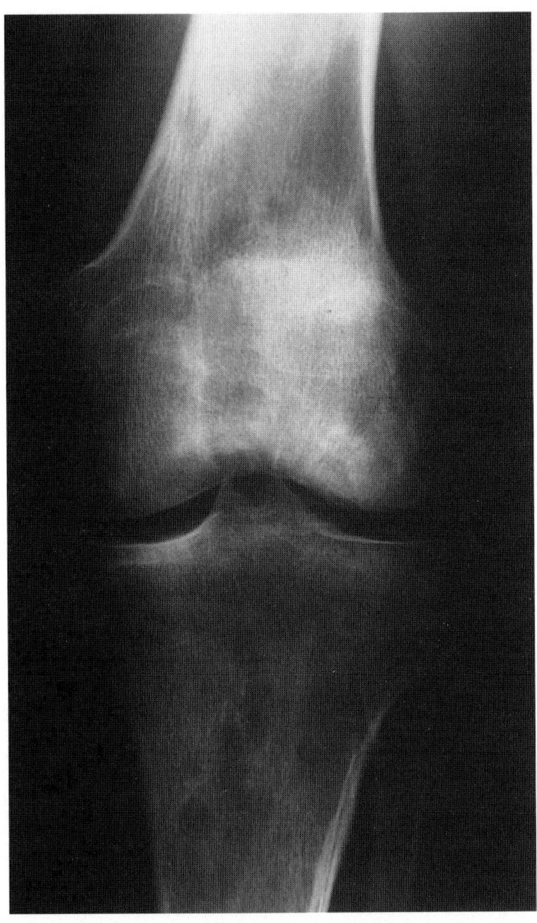

FIGURE 46.25. **Early Bone Infarct.** Patchy demineralization is seen in the distal femur and proximal tibia in this patient with systemic lupus erythematosus. The opposite leg was similarly involved. This is characteristic for early bone infarcts and should not be confused with infection or metastatic disease.

area that does not receive undue stress. In fact, a pseudotumor of the calcaneus is seen in the identical position because of the absence of stress and resulting atrophy of bony trabeculae (Fig. 46.24). These lesions are asymptomatic, only rarely fracture, and should not suffer the same fate as their counterparts in long bones—that is, surgical removal.

Bone Infarction. Early in the course of its development, a bone infarct can have a patchy or mixed lytic-sclerotic pattern or even resemble a permeative process (Fig. 46.25) (16). In a patient with bone pain and a permeative bone lesion, many aggressive disorders head the differential list and a biopsy soon ensues. If this process can be noted to be multiple and in the diametaphyseal region of a long bone, especially if the patient has an underlying disorder such as sickle cell anemia or systemic lupus erythematosus, areas of early bone infarction should be considered. In some cases, the characteristic MR appearance of an infarct may save a patient from biopsy when the plain films are equivocal (Fig. 46.26).

These are but a few of the many examples in skeletal radiology in which the well-trained radiologist can be of invaluable assistance to the clinician and the patient by helping avert a needless biopsy. Dozens of other examples are nicely shown in normal variant textbooks, which are widely available. Because of the potential harm in performing a needless biopsy, the examples described in this chapter are stressed. When these lesions are encountered by the radiologist, a differential diagnosis should not be offered, as it will often lead the surgeon to a biopsy in an attempt to get a diagnosis. A biopsy in many of these entities is not only unnecessary but can be misleading.

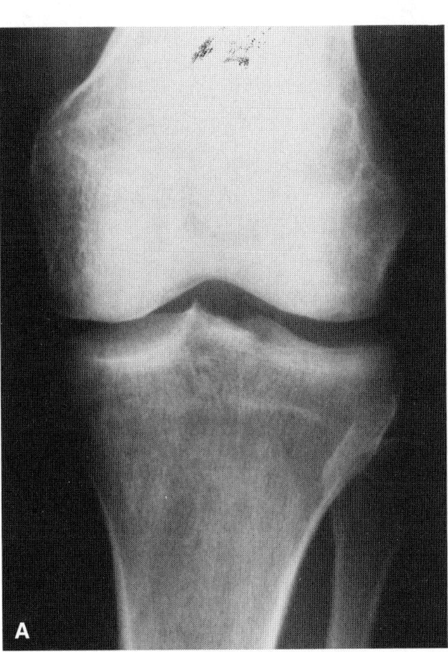

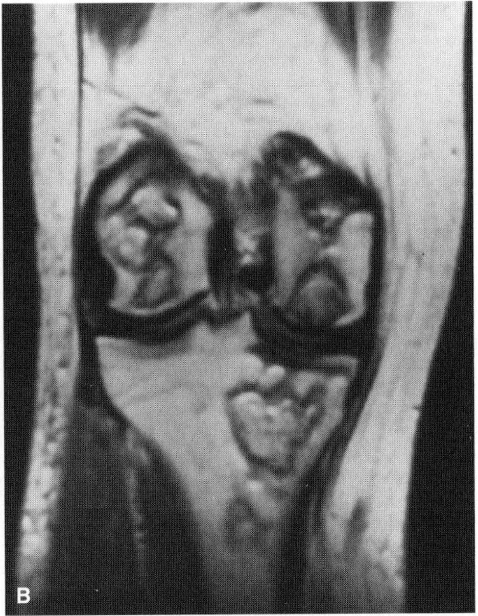

FIGURE 46.26. **Bone Infarct. A.** A plain film of the knee shows a permeative pattern in the proximal tibia, which was thought at first to be infection or a primary tumor. **B.** Coronal T1WI shows the characteristic serpiginous border seen with bone infarct in the tibia and in the femur. MR can on occasion better characterize the ill-defined early bone infarct, as in this example. This patient has systemic lupus erythematosus.

REFERENCES

1. Murray R, Jacobson H. The Radiology of Skeletal Disorders. 2nd ed. New York: Churchill Livingstone, 1977:603.
2. Wootton J, Cross M, Holt K. Avulsion of the ischial apophysis. J Bone Joint Surg 1990;72B:625–627.
3. Schneider R, Kaye J, Ghelman B. Adductor avulsive injuries near the symphysis pubis. Radiology 1976;120:567–569.
4. Barnes G, Gwinn J. Distal irregularities of the femur simulating malignancy. AJR Am J Roentgenol 1974;122:180–185.
5. Ostlere S, Seeger L, Eckardt J. Subchondral cysts of the tibia secondary to osteoarthritis of the knee. Skeletal Radiol 1990;19: 287–289.
6. Resnick D, Niwayama G, Coutts R. Subchondral cysts (geodes) in arthritic disorders: pathologic and radiographic appearance of the hip joint. AJR Am J Roentgenol 1977;128:799–806.
7. Martel W, Seeger J, Wicks J, et al. Traumatic lesions of the discovertebral junction in the lumbar spine. AJR Am J Roentgenol 1976;127:457–464.
8. Lipson S. Discogenic vertebral sclerosis with calcified disc. New Engl J Med 1991;325:794–799.
9. Helms C, Richmond B, Sims R. Pseudodislocation of the shoulder: a sign of an occult fracture. Emerg Med 1986;18:237–241.
10. Johnson JF, Brogdon BG. Dorsal effect of the patella: incidence and distribution. AJR Am J Roentgenol 1982;139:339–340.
11. Helms C. Pseudocyst of the humerus. AJR Am J Roentgenol 1979;131:287–292.
12. Resnick D, Cone R. The nature of humeral pseudocysts. Radiology 1984;150:27–28.
13. Minderhoud J, Braakman R, Penning L. Os odontoideum: clinical, radiological, and therapeutic aspects. J Neurol Sci 1969;8:521–544.
14. Holt RG, Helms CA, Munk PL, et al. Hypertrophy of C-1 anterior arch: useful sign to distinguish os odontoideum from acute dens fracture. Radiology 1989;173:207–209.
15. Onitsuka H. Roentgenologic aspects of bone islands. Radiology 1977;124:607–612.
16. Munk PL, Helms CA, Holt RG. Immature bone infarcts: findings on plain radiographs and MR scans. AJR Am J Roentgenol 1989;152:547–549.

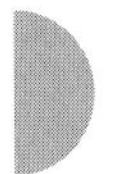

Chapter 47

Miscellaneous Bone Lesions

Clyde A. Helms

Achondroplasia
Avascular Necrosis (Osteonecrosis)
Hypertrophic Pulmonary Osteoarthropathy
Melorheostosis
Mucopolysaccharidoses (Morquio, Hurler, and Hunter Syndromes)
Multiple Hereditary Exostosis
Osteoid Osteoma
Osteopathia Striata
Osteopoikilosis
Pachydermoperiostosis
Sarcoidosis
Transient Osteoporosis of the Hip

There are a host of bony conditions, diseases, and syndromes that do not fit conveniently into any of the preceding chapters, yet should be given some mention in an attempted overview of musculoskeletal radiology. These are listed alphabetically for lack of a more scientific basis.

Achondroplasia

The most common cause of dwarfism is achondroplasia, a congenital, hereditary disease of failure of endochondral bone formation. The femurs and humeri are more profoundly affected than the other long bones, although the entire skeleton is abnormal. A characteristic finding is that the spine typically has narrowing of the interpedicular distances in a caudal direction (Fig. 47.1), the opposite of normal, in which the interpedicular distances get progressively wider as one proceeds down the spine. The long bones are short but have normal width, giving them a thick appearance.

Avascular Necrosis (Osteonecrosis)

The terms *avascular necrosis* (AVN) and *osteonecrosis* refer to a lack of blood supply with subsequent bone death and ensuing bony collapse in an articular surface. The etiology of AVN is an extensive differential that most commonly includes *trauma, steroids, aspirin, collagen vascular diseases, alcoholism,* and *idiopathic causes* (Table 47.1) (1). The radiographic appearance ranges from patchy sclerosis (Fig. 47.2A) to articular surface collapse and fragmentation (Fig. 47.3). Just before collapse, a subchondral lucency is occasionally seen (Fig. 47.4); however, this is a late and inconstant sign of AVN. MR is extremely valuable in demonstrating the presence and extent of AVN (Fig. 47.2B), even when plain films are apparently normal. MR is currently considered the most efficacious means to evaluate a joint for AVN (2). It is useful not only in AVN of the hip but also in the knee, wrist, foot, and ankle.

Hypertrophic Pulmonary Osteoarthropathy

Hypertrophic pulmonary osteoarthropathy is manifested by clubbing of the fingers and periostitis, usually in the extremities (Fig. 47.5), which might or might not be associated with bone pain. It is most commonly seen in patients with lung cancer, but many other etiologies have been reported, including bronchiectasis, GI disorders, and liver disease. The actual mechanism of formation of periostitis secondary to a distant malignancy or other process is unknown. The differential diagnosis for periostitis in a long bone without an underlying bony abnormality would include *hypertrophic pulmonary osteoarthropathy, venous stasis, thyroid acropachy, pachydermoperiostosis*, and *trauma* (Table 47.2).

Melorheostosis

Melorheostosis is a rare, idiopathic disorder characterized by thickened cortical new bone that accumulates near the ends of long bones, usually only on one side of the bone,

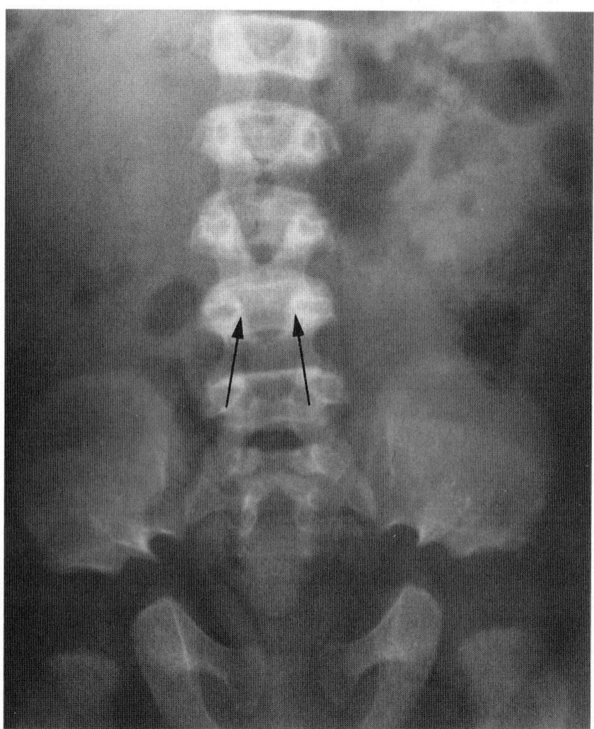

FIGURE 47.1. Achondroplasia. An anteroposterior plain film of the spine in this patient with achondroplasia demonstrates narrowing of the interpedicular distance (*arrows*) in a caudal direction, which is characteristic of this disorder. Ordinarily, the interpedicular distance widens in each vertebra in a caudal direction.

TABLE 47.1 Common Causes of Avascular Necrosis

Trauma
Steroids
Collagen vascular diseases
Alcoholism
Idiopathic causes

and has an appearance likened to "dripping candle wax" (Fig. 47.6). It can affect several adjacent bones and can be symptomatic.

Mucopolysaccharidoses (Morquio, Hurler, and Hunter Syndromes)

The mucopolysaccharidoses are a group of inherited diseases characterized by abnormal storage and excretion in the urine of various mucopolysaccharides, such as keratan sulfate (Morquio) and heparan sulfate (Hurler). These patients have short stature, primarily from shortened spines, and characteristic plain film findings. In the spine, patients with Morquio have platyspondyly (generalized flattening of the vertebral bodies) with a central anterior projection or "beak" off the vertebral body, as viewed on a lateral plain film (Fig. 47.7). Hurler and Hunter syndromes show

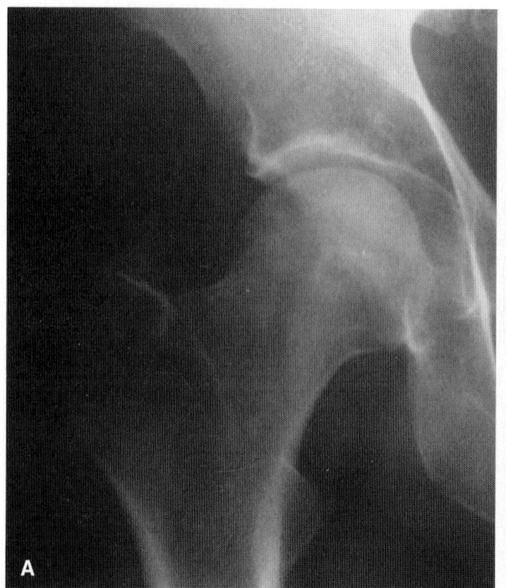

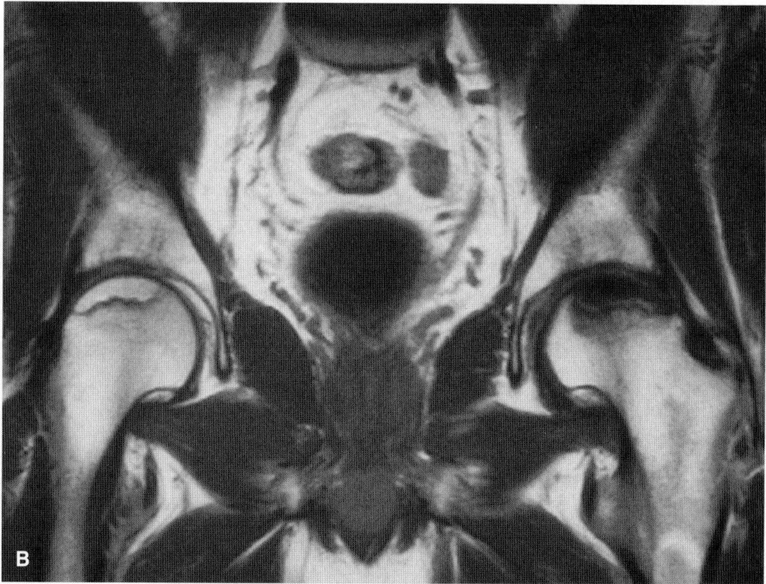

FIGURE 47.2. Avascular Necrosis (AVN). A. A plain film of the hip in this patient with AVN shows faint, patchy sclerosis throughout the femoral head. This is a relatively early plain film finding for AVN. **B.** Coronal T1WI shows typical findings in AVN. Diffuse low signal in the left hip is noted, which has more extensive involvement than the right. The right hip has a low signal serpiginous rim which is characteristic for AVN.

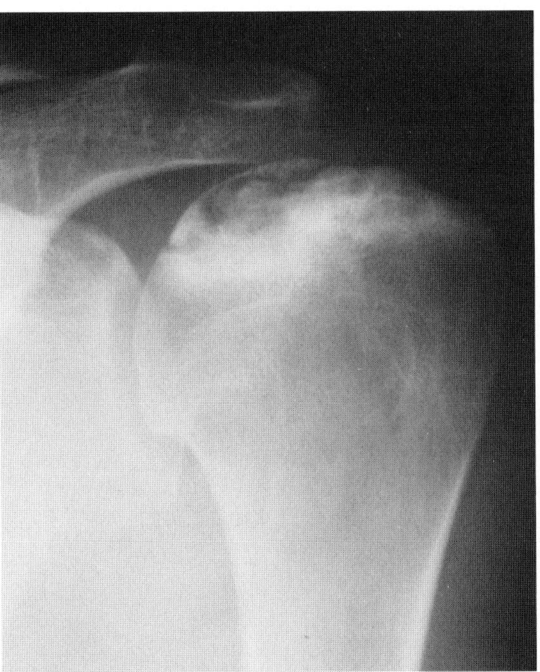

FIGURE 47.3. **Avascular Necrosis (AVN).** An anteroposterior plain film of the shoulder reveals articular surface collapse in this patient who was treated with steroids for systemic lupus erythematosus. This is an advanced stage of AVN.

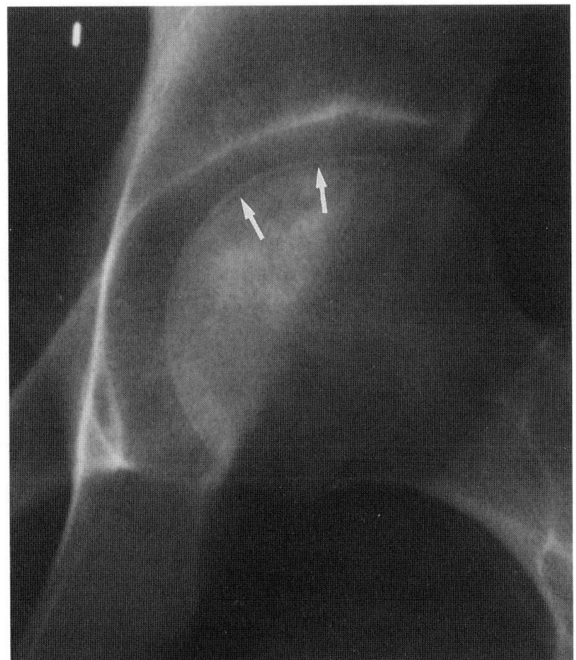

FIGURE 47.4. **Avascular Necrosis (AVN).** An anteroposterior frog-leg lateral view of the hip in this patient with sickle cell disease shows a subchondral lucency (*arrows*) and patchy sclerosis in the femoral head, indicative of AVN. This is a relatively advanced stage of AVN. The subchondral lucency is often better demonstrated with the frog-leg lateral view.

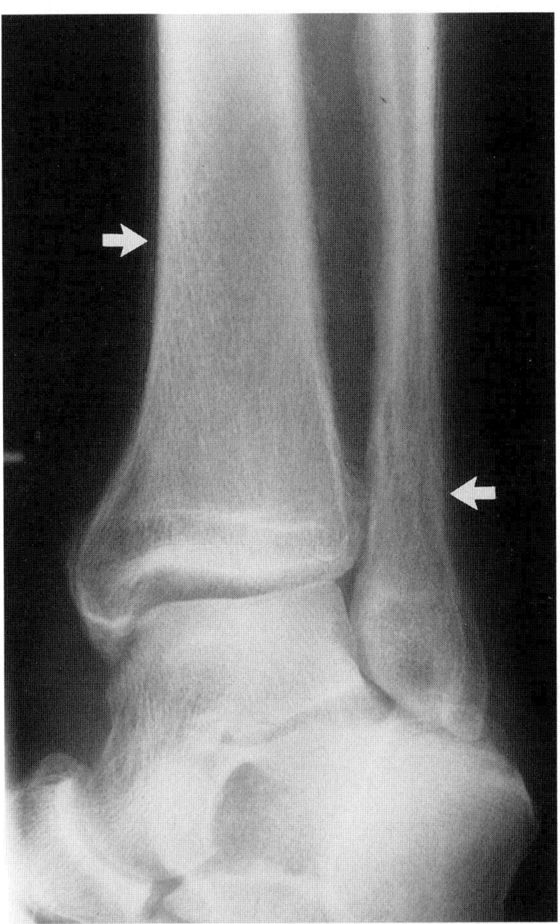

FIGURE 47.5. **Hypertrophic Pulmonary Osteoarthrosis.** Periostitis can be seen along the shafts of the distal tibia and fibula (*arrows*) in this patient with bronchogenic carcinoma and leg pain. This is characteristic for hypertrophic pulmonary osteoarthrosis.

platyspondyly, with a beak that is anteroinferiorly positioned (Fig. 47.8). The pelvis in these disorders is similar in appearance to that seen in patients with achondroplasia, with wide, flared iliac wings and broad femoral necks. A characteristic finding in the hands is a pointed proximal fifth metacarpal base that has a notched appearance to the ulnar aspect (Fig. 47.9).

TABLE 47.2 Differential Diagnosis for Periostitis Without Underlying Bony Lesions

Trauma
Hypertrophic pulmonary osteoarthropathy
Venous stasis
Thyroid acropachy
Pachydermoperiostosis

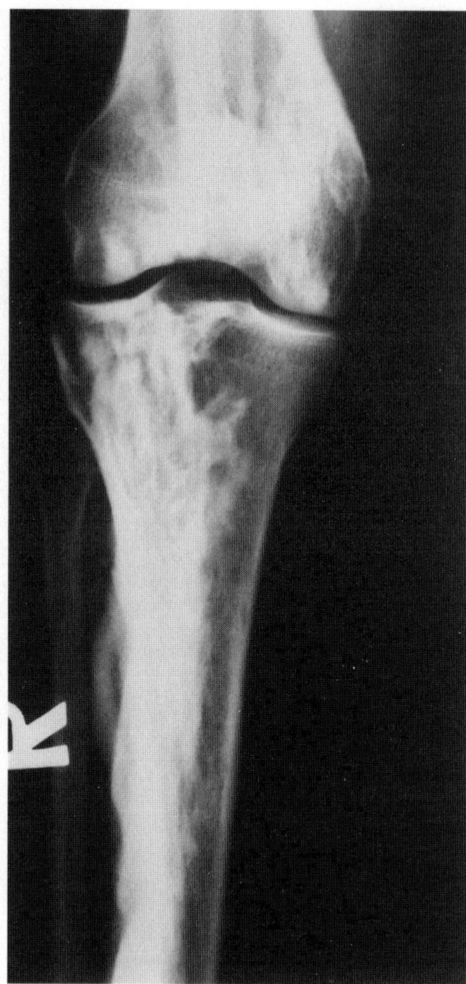

FIGURE 47.6. **Melorheostosis.** Dense, wavy, new bone is seen adjacent to the lateral tibial cortex, which has a dripping candle wax appearance, which is classic for melorheostosis. A similar pattern can be seen in the medial aspect of the distal femur.

Multiple Hereditary Exostosis

Also known as *diaphyseal aclasia*, this is a not uncommon hereditary disorder that seems to affect multiple members of a family with multiple osteochondromas, or exostoses. An osteochondroma is a cartilage-capped bone outgrowth that may be pedunculated or sessile in appearance. In the multiple hereditary form, the knees are virtually always involved (Fig. 47.10). Undertubulation (a widened diameter of the bone) is invariably present at the site of the exostosis. The incidence of malignant degeneration in this population has been reported to be as high as 20%, but this is a gross overestimation; malignant degeneration is in fact extremely rare. As with solitary osteochondromas, the more axially situated lesions are more prone to undergo malignant degeneration, whereas the more peripheral lesions are less likely to do so. The proximal femurs are

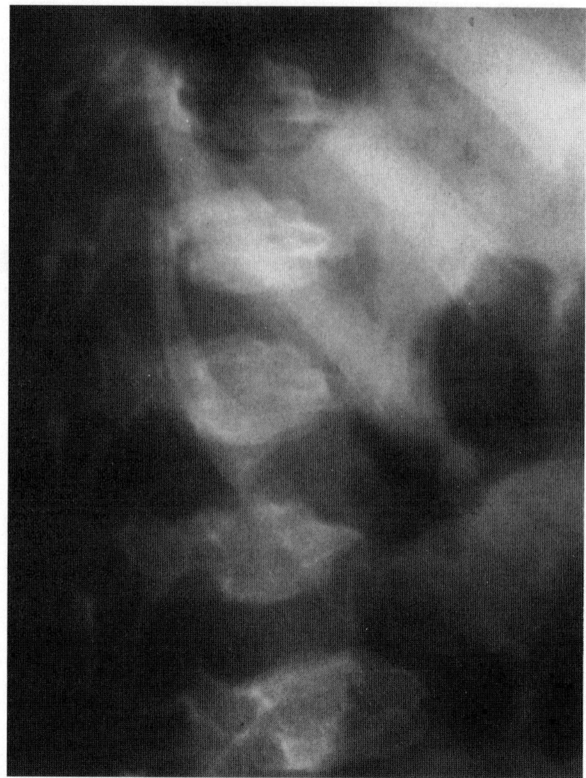

FIGURE 47.7. **Morquio Syndrome.** A lateral plain film of the spine reveals a central beak or anterior bony projection off the vertebral bodies in this patient with Morquio syndrome.

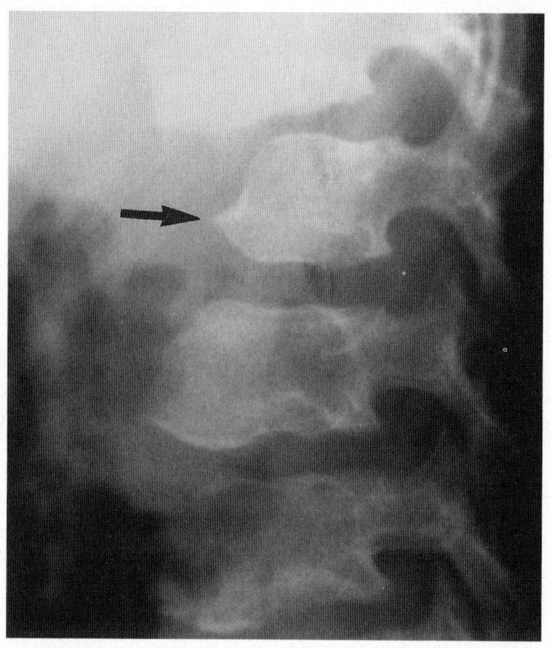

FIGURE 47.8. **Hurler Syndrome.** A lateral plain film of the spine in this patient with Hurler syndrome shows an inferiorly placed bony projection extending anteriorly off the vertebral bodies (*arrow*).

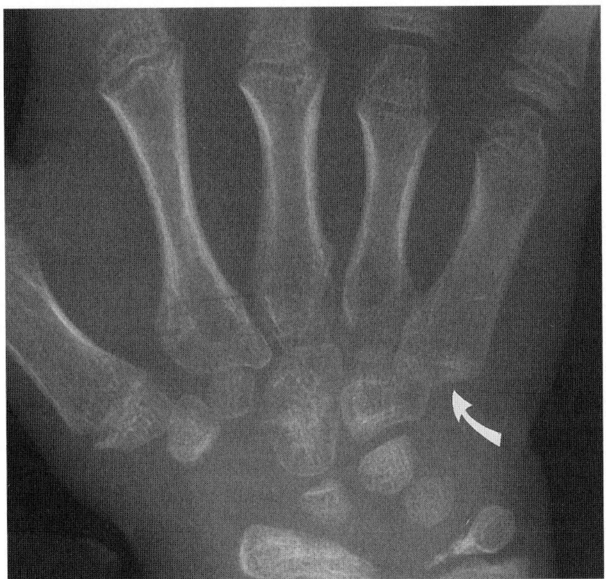

FIGURE 47.9. **Hurler Syndrome.** An anteroposterior plain film of the hand in this patient with Hurler syndrome shows a notch (*arrow*) at the base of the fifth metacarpal, which is a characteristic finding in all of the mucopolysaccharidoses.

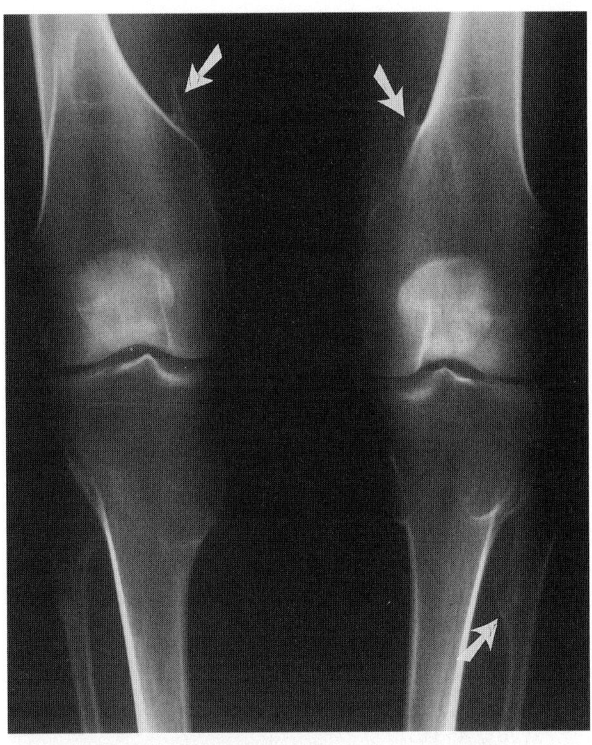

FIGURE 47.10. **Multiple Hereditary Exostosis.** The knees are involved in virtually every case of multiple hereditary exostosis. They typically show not only multiple exostoses (*arrows*) but marked undertubulation in the metaphyses.

frequently involved and have a characteristic appearance (Fig. 47.11).

Osteoid Osteoma

The etiology of osteoid osteoma is unknown. It is a painful lesion that occurs almost exclusively in patients younger than 30 years of age and is treated successfully with surgical excision or thermal ablation.

Radiographically, an osteoid osteoma is said to have a classic appearance, but it has many different appearances, which can make diagnosis difficult (3). The classically described radiographic appearance is a cortically based sclerotic lesion in a long bone that has a small lucency within it called the nidus (Fig. 47.12A). It is the nidus that causes the pain and the surrounding reactive sclerosis. If the nidus is surgically removed or thermally ablated,

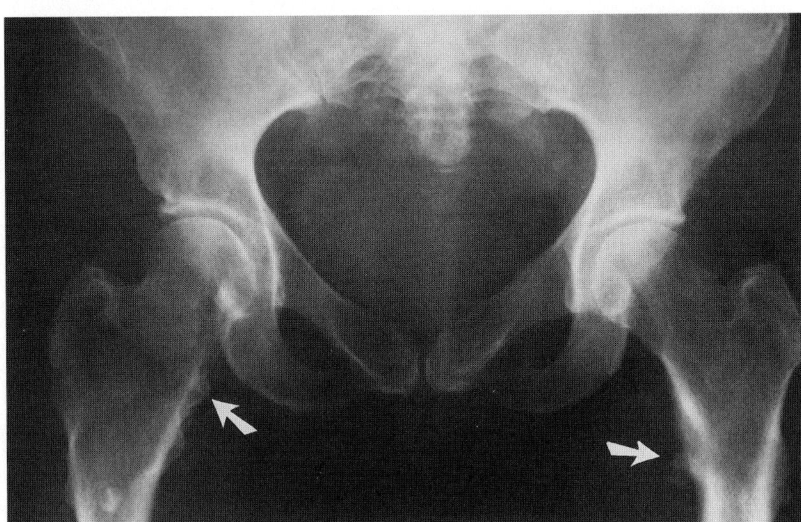

FIGURE 47.11. **Multiple Hereditary Exostosis.** The femoral necks are often involved in multiple hereditary exostosis. They will show undertubulation, as in this example, and usually have one or more exostoses (*arrows*).

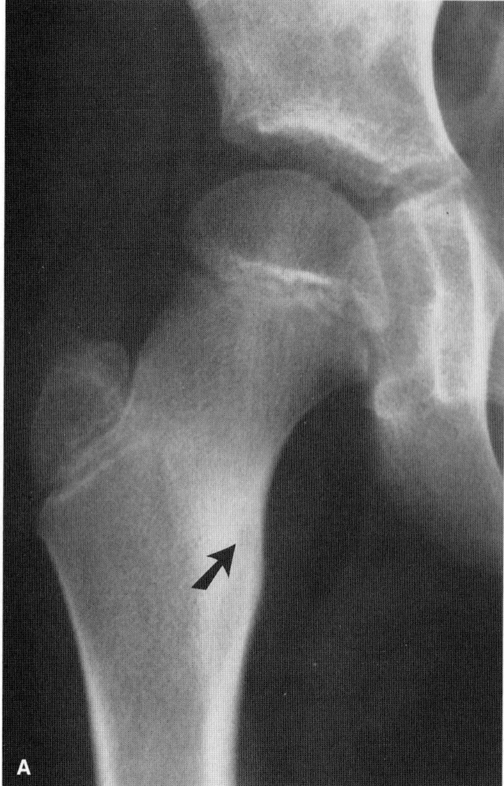

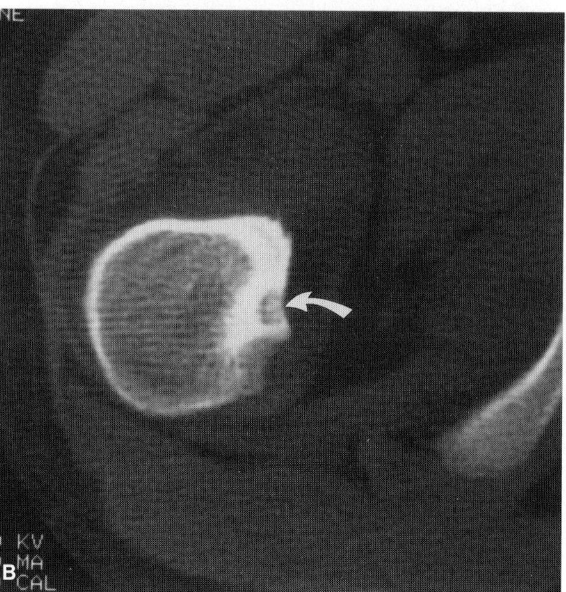

FIGURE 47.12. **Osteoid Osteoma. A.** An anteroposterior plain film of the femur in a child with hip pain shows an area of sclerosis medially near the lesser trochanter with a small lucency (*arrow*), which is the nidus of an osteoid osteoma. Osteomyelitis could have this identical appearance. **B.** CT scan of the femur shows the sclerosis medially and the lucent nidus (*arrow*) to better advantage. The CT scan gives the surgeon a more precise anatomic location of the nidus than the plain film.

complete cessation of pain is the rule. CT is often very helpful in demonstrating the exact location of the nidus (Fig. 47.12B).

If the nidus of an osteoid osteoma is located in the medullary rather than the cortical portion of a bone, or if it is located in a joint, there is much less reactive sclerosis present. This gives the lesion a different overall appearance than the more common cortical lesion, in that it does not appear as sclerotic. Up to 80% of osteoid osteomas are located intracortically, with the remainder located in the intramedullary part of a bone. Rarely, an osteoid osteoma will present in the periosteum, causing exuberant periostitis.

The nidus itself is usually lucent but often develops some calcification within it. It then has the appearance of a sequestrum, as is seen in osteomyelitis. If the nidus calcifies completely, it blends in with the surrounding sclerosis and cannot be seen on most radiographs. Therefore, the diagnosis of an osteoid osteoma should not depend on visualization of a nidus.

Because an osteoid osteoma resembles osteomyelitis, regardless of the appearance of the nidus, it can be difficult to differentiate the two radiographically. It cannot be reliably done with plain films, CT, or MR. However, because the nidus is extremely vascular, it avidly accumulates radiopharmaceutical bone-scanning agents. An osteoid osteoma will have an area of increased uptake corresponding to the area of reactive sclerosis and will additionally demonstrate a second area of increased uptake corresponding to the nidus (Fig. 47.13). This has been termed the double-density sign (4). In contrast, osteomyelitis has a photopenic area corresponding to the plain film lucency that represents an avascular focus of purulent material. The natural history of an osteoid osteoma is presumed to be spontaneous regression, as they are rarely seen in patients over the age of 30.

Osteopathia Striata

Also known as Voorhoeve disease, this disorder is manifested by multiple 2- to 3-mm-thick linear bands of sclerotic bone aligned parallel to the long axis of a bone (Fig. 47.14). It usually affects multiple long bones and is asymptomatic; hence, it is usually an incidental finding.

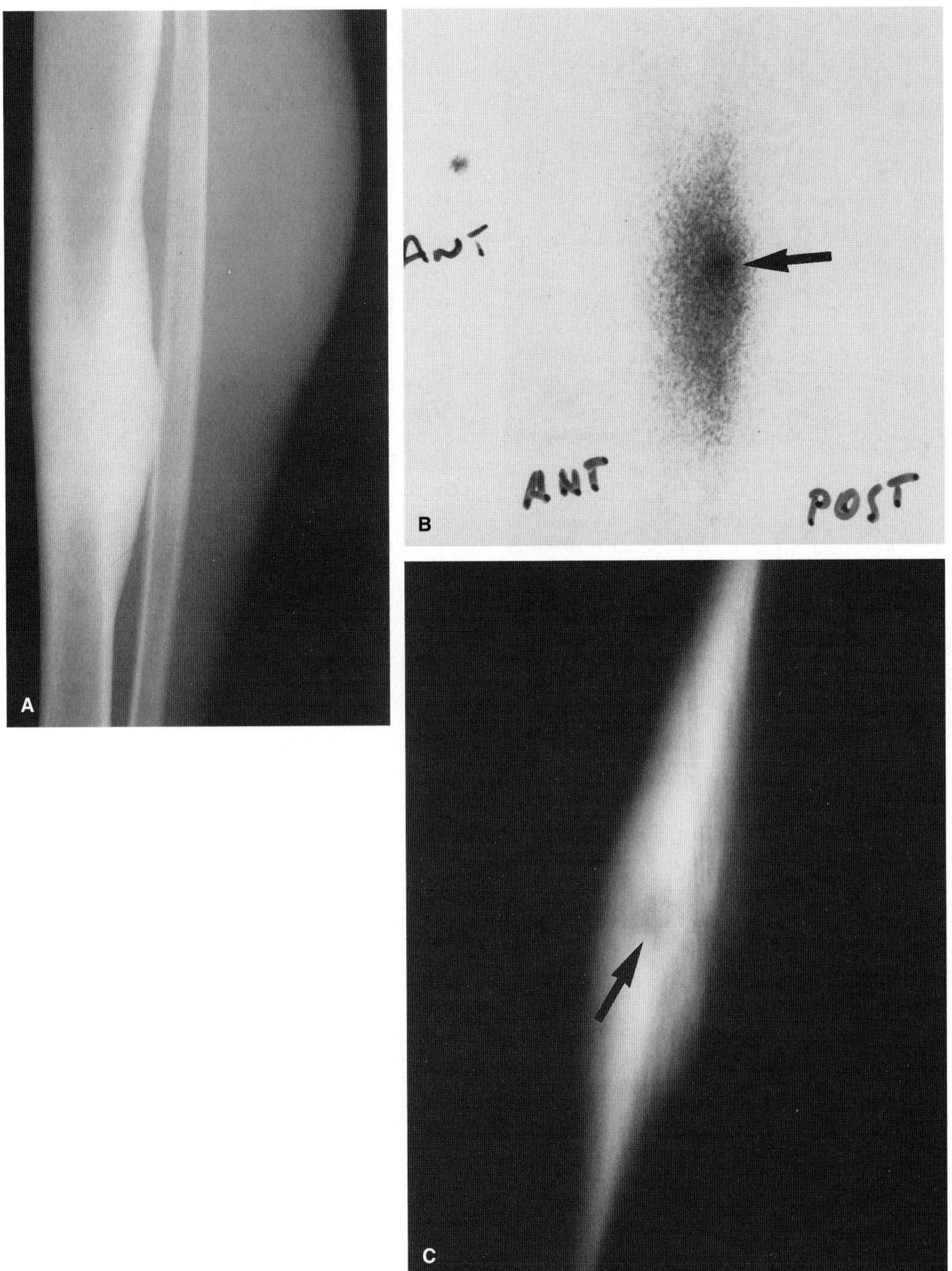

FIGURE 47.13. **Osteoid Osteoma. A.** A lateral plain film of the tibia in this child with leg pain shows cortical thickening in the posterior diaphysis. No lucency in the sclerotic area could be identified. **B.** A radionuclide bone scan reveals uptake corresponding to the area of sclerosis in the tibia, with a more marked area of uptake centrally (*arrow*), which is the double-density sign of an osteoid osteoma. **C.** The surgical specimen shows the nidus (*arrow*) as a faint lucency within the sclerotic bone.

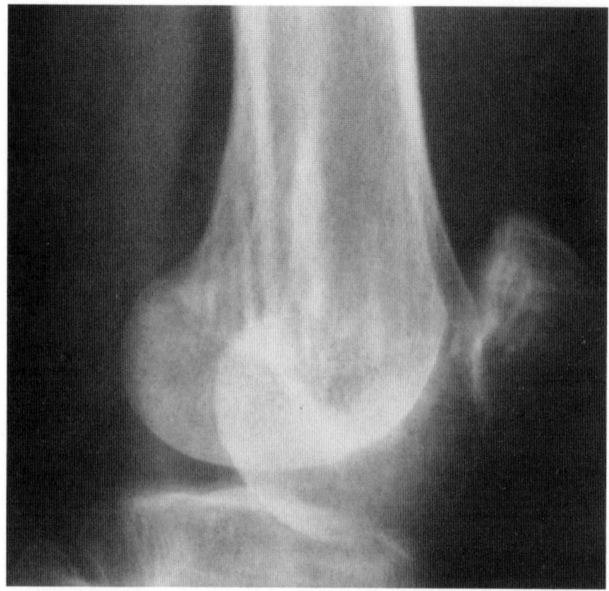

FIGURE 47.14. **Osteopathia Striata.** Multiple dense linear streaks are seen in the distal femur, which are characteristic of osteopathia striata.

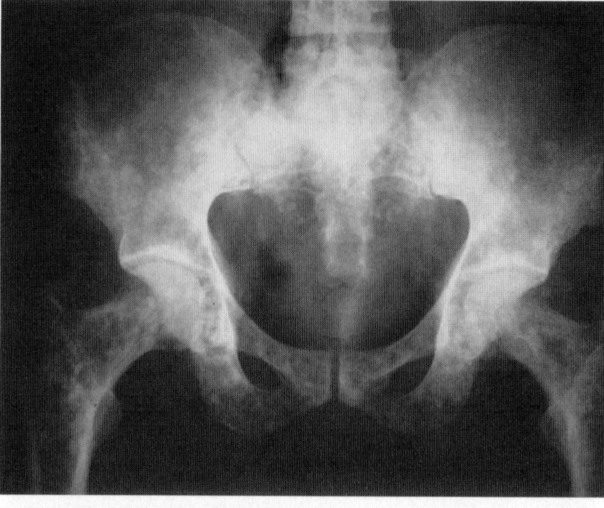

FIGURE 47.15. **Osteopoikilosis.** An anteroposterior view of the pelvis reveals multiple small, round sclerotic foci throughout the pelvis and femurs. This is diagnostic of osteopoikilosis. This is occasionally mistaken for metastatic disease.

Osteopoikilosis

Osteopoikilosis is an hereditary, asymptomatic disorder that is usually an incidental finding of multiple small (3 to 10 mm) sclerotic bony densities affecting primarily the ends of long bones and the pelvis (Fig. 47.15). It has no clinical significance other than that it can be confused for diffuse osteoblastic metastases.

Pachydermoperiostosis

Pachydermoperiostosis is a rare familial disease that is manifested by thickening of the skin of the extremities and face, clubbing of the fingers, and widespread periostitis. It seems to be more common in black patients. The periosteal reaction is similar to that of hypertrophic pulmonary osteoarthropathy, but pachydermoperiostosis is only occasionally painful.

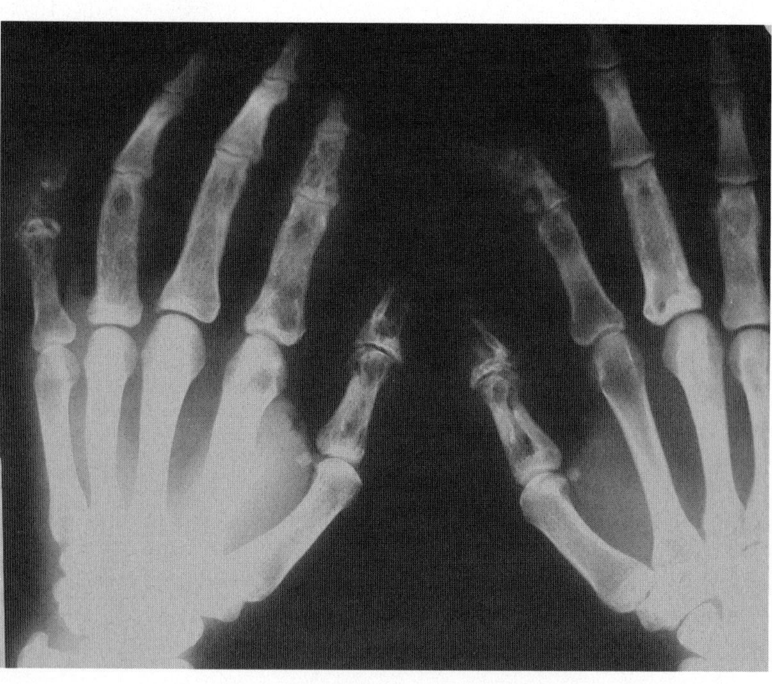

FIGURE 47.16. **Sarcoid.** An anteroposterior plain film of the hands in a patient with sarcoidosis shows multiple lytic lesions, many of which demonstrate a lacelike pattern.

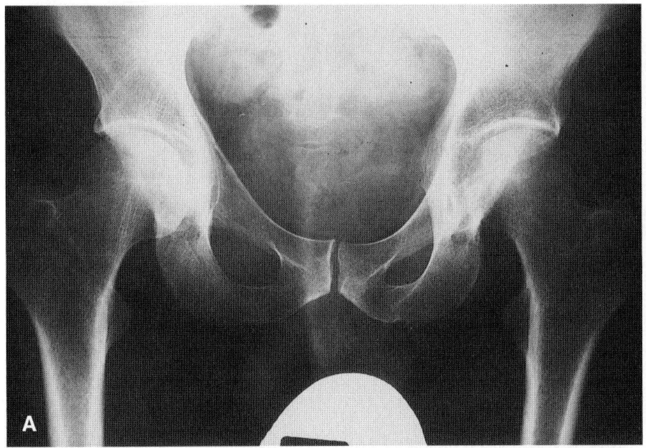

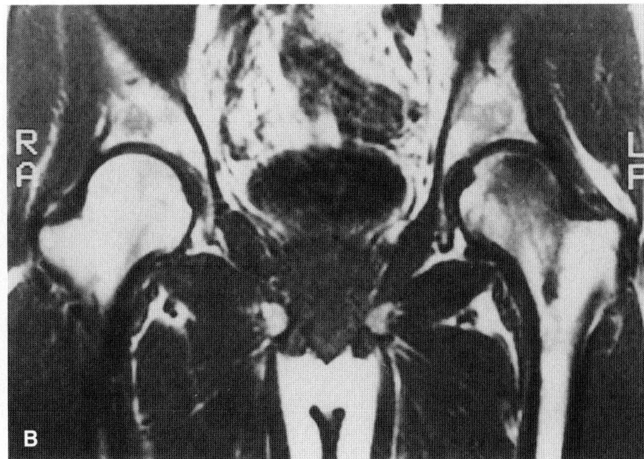

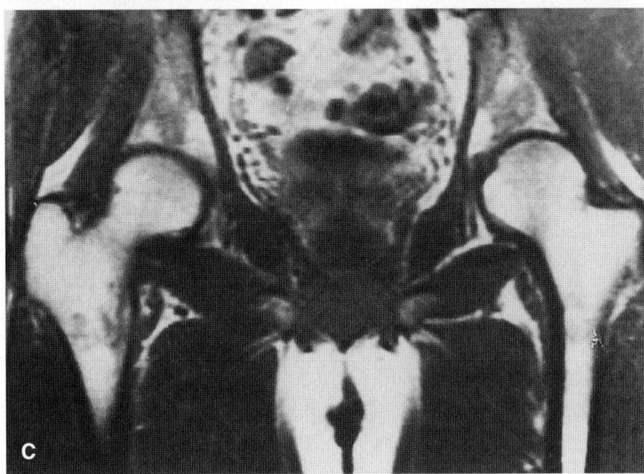

FIGURE 47.17. **Idiopathic Transient Osteoporosis of the Hip. A.** A plain film of a 40-year-old man with left hip pain shows osteoporosis involving the left hip, with no other abnormalities seen. **B.** A coronal T1WI done at the same time as the plain film shows low signal in the superior portion of the left femoral head. This is a characteristic appearance for avascular necrosis (AVN) but is a nonspecific finding. Clinically, this patient had no underlying causes for AVN, and he was treated conservatively. **C.** Seven months later, after near total cessation of the hip pain, a repeat T1WI shows no abnormality in the hip. This is consistent with idiopathic transient osteoporosis of the hip.

Sarcoidosis

Sarcoidosis is a noncaseating granulomatous disease that primarily affects the lungs. When the musculoskeletal system is involved, the hands are most often affected, with the spine and long bones only infrequently involved. Sarcoid causes a characteristic lacelike pattern of bony destruction in the hands (Fig. 47.16). Multiple phalanges are typically affected in either one or both hands. It is so radiographically characteristic that there is almost no differential diagnosis for this pattern.

Transient Osteoporosis of the Hip

This poorly understood disorder is an idiopathic process that begins with a painful hip with no underlying disorder or other findings other than osteoporosis, which is limited to the painful hip. Some believe it is early AVN; however, this has not been proved. Its appearance on MR is similar to that of early AVN (5) in that low signal on T1WIs is seen throughout the femoral head and neck (Fig. 47.17). Transient osteoporosis of the hip invariably is self-limited with full resolution. It tends to occur more often in men.

REFERENCES

1. Mankin H. Nontraumatic necrosis of bone (osteonecrosis). N Engl J Med 1992;326:1473–1479.
2. Mitchell D, Kressel H, Arger P, et al. Avascular necrosis of the femoral head: morphologic assessment by MR imaging, with CT correlation. Radiology 1986;161:739–742.
3. Marcove R, Heelan R, Huvos A, et al. Osteoid osteoma. Diagnosis, localization, and treatment. Clin Orthop 1991;267:197–201.
4. Helms CA, Hattner RS, Vogler JB III. Osteoid osteoma: radionuclide diagnosis. Radiology 1984;151:779–784.
5. Takatori Y, Kokubo T, Ninomiya S, et al. Transient osteoporosis of the hip. Magnetic resonance imaging. Clin Orthop 1991;271: 190–194.

Chapter 48

Magnetic Resonance Imaging of the Knee

Clyde A. Helms

Technique

Menisci

Cruciate Ligaments

Collateral Ligaments

Patella

Bony Abnormalities

Bursae

MR of the knee has developed into one of the most frequently requested examinations in radiology. This is because of its inherent accuracy in depicting internal derangements and its ability to allow orthopaedic surgeons to use it as a road map for subsequent therapeutic arthroscopic procedures. Also, MR has a very high negative predictive value; therefore, a normal MR knee examination is highly accurate in excluding an internal derangement (1,2).

TECHNIQUE

The proper imaging protocol is essential for a high diagnostic accuracy rate. If the appropriate sequences are obtained, an accuracy of 90% to 95% can be expected. A sagittal T1W (or proton-density) sequence is essential for examining the menisci, and 4- or 5-mm-thick slices with a relatively small field of view and at least a 256×192 matrix are recommended. The knee should be imaged using a dedicated knee coil and externally rotated about 5° to 10° (should not exceed 10°) to put the anterior cruciate ligament in the plane of imaging. T2 fast spin-echo (FSE, also called turbo spin echo) or T2* GRASS (gradient-recalled acquisition in the steady state) sagittal images are obtained primarily to examine the cruciate ligaments and cartilage.

FSE sequences are particularly poor for examining the menisci. Even when performed as fast proton-density images with a short echo train length, they have too much blurring to provide an accurate demonstration of meniscal tears. Conventional spin-echo images have consistently given a sensitivity for meniscal tears in the 90% to 95% range, whereas FSE proton-density sequences have been reported in multiple papers to be only around 80% sensitive for meniscal tears.

Coronal images are obtained to examine the collateral ligaments and cartilage and to look for meniscocapsular separations. These abnormalities can generally only be seen with T2WIs. Coronal T1WIs are therefore a waste of time, because nothing can be seen on these images that cannot be seen equally as well on the sagittal images or the T2 or T2* coronal images. The coronal images are rarely useful for seeing a meniscal tear that cannot be appreciated on the sagittal images.

Axial images are used for viewing the patellofemoral cartilage, identifying bursal fluid collections, and examining a medial patellar plica. As for the coronal images, to afford an opportunity to see any pathology, T2WIs must be obtained.

MENISCI

The normal meniscus is a fibrocartilaginous, C-shaped structure that is uniformly low in signal on both T1WIs and T2WIs. Many centers have found that the menisci are more easily examined if they fat-suppress the T1 or proton-density sequences (Fig. 48.1). With T2* sequences, the menisci will usually demonstrate some internal signal. With T1WIs, any signal within the meniscus is abnormal,

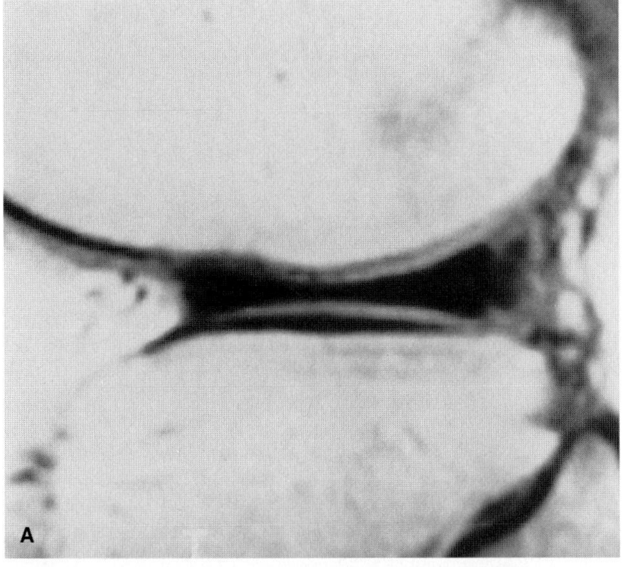

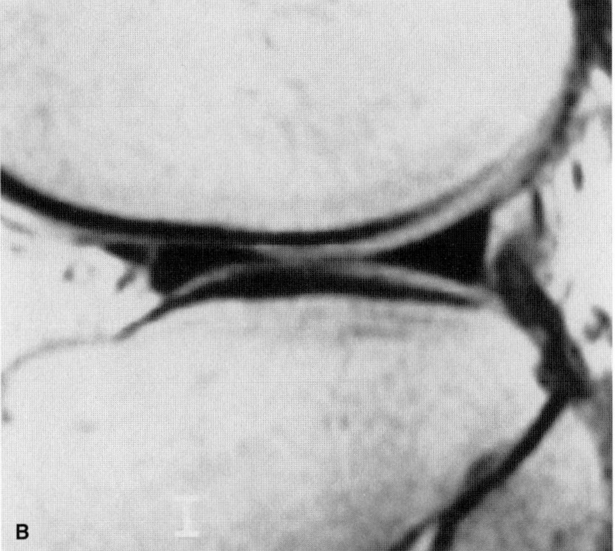

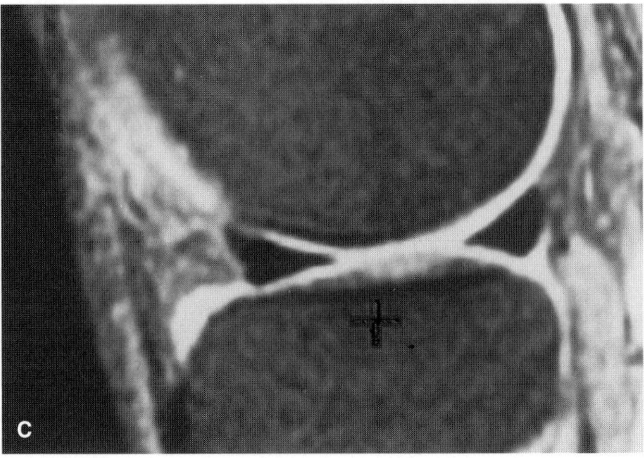

FIGURE 48.1. **Normal Meniscus. A.** A sagittal T1WI (time of repetition [TR] 600; time of echo [TE] 30) through a normal lateral meniscus demonstrates uniform low signal in the meniscus. This is a section through the body of the meniscus, as it has a bow-tie configuration. With 4- or 5-mm-thick slices, two sections of the body should be seen in each meniscus. **B.** In the same T1W sequence, this sagittal image demonstrates uniform low signal in the anterior and posterior horns of this normal lateral meniscus. **C.** This sagittal proton-density image (TR 2,000; TE 20) shows how fat suppression accentuates the menisci.

except in children, in whom some signal is normal and represents normal vascularity.

Meniscal Degeneration. Meniscal signal that does not disrupt an articular surface is representative of intrasubstance degeneration (Fig. 48.2), which is myxoid degeneration of the fibrocartilage. It most likely represents aging and normal wear and tear. It is not thought to be symptomatic and cannot be diagnosed clinically or with arthroscopy. Some choose, therefore, not to mention intrasubstance degeneration in the radiology interpretation. A grading scale for meniscal signal that is widely used is the following (Fig. 48.3): grade 1, rounded or amorphous signal that does not disrupt an articular surface; grade 2, linear signal that does not disrupt an articular surface; and grade 3, rounded or linear signal that disrupts an articular surface. Grades 1 and 2 are intrasubstance degeneration and should not be reported as "grade 1 or 2 tears," since the term "tear" can lead to unnecessary arthroscopy (arthroscopy is not indicated for intrasubstance degeneration). Grade 3 is a meniscal tear.

Meniscal Tear. When high signal in a meniscus disrupts the superior or inferior articular surface, a meniscal tear is diagnosed (Fig. 48.4). Meniscal tears have many different configurations and locations; an oblique tear extending to the inferior surface of the posterior horn of the medial meniscus is the most common type. In a small but significant percentage of cases, it can be virtually impossible to be certain whether meniscal high signal disrupts an articular surface. In these cases it is recommended that the surgeon be advised that it is too close to call. The surgeon can then rely on his or her clinical expertise to decide if arthroscopy is warranted, and if it is, the MR will guide the surgeon to the location of the questionable tear. If these equivocal cases are excluded, the remaining cases will have an extremely high accuracy rate.

It has been shown that MR imaging sensitivity for meniscal tears decreases significantly when the anterior cruciate ligament (ACL) is torn (3). These frequently overlooked tears occur in the periphery of the meniscus and in the posterior horn of the lateral meniscus. Hence, great

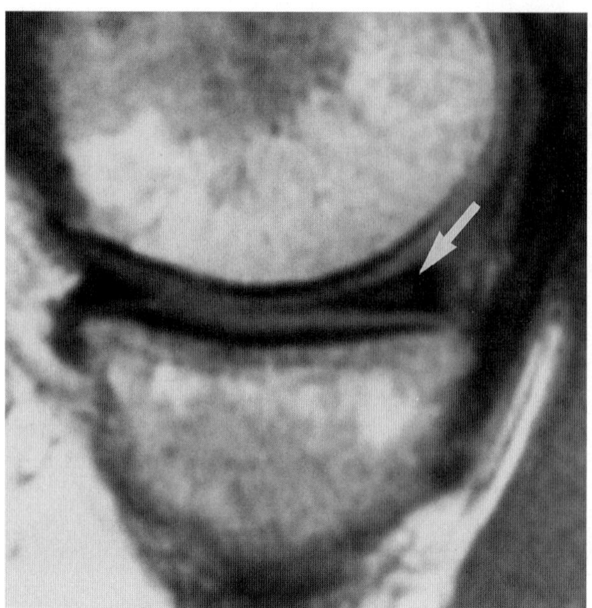

FIGURE 48.2. **Intrasubstance Degeneration.** Faint intermediate signal can be seen in the posterior horn of this meniscus (*arrow*) that does not disrupt the articular surface of the meniscus. This is intrasubstance degeneration.

care must be used in examining these areas of the menisci in patients with ACL tears.

Bucket-Handle Tear. Another very common meniscal tear is a bucket-handle tear. This is a vertical longitudinal tear that can result in the inner free edge of the meniscus becoming displaced into the intercondylar notch (Fig. 48.5). It is most easily recognized by observing on the sagittal images that only one image is present that has the bow-tie appearance of the body segment of the meniscus (4) (Fig. 48.6). Normally, two contiguous sagittal images with a bow-tie shape are seen, because the normal meniscus is 9 to 12 mm wide and the sagittal images are 4 to 5 mm in thickness. On the coronal images, a bucket-handle tear may reveal the meniscus to be shortened and truncated; however, the torn meniscus often remodels and truncation cannot be appreciated. The displaced inner edge of the meniscus (the "handle" of the bucket) is often seen in the intercondylar notch on sagittal or coronal views (Fig. 48.7).

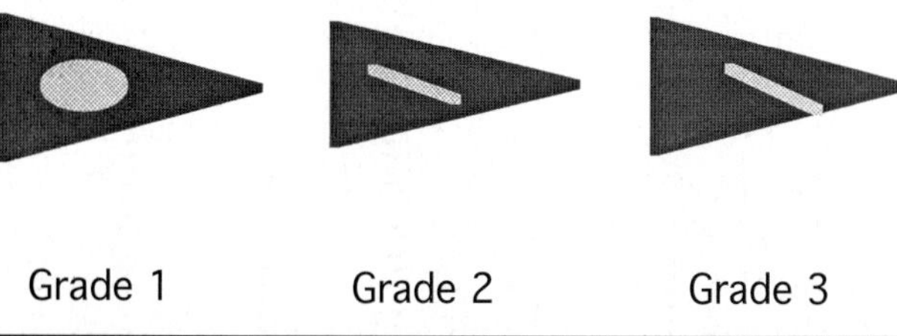

FIGURE 48.3. **Grading Scale for Menisci.** A schematic of the MR grading scale for meniscal abnormalities. Grade 1 is rounded or amorphous signal in the meniscus that does not disrupt an articular surface. Grade 2 is linear signal that does not disrupt an articular surface. Grades 1 and 2 represent intrasubstance degeneration. Grade 3 is signal that does disrupt an articular surface and indicates a meniscal tear.

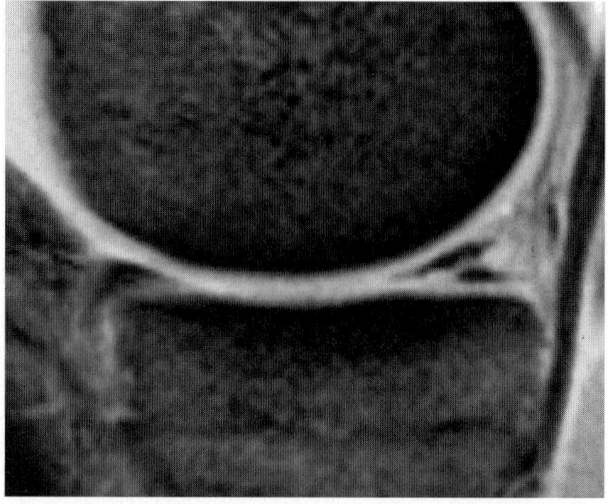

FIGURE 48.4. **Meniscal Tear.** This T1W sagittal image (time of repetition 600; time of echo 30) shows linear high signal in the posterior horn of the meniscus that disrupts the inferior articular surface. This is the appearance of a meniscal tear.

Discoid Meniscus. A discoid meniscus is a large meniscus that can have many different shapes: lens-shaped, wedged, flat, and others. Whether it is congenital or acquired is not known, but most are found in children and

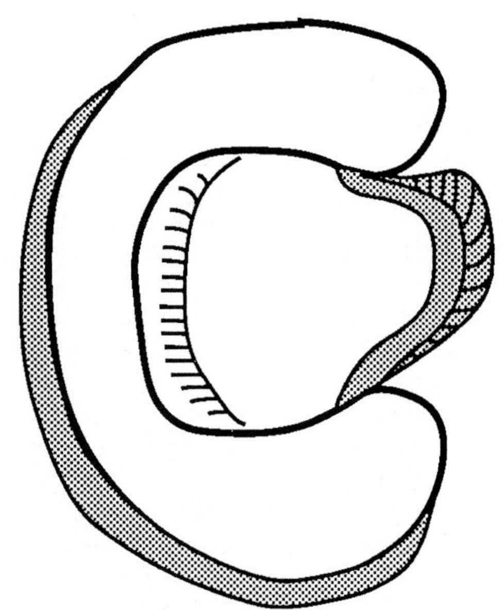

FIGURE 48.5. **Bucket-Handle Tear.** This drawing illustrates a bucket-handle tear, with the torn free edge of the meniscus displaced as the handle of the bucket.

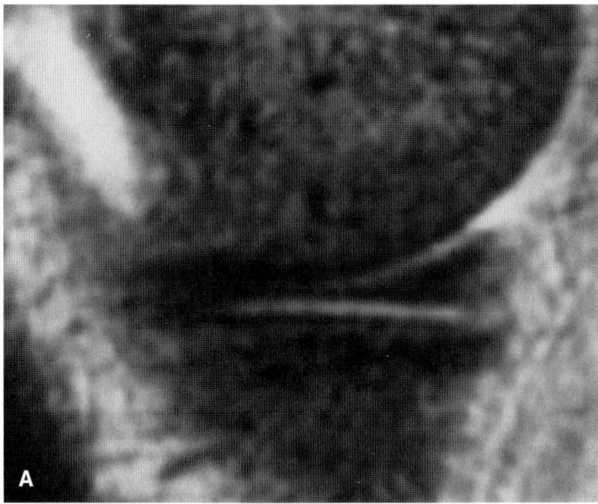

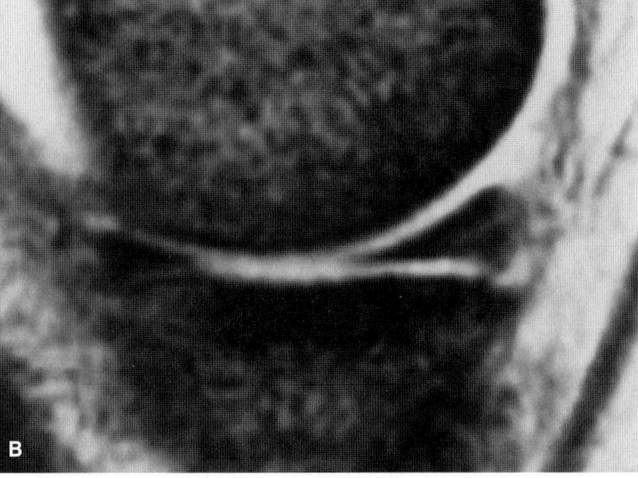

FIGURE 48.6. **Bucket-Handle Tear.** Sagittal T1WIs (time of repetition 600; time of echo 30) through the medial meniscus at its most medial aspect reveal one bow-tie, indicative of the body of the meniscus **(A)**, with the adjacent image **(B)** showing apparently normal anterior and posterior horns. However, since there should be two consecutive sagittal images with a bow-tie configuration, this suggests a bucket-handle tear.

young adults. It is seen laterally in up to 3% of the population, with a discoid medial meniscus being much less common. A discoid meniscus is thought to be more prone to tear than a normal meniscus, and it can be symptomatic even without being torn. Although they are easily identified on coronal images by noting extensions of meniscal tissue into the tibial spines at the intercondylar notch (Fig. 48.8), they are most reliably diagnosed by noting more than two consecutive sagittal images that show the meniscus with a bow-tie appearance (Fig. 48.9) (5).

Meniscal Cysts. Meniscal cysts occur in about 5% of cases and can cause pain even if the meniscus is not torn. The etiology is unknown, but they occur more frequently in discoid menisci. If the meniscus is not torn, the surgical approach used by some is percutaneous decompression and packing, whereas if a meniscal tear is associated with the cyst, it is approached intra-articularly. Hence, accurate diagnosis of a tear is imperative. The intrameniscal portion of the cyst typically does not get as bright as fluid in signal on T2 sequences (Fig. 48.10), which has misled many

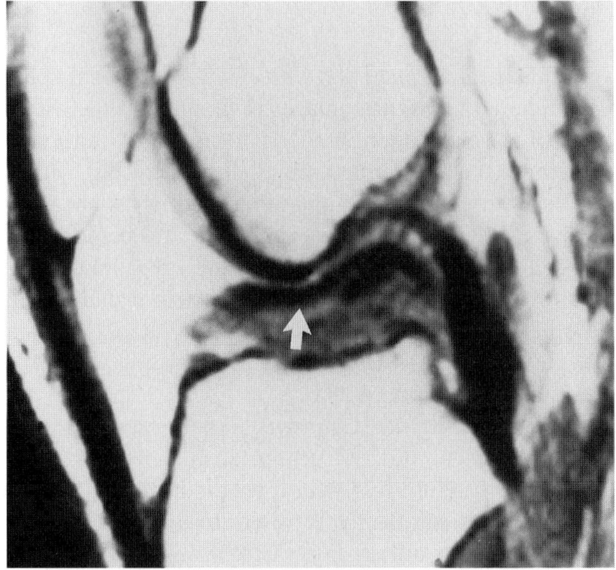

FIGURE 48.7. **Displaced Fragment in Bucket-Handle Tear.** A sagittal T1WI (time of repetition 600; time of echo 30) through the intercondylar notch in a patient with a bucket-handle tear reveals the displaced free fragment or handle (*arrow*) just anterior to the PCL.

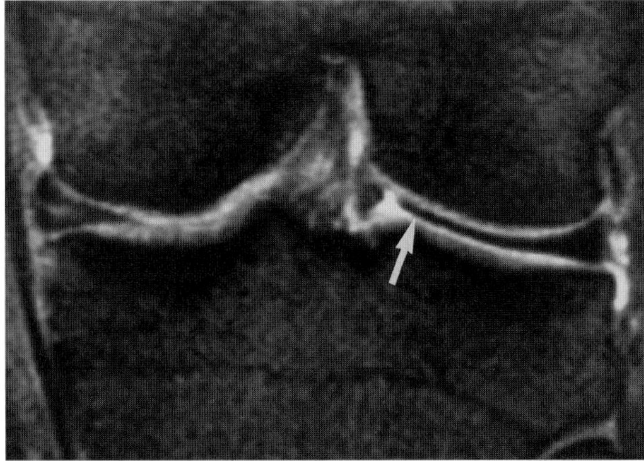

FIGURE 48.8. **Discoid Lateral Meniscus.** A coronal gradient-recalled acquisition in the steady state image (time of repetition 500; time of echo 30; θ 30°) through the intercondylar notch shows a large lateral meniscus with meniscal tissue extending into the notch medially (*arrow*).

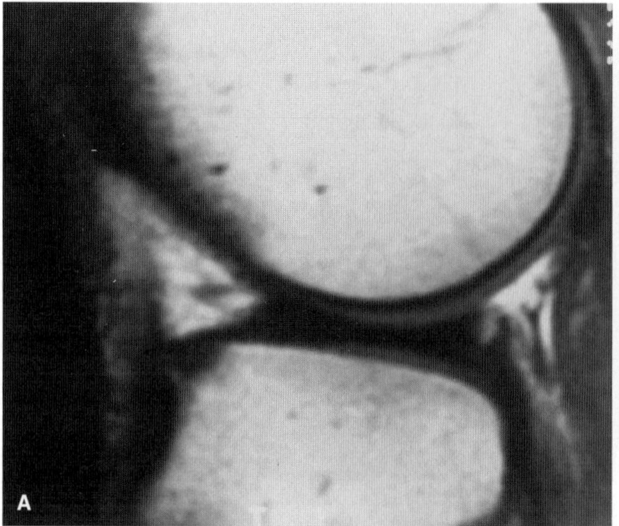

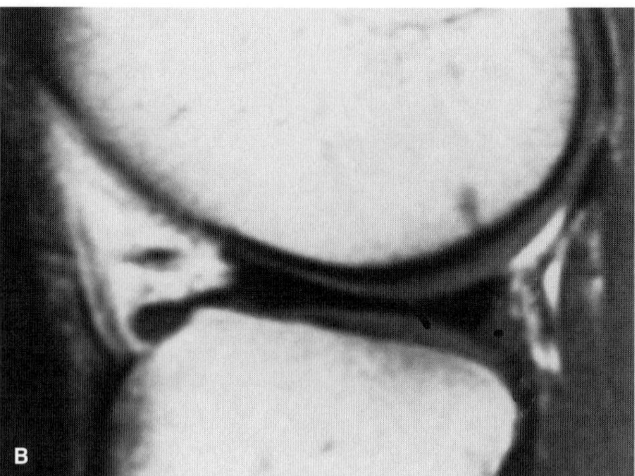

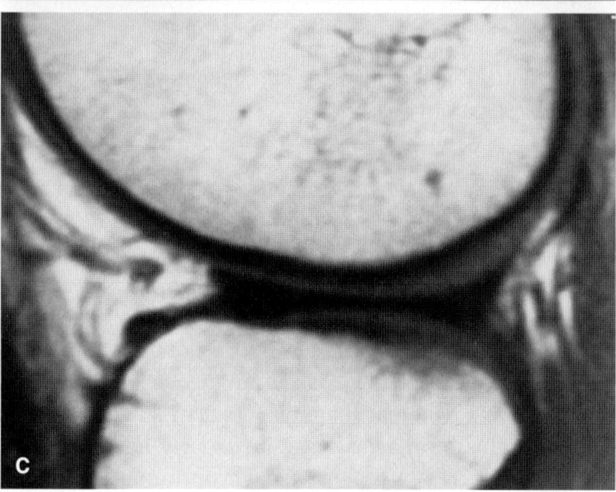

FIGURE 48.9. **Discoid Lateral Meniscus.** Three consecutive 5-mm-thick T1WIs (time of repetition 600; time of echo 30) through the lateral meniscus, beginning with the most lateral **(A)** and extending medially **(B, C)**, each show the meniscus to have a bow-tie configuration. Because only two images should have a bow-tie shape, indicative of the body of the meniscus, this is diagnostic of a discoid lateral meniscus. (Fig. 48.8 is an image of the same knee.)

radiologists into discounting the presence of a cyst. A meniscal cyst will enlarge the meniscus and give it a swollen appearance unless it decompresses into the soft tissues (called a parameniscal cyst) or into the joint via a meniscal tear. Decompression into a parameniscal cyst does not indicate a meniscal tear. A meniscal tear, by definition, has to disrupt the articular surface of the meniscus.

Transverse Ligament. The lateral meniscus often has what appears to be a tear on the anterior horn near its upper margin, which is a pseudotear from the insertion of the transverse ligament (Fig. 48.11). This can easily be differentiated from a real tear by following it medially across the knee in the Hoffa fat-pad, where it inserts into the anterior horn of the medial meniscus.

CRUCIATE LIGAMENTS

Anterior Cruciate Ligament. The normal ACL is seen in the intercondylar notch as a linear, predominantly low-signal structure on T1WIs; it often shows some linear striations near its insertion onto the medial tibial spine when viewed on sagittal images (Fig. 48.12). When torn, the ACL is most often simply not visualized, although sometimes the actual disruption will be seen (Fig. 48.13). T2WIs are imperative for obtaining the highest accuracy in diagnosing ACL tears, because fluid and hemorrhage will often obscure the ligament on T1WIs. Partial tears or sprains of the ACL are manifested by high signal within an otherwise intact ligament. MR is highly accurate in diagnosing a torn ACL, with sensitivities reported in the literature approaching 100%.

Posterior Cruciate Ligament. The normal posterior cruciate ligament (PCL) is a gently curved, homogeneously low-signal structure (Fig. 48.14) that is infrequently torn and even less frequently repaired by surgeons. When torn, it takes on diffuse intermediate signal throughout (Fig. 48.15). This increased signal usually does not get brighter with T2WIs and is therefore often overlooked. Most orthopaedic surgeons do not even inspect the PCL at arthroscopy and do not repair it when torn, because it is rarely a cause of instability.

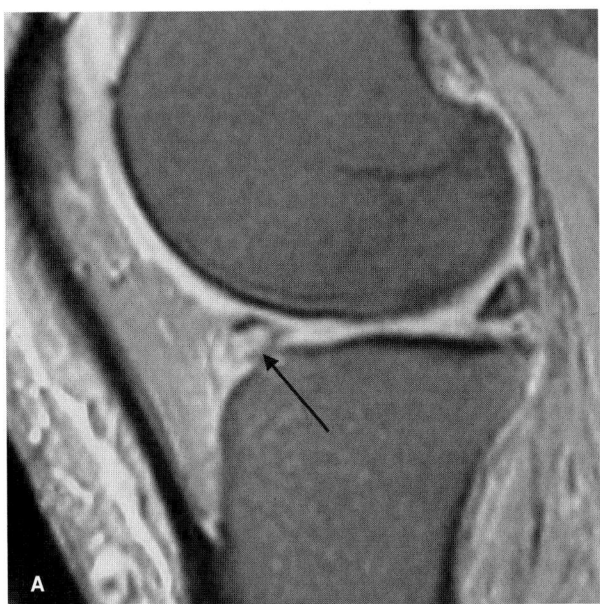

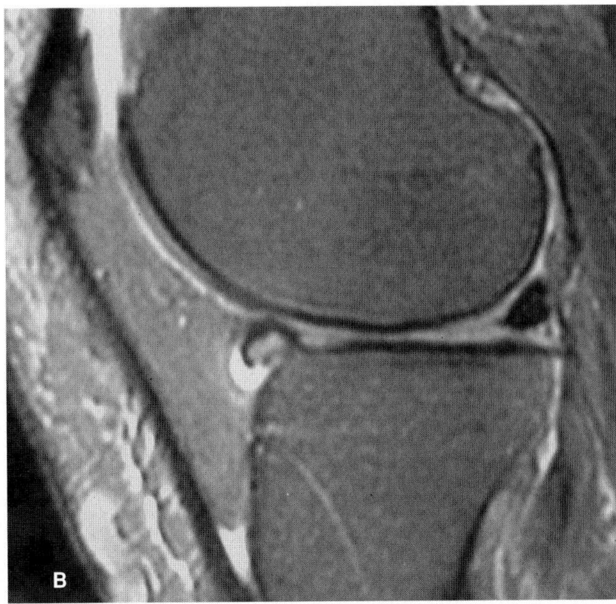

FIGURE 48.10. **Meniscal Cyst.** A sagittal proton-density weighted image **(A)** through the medial meniscus shows a swollen anterior horn filled with increased signal (*arrow*). A T2WI **(B)** shows high signal similar to fluid in the parameniscal portion, whereas the intrameniscal signal is only intermediate.

Meniscofemoral Ligament. A low-signal, round structure is often seen just anterior or posterior to the PCL, as seen in the sagittal views. A loose body or a free fragment of a piece of torn meniscus can have this appearance (Fig. 48.16), but it is most commonly caused by a meniscofemoral ligament that extends obliquely across the knee from the medial femoral condyle to the posterior horn of the lateral meniscus. If it passes in front of the PCL, it is called the ligament of Humphry, and if it passes behind the PCL, it is called the ligament of Wrisberg (Fig. 48.17). Either one of these ligaments is present in up to 72% of all knees.

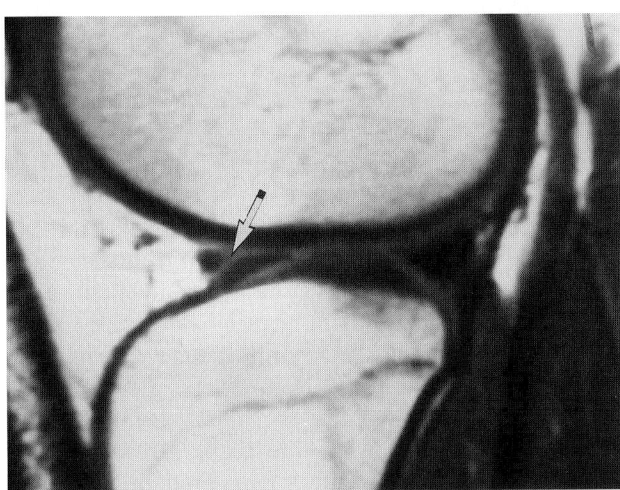

FIGURE 48.11. **Pseudotear From a Transverse Ligament.** A sagittal T1WI (time of repetition 600; time of echo 30) through the lateral meniscus shows linear high signal through the upper anterior horn (*arrow*), which resembles a tear. This is the insertion of the transverse ligament onto the meniscus.

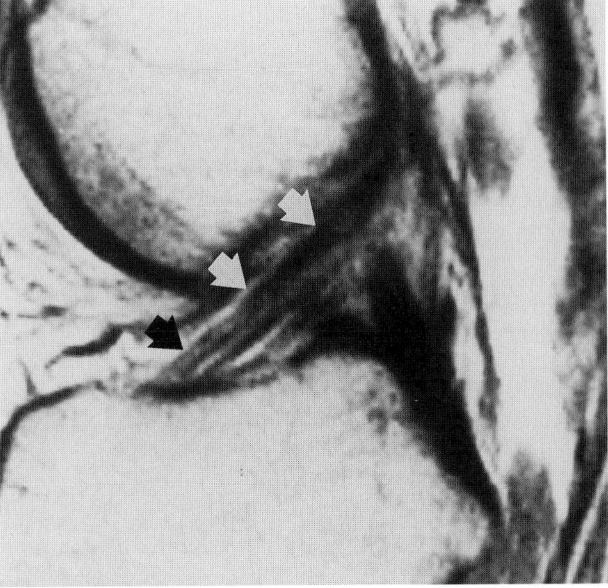

FIGURE 48.12. **Normal Anterior Cruciate Ligament (ACL).** A sagittal T1WI (time of repetition 600; time of echo 30) through the intercondylar notch shows the normal appearance of the ACL (*arrows*).

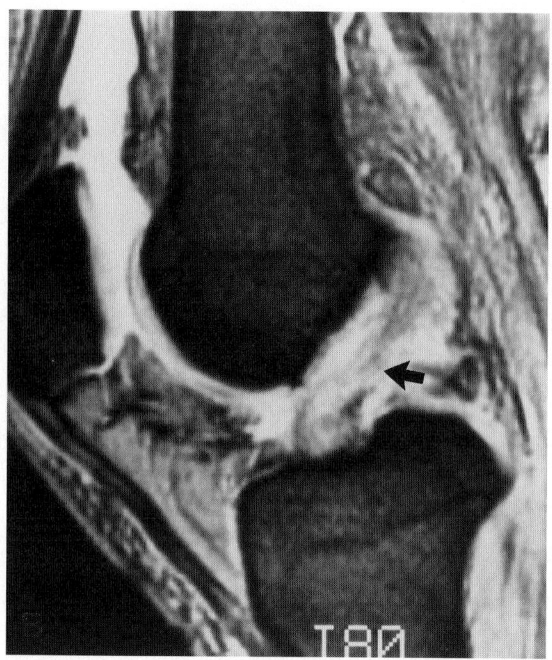

FIGURE 48.13. **Torn Anterior Cruciate Ligament (ACL).** A sagittal T2WI through the intercondylar notch shows fibers of the ACL that are disrupted centrally (*arrow*).This is a common MR appearance of a torn ACL.

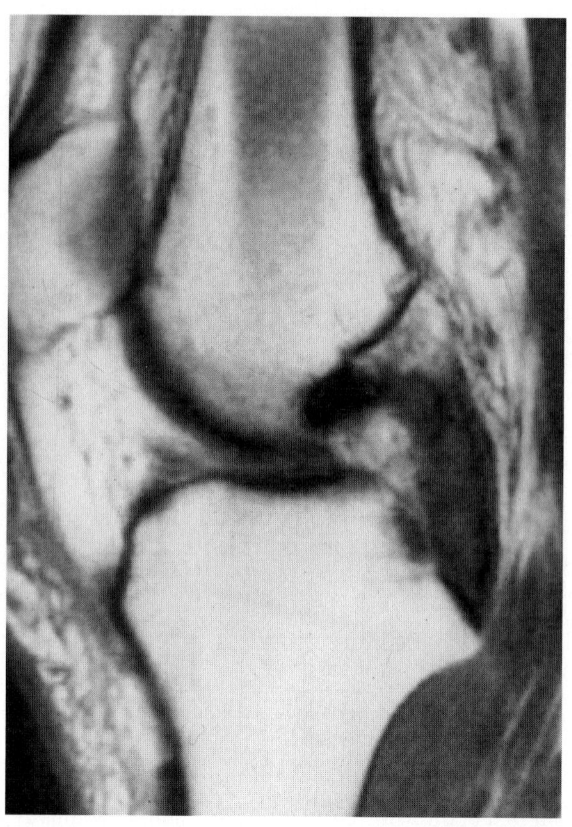

FIGURE 48.15. **Torn Posterior Cruciate Ligament (PCL).** A sagittal T1WI (time of repetition 600; time of echo 30) through the intercondylar notch reveals the PCL to have diffuse intermediate signal throughout. This is typical for a torn PCL.

The insertion of the ligament of Humphry or Wrisberg onto the lateral meniscus can produce a pseudotear similar to that caused by the transverse ligament on the anterior horn of the lateral meniscus (Fig. 48.18). Prior to diagnosing a tear on the upper aspect of the posterior horn of the lateral meniscus, care must be taken to look for a meniscofemoral ligament to be certain it is not a pseudotear from the ligament's insertion. Similarly, prior to diagnosing a loose body in front of or behind the PCL, care must be taken to try to follow the structure across to the lateral meniscus to determine whether it is a meniscofemoral ligament.

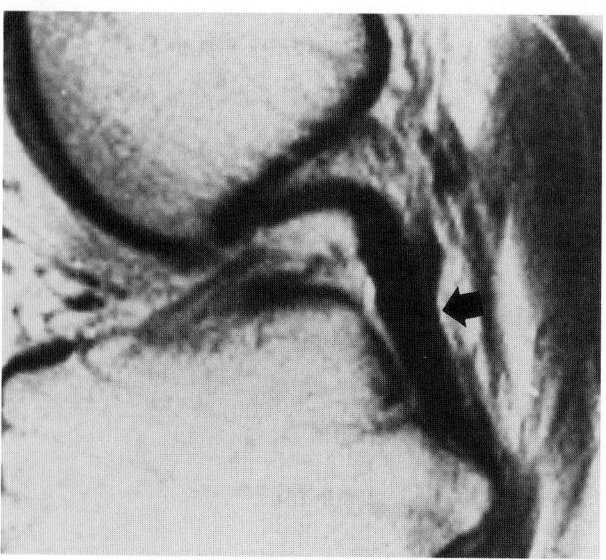

FIGURE 48.14. **Normal Posterior Cruciate Ligament (PCL).** A sagittal T1WI (time of repetition 600; time of echo 30) through the intercondylar notch shows the appearance of the normal PCL, with its characteristic uniform low signal (*arrow*).

COLLATERAL LIGAMENTS

Medial Collateral Ligament. The medial collateral ligament (MCL) originates on the medial femoral condyle and inserts on the tibia. It is closely applied to the joint and is intimately associated with the medial joint capsule and the medial meniscus. The MCL is uniformly low in signal on T1 and T2 or T2* sequences. Injuries to the MCL usually occur from a valgus stress to the lateral part of the knee (such as a "clipping" injury in football). A grade 1 injury represents a mild sprain and is diagnosed on MR by the presence of fluid or hemorrhage in the soft tissues medial to the MCL. The ligament is otherwise normal. A grade 2 injury is a partial tear and is seen as high signal in and around the MCL on T2 or T2* coronal sequences. The ligament is intact, although the deep or superficial fibers may

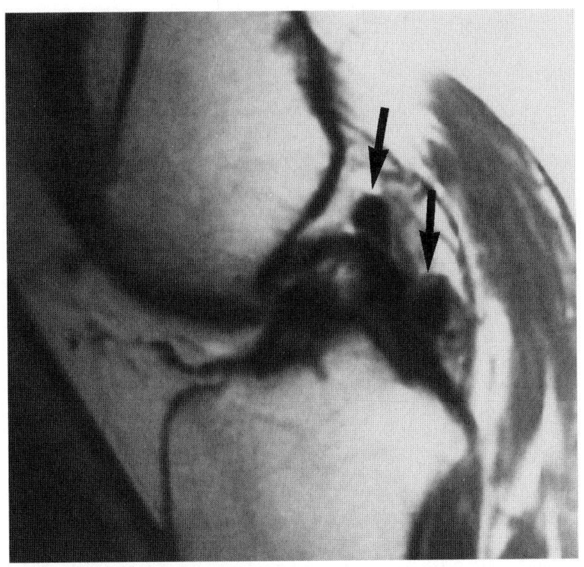

FIGURE 48.16. **Free Fragment of a Torn Meniscus.** A sagittal T1WI (time of repetition 600; time of echo 30) through the intercondylar notch in this patient with a torn meniscus shows two rounded, low-signal structures (*arrows*) that are free fragments of meniscal tissue. A meniscofemoral ligament of Wrisberg could have the appearance of either of these loose bodies.

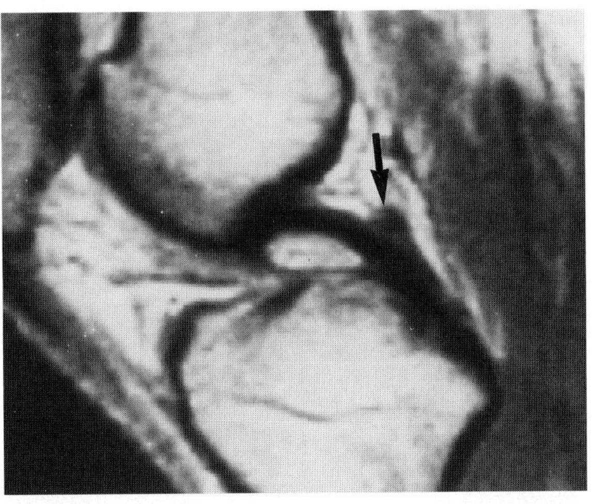

FIGURE 48.17. **Ligament of Wrisberg.** A sagittal T1WI (time of repetition 600; time of echo 30) through the intercondylar notch shows a rounded, low-signal structure posterior to the posterior cruciate ligament, which is the meniscofemoral ligament of Wrisberg (*arrow*).

show minimal disruption (Fig. 48.19). A grade 3 injury is a complete disruption of the MCL. It is best appreciated on T2 or T2* images (Fig. 48.20).

A meniscocapsular separation occurs when the medial meniscus is torn from its attachment to the joint capsule. This occurs most commonly at the site of the MCL and often occurs concomitantly with an MCL injury. It is easily recognized on a T2 or T2* coronal image by noting joint fluid extending between the medial meniscus and the capsule (Fig. 48.21). It is essential to use T2 or T2* sequences, as a T1WI will not detect the fluid between the meniscus and the capsule.

Lateral Collateral Ligament. The lateral collateral ligament (LCL) consists of three parts. The most posterior

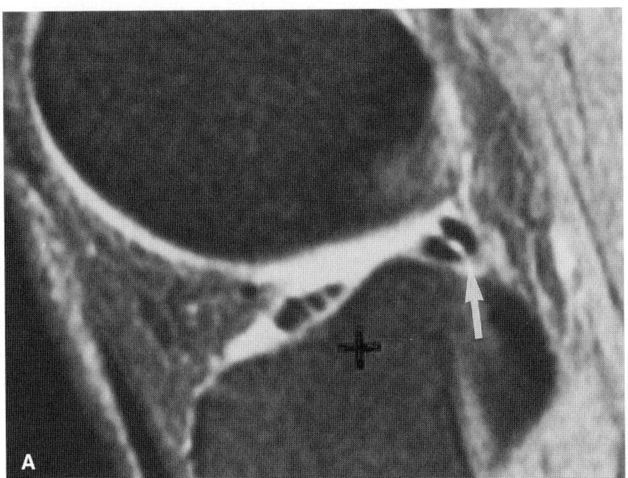

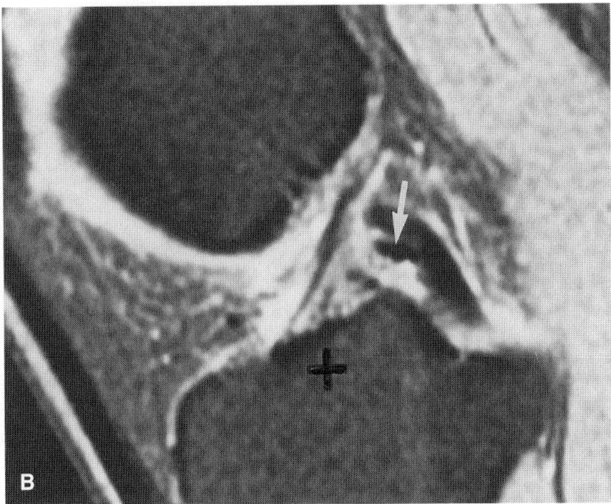

FIGURE 48.18. **Pseudotear From Ligament of Humphry Insertion. A.** A sagittal proton-density fat-suppressed image (time of repetition 2,000; time of echo 20) through the lateral meniscus reveals an apparent tear of the posterior horn (*arrow*). (The "speckled" appearance in the anterior horn of the lateral meniscus is a frequently seen normal variant and should not be confused for a torn meniscus.) **B.** On the image through the intercondylar notch, a ligament of Humphry (*arrow*) is seen anterior to the posterior cruciate ligament (PCL). The ligament of Humphry could be followed on adjacent images, from anterior to the PCL to its insertion on the posterior horn of the lateral meniscus.

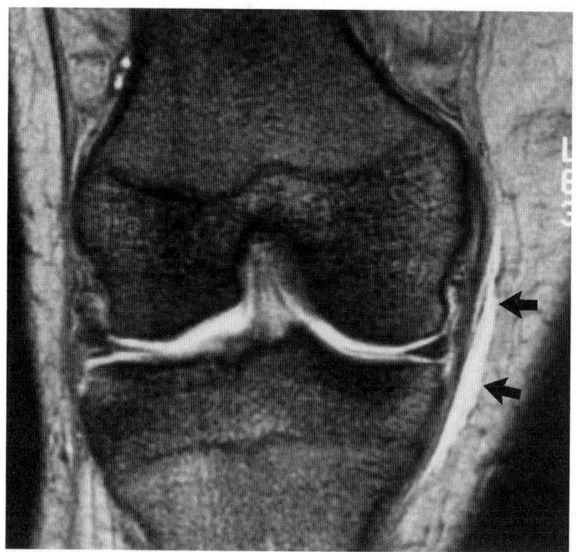

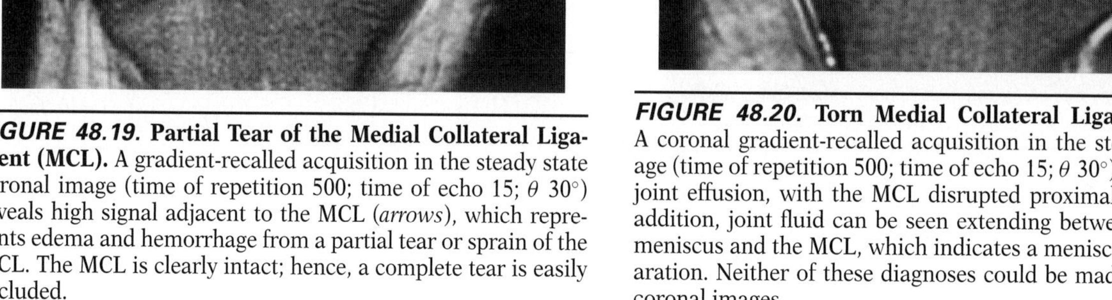

FIGURE 48.19. **Partial Tear of the Medial Collateral Ligament (MCL).** A gradient-recalled acquisition in the steady state coronal image (time of repetition 500; time of echo 15; θ 30°) reveals high signal adjacent to the MCL (*arrows*), which represents edema and hemorrhage from a partial tear or sprain of the MCL. The MCL is clearly intact; hence, a complete tear is easily excluded.

FIGURE 48.20. **Torn Medial Collateral Ligament (MCL).** A coronal gradient-recalled acquisition in the steady state image (time of repetition 500; time of echo 15; θ 30°) shows a large joint effusion, with the MCL disrupted proximally (*arrow*). In addition, joint fluid can be seen extending between the medial meniscus and the MCL, which indicates a meniscocapsular separation. Neither of these diagnoses could be made on the T1W coronal images.

structure is the tendon of the biceps femoris, which inserts onto the head of the fibula. Next, anterior to the biceps, is the true lateral collateral ligament, also called the fibular collateral ligament, which extends from the lateral femoral condyle to the head of the fibula. The biceps and the fibular collateral ligament usually join and insert onto the head of the fibula in a conjoined fashion. Anterior to the fibular collateral ligament is the iliotibial band, which extends into the fascia more anteriorly and blends into the lateral retinaculum on the patella. The LCL is torn

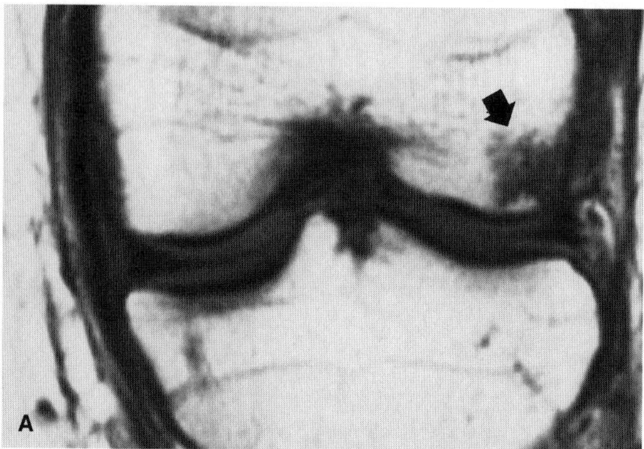

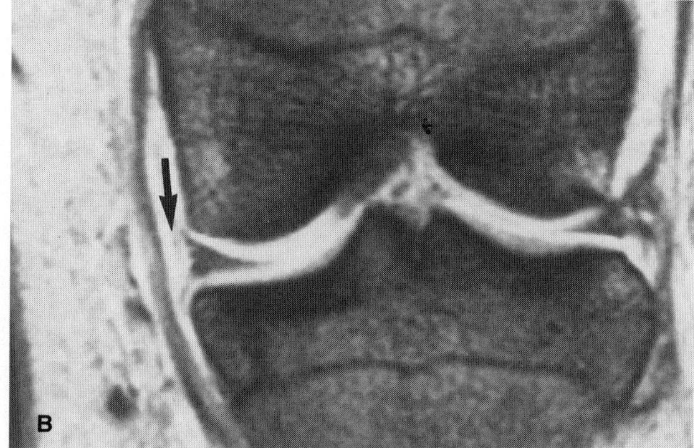

FIGURE 48.21. **Meniscocapsular Separation. A.** A T1W coronal image (time of repetition [TR] 600; time of echo [TE] 30) reveals a contusion of the lateral femoral condyle (*arrow*), indicative of a valgus strain, which is often associated with a medial collateral ligament (MCL) tear. The MCL appears normal on this image; however, the linear low signal in the soft tissues just adjacent to the MCL is suggestive of fluid. This would indicate a partial tear or sprain of the MCL. **B.** A coronal gradient-recalled acquisition in the steady state image (TR 500; TE 15; θ 30°) in the same knee reveals fluid between the medial meniscus and the MCL (*arrow*), which is diagnostic for a meniscocapsular separation. Faint high signal in the MCL and adjacent to it indicates a partial tear. A T2 or T2* sequence in the coronal plane is necessary to see these abnormalities.

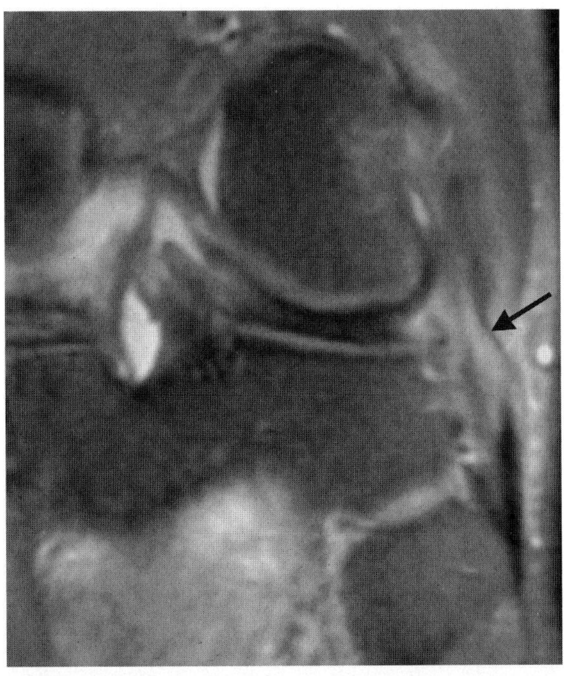

FIGURE 48.22. **Lateral Collateral Ligament Tear.** A coronal fast spin-echo T2WI with fat suppression reveals a tear of the lateral collateral ligament (fibular collateral ligament) (*arrow*). The normal ligament should be a low-signal structure between the femur and the fibula.

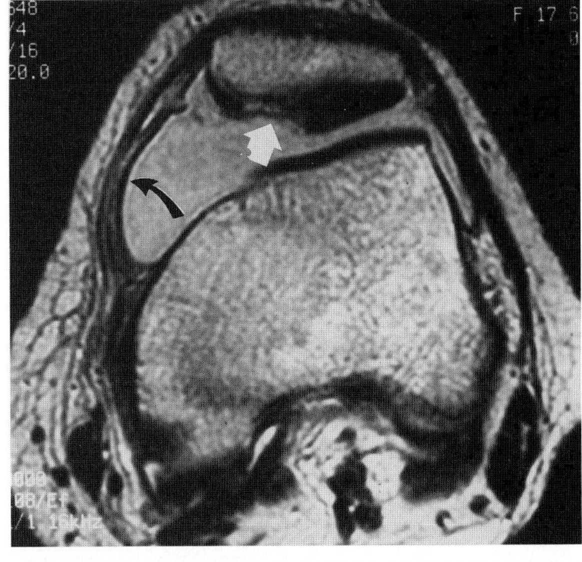

FIGURE 48.23. **Chondral Defect in Patella.** An axial fast spin-echo T2WI (time of repetition 3,000; time of echo 108) through the patella shows a large cartilage defect on the apex and medial facet of the patella (*white arrow*) in this patient who suffered a dislocated patella. Note the high signal throughout the medial retinaculum (*curved arrow*), a frequent finding after a patella dislocation.

infrequently in comparison to the MCL, but a tear can require surgery if instability is present. A torn LCL is seen as disruption of the ligamentous fibers on coronal images (Fig. 48.22).

PATELLA

Chondromalacia Patella. The patellar cartilage commonly undergoes degeneration, causing exquisite pain and tenderness. This is called chondromalacia patella. It can be diagnosed on sagittal images but is more easily identified on axial images. Because hyaline articular cartilage has the same signal intensity as joint fluid on T1W sequences, T2 or T2* sequences are necessary to diagnose chondromalacia patella in most instances.

Chondromalacia patella begins with focal swelling and degeneration of the cartilage. This can be seen as low- or high-signal foci in the cartilage. Its progression causes thinning and irregularity of the articular surface of the cartilage; finally, underlying bone is exposed. This final stage occurs more commonly from trauma than from wear and tear. A frequent cause of a patellar cartilage defect is dislocation of the patella, in which the patella strikes the lateral femoral condyle and displaces a piece of patellar articular

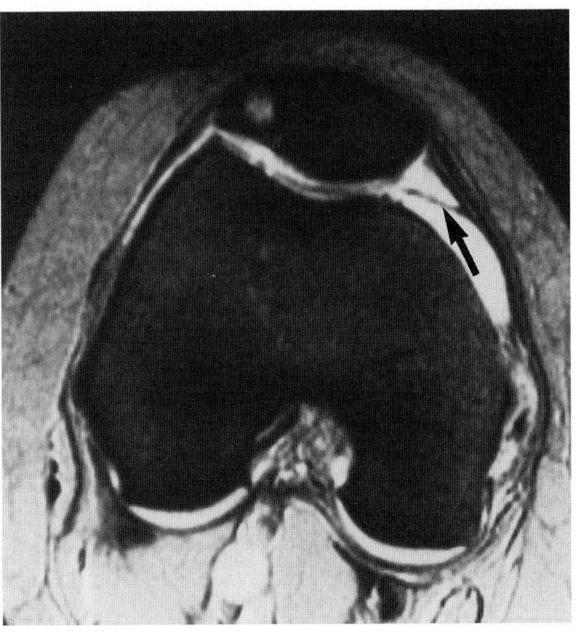

FIGURE 48.24. **Plica.** An axial gradient-recalled acquisition in the steady state image (time of repetition 500; time of echo 15; θ 30°) through the patella shows a low-signal linear structure (*arrow*) extending from the medial capsule toward the medial facet of the patella. This is a medial patellar plica that is not abnormally thickened. Without the joint effusion or the T2WI, the plica would not be visualized.

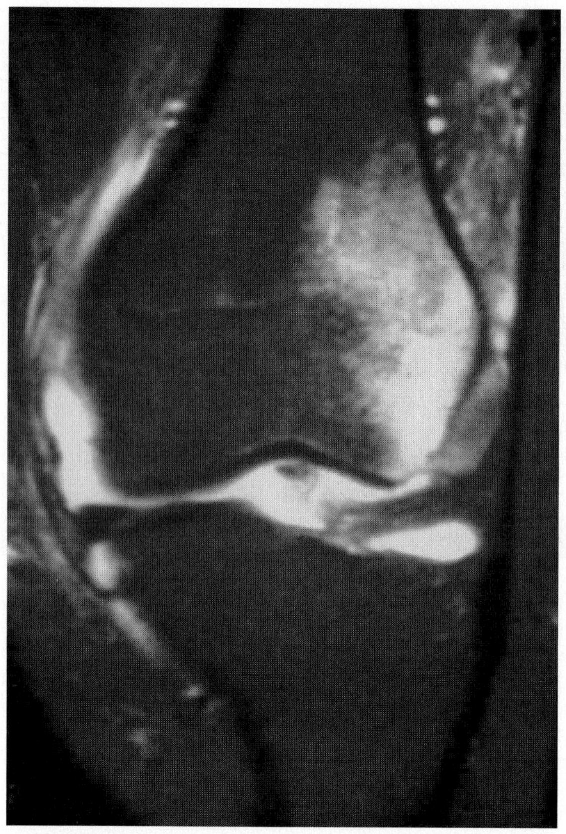

FIGURE 48.25. **Contusion.** A coronal fast spin-echo T2WI with fat suppression shows a focus of high signal in the lateral femoral condyle, which is a characteristic appearance for a severe bone contusion. This occurred from a patella dislocation.

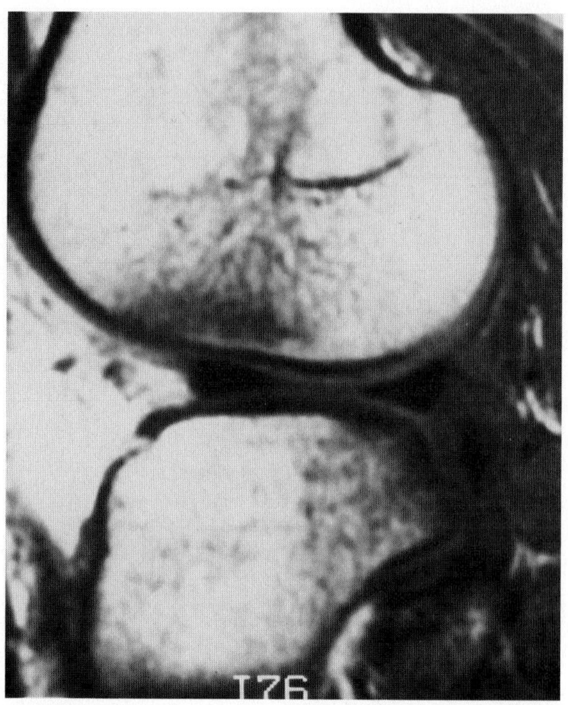

FIGURE 48.26. **Contusion.** A sagittal T1WI through the lateral compartment shows irregular low signal in a subarticular location of the posterior tibial plateau and in the anterior part of the lateral femoral condyle. These findings are characteristic for bone contusions. This distribution of contusions in the posterior lateral tibial plateau and anterior in the lateral femoral condyle is almost always associated with a torn anterior cruciate ligament.

cartilage (Fig. 48.23). The lateral femoral condyle invariably has a contusion following a dislocated patella.

Patellar Plica. A normal structure seen in over half of the population is the medial patellar plica. It is an embryologic remnant from when the knee was divided into three compartments. It is a thin, fibrous band that extends from the medial capsule toward the medial facet of the patella (Fig. 48.24). Suprapatellar and infrapatellar plicae also exist. The medial patellar plica can, on rare occasions, thicken and cause clinical symptoms that are indistinguishable from those of a torn meniscus; this has been termed "plica syndrome." An abnormal plica can be removed arthroscopically quite easily.

BONY ABNORMALITIES

Contusions. The most frequently encountered bony abnormality seen with MR is a contusion. A contusion represents microfractures from trauma (6). They are also called bone bruises. They are easily identified on T1WIs

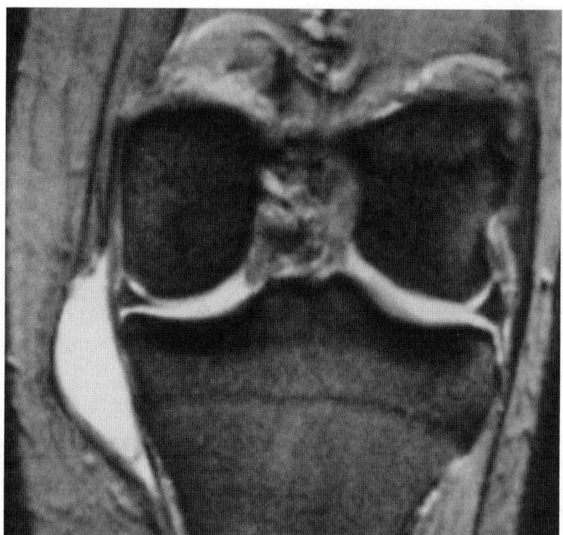

FIGURE 48.27. **Pes Anserinus Bursitis.** A coronal T2* gradient-echo image shows a fluid collection below the medial joint line near the insertion of the pes anserinus tendons. This is pes anserinus bursitis.

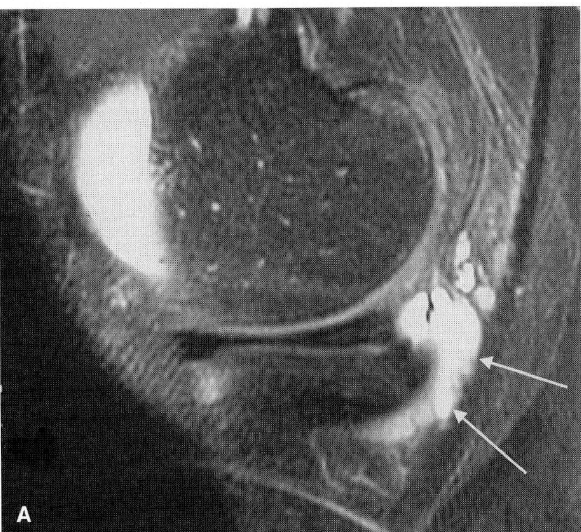

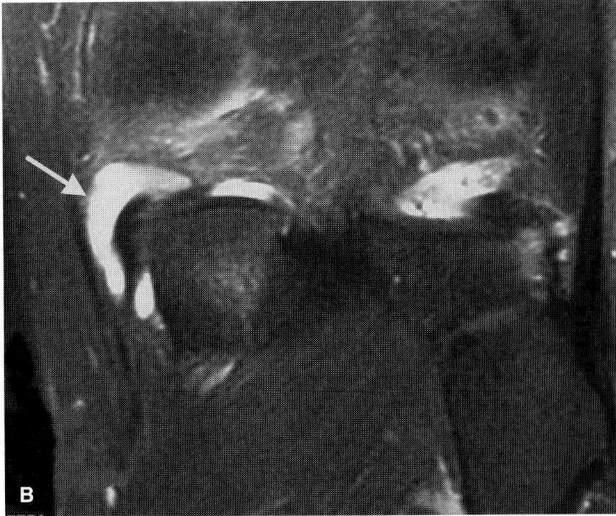

FIGURE 48.28. **Semimembranosus Tibial Collateral Ligament Bursa. A.** A sagittal fast spin-echo (FSE) T2WI with fat suppression through the medial aspect of the knee shows a fluid collection (*arrows*) at the joint line that is adjacent to the posterior horn of the medial meniscus. This is characteristic of a semimembranosus medial collateral ligament bursa. **B.** A coronal FSE T2WI with fat suppression shows that this bursa has a comma-shaped appearance at the joint line (*arrow*).

as subarticular areas of inhomogeneous low signal. With T2 weighting, a contusion will show increased signal for several weeks, depending on its severity (Fig. 48.25). Visualization of increased signal with T2* images can be difficult because of the susceptibility artifacts of the bone seen with T2* images. Contusions can progress to osteochondritis dissecans if they are not treated with decreased weight bearing; hence, an isolated bone contusion, with no other internal derangement, is a serious finding that requires protection.

A commonly seen contusion is one that occurs on the posterior part of the lateral tibial plateau (Fig. 48.26). It is invariably associated with a torn ACL. Acute ACL tears have been reported to have this type of contusion in over 90% of cases (7).

Fractures. MR is useful in examining fractures about the knee. Tibial plateau fractures can be imaged precisely with CT; however, MR allows the soft tissues to be seen in addition to any bony abnormalities. A fracture that is almost always associated with an internal derangement is the Segond fracture. A small, bony fragment pulled off the posterior lateral tibial joint line by an avulsion of the lateral joint capsule, it is almost always associated with an ACL tear.

BURSAE

An abnormality that can cause joint pain and clinically mimic plica syndrome or a torn meniscus is bursitis. Two bursae typically are identified medially that can become symptomatic. The first is the pes anserine bursa, which is somewhat uncommon. Three tendons—the sartorius, the gracilis, and the semitendinosus—insert onto the anteromedial aspect of the tibia in a fan-shaped manner that has been likened to a goose's foot, hence the name pes anserinus. A bursa lies beneath the insertion site, which can become inflamed and cause medial joint line or patellar pain; this can be confused with plica syndrome or a torn medial meniscus (Fig. 48.27). A second and much more common medial bursa is the semimembranosus tibial collateral ligament bursa. It occurs at the medial joint line and often mimics a meniscal cyst. It has a characteristic comma shape as it drapes over the semimembranosus tendon (Fig. 48.28). Making the diagnosis of pes anserinus or semimembranosus tibial collateral ligament bursitis with MR imaging can prevent an unnecessary arthroscopy procedure—one in which the bursae would be overlooked, since they are extracapsular structures.

REFERENCES

1. Crues JI, Mink J, Levy T, et al. Meniscal tears of the knee: accuracy of MR imaging. Radiology 1987;164:445–448.
2. Mink JH, Deutsch AL. Magnetic resonance imaging of the knee. Clin Orthop 1989;244:29–47.
3. De Smet A, Graf B. Meniscal tears missed on MR imaging: relationship to meniscal tear patterns and anterior cruciate ligament tears. AJR Am J Roentgenol 1994;162:905–911.

4. Helms CA, Laorr A, Cannon WD Jr. The absent bow tie sign in bucket-handle tears of the menisci in the knee. AJR Am J Roentgenol 1998;170(1):57–61.
5. Silverman J, Mink J, Deutsch A. Discoid menisci of the knee: MR imaging appearance. Radiology 1989;173:351–354.
6. Mink JH, Deutsch AL. Occult cartilage and bone injuries of the knee: detection, classification, and assessment with MR imaging. Radiology 1989;170:823–829.
7. Murphy B, Smith R, Uribe J, et al. Bone signal abnormalities in the posterolateral tibia and lateral femoral condyle in complete tears of the anterior cruciate ligament: a specific sign? Radiology 1992;182:221–224.

Chapter 49

Magnetic Resonance Imaging of the Shoulder

Clyde A. Helms

Anatomy

Rotator Cuff

Bony Abnormalities

Glenoid Labrum

Biceps Tendon

Suprascapular Nerve Entrapment

Quadrilateral Space Syndrome

Parsonage-Turner Syndrome

MR of the shoulder is well accepted for its diagnostic utility for abnormalities of the rotator cuff and the glenoid labrum. It has been shown to have a high degree of accuracy (1–4). MR of the shoulder has replaced standard arthrography and CT arthrography for examining the rotator cuff and the glenoid labrum in the vast majority of diagnostic imaging centers.

ANATOMY

The rotator cuff is comprised of the tendons of four muscles that converge on the greater and lesser tuberosities of the humerus: the supraspinatus, infraspinatus, subscapularis, and teres minor (Fig. 49.1). Of these, the supraspinatus most commonly causes clinically significant problems, and it is the most commonly surgically treated. The supraspinatus tendon lies just superior to the scapula and inferior to the acromioclavicular (AC) joint and acromion. It inserts onto the greater tuberosity of the humerus. Two to three centimeters proximal to its insertion is a section of the tendon called the "critical zone." This area is reported to have decreased vascularity and is therefore less likely to heal following trauma. The critical zone of the supraspinatus tendon is a common location for rotator cuff tears. Most cuff tears, however, begin at the bone/tendon interface on the greater tuberosity.

The glenoid labrum is a fibrocartilaginous ring that surrounds the periphery of the bony glenoid of the scapula. It serves as an attachment site for the capsule and broadens the base of the glenohumeral joint to allow increased stability. Tears or detachments of the glenoid labrum most commonly occur from, and result in, dislocations or instability of the humerus.

ROTATOR CUFF

The rotator cuff commonly suffers from what has been termed *impingement syndrome*. Impingement of the supraspinatus tendon occurs from abduction of the humerus, which allows the tendon to be impinged between the anterior acromion and the greater tuberosity. The tendon can also be impinged by the undersurface of the AC joint if downward-pointing osteophytes or a thickened capsule are present. Other theories exist for rotator cuff disease, including natural degeneration from aging and a predisposition for the cuff to undergo degeneration as a result of decreased blood supply. Most investigators agree that whatever the cause, the natural course of impingement syndrome or cuff degeneration is a complete, or full-thickness, tear of the rotator cuff.

The rotator cuff is best seen on oblique coronal images that are aligned parallel to the supraspinatus muscle (Fig. 49.2) and on oblique sagittal images (Fig. 49.3). Both T1W (or proton-density) and T2W sequences are typically performed, although little diagnostic information is

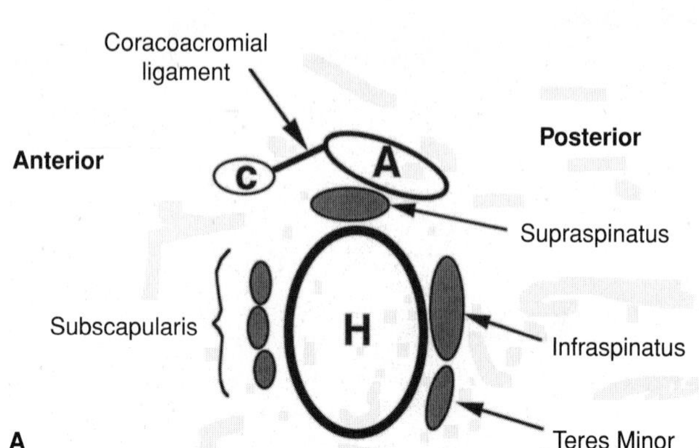

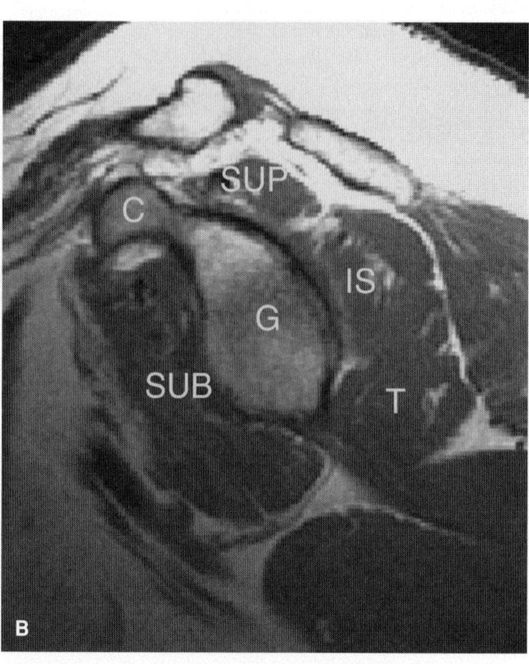

FIGURE 49.1. **Normal Shoulder Anatomy. A.** Drawing showing the rotator cuff muscles in a sagittal plane (anterior is on the left). C, Coracoid; A, acromion; H, humeral head. **B.** This sagittal T1WI through the glenoid shows the normal cuff musculature. SUB, Subscapularis; SUP, supraspinatus; IS, infraspinatus; T, teres minor; C, coracoid process; G, glenoid.

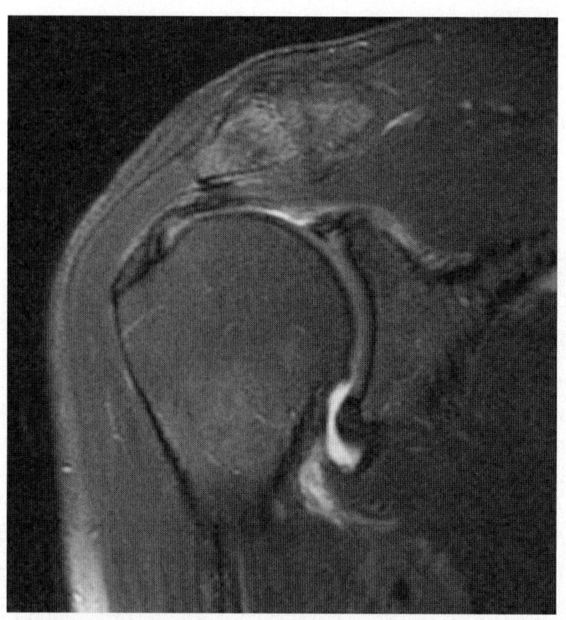

FIGURE 49.2. **Oblique Coronal Image of Normal Rotator Cuff.** This oblique coronal fast spin-echo T2WI with fat suppression through the supraspinatus shows a normal supraspinatus with a broad footprint where the tendon inserts onto the greater tuberosity.

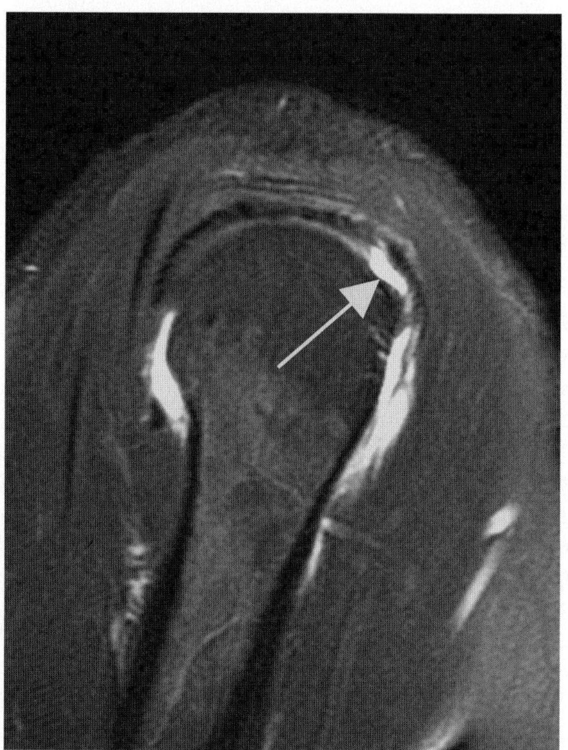

FIGURE 49.3. **Oblique Sagittal Image of a Torn Rotator Cuff.** An oblique coronal image fast spin-echo T2WI with fat suppression shows the rotator cuff inserting onto the greater tuberosity in a normal fashion, except at the far anterior portion (*arrow*). This indicates a partial tear of the articular surface fibers of the cuff.

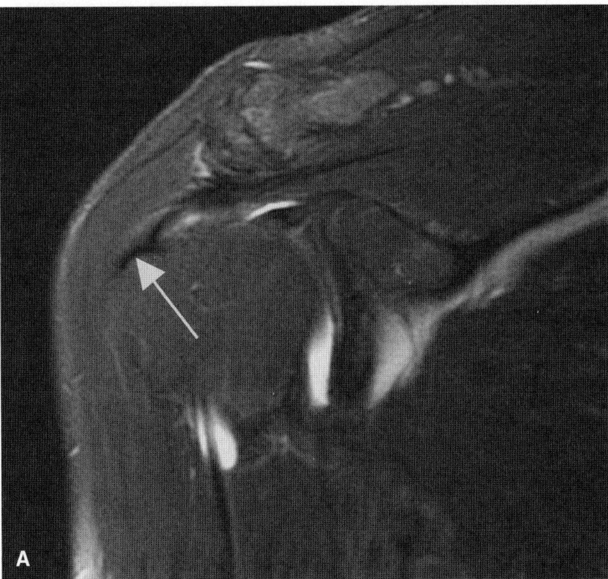

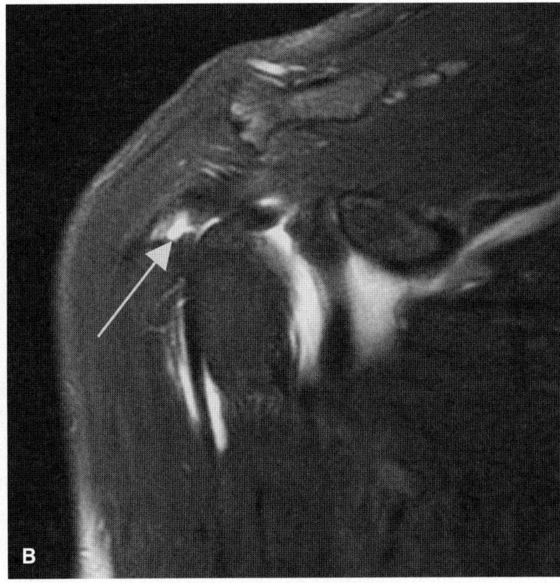

FIGURE 49.4. **Internal Rotation Hiding Partial Tear of the Supraspinatus Tendon. A.** An oblique coronal fast spin-echo T2WI with fat suppression shows an apparently normal supraspinatus inserting onto the greater tuberosity (*arrow*). **B.** One slice anterior to that shown in **(A)**, the bicipital groove can be identified, with the fibers of the supraspinatus just lateral to the groove lifted off of the greater tuberosity (*arrow*). This is a partial tear of the rotator cuff at its anteriormost portion.

present on the T1WIs and they are not obtained by many radiologists. Multiple acceptable variations of imaging sequences are available to demonstrate normal and abnormal structures. A fat-suppressed fast spin-echo (FSE) T2W oblique coronal sequence is gaining popularity as the primary sequence for imaging the rotator cuff in many imaging centers. The slice thickness should be no greater than 5 mm, and 3 mm is preferable. As with most joint imaging, a small field of view (16 to 20 cm) is recommended. A dedicated shoulder coil or a surface coil placed anteriorly over the shoulder is necessary.

In examining the rotator cuff, the most anterior oblique coronal images will show the supraspinatus tendon. A useful landmark for noting the anterior portion of the supraspinatus tendon is the bicipital groove, which has the anteriormost fibers of the supraspinatus immediately lateral to the groove. This is where most cuff tears begin and can be overlooked if the patient's shoulder is internally rotated, which is common (Fig. 49.4). The infraspinatus tendon is seen on the more posterior images and can easily be mistaken for the tendon of the supraspinatus. The supraspinatus tendon can be differentiated from that of the infraspinatus by noting the more horizontal course of the supraspinatus as compared with the infraspinatus, which runs obliquely inferiorly to superiorly.

The normal supraspinatus tendon is said to be uniformly low in signal on all pulse sequences. Unfortunately, this is not always the case. In fact, it usually has some intermediate to high signal in the tendon, which causes much confusion. If the signal in the tendon gets brighter on T2WIs, it is abnormal and represents either tendonitis (many investigators prefer the terms *tendinosis* or *tendinopathy* over *tendonitis,* as no inflammatory cells are found histologically) or a partial tear. A partial tear can be diagnosed by noting thinning of the tendon itself (Fig. 49.5). However, if it disappears or has the same signal

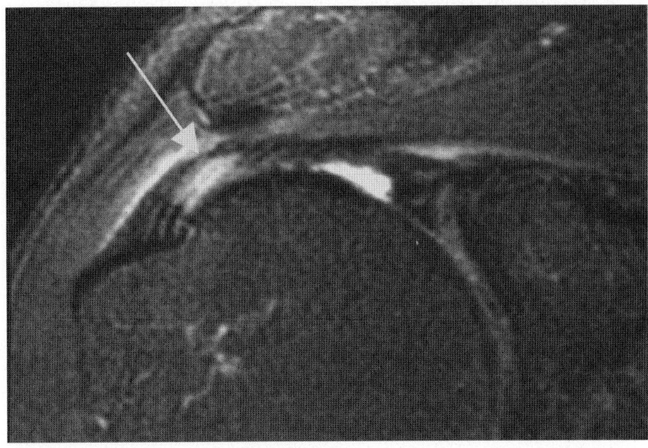

FIGURE 49.5. **Partial Cuff Tear.** An oblique coronal fast spin-echo T2 image with fat suppression shows thinning of the supraspinatus tendon (*arrow*), which is a partial tear of the articular side of the cuff.

intensity as the adjacent muscle on T2WIs, it may represent one of many different processes:

1. Partial volume averaging of peritendinous fat can cause some high signal in the supraspinatus tendon on the oblique coronal images; this does not get brighter on T2WIs.
2. If the plane of the oblique coronal images is slightly off of the plane of the tendon, muscle slips can be partially volume averaged, which may appear as relatively high signal on T1WIs but will not get brighter with T2WIs.
3. The so-called "magic angle" effect can cause apparent high signal in a tendon that lies at 55° to the bore of the magnet (as does the critical zone of the supraspinatus tendon) (5). This high signal will not be seen on T2WIs (or any sequence with a long time of echo). This is believed to be a common cause of high signal in the critical zone on T1WIs.
4. Myxoid and fibrillar degeneration of the supraspinatus tendon are commonly found in autopsy specimens in older patients. The majority of asymptomatic shoulders in patients over the age of 50 are believed to have some degeneration of the supraspinatus; this has been termed *tendinopathy*. This is seen as high signal in the critical zone on T1WIs that does not increase with T2 weighting (6).

Myxoid degeneration is felt by many surgeons to be more significant than anatomic impingement as a source of cuff pathology (7). Rather than decompressing the coracoacromial arch by removing bony structures and the coracoacromial ligament, which might be sources of impingement, these surgeons resect the areas of myxoid degeneration in the cuff tendons.

Tendon degeneration (tendinopathy) can be seen in asymptomatic shoulders of all ages; hence, it needs to be correlated with the clinical picture. If the signal gets brighter on T2WIs, it must be considered pathologic—either tendonitis or a partial tear.

If disruption of the supraspinatus tendon is seen, obviously a full-thickness tear is present. In these cases, fluid is invariably present in the subacromial bursa (Fig. 49.6). It should be noted that fluid in the subacromial bursa can also occur from isolated subacromial bursitis or for several days following a therapeutic injection into the bursa. Care should be made to look for retraction of the supraspinatus muscle, as marked retraction will obviate some types of surgery.

Three basic categories exist for the appearance of the supraspinatus tendon:

1. *Normal*—high signal on T1WIs that does not get brighter on T2WIs. This can represent one of several processes in a normal tendon or myxoid degeneration, also called tendinopathy. This should basically be considered "normal" unless it is an inordinate amount, as it has not been proved that tendinopathy is symptomatic.
2. *Tendonitis (or tendinosis)*—high signal on T1WIs that gets brighter on T2WIs. This represents tendonitis or a partial tear.
3. *Cuff tear*—tendon disruption; a gap must be seen to call a full-thickness cuff tear.

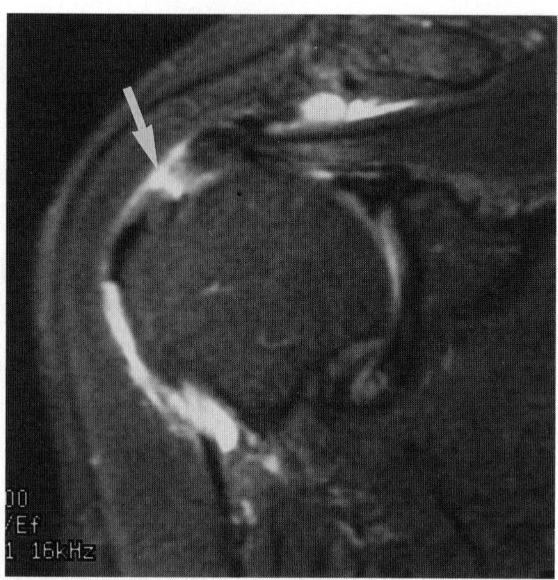

FIGURE 49.6. **Complete Tear of the Supraspinatus Tendon.** An oblique coronal fast spin-echo T2WI with fat suppression shows disruption of the supraspinatus tendon (*arrow*) with fluid in the torn tendon.

It is generally easy to place the MR appearance of the rotator cuff into one of these three categories, and a high degree of accuracy in diagnosing the state of the rotator cuff can be expected.

Partial cuff tears have marked clinical significance, since most agree that they will not heal on their own if they are greater than 25% of the cuff thickness (8). Although we generally cannot be so precise as to what percentage of the cuff is involved, we can usually identify partial cuff tears. If there is an irregularity or thinning of the cuff on either the bursal side of the cuff (Fig. 49.5) or on the joint side I will describe it as small, medium, or large (near full thickness).

A particular type of articular-sided partial tear has been described that is commonly seen. This has been termed a "rim rent" tear (Fig. 49.7). It occurs at the insertion of the fibers of the cuff onto the greater tuberosity. It most commonly occurs anteriorly, at the insertion of the supraspinatus, and, as mentioned previously, can be easily overlooked if the patient's arm is internally rotated.

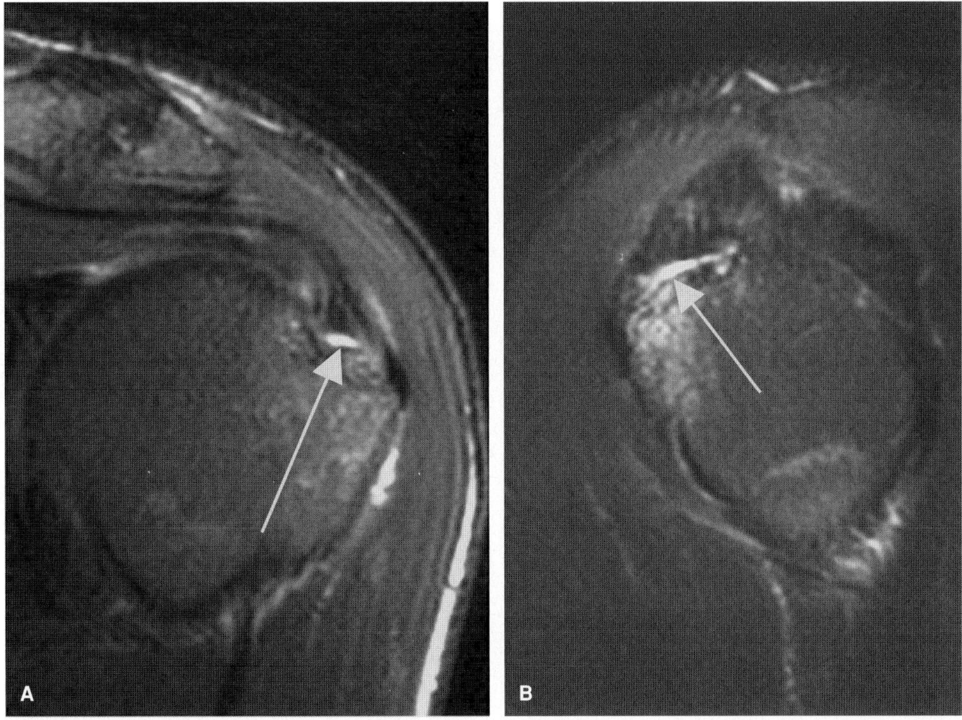

FIGURE 49.7. **Rim Rent Tear. A.** An oblique coronal fast spin-echo (FSE) T2 image with fat suppression shows increased signal at the insertion of the supraspinatus onto the greater tuberosity (*arrow*). **B.** An oblique sagittal FSE T2 image with fat suppression shows linear high signal anteriorly between the cuff fibers and the greater tuberosity (*arrow*). This is an articular-sided partial tear called a rim rent tear.

BONY ABNORMALITIES

The undersurface of the anterior acromion and the AC joint should be examined for osteophytes or irregularities that can be responsible for impingement syndrome (Fig. 49.8). In the proper clinical setting, an anterior acromioplasty will relieve the symptoms of impingement syndrome and prevent a more serious full-thickness rotator cuff tear. Many believe it is imperative that the surgeon also remove any AC joint undersurface irregularity, if present, or failed surgery can occur, although more recently this theory has been challenged (7).

Abnormalities of the humeral head include sclerosis and cystic changes about the greater tuberosity, which are commonly present in patients with impingement syndrome and rotator cuff tears. Bony impaction on the posterosuperior aspect of the humeral head can be seen in patients with anterior instability of the humeral head. This is called a Hill-Sachs lesion and is best identified on the two or three superiormost axial images (Fig. 49.9). The normal humeral head should be round on the superior slices; any irregularity seen posteriorly is abnormal.

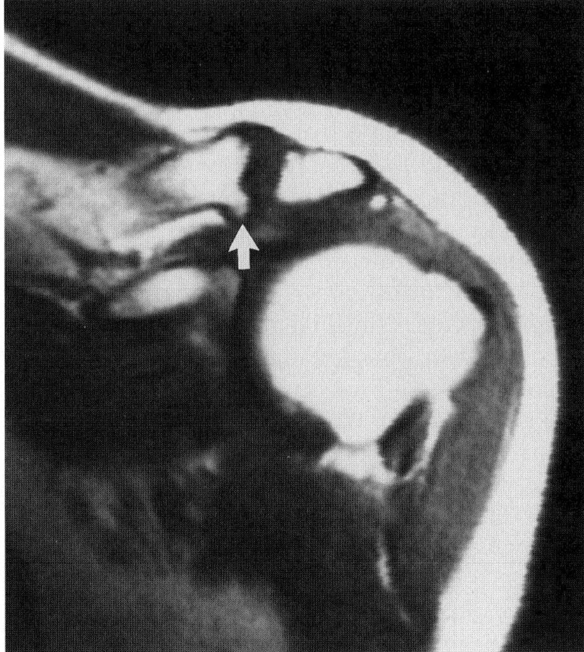

FIGURE 49.8. **Acromioclavicular Joint Osteophytes.** An oblique coronal T1WI (time of repetition 600; time of echo 30) reveals osteophytes extending inferiorly off the acromioclavicular joint (*arrow*). This is a common source of impingement on the supraspinatus tendon.

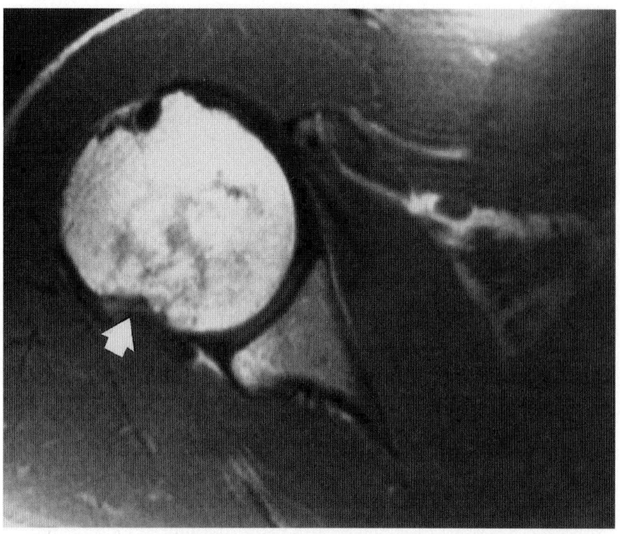

FIGURE 49.9. **Hill-Sachs Lesion.** An axial T1WI (time of repetition 600; time of echo 30) through the superior portion of the humeral head shows a posterior impaction (*arrow*) caused by the glenoid labrum during an anterior dislocation of the humerus. This has been termed a Hill-Sachs lesion.

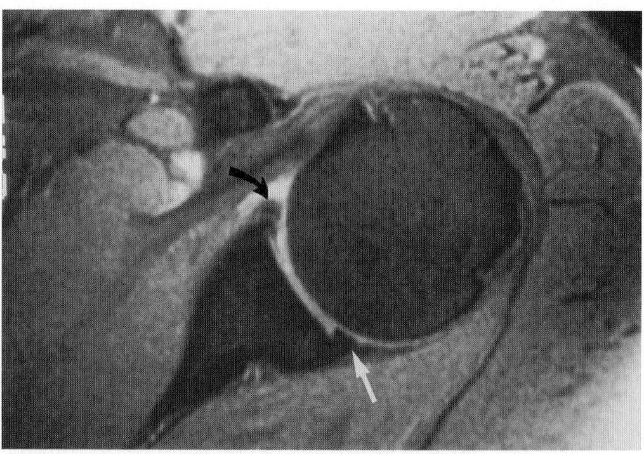

FIGURE 49.10. **Normal Labrum.** An axial T2* gradient-recalled acquisition in the steady state (GRASS) image (time of repetition 600; time of echo 30; θ 20°) shows a normal anterior (*black arrow*) and posterior (*white arrow*) glenoid labrum. The anterior labrum is usually larger than the posterior labrum.

GLENOID LABRUM

Tears or detachments of the glenoid labrum cause glenohumeral joint instability. They are commonly caused by dislocations, but less traumatic episodes, such as repeated trauma from throwing, can also result in labral tears. Torn or detached labra are often repaired arthroscopically with good results.

The glenoid labrum is best imaged on axial T2WIs or T2*WIs. Axial T1WIs are not necessary to diagnose labral abnormalities and can be omitted from the shoulder protocol. Fluid in the joint makes for easier assessment of the labrum; hence, MR arthrography has evolved into a routine exam in many centers. It is performed by injecting a 1:200 dilution of gadolinium/diethylenetriamine pentaacetic acid with saline into the joint using fluoroscopic guidance.

The normal labrum is a triangular-shaped, low-signal structure as viewed on an axial image, with the anterior labrum usually larger than the posterior labrum (Fig. 49.10). The anterior labrum is much more commonly involved with tears than the posterior, and the superior labrum is even less commonly involved. The superior labrum is evaluated on the oblique coronal views.

If no joint effusion is present, a labral tear can be difficult to see unless it is quite severe. If joint fluid extends between the bony glenoid and the base of the labrum, a detached labrum is present. Tears or detachments of the labrum are diagnosed by noting fluid extending between the labrum and the bony glenoid or by truncation of the labrum (Fig. 49.11). Superior labral tears are called SLAP lesions (*s*uperior *l*abrum *a*nterior to *p*osterior) (Fig. 49.12). They are seen most frequently in throwing athletes secondary to the pull of the long head of the biceps, which inserts on the superior labrum. They are also seen in older patients in association with cuff tears.

Several normal variants in the labrum that can mimic a torn or detached labrum have been described. Two

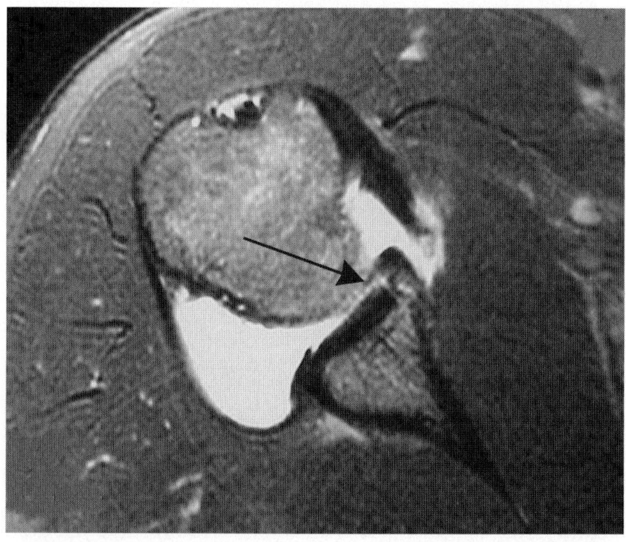

FIGURE 49.11. **Torn Labrum.** An axial fast spin-echo T2WI with fat suppression shows a tear of the anterior labrum (*arrow*).

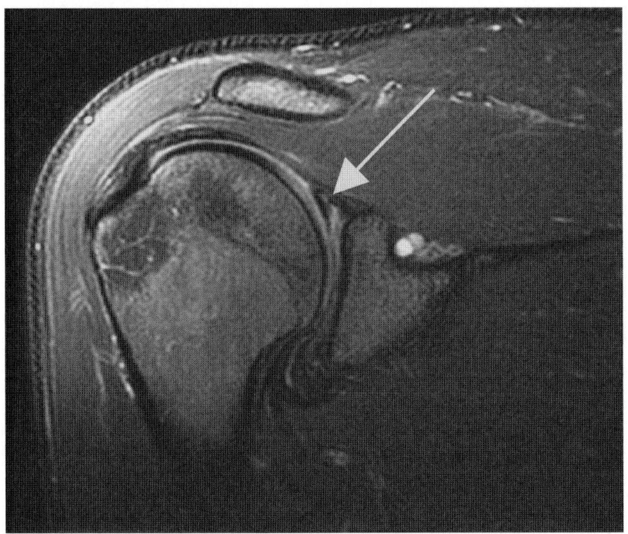

FIGURE 49.12. **SLAP (Superior Labrum Anterior to Posterior) Lesion.** An oblique coronal T2WI with fat suppression shows a torn superior labrum (*arrow*).

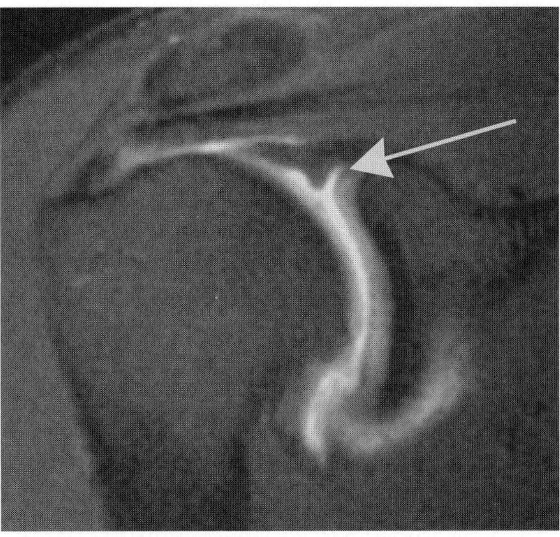

FIGURE 49.14. **Sublabral Recess.** A coronal T1W gadolinium arthrogram with fat suppression shows fluid between the superior labrum and the cartilage of the bony glenoid (*arrow*), which is thin and smooth. This is a sublabral recess.

occur solely in the anterosuperior portion of the labrum, an area in which tears are uncommon. The first is a *sublabral foramen,* which is an opening beneath the anterosuperior labrum and the bony glenoid that mimics a detachment (Fig. 49.13). This is seen in up to 20% of the population. A second variant is called a *Buford complex.* It consists of an absent anterosuperior labrum in association with a thickened, cordlike middle glenohumeral ligament. This is seen in about 3% of the population (9). A sublabral recess is often seen on the oblique coronal images, which can mimic a SLAP tear. It is found in up to 70% of shoulders. A sublabral recess should be seen only on the anterior part of the superior labrum, should be thin and smooth (Fig. 49.14), and extends medially, whereas a SLAP tear is typically more irregular and extends superiorly or laterally.

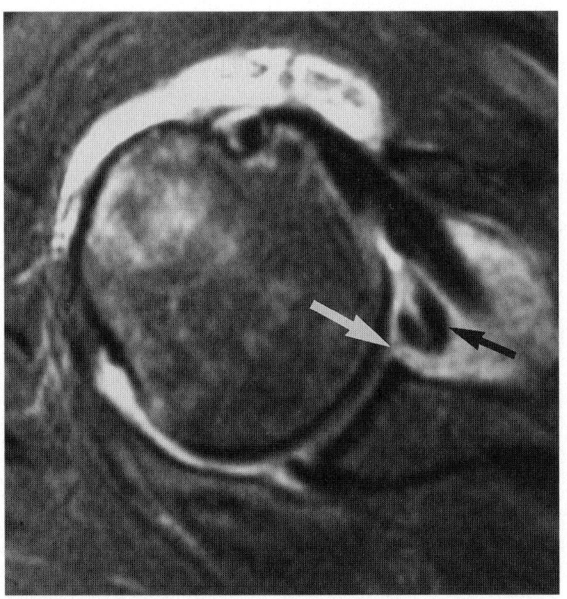

FIGURE 49.13. **Sublabral Foramen.** This axial fast spin-echo T2WI with fat suppression reveals fluid between the glenoid and the anterior labrum (*white arrow*), which appears to be a detached labrum; however, this is a sublabral foramen, which is a normal variant seen only in the anterosuperior labrum. Note the normal middle glenohumeral ligament (*black arrow*) anterior to the labrum.

BICEPS TENDON

The long head of the biceps tendon runs in the bicipital groove between the greater and lesser tuberosities and inserts onto the superior labrum. It can be impinged by an abnormal acromion in the same way the supraspinatus tendon is impinged, resulting in tenosynovitis or tendonitis. In tenosynovitis, fluid can be seen in the tendon sheath surrounding an otherwise normal tendon. Because fluid in the glenohumeral joint can normally fill the biceps tendon sheath, this diagnosis is difficult to make with MR alone. If the tendon is enlarged and/or has signal within it, tendonitis or a partial tear is present (Fig. 49.15). If the tendon is not seen on one or more of the axial images, it is disrupted or dislocated. Dislocation is uncommon, but when it occurs, the tendon can be seen to lie anteromedial to the joint. A subscapularis tear must be present if the biceps is dislocated.

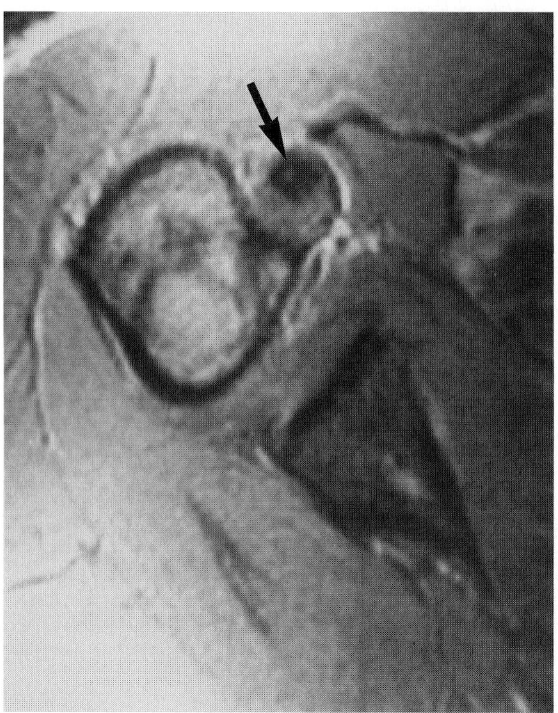

FIGURE 49.15. **Biceps Tendonitis.** An axial T2* gradient-recalled acquisition in the steady state (GRASS) image (time of repetition 600; time of echo 30; θ 30°) shows the biceps tendon (*arrow*) to be swollen and filled with high signal, indicating tendonitis.

SUPRASCAPULAR NERVE ENTRAPMENT

The suprascapular nerve is made up of branches from the C4, C5, and C6 roots of the brachial plexus. It runs superior to the scapula, from anterior to posterior, just medial to the coracoid process. It gives off a branch that innervates the supraspinatus muscle as it courses posteriorly in the suprascapular notch, and then innervates the infraspinatus muscle after it runs through the spinoglenoid notch in the posterior scapula. It can easily be entrapped by a tumor or a ganglion as it runs above the scapula, because it is bounded superiorly by a transverse ligament both anteriorly and posteriorly. A fairly common finding is a ganglion in the spinoglenoid notch that impresses the infraspinatus portion of the nerve, with resultant pain and atrophy of the infraspinatus muscle (Fig. 49.16). This is most commonly seen in men who are athletic, particularly weightlifters. The ganglion can be percutaneously drained with CT guidance or surgically removed. They can also spontaneously rupture, which results in cessation of symptoms (10). There is a 100% association of a torn posterior labrum with these cysts.

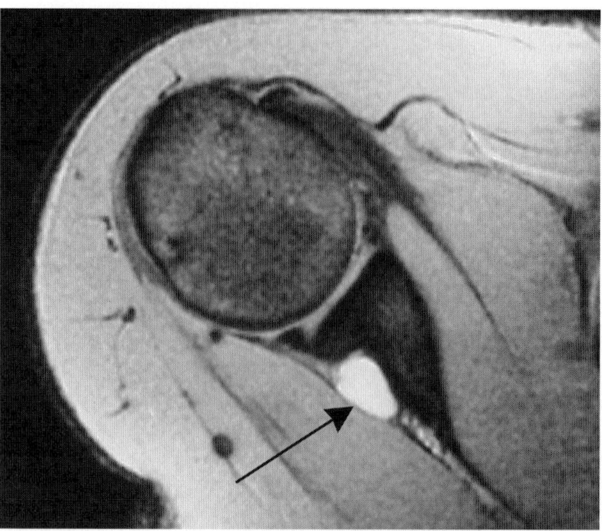

FIGURE 49.16. **Ganglion in Spinoglenoid Notch.** An axial T2WI reveals a high-signal mass posterior to the scapula in the spinoglenoid notch (*arrow*). This is a ganglion that has impressed the suprascapular nerve, causing shoulder pain and atrophy of the infraspinatus muscle.

QUADRILATERAL SPACE SYNDROME

Oblique sagittal T1WIs are useful to observe fatty atrophy in any of the cuff muscles. If the infraspinatus is smaller than the other muscles and/or has fatty infiltration,

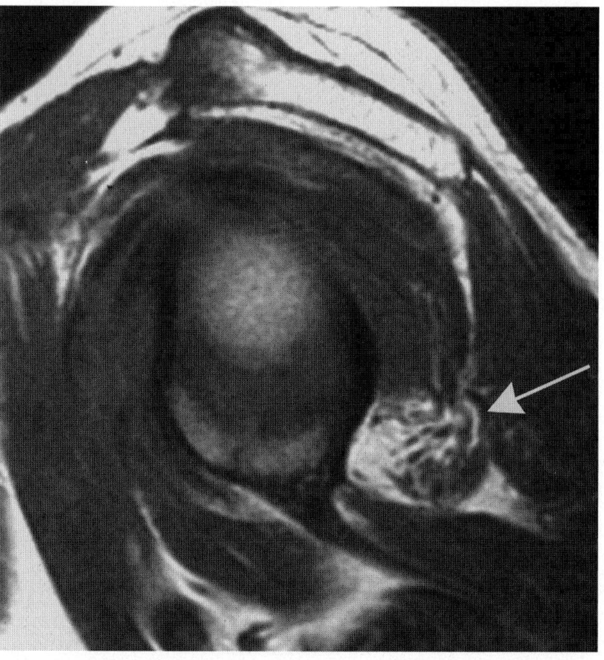

FIGURE 49.17. **Quadrilateral Space Syndrome.** This oblique sagittal T1WI shows fatty atrophy of the teres minor muscle (*arrow*), which is diagnostic of quadrilateral space syndrome.

the aforementioned suprascapular nerve entrapment secondary to a ganglion in the spinoglenoid notch is the likely diagnosis. If the teres minor has fatty atrophy (Fig. 49.17), the diagnosis is quadrilateral space syndrome. This most commonly occurs from fibrous bands or scar tissue in the quadrilateral space impinging on the axillary nerve. The quadrilateral space lies between the teres minor superiorly, the teres major inferiorly, the long head of the triceps medially, and the diaphysis of the humerus laterally. The axillary nerve traverses the quadrilateral space and innervates the teres minor and deltoid muscles; however, the deltoid is rarely involved in quadrilateral space syndrome. Quadrilateral space syndrome is found in about 1% of shoulder MR images. The presentation of these patients is clinically similar to that of a rotator cuff tear, and many patients have had needless surgery for presumed cuff pathology when the real problem was quadrilateral space syndrome. Generally no surgery is necessary, as physical therapy is usually successful in breaking up the fibrous bands or scar tissue that cause this entity.

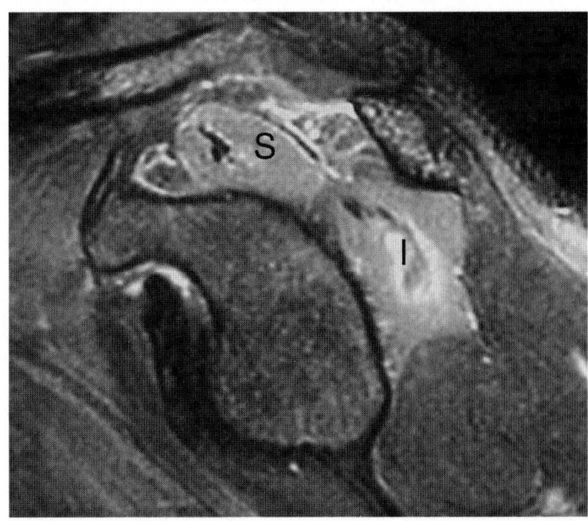

FIGURE 49.18. **Parsonage-Turner Syndrome.** An oblique sagittal T2WI with fat suppression shows edema in the supraspinatus (S) and the infraspinatus (I) muscles, consistent with involvement of the suprascapular nerve. The sudden onset with no history of trauma is characteristic for Parsonage-Turner syndrome.

PARSONAGE-TURNER SYNDROME

Oblique sagittal FSE T2W fat-suppressed images are useful for identifying muscle edema. In about 1% of cases, neurogenic edema is found in muscle groups that corresponds to a particular nerve (i.e., supraspinatus/infraspinatus = suprascapular nerve; teres minor/deltoid = axillary nerve). This is characteristic for Parsonage-Turner syndrome (Fig. 49.18) but not pathognomonic, because a traumatic nerve injury (such as a brachial plexus injury) could have a similar appearance. It becomes pathognomonic once the clinical presentation is provided. If there is no history of trauma or of an insidious onset, and if the onset is sudden, with severe pain followed in a day or two by profound weakness, the edema pattern is virtually pathognomonic for Parsonage-Turner syndrome.

The etiology of Parsonage-Turner syndrome is unknown, but it seems to have an association with prior vaccinations, viral illness, or general anesthesia in about one third of cases. It is bilateral in about 10% to 15% of cases. It affects all ages of both sexes and is self-limited. It can affect either the axillary or suprascapular nerves, or both simultaneously. Unnecessary shoulder, brachial plexus, and cervical spine surgeries have been performed on patients with Parsonage-Turner syndrome before the correct diagnosis was made.

Parsonage-Turner syndrome was first described in the radiology literature in 1998 (11), indicating that we all missed it on MR for over 15 years. This is because fat suppression on shoulder images was not routinely done until the early 1990s, and the edema in the muscles was not conspicuous enough to be picked up on non–fat-suppressed sequences.

REFERENCES

1. Palmer W, Brown J, Rosenthal D. Rotator cuff: evaluation with fat-suppressed MR arthrography. Radiology 1993;188:683–688.
2. Singson RD, Hoang T, Dan S, Friedman M. MR evaluation of rotator cuff pathology using T2-weighted fast spin-echo technique with and without fat suppression. AJR Am J Roentgenol 1996;166(5):1061–1065.
3. Rafii M, Firooznia H, Sherman O, et al. Rotator cuff lesions: signal patterns at MR imaging. Radiology 1990;177(3):817–823.
4. Zlatkin MB, Iannotti JP, Roberts MC, et al. Rotator cuff tears: diagnostic performance of MR imaging. Radiology 1989;172:223–229.
5. Erickson S, Cox I, Hyde J, et al. Effect of tendon orientation on MR imaging signal intensity: a manifestation of the "magic angle" phenomenon. Radiology 1991;181:389–392.
6. Kjellin I, Ho CP, Cervilla V, et al. Alterations in the supraspinatus tendon at MR imaging: correlation with histopathologic findings in cadavers. Radiology 1991;181:837–841.
7. Budoff JE, Nirschl RP, Guidi EJ. Debridement of partial-thickness tears of the rotator cuff without acromioplasty. Long-term follow-up and review of the literature. J Bone Joint Surg Am 1998;80:733–748.
8. Fukuda H. The management of partial-thickness tears of the rotator cuff. J Bone Joint Surg Br 2003;85:3–11.
9. Carroll KW, Helms CA. Magnetic resonance imaging of the shoulder: a review of potential sources of diagnostic errors. Skeletal Radiol 2002;31(7):373–383.
10. Fritz R, Helms CA, Steinbach L, Genant H. Suprascapular nerve entrapment: evaluation with MR imaging. Radiology 1992;182:437–444.
11. Helms CA, Martinez S, Speer KP. Acute brachial neuritis (Parsonage-Turner-syndrome): MR imaging appearance—report of three cases. Radiology 1998;207:255–259.

Magnetic Resonance Imaging of the Foot and Ankle

Clyde A. Helms

Tendons

Ligaments

Avascular Necrosis

Bony Abnormalities

Tumors

MR is playing an increasingly important role in the examination of the foot and ankle (1). Orthopaedic surgeons and podiatrists are learning that critical diagnostic information can be obtained in no other way and are relying on MR for many therapeutic decisions.

TENDONS

One of the more common reasons to perform MR of the foot and ankle is to examine the tendons. Although multiple tendons course through the ankle, only a few are routinely affected pathologically. These are primarily the flexor tendons, located posteriorly in the ankle. The extensor tendons, located anteriorly, are rarely abnormal. Only those tendons that are more commonly seen to be abnormal will be discussed in detail.

Tendons can be traumatized directly or be injured from overuse. Either etiology can result in (*1*) *tenosynovitis,* which is seen on MR as fluid in the tendon sheath with the underlying tendon appearing normal; (*2*) *tendonitis* or a partial tear, which is seen as focal or fusiform swelling of the tendon with signal within the tendon that gets bright on T2W or T2*W images; thinning or attenuation of the tendon is a more severe form of tendonitis that can be recognized on MR; *tendinosis* is seen as increased signal within a tendon that does not get fluid-bright on T2WI and represents myxoid degeneration; and (*3*) *tendon rupture,* which is best identified on axial images by noting the absence of a tendon on one or more images. Complete tendon disruption can be difficult to see on sagittal or coronal images because of the tendency for tendons to run oblique to the plane of imaging. An exception to this is the Achilles tendon, which is usually best seen on a sagittal image (2).

It is important to distinguish between tendonitis (or partial tear) and a complete disruption, because surgical repair is often warranted for the latter and not for the former. Making the distinction clinically is often difficult.

Achilles Tendon. The Achilles tendon does not have a sheath associated with it; therefore, tenosynovitis does not occur. Tendonitis (or a partial tear) is commonly seen in the Achilles tendon; however, it is such an easy clinical diagnosis that MR is usually not necessary. Complete disruption is commonly seen in athletes and in men who are approximately 40 years of age. It is also commonly associated with other systemic disorders that cause tendon weakening, such as rheumatoid arthritis, collagen vascular diseases, crystal deposition diseases, and hyperparathyroidism.

Achilles tendon disruption can be treated surgically or by placing the patient in a cast with equinus positioning (marked plantar flexion) for several months. Which treatment is superior is a controversial issue, with both methods of treatment seemingly working well. MR is used by many surgeons to help decide whether surgery should be performed. If a large gap is present (Fig. 50.1), some surgeons feel that surgery should be performed for reapposition of the torn ends of the tendon; on the other hand, if the ends of the tendon are not retracted, nonsurgical

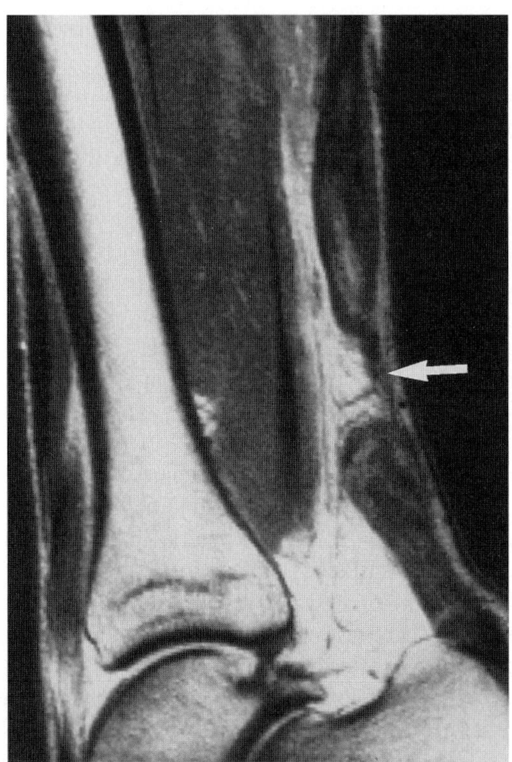

FIGURE 50.1. **Torn Achilles Tendon.** A sagittal T1WI (time of repetition 600; time of echo 30) reveals the Achilles tendon to be torn, with a 2-cm gap. Only a thin remnant of the tendon remains intact across the gap (*arrow*). Note the high signal in the swollen ends of the separated tendon, indicative of hemorrhage and edema.

treatment is preferred. However, no published papers have shown that this is, in fact, valid.

Posterior Tibial Tendon. The flexor tendons are easily remembered and identified by using the mnemonic "Tom, Dick, and Harry," with Tom representing the posterior tibial tendon, Dick the flexor digitorum longus tendon, and Harry the flexor hallucis longus tendon. The posterior tibial tendon (PTT) is the most medial and the largest, except for the Achilles, of the flexor tendons (Fig. 50.2). The posterior tibial tendon inserts onto the navicular, second and third cuneiforms, and the bases of the second to fourth metatarsals. As it sweeps under the foot, it provides some support for the longitudinal arch; hence, problems in the arch or plantar fascia can sometimes lead to stress on the posterior tibial tendon, with resulting tendonitis or even rupture. Posterior tibial tendonitis and rupture are commonly encountered in patients with rheumatoid arthritis.

Differentiation of tendonitis from tendon rupture can be difficult, and MR has become very valuable for making this distinction (3). Most surgeons will operate on a disrupted posterior tibial tendon; however, nonoperative therapy is usually preferred for tendonitis.

Posterior tibial tendinosis is seen on axial T1WIs as swelling and/or signal within the normally low-signal tendon on one or more images (Fig. 50.3). T2WIs or T2*WIs show the signal in the tendon getting brighter but not fluid-bright. Tendon disruption is diagnosed by noting the absence of the tendon on one or more axial images (Fig. 50.4).

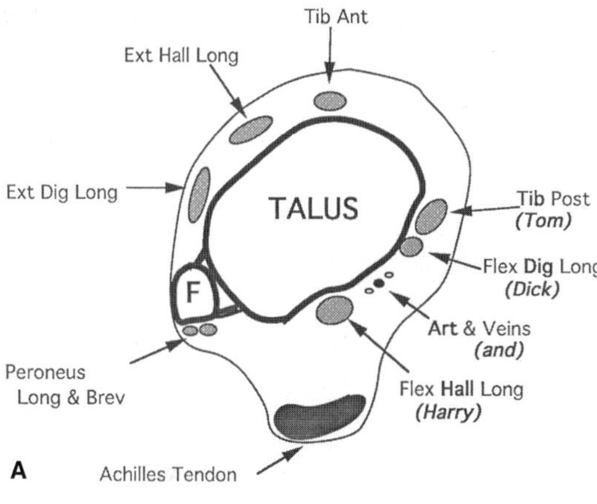

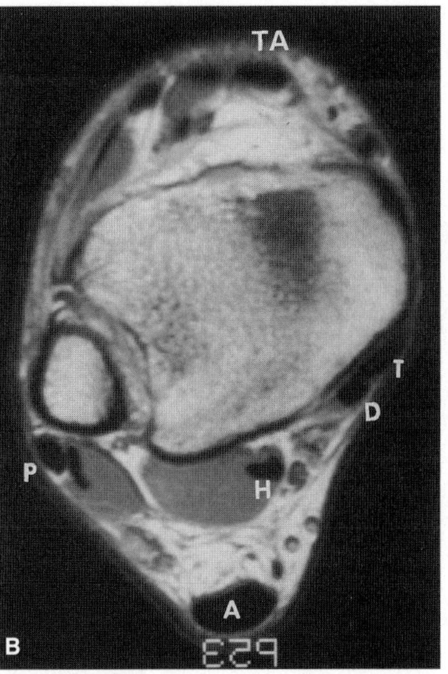

FIGURE 50.2. **Normal Ankle Anatomy. A.** This drawing of the tendons around the ankle at the level of the tibiotalar joint shows the relationship of the flexor tendons posteriorly and the extensor tendons anteriorly. **B.** An axial T1WI through the ankle just above the tibiotalar joint shows the normal anatomy. A, Achilles tendon; T, posterior tibial tendon; D, flexor digitorum tendon; H, flexor hallucis tendon; P, peroneus tendons; TA, tibialis anterior tendon.

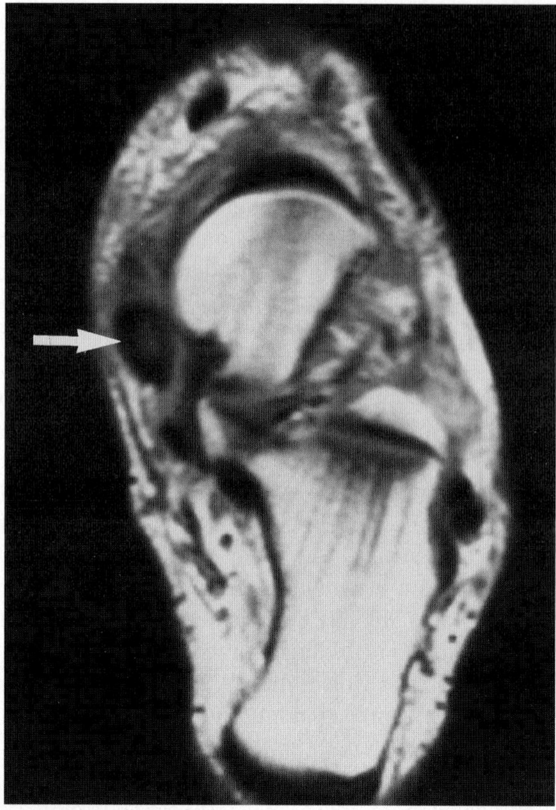

FIGURE 50.3. **Posterior Tibial Tendon Tendinosis.** A proton-density (time of repetition 2,000; time of echo 20) axial image through the ankle at the midlevel of the calcaneus shows the posterior tibial tendon (*arrow*) swollen and containing high signal. This is the appearance of marked tendinosis.

This typically occurs just at or above the level of the tibiotalar joint.

Rupture of the PTT results clinically in a flat foot as a result of the loss of arch support given by this tendon. The spring ligament runs just deep to the PTT and then goes underneath the neck of the talus, which it supports in a sling-like fashion. When the PTT tears, stress is then placed on the spring ligament to support the talus and the arch. The spring ligament has a high incidence of disruption when the PTT tears. The spring ligament is identified on axial and coronal images just deep to the PTT. When it is stressed, it typically gets scarred and thickened (Fig. 50.5). A tear can be diagnosed by noting a gap in the ligament.

After the PTT and the spring ligament tear, the next structures to fail are the subtalar joint ligaments in the sinus tarsi. In a report of 25 patients with PTT tears, it was found that 92% of the cases had abnormal spring ligaments (thickened or torn), and 72% had an abnormal sinus tarsi (4). It's clear that these structures are linked, and injury or stress to one can affect the others.

Flexor hallucis longus tendon (FHL) tendon is easily identified near the tibiotalar joint because it is usually the only tendon at that distal level that has muscle still attached. In the foot, the FHL can be seen beneath the sustentaculum talus, which it uses as a pulley to plantar flex the foot.

The FHL is known as the Achilles tendon of the foot in ballet dancers because of the extreme flexion positions they employ. Ballet dancers often will have tenosynovitis of the FHL, seen on MR as fluid in the sheath surrounding the tendon. Care must be taken to have clinical correlation, because fluid can be seen in the FHL tendon sheath from a connection to the ankle joint, which has an effusion in

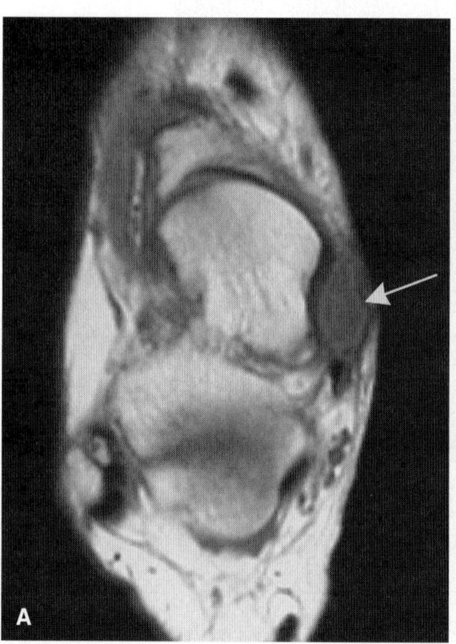

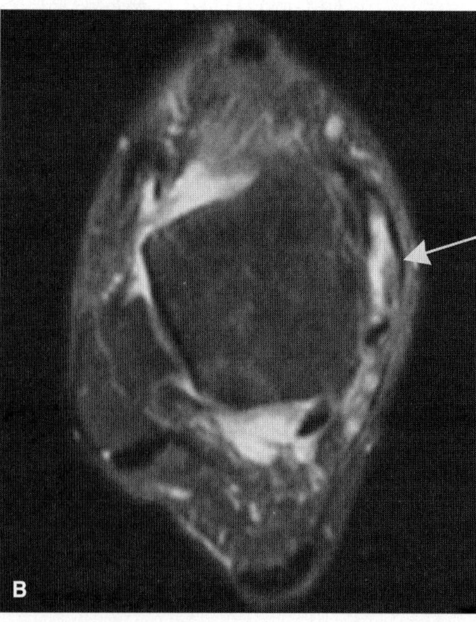

FIGURE 50.4. **Torn Posterior Tibial Tendon.** Axial T1WI **(A)** and T2WI **(B)** through the ankle in this patient with chronic pain reveal a distended posterior tibial tendon sheath (*arrows*), with no low-signal tendon identified within. This is a tear of the posterior tibial tendon.

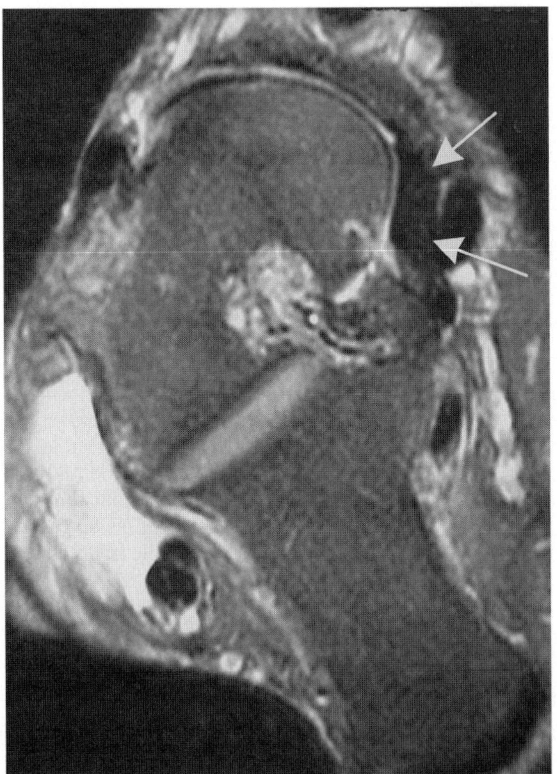

FIGURE 50.5. **Abnormal Spring Ligament.** An axial T2WI through the ankle shows a markedly thickened spring ligament (*arrows*) just deep to the posterior tibial tendon.

as many as 20% of normal patients. Rupture of the FHL is rare.

Peroneus Tendons. The peroneus longus and peroneus brevis tendons can be seen posterior to the distal fibula, to which they are bound by a thin fibrous structure, the superior retinaculum. The fibula serves as a pulley for the tendons to work as the principal everter of the foot. The tendons course close together adjacent to the lateral aspect of the calcaneus until a few centimeters below the lateral malleolus, where they separate, with the peroneus brevis tendon inserting onto the base of the fifth metatarsal and the peroneus longus tendon crossing under the foot to the base of the first metatarsal. Avulsion of the base of the fifth metatarsal from a pull by the peroneus brevis tendon is known as a "dancer's fracture" or a Jones fracture.

Disruption of the superior retinaculum, often seen in skiing accidents (5), can result in displacement of the peroneus tendons (Fig. 50.6) and must be surgically corrected.

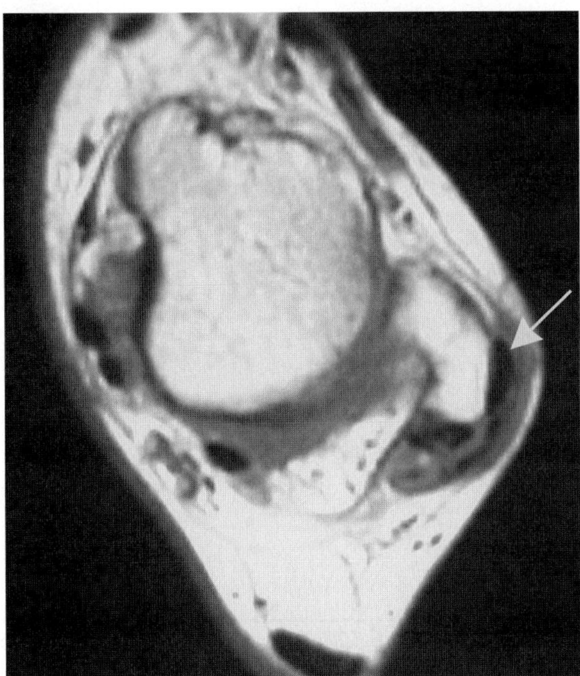

FIGURE 50.6. **Dislocated Peroneus Longus Tendon.** An axial T1WI in this rock climber who injured his ankle in a fall shows a low-signal rounded structure (*arrow*) lateral to the lateral malleolus. This is a dislocated peroneus longus tendon.

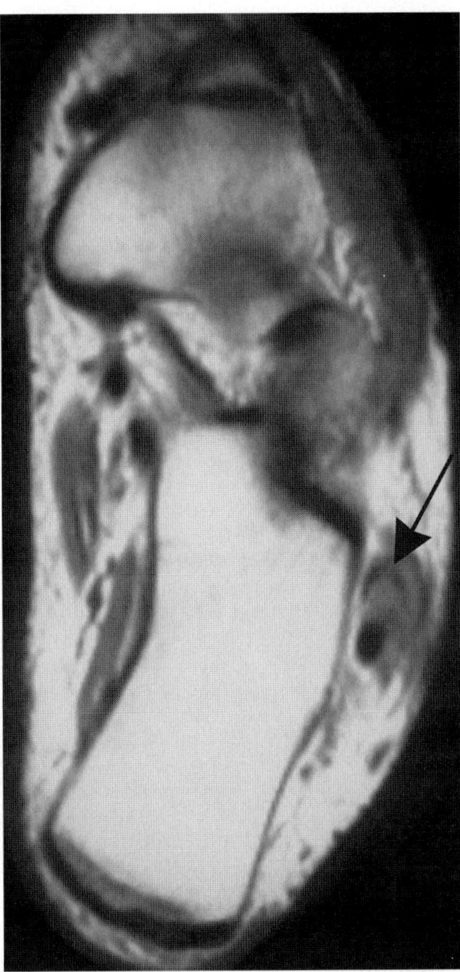

FIGURE 50.7. **Longitudinal Split Tear of the Peroneus Brevis.** This axial T1WI shows the peroneus brevis (*arrow*) with a "V" or chevron shape, which is characteristic for a longitudinal split tear of the brevis.

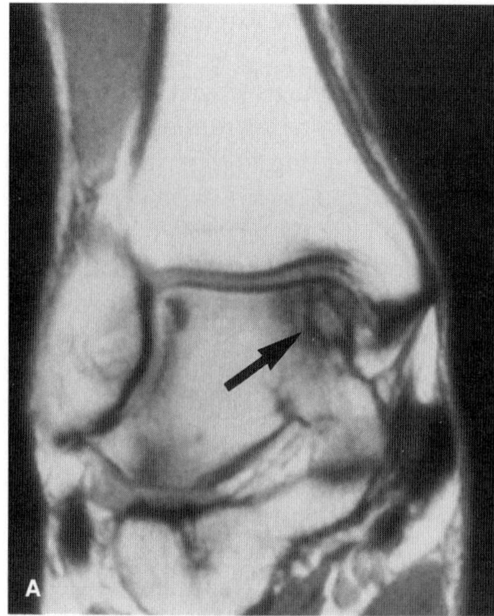

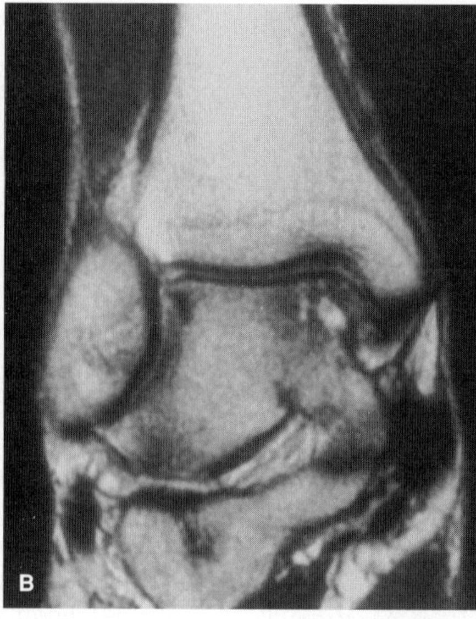

FIGURE 50.8. **Unstable Osteochondral Lesion of the Talus. A.** A proton-density (time of repetition [TR] 2,000; time of echo [TE] 20) coronal image through the talus shows a focus of low signal in the medial subarticular part of the talus (*arrow*). This is a characteristic appearance for an osteochondral lesion. **B.** A T2WI (TR 2,000; TE 80) shows high signal throughout the focus of the osteochondral lesion, which indicates an unstable fragment.

It often occurs with a small bony avulsion, called a flake fracture, off the fibula.

Entrapment of the peroneus tendons in a fractured calcaneus or fibula can occur and is easily diagnosed with MR. This can be a difficult diagnosis to make clinically. Complete disruption of the peroneus tendons is uncommon but is easily noted with MR.

Longitudinal split tears of the peroneus brevis are commonly seen in patients following an inversion ankle sprain with associated dorsiflexion. The peroneus brevis gets trapped against the fibula by the peroneus longus, and a longitudinal split tear of the peroneus brevis results. These patients have chronic lateral ankle pain, often associated with ankle instability because of the lateral collateral ligament disruption that also occurs with the inversion trauma. A split tear of the peroneus brevis is easily identified on MR images by noting either a chevron or "V" shape to the tendon distal to the fibula (Fig. 50.7), or by noting a division of the tendon into two parts. There is an 80% association with lateral ligament tears, so close attention should be paid to the ligaments when a split tear of the peroneus brevis is found.

AVASCULAR NECROSIS

Avascular necrosis commonly occurs in the foot and ankle. The talar dome is the second most common location for an osteochondral lesion (OCL), formerly called osteochondritis dissecans. (The knee is the most common site.) MR is useful in identifying and staging an OCL. Even when not apparent on plain films, MR can show an OCL as a

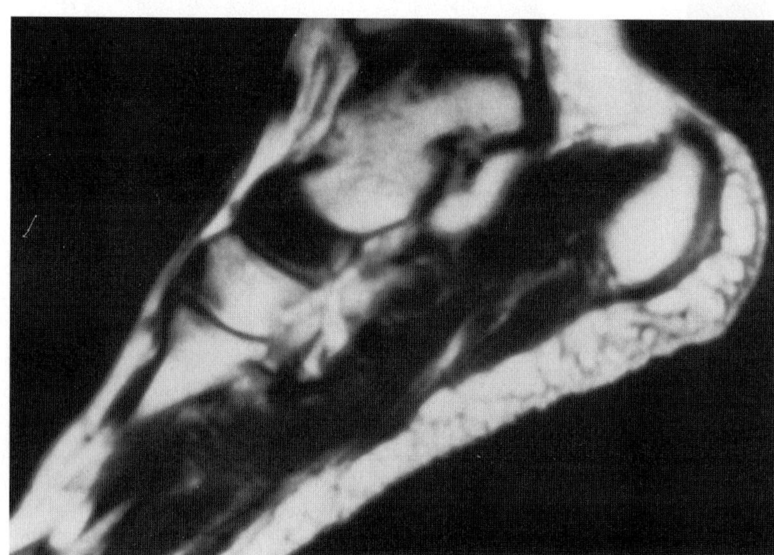

FIGURE 50.9. **Avascular Necrosis of the Tarsal Navicular.** A T1W (time of repetition 600; time of echo 30) sagittal image of the ankle in this patient with pain on the dorsum of the foot shows diffuse low signal throughout the tarsal navicular. This is a characteristic appearance for avascular necrosis and will often precede any plain film findings.

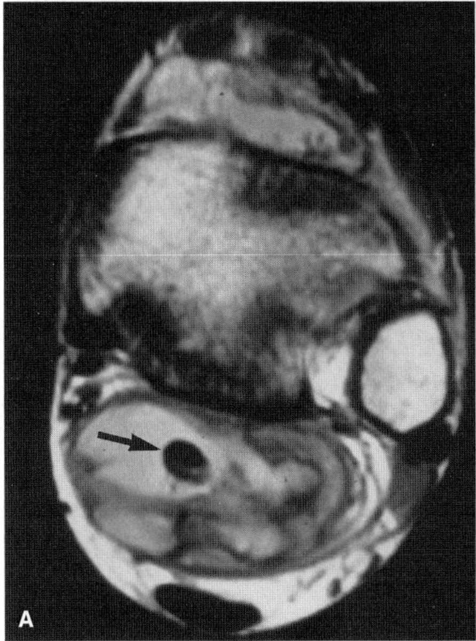

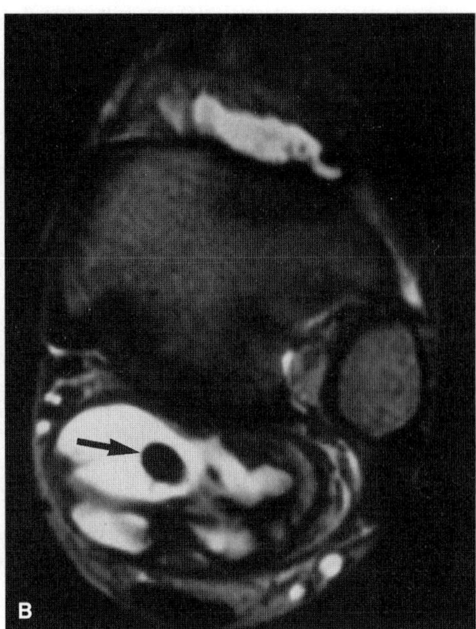

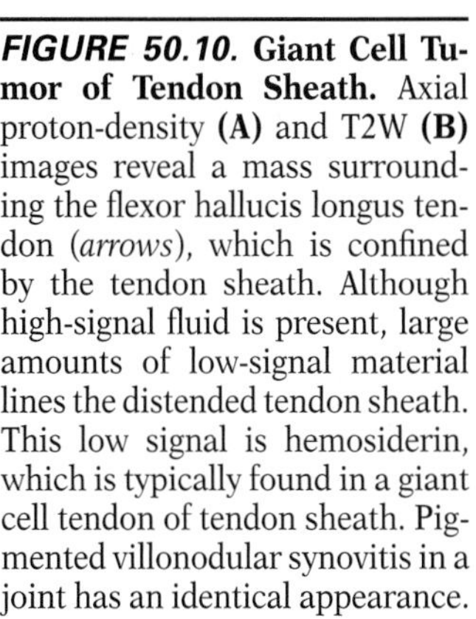
FIGURE 50.10. **Giant Cell Tumor of Tendon Sheath.** Axial proton-density **(A)** and T2W **(B)** images reveal a mass surrounding the flexor hallucis longus tendon (*arrows*), which is confined by the tendon sheath. Although high-signal fluid is present, large amounts of low-signal material lines the distended tendon sheath. This low signal is hemosiderin, which is typically found in a giant cell tendon of tendon sheath. Pigmented villonodular synovitis in a joint has an identical appearance.

focal area of low signal in the subarticular portion of the talar dome on T1WIs. On T2WIs or T2*WIs, if high signal is seen surrounding the dissecans fragment in the bone at the bed of the fragment or throughout the fragment (Fig. 50.8), the fragment is most likely unstable. If the fragment has become displaced and lies in the joint as a loose body, MR can sometimes be useful to localize it; however, loose bodies in any joint can be exceedingly difficult to find.

Diffuse low signal throughout a tarsal bone on a T1WI is typical for avascular necrosis. If the signal is increased on T2WIs, it may or may not be reversible. This occasionally occurs in the tarsal navicular (Fig. 50.9). MR can be useful in making this diagnosis when plain films are normal or equivocal.

TUMORS

A few tumors have a predilection for the foot and ankle (6). Up to 16% of synovial sarcomas occur in the foot. Desmoid tumors are commonly seen in the foot. Giant cell tumors of tendon sheath are often found in the tendon sheaths of the foot and ankle (Fig. 50.10). They are characterized by marked low signal in the synovial lining and in the tendons on T1WIs and T2WIs, just as pigmented villonodular synovitis appears in a joint.

The differential diagnosis for calcaneal tumors is similar to that of the epiphyses—giant cell tumor, chondroblastoma, and infection—with a unicameral bone cyst added.

Soft tissue tumors in the medial aspect of the foot and ankle can press on the posterior tibial nerve, resulting in tarsal tunnel syndrome (7). Clinically, patients with tarsal tunnel syndrome present with pain and paresthesia in the plantar aspect of the foot. In the aforementioned

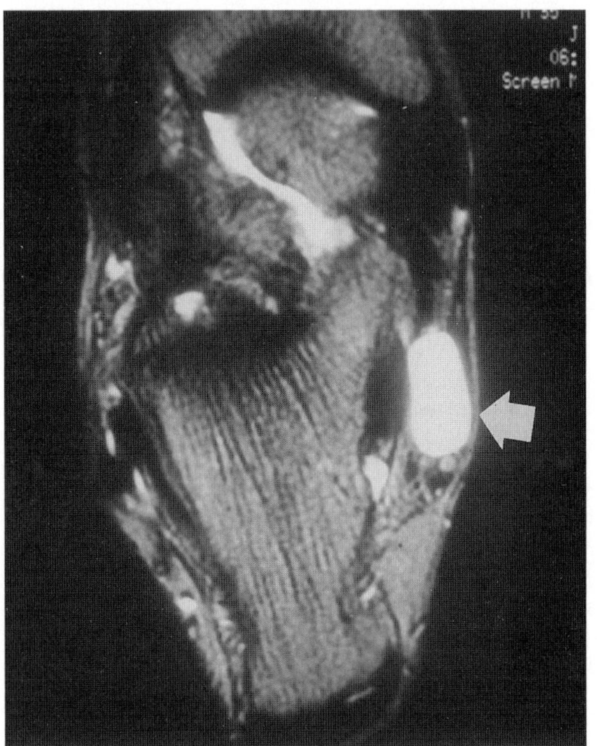

FIGURE 50.11. **Ganglion Causing Tarsal Tunnel Syndrome.** A fast spin-echo T2W axial image of the ankle in a patient complaining of pain and paresthesia on the plantar aspect of the foot shows a homogeneous, high-signal mass (*arrow*) lying adjacent to the flexor hallucis longus tendon. This is the position of the tarsal tunnel, which contains the tibial nerve, that can be impinged by a mass, such as in this case, resulting in tarsal tunnel syndrome. This was a ganglion.

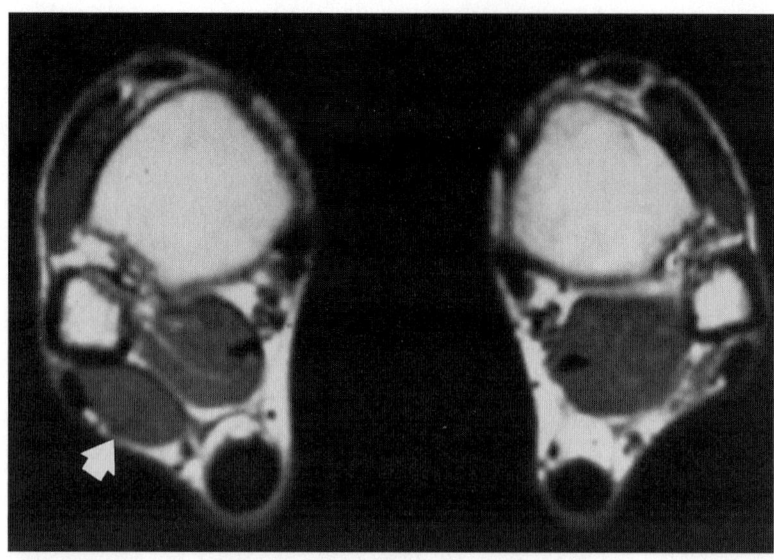

FIGURE 50.12. **Anomalous Muscle.** An axial T1WI of both ankles in this patient complaining of a mass in the right ankle shows an anomalous muscle (*arrow*) lateral to the flexor hallucis longus muscle that is responsible for the mass the patient feels.

mnemonic, "Tom, Dick, and Harry," the "and" is for artery, nerve, and vein. It is the position of the posterior tibial nerve. The nerve is easily compressed in the tarsal tunnel, which is bounded medially by the flexor retinaculum, a strong fibrous band that extends across the medial ankle joint for approximately 5 to 7 cm in a superior-to-inferior direction. Ganglions and neural tumors, which can look similar on T1WIs and T2WIs, often lie in the tarsal tunnel (Fig. 50.11) and compress the posterior tibial nerve, resulting in pain and paresthesia on the plantar aspect of the foot, extending into the toes. Tarsal tunnel syndrome often occurs secondary to trauma or fibrosis, or it can occur idiopathically. Regardless, this syndrome may not respond to surgical intervention; hence, MR is valuable in delineating a treatable lesion in many cases.

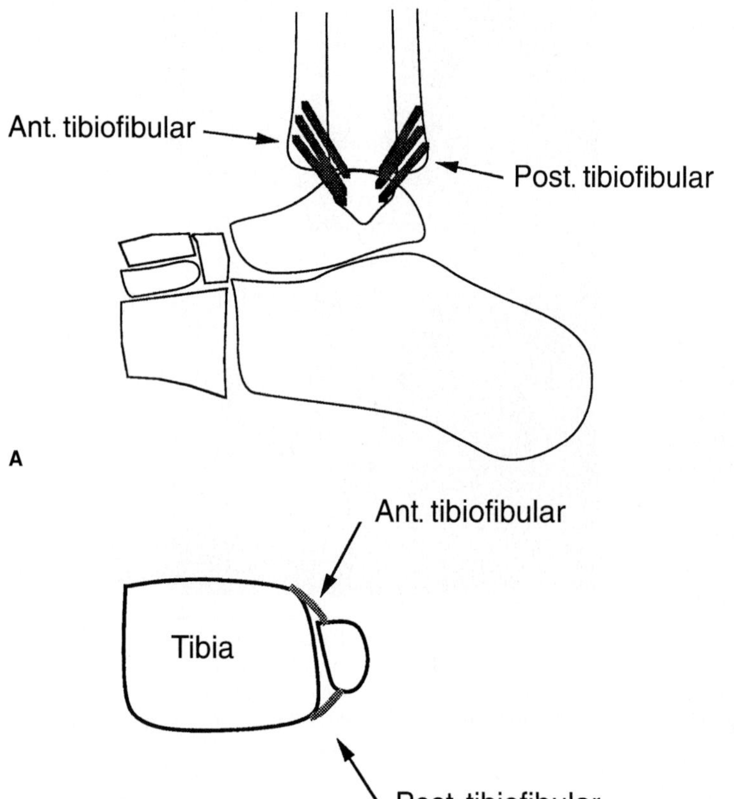

FIGURE 50.13. **Schematic of Lateral Collateral Ligaments. A.** This drawing of the ankle in a lateral view shows how the anterior (ant.) and posterior (post.) tibiofibular ligaments extend off the fibula and course superiorly to the tibia. **B.** A drawing in the axial plane shows that the fibula has a flat or convex surface at the origin of these ligaments.

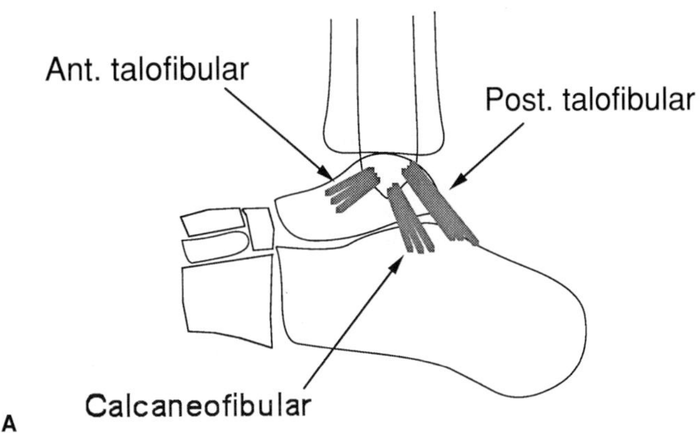

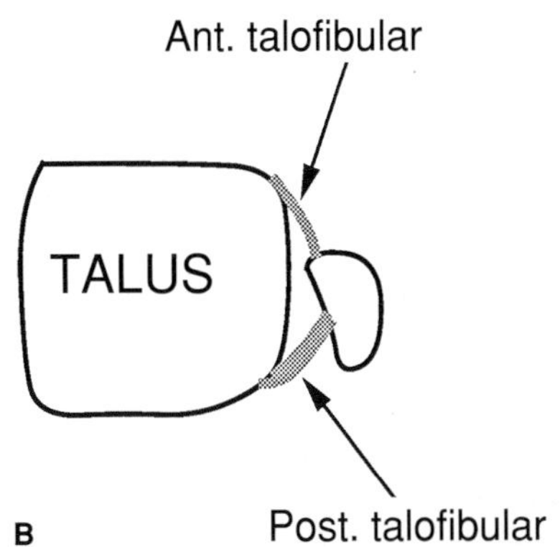

FIGURE 50.14. **Schematic of Lateral Collateral Ligaments. A.** This drawing of the ankle in a lateral view shows how the anterior (ant.) and posterior (post.) talofibular ligaments and the calcaneofibular ligament extend off the fibula and course inferiorly. These ligaments arise off of the fibula more distally than the anterior and posterior tibiofibular ligaments. **B.** A drawing in the axial plane shows that the anterior and posterior talofibular ligaments arise from the level of the distal fibula, which has a concave medial surface, the malleolar fossa.

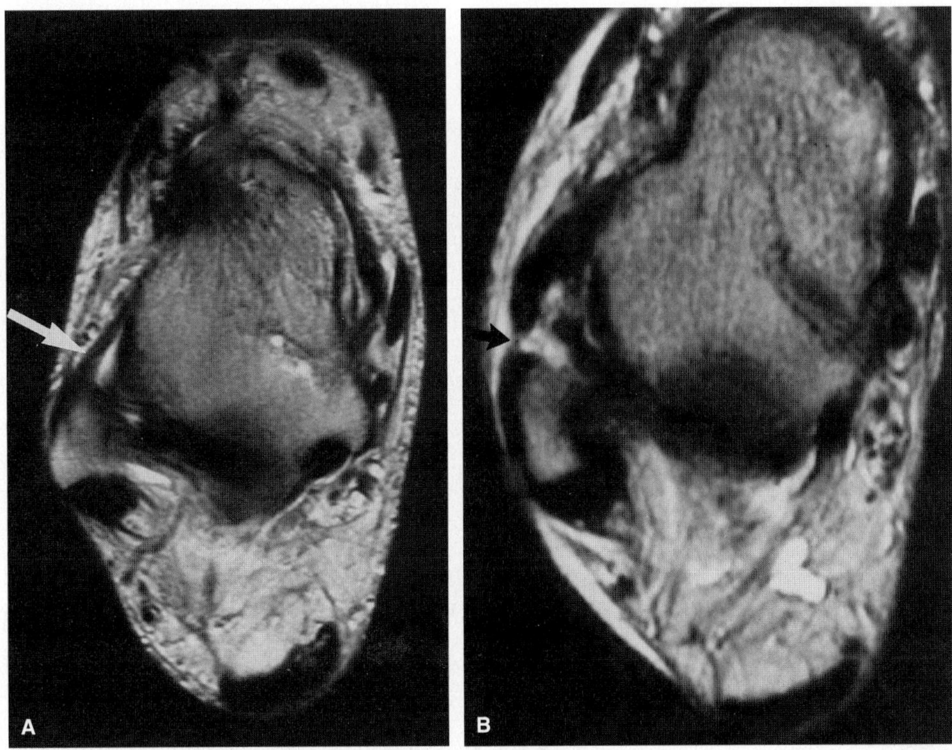

FIGURE 50.15. **Anterior Talofibular Ligament. A.** An axial T2WI (time of repetition [TR] 4,000; time of echo [TE] 76) through the distal fibula at the level of the malleolar fossa (the concave medial surface of the fibula) shows an intact anterior talofibular ligament (*arrow*) that makes up part of the joint capsule at this level. Note the high-signal joint fluid adjacent to the ligament. **B.** This axial T2WI (TR 3,200; TE 100) at the level of the malleolar fossa reveals a thickened anterior talofibular ligament that has a disruption (*arrow*). The marked thickening of the ligament indicates a chronic process.

Anomalous muscles in the foot or ankle are reported to be present in up to 6% of the population. These can be mistaken for a tumor and biopsy may be performed unnecessarily. MR will show these "tumors" to have imaging characteristics identical to those of normal muscle (Fig. 50.12) and to be sharply circumscribed. Accessory soleus and peroneus quartus muscles are the most common accessory muscles encountered around the foot and ankle.

LIGAMENTS

MR is not the best way to diagnose acute ankle ligament abnormalities. The clinical evaluation is usually straightforward and no diagnostic imaging of any type is necessary. Nevertheless, in clinically equivocal cases or when the examination is ordered for other reasons, the ligaments can be clearly evaluated with high-quality MR in most instances (8).

The deltoid ligament lies medially as a broad band beneath the tendons. Although often seen on coronal images deep to the posterior tibial tendon, it has a variable anatomic appearance. Injury to the deltoid ligament accounts for only 5% to 10% of ankle ligament sprains.

The lateral ligaments are injured in more than 90% of ankle sprains. The lateral complex is made up of two parts:

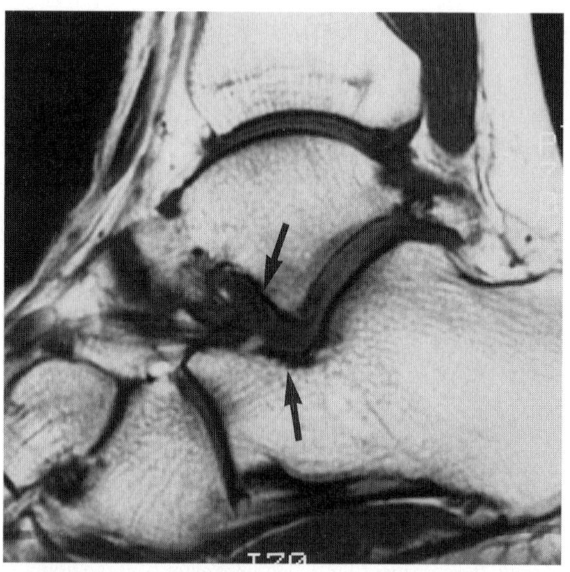

FIGURE 50.16. **Sinus Tarsi Syndrome.** A sagittal T1WI in a patient with chronic lateral ankle pain shows absence of the normal fat in the sinus tarsi (*arrows*). This is virtually diagnostic of sinus tarsi syndrome, except in the setting of an acute ankle sprain.

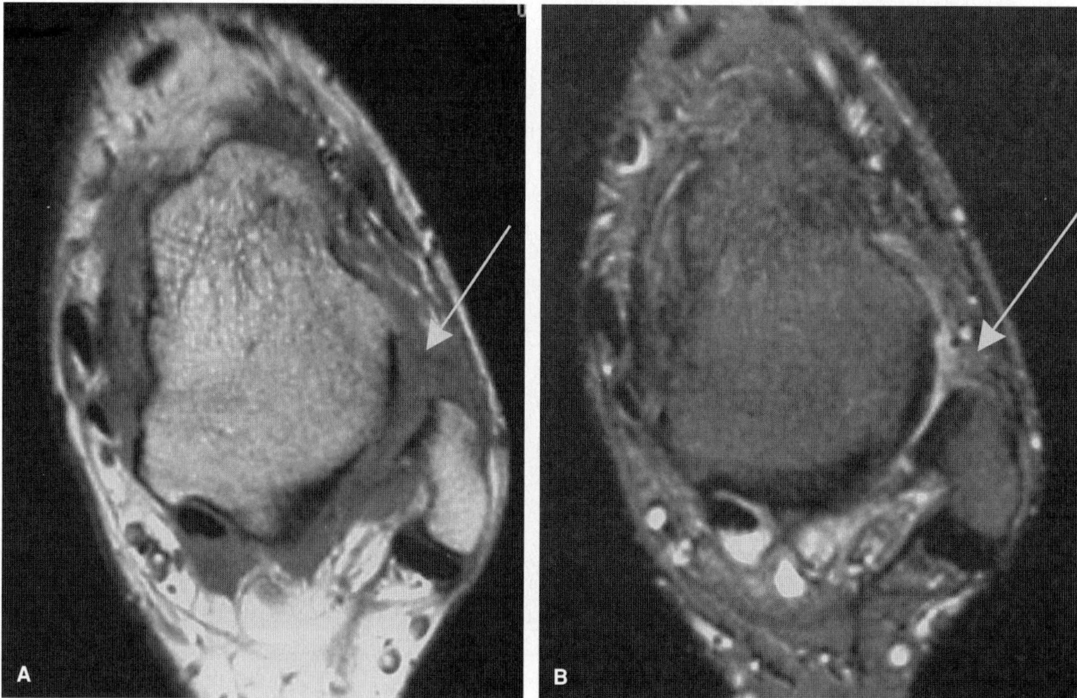

FIGURE 50.17. **Anterolateral Impingement Syndrome.** This axial T1WI **(A)** through the ankle reveals absence of the anterior talofibular ligament (*arrow*). The corresponding T2WI **(B)** shows low-signal scar tissue deep to the expected location of the anterior talofibular ligament (*arrow*), which indicates anterolateral impingement syndrome.

a superior group, i.e., the anterior and posterior tibiofibular ligaments that make up part of the syndesmosis (Fig. 50.13); and an inferior group, i.e., the anterior and posterior talofibular ligaments and the calcaneofibular ligament (Fig. 50.14). The anterior and posterior tibiofibular ligaments can be seen on axial images at or slightly below the tibiotalar joint. The anterior and posterior talofibular ligaments are seen on axial images just below the tibiotalar joint and emanate from a concavity in the distal fibula called the malleolar fossa (Fig. 50.14B). The most commonly torn ankle ligament is the anterior talofibular ligament. It is easily identified when a joint effusion is present, because it makes up the anterior capsule of the joint (Fig. 50.15). The anterior talofibular ligament is usually torn without other ligaments being involved; however, if the injury is severe enough, the next ligament to tear is the calcaneofibular ligament. Even with very severe trauma, the posterior talofibular ligament will rarely tear.

Several entities have a high association with chronic tears of the lateral ligaments. These include chronic lateral ankle instability, sinus tarsi syndrome, and anterolateral impingement syndrome.

Patients with sinus tarsi syndrome present with lateral ankle pain and tenderness and a perception of hindfoot instability. The sinus tarsi is the cone-shaped space between the talus and the calcaneus that opens up laterally. It is a fat-filled space through which traverse several important ligaments that provide subtalar stability. In sinus tarsi syndrome, these ligaments are torn and the fat is replaced with granulation tissue or scar tissue. Hence, on T2WIs there may be high signal (granulation tissue) or low signal (scar), but on T1WIs there is low signal in the sinus tarsi (Fig. 50.16). In the acutely sprained ankle, the sinus tarsi may undergo replacement of the fat because of hemorrhage and edema, which will resolve.

Anterolateral impingement syndrome results from hypertrophy and scarring of the synovium in the lateral

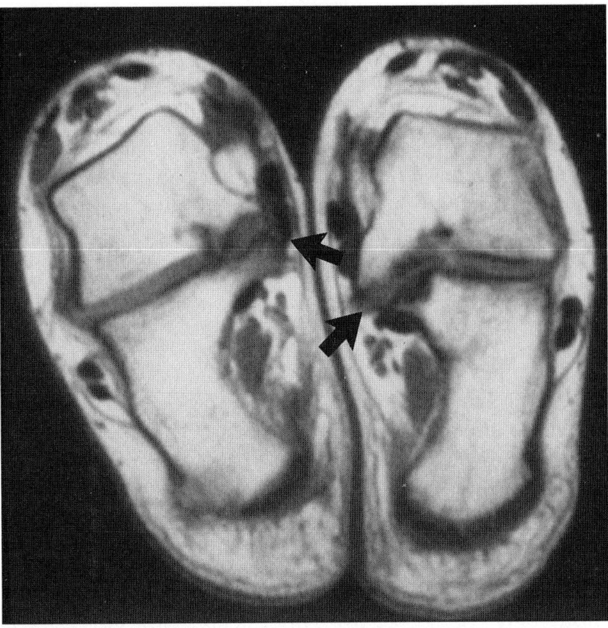

FIGURE 50.18. **Tarsal Coalition.** An axial T1WI in a patient with painful flat feet shows bilateral talocalcaneal coalition (*arrows*), which is primarily fibrous. The normal joint space is irregular and widened bilaterally. In cases of suspected coalition, both ankles should be imaged, as coalition often occurs bilaterally.

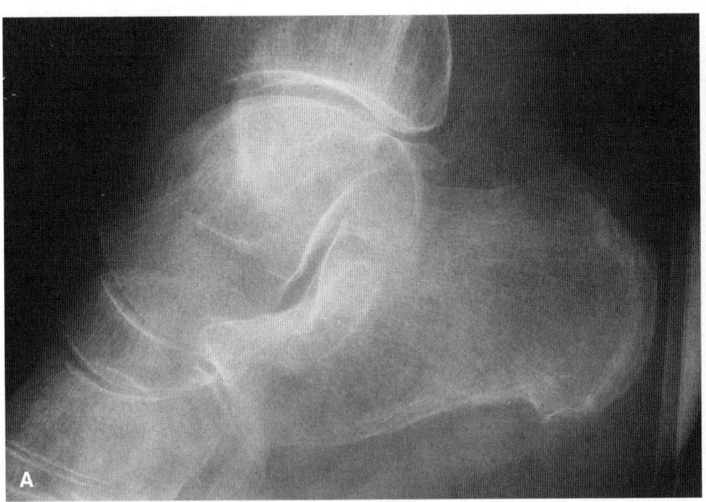

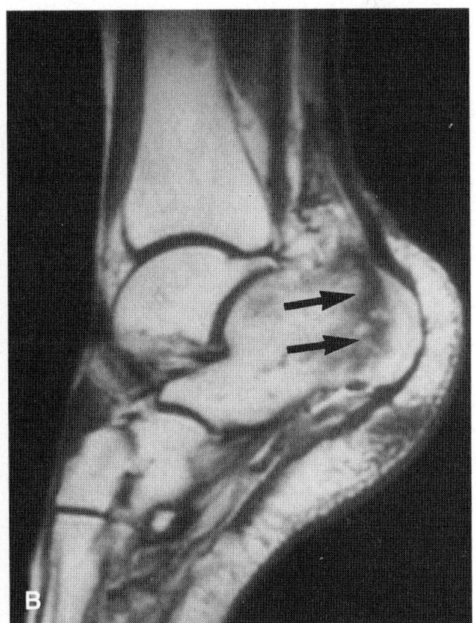

FIGURE 50.19. **Calcaneal Stress Fracture. A.** A 70-year-old patient with a prior history of lung cancer presented with heel pain and a normal plain film. A bone scan showed diffuse increased radionuclide uptake throughout the posterior calcaneus. **B.** A sagittal T1WI revealed a linear area of low signal (*arrows*), which is characteristic for a stress fracture. Metastatic disease would not have this appearance.

gutter of the ankle. The lateral gutter is the space between the tibia and fibula and is bound by the lateral ankle ligaments. Patients with anterolateral impingement syndrome present with lateral ankle pain and inability to dorsiflex normally. They often have a click on dorsiflexion. Arthroscopic resection of the scar tissue has been reported, with good results. T2WIs show low-signal tissue in the lateral gutter (Fig. 50.17). The anterior talofibular ligament is commonly torn or fibrosed in this condition.

BONY ABNORMALITIES

Tarsal coalition is a common cause of a painful flatfoot. It occurs most commonly at the calcaneonavicular joint and the middle facet of the talocalcaneal joint (Fig. 50.18). Up to 50% of patients with tarsal coalition have bilateral coalition. It can be difficult (or impossible) to see the coalition on plain films; however, CT and MR will show bony coalition with a high degree of accuracy. The coalition can also be fibrous or cartilaginous. In these cases, secondary findings, such as joint space irregularity at the affected joint or degenerative joint disease at nearby joints that are subjected to accentuated stress, can be seen.

Fractures of the foot and ankle are usually well documented with plain films. Stress fractures, however, can be difficult to diagnose radiographically or clinically, and they can mimic more sinister abnormalities. MR will show stress fractures as linear low signal on T1WIs and high signal on T2WIs (Fig. 50.19).

MR has had mixed reviews when used for diagnosing osteomyelitis in the foot. In diabetic patients with foot infections, diagnosing osteomyelitis is important because the treatment is often much more aggressive—including amputation—than if the bone is not involved. If the marrow appears normal, MR is highly accurate in predicting no osteomyelitis; however, if low signal is present in the marrow around a joint, osteomyelitis may or may not be present. Low signal can be caused by edema or hyperemia without infection. The only definitive MR findings for osteomyelitis are cortical disruption, a bony abscess (not a common finding), or a sinus tract (an even less common finding). MR is therefore very sensitive but not very specific in diagnosing osteomyelitis in the foot and ankle (9).

REFERENCES

1. Anzilotti K, Schweitzer ME, et al. Effect of foot and ankle MR imaging on clinical decision making. Radiology 1996;201:515–517.
2. Quinn S, Murray W, Clark R, Cochran C. Achilles tendon: MR imaging at 1.5 T. Radiology 1987;164:767–770.
3. Rosenberg Z, Cheung Y, Jahss M, et al. Rupture of posterior tibial tendons: CT and MR imaging with surgical correlation. Radiology 1988;169:229–236.
4. Balen PF, Helms CA. Association of posterior tibial tendon injury with spring ligament injury, sinus tarsi abnormality, and plantar fasciitis on MR imaging. AJR Am J Roentgenol 2001;176:1137–1143.
5. Oden R. Tendon injuries about the ankle resulting from skiing. Clin Orthop 1987;216:63–69.
6. Keigley B, Haggar A, Gaba A, et al. Primary tumors of the foot: MR imaging. Radiology 1989;171:755–759.
7. Erickson S, Quinn S, Kneeland J, et al. MR imaging of the tarsal tunnel and related spaces: normal and abnormal findings with anatomic correlation. AJR Am J Roentgenol 1990;155:323–328.
8. Erickson S, Smith J, Ruiz M, et al. MR imaging of the lateral collateral ligament of the ankle. AJR Am J Roentgenol 1991;156:131–136.
9. Erdman W, Tamburro F, Jayson H, et al. Osteomyelitis: characteristics and pitfalls of diagnosis with MR imaging. Radiology 1991;180:533–539.

SECTION XI

Pediatric Radiology

Chapter 51

Pediatric Chest

Susan D. John and Leonard E. Swischuk

Abnormal Lung Opacity
Alveolar Patterns
Peribronchial and Interstitial Patterns

Abnormal Lung Volume
Pulmonary Hypoplasia or Agenesis
Bilateral Lung Hyperinflation
Asymmetric/Unilateral Aeration Abnormalities

Pulmonary Cavities

Lung Disease in the Neonate

Pleural Thickening and Effusions

Lung Masses

Mediastinal and Hilar Masses

Chest Wall Masses

Congenital Heart Disease
Acyanotic Heart Disease With Increased Pulmonary Vascularity
Cyanotic Heart Disease With Increased Pulmonary Vascularity
Decreased Pulmonary Vascularity
Normal Pulmonary Vascularity
Cardiac Malpositions

ABNORMAL LUNG OPACITY

Pulmonary opacities in children are classified in the same way as in adults: as primarily alveolar or interstitial, focal or diffuse, and unilateral or bilateral. Some abnormalities occur in a central or parahilar distribution, whereas others are predominantly peripheral or basal in location. Mixed patterns also occur. An understanding of the causes of these various patterns is necessary to provide a useful interpretation of abnormal lung opacities in children.

Alveolar Patterns

Alveolar consolidation occurs when the alveolar airspace is replaced by a substance, usually fluid. Focal consolidations most often represent exudates associated with bacterial pneumonia (Table 51.1). Bacterial consolidation begins as an oval, round, ill-defined, or fluffy area of solid opacification, often more peripheral than central in location. The pneumonia may progress to involve an entire lobe, but involvement of an entire lung is uncommon. Bacterial pneumonia is a space-occupying process within the lung and, therefore, little or no volume will be lost in the affected lung during the acute stage of infection (Fig. 51.1).

Streptococcus pneumoniae is the most common cause of lobar pneumonia throughout childhood. The incidence of *Haemophilus influenzae* pneumonia has dramatically decreased in the United States and other developed countries because of the use of the *H. influenzae* type b vaccine. *Mycoplasma* infections may also occasionally produce focal consolidating pneumonia.

Consolidations with viral infections are not particularly common but can occur with more serious viral infection, such as adenovirus, influenza, parainfluenza, and respiratory syncytial virus. There is some question as to whether these consolidations represent true airspace consolidations. It is likely that they represent intense interstitial disease causing compression of the alveoli and mimicking the findings of airspace consolidations. The same may be true of *Mycoplasma* infections.

Pneumonia caused by gram-negative bacilli is uncommon in children; it occurs primarily in infants and

TABLE 51.1 Causes of Focal Alveolar Consolidation

Bacterial pneumonia
Streptococcus pneumoniae
Mycobacterium
Staphylococcus
Haemophilus influenzae
Nonbacterial infection
Tuberculosis
Actinomycosis
Pulmonary infarction
Pulmonary contusion

immunocompromised children. Primary tuberculosis should be considered when the infiltrate is accompanied by hilar lymphadenopathy. Other causes of isolated lung consolidation in children include fungal infection, pulmonary infarction, lung contusion, and focal pulmonary hemorrhage.

Atelectasis is a common occurrence in children, especially those with bronchial disease such as acute viral respiratory tract infections, reactive airway disease, and asthma. Atelectasis can sometimes resemble a bacterial consolidation. The findings of volume loss, such as shift of the fissures or the mediastinum, help to distinguish atelectasis from bacterial consolidation. Generally, volume loss will not be seen with a bacterial pneumonia until it begins to resolve. A flattened or linear shape in a pulmonary opacity should also suggest that it represents atelectasis rather than consolidation (Fig. 51.2). Atelectasis is particularly problematic in children with asthma, who are also at increased risk for bacterial pneumonia. Clinical information may be necessary to help distinguish atelectasis from pneumonia in such children. Opacities seen in a child with acute asthmatic exacerbation but without high fever, chest pain, or leukocytosis are much more likely to be caused by atelectasis than pneumonia.

Multiple patchy lung opacities is a pattern seen in a wide variety of conditions (Table 51.2). Such opacities reflect filling of the alveolar space with exudates, edema, or blood. Multiple bilateral alveolar infiltrates suggest bacterial infection (most commonly staphylococcal) (Fig. 51.3) or fungal disease. Opportunistic infections in immunocompromised patients are much more likely to be multiple and bilateral. Aspiration pneumonia also tends to present with multiple patchy pulmonary opacities. The

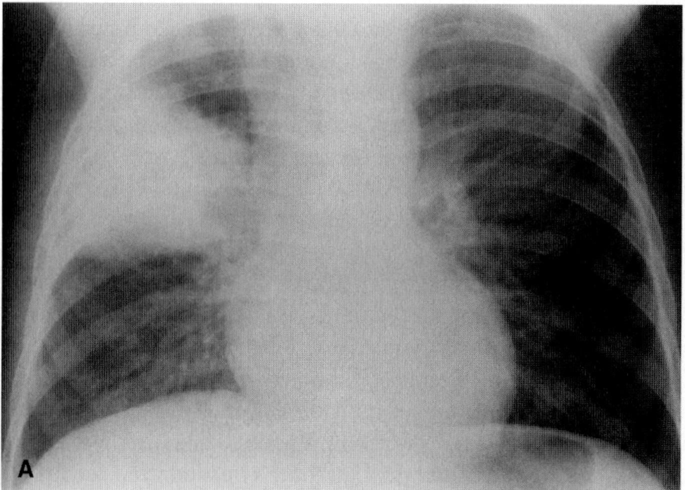

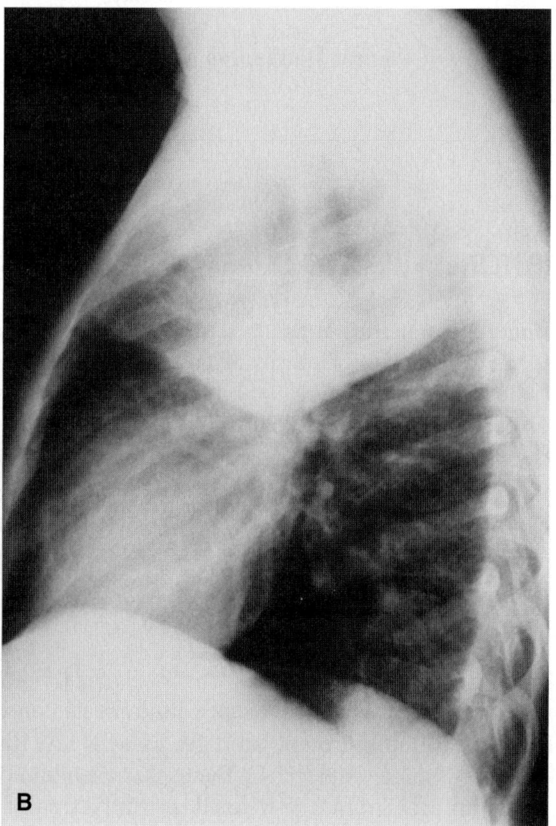

FIGURE 51.1. **Bacterial Pneumonia. A.** Frontal view. **B.** Lateral view. A typical alveolar consolidation in the right upper lobe. Note that the fissures are not displaced, indicating that there is little volume loss. A right pleural effusion is also present.

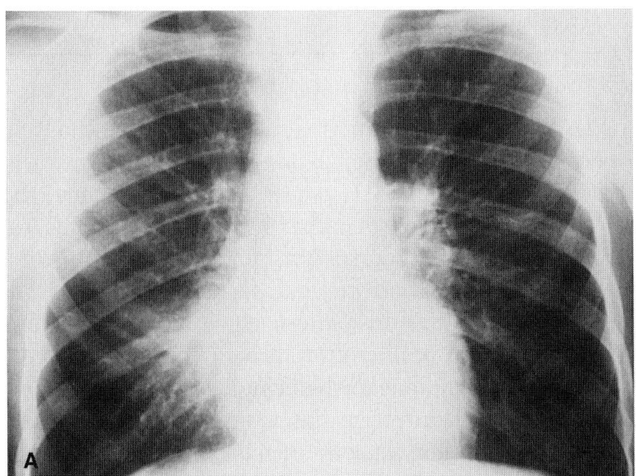

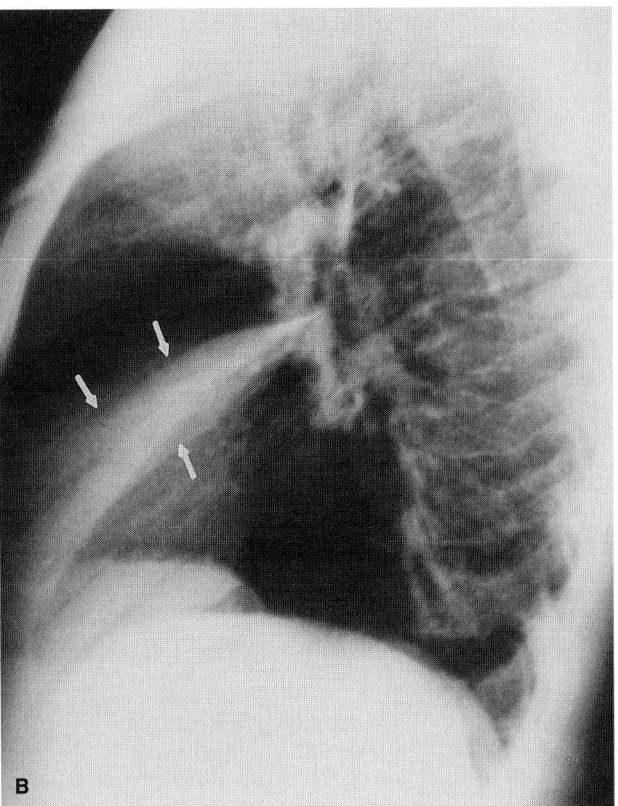

FIGURE 51.2. **Acute Asthma. A.** Opacity silhouettes the right heart border on the posteroanterior view. **B.** Lateral view shows displacement of the horizontal and oblique fissures (*arrows*), indicating right middle lobe atelectasis.

pneumonitis associated with hydrocarbon ingestion typically occurs in the medial portions of the lung bases (Fig. 51.4). Other less common causes of patchy alveolar opacities include milk allergy, hypersensitivity pneumonitis, uremic lung disease, near drowning, and pulmonary hemorrhage (i.e., idiopathic pulmonary hemosiderosis).

TABLE 51.2 Sources of Multiple Patchy Lung Opacities

Infection
Staphylococcus
Mycoplasma
Fungal
Opportunistic organisms
Aspiration
Hydrocarbon ingestion
Near drowning
Immune-mediated pneumonitis
Milk allergy
Hypersensitivity pneumonitis
Pulmonary hemorrhage
Pulmonary edema

Peribronchial and Interstitial Patterns

The vast majority of upper respiratory tract infections in childhood are viral in nature and primarily bronchial in location. Such infections may result in pulmonary opacities that differ significantly from those seen with bacterial pneumonia.

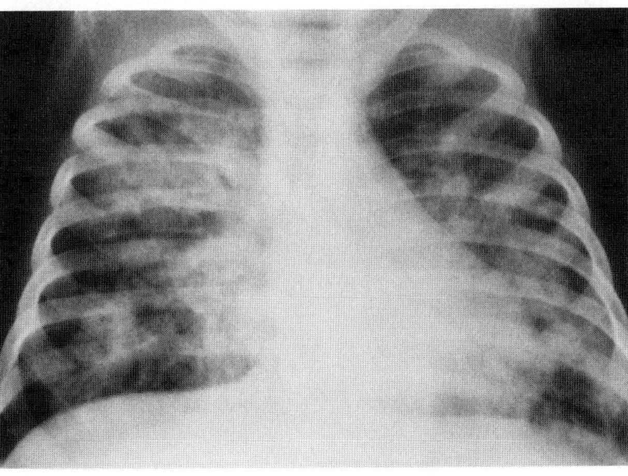

FIGURE 51.3. **Staphylococcal Pneumonia.** Note the typical multiple, bilateral alveolar opacities.

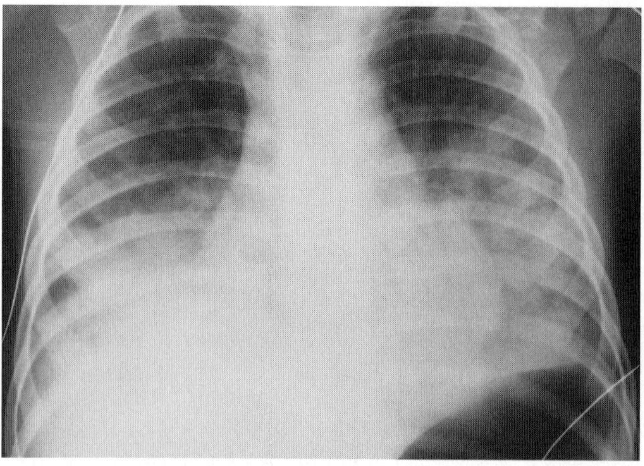

FIGURE 51.4. **Hydrocarbon Aspiration.** Typical patchy alveolar opacities are seen in the lung bases bilaterally in this child who ingested kerosene.

TABLE 51.3 Causes of Parahilar Peribronchial Opacity

Acute (infection)
Viral
Mycoplasma
Chlamydia
Pertussis
Chronic
Asthma
Cystic fibrosis
Immunologic deficiency disease
Chronic aspiration

Parahilar peribronchial opacities are sometimes seen and are the result of peribronchial inflammation and edema associated with bronchitis (Table 51.3) (Fig. 51.5A). The pattern consists of bilateral, ill-defined, hazy soft tissue opacity in the hilar region of the lungs. When extensive, these opacities may cause a "shaggy" appearance to the cardiac borders (Fig. 51.5B). Acute peribronchial opacities are most often caused by viral respiratory infections (1,2). Bilateral hilar adenopathy and scattered areas of subsegmental atelectasis are common associated findings (Fig. 51.6). This pattern is very different from the more peripheral alveolar opacification that is usually seen with bacterial pneumonias. However, it should be noted that a superimposed consolidating bacterial pneumonia can develop later in the course of a viral lower respiratory tract infection. *M. pneumoniae* and pertussis infections also commonly produce this pattern (3). Follicular bronchitis, associated with proliferation of lymphoid follicles along the airways, is indistinguishable radiographically. *Chlamydia trachomatis* infection has a similar appearance and usually occurs just after the newborn period (Fig. 51.7). Chronic bronchial inflammation associated with conditions such as asthma, cystic fibrosis (4) (see Fig. 51.18), immunologic deficiency diseases, and recurrent aspiration may result in persisting patterns of parahilar peribronchial opacity and may eventually lead to bronchiectasis.

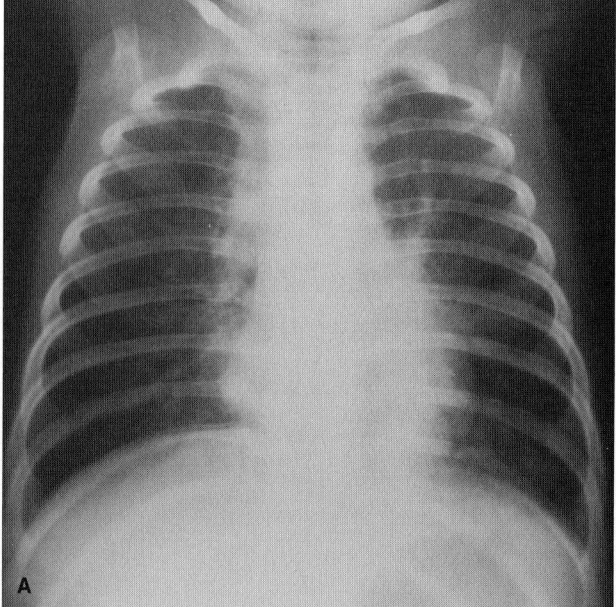

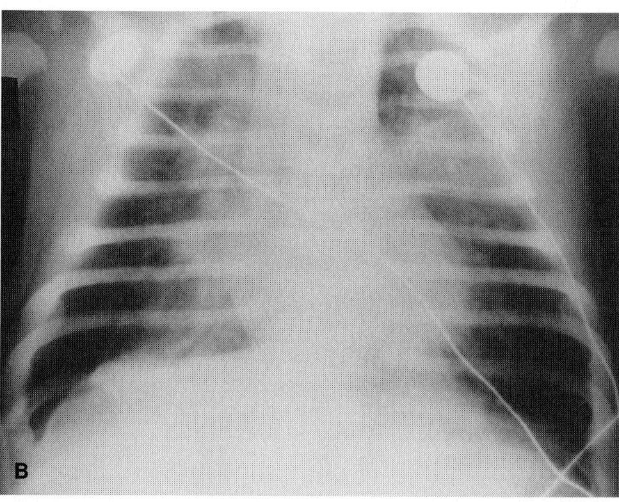

FIGURE 51.5. **Viral Infection. A.** Bilateral parahilar peribronchial opacities are typical of viral lower respiratory tract infections. **B.** More pronounced inflammatory edema produces dense parahilar regions, leading to the "shaggy heart" appearance.

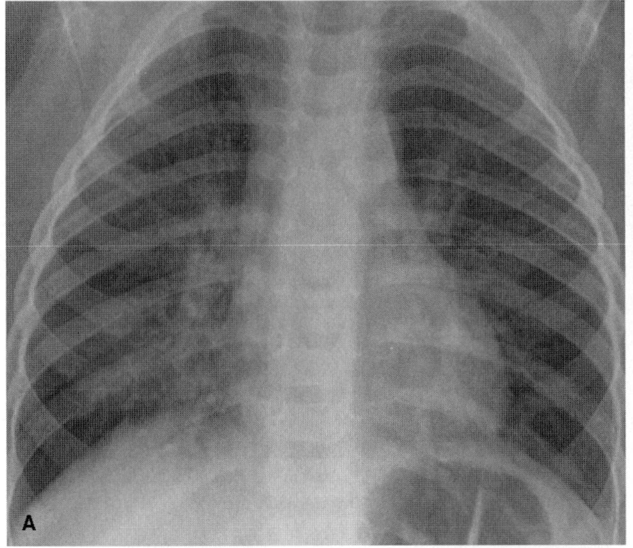

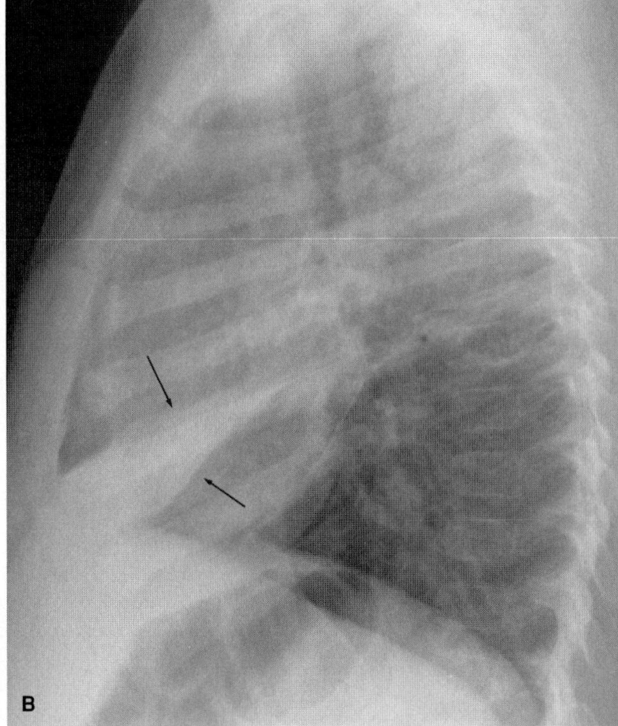

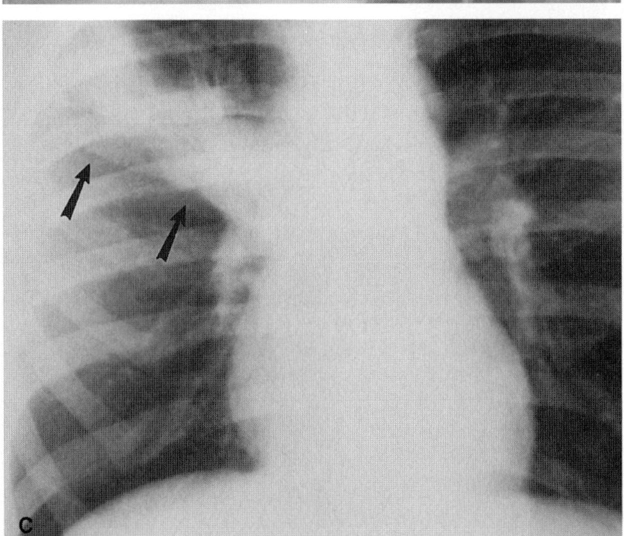

FIGURE 51.6. **Viral Lower Respiratory Tract Infection With Atelectasis. A.** Note the ill-defined bilateral parahilar peribronchial opacities and vague focal opacity at the right heart border. **B.** On the lateral view, shift of the fissures (*arrows*) toward the right middle lobe opacity indicates volume loss (atelectasis) **C.** The common peribronchial opacities are accompanied by elevation of the horizontal fissure (*arrows*).

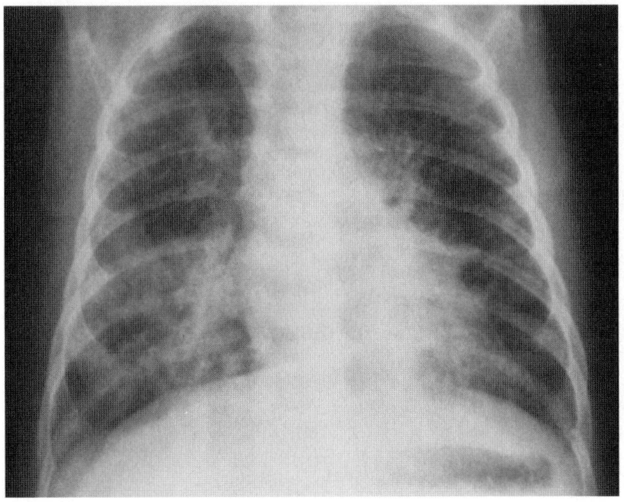

FIGURE 51.7. **Chlamydia Pneumonitis.** Prominent bilateral peribronchial opacities with slight nodularity are seen in the lung bases. The appearance is similar to that seen with viral infections.

Hazy, reticular, or reticulonodular opacities that occur diffusely in the lungs indicate interstitial lung pathology, and the causes include many of the same conditions that cause parahilar peribronchial opacities (Table 51.4). The most common cause of an interstitial pattern in the lungs of a child is viral or *Mycoplasma* infection (Fig. 51.8). In general, bacterial infections of the lung do not have this appearance, except in the neonate, when bacterial pneumonia can present as diffuse haziness or reticulonodularity. Infections with fungi, such as *Histoplasma capsulatum* and *Coccidioides immitis,* can also occasionally result in an interstitial pattern.

Pulmonary edema, when it is confined to the interstitial space, often produces a hazy or reticular pattern in the lungs. Cardiogenic pulmonary edema occurs when the pulmonary venous pressures are elevated because of left-sided myocardial failure or congenital lesions that impede blood flow through the left side of the heart (e.g., pulmonary vein atresia, cor triatriatum, hypoplastic left heart syndrome).

TABLE 51.4 Conditions Causing Hazy, Reticular, or Reticulonodular Patterns

Infection
Viral
Mycoplasma
Fungal
Pulmonary edema
Heart disease
Acute renal failure
Near drowning
Increased intracranial pressure
Inhalation injury
Drug overdose
"Acute" respiratory distress syndrome (ARDS)
Pulmonary lymphangiectasia/hemangiomatosis
Idiopathic pulmonary hemosiderosis
Interstitial pneumonitis
Langerhans cell histiocytosis
Tuberous sclerosis
Connective tissue diseases
Lymphocytic infiltrative disease
Malignancy
Leukemia/lymphoma
Lymphangitic metastasis

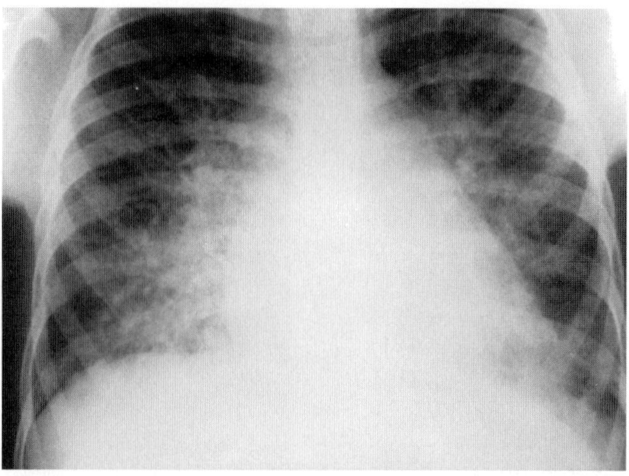

FIGURE 51.9. **Acute Glomerulonephritis.** Note marked bilateral vascular congestion edema. The heart is mildly enlarged.

Noncardiogenic causes of pulmonary edema predominate in children. One of the most common causes of pulmonary edema in children is acute glomerulonephritis (Fig. 51.9). Sodium and fluid retention leads to hypervolemia, which can then result in cardiomegaly and pulmonary vascular

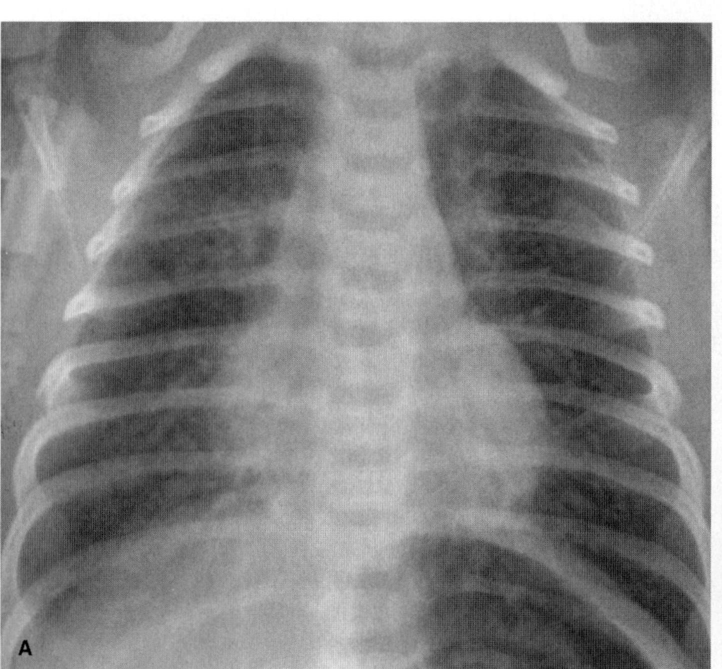

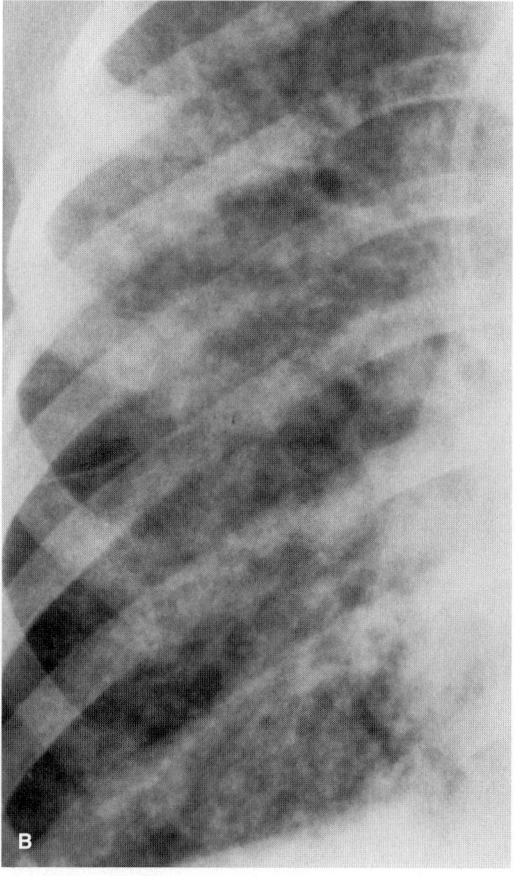

FIGURE 51.8. **Viral Lower Respiratory Tract Infection. A.** A mild, diffuse, reticulonodular pattern is present in this patient with respiratory syncytial virus infection. **B.** Note the prominent reticulonodular pattern caused by herpes pneumonia in an immunosuppressed patient.

congestion with edema. The radiographic appearance can be indistinguishable from that of edema caused by cardiac failure. Other noncardiogenic causes of pulmonary edema in children include near drowning, increased intracranial pressure, inhalation injuries, drug overdose, and ARDS.

Pulmonary lymphangiectasia is a rare condition that consists of dilated lymphatic channels secondary to either abnormal embryonic development of the lymphatic system or obstruction of lymphatic drainage. The dilated lymphatics cause a coarsely nodular or reticular pattern in the lungs, usually developing early in infancy (Fig. 51.10A) (5,6). Pulmonary hemangiomatosis is a similar rare condition. Recurrent hemorrhage into the lungs in patients with idiopathic pulmonary hemosiderosis eventually leads to chronic diffuse haziness or reticula in the lungs, representing pulmonary fibrosis (Fig. 51.10B, C). Langerhans cell histiocytosis (LCH) causes an interstitial pattern that often is more prominent in the upper lung zones. The lung volumes in LCH are normal or increased, which differs from fibrotic conditions, in which lung volumes tend to be decreased. HRCT may show cysts and nodules (7).

Interstitial lung disease that predominates in the lower lobes can be seen with tuberous sclerosis, connective tissue diseases, and primary interstitial pneumonitis. Leukemia, lymphoma, and lymphatic metastases to the lungs can also cause a reticular or reticulonodular infiltrative pattern. *Mycoplasma* pneumonitis sometimes presents as an interstitial pattern confined to one lobe of the lung (3).

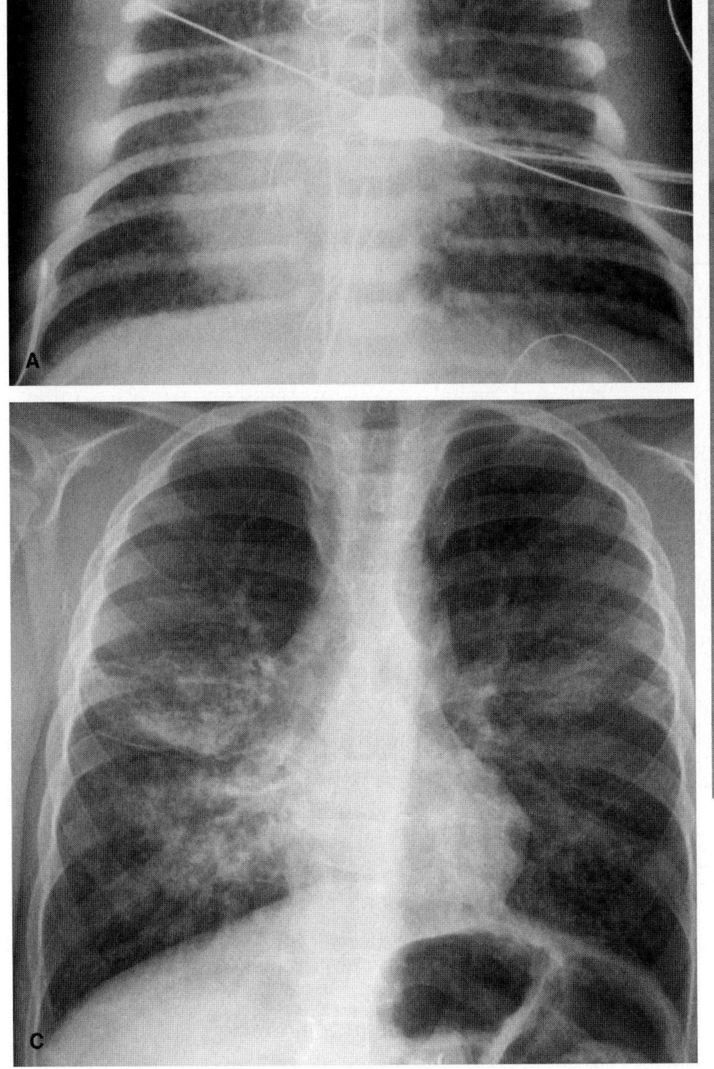

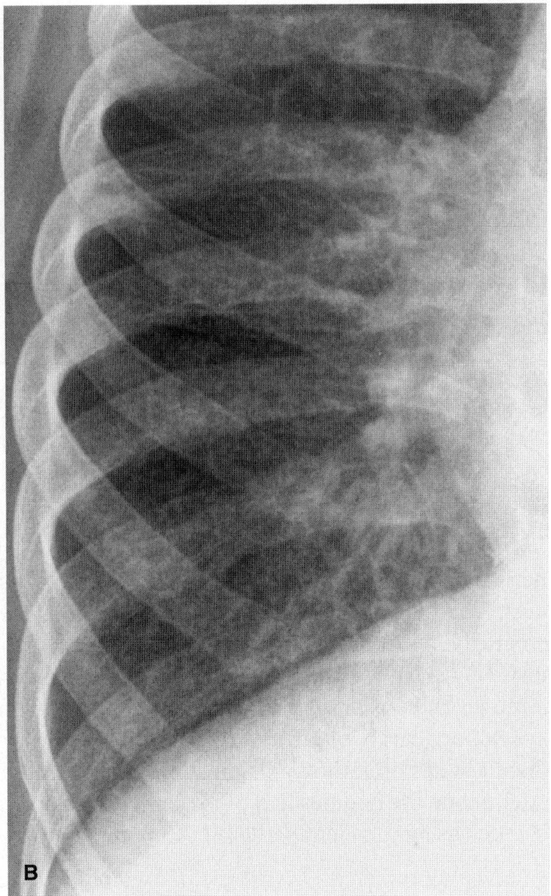

FIGURE 51.10. **Interstitial Patterns. A.** Pulmonary lymphangiectasia. Note the diffuse reticulonodular pattern throughout both lungs caused by dilated lymphatics in the interstitium. Dextrocardia is also present. **B.** Another patient with a fine reticular pattern in the lungs, caused in this case by idiopathic pulmonary hemosiderosis. **C.** The same patient after an episode of acute hemorrhage.

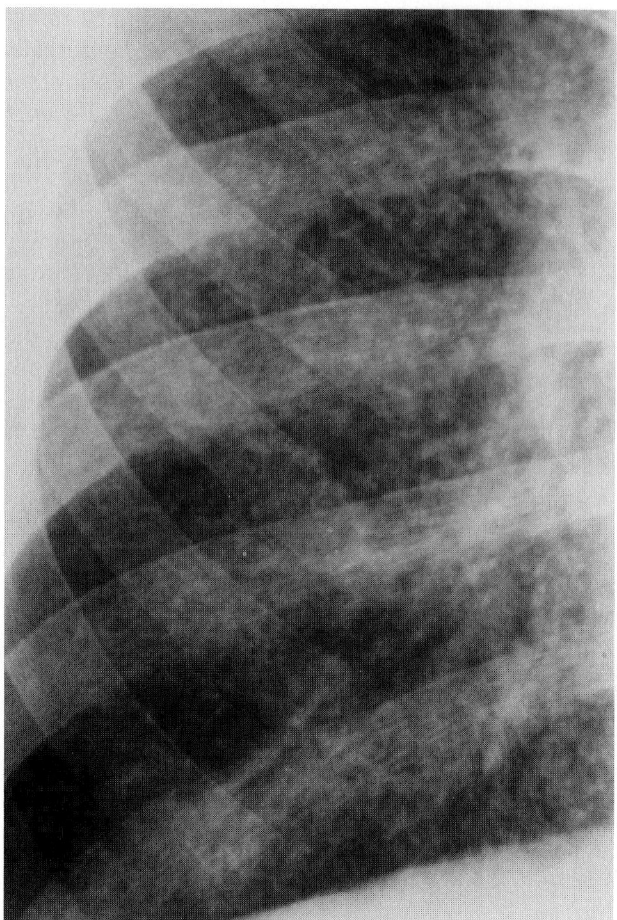

FIGURE 51.11. **Miliary Tuberculosis.** The numerous tiny nodules in the lungs of this immunosuppressed patient represent hematogenous dissemination of tuberculosis.

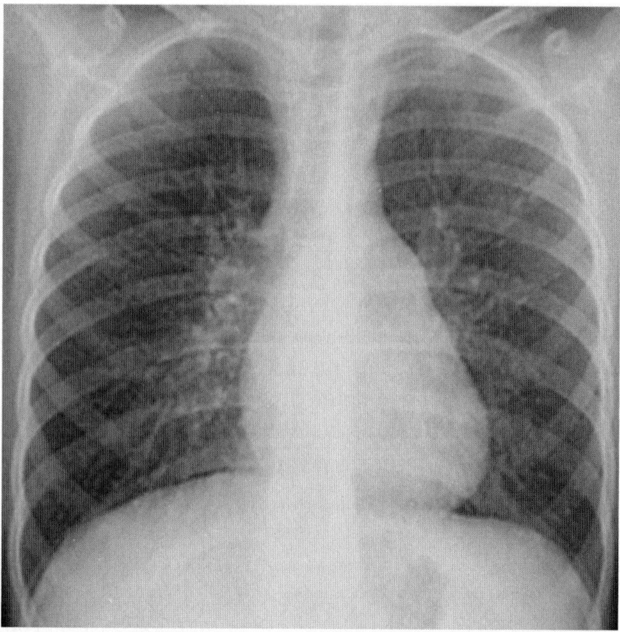

FIGURE 51.12. **Lymphocytic Interstitial Pneumonitis.** Note the diffuse interstitial pattern in the lungs of an HIV-positive child.

Miliary nodules usually consist of tiny nodules (smaller than 5 mm) that are randomly distributed throughout the lungs. This pattern in children is most often caused by hematogenous dissemination of tuberculosis or histoplasmosis (Fig. 51.11), although viral pneumonitis, idiopathic pulmonary hemosiderosis, and metastatic disease can also have this appearance (Table 51.5). The tiny nodules can be difficult to see on radiographs in some cases, and CT can better define the nodules and other associated abnormalities, such as lymphadenopathy (8). Acute disseminated tuberculosis in infants and young children can sometimes produce larger nodules, and CT may show larger areas of opacity caused by coalescent nodules and interstitial thickening.

TABLE 51.5 Causes of Miliary Nodules

Infection
Tuberculosis
Histoplasmosis
Viral
Idiopathic pulmonary hemosiderosis
Metastatic disease

Opportunistic infections may occur in children with HIV infection and other forms of congenital or acquired immunodeficiency. Infection with common viral, bacterial, and fungal organisms creates a pattern similar to that seen in immunocompetent children, but the findings tend to be more rapidly progressive and more pronounced. Lymphocytic infiltrative disease (LIP) produces a reticulonodular pattern that is indistinguishable from infection (Fig. 51.12), except for its chronicity.

ABNORMAL LUNG VOLUME

Pulmonary aeration abnormalities are best evaluated on the chest radiograph by observing the following criteria: (*1*) the relative size of a lung or hemithorax, (*2*) the degree of radiolucency of the lung, and (*3*) the pulmonary vascularity or blood flow to the lung. Bilateral smallness of the lungs is commonly caused by less than complete inspiration. The technical difficulties of obtaining good inspiratory chest films in children are significant. The lungs may appear small if the diaphragm is elevated, because of either neuromuscular abnormality or the presence of large masses, fluid collections, or bowel distension in the abdomen. Infrequently, inspiratory obstruction of the trachea can lead to bilateral underaeration of the lungs. Causes of such obstruction include intratracheal masses or foreign bodies, or extrinsic compression of the trachea by anomalous vascular structures. A hyperlucent but small hemithorax usually signifies some degree of pulmonary hypoplasia, either congenital or acquired.

Pulmonary Hypoplasia or Agenesis

Congenital pulmonary hypoplasia is associated with hypoplasia or absence of the ipsilateral pulmonary artery (9); thus, pulmonary vascular markings will be diminished in size on radiographs. Congenital lung hypoplasia is sometimes associated with congenital heart disease, most often tetralogy of Fallot or persistent truncus arteriosus. In cases of tetralogy of Fallot, the left lung is hypoplastic. A hypogenetic lung is one of the features of congenital pulmonary venolobar (scimitar) syndrome. Other variable components of this syndrome include partial anomalous venous return, hypoplasia or absence of the pulmonary artery, pulmonary sequestration, systemic arterialization of the lungs, accessory diaphragm, and absent inferior vena cava (10). Pulmonary agenesis is a rare anomaly that results from an insult during the fourth week of fetal life. The right and left lung are affected with equal frequency. Right pulmonary agenesis has an increased association with other congenital malformations involving the heart, skeleton, GI tract, and genitourinary tract. Chest radiographs or CT demonstrate severe volume loss and opacity on the side of agenesis, often with close spacing of the ribs. The bronchus and pulmonary artery to the affected lung are absent.

Pulmonary hypoplasia in the neonate can be unilateral or bilateral. Bilateral pulmonary hypoplasia is most often the result of compression of the lungs during fetal development. Congenital dysplasias and syndromes associated with short ribs and a small thoracic cage (asphyxiating thoracic dystrophy, thanatophoric dwarfism, Ellis–van Creveld syndrome) compress the lungs and cause hypoplastic lungs (Fig. 51.13). The degree of hypoplasia is often severe and leads to the demise of these infants. Chromosomal abnormalities such as the trisomies are associated with hypoplastic lungs, and in some infants, hypoplasia is "primary" and unexplained.

The most common cause of intrathoracic compression of the fetal lungs is congenital diaphragmatic hernia. Although the hernia itself is most often unilateral, the increased volume of the thorax on the side of the hernia causes compression of the contralateral lung, resulting in bilateral and asymmetric lung hypoplasia (Fig. 51.14). The degree of hypoplasia varies in severity; the earlier in gestation that the hernia occurs, the more severe the lung hypoplasia. Pulmonary insufficiency is the most significant cause of morbidity and mortality in these infants. Infants with less severely hypoplastic lungs can be supported with artificial ventilation or extracorporeal membranous oxygenation (ECMO) until their lungs develop enough to permit survival. Other causes of intrathoracic compression leading to bilateral pulmonary hypoplasia include bilateral chylothorax, large intrathoracic cysts or tumors (neuroblastoma, teratoma, cystic adenomatoid malformation), or marked cardiomegaly.

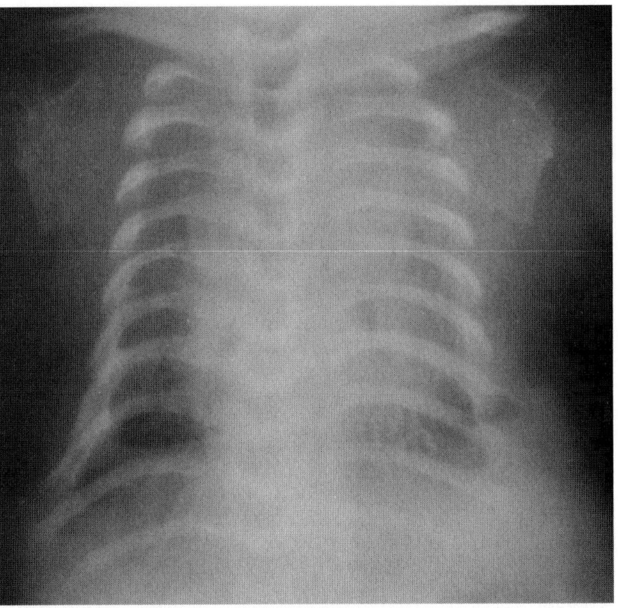

FIGURE 51.13. **Lung Hypoplasia.** The very small thoracic cage caused by rib shortening in this thanatophoric dwarf is associated with marked lung hypoplasia.

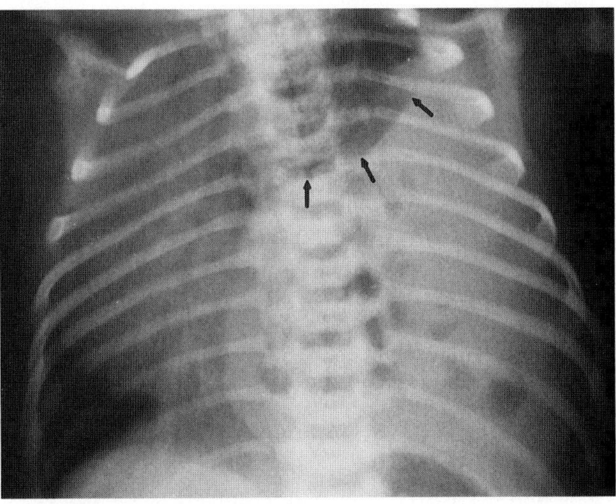

FIGURE 51.14. **Congenital Diaphragmatic Hernia.** Multiple air- and fluid-filled loops of bowel in the left hemithorax displace the mediastinum into the right hemithorax. Note the small, hypoplastic left lung (*arrows*).

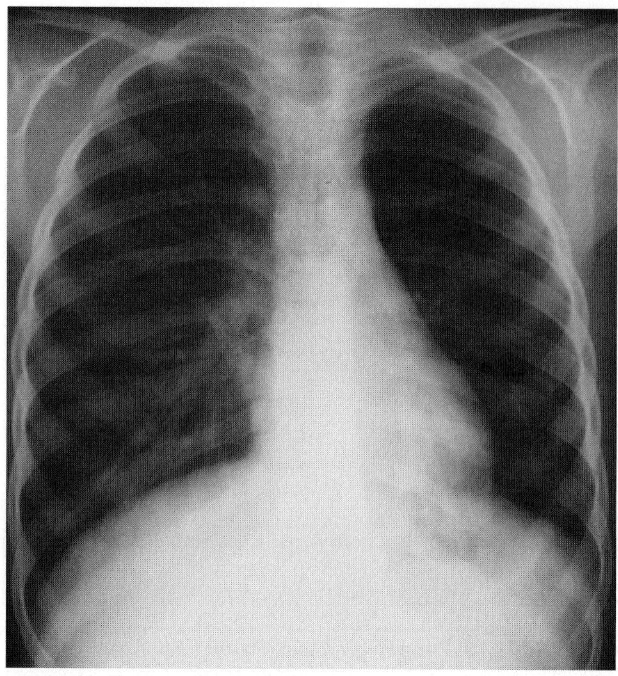

FIGURE 51.15. **Swyer-James Lung.** Note that the left lung is small and relatively hyperlucent when compared with the right lung. The left pulmonary vascularity is decreased.

Extrathoracic compression of the fetal lungs is most often caused by oligohydramnios secondary to fetal urinary tract abnormalities or by abnormal amniotic fluid production or leakage. Potter syndrome, associated with bilateral renal agenesis, congenital renal cystic disease, or obstructive uropathy (posterior urethral valves, prune belly syndrome), commonly results in hypoplastic lungs. Additional causes include neuromuscular abnormalities with persistent elevation of the diaphragm or prolonged distension of the abdomen by large abdominal masses or ascites.

Swyer-James Syndrome is an acquired hypoplastic lung that develops following severe obliterative bronchiolitis, leading to bronchiolar obstruction, bronchiectasis, and distal airspace destruction (Fig. 51.15). Bronchiectasis is not present in all cases (11). Air enters the lung by air drift phenomenon but becomes trapped because of the bronchiolar obstruction. Air trapping results in a lung that changes very little in size between inspiration and expiration. This important feature helps to distinguish the hypoplastic Swyer-James lung from the congenitally hypoplastic lung. Radionuclide ventilation/perfusion studies can be used to verify the expiratory airway obstruction as well as the diminished perfusion of the hypoplastic lung. CT is more sensitive than radiographs in detecting areas of air trapping and helps to exclude other causes of central bronchial obstruction (12). Although the Swyer-James lung is classically clear and hyperlucent, some patients show a fibrotic reticular pattern in the hypoplastic lung.

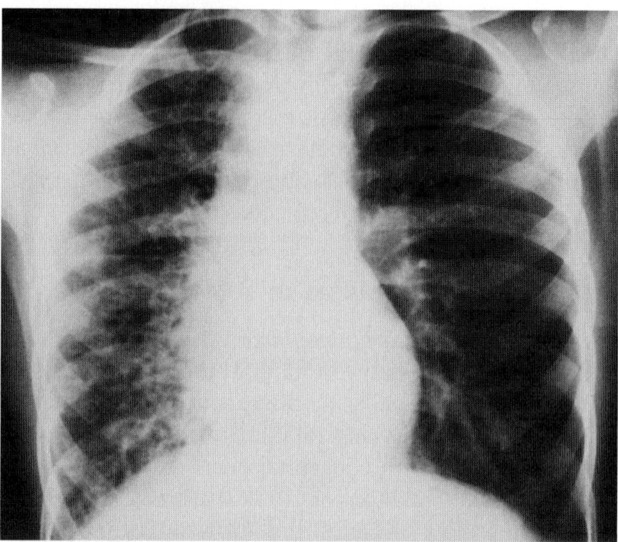

FIGURE 51.16. **Unilateral Pulmonary Vein Atresia.** The right lung is small with diffuse reticula, very likely caused by fibrosis from prolonged pulmonary edema and/or infection in this patient with pulmonary vein atresia on the right.

Other causes of a unilateral small reticular lung include scarring after radiation therapy or congenital unilateral pulmonary vein atresia or stenosis (Fig. 51.16). The reticula of the lung in pulmonary vein atresia are caused by a combination of interstitial pulmonary edema, fibrosis, and dilated interstitial lymphatics.

Bilateral Lung Hyperinflation

Bilateral overaeration of the lungs is most often caused by airway obstruction that can be central or diffuse and peripheral (Table 51.6).

Small Airway Obstruction. Widespread obstruction of the peripheral airway is a common cause of obstructive emphysema and is most often the result of viral bronchitis and bronchiolitis or asthma. Acute bronchiolitis in infants often is accompanied by severe air trapping and overinflation of the lungs, with little or no other visible pulmonary abnormality. Hyperinflation tends to be less severe in older children with viral lower respiratory tract infections, but the mechanism (i.e., mucosal edema and bronchospasm secondary to inflammation) is the same. Infants with cystic fibrosis can present with an appearance identical to that of bronchiolitis. Cystic fibrosis should be considered in any infant who presents with multiple episodes of bronchiolitis (Fig. 51.17). Peripheral small airway obstruction with parahilar peribronchial opacities is seen with certain immunologic deficiency diseases, chronic aspiration, and graft versus host disease.

Central airway obstruction leading to bilateral overaeration of the lungs is less common than peripheral

TABLE 51.6 Possible Causes of Bilateral Lung Hyperinflation

Diffuse peripheral obstruction
Viral bronchitis/bronchiolitis
Asthma
Cystic fibrosis
Immunologic deficiency diseases
Chronic aspiration
Graft versus host disease
Central obstruction
Extrinsic
Vascular anomalies
Mediastinal masses
Intrinsic
Tracheal foreign body
Tracheal neoplasm/granuloma

obstruction. Intratracheal foreign bodies, neoplasms, granulomas, and intrinsic stenoses of the trachea are all rather rare. More commonly, tracheal obstruction is the result of extrinsic compression caused by cysts, neoplasms, adenopathy, and congenital vascular abnormalities.

A right-sided aortic arch is the key radiographic clue to the presence of an obstructing vascular ring (Fig. 51.18). Most cases of double aortic arch consist of a large posterior, right-sided arch and a small anterior, left-sided arch that encircle the esophagus and trachea. The diagnosis may be verified by barium esophagram, which shows a reverse S configuration caused by the bilateral vascular impressions on the esophagus (Fig. 51.19). Lateral radiographs demonstrate increased retrotracheal opacity, tracheal narrowing, and anterior tracheal bowing (13). Similar radiographic abnormalities are seen when the vascular ring consists of a right ascending aortic arch, an aberrant left subclavian artery that passes posterior to the esophagus, and a ligamentum arteriosum or persistent ductus arteriosus stretching from the left subclavian artery to the pulmonary artery anterior to the trachea. Definitive evaluation of the vascular anatomy is best accomplished with MR or helical CT (14,15) (see Fig. 51.18).

The pulmonary sling anomaly is a rare condition that may also result in tracheal compression and bilateral hyperaeration of the lungs. The left pulmonary artery arises from the right pulmonary artery, and as it courses to the left lung, the left pulmonary artery passes between the trachea and esophagus and compresses the trachea posteriorly (Fig. 51.20). The right lung may be either underaerated or overaerated.

Asymmetric/Unilateral Aeration Abnormalities

Pulmonary aeration abnormalities are frequently asymmetric or unilateral. A large, hyperlucent hemithorax most often indicates overinflation of an entire lobe or lung. Such hyperaeration may represent obstructive emphysema (Table 51.7) or compensatory overinflation resulting from decreased volume of the contralateral lung. Pulmonary vascularity is the key to differentiation. Obstructive emphysema generally results in diminished size of the pulmonary vessels because of compression and hypoxia-induced

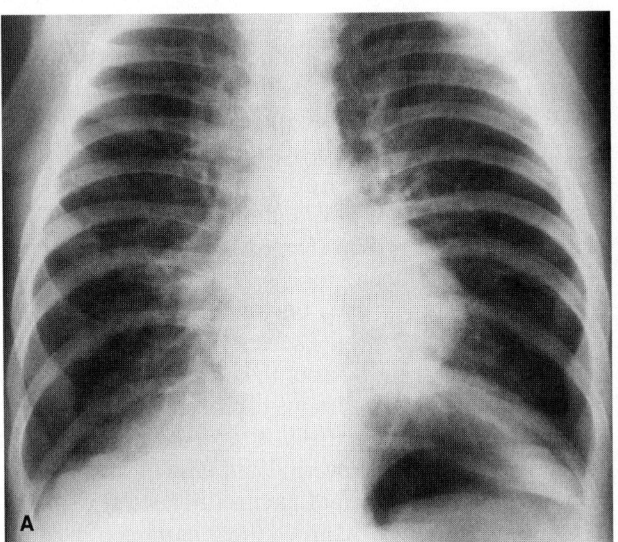

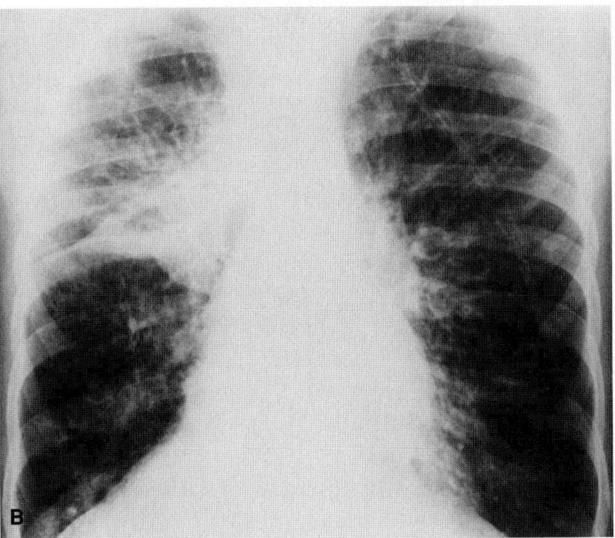

FIGURE 51.17. **Cystic Fibrosis. A.** The early stages of this disease are often manifest only by bilateral peribronchial opacities and hyperinflation of the lungs. This appearance resembles that seen with viral lower respiratory tract infections or bronchiolitis. **B.** Here, the characteristic changes of late-stage cystic fibrosis are seen, including bronchial wall thickening, bronchiectasis, and persistent atelectasis.

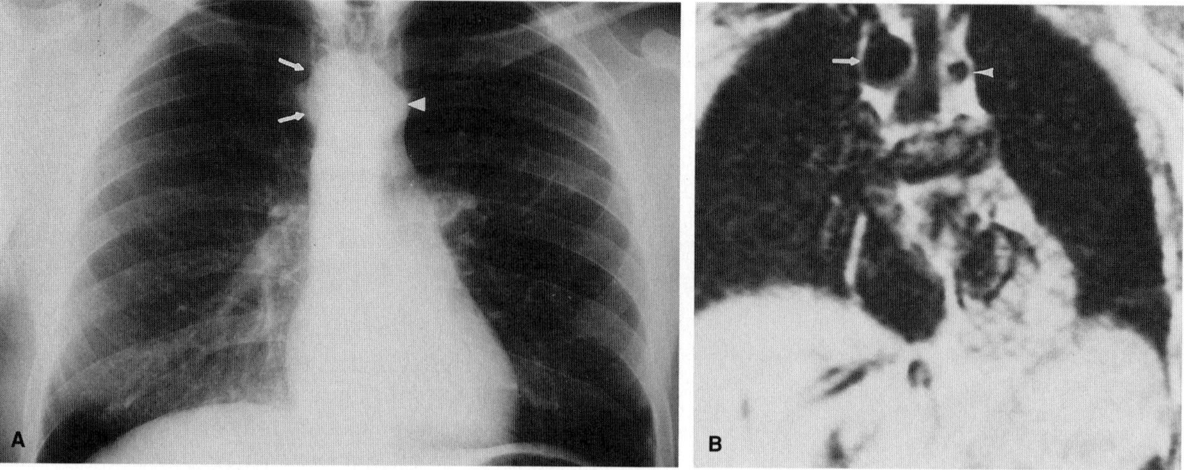

FIGURE 51.18. **Double Aortic Arch. A.** Note the large right-sided aortic arch displacing the trachea to the left (*arrows*). A smaller nodular opacity is seen to the left of the tracheal shadow. **B.** Coronal MR clearly defines the large right aortic arch (*arrow*) and the smaller left arch (*arrowhead*), which encircle and compress the trachea.

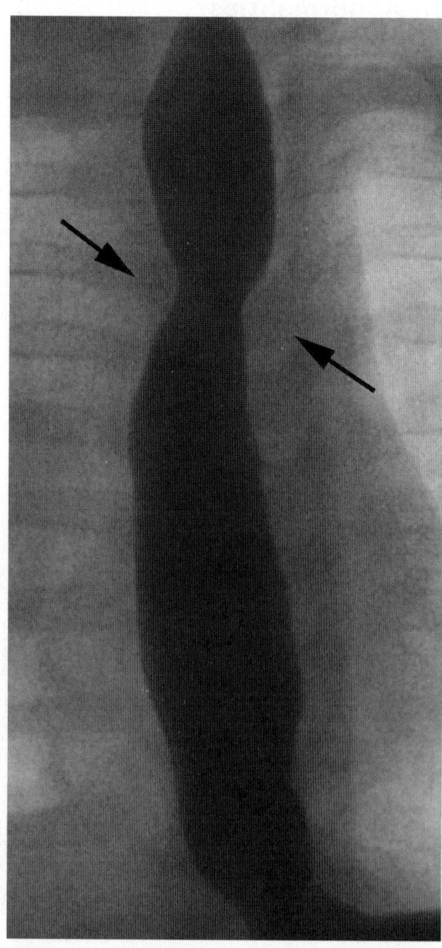

FIGURE 51.19. **Double Aortic Arch.** The encircling aortic arches compress the esophagus, creating a reverse S configuration (*arrows*). Note that the right arch is higher and more prominent than the left arch.

reflex arterial spasm. With compensatory hyperinflation, the pulmonary vessels are normal or even increased in size. If doubt remains, inspiratory and expiratory frontal views of the chest or fluoroscopy can be helpful. The lung that changes the least in volume between inspiration and expiration is the abnormal lung (Fig. 51.21). This holds true whether the lung is obstructed and overinflated or is small because of atelectasis or hypoplasia. The only exception to this rule is mild congenital pulmonary hypoplasia, which is associated with relatively normal lung dynamics.

Congenital lobar emphysema consists of obstructive emphysema of a single lobe of the lung, most commonly the left upper, right middle, or right upper lobe. Usually emphysema is the result of underdevelopment of the segmental bronchial cartilage, which leads to expiratory airway collapse and a ball valve type of obstruction. Early in the newborn period, the obstructed lobe may be opaque because of delayed clearance of fluid distal to the obstruction. Gradually, the fluid clears, and the involved lobe is filled with air and overinflated (Fig. 51.22). A severely enlarged emphysematous lobe can occupy the entire hemithorax and erroneously suggest a pneumothorax or emphysema of the entire lung. Careful inspection reveals the collapsed, compressed adjacent lobes of the lung, confirming the diagnosis. A similar appearance can occur in the rare case of bronchial stenosis or atresia. Classically, an oval opacity is seen adjacent to the overinflated lung, near the hilum, representing a collection of mucus (mucocele) within the obstructed bronchus. Acquired lobar emphysema can occur as a result of bronchial damage associated with inflammatory conditions or bronchopulmonary dysplasia (BPD) (Fig. 51.23).

Endobronchial Lesions. In older infants and children, obstructive emphysema is most often caused by an

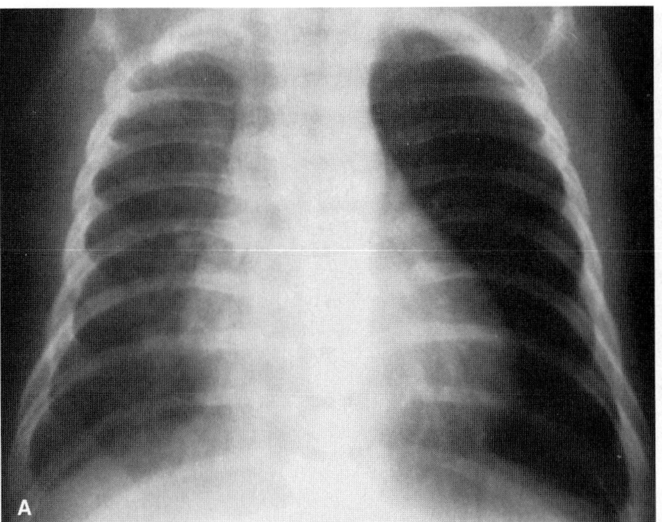

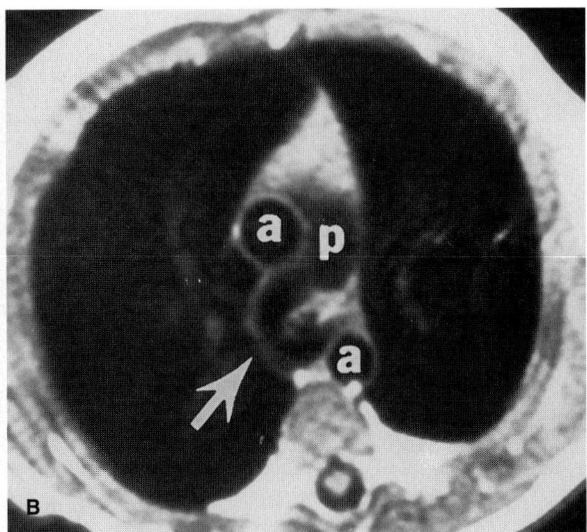

FIGURE 51.20. **Aberrant Left Pulmonary Artery (Pulmonary Sling). A.** Note slight smallness of the right lung. **B.** MR study demonstrates the typical course of the aberrant left pulmonary artery (*arrow*). Ascending and descending aorta (a), pulmonary artery (p). (From Swischuk LE. Imaging of the Newborn, Infant, and Young Child. 5th ed. Baltimore: Williams & Wilkins, 2004:315; used with permission.)

endobronchial foreign body or a mucous plug (see Fig. 51.21). Mucous plugs occur most commonly in asthmatics and in children with viral lower respiratory tract infections. Other less common causes of unilateral obstructive emphysema include endobronchial masses such as tuberculous granulomas (Fig. 51.24) and extrinsic compressing lesions such as anomalous blood vessels and mediastinal tumors and cysts. Pneumothorax may cause a large hyperlucent hemithorax that mimics obstructive emphysema. In supine patients, the pleural air may lie entirely along the anterior surface of the lung and no free lung edge will be visible. Clues to the presence of an anterior pneumothorax include increased radiolucency of the hemithorax and increased sharpness of the mediastinal border (Fig. 51.25). In newborns, a pneumothorax can compress the normal thymus gland, creating a mediastinal "pseudomass." Rarely, an air-filled lung cyst or pneumatocele, or a markedly dilated stomach in a diaphragmatic hernia, can occupy an entire hemithorax, rendering it hyperlucent.

TABLE 51.7 Causes of Unilateral Obstructive Emphysema

Bronchial foreign body
Mucous plug
Congenital lobar emphysema
Bronchial stenosis/atresia
Tuberculosis
Vascular anomalies
Mediastinal masses

PULMONARY CAVITIES

Cavities in the lungs of children are most often inflammatory or postinflammatory.

Lung abscesses usually develop as a complication of a bacterial pneumonia and can be solitary or multiple. The wall of an abscess is thick and irregular, and some contain air–fluid levels (Fig. 51.26). CT is valuable for distinguishing intrapulmonary abscess from loculated empyema in the pleural space (Fig. 51.27). An abscess may form distal to a bronchial obstruction, which in children is often caused by a retained foreign body. Cavitary tuberculosis is rare in childhood, and echinococcal cysts are rare outside of endemic areas.

Pneumatoceles are thin-walled lung cavities that commonly occur with pulmonary infections in children. Staphylococcal pneumonia is classically associated with pneumatocele formation, although they can occur with other infections, including tuberculosis (Fig. 51.28). Pneumatoceles develop from a bronchiolar obstruction that leads to air trapping and alveolar rupture. Pneumatoceles can become large and cause significant mass effect. More often, the pneumatoceles remain relatively small and resolve spontaneously. Occasionally, pneumatoceles rupture, leading to pneumothorax or pneumomediastinum. Other causes of pneumatoceles in children include blunt chest trauma, hydrocarbon pneumonitis, and LCH.

Congenital lung cysts are uncommon and may be indistinguishable from pneumatoceles. Congenital cysts are usually thin walled and more commonly occur in the lower lobes. Most are asymptomatic unless they become infected

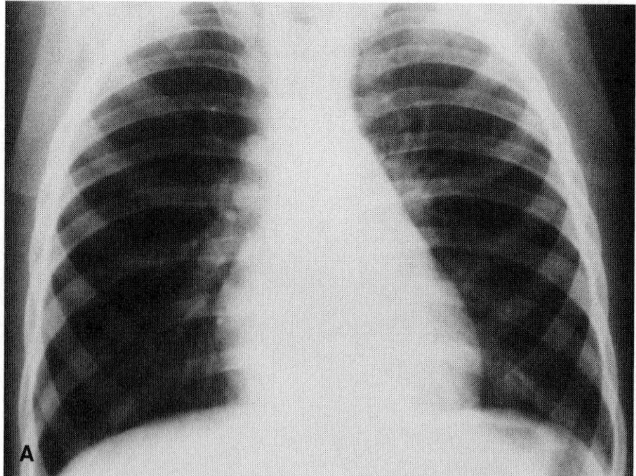

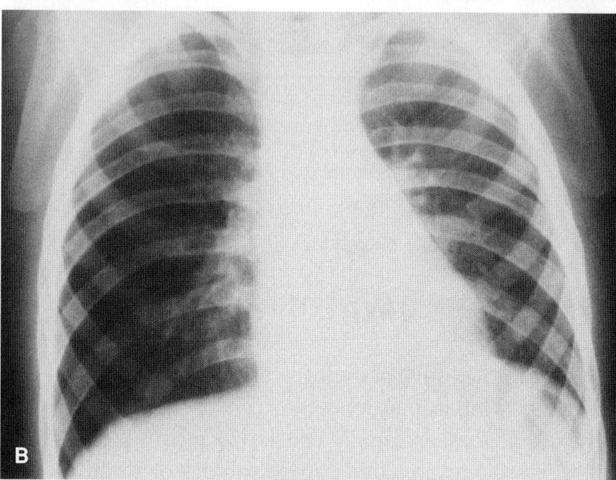

FIGURE 51.21. **Bronchial Foreign Bodies on the Right. A.** On inspiration, the right lung is slightly larger and more radiolucent than the left lung. **B.** With expiration, the left lung decreases in size, but the right lung remains overinflated. This indicates obstructive emphysema on the right, in this case caused by pieces of walnut lodged in the right mainstem bronchus.

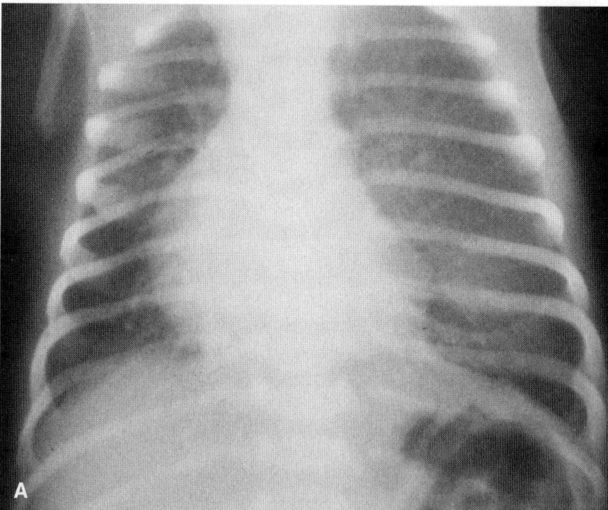

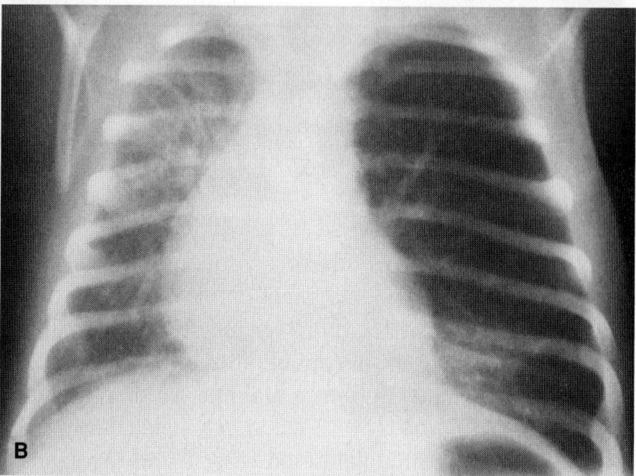

FIGURE 51.22. **Congenital Lobar Emphysema. A.** Initially, the left upper lobe was large and hazy because fluid was trapped in the obstructed lung. **B.** A later film shows that the fluid has cleared, leaving a typical overinflated left upper lobe, with compressive atelectasis of the left lower lobe.

or undergo rapid expansion with the development of a tension phenomenon.

Cystic adenomatoid malformation is a congenital lesion of the lung characterized by abnormal lung tissue containing dysplastic adenomatous tissue within communicating cysts of variable sizes. The radiographic appearance can vary from a predominantly solid lesion with multiple tiny cysts to multiple, large, thin-walled cysts that mimic congenital lobar emphysema (Fig. 51.29) (16). In the first days of life, the cysts are fluid filled and the lesion has the appearance of a solid mass. With time, air replaces the fluid, and small radiolucent cysts become apparent. The cysts gradually enlarge and can cause enough mass effect to lead to respiratory distress. The malformation is usually unilateral and can affect any portion of the lung.

Congenital Diaphragmatic Hernia. Air-filled loops of bowel in a congenital diaphragmatic hernia can resemble the multiple cysts of cystic adenomatoid malformation. An important clue to the correct diagnosis of diaphragmatic hernia is the absence or paucity of gas-filled bowel loops within the abdomen (Fig. 51.30). Congenital diaphragmatic hernias most often occur through the foramen of Bochdalek, which lies posteriorly and medially in each hemidiaphragm. Left-sided hernias are more common and more frequently involve bowel herniation. Solid abdominal viscera are more likely to herniate into the chest through right-sided hernias (Fig. 51.30B). Hernias through the foramen of Morgagni, which lies anteriorly, are less common and usually are less severe.

Infants with large diaphragmatic hernias usually present with severe respiratory distress immediately after birth. Compression of the ipsilateral lung in utero causes it to be hypoplastic, and often the contralateral lung is also

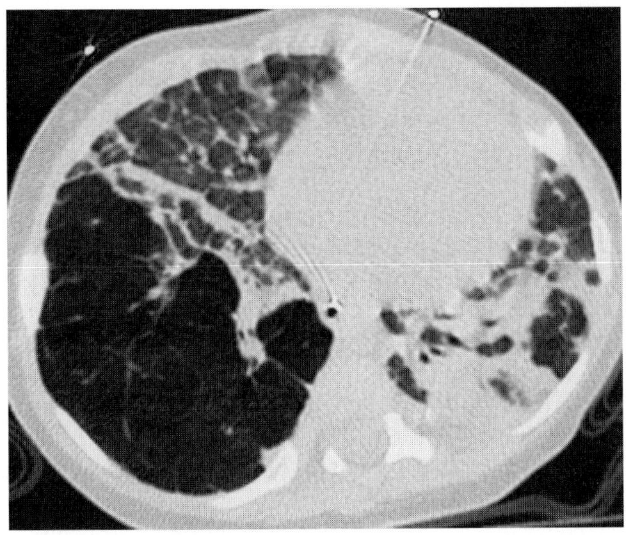

FIGURE 51.23. **Acquired Lobar Emphysema.** CT shows marked hyperinflation of the right lower lobe secondary to severe bronchopulmonary dysplasia. The infant was able to be extubated after lobectomy.

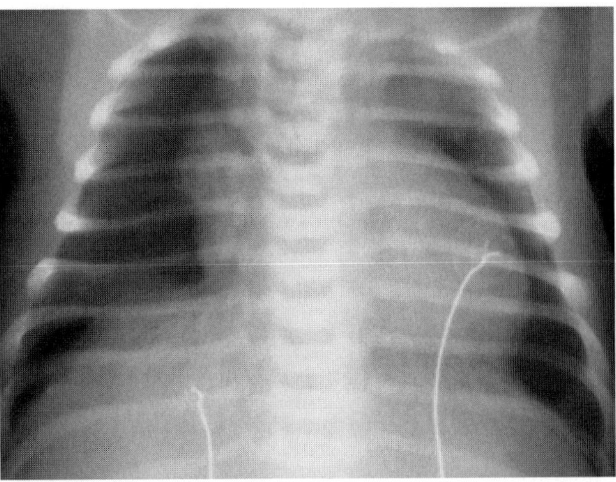

FIGURE 51.25. **Bilateral Pneumothorax in a Neonate.** The anterior pneumothoraces cause increased radiolucency along the mediastinum and increased sharpness of the heart border.

small. The patients are profoundly hypoxic, and persistent fetal circulation caused by hypoxia-induced pulmonary hypertension usually further compromises the infant's condition. Even with early diagnosis and surgery, the mortality of this condition remains high. ECMO has improved the survival of some patients by circumventing the problem of pulmonary hypertension and the right-to-left shunting of blood away from the lungs. Congenital diaphragmatic hernia may be minimally symptomatic at birth and can present later in life.

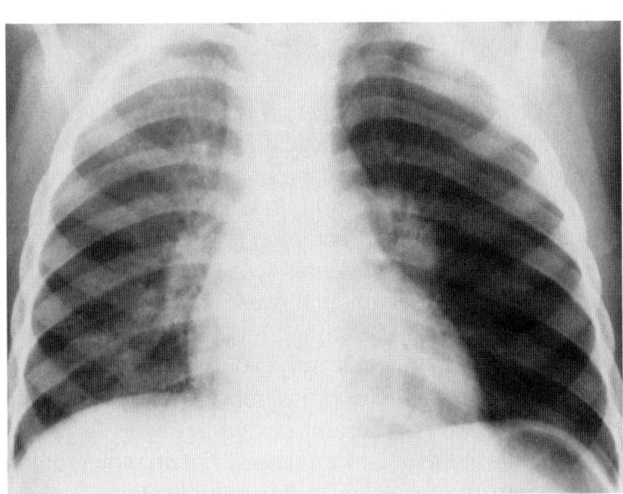

FIGURE 51.24. **Primary Tuberculosis.** Note the left hilar adenopathy and obstructive emphysema of the left lung, caused by tuberculous granulomas of the left main bronchus.

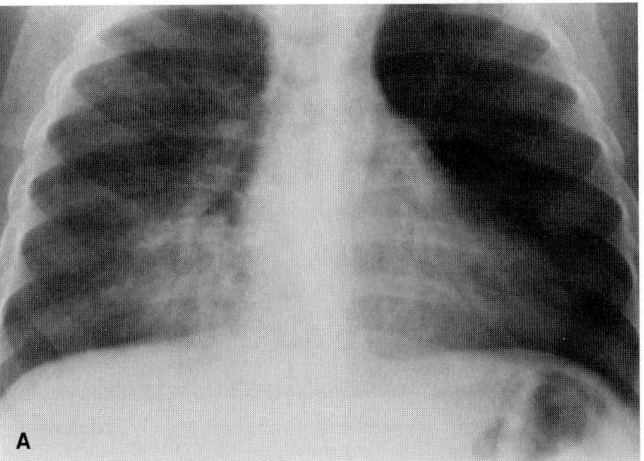

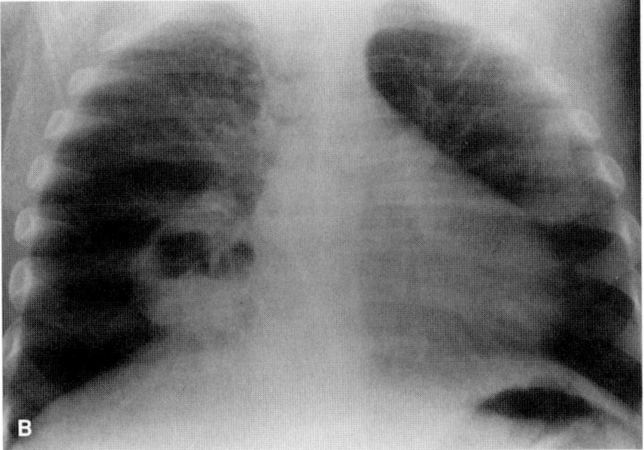

FIGURE 51.26. **Pulmonary Abscess. A.** A typical bacterial pneumonia is seen in the right middle lobe. **B.** Later, cavitation has developed in the central portion of the pneumonia, and an air–fluid level is evident. This is a typical appearance for a lung abscess.

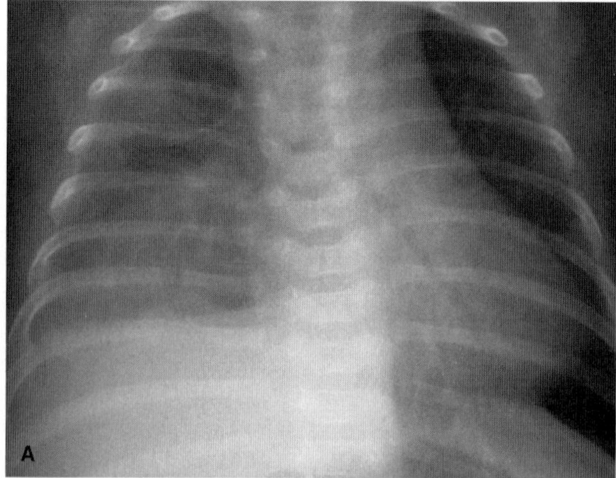

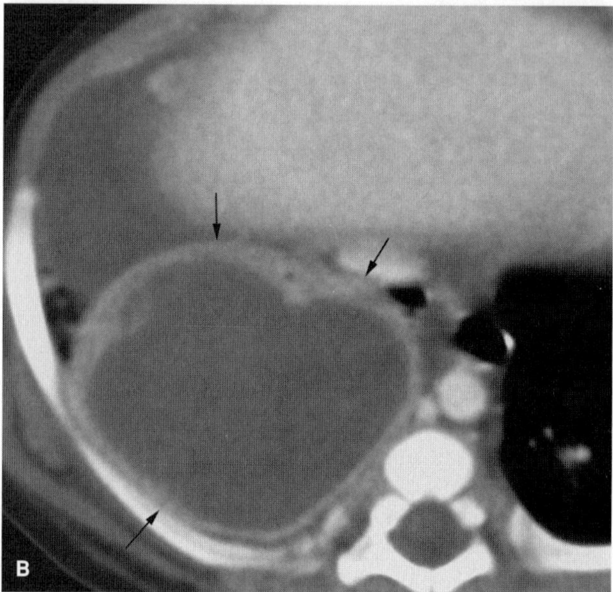

FIGURE 51.27. **Pulmonary Abscess. A.** Radiograph shows a solid-appearing mass in the right lower lobe. **B.** CT demonstrates the intrapulmonary location of this large abscess (*arrows*).

LUNG DISEASE IN THE NEONATE

The conditions leading to respiratory distress in the newborn infant are numerous and can be divided into those that can be treated medically and those that require surgical intervention. Surgical conditions consist primarily of congenital and developmental abnormalities that result in a space-occupying lesion within the chest (diaphragmatic hernia, congenital lobar emphysema, chylothorax, pneumothorax, cystic adenomatoid malformation). This section will deal with diffuse pulmonary disease of the newborn.

Surfactant deficiency disease (hyaline membrane disease) is one of the most common causes of respiratory distress in the newborn (17,18). It is most common in premature infants; however, it occasionally occurs in full-term infants of diabetic mothers. In both cases, lung immaturity is the main predisposing factor. The primary abnormality is a lack of surfactant normally produced by the type II alveolar cells. This substance is responsible for decreasing the surface tension of the alveoli. When absent, the alveoli are poorly distensible and remain collapsed. A cycle of hypoxia, acidosis, and diminished perfusion results. Clinically, these infants present with respiratory distress within the first few hours after birth. The classic radiographic findings of surfactant deficiency disease consist of lungs that are small in volume and have a finely granular pattern, with air bronchograms that extend into the lung periphery (Fig. 51.31). The granular pattern reflects the histologic findings of distended alveolar ducts and terminal bronchioles superimposed over generalized alveolar collapse. When the alveoli and terminal bronchioles overdistend, small, round, 1- to 2-mm bubbles result. During expiration, the air bronchograms and granular pattern disappear and the lungs become totally opaque. With surfactant therapy, these changes are very transient.

Similar lung opacities can be seen with neonatal pneumonia, pulmonary lymphangiectasia, neonatal retained fluid syndrome, and congenital heart abnormalities associated with severe pulmonary venous obstruction. However, unlike patients with hyaline membrane disease, the lung volumes in these conditions are normal to increased (Fig. 51.32). In a few cases of neonatal pneumonia, the lung pattern is indistinguishable from that seen in surfactant deficiency. Until recently, the primary form of therapy of this condition consisted of positive pressure–assisted ventilation, which attempts to force air deeper into the respiratory tree and alveoli. Although in some patients the use of assisted ventilation significantly improves oxygenation, in others, the elevated airway pressures result in complications caused by air leakage from the distended terminal airways. Air dissects through the interstitium and lymphatics (pulmonary interstitial emphysema), creating a radiographic pattern of serpiginous bubbles that extends all the way to the lung periphery (Fig. 51.33). Unlike the air bronchograms of uncomplicated hyaline membrane disease, the bubbles of pulmonary interstitial emphysema do not collapse upon expiration. Pneumomediastinum and pneumothorax are other common complications of positive pressure ventilation. Air also can dissect into the pericardium and peritoneum, and occasionally air embolism can develop, with devastating consequences. Early surfactant therapy has significantly reduced the incidence of these complications. The hypoxemia associated with the respiratory distress syndrome sometimes leads to persistent patency of the ductus arteriosus. Often, radiographic changes are the first clue to this complication. Suggestive findings include lungs that are large and increasingly opaque with loss of the granular pattern, cardiomegaly, and pulmonary vascular congestion (Fig. 51.34). The

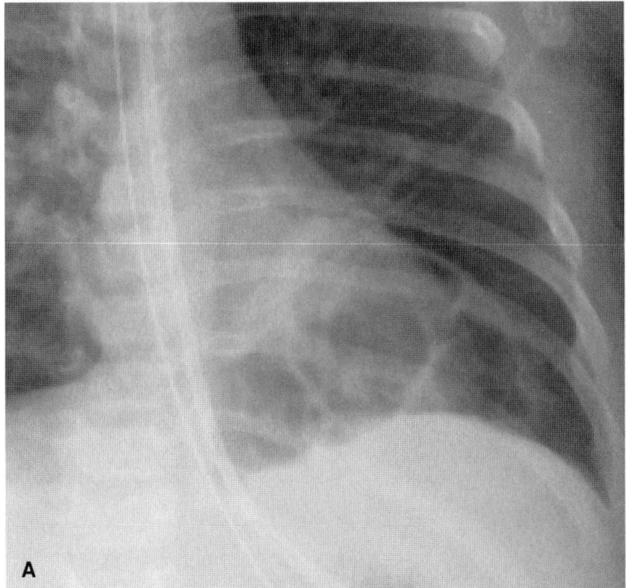

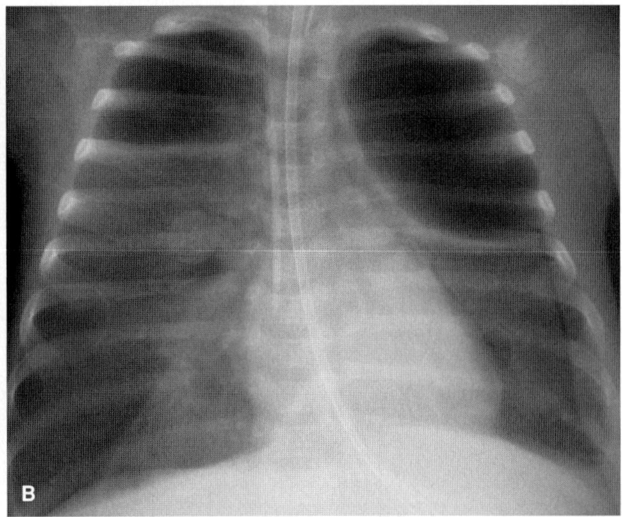

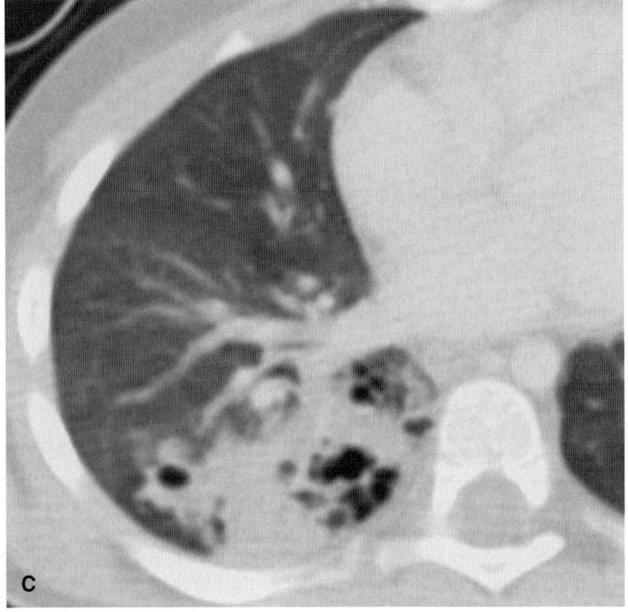

FIGURE 51.28. **Postinflammatory Pneumatocele. A.** Note the multiple thin-walled cysts within this nearly resolved pneumococcal pneumonia. **B.** Multiple large pneumatoceles followed a viral infection in this HIV-positive child. **C.** Multiple small pneumatoceles are seen within this resolving pneumonia.

increased lung opacity represents pulmonary edema. Poor renal function and neurogenic pulmonary edema resulting from cerebral hypoxic injury and hemorrhage are common noncardiac causes of pulmonary edema in the premature infant.

Bronchopulmonary Dysplasia. Continued use of positive pressure–assisted ventilation and high oxygen concentration damages the lung parenchyma and results in the condition known as BPD. Inflammation probably also plays a role in the development of BPD. Initially described in four stages, now most authors recognize an edematous phase and a bubbly phase. The initial edematous phase results from oxygen toxicity and hypoxia. Damage to the basement membrane of the capillaries causes them to leak fluid into the interstitium of the lungs. The lungs become hazy and in some cases even reticular (Fig. 51.35). The hazy pattern is the most common pattern encountered in premature infants and may persist for weeks or months. Because there is no dysplasia in this phase, it has been suggested that this phase be termed "leaky lung syndrome" (17,18). Pathophysiologically, this phase of the disease resembles ARDS.

The pulmonary edema pattern can precede or occur simultaneously with the bubbly phase of BPD. However, in most cases, the conditions are somewhat separated. The bubbly phase results from the overdistension of some alveolar groups, while others remain atelectatic. Originally believed to be exclusively a late stage, it is now known that

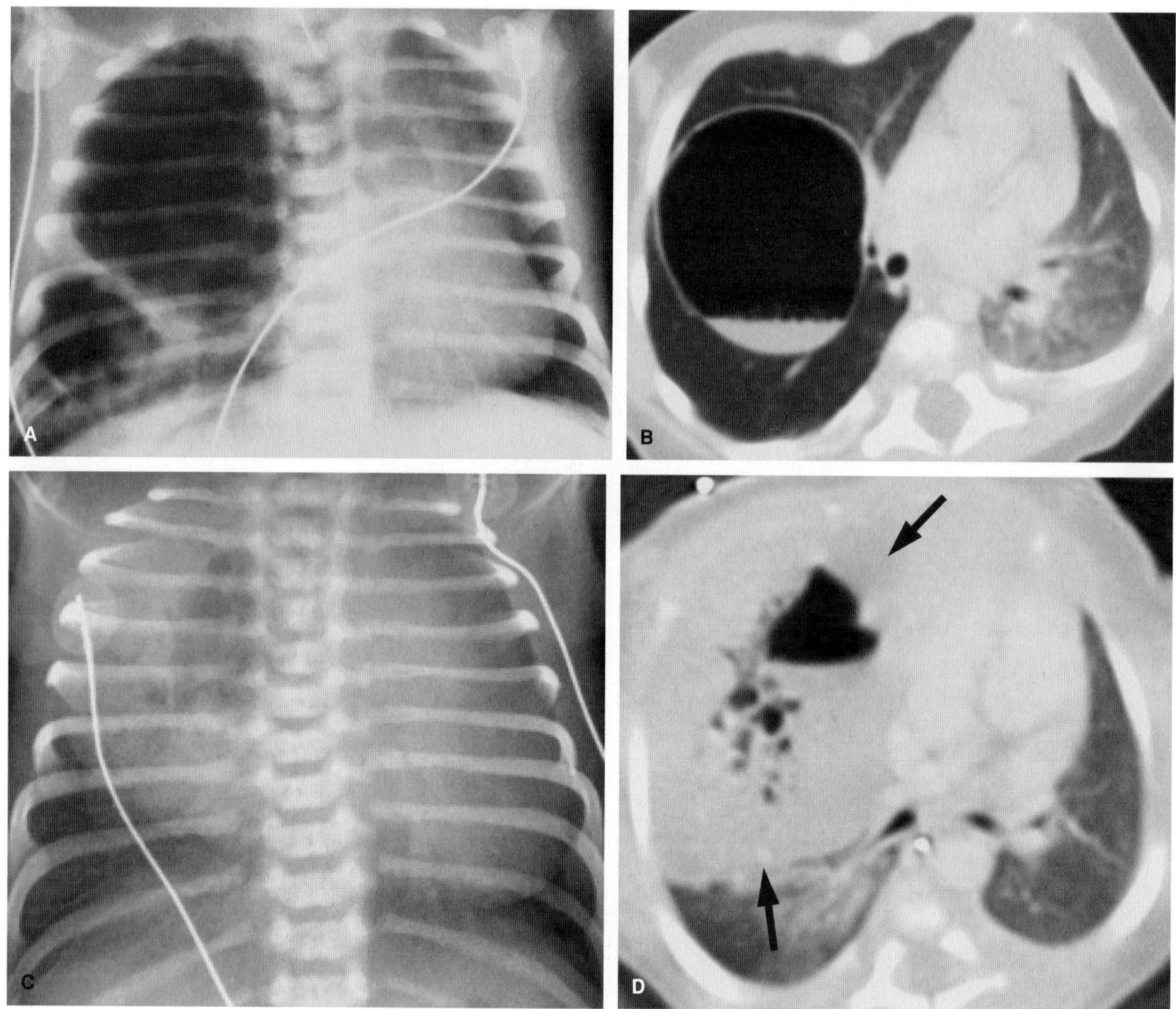

FIGURE 51.29. **Cystic Adenomatoid Malformation. A.** Multiple air-filled cysts of widely variable size expand the right lung and shift the mediastinum to the left. **B.** Another malformation that consists of a single thin-walled cyst is seen on CT. **C.** and **D.** Chest radiograph and CT in another patient reveal that the congenital malformation is predominantly solid or fluid filled, with multiple, small, air-filled cysts of varying sizes.

bubbly lungs can occur early, even within days after birth (19). The problem can be seen even in patients who are born with clear lungs and who do not have surfactant deficiency disease. BPD is generally considered to be a result of damage to the structurally immature lung by oxygen and positive pressure ventilation.

The edematous phase of BPD is treated with fluid restriction and diuretics. Vitamin A supplementation and low-dose dexamethasone may also decrease BPD; however, routine use of steroids is not advocated because of the potential risk of neuromotor and cognitive dysfunction later in life. The major predisposing factors for BPD are sepsis, very low birth weight, and young gestational age. The radiographic findings of advanced BPD consist of overaerated lungs with bubbles of varying sizes (Fig. 51.36). In other cases, the bubbly pattern is less pronounced, but pulmonary fibrosis and scattered areas of segmental atelectasis are seen. CT findings include reticular opacities, air trapping, and architectural distortion (20) (see Fig. 51.23).

Retained fetal lung fluid is the result of delayed clearance of the fluid normally present in the fetal lung. This condition, also known as wet lung disease, transient tachypnea of the newborn, and transient respiratory distress of the newborn, causes grunting and tachypnea in otherwise healthy term infants. The condition is particularly common in infants delivered by cesarean section, presumably caused by the lack of squeezing of the chest as it passes through the vaginal canal. In some cases,

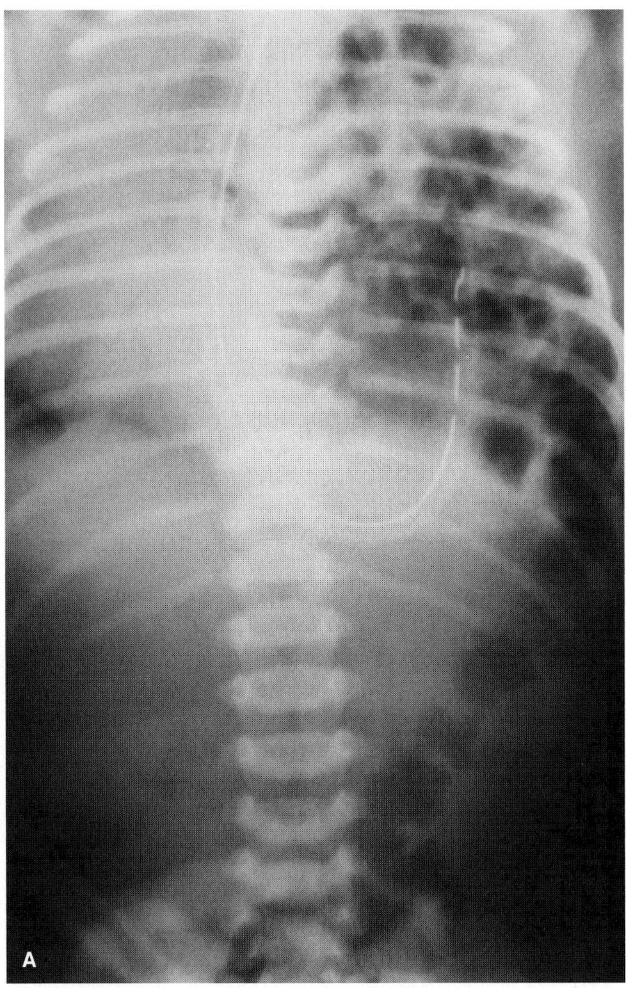

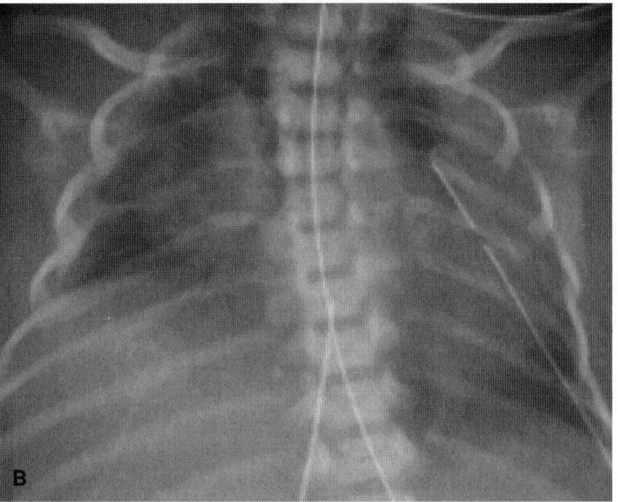

FIGURE 51.30. **Congenital Diaphragmatic Hernia. A.** The left hemithorax is filled with multiple air-filled loops of bowel, displacing the mediastinum to the right. The course of the nasogastric tube and the absence of normal bowel loops in the abdomen are additional clues to the diagnosis. **B.** Another infant with right-sided diaphragmatic hernia. What appears to be an elevated right hemidiaphragm is actually the liver extending into the chest.

the radiographic findings of retained fetal lung fluid are minimal, but commonly diffuse haziness or reticula is seen within the lungs. The symptoms and radiographic findings are transient and resolve within 24 to 48 hours (Fig. 51.37).

Other conditions can produce these patterns (Table 51.8). A streaky parahilar appearance can occur with retained fluid that is similar to that seen with neonatal pneumonia; however, pneumonia characteristically progresses during the first few days of life. In other cases, the lung fluid may cause a granular pattern in the lungs that resembles surfactant deficiency disease. However, the lung volumes are generally normal to large with retained lung fluid, versus the small lung volumes seen with surfactant deficiency.

Meconium Aspiration. Intrauterine fetal distress can lead to the passage of meconium, which can be aspirated into the tracheobronchial tree. Aspirated meconium particles cause obstruction of small peripheral bronchioles, resulting in unevenly distributed areas of subsegmental atelectasis with alternating areas of overdistension. This creates a coarse reticulonodular or nodular appearance of the lungs (Fig. 51.38). In severe cases, progressive air trapping results in complications such as pneumothorax and pneumomediastinum. The resultant hypoxia can lead to persistent fetal circulation, with right-to-left shunting across the foramen ovale. Treatment consists of endotracheal suctioning and the administration of humidified oxygen. ECMO may be required in severe cases.

Pulmonary lymphangiectasia is a rare condition that can occur as an isolated abnormality or be associated with congenital heart disease or generalized lymphangiectasia. The isolated form is caused by abnormal pulmonary lymphatic development, resulting in dilated and obstructed lymphatic channels. Lymphangiectasia associated with congenital heart disease usually occurs with conditions leading to severe pulmonary venous obstruction (e.g., hypoplastic left heart syndrome, total anomalous pulmonary venous return type III, or pulmonary vein atresia). In both forms of the condition, the dilated lymphatics course through the lung interstitium, causing a diffuse reticular or reticulonodular pattern on radiographs (see Fig. 51.10). The lungs often are hyperinflated and pleural effusions may occur.

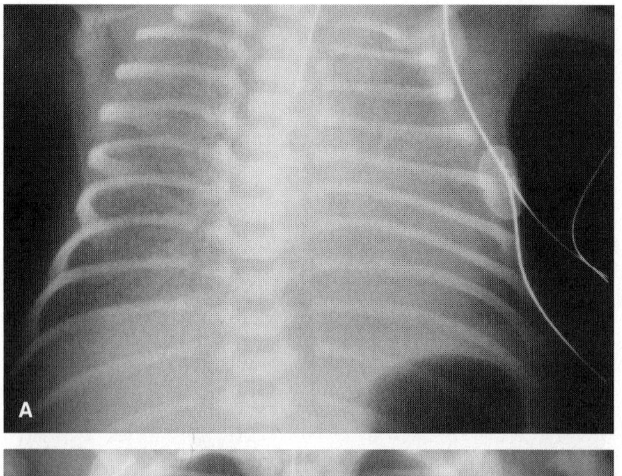

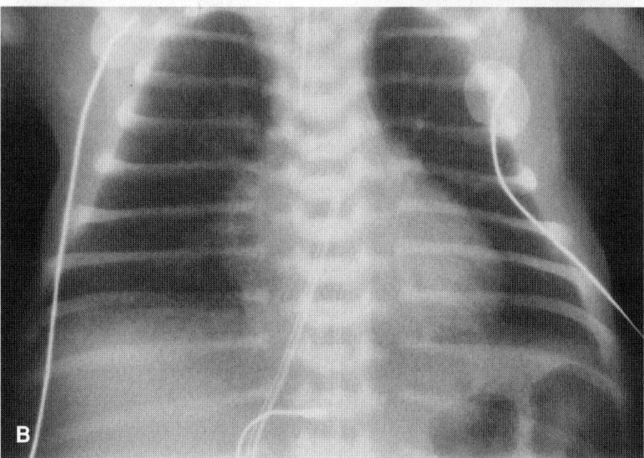

FIGURE 51.31. **Surfactant Deficiency Disease. A.** Shortly after birth, the lungs are small and diffusely opaque with air bronchograms that extend into the periphery of the lung. This is a typical appearance for surfactant deficiency disease. **B.** After treatment with endotracheal surfactant, lung volumes have dramatically improved and lung opacity has virtually disappeared.

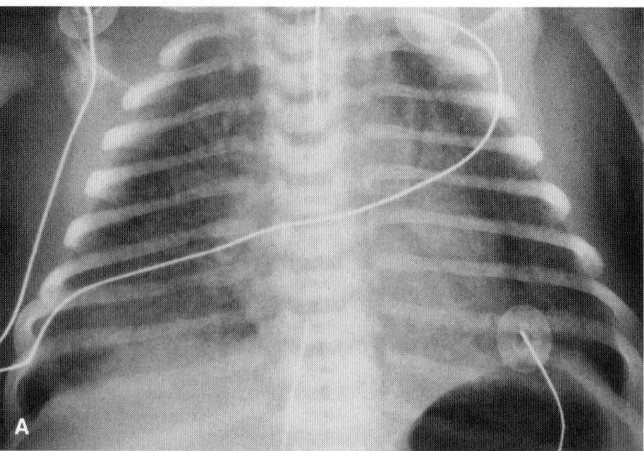

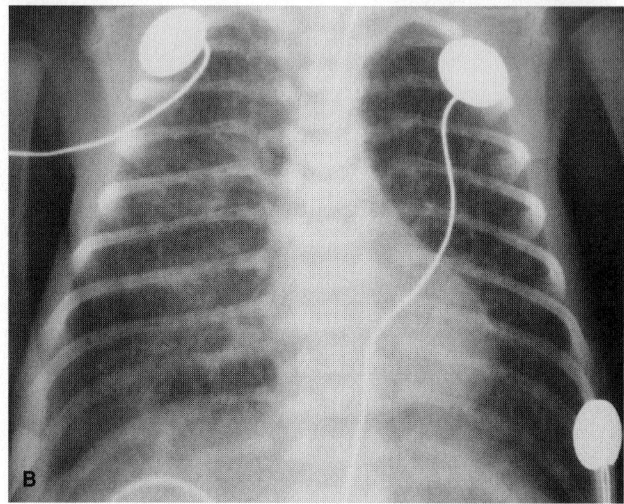

FIGURE 51.32. **Neonatal Pneumonia. A.** The lungs are diffusely hazy, with a granular appearance that is similar to that seen with hyaline membrane disease. Note, however, that the lungs are normal in volume. **B.** Pneumonia in a different neonate has a more reticular appearance, with central alveolar opacities.

Extracorporeal membranous oxygenation is a widely used therapy to support infants with life-threatening respiratory disease. The technique consists of a bypass of the pulmonary blood flow through a semipermeable silicon membrane. The procedure interrupts the cycle of pulmonary hypertension and persistent fetal circulation (right-to-left shunting) and diminishes the damaging effect of high oxygen concentrations and barotrauma to the lungs. ECMO is commonly used in patients with congenital diaphragmatic hernia, meconium aspiration syndrome, neonatal sepsis, and pneumonia. Premature infants with surfactant deficiency disease are often too small for the large-caliber ECMO catheters; therefore, use of ECMO is limited for this condition. While on the extracorporeal circuit, the lungs invariably become opaque because the ventilator settings are reduced, allowing the lungs to collapse. Often, pleural effusions are present but may be obscured on chest radiographs by the opacity of the lungs. In such cases, the lungs often fail to re-expand despite increasing ventilator pressures. Shifting of the position of the ECMO catheters on radiographs should suggest an increased pleural fluid collection (21). US can be used to identify the pleural fluid and help distinguish blood from serous fluid.

PLEURAL THICKENING AND EFFUSIONS

Generalized thickening of the pleural space because of the accumulation of fluid has the same configurations in children as in adults. The most easily recognized pattern is thickening along the lateral and apical portions of the lung. Subpulmonic collections can mimic an elevated diaphragm, but characteristic flattening and laterally displaced curvature of the dome are clues to the presence of subpulmonic pleural fluid (Fig. 51.39). A totally opaque hemithorax of normal or increased volume nearly always

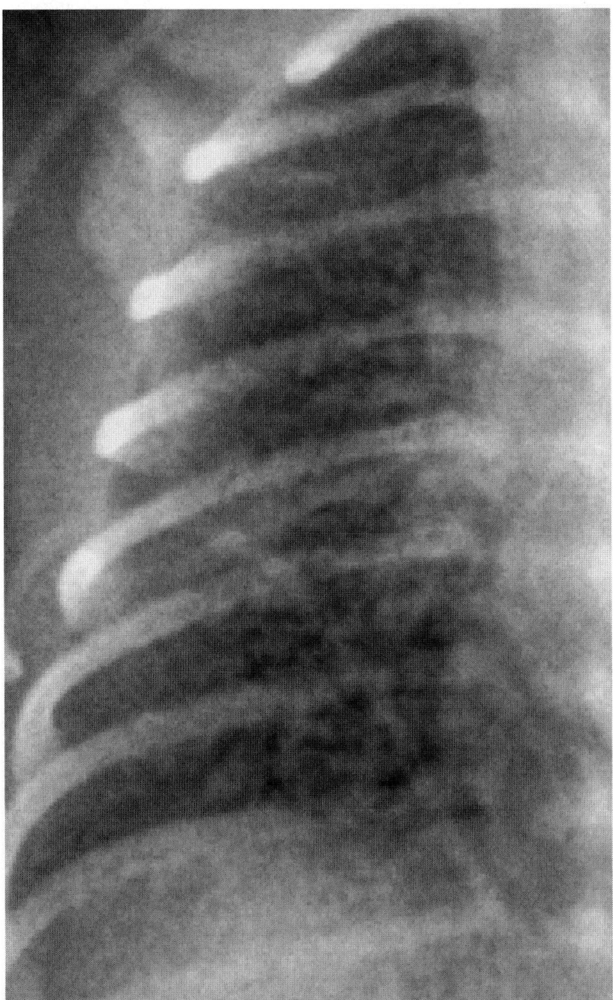

FIGURE 51.33. **Pulmonary Interstitial Emphysema.** Serpiginous bubbles of interstitial air extend to the periphery of the left lung. The interstitial air causes the lung to be stiff and hyperexpanded, even during expiration.

indicates a large collection of pleural fluid. Opacification of an entire lung by pneumonia is very unusual in children. However, occasionally a large cyst or intrathoracic mass can occupy most of the hemithorax. In such cases one should look for residual radiolucency in the costophrenic angle, which is not present when pleural fluid is the cause of total opacification of a hemithorax. The presence of pleural fluid is easily verified by US. The type of fluid in the pleural space (serous effusion, inflammatory exudate, chyle, or blood) cannot be reliably determined radiographically.

Unilateral pleural effusions are most commonly associated with pneumonia in the ipsilateral lung (Table 51.9). Such effusions are often transudates, but empyema is likely if the collection is large. Empyemas most often occur with staphylococcal, *Haemophilus*, and pneumococcal pneumonias. Empyema is characteristically loculated,

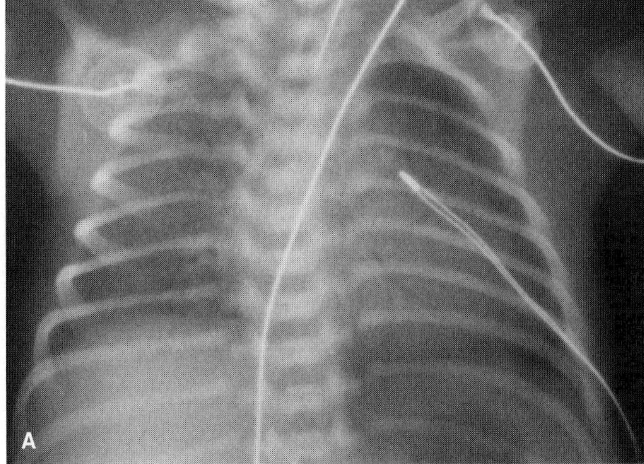

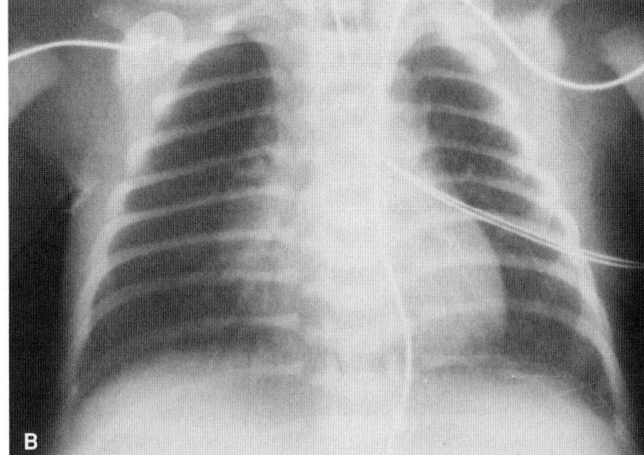

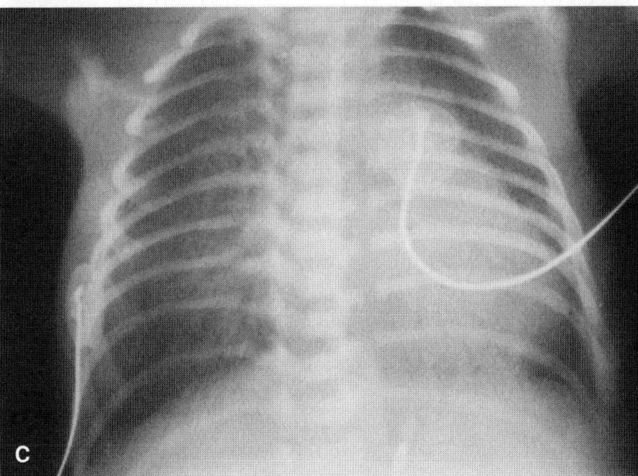

FIGURE 51.34. **Patent Ductus Arteriosus in a Premature Infant With Hyaline Membrane Disease. A.** Early films showed the typical small granular lungs seen in hyaline membrane disease. **B.** Following surfactant therapy, the lungs increased in volume and became clear. **C.** A few days later, the heart has enlarged and, although the lungs have increased in volume, they have also become more opaque. The lung opacity represents pulmonary edema because of the development of a patent ductus arteriosus.

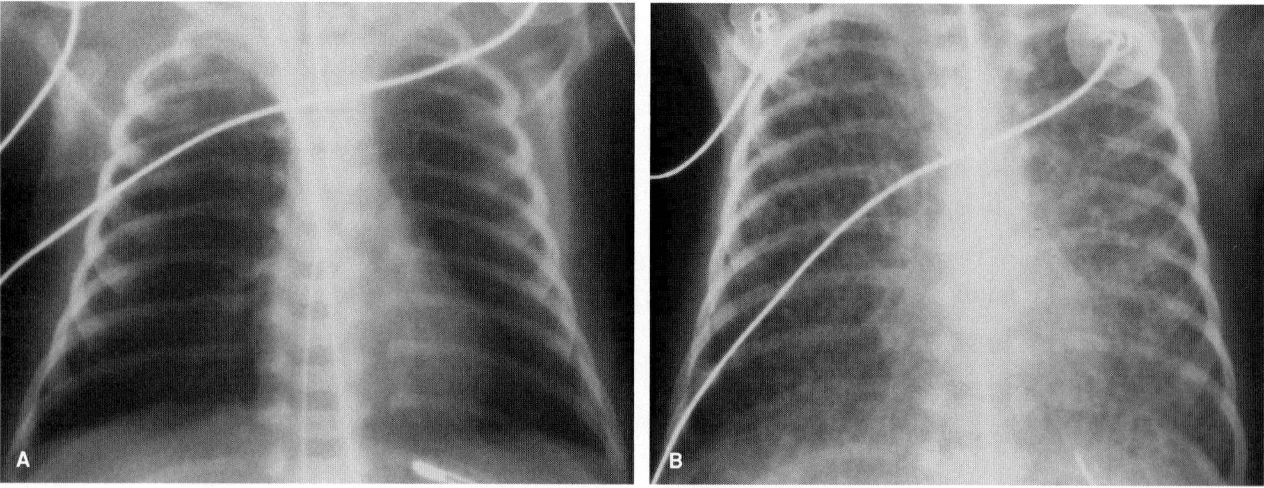

FIGURE 51.35. **"Leaky Lung" Syndrome. A.** This premature infant was born with clear lungs. **B.** A few days later the lungs, although well expanded, are hazy to opaque. The opacity represents capillary leak pulmonary edema.

and the internal septations are easily verified with US (Fig. 51.40). Prompt diagnosis of loculated empyema is important for successful treatment by video-assisted thoracoscopic surgery (VATS). Serous effusions may be seen with a variety of infections, including *Mycoplasma*. Inflammation below the diaphragm, particularly abscesses or pancreatitis, can also result in pleural effusions. Rarely, a unilateral effusion will accompany an intrathoracic tumor that involves the pleura (Fig. 51.41; see Fig. 51.50).

Bilateral serous pleural effusions are most commonly seen in patients with renal diseases such as acute glomerulonephritis or nephrotic syndrome, lymphoma (usually non-Hodgkin), or neuroblastoma. Congestive heart failure, collagen vascular diseases, and fluid overload may also result in pleural effusions.

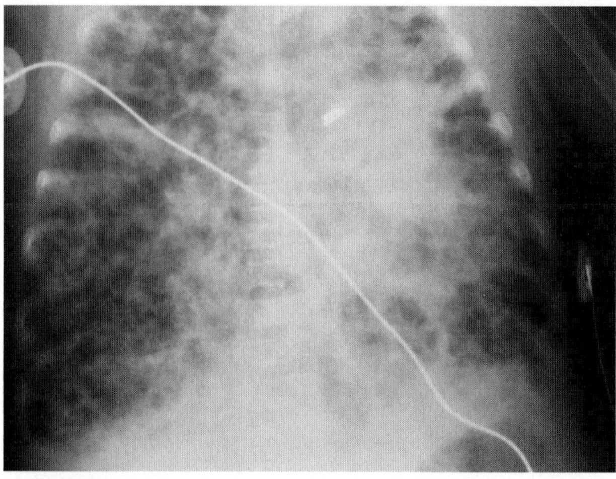

FIGURE 51.36. **Bronchopulmonary Dysplasia.** Typical bubbly appearance with bubbles of various sizes is seen in advanced bronchopulmonary dysplasia.

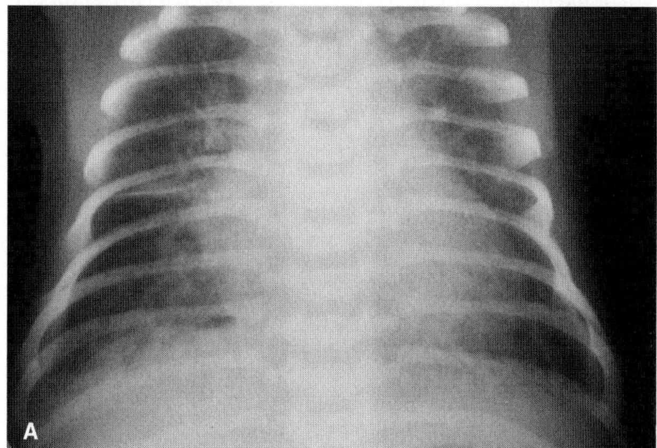

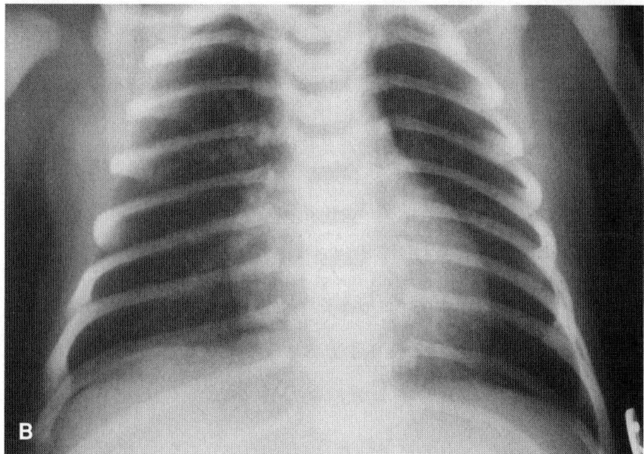

FIGURE 51.37. **Retained Fluid Syndrome. A.** On the first day of life, the lungs of this term newborn show diffuse haziness, streaky parahilar opacities, and bilateral pleural effusions. **B.** The following day, all the abnormalities have resolved, which is the typical sequence of events in an infant with retained lung fluid.

TABLE 51.8 Sources of Diffusely Hazy or Reticular Lungs in the Neonate

Decreased lung volumes
Poor inspiration
Hyaline membrane disease
Normal to increased lung volumes
Retained fluid
Aspiration (amniotic fluid/meconium)
Pneumonia
Pulmonary edema
Pulmonary lymphangiectasia

Hemothorax is usually the result of trauma, either direct chest wall trauma with or without rib fractures or aortic rupture from deceleration injury. Occasionally, bleeding disorders can result in hemothorax. Rarely, an aneurysm of the ductus arteriosus can rupture and bleed into the pleural space.

Chylothorax is the most common cause of massive pleural effusion in the neonate. Chylous effusions are usually unilateral and are somewhat more common on the right (Fig. 51.42). The cause of chylothorax is uncertain, but hypotheses include traumatic tear or congenital defect of the thoracic duct. Chylous effusions that occasionally result from superior vena cava thrombosis are more difficult to manage. Pulmonary lymphangiectasia is a rare cause of chylothorax. Most chylothoraces resolve following thoracentesis, although occasionally chest tube drainage or pleuroperitoneal shunting is required.

Complications of indwelling catheters in thoracic vessels are a relatively common iatrogenic cause of pleural fluid (22).

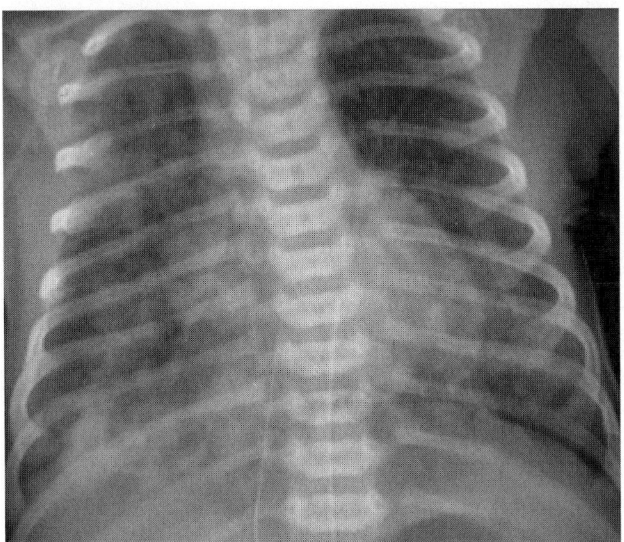

FIGURE 51.38. **Meconium Aspiration.** A coarse, reticulonodular pattern throughout both lungs is typical of meconium aspiration.

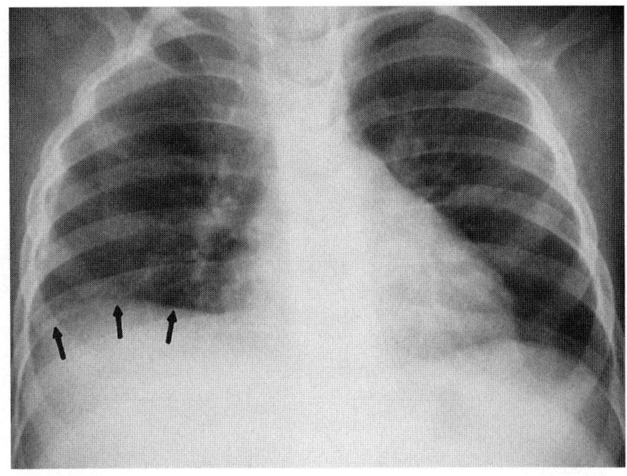

FIGURE 51.39. **Right Pleural Effusion in a Patient With Nephrotic Syndrome.** The flattened and laterally displaced curvature of the right hemidiaphragm (*arrows*) indicates the presence of subpulmonic pleural fluid.

LUNG MASSES

The most common pulmonary "mass" in children is a pseudomass caused by a spherical pneumonia (Fig. 51.43). Such an appearance is not uncommon at certain stages of pneumonia in children. Pulmonary abscess has a similar masslike appearance but usually contains central cavitation with air–fluid levels. Postinflammatory granulomas caused by tuberculosis or fungal infections are the most common true lung masses. Such granulomas are usually small and are very often calcified (Fig. 51.44). Plasma cell granuloma, or postinflammatory pseudotumor, is a reactive lesion that develops from a healing pneumonia. Calcification is uncommon, and the lesion gradually resolves over a period of years.

TABLE 51.9 Possible Causes of Pleural Effusions

Unilateral
Pneumonia/empyema
Chylothorax
Iatrogenic
Trauma
Intra-abdominal inflammation
Intrathoracic neoplasm
Ruptured aneurysm of ductus arteriosus
Bilateral
Renal disease
Lymphoma
Neuroblastoma
Congestive heart failure
Collagen vascular diseases
Fluid overload

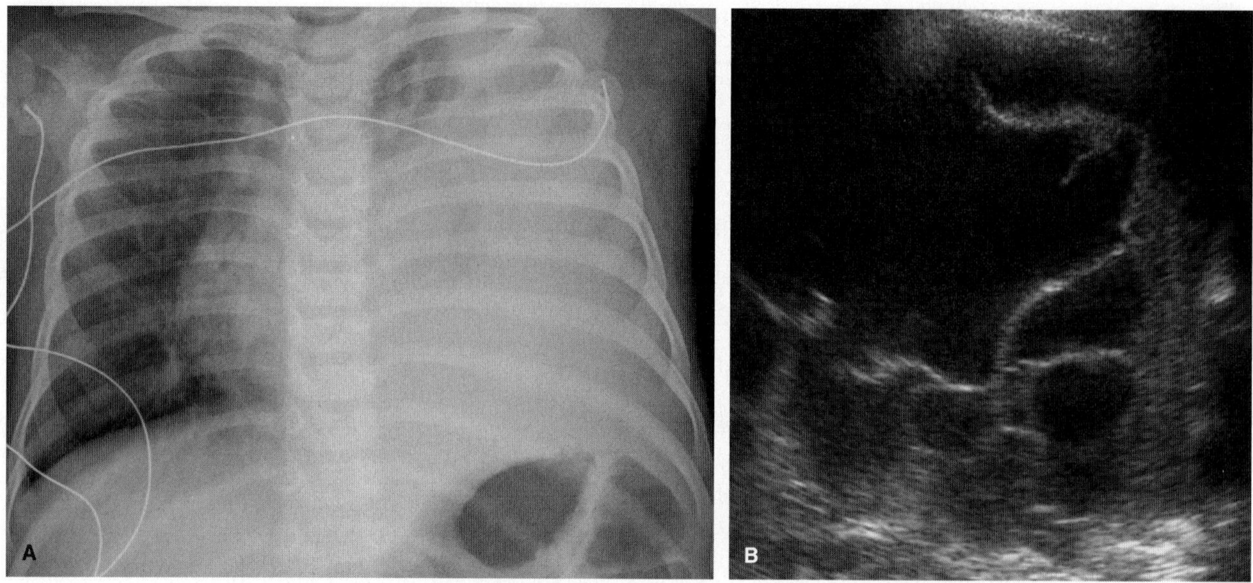

FIGURE 51.40. **Empyema. A.** Radiograph of an 18-month-old child shows a large area of opacity in the left lung. **B.** US localizes the fluid to the pleural space and shows multiple septations, which is characteristic of empyema.

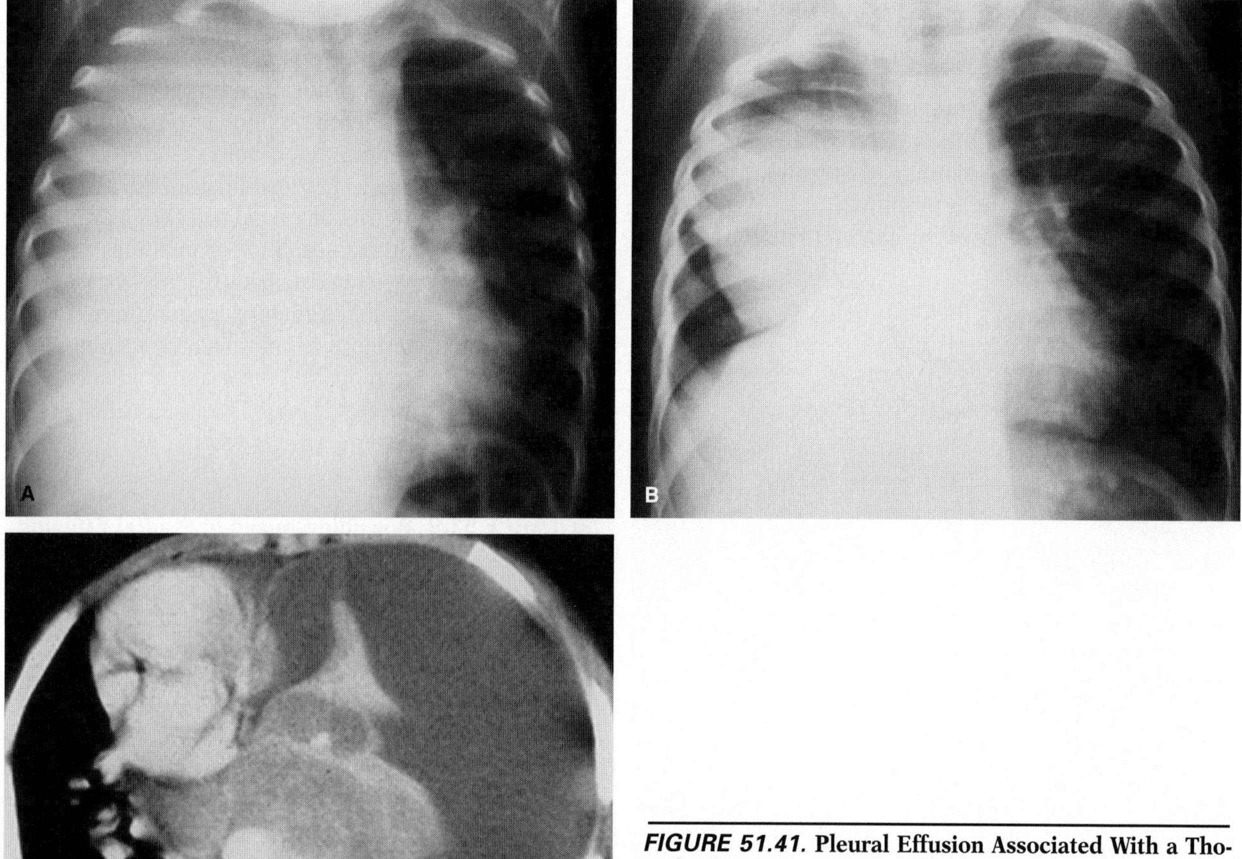

FIGURE 51.41. **Pleural Effusion Associated With a Thoracic Neoplasm. A.** Pleural fluid causes complete opacification of the right hemithorax and shift of the mediastinum to the left. **B.** Upon drainage of the effusion, a large right intrathoracic mass (teratoma) becomes apparent. **C.** CT of another child shows a large pleural effusion associated with mediastinal neuroblastoma.

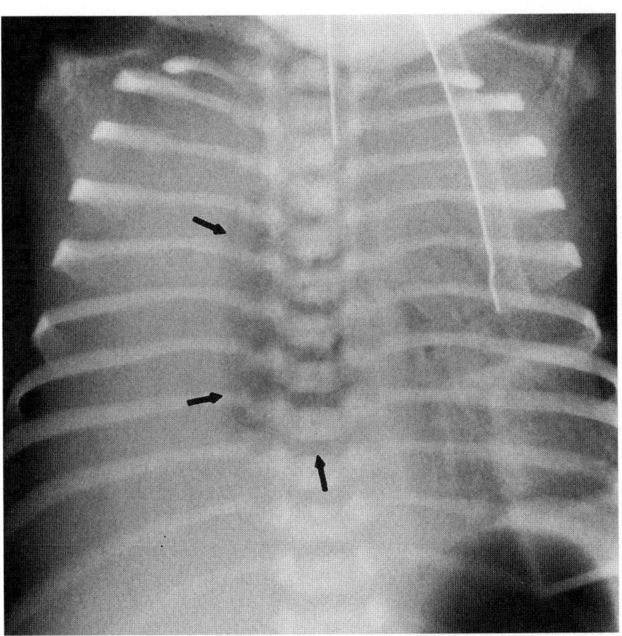

FIGURE 51.42. **Chylothorax in Newborn Infant.** A large right pleural fluid collection compresses the right lung (*arrows*) and displaces the mediastinum to the left.

Bronchogenic cysts are lined with respiratory epithelium and filled with mucoid liquid. They occur in the lung parenchyma or in the mediastinum. A subcarinal location is very common. Some are connected to the bronchial tree and are air filled. The cystic nature of these lesions is readily demonstrable with CT or MR (Fig. 51.45).

Pulmonary sequestration is a mass of lung tissue that lacks a connection to the bronchial tree and is supplied by abnormal vessels from the descending aorta. Sequestrations are classified as extralobar (covered by their own pleura) or intralobar (covered by the pleura of the adjacent normal lung). Most appear as a triangular or oval-shaped mass in the medial and basal portions of a lung, more commonly on the left (Fig. 51.46A). Air is sometimes present within sequestrations because of collateral air drift. Most are clinically silent until they become infected and present as pneumonia. The diagnosis is made by demonstrating the abnormal blood supply with US (23), CT (24), or MR angiography (Fig. 51.46B) (25,26).

Rare Pulmonary Masses. Other rare causes of a pulmonary mass usually have few distinguishing features. A mass connected to an unusually large vessel is likely to be a pulmonary arteriovenous malformation. A central, oval-shaped nodule associated with overaeration of the involved lobe suggests the diagnosis of a mucocele in a patient with bronchial atresia. Primary lung tumors are rare, and the majority are benign. Pulmonary hamartoma is a benign congenital tumor that occasionally contains characteristic flocculent calcifications. Rarely, laryngeal papillomas can spread into the trachea and the lungs.

Primary pulmonary malignancies are very rare and include sarcomas, primitive neuroectodermal tumors, and squamous cell carcinoma. Pleuropulmonary blastoma is a rare neoplasm composed of both epithelial and mesenchymal elements. These neoplasms often arise from a congenital lung cyst. Pleuropulmonary blastoma can be either solid or cystic and is usually accompanied by a pleural effusion (27).

Multiple Nodules. By far the most common malignant neoplasm in the lung during childhood is metastasis, whether single or multiple. The most common childhood tumors to metastasize to the lungs are Wilms tumor, Ewing sarcoma, osteosarcoma, and rhabdomyosarcoma. Other masses and nodules that can be multiple include granulomas (most often fungal), abscesses, hemangiomas, and Wegener granulomatosis. Cavitary nodules are characteristic of septic emboli, Wegener granulomatosis, laryngeal papillomatosis, sarcoidosis, and metastases. Staphylococcal pneumonia can also be associated with multiple cavitating lesions (Fig. 51.47).

MEDIASTINAL AND HILAR MASSES

The division of the mediastinum into anterior, middle, and posterior compartments is the most useful scheme for categorizing mediastinal masses in both children and adults. This discussion will use an arbitrary system based on the division of the chest into rough thirds on the lateral view.

The ***thymus gland*** is the primary normal structure in the anterior mediastinum and is also the most common cause of an apparent anterior mediastinal mass. The normal thymus gland varies widely in its appearance, sometimes causing considerable confusion during the interpretation of an infant or young child's chest radiograph. The gland is commonly very prominent at birth, remains easily visible up to about 2 years of age, and may be seen in an older child. On posteroanterior chest radiographs, the thymus gland causes smooth bilateral widening of the superior mediastinum. The gland overlies and silhouettes the upper cardiac borders, and sometimes a small notch is visible at the junction between the thymus and the heart (Fig. 51.48A, B). The border of the thymus gland may have a wavy contour caused by compression by the overlying ribs (Fig. 51.48C). One thymic lobe may appear more prominent than the other and have a triangular configuration called the "sail" sign (Fig. 51.48D). This appearance is more commonly seen on the right and may be mistaken for lung consolidation, particularly if the patient is in a slightly right-sided rotated position. On the lateral view of the chest, the thymus lies over the anterosuperior portion of the cardiac silhouette in the retrosternal space (Fig. 51.48E). The normal thymus gland can have more unusual configurations, such as extensions high into the superior

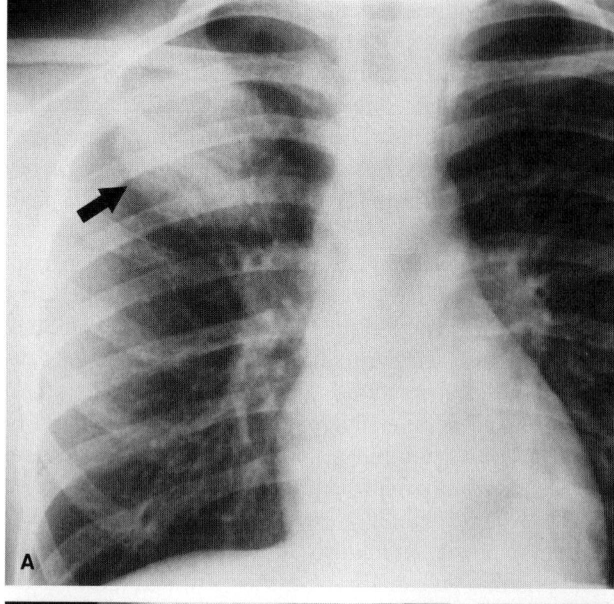

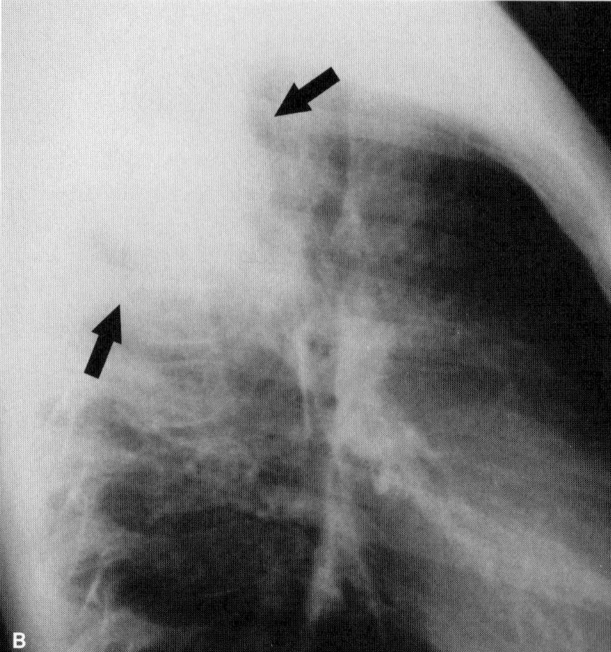

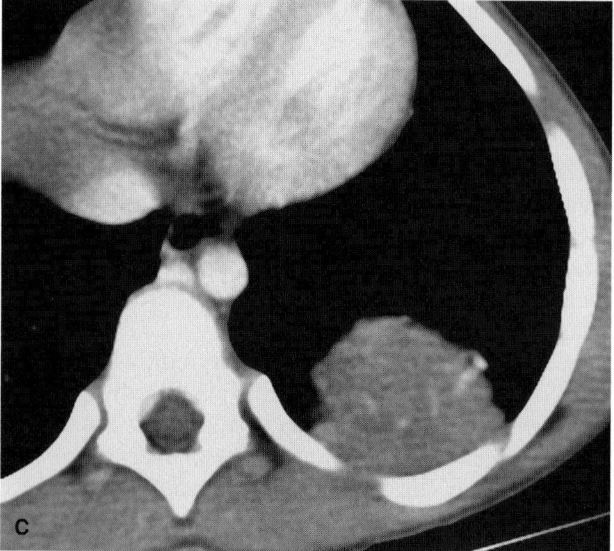

FIGURE 51.43. **Round Pneumonia. A.** and **B.** This pneumonia (*arrows*) of the right upper lobe has a round, masslike configuration on frontal and lateral views. **C.** Another child with left lower lobe pneumonia that has a round configuration on CT.

mediastinum, the lower neck, or posteriorly between the innominate and left brachiocephalic arteries. Only rarely do these atypical positions result in symptoms.

Stress atrophy of the thymus is an interesting phenomenon that occurs secondary to almost any type of illness or to the use of steroids. The thymus rapidly shrinks in size during illness, only to return to normal size after the infant has recovered. Occasionally, rebound hypertrophy follows stress atrophy. When stress atrophy is severe, the mediastinum appears very narrow, suggesting absence or hypoplasia of thymus gland (Fig. 51.49). The distinction between thymic atrophy and aplasia becomes important in infants who are suspected of having certain immunologic disorders. The best known of these is the DiGeorge syndrome, which consists of thymic aplasia, absence of the parathyroid glands, and cardiovascular anomalies. This syndrome is caused by faulty development of the third and fourth pharyngeal pouches. US is helpful in identifying a small thymus gland that is not apparent radiographically. Thymic tissue has a characteristic texture on US, with multiple linear connective tissue septa (28). Ectopic cervical thymic tissue can mimic a neck mass but can be distinguished from other neck masses sonographically (29,30).

A large thymus gland is nearly always a normal gland in an infant. Leukemia or lymphoma can infiltrate the thymus gland, sometimes causing massive enlargement (Fig. 51.50). Thymic cysts are uncommon developmental lesions that can be seen with US, appearing as well-defined, round lesions that are anechoic unless complicated by hemorrhage or infection. Spontaneous hemorrhage into the thymus gland has been described in newborn infants. When pneumothorax is present in a neonate, the thymus

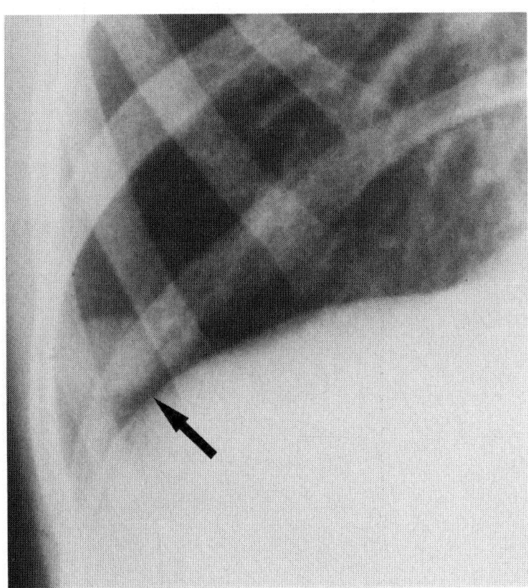

FIGURE 51.44. **Histoplasma Granuloma.** The small, round, well-defined mass in the right costophrenic angle (*arrow*) is a granuloma.

gland can become compressed and elevated by the free air, creating a pseudomass in the superior mediastinum (Fig. 51.51). This masslike compression of the thymus gland may be a clue to a subtle anterior pneumothorax.

On cross-sectional imaging, the lobes of the normal thymus gland have a smooth, somewhat triangular shape with homogeneous texture. Bulging or convexity of the borders of the thymus gland suggests pathologic enlargement, particularly if the trachea or the great vessels are displaced or compressed. Primary neoplasms and cysts produce focal alterations of attenuation or signal intensity, whereas infiltration by leukemia or lymphoma or hemorrhage results in a more diffuse and heterogenous parenchymal pattern. Overall, MR probably is the best examination for defining whether thymic tissue is normal or abnormal.

Anterior Mediastinal Masses. The majority of pathologic masses in the anterior mediastinum in children are neoplasms. Benign germ cell tumors (i.e., teratoma, dermoid) are common in this location. Dermoids are benign tumors comprised only of ectodermal elements, whereas teratomas contain elements from all dermal layers. Mature teratomas characteristically contain calcifications, fluid, and fat, which are best demonstrated by CT (Fig. 51.52) (31). Malignant germ cell tumors also occur in the anterior mediastinum (32). Other neoplasms in the anterior mediastinum include thyroid tumors, hemangiomas, and cystic hygromas. Cystic hygroma is a congenital malformation of lymphatic origin that commonly arises in the neck. Cystic hygroma tends to be locally invasive and often extends into the mediastinum. US reveals the multiloculated, cystic nature of this mass (Fig. 51.53). MR is usually used to evaluate the extent of cystic hygroma prior to resection. Hemangiomas tend to be solid and echogenic, with small cystic areas representing vascular lakes in the cavernous type of hemangioma. Blood flow is demonstrable with color Doppler imaging.

Middle Mediastinal Masses. Normal structures in the middle mediastinum from which masses can arise include lymph nodes, the airway, the esophagus, and the heart and great vessels. Lymphadenopathy is by far the most common middle mediastinal mass. Inflammatory lymphadenopathy is much more common than neoplastic disease, but when massive adenopathy is seen, lymphoma or leukemia should be considered (Fig. 51.54). Hilar lymph node enlargement may accompany mediastinal adenopathy or may occur alone. Bilateral hilar adenopathy commonly is the result of viral lower respiratory tract infections in children, but mycoplasmal, fungal, and tuberculous infections are also common causes. Other causes of lymphadenopathy include LCH, metastatic disease, sarcoidosis, and Wegener granulomatosis.

Unilateral lymphadenopathy is a common radiographic finding of primary tuberculosis in children (33) and is often associated with a small area of opacity in the ipsilateral lung (the Ghon complex) (Fig. 51.55A) (23). Unilateral lymphadenopathy is seen frequently with mycoplasma or fungal infections of the lung and occasionally with a bacterial pneumonia (Fig. 55B). Unilateral lymphadenopathy is uncommon with viral infections. Neoplastic lymph node enlargement can be unilateral or bilateral.

Cystic masses in the middle mediastinum can be associated with the airway or the esophagus. Bronchogenic cysts are sharply marginated, fluid-filled masses that may be lobulated and commonly occur around the carina (see Fig. 51.45) (34). Occasionally, the cysts will appear solid on CT, and MR may better demonstrate the cystic nature of the lesion. GI duplication cysts are caused by abnormal development of the posterior division of the primitive foregut. Duplication cysts that reside in the thorax tend to arise from the esophagus, the stomach, or the duodenum (Fig. 51.56). These cysts usually do not communicate with the esophagus, but they displace and compress the esophagus on contrast studies. In some cases, gastric mucosa will be present in the cyst lining, leading to ulceration and hemorrhage.

Enlarged vascular structures may present as a middle mediastinal mass. Aortic aneurysms are rare in childhood, except for those associated with trauma or with connective tissue disorders such as the Marfan or Ehlers-Danlos syndromes. In the newborn infant, a small bump may be visible along the upper descending aorta, caused by a dilated infundibulum of the ductus arteriosus after closure (Fig. 51.57). Normally this "ductus bump" disappears in the first weeks of life. Enlargement or persistence of this bump in later infancy suggests an aneurysm of the ductus arteriosus. Enlargement of the aorta and the main pulmonary artery may occur with congenital cardiac anomalies (see "Congenital Heart Disease").

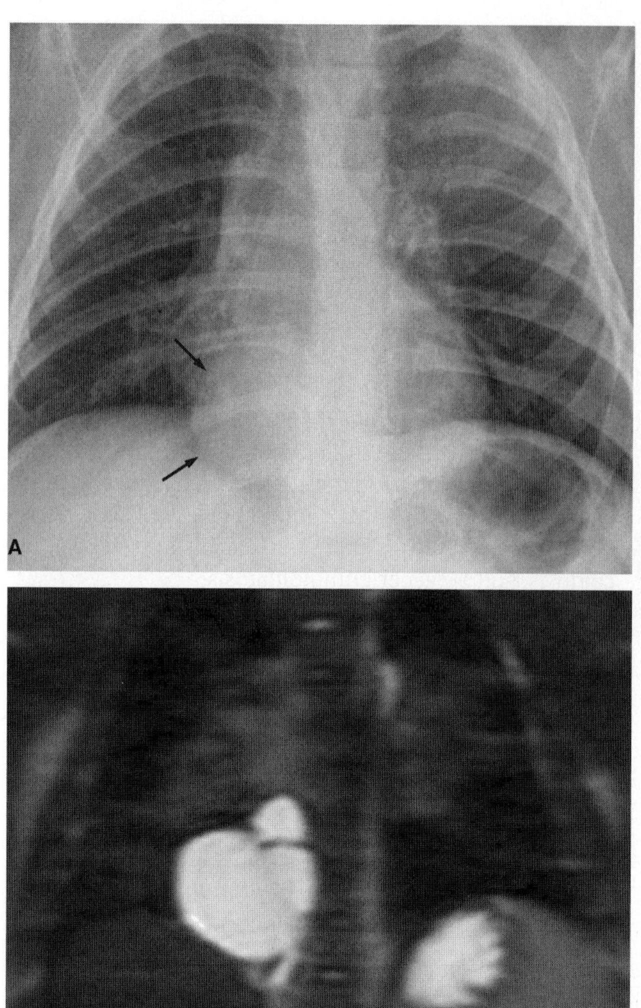

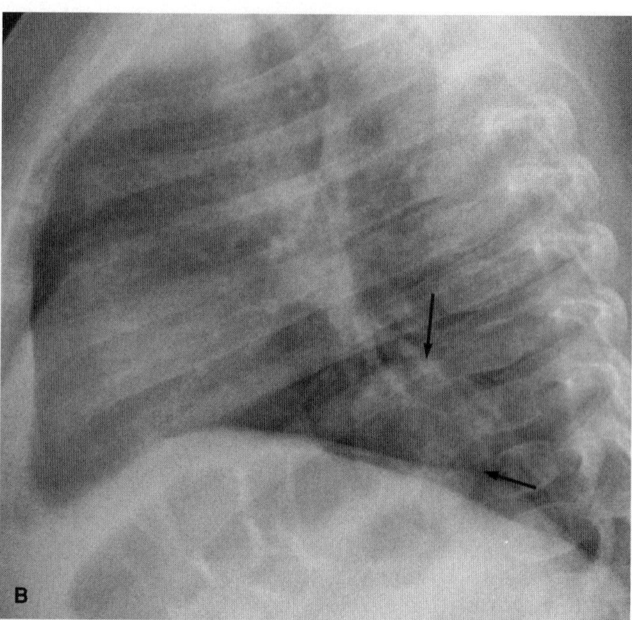

FIGURE 51.45. Bronchogenic Cyst. A. A rounded opacity peeks out from behind the right heart border (*arrows*). **B.** A lateral view more clearly shows the round, well-defined cyst (*arrows*). **C.** Coronal T2WI shows the high-intensity bronchogenic cyst in a right paraspinal location.

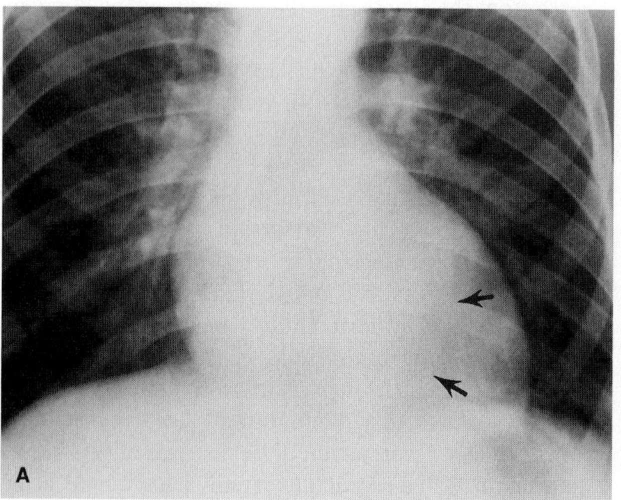

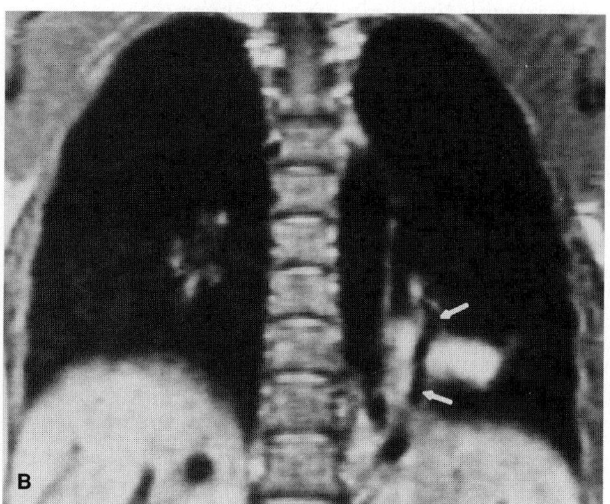

FIGURE 51.46. Pulmonary Sequestration. A. A poorly defined opacity is seen through the cardiac silhouette on the left (*arrows*). **B.** Coronal MR image in another patient shows a left lower lobe sequestration. The sequestration appears as a high-intensity mass associated with a large abnormal vessel (*arrows*).

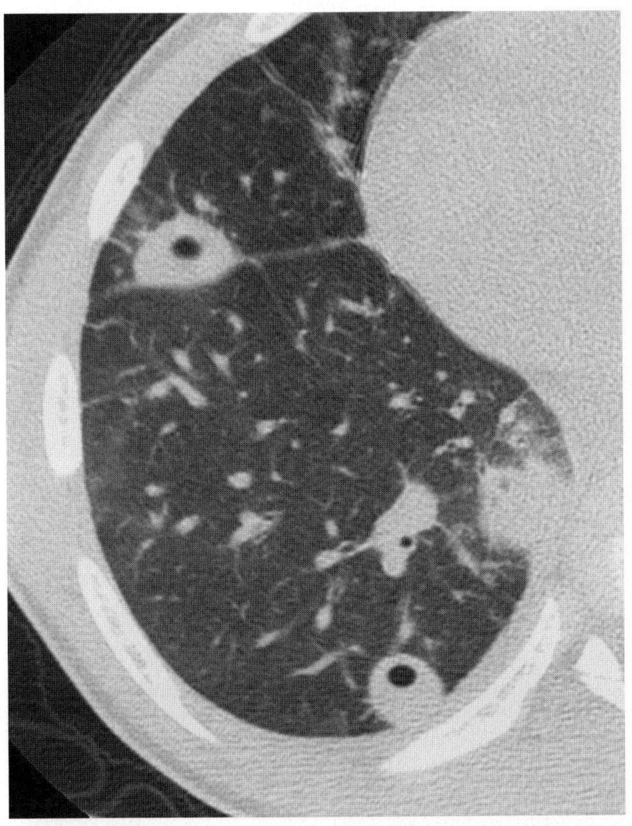

FIGURE 51.47. **Staphylococcal Pneumonia.** Multiple cavitary nodules are seen on CT.

A mass along the upper left cardiac border can be caused by herniation of the left atrial appendage through a partial pericardial defect or by a coronary artery aneurysm. Coronary artery aneurysms occur in children with periarteritis nodosa or the mucocutaneous lymph node syndrome. Enlargement of the azygos vein presents as a mass in the right paratracheal region. In children, this most often occurs with total anomalous pulmonary venous return to the azygos vein or absence of the inferior vena cava with azygos continuation.

Posterior mediastinal masses are largely of neurogenic origin (35). Close inspection of the vertebra and posterior ribs may reveal pedicle erosion, interpedicular or rib space widening, or bone erosions, which are clues to a mass extending into the spinal canal. In such cases, the mass is most often a neoplasm of the neuroblastoma-ganglioneuroma group (Fig. 51.58). These tumors are probably congenital in origin and arise in paraspinal sympathetic nerve tissue. Primary thoracic neuroblastoma has a more favorable prognosis than neuroblastoma that originates in the abdomen. Ganglioneuroma is the benign counterpart of neuroblastoma, and the two lesions cannot be reliably distinguished from one another radiologically. Calcifications may be seen in both lesions, and it is believed that some neuroblastomas can mature to ganglioneuromas. MR is valuable to assess the extent of tumor, especially intraspinal extension (36,37).

Neurofibromas also occur in the posterior mediastinum and cause widening of intervertebral foramina. These tumors can be solitary but more often occur with the neurofibromatosis syndromes. Anterior thoracic meningoceles also occur in patients with neurofibromatosis and have a similar radiographic appearance. Neurenteric cysts are a form of enteric duplication cysts that communicate with the spinal canal. The cysts lie in the posterior mediastinum and are almost always associated with vertebral anomalies (Fig. 51.59). Spinal cord anomalies may also be present. MR is the procedure of choice for evaluating this condition. A posterior mediastinal inflammatory mass occasionally accompanies inflammatory conditions of the spine. Rare causes of a posterior mediastinal mass include lymphangioma, teratoma, lymphoma, and sarcoma. Diaphragmatic hernias through the foramen of Bochdalek and pulmonary sequestration often present as masses in the inferior portion of the posterior mediastinum, adjacent to the diaphragm.

CHEST WALL MASSES

Most masses that involve the chest wall of children arise from the cartilage or bones of the thoracic cage. Many such lesions are malignant and are often quite large at the time of presentation (Fig. 51.60A). Ewing sarcoma and primitive neuroectodermal tumor (Askin tumor) are the most common malignancies to involve the chest wall in children. Radiologically, both lesions appear as large extrapleural soft tissue masses, usually with evidence of rib destruction and ipsilateral pleural effusion. CT is the most helpful way to characterize the extent of these tumors (38). Rhabdomyosarcoma may also involve the chest wall. Chondrosarcoma is rare in childhood. Metastatic rib lesions are common in infants and children with neuroblastoma. Chest wall involvement in leukemia and lymphoma is also common. Pleural thickening adjacent to such lesions can help identify subtle metastases.

A variety of benign masses may occur in the chest wall (Table 51.10). Osteochondromas of the ribs are common. Mesenchymal hamartoma is a rare benign neoplasm of the ribs that occurs primarily in infants under 1 year of age (39). The neoplasm is composed of solid elements of proliferating cartilage, bone, and fibroblasts. Cystic areas of hemorrhage are commonly seen within the mass. These tumors are noninvasive, but they often cause erosion of adjacent ribs and compression of other adjacent tissues. Complete resection is curative. Intrathoracic infection (empyema) may extend to involve the chest wall, creating the appearance of a mass (Fig. 51.60B). *Staphylococcus* and *Fusobacterium* are common organisms.

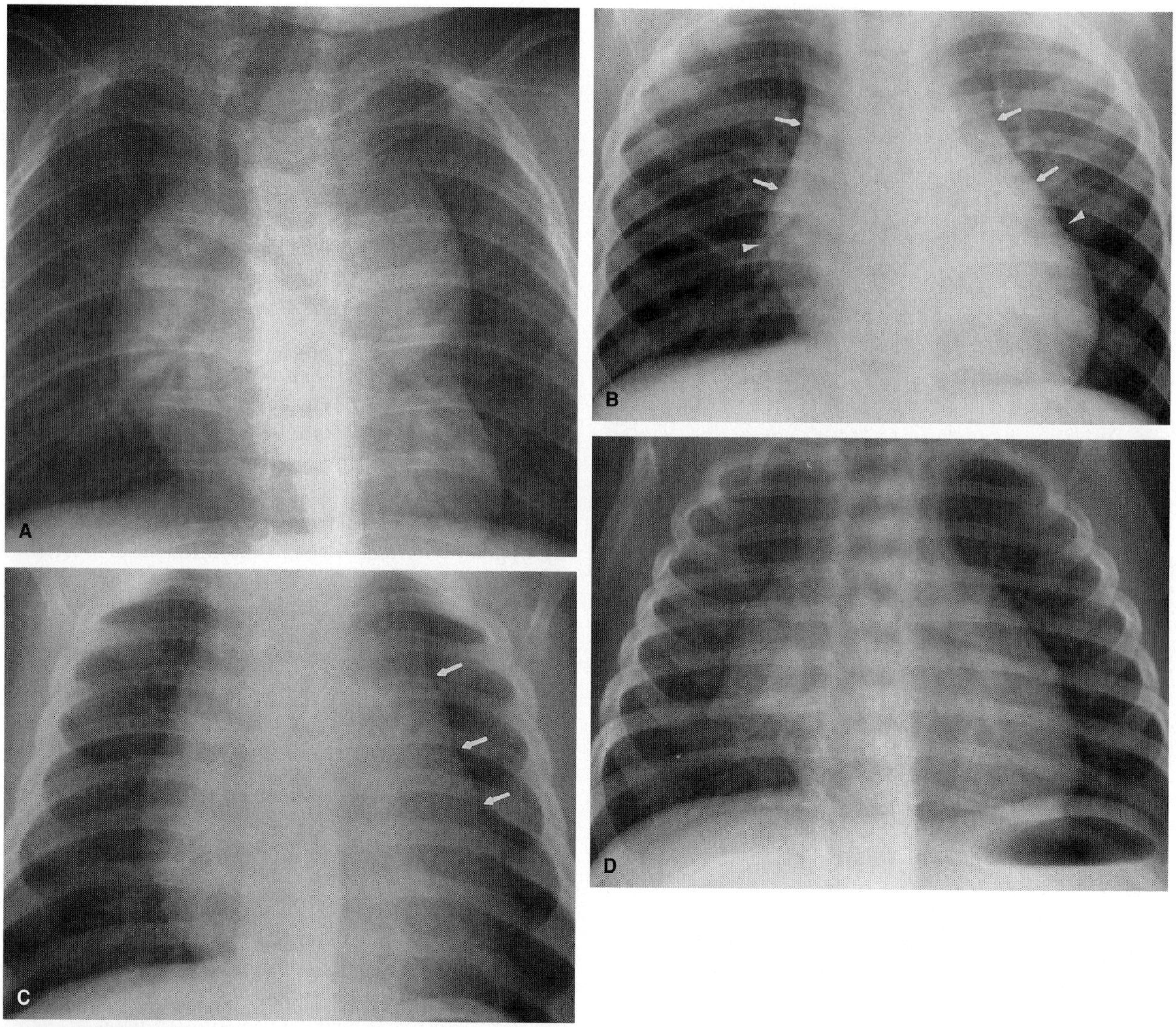

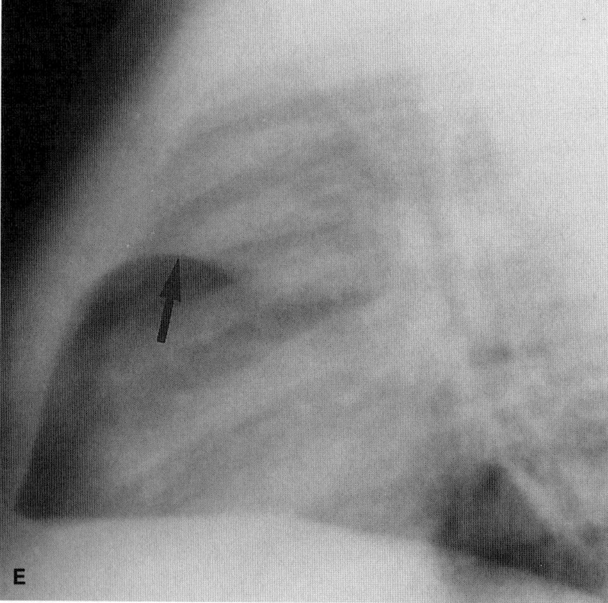

FIGURE 51.48. **Normal Thymus Configurations. A.** In a young infant, the thymus is often quite prominent, causing bilateral superior mediastinal widening. Note the right-sided buckling of the trachea, which is a normal finding during expiration in infants and should not be mistaken for mass effect. **B.** In older infants and young children, the lobes of the thymus gland become less prominent (*arrows*). Note the subtle notch at the junction of the thymic and cardiac shadows (*arrowheads*). **C.** The wavy thymic contour on the left is caused by rib compression (*arrows*). **D.** The right thymic lobe is prominent in this patient, with a configuration that has been likened to a sail. **E.** The straight inferior border of the thymus gland, which lies in the retrosternal space, is seen on the lateral view.

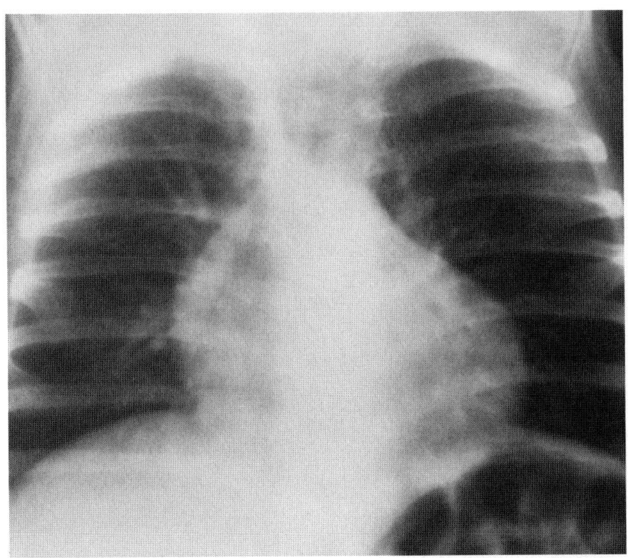

FIGURE 51.49. **Stress Atrophy of the Thymus.** The narrow superior mediastinum is caused by absence of a thymic shadow in this infant suffering from failure to thrive.

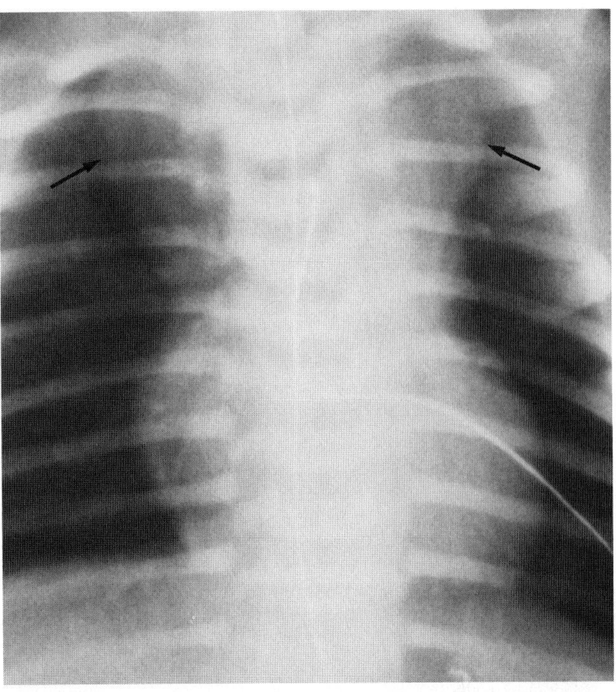

FIGURE 51.51. **Thymic Pseudomass.** The thymus gland is elevated and compressed by the bilateral anterior pneumothoraces, creating the appearance of a superior mediastinal mass (*arrows*).

CONGENITAL HEART DISEASE

A wide variety of imaging modalities is now available for evaluation of congenital heart disease in children. Many congenital cardiac abnormalities that previously required angiocardiography can now be diagnosed noninvasively by echocardiography, MR, and helical CT (40–43). Radiographs continue to play a role in the initial evaluation for congenital cardiac anomalies in infants and children. Although the specific diagnosis often will not be apparent on the plain films, a systematic approach to plain film interpretation will allow categorization into one of several groups of disorders. This section will provide a framework for an organized scheme for radiographic evaluation of congenital heart disease.

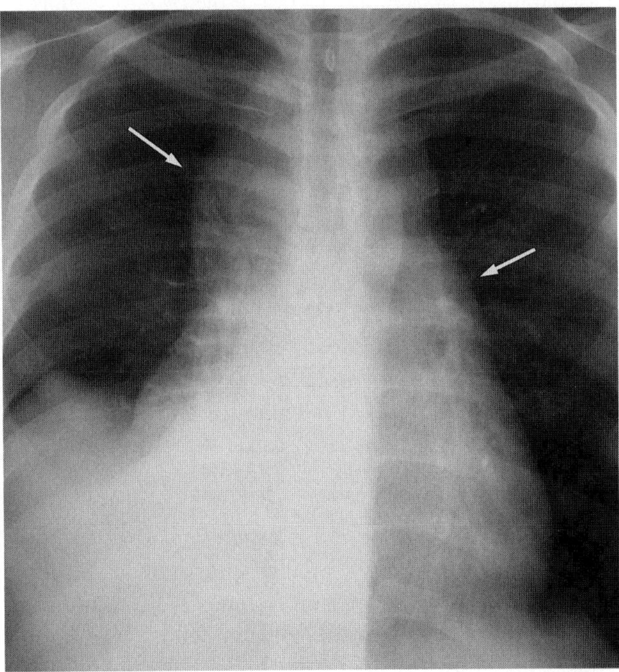

FIGURE 51.50. **Hodgkin Lymphoma.** The mediastinal enlargement is caused by lymphomatous involvement (*arrows*) of mediastinal lymph nodes. A right pleural effusion is present.

Assessment begins with the pulmonary vascularity. Vascular patterns are placed in one of three broad groups: increased (congested), decreased, and normal (Table 51.11). If the vascularity is increased, one should attempt to distinguish active congestion from passive congestion.

Active congestion occurs whenever the amount of blood flowing through the pulmonary vasculature has increased. This occurs in conditions with left-to-right shunts and with preferential blood flow into the lower-pressure pulmonary circulation. Left-to-right shunts do not become radiographically apparent until the output of the RV is approximately two and a half times greater than that of the LV. At this point, the pulmonary vessels become increased in diameter and are visible farther than usual into the periphery of the lungs (Fig. 51.61A). The vessels may appear tortuous, but their margins remain relatively distinct. In borderline cases, if the diameter of the right descending pulmonary artery (PA) is less than that of the trachea, a left-to-right shunt is unlikely.

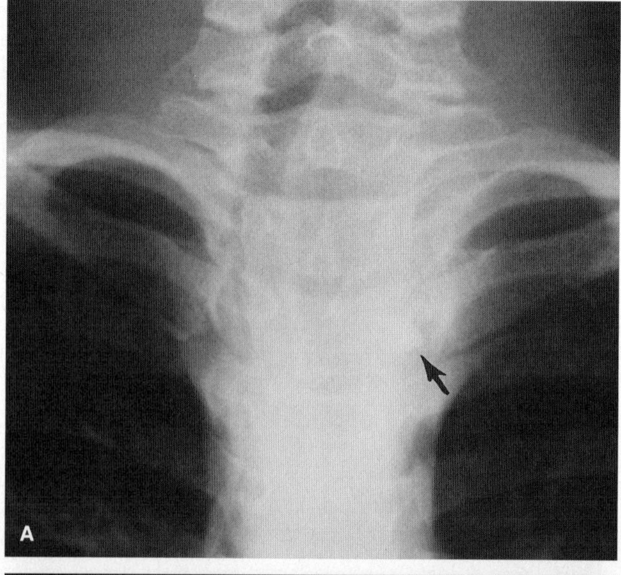

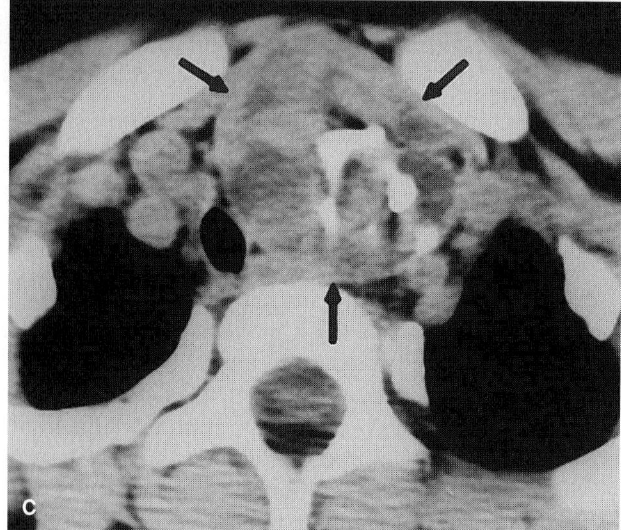

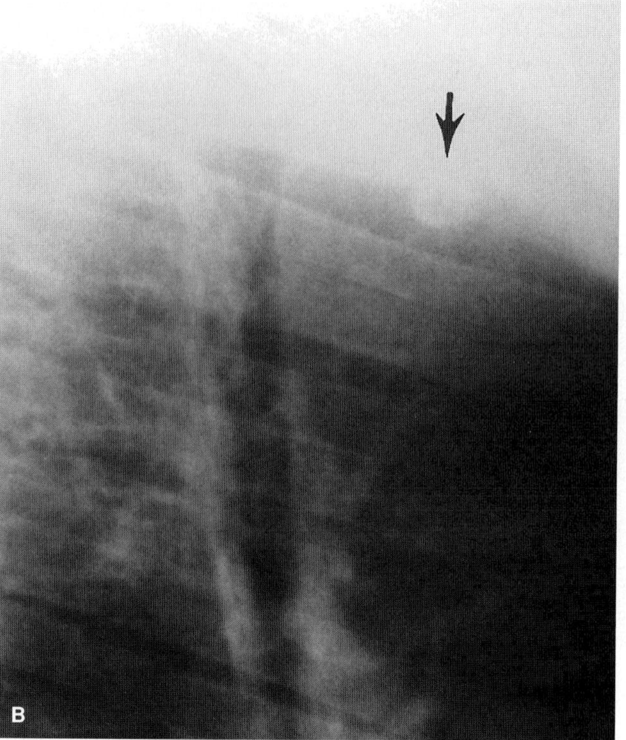

FIGURE 51.52. **Mediastinal Teratoma. A.** A superior mediastinal mass displaces the trachea to the right. A toothlike calcification (*arrow*) is seen within the mass. **B.** Lateral view shows the anterior location of the mass and the calcification (*arrow*). **C.** A CT scan reveals the heterogeneous nature of this teratoma (*arrows*), which contains dense calcifications and hypodense areas representing fat.

Passive congestion reflects elevation of pulmonary venous pressure, which can result from obstruction or dysfunction of the left side of the heart. As venous pressure increases and the veins dilate, edema fluid leaks into the perivascular interstitial tissues, causing the margins of the vessels to become less distinct on the chest radiograph (Fig. 51.61B). As pulmonary venous hypertension increases, alveolar pulmonary edema and pleural effusions develop. In patients with large left-to-right shunts and left heart failure, a mixed pattern of passive and active congestion occurs.

Decreased pulmonary vascularity indicates diminished blood flow to the lungs, most often caused by obstruction of the right ventricular outflow tract and associated right-to-left shunts. Oligemia causes the lungs to appear more radiolucent, and the vessels appear uniformly thin and wispy (Fig. 51.61C). A diminished caliber of the peripheral two thirds of the PAs combined with prominence of the central PAs is characteristic of pulmonary arterial hypertension and increased pulmonary vascular resistance.

Normal pulmonary vascularity is usually seen in patients with uncomplicated valvular disease, coarctation of the aorta, and mild forms of cardiomyopathy. The vessels retain a normal contour and diameter until congestive heart failure develops.

Asymmetry of pulmonary blood flow is most commonly seen in tetralogy of Fallot, persistent truncus arteriosus, and valvular pulmonic stenosis. In tetralogy of Fallot, the blood flow to the left lung tends to be diminished. Blood flow to either lung, or occasionally only one lobe, can be decreased in persistent truncus arteriosus. In valvular pulmonic stenosis, the abnormal valve tends to direct the blood flow preferentially into the left pulmonary

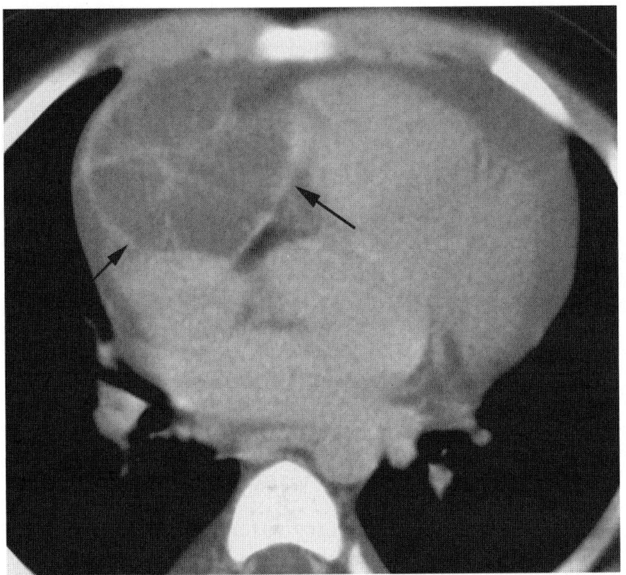

FIGURE 51.53. **Pericardial Lymphangioma.** The pericardial mass has the characteristic multiseptated, cystic appearance of lymphangioma on contrast-enhanced CT (*arrows*).

arterial system, although an enlarged left PA and increased blood flow to the left lung is seldom apparent on the radiographs of children. Unilateral or asymmetric decreased pulmonary vascularity can also be seen in association with obstructive emphysema of the lungs. The next step in radiographic interpretation of congenital heart disease is assessment of the main PA and the aorta.

Pulmonary Artery. An enlarged PA may represent generalized increased pulmonary blood flow, poststenotic dilation caused by valvular pulmonic stenosis (Fig. 51.62), or pulmonary valve insufficiency caused by increased right

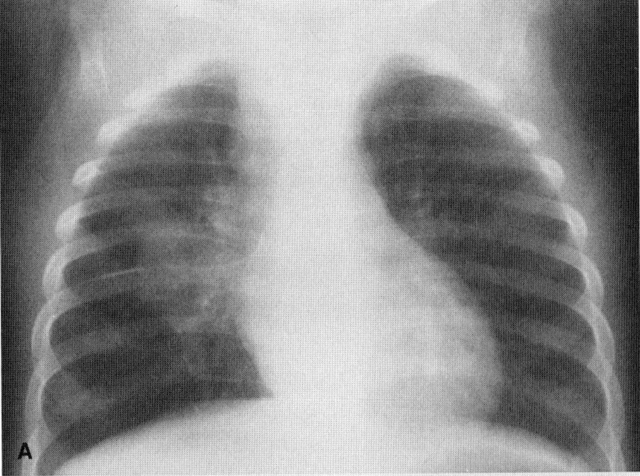

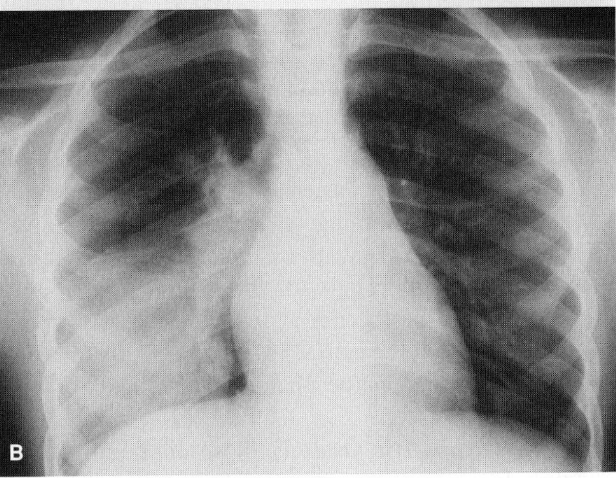

FIGURE 51.55. **Unilateral Hilar Adenopathy. A.** Right hilar adenopathy and adjacent parenchymal opacity comprise the typical Ghon complex of primary tuberculosis. **B.** Right hilar adenopathy is associated with a bacterial pneumonia.

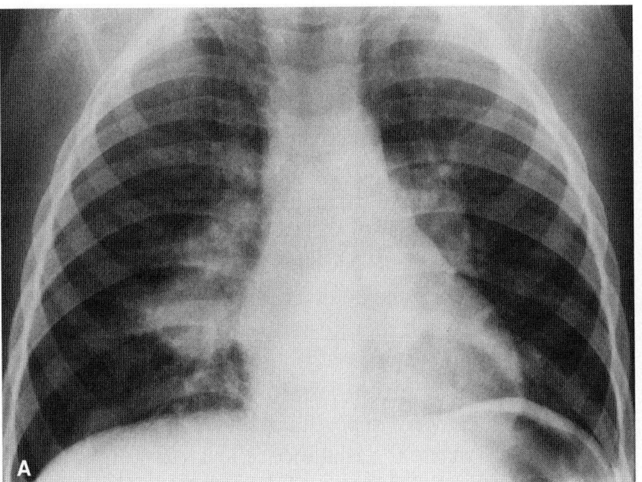

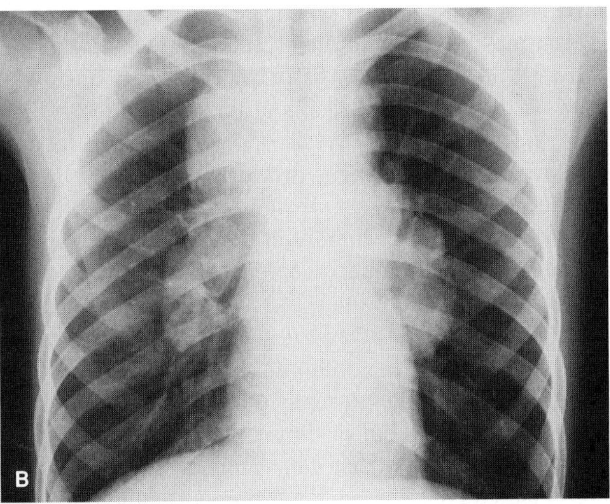

FIGURE 51.54. **Bilateral Hilar Adenopathy. A.** The prominent nodular hilar opacities represent lymph nodes in this patient with primary tuberculosis. **B.** The bilateral hilar and paratracheal masses represent lymphadenopathy caused by Hodgkin lymphoma.

ventricular output. An enlarged PA will often be higher in position than a normal PA and can be mistaken for a large aortic knob. A small or absent PA shadow occurs with decreased blood flow caused by pulmonary outflow obstruction or with an abnormal position of the PA, such as with persistent truncus arteriosus or transposition of the great vessels.

Aorta. Evaluation of the aorta includes estimation of size, position, and contour abnormalities. The size of the aorta is assessed in the region of the aortic knob. The aorta may appear small because of hypoplasia (as in hypoplastic left heart syndrome) and with certain left to-right shunts (e.g., atrial septal defect [ASD], ventricular septal defect [VSD]). Because the aorta in children is normally small relative to adults, a truly small aorta may be difficult to recognize. Enlargement of the ascending aorta and the aortic knob most often represents poststenotic dilation resulting from valvular aortic stenosis; it may also be caused by increased aortic blood flow seen with aortic valve insufficiency, left-to-right shunting at the great vessels level (patent ductus arteriosus, persistent truncus arteriosus), or severe tetralogy of Fallot. Generalized aortic enlargement can occur with systemic hypertension. The most common abnormality of the contour of the aorta is the notching that occurs at the site of coarctation of aorta. Dilation of the aorta proximal and distal to the coarctation results in the characteristic "figure 3" sign (Fig. 51.63).

Right-sided aortic arch is most often an isolated anomaly. However, it can also accompany congenital heart disease, especially persistent truncus arteriosus or tetralogy of Fallot. A right aortic arch is seen as a bulge or fullness in the right paratracheal region, slightly above the usual level of a left-sided aortic arch. The trachea will be displaced to the left by a right aortic arch (see Fig. 51.61C). In addition, a right descending aorta can be visualized just to the right of the spine in many cases. A right-sided aortic arch may be a clue to the presence of a vascular ring, such as a double aortic arch or aberrant left subclavian artery with an encircling ligamentum arteriosum. In such cases, barium swallow reveals opposing indentations in the barium-filled esophagus in a reverse S configuration (see Fig. 51.20).

Cardiomegaly is an important indicator of cardiac disease in children and often accompanies congenital heart disease. Unfortunately, the estimation of cardiac enlargement in children is somewhat subjective, and measurements such as the cardiothoracic ratio are usually not helpful. Beware of the normally prominent thymus gland overlying the heart and of films obtained during a poor degree of inspiration that can erroneously suggest cardiac enlargement. The configurations of enlargement of specific cardiac chambers are the same as those seen in adults. Generalized cardiomegaly with a globular appearance suggests pericardial fluid, which can easily be confirmed with US (Fig. 51.64). Pericardial effusions in children commonly accompany viral infections or rheumatic fever. Other causes include acute or chronic renal failure, collagen vascular diseases, bacterial infections, and, rarely, tuberculosis, fungal infections, and pericardial metastases. Blood in the pericardial space is usually the result of trauma. Generalized cardiac enlargement also occurs with conditions that cause increased blood volume and elevated cardiac outputs, including renal diseases, inappropriate secretion of antidiuretic hormone, large arteriovenous fistulae, chronic anemias (especially sickle cell disease and thalassemia), and hyperthyroidism.

Acyanotic Heart Disease With Increased Pulmonary Vascularity

Actively increased pulmonary vascularity in the absence of cyanosis most often occurs when a defect allows oxygenated blood from the left side of the heart or the aorta to be shunted back to the right side of the heart or the pulmonary circulation. Because no desaturated blood is shunted into the systemic circulation, cyanosis does not occur. The increased blood volume recirculating through the right heart and pulmonary circulation results in cardiac enlargement and increased size of the pulmonary vessels. The most common conditions in this category are VSD, ASD, and patent ductus arteriosus (PDA).

Ventricular septal defect is the most common congenital heart abnormality after bicuspid aortic valve. VSD occurs frequently as an isolated anomaly, although it may accompany many of the cyanotic forms of congenital heart disease. The defect is categorized according to its location within the ventricular septum. Most are perimembranous defects in the portion of the septum near the fusion of the membranous and muscular portions. Defects in the muscular septum are less common and tend to be smaller and less hemodynamically significant than a perimembranous defect. The third type of defect is uncommon and develops high in the membranous septum because of abnormal development of the conus portion of the truncus arteriosus. This type is most often seen with persistent truncus arteriosus or tetralogy of Fallot.

Newborns with VSD are usually asymptomatic. A murmur will often not be detected until after the newborn period. This delay in manifestation of left-to-right shunting is the result of the normal phenomenon of postnatal pulmonary vascular involution. In the fetus, the walls of the PAs are thicker than in postnatal life, resulting in increased pulmonary vascular resistance. Elevated pulmonary vascular pressure inhibits blood flow through the lungs and through the septal defect. During the early postnatal period, the pulmonary vascular resistance diminishes, allowing left-to-right shunting through the septal defect. In patients with moderate to large VSDs, symptoms usually

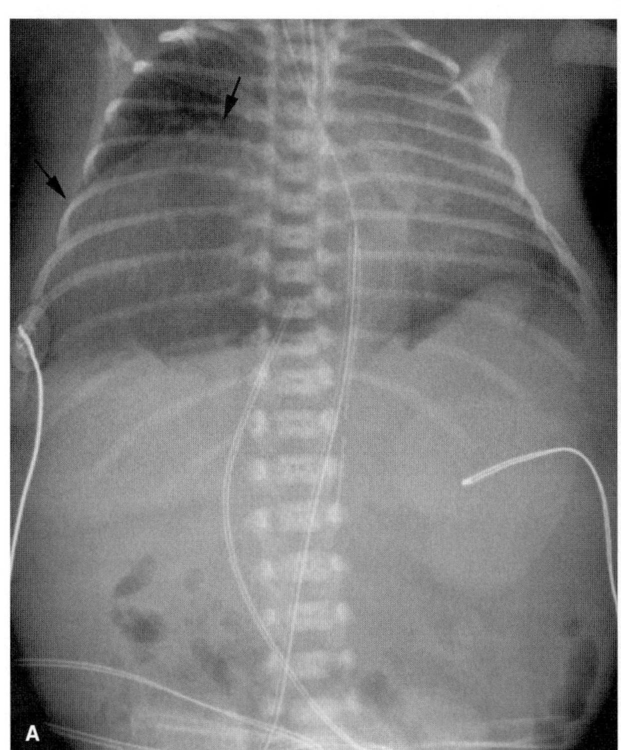

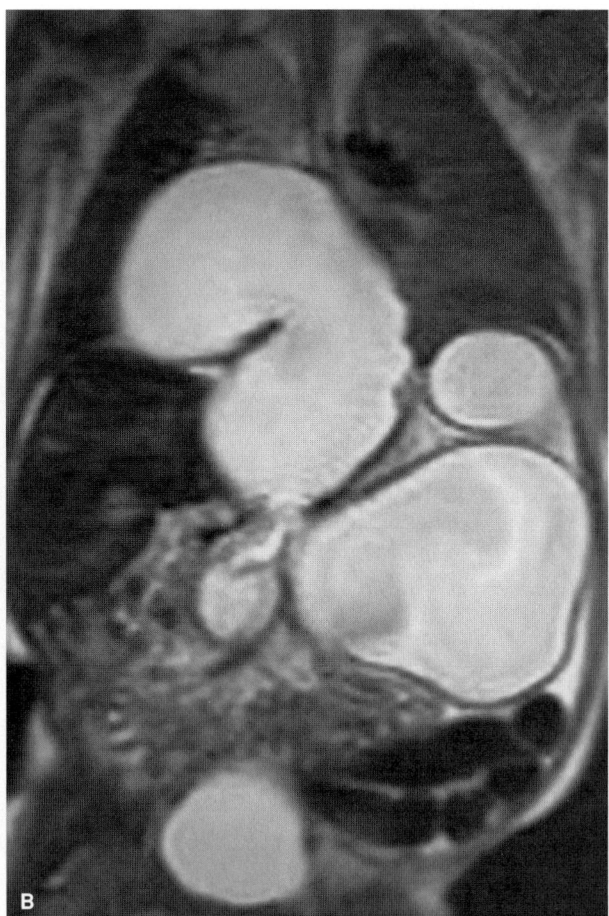

FIGURE 51.56. **Intestinal Duplication Cyst. A.** Radiograph of this newborn infant shows a large soft tissue mass in the right chest (*arrows*), displacing the mediastinum to the left. **B.** Coronal T2WI shows the cystic nature of the mass, which arises from the duodenum.

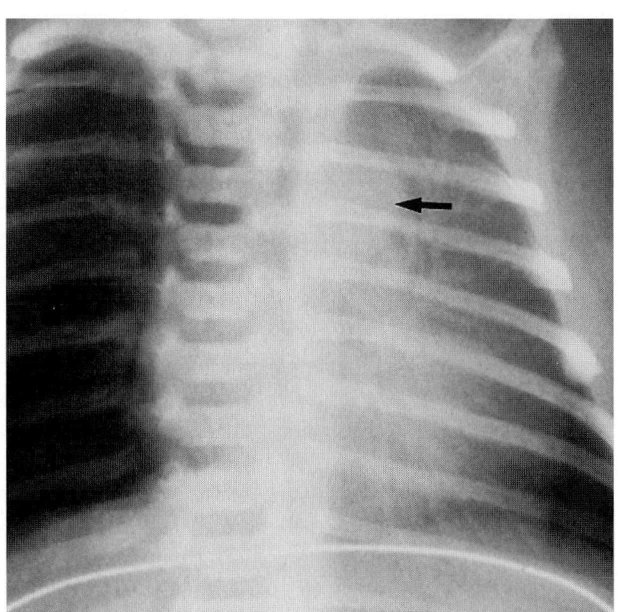

FIGURE 51.57. **Ductus Bump.** The prominent "bump" that is seen along the upper descending aorta represents the dilated infundibulum of the ductus arteriosus in this newborn infant.

develop within the first 2 years of life. Small defects can close spontaneously.

The characteristic findings in VSD are PA enlargement, increased pulmonary vascularity, and cardiomegaly that is predominantly left-sided (Fig. 51.65). Increased pulmonary venous return results in volume overload of the LA and LV, leading to dilation. LV dilation causes a "drooping" shape of the left cardiac border. LA enlargement is best seen on the lateral or left anterior oblique view as a bulge along the upper posterior cardiac border that causes posterior displacement of the esophagus and the left mainstem bronchus. If the shunt is large, biventricular enlargement occurs.

Atrial septal defect is much less common than VSD. The most common type of ASD occurs centrally at the foramen ovale, the ostium secundum defect. Because ASD is associated with a low-pressure shunt, these children seldom develop symptoms in infancy or early childhood. If the shunt persists as the child grows older, the risk of developing pulmonary hypertension increases. As the pressure in the right side of the heart rises, the shunt becomes balanced and eventually reverses. This phenomenon is

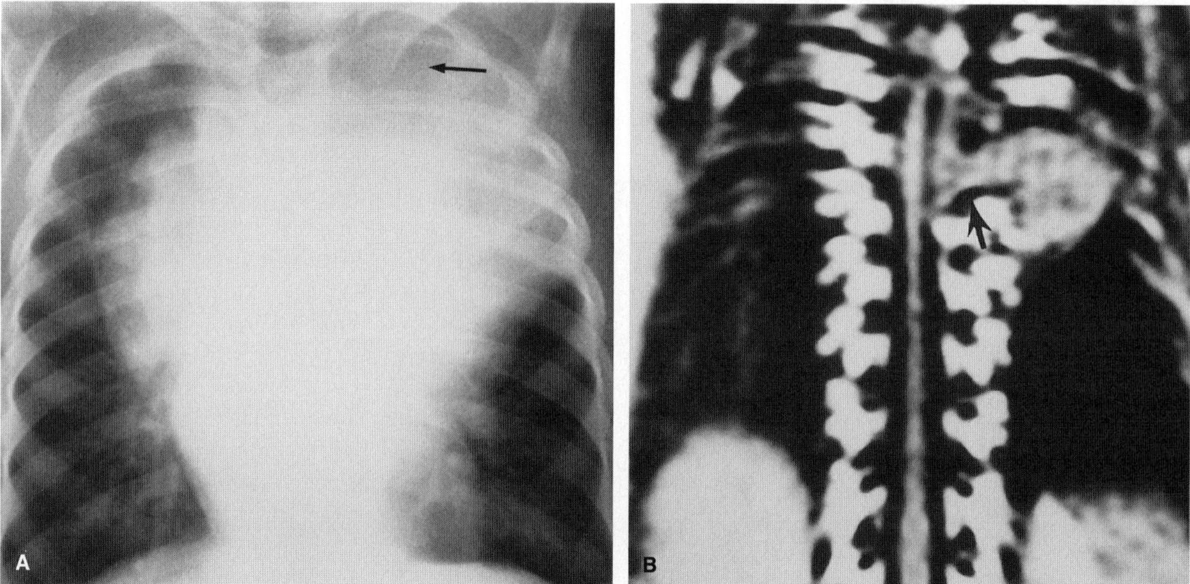

FIGURE 51.58. **Thoracic Neuroblastoma. A.** Note the large mediastinal mass. Thinning of the posterior and medial portion of the left second rib and widening of the T2-T3 rib space (*arrow*) localizes this mass to the posterior mediastinum and suggests possible intraspinal extension. **B.** Coronal MR of a different patient with a left posterior mediastinal mass demonstrates extension of the tumor into the spinal canal (*arrow*).

referred to as Eisenmenger physiology and can be seen with any left-to-right shunt.

The LA is not enlarged with ASD because of rapid shunting of blood away from the LA into the right side of the heart. Typically, the RA is enlarged, causing prominence of the right cardiac border on the frontal view (Fig. 51.66). On the lateral view, RV enlargement produces fullness in the retrosternal space. In both ASD and VSD, the aorta is rather small, as the shunt is below the level of the great vessels.

The ostium primum type of ASD (endocardial cushion defect) is caused by abnormal development of the primitive endocardial cushions that form the interatrial and interventricular septa and atrioventricular valves. This condition commonly occurs in trisomy 21. The specific malformation ranges from two separate atrioventricular valves with a low ASD and a VSD to the complete form, with a common atrioventricular ring and a five-leaflet valve. The mitral valve is clefted and abnormally positioned, resulting in elongation of the left ventricular outflow tract, which creates a "gooseneck" appearance on angiography (Fig. 51.67). The partial form behaves hemodynamically as a simple atrial left-to-right shunt, with only mild degrees of mitral or tricuspid insufficiency. The clinical course of the complete form is much more severe. The shunts are large and usually bidirectional because of the abnormal valve development. The patients are cyanotic and tend to develop pulmonary hypertension and congestive heart failure early. Radiographically, these patients present with marked cardiomegaly with right atrial and right ventricular predominance and pulmonary vascular engorgement (Fig. 51.68).

Patent Ductus Arteriosus. The ductus arteriosus connects the PA and aorta in fetal life. Normally, this structure begins to close immediately after birth, but in some infants, closure is delayed. Prolonged patency is a common complication of hypoxia in the premature infant. In many infants, the cause of persistent patency is unknown. Symptoms develop within the first 2 years of life. Blood is shunted from the aorta through the ductus to the PA, resulting in increased blood volumes flowing through the lungs and the left side of the heart. Consequently, the LA, LV, and PA become dilated with active pulmonary vascular engorgement. An enlarged proximal aorta differs from the small aorta that is seen with ASD and VSD (Fig. 51.69). In young infants with large shunts, cardiomegaly tends to be more generalized, and the size of the aorta is difficult to evaluate because of overlying thymus gland. PDA is easily diagnosed by echocardiography or angiography.

Aortopulmonary window is a rare condition that is very similar to PDA, both hemodynamically and radiographically. The abnormality results from failure of complete division of the primitive truncus arteriosus, which leaves a communication between the aorta and the PA just above the valves. Other rare conditions that result in shunting of blood from the aorta to the PA include rupture of an aneurysm of the sinus of Valsalva and fistulas between the coronary arteries and the coronary sinus, PA, or right cardiac chambers.

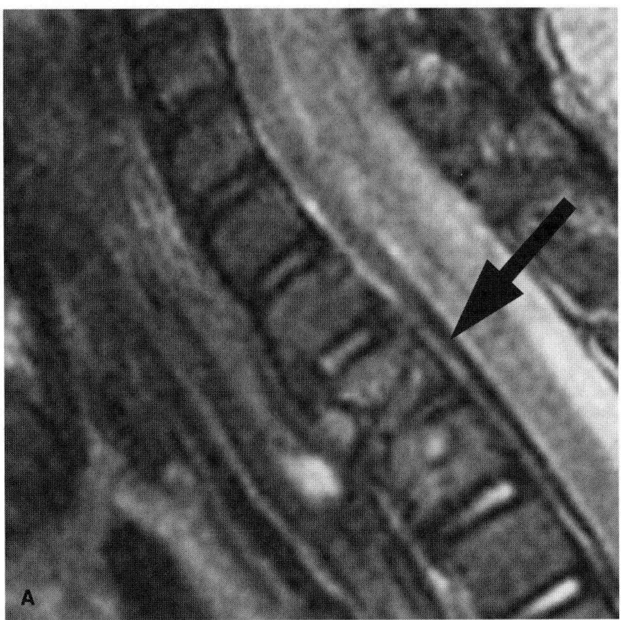

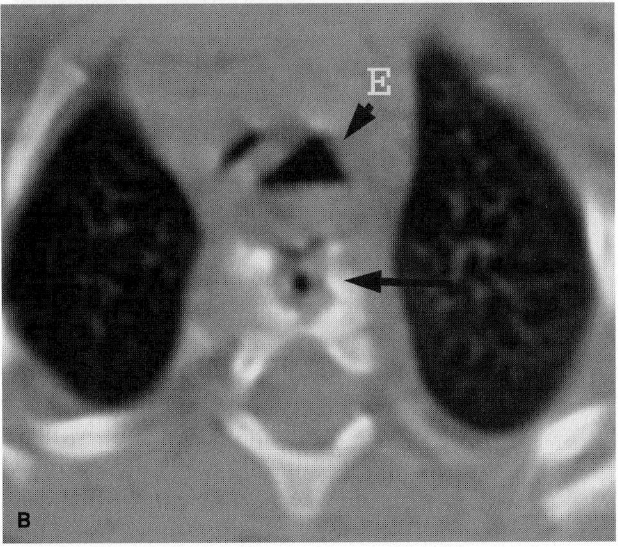

FIGURE 51.59. **Neurenteric Fistula. A.** Sagittal T2WI shows a small anterior cyst with a fistula extending into the T2 vertebra (*arrow*). **B.** Axial CT image shows the obstructed esophagus (E) and the air-filled fistula (*arrow*) extending into a defect in the vertebral body.

Cyanotic Heart Disease With Increased Pulmonary Vascularity

This category consists of a group of complex heart abnormalities whose common feature is the admixture of oxygenated and deoxygenated blood that is circulated systemically, resulting in cyanosis.

Transposition anomalies of the great vessels are lesions with abnormal anteroposterior positioning of the aorta and PA and with abnormalities of the relationship between the atria and ventricles and their connections to the great vessels.

Complete transposition of the great vessels (D-transposition) is the most common form of cyanotic congenital heart disease with increased pulmonary blood flow. In this condition, the positions of the aorta and PA are reversed. The ventricles lie in their normal positions, so that the aorta arises anteriorly from the RV and the PA arises posteriorly from the LV. This results in two separate circulations, one through the pulmonary circulation and the other systemic. Communications that allow the infant to survive are most commonly a VSD, an ASD, or PDA. Bidirectional shunting through these communications allows adequate mixing of the blood if the shunts are large enough. If pulmonary stenosis is not present, blood flows preferentially into the low-resistance pulmonary circulation, resulting in increased pulmonary venous return and pronounced volume overloading. Congestive heart failure develops in the first weeks of life. The prognosis is more favorable with associated pulmonary stenosis.

Cardiomegaly with an oval configuration develops in the first few days of life (Fig. 51.70A). The superior mediastinum and base of the heart are narrow because of thymic atrophy and the abnormal alignment of the aorta and PA. Both active and passive pulmonary vascular congestion can be seen. On lateral views of the chest, the anteriorly placed aorta causes increased opacity in the retrosternal region (Fig. 51.70B). The corrective arterial switch procedure is performed early in many infants, and therefore, the classic radiographic findings may not develop.

Corrected transposition of the great vessels (L-transposition). In L-transposition, ventricular inversion (left to right reversal) accompanies the transposed positions of the aorta and PA, resulting in functional correction of the transposition. Blood circulates through the RA to LV to PA to the pulmonary circulation, and LA to RV to aorta to the systemic circulation. The anatomic RV functions as an LV and vice versa. Because the aorta lies anteriorly and to the left, this condition is often called L-transposition, while complete transposition is called D-transposition. Patients with the simple form of corrected transposition tend to be asymptomatic, but patients with coexisting cardiac defects (VSD, pulmonary stenosis, conduction defects) have an unfavorable prognosis. The diagnosis is suggested radiographically by a characteristic prominence along the upper left cardiac border that represents the right ventricular outflow tract and the left-sided aorta (Fig. 51.70C).

Double-outlet right ventricle is characterized by an aorta that is anterior to or lateral to the PA and arises from the RV (Fig. 51.71). The PA also empties the RV, originating entirely from the RV (type I), or overriding a high VSD and draining both the LV and RV (type II or the Taussig-Bing anomaly). The hemodynamics are similar to complete transposition of the great vessels. Radiographic findings are also similar. However, because the aorta and PA are oriented in a more side-to-side fashion in some cases, the

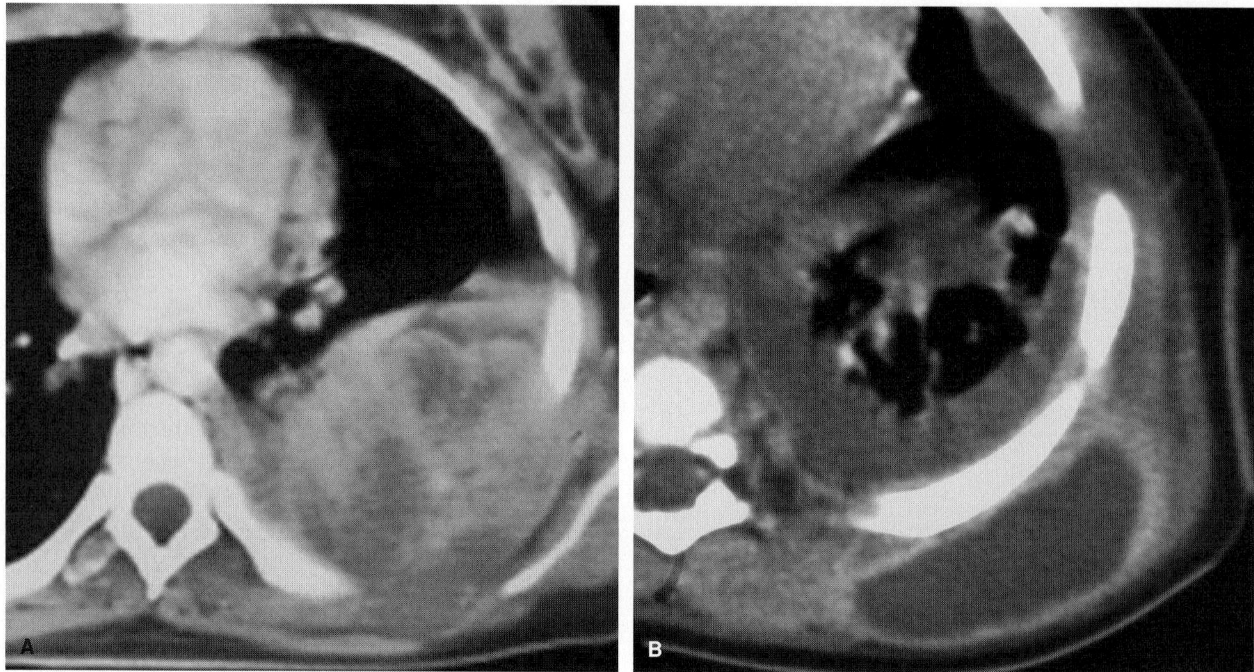

FIGURE 51.60. **Chest Wall Masses. A.** A Ewing sarcoma arises from a posterior rib in a child. Note the rib destruction. **B.** CT shows a large posterior chest wall abscess that arose following staphylococcal empyema (empyema necessitatis).

cardiac waist may be of normal or even increased width, unlike the narrow waist seen in transposition.

Total anomalous pulmonary venous return (TAPVR) is a condition in which the pulmonary veins, instead of emptying into the LA, return blood to the right side of the heart via the RA, coronary sinus, or a systemic vein. This anomaly can occur in conjunction with other major cardiac defects, but this discussion will refer only to the isolated form. The best known classification of the types of TAPVR was described by Craig et al (44). In all types, the pulmonary veins converge into a single common vein before emptying into the anomalous site. In type 1 TAPVR, the most common form, the abnormal vein empties into a large supracardiac vein (a persistent left superior vena cava, the left brachiocephalic vein, the right superior vena cava, or the azygos vein). In the type 2 anomaly, the common vein drains into the coronary sinus or directly into the RA. In the type 3 anomaly, the common vein travels through the esophageal hiatus to empty into the portal vein or, less commonly, an abdominal systemic vein.

TAPVR types 1 and 2 overload the right side of the heart, causing dilation of the RA, RV, and PA and engorgement of the pulmonary vessels. Communication with the left side of the heart is mandatory for survival and usually occurs as an ASD or patent foramen ovale. The classic radiographic configuration of the type 1 anomaly is the "snowman" heart, so named because of prominence of the superior mediastinum caused by a large, inverted U-shaped vessel that empties into the superior vena cava (Fig. 51.72). This configuration is only present when the abnormal common pulmonary vein enters the persistent left superior vena cava or vertical vein. In the other forms of the type 1 anomaly and in the type 2 anomaly, the cardiac configuration is less specific. Type 2 findings resemble

TABLE 51.10 Chest Wall Masses

Malignant
Ewing sarcoma
Primitive neuroectodermal tumor (Askin tumor)
Neuroblastoma
Leukemia
Lymphoma
Rhabdomyosarcoma
Benign
Osteochondroma
Aneurysmal bone cyst
Mesenchymal hamatoma
Langerhans cell histiocytosis
Fibrous dysplasia
Hemangioma
Lymphangioma
Teratoma
Abscess
Calcifying fibrous pseudotumor
Osteoid osteoma

TABLE 51.11 Pulmonary Vascular Patterns

Increased vascularity (active) without cyanosis
- Atrial septal defect
- Ventricular septal defect
- Patent ductus arteriosus
- Aortic-pulmonary window
- Ruptured aneurysm of sinus of Valsalva
- Coronary artery fistula
- Partial anomalous pulmonary venous return

Increased vascularity (active) with cyanosis
- Total anomalous pulmonary venous return (types 1, 2)
- Persistent truncus arteriosus
- Complete endocardial cushion defect
- Transposition of the great vessels complex
- Single ventricle (without pulmonary stenosis)

Increased vascularity (passive)
- Total anomalous pulmonary venous return (type 3)
- Pulmonary vein atresia
- Hypoplastic left heart syndrome (in failure)
- Cor triatriatum

Decreased vascularity
- Tetralogy of Fallot
- Pseudotruncus arteriosus
- Hypoplastic right heart syndrome (right-to-left shunt)
  - Tricuspid atresia
  - Pulmonary atresia
  - Tricuspid stenosis
  - Hypoplastic RV
- Ebstein anomaly
- Uhl anomaly
- Trilogy of Fallot
- Single ventricle or transposition of great vessels with pulmonary stenosis or atresia
- Tricuspid or pulmonary insufficiency with right-to-left shunt

Normal vascularity
- Left heart lesions
  - Coarctation of the aorta
  - Interrupted aortic arch
  - Hypoplastic left heart syndrome (before failure develops)
  - Endocardial fibroelastosis
  - Cardiomyopathy
  - Aberrant left coronary artery
  - Mitral stenosis and insufficiency
  - Aortic stenosis and insufficiency
  - Cor triatriatum
- Right heart lesions (without right-to-left shunt)
  - Pulmonary stenosis or insufficiency
  - Tricuspid insufficiency

those of the transposition complex of lesions. In the type 1 anomaly, when the abnormal vein empties into the azygos vein, the azygos vein will be dilated.

Type 3 TAPVR is hemodynamically and radiographically distinct from the other forms. Like the other forms of TAPVR, blood is directed incorrectly to the right side of the heart. However, the length and small caliber of the common vein with type 3 TAPVR increases the resistance to flow and creates pulmonary venous obstruction. The pulmonary vessels appear thin, with hazy margins caused by pulmonary interstitial edema and passive vascular engorgement (Fig. 51.73). The heart does not enlarge. The differential diagnosis includes hypoplastic left heart syndrome and pulmonary vein atresia. These three diagnoses are the most common causes of passive vascular congestion in the first 3 days of life.

Persistent truncus arteriosus occurs when the primitive truncus arteriosus fails to divide normally into the aorta and PA. Both vessels are fed by a single vessel that overrides a high VSD. The Collett-Edwards classification is based on the site of origin of the PA (Fig. 51.74). The degree of cyanosis is variable and symptoms depend largely on the amount of pulmonary blood flow. Most often, the chest radiograph shows cardiomegaly and active pulmonary vascular congestion. In most forms of persistent truncus, concavity is seen at the usual site of the main PA and strongly suggests the diagnosis. A right aortic arch is present in 30% of the cases (Fig. 51.75). The aorta (truncus) is often dilated, with a high arch and an elevated left PA.

Single ventricle refers to a group of anomalies in which one ventricle is rudimentary, leaving the other large ventricle as the only functional ventricle. An underdeveloped RV is most common. The connections between ventricles and the atrioventricular valves, aorta, and PA are variable. Associated lesions include pulmonary valve stenosis, PA atresia, and transposition of the great vessels. If pulmonary stenosis is not present, mixing of saturated and unsaturated blood occurs in the single chamber, and the radiographs show cardiomegaly and pulmonary vascular engorgement. When pulmonary stenosis is present, blood flow to the lungs is diminished and cyanosis is more severe. Echocardiography is usually diagnostic; however, angiocardiography or MR is sometimes needed for complete demonstration of the anatomy.

Decreased Pulmonary Vascularity

A decreased pulmonary vascular pattern usually indicates a condition in which the flow through the right side of the heart is obstructed. This obstruction can occur anywhere from the tricuspid valve to the PA. Often, an intracardiac right-to-left shunt, which varies with the severity of right ventricular outflow obstruction, is also present.

Tetralogy of Fallot is the most common anomaly to cause diminished pulmonary vascularity and is the most common cause of cyanotic congenital heart disease. The classic components are (*1*) a high VSD, (*2*) pulmonary stenosis (usually infundibular, with or without valvular stenosis), (*3*) right ventricular hypertrophy, and (*4*) an aorta that overrides the VSD. A right aortic arch occurs in 25% of cases, and PA coarctation, hypoplasia, or absence are common.

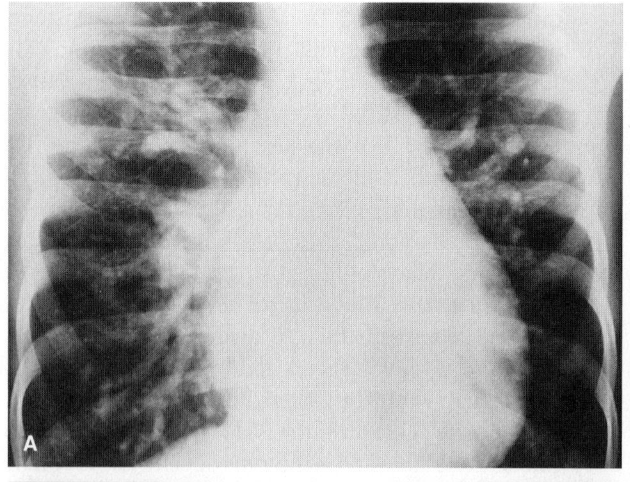

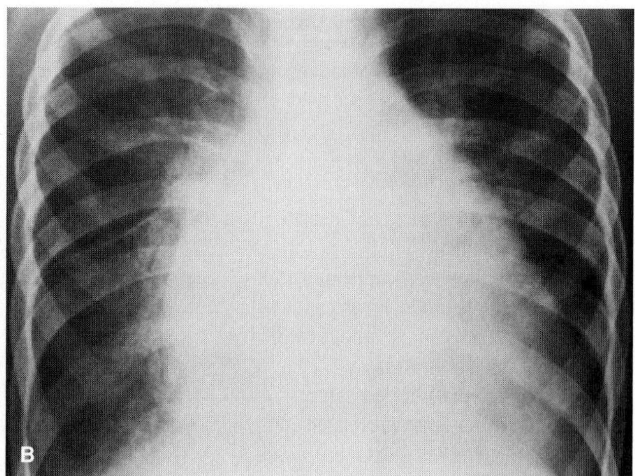

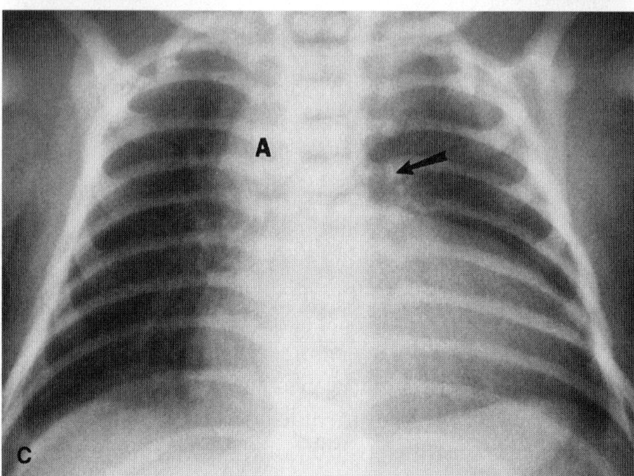

FIGURE 51.61. **Pulmonary Vascular Patterns. A. Active congestion.** Large but distinct pulmonary vessels extend into the periphery of the lung as the result of left-to-right shunting in a patient with a large ventricular septal defect. **B. Passive congestion.** Passive vascular congestion is caused by mitral insufficiency and results in indistinctness of the pulmonary vascular markings. **C. Decreased vascularity** in a patient with tetralogy of Fallot. Note the right aortic arch (A), concave pulmonary artery segment (*arrow*), and the characteristic "boot" cardiac configuration caused by right ventricular hypertrophy.

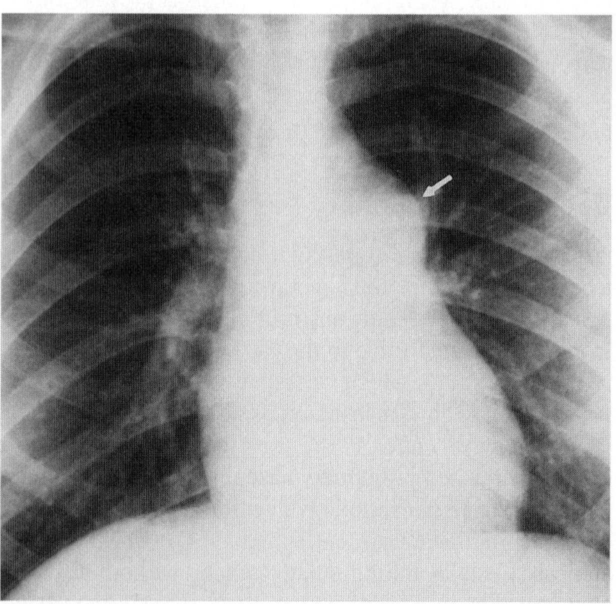

FIGURE 51.62. **Pulmonary Artery Enlargement.** Poststenotic dilation of the pulmonary artery is seen in this patient with valvular pulmonic stenosis (*arrow*).

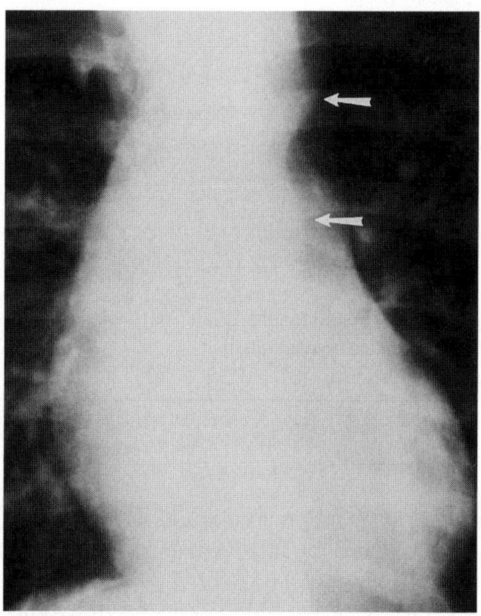

FIGURE 51.63. **Coarctation of the Aorta.** Prestenotic and poststenotic dilation of the aorta creates the characteristic figure-3 sign (*arrows*).

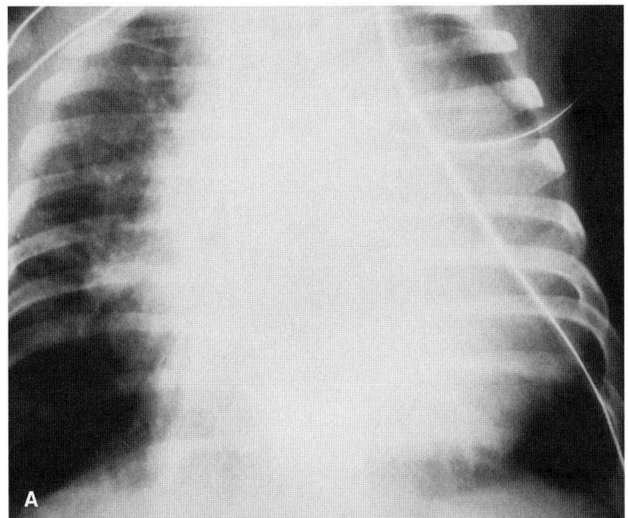

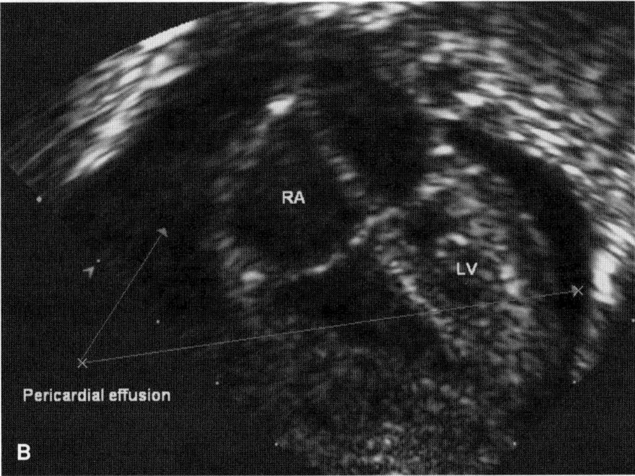

FIGURE 51.64. **Pericardial Effusion. A.** The cardiac silhouette is markedly enlarged and has a rounded, globular appearance caused by a pericardial effusion that developed following open heart surgery. **B.** US is the best method for verifying a pericardial effusion.

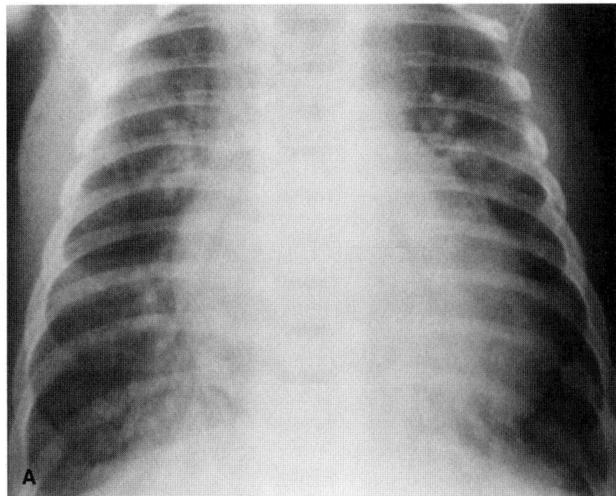

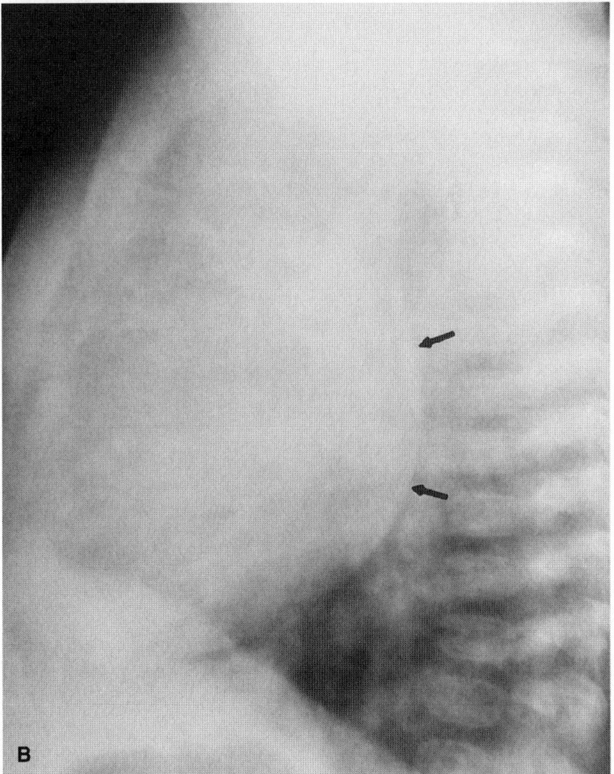

FIGURE 51.65. **Ventricular Septal Defect (VSD). A.** Cardiac enlargement that is predominantly left-sided and increased pulmonary vascularity are characteristic of a VSD. **B.** Lateral view demonstrates left atrial enlargement (*arrows*).

The degree of pulmonary stenosis is the most critical component of this anomaly. Severe stenosis leads to marked right-to-left shunting and aortic enlargement, causing greater overriding. Greater right-to-left shunting results in more severe cyanosis. Patients with mild pulmonary stenosis are usually acyanotic and asymptomatic ("pink" or "balanced" tetralogy of Fallot).

Patients with moderate to severe forms of tetralogy of Fallot have a characteristic radiographic appearance. The pulmonary vascularity is decreased, with a shallow or concave PA shadow. Right ventricular hypertrophy causes lateral and superior displacement of the cardiac apex without overall enlargement of the cardiac silhouette, creating the classic "boot-shaped heart" (Fig. 51.76). Unequal pulmonary blood flow caused by PA hypoplasia or atresia (usually on the left) is a common finding. The combination of a right aortic arch and decreased pulmonary vascularity is highly suggestive of tetralogy of Fallot or persistent truncus arteriosus.

Hypoplastic right heart syndrome consists of tricuspid atresia, usually with pulmonary atresia or stenosis and an underdeveloped RV. Isolated hypoplasia of the RV is rare. The common features are a small RV with right-to-left shunting through an ASD, resulting in cyanosis. A VSD

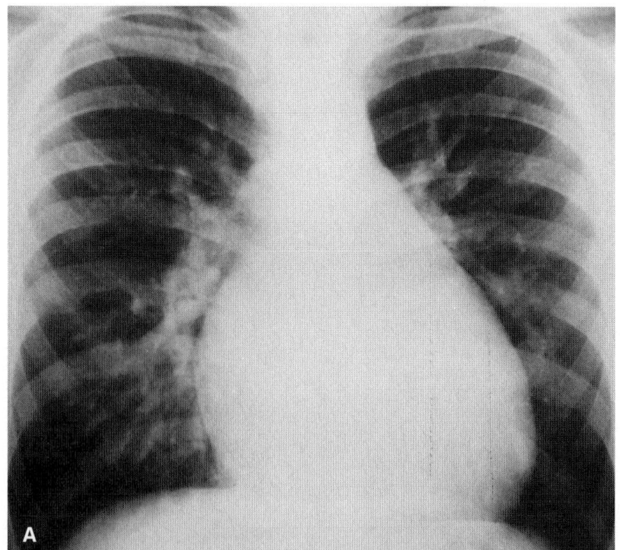

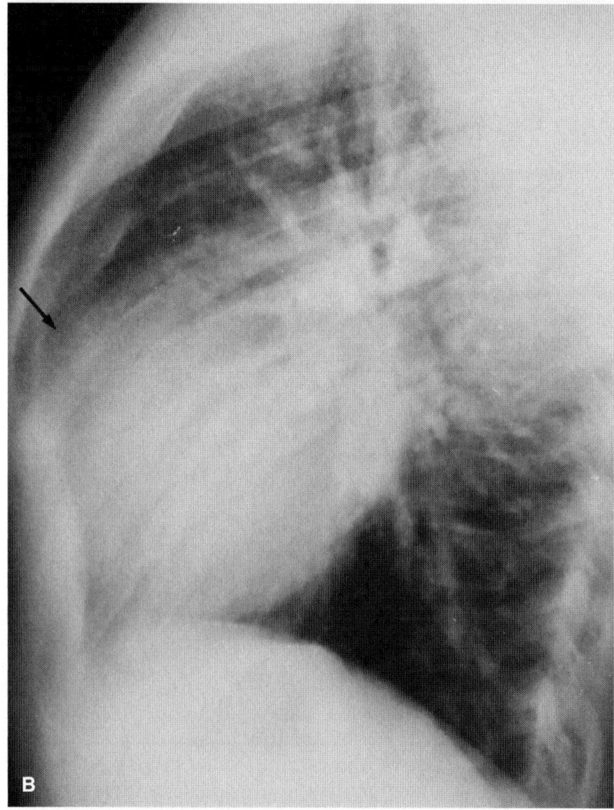

FIGURE 51.66. **Atrial Septal Defect (ASD). A.** Cardiomegaly, mild right atrial enlargement, and increased pulmonary vascularity are characteristic of an ASD. **B.** Lateral view shows a normal LA and fullness in the retrosternal region (*arrow*) caused by right ventricular enlargement.

or PDA can also be present. Nonspecific cardiomegaly and diminished pulmonary vascularity are seen radiographically. The PA shadow is flat or concave, and the RA is enlarged (Fig. 51.77). The smaller the ASD, the larger the RA. Tricuspid atresia may be accompanied by transposition of the great vessels. When this occurs, the PA drains the LV and, if no pulmonary stenosis is present, the pulmonary vascularity is engorged.

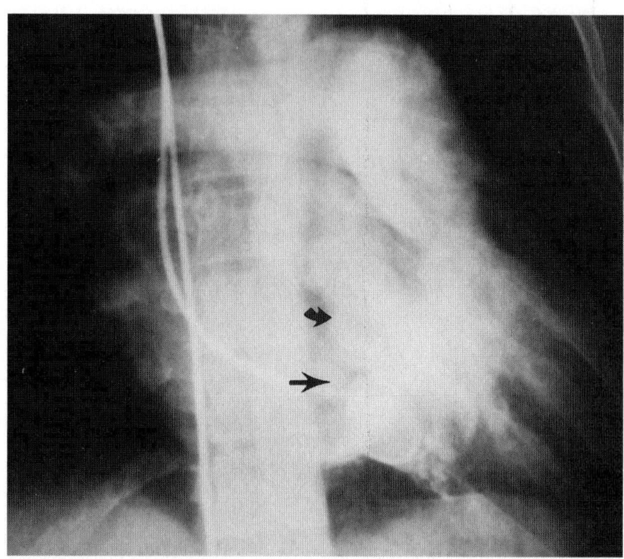

FIGURE 51.67. **Endocardial Cushion Defect.** Angiocardiography demonstrates the cleft mitral valve (*straight arrow*) and the elongated left ventricular outflow tract (gooseneck deformity) (*curved arrow*).

Pulmonary atresia is considered a part of the hypoplastic right heart syndrome when accompanied by an intact ventricular septum. In most cases, the pulmonary valve is atretic and the RV and tricuspid valve are hypoplastic. Less commonly, the RV and tricuspid valve are nearly normal, and blood that enters the RV is regurgitated back into the RA, resulting in marked RA enlargement (Fig. 51.78). In either case, survival requires a PDA to shunt blood into the

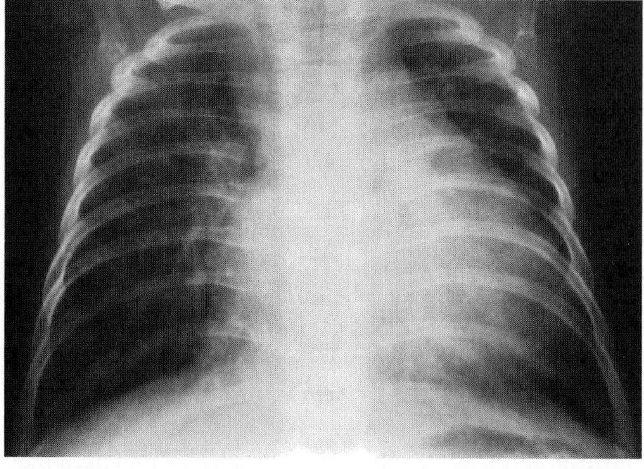

FIGURE 51.68. **Endocardial Cushion Defect.** Marked cardiomegaly, right atrial enlargement, and increased pulmonary vascularity are typical of this condition.

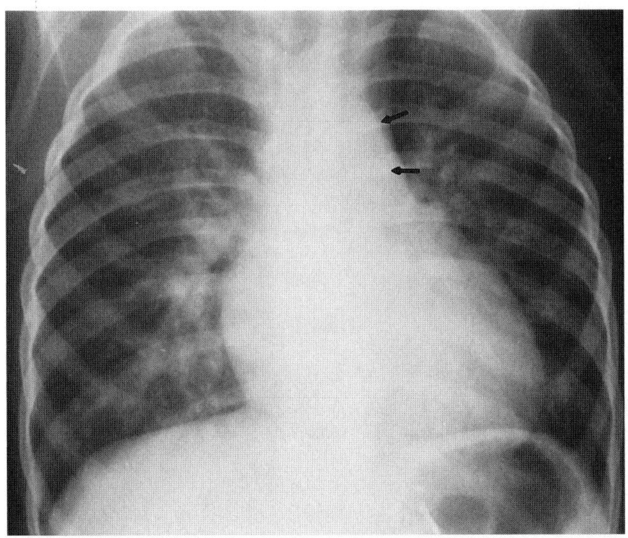

FIGURE 51.69. **Patent Ductus Arteriosus.** The heart is enlarged, with left-sided prominence and increased pulmonary vascularity. Note the prominent aorta (*arrows*).

pulmonary circulation. Prostaglandin E1 is used to help maintain ductal patency until surgery can be performed.

In patients with pulmonary atresia with a VSD, the RV is not hypoplastic. This situation occurs in severe tetralogy of Fallot and in pulmonary atresia with VSD and systemic collaterals (the Collett-Edwards type IV truncus arteriosus). The most significant difference between these two conditions is the derivation of pulmonary blood flow. In severe tetralogy of Fallot, blood reaches the lungs through a long, tortuous, "wandering" PDA. The other form of pulmonary atresia with VSD relies on primitive systemic collaterals that transport blood from the aorta to the PA branches.

Ebstein anomaly consists of a malformed, enlarged tricuspid valve that is displaced downward, resulting in atrialization of a large portion of the RV. The remaining RV is very small. The atrialized portion has abnormal musculature, contracts ineffectively, and causes functional obstruction of RA emptying. Atrial right-to-left shunting results in cyanosis in the more severely affected patients. Clinical symptoms and radiographic findings depend on the degree of downward displacement of the tricuspid valve. Cardiomegaly is mainly right-sided, with decreased pulmonary vascularity and a flattened PA shadow (Fig. 51.79). The right atrial contour is often very prominent. Occasionally, the small displaced RV is seen as a bulge along the upper left cardiac border, causing a squared cardiac appearance.

Uhl anomaly is rare and consists of focal or complete absence of the RV myocardium. The very thin, poorly contractile RV functionally impairs the flow of blood through the right side of the heart. The clinical and radiographic findings are similar to those of the Ebstein anomaly.

Normal Pulmonary Vascularity

Congenital cardiac anomalies with normal pulmonary vascularity are predominantly abnormalities of the cardiac valves and great vessels. Most have left-sided obstruction. When a concomitant left-to-right shunt is present, cardiac failure develops early and the pulmonary vascularity becomes congested. In the absence of a left-to-right shunt, patients can live for many years without left ventricular failure.

Congenital cardiac valve stenosis most commonly affects the aortic or pulmonary valves. The radiographic findings in children are similar to those seen in adults and consist of hypertrophy of the ventricle that ejects blood through the stenotic valve and poststenotic dilation of the affected artery (Fig. 51.80). Ventricular hypertrophy alters the shape of the heart, with little change in the size of the heart. LV hypertrophy causes a more rounded appearance of the left cardiac border. RV hypertrophy produces fullness in the retrosternal region on the lateral view and upward displacement of the cardiac apex on the posteroanterior view. In valvular pulmonic stenosis, poststenotic dilation of the main PA is often accompanied by prominence of the left PA and increased pulmonary blood flow to the left lung. This phenomenon most likely results from preferential flow through the stenotic valve into the left PA. However, it is less commonly observed on the radiographs of children than on those of adults because the findings take time to develop.

Aortic and pulmonary stenosis may also occur above or below the valve. Subvalvular aortic stenosis is more common than supravalvular stenosis, and the subvalvular narrowing can be caused by a discrete diaphragm or disproportionate hypertrophy of the intraventricular septum in the subaortic region. Supravalvular aortic stenosis is most often associated with Williams syndrome (idiopathic hypercalcemia of infancy) (Fig. 51.81) The features of this syndrome include supravalvular aortic stenosis and other systemic and pulmonary vascular stenoses, facial dysmorphism, mental and growth retardation, and hypercalcemia that may be the result of abnormal regulation of vitamin D metabolism. Subvalvular (infundibular) pulmonary stenosis is the most frequently seen form of stenosis in tetralogy of Fallot. Supravalvular pulmonary stenosis usually consists of multiple areas of narrowing in the peripheral pulmonary artery. Unlike the valvular forms of aortic and pulmonary stenosis, the subvalvular and supravalvular forms are usually not associated with poststenotic dilation of the vessel.

Congenital Valvular Insufficiency. Isolated congenital insufficiency of any of the cardiac valves is a very rare occurrence; however, sometimes valvular insufficiency accompanies other cardiac anomalies. In general, valvular insufficiency causes dilation of the cardiac chambers or vessels on both sides of the involved valve. The resulting

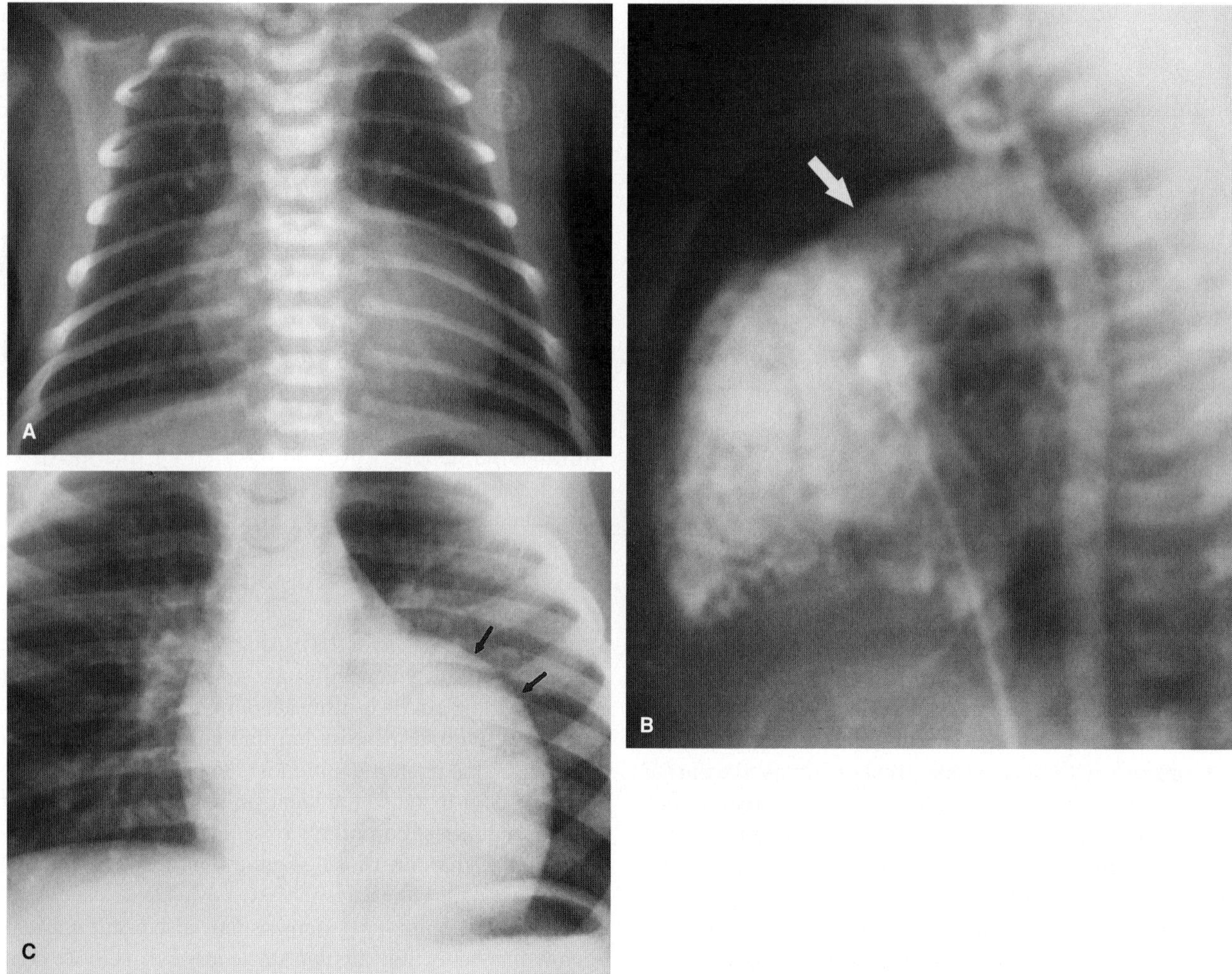

FIGURE 51.70. **Transposition of the Great Vessels. A.** In the more common D-transposition, the heart is enlarged and has an oval "egg" shape. Note the narrow superior mediastinum and increased pulmonary vascularity. **B.** Angiocardiography in lateral projection shows the aorta (*arrow*) arising anteriorly from the RV. **C.** L-transposition. The transposed aorta arising from the inverted RV on the left causes characteristic prominence along the upper left cardiac border (*arrows*).

cardiac configurations are the same as those seen in adults with valvular insufficiency.

Coarctation of the aorta occurs in two distinct forms: the juxtaductal (adult) type, which lies at or just distal to the level of the ductus arteriosus, and the rarer preductal (infantile) form, which generally is a long-segment narrowing. Coarctation of the aorta often is associated with other cardiac anomalies, most commonly bicuspid aortic valve, PDA, or a VSD. Patients with the preductal form of coarctation undergo a more severe clinical course, frequently developing congestive heart failure during the first month of life. Patients with the juxtaductal form usually remain asymptomatic until later in childhood, except in those cases with an associated left-to-right shunt. Older children usually present with hypertension, discrepancies between blood pressure in the upper and lower extremities, or a heart murmur. In juxtaductal coarctation of the aorta, the aortic narrowing leads to pressure overloading and hypertrophy of the LV. Usually the heart is normal in size; however, eventually some rounding and prominence of the left cardiac border can develop. Prestenotic and poststenotic dilation of the aorta commonly occurs and is responsible for the "figure-3" sign (see Fig. 51.63). In some cases, the poststenotic dilatation can extend along the entire thoracic portion of the descending aorta. Progressive collateral circulation develops, usually involving the intercostal arteries. It is the dilation of these arteries that eventually causes a notching along the inferior edge of the posterior ribs, most often from T4 to T8 (Fig. 51.82A). This finding usually is not visible until the patient is at least 7 or 8 years of age. Coarctation of the aorta is now frequently diagnosed by echocardiography,

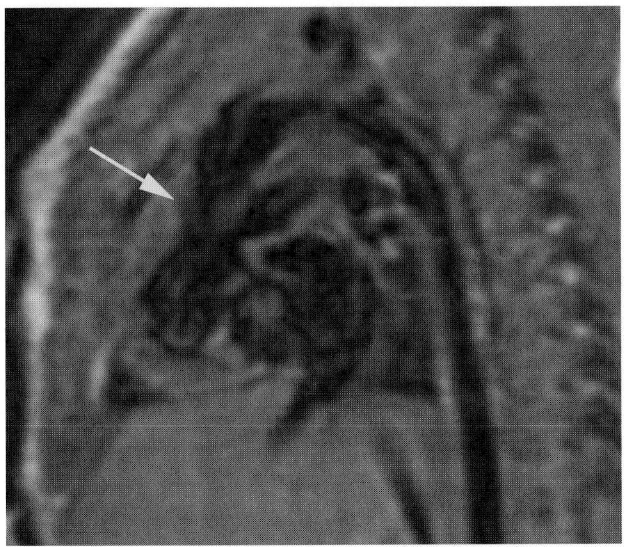

FIGURE 51.71. **Double-Outlet RV With D-Transposition.** Sagittal MR shows that both the aorta and pulmonary artery arise from the RV, with the aorta anterior (*arrow*).

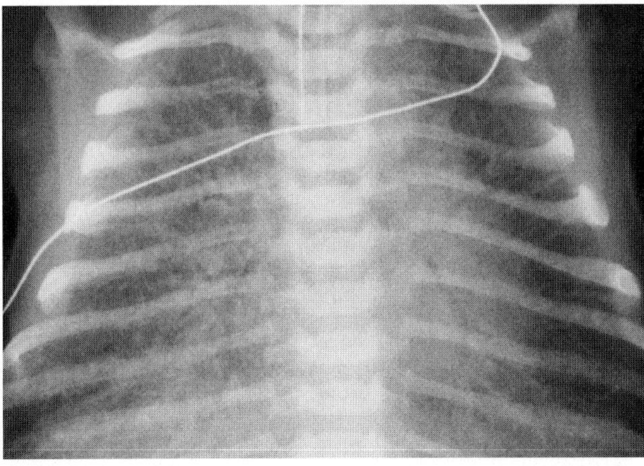

FIGURE 51.73. **Total Anomalous Pulmonary Venous Return, Type 3.** The heart is normal in size, with thin and somewhat indistinct pulmonary vessels owing to passive vascular congestion. A prominent interstitial pattern in the lungs represents pulmonary edema.

and further definition of the anatomy is achieved by MR (Fig. 51.82B).

Hypoplastic left heart syndrome consists of a variety of lesions characterized by some degree of underdevelopment of the left side of the heart. The anomalies range from isolated atresia of the ascending aorta or aortic or mitral valves, to aortic and mitral valve atresia combined with marked hypoplasia of the LA, LV, and ascending aorta. In all cases, blood flow through the left heart is severely impaired and a PDA is necessary to allow blood to reach the systemic circulation. Although the heart size and pulmonary vascularity can appear normal in the first few hours of life, cardiomegaly and congestive heart failure usually develop within the first 2 days. At this point, the pulmonary vasculature becomes passively congested and often a diffusely hazy or reticular pattern develops in the lungs (Fig. 51.83). This pattern signifies interstitial pulmonary edema and resembles that which is seen in other causes of severe pulmonary venous obstruction such as

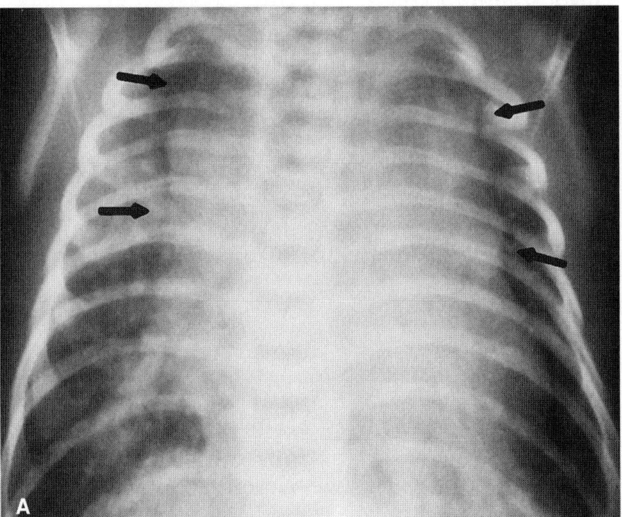

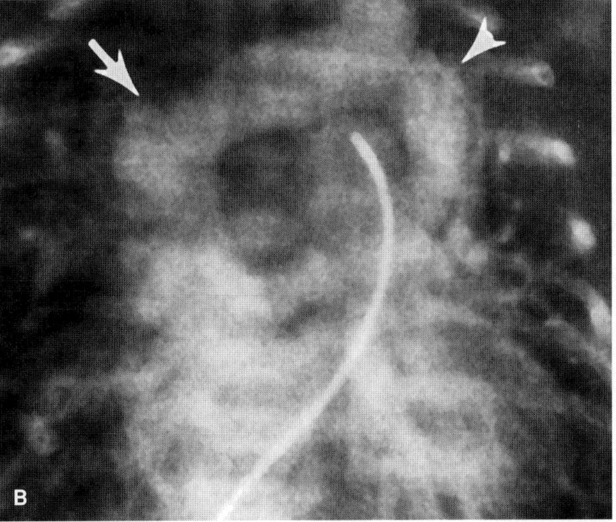

FIGURE 51.72. **Total Anomalous Pulmonary Venous Return, Type 1. A.** The characteristic snowman (*arrows*) or figure 8 configuration results from cardiomegaly combined with prominence of the superior mediastinum because of the anomalous pulmonary vein. **B.** Cardioangiogram demonstrates the inverted, U-shaped vessel (*arrows*), which constitutes the upper portion of the snowman.

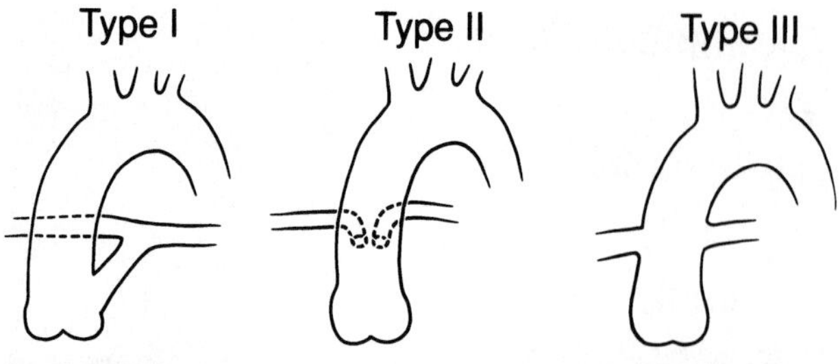

FIGURE 51.74. **Persistent Truncus Arteriosus.** These diagrams illustrate the basic forms of the original Collett-Edwards classification of persistent truncus arteriosus.

pulmonary vein atresia and TAVPR type 3. The diagnosis can usually be accomplished by echocardiography.

Cor triatriatum is a rare anomaly that also presents in early infancy with pulmonary venous obstruction. In this anomaly, the pulmonary veins empty into a common vein, which is abnormally incorporated into the LA. A partial membrane at this site creates an extra chamber along the superior and dorsal aspect of the LA and variably obstructs venous emptying into the LA. The usual radiographic findings consist primarily of cardiomegaly and passive venous congestion without evidence of left atrial enlargement.

Primary abnormalities of the myocardium can also present with a normal pulmonary vascular pattern. Cardiomyopathies may accompany a variety of conditions in children. These include bacterial or viral infections, autoimmune diseases, toxic insults, and hereditary neuromuscular diseases. Asymmetric septal hypertrophy is an unusual form of cardiomyopathy that is associated with subvalvular hypertrophic aortic stenosis. Radiographic findings of cardiomyopathy include cardiomegaly that may be generalized or predominantly left sided (Fig. 51.84). The pulmonary vascularity remains normal until congestive heart failure develops. Endocardial fibroelastosis is a condition in which the left ventricular myocardium becomes markedly thickened and contains increased amounts of elastic and fibrous tissue, resulting in marked enlargement of the LV and LA. Radiographically, the heart has a rounded configuration because of the thickened myocardium (Fig. 51.85). The enlarged LV often encroaches on the RV and impairs right ventricular function as well. The LV also can cause left lower lobe atelectasis by compression of the left lower lobe bronchus. Congestive heart failure usually occurs early in infancy in these patients.

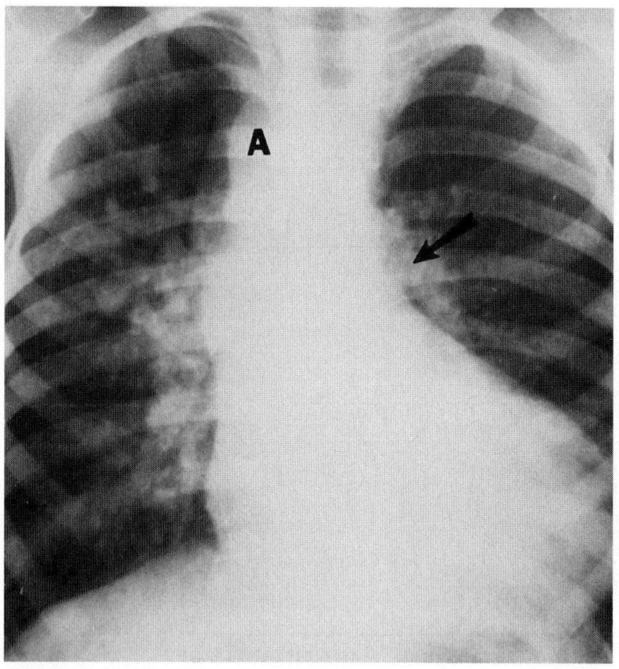

FIGURE 51.75. **Persistent Truncus Arteriosus.** Note oval cardiomegaly, increased pulmonary vascularity, a concave pulmonary artery segment (*arrow*), and a right aortic arch (A).

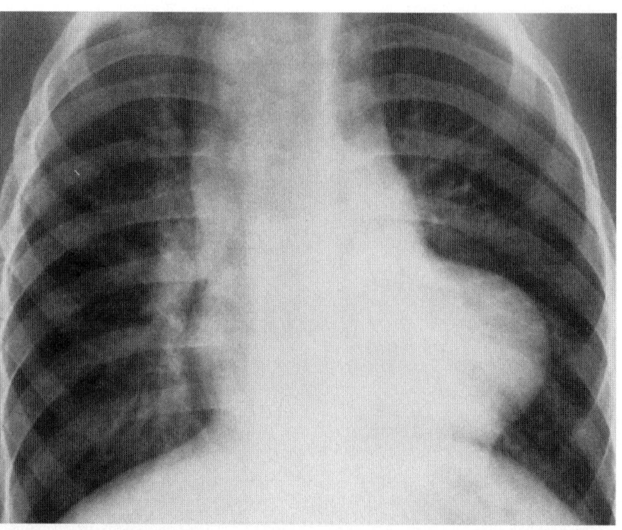

FIGURE 51.76. **Tetralogy of Fallot.** The upwardly displaced cardiac apex caused by right ventricular hypertrophy and the concave pulmonary artery shadow are characteristic of Tetralogy of Fallot.

Cardiac Malpositions

Cardiac malpositions are a confusing group of abnormalities, and a detailed description of these conditions will not be attempted here. Nevertheless, mastery of the terminology used to describe these conditions can help provide a basic understanding of the anatomy involved. Dextrocardia implies a cardiac apex that lies to the right of the spine because of primary malpositioning during development. Levocardia is the normal position of the cardiac apex, to the left of the spine. When faced with cardiac

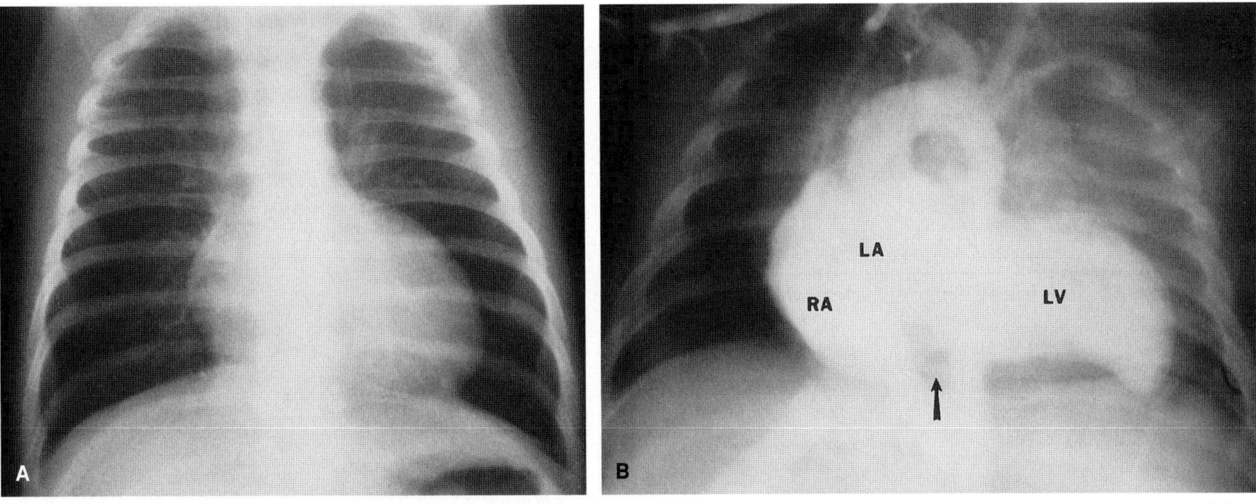

FIGURE 51.77. **Tricuspid Atresia. A.** Typical findings of left ventricular and right atrial enlargement with a concave pulmonary artery segment and decreased pulmonary vascularity are present. **B.** Angiocardiography shows contrast in the RA, LA, and enlarged LV. A bare area is seen because of lack of filling of a normal RV (*arrow*).

malpositioning, one must then determine the position of the abdominal organs (i.e., the abdominal situs). In general, the RA will lie on the same side as the liver and the left atrium will lie on the side opposite the liver. Situs solitus refers to the "normal" position of the viscera—that is, the liver on the right and the stomach on the left. The reversed position is referred to as visceral situs inversus.

Inversion refers to positioning of anatomic structures, usually from right to left and vice versa. The cardiac chambers of a dextroposed heart can be inverted or not. The atria and ventricles can be inverted simultaneously or separately and are referred to as concordant if they remain normally related to each other (i.e., the LA is connected to the LV and the RA to the RV). If the LA is connected to the RV or vice versa, the condition is referred to atrioventricular discordance.

Mirror-Image Dextrocardia. The most common type of cardiac malposition is referred to as mirror-image dextrocardia. In these patients, the cardiac chambers are completely inverted and the cardiac apex points to the right.

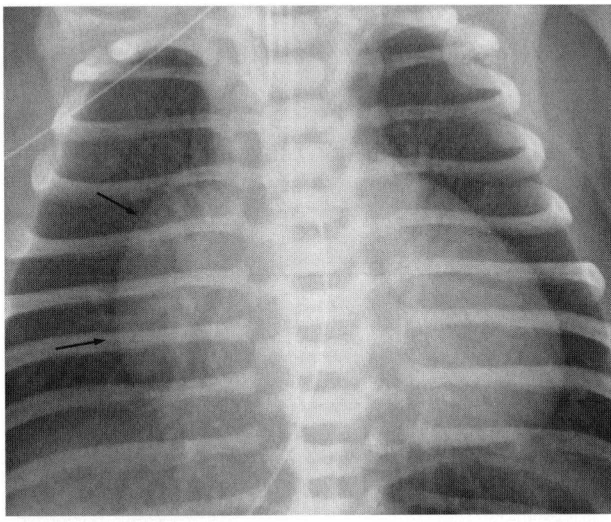

FIGURE 51.78. **Pulmonary Atresia With Intact Ventricular Septum.** In this patient, a nearly normal-sized RV is present. Regurgitation of blood from the RV results in marked right atrial enlargement (*arrows*).

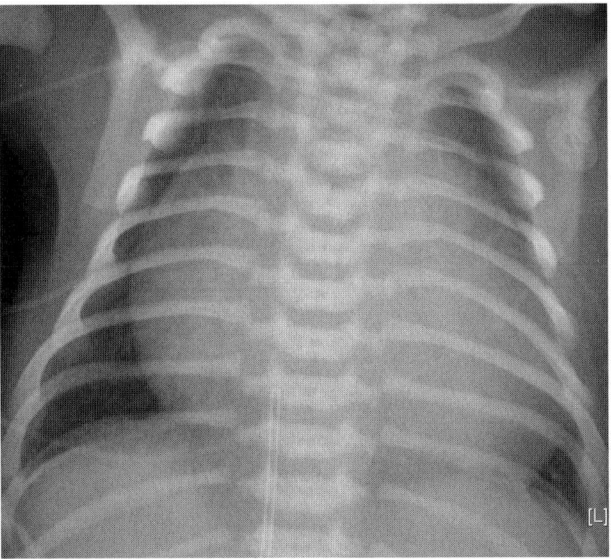

FIGURE 51.79. **Ebstein Anomaly.** Note the severe cardiomegaly with marked right atrial enlargement. Pulmonary vascularity typically is decreased.

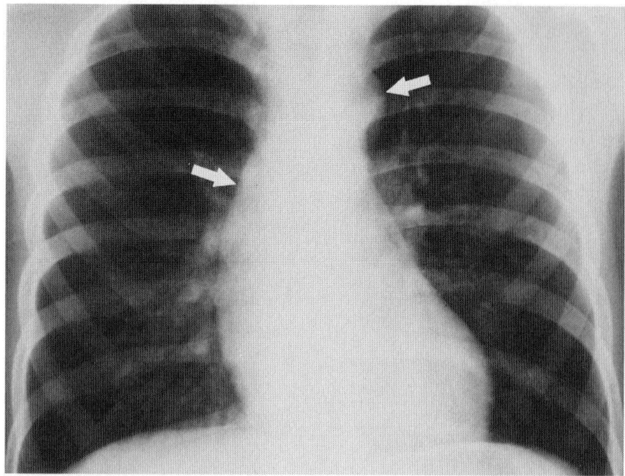

FIGURE 51.80. **Aortic Valve Stenosis.** The ascending aorta and aortic arch are prominent (*arrows*) in this 5-year-old child with congenial aortic stenosis.

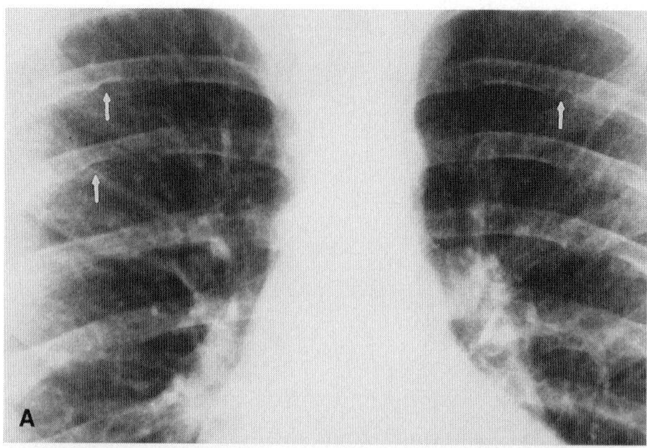

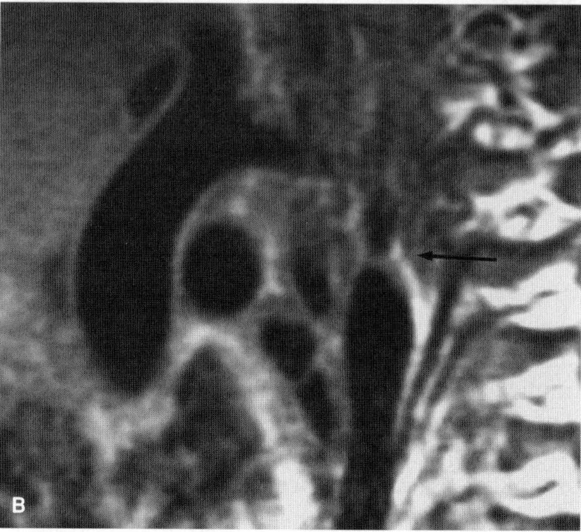

FIGURE 51.82. **Coarctation of the Aorta. A.** The small notches (*arrows*) along the inferior edges of some of the upper ribs bilaterally are caused by enlarged collateral vessels. **B.** A slightly oblique sagittal MR image clearly shows the area of coarctation (*arrow*).

Normal anteroposterior chamber relationships are preserved and there is no discordance. Visceral situs inversus is present, and the incidence of congenital heart disease in such patients is only slightly greater than that in patients with complete situs solitus.

Dextroversion refers to right-sided rotation of the cardiac position so that the RA and RV become more posterior and the LA and LV lie anterior. Chamber inversion does not occur in this condition. Visceral situs solitus or inversus can be present, and in either case congenital cyanotic heart disease is frequent. Other variations of dextroposition are relatively rare.

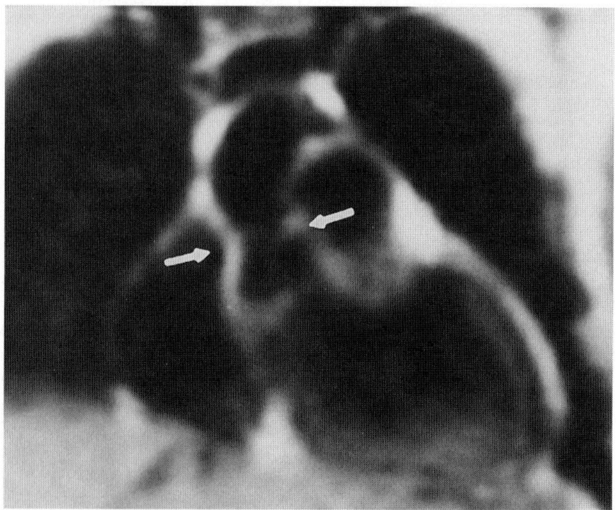

FIGURE 51.81. **Supravalvular Aortic Stenosis (Williams Syndrome).** Coronal MR demonstrates the short-segment narrowing of the aorta (*arrows*) just above the sinus of Valsalva.

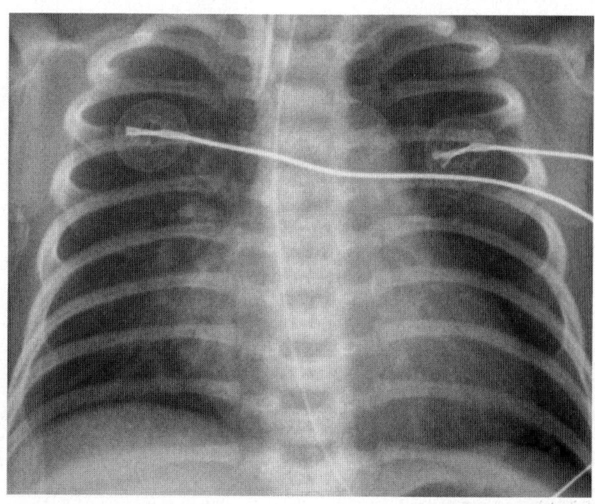

FIGURE 51.83. **Hypoplastic Left Heart Syndrome.** Cardiomegaly and passive pulmonary vascular congestion usually develop within the first few days of life.

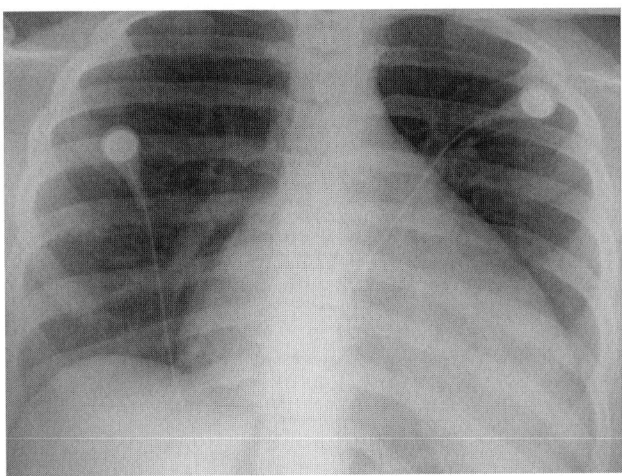

FIGURE 51.84. Cardiomyopathy. Note the marked cardiomegaly with left-sided predominance and early passive vascular congestion in this child with idiopathic cardiomyopathy.

Asplenia-Polysplenia Syndromes. Visceral heterotaxia and congenital heart disease are common components of the cardiosplenic (asplenia or polysplenia) syndromes. Asplenia (Ivemark) syndrome is usually associated with more severe forms of congenital heart disease than the polysplenia syndrome. The liver often lies in the midline, and intestinal malrotation commonly occurs. For simplicity's sake, the asplenia syndrome can be thought of as bilateral right-sidedness (i.e., absent spleen, bilateral three-lobed lung, bilateral superior vena cava) (Fig. 51.86), and polysplenia resembles bilateral left-sidedness (i.e., multiple spleens, bilateral bilobed lungs, interrupted inferior vena cava with azygos continuation, biliary atresia). Situs inversus with levocardia is an uncommon occurrence.

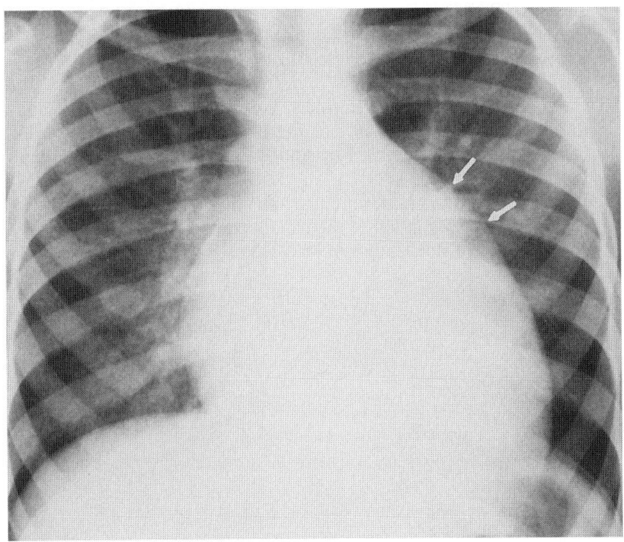

FIGURE 51.85. Endocardial Fibroelastosis. Both the LA (*arrows*) and LV are enlarged.

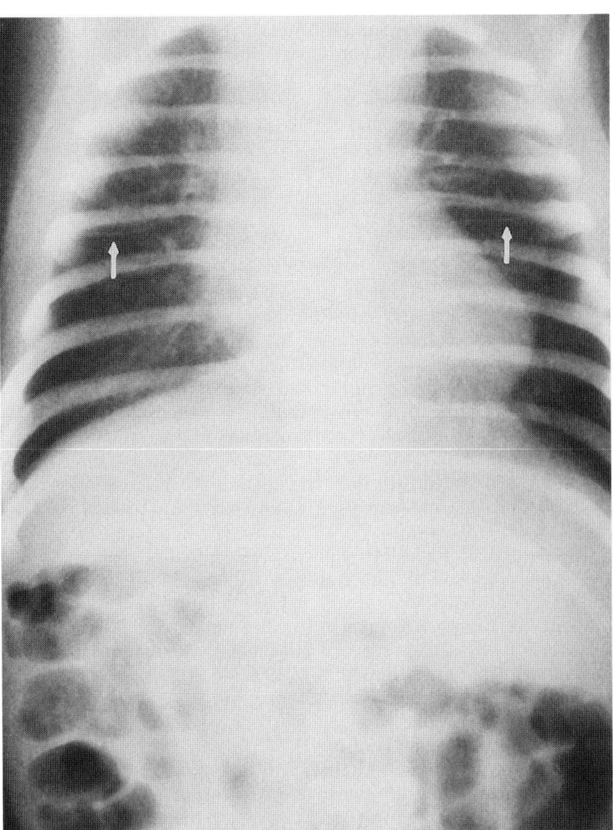

FIGURE 51.86. Asplenia Syndrome. The liver has a midline configuration and bilateral horizontal lung fissures are faintly seen (*arrows*).

Systemic venous abnormalities and congenital heart disease with right ventricular outflow tract obstruction are common associated abnormalities. US is useful to verify the presence or absence of splenic tissue and to evaluate venous anatomy (45).

Positional abnormalities of the aorta and great vessels are common, and the components of these anomalies are highly variable. The most important vascular anomalies are those that produce symptoms, mainly those of airway obstruction. These conditions were discussed previously.

REFERENCES

1. Swischuk LE, Hayden CK Jr. Lower respiratory tract infection in children (Is roentgenographic differentiation possible?). Pediatr Radiol 1986;16:278–284.
2. Khamapirad RT, Glezen WP. Clinical and radiographic assessment of acute lower respiratory tract disease in infants and children. Semin Respir Infect 1987;2:130–151.
3. John SD, Ramanathan J, Swischuk LE. The clinical and radiological spectrum of mycoplasma pneumonia. Radiographics 2001;21: 121–131.
4. Brody AS, Klein JS, Molina PL, et al. High-resolution computed tomography in young patients with cystic fibrosis: distribution of abnormalities and correlation with pulmonary function tests. J Pediatr 2004;145:6–7.

5. Scalzetti EM, Heitzman ER, Groskin SA, et al. Developmental lymphatic disorders of the thorax. Radiographics 1991;11:1069–1085.
6. Nobre LF, Muller NL, de Souza AS Jr, et al. Congenital pulmonary lymphangiectasia: CT and pathologic findings. J Thorac Imaging 2004;19:56–59.
7. Lynch DA, Hay T, Newell JD Jr, et al. Pediatric diffuse lung disease: diagnosis and classification using high-resolution CT. AJR Am J Roentgenol 1999;173:713–718.
8. Kim WS, Moon WK, Kim IO, et al. Pulmonary tuberculosis in children: evaluation with CT. AJR Am J Roentgenol 1997;168:1005–1009.
9. Daltro P, Fricke BL, Kuroki I, et al. CT of congenital lung lesions in pediatric patients. AJR Am J Roentgenol 2004;183:1497–1506.
10. Konen E, Raviv-Zilka L, Cohen RA, et al. Congenital pulmonary venolobar syndrome: spectrum of helical CT findings with emphasis on computerized reformatting. Radiographics 2003;23:1175–1184.
11. Lucaya J, Gartner S, Garcia-Pena P, et al. Spectrum of manifestations of Swyer-James-MacLeod syndrome. J Comput Assist Tomogr 1998;22:592–597.
12. Moore AD, Godwin JD, Dietrich PA, et al. Swyer-James syndrome: CT findings in eight patients. AJR Am J Roentgenol 1992;158:1211–1215.
13. Pickhardt PJ, Siegel MJ, Gutierrez FR. Vascular rings in symptomatic children: frequency of chest radiographic findings. Radiology 1997;203:423–426.
14. Katz ML, Konen E, Rozenman J, et al. Spiral CT and 3D image construction of vascular rings and associated tracheobronchial anomalies. J Comput Assist Tomogr 1995;19:564–568.
15. Beckman RP, Hazekamp MG, Sobotka MA, et al. A new diagnostic approach to vascular rings and pulmonary slings: the role of MRI. Magn Reson Imaging 1998;16:137–145.
16. Rosado-de-Christenson ML, Stocker JT. From the archives of the AFIP congenital cystic adenomatoid malformation. Radiographics 1991;11:865–886.
17. Swischuk LE, Shetty B, John SD. The lungs in immature infants; how important is surfactant therapy in preventing chronic lung problems?. Pediatr Radiol 1996;26:508–511.
18. Swischuk LE, John SD. Immature lung problems: can our nomenclature be more specific? AJR Am J Roentgenol 1996;166:917–918.
19. Fitzgerald P, Donoghue V, Gorman W. Bronchopulmonary dysplasia: a radiographic and clinical review of 20 patients. Br J Radiol 1990;63:514–517.
20. Aquino SL, Schechter MS, Chiles C, et al. High-resolution inspiratory and expiratory CT in older children and adults with bronchopulmonary dysplasia. AJR Am J Roentgenol 1999;173:963–967.
21. Gross GW, Cullen J, Kornhauser MS. Thoracic complications of extracorporeal membrane oxygenation: findings on chest radiographs and sonograms. AJR Am J Roentgenol 1992;158:353–358.
22. Amodio JB, Abramson SJ, Berdon WE, Solar C, Markowitz R, Kasznica J. Iatrogenic causes of large pleural fluid collections in the premature infant: ultrasonic and radiographic findings. Pediatr Radiol 1987;17:104–108.
23. West MS, Donaldson JS, Shkolnik A. Pulmonary sequestration: diagnosis by ultrasound. J Ultrasound Med 1989;8:125–130.
24. Lee EY, Siegel MJ, Sierra LM, et al. Evaluation of angioarchitecture of pulmonary sequestration in pediatric patients using 3D MDCT angiography. AJR Am J Roentgenol 2004;183–188.
25. Berrocal T, Madrid C, Novo S, et al. Congenital anomalies of the tracheobronchial tree, lung, and mediastinum: embryology, radiology, and pathology. Radiographics 2004;24:e17. Epub 2003 Nov 10.
26. Lehnhardt S, Winterer JT, Uhrmeister P, et al. Pulmonary sequestration: demonstration of blood supply with 2D and 3D MR angiography. Eur J Radiol 2002;44:28–32.
27. Naffaa LN, Donnelly LF. Imaging findings in pleuropulmonary blastoma. Pediatr Radiol 2005;35:387–391.
28. Han BK, Suh YL, Yoon HK. Thymic ultrasound. I. Intrathymic anatomy in infants. Pediatr Radiol 2001;31:474–479.
29. Han BK, Yoon HK, Suh YL. Thymic ultrasound. II. Diagnosis of aberrant cervical thymus. Pediatr Radiol 2001;31:480–487.
30. Koumanidou C, Vakaki M, Theophanopoulou M, et al. Aberrant thymus in infants: sonographic evaluation. Pediatr Radiol 1998;28:987–989.
31. Moeller KH, Rosado-de-Christenson ML. Mediastinal mature teratoma: imaging features. AJR Am J Roentgenol 1997;169:985–990.
32. Ueno T, Tanaka YO, Nagata M, et al. Spectrum of germ cell tumors: from head to toe. Radiographics 2004;24:387–404.
33. Leung AN, Müller NL, Pineda PR, et al. Primary tuberculosis in childhood: radiographic manifestations. Radiology 1992;182:87–91.
34. McAdams HP, Kirejczyk WM, Rosado-de-Christenson ML, et al. Bronchogenic cyst: imaging features with clinical and histopathologic correlation. Radiology 2000;217:441–446.
35. Saenz NC, Schnitzer JJ, Eraklis AE, et al. Posterior mediastinal masses. J Pediatr Surg 1993;28:172–176.
36. Lonergan GJ, Schwab CM, Suarez ES, et al. Neuroblastoma, ganglioneuroblastoma, and ganglioneuroma: radiologic-pathologic correlation. Radiographics 2002;22:911–934.
37. Slovis TL, Meza MP, Cushing B, et al. Thoracic neuroblastoma: what is the best imaging modality for evaluating extent of disease? Pediatr Radiol 1997;27:273–275.
38. Sallustio G, Pirronti T, Lasorella A, et al. Diagnostic imaging of primitive neuroectodermal tumour of the chest wall (Askin tumour). Pediatr Radiol 1998;697–702.
39. Groom KR, Murphey MD, Howard LM, Lonergan GJ, Rosado-de-Christensen ML, Torop AH. Mesenchymal hamartoma of the chest wall: radiologic manifestations with emphasis on cross-sectional imaging and histopathologic comparison. Radiology 2002;205–211.
40. Boxt LM. Magnetic resonance and computed tomographic evaluation of congenital heart disease. J Magn Reson Imaging 2004;19:827–847.
41. Gutierrez FR, Siegel MJ, Fallah JH, et al. Magnetic resonance imaging of cyanotic and noncyanotic congenital heart disease. Magn Reson Imaging Clin North Am 2002;10:209–235.
42. Haramati LB, Glickstein JS, Issenberg HJ, et al. MR imaging and CT of vascular anomalies and connections in patients with congenital heart disease: significance in surgical planning. Radiographics 2002;22:337–347.
43. Choe YH, Kim YM, Han BK, et al. MR imaging in the morphologic diagnosis of congenital heart disease. Radiographics 1997;17:403–422.
44. Craig JM, Darling RC, Rothney WB. Total pulmonary venous drainage into the right side of the heart: report of 17 autopsied cases not associated with other major cardiovascular anomalies. Lab Invest 1957;6:44–65.
45. Hernanz-Schulman M, Ambrosino MM, Genieser NB, et al. Pictorial essay. Current evaluation of the patient with abnormal visceroatrial situs. AJR Am J Roentgenol 1990;797–802.

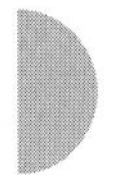

Chapter 52

Pediatric Abdomen and Pelvis

Susan D. John and Leonard E. Swischuk

Gastrointestinal Tract
Gastrointestinal Obstruction
Inflammation and Infection
Gastrointestinal Bleeding

Genitourinary Tract
Renal Abnormalities
Bladder and Urethral Abnormalities
Genital Abnormalities

Abdominal Masses
Renal and Adrenal Masses
Hepatobiliary Masses
Splenic Lesions
Gastrointestinal and Pancreatic Masses
Masses of the Reproductive Organs
Presacral Masses

GASTROINTESTINAL TRACT

Gastrointestinal Obstruction

GI obstruction is a relatively common problem in infants and children and must be distinguished from numerous other causes of vomiting and abdominal distension. The causes of intestinal obstruction in children are widely varied in urgency and management implications, and imaging plays a critical role in the appropriate treatment of such conditions. The most likely causes of obstruction in children shift in importance according to age; therefore, it is helpful to consider the various causes of obstruction within four age-group categories (Table 52.1). Determination of the level of obstruction also helps to infer the possible etiology. Abdominal radiographs continue to be a useful initial screening examination for assessing the site of obstruction and determining the need for further imaging.

Hypopharyngeal/upper esophageal obstruction is uncommon in infants and children but may be caused by a spasm of the cricopharyngeus muscle. Cricopharyngeal spasm may be related to neurologic dysfunction (e.g., Chiari malformation, cerebral palsy) or inflammation resulting from gastroesophageal reflux (GER). Lack of normal cricopharyngeus muscle relaxation disturbs the well-coordinated swallowing mechanism and can lead to aspiration. In refractory cases, surgical division of the muscle may be required.

Difficulties with swallowing can also occur with inflammatory processes such as epiglottitis, retropharyngeal abscess, tonsillar abscess, or a number of tumors or cysts that occur in this area. A large pharyngeal diverticulum may produce obstruction. These diverticula can be congenital or iatrogenic owing to perforation of the hypopharynx during intubation. They are best demonstrated with barium swallow.

Esophageal Obstruction

Esophageal Atresia and Tracheoesophageal Fistula. The most common congenital obstruction of the esophagus is esophageal atresia (Table 52.2). This anomaly is a result of faulty development and separation of the embryonic foregut early in gestation. The site of atresia is usually in the upper third of the esophagus. The air-filled upper esophageal pouch is often visible on radiographs (Fig. 52.1). The distended proximal esophageal pouch may cause pressure on the trachea during fetal development, resulting in focal tracheomalacia.

Esophageal atresia is frequently associated with tracheoesophageal fistula. Most commonly, the fistula extends obliquely from the trachea, just above the carina, to the distal esophageal pouch. The fistula allows air to enter the stomach and intestines, in some cases in large volumes. Air in the GI tract differentiates this type of esophageal

TABLE 52.1 Most Common Causes of GI Tract Obstruction by Age

Age	Cause of Obstruction
0–1 month	Congenital anomalies
	Atresia/stenosis
	Malrotation/volvulus
	Hirschsprung disease
	Meconium plug/small left colon syndrome
	Meconium ileus
1–5 months	Hernias
5 months–3 years	Intussusception
3 years and older	Perforated appendicitis
	Adhesions
	Regional enteritis

TABLE 52.2 Causes of Esophageal Obstruction

Congenital atresia/stenosis
Web/diverticulum
Foreign body
Stricture (peptic, caustic)
Extrinsic compression (cysts, neoplasms, vascular)
Achalasia

atresia from isolated esophageal atresia without tracheoesophageal fistula, in which the stomach and intestines remain gasless. The tracheoesophageal fistula may also develop without esophageal atresia. Such fistulas should be carefully sought on esophagrams performed on infants with choking or respiratory difficulty during feeding (Fig. 52.2). Much less commonly, esophageal atresia may be accompanied by a fistula from the proximal esophageal pouch to the trachea. A small amount of barium may be placed in the proximal esophageal pouch with an end-hole catheter to demonstrate such fistulas.

Esophageal atresia is more common in infants with trisomy 21 and may be associated with vertebral anomalies, duodenal atresia, anal rectal malformations, and other features of the VACTERL syndrome. The prognosis of infants with esophageal atresia depends primarily on the severity of associated anomalies and on the length of the atretic segment. Surgical repair is more challenging with long gap atresia. Common complications of esophageal atresia repair include anastomotic strictures (40%), anastomotic leakage (14% to 21%), and recurrent fistula (3% to 14%). Esophageal peristalsis is abnormal in patients with esophageal atresia, and GER is very common.

A variety of communications may exist between the esophageal pouch and the spine, ranging from fibrous bands to actual fistulae. If the communication involutes at both ends and only the central portion remains, a neurenteric cyst results. In other cases, an esophageal communication persists and a diverticulum is formed that extends into the spine or spinal canal (see Fig. 51.59). Faulty separation of the trachea and esophagus may also result in fistulae, fibrous bands, or diverticula. Tracheoesophageal fistula located high in the esophagus without esophageal atresia is the third most common abnormality in this group of lesions, following esophageal atresia with a distal tracheoesophageal fistula, and isolated esophageal atresia. The fistula is usually identified with barium swallow (Fig. 52.2).

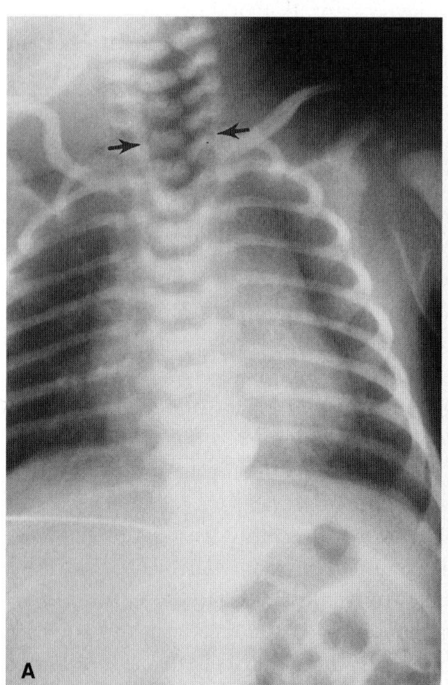

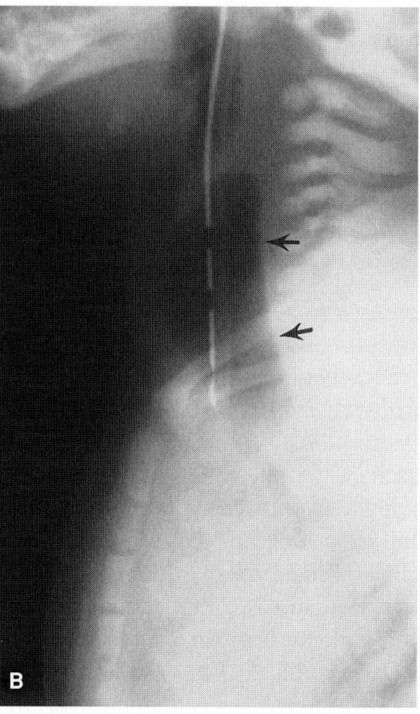

FIGURE 52.1. **Esophageal Atresia. A.** Frontal chest radiograph demonstrates the blind, air-filled upper esophageal pouch (*arrows*). Note the gas within the stomach and intestines, which indicates the presence of an associated lower tracheoesophageal fistula. **B.** Lateral view in another patient demonstrates the typical air-filled proximal esophageal pouch (*arrows*). Esophageal atresia prevents passage of the catheter beyond the pouch. The trachea is compressed and displaced by the dilated pouch.

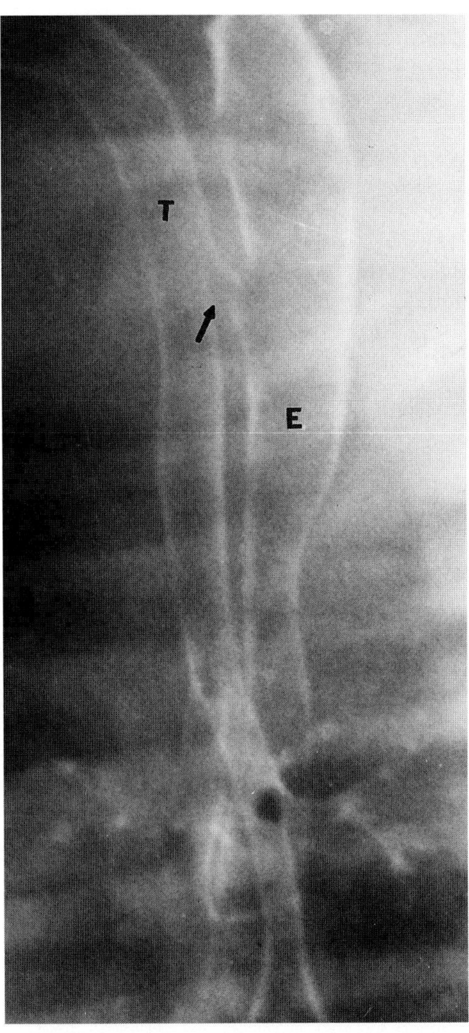

FIGURE 52.2. **Tracheoesophageal Fistula.** The trachea (T) and esophagus (E) are connected by a fistula (*arrow*).

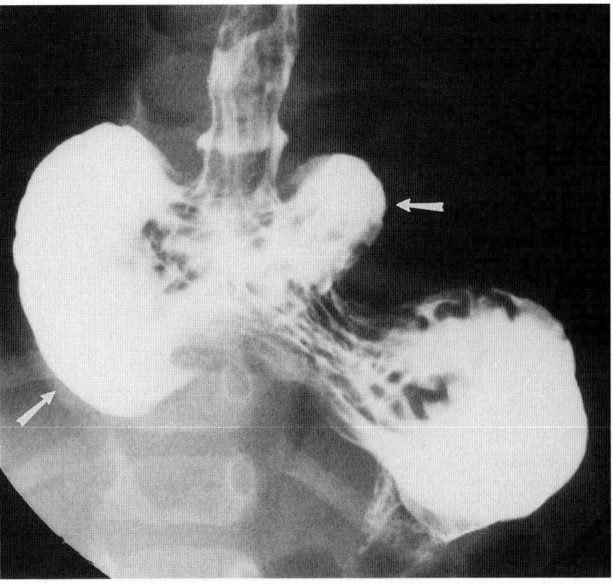

FIGURE 52.3. **Intrathoracic Stomach.** A large portion of the stomach lies above the diaphragm (*arrows*). Note reflux into a dilated, shortened esophagus with thickened mucosa, suggestive of inflammation.

Congenital esophageal stenosis is a far less common cause of congenital esophageal obstruction. As in esophageal atresia, esophageal stenosis arises from faulty tracheal and esophageal separation, where tracheobronchial cartilage remnants remain in the wall of the esophagus. On barium swallow, small diverticula (mucous glands) can be seen in the areas of stenosis.

Congenitally short esophagus with intrathoracic stomach is not a truly congenital lesion. Although it is seen at birth, this condition more likely represents the aftermath of chronic hiatal hernia during fetal life, with GER and subsequent esophageal stricture leading to shortening (Fig. 52.3).

Other uncommon congenital causes of esophageal obstruction include esophageal webs and diverticula.

Esophageal obstruction can also result from a variety of extrinsic lesions that produce pressure on the esophagus. Acquired esophageal obstructive lesions are primarily strictures or foreign bodies. Esophageal neoplasms are extremely rare in infants and children, and malignant neoplasms are virtually nonexistent.

Peptic esophagitis is associated with GER and can be seen with or without hiatus hernia. Although GER is very common in infants, peptic esophagitis with stricture is a relatively uncommon complication. GER may be primary (chalasia), caused by a lax gastroesophageal sphincter, or secondary to a gastric outlet obstruction. Causes of gastric obstruction (pylorospasm, pyloric stenosis, gastric diaphragm, gastric ulcer disease) must be excluded in infants with severe GER. GER is most reliably identified with 24-hour esophageal pH monitoring, but this procedure can be cumbersome and gives no direct information about obstruction. Nuclear gastric reflux studies are also quite sensitive, but barium upper GI series give more anatomic information and are often preferred. US with color Doppler can be used to detect GER, but the technique has not gained widespread popularity (1).

Usually, peptic esophageal strictures are short and located in the distal third of the esophagus. The occasional case of Barrett esophagus with a high stricture may also be encountered. Peptic strictures may be irregular or surprisingly smooth, mimicking the findings of achalasia (Fig. 52.4). Achalasia is uncommon as a cause of distal esophageal obstruction in children.

Caustic esophagitis with stricture usually results from accidental ingestion of alkaline substances such as sodium hydroxide, potassium hydroxide (lye), or alkaline disk batteries. Disk batteries can become lodged in the

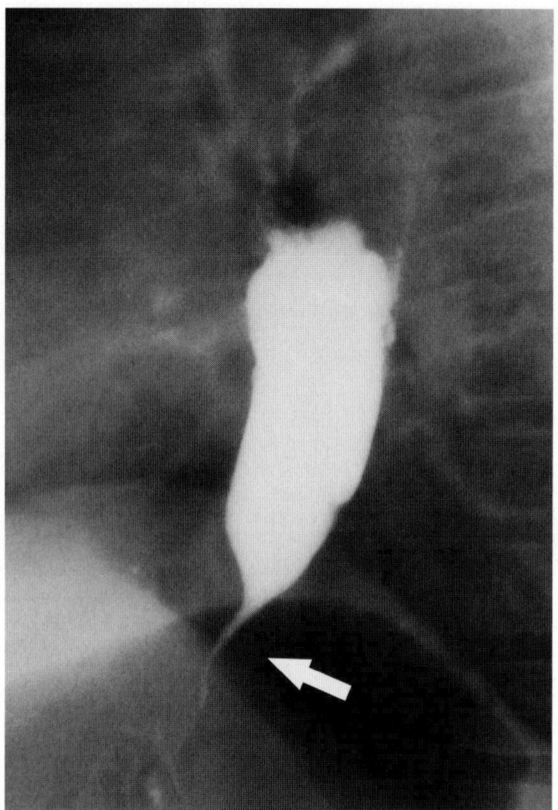

FIGURE 52.4. **Peptic Stricture.** The beaklike narrowing of the distal esophagus (*arrow*) caused by gastroesophageal reflux and stricture mimics achalasia.

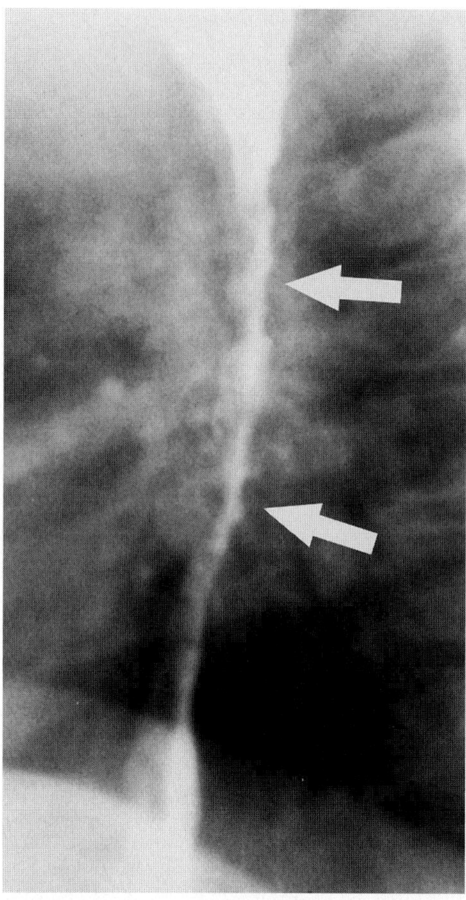

FIGURE 52.5. **Caustic (Lye) Stricture.** The long-segment, irregular configuration of the stricture (*arrows*) is characteristic of caustic ingestion.

esophagus and leak their alkaline contents, producing deep burns of the mucosa and submucosa. All alkaline burns cause deep penetrating injury that commonly results in stricture. Acids, even when swallowed in significant quantities, produce more superficial burns. While mucosal injury may be extensive, deep mural injury with fibrotic stricture is less common. Lye strictures lead to long areas of irregular narrowing (Fig. 52.5). Esophageal burns caused by an ingested battery or medication (aspirin, tetracycline, Clinitest tablets) result in a more focal stricture.

Epidermolysis bullosa is a hereditary condition characterized by inflammatory skin and mucosal lesions that can heal with fibrosis, resulting in esophageal stricture.

Acute Esophagitis. Other forms of esophageal inflammation are uncommon in children. Acute inflammation with spasm occurs with infectious esophagitis, caused by organisms such as *Candida* or herpes. These types of esophagitis are more common in immunocompromised children. Eosinophilic esophagitis is thought to be allergic in nature and is most commonly seen in children with asthma.

Gastric Obstruction

Congenital obstructing lesions of the stomach are far less common than congenital obstructing lesions elsewhere in the GI tract (Table 52.3). Gastric distension on radiographs does not always indicate obstruction in infants. A large, gas-filled stomach is commonly seen in normal infants, and persistent asymptomatic gastric distention occurs in infants receiving prostaglandins for ductal-dependent congenital heart disease (2).

TABLE 52.3 Causes of Gastric Obstruction

Atresia/antral diaphragm
Duplication cyst
Pylorospasm
Hypertrophic pyloric stenosis
Gastritis/ulcer disease
Volvulus
Microgastria

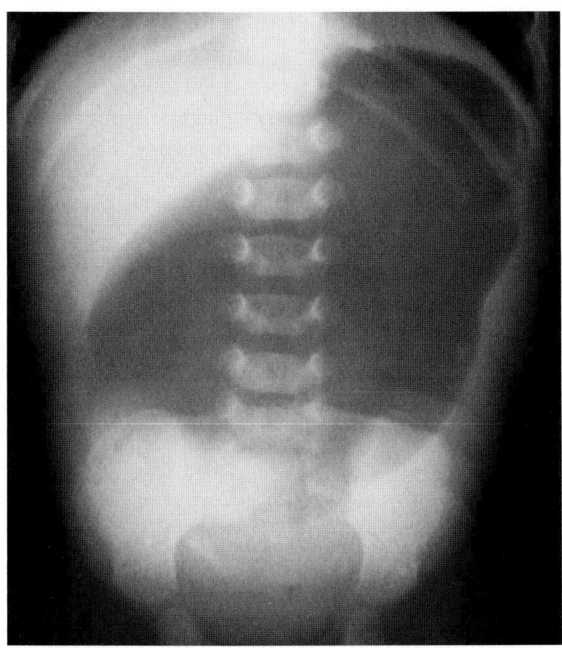

FIGURE 52.6. **Gastric Atresia.** Typical findings consist of a dilated, air-filled stomach, with no air distal to the pylorus.

Gastric atresia is believed to result from a vascular insult to the stomach in utero. In the newborn infant, if obstruction of the stomach is complete, radiographs show no air distal to the stomach (Fig. 52.6). Gastric atresia usually occurs at the level of the pylorus. In some cases, atresia takes the form of a gastric diaphragm or membrane, which if incomplete, will allow some gas distal to the obstructing web. US or an upper GI series can be used to identify the incomplete diaphragm.

Gastric atresia may occur in infants with congenital epidermolysis bullosa because of inflammatory stricture. *Microgastria* occurs with other GI atresias or VACTERL syndrome and is commonly associated with the polysplenia/asplenia syndromes.

Gastric duplications must be critically located in the antrum or be very large to result in obstruction. They are best demonstrated with US, where they appear sonolucent with a wall that demonstrates both mucosal and muscular layers (see Fig. 52.68).

Gastric volvulus is an uncommon cause of gastric obstruction in children. The volvulus may be idiopathic or may be associated with congenital conditions that involve abnormal position of the stomach, such as diaphragmatic hernia, diaphragmatic eventration, or asplenia syndrome. Gastric volvulus may be classified as organoaxial, in which the stomach rotates along its longitudinal axis, or mesoaxial, in which it rotates about a line perpendicular to the cardiopyloric line. Gastric volvulus should be considered an acute surgical emergency; however, in some children volvulus may be chronic.

Pylorospasm is a reactive problem secondary to insult to the gastric mucosa or muscle contraction from other causes of stress. Mucosal inflammation may be caused by milk allergy or peptic disease with ulceration. Real-time US demonstrates persistent contraction of the antropyloric region and poor emptying of liquids from the stomach. Mild (<3 mm) thickening of the outer circular muscle occasionally can be seen (Fig 52.7). Muscle

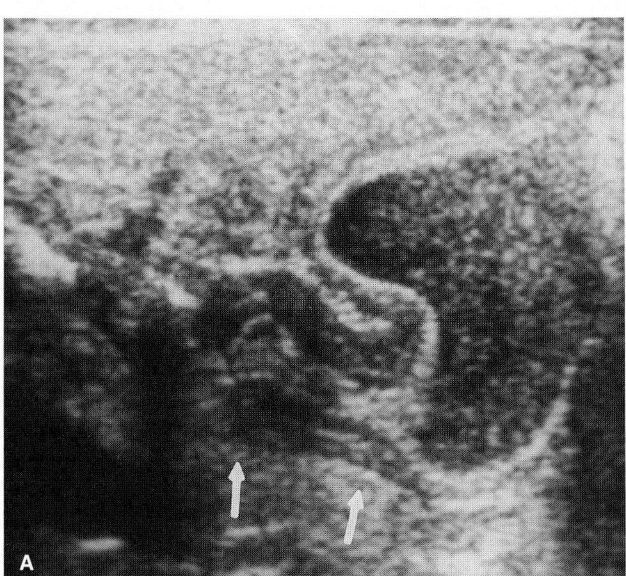

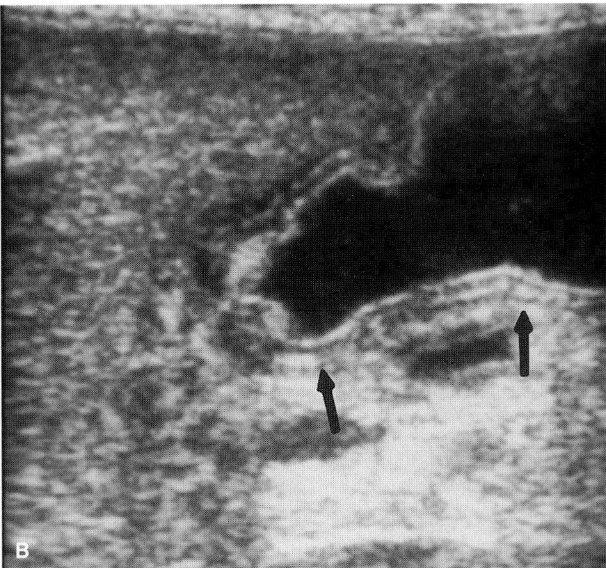

FIGURE 52.7. **Pylorospasm US Features. A.** The antrum is contracted. The muscle is slightly thickened but measures less than 3 mm (*arrows*). **B.** After treatment with antispasm medication, the antrum opens, peristaltic activity is present, and the muscle has returned to normal thickness (*arrows*).

thickening greater than 3 mm is only a transient phenomenon in pylorospasm (3). During sonography, the antropyloric muscle relaxes, causing the muscle thickness to return to normal and allowing gastric contents to pass into the duodenum. The findings can be demonstrated with upper GI series, but US usually suffices.

Hypertrophic pyloric stenosis is now generally considered to be an acquired condition that, in some cases, may be related to prolonged pylorospasm. The abnormal muscle has been shown to be depleted of various components, which may lead to uninhibited muscle contraction, and blood flow is increased on color Doppler US in both muscle and mucosa (4). The condition most often develops between 2 and 10 weeks of age and is characterized by hypertrophy of the pyloric muscle. US is the preferred examination because of its ability to directly assess the thickness of the pyloric muscle and to provide real-time evaluation of contraction of the pyloric canal (5). The hypertrophied pyloric muscle measures 3 mm or more in thickness, and the pyloric canal is elongated beyond 14 mm (Fig. 52.8). The pylorus is in fixed spasm and very little fluid passes through it. In atypical cases the pyloric canal is fixed in spasm, but the muscle measures 2 to 3 mm in thickness, whereas normal muscle measures no more than 1.5 mm in thickness. These patients may be treated medically but should be followed closely, as some may progress to classic pyloric stenosis.

Tangential imaging of the normal, but contracted, pyloric canal may result in an erroneous impression of muscle thickening. Furthermore, it has been demonstrated in pyloric stenosis that at the 6:00 and 12:00 positions, the pyloric muscle may not be as hypoechoic as it is at the 3:00 and 9:00 positions. As the circular muscle passes over the 6:00 and 12:00 positions, more acoustic interfaces are encountered and more echogenicity results. Finally, if the stomach is overfilled, the pyloric muscle mass can assume a posterior, upwardly curving position, making it more difficult to identify (6).

Gastric tumors are quite uncommon but produce the same findings as in adults. Gastric teratomas can occur in the neonate and can be quite large at presentation.

Gastric bezoars are masses or retained gastric solid contents that may result in gastric outlet obstruction. Bezoars may consist of hair (trichobezoar), milk products (lactobezoar), vegetable material (phytobezoar), or cloth that is chronically chewed and swallowed, especially by developmentally delayed children. Air or barium outlining the bezoar is diagnostic (Fig. 52.9). On US, an echogenic arc over the bezoar is characteristic (7,8). The arc is caused by echoes from the layer of air trapped between the bezoar and the gastric wall. CT shows an air-containing mass that is not attached to the gastric wall.

Duodenal Obstruction

Congenital duodenal obstructions are more common than acquired obstructions in pediatric patients (Table 52.4). Radiographs localize the level of obstruction, which determines whether further imaging is required.

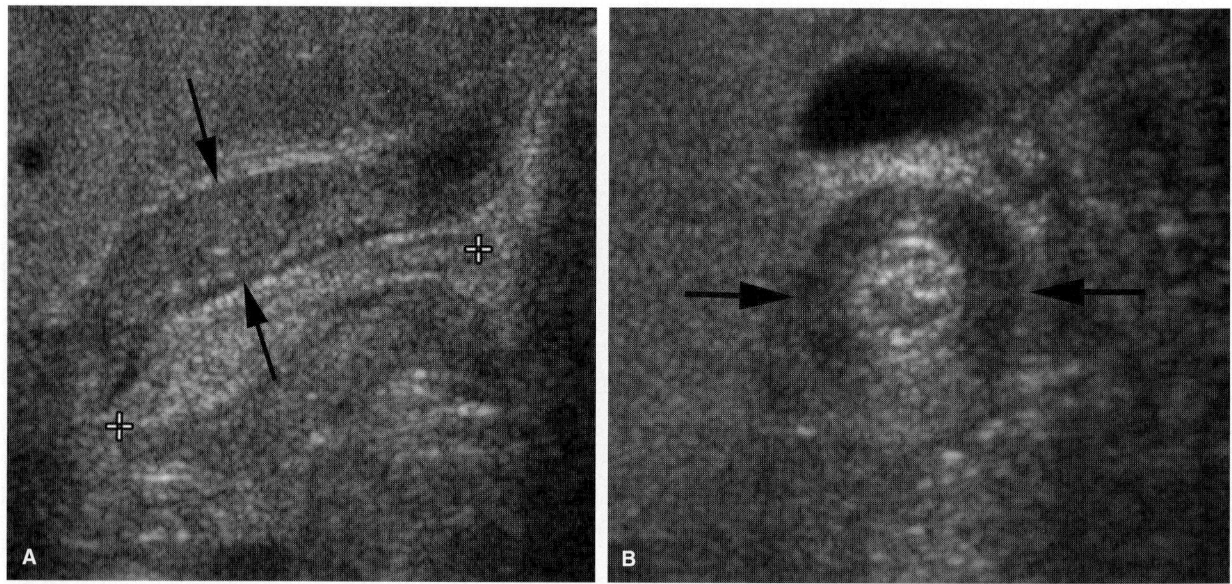

FIGURE 52.8. **Pyloric Stenosis. A.** Longitudinal view through the pylorus demonstrates the classic elongated pyloric canal (*arrows*) with thick outer hypoechoic muscle (*arrows*) exceeding 4 mm in thickness. Note the echogenic layers of mucosa and the linear collections of fluid in the lumen. The canal measures 2.04 cm in length (*between cursors*). **B.** Cross-sectional view demonstrates the typical sonolucent donut configuration (*arrows*).

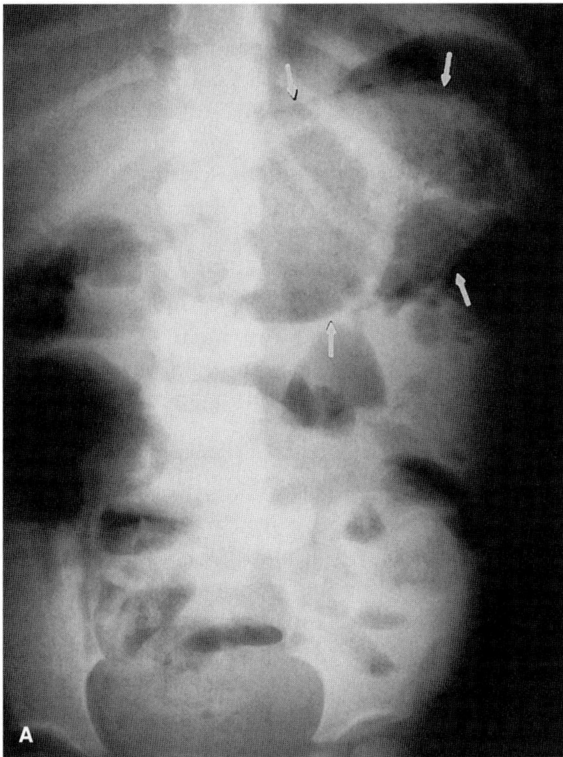

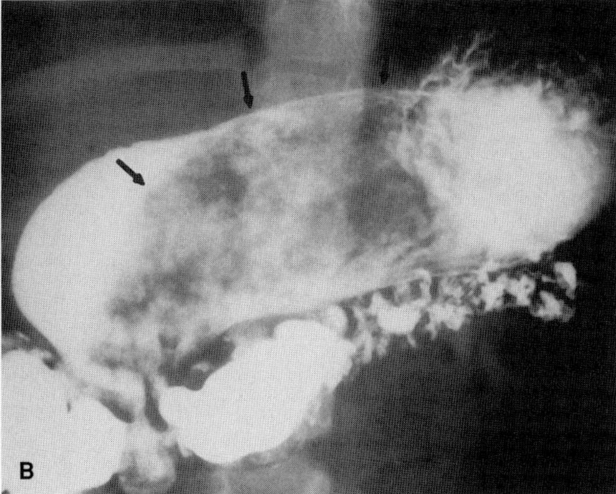

FIGURE 52.9. **Bezoar. A.** A filling defect (*arrows*) is seen in the stomach. **B.** Upper GI series demonstrates barium in the interstices of the intraluminal mass (*arrows*), characteristic of a bezoar.

Duodenal Atresia/Annular Pancreas. In a normal infant, gas passes from the stomach into small bowel during the first hours of life. When the stomach and duodenal bulb are distended with gas ("double bubble" sign) and no gas is present distally (Fig. 52.10), the best diagnostic possibilities are duodenal atresia or annular pancreas. No further imaging is required. Rarely, a small amount of air may be seen in the distal GI tract in duodenal atresia, with an anomalous Y configuration of the hepatopancreatic duct. The upper limb connects to the pre-atretic duodenum, while the lower limb connects to the post-atretic duodenum, allowing air to pass into the distal small bowel. Air distal to a double-bubble obstructive pattern also can be seen with duodenal stenosis or duodenal web with a central perforation. Contrast studies are indicated in these cases to distinguish them from midgut volvulus (Fig. 52.11). US can demonstrate the dilated duodenal bulb with any cause of duodenal obstruction when the duodenum is filled with fluid.

TABLE 52.4 Causes of Duodenal Obstruction

Atresia/stenosis/diaphragm
Annular pancreas
Duodenal band
Midgut volvulus
Hematoma
Neoplasm (duodenum, pancreas, liver)
Peptic ulcer disease

Midgut Volvulus. When the obstruction of the duodenum is located at the third or fourth portions of the duodenum, the most likely causes are duodenal diaphragm or intestinal malrotation with midgut volvulus or an obstructing peritoneal band. Midgut volvulus is a complication of intestinal rotational anomalies that are accompanied by abnormal positions and poor fixation of the duodenum and small bowel. Rotational abnormalities of the intestines are

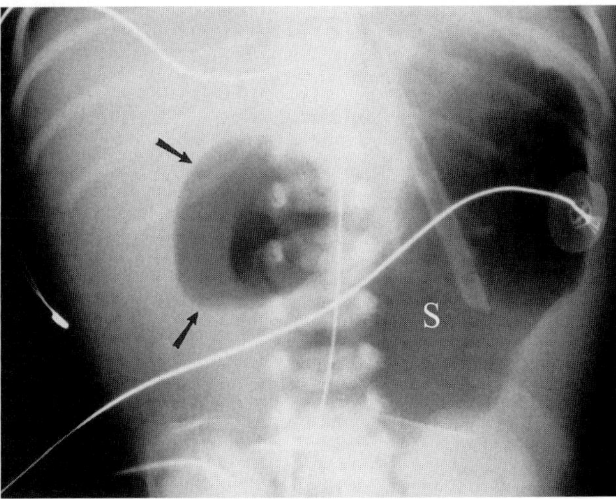

FIGURE 52.10. **Duodenal Atresia.** The classic double-bubble sign consists of a distended duodenal bulb (*arrows*) and a distended stomach (S).

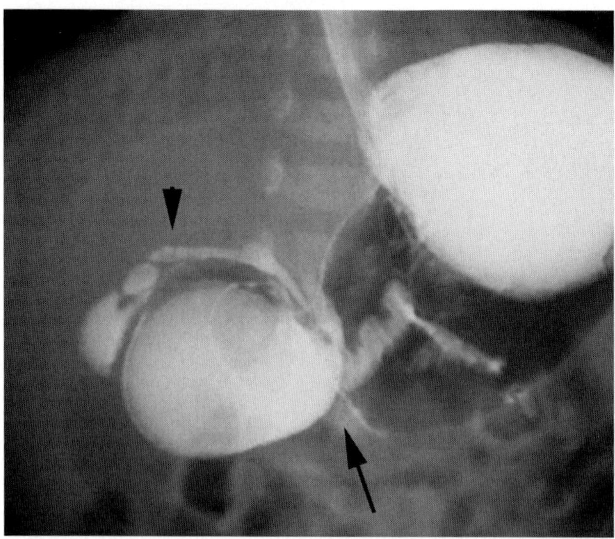

FIGURE 52.11. **Duodenal Diaphragm.** Partial obstruction in the descending duodenum is caused by an incomplete diaphragm (*arrow*). Note retrograde filling of the bile ducts with contrast (*arrowhead*).

developmental abnormalities that may vary from isolated poor fixation of the duodenum to complete nonrotation of the intestine with the colon residing in the left abdomen and small bowel on the right (9,10). A narrow peritoneal attachment in such patients may allow the small bowel to become twisted by active peristalsis. The site of most proximal obstructions usually resides in the midportion of the duodenum. The stomach and duodenum may appear dilated on radiographs, and gas is usually present in the distal bowel (Fig. 52.12). In the supine position, the distended

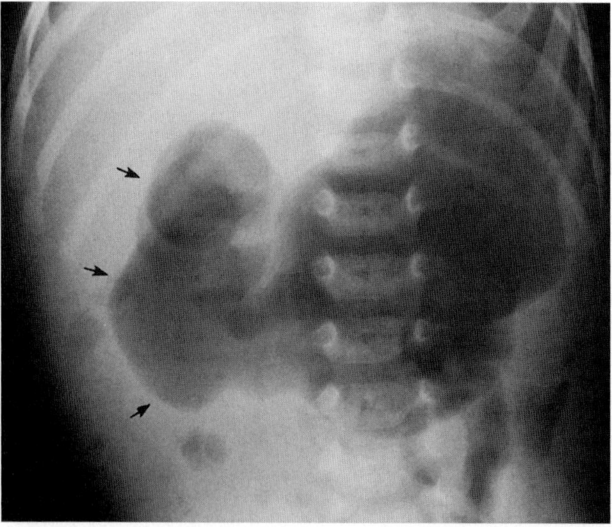

FIGURE 52.12. **Midgut Volvulus.** The stomach, duodenal bulb, and descending duodenum (*arrows*) are distended, but the remainder of the intestine shows sparse gas.

duodenum may contain fluid rather than air, erroneously suggesting a gastric obstruction. In other patients, the abdominal radiograph may appear normal.

A contrast study is mandatory to determine whether volvulus is present. In the past, the barium enema was commonly used to show the cecum displaced high into the midabdomen, just under the transverse colon (Fig. 52.13A). However, because the cecum tends to be mobile in normal infants, any position lower than the transverse colon cannot be interpreted as representative of midgut volvulus. The upper GI series is most commonly used to directly demonstrate obstruction of the duodenum. If midgut volvulus is present, a characteristic beaklike deformity is seen at the point of obstruction, usually just before the duodenum crosses the midline (Fig. 52.13B). US demonstrates these findings along with reversal of the position of the superior mesenteric artery and vein, which is indicative of intestinal malrotation (Fig. 52.13C). Normally the superior mesenteric vein lies to the right of the artery, but with malrotation the vein sits anterior or to the left of the artery. A spiral "whirlpool" appearance on US is highly suggestive of volvulus (11,12). Contrast-enhanced CT shows the abnormal vascular position in addition to findings of bowel infarction when present (13).

Total obstruction at the third portion of the duodenum also can be seen with peritoneal bands (Ladd bands) that frequently accompany rotational abnormalities of the intestines. These bands produce an oblique indentation of the third or fourth portion of the duodenum. With a little time (5 to 10 minutes), some barium may pass through the obstruction and outline a corkscrew appearance of the small bowel when volvulus is present (Fig. 52.13D). The small bowel is malpositioned in the right or midabdomen rather than in its usual left upper quadrant position. Bowel edema caused by venous stasis may also be encountered. Other congenital abnormalities leading to obstruction at this level are duodenal webs and diaphragms, enteric duplication cysts, and, rarely, a preduodenal portal vein.

Duodenal hematoma is perhaps the most common acquired cause of duodenal obstruction. Hematomas usually result from blunt abdominal trauma, commonly caused by motor vehicle collisions or battered child syndrome. CT or US may demonstrate asymmetric or concentric thickening of the duodenal wall at the site of the hematoma. The findings may be confirmed by contrast duodenography (Fig. 52.14). Findings suggestive of duodenal laceration on CT include retroperitoneal air or fluid (14). Intramural hematomas may also occur in children with hemophilia or Henoch-Schönlein purpura.

Obstruction of the duodenum secondary to peptic ulcer disease is rare in children. Duodenal tumors are also rare; however, extrinsic masses occur and may cause obstruction. The duodenum is a common site of origin for intestinal duplication cysts.

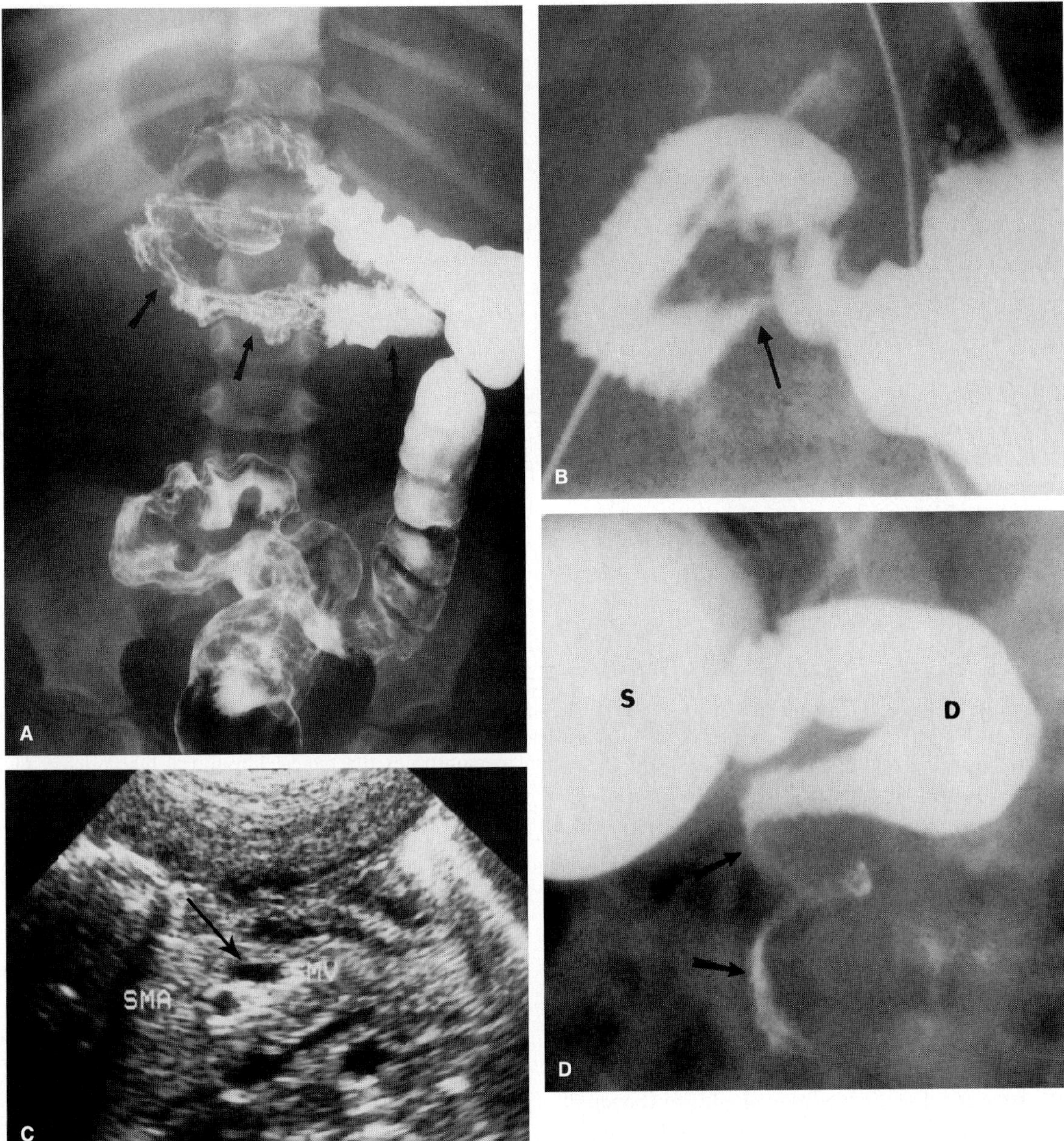

FIGURE 52.13. **Midgut Volvulus. A.** Barium enema demonstrates the typical high medial position of the ascending colon and cecum (*arrows*) with a twisted loop of hepatic flexure. **B.** Upper GI series demonstrates the typical beaklike obstruction (*arrow*) of the third portion of the duodenum, secondary to volvulus. The beak characteristically lies at or just to the right of the spine. **C.** US demonstrates the superior mesenteric vein (SMV, *arrow*) in an abnormal position to the left of the superior mesenteric artery (SMA). **D.** Upper GI series demonstrates typical spiraling of the small bowel (*arrows*). D, descending duodenum; S, stomach.

Small Intestinal Obstruction

Small intestinal obstruction in the neonate and young infant is more likely to be congenital, whereas in the older child, acquired problems are more common (Table 52.5). In the neonate it is difficult to distinguish distal small bowel obstruction from colonic obstruction on plain radiographs. Obstruction anywhere between the ileum and the rectum can produce a similar pattern of numerous dilated loops of intestine. A contrast enema must be performed to better evaluate the location of obstruction.

Jejunal Atresia. Jejunal and ileal atresia are caused by interruption of mesenteric blood supply during fetal development. Radiographs demonstrate a variable number of dilated loops of jejunum, depending on the level of atresia, with no gas distally (Fig. 52.15). Often, no further contrast

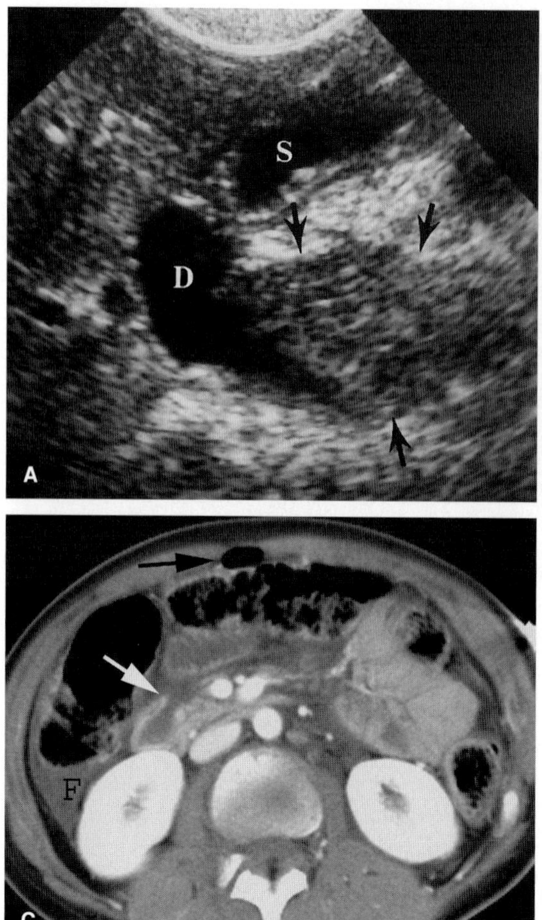

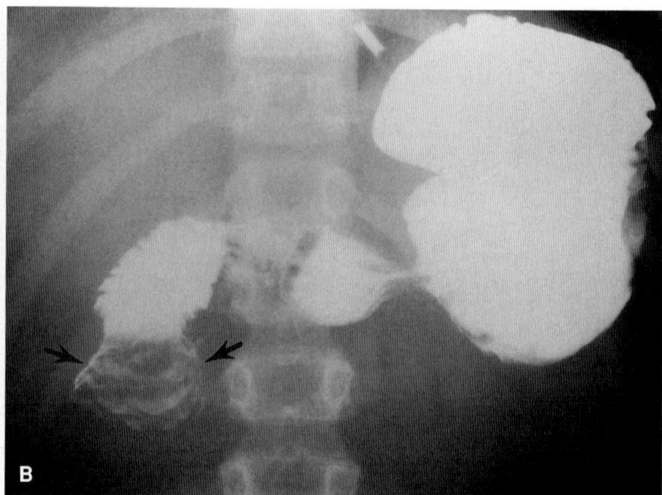

FIGURE 52.14. **Duodenal Injuries. A.** US demonstrates an echogenic hematoma (*arrows*) causing obstruction of the duodenum (D). S, stomach. **B.** Upper GI series in another patient demonstrates the typical intramural filling defect of the hematoma (*arrows*). **C.** CT of a child injured in a motor vehicle collision shows free fluid adjacent to the right kidney (F) and free intraperitoneal air anteriorly (*black arrow*). The duodenal wall enhances and there is a possible disruption of the duodenal wall (*white arrow*).

studies are required. A variation of intestinal atresia, described as *apple peel small bowel*, consists of diffuse atresia of the small bowel with multiple sites of severe stenosis and a spiral configuration of the atretic segment. This condition tends to be familial. Segmental volvulus of the small bowel can occur anywhere along its length, but is an uncommon cause of jejunal obstruction. Similarly, internal hernias are rare.

Ileal atresia and meconium ileus are the most common causes of distal small bowel obstruction in the neonate. In both conditions, contrast studies reveal a characteristic generalized microcolon, indicating that

TABLE 52.5 Causes of Small Intestinal Obstruction

Causes
Atresia/stenosis
Meconium ileus
Incarcerated hernia
Intussusception
Perforated appendicitis
Regional enteritis
Posttraumatic hematoma/stricture

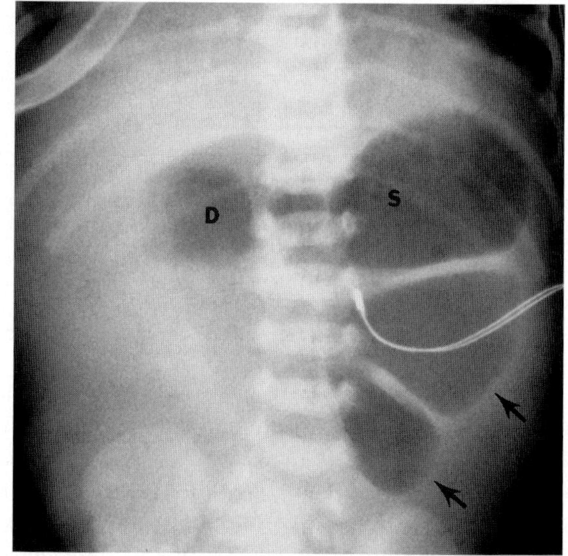

FIGURE 52.15. **Jejunal Atresia.** Plain film shows distention of the stomach (S), duodenum (D), and loops of the upper intestine (*arrows*). No air is present distal to the proximal jejunum.

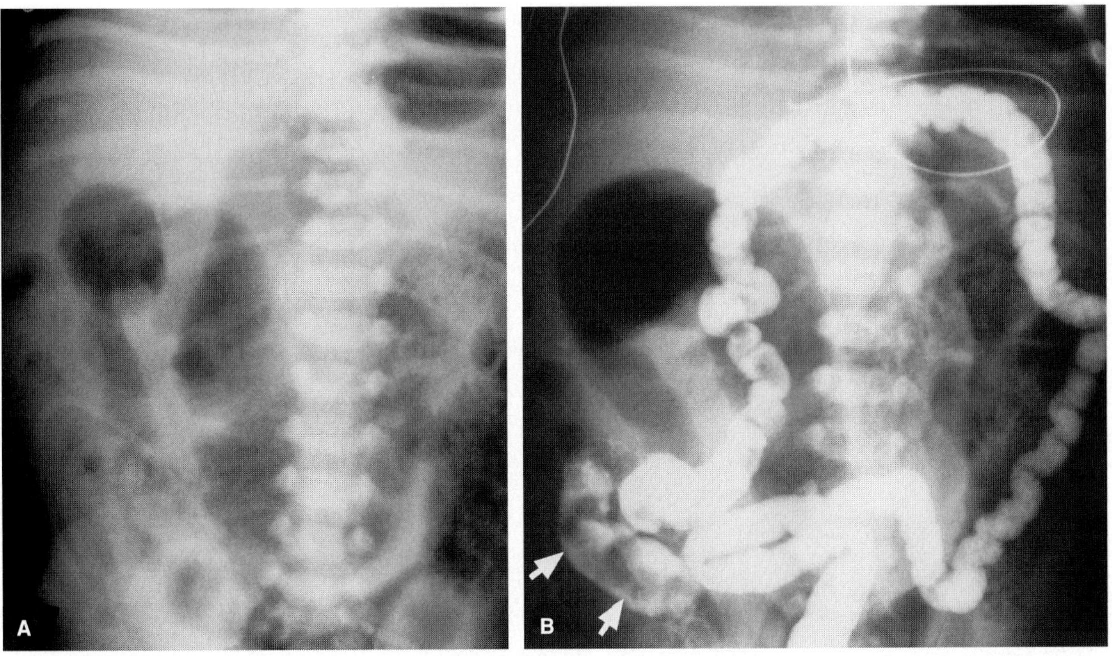

FIGURE 52.16. **Meconium Ileus. A.** Plain film shows the "soap-bubble" effect of air mixed with meconium in the numerous distended loops of intestine. **B.** Contrast enema demonstrates a typical microcolon with reflux into the terminal ileum, which is filled with pellets of meconium (*arrows*).

meconium has not passed normally into the colon during fetal life. Meconium ileus is usually the earliest manifestation of cystic fibrosis (15). It results from abnormally thick meconium, which forms plugs that cannot pass through the ileocecal valve. Plain radiographs demonstrate multiple dilated loops of small intestine, with bubbly intestinal contents representing retained meconium (Fig. 52.16A). When air–fluid levels are present in the dilated small bowel, ileal atresia is the more likely diagnosis. It is important to distinguish between the two conditions, because ileal atresia is corrected surgically whereas meconium ileus is often treated with water-soluble contrast enema. When performing such an enema, contrast material should reflux into the terminal ileum to outline, as well as lubricate, the inspissated meconium (Fig. 52.16B). This procedure should be performed carefully because of the increased risk of perforation of a microcolon. If contrast does not reflux into the terminal ileum, surgery is required for definitive diagnosis as well as treatment.

Meconium plug syndrome is a misleading name for a condition caused by functional immaturity and abnormal peristalsis of the distal colon. Also known as *small left colon syndrome*, this condition should not be confused with meconium ileus. In meconium plug syndrome, a normal to dilated proximal colon filled with meconium and an empty distal descending colonic segment are characteristic (Fig. 52.17). The meconium in infants with this condition is normal and is not the cause of obstruction. This condition is more common in normal large infants and infants of diabetic mothers. The functional obstruction is transient and can often be treated by rectal stimulation or saline enemas. In more persistent cases, an enema using contrast that contains Tween 80 (such as Gastrografin [diatrizoate meglumine and diatrizoate sodium solution]) can be used to irritate the colon and stimulate defecation. Normal ganglion cells are present in these infants, and once the meconium has passed, the patient will defecate normally.

Hirschsprung disease can resemble meconium plug syndrome radiologically, but the cause and prognosis are very different. In meconium plug syndrome, the obstruction usually resolves rapidly after the enema examination, whereas the obstruction generally persists in children with Hirschsprung disease.

Incarcerated inguinal hernia is a common cause of low intestinal obstruction between 1 and 6 months of age. The findings of intestinal obstruction on radiographs are characteristic, and the key to radiologic diagnosis is visualization of a unilaterally prominent inguinal fold or loops of air-filled bowel in the scrotum (Fig. 52.18A). US can identify the incarcerated intestine in the inguinal canal or scrotum and can differentiate a hernia from other causes of scrotal swelling (Fig. 52.18B).

Intussusception. After 6 months of age, intussusception becomes an increasingly important acquired cause of intestinal obstruction. In young children, most intussusceptions are ileocolic and the cause is idiopathic.

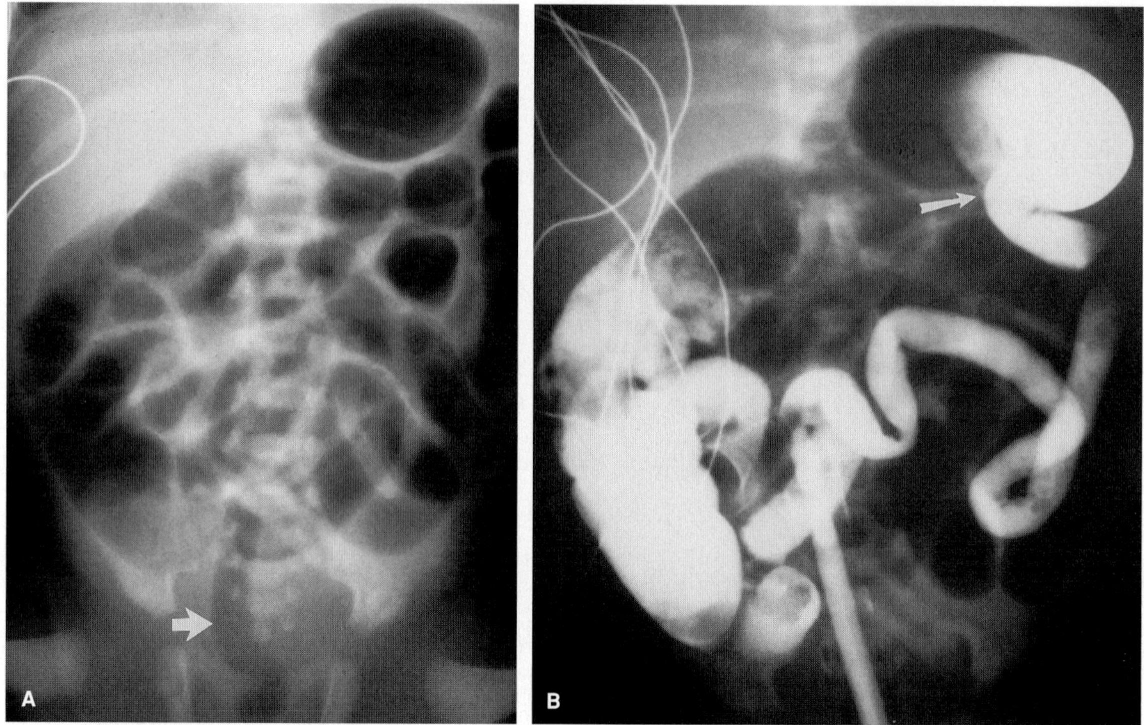

FIGURE 52.17. **Meconium Plug Syndrome (Small Left Colon Syndrome). A.** Numerous loops of intestine are distended with air. Also, note air in the relatively narrow rectosigmoid colon (*arrow*). **B.** Contrast enema demonstrates a small left colon with the characteristic transition zone (*arrow*). These findings mimic those of Hirschsprung disease.

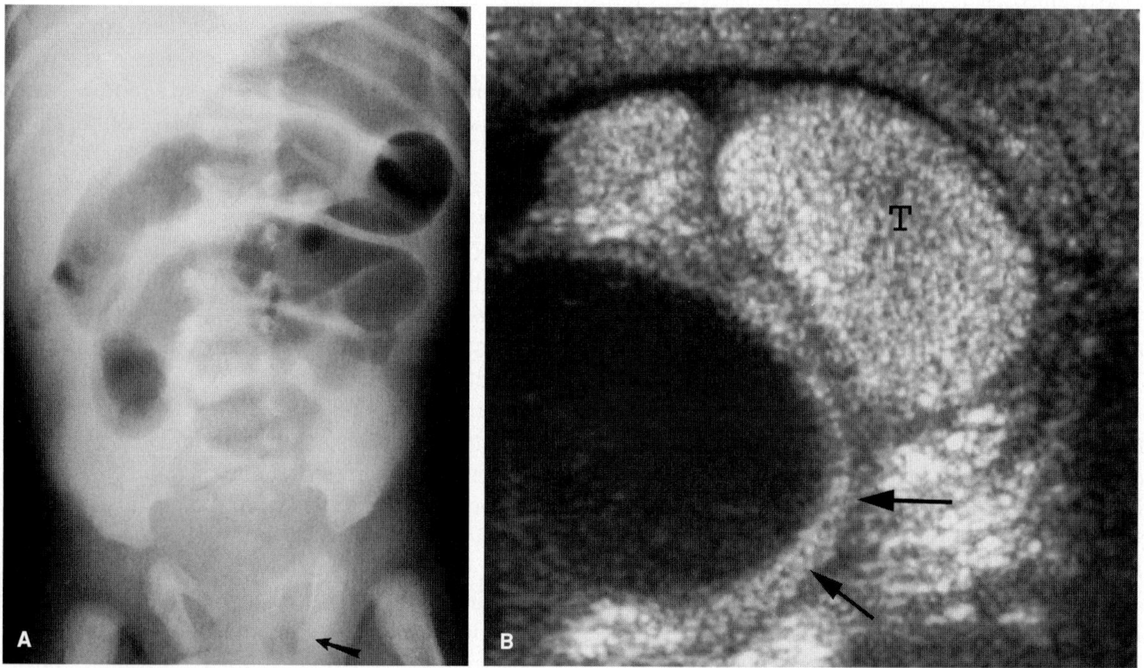

FIGURE 52.18. **Inguinal Hernia. A.** Numerous loops of intestine are distended, signifying the presence of intestinal obstruction on this radiograph. Air is seen in the hernia in the left inguinal region (*arrow*). **B.** US in a different infant shows a fluid-filled, dilated loop of bowel (*arrows*) in the scrotum compressing the testis (T) inferiorly in this incarcerated hernia.

Redundant, inflamed mucosa or lymph nodes may act as the lead point. Definable lead points such as diverticula, polyps, or tumors are more commonly encountered in neonates and in older children.

Abdominal radiographs may be normal or may demonstrate intestinal obstruction (16). In approximately half of cases, the head of the intussusceptum is visible on radiographs as soft tissue mass effect along the course of the colon (Fig. 52.19A). Fat trapped within the intussusceptum may be visible on radiographs. US is a very effective and reliable imaging modality for the demonstration of intussusception (17). Characteristically, a cylindric mass is seen, consisting of an outer hypoechoic ring surrounding tissues of variable echogenicity. Concentric rings may be seen

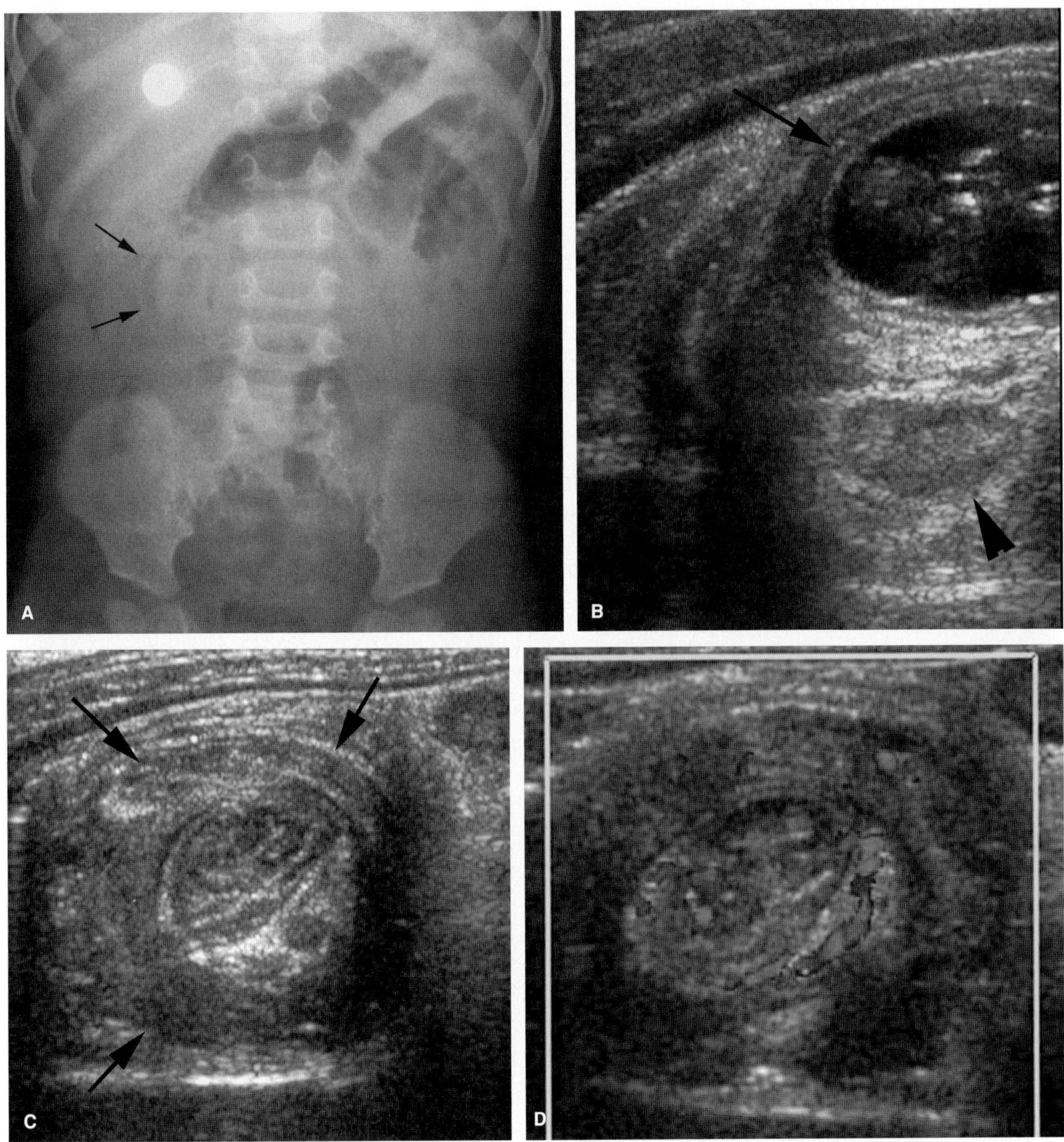

FIGURE 52.19. **(Color Plates) Intussusception. A.** Plain radiograph suggests a soft tissue mass with internal fat in the right upper quadrant (*arrow*). **B.** Transverse US through the intussusception shows a fluid-distended loop of bowel (*arrow*), a mesenteric lymph node (*arrowhead*), and intervening echogenic fat. **C.** Intussusception in another patient shows a thicker rim of edematous bowel (*arrows*). **D.** Color Doppler imaging reveals evidence of flow within the thickened intussusceptum.(*continued*)

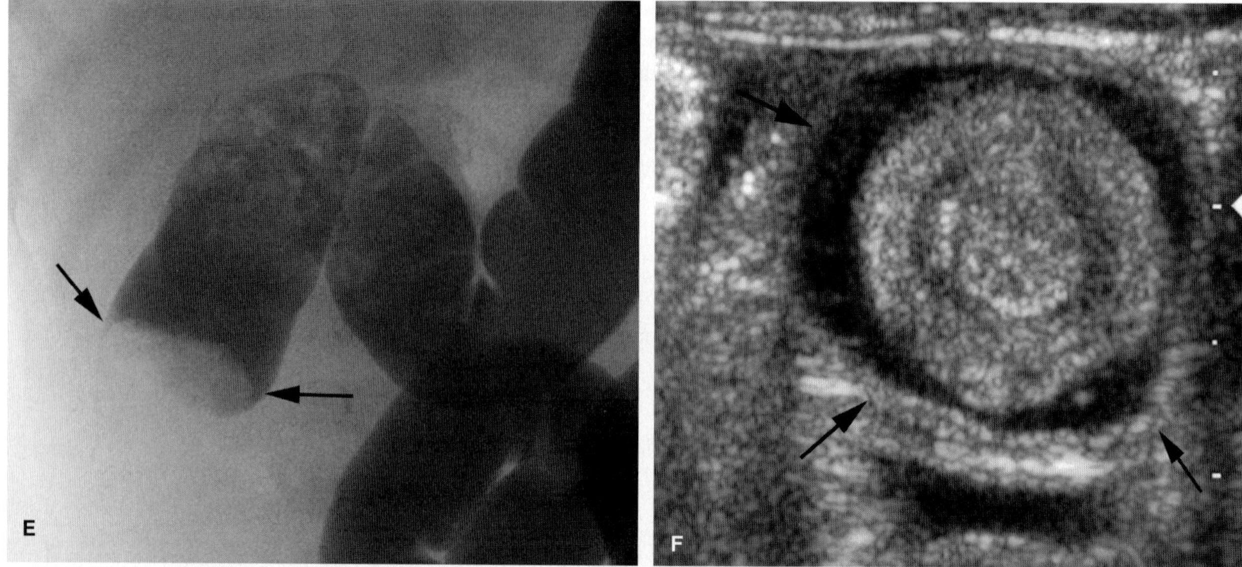

FIGURE 52.19. **(Color Plates)** *(Continued)* **E.** Image obtained during hydrostatic reduction using water-soluble contrast material reveals the typical defect caused by the head of the intussusceptum *(arrows)*. **F.** US of a child with eosinophilic gastroenteritis revealed a transient small bowel intussusception. The bowel within the intussusception *(arrows)* was thin-walled and echogenic, and the intussusception resolved during the examination.

representing layers of edematous intestine alternating with layers of mesentery (18). Often anechoic fluid, echogenic mesentery, mesenteric fat, and small lymph nodes can be identified in the center of the intussusception (Fig. 52.19B, C). Color Doppler US has been utilized to assess viability of the involved intestine (19,20) (Fig. 52.19D). Nonsurgical reduction should be attempted in any case with no evidence of free air or peritonitis (Fig. 52.19E). Small amounts of free fluid are commonly seen with US and do not necessarily indicate perforation.

Enema reduction is performed using either water-soluble contrast or air under pressure. Air enema reduction has been favored by many pediatric radiologists in recent years because the procedure allows generation of higher pressures, which results in faster reduction time and an improved reduction rate (21,22). Pressures must be monitored with a monometer during the procedure, and the intraluminal pressure should not exceed 120 mm Hg. Hydrostatic reduction using water-soluble contrast material, such as a 1-to-5 dilution of Gastrografin, remains a viable alternative to air reduction. The contrast column needs to be elevated to a height of 4 to 5 feet of water-soluble contrast to generate comparable pressures to the air pumps. When appropriate pressures are generated with either procedure, reduction rates are in the range of 80% to 90%. US-guided hydrostaticor air reduction is advocated by some, but this procedure has not gained wide acceptance in the United States (23–26).

When intussusception is initially refractory to reduction, repeated attempts are often helpful (27). Avoiding the use of sedation improves reduction rates by permitting the patients to increase intra-abdominal pressure via Valsalva maneuver (28). The only contraindications to nonsurgical reduction of intussusception are the presence of free air or signs and symptoms of peritonitis. The duration of symptoms and the presence of small bowel obstruction are not generally considered deterrents. Recurrent intussusception occurs in approximately 5% to 10% of cases. When repeated occurrences of intussusception occur in a given patient, the possibility of a fixed lead point is increased, and surgery should be considered.

Transient, spontaneously reducing intussusceptions are increasingly common findings as the use of abdominal CT and US becomes more prevalent. Transient intussusception most commonly involves the small bowel. The intussusception is typically short in length, slightly echogenic at US, and smaller in diameter than the typical ileocolic intussusception (29,30) (Fig. 52.19F). Intussusception can also occur along the course of a gastrojejunostomy tube (31).

Appendicitis. After approximately 2 years of age, perforated appendicitis becomes an increasingly common cause of an obstructive pattern on radiographs. Radiographs tend to be normal or show diminished intestinal gas with acute nonperforated appendicitis. After appendiceal rupture occurs, small bowel dilatation gradually develops because of a combination of decreased small bowel peristalsis and partial bowel obstruction in the region of abscess formation. Symptoms may temporarily improve following perforation. Because of the intense inflammatory response

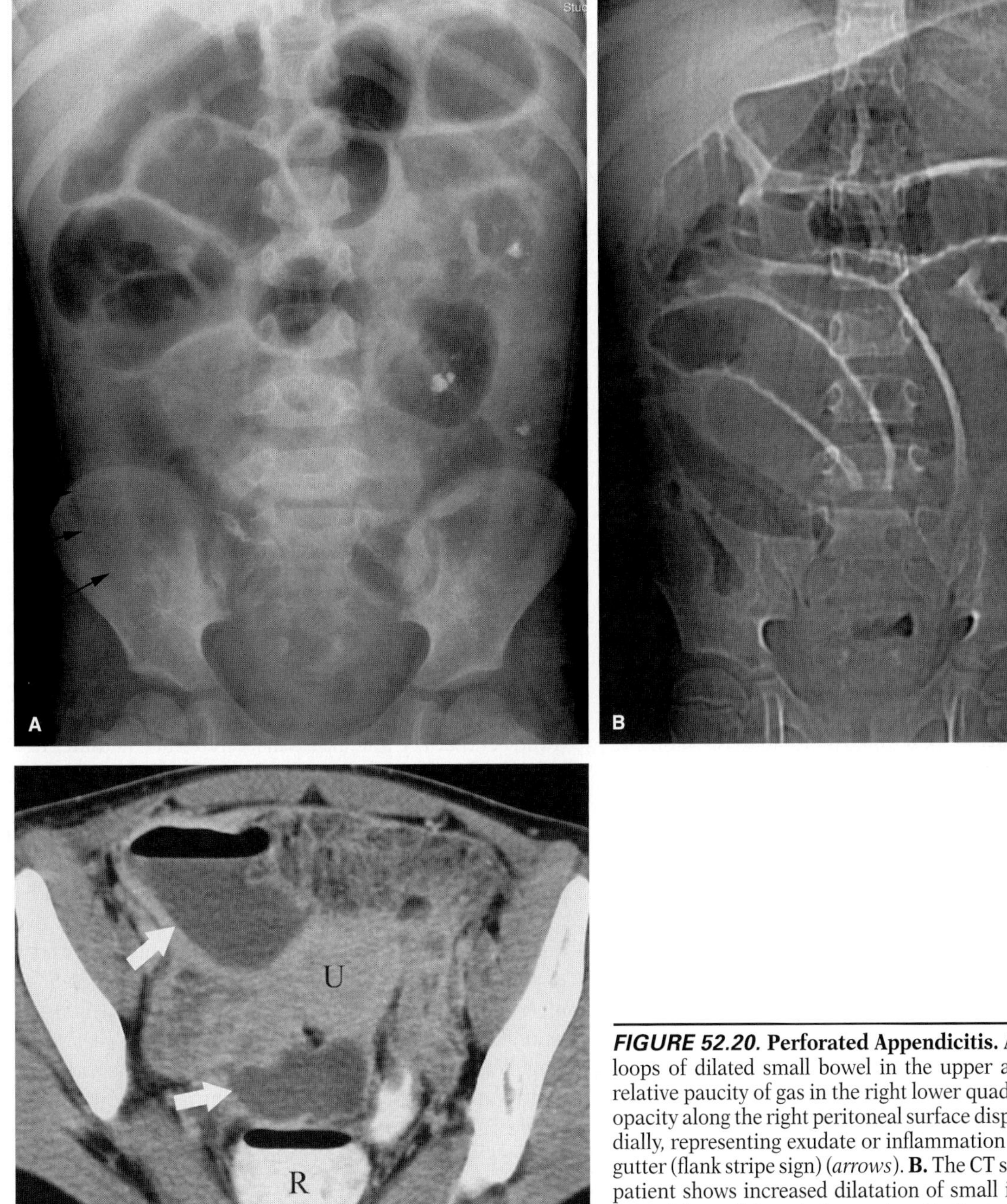

FIGURE 52.20. **Perforated Appendicitis. A.** Note multiple loops of dilated small bowel in the upper abdomen with a relative paucity of gas in the right lower quadrant. Soft tissue opacity along the right peritoneal surface displaces bowel medially, representing exudate or inflammation in the paracolic gutter (flank stripe sign) (*arrows*). **B.** The CT scout in the same patient shows increased dilatation of small intestine consistent with small bowel obstruction. **C.** Contrast-enhanced CT in a 14-year old girl shows loculated collections of fluid (*arrows*) in the right lower quadrant and cul-de-sac resulting from perforated appendicitis. R, rectum. U, uterus.

that occurs around the appendiceal perforation, free intra-abdominal air may be detected on CT but is rarely seen radiographically. As an abscess develops, radiographs may show a right lower quadrant mass. Once the appendix perforates, obstruction gradually develops owing to a combination of functional obstruction and abscess formation (Fig. 52.20).

Abscesses are best detected with US or CT. Sonographically, appendiceal abscesses vary from anechoic to solid in appearance.

Regional enteritis patients clinically mimic those with chronic appendiceal abscess. US shows the thickened wall of the involved small bowel, but contrast studies better evaluate the extent of involvement and provide the

TABLE 52.6 Causes of Colonic Obstruction

Meconium plug syndrome (small left colon)
Hirschsprung disease
Functional megacolon
Ectopic (imperforate) anus
Colon atresia/stenosis
Inflammatory stricture
Volvulus
Trauma
Neoplasm

definitive findings. Other diseases, such as tuberculosis, lymphoma, and *Yersinia* colitis, are much less common but produce findings that may be difficult to differentiate from regional enteritis.

Colonic Obstruction

Congenital obstructions of the colon are more common than acquired obstructions (Table 52.6).

Hirschsprung disease is the result of absence of ganglion cells in the distal colon, resulting in abnormal peristalsis and inability to effectively evacuate the colon. In Hirschsprung disease, functional colonic obstruction is caused by congenital absence of ganglion cells in the distal colon, resulting in abnormal peristalsis. The rectum is always involved but the extent of proximal involvement varies. The aganglionic segment is characteristically contracted. A well-defined change in caliber at the zone of transition is characteristic in older infants (Fig. 52.21A) but is frequently not present in neonates (Fig. 52.21B). Tortuosity or corrugation of the narrowed aganglionic segment of the colon is commonly seen (Fig. 52.21C). Barium evacuation is delayed, usually well beyond 24 hours. Diagnosis of Hirschsprung disease is definitively made with rectal biopsy. Necrotizing enterocolitis is an uncommon but serious complication of Hirschsprung disease caused by stasis colitis.

Functional megacolon is a common condition in childhood that is associated with spasm of the puborectalis muscle. In many instances, the muscle spasm is secondary to anal fissures; in other cases it is idiopathic and probably multifactorial. The rectum is normal to large in caliber. Prominence of the puborectalis sling provides the major clue to diagnosis. These patients can hold considerable volumes of stool in their colon.

Imperforate or ectopic anus is a common cause of obstruction in the neonate. Anatomic deficits range from simple membranous anal atresia to arrest of the colon as it descends through the puborectalis sling, with fistula formation from the blind-ending rectal pouch to some part of the genital or urinary tract (Fig. 52.22). In girls, the fistula may empty into the bladder, uterus, or vagina. In boys, it tends to enter into the urethra or bladder. In both sexes it can enter the perineum. Sacral and urinary tract anomalies, hydrometrocolpos, and persistent cloaca are associated. When sacral abnormalities are present, the spinal cord and canal should be screened with US for abnormalities such as tethering or masses (32). Virtually all of these patients have neurogenic bladder dysfunction (33).

All associated anomalies should be demonstrated, along with the location of the fistula. US can demonstrate the distal end of the pouch. The fistula may be injected directly or it may opacify during retrograde voiding cystourethrography. In girls, flush retrograde vaginography may be required. If the fistula empties above the puborectalis sling, it can be presumed that the puborectalis muscle is hypoplastic and that continence will be difficult to accomplish with any surgical procedure. If the fistula empties below the puborectalis sling, the puborectalis muscle is usually better developed, and achievement of continence is more likely. The "M" line of Cremin has been utilized to determine the level at which the blind pouch ends (Fig. 52.23). This line is drawn perpendicular to the long axis of the ischia on lateral view and passes through the junction between the middle and lower third of the ischia. If the blind pouch and fistula end above the line, the fistula is considered high. If they end below the line, it is considered low, and if they end at the line, it is considered intermediate. Intermediate fistulae usually pose the same problems as high fistulae.

Colon atresia is relatively rare and is evident in the neonatal period. Massive distension of the colon is seen proximal to the area of atresia or stenosis (Fig. 52.24).

Acquired causes of colonic obstruction are relatively uncommon, except for perforated appendicitis and regional enteritis. Inflammatory strictures associated with ulcerative colitis and necrotizing enterocolitis tend to be smooth and appear similar to those in adults. They may be single or multiple (Fig. 52.25). Colonic strictures can also be found in children with cystic fibrosis (15,34). Tumors of the colon are uncommon and the findings are similar to those seen in adults. Trauma to the colon, producing obstruction, is seen with motor vehicle accidents or, more commonly, in battered child syndrome. Sigmoid and cecal volvulus are much less common in children than in adults, but the imaging findings are the same. Volvulus occurs more frequently in bedridden patients and in neurologically impaired children.

Inflammation and Infection

Gastrointestinal Tract

Esophagitis in children is commonly caused by peptic disease, caustic ingestion, and viral and monilial infection. Peptic esophagitis tends to involve the lower third of the esophagus, but with severe reflux, it may involve

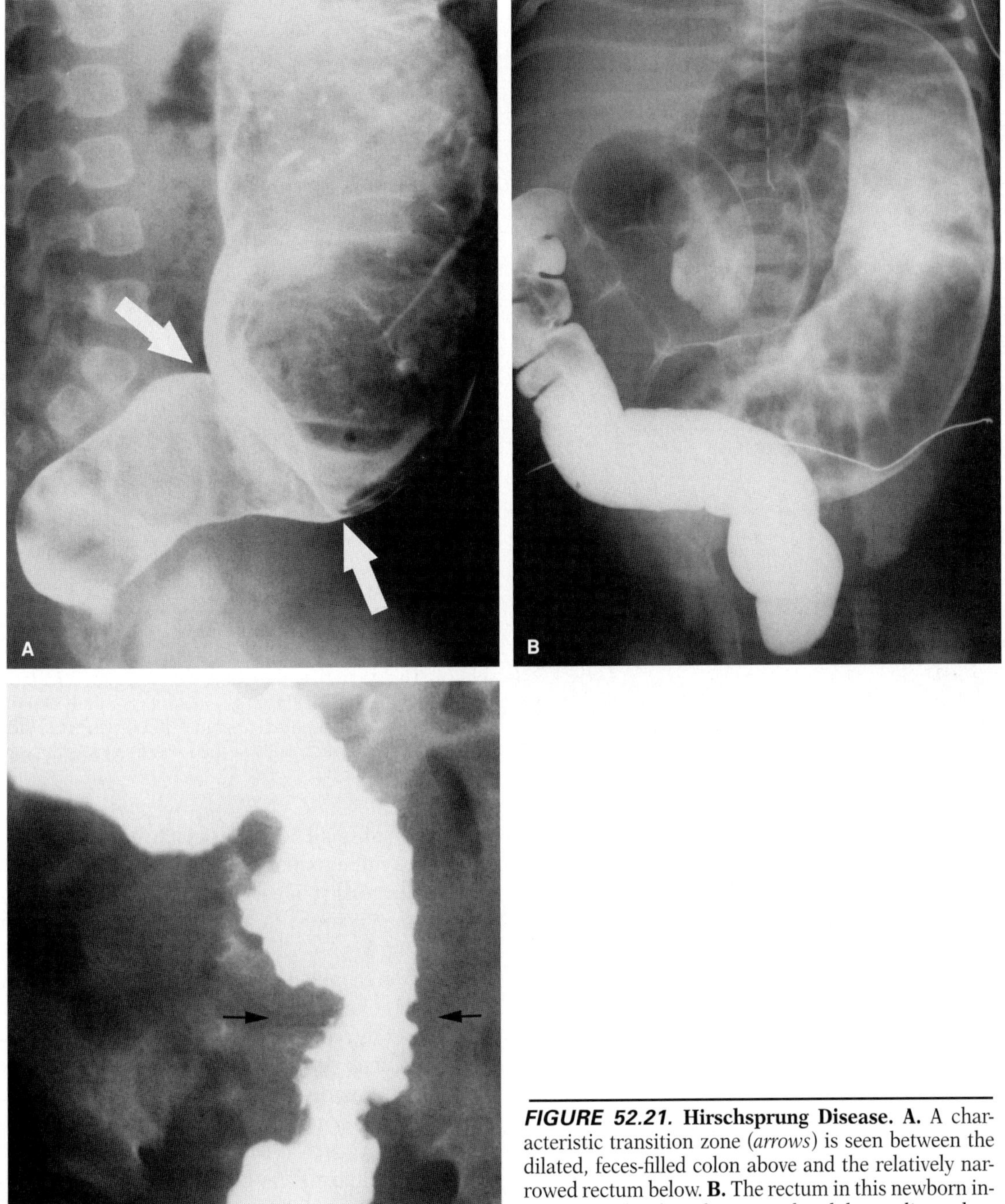

FIGURE 52.21. **Hirschsprung Disease. A.** A characteristic transition zone (*arrows*) is seen between the dilated, feces-filled colon above and the relatively narrowed rectum below. **B.** The rectum in this newborn infant is smaller than the sigmoid and descending colon, but a well-defined transition zone is not present. **C.** A contrast enema in another infant shows spasm and irregularity of the aganglionic segment (*arrows*).

the entire esophagus. Findings consist of thickening of the esophageal wall, lack of normal peristalsis, tertiary contractions in the esophagus, and ulcers that may be superficial or deep. Incomplete relaxation of the cricopharyngeal muscle during swallowing can be a clue to the presence of GER on swallowing studies. With caustic ingestion, extensive esophageal burns are the rule. Perforation into the mediastinum can occur. Contrast studies generally are not performed acutely following caustic ingestion, but such studies are useful later to demonstrate strictures. Viral esophagitis (e.g., herpes) causes small superficial ulcers, which are best demonstrated with double-contrast studies. The ulcers can be diffuse or focal and may result in intense spasm with severe dysphagia. Monilial

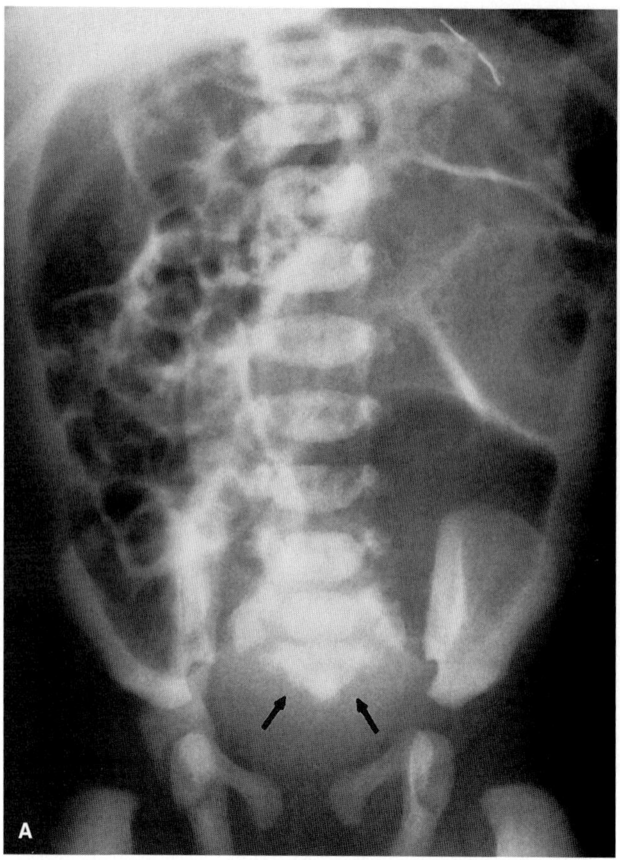

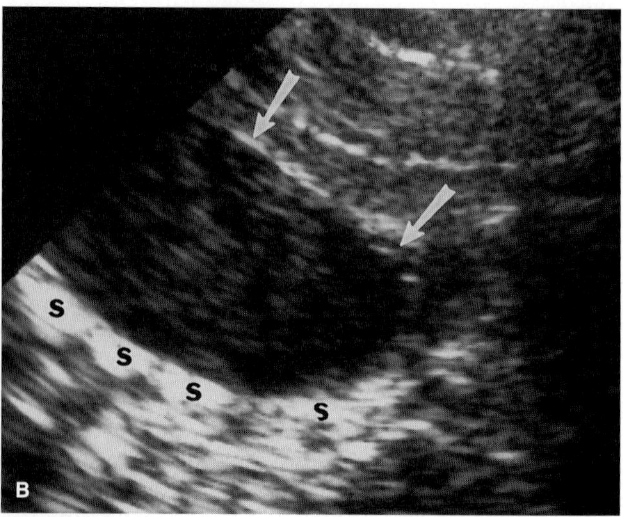

FIGURE 52.22. **Imperforate Anus. A.** Loops of colon are distended in the upper abdomen with gas evident in the small bowel. The rectum is not visualized. The sacrum (*arrows*) is underdeveloped. **B.** Sagittal US in another infant demonstrates the distended distal pouch (*arrows*) that overlies the sacral segments (S). The pouch ends at the lowermost sacral segment.

esophagitis causes mucosal irregularities with intense spasm of the esophagus, leading to pseudodiverticula.

Gastritis is commonly caused by peptic disease or *Helicobacter* and *Campylobacter* infection in infants and children. The findings resemble those seen in adults; superficial ulcerations and a delicate, edematous, cobblestone appearance of the mucosa can occur. Milk allergy is a common cause of gastritis in infants that leads to vomiting and bleeding. Upper GI series in such infants may demonstrate intense antropyloric muscle spasm. US may show thickening of the mucosa in any cause of gastritis. Prominent mucosal inflammation and thickening may lead to gastric outlet obstruction in children with chronic granulomatous disease.

Duodenitis is usually caused by peptic disease, which is more common in children than is often recognized. Ulcer craters are sometimes visualized. Children tend to present with bleeding more often than adults.

Viral gastroenteritis is the most common inflammatory condition of the small bowel in children. US often shows fluid-filled loops of bowel or mildly thickened intestinal mucosa (Fig. 52.26). Abdominal radiographs may show extensive gaseous distension of the GI tract, which may erroneously suggest mechanical obstruction.

Regional enteritis usually affects the terminal ileum as the primary site of involvement. Regional enteritis of the proximal small bowel, stomach, or esophagus is rather rare. The radiographic findings are identical to those in adults and consist of variable lengths of narrowed, irregular terminal ileum with or without linear ulcers and sinus tracts (Fig. 52.27). The transmural bowel wall thickening common in these patients is readily demonstrable with US (35), and color Doppler US reveals increased vascularity in affected intestinal loops (36,37). Gadolinium-enhanced MR is an emerging technique for assessing disease activity in inflammatory bowel disease (38). Chronic ileocolitis and esophagitis have also been described in patients with glycogen-storage disease type 1B.

Colitis. Almost every condition that produces colitis in the adult can produce colitis in infants and children. Almost any form of colitis manifests thickening of the colonic wall or mucosa on US. The pattern of bowel wall thickening can be used to suggest the diagnosis in some cases.

Necrotizing enterocolitis (NEC) is seen almost exclusively in premature and newborn infants. The etiology of this inflammatory bowel condition includes hypoperfusion and hypoxia of the gut. The clinical findings tend to mimic those of sepsis; however, the passage of blood per rectum is more common with NEC. Initial radiographs may demonstrate only dilated loops of small bowel and colon. The hallmark of the disease is pneumatosis cystoides intestinalis (Fig. 52.28). Pneumatosis results from

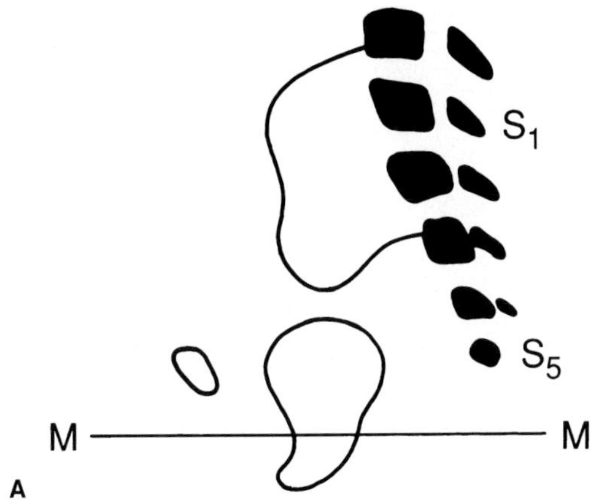

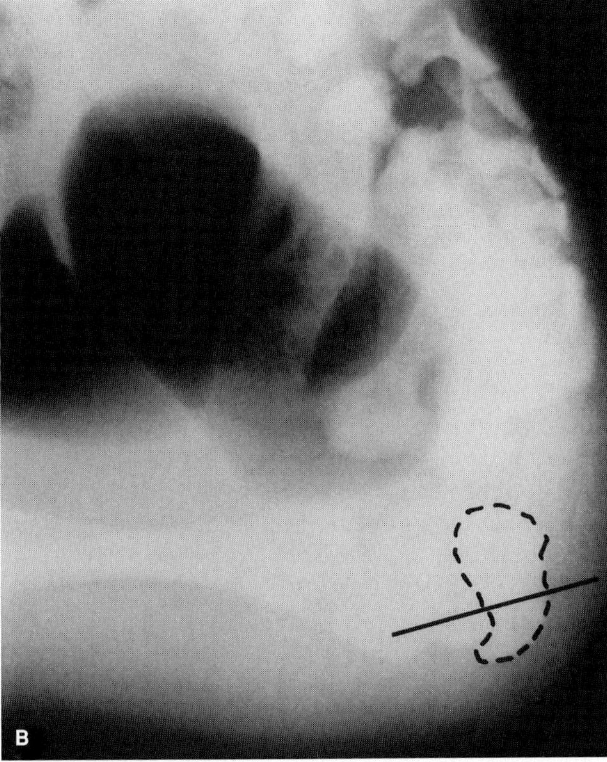

FIGURE 52.23. **Imperforate Anus: Cremin's M Line. A.** The M line is drawn horizontally through the junction of the middle and lower thirds of the ischium (M). The line demarcates the level of the puborectalis sling. S1, S5, sacral segments. **B.** Cross-table lateral film of an infant with the buttocks elevated demonstrates the distal air-filled pouch or the hindgut. Note the position of the M line. The pouch ends well above the M line, indicating a high imperforate anus.

destruction of the mucosa with passage of gas produced by bacteria (*Escherichia coli*) into the bowel wall and, in some cases, into the portal venous system (Fig. 52.28C). Pneumatosis cystoides intestinalis appears as linear, curvilinear, or bubbly to granular collections of air. Small bubbles of intramural and portal vein gas that are not visible radiographically can be detected with US as echogenic punctate foci in the liver vessels and bowel wall. Thickening of the bowel wall and decreased blood flow within the bowel wall with color Doppler imaging suggest bowel necrosis (39). The presence of portal venous gas on the initial radiograph is associated with an increased incidence of perforation (40). Many patients develop strictures, most commonly in the colon. NEC is treated by withholding feedings, administering antibiotics, and blood transfusions. Surgical intervention is necessary when perforation or peritonitis occurs. Free air, indicating intestinal perforation, is best demonstrated with cross-table lateral or left lateral decubitus views of the abdomen. Fixed dilated bowel loops are presumed to be ischemic and nonviable and can be an indication for surgical intervention.

Typhlitis (neutropenic colitis) is a localized necrotizing colitis, usually involving the cecum, that develops in patients with leukemia or other malignancies when they are severely neutropenic. Findings mimic those of acute appendicitis or acute regional enteritis. The clinical setting suggests the correct diagnosis. On US, the affected bowel wall is echogenic and thickened (41) (Fig. 52.29A). Barium enema shows cecal abnormalities, including thumbprinting, spasm, and mucosal irregularity (Fig. 52.29B). Hemolytic-uremic syndrome caused by *E. coli* can be preceded by a hemorrhagic colitis that has similar findings.

Appendicitis. In nonperforated appendicitis the abdomen often is relatively airless, with one or two loops of air-filled small bowel or cecum in the right lower quadrant. Scoliosis with concavity to the right frequently is associated with spasm and indistinctness of the lateral edge of the right psoas muscle. Fecaliths, seen in 50% of cases, are strong presumptive evidence of appendicitis in a patient with an acute abdomen.

US is an excellent screening modality for appendicitis in children, potentially avoiding the higher radiation exposures associated with multidetector CT (42). The dilated, fluid-filled appendix is often surprisingly superficial (Fig. 52.30), and compression of the appendix with a transducer elicits characteristic local tenderness. The abnormal appendix measures greater than 6 mm in diameter (43). Intraluminal fecalith, lack of compressibility, and thickening and increased echogenicity of the periappendiceal fat are secondary findings that support the diagnosis of appendicitis on US. Posterior manual compression and left oblique decubitus body position during scanning may improve detectability of the appendix (44).

When perforation occurs, the appendix decompresses and can be more difficult to detect with US (45). Color Doppler US may show hyperemic periappendiceal soft tissues or fluid collections (46).

CT is increasingly used for appendicitis in children, particularly in those cases in which US findings are indeterminate or the appendix cannot be identified because of large amounts of intestinal gas (47–50). The use of contrast

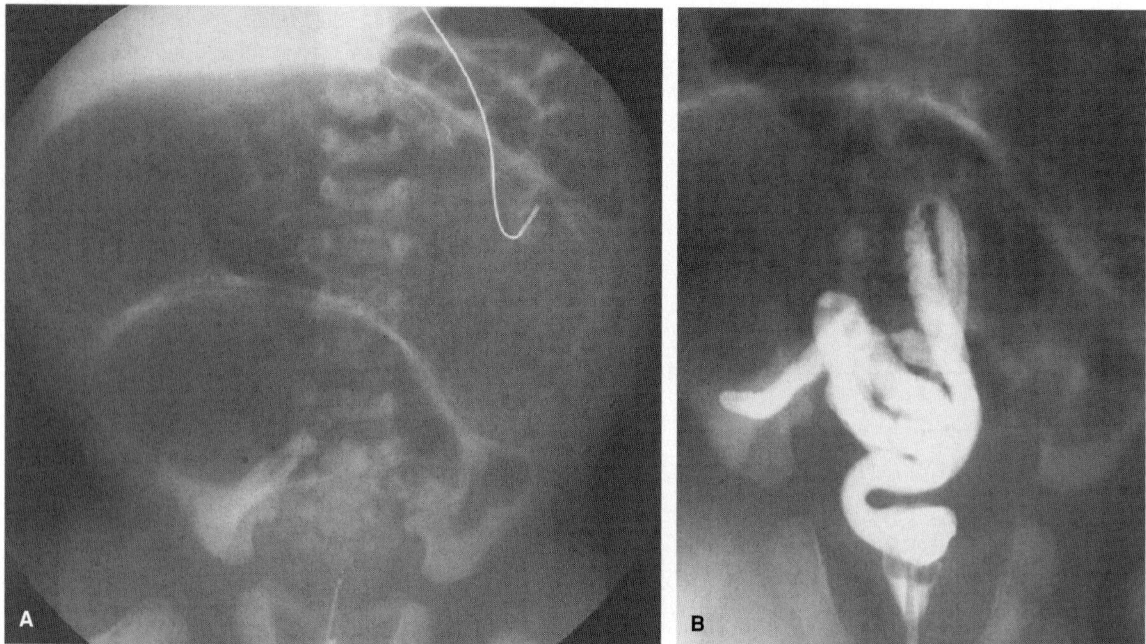

FIGURE 52.24. **Colon Atresia. A.** Plain film demonstrates loops of markedly dilated intestine. **B.** Retrograde contrast study demonstrates the blind-ending microcolon. The proximal colon is air filled and dilated.

for appendicitis in children remains controversial. Some authors advocate unenhanced CT (51,52), but more commonly some combination of IV, oral, and/or rectal contrast is suggested (53–55). Prominent periappendiceal fat stranding is a good predictor of perforation on CT (56). However, the appendix can be difficult to identify on CT in children with intra-abdominal fat (Fig. 52.31). Free intraperitoneal air is occasionally seen. *Omental infarction* mimics appendicitis clinically but can be distinguished from appendicitis on US and CT. The infracted omental segment has the appearance of a heterogeneous mass that is usually located between the anterior abdominal wall and the colon (57) (Fig. 52.32).

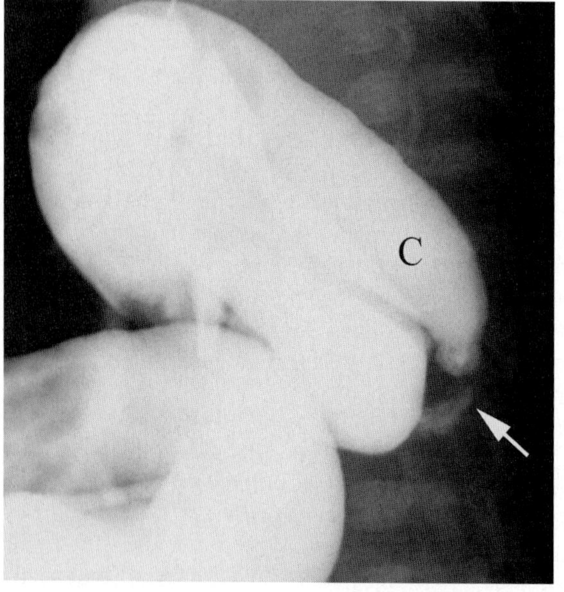

FIGURE 52.25. **Colonic Stricture.** A short stricture (*arrow*) was found in the region of the cecum (C) in this premature infant with a previous history of necrotizing enterocolitis.

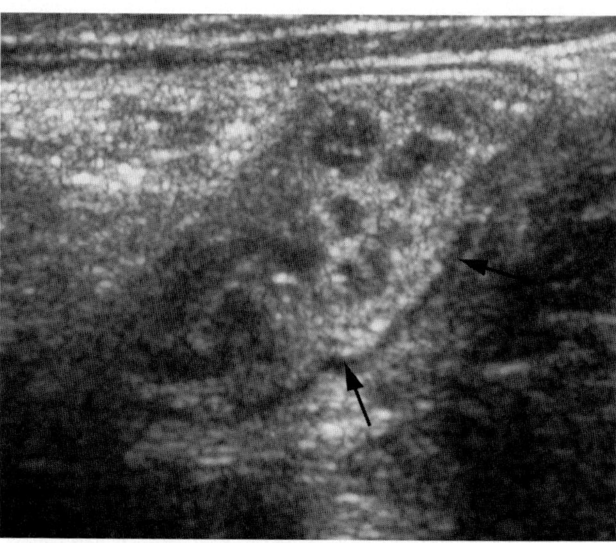

FIGURE 52.26. **Viral Gastroenteritis.** Mild thickening of the echogenic mucosa was seen in the small bowel (*arrows*).

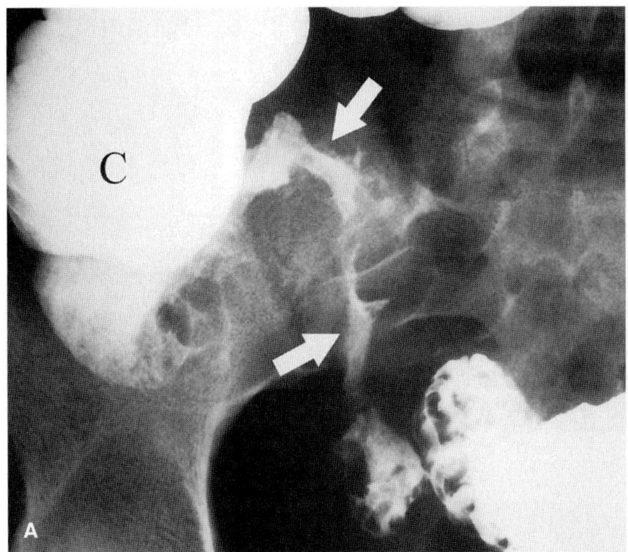

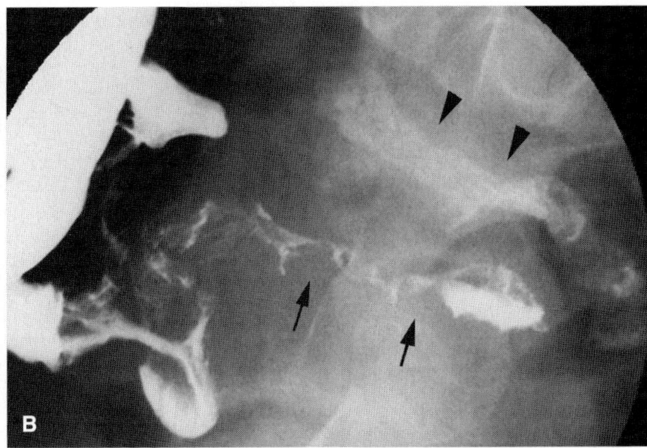

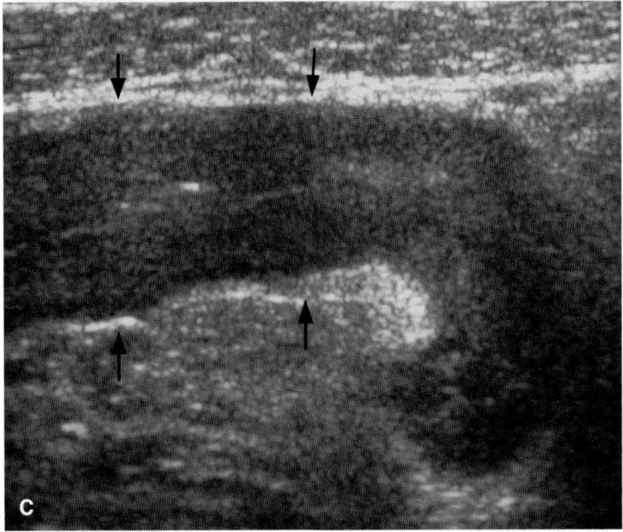

FIGURE 52.27. **Regional Enteritis. A.** Barium enema demonstrates the markedly narrowed and irregular terminal ileum (*arrows*). Note that the tip of the cecum (C) is also involved. **B.** Barium enema in another patient reveals a markedly narrow and irregular segment of ileum (*arrows*). Contrast appeared in the rectum prematurely (*arrowheads*), indicating the presence of an ileorectal fistula. The fistula was difficult to identify. **C.** US reveals transmural hypoechoic thickening of the wall of the terminal ileum (*arrows*).

Mesenteric adenitis is a self-limiting inflammatory condition involving mesenteric lymph nodes and is frequently viral in etiology. US usually demonstrates a cluster of enlarged lymph nodes in the right lower quadrant (Fig. 52.33) and a normal appendix. Enlarged lymph nodes show increased blood flow with color Doppler US. Mild thickening of the mucosa in the distal ileum and cecum is occasionally seen, indicating a mild ileocolitis. Giant mesenteric adenitis can produce a masslike lesion in the right lower quadrant with considerable distortion of the terminal ileum and cecum.

Bacterial peritonitis in children is caused by perforated appendicitis and generalized sepsis. Children with nephrotic syndrome are more prone to develop generalized bacterial peritonitis. Free fluid in the abdomen is the main imaging finding.

Meconium peritonitis results from intrauterine intestinal perforation that occurs as a result of a fetal bowel obstruction or ischemia. In some patients, active perforation remains after birth, and the patient presents with a clinical picture of peritonitis. In other cases, the perforation heals in utero, and the extruded meconium is palpated as an abdominal mass. This meconium sometimes calcifies and is identified on plain radiographs or US. Calcified meconium appears as scattered amorphous or curvilinear calcifications throughout the peritoneal cavity (Fig. 52.34A). Free meconium may enter the scrotum through a patent processus vaginalis. Residual masses of meconium and cystic areas can be identified sonographically (Fig. 52.34B). Calcifications create multiple scattered, bright echoes that have been likened to a "snowstorm." Infants with calcifications but no evidence of obstruction or active peritonitis can be managed nonsurgically. The calcifications slowly disappear. Some patients may develop bowel obstruction because of adhesions later in childhood.

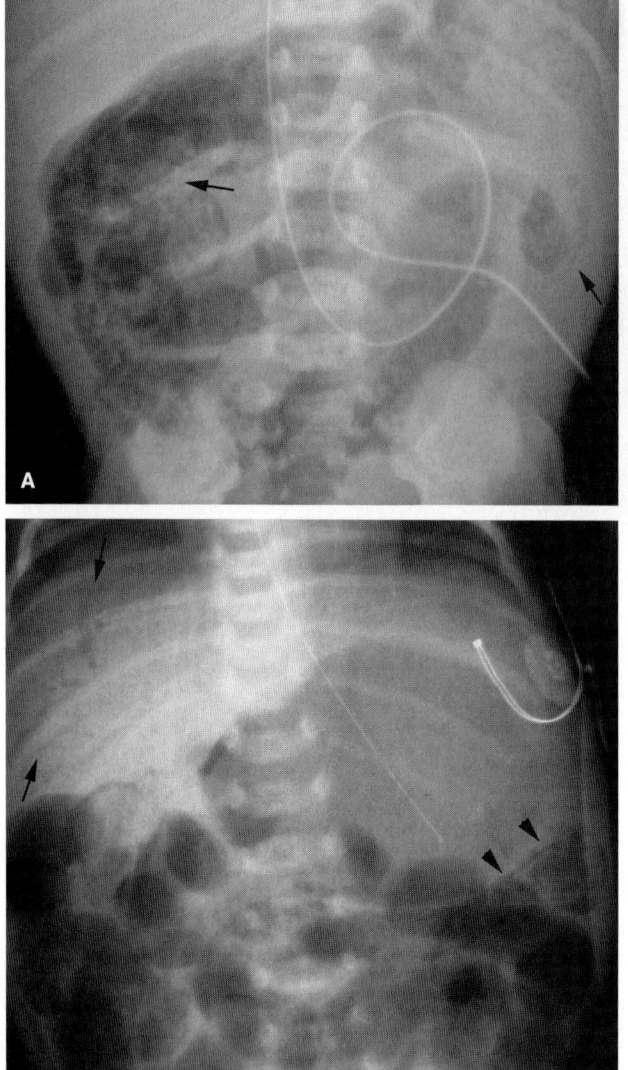

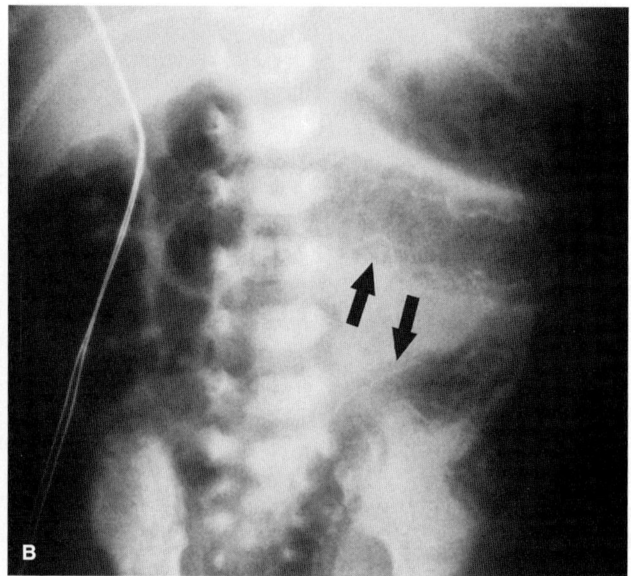

FIGURE 52.28. **Necrotizing Enterocolitis. A.** Multiple loops of distended bowel have bubbly and linear radiolucencies in the bowel wall, representing pneumatosis intestinalis (*arrows*). **B.** Another patient with marked pneumatosis of the wall of the colon (*arrows*). **C.** Another infant showing pneumatosis intestinalis (*arrowheads*) and branching radiolucencies within the liver representing air within the portovenous system (*arrows*).

Hepatobiliary

Cholecystitis is probably more common than is generally appreciated in the pediatric population. The US findings are the same in children as in adults. The inflamed gallbladder is distended, shows a thickened wall, and may show surrounding edema. Cholecystitis occurs in otherwise healthy children but is also seen in HIV-positive patients. Gallstones can occur in infants and children. The most common cause of cholelithiasis in children include sickle cell disease, congenital obstructive anomalies of the biliary tract, total parenteral nutrition, furosemide treatment, dehydration, hemolytic anemia, and short gut syndrome.

Biliary atresia and neonatal hepatitis account for most cases of cholestatic jaundice in the neonate. Hepatitis in the newborn can be related to infection with a specific virus (hepatitis B virus, Cytomegalovirus) or associated with familial or metabolic conditions that result in cholestatic jaundice (alpha-1-antitrypsin deficiency, Byler disease). Diffuse extrahepatic bile duct atresia is believed to result from chronic viral cholangiohepatitis. Less common are intrahepatic ductal atresia and focal atresia of the bile ducts, which are presumably caused by an intrauterine vascular insult.

Neonatal hepatitis is treated medically, whereas extrahepatic bile duct atresia requires prompt surgical correction. US is used primarily to exclude other causes of obstructive jaundice such as choledochal cysts, inspissated bile syndrome, or obstructing masses or gallstones. The gallbladder is small or absent in most patients with extrahepatic biliary atresia, although a normal gallbladder may

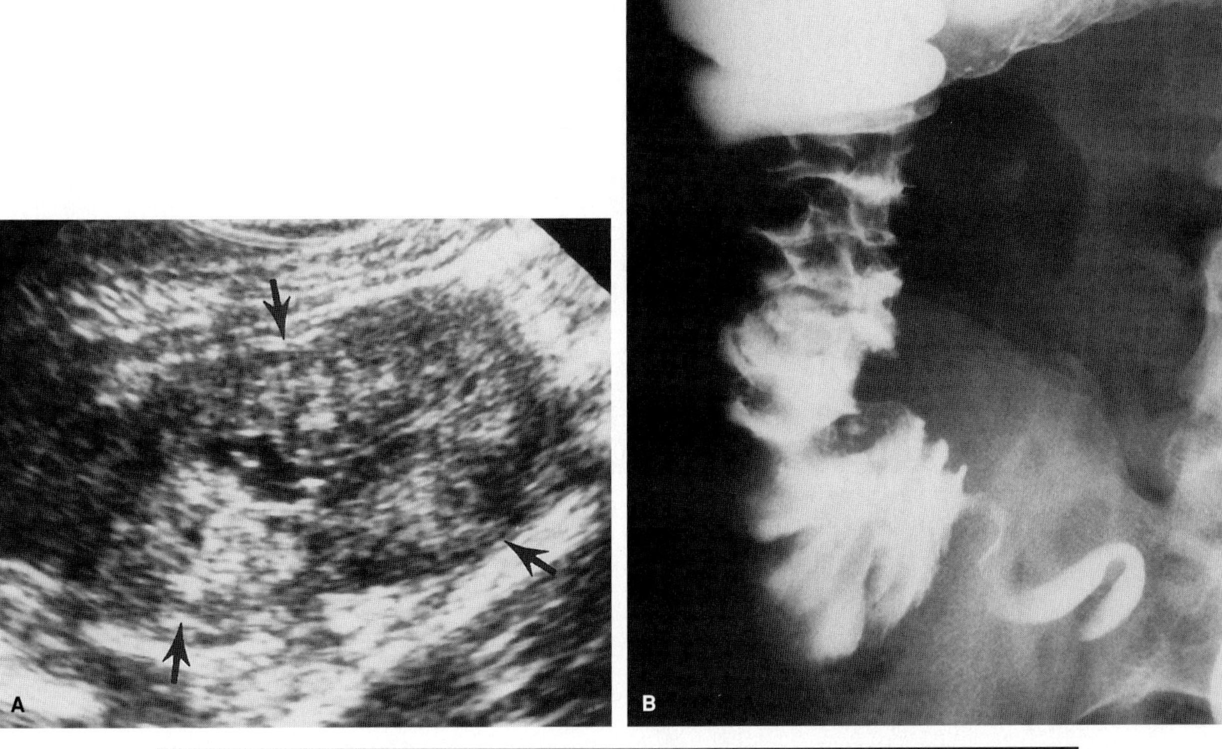

FIGURE 52.29. **Typhilitis. A.** US demonstrates marked echogenic thickening of the cecal wall (*arrows*). **B.** Note the spasm, thumbprinting, and mucosal thickening involving the cecum on barium enema.

be seen in 20% of patients. An echogenic, triangular focus representing the atretic biliary plate has been described as a diagnostic sonographic finding. The triangular cord consists of echogenicity along the anterior wall of the right portal vein of greater than 4 mm in thickness and is thought to be more reliable for the diagnosis of biliary atresia than gallbladder size (58,59). A similar finding may be visible on MR cholangiography (60). Hepatobiliary scintigraphy shows normal hepatic tracer uptake but no excretion into the bile ducts or GI tract (30,31). Tracer activity within the

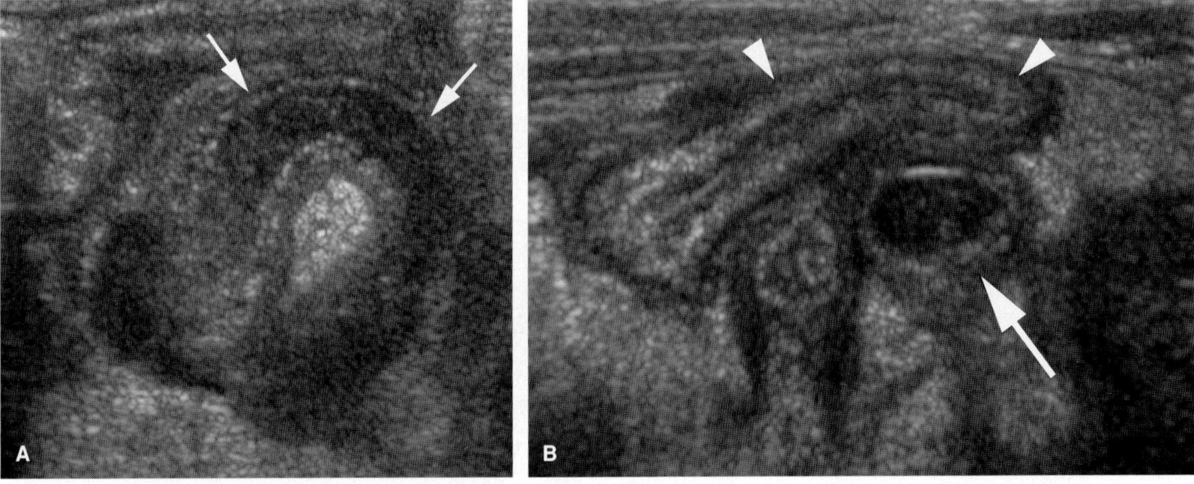

FIGURE 52.30. **Acute Appendicitis A.** A longitudinal US image of the appendix demonstrates the fluid-filled lumen and slight irregularity of the echogenic mucosal lining (*arrows*). **B.** The dilated appendix is shown in cross section (*arrow*). Note mucosal thickening in the adjacent intestinal loop (*arrowheads*) and echogenic thickening of surrounding periappendiceal fat.

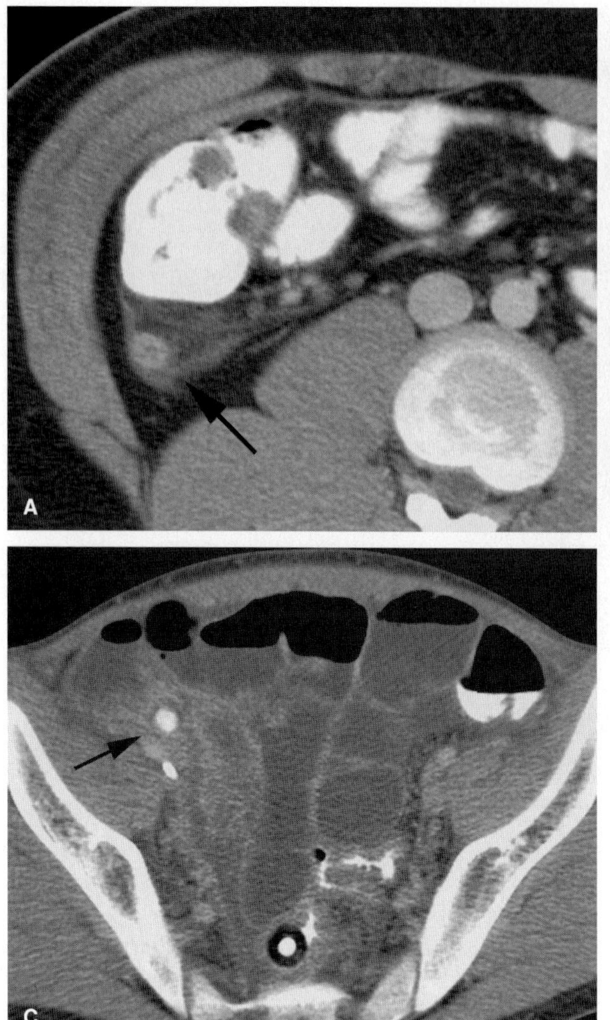

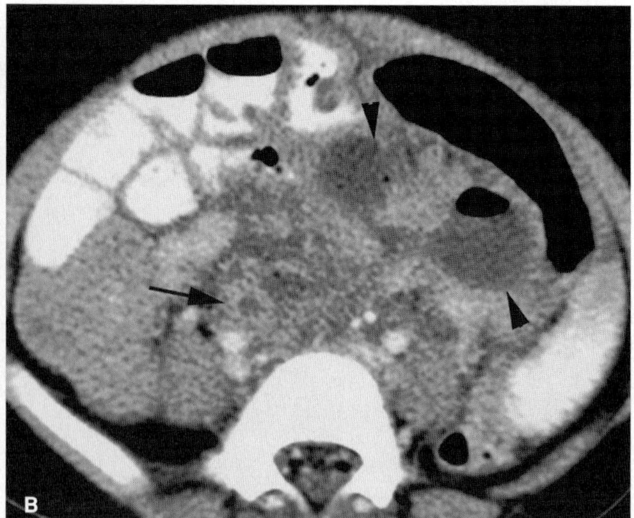

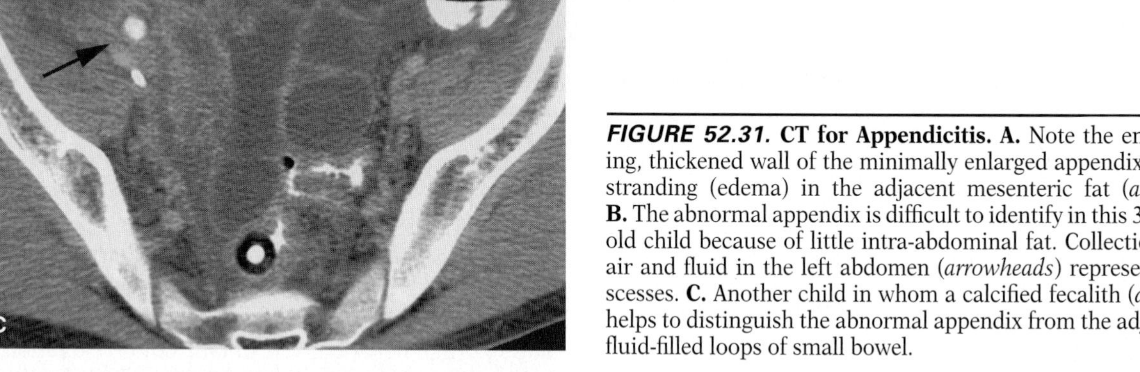

FIGURE 52.31. **CT for Appendicitis. A.** Note the enhancing, thickened wall of the minimally enlarged appendix, with stranding (edema) in the adjacent mesenteric fat (*arrow*). **B.** The abnormal appendix is difficult to identify in this 3-year-old child because of little intra-abdominal fat. Collections of air and fluid in the left abdomen (*arrowheads*) represent abscesses. **C.** Another child in whom a calcified fecalith (*arrow*) helps to distinguish the abnormal appendix from the adjacent fluid-filled loops of small bowel.

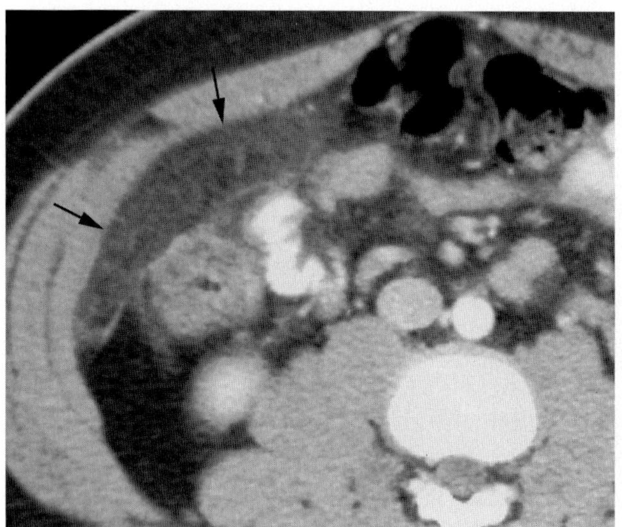

FIGURE 52.32. **Omental Infarction.** The infarcted portion of the omentum gives the appearance of a focal, masslike area of edema within the omental fat, anterior to the right colon (*arrows*).

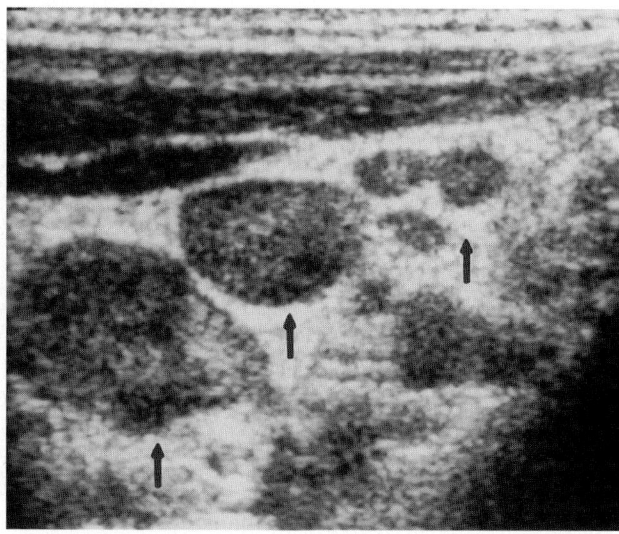

FIGURE 52.33. **Mesenteric Adenitis.** Multiple enlarged, hypoechoic lymph nodes (*arrows*) are seen on US of the right lower quadrant.

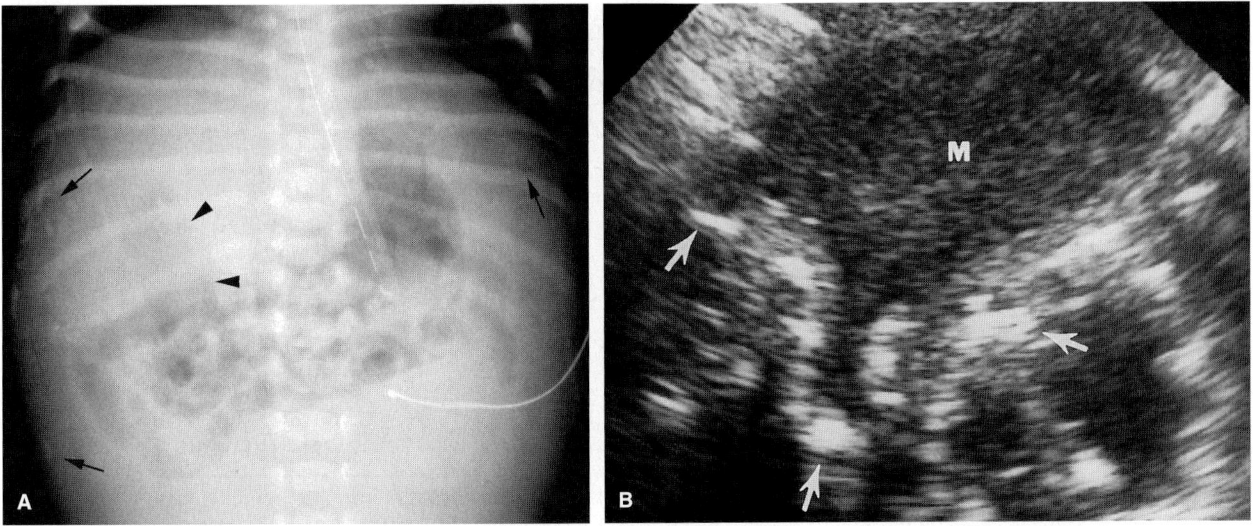

FIGURE 52.34. **Meconium Peritonitis. A.** Numerous linear and amorphous calcifications are seen scattered throughout the peritoneal cavity (*arrows*). A small collection of free intraperitoneal air (*arrowheads*) indicates persistent intestinal perforation. **B.** US in a different infant reveals a hypoechoic mass (M), representing residual meconium in the peritoneal cavity. Note the scattered echogenic calcifications adjacent to the mass (*arrows*).

GI tract strongly supports the diagnosis of neonatal hepatitis and virtually excludes extrahepatic biliary atresia. Phenobarbital is often administered prior to the examination to enhance biliary excretion of the isotope and improve the discriminatory value of the examination. The definitive diagnosis of biliary atresia is made by liver biopsy and intraoperative cholangiography.

Pancreatitis is uncommon in childhood and is most often caused by viral infections or blunt trauma. Pancreatitis can result from functional stenosis of the pancreatic duct due to anomalous development. Pancreas divisum is the most common variant, consisting of abnormal fusion of the ducts of Santorini and Wirsung (61). Such ductal anomalies are best evaluated with MR cholangiopancreatography. Other causes of pancreatitis in children include systemic diseases such as vasculitides or sepsis, hemolytic uremic syndrome, steroid use, metabolic diseases such as hyperlipidemia or hypercalcemia, and gallstones. A familial form of pancreatitis can occur and is accompanied by characteristic pancreatic calcification. However, imaging findings in most cases of pancreatitis in children are minimal. Sonographically, the pancreas may appear normal or enlarged and hypoechoic. In some cases, the pancreatic duct may be enlarged. In severe cases, peripancreatic extravasation of lipase causes lipolysis and increased echogenicity of otherwise undetectable peripancreatic fat. US and CT are useful for detection and follow-up of peripancreatic fluid collections, which commonly resolve spontaneously in children (Fig. 52.35) (62). Pancreatic pseudocyst may complicate either acute or chronic pancreatitis and is the most common cystic lesion of the pancreas. Chronic pancreatitis and pancreatic insufficiency can occur in children with cystic fibrosis and may result in fatty replacement of the pancreatic tissue.

Gastrointestinal Bleeding

The causes of GI bleeding in patients in the pediatric age group are numerous and depend upon the age of the patient (Table 52.7).

In the neonate, common causes include necrotizing enterocolitis, milk allergy, and the enterocolitis that sometimes accompanies Hirschsprung disease. NEC is a form of intestinal inflammation and necrosis that primarily occurs in premature infants but can also be seen in the term neonate. NEC can be triggered by multiple factors, but ischemia and infection are thought to be the most important causative factors. On radiographs, the involved intestinal loops become dilated, and bowel wall thickening may be apparent. Pneumatosis intestinalis is a common and pathognomic finding consisting of linear or bubbly collections of gas that lie within the intestinal wall (see Fig. 52.28). Necrotic loops may remain fixed and distended, even as the other dilated intestinal loops become decompressed. A dilated, fixed loop may be a harbinger of impending intestinal perforation and should be evaluated with left lateral decubitus or crosstable lateral views (Fig. 52.36). Ulcer disease and hemorrhagic gastritis may also be associated with hypoxia or sepsis. Anal fissures are a common cause of rectal bleeding in infants.

In older infants and children, peptic ulcer disease is an important cause of upper GI tract bleeding.

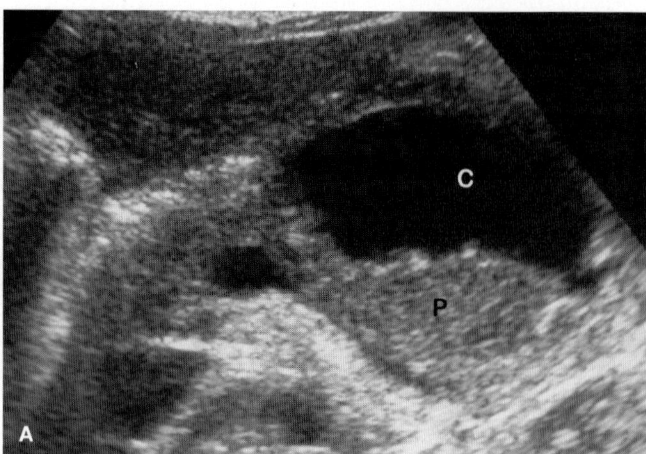

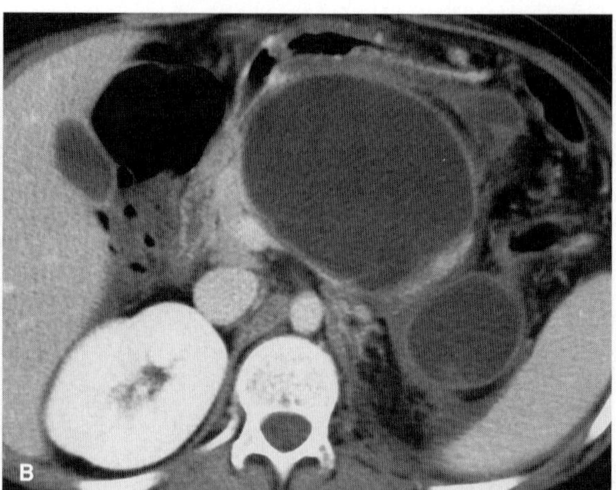

FIGURE 52.35. **Pancreatitis. A.** Posttraumatic pancreatitis in a child following motor vehicle collision was complicated by the development of a large, lobulated pseudocyst (C). P, pancreas. **B.** CT of the same child shows the well-defined, enhancing rim of the pseudocyst collections and inflammation in the adjacent mesenteric fat.

Coagulopathies can result in intestinal hematomas. Bloody diarrhea is a common component of *E. coli*–associated hemolytic uremic syndrome in young children. GI bleeding may be the presenting symptom of unsuspected portal vein thrombosis. Henoch-Schönlein purpura is a vasculitis of unknown etiology that affects the skin, GI tract, joints, and kidneys. In half of cases, crampy abdominal pain and intestinal bleeding occur. The transmural bowel wall thickening that is common in these patients is readily demonstrable with US (35), and color Doppler US reveals increased vascularity in affected intestinal loops (36). Gadolinium-enhanced MR is an emerging technique for assessing disease activity in inflammatory bowel disease (38).

TABLE 52.7 Causes of GI Bleeding

Peptic ulcer disease
Enterocolitis
- Necrotizing enterocolitis
- Milk allergy
- Hirschsprung disease
- Regional enteritis
- Ulcerative colitis

Hemorrhagic gastritis of the newborn
Anal fissures
Bleeding disorders
Henoch-Schönlein purpura
Hemolytic uremic syndrome
Juvenile polyps
Meckel diverticulum
Intussusception
Portal vein thrombosis
Duplication cysts
Colonic vascular malformations

Abdominal symptoms may precede the characteristic skin rash. US demonstrates segmental and circumferential echogenic thickening of the bowel wall (Fig. 52.37) (63). Findings on CT include multifocal areas of bowel wall thickening, mesenteric edema, and lymphadenopathy (64).

Rectal bleeding in older children is most often caused by juvenile inflammatory polyps, which are most common in the sigmoid and rectum. Painless, sometimes profuse, rectal bleeding may occur with Meckel diverticulum. Meckel diverticulum arises from the ileum approximately 80 cm from the ileocecal valve. Ectopic gastric or pancreatic

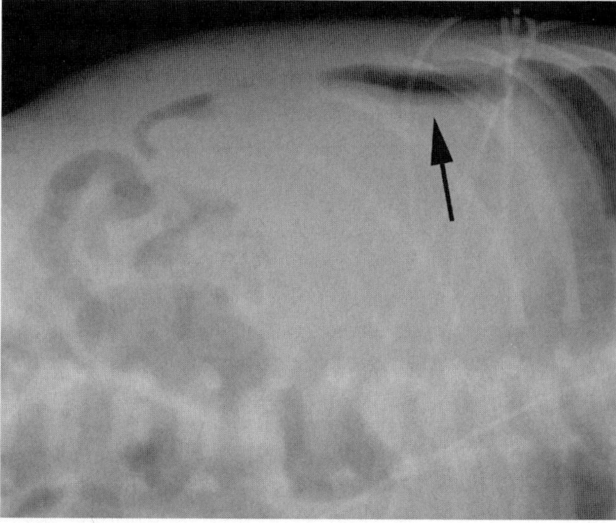

FIGURE 52.36. **Necrotizing Enterocolitis.** Perforation. A left lateral decubitus view shows a sliver of free intraperitoneal air between the liver and abdominal wall (*arrow*).

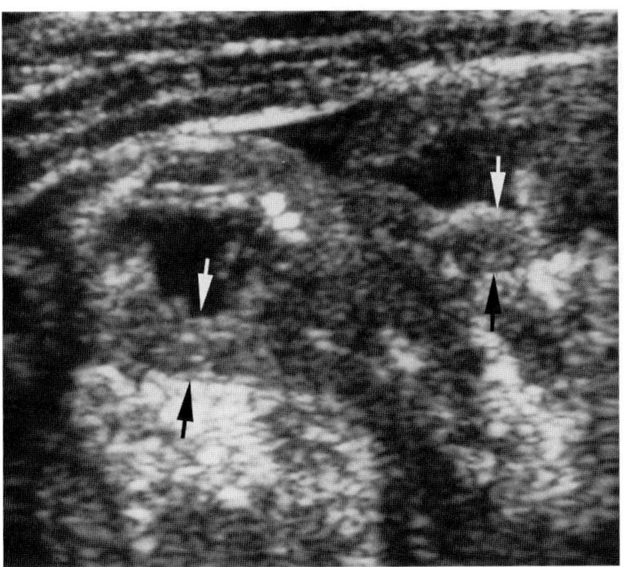

FIGURE 52.37. **Henoch-Schönlein Purpura.** The bowel wall (*arrows*) is echogenic and thickened as a result of mucosal and submucosal edema and hemorrhage.

tissue, found in 20% to 30% of Meckel diverticula, is a site for ulceration, hemorrhage, and perforation. The best initial examination to identify a bleeding Meckel diverticulum is a technetium-99m-pertechnate scan (see Chapter 59). The tracer localizes in the ectopic gastric mucosa (Fig. 52.38). Meckel diverticulum may act as a lead point for intussusception, which is an important cause of painful hematochezia in young children. The diverticulum may also become inflamed or mimic appendicitis. Vascular malformations of the colon are uncommon and may present confusing imaging findings (65).

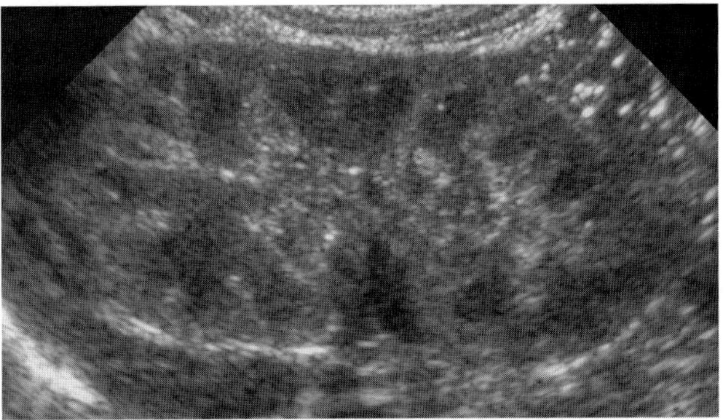

FIGURE 52.39. **Normal Neonatal Kidney.** Note the mildly echogenic cortex and the sonolucent medullary pyramids, which are often mistaken for cysts. The echogenicity of the cortex is similar to that of the liver and is normal.

GENITOURINARY TRACT

Normal Anatomy. Neonatal kidneys are proportionately larger and more lobulated than the kidneys of older children and adults. On US, the renal cortex in infants under 2 or 3 months of age is normally echogenic, whereas the medullary pyramids are prominent and hypoechoic (Fig. 52.39). The appearance should not be mistaken for hydronephrosis or renal cysts. Newborn female infants have a prominent uterus owing to stimulation by maternal estrogen. The uterus remains enlarged for 2 or 3 months and then involutes and remains small until puberty. The epididymis in male neonates and young infants is larger than in older children and adults.

Renal Abnormalities

Urinary tract infection is a common problem in infants and children, especially in girls. Ascending infection from

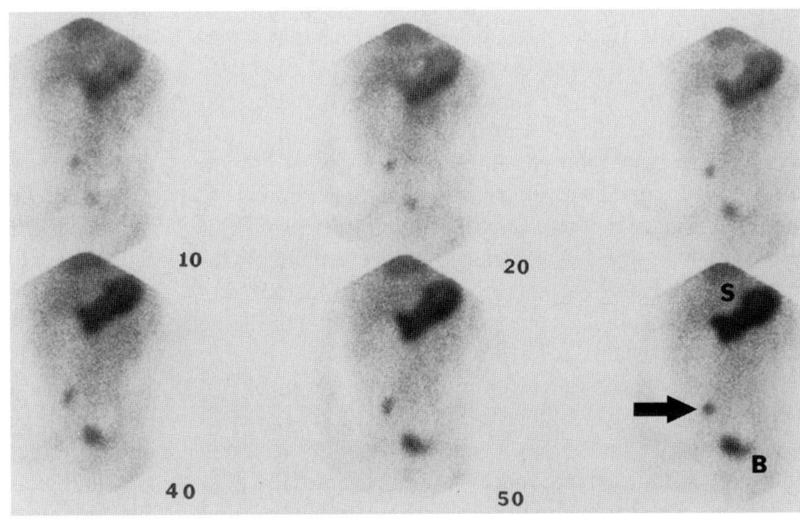

FIGURE 52.38. **Meckel Diverticulum.** A scan performed with technetium-99m-pertechnate shows an abnormal collection of tracer in the right lower quadrant (*arrow*), whose intensity parallels that of the stomach (S). Gastric mucosa within the Meckel diverticulum is responsible for the tracer localization. B, bladder.

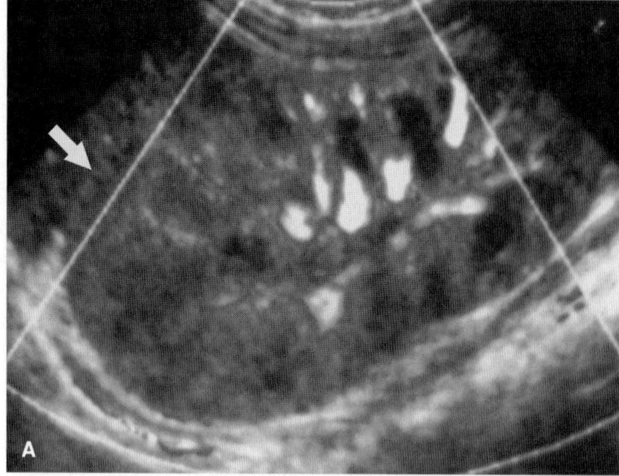

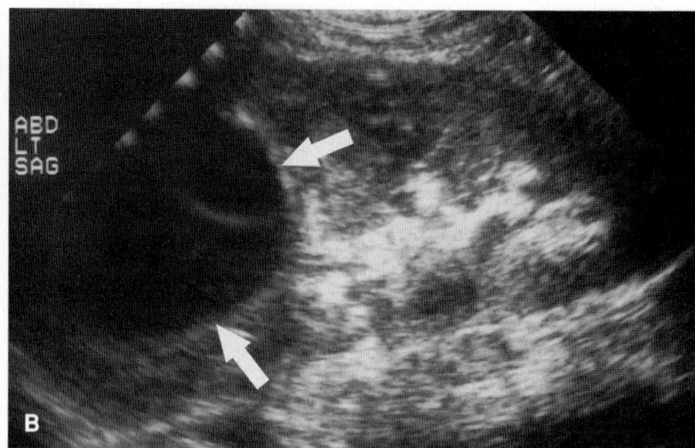

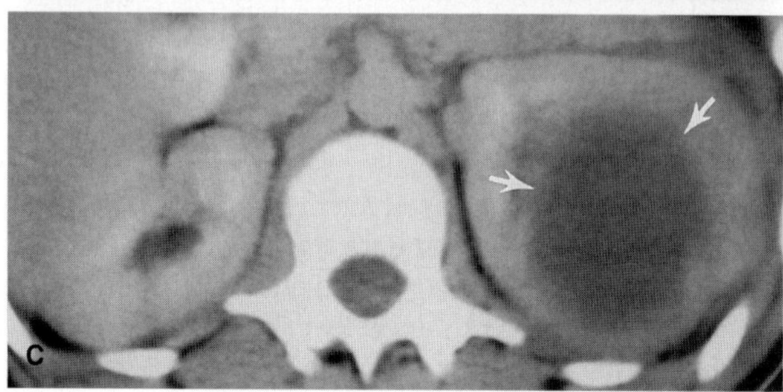

FIGURE 52.40. **(Color Plates) Renal Abscess. A.** Color flow Doppler shows decreased blood flow in the slightly enlarged and echogenic upper pole (*arrow*) of the kidney caused by pyelonephritis.**B.** US shows an anechoic abscess (*arrows*) in the upper pole of the left kidney. **C.** CT study with contrast enhancement also demonstrates the abscess (*arrows*) in the enlarged left kidney. Compare with the normal right kidney.

the bladder can lead to chronic reflux, scarring, and growth impairment of the kidneys. In neonates, urinary tract infection is usually hematogenous and accompanies generalized sepsis. Obstructive uropathy can lead to urinary tract infection. Isolated cystitis may be bacterial or viral and is manifest by thickening of the mucosa of the bladder, demonstrated by US or cystourethrography. Renal US is an important component of the diagnostic evaluation of children with urinary tract infection and has largely replaced IV pyelography for evaluation of the kidneys in children. Renal sonography allows assessment of renal size and parenchymal architecture and allows identification of hydronephrosis, renal cysts, and other lesions that might predispose the patient to develop urinary tract infection. Pyelonephritis is the most common cause of renal scarring in children, and the scarring appears to occur independently from vesicoureteral reflux (VUR) (66). Children are usually treated for pyelonephritis based on clinical parameters. Color or power Doppler sonography may show altered vascularity in the region of acute pyelonephritis (Fig. 52.40A). Renal cortical scintigraphy or MR may provide useful information about renal scarring after the acute infection has resolved (67,68).

Renal abscess is an uncommon complication of urinary tract infection in children. The abscess can be demonstrated with US and CT as a round or oval cystic lesion that may contain debris and enhances peripherally (Fig. 52.40B, C). Premature infants and immunocompromised children are prone to fungal infection, in which echogenic clusters of hyphae can become impacted in the renal collecting structures and result in hydronephrosis.

Vesicoureteral reflux is a common disorder in children that lead to ascending infection, renal growth impairment, and parenchymal scarring. VUR may occur in an otherwise normally functioning bladder or may be secondary to poor bladder emptying because of bladder outlet obstruction or neurogenic bladder. Primary VUR is caused by a short, submucosal tunnel of the distal ureter at the ureterovesical junction, compromising the valve mechanism at this site that normally prevents urine from refluxing into the ureters and kidneys. Experiments have shown that sterile reflux does not result in renal damage beyond fetal life and that most renal scarring is the result of infection transmitted from the bladder to the kidneys during VUR. Children with siblings or parents who have VUR have a higher incidence of reflux than the general population and should be screened with voiding cystourethrography (VCUG).

VUR and bladder and function can be evaluated with contrast or radioisotope VCUG. Nuclear scintigraphy is more sensitive for VUR but provides poor anatomic detail. Contrast VCUG provides better definition of urethra, bladder, and ureteropelvic anatomy (Fig 52.41). Structural abnormalities at the ureterovesical junction, such as congenital Hutch diverticulum, may alter the ureteral insertion and predispose the patient to VUR and infection. Dysfunctional voiding may also be recognized with VCUG in

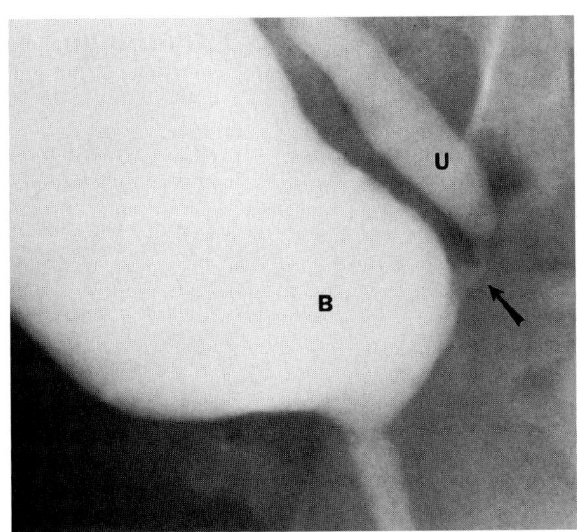

FIGURE 52.41. **Horizontal Ureteral Insertion With Reflux.** Voiding cystourethrogram reveals reflux of contrast from the bladder (B) that opacifies and dilates the left ureter (U). Note the horizontal orientation of the distal ureter (*arrow*).

otherwise healthy children. Contraction of the external urinary sphincter in the presence of muscular bladder contractions results in increased intervesicular pressures and predisposes to VUR. Contrast-enhanced US for evaluation of the urethra and VUR is shown to be feasible but has yet to be widely accepted (69,70).

VUR is graded from I through IV (Fig. 52.42). Grade III reflux causes mild dilatation of the ureter and renal collecting structures, while grade IV reflux is characterized

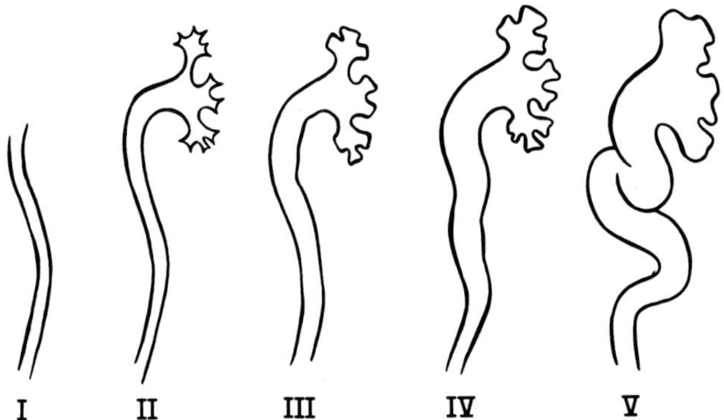

FIGURE 52.42. **Classification of Reflux.** Reflux into the distal ureter is grade I. Reflux into the upper collecting system with no dilation of the upper tract is grade II. Grade III reflux shows similar findings, but with mild blunting of the calices. All of these findings are exaggerated in grade IV reflux, with marked hydroureter and caliceal dilatation. When the ureter is massively dilated and tortuous and the upper tract is markedly dilated, grade V reflux is present. (International classification modified after: Medical versus surgical treatment of primary vesicoureteral reflux: report of the International Reflux Study Committee. Pediatrics 1981;67:392–400.)

by greater dilatation of the renal pelvis, calices, and ureter and blunting of the renal calices. Severe hydronephrosis with marked tortuosity and dilatation of the ureter indicates grade V reflux. VUR grades I through III commonly resolves spontaneously as the child grows and usually is treated medically with low-dose prophylactic antibiotics. Surgical correction is usually reserved for children with the more severe grades of reflux (IV and V) or children who develop urinary tract infections despite prophylactic antibiotics. Surgical correction involves reimplantation of the ureter to create a longer submucosal tunnel for the distal ureter. Laparoscopic injection of synthetic substances at the ureterovesical junction can be performed in some children.

Hydronephrosis can result from obstructive uropathy or VUR. Not all patients with VUR show hydronephrosis at US, especially when the urinary bladder is not fully distended. Therefore, renal US cannot be used to reliably screen children for VUR. The addition of color Doppler to US imaging improves visualization of retrograde flow of urine from the bladder into the ureters and renal collecting structures. With experience, cystoscopy utilizing color Doppler US may become a sufficiently sensitive screening modality for VUR, with considerable savings in radiation dosage. Hydronephrosis may also be seen in conditions associated with increased urine output and overload of the renal collecting system. Such high-output hydronephrosis is rare but may be seen with Bartter syndrome, diabetes insipidus, and psychogenic water drinking.

Urinary tract obstruction in infants and children is predominantly the result of a variety of congenital and developmental abnormalities. Urinary tract obstruction may develop at any point along the course of the urinary tract, but the most common sites are the ureteropelvic junction, the ureterovesical junction, and the bladder outlet and ureter. Congenital ureteropelvic junction obstruction may be caused by inadequate recanalization of the ureteral lumen during fetal development, kinking of the ureteropelvic junction, or extrinsic compression by bands or aberrant vessels. Dilatation of the renal pelvis and calices can become severe during fetal life and is often detected at prenatal US. Typically, with ureteropelvic junction obstruction, the renal pelvis and calices are dilated but the ureter is normal in caliber (Fig. 52.43A). The severity of obstruction can only be implied by the degree of hydronephrosis on US and is more precisely evaluated using renal scintigraphy with furosemide washout (Fig. 52.43B to D). MR urography is a developing technique that may allow detailed evaluation of renal anatomy and function (71).

Hydronephrosis accompanied by ureteral dilatation can be seen with severe VUR or obstruction at the ureterovesical junction. Primary megaureter is an uncommon form of congenital obstruction of the distal ureter that results from abnormal development of the muscular layers of the distal ureter. Passage of urine through the abnormal

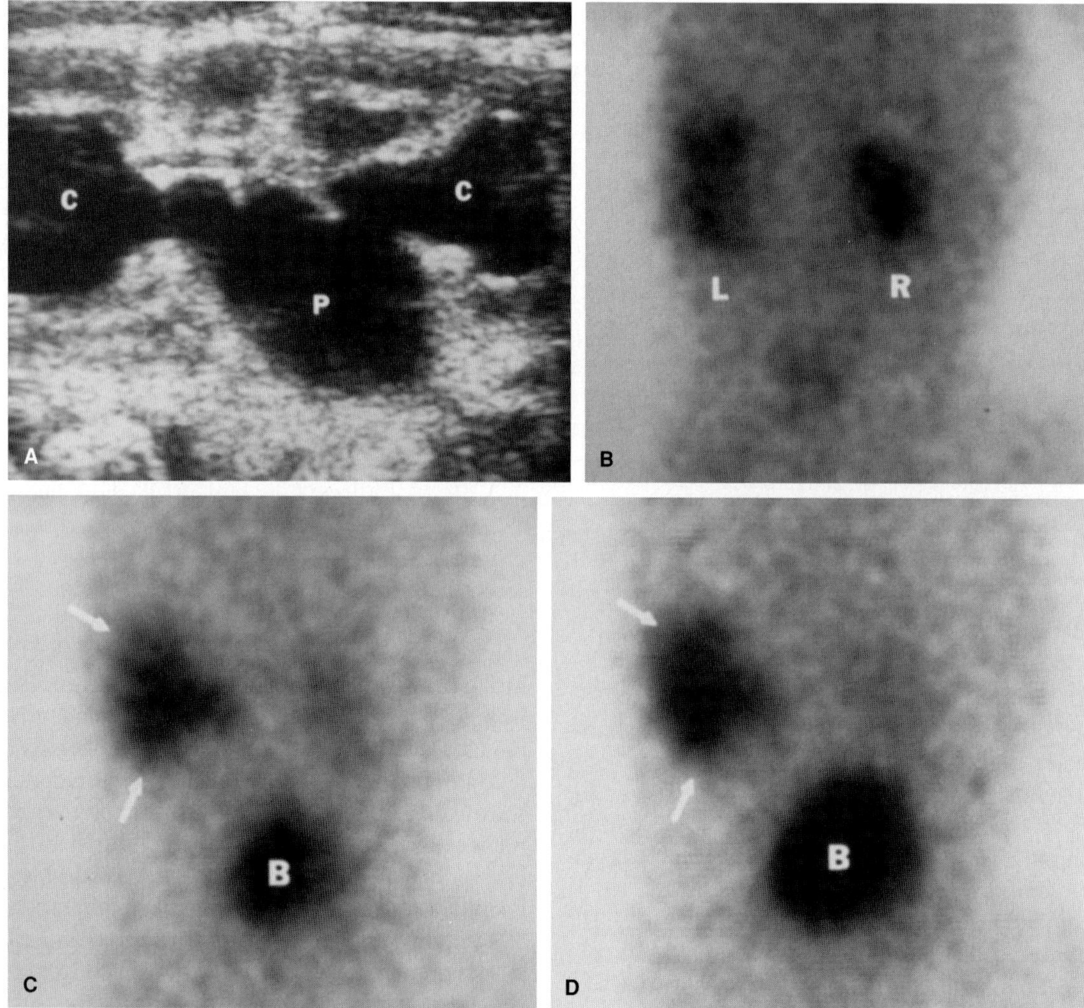

FIGURE 52.43. **Ureteropelvic Junction Obstruction. A.** Sonogram demonstrates a dilated renal pelvis (P) and markedly dilated renal calices (C). **B.** Nuclear scintigraphy, early phase, demonstrates activity in both the right (R) and left (L) kidneys. Note that less activity is seen in the left kidney. **C.** Fifteen minutes later, there is marked accumulation of radioactive tracer in the left kidney (*arrows*); some is now accumulating in the bladder (B). The right kidney has emptied and is normal. **D.** After the administration of furosemide, no activity is seen in the right kidney, increased activity is seen in the bladder (B), and marked activity has persisted in the obstructed left kidney (*arrows*).

distal ureteral segment is ineffective because of diminished peristalsis, resulting in functional obstruction and dilatation of the more proximal portions of the normal ureter (Fig. 52.44). Antegrade pyelograms reveal a contracted juxtavesical portion of the ureter with primary megaureter, in comparison to a widely patent ureterovesical junction that occurs with refluxing megaureter. Functional obstruction of the distal ureter may also occur when intravesical pressures are elevated because of poor bladder emptying (e.g., neurogenic bladder, urethral obstruction).

Ureteral Duplication and Ectopic Ureterocele. Duplication anomalies of the renal collecting structures and ureters are common in children but are only clinically significant when accompanied by VUR or obstruction. In those children with complete ureteral duplications, the ureter that drains the upper pole collecting system of the kidney typically exerts in an ectopic location, often the bladder neck or urethra. Ureterocele is a saccular dilated segment of the distal ureter that invaginates into the bladder lumen and impedes the flow of urine from the ureter into the bladder. Ureteroceles may also occur with single ureters and may arise in an orthotopic position within the urinary bladder. Ectopic ureterocele is more common in girls, and approximately 10% are bilateral. The upper pole moiety of the kidney may be hydronephrotic (Fig. 52.45A) or atrophic and difficult to visualize. The urine-filled

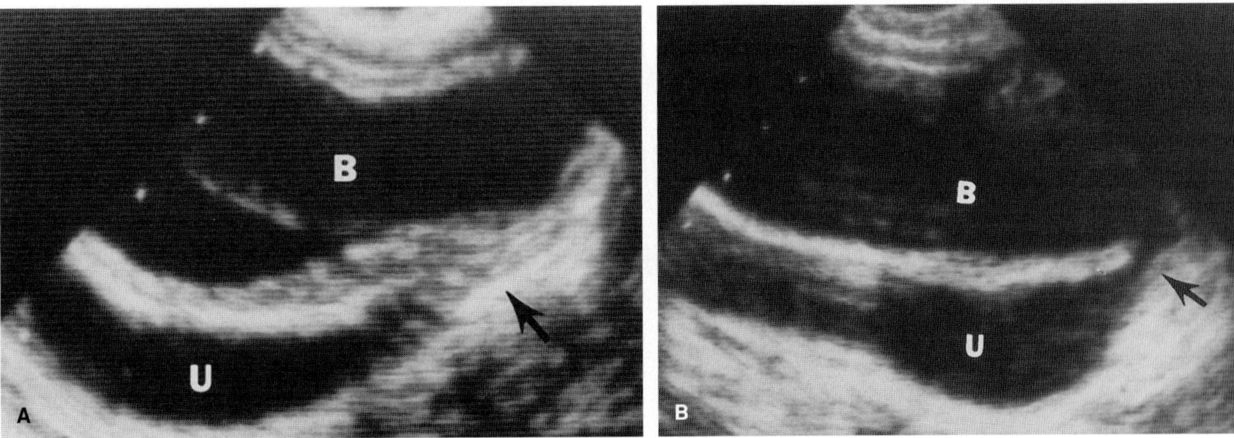

FIGURE 52.44. **Megaureter Versus Refluxing Ureter. A.** Primary megaureter is diagnosed when the dilated ureter (U) demonstrates a persistently spastic distal segment (*arrow*). B, urinary bladder. **B.** Refluxing ureter (U) demonstrates similar dilation, but the distal end is open (*arrow*). B, urinary bladder. (From Hayden CK Jr, Swischuk LE. Pediatric Ultrasonography. 2nd ed. Baltimore: Williams & Wilkins, 1992; reprinted with permission.)

ureterocele has a round or oval configuration and is easily visible with US (Fig. 52.45B). Ureteroceles are sometimes visible as filling defects in the lower bladder with cystourethrography; however, the pressures generated within the bladder during this procedure may compress the ureterocele, making it more difficult to visualize. Hydronephrosis of the lower pole moiety of the kidney is also common, usually the result of VUR. Single-system ureteroceles are much less common than those associated with ureteral duplication. Single-system ureteroceles tend to be small and tend to event during VCUG, giving the appearance of a paravertebral diverticulum (72).

Renal Agenesis. Agenesis of one or both kidneys may be an isolated anomaly or may be associated with autosomal dominant transmission. Unilateral renal agenesis is frequently detected on prenatal US. Anomalies of the male or female reproductive system are commonly associated with unilateral absence of the kidney. Renal agenesis results from the lack of induction of the primitive renal tissue (i.e., metanephric blastema) by the ureteral butt. Bilateral renal agenesis leads to oligohydramnios and compression of the fetus. Fetal compression leads to abnormal facial features, skeletal abnormalities, and severe hypoplasia. Bilateral pneumothoraces often occur at birth and tend to be refractory. The absence of renal tissue should be verified with US postnatally, because other congenital conditions that cause decreased urine output (e.g., polycystic kidney disease, posterior urethral valves) may also lead to Potter

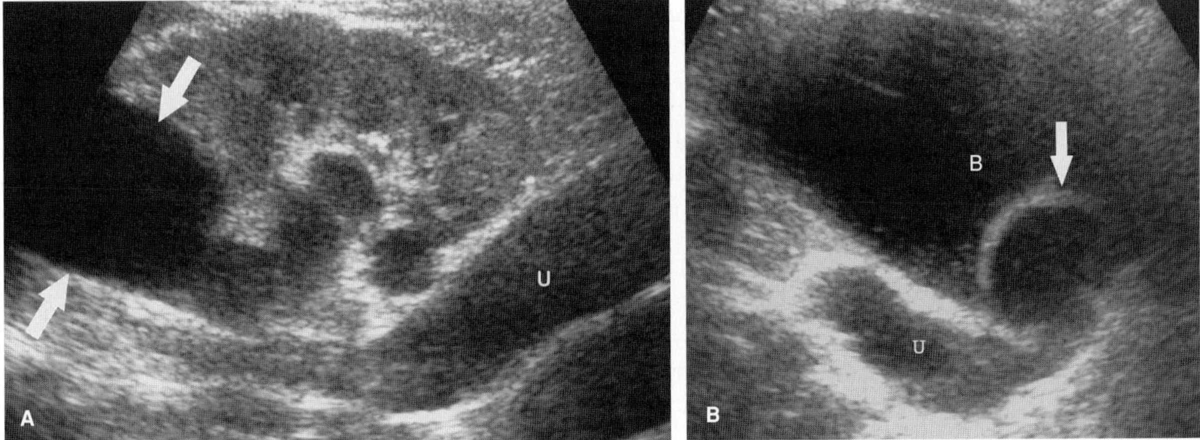

FIGURE 52.45. **Ectopic Ureterocele. A.** Sagittal US of the left kidney demonstrates a hydronephrotic upper pole (*arrows*) and a dilated distal ureter (U). **B.** Sagittal US through the urinary bladder (B) demonstrates the distended ureterocele (*arrow*) projecting into the bladder base. The distal ureter (U) is dilated as it inserts into the ureterocele.

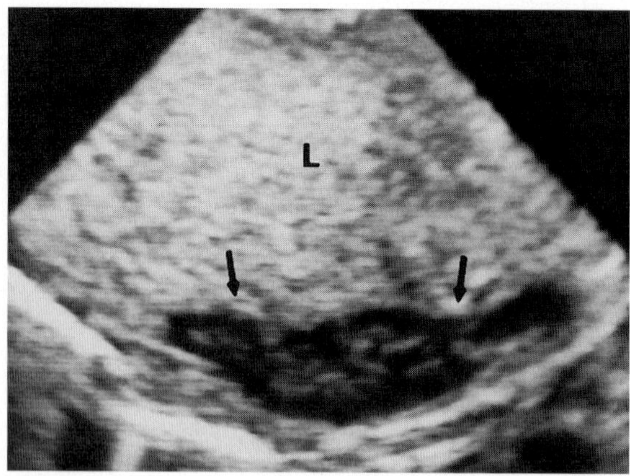

FIGURE 52.46. **Renal Agenesis.** In this patient with bilateral renal agenesis (Potter syndrome), the large but normal adrenal gland (*arrows*) may erroneously suggest the presence of a kidney. L, liver.

syndrome. When renal tissue is absent, the adrenal glands often appear large and elongated, but they should not be mistaken for kidneys (Fig. 52.46).

Renal cystic disease is reviewed in detail in Chapter 33. High-resolution US technology has improved the ability to distinguish between the various types of renal cystic disease, especially the autosomal dominant and autosomal recessive forms of polycystic kidney disease (Fig. 52.47). Simple renal cysts are less common in children than in adults and more commonly benign in nature (Table 52.8).

Renal calcifications may lie within the collecting structures (nephrolithiasis) or within the renal parenchyma (nephrocalcinosis). Nephrolithiasis is relatively rare in children, and the imaging evaluation is the same as that in adults. Nephrolithiasis can be seen in children without underlying metabolic disease. Nephrocalcinosis, on the other hand, is seen in a variety of metabolic conditions. The calcifications frequently reside in the medullary portion of the kidney, giving the appearance of punctate or diffuse increased echogenicity in the renal pyramids on US (Fig. 52.48). The most common causes of nephrocalcinosis in children are listed in Table 52.9. Transient increased echogenicity is often seen in the tips of medullary pyramids in normal newborns.

Bladder and Urethral Abnormalities

Bladder Dysfunction. Abnormal bladder function and voiding may be a primary abnormality or may result from central or peripheral neurologic disease such as myelodysplasia, hydrocephalus, cerebral infarcts, or brain or spinal cord neoplasms. Upper motor neuron abnormalities, which occur above the level of the pons, result in loss of voiding control and spastic bladder (detrusor hyperreflexia). Spinal cord lesions or injuries between the pons

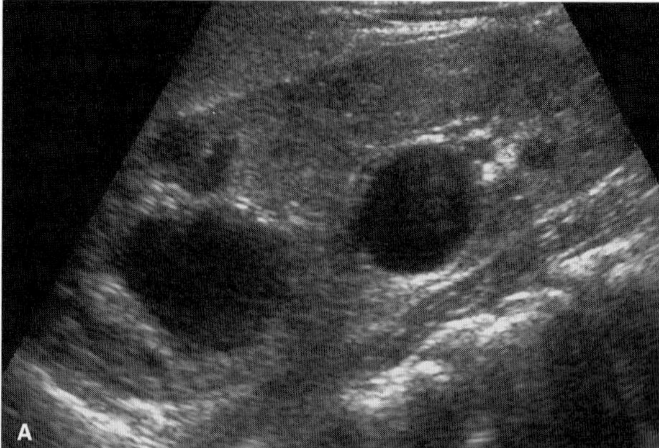

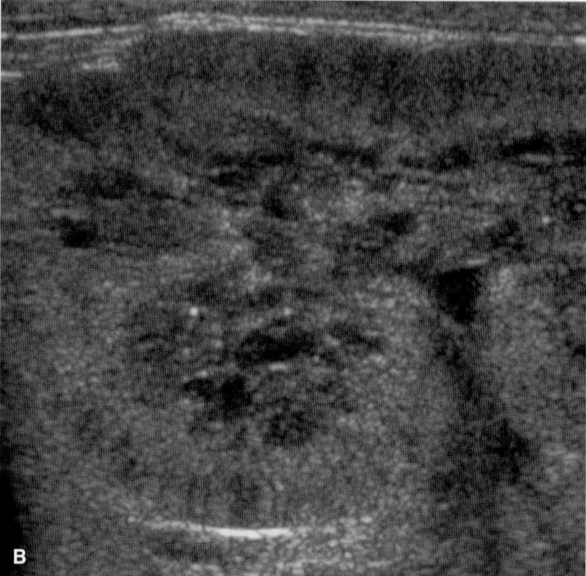

FIGURE 52.47. **Polycystic Kidney Disease. A.** Autosomal dominant polycystic kidney disease characteristically shows round cysts of varying sizes. The kidneys may be enlarged bilaterally, but the presence of cysts is often asymmetric. **B.** Autosomal recessive polycystic kidney disease is characterized by small, more uniformly sized cysts with a tubular appearance with high-resolution US. These cysts may predominate in the medullary portion of the kidney or may extend to the cortex.

and the sacral cord also result in a spastic bladder. In some patients, abnormal external sphincter contraction occurs during contraction of the detrusor muscle, preventing urination and increasing the pressure within the bladder. This condition, known as *detrusor-sphincter dyssynergy,* is common in children with myelodysplasia and often results in VUR. Cystography of those patients reveals a small, often markedly trabeculated bladder. Disorders of the sacral spinal cord or peripheral nerves lead to an overdistended bladder because of lack of bladder contraction (detrusor areflexia). The bladder in such patients appears large but smooth in contour.

Bladder diverticula may be solitary or multiple. Solitary bladder diverticula are usually congenital in nature.

TABLE 52.8 Causes of Renal Cysts

Single
Simple cyst
Caliceal diverticulum
Abscess
Multilocular cystic nephroma
Multiple
Multicystic dysplastic kidney
Polycystic kidney disease
Glomerulocystic disease
Medullary cystic disease (juvenile nephronophthisis)
Tuberous sclerosis
Turner syndrome
von Hippel-Lindau disease
Zellweger syndrome
Beckwith-Wiedemann syndrome
Meckel-Gruber syndrome

TABLE 52.9 Causes of Echogenic Renal Pyramids

Normal neonate
Tamm-Horsfall proteinuria
Sickle-cell disease
Hypercalciuria
Renal tubular acidosis
Medullary sponge kidney
Hyperparathyroidism
Drugs (furosemide, steroids, vitamin D)
Prolonged immobilization
Bartter syndrome
Williams syndrome
Autosomal recessive polycystic kidney disease
Storage diseases
Glycogen-storage disease type 1A
Hurler mucopolysaccharidosis
Lesch-Nyhan syndrome
Oxalosis

The congenital Hutch diverticulum lies adjacent to the ureterovesical junction (Fig. 52.49) and is associated with an increased incidence of VUR. Multiple bladder diverticula are commonly the result of neurogenic bladder or chronic bladder outlet obstruction in children. The bladder diverticula are usually numerous. Multiple bladder diverticula may also be seen with such syndromes as Ehlers-Danlos syndrome, Williams syndrome, Menkes syndrome, and prune belly syndrome (73). Urachal remnants arise from the dome of the bladder at the midline. Urachal anomalies include asymptomatic vesicourachal diverticula, with obliteration of the urachus on each end, or the urachal sinus consisting of a persistently patent urachus extending from the urinary bladder to the umbilicus.

Megacystis (marked enlargement of the urinary bladder) is a prominent feature in two syndromes.

Prune belly (Eagle-Barrett) syndrome is a condition that is seen almost exclusively in males. Features include absent or deficient abdominal musculature; a large, vertically oriented urinary bladder; severe hydronephrosis

FIGURE 52.48. **Nephrocalcinosis.** Punctate areas of increased echogenicity are present in the medullary pyramids (*arrows*), representing calcifications. Nephrocalcinosis occurred in this infant as a result of chronic furosemide therapy.

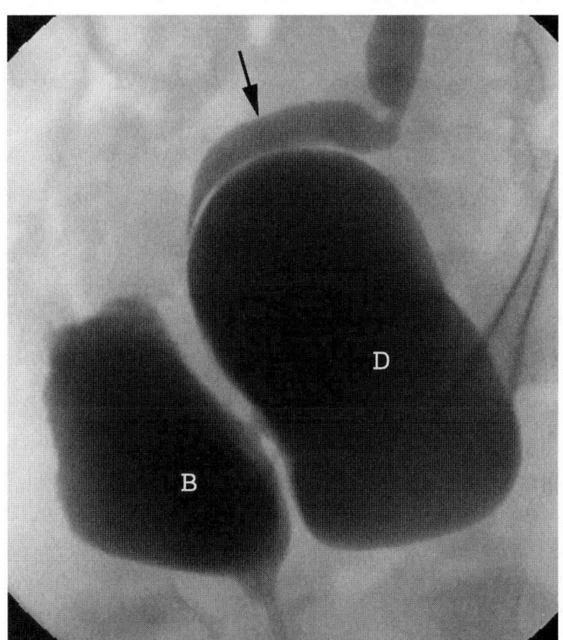

FIGURE 52.49. **Hutch Diverticulum.** An unusually large paraureteral (Hutch) diverticulum (D) arises from the region of the left ureterovesical junction and is associated with reflux into the left ureter (*arrow*). B, bladder.

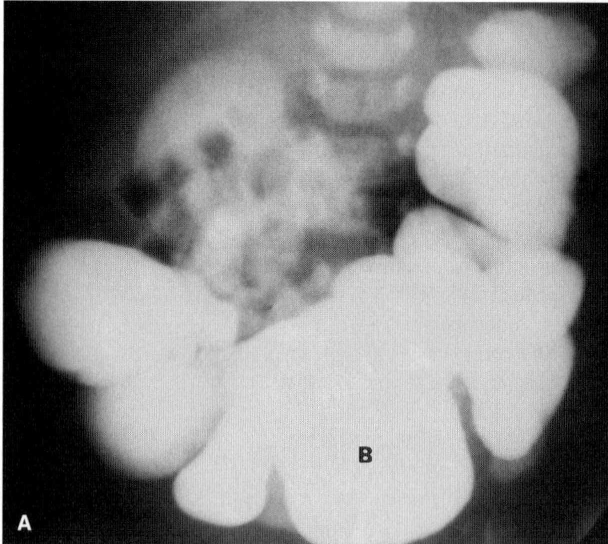

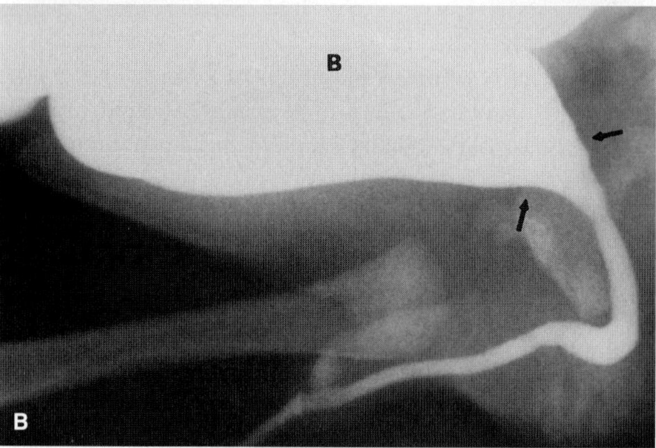

FIGURE 52.50. **Prune Belly Syndrome (Eagle-Barrett Syndrome). A.** Note the large bladder (B) and massive reflux into the grossly dilated ureters and upper collecting systems on both sides. **B.** Lateral view of the bladder (B) during voiding demonstrates the characteristic cone-shaped posterior urethra-bladder neck region (*arrows*).

and ureterectasis; cryptorchidism; and urethral dysfunction leading to functional bladder obstruction (Fig. 52.50). Urachal remnants are also common.

Megacystis-microcolon-hypoperistalsis (MMH) syndrome results from a disorder of smooth muscle in the urinary and GI tract. This condition occurs almost exclusively in girls. Insufficiency of the abdominal musculature is also seen in the MMH syndrome. The bladder is very large and dysfunctional. Decreased intestinal peristalsis leads to poor evacuation of the colon in infants who survive. Bladder exstrophy occurs when the bladder is exposed through a large defect in the anterior abdominal wall. Marked widening of the symphysis pubis and splaying of the pelvic bones are noted on radiographs in these infants.

Cloacal anomalies represent persistence of a primitive common channel that includes the rectum, vagina, and urethra. The anatomy of these malformations is quite variable and requires injection of contrast into all available orifices for complete evaluation. Cloacal exstrophy is caused by failed closure of the lower abdominal wall and represents a severe form of bladder exstrophy.

Rhabdomyosarcoma is the most common tumor to affect the lower urinary tract in children. The neoplasm most often arises from the prostate gland in boys and from the vagina in girls. The mass is usually quite large at the time of presentation and is detected early in infancy. Imaging findings include a polypoid or grapelike mass causing elevation of the bladder and obstruction of the bladder neck.

Posterior urethral valve is the most common cause of urethral obstruction in male infants. Abnormal migration and insertion of the urethrovaginal folds result in sail-like flaps of tissue that arise at the base of the prostatic urethra below the verumontanum, known as type I valves. The valves cause obstruction to antegrade flow of urine, leading dilatation of the posterior urethra, bladder wall thickening and trabeculation, and VUR (Fig. 52.51A, B). Type III posterior urethral valves consist of a membrane caused by incomplete canalization in the region of the urogenital diaphragm (Fig. 52.51C). The type II "valve" actually consists of a nonobstructive mucosal fold rather than an obstructing membrane. Anterior urethral valves are rare obstructive lesions of uncertain etiology. The valve may appear as a linear filling defect or simply an abrupt change of caliber within the anterior urethra.

Genital Abnormalities

Ambiguous genitalia result from a variety of congenital abnormalities of sexual differentiation. Congenital adrenal hyperplasia is the cause of approximately 60% of cases of ambiguous genitalia. Most often the infant is genotypically female with two ovaries. Virilization is most often the result of 21-hydroxylase deficiency leading to buildup of androgens. Male pseudohermaphrodism is often caused by androgen insensitivity. The male gonads are underdeveloped and the Müllerian structures are absent. Mixed gonadal dysgenesis is characterized by a testis plus a gonadal streak, and pure gonadal dysgenesis consists of bilateral streak, dysgenetic gonads. Both ovarian and testicular tissues are present in true hermaphrodism, which accounts for fewer than 10% of intersex abnormalities. Imaging is used to demonstrate the presence or absence of a vagina and uterus and to aid with gender assignment. US is usually adequate, but retrograde vaginography may be required in some cases. US may reveal enlarged, undulating, "cerebriform adrenal" glands in infants with congenital adrenal hyperplasia. Contrast injected into the urethra may fill an enlarged utricle in boys or confluence of the vagina and urethra into a urogenital sinus in girls

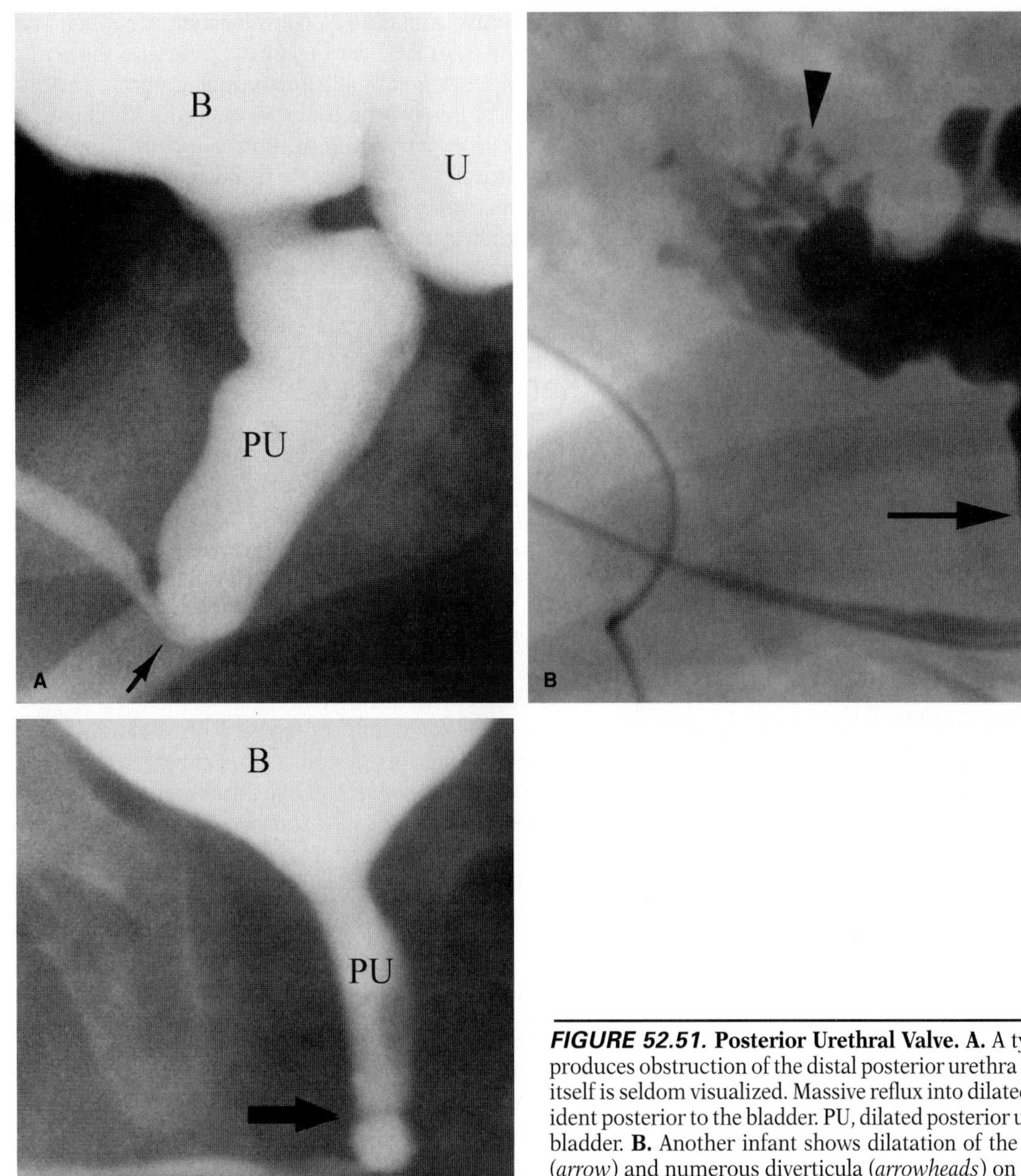

FIGURE 52.51. **Posterior Urethral Valve. A.** A typical type I valve produces obstruction of the distal posterior urethra (*arrow*). The valve itself is seldom visualized. Massive reflux into dilated ureters (U) is evident posterior to the bladder. PU, dilated posterior urethra; B, urinary bladder. **B.** Another infant shows dilatation of the posterior urethra (*arrow*) and numerous diverticula (*arrowheads*) on the small, chronically obstructed bladder. **C.** The thin diaphragm (*arrow*) in the distal posterior urethra (PU) is characteristic of a type III valve. B, bladder.

(Fig. 52.52). The length of the urogenital sinus determines the type of surgical repair.

Testicular abnormalities are reviewed in chapters 35 and 37. The most common cause of a scrotal mass in children is congenital hydrocele. Peritoneal fluid passes into the scrotum through a patent processus vaginalis (Fig. 52.53). The defect usually closes spontaneously, and most hydroceles resolve by 2 years of age. Acquired hydroceles may develop in association with testicular inflammation, trauma, or torsion. The identification of blood flow within the testis with color Doppler imaging helps to differentiate inflammation from acute testicular torsion. With torsion, blood flow within the testis is decreased or absent (Fig. 52.54), but with epididymitis or orchitis, blood flow is increased within the testis (74). The spermatic cord should be evaluated during color Doppler US to identify a spiral configuration indicating torsion (75).

Cryptorchidism (undescended testis) is common, occurring in approximately 4% of term newborn boys. The majority of undescended testes will spontaneously descend into the scrotal sac by 1 year of age. Most undescended testes can be found in the inguinal region and are easily identified by US. MR is better suited for detection of testes that reside in the pelvis.

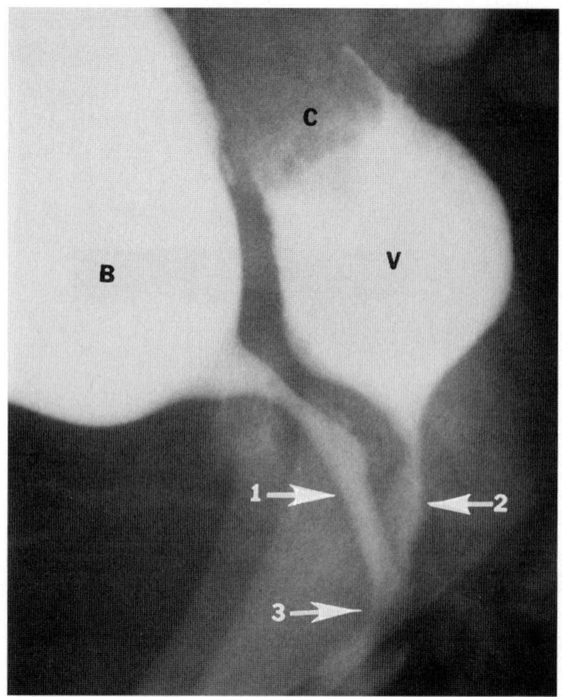

FIGURE 52.52. **Urogenital Sinus.** A short urogenital sinus (3) receives drainage from the vagina (V) via a fistula (2) and from the urinary bladder (B) via the urethra (1). The cervix (C) is seen as a filling defect in the contrast-filled vagina.

Testicular tumors are uncommon in childhood. The most common testicular neoplasm before puberty is the yolk sac tumor. Non–germ cell tumors that occur in children include the Leydig cell tumor, which occurs most commonly at 4 to 5 years of age, and the Sertoli cell tumor, which is most often seen in infants under 6 months of age. Gonadoblastoma is a neoplasm that occurs in children with intersex disorders, usually arising in the gonadal streaks or intra-abdominal testes of phenotypic females.

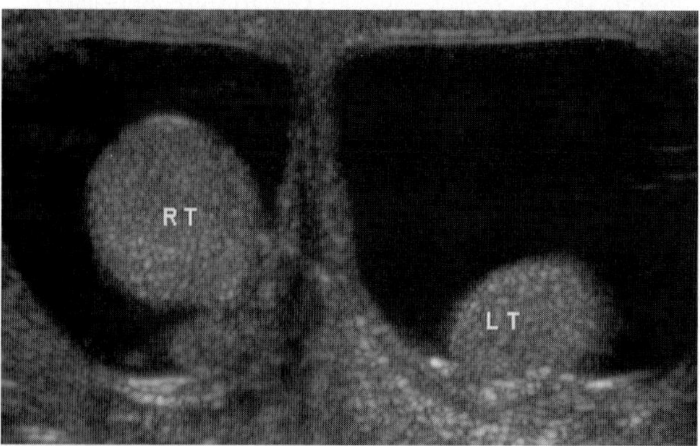

FIGURE 52.53. **Bilateral Hydroceles.** Transverse US demonstrates large, intrascrotal fluid collections that surround the right (RT) and left (LT) testes anchored to the posterior scrotal wall.

Rhabdomyosarcoma is a paratesticular neoplasm arising from the spermatic cord and extending into the scrotum. Leukemia and lymphoma are the most common metastatic tumors to involve the testes in children. Malignant neoplasms of the testis and scrotum are often accompanied by hydrocele. US verifies the solid nature of a testicular mass but cannot differentiate the type of tumor (76). Small, hypoechoic nodules representing adrenal rests can occur with congenital adrenal hyperplasia and should not be mistaken for malignancy (77,78).

ABDOMINAL MASSES

Abdominal masses are common in infants and children, and imaging plays an important role in their diagnosis and management. Plain radiographs provide clues to the location of the mass and the presence of calcifications. US is generally the most valuable procedure for the initial evaluation. US differentiates cystic from solid masses, indicates the organ of origin, and commonly suggests the diagnosis. CT or MR may be needed when the mass is large, poorly defined, or obscured by bowel gas.

Pseudomasses may be caused on abdominal radiographs by a fluid-filled stomach, urinary bladder, or a loop of intestine. Structures outside the abdomen, such as large skin lesions, umbilical hernias, and meningomyelocele, can also mimic an abdominal mass. The most common abdominal masses in infants and children are enlarged kidneys caused by hydronephrosis or cystic renal disease.

Renal and Adrenal Masses

Large Kidneys. Unilateral enlargement of a kidney results from hydronephrosis, multicystic dysplastic kidney, renal vein thrombosis, or renal tumors (Table 52.10). Bilateral renal enlargement can be seen with hydronephrosis, polycystic kidney disease, storage diseases, and glomerulonephropathies, including nephrotic syndrome. Bilateral renal enlargement caused by neoplasms is less common, although leukemia or lymphoma may infiltrate the renal parenchyma bilaterally.

Nephroblastomatosis. Small islands of primitive metanephric blastema, which are thought to be a precursor of Wilms tumor, commonly exist in the kidneys of the normal newborn infant. These primitive cells usually spontaneously regress by 4 months of age. A diffuse and proliferative form of persistent renal blastoma is referred to as nephroblastomatosis. The abnormal tissue can form as multiple discrete nodules within the renal parenchyma or may completely replace the renal cortex. Nephroblastomatosis appears on CT or IV pyelogram as bilateral lobulated and enlarged kidneys with marked compression, stretching, and distortion of the pelvicaliceal structures (Fig. 52.55). On US, the kidneys are enlarged, lobular, and

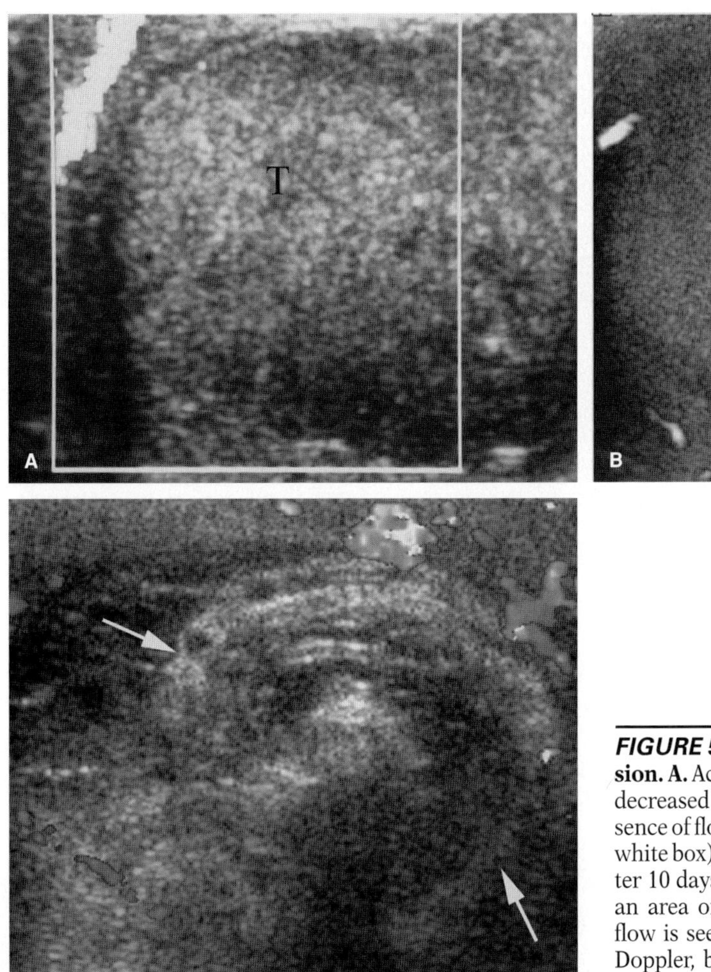

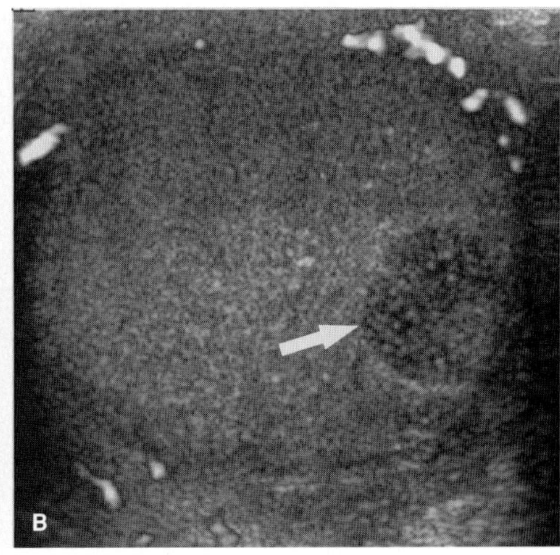

FIGURE 52.54. **(Color Plates) Testicular Torsion. A.** Acute torsion is accompanied by slightly decreased echogenicity of the testis (T) and absence of flow with color Doppler (area within the white box). **B.** Another patient who presented after 10 days of pain has a hypoechoic testis with an area of central necrosis (*arrow*). Increased flow is seen surrounding the testis with power Doppler, but no intratesticular flow is present. **C.** Note the spiral appearance of the spermatic cord, indicative of torsion (*arrows*).

TABLE 52.10 Causes of Renal Enlargement

Bilateral
- Diffuse renal disease (e.g., nephrotic syndrome, glomerulonephritis)
- Diabetic mother
- Autosomal recessive or autosomal dominant polycystic kidney disease
- Leukemia, lymphoma
- Hemolytic uremic syndrome
- Henoch-Schönlein purpura
- Beckwith-Wiedemann syndrome
- Glycogen-storage disease
- Tuberous sclerosis
- Nephroblastomatosis

Unilateral
- Hydronephrosis
- Duplication anomaly
- Compensatory hypertrophy
- Crossed fused ectopia
- Multicystic dysplastic kidney
- Renal abscess
- Renal neoplasm
- Renal vein thrombosis

echogenic, or enlarged with diffuse hypoechoic thickening of the cortex. In such cases, Wilms tumor should be suspected. Nephrogenic rests are more likely to appear cortical, tend to be homogeneous, and are of low echogenicity on US, low attenuation on CT, and low signal intensity on T1WIs (79,80). Small, focal nephrogenic rests smaller than 1 cm are difficult to visualize by US and are better evaluated with contrast-enhanced CT or T1WI.

Wilms tumor is the most common renal neoplasm of childhood (81). It arises from the primitive metanephric epithelium and demonstrates varied histologies, which are classified into favorable and unfavorable groups. The prognosis is dependent on tumor histology and resectability, with survival above 90% for tumors with favorable histology. Wilms tumor presents as a nontender, rapidly growing, unilateral abdominal mass in a young child. The mean age of presentation is 3 years. Bilateral tumors are found in 10% of patients—more commonly in children with associated congenital anomalies or nephroblastomatosis.

On US, Wilms tumor characteristically is a well-defined, predominantly solid mass arising from the kidney

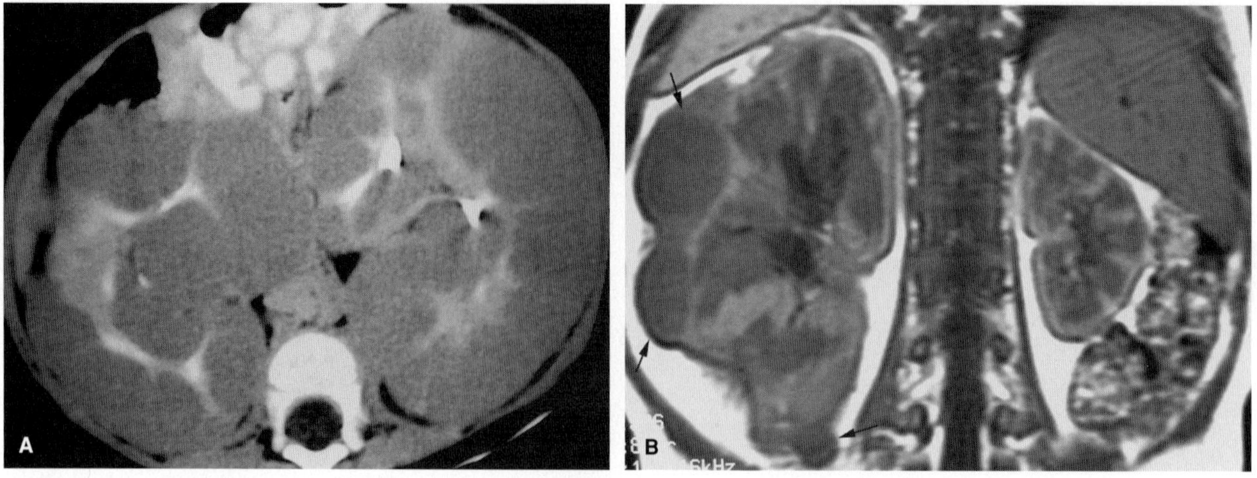

FIGURE 52.55. **Nephroblastomatosis. A.** The kidneys are massively enlarged, with lobulated thickening of the parenchyma and stretching and compression of the collecting structures. **B.** T1WI in another patient shows multiple peripheral Wilms tumors (*arrows*) in a child with nephroblastomatosis.

(Fig. 52.56A). Hypoechoic or anechoic areas within the tumor represent necrosis. Hydronephrosis is commonly present. Wilms tumor has a propensity to extend into the renal vein, inferior vena cava, and RA; all of these structures must be evaluated preoperatively (Fig. 52.56B). CT is used to evaluate large tumors and the lungs, which are a common site of metastasis. Either CT or MR can be used to exclude small masses in the contralateral kidney, which can be difficult to identify with US (Fig. 52.56C). Calcification is uncommon in Wilms tumor.

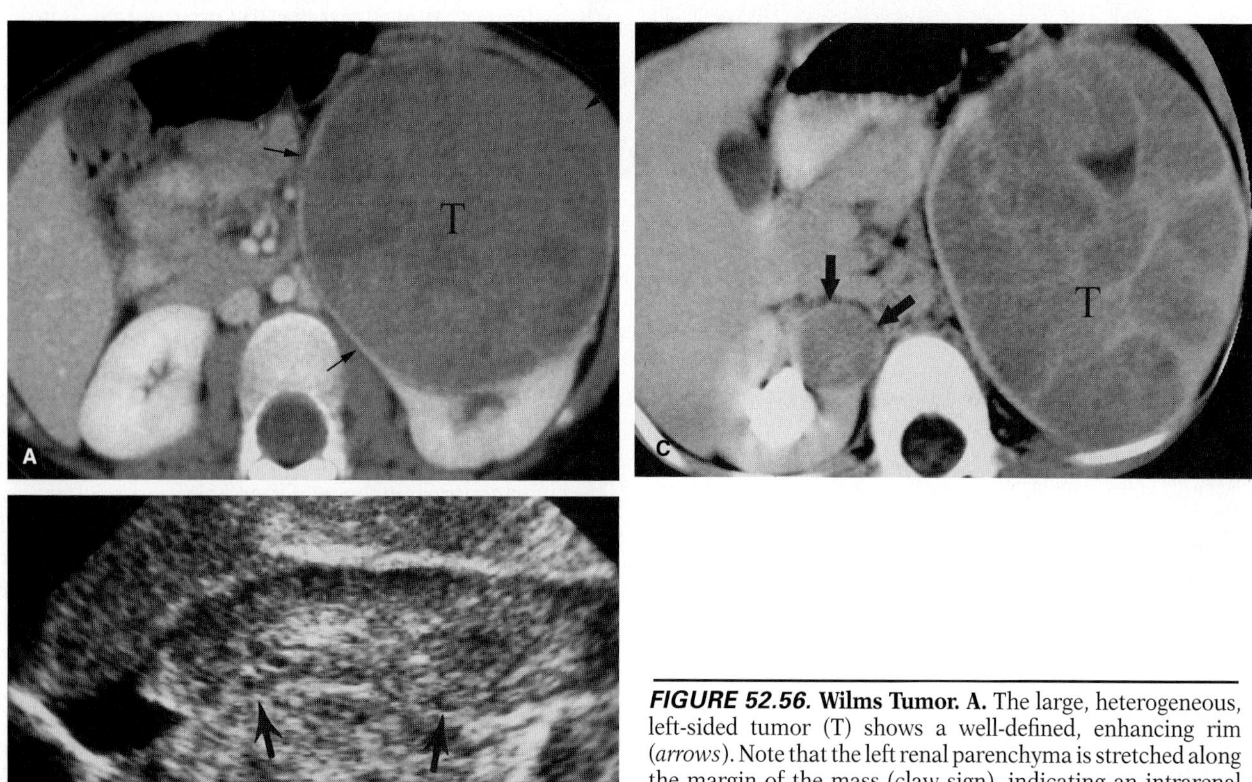

FIGURE 52.56. **Wilms Tumor. A.** The large, heterogeneous, left-sided tumor (T) shows a well-defined, enhancing rim (*arrows*). Note that the left renal parenchyma is stretched along the margin of the mass (claw sign), indicating an intrarenal mass. **B.** Tumor extension into the inferior vena cava (*arrow*) in another patient is seen with US. **C.** CT scan in a different child shows a large, partially cystic Wilms tumor (T) on the left and identifies a smaller Wilms tumor mass in the contralateral kidney (*arrows*).

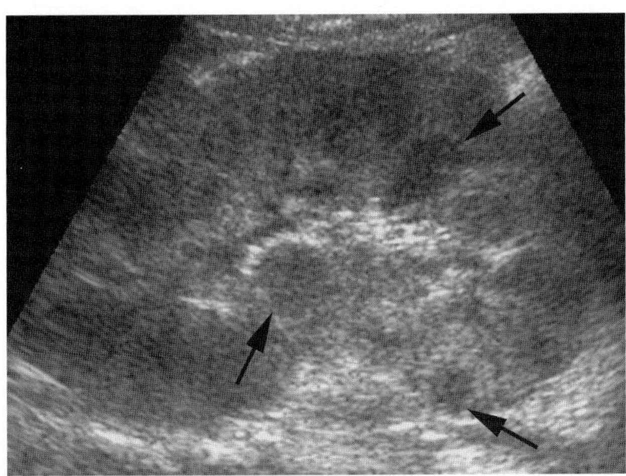

FIGURE 52.57. **Renal Lymphoma.** Multiple nodular tumor masses (*arrows*) are visible within the enlarged kidney on US.

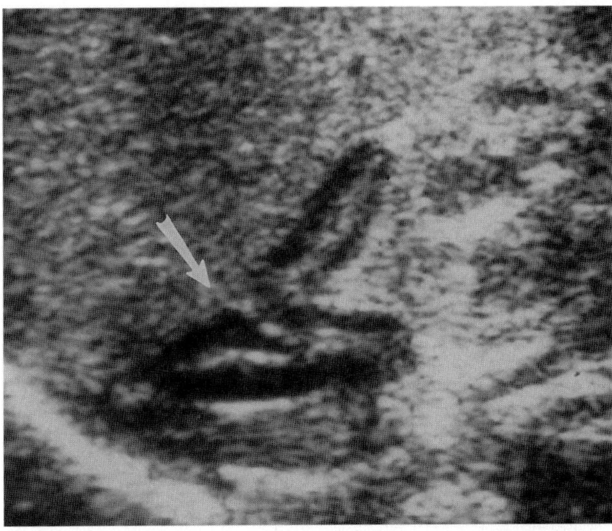

FIGURE 52.58. **Normal Adrenal Gland.** Note the characteristic "Y" shape (*arrow*) of the normal adrenal gland sitting astride the kidney.

Renal cell carcinoma is very rare in young children but sometimes occurs in older children and adolescents. Like Wilms tumor, renal cell carcinoma usually presents as an asymptomatic abdominal mass, although hematuria is sometimes present. Hypertension is less common with renal cell carcinoma than with Wilms tumor. The imaging characteristics of renal cell carcinoma are indistinguishable from those of Wilms tumor.

Other malignant tumors are rare in children. Clear-cell sarcoma and rhabdoid tumor of the kidney are highly aggressive neoplasms that were once considered variants of Wilms tumor. They are distinguished by a very poor prognosis and different metastatic patterns. The primary tumors have an imaging appearance identical to that of Wilms tumor, but bone metastases are common in clear-cell sarcoma, and rhabdoid tumor is associated with brain metastases and second intracranial primaries. Metastatic disease to the kidneys is uncommon. The kidneys may be infiltrated by leukemia or lymphoma, causing diffuse enlargement or multiple masses (Fig. 52.57).

Mesoblastic nephroma is the most common renal tumor of the neonate. Like Wilms tumor, mesoblastic nephroma arises from the metanephric blastema, and these tumors are indistinguishable on US. Although mesoblastic nephroma is usually considered benign, metastasis occasionally occurs (82,83).

Adrenal Hemorrhage. Adrenal masses characteristically cause downward and outward displacement of the kidney. In the newborn, the most common cause of adrenal enlargement is adrenal hemorrhage. Predisposing factors include large babies, obstetric trauma, neonatal sepsis, and hypoxia. The infants may present with an abdominal mass, jaundice, hypotension, or anemia, but small hemorrhages may go unnoticed. Hemorrhage occurs more frequently on the right and is occasionally bilateral. Older children develop adrenal hemorrhage as a result of accidental trauma, child abuse, meningococcemia, or anticoagulant therapy.

US is an ideal modality for evaluating adrenal hemorrhage. The normal adrenal gland in the newborn is larger and more easily visualized than that of the adult. The gland appears as an inverted V–shaped structure with an echogenic central region and a peripheral hypoechoic zone (Fig. 52.58). Hemorrhage enlarges the gland and causes loss of the V shape. Initially, the hematoma resembles a solid, echogenic mass (Fig. 52.59A). As the hemorrhage resolves, it becomes increasingly hypoechoic, starting in the central region and progressing peripherally (Fig. 52.59B). The hematoma decreases in size within the first week and sometimes calcifies. The calcifications begin around the rim of the gland, but eventually a small, completely calcified gland remains. Adrenal insufficiency rarely develops. Adrenal hemorrhage may be complicated by compression of the kidney, renal vein thrombosis, or infection.

Neuroblastoma belongs to a group of neural crest origin tumors that range from the benign ganglioneuroma to the highly malignant neuroblastoma. Neuroblastoma arises from the adrenal gland or from sympathetic ganglia in the retroperitoneum, posterior mediastinum, neck, or pelvis. It is a neoplasm of early childhood, presenting in children younger than 5 years of age. Most children present with advanced disease and large abdominal masses. Symptoms are often related to bone metastases or intraspinal extension. In contrast to Wilms tumor, neuroblastoma is a poorly marginated mass that frequently extends across the midline and into the chest. The kidney may be invaded, causing the tumor to be mistaken for an intrarenal mass (Fig. 52.60A). Calcifications are much more common in

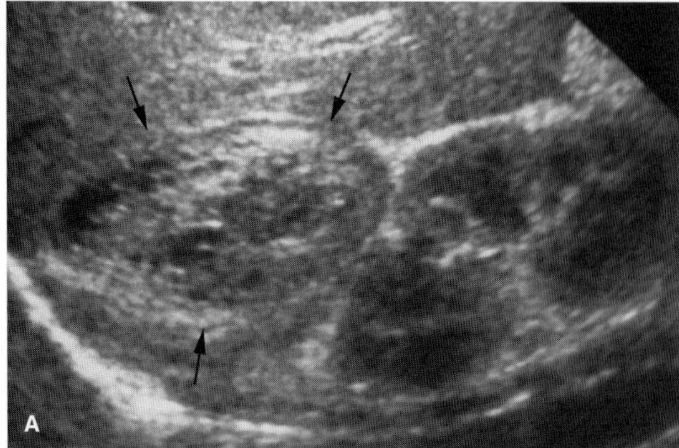

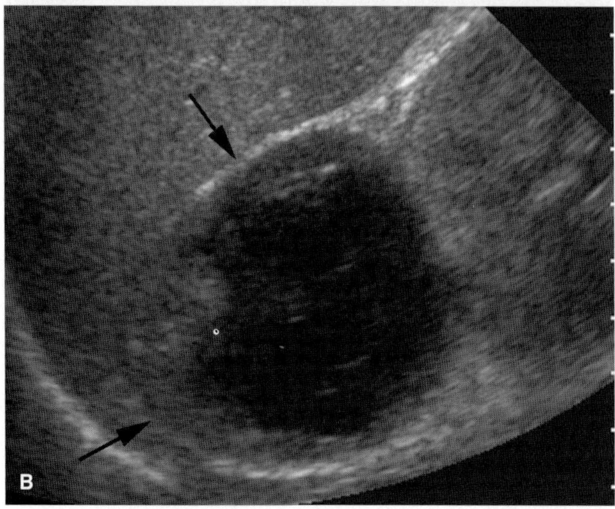

FIGURE 52.59. **Adrenal Hemorrhage. A.** In the early stages, hemorrhage into the adrenal gland presents as an echogenic suprarenal mass (*arrows*). **B.** A resolving adrenal hemorrhage in a different infant appears cystic centrally on US (*arrows*).

neuroblastoma than in Wilms tumor, with an incidence as high as 50% to 75% (Fig. 52.60B).

Most neuroblastomas appear echogenic and heterogeneous. In some cases, a characteristic echogenic nodule can be identified within the larger part of the tumor mass. CT and MR can be used to better define the extent of involvement of large tumors and to detect metastatic deposits (Fig. 52.60C). Neuroblastoma metastasizes to the liver, lymph nodes, and bone marrow. MR demonstrates intraspinal extension (Fig. 52.60D), bone marrow infiltration, and encasement of blood vessels without using IV contrast. Skeletal metastases are shown with technetium bone scintigraphy. Iodine-131-meta-iodobenzylguanidine is a tracer that resembles norepinephrine and is metabolized by neuroblastoma, pheochromocytoma, and other catecholamine-producing tumors. Octreotide is a ligand for G-protein receptor cell membranes. These two tracers have improved detection of primary tumor and metastases in some cases (84–86).

Other tumors of the adrenal gland are quite rare in children. Adrenocortical carcinoma is highly malignant and locally invasive, with CT and US characteristics similar to those of neuroblastoma. Adrenocortical carcinoma metastasizes to the lungs, liver, and regional lymph nodes. The tumor frequently causes endocrine symptoms, such as virilization and Cushing syndrome. Hypercortisolism may cause an increase in retroperitoneal fat that is visible on CT and MR and is a clue to the diagnosis (87,88). Benign adenomas, pheochromocytomas, and congenital adrenal cysts are uncommon in children.

Diffuse adrenal enlargement occurs with adrenocortical hyperplasia, which causes adrenogenital syndrome. The enlarged adrenals may have an undulating configuration, described as cerebriform (Fig. 52.61) (89). Marked, reversible adrenal enlargement is seen in infants treated with adrenocorticotropic hormone for infantile spasm (90).

Wolman disease is a rare lipidosis that results in enlarged, densely calcified adrenal glands. Plain films are usually diagnostic. Wolman disease is usually fatal at an early age.

Hepatobiliary Masses

A variety of cystic and solid masses may arise from the liver and biliary tract in children (Table 52.11). Most conditions can be differentiated with US.

Acute hydrops of the gallbladder is a poorly understood condition probably caused by transient obstruction of the cystic duct. It has been associated with the mucocutaneous lymph node syndrome (Kawasaki disease); however, in many cases the cause is unknown. US shows a markedly enlarged, tender gallbladder with a thin wall. Acute acalculous cholecystitis causes similar gallbladder enlargement, but the gallbladder distension is less pronounced and gallbladder wall thickening is present. Transient distension of the gallbladder sometimes occurs in the neonate, particularly in premature infants. Prolonged total parenteral nutrition and sepsis have been implicated as possible etiologic factors.

Choledochal cysts are congenital malformations of the intrahepatic or extrahepatic bile ducts. Multiple factors probably lead to the development of choledochal cysts, but the majority of cysts are associated with an anomalous junction of the common bile duct and pancreatic duct (abnormal pancreatobiliary junction [APBJ]). The APBJ allows pancreatic enzymes to reflux into the common bile duct, which may lead to inflammation and weakening of the bile duct wall. Jaundice, pain, and a right upper quadrant mass comprise the classic triad of findings seen with a choledochal cyst. Young infants more commonly present with fluctuating jaundice, pain, and fever. The most common type of choledochal cyst (type 1) is a localized, fusiform or saccular dilation of the common

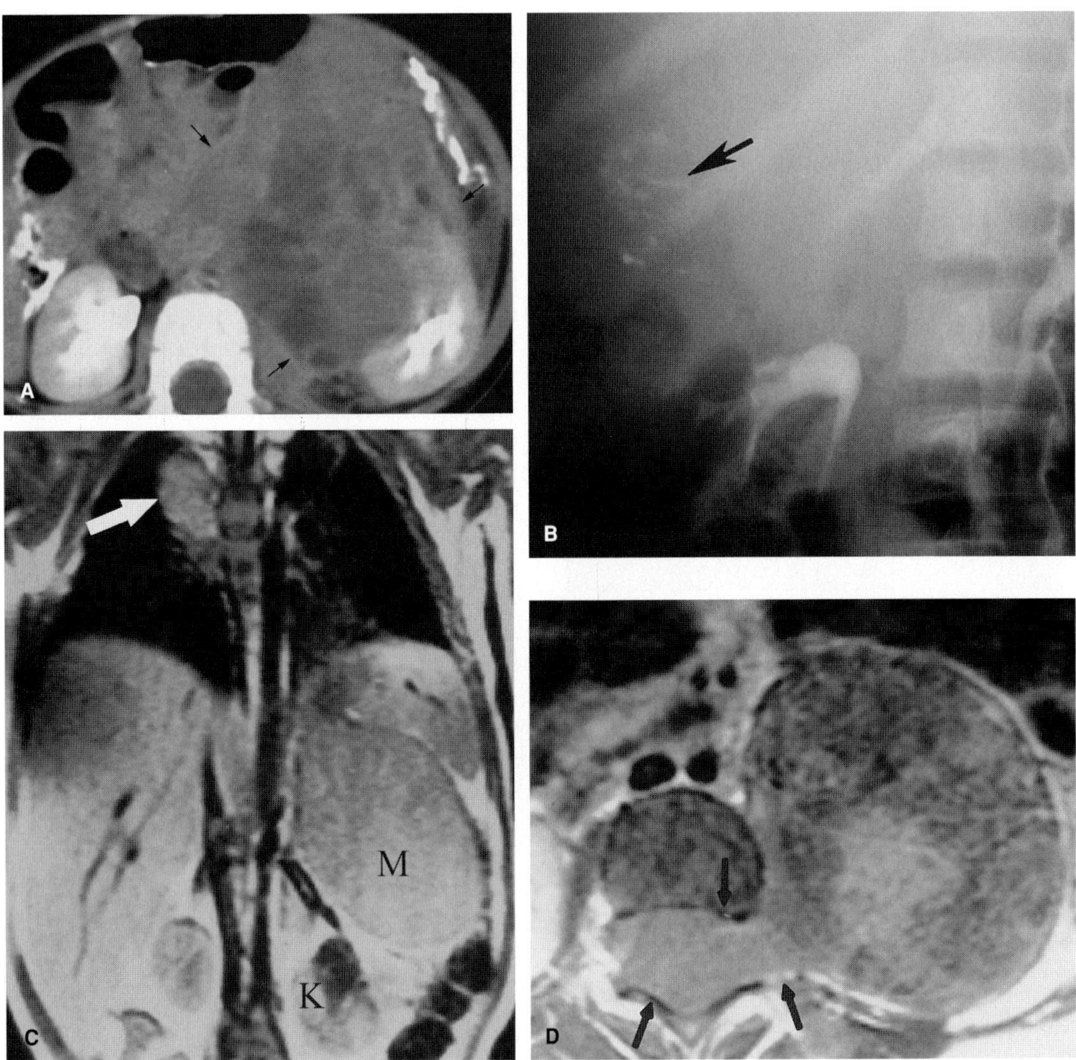

FIGURE 52.60. **Neuroblastoma. A.** Note the large, ill-defined, heterogeneous left abdominal mass (*arrows*). The mass crosses the midline and secondarily invades the left kidney. **B.** Radiograph shows a large soft tissue mass that displaces the right kidney inferiorly. Irregular, amorphous calcifications are seen within the mass (*arrow*). **C.** MR in a different patient shows a large mass (M) displacing the left kidney (K). A second tumor mass is identified adjacent to the spine in the right upper hemithorax (*arrow*). **D.** Axial T1WI in another patient clearly shows tumor extension into the spinal canal (*arrows*).

bile duct below the cystic duct. Choledochal cysts are usually diagnosed by US, appearing as a cystic mass in the porta hepatis, separate from the gallbladder and associated with dilated intrahepatic ducts (Fig. 52.62). Hepatobiliary scintigraphy confirms that the cyst communicates with the biliary tract, aiding in differentiation from other cystic abdominal masses (Table 52.8). MR cholangiopancreatography may provide more detailed information about bile duct anatomy and anatomic relationships to adjacent structures (91).

Hepatic cysts are less common in infants and children than in adults. Solitary congenital cysts of the liver are usually encountered as an incidental finding at US or CT. The cyst walls are thin and the fluid is anechoic on US. Some cysts are very large and pedunculated, and their hepatic origin may be difficult to ascertain. Multiple hepatic cysts occur in patients with autosomal dominant polycystic disease. Acquired hepatic cysts may be solitary or multiple and are most commonly of infectious origin (Fig. 52.63). Resolving hematoma of the liver may also appear as a well-defined cystic lesion.

Hemangioendothelioma is the most common benign liver tumor encountered in infancy (92). This vascular lesion may be solitary or multiple and is associated with cutaneous hemangiomas in 40% of cases. Hemangioendothelioma may be complicated by high-output cardiac failure,

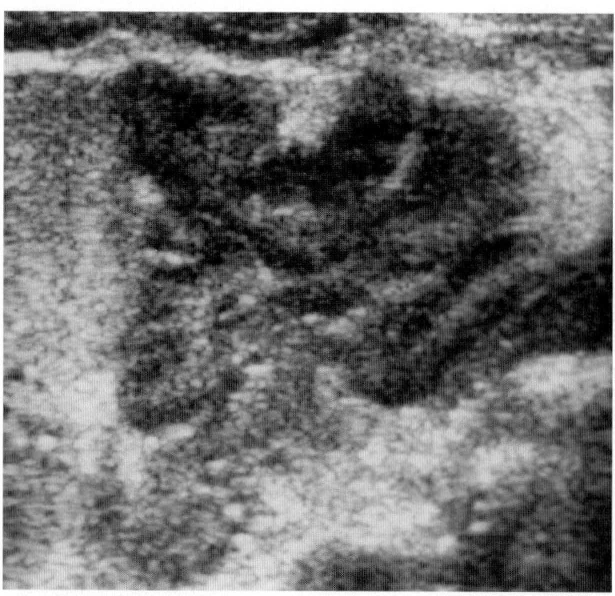

FIGURE 52.61. **Congenital Adrenal Hyperplasia.** Note the undulating configuration of the enlarged adrenal gland.

TABLE 52.11 Cystic Abdominal Masses

Renal/adrenal
Hydronephrosis
Renal cysts (see Table 52.9)
Multicystic dysplastic kidney
Adrenal hemorrhage (resolving)
Hepatobiliary
Gallbladder hydrops
Choledochal cyst
Mesenchymal hamartoma
Abscess/parasitic cyst
Pancreatic
Pseudocyst
Solid-cystic papillary tumor
Splenic
Congenital cyst
GI
Duplication cyst
Mesenteric cyst
Meconium pseudocyst
Lymphangioma
Appendiceal abscess
Genitourinary
Ovarian cyst
Abdominoscrotal hydrocele
Hydrometrocolpos
Urachal cyst
Teratoma/dermoid cyst
Miscellaneous
CSF pseudocyst

hemorrhage, jaundice, hemolytic anemia, or thrombocytopenia because of sequestration of platelets within the tumor. The typical sonographic appearance is a solid or complex mass associated with large feeding and draining vessels, seen best with color Doppler US (Fig. 52.64). The mass is well circumscribed and low in attenuation on CT and shows predominantly peripheral contrast enhancement. High signal intensity is seen on T2WIs, with multiple flow voids throughout the lesion representing vessels. The tumor may be treated with steroids, but arterial embolization or surgery may be needed in more symptomatic cases.

Mesenchymal hamartoma is an uncommon benign tumor seen most often in infants and young children. Hamartomas are usually solitary and predominantly cystic, with multiple thin septations and intervening nodules of solid tissue apparent on US. CT shows multiple areas of low attenuation within the tumor mass.

Hepatic adenomas are rare in childhood but have been reported in association with Fanconi anemia, glycogen-storage disease type 1, Hurler disease, and severe combined immunodeficiency.

Focal nodular hyperplasia presents as a masslike lesion that most likely represents a hyperplastic response to a congenital arteriovenous malformation. Scintigraphy using sulfur colloid demonstrates normal to increased tracer uptake in many cases, differentiating it from adenomas that do not concentrate the tracer. On CT, the lesions show early phase enhancement but become isoattenuating with the liver on delayed images. An enhancing central scar may be seen.

Metastatic Disease. Neuroblastoma is the most common childhood tumor to metastasize to the liver, followed by lymphoma, leukemia, and Wilms tumor. Metastatic lesions are usually multiple, and their imaging appearance is generally nonspecific.

Hepatoblastoma is a tumor of early childhood, presenting before 3 years of age (Fig. 52.65). The tumor is more common in children with Beckwith-Wiedemann syndrome and familial adenomatous polyposis.

Hepatocellular carcinoma is more commonly seen in older children and adolescents. Sonographically, these tumors appear as single or multiple hyperechoic lesions, sometimes containing hypoechoic or anechoic areas because of hemorrhage or necrosis. Invasion of the hepatic or portal veins may be identified. On CT, the tumors appear as low-attenuation lesions with variable contrast enhancement. MR is comparable with CT for the initial diagnosis of these tumors; however, MR is more sensitive in the detection of postoperative tumor recurrence (65). MR angiography with three-dimensional reconstruction helps to evaluate tumor blood supply for surgical planning. Complete resection is required for survival, and orthotopic liver transplantation has been successful in some advanced cases of hepatoblastoma that would otherwise be unresectable. PET-CT promises to be a more sensitive

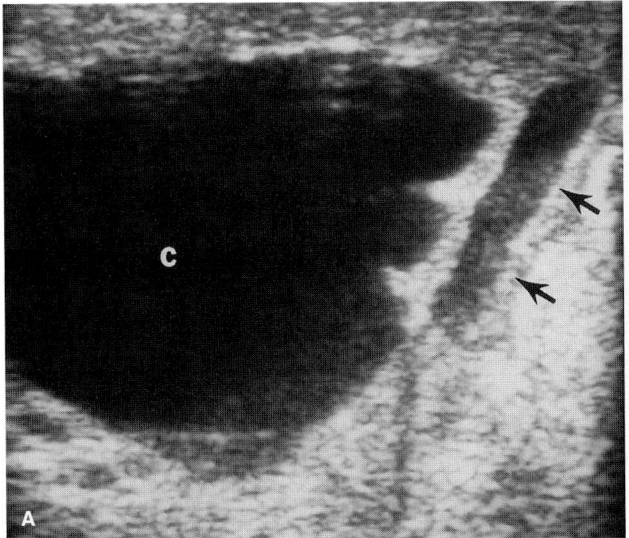

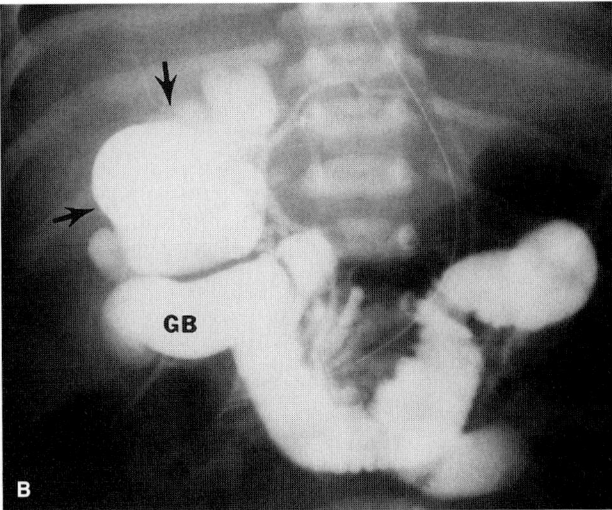

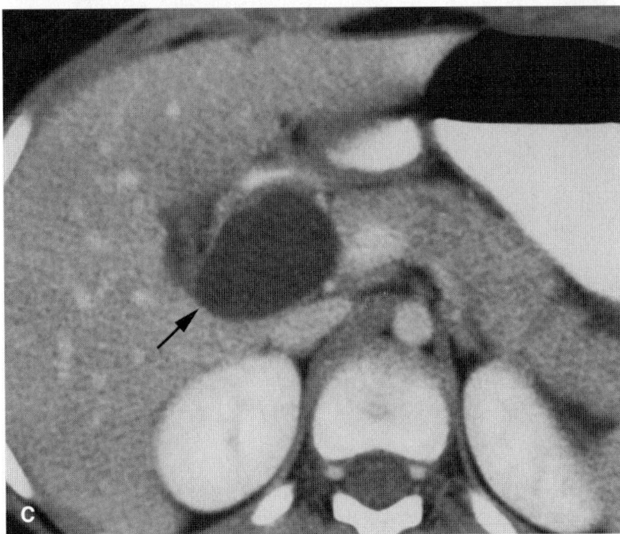

FIGURE 52.62. Choledochal Cyst. A. US shows a large, multilobulated anechoic cyst (C) that is adjacent to, but separate from, the gallbladder (*arrows*). **B.** Cholangiography confirms the presence of a large intrahepatic choledochal cyst (*arrows*) involving the right hepatic duct. GB, gallbladder. **C.** CT scan of a different child shows a well-defined cyst in the porta hepatis (*arrow*) associated with dilated central hepatic ducts.

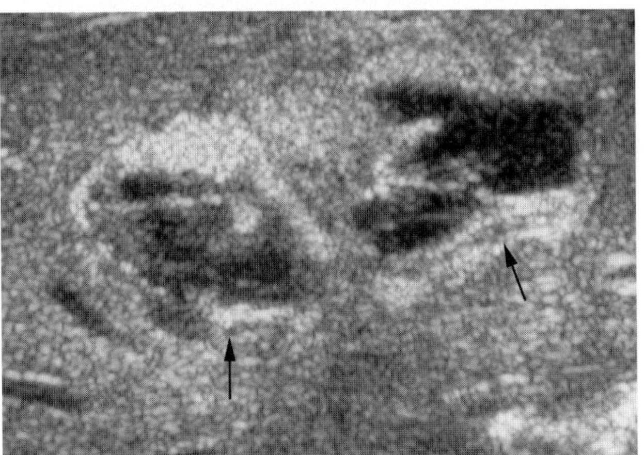

FIGURE 52.63. *Candida* Abscess of the Liver. Two irregular cystic collections with peripheral echogenicity are liver abscesses in this newborn infant with *Candida* sepsis.

modality for identifying tumor metastases and local recurrence (93).

Other less common primary malignant tumors in children include undifferentiated (embryonal) sarcoma and embryonal rhabdomyosarcoma of the biliary ducts. The latter tumor typically occurs in children between 2 and 5 years of age. When the tumor originates in a major bile duct, the patient presents with jaundice. Those tumors that originate within the intrahepatic ducts cannot be differentiated from other primary malignancies of the liver.

Splenic Lesions

Splenomegaly is a relatively common cause of a left upper quadrant mass in children. Splenic enlargement is most often secondary to a systemic illness. Common causes include hematologic diseases, infections, portal hypertension, and infiltrative diseases (mucopolysaccharidoses, reticuloendothelioses, leukemia, and lymphoma).

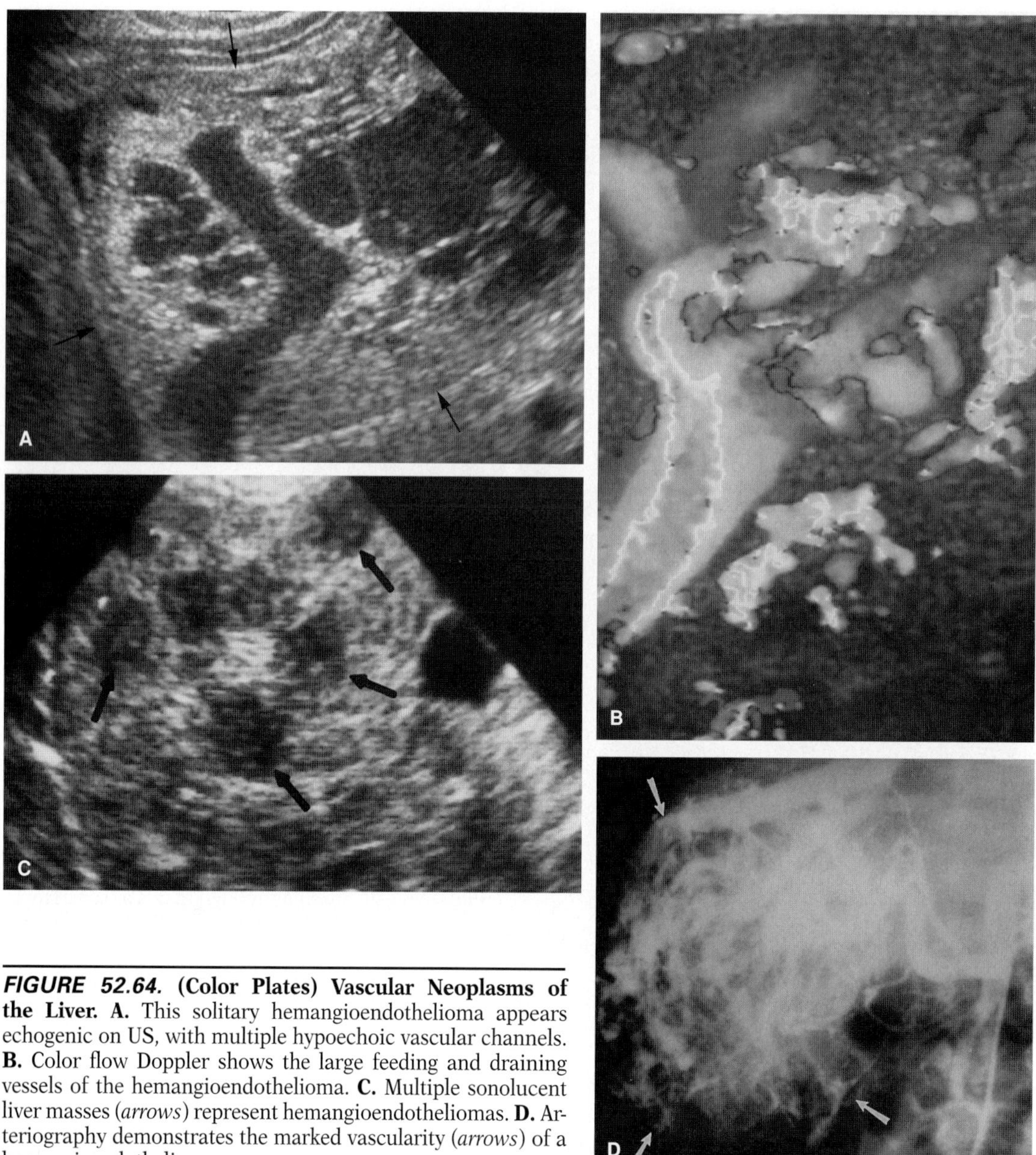

FIGURE 52.64. **(Color Plates) Vascular Neoplasms of the Liver. A.** This solitary hemangioendothelioma appears echogenic on US, with multiple hypoechoic vascular channels. **B.** Color flow Doppler shows the large feeding and draining vessels of the hemangioendothelioma. **C.** Multiple sonolucent liver masses (*arrows*) represent hemangioendotheliomas. **D.** Arteriography demonstrates the marked vascularity (*arrows*) of a hemangioendothelioma.

The imaging characteristics are usually nonspecific and insufficient for diagnosing the cause of splenomegaly.

In the newborn and young infant, splenomegaly most often occurs because of bacterial sepsis and infection. Hepatomegaly is generally also present. In older children, infections such as infectious mononucleosis, typhoid fever, and catscratch fever are more common. Multiple small, poorly defined hypoechoic lesions (Fig. 52.66) can be seen with US in granulomatous splenic infection such as *Bartonella* (catscratch fever), tuberculosis, or fungal infection. Splenic abscess is uncommon in children and is most often associated with an impaired immune system.

Cystic masses of the spleen are uncommon and include congenital epidermoid cysts, posttraumatic pseudocysts, and echinococcal cysts (see Chapter 28). Cystic lymphangiomatosis is a benign lymphatic malformation with a characteristic multiloculated cystic appearance. The lesion may contain calcification and enhances on CT.

Splenic Neoplasms. Primary neoplasms of the spleen (hemangioma, hamartoma, angiosarcoma) are rare. Lymphoma and leukemia commonly involve the spleen. However, splenic involvement with lymphoma does not necessarily result in splenic enlargement. Conversely, children with leukemia or lymphoma may have an enlarged spleen without neoplastic involvement. Hemophagocytic lymphohistiocytosis (HLH) is a rare disease that consists of overactive histocytes and macrophages that phagocytize the normal cellular structures of the blood. This condition

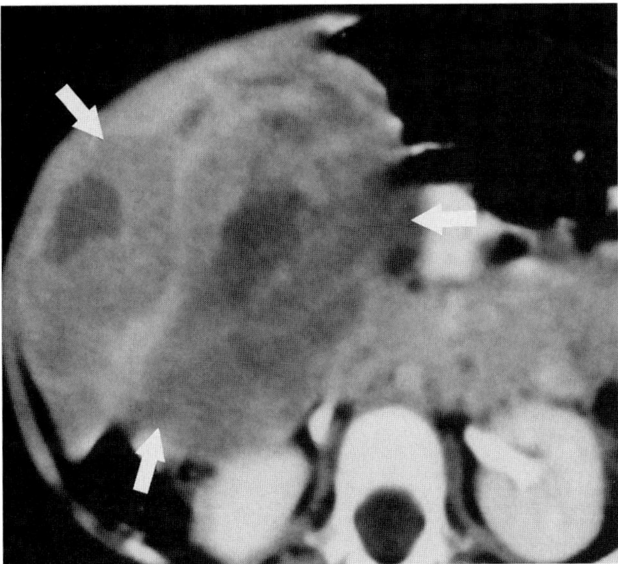

FIGURE 52.65. **Hepatoblastoma.** A CT scan demonstrates a large inhomogeneous tumor within the right lobe of the liver (*arrows*).

is not truly malignant and is probably caused by an inappropriate immune reaction. HLH usually occurs in infants under 1 year of age and is characterized by hepatosplenomegaly, ascites (Table 52.12), gallbladder wall thickening, lymphadenopathy, and pleural effusion (94).

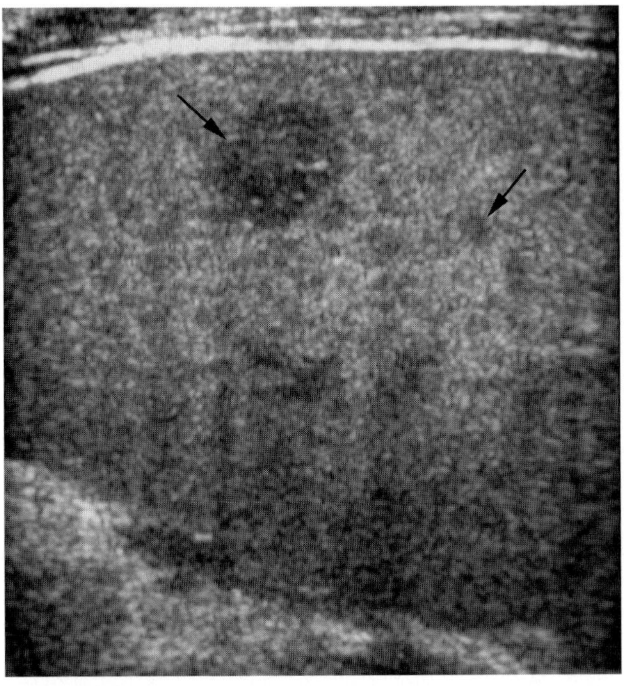

FIGURE 52.66. **Catscratch Disease.** US demonstrates the multiple hypoechoic nodules in the spleen (*arrows*) that are characteristic of this infection.

TABLE 52.12 Causes of Ascites

Newborn
Hydrops fetalis
Chylous ascites
Urinary tract obstruction
Iatrogenic (line perforation)
Intestinal perforation (necrotizing enterocolitis)
Older infants and children
Liver disease
Nephrotic syndrome
Portal vein obstruction
Traumatic intestinal injury
Peritonitis
Hypoproteinemia
Pancreatitis
Ruptured abdominal cyst
Intestinal lymphangiectasia
GI ischemia
Bile duct perforation

Splenic Infarction. In children, infarction of the spleen occurs most often as a complication of sickle cell anemia, leukemia, Gaucher disease, or cardiac valvular disease. Acute splenic infarction results in decreased echogenicity on US and diminished or mottled enhancement on CT. Rarely, a poorly fixed ("wandering") spleen may undergo torsion, leading to infarction (Fig. 52.67).

Gastrointestinal and Pancreatic Masses

Enteric Duplication Cysts. A majority of abdominal masses that arise from the GI tract or pancreas are cystic. GI duplication cysts most commonly arise from the small bowel (approximately 44% of cases) or colon (15% of cases). Most are asymptomatic, but those that contain ectopic gastric or pancreatic tissue may ulcerate or hemorrhage. The cyst can act as a lead point for intussusception or volvulus. Diagnosis is usually best accomplished by US (95,96). The cysts appear as simple, anechoic, round to oval masses with a characteristic two-layered wall (66) consisting of inner echogenic mucosa and peripheral hypoechoic muscle (Fig. 52.68). Because most enteric duplication cysts do not communicate with the intestinal lumen, GI contrast studies are of little value. Cysts that contain gastric mucosa are detectable by scintigraphy using technetium-99m-pertechnate.

Mesenteric and omental cysts are occasionally seen in the first decade of life and are thought to represent benign lymphatic malformations. These cysts are thin walled and unilocular or may contain multiple internal septations. The wall of the cyst has a single layer rather than the double layer seen with duplication cysts.

Pseudocysts are acquired, loculated fluid collections that most commonly result from various inflammatory

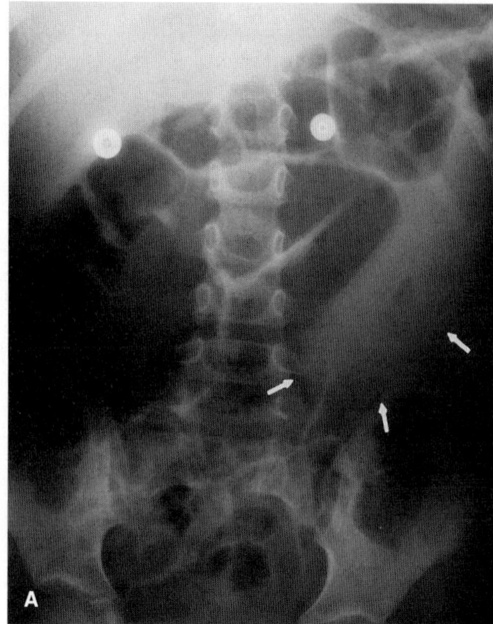

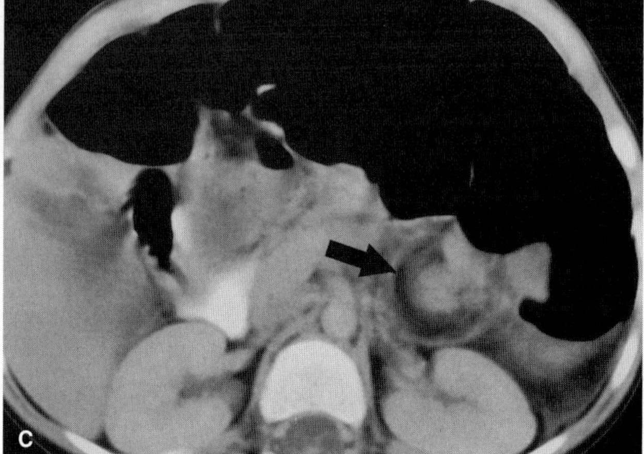

FIGURE 52.67. **Splenic Torsion. A.** Plain radiograph shows a soft tissue mass in the left abdomen (*arrows*). A normal splenic shadow is not seen. **B.** A CT scan confirms absence of the spleen in the usual location in the left upper quadrant. **C.** A more caudal image demonstrates a donut appearance, which represents the torsed splenic pedicle (*arrow*).

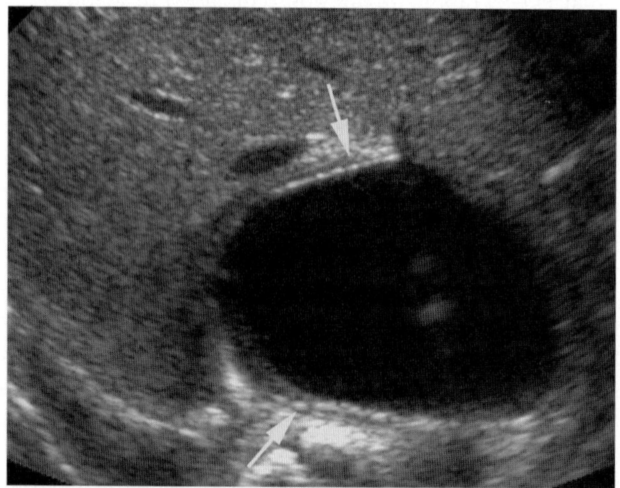

FIGURE 52.68. **Enteric Duplication Cyst.** US reveals an anechoic cyst in the right upper quadrant of a young infant. The cyst shows a well-defined, two-layered wall that consists of an inner echogenic mucosal layer and a thin outer muscular layer (*arrows*), characteristic of intestinal wall.

conditions in the abdomen. The pancreas is the most common site of origin of pseudocysts secondary to pancreatitis or blunt abdominal trauma (see Fig. 52.35). True congenital cysts of the pancreas are rare and occur chiefly in association with autosomal dominant polycystic kidney disease or von Hippel-Lindau syndrome. CSF pseudocyst is a complication of the use of a ventriculoperitoneal shunt for the treatment of hydrocephalus. Adhesions developing in the region of the intraperitoneal shunt trap the draining fluid in a closed space and can lead to shunt malfunction. US clearly defines the cystic mass surrounding the shunt tip (Fig. 52.69).

Pancreatic neoplasms are rare in children. The most common endocrine tumor is the benign islet cell adenoma (insulinoma), which is usually small and difficult to demonstrate by imaging. Solid-cystic papillary tumor of the pancreas is an uncommon tumor that contains variable amounts of cystic and solid tissue. Rare pancreatic neoplasms include adenocarcinoma, hamartoma, lymphangioma, pancreatoblastoma, and cystadenoma (97).

Tumors of the GI tract are uncommon in infants and children. Non-Hodgkin lymphoma is the most common malignant tumor of the small intestine. Inflammatory polyps or polyps associated with one of the colonic

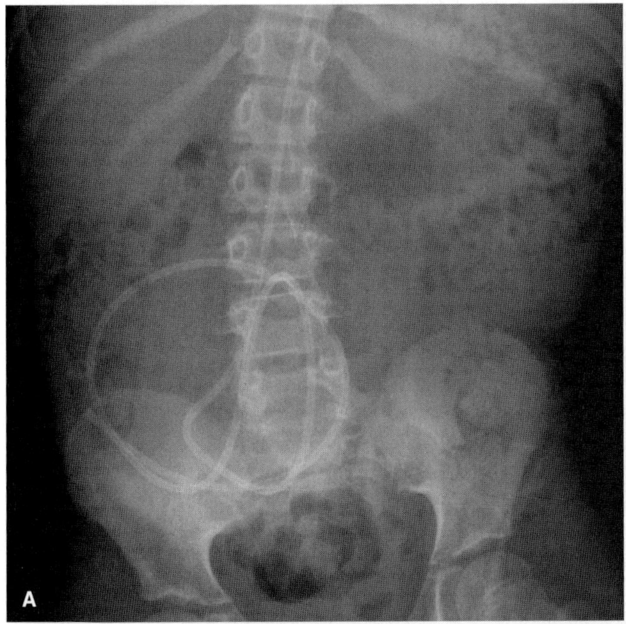

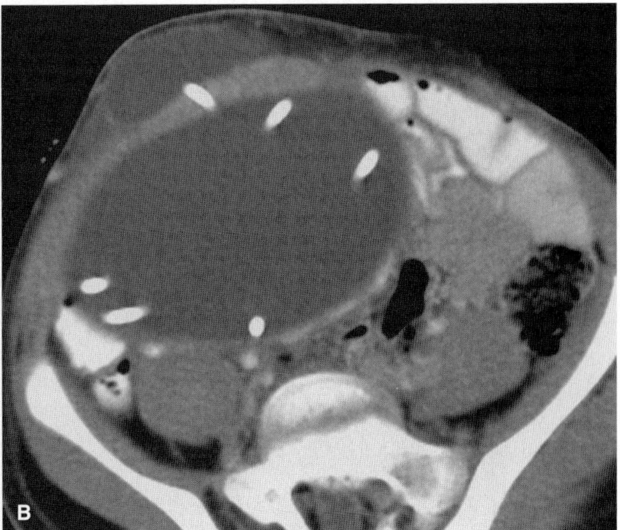

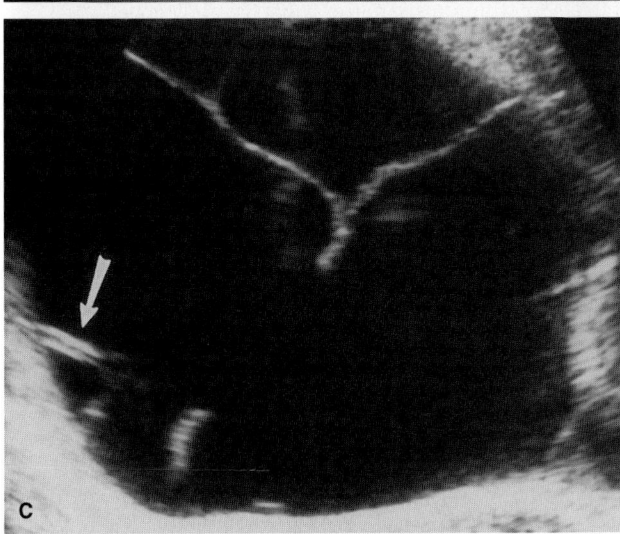

FIGURE 52.69. **CSF Pseudocyst. A.** Note the absence of gas in the region of the coiled distal ventriculoperitoneal shunt on abdominal radiography. **B.** CT of the patient shows a well-defined cyst surrounding the distal portion of the shunt and extending into the abdominal wall. **C.** US in a different child clearly identifies the shunt tip (*arrow*) surrounded by a loculated pseudocyst.

polyposis syndromes are the most common colon lesions. Colon tumors in infancy are likely to be leiomyoma, leiomyosarcoma, or lymphoma. Tumors of the mesentery and omentum are primarily Burkitt lymphoma or metastases. Benign tumors include neurogenic tumors, inflammatory pseudotumor, hemangioma, and teratoma.

Masses of the Reproductive Organs

Abdominal and pelvic masses that arise from the reproductive system are very common in young girls.

Ovarian cysts in children and adolescents are usually simple follicular or corpus luteum cysts (98). These cysts are common in neonates because of maternal hormonal stimulation. Most remain asymptomatic and spontaneously resolve without surgical intervention. Those cysts that are very large (>5 cm) or that are complicated by hemorrhage or torsion require aspiration or removal. Simple ovarian cysts appear on US as round or oval anechoic masses with a thin rim (Fig. 52.70A). In adolescents, hemorrhage into ovarian cysts is a common cause of pelvic pain. When hemorrhage occurs, the cyst appears more echogenic and complex (Fig. 52.70B, C).

Complex adnexal masses must generally be differentiated on clinical grounds rather than imaging characteristics (99). Infection and abscess caused by pelvic inflammatory disease are common in adolescents. Ectopic pregnancy must always be considered in postmenarchal females. The most common ovarian tumor is the benign teratoma. On US, teratomas vary from an entirely cystic mass to a predominantly solid mass with internal cystic components (Fig. 52.71A, B). A recognizable tooth within

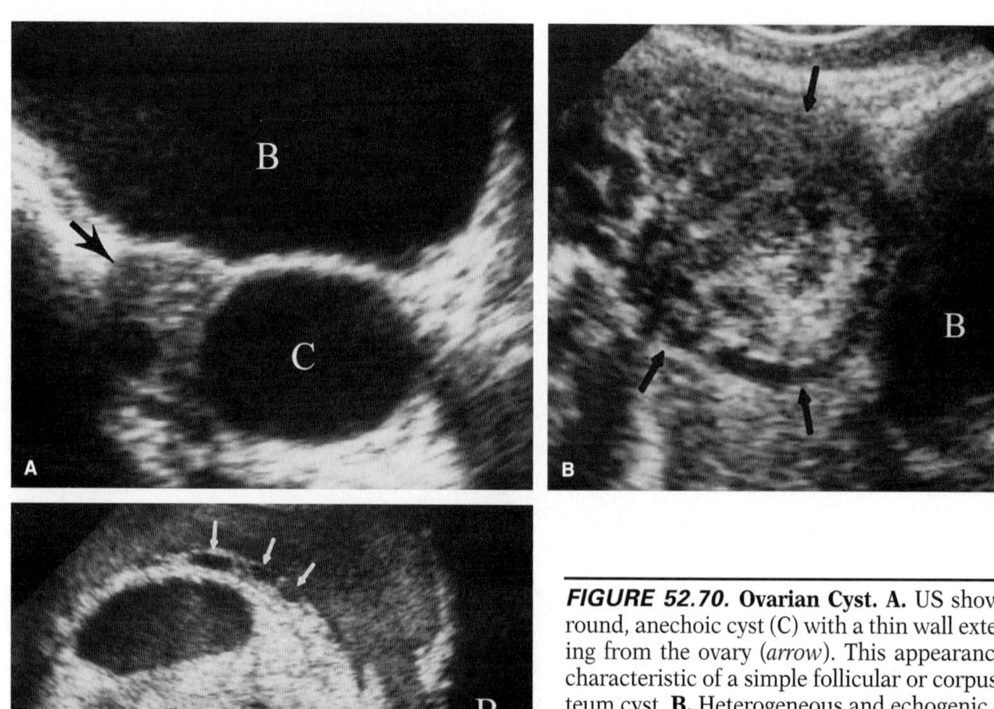

FIGURE 52.70. **Ovarian Cyst. A.** US shows a round, anechoic cyst (C) with a thin wall extending from the ovary (*arrow*). This appearance is characteristic of a simple follicular or corpus luteum cyst. **B.** Heterogeneous and echogenic clot is seen within an ovarian cyst that has undergone hemorrhage (*arrows*). **C.** A large hemorrhagic corpus luteum cyst (C) is seen in a patient on Coumadin (warfarin). Note the blood–fluid level within the cyst and several small follicles within the compressed and displaced ovary (*arrows*). B, bladder.

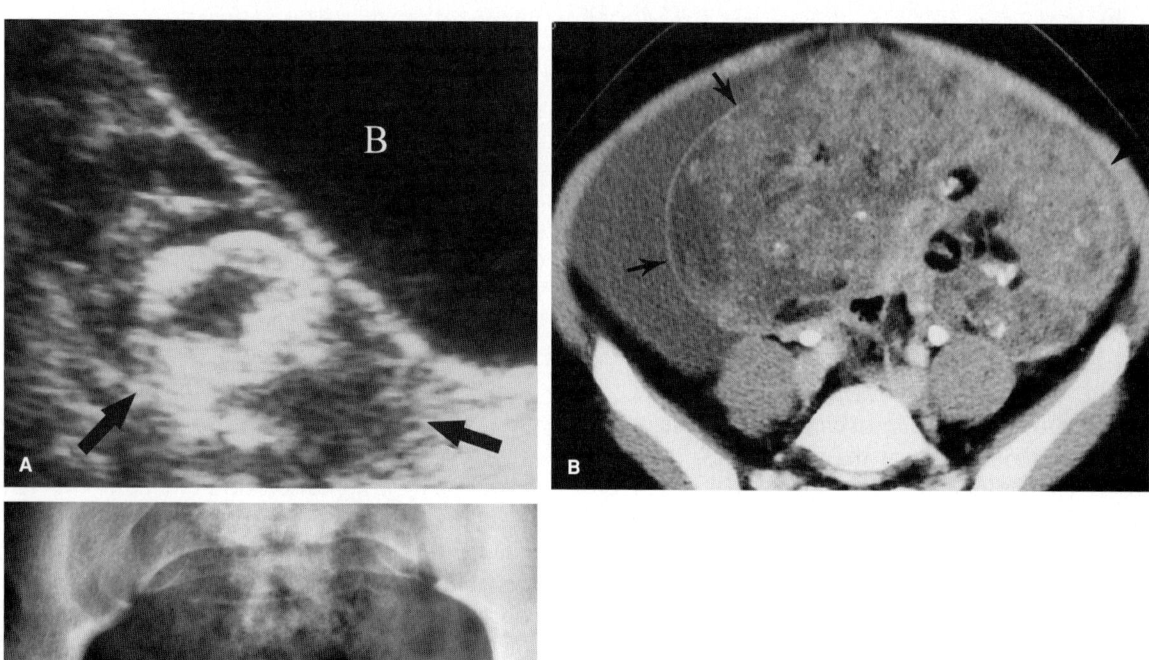

FIGURE 52.71. **Ovarian Teratoma. A.** US demonstrates a complex adnexal mass that contains both cystic and solid components as well as intensely echogenic areas of calcium and fat (*arrows*). B, bladder. **B.** A CT scan of a different patient shows a very large ovarian teratoma. The mass (*arrows*) is heterogenous, with scattered calcifications and areas of fat density. **C.** Plain film of the pelvis reveals a formed calcification that closely resembles a tooth (*arrow*).

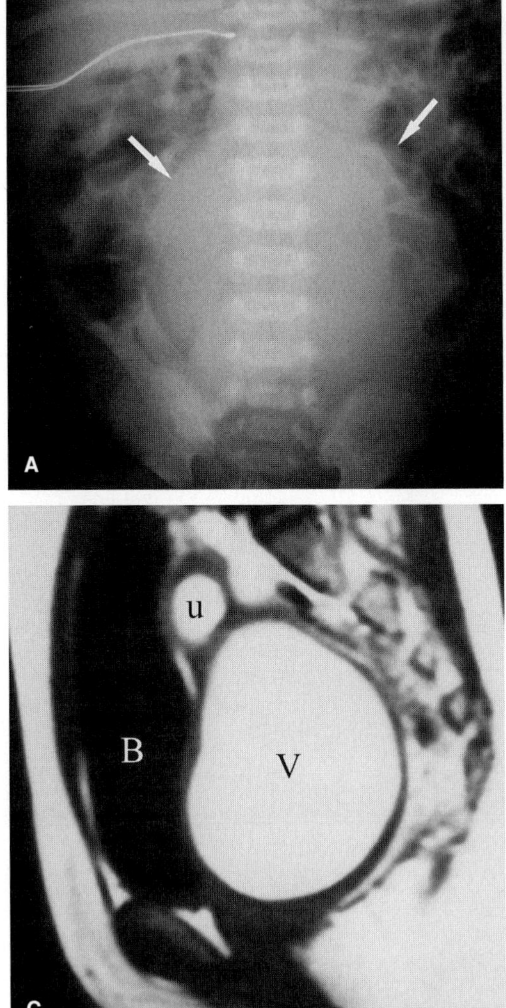

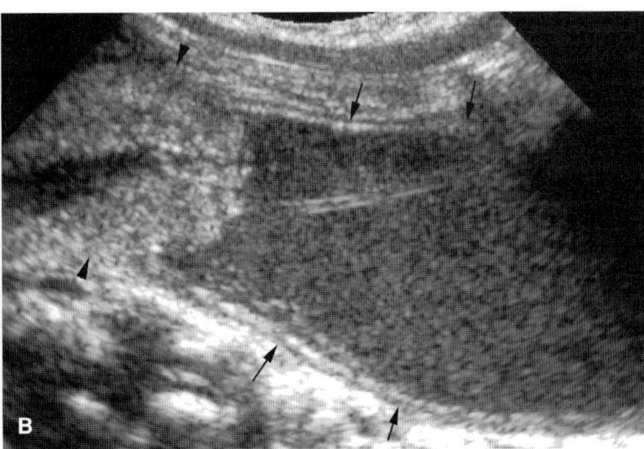

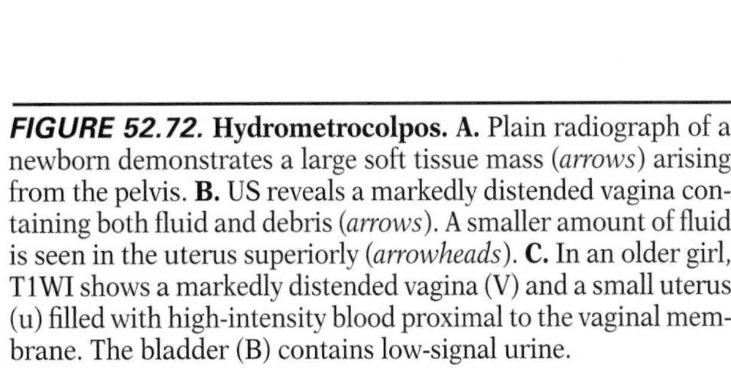

FIGURE 52.72. **Hydrometrocolpos. A.** Plain radiograph of a newborn demonstrates a large soft tissue mass (*arrows*) arising from the pelvis. **B.** US reveals a markedly distended vagina containing both fluid and debris (*arrows*). A smaller amount of fluid is seen in the uterus superiorly (*arrowheads*). **C.** In an older girl, T1WI shows a markedly distended vagina (V) and a small uterus (u) filled with high-intensity blood proximal to the vaginal membrane. The bladder (B) contains low-signal urine.

the mass is a pathognomonic finding (Fig. 52.71C). Malignant teratomas are accompanied by ascites, evidence of intraperitoneal spread, and metastasis to the liver. The larger the component of solid tissue, the more likely the tumor is malignant. Less common ovarian neoplasms of childhood include dysgerminoma, cystadenoma and cystadenocarcinoma, and granulosa cell tumor.

Enlarged uterus is sometimes the cause of a palpable abdominal mass. Pregnancy must be considered in adolescents. Congenital vaginal obstruction with hydrometrocolpos or hematometrocolpos presents in the newborn period or at puberty. In most cases, US identifies the enlarged uterus as being filled with anechoic fluid in the newborn or echogenic blood in the adolescent (Fig. 52.72A, B). MR is useful for classifying the vaginal abnormality in older patients (Fig. 52.72C).

Rhabdomyosarcoma arises from the anterior wall of the vagina, or in boys, from the prostate or bladder trigone (100). Since rhabdomyosarcoma frequently infiltrates the pelvic floor and surrounding structures, CT or MR is usually preferable to US for determining the extent of the disease.

Presacral Masses

Sacrococcygeal teratoma is the most common tumor in newborns. Prenatal complications include polyhydramnios and hemorrhage, which can lead to fetal hydrops. The tumors may be associated with congenital malformations of the hindgut and cloacae. Neonatal tumors are often benign, but malignant components may be present in up to 30% of cases. Sacrococcygeal teratomas are often large and extend externally from the region of the coccyx. Deformity of the sacrococcyx is usually present. The mass frequently contains calcifications, which may be amorphous or formed (e.g., teeth) (Fig. 52.73A). Cystic components are also common within a teratoma (Fig. 52.73B).

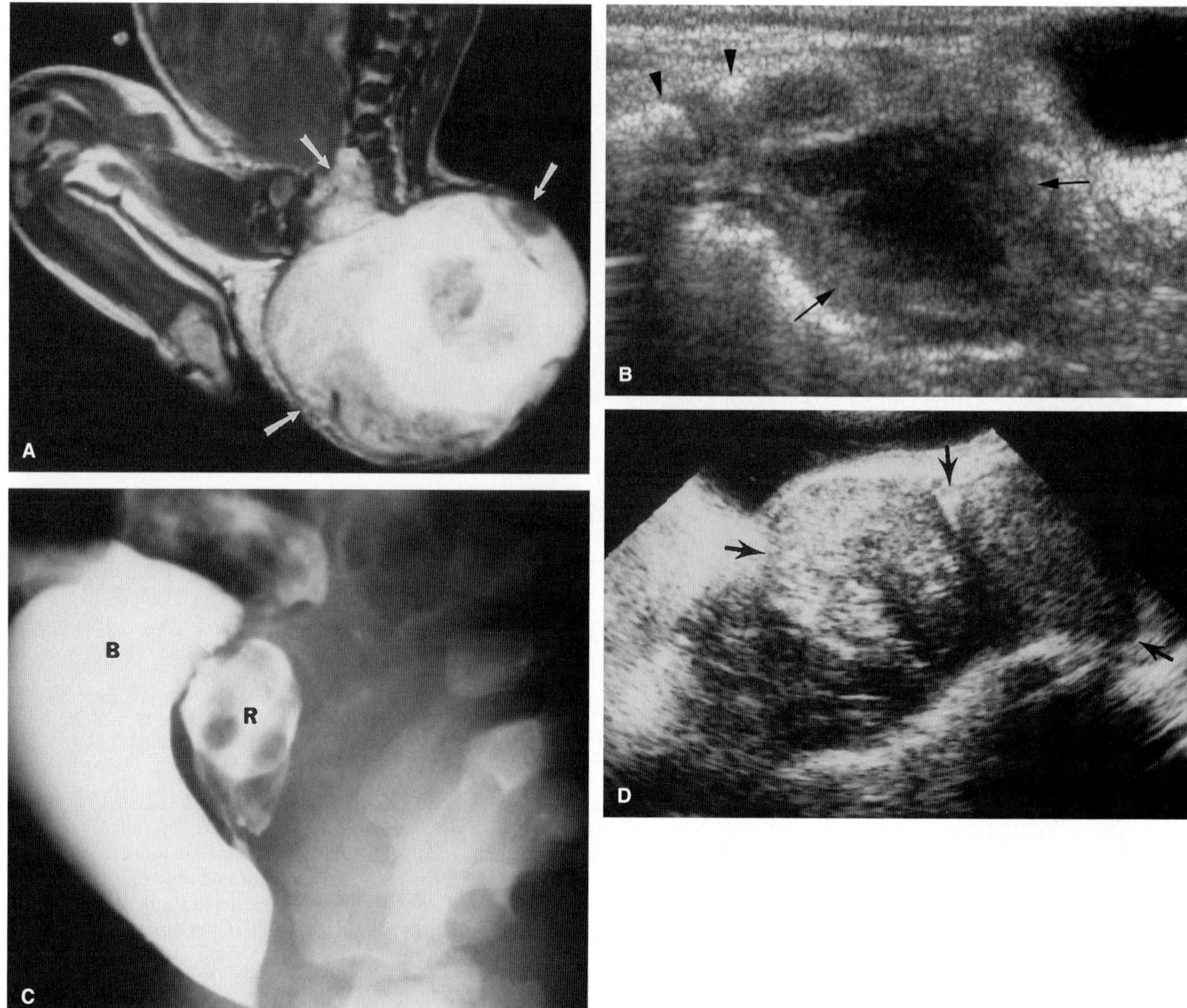

FIGURE 52.73. **Presacral Masses. A.** Sagittal plane T1WI shows a large complex mass (*arrows*) extending from the presacral region, representing a sacrococcygeal teratoma. **B.** US of a smaller presacral teratoma shows a predominantly cystic mass (*arrows*) anterior to the sacrum (*arrowheads*). **C.** A neuroblastoma in the presacral space displaces the bladder (B) and rectum (R) anteriorly. **D.** US shows a homogeneous, moderately echogenic mass in the presacral space (*arrows*) caused by neuroblastoma.

Neuroblastoma can rarely develop as a primary tumor in the presacral space, comprising only 5% of cases of neuroblastoma. Amorphous, irregular calcifications are common and characteristic of this tumor (Fig. 52.73C). Presacral neuroblastomas carry a better prognosis than those that arise from the upper abdomen.

Rhabdomyosarcoma commonly arises from the genitourinary tract in children and may appear in a presacral location.

Sacral chordoma is a rare tumor that originates from remnants of the primitive nota cord. Plain radiographs demonstrate destruction and expansion of the sacrum associated with a presacral or sacrococcygeal soft tissue mass. Typical flocculated calcifications are often visible on radiographs or CT. MR shows a lobulated mass arising from the sacrum, with heterogeneous contrast enhancement.

Anterior sacral meningoceles develop when a portion of the thecal sac protrudes anteriorly into the presacral space through a sacral defect. The meningoceles are typically associated with a crescent-shaped deformity of the sacrum (scimitar sacrum). US, CT, or MR shows the cystic meningocele, which may be unilocular or multilocular, with associated sacral deformity. MR best defines the spinal origin of the mass and any associated tumor or spinal cord anomalies, such as cord tethering. Anterior sacral meningocele may be a part of the Currarino triad (partial sacral agenesis, anorectal stenosis, presacral mass). Anterior meningoceles may also occur in patients with neurofibromatosis.

Neuroenteric cysts are also occasionally seen in the presacral space and can also be associated with anterior sacral defects.

REFERENCES

1. Hirsch W, Kedar R, Preiss U. Color Doppler in the diagnosis of the gastroesophageal reflux in children: comparison with pH measurements and B-mode ultrasound. Pediatr Radiol 1996;26:232–235.
2. Kriss WM, Desai NS. Relation of gastric distention to prostaglandin therapy in neonates. Radiology 1997;203:219–221.
3. Cohen HL, Zinn HL, Haller JO, et al. Ultrasonography of pylorospasm: findings may simulate hypertrophic pyloric stenosis. J Ultrasound Med 1988;17:705–711.
4. Hernanz-Schulman M, Zhu Y, Stein SM, et al. Hypertrophic pyloric stenosis in infants: US evaluation of vascularity of the pyloric canal. Radiology 2003;229:389–393.
5. Hernanz-Schulman M, Sells LL, Ambrosino MM, et al. Hypertrophic pyloric stenosis in the infant without a palpable olive: accuracy of sonographic diagnosis. Radiology 1994;193:771–776.
6. Swischuk LE, Hayden CK Jr, Stansberry SD. Sonographic pitfalls in imaging of the antropyloric region in infants. Radiographics 1989;9:437–447.
7. Ripolles T, Garcia-Aguayo J, Martinez MJ, et al. Gastrointestinal bezoars: sonographic and CT characteristics. AJR Am J Roentgenol 2001;177:65–69.
8. Newman B, Girdany BR. Gastric trichobezoars—sonographic and computed tomographic appearance. Pediatr Radiol 1990;20:526–527.
9. Strouse PJ. Disorders of intestinal rotation and fixation ("malrotation"). Pediatr Radiol 2004;34:837–851.
10. Long FR, Kramer SS, Markowitz RI, et al. Radiographic patterns of intestinal malrotation in children. Radiographics 1996;16:547–556.
11. Pracros JP, Sann L, Genin G, et al. Ultrasound diagnosis of midgut volvulus: the "whirlpool" sign. Pediatr Radiol 1992;22:18–20.
12. Patino MO, Munden MM. Utility of the sonographic whirlpool sign in diagnosing midgut volvulus in patients with atypical clinical presentations. J Ultrasound Med 2004;23:397–401.
13. Aidlen J, Anupindo SA, Jaramillo D, et al. Malrotation with midgut volvulus: CT findings of bowel infarction. Pediatr Radiol 2005; 35:529–531.
14. Desai KM, Dorward IG, Minkes RK, et al. Blunt duodenal injuries in children. J Trauma 2003;54:640–645; discussion 645–646.
15. Agrons GA, Corse WR, Markowitz RI, et al. Gastrointestinal manifestations of cystic fibrosis: radiologic-pathologic correlation. Radiographics 1996;16:871–893.
16. Hernandez JA, Swischuk LE, Angel CA. Validity of plain films in intussusception. Emerg Radiol 2004;10:323–326.
17. Verschelden P, Filiatrault D, Garel L, et al. Intussusception in children: reliability of US in diagnosis—a prospective study. Radiology 1992;184:741–744.
18. del-Pozo G, Albillos JC, Tejedor D. Intussusception: US findings with pathologic correlation—the crescent-in-doughnut sign. Radiology 1996;199:688–692.
19. Lam AH, Firman K. Value of sonography including color Doppler in the diagnosis and management of long standing intussusception. Pediatr Radiol 1992;22:112–114.
20. Kong M-S, Wong H-F, Lin S-L, et al. Factors related to detection of blood flow by color Doppler ultrasonography in intussusception. J Ultrasound Med 1997;16:141–144.
21. Shiels WE II, Maves CK, Hedlung GL, Kirks DR. Air enema for diagnosis and reduction of intussusception: clinical experience and pressure correlates. Radiology 1991;181:169–172.
22. Daneman A, Navarro O. Intussusception. Part 2: An update on the evolution of management. Pediatr Radiol 2004;34:97–108.
23. Wood SK, Kim JS, Suh SJ, et al. Childhood intussusception: US-guided hydrostatic reduction. Radiology 1992;182:77–80.
24. Riebel TW, Nasir R, Weber K. US-guided hydrostatic reduction of intussusception in children. Radiology 1993;188:513–516.
25. Rohrschneider WK, Troger J. Hydrostatic reduction of intussusception under US guidance. Pediatr Radiol 1995;25:530–534.
26. Yoon CH, Kim HJ, Goo HW. Intussusception in children: US-guided pneumatic reduction—initial experience. Radiology 2001;8:85–88.
27. Navarro OM, Daneman A, Chae A. Intussusception: the use of delayed, repeated reduction attempts and the management of intussusception due to pathologic lead points in pediatric patients. AJR Am J Roentgenol 2004;182:1169–1176.
28. Shiels WE II, Kirks DR, Keller GL, et al. Colonic perforation by air and liquid enemas: Comparison study in young pigs. AJR Am J Roentgenol 1993;160:931–935.
29. John SD. The value of ultrasound in children with suspected intussusception. Emerg Radiol 1998;5(5):297–305.
30. Strouse PJ, DiPietro MA, Saez F. Transient small-bowel intussusception in children on CT. Pediatr Radiol 2003;33:316–320.
31. Hui GC, Gerstle JT, Weinstein M, et al. Small-bowel intussusception around a gastrojejunostomy tube resulting in ischemic necrosis of the intestine. Pediatr Radiol 2004;34:916–918.
32. Tsakayannis DE, Shamberger RC. Association of imperforate anus with occult spinal dysraphism. J Pediatr Surg 1995;30:1010–1012.
33. Boemers TM, Beek FJ, van Gool JD, et al. Urologic problems in anorectal malformations. Part 1. Urodynamic findings and significance of sacral anomalies. J Pediatr Surg 1996;31:407–410.
34. Zerin JM, Kuhn-Fulton J, White SJ, et al. Colonic strictures in children with cystic fibrosis. Radiology 1995;194:223–226.
35. Sarrazin J, Wilson SR. Manifestations of Crohn disease at US. Radiographics 1996;16:499–520.
36. Spalinger J, Patriquin H, Miron MC, et al. Doppler US in patients with Crohn disease: vessel density in the diseased bowel reflects disease activity. Radiology 2000;217:787–791.
37. Baud C, Saguintaah M, Veyrac C, et al. Sonographic diagnosis of colitis in children. Eur Radiol 2004;14:2105–2119.
38. Maccioni F, Colaiacomo MC, Parlanti S. Ulcerative colitis: value of MR imaging. Abdom Imaging 2005 Sep–Oct;30(5):584–592.
39. Faingold R, Daneman A, Tomlinson G, et al. Necrotizing enterocolitis: assessment of bowel variability with color Doppler US. Radiology 2005;235:587–594.
40. Ping AJ, Blane CE, Garver KA. Current prognosis in necrotizing enterocolitis with portal vein gas. Can Assoc Radiol J 1998;49:237–240.
41. McCarville MB, Adelman CS, Li C, et al. Typhlitis in childhood cancer. Cancer 2005;104:380–387.
42. Hernandez JA, Swischuk LE, Angel CA, Chung D, Chandler R, Lee S. Imaging of acute appendicitis: US as the primary imaging modality. Pediatr Radiol 2005 Apr;35(4):392–395.
43. Kao SC, Smith WL, Abu-Yousef MM, et al. Acute appendicitis in children: sonographic findings. AJR Am J Roentgenol 1989;153: 375–379.
44. Lee JH, Jeong YK, Park KB, et al. Operator-dependent techniques for graded compression sonography to detect the appendix and diagnose acute appendicitis. AJR Am J Roentgenol 2005;184: 91–97.
45. Hayden CK Jr, Kuchelmeister J, Lipscomb TS. Sonography of acute appendicitis in childhood: perforation versus non-perforation. J Ultrasound Med 1992;11:209–216.
46. Patriquin HB, Garcier J-M, Lafortune M, et al. Appendicitis in children and young adults: Doppler sonographic-pathologic correlation. AJR Am J Roentgenol 1996;166:629–633.
47. Kaiser S, Frenckner B, Jorulf HK. Suspected appendicitis in children: US and CT—a prospective randomized study. Radiology 2002;223:633–638.
48. Poortman P, Lohle PN, Schoemaker CM, et al. Comparison of CT and sonography in the diagnosis of acute appendicitis: a blinded prospective study. AJR Am J Roentgenol 2003;181:1355–1359.
49. Garcia Pena BM, Cook EF, Mandl KD. Selective imaging strategies for the diagnosis of appendicitis in children. Pediatrics 2004;113: 24–28.
50. Sivit CJ. Controversies in emergency radiology: acute appendicitis in children—the case for CT. Emerg Radiol 2004;10:238–240.
51. Lowe LH, Penney MW, Stein SM, et al. Unenhanced limited CT of the abdomen in the diagnosis of appendicitis in children: comparison with sonography. Am J Roentgenol AJR 2001;176:31–35.

52. Hoecker CC, Billman GF. The utility of unenhanced computed tomography in appendicitis in children. J Emerg Med 2005;28: 415–421.
53. Fefferman NR, Roche KJ, Pinkney LP, et al. Suspected appendicitis in children: focused CT technique for evaluation. Radiology 2001;220:691–695.
54. Callahan MJ, Rodriguez DP, Taylor GA. CT of appendicitis in children. Radiology 2002;224:325–332.
55. Kaiser S, Finnbogason T, Jorulf HK. Suspected appendicitis in children: diagnosis with contrast-enhanced versus nonenhanced helical CT. Radiology 2004;231:427–433.
56. Foley TA, Earnest F IV, Nathan MA, Hough DM, Schiller HJ, Hoskin TL. Differentiation of nonperforated from perforated appendicitis: accuracy of CT diagnosis and relationship of CT findings to length of hospital stay. Radiology 2005 Apr;235(1):89–96.
57. Grattan-Smith JD, Blews DE, Brand T. Omental infarction in pediatric patients: sonographic and CT findings. AJR Am J Roentgenol 2002;178:1537–1539.
58. Lee HJ, Lee SM, Park WH, et al. Objective criteria of triangular cord sign in biliary atresia on US scans. Radiology 2003;229:395–400.
59. Kanegawa K, Akasaka Y, Kitamura E, et al. Sonographic diagnosis of biliary atresia in pediatric patients using the "triangular cord" sign versus gallbladder length and contraction. AJR Am J Roentgenol 2003;181:1387–1390.
60. Kim MJ, Park YN, Han SJ, et al. Biliary atresia in neonates and infants: triangular area of high signal intensity in the porta hepatic at T2-weighted MR cholangiography with US and histopathologic correlation. Radiology 2000;215:395–401.
61. Nijs E, Callahan MJ, Taylor GA. Disorders of the pediatric pancreas: imaging features. Pediatr Radiol 2005;35:358–373.
62. King LR, Siegel MJ, Balfe DM. Acute pancreatitis in children: CT findings of intra- and extrapancreatic fluid collections. Radiology 1995;195:196–200.
63. Couture A, Veyrac C, Baud C, et al. Evaluation of abdominal pain in Henoch-Schonlein syndrome by high frequency ultrasound. Pediatr Radiol 1992;22:12–17.
64. Jeong YK, Ha HK, Yoon CH, et al. Gastrointestinal involvement in Henoch-Schonlein syndrome: CT findings. AJR Am J Roentgenol 1997;168:965–968.
65. Defreyne L, Meersschaut V, van Damme S, et al. Colonic arteriovenous malformation in a child misinterpreted as an idiopathic colonic varicosis on angiography: remarks on current classification of childhood intestinal vascular malformations. Eur Radiol 2003;13(suppl 4):L138–141.
66. Taskinen S, Ronnholm K. Post-pyelonephritic renal scars are not associated with vesicoureteral reflux in children. J Urol 2005;173:1345–1348.
67. Lonergan GJ, Pennington DJ, Morrison JC, et al. Childhood pyelonephritis: comparison of gadolinium-enhanced MR imaging and renal cortical scintigraphy for diagnosis. Radiology 1998;207:377–384.
68. Kavanagh EC, Ryan S, Awan A, et al. Can MRI replace DMSA in the detection of renal parenchymal defects in children with urinary tract infections? Pediatr Radiol 2005;35:275–281.
69. Bosio M. Cystosonography with echocontrast: a new imaging modality to detect vesicoureteral reflux in children. Pediatr Radiol 1998;28:250–255.
70. Berrocal T, Gaya F, Arjonilla A. Vesicoureteral reflux: can the urethra be adequately assessed by using contrast-enhanced voiding US of the bladder? Radiology 2005;234:235–241.
71. Jones RA, Perez-Brayfield MR, Kirsch AJ, et al. Renal transit time with MR urography in children. Radiology 2004;233:41–50.
72. Zerin JM, Baker DR, Casale JA. Single-system ureteroceles in infants and children: imaging features. Pediatr Radiol 2000;30:139–146.
73. Blane CE, Zerin JM, Bloom DA. Bladder diverticula in children. Radiology 1994;190:695–697.
74. Aso C, Enriquez G, Fite M, et al. Gray-scale and color Doppler sonography of scrotal disorders in children: an update. Radiographics 2005;25:1197–1214.
75. Baud C, Veyrac C, Couture A, et al. Spiral twist of the spermatic cord: a reliable sign of testicular torsion. Pediatr Radiol 1998;28:950–954.
76. Aragona F, Pescatori E, Talenti E, Toma P, Malena S, Glazel GP. Painless scrotal masses in the pediatric population: prevalence and age distribution of different pathologic conditions—a 10-year retrospective multicenter study. J Urol 1996;155:1424–1426.
77. Avila NA, Premkumar A, Shawker TH, et al. Testicular adrenal rest tissue in congenital adrenal hyperplasia: Findings at Gray-scale and color Doppler US. Radiology 1996;198:99–104.
78. Avila NA, Premkumar A, Merke DP. Testicular adrenal rest tissue in congenital adrenal hyperplasia: comparison of MR imaging and sonographic findings. AJR Am J Roentgenol 1999;172:1003–1006.
79. Rohrschneider WK, Weirich A, Rieden K, et al. US, CT and MR imaging characteristics of nephroblastomatosis. Pediatr Radiol 1998;28:435–443.
80. Lonergan GJ, Martinez-Leon MI, Agrons GA, et al. Nephrogenic rests, nephroblastomatosis, and associated lesions of the kidney. Radiographics 1998;18:947–968.
81. Lowe LH, Isuani BJ, Heller RM, et al. Pediatric renal masses: Wilms tumor and beyond. Radiographics 2000;20:1585–1603.
82. Heidelberger KP, Ritchey ML, Dauser RC, et al. Congenital mesoblastic nephroma metastatic to the brain. Cancer 1993;72: 2499–2502.
83. Schlesinger AE, Rosenfield NS, Castle VP, Jasty R. Congenital mesoblastic nephroma metastatic to the brain: a report of two cases. Pediatr Radiol 1995;25(suppl 1):–S73-S75.
84. Lonergan GJ, Schwab CM, Suarez ES, et al. Neuroblastoma, ganglioneuroblastoma: radiologic-pathologic correlation. Radiographics 2002;22:911–934.
85. Pashankar FD, O'Dorisio MS, Menda Y. MIBG and somatostatin receptor analogs in children: current concepts on diagnostic and therapeutic use. J Nucl Med 2005;46(suppl 1):–55S-61S.
86. Kushner BH. Neuroblastoma: a disease requiring a multitude of imaging studies. J Nucl Med 2004;45:1172–1188.
87. Ribeiro J, Ribeiro RC, Fletcher BD. Imaging findings in pediatric adrenocortical carcinoma. Pediatr Radiol 2000;30:45–51.
88. Agrons GA, Lonergan GJ, Dickey GE, et al. Adrenocortical neoplasms in children: radiologic-pathologic correlation. Radiographics 1999;19:989–1008.
89. Avni EF, Rypens F, Smet MH, Galetty E. Sonographic demonstration of congenital adrenal hyperplasia in the neonate: the cerebriform pattern. Pediatr Radiol 1993;23:88–90.
90. Liebling MS, Starc TJ, McAlister WH, et al. ACTH-induced adrenal enlargement in infants treated for infantile spasms and acute cerebellar encephalopathy. Pediatr Radiol 1993;23:454–456.
91. Kim MJ, Han SJ, Yoon CS, et al. Using MR cholangiopancreatography to reveal anomalous pancreaticobiliary ductal union in infants and children with choledochal cysts. AJR Am J Roentgenol 2002;179;209–214.
92. von Schweinitz D. Neonatal liver tumours. Semin Neonatol 2003; 8:403–410.
93. Figarola MS, McQuiston SA, Wilson F, Powell R. Recurrent hepatoblastoma with localization by PET-CT. Pediatr Radiol 2005 Dec;35(12):1254–1258.
94. Schmidt MH, Sung L, Shuckett BM. Hemophagocystic lymphohistiocytosis in children: abdominal US findings within 1 week of presentation. Radiology 2004;230:685–689.
95. Barr LL, Hayden CK Jr, Stansberry SD, Swischuk LE. Enteric duplication cysts in children: are their ultrasonographic wall characteristics diagnostic? Pediatr Radiol 1990;20:326–328.
96. Cheng G, Soboleski D, Daneman A, et al. Sonographic pitfalls in the diagnosis of enteric duplication cysts. AJR Am J Roentgenol 2005;184:521–525.
97. Konen O, Rathaus V, Dlugy E, et al. Childhood abdominal cystic lymphangioma. Pediatr Radiol 2002;32:88–94.
98. Surratt JT, Siegel MJ. Imaging of pediatric ovarian masses. Radiographics 1991;11:533–548.
99. Garel L, Dubois J, Grignon A, et al. US of the pediatric female pelvis: a clinical perspective. Radiographics 2001;21:1393–1407.
100. Agrons GA, Wagner BJ, Lonergan G, et al. Genitourinary rhabdomyosarcoma in children: Radiologic-pathologic correlation. Radiographics 1997;17:919–937.

SECTION XII

Nuclear Radiology

Section Editor: David K. Shelton

Chapter 53

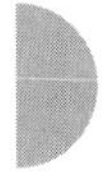

Introduction to Nuclear Radiology

David K. Shelton

An Approach to Image Interpretation

Section Overview

Nuclear radiology encompasses both therapeutic and diagnostic modalities that support practically every field of medical endeavor. Despite changes in referral patterns and the advent of managed care, nuclear medicine studies remain among the most cost-effective for the diagnosis and management of a variety of diseases. Radiographic, ultrasonographic, and MR studies provide high spatial resolution and important anatomic or structural information from which pathologic processes are inferred. On the other hand, nuclear medicine studies provide high functional resolution and provide physiologic and functional information not otherwise available. Anatomic imaging can measure the dimensions of a spot, but functional imaging can show whether it is active and whether it is malignant (Fig. 53.1). Many new, important techniques have become commonplace in the clinical environment. PET, PET-CT, and now SPECT have improved sensitivity and specificity for neural, cardiac, and oncologic imaging. PET-CT has greatly improved patient throughput, tumor staging, and evaluation of tumor response to therapy (Fig. 53.2). Molecular medicine and molecular imaging promise to bring applications of genomics and protein messaging quickly into the clinical arena. We now have the ability to follow gene therapy as well as stem cell therapy beginning with their introduction into the subject. Lymphoscintigraphy is helping surgeons to better stage melanoma and breast cancer and has significantly decreased patient morbidity following nodal staging procedures. Handheld probes allow better localization of sentinel nodes as well as small, difficult lesions identified on PET fluorodeoxyglucose scans. New therapies include antibody therapy for lymphoma, and research is being advanced for breast cancer antibody therapy, iodine-131 (I-131) metaiodobenzylguanidine (MIBG), and yttrium (Y) -labeled octreotide.

The material in this section is intended to provide an overview of the specialty and at the same time serve as the basis of review for those residents preparing for board examinations. The information should also be useful to those who may not practice nuclear radiology regularly or may not have done so recently.

Imaging Principles. The basic principles of diagnostic nuclear radiology are simple to grasp yet somehow seem to elude first-year residents as they are overwhelmed with information at the outset of their training. The concept of nuclear imaging is based on the external detection and mapping (image formation) of the biodistribution of radiotracers that have been administered to a patient. The knowledge of the normal patterns of uptake, distribution, and excretion permits us to make decisions concerning the presence or absence of disease.

Sometimes a radionuclide or radioisotope of a naturally occurring element essential to normal biologic function (e.g., I-123) or an analog (e.g., technetium-99m pertechnetate [Tc-99m-O_4]) is used without additional chemical alteration (Fig. 53.3). More commonly, a radioactive isotope is combined with a physiologically "active" compound to create a radiopharmaceutical, which can be administered intravenously, orally, or via direct injection. Thus, Tc-99m-O_4 may be combined with a diphosphonate compound for skeletal imaging. If the same radioactive compound is combined with an iminodiacetic acid derivative, the biologic distribution reflected by the images will be that of a biliary scan. This simple concept is the foundation for imaging the biodistribution of radiolabeled blood cells, monoclonal antibodies, peptides, and energy substrates such as glucose and fatty acids. If this unifying principle can be kept in mind while reading the various sections on nuclear imaging, the diverse number and types of studies may seem somewhat less bewildering.

Radiotherapy is an extremely important arm of nuclear medicine and is critical to several areas of clinical medicine. Most of the therapeutic radioisotopes and

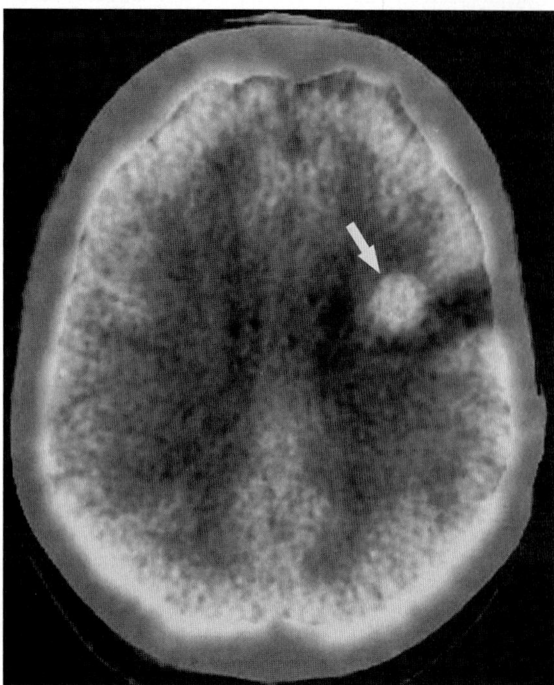

FIGURE 53.1. **PET-CT Scan of Brain.** PET scan of the brain with fluorodeoxyglucose (FDG) is fused onto a CT scan and shows increased FDG metabolic activity (*arrow*), confirming recurrence of glioblastoma after previous surgery and radiotherapy.

radiopharmaceuticals are particulate emitters, most commonly beta particles. Beta particles only travel a short distance through tissues, depositing most of their energy within a couple of millimeters. I-131 is utilized for benign thyroid conditions such as Graves disease, toxic hot nodules, and toxic multinodular goiter (Fig. 53.3). I-131 is also the primary treatment of choice for thyroid remnant ablation and metastatic thyroid cancer. Phosphorus-32 can be utilized for hematologic disorders such as essential thrombocytosis, in colloidal form for localized installation in arthritic joints for radiosynovectomy, in cystic tumors, or in malignant fluid collections. Strontium-89 and samarium-153 have proven effective in palliative pain management for patients with osteoblastic bone metastases. Radioimmunotherapy with monoclonal antibodies is now being utilized for refractory lymphoma treatment and studied for refractory metastatic breast cancer (Fig. 53.4). I-131 MIBG and Y-90 octreotide are being studied for treatment of metastatic neuroendocrine tumors.

AN APPROACH TO IMAGE INTERPRETATION

Obviously a basic foundation of anatomic, physiologic, and nuclear imaging knowledge is necessary to make intelligent diagnoses and differential diagnoses based on nuclear medicine images. The suggested approach to image interpretation provided here will make more sense after reading the remainder of the nuclear medicine section; for the resident, it will be of greater value after the second or third nuclear medicine rotation.

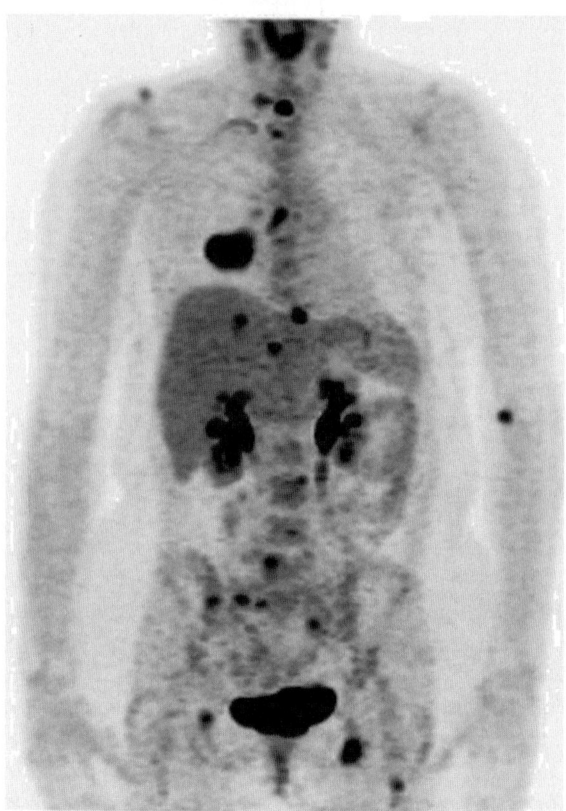

FIGURE 53.2. **Myocardial Isotopic Perfusion Scan Projection Image From Whole-Body PET Fluorodeoxyglucose Scan.** Whole body PET-CT scan was done for initial staging in this breast cancer patient and demonstrates multiple areas of abnormal hypermetabolic foci, consistent with diffuse metastatic breast cancer.

When preparing to discuss a case, it is first important to determine the radiopharmaceutical and therefore the type of study, which may be as simple as reviewing the film margins or paperwork for textual information. It is poor form to ask, "What type of study is this?" when the information is readily at hand. At the same time one may also glean important information about the age and sex of the patient, the site of injection, the temporal sequence when multiple images are present, the type of images (planar or tomographic, static, or dynamic), and patient orientation during imaging (e.g., right/left, oblique, posterior, upright/supine).

If the radiopharmaceutical information is not known, then the first step in analysis is based on determining the relative count density of the images. Typically, images of Tc-99m-O_4–labeled radiopharmaceuticals have a relatively high count density. Many medium- and higher-energy

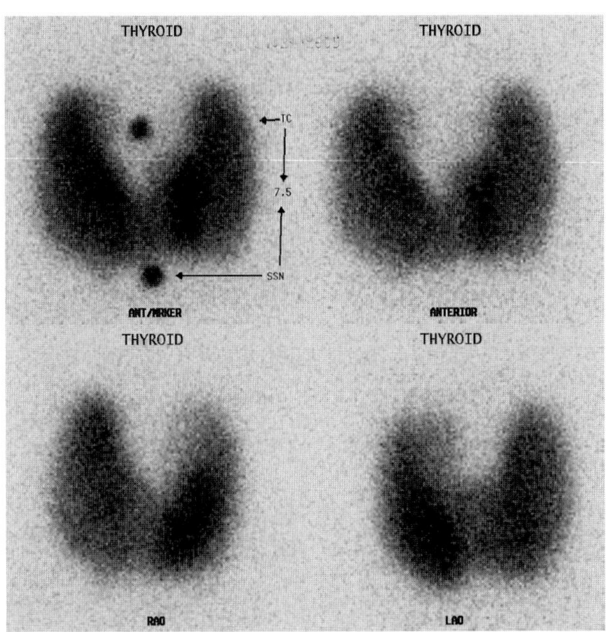

FIGURE 53.3. **Iodine-123 Thyroid Scan.** The patient presented with symptoms and laboratory findings of hyperthyroidism. The scan shows diffuse, homogeneous enlargement and an increased uptake of 77%. She was then successfully treated with iodine-131.

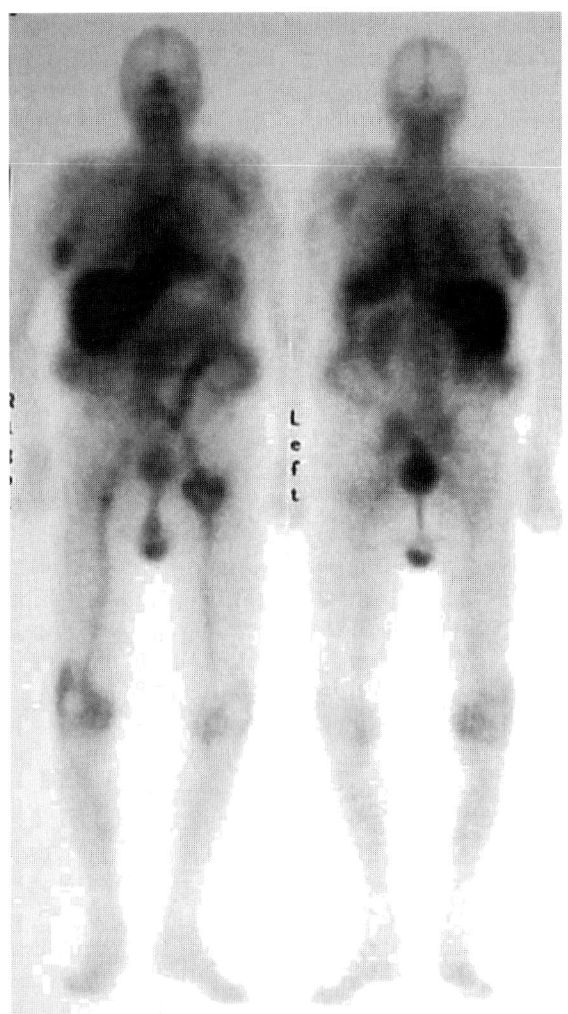

FIGURE 53.4. **Indium-111 Zevalin (Ibritumomab Tiuxetan) Antibody Scan.** Whole-body scan demonstrates normal biodistribution of the antibody agent and multiple foci of increased uptake, consistent with known B-cell lymphoma. The patient was then successfully treated with yttrium-90 Zevalin radioimmunotherapy with good clinical and CT response.

isotopes (indium-111, gallium-67, I-131, etc.) have lower count density based on longer half-lives and therefore lower administered doses. This often results in relatively noisy images. A notable exception to this generalization is arterial flow studies performed with Tc-99m–labeled radiopharmaceuticals. Because these studies are performed as dynamic acquisitions at a typical rate of 1 to 5 seconds per frame, they too will have a low count density.

The number and type of images presented and type of acquisition (e.g., PET, SPECT, or planar) should be noted. If a series of frames is provided, the study is either a dynamic acquisition with the typical timing of seconds or minutes per frame, or possibly a series of SPECT image slices that will usually have more counts and appear somewhat smoothed because of the processing algorithms employed.

Next, study the biodistribution of activity and anatomy in the images: Is there evidence of cardiac or great vessel blood pool activity? Is skeletal activity present? What organs or structures are visualized? Are there obvious focal abnormalities? From a knowledge of the biodistribution evident on the images and a reasonable assumption about the likely radioisotope, one may make some conjecture as to the most likely radiopharmaceutical in use.

After the radiopharmaceutical and type of study are determined, proceeding with the rest of the analysis is fairly straightforward. Again, a basic knowledge of the normal biodistribution of the radiopharmaceutical and the usual indications for performing the study is required. Given these, plus a relatively rudimentary understanding of anatomy and physiology, one can "make the finding(s)" with relative certainty. A word of caution is in order, however. Two common errors continue to cause problems for each new generation of residents. First, it is extremely difficult to "see what is not there." Always "take attendance" and be certain that all organs and structures that should be "present" on a given study are visualized with their normal pattern and relative uptake of radiopharmaceutical. Next, frequently more than one finding of importance will exist. It is easy to suffer from "search satisfaction" and quit looking for additional abnormalities after one is found. A rigid approach to image analysis is required to prevent both of these errors.

When studying dynamic series such as arterial flow studies, Tc-99m–labeled red blood cell studies for GI hemorrhage localization, renal function images, and so forth, it is important to note the time per frame because you will need to make comments concerning the timing of the arrival of the radiopharmaceutical in various structures. This information may be critical to image interpretation and is frequently overlooked by neophytes. Identifying changes from one frame to the next may be difficult. One approach to enhance and speed detection of abnormalities and asymmetries is to study the first frame or two relatively closely and then move directly to the last frame. Direct comparison of early and late images will demonstrate changes between the two most dramatically and will allow you to direct your attention to the appropriate areas on the intervening images and define the correct timing of events. It is helpful to "back through" the images from last to first after identifying any abnormalities on the later images. This approach will rapidly identify with great temporal and anatomic accuracy the exact time of appearance and location of GI hemorrhage, for example.

An orderly approach to image analysis for static images is also required but will vary based on the type of study in question. Here are specific techniques for some common studies that may be helpful.

Skeletal Imaging. Review the images provided with a "top-down" approach, addressing skeletal structures first on the anterior view, then on the posterior view (Fig. 53.5). Note areas of increased or decreased activity without attaching strong clinical significance to them initially. Always comment on the renal activity that should normally be present, and use this as a reminder to evaluate soft tissue activity for abnormal increases, decreases, and asymmetry. This type of approach works well with many of the whole-body imaging studies, although the biodistribution will vary.

SPECT Myocardial Perfusion Imaging. Always view the raw data images first, if available, and evaluate for quality control issues, artifacts, and ancillary or incidental findings (e.g., breast attenuation, motion, pacemaker artifact, pulmonary uptake, breast tumor). Always review the exercise data to confirm adequacy of stress or determine what, if any, pharmacologic agent was employed. Next review the short-axis slices, then the vertical long-axis slices, and finally the horizontal long-axis slices. Note the presence or absence of areas of increased or decreased perfusion and whether they appear fixed or seem to change between stress and rest images. Note chamber size and whether or not it is more dilated at stress than rest. Attempt to confirm the presence of any defects in two planes. Then evaluate the wall motion, brightening, and thickening. Check the end-diastolic and end-systolic volumes. Evaluate the stress and rest data, including the ejection fractions. Formulate a working hypothesis to explain the constellation of findings present.

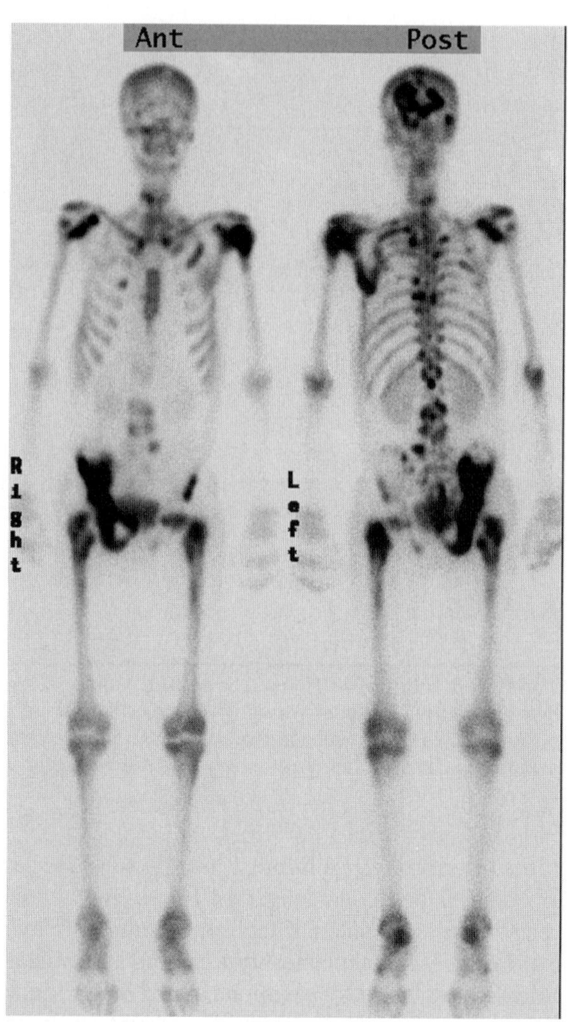

FIGURE 53.5. **Whole-Body Bone Scan With Tc-99m Methylene Diphosphonate.** The scan demonstrates multiple areas of increased uptake caused by diffuse bony metastatic disease in this patient with prostate cancer.

Ventilation/Perfusion Imaging for Pulmonary Embolus. Always review a chest radiograph or chest CT first, if provided. If not initially available, comment that review of the radiograph is essential prior to making a definitive statement about the likelihood of pulmonary embolus. Review the perfusion study in its entirety first. Note the presence of any defects; their relative sizes (lobar, segmental, subsegmental); and their locations. Attempt to confirm the findings in more than one view. Once the number and location of the defects are known, attempt to match these defects in the corresponding areas on the ventilation study. Summarize the findings and segmental anatomy, verbally reciting the number and size of matched and mismatched defects. Offer a probability of pulmonary embolus based on the findings, and determine whether another study such as CT angiography is needed.

Hepatobiliary Imaging. For this and any other study in which flow studies and dynamic imaging are performed, studying the images in the order in which they were acquired is best: flow study first, then dynamic images using the approach outlined previously, and, finally, static images (right lateral or left anterior oblique views would be typical), if any. Note the temporal sequence of the arrival of the arterial bolus in the kidneys, spleen, and, finally, liver if an arterial flow study of the abdomen is provided. With approximately 80% of hepatic blood flow arriving via the portal system, the liver should appear later than the other organs; if it does not, portal hypertension may be present. Early flow to the gallbladder fossa implies significant inflammation. On the dynamic series, note the appearance of the early images, then study the later images: Are gallbladder and bowel activity present? If so, "back through" the images and note their first appearance. Is activity visualized in the normal sequence of intrahepatic ducts, common hepatic duct, gallbladder, common bile duct, and duodenum? Is there activity in any areas other than expected—stomach, esophagus, or free spill into the peritoneum? Are there any focal accumulations of labeled bile in the liver, gallbladder fossa, or elsewhere?

VINDICATE. For a situation in which a finding has been made but no explanation is readily apparent, it is helpful to contemplate the finding while considering a standard list of generic causes as well as mechanisms that might lead to the finding. One such generic list uses the mnemonic VINDICATE as follows: **V**ascular (any cause of increased/decreased blood flow, collagen vascular diseases); **I**nfectious (always include tuberculosis, fungal, HIV); **N**eoplastic (benign or malignant, primary or metastatic); **D**rug-induced (radiopharmaceutical preparation and quality control, recent prior radiopharmaceutical administration or contrast study, thyroid hormone ingestion); **I**diopathic (sarcoidosis, amyloidosis); **C**ongenital; **A**rtifact (related to patient, clothing, imaging equipment, computer processing, or film processing); **T**rauma; or **E**ndocrine/metabolic (Paget disease, hyperparathyroidism, etc.).

If the physiologic mechanisms of radiopharmaceutical localization are understood, then mechanistic explanations for findings allow another route to a solution. Thus, from a mechanistic standpoint, increased activity on a bone scan is caused by either increased delivery of radiopharmaceutical to the bone or increased incorporation owing to either increased osteoblastic activity or increased dwell time for extraction by normally functioning osteoblasts. Reasons for increased delivery include the following: arterial injection, arteriovenous malformation, infection, tumor, localized inflammation caused by trauma, increased use of a limb, neurologic reflex increased flow, and apparent increased uptake with actual reduced uptake in the contralateral body part. Reasons for increased osteoblastic activity include the following: normal growth in epiphyseal bone and enhanced repair in response to fracture, infection, and benign or malignant tumors. Increased dwell time may be caused by constricting clothing, tourniquets, venous obstruction, and lymphatic obstruction.

When taking a case it is best to follow your initial comments concerning the findings with a final image review as you verbally summarize what you believe to be pertinent to the diagnosis. It is not uncommon to realize only as the summary is presented aloud that a specific diagnosis is indicated or that the findings significantly limit the differential diagnosis.

The foregoing discussion is not meant to be all encompassing and does not do justice to the entire spectrum of studies and diseases that will be encountered. However, it should provide a starting point for the development of one's own approach to image analysis and case-discussion skills. Consider using the images in each of the subsequent chapters as sample unknown cases and attempt to analyze them before reading the captions. This sort of practice will undoubtedly enhance one's ability to take unknown cases with greater confidence and accuracy.

SECTION OVERVIEW

For this edition of the text, the nuclear radiology section has been thoroughly revised and updated with multiple new images and current references as needed. The inflammation and infection chapter has been completely rewritten. The oncology chapter has been rewritten to incorporate the new approach of molecular imaging. A separate chapter on the rapidly expanding area of PET and PET-CT has been added. In every case, the authors have attempted to provide clear, concise, current, and useful information. I have no doubt that you will find that they have succeeded.

Chapter 54

Essential Science of Nuclear Medicine

Ramsey D. Badawi, Linda A. Kroger, and Jerrold T. Bushberg

Relevant Aspect of Radiation Physics

Radiation Safety

Radiopharmaceuticals

Imaging Systems and Radiation Detectors
Gamma Camera Quality Control
Positron Emission Tomography Scanner Quality Control
Nonimaging Detector Systems

RELEVANT ASPECTS OF RADIATION PHYSICS

Types of Radiation in Nuclear Medicine. The electromagnetic spectrum of radiation can be divided into nonionizing and ionizing radiation. Nonionizing radiation includes commonly encountered forms of electromagnetic radiation such as visible light, microwave, and radiofrequencies (used in radio transmissions and in MR). The ionizing radiation used in diagnostic medical imaging includes x-rays, γ rays, and annihilation radiation. The difference between these forms of radiation lies in their origin. X-rays are extranuclear in origin and can be produced by bombarding an atom with photons or electrons; in diagnostic radiology this is achieved with an x-ray tube, which produces x-rays with energies at and below 140 keV. γ rays are produced from within the atomic nucleus as unstable nuclei transition to a more stable state. In diagnostic radiology, γ-ray energies lie typically in the 80- to 350-keV range (Table 54.1). Annihilation radiation is produced when a particle and its antiparticle interact and annihilate each other; this is the type of radiation detected in PET. When positrons annihilate, the resulting radiation has a fixed energy of 511 keV.

Ionizing radiation need not be part of the electromagnetic spectrum; it can also come in a particulate form. The particle of most common medical interest is the β particle, which is an electron that has its origin within the unstable nucleus. As opposed to x-rays, γ rays, or annihilation radiation, β particles interact quite easily with matter, traveling only a few millimeters in tissue as they transfer their energy to their surroundings. This energy-transferring property produces a high dose within a short range and provides therapeutic usefulness in such entities as Graves disease and thyroid cancer with iodine-131 (I-131). β antiparticles ($\beta+$) are the positrons used in PET imaging; they interact in and deliver radiation to human tissue in a similar way to ordinary β particles prior to annihilating.

A form of radiation that is generally not of interest for imaging but that can be important when considering radiation safety is *bremsstrahlung* ("braking radiation"). Bremsstrahlung can be generated when high-energy electrons or positrons interact with an atomic nucleus. Bremsstrahlung events become more likely as particle energy increases and as the effective atomic number of the nucleus increases. Surrounding the source with material such as plastic, which has a low effective atomic number, will stop the particles and minimize the radiation hazard. If necessary, any additional photon radiation can be reduced by surrounding the plastic shielding layer with a denser material, such as lead.

Photon Interactions With Matter. There are two primary interactions of photons with matter at the energies of interest for nuclear medicine. These are *photoelectric interactions* and *Compton interactions*. In a photoelectric interaction, a photon interacts with an atom and transfers all of its energy to an orbital electron (Fig. 54.1A, *right* Fig 54.1), disappearing in the process. The electron is ejected, ionizing the target atom. The ejected electron may

TABLE 54.1 Radionuclides

Radionuclide (Symbol)	*Method of Production*	*Mode of Decay (%)*	*Principal Imaging Photons keV (Abundance)*	*Physical Half-life*	*Comments*
Chromium-51 (Cr-51)	Nuclear reactor (neutron activation)	EC (100)	320 (9)	27.8 d	Used for in vivo red cell mass determinations, not for imaging; samples counted in sodium iodide well counter
Cobalt-57 (Co-57)	Cyclotron	EC (100)	122 (86) 136 (11)	271 d	Primarily used as a uniform flood field source for gamma camera quality control
Fluorine-18 (F-18)	Cyclotron	$\beta+$ (97), EC (3)	511 (AR)	110 mo	This radionuclide accounts for more than 80% of all clinical PET use; typically formulated as fluorodeoxyglucose
Gallium-67 (Ga-67)	Cyclotron	EC (100)	93 (40) 184 (20) 300 (17) 393 (4)	78 hr	In practice, the 93-, 184-, and 300-keV photons are used for imaging
Indium-111 (In-111)	Cyclotron	EC (100)	171 (900) 245 (94)	2.8 d (67.2 hr)	Principally utilized when optimal imaging occurs more than 24 hr after injection; both photons used in imaging
Iodine-123 (I-123)	Cyclotron	EC (100)	159 (83)	13.2 hr	Replaced I-131 for most diagnostic imaging applications to reduce radiation dose
Iodine-125 (I-125)	Nuclear reactor (neutron activation)	EC (100)	35 (6) 27 (39) 28 (76) 31 (20)	60.2 d	Used as I-125 albumin for in vivo blood/plasma volume determinations; not utilized for imaging, samples counted in well counter
Iodine-131 (I-131)	Nuclear reactor (U-235 fission)	$\beta-$(100)	284 (6) 364 (81) 637 (7)	8.0 d	Typical use now reserved for therapeutic applications; imaging is limited by high-energy photon (364 keV) and high patient dosimetry, mostly from β particles
Krypton-81m (Kr-81m)	Generator product	IT (100)	190 (67)	13 s	Ultrashort-lived parent (rubidium-81, 4.6 hr) and high expense limit the use of this agent
Molybdenum-99 (Mo-99)	Nuclear reactor (U-235 fission)	$\beta-$(100)	181 (16) 740 (12) 780 (4)	67 hr	The source (parent) for Mo/Tc generators; not used directly; 740- and 780-keV photons used to identify contamination of Tc-99m elution as "Moly breakthrough"
Phosphorus-32 (P-32)	Nuclear reactor (neutron activation)	$\beta-$(100)		14.3 d	Used in treatment of polycythemia vera, metastatic bone disease, and serous effusions
Samarium-153 (Sm-153)	Nuclear reactor (U-235 fission)	$\beta-$(100)	103 (28)	46 hr	Used for palliative treatment of metastatic bone pain
Strontium-89 (Sr-89)	Nuclear reactor (U-235 fission)	$\beta-$(100)	910 (.02)	50.5 d	Used for palliative treatment of metastatic bone pain
Technetium-99m (Tc-99m)	Generator product	IT (100)	140 (90)	6.02 hr	This radionuclide, typically in kit form, accounts for more than 70% of all imaging studies
Thallium-201 (Tl-201)	Cyclotron	EC (100)	69–80 (94) 167 (10)	73.1 hr	Majority of photons are low-energy x-rays (69–80 keV) from mercury 201 (Hg-201), the daughter of Tl-201
Xenon-133 (Xe-133)	Nuclear reactor (U-235 fission)	$\beta-$(100)	81 (37)	5.3 d	Xe-133 is a heavier-than-air gas; low abundance and energy of photon reduce image resolution

AR, annihilation radiation; $\beta-$, beta minus decay; $\beta+$, beta plus decay; EC, electron capture; IT, isomeric transition (i.e., gamma ray emission); U-235, uranium-235.

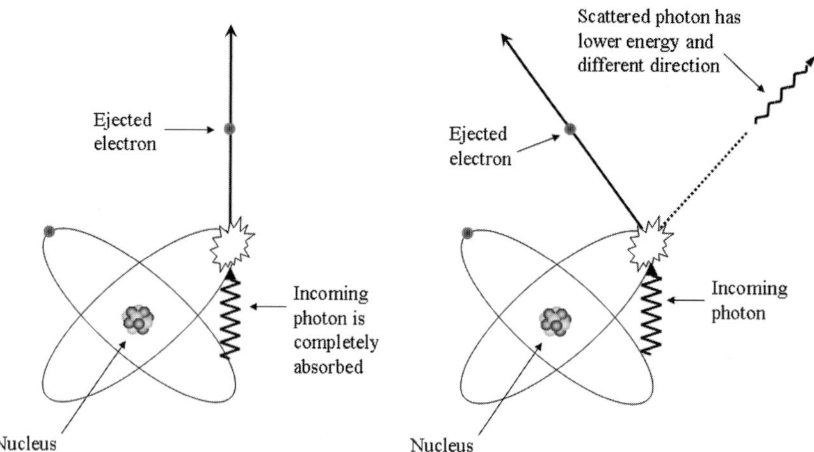

FIGURE 54.1. **Relevant Photon Interactions With Matter.** Left: Photoelectric interaction. Right: Compton scatter.

have sufficient energy to subsequently ionize other atoms with which it interacts. In a Compton interaction, also known as a scattering event, the incident photon interacts with an atom and imparts part of its energy to an orbital electron. The electron recoils, and the photon, now with lower energy, continues to propagate along a path at an angle to its original path (Fig. 54.1A, *left*). This scattering angle is dependent upon the amount of energy lost to the electron. Small angles are associated with small transfers of energy to the electron, and the maximum scattering angle, 180°, is associated with the maximum transfer of energy.

When a photon interacts with an atom, the relative likelihood of a photoelectric or a Compton interaction is dependent on the photon energy and on the density and effective atomic number of the target material. For typical nuclear medicine photon energies in human tissue, the Compton scattering interaction is the most prevalent, becoming completely dominant at the higher end of the range (e.g., for gallium-67 [Ga-67] or PET imaging). However, the detector materials used for nuclear medicine are much denser than tissue, and for these, both photoelectric and Compton interactions are important.

Units. Various units to describe radiation and its effects have been established. Because the scientific community is in transition between conventional units and the Système Internationale (SI), a table of both units with their conversion factors is provided in Table 54.2. *Activity* is used to describe the quantity of the radionuclide being administered and represents the rate of nuclear transformations, denoted by *curies* (Ci) in conventional units and *becquerels* (Bq) in SI units. The *roentgen* is the unit utilized to express radiation exposure and is a measure of the ability of x-rays and γ rays to produce a given amount of ionization in a given volume of air. From a biologic point of view, the important consideration is how much of the radiation exposure is deposited in an individual at a particular location. *Absorbed dose* is the amount of energy deposited by ionizing radiation per unit mass in joules per kilogram; the conventional unit is the *radiation-absorbed dose* (rad) and the SI unit is the *gray* (Gy). Because certain types of radiation are more biologically damaging than others, a radiation weighting factor (also called quality factor) is multiplied by the absorbed dose to yield the *dose equivalent*, which is measured in *rem* (roentgen equivalent man)

TABLE 54.2 Conventional and SI Radiologic Units and Conversion Factors

	Conventional Units		Multiply by Conventional Units to Obtain SI Units	SI Units		
Quantity	Name	Symbol		Name	Symbol	Example
Activity	Curie	Ci	3.7×10^{10}	Becquerel[b]	Bq	10 mCi = 370 mBq
Exposure	Roentgen	R	2.58×10^{-4}	Coulomb per kilogram	C/kg	
Absorbed dose	Radiation-absorbed dose	rad[a] (acronym)	10^{-2}	Gray[c]	Gy	100 rad = 1 Gy
Dose equivalent	Roentgen-equivalent man	rem (acronym)	10^{-2}	Sievert	Sv	100 rem = 1 Sv

[a]1 rad = .01 joule/kg.
[b]1 Bq = 1 disintegration/s.
[c]1 Gy = 1 J/kg.

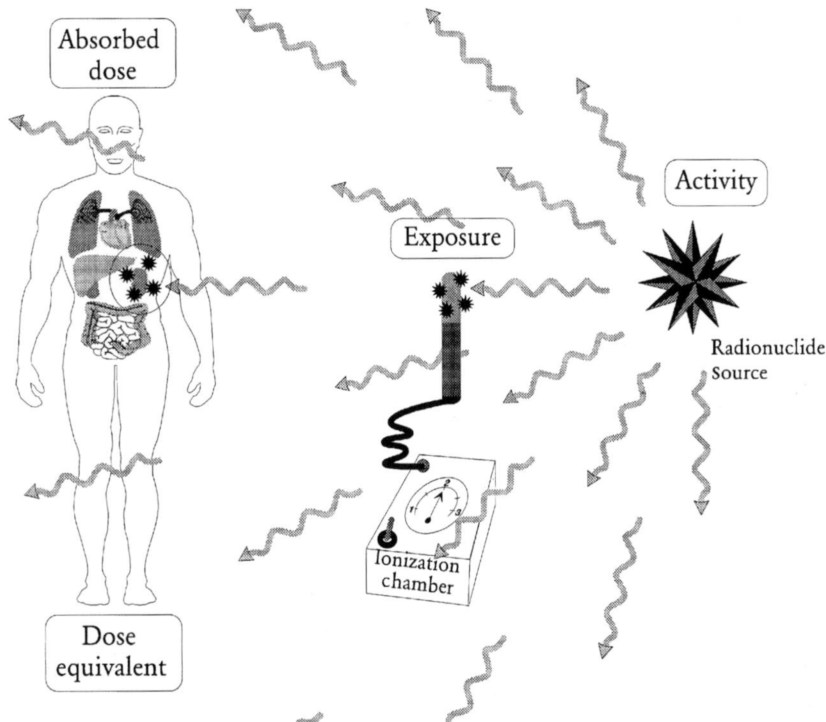

FIGURE 54.2. **Graphic Representation of Radiation Units.** The unit of measurement that is used to measure radioactivity is determined by where radioactivity is measured. Activity (curie/becquerel), whether occurring outside the body or inside, is measured at the source. Exposure (roentgens or coulomb per kilogram) is measured by an ionization chamber of the radioactivity as it transits air. Absorbed dose (rad/gray) is a measure of radioactivity that has interacted with the tissue where it deposits its energy. Dose equivalent (rem/Sievert) compares the effects on tissue by different types of radioactivity: α particles, β particles, and photons. The particles deposit more energy to the tissue than photons.

in conventional units and the *sievert* (Sv) in SI units. The dose-equivalent unit allows comparison between the various ionizing radiation sources (photons, β particles, α particles). Because the quality factor is equal to 1 for photons and electrons, 1 R approximately equals 1 rad in the diagnostic energy range for soft tissue, which approximately equals 1 rem (Fig. 54.2). That is, 1 R $\approx$ 1 rad (0.01 Gy) $\approx$ 1 rem (0.01 Sv).

RADIATION SAFETY

Radiation Exposure to the Worker. The total average exposure for a radiology technician results in an annual dose equivalent of only 100 to 150 mrem, whereas for the nuclear medicine technologist it is 200 to 300 mrem. Occupational exposure to nuclear medicine technologists who perform PET procedures can be two to four times higher because of high-energy γ rays. The majority of whole-body radiation to the nuclear medicine worker comes from exposure to the dosed patient during imaging. Localized extremity exposure doses from radiopharmaceutical preparation and injection can be higher.

The Nuclear Regulatory Commission (NRC) limits for radiation exposure (total effective dose equivalent) are 5,000 mrem/yr for designated occupationally exposed workers and 100 mrem/yr for members of the public.

The primary risk from any increased radiation exposure is an increased risk for cancer. For each additional rem, the lifetime increased risk of cancer is approximately 5×10^{-4} (5% per Sv). With the cancer incidence risk in the general population at 33%, each additional rem will increase the risk by 0.05%. Therefore, a lifetime occupational whole-body dose of 5 rem (e.g., 250 mrem/yr $\times$ 20 years) will increase the risk of developing cancer from 33% to 33.25%. With these numbers, several caveats to radiation exposure need to be remembered: any increased risk is spread over a lifetime; increased risks from exposure are additive; and the minimum latency of cancer is 5 to 8 years, with the mean for solid tissue tumors being closer to 20 to 25 years.

Because contamination in the workplace also increases radiation exposure to the worker, several guidelines should be followed to minimize contamination: (*1*) follow universal precautions by wearing protective clothing; (*2*) use plastic-backed absorbent to restrict any spills; (*3*) wash hands frequently; (*4*) use covers over collimators that can be discarded if contaminated; (*5*) monitor and wipe test frequently (see following); and (*6*) avoid smoking, eating, or drinking when handling radioactive materials.

Radiation Exposure to the Patient. The average total annual radiation dose to the population in the United States is 370 mrem/yr. Natural background radiation from atmospheric and terrestrial sources contributes 300 mrem/yr (~80%), whereas manmade sources, primarily from medical procedures, provide the other 60 mrem/yr (~20%).

Because nuclear medicine procedures involve radionuclides and radiopharmaceuticals that are variably transient in the human body, dosimetric considerations include not only the initial activity administered, but the biodistribution, the physical and biologic half-lives, and the possible pathologic processes. The physical half-life is defined as the time required for the number of radioactive atoms in a sample to decrease by half, and the biologic half-life is the time required for half of the radionuclide to be eliminated by biologic processes. On a relative scale, the dose to the whole body from most nuclear medicine diagnostic procedures is equivalent to half to six times the average annual dose equivalent from natural background. That is, the whole dose for nuclear medicine examinations range from 150 mrem for a technetium (Tc)-99m–macroaggregated albumin lung perfusion study to 2 rem for a tumor imaging study with 5 mCi of Ga-67 citrate. An additional dose might be received during a PET study from the x-ray component of the CT if patient is scanned on a combined PET-CT device. As of 2005, there were no standard scanner parameters for the CT component of a PET-CT procedure, so this additional dose can vary widely.

An additional dosimetry term that relates directly to the patient is the concept of "critical organ." The critical organ is identified as the organ or tissue that receives the largest dose of radiation or that has the highest radiosensitivity to a radiopharmaceutical. The dose to the critical organ depends on the radionuclide concentration by the organ, geometric factors, the effective retention in that organ, and the relative radiosensitivity of the organ. Interestingly, in many cases the dose to any organ (the target organ) comes as much from the organ itself as it does from the surrounding tissue (the source).

It is a common problem to see a pregnant patient in need of a nuclear medicine procedure. There are no absolute contraindications regardless of the nuclear medicine exam being considered. Risk-versus-benefit evaluation determines the indication for the exam. If the radionuclide exam is indicated and cannot be postponed until after term, measures to minimize the dose can be employed, such as halving the adult dose (and doubling the imaging time) and increasing hydration to enhance excretion. For PET-CT scans, the CT tube current may be reduced to about 40 mA without significantly impacting the PET portion of the study; however, this will compromise the quality of the resulting CT images.

A lactating woman who is administered a radiopharmaceutical requires counseling to proscribe feeding her infant for a specified length of time. The guidelines for these lengths of time are based on the physical and biologic half-lives of the radionuclides (called *effective half-lives*), which, in turn, predict when the breast milk is safe to drink. The recommended times for cessation of feeding are listed in Table 54.3. If the radiopharmaceutical is not listed on Table 54.3, refer to the package insert provided by the radiopharmaceutical manufacturer for their recommendation.

Radiation Safety in the Workplace: General Guidelines. The common goals of radiation safety are to minimize exposure to radiation, whether to the worker, the patient, or the public. Individuals exposed to radiation can limit their exposure by observing three very basic principles: time, distance, and shielding. Specifically, (*1*) limit the time of exposure, which, for the worker, can translate into being familiar enough with procedures that it is performed efficiently, thus minimizing exposure; (*2*) maximize the distance of exposure, observing that the exposure rate from a point source of radiation decreases as the distance from the source is squared (the inverse square law); and (*3*) use shielding when possible. Shielding with thin lead aprons in diagnostic radiology is quite effective in stopping the low-energy scatter photons. In nuclear medicine, because of the higher-energy photons, shielding is confined to containers for the source activity, such as preparation vials and syringe shields.

Regulations. The NRC governs nuclear material and its byproducts. Byproducts include reactor-produced radionuclides, such as molybdenum-99 and I-131. The NRC does not regulate accelerator-produced radioactive material; individual states govern the possession and use of these. The NRC licenses users (individuals or institutions) and governs many aspects of nuclear medicine operations, including the standards for protection against radiation (radiation protection program), waste disposal, licensing, surveys, instrumentation, and training requirements. Many states, after accepting the responsibility to regulate radioactive materials, become "agreement states" and license users and enforce regulations compatible with those of the NRC.

The central goal of a radiation protection program is called ALARA, which promotes efforts to keep radiation exposures *as low as reasonably achievable*. As a requirement of the NRC, ALARA represents an administrative philosophy to encourage, enforce, teach, and observe all reasonable ways to minimize radiation doses and exposure. The ALARA program extends into personnel exposure (workers), misadministrations (medical events) (patients), and environmental releases (general public) to achieve this dose minimization goal.

The NRC regulations that cover nuclear medicine are covered in the Code of Federal Regulations parts 19, 20, and 35. Part 19 covers the rights and responsibilities of workers to maintain a safe environment, and employers to educate their workers. Part 20 discusses regulations of radiation protection for facilities to include dose limits for personnel and the environment. Part 35 focuses on medical utilization of radiation sources, listing medical event definitions (formerly referred to as *misadministrations*) and training requirements for authorized users. Board certification in diagnostic radiology or nuclear medicine

TABLE 54.3 Recommendations for Cessation of Breastfeeding After Administration of Radiopharmaceuticals to Mothers

Radiopharmaceutical	*Administered Activity*	*Imaging Procedure*	*Recommended Duration of Interruption of Breastfeeding*[a]
Tc-99m sodium pertechnetate	30 mCi	Thyroid scan, Meckel scan	24 hr
Tc-99m kits (general rule)	5 to 25 mCi	All	24 hr
Tc-99m DTPA	10 to 15 mCi	Renal scan	None
Tc-99m MAA	3 to 5 mCi	Lung perfusion scan	12 hr
Tc-99m SC	5 mCi	Liver/spleen scan	6 hr
Tc-99m MDP	15 to 25 mCi	Bone scan	None
Tc-99m sestamibi/ tetrofosmin[b]	10 to 30 mCi	Cardiac studies	None
Fluorine-18 FDG	10 to 20 mCi	Tumor, neuro, or cardiac PET scan	12 hr
Gallium-67 citrate	6 to 10 mCi	Infection and tumor scans	4 wk
Thallium-201 chloride	3 mCi	Myocardial Perfusion	2 wk
Sodium iodine-123	30 μCi	Thyroid uptake only	None
Sodium iodine-123	200 to 400 μCi	Thyroid scan	None
Sodium iodine-131	5 μCi	Thyroid uptake	Discontinue[c]
Sodium iodine-131	10 mCi	Thyroid cancer Metascan or Graves therapy	Discontinue[c]
Sodium iodine-131	33 mCi	Outpatient therapy for hyperfunctioning nodule	Discontinue[c]
Sodium iodine-131	100 mCi or more	Thyroid cancer treatment (ablation)	Discontinue[c]

[a] Adapted from Nuclear Regulatory Commission Regulatory Guide 8.39, 1997. See Romney et al for derivation of milk concentration values for radiopharmaceuticals. U.S. Government Printing Office Washington DC.
[b] Minimal F-18 FDG in breast milk (Hicks et al, J Nucl Med 2001;42(8):1238–1242). Waiting six half-lives (12 hr) lowers the exposure to the infant from the mother.
[c] Discontinuance is based not only on the excessive time recommended for cessation of breastfeeding but also on the high dose the breasts themselves would receive during the radiopharmaceutical breast transit.
DTPA, Diethylenetriaminepentaacetic acid; FDG, fluorodeoxyglucose; MAA, macroaggregated albumin; MDP, methylene diphosphonate; SC, sulfur colloid; Tc, technetium.

suffices to qualify an individual as an authorized user in most states.

Radiation Safety Instruments. Two types of radiation detectors are commonly used for radiation safety in nuclear medicine departments. The Geiger-Müller (GM) detector is a gas-filled survey meter that measures radiation in counts per minute. The GM meter is a very sensitive radiation detector that is useful for localizing very small quantities of activity but will not accurately quantify it. Its primary use, therefore, is as a lab survey instrument looking for contamination. The ion chamber, another gas-filled detector, is used to accurately measure radiation exposure, especially at high levels. The ion chamber has several uses, including quantification of exposure levels, estimation of doses prior to administration (dose calibrator; see later discussion), and inspection of packages for compliance with transportation regulations.

Radiopharmaceutical Possession and Handling. In general, compliance regulations require "cradle-to-grave" documentation of all radioactive substances. These requirements begin with ordering of the radiopharmaceuticals by an authorized individual, then setting standards for packaging and shipping, followed by procedures for the receipt of the package, and finally demonstrating documentation of its use (patient or research) and disposal. Meticulous records of each step are imperative for adequate documentation of the "life" of a radioactive substance.

Radiation Monitoring. In a personnel monitoring program, designated workers exposed to radiation wear dosimetry, commonly either a thermoluminescent dosimeter or a film badge. For the film badge, the film is processed and the optical density is related to the radiation exposure. Depending on the magnitude of the potential exposure, reporting programs for personnel dosimeters can be established (e.g., monthly, quarterly).

The nuclear medicine workplace requires frequent monitoring for contamination. A typical monitoring program is as follows:

Daily. A GM survey meter is used to check over all work surfaces and trash. As a general rule, if any reading is greater than two times background, then the area should be decontaminated (wash area) and resampled until readings are less than twice background. In an unrestricted area (general public area), all readings should be lower than two times background. Label all contaminated trash as radioactive and store for decay (typically 10 physical half-lives).

Weekly. Perform a radiation field survey using an ion chamber to survey controlled areas within the workplace. Dose rates in unrestricted areas must be less than 2 mrem in any one hour and less than 100 mrem/year; however, all potential exposures should be kept ALARA.

Weekly. Wipe test multiple sample areas of the workplace. Count in a sodium iodide thallium gamma well counter using a wide energy window for 1 minute. An acceptable threshold is 200 disintegrations per minute per 100 square centimeters of surface area. If this is exceeded, then decontaminate and resample until within limits.

RADIOPHARMACEUTICALS

Mechanism of Localization of Radiopharmaceuticals. A radiopharmaceutical (which in an imaging context may be known as a *radiolabeled tracer* or *radiotracer*) is a specific compound containing a radionuclide. The compound dictates the biodistribution of the radiopharmaceutical. Many radiopharmaceuticals act like analogs of natural biologic compounds and thus localize by means of some physiologic process. For example, Tc-99m-pertechnetate is analogous to the iodide molecule and distributes to the thyroid, salivary glands, stomach, and kidneys. Tc-99m sulfur colloid acts like a colloid particle of approximately 1 μm and distributes throughout the reticuloendothelial system (liver, spleen, and bone marrow). Substituted iminodiacetic acid Tc-99m agents are analogous to bilirubin and are actively transported into hepatocytes and excreted into the biliary tree. Fluorine-18 fluorodeoxyglucose (FDG) acts as a glucose analogue, but after transport into the cell and phosphorylation it is physiologically trapped; thus after an uptake period of 45 to 90 minutes, the concentration of FDG in tissue gives an indication of glucose utilization. See Table 54.4 for other examples.

Generation of Radiopharmaceuticals. Nuclear medicine procedures are best served by tracers labeled with a radionuclide that has a physical half-life that is long enough to allow for imaging in a reasonable amount of time, but not so long as to continue to irradiate the patient much beyond that imaging. Thus radiotracers cannot be stored but must be generated daily for immediate use. To provide for tracers labeled with short-lived radionuclides, generators containing the parent material are constructed to provide an extended source of the daughter; alternatively, the radionuclide may be generated in a medical cyclotron, used to label a tracer, and the tracer shipped to the nuclear medicine department for use. This latter method is generally employed for positron-emitting radionuclides, the exception being rubidium-82, a blood flow PET tracer produced in a generator. The most commonly used radionuclide in nuclear medicine procedures is Tc-99m, and the generation of this radionuclide is described in detail below.

Moly Generator. Tc-99m comes from a generator, named for this parent-daughter relationship, the molybdenum-99 (Mo-99)-Tc-99m generator or Moly generator. Mo-99 decays with a physical half-life ($T_{1/2}$) of 67 hours, while Tc-99m decays with a 6-hour $T_{1/2}$ (Fig. 54.3). The Mo-99 is adsorbed to an alumina column. As the Tc-99m evolves on the column, it is easily removed by elution, as needed, by passing normal saline over the column, exchanging chloride for Tc-99m, in the form of sodium pertechnetate (Na-Tc-99m-O_4). Two types of Moly generators are commercially available (Fig. 54.4). The wet generator has a large reservoir of saline attached to one end of the column with which a vacuum bottle, attached to the other end, can extract the Tc-99m pertechnetate. The column is always "wet." The dry generator requires that a small saline vial be attached to one end, and the vacuum extraction vial is attached to the other. The column is left "dry" after the elution.

After eluting (also known as milking) the Moly generator, the shorter-lived daughter, Tc-99m, begins immediately to reaccumulate on the column. This regrowth occurs at a predictable rate and dictates the yield at the subsequent elution (Fig. 54.5). The key times for regrowth and their yields include 6 hr = 50% of activity, 23 hr = maximum activity. It can be readily appreciated from an inspection of the generator elution curve that eluting every 24 hours is both convenient and efficacious with respect to yield.

Quality control (QC) for the Moly generator consists of checking every elution for Mo-99 and aluminum breakthrough—that is, escape from the column. Although uncommon, the consequences of Moly breakthrough are important enough to mandate this QC procedure for each elution. The assay for Moly breakthrough looks for the very high-energy photons (740 and 780 keV) emitted by Mo-99. The entire eluate is placed in a lead container, called a Moly pig, that absorbs the majority of the 140-keV Tc-99m photons, but allows the higher-energy Mo-99 photons to pass. This pig is then assayed in a dose calibrator with the Mo-99 button selected. The NRC limits are 0.15 mCi of Mo-99 per millicurie of Tc-99m at the time of administration.

Aluminum breakthrough will cause Tc-99m kits to flocculate. These colloid particles will cause increased lung uptake on a sulfur colloid liver/spleen scan and increased liver uptake on a bone scan. The QC procedure to check for aluminum breakthrough is the colorimetric spot test, in which a drop of eluate is placed on the colorimetric paper and compared with a standard. The maximum permissible amount of aluminum is 10 μg/mL of eluate.

TABLE 54.4 Biodistribution: Mechanism of Localization of Radiopharmaceuticals

Imaging Procedure	*Radiopharmaceuticals*	*Mechanism of Localization*	*Closest Biochemical Analog*	*Critical Organ (rad/mCi)*
Lung perfusion scan	Tc-99m MAA	Capillary blockade	Thromboembolus	Lungs (0.15–0.48)
Lung ventilation scan	Xenon-133 gas	Compartment localization	Air	Trachea (0.64)
Bone scan	Tc-99m MDP	Chem-adsorption onto bone crystal	Phosphate	Bladder (0.1–0.2)
Hepatobiliary scan	Tc-99m IDA	Active hepatocyte cellular transport	Bilirubin	Gallbladder (0.12–0.18)
Myocardial perfusion scan	Thallium-201 chloride	Adenosine triphosphate transport system	Potassium	Kidneys (0.4–0.9)
Labeled white blood cell scan	Indium-111 WBC Tc-99m HMPAO	Active migration of leukocyte to site of infection or inflammation after binding of radionuclide to intracellular component	Migratory leukocyte	Spleen (8.4–18.0) (0.79)
Renal scan	Tc-99m DTPA Tc-99m MAG3	Glomerular filtration Glomerular filtration and tubular secretion	Inulin p-aminohippurate (PAH)	Bladder (0.07–0.6)
Thyroid	Iodine-123	Active transport	Iodine	Thyroid (11.0–20.0)
Brain scan	Tc-99m HMPAO	Lipophilic passive transport	Fatty acid	Lachrymal gland (5.16)
Gated equilibrium blood pool scan	Tc-99m-labeled RBCs	Compartment localization of RBC after Tc-99m binds to intracellular hemoglobin	RBC	Spleen (2.2)
Tumor imaging	Fluorine-18 FDG	Cellular uptake via glucose transporters followed by metabolic trapping of FDG-6-phosphate	Glucose	Bladder (0.4)
	Gallium-67 citrate	Unknown; iron receptor theory	Ferric ion	Colon (0.6–0.9)
	Indium-111 OncoScint monoclonal antibody (satumomab pendetide)	Antibody-antigen complex	Antibody	Spleen (3.2)
Meckel scan	Tc-99m pertechnetate	Active ion transport	Iodide	Thyroid (0.12–0.18)
Liver/spleen scan	Tc-99m colloid	Reticuloendothelial phagocytosis	Colloid particle	Liver (0.2–0.4)

DTPA, diethylenetriaminepentaacetic acid; FDG, fluorodeoxyglucose; HMPAO, hexametazime; IDA, iminodiacetic acid; MAA, macroaggregated albumin; MAG-3, mertiatide; MDP, methylene diphosphonate; RBC, red blood cell; Tc, technetium.

Radiochemical Purity. Many of the Tc-99m–based radiopharmaceuticals are produced by adding the generator elute, the "free" or unbound Tc-99m pertechnetate (TcO_4), to a "cold" kit containing the chelate (e.g., methylene diphosphonate [MDP], diethylenetriaminepentaacetic acid [DTPA], diisopropyl iminodiacetic acid) and a reducing agent, usually stannous chloride. The reducing agent enables the stable Tc-99m with a valence of +7 to react with the chelate. Occasionally, a kit will require heat, such as sulfur colloid and MAG-3, to allow for the chelation to occur. Aside from the desired Tc-99m chelate, several radiochemical impurities can occur as a result of the introduction of either air or water into the kit vial. Air, which can be inadvertently introduced at the time of kit preparation, causes the oxidation of stannous chloride (Sn^{+2} to Sn^{+4}). This inhibits the reduction of Tc-99m, thus

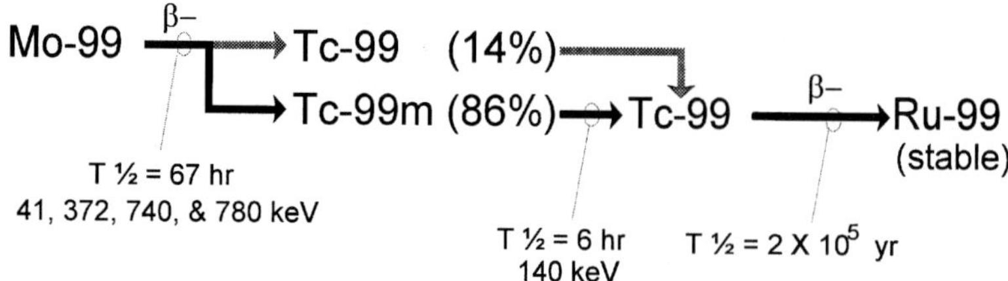

FIGURE 54.3. **Molybdenum-99 (Mo-99)/Technetium-99m (Tc-99m) Decay Scheme.** The Mo-99 decays with both high-energy photons and β particles (electrons). Fourteen percent of Mo-99 decays directly to Tc-99, while the other 86% produces metastable Tc-99m. Tc-99m gives up its 140-keV photon and reaches Tc-99. $T_{1/2}$, physical half-life; Ru-99, rubidium-99.

interfering with the complexation of the radiopharmaceutical. Water, which can be introduced prior to kit preparation, will hydrolyze stannous chloride to stannous hydroxide, a colloid. Another impurity formed after kit preparation is the production of hydrolyzed reduced Tc-99m, also known as Tc-99m dioxide.

Radiochemical purity is defined as the percentage of total radioactivity in a source that is present in the form of the desired chemical (i.e., the radiopharmaceutical). The Food and Drug Administration mandates testing of radiopharmaceuticals for radiochemical purity prior to commercial release of a new product. The procedure to test for impurities involves separating the different species based on solubility using appropriate solvents. Various solvents and media are used in the separation method, but the most common method is thin-layer chromatography, which consists of glass fiber strips impregnated with silica gel. After a drop of the radiopharmaceutical is placed on the end (origin) of a thin-layer chromatography strip, the strip is placed, origin end down, in a shallow pool of solvent until the solvent front reaches the top. Because free Tc-99m is soluble in acetone and saline, it migrates with the solvent front, leaving behind the insoluble species for that particular solvent. In saline, both Tc-99m dioxide and Tc-99m tin colloid are insoluble and remain at the origin, whereas the Tc-99m radiopharmaceutical migrates with any free Tc-99m to the top. In acetone, only the free Tc-99m migrates to the top, leaving behind all other species. By cutting the strips into an origin half and a solvent front half, each part of the total strip can be counted in a sodium iodide well counter. The total value of radiochemical impurities is calculated by subtracting from 100% the sum of the percentage of the various impurities present (free Tc-99m, Tc-99m tin colloid, and Tc-99m dioxide). No NRC limits are set for radiochemical purity, but the United States Pharmacopoeia, which sets standards for pharmacies, defines the lower limit of acceptability for purity for most radiopharmaceuticals as 90%, with a few exceptions. The manufacturer's package insert will provide specific information for each radiopharmaceutical.

Medical Events. The NRC defines certain errors in the administration of radiopharmaceuticals as medical events, formerly called misadministrations. The current NRC definition of a medical event is as follows:

- The administration of byproduct material that results in one of the following conditions unless its occurrence was as the direct result of patient intervention (e.g., I-131 therapy in which patient takes only half of the prescribed dose then refuses to take the balance).
- A dose that differs from the prescribed dose by more than 0.05 Sv (5 rem) effective dose equivalent, 0.5 Sv (50 rem) to an organ or tissue, or 0.5 Sv (50 rem) shallow dose equivalent to the skin; and one of the following conditions had also occurred.
- The total dose delivered differs from the prescribed dose by 20% or more.

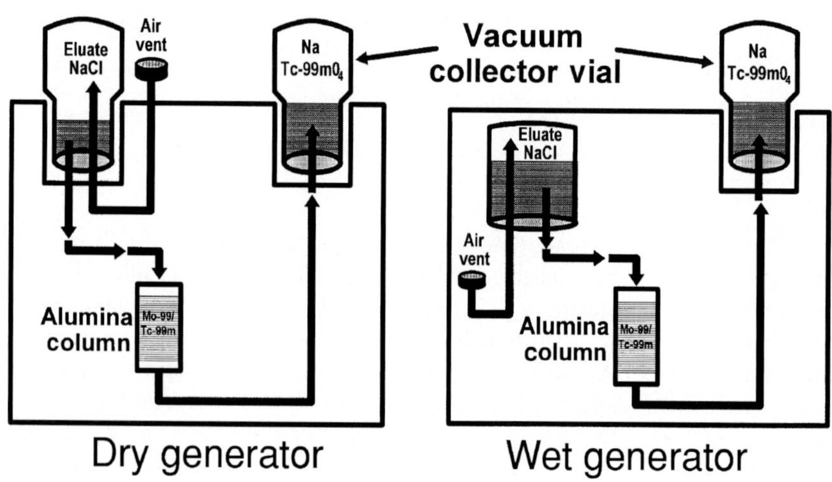

FIGURE 54.4. **Wet/Dry Generators.** Both dry and wet generators use a vacuum collection vial; the difference is in the source of the sodium chloride (NaCl) eluate. The dry generator has a replaceable vial, whereas the wet generator has a fixed one. Both types of generators use the alumina column and are therefore susceptible to aluminum and molybdenum-99 (Moly) breakthrough. The end product is also the same: sodium pertechnetate (Na Tc-99mO_4).

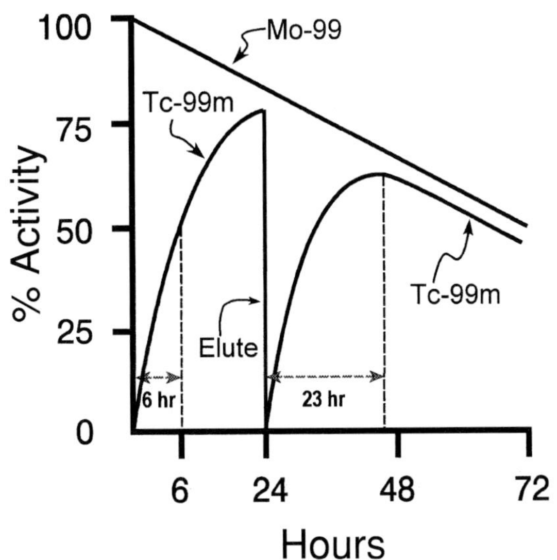

FIGURE 54.5. **Molybdenum-99/Technetium-99 (Mo-99/Tc-99m) Generator Elution Curves.** The regrowth of the daughter (Tc-99m) on the column takes a predictable course after each elution. Inspection of the curves reveals that approximately 50% of the activity will be present 6 hours after an elution and that maximum activity is achieved at 23 hours after elution. This is convenient for a daily morning-scheduled elution and allows for an unplanned elution by midday if needed.

- The total dosage delivered differs from the prescribed dosage by 20% or more or falls outside the prescribed dosage range. Falling outside the prescribed dosage range means the administration of activity that is greater or less than a predetermined range of activity for a given procedure that has been established by the licensee (e.g., 370 to 1,100 MBq [10 to 30 mCi] Tc-99m-MDP for an adult bone scan).
- The fractionated dose delivered differs from the prescribed dose, for a single fraction, by 50% or more.
- A dose that exceeds 0.05 Sv (5 rem) effective dose equivalent, 0.5 Sv (50 rem) to an organ or tissue, or 0.5 Sv (50 rem) shallow dose equivalent to the skin from any of the following:
- An administration of a wrong radioactive drug containing byproduct material;
- An administration of a radioactive drug containing byproduct material by the wrong route of administration;
- An administration of a dose or dosage to the wrong individual or human research subject;
- An administration of a dose or dosage delivered by the wrong mode of treatment; or
- A leaking sealed source.
- Any event resulting from intervention of a patient or human research subject in which the administration of byproduct material results or will result in unintended permanent functional damage to an organ or a physiological system, as determined by a physician. Patient intervention means actions by the patient, whether intentional or not, that affect the radiopharmaceutical administration.

Federal law requires that medical events be reported to the NRC no later than the next calendar day after the discovery of the event. This must be followed by a written report within 15 days that details a number of items, including the cause of the medical event, the effect (if any) on the individual involved, and proposed corrective actions. Other reporting requirements can be found in 10CFR35 (U.S. Nuclear Regulatory Commission; Title 10, Code of Federal Regulations; Part 35—Medical Use of Byproduct material). It should be noted that Agreement States may have different, and possibly more restrictive, definitions of medical events (misadministrations) and reporting requirements.

IMAGING SYSTEMS AND RADIATION DETECTORS

Image Content. Most x-ray, MR, and US images carry a predominance of anatomic information (although this is less true for Doppler US and dynamic flow MR). For nuclear medicine images, anatomic information is secondary to the functional content. Currently there is an increasing tendency to interpret nuclear medicine images in correlation with roughly contemporaneous anatomic images; this tendency reaches its apogee with combined imaging modalities such as PET-CT or SPECT-CT. In the absence of combined scanning devices, functional and anatomic images may be digitally reoriented or coregistered ("fused") with each other prior to display and interpretation; this process is becoming increasingly common in clinical practice, particularly in neuroimaging.

Nuclear medicine images reflect not only the biodistribution of the radiopharmaceutical but also the anatomic, pathologic, and artifact overlays present at the time of imaging. Thus their interpretation must be tempered with a knowledge of not only the patterns of the normal and pathologic processes, but also with a knowledge of the influence of the individual patient's physiology, habitus, and positioning, as well as the technical aspects of the exam. In nuclear medicine, technical aspects may take an overriding, and sometimes dangerously subtle, dominance in their contribution to the final image output. A mastery of the basic details of image acquisition combined with an awareness of the artifactual patterns will enable the interpreting physician to avoid erroneous conclusions caused by the myriad interplay of physiologic, anatomic, and technical factors.

Scintillation Detectors. Almost all nuclear medicine imaging devices available today are based on scintillation

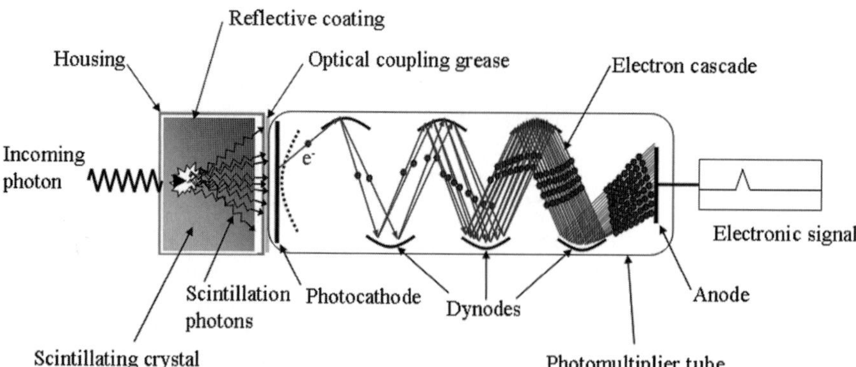

FIGURE 54.6. **Components of a Scintillation Detector.**

detector technology. Such detectors consist of a scintillating crystal that emits visible-light photons on interaction with a γ ray or annihilation photon. These visible-light photons are then converted into an electric signal by photomultipliers that are optically coupled to the scintillation crystal (Fig. 54.6). In most imaging systems a scintillation crystal is coupled to an array of photomultipliers. When an incoming photon interacts with the crystal, the resulting light distribution is most intense nearest to the interaction point and decreases with distance; by examining the ratio of signals from the photomultiplier array it is therefore possible to pinpoint the interaction point to within a few millimeters (Fig. 54.7). The earliest form of such an imaging detector was called the Anger camera after its inventor, Hal Anger; very similar devices, more commonly known as gamma cameras, are the most widely used imaging tools in nuclear medicine today.

The faces of the photomultipliers in the array cover a significant fraction of the crystal to maximize light collection. Direct readout of the photomultiplier signals would generate a distorted distribution of events, because photomultipliers do not have a perfectly linear response with respect to the distance from their center. The signals are therefore adjusted by means of a stored correction matrix. This correction matrix is dependent on the energy of the incoming photons and may also vary with time as the photomultiplier tube gains drift or as the crystal ages. An important part of imaging scintillation detector QC is to ensure that this correction matrix is kept accurate. This is particularly true for rotating gamma cameras, where a fault in one part of the detector can affect a large fraction of the final image and may produce ring artifacts. The correction matrix may consist of several components, including uniformity, energy, and linearity.

The thickness of the scintillator material is an important design consideration. Thicker crystals are more likely to stop the incoming photons, resulting in greater sensitivity. This is crucial in high-energy applications such as PET imaging. However, there is more light spreading in thicker crystals, which reduces spatial resolution. For low-energy photon imaging, then, thinner crystals are preferred.

The optimal scintillator material is also dependent on the application. Important material parameters are stopping power, scintillation light output, speed of scintillation light decay, and cost. For single-photon imaging with gamma cameras, sodium iodide (NaI), which is cheap and

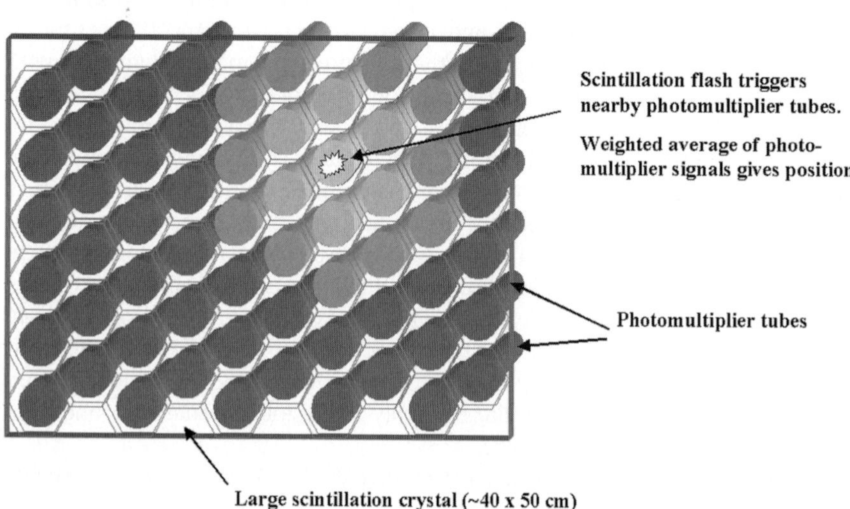

FIGURE 54.7. **Components of a Gamma Camera Detector.**

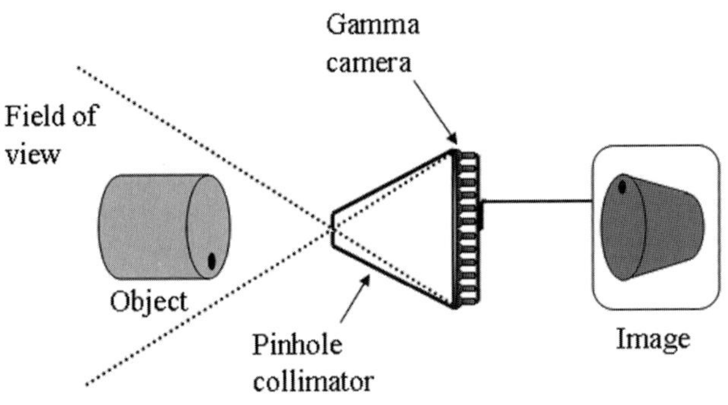

FIGURE 54.8. **Pinhole Collimation.** The image is inverted, and because the magnification increases as the distance to the pinhole decreases, it is distorted.

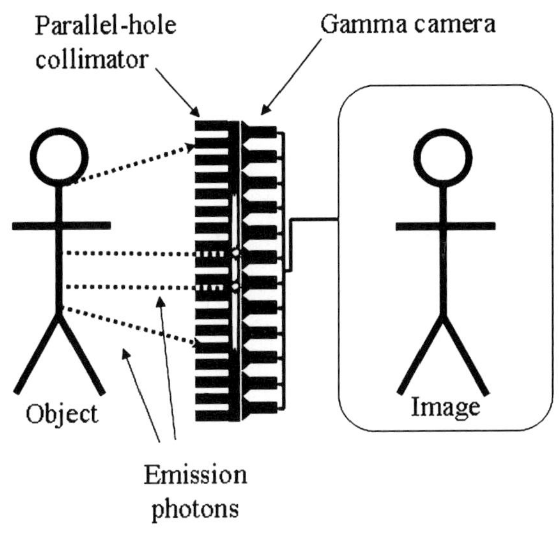

FIGURE 54.9. **Parallel-Hole Collimation.** Only photons traveling parallel to the collimator holes may hit the detector. The image is not inverted, and there is no magnification.

produces a large number of scintillation light photons for a given amount of deposited interaction energy, is the material of choice. For PET applications, the high-energy annihilation photons require materials of greater stopping power. As will be explained below, PET detectors must operate at very high data rates, so the speed of scintillation light decay is also important. Current materials of choice are bismuth germanate (BGO), lutetium oxy-ortho-silicate (LSO), and gadolinium silicate (GSO). BGO has the greatest stopping power, but LSO and GSO produce scintillation light more quickly and can operate at greater data rates.

Collimation. Determination of the interaction point alone is insufficient to generate an image. It is also necessary to determine (or constrain) the direction from which the incoming photon impinges upon the detector. In an optical imaging device, such as a photographic camera, this is achieved with a lens. In nuclear medicine, where the photon wavelengths are too short for lens-based refraction to be effective, this is achieved either with an absorbing collimator in the case of single-photon imaging or with coincidence circuitry (also known as "electronic collimation") in the case of PET imaging.

Pinhole Collimators. The simplest form of absorbing collimator is the pinhole collimator, made of a hollow cone of lead or tungsten with a small hole at the apex (Fig. 54.8). This results in a low-sensitivity device, because the object subtends only a very small solid angle at the detector face. Sensitivity can be increased by enlarging the collimator hole, but this reduces the spatial resolution of the image. A pinhole collimator has the property that objects that are closer to the pinhole than the detector are magnified in the image. The degree of magnification is given simply by the ratio of the distances from the pinhole to the object and from the pinhole to the detector. This magnification property renders it particularly useful for imaging small structures such as the thyroid or focal areas of the skeleton. In sequential studies, care must be taken to ensure that the pinhole-organ distance is constant, or variations in the degree of magnification will render size comparisons impossible.

Parallel-hole collimators consist of a lattice of lead or tungsten that is constructed to form an array of closely-spaced small parallel holes (Fig. 54.9). Placing such a device in front of a scintillation camera prevents photons that are not parallel to the holes from impinging on the crystal. As a result, there is a one-to-one correspondence between the number of photons hitting a given area of the crystal and the number of photons being emitted from a given part of the patient, and this is how the image is formed. There is no magnification or minification in an image generated with a parallel-hole collimator. However, the spatial resolution of the image falls off as the distance from the object to the collimator face increases; it is therefore desirable to place the patient as close as possible to the collimator face.

The absorbing lattice forms what are known as the collimator "septa," and the geometry of the septa has important effects on the image. The primary parameters are septal length, septal thickness, and hole diameter. Longer septa and narrower holes result in increased resolution at the expense of sensitivity. Longer and thicker septa result in reduced septal penetration by incoming photons, which is important for high-energy photon imaging, but also result in reduced sensitivity. There is thus a design trade-off between septal parameters that depends on the application. For Ga-67 imaging (maximum photon energy 300 keV), high-energy collimators should be utilized. These have long, thick septa to reduce penetration. For most other single-photon applications, low-energy high-resolution (LEHR) collimators are used. In some circumstances greater sensitivity is desired, and low-energy general-purpose (LEGP) collimators might be chosen. Inappropriate use of LEHR collimators with

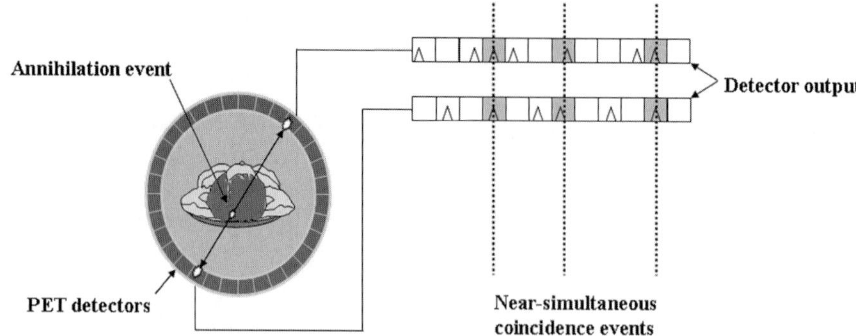

FIGURE 54.10. **The Principle of Coincidence Detection.** When pulses from separate detector elements occur together in a short space of time, it is assumed that the photons that gave rise to those pulses arose from a single annihilation event.

high-energy photon emitters results in substantial degradation of the image and must be guarded against.

Converging and Diverging Collimators. A converging collimator can be used rather than a pinhole collimator to obtain a magnified image with greater sensitivity. Reversing the orientation of such a device results in a diverging collimator. This minifies the image but results in a larger field of view, allowing more of the body to be imaged without moving the patient.

Electronic Collimation or Coincidence Detection. Imaging of the 511-keV annihilation radiation resulting from positron emission can be performed using collimators designed for ultrahigh-energy use. Such collimators can be purchased commercially, but in practice there is no septal design that can achieve an appropriate trade-off between septal penetration, sensitivity, and resolution at such high energies, and image quality is generally poor. However, it is possible to take advantage of the fact that each annihilation event results in two annihilation photons travelling in almost exactly opposite directions to obtain directional information on the photon flight (Fig. 54.10). It takes approximately 3 ns for a photon to travel about 1 m, which is approximately the field of view of a medical tomograph. If two opposing detectors are set up to measure the time of arrival of the photons as well as their position, it is possible to examine the data for pairs of detection events that occur within such a short time window—that is, for pairs of events that are "coincident." These can then be considered to have arisen from the same annihilation event, which, in turn, must have occurred along the line joining the locations of the two detection events. In practice, current PET systems consider events to be coincident if they occur within 6 to 12 ns of each other. In this way, the flight direction of the photons can be constrained without the use of an absorbing collimator, and images can be generated from the resulting data. This process is known as electronic collimation, or more commonly as coincidence detection.

False or "random" coincidences can be detected if two photons from unrelated annihilations happen to interact with the detectors within the coincidence time window. Random coincidences can be corrected for but always result in increased noise in the image. The rate of random coincidences increases roughly in proportion to the square of the activity in the field of view, and this places an upper limit on the activity concentration within the patient at the time of imaging.

Removal of the absorbing collimators results in a significant increase in sensitivity but also has an impact on detector design. The absence of the shielding effect of the collimators means that coincidence detectors must be able to operate at very high data rates without suffering from significant data loss or event malpositioning. Such negative consequences arise when light pulses from photons interacting with the detector in a short space of time mix and "pile up" on each other. Most PET scanners achieve high rate capability by detector segmentation—that is, the scanner consists of an array of small detectors (typically 100 to 300), rather than a small number of large detectors (typically two or three in a collimated design). Thus if one small detector is busy processing a signal, the others are free to continue obtaining data. Unfortunately, this design option increases the complexity and cost of the resulting scanner. A diagram of a typical PET "block" detector is shown in Fig. 54.11.

Energy Analysis. Although each radionuclide has one or more imaging photon energies (Table 54.1), Compton interactions between the original photon and the patient and camera produce a wide range of energies that may be detected (Fig. 54.12). These various energies can be

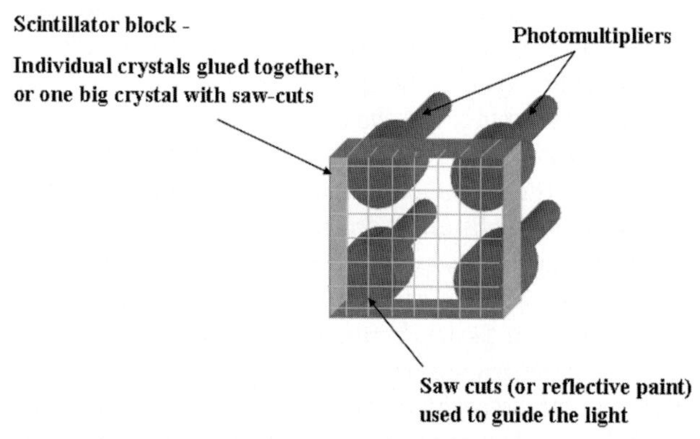

FIGURE 54.11. **A Block Detector for PET Imaging.**

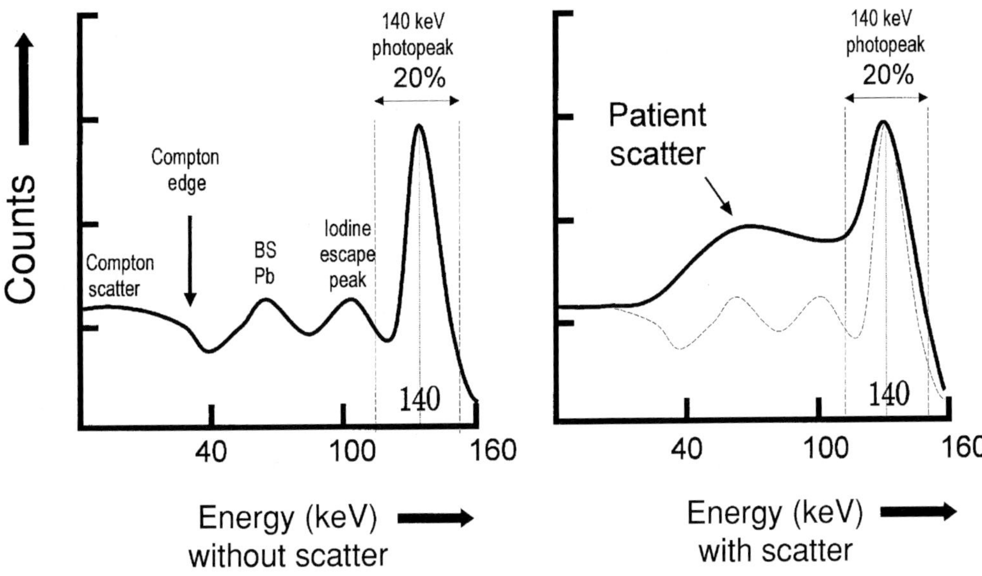

FIGURE 54.12. **Technetium-99m Photospectra.** The left photospectrum describes the energies present from the radionuclide imaged by itself (without scatter), while the right photospectrum is from the radionuclide imaged from inside a patient (with scatter). The primary energies of the curve include: (*a*) **Compton scatter** (0 to 50 keV); (*b*) **Compton edge** at 50 keV: note that in the patient, scatter contributes to a broad increase in the 90- to 140-keV level; (*c*) **Backscatter** (BS): primary gamma undergoes 180° scatter from behind the crystal and upon reentering the crystal they are completely absorbed; (*d*) **Lead x-ray peak** (Pb): photoelectric absorption in lead shielding of camera housing causes 75- to 90-keV x-ray photons; (*e*) **Iodine escape peak** (112 keV): Iodine K-shell electrons escape the sodium iodide crystal with an energy of 28 keV; therefore an incoming gamma of, say, 140 keV would lose this much energy before it was registered by the photomultiplier tubes (140 – 28 = 112 keV); (*f*) **Photopeak**: for imaging purposes, a 20% window over the 140-keV photopeak defines the limits of acceptance of detected energies. Note that some of the scatter photons from the patient are accepted, contributing to decreased image quality (loss of resolution).

displayed by most gamma cameras using a multichannel analyzer function, which plots frequency of event against photon energy. The desired photon energy range is that which contains those events where the incident photons deposit all their energy and is known as the *full-energy peak* or *photopeak*. The energies outside the photopeak arise from Compton scattering events, either within the patient or within the detector itself. A line back-projected along the path of a photon that has scattered within the patient will not intersect the original emission point. Such events are undesirable because they do not reflect the source distribution in the patient and result in reduced contrast and, in some circumstances, artifacts in the final image.

On a gamma camera, the multichannel analyzer function can be used to select the desired photon energy by placing a "window" of acceptance of plus and minus 10% around the photopeak, thereby limiting the contribution of scatter to the image. Multiple windows can be simultaneously acquired in this manner, as would be needed, for example, by Ga-67 (93, 184, and 300 keV) and indium-111 (172 and 245 keV). PET scanners, which, because of design trade-offs, tend to have poorer energy resolution than gamma cameras, also have the ability to set energy windows, but these are wider—usually ±20% to 30% of the 511-keV photopeak. Depending on patient size and detector configuration, scatter can be a very significant problem in PET.

Planar and Tomographic Imaging. A gamma camera with parallel-hole collimators collects data as sets of projections through the patient. That is, the number of events accumulated in the camera's computer corresponding to the detector position lying behind a particular hole in the collimator consists of the sum of all detected photons arising from activity along the line of sight from the detector, along the collimator hole and through the patient. Such a set of projections forms an image directly; this is known as planar imaging and is commonly used in the clinic. It is analogous to plain-film x-ray imaging, with the primary difference that the detected radiation is emitted from inside the patient rather than transmitted through the patient from an external source.

A disadvantage of planar imaging is that features that overlay each other along the line of sight are difficult to distinguish. This problem may be reduced by taking planar images from more than one view angle, allowing the reader to make some attempt to gauge depth effects. If a sufficient number of views is acquired, then it is mathematically possible to recover the entire three-dimensional structure of the original object, which may then be viewed as, for example, a series of adjacent and parallel slices through the body. This image reconstruction process is known as *computed tomography* (CT) and has become eponymous with the term *x-ray computed tomography*. In nuclear medicine there are two forms: *single-photon emission computed tomography* (SPECT), which may be undertaken with a rotating gamma camera, and *positron emission tomography* (PET), usually undertaken with a dedicated PET scanner or combined PET-CT scanner.

With a few exceptions, PET scanners consist of a complete ring of detectors and can therefore simultaneously acquire all the projections necessary for reconstruction. With the exception of one or two specialized devices, gamma cameras consist of one, two, or three flat detectors, and, since they are collimated, they must be rotated to acquire the necessary projection sets for SPECT imaging. Because the detectors must rotate around the patient, the average distance between the patient and the collimator is greater than that achievable in planar imaging; this results in a resolution penalty, but this is offset by the much-improved depth information gained. Some cameras are capable of noncircular orbits to reduce the average distance to the patient and thus improve resolution.

A typical SPECT study might consist of 60 stops or projection angles, with each stop consisting of 5 seconds of acquisition time. Increasing the acquisition time results in a larger number of counts, but it also increases the likelihood of patient discomfort and motion. This trade-off between total signal intensity and patient motion must also be made in PET imaging. SPECT data are usually reconstructed into a 64 × 64 image matrix; if the data are very rich in counts, this may be increased to 128 × 128. PET data is acquired with between roughly 100 and 250 projection angles (depending on the system design), and is usually reconstructed on a 128 × 128 image matrix. Pixel sizes for PET images would typically be approximately 5 mm on a side for body imaging and 2 mm on a side for brain imaging.

Image Reconstruction. There are many ways to reconstruct an image volume from a set of projections. Filtered back-projection is an analytic approach that will generate an exact replica of the object in the limit of an infinite number of projection angles and noise-free data and was the main reconstruction algorithm used in nuclear medicine until the end of the 20th century. The major disadvantage of filtered back-projection is that it gives equal weight to all projections in the raw data, even those with very few counts that are therefore statistically untrustworthy. This results in streak artifacts in the image. In recent years, iterative reconstruction methods that apply weighting factors to the data based on statistical considerations have gained favor. These can be very computationally expensive, but accelerated methods that approximate the full algorithms have been introduced. Currently the most popular of these is the ordered subsets-expectation-maximization (OSEM) method developed by Hudson and Larkin. These iterative methods are more robust to noisy data, but when the number of acquired counts is low, they will tend to produce mottled or "blobby" images, which can render image interpretation difficult.

Image properties are dependent not just on the quality of the acquired data but also on the choice of reconstruction parameters. The relationship is complex, but loosely speaking, more iterations and/or subsets will result in images that are higher in resolution but noisier. With too few iterations and/or subsets, poor resolution will interfere with the detection of small features and lesions. All images, regardless of reconstruction method, can be filtered to reduce noise. Many different filters are available, and filter optimization is an extremely complex (and task-dependent) problem, so the choice will often be guided by the manufacturer. Again, filtration always reduces noise at the expense of spatial resolution.

Attenuation Correction. The thickness of material required to reduce the intensity of a narrow beam of radiation by 50% is known as the half-value layer. The half-value layer for 511-keV photons traversing water or human tissue is approximately 7 cm. For lower-energy photons it is thinner. Clearly, then, a very significant fraction of the photons emitted from the center of a patient will not emerge from the patient without undergoing some kind of interaction and losing their directional information. This effect is known as *attenuation*. The degree of attenuation is dependent on depth; it is a smaller effect at the surface of the patient than at the center. In planar imaging, attenuation can sometimes be helpful, as it reduces the amount of interference from organs that overlie each other along the line of sight. In tomographic imaging, however, it always introduces significant image distortions. In particular, deep structures are poorly visualized, whereas superficial structures are overintense. The lungs, which are less dense and therefore less attenuating than soft tissue, can also be represented with falsely high intensity. This may sometimes help with lesion detection in the lung, but in general, attenuation effects render images more difficult to interpret and interfere with lesion detection. In cardiac imaging in particular, attenuation artifacts can mimic myocardial defects.

Many different attenuation correction schemes have been implemented in clinical systems. Of these, the most effective are based on transmission scanning, which directly measures the amount of attenuation along a particular line of response. Accurate attenuation correction is mathematically complex for single-photon imaging, because the amount of attenuation along a particular line of response varies with depth. This is not so in PET, because the requirement that both annihilation photons be detected means that the degree of attenuation for a given line of response is dependent on only the total amount of attenuating material along it.

Conventionally, transmission measurements have been made with radioactive sources that emit photons of similar energy to those arising from within the patient. However, the recent trend toward combined PET-CT and SPECT-CT devices has encouraged the development of schemes that process the CT data to generate attenuation correction matrices. Because CT transmission scans are usually much faster than radionuclide transmission scans, this has the very important benefit of substantially reducing the scanning time per patient. However, there are some difficulties with the technique. In particular, CT tends to acquire a snapshot of lung motion, whereas emission imaging, because it takes minutes rather than seconds, represents a time-average of tidal lung motion. The resulting mismatch between the emission and transmission data very frequently leads to image artifacts and misregistrations at the lung/liver boundary. Also, the use of CT contrast can lead to erroneous estimates of attenuation factors and can sometimes result in artifacts in the emission image that may mimic lesions. This is particularly true for PET, where the disparity between the emission photon energy (511 keV) and the transmission photon energy (70 to 140 keV for CT) is very large. Care must also be taken with dental and orthopedic prostheses and surgical clips, which can all contribute to erroneous focal artifacts in the emission data. In these circumstances, dual reading of attenuation-corrected and non–attenuation-corrected images can be helpful.

Where attenuation correction is applied, data should also be corrected for scattered photons that fall within the accepted energy window. Failure to account for scatter prior to attenuation correction can lead to focal artifacts in dense regions and will interfere with quantitative measurements. Scatter correction can also be helpful in planar imaging.

Imaging Moving Organs. Radionuclide imaging takes place over several minutes, which creates a challenge when trying to image organs that move on a time scale of seconds or less. Thus, both cardiac and respiratory motion result in blurring of the image. Whereas respiratory motion itself is not of particular clinical interest, cardiac motion is, and this has led to schemes for imaging it. Such schemes involve a process known as "gating," in which electrocardiographic signals are used as triggers to the acquisition system. This allows the computer to sort the incoming data into several "bins," with each one corresponding to a particular part of the cardiac cycle. Over many cycles, enough data are collected to allow each bin to be reconstructed separately, and a movie of the cardiac motion can be constructed.

Similar methods may be applied to respiratory motion, although this is more problematic because respiratory motion is not as regular as cardiac motion. Respiratory gating may be employed to reduce motion blurring (which can be very significant at the lung base) and thus to enhance detection of small lesions.

Quality Control for Imaging Systems. The QC program of a nuclear medicine department must cover instrumentation (Table 54.5) as well as radiopharmaceutical preparation. The goal of the QC of a gamma camera is to assure both the uniform response of the detectors and the correct location of the scintillation events occurring in the crystal; for a PET scanner, the goal also includes ensuring good calibration for quantitative accuracy.

In addition to the specific procedures described below, total imaging performance may be assessed using commercially available phantoms. These phantoms are filled by the operator with an appropriate radionuclide in aqueous solution and are designed so that areas of cold and hot activity are present in varying dimensions. A subsequent acquisition, reconstruction, and display of the phantom can test the imaging system's contrast, resolution, field uniformity, and attenuation correction.

Gamma Camera Quality Control

Intrinsic Flood. The quickest and easiest check of a gamma camera is by the daily acquisition of an intrinsic (no collimator) flood field image. An intrinsic flood field image is obtained by exposing the entire crystal to either a uniform source of radioactivity, typically from a point source, Tc-99m, or a commercially prepared sheet source, cobalt-57 (Co-57). Regardless of the source used, it must deliver count rates with less than 1% variation across the surface of the crystal. This is accomplished by positioning the point source at least four collimator crystal widths from the detector; the sheet source, which is placed on the detector face during the acquisition of the flood, is purchased with the manufacturer's guarantee that there is less than 1% inherent variation. A visual inspection of the flood will give an adequate qualitative assessment of nonuniformities. The human eye can detect significant nonuniformities of 5% or more. Results from quantitative analysis, performed by flood field–specific software, along with the flood image itself, can be logged into a computer-based database for detection of subtle changes over time. If the pattern is abnormal, remedies include reloading correction matrices, replacing photomultiplier tubes, and addressing other electronic or mechanical problems (Fig. 54.13).

In a similar vein, a quantitative value of general camera performance can be obtained by comparing the uniformity flood field image acquired with and without the uniformity correction. This difference value, termed "data loss," represents additional processing time imposed by the correction circuits to reach a set number of counts. Using a 1- to 2-million count flood, the data loss can be calculated as the

TABLE 54.5 Planar and SPECT Camera Recommended Quality Control Procedures

Procedure	*Frequency*	*Camera System*	*Comment*
Flood field	Daily	Planar	Intrinsically or extrinsically; intrinsic flood is acquired for 1 to 2 million counts with and without uniformity correction; percent difference should be less than 15% for most systems
Sensitivity	Weekly	Planar	Intrinsically or extrinsically; result is in counts per minute per microcurie
Spatial resolution	Weekly	Planar	Intrinsic or extrinsic; use bar phantom
Linearity	Weekly	Planar	Bar phantom or multi-holed phantom
High-count collimator flood	Weekly	SPECT	30 million counts for 64 × 64 matrix; 90 million counts for 128 × 128 matrix
Center of rotation (COR)	Weekly	SPECT	Corrected to less than 0.5 pixel for 64 × 64 matrix, less than 1.0 pixel for 128 × 128 matrix
Pixel calibration	Monthly	SPECT	Measurement of pixel size in both x and y directions; used for attenuation correction
Jaszczak or Carlson phantom	Quarterly	SPECT	Commercially available phantoms that test total system performance

percentage difference between the time required to obtain an intrinsic flood with and without the uniformity correction turned on. Typically, differences under 15% are normal for most recent gamma camera systems. Greater differences significantly prolong imaging times and require either a reacquisition of the uniformity or other correction matrix or implicate a hardware electronic problem requiring a service call.

Resolution and Linearity. Two basic QC procedures performed to assure correct positioning of events are spatial resolution and linearity (Fig. 54.14). These are generally performed weekly by acquiring a flood with a

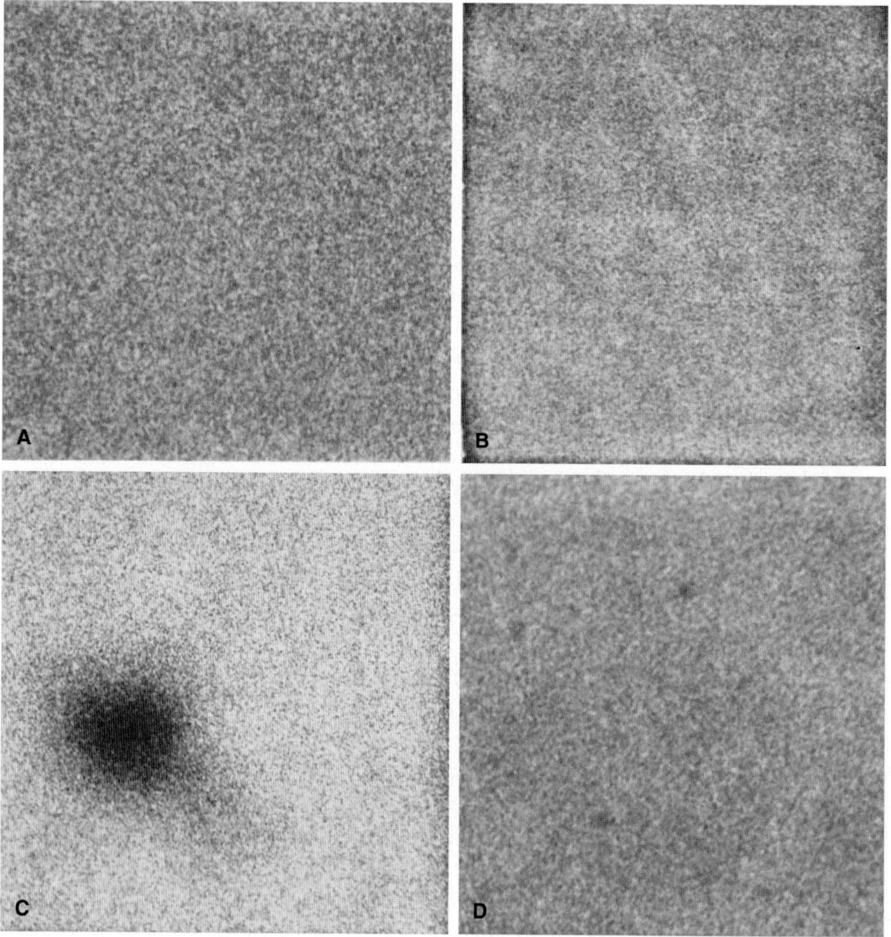

FIGURE 54.13. **Intrinsic Floods. A.** Normal uniform flood, with correction matrices applied. **B.** Same camera as in **A.**, but with the correction matrices turned off. The correction matrices are able to compensate sometimes for striking nonuniformities in the flood field. These corrections are acceptable as long as they do not represent too great a data loss and prolong imaging times. **C.** Uncorrectable off-peak photomultiplier (PM) tube. The photopeak for this PM tube had drifted down and was accepting more counts than its neighboring PM tubes. **D.** Uncorrectable crystal hydration ("measles"). The dark spots are areas in the crystal where water has breached the manufacturer's watertight seal to gain access to a hygroscopic sodium iodide crystal. The expensive crystal had to be replaced.

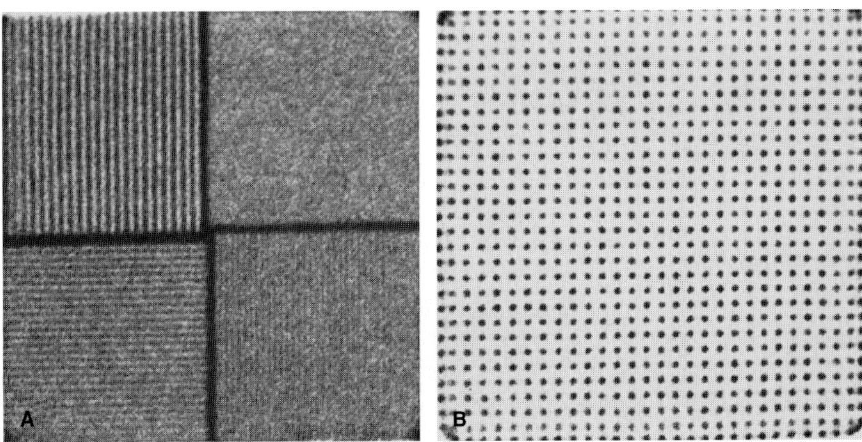

FIGURE 54.14. **Spatial Resolution and Linearity of a Gamma Camera.** Both of these floods were acquired without the collimator using a cobalt-57 sheet source over the phantom. **A.** Four-quadrant bar phantom. The distance between bars is equal within a quadrant but progressively diminishes between quadrants. This bar flood demonstrates lack of visibility of the bars in the quadrant with the narrowest bars. Rotating the bars 90° will allow the entire crystal to be checked. Linearity can also be assessed with this phantom. **B.** Orthogonal holed phantom. Pincushion (inward) and barrel (outward) distortion can easily be evaluated by visual inspection of this flood. Both are absent here.

specially designed phantom sandwiched between a Co-57 sheet source and the camera, with or without the collimator. Alternatively, a Tc-99m point source at a distance of four collimators can be substituted for the sheet source. Several commercial bar phantoms, such as PLES (parallel lines equally spaced) and four quadrant, are available to assess spatial resolution using a series of equally spaced lead bars. Linearity can also be assessed by visual inspection of any of these straight bar phantoms, or it can be individually assessed by a dedicated phantom such as an orthogonal (perpendicular to crystal) holed phantom. Generally, inspection of these types of floods will reveal any linearity distortion such as pincushion or barreling.

Collimator Quality Control. The QC for collimators is directed at assessing the integrity of the collimator. Imperfections from damaged septa in the collimator will introduce nonuniformities, causing image degradation. The effect of these collimator imperfections can be minimized by mathematically applying a statistically high-count extrinsic collimator flood to each individual raw planar image prior to reconstruction. This extrinsic collimator flood is computer acquired using a Co-57 sheet source for 30 million counts when using a 64 × 64 matrix and for 90 million when using a 128 × 128 matrix.

Center of Rotation. In addition to the routine planar camera quality control, several SPECT-specific QC procedures are necessary to minimize artifact formations (Table 54.5). The most important of these relates to the camera's mechanical center of rotation (COR), which must be calibrated with the center of the computer's matrix as it is projected from the face of the crystal (Fig. 54.15). For various mechanical and electronic reasons, these are not perfectly aligned. An offset greater than half a pixel for a 64 × 64 matrix will result in loss of contrast, loss of resolution, and distortion in the tomographic images. The COR calibration is performed by imaging a point or line source at multiple opposing intervals over 360°. The COR is then calculated by averaging the difference in the sets of offset of the source from the matrix center as seen by the opposing pairs of images. The COR value is stored by the computer for use during the ensuing reconstruction of the three-dimensional images. When this calibration factor is applied during reconstruction, the matrix centers are shifted to align with the mechanical rotational center. This COR calibration must be performed for each collimator, zoom factor, and matrix size used for SPECT acquisitions.

Pixel size calibration prior to attenuation correction is a necessary QC procedure to match the matrix size with the physical dimensions of the body part being imaged. Pixel calibration is easily performed by acquiring two point or line sources separated by a known distance; the computer calculates and stores the pixels-per-millimeter calibration factor for subsequent attenuation corrections.

Positron Emission Tomography Scanner Quality Control

Most PET scanners consist of a full ring of detectors, obviating the need for rotation. This changes the way that detector nonuniformities manifest in the images; in particular, a problem with a single detector is unlikely to reinforce and create ring artifacts. Additionally, since there are many detectors in a system, the impact of a single detector

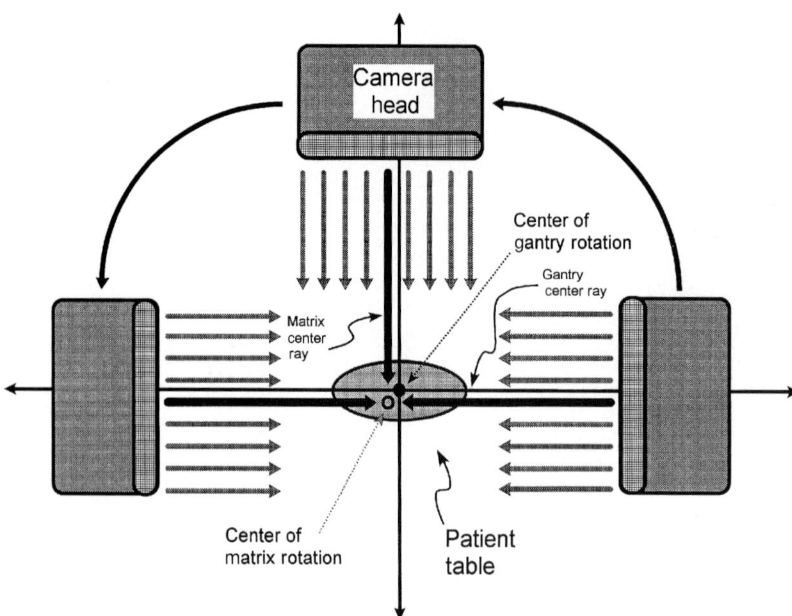

FIGURE 54.15. **Center of Rotation (COR).** This illustration is diagrammatically exaggerated for clarity. The COR represents the difference between the mechanical center of rotation (*black dashed arrow/black dot*) and the center of the projected image matrix (*gray dashed arrow/black circle*). This difference must be adjusted to less than half a pixel for a 64 × 64 matrix and 1 pixel for a 128 × 128 matrix, to avoid SPECT reconstruction defects.

failure may not be so great that imaging must cease until repair. However, since there are so many detectors in a system, the chance of a component failure becomes statistically greater. There are also downstream components that can impact large numbers of detectors at once if they fail, producing an immediate impact on image quality. The segmented nature of most PET detectors removes the need for pixel-size calibration, but for combined PET-CT systems, it is necessary to check the alignment of the PET and CT components.

Daily Check. Every day the detectors are illuminated by a rotating source of high-energy photons (usually a positron emitter), and the results are compared with a high-quality reference scan. The comparison is usually automated and examines the data, both for overall drift and for specific variations for detector performance, such as a failed, or failing, detector.

Timing Alignment and Photomultiplier Gain Adjustment. In a PET scanner, timing signals from the detectors must be well synchronized or coincidence sensitivity will be compromised. Also, just as in a gamma camera, the photomultipliers have a tendency to drift, and gains must be adjusted to keep the responses in range. The frequency with which these adjustments are carried out is dependent on the hardware; some manufacturers recommend weekly updates, while others design the system so that these procedures are carried out at normalization time (see following).

Normalization and Calibration. The sensitivity of detectors in a PET system is quite variable, and in addition, geometric considerations mean that there are systematic variations in sensitivity across the field of view. To account for these, a high count-density acquisition using a rotating radioactive source is performed, and a sensitivity correction matrix is computed from it. This process is known as detector normalization. It is usually supplemented with a scan of a cylindric source containing a known amount of activity. The source concentration is determined using the dose calibrator that is used for measuring patient doses; this way, the scanner can be calibrated appropriately for quantitatively accurate imaging. Care must be taken to ensure that the cylindric source is placed centrally in the field of view, with no additional attenuating material obscuring the detectors. Depending on the implementation of the software, placement of the source off center or with additional attenuating media can negatively impact the normalization.

Normalization should be performed not less frequently than once per quarter; once per month is common. After normalization, the baseline reference scan is set, against which the daily check will be performed.

Phantoms and Acceptance Testing. Total imaging performance may be assessed using commercially available phantoms. Examples of these include the Derenzo phantom, the Jaszczak phantom, the Rollo phantom, the Hoffman brain phantom, and the International Electrotechnical Commission (IEC) chest phantom. These phantoms are filled by the operator with an appropriate radionuclide in aqueous solution and are designed so that areas of cold and hot activity are present in varying dimensions. A subsequent acquisition, reconstruction, and display of the phantom can test the imaging system's contrast, resolution, field uniformity, and attenuation correction. The National Equipment Manufacturer's Association (NEMA) has issued standard performance tests for nuclear medicine imaging equipment, and these are frequently used as part

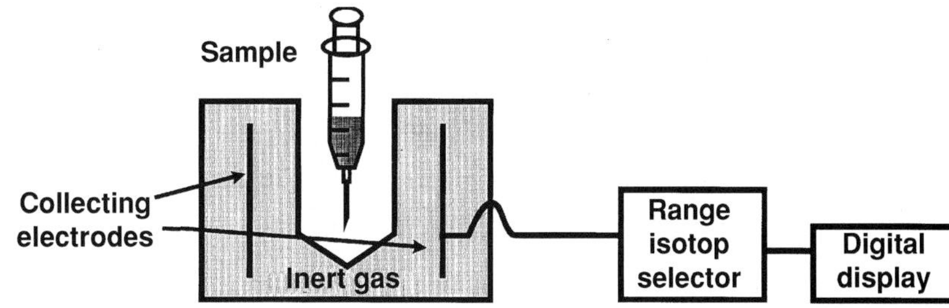

FIGURE 54.16. **Dose Calibrator.**

of acceptance testing of new scanners. See the reading list for full details.

Nonimaging Detector Systems

Dose Calibrator. All diagnostic and therapeutic doses are required by the NRC to be calibrated prior to administration. (See "Medical Events" for prescription limits.) The dose calibrator is an ionization chamber, not a sodium iodide crystal. It is a cylinder that holds a defined volume of inert gas and a cylindric collecting electrode (Fig. 54.16). A voltage applied across the electrodes will not pass current until the gas is ionized by radiation emitted from a radiopharmaceutical in the well. The measurement of the current is proportional to the activity for a given radionuclide. By calibrating to known radionuclides and known amounts of activity, the current can be equated to dose activity. A series of buttons imprinted with the radionuclide names resides on the face of the control unit. A calibration factor is assigned to each button, unique for that particular radionuclide, to adjust the correct proportionality between current and activity. The dose calibrator will read activity with any button selected, but it is only accurate for the isotope for which the button has been calibrated. As opposed to the well counter, which measures only in the microcurie range, the dose calibrator is capable of measuring quantities in the curie, millicurie, and microcurie ranges. The well counter, therefore, cannot act as a substitute for a dose calibration.

QC for the dose calibrator consists of periodic checks on its performance. Checks of constancy, performed daily, measure the activity of long-lived reference sources to look for deviations from expected values. Using isotopes with long physical half-lives, such as Co-57 (120 keV) in the Tc-99m channel and Cs-137 (662 keV) in the Mo-99 channel, the measured activity must agree with calculated activity $\pm 5\%$. Checks of linearity, performed quarterly, assess the accuracy of measurements over a wide range of activity, usually from 10 mCi to the maximum administered dose, which in most labs is around 200 mCi. With a high-activity Tc-99m source, a series of measurements is collected either over a 48-hour period of time or by using commercially available simulated decay (leaded) cylinders. These measurements, compared with calculated (using decay factors) measurements, should agree within $\pm 10\%$. A check of accuracy, performed annually, measures certified sources of different photon energies, typically Co-57 and cesium-137, obtained from the National Institute of Standards and Technology (formerly the National Bureau of Standards). The measurements must agree with the known source activity within $\pm 10\%$. At installation and after repairs, geometry is evaluated to compensate for measurements made of sources in different volume dilutions or in different containers. Glass and plastic syringes can affect readings significantly. The operator applies these calculated correction factors to activity measurements (e.g., 2% is added for volumes greater than 20 mL).

Sodium Iodide Well Counter. The sodium iodide well counter is used to quantify small amounts of activity in examinations such as an in vitro Schilling test or survey wipe tests. Constructed of a sodium iodide cylinder with a hole drilled in it, sitting on a single photomultiplier tube, and surrounded by lead on all sides, the design provides for good geometric and detection efficiency (Fig. 54.17).

The QC for the sodium iodide well counter consists of daily assessment of the high voltage and sensitivity. Additionally, resolution, chi-square, and linearity are checked quarterly.

Thyroid Uptake Probe. The thyroid uptake probe is used to quantitate the percentage of radioactive iodine taken up by the thyroid and to survey workers (called bioassay) for possible radioiodine contamination, most notably after therapeutic administrations of radioiodine

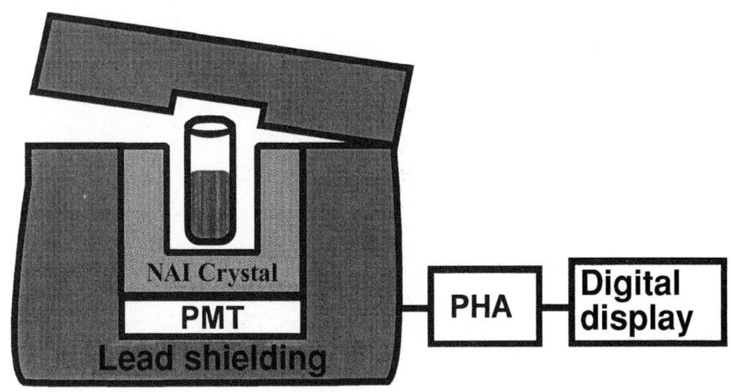

FIGURE 54.17. **Sodium Iodide Well Counter.** PMT, photomultiplier tube.

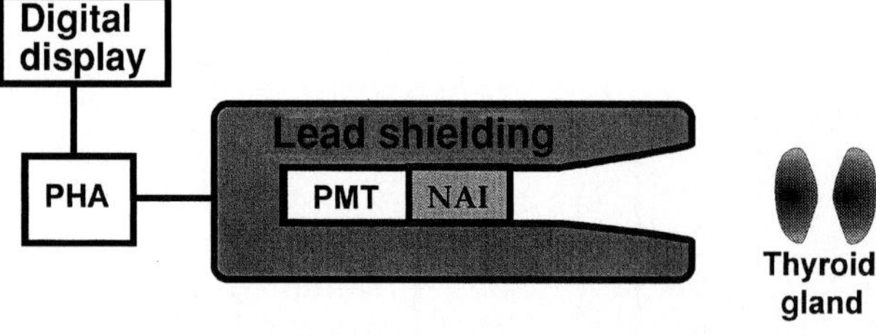

FIGURE 54.18. **Thyroid Uptake Probe.** PMT, photomultiplier tube.

that may have resulted in some of the radioiodine entering the body (called internal contamination). Constructed of a single 2- or 3-inch-thick sodium iodide crystal, 5 cm in diameter, juxtaposed to a single photomultiplier, the field of view is defined by a cone-shaped, flat-field collimator (Fig. 54.18). No imaging is performed with this probe, only quantitative count measurements performed at a fixed crystal-to-patient distance. QC for the thyroid uptake probe is identical to that of the sodium iodide well counter.

SUGGESTED READINGS

Alazraki NP, Mishkin FS. Fundamentals of Nuclear Medicine. 2nd ed. New York: The Society of Nuclear Medicine, 1988:3–20.

Brown ML, David Collier B, eds. Syllabus: A Categorical Course in Nuclear Medicine. Oak Brook: SNA Publications, 1996.

Bushberg JT, Seibert JA, Leidholdt EM, Boone JM. The Essential Physics of Medical Imaging. 2nd ed. Philadelphia: Lippincott Williams & Wilkins, 2002.

Cherry SR, Sorensen JA, Phelps ME. Physics in Nuclear Medicine. 3rd ed. Philadelphia: WB Saunders Co, 2003.

English RJ, Brown SE. SPECT Single-Photon Emission Computed Tomography: A Primer. 2nd ed. New York: The Society of Nuclear Medicine, 1990.

Graham LS. Quality assurance for SPECT. In: Freeman LM, Weissmann HS, eds. Nuclear Medicine Annual 1989. New York: Raven Press, 1989:81–108.

IAEA-TECDOC-602. Quality Control of Nuclear Medicine Instruments, May 1991. Vienna: Nuclear Medicine Section, Division of Life Sciences, International Atomic Energy Agency, 1991.

Kowalsky RJ, Perry JR. Radiopharmaceuticals in Nuclear Medicine Practice. Norwalk, CT: Appleton & Lange, 1987.

Mettler FA, Guiberteau MJ. Essentials of Nuclear Medicine Imaging. 3rd ed. Philadelphia: WB Saunders Co, 1991.

NEMA Standards Publication No. NU-1 1994. Performance Measurements of Scintillation Cameras. Washington, DC: National Electrical Manufacturers Association, 1994.

NEMA Standards Publication NU-2 1994. Performance Measurements for Positron Emission Tomographs. Washington, DC: National Electrical Manufacturers Association, 1994.

NEMA Standards Publication NU-2 2001. Performance Measurements for Positron Emission Tomographs. Washington, DC: National Electrical Manufacturers Association, 2001.

Romney BM, Nickloff EL, Esser PD, et al. Radionuclide administration to nursing mothers: mathematically derived guidelines. Radiology 1986;160:549–554.

Simmons GH, ed. The Scintillation Camera. New York: The Society of Nuclear Medicine, 1988.

U. S. National Academy of Sciences. Report by the Committee on the Biological Effects of Ionizing Radiations ("BEIR-V"). Washington, DC: National Academy of Sciences/National Research Council, 1989.

Valk PE, Bailey DL, Townsend DW, Maisey MN, eds. Positron Emission Tomography: Basic Science and Clinical Practice. London: Springer-Verlag, 2003.

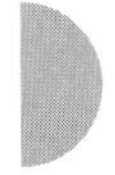

Chapter 55

Skeletal System Scintigraphy

David K. Shelton and Michael F. Hartshorne

Interpretation

Bone Mineral Densitometry

Musculoskeletal imaging studies performed with gamma cameras and technetium-99m (Tc-99m)–labeled diphosphonates are a staple of nuclear medicine. The bone scan is a map of osteoblastic activity that occurs in response to a variety of benign and malignant conditions. It is an excellent complement to anatomic studies of the skeletal system but is usually far more sensitive in detecting bony abnormalities, such as osteomyelitis or bony metastatic disease. After injection, blood flow is required to deliver the radiopharmaceutical to the extracellular space around functioning osteoblasts. Within minutes, they begin to assemble labeled diphosphonates into the hydration shell of hydroxyapatite crystals as they are formed and modified. Osteoclastic function is not measured by this technique.

Radiopharmaceuticals. The primary radiopharmaceuticals utilized for skeletal scintigraphy have been technetium pyrophosphate and most recently the Tc-based diphosphonates, primarily Tc-99m-MDP (methylene diphosphonate). Because it is Tc-based, Tc-MDP has a half-life of 6 hours and an energy of 140 KeV (Table 55.1). The usual adult dose is 20 mCi intravenously; however, up to 30 mCi may be utilized in heavy patients or for better detail.

Fluorine-18 (F-18) is a positron-emitting radionuclide used for PET bone scanning or PET-CT scanning. The usual dose given is 5 to 15 mCi intravenously and it has an energy of 511 KeV with a 110-minute half-life.

Two radionuclides are utilized for internal radiotherapy of painful bony metastatic disease. Strontium-89 (Metastron) is a pure beta emitter with an energy of 1.46 MeV and a 50.5-day half-life. It is given intravenously with a typical dose between 2 and 4 mCi. Samarium-153 (Quadramet) is a beta emitter with 0.81 MeV of energy and has a gamma photon of 103 KeV, which can be used for imaging. The usual dose is 1 mCi/kg intravenously and it has a half-life of 1.9 days.

Biodistribution and Physiology. Tc-99m-MDP is administered intravenously and is delivered to the skeletal system based on vascular distribution. Vigorous osteoblastic activity in the growth plates of juvenile skeletons, healing fractures, pathologic conditions stimulating skeletal blood flow, and bone repair increase the bone labeling. The Tc agents are excreted by glomerular filtration from the kidneys. In a normal subject, 50% is excreted by 4 hours, and up to 80% of the injected diphosphonate will be excreted by 24 hours. Normal renal function clears soft tissue activity, thus improving the quality of bone images because of improved target-to-background ratios. Decreased renal function from any cause degrades image quality. Waiting 3 to 4 hours before delayed skeletal imaging is a compromise between radiotracer decay and the clearance of background activity around the skeleton. Three-phase and four-phase skeletal scintigraphy techniques have proven clinically useful in determining the vascular nature of lesions as well as in separating soft tissue injury or infection such as cellulitis from a focal skeletal disease such as osteomyelitis. *Phase one* is the dynamically acquired arterial phase. *Phase two* is a set of static images, which can be acquired in multiple views, representing the blood pool and soft tissue phase. *Phase three* is acquired 3 to 4 hours later and represents the delayed skeletal uptake. *Phase four* can be acquired the following morning if better skeletal detail is needed, usually when the patient has poor renal function, such as in the diabetic foot.

The mechanism of Tc-MDP tracer localization is by chem-adsorption to the mineral phase of bone, primarily in the areas of increased osteogenic activity. The bladder is the critical organ for Tc-MDP, with 2.6 rads per 20 mCi, and the whole-body radiation-absorbed dose is 0.13 rads per 20 mCi. Strontium is a calcium analog and binds avidly to the hydroxyapatite crystals of bone. F-18 is a hydroxyl ion analog, which also binds to the hydroxyapatite crystals in

TABLE 55.1 Radionuclides Used to Evaluate the Skeletal System

Radionuclide	Dosage	Half-life	Energy	Decay
Tc-pyrophosphate	15–25 mCi	6 hr	140 KeV	Isomeric transition
Tc-MDP	20–30 mCi	6 hr	140 Kev	Isomeric transition
Fluorine-18	5–15 mCi	110 min	511 Kev	Positron
Strontium-89	2–4 mCi	50.5 days	1.46 MeV	Beta only
Samarium-153	1 mCi/kg	1.9 days	0.81 MeV 103 Kev	Beta and gamma

MDP, methylene diphosphonate; Tc, technetium.

bone. F-18-fluorodeoxyglucose (FDG) is a glucose analog radiopharmaceutical, which is a tumor-avid agent, also capable of identifying malignant tumors and bony metastatic disease.

Technical Issues. Skeletal scintigraphy has a resolution of about 5 mm in the best conditions. Adult IV doses of 20 mCi (740 mBq) or more for Tc-MDP are usually adequate for static imaging 3 to 4 hours after injection. Flow images are typically acquired in the anterior and posterior plane or as plantar/palmar views of the area in question. Blood pool images can be obtained in multiple views, similar to "spot-view" images. Whole-body delayed images are typically acquired in the anterior and posterior plane with oblique, lateral, or other spot views as required. The static spot views usually have better resolution than the table-feed, whole-body images. SPECT imaging may be utilized for improved contrast resolution and better anatomic depiction in such areas as the spine, skull, knees, or ankles. High-resolution, low-energy collimation is most commonly used for good-quality images. Ultrahigh-resolution collimation will produce a minor improvement in image quality but at the price of a geometric increase in imaging time. A pinhole collimator can be utilized to produce exquisite images of limited areas such as the wrist. The completed bone scan should be interpreted "online" and tailored as necessary to answer the specific clinical question.

INTERPRETATION

Normal Skeletal Scintigram. In the normal adult, skeletal tracer uptake is fairly uniform and symmetric. Uptake is greater in the axial skeleton (pelvis, spine) than in the appendicular skeleton (skull and extremities). Mild, uniform soft tissue uptake is noted in the background. The kidneys should be slightly hotter than the soft tissues and should be symmetric and normal anatomically. The renal collecting system, ureters, and bladder activity appear very intense. Children will demonstrate intense, symmetric activity in their growth plates, which needs to be evaluated carefully, preferably on a workstation.

Trauma to the skeleton may be undetectable on standard radiographic examinations. The classic stress fracture may be caused by overuse of the normal skeleton, or an insufficiency fracture may result from normal use of weakened bone. Scintigraphically demonstrated trauma precedes radiographically detectable fracture healing by approximately 10 days. Decreased or normal osteoblastic activity is seen at the fracture site in this first phase of repair. The subsequent osteoblastic activity then shows as a "hot spot" weeks before the calcified callus appears on a radiograph (Figs. 55.1, 55.2). In an uncomplicated fracture, repaired bone returns to normal appearance as the callus at the fracture site remodels over a period of months (Fig. 55.3). A complicated fracture in a weight-bearing bone that is healing with angulation may take many years to return to normal bone scan activity. Some fractures may show remodeling on bone scans for life. Bone scans or SPECT of the spine are frequently useful in osteoporotic vertebral fractures, prior to vertebroplasty. The scan evaluates for a metastatic pattern and for the acuteness and level of the fracture.

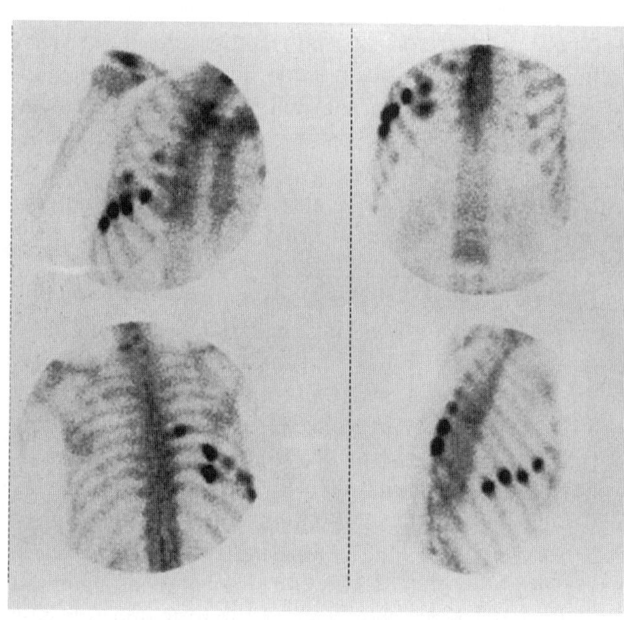

FIGURE 55.1. **Multiple Rib Fractures.** Vigorous osteoblastic repair activity is seen in two rows of fractures, which were not visible on radiographs. Note the "linear array" distribution, which is not seen with the metastases in scans of Figs. 55.13 and 55.14.

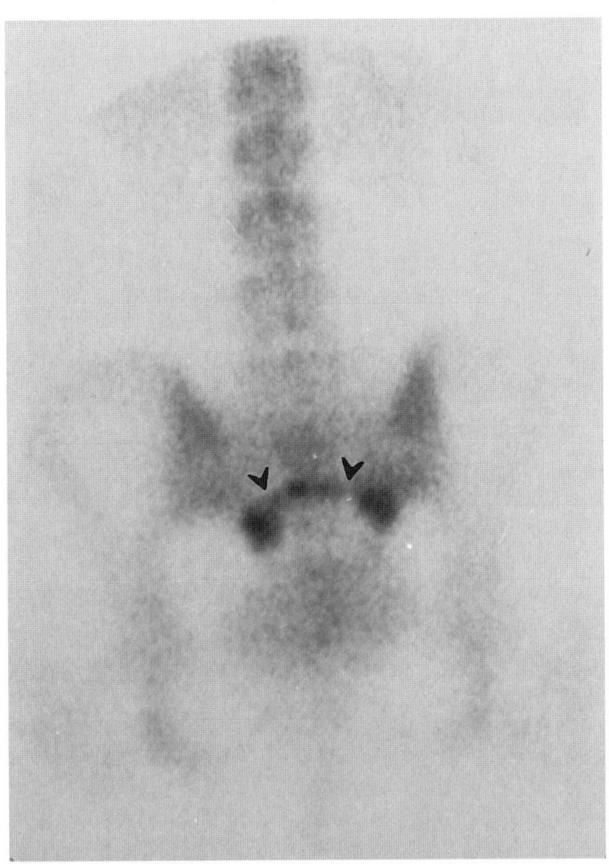

FIGURE 55.2. **Occult Sacral Fracture.** A posterior image of the pelvis shows a horizontal line of increased uptake (*arrowheads*) across the sacrum, which marks healing along a painful fracture that is invisible on radiographs. This can take the shape of an H, called the "Honda sign."

The three-phase bone scan can accurately diagnose shin splints and discriminate them from the more serious stress fracture. Shin splints demonstrate superficial, vertically oriented uptake in the tibia, usually posteromedially. Stress fractures are more localized and run horizontally. Recent studies have shown that a pinhole bone scan is more sensitive than plain film or CT for scaphoid and other fractures of the wrist. Whole-body bone scans are useful in detecting unsuspected fractures following severe cases of multiple trauma.

Prosthetic joint replacements may loosen and/or become infected. For about 6 months after hip replacement surgery, the bone around the prosthesis is expected to have increased osteoblastic activity. Thereafter, increased labeling correlates with infection, loosening, and heterotopic bone formation, depending upon the pattern of localization. The **toggle sign** is indicative of prosthetic loosening and refers to a hot spot at the tip of a prosthesis and two areas of increased uptake at the proximal end, like a toggle switch. Radiographs and, occasionally, radiolabeled white blood cell scans may be required to further diagnose abnormal findings (Fig. 55.4).

Arthropathies and Arthritides. Inflammation of a joint creates increased blood flow and increases the amount of radiopharmaceutical supplied to those portions of the bone bounded by the synovial capsule. Increased bone labeling is seen in toxic synovitis, septic joints, inflammation associated with early degenerative conditions, and connective tissue arthropathies. In early osteoarthropathy, high-resolution bone scan images can detect increased

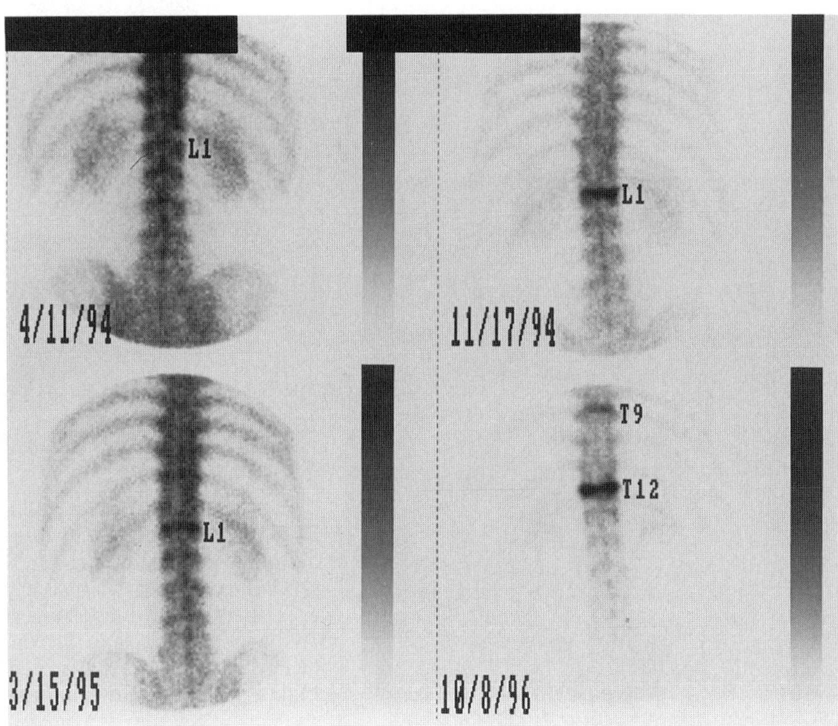

FIGURE 55.3. **Fracture Healing.** Serial bone scans of the lower thoracic and lumbar spine at intervals of months show a normal spine followed by a compression fracture of L1, which gradually heals, only to be replaced by new fractures at T9 and T12. Note the horizontal, linear pattern of a simple vertebral compression fracture.

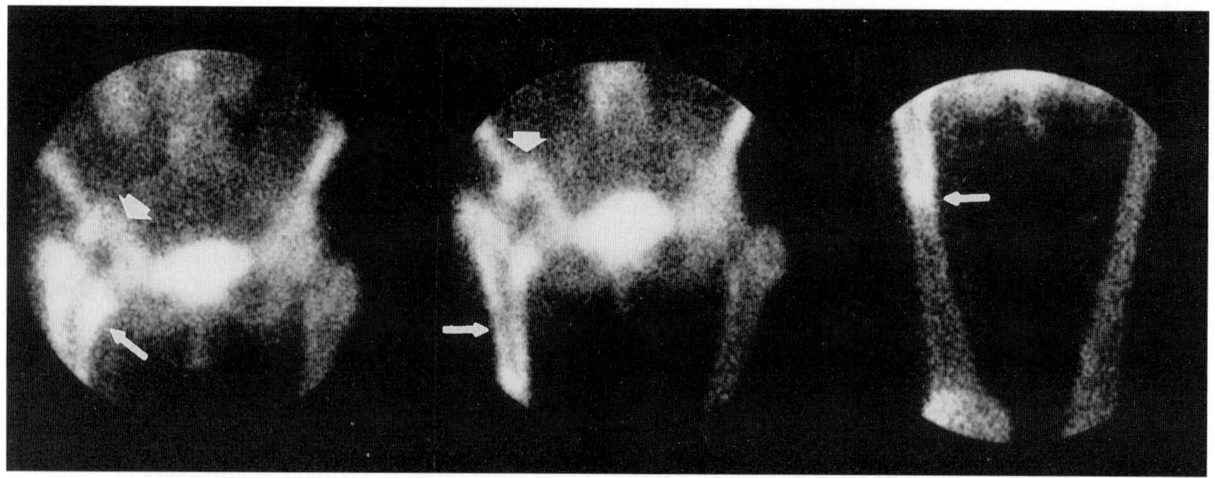

FIGURE 55.4. **Hip Prosthesis Loosening.** Anterior images of the pelvis, hips, and femurs show intense labeling around the femoral (*long arrows*) and acetabular (*wide arrows*) components of a 2-year-old total hip arthroplasty. Both had loosened without infection.

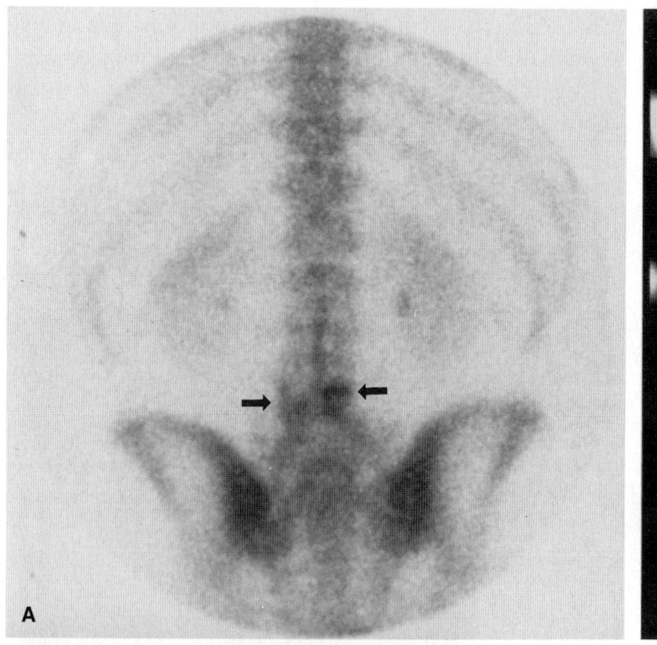

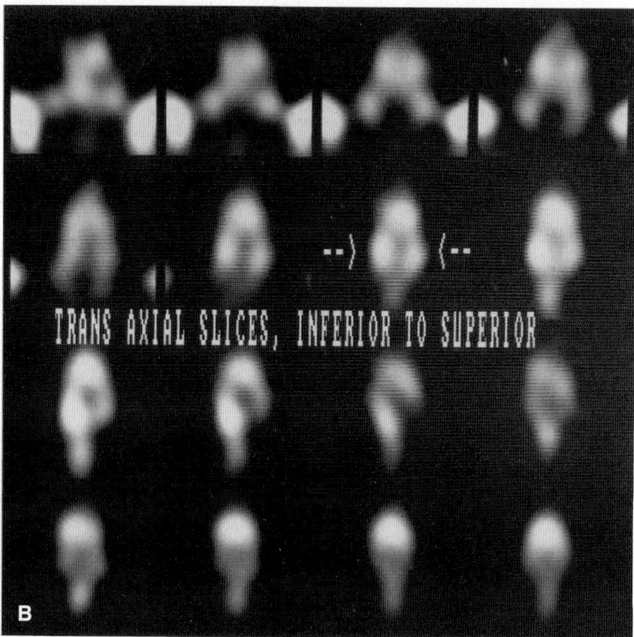

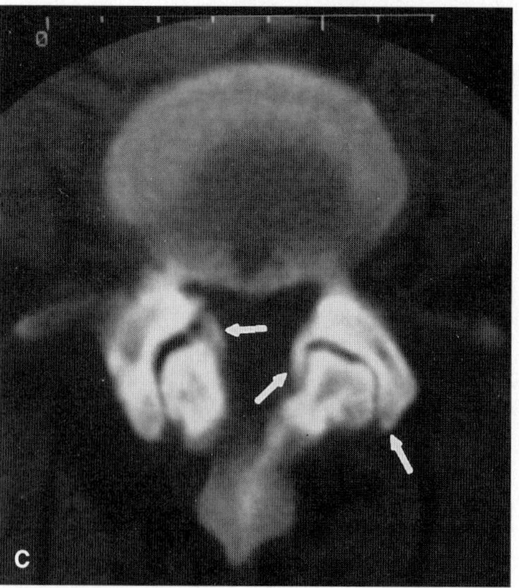

FIGURE 55.5. **L4–L5 Facet Degenerative Arthropathy. A.** A planar, posterior image of the lumbar spine shows small areas of increased activity (*arrows*) in the lower lumbar spine in a patient with chronic low back pain. **B.** Transaxial SPECT images of the same lumbar spine start at the L5–S1 facet joint level and continue up to the L3–L4 level. Note the conspicuity of the abnormality. Areas of increased bone labeling at the L4–L5 facet joints are marked by arrows. **C.** CT of the same level shows hypertrophic spurs (*arrows*) embracing the facet joints.

subchondral bone labeling long before there are radiographic findings. Intense, abnormal labeling also is seen in neuropathic joints long before the abnormality is detected by radiographs (Fig. 55.5).

Osteomyelitis. In a large bone such as a tibia, acute hematogenous infection of bone that precedes radiographic abnormality can be sensitively and specifically diagnosed by three-phase bone scans. Early arterial flow seen seconds after injection (first phase); increased blood pool (second phase), seen for a few minutes before bone labeling begins; and intense delayed labeling 3 or more hours after injection (third phase) are characteristic of early infection. This phenomenon requires several days of symptoms before it develops. Radiographic changes may not be seen for 10 to 14 days. The scan is more difficult to read and not as specific when the target is small (e.g., the bones of the foot) in comparison with the resolving power of the camera (Figs. 55.6, 55.7). False-negative examinations have been reported in children when the duration of clinical illness is brief.

Cellulitis adjacent to bone is seen as a soft tissue area of increased activity in the arterial and immediate blood pool phases, with little or no focally increased activity in the bone on the third phase. In the peripheral skeleton where bones are small, it is frequently more difficult to tell the difference between an infection adjacent to a bone with increased soft tissue and increased periosteal labeling from an infection within the bone. Bone scans may take months to normalize after infections of bone are sterilized, and thus a white blood cell scan may be useful for follow-up.

Vascular Phenomena. There is a strong vascular influence on the labeling of bones. Increased blood flow stimulates increased osteoblastic and osteoclastic activity. Increased flow and presentation of radiotracer usually result in increased deposition. Common pathologic conditions, such as tumor and trauma, cause hyperemia and increased blood pooling, with increased delivery of radiopharmaceuticals to the bone's osteoblasts. This is an appropriate response to injury. Reflex sympathetic dystrophy is an

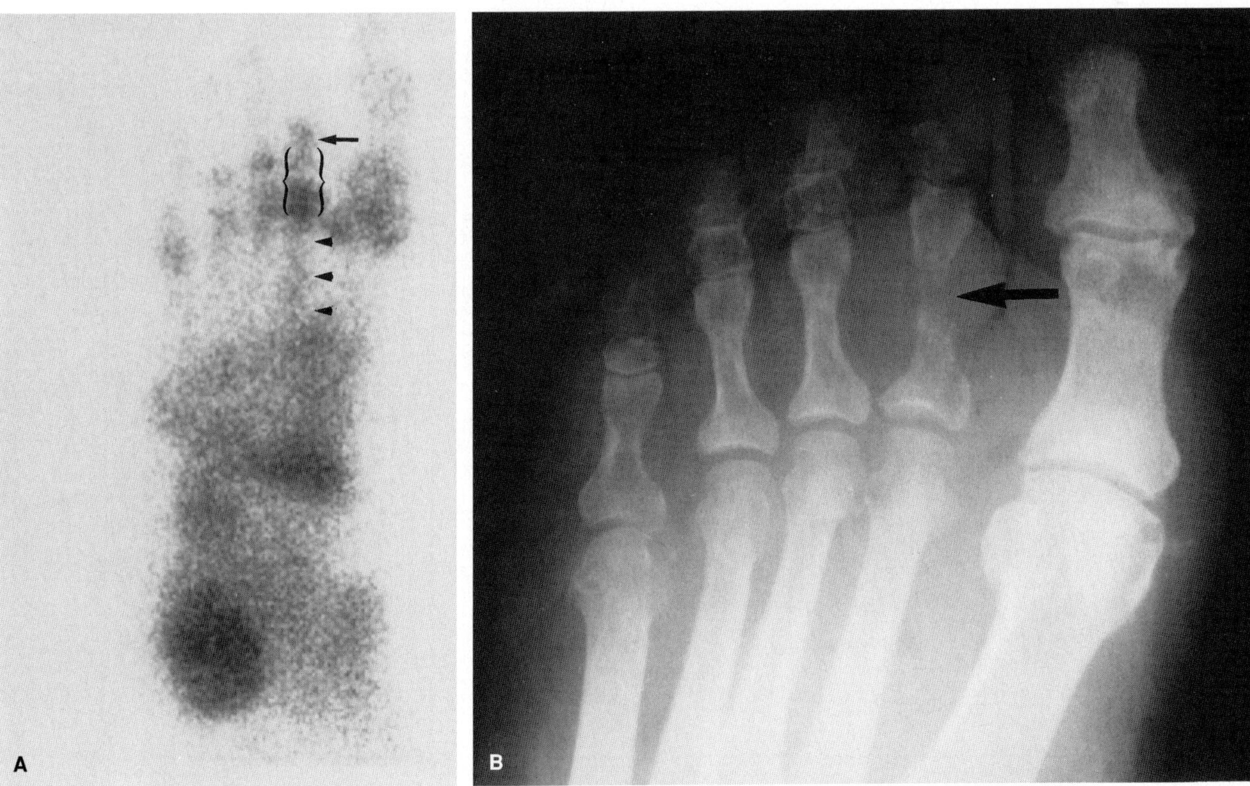

FIGURE 55.6. **Osteomyelitis of the Second Toe and Metatarsal and Septic Second Metatarsal Phalangeal Joint. A.** A plantar bone scan shows increased activity in the second proximal phalanx (*arrow*), metatarsal phalangeal joint (*brackets*), and second metatarsal (*arrowheads*), indicating reactive bone stimulated by the infection. Decreased activity distal to that point corresponds with necrotic tissue. **B.** A radiograph shows destructive changes in the second proximal phalanx (*arrow*), but the foot appears normal in the second metatarsal phalangeal joint and metatarsal phalangeal shaft.

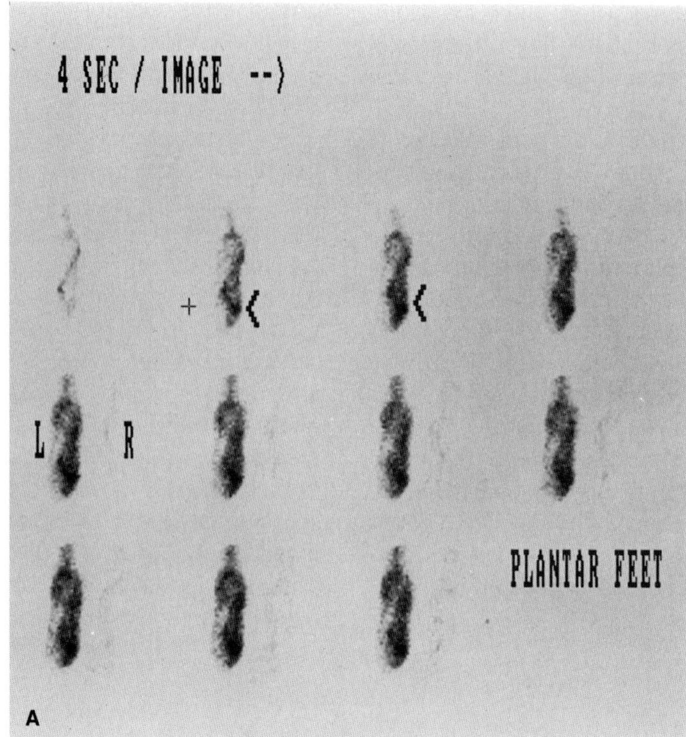

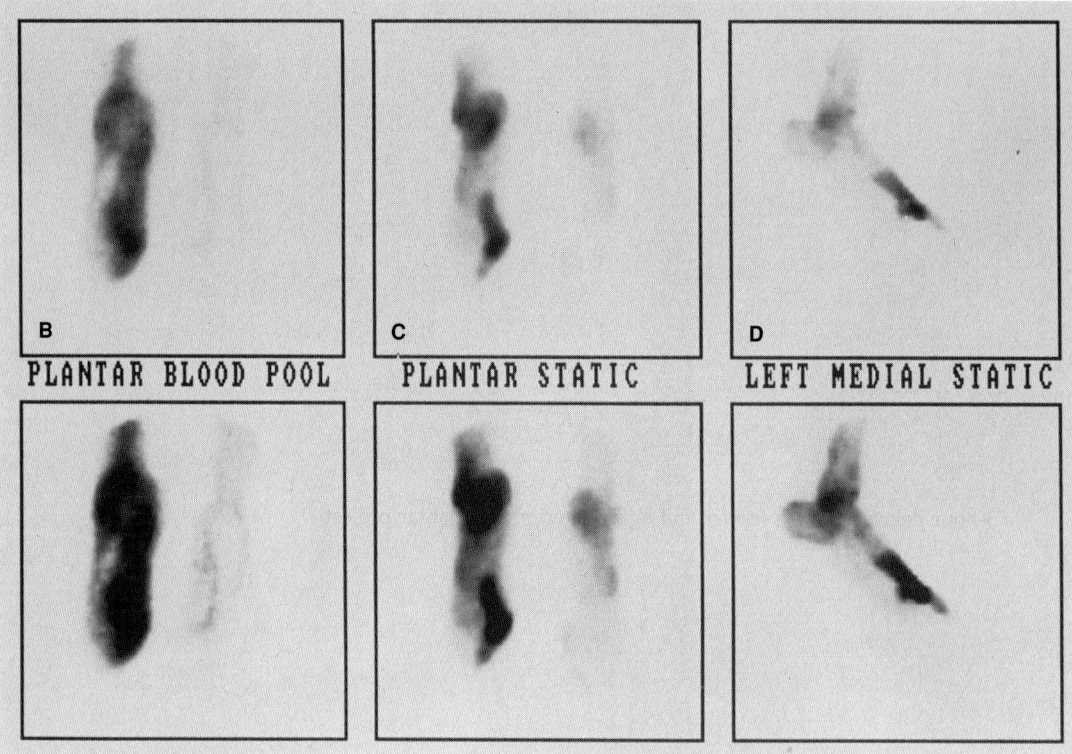

FIGURE 55.7. **First Metatarsal Osteomyelitis and Septic First Metatarsal Phalangeal Joint.** The plantar flow study **(A)** shows intense, early flow to the left foot and first metatarsal head (*arrowheads*). The plantar blood pool images **(B)** show diffuse increased blood pooling in the same areas. The plantar **(C)** and left medial **(D)** views of the static bone scan show intense osteoblastic activity in the entire first metatarsal and in the first metatarsal joint.

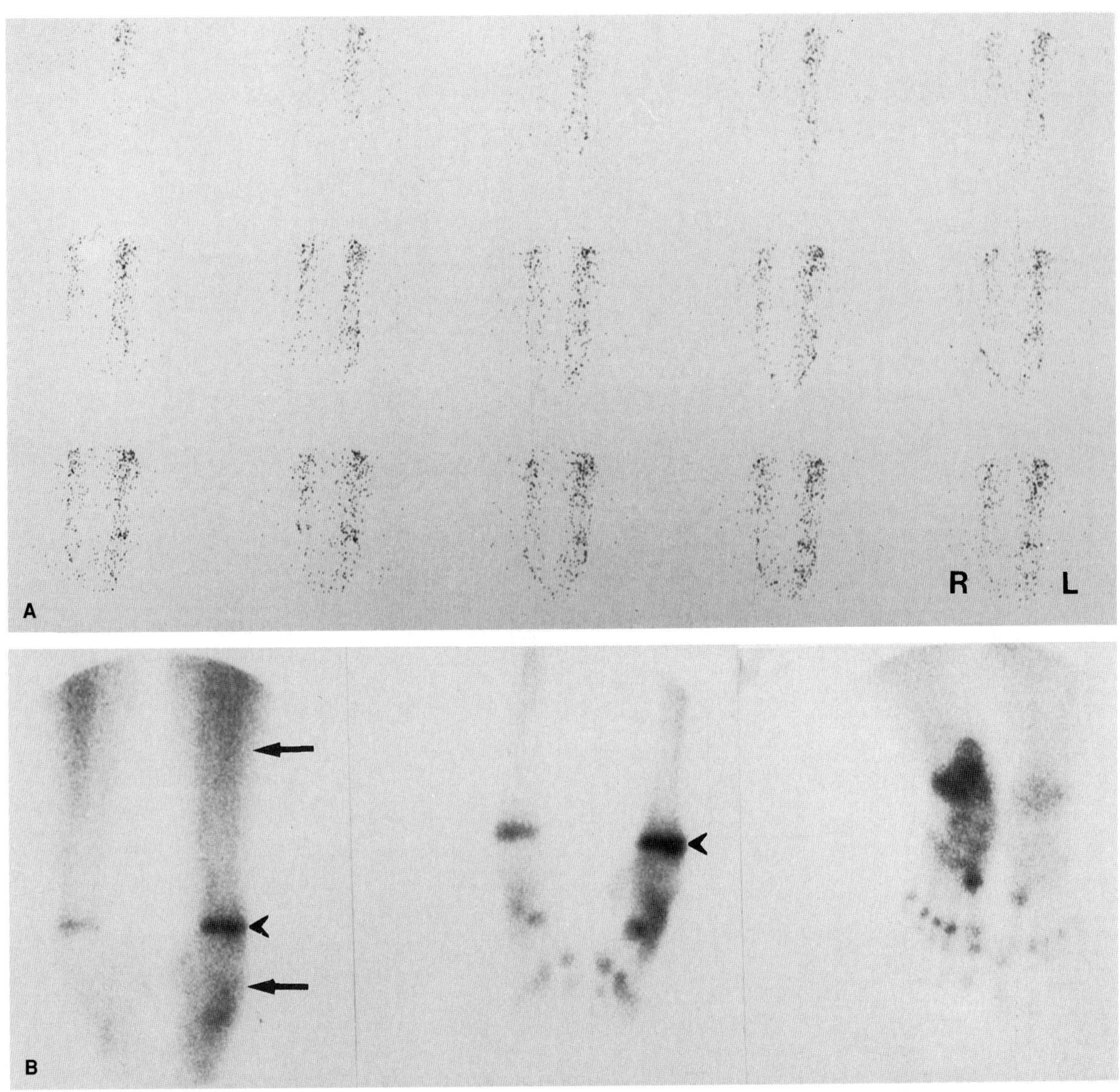

FIGURE 55.8. **Reflex Sympathetic Dystrophy.** Three-phase bone scan in a 13-year-old boy with a painful left ankle and foot. **A.** The initial bolus, filmed at 1 second per frame in the anterior projection with heels together, arrives in the left foot (L) and ankle earlier than the right foot (R). **B.** The early blood pool image (*left*) shows greater blood pooling (*arrows*) in the same area. The 3-hour delayed images (*center* and *right,* anterior and plantar projections, respectively) show a generalized increase in bone labeling. Note the preferential labeling of the physeal plates, which is expected in a juvenile patient.

example of an inappropriately increased vascular response, where one extremity will usually be "hotter" than the other. The release of sympathetic vascular tone causes arteries to dilate (Fig. 55.8). However, "atypical reflex sympathetic dystrophy" occurs in about 10% of cases and demonstrates vasospasm with decreased flow and decreased uptake on the affected side. A bone scan is also a simple test of the vascular status of a bone or bone graft. If osteoblasts are labeled, the blood supply must be intact. Acute avascular necrosis shows no labeling of the affected bone but in later phases will be "hot." Bone subjected to radiation therapy may lose blood supply and osteoblastic activity. Square-edged radiation portals produce typical areas of decreased labeling (Fig. 55.9).

Abnormal Soft Tissue Uptake. Areas of increased soft tissue uptake may be seen with tumors such as breast carcinoma or as normal symmetric, physiologic breast uptake. Atherosclerotic uptake can be seen in the femoral and carotid arteries. Diffuse liver uptake may be seen with diffuse liver disease or with technical problems, such as

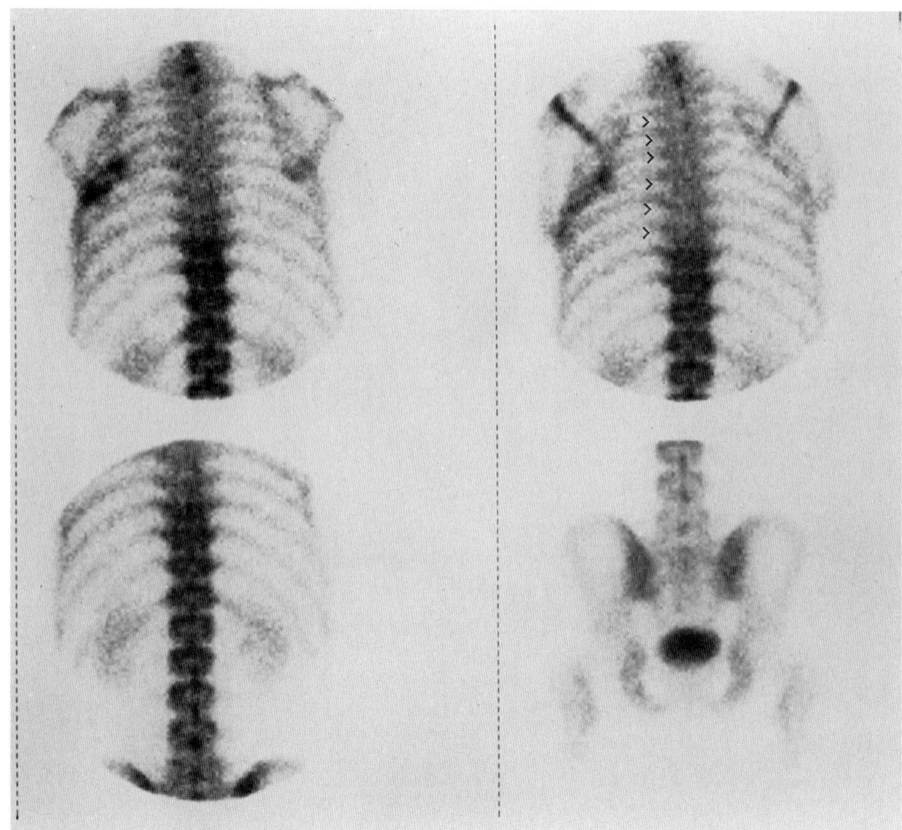

FIGURE 55.9. **Radiation Therapy Changes.** Decreased uptake is seen in the thoracic spine (*arrowheads*) within the radiotherapy portal. Note reactive changes in the lateral left ribs, where a lateral thoracotomy was performed in this patient with bronchogenic carcinoma of the lung.

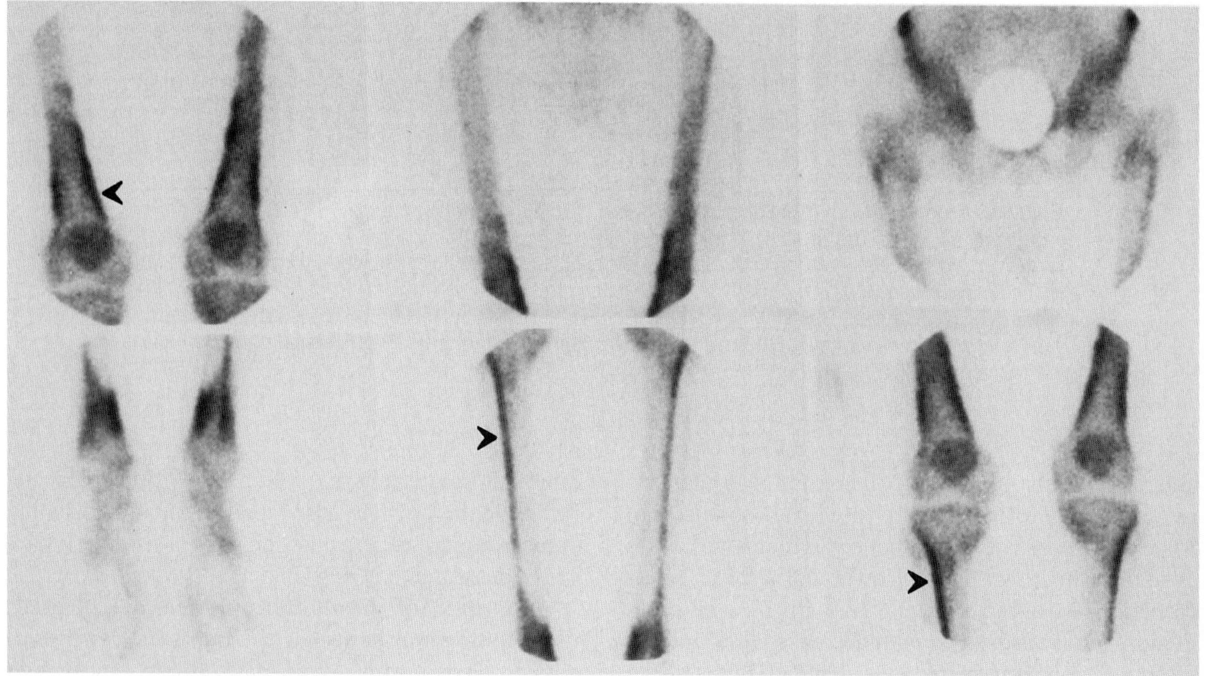

FIGURE 55.10. **Hypertrophic Osteoarthropathy.** A scan done to evaluate for metastases in a patient with carcinoma of the lung shows increased periosteal labeling (*arrowheads*), principally in the metaphyses of the lower extremity. The patient does not have metastases.

colloid formation in the radiotracer as a result of aluminum contamination. Focal abnormal uptake in the liver is usually seen with mucinous metastatic disease such as colon or breast cancer. Soft tissue trauma, cellulitis, bursitis, and rhabdomyolysis will also demonstrate abnormal soft tissue uptake.

Heterotopic Bone. Repair of soft tissue injuries sometimes leads to the formation of heterotopic bone. Histologically normal bone may form from differentiating fibroblasts after trauma. Muscle crush injuries healing with the formation of heterotopic bone (myositis ossificans) are readily labeled on bone scans, weeks before a plain film will show signs of calcification. The restricting area may be safely released or resected after the blood pool phase becomes inactive. Soft tissues around joint prostheses, in paralyzed limbs, and in burn injuries are common sites of heterotopic bone formation.

Metabolic Conditions. Increased parathormone levels (or the presence of tumor-produced parathormone-like substances) simultaneously increase serum calcium and phosphate. Hyperparathyroidism causes calcium/phosphate complexes to precipitate in the lungs and stomach. This "metastatic calcification" is rarely seen on radiographs but is routinely visible as increased uptake on bone scans. Other generalized skeletal abnormalities, such as tumoral calcinosis, hypertrophic osteoarthropathy, systemic mastocytosis, and many other diseases with calcification or ossification of tissues, may be shown with bone scans (Fig. 55.10).

Bone dysplasias frequently show the expected increase in labeling on bone scans. Paget disease of bone, fibrous dysplasia, enchondromas, exostoses, and many other benign conditions of bone are detected by bone scan. Comparison with skeletal radiographs will clarify these multicentric diagnoses. An efficient way to screen the whole skeleton for polyostotic disease is the bone scan. In the osteolytic phase of Paget disease of bone, the radiographic changes are accompanied by marked increases in bone labeling. This repair continues with increased labeling during the radiographic stage of sclerotic, expansile, pagetic bone. The increased activity on bone scans may eventually disappear, because repair is complete (Fig. 55.11). Fibrous

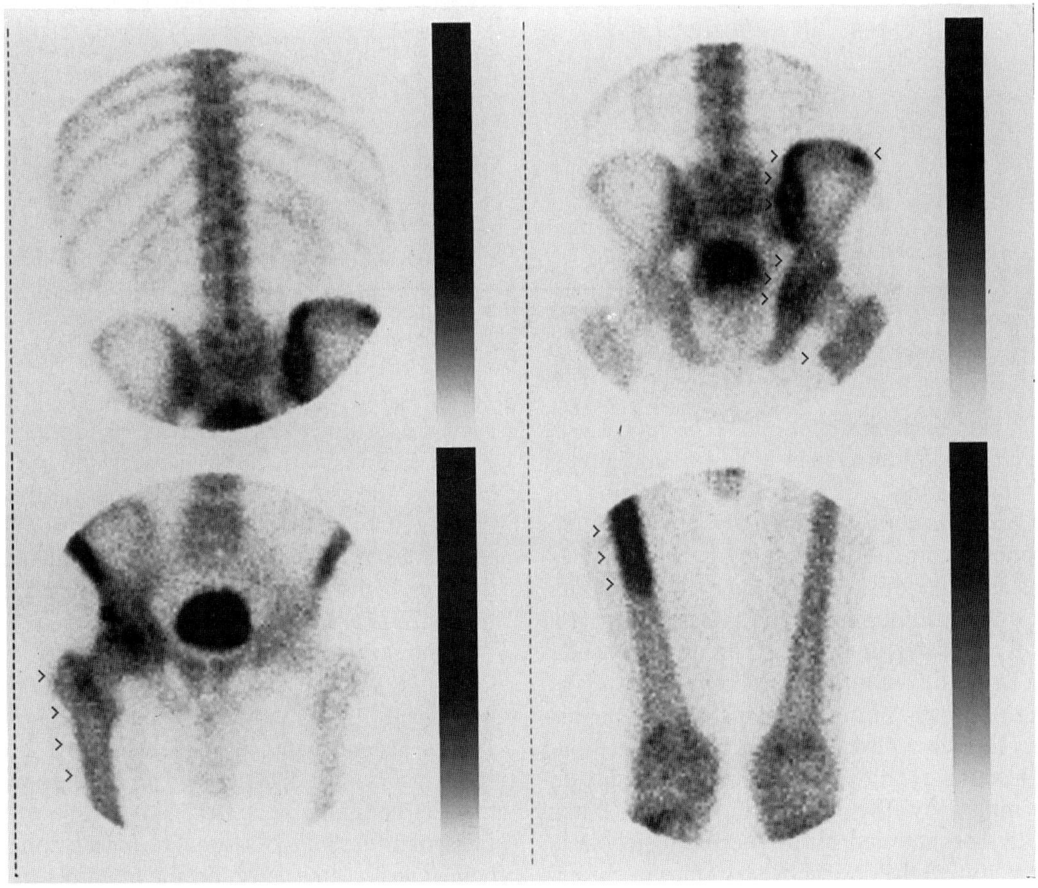

FIGURE 55.11. **Paget Disease of Bone.** Image of the pelvis and femurs of a 60-year-old man with carcinoma of the prostate. There is abnormal, increased uptake in the right hemipelvis and proximal right femur (*arrowheads*), which is characteristic of pagetic bone. Note the distal "flame edge" of the pagetic portion of the femur. The patient does not have bony metastatic disease.

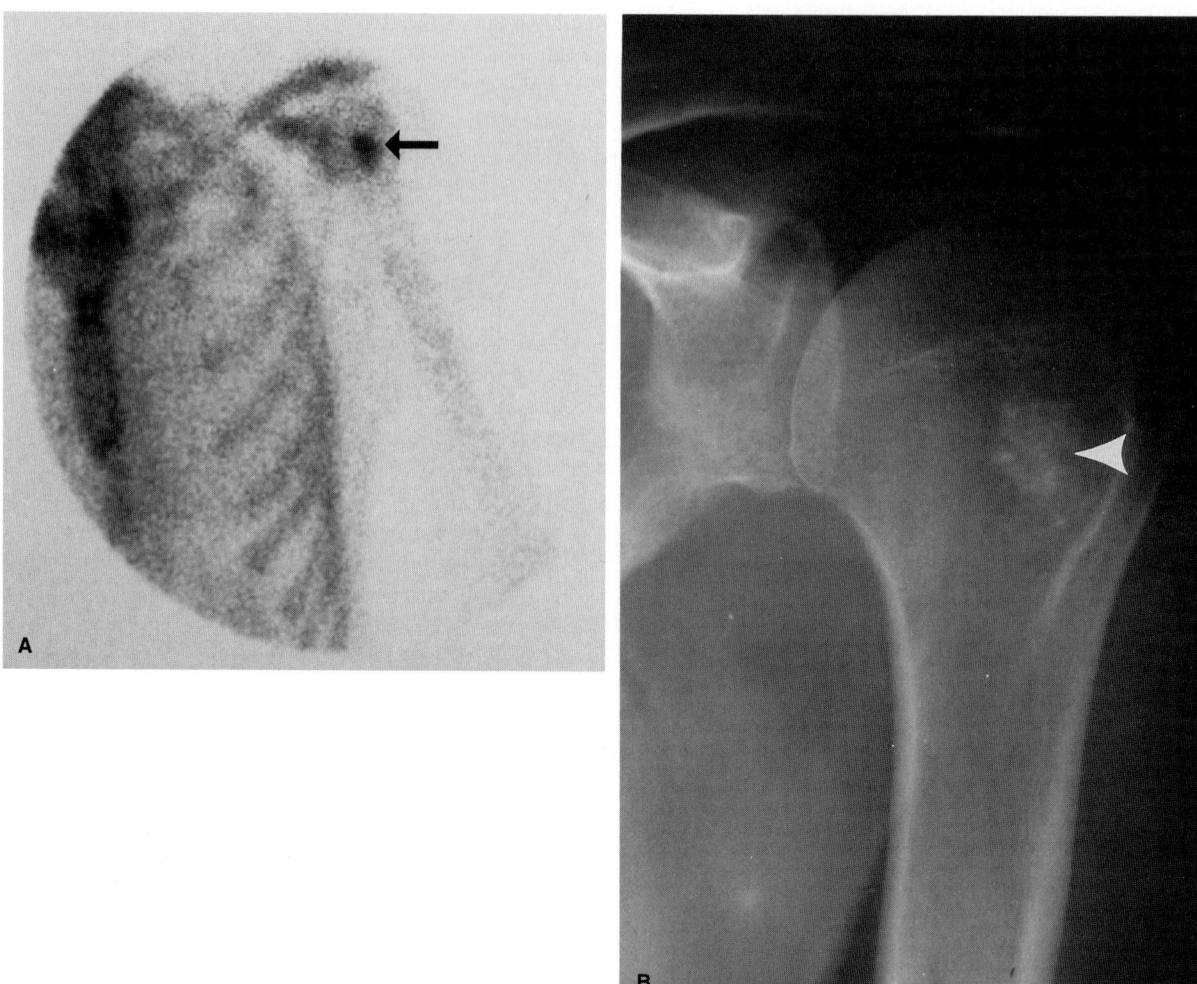

FIGURE 55.12. **Low-Grade Chondrosarcoma. A.** An area of reactive bone (*arrow*) is seen in the proximal left humeral metaphysis. **B.** A radiograph shows the calcified cartilaginous matrix (*arrowhead*) of this tumor.

dysplasia is a benign condition of bone that may also be polyostotic. It is readily detected by bone scans because of its intense bone labeling.

Primary Bone Tumors. There are two principal ways in which bone tumors are detected by bone scans. Osteosarcomas and chondrosarcomas may have abnormal osteoblastic or chondroblastic activity associated with the production of abnormal tumor calcification. This is a malignant process, with the tumor itself being "hot" (Figs. 55.12, 55.13). Metastases from calcifying or ossifying primary tumors to other nonskeletal sites may also take up Tc-99m diphosphonates directly, making them readily detected by scintigraphy. The Tc-99m diphosphonate may also be avidly concentrated by the normal osteoblasts, which are reacting to the destructive presence of the primary tumor. This process makes the bone adjacent to tumors much more intense than the surrounding bone. Some malignancies may arise in the soft tissues adjacent to bone and invade through periosteum into the bone. In either case, the resulting reactive osteoblastic changes show the extent of invasion without showing the tumor itself. An extremely destructive bone tumor may destroy bone more quickly than repair can be effected. Thus, a "cold" defect in a bone with a primary malignancy is an indication of a very aggressive tumor. High-grade sarcomas usually show this phenomenon.

Bone scans may also be useful in benign bone tumors. Osteomas or bone islands may be neutral or not seen on bone scans, even though they appear sclerotic on radiographs. Osteoid osteomas are typically very hot and will show the "double-density" sign on a bone scan because of the very hot nidus.

Metastatic Bone Disease. The most common use of the bone scan is for the detection and monitoring of metastatic tumor involving the skeleton. The tumors monitored include prostate, lung, breast, thyroid, and renal carcinoma, among many others. The majority of metastases affect the axial skeleton in a pattern that reflects the distribution of

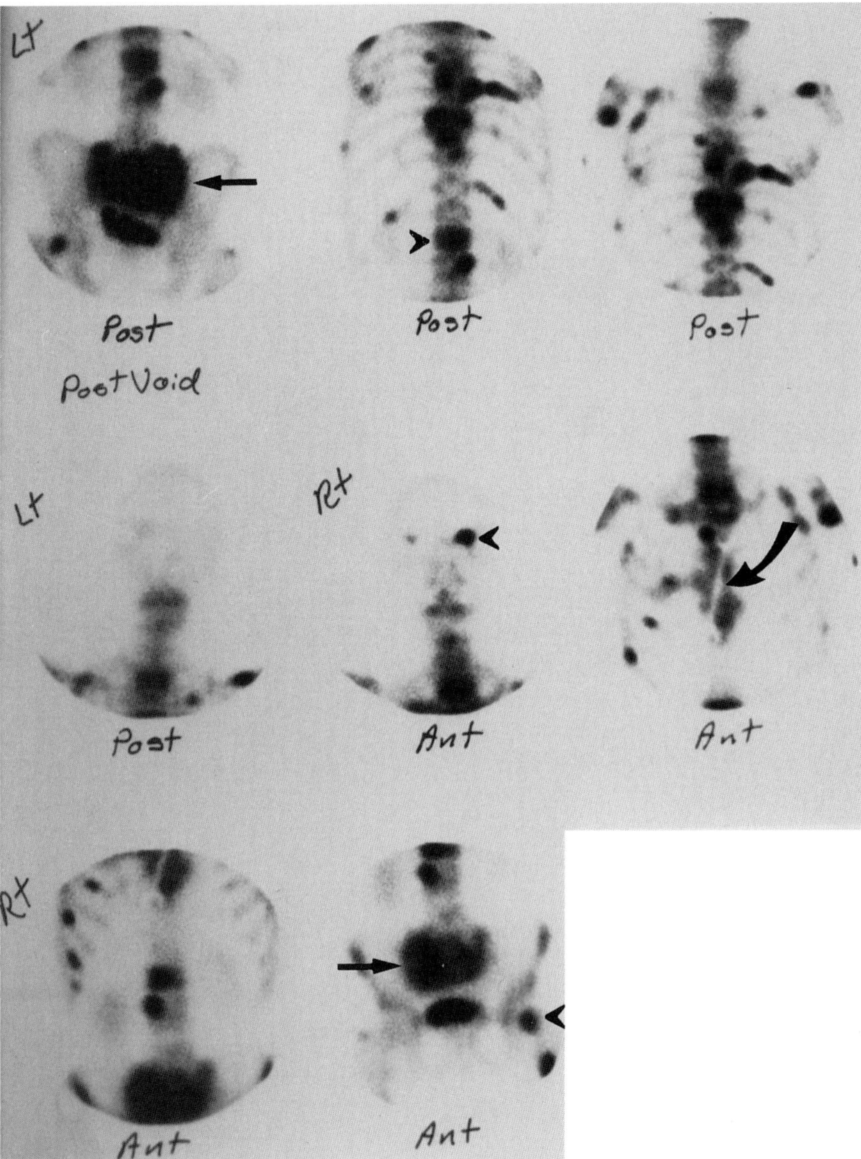

FIGURE 55.13. **Osteogenic Sarcoma and Metastases.** A 65-year-old man with a bone marrow burden of plutonium. A large primary tumor replaced the sacrum (*arrows*) and is seen as the most intense area of uptake. The balance of the skeleton shows multiple metastases (*arrowheads*), which have similarly intense labeling. There is a wrench (*curved arrow*) projecting over the sternum. The patient kept it to adjust a mechanical collar he wore for the last 6 months of his life because of extensive cervical vertebral metastases that threatened quadriplegia.

the erythropoietic marrow. The likelihood of a metastasis peripheral to erythropoietic marrow is low. Most metastases are multiple at the time of discovery. Thus, a solitary hot spot in the skull or a rib has a low probability (<10%) of being a metastatic lesion. Comparison bone scans at intervals of 3 to 6 months allow an accurate assessment of tumor spread (Fig. 55.14). Because of its sensitivity, the bone scan can be utilized when a cancer patient has new back pain or bone pain. Likewise, a bone scan is helpful when a sclerotic lesion (e.g., bone island) or lytic lesion (e.g., venous lake in skull) in seen on an anatomic study.

Knowledge of a given primary tumor's propensity to metastasize to the skeleton is helpful for scan interpretation. Confusion arises if an inexperienced observer cannot distinguish between common degenerative or post-traumatic changes and metastases. Merely counting the hot spots is of little value in the management of oncologic problems. Experience is necessary to judge metastatic disease in the skeleton. As metastases progress or regress, increases in labeling reflect the status of bone repair, not the status of the metastases. Increased numbers and size of individual lesions usually indicate that the tumor load of the skeleton is expanding. Increased *intensity* of the individual lesions (in the absence of new lesions) frequently means that the tumor has become static and that the osteoblasts around it are engaged in vigorous repair. This "flare" response early after institution of chemotherapy is usually a good indicator that tumor has been checked by therapy and should not be misinterpreted as worsening of the metastatic disease.

Aggressive metastases may destroy bone so quickly that there is no repair (Fig. 55.15). Special attention and anatomic imaging should be obtained for those metastases in a critical, weight-bearing bone such as the femur. Early

(*text continues on p.1370*)

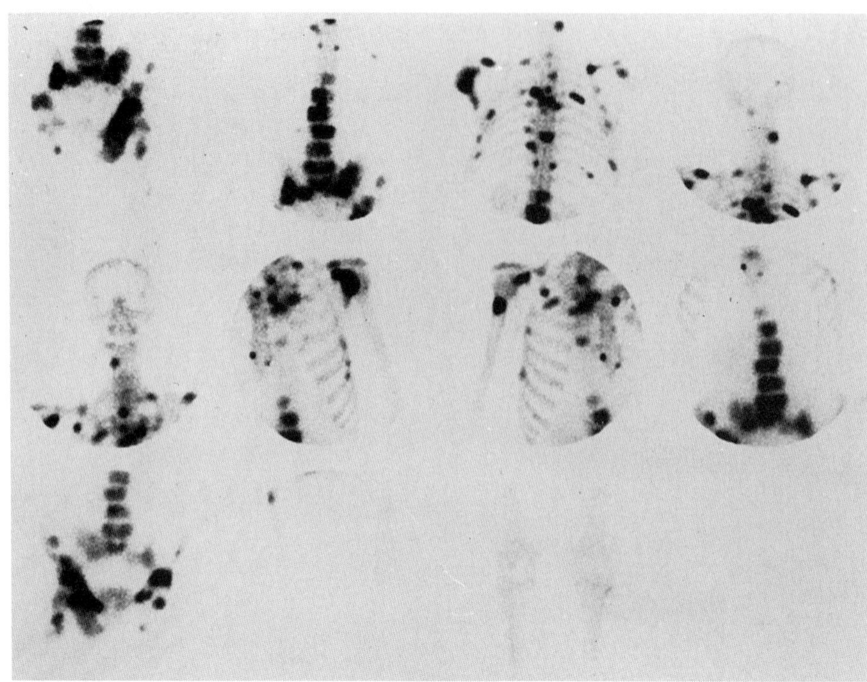

FIGURE 55.14. **Superscan.** Numerous prostate cancer metastases produce "hot" spots of intense isotope accumulation that leave little or none of the radiopharmaceutical for renal excretion or soft tissue uptake.

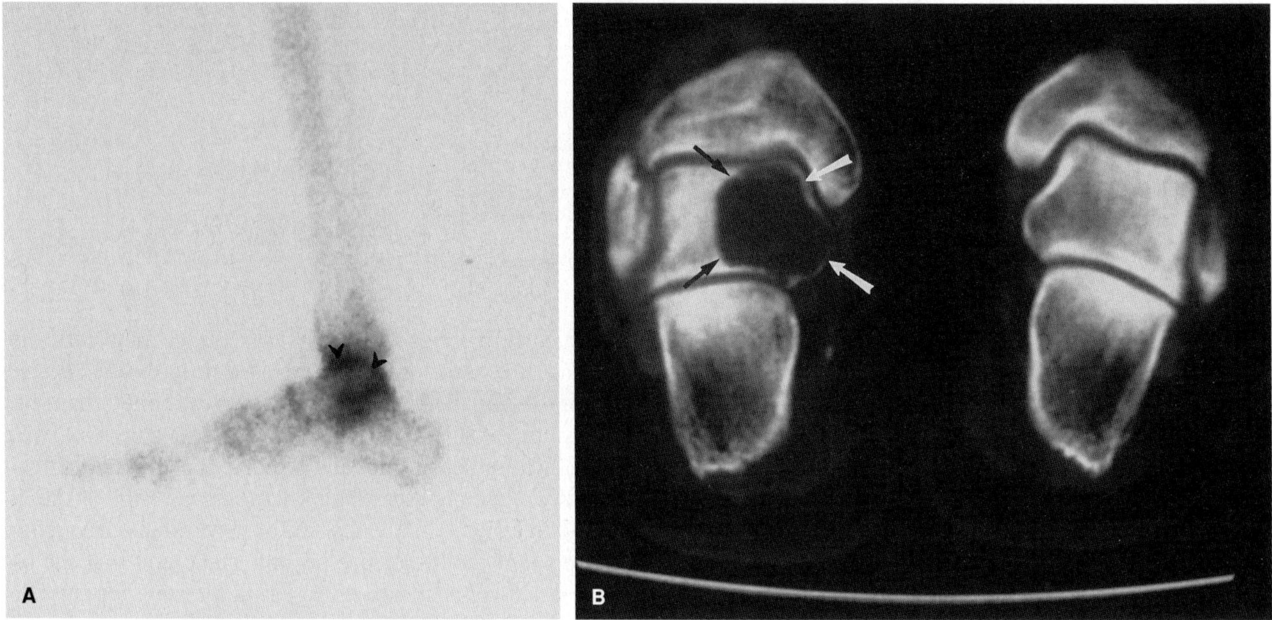

FIGURE 55.15. **Aggressive Metastasis. A.** A medial projection bone scan of the ankle and foot of a patient with renal cell carcinoma shows a halo of increased activity (*arrowheads*) around the ankle joint. **B.** A CT scan of the ankle shows a scooped-out lesion (*arrows*) of the right talus, where the metastasis has destroyed bone so fast that bone repair has had no chance to take place. The talus does not show a hot spot. The bone scan is abnormal because of hemarthrosis irritation of the synovium. Increased blood supplied to the inflamed synovium brings with it increased radiopharmaceutical, which labels all of the bones of the joint.

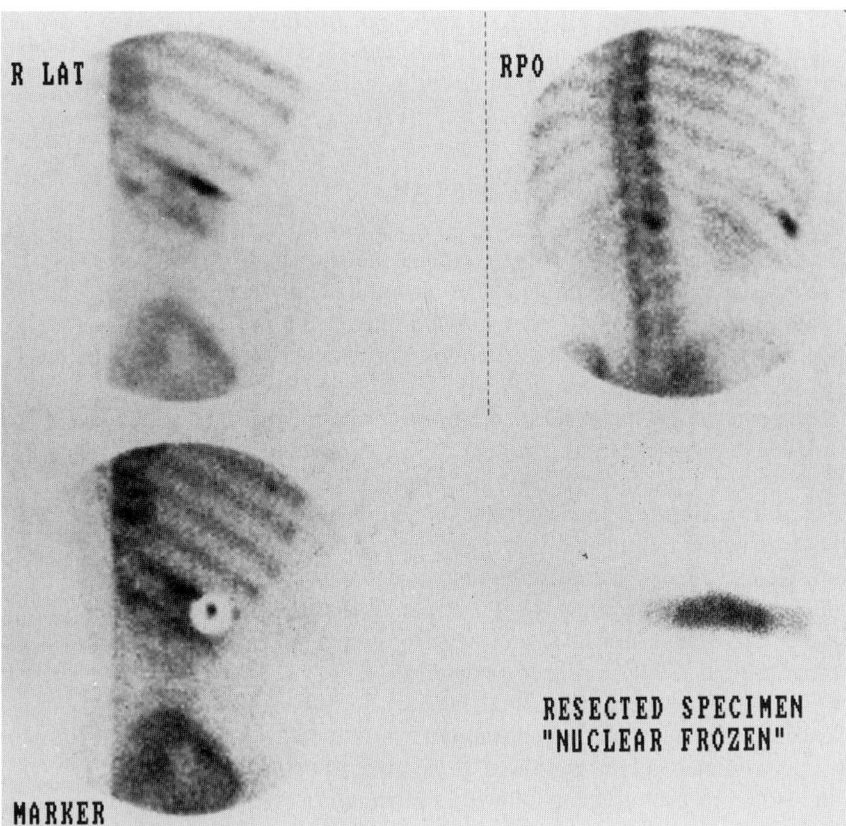

FIGURE 55.16. **Resection of a Solitary Metastasis.** A solitary metastasis from an adenocarcinoma of unknown origin is located with a "cold" lead ring maneuvered over the right lateral rib lesion before surgery to locate the correct rib for resection. On the way to the surgical pathologist, the resected rib was imaged to confirm that the correct rib had been resected.

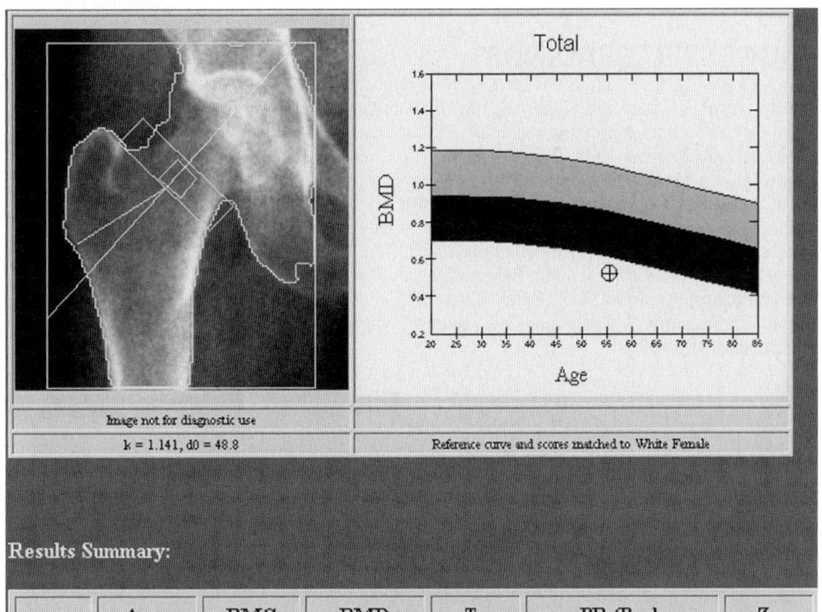

Region	Area [cm²]	BMC [(g)]	BMD [g/cm²]	T - Score	PR (Peak Reference)	Z - Score
Neck	5.04	1.93	0.382	-4.2	45	-3.1
Troch	9.81	3.70	0.377	-3.2	54	-2.5
Inter	24.09	14.70	0.610	-3.2	55	-2.7
Total	**38.94**	**20.33**	**0.522**	**-3.4**	**55**	**-2.7**
Ward's	1.06	0.25	0.238	-4.2	32	-2.5

FIGURE 55.17. **Bone Mineral Densitometry With Dual-Energy X-Ray Absorptiometry (DEXA) Scan.** DEXA scan of the right hip in a 55-year-old woman demonstrates low bone mineral density (BMD), low Z scores, and low T scores, consistent with significant osteoporosis. Her spine showed similar changes, indicating a high risk of fracture.

detection and treatment can prevent pathologic fractures, which add to the suffering with a terminal illness. The bone scan can also guide biopsy in cases where pathologic diagnosis of a bone lesion is required (Fig. 55.16).

BONE MINERAL DENSITOMETRY

Bone mineral densitometry (BMD) is one of the few health care screening tests in radiology. It is also utilized to accurately follow patients after institution of therapy for osteoporosis or osteopenia. Dual-energy x-ray absorptiometry (DEXA) utilizes two x-ray energies that have different attenuation coefficients for dense bone, muscle, and fat. The measured bone mineral density is compared to a database of normal values for age and sex to give a *Z score* (Fig. 55.17). The Z score is stated in standard deviations above or below the normal average for the patient's age and sex. The *T score* compares the individual against peak young normals of the same sex in standard deviations. A T score between –1 and –2.5 is considered *osteopenia.* A T score of –2.5 or worse is defined as *osteoporosis.* A T score of –1 or better is considered normal. For each T score standard deviation below normal, the fracture risk is increased by approximately a factor of three. Bone mineral density can also be measured using CT with a phantom or with smaller US units for peripheral measurements of the heel or wrist.

SUGGESTED READINGS

Batt ME, Ugalde V, Anderson MW, Shelton DK. A prospective controlled study of diagnostic imaging for acute shin splints. Med Sci Sports Exerc 1998;30:1564–1571.

Brown ML, Collier BD, Fogelman I. Bone scintigraphy: part 1. Oncology and infection. J Nucl Med 1993;34:2236–2240.

Brunader R, Shelton DK. Radiologic bone assessment in the evaluation of osteoporosis. Am Fam Physician 2002;65:1357–1364.

Collier BD, Fogelman I, Brown ML. Bone scintigraphy: part 2. Orthopedic bone scanning. J Nucl Med 1993;34:2241–2246.

Collier BD, Fogelman I, Rosenthal I, eds. Skeletal Nuclear Medicine. St. Louis: Mosby, 1996.

Collier BD, Hellman RS, Krasnow AZ. Bone SPECT. Semin Nucl Med 1987;17:247–266.

Connolly LP, Connolly SA. Skeletal scintigraphy in the multimodality assessment of young children with acute skeletal symptoms. Clin Nucl Med 2003;28(9):746–754.

Corcoran RJ, Thrall JH, Kyle RW, et al. Solitary abnormalities in bone scans of patients with extraosseous malignancies. Radiology 1976;121:663–667.

Evan-Sapir E. Imaging of malignant bone involvement by morphologic, scintigraphic, and hybrid modalities. J Nucl Med 2005; 46(8):1356–1367.

Freeman LM, Blaufox MD, eds. Metabolic bone disease. Semin Nucl Med 1997;27:195–305.

Freeman LM, Blaufox MD, eds. Orthopedic nuclear medicine (part I). Semin Nucl Med 1997;27:307–389.

Freeman LM, Blaufox MD, eds. Orthopedic nuclear medicine (part II). Semin Nucl Med 1998;28:1–131.

Groves AM, Cheow H, Balan K, et al. 16-MDCT in the detection of occult wrist fractures: a comparison with skeletal scintigraphy. AJR Am J Roentgenol 2005;184:1470–1474.

Kozin F, Soin JS, Ryan LM, et al. Bone scintigraphy in the reflex sympathetic dystrophy syndrome. Radiology 1981;138:437–443.

Maeseneer MD, Lenchik L, Everaert H, et al. Evaluation of lower back pain with bone scintigraphy and SPECT. Radiographics 1999;19: 901–912.

Matin P. Bone scintigraphy in the diagnosis and management of traumatic injury. Semin Nucl Med 1983;8:108–122.

Pandit-Taskar N, Batraki M, Divgi CR. Radiopharmaceutical therapy for palliation of bone pain from osseous metastases. J Nucl Med 2004;45(8):1358–1365.

Ryer JS, Kim JS, Moon DH, et al. Bone SPECT is more sensitive than MRI in the detection of early osteonecrosis of femoral head after renal transplantation. J Nucl Med 2002;43:1006–1011.

Savelli G, Maffioli L, Maccauro M, et al. Bone scintigraphy and the added value of SPECT (single photon emission tomography) in detecting skeletal lesions. Q J Nucl Med 2001;45:27–37.

Schauwecker DS. The scintigraphic diagnosis of osteomyelitis. AJR Am J Roentgenol 1992;158:9–18.

Schirrmeister H, Glatting G, Hetzel J, et al. Prospective evaluation of the clinical values of planar bone scans, SPECT, and F-18-labelled Na F PET in newly diagnosed lung cancer. J Nucl Med 2001;42:1800–1804.

Shehab D, Elgazzar AH, Collier BD. Heterotopic ossification. J Nucl Med 2002;43(3):346–353.

Sutter CW, Shelton DK. Three phase bone scan in osteomyelitis and other musculoskeletal disorders. Am Fam Physician 1996;54:1639–1647.

Treves ST, ed. Pediatric Nuclear Medicine. New York: Springer, 1998.

Vande Streek P, Carretta RF, Weiland FL, Shelton DK. Upper extremity radionuclide bone imaging: the wrist and hand. Semin Nucl Med 1998;28:14–24.

Weiss PE, Mall JC, Hoffer PB, et al. 99mTc-methylene diphosphonate bone imaging in the evaluation of total hip prosthesis. Radiology 1979;133:727–729.

Chapter 56

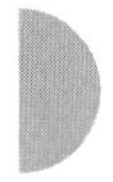

Pulmonary Scintigraphy

David K. Shelton and Rhonda A. Wyatt

Anatomy and Physiology

Ventilation Lung Scan
Radiopharmaceuticals
Ventilation Scan Technique

Perfusion Lung Scan
Radiopharmaceuticals
Perfusion Scan Technique

Ventilation/Perfusion Scans

Pulmonary Embolism

Ventilation/Perfusion Scan Interpretation

Nonthromboembolic Pulmonary Disease

Although CT angiography (CTA) has taken a central role in diagnosing pulmonary embolism (PE), ventilation perfusion (V/Q) scans remain important. A scintigraphic lung scan is a physiologic map that evaluates the primary functions of the lung, pulmonary vasculature perfusion, and segmental bronchioalveolar tree ventilation. Most commonly, V/Q scans are used to evaluate patients suspected of having PE. In an attempt to provide more accurate results, the criteria for interpreting V/Q studies have been constantly revised. Different schema that compare defects present on the perfusion scan with those found on the ventilation scan and/or chest radiograph (CXR) have been developed to estimate the probability of PE. This chapter describes radiopharmaceuticals used, examination technique, imaging protocols, and criteria for the interpretation of V/Q scans.

ANATOMY AND PHYSIOLOGY

An understanding of the segmental anatomy of the lungs (Fig. 56.1) is vital to the interpretation of lung scans. The three-dimensional location of ventilation or perfusion defects must be determined individually and correlated with the segmental or subsegmental anatomy of the lung. PE will have a segmental or subsegmental distribution pattern, usually peripheral and wedge shaped in nature.

Although pulmonary ventilation occurs primarily via the branching bronchial system, other pathways exist by which distal alveoli can be aerated. The pores of Kohn connect adjacent alveoli, and the canals of Lambert connect alveoli with respiratory, terminal, and preterminal bronchioles. These canals and pores permit collateral ventilation of alveoli whose conducting airways have become blocked. Collateral air drift is dynamic and is mediated by neurohormonal control, which can be altered by pathologic events, atmospheric/alveolar gas tension, and drugs.

Ventilation and pulmonary blood flow both demonstrate marked gravity effects. When a patient is in an upright posture, the gradient for blood flow is from the apices to the lung bases; the apex receives only one third of the blood volume that the base receives. A corresponding ventilation gradient exists when the patient sits upright. Because intrapleural pressure is greater at the bases, the differential negative intrapleural pressure at the apices causes alveoli there to remain more open at expiration than the basilar alveoli. Therefore, basilar alveoli undergo greater respiratory cycle changes in size. This results in greater gas exchange occurring in the base and greater oxygen tension in the apices. On average, ventilation at the base is 1.5 to 2 times that at the apex. When a patient is supine, the ventilation gradient shifts from superoinferior to anteroposterior, and perfusion is increased to the dependent posterior portions of the lungs.

Normally, capillary perfusion and alveolar ventilation are matched to maximize gas exchange. Diseases that produce localized hypoxia invoke autoregulatory mechanisms that divert blood flow away from the hypoxemic pulmonary segments. These dynamic changes prevent

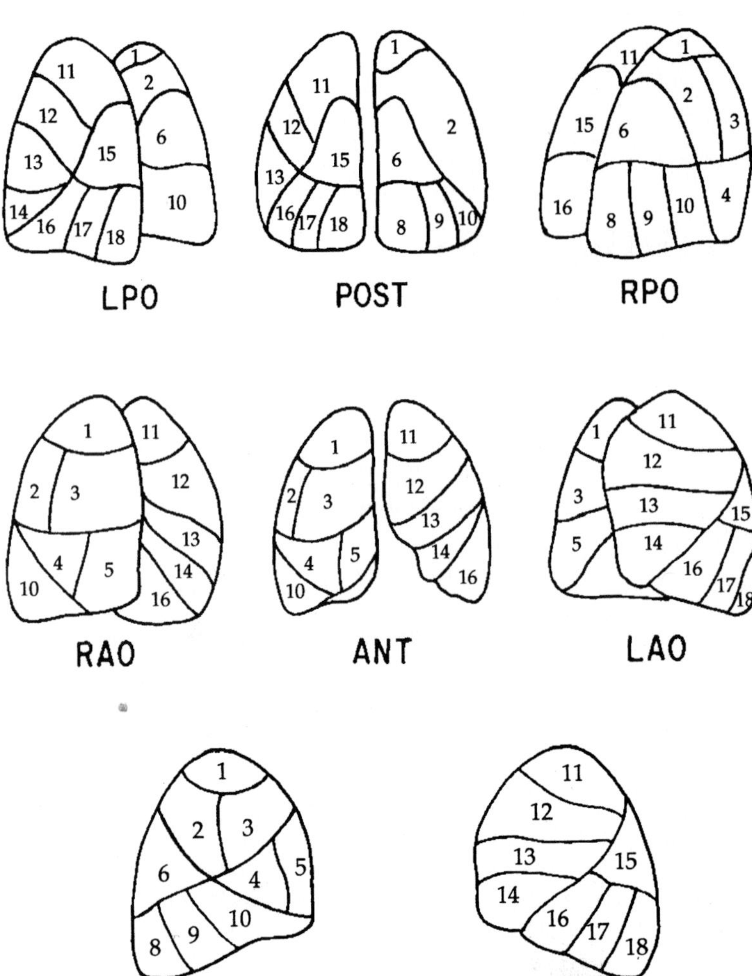

FIGURE 56.1. **Pulmonary Segment Anatomy.** Bronchopulmonary segments of the right lung: 1, apical; 2, posterior; 3, anterior; 4, lateral; 5, medial; 6, superior; 7, medial basal; 8, posterior basal; 9, lateral basal; 10, anterior basal. Bronchopulmonary segments of the left lung: 11, apical posterior; 12, anterior; 13, superior lingual; 14, inferior lingual; 15, superior; 16, anterior medial basal; 17, lateral basal; 18, posterior basal. LPO, left posterior oblique; POST, posterior; RPO, right posterior oblique; RAO, right anterior oblique, ANT, anterior; LAO, left anterior oblique; RLAT, right lateral; LLAT, left lateral. (Adapted with minor modifications from Sostman HD, Gottschalk A. Diagnostic Nuclear Medicine. 2nd ed. Baltimore: Williams & Wilkins, 1988:513; used with permission.)

nonventilated lung segments from being perfused. Conversely, localized hypoperfusion rarely induces localized bronchoconstriction. Primary vascular disorders such as PE, if unassociated with parenchymal consolidation or pulmonary infarction, usually have normal ventilation. Thus an anatomic perfusion deficit with normal ventilation is referred to as a *V/Q mismatch* and is the hallmark of PE diagnosis.

VENTILATION LUNG SCAN

Radiopharmaceuticals

Xenon-133 (Xe-133) is a radioisotope widely used to perform ventilation lung scans. A noble gas produced by fission of uranium-235 in a nuclear reactor, Xe-133 has a half-life of 5.3 days and is a beta emitter. The principle photon energy is 81 keV, which results in significant attenuation effects. Xe-133 ventilation scans should be performed before perfusion lung scans, because Compton scatter from the higher-energy technetium-99m (Tc-99m) macroaggregated albumin (MAA) (140 keV) down-scatters into the region of the 81-keV photopeak of the Xe-133 and would thus interfere with ventilation images. The usual adult dose of Xe-133 for a ventilation scan is 10 to 20 mCi (370 to 540 MBq).

Xenon-127 (Xe-127) is a cyclotron-produced isotope with a physical half-life of 36.4 days and principle photon energies of 203 keV, 172 keV, and 365 keV. Because it has higher-energy photons, Xe-127 ventilation scans can be performed, if needed, after the perfusion scan, since down-scatter image deterioration is not a significant problem. Unfortunately, because Xe-127 is cyclotron-produced, it is both expensive and of limited availability. The usual adult dose is 8 to 15 mCi (296 to 555 MBq).

Krypton-81m (Kr-81m) is the other noble gas used for ventilation scans. With an extremely short half-life of only 13 seconds, Kr-81m is produced from a rubidium-81-Kr-81m generator. Kr-81m decays by isomeric transition and has a photon energy of 191 keV. The higher energy allows the ventilation scan to be acquired, if needed, after an abnormal perfusion scan. Unfortunately, the generator is expensive and therefore Kr-81 is limited in use. The usual adult dose is 10 to 20 mCi (370 to 740 MBq).

Technetium-99m Aerosols. Ventilation scans can be performed using aerosolized rather than gaseous agents. Radioisotope-labeled aerosols are produced by nebulizing radiopharmaceuticals into a fine mist that is inhaled. Tc-99m diethylenetriaminepentaacetic acid (DTPA) is the most commonly used radioaerosol. The advantages of Tc-99m aerosols are that they are widely available and inexpensive, and they have a 140-keV photopeak, which is ideal for gamma camera imaging. The nebulizer-produced mist is passed through a settling bag, which traps larger particles. The mist is delivered to the patient via a nonrebreathing valve and is inhaled. The process is inefficient; only 2% to 10% of the aerosolized radioisotope is deposited within the lungs. Of 30 mCi of nebulized Tc-99m DTPA, only 1 to 2 mCi actually are deposited within the lungs.

The site of deposition of the aerosolized particles depends on the size of the inhaled particle. The larger the particle, the greater the gravitational effect, which results in more central deposition. Particles larger than 2 μm localize in the trachea and pharynx. Current aerosol nebulizers can produce microaerosols of less than 0.5 μm. Thus, microaerosol particles are small enough to reach the distal tracheobronchial tree and reflect regional ventilation. Patients with narrowed airways caused by asthma, bronchitis, or chronic obstructive pulmonary disease (COPD) have more central deposition of the particles than normal patients because of airway turbulence. This results in poor visualization of the peripheral lung fields. The deposited Tc-99m DTPA is absorbed across the alveolar membrane, with a clearance half-life of 60 to 90 minutes. The half-life is approximately 20 minutes shorter in tobacco smokers, owing to their increased alveolar permeability.

Dosimetry. The critical organ for Xe-133 is the trachea, which receives a dose of 0.64 rad/mCi. The lung dose is 0.01 to 0.04 rad/mCi, whereas the whole-body absorbed dose is 0.001 rad/mCi. For Tc-99m aerosols, the lungs receive an absorbed dose of 0.1 rad/mCi, the bladder wall a dose of 0.18 rad/mCi, and the entire body a dose of 0.01 rad/mCi.

Ventilation Scan Technique

Ventilation scanning using radioactive gases requires special equipment to prevent leakage of the gas into the imaging room. Gas delivery systems consist of a shielded spirometer, oxygen delivery system, and a Xe charcoal trap to capture most of the exhaled Xe. Because Xe is heavier than air, loose Xe pools at floor level; thus the room should be well ventilated and have negative pressure flow.

Xenon-133 Ventilation Scanning. The patient is initially fitted with an airtight facemask. While the patient takes a maximal inspiration, Xe-133 is injected into the mask intake tubing. The patient is instructed to hold his or her breath as long as possible. A posterior-projection, 100,000-count, first-breath image of the lungs is then obtained. The ventilation system is then switched so that the patient rebreathes the air/Xe-133 mixture. After 5 minutes of rebreathing, a posterior 100,000-count equilibrium image is obtained. The distribution of Xe-133 activity on the equilibrium image represents aerated lung volume. The ventilation system is then readjusted so that the patient breathes in fresh air and exhales the Xe-133 mixture into the trap. Serial posterior 30-second washout images are obtained over a 5-minute interval. The Xe-133 normally washes out of the lungs within 3 to 4 minutes. Because the lung bases are better ventilated than the apices, the Xe-133 washes out of the bases faster than the apices in a normal patient. If possible, all images should be performed with the patient in an upright position.

Xenon-127 Ventilation Scanning is performed in the same manner as Xe-133 ventilation lung scans. The Xe-127 ventilation scan need be performed only if the perfusion scan is abnormal.

Krypton-81m Ventilation Scanning. The high-photon energy of Kr-81m allows ventilation scans to follow perfusion scans. Immediately after each perfusion image and without moving, the patient inhales Kr-81m and the corresponding ventilation image is obtained. This process is repeated until ventilation and perfusion images are obtained in all six matching positions.

Technetium-99m Aerosol Ventilation Scanning. The patient inhales the nebulized aerosol while in the supine position to avoid the normal apex-to-base gravity gradient. After inhaling the Tc-99m aerosol for 3 to 5 minutes, the patient sits upright and is imaged in the same projections as for the perfusion lung scan. The exhaled aerosol is trapped in a filter that is stored until decay is sufficient for safe disposal.

A Tc-99m aerosol ventilation lung scan can be performed either before or after the perfusion lung scan. If the perfusion scan is performed first, a small dose (0.5 mCi) of Tc-99m MAA is used with a large dose (30 mCi) of Tc-99m DTPA. If the ventilation scan is performed first, 5 to 10 mCi of Tc-99m DTPA and 5 mCi of Tc-99m MAA are administered.

PERFUSION LUNG SCAN

Radiopharmaceuticals

Perfusion lung scanning is based on the principle of capillary blockade. Particles slightly larger than the pulmonary capillaries (>8 μm) are injected intravenously and travel to the right heart, where venous blood is uniformly mixed. Radiolabeled particles in the pulmonary arterial blood pass into the distal pulmonary circulation. Because the radioactive particles are larger than the capillaries, they lodge in the precapillary arterioles. Their distribution in the lung reflects the relative blood flow to pulmonary segments. Pulmonary segments with decreased or absent blood flow show diminished radioactivity.

Tc-99m-MAA is the radiopharmaceutical used to perform most perfusion lung scans. MAA is prepared by heat denaturation of human serum albumin. The MAA particles are irregularly shaped molecules, with the size range and number of particles in commercially available kits tightly controlled. Most particles are in the 20- to 40-μm size range, with 90% of the particles between 10 and 90 μm. Particles larger than 150 μm should not be injected, because they can obstruct arterioles. The size and number of particles in a kit are checked by counting a sample volume in a light microscopy hemocytometer. Tc-99m-MAA is prepared by adding Tc-99m-pertechnetate (Tc-99mO_4) to the MAA kit. The MAA leaves the lungs by breaking down into smaller particles that pass through the alveolar capillaries into the systemic circulation, where they are removed by the reticuloendothelial system. The biologic half-life of MAA particles in the lung is 2 to 9 hours. The physical half-life of Tc-99m-MAA is 6 hours.

A minimum of 60,000 Tc-99m MAA particles must be injected to ensure reliable count statistics and image quality. Typically, 200,000 to 500,000 particles are injected, and fewer than 0.1% of capillaries are temporarily and safely occluded. However, several types of patients should receive a reduced number of particles during a perfusion scan. Patients with pulmonary hypertension and right-to-left shunts should be given only 100,000 particles. Children should also be injected with only 100,000 particles because they have fewer pulmonary arterioles. To perform reduced-count imaging, each perfusion view is imaged for a longer time interval, allowing for nearly equivalent count statistics. Alternatively, the kit can be reconstituted with higher-than-usual Tc-99m activity per particle. The normal 5-mCi dose can be administered but with fewer particles. Contraindications to perfusion lung scanning include severe pulmonary hypertension and allergy to human serum albumin products.

Dosimetry. The normal adult dose is 3 to 5 mCi (111 to 185 MBq). The lung is the critical organ and receives an absorbed dose of 0.15 to 0.5 rad/mCi. The whole-body and gonadal absorbed dose is 0.15 rad/mCi.

Perfusion Scan Technique

The syringe containing the Tc-99m MAA should be gently agitated prior to injection to resuspend all particles. The patient is injected in the supine position while taking slow, deep breaths to minimize the pulmonary perfusion gravitational gradient. Blood should not be drawn into the syringe because aspirated blood may form clots, which then become labeled by the Tc-99m MAA. Injection of clumped Tc-99m MAA particles or labeled clot can result in multiple small focal hot spots scattered through the lungs.

The patient is usually imaged in the upright position using a large field of view and a high-resolution gamma camera. Images (500,000 count) are obtained in the anterior, posterior, right lateral, left lateral, right posterior oblique, left posterior oblique, right anterior oblique, and left anterior oblique positions. Supplemental or decubitus views can be added to clarify findings on the standard views.

VENTILATION/PERFUSION SCANS

Indications. The most common indication for V/Q scans is diagnosis of suspected PE. This examination has also been used to monitor pulmonary function of lung transplants, to provide preoperative estimates of lung function in lung carcinoma patients in whom pneumonectomy is planned (split lung function study), to evaluate right-to-left shunts, and to conduct serial assessment of inflammatory lung disease. The CXR should be evaluated prior to obtaining a V/Q scan. Infiltrates, effusions, pulmonary edema, or pneumothorax may explain sudden respiratory deterioration and eliminate the need for a V/Q scan.

CT Angiography Versus Ventilation/Perfusion Scans. There are situations in which a V/Q scan should be the first option to diagnose PE and times when CTA should be the first option. The sensitivity and accuracy of CTA have increased with the use of thin-cut helical CT and multidetector CT (Fig. 56.2). It should be considered when the patient is in intensive care or has an abnormal CXR, high clinical probability for PE, or a relative contraindication for anticoagulation. A V/Q scan is highly sensitive and avoids the use of iodinated contrast. It should be considered when

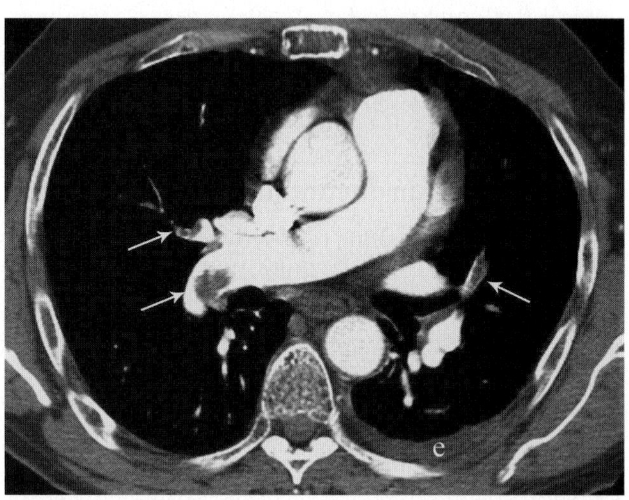

FIGURE 56.2. **Pulmonary Emboli on MDCT Pulmonary Angiogram.** Scan demonstrates multiple bilateral pulmonary emboli (*arrows*) and a left pleural effusion (e).

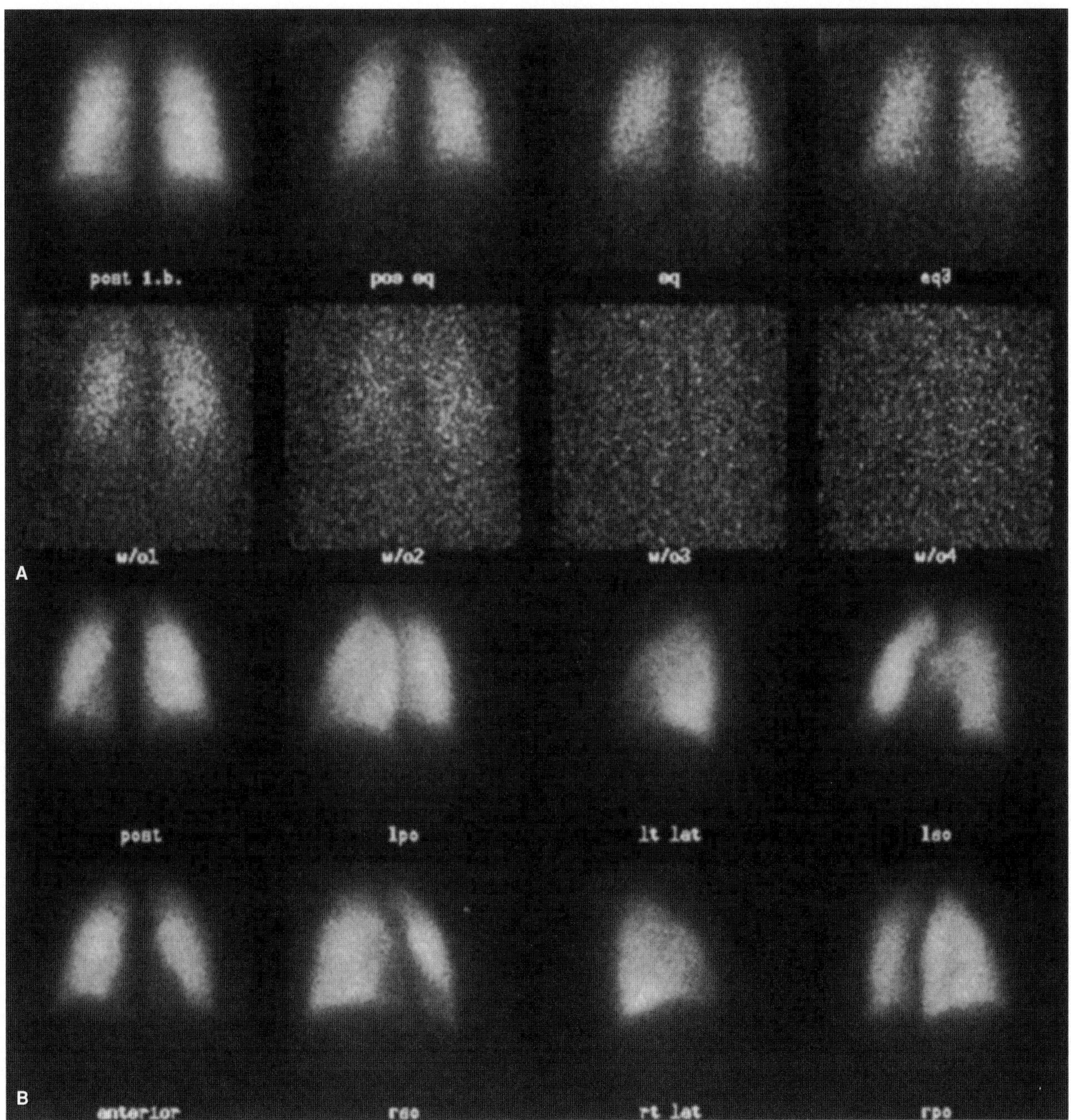

FIGURE 56.3. **Normal Ventilation/Perfusion Scan. A. Normal Xenon-133 ventilation lung scan** (top two rows). post 1b, posterior initial breath; pos eq, posterior equilibrium; eq, equilibrium; eq3, equilibrium after 3 minutes; wo/1, 1 minute after start of washout; wo/2, 2-minute washout; wo/3, 3-minute washout; wo/4, 4-minute washout. **B. Normal Technetium-99m macroaggregated albumin perfusion lung scan** (bottom two rows). post, posterior; lpo, left posterior oblique; lt lat, left lateral; lao, left anterior oblique; rao, right anterior oblique; rt lat, right lateral; rpo, right posterior oblique.

the clinical probability is low, the CXR is normal, and the patient is pregnant or has a relative contraindication for iodinated contrast.

Normal ventilation scans (Fig. 56.3A) have homogeneous radiopharmaceutical distribution throughout all lung fields on all three phases of the scan (initial breath, equilibrium, and washout). A subtle base-to-apex gradient may be seen because more lung parenchyma is located at the base than the apex. The first-breath Xe-133 image is often grainy because it has relatively poor count statistics. However, it still reflects regional lung volume. The equilibrium images have greater activity and will fill in areas of restricted lung disease. The washout phase of the study demonstrates rapid clearance of the Xe-133 from the lungs. Normal half-time for xenon washout is less than 1 minute. Washout is complete within 3 minutes. Retention (trapping) of xenon in the lungs in a focal or diffuse pattern is an indication of obstructive lung disease.

Normal Tc-99m DTPA aerosol scans resemble normal Tc-99m MAA perfusion scans. However, activity is frequently present within the trachea and mainstem bronchi, especially in smokers. Swallowed Tc-99m DTPA aerosol is sometimes seen within the esophagus and stomach.

Normal perfusion scans show well-defined margins of both lungs on all views, with sharply defined costophrenic angles. A mild base-to-apex count activity gradient is present because of the physical differences in lung thickness of the base compared to the apex. Tracer distribution should otherwise be homogeneous (Fig. 56.3B).

The heart causes a smoothly defined defect along the left medial lung border that is curvilinear in all projections. A prominent, focal triangular margin suggests the presence of a perfusion defect abutting the heart. The hila are usually seen, even in normal patients. Focal asymmetric hilar perfusion defects are abnormal. Cardiomegaly, tortuosity of the aorta, and mediastinal or hilar enlargement cause defects along the medial border of the lung associated with less well-defined corresponding defects on the ventilation scan. The size and shape of any mediastinal structure on the V/Q scan should match its appearance on the CXR.

Abnormal Scans. Focal defects or inhomogeneous tracer distribution are abnormal on either ventilation or perfusion scans. Focal perfusion defects should be compared with corresponding areas on the ventilation scan and vice versa. The relative size and shape of V/Q defects should then be correlated with corresponding areas on a recent CXR. Ideally, the correlative CXR should have been performed no more than 6 to 12 hours prior to the V/Q scan since acute findings may change rapidly.

Ventilation scans are abnormal if areas of delayed Xe wash-in or washout are present. Restrictive changes or defects on the single-breath image may disappear on the equilibrium images when Xe bypasses obstructed pulmonary bronchioles through the pores of Kohn and canals of Lambert. Movement by collateral air drift proceeds more slowly than through the bronchioles, resulting in delayed wash-in and washout. Focal areas of abnormal retention therefore suggest obstructive lung disease (Fig. 56.4).

PULMONARY EMBOLISM

PE is a common cause of death in the United States. Dahlen and Alpert estimated that 30% of untreated patients with PE die as a consequence of their emboli, in comparison to 10% to 16% mortality for patients treated with anticoagulant therapy. Anticoagulants, however, place patients at significant risk for life-threatening bleeding and should not be prescribed without high probability for the diagnosis of venous thrombosis or PE.

PE usually originate from thrombi within the deep venous system of the legs and pelvis. Predisposing factors include prolonged immobilization, surgery (particularly intrapelvic or hip surgery), history of prior PE, preexisting cardiac disease, estrogen therapy, smoking, hypercoagulable states such as cancer, and congenital defects of thrombolysis.

PE can be difficult to diagnose clinically. In 70% of patients who survive PE, the emboli may not be clinically suspected. The classic triad of dyspnea, hemoptysis, and pleuritic chest pain occurs in fewer than 20% of patients with PE. Larger emboli increase the likelihood of symptoms. Symptoms associated with PE, however, are nonspecific. Pulmonary infection or inflammation, pneumothorax, cancer, and cardiac disease may produce similar symptoms. An electrocardiogram should be performed in patients suspected of having PE to detect cardiac causes for chest pain or dyspnea. If a patient develops acute cor pulmonale because of pulmonary emboli, the electrocardiogram will show signs of right heart strain.

Radiographic Findings of Pulmonary Embolism. The CXR is normal in 12% of patients with PE. The classic findings are a wedge-shaped, pleural-based infarct (Hampton hump) or a wedge-shaped area of oligemia (Westermark sign). The most common but nonspecific CXR finding of PE is atelectasis or opacities in the region with emboli. An elevated diaphragm, small pleural effusion, and/or prominent hilum are also frequently seen.

Recently, spiral CT and MR have been used to diagnose pulmonary emboli. The sensitivity of spiral CT is 73% to 95%, with a specificity of 87% to 97%. Spiral CT and MR accurately detect emboli in the segmental or larger pulmonary arteries but may not display more peripheral emboli.

Scintigraphic Findings of Deep Venous Thrombosis. A radionuclide venogram may be performed in conjunction with a perfusion lung scan. Tc-99m MAA is divided between two syringes and injected into the veins on the dorsa of the feet instead of into the arm. The nuclear venogram is most sensitive for thrombi occurring above the knees. Deep venous thrombosis (DVT) is indicated by obstruction of the veins, which show cutoff of activity and multiple collateral vessels.

Tracers are also utilized to detect acute DVT, such as antifibrin monoclonal antibodies and Tc-99m–labeled peptides. Acute thrombi demonstrate focal areas of asymmetric increased uptake within the deep venous system and could be helpful in differentiating chronic from acute DVT.

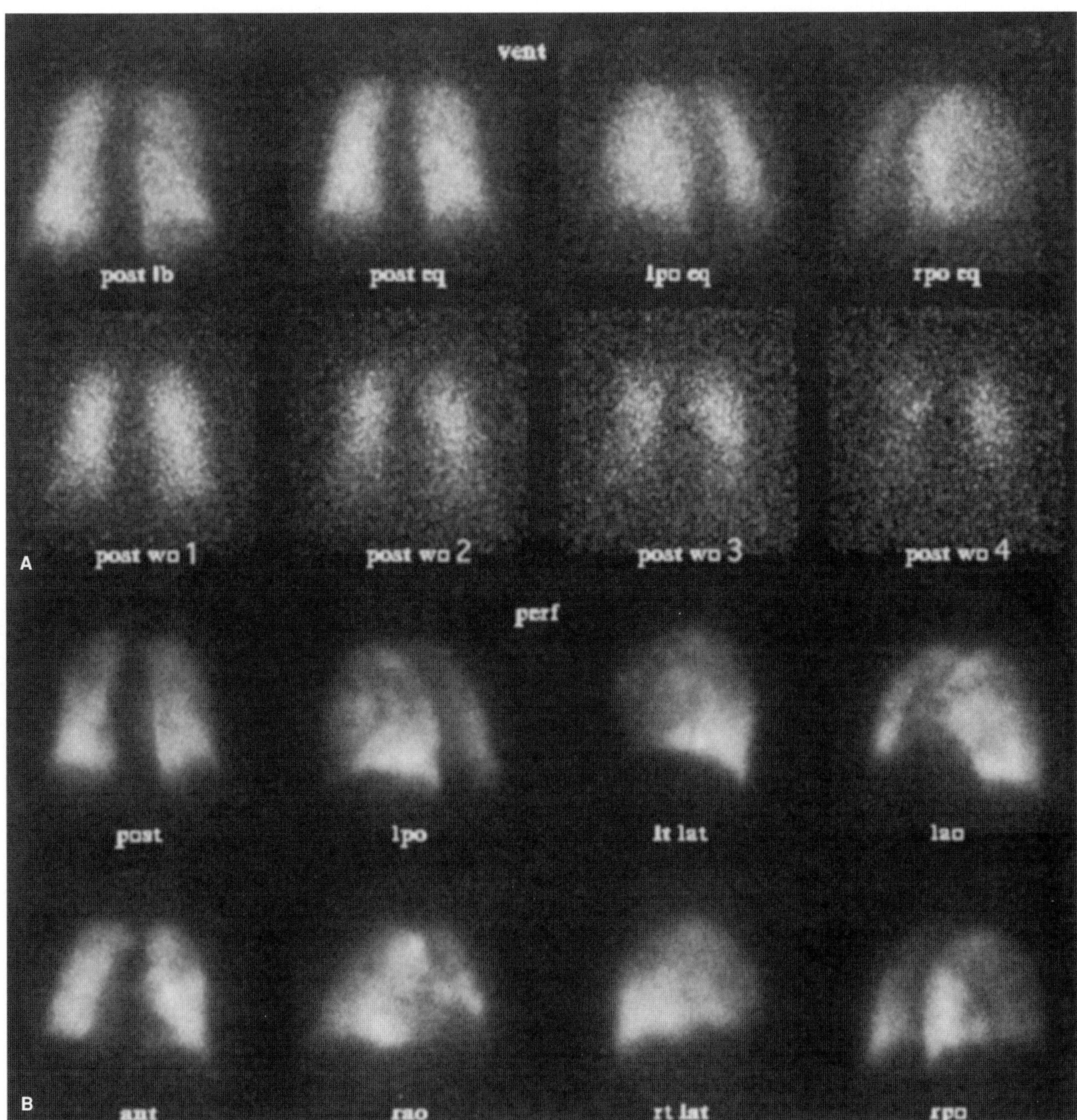

FIGURE 56.4. **Chronic Obstructive Pulmonary Disease. A. Ventilation scan,** posterior projection (top two rows). Obstructive changes in middle and upper lobes cause retention of xenon-133 on 4- minute washout image (post wo/4). post 1b, posterior initial breath; post eq, posterior equilibrium; lpo eq, left posterior oblique equilibrium; rpo eq, right posterior oblique equilibrium; second row: post-washout images at 1 to 4 minutes. **B. Technetium-99m macroaggregated albumin perfusion scan** (bottom two rows). Labeling is the same as in Fig. 56.3. Patchy, inhomogeneous uptake is seen primarily in the middle and upper lung zones. Perfusion defects match those seen on the initial-breath image of the ventilation scan.

VENTILATION/PERFUSION SCAN INTERPRETATION

Multiple, bilateral perfusion defects with a normal ventilation scan are the classic diagnostic findings of PE (Fig. 56.5). Pulmonary emboli that occlude pulmonary arteries produce segmental perfusion defects that extend to the pleural surface. However, pneumonia, COPD, tumors, and prior infarcts may also produce perfusion defects. The ventilation scan is performed to improve the low specificity

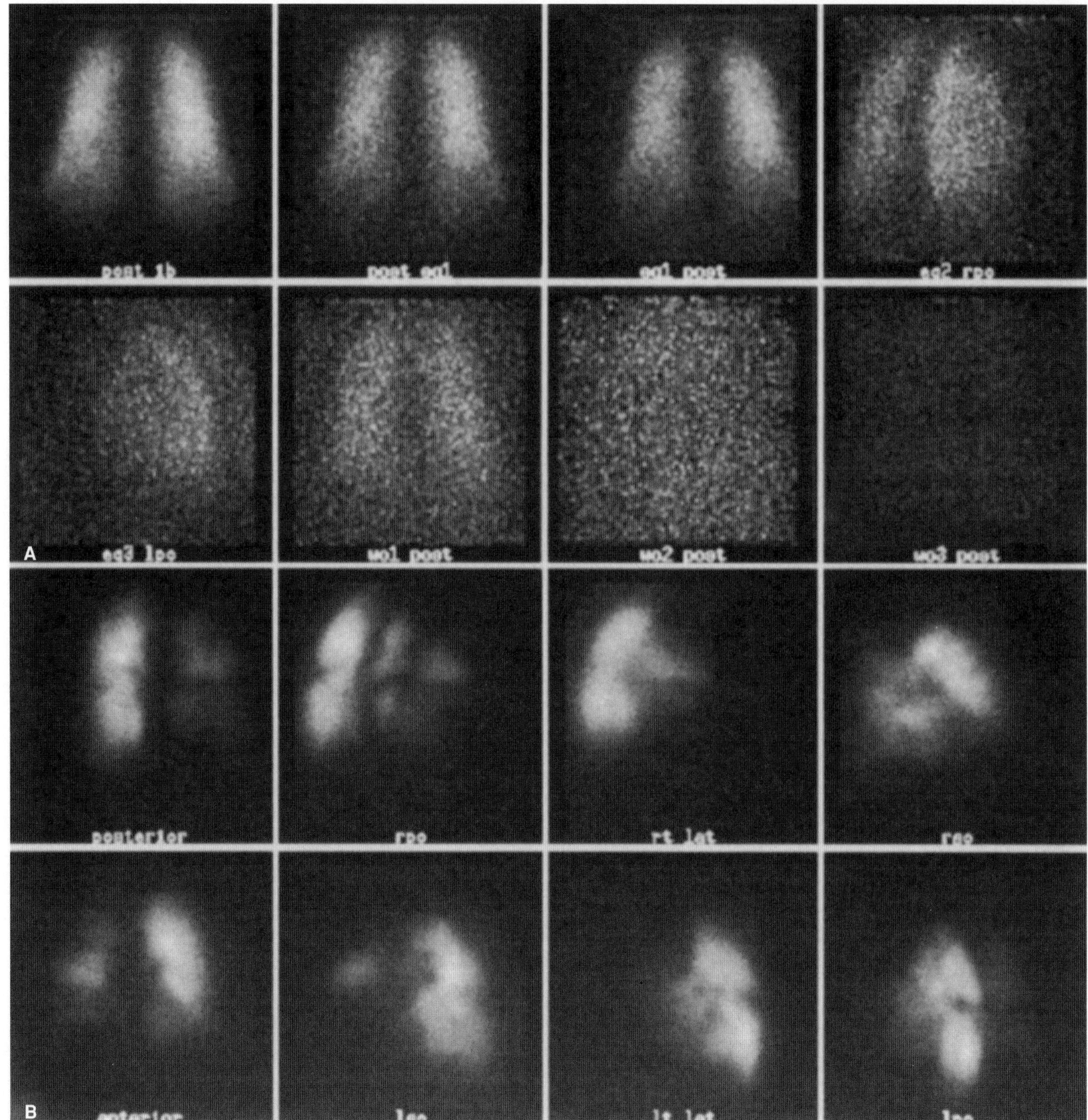

FIGURE 56.5. **High-Probability Ventilation/Perfusion Scan. A. Xenon-133 ventilation scan** (top two rows) is normal. **B. Technetium-99m macroaggregated albumin perfusion scan** (bottom two rows). The perfusion scan demonstrates absence of perfusion to most segments of the right lung with multiple subsegmental defects in the left lung. Labeling is the same as in Fig. 56.3.

of the perfusion scan. The bronchial tree is unaffected by vascular embolization; thus, ventilation of the embolized region remains normal. Most nonembolic lung diseases have both ventilation and perfusion abnormalities, which are typically matched defects. Pulmonary emboli are more common in the lower lobes because more pulmonary blood flow goes to the basilar pulmonary segments.

V/Q scan findings are categorized according to the likelihood that emboli will be demonstrated on pulmonary angiography. All interpretation schemas are based on careful analysis of perfusion scan defects to determine whether they correspond to anatomic segments or subsegments of the lung. An understanding of the segmental anatomy of the lung is essential. The shape, location, and size of any defect are analyzed for fit to a specific pulmonary segment on all views.

The size of a segmental defect must be assessed. By definition, a defect of less than 25% of a pulmonary

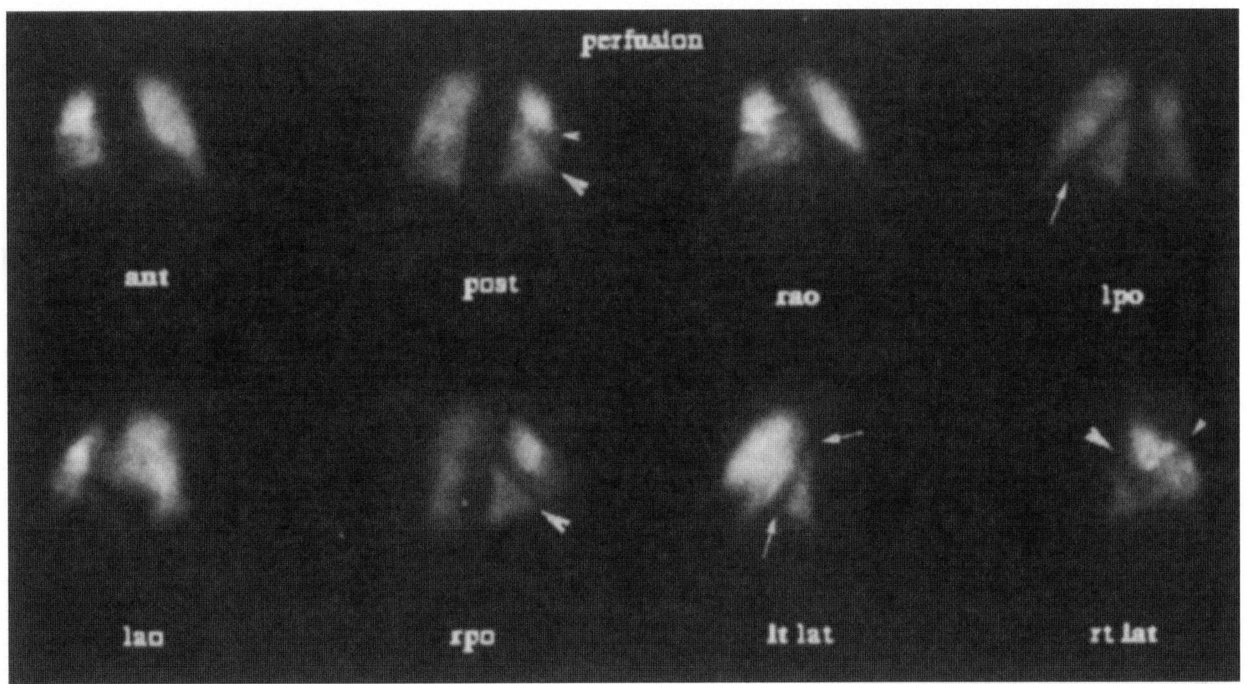

FIGURE 56.6. **Low-Probability Perfusion Scan With Bilateral Pleural Effusions.** Scan demonstrates bilateral wedge-shaped defects that correspond to pleural effusions within the major fissures bilaterally (*open arrows*) and the minor fissure on the right (*closed arrow*). Ant, anterior; post, posterior, rao, right anterior oblique; lpo, left posterior oblique, lao, left anterior oblique; rpo, right posterior oblique; lt lat, left lateral; rt lat, right lateral.

segment is a small defect, 25% to 75% is a moderate defect, and greater than 75% is a large defect. Subsegmental defects are summed to provide full-segment equivalents. Two moderate or four small perfusion defects are equivalent to a full-segment defect. Even experienced readers tend to underestimate the size of segmental defects.

Interpretation schemes compare defects visualized on the perfusion scan with corresponding regions of the ventilation scan and CXR. A perfusion defect that demonstrates normal ventilation is termed a *mismatched defect.* A perfusion defect the same size and location as a ventilation defect is called a *matched defect.* Perfusion defects that match ventilation and CXR abnormalities in size and location are called *triple match defects.* The size and number of matched and/or mismatched segmental defects are used to estimate the likelihood that the defects represent emboli.

Nonsegmental defects should be compared to CXRs to determine whether a mass, an effusion, or a mediastinal or hilar structure is responsible for the perfusion scan finding. Non–wedge-shaped defects, or wedge-shaped defects that do not correspond to segmental anatomy, are usually not caused by pulmonary emboli. Common nonsegmental defects include cardiomegaly, pleural effusions (Fig. 56.6), adenopathy, hilar and parenchymal masses, cardiac pacemakers (Fig. 56.7), pneumonia, large bullae, atelectasis, pulmonary hemorrhage, and aortic aneurysm or tortuosity.

Diagnostic Criteria. The Biello criteria originally categorized V/Q scans as normal, low probability, intermediate, or high probability. The PIOPED (Prospective Investigation of Pulmonary Embolism Diagnosis) study used a modified Biello schema, with more detailed categorizations of V/Q scan patterns. The PIOPED classification has undergone several revisions after retrospective analysis of the data pointed out subcategories of incorrectly classified scan patterns. The amended PIOPED criteria are listed in Table 56.1, with examples provided in Figs. 56.3, 56.6, 56.7, and 56.8.

Stripe and Fissure Signs. Two types of perfusion defects not listed in either the original PIOPED or Biello criteria have been found to strongly correlate with a normal pulmonary angiogram. Central perfusion defects that have a rim or stripe of increased activity around them have a less than 10% probability of being caused by PE. The defect should be seen in different views to not extend to the pleural surface. The surrounding stripe of perfused lung is called the *stripe sign.* PE perfusion defects extend to the pleural surface and have no overlying stripe of perfused lung.

Perfusion defects that match the location and shape of the major or minor fissures of the lung usually represent

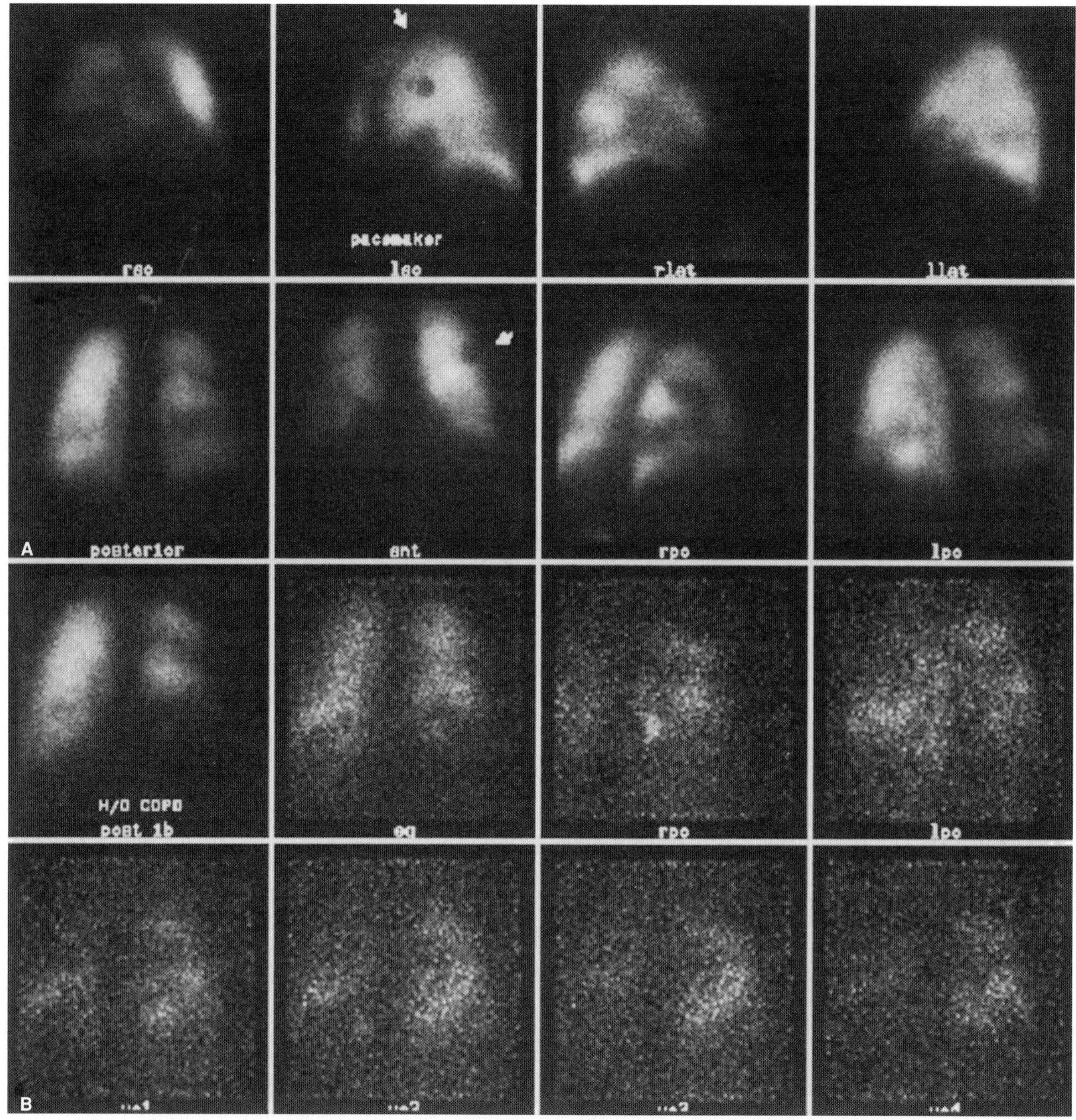

FIGURE 56.7. **Chronic Obstructive Pulmonary Disease. A. Technetium-99m macroaggregated albumin perfusion** (top two rows). Moderate to large bilateral perfusion defects match the ventilation scan defects. A nonsegmental defect is also present over the left upper lobe, representing an artifact secondary to a cardiac pacemaker (*arrow*). **B. Xenon-133 ventilation scan** (bottom two rows). Patchy defects are seen in the mid and lower lung zones on the right on the initial breath image (post 1b). The defects partially fill in on the equilibrium images (eq, rpo, lpo). Persistent retention of xenon-133 is seen in these same regions on the washout images (wo/1, wo/2, wo/3, wo/4). Labeling is the same as in Fig. 56.3.

pleural effusions tracking up the fissures (Fig. 56.6). When this defect is seen, the lateral view can be repeated with the patient in the supine or decubitus position to demonstrate layering of the fluid. The *fissure sign* usually correlates with the presence of a pleural effusion on CXR.

PIOPED Findings. The PIOPED study was designed to evaluate the usefulness of V/Q scans for diagnosing acute PE. In the original study, 13% of patients had high-probability V/Q scans, 39% had intermediate-probability scans, 34% had low-probability scans, and 14% showed

TABLE 56.1 Amended PIOPED Criteria

V/Q Scan Category	*Criteria*	*Likelihood of PE*	*Prevalence of PE*
High	Two or more mismatched perfusion segments or segmental equivalents without corresponding ventilation or CXR abnormalities: a. ≥2 large segmental perfusion defects b. 1 large and 2 moderate segmental defects c. ≥4 moderate segmental defects	≥80%	87%
Intermediate	1. One moderate to ≤2 large mismatched segments or segmental equivalents without corresponding ventilation or CXR abnormalities 2. Triple matched defects in the lower lung zone 3. Single moderate matched V/Q defects with normal CXR 4. Corresponding V/Q defects and small pleural effusion 5. Findings difficult to classify as normal, high, or low	20%–79%	35%
Low	1. Multiple matched V/Q defects with a normal CXR 2. Corresponding V/Q defects and CXR opacities (triple matched defects) in the middle or upper lung zones 3. Corresponding V/Q defects and large pleural effusions (more than one third of the hemithorax) 4. Any perfusion defect with substantially larger CXR abnormality 5. Any defect with a rim of surrounding normally perfused lung (stripe sign) 6. >3 small perfusion defects with normal CXR 7. Nonsegmental perfusion defects	≤19%	12%
Very low	<3 small perfusion defects with a normal CXR		2.5%
Normal	No defects present on the perfusion scan, or they exactly match the shape of the lungs on CXR		0

CXR, chest radiograph; V/Q, ventilation/perfusion.

normal or near-normal scans. The interobserver agreement in classifying scans was very good (92% to 95%) for normal/near-normal scans and high-probability scans, but it was significantly worse for low- and intermediate-probability scans (25% to 30%). The prevalence of thromboembolism in patients who underwent angiography was 33%. The sensitivity of a high-probability scan was 41%, with a specificity of 97%.

The positive predictive value for a high-probability scan was 91% in patients with no prior history of PE but fell to 74% in those who had previously documented PE. Prior PE may leave residual perfusion defects that cannot be distinguished from acute emboli unless comparison scans are available. Use of two segmental equivalents as the criteria for high probability yielded a likelihood for PE of 71%. Use of 2.5 segmental equivalent mismatched defects was 100% predictive of PE.

The negative predictive value of a normal/near-normal scan was 91% to 96%, whereas that of a low-probability scan was 84% to 88%. Patients with normal or nearly normal V/Q scans are highly unlikely to have clinically significant PE.

Clinical Assessment and Ventilation/Perfusion Scan Interpretation. The V/Q scan should not be interpreted in a clinical vacuum. The PIOPED study demonstrated that the addition of the clinical assessment to V/Q scan interpretation improved the chance of correctly evaluating the patient's risk of having PE. Of patients with high-probability scans and a high clinical suspicion, 96% had emboli on pulmonary angiography. Of patients with low-probability scans and low clinical suspicion, 96% had no evidence of PE on angiography. Patients with high-probability scans but intermediate clinical suspicion had an 88% positive PE rate, whereas those with high-probability scans and low clinical suspicion had a 56% positive PE rate. Patients with high-probability scans and high or intermediate clinical suspicion have a high risk of PE, which justifies treatment with anticoagulants. Patients with low-probability scans and low clinical suspicion have a very low chance of having PE.

Ventilation/Perfusion Scans and Pulmonary Angiography. Patients with intermediate-probability scans have a significant risk of PE. However, the V/Q scan alone is insufficient in determining which of these require anticoagulation therapy. Patients with intermediate-probability scans (Fig. 56.9) and multiple risk factors or clinical findings suggestive of DVT should undergo another examination such as Doppler US or CTA. If DVT is diagnosed, the patient can be placed on anticoagulants that would treat the DVT and serendipitously treat any PE. If the noninvasive search for DVT is negative, then CTA or pulmonary angiography should be performed. The location of mismatched defects on the perfusion scan would be the most likely sites for PE. CTA or pulmonary angiography should

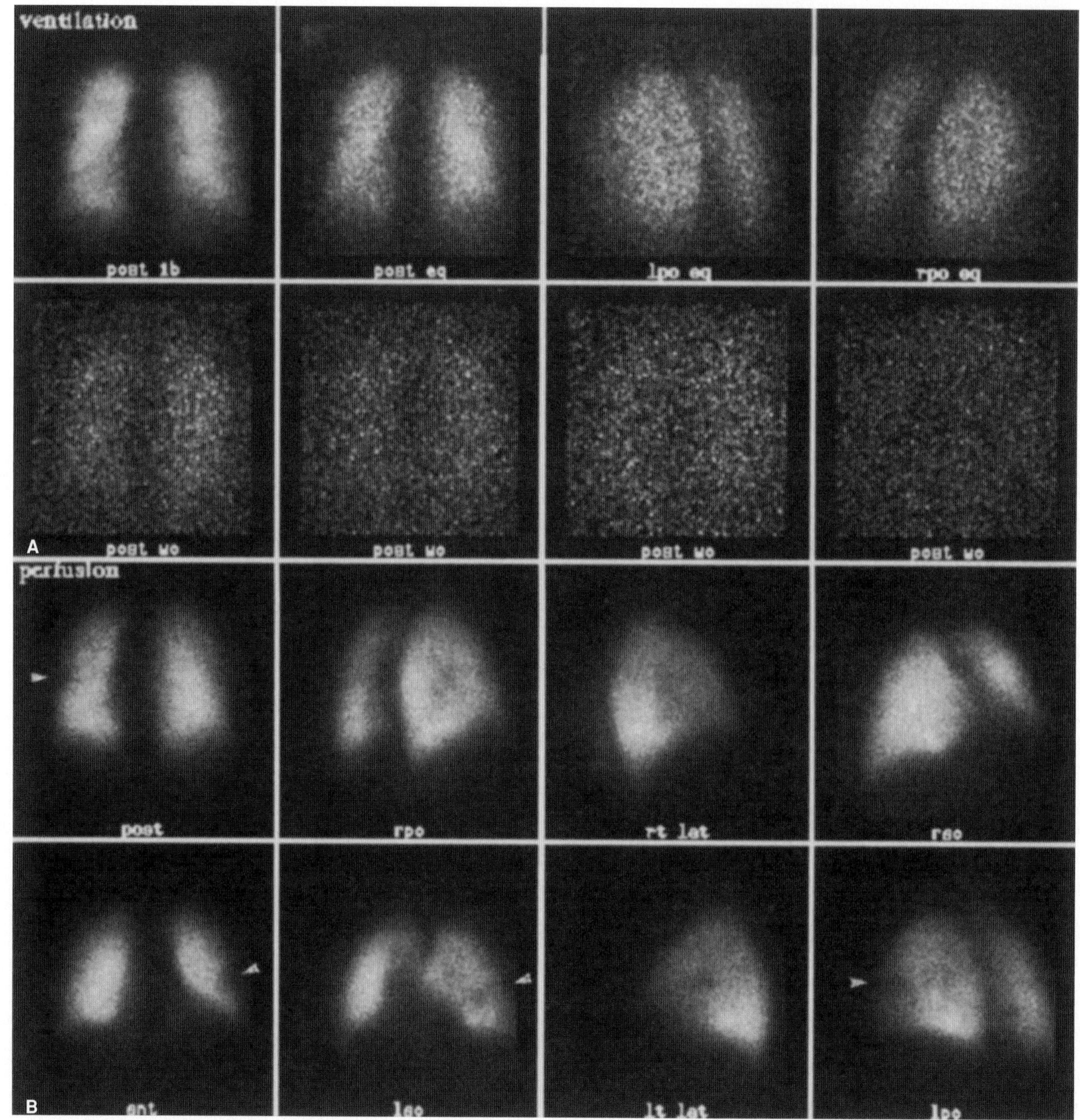

FIGURE 56.8. **Intermediate-Probability Ventilation/Perfusion Scan. A. Xenon-133 ventilation scan** (top two rows) demonstrates a moderate-sized defect in the anterior medial basal segment of the left lower lobe (*open arrow*). **B. Technetium-99m macroaggregated albumin perfusion lung scan** (bottom two rows). A single, moderate-sized matched perfusion defect is seen in the anterior medial basal segment of the left lower lobe (*arrowheads*).

also be strongly considered to confirm the diagnosis of PE in patients with high-probability scans when anticoagulation is risky. It also may be indicated in patients with low-probability scans but high clinical suspicion for having PE.

Follow-up Ventilation/Perfusion Scans Following Anticoagulation. Most patients with PE show a gradual reduction in the size of perfusion defects, with normalization of their scans within 3 months. Defects that are still present after 3 months of anticoagulation will usually remain as permanent abnormalities. The larger the initial defect, the less likely it is to completely resolve. Perfusion scan defects are thought to last longer than filling defects detectable on CTA and pulmonary angiography.

Follow-up scans done within 2 weeks of the initiation of anticoagulation therapy may show new defects that do

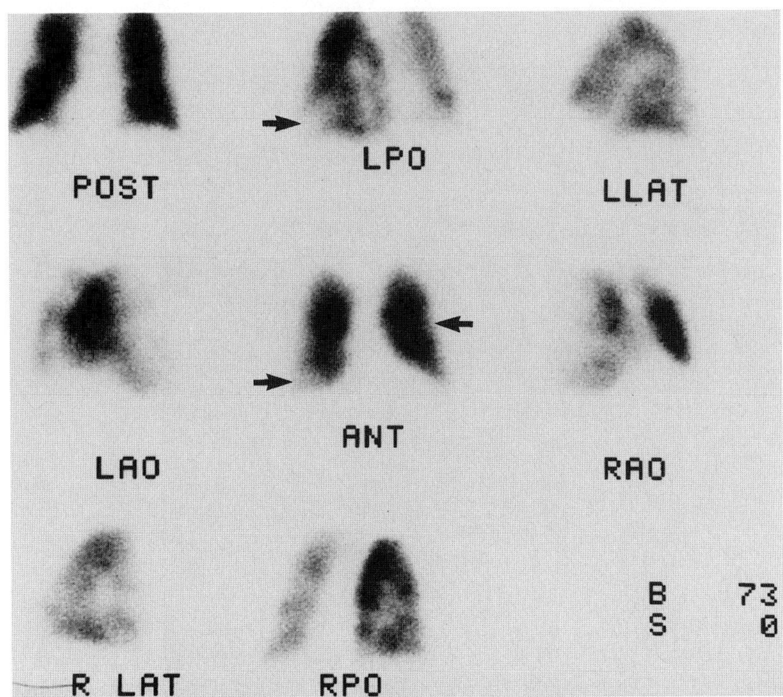

FIGURE 56.9. **Intermediate-Probability Ventilation/Perfusion Scan.** Technetium-99m macroaggregated albumin perfusion scan demonstrates multiple bilateral small and moderate defects (*arrows*). The xenon-133 ventilation scan was normal.

not represent recurrent emboli. Large central thrombi may fragment and produce small distal thrombi. Thus, emboli that were previously nonocclusive may become obstructive and show as new defects. The diagnosis of recurrent PE is more likely if multiple new large or moderate defects are present in areas that were previously normal (Fig. 56.10).

False-Positive Ventilation/Perfusion Scans. Mismatched perfusion defects can represent chronic pulmonary emboli in patients with a remote history of PE. Follow-up V/Q scans after patients have been placed on oral anticoagulants are useful as baselines in this patient population. If old scans are available, it is possible to determine which emboli are old and which are new. Patients with a history of PE are at higher risk of another PE than patients without such a history. Mismatched perfusion defects can also be produced by extrinsic compression of the pulmonary vessels, such as mass lesions or adenopathy. The pulmonary vessels may also become obstructed by mediastinal fibrosis, intraluminal metastases, sarcomas, and lymphangitic carcinomatosis. Radiation therapy and vasculitides, such as Takayasu arteritis and systemic lupus erythematosus, can also cause false-positive scans.

False-Negative Ventilation/Perfusion Scans. V/Q scans may be falsely negative if the emboli are only partially occlusive. Very small emboli may produce perfusion defects that are too small to be visualized on a perfusion scan, but are thought to be clinically insignificant.

NONTHROMBOEMBOLIC PULMONARY DISEASE

Asthma produces bronchospastic narrowing of the airways, resulting in decreased ventilation. Focal segmental or subsegmental ventilation defects are present on the first-breath image during an acute asthma attack. These defects may wash in later on the equilibrium images. Defects associated with mucous plugs may persist. Bronchospasm induces localized hypoxia, which in turn produces localized vasoconstriction and perfusion scan defects that match the ventilation defects. This can result in an intermediate- or low-probability scan. Most V/Q defects caused by asthma will resolve with 24 hours of bronchodilator therapy.

Lung neoplasms may produce V/Q scan abnormalities. Focal parenchymal masses and extrinsic mediastinal or chest wall tumors that displace lung parenchyma tend to produce matching V/Q defects, which correspond to the size and shape of the mass on CXR. The V/Q defects do not correspond to segmental anatomy unless the mass has invaded or compressed a local branch of the bronchovascular tree. This may result in a perfusion defect, a ventilation defect, or a matched defect.

Quantitative Perfusion Lung Scan. Perfusion lung scans are useful in preoperatively estimating a lung carcinoma patient's postsurgical pulmonary function. The quantitative perfusion scan is performed in the same manner as a regular perfusion lung scan, except that a single posterior image is obtained. Regions of interest are drawn

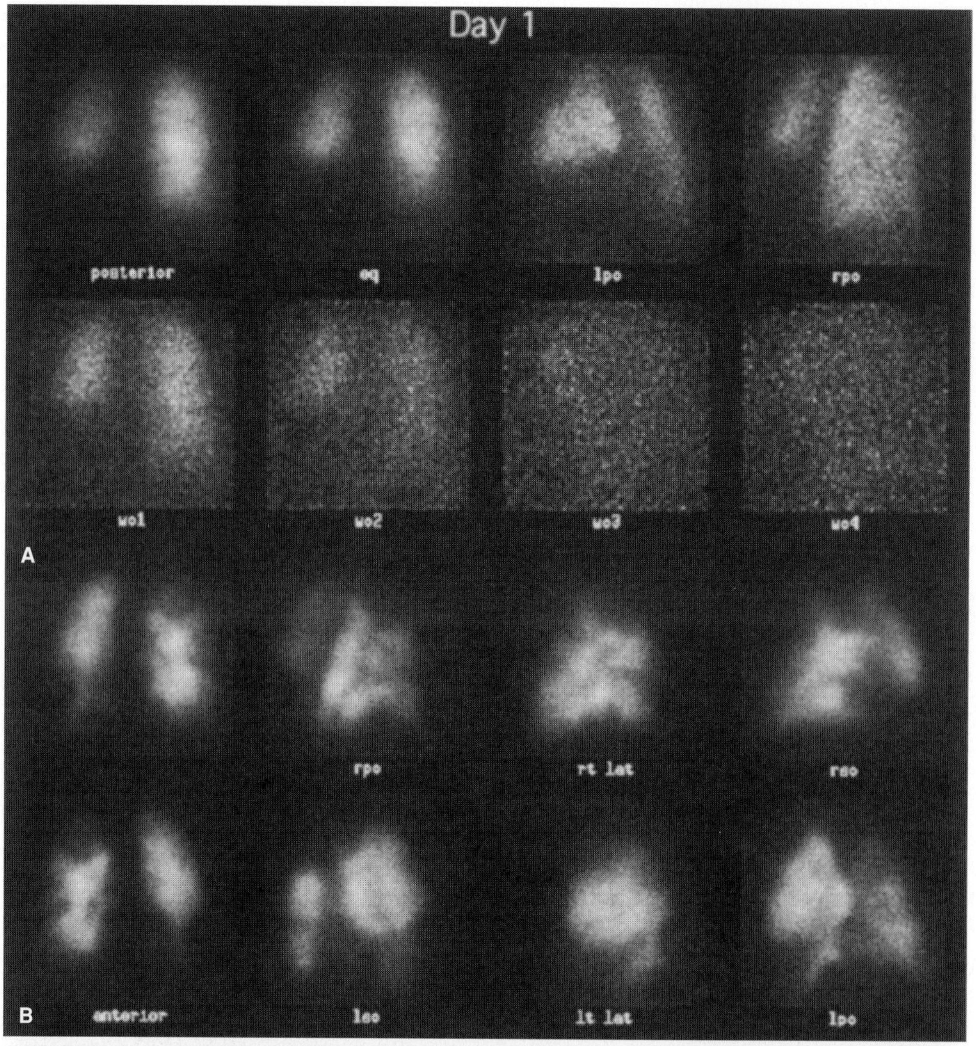

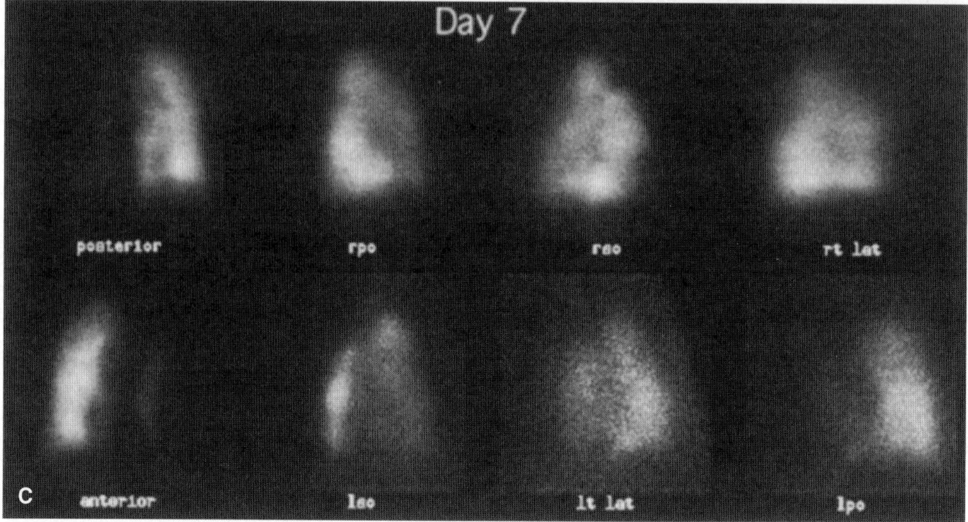

FIGURE 56.10. **Recurrent Pulmonary Emboli. A. Xenon-133 ventilation scan** (top two rows) demonstrates lack of ventilation of most of the left lower lobe owing to a pleural effusion. **B. Technetium-99m macroaggregated albumin perfusion scan** (third and fourth rows) demonstrates multiple moderate and large mismatched perfusion defects in the right lung. **C. Repeat technetium-99m macroaggregated albumin perfusion scan** was performed 1 week later. The patient had recurrent symptoms while being treated with heparin. Marked improvement is seen in the perfusion defects previously noted in the right lung, indicating resolution of some of the emboli with therapy. The left lung on the new scan shows almost complete absence of perfusion, indicative of new emboli to the lungs despite anticoagulation.

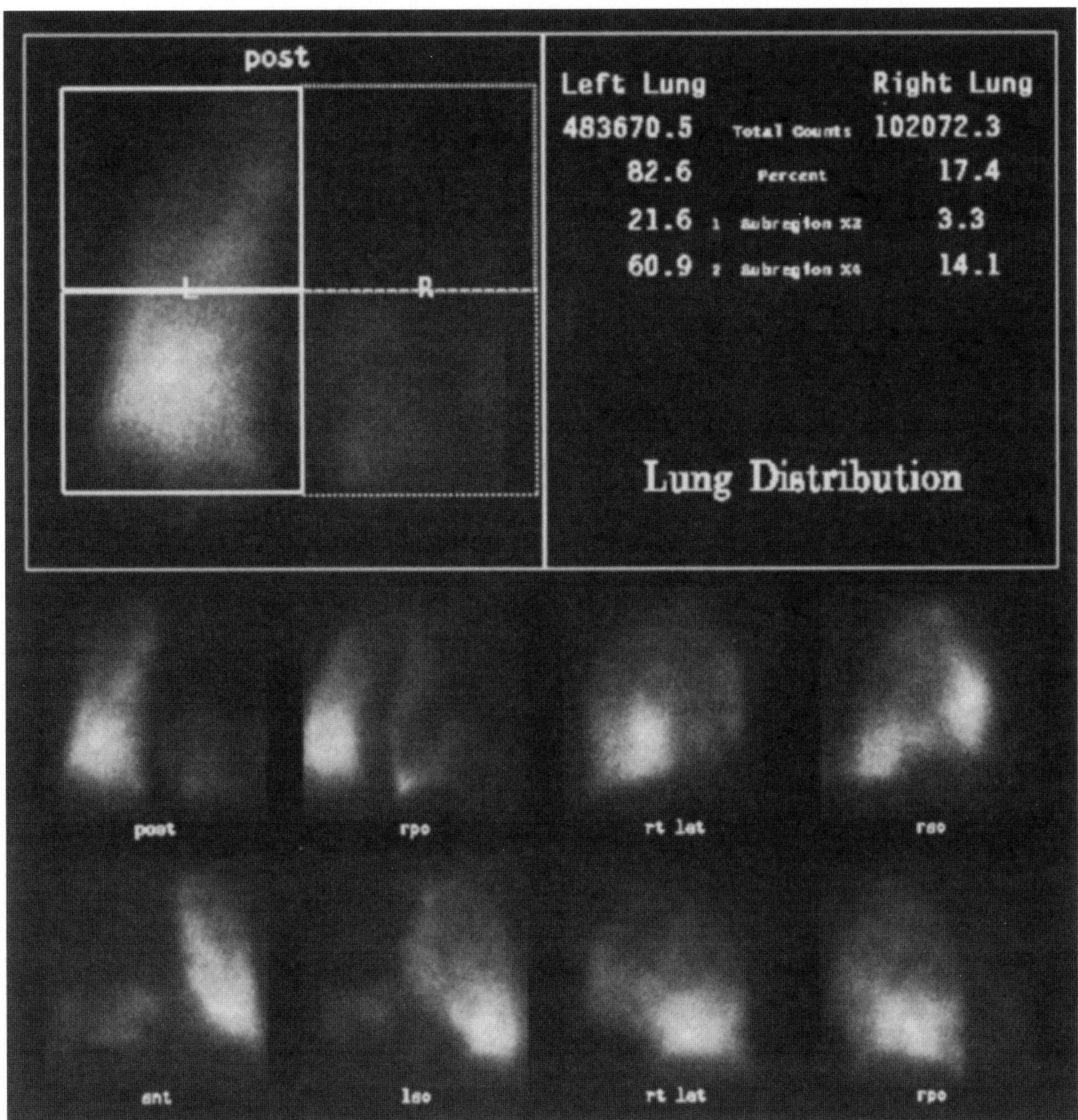

FIGURE 56.11. **Quantitative Technetium-99m Macroaggregated Albumin Perfusion Scan.** The percentage of the pulmonary perfusion to each lung is calculated based on the relative counts over each lung on the posterior image.

around each lung, and the counts over each lung are obtained. The percentage of the total count that each lung contributes is calculated (Fig. 56.11). The postoperative FEV1 (forced expiratory volume in 1 second) is estimated by multiplying the preoperative FEV1 by the percent perfusion going to the lung that will remain after pneumonectomy. With SPECT acquisition or a lateral projection, outcomes for an upper or lower lobectomy can also be estimated. A patient needs to have a postoperative FEV1 of 800 to 1,000 mL to have adequate lung function.

Chronic Obstructive Pulmonary Disease. The narrowed airways associated with COPD reduce ventilation. Xe scans demonstrate delayed wash-in and delayed washout. First-breath images may have defects that gradually fill in on the equilibrium phase. Xe washes out of the affected area more slowly than the rest of the lung and may still be visible on images more than

3 minutes after the patient was switched to breathing room air.

Perfusion lung scans are also frequently abnormal. Localized hypoxia in the lung induces localized vasoconstriction. Destruction of lung tissue and inflammatory narrowing of blood vessels produce areas of reduced perfusion. Regions of the lung that demonstrate obstructive changes on the ventilation scan usually have corresponding abnormalities on the perfusion scan (Figs. 56.3, 56.6). When the ventilatory changes are widespread, the perfusion scan has a mottled appearance. Perfusion scans may be normal if the ventilatory obstructive changes produce little hypoxia or vascular damage. Because COPD tends to affect the lung apices more than the bases, V/Q abnormalities are usually more pronounced at the apices. However, a-1-antitrypsin deficiency produces more pronounced emphysematous changes in the lower lobes, which are reflected on the V/Q scan.

Inflammatory/Infectious Disease of the Lung. Areas of consolidation on CXR will be abnormal on a V/Q scan. Consolidated areas do not ventilate well and will produce defects on ventilation scans. The resulting local hypoxia produces reflex vasoconstriction and may cause perfusion defects in the consolidated region. Perfusion defects that are significantly smaller than the consolidated region on CXR are low probability for PE. Perfusion defects that are significantly larger than the CXR abnormality are high probability for PE.

Tc-99m aerosol clearance from the lung has also been used to evaluate inflammatory diseases of the lung. Normal lungs have a Tc-99m aerosol lung clearance half-life of approximately 60 minutes. Increased permeability of inflamed pulmonary epithelium shortens the clearance time. Alveolitis and ARDS have rapid Tc-99m aerosol lung clearance. Smokers also have faster-than-normal aerosol clearance. Conversely, processes that thicken the alveolar membranes or cause fibrosis will have prolonged Tc-99m aerosol clearance. Abnormal aerosol clearance is a very sensitive but nonspecific indicator of inflammation.

Smoke Inhalation. Many patients with serious burns also have inhalation injury of the lungs. Of patients admitted to a hospital for burns, 20% to 30% develop pulmonary complications; 70% to 75% of these patients die. Smoke consists of a mixture of toxic gases and particles. Inhalation of these toxins combines with thermal injury to produce severe pulmonary damage. A CXR is insensitive in detecting early inhalation injury, with a lag period of 12 to 48 hours before the radiograph becomes abnormal. Xe-in-saline ventilation scans have proven useful in detecting inhalation lung injury. Xe-133 under pressure will dissolve in saline; when injected intravenously, the Xe remains in solution until it reaches the lungs. In the alveolar capillaries, the Xe diffuses across the capillary membrane into the alveoli and is exhaled. Normally, the Xe washes out of the lungs in less than 2 minutes. Areas of inhalational injury demonstrate retention of Xe. The Xe-in-saline study is 92% accurate in detecting lung injury.

SUGGESTED READINGS

Cham MD, Yankelevitz DF, Henschke CI. Thromboembolic disease detection at indirect CT venography versus CT pulmonary angiography. Radiology 2005;234:591–594.

Dahlen JE, Alpert JS. Natural history of pulmonary embolism. Prog Cardiovasc Dis 1975;17:259–270.

Eng J, Krishnah JA, Segal JB, et al. Accuracy of CT in the diagnosis of pulmonary embolism: a systematic literature review. AJR Am J Roentgenol 2004;183:1819–1827.

Eyer BA, Goodman LR, Washington L. Clinicians response to radiologists' reports of isolated subsegmental pulmonary embolism or inconclusive interpretation of pulmonary embolism using MDCT. AJR Am J Roentgenol 2005;184:623–625.

Fraser RS, Muller NL, Coleman N, Pare PD. Diagnosis of Diseases of the Chest. 4th ed. Philadelphia: WB Saunders, 1999.

Goldberg SN, Richardson DD, Palmer EL, et al. Pleural effusion and ventilation/perfusion scan interpretation for acute pulmonary embolus. J Nucl Med 1996;37:1310–1313.

Gottschalk A, Sostman HD, Coleman RE, et al. Ventilation-perfusion scintigraphy in the PIOPED study. Part II. Evaluation of the scintigraphic criteria and interpretations. J Nucl Med 1993;34:1119–1126.

Gottschalk A, Stein PD, Henry JW, et al. Matched ventilation, perfusion and chest radiographic abnormalities in acute pulmonary embolism. J Nucl Med 1996;37:1636–1638.

Henry JW, Stein PD, Gottschalk A, et al. Pulmonary embolism among patients with a nearly normal ventilation/ perfusion lung scan. Chest 1996;110:395–398.

Juni JE, Alavi A. Lung scanning in the diagnosis of pulmonary embolism: the emperor redressed. Semin Nucl Med 1991;21:281–296.

Kipper MS, Moser KM, Kortman KE, et al. Long term follow-up of patients with suspected pulmonary embolism and a normal lung scan. Chest 1982;82:411–415.

Muto P, Lastoria S, Varrella P, et al. Detecting deep venous thrombosis with technetium-99m-labeled synthetic peptide P280. J Nucl Med 1995;36:1384–1391.

Parker JA, Coleman RE, Siegel BA, et al. Procedure guideline for lung scintigraphy: 1.0. J Nucl Med 1996;37:1906–1910.

The PIOPED Investigators. Value of the ventilation/perfusion scan in acute pulmonary embolism. Results of the Prospective Investigation of Pulmonary Embolism Diagnosis (PIOPED). JAMA 1990;263:2753–2759.

Sostman HD, Coleman RE, DeLong DM, et al. Evaluation of revised criteria for ventilation-perfusion scintigraphy in patients with suspected pulmonary embolism. Radiology 1994;193:103–107.

Wittram C, Maher MM, Yoo AJ, et al. CT angiography of pulmonary embolism: diagnostic criteria and causes of misdiagnosis. Radiographics 2004;24:1219–1238.

Worsley DF, Alavi A. Comprehensive analysis of the results of the PIOPED study. J Nucl Med 1995;36:2380–2387.

Worsley DF, Alavi A. Radionuclide imaging of acute pulmonary embolism. Radiol Clin North Am 2001;39:1035–1052.

Chapter 57

Cardiovascular System Scintigraphy

David K. Shelton and Michael F. Hartshorne

Myocardial Perfusion Scans
Technique
Radiopharmaceuticals
Interpretation
Positron Emission Tomography

Gated Blood Pool Scans
Technique
Interpretation

Right Ventricular Studies
First-Pass Function Studies
First-Pass Flow Studies

Nuclear medicine applications in the cardiovascular system include gated or nongated myocardial perfusion imaging, myocardial viability studies, infarction imaging, gated ventricular function studies of the blood pool in the ventricles, and detection and quantitation of intracardiac shunts.

MYOCARDIAL PERFUSION SCANS

Technique

Each of the perfusion agents may be imaged with planar techniques or with SPECT. Meticulous quality control of the stress and rest images is essential. The comparison of images between stress and rest requires identical repositioning so that the same areas of myocardium are visualized. Poor positioning will lead to false-positive interpretations of ischemia and infarct.

The three principle coronary artery distributions of the LV are the left anterior descending artery (LAD), the left circumflex artery (LCX), and the posterior descending artery (PDA). Each artery normally provides an equal intensity of myocardial labeling at any given level of cardiac work. Perfusion of the thinner right ventricular wall is considerably less than that of the LV, but it can be imaged using the same techniques (Figs. 57.1 to 57.3).

Exercise on a treadmill, or simulation of exercise by infusion of dipyridamole or adenosine, is used in conjunction with perfusion agents to increase radionuclide delivery to the normal myocardium. Stepwise increases in physical exercise are monitored by sequential electrocardiogram (ECG) and blood pressure and pulse measurements while the patient is queried for symptoms of angina. The radiopharmaceutical is injected under conditions of maximal exercise, which should be continued for 30 to 60 seconds after injection to obtain optimal mapping of stress perfusion. Exercise should reach at least 85% of the maximum predicted heart rate to achieve adequate stress. Exercise may also be stopped because of chest pain and ischemic changes on the ECG. Adequacy of the exercise challenge can be more thoroughly estimated simply from a calculation of the "double product" (DP) (systolic pressure × heart rate = DP). The DP correlates with an individual's myocardial work performed, whereas the duration of exercise and heart rate alone may not. For exercise to be judged as adequate, the DP should double, or preferably triple, from rest to peak exercise and should rise to above 20,000.

For those patients who cannot perform physical exercise, coronary vasodilatation can be pharmacologically induced. IV dipyridamole or adenosine will vasodilate normal coronary arteries but does not effectively increase flow through vessels with 50% stenosis or greater. Those areas, which cannot dilate normally, will appear to have decreased myocardial perfusion when compared with the rest of the myocardium.

IV dobutamine can also be used when dipyridamole or adenosine are contraindicated, such as active bronchospasm. Dobutamine has direct inotropic and chronotropic effects that result in increased coronary flow

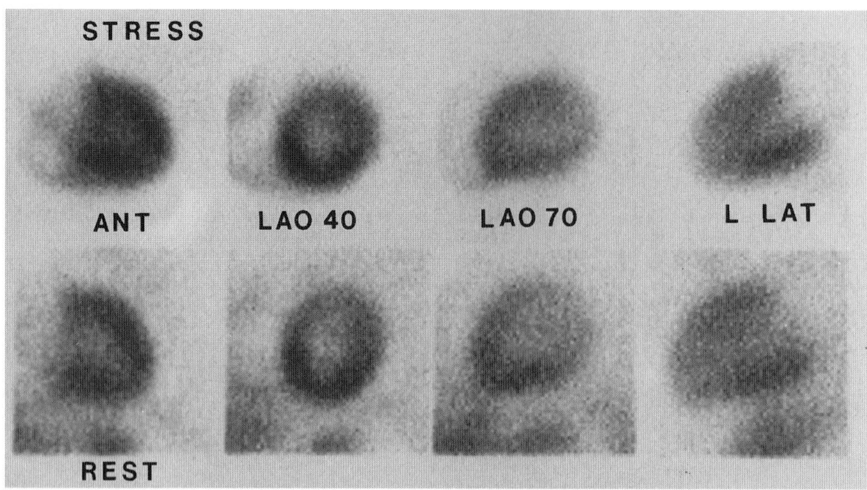

FIGURE 57.1. **Normal Exercise/Rest Planar Technetium-99m Sestamibi Myocardial Scan.** Anterior (ANT), left anterior oblique (LAO 40, LAO 70), and left lateral (L LAT) planar views of a 380-pound patient, with the upper row representing stress and the lower row representing rest injections of the radiopharmaceutical. Note the superb image quality in spite of the patient's large size.

similar to true exercise. Areas of relative hypoperfusion result from coronary stenosis.

Image Acquisition. Planar imaging has largely been replaced by SPECT imaging with reconstruction of the LV myocardium into short-axis, vertical long-axis, and horizontal long-axis planes. A 180° acquisition is generally preferred over 360° acquisition because of the asymmetry of the heart in the thorax and owing to spine attenuation effects in the posterior projections. ECG gated acquisitions are readily accomplished for technetium and thallium radiotracers, allowing evaluation of wall motion, brightening, and thickening from diastole to systole. Functional data acquisition has also become routine, allowing accurate calculations of end-diastolic volume, end-systolic volume, and left ventricular ejection fraction (LVEF). ECG gated planar imaging can still be accomplished for patients who cannot be imaged on the SPECT table (often because of weight).

The tomographic images from SPECT have improved the accuracy of myocardial perfusion imaging (MPI) and provide better correlation to other imaging modalities such as echocardiography, CT, and MR. The addition of ECG gated SPECT allows wall motion analysis and functional information, which has improved interpretation and made MPI a more complete examination.

Prone imaging is frequently accomplished after the standard supine, post–stress acquisition, and may help reduce false-positive results caused by breast or diaphragm attenuation, hot bowel loops, or motion artifacts. Attenuation correction can also be accomplished with emission

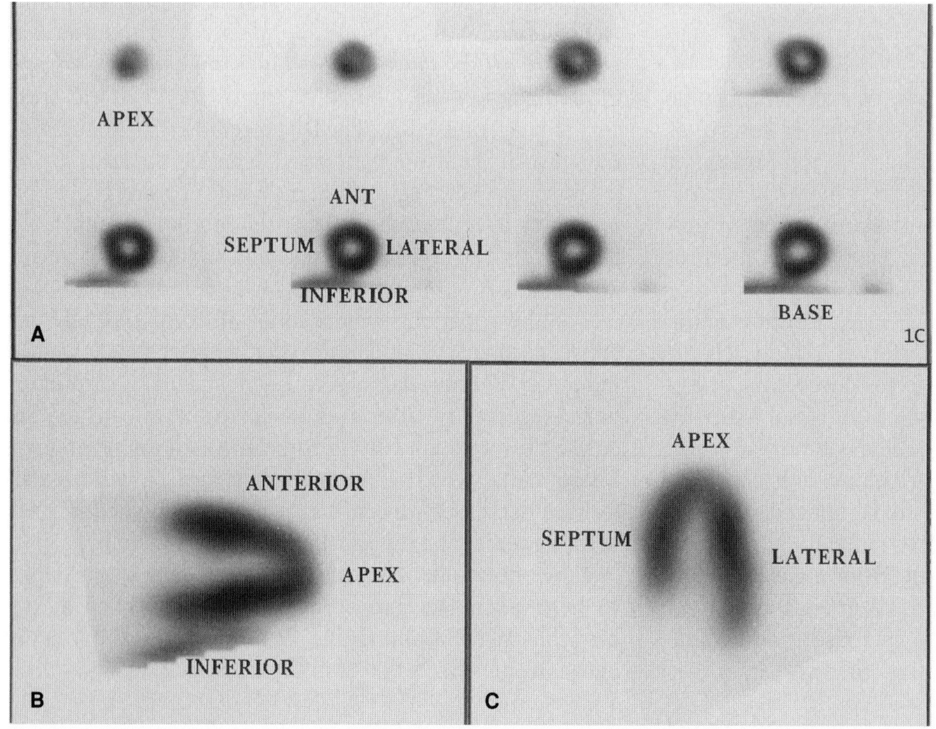

FIGURE 57.2. **Normal SPECT Projections.** Short-axis **(A)**, vertical long-axis **(B)**, and horizontal long-axis **(C)** images in standard projections show the walls of the LV. In the short-axis images, an apical "button" starts the series, which extends back to the base of the ventricle. The names of the walls for the short-axis images are best given by the diagram in Fig. 57.3. In the vertical long-axis images, the anterior and inferior (or posterior) walls are seen. In the horizontal long-axis images, the short septum and long lateral or "free" walls are well seen. The long-axis images also show the apex very well.

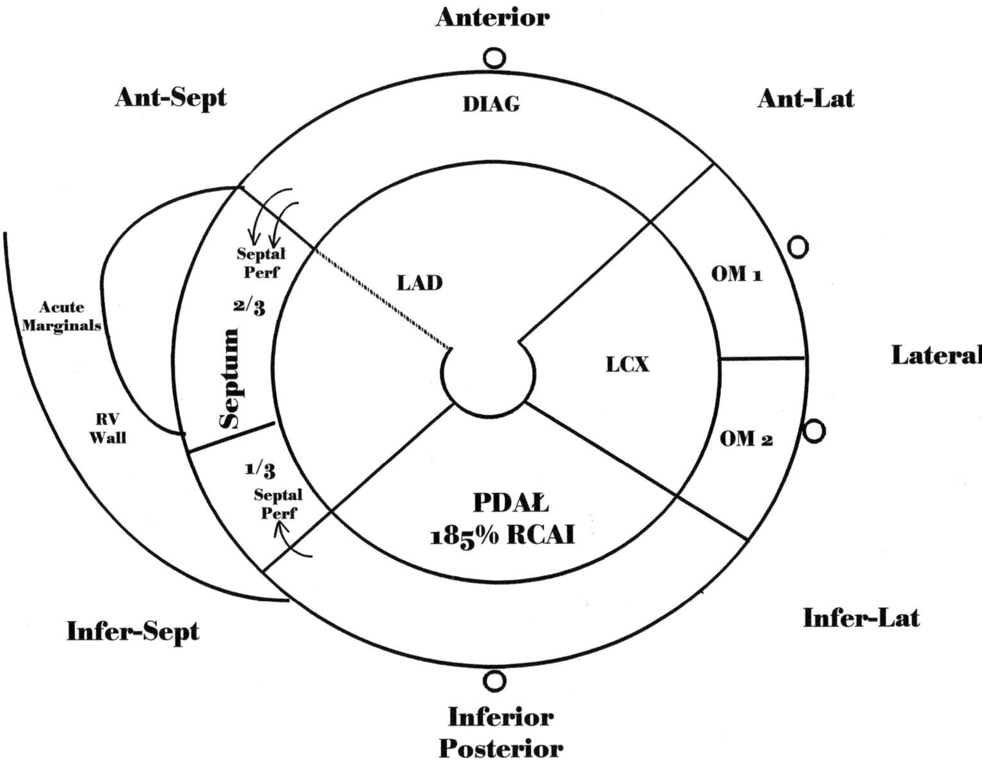

FIGURE 57.3. **LV Short Axis Vascular Distributions and Wall Names.** The schematic diagram locates the expected position of the principle coronary arteries. The left anterior descending artery (LAD) usually serves the apex. The names of the wall segments are listed in a clockwise fashion as anterior, anterior-lateral, lateral, inferior-lateral, inferior, inferior-septal, septal, and anterior-septal. The LAD sends diagonal vessels (numbered with digits in the order in which they leave the LAD, e.g., D1, D2, etc.) onto the anterior and anterior-lateral walls and septal perforators down into the septum. The left circumflex (LCX) sends obtuse marginal (OM) branches along the free wall, numbered in sequence (OM1, OM2, etc.) The posterior descending artery (PDA) arises from the right coronary artery (RCA) 85% of the time and serves the inferior wall and the inferior-septal wall.

sources or on the new SPECT-CT devices. The SPECT camera itself can be a single-, dual-, or triple-headed camera.

Radiopharmaceuticals

Three gamma-emitting radiopharmaceuticals are readily available for mapping the flow of blood to the myocardium. Each has advantages and some disadvantages.

Thallium-201 (Tl-201), an analog of the potassium ion (K^+), is delivered to capillary beds by regional blood flow and is actively pumped into viable cells by the sodium/potassium (Na^+/K^+) adenosine triphosphatase pump. Cyclotron production at a remote site (requiring shipping); a long physical half-life (73 hours); low-energy, poorly penetrating photons (mostly 69- to 83-keV γ rays); and a relatively high absorbed dose (0.24 rad/mCi for the whole body at the usual dose of 2 to 5 mCi) combine to make Tl-201 a less-than-ideal agent for imaging. However, because of its active transport into cells, it is a more physiologic radionuclide than the technetium-99m (Tc-99m)–labeled agents.

A widely used technique utilizes Tl-201 with exercise stress or a pharmacologic challenge. Images are usually acquired as soon after injection as possible. However, some authors advocate waiting for 5 to 10 minutes to allow the exercised patient to stop breathing heavily so that movement of the heart heaving up and down with the diaphragm will be minimized. This slight delay also limits an artifact caused by the "upward creep" of the heart. As the lungs decrease in volume slowly after exercise, the average level of the diaphragm is raised, shifting the heart upward. This shift in location of the heart produces an artifactual shift in radionuclide activity that may be misinterpreted as ischemia.

The effective half-life, or 50% washout, of Tl-201 from the normal myocardium is about 4 hours. A complex "redistribution" of the isotope within the myocardium is governed by rates of washout from myocardial cells, renal

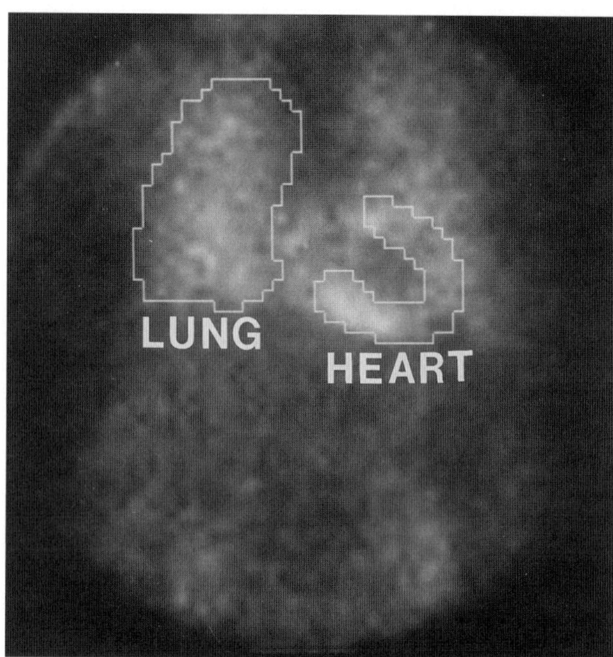

FIGURE 57.4. **Abnormal Thallium-201 Lung/Heart Ratio.** This frame is an anterior projection acquired immediately after the start of a stress SPECT study. The lung:heart ratio of 0.77 is markedly elevated, indicating that the patient experienced heart failure during exercise.

excretion, and shifts of the isotope between muscle, viscera, and other compartments. Rest or redistribution imaging is usually done 3 to 4 hours after the stress injection. Because Tl-201 has significant blood pool activity, it can slowly redistribute into the myocardium and thus slowly fill in ischemic-type defects. In addition to clinical data (ECG, angina, etc.), the initial Tl-201 images of the chest and heart may help assess the heart's performance. High lung activity immediately after exercise usually indicates that left ventricular failure occurred during exercise. Poststress dilation of the heart compared to the resting images is another indicator of failure. Both phenomena have a severe prognosis for subsequent cardiac events (angina, infarction, arrhythmia, and sudden death) (Fig. 57.4). Another imaging strategy for improving the visual detection of ischemic myocardium by Tl-201 scintigraphy calls for a "reinjection" of 1 mCi of Tl-201 just before delayed rest imaging. This technique is especially important to view defects caused by very high-grade stenoses, resulting in more accurate diagnosis of ischemia versus infarction.

Tc-99m is used to label two commercially available myocardial perfusion agents.

Tc-99m Sestamibi (trade name Cardiolite) is taken up by the perfused myocardium by passive diffusion and is bound in the myocyte, mostly within myocardial mitochondria. There is no significant redistribution effect with this agent. Washout is negligible. Imaging of the 15- to 20-mCi dose is delayed for 30 minutes to 1 hour after stress to allow for biliary and background clearance. Because there is neither redistribution nor significant washout of Tc-99m sestamibi, a repeat injection of 15 to 20 mCi for resting images is commonly performed on a different day. With this 2-day protocol, stress imaging is usually done first. An alternative 1-day approach uses a small dose (8 mCi) for the initial rest scan, followed 4 hours later by the stress scan, with a larger dose of 20 to 25 mCi.

Tc-99m Tetrofosmin (trade name Myoview) is rapidly extracted from the blood by perfused myocardium in a fashion that resembles Tc-99m sestamibi. The manufacturer claims that it clears background faster and therefore can be imaged sooner than Tc-99m sestamibi. The two agents have proven to act clinically in a very similar manner, but availability and pricing make important considerations.

Both of the Tc-99m–labeled agents are prepared from Tc-99m pertechnetate and stocked pharmaceutical kits. Both are easy-to-image radiopharmaceuticals with good soft tissue penetration (140 keV gamma energy) and a high photon flux from typical doses of 8 to 25 mCi. In addition, the Tc-99m agents also provide perceptibly improved image quality and an opportunity with the same injection to better perform gated first-pass or gated SPECT studies, which can be used to evaluate wall motion, and left ventricular functional parameters such as LVEF.

Dual-Isotope Myocardial Scans. An innovative way to maximize the logistical patient throughput involves the use of a Tl-201 and a Tc-99m agent for sequential scans. The most widely used dual-isotope scan technique uses a resting Tl-201 scan, which can be immediately or subsequently followed by a Tc-99m (sestamibi or tetrofosmin) stress scan. Because the energy and photon flux of the subsequent Tc-99m scan are higher than those of the Tl-201 scan there is no problem with cross talk between the rest and stress images. Excellent scan quality can be combined with 1-day convenience, or a delayed 24-hour thallium scan can be accomplished if needed.

Interpretation

Myocardial Ischemia. Interpretation of myocardial perfusion scans is difficult but important. Subtle abnormalities can signal serious coronary artery disease. Observer knowledge and experience are essential for an accurate diagnosis. Parametric methods of perfusion image analysis have been employed in attempts to standardize diagnosis. Circumferential profiles of isotope distribution and analyses of regional rates of Tl-201 washout, compared with normal databases, make interpretation more sensitive in the detection of ischemia. Displayed as graphic data, "bull's-eye" maps of SPECT images, and three-dimensional reconstruction of SPECT data, these aids in interpretation may be overly sensitive. If an abnormality is truly present, it should also be visible in the planar or SPECT images. Depending on the statistical assumptions used and the population studied, the sensitivity and specificity for detecting myocardial ischemia are in the percent range of the high 80s or low 90s. It is important to remember that according to Bayes theorem, the positive and negative predictive values of a test will vary according to the prevalence of disease in the population being tested. The myocardial perfusion scan also detects other causes of ischemia (including left bundle branch block, coronary vasculitis, and small vessel disease) that cannot be seen on coronary arteriography and thereby reduces its apparent specificity. In addition to detecting significant coronary artery disease, the presence and severity of ischemic myocardium correlates strongly with the prognosis for adverse cardiac events, including angina and cardiac death (Fig. 57.5).

Myocardial perfusion imaging demonstrates relative regional perfusion. Areas of myocardium with poor blood supply, usually because of atherosclerosis, fail to increase radiotracer uptake during the stress component. The most important feature of the myocardial perfusion test is comparison of the stress and rest images to detect areas of ischemia that are inadequately perfused at exercise yet still viable. These areas are redundantly called *reversibly ischemic*. Ischemia detected by exercise or pharmacologic dilation of normal vessels usually corresponds with angiographic abnormalities in coronary arteries. Correction of the anatomic abnormality by angioplasty, laser atherectomy, or coronary artery bypass surgery is expected to relieve the ischemia. A frequent location of ischemic tissue is immediately adjacent to an area of infarct. This is called *peri-infarct ischemia* and does not portend the same clinical significance as an ischemic or reversible zone.

Some patients will have naturally recruited coronary collaterals or bypass grafts that produce apparent discrepancies between angiographic and scintigraphic studies. Abnormal anatomy in a coronary artery may not produce hemodynamically significant changes in blood flow to the myocardium, and not all ischemia is produced by large vessel atherosclerosis. Capillary disease in diabetics, left bundle branch block, vasospasm, vasculitis, or cardiomyopathy (dilated or hypertrophic) may produce ischemic myocardium even with normal arteries. Ischemia may not

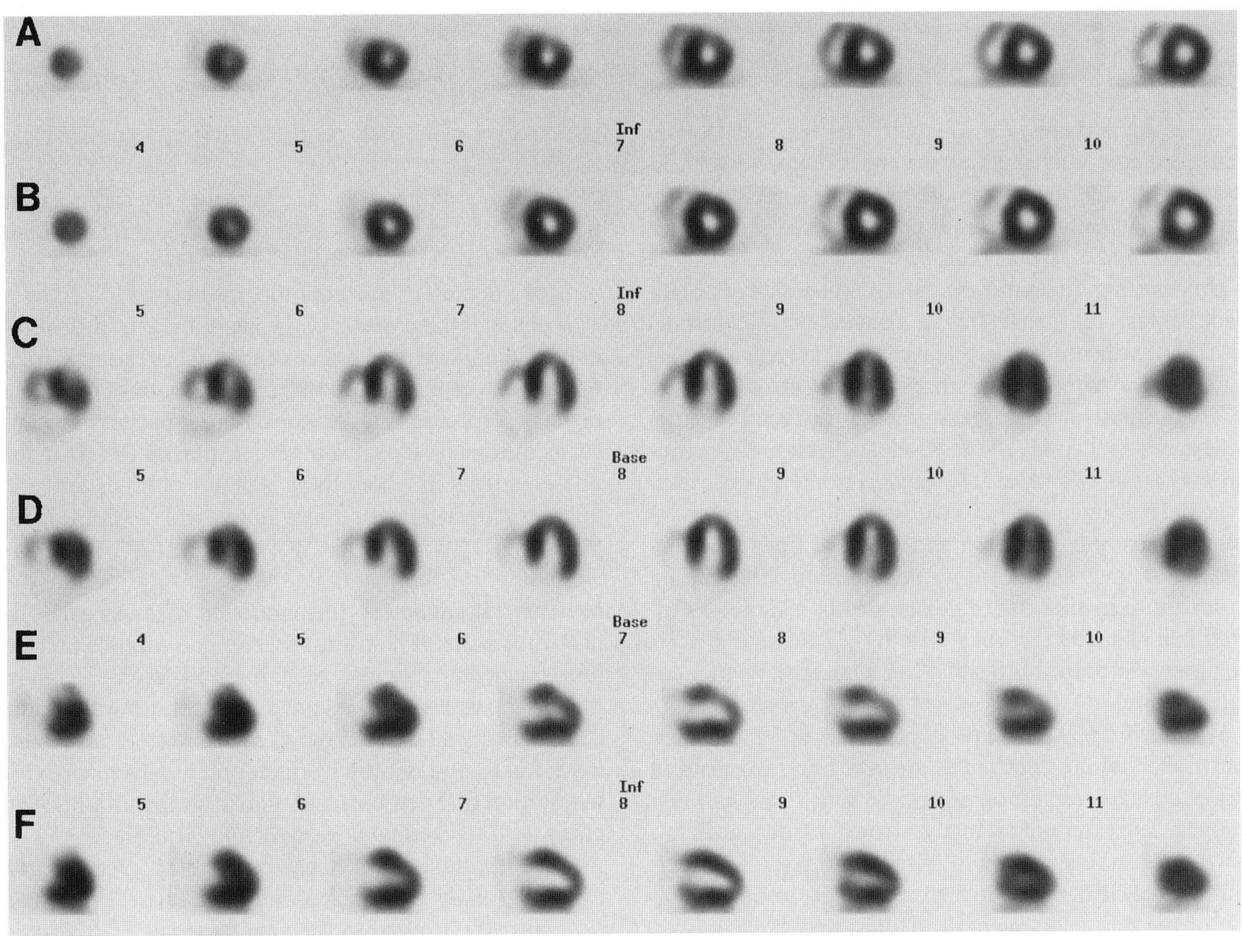

FIGURE 57.5. **SPECT of Left Anterior Descending Artery Reversible Ischemia.** The row of short-axis stress images **(A)** has a perfusion defect in the anterior wall, which perfuses normally in the rest of the short-axis images **(B).** This is also visible in the horizontal long-axis stress **(C)** and vertical long-axis stress images **(E)**, which have the same perfusion defect. At rest the matched images **(D, E, F)** show normal perfusion.

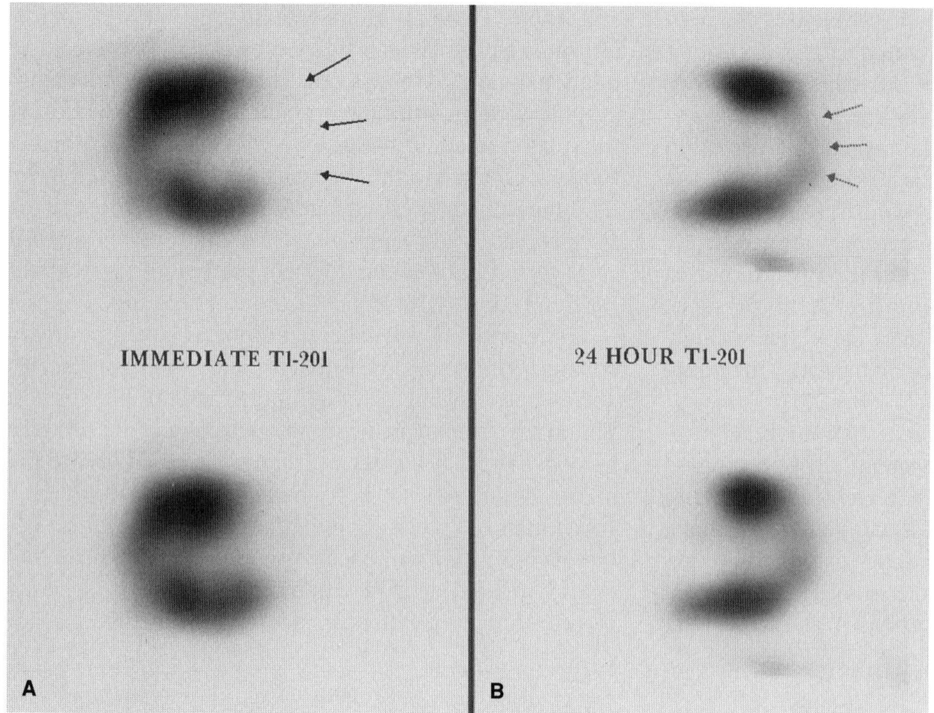

FIGURE 57.6. **Hibernating Myocardium.** Two vertical long-axis thallium-201 images at rest **(A)** are compared with matched images at 24 hours **(B).** The large anteroapical defect (*arrows*) partly fills in over time, indicating that some hibernating (viable) myocardium is present in the midst of what looked initially to be infarcted tissue.

be detected if there is inadequate exercise, inadequate pharmacologic challenge, or balanced triple-vessel disease. Fortunately, it is uncommon for all three coronary arteries to be hemodynamically compromised equally, and poststress dilation will usually be present.

Hibernating Myocardium. Severe ischemia with high-grade stenosis may be so slow to "reverse" on Tl-201 imaging that it will not be detected by rest or redistribution images at 3 to 4 hours after stress. Imaging at 24 hours, or a Tl-201 second injection rest study, may be required to detect extreme ischemia. The Tc-99m–labeled agents are routinely given as two separate injections, but evidence suggests that rest-injected Tl-201 with delayed imaging may be best for detecting the severe ischemia that leads to a phenomenon known as *hibernating myocardium.* Hibernating myocardium is important to diagnose, as it simulates infarction by not contracting at rest. It remains viable, however, and will return to normal function after revascularization (Fig. 57.6).

Myocardial infarction produces layers of nonperfused scar tissue that are detected as areas of thin myocardium with decreased radiotracer uptake at *both* stress *and* rest imaging. The extent of an infarct, from subendocardial to transmural, is reflected by the size and degree of the perfusion defect (Fig. 57.7). Technical artifacts from attenuation of the perfusion agent's radiation may be produced by SPECT tables, breast tissue, and subdiaphragmatic structures. These may appear as fixed defects superimposed on planar or SPECT images, which may lead to a false-positive reading of infarction. A false-positive interpretation of ischemia should not occur as long as the artifact does not change between stress and rest imaging.

Three techniques are in use to reduce the artifactual appearance of fixed defects seen with myocardial perfusion scanning. The simplest relies on repeat poststress scanning of the patient in the prone position with a Tc agent. This changes the position of the heart, breasts, diaphragm, and subdiaphragmatic organs and reduces the appearance of fixed defects in the appropriate distribution, which may be misinterpreted as infarctions. Repeat prone positioning scans may also help with motion artifacts. Unfortunately, obese patients in whom there is plenty of breast or subdiaphragmatic attenuation may not be able to lie prone for this scan (Fig. 57.8).

Another technique that avoids misinterpretation of fixed artifactual defects as infarctions relies on gating the acquisition. It is a very simple technique with planar scans and somewhat more involved with SPECT scans. A cine replay of the gated study allows assessment of wall motion. The normal wall moves inward during systole, thickens as it contracts, and becomes brighter on the display. An area in question that demonstrates normal wall motion, brightening, and thickening is probably not infarcted.

The elegant solution to the problem of attenuation artifacts has only recently become available. This attenuation correction relies on the simultaneous SPECT acquisition of an emission scan *and* a transmission scan performed with a radioactive source of a different energy than that used for the emission scan. The transmission scan can also be acquired with the CT component of SPECT-CT. With a transmission scan, allowance for the emission

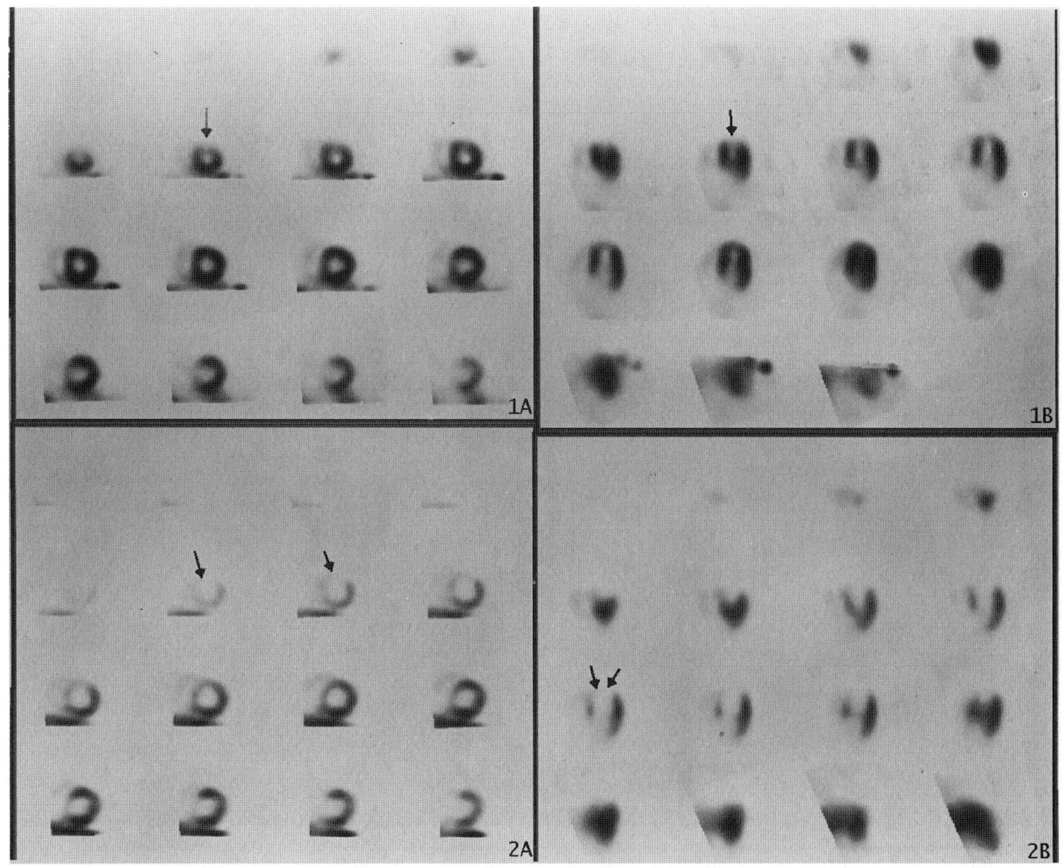

FIGURE 57.7. **Resting Images of Infarcts of the Left Anterior Descending Artery (LAD).** Short-axis **(1A)** and horizontal long-axis **(1B)** SPECT images show a small anterior LAD infarct (*arrows*). This is compared with another patient who has a much larger LAD infarct **(2A, 2B)** in the same vascular distribution (*arrows*). Note that the second patient's infarct extends from the anterolateral wall to and including the septum. The ventricle is also dilated at rest.

photons lost because of attenuation can be made, and the resulting SPECT scans are surprisingly free of artifacts. A related improvement on this scheme incorporates correction for photons scattered from the emission source but still accepted by the imaging system. A combination of attenuation and scatter correction promises truly quantitative imaging in the future (Fig. 57.9).

Stunned Myocardium. A single myocardial perfusion scan cannot determine the age of an infarct. Acute infarcts usually appear larger than old infarcts when imaged with Tl-201. Temporarily damaged cells around infarcted cells, referred to as "stunned myocardium," will be hypokinetic or akinetic and will not hold on to the Tl-201 until recovery several weeks later. Thus the defect can appear worse on the rest imaging compared to the stress imaging, in a so-called "reverse redistribution." The abnormality may revert to normal or shrink as repair occurs.

Infarct-Avid Scans. Acute infarcts may also be detected with Tc-99m pyrophosphate labeling. Ionized calcium released from myocytes forms dystrophic calcifications with phosphates, and a "hot spot" is formed, marking the infarcted tissue. Antimyosin antibodies labeled with Tc-99m or indium-111 also localize on the fringes of acute infarctions. The need for imaging of acute infarction is clinically infrequent, usually when the patient has left bundle branch block. Contused myocardium is also detected with these techniques.

Positron Emission Tomography

Technique. PET is more expensive than standard myocardial perfusion imaging but offers the advantages of coincidence imaging, higher-energy photons, efficient attenuation correction, and different radiopharmaceuticals. PET agents can also be imaged on hybrid SPECT cameras or SPECT cameras with heavy collimators. PET scanning with coincidence detection allows high photon flux because collimators are not required. PET scans have higher-resolution images and fewer attenuation artifacts than standard MPI. Thus, PET scans may be the gold standard for MPI.

Radiopharmaceuticals. For PET scans, stress testing is usually done with pharmacological agents. Perfusion is usually evaluated with rubidium-82 or ammonia-13

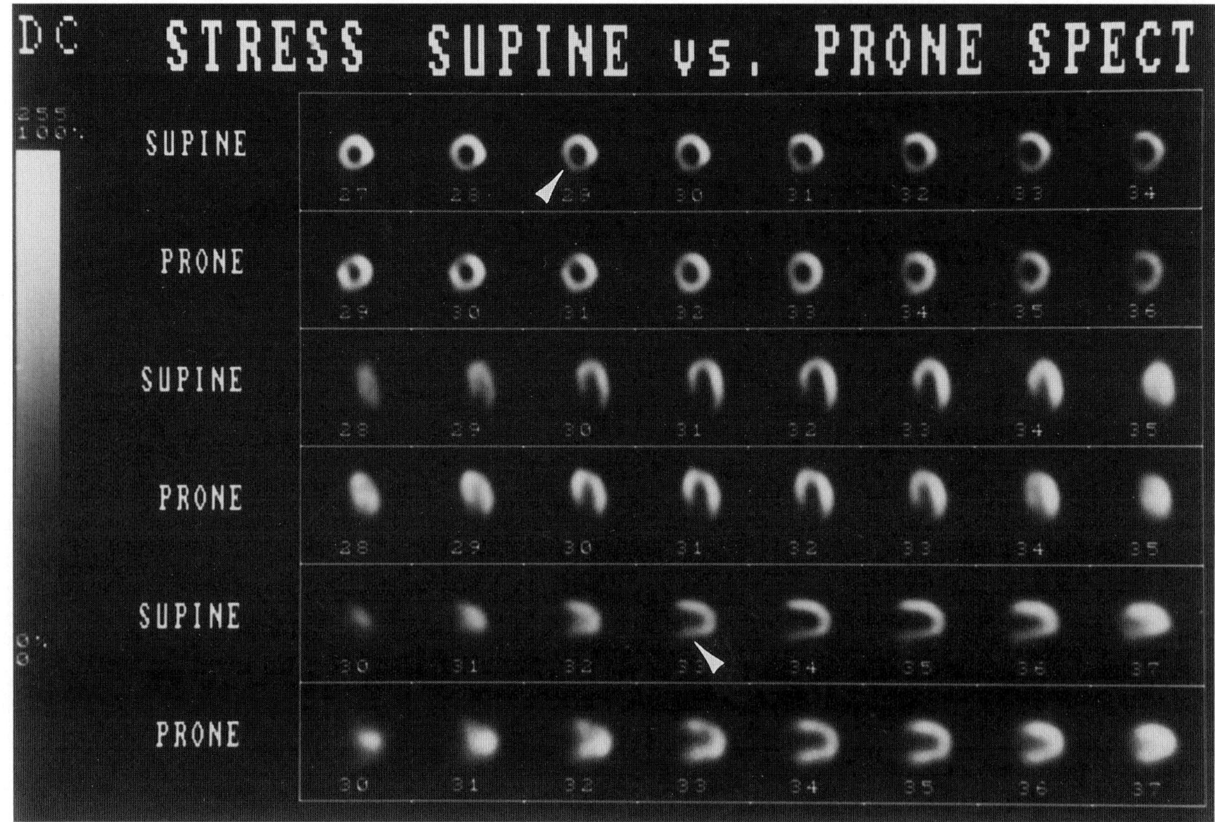

FIGURE 57.8. **Stress Versus Prone Imaging.** Technetium-99m sestamibi imaging with a single headed SPECT camera shows a defect in the inferior wall during stress imaging (*arrowheads*), which is not present when the patient is imaged again in the prone position.

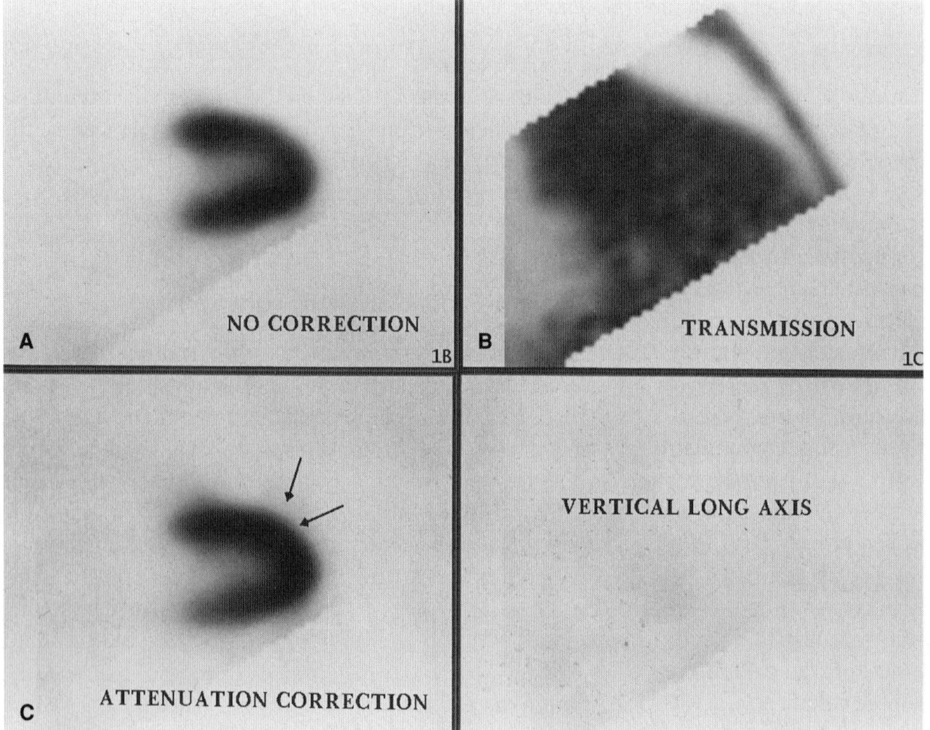

FIGURE 57.9. **Attenuation Correction.** An apparent anterior wall defect caused by large breasts is corrected by simultaneous transmission and emission scans. An uncorrected vertical long-axis scan **(A)** shows an apparent anterior wall defect, which disappears when the transmission scan **(B)** is used to correct for the asymmetric attenuation **(C)**. The anterior wall (*arrows*) is normal.

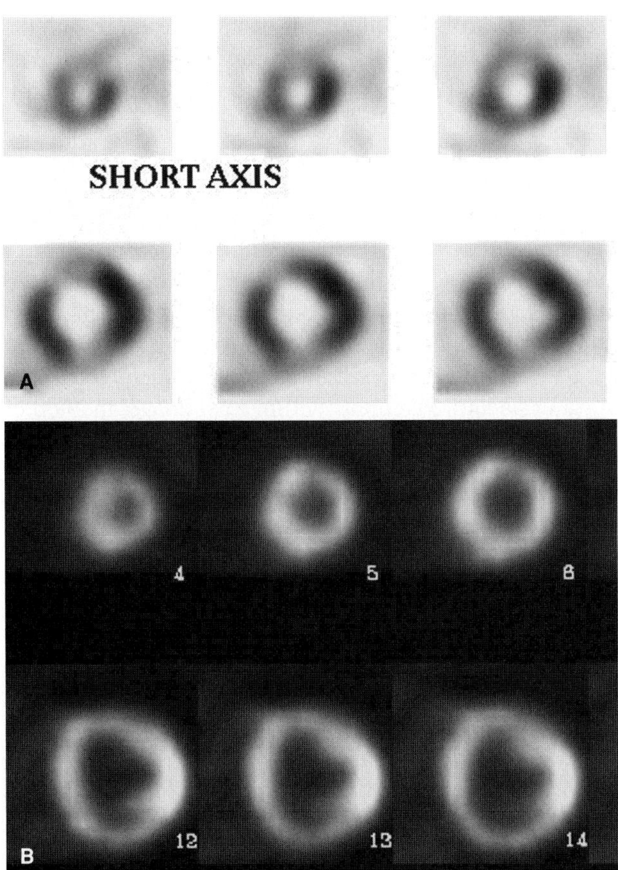

FIGURE 57.10. **Fluorodeoxyglucose (FDG) PET Myocardial Viability Scan.** Tc-tetrofosmin resting scan **(A)** shows defects in the anterior and inferior walls on male for potential bypass surgery. Fluorine-18 FDG resting PET scan **(B)** demonstrates normal uptake consistent with fully viable, hibernating myocardium.

($^{13}NH_3$), with comparisons of rest imaging with stress imaging, as in standard MPI. Viability or hibernating myocardium is evaluated with resting injection of fluorine-18 fluorodeoxyglucose (FDG).

Interpretation. In evaluation of coronary artery disease, rubidium or ammonia-13 pharmacologic stress imaging is accomplished, and defects, which reverse on rest imaging, are indicative of coronary stenosis. Fixed defects on stress and rest usually identify infarcted myocardium or hibernating myocardium. With FDG imaging, hibernating myocardium will show normal or even relatively increased FDG uptake as the result of a shift from free fatty acid metabolism to glucose metabolism (Fig. 57.10). True infarction will show no significant FDG uptake.

GATED BLOOD POOL SCANS

The radionuclide ventriculogram (RVG) is a study that uses circulating, Tc-99m–labeled red blood cells to evaluate the size, wall motion, and functional parameters of the LV. RV evaluation is better accomplished by the first-pass study, to be discussed later.

Technique

The red blood cells are labeled with Tc-99m, utilizing one of several techniques, and make an excellent blood pool imaging agent. Doses of 20 to 30 mCi are commonly used for typical adult patients. ECG leads are placed to obtain a suitable gating signal (the R wave) for the computer. With the ECG as a measure of the cardiac cycle length, the cardiac cycle is divided into a minimum of 16 frames for analysis of systolic function. Higher temporal resolution of 32 frames per cardiac cycle is required for good measurement of diastolic function. The result of this acquisition is a composite, "averaged" series of images representing the patient's cardiac cycle. Data from a sufficient number of cardiac cycles (several hundred) must be obtained to make the images statistically significant for analysis. Typical acquisition time is 5 to 20 minutes per view (Fig. 57.11).

Analysis of the functional parameters of the LV, including the LVEF and first derivative (dV/DT; where V is LV volume and T is time) of the LV volume curve, is most accurate from images obtained in the "best septal" left anterior oblique view. This view produces the greatest separation of the activity of the LV from that of the RV.

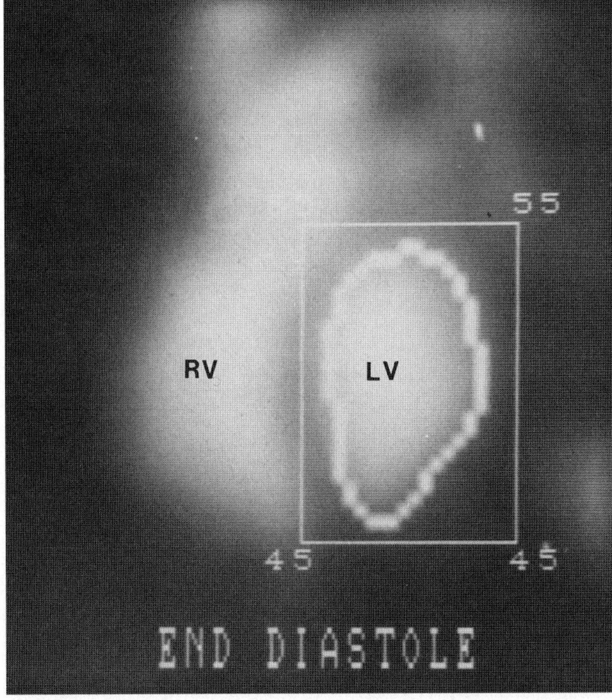

FIGURE 57.11. **Normal Gated Blood Pool Image.** An end-diastolic image is shown with a computer-generated region of interest around the LV blood pool. The RV is adjacent.

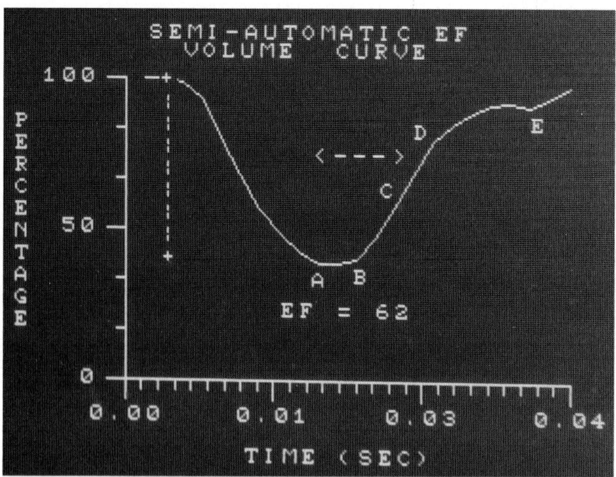

FIGURE 57.12. **Left Ventricular Time Activity Curve.** The graph shows this curve (from the patient in Fig. 57.11) that displays the ventricle's relative volume during the cardiac cycle. The vertical dashed line represents the relative stroke volume, expressed as an ejection fraction of 62%. The curve begins at end diastole, A marks end systole, B marks the start of diastolic filling, C marks the peak filling rate, D is the end of rapid filling, and E represents the beginning of the atrial "kick." The horizontal dashed line shows the interval of the first third of diastole, during which more than half of the stroke volume is recovered.

Computer processing of the image data by spatial and temporal smoothing algorithms improves both the visual analysis of wall motion and the accuracy and precision of the derived functional parameters. Outlining the edge of the ventricular blood pool in each frame of the study with computerized second-derivative edge detection methods is superior to threshold detection or manually drawn regions of interest. The volume curve is generated by plotting the number of counts in the ventricle versus time during the cardiac cycle. This curve generates the LVEF, which measures the change in volume between end diastole and end systole. The LVEF is the single best parameter of LV function (Fig. 57.12).

Arrhythmias such as frequent premature beats and atrial fibrillation tend to falsely lower the LVEF. The R-R (R-wave) interval histogram from the ECG can demonstrate the presence of arrhythmias. Most nuclear medicine computer systems allow analysis of selected populations of beats of the same R-R interval to yield a more accurate LVEF.

Additional functional parameters are easily obtained. The dV/DT of the LV volume curve gives important information on the rates (average or maximal) of systolic emptying and diastolic filling.

Cardiac output (CO) in liters per minute may be calculated if the heart rate, the LVEF, and the left ventricular end-diastolic volume (LVEDV) are known. The product of all three is CO. The LVEDV can be measured by comparing the count rate of a blood sample of known volume with the count rate of the ventricle at end diastole and end systole.

Another simpler method to measure CO uses a count-based ratio method. The ratio of the total counts to the maximum counts in the diastolic frame is entered into an equation that also requires a calibration of the voxel size for the acquisition and depends on constants derived from the formula for a sphere. The resulting measurement of the LVEDV has about the same error as more complicated methods and allows a rapid estimate of CO (Fig. 57.13).

The exact range of normal for functional parameters of the RVG will depend on multiple factors, such as number of frames acquired, counts within each image, method of computer filtering of the data, and methods of background correction and edge detection. In general, the clinically established normal resting LVEF is approximately 65%, with a standard deviation of 5%. (The normal range of 2 standard deviations is 55% to 75%.)

Interpretation

Left Ventricular Ejection Fraction. The most common causes of elevated LVEF values include mitral or aortic valvular regurgitation, hypertrophic cardiomyopathy, and high cardiac output states such as those found in hyperthyroidism. Low LVEF values are usually seen in patients with prior myocardial infarction, ischemia (with congestive heart failure), or cardiomyopathy of any cause. A common application of the RVG is monitoring for the development of cardiotoxicity from chemotherapeutic drugs.

End-Diastolic Volume. The relative end-diastolic size and shape of the RV and LV chambers (RVEDV and LVEDV) should be always noted. Although they appear roughly equal in a normal best-septal left anterior oblique view, the RVEDV is normally greater than the LVEDV. If no intracardiac shunts are present, the stroke volumes of the ventricles are equal because the RV ejection fraction is smaller than the LVEF. As the LV fails for any reason, it dilates and usually becomes rounder in shape. (See Fig. 57.13 for an example of a dilated LV.)

Wall motion of various regions of the LV can be assessed from an overlay of end-diastolic and end-systolic edge images. This is best evaluated by visually observing a cine display of the beating heart in orthogonal views. The left anterior oblique or best septal view is the critical view, but the anterior and left posterior oblique views are complementary.

As the ventricular wall is damaged or infarcted, the progression of wall motion abnormality is from normal to hypokinetic to akinetic. If an aneurysm forms, the wall will become dyskinetic. This analysis is true for gated SPECT as well as RVG. To determine the degree of abnormality, it is important to concentrate on the margins of the LV chamber, which is the interface of the endocardial surface and blood. The observer should attempt to correlate a

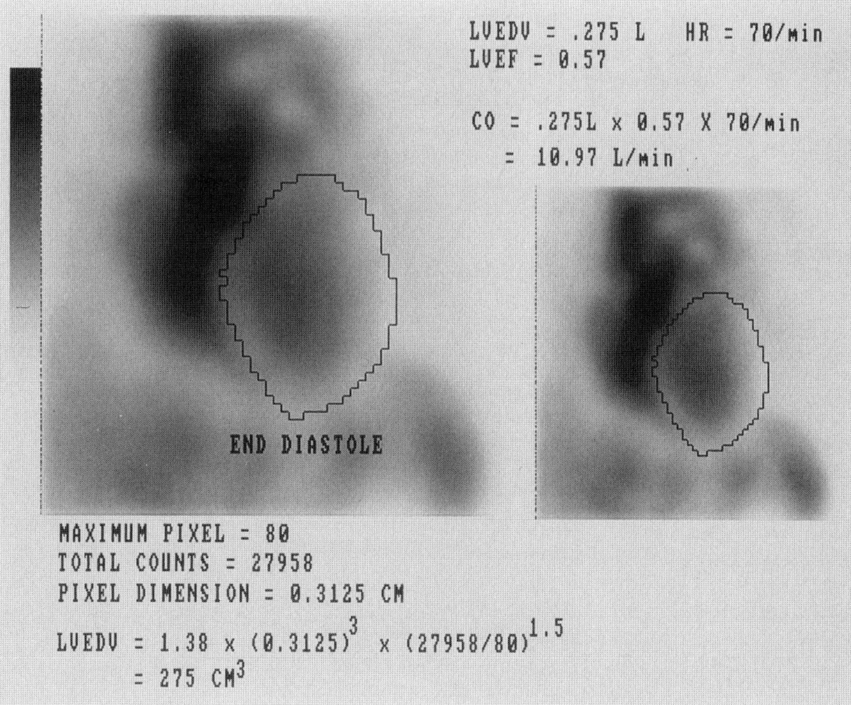

FIGURE 57.13. **Sample Calculations of Cardiac Output (CO).** Calculation of left ventricular end-diastolic volume (LVEDV) can be done using the count-based ratio method, which requires measurement of the total counts in the end-diastolic region of interest, the maximum pixel counts in the same region of interest, and measurements of the size of a pixel in centimeters. In this case, the dilated LV has a LVEDV of 275 cm^3. Multiplication of the LVEDV by the LVEF and heart rate gives a global CO of 10.97 L/min.

suspicion of abnormal wall motion in one view with this same area on the orthogonal view. Color computer displays that enhance the margins of the chambers may make subtle wall motion abnormalities more easily detectable.

Fourier phase analysis provides powerful additional information on the amount of motion (amplitude) of various LV wall segments and also their relative timing (phase). The amplitude image is especially useful for confirming areas suspected to be hypokinetic or akinetic on the cine display. Damaged areas of myocardium contract with less vigor than normal areas. The phase display may help detect such areas because damaged areas contract slowly (tardive kinesis). Dyskinetic, aneurysmal areas are dramatically displayed using Fourier amplitude and phase images. There is wall motion of the segment displayed on the amplitude image, but it is opposite (180° out of phase) compared with undamaged areas (Figs. 57.14, 57.15).

Valvular Regurgitation. Another use of Fourier amplitude images is in the calculation of valvular regurgitation. Each pixel in an amplitude image is coded with a number proportional to the blood volume change under that pixel during the cardiac cycle. A simple total of the pixel values in all the LV and RV pixels outlined with region-of-interest markers will produce a ratio of the LV-to-RV stroke volume. The ratio can be used to calculate the regurgitant fraction. This method works only when there are regurgitant valves on one side of the septum. It cannot distinguish aortic regurgitation from mitral regurgitation, however (Fig 57.16).

Exercise Radionuclide Ventriculogram. The RVG study can also be done repeatedly while the patient is exercising on a bicycle ergometer at various workload levels. This is an excellent method to monitor cardiac functional response to exercise. The 2- to 3-minute periods for each exercise level usually supply a minimally acceptable amount of statistical counts in the gated images. Finally, a large amount of data must be processed and reviewed because each stage of the study is compared with the resting study (Table 57.1).

The relative cardiac output can be measured from one stage to another and rises with increasing workload. Normal patients increase or augment their LVEF and dV/DT significantly while decreasing their LV end-systolic volume. Abnormal exercise RVG response can be seen in several ways, such as an increase of LVEDV by more than 10%, lack of increase or even a fall in LVEF with greater workloads, and development of wall motion abnormalities caused by ischemia brought on by the exercise.

RIGHT VENTRICULAR STUDIES

First-Pass Function Studies

Right ventricular function is more difficult to assess by the RVG study than is LV function. This is because labeled activity in the RV cannot be isolated as well from other chambers as can LV activity. RV function is best assessed by analyzing images from the first pass of a radionuclide

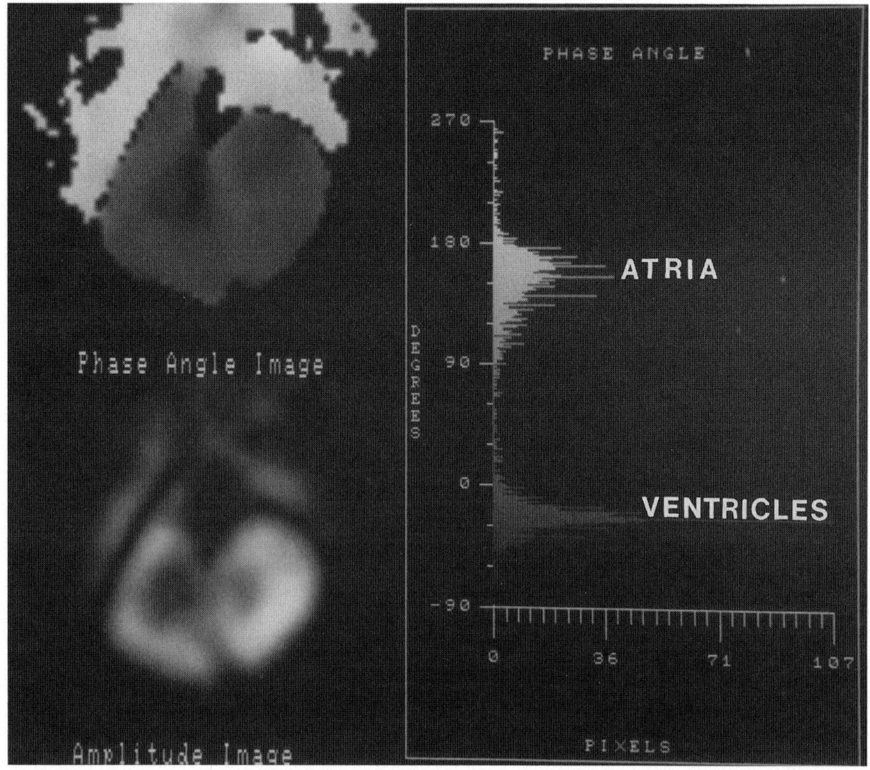

FIGURE 57.14. Normal Fourier Phase and Amplitude Images. These are from the same patient shown in Figs. 57.11 and 57.12. The lower (amplitude) image shows the relative displacement of blood in each chamber of the heart. The pixel brightness depicts the relative degree of motion. The upper (phase) image shows the relative timing of contraction of each chamber. The histogram summarizes the number of pixels with a given phase angle. The cardiac cycle is represented on an arbitrary scale of –90° to 270°. Note that the gray pixels representing ventricular motion are tightly grouped around –30°, indicating synchronous contraction. Approximately 180° up the time scale, there is a cluster of white pixels corresponding to atrial motion.

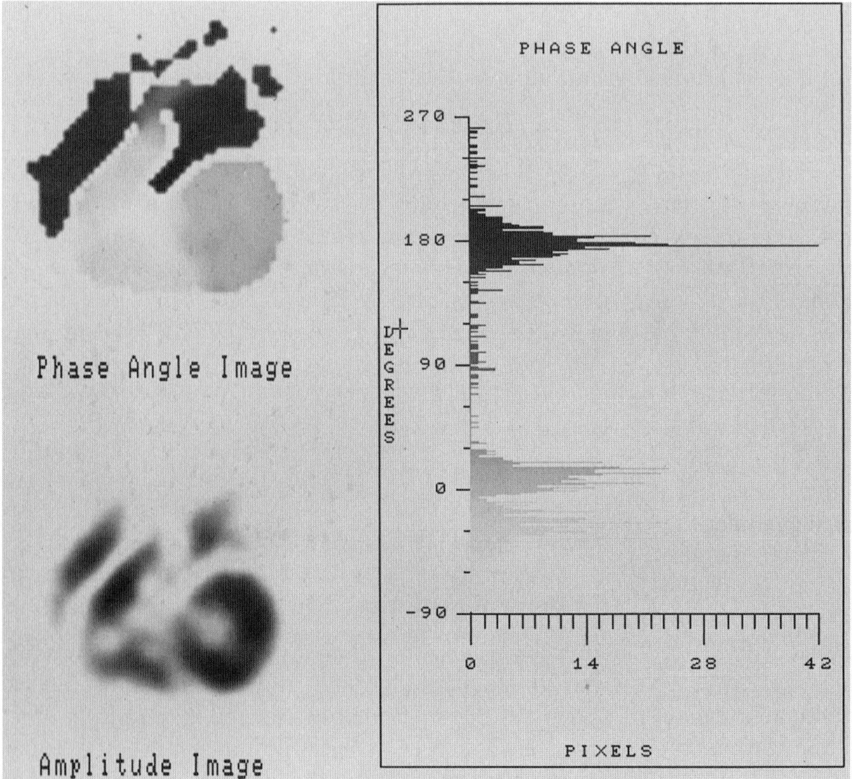

FIGURE 57.15. Fourier Phase and Amplitude in Left Bundle Branch Block. Two separate populations of phase values are seen in the RV and LV. The lighter-colored RV contracts before the darker-colored LV. This is much easier to see in color.

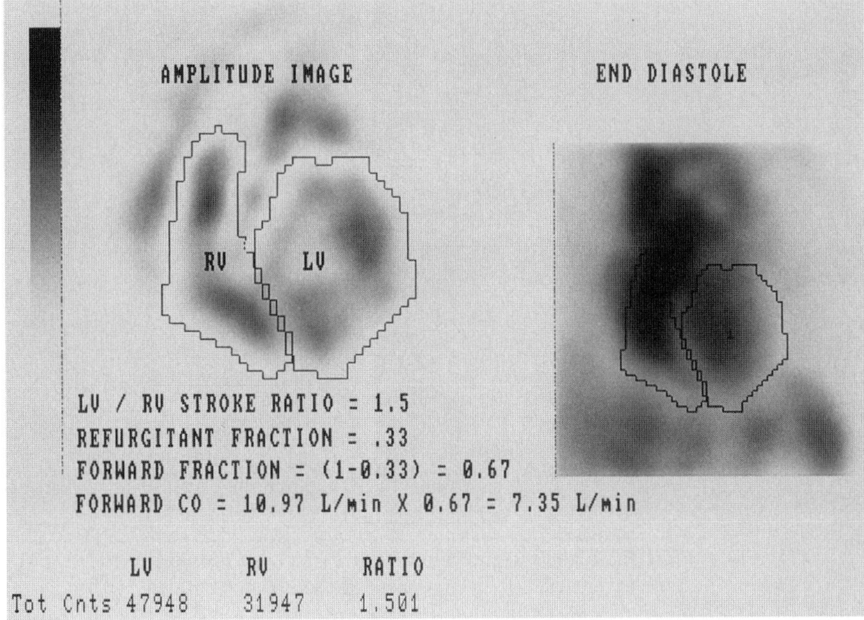

FIGURE 57.16. **Mitral Regurgitation Calculated From a Fourier Amplitude Image.** The total counts in the LV and RV regions of interest yield a 1.5:1 LV/RV stroke ratio with a 0.33 regurgitant fraction. This is the same patient imaged in Fig. 57.12. The global cardiac output (CO) of 10.97 is multiplied by the complement of the regurgitant fraction (0.67) to generate a forward CO of 7.35 L/min.

bolus through the right-sided chambers and lungs before the overlapping left-sided chambers are seen. The patient is usually imaged in the right anterior oblique projection. A bolus of up to 30 mCi of high-specific-activity isotope must be very rapidly injected, followed immediately by a nonradioactive flush dose. This activity will pass through the RV in three to eight heartbeats. A region of interest is established around the RV and a time-activity curve allows an RV ejection fraction to be measured for each beat. An average RV ejection fraction is then calculated (Fig. 57.17).

Another good RVEF technique uses xenon-133 in saline solution for injection. During a slow venous infusion, the xenon-133 passes through the right side of the heart and into the lungs, where it immediately fills the alveoli and is exhaled. In this way, overlapping activity never enters the left side of the heart. A gated study over many seconds is acquired and processed in a manner identical to the standard RVG of the LV. In general, an average RVEF is 42%, with a standard deviation of 5% and a normal range of 32% to 52% (Fig. 57.18).

First-Pass Flow Studies

The first-pass study in an anterior projection can also be used to detect abnormalities of blood flow to one lung compared with the other. The effect of extrinsic compression on a pulmonary artery by a mediastinal or hilar mass can be easily detected. Abnormal blood flow to a lung segment

TABLE 57.1 Example of Poor Diastolic Function as Measured by Exercise Radionuclide Ventriculogram-Relative Volumes and Cardiac Output

Level	*HR*	*BP*	*DP (× 1,000)*	*LVEF*	*rLVEDV*	*rLVESV*	*rLVSV*	*rCO*
Rest	78	150	11.7	0.56	1.00	1.00	1.00	1.00
EX1	101	152	15.4	0.60	0.83	0.76	0.89	1.16
EX2	102	158	16.1	0.64	0.90	0.74	1.03	1.35
EX3	106	158	16.7	0.64	0.96	0.79	1.10	1.50
EX4	115	170	19.6	0.68	0.91	0.66	1.11	1.63
EX5	133	190	25.3	0.72	0.77	0.49	1.00	1.70
EX6	153	192	29.4	0.71	0.59	0.39	0.75	1.47
Post-EX	162	162	26.2	0.70	0.69	0.47	0.86	1.79

This exercise radionuclide ventriculogram shows that the patient worked hard during six levels of bicycle exercise (EX1 to EX6) as the heart rate (HR) rose from 78 to 153, while systolic blood pressure (BP) rose from 150 to 192, with a resultant rise in double product (DP) from 11,700 to 29,400. The left ventricular ejection fraction (LVEF) rose appropriately from 0.56 to 0.71 at peak exercise. However, the ventricle filled poorly during exercise as relative end-systolic volume (rLVESV) went progressively down (normal) and relative end-diastolic volume (rLVEDV) also declined (abnormal). The stroke volume (rLVSV) changed little and the only improvement in relative cardiac output (rCO) was the result of increased heart rate. Poor diastolic function (poor compliance) limited exercise endurance in this otherwise healthy individual. This is a superb example of the quantitative data inherent in nuclear medicine images.

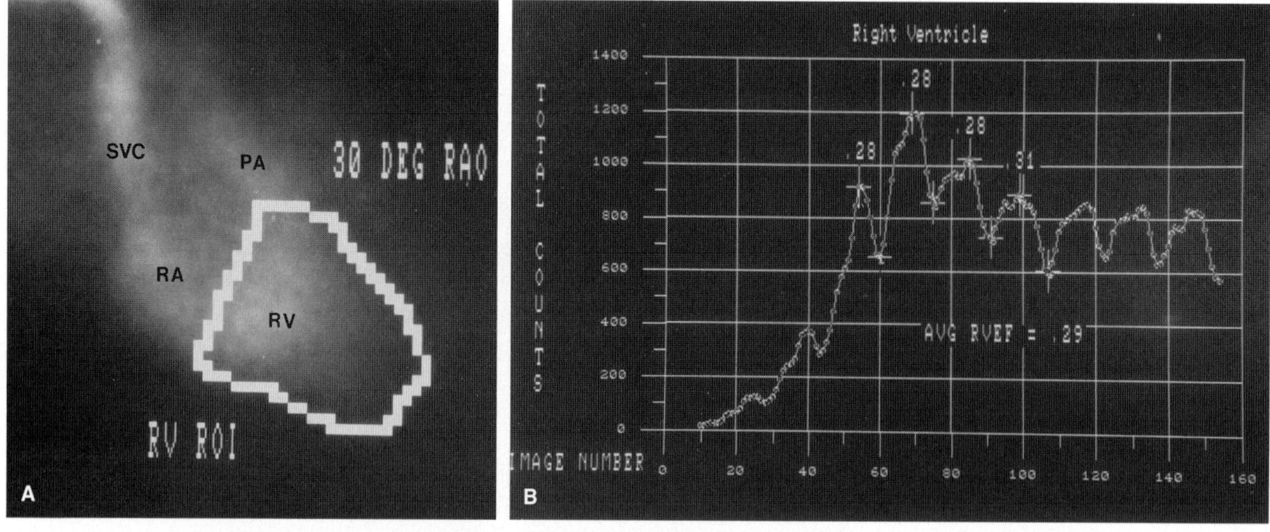

FIGURE 57.17. **Right Ventricular First-Pass Function Study. A.** Fast dynamic right ventricular ejection fraction by first pass. The acquisition totaled 512 frames taken at 40-ms intervals in the right anterior oblique (RAO) projection as a radioactive bolus traversed the RA and RV. An image of the RV is made by summing dozens of individual frames. A fixed region of interest (ROI) is drawn around the RV. SVC, Superior vena cava; PA, pulmonary artery. **B.** A time-activity curve from the ROI in **(A)** shows the relative volume of the ventricle rising and falling with diastole and systole. Peaks and valleys in the curve are flagged, and beat by beat ejection fractions are averaged.

such as is seen in pulmonary sequestration can be detected. The first-pass study can be used to measure the transit time of an injected bolus between ventricles. There is a delay in the passage of blood from the RV to the LV, which typifies congestive heart failure. Obstruction of the superior vena cava is also easily diagnosed in a matter of seconds (Fig. 57.19).

Left-to-right intracardiac shunts can be detected and quantified using a first-pass imaging technique. Instead of using a region of interest over the RV for analysis, an area

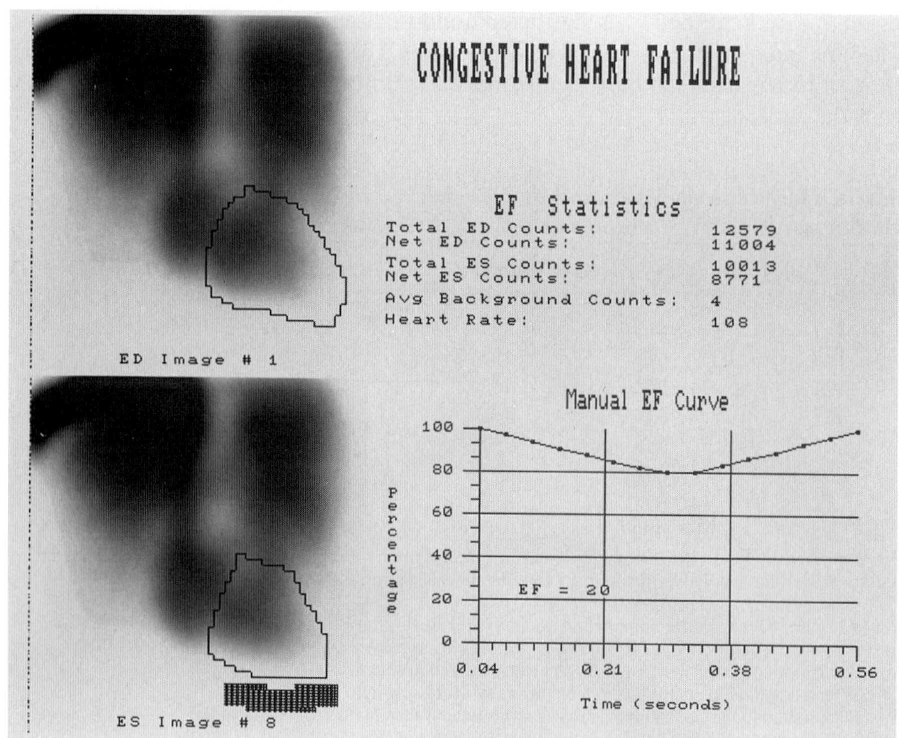

FIGURE 57.18. **Xenon-133 Right Heart Gated First-Pass Study.** Xenon-133 in saline is slowly infused for a gated first-pass study. It is shown with right anterior oblique end-diastolic and end-systolic frames and their respective regions of interest around the RV blood pool. The RV ejection fraction in this patient with congestive heart failure is only 20%.

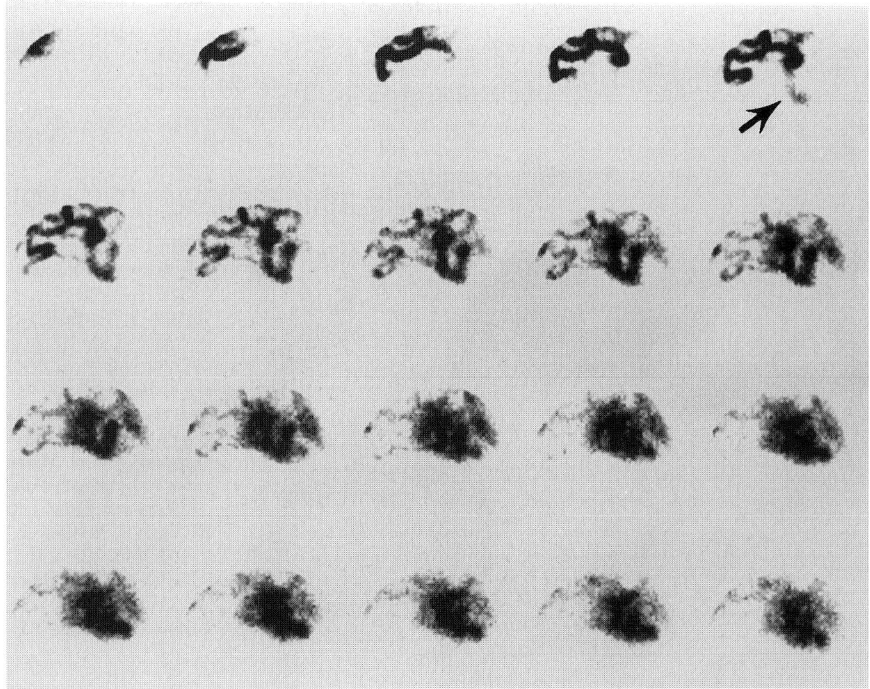

FIGURE 57.19. **Superior Vena Cava (SVC) Obstruction.** A first-pass study with 1-second frames is shown in the anterior projection after injection in the right antecubital vein. Serpiginous collateral veins on the chest wall probably communicate with the intercostal and azygos veins. Very little flow courses through the SVC into the RA and RV (*arrow*). The patient required stenting of the SVC to relieve obstruction caused by an encircling tumor.

of lung is used. In a normal person, the bolus of activity passes into and out of the lung exponentially in a way that can be mathematically described by a gamma function. If a left-to-right shunt is present, some blood that has gone through the lungs to the left side of the heart reenters the right side of the heart and is pumped back into the lungs. This causes a prolongation of the washout of activity from the lung region of interest. A gamma-variate curve-fitting method can be used to detect and quantify the amount of the left-to-right shunt. The method is sensitive to detect

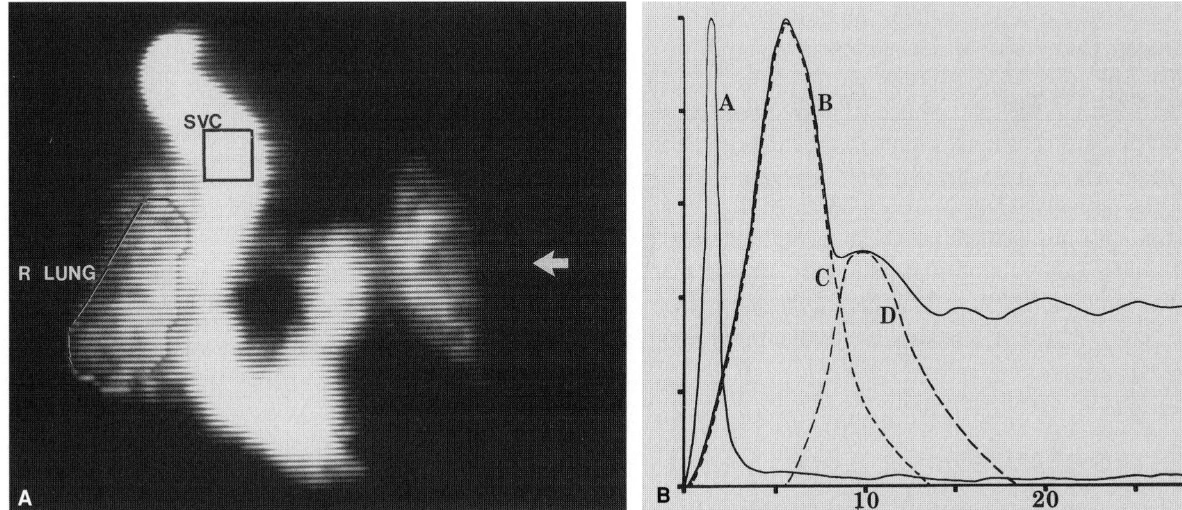

FIGURE 57.20. **Abnormal Left-to-Right Shunt Study. A.** Regions of interest are drawn around the superior vena cava (SVC, *square box*) and the right lung (R lung) on image data from a first-pass flow study. Note lack of activity in the LV (*arrow*) in this summary of images from the right heart phase of the flow. **B.** Graph showing time-activity curve of the activity within the two regions shown in **(A).** A is the sharp bolus injection passing through the superior vena cava. B is the right lung time activity curve, which rises exponentially but does not follow the fitted gamma variate curve (C) on the way down. This indicates early recirculation owing to a left-to-right shunt. The shunt is quantified by comparing the area under C with the area under the fitted recirculation gamma variate (D).

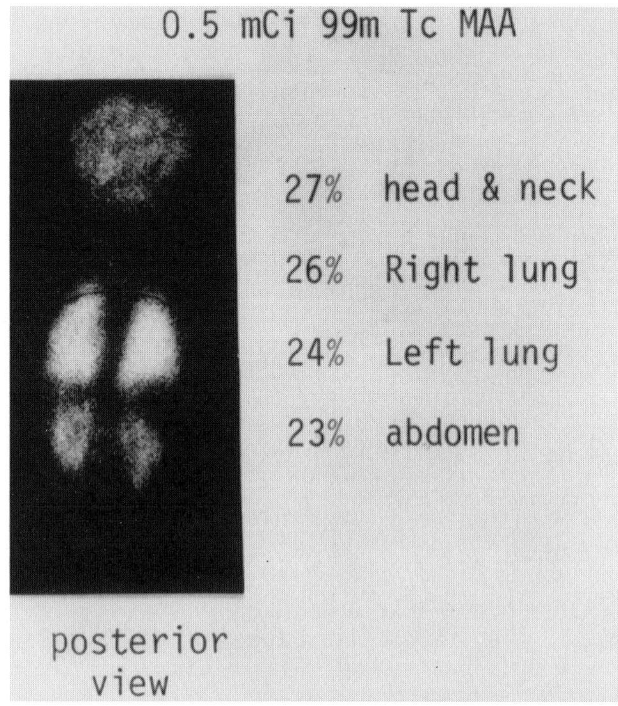

FIGURE 57.21. **Abnormal Right-to-Left Shunt Study.** A significant portion of the injected technetium-99m macroaggregated albumin (MAA) particles are seen in capillary beds outside the lungs in the brain and kidneys. This indicates and measures the amount of shunted blood.

shunts with a ratio as low as 1.2:1, far below the 2:1 shunt that can be detected by chest radiograph (Fig. 57.20).

Right-to-left shunts can be detected by using an IV injection of macroaggregated albumin particles. In a normal person, less than 10% of the injected dose should pass through normal arteriovenous shunts in the lungs and be found in the systemic circulation. After injection, static images of the patient's whole body are obtained. Regions of interest are taken over the lungs, head, neck, abdomen, and extremities. The amount of radioactivity outside the lungs in the systemic circulation is then quantified. The study can be repeated at a later date to check progression (Fig. 57.21).

SUGGESTED READINGS

Anagnostopoulos C, Harbinson M, Kelion A. et al. Procedure guidelines in radionuclide myocardial perfusion imaging. Heart 2004;90:1–10.

Bax JJ, Cornell JH, Visser FC, et al. Comparison of fluorine-18-FDG with rest-redistribution thallium SPECT to delineate viable myocardium and predict functional recovery after revascularization. J Nucl Med 1998;39:1481–1486.

Bax JJ, Patton JA, Poldermans D, et al. 18-Fluorodeoxyglucose imaging with position emission tomography and single photon emission computer tomography: cardiac applications. Semin Nucl Med 2000;30:281–298.

Beller GA. Clinical value of myocardial perfusion imaging in coronary artery disease. J Nucl Cardio 2003;10:529–542.

Berman DS, Kiat H, Friedman J, et al. Separate acquisition rest-thallium-201/stress Tc-99m sestamibi dual isotope myocardial perfusion SPECT: a clinical validation study. J Am Coll Cardiol 1993;23:1455–1464.

Berman DS, Kiat H, van Train K, et al. Myocardial perfusion imaging with technetium-99m-sestamibi: comparative analysis of available imaging protocols. J Nucl Med 1994;35:683–688.

Bolli R. Myocardial "stunning" in man. Circulation 1992;86:1671–1691.

Bonow RO. Identification of viable myocardium. Circulation 1996; 94:2674–2680.

Crean A, Dutka D, Coulder R. Cardiac imaging using nuclear medicine and position emission tomography. Radiol Clin North Am 2004;42(3):619–634.

Demer LL, Gould KL, Goldstein RA, et al. Assessment of coronary artery disease severity by positron emission tomography. Comparison with quantitative arteriography in 193 patients. Circulation 1989;79:825–835.

DePuey EG, Berman DS, Garcia EV. Cardiac SPECT Imaging. 2nd ed. Philadelphia: Lippincott Williams and Wilkins, 2001.

Dilsizian V, et al. Myocardial viability in patients with chronic coronary artery disease. Comparison of 99mTc-sestamibi with thallium reinjection and [18F] fluorodeoxyglucose. Circulation 1994;89:578–587.

Eitzman D, Al-Aouar Z, Kanter H, vom Dahl J, et al. Clinical outcome of patients with advanced coronary artery disease after viability studies with positron emission tomography. J Am Coll Cardiol 1992;20:559–565.

Gibbons RJ, Balady GJ, Bricker JT, et al. ACC/AHA 2002 guidelines update for exercise testing. Circulation 2002;106;1883–1892.

Go RT, Marwisk TH, MacIntyre WJ, et al. A prospective comparison of rubidium-82 PET and thallium-201 SPECT myocardial perfusion imaging utilizing a single dipyridamole stress in the diagnosis of coronary artery disease. J Nucl Med 1990;31:1899–1905.

Green MV, Bacharach SL. Functional imaging of the heart: methods, limitations, and examples from gated blood pool scintigraphy. Prog Cardiovasc Dis 1986;28:319–348.

Hayes SW, De Lorenzo A, Hachamovitch R, et al. Prognostic implications of combined prone and supine acquisitions in patients with equivocal or abnormal supine myocardial perfusion SPECT. J Nucl Med 2003;44:1633–1640.

He ZX, Iskandrian AS, Gupta NC, et al. Assessing coronary artery disease with dipyridamole technetium-99m tetrofosmin SPECT: a multicenter trial. J Nucl Med 1997;38:44–48.

Jones RH. Use of radionuclide measurements of left ventricular function for prognosis in patients with coronary artery disease. Semin Nucl Med 1987;17:95–103.

Kapur A, Latus KA, Davies G, et al. A comparison of three radionuclide myocardial perfusion tracers in clinical practice: the ROBUST study. Eur J Nucl Med 2002;29:1608–1616.

Kiat H, Berman DS, Maddahi J. Myocardial perfusion imaging using technetium-99m radiopharmaceuticals. Radiol Clin North Am 1993;31:795–815.

Kiat H, Van Train KF, Friedman JD, et al. Quantitative stress-redistribution thallium-201 SPECT using prone imaging: methodologic development and validation. J Nucl Med 1992;33:1509–1515.

Leppo JA. Dipyridamole myocardial perfusion imaging. J Nucl Med 1994;35:730–733.

Lette J, Lapointe J, Waters D, Cerino M, Picard M, Gagnon A. Transient left ventricular cavitary dilation during dipyridamole-thallium imaging as an indicator of severe coronary artery disease. Am J Cardiol 1990;66:1163–1170.

Loong CY, Anagnostopoulos C. Diagnosis of coronary artery disease by radionuclide myocardial perfusion imaging. Heart 2004;90(suppl V):V2–V9.

Miller DD, Younis LT, Chaitman BR, et al. Diagnostic accuracy of dipyridamole technetium-99m-labeled sestamibi myocardial tomography for detection of coronary artery disease. J Nucl Cardiol 1997;4: 18–24.

Parker DA, Karvelis KC, Thrall JH, Froelish JW. Radionuclide ventriculography: methods. In: Gerson MC, ed. Cardiac Nuclear Medicine. New York: McGraw Hill,1991:81–125.

Robinson VJB, Corley JH, Marks DS, et al. Causes of transient dilatation of the left ventricle during myocardial perfusion imaging. AJR Am J Roentgenol 2000;174:1349–1352.

Rozanski A. Referral bias and the efficacy of radionuclide stress tests: problems and solutions. J Nucl Med 1992;33:2074–2079.
Santoro GM, Sciagra R, Buonamici P, et al. Head-to-head comparison of exercise stress testing, pharmacologic stress echocardiography and perfusion tomography as first-line examination for chest pain in patients without history of coronary artery disease. J Nucl Cardiol 1998;5:19–27.
Schelbert HR. Assessment of myocardial viability with positron emission tomography. In: Iskandrian AE, Van der Wall EE, eds. Myocardial Viability. Dordrecht: Kluwer Academic Publishers, 2000:47–72.
Sharir T, Germano G, Kavanagh PB, et al. Incremental prognostic value of post-stress left ventricular ejection fraction and volume by gated myocardial perfusion single photon emission computed tomography. Circulation 1999;100:1035–1042.
Schwaiger M. Myocardial perfusion imaging with PET. J Nucl Med 1994;35:693–698.
Smanio OE, Watson DD, Segalla DL, et al. Value of gating of technetium-99m sestamibi single-photon emission computed tomographic imaging. J Am Coll Cardiol 1997;30:1687–1692.
Stewart R. Schwaiger M, Molina E, et al. Comparison of rubidium-82 positron emission tomography and thallium-201 SPECT imaging for detection of coronary artery disease. Am J Cardiol 1991;67:1303–1310.
Tamaki N, Ohtani H, Yamashita K, et al. Metabolic activity in the areas of new fill-in after thallium-201 reinjection: comparison with positron emission tomography using fluorine-18 deoxyglucose. J Nucl Med 1991;32:673–678.
Tamaki N, Takahashi N, Kawamoto M, et al. Myocardial tomography using technetium-99m tetrofosmin to evaluate coronary artery disease. J Nucl Med 1994;35:594–600.
Treves S, Parker JA. Detection and quantification of intracardiac shunts. In: Strauss HW, Pitt B, eds. Cardiovascular Nuclear Medicine. St. Louis: CV Mosby, 1979:148–161.
Van Train KF, Garcia EV, Maddahi J, et al. Multicenter trial validation for quantitative analysis of same-day rest-stress technetium-99m-sestamibi myocardial tomograms. J Nucl Med 1994;35:609–618.
Watanabe K, Sekiya M, Ikeda S, et al. Comparison of adenosine triphosphate and dipyridamole in diagnosis by thallium-201 myocardial scintigraphy. J Nucl Med 1997;38:577–581.
Wijns W, Vatner S, Camici P. Hibernating myocardium. N Engl J Med 1998;339:173–181.
Williams B, Millani N, Jansen D, Anderson B. A retrospective study of the diagnostic accuracy of a community hospital-based PET center for the detection of coronary artery disease using rubidium-82. J Nucl Med 1994;35:1586–1592.
Yamagishi H, Shirai A, Yoshiyama M, et al. Incremental value of left ventricular ejection fraction for detection of multivessel coronary artery disease in exercise ^{201}Tl gated myocardial perfusion imaging. J Nucl Med 2002;43:131–139.
Zaret BL, Beller GA. Clinical Nuclear Cardiology. 3rd ed. Philadelphia: Elsevier Mosby, 2005.
Zaret BL, Wackers FJT. Nuclear cardiology (1). N Engl J Med 1993;329: 775–783.
Zaret BL, Wackers FJT. Nuclear cardiology (2). N Engl J Med 1993;329: 855–863.

Chapter 58

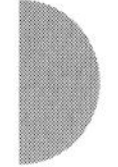

Endocrine Gland Scintigraphy

Marc G. Cote

Thyroid
Thyroid Nodules

Parathyroid

Adrenal

THYROID

Imaging Methods. Diagnosis and treatment of thyroid disease require the evaluation of thyroid function, anatomy including palpatory findings with or without thyroid US, and tissue characterization of thyroid lesions. Radionuclide scintigraphy and measurement of radioactive iodine uptake (RAIU) form the basis of functional assessment of the thyroid.

Radionuclide scintigraphy is used to assess the physiologic function of the gland and to determine the presence or functional status of thyroid nodules post–fine-needle aspiration (FNA). Thyroid imaging is most commonly indicated to evaluate hyperthyroidism. Solitary palpable thyroid nodules are best evaluated initially with FNA. Radionuclide scintigraphy utilizing iodine-123 (I-123) is useful in differentiating substernal thyroid from thymus glands.

Normal thyroid parenchyma appears relatively homogeneous with technetium-99m-pertechnetate (Tc-99m-O_4) or I-123 scintigraphy. Iodine is trapped via active transport and organified onto the tyrosine contained in intrathyroidal thyroglobulin within thyroid follicles. Tc-99m-O_4 is only trapped and will subsequently wash out of the gland since it is not organified. I-123 is the agent of choice for thyroid imaging, especially when imaging nodules (Table 58.1). Tc-99m-O_4 is best reserved for imaging hyperthyroid patients in conjunction with an I-131 RAIU measurement, in which the percentage of the administered dose present in the thyroid gland is measured at a specific time after oral administration, usually at 4 and 24 hours.

The functional status of a thyroid nodule may be categorized as hyperfunctioning (“hot”), hypofunctioning (“cold”), or indeterminate (sometimes called “warm”) relative to the normal parenchymal uptake of radioiodine. The term “warm” is misleading to clinicians and should not be used. Hot nodules usually represent hyperfunctioning adenomatous tissue and are rarely malignant. Although solitary cold nodules are hypofunctioning adenomatous tissue in approximately 40% of cases, they may harbor malignancy in up to 15% of cases. Indeterminate nodules have the same significance as cold nodules. The term “warm” should be avoided since it is easily misunderstood by the referring physician to have the same clinical significance as a “hot” nodule. Indeterminate nodules are caused by normal activity overlying or surrounding a hypofunctioning cold nodule.

Tc-99m-O_4 is inexpensive but has the disadvantage of a lower target-to-background ratio. Also, if a nodule is hot with Tc-99m-O_4, an additional I-123 study must be performed to exclude a discordant nodule. A discordant nodule demonstrates increased Tc-99m-O_4 uptake but decreased I-123 uptake and thus potentially harbors malignancy. Discordant nodules still have the ability to trap Tc-99m-O_4 but have lost their ability to organify iodine. Because pertechnetate imaging is performed 4 to 6 hours after administration, initial trapping of the radiopharmaceutical may reveal uptake that is isointense or increased relative to normal parenchyma. Imaging of I-123 is performed at 18 to 24 hours after administration; therefore, any iodine that may have been trapped has time to wash out of the gland prior

TABLE 58.1 Radiopharmaceuticals Used for Thyroid Imaging

Isotope	*Half-life*	*Principal γ ray (keV)*	*Advantages*	*Disadvantages*	*Comments*
I-123	13 hr	159	Physiologic Good organ-to-background ratio Same dose can be used for imaging and uptake	Expensive Image 4 hours after administration	
I-131	8 days	364	Inexpensive Widely available Long half-life	High radiation dose per mCi High-energy photon Unsuitable for gamma camera imaging	Whole-body scans used for evaluation of residual thyroid and metastatic disease in patients with thyroid cancer
Tc-99m	6 hr	140	Inexpensive Excellent imaging qualities	Requires separate dose of I-123 or I-131 for uptake measurements Must repeat imaging with I-123 if hot nodule found	

I, Iodine; Tc, technetium.

to imaging, thereby revealing the true nature of the nodule.

It is possible to detect nonpalpable abnormalities using a gamma camera with a pinhole collimator. Abnormalities smaller than 1 cm cannot be reliably resolved because of the inherent limitations of the Anger camera. Thyroid US is rapidly replacing this use of scintigraphy because studies that compared palpation of the gland to US have demonstrated the relative insensitivity of palpation to small nodules.

RAIU measurement served as a measure of thyroid function for many years prior to the development of laboratory assays. The development of accurate serologic methods of measuring serum levels of thyroid hormones and ultrasensitive third- and fourth-generation thyroid-stimulating hormone (TSH) assays has provided superior methods of evaluating thyroid function. Serum TSH is the single best test for screening thyroid function. Only in cases of suspected pituitary or hypothalamic disease is the TSH assay alone insufficient for screening thyroid functional status. Measurement of the RAIU is usually indicated for one of three reasons: (*1*) differentiation of Graves disease (uptake high, usually >35% at 24 hours) from subacute or factitious hyperthyroidism (uptake usually <2%), (*2*) assisting in the calculation of radioactive iodine dose for treatment of Graves disease, and (*3*) assessment of suspected toxic multinodular goiters.

If the 24-hour RAIU is to be performed with I-131, 5 to 10 uCi are administered orally, and no imaging is possible at this dose. I-123 administered orally may be used to perform both the imaging and uptake studies in doses of 200 to 400 uCi. For the uptake, a nonimaging uptake probe is used to obtain counts in a neck phantom standard. At 24 hours, counts are obtained of the patient's neck, thigh, and background activity. Many laboratories also count the patient at 4 to 6 hours so that rapid-turnover patients are not missed. Rapid-turnover patients show a markedly elevated 4- to 6-hour RAIU (25% to 50%) but a lower if not normal 24-hour RAIU. Rapid turnover is seen in the setting of Graves disease when the small dose of radioactive iodine is rapidly organified and released into the blood stream as thyroid hormone and subtracted with the thigh background counts.

$$\%\,\text{Uptake} = \frac{\text{Neck} - \text{thigh cpm} \times 100}{\text{Standard} - \text{background cpm}}$$

where cpm = counts per minute. A normal reading = 10% to 30% at 24 hours (highly dependent on iodine intake).

Anatomy, Physiology, and Embryology. The thyroid is located in the lower part of the neck. It consists of two lobes of approximately equal size (5 × 2 cm) positioned on either side of the trachea and connected across the midline by the thin thyroid isthmus inferiorly (Fig. 58.1). A mild degree of asymmetry in the size of the lobes is common. The lobes of the thyroid lie between the carotid artery and jugular vein laterally and the trachea medially. They rest on the longus colli muscles posteriorly and are covered by the sternohyoid, sternothyroid, and prominent sternocleidomastoid muscles anteriorly. A pyramidal lobe (normal variant) extends upward from the isthmus or most commonly from the left lobe in as many as 40% of individuals and represents a lower thyroglossal duct remnant. Histologically, the thyroid gland is composed of thyroid hormone–secreting follicular cells arranged in acini, with central collections of colloid. Embryologically, follicular cells originate from endoderm at the base of the tongue (foramen ovale) that descends to its usual position in the

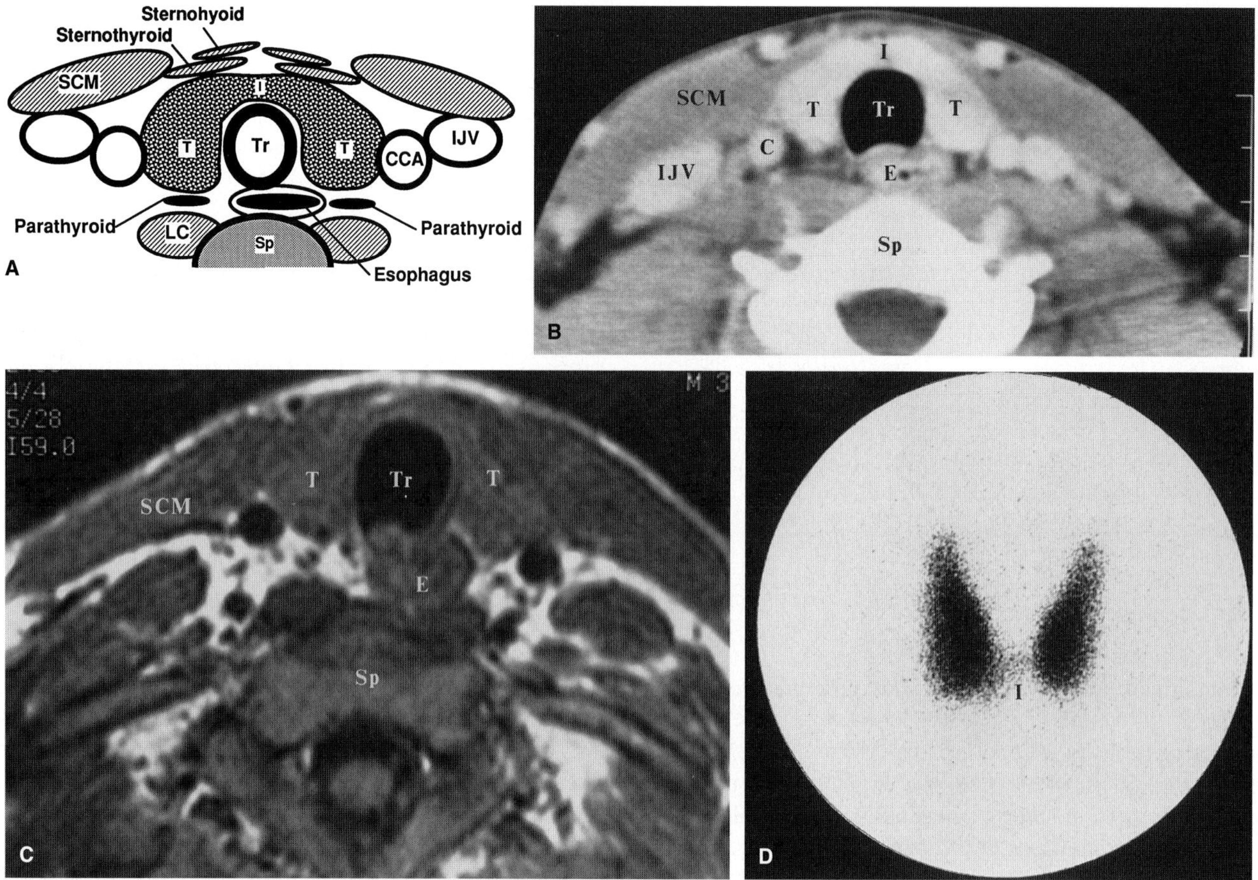

FIGURE 58.1. **Normal Thyroid.** Diagram **(A)**, CT image **(B)**, and T1WI **(C)** of the thyroid gland in cross section. **D.** Normal iodine-123 thyroid scan. T, thyroid gland; I, isthmus of thyroid gland; Tr, trachea; CCA, common carotid artery; IJV, internal jugular vein; E, esophagus; SCM, sternocleidomastoid muscle; LC, longus colli muscle; Sp, spine.

neck. Failure of the thyroid to descend may result in a lingual thyroid. Lingual thyroid pediatric patients are at high risk of developing hypothyroidism, with an estimated risk of ~30%. Thyroglossal duct persistence beyond the second gestational month of the thyroid's descent tract may occur and result in a persistent thyroglossal duct. Perifollicular cells ("C cells"), which produce calcitonin, comprise a small proportion of the cell population. Embryologically, perifollicular "C" cells are of ectodermal origin from the fourth pharyngeal pouch and descendants of the amine precursor uptake and decarboxylation (APUD) system.

The role of the thyroid gland is the production, storage, and release of thyroid hormones. TSH, produced by the anterior portion of the pituitary gland, regulates the production and release of thyroid hormones. TSH secretion is regulated by hypothalamic thyrotropin–releasing hormone (TRH) and suppressed by circulating thyroxine (T4) and triiodothyronine (T3). Dietary iodine is absorbed in the stomach and upper small bowel, where it is rapidly reduced to iodide. It is trapped by active transport from the bloodstream by the follicular cells of the thyroid, where it is incorporated (organified) onto the tyrosine contained in the intrathyroidal thyroglobulin in the production of T4 and T3. Depending upon dietary content, about 25% of ingested iodine is taken up by the thyroid and 75% is excreted in the urine. The recommended daily adult allowance for iodine is 100 to 150 mg. This is greatly exceeded in most developed countries such as the United States, where the daily intake of iodine may be as high as 500 mg from some of the rich sources in the American diet: commercial breads, seafood, and dairy products. However, iodine deficiency is still endemic in certain parts of the world, particularly the Andes, Himalayas, and inland areas of Europe and Africa. Iodine uptake competes with the monovalent anion of pertechnetate, perchlorate, and thiocyanates. Thiocyanates are found in vegetables such as cabbage and turnips.

Hypothyroidism. In endemic areas, hypothyroidism is usually caused by dietary iodine deficiency (with a goiter [enlarged gland] present), whereas in iodine-replete areas, the commonest noniatrogenic cause is chronic thyroiditis (Hashimoto disease), in which a goiter is also usually present. Prior treatment of hyperthyroidism with radioactive iodine is another common cause (no goiter). Neonatal hypothyroidism is caused by thyroid dysgenesis (agenesis, hypoplasia, or ectopia). Pediatric lingual thyroid has a 30% chance of developing hypothyroidism. Hypothyroidism's usual clinical features include weight gain, cold intolerance, sluggishness, fatigue, and dry skin. Laboratory findings include elevated serum TSH and low serum T4.

Hyperthyroidism. Graves disease (diffuse toxic goiter) is the most common cause of hyperthyroidism. Other causes include subacute or painless thyroiditis, toxic nodular goiter, and factitious hyperthyroidism caused by ingestion of thyroid hormone tablets. Clinical features of hyperthyroidism include weight loss, increased appetite, tremor, heat intolerance, palpitations, muscle weakness, goiter, exophthalmus, and mood changes or irritability. Laboratory findings include a markedly decreased (suppressed) serum TSH and an elevated serum T4.

Goiter refers to the clinical finding of generalized thyroid enlargement. Goiter may be associated with increased, decreased, or normal thyroid hormonal function. Thyroid enlargement may be suspected by physical exam and its accurate extent determined by a variety of imaging techniques. Goiters extending into the thorax may be imaged with the use of I-123. Tc-99m-O_4 is not useful with substernal goiter because of the large amount of blood pool activity within the chest.

Multinodular goiter is a commonly used clinical term for adenomatous hyperplasia. Imaging studies reveal a diffusely abnormally enlarged nodular gland, with heterogeneous uptake of the radiopharmaceutical or a pattern of multiple, discrete hot nodules on a background of normal or "cool" parenchyma. Photopenic regions should be palpated and dominant palpable nodules should be marked to ensure that they do not represent a dominant cold nodule. A recent study reported a 4.1% rate of malignancy in patients with a dominant palpable cold nodule in the setting of multinodular goiter. The hot nodules represent autonomously functioning thyroid adenomas, which are usually benign (Fig. 58.2).

Nontoxic goiter may be related to iodine deficiency, goitrogens in the diet, medications, or a thyroid enzyme deficiency. The gland is usually soft and symmetric but may appear multinodular with age.

Thyroiditis. All types of thyroiditis are characterized by rapid, asymmetric glandular enlargement with or without nodularity. Inflammatory changes may fixate the gland to adjacent structures and simulate malignancy. Infection of the thyroid gland may be acute and suppurative because of gram-positive bacteria or subacute because of viral infection, which may involve only a portion of the gland. Immunocompromised patients (e.g., diabetics with multinodular goiters) have a greater risk of developing suppurative infections. Suppurative infection is associated with hemorrhage, necrosis, and abscess formation and is a medical emergency, because it may transcend into the mediastinum. Subacute viral infection usually causes focal edematous enlargement of the gland. Subacute viral infection may have a protean presentation that mimics some of the clinical features of Graves disease because of release of all preformed thyroid hormone as a response to the inflammation. The RAIU test allows for differentiation of this syndrome from Graves disease. Unlike Graves disease, with its high RAIU and intense thyroid scan appearance, subacute viral patients have a very low RAIU, such that scintigraphy of the thyroid gland is rarely indicated. The majority of patients with subacute thyroiditis will resolve and return to a euthyroid state after a transient period of hypothyroidism and elevation of RAIU as the gland returns to normal.

Graves disease is the most common cause of hyperthyroidism. It is an autoimmune disorder in which thyroid-stimulating antibodies cause hyperplasia and hyperfunction of the thyroid gland. The gland is usually enlarged by two to three times, homogeneous on thyroid scan, and free of palpable nodules (Fig. 58.3). The treatment of choice for nonpregnant, nonlactating adults with Graves disease is oral I-131 in conjunction with β-blockers such as propranolol to control symptoms during therapy. Treatment options include subtotal thyroidectomy or antithyroid drugs such as propylthiouracil, methimazole, and carbimazole.

I-131 in the form of sodium iodide has been in use for many years. It is given by mouth either as a capsule or as a liquid. After uptake by the gland, the high-energy β particles (mean energy of 0.19 MeV) deliver an average of 1 rad/μCi (1,000 rads/mCi) to the thyroid cells. There is

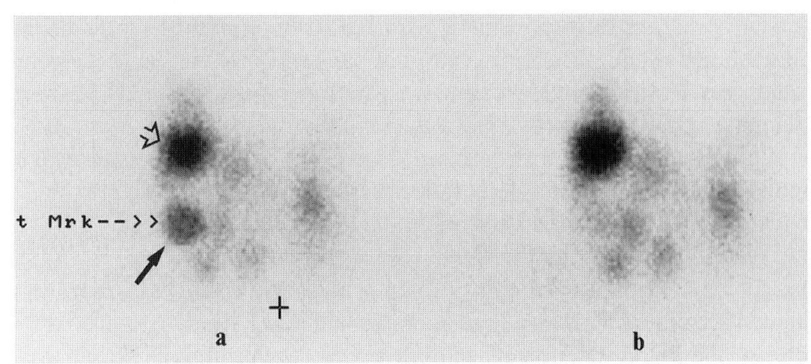

FIGURE 58.2. **Thyroid Nodules.** Two images from an iodine-123 thyroid scan. A radioactive marker (*closed arrow*) was placed over a 2-cm palpable nodule in the right thyroid lobe for the image on the left (a). The image on the right (b), without the marker, demonstrates the palpable nodule to be cold. A second palpable nodule in the right upper lobe (*open arrow*) is shown to be hot. Biopsy confirmed a papillary thyroid cancer with multinodular goiter. This case illustrates the importance of palpating and marking nodules.

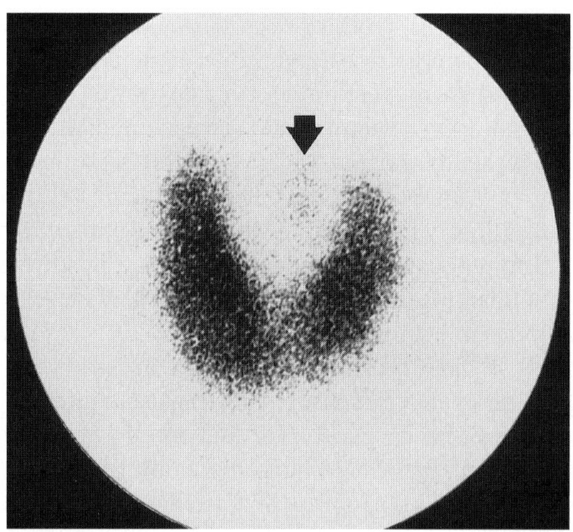

FIGURE 58.3. **Graves Disease.** This iodine-123 scan demonstrates diffuse thyroid enlargement without nodules. A pyramidal lobe is visualized *(arrow)*.

very little radiation dose to structures outside the thyroid gland, since the average range of the β particles is 0.8 to 1.0 mm in soft tissue. Most patients will become euthyroid or hypothyroid after a single dose. Ten percent to 20% of patients require a second or third dose. Patients generally become euthyroid by 10 to 12 weeks after therapy and frequently become hypothyroid by 6 to 12 months. Estimation of the dose of I-131 is empiric. A commonly used formula is:

$$\text{Dose in mCi} = \frac{100 - 150\,\text{uCi/g} \times \text{wt of the gland in grams}}{\text{24-hr RAIU \% uptake} \times 10}$$

This results in a typically administered oral dose of approximately 5 to 20 mCi of I-131. The higher the dose, the quicker the response and the sooner the patient becomes hypothyroid. The smaller the dose, the longer it takes to become euthyroid and the later the development of hypothyroidism. However, it appears that hypothyroidism cannot be avoided but only delayed by using small doses of I-131. Therefore it has become a common policy in many centers to give larger doses of I-131 in the range of 15 to 25 mCi with the understanding that hypothyroidism is inevitable and is easily treated with daily replacement levothyroxine. It is important to document with laboratory testing that women of childbearing age are not pregnant prior to treatment with radioactive iodine, since iodine crosses the placental barrier and will damage the fetal thyroid.

Complications are uncommon. However, transient worsening of thyrotoxicosis is fairly common. It occurs a few days to 2 to 3 weeks after treatment and is caused by the release of preformed thyroid hormone from disrupted follicles. Occasionally patients develop symptoms of subacute thyroiditis, with pain and tenderness in the thyroid, often radiating to the ears or jaw. Temporary hypoparathyroidism and recurrent laryngeal nerve damage have been reported after radioactive iodine treatment, but both are exceedingly rare. Though serious and life threatening, thyroid storm is a very rare complication that is more often seen after surgery in inadequately prepared patients. The patient's risk of genetic damage to a fetus is no greater than the baseline pretreatment risk, provided the patient waits 6 months prior to conception. Carcinogenesis is not statistically increased over baseline.

All forms of thyroiditis may be mistaken for tumor because of rapid asymmetric enlargement and nodularity.

Acute (suppurative) thyroiditis is secondary to bacterial infections caused by *Streptococcus, Staphylococcus,* or *Pneumococcus*. The condition presents with fever, severe sore throat, and asymmetric swelling and may result in sepsis from hematogenous spread or extend into the mediastinum via fascial planes. Other clinical complications include airway compromise and vascular thrombosis of neighboring vessels. Surgical drainage, antibiotics, and medical management with attention to the airway may be required in these acutely ill patients.

Subacute (viral) thyroiditis has many eponyms but is commonly known as de Quervain or granulomatous thyroiditis. Subacute thyroiditis presents with thyroid pain and hyperthyroidism following an upper respiratory infection as the gland is disrupted and releases its thyroid hormone into the bloodstream. Iodine uptake is usually decreased or absent in the acute stages. The disease runs a subacute course of a few weeks to a few months before healing and returning back to a euthyroid state.

Hashimoto thyroiditis is the most common cause of goiter and primary hypothyroidism in adults in developed countries. It is an autoimmune disorder with circulating antithyroid antibody. Histology demonstrates diffuse lymphocytic infiltration of the gland. The thyroid is diffusely enlarged with a rubbery, palpable texture. Its early phase is a hyperthyroid-like picture that subsequently evolves into its final hypothyroid sine qua non.

Riedel thyroiditis is a rare inflammatory fibrosing process that involves the thyroid and commonly extends into the neck. Radionuclide uptake is absent (cold) in the involved areas.

Secondary hyperthyroidism may develop in patients with hydatidiform moles or choriocarcinoma. A subunit of the human chorionic gonadotropin produced by these conditions demonstrates considerable similarity to TSH, thereby directly stimulating the thyroid. Clinical history and serum determination of human chorionic gonadotropin should be performed if this is a consideration.

Thyroid Nodules

Thyroid nodules are extremely common, whereas thyroid cancer is relatively rare. Nodules can be palpated in 4% to 7% of American adults who are asymptomatic for thyroid disease. Autopsy studies demonstrate thyroid nodules in 50% of patients with clinically normal thyroid glands. US studies can detect thyroid nodules in 36% to 41% of middle-aged adults, with some studies reporting even higher rates of 67%. Thyroid cancer, on the other hand, affects only 0.1% of the population. The incidence of thyroid cancer is ~20,000 new cases each year. Thyroid cancer represents less than 1% of all cancers and is responsible for <0.5% of all cancer deaths. The challenge of clinical evaluation and imaging studies is to establish the likelihood of malignancy and to select for surgery only those patients at high risk for thyroid malignancy.

US is highly sensitive for the detection of thyroid nodules, but its specificity for determining malignancy is low. Recent consensus panels have discouraged the routine use of US for screening. Neither MR nor CT improves specificity. This is not surprising, since the histologic differentiation of benign follicular adenoma from well-differentiated follicular carcinoma is based solely on identification of vascular invasion.

On the basis of radioiodine or Tc-99m-O_4 uptake during imaging, nodules may be classified as hypofunctioning (cold) (Fig. 58.4), relative to the rest of the gland, hyperfunctioning (hot) (Fig. 58.5), or indeterminate. In a patient with a nodular goiter, the main concern is whether or not thyroid carcinoma is present. Single cold nodules have a 10% to 15% incidence of malignancy, whereas malignancy is exceedingly rare in hot nodules. A multinodular gland with one or more cold nodules may harbor cancer in up to 5% of patients. If Tc-99m-O_4 is used for imaging and a hot nodule is discovered, imaging must be repeated with I-123, as thyroid carcinoma may occasionally trap Tc-99m-O_4, resulting in a hot nodule. This nodule would be cold with I-123.

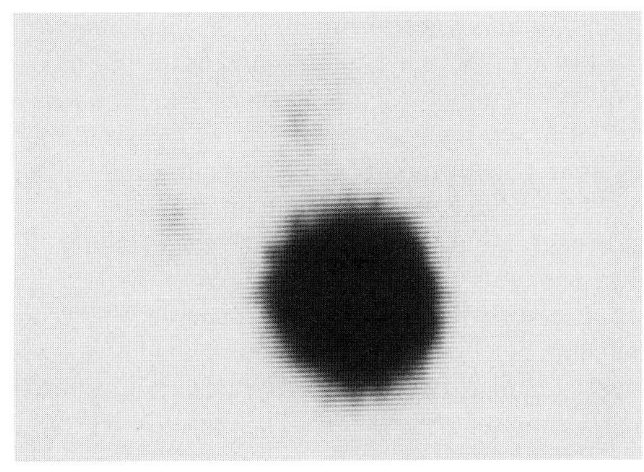

FIGURE 58.5. **Hot Nodule: Hyperfunctioning Adenoma.** A hyperfunctioning adenoma demonstrates intense radionuclide activity with suppression of function of the remainder of the gland.

The differential diagnosis of thyroid nodules is as follows:

Follicular adenoma is the most common benign neoplasm of the thyroid and represents about 20% of thyroid nodules. There are many subtypes based upon histologic criteria, including Hürthle cell adenoma, colloid adenoma, and others. Most are solitary, round or oval, and well encapsulated. Regressive changes are extremely common and greatly affect a nodule's imaging appearance. These include focal necrosis, hemorrhage, edema, infarction, fibrosis, and calcification.

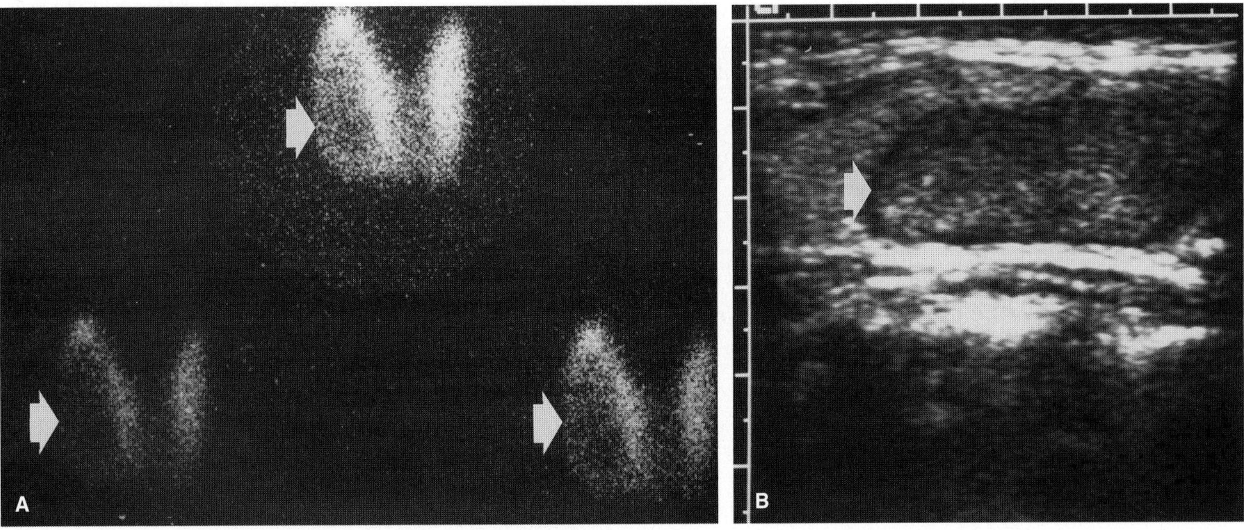

FIGURE 58.4. **Cold Nodule: Follicular Adenoma. A.** An iodine-123 scan photographed at three different intensities demonstrates a large hypofunctioning nodule (*arrows*) in the right thyroid lobe. **B.** Longitudinal US image of the right thyroid lobe reveals a well-defined solid nodule (*arrow*) with a hypoechoic rim. Pathology confirmed a follicular adenoma.

Adenomatous hyperplasia is responsible for up to 50% of thyroid nodules. Adenomatous nodules, also called *colloid nodules*, are not true neoplasms but are the result of cycles of hyperplasia and involution of a thyroid lobule. They are frequently multiple, but one nodule may be dominant. Regressive changes are common, including necrosis, hemorrhage, cystic degeneration, and calcification.

Thyroid cysts are extremely rare. Most cystic nodules found in the thyroid are actually cystic degeneration of an adenomatous nodule or a follicular adenoma. The incidence of malignancy within a thyroid cyst is reported to be in the range of 0.5% to 3.0%. Therefore, fluid should be submitted for cytology and the area aspirated should have adequate sampling.

Hemorrhagic cysts also usually represent hemorrhage into an adenomatous nodule or a follicular adenoma. Hemorrhage into normal parenchyma also may produce a hemorrhagic cyst.

Thyroid Cancer. It is estimated that 20,000 new thyroid cancer cases occur each year resulting in more than 1400 deaths per year in the U.S. Thyroid cancer's annual incidence is ~7/100,000 population. Malignant nodules cannot be reliably differentiated from benign nodules by any imaging method. FNA with good sampling technique and good cytologic support is essential in every suspicious case. However, a number of criteria can be used to assess the relative risk of malignancy (Tables 58.2, 58.3). Every assessment of thyroid nodules must consider all clinical and imaging features. A nodule that is hot on radioiodine scan is extremely unlikely to be malignant. A nodule that is solitary and cold on scintigraphy has a 6% to 10% chance of being malignant. A history of neck irradiation, particularly in childhood, increases the risk of malignancy by 5 to 10 times (0.3 to 12.5/10,000 person-years). Nodules with an extensive cystic component (>50% cystic) or well-defined peripheral calcification as seen at US are unlikely to be malignant. Regression of nodule size following thyroid hormone therapy is a sign of a benign nodule. Large, predominantly solid nodules with irregular contour and poor margination on US examination are likely to be malignant. Five-year survival rates with treatment are ~90% to 95%. The histologic types of thyroid malignancy are as follows:

TABLE 58.2 Signs Suggesting Benign Etiology of Thyroid Nodules

Extensive cystic component
Multiple nodules
Hot on radionuclide scan
Peripheral calcification
Shrinkage in size following levothyroxine suppression hormone therapy
Sudden onset
Female gender
Older patient

TABLE 58.3 Signs Suggesting Malignancy of Thyroid Nodules

Imaging findings
Solid nodule
Cold on radionuclide scan
Irregular contour
Poor margination
Size >4 to 5 cm
Clinical findings
Hard on palpation
History of neck irradiation
Age <20 yr
Male
Familial history of thyroid cancer

Papillary carcinoma is the most common type and is responsible for 75% of cases. Patients are predominantly female (female:male = 4:1), with an average age of 45. The major route of spread is lymphatic to regional nodes, followed by hematogenous dissemination to lungs and bone (Fig. 58.6).

Follicular carcinoma represents 15% of cases and is also more common in women. The primary route of spread is hematogenous to lung and bone. The prognosis is not as good as for papillary carcinoma.

Medullary carcinoma arises from perifollicular cells (C cells) and is associated with multiple endocrine neoplasia (MEN II) in some cases. Calcitonin is a useful tumor marker. The prognosis is worse than for papillary or follicular carcinoma. The tumor spreads by both lymphatic and hematogenous routes. Although the tumor does not concentrate I-131, metastases can be detected by thallium-201 (Tl-201), Tc-99m dimercaptosuccinic acid, pentavalent form, and I-123/131-metaiodobenzylguanidine (MIBG). I-131-MIBG has also been used for treatment.

Anaplastic carcinoma is an extremely lethal malignancy with no effective treatment and a 5-year survival rate of less than 4%. The tumor invades locally very aggressively, spreads early to distant sites, and generally occurs in an older population.

The initial postthyroidectomy I-131 whole-body scan with its 72-hour RAIU, the surgical pathology report of the thyroid tumor, its size, presence of contralateral lobe involvement or noninvolvement, and lymph node status determination allow for initial staging of the tumor and treatment planning. One must consider the common routes of spread for the specific type of malignancy to optimally plan the imaging study and subsequent treatment. For non–iodine-avid tumors, lymph node involvement is determined primarily by size criteria with subsequent pathologic confirmation. Normal lymph nodes in the neck

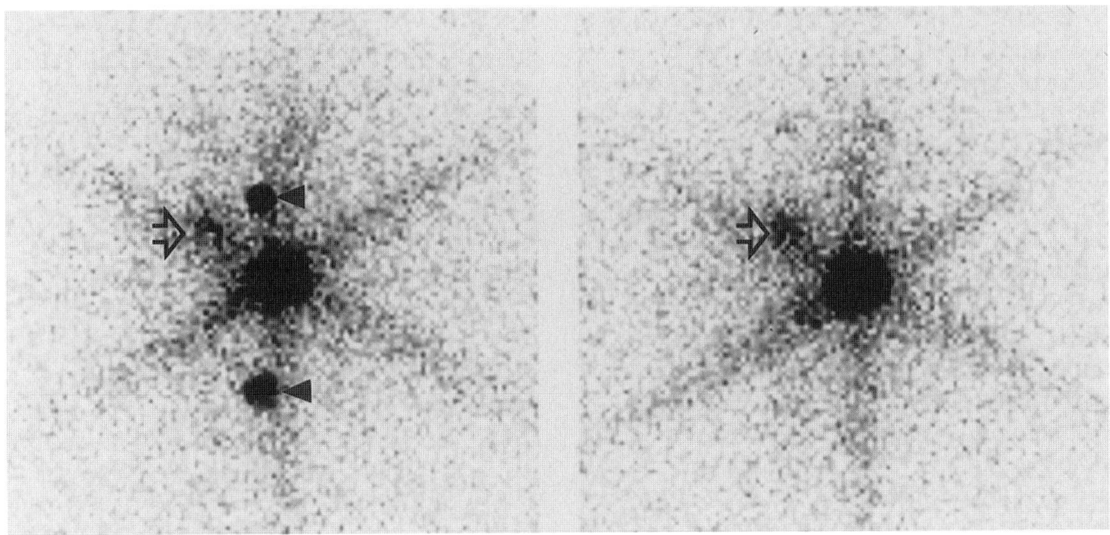

FIGURE 58.6. **Thyroid Cancer Metastasis.** Iodine-131 scan of the neck in patient who has undergone near-total thyroidectomy for thyroid cancer. Radioactive markers of the chin and suprasternal notch are seen on the first scan (*arrowheads*). The large star artifact is caused by septal penetration of the collimator. The center of the star represents the original thyroid bed. A lymph node metastasis is evident in the right upper neck (*open arrows*).

are smaller than 10 mm in diameter. Som provides an excellent review of the anatomy and description of cervical lymph nodes.

Whole-body radionuclide scans using I-131 are effective in demonstrating thyroid metastases and tumor recurrence following thyroidectomy for papillary carcinoma (Fig. 58.7). However, radionuclide whole-body scans are ineffective in medullary and anaplastic carcinoma because of the lack of iodine uptake by the tumor.

Radioiodine (I-131) scans of the whole body, neck, and chest are performed to determine the completeness of surgery and to evaluate the response to treatment. Uptake of I-131 in the thyroid bed frequently represents residual thyroid tissue. Salivary, stomach, bowel, and bladder activity represents physiologic traces of iodine distribution. Focal activity in the lungs, skeleton, or in the neck remote from the thyroid bed is pathologic. Nasal secretions may contain radioiodine. A contaminated pocket handkerchief should not be mistaken for a metastasis. Similarly, some breast uptake may occur. This should not be confused with lung metastasis. Unfortunately, some patients may have non–I-131-avid thyroid tumor but demonstrate persistent disease, as noted by elevated serum thyroglobulin. Tl-201 and more recently Tc-99m-sestamibi (Tc-99m-MIBI) and Tc-99m-tetrofosmin (Tc-99m-Tfos) have shown some utility in imaging non–I-131-avid thyroid tumor.

Postablation Imaging of Thyroid Cancer Patients. The use of recombinant human thyroid stimulating hormone treatment (rhTSH) to image postablation patients for follow-up screening is an option that does not require withdrawal of levothyroxine replacement. Serum thyroglobulin is a sensitive serum marker of recurrent differentiated thyroid cancer. On day 1, baseline serum thyroglobulin levels are obtained, and an intramuscular injection of 0.9 mg of rhTSH is administered on day 1 and

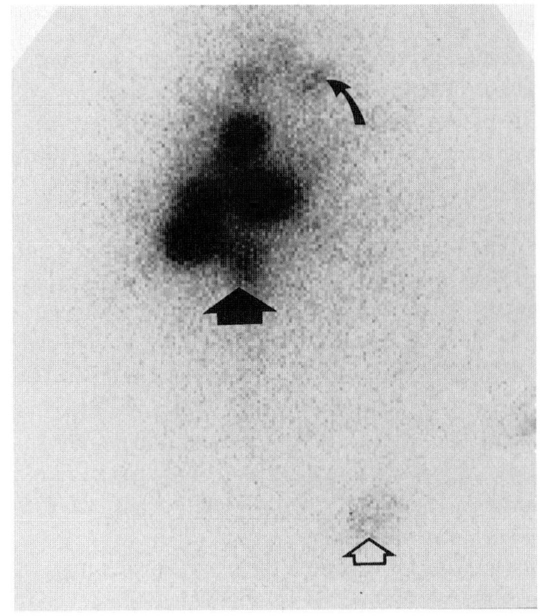

FIGURE 58.7. **Lymph Node Metastases.** Iodine-131 whole-body scan postthyroidectomy shows intense radionuclide activity in papillary carcinoma lymph node metastases in the neck (*solid arrow*). Normal activity is present in the stomach (*open arrow*) and submandibular salivary glands (*curved arrow*).

day 2. Serum thyroglobulin levels are obtained on days 3 and 5. Low or undetectable baseline thyroglobulin levels ≥2 ng/mL following rhTSH stimulation are suggestive of recurrent thyroid cancer. I-131 or I-123 is given 24 hours after the second rhTSH dose, and imaging can be performed at 48 hours after I-131 administration or at 24 hours for I-123. In the future, rTSH may be useful in preparation for ablation therapy for thyroid remnants following surgery, based on preliminary data, but studies are still underway to validate this general use.

Radioiodine Therapy. Most authorities agree with postthyroidectomy ablation in primary thyroid tumors >1.5 cm. Some disagreement now exists in the literature on the treatment of patients with I-131 if the primary tumor is <1 cm.

According to the Nuclear Regulatory Commission (NRC) (NUREG-1556, vol. 9) patients receiving 33 mCi or more of I-131 require hospitalization until the residual amount of I-131 falls below 33 mCi or a rate meter reading of <7 mR/hr at 1 m, unless it can be shown that it is unlikely that releasing the patient would result in a member of the public receiving a dose greater than 500 mrem. Doses close to 33 mCi of I-131 are frequently used on an outpatient basis to ablate residual thyroid postthyroidectomy. Revised NRC rules for doses greater than 33 mCi I-131 as an outpatient require extensive regulatory documentation and calculations. Some authors advocate larger doses on the grounds that 33 mCi I-131 are inadequate to ablate thyroid cancer and may cause a stunning effect that makes the thyroid more radioresistant on subsequent treatment. Doses of 100 to 200 mCi I-131 are frequently used, depending on the tumor cytology, its size, and the presence of capsular, vascular, or lymph node involvement.

The patient should be hypothyroid with a serum TSH greater than 40 IU/mL prior to whole body I-131 imaging or ablation, because elevated TSH is the strongest determinant in activating active transport of the iodine into the thyroid cell. This is to ensure maximal stimulation of residual thyroid and/or thyroid cancer and thereby promote appropriate localization of the radioiodine. Iodine-rich foods such as shellfish, bread, and kelp should be avoided at least 1 week prior to therapy. Dairy products should also be limited because they are a rich source of "cold" iodine that can inhibit uptake of the I-131. A radiographic study with iodinated contrast will delay therapy by at least 2 to 3 months unless clinical maneuvers to deplete the patient of the exogenous iodine is performed.

The frequency of side effects varies directly with the dose of radioiodine administered. Doses greater than 100 mCi may cause sialoadenitis, which may lead to permanent xerostomia. For this reason, patients should be strongly encouraged to drink copious amounts of water and suck on sialogogues such as lemon drops or sour candy for 3 to 7 days after therapy. Pulmonary fibrosis has been reported in patients who have received multiple doses of radioiodine therapy for extensive pulmonary disease. Leukemia has been reported in patients who have received cumulative doses in excess of 600 to 800 mCi.

Metastases to the thyroid gland are rare. The most common primary tumors to metastasize to the thyroid are breast, lung, kidney, malignant melanoma, and lymphoma.

PARATHYROID

Parathyroid disorders are classified in terms of function: excessive parathyroid hormone (PTH) production or hyperparathyroidism, and insufficient PTH production or hypoparathyroidism. Imaging studies of the parathyroid glands are performed to localize parathyroid abnormalities in patients with hyperparathyroidism that has been confirmed clinically. There is no role for imaging in hypoparathyroidism. The causes of hyperparathyroidism are listed in Table 58.4.

Imaging Methods. Approximately 80% to 85% of abnormal parathyroid glands are located near the thyroid. Ectopic locations for abnormal parathyroid tissue include: thymus (10% to 15%), posterior mediastinum (5%), retroesophageal (1%), within the carotid sheath (1%), and parapharyngeal (0.5%). US, scintigraphy with Tl-201, Tc-99m-MIBI, CT, and MR have various sensitivities and specificities that depend on whether the patient has had prior surgery. At centers with very experienced surgeons, surgery is curative in 92% to 98% of patients with previously unoperated hyperparathyroidism, but reoperation success decreases to 62% in patients who require a repeat surgery. Localization procedures are indicated in patients

TABLE 58.4 Causes of Hyperparathyroidism

Primary hyperparathyroidism
- Solitary parathyroid adenoma, 85%
- Parathyroid hyperplasia, 10%
- Multiple parathyroid adenomas, 4%
- Parathyroid carcinoma, 1%

Secondary hyperparathyroidism
- Diffuse or adenomatous parathyroid hyperplasia caused by calcium-losing renal disease

Tertiary hyperparathyroidism
- Autonomous parathyroid function resulting from long-standing secondary hyperparathyroidism

Paraneoplastic syndromes
- Ectopic parathormone production
- Bronchogenic carcinoma
- Renal cell carcinoma

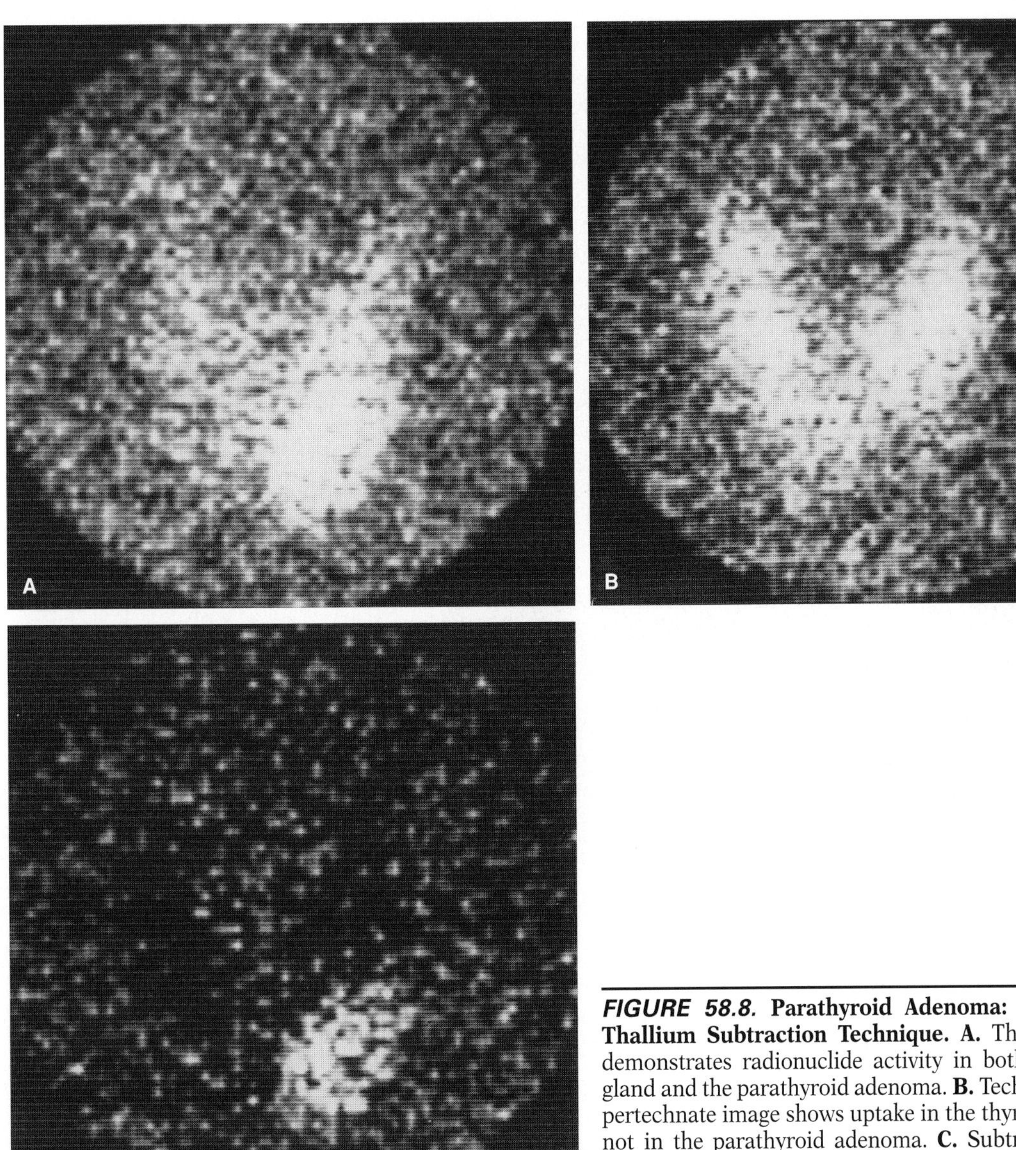

FIGURE 58.8. **Parathyroid Adenoma: Technetium-Thallium Subtraction Technique. A.** Thallium image demonstrates radionuclide activity in both the thyroid gland and the parathyroid adenoma. **B.** Technetium-99m-pertechnate image shows uptake in the thyroid gland but not in the parathyroid adenoma. **C.** Subtraction image shows a residual focus of activity, identifying a parathyroid adenoma at the lower pole of the left thyroid lobe.

who are surgical failures requiring a second surgery and may be helpful prior to a first operation when the local surgical experience is limited.

Technetium-99m-pertechnate/thallium-201 radionuclide subtraction imaging has been used to detect parathyroid adenomas with a sensitivity of about 75% and a specificity of 90%. Thyroid tissue concentrates both Tc-99mO_4 and Tl-201 (Fig. 58.8). Parathyroid adenomas take up Tl-201 but not Tc-99mO_4. This is the basis for dual-isotope imaging. First the Tl-201 images are acquired; then, without moving the patient, Tc-99mO_4 is administered and imaging is performed at the Tc peak. The Tc-99mO_4 images are subsequently subtracted from the Tl-201 images. A residual focus of activity indicates the presence of a parathyroid adenoma. It is vital that the patient does not move at all; otherwise, erroneous results will be obtained. False-positive results can be seen with Tl-201 uptake in thyroid nodules, sarcoid-containing lymph nodes, or metastases to the neck, because the technique is predicated on the presence of an underlying normal thyroid gland.

Sestamibi and Tetrofosmin Imaging. Recently Tc-99m-MIBI and Tc-99m-Tfos have virtually replaced Tc-99mO_4/Tl-201 subtraction imaging at most centers. Both of these agents have similar sensitivities and specificities to other imaging methods. When Tc-99m-MIBI or Tc-99m-Tfos is used for parathyroid imaging, immediate and delayed images of the neck and mediastinum are performed. Parathyroid adenomas may or may not be visualized on initial imaging, but they tend to retain the radiopharmaceutical on delayed (1- to 2-hour) images (Fig. 58.9) whereas the normal thyroid gland washes out (Fig. 58.9). Retention occurs in the mitochondria-rich cells

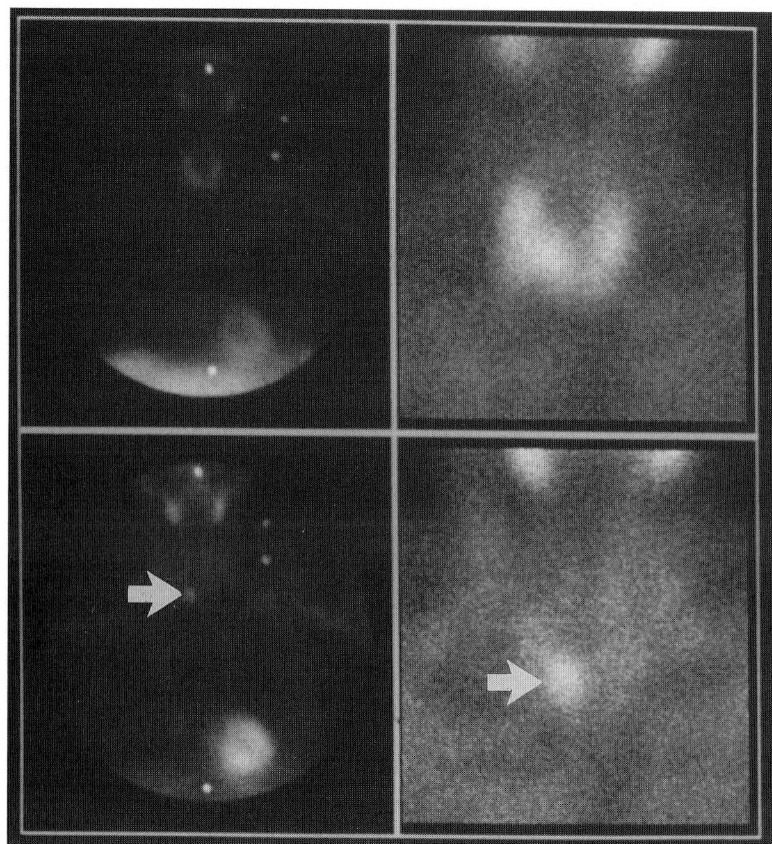

FIGURE 58.9. Parathyroid Adenoma: Technetium-Sestamibi Scan. A focus of radionuclide activity is seen in the lower pole of the right lobe of the thyroid (*arrows*). Surgery confirmed a parathyroid adenoma.

of the adenoma. False-negative results may be seen in clear cell adenomas, which histologically contain a paucity of mitochondria.

Anatomy. Most people (80%) have four parathyroid glands, two superior and two inferior. However, autopsy studies have demonstrated that 20% of individuals have three, five, or six parathyroid glands. The superior parathyroid glands arise from the fourth branchial pouch along with the thyroid gland and are seldom ectopic. The inferior parathyroid glands arise from the third branchial pouch along with the thymus and are more commonly ectopic, usually in the mediastinum. Normal glands measure 5 × 3 × 1 mm in size and average 10 to 80 mg. Because they are so small and flat, normal glands are not usually demonstrated by any imaging method. The normally located parathyroid glands are found posterior to the thyroid lobes, superficial to the longus colli muscles (Fig. 58.1), and between the trachea and carotid sheath.

Parathyroid adenomas are characteristically oval in shape and 8 to 15 mm in greatest diameter. Their cellularity is homogeneous, giving a uniform internal appearance on all imaging modalities.

Multiple Gland Disease. Parathyroid hyperplasia cannot be differentiated from multiple parathyroid adenomas by imaging methods. Hyperplasia affects all of the parathyroid glands but is frequently asymmetric. The individual glands have the same imaging appearance as parathyroid adenomas.

Parathyroid carcinomas are usually larger than adenomas (at least 2 cm in size). The internal architecture is much more heterogeneous, with cystic degeneration more common. Invasion of adjacent muscle or vessels may be demonstrated. The differentiation of parathyroid carcinoma from a large adenoma can usually be made only histologically.

Ectopic parathyroids are most common in the anterosuperior mediastinum or low in the neck. Immediate and delayed imaging of the neck and mediastinum with Tc-99m-MIBI or Tc-99m-Tfos has a diagnostic sensitivity of 75%. Tc-99m-MIBI or Tc-99m-Tfos imaging currently seems to be the modality of choice for identifying ectopic parathyroids, in view of the improved target-to-background visualization when compared to Tl-201. CT, MR, and scintigraphy all have reported sensitivities of approximately 75%.

ADRENAL

High-resolution anatomic imaging of the adrenal glands is performed by CT, MR, or US and is discussed in Chapter 33. Functional imaging of hyperplastic or neoplastic adrenal disorders can be performed with the following radiopharmaceuticals: I-131-6-iodomethyl-19-norcholesterol (NP59), or I-131-MIBG. NP59, a cholesterol analogue, is taken up by adrenal cortical tissue. Cholesterol is a common precursor of mineralocorticoids, glucocorticoids, and androgens. MIBG is taken up by cells of adrenal medullary origin such as pheochromocytoma. In addition, tumors of neural crest origin such as neuroblastoma and medullary thyroid cancer often concentrate MIBG. MIBG detects neuroblastomas and their metastases in >90% of cases. Note that NP59 is available only for investigational use in the United States, although it is available commercially in many other countries.

Indium-111 pentetreotide is a synthetic somatostatin analogue with a longer plasma half-life than native somatostatin. This radiopharmaceutical is useful in imaging a wide variety of neuroendocrine tumors. Sensitivities vary according to tumor type, with carcinoid and paraganglioma having fairly high sensitivities.

SUGGESTED READINGS

Code of Federal Regulations, Title 10, Part 35, Subpart C, Section 35.75, 24 April 2002.

David A, Blotta A, Bondanelli M, et al. Serum thyroglobulin concentrations and I-131 whole-body scan results in patients with differentiated thyroid carcinoma after administration of recombinant human thyroid-stimulating hormone. J Nucl Med 2001;42:1470–1475.

Ezzat S, Sarti DA, Cain DR, et al. Thyroid incidentalomas: prevalence by palpation and ultrasonography. Arch Intern Med 1994;154:1838–1840.

Fjeld JG, Erichsen K, Pfeffer PF, et al. Technetium-99m-tetrofosmin for parathyroid scintigraphy: A comparison with sestamibi. J Nucl Med 1997;38:831–834.

Freitas JE, Freitas AE. Thyroid and parathyroid imaging. Semin Nucl Med 1994;24:234–245.

Hall P, Holm LE, Lundell G, et al. Cancer risks in thyroid cancer patients. Br J Cancer 1991;64:159–163.

Haugen BR, Pacini F, Reiners C, et al. A comparison of recombinant human thyrotropin and thyroid hormone withdrawal for the detection of thyroid remnant or cancer. J Clin Endocrinol Metab 1999;84:3877–3885.

McBiles M, Lambert AT, Cote MG, Kim SY. Sestamibi parathyroid imaging. Sem Nucl Med 1995;25:221–234.

McDougall IR. Thyroid Diseases in Clinical Practice. New York: Oxford University Press, 1992.

Sandler MP, Patton JA, Gross MD, et al. Endocrine Imaging. Norwalk: Appleton & Lange, 1992.

Som PM. Lymph nodes of the neck. Radiology 1987;165:593–600.

Takahashi T, Trott KR, Fujimori K, et al. An investigation into the prevalence of thyroid disease on Kwajalein Atoll, Marshall Islands. Health Phys 1997 Jul;73(1):199–213.

Wiest PW,, Hartshorne MF, Inskip PD, et al. Thyroid palpation versus high-resolution thyroid ultrasonography in the detection of nodules. J Ultrasound Med 1998;17:487–496.

Chapter 59

Gastrointestinal, Liver/Spleen, and Hepatobiliary Scintigraphy

David K. Shelton and Michael F. Hartshorne

Gastrointestinal Studies

Liver and Spleen Studies

Hepatobiliary Imaging

Hepatic Blood Pool Scintigraphy

PET Fluoroxydeglucose in Gastrointestinal Cancers

GASTROINTESTINAL STUDIES

Nuclear medicine imaging studies can provide considerable information in the functional evaluation of the GI system. Routine studies include hepatobiliary, GI bleeding studies, and gastric emptying measurements. Other procedures that are less frequently ordered provide clinically valuable information.

Salivary Scanning. A quick look at the salivary glands of the mouth is frequently performed in conjunction with the technetium-99m pertechnetate (Tc-99mO_4) scan of the thyroid gland. The salivary glands can be scanned intentionally with Tc-99mO_4. A 5- to 10-mCi dose is injected intravenously with planar images performed immediately and after a delay, during which lemon juice is washed around the mouth. In the past, this study has been used to grade the severity of Sjögren syndrome, as inflammation degrades the secretory function of the glands. The salivary scan can demonstrate salivary obstruction and can be used as an adjunct to or replacement for sialography. Stimulation of the glands with lemon juice is important to document the drainage of saliva through the duct system to the mouth (Fig. 59.1). A *salivagram* can also be accomplished by swabbing a child's mouth with radiotracer. Delayed images of the lungs can be used to check for aspiration in children suspected of swallowing disorders.

Esophageal Imaging. The esophageal transit study, performed with swallowed solutions or solid boluses labeled with Tc-99m sulfur colloid (Tc-SC), is an examination that can be done in lieu of esophageal manometry. It has been reported to detect esophageal dysmotility in 50% of symptomatic patients with an otherwise normal evaluation for dysphagia.

In the supine or upright position with a gamma camera placed in the anterior projection, the patient swallows a radiolabeled bolus, and dynamic data are obtained via computer. The esophagus is divided into three regions of interest (ROIs): upper, middle, and lower. Transit times are then calculated from time-activity curves representing the ROIs. The normal esophagus demonstrates sequential activity from proximal to distal, with no visualized esophageal activity remaining after 10 seconds. Regional analysis may differentiate between achalasia and scleroderma. It is important to remember that esophageal scintigraphy is functional and does not provide detailed anatomic information. A barium or endoscopic study is necessary to exclude the possibility of neoplasm or infection as the cause of impaired esophageal function (Fig. 59.2).

Gastroesophageal Reflux. The evaluation of heartburn and atypical chest pain in the adult commonly raises the clinical question of gastroesophageal reflux (GER) disease. In the pediatric population, failure to thrive and recurrent pneumonia often elicit the same question. A common diagnostic tool currently used in the diagnosis of GER disease is acid reflux monitoring. This examination unfortunately

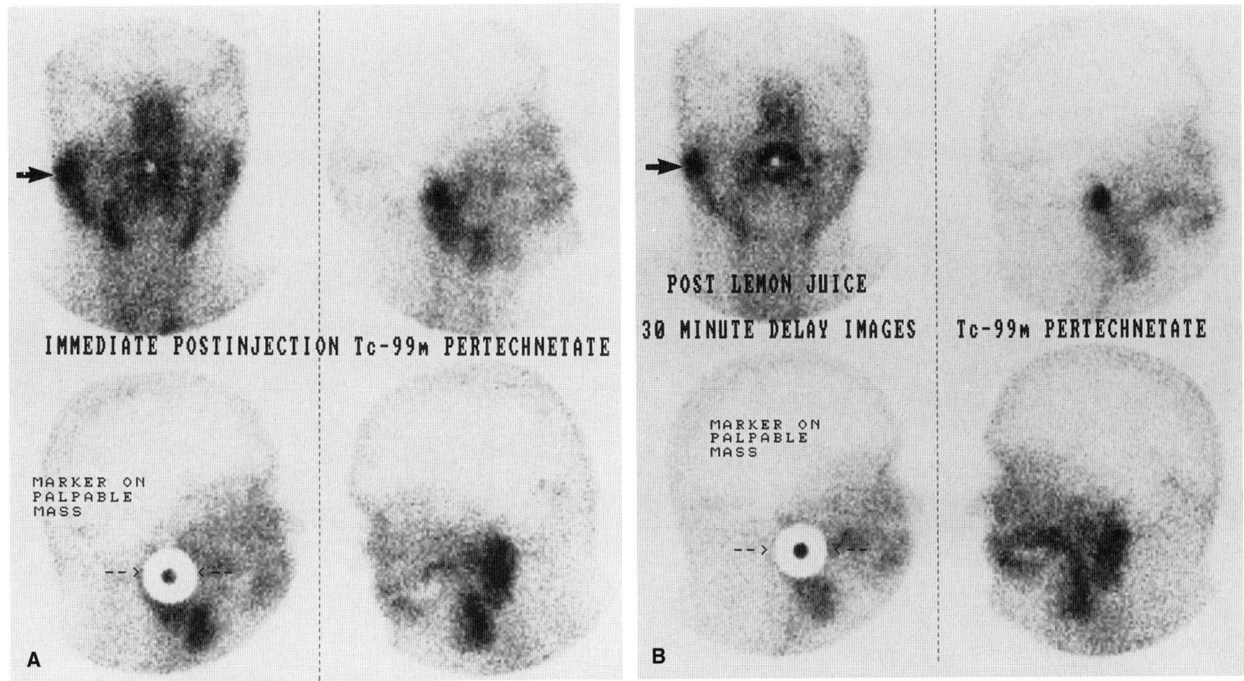

FIGURE 59.1. **Warthin Tumor by Salivary Scan.** Immediate **(A)** and delayed **(B)** images after IV administration of technetium-99m pertechnetate show extra uptake in a palpable mass in the right parotid gland. Retention of the pertechnetate is prolonged in the mass (*arrows*), even after lemon juice stimulation of the salivary glands. This finding is characteristic of a functioning Warthin tumor, which is not drained by salivary ducts.

requires nasoesophageal intubation and 24-hour continuous recording. It is invasive and unwieldy, especially in the pediatric age group.

GER scintigraphy is performed with acidified orange juice mixed with Tc-SC. The acid decreases the lower esophageal sphincter pressure and also delays gastric emptying. ROIs are established via computer to correspond to the stomach and the segments (upper, middle, and lower) of the esophagus. In the pediatric population, ROIs over the lungs detect aspiration by the end of the study or on delayed imaging 1 to 3 hours later. Images may be recorded in adults with an abdominal binder that increases abdominal

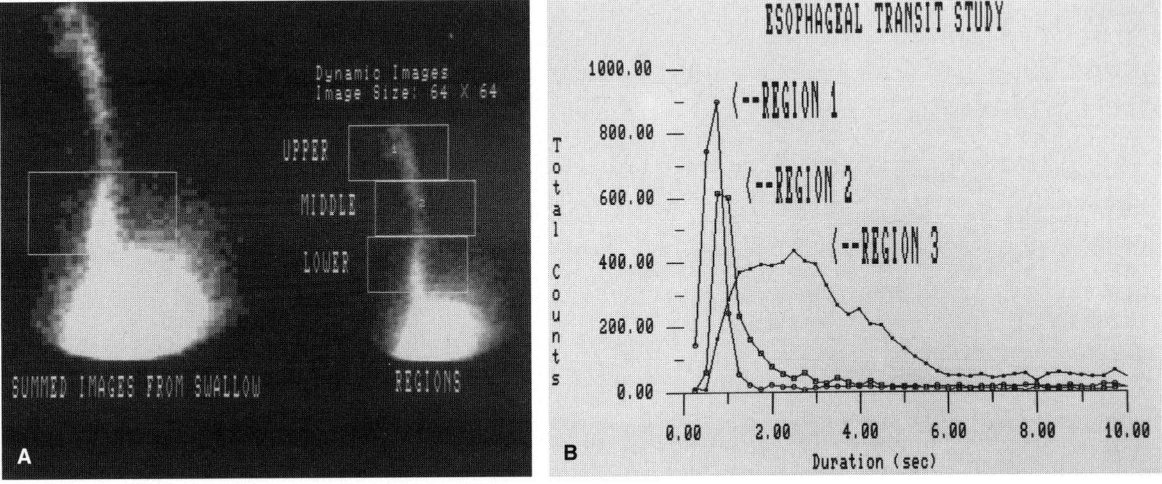

FIGURE 59.2. **Normal Esophageal Transit Study. A.** A composite image of the esophagus and stomach is used to generate regions of interest around the upper, middle, and lower esophagus. **B.** Time-activity curves for each region are displayed for 10 seconds after the swallow. Inspection of the curves allows calculation of the transit time.

pressure sequentially in 10-mm Hg increments to a maximum of 100 mm Hg. Normal patients have no detectable GER activity. This examination is reported to have a 90% sensitivity in the detection of GER (Fig. 59.3).

Gastric emptying is a complex physiologic process directed not only by neuroendocrine processes but also by a host of local factors. Food type, pH and fatty content, as well as food osmolality affect the rate of gastric emptying. Impaired gastric emptying can be caused by many disease states, such as diabetes mellitus, electrolyte disturbances, postvagotomy syndromes, and by some medications.

Exclusion of mechanical obstruction is important in diagnosing the cause of the patient's symptoms. Endoscopy or barium studies are superior in the detection of gastric ulcers, tumors, or bezoars. Gastric emptying scintigraphy has become the gold standard in the clinical evaluation of gastric motility. It is a simple test to perform, although interpretation is based upon complicated mathematical models. Solid food, liquids, or both are labeled with a radiotracer and consumed by the patient. Digital images of the stomach are acquired, and a time-activity curve is generated for graphic analysis of the rate of emptying (Fig. 59.4).

The normal half-emptying time ($T_{1/2}$) of radioactive solids and liquids varies with the technique employed. In general, the normal $T_{1/2}$ is less than 90 minutes for solids and less than 60 minutes for liquids. Each laboratory should establish its own normal $T_{1/2}$ values. Liquid gastric emptying usually follows an exponential curve, whereas

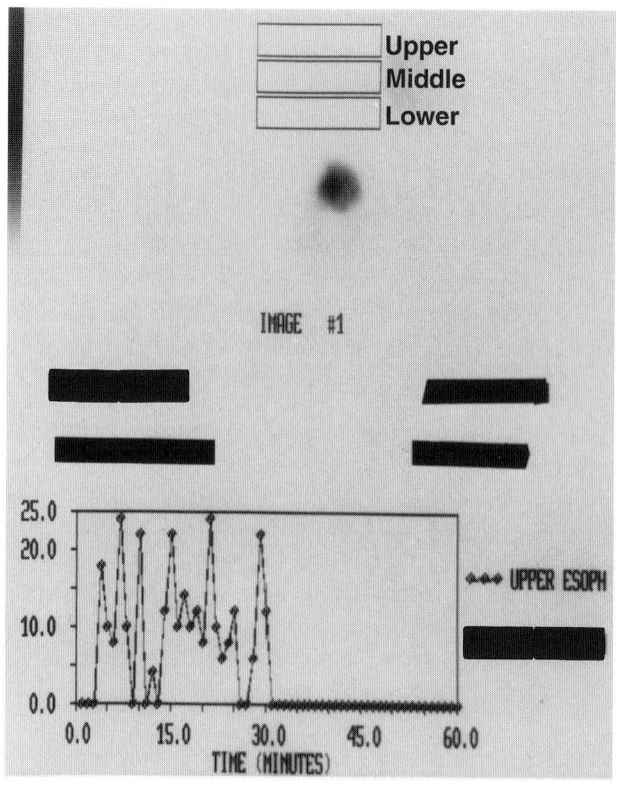

FIGURE 59.3. **Abnormal Gastroesophageal Reflux Study.** Three regions of interest (ROIs) are established over the esophagus. A time-activity curve corresponding to the upper ROI for 60 minutes shows refluxed activity after 3 minutes, which continues for about 30 minutes.

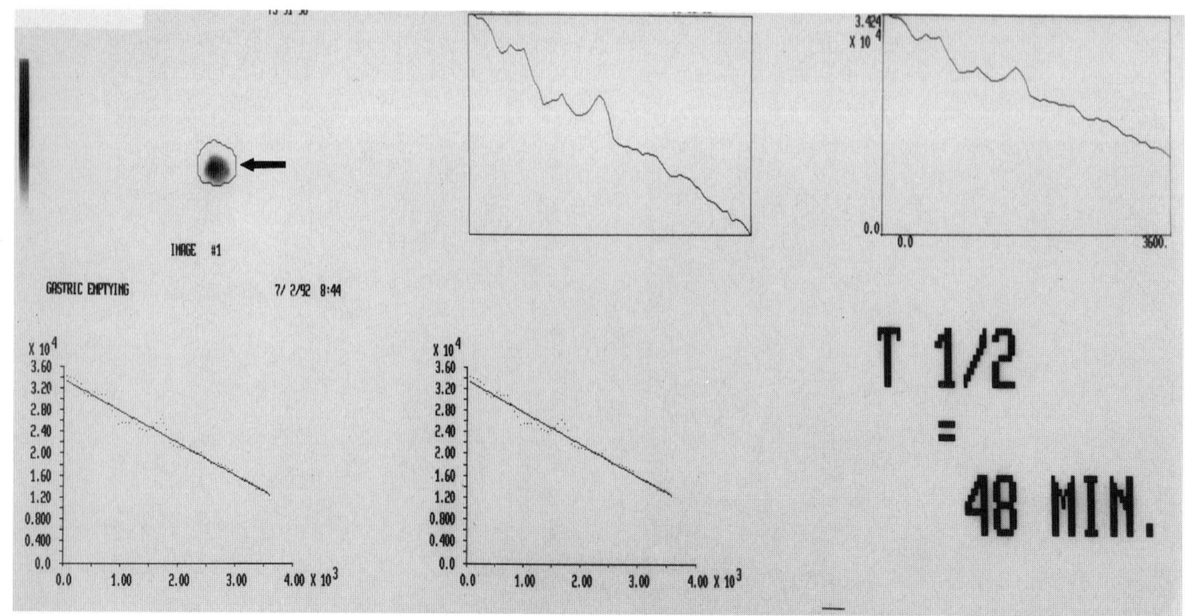

FIGURE 59.4. **Normal Solid Gastric Emptying Study.** In the image at upper left, a region of interest (*arrow*) is established around the stomach. The next two graphics show the stomach's time-activity curve. The bottom two graphics show the linear best-fit to this data. The slope of the curve allows calculation of the half-emptying time ($T_{1/2}$) of 48 minutes.

solid emptying is biphasic, with an initial lag phase followed by a linear curve. Visual interpretation of the stomach images is invaluable in understanding the "number" generated for $T_{1/2}$. The gastric emptying technique can be extended to study and time the transit between stomach and colon to characterize disorders of the bowel's smooth muscle or enteric nervous system.

Carbon-14 Urea Breath Test. The carbon-14 urea breath test (C-14 UBT) is an inexpensive, accurate, noninvasive test for active infection with *Helicobacter pylori*. *H. pylori* is a gram-negative, spiral-shaped bacterium that is found in the gastric mucosa or adherent to the epithelial lining of the stomach. *H. pylori* is known to cause more than 90% of duodenal ulcers and up to 80% of gastric ulcers. It has also been associated with an increased incidence of gastric carcinoma and gastric lymphoma. For the UBT, a patient needs to be fasting and off antibiotics, bismuth, and proton pump inhibitors. A 1-μCi capsule of C-14–labeled urea is administered by mouth, and 10 minutes later a breath sample is collected. *H. pylori* contains an enzyme, urease, which hydrolyzes the urea into ammonia and C-14–labeled carbon dioxide, which is subsequently detected in the breath sample using liquid scintillation techniques. This can be accomplished locally, or the sample can be sent into a central laboratory. The UBT has a sensitivity and specificity of 94% to 98%. Alternative tests include endoscopic biopsy to identify the bacterium or serology titers, which will remain positive even after treatment.

Gastrointestinal Bleeding Scintigraphy. Patients who present with clinically suspected upper GI bleeding are usually evaluated and often treated by endoscopy. Scintigraphy is not usually needed. The patient with suspected lower GI bleeding presents different problems in diagnosis and therapy. Proctosigmoidoscopy can exclude hemorrhoidal bleeding, and colonoscopy may identify the cause. An emergent GI bleeding study with in vitro Tc-99m–tagged red blood cells is very sensitive and can locate the bleeding site. Continuous 1-minute dynamic frames are acquired over the abdomen and pelvis in the anterior projection for at least 90 minutes or until the patient has bled enough to locate the source of hemorrhage. This technique can detect bleeding rates as low as 0.1 mL/min versus contrast angiography, which detects 1 mL/min of GI bleeding.

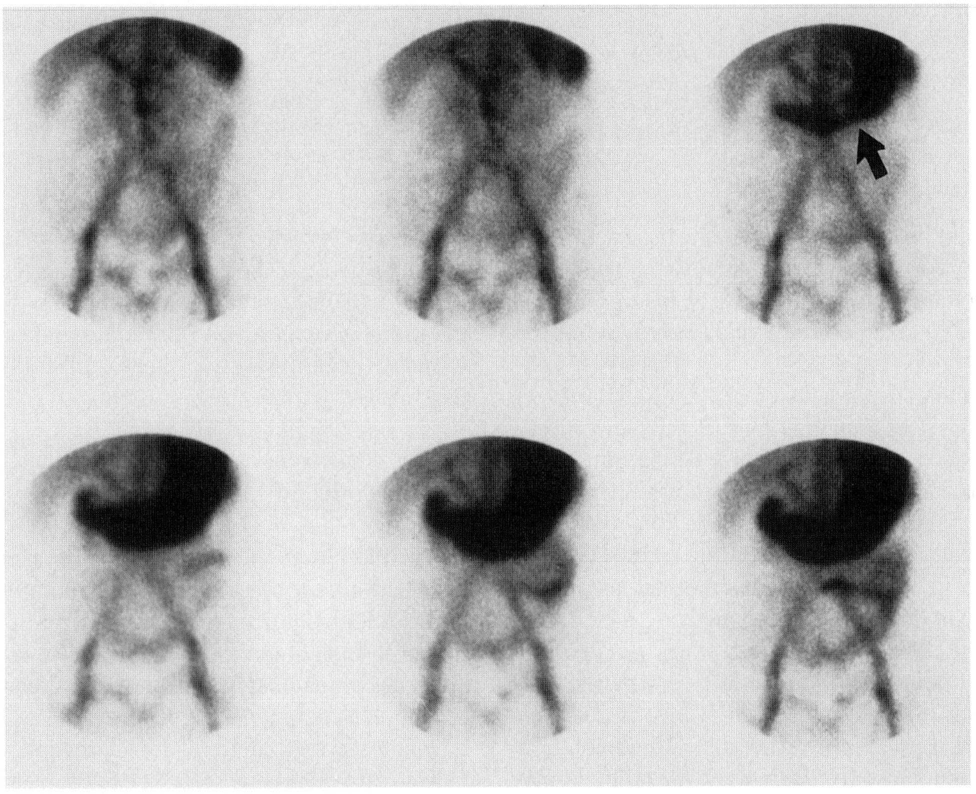

FIGURE 59.5. **Upper GI Bleeding Caused by Gastric Varices.** Sequential 5-minute images of the abdomen, in a patient with negative endoscopy, show tagged red cells filling the lumen of the stomach (*arrow*). This diagnosis cannot be made if there is free technetium-99-pertechnetate (Tc-99mO_4) mixed with the red cells; Tc-99mO_4 is excreted physiologically in the stomach. The tagged red blood cells used had no free Tc-99mO_4.

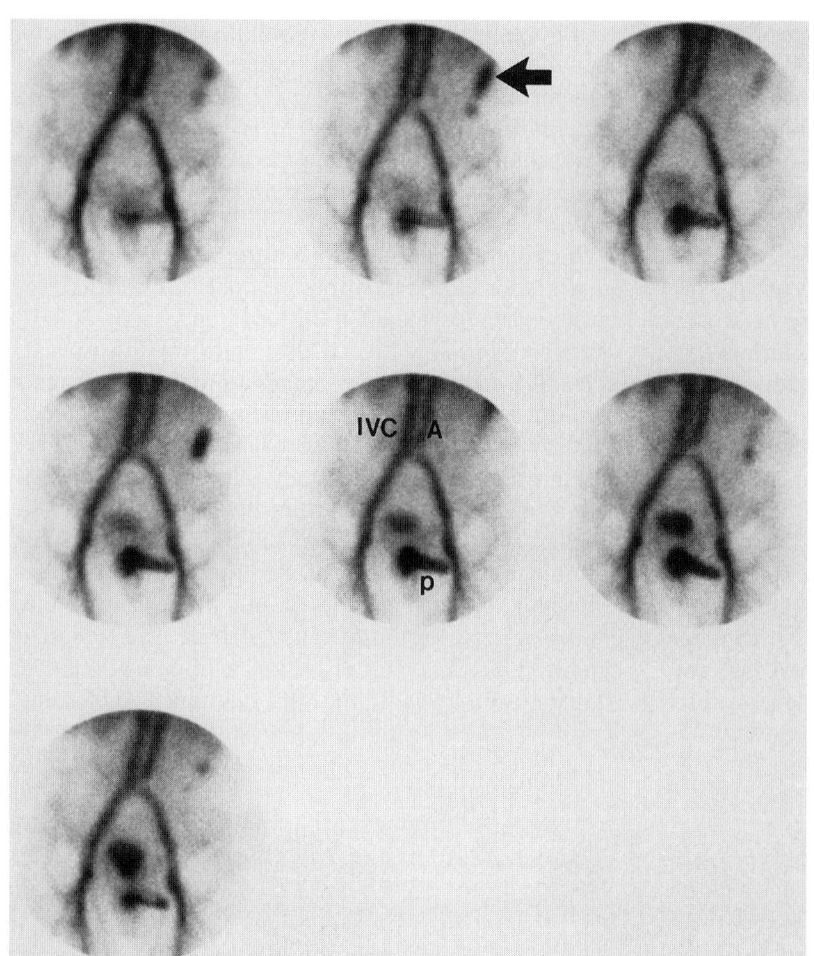

FIGURE 59.6. **Splenic Flexure Bleeding in the Colon Caused by Diverticular Disease.** Sequential 5-minute images show a small focus of bleeding (*arrow*) in the left upper quadrant that varies with intensity as it accumulates and moves through the colon. Note that the patient has a large, static blood pool in the penis. Unchanging blood pools such as the aorta (A), the inferior vena cava (IVC), and penis (P) should not be misinterpreted as hemorrhage.

The study should be done emergently during the clinical period of suspected active bleeding. Repeated imaging can be done at any time up to 24 hours after red cell labeling, but care should be taken because blood may have moved into the colon.

Accurate hemorrhage localization is required for resection of a bleeding site. If angiographic therapy for a bleeding site is proposed, the more sensitive GI bleeding study should be done first. The GI bleeding study will guide selection of appropriate vessels for embolization or infusion of vasoactive drugs. Positive GI bleeding studies demonstrate three cardinal findings: (*1*) an abnormal hot spot of radiotracer activity appears "out of nowhere" as it enters the bowel lumen; (*2*) this activity persists and may increase with time; and (*3*) the activity moves with peristalsis antegrade, retrograde, or in both directions (Figs. 59.5–59.7).

Meckel Scan. A Meckel diverticulum, which contains ectopic gastric mucosa, may ulcerate and bleed. Tc-99mO_4 is given intravenously and the abdomen is imaged immediately and for 1 hour's worth of dynamic images. Tc-99mO_4 localizes in the gastric mucosa and can be used to detect the acid-producing mucosa in the diverticulum. A focus of activity representing the ectopic gastric mucosa in the middle or right lower quadrant of the abdomen is detected as it concentrates the Tc-99mO_4 in synchrony with the stomach. Detection may be enhanced by the use of pentagastrin to stimulate uptake or cimetidine to block the outflow of Tc-99m-O_4 from the diverticulum (Fig. 59.8).

LIVER AND SPLEEN STUDIES

Liver/Spleen Scan. Liver/spleen scanning is performed by IV injection of Tc-99m–radiolabeled albumin or sulfur colloid. Colloid imaging provides information based upon organ perfusion and the distribution of reticuloendothelial cells, which phagocytize the colloid particles. Kupffer cells in the liver and reticuloendothelial cells in the spleen are normally imaged. Reticuloendothelial cells in the bone marrow are minimally seen. The liver/spleen scan is an inexpensive and easy means to evaluate for focal or diffuse hepatic disease, but it lacks disease specificity. Radiotracer uptake may be abnormal in a multitude of diseases. To make matters worse, hepatic lesions smaller than 1 cm in diameter are routinely missed, even with SPECT. MR, CT,

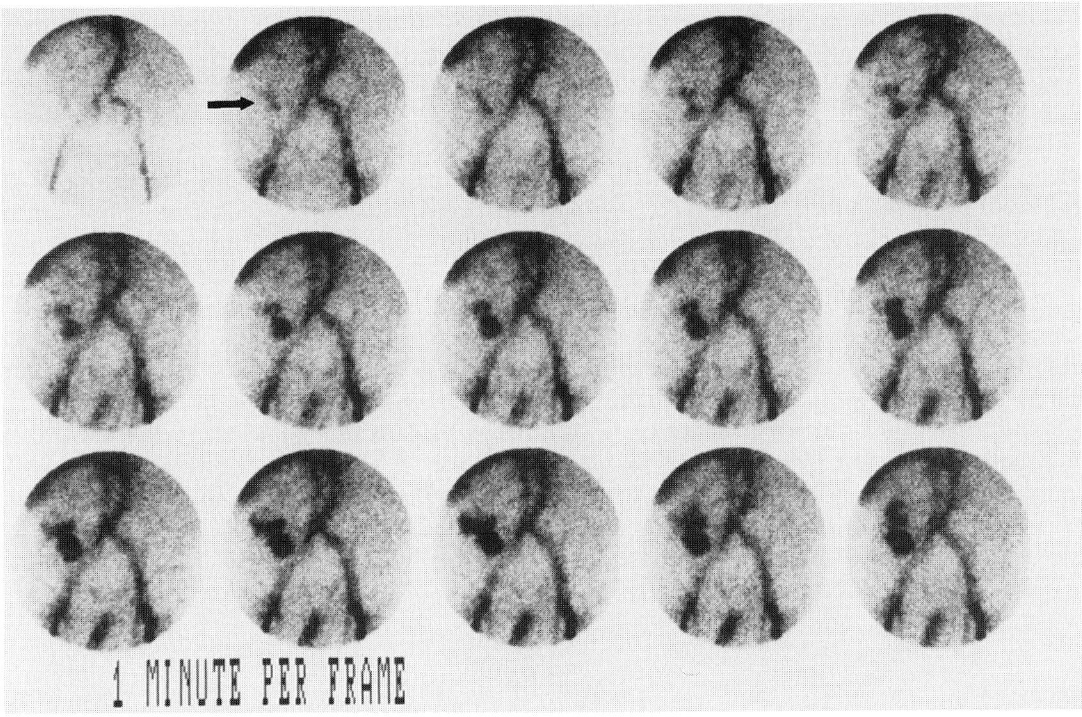

FIGURE 59.7. **Cecal Bleeding Caused by Angiodysplasia.** Images show a right lower quadrant hemorrhage (*arrow*).

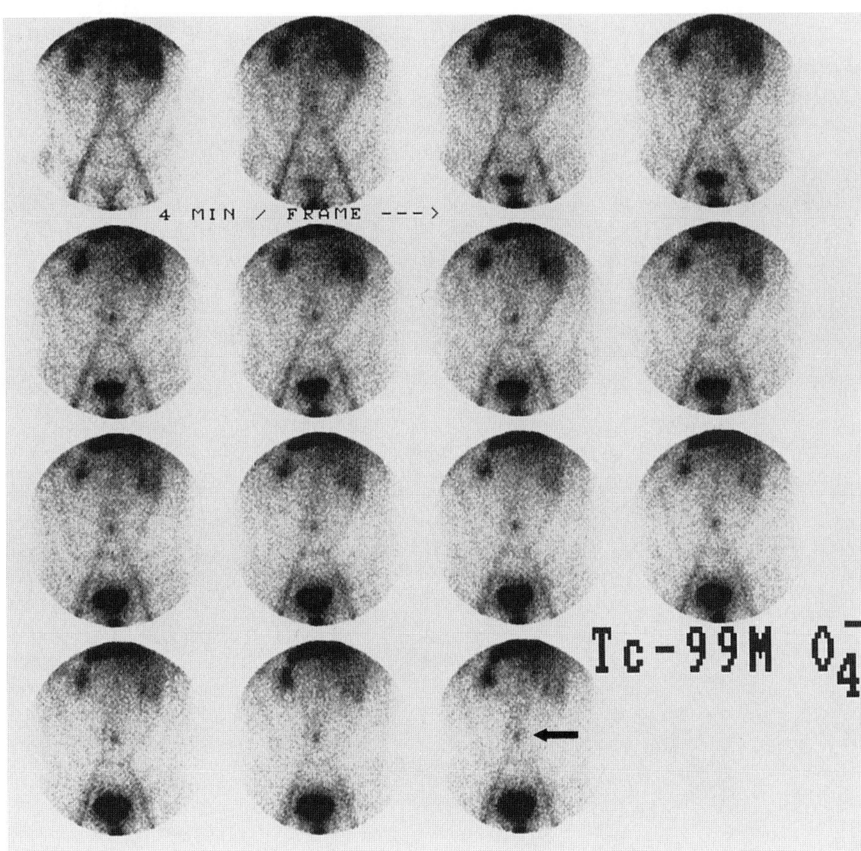

FIGURE 59.8. **Meckel Diverticulum.** A small focus (*arrow*) of technetium-99-pertechnetate uptake gradually becomes visible in the ectopic gastric mucosa of a Meckel diverticulum in the midabdomen.

and US have better resolution for hepatic masses. Tc-SC liver SPECT, however, can be very specific in diagnosing focal nodular hyperplasia (FNH). Lesions that are large enough to be identified on SPECT and are isointense or hotter than liver parenchyma on uptake may be confidently diagnosed as FNH. This is because of the presence or increased concentration of reticuloendothelial cells within the lesion. Tc-SC scanning can also be useful in diagnosing masses outside of the liver as myelolipomas or extramedullary hematopoiesis.

Liver/spleen radionuclide imaging remains accurate and easy for evaluation of liver and spleen size, configuration, and position. This helps in the evaluation of suspected hepatomegaly in patients with obstructive lung disease causing diaphragmatic flattening or in patients with anatomic variants, such as a large left liver lobe or a Riedel lobe on the right (Fig. 59.9). Alterations in perfusion and reticuloendothelial system function caused by cirrhosis and hepatitis are seen as a "shift" of activity to the spleen, bone marrow, and lungs. The liver/spleen scan provides information that helps monitor the disease process and efficacy of therapy (Fig. 59.10).

Liver/spleen scans can be "subtracted" from other nuclear medicine studies to provide spatial information about the liver or spleen in relation to a suspected abnormality. Indium-111 leukocyte scans (for infection); gallium-67 scans (for inflammation, lymphoma, or hepatoma); indium-111 octreotide scans (for neuroendocrine tumors); and labeled antibody scans have physiologic uptake in the liver and/or spleen. Subtracting the liver/spleen scan from any of these scans confirms "hot" abnormalities adjacent to the liver or spleen (Fig. 59.11). This may be particularly useful in cirrhotic livers with regenerating nodules.

Heat-Damaged Red Blood Cell Scan for Splenic Tissue. Tc-99m–labeled red blood cells that have been damaged by heating are preferentially extracted from circulation by splenic tissue. Applications include diagnosis

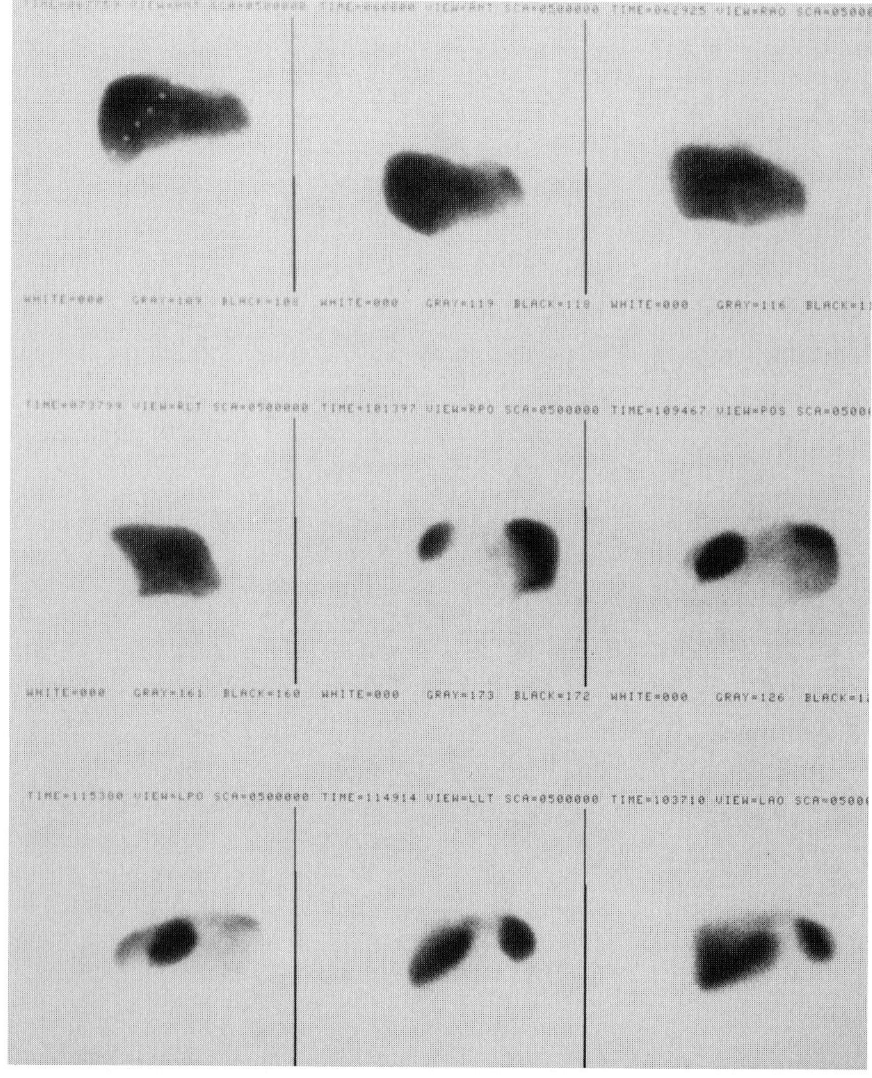

FIGURE 59.9. **Normal Liver/Spleen Scan.** Sequential images begin with an anterior projection with a lead marker (*row of cold dots*) on the right costal margin. Subsequent images are anterior, right anterior oblique, right lateral, right posterior oblique, posterior, left posterior oblique, left lateral, and left anterior oblique from left to right, top to bottom. Note the homogeneous labeling of the liver and spleen and the relative size and position of these two organs in various projections.

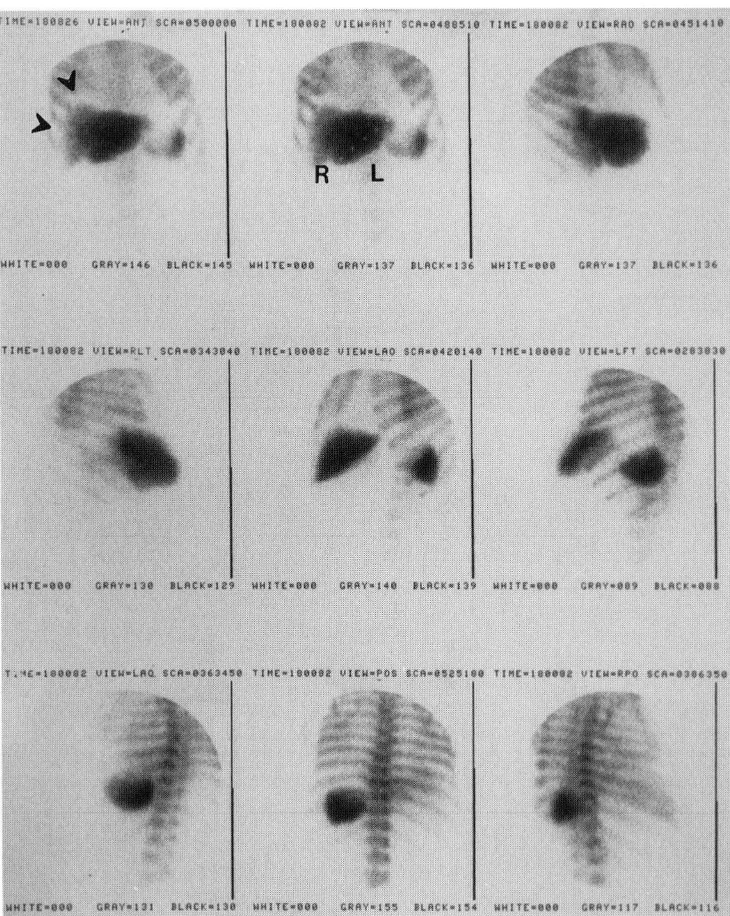

FIGURE 59.10. **Abnormal Liver/Spleen Scan in a Patient With Cirrhosis.** The liver is small and labels poorly. The left lobe of the liver (L) is better seen than the right lobe (R). Note the "colloid" shift of the radiopharmaceutical to the bone marrow and spleen. Ascites separate the liver from the right ribs (*arrowheads*). Compare these images with Fig. 59.9.

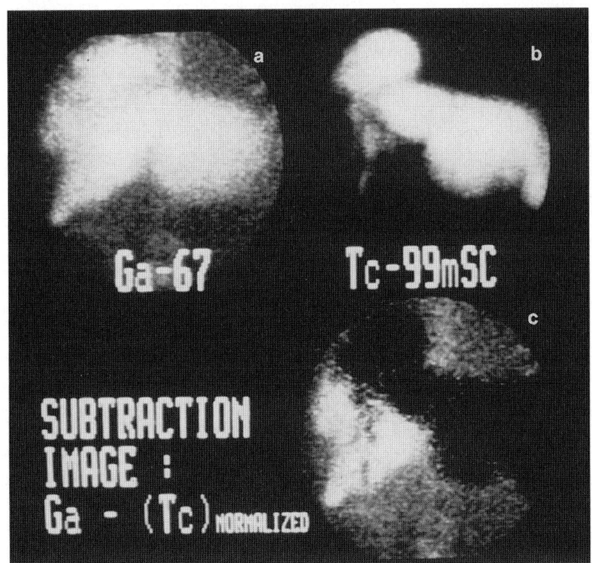

FIGURE 59.11. **Liver/Spleen Subtraction From a Gallium-67 Scan in a Patient With a Hepatoma. A.** Image of gallium-67 (Ga-67) distribution in the anterior projection at 48 hours. **B.** Matched image of colloid distribution (Tc-99mSC). Careful selection of the gamma camera energy windows allows simultaneous imaging of the two radiopharmaceuticals. **C.** The subtraction image shows the gallium-avid hepatoma, which does not label with the colloid.

of polysplenia and splenosis and confirmation of accessory splenic tissue.

HEPATOBILIARY IMAGING

Nuclear imaging of the gallbladder and biliary system is easily performed with Tc-99m–labeled iminodiacetic acid compounds. Only two of the numerous iminodiacetic acid radiotracers that have been developed are still commercially available: Tc-disofenin and Tc-mebrofenin. Tc-HIDA (lidofenin) is actually no longer commercially available. These radiopharmaceuticals are excreted unchanged into the biliary system and work even in the presence of elevated serum bilirubin.

Acute Cholecystitis. Hepatobiliary scans are most commonly used to evaluate suspected acute cholecystitis. A minimum of 2 hours' fasting is recommended in preparation for this scan. The anterior dynamic images of normal hepatobiliary scans show prompt and homogeneous uptake of the radiopharmaceutical by the liver. Liver activity decreases progressively as the radiotracer is excreted into the biliary system and drains into the small bowel. The activity should be seen in the major extrahepatic ducts,

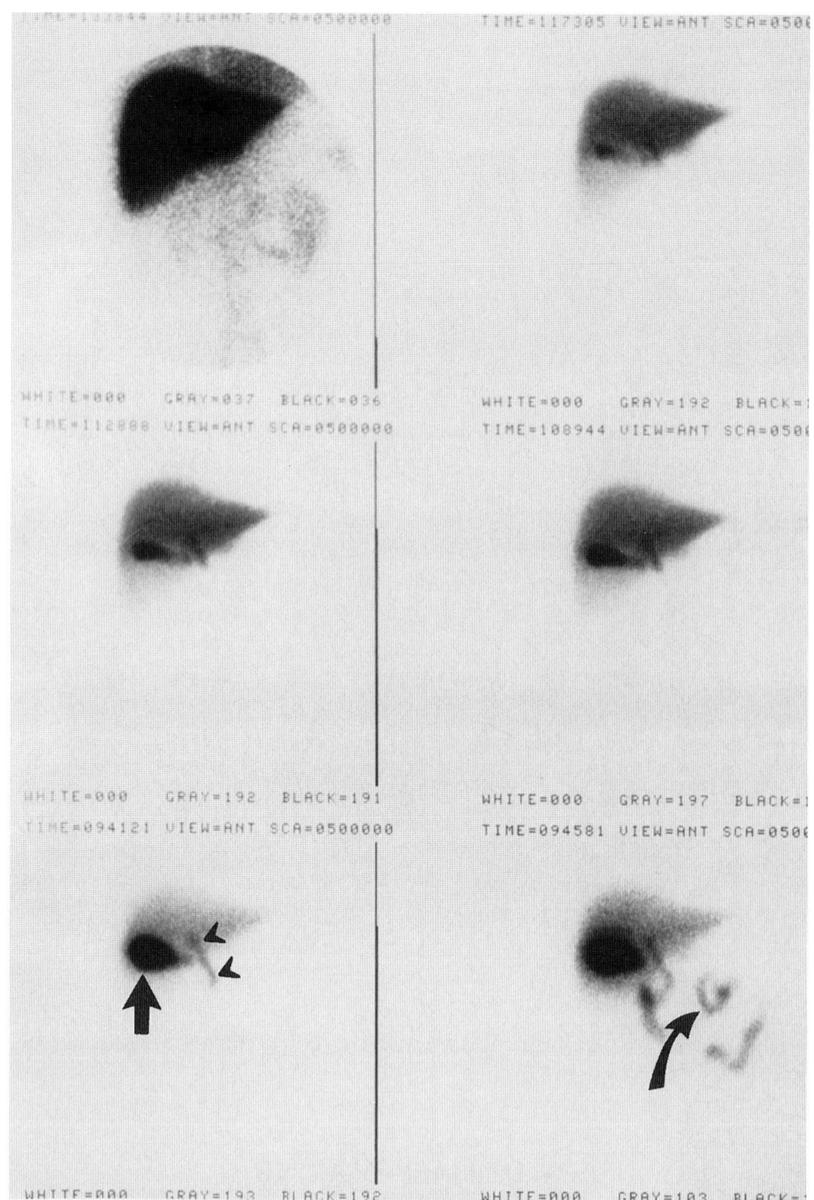

FIGURE 59.12. **Normal Hepatobiliary Scan.** Images of the liver immediately after injection and at subsequent 5-minute intervals show rapid clearance of the blood pool followed promptly by central biliary duct and gallbladder (*straight arrow*) activity. Activity continues to fill the common bile duct (*arrowheads*) at 20 minutes and the small bowel (*curved arrow*) at 25 minutes.

gallbladder, and small bowel within 1 hour (Fig. 59.12). Most patients with acute cholecystitis have a stone or stones obstructing the cystic duct. A small minority of patients, usually the chronically ill, have acalculous cholecystitis. The hallmark of acute cholecystitis by cholescintigraphy is nonvisualization of the gallbladder at both 1- and 4-hour intervals after IV injection of the biliary agent, or 30 minutes after morphine administration.

Chronic cholecystitis is diagnosed when the gallbladder is not visualized at 1 hour but is seen by 4 hours. When properly done, the nuclear medicine hepatobiliary examination has a sensitivity and specificity of 98% and better than a 95% accuracy rate in the diagnosis of acute cholecystitis. Small doses of IV morphine (1 to 2 mg) can be used during the scan to raise the pressure on the sphincter of Oddi. This helps push radiolabeled bile into the gallbladder. It is a handy way to speed up a "normal scan," because the diagnosis of acute cholecystitis is excluded as soon as the gallbladder is seen. Morphine administration may also allow true negative scans to be performed in patients who have stimulated their gallbladders to contract by eating before the scan.

Increased blood flow on radionuclide angiograms of the gallbladder fossa aids in the diagnosis of acute cholecystitis. A "rim sign" on hepatobiliary scan images is seen as a band of increased activity around the gallbladder fossa, which represents poor excretion of radiotracer from inflamed hepatocytes. The rim sign is usually associated with gangrenous cholecystitis (Fig. 59.13). A pitfall in interpretation of acute cholecystitis may be caused by prolonged

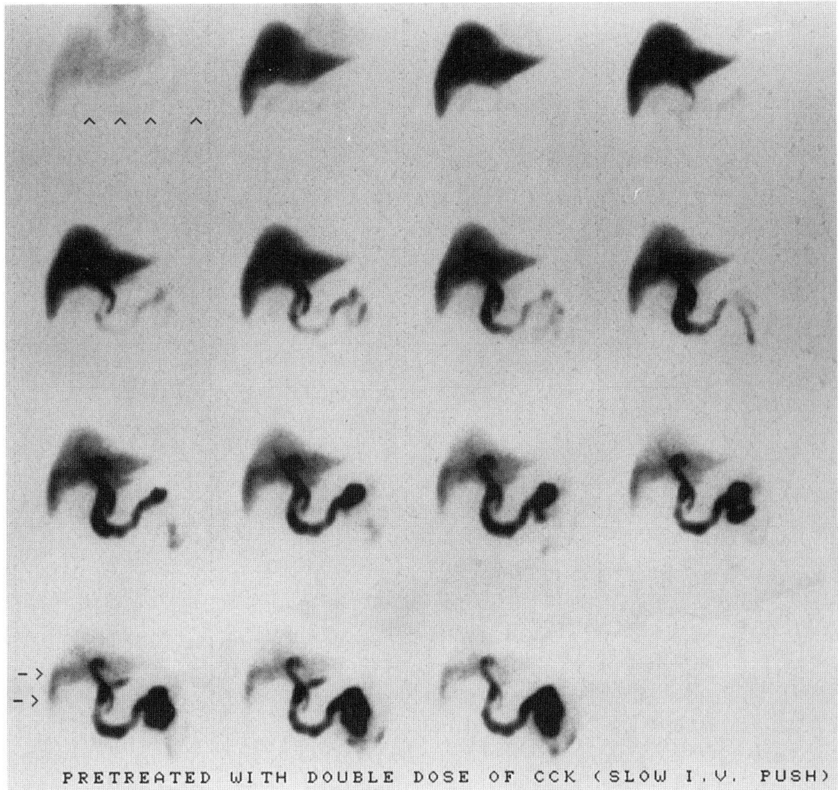

FIGURE 59.13. **Acute Cholecystitis Diagnosed by Hepatobiliary Scan.** The first hepatobiliary scan in this patient was positive for acute cholecystitis but the referring service did not believe the diagnosis. The scan was repeated on the next day. In it, the first image shows radioisotope left over from that first scan. A dim line of activity in the transverse colon is marked (*arrowheads*). Cholecystokinin (CCK) was used as a pretreatment for the second scan. Starting with the second image, the dose is rapidly concentrated and excreted by the liver into bile ducts and small bowel. The gallbladder never fills. As the liver clears, a "hot rim" of activity is seen around the gallbladder fossa (*arrows*), which indicates inflammation caused by the severe acute cholecystitis.

fasting with gallbladder distension. The radiopharmaceutical will not enter the completely full, atonic gallbladder. This can be avoided by pretreating the patient with analogs of cholecystokinin (CCK). CCK is a short-acting, natural hormone that causes prompt gallbladder contraction. After emptying, the gallbladder refills, allowing entry of the biliary agent. A false-positive diagnosis of acute cholecystitis may also occur with previous cholecystectomy, tumor obstructing the cystic duct, and agenesis of the gallbladder. *Mirizzi syndrome* can be suspected when there is evidence of acute cholecystitis (nonvisualization of gallbladder) and common bile duct obstruction.

Acalculous biliary disease includes chronic acalculous cholecystitis, cystic duct syndrome, and gallbladder dyskinesis. These patients present with similar complaints of right upper quadrant pain, fatty food intolerance, and epigastric distress. Routine cholescintigraphy and US may be normal. CCK-assisted cholescintigraphy in acalculous biliary disease demonstrates decreased gallbladder contraction and decreased gallbladder ejection fraction. The normal gallbladder ejection fraction is greater than 35%.

Other uses for the hepatobiliary scan include the detection of postoperative complications and bile leaks in trauma (Fig. 59.14). The excretion phase of the scan is important in evaluating hepatic and common bile duct patency. A delay of more than 1 hour in visualization of the bile ducts suggests obstruction. Caution must be exercised to differentiate severe hepatocellular disease from obstruction, as both present with delays in biliary visualization. The hepatobiliary scan maintains a niche in differentiating neonatal hepatitis from *biliary atresia.* In the latter case, radiolabeled bile will never enter the bowel or gallbladder. Unfortunately, if the hepatitis is bad enough, the radiopharmaceutical may not leave the liver. When bowel activity is seen (and this may take 4 to 24 hours), the diagnosis of biliary atresia is excluded.

HEPATIC BLOOD POOL SCINTIGRAPHY

Cavernous hemangioma is the most common benign hepatic tumor and the second most common hepatic tumor after metastatic disease. Frequently subcapsular in location, this tumor is often found incidentally by US, CT, or MR. Although there are specific criteria for diagnosis of hepatic hemangioma by these techniques, no study is 100% specific. Because a significant risk of hemorrhage exists with biopsy, a noninvasive diagnostic approach is preferred. Scintigraphy with Tc-99m–labeled red blood cells using an in vitro labeling technique has proved both sensitive and specific for cavernous hemangioma. A flow study should be performed initially and will demonstrate normal or decreased early uptake if the suspected lesion is a hemangioma. Tumors and inflammatory lesions tend to have increased arterial flow. Subsequent delayed SPECT imaging will reveal foci of increased activity within the

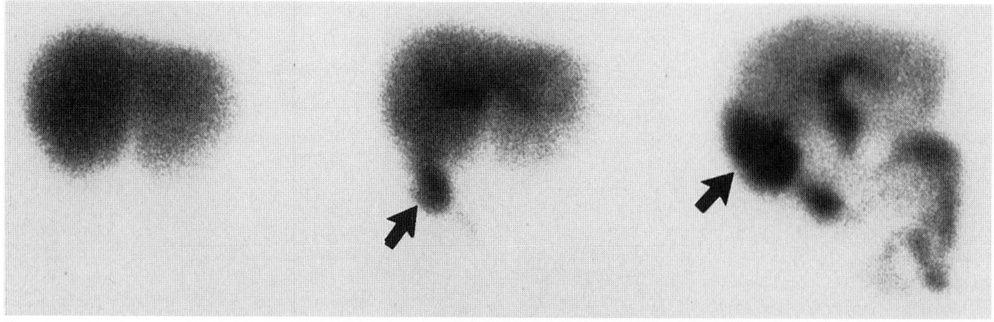

FIGURE 59.14. **Biliary Leak After Cholecystectomy Detected by a Hepatobiliary Scan.** Images (*left to right*) obtained immediately, 30 minutes, and 1 hour after administration of the biliary agent show accumulation of bile in the area around the right lobe of the liver (*arrows*).

liver that are hotter than surrounding parenchyma. Sensitivity decreases with lesions smaller than 1.5 cm, greater organ depth, and single-detector SPECT as opposed to multidetector SPECT. Correlation with a second imaging technique is always advised because these lesions may be seen concomitant with malignancy. Specificity is generally high, although isolated cases of increased activity on delayed imaging with both colon and lung carcinoma metastases have been reported. In general, if two of the four imaging techniques demonstrate characteristic features of cavernous hemangioma, no further evaluation is warranted (Fig. 59.15).

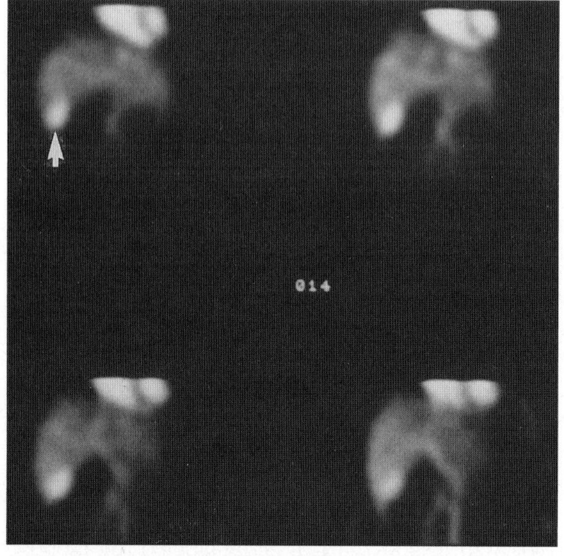

FIGURE 59.15. **Hepatic Hemangioma.** At first glance, this study could be confused with a biliary scan. However, note the vascular blood pool and that these are four coronal slices from a SPECT study of the liver performed 1 hour after the injection of 25 mCi of technetium-99m-pertechnetate–labeled red blood cells. The area of increased activity (*arrow*), which simulates a gallbladder, is actually a hemangioma in the liver of this hepatic transplant recipient.

PET FLUOROXYDEGLUCOSE IN GASTROINTESTINAL CANCERS

PET with fluorodeoxyglucose (FDG) is an extremely powerful tool in the evaluation and staging of GI tumors but is covered more fully in chapter 64. It has a higher sensitivity (95% to 100%) than CT (81% to 92%) for detecting esophageal cancer and helps in radiotherapy planning. Likewise, PET has better sensitivity and specificity in nodal staging and in detecting distant metastatic disease. PET has also been approved for the initial staging and restaging of colorectal carcinoma, with sensitivity and specificity of 95% to 99% for recurrent colorectal cancer. It may prove useful in pancreatic and gastric carcinoma evaluation as well. PET-CT has the ability to improve the anatomic mapping of functional data and improves the accuracy of detection of metastatic abdominal adenopathy, adrenal lesions, and hepatic involvement. In general, the positive predictive value of PET-CT for metastatic disease in the liver is so high as to militate against the necessity for biopsy in most cases. "Incidental" findings of focal uptake in the colon on other PET studies usually indicate cancerous lesions or premalignant lesions such as adenomatous polyps, which require further evaluation.

SUGGESTED READINGS

Balon HR, Fink-Bennett DM, Brill DR, et al. Procedure guideline for hepatobiliary scintigraphy. Society of Nuclear Medicine. J Nucl Med 1997;38:1654–1657.

Charron M. Pediatric inflammatory bowel disease imaged with Tc-99m white blood cells. Clin Nucl Med 2000;25:708–715.

Charron M, Di LC, Kocoshis S. CT and 99mTc-WBC vs colonoscopy in the evaluation of inflammation and complications of inflammatory bowel diseases. J Gastroenterol 2002;37:874–875.

Chatziioannou SN, Moore WH, Ford PV, Dhekne RD. Hepatobiliary scintigraphy is superior to abdominal ultrasonography in suspected acute cholecystitis. Surgery 2000;127:609–613.

Connolly LP, Treves St, Bozorgi F, O'Connor SC. Meckel's diverticulum: demonstration of heterotopic gastric mucosa with technetium-99m-pertechnetate SPECT. J Nucl Med 1998;39:1458–1460.

Donohoe KJ, Maurer AH, Ziessman HA, Urbain JL, Royal HD. Procedure guideline for gastric emptying and motility. Society of Nuclear Medicine. J Nucl Med 1999 Jul;40:1236–1239.

Ford PV, Bartold SP, Fink-Bennett DM, et al. Procedure guideline for gastrointestinal bleeding and Meckel's diverticulum scintigraphy. Society of Nuclear Medicine. J Nucl Med 1999 Jul;40(7):1226–1232.

Hustinx R. PET imaging in assessing gastrointestinal tumors. Radiol Clin North Am 2004;42:1123–1139.

Kamel EM, Thumshirn M, Truninger K, et al. Significance of incidental 18F-FDG accumulations in the gastrointestinal tract in PET/CT: correlation with endoscopic and histopathologic results. J Nucl Med 2004;45:1804–1810.

Klein HA. Esophageal transit scintigraphy. Semin Nucl Med 1995;25:306–317.

Krishnamurthy S, Krishnamurthy GT. Cholecystokinin and morphine pharmacological intervention during ^{99m}Tc-HIDA cholescintigraphy: a rational approach. Semin Nucl Med 1996;26:16–24.

Mariani G, Boni G. Barreca M, et al. Radionuclide gastroesophageal motor studies. J Nucl Med 2004;45:1004–1028.

Mauree AH, Krevsky B. Whole-gut transit scintigraphy in the evaluation of small-bowel and colon transit disorders. Semin Nucl Med 1995;25:326–338.

Maurer AH. Gastrointestinal bleeding and cine-scintigraphy. Semin Nucl Med 1996;26:43–50.

Nadel HR. Hepatobiliary scintigraphy in children. Semin Nucl Med 1996;26:25–42.

Szepes A. Bertalan V, Varkonyi T, et al. Diagnosis of gallbladder dyskinesia by quantitative hepatobiliary scintigraphy. Clin Nucl Med 2005;30:302–307.

Tripathi M, Chandrashekar N, Kumar R, et al. Hepatobiliary scintigraphy: an effective tool in the management of bile leak following laparoscopic cholecystectomy. Clin Imaging 2004;28:40–43.

Urbain J-L, Charkes ND. Recent advances in gastric emptying scintigraphy. Semin Nucl Med 1995;25:318–325.

Zuckier LS, Freeman LM. Selective role of nuclear medicine in evaluating the acute abdomen. Radiol Clin North Am 2003;41:1275–1288.

Chapter 60

Genitourinary System Scintigraphy

Mike McBiles and Peter W. Blue

Renal Imaging
Clinical Applications

Testicular Imaging

Prostate Cancer Imaging

RENAL IMAGING

Renal radionuclide imaging has always been an important part of the practice of nuclear medicine. US, CT, and MR have the clear advantage of superior anatomic images. Despite advances in US functional imaging with the refinement of Doppler techniques, and in MR with newer dynamic protocols, there remain many areas in which scintigraphy remains the easiest, least expensive, most accurate test, or the least radiation-burdensome test available. Radiopharmaceuticals are well suited for evaluating blood flow, nephron function and mass, and collecting system excretory function and drainage.

Radionuclide renal studies are safe, minimally invasive, and expose patients to radiation doses comparable to or lower than those used in competing radiologic procedures. They are used to study such disorders as renal collecting system obstruction, vesicoureteral reflux, renovascular hypertension, renal masses, and pyelonephritis. Renal function parameters such as renal flow, differential function, glomerular filtration rate (GFR), and effective renal plasma flow (ERPF) can be determined with radioisotopes. In patients with radiographic contrast sensitivity or contraindications to MR, radionuclide studies can frequently answer the clinical question, despite their limited spatial resolution.

Radiopharmaceuticals. Radionuclide renal imaging involves the assessment of the four major renal functions: blood flow, glomerular filtration, tubular function, and excretory system function. The nuclear physician will choose a radiopharmaceutical tailored for the specific function or combination of functions to be studied. Only with an understanding of the sequential dynamic movement of the tracer from the blood to the bladder is accurate interpretation possible.

The following radiopharmaceutical doses should be adjusted for body surface area for pediatric patients, with minimum doses as per published recommendations.

Blood Flow. Renal perfusion can be assessed using any radioisotope that is given intravenously in sufficient dosage to acquire a usable series of 3- to 5-second images. Flow images are usually obtained using the commonly accepted doses of technetium-99m (Tc-99m) renal agents: diethylenetriamine pentaacetic acid (Tc-99m-DTPA) (380 to 860 MBq), mercaptoacetyltriglycine (Tc-99m-MAG_3) (380 to 570 MBq), or glucoheptonate (Tc-99m-GH) (570 to 860 MBq).

Glomerular filtration is a passive pumping of plasma components through the semipermeable glomerular membrane into the Bowman space. Plasma water and those molecules small enough to pass the membrane (e.g., electrolytes, creatinine, urea, etc.) are filtered and, if not fully reabsorbed, reach the renal collecting system. In general, proteins are too large to be filtered. Tc-99m-DTPA is small enough and not significantly protein bound (5% to 10%) and so is almost completely filtered. Its lack of protein binding increases its extravascular distribution and consequently its "background" presence, causing a lower target-to-background ratio than Tc-99m-MAG_3 or Tc-99m-dimercaptosuccinic acid (Tc-99m-DMSA), especially at lower levels of renal function. Because there is no significant reabsorption of Tc-99m-DTPA, and because Tc-99m-DTPA does not reach the urine by any other mechanism than glomerular filtration, it traces this function well and can be used to accurately measure the GFR. Although diffusion across the glomerulus is passive, the glomerular permeability and preglomerular pressure must be maintained for filtration to continue. Renal artery stenosis, microvascular disorders, and cardiac pump failure decrease the preglomerular pressure. Renal obstruction and acute tubular necrosis increase the postglomerular (Bowman space) pressure. In either case, the net pressure across the glomerulus drops, decreasing the GFR and the amount of tracer (Tc-99m-DTPA) passing through the kidney. Intrinsic diseases such as glomerulonephritis (chronic renal failure) disrupt glomerular membrane permeability, resulting in diminished filtration and tracer movement.

Tc-99m-GH is a glucose analog that is mostly glomerularly filtered; 90% of the total dose reaches the urine, whereas 10% is retained by the proximal tubular cell, allowing for delayed cortical imaging and some functional imaging.

Tubular secretion is an active process by which certain molecules are removed from the peritubular capillaries and secreted into the glomerularly filtered tubular urine that is passing by. For a radionuclide to effectively trace tubular function, most or all of the tracer must be removed in one pass by the tubule; that is, it must be secreted into the urine and not be reabsorbed. Until recently, iodine-131-orthoiodohippurate (I-131-OIH) was used because of its high tubular extraction efficiency and lower protein binding, and there is an extensive literature on its use. However, because of inferior spatial resolution owing to its I-131 component, and its high kidney dosimetry in situations of prolonged cortical retention, it has been replaced by Tc-99m-MAG_3. Tc-99m-MAG_3, with a 5% glomerular/55% tubular extraction efficiency, a high (90%) protein binding, which limits extravascular distribution, and relatively high target-to-background ratio, has become the agent of choice for most tubular functional imaging.

Because the clearance of Tc-99m-MAG_3 (300 to 400 mL/min) (extraction efficiency = 60%) is so much greater than that of Tc-99m-DTPA (80 to 140 mL/min) (extraction efficiency = 20%), Tc-99m-MAG_3 is the agent of choice for imaging kidneys in moderate to severe renal failure, immature kidneys, and transplant kidneys, in which renal function is often in flux. In practice, because glomerular function and tubular function generally parallel each other, Tc-99m-MAG_3 has replaced Tc-99m-DTPA in many clinics, unless glomerular function analysis is specifically requested or comparison with legacy Tc-99m-DTPA exams is needed.

Cortical Imaging. While both Tc-99m-GH and Tc-99m-DMSA can be used, Tc-99m-DMSA has minimal urinary excretion (<5%) and high cortical binding (50% of the dose at 4 hours postinjection) and is the cortical agent of choice. When the usual dose of 190 MBq for Tc-99m-DMSA is used, this results in excellent target-to-background ratio and minimal interference of excreted radiopharmaceutical with analysis of the kidney cortex.

Collecting System and Ureters. Isotopes for examining the collecting system include Tc-99m-DTPA, Tc-99m-GH, and Tc-99m-MAG_3. Because Tc-99m-MAG_3 has the highest extraction ratio and least interference by background activity of the Tc-99m agents, it is the agent of choice for studies directed specifically at the evaluating collecting system and ureters. For direct instillation into the bladder, Tc-99m-pertechnetate (Tc-99m-O_4) (38 MBq) is used.

Miscellaneous. Gallium-67 (Ga-67) citrate (200 to 380 MBq) is useful in evaluating infectious and neoplastic processes of the kidneys and perinephric spaces. Indium-111–labeled white blood cells (In-111-WBCs) (19 MBq) are even more specific for the detection of focal inflammatory and acute infectious processes. Tc-99m-O_4 (190 to 380 MBq) is used in scrotal imaging. If possible, the thyroid should be blocked with oral potassium perchlorate prior to Tc-99m-O_4 injection.

Imaging Techniques. Recent advances in gamma camera technology and the increasing availability of SPECT allow for the acquisition and processing of good resolution images. The image acquisition matrix (64 × 64 or 128 × 128) and the computer or camera zoom should be chosen such that the resultant images include all desired structures and the pixel size is approximately half the resolving capacity of the system at the distance of the organ of interest from the camera. Recent advances in computer technology and commercial processing packages allow for the acquisition and rapid processing of large volumes of dynamic functional data and curve generation, which are essential in the evaluation of renovascular hypertension and the assessment of collecting system obstruction.

The consensus reports on both diuretic renography and the scintigraphic evaluation of renovascular hypertension should be read by those unfamiliar with these studies, as their advice on study performance and interpretation, avoiding artifacts, performance, and interpretation pitfalls is sound, and because of their excellent explanations of patient preparation, pathology, and physiology.

In all renal studies it is critical that the patient be immobilized during acquisition. Although this is challenging in pediatric patients, with judicious use of immobilization devices and patient and parent reassurance, skilled technologists only occasionally require either sedation or the need for image reregistration because of patient movement. The supine position is used routinely. The more physiologic upright sitting position or semiupright positions may be used, especially when ureteral drainage is evaluated or where renal pelvic activity might interfere with the study (e.g., evaluation for renovascular hypertension and the assessment of collecting system obstruction). The main drawback to nonsupine positions is that differential function determinations may be inaccurate because mobile kidneys may move from nearly the same depth when the patient is supine to different depths when not supine. Renal transplants and some renal variants (e.g., horseshoe kidney) and the urinary bladder are best imaged anteriorly. When dynamic imaging studies are performed, the injection site should be imaged, since even a small amount of infiltrated dose can affect quantitative analysis of excretion and uptake.

Adequate hydration is mandatory to avoid false-positive renovascular hypertension and collecting system obstruction studies and to give reproducible results for quantitative washout parameters in follow-up studies. Many departments perform IV hydration and supplemental oral hydration routinely on all children and many adults because of the wide variability in the state of hydration upon presentation for the procedure.

For vascular flow studies, an IV bolus of tracer is injected and a set of sequential 1- to 3-second images is obtained. Tracer normally arrives at the kidney 1 to 2 seconds after the bolus has reached the adjacent aorta. Although flow studies are routinely performed for all dynamic renal studies in many clinics, some clinics perform them only in acute renal failure, when there is a probability of rapidly changing renal function, such as in transplantation, or in the evaluation of renal masses.

For the uptake and excretion phases of dynamic Tc-99m-DTPA and MAG_3 imaging, a series of 15- to 60-second dynamic images are acquired over the following 20 to 30 minutes. In collecting system obstruction studies, an indwelling bladder catheter may be inserted to ensure bladder decompression and to monitor urine output, and furosemide (20 to 40 mg IV) is given either 15 minutes before, at the time of, or 20 minutes after radiopharmaceutical injection; imaging then continues for another 20 to 30 minutes. Maximum effect of furosemide is 15 minutes after injection, so injecting 15 minutes prior to radiopharmaceutical injection should be strongly considered when the collecting system is known to be markedly dilated.

For evaluation of renal vascular hypertension, an angiotensin-converting enzyme inhibitor (ACEI) is given in conjunction with either Tc-99m MAG_3 or Tc-99mDTPA dynamic scintigraphy. This is accomplished either with enalaprilat 2.5 mg IV over 5 minutes beginning 15 minutes prior to radiopharmaceutical bolus, or with oral captopril 25 to 50 mg given 1 hour prior to the radiopharmaceutical. Blood pressures are recorded before ACEI administration and at various times during the study. Many protocols require a baseline renal study without ACEI, which can be accomplished either on a separate day or on the same day with a smaller dose of radiopharmaceutical.

When using Tc-99m-DMSA or Tc-99m-GH for cortical imaging, static images are usually obtained 4 hours after injection (to allow time for radiopharmaceutical in the collecting system to wash out) with both posterior planar and pinhole collimator images in the posterior and posterior oblique position for each kidney. Alternatively, high-resolution SPECT images can be obtained at that time.

Except in infants when supine imaging is obtained, vesicoureteral reflux studies (direct radionuclide cystography) are usually obtained posteriorly in the upright position as 1-minute dynamic acquisitions during retrograde filling to maximum bladder volume through a bladder catheter and during voiding after catheter removal.

Dynamic Imaging. The approach to interpreting dynamic renal studies can be divided into phases, and sequential attention to each phase allows for a methodic evaluation of pertinent positive and negative findings so that a reasonable differential diagnosis can be reached (Fig. 60.1).

The flow phase lasts for the first minute after injection, when arterial flow to the kidney can be analyzed semiquantitatively. Radiotracer is normally seen arriving at the kidneys within 1 to 2 seconds after appearance in the adjacent aorta and appears at least as intense as the spleen. With Tc-99m-DTPA and Tc-99m-GH, peak activity in the kidney is reached 6 seconds later and declines, because of only 20% first-pass extraction, until recirculation of the systemic bolus. With Tc-99m-MAG_3, the decline in intensity is less evident visually because of 60% first-pass extraction. Areas of hyperperfusion and hypoperfusion are noted and correlated to delayed images.

The uptake or cortical phase continues until radiotracer begins to leave the parenchyma 3 to 4 minutes after radiopharmaceutical injection. Radiopharmaceutical time to collecting system appearance and areas of increased or decreased uptake should be noted. Differential function is computed by drawing regions of interest (ROIs) and obtaining background subtracted 1- to 2-minute integrated unilateral whole kidney counts and expressing them as a percentage of total kidney counts. This parameter is a crucial piece of information, so careful examination of ROIs for proper position and artifacts is very important. Differential function can also be obtained on 4-hour delayed static images of Tc-99m-GH and Tc-99m-DMSA, with excellent intrapatient and inter-radiopharmaceutical reproducibility above 95%. Differential function values for each kidney should be 45% to 55%.

The excretory phase begins after the uptake phase, although both continue to occur simultaneously. Time of arrival of the radiopharmaceutical to the renal pelvis should be noted, as well as any areas of prolonged or diminished cortical retention, which should be correlated with abnormalities in the uptake phase and their relation to the calices. Although the calices, renal pelvis, and ureters may be seen in a normal study, prolonged or intense accumulations, structural displacement, or unusual contours should be noted. Background subtracted time-activity curves for whole kidney, renal cortex, collecting system, or renal pelvis (depending on the clinical question) are usually generated. Various parameters to quantitatively evaluate

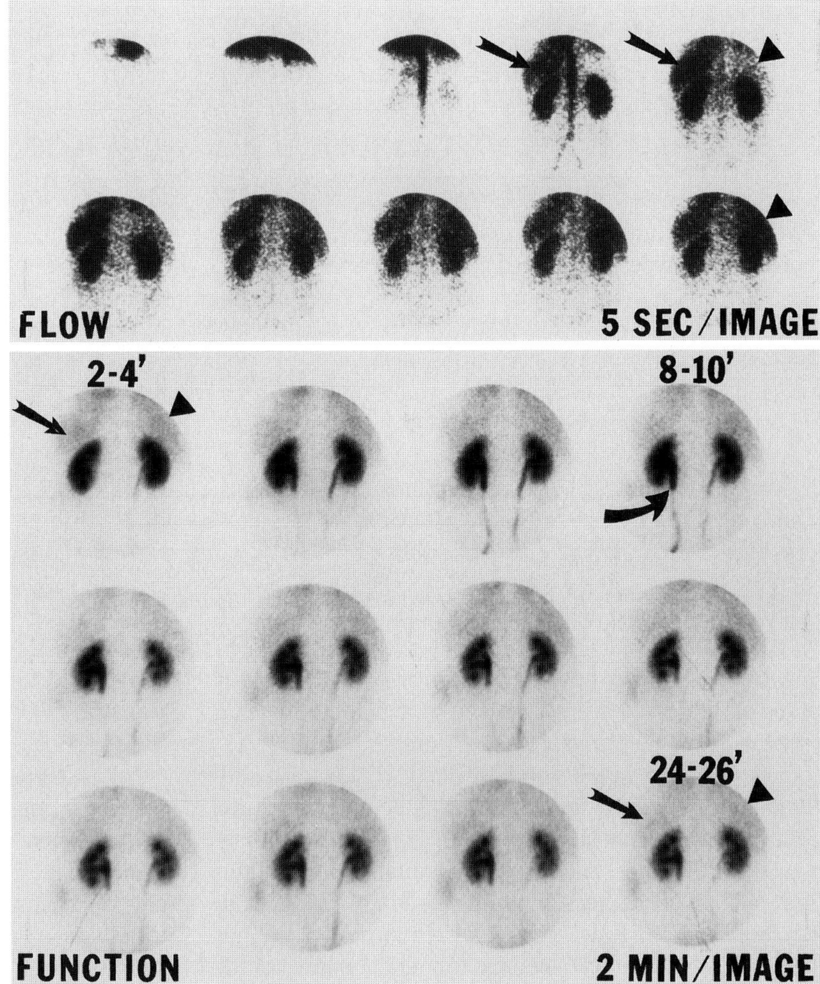

FIGURE 60.1. **Normal Technetium-99m-Diethylenetriamine Pentaacetic Acid Study. Posterior projection renal blood flow** (FLOW, *at top*): The bolus reaches the aorta (third image) and, within 2 seconds, the kidneys. The kidneys should be as hot or hotter than the spleen (*arrows*) on the image following the aorta bolus image. Hepatic activity (*arrowheads*) appears later than splenic activity because hepatic perfusion is predominantly from the portal vein. **Uptake** (FUNCTION, *at bottom*): Tracer is rapidly cleared by the kidneys, resulting in peak cortical activity in the 2- to 4-second (2-4′) image. Intense cortical uptake in the 2- to 4-second image and rapid decrease of blood pool, liver (*arrowheads*) and spleen (*arrows*) activity is evidence of normal glomerular filtration rate. **Cortical uptake and excretion:** This patient, who was allergic to iodinated contrast, was imaged after a renal stone had passed. Because tracer passes rapidly from an undilated collecting system to the bladder, there is no obstruction. The small column of tracer (*curved arrow*) represents ureteral spasm, where the stone had probably impacted.

washout from these curves have been proposed, but the most common are the $T_{1/2}$ and the residual cortical or kidney activity. The $T_{1/2}$ is defined as the time from either radiopharmaceutical injection or furosemide injection to half maximum activity. A normal value is less than 10 minutes, but in poor renal function or in collecting system dilation, this parameter may not be determinable within the constraints of the usual 20- to 30-minute exam. The residual cortical or kidney activity is the ratio of the 20-minute activity to the maximum activity. A normal value is less than 0.3.

Knowledge of the exact clinical question, results of other imaging modalities, laboratory results, and patient history markedly narrows the differential diagnosis, allows for selection of the appropriate radiopharmaceutical and imaging protocol, allows for the proper evaluation of artifacts, and increases the clinical usefulness of the scan. Every effort should be made, especially in transplant evaluations, to correlate the nuclear medicine images with available clinical, imaging, and laboratory data.

Absolute Function Quantitation. Renal tracer clearance (GFR with Tc-99m-DTPA or ERPF with Tc-99m-MAG_3) can be estimated by assessing the rate of disappearance of tracer from the blood (cardiac blood pool and/or background), the rate of appearance of renal cortical activity, or the rate of appearance of urine (usually bladder) activity. It is beyond the scope of this chapter to cover the myriad of camera-based or blood and/or urine activity counting techniques available for estimating absolute tubular or glomerular function. In general, the simpler gamma camera–based techniques are highly reproducible but less accurate than the more complicated techniques that supplement gamma camera counting with urine or blood activity.

Clinical Applications

Anatomic Variants. Nuclear renal imaging is of use in evaluating anatomic variants when other imaging modalities have not fully defined an abnormality. The ability to assess function makes scintigraphy even more valuable. A dromedary hump, a fetal lobulation, or a renal column of Bertin may appear as a mass on US or CT. Tc-99m-DMSA or Tc-99m-GH images (pinhole and/or SPECT) will

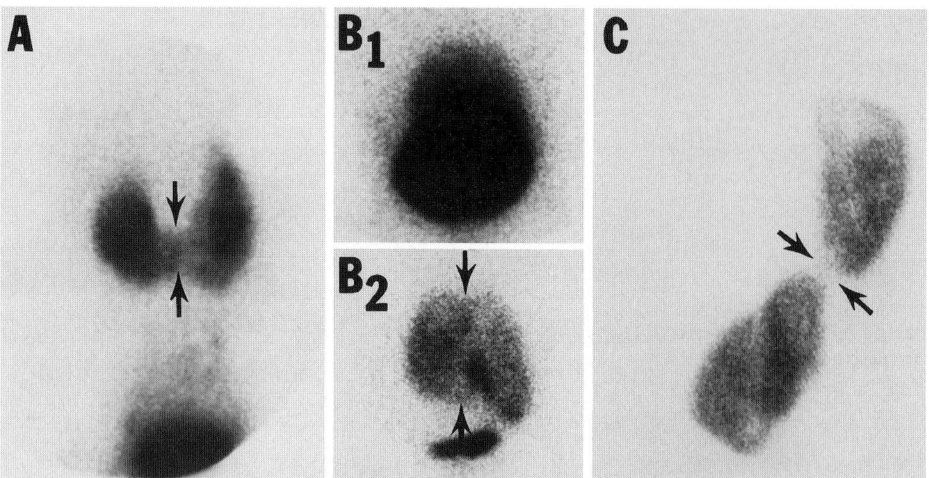

FIGURE 60.2. **Congenital Renal Abnormalities. A.** Horseshoe kidney (imaged with technetium-99m-diethylenetriamine pentaacetic acid [Tc-99m-DTPA]). The medial angulation of the inferior renal poles and the connecting bridge characteristic of horseshoe kidney are best seen in this anterior view (*arrows*). Collecting system obstruction, a possible complication, is not seen. **B.** Lump or cake kidney (Tc-99m-DTPA). Anterior image of the bladder (B1) demonstrates no appreciable renal activity. After voiding (B2), the fused pelvic kidney was easily seen. The line of fusion (*arrows*) is apparent. **C.** Crossed-fused ectopia (Tc-99m-dimercaptosuccinic acid [DMSA]). The bridge of fusion (*arrows*) was best seen on this anterior Tc-99m-DMSA image.

demonstrate the questionable tissue to be normally functioning and rule out a pathologic lesion. Nuclear imaging is particularly useful in congenital abnormalities (Fig. 60.2) such as horseshoe kidney, lump or cake kidney, and crossed-fused ectopia when other modalities have not located or explained the functional nature of the abnormality.

Mass Lesions. Although radionuclide studies are not generally used to detect solid intrarenal masses, they may be of value in investigating cystic lesions or hydronephrosis (HN) as a possible cause of a mass and in demonstrating functioning tissue associated with a mass (Fig. 60.3). In the neonate, multicystic dysplastic kidney and HN both present as fluid-filled masses. They can be differentiated by the presence (in HN) or the absence (in multicystic dysplastic kidney) of tracer in the fluid. On Tc-99m-DTPA or Tc-99m-MAG$_3$ imaging, urine collections such as HN or urinoma increase tracer concentration with time. Except in differentiating the nature of these fluid-filled lesions, it is axiomatic that renal masses never accumulate the technetium radiopharmaceuticals. Occasionally, a hypertrophied column of Bertin can mimic a mass, and demonstration of normal Tc-99m-DTPA, Tc-99m-GH, Tc-99m-DMSA, or Tc-99m-MAG$_3$ accumulation in the area in question confirms the benign nature of this finding seen on other radiographic studies.

Acute Renal Failure. The differential diagnosis of acute renal failure includes acute vascular occlusion, venous thrombosis, acute collecting system or bladder outlet obstruction, acute tubular necrosis, and, in transplant patients, cyclosporine toxicity and transplant rejection. A renal perfusion (flow) study can demonstrate absent perfusion of one or both kidneys and may define the level of aortic cutoff from a dissecting aneurysm. In renal vein thrombosis (Fig. 60.4), decreased perfusion of an enlarged kidney with prolonged cortical retention of tracer is seen. Delayed images (Tc-99m-MAG$_3$) demonstrating tracer in a dilated collecting system suggest a high-grade obstruction. In acute tubular necrosis (ATN) (Fig. 60.5) and acute high-grade urinary obstruction, arterial flow is relatively well maintained despite almost absent transit of tracer in the urinary collection system. In both these situations, although glomerular filtration drops to near zero and Tc-99m-DTPA studies reveal no uptake, tubular cell uptake of Tc-99m-MAG$_3$ continues as long as the cells are viable. This combination is relatively specific for these entities, which can then be differentiated by anatomic imaging of presence or lack of a dilated collecting system.

Renal Transplantation. Renal imaging of the anuric or oliguric transplanted kidney is performed to help distinguish acute tubular necrosis from transplant rejection as well as to detect other posttransplant complications. Differential diagnosis includes all of the diseases of concern in acute renal failure, with several others that are unique to transplantation. As a complementary modality to Doppler US, dynamic functional imaging can assist in situations in which oliguric renal failure is a contraindication to nephrotoxic contrast agents. The findings in ATN were described previously. Acute or chronic rejection results in a more balanced loss of perfusion and function

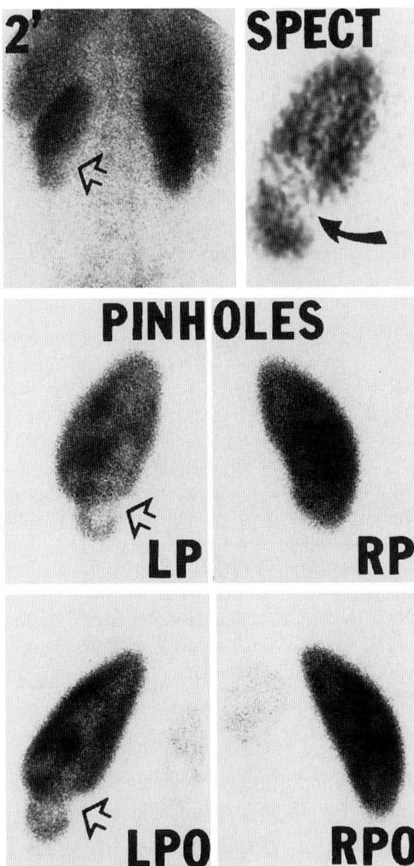

FIGURE 60.3. **Renal Mass.** Technetium-99m (Tc-99m)-diethylenetriamine pentaacetic acid posterior image (2′, *upper left*) and Tc-99m-dimercaptosuccinic acid pinhole images (*middle and below*) demonstrate a renal contour abnormality (*open arrows*) of the lower pole of the left kidney. The SPECT image (*upper right*) demonstrates the true cortical defect (*curved arrow*), which corresponds to a renal tumor. LP, left posterior; RP, right posterior; LPO, left posterior oblique; RPO, right posterior oblique.

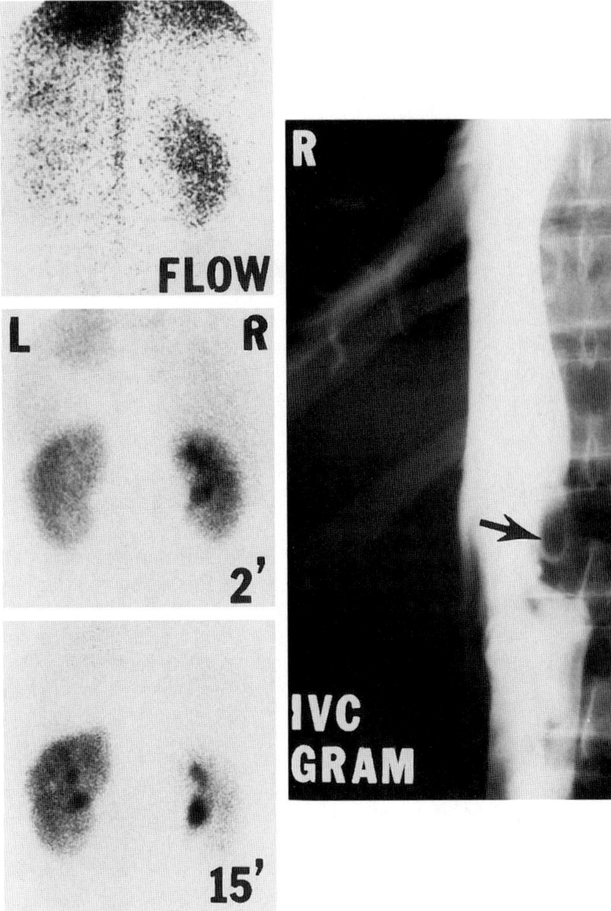

FIGURE 60.4. **Renal Vein Thrombosis.** Technetium-99m-mercaptoacetyltriglycine posterior scintigrams (*left*) demonstrate normal flow, cortical uptake, and excretion for the right kidney. The left kidney is enlarged, with severely diminished flow and a progressive rise in cortical tracer through 15 minutes. The contrast inferior vena cavagram (IVC GRAM) (*right*) confirms thrombus in the left renal vein (*arrow*).

because the damage is to small vessels, with secondary and equivalent loss of function. The scintigraphic pattern of cyclosporine toxicity is variable. A myriad of additional postoperative complications is seen following transplantation. Although Doppler US and biopsy have assumed the major role in evaluating the failing transplant kidney, renal scintigraphy can detect renal infarction and infection (demonstrated by photopenic defects on functional or cortical imaging), characterize fluid collections as urinomas or lymphoceles by the respective presence or lack of accumulation of excreted radiopharmaceuticals, and noninvasively determine whether the common posttransplant findings of hydroureter and hydronephrosis are caused by urinary obstruction (see following).

Correlation of dynamic imaging with US studies with the known time course of common transplant pathology can strongly suggest a diagnosis. ATN usually occurs during the first week and acute rejection between the second and the fourth weeks following transplantation. Cyclosporine toxicity occurs later and only in patients taking cyclosporine. Chronic rejection is a late phenomenon that eventually occurs to some degree in all transplants. Urinomas tend to occur early, whereas lymphoceles usually occur several weeks after transplantation (Fig. 60.6).

Renovascular Hypertension. Standard renal scintigraphy is neither sensitive nor specific in investigating hypertensive patients for renal artery stenosis (RAS) (Fig. 60.7). The accuracy of scintigraphy is markedly enhanced by incorporating an ACEI (captopril or enalaprilat) into the study. Hemodynamically significant RAS, manifested as renovascular hypertension, decreases the blood pressure in the *afferent* glomerular arteriole, resulting in an increase in renin production by the juxtaglomerular apparatus. Renin stimulates the conversion of angiotensin I

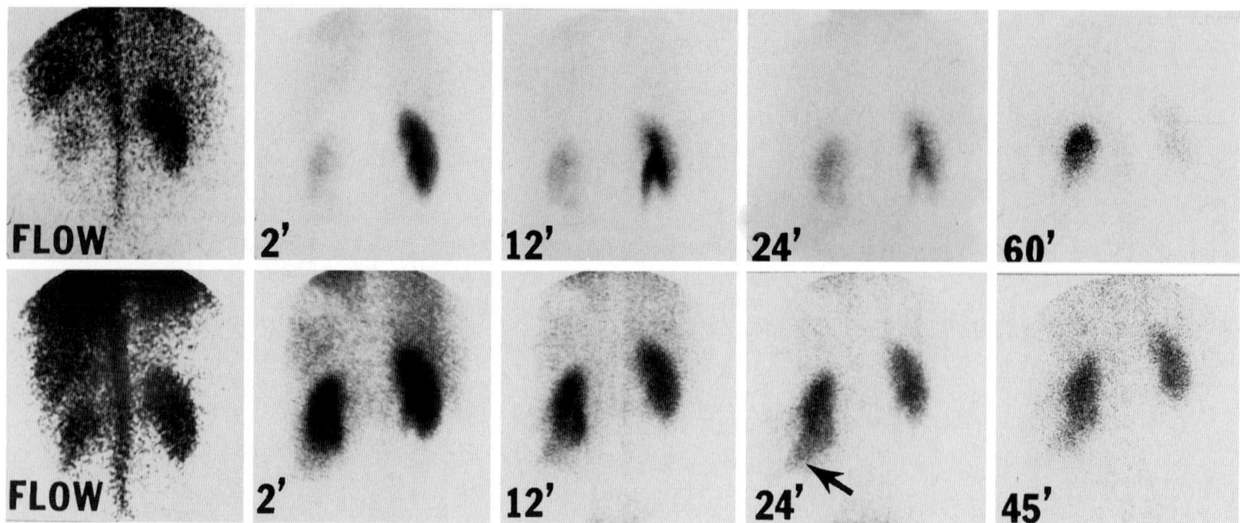

FIGURE 60.5. **Acute Tubular Necrosis (ATN). A.** Posterior technetium-99m-mercaptoacetyl-triglycine renal scintigrams 48 hours after left renal ischemia during a surgical procedure reveal diminished left renal flow that is relatively well preserved compared to initial cortical uptake, with slowly increasing cortical tracer retention through 60 minutes. **B.** A study performed 1 month later reveals almost complete resolution of the unilateral ATN. Extrarenal tracer activity (*arrow*) indicates a urine leak along a postoperative nephrostomy tract.

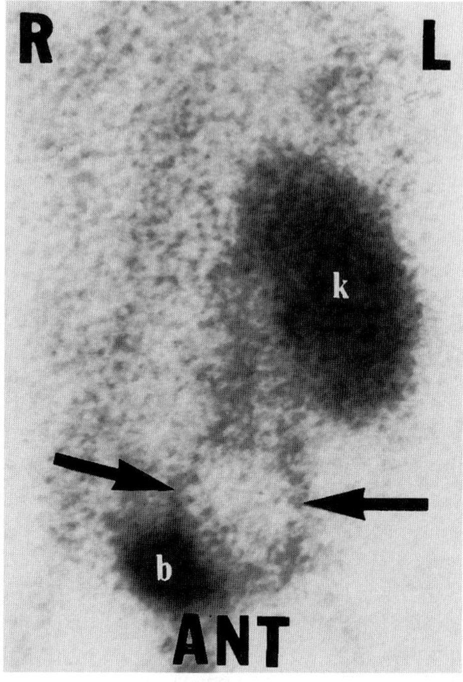

FIGURE 60.6. **Lymphocele in a Renal Transplantation Patient.** Anterior scintigram shows a photopenic area (*arrows*) adjacent to the bladder (b) representing a lymphocele, confirmed by US examination. Because it is not obstructing the transplant ureter, it is probably not clinically significant. k, transplant kidney.

to angiotensin II. This local rise in angiotensin II causes constriction of the *efferent* arteriole, which maintains the glomerular perfusion pressure and thus the GFR. The ACEIs block the production of angiotensin II and, in compensated RAS, cause relaxation of the constricted efferent arteriole. The glomerular perfusion pressure and GFR drop and the transit of filtrate from glomerulus to renal pelvis is prolonged. In an unaffected kidney, the efferent arteriole is not constricted, so ACEIs have little or no effect. Changes induced in the renogram curves with ACEIs, as manifested by prolonged cortical retention and washout, are best documented by performing renography with Tc-99m-MAG_3 before and after the administration of enalaprilat or captopril (Fig. 60.6). Renogram changes are less apparent with Tc-99m-DTPA and Tc-99m-GH, and differential function changes are more reliable indicators with these radiopharmaceuticals. Sensitivity and specificity for renovascular hypertension, as determined by response to lesion treatment, are both approximately 90%, which is as good or better than US, MR, and CT protocols.

Urinary Tract Obstruction. Because radiopharmaceuticals such as Tc-99m-DTPA and Tc-99m-MAG_3 are rapidly cleared through the kidneys, they are useful for the detection of both acute and chronic urinary tract obstruction (Figs. 60.8, 60.9). These agents are also used to measure differential function in evaluation of stability and/or salvageability of obstructed kidneys. The gold standard for determining obstruction ultimately is retrospective: decreasing renal function in the face of qualitative evidence (symptoms) or quantitative evidence (objective imaging criteria). In the case of equivocal or absent symptoms,

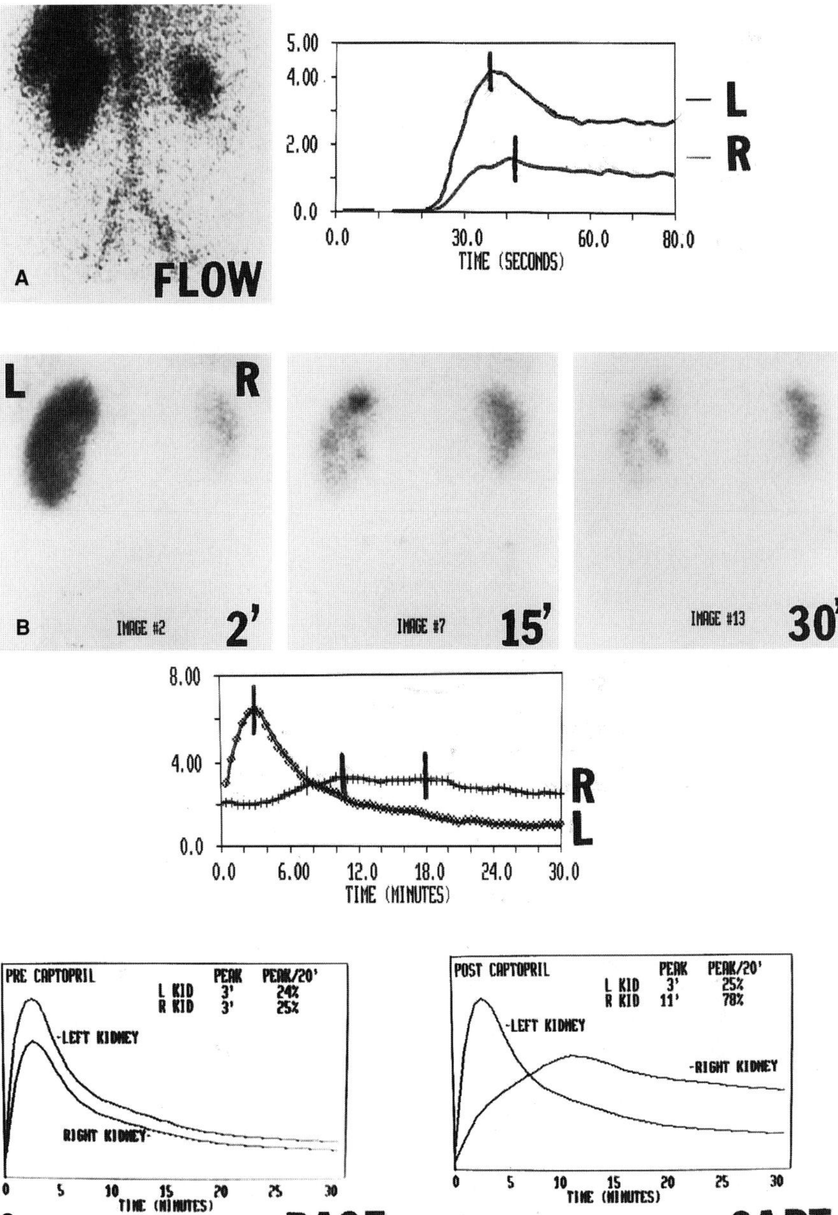

FIGURE 60.7. **Renal Artery Stenosis (RAS).** Posterior scintigrams after captopril. **A.** Technetium-99m-mercaptoacetyltriglycine (Tc-99m-MAG_3) arterial flow study. Flow to the small right kidney is decreased (image) and delayed (curve). **B.** Right cortical Tc-99m-MAG_3 activity continues to rise during the first 12 minutes of the study. Tc-99m-MAG_3 reveals the characteristic of a severe RAS. **C.** Typical Tc-99m-MAG_3 captopril curves of a patient with compensated right RAS. Both curves are normal in the baseline study. This is because efferent arteriolar constriction is maintaining glomerular perfusion pressure and glomerular filtration rate (GFR) (see text). After captopril, the right GFR has dropped and the cortical-glomerular-to-pelvis transit time has become prolonged. This is demonstrated by a prolonged time to peak and a delayed washout on the stenotic side.

imaging studies must prospectively determine the presence of obstruction, and some controversy exists concerning the relative utility of many imaging studies. While this is also the case with renal scintigraphy, it is generally well accepted as the noninvasive procedure of choice in evaluating clinically equivocal obstruction.

When collecting system obstruction occurs, the post-glomerular (Bowman space) pressure rises and the GFR drops. Tubular damage occurs later than glomerular damage and takes significantly longer to reverse. Renal imaging with Tc-99m-MAG_3 or Tc-99m-DTPA reliably detects unilateral or bilateral urinary tract obstruction by demonstrating a dilated pelvicaliceal system and/or ureter with delayed drainage. However, because large but unobstructed collecting systems or decreased urine production in renal failure can mimic these obstructive patterns, the routine study is frequently augmented with furosemide. Analysis of the cortical and whole-kidney renogram curves should always occur in conjunction with inspection of dynamic images and regions of interest chosen, and the time of arrival of the radiopharmaceutical to renal pelvises and calices should be noted. In the absence of renal failure, the post–furosemide lack of disappearance of tracer from the collecting system correlates with the severity of obstruction. In such cases in the adult, a $T_{1/2}$ of 15 minutes or less is interpreted as unobstructed, and a $T_{1/2}$ greater than

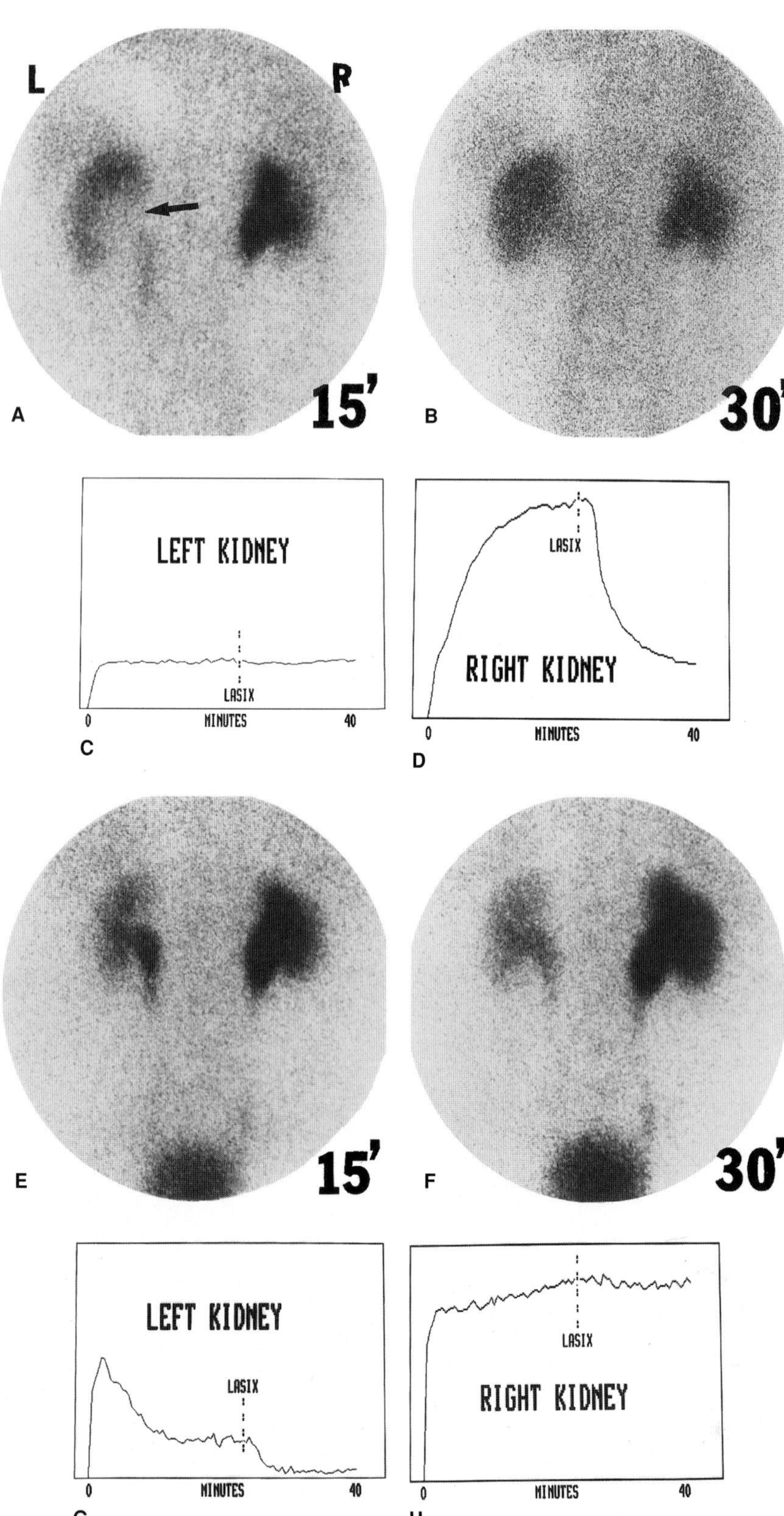

FIGURE 60.8. **Furosemide Renography.** Posterior scintigrams, with furosemide (Lasix) administered at 15 minutes. A high-grade obstruction is seen on the left **(A, B, C)**, with little tracer reaching the renal pelvis (*arrow*) and an absent furosemide response. On the right **(A, B, D)**, a dilated but unobstructed renal pelvis empties rapidly following furosemide administration. A follow-up study performed many months later **(E to H)** demonstrates that, following surgery, the left kidney has returned to normal. However, the right kidney has developed a high-grade obstruction with poor furosemide response.

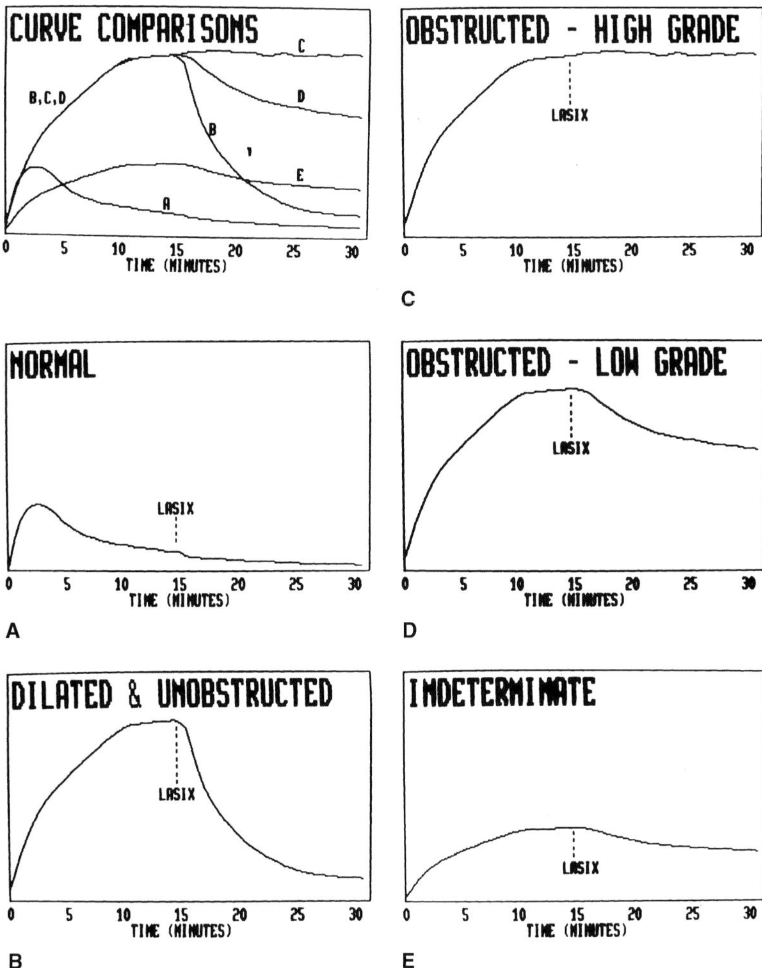

FIGURE 60.9. **Furosemide Curve Patterns. A.** Normal kidney. **B.** Dilated and unobstructed kidney. **C.** High-grade obstruction (no Lasix response). In a complete obstruction, no tracer would arrive at the renal pelvis. **D.** Low-grade obstruction. A partial response between that of curves **(B)** and **(C)** is seen. This pattern may be difficult to distinguish from an indeterminate study. If this pattern is seen with relatively good unilateral renal function, and if the collecting system is not markedly dilated, then low-grade or partial obstruction can be confidently diagnosed. **E.** Indeterminate study. In a patient with a very large dilated collecting system or poor function in the kidney of interest, the furosemide dose may be insufficient to wash tracer from the collecting system. This curve represents a failed kidney that did not respond to furosemide.

20 minutes generally confirms obstruction, although there is disagreement over using these parameters as diagnostic absolutes. Therefore, positive obstructive renogram curves in the presence of compromised renal function, marked collecting system dilation, full bladder, radiopharmaceutical infiltration, and poor patient hydration should be interpreted with caution. The degree of renal compromise at which renogram curves become unreliable is unknown and probably varies from patient to patient, but some authors use a unilateral GFR of less than 15 mL/min (as estimated from the differential function and clinical or measured estimates of total renal function) as a point at which positive curves are unreliable. Such curves should be interpreted as indeterminate and not as partial obstruction. Also, in neonates and infants, obstructive curves are unreliable, probably because of immature kidney function. It has been shown that, even in the presence of significantly decreased single kidney function, obstructive curves do not predict kidney deterioration, and these children may spontaneously improve in such cases. It is worth stressing, however, that at any age, level of renal function, or collecting system dilation, a nonobstructive curve effectively rules

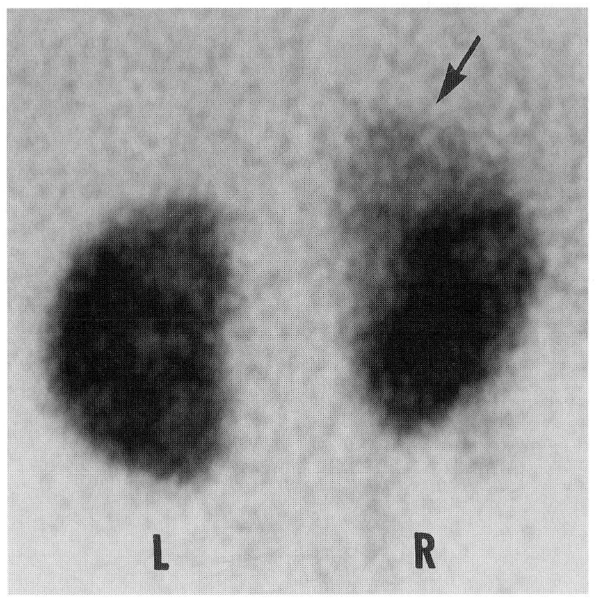

FIGURE 60.10. **Acute Pyelonephritis.** Posterior scintigrams show a photopenic area in the upper pole of the right kidney (*arrow*). Chronic pyelonephritis cannot be distinguished from acute pyelonephritis unless prior scans are available and show that the pattern is unchanged.

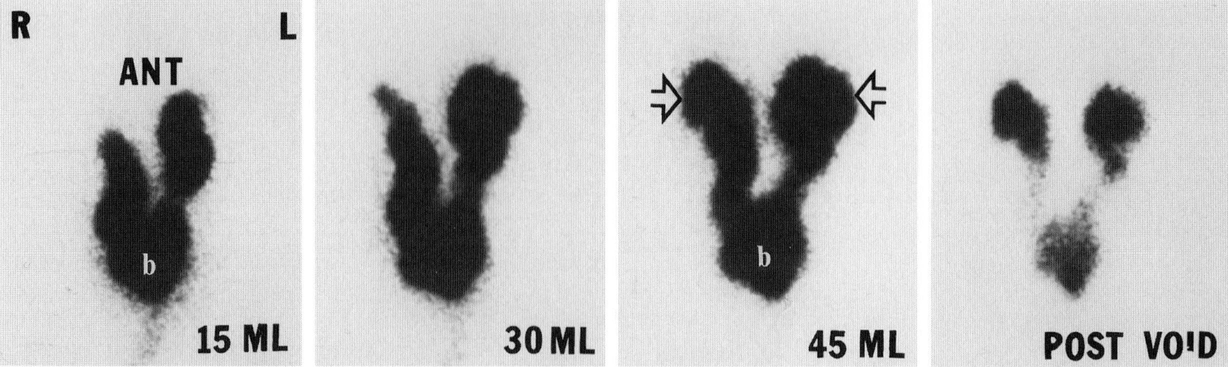

FIGURE 60.11. **Ureteral Reflux.** Anterior scintigrams demonstrate reflux of tracer to the renal pelvis (*arrows*) immediately on the left and at 45-mL bladder volume on the right. b, bladder.

out obstruction and does so more reliably than any other modality.

Infection. Imaging with Tc-99m-DMSA or Tc-99m-GH is still the most sensitive modality for detecting pyelonephritis, despite recent advances in MR, US, and CT. Scintigraphy has the additional advantage that neonates and infants rarely require sedation. In acute pyelonephritis, decreased parenchymal uptake of Tc-99m-DMSA or Tc-99m-GH is seen either focally or diffusely within the normal renal contours (Fig. 60.10). In chronic pyelonephritis, scarring occurs and results in renal contour abnormalities with foci of diminished uptake. Renal or perinephric abscess and infected renal cysts may be imaged with Ga-67 or In-111-WBC.

Ureteral Reflux. Direct radionuclide cystography is the most sensitive of any imaging method for detecting ureteral reflux (Fig. 60.11), probably because even the smallest amount of transient reflux can be seen and the entire filling and voiding process is evaluated during radionuclide studies, whereas transient reflux is missed during contrast cystograms. The bladder volume is reported when reflux occurs. The very low radiation dose, in comparison with contrast cystography, is especially desirable in pediatric screening or when multiple studies are needed to evaluate progression of disease and response to therapy.

TESTICULAR IMAGING

Radionuclide testicular imaging (Fig. 60.12) has been largely replaced by Doppler US studies. Nevertheless, it remains a robust, non–operator-dependent procedure with an extremely high sensitivity and specificity for acute torsion. Testicular torsion presents as a central hypovascular defect. As time passes, a hypervascular rim develops

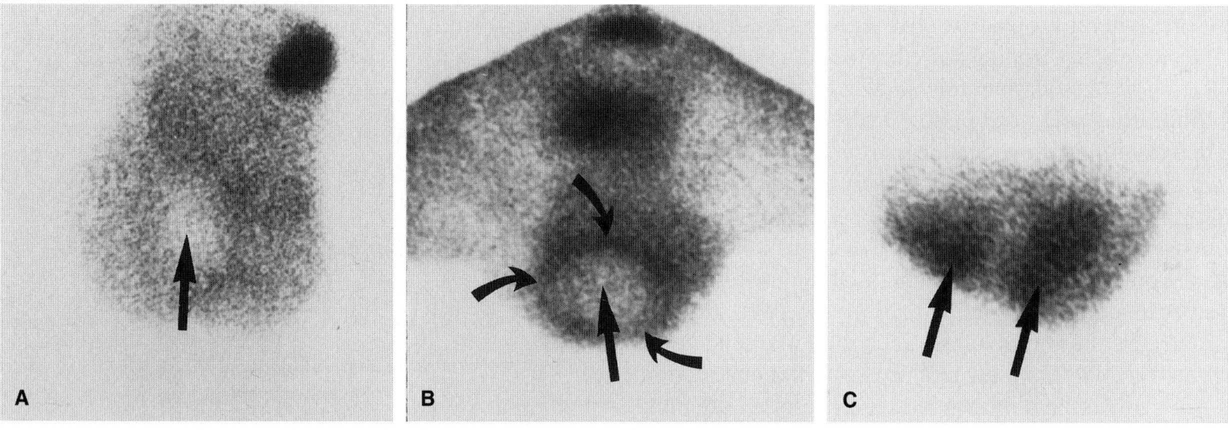

FIGURE 60.12. **Imaging of the Painful Testis.** Anterior scintigrams. **A.** Testicular torsion is seen as a photon-deficient testis on arterial flow imaging (*arrow*). **B.** The hyperemic rim (*curved arrows*) surrounding the photon-deficient testis (*straight arrow*) occurs when the diagnosis of torsion is delayed ("missed") and correlates well with loss of testicular viability. **C.** Hyperemic inflammation occurs with epididymitis, resulting in increased radionuclide accumulation in the epididymis, in this case bilaterally (*arrows*).

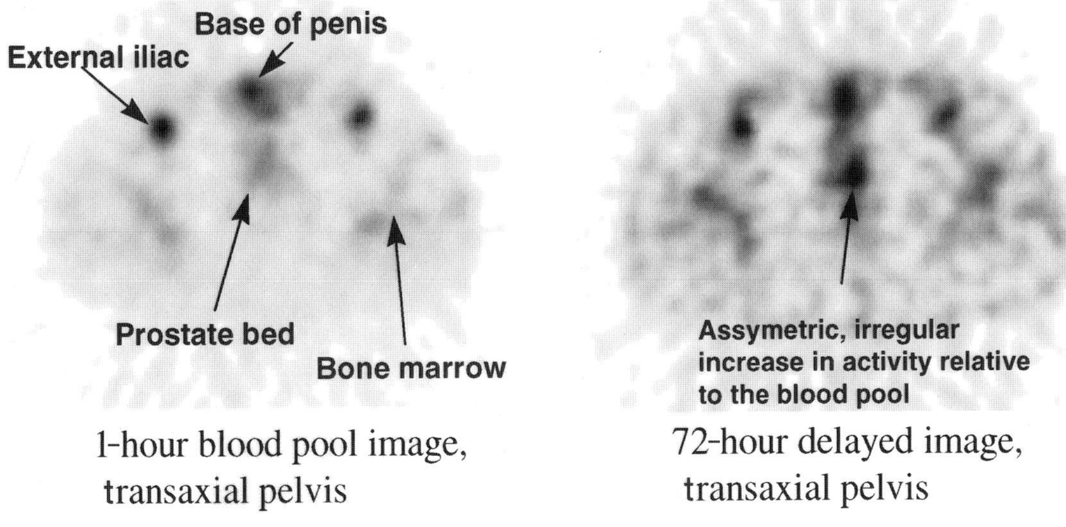

FIGURE 60.13. **Prostate Cancer.** Transaxial SPECT scintigrams using indium-111 capromab pendetide. Early (1-hour) and late (72-hour) images through the prostate in a patient with rising prostate-specific antigen (PSA) 3 years after radical prostatectomy. US-guided biopsy of the prostate bed nodules was negative for cancer. This study shows an unequivocal abnormality in the prostate bed on the late images. The patient was treated with external beam therapy to the prostate bed, and the PSA fell to an undetectable level. This implies that the prostate nodule biopsy was a false-negative result, a common scenario.

around the torsed testis, indicating loss of viability (delayed torsion). This rim may also be seen in abscess and hematoma. Epididymitis and epididymoorchitis manifest as increased flow to the affected testes. Masses and other testicular lesions are best evaluated with other modalities.

Scrotal imaging for testicular torsion is performed as a dynamic arterial flow study after Tc-99m-O_4 injection with sequential 1-second anterior images centered on the scrotum, followed by a 3- to 5-minute blood pool static image.

PROSTATE CANCER IMAGING

Prostate cancer spread is notoriously difficult to image, with all other imaging modalities demonstrating less than 50% sensitivity and specificity. Therapy depends on whether the patient has local disease versus distant metastasis. In-111 capromab pendetide (190 MBq) is a monoclonal antibody directed against cytoplasmic membrane antigens expressed only by prostate cancer. It has a sensitivity and specificity of 75% in detecting local disease and distant metastases. It is helpful when positive for distant spread in patients with a reasonable preprostatectomy possibility of metastasis and in patients with rising postprostatectomy prostate-specific antigen counts to determine local recurrence or distant spread (Fig. 60.13). However, imaging with this agent requires exquisite attention to imaging protocol detail, knowledge of the normal scintigraphic distribution of the agent in the abdomen and pelvis, and a SPECT camera, preferably with multiple-energy acquisition capabilities. On SPECT imaging 3 to 4 days postinjection, significant radiopharmaceutical remains in the blood pool; therefore, comparison with early 1-hour postinjection blood pool images, with simultaneously or sequentially acquired SPECT blood pool imaging with Tc-O_4–labeled red blood cells (960 MBq) on day 3 or 4, or with CT scan with or without SPECT-CT fusion is necessary to delineate abnormal foci.

SUGGESTED READINGS

Ell PJ, Gambhir SS. Nuclear Medicine in Clinical Diagnosis and Treatment. 3rd ed. Edinburgh: Churchill Livingstone, 2004:1497–1684.

Sandler MP, Coleman RE, et al, eds. Diagnostic Nuclear Medicine. 4th ed. Philadelphia: Lippincott Williams & Wilkins, 2002.

Freeman I, Blaufox MD. Renal nuclear medicine including consensus reports. Semin Nucl Med 1999;29(4):146–188.

Scintigraphic Diagnosis of Inflammation and Infection

Christopher J. Palestro and Charito Love

Gallium-67

Radiolabeled Leukocytes

Technetium-99M-Fanolesomab

Fluorine-18-Flurodeoxyglucose

The scintigraphic evaluation of infection and inflammation is extremely broad in scope, encompassing numerous radiopharmaceuticals, imaging techniques, and diseases. In addition to reviewing the roles of gallium-67 (Ga-67) citrate and radiolabeled leukocytes (WBC), this chapter also addresses the potentials of the recently approved antigranulocyte antibody, technetium-99m (Tc-99m) -fanolesomab, and of fluorine-18-fluorodeoxyglucose PET (F-18-FDG-PET) for imaging inflammation and infection.

GALLIUM-67

Ga-67, which has been used for localizing infection for more than three decades, is produced with a cyclotron. Decay is by electron capture and the half-life is 78.1 hours. With principal photon energies of 93, 184, and 296 keV used for imaging and a poor photon yield per disintegration, Ga-67 is a suboptimal imaging agent (1).

Several factors govern uptake of this tracer in inflammation and infection. About 90% of circulating Ga-67 is in the plasma, nearly all transferrin bound. Increased blood flow and increased vascular membrane permeability result in increased delivery and accumulation of transferrin-bound Ga-67 at inflammatory foci. Ga-67 also binds to lactoferrin, which is present in high concentrations in inflammatory foci. Direct bacterial uptake may also account for some Ga-67 accumulation in infection. Siderophores, low-molecular-weight chelates produced by bacteria, have a high affinity for Ga-67. The siderophore–Ga-67 complex is presumably transported into the bacterium, where it eventually is phagocytosed by macrophages. Although some Ga-67 may be transported bound to leukocytes, it is important to note that, even in the absence of circulating leukocytes, Ga-67 accumulates in infection (1).

Imaging is usually performed 18 to 72 hours after injection of 185 to 370 MBq (5 to 10 mCi) of Ga-67 citrate. A gamma camera equipped with a medium-energy collimator and capable of imaging multiple energy peaks is used. The normal biodistribution of Ga-67 is variable and includes bone, bone marrow, liver, genitourinary and GI tracts, and soft tissues (2) (Fig. 61.1). Nasopharyngeal and lacrimal gland activity can be very prominent, even in the absence of disease. Intense breast uptake is associated with hyperprolactinemic states, including pregnancy, lactation, certain drugs, and hypothalamic lesions. In patients who have undergone multiple transfusions, increased renal, bladder, and bone/marrow activity, together with decreased hepatic and colonic activity, is often observed, presumably because of iron receptor saturation by exogenous iron from the transfused cells. The MR contrast agent gadolinium can cause similar alterations in the biodistribution of Ga-67 (3–8).

Although labeled leukocyte imaging is generally considered the radionuclide test of choice for imaging infection in the immunocompetent population, Ga-67 imaging remains both popular and useful, providing information that is complementary to, and at times not available from, other tests. Indications for gallium imaging include the following.

Opportunistic Infection. Nuclear medicine plays an important role in the detection of infections unique to the immunocompromised patient, and for most of these,

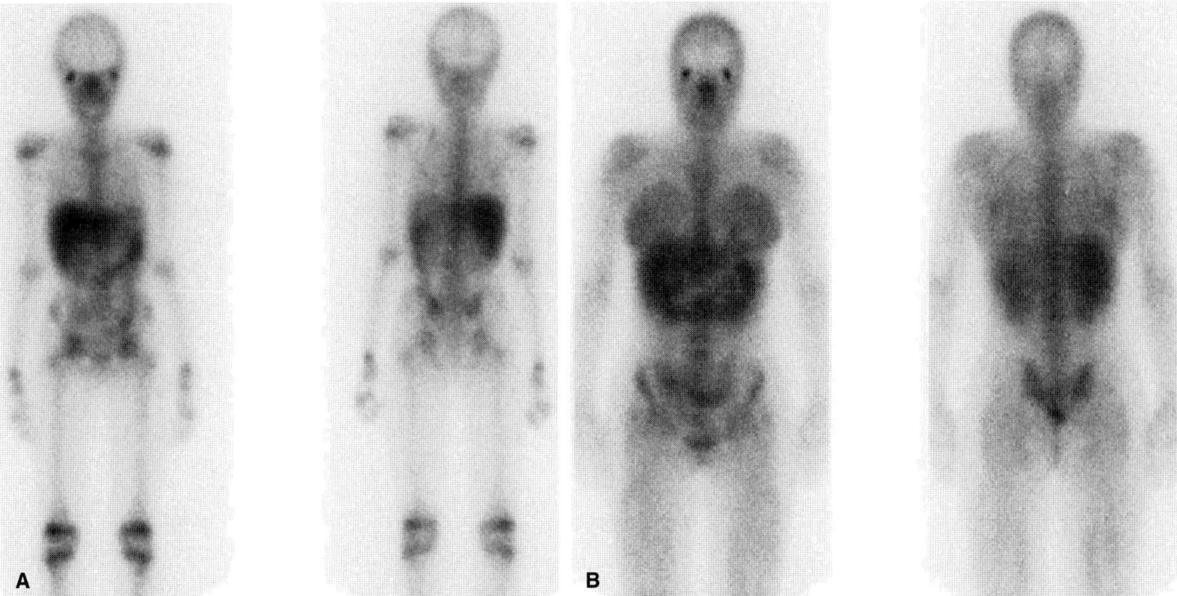

FIGURE 61.1. **Normal Pediatric and Adult Gallium Studies. A.** Anterior and posterior whole-body gallium-67 (Ga-67) images performed on an 11-year-old child. Prominent skeletal uptake is normal in children. The distal femoral and proximal tibial growth plates are easily identified. **B.** Anterior and posterior whole-body Ga-67 images performed on a 20-year-old woman. In this patient there is more soft tissue and less skeletal activity than in the patient illustrated in **A.** Note the physiologic breast activity, which can be confused with abnormal pulmonary uptake. This can be resolved by obtaining oblique and lateral views, or by SPECT.

Ga-67 imaging is the radionuclide procedure of choice. Many opportunistic infections affect the lungs, and a normal Ga-67 scan of the chest excludes infection with a high degree of certainty, especially in the setting of a negative chest radiograph. In the HIV-positive patient, lymph node uptake of Ga-67 is most often caused by mycobacterial disease or lymphoma. Focal, or localized, pulmonary parenchymal Ga-67 uptake is usually associated with bacterial pneumonia. Diffuse pulmonary gallium uptake is indicative of *Pneumocystis jiroveci* pneumonia, especially when the uptake is intense (Fig. 61.2). In addition to its value for diagnosis, Ga-67 can be used for monitoring response to therapy. Kaposi sarcoma, a malignancy often found in patients with AIDS, is not Ga-67 avid (1,9,10).

Interstitial Lung Disease. Ga-67 is an extremely sensitive indicator of pulmonary inflammation. Uptake of this tracer occurs in sarcoidosis, interstitial pneumonitis in virtually all its forms and etiologies, drug reactions, collagen vascular disease, and pneumoconioses. Although the degree of activity generally correlates with the severity of the underlying illness, a normal study does not exclude very mild inflammation. Furthermore, neither the intensity nor the pattern of uptake is diagnostic of specific illnesses (11,12).

In sarcoidosis, pulmonary uptake of Ga-67 correlates with disease activity and response to therapy. Ga-67 scintigraphy has been reported to be up to 97% sensitive

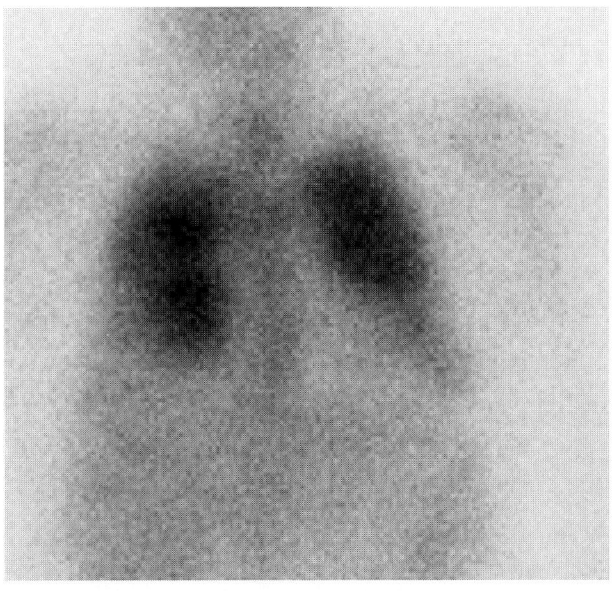

FIGURE 61.2. ***Pneumocystis jiroveci*** **Pneumonia.** Gallium-67 image of the chest demonstrates intense diffuse bilateral pulmonary activity that, in an AIDS patient with a normal chest radiograph, strongly suggests *P. jiroveci* pneumonia.

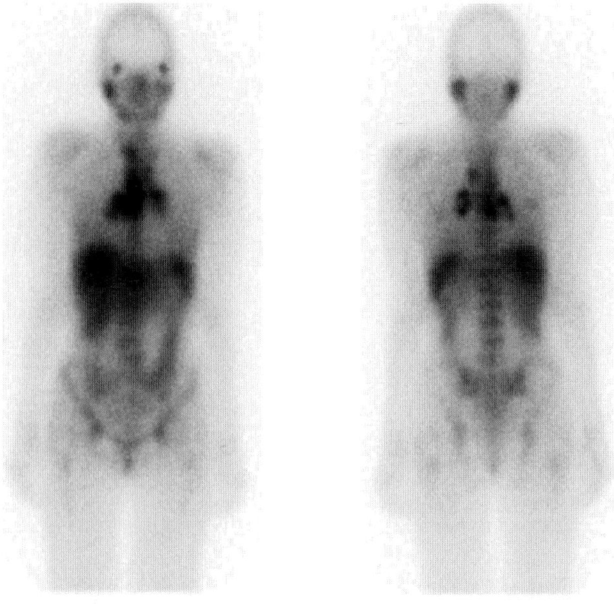

FIGURE 61.3. **Sarcoidosis.** Anterior and posterior whole-body gallium-67 images demonstrate bilateral hilar activity, a pattern that is characteristic for sarcoidosis. Prominent parotid and submandibular gland activity is often seen in sarcoidosis as well. Moderately intense activity in the descending colon is normal.

for detection of active sarcoidosis when considering both pulmonary and extrapulmonary sites (Fig. 61.3). Whether Ga-67 imaging can provide prognostic information or therapeutic insight for other inflammatory lung diseases is not known.

Because the determination of relative pulmonary Ga-67 activity may be helpful for assessing the level of inflammatory activity present, an objective index of Ga-67 activity has been sought. Some authors have chosen to compare pulmonary activity with sternal activity, others have compared pulmonary activity with hepatic activity, and still others have used semiquantitative techniques involving computer acquisitions, SPECT, and whole-body imaging to report activity ratios. As a result, there is no standard method for quantifying Ga-67 pulmonary activity. Therefore, when reporting Ga-67 activity, the specific scale and reference standard should be stated. We use a scale of 0 to 4, in which pulmonary activity is compared to liver activity. In this schema, 0 (normal) represents pulmonary activity that is indistinguishable from background, and 1 represents equivocally increased activity. Grades 2, 3, and 4 represent definitely abnormal pulmonary activity; grade 2 is less than, grade 3 is equal to, and grade 4 is greater than, hepatic activity. A photopenic or "cold" cardiac silhouette is present in patients with grades 2, 3, and 4 uptake (Fig. 61.4) (1).

Interstitial nephritis, a well-recognized cause of acute renal failure, is characterized by interstitial edema and a mononuclear cellular infiltrate. Although definitive diagnosis is by biopsy, Ga-67 can be helpful in differentiating interstitial nephritis from acute tubular necrosis in the acute setting. Interstitial nephritis is characterized by renal uptake of Ga that is more intense than spinal uptake, while acute tubular necrosis is characterized by little or no renal uptake. The test is less reliable in patients with chronic renal failure (Fig. 61.5) (13).

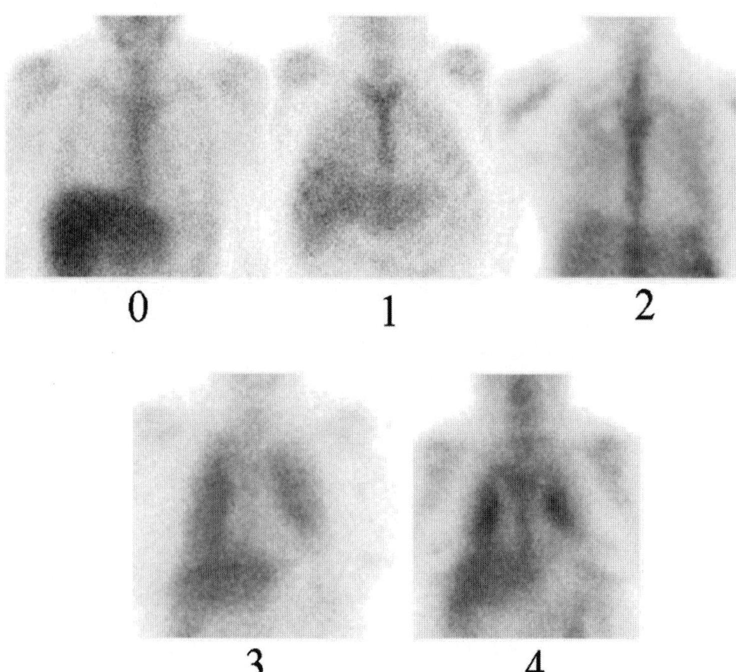

FIGURE 61.4. **Diffuse Pulmonary Uptake of Gallium-67 (Ga-67).** Pulmonary uptake of Ga-67 is often compared to hepatic activity and here is graded on a numeric scale from 0 (normal) to 4 (abnormal, with pulmonary activity more intense than hepatic activity). Details are provided in the text.

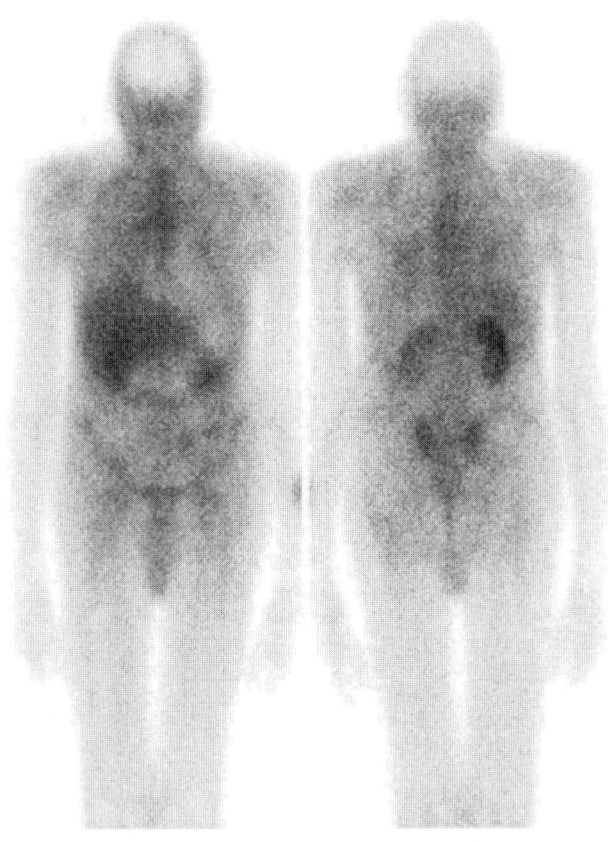

FIGURE 61.5. **Interstitial Nephritis**. Anterior and posterior whole-body gallium-67 images. Renal activity is more intense than adjacent lumbar spine activity, which is a pattern typical of interstitial nephritis.

Fever of undetermined origin (FUO) is an illness of at least 3 weeks' duration with several episodes of fever exceeding 38.3°C and no diagnosis after an appropriate inpatient or outpatient evaluation. There are numerous causes of FUO, and infection accounts for only about 20% to 30% of them. Neoplasms are responsible for about 15% to 25%. Other etiologies include collagen vascular disease, vasculitis, granulomatous diseases, pulmonary emboli, cerebrovascular accidents, and drug fever. Radionuclide imaging is typically reserved for those situations in which other imaging tests fail to localize the source of the fever. Nearly 80% of FUOs are caused by an entity other than infection, and therefore Ga-67, which accumulates in infection, inflammation, and tumor, is often preferred over WBC imaging for this indication (Fig. 61.6) 1,2).

Spinal Osteomyelitis. Although it has been replaced by labeled leukocyte imaging for evaluation of osteomyelitis in most regions of the skeleton, Ga-67 remains the radionuclide procedure of choice for diagnosing spinal osteomyelitis. Ga-67 imaging is frequently performed in conjunction with bone scintigraphy, and over the years, criteria have been established for the interpretation of bone/Ga-67 imaging. These criteria are used regardless of the area of the skeleton being evaluated (14). The combined test is:

Positive for osteomyelitis when distribution of the two tracers is spatially incongruent, or when the distribution is spatially congruent and the relative intensity of uptake of Ga-67 is greater than that of the bone agent (Fig. 61.7)

Equivocal for osteomyelitis when the distribution of the two radiotracers is congruent, both spatially and in terms of intensity (Fig. 61.8)

Negative for osteomyelitis when the Ga-67 images are normal, regardless of the bone scan findings, or when the distribution of the two tracers is spatially congruent and the relative intensity of uptake of Ga-67 is less than that of the bone agent (Fig. 61.9).

RADIOLABELED LEUKOCYTES

Although a variety of in vitro leukocyte labeling techniques have been investigated, the only approved methods in the United States employ the lipophilic compounds indium-111 (In-111) oxyquinoline and ^{99m}Tc-HMPAO (exametazine hexamethyl propyleneamine oxime). The labeling procedure takes about 2 to 3 hours. Approximately 40 to 60 mL of whole blood is withdrawn from the patient into an anticoagulant-containing syringe. All of the cellular components of the blood can be labeled, and the leukocytes must be separated from erythrocytes and platelets. After withdrawal, therefore, the syringe containing the blood is kept in an upright position for about 1 to 2 hours to promote erythrocyte sedimentation, a process facilitated by the addition of hydroxyethyl starch. This process can also be accelerated by substituting hypotonic lysis of the red cells for gravity sedimentation. After they are separated from the erythrocytes, the leukocytes are separated from platelets via centrifugation, and the leukocyte "pellet" that forms at the bottom of the tube is incubated with the radiolabel, washed, and reinjected into the patient (2).

Indium-111–Labeled Leukocytes. The imaging characteristics of In-111 are superior to those of Ga-67, with photopeaks of 173 keV and 247 keV. It decays by electron capture with a half-life of 67 hours. These energies require the use of a medium-energy collimator and a gamma camera capable of imaging multiple energy peaks. Energy discrimination is accomplished by using a 15% window centered on the 174-keV photopeak and a 20% window centered on the 247-keV photopeak of In-111. High target (abscess)–to-background ratios provide excellent image contrast. The spleen is the critical organ, receiving up to 20 rads per mCi of injected cells. As a result, the adult dose of In-111–labeled leukocytes is limited to about 18.5 MBq (500 μCi). Images obtained shortly after injection are characterized by intense pulmonary activity. This activity, which clears rapidly, is probably caused by

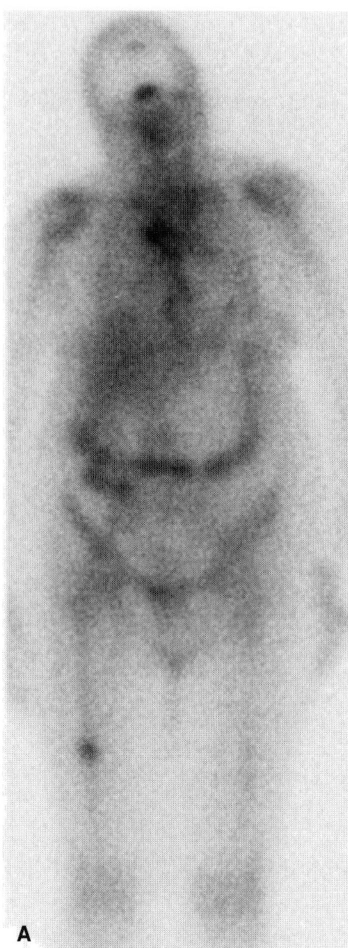

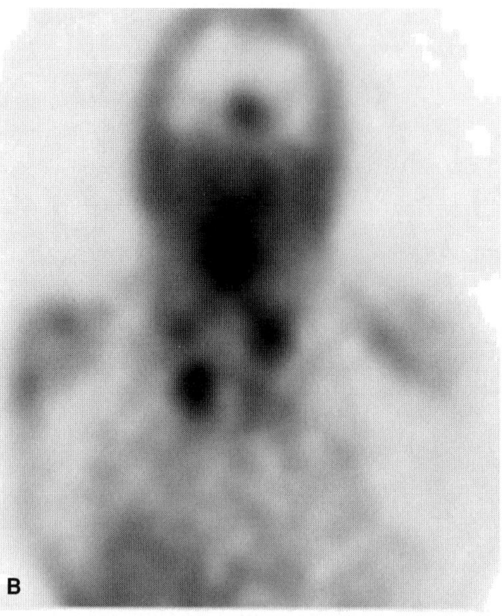

FIGURE 61.6. **Fever of Undetermined Origin in a Patient With Metastatic Renal Cell Carcinoma.** Anterior whole-body **(A)** and coronal SPECT **(B)** images from a gallium-67 study, performed on an 81-year-old woman with a history of renal cell carcinoma, persistent fevers, and no localizing signs, demonstrate focally increased activity in the mediastinum, left supraclavicular region, brain, and distal right femur. Mediastinal lymph node biopsy confirmed involvement by metastatic renal cell carcinoma. Brain and femoral metastases were radiographically confirmed.

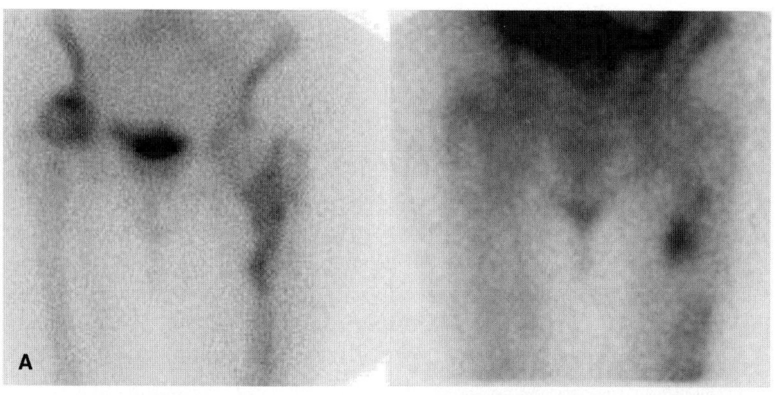

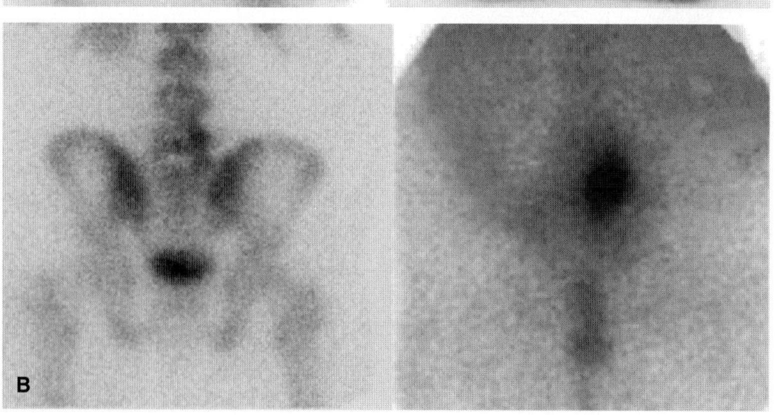

FIGURE 61.7. **Positive Bone/Gallium-67 (Ga-67) Study. A.** The distribution of activity in the bone (*left*) and Ga-67 (*right*) images of the pelvis and upper thighs is spatially incongruent. Irregularly increased activity in the proximal left femur is present on the bone scan, while the abnormal Ga-67 activity occupies a much smaller area. **B.** The distribution of activity on the bone (*left*) and Ga-67 (*right*) images of the lumbar spine is spatially congruent; increased activity involving the right pedicular region of L5 is present on both studies. The intensity of this uptake is greater on the Ga-67 image than on the bone image.

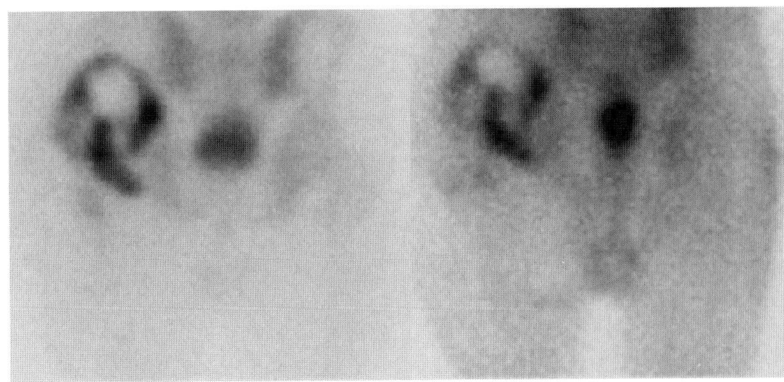

FIGURE 61.8. **Equivocal Bone/Gallium-67 (Ga-67) Study.** Posterior bone (*left*) and Ga-67 (*right*) images from a study performed on a patient with a failed left hip arthroplasty. The spatial distribution and intensity of uptake of both tracers are virtually identical, and hence the study is equivocal for infection.

leukocyte activation during labeling, which impedes their movement through the pulmonary vascular bed, prolonging their passage through the lungs. At 24 hours after injection, the usual imaging time for In-WBCs, the normal distribution of activity is limited to the liver, spleen, and bone marrow (2).

Advantages of the In-111 label are its stability and a virtually constant normal distribution of activity limited to the liver, spleen, and bone marrow. The 67-hour physical half-life of In-111 permits delayed imaging, which is particularly valuable for musculoskeletal infection. There is another advantage to the use of In-WBCs in musculoskeletal infection. Patients undergoing this test often require bone or marrow scintigraphy, which can be performed while the patient's cells are being labeled, or as simultaneous dual-isotope acquisitions, or immediately after completion of the In-WBC study. If Tc-WBCs are used, an interval of at least 48 hours is required between the white cell and bone or marrow scans (2).

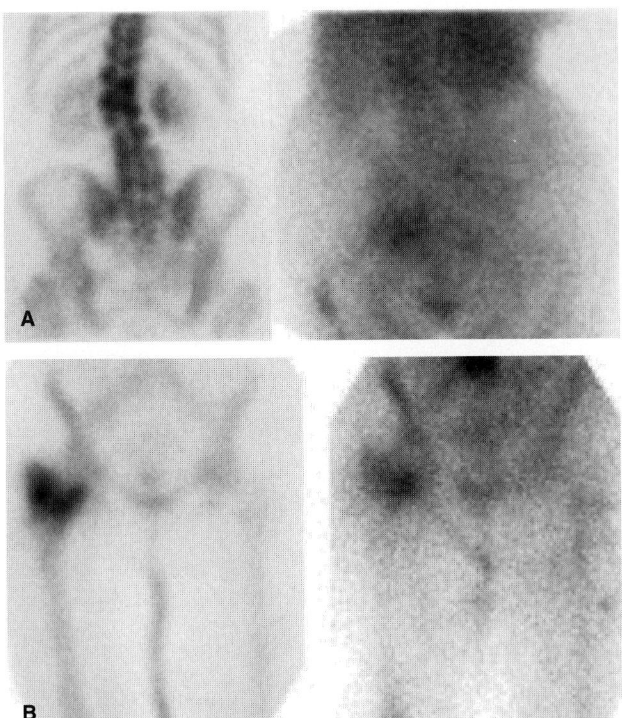

FIGURE 61.9. **Negative Bone/Gallium-67 (Ga-67) Studies. A.** Increased activity involving contiguous lower thoracic/upper lumbar vertebrae is present on the bone scan (*left*). The Ga-67 image is normal. **B.** The distribution of activity on the bone (*left*) and Ga-67 (*right*) images of the pelvis and femurs is spatially congruent; there is increased activity in the intertrochanteric region on both studies. The uptake, however, is less intense on the Ga-67 image than on the bone image.

Disadvantages of the In label include a low photon flux, less-than-ideal photon energies, and the fact that a 24-hour interval between injection and imaging is generally required (2).

Technetium-99m–Labeled Leukocytes. For Tc-WBC studies, a high-resolution, low-energy parallel hole collimator is used with a 15% to 20% window centered on the 140-keV photopeak of Tc-99m. The usual adult dose of Tc-WBCs is 185 to 370 MBq (5 to 10 mCi). The normal biodistribution of Tc-WBCs is more variable than that of In-WBCs. In addition to the reticuloendothelial system and pulmonary activity seen soon after injection, activity is also normally present in the genitourinary tract, large bowel (within four hours after injection), blood pool, and occasionally, the gallbladder (Fig. 61.10). The time interval between injection of Tc-WBCs and imaging varies with the indication; in general, imaging is usually performed within a few hours after injection (2).

Advantages of Tc-99m-WBCs include a photon energy that is optimal for imaging using current instrumentation, a high photon flux, and the ability to detect abnormalities within a few hours after injection. Disadvantages include genitourinary tract activity, which appears shortly after injection, and colonic activity, which appears by 4 hours after injection. The instability of the label and the 6-hour half-life of Tc-99m are disadvantages when delayed 24-hour imaging is needed. This occurs in those infections that tend to be indolent in nature and for which several hours may be necessary for accumulation of a sufficient quantity of labeled leukocytes to be successfully imaged (2).

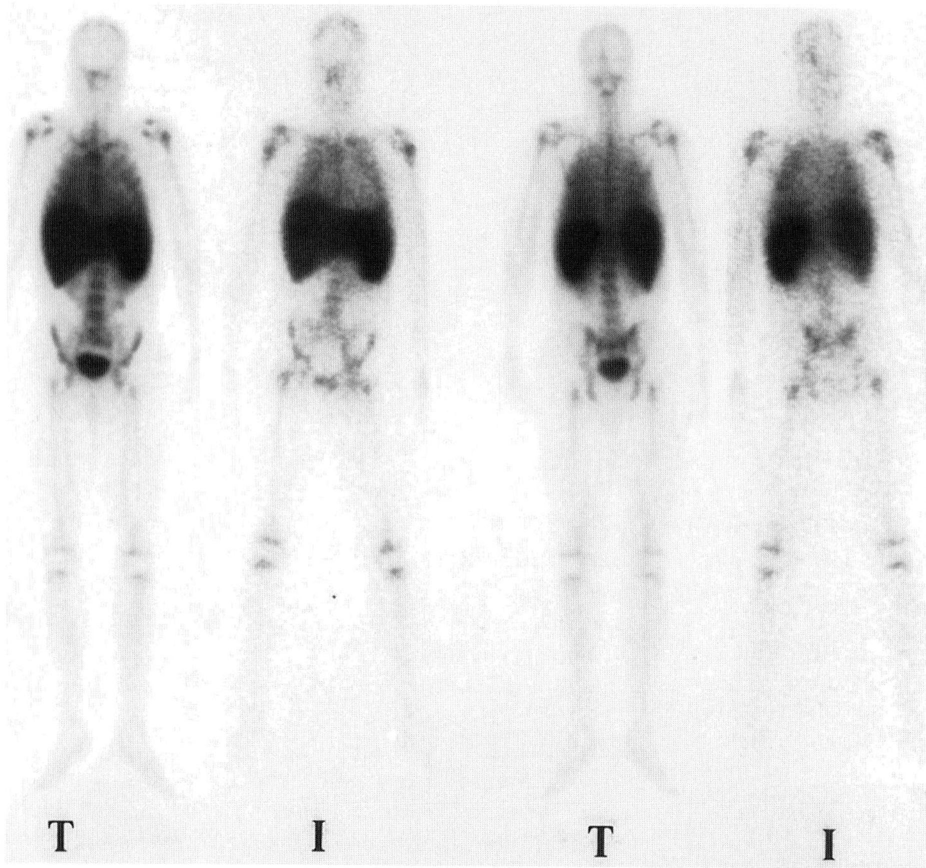

FIGURE 61.10. **Normal White Blood Cell (WBC) Studies** in the same adolescent male patient, approximately 2 weeks apart. Anterior images on the left and posterior images on the right. Compare the biodistribution of technetium (Tc)-WBCs at 90 minutes postinjection with that of indium (In)-WBCs at 18 hours postinjection. Note the cardiac, femoral vessel, renal, and bladder activity on the Tc-WBC images, which is not seen on the In-WBC images. Faint early intestinal activity is superimposed on the sacrum in the anterior Tc-WBC image. Physeal plate marrow activity on both studies is normal for the patient's age. T, Tc-WBC; I, In-WBC.

General Observations. Regardless of the radiolabel used, uptake of labeled WBCs depends on intact chemotaxis, the number and types of cells labeled, and the cellular component of a particular inflammatory response. Labeling of WBCs, now a routine procedure, does not affect their chemotactic response. A total white count of at least 2,000/μL is needed to obtain satisfactory images. Because the majority of leukocytes labeled are neutrophils, the procedure is most useful for identifying neutrophil-mediated inflammatory processes, such as bacterial infections. The procedure is less useful for those illnesses in which the predominant cellular response is not neutrophilic e.g., opportunistic infections, tuberculosis, and sarcoidosis (Fig. 61.11) (2,9,15).

Although pulmonary uptake of WBCs during the first few hours after injection is a normal physiologic event, by 24 hours such uptake is abnormal. Focal pulmonary uptake that is segmental or lobar in appearance is usually associated with bacterial pneumonia (Fig. 61.12). This pattern is also seen in patients with cystic fibrosis and is caused by WBC accumulation in pooled secretions in bronchiectatic regions of the lungs. Nonsegmental focal pulmonary uptake is caused by technical problems during labeling or reinfusion and is not usually associated with infection (16).

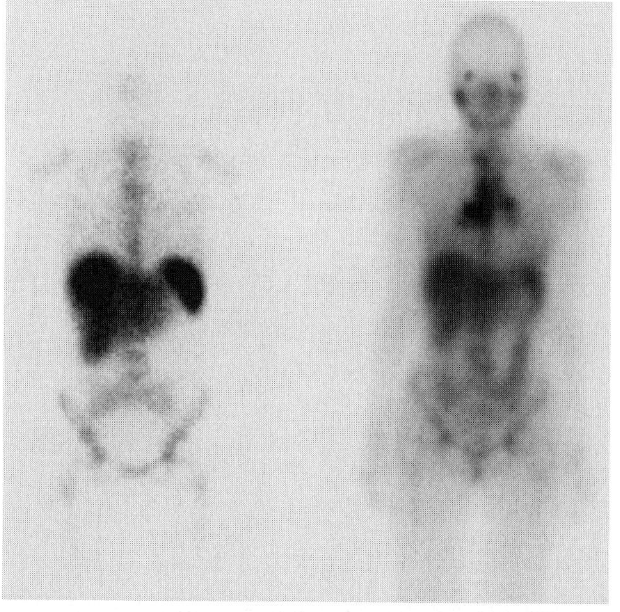

FIGURE 61.11. **Sarcoid.** Anterior indium–white blood cell (In-WBC) (*left*) and gallium-67 (Ga-67) (*right*) whole-body images of a patient with sarcoid (same patient as illustrated in Fig. 61.3). Compare the normal In-WBC image to the obviously abnormal Ga-67 image. Radiolabeled WBC studies are not useful for detecting inflammations and infections in which neutrophils are not the predominant cellular response.

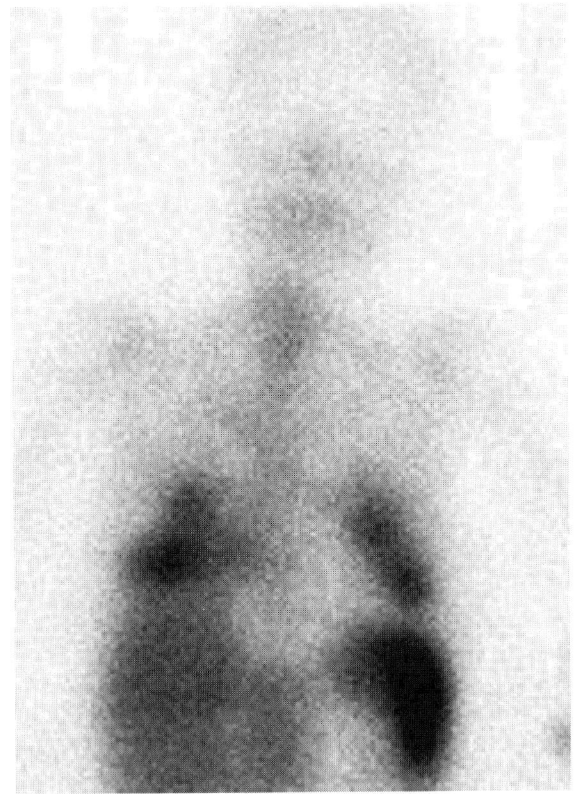

FIGURE 61.12. **Focal White Blood Cell (WBC) Pulmonary Activity.** Focal pulmonary activity that is segmental or lobar in appearance, as shown in this indium-WBC image, is usually associated with bacterial pneumonia.

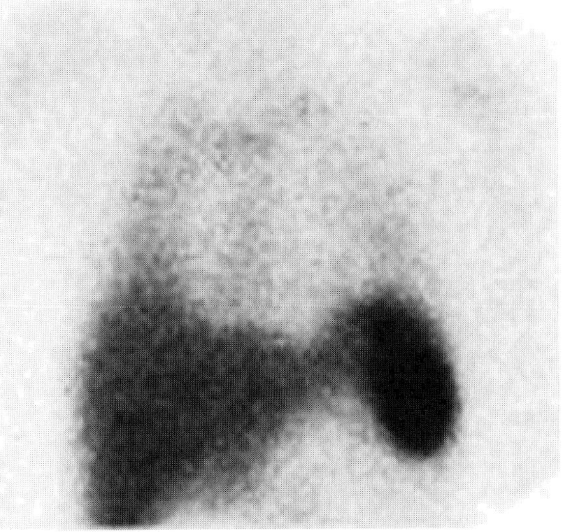

FIGURE 61.13. **Diffuse White Blood Cell (WBC) Pulmonary Activity.** There is mild, diffuse bilateral pulmonary activity on this indium-WBC image. While this is a normal finding on images performed shortly after injection, this is an abnormal finding on later images and is associated with many entities, but not with bacterial pneumonia.

Diffuse pulmonary uptake on images obtained more than 4 hours after reinjection of labeled cells is associated with opportunistic infection, radiation pneumonitis, pulmonary drug toxicity, and ARDS (Fig. 61.13). This pattern is almost never seen, however, in bacterial pneumonia (16).

Diffuse pulmonary uptake of WBCs is also seen in septic patients with normal chest radiographs and who have no clinical evidence of respiratory tract inflammation or infection. It is believed that the circulating neutrophils, activated by cytokines, pool in the pulmonary circulation because it is more difficult for them to undergo the cytoskeletal deformation required to maneuver through the pulmonary circulation. The cytokines presumably also activate pulmonary vascular endothelial cells, causing increased adherence of leukocytes to the cell walls (16).

In-WBCs do not accumulate in normal bowel. Such activity is always abnormal and is seen in antibiotic-associated or pseudomembranous colitis, infectious colitis, inflammatory bowel disease, ischemic colitis, and GI bleeding (Fig. 61.14) (2,9).

Radiolabeled WBCs do not accumulate in normally healing surgical wounds, so the presence of such activity indicates infection—although there are certain exceptions. Granulating wounds, which heal by secondary intention, can appear as areas of intense activity on WBC images even in the absence of infection. Examples include "ostomies" (tracheostomies, ileostomies, feeding gastrostomies, etc.) and skin grafts (Fig. 61.15). Vascular access lines, dialysis catheters, and even lumbar punctures can all produce false-positive results in the absence of appropriate clinical history (17). Indications for In-labeled leukocyte imaging include the following.

Fever of Undetermined Origin. As mentioned previously, because of its diverse etiologies, it can be argued that the nonspecific tracer Ga-67 is the preferred radionuclide test for FUO. However, the data suggest that In-WBC imaging is more sensitive early in the course of an illness, whereas Ga-67 is more sensitive later in the illness, and thus the selection of the procedure might be governed by the duration of the illness. We prefer to begin with an In-WBC study and follow with Ga-67 if needed (Fig. 61.16). Our rationale is as follows. The energies of the photons emitted by, and the physical half-lives of, these two tracers are similar. The amount of activity injected for Ga-67 is typically 10 or more times the amount of activity injected for an In-WBC study. Should the In-WBC study fail to provide a diagnosis, the patient can be injected with Ga-67 and scanned 48 to 72 hours later. If In-WBC is performed after Ga-67, however, it is necessary to wait a minimum of 1 week to obtain diagnostically useful images (2).

Postoperative Infection. Radionuclide tests are an adjunct to anatomic imaging modalities and facilitate the

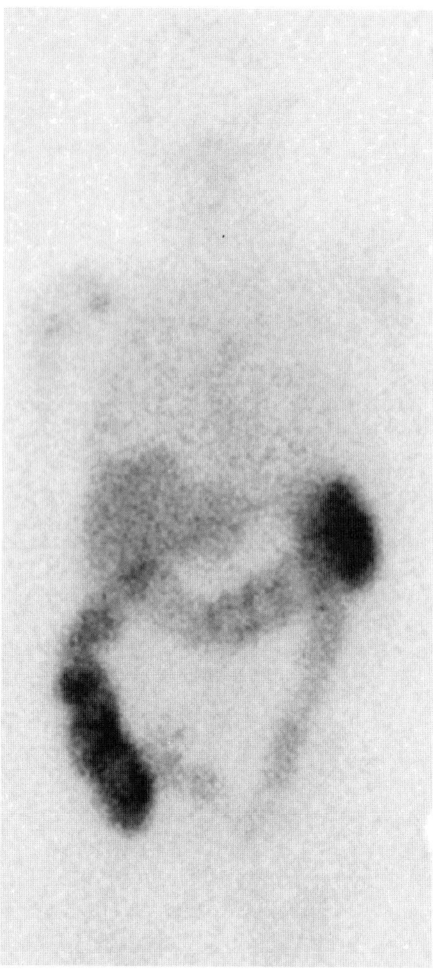

FIGURE 61.14. **Colitis.** Anterior whole body indium–white blood cell image demonstrates intense pancolonic activity. The differential diagnosis includes antibiotic-associated (pseudomembranous) colitis, infectious colitis, ischemic colitis, and inflammatory bowel disease. No conclusions about the extent of bowel involvement can be drawn from a single 24-hour image, because activity in the bowel lumen is redistributed over time by normal peristalsis.

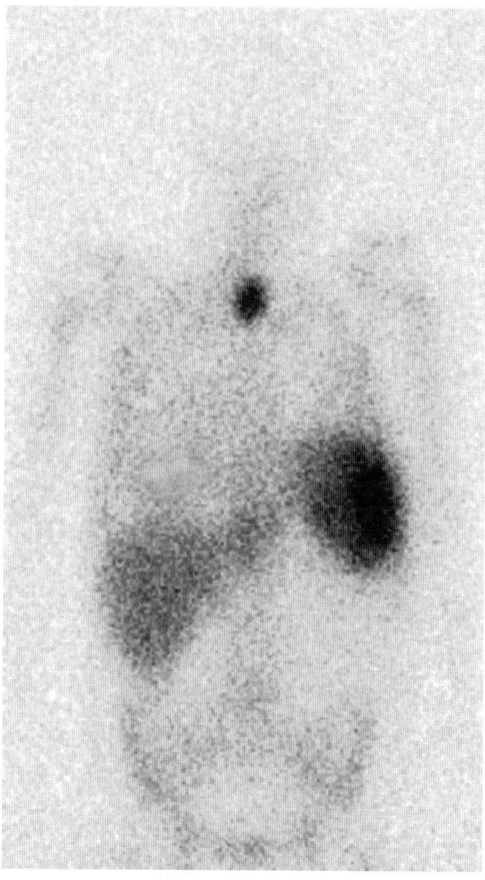

FIGURE 61.15. **White Blood Cell (WBC) Activity at a Tracheostomy Site**. Focally increased activity around a tracheostomy site can be seen on this anterior whole-body indium-WBC image. "Ostomies" are granulating wounds and as such recruit granulocytes. Thus WBC activity around an ostomy is normal finding. As this case illustrates, normal "ostomy" uptake can be intense.

differentiation of abscess from other fluid collections, from tumor, and even from normal postoperative changes. Ga-67 can detect intra-abdominal infection, but the presence of large bowel activity can obscure foci of infection, and the need to often wait 48 hours or more between injection and imaging is another disadvantage. Furthermore, Ga-67 accumulates in both infection and tumor, as well as in normally healing surgical incisions. Labeled WBCs, in contrast, rarely accumulate in uninfected neoplasms, and do not, with the exceptions already mentioned, accumulate in normally healing surgical incisions. For these reasons, WBC imaging is the preferred radionuclide study for the evaluation of postoperative infection (Fig. 61.17) (17).

Cardiovascular and CNS Infections. Echocardiography is a readily available and accurate method for diagnosing bacterial endocarditis, and radionuclide methods play a very limited role in the diagnostic workup of this entity. Echocardiography is less sensitive, however, for detecting one of the complications of bacterial endocarditis: the myocardial abscess. Both Ga-67 and WBC imaging detect myocardial abscesses in patients with infective endocarditis (2). WBC imaging is the radionuclide procedure of choice for diagnosing prosthetic vascular graft infection, with a sensitivity of more than 90% (Fig. 61.18). Neither duration of symptoms nor pretreatment with antibiotics adversely affects the study. The specificity of WBC imaging is more variable, however, ranging from 53% to 100%. Causes of false-positive results include perigraft hematoma, bleeding, graft thrombosis, pseudoaneurysms, and graft endothelialization, which occurs within the first 1 to 2 weeks after placement (2,9).

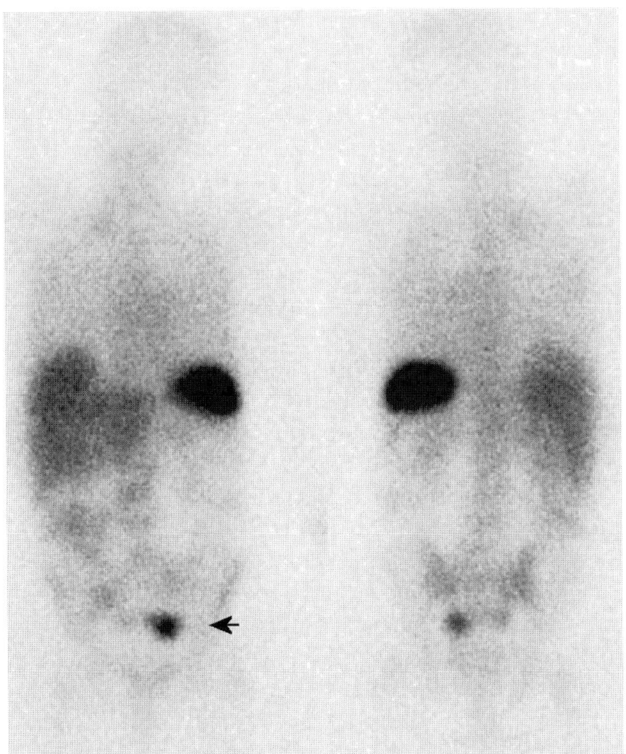

FIGURE 61.16. **Pelvic Abscess in a Patient With Fever of Unexplained Origin.** Anterior and posterior whole-body indium-WBC images demonstrate a focus of intense activity in the left lower quadrant of the abdomen (*arrow*). A subsequent CT scan (not shown) confirmed a pelvic abscess. Faint ascending and transverse colonic activity was attributed to antibiotic-associated colitis.

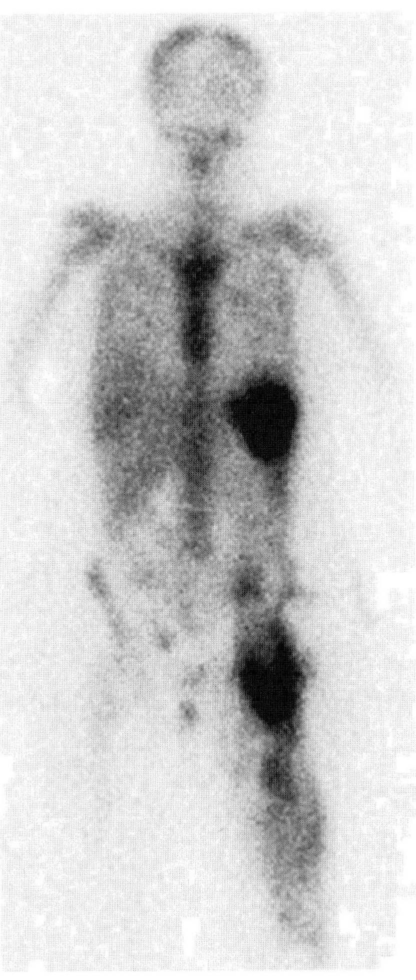

FIGURE 61.17. **Postoperative Infection.** A patient with a history of multiple abdominal surgeries was noted to have a mass on CT scan of the abdomen and pelvis (not shown). The differential diagnosis included postoperative changes and tumor. On the anterior whole-body indium–white blood cell (WBC) image, abnormal accumulation of labeled leukocytes extends from the left abdomen into the thigh. Multiple abscesses were subsequently drained. WBC imaging is a useful adjunct to CT in the evaluation of postoperative infection.

The differential diagnosis of a contrast-enhancing brain lesion identified on CT or MR includes abscess, tumor, cerebrovascular accident, and even multiple sclerosis. WBC scintigraphy provides valuable information about contrast-enhancing brain lesions. A positive study indicates that the origin of the brain lesion is almost assuredly infectious; a negative result rules out infection with a high degree of certainty. Faint uptake in brain tumors has been observed, and false-negative results in patients receiving high-dose steroids have been reported (18,19).

Osteomyelitis. Three-phase bone scintigraphy is the radionuclide procedure of choice for diagnosing osteomyelitis in bones not affected by underlying conditions. Focal hyperperfusion, focal hyperemia, and focally increased bony uptake on delayed (2 to 4 hours postinjection) images are the classic presentation of osteomyelitis (Fig. 61.19). Bone scan abnormalities reflect the rate of new bone formation in general; consequently, fractures, orthopedic hardware, and the neuropathic joint can all produce a positive three-phase bone scan, even in the absence of infection. In these situations, often described as "complicating osteomyelitis," the bone scan, because of decreased specificity, is less reliable (20,21).

Except in the spine, In-WBC scintigraphy is the procedure of choice for diagnosing complicating osteomyelitis. To maximize accuracy, the test is frequently performed in conjunction with Tc-99m sulfur colloid marrow imaging. Although labeled leukocytes do not usually accumulate at sites of increased bone mineral turnover in the absence of infection, they do accumulate in the bone marrow. The normal distribution of hematopoietically active bone marrow in adults is limited to the axial and proximal appendicular skeleton, and WBC activity outside this normal distribution is indicative of infection. Unfortunately, the "normal" distribution of hematopoietically active bone

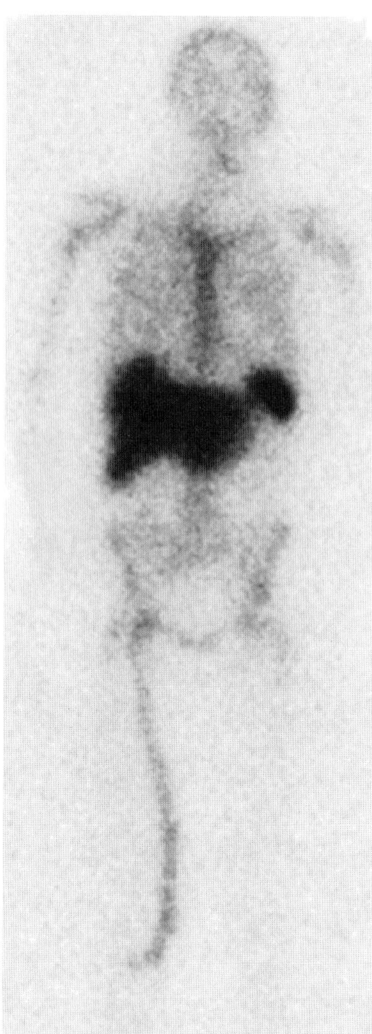

FIGURE 61.18. **Vascular Graft Infection.** Indium–white blood cell study demonstrates linearly increased activity along the medial aspect of the right thigh, from the groin to the knee, in a patient with an infected femoral popliteal prosthetic graft.

marrow is variable. Systemic conditions such as sickle cell and Gaucher diseases produce generalized alterations in marrow distribution, whereas fractures, orthopedic hardware, and the neuropathic joint cause localized alterations. The normal distribution of hematopoietically active marrow in children varies with age. Consequently, it may not be possible to determine if an area of activity on a WBC image represents infection or marrow. Performing complementary bone marrow imaging with Tc-99m sulfur colloid overcomes this problem. Both labeled leukocytes and sulfur colloid accumulate in the bone marrow. Leukocytes also accumulate in infection; sulfur colloid, however, does not. The combined study is positive for infection when activity is present on the WBC image without corresponding activity on the sulfur colloid marrow image. Any other pattern is negative for infection (Figs. 61.20, 61.21). The overall accuracy of combined WBC/marrow imaging is approximately 90% (21).

In contrast to other areas in the skeleton, WBC imaging with or without marrow imaging is not useful for detecting spinal osteomyelitis. Although increased uptake is virtually diagnostic of this entity, 50% or more of all cases of vertebral osteomyelitis present as areas of decreased or absent activity on WBC images. This photopenia is not specific for vertebral osteomyelitis and is associated with other entities such as tumor, infarction, and Paget disease (Fig. 61.22) (21,22).

Inflammatory Bowel Disease. Although early studies were performed with In-WBCs, it is now agreed that Tc-WBC is the radionuclide study of choice for inflammatory bowel disease, a group of idiopathic chronic disorders that includes Crohn disease and ulcerative colitis. WBC imaging is very sensitive for detecting inflammatory bowel disease and can be used as a screening test to determine which patients need to undergo more invasive investigation. In patients thought to have ulcerative or indeterminate colitis, skip areas of activity in the colon or the presence of small bowel activity support the diagnosis of Crohn disease (Fig. 61.23). The radionuclide study is also useful in patients who refuse endoscopy or contrast radiography, as well as in those in whom these studies cannot be satisfactorily performed because of narrowing of the bowel lumen. The ability of the radionuclide study to differentiate active inflammation, which may respond to medical therapy, from scarring, which may require surgery, can have a significant impact on patient management. WBC imaging can also be used to monitor patient response to therapy. Decreasing bowel uptake on serial studies confirms that the patient is responding to treatment, whereas persistent or recurrent uptake indicates residual disease or relapse (23–25).

Imaging at multiple time points and SPECT increase the sensitivity of the test. The caudal, or pelvic outlet, view facilitates detection of rectal disease that might otherwise be masked by urinary bladder activity. Physiologic bowel activity, probably caused by hepatobiliary excretion of Tc-99m–labeled hydrophilic complexes, frequently appears on delayed images and must be differentiated from activity secondary to inflammation. Physiologic activity appears in the distal small bowel no sooner than 3 hours after injection, is diffuse and mild in intensity, and migrates into the cecum by 4 hours. There must be no accumulation in other bowel segments (26).

There are limitations to WBC imaging. It cannot be the only imaging test used for inflammatory bowel disease. It cannot define anatomic changes such as strictures, which are best delineated with endoscopy and contrast radiography. The test is less sensitive for disease of the upper GI tract versus the lower GI tract. The sensitivity of the test also may be affected adversely by concomitant administration of corticosteroids (24,27).

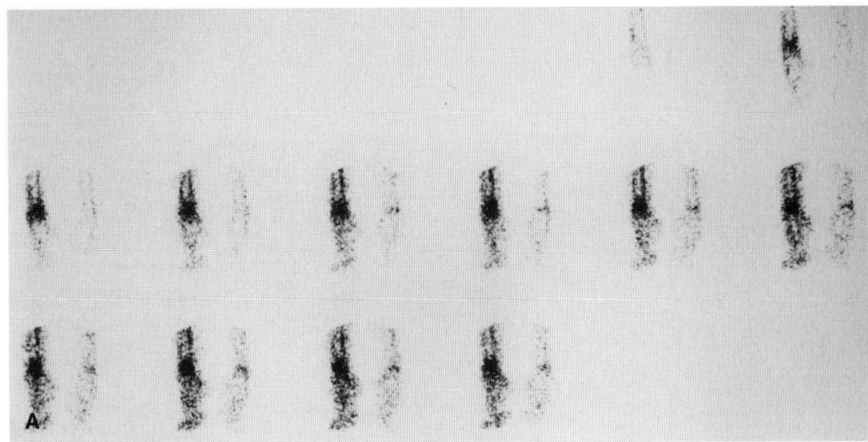

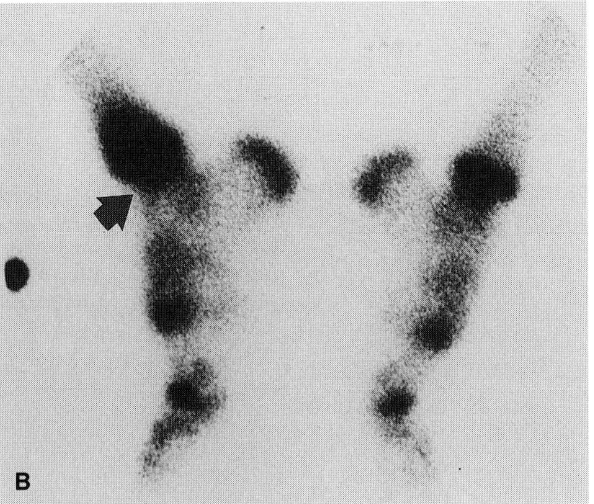

FIGURE 61.19. **Acute Osteomyelitis.** Three-phase bone scan in a 13-year-old girl. Radiographs were normal. **A.** Anterior view of flow study of the feet and ankles with technetium-99m methylene diphosphonate, 2 seconds per frame. Note the early and increased flow to the right foot and ankle. **B.** Blood pool image, with a marker indicating the right side. Note the markedly increased activity in the distal tibia (*arrow*) extending to the physeal plate.

TECHNETIUM-99M-FANOLESOMAB

Tc-99m-fanolesomab, a monoclonal murine M-class immunoglobulin, binds to CD15 receptors present on leukocytes. This agent presumably binds to circulating neutrophils that eventually migrate to the focus of infection, as well as to neutrophils or neutrophil debris containing CD15 receptors, already sequestered in the area of infection. About 370 to 740 MBq (10 to 20 mCi) of the radiolabeled compound, containing 75 to 125 μg of antibody is injected. In contrast to in vitro labeled leukocytes, there is no increased retention of activity in the lungs. The normal distribution includes liver, spleen, bone marrow, and genitourinary tract. Blood pool activity, present on images obtained shortly after injection, decreases over time. Large bowel activity normally appears as early as 4 hours

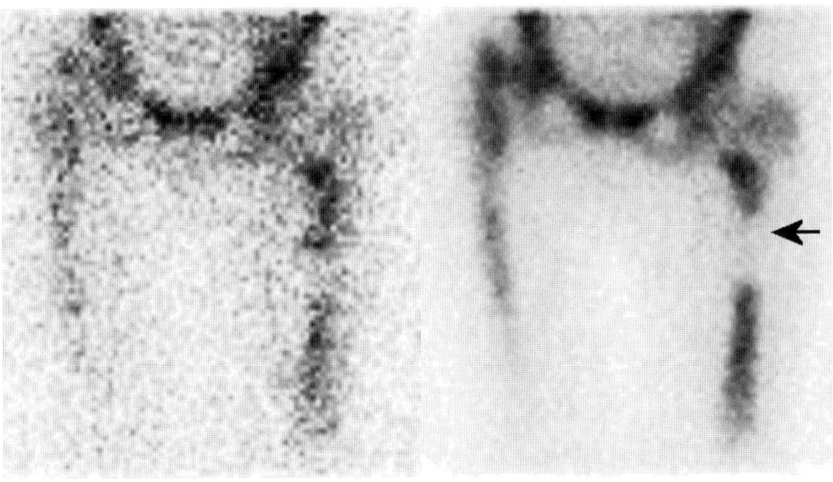

FIGURE 61.20. **Infected Orthopedic Hardware.** There is slightly increased left femoral activity on the indium–white blood cell (In-WBC) image (*left*) performed on a patient with an intramedullary rod in the left femur. There is a photopenic area (*arrow*) on the marrow image (*right*), and the study is positive for infection. Notice also, however, that most of the left femur activity on the In-WBC image is caused by marrow, not infection.

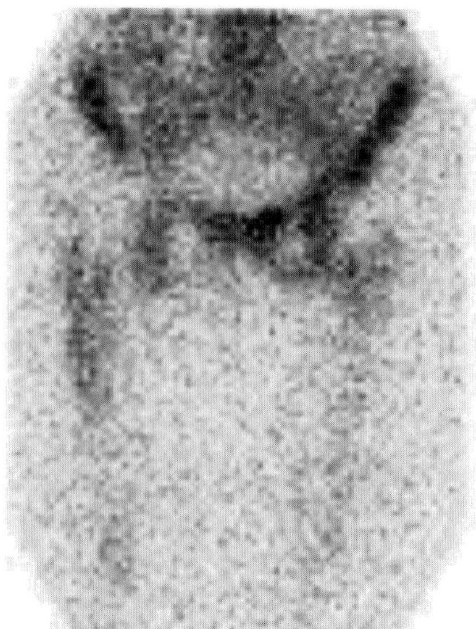

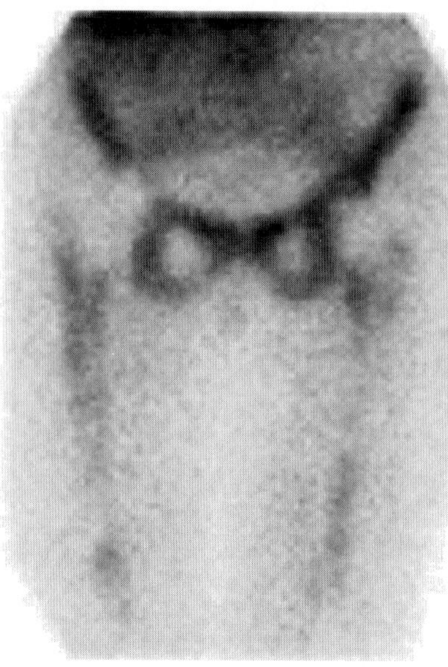

FIGURE 61.21. **Aseptic Loosening of Right Total Hip Replacement.** Indium–white blood cell (In-WBC) image (*left*) in a patient with bilateral total hip arthroplasties shows increased activity around the femoral component of a right total hip replacement. Infection cannot be excluded. The distribution of activity on the marrow image (*right*) is identical to that on the In-WBC image. Therefore the combined study is negative for infection.

after injection and is usually present on images obtained at 24 hours. Small bowel activity is also occasionally seen (Fig. 61.24). The dose-limiting organ is the spleen, which receives an estimated 0.064 mGy/MBq (0.24 rads/mCi), considerably lower than the estimated 5 mGy/MBq (18 rads/mCi) for In-WBCs. Within 20 minutes after injection, there is a transient decrease in the number of circulating WBCs. There have been no clinical complaints associated with this phenomenon, and recovery usually occurs within 45 minutes. Based on available data, the agent is safe, with little toxicity (28,29).

At the present time, Tc-99m-fanolesomab is approved for diagnosis of equivocal appendicitis in patients older

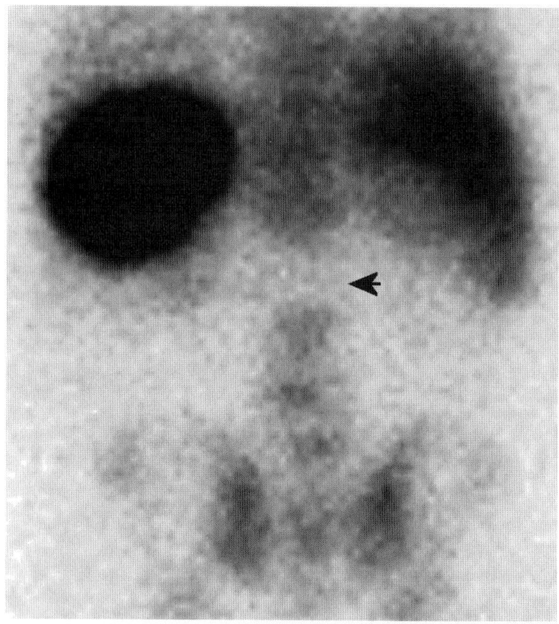

FIGURE 61.22. **Spinal Osteomyelitis.** Posterior indium–white blood cell image of the abdomen demonstrates absent activity in a midlumbar vertebra (*arrow*). Photopenia is seen in more than 50% of all cases of spinal osteomyelitis. Although decreased activity is consistent with spinal osteomyelitis, it is not specific for it, and is also associated with numerous other entities, including tumor, infarction, compression fracture, and Paget disease.

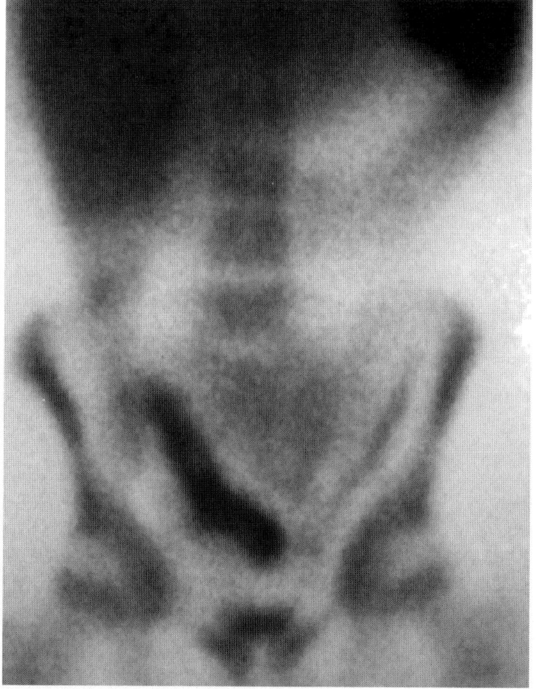

FIGURE 61.23. **Crohn Disease.** Technetium–white blood cell activity is present in the distal jejunum/proximal ileum, distal ileum, and colon. Small bowel activity in a patient with colitis supports the diagnosis of Crohn disease. (Courtesy of Dr. Martin Charron.)

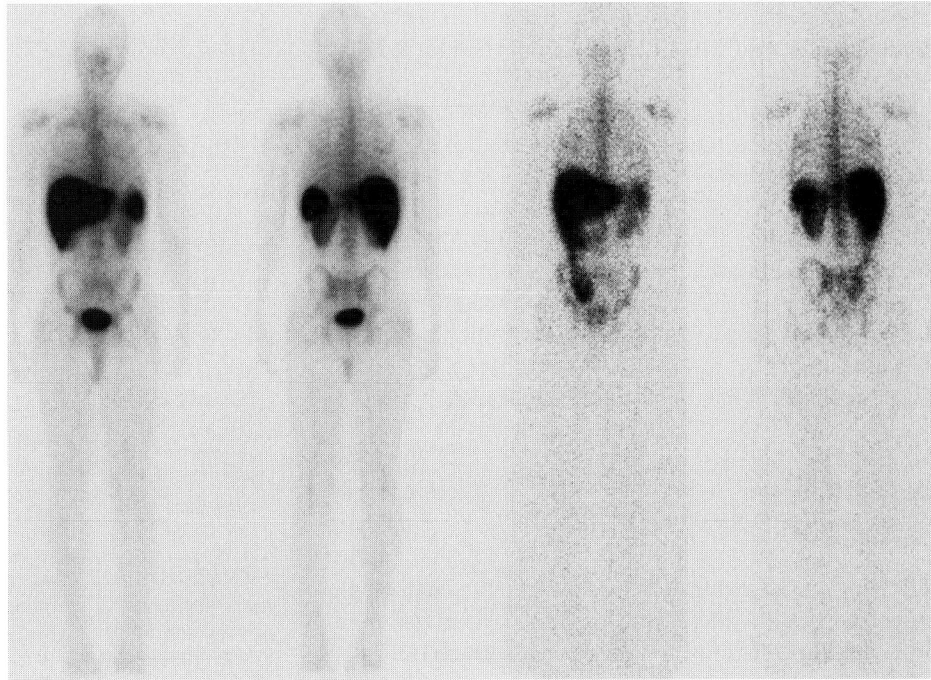

FIGURE 61.24. **Whole-Body Technetium-99-Fanolesomab Images.** Anterior and posterior images were acquired about 2 (*left*) and 24 (*right*) hours after injection. In addition to reticuloendothelial activity, genitourinary tract activity appears soon after injection. Colonic activity may be seen as early as 4 hours after injection and is usually present at 24 hours.

than 5 years. A large multicenter trial involving 200 patients between 5 and 86 years old was conducted to assess the efficacy of fanolesomab for diagnosing acute appendicitis in patients with an equivocal presentation to evaluate its safety and to assess its potential impact on the clinical management of these patients. Fifty-nine patients had histopathologically confirmed acute appendicitis. The diagnosis of appendicitis was made in all cases within 90 minutes after injection. Images became positive within 8 minutes in 50% of patients with acute appendicitis and within 50 minutes in 90% (Fig. 61.25). Sensitivity, specificity, and accuracy were 91%, 86%, and 87%, respectively. Positive and negative predictive values of the test were 73% and 96%, respectively. The high negative predictive value

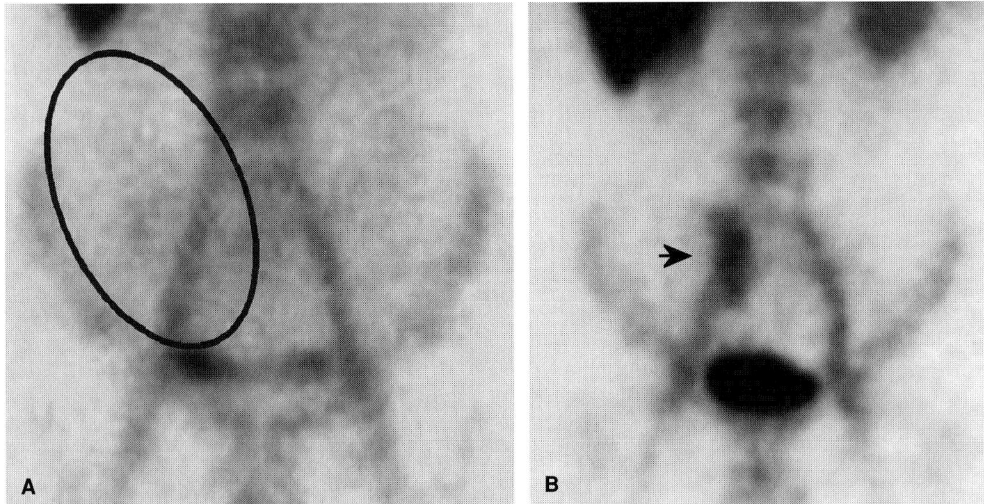

FIGURE 61.25. **Appendicitis. A.** The "appendicitis zone" (*oval*) extends approximately from the pubic symphysis to the lower pole of the right kidney. Any activity in this region is considered indicative of appendicitis (courtesy of Dr. Samuel Kipper). **B.** Image in another patient, taken about 30 minutes after injection of technetium-99-fanolesomab, shows a linear area of increased activity overlying the right iliac vessels (*arrow*) indicative of appendicitis. The diagnosis was confirmed at surgery.

is especially important, because a negative result means that acute appendicitis is very unlikely, thereby reducing unnecessary time in the hospital for observation as well as unnecessary surgery. Finally, there was a significant improvement in making the appropriate management decision, in both patients with and without appendicitis, after the scan (30).

Planar imaging is carried out over 90 minutes. Abnormal right lower quadrant activity in the "appendicitis zone" that persists is considered positive for appendicitis (30).

Preliminary investigations suggest that Tc-99m-fanolesomab may be a satisfactory alternative to In-WBC imaging for diagnosis of osteomyelitis (31,32).

FLUORINE-18-FLUORODEOXYGLUCOSE

FDG, a glucose analogue, is transported into cells via glucose transporters. Increased uptake of FDG in inflammation is related—at least in part—to an increased number of glucose transporters. In addition, the affinity of glucose transporters for deoxyglucose presumably is increased by various cytokines and growth factors. The normal distribution of FDG includes brain, myocardium, and genitourinary tract. Bone marrow, gastric, and bowel activity are variable. Thymic uptake, especially in children, can be prominent. Liver and spleen uptake are generally low-grade and diffuse, although in infection, splenic uptake may be intense. Imaging is performed about 1 hour after injection of 370 to 740 MBq (10 to 20 mCi) F-18-FDG (33).

Although it is not approved for evaluation of inflammation and infection, FDG-PET is an intriguing and exciting alternative to the conventional radionuclide approach to the FUO. FDG is similar to Ga; i.e., although it is not specific, it is exquisitely sensitive, ideally suited to the evaluation of an entity with diverse etiologies. The short half-life of F-18, moreover, does not delay the performance of any additional radionuclide studies that might be contemplated (Fig. 61.26). Recent investigations have found that the test is sensitive and compares favorably to and could potentially replace Ga-67 for the evaluation of patients with FUO (33,34). The value of FDG-PET is further enhanced by data that suggest that vasculitis and bacterial endocarditis, both of which can be the source of an FUO and which are not amenable to detection with other radionuclide studies, may be identified with this test. Other entities including thromboembolic disease, sarcoidosis, and chronic granulomatous disease, which can all present as an FUO, are also associated with increased FDG uptake (33).

The negative predictive value of FDG-PET in the patient with an FUO is apparently very high; i.e., a negative test makes it very unlikely that a morphologic origin of the fever will be identified. If confirmed in future investigations, FDG-PET, by reducing the number of imaging studies performed, may prove to be a very cost-effective method of investigating the FUO (34).

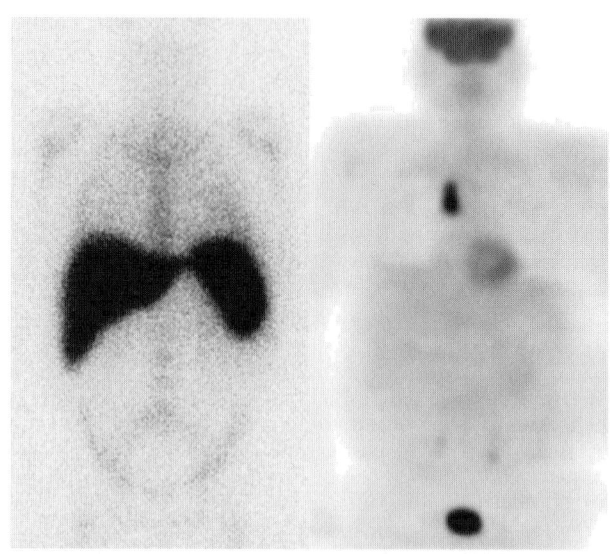

FIGURE 61.26. **Recurrent Lung Carcinoma.** An 81-year-old man with chronic lymphocytic leukemia and a remote history of lung carcinoma presented with fever of unknown origin and an elevated leukocyte count. The indium–white blood cell study (In-WBC) (*left*) was negative. The fluorodeoxyglucose (FDG) PET study (*right*) demonstrated focal hypermetabolism in the right paratracheal region that corresponded to lymph nodes identified on CT (not shown). The final diagnosis was recurrent lung carcinoma. This case demonstrates the importance of sensitivity when evaluating patients with fever of undetermined origin (FUO). In-WBC correctly excluded infection as the source of the fever, but provided no information about what the source of the fever was. Although FDG did not provide a diagnosis, it did correctly localize the source of the FUO, facilitating the diagnosis with other studies.

FDG-PET also appears to be a potentially useful test for spinal osteomyelitis. Although most of the series reported

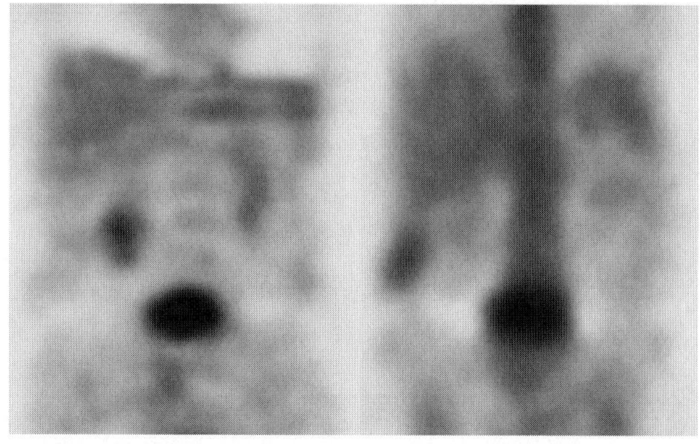

FIGURE 61.27. **Spinal Osteomyelitis.** Intense fluorodeoxyglucose accumulation in the lower lumbar spine is seen in this patient with spinal osteomyelitis (*left*), similar to the abnormality on the coronal gallium SPECT image (*right*).

to date involve small patient samples, this test accurately diagnoses spinal osteomyelitis, with an accuracy comparable to that of Ga-67 (Fig. 62.27) (33,35).

Radionuclide imaging plays a pivotal role in the diagnosis of infection and inflammation and will continue to do so for the foreseeable future. Optimal diagnosis requires careful consideration of the patient, indications for the study, and the imaging modalities at one's disposal.

REFERENCES

1. Palestro CJ. The current role of gallium imaging in infection. Semin Nucl Med 1994;24:128–141.
2. Love C, Palestro CJ. Radionuclide imaging of infection. J Nucl Med Technol 2004;32:47–57.
3. Palestro CJ, Malat J, Collica CJ, et al. Incidental diagnosis of pregnancy on bone and gallium scintigraphy. J Nucl Med 1986;27:370–372.
4. Lopez OL, Maisano ER. Ga-67 uptake post cesarean section. Clin Nucl Med 1984;9:103–104.
5. Desai AG, Intenzo C, Park C, et al. Drug-induced gallium uptake in the breasts. Clin Nucl Med 1987;12:703–704.
6. Vasquez R, Oates E, Sarno RC, et al. Gallium-67 breast uptake in a patient with hypothalamic granuloma (sarcoid). J Nucl Med 1998;19:118–121.
7. Engelstad B, Luks S, Hattner RS. Altered ^{67}Ga citrate distribution in patients with multiple red blood cell transfusions. AJR Am J Roentgenol 1982;139:755–759.
8. Hattner RS, White DL. Gallium-67/stable gadolinium antagonism. MRI contrast agent markedly alters the normal biodistribution of Gallium–67. J Nucl Med 1990;31:1844–1846.
9. Palestro CJ, Torres MA. Radionuclide imaging of nonosseous infection. Q J Nucl Med 1999;43:46–60.
10. Palestro CJ, Goldsmith SJ. The use of gallium and labeled leukocyte scintigraphy in the AIDS patient. Q J Nucl Med 1995;39:221–230.
11. Waxman AD. An update on the role of nuclear medicine in pulmonary disorders. In: Freeman LM, Weissman HS, eds. Nuclear Medicine Annual 1985. New York: Raven Press,1985:199–231.
12. Kramer EL, Divgi CR. Pulmonary applications of nuclear medicine. Clin Chest Med 1991;12:55–75.
13. Linton AL, Richmond JM, Clark WF, et al. Gallium^{67} scintigraphy in the diagnosis of acute renal disease. Clin Nephrol 1985;24:84–87.
14. Palestro CJ, Torres MA. Radionuclide imaging in orthopedic infections. Semin Nucl Med 1997;27:334–345.
15. Fineman DS, Palestro CJ, Kim CK, et al. Detection of abnormalities in febrile AIDS patients with In-111-labeled leukocyte and Ga-67 scintigraphy. Radiology 1989;170:677–680.
16. Love C, Opoku-Agyemang P, Tomas MB, et al. Pulmonary activity on labeled leukocyte images: physiologic, pathologic, and imaging correlation. Radiographics 2002;22:1385–1393.
17. Palestro CJ, Love C, Tronco GG, et al. Fever in the postoperative patient: role of radionuclide imaging in its diagnosis. Radiographics 2000;20:1649–1660.
18. Schmidt KG, Rasmussen JW, Frederiksen PB, et al. Indium-111-granulocyte scintigraphy in brain abscess diagnosis: limitations and pitfalls. J Nucl Med 1990;31:1121–1127.
19. Palestro CJ, Swyer AJ, Kim CK, et al. Role of In-111 labeled-leukocyte scintigraphy in the diagnosis of intracerebral lesions. Clin Nucl Med 1991;16:305–308.
20. Schauwecker DS. The scintigraphic diagnosis of osteomyelitis. AJR Am J Roentgenol 1992;158:9–18.
21. Palestro CJ, Torres MA. Radionuclide imaging in orthopedic infections. Semin Nucl Med 1997;27:334–345.
22. Palestro CJ, Kim CK, Swyer AJ, et al. Radionuclide diagnosis of vertebral osteomyelitis: indium-111-leukocyte and technetium-99m-methylene diphosphonate bone scintigraphy. J Nucl Med 1991;32:1861–1865.
23. Martin-Comin J, Prats E. Clinical applications of radiolabeled blood elements in inflammatory bowel disease. J Nucl Med 1999;43:74–82.
24. Del Rosario MA, Fitzgerald JF, Siddiqui AR, Chong SK, Croffie JM, Gupta SK. Clinical applications of technetium Tc 99m hexamethyl propylene amine oxime leukocyte scan in children with inflammatory bowel disease. J Pediatr Gastroenterol Nutr 1999;28:63–70.
25. Charron M. Pediatric inflammatory bowel disease imaged with Tc-99m white blood cells. Clin Nucl Med 2000;25:708–715.
26. Charron M, Del Rosario JF, Kocoshis S. Comparison of the sensitivity of early versus delayed imaging with Tc-99m HMPAO WBC in children with inflammatory bowel disease. Clin Nucl Med 1998;23:649–653.
27. Granquist L, Chapman SC, Hvidsten S, et al. Evaluation of ^{99m}Tc-HMPAO leukocyte scintigraphy in the investigation of pediatric inflammatory bowel disease. J Pediatr 2003;143:48–53.
28. Thakur ML, Marcus CS, Henneman P, et al. Imaging inflammatory diseases with neutrophil-specific technetium-99m-labeled monoclonal antibody anti-SSEA-1. J Nucl Med 1996;37:1789–1795.
29. Love C, Palestro CJ. 99mTc-fanolesomab. IDrugs 2003;6:1079–1085.
30. Rypins EB, Kipper SL, Weiland F, et al. ^{99m}Tc anti-CD15 monoclonal antibody (LeuTech) imaging improves diagnostic accuracy and clinical management in patients with equivocal presentation of appendicitis. Ann Surg 2002;235:232–239.
31. Palestro CJ, Kipper SL, Weiland FL, et al. Osteomyelitis: diagnosis with ^{99m}Tc-labeled antigranulocyte antibodies compared with diagnosis with indium-111-labeled leukocytes—initial experience. Radiology 2002;223:758–764.
32. Palestro CJ, Caprioli R, Love C, et al. Rapid diagnosis of pedal osteomyelitis in diabetics with a technetium-99m-labeled monoclonal antigranulocyte antibody. J Foot Ankle Surg 2003;42:2–8.
33. Love C, Tomas MB, Tronco GG, Palestro CJ. FDG-PET of infection and inflammation. Radiographics 2005 Sep–Oct;25(5):1357–1368.
34. Bleeker-Rovers CP, de Kleijn EMHA, Corstens FHM, et al. Clinical value of FDG PET in patients with fever of unknown origin and patients suspected of focal infection or inflammation. Eur J Nucl Med Mol Imaging 2004;31:29–37.
35. Stumpe KDM, Zanetti M, Weishaupt D, et al. FDG positron emission tomography for differentiation of degenerative and infectious endplate abnormalities in the lumbar spine detected on MR imaging. AJR Am J Roentgenol 2002;179:1151–1157.

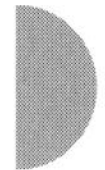

Chapter 62

Molecular Imaging of Tumors

James H. Timmons

When Physiology Matters

Imaging Physiologic Processes

Classes of Imaging Isotopes

Radioiodine: The Index Agent for Tumor Imaging

The Ideal Tumor Imaging Agent

Blood Flow and Capillary Permeability: A Caveat

Classes of Non-PET Tumor Imaging Radiopharmaceuticals

Dual-Agent Scintigraphy, Hybrid Imaging, and Fusion Imaging

Tumor Therapy With Radiopharmaceuticals

A Complete Oncology Imaging Approach

WHEN PHYSIOLOGY MATTERS

Radiologists tend to be intellectually oriented toward pathologic anatomy. This partially results from the historical development of the field. Anatomic imaging methods have been dominant in the field of radiology. Nuclear medicine developed originally from a confluence of the interests of internal medicine, pathology, and radiology physicians in investigating the physiology of disease. Imaging moved only gradually to the forefront of nuclear medicine, with evolution from radiotracers and radioimmunoassay to single- or dual-probe studies, then Anger camera imaging, and then SPECT. From the standpoint of a radiologist, nuclear medicine is often viewed as unappealing because the images generally have poorer resolution and less anatomic detail than traditional radiographs. This disadvantage is even more apparent when comparisons are made to CT, US, or MR.

It is important for the modern radiology resident to overcome this anatomic bias. The recent rapid evolution of PET from a research tool to the dominant imaging modality in oncology stems from its ability to distinguish physiologically active masses from mere masses. Although advances continue in anatomic imaging (such as MR white matter tractography), technical advances in imaging physiology are likely to dwarf those in imaging of anatomy in the next decade. This will likely be true even without nuclear medicine, as evident from development of functional contrast agents for MR and of functional MR imaging of brain activity. At the same time, the development of hybrid devices such as PET-CT and SPECT-CT imagers has largely overcome the "unclear medicine" reputation of the nuclear image. Coregistered images obtained at a single setting allow simultaneous investigation of anatomy and physiology.

There has been remarkable growth in the availability of scintigraphic methods for tumor imaging over the past few years. Many of these agents provide information that was not previously available. Dramatic improvements in both sensitivity and specificity for detection and staging of tumors have been made. These agents are unique because they provide physiologic information concerning the imaged tumor, such as metabolic activity (and by extension viability), presence of specific cell surface receptors, and presence of multidrug resistance apparatus. The development of these agents has depended heavily on the use of tracer techniques that do not significantly alter the physiologic activity of the substance being employed for imaging. Development has also been made possible by extensive basic science investigations into polypeptide chemistry and monoclonal antibodies and by serendipitous clinical observations.

It is important to note that the recent rapid evolution of clinical PET resulted entirely from a change in the regulatory climate. There was no fundamental technologic leap that opened the floodgates. Rather, the already mature imaging technology began to be applied clinically when Food and Drug Administration (FDA) rules were changed to allow regional fluorine-18 fluorodeoxyglucose (F-18-FDG) production in a cost-effective manner and when the Center for Medicare Studies recognized F-18-FDG scanning as both clinically effective and cost competitive. Hundreds of PET radiotracers and SPECT radiotracers for basic physiologic processes have been developed and clinically proven over the past two decades. What stands between these agents and rapid clinical diffusion is political recognition of the very low toxicologic risk represented by the use of tracer imaging and of the cost-effectiveness of tracer use. At the doses employed, only substances such as botulinum toxin and cyanide retain any toxicity. The gram quantities of material actually employed in scanning are lower than the accepted levels of known toxins in drinking water (Table 62.1). Monoclonal antibodies are an exception to the rule, because of larger material quantities and because of the inclusion of foreign proteins.

Only political decisions prevent widespread adoption of multiple molecular targeted agents. The clear choice is for radiology residents to become comfortable with physiologic imaging or become competitively disadvantaged. Fortunately, the average radiology resident is well prepared for imaging physiology. Preparedness requires mainly a shift in emphasis.

PET has become important enough for tumor imaging to require a separate chapter. The current chapter is devoted to single-photon agents for imaging tumors. Whereas these agents are relatively less important than PET in oncologic diagnosis, the therapeutic applications of these agents are now beginning to become significant. There are literally hundreds of agents currently under academic investigation for possible clinical use. Unfortunately, whereas physicians would generally prefer the most specific agent available, economic considerations currently favor nonspecific but generally applicable agents like F-18-FDG. It is therefore quite difficult to predict which agents may be used routinely a few years hence. Specific agents are discussed herein only as examples. It is much more important to understand the general principles behind imaging and therapy with the various classes of agents, along with their potential benefits and limitations, than to understand the specific imaging appearances for any individual agent.

IMAGING PHYSIOLOGIC PROCESSES

Physiology covers a broad range of activities distinguished primarily by scale. Processes such as blood flow, excretion, and motion are physiologic and are amenable to imaging. Blood flow principles applicable to time-of-flight MR, Doppler US, and timing of the liver bolus in CT are similar to those involved in three-phase bone scintigraphy. Excretion principles are identical in excretory urography and the nuclear medicine renal scan. Motion analysis is common to echocardiography, MR cardiography, and SPECT cardiac stress/rest perfusion scanning. The recent paradigm shift toward "molecular imaging" indicates imaging of biologic processes in living beings at the biochemical or molecular level. Our ability to do this is rapidly growing, but it is in no sense new. This potential is also developing in more traditionally anatomic imaging. Examples include MR spectroscopy, the blood oxygenation level-dependent (BOLD) technique in MR, and MR contrast agents that assess bile excretion or Kupffer cell function. A radiology resident should not allow themselves to be cowed simply by the concept of imaging physiology.

Imaging of molecular physiology is of particular value in oncology. Tumors tend to be dedifferentiated relative to their cell of origin. This has implications for loss of contact inhibition, alteration of cell surface receptors, failure of apoptosis, disordered vessel growth with relative hypoxia, alterations in transport systems for metabolically significant substances, and unregulated energy use. The rapidly growing, relatively hypoxic tumor cell has a high rate of glucose utilization, allowing FDG PET images to detect and gauge the metabolic rate of malignancies. Because

TABLE 62.1 Monoclonal Antibody Imaging Agents

Name	*Trade Name*	*Antigen*	*Ab Type*	*Label*	*Source*
Satumomab	OncoScint	TAG-72	Whole	Indium-11	Cytogen Corp.
Nofetumomab	Verluma	40-kD glycoprotein	Fab	Technetium-99m	DuPont Pharma
Arcitumomab	CEA-Scan	CEA	Fab′	Technetium-99m	Immunomedics, Inc.
Capromab pendetide	ProstaScint	Prostate-specific membrane antigen	Whole	Indium-111	Cytogen Corp.

CEA, carcinoembryonic antigen; Fab, fragment of IgG involved in antigen binding; Fc, fragment of IgG in effector mediator region; TAG-72, tumor-associated glycoprotein-72.

all of the underlying processes (receptor display, apoptosis, hypoxia, transport systems, and symporters) can currently be effectively imaged in vivo, any of the underlying imaging technologies may potentially spring full-grown into clinical imaging practice with little forewarning. Each physiologic alteration in a tumor cell also provides a potential target for the therapeutic application of a radiopharmaceutical attached to an appropriate ligand. All radiology residents should be forewarned to think physiologically while they continue to image anatomically.

CLASSES OF IMAGING ISOTOPES

Isotopes suitable for tumor imaging may be divided into positron emitters and isotopes that emit single γ photons. The former are the basis for an imaging technology known as PET. The latter are employed in standard gamma camera imaging and in SPECT. Typical γ-emitting isotopes are technetium-99m (Tc-99m) and iodine-123 (I-123).

γ-Emitting isotopes are advantageous because they are available with a variety of half-lives, suitable to any purpose. Several generator systems are obtainable for convenient production of the desired isotope at the point of consumption, the most common being the molybdenum-99 (Mo-99)/Tc-99m generator system. The cost of the gamma camera and generator is significantly lower than the cost of a PET scanner and cyclotron and is similar to the cost for competing technologies such as CT and MR.

PET radiopharmaceuticals are very similar chemically to an unlabeled substrate molecule. γ emitters are disadvantageous in that they are not easily incorporated into molecules without disrupting their biologic function. The "atoms of life" generally do not have γ-emitting isotopes, although γ isotopes are available for some less common biometallic elements, such as selenium-75. Incorporation of γ emitters into biomolecules generally involves addition of significant bulk. It is difficult to produce a γ-labeled molecule that exhibits biologic behavior identical to that of the original molecule.

Positron-emitting isotopes have the disadvantage of short half-life, which makes the synthesis and use of a positron emitter–labeled substance a race against time. This does not merge well with "best manufacturing practice," at least as currently understood by the FDA. It is possible to make PET agents with gallium-68 (Ga-68), available as a generator system product. Unfortunately, the limitations that apply to single-photon agents apply equally to Ga-68.

RADIOIODINE: THE INDEX AGENT FOR TUMOR IMAGING

The first radiopharmaceutical identified as having clear medical potential was radioiodine. The natural trapping of iodine by the thyroid made radioiodine a potentially ideal agent for imaging and therapy. We examine thyroid tumor imaging here briefly because it is paradigmatic of the choices involved in the development and use of tumor imaging agents generally.

Iodine is trapped within the thyroid by conversion to thyroxine, which is stored within the colloid cells of thyroid tissue. Uptake is proportional to metabolic activity. Some thyroid tumors also trap iodine by the same mechanism. However, because their metabolism is disordered, they trap iodine at a much lower rate. This leads to an interesting phenomenon: thyroid tumors typically appear as cold spots in the thyroid gland on radioiodine imaging of the intact gland but as hot spots in the body when metastases are imaged after thyroid removal or ablation. Thyroid tumors arising from cells that do not trap and metabolize iodine, such as medullary carcinoma of the thyroid, will not take up radioiodine.

Multiple isotopes of iodine are available. Each is suitable for a particular purpose. Reactor-produced I-131 is relatively inexpensive. It has photons that can be imaged but extensive β particle emission. It thus images and destroys thyroid tissue and can be used to ablate both malignant and benign thyroid tissue. The location of the tissues being ablated and the extent of uptake within those tissues can be determined simultaneously. I-131 is suboptimal when only imaging is desired, however, because the significant β radiation increases the risk of development of benign and malignant tumors. Cyclotron-produced I-123 has no β radiation and is safer for routine imaging. It also has a nearly ideal γ energy of 159 keV. Cyclotron production means this agent is more expensive than I-131, and its relatively short half-life means that I-123 is limited to use at scheduled times.

Every imaging prescription involves issues of cost, likely tumor type, adequacy of the agent for the available equipment, availability of the agent, metabolic rate and route and their effect on timing of imaging, and patient radiation dose and safety. Every therapeutic dose must be planned to achieve adequate dose to the tissue to be ablated while minimizing whole-body and nontarget organ radiation. The choices involved are typical of those in other areas of oncologic scintigraphy.

THE IDEAL TUMOR IMAGING AGENT

What are the characteristics of an ideal tumor imaging agent? Foremost is specificity for the target tissue. In practice, this is never fully realized. Radioiodine is secreted by the salivary glands and swallowed. Because bowel clearance is slow, whole-body images for metastases may be problematic in the abdomen, where swallowed radioiodine in the bowel may mimic or obscure tumor. Similarly, FDG localizes in metabolically active cardiac tissue, monoclonal antibodies are bound nonspecifically to liver tissue, and Ga-67 is bound to metabolically active bone and also taken up by normal liver. When uptake by normal tissue occurs, it is preferable that the tissue be one that is less frequently involved by the primary tumor or by metastatic disease. Because cardiac metastases and malignant pericardial effusion are much less common than liver metastases, the normal distribution of FDG is preferable, in terms of imaging sensitivity, to that of a monoclonal antibody.

Rapid clearance of background activity is essential for short-lived isotopes such as pertechnetate, which must be imaged within a few hours of administration. Clearance need not be as rapid for longer-lived isotopes. For whole-body I-131 scans, imaging of the abdomen may be delayed for a day to allow administration of a cathartic to purge nonspecific bowel radioactivity. Similarly, agents that clear rapidly, such as by renal excretion, are preferable to those that clear more slowly, such as by hepatic excretion. "Metabolic trapping" of an imaging agent within a tumor by any mechanism increases conspicuity and thus imaging sensitivity by increasing target activity over background. Trapping of radioiodine, for example, leads to increasing activity in tumor relative to background over time. An agent that is metabolically trapped, such as Tc-99m-sestamibi (Tc-99m-MIBI), will generally be more sensitive than an agent that is easily washed out, such as thallium-201 (Tl-201). In general, the higher the target-to-background ratio at the time of imaging, the higher the sensitivity for detection of tumor.

An additional desirable trait is the ability of an imaging agent to predict the effectiveness of therapy. This may be inherent in the localization of the agent. Iodine avidity indicates greater likelihood of effective radioiodine therapy, and somatostatin receptor avidity increases the likelihood of successful therapy with "cold" somatostatin in carcinoid tumors. Repeat scanning after therapy may differentiate patients who responded from those who require further therapy. Thus, increased bone scan activity suggests effective therapy for bone metastases (the flare phenomenon), and decreased glucose localization on FDG PET scans indicates improved outcome after chemotherapy for lymphoma.

BLOOD FLOW AND CAPILLARY PERMEABILITY: A CAVEAT

Tumor imaging based on differential blood flow or capillary permeability is of incidental interest only, since these methods lack tissue specificity. Nevertheless, it is important to consider agents that localize in tumors by these mechanisms, because the potential for differential labeling on the basis of these mechanisms exists with any imaging tracer. Tc-99m-methylene diphosphonate (Tc-99m-MDP) is a typical example of a blood flow imaging agent, and Tc-99m-glucoheptonate is a typical example of a capillary permeability agent.

During the flow and immediate static phases of a bone scan, it is occasionally possible to detect a hypervascular tumor because of increased blood flow to the tumor and a vascular blush within the tumor. On delayed static images, increased activity in bone usually is a result of increased osteoblast activity. However, the bone may have increased activity solely on the basis of increased blood flow to that bone, whatever the underlying cause. Similarly, a cold defect on a bone scan can indicate an absence of osteoblast activity caused by rapid tumor growth, or it may point to an absence of blood flow caused by tissue necrosis or vascular obstruction. These findings based on alterations of blood flow may result in either unintentional or intentional detection of tumor but are entirely nonspecific.

In the classic but obsolete brain scan, Tc-99m glucoheptonate or Tc-99m diethylenetriamine pentaacetic acid (DTPA) were used to detect areas of increased capillary permeability. This breakdown of the blood-brain barrier may be caused by a number of disease processes, including primary or metastatic tumors. When positive, these studies provided excellent "hot-spot" images, which allowed detection of the tumor. Again, though, the mechanism is nonspecific, and diagnosis is limited to what can be determined through pattern recognition and clinical scenario.

It is important to realize that these mechanisms still apply when using modern imaging agents. A hypervascular structure may have activity that exceeds background because of high blood flow and nonspecific binding of the antibody. A tumor with high antibody affinity but poor blood flow can incidentally display activity similar or equal to background when imaged with a monoclonal antibody imaging agent. A tumor with high blood flow can appear to have high affinity for a radiolabeled antibody on the basis of preferential exposure to the imaging agent, without having specific affinity for that agent. If a brain tumor demonstrates increased activity after administration of Tc-99m-hexametazime, for example, it is difficult a priori to determine if the localization is caused by increased blood flow, diffusion across a damaged blood-brain barrier, or specific localization within the tumor. With all agents discussed in this review, the reader is urged to consider possible mechanisms for nonspecific localization when interpreting images.

CLASSES OF NON-PET TUMOR IMAGING RADIOPHARMACEUTICALS

Markers of Metabolism. Tc-99m-MIBI and Tc-99m-tetrofosmin (Tc-99m-TFos) are typical metabolic agents for gamma camera imaging. Both were developed for myocardial perfusion imaging. In oncology, they are of greatest potential interest for scintimammography. These agents were initially designed to substitute for Tl-201 in evaluating myocardial viability. Tl-201 had been serendipitously observed to localize within some tumors. Evaluation of Tc-99m-MIBI for tumor localization was a logical extension of this prior work. While the mechanism of localization is quite different, these agents fill a niche similar to that of FDG. These agents are lipophilic, cationic materials whose uptake is dependent, in part, on cellular and mitochondrial membrane potentials. Malignant tumors have negative membrane potentials and high mitochondrial content to support their high metabolic rate. Thus, unlike FDG, these agents are indirect markers of metabolic activity. Both agents also bind to P glycoprotein (P-gp), a mediator of multidrug resistance in breast cancer cells. When the multidrug resistance gene is present and active in a cell, P-gp is manufactured by the cell. P-gp traps cancer drugs by the same mechanism employed to trap these imaging pharmaceuticals: both are actively transported out of the cell. Thus, a breast cancer that localizes Tc-99m-MIBI or Tc-99m-TFos is likely to be responsive to chemotherapy. Alternatively, a breast cancer that does not localize these agents is likely to express multidrug resistance. Tl-201 apparently is not transported out of the cell by P-gp. This is reasonable, because Tl-201 is a simple ion and is not representative of the types of large molecules (anthracyclines, vinca alkaloids, actinomycin D) that are usually transported by P-gp.

The greatest advantage of metabolic agents for staging is their ability to detect small or diffuse foci of primary or metastatic disease that are not detectable on anatomic images or are not pathologic by size criteria. They are also very useful for determining the presence or absence of recurrence in the bed of a treated tumor. The major disadvantage of these agents is that they are nonspecific: They image high metabolic activity rather than tumor per se. For example, FDG may localize in an active tuberculous granuloma. With firm clinical acceptance of FDG, the role of γ-emitting agents in this arena has faded rapidly. They remain one good reason to look at the projection images on myocardial perfusion studies (Fig. 62.1)

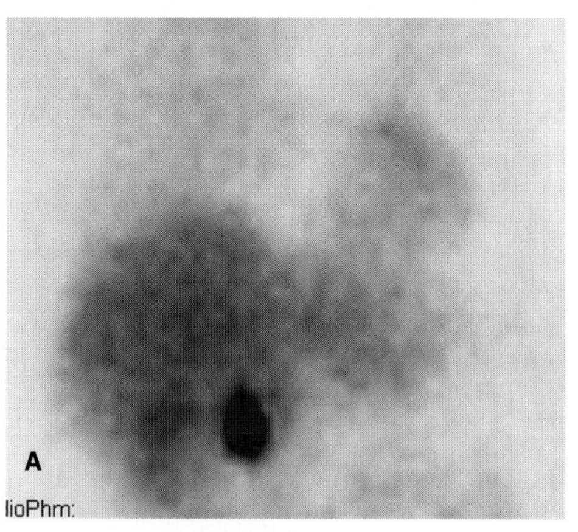

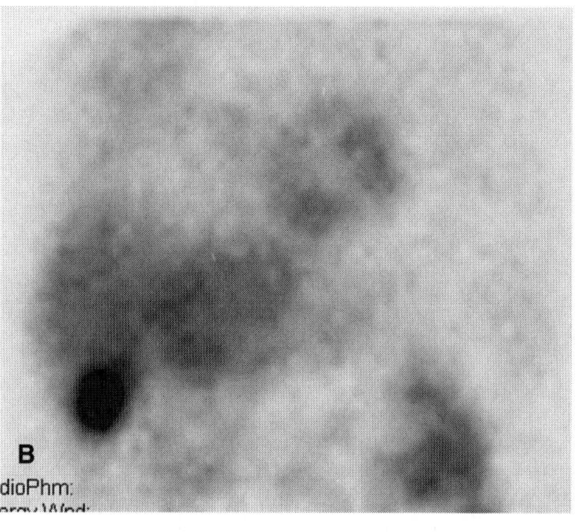

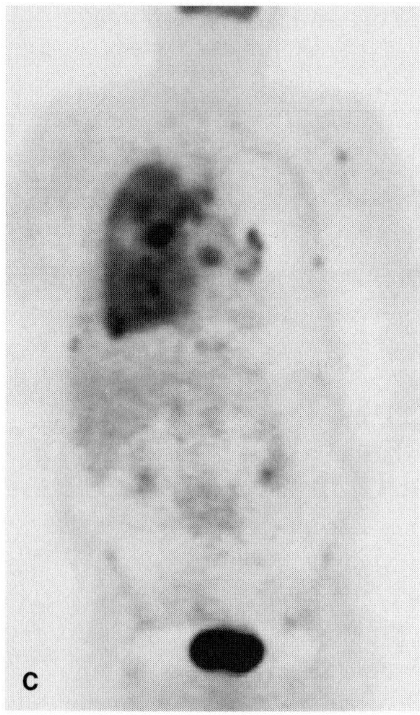

FIGURE 62.1. **Lung Cancer on Myocardial Perfusion Study.** Frontal **(A)** and left anterior oblique **(B)** views from acquisition for technetium-99m-sestamibi (Tc-99m-MIBI) myocardial perfusion study. A diffuse, mild, and unilateral increase in lung activity with vague focal uptake in right hilum is apparent. **C.** Coronal image from PET scan in same patient. The Tc-99m-MIBI was localizing in the right retrohilar area (non–small cell lung cancer) and throughout the lung because of lymphangitic spread of tumor.

Monoclonal Antibodies. *Polyclonal antibodies* are formed in response to an antigenic stimulus. The polyclonal antibody formed is really a set of chemically different substances that share the basic antibody structure but have widely variant affinities for the intended target of the antigenic response. The variations occur because a large number of different cells respond with rapid division and antibody secretion when they are stimulated by an antigen. Each activated cell divides rapidly to form a clone of identical cells that produce one of the antibodies in the set. The set of antibodies produced by the many activated cell lines is thus termed *polyclonal.* Polyclonal antibodies have variable affinities for nontarget tissues. For an imaging agent, it is clearly desirable to have a single antibody of known and reliable affinity. A single antibody has the additional advantage of decreased nonspecific cross-reactivity with tissues other than the intended target. Such antibodies must be produced by a single clone, the descendants of a single cell. It is thus termed a monoclonal antibody.

Monoclonal antibodies have three important advantages over polyclonal antibodies for imaging: maximum specificity, maximum sensitivity, and predictable nontarget binding. By providing a high affinity, the monoclonal antibody reduces the dose of labeled antibody necessary to produce an acceptable target (tumor)-to-background ratio. By selecting a monoclonal antibody with high affinity, one simultaneously selects for greater specificity for that target. Nevertheless, some cross-reactivity may be inevitable, especially if the target tumor is very similar to a tissue normally present in the body. These cross-reactions need to be constant so that the appearance of a normal scan may be determined with a high degree of certainty.

Basic Antibody Structure. A variety of antibody fragments and modified antibodies are employed for both imaging and therapy. Imaging agents to date have generally been based on the IgG antibody. This discussion will be limited to IgG for the sake of brevity, although there is no intrinsic reason that other antibody classes (IgA, IgE, IgD or IgM) could not be employed for imaging.

Each IgG molecule has two binding regions for antigen (Fig. 62.2). An additional host binding region mediates effector functions such as blood clearance and nonspecific liver binding. When separated from the remainder of the antibody, the antigen-binding regions are termed *Fab fragments* and the effector mediator region is termed an *Fc fragment.* In the intact antibody, two Fab fragments are bound together by disulfide bonds. The Fc fragment is bound to each Fab fragment by covalent bonds. It is possible to remove the Fc region while retaining the disulfide bonds between Fab regions. The resulting fragment is termed Fab_2. The antibody also consists of constant, variable, and hypervariable regions. The constant regions are the same from antibody to antibody for a given antibody class and species of organism. The variable regions differ between antibodies within a class and contain the binding sites for antigen. The hypervariable regions have the greatest effect on antibody affinity and are those portions of the variable region that are most exposed at the antigen-binding site.

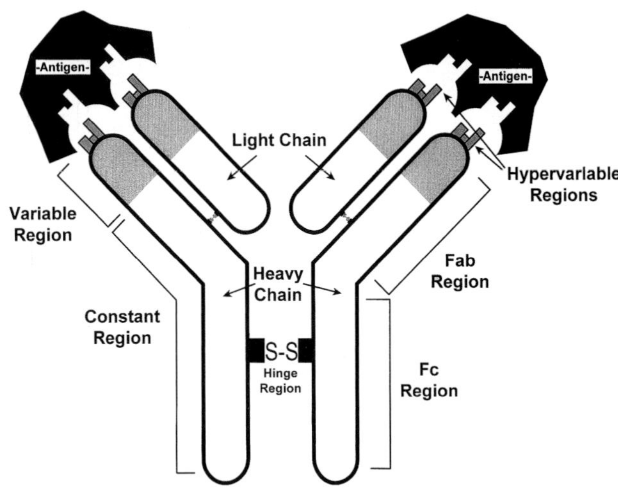

FIGURE 62.2. **Monoclonal Antibody Structure.** The basic antibody glycoprotein molecule consists of two identical heavy and light chains linked by a disulfide bridge. Each chain has a variable region that is responsible for antigenic binding and a constant region that is involved in complement fixation and antibody-dependent cell toxicity. Each variable region, in turn, contains three hypervariable regions that form unique antigen-binding sites. The antibody can be fragmented into smaller units, depending on the cleavage plane. Enzymatic digestion produces either a Fab_2 fragment or two smaller Fab fragments and an Fc fragment. Fragment size dictates blood pool clearance rates, with the smaller ones clearing faster.

The behavior of antibody fragments in biologic systems is predictable in part on the basis of molecular weight alone. Smaller fragments partition more rapidly into various cellular and extracellular tissues because of their smaller size. They are also metabolized and cleared from the bloodstream more rapidly for the same reason. A small fragment is thus maximally exposed to the target tissue earlier but for a shorter period of time. Smaller fragments will be favored for imaging when binding is rapid and strong, as this will result in rapid target labeling and rapid background clearance. Local recurrences, nodal metastases, and peritoneal metastases may be better detected with fragments because their intact vasculature will insure that antigen will be exposed to the antibody. Smaller fragments will be advantageous, and are often required, for isotopic labels with relatively short half-lives. The Tc-99m label, with a 6-hour half-life, requires rapid localization and background clearance, so imaging can be performed within a day. Smaller fragments are also less immunogenic and thus less likely to induce an undesirable immune response. Larger fragments or intact antibody may be preferable when a long reaction time is required, such as when binding is weak or slow, or for therapeutic applications in which extended residence time in the target tissue is required to maximize radiation dose to the tumor. Because larger fragments and intact antibodies are cleared more slowly from the background, target-to-background ratios are lower. However, absolute uptake in tumor is higher with intact antibody. Slow background clearance increases whole-body and nontarget dose in both imaging and therapeutic applications. Larger fragments allow, and may require, use of isotopes with longer half-lives.

Biochemical differences between fragments also affect biodistribution. The Fc region is of greatest interest because it mediates nonspecific binding to the liver. For imaging agents, nonspecific liver binding significantly decreases sensitivity for detection of liver metastases. Metastases may even appear as photopenic rather than photo-enhanced areas. High activity in the liver may also obscure activity in adjacent structures unless a lead shield is employed to cover the liver. Unfortunately, use of a shield also carries the risk of obscuring an area of tumor activity. Dual-isotope imaging with simultaneous acquisition of planar or SPECT data may allow digital subtraction of normal tissue or comparison of the biologic distributions of an organ imaging agent (e.g., Tc-99m sulfur colloid [Tc-99m-SC]) with that of the labeled antibody to increase diagnostic accuracy. Finally, sequestration of an antibody or fragment in the liver reduces bioavailability of the agent for binding to the intended target. For a target outside the liver, rapid clearance of the background through nonspecific liver binding could improve imaging sensitivity. In practice, this advantage seldom outweighs the disadvantages listed. The use of antibody fragments for imaging began as an attempt to address the problem of nonspecific liver binding. Other techniques, such as pretreatment with Fc fragment to reduce nonspecific binding, have variable success.

The use of smaller fragments for imaging results in significantly increased renal activity. This can be addressed by administration of unlabeled leucine, which saturates the renal binding sites for the fragments and reduces their residence time in the kidneys. Mixtures of amino acids, commercially available for total parenteral nutrition, appear to work just as well. Another approach to limiting renal activity is to use smaller fragments consisting only of the active binding site or even of fragments of this active site.

It is important to recognize that monoclonal antibodies for imaging are usually produced from mouse hybridoma cells. These cells result from the fusion of antibody-producing B lymphocytes with "immortal" myeloma cells. From the numerous fusion products that result, a single clone that produces high-affinity antibody is selected. This cell line is then grown to produce the antibody. Because the mouse antibody is a foreign protein in the human bloodstream, it may incite an immune response. This results in production of human antimouse antibody (HAMA), which can cause mild to severe symptoms. Of greater concern, subsequent administrations of mouse antibody can result in mild to fatal (anaphylactic) reactions. This problem could limit the repeat use of monoclonal imaging or of therapeutic agents based on murine antibodies.

A variety of attempts have been made to reduce the antigenicity of the monoclonal imaging agents. Chimeric antibodies are formed from the variable regions of mouse antibodies and the constant regions of human antibodies. Humanized antibodies are formed by inserting the hypervariable region of the mouse antibody into a human antibody using recombinant DNA techniques. These modifications improve product safety at the cost of increased complexity and expense of production.

Clearly, monoclonal antibody imaging carries a significant risk of side effects. Before using these agents, physicians should thoroughly familiarize themselves with the side effect profile for the agent and be prepared to deal with any complications. Prior to administration, the risk of HAMA reaction should be assessed in those patients who have previously undergone monoclonal antibody imaging or therapy.

Some current agents of interest are available with either a diagnostic or a therapeutic label (or a label suitable for both), so that the likelihood of successful therapy can be assessed in advance of administration of the therapeutic agent. The agents of greatest current interest are CD20 antibodies for therapy of lymphoma (discussed later). Figure 62.3 illustrates a normal antibody fragment scan. Figure 62.4 illustrates a positive scan.

Peptide Receptor Scintigraphy. Regulatory peptides are a group of polypeptides that serve as internal messengers. They bind to targets on multiple tissues, most notably those of the brain and GI system. They are expressed variably on the surfaces of a variety of human tumor cell lines. In patients in whom a stable radioactive label can be achieved without significantly decreasing the affinity of the receptors for the polypeptide, imaging and therapy are possible for specific tumor cells. The index compound, and the only one commercially available at the time of this writing, is indium-111-DTPA-D-Phe^1-octreotide (In-111-OCT). This protein binds with high affinity to the sst2 somatostatin receptor and with lesser affinity to two of the remaining five receptors for somatostatin.

Somatostatin receptors are expressed by neuroendocrine tumors, some neural tumors (meningiomas, medulloblastomas, most astrocytomas and neuroblastomas), and small cell lung carcinomas. They are also highly expressed on the cell surfaces of carcinoid tumors and by cells in some nonmalignant conditions such as Wegener granulomatosis, rheumatoid arthritis, and tuberculosis. The sst2 receptor with the attached ligand is internalized by the cell, resulting in effective metabolic trapping of the radioligand within the tumor cell. In-111-OCT has >90% sensitivity for detection of carcinoid tumors. It can also be used to detect gastrinomas, insulinomas, glucagonomas, and other (or unclassified) APUDomas (Fig. 62.5). It also has fair sensitivity for medullary thyroid carcinoma (65%).

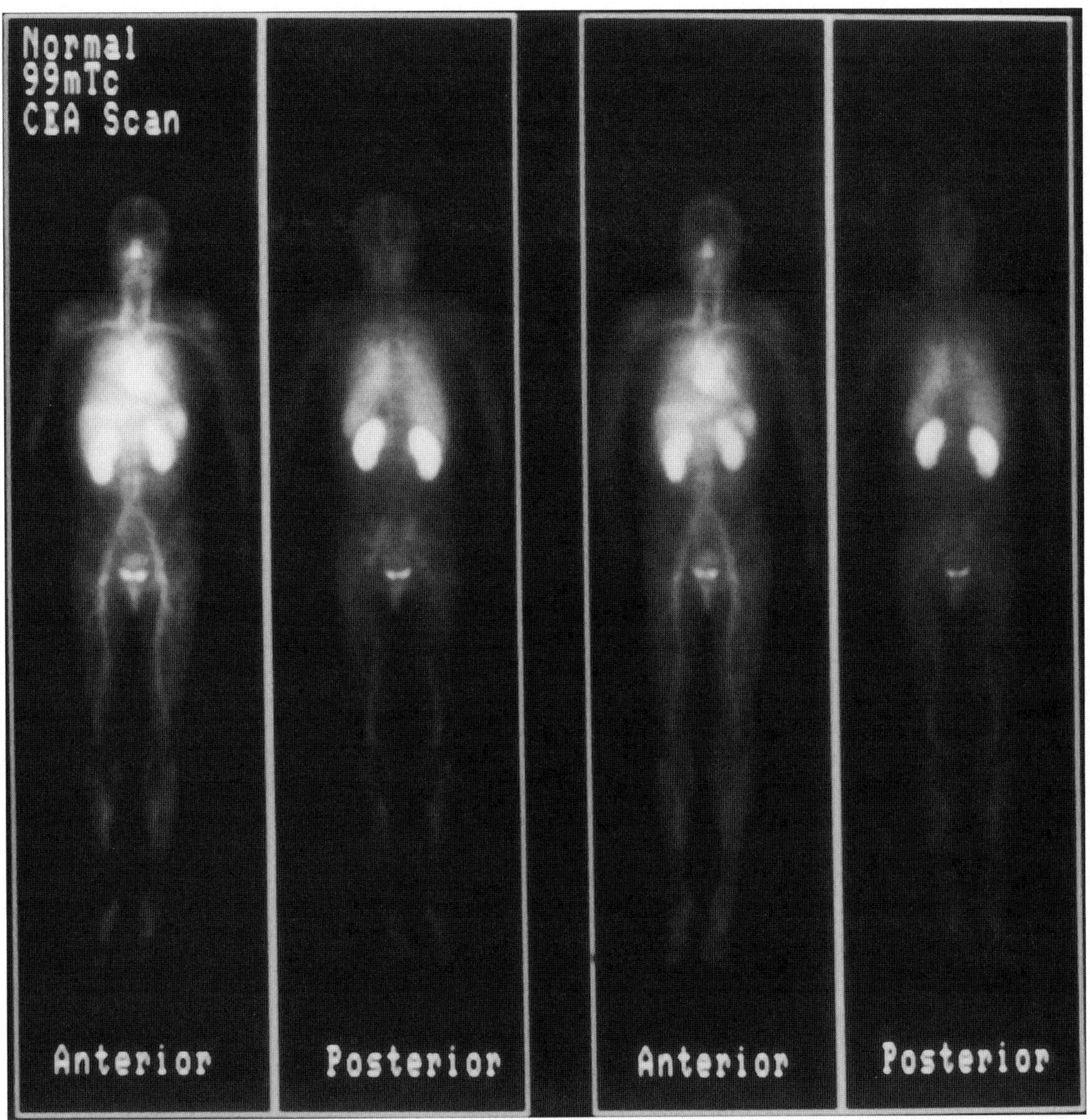

FIGURE 62.3. **Normal Carcinoembryonic Antigen Scan (Arcitumomab).** Whole-body anterior and posterior images.

It detects primary small cell lung carcinoma with 90% sensitivity and nonliver metastases from small cell lung carcinoma with 70% sensitivity. It has successfully detected recurrent small cell lung carcinoma in patients who were in complete remission by standard criteria. The agent is rapidly cleared by renal excretion, with 90% excretion at 24 hours. It should be clear that the agent lacks specificity, but this is not significant in most tumor imaging applications. The agent will also image active granulomas, which are a potential source of false-positive scans.

Tc-99m depreotide became an important agent during the relatively brief period it was available. This agent has affinity for three of the five types of somatostatin receptors and was an excellent agent for imaging non–small cell lung cancer. SPECT imaging with this agent remains the most cost-effective method for assessing solitary pulmonary nodules that are equivocal for tumor. Depreotide was achieving significant clinical acceptance when manufacturing problems resulted in a drop in chemical and radiochemical purity, causing the agent to be removed from the market. Although the "impure" product was essentially equally useful for diagnostic purposes and clearly harmless, it was removed from the market to protect the public. The irony in this age of revelations about the dangers of (for example) cyclooxygenase-2 inhibitors could not be more stark. The equivalent assessment with FDG is significantly more expensive, although the FDG scan has decreased background and improved resolution (Fig. 62.6). Unfortunately, past experience indicates that an agent is unlikely to again achieve wide acceptance once taken off the market. The extensive replacement of synthetic cholecystokinin with fatty meal for gallbladder ejection fraction,

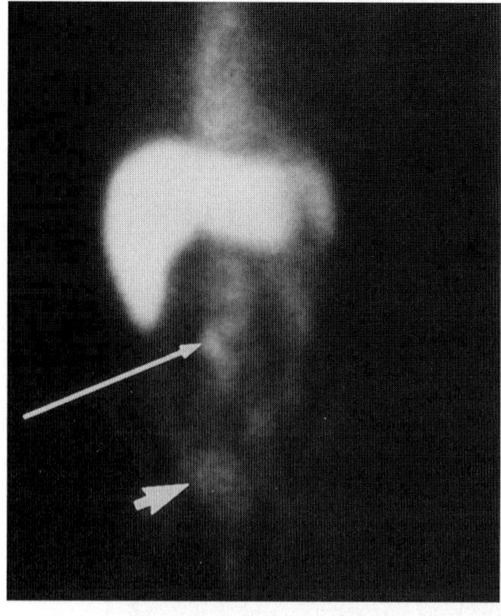

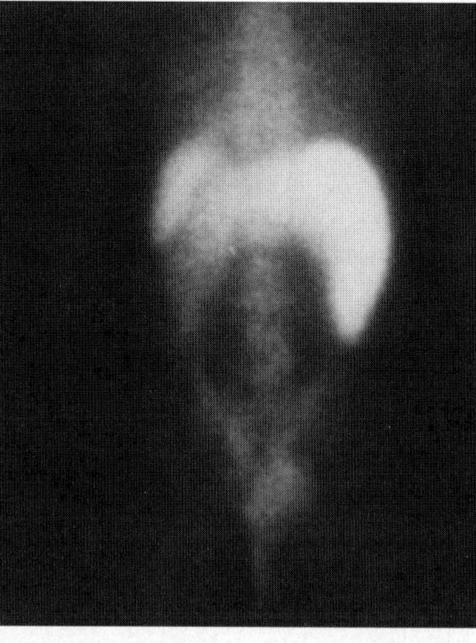

FIGURE 62.4. **Metastatic Colon Carcinoma.** Indium-111-OncoScint study, anterior **(A)** and posterior **(B)** views. Patient is status postresection of colon carcinoma with rising carcinoembryonic antigen. Study demonstrates paraspinous adenopathy (*long arrow*). Less obvious is the fixed uptake in the pelvis (*short arrow*), which remained unchanged over several days of imaging and was proven to be locally recurrent carcinoma.

resulting from temporary unavailability of the agent because of manufacturing problems, is instructive in this regard. An interesting case of depreotide labeling in an early mesothelioma is illustrated in Fig. 62.7.

Mixed Mechanisms. The traditional gamma camera imaging agent Ga-67 depends on receptor binding but also falls within the category of metabolic marker agents. The metabolic activity imaged by Ga, at least in part, is the cellular competition for nutrient iron. Ga-67 ion, administered as the citrate salt, mimics free iron. It is rapidly bound to transferrin receptors on tumor cells, which are overexpressed in an attempt to maximize this scarce

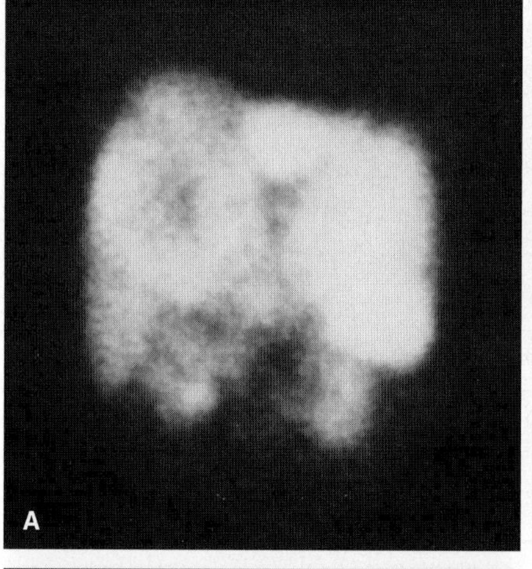

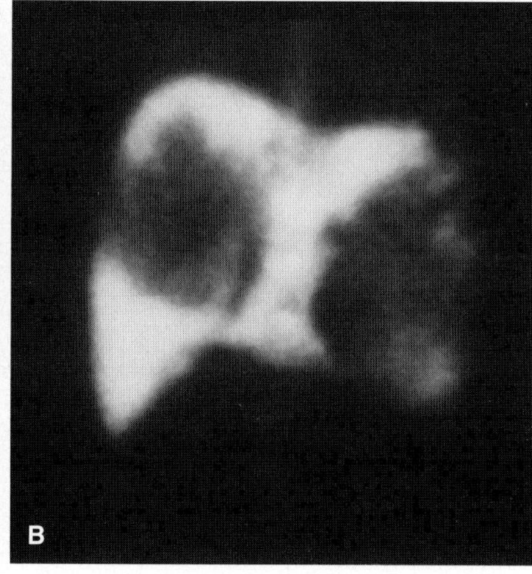

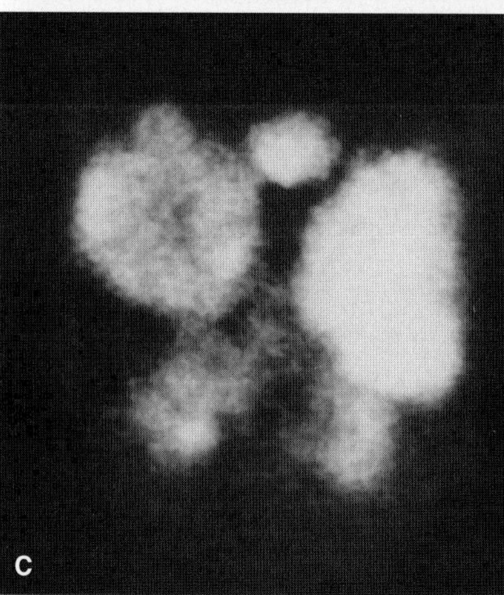

FIGURE 62.5. **Metastatic Islet Cell Tumor.** Patient with known metastatic islet cell tumor was evaluated for receptor status. **A.** The anterior liver and spleen were imaged with indium-111-octreotide. **B.** Technetium-99m sulfur colloid liver-spleen scan shows multiple defects corresponding to the tumor. **C.** Subtraction study shows uptake by the tumor receptors.

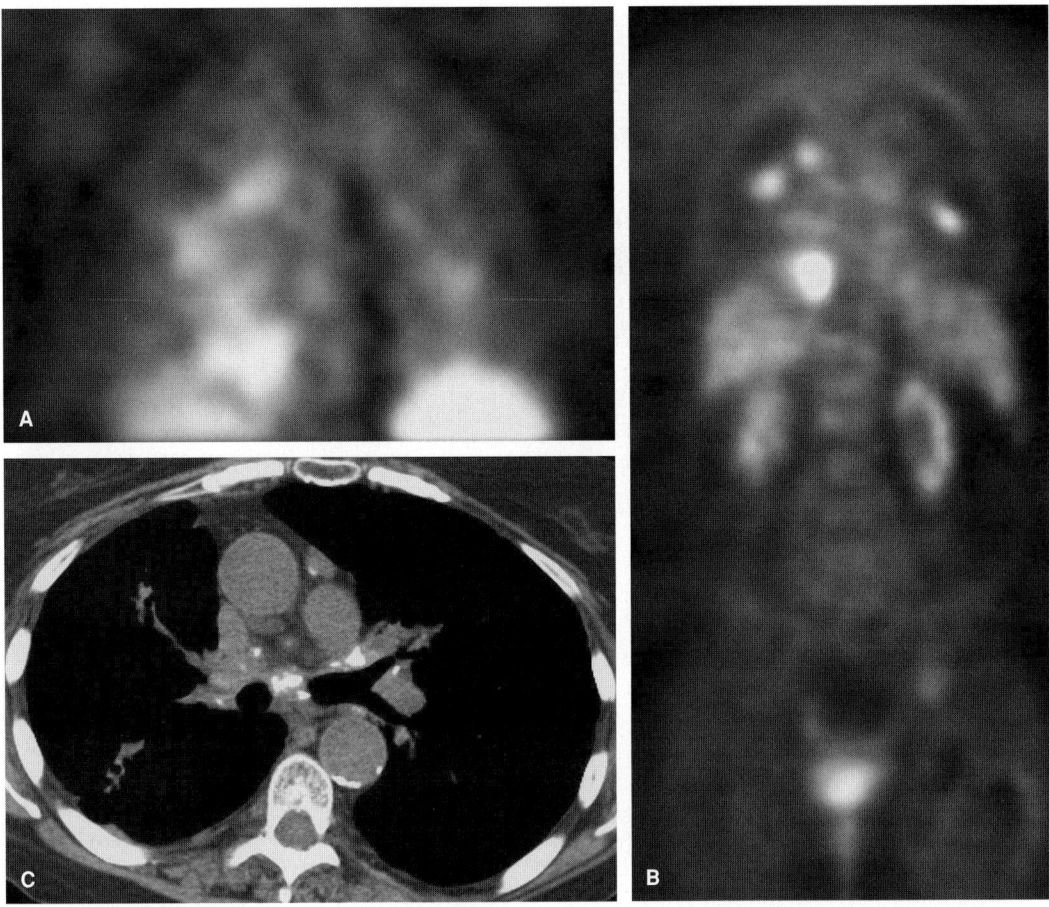

FIGURE 62.6. **False-Positive Depreotide and Fluorodeoxyglucose (FDG) Scans.** Coronal image **(A)** from technetium-99m-depreotide SPECT lung scan and coronal image **(B)** from FDG PET scan in a patient with diffuse pulmonary abnormalities. These were felt to represent granulomatous disease radiographically, based on the CT scan **(C)**. Granulomas were subsequently demonstrated on biopsy, and stability was demonstrated on long-term clinical and imaging follow-up. The exact etiologic factor remains unknown. Note the nearly identical pathologic distribution of the radiopharmaceutical in the two scintigraphic scans. The high lung background on the depreotide scan makes it less appealing, but the information content is identical for the two scans.

resource required for rapid growth. Limitation of free iron is a major defense mechanism of the body, although this is directed primarily at defense from pathogens. It is mediated by free transferrin protein in serum and by transferrin receptors on white cells. Pathogens also compete for free iron through production of soluble iron chelators termed *siderophores*. Ga tumor activity thus depends both on the availability of transferrin receptors on the tumor and the metabolic activity of the tumor, which determines the extent to which these receptors will be expressed. Tumors for which Ga-67 imaging was historically useful are now generally evaluated with other techniques (FDG PET for lymphomas and MR or multiphase CT for hepatocellular carcinoma). The high-energy γ emissions of Ga-67 result in "fuzzy" images that were instrumental in creating the "unclear" medicine reputation (Fig. 62.8). Tumor localization by Ga is now more significant as a confounding factor when Ga-67 is employed for infection imaging.

Lymphoscintigraphy has undergone a revival as the result of the sentinel node concept. Cutaneous melanoma and breast cancer tend to migrate to the nearest draining node without skip lesions in nodes further along the drainage chain. Absence of tumor within the first draining lymph node makes presence of other metastatic disease highly unlikely. If the sentinel node can be located and demonstrated to be free of disease, more extensive lymph node dissection can be avoided. This approach is now the standard of care in breast cancer in most localities because it reduces the morbidity of surgical therapy, especially postoperative lymphedema. Sentinel node biopsy is more accurate than FDG PET. This fact has limited the use of FDG PET in breast cancer role to restaging of recurrent tumor. PET retains a primary role in the diagnosis and staging of melanoma. Sentinel node biopsy is less useful in melanoma because of the relatively poor success of current melanoma therapies other than resection of an

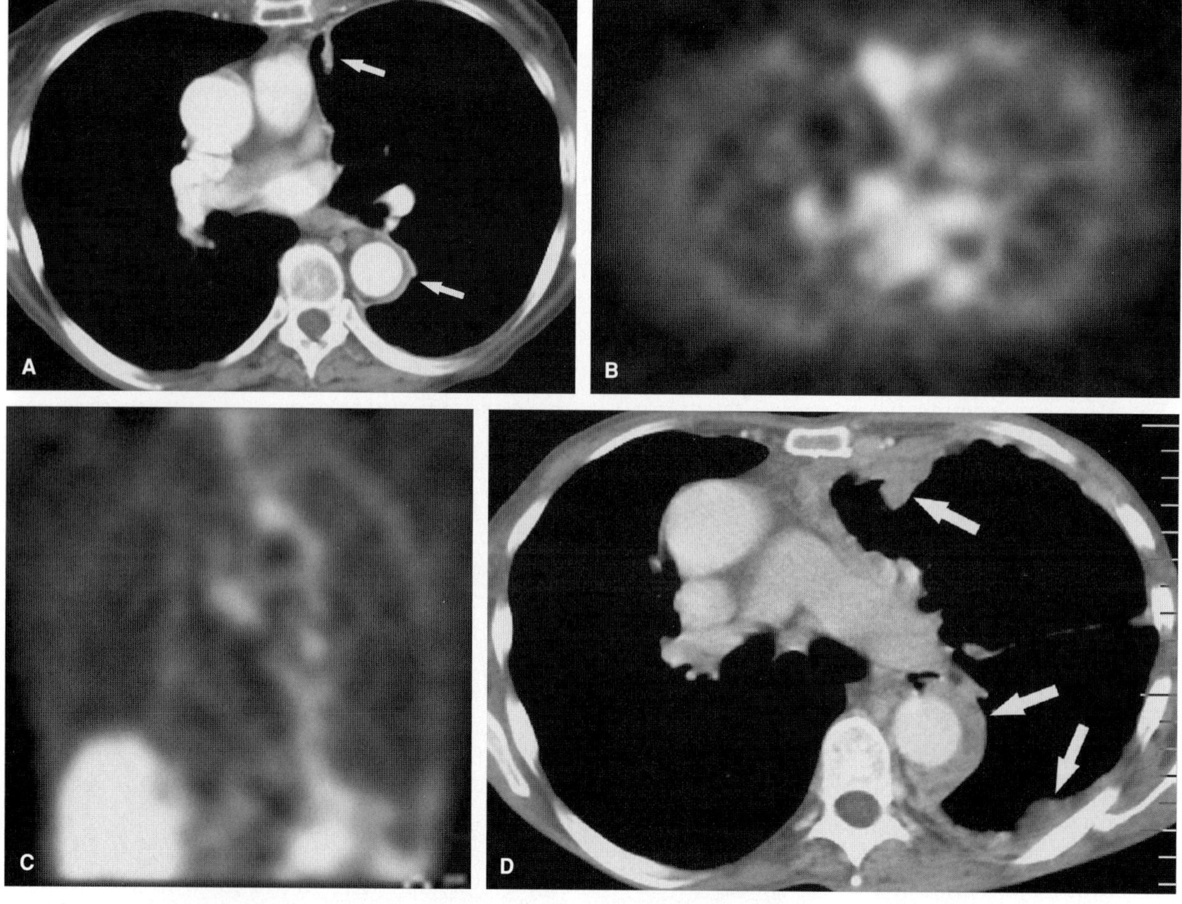

FIGURE 62.7. **Technetium-99m-Depreotide Scan in Mesothelioma.** Axial CT image **(A)** 3 weeks prior to depreotide scan shows pleural thickening (*arrows*) in the left thorax caused by mesothelioma. Axial depreotide image at the approximate location of CT slice **(B)** and coronal **(C)** depreotide image both show diffuse uptake in the pleura, indicating that tumor involvement is more widespread than indicated by CT. **D.** Axial slice from CT scan 3 months later shows marked progression (*arrows*).

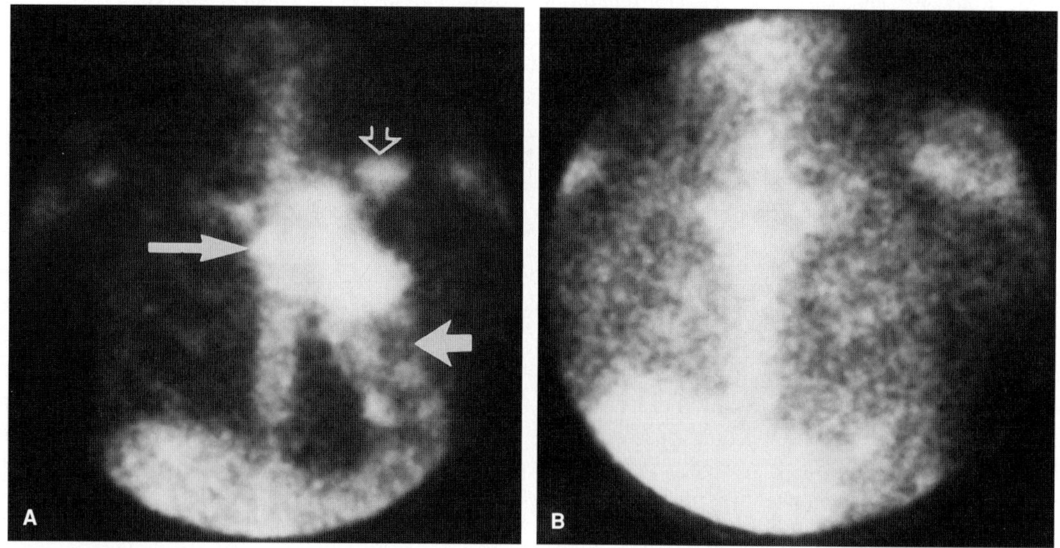

FIGURE 62.8. **Lymphoma.** Anterior chest images from gallium-67 studies pretreatment **(A)** and posttreatment **(B)** for lymphoma demonstrate the complete resolution of mediastinal (*long arrow*), parenchymal (*short arrow*), and left supraclavicular nodal (*open arrow*) disease.

isolated primary tumor for cure. The role of sentinel node biopsy in other tumors, especially head and neck tumors, remains in flux.

Any colloidal agent can in principle be employed for lymphoscintigraphy. Agents with particle sizes smaller than 50 nm are ideal. Reasonable agents are Tc-99m-SC and Tc-99m human serum albumin (Tc-99m-HSA). Tc-99m-SC is somewhat suboptimal because of its large particle size, which results in significant retention at the injection site. This problcm is partially ovcrcomc by filtration to obtain only the smaller particles. Tc-99m-HSA immediately enters the lymphatic system and allows rapid dynamic imaging of lymphatic channels with reduced overall imaging time. However, retention in lymph nodes is significantly less than with Tc-99m-SC, which may make Tc-99m-HSA less optimal for use of an intraoperative gamma probe to localize the sentinel node. In general, Tc-99m-HSA is probably preferable for imaging and Tc-99m-SC for intraoperative use, but either can be used effectively. Only Tc-99m-SC is currently available in the United States.

Technical factors can significantly affect the outcome of the study. There has been extensive debate on the best method of injection; some favor axillary subdermal, some periareolar subdermal, and some intratumoral injection. At the current time, it appears that the periareolar approach is both most accurate and best tolerated.

A transmission scan or other body image scan (i.e., bone scan) is required to allow effective interpretation of node location (Fig. 62.9). Head and neck lesions have especially short drainage chains. Since these lesions drain inferiorly, injection should occur above (cranial to) the level of the lesion to ensure that activity at the injection site does not obscure the sentinel node. Body wall lymphatics are highly variable. Both ipsilateral and contralateral imaging is required with body wall injections to ensure that all nodal groups draining the lesion are detected.

The need for imaging in breast cancer sentinel node lymphoscintigraphy is hotly debated. Imaging will reveal drainage to nodes outside the axilla. This is important only in those centers in which surgeons are willing to sample the extra-axillary nodes when present. Currently, these centers are in the minority. Imaging is still mandatory for nonextremity melanoma, which can drain to multiple sentinel node sites, whereas imaging is useful, but not necessarily mandatory, for extremity melanomas. These always drain first to the axilla or groin, but the intraoperative search is facilitated by imaging. Head and neck sentinel node imaging clearly requires meticulous high-resolution imaging for success because of the complex and densely packed anatomy. Hybrid or fusion imaging is of great potential interest to provide additional anatomic information in this setting.

Other Tumor Imaging Agents. Metaiodobenzylguanidine can be used for detection and therapy of neuroblastoma and pheochromocytoma (Fig. 62.10), and iodinated cholesterol derivatives can be used for adrenal cortical carcinoma. Bone imaging agents for both primary bone tumors and metastatic disease are discussed in Chapter 55. In addition to localizing areas of increased or absent bone repair ("hot" and "cold" lesions, respectively), these agents have a tendency to localize within malignant effusions and

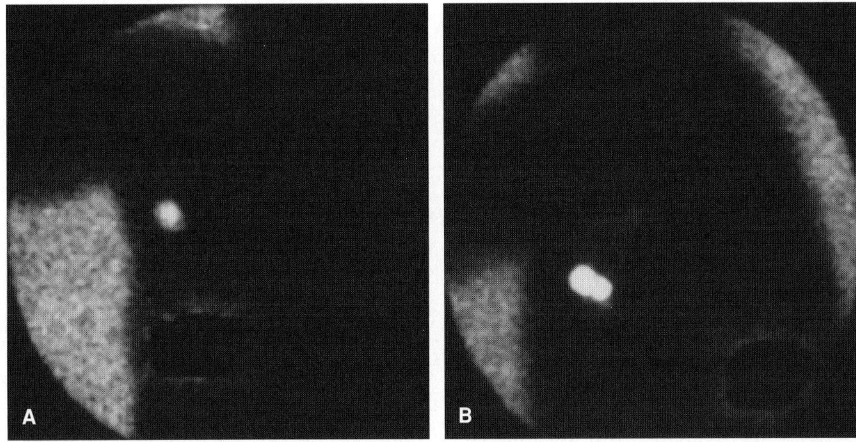

FIGURE 62.9. **Malignant Melanoma.** Example of lymphoscintigraphy, with filtered technetium-99m sulfur colloid (Tc-99m-SC) injected intradermally in four locations around the site of malignant melanoma located on the back at the inferior aspect of the left clavicle. Transmission imaging is performed with a Tc-99m flood source, causing the patient to cast a "shadow" for positioning information. **A.** Image is slightly off center, true posterior with left arm held out to the side. **B.** A left lateral image. In both images the injection sites have been digitally subtracted (a "halo" remains in the lower portion of each image) so that axillary nodal activity is more readily apparent. Imaging of the remainder of the trunk failed to demonstrate drainage elsewhere.

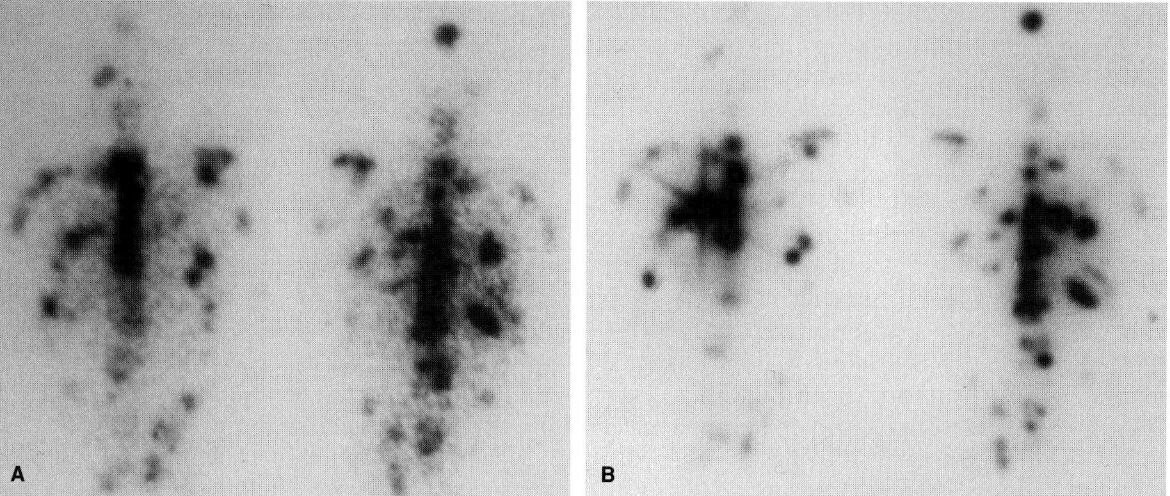

FIGURE 62.10. **Metastatic Pheochromocytoma.** Anterior **(A)** and posterior **(B)** whole-body images with iodine-131-metaiodobenzylguanidine in a patient with widely metastatic pheochromocytoma. (Courtesy of Dr. Peter Blue, Columbia, South Carolina.)

malignant ascites. The mechanism for this localization has yet to be fully explained. The use of Tc-99m-MIBI for localization of benign but clinically significant parathyroid tumors is also discussed elsewhere.

Pretreatment with agents designed to improve target-to-background ratios may become more common in the future. These agents may increase binding of the imaging agent to the intended target or they may decrease binding of the agent to nontarget tissues. The best current example is the use of "cold" rituximab to saturate nonspecific binding sites prior to imaging with In-111-ibritumomab prior to yttrium-90-ibritumomab tiuxetan therapy.

DUAL-AGENT SCINTIGRAPHY, HYBRID IMAGING, AND FUSION IMAGING

Dual-agent imaging may improve sensitivity for detection of metastases from certain classes of tumors in which the metastatic foci have variable receptor expression because of dedifferentiation or origin from different cell clones. FDG and I-131 may be used in combination to simultaneously or sequentially image differentiated (I-131) and dedifferentiated (FDG) metastases from thyroid cancer. The combination of Tc-99m-MIBI and In-111-OCT has also been suggested as a means for determining multiple drug resistance in small cell lung carcinoma. Presumably, FDG or Tl-201 in combination with any of the MIBI-like agents could achieve the same effect in tumors that do not have somatostatin receptors.

Fusion imaging is the exact superimposition of the physiologic information from a nuclear medicine study with the anatomic information from CT or MR using fiduciary markers. ***Hybrid imaging*** achieves the same goal more elegantly by performing both an anatomic and a functional study on a single system without patient movement between scans. PET-CT hybrid scanners have captured nearly all of the recent PET scanner market. Current research would tend to favor this approach over visual or fusion imaging of separate anatomic and functional studies. My own experience and reading of this literature suggest there is significant bias resulting from comparison of hybrid imaging to either anatomic or functional images alone. Those studies that have compared hybrid to fused or visual comparison of anatomic and functional images have not tended to use interpreters who are significantly experienced in both the anatomic and the functional technique employed—a nearly unavoidable bias in academic centers where radiology and nuclear medicine tend to be separate endeavors. It is likely that a properly performed, definitive study will be moot before it is available (if ever). Just as the speed and convenience of CT angiography for assessment of pulmonary embolus resulted in a large-scale conversion to this technique before the comparisons with ventilation/perfusion lung scanning were published, the simplicity of reading hybrid images is selling the technique long before the intellectual justification is available. The issue has already been settled de facto by sales of hybrid scanners.

Conversely, hybrid scanners have the potential to salvage some γ-emitting agents that have been too difficult for general use. Especially notable is the improvement in sensitivity and specificity for imaging with the monoclonal antibody In-111 capromab pendetide when SPECT-CT hybrid scanners are employed (Fig. 62.11). Without reliable anatomic coregistration, this agent is extremely unreliable.

A resident being shown a tumor imaging case in nuclear medicine at the current time may expect that anatomic

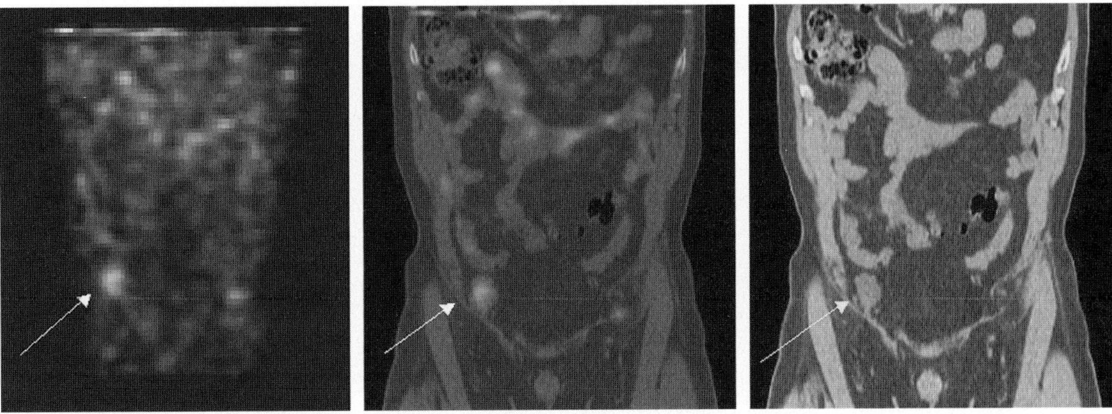

FIGURE 62.11. **(Color Plates) SPECT-CT of Metastatic Prostate Carcinoma With ProstaScint.** Coronal images presented in standard sequence (scintigram, fusion, CT). (Courtesy of Dr. Milton Gross, VA Hospital and University of Michigan, Ann Arbor, Michigan.)

imaging for comparison will be provided if hybrid or fusion images are not provided. The current standard of care requires correlation of functional and anatomic imaging by some method. The resident has a right to expect that the test cases will allow him or her to work at the standard of care.

TUMOR THERAPY WITH RADIOPHARMACEUTICALS

A complete discussion of therapy with radiopharmaceuticals is beyond the scope of this text, which is intended primarily to help residents learn and review information important in the board examination in radiology. The discussion will be limited to the example provided by two anti-CD20 monoclonal antibodies for lymphoma therapy: I-131 tositumomab (trade name Bextra) and Y-90 ibritumomab tiuxetan (trade name Zevalin). These agents exemplify the general principles involved in tumor therapy with radiopharmaceuticals. Radiology residents should be aware that therapeutic radiopharmaceuticals are available for treatment of bone metastases (commonly 89-strontium chloride [$SrCl_2$] or samarium-153 ethylenediamine tetramethylene phosphoric acid). These are essentially bone scan agents with β emitters. I-131 metaiodobenzylguanidine is employed to treat neuroblastoma. Somatostatin-avid polypeptides with β-emitter labels are available to treat neuroendocrine tumors, at least under protocol. Agents are under development for most tumor types that will clearly be part of nuclear medicine and radiation oncology practice. Most radiologists will not be directly involved in administering these therapies, but most radiologists will be involved in determining the correct therapy.

Both Bextra and Zevalin were developed because of the success of rituximab (Rituxan) in treating low-grade B-cell non-Hodgkin lymphoma. This anti-CD20 antibody has been remarkably successful in palliating low-grade lymphoma, for which a cure is seldom achieved because of the slow growth rate. Generally, tumor therapy other than resection is only effective for growing cells. Since rituximab can be used repeatedly in the same individual, long-term therapy selects for cells with reduced cell surface CD20 receptors that are not killed by rituximab.

Radiopharmaceuticals can overcome the increasing chemoresistance of these tumors through the process of crossfire. A monoclonal agent with a β emitter attached will deliver radiation to cells with the CD20 receptor. By choosing a β emitter with a mean free path that is greater than a typical cell radius, the radiation damage can be extended to a few tumor cells distant to the target. This crossfire from cells retaining CD20 receptors and adequate blood supply can kill tumor cells that have dedifferentiated to lose the CD20 receptor and cells whose blood supply is partially disrupted. The therapy treats tumors that have become resistant to standard therapy. It also renews the therapeutic effectiveness of the unlabeled monoclonal antibody by increasing the relative number of CD20-expressing cells in the tumor population.

Bextra is labelled with I-131. Because this isotope is also a γ emitter, it can be imaged and provides its own dosimetry scan. The major disadvantage of the agent is the need to hospitalize the patient as a radiation safety precaution for bystanders. Zevalin relies on Y-90, a pure β emitter with no γ component. A patient receiving this agent does not have to be hospitalized. However, to visualize biodistribution, it is necessary to scan with antibody labeled with the γ emitter In-111 in the week prior to the therapeutic dose (Fig. 62.12). Bextra and Zevalin have roughly equivalent efficacy. It is likely that only one of these agents will survive the marketplace. It is also likely that the outcome will depend more on cost, convenience, and marketing than on any absolute advantage in outcome, even if such an advantage is ultimately established.

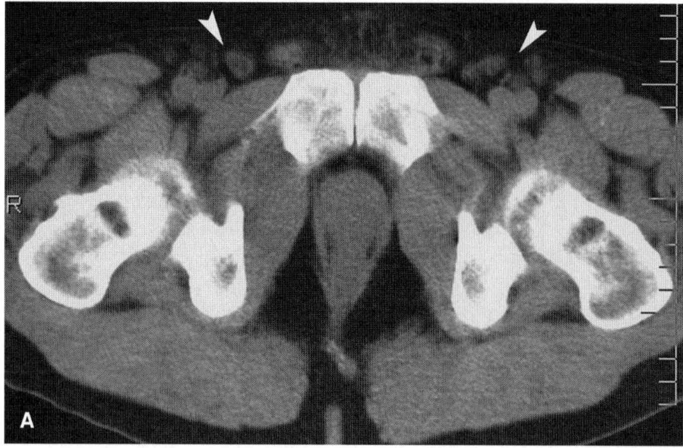

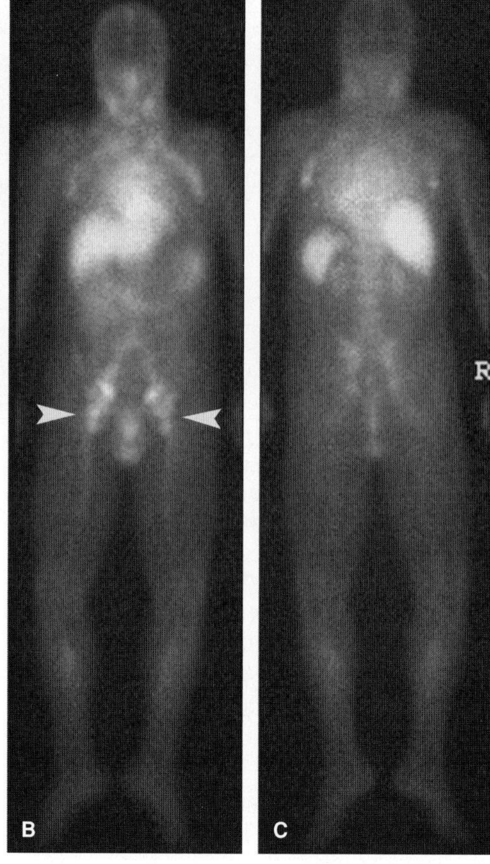

FIGURE 62.12. **Zevalin Therapy of Low-Grade Non-Hodgkin Lymphoma.** Pretreatment axial CT image **(A)** shows innocuous-appearing groin nodes (*arrowheads*). Anterior **(B)** and posterior **(C)** pretreatment scans with indium-111-ibritumomab showed extensive uptake in the groin nodes (*arrowheads*). Biopsy of a groin node confirmed recurrent disease. After treatment, the patient was free of recurrence for more than a year.

A COMPLETE ONCOLOGY IMAGING APPROACH

In addition to primary diagnosis, staging, and therapy, radiology residents should remain attuned to the value of ancillary nuclear medicine techniques in the oncology setting. Pretherapy and posttherapy assessment of cardiac function with tagged red blood cell equilibrium ventriculography remains important for patients receiving cardiotoxic chemotherapy. Ga scanning, tagged white blood cell agents, and the newer monoclonal antibody agent for infection imaging (Tc-99m fanolesomab; trade name NeutroSpec) will remain important to assess posttherapy infectious complications. Ga-67 may also be useful to assess lung toxicity from chemotherapeutic agents such as bleomycin. Ga-67 is especially useful to assess fever of unknown origin, when both recurrent tumor and infection are in the differential diagnosis.

Effective tumor screening remains the holy grail of imaging, but successful examples in nuclear oncology are limited. Scintimammography of the dense breast, for all of its theoretical advantages, has made little headway in most practices. If the economics are right, newer breast-specific cameras may increase the use of scintimammography. Bone scan for bony metastatic disease is the only widely employed nuclear medicine screening method in oncology. The concept that bone scan is unnecessary in the absence of bone pain, while likely true for some tumors like prostate cancer, is not universally true for all tumors.

Familiarity with molecular imaging as a research tool for understanding basic molecular biologic processes is valuable. The resident should also be alerted to techniques of preclinical development imaging employed by drug manufacturers. An occasional foray into the literature in these areas is of great value to maintain enthusiasm for the potential of molecular imaging, however remote the clinical applications may seem. Tumor imaging with PET, for example, labored in research laboratories for many years but has now become the standard of care.

This list is not intended to be inclusive. During the board examination, as in real life, expertise in handling problems at the fringe of a field of practice often distinguishes the proficient practitioner. Oncology should be approached with a combination of all available radiologic and nuclear medicine techniques to achieve the best outcome for the patient. Residents should seek to become proficient in comparing the effectiveness of all modalities available to them. Your clinical colleagues will ultimately show their appreciation for this effort through consultation and referral.

Summary. Oncologic nuclear medicine is an expanding field. The indications for radiopharmaceuticals in the detection and treatment of primary and metastatic cancer will doubtless increase. The advances in cost-effective PET imaging technology have greatly strengthened the position of nuclear radiology in the cost-conscious care environment. Radiologists will need to understand not only the indications, contraindications, and pitfalls of this new imaging technology but also its position in the cost-effective delivery of care.

SUGGESTED READINGS

Aboagye EO. Positron emission tomography imaging of small animals in anticancer drug development. Mol Imaging Biol 2005;7:53–58.

Barrio J, Marcus C, Hung JC, Keppler JS. A rational regulatory approach for positron emission tomography imaging probes: from "first in man" to NDA approval and reimbursement. Mol Imaging Biol 2004;6:361–367.

Baulieu F, Bourlier P, Scotto B, et al. The value of immunoscintigraphy in the detection of recurrent colorectal cancer. Nucl Med Commun 2001;22:1295–1304.

Britz-Cunningham SH, Adelstein S. Molecular targeting with radionuclides: state of the science. J Nucl Med 2003;44:1945–1961.

Burak Z, Moretti JL, Ersoy O, et al. ^{99m}Tc-MIBI imaging as a predictor of therapy response in osteosarcoma compared with multidrug resistance-associated protein and p-glycoprotein expression. J Nucl Med 2003;44:1394–1401.

Carlisle MR, Lu C, McDougall IR. The interpretation of ^{131}I scans in the evaluation of thyroid cancer, with an emphasis on false positive findings. Nucl Med Commun 2003;24:715–735.

Dadachova E, Carrasco N. The Na^{+}/I^{-} symporter (NIS): imaging and therapeutic applications. Semin Nucl Med 2004;34:23–31.

Danthi SN, Pandit SD, Li KCP. A primer on molecular biology for imagers: VII. Molecular imaging probes. Acad Radiol 2004;11:S77–S84.

Debray MP, Geoffroy O, Laissy JP, et al. Imaging appearances of metastases from neuroendocrine tumours of the pancreas. Br J Radiol 2001 Nov;74:1065–1070.

Duet M, Sauvaget E, Petelle B, et al. Clinical impact of somatostatin receptor scintigraphy in the management of paragangliomas of the head and neck. J Nucl Med 2003;44:1767–1774.

Fuster D, Munoz M, Pavia J, et al. Quantified ^{99m}Tc-MIBI scintigraphy for predicting chemotherapy response in breast cancer patients: factors that influence the level of ^{99m}Tc-MIBI uptake. Nucl Med Commun 2002;23:31–38.

Higuchi T, Taki J, Sumiya H, et al. Intense ^{201}Tl uptake in giant-cell tumor of bone. Nucl Med Commun 2002;23:595–599.

Hutton BF, Braun M. Software for image registration: algorithms, accuracy, efficiency. Semin Nucl Med 2003;33:180–192.

Ilias I, Pacak K. Current approaches and recommended algorithm for the diagnostic localization of pheochromocytoma. J Clin Endocrinol Metab 2004;89:479–491.

Jani AB, Spelbring D, Hamilton R, et al. Impact of radioimmunoscintigraphy on definition of clinical target volume for radiotherapy after prostatectomy. J Nucl Med 2004;45:238–246.

Keidar Z, Israel O, Krausz Y. SPECT/CT in tumor imaging: technical aspects and clinical applications. Semin Nucl Med 2003;33:205–218.

Krausz Y. Normal SPECT/CT scans: artifacts and pitfalls in iodine, iodine-MIBG, and indium octreotide imaging. In von Schultess G, ed. Clinical Molecular Anatomic Imaging. Philadelphia: Lippincott Williams & Wilkins, 2003:441–446.

Kushner BH. Neuroblastoma: a disease requiring a multitude of imaging studies. J Nucl Med 2004;45:1172–1188.

Lewington VJ. Bone-seeking radionuclides for therapy. J Nucl Med 2005;46:38S–47S.

Li, KCP. A primer on molecular biology for imagers: IX. How to become a "molecular imager." Acad Radiol 2004;11:S97–S100.

Machac J, Krynyckyi B, Kim C. Peptide and antibody imaging in lung cancer. Semin Nucl Med 2002;32:276–292.

Meier DA, Kaplan MM. Radioiodine uptake and thyroid scintiscanning. Endocrinol Metab Clin 2001;30:291–313.

Menda Y, Kahn D. Somatostatin receptor imaging of non-small cell lung cancer with ^{99m}Tc depreotide. Semin Nucl Med 2002;32:92–96.

Mozley P. Weaving single photon imaging into new drug development. Mol Imaging Biol 2005;7:30–36.

Pashankar FD, O'Dorisio M, Menda Y. MIBG and Somatostatin receptor analogs in children: current concepts on diagnostic and therapeutic use. J Nucl Med 2005;46:55S–61S.

Pelosi E, Bello M, Giors M, et al. Sentinel lymph node detection in patients with early-stage breast cancer: comparison of periareolar and subdermal/peritumoral injection techniques. J Nucl Med 2004;45: 220–225.

Reubi JC, Macke HR, Krenning EP. Candidates for peptide receptor therapy today and in the future. J Nucl Med 2005;46:67S–75S.

Robbins RJ, Schlumberger MJ. The evolving role of ^{131}I for the treatment of differentiated thyroid carcinoma. J Nucl Med 2005;46: 28S–37S.

Schettino CJ, Kramer EL, Noz ME, Taneja S, Padmanabhan P, Lepor H. Impact of fusion of indium-111 capromab pendetide volume data sets with those from MRI or CT in patients with recurrent prostate cancer. AJR Am J Roentgenol 2004;183:519–524.

Schirrmeister H, Arslandemir C, Glatting G, et. al. Omission of bone scanning according to staging guidelines leads to futile therapy in non-small cell lung Cancer. Eur J Nucl Med Mol Imaging 2004;31: 964–968.

Sharkey RM, Goldenberg DM. Perspectives on cancer therapy with radiolabeled monoclonal antibodies. J Nucl Med 2005;46:115S–127S.

Silverman DH, Delpassand ES, Torabi F, Goy A, McLaughlin P, Murray JL. Radiolabeled antibody therapy in non-Hodgkins lymphoma: radiation protection, isotope comparison and quality of life issues. Cancer Treat Rev 2004;30:165–172.

Stokking R, Zubal IG, Viergever MA. Display of fused images: methods, interpretation and diagnostic improvements. Semin Nucl Med 2003;33:219–227.

Taillefer R. Clinical applications of ^{99m}Tc-sestamibi scintimammography. Semin Nucl Med 2005;35:100–115.

Thomasson DM, Gharib A, Li KCP. A primer on molecular biology for imagers: VIII. Equipment for imaging molecular processes. Acad Radiol 2004;11:S85–S96.

Torabi M, Aquino SL, Harisinghani MG. Current concepts in lymph node imaging. J Nucl Med 2004;45:1509–1518.

Wagner JD, Evdokimow DZ, Weisberger E, et al. Sentinel node biopsy for high-risk nonmelanoma cutaneous malignancy. Arch Dermatol 2004;140:75–79.

Wahl RL. Tositumomab and ^{131}I therapy in non-Hodgkin's lymphoma. J Nucl Med 2005;46:128S–140S.

Wilczek B, Sandelin K, Eriksson S, Larsson SA, Jacobsson H. Sentinel node scintigraphy in breast cancer using a dual tracer technique. Nucl Med Commun 2004;25:135–138.

Willkomm P, Bender H, Bangard M, Decker P, Grunwald F, Biersack HJ. FDG PET and immunoscintigraphy with ^{99m}Tc-labeled antibody fragments for detection of the recurrence of colorectal carcinoma. J Nucl Med 2000;41:1657–1663.

Yuksel M, Cermik TF, Doganay L, et al. ^{99m}Tc-MIBI SPET in non-small cell lung cancer in relationship with Pgp and prognosis. Eur J Nucl Med 2002;29:876–881.

Chapter 63

Central Nervous System Scintigraphy

David H. Lewis and Vivek Manchanda

Two-Dimensional (Planar) Brain Scans

Cerebrospinal Fluid Studies

Functional Brain Imaging in Three Dimensions (Tomographic Brain Scans)
Positron Emission Tomography
Single-Photon Emission Computed Tomography

TWO-DIMENSIONAL (PLANAR) BRAIN SCANS

Before the advent of CT, the planar nuclear medicine brain scan, using radiopharmaceuticals like technetium-99m diethylenetriaminepentaacetic acid (Tc-99m-DTPA) or Tc-99m glucoheptonate (Tc-99m-GH), was used to detect a breakdown in the blood-brain barrier (BBB). Currently, a similar study using agents that cross the intact BBB, such as Tc-99m hexamethylpropyleneamine oxime (Tc-99m-HMPAO) or Tc-99m ethyl cysteinate dimer (Tc-99m-ECD), can detect absence of cerebral blood flow, which is characteristic of brain death. The normal BBB protects the CNS by preventing entry of harmful substances. Most materials are excluded from the CNS on the basis of molecular size and chemical characteristics. Active transport mechanisms are present for certain key nutrients such as glucose.

Radiopharmaceuticals. Planar brain scanning for the detection of the BBB breakdown is typically performed with Tc-99m bound to either DTPA or GH. Any agent that does not normally cross the BBB can potentially be employed, although agents of cellular size (radiolabeled red blood cells, for example) will be excluded even by a damaged BBB.

Technique. A dose of 15 to 20 mCi of Tc-99m-DTPA or Tc-99m-GH is injected into an arm vein. Flow images are typically obtained at a rate of one image every 3 seconds for a total of 60 seconds, with the camera anterior to the head. Anterior, posterior, and lateral static images are subsequently obtained; vertex images, obtained by placing the camera at the vertex of the skull, are often useful. A lead collar is employed to exclude radiation from the radiopharmaceutical localized below the neck. Immediate static images are useful to evaluate blood pool abnormalities, while delayed static images after clearance of the background activity are of greater value to detect breakdown of the BBB.

Interpretation. Interpretation of the static images depends primarily upon detection or exclusion of radiopharmaceutical localization within the brain parenchyma. Some activity is invariably present from the radiopharmaceutical within the soft tissues of the scalp and within intracerebral blood vessels. Increased or asymmetric localization indicates breakdown of the BBB. This finding is entirely nonspecific; it is present in conditions as diverse as cerebral infarction, primary or metastatic tumor, and infectious processes. For this reason, clinical information is essential for interpretation. The presence of a lenticular photo-enhanced (or occasionally photopenic) rim can be used to diagnose subdural hematoma.

The normal radionuclide angiogram is characterized by prompt symmetric perfusion. Asymmetric flow in the carotid arteries may indicate occlusive disease. The so-called "flip-flop sign" (decreased activity in the arterial phase and increased activity in the venous phase) may be seen in carotid occlusion. Vascular malformations, high-grade or vascular tumors (e.g., glioblastoma multiforme and meningioma), and inflammatory processes have increased flow. Low-grade or benign tumors, areas of porencephaly or edema, and occlusive processes have decreased flow. The complete absence of brain activity in the presence of prompt common carotid and scalp flow indicates brain death.

The traditional brain scan with Tc-99m-DTPA or Tc-99m-GH has largely been superseded by planar perfusion brain scans in clinical practice to corroborate the impression of brain death. There is little doubt that modern brain radiopharmaceuticals such as Tc-99m-HMPAO or

Tc-99m-ECD provide, with greater assurance, the status of cerebral blood flow. These scans are also much easier to interpret, although they are more costly to perform because of the higher expense of the radiopharmaceuticals employed. Total cessation of cerebral blood flow including posterior fossa structures can be demonstrated with this technique, which is required by the Uniform Determination of Death Act (passed by the U.S. Congress in 1981).

CEREBROSPINAL FLUID STUDIES

CSF is formed in the choroid plexus as an ultrafiltrate of plasma. It flows from the ventricles through the foramina of the fourth ventricle and ascends over the convexities of the brain to be absorbed by the arachnoid villa. Processes that impede flow over the convexities or absorption of the fluid by the villi result in communicating hydrocephalus. Tracer techniques are ideal for imaging of this process, because they are injected in small amounts and do not alter CSF flow. Processes that obstruct the outflow from a ventricle are more difficult to assess by these techniques because injection can be made directly into the ventricle. Patency and flow in therapeutic shunts and reservoirs can easily be evaluated by injecting the tracer directly into the device.

Radiopharmaceuticals and Technique. The standard cisternogram is performed by intrathecal injection of a sterile, pyrogen-free radiopharmaceutical. The only approved agent currently marketed for this purpose is indium-111-DTPA (half-life = 2.8 days). The injection of 0.5 mCi follows a spinal tap performed in the standard manner. Initial images may be obtained to ensure intrathecal injection. Subsequently, the radiopharmaceutical ascends to the basilar cisterns in approximately 4 hours and flows over the convexities within 24 hours in a normal individual. Images of the basilar cisterns are obtained at 4 to 6 hours. If images at 24 hours show ascent over the convexities with activity in the interhemispheric fissure and relative clearance of the basilar cisterns, imaging may be terminated. Otherwise, images should be obtained at 48 and 72 hours.

CSF shunt and reservoir studies are performed by direct injection of the device with radiopharmaceutical in a small volume. Maintenance of sterile techniques during the injection is critical. It is also critical to understand the specific device being evaluated, as shunts often contain check valves and reservoir capacities are limited. A patient may also have several shunt tubes, some of which may be known to be occluded. In general, it is best to have direct input from the neurosurgeon involved in the case to ensure that the maximum amount of information is obtained. A small amount of CSF, up to 1 mL, may be withdrawn for lab studies prior to the tracer injection. Dynamic gamma camera imaging for 10 minutes is usually first performed in the supine position. If radiotracer drains from the reservoir, then in cases of ventriculoperitoneal shunts, an abdominal image is obtained. If the shunt leads elsewhere, such as the atrium, imaging of the thyroid and chest is performed.

Application to Hydrocephalus. Standard cisternography is performed primarily to evaluate for normal-pressure hydrocephalus and for CSF leak. Normal-pressure hydrocephalus is a form of communicating hydrocephalus clinically associated with ataxia, dementia, and urinary incontinence. Cisternography demonstrates early localization of activity within the lateral ventricles persisting beyond 24 hours and delayed clearance over the convexities (Fig. 63.1). While these findings indicate an increased likelihood of a clinical response to shunting, they are not univariate predictors of outcome. Other forms of communicating hydrocephalus (such as might result from radiation therapy or intrathecal chemotherapy) can also be evaluated with cisternography.

Application to Cerebrospinal Fluid Leak. Cisternography has high sensitivity for CSF leak and remains the procedure of choice for this condition. Its sensitivity results from the ability of tracer technique to detect very small amounts of activity that may be intermittently leaking. Imaging is performed between 1 and 3 hours after injection and also at 24 hours and perhaps 48 hours. Patient and camera positions are chosen to maximize the likelihood of detection, with lateral views for CSF rhinorrhea and anterior views for CSF otorrhea. Cotton pledgets should be placed in the nostrils after intrathecal injection of tracer. These are counted at 4 to 6 hours in a well counter. A serum sample from peripheral blood drawn concurrently is also counted. Pledget activity exceeding 1.5 times the serum concentration is evidence for CSF rhinorrhea. However, because this method does not give morphologic information about the leakage, DiChiro et al. suggested the use of imaging as well.

Application to Shunts and Reservoirs. Shunts are evaluated primarily for patency. If the proximal portion is occluded manually (or contains a check valve), flow through the distal limb can be evaluated. The tracer should flow freely into the peritoneum (for ventriculoperitoneal shunts). Delayed flow or persistent activity at the shunt tip suggests malfunction. Diffusion will typically allow determination of the level of obstruction, even when the flow is absent. Reservoir injection tests for proper placement, patency, and proper functioning of the reservoir. If the reservoir empties directly into the ventricle (such as an Omaya shunt placed for intrathecal chemotherapy), noncommunicating hydrocephalus may be excluded by normal progression of activity to the basilar cisterns and over the convexities. Ventricular spinal shunts may be evaluated only by direct injection of radiopharmaceutical into the ventricle. The half-time to clearance from the reservoir can be

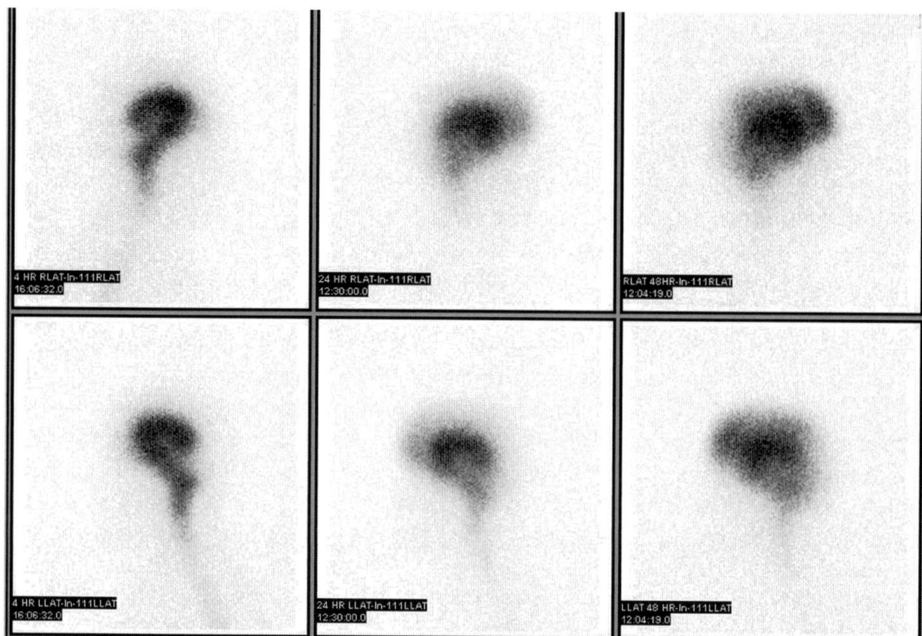

FIGURE 63.1. **Normal-Pressure Hydrocephalus on Cisternogram.** Selected images from an indium-111 diethylenetriaminepentaacetic acid cisternogram in lateral views shown at 4 to 6 hours, 24 hours, and 48 hours. Abnormal uptake is seen in lateral ventricles that persists through 48 hours.

calculated and should usually be less than 8 minutes. If the CSF flow is disturbed and opening pressure is low, the blockage is in the proximal limb. If opening pressure is high (more than 20 cm H_2O), the obstruction is distal to the reservoir.

In instances of distal malfunction of the shunt system, the clearance curve is flat and the half-time to clearance of the reservoir indicates infinite values. For complete distal obstruction or rupture of abdominal catheter, the isotope fails to migrate through the tubing, whereas in partial distal obstruction caused by relatively high abdominal pressure or obstruction of the valve, extremely low radionuclide clearance is encountered. Peritoneal loculations are typically characterized by stagnation of radioactivity at the initial site of appearance within the abdominal cavity and absence of uniform diffusion in the peritoneum.

Clearance studies of isotope are not of much help in proximal obstruction, as the time required for isotope to reach distal site of shunt depends on many factors, including the patient's CSF production, the proportion of CSF circulating through normal pathways, resting intraventricular pressure, the patient's position prior to the test, opening pressure of the shunt system, length of the tubing, and variations of intraventricular pressure caused by coughing, straining, or crying.

Conversely, absence of ventricular reflux seems to be a highly reliable scintigraphic feature in proximal obstruction. Inability to measure intraventricular pressure, to aspirate CSF freely, or to inject the isotope into the ventricle were considered of some help in assessing proximal shunt obstruction. Vernet et al suggest that a shuntogram exhibiting good opacification of the distal shunt system and normal clearance of the isotope, but no ventricular reflux, cannot be considered as normal but rather as inconclusive.

FUNCTIONAL BRAIN IMAGING IN THREE DIMENSIONS (TOMOGRAPHIC BRAIN SCANS)

Radiotracer techniques may be employed to evaluate blood flow in the cerebral microvasculature. Suitable for this purpose are diffusible radiotracers such as xenon-133, tracers that are passively taken up by neural tissues as lipophilic substances, and tracers that effectively function as "chemical microspheres." True microspheres that lodge in and thus obstruct capillaries are contraindicated because they could cause a stroke. Therefore, these radiopharmaceuticals must cross the BBB, enter, and be retained in cells. Glucose consumption and blood flow are linked in normally functioning brain tissues and in most pathologic processes. Therefore, the relative localization of SPECT blood flow or PET metabolic tracers in various cortical tissues gives a reasonable qualitative indication of relative function.

Positron Emission Tomography

Receptor Imaging. The paradigmatic technique for performance of in vivo biochemical and functional evaluation of the brain is PET. This technique allows qualitative and quantitative evaluation of receptor systems within the brain. Adrenergic, cholinergic, dopaminergic, serotonergic, benzodiazepine, and opioid receptors have been evaluated extensively. PET allows true biochemical assessment of the properties of these receptor systems, such as affinity, saturation, and nonspecific bindings, as well as more general information about distribution and uptake kinetics. These unique capabilities of the PET technique provide an extremely valuable research tool for evaluation of brain biochemistry and development of both imaging agents and therapeutic pharmaceuticals. However, these studies are expensive, experimental, and time consuming. Experimental uses should be clearly differentiated from proven clinical indications; the associated ethical issues have been assessed and summarized by the Brain Imaging Council of the Society of Nuclear Medicine.

Metabolic Imaging With Fluorine-18-Fluorodeoxyglucose (F-18-FDG). Clinical indications for PET almost exclusively involve F-18-FDG, although a tailored examination with other agents may be warranted in evaluating the status of some brain tumors. The primary clinical indications for PET are evaluation of epilepsy, dementia, and glioma. PET use in epilepsy is predominantly in the presurgical evaluation of mesial temporal lesions resulting in partial complex seizures. Approximately 85% of these can be cured surgically if the focus of the abnormal brain is limited to a single temporal lobe. F-18 scanning must be performed interictally in seizure patients, as the 1.83-hour half-life of F-18 does not allow it to be held available for ictal scanning. Interictally, the seizure focus is usually hypometabolic. This is now thought to be caused by interruptions with adjacent neurons, which reduce neural activity and thus metabolism. Loss of neural connections can also result in decreased metabolism in more distant sites (diaschisis). Sites of temporal epilepsy are identified as hypometabolic foci in 70% of interictal scans, with a false-positive rate of only 5%. Dementia evaluation is performed predominantly to distinguish Alzheimer-type dementia from other types of dementia and from pseudodementia caused by depression. While the only unequivocal test remains brain biopsy, detection of Alzheimer disease (AD) is very reliable when applied to an appropriate population at risk. Patterns of activity with F-18-FDG are similar to those described for SPECT agents subsequently in this review.

The role of PET and SPECT scanning in evaluation of brain tumors has been discussed elsewhere and will not be repeated here. While PET is certainly a useful technique in each of these considerations, there are techniques available for SPECT imaging in each of these conditions that have similar sensitivity and specificity at decreased cost. Because both SPECT cameras and the appropriate imaging pharmaceuticals are more likely to occupy the predominant role in routine clinical application of functional brain imaging, with PET reserved for special circumstances. For this reason, the technique and interpretation of these studies are not discussed in detail. The interested reader is referred to one of the many excellent reviews available for PET brain imaging.

Single-Photon Emission Computed Tomography

Radiopharmaceuticals. Much of the early work in this area was performed with xenon-133. This inhaled gas dissolves in blood to an extent adequate for imaging. The rapidity of perfusion and diffusion of this agent makes rapid imaging essential. Therefore, multiple probe–type cameras have predominantly been employed. This tracer is not well suited to the rotating camera SPECT technique. For this reason, and because of difficulties in handling and recovering a gaseous agent, this agent has largely been superseded by other radiopharmaceuticals.

Iodinated amphetamines tagged with iodine-123 replaced radioxenon for a time. These agents readily cross the BBB. Both uptake and BBB diffusion are reversible. This agent, therefore, will slowly redistribute over time. Iodoamphetamine is also immediately sequestered by and slowly released from the lung. This effectively yields slow intra-arterial injection over a period of hours. Because of these phenomena, iodoamphetamine images represent integration of all brain activity from the time of injection until completion of imaging. Because iodine-123 is cyclotron produced and has a relatively short half-life (13.2 hours), availability has proven problematic. This agent also has been largely superseded and is no longer commercially available in the United States. Agents currently in widespread use include Tc-99m-HMPAO and Tc-99m-ECD.

Tc-99m-HMPAO is an agent of the chemical microsphere type. This agent crosses the BBB and is trapped within the brain substance. The mechanisms proposed for trapping have included change in the ionic state, binding to glutathione, and chemical decomposition. For purposes of scan interpretation, it is necessary to understand only that this agent essentially crosses the BBB irreversibly. Unlike iodinated amphetamine, this agent provides a "snapshot" of brain activity for a short period after injection (less than 10 minutes, with peak activity usually within 1 minute after IV injection). The HMPAO is available as a kit that is combined with the generator-produced, freshly eluted pertechnetate prior to use. Availability is thus not problematic. The initial form of this agent was unstable in aqueous solution. It had to be used within 30 minutes after preparation, which made quality control procedures difficult. A stabilized form is now available that can be used for 4 hours after aqueoust preparation.

Tc-99m-ECD is also an agent of the "chemical microsphere" type. This agent, unlike Tc-99m-HMPAO, does not localize in areas of luxury perfusion (Fig. 63.2). While there are a number of subtle differences between Tc-99m-ECD and Tc-99m-HMPAO, the remaining differences are not of routine clinical relevance. Tc-99m-ECD is stable in

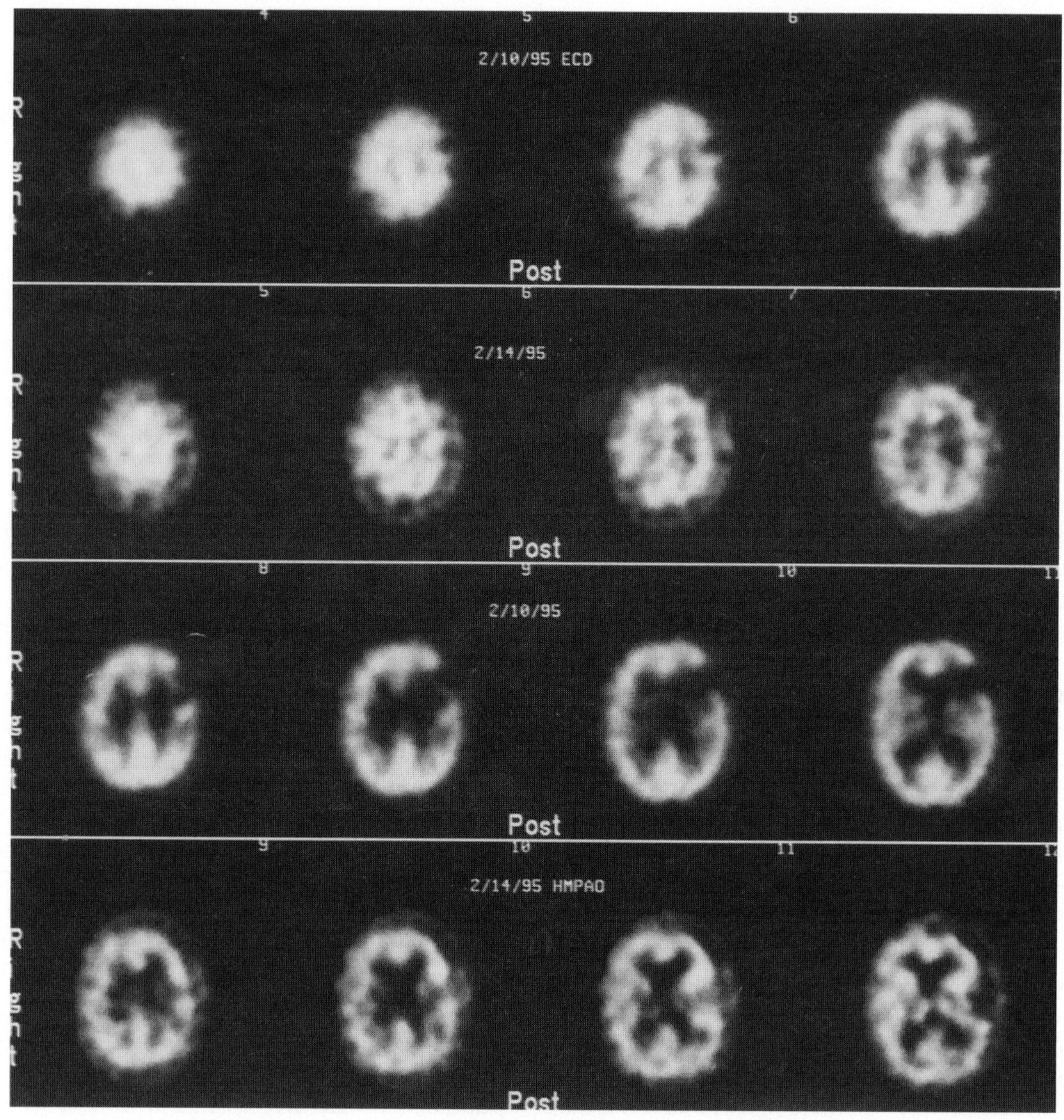

FIGURE 63.2. **(Color Plates) Ethyl Cysteinate Dimer (ECD) Versus Hexamethylpropyleneamine Oxime (HMPAO) in Luxury Perfusion.** Transverse axial images of technetium-99m (Tc-99m)-ECD on rows 1 and 3 and Tc-99m-HMPAO on rows 2 and 4. The photopenic defect in left frontal lobe on ECD imaging shows uptake on HMPAO imaging. This was a subacute stroke.

aqueous solution for at least 6 hours and is therefore preferable when attempting ictal injection and scanning of seizure disorders. This advantage is somewhat offset by a higher pharmaceutical cost. Both agents have their proponents and are in common use.

Technique. Brain-perfusion SPECT scans are preferably performed with a multi-detection rotating camera. A dual-head rotating camera can be employed, but single-head cameras are not generally recommended at this time. Cameras limited to brain work are not generally necessary because of improvements in equipment since the first edition of this book, although they may be useful in practices with a large brain scanning referral base. High-resolution collimators should be employed. The key issues for dual imaging are distance from the brain to the detector head and total counts acquired. One should try to achieve the smallest possible radius of rotation camera while remaining cognizant of patient comfort and safety.

Prior to the procedure, the physician should review history, the recorded neurologic physical examination, and the mini mental status examination if available. Historical data of importance include symptoms and duration; history of stroke, head injury, or seizure; any medications (especially psychotropic anticonvulsants); and whether CT or MR scans have been performed. The neurologic examination should include cognitive and motor examination and cranial nerve examination. The mental status examination should address orientation, registration, attention, recall and language functions.

The scanning agent is injected with a patient in a controlled resting state. This usually involves a supine, resting patient with closed eyes in a quiet room (or a room with white noise) and indirect lighting (see procedure guidelines). Alternatively, tracer can be injected during seizure ictus or acute stroke. The IV line should be established in advance, and all instructions and questions should be dealt with prior to injection to avoid unintended stimulation of brain activity. The patient should remain in this controlled environment for at least 5 minutes after injection. Injection of 15 to 30 mCi of Tc-99m-HMPAO or Tc-99m-ECD should be employed (0.2 to 0.3 mCi/Kg in pediatric patients). A delay after injection of no less than 60 minutes and preferably 90 minutes should be employed with Tc-99m-HMPAO to allow for background clearance. No less than 10 minutes and preferably 60 minutes should elapse before Tc-99m-ECD imaging with SPECT. Quality control on the radiopharmaceutical should be performed prior to injection, according to the package insert. Careful patient monitoring is mandatory throughout the scan, since patients considered for the study often have dementia, neurologic dysfunction, stroke, psychiatric disease, or another condition that requires monitoring.

If sedation is required, it should be given after injection of the radiopharmaceutical if at all possible. Attention to medications is critical, since both the presence of and withdrawal from (prescription and illicit) drugs can affect biodistribution of the tracer within the brain. ECD or stabilized HMPAO should be prepared in advance if ictal scanning is to be attempted. The patient must be monitored carefully and continuously with IV catheter in place and ready availability of agent nearby and injected very rapidly after seizure onset, since generalization of seizure focus can occur very rapidly. To deploy properly, the nursing staff need to perform the injection and thus must be trained in radiation safety and proper handling of radiopharmaceuticals.

Acetazolamide (Diamox) is employed to assess vasodilatory reserve, as it is a cerebrovascular-specific vasodilator. It should be given as a slow IV push over 5 minutes at about 20 minutes prior to radiotracer injection. The typical dosage is 1,000 mg for adults and 14 mg/kg for children. This agent is contraindicated for patients with known sulfa drug allergy, history of complicated migraine headache, or within 3 days of acute stroke. It rarely may cause postural hypotension, increasing the need for monitoring when arising from the scanning table. Dipyridamole and adenosine have also been used to assess vascular reserve but are not in routine use. All patients should void immediately prior to imaging to improve comfort. This is especially important when using acetazolamide, which is a mild diuretic.

Processing and Interpretation. Filtering should be performed in all three dimensions. A low-pass filter is generally recommended, typically a Butterworth. Other filters can be used, but spatially varying filters may create artifacts, particularly in low-count studies. The whole brain should be reconstructed, taking care to include the vertex and cerebellum. Any summing of data should occur only after reconstruction at single pixel slices. Attenuation correction should always be performed in intact skulls and the data should be evaluated in three orthogonal planes. It is also important to evaluate the raw data for acquisition errors. These should be evaluated on rotating display to check for patient motion during acquisition, which can also create serious artifacts. Rigorous quality control is required for all these as well as other SPECT studies. Averaged slices should approach the full width at half maximum of the device. It is worthwhile to reconstruct the transaxial plane images along the anterior/posterior commissural line. A typical normal study is demonstrated in Fig. 63.3.

In interpretation, it is important that background subtraction not be excessive and that a continuous color scale (or a continuous gray scale) be employed to avoid artifactual edges. The range of normal should be considered in rendering an opinion, and one should use a normal database that is specific to the radiopharmaceutical employed. Correlation with clinical data is required. Any regional perfusion defects should also be correlated with the locations of any CT or MR abnormalities. This is substantially easier if some type of fusion imaging (overlay of anatomic and functional images with or without the use of fiduciary markers) is employed, but it can be performed visually. The extent and severity of defects should be reported.

The recommendations for image acquisition, processing, and interpretation conform generally and specifically to the recommendations of the Brain Imaging Council of the Society of Nuclear Medicine in place at the time this chapter was written. Readers are encouraged to check the current guidelines prior to initiating a brain imaging program (www.snm.org).

Indications. According to the American Academy of Neurology (AAN), the established indications for these techniques are confirmation of AD, presurgical ictal identification of seizure foci, and evaluation of acute brain ischemia. Most nuclear medicine physicians in clinical practice would consider brain death evaluation to be an established indication for planar brain scans. Areas considered promising by the AAN are determination of stroke subtypes, assessment of vasospasm following subarachnoid hemorrhage, and (nonictal) localization of seizure foci. Therapeutic options for these disorders, including medical or interventional, are available. The expansion of research into use of brain SPECT in psychiatric disorders, where therapeutic options are broad but objective

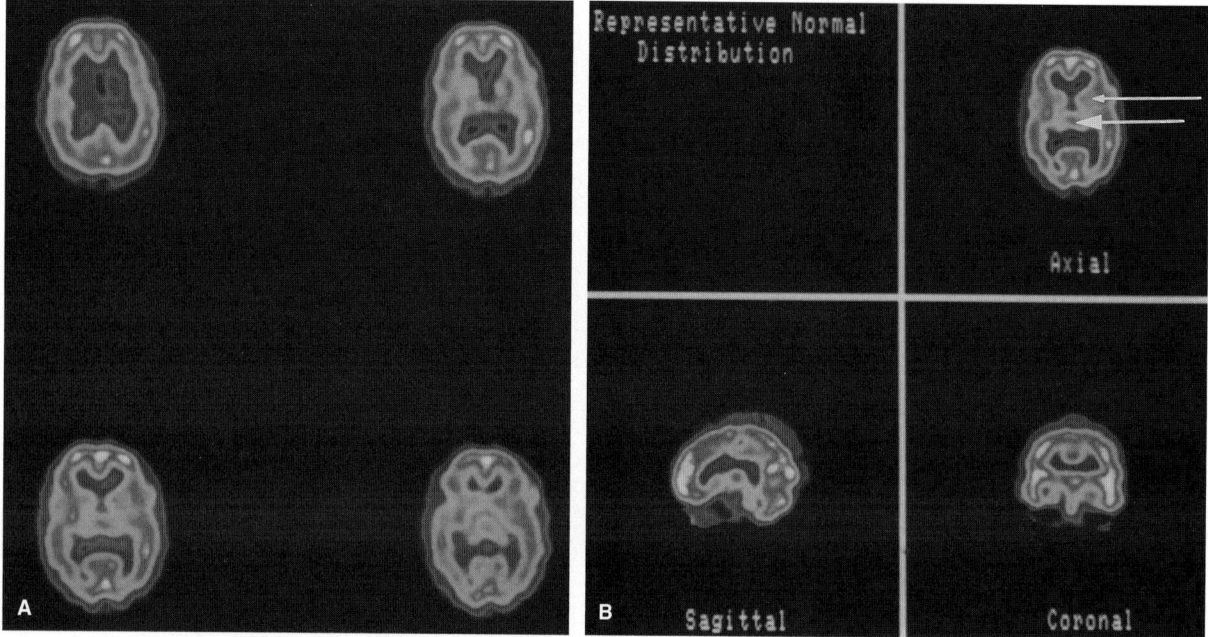

FIGURE 63.3. **(Color Plates) Normal Hexamethylpropyleneamine Oxime (HMPAO) Study.** Selected images from a normal technetium-99m-HMPAO study. **A.** Axial images. **B.** Representative central images in three standard planes (axial, sagittal, and coronal to the long axis of the brain). The large arrow indicates the brainstem; the small arrow indicates the basal ganglia. With modern equipment, it should be possible to routinely obtain scans that resolve the gyri, basal ganglia, and brainstem. Interpreters should consult an atlas to familiarize themselves with the normal distribution of radiotracer in the brain structures.

evaluation of biologic aspects of the diseases is extremely weak, is promising but as yet not validated. The remainder of the discussion will be limited primarily to the accepted indications, with brief discussion of other applications considered promising, applications to presurgical planning (balloon occlusion test and Wada test), and testing of vascular reserve.

Applications for brain SPECT include the following.

Stroke and Ischemia. The extent of stroke can be determined a short time after its occurrence with functional brain scanning (Figs. 63.4, 63.5). Imaging with Tc-99m-ECD has demonstrated a specificity of 98% and sensitivity of 86% for localization of acute strokes. This contrasts with several hours for standard MR and CT, although MR molecular diffusion imaging has allowed improved assessment of strokes acutely. Therapeutic administration of tissue plasminogen activator is effective, but the time between initial onset and therapy is critical. The time of onset must be established and hemorrhagic stroke excluded prior to administration of tissue plasminogen activator. CT is employed to rapidly exclude hemorrhage, and administration is begun as soon thereafter as possible. Functional imaging has not been widely employed on the theoretical basis that it would delay therapy when stroke has already been confirmed clinically. Therapy of acute stroke has otherwise been limited to anticoagulation and supportive care. Anticoagulation requires only exclusion of hemorrhage, which is best accomplished with CT.

The use of functional imaging to evaluate for ischemia caused by vasospasm after subarachnoid hemorrhage is in widespread use. Vasospasm of clinical impact occurs in 30% of patients with subarachnoid hemorrhage (Fig. 63.6). SPECT brain imaging in association with neurologic examination and transcranial Doppler artery narrowing assessment allows effective noninvasive monitoring and early intervention. Because there are multiple potential therapies (hyperdynamic hypertension, hemodilution and hypovolemia, calcium-channel blockers, microballoon cerebral angioplasty, intra-arterial papaverine), which require definitive diagnosis, this technique has significant clinical use.

In patients with ischemic stroke, a nearly normal brain SPECT study may be an indication of lacunar infarction. Using this criterion, SPECT was 69% sensitive and 100% specific in identifying a lacunar stroke. High-resolution SPECT has the potential to image lacunar strokes as well. Early differentiation of the mechanism is important, since embolic disease should prompt cardiac evaluation for a source and consideration of anticoagulant therapy. Prediction of prognosis after stroke or transient ischemic attack (TIA) is another area of likely application. Lesion volume correlates with early outcome in acute stroke, and large,

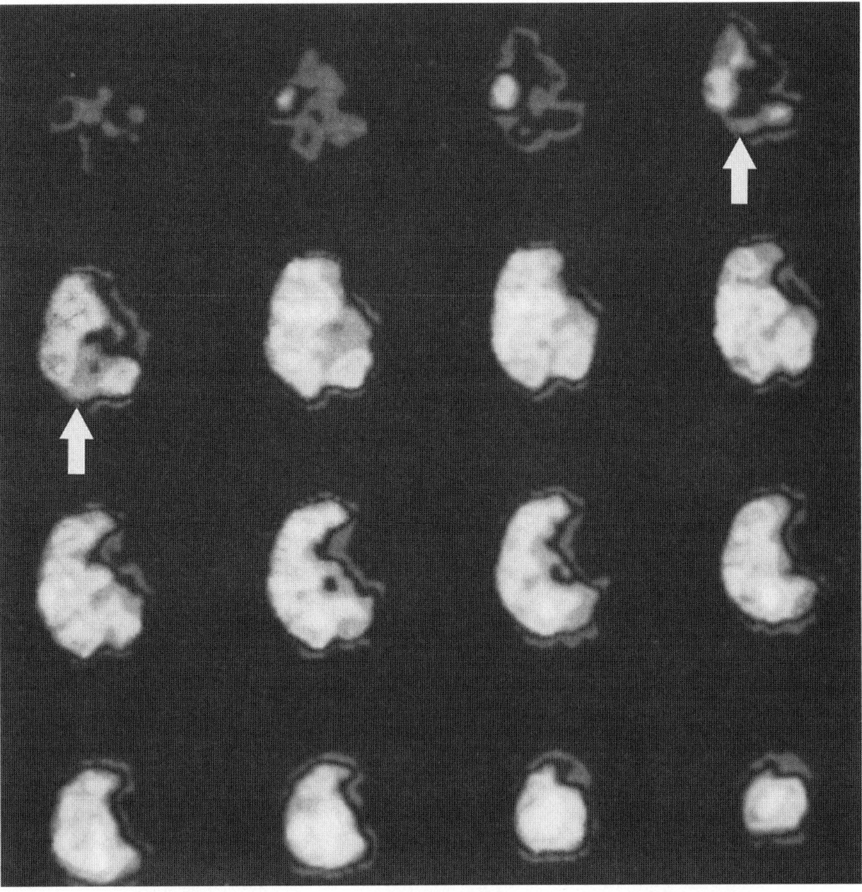

FIGURE 63.4. **(Color Plates) Cerebral Infarction.** Transaxial images reformatted into the plane of the orbitomeatal line (standard CT format) from a iodine-123-iofetamine scan show a large region of absent perfusion (*arrows*) in the distribution of the left middle cerebral artery after cerebral infarction. Note the decreased cerebellar activity on the side opposite the infarct (*arrow*), an example of crossed cerebellar diaschisis. This phenomenon results from decreased right cerebellar metabolism caused by decreased neuronal communication between the right cerebellum and the infarcted portion of the left cerebral hemisphere. (All iofetamine images in this chapter were obtained during phase III trials of the agent under approved protocol. Modern equipment allows significant improvement in resolution.)

severe perfusion defects are predictive of nonnutritive perfusion. After TIA, a prolonged deficit on functional scanning with brain SPECT predicts a high likelihood of ischemic stroke in the period following the TIA.

In the early phase of cerebrovascular compromise, blood flow is maintained through autoregulated vasodilatation, leading to an increase in blood volume. As the compensatory capacity of autoregulation is exceeded, blood flow falls, while oxygen metabolism is maintained, corresponding to an increase in oxygen extraction fraction (the beginning of misery perfusion). Once oxygen extraction fraction has increased maximally, continued decline in blood flow leads to a decline in oxygen delivery and metabolism (the onset of ischemia). Severe and prolonged compromise results in infarction of brain tissue, with decreased demand for oxygen metabolism, while vasodilatation persists, leading to a decline in oxygen extraction fraction (and onset of "luxury perfusion"). As revascularization occurs, blood flow to the region increases and the infarcted area typically remains in a state of luxury perfusion for days to weeks.

By judicious use of acetazolamide to test vasodilatory reserve of the cerebral vessels, it is possible to perform the equivalent of pharmacologic coronary stress imaging for cerebral vessels. Studies with and without acetazolamide may provide information on the mechanism of ischemia. These studies may also be useful in presurgical planning when carotid surgery or intracranial/extracranial bypass surgery is contemplated, because they can indicate the physiologic significance of an anatomic vascular lesion. Interpretation of these studies depends on identification of a significant area of relatively decreased perfusion (actually indicating increased perfusion in the unaffected portions of the brain) after stimulation that was not present on the study without stimulation, which would indicate impaired vasodilatory reserve (Fig. 63.7). This is exactly analogous to evaluation of coronary artery reserve with dipyridamole or adenosine stress imaging, as discussed in Chapter 57. Ramsay et al used a combination of acetazolamide and cerebral Tc-99m-HMPAO to demonstrate reduction in cerebral blood flow reserve, which improved after carotid endarterectomy in 45% of selected patients with unilateral ICA stenosis.

As with coronary studies, evaluation of clinical data, accurate registration of images, and comparison to a radiopharmaceutical-specific normal database are important.

Injection during vascular occlusion of a carotid artery can test cross-circulation across the circle of Willis, demonstrating the precise areas of decreased perfusion

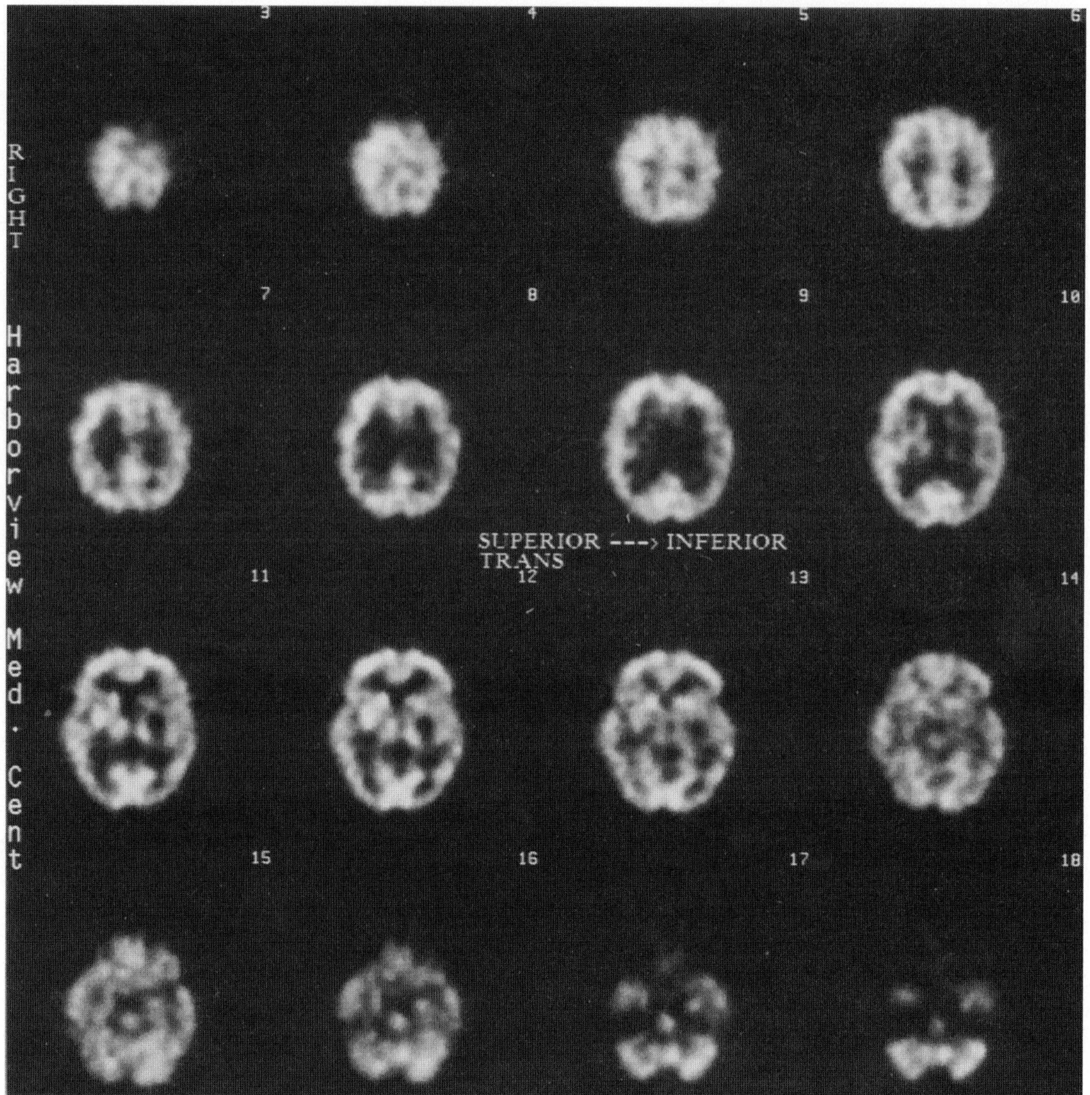

FIGURE 63.5. **(Color Plates) Subcortical Cerebral Infarct.** Transverse axial images of technetium-99m ethyl cysteinate dimer in patient with acute stroke shows absence of uptake in the left lenticular nucleus.

during occlusion. This is the nuclear medicine version of the Matas test (Fig. 63.8). The distribution of amobarbital injected for localization of speech and memory functions (the Wada test) may also be assessed accurately using functional agents as tracers.

Dementia. The most important use for PET imaging in the workup of the dementia patient is to aid in making an accurate diagnosis as early in the course of AD as possible and, a review by Silverman concluded that F-18-FDG PET appears to supersede SPECT in this area. It can be diagnosed with an accuracy of approximately 80% with functional SPECT brain scans. In patients with AD of varying severity, the magnitude and extent of hypometabolism correlate with the severity of the dementia symptoms. Usually, there are only minor decreases in the parietal lobes in patients with early mild AD. Moderately affected patients show significantly decreased metabolism in the left midfrontal lobes, bilateral parietal lobes, and the superior temporal regions. In patients with severe AD, the same regions are affected, but the hypometabolism is much more pronounced, with sparing only of the sensorimotor, visual, and subcortical areas. The typical pattern is decreased activity in parietal and posterior temporal regions bilaterally but often asymmetrically (Fig. 63.9). The characteristic AD radiotracer distribution pattern is similar for SPECT and PET imaging. The classic bilateral temporoparietal defect of AD can also be seen in other conditions, including carbon monoxide poisoning, hypoglycemia, mitochondrial encephalomyelopathy, severe Parkinson disease, and diffuse Lewy body dementias (DLBD). The relatively recent development of several pharmaceuticals for AD provides an important area for PET imaging. For example, patients

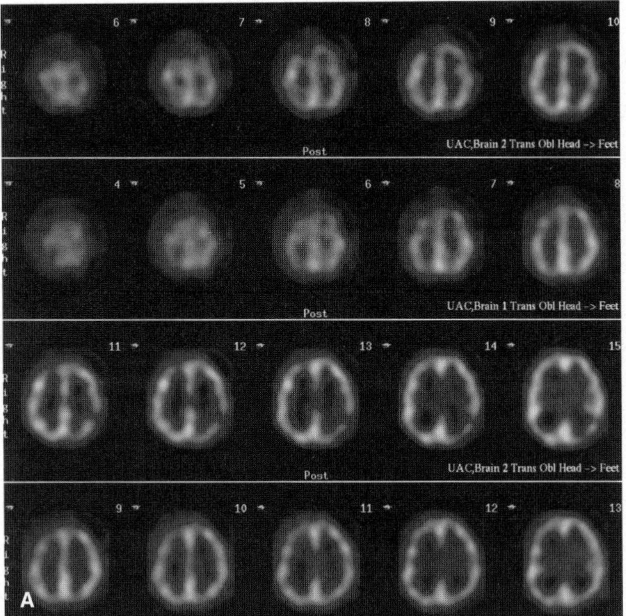

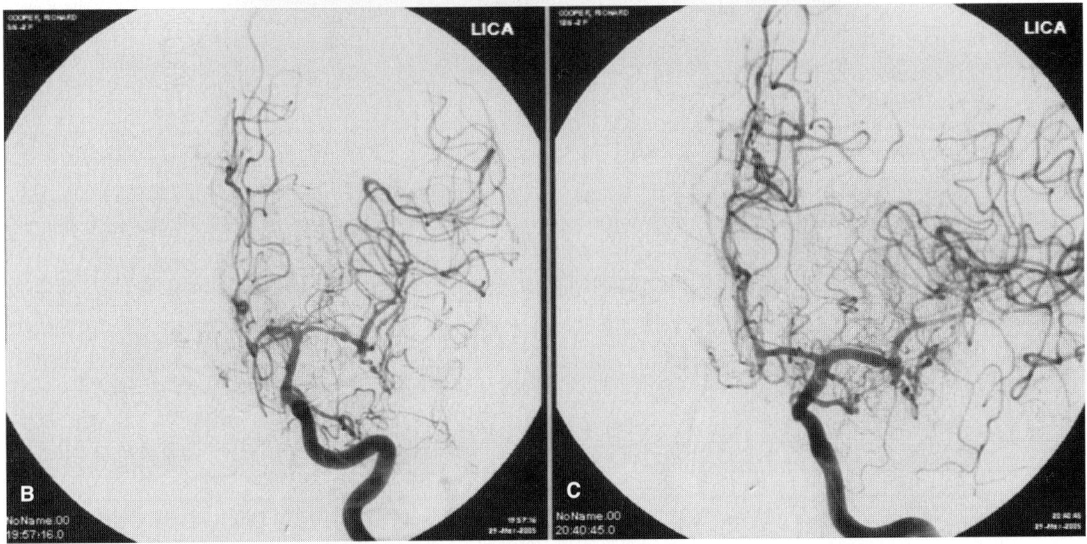

FIGURE 63.6. **(Color Plates) Subarachnoid Hemorrhage and Cerebral Vasospasm. A.** Transverse axial images of technetium-99m ethyl cysteinate dimer show baseline scan on rows 2 and 4 and scan during vasospasm on rows 1 and 3. New defect is seen in left hemisphere in the posterior frontoparietal cortex corresponding to ischemia from vasospasm. **B.** Angiogram of left internal carotid artery shows vasospasm in the midportion of the left middle cerebral artery. **C.** Angiogram of left internal carotid artery shows resolution of vasospasm after percutaneous transluminal micro-balloon angioplasty.

treated with donepezil were found to have relatively stable cerebral metabolism at 24 weeks compared with a placebo group, which showed a 10% decline.

Frontotemporal lobe degeneration (including the subtype Pick disease, which is associated with cognitive and language dysfunction and behavioral changes) can generally be differentiated from AD. Frontotemporal lobe degeneration is classically associated with frontotemporal perfusion defects on brain SPECT. Again, the pattern is not specific to this group of diseases (depression, alcoholism, schizophrenia, Pick disease, severe AD, and progressive supranuclear palsy form the differential). Vascular dementias can result in defects in any portion of the brain and can coexist with AD in a proportion of the elderly. Further complicating the picture is an increasing tendency for nonspecific defects to occur in older patients, especially as a result of sulcal enlargement owing to brain atrophy. The evaluation of dementia is, therefore, not a simple task and

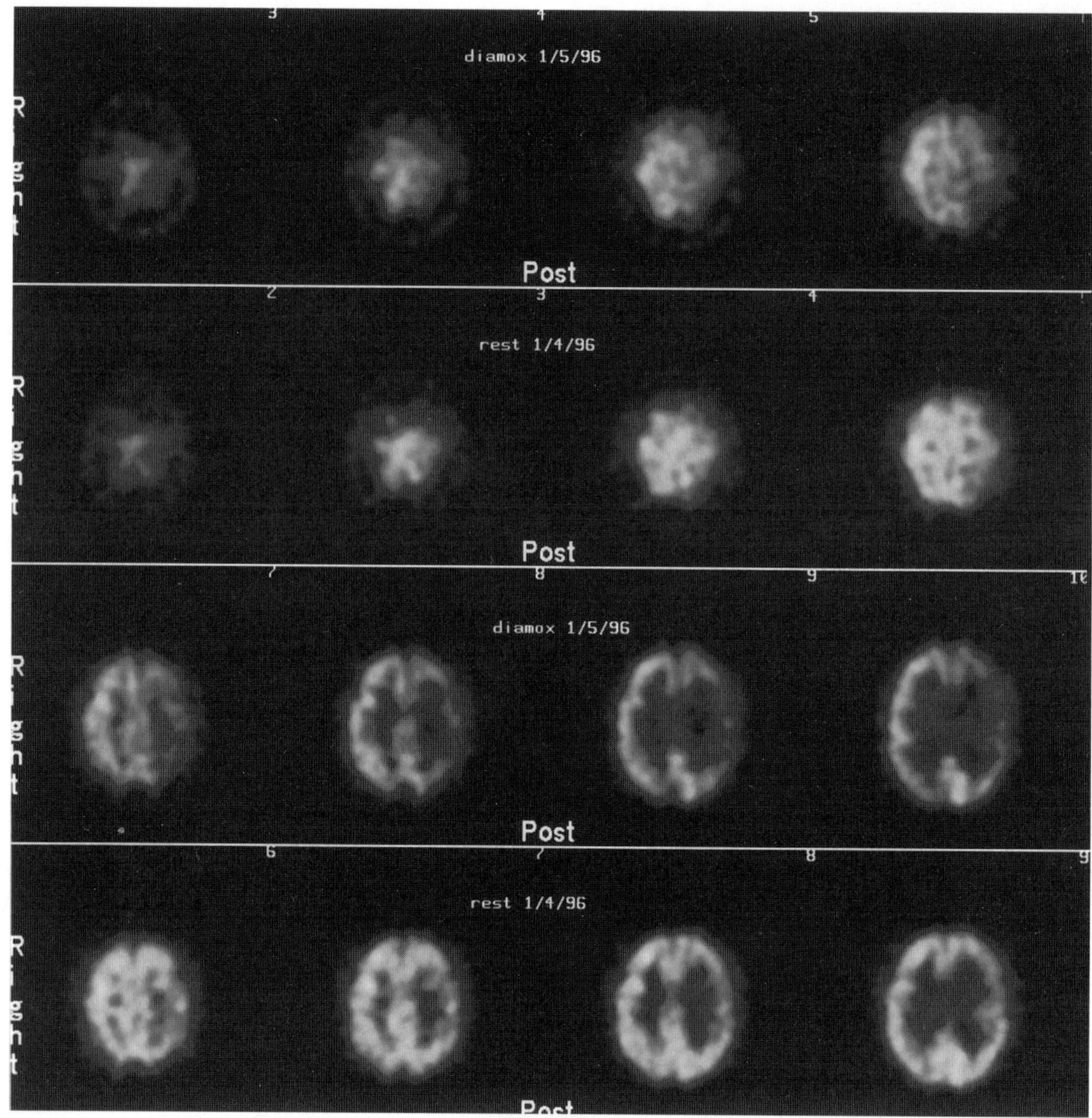

FIGURE 63.7. **(Color Plates) Acetazolamide Vascular Reserve Testing in Occlusive Carotid Disease.** Transverse axial images of technetium-99m ethyl cysteinate dimer with acetazolamide on rows 1 and 3 and at rest on rows 2 and 4. Images show decreased uptake in the left hemisphere with acetazolamide, which improves largely at rest. This finding indicates exhausted vasodilatory reserve in the left hemisphere corresponding to left internal carotid artery occlusion.

should require anatomic as well as functional imaging; it is recommended that quantitative analysis software be employed for corroboration. The use of quantitative software techniques (Fig. 63.10) has aided the visual interpretation and accuracy of dementing diseases and has helped to identify hypoperfusion or hypometabolism of the posterior cingulate gyrus and parietal precuneus as the earliest findings in AD.

A negative PET scan indicated that pathologic progression of cognitive impairment during the mean 3-year follow-up was unlikely to occur. There is substantial clinical overlap between elderly patients with AD, vascular dementia, and pseudodementia caused by depression. Thus, having scans that can help in the differential diagnosis is quite important. The therapeutic options (such as cholinesterase inhibitors in the recent past and now glutamate regulators) for treating AD have been slowly emerging and have had some clinical benefits in the last decade.

DLBD, which is characterized by visual hallucination, fluctuating cognitive decline, and Parkinsonian symptoms, has been reported to be the second most common type of degenerative dementia, accounting for up to 20% of all dementia cases at autopsy. SPECT findings include temporoparietal hypoperfusion similar to that seen in AD patients and occipital lobe hypoperfusion. Occipital hypometabolism (or hypoperfusion)

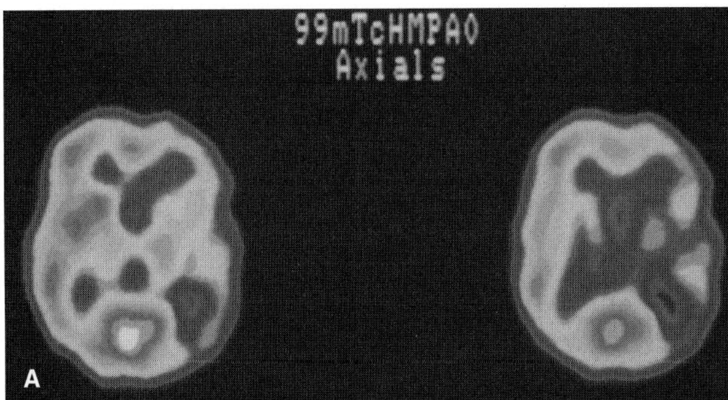

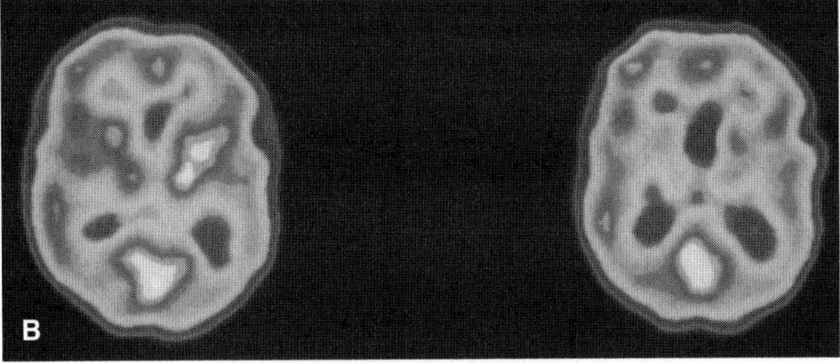

FIGURE 63.8. **(Color Plates) Positive Balloon Occlusion Study.** This patient was asymptomatic after inflation of a left carotid artery balloon, but images show decreased regional blood flow in the left middle cerebral artery distribution **(A).** Baseline study **(B)** shows normal tracer distribution. If occlusion study had been normal, the baseline images would be omitted. The radiopharmaceutical is technetium-99m hexamethylpropyleneamine oxime.

measured by PET and SPECT yielded differential diagnostic accuracy of probable DLBD from probable AD with sensitivity and specificity of 92%. Similarly, hypometabolism in the primary visual cortex differentiated probable DLBD from probable AD with 86% sensitivity and 91% specificity. An MR study indicated that absence of medial temporal atrophy could separate DLBD from AD or vascular dementia with specificities of 100% and 88% respectively, but sensitivity was only 38%.

Vascular disease contributing to dementia, which is potentially reversible, can be unmasked by administration of acetazolamide with SPECT and compared against anatomic imaging, suggesting vascular disease. In multi-infarct dementia, patients typically present abruptly with a history of prior stroke and hypertension. Generally speaking, multiple perfusion deficits are evident that may be equivalent or more extensive than the findings on an MR scan. The likelihood of development of etiologically specific therapies for at least some dementias remains high, making continued investigation of diagnostic techniques of utmost importance. Follow-up scans improve sensitivity and specificity by demonstrating an appropriate pattern of progression in true dementias.

Seizure Disorders. The seizure disorder most commonly referred for medical imaging is the patient with a temporal lobe syndrome, typically complex partial seizures. Interictally, seizure foci tend to have decreased activity, and increased activity is seen with ictus (Fig. 63.11). In simplistic terms, focal neuronal loss or damage results in a local phenomenon similar to diaschisis. Because of secondary activation and spread of the seizure foci, it is difficult to pinpoint the exact seizure focus unless injection can be made early during the seizure. This should be confirmed by video/electroencephalogram (EEG) review. However, ictal SPECT may identify seizure foci, which are not identified by MR, and is especially useful in epileptogenic cortical developmental disorders, where EEG often fails to find the epileptogenic focus. An ictal SPECT study showing an area of increased regional blood flow, which may correspond to an area of decreased regional blood flow on interictal SPECT, is strong evidence for an epileptogenic

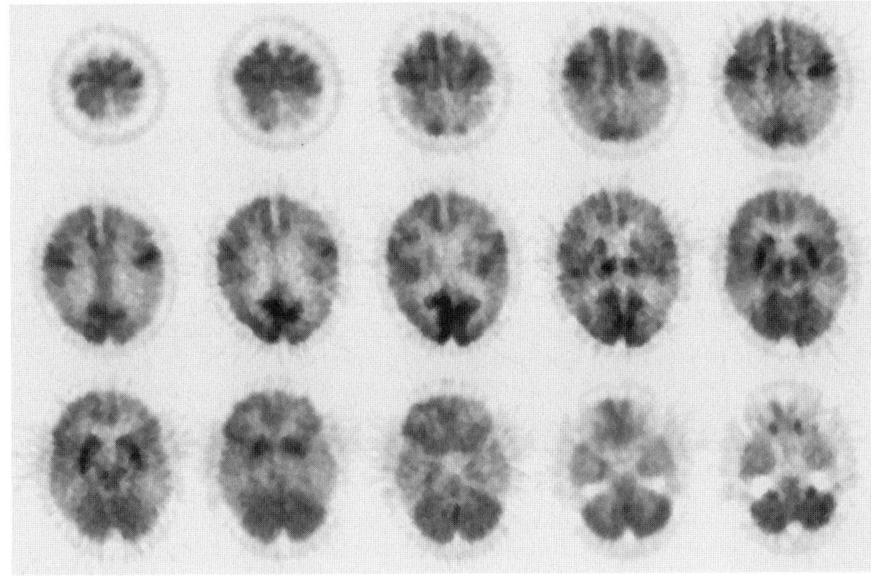

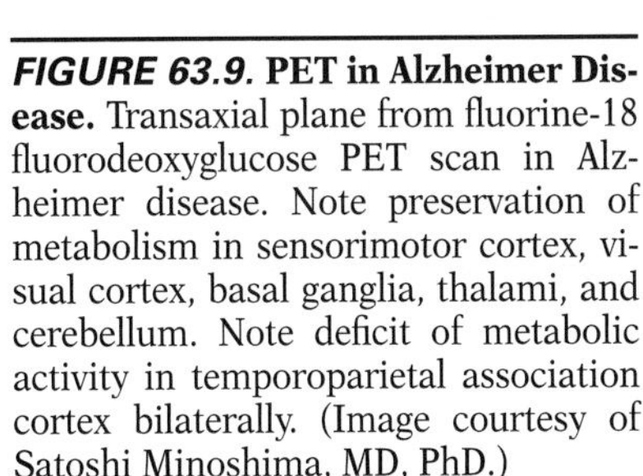

FIGURE 63.9. **PET in Alzheimer Disease.** Transaxial plane from fluorine-18 fluorodeoxyglucose PET scan in Alzheimer disease. Note preservation of metabolism in sensorimotor cortex, visual cortex, basal ganglia, thalami, and cerebellum. Note deficit of metabolic activity in temporoparietal association cortex bilaterally. (Image courtesy of Satoshi Minoshima, MD, PhD.)

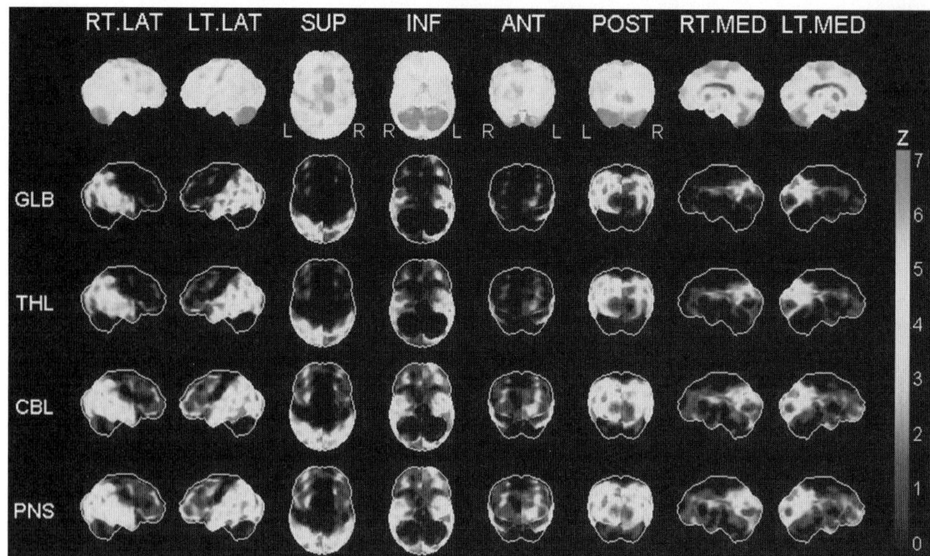

FIGURE 63.10. **(Color Plates) Three-dimensional SSP Display of SPECT in Alzheimer Disease.** Stereotactic three-surface projection display of Z-scores in brain SPECT in Alzheimer disease showing statistically significant decreases in perfusion in bilateral temporoparietal association cortices and also in posterior cingulate. GLB, THL, CBL, and PNS indicate that each corresponding row is normalized to global, thalamic, cerebellar, and pons uptake, respectively.

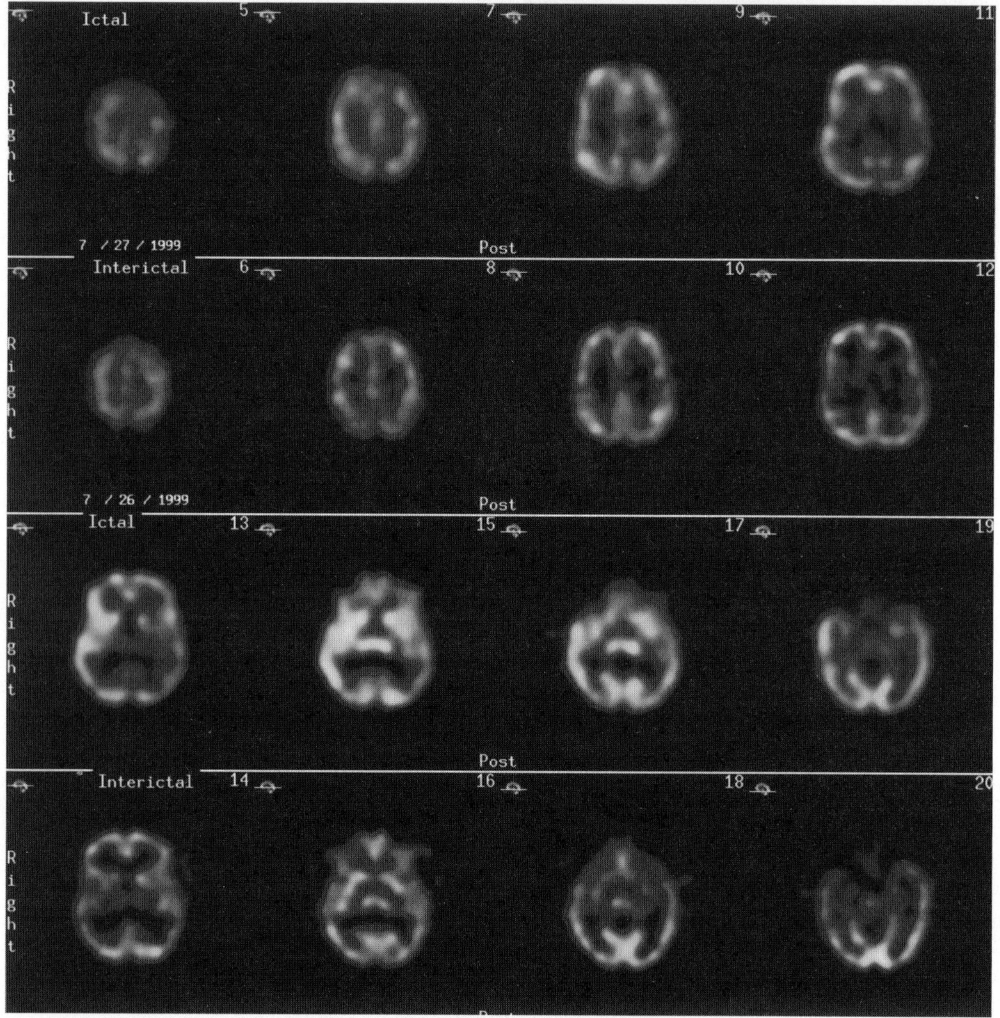

FIGURE 63.11. **(Color Plates) Ictal and Interictal SPECT Scans in Complex Partial Epilepsy.** Transverse axial images of technetium-99m ethyl cysteinate dimer injected with seizure ictus on rows 1 and 3 and also injected during interictal time period on rows 2 and 4. Ictal imaging shows increased uptake in the right hemisphere, which is predominantly in the right temporal lobe. Interictal imaging shows relatively decreased uptake in the right temporal lobe.

lesion. Ictal SPECT is reported to be more accurate than interictal SPECT and PET, with overall accuracy rates greater than 90%. In a group with structural lesions, the two techniques were shown to have comparable results. Both ictal SPECT and interictal PET have complementary roles where localization is difficult. If these findings also concur with the EEG findings and or CT/MR evidence of a lesion, the need for more invasive depth electrocorticography or intraoperative electrocorticography may be obviated or more accurately guided. For this indication, the technique will be applied mainly in larger referral centers that perform surgery for removal of the seizure foci.

When newer methods for analyzing PET images such as statistical parametric mapping were used to detect temporal interhemispheric asymmetry, hypometabolism was identified on the side chosen for resection in most cases (sensitivity, 71%; specificity, 100%) and was predictive of favorable postsurgical outcome in 90% of the patients. The findings from some studies have suggested that metabolic dysfunction of the thalamus ipsilateral to the seizure focus becomes more severe with long-standing temporal or frontal lobe epilepsy and also with secondary generalization of seizures.

FDG PET is also a sensitive and specific technique for investigating patients with seizures of probable frontal lobe origin, because many of these seizures begin in the medial or inferior aspects of the frontal lobe and scalp EEG readings do not provide adequate localization of foci. Performance of ictal PET studies is logistically impractical, primarily because of the relatively short half-life of the positron-emitting isotopes, such as F-18 or oxygen-15. Receptor PET imaging with carbon-11-flumazenil, although still investigational, may have a useful clinical role in patients with partial epilepsy who have normal or nondiagnostic FDG PET, in patients with bilateral FDG findings but unifocal seizure activity on EEG, and in patients after surgical resection who continue to have seizures. Excision of well-localized foci can lead to elimination of seizures or significantly improve pharmacologic control in 80% of surgical patients.

Viral encephalopathies can present a diagnostic imaging challenge. Launes et al reported abnormally increased accumulation of Tc-99m-HMPAO in the affected temporal lobe, even at an early stage of herpes simplex encephalopathy, when CT was normal.

Brain Tumors. PET can play an important role in the evaluation and management of patients with brain tumors, including the grading of tumors, determination of prognosis, and differentiation of recurrent tumor from radiation necrosis. The sensitivity for making the determination of radiation necrosis versus tumor recurrence may be as high as 86%, with a specificity as high as 56%. FDG studies have concluded that high-grade tumors are hypermetabolic, whereas low-grade tumors are hypometabolic. One distinction from this typology is

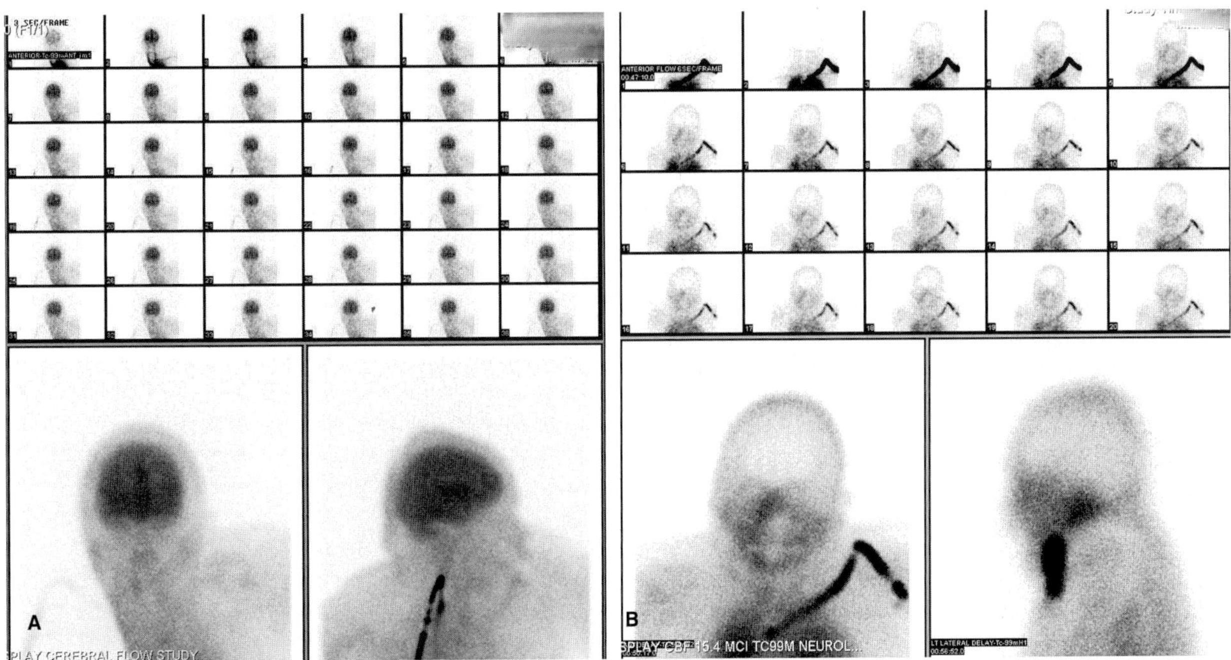

FIGURE 63.12. **Brain Perfusion Planar Scans for Brain Death. A.** Planar scan demonstrates uptake in brain parenchyma and therefore does not meet Society of Nuclear Medicine criteria for the corroboration of the clinical impression of brain death. **B.** Planar scan in another patient shows absence of uptake in brain and therefore does meet criteria for the corroboration of the clinical impression of brain death by total absence of cerebral blood flow.

juvenile pilocytic astrocytomas, which typically have a high glucose metabolism despite their benign nature. It should be noted that PET does not differentiate between primary lymphomas of the CNS, secondary tumors of the brain, or malignant gliomas, because all of these may be hypermetabolic.

Brain Trauma. SPECT brain imaging has been proposed to confirm the presence of a focal or diffuse injury in patients with persistent symptoms after trauma but normal or nondiagnostic anatomic imaging studies. The increased sensitivity of functional SPECT relative to CT or MR favors this use and is supported by the procedure guidelines for SPECT using brain perfusion radiopharmaceuticals (www.snm.org).

Brain Death. Criteria for Tc-99m brain perfusion radiopharmaceutical planar scanning have been retrospectively validated. Brain perfusion agents have advantages over conventional agents such as Tc-99m-GH or Tc-99m-DTPA, are less dependent on the quality of bolus injection, are easier to interpret, and allow evaluation of posterior fossa blood flow. Radionuclide cerebral angiography without brain perfusion radiopharmaceuticals requires rapid acquisition of dynamic images in technically challenging situations, cannot image flow in posterior fossae, and may result in difficult or equivocal interpretation.

Radionuclide scintigraphy is not affected by drug intoxication, hypothermia, or hypovolemia. In the presence of brain death, the radioactive bolus stops at the base of the skull because of increased intracranial pressure. It is important to have a good bolus injection, and if distinct activity is not identified in the common carotid artery, the injection should be repeated. Absence of intracerebral arterial flow and no visualization of major venous sinuses on subsequent static images fit the nuclear medicine criteria for brain death (Fig. 63.12). The "hot nose sign," caused by increased collateral blood flow in the nasal area, could be a secondary sign in brain death.

SUGGESTED READINGS

Alexandrov AV, Black SE, Ehrlich LE, et al. Simple visual analysis of brain perfusion on HMPAO SPECT predicts early outcome in acute stroke. Stroke 1996;27:1537–1542.

Assessment of brain SPECT: report of the Therapeutics and Technology Assessment Subcommittee of the American Academy of Neurology. Neurology 1996;46:278–285.

Bonte FJ, Harris TS, Roney CA, Hynan LS. Differential diagnosis between Alzheimer's and frontotemporal disease by posterior cingulate sign. J Nucl Med 2004;45(5):771–774.

Conti PS. Introduction to imaging brain tumor metabolism with positron emission tomography (PET). Cancer Invest 1995;13:244–259.

Chiro D, Ommaya AK, et al. Isotope cisternography in the diagnosis and follow-up of cerebrospinal fluid rhinorrhea. J Neurosurg 1968;28:522–529.

Drzezga A, Arnold S, Minoshima S, et al. F-18 FDG PET studies in patients with extratemporal and temporal epilepsy: evaluation of an observer-independent analysis. J Nucl Med 1999;40(5):737–746.

Harbert JC. Radionuclide cisternography. Semin Nucl Med 1971;1:90–106.

Hartshorne ME. Positron emission tomography. In Orrison WW, Lewine JD, Sanders JA, Hartshorne MF, eds. Functional Brain Imaging. St. Louis, MO: Mosby, 1995:187–212.

Hustinx R, Pourdehnad M, Kaschten B, Alavi A. PET imaging for differentiating recurrent brain tumor from radiation necrosis. Radiol Clin North Am 2005;43(1):35–47.

Idea RJ, Lewis DH. Timely diagnosis of brain death in an emergency trauma center. AJR Am J Roentgenol 1994;163:927–928.

Launes J, Nikkinen P, Lindroth L, et al. Diagnosis of acute herpes simplex encephalitis by brain perfusion single photon emission computed tomography. Lancet 1988;1(8596):1188–1191.

Lewis DH, Hsu S, Eskridge J, et al. Brain SPECT and transcranial Doppler ultrasound in vasospasm-induced delayed cerebral ischemia after subarachnoid hemorrhage. J Stroke Cerebrovasc Dis 1992;2:12–21.

Messa C, Fazio F, Costa DC, Ell PJ. Clinical brain radionuclide imaging studies. Semin Nucl Med 1995;15:111–143.

Minoshima S, Foster N, Sima AA, Frey KA, Albin RL, Kuhl DE. Alzheimer's disease versus dementia with Lewy bodies: cerebral metabolic distinction with autopsy confirmation. Ann Neurol 2001;50(3):358–365.

Moretti JL, Caglar M, Weinmann P. Cerebral perfusion imaging tracers for SPECT: which one to choose? J Nucl Med 1995;36:359–363.

Mrhac L, Zakko S, Parikh Y. Brain death: the evaluation of semi-quantitative parameters and other signs in HMPAO scintigraphy. Nucl Med Commun 1995;16:1016–1020.

O'Connell RA. Psychiatric disorders. In Van Heertum RL, Tikofsky RS, eds. Cerebral SPECT Imaging. 2nd ed. New York: Raven Press, 1995.

Silverman DH. Brain 18F-FDG PET in the diagnosis of neurodegenerative dementias: comparison with perfusion SPECT and with clinical evaluations lacking nuclear imaging. J Nucl Med 2004;45(4):594–607.

Silverman DH, Alavi A. PET imaging in the assessment of normal and impaired cognitive function. Radiol Clin North Am 2005;43(1):67–77.

Silverman DH, Small GW, Chang CY, et al. Positron emission tomography in evaluation of dementia. JAMA 2001;86(17):2120–2127.

Society of Nuclear Medicine Brain Imaging Council. Ethical clinical practice of functional brain imaging. J Nucl Med 1996;37:1256–1259.

Vernet O, Farmer JP, Lambert R, Montes JL. Radionuclide shuntogram: adjunct to manage hydrocephalic patients. J Nucl Med 1996;37:406–410.

Chapter 64

Positron Emission Tomography

Bijan Bijan, David K. Shelton, and William E. Brant

Oncologic PET Imaging

Neurologic PET Imaging

Cardiac PET Imaging

PET Imaging in Inflammation and Infection

Pitfalls in PET-CT

PET imaging is the basis of molecular imaging in today's clinical practice. The new hybrid imaging instrument, PET-CT (PET plus CT), combines anatomic and physiologic imaging and opens a door to a new era in radiology and nuclear medicine. Currently the clinical applications of PET imaging are focused in four main areas: (*1*) oncology, comprising about 80% of the current practice of clinical PET; (*2*) neurologic applications (Alzheimer disease, epilepsy); (*3*) cardiac applications (coronary artery disease, myocardial viability); and (*4*) infection and inflammation imaging (fever of unknown origin, immunocompromised patients). With the expanding approval of reimbursement of PET for more indications, the number of PET scanners has increased dramatically throughout the United States.

PET Instrumentation. PET imaging is based upon positron emitters, which are used as labelling tracers for metabolic molecules. Positron-emitting radionuclides include fluorine-18 (F-18), nitrogen-13 (N-13), oxygen-15 (O-15), carbon-11 (C-11), and rubidium-82 (Rb-82). Current clinical PET imaging is based on F-18, an unstable radioisotope with a half-life of 109 minutes that is produced in a cyclotron. Its relatively short half-life requires that imaging be performed within relatively short transit proximity to a cyclotron. Other positron emitters have even shorter half-lives (75 seconds to 20 minutes) and must be imaged at the cyclotron site within minutes of their production. F-18 decay releases a positron, which has the same mass as an electron but is positively charged. Within milliseconds of emission, the positron annihilates with a nearby electron to release two high-energy (511 keV) γ-ray photons. These photons move apart in opposite directions (a near 180° angle). Because of their high energy, these photons are highly penetrative in soft tissue and therefore leave the body with limited absorption or deflection.

The PET imaging system consists of a ring of scintillation detectors set to detect coincident photons that strike the detectors within a very narrow time window. Noncoincident, mostly scattered, photons are rejected from the data set. Simultaneous detection of two 511-keV photons by any two detectors indicates that an annihilation event has occurred somewhere in the column of space between the two detectors. These raw data projections are reconstructed into cross-sectional images by algorithms similar to those used in CT and MR. PET scans viewed alone provide limited morphologic detail and can be difficult to interpret. Spatial resolution of current PET systems is 4 to 5 mm. Systems under development improve spatial resolution to 2 mm.

Recently developed hybrid instruments combine PET scanners with CT scanners. CT provides excellent anatomic detail but lacks functional information. PET provides metabolic measurements and functional information but lacks precise morphology. The union of the two allows correlation of complementary findings into a single comprehensive examination. A typical PET-CT scanner consists of a PET scanner immediately adjacent to a multidetector CT scanner. A patient couch, accurately calibrated for position, runs through both scanning assemblies. Scans may be obtained from either instrument independently or from both simultaneously. Computer software is used to fuse the two sets of images into composite images.

Attenuation correction must be applied to PET images. Attenuation of either of the paired photons by absorption or scatter would result in rejection of data and nondetection of annihilation events. Attenuation is increased when the origin of the photons is from deeper within the body because of the greater thickness of intervening soft tissues. Correspondingly, attenuation is less in the thorax because of the air-filled lungs than in the abdomen or pelvis. The CT transmission data is used to create an attenuation map that is applied to the PET images to compensate for attenuation defects. The attenuation correction process increases sensitivity for detection of positron activity, but it may introduce artifacts into the images. Therefore PET interpretation includes viewing of both attenuation-corrected and attenuation-uncorrected PET image.

The F-18 radioisotope is the radiotracer in the molecule 2-[flourine-18]fluoro-2 deoxy-D-glucose (FDG). FDG is an analog of glucose and tends to concentrate in areas of high metabolic activity everywhere in the human body. Tumor cells with a high rate of mitosis are highly metabolically active and have an increased number of glucose transporters, thus concentrating FDG in tumor cells in higher concentrations than in normal tissue. In addition, FDG becomes trapped within cells because, unlike glucose, it is not metabolized in most tissues.

Performing PET-CT. Patients fast for 4 to 6 hours prior to the scan to limit metabolic activity with the GI tract. Blood glucose should be under good control (<150 mg/dL) to limit the competition for FDG uptake by glucose. Strenuous activity should be limited for 24 hours prior to and immediately following radionuclide administration to limit muscle uptake of FDG. Speech should be curtailed after injection, especially in patients being studied for head and neck malignancy to limit FDG uptake in the muscles of the head and neck. The bladder is emptied by voiding or catheterization just prior to scanning. Rinsing the bladder with saline and scanning the pelvis first is helpful in limiting bladder activity that may obscure disease activity in the uterus, ovaries, or pelvic lymph nodes. The usual dose is 10 to 20 mCi (0.22 mCi/kg body weight) given by intravenous injection. Scanning is performed approximately 60 minutes after IV injection of FDG to allow time for cellular uptake of FDG and clearance of FDG from the blood to decrease background activity. The patient lies supine on the scanning table with arms overhead or at the sides. The arms-at-side position is preferred for head and neck scanning, whereas holding the arms overhead is best for body scanning. Because of the long scan time and the discomfort of the arms-overhead position, most patients are scanned with the arms at the sides, generating some beam-hardening artifacts (see Fig. 64.5). Whole-body CT scans from the top or base of the skull through the neck, chest, abdomen, and pelvis are performed, usually without IV administration of CT contrast agents. Some institutions prep the bowel with oral contrast as part of patient preparation. While administration of IV and/or oral iodinated contrast agents would make the CT more diagnostic, it introduces artifacts in attenuation correction for the PET images. Multidetector CT scanning generally takes less than 2 minutes. PET scanning is performed over 30 to 60 minutes, depending upon the area covered. CT and PET images are reconstructed separately and then fused into composite images utilizing table position calibrations.

PET-CT Interpretation. Axial, coronal, and sagittal reformatted CT; attenuation-corrected PET; attenuation-uncorrected PET; and fused PET-CT images are viewed interactively on a workstation (Fig. 64.1). Software allows rotation of maximum intensity projection images to aid in localization of FDG activity. Window width and level settings are optimized interactively. Assessment of normal and pathologic radiotracer uptake is made by visual inspection, by the standardized uptake value (SUV), and by glucose metabolic rate calculation.

FDG distributes and is taken up by active glucose transport through the cell membrane exactly like regular glucose. It is subsequently phosphorylated to FDG-6-phosphate. Unlike glucose, FDG is not further metabolized and is thus concentrated in tissues in which it accumulates. The major exception to metabolic trapping is in the liver, where concentrated phosphatase enzymes dephosphorylate FCG-6-phosphate and clear FDG from the liver. FDG accumulation depends on the blood supply of the tissue and the level of the glycolytic metabolic activity of the tissue. Organs with higher metabolic activity, like the brain, will accumulate more FDG. Multiple factors, including blood sugar level, blood insulin level, and muscular activity, affect the biodistribution of FDG. FDG is excreted mainly in the urine, like glucose. However, in contrast to glucose, FDG cannot be reabsorbed in proximal convoluted tubules. Therefore the urinary system shows intense activity. Variable activity of the GI tract, liver, thymus, breast, salivary glands, and bone marrow is also commonly seen. The uptake by myocardium largely depends on the metabolic state of the heart at the time of the injection. Accumulation of FDG is also seen in interstitial body fluids, including pleural, peritoneal, and synovial fluids. Variable excretion from lacrimal, salivary, and sweat glands needs to be recognized as variants on PET images and not mistaken for hypermetabolic lesions.

FDG is an indiscriminate identifier of foci of high metabolic activity within the body. Its usefulness is based on the fact that most malignant tumors are more metabolically active and take up more glucose than normal tissues. Some nonmalignant pathologic processes, such as infections, foci of inflammation, and benign neoplasms, also concentrate FDG on the basis of their metabolic activity. The challenge to PET interpretation is the differentiation of pathologic activity from normal and normal variant FDG activity.

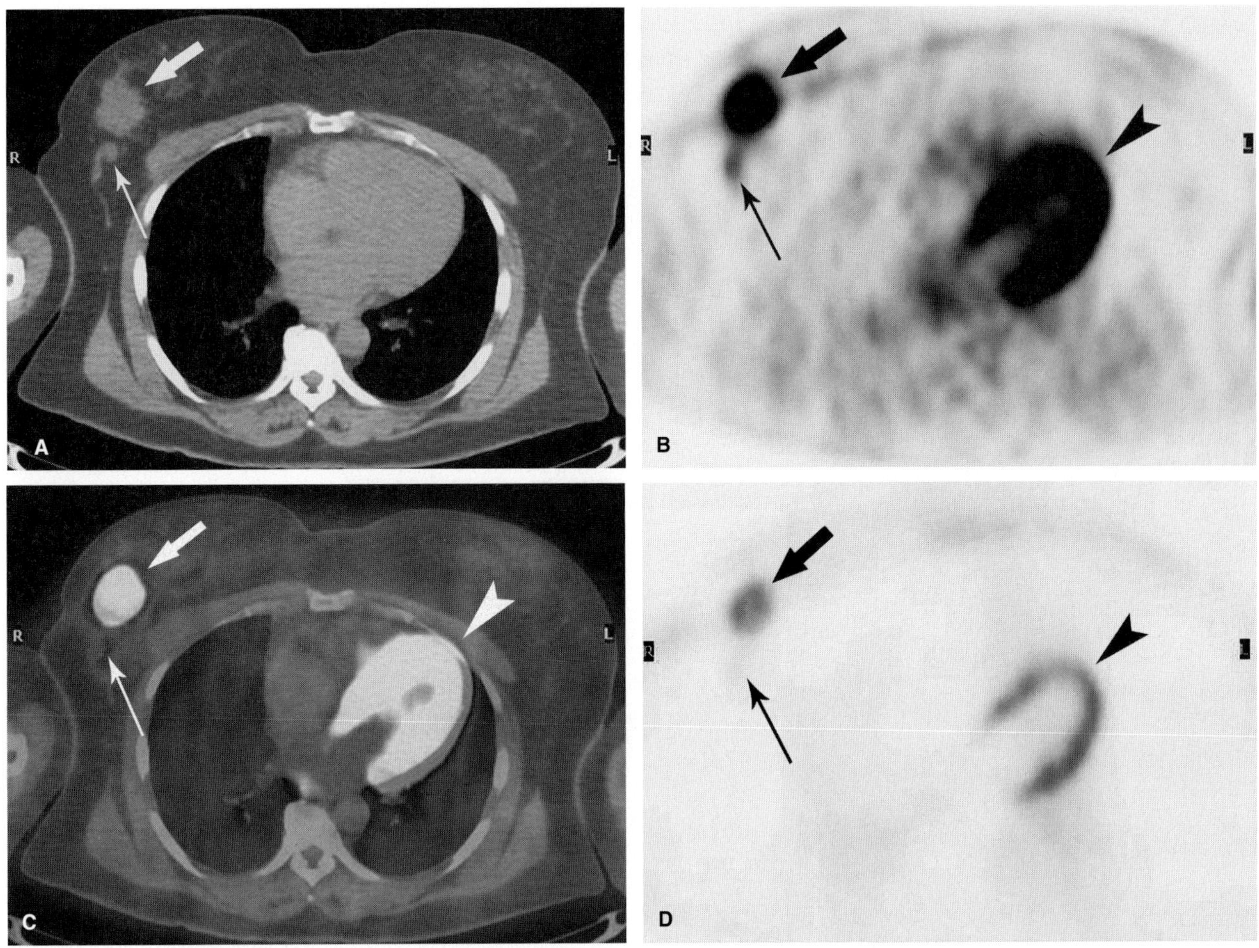

FIGURE 64.1. **(Color Plates) Breast Cancer PET-CT.** Axial images through the thorax demonstrate marked fluorodeoxyglucose (FDG) activity within a carcinoma (*wide arrows*) in the right breast. Activity in a small adjacent lymph node (*thin arrows*) is indicative of metastatic spread of tumor. Normal myocardial FDG activity is seen in the heart (*arrowheads*). **A.** Noncontrast CT. **B.** PET with attenuation correction. **C.** Fused PET-CT. **D.** PET without attenuation correction. FDG activity on the PET with attenuation correction and on the fused PET-CT images is confirmed by identifying activity in the same focus on the PET image without attenuation correction.

Skeletal muscle FDG uptake is dependent on muscle activity. In a resting state, muscle uptake of FDG is negligible. Heavy muscle activity in the 24 hours prior to imaging may result in high FDG uptake. Patients should minimize activity following FDG injection to minimize uptake by skeletal muscles. Patients with breathing difficulty may show prominent uptake in the muscles of the chest wall and diaphragm. Insulin injection by diabetics increases skeletal muscle FDG uptake. Talking and eye movement increase uptake in the ocular muscles, the larynx, and the muscles of mastication (Fig. 64.2).

Brain uptake of FDG is always prominent because the brain uses glucose as its primary energy source (Fig. 64.3). Normal gray matter uptake is particularly avid and difficult to differentiate from malignant brain lesions. Focal low-level activity may be seen in areas that have been radiated or resected.

Cardiac muscle uptake is particularly prominent after eating. Fasting for 4 to 6 hours prior to FDG scanning decreases FDG uptake as the myocardium switches to fatty acid metabolism. Most patients show variable and nonuniform myocardial FDG activity, even after a fast, caused by nonuniform transition to fatty acid metabolism by the myocardium. FDG activity is most variable at the base of the LV (Fig. 64.4).

Liver. The entire liver demonstrates low-level FDG activity in nearly all patients. Most challenging is the fact that uptake often appears heterogeneous, mimicking the appearance of multiple small metastases (Fig. 64.5). Hepatic uptake of FDG is not surprising because the liver is a major site of carbohydrate metabolism, glycolysis, and glycogen storage. However, hepatocytes have high levels of FDG-6-phosphatase, which acts to clear FDG from hepatocytes. Primary liver tumors may demonstrate high

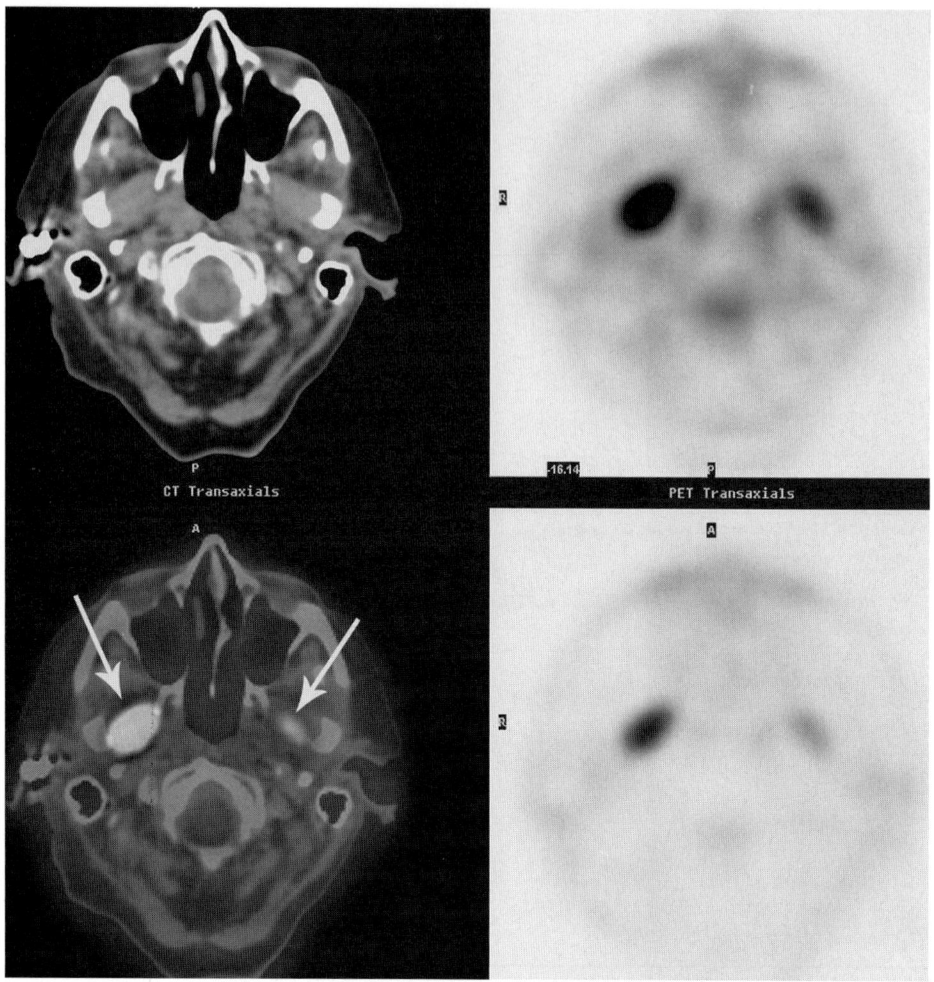

FIGURE 64.2. **(Color Plates) Physiologic Fluorodeoxyglucose (FDG) Activity in Muscle.** Axial CT, PET, and fused PET-CT images demonstrate avid uptake of FDG by the greater pterygoid muscles (*arrows*). This activity is physiologic and is caused by talking and mastication. It should not be confused with malignant lesions.

FDG-6-phosphatase activity, have high rates of clearance of FDG, and be difficult to detect on PET images. In summary, FDG PET is limited in the detection of small liver metastases and small primary liver tumors.

Gallbladder activity is rarely seen. FDG activity in the gallbladder bed suggests acute or chronic cholecystitis, gallbladder cancer, or adjacent liver tumor.

Spleen activity is usually slightly greater than blood pool but slightly less than liver. Spleen uptake is substantially increased by activation of hematopoiesis.

Bone marrow radionuclide activity is mild to moderate, diffuse, and symmetric within the spine, pelvis, ribs, sternum, and proximal femurs. Asymmetric or heterogeneous uptake is caused by skeletal metastases, old fractures, effects of radiation therapy, and activation of hematopoiesis by severe anemia.

Stomach activity is usually low level and best recognized on axial images by its characteristic position and shape. FDG activity is accentuated by stomach muscle contraction. Foci of uptake in the lower thorax may represent inflammation within a hiatal hernia or in the distal esophagus related to reflux.

Colon activity is highly variable and usually more intense than in the small bowel. Intense FDG uptake makes recognition of pathologic sites in the abdomen difficult (Fig. 64.6). Colon activity varies with colon muscle contraction, mucosal inflammation, amount of lymphoid tissue in the colon wall, and possibly uptake by colon bacteria. Multifocal or segmental activity suggests inflammatory bowel disease, while intense focal activity suggests colon carcinoma, malignant peritoneal implants, or adjacent lymph node metastases.

Urinary Tract. FDG is excreted by glomerular filtration without significant renal tubular reabsorption. This results in concentrated radionuclide activity in the urine (Fig. 64.7). The bladder should be emptied prior to PET imaging. Good hydration facilitates FDG clearance and decreases collecting system activity. High (but normal) renal collecting system activity impairs detection of small renal lesions. Partial filling of the ureters resulting from normal peristalsis may show focal high FDG activity anywhere along the course of the ureters. Bladder diverticula commonly retain urine with FDG even after bladder emptying.

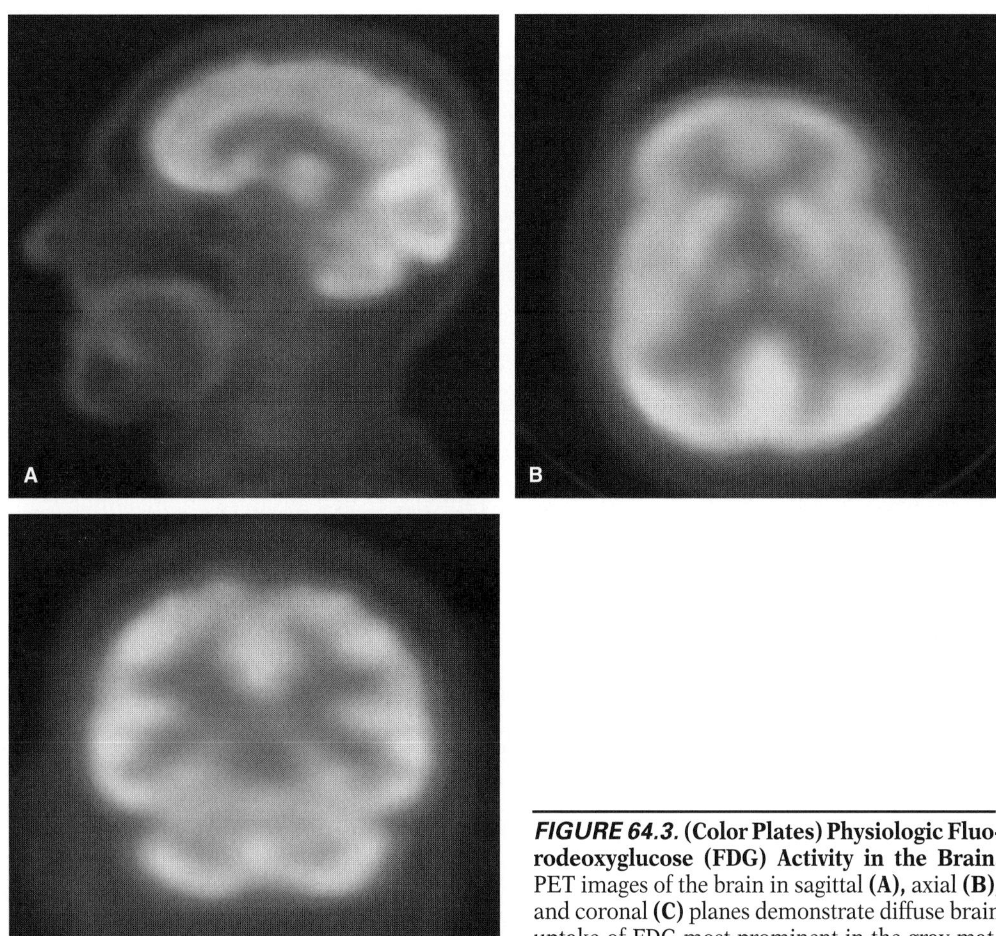

FIGURE 64.3. **(Color Plates) Physiologic Fluorodeoxyglucose (FDG) Activity in the Brain.** PET images of the brain in sagittal **(A),** axial **(B),** and coronal **(C)** planes demonstrate diffuse brain uptake of FDG most prominent in the gray matter. FDG activity reflects the use of glucose as a primary energy source for the brain.

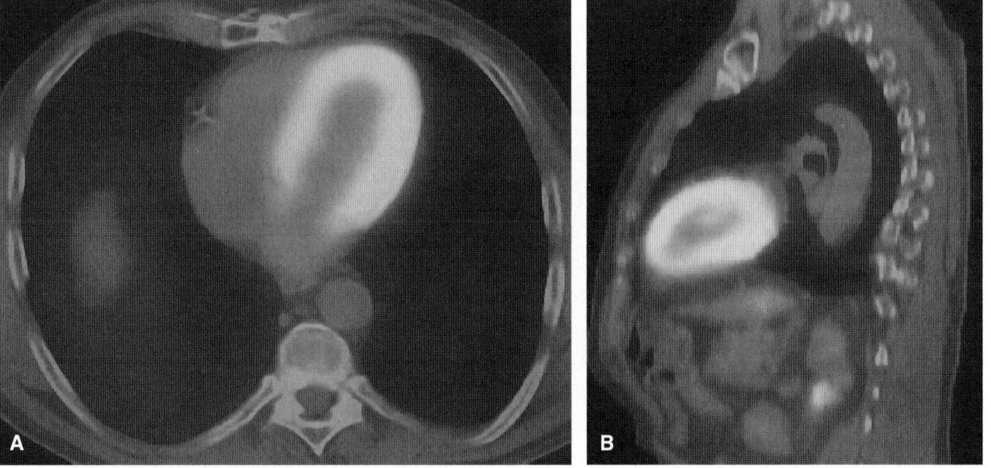

FIGURE 64.4. **(Color Plates) Physiologic Fluorodeoxyglucose (FDG) Activity in the Heart.** Fused PET-CT images in axial **(A)** and sagittal **(B)** planes demonstrate normal prominent myocardial uptake by the LV.

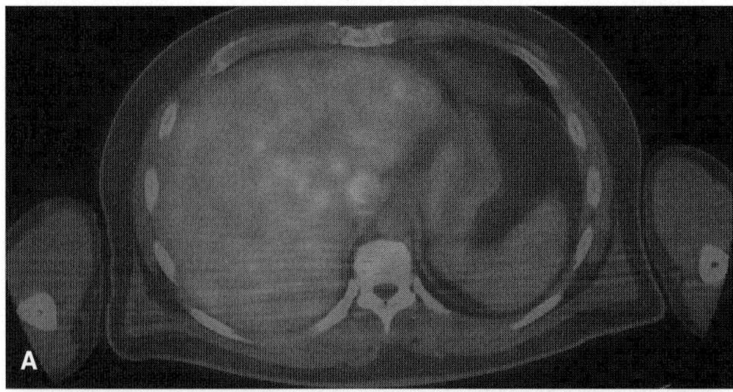

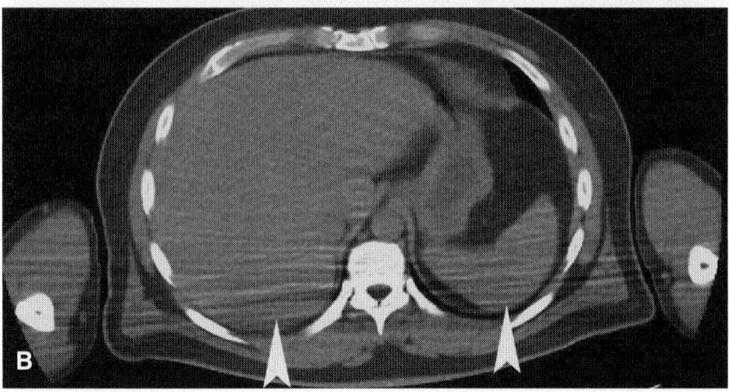

FIGURE 64.5. **Physiologic Fluorodeoxyglucose (FDG) Activity in the Liver. A.** FDG activity is strikingly heterogeneous but normal on the fused PET-CT image. High metabolic activity within the liver combined with variable clearance of FDG from hepatocytes results in this heterogenous pattern, which makes detection of hepatic masses somewhat difficult. **B.** The corresponding CT image demonstrates the streaks (*arrowheads*) of beam-hardening artifact resulting from the patient being in arms-at-side position.

Uterus. The endometrium commonly demonstrates intense radionuclide activity during active menstruation. Activity may also be seen from menstrual blood in vaginal tampons. Pelvic endometriosis is a benign cause of high-activity foci in the pelvis.

Ovaries show uptake in functional ovarian cysts.

Salivary gland uptake is normally minimal to low. Radiation therapy, infection, and inflammation increase FDG activity.

Thyroid gland uptake is normally diffuse and low level. Intense activity is associated with Graves disease or thyroiditis. An asymmetric focus of activity suggests possible thyroid cancer and warrants US evaluation and consideration of biopsy.

Brown Fat. A pattern of symmetric uptake in the paraspinal regions, mediastinum, neck, and supraclavicular area may be localized on the CT images as coming from fat. When a patient is cold or anxious, increased levels of catecholamines increase glycolytic activity in brown fat. This may be very difficult to differentiate from lymphadenopathy. Keeping the scan room warm and sedating anxious patients may diminish this activity.

In attempt to semiquantitatively assess the uptake of radiotracer, the SUV was introduced to take into consideration the weight of the patient as well as the administered dose. Software to calculate SUV is available with most imaging systems. SUV is calculated by placing a region of interest over the lesion to measure tracer activity in microcuries/cubic centimeter. This value is divided by the administered dose (in microcuries) divided by the patient's body weight (in grams).

$$\text{SUV} = \frac{\text{Tracer activity in the focus}}{\text{Administered dose/patient's body weight}}$$

Most malignant tumors have an SUV of 2.5 to 3.0. Physiologic activity usually has an SUV of 0.5 to 2.5. Relying on SUV has limitations. Many factors affect the uptake of radiotracer in a given lesion, including lean body weight, state of hydration, insulin level, blood sugar level, distribution of nontarget organs and space, etc. Taking into consideration only body weight may not be the best way to accurately assess the accumulated activity, especially for purposes of comparison.

ONCOLOGIC PET IMAGING

Currently PET is utilized in oncology for three major indications: *initial staging, evaluation of response to treatment*, and *assessment for recurrence*. Recent literature also cites emerging application of PET for predicting the prognosis of a few malignancies. In addition, primary assessment of single pulmonary nodule by PET is now an acceptable next step in the evaluation of malignancy. Although there have been a few reports of hypometabolic malignancies causing false-negative PET cases, the majority of common cancers are highly metabolically active and glucose avid. In addition, there are a few nonmalignant processes with high metabolic activity, which should be recognized to avoid false-positive results. These include infectious and inflammatory conditions, as well as a few benign neoplastic processes.

Lung Cancer. Traditionally lung cancer has been classified into small cell lung cancer (15%) and non–small cell lung cancer (85%). Non–small cell lung cancer is subdivided into the histologic subtypes adenocarcinoma (including bronchoalveolar cell carcinoma) (50%), squamous cell carcinoma (30%), and large cell carcinoma (5%). PET has been proven to be most useful with non–small cell cancers, most of which are highly avid for FDG. Early detection and accurate staging have immense impact on the survival of all subtypes of lung cancer.

Solitary Pulmonary Nodule. PET is one of the most valuable modalities in the workup of a solitary pulmonary nodule detected by CT or radiographs. Most cancers have high metabolic activity and are hyperintense on PET (Figs. 64.8,

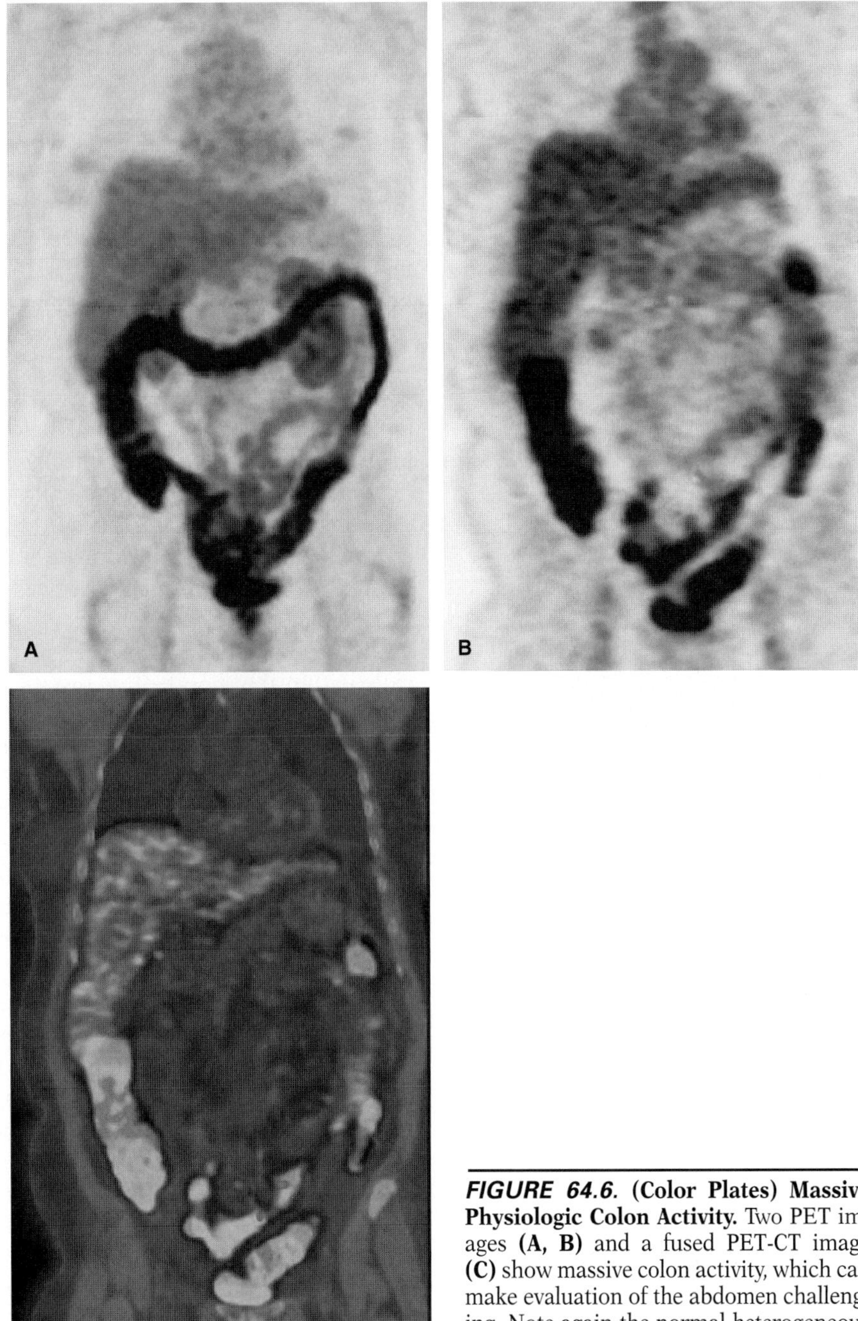

FIGURE 64.6. **(Color Plates) Massive Physiologic Colon Activity.** Two PET images **(A, B)** and a fused PET-CT image **(C)** show massive colon activity, which can make evaluation of the abdomen challenging. Note again the normal heterogeneous fluorodeoxyglucose activity in the liver.

64.9). Most benign lesions, including granulomas, other inflammatory nodules, and hamartomas, do not accumulate FDG and appear hypointense on PET imaging. PET is reported to be 97% sensitive and 78% specific for diagnosis of malignant pulmonary nodules. PET can also be used for assessment of multiple pulmonary lesions (Fig. 64.10) of unknown etiology, although the efficacy of this application is currently under investigation. If a solitary pulmonary nodule is a metastasis, PET can potentially detect the extrapulmonary primary cancer in the same study.

Despite its limitations, SUV is commonly used to estimate the likelihood of malignancy. An SUV of 2.5 or greater is considered indicative of malignancy. An SUV under 1.5 is indicative of a benign nodule. SUV may be artifactually lowered by smearing artifact produced by breathing during the prolonged acquisition of the PET study over several minutes. Respiratory gating and corrective algorithms for the PET data, based on CT images, can be used to further enhance the accuracy of the SUV (cSUV = corrected SUV). With small nodules (<1.5 cm), the partial

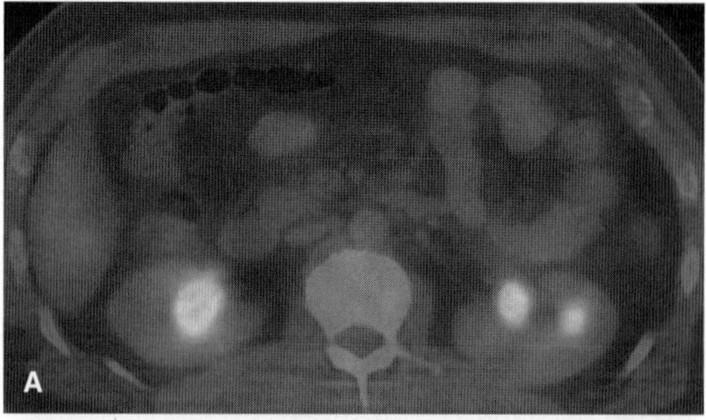

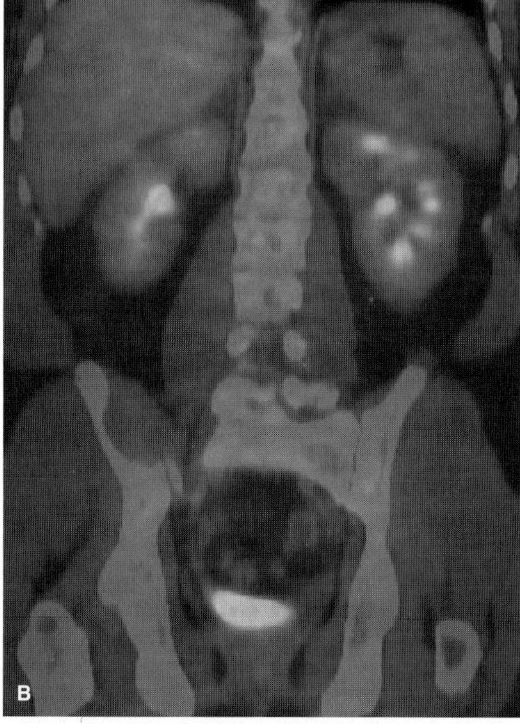

FIGURE 64.7. **(Color Plates) Normal Physiologic Activity in the Urinary Tract.** Axial **(A)** and coronal **(B)** fused PET-CT images show the normal intense fluorodeoxyglucose activity in the urinary tract owing to glomerular filtration and urinary excretion of the radionuclide. Radionuclide activity is more prominent in the renal collecting systems, ureters, and bladder.

volume averaging effect may falsely lower the SUV below 2.5, even though the nodule is malignant. False-positive results occur with tuberculosis, fungal infections, and sarcoidosis. However, most PET-positive nodules are malignant, and hypermetabolic lesions should be considered malignant until proven benign. PET-negative nodules can generally be followed rather than biopsied. The reported false-negative cases are usually hypometabolic malignancies, including bronchoalveolar carcinoma and carcinoid tumor. Analysis of CT characteristics of the nodule is crucial in making the correct diagnosis.

Staging. Lymph nodes that are normal by CT size criteria can still harbor metabolically active malignant cells, which are detectable by PET. PET is 80% to 90% sensitive and 85% to 100% specific for malignancy in mediastinal nodes and 75% sensitive and specific for malignancy in hilar nodes (Fig. 64.11). The negative predictive value of PET for mediastinal involvement is 95%, allowing surgical resection of lung cancer with a high degree of confidence. Inflammatory changes in hilar and mediastinal lymph nodes cause false-positive PET scans. PET demonstration of distant metastases in bones, brain, liver, or adrenal glands precludes surgery for cure. PET may demonstrate sites of tumor involvement not suspected by CT in 11% of patients with non–small cell lung cancer. CT can overestimate the size of the pulmonary lesion because of perilesional inflammation, necrosis, and distal atelectasis. PET is useful in demonstrating the metabolically active tumor within hypometabolic areas of consolidation or atelectasis. Increased FDG activity within a pleural effusion is indicative of malignant pleural effusion, with an accuracy of 92%. Inflammatory changes postpleurodesis may also result in FDG activity.

Detecting Recurrence. Recurrent disease, whether locally within the thorax or as distant metastases, is common in lung cancer. PET serves as a comprehensive imaging modality in screening the whole body for all potential sites of recurrence (see Fig. 64.26). PET accurately differentiates postsurgical changes in the thorax from recurrent malignancy. Radiation pneumonitis is metabolically active in the first 6 months following radiotherapy, making detection of tumor recurrence by PET difficult (Fig. 64.12). Interpretation of FDG activity in a radiation port must be interpreted cautiously and in correlation with CT findings.

Lymphoma. Staging determines therapy in lymphoma (Fig. 64.13). Staging is based on presence of disease above or below the diaphragm, involvement of single or multiple nodal basins, and confinement to lymph nodes or spread to extranodal tissues. Because of its ability to detect disease in nodes that are not enlarged, PET is more sensitive and more specific than CT in lymphoma staging (86% versus 81% sensitive and 96% versus 41% specific). FDG uptake correlates with histologic grade and the degree of the proliferative activity of the lymphomatous tissue. Some cases of malignant lymphoma are not highly metabolically active and therefore produce a false-negative result on PET. Low-grade lymphomas show limited PET activity, and mucosal-associated lymphoid tissue lymphomas are easily overlooked because of background activity of the GI tract. False-positive PET scans occur with hypermetabolic sarcoidosis, tuberculosis, pyogenic abscesses, histoplasmosis and other fungal infections, and discitis. In practice, hypermetabolic lymph nodes are considered malignant until proven benign, usually by biopsy.

Initial Staging. PET is an excellent modality for initial assessment of Hodgkin disease and aggressive non-Hodgkin lymphoma (NHL) but is less useful for low-grade follicular NHL. For nodal disease assessment, PET is

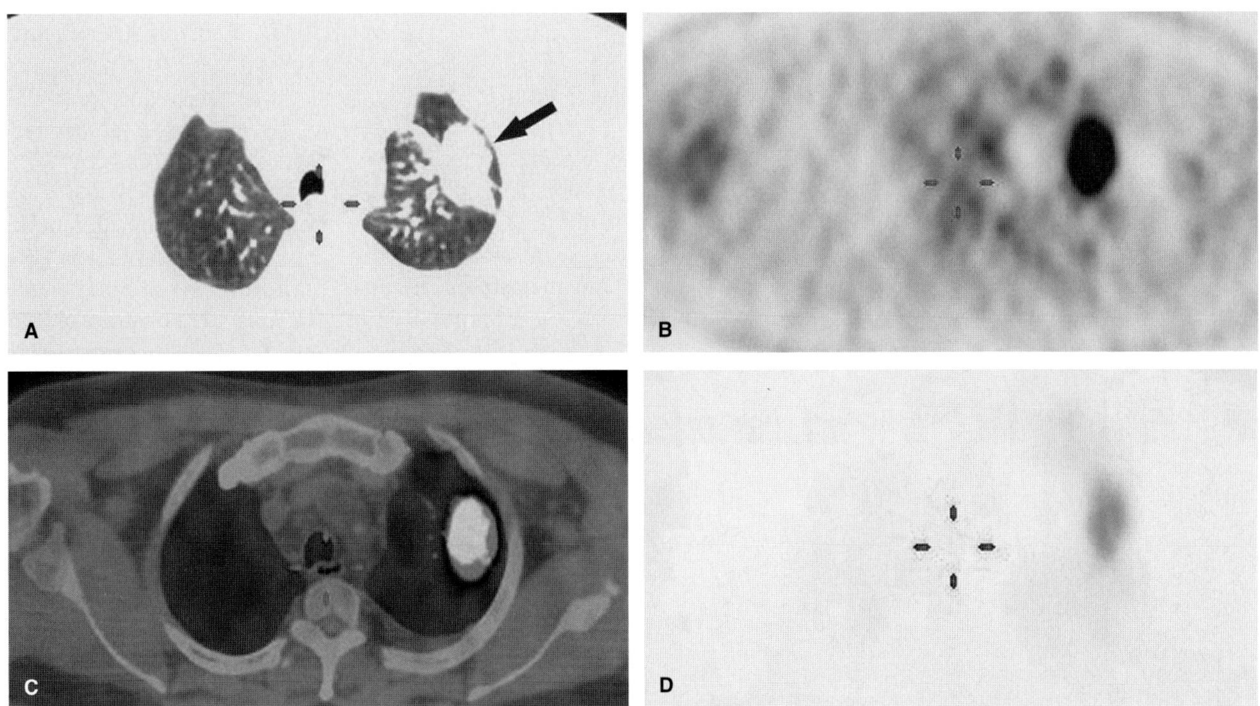

FIGURE 64.8. **(Color Plates) Hot Pulmonary Nodule: Bronchogenic Carcinoma.** Irregular mass (*arrow*) in the left upper lobe on axial CT is shown by PET to demonstrate avid fluorodeoxyglucose uptake, indicating the high metabolic activity that is typical of lung malignancies. **A.** CT. **B.** Corrected PET. **C.** Fused PET-CT. **D.** Uncorrected PET.

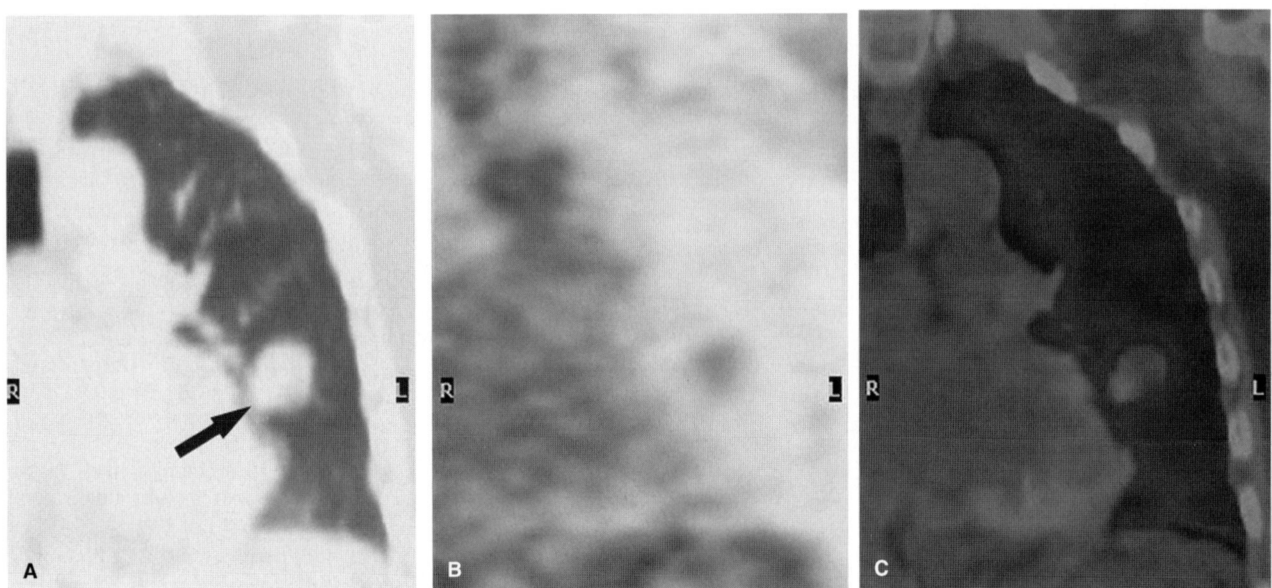

FIGURE 64.9. **(Color Plates) Warm Pulmonary Nodule: Bronchoalveolar Carcinoma.** Mild increased activity is noted on the PET images of this bronchoalveolar cell carcinoma of the lung (*arrow*). Mild activity is compatible with either an inflammatory or a neoplastic process. **A.** CT. **B.** Corrected PET. **C.** Fused PET-CT.

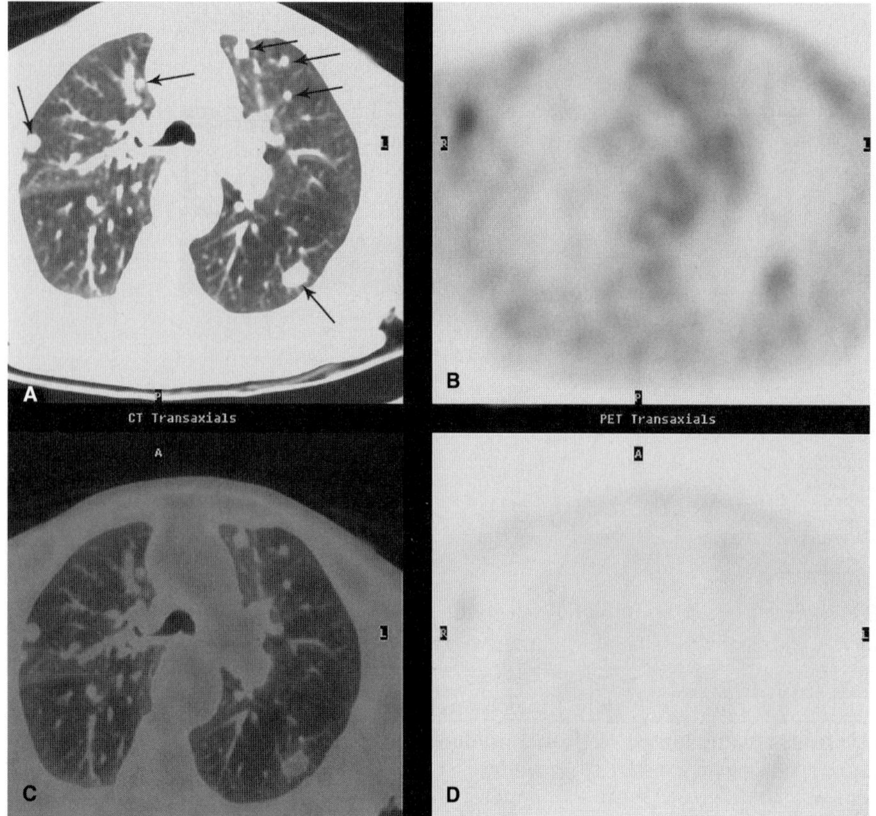

FIGURE 64.10. **(Color Plates) Multiple Pulmonary Nodules.** CT scan **(A)** demonstrates multiple pulmonary nodules in this patient without known malignancy. Corresponding PET images **(B, C)** show very low metabolic activity in the lesions, consistent with benign inflammatory nodules.

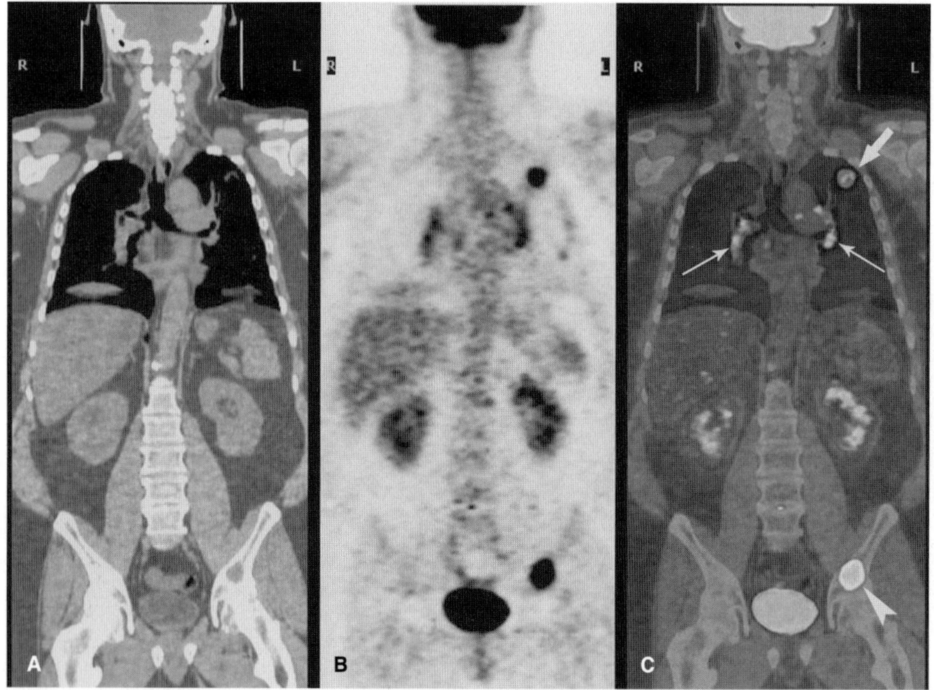

FIGURE 64.11. **(Color Plates) Lung Cancer Staging.** PET-CT demonstrates fluorodeoxyglucose hyperactivity in the primary lung cancer (*wide arrow*) as well as within hilar lymph nodes (*thin arrows*) and the left acetabulum (*arrowhead*), indicating widespread metastatic disease. Heterogeneous activity in the liver, spine, bowel, both kidneys, and bladder is normal. **A.** CT. **B.** Corrected PET. **C.** Fused PET-CT.

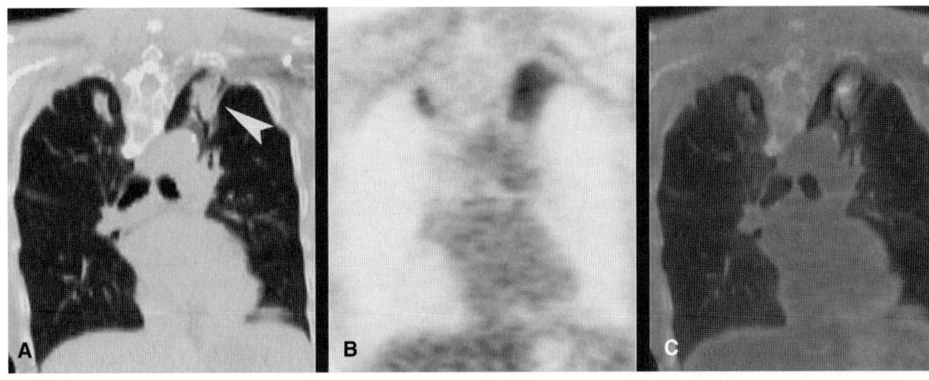

FIGURE 64.12. **(Color Plates) Postradiation Pneumonitis.** Coronal PET-CT images show high fluorodeoxyglucose activity in the left upper lobe (*arrowhead*) in patient who has undergone surgical resection of lung cancer and radiation therapy in the previous 4 months. Focal hyperactivity during this time frame is nonspecific and compatible with either postradiation pneumonitis or tumor recurrence. **A.** CT. **B.** Corrected PET. **C.** Fused PET-CT.

superior to CT in thorax and abdomen. For extranodal disease, which is present in 40% of lymphoma patients, PET is also excellent but has the following limitations. Diffuse lymphomatous involvement of the spleen is a challenge for all imaging modalities, including PET. Diffuse splenic activity greater than that of liver activity is consistent with diffuse lymphomatous infiltration of the spleen. Focal hyperactivity in the spleen suggests focal lymphoma, whether or not a corresponding mass is shown on CT (Fig. 64.14). Focal spleen hyperactivity with SUV >2.3 corresponds to malignant mass in the spleen. Assessment of bone marrow is also limited, as a variable degree of activity is always present in normal marrow spaces. However, PET can provide a map for hypermetabolic marrow foci to increase the yield of marrow biopsy. Hyperactive marrow on PET images could be caused by hyperplasia of normal marrow after chemotherapy, rather than representing lymphomatous tissue. Increased activity in the spleen usually accompanies hyperplasia of the marrow and may provide a clue to the correct diagnosis. An osteolytic bone lesion in NHL may be a cold lesion on radionuclide bone scans. PET can demonstrate significant metabolic activity in cold osteolytic lesions characterizing them accurately as aggressive active disease.

Early Assessment of Treatment Response. Conventionally, the response to the treatment is evaluated by cross-sectional anatomic imaging modalities, using nodal size criteria. PET is able to detect appreciable decreases in FDG activity even before completion of the first course of chemotherapy (Fig. 64.15). This application can save significant time and resources by early confirmation of the effectiveness or failure of applied therapy. SUV measurements before, during, and after treatment provide semiquantitative measurements of the response to therapy.

Posttherapy Residual Mass. If no residual activity is detected on PET after completion of the course of treatment, we can conclude that the patient is in remission with favorable prognosis. Residual masses, demonstrated by CT, are common after completion of therapy. Lack of FDG metabolic activity in these masses is evidence of the absence of viable tumor. However, residual activity needs to be interpreted with caution, as it may represent either residual hypermetabolic neoplastic tissue or active

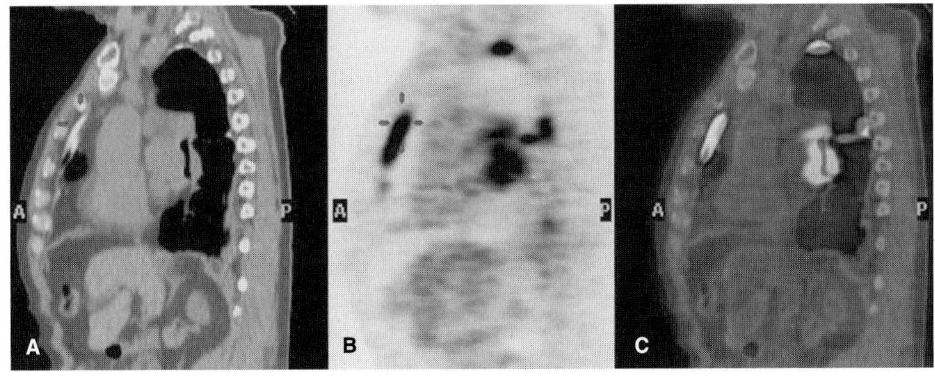

FIGURE 64.13. **(Color Plates) Lymphoma Staging.** PET-CT demonstrates active hilar and mediastinal adenopathy and multiple bony lesions in a patient with lymphoma. Whole-body scanning indicated that all detectable disease was above the diaphragm. Images are in the sagittal plane. **A.** CT. **B.** Corrected PET. **C.** Fused PET-CT.

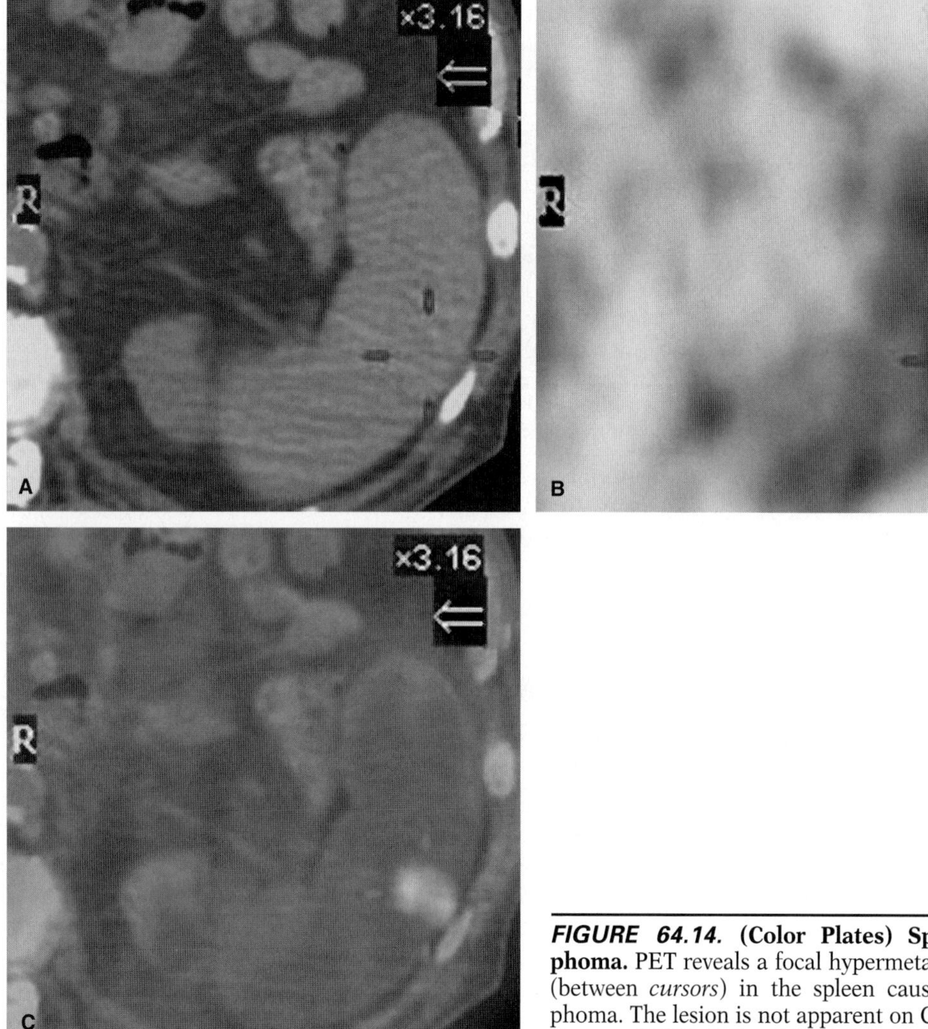

FIGURE 64.14. **(Color Plates) Spleen Lymphoma.** PET reveals a focal hypermetabolic lesion (between *cursors*) in the spleen caused by lymphoma. The lesion is not apparent on CT. **A.** CT. **B.** Corrected PET. **C.** Fused PET-CT.

inflammation with ongoing necrosis. These cases may require biopsy to confirm the diagnosis.

Detection of Recurrence. Periodic PET scanning is reliable for assessment of continuing remission. Comparison with initial (pretherapy) and posttherapy PET and CT scans is of utmost importance. FDG activity is highly indicative of active tumor, whereas absence of FDG activity indicates continued remission.

Sources of error in the use of PET for staging and follow-up of lymphoma include infection, drug toxicity, effects of radiation therapy and surgery, and physiologic activity. Infections are common in bone marrow–suppressed patients, especially in the respiratory and GI tracts. Active infection and inflammation show PET activity that may be mistaken for lymphomatous involvement. Drugs, such as bleomycin, may injure the lungs, resulting in diffuse FDG lung activity. Granulocyte colony-stimulating factor therapy used to stimulate proliferation of granulocytes may cause focal marrow activity, mimicking lymphoma involvement. Inflammatory response and healing induced by radiation therapy or surgical procedures cause PET activity. False-positive FDG uptake in the thymus, associated with thymic enlargement on CT, owing to thymic rebound commonly occurs in children undergoing treatment for lymphoma.

Melanoma. Early stage melanoma (85% of patients) is curable by surgery, whereas 15% of patients have advanced local disease or metastases. Diagnosis is usually made by physical examination and biopsy. It is currently unknown whether PET can differentiate melanoma from atypical nevi or benign pigmented skin lesions. Melanoma is highly avid for FDG, but the volume of tumor in nodal metastases is small, limiting the usefulness of PET for regional staging. Acne and carbuncles show FDG hyperactivity and may mimic melanomas or skin metastases.

Sentinel lymph node (SLN) mapping is safe and accurate in regional node staging of melanoma. A small amount of technetium-99m (Tc-99m)–labelled sulfur colloid is injected intradermally around the tumor. The colloid particles are cleared by the local lymphatics, and the

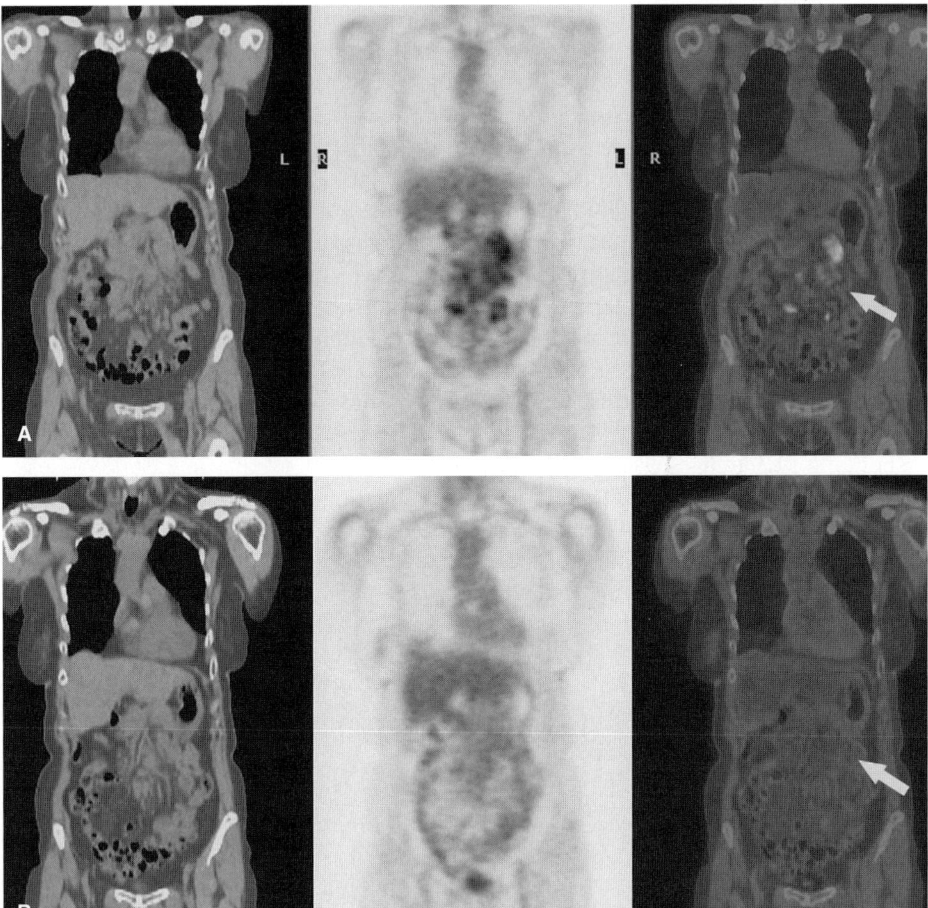

FIGURE 64.15. **(Color Plates) Lymphoma: Early Response to Therapy.** Before an appreciable change in size is detectable by CT, fluorodeoxyglucose (FDG) PET shows an early, favorable response to chemotherapy. **A.** Coronal-plane PET-CT shows hypermetabolic activity in mesenteric adenopathy (*arrow*), indicating involvement by lymphoma. **B.** Follow-up scan obtained after the first course of chemotherapy shows lack of FDG activity within the mesenteric adenopathy (*arrow*) that is not changed on CT.

radioactive colloid is trapped in regional lymph nodes that drain the tumor site. These nodes can be located by a gamma probe and removed at surgery. Although it is highly specific (97%), PET is relatively insensitive for these regional node metastases (as low as 17% sensitivity); thus SLN mapping is preferred. PET is highly useful in the demonstration of distant metastases, which occur most commonly in the lungs, liver, adrenal glands, GI tract, and bone, as well as in unusual sites such as the spleen, thyroid, gallbladder, pancreas, and skin. Whole-body PET is 92% sensitive and 90% specific in detection of distant metastases. Limitations are small lung and brain metastases, which may not be detected.

Melanoma may recur many years after apparent cure and is often widespread before detection. Whole-body FDG PET is highly useful for surveillance, with detection rates for recurrence similar to those of initial staging for distant metastases.

Esophageal Cancer. PET is reported to be highly specific (80% to 92%) for initial diagnosis of primary esophageal cancer, although its sensitivity is as low as 50%. High affinity for FDG is seen in all subtypes of esophageal cancer. Sensitivity is volume dependent. False-negative cases are caused by the small size of the primary lesion. Current PET scanners detect lesions of 3 to 5 mm. No correlation is noted between SUV and depth of invasion. Fasting is recommended to decrease the nearby cardiac activity when PET is customized for esophageal cancer assessment. A cup of water just before scanning can clear the activity from salivary secretions. Care should be taken to avoid attaching too much importance to activity in the distal esophagus, because distal esophagitis, gastric reflux, Barrett's esophagus, hiatal hernia, and retained saliva can mimic carcinoma. Correlation with the CT portion of PET-CT enhances the accuracy significantly. PET is limited in detection of nodal metastases (22% to 57% sensitivity) but is highly specific (>90%) when hyperactivity is present in regional nodes.

PET can be employed for assessment of the response to radiation therapy as well as for restaging after radical treatment. Recurrences occur in the surgical bed (one third of patients), in regional nodes, or distally in liver, lung, or bone. PET is sensitive (~100%) but not specific (57%) for surgical bed recurrence. Distant disease is effectively demonstrated (95% sensitive, 80% specific). Inclusion of PET in the management of esophageal cancer has a significant impact in deciding the best route of treatment and prevents unnecessary surgery by accurately upstaging the disease process.

Stomach Cancer. Stomach mucosa concentrates FDG physiologically. Therefore, detection of a hypermetabolic lesion in a highly active background is of limited accuracy, especially if the lesion is small. PET should not be used as the primary mode of diagnosis. Involvement of regional nodes along the lesser curvature can be overlooked on PET imaging because of the marked nearby gastric activity. Regional disease, including celiac nodal involvement, and distant metastases are assessed with better accuracy. PET images should be correlated closely with corresponding CT images. Prominent nodes on CT need to be assessed on corresponding PET images. Peritoneal surfaces, the greater omentum, and the cul-de-sac need to be assessed meticulously in association with CT images to detect subtle hypermetabolic foci. PET detection of hepatic metastases is limited; therefore contrast-enhanced CT or MR should be added to the staging evaluation.

Pancreatic cancer staging is best accomplished by other cross-sectional imaging modalities, as PET lacks the resolution to assess for subtle features such as vascular invasion. However, distant metastases can be accurately detected using PET imaging if radical treatment of a small, well-localized lesion is considered. Gastric activity can overshadow the pancreatic bed. Intake of water can slightly improve the assessment of this region. PET can assess the response to treatment reliably. Persistent high activity on postradiation cases suggests very poor prognosis. PET is useful in the differentiation of chronic pancreatitis from pancreatic cancer.

Colorectal Cancer. Most (95%) colon cancers are FDG-avid adenocarcinomas. Approximately 20% of patients have metastatic disease at the time of diagnosis. PET provides one-stop accurate assessment for whole-body staging at the time of initial diagnosis (Fig. 64.16). In about 40% of cases, clinical staging is modified by PET results. Accurate up-staging by PET prevents unnecessary surgery in patients with advanced, albeit clinically

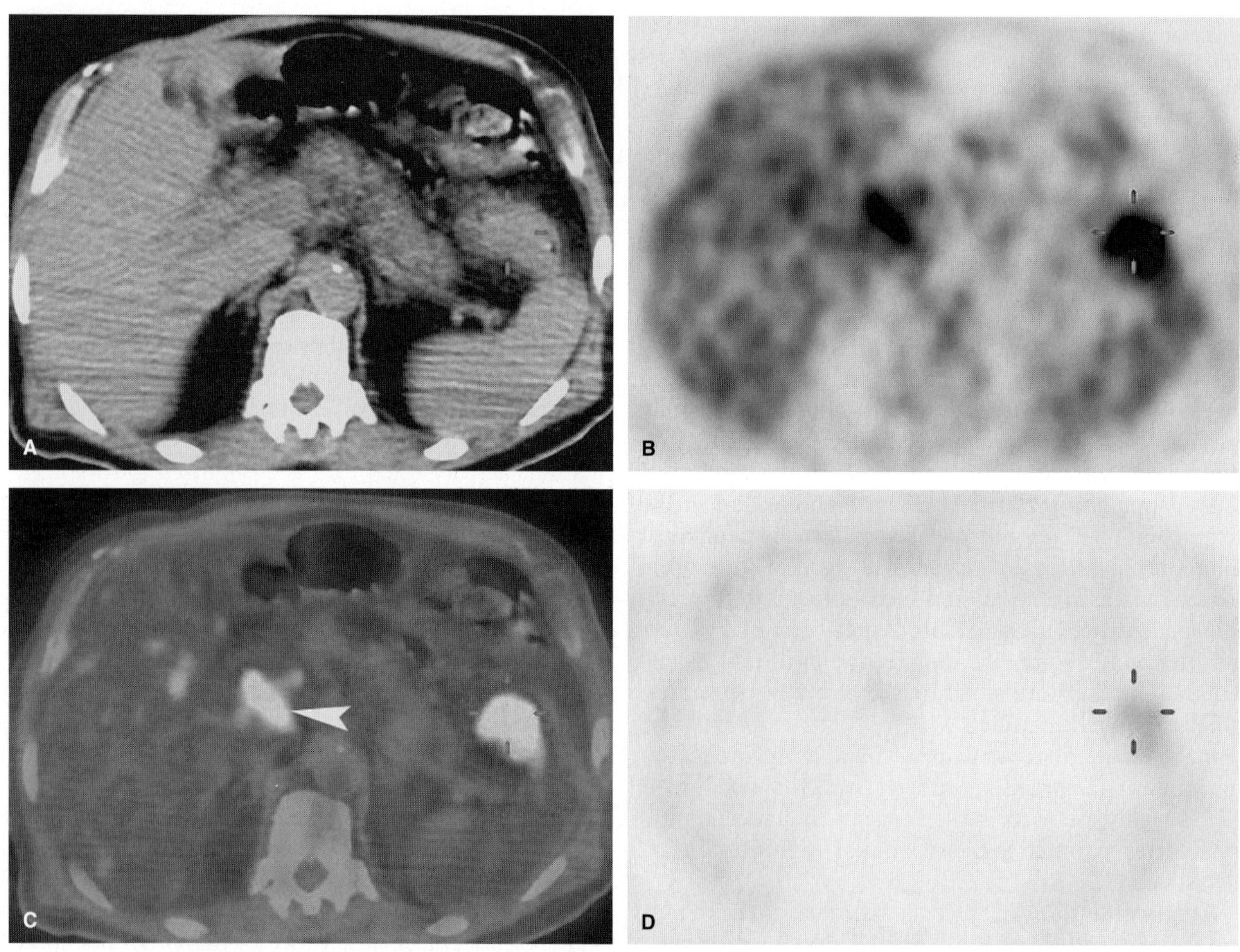

FIGURE 64.16. **(Color Plates) Colon Cancer Staging.** A colon cancer (between *cursors*) in the splenic flexure is hypermetabolic on PET-CT as is metastatic adenopathy in the porta hepatis (*arrowhead*). **A.** CT. **B.** Corrected PET. **C.** Fused PET-CT. **D.** Uncorrected PET.

occult, disease. Currently PET is widely utilized for staging and restaging of patients and for assessment of response to treatment. PET is currently not widely employed for early detection or colon cancer screening. Some groups are using hybrid PET-CT with virtual colonoscopy to offer functional and anatomic imaging for early detection of adenomatous polyps and small colon cancers. Nonspecific colonic activity can be a source of overcalling (Fig. 64.6). Diffuse activity is usually physiologic, especially in the descending and sigmoid colon. Benign conditions, including sigmoid diverticulitis, inflammatory polyps, and fecal material, can accumulate FDG. Any focal activity in the colon should be further evaluated. The rectal region may be obscured by bladder activity. Therefore the bladder should be emptied immediately prior to imaging, and scanning should begin in the pelvis and proceed superiorly.

PET has low sensitivity (29%) for regional node metastases because involved nodes are often small, have a limited number of tumor cells, and are located close to and masked by bowel activity. When pericolic nodes are FDG positive, specificity for malignancy is high (96%). PET sensitivity is equal to or slightly better than CT alone in detection of hepatic metastases, and PET-CT specificity for hepatic metastases approaches 100%. Small lesions (<1 cm) are often not detected, and anatomic localization of lesions within the liver by PET alone is not precise enough for surgical planning of resection of hepatic metastases. However, PET demonstration of extrahepatic metastases (11% to 23% of patients) precludes hepatic resection for cure. The major role of PET is in detection of distant metastases, which preclude surgery for cure. Overall, for the presence of metastatic disease, PET is 97% sensitive and 76% specific.

Recurrence of colon cancer occurs at the anastomotic site, the surgical bed, or distantly, usually in the liver or lung. Activity at the anastomotic site needs to be interpreted with caution, as healing and active granulation tissue present soon after surgery can avidly accumulate FDG (Fig. 64.17). Correlation with CT findings, the time of surgery, and/or radiation therapy is also helpful. Chronic scarring at the surgical site commonly produces nonspecific soft tissue density on CT. In assessing for recurrence more than 6 months after surgery or radiotherapy,

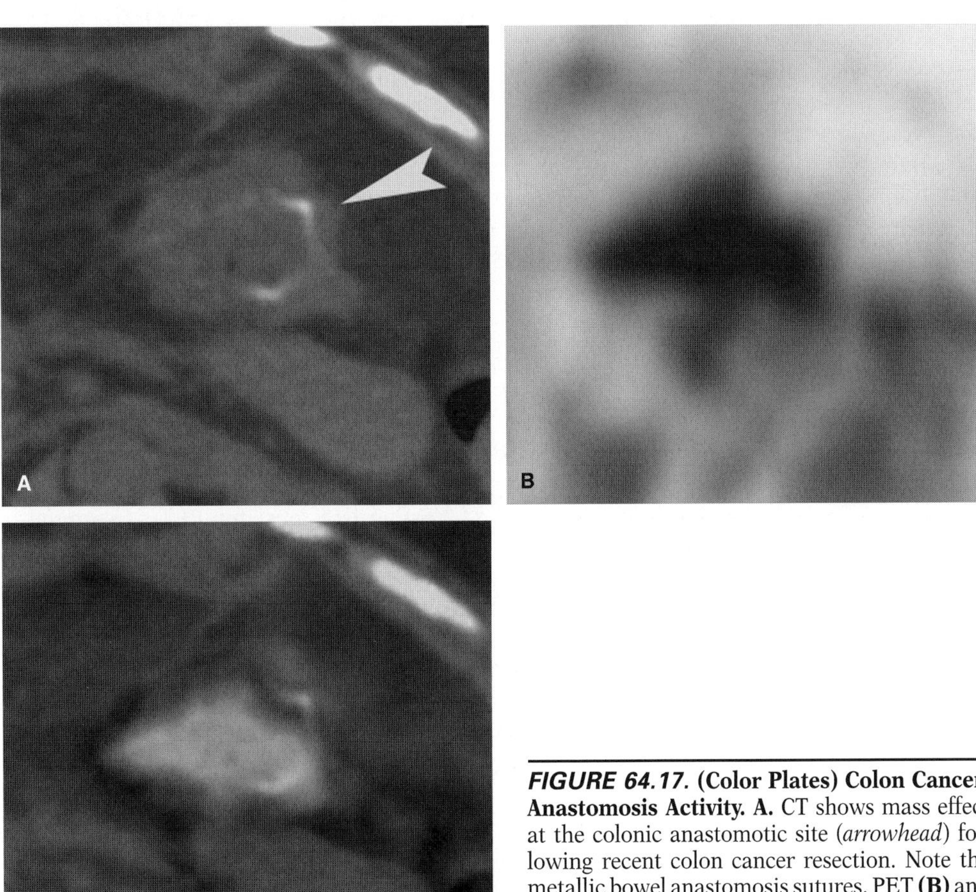

FIGURE 64.17. **(Color Plates) Colon Cancer: Anastomosis Activity. A.** CT shows mass effect at the colonic anastomotic site (*arrowhead*) following recent colon cancer resection. Note the metallic bowel anastomosis sutures. PET **(B)** and fused PET-CT **(C)** images of the same area show marked hypermetabolic activity caused by postoperative inflammation. Recurrent tumor may have a similar appearance.

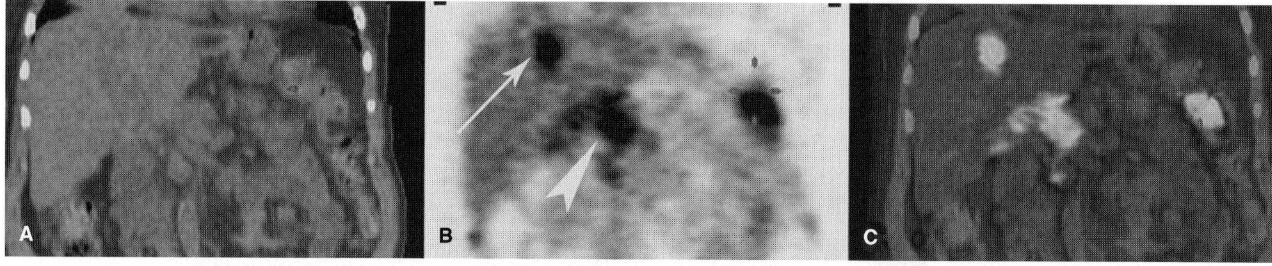

FIGURE 64.18. **(Color Plates) Hepatic Metastasis: Colon Cancer.** Coronal-plane PET images in the same patient shown in Fig. 64.17 reveal a hepatic metastasis (*arrow*) that is barely visible on the corresponding noncontrast CT. Hypermetabolic activity is also evident in metastatic lymph nodes in the porta hepatic (*arrowhead*) and in the primary cancer in the splenic flexure of the colon (between *cursors*). **A.** CT without contrast. **B.** Corrected PET. **C.** Fused PET-CT.

focal FDG hyperactivity is indicative of tumor recurrence, whereas surgical scarring is not hypermetabolic.

Hepatic Malignancies. Owing to physiologic, and commonly heterogeneous, metabolic activity of the background hepatic parenchyma, the detection of small hypermetabolic foci is somewhat limited. FDG uptake by hepatocellular carcinoma (HCC) is inversely related to the degree of tumor differentiation. Well-differentiated HCC shows low FDG accumulation. One should be cautious in utilizing PET as the primary evaluation for HCC. However, once the diagnosis is established, PET can provide valuable regional as well as whole-body assessment of the stage of HCC. The overall sensitivity of PET for detection of primary HCC is around 70%; specificity is limited. Nonmalignant hepatic lesions such as hepatic adenoma may show increased activity and contribute to false-positive results.

PET sensitivity for detection of cholangiocarcinoma (CCA) mainly depends on its morphologic appearance. The nodular (focal) subtype can be detected up to 80% of the time, whereas detection of the infiltrative subtype is below 20%. Inflammation associated with biliary obstruction causes false-positive results. PET is not a first-line modality for detection of CCA, although it can be used for staging of the extrahepatic disease and in detection of recurrence.

Metastases. PET is most accurate for metastases in the liver that are larger than 1 cm (Fig. 64.18). Demonstration of smaller lesions is limited by PET resolution and physiologic liver background activity. Background FDG activity is commonly heterogeneous in the liver, so focal activity must be interpreted with caution. Metastases appear as discrete foci of increased activity, often multiple and varying in size. Large metastases with necrotic centers may appear as rings of increased activity (Fig. 64.19). Occasionally, metastatic lesions, even large ones, do not show increased FDG activity. In patients with colorectal carcinoma, PET may show only 70% of the liver lesions evident on resection specimens.

Gallbladder cancer shows high affinity for FDG and is detected with high sensitivity. Local invasion of liver is more accurately evaluated by CT or MR. PET provides regional and whole-body staging of gallbladder cancers. Hypermetabolic activity in the gallbladder bed is more commonly caused by inflammatory diseases of the gallbladder than by malignancy (Fig. 64.20). Correlation with CT, MR, or US is of great value in minimizing false-positive results. Active hepatic foci near the gallbladder fossa can be misinterpreted as a gallbladder focus. Multiplanar assessment improves the accuracy of localization and should be employed routinely.

Breast Cancer. PET is reliable for assessment of breast lesions larger than 15 to 20 mm (Fig. 64.1). Detection of microscopic cancers is below the current threshold of PET. Overall, the uptake of FDG in breast cancer is less than that of lung cancer. An SUV above 2.0 correlates with malignancy. False-positive uptake occurs with inflammatory breast disease. False-negative rates of up to 60% for invasive lobular cancers and up to 24% for invasive ductal cancers have been reported. Sentinel node lymphoscintigraphy is very valuable and exceeds PET capabilities in preoperative staging of the axillary nodes. However, PET is very accurate in whole-body staging, can reliably assess the response to treatment, and is widely used in the detection of recurrence.

Fasting is a must for PET assessment of breast cancer patients because of the relatively low avidity of breast cancer tissue for FDG. Detailed assessment of axillary and internal mammary nodal chains in coronal and sagittal planes is essential on both PET and CT images (Figs. 64.21, 64.22). The opposite breast is assessed for bilateral disease. Postoperative muscle flaps may contain hypermetabolic muscle tissue. Postradiation pneumonitis mimics transthoracic extension of breast cancer. Knowledge of the site and time of radiation therapy, as well as correlation with radiographic findings, are essential for correct interpretation. PET may detect bone metastases not evident on radionuclide bone scans.

Cervical Cancer. PET is clearly superior to CT and US in regional node assessment at the time of cervical cancer diagnosis. PET has been successfully employed for

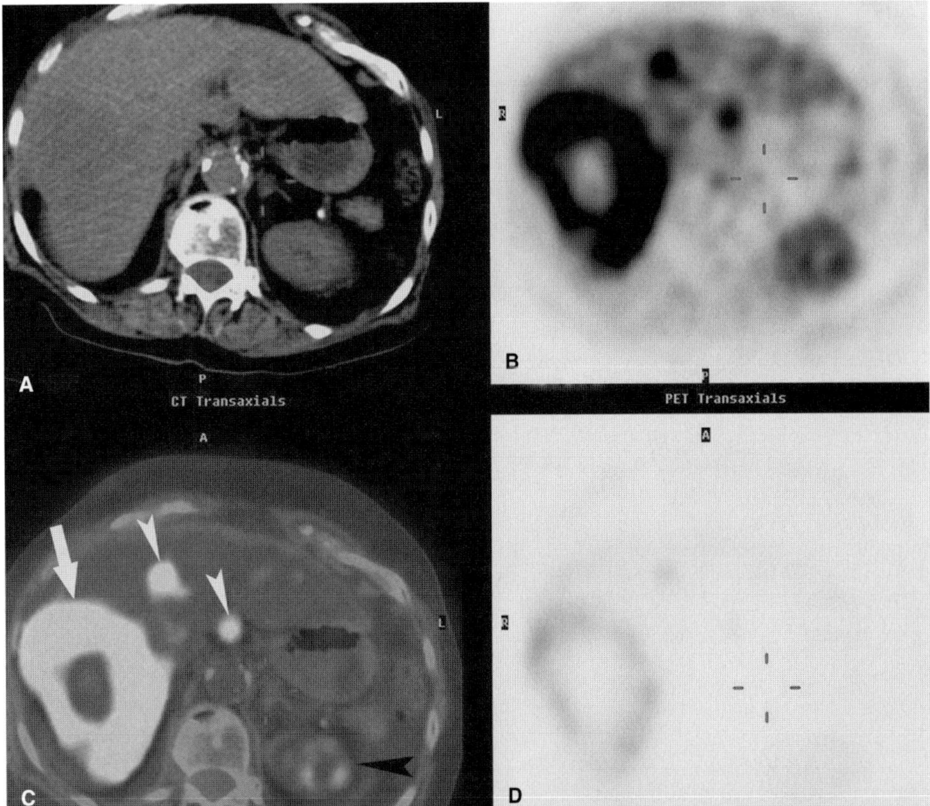

FIGURE 64.19. **(Color Plates) Necrotic Hepatic Metastasis.** PET-CT shows a very large liver metastasis with central necrosis (*arrow*) in a patient with history of colon cancer and poor response to chemotherapy. Two additional smaller metastases (*white arrowheads*) are also evident. Normal physiologic activity is seen the in left kidney (*black arrowhead*). **A.** CT. **B.** Corrected PET. **C.** Fused PET-CT. **D.** Uncorrected PET.

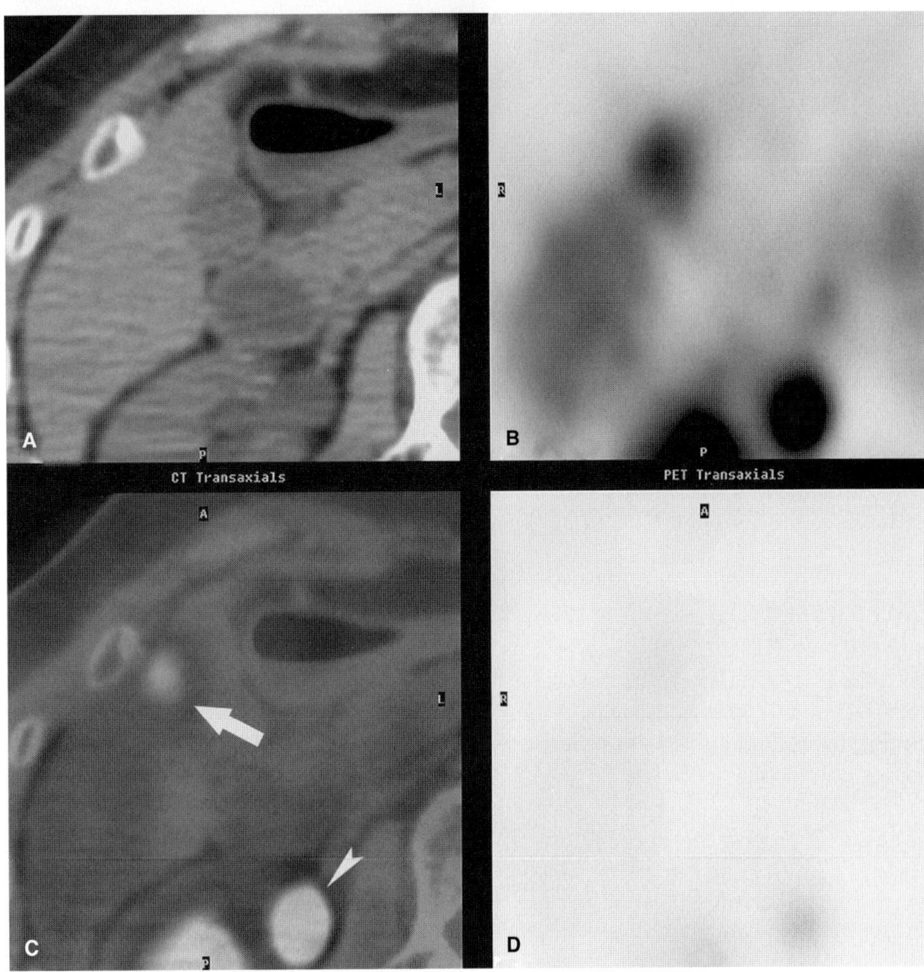

FIGURE 64.20. **(Color Plates) Chronic Cholecystitis.** High metabolic activity in the gallbladder (*arrow*) is caused by chronic cholecystitis. Gallbladder uptake of fluorodeoxyglucose may represent inflammation or tumor. Physiologic activity is seen in the right renal pelvis (*arrowhead*) and right kidney. **A.** CT. **B.** Corrected PET. **C.** Fused PET-CT. **D.** Uncorrected PET.

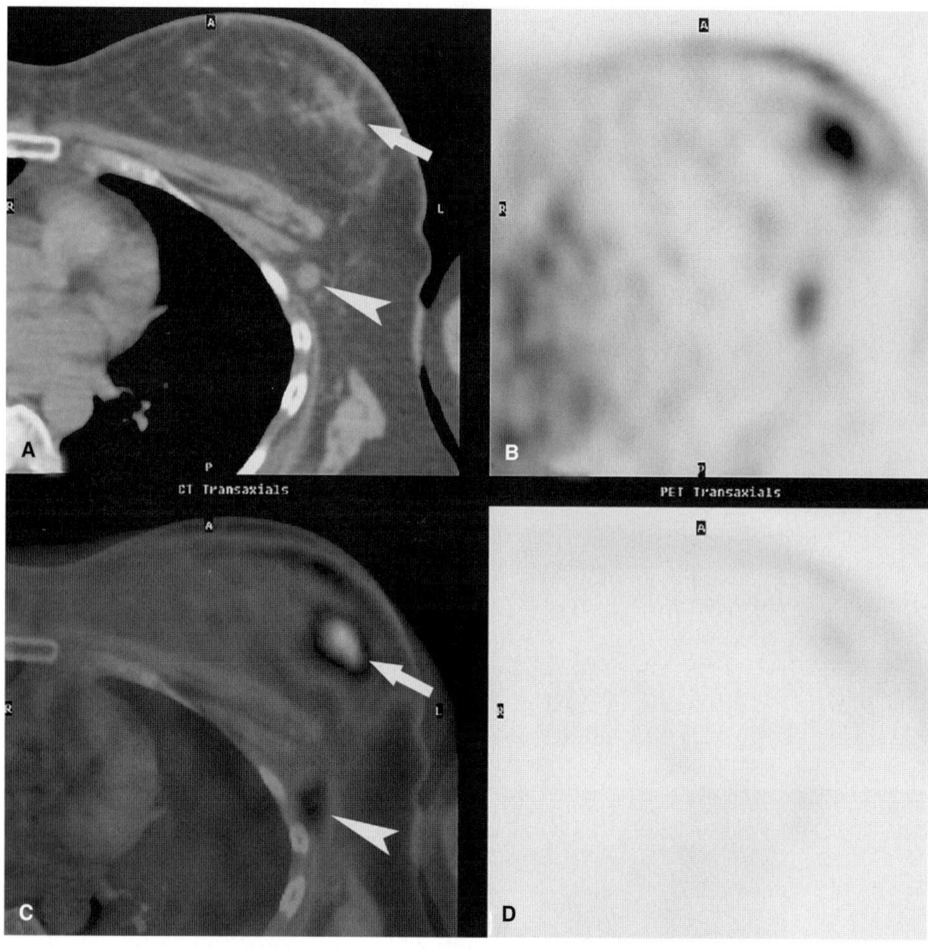

FIGURE 64.21. **(Color Plates) Breast Cancer: Axillary Node Metastasis.** Axial images from PET-CT demonstrate hypermetabolic activity in the cancer (*arrows*) within the left breast and within an axillary lymph node (*arrowheads*) that would be considered benign by CT size criteria. **A.** CT. **B.** Corrected PET. **C.** Fused PET-CT. **D.** Uncorrected PET.

evaluation of response to treatment and is the modality of choice for restaging and detection of recurrence. Placement of a urinary catheter to empty the bladder and rinse it with saline just prior to scanning reduces bladder activity that may obscure subtle disease activity.

Uterine Cancer. PET has limited value in primary detection and in assessing the depth of invasion of endometrial cancer. However, PET is valuable for assessment of regional nodes and the peritoneal cavity, for whole-body screening for distant metastases, and for detection of recurrent tumor (Fig. 64.23). Special attention should be focused on the peritoneal surface to detect subtle peritoneal seeding. Section-by-section correlation with CT is crucial. Uterine fibroids and peri-ovulatory hypermetabolism of the ovary may cause interpretation difficulties.

Ovarian Cancer. Hybrid PET-CT imaging is superior to CT or PET alone in staging and detecting recurrence of ovarian cancer (Fig. 64.24). However, small peritoneal

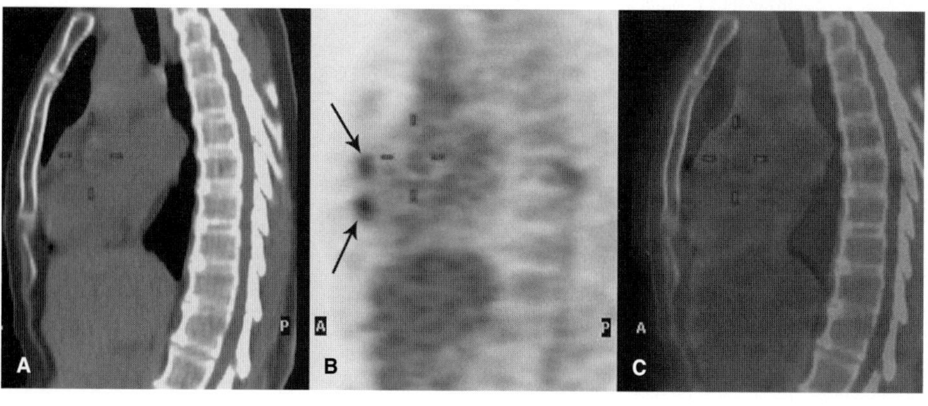

FIGURE 64.22. **(Color Plates) Breast Cancer: Internal Mammary Node Metastases.** Sagittal images from PET-CT in a woman with breast cancer reveal breast cancer recurrence in internal mammary lymph nodes (*arrows*). **A.** CT without contrast. **B.** Corrected PET. **C.** Fused PET-CT.

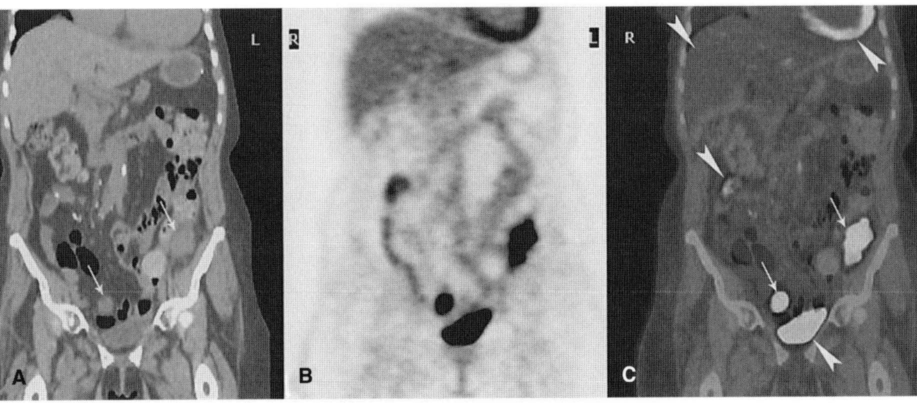

FIGURE 64.23. **(Color Plates) Uterine Cancer Recurrence.** PET-CT images in a woman post–total abdominal hysterectomy and bilateral oophorectomy for uterine cancer reveals recurrence of tumor in two locations (*arrows*). Physiologic activity (*arrowheads*) is seen in the bladder, liver, heart, and bowel. **A.** CT without contrast. **B.** Corrected PET. **C.** Fused PET-CT.

metastases (<5 mm) usually escape detection by PET-CT. PET provides whole-body screening for recurrent disease in patients with elevated cancer antigen 125. Knowledge of the menstrual cycle is recommended, as peri-ovulatory follicles can be hypermetabolic. Multiplanar assessment is useful to follow the track of distal ureters in the pelvis to avoid mistaking ureteral activity for nodal metastases.

Renal Malignancies. Owing to high physiologic activity in the renal parenchyma and in the urinary collecting system, detection of hypermetabolic lesions in the genitourinary tract is challenging. The efficacy of PET for further characterization of renal lesions detected by other modalities is expectedly low. However, PET is outstanding in detection of extrarenal involvement by renal carcinoma. PET is used for detection of normal-sized nodes that harbor malignancy. PET detects metastatic osseous foci and appears to be superior to Tc-99m methylene diphosphonate (MDP) bone scans in detection of lytic lesions, which may be cold on bone scan. PET is employed to detect recurrence in patients after nephrectomy.

Ureter and Urinary Bladder Malignancies. Limitations of PET in detection of bladder tumors are mainly caused by the presence of massive urinary FDG activity in the bladder (Fig. 64.25). PET readily detects extravesical involvement. PET is superior to CT and MR for accurate detection of involved regional nodes and whole-body staging. Aggressive hydration, frequent voiding, and rinsing the bladder prior to PET scanning have been employed with limited success. An obstructed nonfunctional kidney may show ureteral activity originating from a malignancy in the ureter.

Adrenal Malignancy. Limited studies are promising in the use of PET to differentiate benign from malignant lesions (Figs. 64.26, 64.27). Three studies have reported a PET sensitivity of 100% with specificity of 80% to 100%. These small studies need confirmation by larger studies. CT and MR remain the imaging methods of choice to differentiate the common benign adrenal adenoma from adrenal metastases (see Chapter 33).

Testicular Malignancies. PET is superb in the detection of testicular cancer metastatic deposits throughout the body. Seminoma is usually more FDG avid than nonseminoma, but PET is successfully used for both subtypes. Postoperative changes can pose difficulty in interpretation of PET images. Also, urinary bladder activity can overshadow the pelvis. Correlation with corresponding CT images is imperative for initial staging as well as assessment for recurrence.

Prostate Cancer. FDG uptake is low in prostate cancer, especially when the tumor is well differentiated. Because of its variable uptake, the value of PET in the evaluation of prostate cancer has not been established. PET has low sensitivity for detection of osseous metastases caused by prostate cancer.

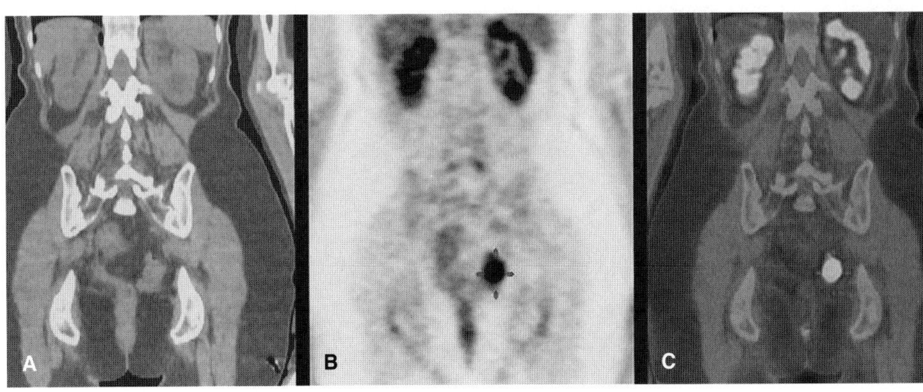

FIGURE 64.24. **(Color Plates) Ovarian Cancer, Stage 1.** PET-CT shows a hypermetabolic focus in the left ovary (between *cursors*). Further evaluation confirmed an ovarian cancer confined to the ovary. Similar FDG activity may be seen in physiologic ovarian cysts. **A.** CT. **B.** Corrected PET. **C.** Fused PET-CT.

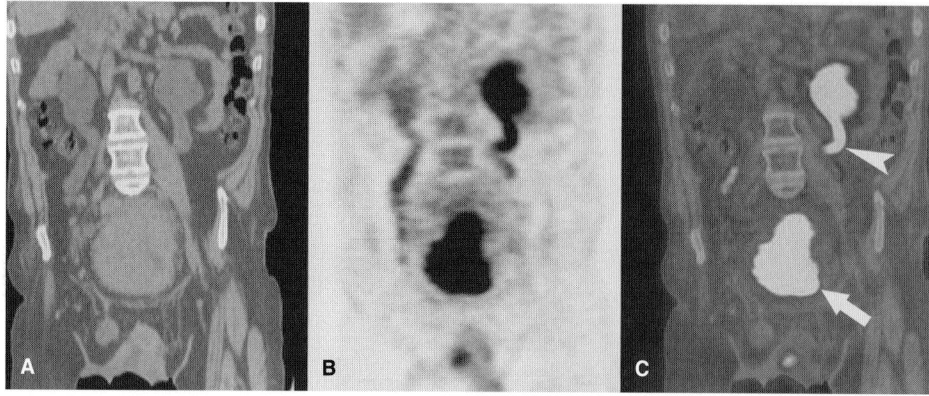

FIGURE 64.25. **(Color Plates) Transitional Cell Carcinoma of the Bladder.** A large bladder tumor (*arrow*) shows fluorodeoxyglucose hyperactivity. Hydronephrosis of the left renal collecting system (*arrowhead*) caused by the obstructing bladder tumor is apparent. **A.** CT. **B.** Corrected PET. **C.** Fused PET-CT.

Head and Neck Malignancies. Head and neck cancers include squamous cell carcinoma of mucosal surfaces and adenocarcinoma of salivary and lacrimal glands (Fig. 64.28). PET is superior to CT and MR for the detection of involved nodes in the neck and distant metastases (Fig. 64.29). PET can detect occult head and neck malignancy reliably. PET by itself is limited in its assessment of the extent of the primary lesion (T-staging). T-staging is greatly improved by hybrid PET-CT imaging. Up to 15% of patients with primary head and neck malignancies develop other malignancies, including lung and esophageal carcinomas, that may be detected by PET during initial staging. Reports show good correlation between the degree of FDG activity and the prognosis of head and neck malignancies. Also, reliable early assessment of the response to radiation and chemotherapy by PET has been reported.

Physiologic activity in the head and neck is best recognized by cross-referencing PET-CT scans. Radionuclide activity may be seen in the salivary glands, from salivary secretions retained in the gingival recesses and

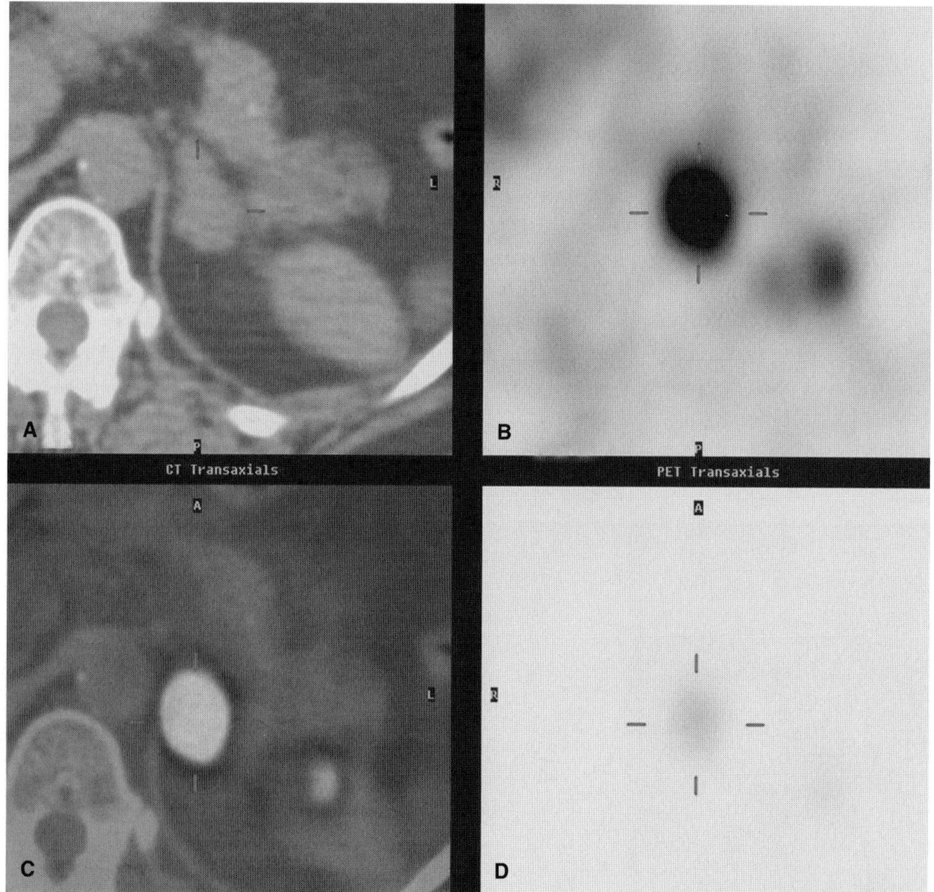

FIGURE 64.26. **(Color Plates) Adrenal Metastasis.** PET-CT of a patient with a history of lung cancer shows a focus of fluorodeoxyglucose activity in the left adrenal gland (between *cursors*). Biopsy confirmed metastatic disease. This was the only site of disease recurrence in this patient. **A.** CT. **B.** Corrected PET. **C.** Fused PET-CT. **D.** Uncorrected PET.

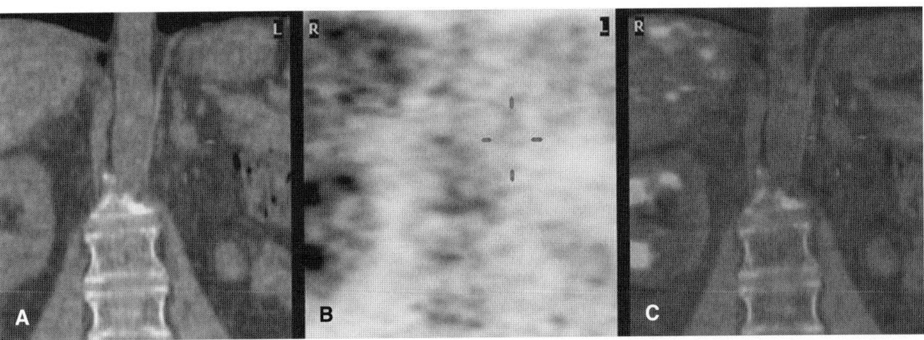

FIGURE 64.27. **(Color Plates) Benign Adrenal Adenoma.** PET-CT of a patient with a history of colon cancer reveals enlargement of the left adrenal gland (between *cursors*). PET shows a hypometabolic lesion compatible with benign adrenal adenoma. Adrenal protocol CT was confirmatory. **A.** CT. **B.** Corrected PET. **C.** Fused PET-CT.

vallecula, in the tonsils and lymphatic tissues of the Waldeyer ring, and in the tongue musculature, masticator muscles, and laryngeal musculature. Swishing the mouth with water prior to scanning can clear retained saliva. Unilateral laryngeal uptake may signify vocal cord paralysis caused by recurrent laryngeal nerve damage or tumor. Dental implants should be removed, if possible, as they may produce artifacts in the attenuation correction algorithm. Infection and inflammatory processes, especially dental disease, recent dental procedures, or tracheotomy sites, can demonstrate FDG activity. Postradiation mucositis, including esophagitis and gingivitis, produces confusing findings. Benign tumors, such as Warthin tumor of the salivary gland (papillary cystadenoma lymphomatosum), can show FDG activity. Posttherapy bone marrow activation can also produce a confusing picture.

PET is excellent for detection of recurrence, but interpretation of postoperative and postradiation changes is challenging. Because inflammation in the treatment bed causes PET activity, posttreatment PET scans are best delayed for 2 to 3 months after treatment.

Sarcomas and Osseous Malignancies. FDG PET and PET-CT are very useful in staging, assessing tumor response to therapy, and restaging of soft tissue sarcomas and primary bony tumors. It is also important to identify all of the metastatic foci, because surgical resection of a limited number of metastatic lesions has been shown to increase survival with these tumors. FDG PET is highly sensitive and specific in detecting and following bony metastatic disease for most cancers (Figs 64.30 to 64.34). Hypermetabolic changes in the bone marrow that occurs as a result of chemotherapy and inflammatory changes related to arthritides must be differentiated from metastatic disease. Because prostate cancer is frequently hypometabolic, osseous metastases are better demonstrated with routing bone scan than with FDG PET.

NEUROLOGIC PET IMAGING

F-18-FDG, reflecting glucose metabolism, is currently the most widely used radiotracer for CNS imaging. Cerebral blood perfusion (CBF) maps can be obtained from O-15 H_2O PET imaging. CBF and FDG images appear very similar, as glucose uptake and cerebral blood flow are tightly coupled in the brain. Cortical gray matter, the putamen, head of the caudate, thalamus, and cerebellum have high glucose metabolic activity, which results in marked activity on FDG imaging. Blood glucose levels markedly affect the degree of FDG activity in the brain, as glucose competes with FDG for uptake. Visual and cognitive activity affect the distribution of FDG owing to activation of certain centers throughout the brain. This serves as the basis for functional mapping of sensomotor centers throughout the CNS. IV injection of FDG is preferably done in a calm and dark room to assure homogenous distribution throughout the cortex.

CNS Malignancies. PET is used for assessment of grade of malignancy, for biopsy guidance, to predict prognosis, to monitor treatment response, and to detect posttherapy recurrence. The degree of malignant differentiation shows direct correlation with the degree of FDG activity, i.e., high-grade gliomas show more FDG activity. A well-known exception to this rule is pilocytic astrocytoma, which is a low-grade malignancy with high metabolic activity on PET imaging. A great deal of research has been focused

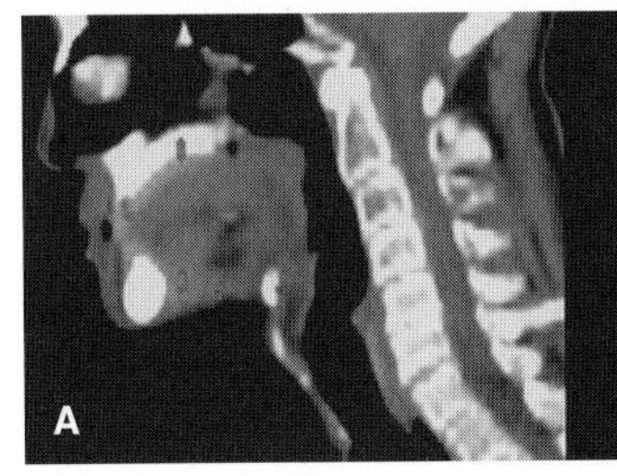

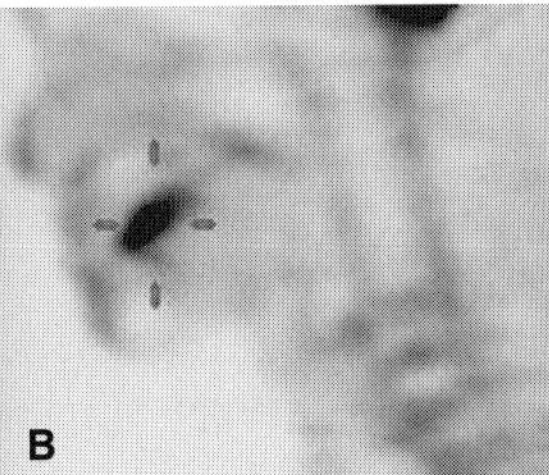

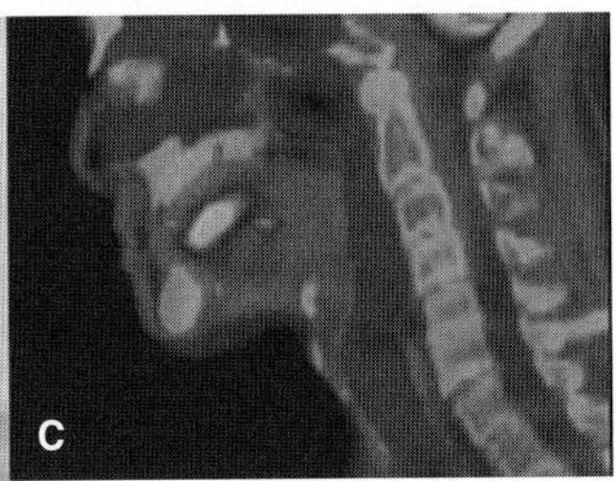

FIGURE 64.28. **Squamous Cell Carcinoma of the Tongue.** PET-CT shows that the tumor is localized to the primary site (between *cursors*) on the tongue without evidence of metastatic disease. **A.** CT. **B.** Corrected PET. **C.** Fused PET-CT.

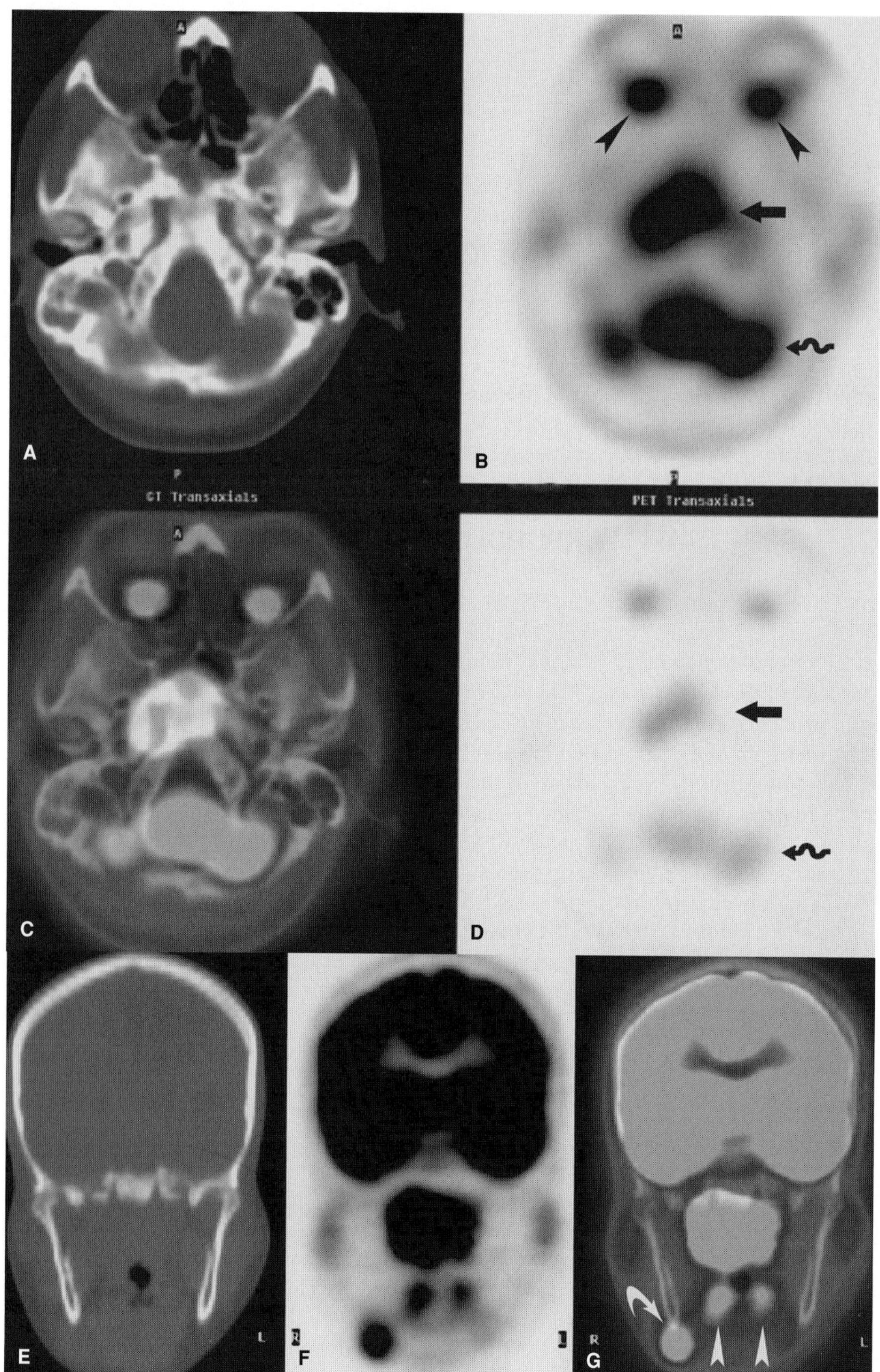

FIGURE 64.29. (Color Plates) Metastatic Squamous Cell Carcinoma of the Nasopharynx. Axial PET-CT images (**A.** CT; **B.** corrected PET; **C.** fused PET-CT; **D.** uncorrected PET) reveal an invasive tumor (*straight arrow*) of the nasopharynx. Fluorodeoxyglucose uptake in the ocular muscles (*black arrowheads*) caused by eye movement is prominent. Note how attenuation correction overestimates the extent of tumor (*straight arrow*), as well as brain activity (*squiggly arrow*) in **B.** and **C.** as compared to the uncorrected PET image **(D)**. Careful correlation with CT and other imaging studies is needed for accurate interpretation. Coronal-plane PET-CT images (**E.** CT; **F.** corrected PET; **G.** fused PET-CT) show metastatic spread of tumor to the nasopharyngeal lymph nodes (*white arrowheads*) and the mandible (*curved arrow*).

on quantification of the activity to enhance the ability of PET to differentiate between benign and malignant CNS masses. Tumor activity more than 1.5 times that of white matter or more than 0.6 times that of gray matter has sensitivity of 94% and specificity of 77% for malignancy (Fig. 64.35). High FDG activity is a poor prognostic factor, independent of the degree of histologic differentiation. Detection of a hypermetabolic lesion in the background of the hypermetabolic cortex is a difficult task; therefore, PET should never be used alone to detect subtle cortical lesions. Slice-by-slice correlation with CT or MR is crucial. A thorough knowledge of cross-sectional neuroanatomy is a must for interpretation of neurologic PET.

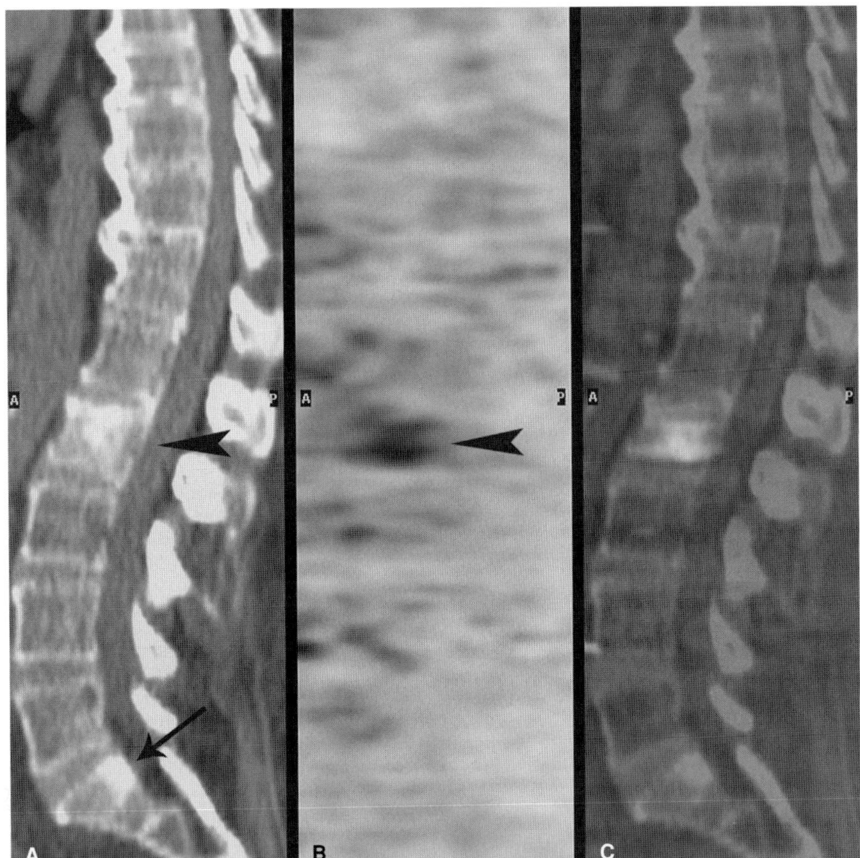

FIGURE 64.30. **(Color Plates) Metastasis to Spine.** PET-CT of the spine in a patient with colon cancer shows fluorodeoxyglucose (FDG) activity corresponding to a lytic and sclerotic destructive lesion (*arrowheads*) in a lumbar vertebral body. Findings are indicative of osseous metastasis. Discogenic sclerosis (*arrow*) in another vertebral body shows no FDG activity. **A.** CT. **B.** Corrected PET. **C.** Fused PET-CT.

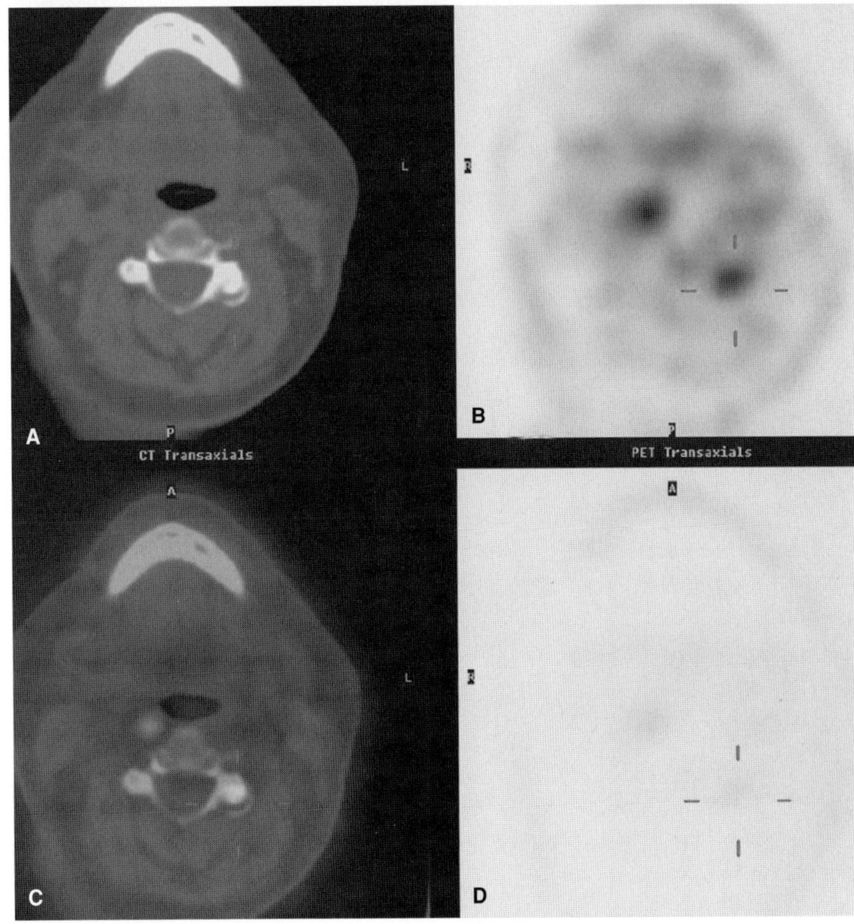

FIGURE 64.31. **(Color Plates) Facet Hypertrophy, Not Metastasis.** PET-CT in a patient with breast cancer demonstrates focal fluorodeoxyglucose activity (between *cursors*) in the cervical spine. Correlation of PET with CT confirms that the activity represents benign inflammation associated with degenerative disease in the facet joint. **A.** CT. **B.** Corrected PET. **C.** Fused PET-CT. **D.** Uncorrected PET.

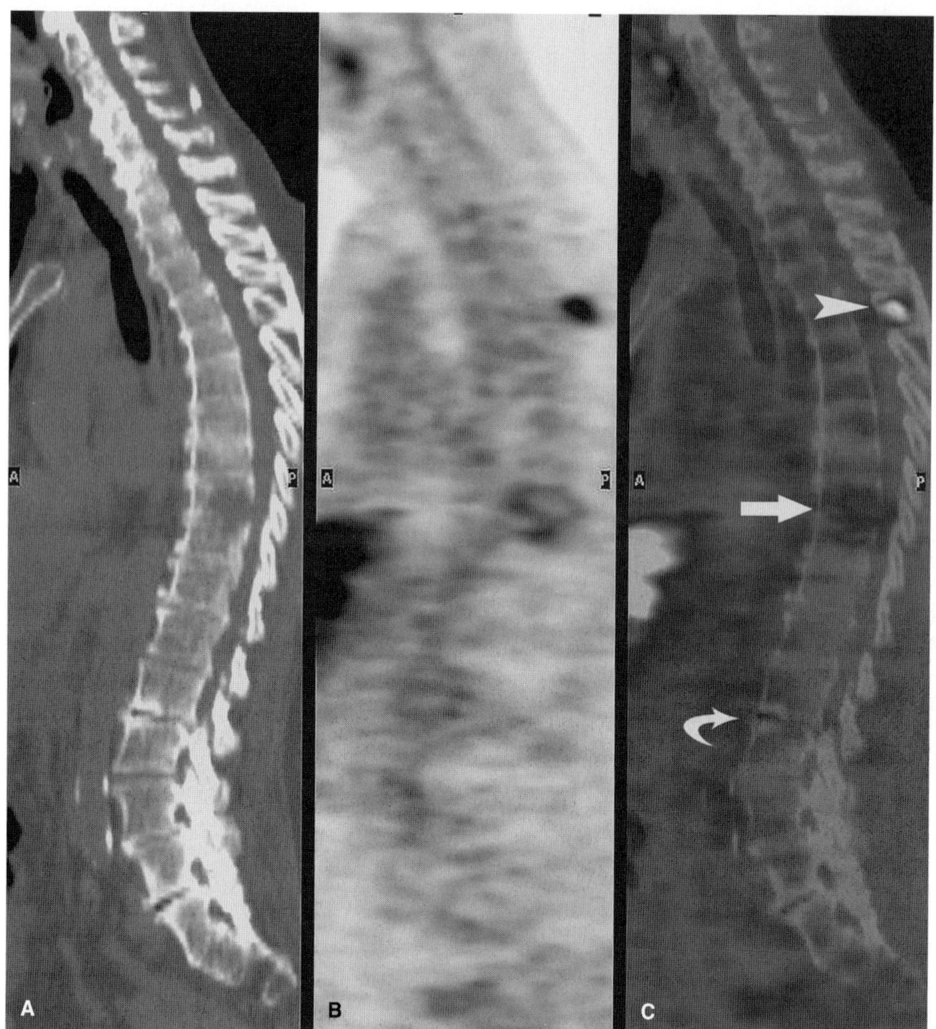

FIGURE 64.32. **(Color Plates) "Hot" and "Cold" Osseous Metastases.** PET-CT of the spine in another patient with breast cancer reveals an osseous metastasis with high fluorodeoxyglucose (FDG) activity (*arrowhead*), a metastasis that is obviously destructive on CT but hypometabolic on PET (*straight arrow*), and degenerative change (*curved arrow*) that shows no FDG uptake. **A.** CT. **B.** Corrected PET. **C.** Fused PET-CT.

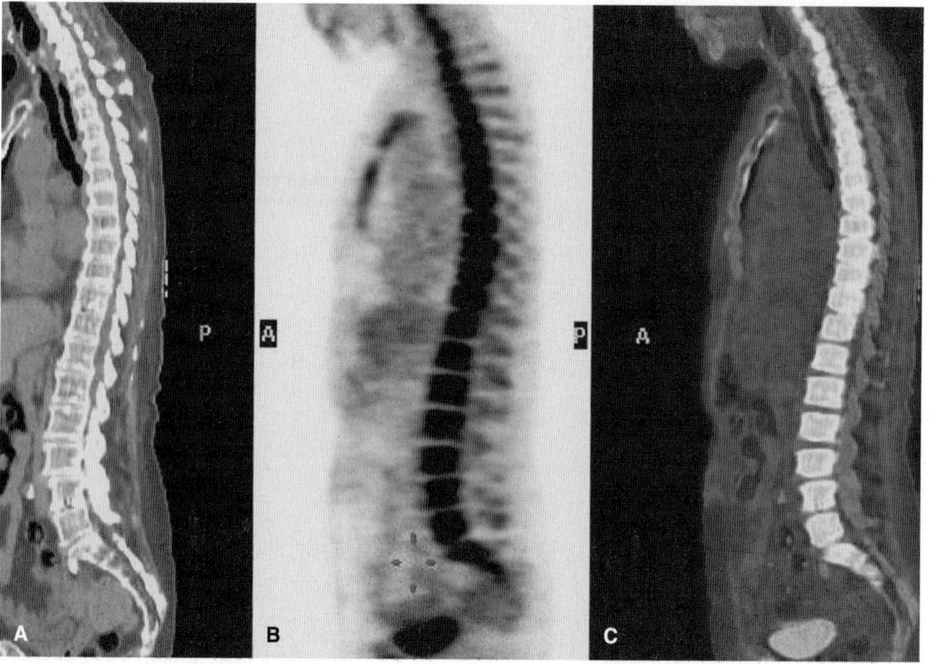

FIGURE 64.33. **(Color Plates) Benign Hypermetabolic Bone Marrow.** Marked diffuse fluorodeoxyglucose uptake is seen throughout the spine on PET in a patient with colon cancer. Correlation with the CT scan shows no evidence of metastatic disease. These findings are indicative of diffuse marrow stimulation related to recovery from chemotherapy or marrow-stimulating drugs. **A.** CT. **B.** Corrected PET. **C.** Fused PET-CT.

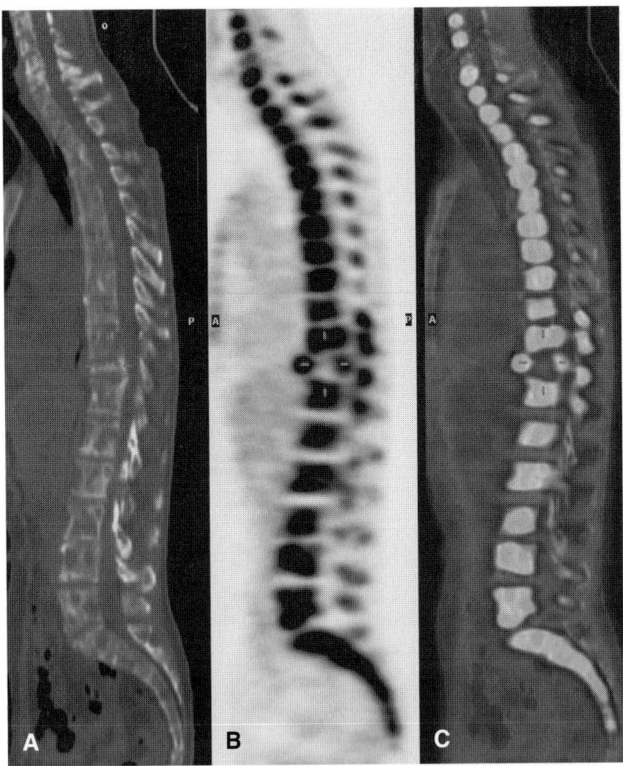

FIGURE 64.34. **(Color Plates) Diffuse Metastatic Disease With Hypermetabolic Bone Marrow.** Compare to Fig. 64.33. In this patient with breast cancer, advanced lytic destructive change is evident throughout the spine on CT. PET shows diffuse marrow hyperactivity, representing both hypermetabolic marrow stimulation and osseous metastatic disease. **A.** CT. **B.** Corrected PET. **C.** Fused PET-CT.

PET can serve as an accurate guide for planning of a brain mass biopsy. It is common for CNS malignancies to contain cells with different degrees of differentiation. Sampling errors occur by biopsy of a well-differentiated portion of the mass, rather than the most malignant component, causing underestimation of the malignant grade. PET localizes the most hypermetabolic portion of the lesion and guides biopsy to the most aggressive portion of the mass. This tremendously enhances the yield of the biopsy.

Multifocal tumors and distant metastases from primary CNS malignancies are detected by whole-body PET. Drop metastases are evident within the spinal canal. Intraperitoneal spread of CNS malignancy via a ventriculoperitoneal shunt may be demonstrated.

Postoperative PET can differentiate between necrotic mass and residual viable tumor (Fig. 64.36). No appreciable activity is usually seen in the surgical bed, even early after the surgery; therefore, focal FDG activity is usually indicative of viable tumor. High-dose, focused radiation therapy induces inflammation, which in its acute phase can be hypermetabolic on PET imaging. It is therefore prudent to wait 2 to 4 months after high-dose radiation therapy. Foci of high FDG activity in patients with brain tumors may represent active seizure centers near the surgical bed and not necessarily residual viable tumor. Slice-by-slice comparison with CT or MR in multiple imaging planes will clarify this finding as a seizure focus lacking the presence of a mass. Intracavitary instillation of radioactive monoclonal antibody results in a rim of high metabolic activity caused by active inflammation induced by radiation necrosis. Nodular rather than rimlike activity may represent residual viable tumor tissue. Steroid therapy in oncology patients may induce hyperglycemia that results in a generalized decrease of normal brain uptake of FDG because of competition with glucose.

Brain Metastases. PET detection of metastases to the brain from non-CNS malignancies has limitations, with reported sensitivity of 75% and specificity of 83%. Metabolic foci with FDG activity greater than that of normal gray matter are considered likely metastatic lesions (Fig. 64.37). PET is clearly inferior to contrast-enhanced MR. The size of a lesion is a significant factor, with only 40% of 1-cm metastases detected by PET alone. Approximately 90% of lesions >1.8 cm are detected. CNS metastases from melanoma are frequently small and poorly detected. Because of limited sensitivity, PET scanning of the brain is commonly not performed as part of whole-body PET staging for non-CNS malignancies.

Epilepsy. Postictal imaging with PET to identify the seizure focus is impractical in routine practice. Currently, ictal studies are usually performed using SPECT imaging with Tc-99m–based tracers such as hexamethylpropyleneamine oxime. These can be injected during an observed seizure, and imaging can be performed after the seizure has stopped. Ictal imaging usually shows a high degree of activity in the seizure focus. In contrast, interictal imaging and PET show a hypometabolic area at this focus. The majority of PET-imaged seizure foci are in the medial temporal lobe medially and often extend laterally, representing functionally related cortex deafferentation. The primary role for PET is to determine the side of temporal lobe seizure for surgical resection. Correlation with morphologic imaging is crucial, as seizure can be caused by anatomic lesions including tumors, ectopic gray matter, gyration anomalies, and tuberous sclerosis. Accessory findings include hypometabolic frontal lobe, basal ganglia, and thalami.

Dementia. In dementia, PET provides functional information early, before the structural changes seen on CT or MR occur. Typical features seen on PET imaging can confirm the presence of certain subtypes of dementia. Accurate early diagnosis is important, as preventive or risk-modification therapy may be instituted to slow down progression of disease.

Alzheimer dementia is difficult to diagnose early in the disease process by anatomic imaging. Characteristic atrophy of frontal, temporal, and parietal lobes is generally a

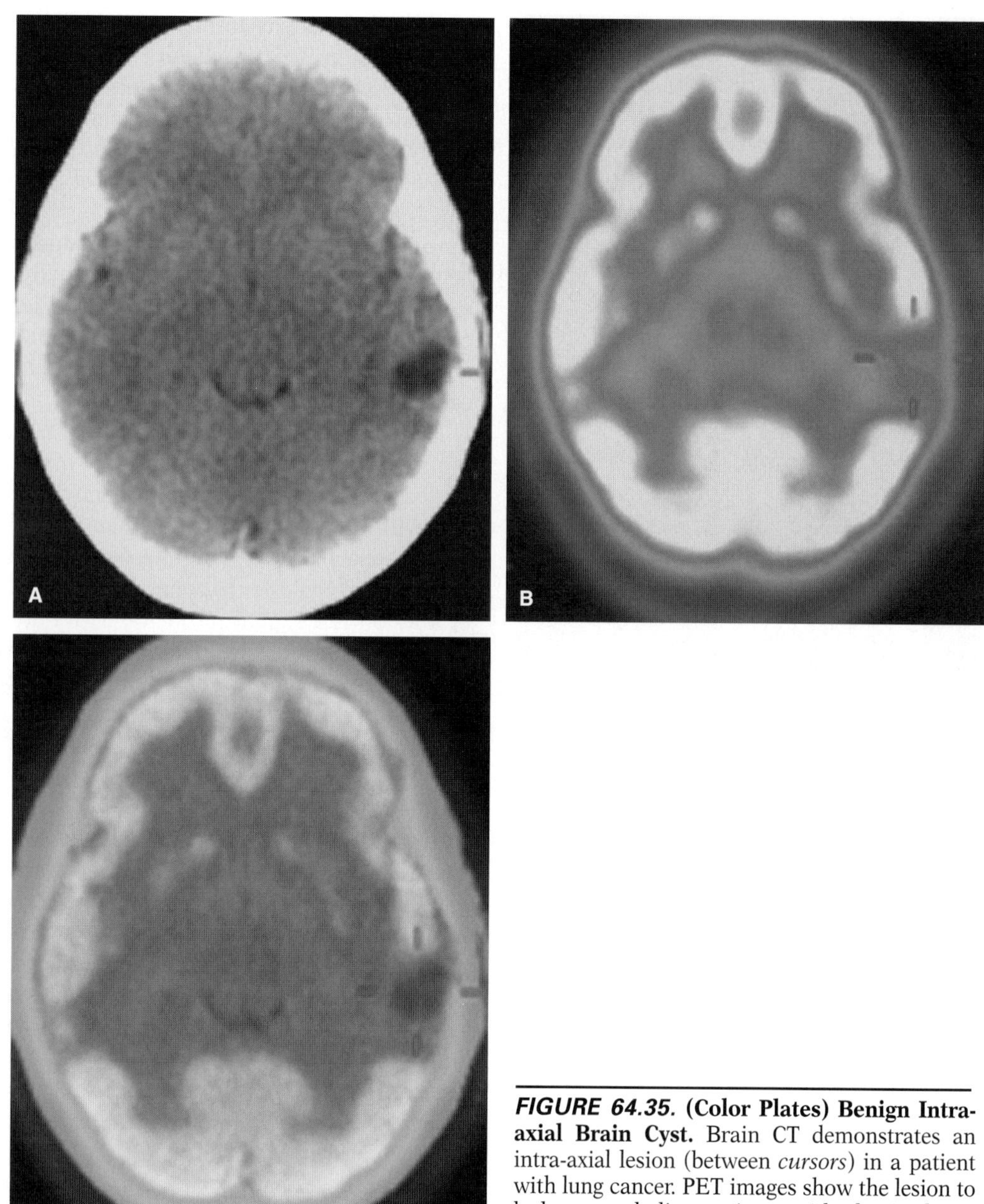

FIGURE 64.35. **(Color Plates) Benign Intra-axial Brain Cyst.** Brain CT demonstrates an intra-axial lesion (between *cursors*) in a patient with lung cancer. PET images show the lesion to be hypometabolic, consistent with a benign brain cyst. **A.** CT. **B.** Corrected PET. **C.** Fused PET-CT.

late finding. PET features of Alzheimer disease are bilateral hypometabolism of the temporal and parietal lobes, with conspicuous sparing of visual and motor cortices (Fig. 64.38). PET findings are 86% sensitive and 86% specific for Alzheimer disease.

Pick disease (a type of frontotemporal dementia) shows hypometabolic areas involving both the frontal and the anterior temporal lobes.

Multi-infarct dementia, in contrast, shows multiple defects throughout the brain parenchyma without sparing the visual and motor cortices. The number and volume of the hypometabolic areas correlate closely to the clinical degree of dementia.

Normal-pressure hydrocephalus characteristically presents clinically with dementia, gait disturbances, and incontinence. The diagnosis is made with radiotracer cisternography, CT, or MR. PET shows diffuse hypometabolism, which may reverse after effective shunting.

Parkinson disease is a common neurodegenerative disease manifest by tremor, rigidity, akinesia, and slow speech. In the long term, up to 30% of patients will also develop dementia. In these patients, PET can help exclude other types of dementia. PET demonstrates high FDG activity in lentiform nuclei and thalami related to lack of dopaminergic inhibition. The caudate nuclei are

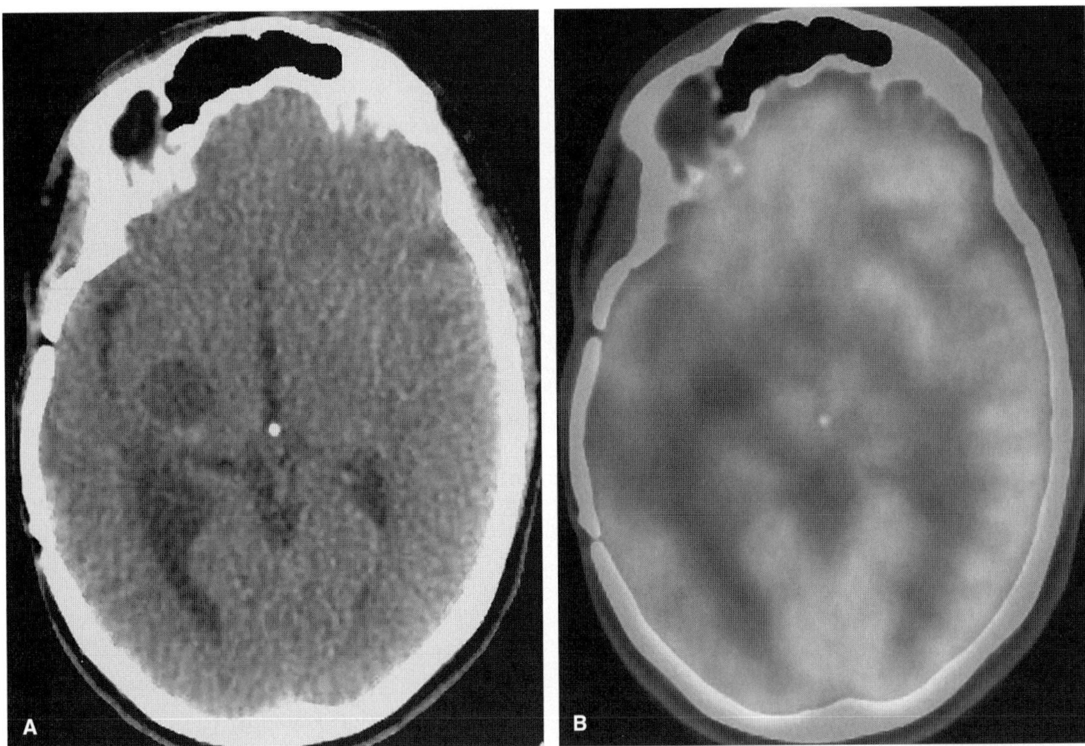

FIGURE 64.36. **(Color Plates) Absence of Residual Brain Tumor.** CT shows postoperative changes on the right related to resection of a malignant brain tumor. PET reveals no hypermetabolic foci in the surgical bed or elsewhere in the brain, indicating the absence of residual viable tumor. **A.** CT. **B.** Fused PET-CT.

characteristically spared. F-11 fluorodopamine has been utilized to identify the dopamine deficiency in the putamen (substantia nigra) and follow these patients for response to therapy.

CARDIAC PET IMAGING

Cardiac PET is accurate in assessing cardiac metabolism with F-18-FDG and in evaluating myocardial perfusion with other positron-emitting radionuclides. Although Tc-99m–based tracers and thallium-201 (Tl-201) chloride are very successfully utilized in daily nuclear cardiology practice (see Chapter 57), FDG PET is considered the gold standard for evaluation of myocardial viability by accurate identification of hibernating viable myocardium. PET is more accurate (93% sensitive, 93% specific) than SPECT in detection of myocardial ischemia.

Myocardial Perfusion PET Imaging. SPECT myocardial perfusion imaging is performed with Tl-201 or Tc-99m

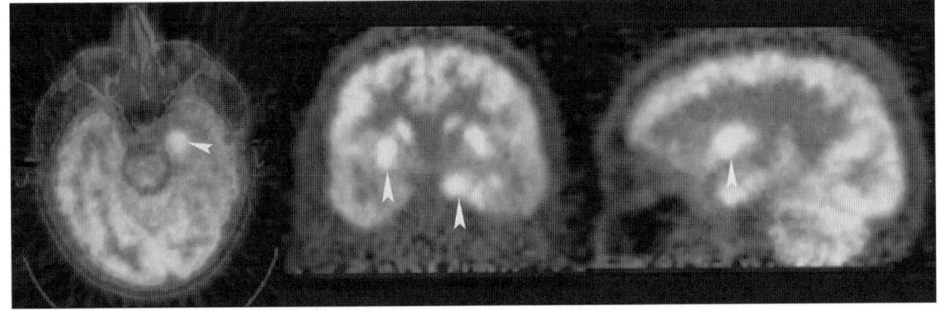

FIGURE 64.37. **(Color Plates) Brain Metastases.** Axial, coronal, and sagittal PET images demonstrate multiple hypermetabolic foci (*arrowheads*) with higher fluorodeoxyglucose activity compared to the gray matter. These findings are compatible with multiple brain metastases in this patient with lung cancer and confused mentation.

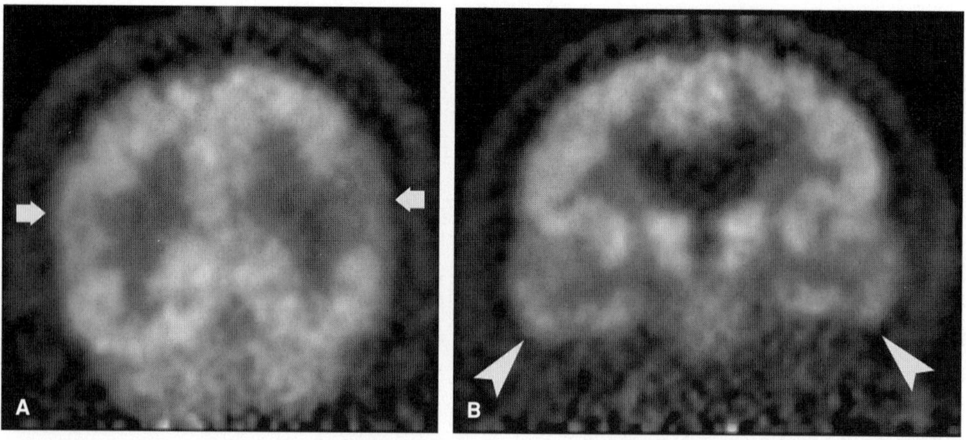

FIGURE 64.38. **(Color Plates) Alzheimer Dementia.** Brain PET images in the coronal plane demonstrate hypometabolism of both parietal lobes (*arrows*, **A**) and both temporal lobes (*arrowheads*, **B**), with normal fluorodeoxyglucose activity elsewhere in the brain.

sestamibi or tetrofosmin. Radiotracers used in PET cardiac perfusion scanning are N-13 NH_3 (ammonia), Rb-82 chloride, and O-15 H_2O (water). The short half-lives of N-13 and O-15 require proximity to a cyclotron. N-13 NH_3 diffuses rapidly into the myocardium and is retained by entering the glutamate pathway. Its accumulation depends on regional perfusion and the presence of viable myocardial tissue. Marked hepatic activity is problematic. Rb-82 is a potassium analog taken up actively by myocardium via the sodium-potassium pump and generates more penetrative positrons than N-13. These travel further before annihilation, resulting in lower spatial resolution than N-13. However, Rb-82 can be drawn from a portable strontium-82/rubidium generator, which can be leased by busy cardiac imaging practices.

As with SPECT perfusion imaging, exercise or pharmacologic stress are used to increase myocardial metabolism and need for blood flow. Simultaneous exercise stress and PET imaging is not practical in most PET suites, which do not accommodate simultaneous exercise and scanning. Pharmacologic stress with inotropes (dobutamine), vasodilators (dipyridamole), or transvenous or transesophageal atrial pacing is usually used for PET perfusion imaging; images acquired after injection of radiotracer at peak stress are compared to images obtained at rest. *Ischemic myocardium* shows transient, reversible, stress-induced perfusion defects. Fixed, nonreversible, perfusion defects are seen with *infarcted myocardium* or with tight, severe, flow-limiting, coronary artery stenosis. *Hibernating myocardium* is viable myocardium with impaired contraction caused by reduced perfusion. Hibernating myocardium will respond to revascularization procedures. *Stunned myocardium* results from repetitive ischemic injury and shows contractile dysfunction despite normalization of perfusion. The critical determination is diagnosis of hibernating myocardium that will respond to revascularization with improved left ventricular contractility and increased ejection fraction. To make this diagnosis most accurately, myocardial perfusion imaging performed with SPECT or PET is compared to myocardial metabolism imaging performed with F-18-FDG.

Myocardial Metabolism PET Imaging. F-18-FDG imaging is used to assess glucose metabolism of the myocardium. Glucose is the fuel of second choice for myocardium, behind fatty acids. Levels of insulin and glucose in the blood markedly affect FDG uptake. Fasting causes a switch of myocardial metabolism toward fatty acid metabolism, thereby hampering FDG uptake into myocardium. Pretreatment with 50 g of glucose is usually performed for FDG imaging. Diabetes poses a major problem in FDG cardiac imaging, as myocardial uptake in diabetic patients is heterogeneous and nonspecific defects are prevalent. In diabetic patients, oral glucose loading with continuous infusion of insulin, glucose, and potassium enhances FDG uptake by the myocardium.

Increased FDG uptake is seen in ischemic myocardium, while reduced or absent FDG uptake is indicative of infarcted myocardium with scar. Myocardial segments with perfusion defects matched with high FDG activity (perfusion-metabolism mismatch) will benefit from revascularization (85% positive predictive value). Perfusion-metabolism mismatch is indicative of hibernating myocardium (Fig. 64.39). Reduced perfusion and reduced metabolism in the same segment (perfusion-metabolism match) indicate nonviable scar tissue in an area of myocardial infarction that will not improve functionally with revascularization (92% negative predictive value). A pitfall is that an acute evolving myocardial infarction may show high FDG activity. FDG metabolism imaging is best performed when the patient is clinically stable.

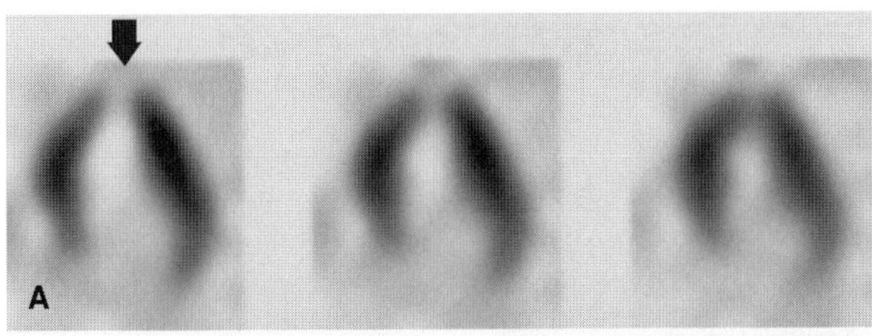

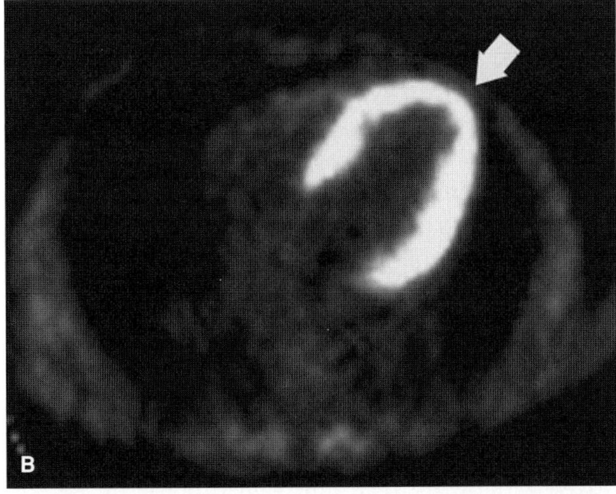

FIGURE 64.39. **Hibernating Myocardium: Perfusion-Metabolism Mismatch. A.** Myocardial perfusion study shows anteroseptal defect (*arrow*) on horizontal long images in this patient with recent infarction. **B.** Subsequent fluorodeoxyglucose (FDG) PET viability imaging demonstrates marked FDG activity throughout the myocardium, including the anteroseptal segment (*arrow*), assuring the viability of this area. These findings confirm that this patient is a good candidate for revascularization.

PET IMAGING IN INFLAMMATION AND INFECTION

FDG PET can be utilized to detect active inflammation or infection and is of particular benefit in fever of undetermined origin (FUO), in immunocompromised patients, and in the diagnosis of sarcoidosis and vasculitis.

FUO is defined as recurrent fevers without apparent cause recurring over a period of at least 3 weeks. A long list of causes have been reported, but indolent infection accounts for 20% to 30% of cases and undiscovered neoplasms for 15% to 25%. Whole-body PET is an ideal screening modality for both categories of lesions (Fig. 64.40). In approximately 40% of cases, PET provides useful diagnostic information. More specific analysis is made on the accompanying CT or other imaging modalities.

Immunocompromised patients, especially those with AIDS, can benefit by whole-body PET localization of unsuspected sites of infection or tumor. Specific diagnosis is usually made by correlation with other imaging and clinical data. Differentiation of CNS toxoplasmosis from CNS lymphoma in AIDS patients is usually not possible by CT or MR findings alone. On PET, CNS lymphoma is hypermetabolic, while toxoplasmosis shows little or no FDG activity.

Sarcoidosis disease activity determines the need for treatment. FDG uptake correlates with disease activity and thus can be used to determine extent of disease, if and when treatment is indicated, and the response to treatment in patients with known sarcoidosis.

Vasculitis commonly lacks specific signs and symptoms. FDG is taken up in blood vessels affected by the inflammation and necrosis that are characteristic of vasculitis. PET demonstrates the extent of active disease with a positive predictive value of 93%. FDG PET excludes active vasculitis with a negative predictive value of 80%.

PITFALLS IN PET-CT

Physiologic activity, reflecting normal glucose metabolism, is seen in numerous organs and muscles as described previously (Figs. 64.2 to 64.7). Any focus of FDG activity must be scrutinized as a possible site of normal physiologic activity.

Inflammatory processes in many locations are metabolically active, take up FDG, and must be considered in the differential diagnosis of hypermetabolic lesions (Fig. 64.20). Correlation with clinical history and CT findings is essential for recognition. Arthritis is a common cause of uptake in the hips, knees, and shoulders (Fig. 64.41) and in the sternoclavicular, acromioclavicular, and spinal facet joints (Fig. 64.31). Pneumonia and radiation pneumonitis show variable FDG activity in the lungs (Fig. 64.12). Sarcoidosis is associated with heterogeneous uptake in areas of involvement. Hemorrhoid uptake is related to acute inflammation. Patients receiving chemotherapy are immunosuppressed and may develop infections in unusual sites.

Benign tumors may also concentrate FDG. FDG hyperactivity is not specific for malignant neoplasia.

Recent Surgery. FDG accumulates in surgical healing sites; this is related to increased metabolism and the inflammation associated with tissue repair. Surgical sites that may be confusing include tracheotomies, sternotomies (activity persists for 6 months), and joint prosthesis healing (which must be differentiated from infection).

Fractures demonstrate FDG hyperactivity for weeks while fracture healing occurs (Fig. 64.42). Uptake is related to hematoma resorption, presence of granulation tissue, callous formation, and growth of new bone. Correlation with CT reviewed on bone windows is usually diagnostic.

Low Uptake by Malignant Tumors. A number of malignant lesions show low FDG activity and may be missed on PET scans. These include lobular carcinoma of the breast, low-grade lymphoma, salivary gland neoplasms, and extensively necrotic primary tumors and lymph nodes.

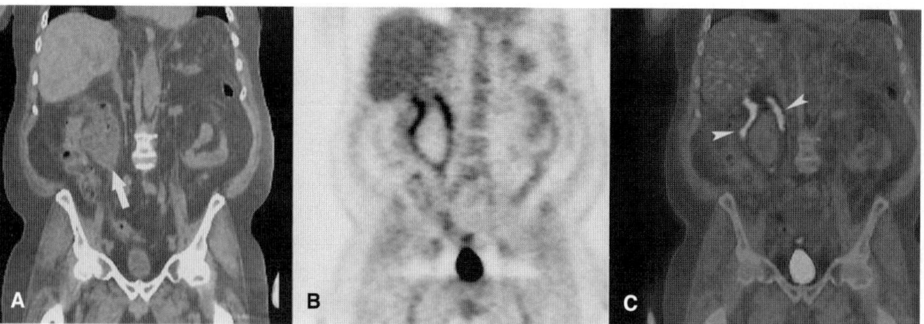

FIGURE 64.40. **(Color Plates) Abdominal Abscess.** An unsuspected postoperative abdominal abscess cavity (*arrow*) was discovered by PET-CT in this patient with colon cancer. Only the inflammatory rim (*arrowheads*) of the abscess shows fluorodeoxyglucose activity. The purulent center of the mass shows no activity. **A.** CT. **B.** Corrected PET. **C.** Fused PET-CT.

Attenuation correction artifacts appear as artifactual foci of apparently increased PET activity on attenuation-corrected PET images. These are induced by any highly attenuating object, including metallic joint prostheses, fracture fixation rods, vertebroplasty sites, cardiac pacemakers, dental devices, concentrations of oral contrast, and contrast-enhanced blood vessels. Attenuation-correction software overcorrects photopenic areas seen on CT adjacent to the highly attenuating objects. The artifact is accentuated when the patient moves between the emission (PET) and transmission (CT) scans. This artifact is recognized by identifying that the high-activity focus appears adjacent to a high-attenuation object shown on the CT scan. Attenuation-uncorrected PET images show a photopenic defect in the same area. The artifact is limited by attenuation-weighted iterative reconstruction algorithms used on some systems.

Misregistration of bowel activity occurs when peristalsis displaces bowel contents between the PET scan and the CT scan. Artifactual foci of increased or decreased activity are seen adjacent to bowel on PET images. This pitfall is recognized by carefully correlating the

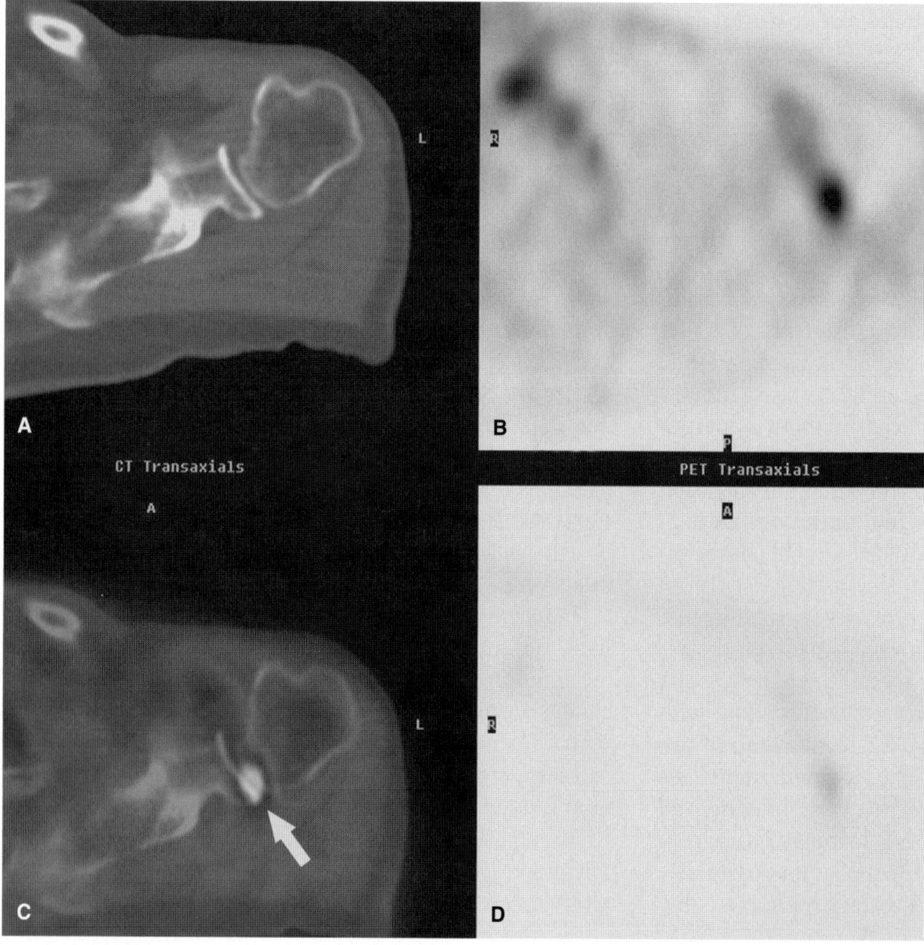

FIGURE 64.41. **(Color Plates) Shoulder Arthritis.** PET-CT shows intense fluorodeoxyglucose activity (*arrow*) confined to the shoulder joint, indicative of inflammation rather than metastatic disease. **A.** CT. **B.** Corrected PET. **C.** Fused PET-CT. **D.** Uncorrected PET.

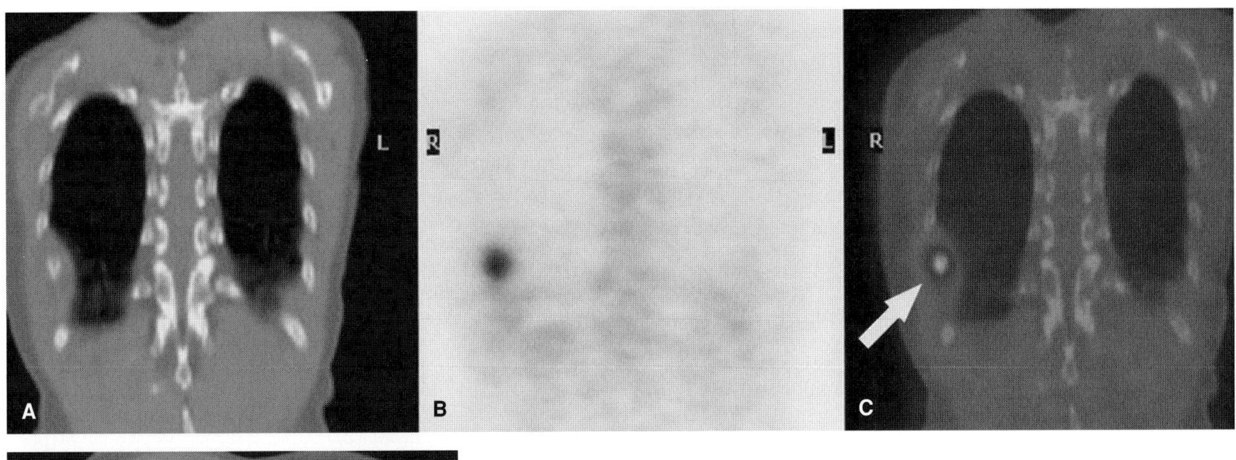

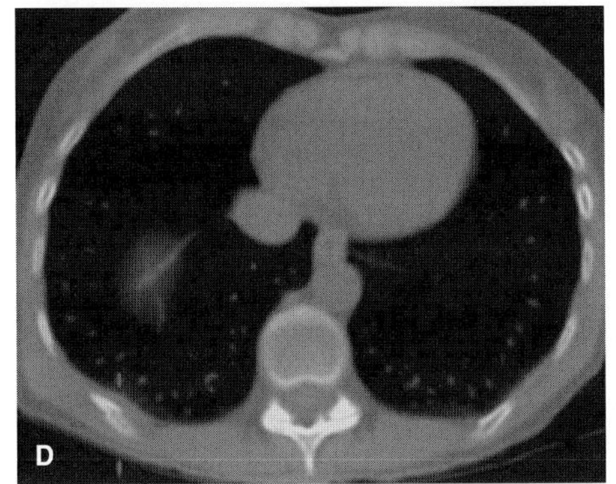

FIGURE 64.42. **(Color Plates) Rib Fracture.** Coronal-plane PET-CT (**A.** CT; **B.** corrected PET; **C.** fused PET-CT) shows a focus of hyperactivity (*arrow*) in a right rib. **D.** Axial CT reveals an acute rib fracture (between *cursors*) as the cause.

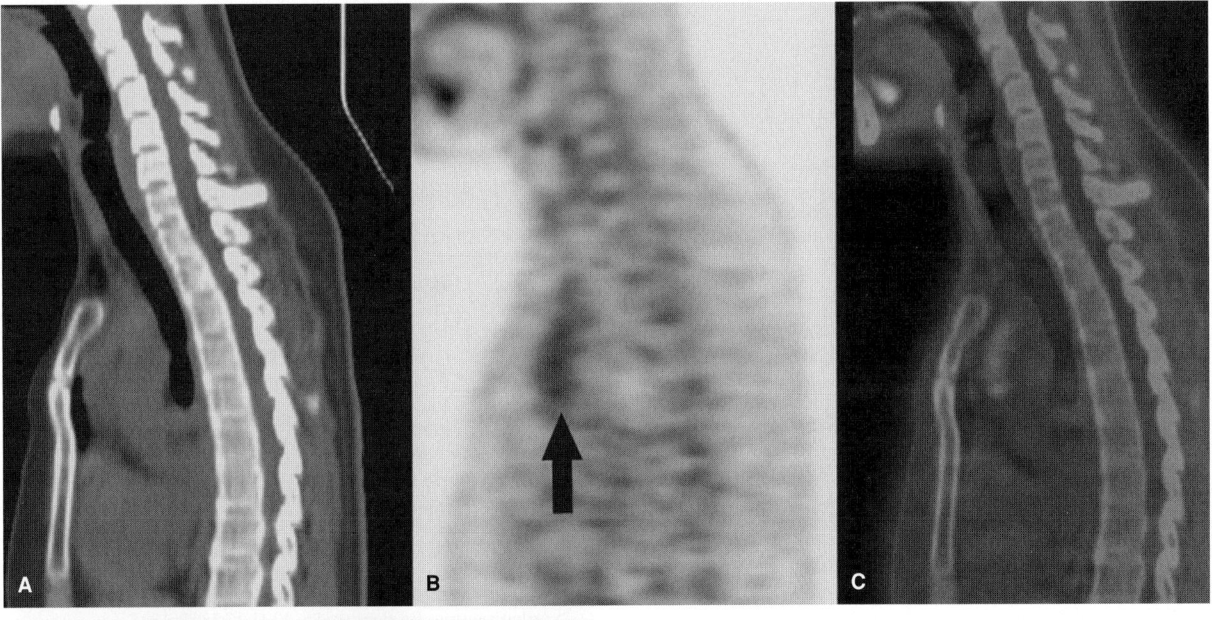

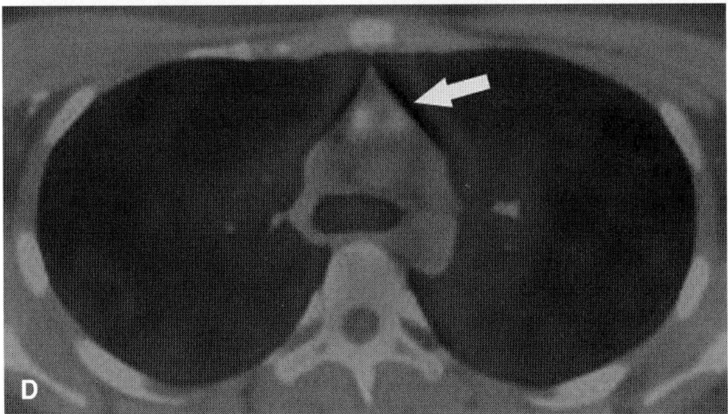

FIGURE 64.43. **(Color Plates) Thymic Rebound.** On this follow-up scan of a patient examined following completion of chemotherapy for colon carcinoma, the thymus (*arrows*) shows fluorodeoxyglucose hyperactivity and has become soft tissue density on CT. This is a common event following chemotherapy. **A.** Sagittal CT. **B.** Sagittal PET, corrected. **C.** Sagittal fused PET-CT. **D.** Axial fused PET-CT.

CT images with the PET images. Patient movement between the CT and PET acquisitions causes misregistration of FDG activity on the fusion images.

CT truncation artifacts occur as a result of objects outside the CT field of view. These appear as a series of dark lines on the attenuation-corrected PET images. This artifact is most commonly seen in obese patients or those who move their arms or legs during the long PET-CT scan time. The attenuation-correction algorithm does not correct for attenuation of CT x-rays by objects or tissues outside the field of view.

Thymic Rebound. The normal thymus regresses during adolescence, becoming diffusely fatty infiltrated. Thymic cell death may be induced by chemotherapy or corticosteroids. Following cessation of therapy, the thymus commonly rebounds, returning to soft tissue density on CT and demonstrating moderate to high FDG activity (Fig. 64.43). This phenomenon should not be confused with lymphoma or nodal metastatic disease.

Osteophytes develop in the vertebral column and from joints. They may be metabolically active and take up FDG, mimicking paravertebral adenopathy.

Injection Leakage. FDG uptake may be seen at the injection site or within lymph nodes that drain the injection site if skin infiltration occurs during FDG injection or if thrombus is present at the tip of an indwelling catheter.

SUGGESTED READINGS

Akhurst T, Ng V, Larson SM, et al. Tumor burden assessment with positron emission tomography with [^{18}F] 2-fluoro 2 deoxyglucose (FDG PET) modeled in metastatic renal cell cancer. Clin Positron Imaging 2000;3:57–65.

Aquino SL, Fischman AJ. Does whole-body 2-[^{18}F]-fluoro-2-deoxy-d-glucose positron emission tomography have an advantage over thoracic positron emission tomography for staging patients with lung cancer? Chest 2004;126:755–760.

Avril N, Rose CA, Schelling M, et al. Breast imaging with positron emission tomography and fluorine-18 fluorodeoxyglucose: use and limitations. J Clin Oncol 2000;18:3495–3502.

Bachor R, Kotzerke J. Reske SN, Hautmann R. Lymph node staging of bladder neck carcinoma with positron emission tomography [in German]. Urologe A 1999;38:46–50.

Blodgett TM, Fufui MB, Snyderman CH, et al. Combined PET-CT in the head and neck. Part 1. Physiologic, altered physiologic, and artifactual FDG uptake. Radiographics 2005;25:897–912.

Blodgett TM, Fufui MB, Snyderman CH, et al. Combined PET-CT in the head and neck. Part 2. Diagnostic uses and pitfalls of oncologic imaging. Radiographics 2005;25:913–930.

Cerfolio RJ, Bryant AS, Winokur TS, Ohja B, Bartolucci AA. Repeat FDG-PET after neoadjuvant therapy is a predictor of pathologic response in patients with non-small cell lung cancer. Ann Thorac Surg 2004;78:1903–1909.

Choi Y, Huang SC, Hawkins RA, et al. Quantification of myocardial blood flow using 13N-ammonia and PET: comparison of tracer models. J Nucl Med 1999;40:1045–1055.

Eubank WB, Mankoff DA, Takasugi J, et al. ^{18}Fluorodeoxyglucose positron emission tomography to detect mediastinal or internal mammary metastases in breast cancer. J Clin Oncol 2001 Aug;19:3516–3523.

Flamen P, Lerut A, Van Cutsem E, et al. Utility of positron emission tomography for the staging of patients with potentially operable esophageal carcinoma. J Clin Oncol 2000;18:3202–3210.

Fogelman I, Cook G, Israel O, Van der Wall H. Positron emission tomography and bone metastases. Semin Nucl Med 2005;35:135–142.

Freeman L, Blaufox MD. Renal nuclear medicine including consensus reports. Semin Nucl Med 1999;29(4):146–188.

Gambhir SS, Hoh CK, Phelps ME, et al. Decision tree sensitivity analysis for cost-effectiveness of FDG-PET in the staging and management of non-small-cell lung carcinoma. J Nucl Med 1996;37:1428–1436.

Goldberg MA, Mayo-Smith WW, Papanicolaou M, et al. FDG PET characterization of renal masses: preliminary experience. Clin Radiol 1997;52:510–515.

Heicappell R, Muller-Mattheis V, Reinhardt M, et al. Staging of pelvic lymph nodes in neoplasms of the bladder and prostate by positron emission tomography with 2-[(18)F]-2-deoxy-D-glucose. Eur Urol 1999;36:582–587.

Himeno S, Yasuda S, Shimada H, Tajima T, Makuuchi H. Evaluation of esophageal cancer by positron emission tomography. Jpn J Clin Oncol 2002;32:340–346.

Hossein J, Strauss HW, Segall GM. SPECT and PET in the evaluation of coronary artery disease. Radiographics 1999;19:915–926.

Hricak H, Yu KK. Radiology in invasive cervical cancer. AJR Am J Roentgenol 1996;167:1101–1108.

Huebner RH, Park KC, Shepherd JE, et al. A meta-analysis of the literature for whole-body FDG PET detection of recurrent colorectal cancer. J Nucl Med 2000;41:1177–1189.

Jadvar H, Strauss HW, Segall GM. SPECT and PET in the evaluation of coronary artery disease. Radiographics 1999;19:915–926.

Kapoor V, Fukui MB, McCook BM. Role of 18F-FDG PET/CT in the treatment of head and neck cancers: posttherapy evaluation and pitfalls. AJR Am J Roentgenol 2005;184:589–597.

Kapoor V, Fukui MB, McCook BM. Role of 18F-FDG PET/CT in the treatment of head and neck cancers: principles, technique, normal distribution, initial staging. AJR Am J Roentgenol 2005;184:579–587.

Kapoor V, McCook BM, Torok FS. An introduction to PET-CT imaging. Radiographics 2004;24:523–543.

Kazama T, Faria SC, Varavithya V, et al. FDG PET in the evaluation of treatment for lymphoma: clinical usefulness and pitfalls. Radiographics 2005;25:191–207.

Koga H, Sasaki M, Kuwabara Y, et al. An analysis of the physiological FDG uptake pattern in the stomach. Ann Nucl Med 2003;17:733–738.

Kostakoglu L, Agress H Jr, Goldsmith SJ. Clinical role of FDG PET in evaluation of cancer patients. Radiographics 2003;23:315–340.

Kostakoglu L, Hardoff R, Mirtcheva R, Goldsmith SJ. PET-CT fusion imaging in differentiating physiologic from pathologic FDG uptake. Radiographics 2004;24:1411–1431.

Kosuda S. Kison PV, Greenough R, et al. Preliminary assessment of fluorine-18 fluorodeoxyglucose positron emission tomography in patients with bladder cancer. Eur J Nucl Med 1997;24:615–620.

Lardinois D, Weder W, Hany TF, et al. Staging of non-small-cell lung cancer with integrated positron emission tomography and computer tomography. N Engl J Med 2003 Jun 19;348:2500–2507.

Lerut T, Flamen P, Ectors N, et al. Histopathologic validation of lymph node staging with FDG-PET scan in cancer of the esophagus and gastroesophageal junction: a prospective study based on primary surgery with extensive lymphadenectomy. Ann Surg 2000;232:743–752.

Love C, Tomas MB, Tronco GG, Palestro CJ. FDG PET of infection and inflammation. Radiographics 2005;25:1357–1368.

Metser U, Goor O, Lerman H, et al. PET-CT of extranodal lymphoma. AJR Am J Roentgenol 2004;182:1579–1586.

Narayan K, Hicks RJ, Jobling T, et al. A comparison of MRI and PET scanning in surgically staged loco-regional advanced cervical cancer: potential impact on treatment. Int J Gynecol Cancer 2001;11:263–271.

Patwardhan MB, McCrory DC, Matchar DB, et al. Alzheimer disease: operating characteristics of PET—a meta-analysis. Radiology 2004;231:73–80.

Rajadhyaksha CD, Parker JA, Barbaras L, Gerbaudo VH. Normal and benign pathologic findings in 18-FDG-PET and PET-CT. An interactive web-based image atlas. Joint Program in Nuclear Medicine, Harvard Medical School, 2005. Available at: http://www.jpnm.org

Ramdave S, Thomas GW, Berlangieri SU, et al. Clinical role of F-18 fluorodeoxyglucose positron emission tomography for detection and management of renal cell carcinoma. J Urol 2001;166:825–830.

Reinhardt MJ, Ehritt-Braun C, Vogelgesang D, et al. Metastatic lymph nodes in patients with cervical cancer: detection with MR imaging and FDG PET. Radiology 2001;218:776–782.

Rohren EM, Turkington TG, Coleman RE. Clinical applications of PET in oncology. Radiology 2004;231:305–332.

Rose PG, Adler LP, Rodriguez M, et al. Positron emission tomography for evaluating para-aortic nodal metastasis in locally advanced cervical cancer before surgical staging: a surgicopathologic study. J Clin Oncol 1999;17:41–45.

Safaei A, Figlin R, Hoh CK, et al. The usefulness of F-18 deoxyglucose whole-body positron emission tomography (PET) for re-staging of renal cell cancer. Clin Nephrol 2002;57:56–62.

Samson DJ, Flamm CR, Pisano ED, Aronson N. Should FDG PET be used to decide whether a patient with an abnormal mammogram or breast finding at physical examination should undergo biopsy? Acad Radiology 2002;9:773–783.

Schiepers C, Penninckx R, De Vadder N, et al. Contribution of PET in the diagnosis of recurrent colorectal cancer: comparison with conventional imaging. Eur J Surg Oncol 1995;21:517–522.

Schöder H, Meta J, Yap C, et al. Effect of whole-body ^{18}F-FDG PET imaging on clinical staging and management of patients with malignant lymphoma. J Nucl Med 2001;42:1139–1143.

Seto E, Segall GM, Terris MK. Positron emission tomography detection of osseous metastases of renal cell carcinoma not identified on bone scan. Urology 2000;55:286.

Silverman DH, Small GW, Chang CY, et al. Positron emission tomography in evaluation of dementia: Regional brain metabolism and long-term outcome. JAMA 2001;286:2120–2127.

Stafford SE, Gralow JR, Schubert EK, et al. Use of serial FDG PET to measure the response of bone-dominant breast cancer to therapy. Acad Radiol 2002;9:913–921.

Subhas N, Patel PV, Pannu HK, et al. Imaging of pelvic malignancies with in-line FDG PET-CT: case examples and common pitfalls of FDG PET. Radiographics 2005;25:1031–1043.

Sugawara Y, Zasadny KR, Kison PV, et al. Splenic fluorodeoxyglucose uptake increased by granulocyte colony-stimulating factor therapy: PET imaging results. J Nucl Med 1999;40:1456–1462.

Valk PE, Abella-Columna E, Haseman MK, et al. Whole-body PET imaging with [^{18}F]fluorodeoxyglucose in management of recurrent colorectal cancer. Arch Surg 1999;134:503–511.

Von Schulthess GK, ed. Clinical Molecular Anatomic Imaging. Philadelphia: Lippincott Williams & Wilkins, 2003.

Vranjesevic D, Filmont JE, Meta J, et al. Whole-body ^{18}F-FDG PET and conventional imaging for predicting outcome in previously treated breast cancer patients. J Nucl Med 2002;43:325–329.

Wahl RL, Siegel BA, Coleman RE, Gatsonis CG. Prospective multicenter study of axillary nodal staging by positron emission tomography in breast cancer: a report of the staging breast cancer with PET study group. J Clin Oncol 2004;22:277–285.

Wallace MB, Nietert PJ, Earle C, et al. An analysis of multiple staging management strategies for carcinoma of the esophagus: computed tomography, endoscopic ultrasound, positron emission tomography, and thoracoscopy/laparoscopy. Ann Thorac Surg 2002;74:1026–1032.

Williams AD, Cousins C. Soutter WP, et al. Detection of pelvic lymph node metastases in gynecologic malignancy: a comparison of CT, MR imaging, and positron emission tomography. AJR Am J Roentgenol 2002;178:762–764.

Yau YY, Chan WS, Tam YM, et al. Application of intravenous contrast in PET/CT: does it really introduce significant attenuation correction error? J Nucl Med 2005;46:283–291.

INDEX

NOTE: Italic *f* indicates figures; *t* indicates tables.

A

AA. *See* Amyloid A
AAAs. *See* Abdominal aortic aneurysms
AAN. *See* American Academy of Neurology
Abciximab, for vascular radiology, 674
ABCs. *See* Aneurysmal bone cysts
Abdomen
  abscess, 1516*f*
  acute, 741–743, 741*t*, 742*f*, 742*t*, 743*t*
  AIDS in, 751–754, 753*t*
  anomalies of, in pregnancy, 997–1000, 998*f*, 999*f*, 1000*f*
  beam-hardening artifact in, 10*f*
  calcifications of, 738–741, 739*f*, 740*f*, 741*f*, 742*f*
  of children, 1277
  compartmental anatomy of, 733–735, 734*f*, 735*f*
  film radiograph of, 4*f*
  foreign bodies in, 751, 752*f*
  gray scale image of, 8*f*
  mirror-image artifact in, 22*f*
  trauma to, 747, 748*f*
  ultrasound, 927–953
Abdominal aortic aneurysms (AAAs), 700–701, 701*f*
  US of, 1036–1038, 1039*t*, 1040*f*, 1041*f*
Abdominal aortic dissection, 702–703
Abdominal aortography, 700–703, 701*f*, 702*f*, 703*f*
Abdominal masses, 1312
Abdominal vessels
  anatomy, 1034–1035, 1039*f*
  aneurysm, 1036–1038, 1039*t*, 1040*f*, 1041*f*
Abnormal lung opacity, 1227–1234
Abnormal pancreatobiliary junction (APBJ), 1316
Abnormal soft tissue uptake, 1363–1364
Abortion, 979
Abscess
  abdominal, 1516*f*
  amebic, 769–770, 770*f*
  of brain, stages of, 156–159
  epidural, 284, 289*f*
  intraperitoneal, 927–928, 928*f*
  of liver, 1319*f*
  of lung, 1239
  pelvic, 1449*f*
  in peritoneal cavity, 751, 752*f*
  prevertebral, 290*f*
  pulmonary, 1241*f*, 1242*f*
  pyogenic, 156, 769, 770*f*
  renal, 1304, 1304*f*
  retropharyngeal, 261*f*
  of spine, 286, 288*f*
  tuberculous, 161–162
  US of, 933, 934*f*
Absolute function quantitation, 1431
AC. *See* Acromioclavicular joint
ACA. *See* Anterior cerebral artery
Acalculous biliary disease, 1425
Acetazolamide (Diamox), 1477, 1479, 1482*f*
Acetylsalicylic acid, 674
Achilles tendon, 1214–1215
  torn, 1215*f*
Achondroplasia, 1183, 1184*f*
ACL. *See* Anterior cruciate ligament
Acoustic enhancement, 21, 21*f*
Acoustic shadowing, 21, 21*f*
"Acoustic windows," 19
Acquired disease, imaging in
  cardiac masses, 645–648, 646*f*, 647*f*
  cardiomyopathies, 636–639, 636*t*, 637*f*, 638*f*
  ischemic heart disease, 629–636, 630*f*, 631*f*, 631*t*, 632*f*, 633*f*, 634*f*, 635*f*
  pericardial disease, 648–650, 648*f*, 648*t*, 649*f*, 650*f*
  pulmonary vascular disease, 639–640, 639*f*, 640*f*, 641*f*, 641*t*
  valvular heart disease, 640–645, 641*t*, 642*f*, 643*f*, 644*f*, 645*f*, 646*f*
Acquired immunodeficiency syndrome. *See* AIDS
Acquired lobar emphysema, 1241*f*
Acquired uremic cystic kidney disease, 881, 881*f*
Acromegaly, 1162, 1162*f*
Acromioclavicular (AC) joint, 1205
  degenerative joint disease and, 1133
  osteophytes and, 1209*f*
Actinomyces israelii, 464
Actinomycosis, 464
Actinomycotic Infections, 156
Acute disseminated encephalomyelitis (ADEM), 159, 174*f*, 194–195, 196*f*
  spinal cord and, 280
Acute inflammatory demyelinating polyradiculopathy. *See* Guillain-Barré syndrome
Acute interstitial pneumonia (AIP), 491, 492, 493*f*
Acute respiratory distress syndrome (ARDS), 420, 489, 1233, 1243
  acute interstitial pneumonia and, 492
  lung stiffness and, 420
Acute tubular necrosis (ATN), 1432, 1434*f*
Acyanotic heart disease, 1260–1262
AD. *See* Alzheimer disease
Adamantinoma, 1066, 1067*f*
Addison disease, 868
ADEM. *See* Acute disseminated encephalomyelitis
Adenocarcinoma, 440
  fetal, 459
  of the small bowel, 834–835, 835*f*
Adenoid cystic carcinoma, 253*f*
Adenoidal hypertrophy, 251*f*
Adenomas
  follicular, 1008, 1008*t*
  hepatic, 767, 769*f*
  pituitary, 147–148, 148*f*, 149*f*
Adenomatous hyperplasia, 1410
Adenomatous nodules, 1008, 1008*t*
Adenomyomatosis, 939, 939*f*
Adenomyosis, 957, 958*f*
  uterine, 917, 917*f*
Adenovirus, 467
Adhesive atelectasis, 367
Adnexa
  in pregnancy, 986
  US of, 958–963, 958*f*, 959*f*, 960*f*, 961*f*, 962*f*, 963*f*
Adnexal torsion, 962
Adrenal adema, 1507*f*
Adrenal glands, 1315*f*, 1414–1415
  anatomy of, 867–868
  calcified, 739, 740*f*, 871, 871*f*
  enlargement of, 1316
  imaging methods for, 867
  lesions of
    benign, 869–871, 869*f*, 870*f*, 871*f*
    malignant, 871–872, 872*f*
    problematic, 872, 873*f*
  US of, 944–945, 945*f*
Adrenal hemorrhage, 1315, 1316*f*
Adrenal leukodystrophy, 203, 205*f*
Adrenal malignancy, 1505

Adrenal mass, characterization of, 452*f*
Adrenal masses, 1312
Adrenal metastasis, 1506*f*
Adrenogenital syndrome, 868
Adult herpes encephalitis, 172*f*
Adynamic ileus, 742, 742*t*
Aeration abnormalities of, of lungs, 1237–1239
AFP. *See* Alpha-fetoprotein
Agnogenic myeloid metaplasia. *See* Myelofibrosis
AICA. *See* Anterior inferior cerebellar arteries
AIDS (Acquired immune deficiency syndrome), 174–183. *See also* HIV
  in abdomen, 751–754, 753*t*
  bacterial pneumonia and, 472–473
  Candida and, 475
  cholangitis, 936
  coccidioidomycosis and, 475
  colitis and, 858
  cryptococcosis and, 475, 476*f*
  cytomegalovirus infection and, 474
  dementia complex, 194
  enteritis, 844
  fungal meningitis and, 178–181
  immunocompromise and, 473*t*
  intracranial mycobacterial infections and, 183
  lymphoma and, 288, 754
  magnetic resonance imaging and, 280
  mycobacterium aviumintracellulare and, 474
  myelopathy and, 280
  parotid cysts and, 255
  pneumonia and, 462, 474
  primary CNS lymphoma and, 183, 183*f*
  progressive multifocal leukoencephalopathy and, 181
  related atrophy and, 180*f*
  renal disease and, 884
  splenomegaly and, 796, 796*t*
  thymic cysts and, 392
  toxoplasmosis and, 177–178
  tuberculosis and, 473
  viral infection and, 181
AIP. *See* Acute interstitial pneumonia
Air bronchograms, 365, 365*f*
Air cyst, 376
Airspace disease, 365, 365*f*, 444
  computed tomography and, 366
  high resolution computed tomography and, 366
  radiographic characteristics of, 364*t*
Airspace opacities, 366*t*
Airway obstruction of, 422, 1236–1237
Airways disease, 511–526
AL. *See* Amyloid L
ALARA. *See* As low as reasonably achievable
Alcoholism, avascular necrosis and, 1183
Alexander disease, 203–205
Alkylating agents, for pulmonary disease, 560
Allergic bronchopulmonary aspergillosis, 518–519, 519*f*
Alobar holoprosencephaly, 225, 226*f*
Alpha-fetoprotein (AFP), 990, 991*t*
Aluminum, pneumoconiosis and, 500
Alveolar interstitium, 479
Alveolar microlithiasis, 509
Alveolar sacs, 342
Alveolar septal amyloidosis, 496–497
Alzheimer disease (AD), 209*f*, 1475, 1482, 1514*f*
  dementia and, 209–210
  Pick disease and, 1481
  positron emission tomography and, 1483*f*
  SPECT and, 1484*f*
Ambiguous genitalia, 1310–1311
Amebiasis, 471, 857
Amebic abscess, 769–770, 770*f*
American Academy of Neurology (AAN), 1477
American Thoracic Society (ATS), 359, 399*f*
Amine precursor uptake and decarboxylation (APUD), 393, 1406
Amiodarone, for pulmonary disease, 560, 561*f*
AML. *See* Angiomyolipoma
Ammonia-13, 1393
Amniotic fluid, 988–989
Amniotic fluid embolism, 422
Amyloid A (AA), 497
Amyloid angiopathy, 119
Amyloid L (AL), 497
Amyloidosis, of small bowel, 843
Anaerobic bacterial infection, 464
Anaplastic carcinoma, 1410–1411
Anencephaly, 993, 993*f*
Aneurysm(s)
  abdominal aortic, 700–701, 701*f*, 1036–1038, 1039*t*, 1040*f*, 1041*f*
  of iliac artery, 903
  mycotic, 701
  peripheral arteries, 1047
  Rasmussen, 466
  renal artery, 705
  ruptured thoracic aortic, 410*f*
  splenic artery, 707, 707*f*
  subarachnoid hemorrhage and, 112–114, 116
  of thoracic aorta, 678–679, 679*f*
Aneurysmal bone cysts (ABCs), 1075, 1077–1078, 1077*f*
Aneurysmal disease, 695–696
Angiodysplasia, 860, 1421*f*
Angiofollicular lymph node hyperplasia, 400
Angiogram
  CT, 9*f*
  noninvasive, 47–48
Angiography
  conventional, 5
  coronary, 619–620
  hepatic, 707–710, 708*f*, 709*f*, 710*f*
  mesenteric, 710–713, 712*f*, 713*f*
  pulmonary, 684–687, 685*f*, 687*f*
  renal, 703–706, 704f, 705*f*, 706*f*
  splenic, 706–707, 707*f*
Angioimmunoblastic lymphadenopathy, 400
Angiomyolipoma (AML), 877–878, 878*f*, 949–950, 950*f*
Angiopathy
  amyloid, 119
  cardiac, 623, 623*f*
  congophilic, 119
Ankle
  anatomy of, 1215*f*
  avascular necrosis of, 1218–1219
  bony abnormalities of, 1224
  ligaments of, 1222–1224
  magnetic resonance imaging of, 1214
  tendons of, 1214–1218
  tumors of, 1219–1222
Ankylosing spondylitis, 491, 1112, 1139*f*
  hips and, 1140*f*
  spine fracture in, 1112*f*
  syndesmophytes in, 1138*f*
Annular pancreas, 829–830, 829*f*, 1283
Annular tear, 324
Anterior cerebral artery (ACA), ischemic stoke and, 97, 100*f*, 101*f*, 102*t*
Anterior (carotid) circulation, ischemic stroke and, 96–97, 98*f*–99*f*, 99–100, 100*f*, 101*f*, 102*f*, 102*t*
Anterior cruciate ligament (ACL), 1193, 1196, 1197*f*
  torn, 1198*f*
Anterior inferior cerebellar arteries (AICA), ischemic disease and, 104
Anterior junction lines, 351*f*, 352*f*
Anterior mediastinal masses, 1253
Anterior pararenal space, 734, 735*f*
Anterior sacral meningoceles, 1326–1327
Anterior talofibular ligament, 1221*f*

Anterior wedge compression fracture, 1110*f*
Anterolateral impingement syndrome, 1222*f*
Anteroposterior (AP) view, 5
Anthrax, 415
Antibiotics
  brain abscesses and, 158
  for vascular radiology, 673
Anticoagulants, for vascular radiology, 673
Anti-neoplastic drugs, 185
Antiphospholipid antibody syndrome, 190*f*
Antiplatelet agents, for vascular radiology, 673–674
Antrochoanal polyp, 243
Anus
  ectopic, 1292
  imperforate, 1292, 1294*f*, 1295*f*
Aorta, 606, 1260
Aortic dissection, 681–684, 683*f*, 684*f*
Aortic hiatus, 364
Aortic knob, 353
Aortic nipple, 353*f*
Aortic stenosis, 642–643, 643*f*
Aortic syndrome, 683–684, 684*f*
Aortic valve stenosis, 1274*f*
Aortography, 676–678
  abdominal, 700–703, 701*f*, 702*f*, 703*f*
Aortoiliac occlusive disease, 701–702, 702*f*
Aortopulmonary window, 353–354, 357, 1262
APBJ. *See* Abnormal pancreatobiliary junction
Appendicitis, 861–862, 862*f*, 863*f*, 1290–1291, 1295–1296, 1299*f*, 1300*f*, 1453*f*
  perforated, 1291*f*
Appendicoliths, 739
Appendix
  anatomy of, 861, 861*f*
  epididymis, 965
  imaging methods of, 860–861
  mucocele of, 862, 863*f*
  tumors of, 862–863
Apple peel small bowel, 1286
APUD. *See* Amine precursor uptake and decarboxylation
Arachnoid cysts, 154, 311, 315*f*
Arachnoidal hyperplasia, 261
Arachnoiditis, 280–281
Arch of azygos vein, 352
Architectural distortion, 486*f*
  of breast, 584, 585*f*
ARDS. *See* Acute respiratory distress syndrome
Arm, fractures of, 1118
Arnold-Chiari malformations, 294
Arrhythmogenic RV cardiomyopathy (ARVC), 662, 662*f*
Arterial puncture, peripheral arteries and, 1044–1047, 1046*f*, 1047*f*, 1048*f*
Arteries
  anatomic structure of, 671
  bronchial, 349
  cerebellar, ischemic stroke and, 103–105, 103*f*, 105*f*
  peripheral
    anatomy, 1041–1042, 1044, 1045*f*
    aneurysm, 1047
    arterial puncture in, 1044–1047, 1046*f*, 1047*f*, 1048*f*
    graft surveillance, 1048–1049, 1049*f*, 1050*f*, 1051*t*
    stenosis and occlusion, 1047–1048
  pulmonary, 347–349, 605, 608*f*, 1259–1260
    bilateral enlargement of, 416
    enlargement of, 414, 414*f*
    with venous returns, 348*f*–349*f*
  vertebral, ischemic stroke and, 100, 103*f*
Arteriography, diagnostic, 340
Arteriomegaly, 696
Arteriovenous fistula (AVF)
  dialysis and, 719–720
  in peripheral arteries, 1047, 1048*f*
Arteriovenous malformations (AVM), 294, 435
  extramedullary, 305–306
  intramedullary, 305, 307*f*
  of spine, 305
Arteriovenous malformations (AVMs), 117–118, 118*f*
  peripheral arterial disease and, 696–697
  pulmonary, 556
Arthritides, 1359
Arthritis, 1132. *See also* Juvenile rheumatoid arthritis; Osteoarthritis; Rheumatoid arthritis
  crystal-induced, 1141–1144
  psoriatic, 1140*f*
    with sacroiliac joint disease, 1139*f*
    syndesmophytes in, 1138*f*
  shoulder, 1516*f*
Arthropathies, 1359
Arthroscopy, meniscal degeneration and, 1193
Artifacts
  CT, 10, 10*f*, 11*f*
  doppler, 1024–1025, 1025*f*
  MR, 15–16, 15*f*, 16*f*
  US, 21, 21*f*, 22*f*
ARVC. *See* Arrhythmogenic RV cardiomyopathy
As low as reasonably achievable (ALARA), 1340
Asbestos, 443
Asbestosis, 497–499, 498*f*
Asbestos-related pleural disease, 538–539, 538*f*, 539*f*, 540*f*
Ascariasis, 838, 838*f*
Ascaris lumbricoides, 507
Ascites, 1321*t*
ASD. *See* Atrial septal defect
Aspergilloma, 471*f*
Aspergillosis, 468, 470
  CNS and, 162
  disseminated, 163*f*
  invasive, 475*f*
    high resolution computed tomography of, 475*f*
Aspergillus, 289, 508
Aspiration, 557–558, 558*f*
Aspirin, avascular necrosis and, 1183
Asplenia syndrome, 1275, 1275*f*
Asthma, 515–516, 516*f*, 1229*f*, 1230, 1383
Astrocytoma, 122, 128–129
  lower-grade, 131–132
Astrocytomas, 293–294, 294*f*
Atelectasis, 366, 366*t*, 1228, 1231*f*
  adhesive, 367
  cicatricial, 367
  combined middle and right lower lobe, 373
  compressive, 366
  left lower lobe, 373
  left upper lobe, 368, 369*f*
  lobar, 367, 367*f*, 367*t*, 369*f*
  middle lobe, 373
  obstructive, 366
  passive, 366
  resorptive, 366
  right lower lobe, 373
  right upper lobe, 368
  round, 368, 368*f*
  segmental, 367
  subsegmental, 367, 368*f*
Atherosclerosis, peripheral arterial, 689–690, 689*f*, 689*t*
Atherosclerotic disease, aneurysms and, 678–679
Atherosclerotic plaque imaging, 659–660, 660*f*
Atherosclerotic renal occlusive disease, 704–705
Atherosclerotic uptake, 1363
Athletes, bones and, 1167
Atlantoaxial joint, rotary fixation of, 1106*f*, 1107
ATN. *See* Acute tubular necrosis
Atrial septal defect (ASD), 1260, 1261, 1268*f*
Atrophy, 180*f*

ATRT. *See* Atypical teratoid/rhabdoid tumor
ATS. *See* American Thoracic Society
Attenuation correction, 1350–1351, 1394*f*
Attenuation pattern, 54
Atypical teratoid/rhabdoid tumor (ATRT), 141
Augmented breast, mammogram of, 586–588, 587*f*, 588*f*, 689*f*
Autoimmune disorders, 507
Autosomal dominant polycystic disease, 880–881, 881*f*
Autosomal recessive polycystic kidney disease, 881–882, 881*f*
Avascular necrosis (AVN), 1117, 1134, 1152–1155, 1155, 1183, 1184*f*, 1185*f*
  causes of, 1184*t*
  of foot and ankle, 1218–1219
  of hip, 1151*f*
  of navicular, 1116*f*
  of shoulder, 1152*f*
  of tarsal navicular, 1218*f*
AVF. *See* Arteriovenous fistula
AVM. *See* Arteriovenous malformations
AVMs. *See* Arteriovenous malformations
AVN. *See* Avascular necrosis
Avulsion
  injuries, 1126
  of nerve root, 317–320, 318*f*, 320*f*
  off ischium, 1125*f*
  rectus femoris, 1125*f*
Avulsion injury, 1168, 1172*f*
Axial interstitium, 479
Axillary adenopathy, mammogram and, 585–586, 586*f*
Azygoesophageal recess, 352

B

BAC. *See* Bronchioloalveolar cell carcinoma
Bacillus anthracis, 462–463. *See also* Anthrax
Back pain, 271
Bacteria
  gram-negative, 463
  gram-positive, 461–462
Bacterial meningitis, 176*f*
Bacterial peritonitis, 1297
Bacterial pneumonia, 461–463
  AIDS and, 472–473
Bacteroides, 464
Bactrim. *See* Co-trimoxazole
BAL. *See* Bronchoalveolar lavage
Balloon catheters, 672
Balloon expandable stents, 672–673
Balloon occlusion test, 1478, 1483*f*
BALT. *See* Bronchus-associated lymphoid tissue
Bankart deformity, 1120
Barium study, of esophagus, 404
Barium sulfate, 24
Barrett esophagus, 1279
Bartonella, 1320
Baseball finger. *See* Mallet finger
Basilar artery, ischemic stroke and, 100–101, 103*f*
"Bat's Wing." *See* Perihilar pulmonary edema
Battered child syndrome, 1292
BBB. *See* Blood-brain barrier
Beam-hardening artifact, in CT, 10, 10*f*
Beckwith-Wiedemann syndrome, 1318
Becquerel (Bq), 1338
Behçet disease, 845–846
Behçet syndrome, 190, 415
Benign cystic teratomas, 960, 960*f*
Benign hepatic cyst, 768–769, 769*f*
Benign postoperative meningeal enhancement, 180*f*
Benign prostate hyperplasia (BPH), 970, 971–972, 972*f*
Bennett fracture, 1112, 1113*f*
Berylliosis, 415, 504
β particle emission, 1458
β-interferon drugs, 185
Bextra. *See* I-131 tositumomab
Bezoar, 1283*f*
BGO. *See* Bismuth germanate
Biceps
  tendon of, 1211
  tendonitis of, 1212*f*
Biello criteria, 1379
Bifid renal pelvis, 889
Bilateral hilar enlargement, 415–416, 415*t*, 1259*f*
Bilateral hydroceles, 1312*f*
Bilateral hyperlucent lungs, 376
Bilateral lung hyperinflation, 1237*t*
Bilateral pleural effusions, 1379*f*
Bilateral pneumothorax, 1241*f*
Bilateral pulmonary artery enlargement, 416
Bilateral serous pleural effusions, 1248
Bile ducts, US of, 934–936, 935*f*, 936*f*
Biliary ascariasis, 936
Biliary atresia, 1298–1301, 1425
Biliary drainage, percutaneous, 725–728, 727*f*, 728*f*
Biliary leak, 1426*f*
Biliary tract, 771–772
Biliary tree
  dilation, 772–776, 772*f*, 773*f*, 773*t*, 774*f*, 775*f*
  gas in, 776, 776*f*, 776*t*
  imaging methods of, 771, 771*f*, 771*t*
  US of, 934, 935, 935*f*
Binswanger disease, 189
Biopsy
  percutaneous, 594–596, 595*f*, 596*f*, 597*f*
  transbronchial, 502
  with transthoracic needle, 340, 437
  US-guided, 450
  Wang, 450
Biphastic blastomas, 459
BI-RADS. *See* Breast Imaging Reporting and Data System
Bismuth germanate (BGO), 1347
"Black blood," 17
Bladder
  anatomy of, 898–899
  carcinoma, 973
  diverticula of, 973, 973*f*
  dysfunction of, 1308
  exstrophy, 898
  fistula of, 904
  imaging methods for, 898
  incontinence of, 271
  outpouchings, 903–904, 904*f*
  pear-shaped, 903
  stones, 973
  trauma to, 904–905, 904*f*
  US anatomy of, 972–973, 973*f*
  wall
    calcified, 900–901, 900*f*
    masses/filling defects of, 901–903, 901*f*, 902*f*, 902*t*, 903*f*
    thickened, 899–900, 899*f*, 900*f*
Bladder diverticula, 1308
Bladder outlet obstruction, 973–974, 974*f*
Blastomyces dermatitidis, 468
Blastomycosis, 470
Bleb, 376
Bleomycin, 560
Block detectors, 1348, 1348*f*
Blood, MR imaging and, 17
Blood clots
  in bladder, 973
  in pelvicaliceal system, 893
Blood flow, imaging and, 1459
Blood-brain barrier (BBB), 1472
"Blown pupil," 123
Blowout fractures, 78–80, 79*f*
BMD. *See* Bone mineral density

BMT. *See* Bone marrow transplant
Bochdalek hernia, 549–550, 549*f*
Body fluids, MR of, 16–17, 17*t*
Boerhaave syndrome, 407, 814
Böhler angle, 1129
  in calcaneus, 1131*f*
BOLD technique, 1457
Bone(s). *See also* Fracture(s)
  aneurysmal cysts of, 1075, 1077–1078, 1077*f*
  in athletes, 1167
  of chest, 351
  contusions of, 1202–1203
  diseases, metabolic, 1156
  infarction of, 1181, 1181*f*
  joints and, trauma to, 1170
  lesions, 1082–1084, 1082*t*, 1083*t*, 1084*t*, 1089*f*, 1090–1091, 1090*f*
  lesions of, 1183
  malignant tumors, 1086–1098
  mineralization of, 1157*f*
  primary lymphoma of, 1096*f*, 1098
  scans of, with nuclear medicine, 278
  solitary cysts of, 1078–1079, 1078*f*, 1079*f*
  temporal fractures of, 56–57, 57*f*
  tumors, 1086–1098, 1366
Bone dysplasias, 1365–1366
Bone grafts, computed tomography and, 329
Bone islands, 1180
Bone marrow, 303
  diffuse metastatic disease and, 1511*f*
  hypermetabolic, 1510*f*
  magnetic resonance imaging and, 304*f*
Bone marrow transplant (BMT), 304*f*, 477
Bone mineral density (BMD), 1369*f*, 1370
Bone scans, with technetium, 303
Bony abnormalities
  of foot and ankle, 1224
  in knee, 1202–1203
  of shoulders, 1209
Bony thorax, 542–547, 543*t*, 544*f*, 545*f*, 546*f*, 547*f*
BOOP. *See* Bronchiolitis obliterans with organizing pneumonia
Borrelia buregdorferi, Lyme disease and, 166
Bowel
  dilated, 741–742
  gas in, 741, 742*f*
  incontinence of, 271
  inflammatory, 1450
  ischemia/infarction, 746–747, 747*f*
  large, 745–746, 745*f*, 745*t*, 746*f*
  mechanical obstruction of, 743
  small. *See* Small bowel
BPD. *See* Bronchopulmonary dysplasia
BPH. *See* Benign prostate hyperplasia
Bq. *See* Becquerel
Brain
  abscesses of, 156–159, 159*f*
  in axial plane CT, 30*f*–31*f*
  basal cisterns of, 29, 44
  calcification in, 238
  cancer, imaging, 51*t*, 52
  common syndromes of, 51–52, 51*t*
  cyst in, 1512*f*
  gadolinium chelates, 49*f*
  herniation of, 69, 70*f*
  imaging of
    abnormalities in, 52–54
    gadolinium-enhanced, 49*f*
    options for, 44, 47–48, 51
    strategies for, 51–52
  metabolism, selective vulnerability and, 87
  metastases and, 1511, 1513*f*
  midline, 29
    anatomy of, 45*f*–46*f*
  migration anomalies in, 228–233
  neonatal, 1012–1018
  positron emission tomography and, 1332*f*
  symmetry of, 29
  trauma to, 1486
  tuberculoma of, 160–161
  tumors in, 1485, 1513*f*
  ventricles, 44
  in weighted axial plane CT, 32*f*–38*f*, 50*f*
  in weighted coronal plane CT, 38*f*–43*f*
Brain death, 1485*f*, 1486
Brain Imaging Council of the Society of Nuclear Medicine, 1477
Brainstem, MS and, 187*f*
Brainstem glioma, 139–140, 140*f*
Brainstem injury, 70–72
  primary, 70, 72, 72*f*
  secondary, 72, 73*f*
Branchial cleft cysts, 267–269, 269*f*
Breast(s). *See also* Mammogram
  architectural distortion of, 584, 585*f*
  augmented, 586–588, 587*f*, 588*f*, 689*f*
  imaging of. *See also* Mammogram
    MR, 590–593, 593*f*, 594*f*
    nonpalpable lesions and, 594–599, 595*f*, 596*f*, 598*f*, 897*f*
    radiologic report/plan in, 593–594
    technical considerations in, 568–572, 570*f*, 571*f*, 572*t*
  male, 588–589, 590*f*, 591*f*
  occult lesions of, 596–597, 598*f*
  radiography of lungs and, 354
  tissue, density of, 584–585, 586*f*
Breast cancer, 565–568, 566*t*, 1502
  axillary node metastasis and, 1504*f*
  internal mammary node metastases and, 1504*f*
  positron emission tomography and, 1489*f*
  screening for, 565–568, 566*t*
Breast Imaging Reporting and Data System (BI-RADS), 593–594
Breastfeeding, radiology and, 1341*t*
Bremsstrahlung, 1336
Bronchi, trauma to, 514, 515*f*
Bronchial arteries, 349
Bronchial arteriography, 687–688, 688*f*
Bronchial atresia, 553
Bronchial carcinoid, 454*f*
Bronchial carcinoma, 455
Bronchial embolotherapy, 688
Bronchiectasis, 517–519, 517*f*, 518*f*, 518*t*, 519*f*, 1230
Bronchiectatic cysts, 376
Bronchioles, 340
  anatomy of, 343*f*
  arteries of, 349
  masses of, 402
  segmental, 341*f*
Bronchiolitis, 524–526, 524*t*, 525*f*
Bronchiolitis obliterans with organizing pneumonia (BOOP), 493
Bronchioloalveolar cell carcinoma (BAC), 440, 444*f*, 445*f*
Bronchitis, chronic, 516–517
Bronchoalveolar carcinoma, 1495*f*
Bronchoalveolar lavage (BAL), 509
Bronchoceles. *See* Mucoid impaction
Bronchogenic carcinoma, 440, 441*t*, 1495*f*
  diagnostic evaluation of, 446
  epidemiology of, 442–443
  nodule metastases with, 450*f*
  radiographic findings and, 443–446
  smoking and, 442
Bronchogenic cysts, 400, 401*f*, 415, 439–440, 1251, 1254*f*
Broncholithiasis, 515, 516*f*
Bronchopneumonia, 460
Bronchopulmonary dysplasia (BPD), 1243–1244, 1248*f*
Bronchovascular interstitium, 479
Bronchus-associated lymphoid tissue (BALT), 438

Brown tumors, 1160. *See also* Hyperparathyroidism
in hyperparathyroidism, 1161*f*
Brunner glands, 827
Bucket-handle tear, 1194, 1194*f*, 1195*f*
Budd-Chiari syndrome, 721, 722*f*, 762–763, 763*f*
Buerger disease, 691, 694*f*
Buford complex, 1211
Bulging annulus fibrosus, 324
Bulla, 376
Bullous edema, 900
Bullous lung disease, 523–524, 523*f*, 524*t*
Burkitt lymphoma, 247, 836, 1323
Bursae, 1203
semimembranosus tibial collateral ligament, 1203
Butterfly glioma, 129–130

C

Calcaneal stress fracture, 1223*f*
Calcaneal tumors, 1219
Calcaneus
fracture of, 1131, 1131*f*
pseudocyst of, 1180
stress fracture of, 1129*f*
Calcifications
of abdomen, 738–741, 739*f*, 740*f*, 741*f*, 742*f*
adrenal, 739, 740*f*, 871, 871*f*
in brain, 238
in breast, 580–584, 581*f*, 582*f*, 583*f*, 584*f*, 585*f*
cardiac, 612–613, 613*f*
concentric, 435
laminated, 435
of lymph nodes, 438, 738
pancreas, 739–740, 740*f*
renal, 1308
soft tissue, 740–741
solitary pulmonary nodule and, 437*f*
in tuberculomas, 161
tumors, 740, 741*f*
Calcium pyrophosphate dihydrate crystal deposition disease (CPPD), 1134, 1143*f*, 1144*f*
diseases and, 1145*t*
locations of, 1145*t*
Caliceal diverticula, 897–898, 897*f*, 898*f*
CAM. *See* Cystic adenomatoid malformation
Campylobacter fetus jejuni, 845
Campylobacter infection, 1294
Canal of Kovalevski, 405
Canals of Lambert, 365, 460, 1371
Canavan disease, 203–205, 207*f*
Cancer
brain, imaging strategies for, 51*t*, 52
breast, 565–568, 566*t*
cervical, 913–914, 914*f*, 914*t*, 1502–1504
colon, 1500–1502, 1500*f*, 1501*f*, 1502*f*
colorectal, 1500–1502
gallbladder, 1502
gastrointestinal, 1426
lung, 447–451, 447*f*, 1460*f*, 1492–1494, 1496*f*
ovarian, 911–913, 912*t*, 913*f*, 1504–1505, 1505*f*
pancreatic, 1500
prostate, 300, 1439*f*, 1505
sophageal, 1499
stomach, 1500
thyroid gland, 1410, 1411f
uterine, 1504, 1505*f*
Candida, 289, 468
abscess of liver, 1319*f*
AIDS and, 475
Capillary hemangioblastomas, 140, 141*f*
Capillary hemangiomas, 262
Capillary permeability, imaging and, 1459
Capsule
early, in brain abscesses, 158
late, in brain abscesses, 158
Carbon monoxide toxicity, 211*f*
Carcinoembryonic antigen scan, 1463*f*
Carcinoma, 143–144. *See also* Adenocarcinoma; Squamous cell carcinoma; Transitional cell carcinoma
adenoid cystic, 253*f*
adrenal, 871–872, 872*f*
anaplastic, 1410–1411
bladder, 973
bronchioloalveolar cell, 440, 444*f*, 445*f*
bronchoalveolar, 1495*f*
bronchogenic, 440–446, 441*t*, 450*f*, 1495*f*
colon, 1463*f*
endometrial, 914–915, 915*f*, 915*t*
fibrolamellar, 767, 769*f*
follicular, 1410
gallbladder, 938–939, 939*f*
hepatocellular, 765–766, 766*f*, 766*t*, 933, 933*f*, 1318–1319
large cell, 442, 442*f*
laryngeal, 453
lung, 302*f*, 1454*f*
medullary, 1410
metastatic, 1164
nasopharyngeal, 250, 252*f*
papillary thyroid, 1009, 1009*f*, 1410
parathyroid glands, 1414
prostate, 921–922, 922*f*, 922*t*, 970–971, 971*f*, 971*t*, 1469
renal cell, 876–877, 876*f*, 877*f*, 878*t*, 1315
small cell, 440–442, 442*f*
urinary bladder, 1506*f*
Carcinomatous meningitis, 300*f*
Cardiac anatomy, 603–607, 604*f*, 605*f*, 606*f*, 607*f*, 608*f*
Cardiac angiopathy, 623, 623*f*
Cardiac calcifications, 612–613, 613*f*
Cardiac catheterization, 607–609, 609*f*, 609*t*
Cardiac circulation, 1385*f*
Cardiac CT, 623–626, 624*f*, 625*f*, 626*f*
Cardiac disease, 418*f*
Cardiac imaging
in acquired diseases, 629–650
methods of, 603
Cardiac malpositions, 1272
Cardiac masses, 645–648, 646*f*, 647*f*
Cardiac MR, 626–627, 626*f*, 627*f*
cardiomyopathies, 660–662, 660*f*, 661*f*, 662*f*
congenital heart disease, 665–666, 665*f*, 666*f*
ischemic heart disease, 652–660, 653*f*, 655*f*, 657*f*, 658*f*, 659*f*, 660*f*, 664*f*
of masses, 666–668, 667*f*
pericardial disease, 662, 663*f*
pulmonary veins, 668, 668*f*
valvular heart disease, 663–665, 663*f*, 664*f*
Cardiac output (CO), 1396, 1397*f*
Cardiac silhouette, 610, 610*f*
Cardiac tamponade, 648
Cardiolite, 1390
Cardiology, nuclear, 617
Cardiomegaly, 1260
Cardiomyopathies, 636–639, 636*t*, 637*f*, 638*f*, 1275*f*
MR, 660–662, 660*f*, 661*f*, 662*f*
Cardiovascular infections, 1448–1449
Cardiovascular system scintigraphy, 1387
interpretation of, 1390–1393
radiopharmaceuticals and, 1389–1390
Caron-14 urea breath test, 1419
Carotid body tumors, 252, 254*f*
Carotid cavernous fistula (CCF), 67, 68*f*, 266*f*
Carotid space, 248, 252–253, 257*f*
Carotid ultrasound
anatomy, 1026–1027, 1027*f*, 1028*f*, 1029*f*, 1029*t*
occlusion, 1032–1033, 1035*f*, 1036*f*, 1037*f*

pitfalls in, 1033–1034, 1038*f*, 1039*t*
plaque evaluation, 1027–1030, 1029*f*, 1030*f*
stenosis, 1030–1032, 1030*f*, 1031*t*, 1032*t*, 1033*f*, 1034*f*
stroke, 1025–1026, 1026*f*
Castleman disease. *See* Angiofollicular lymph node hyperplasia
Cathartic colon, 858
Catheter(s)
retrieval, 715, 716*f*
types of, 672
Catheter drainage, percutaneous, 340
Catheterization, cardiac, 607–609, 609*f*, 609*t*
Catscratch fever, 1320, 1321*f*
Caudal regression syndrome, 311, 314*f*
Caustic esophagitis, 1279
Caustic (lye) stricture, 1280*f*
Cavernous fistula, of carotid, 266*f*
Cavernous hemangiomas, 263, 266*f*, 765, 765*f*, 932, 932*f*, 1425–1426
Cavernous malformations, 118
Cavernous sinus thrombosis, 243*f*
CC. *See* Craniocaudad view
CCF. *See* Carotid cavernous fistula
CCK. *See* Cholecystokinin
Cecal bascule, 746
Cecal bleeding, 1421*f*
Cecal volvulus, 746, 746*f*
Celiac disease, 840–841, 843*f*
Center of rotation (COR), 1353, 1354*f*
Central canal stenosis, 326, 327*f*
Central caseous necrosis, in granuloma, brain infection and, 160
Central herniation, 123
Central nervous system (CNS). *See also* Spine
anomalies of, in pregnancy, 991–995, 991*f*, 992*f*, 993*f*
infections of, 156, 1448–1449
diagnosis of, 156
lymphoma, 133, 134*f*
secondary, 143
malignancies of, 1507–1511
neoplasms
brainstem glioma, 139–140, 140*f*
capillary hemangioblastomas, 140, 141*f*
clinical presentation of, 123, 128, 128*t*
dysplastic cerebellar gangliocytoma, 140–141
extra-axial tumors, 141–143, 142*f*
gliomas, 128–129, 130*f*, 131*f*, 131*t*
imaging protocol, 125, 125*f*
intra-axial tumors, 133–135, 134*f*, 135*t*, 136*f*, 137*f*
intraventricular tumors, 143–145, 143*t*, 144*f*, 145*f*, 145*t*
nerve sheath tumors, 149–151, 151*f*, 152*f*, 153*f*
pineal region masses, 146–147, 146*f*, 147*t*
posterior fossa tumors, 135–141, 137*f*, 138*f*, 139*f*, 140*f*, 141*f*
postoperative patient, 127
follow-up scan of, 127–128, 128*f*
radiographic abnormalities, 123–125, 124*f*
sellar masses, 147–149, 148*f*, 149*f*, 150*f*
Central nervous system scintigraphy, 1472
Central neurocytoma, 144, 145*f*
Central pontine myelinolysis (CPM), 196–197, 198*f*
Central venous catheters, 672
Centrilobular interstitium, 479
Cephaloceles, 228, 993, 993*f*
Cerebellar arteries, ischemic stroke and, 103–105, 103*f*, 105*f*
Cerebellar vermis, lipomas of, 228*f*
Cerebral atrophy, imaging strategies for, 56
Cerebral infarction, 1479*f*
subcortical, 1480*f*
Cerebral vasospasm, 1481*f*
Cerebritis
antibiotics and, 158
early, 156–157, 157*f*
in brain abscesses, 157*f*
late, 158*f*
in brain abscesses, 158
Cerebrospinal fluid
leak of, 1473
studies of, 1473–1474
Cerebrospinal fluid dynamics
ex vacuo ventriculomegaly and, 207
hydrocephalus and, 203, 205–207
normal pressure hydrocephalus and, 207–208
Cerebrovascular disease, 86–120
Cervical cancer, 913–914, 914*f*, 914*t*, 1502–1504
Cervical spine
C1 and C2
dislocation of, 1105*f*
radiograph of, 1104*f*
Jefferson fracture of, 1105*f*
radiograph of, 1104*f*
trauma to, 1102–1112
Chamber enlargement, 610–611, 611*f*
Charcot joint, 1146, 1146*f*
Charcot spine, 1147*f*
CHD. *See* Common hepatic duct
Chemical shift misregistration, 15–16, 16*f*
Chemodectomas, 252
Chemotherapy
bone marrow and, 303
spine and, 281
Chest
anatomy of, 362, 362*f*, 363*f*
anomalies of, in pregnancy, 995–997, 996*f*, 997I
bony abnormalities in, 617
disease of, drug-induced, 558–560, 559*f*, 561*f*
diseases of, 364
radiographic findings with, 364–388
lesions of, 388
pediatric, 1227
pleural space of, 1002, 1003*f*, 1004, 1004*f*
radiographs of, 382*f*
tumors of, 447, 448*f*
Chest radiograph (CXR), 1371
Chest radiography, 335, 609–610
cardiac calcifications, 612–613, 613*f*
cardiac silhouette, 610, 610*f*
chamber enlargement, 610–611, 611*f*
mediastinal contours, 610–611, 611*f*
of pericardium, 615–616, 616*f*
posteroanterior, erect, 6, 6*f*
pulmonary vascularity, 613–615, 614*f*, 615*f*, 615*t*
Chest wall
bony thorax of, 542–547, 543*t*, 544*f*, 545*f*, 546*f*, 547*f*
lesions, 540*t*
masses of, 1255–1256, 1264*t*
soft tissue of, 539–542, 541*f*, 542*f*
Chiari I malformations, 232, 233*f*, 308
Chiari II malformations, 231–232, 232*f*, 233*f*
in spine, 232
Child abuse, head injuries and, 73–75, 75*f*
Children
abdomen and pelvis, 1277
abnormal lung opacity in, 1227–1234
cystic blastomas and, 459
cysts in, 265
head injury of, 73–75
HIV and, 1234
lung masses in, 1249
lungs and, 1227
pediatric neuroimaging for, 213
pleuropulmonary blastomas and, 459
posterior fossa tumors in, 135–136, 137*t*
spinal lesions in, 289
with spine defects, 308–311
Chlamydia pneumonitis, 1231*f*
Chlamydia trachomatis, 1230
Cholangiocarcinoma, 935–936, 936*f*
Cholangitis, AIDS-related, 936

Cholecystitis, 1298, 1423–1424
  acute, 1424, 1425*f*
  chronic, 1424, 1503*f*
  US and, 938, 938*f*
Cholecystokinin (CCK), 1425
Cholecystostomy, 728
Choledochal cysts, 1316–1317, 1319*f*
Choledocholithiasis, US of, 934–935, 935*f*
Cholesteatoma, 246–247
Cholesterol granuloma, 248
Choline, tumors and, 47
Chondroblastoma, 1080–1082, 1081*f*, 1082*f*
Chondrocalcinosis
  in knees, 1142*f*
  in wrist, 1143*f*
Chondromalacia patella, 1201–1202, 1201*f*
Chondromyxoid fibroma, 1082, 1082*f*
Chondrosarcomas, 246, 453, 1093, 1094*f*, 1095, 1254, 1366*f*
Chordoma, 246
Choroid plexus papilloma, 143–144, 144*f*
Chromosome abnormalities, in pregnancy, 990–991
Chronic obstructive pulmonary disease (COPD), 463, 1373, 1377*f*, 1380*f*, 1385
Chronic thromboembolic pulmonary hypertension (CTPH), 431
Chylothorax, 530–531, 531*f*, 1249, 1251*f*
Ci. *See* Curies
Cicatricial atelectasis, 367
Circle of Willis, 278, 1479
Cirrhosis, 760–762, 761*f*, 761*t*, 1423*f*
  US of, 931, 931*f*
Cisternogram, 1474*f*
CJD. *See* Creutzfeldt-Jakob disease
Clavicle, 546
Clay shoveler's fracture, 1107*f*, 1110
Cleft lip, 994–995, 996*f*
Cloacal anomalies, 1310
Clopidogrel, for vascular radiology, 674
Closed-loop obstruction, of small bowel, 744
CNS. *See* Central nervous system
CO. *See* Cardiac output
Coagulopathies, hemorrhage and, 119
Coal worker's pneumoconiosis (CWP), 499–500
Coarctation of aorta, 1266*f*, 1270–1271, 1274*f*
Coats disease, 265
Cocaine, 411
Coccidioides infection, 386*f*, 468, 470*f*, 1231
Coccidioidomycosis, AIDS and, 475
Coccidioidomycosis immitis, 469–470
Coccidioidomycosis meningitis, 178*f*, 289, 290*f*, 400, 413
Coincidence detection, 1348, 1348*f*
"Cold spot" imaging, 634–635, 634*f*
Colitis, 858, 1294, 1448*f*
Collagen, brain abscesses and, 158
Collagen-vascular diseases, 1144–1145
Collapsed lung, 373
Collateral ligaments, 1198–1201
Colles fracture, 1118, 1118*f*
Collett-Edwards type IV truncus arteriosus, 1269
Collimation, 1347
  quality control in, 1353
Colloid cyst, 145, 145*f*, 145*t*
Colon
  anatomy of, 849–850
  diverticular disease of, 858–860, 859*f*, 860*f*
  filling defects/mass lesions of, 850–855, 850*f*, 851*f*, 852*f*, 853*f*, 854*f*
  imaging methods for, 848–849, 849*f*
  inflammatory disease of, 855–858, 855*f*, 855*t*, 856*f*, 857*f*, 858*f*
Colon atresia, 1292, 1296*f*
Colon cancer
  anastomosis activity in, 1501*f*
  hepatic metastasis in, 1502*f*
  recurrence of, 1501
  staging of, 1500*f*
Colon carcinoma, 1463*f*
Colonic diverticula, 711
Colonic obstruction, 1292
  causes of, 1292*t*
Colonic stricture, 1296*f*
Color doppler, 19
Color flow US, 1023–1024, 1024*f*
Colorectal cancer, 1500–1502
Colpocephaly, 227
Coma, imaging strategies for, 51*t*, 52
Combined middle and right lower lobe atelectasis, 373
Comet tail artifact. *See* Ring down artifact
Common hepatic duct (CHD), 771–772
Complex adnexal masses, 1323–1325
Compression fracture, 302*f*
Compressive atelectasis, 366
Compton interactions, 1336–1338
Computed radiography (CR), 3
Computed tomography (CT), 1350. *See also* High resolution computed tomography
  of adrenal mass characterization, 452*f*
  airspace disease and, 366
  artifacts, 10, 10*f*, 11*f*
  bone grafts and, 329
  of brain, 30*f*–31*f*
  cardiac, 623–626, 624*f*, 625*f*, 626*f*
  of cervical spine, 277, 311
  of chest, 362
  of chest wall lesions, 388
  chronic sclerosing mediastinitis and, 408
  with CNS infection, 156
  contrast administration, 10
    in ischemic stroke, 93
  contrast-enhanced, with solitary pulmonary nodule, 436
  of diaphragm, 364*f*
  disk disease and, 324
  emergency checklist for, 44
  of esophagus, 404
  of facial trauma, 75–85
  free fragments and, 324
  for head and neck, 241
  of head trauma, 55–75
  helical, 9, 9*f*
  hemangiomas and, 258
  hilar disease and, 380, 381*f*
  of hilar nodes, 398*t*
  of hypoxic ischemic injury, 220, 220*f*
  inadequate techniques in, 323*f*
  interpretation of, 10–11
  intramedullary masses and, 291
  of lumbar spine, 322
  of lung, 448*f*
  of lymph nodes, 260, 398
  lymphoma and, 395
  of mediastinum, 356
  multidetector helical, 9
  of mycoplasma pneumonia, 465*f*
  with myelography, 272
  nonhelical, 9
  of orbit, 261
  of pancreatic pseudocyst, 406
  pediatric, 213
  pleural effusion and, 384*f*
  principles of, 6–7, 8*f*, 9
  pulmonary edema and, 418, 419*f*
  of pulmonary embolism, 426–429, 426*f*
  of pulmonary hemorrhage, 424*f*
  radiation dose in, 9–10
  sarcoidosis and, 503*f*

of solitary pulmonary nodule, 437*f*
of spinal lymphoma, 306*f*
of spine, 273–275
for thoracic disease, 335, 338, 338*t*
tuberculomas and, 161
Computed tomography angiography (CTA), 1371
vs. ventilation/perfusion lung scanning, 1374
Computed tomography angiography of pulmonary arteries (CTPA), 426–429, 426*f*, 428
Computed tomography venography (CTV), 428
Concentric calcification, 435
Conduction system, 606–607
Confluent fibrosis, 762
Congenital adrenal hyperplasia, 1318*f*
Congenital cardiac valve stenosis, 1269
Congenital diaphragmatic hernia, 1235, 1235*f*, 1240, 1245*f*
Congenital esophageal stenosis, 1279
Congenital heart disease, 1257–1275
MR, 665–666, 665*f*, 666*f*
Congenital lesions, 265–270
agenesis, of corpus callosum, 226–227
cephaloceles, 228
holoprosencephaly, 225
lipomas, of corpus callosum, 227–228
septo-optic dysplasia, 225
Congenital lobar emphysema, 1238, 1240*f*
Congenital lung cysts, 1239–1240
Congenital malformations, of spine, 308–311
Congenital megaureter, 893
Congenital pulmonary hypoplasia, 1235, 1235*f*
Congenital valvular insufficiency, 1269–1270
Congenitally short esophagus, 1279
Congestive heart failure, pleural effusion and, 528
Conglomerate masses, 486
Congophilic angiopathy, 119
Conjoined roots, 325*f*
Conn syndrome, 868
Connective tissue disease, 488
Consolidation, of lung, 1004, 1005*f*
Contrast
enhancement of, 126, 127*f*
in ischemic stroke, 93–94, 94*f*, 95*f*
soft tissue, 16, 16*t*
Contrast agents
administration of, 10
gastrointestinal, 24
iodinated, 22–24
in MR, 14–15, 14*f*
MR intravascular, 24
ultrasound intravascular, 24–25
Contrecoup, 67–68
Contusion(s), 1202, 1202*f*
of spine, 317*f*
Converging collimators, 1348
COP. *See* Cryptogenic organizing pneumonia
COPD. *See* Chronic obstructive pulmonary disease
COR. *See* Center of rotation
Cor triatriatum, 1272
Cord compression, of spine, 274*f*–275*f*
Corona radiata, 435
Coronary anatomy, 620, 620*f*, 621*f*, 622*f*
Coronary angiography, 619–620
Coronary arteriography, 658–659, 659*f*
Coronary artery disease, 629–633, 630*f*, 631*f*, 631*t*, 632*f*, 633*f*
Coronary pathology, 621–622, 622*f*
Corpus callosum
agenesis of, 226–227, 227*f*
lipomas of, 227–228, 228*f*
Cortical contusions, 63–64, 65*f*, 66*f*
Cortical desmoid, 1168–1169, 1172*f*, 1173*f*
Cortical destruction, 1086–1087, 1087*f*, 1088*f*
Cortical nephrocalcinosis, 885, 886*t*
Cortical ring, 84
Corticomedullary phase, 873
Co-trimoxazole, 506
Couinaud segments, of liver, 756–757, 757*f*, 757*t*
Coup, 67–68
Cowden disease, 853
CPM. *See* Central pontine myelinolysis
CPPD. *See* Calcium pyrophosphate dihydrate crystal deposition disease
CR. *See* Computed radiography
Craniocaudad view (CC), 5
of breast, 570–571, 571*f*
Craniocervical junction, 38*f*, 44, 46*f*
Craniofacial dysjunction, 82
Craniofacial trauma, 55–85
Craniopharyngioma, 148–149, 150*f*
Cremin's M line, 1292, 1295*f*
CREST syndrome, 490
Creutzfeldt-Jakob disease (CJD), 171–172, 212
Cricopharyngeal achalasia, 801–802
Cricopharyngeal spasm, 1277
Crohn disease, 1452*f*
of colon, 855–856, 856*f*
of duodenum, 827
of small bowel, 844–845, 845*f*, 846*f*
Cronkhite-Canada syndrome, 853
Cross sectional imaging, principles of, 6–22. *See also* Computed tomography (CT); Magnetic resonance imaging (MR); Ultrasonography (US)
Crossed-fused renal ectopia, 875, 875*f*
Cruciate ligaments, 1196–1198
Cryptococcosis, 182*f*, 289, 400
AIDS and, 475, 476*f*
Cryptococcus, 508
Cryptogenic organizing pneumonia (COP), 486*f*, 489, 493
Cryptorchidism, 1311
Crystal-induced arthritis, 1141–1144
CSF leaks, 70, 71*f*
CT. *See* Computed tomography
CT truncation artifacts, 1518
CTA. *See* Computed tomography angiography
CTPA. *See* Computed tomography angiography of pulmonary arteries
CTPH. *See* Chronic thromboembolic pulmonary hypertension
CTV. *See* Computed tomography venography
Curies (Ci), 1338
Cushing syndrome, 393, 868, 1316
CWP. *See* Coal worker's pneumoconiosis
CXR. *See* Chest radiograph
Cyanotic heart disease, 1263
Cyclophosphamide therapy, 506
Cyst(s), 392. *See also* Geode(s); Pseudocyst(s)
adrenal, 871, 871*f*
air, 376
arachnoid, 154, 311, 315*f*
benign hepatic, 768–769, 769*f*
bone, 1075, 1077–1079, 1077*f*, 1078*f*, 1079*f*
brain, 1512*f*
branchial cleft, 267–269, 269*f*
bronchiectatic, 376
bronchogenic, 400, 401*f*, 415, 439–440, 1251, 1254*f*
calcified, 740, 740*f*
in children, 265
choledochal, 1316–1317, 1319*f*
cholesteatoma, 246–247
classification of, 879–880
echinococcus, 770
enteric, 405
enteric duplication, 1321, 1322*f*
esophageal duplication, 405*f*
foregut, 400
hemorrhagic, 1410
hepatic, 1317
intestinal duplication, 1261*f*

Cyst(s) (*Contd.*)
leptomeningeal, 70
of lung, 477*f*
congenital, 1239–1240
lymphoepithelial, 259*f*
meniscal, 1195–1196, 1197*f*
mesenteric, 1321
mesothelial, 400
mucous retention, 243
nabothian, 917, 957
neurenteric, 405
neuroenteric, 1327
omental, 1321
ovarian, 917, 958–959, 959*f*, 1323, 1324*f*
pericardial, 401, 401*f*
peripheral arterial disease and, 694
peritoneal inclusion, 963, 963*f*
physiologic ovarian, 917
pineal, 147
rathke cleft, 148–149
renal, 879–880, 879*f*, 880*f*, 1309*t*
retention, 249
sacral, 315*f*
of shoulder, 1135*f*
of sinus, 243
of spine, 311
thymic, 392–393
thyroglossal duct, 265, 268*f*
thyroid, 1410
Tornwaldt, 249
unicameral bone, 1180
urachal, 899
US of, 932, 932*f*
Cystic abdominal masses, 1318*t*
Cystic adenomatoid malformation (CAM), 552, 553*f*, 1240, 1244*f*
Cystic blastomas, 459
Cystic fibrosis, 517–518, 1230, 1237*f*
Cystic hygroma, 270, 270*f*
Cystic Lesions, of posterior fossa, 232
Cystic nodal metastasis, 247*f*
Cysticercosis, 165*f*, 166*f*, 289
intraventricular, 164, 167*f*
late stage, 167*f*
meningobasal, 164
parenchymal, 164
racemose, 164, 168*f*
subarachnoid, 168*f*
Cystic/necrotic tumor, 770
Cystitis, 974
of bladder, 900, 900*f*
Cytomegalovirus infection
AIDS and, 474
congenital, 170*f*
Cytosine arabinoside, for pulmonary disease, 560
Cytoxan. *See* Cyclophosphamide therapy

D

DAI. *See* Diffuse axonal injury
Dandy-Walker malformation, 232–233, 234*f*, 994, 995*f*
DeBakey classification, 682
Deep venous thrombosis (DVT), 424, 428, 1376
lower-extremity, 1052–1053, 1053*f*, 1054*f*
noninvasive imaging for, 427
upper-extremity, 1055, 1056*f*, 1057, 1057*f*
Degenerative joint disease (DJD), 326, 329, 1126, 1133, 1133*f*
hallmarks of, 1133*t*
joint space narrowing and, 1232
joints with, 1133*t*
of knees, 1137*f*
osteophytosis and, 1132
sclerosis and, 1132
Dementia, 1479, 1480, 1482, 1511
AIDS and, 194
imaging strategies for, 51*t*, 52
multi-infarct, 1512
Demyelination, 184
age-related, 189
infection-related, 194–195
acute disseminated encephalomyelitis as, 194–195
central pontine myelinolysis as, 196–197
herpes encephalitis as, 195
HIV encephalopathy as, 194
Korsakoff syndrome as, 198–199
Marchiafava-Bignami disease as, 198
posterior reversible encephalopathy syndrome as, 197–198
progressive multifocal leukoencephalopathy as, 194
radiation arteritis as, 199–202
radiation leukoencephalitis as, 199
radiation necrosis as, 199–202
subacute sclerosing panencephalitis as, 195
Wernicke encephalopathy as, 198–199
infections and, 194–199
ischemic, 189–193, 189*f*
metabolic, 196–202
primary, 184
multiple sclerosis and, 184–189
toxic, 196–202
Density
of breast tissue, 584–585, 586*f*
in mammogram, 576–578, 578*f*
Dental infections, 256
pyogenic abscesses and, 156
Depreotide scan, 1465*f*, 1466*f*
Derenzo phantom, 1354
Dermatomyositis, 490
Dermoid, 267*f*
Dermoid mass, 151–153
Desiccated disk, 322*f*
Desmoid tumor, 1096, 1096*f*, 1219
Desquamative interstitial pneumonia (DIP), 485, 494, 495*f*
Detrusor-sphincter dyssynergy, 1308
Developmental venous anomalies, 118
DEXA. *See* Dual-energy X-ray absoprtiometry scan
Dextrocardia, 1272
Dextroposition, 616–617
Diagnostic arteriography, 340
Dialysis
grafts, 1049
venous access for, 719–721, 722*f*
Diamox. *See* Acetazolamide
Diaphragm, 354, 547–552, 548*f*, 548*t*, 549*f*, 550*f*, 551*f*
anatomy of, 364, 364*f*
hernias of, 402
radiographs of, 388
Diaphyseal aclasia. *See* Multiple hereditary exostosis
Diastematomyelia, 316*f*
Diastolic function, 1399*t*
Diethylenetriamine pentaacetic acid (DTPA), 426, 1343, 1459
Diffuse adrenal enlargement, 1316
Diffuse axonal injury (DAI), 62–64, 63*f*–65*f*
Diffuse cerebral swelling, 68–69, 69*f*
in children, 74–75
Diffuse fatty infiltration, 760
Diffuse idiopathic skeletal hyperostosis, 1133*f*
Diffuse Lewy body dementia (DLBD), 1479, 1482
Diffuse lung disease, 479
Diffuse mediastinal widening, 407*t*
Diffuse pleural disease, 536–538, 537*t*
Diffuse pleural thickening, 386
Diffuse pulmonary ossification, 509–510
Diffuse pulmonary uptake, 1442*f*
Diffuse renal parenchymal disease, 947–948, 948*f*, 948*t*
Diffuse thyroid disease, 1009–1011, 1010*f*
Diffusion-weighted imaging (DWI), 158, 300
in acute ischemia, 90, 90*f*
in neuroradiology, 48

Digital radiography (DR), 3, 5
Dilated rete testis, 967, 968*f*
Dilated spinal veins, 309*f*
Diluted small bowel lumen, 839–840, 840*t*
DIP. *See* Desquamative interstitial pneumonia
Diphenhydramine, contrast administration and, 24
Discitis, 282–284
  osteomyelitis and, 286*f*
Discogenic vertebral sclerosis, 1170, 1175*f*
Discoid meniscus, 1194–1195, 1195*f*, 1196*f*
Disk(s)
  annual tear of, 324
  bulging annulus fibrosus, 324
  central canal stenosis, 326, 327*f*
  conjoined root, 325*f*
  desiccated, 322*f*
  free fragments and, 324–325, 325*f*, 326*f*
  herniated nucleus pulposus, 324
  infections and, 330*f*
  lateral, 325, 337*f*
  lateral recess stenosis, 326
  neuroforaminal stenosis, 326
  protrusions of, 323*f*
  spondylolisthesis, 326–329, 328*f*, 329
  spondylolysis, 326–329, 328*f*
  stenosis, facet hypertrophy and, 328*f*
Disuse osteoporosis, 1156, 1157*f*
Diverging collimators, 1348
Diverticula
  bladder, 973, 973*f*
  caliceal, 897–898, 897*f*, 898*f*
  colonic, 711
  duodenal, 828–829, 828*f*
  of small bowel, 846, 846*f*
Diverticular disease, 1420*f*
DJD. *See* Degenerative joint disease
DLBD. *See* Diffuse Lewy body dementia
Don't touch lesions, 1168
DOPA. *See* Levodopa
Dopamine, 210
Doppler US
  artifacts, 1024–1025, 1025*f*
  basics of, 1019–1021, 1020*f*, 1020*t*, 1021*f*
  blood flow and, 1022–1023, 1022*f*, 1023*f*
  color flow, 1023–1024, 1024*f*
  principles of, 19, 21
  spectral waveforms, 1021–1022, 1021*f*, 1022*f*
Dose calibrator, 1355, 1355*f*
Dosimetry, 1374
Double aortic arch, 1238*f*
Double bleb sign, 978, 978*f*
Double bubble, 998, 998*f*
Double decidual sac sign, 977, 977*f*
Double-outlet right ventricle, 1263–1264
  with D-transposition, 1271*f*
Doubling time, 434
Down syndrome, 991
DR. *See* Digital radiography
Drainage catheters, 672
Dressler syndrome, 634
Drop metastases, 297, 299*f*, 300*f*
Drug-induced chest disease, 558–560, 559*f*, 561*f*
Drugs. *See also* Antibiotics; *specific drugs*
  anti-neoplastic, 185
  β-interferon, 185
  non-prescription, 411
DTPA. *See* Diethylenetriamine pentaacetic acid
D-transportation, 1263
Dual-agent imaging, 1468
Dual-energy X-ray absoprtiometry (DEXA) scan, 1369*f*
Dual-isotope myocardial scans, 1390
Duct of Santorini, 1301
Duct of Wirsung, 1301
Ductography, of breasts, 598–599
Ductus bump, 1261*f*
"Dumbbell" schwannoma, 298*f*
Duodenal atresia, 1283, 1283*f*
Duodenal diaphragm, 1284*f*
Duodenal diverticula, 828–829, 828*f*
Duodenal hematoma, 1284
Duodenal injuries, 1286*f*
Duodenal obstruction, 1282
  causes of, 1283*t*
Duodenal ulcers, 827–828, 828*f*
Duodenitis, 827, 827*f*, 1294
Duodenum
  anatomy of, 816–818, 817*f*
  filling defects/mass lesions, 825–827, 826*f*
  imaging methods of, 816
  narrowing of, 829–830, 829*f*, 830*f*
  thickened folds of, 827, 827*f*
Duplex doppler, 19
Dural fistulas, 67
"Dural tail," 141
DVT. *See* Deep venous thrombosis
DWI. *See* Diffusion-weighted imaging
Dysembryoplactic neuroepithelial tumor, 134
Dysmotile cilia syndrome, 518, 518*f*
Dysmyelination, 184
  diseases of, 202–205, 203*t*
    adrenal leukodystrophy, 203
    Alexander disease, 203–205
    Canavan disease, 203–205
    Leigh disease, 203
    metachromatic leukodystrophy, 203
Dysplasia, fibrous, 1064–1067, 1065*f*, 1066*f*, 1067*f*
Dysplastic cerebellar gangliocytoma, 140–141
Dysraphism, of spine, 312*f*

E

Eagle-Barrett syndrome, 1309, 1310*f*
Ebstein anomaly, 416, 1269, 1273*f*
ECD. *See* Ethyl cysteinate dimer
ECG. *See* Electrocardiogram
Echinococcosis, 472
Echinococcus, 289
Echinococcus cyst, 770
Echocardiography, 617, 618*f*, 619
Echogenic bile, 936, 936*f*
Echogenic renal pyramids, 1309*t*
Echo-planar, 13
ECMO. *See* Extracorporeal membranous oxygenation
Ectopic anus, 1292
Ectopic parathyroid adenoma, 392*f*
Ectopic pregnancy, 980–981, 980*t*, 981*f*
Ectopic ureterocele, 973, 974*f*, 1306–1307, 1307*f*
Edema
  high-altitude pulmonary, 422
  hydrostatic, 421
  increased capillary permeability, 420–421
  neurogenic pulmonary, 422
  permeability, 423*f*
  pulmonary, 417, 419*f*
Effective renal plasma flow (ERPF), 1428
EG. *See* Eosinophilic granuloma
Ehlers-Danlos syndrome, 681, 1253, 1309
Eisenmenger syndrome, 429*f*
Ejaculatory duct obstruction, 972
Elbow
  fat-pads
    displaced, 1120*f*, 1121*f*
    normal, 1121*f*
  osteochondritis dissecans of, 1153*f*
Electrocardiogram (ECG), 1387
Electroencephalogram (EEG), 1483
Electronic collimation, 1348

Embolism
peripheral arterial disease and, 690, 691*f*
pulmonary, 685–687, 685*f*
Embolization
agents, 673, 673*t*
hepatic angiography and, 709–710, 709*f*
Emphysema, 519–523, 520*f*, 521*t*, 522*f*
acquired lobar, 1241*f*
congenital lobar, 1238
pulmonary interstitial, 1247*f*
unilateral obstructive, 1239*t*
Emphysematous cholecystitis, 938
Emphysematous pyelonephritis, 883, 883*f*
"Empty" gestational sac, 979–980, 979*f*, 979*t*
Empyema, 528, 529*f*, 529*t*, 1250*f*
Encephalitis, 171
Encephalocele, frontal, 229*f*
Encephalomalacia, 70, 71*f*
Encephalomyelitis, 280
Enchondroma, 1067, 1067*f*, 1068*f*, 1069, 1069*f*
End-diastolic volume, 1396
Endobronchial lesions, 1238
Endocardial cushion defect, 1268*f*
Endocardial fibroelastosis, 1275*f*
Endocarditis, 256
Endocrine glands scintigraphy, 1404
Endocrine system, syndromes of, 868–869, 868*f*, 869*f*
Endometrial atrophy, 956–957, 957*f*
Endometrial carcinoma, 914–915, 915*f*, 915*t*
Endometrial cavity, fluid in, 957, 957*f*
Endometriosis, 917–918, 918*f*, 959, 960*f*
Endometrium, thickened, 956, 956*f*, 957*f*
Endoscopy, of esophagus, 404
Energy analysis, 1348–1349
Entamoeba histolytica, 471
Enteric cysts, 405
Enteric duplication cysts, 1321, 1322*f*
Enteritis, AIDS and, 844
Enteroclysis, 832
Enteroliths, 739
Eosinophilic gastroenteritis, 843
Eosinophilic granuloma (EG), 504, 507*t*, 508*f*, 1069–1070, 1070*f*, 1071*f*
Eosinophilic lung disease, 508
autoimmune diseases and, 508–509
etiology of, 508–509
Ependymitis granularis, 191, 192*f*
Ependymomas, 139, 139*f*, 293, 293*f*
myxopapillary, 294*f*
Epidemiology, 442
Epidermoid mass, 151–152
Epidermolysis bullosa, 1280
Epididymal lesions, 969, 970*f*
Epididymitis, 1439
Epididymo-orchitis, 965, 965*f*, 966*f*, 1439
Epidural abscess, 178*f*, 284, 289*f*
with osteomyelitis and discitis, 287*f*
Epidural hematomas, 57, 58*f*, 317, 319
Epidural tumors, 304
Epilepsy, 1484*f*, 1511
Epiphrenic diverticulum, 805, 806*f*
Epithelial tumors, 960–961, 961*f*
Epstein-Barr virus, 250
Equivocal bone/gallium-67 study, 1445*f*
Erb palsy, 320
Erect view, 6
ERPF. *See* Effective renal plasma flow
Escherichia coli, 286, 463
Esophageal achalasia, 802–803, 802*f*
Esophageal atresia, 1277, 1278*f*
Esophageal cancer, 1499
Esophageal duplication cyst, 405*f*
Esophageal folds, 810–811, 811*f*
Esophageal hiatus, 364
Esophageal imaging, 1416
Esophageal lesions, 404
Esophageal obstruction, 1277
causes of, 1278*t*
Esophageal stricture, 809–810, 809*f*, 810*f*, 811*f*
Esophageal transit study, 1417*f*
Esophagitis, 806–809, 807*f*, 808*f*, 809*f*, 1292–1294
acute, 1280
Esophagus
anatomy of, 798–800, 799*f*, 800*f*
barium study of, 404
Barrett, 1279
computed tomography, 404
congenitally short, 1279
endoscopy of, 404
imaging methods of, 798
magnetic resonance imaging of, 404
motility and, 800–801
perforation/trauma of, 813–814, 814*f*
Esthesioneuroblastoma, 245*f*
in sinus, 245
Ethyl cysteinate dimer (ECD), 1476*f*
Euthyroid ophthalmopathy, 264
Ewing sarcoma, 256, 1093, 1094f, 1251, 1264*f*
osteoporosis and, 1157
Ex vacuo ventriculomegaly and, 207
Excretory urography (XU), 872–873, 874*f*
Exercise radionuclide ventriculogram, 1397
Exstrophy, bladder, 898
Extra-axial tumors, 124, 124*f*
Extracorporeal membranous oxygenation (ECMO), 1235, 1241, 1246
Extradural masses, 297–305
Extramedullary lesions, 273
Extramedullary masses, 295–297
Extramedullary tumors, 277*f*
Extraperitoneal bladder rupture, 904, 904*f*
Extrapleural lesions, 386
Extrinsic allergic alveolitis, 500

F

Fab fragments, 1461
Facet degenerative arthropathy, 1360*f*
Facet hypertrophy, 1509*f*
Facial trauma
imaging strategy for, 75–76, 76*f*
Le Fort, 81–82, 82*f*
mandibular, 83–85, 83*f*, 84*f*
nasal fractures in, 77
nasoethmoidal, 82–83, 83*f*
orbital, 78–80, 79*f*, 80*f*
sinus fractures and, 77–78, 78*f*
soft tissue and, 76–77, 77*f*
zygoma, 80–81, 81*f*
Falciform ligament, 734
Familial adenomatous polyposis syndrome, 852, 853*f*
Fast low-angle acquisition with relaxation enhancement (FLARE), 13
Fast low-angle shot (FLASH), 13
Fast spin-echo (FSE), 13, 186, 250, 260, 1192, 1207
of spine, 275
Fat, imaging techniques of, 13, 14*f*, 17, 17*t*
Fat embolism, 422, 423*f*
Fat-saturation technique, 13
Fatty infiltration
of liver, 758–760, 759*f*, 759*t*, 760*f*
US of, 930, 930*f*
Fc fragments, 1461
FDA. *See* Food and Drug Administration
FDG. *See* Fluorodeoxyglucose scan
Fecal impaction, 746
Fegnomashic, 1063–1064, 1064*t*, 1082–1084, 1082*t*, 1083*t*, 1084*t*

Femoral head, migration of, 1135*f*
Femoral neck, stress fracture of, 1127*f*
Femur, stress fracture of, 1127*f*
Fentanyl, for vascular radiology, 673
Fetal adenocarcinomas, 459
Fetal alcohol syndrome, 270
Fetal cystic hygromas, 269
Fetal hydrops, 990, 990*f*
Fetus
  anomalies of
    abdomen, 997–1000, 998*f*, 999*f*, 1000*f*
    chest and heart, 995–997, 996*f*, 997*f*
    CNS, face and neck, 991–995, 991*f*, 991*t*, 992*f*, 993*f*, 994*f*, 995*f*, 996*f*
    general, 990–991, 991*t*
    skeleton, 1000, 1000*f*
  environment of, 986–990, 986f, 987*f*, 988*f*, 989*f*
  measurements and growth of, 983–986, 983f, 984f, 985f, 985t
  sector transducer image of, 20*f*
Fever of undetermined origin (FUO), 1443, 1444*f*, 1447, 1449*f*, 1515
FFDM. *See* Full-field digital mammography
FHL. *See* Flexor hallucis longus tendon
Fibrillary astrocytoma, 131–132
Fibroadenomas, 581, 583*f*
Fibroblast migration, in brain abscesses, 158
Fibroepithelial polyp, 895, 896*f*
Fibroids, 955–956, 956*f*
  in pregnancy, 986
Fibrolamellar carcinoma, 767, 769*f*
Fibrolipoma, of filum terminale, 313*f*
Fibroma, 438–439
  nonossifying, 1179
Fibromuscular disease (FMD)
  peripheral arterial disease, 693, 696*f*
  renal angiography and, 703–704, 704*f*
Fibrosarcomas, 1094*f*, 1095, 1095*f*
Fibrosis, 389
  retroperitoneal, 750–751
Fibrothorax, 386, 536
Fibrotic neoplasms, 919
Fibrous cortical defect, 1073
Fibrous dysplasia, 1064–1067, 1065*f*, 1066*f*, 1067*f*
Film radiography, 3, 4*f*
Films
  mammogram, 589–590, 592*f*
  plain, 75
  skull, 55–56
Filum terminale, fibrolipoma of, 313*f*
Fine-needle aspiration (FNA), 1404
First-pass flow studies, 1399–1402
First-pass function studies, 1397–1399
FISP. *See* True fast imaging with steady-state precession
Fissures, in lungs, 345–347
Fistula
  arteriovenous, 719–720
  of bladder, 904
  bronchopleural, 531, 533*f*
  carotid cavernous, 67, 68*f*
  vesicocolonic, 904, 904*f*
F-labeled levodopa PET scan, 210*f*
FLAIR. *See* Fluid-attentuated inversion recovery
Flake fractures, 1218
FLARE. *See* Fast low-angle acquisition with relaxation enhancement
FLASH. *See* Fast low-angle shot
Flexion teardrop fracture, 1108*f*, 1110
Flexor hallucis longus tendon (FHL), 1216–1217
Flexural pseudotumors, 828
Floating palate fracture, 81, 82*f*
Flow-related enhancement, 48
Fluid-attenuated inversion recovery (FLAIR), 157, 158, 186
  CNS neoplasms and, 125
  in ischemia, 91
Fluorine-18-fluorodeoxyglucose, 1454–1455
Fluorodeoxyglucose (FDG) scan, 339, 395, 1342, 1465*f*, 1475, 1488, 1490*f*
  brain and, 1491*f*
  heart and, 1491*f*
  liver and, 1492*f*
Fluoroscopy, 5, 5*f*
  chest, 337
  of spine, 272
Fluorosis, 1167
FMD. *See* Fibromuscular disease
fMRI. *See* Functional MR imaging
FNA. *See* Fine-needle aspiration
FNH. *See* Focal nodular hyperplasia
Focal alveolar consolidation, 1227
  causes of, 1228*t*
Focal back pain, 271
Focal bacterial nephritis, 883
Focal fatty infiltration, 760
Focal nodular hyperplasia (FNH), 766–767, 768*f*, 1318, 1423
Focal organizing pneumonia, 440
Focal pleural disease, 535–536, 535*t*, 536*f*, 537*f*
Focal sparing, 760, 760*f*
"Fogging effect," 91
Follicular adema, 1409–1410, 1409*f*
Follicular adenoma, 1008, 1008*t*
Follicular carcinoma, 1410
Food and Drug Administration (FDA), 1457, 1458
Foot
  magnetic resonance imaging of, 1214
  tumor of, 1219
Foramina of Bochdalek, 364, 1240
Foramina of Morgagni, 364, 1240
Foregut cysts, 400
Foreign bodies, in abdomen/pelvis, 751, 752*f*
Fourier phase, 1398*f*, 1399*f*
Fourier transformation, 276
Fracture(s), 1108*f*, 1515. *See also* Stress fractures
  anterior wedge compression, 1110*f*
  of arms, 1118
  Bennett, 1112, 1113*f*
  blowout, 78–80, 79*f*
  of calcaneus, 1131, 1131*f*
  clay shoveler's, 1107*f*, 1110
  Colles, 1118, 1118*f*
  compression, 302*f*
  flake, 1218
  flexion teardrop, 1108*f*, 1110
  floating palate, 81, 82*f*
  Galeazzi, 1119, 1119*f*
  of glenoid, 1123*f*
  of hands, 1112
  hangman's, 1107*f*, 1110
  healing, 1359*f*
  of hips, 1127, 1130*f*
  hook of the hamate, 1114–1115, 1115*f*, 1116*f*
  insufficiency, 1124
  Jefferson, 1105*f*, 1107
  le Fort, 81–82, 82*f*
  of Lisfranc, 1129
  mandibular, 83–85, 83*f*, 84*f*
  maxillary, 77–78, 78*f*
  medial wall, 78
  midface, 81–82, 82*f*
  Monteggia, 1118–1119, 1119*f*
  nasoethmoidal, 82–83, 83*f*
  navicular, 1116
  occult sacral, 1359*f*
  osteomalacia and, 1160*f*
  osteosarcoma and, 1175*f*

Fracture(s) (*Contd.*)
with osteosclerosis, 1170
of patella, 1203
of pelvis, 1123
with periostitis, 1170
pseudo-Bennett, 1112
pyramidal, 81–82
of ribs, 1358*f*, 1517*f*
Rolando, 1112, 1113*f*
of sacrum, 1124, 1124*f*
scaphoid, 1116*f*
seatbelt, 1108*f*, 1110
sinus, 77–78, 78*f*
skull, 56, 56*f*
Smith, 1118, 1118*f*
of spine, 317*f*, 1112, 1112*f*
temporal bone, 56–57, 57*f*
of tibial plateau, 1127–1129, 1130*f*
triquetral, 1117*f*
zygoma, 80–81, 81*f*
Free fragments, 325*f*, 326*f*
in lumbar disks, 324–325
Free radicals, in brain abscesses, 158
Free water, MR and, 16–17, 17*t*
Freiberg infraction, 1154*f*
Frontal lobes, 156
tuberculomas and, 161
Frontal projection, 604
Frontotemporal lobe degeneration, 1481
FSE. *See* Fast spin-echo
Full energy peak, 1349
Full-field digital mammography (FFDM), 569
Functional megacolon, 1292
Functional MR imaging (fMRI), in neuroradiology, 48, 51
Fungal infections. *See* Infection(s), fungal
Fungal meningitis, 173
AIDS and, 178–181
Fungal pneumonia, 468
FUO. *See* Fever of undetermined origin
Furosemide renography, 1436*f*, 1437*f*
Fusion imaging, 1468
Fusobacterium, 464

G

Gadolinium, 277
discitis and, 286
enhanced imaging by, 278*f*
MR and, 157
tuberculomas and, 161
postoperative scar enhancement with, 329
Gadolinium chelates
in brain, 49*f*
in liver, 14–15, 14*f*
MR and, 24
Gadolinium silicate (GSO), 1347
Galeazzi fracture, 1119, 1119*f*
Gallbladder, 776–780, 777*f*, 778*f*, 779*f*, 780*f*
acoustic shadowing in, 21*f*
acute hydrops of, 1316
calcified, 738, 739*f*
cancer of, 1502
carcinoma of, 938–939, 939*f*
US of, 936–939, 936*f*, 937*f*, 938*f*, 939*f*
Gallium scintigraphy, 395, 1441*f*, 1442*f*, 1444*f*, 1445*f*
Gallstone ileus, 745
Gallstones, 738, 777, 777*f*
US of, 937, 937*f*
Gamekeeper's thumb, 1113, 1114*f*
Gamma camera detector, 1351–1353
components of, 1346*f*
resolution and linearity of, 1353*f*
Gangliocytoma, 133–134
Ganglioglioma, 133–134
desmoplastic infantile, 134
Ganglioneuroblastoma, 303*f*
Ganglioneuroma, 403*f*
Gas
abdominal, 741, 742*f*
in biliary tree, US of, 935, 935*f*
in portal venous system, 763–764, 763*f*
Gas agents, contrast imaging and, 24
Gastric atresia, 1281, 1281*f*
Gastric bezoars, 1282
Gastric duplications, 1281
Gastric emptying, 1418–1419
study of, 1418*f*
Gastric folds, 822–824, 823*f*, 824*f*
Gastric obstruction, causes of, 1280*t*
Gastric tumors, 1282
Gastric ulcers, 824–825, 825*f*
Gastric volvulus, 1281
Gastrinomas, 1462
Gastritis, 822–824, 823*f*, 824*f*, 1294
Gastroduodenal artery (GDA), hepatic angiography and, 707–708, 708*f*
Gastroesophageal reflux (GER), 1277, 1279, 1416–1418
study of, 1418*f*
Gastroesophageal reflux disease (GERD), 804–805, 804*f*, 805*f*
Gastrointestinal bleeding, 1301–1303, 1419*f*
causes of, 1302*t*
Gastrointestinal bleeding scintigraphy, 1419–1420
Gastrointestinal cancers, positron emission tomography and, 1426
Gastrointestinal contrast agents, 24
Gastrointestinal hemorrhage
lower, 860, 860*t*
mesenteric angiography and, 711–712, 712*f*
upper, 830
Gastrointestinal masses, 1321–1323
Gastrointestinal obstruction, 1277–1292
causes of, 1278*t*
Gastrointestinal scintigraphy, 1416, 1419–1420
Gastrointestinal tumors, 1322–1323
Gastroschisis, 999, 999*f*
Gated blood pool scans, 1395, 1395*f*
interpretation of, 1396–1397
techniques for, 1395–1396
Gated blood pool scintigraphy, 629
Gaucher disease, 1450
GBM. *See* Glioblastoma multiforme
GCS. *See* Glasgow coma scale
GDA. *See* Gastroduodenal artery
Geiger-Müller (GM) detector, 1341
Gelatinous pseudocysts, 181
γ-Emitting isotopes, 1458
Genital abnormalities, 1310–1312
Genital tract
female
anatomy of, 909–911, 910*f*, 911*f*
benign conditions of, 916–919, 916*f*, 917*f*, 918*f*, 919*f*
congenital anomalies of, 911, 912*f*
gynecologic malignancy and, 911–915, 913*f*, 914*f*, 914*t*, 915*f*, 915*t*, 916*f*
US of, 954–963
male
prostate/seminal vesicles, 920–923, 921*f*, 922*f*, 922*t*, 923*f*
testes/scrotum of, 919–920, 920*f*
US of, 963–972
Genitourinary system, 1303–1312
Genitourinary system scintigraphy, 1428
Geodes, 1081, 1082*f*, 1133, 1174*f*
of hip, 1153*f*

GER. *See* Gastroesophageal reflux
GERD. *See* Gastroesophageal reflux disease
Germ cell neoplasms, 396–397
Germ cell tumors, 146–147, 396*f*, 961
Germinal matrix, 1015*f*, 1016–1017, 1017*f*, 1017*t*
Germinal matrix hemorrhage, 220
Gestation, 977–978, 977*f*, 977*t*, 978*f*, 978*t*
Gestational sac, "empty," 979–980, 979*f*, 979*t*
Gestational trophoblastic disease, 982–983, 982*f*, 983*f*
GFR. *See* Glomerular filtration rate
Ghon lesion, 466, 1253
Ghost tumor, 133
GI stromal tumors (GISTs), 820–821, 821*f*
Giant bone island, 1180*f*
Giant cell arteritis, 691, 693*f*
Giant cell astrocytoma, 131–132
Giant cell tumor, 1070–1073, 1071*f*
  malignant, 1095
Giant cholesterol cyst. *See* Cholesterol granuloma
Giardiasis, 827
GISTs. *See* GI stromal tumors
Glasgow coma scale (GCS), 73, 74*t*
Glenoid, fracture of, 1123*f*
Glenoid labrum, 1210–1211, 1210*f*
"Gliding sign," 1002, 1003*f*, 1004
Glioblastoma multiforme (GBM), 129–131, 131t
Gliomas, 128–129, 130*f*, 131*f*, 131*t*
  butterfly, 129–130
  neurofibromatosis and, 235*f*
Gliomatosis, 261
Gliomatosis cerebri, 131–132
Globe, 265
Glomerular filtration rate (GFR), 1428
Glomerulonephritis, 1232*f*
Glomus jugulare tumor, 255*f*
Glucagonomas, 1463
GM. *See* Geiger-Müller detector
GM-CSF. *See* Granulocyte macrophage-colony-stimulating factor
Goiter, 391*f*, 454, 1010, 1010*f*, 1407
  multinodular, 1407
  nontoxic, 1407
Gonadal stromal tumors, 966
Goodpasture syndrome, 423, 423*f*
Gout, 1141, 1142*f*
  hallmarks of, 1141*t*
Gradient-recalled acquisition in the steady state (GRASS), 13, 1192
Gradient-recalled echo, 13
Graft surveillance, in peripheral arteries, 1048–1049, 1049*f*, 1050*f*, 1051*t*
Gram-negative bacteria, 463
Gram-positive bacteria, 461–462
Granular cell myoblastoma, 438, 453
Granulocyte macrophage-colony-stimulating factor (GM-CSF), 509
Granuloma, as infection, of brain, 160
Granulomatous diseases, 501
GRASS. *See* Gradient-recalled acquisition in the steady state
Graves disease, 391, 1332, 1407–1408, 1408*f*. *See also* Thyroid ophthalmopathy
Gray (Gy), 1338
Gray matter
  diseases of, 53–54
  subcortical, injury of, 64, 67
Greater omentum, 734
Ground glass densities, 485
Growing fracture. *See* Leptomeningeal cyst
GSO. *See* Gadolinium silicate
Guide wires, 672
Guillain-Barré syndrome, 280, 283*f*
Gunshot injury, to head, 73, 74*f*
Gy. *See* Gray

H

HAART. *See* Highly active antiretroviral therapy
Haemophilus influenzae, 172, 177*f*, 463, 1227
Half-fourier acquisition single-shot turbo spin-echo (HASTE), 13
Hallervorden-Spatz disease, 211*f*
HAMA. *See* Human antimouse antibody
Hamartoma, 439*f*
  of tuber cinereum, 155, 155*f*
Hamartomatous polyposis syndrome, 852–853
Hamman-Rich syndrome, 492, 493*f*
Hands, fractures of, 1112
Hangman's fracture, 1107*f*, 1110
Hard metal pneumoconiosis, 500
Hashimoto thyroiditis, 1010, 1010*f*, 1408
HASTE. *See* Half-fourier acquisition single-shot turbo spin-echo
Hazy, reticular, or reticulonodular opacities, 1231–1233
  causes of, 1232*t*
  in neonates, sources of, 1249*t*
Head, injury
  brainstem, 70–72
  in children, 73–75
  classification of, 57
  imaging strategies for, 55–57
  mechanisms of, 67–68
  penetrating, 72–73
  primary, 57–68
  secondary, 68–70
Head and neck
  compartments of, 249
  computed tomography for, 241
  magnetic resonance imaging for, 241
  malignancies of, 1506–1507
  positron emission tomography of, 260
  suprahyoid, 247–259
Headache
  imaging strategies for, 51*t*, 52
  pyogenic abscesses and, 156
Heart. *See also* Cardiac anatomy
  active congestion and, 1257
  anatomy of, 620, 620*f*, 621*f*, 622*f*
  anomalies of, in pregnancy, 995–997, 996*f*, 997I
  decreased pulmonary vascularity and, 1258
  diseases of
    congenital heart disease, 665–666, 665*f*, 666*f*
    congestive heart failure, 528
    ischemic heart disease. *See* Ischemic heart disease
    valvular heart disease, 640–645, 641*t*, 642*f*, 643*f*, 644*f*, 645*f*, 646*f*, 663–665, 663*f*, 664*f*
  passive congestion of, 1258
  pulmonary blood flow and, 1258
Heat-damaged red blood cell scan, 1422–1423
Heel spurs, 1127
Helical computed tomography, 9, 9*f*
Helicobacter infection, 1294, 1419
Helicobacter pylori infection, 818
Hemangioblastomas, 293, 294, 295*f*
Hemangioendothelioma, 1317–1318
Hemangioma, 257, 262*f*, 397, 453
  cavernous, US of, 932, 932*f*
  pseudopermeative process and, 1159*f*
Hemangiopericytoma, 142–143, 439
Hematogenous metastases, 455
Hematologic malignancies, 301
Hematomas
  epidural, 57, 58*f*, 319*f*
  intracerebral, 64, 66*f*
  intramural, 683
  mediastinal, 410*f*
  of spinal cord, 318*f*, 319*f*
  subdural, 57–59, 58*f*, 59*f*, 60*f*, 61*f*

Hemimegalencephaly, 230
Hemochromatosis, 763, 763*f*, 1144, 1146, 1146*f*
Hemolytic-uremic syndrome, 1295
Hemophagocytic lymphohistiocytosis (HLH), 1320
Hemophilia, 1147–1148
Hemoptysis, 688
Hemorrhage
  adrenal, 870, 870*f*, 1315, 1316*f*
  of bladder, 903
  definition of, 86
  drug-associated, 119
  gastrointestinal, 711–712, 712*f*, 830, 860, 860*t*
  germinal matrix, 220
  hemorrhagic neoplasm v., 119, 120*f*, 120*t*
  hemorrhagic transformation of infarction v., 120
  imaging of, 108–110, 112, 112f, 112t, 113f
  intraventricular, 61, 65*f*
  in late capsule stage, in brain abscesses, 158
  liver laceration and, 708*f*
  lower GI, 860, 860*t*
  mediastinal, 408–410
  MR of, 18, 18*t*
  nontumoral, 126
  parenchymal, 116–119, 117*f*, 118*f*, 119*f*
  pulmonary, 422–424, 423*f*
    causes of, 423*t*
    computed tomography of, 424*f*
    idiopathic, 423
  septic embolus and, 159
  subarachnoid, 59, 61, 62*f*, 112–114, 114*f*, 115*f*, 116, 116*f*, 1481*f*
  tumoral, 126
  upper GI, 830
Hemorrhagic cysts, 1410
Hemorrhagic neoplasm, 126
  hemorrhage v., 119, 120*f*, 120*t*
Hemorrhagic ovarian cysts, 959, 959*f*
Hemothorax, 1249
Henoch-Schönlein purpura, 1302, 1303*f*
Heparin, for vascular radiology, 673
Hepatic adenomas, 767, 769*f*, 1318
Hepatic angiography, 707–710, 708*f*, 709*f*, 710*f*
Hepatic blood pool scintigraphy, 1425
Hepatic congestion, 763, 930–931
Hepatic cysts, 1317
Hepatic hemangioma, 1426*f*
Hepatic malignancies, 1502
Hepatitis
  acute, 760
  chronic, 760
Hepatobiliary, 1298–1301
Hepatobiliary imaging, 1334–1335, 1416, 1423–1425, 1424*f*
  acute cholecystitis and, 1425*f*
Hepatobiliary masses, 1316–1319
Hepatobiliary scintigraphy, 1416
Hepatoblastoma, 1318, 1321*f*
Hepatocellular carcinoma, 765–766, 766*f*, 766*t*, 1318–1319
  US of, 933, 933*f*
Hepatomegaly, 758, 759*t*
Hereditary hemorrhagic telangiectasia (HHT), PAVMs and, 686
Hernia(s)
  bochdalek, 549–550, 549*f*
  congenital diaphragmatic, 1235, 1235*f*, 1240, 1245*f*
  of diaphragm, 402
  inguinal, 1287, 1288*f*
  morgagni, 550, 551*f*
  of scrotum, 969, 970*f*
Herniated nuclear pulposus, 324
Herniation
  brain, 69, 70*f*
  central, 123
  subfalcine, 123
  uncal, 123
Herpes encephalitis, 173*f*, 195, 197*f*
Herpes simplex virus (HSV), 169–170, 195
  neonatal, 171*f*
Heterotopic bone, 1365
Heterotopic gray matter, 230, 231*f*
Hexamethylpropyleneamine oxime (HMPAO), 1476*f*, 1478*f*
HHT. *See* Hereditary hemorrhagic telangiectasia
Hibernating myocardium, 1392, 1392*f*, 1515*f*
HIE. *See* Hypoxic ischemic encephalopathy
High intensity zone (HIZ), 324
High resolution computed tomography (HRCT), 338
  airspace disease and, 366
  asbestosis and, 498
  interstitial lung disease and, 480*t*, 481*f*
  of invasive aspergillosis, 475*f*
  LCH and, 506
  lung disease and, 479
    diagnosis of, 482*t*
  of lung fissures, 346*f*
  in lymphangitic carcinomatosis, 456
  of pleura, 362
  pulmonary edema and, 418
  pulmonary interstitium and, 350
  for thoracic disease, 339*t*
High-altitude pulmonary edema, 422
Highly active antiretroviral therapy (HAART), 174, 472, 476
Hila, 389
  small, 416, 416*t*
Hilar
  abnormalities of, 412
  bilateral enlargement of, 415–416, 415*t*
  infection of, 413, 415
  malignancy of, 412
  metastases of, 414*f*
Hilar anatomy, 359–362, 360*f*
  frontal view, 359–361
  left lateral view, 361–362
Hilar disease, 379, 381*f*
  radiographs and, 380
  tumors and, 380
Hilar masses, 1251–1255
Hilar nodes, 398*t*
Hill-Sachs deformity, 1120, 1209, 1210*f*
Hip(s)
  ankylosing spondylitis and, 1140*f*
  avascular necrosis of, 1151*f*
  dislocation of, 1123*f*
  fracture of, 1127, 1130*f*
  loosening prosthesis in, 1360*f*
  osteochondritis dissecans of, 1153*f*
  replacement of, aseptic loosening of, 1452*f*
  rheumatoid arthritis of, 1136
  transient osteoporosis of, 1191, 1191*f*
Hirschsprung disease, 1292, 1293*f*, 1301
Histoplasma capsulatum, 408, 468, 1231
Histoplasma granuloma, 1253*f*
Histoplasmoma, 469
Histoplasmosis granuloma, 162*f*, 400, 409*f*, 413, 468–469
HIV (Human immunodeficiency virus)
  in abdomen, 751–754, 753*t*
  children and, 1234
  encephalopathy and, 175–176, 180*f*, 194, 195*f*
  pneumonia and, 466
  pulmonary infections and, 472
HIZ. *See* High intensity zone
HLA. *See* Human leukocyte antigen
HLH. *See* Hemophagocytic lymphohistiocytosis
HMPAO. *See* Hexamethylpropyleneamine oxime
HN. *See* Hydronephrosis
Hodgkin disease, 394, 395*f*, 398, 413, 1257*f*. *See also* Non-Hodgkin lymphoma
  atelectasis in, 456

Hodgkin lymphoma, 749, 749*f*
Hoffman brain phantom, 1354
Holoprosencephaly, 994, 994*f*
  alobar, 225
  lobar, 226
  semilobar, 225
Homunculus, 97*f*
Honeycomb lung, 484*f*
  rheumatoid, 488*f*
Hook of the hamate fracture, 1114–1115, 1115*f*, 1116*f*
Horner syndrome, 444
Horseshoe kidney, 875, 875*f*
Hot pulmonary nodule, 1495*f*
HPT. *See* Hyperparathyroidism
HRCT. *See* High resolution computed tomography
HSV. *See* Herpes simplex virus
Hughes-Stovins syndrome, 415
Human antimouse antibody (HAMA), 1462
Human immunodeficiency virus. *See* HIV
Human leukocyte antigen (HLA), 1136–1141
Humerus
  pseudocyst of, 1171–1173, 1177*f*
  pseudodislocation of, 1170–1171
Hunter syndrome, 1184
Huntington disease, 211, 211*f*
Hurler syndrome, 1184, 1186*f*, 1187*f*
Hutch diverticulum, 1309, 1309*f*
Hyaline membrane disease. *See* Surfactant deficiency disease
Hybrid imaging, 1468
Hydatid disease, 472
Hydranencephaly, 216–217, 218*f*, 994, 995*f*
Hydrocarbon aspiration, 1230*f*
Hydrocele, 968, 969*f*
Hydrocephalus, 69, 123, 208*f*, 1474*f*
  brain abscesses and, 158
  cerebrospinal fluid studies and, 1473
  communicating, 205
  noncommunicating, 205
Hydrometrocolpos, 1325*f*
Hydromyelia, 294
Hydronephrosis (HN), 891–893, 893*f*, 1305, 1432
Hydrops, acute, of gallbladder, 1316
Hydrosalpinx, 918, 918*f*, 963, 963*f*
Hydrostatic edema, 421
Hypercortisolism, 1316
Hyperdense neoplasms, 126
Hyperemia, 68–69
Hypereosinophilic syndrome, 507
Hyperostosis, skeletal, 1133*f*
Hyperparathyroidism (HPT), 1011, 1012*f*, 1079–1080, 1079*f*, 1144, 1159–1161, 1160*f*, 1161*f*
  metastatic calcification and, 1365
    brown tumors in, 1161*f*
    causes of, 1412*t*
Hypersensitivity pneumonitis, 500
Hypersplenism, 706–707
Hypertension
  pulmonary arterial, 429*f*
  pulmonary arteries and, 430, 431*f*
    causes of, 430*t*
  pulmonary venous, 420*t*
Hypertensive hemorrhage, 116–117, 117*f*
Hyperthyroidism, 1407, 1408
Hypertrophic cardiomyopathy, 637, 637*f*, 661, 661*f*
Hypertrophic osteoarthropathy, 1364*f*
Hypertrophic pulmonary osteoarthropathy, 1183, 1185*f*
Hypertrophic pyloric stenosis, 1282
Hypoattenuating lesions, 770–771, 770*f*
Hypogammaglobulinemia, 391
Hypogenetic lung-scimitar syndrome, 555–556, 556*f*
Hypoparathyroidism, 1161
Hypopharyngeal/upper esophageal obstruction, 1277
Hypoplastic aortic syndrome, 702
Hypoplastic left heart, 1271–1272, 1274*f*
Hypoplastic lung, 554
Hypoplastic right heart, 1267
Hypothenar hammer, 692–693
Hypothyroidism, 1406–1407
Hypoxic ischemic encephalopathy (HIE), 215, 216–225, 221*f*. *See also* Nonhypoxic ischemic encephalopathy
  imaging of, 216*t*
  partial perinatal, 224
  perinatal
    acute, 221*f*
    chronic, 223*f*
Hypoxic ischemic injury, 219*f*
  computed tomography of, 220, 220*f*
  germinal matrix hemorrhage, 220
  hydranencephaly, 216–217
  imaging of, 224*t*
  perinatal, 222*f*
  periventricular leukomalacia, 217, 219*f*
  in premature infants, 217–219
  prenatal, 217
  profound, 220–221
    imaging of, 223*t*
  profound *vs.* partial, 220–225
  prolonged, 220*f*
Hysterosalpingography, 911, 911*f*

I

I-131 tositumomab (Bextra), 1469
ICA. *See* Internal carotid artery
Idiopathic pulmonary fibrosis (IPF), 482, 483*f*, 484, 486*f*, 489
Idiopathic pulmonary hemorrhage, 423
Idiopathic pulmonary hypertension, 431
IEC. *See* International Electrotechnical Commission phantom
Ileal atresia, 1286
Iliac artery, aneurysms of, 903
IMA. *See* Inferior mesenteric artery
Image generation, definition of, 3
Image matrix, of CT, 7, 7*f*
Image reconstruction, 1350
Image wraparound artifact, 16
Imaging
  center of rotation in, 1353
  isotopes for, 1458
  linearity in, 1352
  moving organs, 1351
  of physiologic processes, 1456–1457
  pixel size calibration in, 1353
  quality control in, 1351, 1352*t*
  resolution in, 1352
  stress *vs.* prone, 1394*f*
  systems, 1345–1356
Immunocompromise, 472
  in AIDS patients, 473*t*
  in non-HIV patients, 473*t*
Imperforate anus, 1292, 1294*f*, 1295*f*
Impingement syndrome, 1205
Implantation bleeding, in pregnancy, 981–982
Implanted ports, 672
Incarcerated inguinal hernia, 1287
Inclinometer, 336
Increased capillary permeability edema, 420–421, 421*f*. *See also* Acute respiratory distress syndrome
  etiologies of, 421*t*
Indium-111 pentetreotide, 1415
Indium-111 zevalin antibody scan, 1333*f*
Indium-111-labeled leukocytes, 1443–1445
Infarct imaging of, ischemic heart disease, 634–636, 634*f*, 635*f*
Infarct-avid scans, 1393
Infarction, 69–70
  bone, 1181, 1181*f*
  bowel, 746–747, 747*f*
  brain abscesses and, 158

Infarction (*Contd.*)
definition of, 86
Freiberg, 1154*f*
hemorrhagic transformation of, 91–93, 92*f*
hemorrhage v., 120
myocardial, 633–634, 634*f*
pulmonary, 427*f*
of spinal cord, 305
venous, 106–108, 110*f*, 111*f*
watershed, 105, 106*f*, 107*f*
Infection(s)
actinomycotic, 156
anaerobic bacterial, 464
brain, imaging strategies for, 51*t*, 52
cardivascular, 1448–1449
central nervous system, 156, 1448–1449
coccidioides, 386*f*, 468, 470*f*, 1231
cytomegalovirus
AIDS and, 474
congenital, 170*f*
demyelination and, 194–195
dental, 256
pyogenic abscesses and, 156
of disks, 330*f*
epidural, 174
extra-axial
fungal meningitis, 173
meningitis, 172
racemose cysticercosis, 173
tuberculous meningitis, 172–173
viral meningitis, 174
fungal
aspergillosis, 162
blastomycosis, 162
candidiasis, 162, 163
coccidioidomycosis, 162
cosmopolitan, 162–164
cryptococcosis, 162, 163–164
endemic, 162
histoplasmosis, 162
hydrocephalus and, 162
Mucormycosis, 162
mucormycosis, 162
of spine, 289
toxoplasmosis, 165
in tuberculomas, 161
gam-negative rod, 156
of gastrointestinal tract, 1292
granuloma and, of brain, 160
helicobacter, 1294, 1419
helicobacter pylori, 818
of hilar, 413, 415
HIV and, pulmonary infections and, 472
of kidneys, 1438
listerial, 156
of mediastinum, 407
mucormycosis, 260*f*
mycobacterial, 464–466
in CNS, 160–162
mycoplasma, 1227
Nocardia, 473
nocardial, 156
nonpyogenic, 288
opportunistic, 1440–1441
AIDS and, 754
of orthopedic hardware, 1451*f*
otomastoiditis, temporal lobes and, 156
parasitic
amebic meningoencephalitis, 165
cysticercosis, 164
echinococcosis, 165
of thorax, 471–472
in tuberculomas, 161
parenchymal, 156–159
pneumococcal, 156
pogenic, 286–287
positron emission tomography and, 1515
postoperative, 1447–1448, 1449*f*
pulmonary, 460
renal, 882–884, 883*f*, 884*f*
scintigraphic diagnosis of, 1440
sinus, frontal lobes and, 156
of spine, 281–286
spirochete
Lyme disease, 166–167
neurosyphilis, 165
streptococcal, 156
subdural, 174
urinary tract, 1303–1304
vascular graft, 1450
viral, 167–172
acute disseminated encephalomyelitis (ADEM), 170–171
AIDS and, 181
Creutzfeldt-Jakob disease, 171–172
cytomegalovirus, 168, 170*f*
encephalitis, 171
herpes simplex, 169–170
of lungs, 1230*f*
progressive multifocal leukoencephalopathy (PML), 171
respiratory, 1232*f*
sarcoidosis, 174
subacute sclerosing panencephalitis, 171
varicella zoster, 170
Infectious esophagitis, 807–808, 807*f*
Inferior mesenteric artery (IMA), mesenteric angiography and, 710–711
Inferior pulmonary ligament, 347, 347*f*
Inferior vena cava (IVC), 713–714
filters, 715–716, 717*f*
Infiltrative cardiomyopathies, 661–662, 662*f*
Inflammation
positron emission tomography and, 1515
scintigraphic diagnosis of, 1440
of spine, 278–281
multiple sclerosis and, 278–281
Inflammatory bowel disease, 1450
Inflammatory polyps, in sinus, 243
Influenza, 467
Inguinal hernia, 1288*f*
Inhalational disease, 497
Injection leakage, 1518
In-phase images (IP), 13
Insufficiency fracture, 1124
Insulinomas, 1463
Interlobar fissures, 342–343
of lungs, 340
Internal carotid artery (ICA), ischemic stroke and, 96–97, 98*f*
International Electrotechnical Commission (IEC) phantom, 1354
Interstitial disease, 373
Interstitial lung disease, 1441–1442
high resolution computed tomography and, 481*f*
Interstitial nephritis, 1442, 1443*f*
Interstitial opacity, 374*f*
linear patterns of, 375
Interstitial patterns, lungs and, 1229–1234, 1233*f*
Interstitial pulmonary edema, 419*f*
Interstitium, pulmonary, 350, 350*f*
Intestinal duplication cyst, 1261*f*
Intestinal ischemia, 842, 843*f*
Intra-axial tumors, 124, 124*f*
Intracerebral hematoma, 64, 66*f*
Intracranial lipomas, 153–154, 154*f*
Intracranial mycobacterial infections, 183
Intradecidual sign, 977, 977*f*
Intraductal papillary mucinous tumor (IPMT), 789–790, 790*f*
Intradural masses, 295–297

Intralobular lines, in lung disease, 482
Intraluminal diverticula, 829, 829*f*
Intramedullary lipomas, in spine, 309–311
Intramedullary masses, 291–295
Intramural hematoma, 683
Intraperitoneal abscess, US of, 927–928, 928*f*
Intraperitoneal bladder rupture, 904–905, 904*f*
Intraperitoneal fluid, US of, 927, 928*f*
Intraperitoneal tumor, US of, 928–929, 929*f*
Intrathecal lipoma, 314*f*
Intrathecal (drop) metastases, 297, 299*f*, 300*f*
Intrathoracic stomach, 1279*f*
Intrauterine growth retardation (IUGR), 984–985, 985*t*
Intraventricular hemorrhage, 61, 65*f*
Intraventricular tumors, 143–145, 143*t*, 144*f*, 145*f*, 145*t*
Intrinsic flood, 1351, 1352*f*
Intussusception, 1287, 1289*f*–1290*f*
  of small bowel, 744–745, 744*f*
Inversion recovery (IR), 13
Inverting papilloma, in sinus, 244–245
Iodinated contrast agents, 22–24
Iodine-123 thyroid scan, 1333*f*
Ionic contrast agents, 22, 273
Ionizing radiation, 1336
IP. *See* In-phase images
IPF. *See* Idiopathic pulmonary fibrosis
IPMT. *See* Intraductal papillary mucinous tumor
IR. *See* Inversion recovery
Ischemia, 69–70, 1478
Ischemic brain injury, neonatal, 1015–1018, 1015*f*, 1016*f*, 1017*f*, 1017*t*
Ischemic heart disease
  coronary artery disease, 629–633, 630*f*, 631*f*, 631*t*, 632*f*, 633*f*
  infarct imaging of, 634–636, 634*f*, 635*f*
  MR, 652–660, 653*f*, 655*f*, 657*f*, 658*f*, 659*f*, 660*f*, 664*f*
  myocardial infarction, 633–634, 634*f*
Ischemic stroke
  anterior (carotid) circulation, 96–97, 98*f*–99*f*, 99–100, 100*f*, 101*f*, 102*f*, 102*t*
  contrast in, 93–94, 94*f*, 95*f*
  etiology of, 86–87, 87*t*
  hemorrhagic transformation in, 92–93, 92*f*
  imaging changes in, 87, 88*f*, 89*f*, 90–91, 90*f*, 91*f*
  pattern recognition in, 94, 94*t*, 96, 96*f*
  posterior (vertebrobasilar) circulation, 100–101, 103–105, 103*f*, 104*f*, 105*f*
  small-vessel, 105–106, 107*f*, 108*f*, 109*f*
  venous infarction, 106–108, 110*f*, 111*f*
  watershed (border zone) infarction, 105, 106*f*, 107*f*
Ischium, avulsion off, 1125*f*
Islet cell tumor, 1464*f*
Isotopes, for imaging, 1458
IUGR. *See* Intrauterine growth retardation
IV pyelography (IVP), 872–873, 874*f*
IVC. *See* Inferior vena cava
IVP. *See* IV pyelography

J

Jaszczak phantom, 1354
Jefferson fracture, 1105*f*, 1107
Jejunal atresia, 1285, 1286*f*
Joint(s). *See also* Degenerative joint disease; Sacroiliac joint
  acromioclavicular, 1205
    degenerative joint disease and, 1133
    osteophytes and, 1209*f*
  arthritis and, with sacroiliac joint disease, 1139*f*
  atlantoaxial, rotary fixation of, 1106*f*, 1107
  Charcot, 1146, 1146*f*
  knee, 1151*f*
  Lisfranc Charcot, 1147*f*
  osteoarthritis and, 1126*f*, 1134*f*
  prosthetic replacements for, 1359
  pseudo-Charcot, 1144, 1147
  psoriasis and, 1140*f*
  temporomandibular, 1133
  trauma in, 1170
Joint effusions, 1150–1152
Joint space narrowing, 1132
JRA. *See* Juvenile rheumatoid arthritis
Jugular chain adenopathy, 257*f*
Junction lines, 351*f*, 352*f*
Juvenile nasopharyngeal angiofibromas, in sinus, 245
Juvenile rheumatoid arthritis (JRA), 1147–1148, 1147*f*
  muscular dystrophy and, 1148*f*

K

Kaposi sarcoma (KS), 458–459, 458*f*, 476
  AIDS and, 754
Kartagener syndrome, 616, 616*f*
Kawasaki disease, 1316
Kayser-Fleischer ring, 212
Kearns-Sayre syndrome, 211*f*
Kerley lines, 375, 418, 456, 482
  pulmonary edema and, 417
Kidney(s). *See also* Renal abnormalities
  anatomy of, 874–875
  chemical shift artifact in, 16*f*
  imaging methods for, 872–873, 874*f*
  Infections of, 1438
  large, 1312
    causes of, 1313*t*
  medullary sponge, 882, 882*f*
  neonatal, 1303*f*
  stones, 947, 947*f*
  transplant of, 1432
  tuberculosis of, 900–901
  US of, 945–953, 946*f*, 947*f*, 948*t*, 949*f*, 950*f*, 951*f*, 952*f*
Kienböck malacia, 1117*f*, 1154*f*, 1155, 1155*f*
  trauma and, 1117
Kinetic curves, of breast MR, 592, 593f
Klebsiella, 286, 463
Knee(s)
  bony abnormalities in, 1202–1203
  chondrocalcinosis in, 1142*f*
  degenerative joint disease and, 1137*f*
  magnetic resonance imaging of, 1192
    techniques for, 1192
Knee joint effusion, 1151*f*
Köhler disease, 1154*f*, 1155
Korsakoff syndrome, 198–199
Krypton-81m, 1372
  ventilation scanning, 1373
KS. *See* Kaposi sarcoma
Kulchitsky cells, 393, 441, 454
Kümmel disease, 1111, 1111*f*
Kyphoscoliosis, 296, 406

L

Labrum, 1210, 1210*f*
Lacrimal gland, 264
Lactobezoar, 1282
Lacunes
  internal capsule, 105, 108*f*
  ischemic disease and, 105, 107*f*
  perivascular spaces v., 106, 108*f*
LAD. *See* Left anterior descending artery
LAM. *See* Lymphangioleiomyomatosis
Laminar blood flow, 1022–1023, 1022*f*, 1023*f*
Laminated calcification, 435
Laminectomy, 282*f*
Langerhans cell histiocytosis (LCH), 484, 504–505, 505*f*, 506*f*, 1233
Large cell carcinoma, 442, 442*f*
Large kidneys, 1312
  causes of, 1312*t*

Laryngeal carcinoma, 453
Laryngoceles, 267, 269*f*
Lateral collateral ligament (LCL), 1199
  schematic of, 1220*f*, 1221*f*
  torn, 1201*f*
Lateral disk, 327*f*
Lateral projection, 604
Lateral radiography, of chest, 354–355
Lateral recess stenosis, 326
Lateral thoracic meningoceles, 405
LC. *See* Lymphangitic carcinomatosis
LCH. *See* Langerhans cell histiocytosis
LCL. *See* Lateral collateral ligament
LCX. *See* Left circumflex artery
Le Fort fractures, 81–82, 82*f*
Leaky lung syndrome, 1248*f*
Left anterior descending artery (LAD), 1387, 1391*f*
Left atrium, 605, 608*f*
Left circumflex artery (LCX), 1387
Left lower lobe (LLL), atelectasis, 373
Left middle lobe (LML), 372*f*
Left subphrenic space, 733–734
Left upper lobe (LUL), 344*f*
  atelectasis, 368, 369*f*
  of lung, 342
Left ventricle, 605–606, 607*f*, 608*f*
Left ventricular ejection fraction (LVEF), 1388
Left ventricular end-diastolic volume (LVEDV), 1396
Left-to-right intracardiac shunts, 1400–1402, 1401*f*
Leg(s), 1127
Legg-Perthes disease, 1155
Legionella pneumophilia, 463, 464*f*
LEGP. *See* Low energy general-purpose
LEHR. *See* Low energy high resolution
Leigh disease, 199, 203, 206*f*, 211*f*
Leiomyomas, 397, 438–439, 955–956, 956*f*
  uterine, 916, 916*f*
Leiomyosarcoma, 438–439
Leptomeningeal cyst, 70
Leptomeningeal metastases, 297
Leptomeningeal spread, 135
Lesion(s). *See also* Congenital lesions; Thymomas
  adrenal, 869–872, 869*f*, 870*f*, 871*f*, 872*f*, 873*f*
  bone, 1082–1084, 1082*t*, 1083*t*, 1084*t*, 1089*f*, 1090–1091, 1090*f*, 1097*f*, 1098, 1183
  cephaloceles, 228
  chest wall, 540*t*
  of chest wall, 388
  cold, 1467
  congenital, 225–228, 265–270
  cystic, of posterior fossa, 232
  don't touch, 1168
  endobronchial, 1238
  epididymal, 969, 970*f*
  esophageal, 404
  extramedullary, 273
  extrapleural, 386
  Ghon, 466, 1253
  of globe, 265
  holoprosencephaly, 225
  hot, 1467
  hypoattenuating, 770–771, 770*f*
  of lacrimal gland, 265
  of mucosal space, 249
  multiple sclerosis and, 186*f*, 278
  neurogenic, 402
  nonneoplastic, 235*f*, 236*f*
  obviously benign, 1179–1181
  occult breast, 596–597, 598*f*
  osteochondral, of talus, 1218*f*
  pleural, 386
  posttraumatic, 1168
  pulmonary lucency and, 377*f*
  sclerotic, 1084–1085, 1084*f*
  solitary pulmonary nodule and, 438
  of spine, 273
    in children, 289
    diagnosis of, 276*t*
  spleen, 793–794, 793*f*, 794–796, 794*f*, 794*t*, 795*f*, 796*f*
  vascular, 262–263, 402
  of white matter, 190–191
Lesser omentum, 734
Lesser sac, 734, 735*f*
Leukemia, 301, 398, 457–458
  thymus gland and, 1252
Leukocoria, 265
Leukomalacia, 217
  periventricular, 1017–1018, 1017*f*
Leukoplakia, 896
Levocardia, 1272
Levodopa (DOPA), 210*f*
Leydig cell tumor, 1312
Lhermitte-Duclos disease, 140–141
Ligament(s), 1197, 1199*f*
  anterior cruciate, 1193, 1196, 1197*f*, 1198*f*
  anterior talofibular, 1221*f*
  collateral, 1198–1201
  cruciate, 1196–1198
  of foot and ankle, 1222–1224
  lateral collateral, 1199, 1201*f*, 1220*f*, 1221*f*
  medial collateral, 1198–1199, 1200*f*
  meniscofemoral, 1197
  pericardiophrenic, 347, 347*f*
  posterior cruciate, 1196, 1198*f*
  pulmonary and pericardiophrenic, 347, 347*f*
  spring, 1217*f*
  transverse, 1196, 1197*f*
Ligament of Humphry, 1197, 1199*f*
Ligament of Wrisberg, 1197, 1199*f*
Ligamentum flavum hypertrophy, 326
Lightning, spine and, 281
Linearity, 1352
LIP. *See* Lymphocytic interstitial pneumonitis
Lip, cleft, 994–995, 996*f*
Lipoid pneumonia, 439
Lipomas, 439
  of cerebellar vermis, 228*f*
  of corpus callosum, 227–228, 228*f*
Liposarcoma, 750, 750*f*
Lisfranc Charcot joint, 1147*f*
Lisfranc fracture, 1129, 1131*f*
Lissencephaly, 229, 229*f*
Listeria monocytogenes, 159, 172
Listerial rhombencephalitis, 159
Literial infections, 156
Liver. *See also* Hepatic
  abscess of, 1319*f*
  acoustic enhancement in, 21*f*
  anatomy of, 756–758, 757*f*, 757*t*, 758*f*
  disease of, 758–764
  fat-suppression technique in, 14*f*
  gadolinium chelates in, 14–15, 14*f*
  granulomas, 739
  hemorrhage laceration of, 708*f*
  imaging methods for, 756
  masses, 764–771, 764*t*
  motion artifact in, 16*f*
  perfusion abnormalities of, 758, 758*f*
  US of, 930–934, 930*f*, 931*f*, 932*f*, 933*f*, 934*f*
  vascular neoplasm of, 1320*f*
Liver scintigraphy, 1416
Liver transplantation
  hepatic angiography and, 710, 710*f*
  US of, 934
Liver/spleen scan, 1420–1422, 1423*f*
Lobar atelectasis, 367, 367*f*, 367*t*, 369*f*

Lobar holoprosencephalysis, 226
Lobar hyperinflation, 553, 554*f*
Lobar nephronia, 883
Localized pleural thickening, 386
Locked facets, 1108*f*
Low energy general-purpose (LEGP), 1347
Low energy high resolution (LEHR), 1347
LSO. *See* Lutetium oxy-ortho-silicate
L-transportation, 1263
Ludwig angina, 412
Lumbar spine
 desiccated disks in, 322*f*
 disease of, 322
 disk diseases of, 324
 disk protrusions in, 323*f*
 spondylolisthesis and, 1109*f*
 spondylolysis and, 1109*f*
Lunate dislocation, 1113–1114, 1114*f*, 1115*f*
Lung(s). *See also* Pulmonary agenesis; Ventilation/perfusion (V/Q) lung scanning
 abnormal, capacity, 1227–1234
 abnormal volumes of, 1234–1235
 abscesses of, 1239
 aeration abnormalities of, 1237–1239
 alveolar sacs and, 342
 anatomy of, 340, 1371–1372
 bilateral hyperlucent, 376
 bilateral lung hyperinflation, 1237*t*
 breast and radiography of, 354
 bullous disease of, 523–524, 523*f*, 524*t*
 cancer of, 1460*f*
  with airway involvement, 448
  with lymph node metastases, 449–451
  lymph nodes and, 1494
  with mediastinal invasion, 448
  with metastatic disease, 451
  with multiple tumor nodules in same lobe, 449
  with pleural effusion, 449
  positron emission tomography and, 1492–1494
  with primary tumor, 447–449
  radiologic staging of, 447, 447*f*
  recurrence of, 1494
  staging of, 1496*f*
  TNM classification of, 447
 carcinoma of, 302*f*, 1454*f*
 children and, 1227–1234
 collapse of, 373
 computed tomography of, 448*f*
 consolidation, 1004, 1005*f*
 cysts in, 477*f*
  congenital, 1239–1240
 direct invasion of, 455
 diseases, 479, 502–503
  architectural distortion, 486–487
  chronic interstitial, 487
  congenital, 552–556, 553*f*, 554*f*, 554*t*, 555*f*, 555*t*, 556*f*
  ground glass, 485
  high resolution computed tomography and, 479
  inflammatory/infectious, 1386
  interstitial, 480*t*, 487*t*
  intralobular lines and, 482
  micronodules and, 485
  in neonates, 1242–1246
  parenchymal bands and, 484
  radiation-induced, 560–562, 561*f*
  rheumatoid, 488*f*, 488*t*
  subpleural lines and, 483–484
  thickened fissures and, 482
  thin-walled cysts and, 484
  traction bronchiectasis, 486–487
  traumatic, 556–557, 557*f*
 fissures in, 345–347
  high resolution computed tomography of, 346
 hypoplastic, 554
 interfaces, radiographs of, 355
 interlobar fissures of, 340
 left upper lobe of, 342
 minor fissures in, 345
 opacity of, 354
 paraspinal interface and, 353
 physiology of, 1371–1372
 right middle lobe in, 345
 right upper lobe of, 340
 true unilateral hyperlucent, 376
Lung masses, 1249–1251
Lung neoplasm, 1383
Lung parenchyma, 1004–1005, 1005*f*, 1006*f*
"Lung windows," 11
Lung-mediastinal interfaces, 351, 352*t*
Lupus cerebritis, 190*f*
Lupus erythematosus, 279, 281*f*, 423
Lutetium oxy-ortho-silicate (LSO), 1347
LVEDV. *See* Left ventricular end-diastolic volume
LVEF. *See* Left ventricular ejection fraction
Lymph nodes, 259–261, 379. *See also* Hilar disease; Mediastinum
 calcified, 738
 enlargement of, 397, 502
 Hilar, enlargement of, 379*f*
 hyperplasia of, 400
 masses of, 397
 metastases of, 1411*f*
 stations of, 399*f*
Lymphadenopathy, 748–750, 749*f*, 749*t*
 angioimmunoblastic, 400
 of bladder, 903
 in sarcoidosis, 400*f*
 tuberculous, 400*f*
Lymphangiectasia, 842
Lymphangioleiomyomatosis (LAM), 484, 484*f*, 495, 496, 496*f*
Lymphangiomas, 257, 263, 265*f*, 266*f*, 269, 270, 390, 750
Lymphangitic carcinomatosis (LC), 445, 446*f*, 456, 483*f*
Lymphatics, pulmonary, 349
Lymphocele, in renal transplant, 1434*f*
Lymphocytes, in brain abscesses, 156
Lymphocytic interstitial pneumonitis (LIP), 457, 457*f*, 491, 1234, 1234*f*
Lymphoepithelial cysts, 259*f*
Lymphoid hyperplasia, 826
Lymphoma, 301, 304–305, 305*f*, 394, 456–457, 1466, 1494–1497, 1499*f*. *See also* Pseudolymphoma
 AIDS and, 183, 288
 AIDS-related, 754
 bone, 1096*f*, 1098
 burkitt, 836
 CNS, 133, 134*f*, 143
 computed tomography and, 395
 hodgkin, 749, 749*f*
 of the liver, 767–768, 769*f*, 950–951
 with mucosa, 250
 pseudotumors and, 263–264
 renal, 878–879, 878*f*
 in spinal canal, 306*f*
 staging of, 1497*f*
Lymphomatoid granulomatosis, 457
Lymphoscintigraphy, 1465–1467

M

MAA. *See* Macroaggregated albumin
Mach bands, 379
Macklin effect, 411
Macroaggregated albumin (MAA), 1372
Macrocystic serous cystadenoma, 789, 789*f*
Macrophages, brain abscesses and, 158
Maffucci Syndrome, 1069, 1069*f*
Magnetic resonance imaging (MR or MRI)
 advantages of, 14

Magnetic resonance imaging (MR or MRI) (*Contd.*)
AIDS and, 280
angiograms, 320
artifacts, 15–16, 15*f*, 16*f*
bone lesions and, 1089*f*, 1090–1091, 1090*f*
bone marrow and, 304*f*
bone scans and, 278
of brain, 32*f*–43*f*
of breast, 590–593, 593*f*, 594*f*
cardiac, 626–627, 626*f*, 627*f*
of cervical spine, 277
of chest wall lesions, 388
with CNS infection, 156
contrast administration, 14–15, 14*f*
in ischemic stroke, 93–94, 94*f*, 95*f*
diffusion-weighted, 48
disk disease and, 324
of esophagus, 404
of foot and ankle, 1214
functional, 48, 51
for head and neck, 241
with Hippel-Lindau syndrome, 240
intravascular contrast agents and, 24
of knees, 1192
lesions and, 157
Listeria monocytogenes and, 159
of lumbar spine, 322
of lymph nodes, 260, 398
mediastinal masses and, 390*t*
meningitis and, 286
of metastatic lymph nodes, 263*f*
myelograms, 320
opposed-phase, 13
of orbit, 261
of pediatric brain, 213
postoperative scars and, 329
principles of, 11–12, 16–18, 16*t*, 17*t*, 18*t*
proper technique in, 323*f*
prostate cancer and, 300
of shoulders, 1205
and soft tissue, 275–278
of spine, 272, 275–278, 297
spin-echo, 12–13
for thoracic disease, 335, 338–339, 339*t*
Magnetic resonance spectroscopy (MRS), 200
of hypoxic ischemic injury, 222*f*
proton, 200
Magnetic susceptibility, 15, 15*f*, 109
Magnetization transfer, magnetic resonance imaging and, 157
Magnetization-prepared RAGE (MPRAGE), 13
MAI. *See* Mycobacterium aviumintracellulare
Malacoplakia, 896
Male breast, mammogram of, 588–589, 590*f*, 591*f*
Malignant fibrous histiocytoma, 1095*f*, 1096
Malignant giant cell tumor, 1095
Malignant lesions, of mucosal space, 249
Mallet finger, 1112, 1113*f*
Mallory-Weiss tear, 814
Mammogram
analyzing of
architectural distortion, 584, 585*f*
of augmented breast, 586–588, 587*f*, 588*f*, 689*f*
axillary adenopathy, 585–586, 586*f*
breast tissue density and, 584–585, 586*f*
calcifications, 580–584, 581*f*, 582*f*, 583*f*, 584*f*, 585*f*
film comparisons, 589–590, 592*f*
of male breast, 588–589, 590*f*, 591*f*
masses, 572–580
patient evaluation in, 568
technical considerations in, 568–572, 570*f*, 571*f*, 572*t*
Mandibular fractures, 83–85, 83*f*, 84*f*
Marchiafava-Bignami disease, 198
Marfan syndrome, 680–681, 1253
Margins, in mammogram, 573–576, 574*f*, 575*f*, 576*f*, 577*f*, 578*f*
Marijuana, 411
Markers of metabolism, 1459–1460
Mass lesions, imaging strategies for, 52–54
Masses
cardiac, 645–648, 646*f*, 647*f*, 666–668, 667*f*
liver, 764–771, 764*t*
maldevelopmental, 151–155, 154*f*, 154*t*, 155*f*
mammogram and, 572–580
mediastinal, 1005, 1006*f*, 1251–1255
mediastinum, 377, 378*f*, 389, 393*t*
pelvicaliceal system, 893–896, 894*f*, 895*f*, 896*f*, 896*t*
pineal region, 146–147, 146*f*, 147*t*
renal, 876–879, 876*f*, 877*f*, 878*f*, 878*t*, 879–880, 879*f*, 880*f*
sellar, 147–149, 148*f*, 149*f*, 150*f*
small bowel, 834–839, 835*f*, 836*f*, 838*f*, 839*f*
US of, 933
Masticator space, 255–256
non-Hodgkin lymphoma, 248*f*
Mastocytosis, 1165, 1165*f*
Maxillary fractures, 77–78, 78*f*
Maximum intensity projection (MIP), 47–48
May-Thurner syndrome, 719, 721*f*
MCA. *See* Middle cerebral artery
McCune-Albright syndrome, 1066–1067
MCL. *See* Medial collateral ligament
MDCT. *See* Multidetector helical computed tomography; Multidetector-row computed tomography
MDP. *See* Methylene diphosphonate
Meckel diverticulum, 846, 1302, 1303*f*, 1421*f*
Meckel scan, 1420
Meconium aspiration, 1245, 1249*f*
Meconium ileus, 1286, 1287*f*
Meconium peritonitis, 1297, 1301*f*
Meconium plug syndrome, 1287, 1288*f*
Medial collateral ligament (MCL), 1198–1199
partial tear of, 1200*f*
torn, 1200*f*
Medial wall fractures, 78
Mediastinal contours, 611–612, 612*f*
Mediastinal hematoma, 410
Mediastinal hemorrhage, 408–410
Mediastinal lipomatosis, 410, 411*f*
Mediastinal masses, 1005, 1006*f*, 1251–1255
Mediastinal teratoma, 1258*f*
Mediastinitis
acute, 407
chronic sclerosing, 408, 409*f*
chronic sclerosing (fibrosing), 408, 409*f*
Mediastinum, 1005, 1006*f*
anatomy of, 355–359, 357*f*–358*f*, 359*f*
anterior, 356
compartments of, 356*f*
contents of, 356*t*
infection of, 407–408
malignancy in, 410
masses of, 377, 378*f*, 389
anterior, 393*t*
middle, 356–359
masses of, 397–402, 397*t*
nodes, 398*t*
posterior, 359
masses of, 402–407, 402*t*
widening of, 378, 407*t*
Medical events, 1344–1345
Mediolateral oblique view (MLO), of breast, 569–570, 570*f*
Mediterranean fever, 497
Medullary carcinoma, 1410
Medullary nephrocalcinosis, 885, 886*t*
Medullary sponge kidney, 882, 882*f*
Medulloblastoma, 136–137, 138*f*
Mega cisterna magna, 233
Megacystis, 1309

Megacystis-microcolon-hypoperistalsis (MMH) syndrome, 1310
Megaureter, 1307*f*
Melanoma, 1498–1499
  hilar and, 414*f*
  malignant, 1467*f*
MELAS. *See* Mitochondrial myelopathy, encephalopathy, lactic acidosis, and strokelike episodes
Melorheostosis, 1183–1184, 1186*f*
MEN. *See* Multiple endocrine neoplasia
Meningiomas, 141–142, 142*f*, 237, 295, 296*f*
Meningitis, 286
  bacterial, 176*f*
  carcinomatous, 300*f*
  coccidioidomycosis, 178*f*, 289, 290*f*, 400, 413
  fungal, 173, 178–181
  histoplasmosis and, 162
  Listeria monocytogenes and, 159
  magnetic resonance imaging and, 286
  neonatal, 1014–1015, 1015*f*
  tuberculous, 172–173, 177*f*, 292*f*
    in CNS, 160
Meningoceles, 228
Meningoencephalitis, Listeria monocytogenes and, 159
Meningovascular syphilis, 169*f*
Meniscal cysts, 1195–1196, 1197*f*
Meniscal degeneration, 1193, 1194*f*
Meniscal tear, 1193–1194, 1194*f*
Menisci, 1192–1196, 1193*f*
  grading scale of, 1194*t*
Meniscocapsular separation, 1200*f*
Meniscofemoral ligament, 1197
Menkes syndrome, 1309
MERRF. *See* Myoclonic epilepsy and ragged-red fibers
Mesenchymal hamartoma, 1318
Mesenchymal tumors, 397, 1255
Mesenteric adenitis, 1297, 1300*f*
Mesenteric angiography, 710–713, 712*f*, 713*f*
Mesenteric cysts, 1321
Mesenteric ischemia, 712–713, 713*f*
Mesoblastic nephroma, 1315
Mesothelial cysts, 400
Mesothelioma, 539, 540*f*, 1466
Metabolism, markers of, 1459–1460
Metachromatic leukodystrophy, 203
Metaiodobenzylguanidine (MIBG), 1331
Metastasis
  adrenal, 871, 872*f*
  aggressive, 1368*f*
  brain and, 1511, 1513*f*
  CNS, 135, 137*f*, 135136*f*
  dural, 143
  evaluation of, 301*f*
  in extradural masses, 297
  inversion recovery in, 301*f*
  of kidney, 879
  liver, 764–765, 764*f*, 765*t*
  peritoneal, 750, 750*f*
  US of, 932, 933*f*
Metastatic bone disease, 1366–1370
Metastatic carcinoma, 1164
Metastatic disease, 1075, 1075*f*, 1318
  bone lesions, 1097*f*, 1098
  lung cancer and, 451
  to thorax, 455–456
Metastatic lymph nodes, 257*f*
  magnetic resonance imaging of, 263*f*
Metformin, contrast agents and, 23
Methotrexate, for pulmonary disease, 560
Methylene diphosphonate (MDP), 1343
Methylprednisolone, contrast administration and, 24
MIBG. *See* Metaiodobenzylguanidine
Microcatheters, 672
Microcephaly, 169*f*
Microgastria, 1281
Midazolam, for vascular radiology, 673
Middle cerebral artery (MCA), ischemic stoke and, 97, 99–100, 102*f*
Middle lobe atelectasis, 373
Middle mediastinal masses, 1253–1255
Middle mediastinum, 356
Midesophageal diverticulum, 805, 806*f*
Midface fractures, 81–82, 82*f*
Midgut volvulus, 1283, 1284*f*, 1285*f*
Migration anomalies
  in brain, 228–233
  Chiari I malformations, 232
  Chiari II malformations, 231–232
  heterotopic gray matter, 230
  lissencephaly, 229
  pachygyria/agyria complex, 229–230
  schizencephaly, 230–231
Miliary nodules, 1234
  causes of, 1234*t*
Miliary tuberculosis, 466, 468*f*, 471*f*, 485, 1234, 1234*f*
Mineralizing microangiopathy, 202
Minor fissures, in lungs, 345
MIP. *See* Maximum intensity projection
Mirror-image artifacts, 21, 21*f*
Mirror-image dextrocardia, 1273
Mismatched defect, 1379
Mitochondrial myelopathy, encephalopathy, lactic acidosis, and strokelike episodes (MELAS), 203
Mitral regurgitation, 641–642, 641*t*, 642*f*, 1399*f*
Mitral stenosis, 640–641
Mitral valve prolapse, 642
Mixed tissue disease, 491
MLO. *See* Mediolateral oblique view
MMH. *See* Megacystis-microcolon-hypoperistalsis syndrome
"Moguls of the heart," 610, 610*f*
Molecular imaging, 1456
Moly generator, 1342
Molybdenum-99/technetium-99m decay scheme, 1344*f*
Molybdenum-99/technetium-99m generator elution curves, 1345*f*
Monoclonal antibodies, 1461
  structure of, 1461*f*
Monoclonal antibody imaging agents, 1457*t*
Monteggia fracture, 1118–1119, 1119*f*
Morgagni hernia, 550, 551*f*
Morquio syndrome, 1184–1185, 1186*f*
Motility, 800–801
  disorders, 801–805, 801*f*, 802*f*, 802*t*, 803*f*, 804*f*, 805*f*
Motion artifacts, 15, 16*f*
  in CT, 10, 11*f*
Moyamoya disease, 191*f*, 200
MPRAGE. *See* Magnetization-prepared RAGE
MR. *See* Magnetic resonance imaging
MR cholangiopancreatography (MRCP), 771, 771*f*
MRCP. *See* MR cholangiopancreatography
MRI. *See* Magnetic resonance imaging
MRS. *See* Magnetic resonance spectroscopy
MS. *See* Multiple sclerosis
Mucinous cystic neoplasm, 789, 790*f*
Mucocele, in sinus, 243–244, 244*f*
Mucocutaneous lymph node syndrome, 1316
Mucoid impaction, 375
Mucopolysaccharidoses, 1184–1185
Mucormycosis, 260*f*, 476
Mucosal space, 248–250
Mucous retention cysts, in sinus, 243
Müllerian structures, 1310
Multicystic dysplastic kidney, 882
Multidetector helical computed tomography (MDCT)
  of liver, 756
  principles of, 9
Multidetector-row computed tomography (MDCT), 389, 426
  mediastinal masses and, 390*t*

Multidetector-row computed tomography (MDCT) (*Contd.*)
mediastinitis and, 407
of pulmonary emboli, 1374*f*
for pulmonary embolism, 428*f*
of solitary pulmonary nodule, 434
Multi-infarct dementia, 1512
Multilocular cystic nephroma, 880
Multiloculation, in late capsule stage, in brain abscesses, 158
Multiple endocrine neoplasia (MEN), 1410
Multiple gland disease, 1414
Multiple hereditary exostosis, 1186–1187, 1187*f*
Multiple myeloma, 302*f*, 303
osteoporosis and, 1157
Multiple patchy lung opacities, 1228–1229
sources of, 1229*f*
Multiple pulmonary nodules, 1496*f*
Multiple sclerosis (MS), 184–189, 185*f*, 278, 279*f*, 280*f*
with brainstem involvement, 187*f*
with callosal-septal involvement, 187*f*
with lesion enhancement, 186*f*
signs of, 262
tumefactive, 188*f*
Muscle(s)
anomalous, 1220*f*
cardiac, 1489
skeletal, 1489
Muscular dystrophy, juvenile rheumatoid arthritis and, 1148*f*
Myasthenia gravis, 391, 392
Mycobacterial infection, 464–466
in CNS, 160–162
Mycobacterium aviumintracellulare (MAI), 466, 468*f*, 501
AIDS and, 474
Mycobacterium tuberculosis, 464–466
Mycoplasma, 464, 465*f*, 1227
Mycotic aneurysm, septic embolus and, 159
Mycotic aneurysms, 701
Mycotic aortitis, 680
Myelination. *See also* Demyelination; Dysmyelination
delayed, 215
at eighteen months, 216*f*
at eleven months, 215*f*
landmarks in, 214*t*
in newborn, 214*f*
normal patterns of, 213–216
at six months, 215*f*
at three months, 215*f*
Myelitis, 278, 282*f*
Myelofibrosis, 303, 1163, 1164*f*
Myelography, 272–273
with computed tomography, 272
ionic contrast agents and, 273
lumbar puncture and, 273
Myeloma, 301, 1075, 1076*f*, 1097*f*, 1098
multiple, 302*f*, 303
with permeative process, 1158*f*
Myelomeningocele, 232*f*
Myelopathy, 271
AIDS and, 280
vs. radiculopathy, 272*t*
Myocardial infarction, 1392
Myocardial ischemia, 1390
Myocardial metabolism PET imaging, 1514
Myocardial perfusion scans, 1387–1389, 1388*f*, 1460*f*, 1513
Myocardial viability, 656–658, 658*f*
Myocarditis, 660, 660*f*
Myoclonic epilepsy and ragged-red fibers (MERRF), 203
Myometrium, 910, 910*f*
Myositis ossificans, 1168, 1169*f*, 1171*f*
Myoview, 1390
Myxopapillary ependymoma, 294*f*

N

NAA. *See* N-acetyl aspartate
Nabothian cysts, 917, 957
N-acetyl aspartate (NAA), 177, 200, 207*f*
Nasal cavity, 242–245
Nasal fractures, 77
NASH. *See* Nonalcoholic steatohepatitis
Nasoethmoidal fracture, 82–83, 83*f*
Nasopharyngeal carcinoma, 250, 252*f*
Nasopharynx, 247
squamous cell carcinoma of, 1508*f*
National Equipment Manufacturer's Association (NEMA), 1354
National Institute of Standards and Technology, 1355
Navicular, 1115, 1116*f*
Navicular fracture, 1117
NEC. *See* Necrotizing enterocolitis
Neck. *See* Head and neck
Necrosis. *See also* Avascular necrosis; Radiation necrosis
in brain abscesses, 156
late cerebritis and, 158
Necrotic hepatic metastasis, 1503*f*
Necrotic tumors, brain abscesses and, 158
Necrotizing enterocolitis (NEC), 1294–1295, 1298*f*, 1301, 1302*f*
Necrotizing leukoencephalopathy, 202
Negative bone/gallium-67 study, 1445*f*
Negative ulnar variance, 1117
Neisseria meningitidis, 172
NEMA. *See* National Equipment Manufacturer's Association
Neonatal brain
congenital abnormalities of, 1012, 1014
infection of, 1014–1015, 1015*f*
ischemic injury to, 1015–1018, 1015*f*, 1016*f*, 1017*f*, 1017*t*
US anatomy of, 1012, 1013*f*, 1014*f*
Neonatal hepatitis, 1298–1301
Neonatal herpes, 171*f*
Neonates, lung disease in, 1242–1246
Neoplasms
of central bronchi, 454
classification of, 122, 123*t*
fibrotic, 919
hemorrhagic, 119, 120*f*, 120*t*, 126
hyperdense, 126
mucinous cystic, 789, 790*f*
of nervous system. *See* Central nervous system
pulmonary, 440*t*
retroperitoneal, 750, 750*f*
of spine, 289–291
tracheal, 451–455
Nephroblastomatosis, 1312–1313, 1314*f*
Nephrocalcinosis, 1309*f*
renal, 885, 886*t*
US of, 947, 948*f*
Nephrolithiasis, 889
Nephropathy, contrast-induced, 23
Nephrostomy, for ureteral obstruction, 725, 726*f*, 727*f*
Nerve root avulsion, 317–320, 318*f*, 320*f*
Nerve sheath tumors, 149–151, 151*f*, 152*f*, 153*f*, 296
Neurenteric cysts, 405
Neurenteric fistula, 1263*f*
Neuritic plaques, 209
Neuroblastoma, 303*f*, 1315–1316, 1317*f*, 1326
Neurodegenerative diseases, 184
Neurodegenerative disorders, 208–212
Alzheimer disease, 209–210
Huntington disease, 211
Parkinson disease, 210–211
Wilson disease, 211–212, 1141
Neuroenteric cysts, 1327
Neurofibrillary tangles, 209
Neurofibromas, 150–151, 252, 257, 403*f*, 438–439
Neurofibromatosis, 702
renal angiography and, 705

Neurofibromatosis (NF), 233, 233*t*, 295, 296, 298*f*, 299*f*, 494–496
glioma and, 235*f*
nonneoplastic lesions and, 235*f*, 236*f*
optic glioma and, 235*f*
type 1, 234–236
type 2, 236–237, 236*f*
Neuroforaminal stenosis, 326
Neurogenic bladder, 899
Neurogenic lesions, 402
Neurogenic pulmonary edema, 422
Neurogenic tumors, 402
Neuropathic joint. *See* Charcot joint
Neuroradiology, current options for, 44, 47–48, 51
Neurosarcoidosis, 280, 283*f*
Neutropenic colitis, 1295
Neutrophils, brain abscesses and, 158
NF. *See* Neurofibromatosis
NHL. *See* Non-Hodgkin lymphoma
Nidus, osteoid osteoma and, 1188
Nitrofurantoin, 559–560
Nitroglycerin, for vascular radiology, 673
Nitrous oxide, 411
Nocardial infections, 156, 473, 474*f*, 499, 508
Nodular lymphoid hyperplasia, 457, 836, 837*f*
Nodular opacities, 374
Nodular pulmonary matastases, 456
Nodules, thyroid, 1007–1009, 1007*t*, 1008*f*, 1008*t*, 1009*f*
NOF. *See* Nonossifying fibroma
Nonalcoholic steatohepatitis (NASH), 760
Noncommunicating hydrocephalus, 205
Nonepithelial parenchymal malignancies, 456–459
Nonhelical computed tomography, principles of, 9
Non-Hodgkin lymphoma (NHL), 394, 395*f*, 398, 407, 413, 438, 749, 1494
of masticator space, 248*f*
solitary pulmonary nodule and, 439*f*
Nonhypoxic ischemic encephalopathy, 224*f*
Nonimaging detector systems, 1355–1356
Nonionic contrast agents, 22–23
Nonionizing radiation, 1336
Nonneoplastic intratracheal masses, 454
Nonneoplastic lesions, neurofibromatosis and, 235*f*, 236*f*
Nonossifying fibroma (NOF), 1072*f*, 1073, 1073*f*, 1074*f*, 1075, 1178*f*, 1179–1180, 1179*f*
Nonpyogenic infections, 288
Nonspecific interstitial pneumonia (NSIP), 491, 494, 495*f*
Nonspecific punctuate white matter lesions, 190–191
Nonthromboembolic pulmonary disease, 1383–1386
Nonthrombotic pulmonary embolism, 429
Nontumoral hemorrhage, 126
Nonvascular intervention, 725–728
Noonan syndrome, 270
Normal pressure hydrocephalus (NPH), 207–208, 1512
NPH. *See* Normal pressure hydrocephalus
NRC. *See* Nuclear Regulatory Commission
NSIP. *See* Nonspecific interstitial pneumonia
Nuchal rigidity, pyogenic abscesses and, 156
Nuclear cardiology, 617
Nuclear medicine
bone scans with, 278
essential science of, 1336
Nuclear radiology, 1331
imaging principles of, 1331
Nuclear Regulatory Commission (NRC), 1339, 1412

O

Obstructive arterial disease, 689
Obstructive atelectasis, 366
Obtundation, pyogenic abscesses and, 156
Occlusion
carotid US, 1032–1033, 1035*f*, 1036*f*, 1037*f*
of peripheral arteries, 1047–1048
Occlusive carotid disease, 1482*f*
Occult cerebrovascular malformations, 118–119, 119*f*
Occult vascular malformation, 308*f*
Ochronosis, 1141
OCL. *See* Osteochondral lesion
Oligodendroglioma, 122–123, 132–133, 133*f*, 133*t*
Ollier disease, 1067, 1068*f*, 1069
Omental cysts, 1321
Omental infarction, 1296, 1300*f*
OMU. *See* Ostiomeatal unit
Oncocytoma, 878
OP. *See* Opposed-phase images
Opacity(ies)
airspace, 366*t*
hazy, reticular, or reticulonodular opacities, 1231–1234, 1232*f*, 1249*f*
interstitial, 374*f*
linear patterns of, 375
of lungs, 354
multiple patchy lung, 1228–1234
sources of, 1229*f*
multiple patchy lung opacities, 1228–1229, 1229*f*
nodular, 374
parahilar peribronchial opacities, 1230*f*
parenchymal, 365*t*, 366
pulmonary, 374*t*–375*t*
Opportunistic infections, 1440–1441
Opposed-phase images (OP), 13
Opposed-phase MR, 13
Optic glioma, neurofibromatosis and, 235*f*
Optic nerve glioma, 261, 264*f*
Optic neuritis, 265*f*
Optic neuropathy, head trauma and, 80
Optic sheath meningiomas, 261, 264*f*
Oral cavity, 247
Orbit, 261–265
Orbital trauma, 78–80, 79*f*, 80*f*
Orchitis, 967
Ordered subsets-expectation-maximization (OSEM), 1350
Oriental cholangiohepatitis, 936
Oropharynx, 247
Orthopedic hardware, infection and, 1451*f*
Os odontoideum, 1173–1179, 1178*f*
OSEM. *See* Ordered subsets-expectation-maximization
Osgood-Schlatter disease, 1155
Osseous malignancies, 1507, 1510*f*
Osteoarthritis, 1132–1134, 1133*f*
erosive, 1133
primary, 1133–1134, 1134*f*
of sacroiliac joint, 1126*f*, 1134*f*
of symphysis pubis, 1126*f*
Osteoblastoma, 1074*f*, 1075
Osteochondral lesion (OCL), 1218, 1218*f*
Osteochondritis dissecans, 1153*f*
of elbow, 1153*f*
of talus, 1153*f*
Osteochondromas, 1254
Osteogenic metastases, 1367*f*
Osteogenic sarcoma, 246, 1170*f*, 1367*f*
Osteoid osteoma, 1187–1188, 1188*f*, 1189*f*
Osteomalacia, 1159
looser fractures in, 1160*f*
Osteomyelitis, 282–284, 285*f*, 1080, 1080*f*, 1081*f*, 1361, 1362*f*, 1449–1450
acute, 1451
with discitis, 286*f*
with discitis and epidural abscess, 287*f*
of second toe, 1361*f*
spinal, 1452*f*, 1454*f*
Osteonecrosis. *See* Avascular necrosis
Osteopathia striata, 1188, 1190*f*
Osteopenia, 1370

Osteopetrosis, 1163–1164, 1164*f*
Osteophytes, 1518
  acromioclavicular joint and, 1209*f*
  of sacroiliac, 1126*f*
Osteophytosis, 1132
Osteopoikilosis, 1190, 1190*f*
Osteoporosis, 1112, 1156–1159, 1370
  aggressive, 1158*f*
  disuse, 1156, 1157*f*
  Ewing sarcoma and, 1157
  of hip, 1191, 1191*f*
  multiple myeloma and, 1157
Osteosarcoma, 1091*f*, 1092–1093, 1092*f*, 1093*f*, 1175*f*
Osteosclerosis, 1163–1167
Ostiomeatal unit (OMU), 242, 244*f*
Otomastoiditis, pyogenic abscesses and, 156
Outpouchings, 805–806, 805*f*, 806*f*, 807*f*
  of bladder, 903–904, 904*f*
Ovarian cancer, 911–913, 912*t*, 913*f*, 1504–1505, 1505*f*
Ovarian cysts, 917, 958–959, 959*f*, 1323, 1324*f*
Ovarian teratoma, 1324*f*
Ovaries
  anatomy of, 910
  cysts in, 917, 958–959, 959*f*
  US of, 958–963, 958*f*, 959*f*, 960*f*, 961*f*, 962*f*, 963*f*
Overlap syndromes, 491

P

P glycoprotein (P-gp), 1460
PA. *See* Posteroanterior radiographs
Pachydermoperiostosis, 1190
Pachygyria, 230*f*
Pachygyria/agyria complex, 229–230
PACS. *See* Picture Archiving and Communication System
Paget disease, 246, 1165–1167, 1166*f*
  of bone, 1365*f*
Paget-von Schrötter syndrome, 719
PAN. *See* Polyarteritis nodosa
Pancoast (superior sulcus) tumors, 444, 445*f*
Pancreas
  anatomy of, 782, 784
  annular, 829–830, 829*f*, 1283
  calcified, 739–740, 740*f*
  cystic lesions of, 788–790, 789*f*, 790*f*
  imaging techniques of, 782, 783*f*
  MR sequences of, 12*f*
  solid lesions of, 786–788, 786*f*, 787*f*
  US of, 941–944, 941*f*, 942*f*, 943*f*, 944*f*
Pancreatic cancer, 1500
Pancreatic masses, 1321–1323
Pancreatic neoplasm, 1322
Pancreatic pseudocyst, 406*f*
Pancreatitis, 1301, 1302*f*
  acute, 784, 784*t*, 785*f*
  chronic, 785–786, 785*f*, 786*f*
Panencephalitis, sclerosing, subacute, 171, 195, 280
Pannus, 279
Pantopaque, 280
PAP. *See* Pulmonary alveolar proteinosis
Papaverine, for vascular radiology, 673
Papillary carcinoma, 1410
Papillary cavities, 897–898, 897*f*, 898*f*
Papillary necrosis, 898, 898*f*
  in pelvicaliceal system, 894–895
Papillary thyroid carcinoma, 1009, 1009*f*
Papilledema
  pyogenic abscesses and, 156
  tuberculomas and, 161
Paragangliomas, 252
Paragonimiasis, 472
Paragonimus Westermani, 472
Parahilar peribronchial opacities, 1230, 1230*f*
  causes of, 1230*t*
Parainfluenza virus, 467, 469*f*
Parallel-hole collimation, 1347, 1347*f*
Paralysis, 1147–1148
  radiation myelitis and, 280
Paralysis agitans, 211
Paranasal sinus fractures, 77–78, 78*f*
Paranasal sinuses, 242–245
Parapharyngeal space, 250–252
Parasites, in duodenum, 827
Parasitic infections, 164–166
  of thorax, 471–472
Paraspinal interface, 353
Paraspinous tumor, 301, 304
Parathyroid, 1011, 1012*f*
Parathyroid glands, 1412
  adema of, 1413*f*, 1414
    Technetium-sestamibi scan of, 1414*f*
  adenoma, 392*f*
  anatomy of, 1414
  carcinomas of, 1414
  ectopic, 1414
  imaging methods for, 1412–1414
  masses of, 390
Parathyroid hormone (PTH), 1159, 1412
Paratracheal space, 357
Parenchymal bands, 484
Parenchymal hemorrhage, 116–119, 117*f*, 118*f*, 119*f*
Parenchymal interstitium, 479
Parenchymal lung disease, 431
Parenchymal opacity, 365*t*, 366
Parietal lobes, 156
  tuberculomas and, 161
Parkinson disease, 210–211, 1480, 1512–1513
Parosteal osteosarcoma, 1091*f*, 1092, 1093*f*
Parotid cysts, 255
Parotid space, 253–255
  metastatic lymph nodes and, 257*f*
Parotid tumors, 254
Parsonage-Turner syndrome, 1213, 1213*f*
Passive atelectasis, 366
Patella, 1201–1202
  chondral defect in, 1200*f*
  dorsal defect of, 1171, 1176*f*, 1177*f*
  fractures of, 1203
Patellar plica, 1201*f*, 1202
Patent ductus arteriosus, 1247*f*, 1262, 1269*f*
Patent urachus, 898
PAVMs. *See* Pulmonary arteriovenous malformations
PCA. *See* Posterior cerebral artery
PCH. *See* Pulmonary capillary hemangiomatosis
PCL. *See* Posterior cruciate ligament
PCP. *See* Pneumocystis jiroveci pneumonia
PCWP. *See* Pulmonary capillary wedge pressure
PDA. *See* Posterior descending artery
PDWI. *See* Proton density weighted imaging
PE. *See* Pulmonary embolism
Pear-shaped bladder, 903
Pediatric neuroimaging, 213
Pediatrics. *See* Children
Pelizaeus-Merzbacher disease, 215–216
Pelvic abscess, 1449*f*
Pelvic inflammatory disease, 918–919, 959, 960*f*
Pelvicaliceal system
  anatomy of, 887–888, 888*f*
  congenital anomalies of, 888–889, 888*f*, 890*f*
  filling defects/masses of, 893–896, 894*f*, 895*f*, 896*f*, 896*t*
  hydronephrosis, 891–893, 893*f*
  imaging methods for, 887
  papillary cavities of, 897–898, 897*f*, 898*f*
  renal stone disease, 889–891, 891*f*
  stricture of, 896–897, 897*f*
Pelvis. *See also* Hip(s); Sacrum
  bifid renal, 889

of children, 1277
compartmental anatomy of, 736, 736*f*
foreign bodies in, 751, 752*f*
fractures of, 1123
magnetic susceptibility artifact in, 16*f*
Penetrating aortic ulcer, 683
Penetrating injury, to head, 72–73, 74*f*
Peptic esophagitis, 1279
Peptic stricture, 1280*f*
Peptide receptor scintigraphy, 1462–1464
Percutaneous catheter drainage, 340
Perforated appendicitis, 1291*f*
Perfusion lung scan, 1373–1374
Peribronchial patterns, in lungs, 1229–1234
Pericardial cysts, 401, 401*f*
Pericardial disease, 648–650, 648*f*, 648*t*, 649*f*, 650*f*
MR, 662, 663*f*
Pericardial effusion, 1267*f*
Pericardial lymphangioma, 1259*f*
Pericardiophrenic ligament, 347, 347*f*
Pericardium, 615–616, 616*f*
Perihilar pulmonary edema, 418*f*
Peri-infarct ischemia, 1391
Perilunate dislocation, 1113–1114, 1114*f*, 1115*f*, 1117*f*
Perineum, 736, 737*f*
Perineural disease, 258
Periostitis, diagnosis of, 1185*f*
Peripheral arterial disease
aneurysms in, 695–696
atherosclerosis in, 689–690, 689*f*, 689*t*
cysts/tumors and, 694
embolisms and, 690, 691*f*
fibromuscular disease and, 693, 696*f*
obstructive, 689
thrombosis and, 690
trauma and, 691–693, 695*f*
uterine artery embolization and, 697, 697*f*, 698*f*, 699
vascular compression, 693–694, 696*f*
vasculitis in, 394*f*, 690–691, 693*f*
vasospasm and, 694–695
Peripheral arteries
anatomy, 1041–1042, 1044, 1045*f*
aneurysm, 1047
arterial puncture in, 1044–1047, 1046*f*, 1047*f*, 1048*f*
graft surveillance, 1048–1049, 1049*f*, 1050*f*, 1051*t*
stenosis and occlusion, 1047–1048
Peripheral interstitium, 479
Perirenal space, 735–736, 735*f*
Peritoneal cavity
abscess in, 751, 752*f*
anatomy of, 733–736, 734*f*, 735*f*, 736*f*
calcification in, 741
fluid in, 736–737, 737*f*
US anatomy of, 927
Peritoneal inclusion cysts, 963, 963*f*
Peritoneal mesothelioma, 750
Peritoneal metastases, 750, 750*f*
Periventricular leukomalacia (PVL), 217, 219*f*
Permeative process, in bones, 1157, 1158, 1158*f*
Peroneus brevis tendon, 1217*f*
Peroneus longus tendon, 1217*f*
Persistent truncus arteriosus, 1265, 1272*f*
Pes anserinus bursitis, 1202*f*
PET. *See* Positron emission tomography
Peutz-Jeghers syndrome, 853
P-gp. *See* P glycoprotein
Phagocytes, brain abscesses and, 158
Phakomatoses, 233–240
neurofibromatosis, 233–234
neurofibromatosis type 1, 234–236
neurofibromatosis type 2, 236–237
Sturge-Weber syndrome, 238
tuberous sclerosis, 237
Von Hippel-Lindau syndrome, 239–240
Phantoms, 1354
Pharynx
anatomy of, 798–800, 799*f*, 800*f*
imaging methods of, 798
Pheochromocytoma, 868–869, 868*f*, 944, 945*f*, 1468*f*
Phlegmasia cerulea dolens, 719
Photoelectric interactions, 1336
Photomultiplier gain adjustment, 1354
Photon interactions, 1336–1338, 1338*f*
Photopeak, 1349
Physiologic ovarian cysts, 917
Phytobezoar, 1282
Pica. *See* Posterior inferior cerebellar arteries
Pick disease, 1481, 1512
Picture Archiving and Communication System (PACS), 337
Pigmented villondular synovitis (PVNS), 1149, 1150*f*
Pilocytic astrocytoma, 131–132, 137–139, 138f
Pineal cysts, 147
Pineal region
of brain, 30*f*, 33*f*–35*f*, 44, 45*f*, 46*f*
masses, 146–147, 146*f*, 147*t*
Pineoblastoma, 147
Pineocytoma, 147
Pinhole collimation, 1347, 1347*f*
PIOPED. *See* Prospective Investigation of Pulmonary Embolism Diagnosis
Pitressin, for vascular radiology, 673
Pituitary adenomas, 147–148, 148*f*, 149*f*
Pituitary gland, hyperfunction of, 1162
Pixel size calibration, 1353
Placenta, 986–988, 987*f*, 988*f*, 989*f*
Plague, 415
Plain films, 75. *See* Plain radiographs
Plain radiographs, 272
Planar brain scans
interpretation of, 1472–1473
techniques for, 1472
Planar imaging, 1349–1350
Plaque evaluation, in vascular US, 1027–1030, 1029*f*, 1030*f*
Plasma cell granuloma, 439
Plasma cells, in brain abscesses, 156
Plasmacytomas, 1075
Plastic bowing, of forearm, 1118, 1118*f*
Pleomorphic adenoma, 253*f*, 258*f*
Pleura
anatomy of, 362, 362*f*
bronchopleural fistula, 531, 533*f*
diseases of, 535–539, 535*t*, 536*f*, 537*f*, 537*t*, 538*f*, 539*f*, 540*f*
high resolution computed tomography of, 362
pneumothorax, 532–535, 534*f*, 534*t*, 535*f*, 535*t*
postpneumonectomy space, 532
Pleural effusion, 382, 382*f*, 384*f*, 449, 450*f*, 527–531, 528i, 529*f*, 529*t*, 530*f*, 531*f*, 1246–1249
bilateral subpulmonic, 385*f*
causes of, 1249*t*
detection of, 337
with thoracic neoplasm, 1250*f*
Pleural lesions, 386
Pleural meniscus, 382
Pleural space, of chest, 1002, 1003*f*, 1004, 1004*f*
Pleural thickening, 1246–1249
diffuse, 386
localized, 386
Pleuropulmonary blastomas, 459
Plexogenic pulmonary arteriopathy, 431
Plica, 1201*f*, 1202
PMF. *See* Progressive massive fibrosis
PML. *See* Progressive multifocal leukoencephalopathy
Pneumatoceles, 376, 1239
postinflammatory, 1243*f*
Pneumatosis intestinalis, 746–747, 747*f*

Pneumococcal pneumonia, 461*f*
Pneumoconiosis, 497
  aluminum and, 500
  coal worker's, 499–500
  hard metal, 500
Pneumocystis jiroveci pneumonia (PCP), 476–477, 476*f*, 477*f*, 1441*f*
Pneumocystiscarinii, 340, 458
Pneumomediastinum, 378, 410–412, 411*t*, 412*f*
Pneumonia. *See also* Bronchopneumonia
  acute interstitial, 492
  AIDS and, 462
  aspiration, chronic, 497
  bacterial, 458, 461–463, 1228*f*
  chest radiography in, 6, 6*f*
  eosinophilic, chronic, 507
  focal organizing, 440
  fungal, 468
  HIV and, 466
  lipoid, 439
  mycoplasma, 465*f*
  neonatal, 1246*f*
  parainfluenza virus, 469*f*
  pneumococcal, 461*f*
  pneumocystis jiroveci, 476, 476*f*
  postprimary, 466, 467*f*
  pseudomonas aeruginosa, 462*f*
  round, 1252*f*
  staphylococcus aureus, 463*f*, 1229*f*, 1255*f*
  varicella, 469*f*
  viral, 466
    AIDS and, 474
Pneumonitis, 1497*f*
  hypersensitivity
    acute, 485*f*
    subacute, 484*f*
Pneumopericardium, 378, 616, 616*f*
Pneumoperitoneum, 737–738, 738*f*
Pneumothorax, 383, 385, 386*f*, 387*f*, 1004
Polio virus, 280
Polyarteritis nodosa (PAN), 423
  hepatic angiography and, 710
  renal angiography and, 705, 705*f*
Polyclonal antibodies, 1461
Polycystic kidney disease, 1308*f*
Polycystic ovary syndrome, 962
Polymicrogyria, 229, 230*f*
Polymorphononuclear leukocytes, in brain abscesses, 156
Polymyositis, 490, 491*f*
Polyps, 851–852, 852*f*
  antrochoanal, 243
  fibroepithelial, 895, 896*f*
  inflammatory, in sinus, 243
  US of, 937–938, 938*f*
Polysplenia syndrome, 1275
Pontomedullary separation, 72
Popcorn calcification, 435, 438
Popliteal entrapment, 693–694
Porcelain gallbladder, 939
Porencephaly, 230
Pores of Kore, 365, 460
Portal hypertension
  in liver, 762
  US of, 931, 931*f*
Positive bone/gallium-67 study, 1444*f*
Positron emission tomography (PET), 241, 242*f*, 395, 1350, 1393–1395, 1474–1475, 1487
  bone marrow and, 1490
  of brain, 1332*f*
  brain and, 1489
  brown fat and, 1492
  cardiac muscle and, 1489
  colon and, 1490, 1493*f*
  CT truncation artifacts and, 1518
  as dominant imaging modality, 1456
  with fluorodeoxyglucose, 339
  fractures and, 1515
  gallbladder and, 1490
  of head and neck, 260
  infection and inflammation and, 1515
  injection leakage and, 1518
  instrumentation for, 1487
  interpretation of, 1488–1492
  liver and, 1489
  lungs and, positron emission tomography and, 1492–1494
  mediastinal masses and, 390*t*
  neurologic, 1507
  osteophytes and, 1518
  ovaries and, 1492
  performance of, 1488
  pitfalls of, 1515–1518
  quality control in, 1353–1355
  salivary gland and, 1492
  skeletal muscle and, 1489
  of solitary pulmonary nodule, 436, 437*f*
  spleen and, 1490
  stomach and, 1490
  thyroid and, 1492
  tumors and, 1515
  urinary tract and, 1490, 1494*f*
  uterus and, 1492
Postablation imaging, of thyroid cancer patients, 1411–1412
Posterior cerebral artery (PCA), ischemic stroke and, 101, 103, 104*f*
Posterior (vertebrobasilar) circulation, ischemic stroke and, 100–101, 103–105, 103*f*, 104*f*, 105*f*
Posterior cruciate ligament (PCL), 1196
  normal, 1198*f*
  torn, 1198*f*
Posterior descending artery (PDA), 1387
Posterior fossa, 231
  cystic lesions of, 232
  tumors
    in children, 135–136, 137*t*
    ependymoma, 139, 139*f*
    medulloblastoma, 136–137, 138*f*
    pilocytic astrocytoma, 137–139, 138f
Posterior inferior cerebellar arteries (PICA), ischemic disease and, 104–105, 105*f*
Posterior junction lines, 351*f*, 352*f*
Posterior mediastinal masses, 1255
Posterior mediastinum, 359
Posterior reversible encephalopathy syndrome (PRE), 185, 197–198, 199*f*
Posterior tibial tendon (PTT), 1215–1216
  tendinosis in, 1216*f*
  torn, 1216*f*
Posterior urethral valve, 1310, 1311*f*
Posteroanterior (PA) radiographs, 335, 433
  of anterior and posterior junction lines, 351*f*
  of soft tissues, 350–354
Posteroanterior (PA) view, 5
Postinfectious bronchiectasis, 518
Postmenopausal ovarian cysts, 959
Postoperative infection, 1447, 1449*f*
Postpneumonectomy space, 532
Postprimary tuberculosis, 466, 467*f*
Posttransplant lymphoproliferative disorder, 457, 749–750
Pott disease, 288, 291*f*
Pouch of Douglas, 736*f*
PRE. *See* Posterior reversible encephalopathy syndrome (PRE)
Prednisone, contrast administration and, 24
Pregnancy
  adnexa in, 986
  anomalies of
    abdomen, 997–1000, 998*f*, 999*f*, 1000*f*

CNS, 991–995, 991*f*, 992*f*, 993*f*
heart, 995–997, 996*f*, 997I
chromosome abnormalities in, 990–991
ectopic, 980–981, 980*t*, 981*f*
fibroids, 986
first trimester
abnormal, 979–982, 979*f*, 979*t*, 980*t*, 981*f*
gestational trophoblastic disease in, 982–983, 982*f*, 983*f*
normal gestation in, 977–978, 977*f*, 977*t*, 978*f*, 978*t*
implantation bleeding in, 981–982
skeletal dysplasias in, 1000, 1000*f*
uterus in, 98*f*, 986
vaginal bleeding in, 978, 978*t*
Prenatal hypoxic ischemic encephalopathy, 217
Presacral masses, 1325–1327, 1326*f*
Pretracheal space, 357
Prevertebral abscess, 290*f*
Prevertebral space, 257
Primary bone tumors, 1366
Primary CNS lymphoma, 183, 183*f*
Primary lymphoma of bone, 1096*f*, 1098
Primary malignant neoplasms, in skull base, 246
Primary tuberculosis, 465, 466*f*, 1241*f*
Prion virus, 171
Probst bundles, 227
Progressive massive fibrosis (PMF), 486, 499
Progressive multifocal leukoencephalopathy (PML), 171, 181, 182*f*, 194, 194*f*
Prominent perivascular spaces, 191–192
Prone view, 6
Prospective Investigation of Pulmonary Embolism Diagnosis (PIOPED), 426, 1380–1381, 1381*t*
ProstaScint, 1469*f*
Prostate
anatomy of, 920–921, 921*f*
carcinoma, 921–922, 922*f*, 922*t*, 970–971, 971*f*, 971*t*, 1469
US anatomy of, 371*f*, 969–970
Prostate cancer, 1439*f*, 1505
imaging, 1439
magnetic resonance imaging of, 300
Prostate metastasis, 292*f*
Prostate-specific antigen (PSA), tests for, 970–971, 971*f*, 971*t*
Prostatic hyperplasia, 922–923, 923*f*
Prostatic hypertrophy, 899, 899*f*
Prostatitis, 972, 972*f*
Prosthetic joint replacements, 1359
Proteinaceous fluids, MR and, 17, 17*t*
Proteus, 463
Proton density weighted imaging (PDWI), 188*f*
Proton MR spectroscopy, of brain, 47
Proximal tibia, stress fracture of, 1128*f*
Prune belly syndrome, 893, 1309–1310, 1310*f*
Prussak space, 246
PSA. *See* Prostate-specific antigen
Pseudoaneurysm, 1044–1047, 1046*f*, 1047*f*
Pseudo-Bennett fracture, 1112
Pseudo-Charcot joint, 1144, 1147
Pseudocyst(s), 1321–1322, 1323*f*
of calcaneus, 1180
genatinous, 181
of humerus, 1171–1173, 1177*f*
of pancreas, 406
Pseudodiaphragm, 383
Pseudodislocation
of humerus, 1170–1171
of shoulder, 1176*f*
Pseudodiverticula, 846
Pseudogestational sac, 979*f*, 981
Pseudogout (CPPD), 1141–1143. *See also* Calcium pyrophosphate dihydrate crystal deposition disease
Pseudohypoparathyroidism, 1162, 1162*f*
Pseudolymphoma, 457
Pseudomasses, in carotid space, 252
Pseudomonas, 286
Pseudomonas aeruginosa pneumonia, 462*f*, 463
Pseudomyxoma peritonei, 737, 737*f*
Pseudopermeative process
diagnosis of, 1159*t*
hemangioma and, 1159*f*
Pseudopseudohypoparathyroidism, 1162
Pseudotumors, 267*f*, 383
inflammatory, 439
lymphoma and, 263–264
Psoas muscle, hypertrophy of, 903
Psoriasis
sacroiliac joint and, 1140*f*
with syndesmophytes, 1137*f*
PTH. *See* Parathyroid hormone
PTT. *See* Posterior tibial tendon
Pulmonary acinus, 480
Pulmonary agenesis, 1235–1236
Pulmonary alveolar proteinosis (PAP), 482, 508–509, 509*f*
Pulmonary angiography, 684–687, 685*f*, 687*f*. *See* Computed tomography angiography of pulmonary arteries
Pulmonary arterial hypertension (PAH), 429*f*, 430–432
causes of, 430*t*
chronic, 431*f*
idiopathic, 431
Pulmonary arteriogram, 428*f*
Pulmonary arteriovenous malformations (PAVMs), 686–687, 687*f*
Pulmonary artery, 347–349, 605, 608*f*, 1259–1260
bilateral enlargement of, 416
enlargement, 414, 1266*f*
enlargement of, 414, 414*f*
with venous returns, 348*f*–349*f*
Pulmonary atelectasis, 366*t*
Pulmonary atresia, 1268, 1273*f*
Pulmonary blastoma, 458*f*, 459
Pulmonary blood flow
asymmetry of, 1258–1259
normal, 1258
Pulmonary capillary hemangiomatosis (PCH), 432
Pulmonary capillary wedge pressure (PCWP), 420, 421
Pulmonary cavities, 1239–1241
Pulmonary contusion, 556–557, 557*f*
Pulmonary edema, 417, 419*f*, 420*t*
basic principles of, 418*f*
cardiac disease and, 418*f*
chronic, 487
chronic interstitial, 481
hydrostatic, 419–420
interstitial, 419*f*
perihilar, 418*f*
radiographic findings with, 418*f*
re-expansion, 419
upper lung, 419
Pulmonary embolism (PE), 424–430, 426*f*, 685–687, 685*f*, 1374*f*, 1376
multidetector-row computed tomography for, 428*f*
nonthrombotic, 429
on pulmonary arteriogram, 428*f*
radiographic findings of, 1376
radiologic evaluation of, 424–426
recurrent, 1384*f*
Pulmonary fibrosis, 503
Pulmonary hamartoma, 438, 455
Pulmonary hemorrhage, 422–424, 423*f*
causes of, 423*t*
computed tomography of, 424*f*
idiopathic, 423
Pulmonary hypoplasia, 1235–1236
Pulmonary infarction, 427*f*
Pulmonary infections, 460
mechanisms of, 460–461
radiographic patterns of, 460–461

Pulmonary interstitial emphysema, 1247*f*
Pulmonary interstitium, 350, 350*f*
Pulmonary leukostasis, 457
Pulmonary lobule, 480*f*
Pulmonary lucency, 375. *See also* Unilateral pulmonary hyperlucency
  causes of, 376*t*
  lesions in, 377*f*
Pulmonary lymphangiectasia, 1233, 1245
Pulmonary lymphatics, 349
Pulmonary matastases, nodular, 456*f*
Pulmonary neoplasms, 433, 440*t*
Pulmonary nodule, 375, 455
Pulmonary opacities, 374*t*–375*t*
Pulmonary scintigraphy, 1371
Pulmonary segment anatomy, 1372*f*
Pulmonary sequestration, 1251, 1254*f*
Pulmonary sling, 1239*f*
Pulmonary thromboembolism, 425*f*
Pulmonary tumor emboli, 429–430
Pulmonary vascular disease, 417, 639–640, 639*f*, 640*f*, 641*f*, 641*t*
Pulmonary vascularity, 613–615, 614*f*, 615*f*, 615*t*, 1258
  normal, 1269–1272
  patterns of, 1265–1269, 1265*t*, 1266*f*
Pulmonary veins, 349
Pulmonary venoocclusive disease (PVOD), 431, 432
Pulmonary venous hypertension, 420*t*
Pulsed doppler, 19
PVL. *See* Periventricular leukomalacia
PVNS. *See* Pigmented villondular synovitis
PVOD. *See* Pulmonary venoocclusive disease
Pyelogram phase, 873
Pyelonephritis, 1438
  acute, 1437*f*
  chronic, 883–884, 884*f*
  renal, 882–883, 883*f*
  US of, 951, 951*f*
Pyeloureteritis, 895, 896*f*
Pyknodysostosis, 1164, 1165*f*
Pyloric stenosis, 1282*f*
Pylorospasm, 1281, 1281*f*
Pyogenic abscess, 156, 769, 770*f*
Pyogenic abscesses, 156, 160*f*
Pyogenic infections, 286–287
Pyogenic spondylodiscitis, 284
Pyonephrosis, 892–893, 951, 951*f*
Pyramidal fracture, 81–82

Q

Quadrilateral space syndrome, 1212, 1212*f*

R

RA. *See* Rheumatoid arthritis
Racemose cysticercosis, 173
Rad. *See* Radiation-absorbed dose
Radiation
  bone marrow and, 303
  detectors of, 1345–1356
  dose, in CT, 9–10
  exposure to, 1341–1342
  monitoring of, 1341–1342
  regulations about, 1340–1341
  risk, in breast cancer screening, 567
  safety and, 1341
  safety instruments, 1341
  safety with, 1339
  of spine, effects of, 282*f*
  therapy with, 1364*f*
  units for, 1339*f*
Radiation arteritis, 199–202
Radiation colitis, 858
Radiation esophagitis, 809, 809*f*, 810*f*
Radiation leukoencephalitis, 199, 200*f*
Radiation myelitis, 279–281
Radiation necrosis, 199–202, 200*f*, 202*f*
  acute, 201*f*
  vs. tumor recurrence, 204*f*, 205
Radiation-absorbed dose (rad), 1338
Radiculopathy, 272
  vs. myelopathy, 272
Radioactive iodine uptake (RAIU), 1404
Radiochemical purity, 1343
Radiochemicals, purity of, 1343–1344
Radiographic contrast agents
  gastrointestinal, 24
  iodinated, 22–24
  MR intravascular, 24
  ultrasound intravascular, 24–25
Radiographic views, naming of, 5–6
Radiography, 272
  of airspace disease, 365*t*
  of aortic nipple, 353*f*
  apical lordotic view, 337
  bronchogenic carcinoma and, 443
  of C1 and C2, 1104*f*
  of cervical spine, 1104*f*
  chest, 6, 6*f*, 335, 382*f*, 424, 609–613, 610*f*, 611, 613*f*, 615–616, 616*f*
    interstitial opacity of, 374*f*
  chest fluoroscopy, 337
  of clavicles, 351
  conventional, 3, 4*f*, 5–6
  of diaphragm, 354, 388
  digital *vs.* analog, 337
  expiratory, 337
  hilar disease and, 380
  inclinometer and, 336
  inspiration of, 335
  interpretation principles of, 6
  lateral chest, 350*f*, 354
  lateral decubitus, 337, 337*f*
  of lung interfaces, 355
  of lung-lung interfaces, 351, 352*f*
  of lung-mediastinal interfaces, 351, 353*f*
  of lungs, 354
  motion of, 335
  penetration of, 335
  plain, 272
  for pleural effusion, 337
  pneumothorax and, 385
  portable, 336
  posteroanterior, 335, 336*f*
  posteroanterior chest, 350–354
  pulmonary edema and, 421
  retrocardiac space and, 351
  retrotracheal triangle and, 351
  of ribs, 351
  rotation of, 335
  of scapulae, 351
  of soft tissue, 354
  of spine, 351
  for thoracic disease, 335
  of upper abdomen, 354
  of wrist, 1114*f*
Radioiodine
  therapy with, 1412
  for tumor imaging, 1458
Radiolabeled leukocytes, 1443–1451
Radiolabeled tracer, 1342
Radiologic units, 1338*t*
Radiology
  breastfeeding and, 1341*t*
  vascular, 671–674, 673*t*, 674*t*
Radionuclide imaging, of ischemic heart disease, 634–635, 634*f*
Radionuclide ventriculogram (RVG), 1395

Radionuclides, 1337*t*
  skeletal system and, 1358*t*
Radiopharmaceuticals, 1341, 1342, 1357, 1372
  administration errors of, 1344
  cardiovascular system scintigraphy and, 1389–1390
  cerebrospinal fluid studies and, 1473
  generation of, 1342
  localization of, 1342, 1343*t*
  myocardium and, 1385
  perfusion lung scan and, 1373–1374
  in planar brain scans, 1472
  for positron emission tomography, 1458
  positron emission tomography and, 1393–1395
  renal imaging and, 1428–1429
  single-photon emission computed tomography and, 1475
  for thyroid imaging, 1405*t*
  tumor therapy with, 1469
Radiotherapy, 1331–1332
RAGE. *See* Rapid acquisition with gradient echo
RAIU. *See* Radioactive iodine uptake
Ranke complex, 466
Rapid acquisition relaxation-enhanced (RARE), 13
Rapid acquisition with gradient echo (RAGE), 13
RARE. *See* Rapid acquisition relaxation-enhanced
RAS. *See* Renal artery stenosis
Rasmussen aneurysms, 466
Rathke cleft cyst, 148–149
Raynaud phenomenon, 490
RB-ILD. *See* Respiratory bronchiolitis-associated interstitial lung disease
RCC. *See* Renal cell carcinoma
Recombinant human thyroid stimulating hormone (rhTSH) treatment, 1411
Rectus femoris avulsion, 1125*f*
Re-expansion pulmonary edema, 422
Reflex sympathetic dystrophy, 1363
Reflux nephropathy, 883–884, 884*f*
Regional enteritis, 1291–1292, 1294, 1297*f*
Regions of interest (ROI), 1416
Reiter syndrome, 1137, 1139, 1141*f*
Relapsing polychondritis, 514
Relaxation atelectasis. *See* Passive atelectasis
Rem. *See* Roentgen equivalent man
Renal abnormalities, 1303–1308
Renal abscess, 1304, 1304*f*
Renal agenesis, 1307–1308, 1307*f*, 1308*f*
Renal angiography, 703–706, 704f, 705*f*, 706*f*
Renal anomalies, 875, 875*f*
Renal artery aneurysms, 705
Renal artery stenosis, US of, 952, 952*f*
Renal artery stenosis (RAS), 1433, 1435*f*
Renal blood flow, 1429, 1431*f*
Renal calcifications, 1308
Renal cell carcinoma (RCC), 876–877, 876*f*, 877*f*, 878*t*, 1315
Renal cysts, 1308
  causes of, 1309*t*
Renal disease
  AIDS and, 884
  avascular necrosis and, 1183
Renal failure, acute, 1432
Renal imaging, 1428–1438
Renal infections, 882–884, 883*f*, 884*f*
Renal lymphoma, 1315*f*
Renal malignancies, 1505
Renal masses, 1312, 1433*f*
  cystic, 879–880, 879*f*, 880*f*
  solid, 876–879, 876*f*, 877*f*, 878*f*, 878*t*, 879*f*
Renal osteodystrophy, 1163
Renal parenchymal disease, 884–885, 885*t*
Renal stone disease, 889–891, 891*f*
Renal transplant artery narrowing, 705
Renal transplantation, 1432, 1434*f*
Renal tuberculosis, 884, 884*f*
Renal vein thrombosis, 1433*f*
Renovascular hypertension, 1433
Rent, 72
Reproductive organs. *See also* Ovarian; Testicular
  masses of, 1323–1325
Reservoirs, 1473–1474
Resolution, 1352
Resorptive atelectasis, 366
Respiratory bronchiolitis-associated interstitial lung disease (RB-ILD), 491, 494, 494*f*
Respiratory syncytial virus, 467
Restrictive cardiomyopathy, 637–638, 638*f*
Retained fetal lung fluid, 1244–1245
Retained fluid syndrome, 1248*f*
Retention cysts, 249
Reticular pattern, 373
Reticulin forms, brain abscesses and, 158
Reticulonodular opacities, 375
Retrocardiac space, 351
Retrocaval ureter, 889, 890*f*
Retroperitoneal adenopathy, 929, 929*f*
Retroperitoneal fibrosis, 750–751, 752*f*
Retroperitoneal fluids, 929–930
Retroperitoneal neoplasms, 750, 750*f*
Retroperitoneal tumors, 929
Retroperitoneum, anatomy of, 929
Retropharyngeal abscess, 261*f*
Retropharyngeal space, 256–257
  as danger space, 256
Retrostyloid space, 248
Retrotracheal triangle, 351
Reverberation artifacts, 21
Rhabdomyosarcoma, 1255, 1310, 1325, 1326
Rheumatoid arthritis (RA), 279, 282*f*, 423, 488*t*, 1134, 1135*f*
  hallmarks of, 1135*t*
  of hips, 1136
  of shoulder, 1136*f*
Rheumatoid lung disease, 488–489
RhTSH. *See* Recombinant human thyroid stimulating hormone treatment
Rib(s), 1255
  dysplasia of, 296
  fracture of, 1358*f*, 1517*f*
  notching, 542–543
  ribbon, 495
Ribbon rib, 495
Rickets, 1160*f*. *See also* Osteomalacia
Riedel thyroiditis, 1408
Right atrium, 604, 606*f*
Right lower lobe atelectasis, 373
Right middle lobe (RML), 370*f*, 372*f*
  in lungs, 345
Right posterior (RPO) view, 6
Right sided aortic arch, 1260
Right subphrenic space, 733
Right upper lobe (RUL), 342, 344*f*
  atelectasis, 368
  of lung, 340
Right ventricle, 604–605, 607*f*
Right ventricular studies, 1397–1402
  first-pass function, 1400*f*
Right-to-left shunts, 1402
Rim rent tear, 1208, 1209*f*
Ring down artifact, 21
Rituximab (Rituxan), 1469
RML. *See* Right middle lobe
Roentgen, 1338
Roentgen equivalent man (rem), 1338
ROI. *See* Regions of interest
Rolando fracture, 1112, 1113*f*
Rollo phantom, 1354
Rotary subluxation, of navicular, 1115, 1116*f*

Rotator cuff, 1173
  anatomy of, 1205–1208
  impingement syndrome and, 1205
  normal, 1206*f*
  oblique coronal image of, 1206*f*
  partial tear of, 1207*f*
  torn, 1206*f*
Round atelectasis, 368, 368*f*
Round pneumonia, 1252*f*
Rubella, 415
Rubidium-82, 1393
Rugger jersey spine, 1160
RUL. *See* Right upper lobe
RVG. *See* Radionuclide ventriculogram

S

Saber sheath trachea, 340
Saber-sheath trachea, 513, 513*f*
Sacculations, 805, 807*f*
Sacral chordoma, 1326
Sacral cysts, 315*f*
Sacrococcygeal teratoma, 1325
Sacroiliac joint (SI)
  ankylosing spondylitis and, 1139*f*
  osteoarthritis of, 1126*f*, 1134*f*
  osteophytes of, 1126*f*
  with psoriasis, 1140*f*
Sacroiliac joint disease
  causes of, 1139*t*
  psoriatic arthritis with, 1139*f*
Sacrum
  fracture of, 1124, 1124*f*
  stress fracture of, 1124, 1124*f*, 1125*f*
SAH. *See* Subarachnoid hemorrhage
Salivagram, 1416
Salivary scanning, 1416
  of Warthin tumor, 1417*f*
Salmonella, 286
"Sandwich sign," 749
Sandwich vertebrae, 1165*f*
Sarcoidosis, 174, 415, 501–502, 502*f*, 504, 1145, 1145*f*, 1190*f*, 1191, 1442*f*, 1446*f*, 1515
  bullous changes in, 504*f*
  computed tomography and, 503*f*
  lymphadenopathy in, 400*f*
  radiographic staging of, 504*t*
  in tuberculomas, 161
Sarcomas, 1507
SARS. *See* Severe Acute Respiratory Syndrome
SCA. *See* Superior cerebellar arteries
Scalp injury, 56
Scaphoid fracture, 1116*f*
Scapula, 544–546
Scars, of postoperative disks, 329*f*
Scheuermann disease, 1155*f*
Schistosoma haematobium, 472
Schistosoma japonicum, 472
Schistosoma mansoni, 472
Schistosomiasis, 472, 900, 900*f*
  pelvicaliceal system and, 897
Schizencephaly, 230–231, 231*f*
Schwann cells, 296
Schwannoma, 149–150, 151*f*, 151*t*, 152*f*, 153*f*
Schwannomas, 237, 252, 253, 256*f*, 257, 296, 297*f*
  "dumbbell," 298*f*
Scintigraphy
  cardiovascular system and, 1387–1393
  central nervous system and, 1472
  of endocrine glands, 1404
  endocrine glands and, 1404
  gallium, 395, 1441*f*, 1442*f*, 1444*f*, 1445*f*
  gastrointestinal, 1416, 1419–1420
  gated blood pool, 629
  of genitourinary system, 1428
  genitourinary system and, 1428
  hepatic blood pool and, 1425
  hepatobiliary, 1416
  infection and inflammation and, 1440
  of liver, 1416
  lymphoscintigraphy, 1465–1467
  peptide receptor and, 1462–1464
  pulmonary, 1371
  of skeletal system, 1357
  of spleen, 1416
Scintillation detectors, 1345–1347
  components of, 1346*f*
Scleroderma, 489–490, 490*f*, 803, 803*f*, 1145*f*
  of small bowel, 840, 842*f*
Sclerosis, 1132
Sclerotic lesion, 1084–1085, 1084*f*
Scoliosis, 311, 316*f*
  congenital, 315*f*
Scrotum
  anatomy of, 919–920
  hernia of, 969, 970*f*
  pain in, 964, 965*t*
  US anatomy of, 963–964, 963*f*, 964*f*
SDAFs. *See* Spinal dural arteriovenous fistulas
SE. *See* Spin-echo; Spin-echo
Seatbelt fracture, 1108*f*, 1110
Secondary hyperthyroidism, 1408
Secretory disease, 581, 584*f*
Segmental atelectasis, 367
Seizure(s), 1483
  imaging strategies for, 51*t*, 52
  pyogenic abscesses and, 156
  tuberculomas and, 161
Selective vulnerability, brain metabolism and, 87
Self-expanding stents, 672–673
Sellar masses, 147–149, 148*f*, 149*f*, 150*f*
Semilobar holoprosencephaly, 225, 226*f*
Semimembranosus tibial collateral ligament bursa, 1203*f*
Seminoma, 378*f*
Senescent periventricular hyperintensity, 191
Sentinel loop, 742, 742*f*
Sentinel lymph node (SLN), 1498
Septic embolus, 159
Septo-optic dysplasia (SOD), 225, 225*f*
Sestamibi imaging, 1413
Severe Acute Respiratory Syndrome (SARS), 467–468
Shaken impact injury, 74
Short TI inversion recovery (STIR), 13
Short tau inversion recovery (STIR), 186, 275, 279
Shoulder(s). *See also* Rotator cuff
  anatomy of, 1206*f*
  anterior dislocation of, 1122*f*
  arthritis of, 1516*f*
  avascular necrosis of, 1152*f*
  bony abnormalities of, 1209
  dislocation of, 1103*f*, 1119–1123
    anterior, 1121*f*
  high-riding, 1136*t*
  magnetic resonance imaging of, 1205
  posterior dislocation of, 1122*f*
  pseudodislocation of, 1122*f*, 1176*f*
  radiograph of, 1121*f*
  rheumatoid arthritis of, 1136*f*
  subchondral cyst of, 1135*f*
Shunts, 1473–1474
  left-to-right, 1400–1402, 1401*f*
  right-to-left, 1402
SI. *See* Sacroiliac joint; Système Internationale
Sickle cell disease, 286–287, 1163, 1164*f*, 1450
Siderophores, 1465
Sievert (Sv), 1339
Sigmoid volvulus, 745, 745*f*

Signal intensity, 54
Silicoproteinosis, 498
Silicosis, 415, 485*f*, 498
Silicotic nodules, 498
Simple pulmonary eosinophila, 507
Single ventricle, 1265
Single-photon emission computed tomography
  indications and, 1477–1486
  interpretation of, 1477
  radiopharmaceuticals and, 1475
  techniques for, 1476–1477
Single-positron emission computed tomography (SPECT), 1350, 1388*f*
Sinus(es)
  cysts in, 243
  esthesioneuroblastoma in, 245
  fractures, 77–78, 78*f*
  infections of, frontal lobes and, 156
  inverting papilloma in, 244–245
  juvenile nasopharyngeal angiofibromas in, 245
  malignancies in, 245
  mucocele in, 243–244, 244*f*
  polyps in, 243
Sinus tarsi syndrome, 1222*f*, 1223
Sinusitis, 242–244
  acute, 243*f*
  pyogenic abscesses and, 156
Situs anomalies, 616, 616*f*
Situs solitus, 1273
Sjögren syndrome, 255, 259*f*, 391, 490–491
Skeletal "don't touch" lesions, 1168
Skeletal dysplasias, in pregnancy, 1000, 1000*f*
Skeletal imaging, 1334
Skeletal system, scintigraphy of, 1357
  interpretation of, 1358
  normal, 1358
Skeletal trauma, 1102
Skeleton
  normal variants in, 1171–1179
  trauma to, 1358
Skull
  base of, 245–247
    tumors of, 246
  films, 55–56
  fractures, 56, 56*f*
  temporal bone of, 246–247
SLAP. *See* Superior labral tears
SLE. *See* Systemic lupus erythematosus
SLN. *See* Sentinel lymph node
Slow virus, 172
SMA. *See* Superior mesenteric artery
Small airway disease, 524–526, 524*t*, 525*f*
Small bowel
  adenocarcinoma of, 834–835, 835*f*
  anatomy of, 832–833
  diffuse disease of, 839–844, 839*t*, 840*f*, 840*t*, 841*f*, 841*t*, 842*f*, 843*f*
  diverticula, 846, 846*f*
  erosions/ulcerations of, 844–846, 845*f*, 846*f*
  filling defects/mass lesions of, 834–838, 835*f*, 836*f*, 838*f*
  imaging methods for, 832, 833*f*, 834*f*
  mesenteric masses of, 838–839, 839*f*
  obstruction in, 743–745, 743*f*, 743*t*, 744*f*
Small cell carcinoma, 440–442, 442*f*
Small hila, 416, 416*t*
Small intestinal obstruction, 1285
  causes of, 1286*t*
Small left colon syndrome, 1287, 1288*f*
Small-vessel ischemia, 105–106, 107*f*, 108*f*, 109*f*
Smith fracture, 1118, 1118*f*
Smoke inhalation, 1386
Smoking
  bronchogenic carcinoma and, 442
  LCH and, 504
SOD. *See* Septo-optic dysplasia
Sodium iodide wellcounter, 1355, 1355*f*
Soft tissue
  calcified, 740–741
  of chest wall, 539–542, 541*f*, 542*f*
  contrast, 16, 16*t*
  posteroanterior radiographs of, 350
  radiographs of, 354
  swelling, in facial injury, 76–77, 77*f*
  tumors, 1098*f*, 1099–1101, 1099*f*, 1100*f*
Solitary bone cyst, 1078–1079, 1078*f*, 1079*f*
Solitary metastasis, 1369*f*
Solitary pulmonary nodule (SPN), 433, 438*t*, 455, 1492
  adenocarcinoma and, 436*f*
  border characteristics of, 435
  calcification of, 437*f*
  clinical factors and, 434
  clinical factors with, 434
  density of, 435
  growth pattern of, 434–435
  imaging of, 434*f*
  lesions and, 438
  malignant, 437*f*
  management decisions with, 436–438
  non-Hodgkin lymphoma and, 439*f*
  positron emission tomography of, 437*f*
  size of, 435
  tumors and, 438
Somatostatin receptors, 1462
SPECT. *See* Single-positron emission computed tomography
SPECT myocardial perfusion imaging, 1334
Spectral waveforms, 1021–1022, 1021*f*, 1022*f*
Spina bifida, 993, 994*f*
Spina bifida occulta, 308
Spinal angiography, 278
Spinal contusion, 317*f*
Spinal cord. *See* Spine
Spinal cord infarction, 305
Spinal cord tethering, in adults, 313*f*
Spinal dural arteriovenous fistulas (SDAFs), 306, 310*f*
  anatomy of, 308*f*
Spinal dysraphism, 312*f*
Spinal lipoma, 311*f*
Spinal osteomyelitis, 1443, 1452*f*, 1454*f*
Spinal stenosis, 325–329
Spine. *See also* Cervical spine; Disk(s); Lumbar spine; Thoracic spine
  abscesses of, 286, 288*f*
  acute viral illnesses of, 280
  arachnoid cysts in, 311
  arteriovenous malformations and, 305
  caudal regression syndrome in, 311
  chemotherapy and, 281
  Chiari II malformation in, 232
  collapse of, imaging of, 284*t*
  compression fracture of, 317*f*
  congenital malformations of, 308
  cord compression, 274*f*–275*f*
  CT of, 273–275
  disk herniations of, 272
  extradural masses and, 297
  extramedullary masses and, 295
  fast spin-echo and, 275
  fracture of, with ankylosing spondylitis, 1112
  healing powers of, 272
  hematoma of, 319*f*
  imaging methods for, 272–278
  infections of, 281–286
  inflammation of, 278–281
    lupus erythematosus, 279

Spine (*Contd.*)
multiple sclerosis and, 278–279
radiation myelitis, 279–281
rheumatoid arthritis, 279
intradural masses and, 295
intramedullary lipomas in, 309–311
intrathecal (drop) metastases and, 297
lesions of, diagnosis of, 276*t*
leukemia and, 301
lightning and, 281
lymphoma and, 301, 306*f*
metastasis of, 1509*f*
myeloma and, 301
nondegenerative diseases of, 271
common clinical syndromes and, 271
postoperative changes in, 329–330
radiation of, 282*f*
scoliosis in, 311
strokes and, 305, 307*f*
tethered cord in, 308
thoracic, 546, 546*f*
trauma of, 273, 311
tuberculosis of, 288–289
tumors in, 293
ultrasound and, 278
Spin-echo (SE), 12–13, 186
multiple, 13
Spinoglenoid notch, ganglion in, 1212*f*
Spirochete infections, neurosyphilis, 165–166
Spleen
anatomy, 790–791
cystic lesions of, 793–794, 793*f*, 794*t*
cystic masses of, 1320
granulomas, 739
imaging techniques of, 790
lymphoma of, 1498*f*
motion artifact in, 11*f*
scintigraphy, 1416
solid lesions of, 794–796, 794*f*, 795*f*, 796*f*
US of, 939–941, 940*f*, 941*f*
Splenic angiography, 706–707, 707*f*
Splenic artery aneurysm, 707, 707*f*
Splenic flexure bleeding, 1420*f*
Splenic infarction, 1321
Splenic lesions, 1319–1321
Splenic neoplasm, 1320
Splenic torsion, 1322*f*
Splenomegaly, 792–793, 792*f*, 792*t*, 1319
AIDS and, 796, 796*t*
US of, 939
Splenosis, 791–792
Splenules, 939, 940*f*
SPN. *See* Solitary pulmonary nodule
S-PNET. *See* Supratentorial primitive neuroectodermal tumor
Spondyloarthropathies, 1136
Spondylolisthesis, 326–329, 328*f*, 329, 1109*f*
Spondylolysis, 324, 326–329, 328*f*, 1109*f*, 1110–1111
Spring ligament, 1217*f*
Squamous cell carcinoma, 245, 247*f*, 250, 250*f*, 440, 441*f*, 449*f*, 452
of nasopharynx, 1508*f*
in pelvicaliceal system, 894
of tongue, 259*f*, 1507*f*
of trachea, 453*f*
Squamous cell papilloma, 453, 454*f*
SSFP. *See* Steady-state free precession
Staghorn calculus, 891*f*
Standardized uptake value (SUV), 242, 1493
Stanford classification, 682
Staphylococcus aureus, 286, 287, 462, 463*f*, 467
infection and, 156
Starling forces, 417
Steady-state free precession (SSFP), 652
Stenosis
aortic, 642–643, 643*f*
carotid US, 1030–1032, 1030*f*, 1031*t*, 1032*t*, 1033*f*, 1034*f*
of central canal, 326, 327*f*
facet hypertrophy and, 328*f*
lateral recess, 326
mitral, 640–641
neuroforaminal, 326
of peripheral arteries, 1047–1048
renal artery, 952, 952*f*
of spine, 325–329
tracheal, 511–513
Stents, types of, 672–673
Stereotactic needle aspiration, brain abscesses and, 158
Sternum, 546–547, 547*f*
Steroids, avascular necrosis and, 1183
STIR. *See* Short TI inversion recovery; Short time inversion recovery
Stomach. *See also* Gastric
anatomy of, 816–817, 817*f*
cancer of, 1500
gastric filling defects/mass lesions, 818–822, 818*f*, 819*f*, 819*t*, 820*f*, 821*f*, 822*f*, 822*t*
Helicobacter pylori infection, 818
imaging methods of, 816
intrathoracic, 1279*f*
positron emission tomography and, 1490
Stones
bladder, 973
kidney, 947, 947*f*
"Straddle injury," 908
Strangulation obstruction, of small bowel, 744
Streak artifact, in CT, 10, 11*f*
Streptococcal infections, 156
Streptococcus aureus, 285*f*, 467
Streptococcus pneumoniae, 172, 461, 1227
Streptococcus pyogenes, 462
Stress fractures, 1127
calcaneal, 1223*f*
of femoral neck, 1127*f*
of femur, 1127*f*
of proximal tibia, 1128*f*
of sacrum, 1124, 1124*f*, 1125*f*
of tibia, 1128*f*
Stroke, 1478
carotid US and, 1025–1026, 1026*f*
definition of, 86
imaging strategies for, 51, 51*t*
ischemic. *See* Ischemic stroke
Stromal tumors, 961
Strongyloides stercoralis, 507
Stunned myocardium, 1393
Sturge-Weber syndrome, 238, 238*f*, 239*f*
Subarachnoid hemorrhage (SAH), 59, 61, 62*f*, 112–114, 114*f*, 115*f*, 116, 116*f*, 1481*f*
in pregnancy, 981, 981*f*
Subcortical gray matter, injury to, 64, 67
Subdural effusion, 177*f*
Subdural empyema, 179*f*, 284
Subdural hematomas, 57–59, 58*f*, 59*f*, 60*f*, 61*f*
Subependymal giant cell astrocytoma, 144–145
Subependymoma, 144
Subfalcial herniation, 69
Subfalcine herniation, 123
Sublabral foramen, 1211, 1211*f*
Sublabral recess, 1211*f*
Sublobar septum, 347
Subpleural interstitium, 479
Subpulmonic effusion, 383
Subpulmonic pneumothorax, 385
Subsegmental atelectasis, 367, 368*f*
Sudeck atrophy, 1149–1150, 1151*f*
Superficial mucosal space, 248–250

Superior cerebellar arteries (SCA), ischemic disease and, 103–104
Superior labral tears (SLAP), 1210, 1211*f*
Superior mesenteric artery (SMA), hepatic angiography and, 708, 708*f*
Superior vena cava (SVC), 408, 444, 713–714
  obstruction of, 1401*f*
Superior vena cava syndrome, 719, 720*f*
Superscan, 1368*f*
Supine view, 6
Suprahyoid head and neck, 247–259
Suprascapular nerve entrapment, 1212–1213
Suprasellar cistern, 29, 31*f*, 34*f*, 35*f*, 44
Suprasellar region, of brain, 34*f*, 35*f*, 44, 45*f*, 46*f*
Supraspinatus tendon
  cuff tear and, 1208
  normal, 1208
  tendonitis and, 1208
  torn, 1207*f*, 1208*f*
Supratentorial brain, 231
Supratentorial primitive neuroectodermal tumor (S-PNET), 134–135, 135*t*
Supravalvular aortic stenosis, 1274*f*
Surfactant deficiency disease, 1242–1243, 1246*f*, 1247*f*
Surfer's knees, 1155
SUV. *See* Standardized uptake value
Sv. *See* Sievert
SVC. *See* Superior vena cava
Swallowing. *See* Motility
Swyer-James syndrome, 416, 1236, 1236*f*
Symphysis pubis, 1143
  degenerative joint disease and, 1133
  osteoarthritis of, 1126*f*
Syndesmophytes, 1136
  in ankylosing spondylitis, 1138*f*
  in psoriatic arthritis, 1138*f*
Synovial osteochondromatosis, 1148–1149, 1148*f*
Syphilis, meningovascular, 169*f*
Syphilitic aortitis, 680
Syringohydromyelia, 294–295, 295*f*, 308
Syrinx. *See* Syringohydromyelia
Système Internationale (SI), 1338
Systemic lupus erythematosus (SLE), 279, 489, 493, 1144*f*

T

T1 shortening, 126
Taenia solium, cysticercosis and, 164
Takayasu arteritis, 679–680, 680*f*
Talus
  osteochondral lesion of, 1218*f*
  osteochondritis dissecans of, 1153*f*
TAPVR. *See* Total anomalous pulmonary venous return
Tarsal coalition, 1223*f*, 1224
Tarsal tunnel syndrome, 1219*f*
Taussig-Bing anomaly, 1263
TB. *See* Tuberculosis
TCC. *See* Transitional cell carcinoma
T-cells, in tuberculous abscess, 161
TDI. *See* Tensor diffusion imaging
Technetium-99m aerosols, 1373
  ventilation scanning, 1373
Technetium-99m methylene diphosphonate scan, 1334*f*
Technetium-99m photospectra, 1349*f*
Technetium-99m sestamibi (Cardiolite), 1390
Technetium-99m tetrofosmin (Myoview), 1390
Technetium-99m-fanolesomab, 1451–1454, 1453*f*
Technetium-99m-labeled leukocytes, 1445
Technetium-99m-MDP
  biodistribution of, 1357
  physiology and, 1357
  technical issues with, 1358
Technetium-99m-pertechnate/thallium-201 radionuclide subtraction imaging, 1413, 1413*f*
Telangiectasis, 118
Temporal bone, 246–247
  fractures, 56–57, 57*f*
Temporomandibular joint, degenerative joint disease and, 1133
Tendinopathy, 1207
Tendinosis, 1207, 1214
Tendon(s)
  Achilles, 1214, 1215*f*
  biceps, 1211
  flexor hallucis longus, 1216–1217
  of foot and ankle, 1214–1218
  peroneus brevis, 1217*f*
  peroneus longus, 1217*f*
  posterior tibial, 1215, 1216*f*
  rupture of, 1214
  supraspinatus, 1207*f*, 1208, 1208*f*
Tendonitis, 1207, 1214
  of biceps, 1212*f*
Tenosynovitis, 1214
Tensor diffusion imaging (TDI), in neuroradiology, 48
"Terry Thomas" sign, 1116
Testes
  anatomy of, 919–920
  ruptured, 968, 969*f*
  undescended, 964
  US anatomy of, 963–964, 963*f*, 964*f*
Testicular abnormalities, 1311
Testicular imaging, 1438–1439, 1438*f*
Testicular malignancies, 1505
Testicular microlithiasis, 966–967, 968*f*
Testicular torsion, 1313*f*
Testicular tumors, 1312
Tethered cord, in spine, 308
Tetralogy of Fallot, 377, 416, 1260, 1265, 1267, 1272*f*
Tetrofosmin imaging, 1413
Thallium-201, 1385, 1390*f*
Thoracic aorta
  anatomy of, 674, 675*f*
  aortic dissection of, 681–684, 683*f*, 684*f*
  congenital anomalies of, 674–675, 675*f*
  trauma to, 675–678, 677*f*, 678*f*
  vasculitis, 679–681, 680*f*, 681*f*
Thoracic aortic aneurysm, 410*f*
Thoracic inlet, 357*f*–358*f*, 363*f*
  anatomy of, 355–359
  contents of, 356*t*
  masses of, 389, 390*t*
Thoracic neuroblastoma, 1262*f*
Thoracic outlet syndrome, 693–694, 696*f*, 1057*f*, 1058*f*
Thoracic spine, 546, 546*f*
  anterior wedge compression fracture and, 1110*f*
Thorax
  metastatic disease of, 455–456
  parasitic infections of, 471
Three-dimensional tractography, of head injury, 62
Thrombi, 646, 646*f*, 647*f*
Thrombolysis
  CT screening for, 87, 90
  imaging strategies for, 51–52, 51*t*
Thrombolytic agents, for vascular radiology, 674, 674*t*
Thrombosis
  abdominal, 1038–1039, 1042*f*
  peripheral arterial disease and, 690
  portal vein, 762, 762*f*
    US of, 932, 932*f*
Thymic carcinomas, 390, 393
Thymic cysts, 392–393
Thymic epithelial neoplasms, 390
Thymic hyperplasia, 393–394, 394, 394*f*
Thymic lymphoma, 394
Thymic pseudomasses, 1257*f*
Thymic rebound, 1517*f*, 1518
Thymolipoma, 393

Thymomas, 390, 393*f*
Thymus gland, 1251–1253
  configurations of, 1256*f*
  leukemia and, 1252
  stress atrophy of, 1257*f*
Thyroglossal duct cysts, 265, 268*f*
Thyroid gland, 1404, 1406*f*
  acropachy of, 1163*f*
  anatomy of, 1006–1007, 1006*f*, 1405
  cancer of, 1410
    metastasis of, 1411*f*
  cysts of, 1410
  diseases of, 1009–1011, 1010*f*
  embryology of, 1405
  goiter, 391*f*
  hyperfunction of, 1162, 1404
  hyperfunctioning adema of, 1409*f*
  hyperthyroidism and, 1407, 1408
  hypofunction of, 1163, 1404
  hypothyroidism and, 1406
  imaging of, 1405*t*
  masses of, 389–390, 397
  metastases of, 1412
  nodules, 1007–1008, 1007*t*, 1008*t*
    benign, 1008–1009, 1008*f*
    malignant, 1009, 1009*f*
  nodules of, 1407*f*, 1408–1412
    benign, 1410*t*
    malignancy of, 1410*t*
  physiology of, 1405
Thyroid ophthalmopathy, 264, 267*f*
Thyroid uptake probe, 1355, 1356*f*
Thyroiditis, 389, 1407, 1408
  acute, 1408
  subacute (viral), 1408
  suppurative, 1408
Thyroid-stimulating hormone (TSH), 1405
Thyrotropin-releasing hormone (TRH), 1406
TI. *See* Time of inversion
TIA. *See* Transient ischemic attack
Tibia, stress fracture of, 1128*f*
Tibial plateau, fracture of, 1127–1129, 1130*f*
Ticlopidine, for vascular radiology, 674
Time of inversion (TI), 13
Tissues
  MR of, 16–17, 17*t*
  soft. *See* Soft tissue
TNB. *See* Transthoracic needle biopsy
TNM. *See* Tumor nodal involvement metastases
Toes, 1361*f*
Toggle sign, 1359
Tomographic brain scans, 1474
Tomographic imaging, 1349–1350
Tomography, conventional, 5, 5*f*
Tongue, squamous cell carcinoma of, 259*f*, 1507*f*
Tonsillitis, 256
TORCH. *See* and Herpes; Cytomegalovirus; Other, which includes syphilis; Rubella; Toxoplasmosis
  in neonatals, 1015
Tornwaldt cysts, 249, 251*f*
Total anomalous pulmonary venous return (TAPVR), 1264, 1271*f*
Toulouse-Lautrec syndrome. *See* Pyknodysostosis
Toxic megacolon, 742–743, 743*t*
Toxocara canis, 265
Toxoplasmosis, 133, 177–178, 180*f*, 181*f*, 182*f*, 477
Toxoplasmosis; Other, which includes syphilis; Rubella; Cytomegalovirus; and Herpes (TORCH), 216, 218*f*
Trachea, 342*f*
  anatomy of, 343*f*
  anomalies of, 511, 512*f*
  disease of, 511–514, 512*t*, 513*f*, 513*t*
  masses of, 402
  squamous cell carcinoma of, 453*f*
  trauma to, 514, 515*f*
Tracheal bronchus, 511, 512*f*
Tracheal neoplasms, 451–455
Tracheal stenosis, 511–513
Tracheobronchial tree, 340
Tracheobronchomalacia, 514
Tracheobronchomegaly, 514
Tracheobronchopathia osteochondroplastica, 514
Tracheoesophageal fistula, 1277, 1279*f*
Traction bronchiectasis, 486
Transient ischemic attack (TIA), 1478
  definition of, 86
Transient osteoporosis of hip, 1191, 1191*f*
Transient pseudomasses, 791, 791*f*
Transitional cell carcinoma (TCC)
  of bladder, 901–903, 902*f*, 902t, 903*f*
  in ureter, 893–894, 894*f*, 895*f*
  US of, 950, 951*f*
Transjugular intrahepatic portosystemic shunt (TIPS), 722–723, 723*f*, 724*f*, 725
  US and, 933–934
  vascular US and, 1039–1041, 1043*f*, 1044*f*, 1044*t*, 1045*f*
Transplantation
  liver, 710, 710*f*
    US of, 934
  post, 749–750
  renal, 705
Transposition of great vessels, 1270*f*
Trans-spatial diseases, 257–259
Transtentorial herniation, 69
Transthoracic needle biopsy (TNB), 340, 437
Transverse ligament, 1196
  pseudotear from, 1197*f*
Trauma. *See also* Facial trauma
  to abdomen, 747, 748*f*
  avascular necrosis and, 1183
  to bladder, 904–905, 904*f*
  to brain, 1486
  to bronchi, 514, 514*f*
  intrathecal lipoma and, 314*f*
  in joints, 1170
  Kienböck malacia and, 1117
  of neck, 256
  pyogenic abscesses and, 156
  skeletal, 1102
    diagnosis of, 1102
  to skeleton, 1358
  of spine, 273, 311
TRH. *See* Thyrotropin-releasing hormone
Trichobezoar, 1282
Tricuspid atresia, 1273*f*
Triple match defects, 1379
Triquetral fracture, 1117*f*
Tropical spruce, 841
True fast imaging with steady-state precession (FISP), 13
True unilateral hyperlucent lung, 376
Truncation errors, 16
TSE. *See* Turbo spin-echo
TSH. *See* Thyroid-stimulating hormone
Tubal ring sign, 980, 981*f*
Tuber cinereum, hamartoma of, 155, 155*f*
Tuberculoma, 466
  history of, 160–161
  as infection, of brain, 160–161
  lungs and, 161
  multiple, 161*f*
  posterior fossa and, 161
Tuberculosis (TB), 256, 288–289, 400, 464, 846
  AIDS and, 473
  of kidneys, 900–901
  miliary, 466, 468*f*, 471*f*, 485, 1234, 1234*f*
  mycobacterium, 464

pelvicaliceal system and, 897
postprimary, 466
primary, 465, 466*f*, 1241*f*
progressive primary, 465
renal, 884, 884*f*
of spine, 288
Tuberculous abscess, 161–162
Tuberculous lymphadenopathy, 400*f*
Tuberculous meningitis, 172–173, 177*f*, 292*f*
in CNS, 160
Tuberculous spondylitis, 287
Tuberous sclerosis (TS), 237, 237*f*, 495, 496
Tuberous sclerous, 881
Tumefactive multiple sclerosis, 188*f*
Tumefactive synovial osteochondromatosis, 1149, 1149*f*
Tumor(s). *See also* Lymphangiomas; Pseudotumors
of ankle, 1219–1222
appearance of, 125–126, 127*f*
of appendix, 862–863
astrocytomas, 293–294
atypical teratoid/rhabdoid, 141
benign, 1515
bone, 1086–1098, 1366
brain, 1485, 1513*f*
brown, 1160
in hyperparathyroidism, 1161*f*
calcaneal, 1219
calcified, 740, 741*f*
of carotid space, 252, 254*f*
of central nervous system, 297
of chest, 447, 448*f*
choline, 47
cystic/necrotic, 770
desmoid, 1219
dysembryoplactic neuroepithelial, 134
ependymomas, 293
epidural, 304
epithelial, 960–961, 961*f*
extra-axial, 141–143, 142*f*
extramedullary, 277*f*
fibrosis and, 389
of foot, 1219
gastric, 1282
of gastrointestinal tract, 1322–1323
germ cell, 396*f*
GI stromal, 820–821, 821*f*
giant cell, 1070–1073, 1071*f*
glomus jugulare, 255
gonadal stromal, 966
hilar disease and, 380
imaging agents of, 1467
imaging of, ideals for, 1458–1459
intra-axial, 124, 124*f*, 133–135, 134*f*, 135*t*, 136*f*, 137*f*
intraperitoneal, 928–929, 929*f*
intraventricular, 143–145, 143*t*, 144*f*, 145*f*, 145*t*
islet cell, 1464*f*
Leydig cell, 1312
lung cancer and, 447, 449
lymphoma and, 304–305
malignant, 1515
margin, 124, 124*f*
mesenchymal, 397
molecular imaging of, 1456
necrotic, 158
nerve sheath, 149–151, 151*f*, 152*f*, 153*f*, 296
neurogenic, 402
of optic nerve, 261
pancoast, 444, 445*f*
paraspinous, 301, 304
of parotid space, 254–255
perineural spread of, 262*f*
peripheral arterial disease and, 694
posterior fossa, 135–141, 137*f*, 138*f*, 139*f*, 140*f*, 141*f*
radioiodine and, 1458
radiopharmaceuticals and, 1469
retroperitoneal, 929
schwannomas and, 253
of skull base, 246
soft tissue, 1098*f*, 1099–1101, 1099*f*, 1100*f*
solitary pulmonary nodule and, 438
in spine, 293
stromal, 961
superior sulcus, 444, 445*f*
supratentorial primitive neuroectodermal, 134–135, 135*t*
of tendon sheath, 1219*f*
testicular, 1312
uroepithelial, 897, 897*f*
Warthin, 254, 1417*f*
Tumor nodal involvement metastases (TNM), 447
Tumoral hemorrhage, 126
Tunneled external catheters, 672
Turbo spin-echo (TSE), 13
Turner syndrome, 269
Twins, 989–990
Tyersinia enterocolitis, 845
Typhilitis, 857, 858*f*
Typhlitis, 1295, 1299*f*

U

Uhl anomaly, 1269
UIP. *See* Usual interstitial pneumonia
Ulcerative colitis, 855, 855*f*, 855*t*, 856*f*
Ulcers
duodenal, 827–828, 828*f*
penetrating aortic, 683
Ultrasonography (US)
abdominal, 927–953
artifacts, 21, 21*f*, 22*f*
of bladder, 972–974, 973f, 974*f*
chest, 1002–1006
contrast agents, 24–25
doppler, 19, 21
genital, 954–972
neonatal brain, 1012–1018
obstetric, 976–1000
parathyroid, 1011–1012
principles of, 18–19, 19*f*, 20*f*, 21–22
thyroid, 1006–1011
vascular, 1019–1057
Ultrasound (US)
carotid. *See* Carotid ultrasound
chest, 1000, 1000*f*
pediatric, 213
prenatal, of spine, 308
of spine, 278, 308
for thoracic disease, 339–340
vascular, 1025–1039, 1041–1057
venous. *See* Venous ultrasound
Umbilical cord, 988
Umbilical-urachal sinus, 899
Uncal herniation, 69, 123
Undescended testis, 920
Unicameral bone cyst, 1180
Unilateral hilar enlargement, 412–415, 413*t*, 414*f*, 1259*f*
Unilateral locked facets, 1108*f*, 1110
Unilateral obstructive emphysema, causes of, 1239*t*
Unilateral pulmonary hyperlucency, 376
Unilateral pulmonary vein atresia, 1236, 1236*f*
Urachal cyst, 899
Urachal remnant disease, 898–899
Uremic medullary cystic disease, 882
Ureter
anatomy of, 887–888, 888*f*
congenital anomalies of, 888–889, 888*f*, 890*f*
filling defects/masses of, 893–896, 894*f*, 895*f*, 896*f*, 896*t*
hydronephrosis, 891–893, 893*f*

Ureter (*Contd.*)
imaging methods for, 887
malignancies, 1505
papillary cavities of, 897–898, 897*f*, 898*f*
renal stone disease, 889–891, 891*f*
stricture of, 896–897, 897*f*
Ureteral duplication, 888–889, 888*f*, 1306–1307
Ureteral obstruction, percutaneous nephrostomy and, 725, 726*f*, 727*f*
Ureteral reflux, 1438, 1438*f*
Ureteral strictures, 906–907, 906*f*, 907*f*
Ureterocele, 901, 901*f*
Ureteropelvic junction obstruction, 889, 889*f*, 1306*f*
Urethra
anatomy of, 905–906, 906*f*
imaging methods for, 905, 905*f*
pathology of, 906–908, 906*f*, 907*f*
Urinary bladder carcinoma, 1506*f*
Urinary bladder malignancies, 1505
Urinary calculi, 738–739, 739*f*
Urinary tract infection, 1303–1304
Urinary tract obstruction, 1305–1306, 1434
Uroepithelial tumor, 897, 897*f*
Urogenital sinus, 1312*f*
US. *See* Ultrasonography; Ultrasound
US-guided biopsy, 450
Usual interstitial pneumonia (UIP), 482, 491, 492*f*
Uterine artery embolization, peripheral arterial disease and, 697, 697*f*, 698*f*, 699
Uterine cancer, 1504
recurrence of, 1505*f*
Uterine leiomyomas, 986
Uterine sarcoma, 915, 916*f*
Uterus
anatomy of, 909
enlarged, 1325
in pregnancy, 98*f*, 986
US of, 954–957, 955*f*, 956*f*, 957*f*

V

VACTERL syndrome, 1278
Vagina, anatomy of, 909
Vaginal bleeding, in pregnancy, 978, 978*t*
Valsalva maneuver, 1290
Valvular heart disease, 640–645, 641*t*, 642*f*, 643*f*, 644*f*, 645*f*, 646*f*
MR, 663–665, 663*f*, 664*f*
Valvular regurgitation, 1397
Varicella zoster, 170, 467, 469*f*
Varicoceles, 969, 969*f*
Vascular calcifications, 738, 739*f*
Vascular diseases, 305–308
Vascular graft infection, 1450*f*
Vascular, infectious, neoplastic, drug, idiopathic, congenital, artifact, trauma, endocrine (VINDICATE), 1335
Vascular injury, 67, 67*f*, 68*f*
Vascular lesions, 262–263, 402
of orbit, 265*t*
Vascular malformations, 117
Vascular neoplasm, of liver, 1320*f*
Vascular phenomena, 1361–1363
Vascular radiology
angiographic suite, 671–672
tools for, 672–674, 673*t*, 674*t*
Vascular ultrasound
abdominal, 1034–1039
carotid, 1025–1034
peripheral arteries, 1041–1049
venous, 1050–1057
Vasculitis, 1515
ischemic disease and, 106
peripheral arterial disease and, 394*f*, 690–691, 693*f*
of thoracic aorta, 679–681, 680*f*, 681*f*
Vasoconstrictors, for vascular radiology, 673
Vasodilators, for vascular radiology, 673
Vasogenic edema, brain abscesses and, 158
VATS. *See* Video-assisted thoracoscopic surgery
VCUG. *See* Voiding cystourethrography
Veins
anatomic structure of, 671
arch of azygos, 352
mapping of, 1054
pulmonary, 349
Venous access, methods of, 715
Venous angiomas, 118
Venous infarction, ischemic stroke and, 106–108, 110*f*, 111*f*
Venous malformations, 118
Venous system
diagnosis/intervention of, 713–716, 718–723, 725
portal, gas in, 763–764, 763*f*
Venous thrombolysis, 717–719, 718*f*, 719*f*, 720*f*, 721*f*
Venous ultrasound
lower extremity, 1050–1054, 1052*f*, 1053*f*, 1054*f*, 1055*f*
upper extremity, 1054–1057, 1055*f*, 1056*f*, 1057*f*, 1058*f*
Ventilation/perfusion (V/Q) lung scanning, 340, 424, 425, 426, 1334, 1372–1373
abnormal, 1376
high-probability, 1378*f*
intermediate-probability, 1382*f*, 1383*f*
interpretation of, 1377–1380
low-probability, 1379*f*
normal, 1375–1376
vs. computed tomography angiography, 1374–1375
Ventricular septal defect (VSD), 1260, 1267*f*
Ventriculitis, brain abscesses and, 158
Ventriculomegaly, 992, 993*f*
Vertebral arteries, ischemic stroke and, 100, 103*f*
Vertebral metastasis, restricted diffusion in, 301*f*
Vesical-urachal diverticulum, 899
Vesicocolonic fistula, 904, 904*f*
Vesicoureteral reflux (VUR), 1304–1305, 1305*f*
Vesiocoureteral reflux, 893
Video-assisted thoracoscopic surgery (VATS), 437, 1248
VINDICATE. *See* Vascular, infectious, neoplastic, drug, idiopathic, congenital, artifact, trauma, endocrine
Viral gastroenteritis, 1294, 1296*f*
Viral infections. *See* Infection(s), viral
Viral meningitis, 174
Viral pneumonia, 467
Virchow-Robin spaces, 106, 108*f*, 191, 193*f*
Voiding cystourethrography (VCUG), 1304
Volume averaging, 10
Von Hippel-Lindau disease, 881
Von Hippel-Lindau syndrome, 239–240, 239*f*, 240*f*, 294, 1322
Von Recklinghausen disease, 494
Voorhoeve disease. *See* Osteopathia striata
V/Q. *See* Ventilation/perfusion lung scanning
VSD. *See* Ventricular septal defect
Vulnerable plaque, 629
VUR. *See* Vesicoureteral reflux

W

Wada test, 1478
Wall motion, 1396
Wall-echo-shadow sign, US of, 937, 937*f*
Wang biopsy, 450
Warfarin, for vascular radiology, 673
Warm pulmonary nodule, 1495*f*
Warthin tumor, 254, 1417*f*
"Water-bottle stomach," 818
Watershed (border zone) infarction, 105, 106*f*, 107*f*
Water-soluble iodinated contrast media, 24
Wegener granulomatosis, 423, 505–507, 506*f*, 1251
Wernicke encephalopathy, 198–199
Wernicke-Korsakoff syndrome, 199

West Nile Virus (WNV), 175*f*, 212
Wet/dry generators, 1344*f*
Whipple disease, 843–844
"White blood," 17
White blood cells (WBC)
  pulmonary activity and, 1447*f*
  pyogenic abscesses and, 156
  study of, 1446*f*
  at traceostomy site, 1448*f*
"White matter buckling," 124
White matter diseases, 53–54, 184, 185*t*
  ependymitis granularis, 191
  nonspecific punctuate, 190–191
  prominent perivascular spaces, 191–192
White pupil reflex. *See* Leukocoria
Williams syndrome, 415, 1309
Wilms tumor, 1251, 1313–1314, 1314*f*
Wilson disease, 211–212, 1141
WNV. *See* West Nile Virus
Wolman disease, 1316
World Health Organization, 390
Wrists
  chondrocalcinosis in, 1143*f*
  fractures of, 1112
  radiograph of, 1114*f*

X

Xanthogranulomatous pyelonephritis, 879, 879*f*
  US of, 951–952, 952*f*
Xenon-127, 1372
  ventilation scanning, 1373
Xenon-133, 1372
  right heart gated first-pass study and, 1400*f*
  ventilation scanning, 1373, 1375*f*
Xerorhinia, 491
Xerostomia, 491
X-ray computed tomography, 1350
XU. *See* Excretory urography

Y

Y-90 ibritumomab tiuxetan (Zevalin), 1469
Yersinia pestis, 501. *See also* Plague
Yolk sac, 978, 978*f*

Z

Zenker diverticulum, 805, 805*f*
Zevalin. *See also* Y-90 ibritumomab tiuxetan
  therapy with, 1470*f*
Zollinger-Ellison syndrome, 828
Zone of transition, 1087, 1088*f*, 1089*t*, 1090
Zygoma, fracture of, 80–81, 81*f*

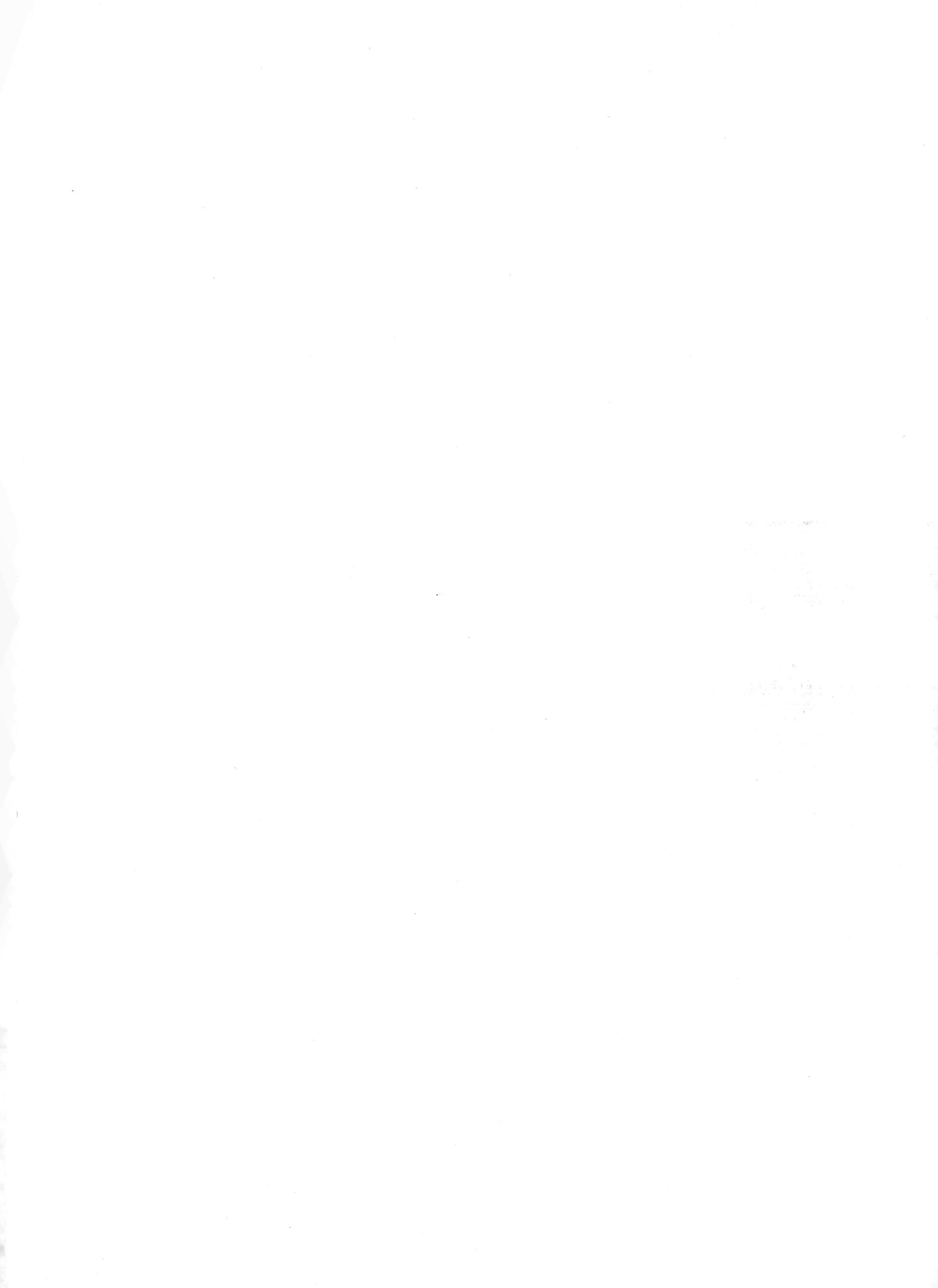